Table 5-3. Neuromuscular Relaxants

Agent	Intubating Dose IV		Onset	Duration	Complications
	Adult	Child			
Succinylcholine*†	1.0–1.5 mg/kg	2.0 mg/kg infant 1–2 mg/kg child	30–60 s	3–12 min	1. Bradyarrhythmias 2. Increased intragastric, intraocular, and intracranial pressure 3. Hyperkalemia 4. Fasciculation-induced musculoskeletal trauma 5. Masseter spasm 6. Malignant hyperthermia 7. Prolonged apnea with pseudocholinesterase deficiency 8. Histamine release
Vecuronium	0.08–0.1 mg/kg	0.1 mg/kg	1.5–4 min	25–40 min	1. Prolonged recovery time in obese or elderly, or if hepatic-renal dysfunction
	0.15–0.28 mg/kg (high-dose protocol)	0.2 mg/kg	1–1.5 min	60–120 min	2. Carbamazepine- and phenytoin-induced resistance
Pancuronium	0.1–0.15 mg/kg	0.1–0.15 mg/kg	1–5 min	30–90 min	1. Vagolytic tachyarrhythmias 2. Prolonged recovery in elderly or if hepatic-renal dysfunction 3. Carbamazepine- and phenytoin-induced resistance
Atracurium	0.4–0.5 mg/kg	0.3–0.4 mg/kg	2–5 min	20–45 min	1. Histamine release 2. Hypotension 3. Bronchospasm

* Pretreat with defasciculating dose of 0.01 mg/kg vecuronium if intracranial hypertension or unstable fractures.

† Pretreat with 0.01 mg/kg atropine in children or vagotonic adults.

Table 14E-2. Pediatric Body Weight Estimation Guidelines

Age	Weight, kg	
Term infant	3.5	Birth weight (BW)
6 months	7	2 × BW
1 year	10	3 × BW
4 years	16	¼ adult weight of 70 kg
10 years	35	½ adult weight

Table 35-9. Guidelines for Intravenous Theophylline in Adults

	Dose
LOADING DOSE*	
No previous theophylline	5 mg/kg IBW
Short-acting theophylline taken < 12 h, or long-acting theophylline taken < 24 h, *and* serum levels therapeutic	None
Oral theophylline as above *and* serum levels subtherapeutic	3 mg/kg *or* ½ (desired level − observed level) mg/kg
MAINTENANCE INFUSION†	
Patients taking oral theophylline *and* serum levels therapeutic	Same dose‡
Patients taking oral theophylline *and* serum levels subtherapeutic	Increase by 25%
Patients not taking oral theophylline:	
Smoking adult	0.8 mg/kg/h
Nonsmoking adult, seriously ill patient	0.5 mg/kg/h
Congestive heart failure, liver disease	0.2 mg/kg/h

* Loading dose should be administered in 50 mL of 5% dextrose in water over 20 to 30 min, *never as a bolus*, and *never through a central venous catheter*.

† Serum theophylline level should be monitored 24–36 h after infusion.

‡ Divide daily dose (mg) by 24 to determine the hourly infusion rate.

Emergency Medicine

A Comprehensive Study Guide

NOTICE

Medicine is an ever-changing science. As new research and clinical experience broaden our knowledge, changes in treatment and drug therapy are required. The editors and the publisher of this work have checked with sources believed to be reliable in their efforts to provide information that is complete and generally in accord with the standards accepted at the time of publication. However, in view of the possibility of human error or changes in medical sciences, neither the editors nor the publisher nor any other party who has been involved in the preparation or publication of this work warrants that the information contained herein is in every respect accurate or complete, and they are not responsible for any errors or omissions or for the results obtained from use of such information. Readers are encouraged to confirm the information contained herein with other sources. For example and in particular, readers are advised to check the product information sheet included in the package of each drug they plan to administer to be certain that the information contained in this book is accurate and that changes have not been made in the recommended dose or in the contraindications for administration. This recommendation is of particular importance in connection with new or infrequently used drugs.

Emergency Medicine

A Comprehensive Study Guide

American College of Emergency Physicians

Third Edition

Editor-in-Chief

Judith E. Tintinalli, M.D., M.S.

Professor and Chairman
Department of Emergency Medicine
University of North Carolina at Chapel Hill

Associate Editors

Ronald L. Krome, M.D.

Visiting Professor, Division of Emergency Health Services
Department of Surgery
University of Michigan Medical School
Ann Arbor, Michigan
Chief, Department of Emergency Medicine
William Beaumont Hospital
Royal Oak, Michigan

Ernest Ruiz, M.D.

Chief, Department of Emergency Medicine
Hennepin County Medical Center
Minneapolis, Minnesota
Assistant Professor
Department of Surgery
University of Minnesota

McGRAW-HILL, INC. **Health Professions Division**

NEW YORK ST. LOUIS SAN FRANCISCO AUCKLAND BOGOTA CARACAS
LISBON LONDON MADRID MEXICO MILAN MONTREAL NEW DELHI
PARIS SAN JUAN SINGAPORE SYDNEY TOKYO TORONTO

EMERGENCY MEDICINE: A Comprehensive Study Guide

ISBN 0-07-004159-8

78910 KPKP 9987654

This book was set in Times Roman by Arcata Graphics/Kingsport; the editors were Edward M. Bolger and Peter McCurdy; the production supervisor was Richard Ruzycka; the cover was designed by N.S.G. Design; Alexandra Nickerson indexed the book.
Arcata Graphics/Halliday was printer and binder.

Library of Congress Cataloging-in-Publication Data

Emergency medicine : a comprehensive study guide / American College of Emergency Physicians ; editor-in-chief, Judith E. Tintinalli ; associate editors, Ronald L. Krome, Ernest Ruiz, —3rd ed.
p. cm.
Includes bibliographical references and index.
ISBN 0-07-004159-8
1. Emergency medicine. I. Tintinalli, Judith E. II. Krome, Ronald L. III. Ruiz, Ernest. IV. American College of Emergency Physicians.
[DNLM: 1. Emergencies. 2. Emergency Medicine. WB 105 E552]
RC86.7.E586 1992
616.85′27—dc20
DNLM/DLC
for Library of Congress

91-28013
CIP

CONTENTS

Contributors *xiii*
Preface *xxv*

Section 1 Resuscitative Problems and Techniques

1 Basic Cardiopulmonary Resuscitation *Raymond Jackson* *1*
2 The Ethics of Resuscitation *Timothy J. Crimmins* *4*
3 MAST *Scott Freeman* *6*
4 Cerebral Ischemia *Blaine C. White, Gary S. Krause* *8*
5 Advanced Airway Support *Daniel F. Danzl* *10*
6 Venous and Arterial Access *William A. Berk, Robert Dailey* *21*
7 Invasive Monitoring and Pacing Techniques *Scott Syverud* *27*
8 Acid-Base Problems *Robert F. Wilson* *35*
9 Blood Gases: Pathophysiology and Interpretation *Robert F. Wilson* *51*
10 Fluid and Electrolyte Problems *Robert F. Wilson* *62*
11 Disturbances of Cardiac Rhythm and Conduction *J. Stephan Stapczynski* *86*
12 Pharmacology of Antiarrhythmic and Vasoactive Medications *David B. Levy, Michael P. Peppers, Michael Ruffing* *109*
13 Life-Threatening Signs and Symptoms in Adults
A. Chest Pain *J. Stephan Stapczynski* *127*
B. Shock *Steven C. Dronen, Patrick Birrer* *132*
C. Cyanosis *Ann L. Harwood-Nuss, Christina Drummond* *140*
D. Syncope *Andrew Wilson* *141*
E. Abdominal Pain *David T. Overton* *144*
F. Gastrointestinal Bleeding *David T. Overton* *147*
G. Coma and Altered States of Consciousness *Gregory L. Henry* *150*
14 Life-Threatening Signs and Symptoms in Children
A. Fever *Carol D. Berkowitz* *159*
B. Fluid and Electrolyte Therapy *Deborah Lubitz, James Seidel* *161*
C. Vascular Access *William H. Spivey, Dee Hodge III* *166*
D. Neonatal Resuscitation and Emergencies *Seetha Shankaran, Eugene E. Cepeda* *171*
E. Pediatric Cardiopulmonary Resuscitation *Robert Luten* *177*
F. Upper Respiratory Emergencies *Nick Relich* *183*

Section 2 Emergency Medical Services

15 Emergency Medical Services *G. Patrick Lilja, Robert Swor* *189*
16 Disaster Medical Services *Brian D. Mahoney* *193*

Section 3 Cardiovascular Diseases

17 Myocardial Ischemia and Infarction *J. Stephan Stapczynski* *199*
18 Acute Interventions in Myocardial Infarction *Steven L. Almany, Cindy L. Grines, William W. O'Neill* *209*
19 Congestive Heart Failure and Pulmonary Edema *J. Stephan Stapczynski* *216*

20 Valvular Heart Disease *J. Stephan Stapczynski* 220
21 The Cardiomyopathies, Myocarditis, and Pericardial Disease *James T. Niemann* 227
22 Pulmonary Embolism *Robert S. Hockberger* 233
23 Hypertensive Emergencies *Raymond Jackson* 237
24 Thoracic and Abdominal Aortic Aneurysms *A. Joel Feldman* 247
25 Mesenteric Ischemia *John L. Glover, Geoffrey B. Blossom* 250
26 Peripheral Vascular Disease and Thrombophlebitis *A. Joel Feldman* 253
27 Cardiovascular Physiology of Aging *Michael Maddens* 257

Section 4 Pulmonary Emergencies

28 Bacterial Pneumonia *Georges C. Benjamin* 263
29 Viral and *Mycoplasma* Pneumonias in Adults *K. P. Ravikrishnan* 267
30 Legionnaires' Disease and *Pneumocystis* Pneumonia *Mark Zwanger* 271
31 Aspiration Pneumonia, Empyema, and Lung Abscess *Georges C. Benjamin* 276
32 Tuberculosis *K. P. Ravikrishnan* 279
33 Spontaneous and Iatrogenic Pneumothorax *Kimberlydawn Wisdom* 284
34 Permeability Pulmonary Edema and the Adult Respiratory Distress Syndrome *Marilyn T. Haupt, Richard W. Carlson* 287
35 Acute Asthma in Adults *Stanley Sherman* 290
36 Chronic Obstructive Pulmonary Disease *Joel C. Seidman* 298

Section 5 The Digestive System

37 Esophageal Emergencies *Richard E. Burney, James R. Mackenzie* 303
38 Swallowed Foreign Bodies *Wade R. Gaasch, Robert A. Barish* 310
39 Peptic Ulcer Disease *Ronald L. Krome* 313
40 Perforated Viscus *W. Kendall McNabney* 316
41 Acute Appendicitis *James A. Catto* 320
42 Intestinal Obstruction *John L. Glover* 322
43 Hernia *Ronald L. Krome* 326
44 Ileitis and Colitis *Howard A. Werman, Hagop S. Mekhjian, Douglas A. Rund* 328
45 Colonic Diverticular Disease *Stephen G. Priest, Steven N. Klein* 333
46 Anorectal Disorders *James K. Bouzoukis* 336
47 Diarrhea and Food Poisoning *James S. Seidel* 347
48 Cholecystitis *John L. Glover* 353
49 Acute Jaundice and Hepatitis *Richard Owen Shields, Jr.* 356
50 Acute Pancreatitis *Donald Weaver* 363
51 Complications of General Surgical Procedures *Geoffrey B. Blossom, John L. Glover* 366

Section 6 Renal and Genitourinary Disorders

52 Emergency Renal Problems *K. Venkateswara Rao* 371
53 Urinary Tract Infections *David S. Howes* 377
54 Male Genital Problems *Robert E. Schneider* 382

Section 7 Gynecology and Obstetrics

55 Gynecologic Emergencies *John R. Musich* 389
56 Vulvovaginitis *Gloria Kuhn* 395

57 Sexual Assault *Marion Hoelzer* 398
58 Toxic Shock Syndrome *Ann L. Harwood-Nuss, Christina Drummond* 403
59 Obstetric Emergencies *Robert P. Lorenz* 406
60 Blunt Abdominal Trauma during Pregnancy *Mark D. Pearlman* 414
61 Emergency Delivery *Paul T. von Oeyen* 418
62 Common Complications of Gynecologic Procedures *Veronica T. Mallett* 422

Section 8 Pediatrics

63 Common Neonatal Problems *Niranjan Kissoon* 425
64 The NICU Graduate *Daniel G. Batton* 431
65 Sudden Infant Death Syndrome *Carol D. Berkowitz* 434
66 Heart Disease *James H. McCrory* 437
67 Otitis and Pharyngitis *David M. Jaffe, Susan Fuchs* 440
68 Skin and Soft Tissue Infections *Gary R. Fleisher* 446
69 Bacteremia, Sepsis, and Meningitis *Joseph A. Zeccardi* 454
70 Viral and Bacterial Pneumonias *Duane D. Harrison* 457
71 Urinary Tract Infections and Vulvovaginitis *Denise J. Fligner* 462
72 Asthma and Bronchiolitis *Stanley H. Inkelis* 466
73 Reye's Syndrome *Carol D. Berkowitz* 475
74 Seizures and Status Epilepticus in Children *Michael A. Nigro* 479
75 Gastroenteritis *Ronald D. Holmes, William M. Belknap* 488
76 Abdominal Emergencies *Robert W. Schafermeyer* 491
77 Child Abuse *Carol D. Berkowitz* 498
78 The Diabetic Child *David A. Poleski* 502
79 Pediatric Exanthems *Michael S. Weinstock, Michael S. Catapano* 505
80 Pediatric Analgesia and Sedation *Roy M. Kulick, Elaine S. Pomeranz* 511

Section 9 Infectious Diseases

81 Sexually Transmitted Diseases *David Nolan* 517
82 HIV Infection and AIDS *Catherine A. Marco* 519
83 Tetanus *Donna L. Carden* 525
84 Rabies *Louis S. Binder* 527
85 Malaria *Jeffrey D. Band* 530
86 Common Parasitic Infections *Harold Osborn* 535
87 Tick-Borne Disease *Bruce S. Auerbach* 540

Section 10 Toxicology

88 General Management of the Poisoned Patient *Michael V. Vance* 545
89 Cyclic Antidepressant Overdose *Michael Callaham* 551
90 Neuroleptics *William P. Kerns II* 555
91 Lithium *P. J. Ryan* 559
92 Barbiturates *P. J. Ryan* 561
93 Phenytoin Toxicity *Brad S. Selden* 563
94 Narcotics *George L. Sternbach* 566

95 Clonidine *E. Martin Caravati* 570
96 Alcohols *William K. Chiang* 572
97 Cocaine *Susi Vassallo* 579
98 Amphetamines and Amphetamine-like Drugs *Donald B. Kunkel* 582
99 Hallucinogens *Robert S. Hoffman* 584
100 Salicylates *Steven C. Curry* 589
101 Acetaminophen Poisoning *Christopher H. Linden, Barry H. Rumack* 593
102 Iron *Steven C. Curry* 598
103 Hydrocarbons *Paul M. Wax* 601
104 Caustic Ingestions *Robert Knopp* 606
105 Organophosphate and Carbamate Poisoning *John Tafuri, James Roberts* 609
106 Theophylline *Charles L. Emerman* 614
107 Digitalis Glycosides *Mark A. Kirk* 617
108 Beta Blockers and Calcium Channel Blockers *Peter Viccellio, Mark Henry* 620
109 Benzodiazepines *George M. Bosse* 624
110 Nonsteroidal Antiinflammatory Agents *Richard F. Clark* 626
111 Cyanide *Kathleen Delaney* 631
112 Anticholinergic Toxicity *Leslie R. Wolf* 636
113 Heavy Metals *Marsha D. Ford* 638

Section 11 Environmental Injuries

114 Frostbite *Barry Heller* 645
115 Hypothermia *Howard A. Bessen* 648
116 Heat Emergencies *Michael V. Vance* 652
117 Insect and Spider Bites *Claude Frazier* 655
118 Reptile Bites and Scorpion Stings *George Podgorny* 660
119 Trauma and Envenomations from Marine Fauna *Paul S. Auerbach* 666
120 High Altitude Medical Problems *Peter H. Hackett* 670
121 Dysbarism *Kenneth W. Kizer* 678
122 Near Drowning *Bruce E. Haynes* 688
123 Burns and Electrical Injuries *Alan R. Dimick* 691
124 Chemical Burns *Marcus L. Martin, Fred P. Harchelroad, Jr.* 695
125 Lightning Injuries *Mary Ann Cooper* 701
126 Carbon Monoxide Poisoning *Earl J. Reisdorff, John G. Wiegenstein* 703
127 Acute Exposure to Toxic Agents *Constance J. Doyle* 707
128 Radiation Injuries *H. Arnold Muller* 711
129 Mushroom Poisoning *Christopher H. Linden, Barry H. Rumack* 716
130 Poisonous Plants *David C. Michener, Rodger Keller, Robert F. Kowalski* 721

Section 12 Endocrine Emergencies

131 Hypoglycemia *Gene Ragland* 727
132 Diabetic Ketoacidosis *Gene Ragland* 735
133 Alcoholic Ketoacidosis *Gene Ragland* 740
134 Nonketotic Hyperosmolar Coma *Gene Ragland* 743
135 Lactic Acidosis *Gene Ragland* 747
136 Thyroid Storm *Gene Ragland* 752
137 Hypothyroidism and Myxedema Coma *Gene Ragland* 755
138 Adrenal Insufficiency and Adrenal Crisis *Gene Ragland* 759

Section 13 Hematologic and Oncologic Emergencies

139 Approach to the Bleeding Patient *Daniel Esposito* 765
140 Acquired Bleeding Disorders *Daniel Esposito* 768
141 Hemophilia *Ronald Sacher* 770
142 Sickle Cell Anemia *Daniel Esposito* 773
143 Blood Transfusion—Components and Practices *Steven J. Davidson* 775
144 Emergency Complications of Malignancy *Daniel Esposito* 780

Section 14 Neurology

145 The Neurological Examination *Gregory L. Henry* 785
146 Headache *Gwendolyn L. Hoffman* 789
147 Stroke Syndromes and Lateralized Deficits *Gregory L. Henry* 793
148 Vertigo and Dizziness *Neal Little* 799
149 Seizures and Status Epilepticus in Adults *Thomas R. Pellegrino* 804
150 Acute Peripheral Neurological Lesions *Gregory L. Henry* 811
151 Demyelinating Diseases *Richard F. Edlich* 817
152 Disorders of Neuromuscular Transmission *Lawrence H. Phillips II, Richard F. Edlich* 822
153 Meningitis, Encephalitis, and Brain Abscess *Charles Rennie III* 827

Section 15 Eye, Ear, Nose, Throat, and Oral Surgery

154 Ocular Emergencies *Roland Clark* 833
155 Otolaryngologic Emergencies in Adults *Frank I. Marlowe* 841
156 Nasal Emergencies and Sinusitis *Frank I. Marlowe* 846
157 Maxillofacial Fractures *Barry H. Hendler* 850
158 General Dental Emergencies *James T. Amsterdam* 860

Section 16 Skin and Soft Tissue Emergencies

159 Toxicodendron Dermatitis *Thomas A. Chapel* 867
160 Exfoliative Dermatitis *Thomas A. Chapel* 869
161 Erythema Multiforme *Thomas A. Chapel* 870
162 Toxic Epidermal Necrolysis *Thomas A. Chapel* 873
163 Cutaneous Abscesses *Harvey W. Meislin* 875
164 Soft Tissue Infections *J. Stephan Stapczynski* 879

Section 17 Rheumatology and Allergy

165 Musculoskeletal Disorders in Adults and Children *Mary Chester Morgan, Carol Godoshian Ragsdale* 883
166 Neck Pain *Myron M. LaBan* 891
167 Thoracic and Lumbar Pain Syndromes *Myron M. LaBan* 896
168 Anaphylaxis and Acute Allergic Reactions *Joseph A. Salomone* 901

Section 18 Trauma

169 Initial Approach to the Trauma Patient *Ernest Ruiz* 905
170 Pediatric Trauma *Gary C. Fifield* 910
171 Head Injury *Gaylan L. Rockswold* 913
172 Spinal Injuries *Brian D. Mahoney* 922
173 Penetrating and Blunt Neck Trauma *Robert Swor* 928
174 Thoracic Trauma *Robert F. Wilson* 932
175 Abdominal Trauma *Arthur L. Ney, Robert C. Andersen* 955
176 Penetrating Trauma to the Posterior Abdomen and Buttock *Mark D. Odland, Arthur L. Ney* 962
177 Trauma to the Genitourinary Tract *Joe Y. Lee, Alexander S. Cass* 964
178 Basic Management of Fractures and Dislocations *Joseph F. Waeckerle* 967
179 Injuries and Infections of the Wrist and Hand *Robert R. Simon* 972
180 Upper Extremity Trauma *John W. Packer* 981
181 Trauma to the Pelvis, Hips, and Femur *Joseph F. Waeckerle, Mark T. Steele* 987
182 Knee Injuries *Joseph F. Waeckerle* 999
183 Leg Injuries *Joseph F. Waeckerle, Mark T. Steele* 1004
184 Ankle Injuries *Joseph F. Waeckerle, Mark T. Steele* 1007
185 Foot Injuries *Joseph F. Waeckerle* 1012
186 Compartment Syndromes *Robert R. Simon, Ernest Ruiz* 1015
187 Wound Ballistics *Jeremy J. Hollerman, Martin L. Fackler* 1019

Section 19 Emergency Wound Management

188 The Evaluation of Wounds in the Emergency Department *Richard F. Edlich, George T. Rodeheaver, John G. Thacker* 1027
189 Local and Regional Anesthesia for Wound Repair *Richard F. Edlich, George T. Rodeheaver, John G. Thacker* 1031
190 Wound Preparation *Richard F. Edlich, George T. Rodeheaver, John G. Thacker* 1037
191 Antibiotics and Drains in Wound Management *Richard F. Edlich, George T. Rodeheaver, John G. Thacker* 1040
192 Puncture Wounds and Mammalian Bites *George Podgorny* 1043
193 Wound Closure *Richard F. Edlich, George T. Rodeheaver, John G. Thacker* 1045
194 Postoperative Wound Care and Tetanus Prophylaxis *Richard F. Edlich, George T. Rodeheaver, John G. Thacker* 1049
195 Soft Tissue Injuries to the Face *Richard F. Edlich* 1052
196 Fingertip Injuries *Richard F. Edlich, Raymond F. Morgan* 1061

Section 20 Behavioral Emergencies

197 Behavioral Disorders: Clinical Features *Stephen C. Olson, Douglas A. Rund* 1067
198 Behavioral Disorders: Emergency Assessment and Stabilization *Jeffrey A. Coffman, Douglas A. Rund* 1074
199 Psychotrophic Medications *Kathy E. Shy, Douglas A. Rund* 1080
200 Anorexia Nervosa and Bulimia Nervosa *Alexander H. Sackeyfio, Susan J. Gottlieb* 1085
201 Panic Disorder *Suck Won Kim* 1088
202 Conversion Reactions *Gregory P. Moore, Kenneth C. Jackimczyk* 1090
203 Crisis Intervention *Zigfrids T. Stelmachers* 1092

Section 21 Emergencies in the Disabled Patient

204 Injury in the Elderly and Elder Abuse *John F. Brown, Daniel W. Spaite* *1097*

205 Assessment of the Neurologically Impaired Patient *David C. Anderson* *1100*

Section 22 The High Technology Patient

206 Patients with Organ Transplants *Leslie Rocher* *1103*

207 Complications of Common Medical Devices *Robert A. Rusnak* *1107*

Section 23 Newer Imaging Modalities

208 Noninvasive Vascular Studies *Phillip J. Bendick* *1113*

209 Emergency Use of Pelvic Ultrasonography *Christine Comstock* *1115*

210 Emergency Applications of Abdominal Sonography *Beatrice L. Madrazo* *1120*

211 Cardiac Ultrasound in the Emergency Department *Andrew M. Hauser* *1123*

212 Computed Tomography *Jeremy J. Hollerman* *1126*

Index *1137*

A-a - alveolar arterial gradient

$A\text{-}a = 150 - (PaO_2 + PaCO_2)$ - Room air

$A\text{-}a = (700)(FIO_2 - (PaO_2 + PaCO_2)$ - O oxygen

FIO_2 - fraction of O_2 in inspired air

Normal - 10-15 mmHg

CONTRIBUTORS

Steven L. Almany, M.D. [*18*]
Department of Medicine
Division of Cardiology
William Beaumont Hospital
Royal Oak, Michigan

James T. Amsterdam, D.M.D., M.D. [*158*]
Chairman, Department of Emergency Medicine
Western Reserve Care System
Northside Medical Center
Youngstown, Ohio

Robert C. Andersen, M.D. [*175*]
Associate Professor of Surgery
University of Minnesota School of Medicine;
Head, Renal Transplant Service
Hennepin County Medical Center
Minneapolis, Minnesota

David C. Anderson, M.D. [*205*]
Department of Neurology
Hennepin County Medical Center
Minneapolis, Minnesota

Bruce S. Auerbach, M.D. [*87*]
Vice President and Chief, Emergency and Ambulatory Services
Sturdy Memorial Hospital
Attleboro, Massachusetts;
Assistant Clinical Professor
Department of Community Medicine
Tufts University Medical School
Boston, Massachusetts;
Clinical Instructor, Department of Medicine
Division of Emergency Medicine
University of Massachusetts Medical School
Wooster, Massachusetts

Paul S. Auerbach, M.D., M.S. [*119*]
Chief, Division of Emergency Medicine
Vanderbilt University
Nashville, Tennessee

Jeffrey D. Band, M.D. [*85*]
Chief, Division of Infectious Diseases and International Medicine
William Beaumont Hospital
Royal Oak, Michigan;
Associate Clinical Professor of Medicine
Wayne State University School of Medicine
Detroit, Michigan

The numbers in brackets following the contributors' names refer to the chapters written or co-written by the contributor.

Robert A. Barish, M.D. [*38*]
Director, Emergency Medical Services
University of Maryland Medical System/Hospital;
Assistant Professor of Surgery and Medicine
Division of Emergency Medicine
Department of Surgery
University of Maryland School of Medicine
Baltimore, Maryland

Daniel G. Batton, M.D. [*64*]
Director of Newborn Medicine
Department of Pediatrics
William Beaumont Hospital
Royal Oak, Michigan

William M. Belknap, M.D. [*75*]
Staff Physician, Pediatric Gastroenterologist
William Beaumont Hospital;
Teaching Attendant, Pediatric Gastroenterologist
Hurley Hospital/Michigan State University
Flint, Michigan

Phillip J. Bendick, Ph.D. [*208*]
Director, Peripheral Vascular Diagnostic Center
William Beaumont Hospital
Royal Oak, Michigan

Georges C. Benjamin, M.D. [*28, 31*]
Acting Commissioner of Public Health
District of Columbia;
Assistant Professor of Medicine
Howard University
Washington, D.C.;
Associate Professor of Military Medicine
Uniformed Services University of the Health Sciences
Bethesda, Maryland;
Clinical Instructor of Emergency Medicine
Georgetown University
Washington, D.C.

William A. Berk, M.D. [*6*]
Assistant Professor, Department of Emergency Medicine
Wayne State University;
Attending Physician, Department of Emergency Medicine
Detroit Receiving Hospital/University Health Center
Detroit, Michigan

Carol D. Berkowitz, M.D. [*14A, 65, 73, 77*]
Acting Chair, Department of Pediatrics
Harbor-UCLA Medical Center;
Professor of Clinical Pediatrics
UCLA School of Medicine
Los Angeles, California

Howard A. Bessen, M.D. [*115*]
Residency Director, Department of Emergency Medicine
Harbor-UCLA Medical Center
Torrance, California;
Associate Clinical Professor of Medicine, UCLA School of Medicine
Los Angeles, California

Louis S. Binder, M.D. [*84*]
Assistant Professor, Department of Emergency Medicine
Texas Tech University Health Sciences Center
El Paso, Texas

Patrick Birrer, M.D. [*13B*]
Department of Emergency Medicine
University of Cincinnati Medical Center
Cincinnati, Ohio

Geoffrey B. Blossom, M.D. [*25, 51*]
Department of Surgery
William Beaumont Hospital
Royal Oak, Michigan

George M. Bosse, M.D. [*109*]
Assistant Professor of Emergency Medicine
University of Louisville School of Medicine
Louisville, Kentucky

James K. Bouzoukis, M.D. [*46*]
Department of Emergency Medicine
Medical Center of Delaware
Wilmington, Delaware

John F. Brown, M.D. [*204*]
Arizona Emergency Medicine Research Center
University of Arizona College of Medicine
Tucson, Arizona

Richard E. Burney, M.D. [*37*]
Acting Chief, Emergency Services
Associate Professor of Surgery
University of Michigan Medical Center
Ann Arbor, Michigan

Michael Callaham, M.D. [*89*]
Professor of Medicine
Division Chief, Emergency Medicine
The Medical Center at the University of California
San Francisco, California

E. Martin Caravati, M.D. [*95*]
Assistant Professor, Division of Emergency Medicine
Department of Surgery
University of Utah School of Medicine;
Associate Medical Director,
Intermountain Regional Poison Control Center
Salt Lake City, Utah

Donna L. Carden, M.D. [*83*]
Department of Physiology and Biophysics
Louisiana State University Medical Center
Shreveport, Louisiana

Richard W. Carlson, M.D. [*34*]
Professor of Medicine
Wayne State University School of Medicine
Detroit, Michigan

Alexander S. Cass, M.B.B.S. [*177*]
Associate Professor, Urologic Surgery
University of Minnesota School of Medicine;
Head, Division of Urology
Hennepin County Medical Center
Minneapolis, Minnesota

Michael S. Catapano, M.D. [*79*]
Assistant Director, Emergency Medical Services
North Shore University Hospital;
Clinical Instructor, Department of Surgery
Cornell University Medical College
Manhasset, New York

James A. Catto, M.D. [*41*]
Department of Surgery
William Beaumont Medical Center
Royal Oak, Michigan

Eugene E. Cepeda, M.D. [*14D*]
Associate Neonatologist
St. John Hospital
Detroit, Michigan

Thomas A. Chapel, M.D. [*159–162*]
Clinical Professor of Dermatology
Wayne State University
Dearborn, Michigan

William K. Chiang, M.D. [*96*]
Clinical Instructor, Department of Surgery/Emergency Medicine
Bellevue Hospital Center
New York University School of Medicine;
Medical Consultant
New York City Poison Control Center
New York, New York

Roland Clark, M.D. [*154*]
Medical Director, Emergency Department
Santa Monica Medical Center
Santa Monica, California

Richard F. Clark, M.D. [*110*]
Department of Medical Toxicology
Good Samaritan Regional Medical Center
Phoenix, Arizona

Jeffrey A. Coffman, M.D. [*198*]
Department of Psychiatry
Veterans Administration Hospital
Lincoln, Nebraska

Christine Comstock, M.D. [*209*]
Assistant Professor, Obstetrics and Gynecology
Wayne State University School of Medicine;
Division of Fetal Imaging
William Beaumont Hospital
Royal Oak, Michigan

Mary Ann Cooper, M.D. [*125*]
Assistant Professor, Division of Surgery (Emergency Medicine)
University of Illinois
Chicago, Illinois

Timothy J. Crimmins, M.D. [*2*]
Department of Emergency Medicine
Hennepin County Medical Center
Minneapolis, Minnesota

Steven C. Curry, M.D. [*100, 102*]
Department of Medical Toxicology
Good Samaritan Medical Center
Phoenix, Arizona

Robert H. Dailey, M.D. [*6*]
Clinical Professor of Medicine
University of California at San Francisco;
Chief, Emergency Medicine
Highland Hospital
Oakland, California

Daniel F. Danzl, M.D. [*5*]
Professor and Chairman, Department of Emergency Medicine
University of Louisville School of Medicine
Louisville, Kentucky

Steven J. Davidson, M.D. [*143*]
Associate Professor of Emergency Medicine
Medical College of Pennsylvania
Philadelphia, Pennsylvania

Kathleen Delaney, M.D. [*111*]
Department of Surgery/Emergency Medicine
University of Texas/SW Medical School
Dallas, Texas

Alan R. Dimick, M.D. [*123*]
Professor of Surgery
Director, Burn Center
Division of General Surgery/Section of Burns and Trauma
The University of Alabama at Birmingham
Birmingham, Alabama

Constance J. Doyle, M.D. [*127*]
Clinical Instructor, Emergency Services
University of Michigan Medical Center;
Emergency Department
Foote Hospital
Jackson, Michigan

Steven C. Dronen, M.D. [*13B*]
Associate Professor, Department of Emergency Medicine
University of Cincinnati Medical Center
Cincinnati, Ohio

Christina Drummond, M.D. [*13C, 58*]
Division of Emergency Medicine
University Medical Center
Jacksonville, Florida

Richard F. Edlich, M.D. [*151, 152, 188–191, 193–196*]
Distinguished Professor of Plastic Surgery and Biomedical Engineering
Department of Plastic Surgery
University of Virginia School of Medicine
Charlottesville, Virginia

Charles L. Emerman, M.D. [*106*]
Director, Emergency Medicine
MetroHealth Medical Center
Cleveland, Ohio

Daniel Esposito, M.D. [*139, 140, 142, 144*]
Assistant Clinical Professor of Medicine
Georgetown University School of Medicine
Washington, D.C.

Martin L. Fackler, M.D. [*187*]
Director, Wound Ballistics Laboratory
Military Trauma Research
Letterman Army Institute of Research
San Francisco, California

A. Joel Feldman, M.D. [*24, 26*]
Department of Vascular Surgery, St. Vincent Hospital and Health Care Center
Indianapolis, Indiana

Gary C. Fifield, M.D. [*170*]
Assistant Professor of Pediatrics
University of Minnesota School of Medicine;
Department of Pediatrics and Emergency Medicine
Hennepin County Medical Center
Minneapolis, Minnesota

Gary R. Fleisher, M.D. [*68*]
Chief, Division of Emergency Medicine
Department of Medicine
Children's Hospital;
Associate Professor of Pediatrics
Department of Pediatrics
Harvard Medical School
Boston, Massachusetts

Denise J. Fligner, M.D. [*71*]
Assistant Professor, Department of Family Practice
Rush Medical College
Chicago, Illinois;
Research Director, Department of Emergency Medicine
Christ Hospital and Medical Center
Oak Lawn, Illionis

Marsha D. Ford, M.D. [*113*]
Director, Division of Toxicology;
Assistant Chairman, Department of Emergency Medicine
Carolinas Medical Center
Charlotte, North Carolina

Claude Frazier, M.D. [*117*]
Private Practice of Allergy and Immunology
Asheville, North Carolina

Scott Freeman, M.D. [*3*]
Assistant Professor, Emergency Medicine
Wayne State University School of Medicine;
Program Director, Emergency Medicine Residency
Detroit Receiving Hospital
Detroit, Michigan

Susan Fuchs, M.D. [*67*]
Emergency Department
Children's Hospital of Pittsburgh;
Assistant Professor of Pediatrics
University of Pittsburgh School of Medicine
Pittsburgh, Pennsylvania

Wade R. Gaasch, M.D. [*38*]
Clinical Instructor, Division of Emergency Medicine
Department of Surgery
University of Maryland School of Medicine
Baltimore, Maryland

John L. Glover, M.D. [*25, 42, 48, 51*]
Department of Surgery
William Beaumont Hospital
Royal Oak, Michigan

Susan J. Gottlieb, M.A. [*200*]
Department of Psychiatry
William Beaumont Hospital
Royal Oak, Michigan

Cindy L. Grines, M.D. [*18*]
Department of Medicine
Division of Cardiology
William Beaumont Hospital
Royal Oak, Michigan

Peter H. Hackett, M.D. [*120*]
Affiliate Associate Professor, College of Health Sciences
University of Alaska;
Affiliate Associate Professor
Department of Medicine
University of Washington School of Medicine
Seattle, Washington;
Director, Air Ambulance and Staff Physician
Emergency Department
Humana Hospital
Anchorage, Alaska

Fred P. Harchelroad, Jr., M.D. [*124*]
Director, Quality Assurance and Research
Assistant Professor, Emergency Medicine
Medical College of Pennsylvania—Allegheny Campus
Allegheny General Hospital
Pittsburgh, Pennsylvania

Duane D. Harrison, M.D. [*70*]
Chief, Pediatric Infectious Diseases
Medical Director, Pediatric Intensive Care Unit
Department of Pediatrics
William Beaumont Hospital
Royal Oak, Michigan

Ann L. Harwood-Nuss, M.D. [*13C, 58*]
Associate Professor, Division of Emergency Medicine
University of Florida
Health Science Center
Jacksonville, Florida

Marilyn T. Haupt, M.D. [*34*]
Assistant Professor of Medicine
Wayne State University School of Medicine;
Director, Medical Intensive Care Unit
Detroit Receiving Hospital
Detroit, Michigan

Andrew M. Hauser, M.D. [*211*]
Director, Cardiac Ultrasound Laboratory
William Beaumont Hospital
Royal Oak, Michigan

Bruce E. Haynes, M.D. [*122*]
Director, EMS Authority
State of California
Sacramento, California

Barry Heller, M.D. [*114*]
Emergency Department
St. Mary's Medical Center
Long Beach, California

Barry H. Hendler, M.D., D.D.S. [*157*]
Director, Post Graduate Oral and Maxillofacial Surgery
University of Pennsylvania School of Dental Medicine and Affiliated Hospitals;
Director of Oral and Maxillofacial Surgery;
Clinical Professor of Medicine and Surgery
Medical College of Pennsylvania
Philadelphia, Pennsylvania

Gregory L. Henry, M.D. [*13G, 145, 147, 150*]
Clinical Assistant Professor, Section of Emergency Medicine
University of Michigan Medical Center;
Chief, Department of Emergency Medicine
Beyer Memorial Hospital
Ypsilanti, Michigan;
Vice President, Emergency Physicians Medical Group
Ann Arbor, Michigan

Mark Henry, M.D. [*108*]
Department of Emergency Medicine
School of Medicine
SUNY at Stony Brook
Stony Brook, New York

Robert S. Hockberger, M.D. [*22, 59*]
Associate Clinical Professor, Emergency Medicine
UCLA School of Medicine;
Chairman, Department of Emergency Medicine
Harbor-UCLA Medical Center
Torrance, California

Dee Hodge III, M.D. [*14C*]
Assistant Professor of Pediatrics and Emergency Medicine
UCLA Medical School;
Director of Pediatric Emergency Medicine
Children's Hospital of Los Angeles
Los Angeles, California

Marion Hoelzer, M.D. [*57*]
Attending Physician, Department of Emergency Medicine
William Beaumont Hospital
Royal Oak, Michigan

Gwendolyn L. Hoffman, M.D. [*146*]
Assistant Professor of Medicine
Michigan State University College of Human Medicine
Ann Arbor, Michigan;
Program Director, Emergency Medicine
Butterworth Hospital
Grand Rapids, Michigan

Robert S. Hoffman, M.D. [*99*]
Associate Medical Director
New York City Poison Control Center;
Clinical Instructor
Department of Surgery/Emergency Medicine
New York University School of Medicine;
Attending Physician
Department of Emergency Medical Services
Bellevue Hospital Center
New York, New York

Jeremy J. Hollerman, M.D. [*187, 212*]
Department of Medical Imaging
Hennepin County Medical Center;
Assistant Professor of Radiology
University of Minnesota
Minneapolis, Minnesota

Ronald D. Holmes, M.D. [*75*]
Department of Pediatrics
University of Michigan Medical Center
Ann Arbor, Michigan

David S. Howes, M.D. [*53*]
Residency Program Director
University of Chicago
Emergency Medicine Residency;
Assistant Professor of Medicine
University of Chicago
Chicago, Illinois

Stanley H. Inkelis, M.D. [*72*]
Associate Director, Pediatric Emergency Medicine
Harbor-UCLA Medical Center
Torrance, California

Kenneth C. Jackimczyk, M.D. [*202*]
Director, Emergency Medicine Residency
Maricopa Medical Center
Phoeniz, Arizona

Raymond Jackson, M.D. [*1, 23*]
Chief, Emergency Medicine
South Chicago Hospital
Chicago, Illinois

David M. Jaffe, M.D. [*67*]
Director, Division of Emergency Medicine
St. Louis Children's Hospital;
Associate Professor of Pediatrics
Washington University School of Medicine
St. Louis, Missouri

Rodger Keller, Ph.D. [*130*]
Horticulturist, Matthaei Botanical Gardens
University of Michigan
Ann Arbor, Michigan

William P. Kerns II, M.D. [*90*]
Clinical Instructor
Department of Emergency Medicine
Carolinas Medical Center
Charlotte, North Carolina

Suck Won Kim, M.D. [*201*]
Assistant Professor, Department of Psychiatry
University of Minnesota and Hennepin County Medical Center
Minneapolis, Minnesota

Mark A. Kirk, M.D. [*107*]
Division of Clinical Toxicology
Department of Emergency Medicine
Carolinas Medical Center
Charlotte, North Carolina

Niranjan Kissoon, M.D. [*63*]
Director, Pediatric Emergency Department
Staff Physician, Pediatric Critical Care Unit
Children's Hospital of Western Ontario;
Associate Professor of Pediatrics
University of Western Ontario
London, Ontario, Canada

Kenneth W. Kizer, M.D., M.P.H. [*121*]
Chairman, Department of Community Health
University of California at Davis
Davis, California

Steven N. Klein, M.D. [*45*]
Staff Physician, Department of Surgery, William Beaumont Hospital
Royal Oak, Michigan

Robert Knopp, M.D. [*104*]
Associate Clinical Professor of Medicine
University of California, San Francisco, School of Medicine;
Chief, Emergency Department
Valley Medical Center
Fresno, California

Robert F. Kowalski, M.D. [*130*]
Department of Emergency Medicine
William Beaumont Hospital
Royal Oak, Michigan

Gary S. Krause, M.D. [*4*]
Assistant Professor
Department of Emergency Medicine
Wayne State University School of Medicine
Detroit, Michigan

Ronald L. Krome, M.D. [*39, 43*]
Visiting Professor, Division of Emergency Health Services
Department of Surgery
University of Michigan Medical School
Ann Arbor, Michigan;
Chief, Department of Emergency Medicine
William Beaumont Hospital
Royal Oak, Michigan

Gloria Kuhn, D.O [*56*]
Program Director, W.S.U./B.M.C./Grace Hospital
Emergency Medicine Residency Program;
Assistant Professor of Emergency Medicine
Wayne State University
Detroit, Michigan

Roy M. Kulick, M.D., M.S. [*80*]
Assistant Professor of Pediatrics
University of Cincinnati School of Medicine;
Associate Director, Division of Emergency Medicine
Children's Hospital Medical Center
Cincinnati, Ohio

Donald B. Kunkel, M.D. [*98*]
Medical Director, Department of Medical Toxicology
Good Samaritan Medical Center
Phoenix, Arizona

Myron M. LaBan, M.D. [*166, 167*]
Director, Department of Physical Medicine and Rehabilitation
William Beaumont Hospital
Royal Oak, Michigan

Joe Y. Lee, M.D. [*177*]
Division of Urology
Hennepin County Medical Center
Minneapolis, Minnesota

David B. Levy, Pharm.D. [*12*]
Clinical Specialist—Emergency Care
Department of Pharmacy Services
Detroit Receiving Hospital and University Health Center
Detroit, Michigan

G. Patrick Lilja, M.D. [*15*]
Clinical Assistant Professor
University of Minnesota School of Medicine;
Director, Emergency Department
North Memorial Medical Center
Minneapolis, Minnesota

Christopher H. Linden, M.D. [*101, 129*]
Assistant Professor of Medicine
Department of Medicine
University of Massachusetts Medical Center;
Director, Regional Poisoning Treatment Center

Neal Little, M.D. [*148*]
Clinical Instructor
Department of Surgery
University of Michigan Medical School;
Attending Emergency Physician
St. Joseph Mercy Hospital
Ann Arbor, Michigan

Robert P. Lorenz, M.D. [*59*]
Assistant Professor, Department of Obstetrics and Gynecology
Wayne State University School of Medicine;
Director, Division of Maternal-Fetal Medicine
Department of Obstetrics and Gynecology
William Beaumont Hospital
Royal Oak, Michigan

Deborah Lubitz, M.D. [*14B*]
Division of Pediatric Emergency Medicine
Rainbow Babies and Children's Hospital
Cleveland, Ohio

Robert Luten, M.D. [*14E*]
Assistant Professor, University of Florida;
Department of Emergency Medicine
University Hospital of Jacksonville
Jacksonville, Florida

James R. Mackenzie, M.D. [*37*]
Northville, Michigan

Michael E. Maddens, M.D. [*27*]
Division of Geriatric Medicine
William Beaumont Hospital
Royal Oak, Michigan

Beatrice L. Madrazo, M.D. [*210*]
Head, Section of Diagnostic Ultrasound
William Beaumont Hospital
Royal Oak, Michigan

Brian D. Mahoney, M.D. [*16, 172*]
Department of Emergency Medicine
Hennepin County Medical Center
Minneapolis, Minnesota

Veronica T. Mallett, M.D. [*62*]
Department of Obstetrics and Gynecology
Hutzel Hospital
The Detroit Medical Center
Detroit, Michigan

Catherine A. Marco, M.D. [*82*]
Instructor of Emergency Medicine
Department of Emergency Medicine
The Johns Hopkins Hospital and School of Medicine;
Attending Physician, Emergency Medicine
Francis Scott Key Medical Center
Baltimore, Maryland

Frank I. Marlowe, M.D. [*155, 156*]
Professor and Chief, Department of Otolaryngology
Medical College of Pennsylvania
Philadelphia, Pennsylvania

Marcus L. Martin, M.D. [*124*]
Emergency Medicine Residency Director;
Associate Professor, Emergency Medicine
Medical College of Pennsylvania—Allegheny Campus
Allegheny General Hospital
Pittsburgh, Pennsylvania

James H. McCrory, M.D. [*66*]
Pediatric Critical Care Center
St. John's Regional Health Center
Springfield, Missouri

W. Kendall McNabney, M.D. [*40*]
Director of Trauma Services, Truman Medical Center;
Professor and Assistant Dean for Clinical Affairs
University of Missouri—Kansas City School of Medicine
Kansas City, Missouri

Harvey W. Meislin, M.D. [*163*]
Chief, Section of Emergency Medicine
Professor, Department of Surgery
University of Arizona Health Sciences Center
Tucson, Arizona

Hagop S. Mekhjian, M.D. [*44*]
Professor of Medicine
Ohio State University School of Medicine
Medical Director and Associate Dean for Clinical Affairs
Ohio State University Hospital

David C. Michener, Ph.D. [*130*]
Assistant Curator, Matthaei Botanical Gardens
University of Michigan
Ann Arbor, Michigan

Gregory P. Moore, M.D. [*202*]
Associate Director, Emergency Medicine Residency
Maricopa Medical Center
Phoeniz, Arizona

Mary Chester Morgan, M.D. [*165*]
Division of Rheumatology
Department of Internal Medicine
University of Pittsburgh
Pittsburgh, Pennsylvania

Raymond F. Morgan [*196*]
Professor and Chairman, Department of Plastic Surgery;
Professor of Orthopaedic Surgery
University of Virginia School of Medicine
Charlottesville, Virginia

H. Arnold Muller, M.D. [*128*]
Professor of Medicine
Emergency Medicine Division
Medical College of the Pennsylvania State University
Hershey, Pennsylvania

John R. Musich, M.D. [*55*]
Clinical Associate Professor of Obstetrics and Gynecology
Wayne State University School of Medicine;
Chairman, Department of Obstetrics and Gynecology
William Beaumont Hospital
Royal Oak, Michigan

Arthur L. Ney, M.D. [*175, 176*]
Department of Surgery
Hennepin County Medical Center
Minneapolis, Minnesota

James T. Niemann, M.D. [*21*]
Director of Research, Department of Emergency Medicine
Harbor-UCLA Medical Center
Torrance, California

Michael A. Nigro, D.O. [*74*]
Associate Professor, Departments of Pediatrics and Neurology
Wayne State University School of Medicine;
Chief, Division of Neurology
Children's Hospital of Michigan
Detroit, Michigan

David Nolan, M.D. [*81*]
Medical Director, Western Michigan Associated Health Departments
Big Rapids, Michigan

Mark D. Odland, M.D. [*176*]
Department of Surgery
Hennepin County Medical Center
Minneapolis, Minnesota

Paul T. von Oeyen, M.D. [*61*]
Assistant Professor, Obstetrics and Gynecology
Wayne State University School of Medicine;
Assistant Director, Maternal-Fetal Medicine
Department of Obstetrics and Gynecology
William Beaumont Hospital
Royal Oak, Michigan

Stephen C. Olson, M.D. [*197*]
Assistant Professor of Psychiatry
Ohio State University School of Medicine
Columbus, Ohio

William W. O'Neill, M.D. [*18*]
Department of Medicine
Division of Cardiology
William Beaumont Hospital
Royal Oak, Michigan

Harold Osborn, M.D. [*86*]
Director, Department of Emergency Medicine;
Professor, Clinical and Community Preventive Medicine
New York Medical College
Bronx, New York

David T. Overton, M.D. [*13E, 13F*]
Assistant Research Director
Department of Emergency Medicine
William Beaumont Hospital
Royal Oak, Michigan

John W. Packer [*180*]
Associate Professor of Surgery (Orthopaedics)
University of North Carolina School of Medicine, Chapel Hill;
Co-Director, Orthopaedic Residency Program
Wake Medical Center
Raleigh, North Carolina

Mark D. Pearlman, M.D. [*60*]
University of Michigan Medical Center
Department of Obstetrics & Gynecology
Ann Arbor, Michigan

Thomas R. Pellegrino, M.D. [*149*]
Professor and Chairman, Department of Neurology
Eastern Virginia Medical School
Norfolk, Virginia

Michael P. Peppers, Pharm. D. [*12*]
Clinical Coordinator
Mineral Area Regional Medical Center
Farmington, Missouri

Lawrence H. Phillips II, M.D. [*152*]
Associate Professor of Neurology
University of Virginia Health Sciences Center
Charlottesville, Virginia

George Podgorny, M.D. [*118, 192*]
Associate Professor of Clinical Surgery
Bowman Gray School of Medicine
Wake Forest University
Winston-Salem, North Carolina

David A. Poleski, M.D. [*78*]
Attending Physician, Pediatrics and Emergency Medicine
William Beaumont Hospital
Royal Oak, Michigan

Elaine S. Pomeranz, M.D. [*80*]
Clinical Instructor, Department of Pediatrics
Acting Director, Pediatric Emergency Services
University of Michigan Medical Center
Ann Arbor, Michigan

Stephen G. Priest, M.D. [*45*]
Staff Physician, Department of Surgery
William Beaumont Hospital
Royal Oak, Michigan

Gene Ragland, M.D. [*131–138*]
Chief, Emergency Medicine
St. Joseph Mercy Hospital
Ann Arbor, Michigan

Carol Godoshian Ragsdale, M.D. [*165*]
Associate Professor, Department of Pediatrics and Communicable Diseases
University of Michigan
Detroit, Michigan

K. Venkateswara Rao, M.D. [*52*]
Associate Professor, Department of Medicine
Division of Nephrology
Hennepin County Medical Center
Minneapolis, Minnesota

K. P. Ravikrishnan, M.D. [*29, 32*]
Director, Pulmonary Disease Section and Medical Critical Care
William Beaumont Hospital
Royal Oak, Michigan

Earl J. Reisdorff, M.D. [*126*]
Department of Emergency Medicine
Ingham Medical Center
Lansing, Michigan

Nick Relich, M.D. [*14F*]
Co-Director, Neonatal Intensive Care Unit
Department of Pediatrics
St. John Hospital
Detroit, Michigan

Charles Rennie III, M.D. [*153*]
Assistant Professor of Surgery
UCLA School of Medicine;
Director, Acute Care
Department of Emergency Medicine
Harbor-UCLA Medical Center
Torrance, California

James Roberts, M.D. [*105*]
Associate Professor, Emergency Medicine
University of Cincinnati College of Medicine
Cincinnati, Ohio

Leslie Rocher, M.D. [*206*]
Director, Division of Nephrology and Transplantation Programs
William Beaumont Hospital
Royal Oak, Michigan

Gaylan L. Rockswold, M.D. [*171*]
Associate Professor, Department of Neurosurgery
University of Minnesota School of Medicine;
Head, Section of Neurosurgery
Hennepin County Medical Center
Minneapolis, Minnesota

George T. Rodeheaver, Ph.D. [*188–191, 193, 194*]
Research Professor of Plastic Surgery
University of Virginia School of Medicine;
Director of Plastic Surgery Research
University of Virginia
Charlottesville, Virginia

Michael J. Ruffing, Pharm. D. [*12*]
Department of Pharmaceutical Services
Detroit Receiving Hospital
Detroit, Michigan

Ernest Ruiz, M.D. [*169, 186*]
Chief, Emergency Medicine
Hennepin County Medical Center;
Assistant Professor, Department of Surgery
University of Minnesota
Minneapolis, Minnesota

Barry H. Rumack, M.D. [*101, 129*]
Professor of Pediatrics
University of Colorado Health Sciences Center;
Director, Rocky Mountain Poison Center
Denver, Colorado

Douglas A. Rund, M.D. [*144, 197–199*]
Professor and Chairman, Department of Emergency Medicine
Ohio State University
Columbus, Ohio

Robert A. Rusnak, M.D. [*207*]
Associate Physician, Department of Emergency Medicine
Hennepin County Medical Center
Minneapolis, Minnesota

P. J. Ryan, M.D. [*91, 92*]
Medical Director, Emergency Department
St. Luke's Medical Center
Phoenix, Arizona

Ronald Sacher, M.D. [*141*]
Professor of Medicine and Pathology
Director, Transfusion Medicine
Georgetown University Medical Center
Washington, DC

Alexander H. Sackeyfio, M.D. [*200*]
Director, Eating Disorders Unit
William Beaumont Hospital
Royal Oak, Michigan

Joseph A. Salomone III, M.D. [*168*]
Associate Director, Emergency Medicine Residency Program
Department of Emergency Health Services
Truman Medical Center;
Assistant Professor, University of Missouri—Kansas City School of Medicine
Kansas City, Missouri

Robert W. Schafermeyer, M.D. [*76*]
Program Director, Department of Emergency Medicine
Carolinas Medical Center;
Clinical Associate Professor of Pediatrics
University of North Carolina Medical School
Chapel Hill, North Carolina

Robert E. Schneider, M.D. [*54*]
Department of Emergency Medicine
Carolinas Medical Center
Charlotte, North Carolina

James S. Seidel, M.D., Ph.D. [*14B, 47*]
Associate Professor of Pediatrics
Chief, Ambulatory Pediatrics
Departments of Pediatrics and Emergency Medicine
Harbor-UCLA Medical Center
UCLA School of Medicine
Torrance, California

Joel C. Seidman, M.D.
Chief, Pulmonary Division
William Beaumont Hospital
Royal Oak, Michigan

Brad S. Selden, M.D.
Department of Medical Toxicology
Good Samaritan Regional Medical Center;
Department of Emergency Medicine
Maricopa Medical Center
Phoenix, Arizona

Seetha Shankaran, M.D. [*14D*]
Associate Professor of Pediatrics
Wayne State University School of Medicine;
Director, Neonatal-Perinatal Medicine
Children's Hospital of Michigan
Detroit, Michigan

Stanley Sherman, M.D. [*35*]
Pulmonary and Critical Care Medicine
William Beaumont Hospital
Royal Oak, Michigan

Richard Owen Shields, Jr. [*49*]
Medical Director, Emergency Center
Memorial Medical Center, Inc.
Savannah, Georgia

Kathy E. Shy, M.D. [*199*]
Assistant Professor of Psychiatry
Ohio State University School of Medicine
Columbus, Ohio

Robert R. Simon, M.D. [*179, 186*]
Chairman, Department of Emergency Medicine
Cook County Hospital
Chicago, Illinois

Daniel W. Spaite, M.D. [*204*]
Associate Professor, Arizona Emergency Medicine Research Center
University of Arizona College of Medicine
Tucson, Arizona

William H. Spivey, M.D. [*14C*]
Associate Professor of Emergency Medicine
Chief, Division of Research
Medical College of Pennsylvania
Philadelphia, Pennsylvania

J. Stephan Stapczynski, M.D. [*11, 13A, 17, 19, 20, 164*]
Chairman, Department of Emergency Medicine
University of Kentucky Medical Center
Lexington, Kentucky

Mark T. Steele, M.D. [*181, 183–184*]
Associate Professor
University of Missouri—Kansas City School of Medicine
Kansas City, Missouri

Zigfrids T. Stelmachers, Ph.D. [*203*]
Clinical Associate Professor of Psychology
University of Minnesota School of Medicine;
Director, Crisis Intervention Center
Hennepin County Medical Center
Minneapolis, Minnesota

George L. Sternbach, M.D. [*94*]
Emergency Physician
Clinical Associate Professor of Surgery
Stanford Medical Center
Stanford, California;
Emergency Physician, Seton Medical Center
Daly City, California

Robert Swor, D.O. [*15, 173*]
Department of Emergency Medicine
William Beaumont Hospital
Royal Oak, Michigan

Scott Syverud, M.D. [*7*]
Assistant Professor, Department of Emergency Medicine
University of Cincinnati College of Medicine
Cincinnati, Ohio

John Tafuri, M.D. [*105*]
Department of Emergency Medicine
University of Cincinnati Hospital
Cincinnati, Ohio

John G. Thacker, M.D. [*188–191, 193, 194*]
Professor of Mechanical and Aerospace Engineering
University of Virginia
Charlottesville, Virginia

Michael V. Vance, M.D. [*88, 116*]
Associate Director, Samaritan Regional Poison Center;
Department of Medical Toxicology
Good Samaritan Medical Center
Phoenix, Arizona

Susi Vassallo, M.D. [*97*]
Senior Consultant, New York Regional Poison Control Center;
Clinical Instructor
Department of Surgery/Emergency Medicine
New York University School of Medicine;
Attending Physician, Department of Emergency Medical Services
Bellevue Hospital Center
New York, New York

Peter Viccellio, M.D. [*108*]
Vice Chairman and Residency Program Director
Department of Emergency Medicine
School of Medicine
SUNY at Stony Brook
Stony Brook, New York

Joseph F. Waeckerle, M.D. [*178, 181–185*]
Clinical Associate Professor
University of Missouri at Kansas City School of Medicine;
Chairman, Department of Emergency Medicine
Baptist Medical Center
Kansas City, Missouri

Paul M. Wax, M.D. [*103*]
Medical Toxicology
New York City Poison Control Center;
Attending Physician, Emergency Services
Bellevue Hospital Center
New York, New York

Donald W. Weaver, M.D. [*50*]
Associate Professor of Surgery, Wayne State University;
Chief, Section of General Surgery
Harper Hospital
Detroit, Michigan

Michael S. Weinstock, M.D. [*79*]
Director, Emergency Medical Services
North Shore University Hospital;
Assistant Professor of Surgery
Cornell University Medical College
Manhasset, New York

Howard A. Werman, M.D. [*44*]
Assistant Professor, Division of Emergency Medicine
Ohio State University
Columbus, Ohio

Blaine C. White, M.D. [*4*]
Associate Professor, Department of Surgery
Wayne State University School of Medicine;
Research Director, Department of Emergency Medicine
Detroit Receiving Hospital
Detroit, Michigan

John G. Wiegenstein, M.D. [*126*]
Professor, Department of Medicine
Michigan State University;
Chairman, Department of Emergency Medicine
Ingham Medical Center
Lansing, Michigan

Andrew Wilson, M.D. [*13D*]
Director, Emergency Department
Troy Beaumont Hospital
Rochester, Michigan

Robert F. Wilson, M.D. [*8–10, 174*]
Professor of Surgery
Director, Thoracic and Cardiovascular Surgery
Wayne State University School of Medicine;
Chief, Department of Surgery
Detroit Receiving Hospital
Detroit, Michigan

Kimberlydawn Wisdom, M.D., M.S. [*33*]
Staff Physician, Department of Emergency Medicine, Henry Ford Medical Center
Dearborn, Michigan

Leslie R. Wolf, M.D. [*112*]
Toxicology Fellow
Department of Emergency Medicine
University of Cincinnati
Cincinnati, Ohio

Joseph A. Zeccardi, M.D. [*69*]
Clinical Associate Professor of Surgery (Emergency Medicine)
Director, Division of Emergency Medicine
Thomas Jefferson University Hospital
Philadelphia, Pennsylvania

Mark Zwanger, M.D. [*30*]
Director, Emergency Medicine Residency Program
Division of Emergency Medicine
Thomas Jefferson University Hospital
Philadelphia, Pennsylvania

PREFACE

The third McGraw-Hill edition of *Emergency Medicine: A Comprehensive Study Guide* appears 13 years after the original American College of Emergency Physicians edition. The term "Study Guide" was originally selected as part of the title because the basic elements of emergency medicine cognitive and technical skills were still being defined. The initial purpose of the Study Guide was to serve as a framework for preparation for the American Board of Emergency Medicine certification examination. Today's *Study Guide* is much more ambitious and is designed to serve as a readable clinical reference for use in the Emergency Department and wherever emergency health care is provided.

Expansion of the sections on pediatrics, infections, toxicology, and wound care reflect the importance of these areas to the clinical practice of emergency medicine. New sections on the disabled patient and the high technology patient reflect the rapidly changing demographics of emergency medicine. The increasing emphasis on outpatient surgery and rapid hospital discharge requires more depth and breadth of knowledge of the emergency physician. The section on newer imaging modalities and the chapters on postoperative surgical complications were devised to meet these needs.

Finally, the *Study Guide* represents the pride, professionalism, and scholarly accomplishments of the newest and most contemporary specialty, emergency medicine.

Judith E. Tintinalli

SECTION 1
Resuscitative Problems and Techniques

1
BASIC CARDIOPULMONARY RESUSCITATION

Raymond Jackson

Basic cardiopulmonary resuscitation (CPR) encompasses the concepts and techniques which form the foundation for effective emergency care. The purpose of cardiopulmonary resuscitation is to provide artificial circulation of oxygenated blood to the vital organs, especially the heart and brain, in an attempt to halt the degenerative processes associated with ischemia and anoxia until spontaneous circulation can be restored. Basic life support alone may in some instances be lifesaving, but in most cases, advanced interventions are essential for the resuscitation of the patient. The critical factor in determining the success of resuscitative efforts is the time elapsed before successful restoration of effective spontaneous circulation. This, for the most part, is dependent upon use of advanced life-support techniques such as defibrillation.

This chapter discusses the physiology of blood flow during closed-chest compression, reviews the basic closed-chest compression technique, and summarizes the initial management of the obstructed airway.

PHYSIOLOGY OF BASIC CLOSED-CHEST COMPRESSION

Hemodynamics

Closed-chest compression produces, in the vast majority of cases, a severe low flow state. With experimental animals, cardiac outputs have ranged from 17 to 27 percent of prearrest values. The mean cardiac index in a small number of patients who had determinations during closed-chest compression was 0.76 L/min per m^2, which is approximately 25 percent of the normal resting cardiac index in humans and is even less than found in cases of severe cardiogenic shock.

Successful resuscitation from experimental ventricular fibrillation is dependent upon myocardial perfusion. Coronary diastolic pressure, which is the driving force for coronary blood flow during closed-chest compression, may be as high as 20 to 40 mmHg immediately after the onset of arrest, but rapidly falls to below 20 mmHg. The likelihood of a successful resuscitation attempt is low when diastolic pressure is below 40 mmHg because coronary blood flow and myocardial perfusion are extremely low during closed-chest compression, typically around 5 percent of prearrest values. There is a strong positive linear correlation between diastolic blood pressure and myocardial perfusion. Cerebral blood flow is also very low during closed-chest compression. In general, if closed-chest compression begins on collapse of the victim, hemodynamic parameters are not as poor as depicted, but rapidly deteriorate without adrenergic support.

Mechanism of Flow Generation

How the application of force onto the thoracic cage reduces movement of blood is a subject of great interest. Liquids flow in closed systems when pressure gradients develop in them. Flow does occur during closed-chest compression, therefore a pressure gradient must be created by this maneuver. Two theories have been formulated to explain where the pressure gradient may develop during chest compressions: the cardiac pump and the thoracic pump.

The "cardiac pump theory" was first formulated by Kouwenhoven and states that the pressure gradient is developed within the heart across the valves by direct compression of the heart. Therefore, a pressure gradient from the aorta to the right atrium would be evident during the actual compression of the chest. Competent cardiac valves are an essential component of this theory. Evidence for this theory has been limited to high-impulse CPR. This form of CPR uses a higher force than normally applied at a higher rate resulting in augmented cardiac output and coronary blood flow.

The lack of an aortic to right atrial pressure gradient observed by many investigators led to the theory that forward flow is generated by an intrathoracic to extrathoracic pressure gradient, the thoracic pump mechanism. During the compression (systolic) phase of standard closed-chest compression, all intrathoracic pressures are equal, while there is a pressure gradient from the intrathoracic to the extrathoracic arterial vessels. Only during the relaxation (diastolic) phase of the cycle does an aortic to right atrial pressure gradient develop. This pressure gradient is the diastolic coronary perfusion pressure, which is the major determinant of coronary blood flow.

Further evidence supporting the thoracic pump mechanism is obtained from observations with two-dimensional echocardiography in humans during closed-chest compression showing that the ventricular dimensions do not change with compression and the mitral and aortic valves remain open during compression. Cineangiography in animal models shows that the mitral and aortic valves are incompetent during compression, with no evidence of ventricular compression. Aortic blood flow occurs during compression, while pulmonary and coronary blood flow take place during the relaxation phase.

The existence of an intrathoracic-extrathoracic pressure gradient is most evident with cerebral blood flow. Valves in the jugular venous system prevent the transmission of the intrathoracic pressure to the venous side of the central nervous system (CNS) vasculature during compression. Maneuvers which increase systolic intrathoracic pressures should, in theory, increase carotid to jugular pressure gradient and, subsequently, cerebral blood flow.

The relative roles of the thoracic pump and direct cardiac compression mechanisms in the generation of blood flow probably vary from patient to patient. Regardless of what mechanism is operating, increasing the rate and depth of compressions augments forward flow.

COUGH-CPR

The form of cardiopulmonary resuscitation which takes most dramatic advantage of the thoracic pump mechanism is cough-CPR. This method consists of rhythmic coughing (every 1 to 3 s) by the patient at the onset of an arrhythmia. Consciousness during ventricular fibrillation has been maintained for up to 92 s by this method. Cineangiograms during cough-CPR show that blood flow is primarily cephalad, starting from the descending aorta and then from the left ventricle, with no changes in left ventricular dimensions. The aortic valve remains incompetent. Cough-CPR should be taught to all patients at risk for lethal arrhythmias.

BASIC CLOSED-CHEST COMPRESSION: AN OVERVIEW OF TECHNIQUE

The application of effective CPR demands a methodical approach. The performance of the following eight maneuvers in order enables the care provider to quickly evaluate the patient's condition, determine the intensity of intervention required, and assure effective care delivery.

1. Establish unresponsiveness
2. Obtain assistance. Activate EMS system
3. Properly position the patient
4. Open the airway
5. Establish breathlessness
6. Ventilate the patient
7. Establish presence or absence of pulse
8. Perform closed-chest compression

Establish Unresponsiveness and Obtain Assistance

The first step in assessing an individual who has collapsed is to establish the level of responsiveness by administering some sort of noxious stimulus.

If the victim is unresponsive, the initial rescuer should call for help and activate the EMS system if outside the hospital. This step is critical, since the time to the institution of advanced life support procedures is the most important determinant of ultimate outcome.

Open the Airway

With loss of muscle tone in the obtunded patient, the tongue may fall back into the oropharynx and cause upper airway obstruction. The negative pressure generated during inspiratory efforts can force the tongue back into the oropharynx, creating a one-way valve effect and occluding the airway during inspiration. This will manifest as stridor. Three simple maneuvers are initially used to open the airway and to relieve upper airway obstruction.

The *head tilt* is the first maneuver which should be attempted. It is accomplished by placing one hand beneath the victim's neck and the other hand on the forehead. The neck is then flexed in relation to the thorax and the head extended in relation to the neck (the so-called sniffing position). If this maneuver is unsuccessful, the chin lift or jaw thrust should be applied. Both of these maneuvers, which should be executed along with the head tilt, effectively lift the tongue out of the oropharynx by displacing the mandible, to which the tongue is connected.

In the *chin lift,* the hand which had been supporting the neck is placed under the symphysis of the mandible, with the mandible lifted forward and up until the teeth barely touch. The other hand remains on the forehead. The soft tissues at the base of the tongue should not be compressed; this can increase the obstruction. If the victim has dentures, the chin lift is more effective if they remain in place.

In the *jaw thrust,* the rescuer, who is positioned at the head of the patient, places the hands at the sides of the victim's face, grasping the angles of the mandible and lifting the mandible forward. The rescuer's elbows may rest on the surface on which the patient lies. The jaw thrust, with use of the head tilt, is the safest method for opening an airway in a patient while maintaining the integrity of the cervical spine.

Establish Breathlessness and Begin Ventilation

Without evidence of air movement or chest expansions, artificial ventilations should be immediately instituted. Occasionally patients who have just lost spontaneous perfusion may have a period of agonal respirations, characterized by a rhythmic sighing. These respirations should not be mistaken for adequate ventilatory efforts, and rescue breathing should ensue.

The mouth-to-mouth method of rescue breathing is initiated by gently pinching the patient's nostrils with the thumb and forefinger. Then, after taking a deep breath, the rescuer, with open mouth around the victim's mouth making an airtight seal, forcibly exhales air into the patient's airway. The volume delivered should not exceed 1200 mL. Larger tidal volumes, and rapid insufflation, should be avoided because of the danger of creating gastric distension and subsequent regurgitation and aspiration. Two breaths are delivered initially, allowing adequate time for exhalation. The rescuer's expired air has an FI_{O_2} of 16 to 17 percent, so resources able to deliver higher oxygen concentrations are needed as soon as possible. The rescuer watches the victim's chest to see that it rises with each forced inhalation and falls with the end of forced inhalation. Any observed impairment to air flow during rescue breathing may indicate either an obstruction in the upper airway or a serious restriction to lung expansion such as a tension pneumothorax. If lack of chest wall motion is noted or there is a large amount of resistance to flow, the oropharynx must be reinspected for an obstruction and efforts to relieve the obstruction should be executed.

With severe maxillofacial trauma, mouth-to-nose ventilation may be more effective than mouth-to-mouth. This is done by using the jaw thrust maneuver in an attempt to lift the tongue from the posterior oropharynx and sealing the mouth shut with the thumb and forefinger during inhalation. The patient's mouth is opened during exhalation to diminish the resistance to airflow. Patients with stomas or tracheostomies are ventilated by placing the mouth over the stoma or tracheostomy tube.

Relieve Foreign-Body Obstruction

Foreign bodies may cause either partial or complete airway obstruction. With partial obstruction, the patient may be capable of air exchange. With sufficient air exchange, the patient may cough, although there may be wheezing or stridor between coughs. As long as good air exchange continues, spontaneous coughing and breathing should be encouraged. The rescuer should not interfere with attempts to expel the foreign body. The child with partial airway obstruction and good airway exchange should not be turned upside down because this may impact a tracheal foreign body against the vocal cords.

Poor air exchange is characterized by a weak, ineffective cough, marked respiratory stridor, and respiratory distress. A patient who exhibits poor air exchange should be managed as a case of complete obstruction. With complete airway obstruction, the patient is unable to speak, breathe, or cough. If still conscious, the patient may clutch his or her neck; this is the *universal distress signal.* In an unconscious victim, a complete obstruction is identified by resistance to artificial ventilation and failure of the chest to rise and fall with each attempted ventilation.

Maneuvers for Relieving Obstruction

The maneuvers recommended for relieving foreign-body obstruction are the finger sweep, back blows or chest thrusts, and manual removal of the object. The sequence in which these maneuvers should be executed is as follows: check the oropharynx by performing finger sweep, apply back blows, and apply manual thrusts. The cycle is repeated until the obstruction is cleared. If at any time the object appears in the oropharynx, it is removed manually. Back blows produce an instantaneous increase in airway pressure, which may result in either partial or complete dislodgement of the foreign body. Manual thrusts develop a lower but more sustained increase in pressure and may further assist in dislodging the object. Combining these techniques appears to be more effective than using one alone.

The back blow technique is a series of four rapid, sharp and forcible blows delivered over the spine and between the scapulae with the heel of the hand. They may be given with the victim standing, sitting, or lying. Whenever possible, the patient's head should be lower than the chest to take advantage of gravity.

The manual thrust method (Heimlich maneuver) consists of four thrusts to the upper abdomen or lower chest. The low chest thrust develops somewhat higher flows and peak pressure. The abdominal thrust can be performed with the patient sitting or standing. The rescuer should be positioned behind the patient with arms wrapped around the victim's waist. Making a fist with one hand and placing the thumb side of the fist into the epigastrium and grasping the fist with the other hand, the rescuer delivers four quick upward thrusts. A patient who is lying prone must be placed in the supine position and the airway opened. The rescuer can be either astride or alongside the patient. The heel of one hand is placed in the epigastrium and covered with the heel of the other hand. A quick upward thrust may then be delivered. This maneuver may be self-administered by delivering a quick upward thrust to the abdomen with a fist or by leaning forward on any firm object. Complications of abdominal thrusts include rupture or laceration of abdominal viscera.

Chest thrusts are performed in a similar manner when the patient is lying or sitting, with the fist placed directly on the sternum. When the patient is supine, the hands should be placed over the sternum as in closed-chest compression and compressed four times. The chest thrust is useful when the rescuer's arms cannot fully reach around the patient's abdomen or when direct abdominal pressure is likely to cause complications, as in advanced pregnancy.

Establish Pulselessness and Begin Compressions

After the initial two ventilations, the presence of a pulse is determined by placing two fingers on the carotid artery, which is located by placing the index and middle fingers on the trachea and then sliding them between the trachea and the sternocleidomastoid muscles. If there is no pulse or if the pulse is slow or weak, closed-chest compression should be started immediately. With the patient supine on a firm surface, the rescuer places two fingers of one hand over the xiphoid process and the heel of the other hand on the sternum 1 to 2 in cephalad to the xiphoid. The first hand is brought to rest on top of the hand that is on the sternum. The rescuer, positioned over the sternum with the arms straight and the elbows locked, forces the sternum straight downward 1.5 to 2 in at a rate of 80 to 120 compressions per minute. The optimum ratio of the compression phase to the relaxation phase is 1:1. With two rescuers, a ventilation is delivered after every fifth compression; with one rescuer two ventilations are delivered after every fifteen compressions.

COMPLICATIONS OF CLOSED-CHEST MASSAGE

Complications of closed-chest compression include sternal and rib fractures, pulmonary contusion, and pneumothorax. Myocardial contusions, primarily of the right ventricle, may result in acute right ventricular failure. Hemorrhagic pericardial effusions have also been observed. Gastric distension, erosions, and rupture have occurred. The incidence of liver laceration is approximately 2 percent. Regurgitation and aspiration pneumonia are frequent complications. Careful performance of basic closed-chest technique can diminish, but not totally abolish, many of these complications.

Late complications include development of pulmonary edema, electrolyte abnormalities, gastrointestinal hemorrhage, pneumonia, and recurrent cardiopulmonary arrest. Anoxic encephalopathy is the major cause of death in resuscitated patients.

TERMINATING RESUSCITATIVE EFFORTS

Resuscitative efforts should be continued until ventilation and circulation are restored, the patient is transported to a hospital setting, the rescuer becomes exhausted, or a physician assumes responsibility for the patient. Success in resuscitation is time-dependent, with a dismal long-term outcome in efforts which last longer than 20 min in normothermic adults.

BIBLIOGRAPHY

Berkowitz I, Rogers M: The physiology of cerebral blood flow during cardiopulmonary resuscitation. *Can J Anaesth* 35:S23, 1988

Bjork R, Snyder B, Campion B, et al: Medical complications of cardiopulmonary arrest. *Arch Intern Med* 142:500, 1982.

Criley J, Blaufuss A, Kissel G: Cough induced cardiac compression: Self administered form of cardiopulmonary resuscitation. *JAMA* 136:1246, 1976.

Deshmukh H, Weil M, Gudipati C, et al: Mechanism of blood flow generated by precordial compression during CPR: I. Studies on closed-chest precordial compression. *Chest* 95:1092, 1989.

Einagle V, Bertrand F, Wise R, et al: Interposed abdominal compressions and carotid blood flow during cardiopulmonary resuscitation: Support for a thoracoabdominal unit. *Chest* 93:1206.

Fitzgerald K, Babbs C, Frissura H, et al: Cardiac output during cardiopulmonary resuscitation at various compression rates and durations. *Am J Physiol* 241:H442, 1981.

Jackson R, Freeman S: Hemodynamics of cardiac massage. *Emerg Clin North Am* 1:501, 1983.

Maier G, Tyson G, Colsen C, et al: The physiology of external cardiac massasge: High impulse cardiopulmonary resuscitation. *Circulation* 70:86, 1984.

Ornato J, Levine R, Young D, et al: The effect of applied chest compression force on systemic arterial pressure and end-tidal carbon dioxide concentration during CPR in human beings. *Ann Emerg Med* 18:732, 1989.

Paradis MA, Martin GB, Rivers EP, et al: Coronary perfusion pressure and the return of spontaneous circulation in human cardiopulmonary resuscitation. *JAMA* 263:1166, 1990.

Paradis MA, Martin GB, Goetting ML, et al: Simultaneous aortic, jugular bulb, and right atrial pressures during cardiopulmonary resuscitation in humans. *Circulation* 80:361, 1989.

Redding J: The choking controversy. Critique and evidence on the Heimlich maneuver. *Crit Care Med* 7:475, 1979.

Redding J: Cardiopulmonary resuscitation: An algorithm and some pitfalls. *Am Heart J* 98:788, 1979.

Rudikoff M, Maughan W, Effron M, et al: Mechanism of blood flow during cardiopulmonary resuscitation. *Circulation* 61:345, 1980.

Standards and guidelines for cardiopulmonary resuscitation and emergency care. *JAMA* 255:2905, 1986.

2
THE ETHICS OF RESUSCITATION

Timothy J. Crimmins

INTRODUCTION

Ethics is the branch of philosophy that asks "What is right?" Medical ethics encompasses more than this, providing a standard of moral conduct that requires of physicians the highest level of professional integrity and social responsibility. The American Medical Association's Code of Ethics begins, "The physician shall be dedicated to providing competent medical services with compassion and respect for human dignity." The emergency physician should adhere to the highest standards of moral conduct, to protect and preserve life, prevent disability, and relieve suffering. The physician should be the patient's advocate and provide treatment that is in the patient's best interest.

Despite a desire to live and practice according to these laudable ethical standards, the emergency physician is often faced with dilemmas in patient care decisions when it is difficult to determine what is "right." The legal and legislative systems have provided ample guidelines in the areas of consent, confidentiality, contract, and liability. Still, the emergency physician has unique ethical challenges in the areas of resuscitation, patient autonomy, and triage that are evolving from the interface between the emergency medical care system and a sometimes unwilling or suffering patient.

RESUSCITATION

Nothing in emergency medicine arouses as much emotional turmoil as the confrontation with death and dying. In previous times death was considered as the natural outcome of disease. Now emergency physicians strive to forestall the moment of death by employing many vigorous, if not invasive, techniques. Physicians think in terms of medical indications and contraindications to the application of these techniques, yet because of many possible ramifications of resuscitation, such decisions may not be the physician's sole prerogative. Often the ethical mandate of the emergency physician to preserve life may conflict with the obligations to relieve suffering and prevent disability.

The emergency physician should promptly institute cardiopulmonary resuscitation and advanced life support procedures for individuals who suffer sudden cardiac arrest or other medical emergencies in the absence of advance directives (to be described later). Emergency personnel should not withhold resuscitation on the basis of age of the patient, cost of care, preexisting mental or physical disability, or the circumstances surrounding the event. However, cardiopulmonary resuscitation may be ethically withheld or discontinued if there is irreversible cessation of cardiac function, brain death, imminently terminal illness (futility), or patient refusal.

Determination of Death

Cardiopulmonary resuscitation need not be instituted if the patient is "dead." The difficulty arises in differentiating this from reversible "cardiac arrest." If dependent lividity, rigor mortis, decapitation, or decomposition is present, the determination is easy. The Uniform Determination of Death Act adopted in 1981 by the American Medical Association and American Bar Association states: "An individual who has sustained either (1) irreversible cessation of circulatory and respiratory functions, or (2) irreversible cessation of all functions of the entire brain, including the brainstem, is dead."

The first alternative can be met if a patient fails to respond to a reasonable trial of resuscitation as outlined in the 1985 National Conference on Standards and Guidelines for Cardiopulmonary Resuscitation and Emergency Cardiac Care. There is often no way of predicting irreversibility short of carrying out resuscitation, with the result that many patients are transported to hospital emergency departments for such a trial. Where emergency medical services systems have advanced life support capability, some patients can be "declared dead" in the field after a suitable trial at resuscitation.

The second alternative, brain death, cannot be invoked as readily. Although state statutes vary regarding the determination of brain death, most require serial examinations over many hours and the exclusion of the presence of certain drugs and hypothermia. These criteria are difficult to meet in the emergency department. Therefore, aggressive resuscitation of patients with apparently severe brain trauma or global ischemic injury is in order.

Terminal Illness

Cardiopulmonary resuscitation is not indicated when the patient's death is predicted within days as the result of irreversible and imminently terminal illness. Such a decision is an exercise of good medical judgment. A physician may ethically direct that resuscitation be withheld if there is no hope of a successful outcome, but this requires extensive knowledge of the patient's prior medical condition. In an emergency, resuscitation should be instituted until such time that the patient's diagnosis and prognosis are known and it can be ascertained that treatment is futile.

PATIENT AUTONOMY

Increasingly, physicians are faced with requests for "death with dignity" and "no heroics." The basis for the physician-patient relationship is the patient's consent for treatment. Competent patients may refuse medical treatment, but the emergency physician is often faced with situations involving incompetent or questionably competent patients, vague directives, ambivalent or absent family members, or a change of mind at the time of the actual "moment of truth." Aggressive medical treatments should be instituted in the absence of clear evidence of competent patient refusal.

Advance Directives

The concept of *advance directives* has been implemented in the metropolitan Minneapolis area as a strictly defined and documented process to serve both suffering patients and rescue personnel. This use of advance directives to provide treatment guidelines for terminally ill or severely incapacitated patients to emergency medical services providers is rapidly spreading across the country. These directives may be in the form of physicians' orders, living wills, or designation of surrogate decision-makers (guardians, conservators, or durable powers of attorney). When these directives are present with the patient, rescue personnel and their physician medical directors and radio control providers can ethically refrain from aggressive resuscitation as specified. State laws governing this matter vary.

Physicians' orders for advance directives commonly use the terminology: do not resuscitate (DNR); do not intubate (DNI); hospice care; and limited treatment plans. DNR or "no-code" orders have been defined as: "in the event of an acute cardiac or respiratory arrest, no cardiopulmonary resuscitative efforts will be instituted" by the President's Commission for the Study of Ethical Problems in Medicine in 1983. This order does not necessarily imply terminal illness, nor is it a refusal of all medical care. Other treatments may be provided prior to cardiac or respiratory arrest. More extensive limitations of treatment can be accomplished by invoking hospice care or limited treatment plans whereby specific treatments can be refused. Patients with limited treatment orders are unique and require thoughtful consideration at critical times. An evaluation and diagnostic workup of a new problem may still be warranted. These patients certainly need ongoing medical and nursing care, as Jonsen writes: "to cure sometimes, relieve occasionally, comfort always."

Living will statutes and laws governing decision-making for the incompetent patient provide mechanisms by which people can direct their medical care or designate a decision-maker prior to their illness. Emergency physicians should be familiar with the laws governing these matters in the state in which they practice. All advance directives should be made prior to the emergency event, and appropriate justification, counseling, and documentation should be provided by the patient's personal physician. These directives should also be updated at frequent intervals for obvious reasons.

The emergency physician has an obligation to aggressively resuscitate the victim of an attempted suicide and should restrain and treat those who pose an imminent danger to themselves or others, even against their will—particularly incompetent, intoxicated, or psychotic patients.

TRIAGE

Medical triage has long been a necessity in the emergency setting. However, new constraints, primarily financial, face the physician making emergency treatment decisions. Institutions may pressure physicians to restrict appropriate care. The emergency physician's position is unique in that this physician must evaluate all individuals presenting to the emergency department but is not obligated to treat nonemergency patient conditions. The emergency physician is sometimes forced to limit treatments (triage) when immediately available resources are limited but should not restrict treatments based on arbitrary determinations of "the cost to society" or a patient's "worth to society."

Restrictions in treatment for financial reasons must be made at a public policy level, with the development of guidelines to limit medical care based on specific criteria that are applied to all individuals. The AMA Council on Ethical and Judicial Affairs has stated: "The organized medical staff has an obligation to avoid wasteful practices and unnecessary treatment that may cause the hospital needless expense. In a situation where the economic interests of the hospital are in conflict with patient welfare, patient welfare takes priority."

Emergency physicians should not transfer unstable patients because of financial considerations when transport may endanger the patient's well-being. This principle should prevail even when Health Maintenance Organization (HMO) patients are involved. Federal law should be consulted regarding patient transfers.

SUMMARY

The emergency physician is often faced with ethical dilemmas when instituting cardiopulmonary resuscitation. Aggressive medical treatments should be used unless the patient is clinically dead or proven brain dead or unless there is compelling evidence that no therapeutic benefit can be gained from resuscitation. Medical treatments may be withheld in the presence of properly executed advance directives in communities that have established this process for the benefit of patients and the emergency medical services system.

Emergency physicians are often obliged to triage patients in an effort to most effectively utilize available resources. This limitation of treatment to patients is ethical when there is a scarcity of immediately available medical resources. Triage for any other consideration is problematic for the emergency physician and the patient. Public policy may dictate triage on the basis of financial considerations, especially with HMOs, but any such policy should be drafted to prevent discrimination and to protect the incompetent and without compromising the patient's health.

BIBLIOGRAPHY

AMA Council on Ethical and Judicial Affairs: Recent opinions of the council on ethical and judicial affairs. *JAMA* 256:2241, 1986.

Deciding to Forego Life-Sustaining Treatment, President's Commission for the Study of Ethical Problems in Medicine and Biomedical and Behavioral Research. Washington, DC, U.S. Government Printing Office, 1983.

Jonsen A, Seigler M, Winslade W: *Clinical Ethics.* New York, Macmillan, 1982.

Miles SH, Crimmins TJ: Orders to limit emergency treatment for an ambulance service in a large metropolitan area. *JAMA* 254:525, 1985.

National Conference on Cardiopulmonary Resuscitation and Emergency Cardiac Care: Standards and guidelines for cardiopulmonary resuscitation and emergency cardiac care: VIII. Medicolegal considerations and recommendations. *JAMA* 255:2979, 1986.

3
MAST

Scott Freeman

The military antishock trouser (MAST) garment, a one-piece layered device made of polyvinyl fabric, is capable of sustaining internal air pressures of up to 104 torr and is used to reverse the signs of shock. It encloses the body from the lower rib cage to, but not including, the feet. The lower extremities are each enclosed separately, allowing access to the perineal area. Three compartments cover the abdomen and two extremities and are fastened with Velcro fasteners. Some versions of the garment allow separate inflation and deflation of these compartments. Most are inflated with a foot pump and are equipped with an interposed inflation pressure monitoring device. Internal pressures of the suit are limited by a pressure relief valve and the ability of the Velcro fastener to withstand stress.

MAST effects appear to include at least four mechanisms: (1) tamponade of bleeding in the lower body, (2) increase in peripheral resistance in the lower body, (3) selective perfusion of the upper body, and (4) an initial increase of venous return (preload) from the lower body. The fourth mechanism plays a minor role in reversing hypotension.

PHYSIOLOGICAL EFFECTS

Vascular Resistance

The effect of the MAST suit on hypotension was attributed to an increase in peripheral vascular resistance by George Crile, who invented the device in 1903. Numerous authors have demonstrated increases in vascular resistance in the areas covered by the device. Some studies suggest that systemic vascular resistance increases when MAST suits are applied, and this is consistent with the observed elevation of blood pressure.

Regional Blood Flow

Redistribution of blood flow has been demonstrated in animal experiments. In a nonshock model, flows in the carotid artery increased, while femoral artery blood flow decreased.

Blood Pressure

The degree of blood pressure elevation is related to blood volume and inflation pressure. Blood pressure rises more with hypovolemia than with normovolemia. Several studies suggest that MAST pressures up to 60 torr produce the most significant increases in blood pressure and inflation pressures above this have less effect.

Hemorrhage Control

Direct pressure is one of the traditional methods for controlling hemorrhage, and MAST slows blood loss in the areas covered by the suit. This has been attributed to decreases in vessel size and decreases in the open area of wounds. Pressure from pneumatic enclosures is also transmitted to the tissues. The pressure in the perinephric space of dogs with inflated MAST suits has been observed to be 80 percent of the suit pressure. In a shock animal model an increase in lactate was observed in the structures covered by the suit when it was inflated above systolic pressure. Centrally obtained lactate levels rose in this setting on deflation of the garment.

Cardiac Preload

Early reports suggested that volume was displaced to the thorax when the antigravity suit was inflated. Despite this work and the earlier suggestion that MAST suits functioned because of alterations in vascular resistance, many subsequent reports persisted in reporting that the effect of MAST suits was due primarily to an increase in preload or autotransfusion. This presumed mechanism of action was probably based on observations of the amount of fluid required to maintain blood pressure as the garment was deflated.

In an attempt to simulate the usual setting in which the MAST device is used, Bivins et al. phlebotomized human volunteers and measured their blood volumes by isotope scanning before and after application of MAST. Isotope scanning allowed evaluation of the blood volume in a compartmental manner. Although the phlebotomy in this experiment amounted to 17 percent of the total blood volume, the amount displaced to the upper body was measured as less than 5 percent. The mean blood volume after phlebotomy was 4434 mL, rendering the autotransfused amount less than 222 mL for this group. Lee et al. induced shock by phlebotomy and obtained direct measurements of the inferior vena cava flow as MAST inflation occurred. The volume of autotransfused blood in this setting was about 4 mL/kg, which, if extrapolated to humans, agrees with volumes determined to have autotransfused by noninvasive techniques. The degree of preload augmentation suggests that it is not the dominant factor in elevating blood pressure.

Pulmonary Function

Pulmonary function can be restricted by MAST, probably because it limits diaphragmatic excursion. In normal human volunteers, Gilbert showed that inflation to 100 torr decreased vital capacity by 13.8 percent. A case report of a patient with traumatic quadriplegia demonstrated a larger decrease in vital capacity. At 100 torr MAST inflation pressure, vital capacity was decreased 42 percent with preservation of the forced expiratory volume/forced vital capacity (FEV/FVC) ratio. In one retrospective study by Ransom of 25 patients requiring MAST for shock, only those with head injury (4 out of 5) showed evidence of hypercarbia.

CNS

The effect of MAST on intracranial pressure has been examined in animal models. Even in the presence of experimentally created intracranial mass lesions, no significant changes in intracranial pressure were observed when the MAST suit was inflated. Cerebral perfusion pressure in a shock model improved after MAST inflation.

BENEFITS AND EFFICACY

Mattox et al. prospectively evaluated the prehospital use of MAST in 911 patients. MAST suits were applied to victims of blunt or penetrating trauma with a systolic blood pressure less than 90 mmHg. Contrary to expectations, mortality was increased in the group that had MAST suits applied, especially in those with thoracic injury. Clearly, further evaluation of indications for use and benefits in trauma patients is needed.

Control of hemorrhage secondary to pelvic fracture, gynecologic hemorrhage, and gastrointestinal hemorrhage, and stabilization of fractures of the pelvis and femur have been indications for the use of MAST. Although many authors have reported use of the garment for such indications on a case-report basis, little is known about actual efficacy in these situations.

INDICATIONS AND CONTRAINDICATIONS

It is difficult to cleary describe the indications for the use of MAST. Contemporary studies are challenging once established views of the importance of elevating blood pressure with this device in the setting of shock. A list of relative and absolute indications and contraindications may expand as we reach a better understanding of the garment's effects. General indications for application are (1) to correct hypotension if the systolic blood pressure is below 100 in the presence of clinical shock, (2) to control pelvic or intraabdominal hemorrhage, and (3) to stabilize pelvic or femur fractures. Increases in systolic blood pressure with decreases in pulse rate have been reported when the MAST garment has been applied for treatment of septic, anaphylactic, or neurogenic shock.

Reports of termination of paroxysmal supraventricular tachycardia in both adults and children exist. When to apply MAST instead of conventional therapy is unclear.

An absolute contraindication for the use of MAST is the presence of pulmonary edema. Relative contraindications for MAST use are pregnancy, impaled objects, evisceration of the abdominal contents, and thoracic and diaphragmatic injuries. Use of MAST suits results in an increase in the vascular resistance of the lower extremities, and this may not be well tolerated by all patients.

Compartment syndromes in the lower extremity have been attributed to the use of MAST on numerous occasions. This is not a frequent complication of their use but one that is potentially serious. The length of time that MAST may be applied without the risk of developing compartment syndrome is not clear. Reports exist of compartment syndrome in untraumatized lower extremities after 140 minutes of MAST application.

APPLICATION AND REMOVAL

The MAST garment is designed to be applied with the patient supine. The leg compartments are inflated first, then the abdominal compartment. Inflation should stop when systolic blood pressure reaches 100 torr or when the device itself limits further inflation. Application of the device for more than 2 h should raise concern about the development of compartment syndrome in the lower extremities. Deflation should be done in a stepwise manner that is the reverse of the inflation sequence. Deflation should be discontinued if the blood pressure falls more than 5 torr, and volume expansion with crystalloid or blood is necessary before further deflation. Deflation of MAST is associated with an increase in metabolic acidosis, but this should not become clinically significant.

Changes in temperature and attitude can cause pressure changes in the garment. For instance, if the garment were applied in an environment where the temperature was 38°C (100°F) and the patient were transported in an air-conditioned environment of 24°C (75°F), the suit could lose as much as 28 torr of pressure. Pressure within the suit rises as altitude increases and falls as altitude decreases. Extrapolation from experimental data reveals that MAST pressure changes by approximately 1.8 torr for each 1000 ft change in altitude.

BIBLIOGRAPHY

Aprahamian C, Gessert G, Bandyk D, et al: MAST-associated compartment syndrome (MACS): A review. *J Trauma* 29(5):549, 1989.

Bivins HG, Knopp R, Tiernan C, et al: Blood volume displacement with inflation of antishock trousers. *Ann Emerg Med* 11:409, 1982.

Gilbert R: *Ann Emerg Med* 12:6, 1983.

Hauswald M, Greene E: Aortic blood flow during sequential MAST inflation. *Ann Emerg Med* 15(11):1297, 1986.

Johnson G, Bond R, Stack L, Class C, et al: Efficacy of military antishock trousers in compensatory and decompensatory hemorrhagic hypotension. *Circ Shock* 21:233, 1987.

Lee HR, Blank WF, Massion WH, et al: Venous return in hemorrhagic shock after application of military anti-shock trousers. *Am J Emerg Med* 1:7, 1983.

Mattox K, Bickell W, Pepe P, et al: Prospective MAST study in 911 patients. *J Trauma* 29(8):1104, 1989.

McSwain NE: Pneumatic anti-shock garment: State of the art 1988. *Ann Emerg Med* 17(5):506, 1988.

Niemann J, Stapczynski J, Rosborough J, et al: Hemodynamic effects of pneumatic external counterpressure in canine hemorrhagic shock. *Ann Emerg Med* 12:661, 1983.

Randall PE: Medical antishock trousers (MAST): A review. *Injury* 17:395, 1986.

Ransom K, McSwain N: *JACEP* 7:297, 1978.

Walker L, MacMath T, Chipman H, et al: MAST application in the treatment of paroxysmal supraventricular tachycardia in a child. *Ann Emerg Med* 17(5):529, 1988.

Wayne MA, MacDonald SC. Clinical evaluation of the antishock trouser: Retrospective analysis of five years of experience. *Ann Emerg Med* 12:342, 1983.

4
CEREBRAL ISCHEMIA

Blaine C. White
Gary S. Krause

The widespread availability of emergency medical services across the United States now results in about 200,000 cardiac resuscitation attempts yearly, with approximately 70,000 successful cardiac resuscitations. Only about 10 percent of the patients recover completely and are able to resume their former lifestyles. The major cause of this poor outcome is permanent neurologic injury (Krause et al., 1986). To date, there are no effective pharmacologic tools for amelioration of brain damage by ischemia and reperfusion.

The injury resulting from global brain ischemia appears to be initiated by the loss of homeostasis of two ions: calcium and iron (Krause et al., 1988). We will outline the crucial role of calcium and iron in the injury mechanism and then suggest possible therapies to ameliorate brain injury following an ischemic insult. Cardiac arrest resulting in ischemic-anoxic brain injury is characterized by three phases: (1) ischemic, (2) early reperfusion, and (3) late reperfusion.

ISCHEMIC PHASE

With the onset of cardiac arrest there is precipitous decline in brain oxygen content, which approaches zero within 6 to 12 s. The brain has very limited reserves of glucose, glycogen, or phosphocreatine; therefore, oxygen depletion leads to a sharp decline in tissue adenosine triphosphate (ATP) levels, which approach zero within 4 min. Anaerobic glycolysis and ATP depletion lead to lactic acidosis and hypoxanthine accumulation, respectively, during the ischemic phase. Since about 80 percent of the brain's ATP is used to maintain transmembrane ionic gradients for potassium, sodium, and calcium, these ionic gradients also decay rapidly. During complete ischemic anoxia these ions equilibrate between the extra- and intracellular fluid within 5 to 10 min of the insult.

The cytosolic accumulation of calcium is now widely thought to be a major initiating event leading to cell death (Siesjo et al., 1989). The high cytosolic calcium causes three key events: the activation of membrane phospholipase A_2, proteolytic cleavage of xanthine dehydrogenase, and release of excitatory neurotransmitters. Phospholipase A_2 cleaves a fatty acid, primarily arachidonate, from the cell membrane, yielding a free fatty acid (FFA) and in the process destroying the membrane's structure. The conversion of xanthine dehydrogenase in brain endothelial cells produces xanthine oxidase, which will react with hypoxanthine to produce the oxygen free radical superoxide (O_2^-) upon reperfusion.

Ultrastructural injury is seen in the brain during complete ischemia. Some margination and clumping of nuclear chromatin is seen by 10 to 15 min of complete ischemia. Mitochondria may be slightly swollen, but their structure does not show major degenerative alterations for up to 30 min of complete ischemia. Similarly, some swelling of the endoplasmic reticulum (ER) may be seen during ischemia, but the polyribosomes remain appropriately associated with the ER, and disaggregation of polyribosomes does not occur during complete ischemia. Nuclear and plasma membranes show a normal, well-defined bilaminar structure without evidence of holes or general structural disintegration.

Thus, the situation at the end of 15 to 30 min of complete ischemic anoxia includes (1) ATP levels near 0; (2) elevated hypoxanthine levels; (3) moderate lactic acidosis; (4) loss of transmembrane ionic gradients; (5) activated phospholipase with elevated FFA, especially arachidonic acid; (6) the presence of the abnormal enzyme xanthine oxidase; (7) release of excitatory neurotransmitters; (8) minimal injury to the high-energy capability of mitochondria; and (9) moderate and homogenous ultrastructural changes.

EARLY REPERFUSION

ATP levels and total adenylate charge recover rapidly during early reperfusion. If the ischemic insult has been less than 20 min, the membrane ionic gradients also recover quickly. After much longer insults of 1 to 3 h, total tissue calcium loads actually increase during reperfusion. It is felt that this reflects extensive and irreversible cell membrane injury during these very prolonged periods of ischemia.

Arachidonate is rapidly oxidized by both cyclo-oxygenase and lipoxygenase, and returns to preischemic levels within 30 min of reperfusion. Several vasoactive substances are produced by the metabolism of arachidonate. The prostaglandins are the products of cyclo-oxygenase, and the leukotrienes are the products of lipoxygenase. The production of the vasodilatory prostaglandin, prostacyclin, is severely inhibited during early reperfusion. Thus, vasospastic compounds predominate in the leukotriene and prostaglandin products. While the free arachidonic acid levels rapidly return to baseline during reperfusion, leukotrienes remain markedly elevated for at least 24 h. The time course of leukotriene elevation may explain the alterations in blood flow seen in the postischemic brain.

Restoration of normal or mildly hypertensive systemic arterial pressure produces an initial brain hyperperfusion. However, within 1 h, global brain perfusion has dropped to levels of 20 to 40 percent of normal, where it remains for up to 1 to 2 days. This phenomenon is inhibited by postresuscitation treatment with calcium antagonists such as flunarizine and nimodipine or the iron chelator deferoxamine.

Oxygen-based free radicals produced upon reperfusion may also contribute to neuronal injury. Availability of a transition metal, such as iron, is required for oxygen radical reactions, including lipid peroxidation. There is a massive shift of iron from storage proteins to species weighing less than 30,000 daltons (low-molecular-weight iron) during the first 2 h of reperfusion following a 15-min cardiac arrest. Iron is rapidly delocalized by reduction out of ferritin by a number of different radical species, including O_2^-. There is reason to believe that excessive O_2^- is present during early reperfusion. Xanthine oxidase and cyclo-oxygenase, whose substrates are hypoxanthine and arachidonate, respectively, produce O_2^- as a side product.

Fe^{2+} that has been released from normal storage sites may then participate in the Fenton reaction to produce hydroxyl radical (OH*) or reactive iron-oxygen complexes (perferryl species). Both these species can initiate lipid peroxidation in biological membrane systems.

Evidence of lipid peroxidation may be measured by assay of malondialdehyde or demonstration of a loss of unsaturated fatty acids. In an animal model of cardiac arrest and resuscitation, there was no increase in low-molecular-weight iron after 15 min of ischemia. After 2 h of reperfusion, the level of free iron had tripled. After 8 h of reperfusion, brain tissue malondialdehyde levels had increased fivefold, and there was a 30-percent loss of unsaturated membrane lipids and transmembrane ionic gradients.

Excitatory neurotransmitter uptake is inhibited by arachidonate and products of lipid peroxidation. Continued stimulation of receptors may contribute to neuronal damage by an as yet unidentified mechanism.

Therapy with calcium antagonists or iron chelators has produced mixed results. In a 10-min cardiac arrest model in rats, deferoxamine therapy produced a dramatic 100-percent increase in 10-day intact neurological survival. However in a 15-min cardiac arrest model in dogs, we were unable to demonstrate significant effects of therapy with deferoxamine and the calcium antagonist lidoflazine on either neurological deficit scores or histopathological evidence of cell death. Both deferoxamine and exogenously administered superoxide dismutase (the scavenger enzyme for superoxide) significantly inhibit malondialdehyde accumulation by 8 h of reperfusion. Deferoxamine retarded the loss of unsaturated fatty acids and protected tissue Na/K ratios. The calcium antagonist flunarizine has no effect on products of lipid peroxidation, ultrastructural injury, or ionic gradient decay.

Protein synthesis in the selectively vulnerable zones is suppressed about 90 percent early in reperfusion and does not recover significantly. Since proteins are intimately involved in cellular processes such as synthesis, catabolism, and regulation, loss of protein synthesis during brain reperfusion must be viewed as a major phenomenon. Failure of protein synthesis must involve damage along the transcription-translation system. Following a 20-min arrest and up to 8 h of reperfusion, neither brain nuclear DNA nor mitochondrial DNA show evidence of damage. We also conducted specific studies for radical-induced formation of transcription-terminating damage to thymine bases and found that neither thymine glycols nor thymine dimers are formed during brain reperfusion. Not only is the DNA intact, but active transcription of new RNA message is occurring during reperfusion (Nowak et al., 1990). This evidence shows that the mechanism for message transcription survives brain ischemia and is active during early reperfusion; therefore, transcriptional failure cannot be the cause of suppressed protein synthesis. The suppression of protein synthesis is likely to be at the translation step. Potential mechanisms include ribosomal structural damage or inhibition by products elaborated in a stereotypic "heat shock" response.

LATE EVENTS DURING REPERFUSION

Brain tissue ionic concentrations are indistinguishable from normal after 4 h of reperfusion following a 15-min cardiac arrest. The tissue iron has been recovered into high-molecular-weight species by 8 h of reperfusion. However, after 8 h large shifts of the concentrations of calcium, potassium, and sodium are observed. These shifts most likely reflect equilibration between the cytosol and the interstitial fluid for these ions. Electron microscopic examination of brains fixed in vivo reveals an obvious general degradation of membrane structure and large holes in the nuclear and cytoplasmic membranes. Nuclear chromatin is densely clumped, with grossly abnormal nuclear architecture. Mitochondrial architecture is well preserved. The endoplasmic reticulum is dilated and ragged, and normally arranged polyribosomes are virtually nonexistent. This picture is consistent with ongoing membrane injury during reperfusion by mechanisms such as lipid peroxidation. This would produce degradation of membrane structure to the point that the membrane becomes freely permeable to ions and the cell is irreversibly injured.

CLINICAL IMPLICATIONS

Optimum therapy to obviate continuing injury and salvage viable brain tissue is unknown. Most therapeutic studies use animal models, use pretreatment, or contain small numbers of patients. However, a few general principles can be stated. Perfusion should be maintained at normal levels. It does not appear that intracranial pressure is increased in the postresuscitation period, and therefore therapies directed at increased intracranial pressure (hyperventilation and osmotic agents) are unneeded. Hypotension should be avoided for the obvious reasons. Oxygenation should be maintained at or near normal levels. Hyperoxia should be avoided, since it is toxic to the lungs and may increase brain damage. Pre-arrest hyperglycemia is associated with poor neurologic outcome (Calle et al., 1989), and although glucose administered postinsult has not been adequately studied, hyperglycemia should probably be avoided.

Several other therapies have been advocated, but human studies have failed to show efficacy. These therapies include pentobarbital coma (Brain Resuscitation . . . Study Group, 1986), calcium antagonists (both pre- and post-arrest), and glucocorticoids (Jastremski et al., 1989; Grafton and Longstreth, 1988).

Ischemic injury of the brain is complex, as indicated in this chapter. The pattern of ATP and ionic recovery and DNA transcription during reperfusion shows that several cellular systems are intact following prolonged ischemia and reperfusion. Effective therapeutic response will be identified only by continued studies.

BIBLIOGRAPHY

Brain Resuscitation Clinical Trial I Study Group: Randomized clinical study of thiopental loading in comatose survivors of cardiac arrest. *N Engl J Med* 314:397, 1986.

Calle PA, Buylaert WA, Vanhaute OA: Glycemia in the post-resuscitation period. *Resuscitation* 17(suppl):S181, 1989.

Grafton ST, Longstreth WT Jr: Steroids after cardiac arrest: A retrospective study with concurrent, nonrandomized controls. *Neurology* 38:1315, 1988.

Jastremski M, Sutton-Tyrrell K, Vaagenes P, et al: Glucocorticoid treatment does not improve neurological recovery following cardiac arrest. Brain Resuscitation Clinical Trial I Study Group. *JAMA* 262:3427, 1989.

Krause, GS, Kumar K, White BC, et al: Ischemia, resuscitation, and reperfusion: Mechanisms of tissue injury and prospects for protection. *Am Heart J* 111:768, 1986.

Krause GS, White BC, Aust SD, et al: Brain cell death following ischemia and reperfusion: A proposed biochemical sequence. *Crit Care Med* 16:714, 1988.

Nowak TS, Bond U, Schlesinger MJ: Heat shock RNA levels in brain and other tissues after hyperthermia and transient ischemia. *J Neurochem* 54:451, 1990.

Siesjo BK, Bengtsson F, Grampp W, et al: Calcium, excitotoxins, and neuronal death in the brain. *Ann NY Acad Sci* 568:234, 1989.

5 ADVANCED AIRWAY SUPPORT

Daniel F. Danzl

This chapter reviews those techniques available to establish an airway and ventilate a patient after basic maneuvers have been utilized. The uses of oral and nasal airways, the bag-valve-mask (BVM) unit, and various esophageal obturator airways are discussed. The techniques of orotracheal and nasotracheal intubation, translaryngeal insufflation, fiberoptic laryngoscopy, retrograde tracheal intubation, and cricothyrotomy are presented. Neuromuscular blockade and the role of respiratory support in cerebral resuscitation are discussed. Finally, suctioning, extubation, and the use of ventilators in the emergency department are reviewed.

ORAL AND NASAL AIRWAYS

The oral airway, or oropharyngeal tube, lifts the base of the tongue off the hypopharynx. Adult, child, and infant sizes should be available. The oral airway should be used only in patients without protective airway reflexes since it stimulates the gag reflex. In the emergency department, a short oral airway functions as a bite block and helps to prevent trismic airway occlusion of an orotracheal tube. Two components of the triple airway maneuver, mouth opening and the jaw thrust, are accomplished with the oral airway. The third, head extension, is occasionally necessary to free the base of the tongue from the posterior pharyngeal wall.

The tube is placed over the tongue after the mouth is opened. One technique is to insert it after depressing the tongue with a tongue blade. Another method is to insert the tube with the convexity caudad. It is then rotated back after insertion. Improper insertion will increase airway resistance by pushing the base of the tongue backward.

A variation of the oropharyngeal tube is the S tube. It is inserted like an oral airway, and then the victim's head is extended. Ventilation is initiated after the nose is pinched and the flange sealed against the lips. A variety of mouth-to-mask with tubing devices are available.

Nasal airways, or nasopharyngeal tubes, are easier to insert than oral airways and are better tolerated by patients not deeply comatose and with active gag reflexes. Epistaxis is minimized by using a lubricated soft tube with good technique. Insertion of a nasal airway may be a useful temporizing maneuver in patients with seizures, trismus, or cervical spine injuries prior to nasotracheal intubation. In addition, a nasogastric tube passed through it will prevent intracranial placement in patients with cribriform plate fractures.

Plastic or soft rubber nasopharyngeal tubes, lubricated with a vasoconstrictor-anesthetic agent, are inserted into the nares parallel to the palate, into the hypopharynx. The tube is advanced until maximal airflow is heard. If inserted too deeply, the tip may stimulate laryngospasm or enter the esophagus. Patients can be ventilated by bag and mask with the nasal airway in place.

THE BAG-VALVE-MASK UNIT

The BVM unit includes a self-inflating bag, a nonrebreathing valve, and a face mask. The unit is not easy to use effectively. The operator should check for adverse anatomic or pathologic facial conditions (Table 5-1). Depending on the operator's expertise, mouth-to-mask ventilation may be superior. The BVM can allow oxygen delivery during both artificial and spontaneous ventilation.

For delivery of 100% oxygen, there must be a reservoir as large as the bag volume and an oxygen flow rate equaling the respiratory minute volume. The nonrebreathing valve at the mask or endotracheal (ET) tube allows air entry into the lungs with bag compression, while exhaled air exits through a separate port. Various sizes of transparent masks should be made available.

Corrugated tubing reservoirs may be sensitive to variations in ventilatory technique and not deliver 100% oxygen. There are two more effective equipment options. Use a 2.5-L reservoir bag with an oxygen inflow of 15 L/min, or attach a demand valve to the reservoir port of the ventilating bag (Campbell et al., 1988).

Before ventilating the patient, the operator should insert an oropharyngeal or nasopharyngeal tube and extend the stable neck. Then the mask is clamped snugly to the face with the thumb and index finger on the mask, with the other fingers pulling the chin upward.

A major advantage of initially using a bag to ventilate via an ET tube is that the operator can better judge pulmonary compliance. Common errors in technique include allowing air leaks around the mask and inadequate tidal volume delivery. Bag-mask ventilation can provide adequate ventilatory support in neurologically uncompromised injured patients.

Some alert patients with mild respiratory insufficiency who do not meet intubation criteria can be temporarily managed with continuous positive airway pressure (CPAP) by means of a snug-fitting face mask. The functional residual capacity and work of breathing is reduced. Mask-CPAP may delay or reduce the need for intubation. It should be avoided in patients with severe maxillofacial trauma and potential basilar skull fractures. Pneumocephalus is a hazard.

ESOPHAGEAL OBTURATOR AIRWAYS

The esophageal obturator airway (EOA) is an additional ventilatory adjunct when endotracheal intubation is not a viable prehospital option. It helps to prevent gastric insufflation and regurgitation during positive pressure ventilation but is not a substitute for tracheal intubation.

The major advantage of the EOA is that insertion does not require laryngeal visualization; thus it can be placed quickly by trained personnel. When necessary, the cervical spine can be held motionless.

The tube should be inserted only in apneic, comatose patients over 16 years of age. Patients with upper airway obstruction, known esophageal disease, or caustic ingestions require different airway management, as do patients with massive nasal or intraoral hemorrhage.

The original EOA is a large-bore 34-cm tube with a rounded, occluded distal tip. A snap lock connects the tube through the center of a clear plastic oronasal mask. There are multiple openings in the proximal half of the tube below the mask at the hypopharyngeal level.

After attaching the mask to the proximal end of the tube, the patient's mandible and tongue are pulled forward with the head held in a neutral position. If a neck injury is excluded, slight neck flexion will decrease the incidence of inadvertent tracheal intubation. The tube is inserted after the distal tip is lubricated. The tube should not be forced against an obstruction.

Once the mask is carefully sealed by hand to the patient's face, ventilation is initiated by mouth or bag-valve unit. This forces air into the trachea, the only unobstructed orifice. Ausculation for bilateral breath sounds ensures esophageal placement of the tube. Then the cuff is inflated with 30 mL of air. The cuff must lie below the level of the carina, or partial compression of the trachea will obstruct ventilation.

Table 5-1. Mask Ventilation Impediments

Beard ± mustache
Cervical arthritis
Edentulous
Facial fractures
Macroglossia
Mandibular surgery
Obesity
Oropharyngeal infections
Prognathism
Temporomandibular arthritis
Upper airway obstructions

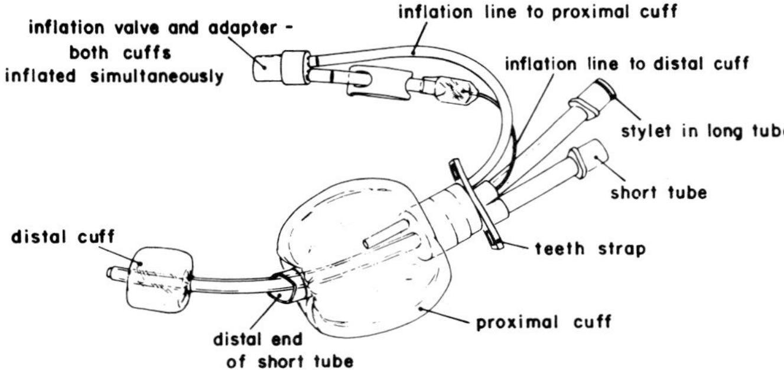

Fig. 5-1. Pharyngeotracheal lumen airway. The distal cuff occludes the esophagus. The proximal cuff occludes the upper airway.

One variation of the original EOA is the esophageal gastric tube airway (EGTA). There are two holes in the mask. The esophageal obturator attaches to one, and a nasogastric tube can be passed down the tube through a valve into the stomach. The unit allows ventilation through the second hole.

Another modification of the EOA, the tracheoesophageal airway, uses a standard ET tube. The ET tube, with a high-volume, low-pressure cuff, is positioned in the esophagus. The modified face mask has two openings, one for the ET tube and the second for oropharyngeal ventilation. The ET tube in the esophagus vents the stomach and facilitates gastric decompression. This should decrease the incidence of esophageal rupture. If the tube is accidentally inserted into the trachea, it is left as a functional ET tube. Neck extension while applying cricoid pressure (Sellick's maneuver) facilitates tracheal placement of a functional ET tube. The EOA does not protect the airway if upper airway hemorrhage occurs.

In the field, a pharyngeotracheal lumen airway (PTL) could prove useful when endotracheal intubation fails (Fig. 5-1). This two-tube two-cuff airway has a large low-pressure cuff that seals the oropharynx at the proximal airway. This might help tamponade an intraoral hemorrhage. Discrimination between esophageal and endotracheal placement can be difficult.

A further variation is the esophageal tracheal combitube. This is a plastic twin-lumen tube, with one lumen resembling an EOA and the other an endotracheal airway. The combitube has a pharyngeal sealing balloon that in effect replaces the EOA mask. Potential advantages of a pharyngeal cuff (combitube) over an oral cuff (PTL) include consistent inflation volume (100 mL) to achieve a seal and less dental trauma to the cuff.

The amount of initial oxygenation possible with the EOA using a FI_{O_2} of 100 percent is theoretically similar to that provided with an ET tube. The P_{CO_2}, with EOA ventilation, will often be higher. In some field evaluations of EOA and EGTA, a marked improvement in both oxygenation and ventilation after ET intubation was noted. In others, the EGTA or EOA when used with an oxygen-powered breathing device achieved adequate ventilation (Geehr et al., 1985).

The most common complication, seen in about 10 percent of EOA insertions, is inadvertent tracheal intubation. Subsequent asphyxia will occur unless this complication is quickly recognized.

The incidence of esophageal rupture is unknown as many patients do not receive postmortem examinations. The probable cause of esophageal tears distal to the cuff is increased intragastric pressure against an occluded esophagus during CPR.

Esophageal tears or perforation may result from direct trauma of the tube or postemesis (Mallory-Weiss syndrome). If conscious, patient symptoms may include shortness of breath, chest pain, and dysphagia. Signs include subcutaneous emphysema, pneumomediastinum, Hamman's crunch, and gastrointestinal hemorrhage.

There will be an increased incidence of complications in patients who are not apneic or deeply comatose. They may vomit, aspirate, or develop laryngospasm or supraglottic obstruction.

After the patient arrives in the emergency department, the operator should intubate the trachea with a cuffed ET tube prior to removal of the EOA. Suctioning equipment and assistants should be nearby for the procedure. A patient with an EOA in place who suddenly becomes responsive, with protective airway reflexes, should be rolled to the side, with the cuff deflated and the tube removed.

OROTRACHEAL INTUBATION

Although adequate oxygenation is usually obtainable with the preceding techniques, the most reliable means to ensure a patent airway, provide ventilation and oxygenation, and prevent aspiration is endotracheal intubation. In the emergency department, endotracheal intubation is indicated in all patients without intact protective airway reflexes.

In addition, many conscious patients require emergency intubation. They may be unable to spontaneously clear the airway of secretions, require mechanical ventilation, have aspirated, or have poor laryngeal reflexes. Most are lying supine on gurneys. The World War I aphorism "He who looks at heaven will soon be there" still holds. In apneic or arrested patients with stable cervical spines, orotracheal intubation is the most rapid method to secure the airway.

A more conservative initial airway approach is indicated in some patients with, for example, chronic pulmonary disease or blunt chest trauma. Deterioration in vital signs or arterial blood gases would direct treatment.

Hypoxemia rather than hypercarbia is the real threat. Given a baseline oxygen consumption of 250 mL/min, ventilatory support is mandated when the Pa_{O_2} falls below 40 to 50 mmHg despite supplementation. Clinical judgment is more critical with hypercarbia or with evidence of excessive work of breathing.

Technique

Evaluate the upper airway anatomy. Brief examination of the teeth, oral cavity size, mentum-cricoid distance, mobility and posterior depth of the mandible, and neck length mobility may clue the operator to anticipate a difficult airway.

While calling for an assistant, the operator should check and arrange the necessary equipment. The appropriate-size tube and an additional tube 0.5 to 1 mm in size smaller should be selected and the cuff checked for air leaks. Selecting a tube with the proper diameter is essential (Table 5-2). Most tubes will require cutting after orotracheal intubation, or they will gradually creep toward the carina.

Tubes with low-pressure high-volume cuffs are best for children over 6 years old and adults. In patients below age 6, the operator should use uncuffed tubes. Thin-walled cuffs prevent aspiration when properly inflated better than medium-walled cuffs. Since microcirculation to the tracheal mucosa is not impaired until cuff pressures exceed 40 cm of water, the operator should attempt to maintain the cuff pressure between 25 and 34 cm of water. After nasogastric decompression, the cuff pressure should be deflated to 15 to 20 cm of water, or just to the point of eliminating audible air leaks. Cuff overinflation can compromise the ET tube lumen.

The light on the size and type laryngoscope desired should be tested. The straight Magill blade directly lifts the epiglottis. The curved Mac-

Table 5-2. Approximate Adult Sizes for Endotracheal Tubes and Suction Catheters

Patient	Endotracheal Tube Inner Diameter (mm)*	Suction Catheter Size (French) Outer Diameter
Adult female	7.5–8.0	12–14
Adult male	8.0–8.5	14

* Tubes of 0.5 to 1 mm smaller inner diameter are used for nasotracheal intubation.

intosh blade rests in the vallecula above the epiglottis and indirectly lifts it off the larynx by traction on the frenulum. Expertise at intubation with both blades is desirable, since they offer differing advantages, depending on the clinical setting and body habitus. The curved blade may be less traumatic and reflex-stimulating since it does not directly touch the larynx, while allowing more room for adequate visualization during tube placement. The straight blade is mechanically easier to insert in many patients without large central incisors. Selecting the proper size blade greatly facilitates intubation.

When all equipment is in order, the patient should be placed in the sniffing position. (*Note:* The novice laryngoscopist's most common reasons for failure—inadequate equipment preparation and poor patient positioning—occur prior to the use of the laryngoscope.)

Flexion of the lower neck with extension at the atlantooccipital joint (sniffing position) aligns the oropharyngeolaryngeal axis, allowing a direct view of the larynx. Placing a folded towel or small pillow under the occiput is often helpful.

If possible, the patient should be oxygenated by mask with 100% oxygen prior to intubation. The operator begins with the laryngoscope in the left hand and an ET tube or tonsil suction catheter in the right hand. After removal of dentures and any obscuring blood, secretions, or vomitus, the suction catheter is exchanged for the endotracheal tube and inserted during the same laryngoscopy.

The blade is inserted into the right corner of the patient's mouth. If a curved Macintosh blade is used, the flange will push the tongue to the left side of the oropharynx. If the blade is inserted down the middle, the tongue forces the line of sight posteriorly, resulting in an apparent "anterior larynx."

After visualization of the arytenoids and the epiglottis, the epiglottis is lifted directly with the straight blade or indirectly with the curved blade. The larynx is exposed by pulling on the handle in the direction it points, that is, 90° to the blade. Cocking the handle back, especially with the straight blade, will fracture incisors.

If the arytenoid cartilages are recognized, one can avoid the most common error, overly deep insertion of the blade. If only the posterior commissure is visible, having an assistant apply pressure on the cricoid (Sellick's maneuver) is helpful. Analogous to fielding a baseball, watch the cuff as it passes completely through the cords to avoid an error. Attempts at blind passage only invite anoxia. Always be willing to abort the attempt if visualization of the larynx is not successful, and resume mask ventilation.

With proper technique and practice, malleable blunt-tipped metal or plastic stylets are rarely necessary. If the patient's anatomy requires it, the proximal end of the stylet may be bent 45°, but the tip should not extend beyond the end of the endotracheal tube. Thin, flexible intubation stylets are commercially available and should be on hand for the unusually difficult intubation.

Visualization of the larynx before the cervical spine is cleared is difficult, since alignment of the oropharyngeolaryngeal axis is not possible. One method of moving the tip of the tube anteriorly is to use a slightly flexed directional-tip tube (Endotrol) coupled with a Sellick maneuver. Another is to aim the tip anteriorly with a Magill forceps while an assistant advances the tube.

Some awake patients in respiratory distress may be easier to intubate orally or nasally in a semi-sitting position.

Blind orotracheal intubation has been studied by a transillumination technique with a lighted stylet which may prove useful. However, this requires optimal body habitus and room illumination. Tactile blind digital intubation has been effective in the field as an alternative to standard oral or nasal intubation.

The tube is positioned by palpating its tip at the suprasternal notch and advancing it 2 to 3 cm. Correct tube placement is about 2 cm above the carina. From the corner of the mouth, this is approximately 23 cm in men and 21 cm in women.

After cuff inflation, insert an oropharyngeal airway or bite block and auscultate to verify bilateral lung expansion. Inadvertent endobronchial intubation is usually on the right side. Cut and secure the tube, being careful not to impede cervical venous return with the umbilical tape. Confirm placement with a chest x-ray.

If the cuff leaks, tube replacement is possible with or without direct visualization. A length of nasogastric tubing two and one-half to three times the length of the ET tube can be inserted as a guide.

Complications

Acute complications, in addition to hypoxia and hypercarbia, include lack of recognition of endobronchial or esophageal intubation. Disposable CO_2 detection devices can confirm endotracheal tube placement, independent of the potential prediction of outcome in cardiac arrest. The tube may be obstructed by a bulging cuff, secretions, kinking, or biting. Subsequent neck movement can also displace the tube.

Deleterious cardiovascular and intracranial pressure changes are occasionally associated with endotracheal intubation. Conflicting data suggest a possible benefit from intravenous or topical lidocaine. Intravenous magnesium sulfate reportedly attenuates catecholamine release. Dental trauma, soft tissue injury, temporomandibular dislocation, and cervical spine subluxation can occur.

Although they are uncommon, chronic complications of endotracheal intubations done under emergency conditions do occur and may be quite debilitating. Arytenoid cartilage displacement, usually on the right, prevents the patient from phonating properly. Chordal synechiae may develop anteriorly or commissural stenosis posteriorly. Subglottic stenosis is the most disastrous complication.

Chemical and ischemic mucosal damage may be minimized by using plastic tubes with cuffs properly inflated. Tube motion in the larynx and trachea should be prevented. This usually occurs in combative patients or those on ventilators.

NASOTRACHEAL INTUBATION

Nasotracheal intubation is an essential skill allowing a flexible approach to airway management. The success rate for a prospective series of 300 patients managed with blind nasotracheal intubation in the emergency department was 92 percent (Danzl and Thomas, 1980). In one field study, the success rate was 95.1 percent.

Technique

Spray both nares with a topical vasoconstrictor-anesthetic, then select a cuffed endotracheal tube 0.5 to 1 mm in size smaller than that optimal for oral intubation. Advance the tube, lubricated with a water-soluble (2% lidocaine, K-Y) jelly, along the nasal floor on the more patent side. If the nares appear equal, initially try the right side. Having the bevel face the septum helps to prevent abrasions of Kiesselbach's plexus. Steady, gentle pressure or slow rotation of the tube usually bypasses small obstructions. If the right side is impassible, attempt the other side before selecting a tube 0.5 mm narrower in inner diameter.

In patients with intact protective airway reflexes, translaryngeal or directed transoral anesthesia may facilitate intubation. After palpating the superior border of the cricoid cartilage in the midline, puncture the cricothyroid membrane with a 22- to 25-gauge 0.5- to 1-in needle on a 3- to 5-mL syringe (Fig. 5-2A,B). The needle should be perpendicular to the membrane in the midline, with the point of injection just cranial to the cricoid cartilage. After aspirating air, swiftly inject 1.5 to 2.0 mL of 4% lidocaine (sterile for injection) and press the site firmly with a finger for a few seconds. If local compression is not done in trauma patients, the small amount of subcutaneous emphysema would erroneously suggest laryngeal injury. In a published review of 17,500 cricothyroid punctures with small-gauge needles, eight minor complications were reported.

An assistant can apply cervical traction to the patient's head and

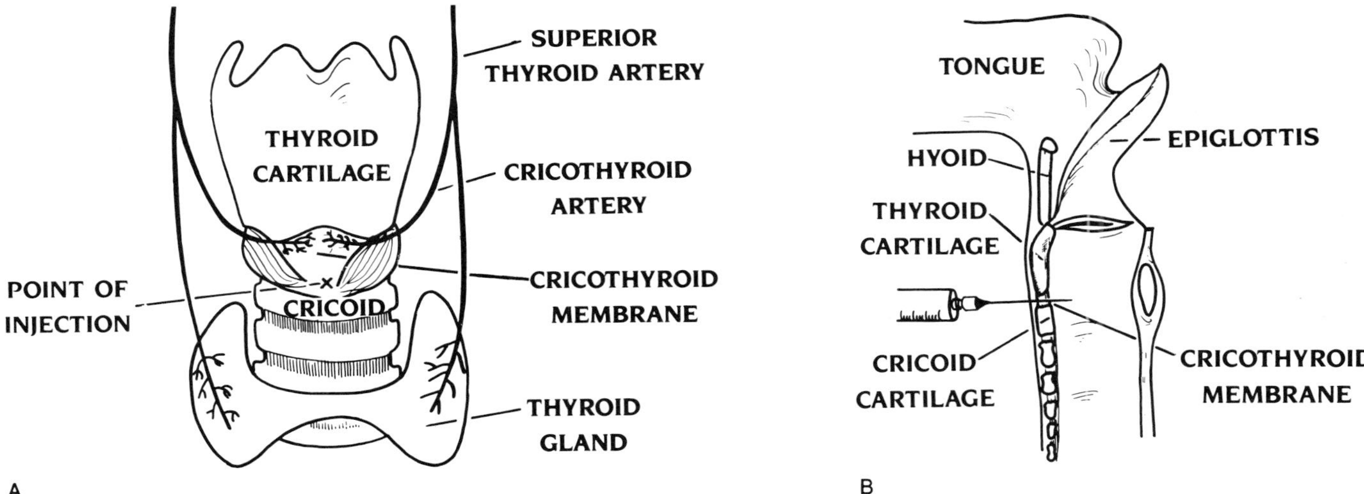

Fig. 5-2. Translaryngeal anesthesia via cricothyroid puncture. **A.** Anatomy—anterior view. **B.** Anatomy—cross-sectional view.

initially maintain it in a neutral or slightly extended position. Stand to the side of the patient, with one hand on the tube and with the thumb and index finger of the other hand straddling the larynx (Fig. 5-3). Advance the tube while rotating it medially 15° to 30° until you hear maximal airflow through the tube. Then gently but swiftly advance the tube during early inspiration. Entrance into the larynx may initiate a slight cough, and most expired air should exit through the tube even though the cuff is uninflated. "Fogging" of the tube may be seen. Most upright patients in severe respiratory distress tolerate intubation in this position. Voluntary tongue extrusion in cooperative patients is helpful. In uncooperative patients, the tongue can be wrapped with gauze and pulled forward.

Advancement toward the carina can be observed externally. Auscultate to verify bilateral lung expansion and cuff inflation. Secretions or blood in the tube should be removed prior to positive pressure ventilation. Secure the tube with umbilical tape or commercial fixaturs rather than adhesive tape.

If intubation is unsuccessful, carefully inspect the neck to determine the malposition of the tube. Most commonly, it is in the pyriform fossa on the same side as the nares used. A bulge will be seen and palpated laterally. Withdraw the tube into the retropharynx until breath sounds are again heard. Redirect while manually displacing the larynx toward the bulge. If there is no contraindication, flexion and rotation of the neck to the ipsilateral side often helps while rotating the tube medially.

The other common tube misplacement is posteriorly, in the esophagus. There will be no breath sounds through the tube, and the trachea will be elevated slightly. Attempt redirection after extending the patient's head and performing Sellick's maneuver. If occult cervical spine pathology is suspected, use a tube with directional tip control (Endotrol) or a fiberoptic laryngoscope. Another aid during neck immobilization is temporary cuff inflation, which can force the tip of the tube anteriorly. Advance slightly (2 cm) before cuff deflation and further passage.

Rarely, the tip of the tube lies anteriorly between the epiglottis and the base of the tongue. A supralaryngeal bulge will be visible. Redirect after flexing the stable neck. If the tube rests on the vocal cords, shrill, turbulent air noises will be heard. Rotate the tube slightly to realign the bevel with the cords, or squirt 2 mL of 4% lidocaine (80 mg) down the tube onto the cords if translaryngeal anesthesia was omitted.

Congenital abnormalities in the nasopharynx, including pharyngeal bursae, may be anatomical causes of tube misplacement. With gentle technique, the obstruction can be felt and guided intubation accomplished. Hypertrophic adenoid tissue, polyps, and neoplastic lesions can divert the tube.

Indications

Nasal intubation is helpful in situations where laryngoscopy is difficult, neuromuscular blockade hazardous, or cricothyrotomy unnecessary.

Emergency department patients may present with trismus from seizures, facial trauma, infection, tetanus, or decorticate-decerebrate rigidity. It may be impossible to align the oropharyngeolaryngeal axis in patients with arthritis, masseter spasm, temporomandibular dislocation, or prior oral surgical procedures. Agitated patients or those with a peculiar body habitus may be impossible to intubate orally.

Nasal intubation with a fiberoptic laryngoscope may be required for neoplastic lesions obstructing the pharynx, Ludwig's angina, peritonsillar abscess, and epiglottitis. If the radiographic status of the neck in a traumatized patient is unknown, the nasal route is one of the noninvasive alternatives to cricothyrotomy or translaryngeal ventilation.

Nasotracheal tubes, in addition to being better tolerated by patients than oral tubes, are less traumatic to the tracheal mucosa since there is less intratracheal tube movement with head motion.

Contraindications

Complex nasal and massive midfacial fractures, and bleeding disorders, are relative contraindications to nasotracheal intubation. How-

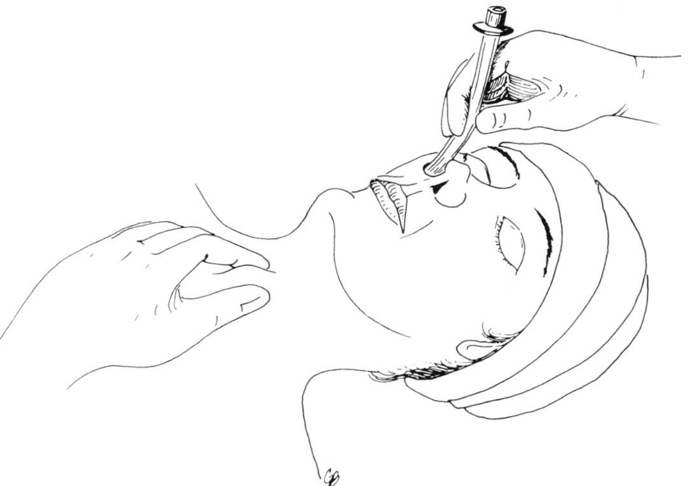

Fig. 5-3. Blind nasotracheal intubation while displacing the larynx to the patient's right.

ever, oral intubation impedes prompt reduction and stabilization of some maxillary fractures. Since a LeFort I fracture does not extend to the cribriform plate, it is not a contraindication. Fiberoptic guidance is preferable when feasible for LeFort II and III fractures.

Unlike nasogastric tube insertion, the risk of inadvertent intracranial passage of a nasotracheal tube seems low. There is only one reported case of intracranial intubation with a nasotracheal tube in the literature. Extremely poor technique in the setting of obvious massive head trauma would be required.

Severe traumatic nasal or pharyngeal hemorrhage may necessitate orotracheal intubation or cricothyrotomy. Nasotracheal intubation should not be done blindly in patients with acute epiglottis. Contamination is a hazard with some basilar skull fractures.

Translaryngeal anesthesia is contraindicated if the landmarks are obscured by thyroid or tumor impingement on the cricothyroid membrane, or in obese or combative patients.

Complications

Serious complications of nasotracheal intubation are quite rare. In a series of 1187 patients, there was no permanent laryngeal damage.

Epistaxis is seen with inadequate topical vasoconstriction, excessive tube size, poor technique, or anatomic defects. Excessive force can damage the nasal septum or turbinates. Recheck the cuff for a potential puncture by a turbinate.

Frequent suctioning, especially if epistaxis or other upper airway hemorrhage is present, will help to prevent thrombotic occlusion of the tube or a mainstem bronchus. Retropharyngeal lacerations, abscesses, and nasal necrosis have been reported.

Paranasal sinusitis, especially occurring with prolonged nasotracheal intubation or severe cranial trauma, can be an unrecognized source of sepsis. Mucopurulent nasal drainage need not be present. The risk of postintubation sinusitis correlates with the duration of intubation, which often reflects the neurologic insult. In the setting of craniofacial trauma, serial CT scans should include views of the paranasal sinuses. Other factors causing sinusitis include the nasogastric tube, sinus hemorrhage or fracture, and corticosteroids. With any route of intubation, one may observe stridor on extubation, tube obstruction or displacement, subglottic stenosis or edema, cuff overinflation, or tracheobronchitis.

TRANSLARYNGEAL VENTILATION

Percutaneous translaryngeal ventilation (PTV) offers a temporizing alternative approach to airway management. It does not substitute for airway control with a cuffed tube. PTV may prove valuable in the initial stabilization of patients not able to be intubated nasotracheally or endotracheally. In those with severe maxillofacial trauma and unknown cervical spine status, PTV can be initiated until cricothyrotomy is completed.

The equipment required for this technique is readily available in emergency departments. The required high-pressure oxygen source can be provided by either a 50-psi wall source with the flow meter set on flush or an oxygen cylinder without a secondary regulator valve. Demand valve devices limited to 50 cm water pressure (70 cm water = 1 psi) do not deliver sufficient tidal volume through large-bore IV catheters (Yealy et al., 1989).

This technique involves puncture of the inferior aspect of the cricothyroid membrane at a *caudal* angle with a 12- to 14-gauge kink-resistant over-the-needle plastic catheter. Cannulae with side holes are preferable and lessen the risk of tracheal mucosal damage. After removing the needle, advance the catheter toward the carina (Fig. 5-4).

The IV catheter and three-way stopcock can be directly attached to high-pressure oxygen tubing if the edges of the stopcock are trimmed. Another convenient way to allow exhalation is to interpose a section of an 18 to 20 French suction catheter with control vent between the stopcock and the tubing.

The patient is ventilated for approximately 2 full seconds or until the chest begins to rise. The valve is then released for 4 to 5 s. This simulates an I:E ratio of 1:2. If exhalation is inadequate, a second venting catheter should be inserted through the cricothyroid membrane next to the first one. Intermittently uncover the second catheter with a finger to allow exhalation. Initially ventilate at 25 psi until correct catheter position is verified. Then increase to 50 psi. Adequate ventilation can be maintained for over an hour.

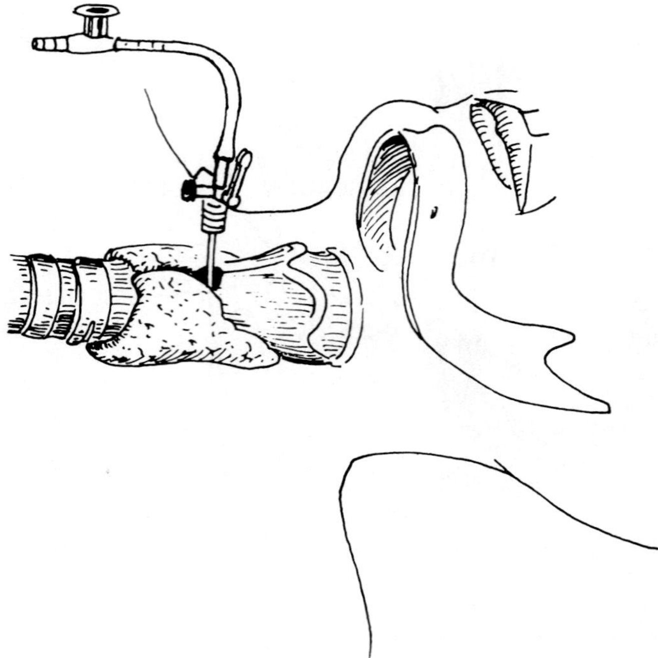

Fig. 5-4. Translaryngeal ventilation. A plastic IV catheter is inserted through the cricothyroid membrane. A three-way stopcock and suction catheter tubing has been attached.

Complications

Complete expiratory obstruction of the airway complicates PTV. Barotrauma, including air embolism, has been an experimental concern. Temporizing lower flow rates might help. Similarly, the use of a large infusion catheter introducer was safe in an airway obstruction model. Avoid attempts to intentionally disimpact an obstruction from below. Other complications of this technique include those reviewed with puncture of the cricothyroid membrane. If the catheter is misplaced or if exhalation is inadequate, massive subcutaneous emphysema from interstitial oxygen insufflation into tissue planes is possible. Esophageal laceration or rupture, pneumomediastinum, or pneumothorax can also occur as a result of excessive insufflation pressures.

FIBEROPTIC LARYNGOSCOPY

The flexible fiberoptic laryngoscope is a valuable adjunct in airway management (Delaney and Hessler, 1988). It is designed to allow visualization of laryngeal structures and can enable difficult intubations, including those around expanding hematomas (Fig. 5-5).

Directed transoral or transnasal and translaryngeal topical anesthesia is essential. Dual suctioning capability is needed; attach one to a tonsil suction catheter for oral blood and secretions, and attach the other to the fiberoptic laryngoscope tubing to aid cord visualization. Intermittent high-flow oxygen helps disperse secretions or vomitus but is less useful with ongoing hemorrhage. Tongue extrusion and anterior mandibular displacement may be helpful if the oral route is chosen. Fragile equipment is more frequently damaged transorally.

Begin by focusing the eyepiece and lubricating the flexible shaft.

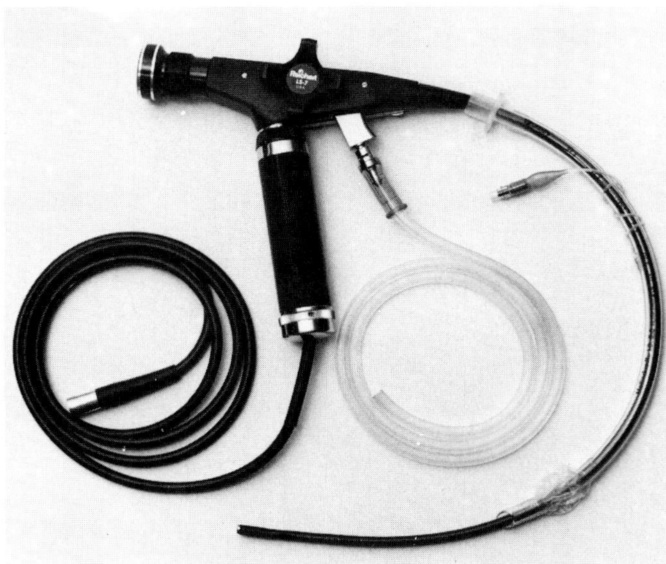

Fig. 5-5. Fiberoptic laryngoscope. An ET tube covers the shaft; suction tubing is attached.

Immerse the lens at the tip of the laryngoscope in warm water to prevent fogging.

To intubate with the flexible laryngoscope, first remove the adapter from an ET tube of 7.0 mm inner diameter or larger. Then slip the lubricated ET tube over the shaft up to the handle. The distal end of the laryngoscope must extend beyond the end of the ET tube. Hold the laryngoscope with your left hand, and control the tip deflection while advancing it through the cords. The laryngoscope will function as a stylet for the tube. After the laryngoscope is in the trachea, advance the ET tube and remove the laryngoscope.

RETROGRADE TRACHEAL INTUBATION

Retrograde tracheal intubation (RTI) is not impeded by the blood that obscures fiberoptically guided intubation. Insertion of a retrograde translaryngeal catheter is a less invasive option than cricothyrotomy when the neck is immobilized and nasotracheal intubation fails. This technique can be time-consuming and must be avoided in apneic patients.

Administer translaryngeal anesthesia (Fig. 5-2) via an 18-gauge needle through the *caudal* aspect of the membrane. After angling the needle 30° to 45° cephalad, advance a 70-cm flexible-tip guide wire. Grasp it in the oropharynx with forceps unless, with luck, it exits spontaneously.

Then thread the end of the guide wire through the distal *side* hole on the ET tube. Clasp the guide wire securely with a hemostat at the neck while advancing the tube. An option is to slide a plastic sheath over the wire and use that as the stylet.

CRICOTHYROTOMY

Cricothyrotomy is an emergency procedure which may be life-saving as a last resort in establishing an airway. This procedure carries far fewer and less serious complications than does emergency tracheostomy, which is indicated only with laryngeal injuries (Mace, 1988).

Cricothyrotomy was initially condemned in 1921 by Chevalier Jackson for its allegedly high incidence of subglottic stenosis. Most of the patients in this preantibiotic-era study had high-pressure tubes placed in the setting of acute laryngeal disease. The technique was reevaluated in 1976. In a series of 655 patients with cricothyrotomy for respiratory management, the complication rate was 6.1 percent. During the last decade at the same center, the complication rate for mostly elective procedures on 78 patients was 28 percent. There were two cases of subglottic stenosis.

The complication rate for patients with emergency cricothyrotomies varies widely. In a series of 147 patients undergoing the procedure, the complication rate was 8.6 percent. In another series of 38 cricothyrotomies performed in the emergency department, the complication rate was 40 percent. Technical changes dropped this rate to 23 percent at the same site in a follow-up series. Nevertheless, in several large series of tracheostomies, the complication rate ranges from 28 to 65 percent, and they are of greater severity.

Indications

Indications for immediate cricothyrotomy include severe, ongoing tracheobronchial hemorrhage, massive midfacial trauma, and inability to control the airway with the usual less invasive maneuvers. Less invasive procedures may be contraindicated or impossible with mechanical upper airway obstruction, facial or cervical trauma, or uncontrollable oral hemorrhage.

Further clinical situations requiring cricothyrotomy include oral or pharyngeal edema from infection, anaphylaxis, or chemical inhalation injuries. Patients with anatomic variants, occult foreign bodies, or obstructing lesions may be impossible to intubate.

Removal of blood or vomitus may not be possible in patients with trismus or masseter spasm. In addition, cricothyrotomy may be required if blind or fiberoptic nasotracheal intubation is unsuccessful.

Contraindications

This technique should not be used on patients who can be safely intubated orally or nasally.

Emergency cricothyrotomy is relatively contraindicated in the presence of acute laryngeal disease due to trauma or infection. It should also be avoided if the patient has very recently been intubated for several days. Tracheostomy may be required in patients who develop airway obstruction after removal of an endotracheal tube in place for over 72 h.

In small children under 10 years of age, the small larynx lies much higher than in adults. A 12- to 14-gauge catheter over the needle is safer than a formal cricothyrotomy or tracheostomy.

Since this is a technique of last resort, a hemorrhagic disorder is not an absolute contraindication. Hemostasis is certainly easier to achieve than with a tracheostomy.

The patient must be completely immobilized because the incision site is 1.5 to 2 cm below the vocal cords and above the vascular thyroid isthmus. The esophagus is posterior and the carotid and jugular vessels lateral to the incision.

Cricothyrotomy, like blind nasotracheal intubation, is contraindicated in patients with laryngotracheal injuries. Retraction of the distal trachea into the superior mediastinum can occur. The management decision depends on operator experience and degree of respiratory distress. Airway options include formal tracheostomy, endotracheal intubation over a flexible fiberoptic bronchoscope, insertion of a small (inner diameter 6.0 to 7.0 mm) orotracheal tube under direct vision, or low transtracheal insufflation.

Technique

Instruments required for emergency cricothyrotomy include a curved Mayo scissors, a dilator, a tracheal hook, and a scalpel blade.

Manual cervical immobilization is applied to the patient by an assistant. After identification of the anatomic landmarks and palpation of the cricothyroid membrane, digitally stabilize the larynx. A vertical 3- to 4-cm incision is made through the skin. Some authors recommend puncturing the membrane caudally with only a needle, which may provide a temporizing airway and guide for the incision. The blade is then rotated to make a horizontal stab through the inferior aspect

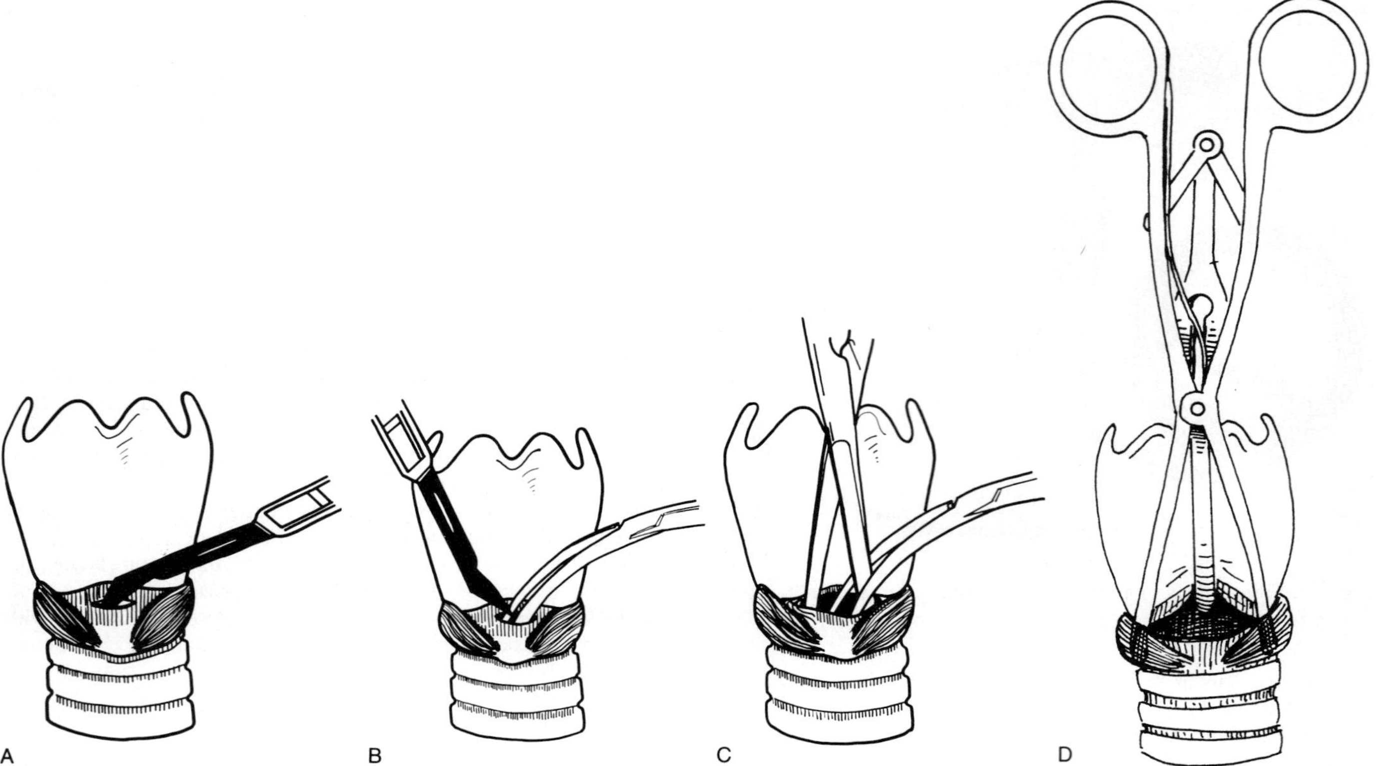

Fig. 5-6. Cricothyrotomy. **A.** Horizontal stab of the cricothyroid membrane following a vertical skin incision. **B** and **C.** Dilation with hemostat and scissors. **D.** Dilation with LaBorde dilator.

of the membrane after it has been repalpated. With the blade tip left in the larynx, scissors points or a hemostat is inserted beside the blade and spread horizontally. Then the scalpel is removed and a dilator (LaBorde, Trousseau) or hemostat is inserted and opened (Fig. 5-6). If blunt scissors are unavailable, the blunt end of the scalpel is used. The scissors are then removed. The largest tracheostomy tube that does not injure the larynx is placed, usually a no. 4 Shiley in adults (outer diameter 8.5 mm). The average fibroelastic adult cricothyroid membrane measures 9 to 10 mm by 22 to 30 mm. Uplifting the larynx with a tracheal hook simplifies tube insertion if the larynx keeps slipping posteriorly.

The cuff is then inflated and the tube securely tied. Alternatively, a small-cuffed (5-mm) endotracheal tube may be cut short and inserted. It should be removed after location of a curved tracheostomy tube, which is less traumatic to the posterior tracheal wall.

A vertical midline skin incision is felt to decrease the incidence of marginal vessel hemorrhage and certainly seems to help with exposure of landmarks. A vertical incision can always be extended. Horizontal incisions have not been reported to produce vascular injury in the prehospital arena. The cricothyroid membrane should be punctured inferiorly and at a caudal angle, since the cricothyroid arteries anastomose superiorly over the membrane. Several "can-opener" cricothyrotomy and percutaneous dilatational devices are available, but there is insufficient clinical experience reported to comment on their safety.

In patients with massive neck swelling, the hemorrhage, subcutaneous emphysema, edema, or fat may make identification of normal landmarks impossible. In such cases, more formal exposure or tracheostomy may be necessary. One approach involves location of the hyoid bone. Measure the distance from the angle of the mandible to the chin. Insert a blade in the midline of the neck down half of that distance from the chin. Attach a skin hook to the hyoid and vertically incise inferiorly.

COMPLICATIONS

Immediate complications of emergency cricothyrotomy include prolonged execution time, excessive hemorrhage, aspiration, and unsuccessful or incorrect tube placement. The most common misplacement is superior to the thyroid cartilage through the thyroid membrane. Inferior tracheotomy placement has also been reported.

Other potential complications include mediastinal or subcutaneous emphysema or creation of a false passage into the trachea. Adjacent vascular, neural, endocrine, esophageal, or pulmonary structures may be injured.

Long-term complications include dysphonia from thyroid cartilage fractures, transient dysphagia, or voice changes. Infection and perichondritis may occur. Innominate artery erosion or pneumothorax, a serious complication of tracheostomy, has not been reported with this technique.

Intubation in Cervical Spinal Injury

There is no single best method of airway management in patients with actual or potential cervical spine injury. At some trauma centers, large numbers of suspected cervical cord injury patients are orally intubated each year without incident. In addition, patients with proven unstable cervical fractures are often electively intubated orally before fusion. In one series of 133 patients with unstable cervical spine fractures, no neurologic complications resulted from 30 oral and 103 nasal intubations (Holley and Jorden, 1989). However, until more data are available, nasotracheal intubation or invasive methods of airway stabilization should generally be selected over orotracheal intubation in the cervical-spine-injured patient.

NEUROMUSCULAR BLOCKADE

Neuromuscular blocking agents facilitate management of selected critical patients in the emergency department. The most commonly used

Table 5-3. Neuromuscular Relaxants

	Intubating Dose IV				
Agent	**Adult**	**Child**	**Onset**	**Duration**	**Complications**
Succinylcholine*†	1.0–1.5 mg/kg	2.0 mg/kg infant 1–2 mg/kg child	30–60 s	3–12 min	1. Bradyarrhythmias 2. Increased intragastric, intraocular, and intracranial pressure 3. Hyperkalemia 4. Fasciculation-induced musculoskeletal trauma 5. Masseter spasm 6. Malignant hyperthermia 7. Prolonged apnea with pseudocholinesterase deficiency 8. Histamine release
Vecuronium	0.08–0.1 mg/kg	0.1 mg/kg	1.5–4 min	25–40 min	1. Prolonged recovery time in obese or elderly, or if hepatic-renal dysfunction
	0.15–0.28 mg/kg (high-dose protocol)	0.2 mg/kg	1–1.5 min	60–120 min	2. Carbamazepine- and phenytoin-induced resistance
Pancuronium	0.1–0.15 mg/kg	0.1–0.15 mg/kg	1–5 min	30–90 min	1. Vagolytic tachyarrhythmias 2. Prolonged recovery in elderly or if hepatic-renal dysfunction 3. Carbamazepine- and phenytoin-induced resistance
Atracurium	0.4–0.5 mg/kg	0.3–0.4 mg/kg	2–5 min	20–45 min	1. Histamine release 2. Hypotension 3. Bronchospasm

* Pretreat with defasciculating dose of 0.01 mg/kg vecuronium if intracranial hypertension or unstable fractures.

† Pretreat with 0.01 mg/kg atropine in children or vagotonic adults.

agents are succinylcholine (Anectine), and vecuronium bromide (Norcuron) and pancuronium (Pavulon). Succinylcholine allows persistent depolarization to occur at the neuromuscular endplate, mimicking acetylcholine. In contrast, vecuronium and pancuronium are nondepolarizing curariform agents. They compete with acetylcholine at the myoneural endplate receptors. The blockade is reversible with acetylcholinesterase inhibitors (Table 5-3).

The most common indication for emergency department neuromuscular blockade should be to improve mechanical ventilation or to control intracranial hypertension. Paralysis improves oxygenation and decreases required peak pressures in a variety of disorders, including refractory pulmonary edema and the adult respiratory distress syndrome. Patients with refractory status asthmaticus; status epilepticus; or tetanic spasms resulting from clostridial infections or a variety of toxins, including strychnine, may improve with blockade.

In addition, extremely violent, agitated patients who jeopardize aeromedical personnel or their own airway security, spinal cord integrity, or fracture stability may require pharmacologic restraint. Be certain to maintain attempts to correct hypoxia and hypovolemia, coupled with physical restraints (Hedges et al., 1988).

For the conditions mentioned above, nondepolarizing agents are preferable to succinylcholine. Although the onset of action is delayed, there are fewer adverse cardiovascular and histaminic effects coupled with a longer duration of paralysis.

The dosage of pancuronium is 0.10 to 0.15 mg/kg IV. After documentation of the neurologic examination, including pupil size, presedation is advised unless there is a significant head injury. Muscle relaxants are neither anxiolytics nor analgesics. Omission of sedation is a common error in patients who remain aware of their paralysis. An increased sympathetic tone can exacerbate arrhythmias. Pancuronium is useful to consider in irreversible status asthmaticus.

Vecuronium bromide (Norcuron) is another nondepolarizing agent. This curariform drug is approximately one-third more potent than pancuronium. The duration of action is one-third to one-half as long. Vecuronium does not cause the degree of tachycardia commonly seen after pancuronium, since it has one-twentieth the vagolytic effect. This simplifies interpretation of a tachycardia developing in the trauma patient. Hypersensitivity reactions are rare, doses are only minimally cumulative, and excretion is biliary. Despite the lack of histamine release, hypotension may occur through two other mechanisms. Sympathetic ganglia blockade occurs, and venous return is decreased from both absent muscle tone and the positive-pressure ventilation.

The usual dose of vecuronium is 0.08 to 0.1 mg/kg IV. Maximal paralysis occurs within 3 to 5 min, with full blockade lasting for 25 to 40 min.

Atracurium is another intermediate-acting agent more suited for patients with hepatic or renal failure. Elimination is via ester hydrolysis and Hoffman degradation, a nonenzymatic process. Atracurium offers advantages when continuous infusion is essential to precisely maintain a required level of neuromuscular blockade. The risk with prolonged infusion is accumulation of laudanosine, a neuroexcitatory metabolic byproduct.

The reversal of nondepolarizing muscle relaxants should not be attempted prior to some sign of motion or spontaneous recovery. Ideally, a "train of four" twitches should be elicited with a neuromuscular stimulator. Reversal requires 0.01 mg/kg of atropine IV, followed by 0.5 to 1.0 mg/kg of edrophonium IV. The onset of action is 30 to 60 s, with a duration of 10 to 30 min. This reversal may be shorter than the duration of the muscle relaxant. Edrophonium is an acetylcholinesterase inhibitor with a faster onset and fewer muscarinic side effects than the longer-acting neostigmine. Prophylactic atropine given before the cholinergic agonist edrophonium helps prevent muscarinic side effects.

When the indication for blockade is tracheal intubation, succinylcholine is the most commonly used agent. It has a more rapid onset (30–60 s) and shorter duration of action (average 5–6 min) than does vecuronium or pancuronium. After a brief fasciculation, complete relaxation occurs at 60 s with maximal paralysis at 2 to 3 min.

The dosage of succinylcholine is 1.0 mg/kg IV for adults and 2.0 mg/kg for children under 12 years. Be prepared to surgically obtain an airway if intubation attempts fail. Succinylcholine appears to produce adequate intubation conditions in the emergency department despite some significant risks (Table 5-3).

The other alternatives for decreasing the time to intubation involve administration of a small "priming" dose (0.10 of actual dose) of vecuronium or high-dose (0.15–0.28 mg/kg) vecuronium. These may prove viable alternatives in the emergency department despite their intermediate duration of action.

Approximately 2 to 3 percent of intubations prove impossible with standard techniques. Emergency physicians selecting neuromuscular blockade must anticipate difficult intubations despite time-limited assessment of the patient's physiognomy.

Before injection of succinylcholine, 0.01 mg/kg of atropine IV may attenuate the muscarinic vagal effects, especially in children and vagotonic adults. Serious arrhythmias are not rare. A desensitization block may develop with prolonged depolarization from repeated doses. An additional pretreatment to consider is a subparalytic dose of 0.01 mg/kg vecuronium to prevent the initial muscle fasciculations that may cause long-bone fractures to become displaced. This is most pronounced in muscular adolescents.

Intraocular pressures also increase. In addition, increased intragastric pressure predisposes to aspiration. Intracranial pressure (ICP) increases are another concern with succinylcholine. This increase in ICP is greater in patients with CNS neoplasms than in those with acute CNS hemorrhage or trauma. If the intubation is rapid, immediate hyperventilation may compensate. Pretreatment with vecuronium and a short-acting barbiturate can attenuate transitory intracranial hypertension, which occurs during tracheal intubation of some patients with significant head trauma.

Avoid barbiturates, including thiopental, unless the cranial trauma is isolated. There is the potential for hypotension with associated injuries. Although there are conflicting data, topical laryngeal or IV lidocaine (1 mg/kg) may minimize the increase in the ICP.

There are other, less preventable side effects of succinylcholine. The serum potassium will transiently rise an average 0.5 mEq/L with succinylcholine. Hyperkalemia is even more pronounced hours after muscle trauma or burns. Avoid depolarizing agents in patients with burns, muscle trauma, myopathies, rhabdomyolysis, narrow-angle glaucoma, renal failure, or neurologic disorders. Any patients with "denervated musculature" (e.g., Guillain-Barré syndrome) are particularly at risk. Genetically susceptible individuals may develop acute malignant hyperthermia. Have dantrolene sodium available.

Patients with an atypical pseudocholinesterase will require prolonged ventilatory support, as will those with burns, cirrhosis, or carcinomas who have low plasma pseudocholinesterase levels.

Effective oxygenation and ventilation during cerebral resuscitation may also require neuromuscular blockade. Cerebral autoregulation of blood flow (CBF) over a range of perfusion pressures may be impaired. As a result, CBF becomes pressure-dependent ($CBF = CPP/CVR$, where *CPP* is cerebral perfusion pressure and *CVR* is cerebral vascular resistance).

Therefore, respiratory support of the bucking or posturing patient becomes critical. After blockade, select an FI_{O_2} sufficient to maintain an arterial P_{O_2} of 100 mmHg, fully saturating hemoglobin. Atelectasis prophylaxis with a positive end-expiratory pressure (PEEP) of up to 5 cm H_2O may be useful. Higher levels impair cerebral venous drainage because of the elevated intrathoracic pressure. Avoid other modalities which also increase the intracranial pressure (ICP), including excessively tight endotracheal tube straps, tight cervical collars, or Trendelenburg positioning.

The optimal Pa_{CO_2} following blockade for the individual patient with intracranial hypertension is frequently unknown. Hyperventilation will decrease cerebral blood volume while cerebral vasoconstriction is intact. Postresuscitation, cerebral vasospasm may decrease CBF, and thus overzealous hyperventilation could be harmful. Always avoid hypercapnia, generally maintaining a Pa_{CO_2} of around 28 to 30 mmHg.

RAPID SEQUENCE INDUCTION

Complex airway emergencies in select nonfasted patients may require rapid sequence induction (RSI), which couples sedation to induce unconsciousness (induction) with muscular paralysis. Intubation follows laryngoscopy while maintaining cricoid pressure to prevent aspiration (Yamamoto, 1990). The principle contraindication is any condition preventing mask ventilation or intubation (Table 5-4).

Thiopental is an ultrashort-acting barbiturate sedative that induces unconsciousness in 10 to 40 s. A dose of 2.0 to 5.0 mg/kg injected at 40 mg/min lasts 10 to 30 min. Another such drug is methohexital (Brevital). Avoid these cerebroprotective agents if hypotension is a problem. Thiopental and methohexital are contraindicated in status asthmaticus.

Fentanyl (Sublimaze) is a potent reversible short-acting narcotic. The dose is 20 to 150 μg/kg, with an onset of action in 1 to 2 min. Rapid injection may cause chest wall rigidity. The optimal dose required for RSI is highly variable, and emergency department experience for this indication is limited. Sufentanil (Sufenta), which is 5 to 10 times as potent as fentanyl, has a more immediate onset at a dose of 8 to 30 μg/kg.

Anothert pharmacologic alternative is a short-acting benzodiazepine. Midazolam (Versed) at a dose of 0.1 mg/kg will probably become the

Table 5-4. Rapid Sequence Induction

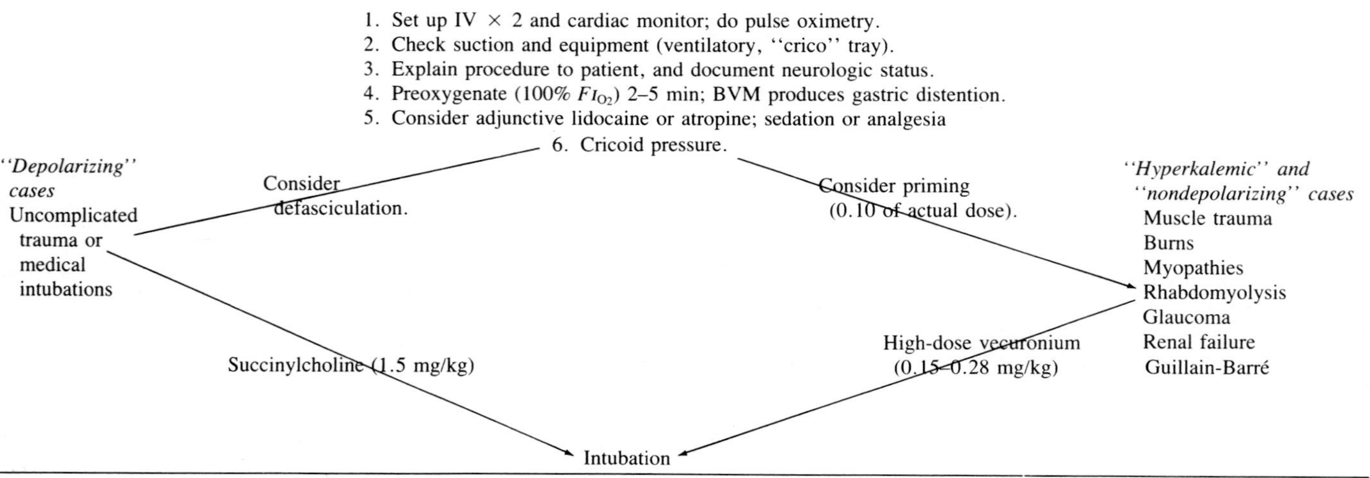

drug of choice if the antagonist flumazenil becomes available. Ketamine is the final consideration in difficult hypotensive or bronchospastic patients. It will increase the ICP in head trauma patients.

Following induction, a full dose of a muscle relaxant is administered. Defasciculation may be desirable when succinylcholine is chosen. A priming dose helps shorten the time to intubation with standard doses of a nondepolarizing agent. High doses without priming are also effective. As mentioned, other adjunctive agents to consider include lidocaine and atropine.

SUCTIONING

Numerous conditions render patients unable to clear tracheal secretions. A rigid-tip plastic tonsil suction catheter should be used for large quantities of oropharyngeal secretions, including blood and vomitus. To suction the nasopharynx and tracheobronchial tree, use a well-lubricated, soft, curved-tip catheter. Straight catheters will usually pass into the right mainstem bronchus. If a curved-tip catheter is available, turning the head to the right in addition to catheter rotation will facilitate passage into the left bronchus.

Select a suction catheter of a size no larger than half the diameter of the tube to be suctioned (Table 5-2). This will prevent pulmonic collapse from insufficient ventilation during suctioning. Oxygenate the patient before and after suctioning to avoid transient desaturation. Insert the catheter without suctioning, and then remove, suctioning with rotation, over 10 to 15 s.

Complications of suctioning include hypoxia, cardiac arrhythmias, hypotension, pulmonic collapse, and direct mucosal injury. The magnitude of the intracranial pressure increase during endotracheal suctioning may be related to the increase in intrathoracic pressure with coughing. Success with topical laryngeal or intravenous lidocaine has been mixed.

Continued airway patency is not assured after endotracheal tube insertion. Suctioning clears clotted blood or inspissated secretions. In addition, mechanical obstruction from tumors or vascular malformations may be detected.

Cuff displacement or overinflation has resulted in ball-valve obstruction of the airway. Cuffs inflated in the field during frigid conditions will expand with warming.

Endobronchial ball-valve obstruction can occur with a clot. This will impair ventilation and produce hyperinflation of individual lobes. Recheck for unequal breath sounds or asymmetrical chest expansion. Elevated inspiratory pressures develop and exhalation is prevented, ultimately resulting in tension pneumothorax.

Deflate the cuff when tracheal ball-valve obstruction is suspected. If the tube is blocked, deflation will allow exhalation. Specific diagnosis and relief of endobronchial obstruction requires bronchoscopy.

EXTUBATION

Emergency department extubations are potentially hazardous. While patients are recovering their protective airway reflexes, they may "fight" the tube. Injecting 1 to 2 mL of 4% lidocaine (sterile for injection) down the endotracheal tube will decrease bucking. Absorption of lidocaine via the airway yields sustained levels, while the maximum serum level is slightly lower than that from an equivalent intravenous dose.

Prior to extubation, rule out metabolic or circulatory abnormalities. Check for respiratory insufficiency. On command, the patient should have an inspiratory capacity of 15 mL/kg. There should be no intercostal or suprasternal retractions, and the patient's grip should be firm. Prior nasogastric decompression is advised.

Arrange all necessary equipment and personnel to treat any acute complications. After suctioning secretions, assure adequate oxygenation of the patient with 100% oxygen. Explain the procedure to the patient. Ventilate with positive pressure, using the BVM unit to exsufflate secretions while the cuff is deflated. At the end of a deep inspiration, to prevent secretory reaccumulation, remove the tube and oxygenate by mask.

Observe the patient closely for stridor. Postextubation laryngospasm is initially treated with oxygen by positive pressure. If necessary, nebulized racemic epinephrine (0.5 mL 2.25% in 4-mL saline) often helps. Rarely, neuromuscular blockade to facilitate reintubation or cricothyrotomy is necessary.

HIGH-FREQUENCY VENTILATION

High-frequency ventilation (HFV) through percutaneous translaryngeal catheters has been used for emergency ventilation with pulmonary dysfunction. There are several forms of HFV, all characterized by rapid rates of ventilation (>60 respirations/min), tidal volumes less than the dead space volume, and low peak airway pressure. These characteristics increase the functional residual capacity and improve oxygenation.

MECHANICAL VENTILATORY SUPPORT

Decisions regarding mechanical ventilatory support in the emergency department include the ventilator type, mode, $F_{I_{O_2}}$, minute ventilation, and use of positive end-expiratory pressure (PEEP) or continuous positive airway pressure (CPAP) (Schuster, 1990).

There are three common ventilator modes or methods of providing the tidal volume: control, assist-control (A/C), and intermittent mandatory ventilation (IMV). Use the control mode for apneic patients. The A/C mode allows the patient to trigger a cycle by inhaling and lowering the airway pressure, which can be adjusted by the ventilator's trigger "sensitivity" (1–3 cmH_2O). The ventilator will provide a nontriggered "controlled" breath unless one is triggered during the selected time cycle. Finally, a predetermined number of ventilator-generated tidal volumes can be assured either unsynchronized (IMV) or synchronized to patient effort (SIMV). In the emergency department, the A/C is the preferred initial mode except with an apneic patient.

Set the initial $F_{I_{O_2}}$ at 1.0 until the results of the first set of arterial blood gases (ABGs) are available. Follow the finger pulse oximetry.

Initially aim for a minute ventilation of 10 L/min. Set the tidal volume at 10 mL/kg ideal body weight and adjust the rate accordingly. Maintain the *peak* airway pressure (PAP) below 40 to 45 cmH_2O to prevent barotrauma. The tidal volume can be increased up to 15 mL/kg to adjust the Pa_{CO_2} unless it elevates the PAP.

PEEP or CPAP should be considered if the decreased pulmonary compliance prevents delivery of an adequate tidal volume. Even low levels (3–5 cmH_2O) of PEEP/CPAP usually render ventilator "sighs" (1.5 × tidal volume) unnecessary. If hypotension develops, adjust the respiratory rate and PEEP to lower the *mean* airway pressure.

BIBLIOGRAPHY

Campbell TP, Stewart RD, Kaplan RM, et al: Oxygen enrichment of bag-valve-mask units during positive-pressure ventilation: A comparison of various techniques. *Ann Emerg Med* 17:232, 1988.

Danzl DF, Thomas DM: Nasotracheal intubations in the emergency department. *Crit Care Med* 8:677, 1980.

Delaney KA, Hessler R: Emergency flexible fiberoptic nasotracheal intubation: A report of 60 cases. *Ann Emerg Med* 17:919, 1988.

Geehr EC, Bogetz MS, Auerbach PS: Pre-hospital tracheal intubation versus esophageal gastric tube airway use: A prospective study. *Am J Emerg Med* 3:381, 1985.

Hedges JR, Dronen SC, Feero S, et al: Succinylcholine-assisted intubations in prehospital care. *Ann Emerg Med* 17:469, 1988.

Holley J, Jorden R: Airway management in patients with unstable cervical spine fractures. *Ann Emerg Med* 18:1237, 1989.

Mace SE: Cricothyrotomy. *J Emerg Med* 6:309, 1988.

Schuster DP: A physiologic approach to initiating, maintaining, and withdrawing mechanical ventilatory support during acute respiratory failure. *Am J Med* 88:268, 1990.

Yamamoto LG, Yim GK, Britten AG: Rapid sequence anesthesia induction for emergency intubation. *Ped Emerg Care* 6:200, 1990.

Yealy DM, Stewart RD, Kaplan RM: Myths and pitfalls in emergency translaryngeal ventilation: Correcting misimpressions. *Ann Emerg Med* 17:690, 1988.

6
VENOUS AND ARTERIAL ACCESS

William A. Berk
Robert Dailey

Immediate access to the venous and arterial circulation is crucial to effective treatment of the critically ill or injured patient. Success facilitates drug, crystalloid, and blood product administration, as well as patient assessment through measurement of central venous and arterial pressures. This chapter discusses indications, techniques, and potential complications of establishing circulatory access.

VENOUS ACCESS

Sites

The normal human anatomy has abundant peripheral veins (Figs. 6-1 and 6-2). In the arms these usually allow ready access. Leg veins are less advantageous due to the risk of precipitating phlebitis and greater technical difficulty. Internal jugular, subclavian, or femoral vein catheterization is performed when peripheral access is impossible or when central venous pressure measurement is desired.

The cephalic vein, in both the forearm and the upper arm, is large, constant, and straight; easily catheterized, it is the time-honored chôice for peripheral access. Veins of the hand are usually accessible even in obese persons but are short, tortuous, and difficult to stabilize—and thus unreliable. Veins in the antecubital fossa are excellent in emergency situations, but an armboard is necessary to prevent catheter kinking or dislodgment with movement. The large basilic vein in the upper arm is usually not visible but with practice can be catheterized by palpating the brachial artery and searching "blindly" for the medially placed vein. Puncture of the brachial artery is common but rarely of clinical significance if care is taken to prevent hemorrhage or hematoma formation.

Veins in the legs often require cutdown for catheter placement. The superficial saphenous vein at the ankle is large, constant, and easy to isolate and cannulate. The proximal great saphenous vein in the thigh may be found reliably 5 cm below the inguinal ligament at the junction of the medial and middle third of the thigh in the supine patient. The deep femoral vein is accessible percutaneously, just medial to the femoral artery; in the pulseless patient the landmark is the junction of the median and middle third of the inguinal ligament. From the great saphenous and deep femoral veins advancement of catheters into the right atrium for central venous pressure measurement is possible.

The external jugular vein can provide reliable access in both adults and children. Although readily distended by Valsalva's or Trendelenburg's maneuvers, scant subcutaneous support can make it difficult to catheterize. Access to central veins without the risk that attends direct internal jugular and subclavian puncture is a major advantage.

In young children intraosseous infusion provides rapid and reliable access in emergencies. A 20-gauge spinal or bone marrow needle is placed in the proximal anterior tibial or distal femur bone marrow to provide emergency access.

Technique Considerations

Care must be taken to minimize the risk of local infectious complications—occurring in up to one-third of patients undergoing venous catheterization—which can rarely result in septicemia. Insertion of peripheral venous catheters should be preceded by a surgical prep and followed routinely by placement of a sterile dressing. Consideration of the indications for venous access and what constitutes appropriate and adequate access in individual patients will minimize risk and facilitate management of emergencies when they occur. If peripheral veins are small, size and visibility can be enhanced by application of hot, moist compresses for 5 min. A gentle circumferential occlusive taping may be necessary if stability of the site is tenuous, with the intravenous line looped and secondarily secured to prevent traction at the point at which the line penetrates the skin. The size of the catheter should be written on the tape dressing.

Catheter-over-needle assemblies are now in common use and provide stable, reliable access in comparison to the steel needles they replaced. Microparticulate matter in intravenous solutions is removed by in-line micropore filters.

Flow Rates

Infusion rate is a crucial issue in resuscitation of patients with severe hypovolemia or progressive hemorrhage. Since flow is a function of the fourth power of the radius of the tube lumen, the internal catheter diameter is a limiting factor. Rate of infusion is also directly proportional to catheter length, which is why a long central catheter will have a slower infusion rate than a shorter catheter of the same caliber in a peripheral vein. Placement of two large-bore—16-gauge or greater—catheters is indicated in stable trauma patients whose injuries could cause potentially life-threatening hemorrhage or for initial therapy of medical patients with hypovolemic shock. Management of exsanguination with an 8.5 French catheter with a pressure infusion cuff around the intravenous bag delivers almost a liter of crystalloid per minute. A single catheter of this type is adequate for preoperative care of almost all surgically remediable injuries. Rapid infusion of larger volumes of fluid should be attended by careful monitoring for clinical signs of volume overload, especially in older patients and those with cardiovascular disease.

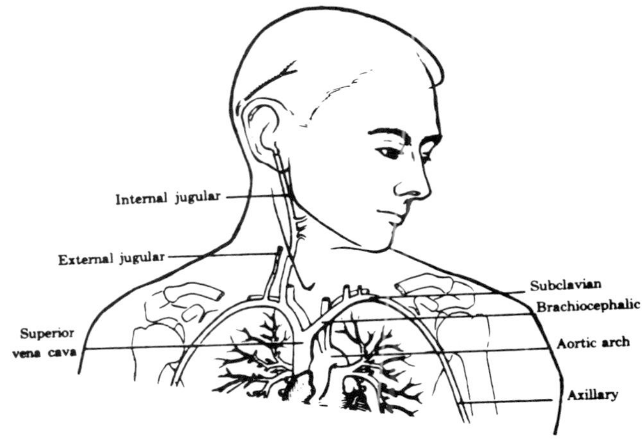

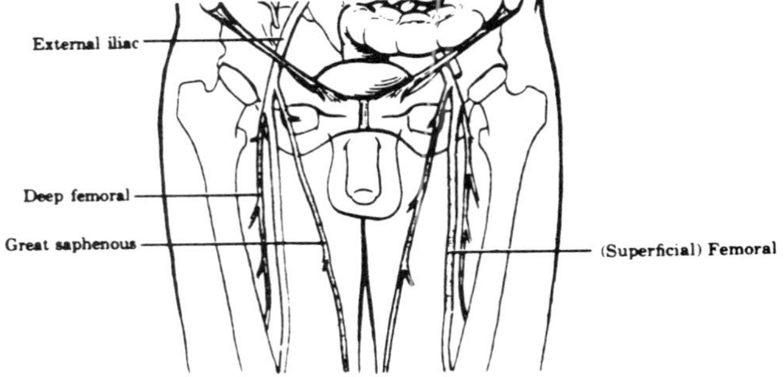

Fig. 6-1. Veins of torso and lower extremities.

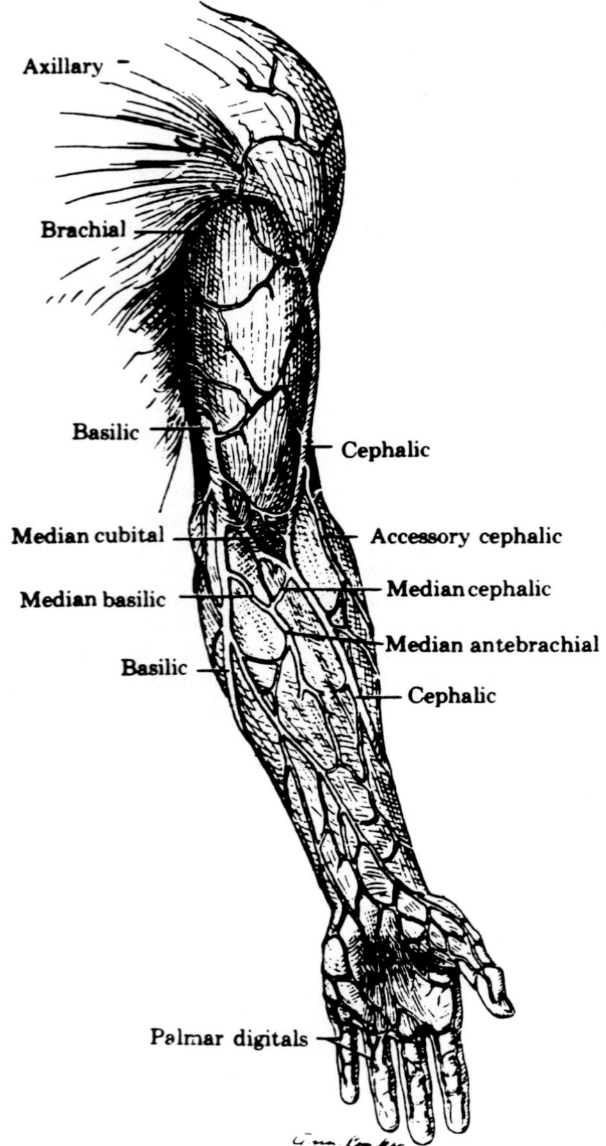

Fig. 6-2. Veins of upper extremity.

Volume repletion and central venous pressure measurement can be accomplished by a Y-arm catheter sheath passed percutaneously into the femoral vein. An 8.5 French catheter can then be used for volume repletion, while a smaller catheter can simultaneously be inserted through the diaphragm into the right atrium for central venous pressure measurement. Femoral catheters should be left in place no longer than 48 h, since iliofemoral thrombophlebitis can result. However, with sterile technique and the use of Silastic catheters, the deep femoral system may be safely employed for a longer duration.

Pressure infusion increases flow two to three times over gravity and is superior to on-line hand-pumped bulbs. Pressure devices are now available for administration of packed red blood cells. Use of a standard urologic Y irrigation set augments flow rates by reducing resistance in the tubing leading to the catheter site. For maximum infusion rates of either blood or crystalloid, use of blood administration set tubing eliminates on-line micropore filters, stopcocks, and one way valves, which increase resistance. Addition of saline to packed red blood cell infusions decreases viscosity, increasing the speed of transfusion.

Volume repletion is effective through intravenous catheters placed distal to an inflated military antishock trouser (MAST) suit. In patients with abdominal hemorrhage, lines in the legs, as well as those in the arms, augment volume.

Warming crystalloid and blood before infusion is essential when volume resuscitation is massive. Crystalloid may be stored in a heating bath or oven, may be safely microwaved, or may be warmed with a heating coil or heat packs. Blood warming coils that allow transfusion rates of up to 500 mL/min are now available. Alternatively, cold-packed red blood cells may be warmed by diluting with an equal amount of hot saline (up to 60°C). Significant hemolysis occurs with microwaving of blood but not with hot saline mixing.

CENTRAL VENOUS PRESSURE CATHETERIZATION AND MONITORING

Central venous catheterization should be performed (1) when rapid delivery of cardiac medications to the coronary circulation is required during CPR; (2) for access when peripheral veins are inadequate; and (3) when central venous pressure measurement is desired. Determination of central venous pressure is indicated (1) when massive volume repletion is administered to elderly patients or those with heart disease, (2) when monitoring fluid administration in patients with visceral trauma and severe head injuries, and (3) when pericardial tamponade is suspected.

Sites and Techniques for Central Venous Pressure Catheter Insertion

Peripheral Sites

Use of peripheral veins to access the central circulation and measure central venous pressure has the indisputable advantage of avoiding the risk associated with direct puncture of the subclavian and internal jugular veins. However, low flow is inevitable, due to the long course of the catheter from extremity to superior vena cava. Peripheral sites also fail frequently due to catheter malposition and kinking. In the arm the brachial-basilic system must be used, since catheters in the cephalic system often become "lost" in the plexus of veins at the shoulder. Smooth passage and correct tip positioning are more likely if the patient is sitting with his or her head angulated sharply toward the catheterized arm, the arm is held abducted, and the catheter is wire-guided. In emergency situations, however, this time-consuming approach to the central circulation is often impractical.

The external jugular vein provides ready central access, since J-wire-guided catheters pass in 75 to 90 percent of cases. Success is enhanced by introducing the wire through a 16-gauge catheter rather than through a needle; using a J-tip with no greater than a 3-mm radius; exaggerating head tilt with marked traction on the skin of the neck; and, when initial attempts with wire through needle techniques are met with resistance at the level of the clavicle, twisting the tip of the J wire 180° before making a second attempt.

The femoral vein can also provide central access, as mentioned above.

Central Venous Puncture

Anatomy

A brief review of anatomy is warranted (Figs. 6-1 and 6-3). The major veins of the upper thorax are deeply and centrally placed and well protected by the clavicles, sternum, and strap muscles. The internal jugular veins join the subclavian veins to form the brachiocephalics (innominates), which in turn join to become the superior vena cava. The sternocleidomastoid muscle attaches separately by two heads to the sternum and clavicle; the triangle formed by these two heads and the clavicle is just above the internal jugular vein. The right internal jugular has a straight path into the superior vena cava, whereas all the other major tributaries curve. Both external jugular veins enter the subclavian veins at close to right angles. The subclavian veins lie

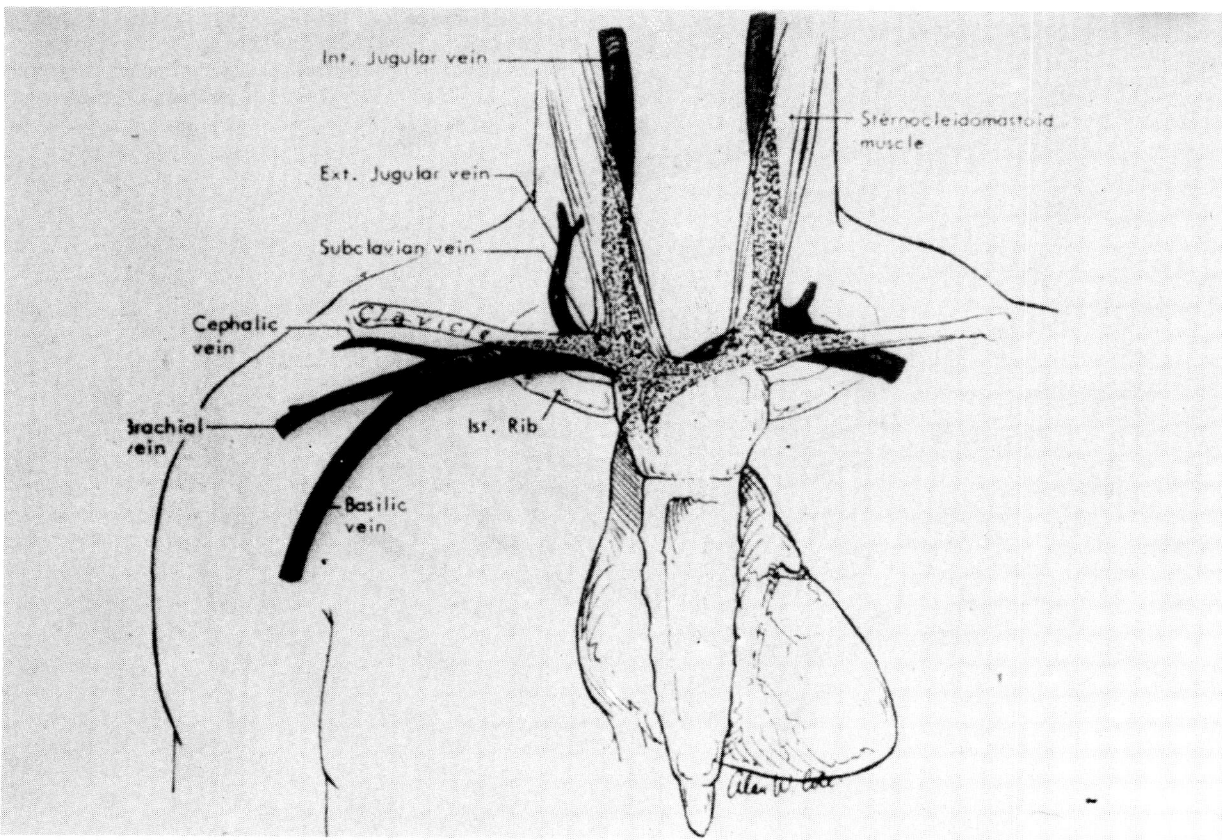

Fig. 6-3. Relationships of major torso veins to other anatomy.

immediately posterior to the junction of the medial and middle third of the clavicle, and are anterior and inferior to the artery; the pleura are immediately posterior and inferior to the subclavian vessels (Fig. 6-4). The internal jugular vein usually lies anterolateral to the carotid.

Equipment

Catheter-through-needle devices, whose large 14-gauge insertion needles are prone to complications and whose 16-gauge catheters allow maximum gravity-assisted flow of 50 mL/min, have been largely supplanted by wire-guided (Seldinger) catheters. An 18-gauge needle is inserted into the vein (Fig. 6-5A), a flexible wire is passed (Fig. 6-5B), and the needle is removed (Fig. 6-5C), leaving just the wire in the vein. The catheter is threaded over the wire and into the vein with a twisting motion (Fig. 6-5E). The wire is then removed, leaving only the catheter in place. If a large-bore catheter is necessary, the apparatus is used with a venodilator, which necessitates a stab for smooth skin penetration. (Fig. 6-5D). In this situation the venodilator is removed with the wire, leaving the large-bore 8.5 French catheter sheath in place (Fig. 6-5F).

The principal advantages of wire-guided catheters are (1) use of a small (and thus safer) needle for insertion; (2) the step-up capability with a venodilator, allowing for higher flow rates often required in trauma resuscitation; (3) the flexibility of exchanging standard intravenous catheters, central venous catheters, and Swan-Ganz catheters without repeated stabs; and (4) the use of J wires to access the central circulation from the external jugular vein.

Preparation—General Aspects

Before central catheterization is implemented, the physician should consider whether the situation actually requires central venous access. Many patients who require volume resuscitation can be managed with large-bore peripheral lines.

All equipment should be at the bedside, including central venous pressure manometer. The patient should be placed in Trendelenburg's position, and the entire route of the neck should be prepped so that all three approaches are possible in case the primary approach fails. The right side is preferred over the left, since (1) the lung apex is slightly lower; (2) there is a straight relationship between the right internal jugular vein and the superior vena cava, and (3) the left-sided

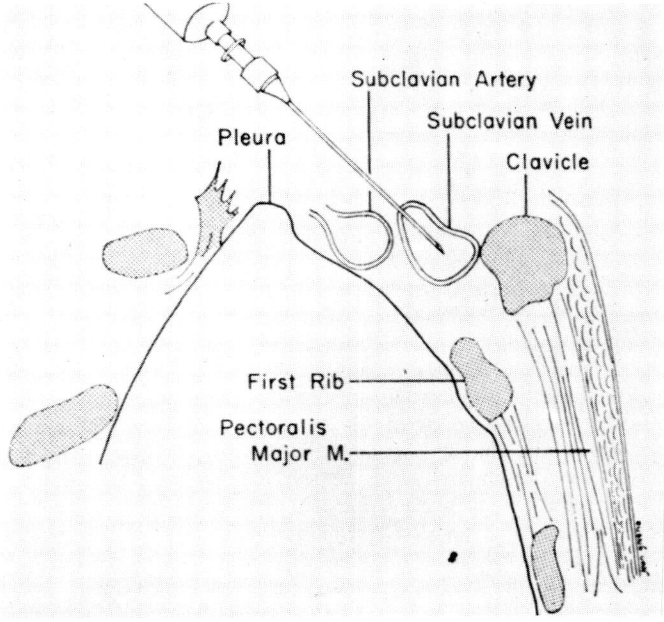

Fig. 6-4. Coronal section through midclavicle.

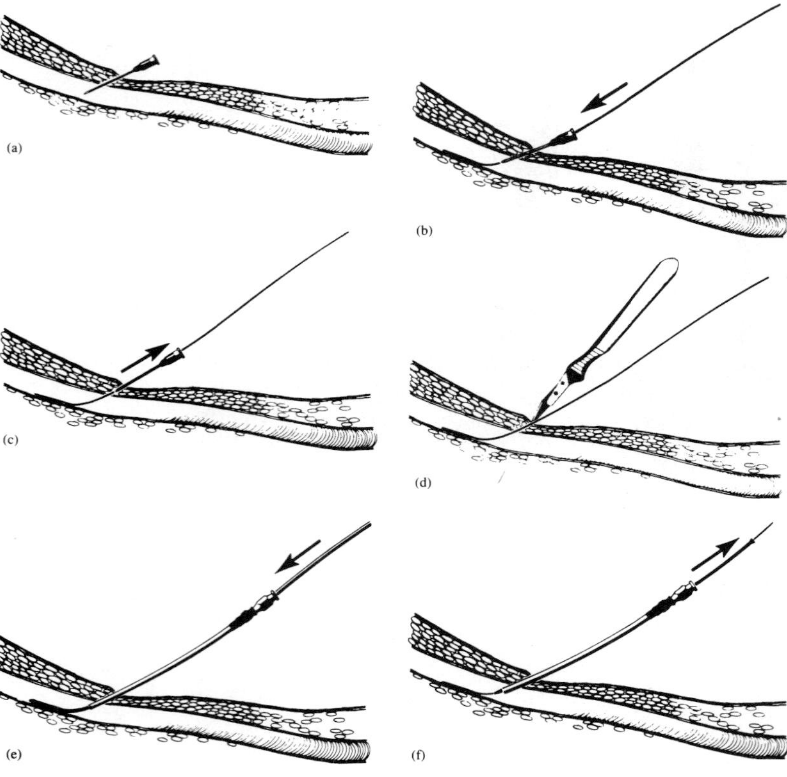

Fig. 6-5. Seldinger technique of catheter insertion (wire-guided). (From Conahan TJ III, Schwartz AJ, Geer RT: Percutaneous catheter introduction: The Seldinger technique. *JAMA* 237:446, 1977. Used by permission.)

thoracic duct cannot be injured. With unilateral chest trauma, the attempt should be on the injured side in order to protect the uninjured hemithorax in the event of complications from the procedure. A local anesthetic should be employed in conscious patients when time permits.

After landmarks are indentified, a 5- to 10-mL syringe attached to a hollow-bore needle appropriate to the size of the guidewire should be inserted. Gentle, continuous negative pressure on the syringe should be maintained. When free flow of blood is obtained, the syringe is removed and a fingertip used to occlude the hub before wire insertion. When the catheter has been advanced over the wire to the proper depth and the wire is removed, the catheter should be sutured to the chest wall, providone-iodine ointment placed at the needle puncture site, and a surgical dressing applied. If one approach fails, another should be performed on the same side, since a contralateral attempt could result in iatrogenic bilateral pneumothorax. A chest film should be performed immediately to verify correct catheter position to rule out complications from the procedure.

Technique of Commonly Utilized Approaches

The internal jugular and subclavian veins may be reliably cannulated by any of several tested approaches. Emergency physicians should become adept with at least two and adopt these for use as primary and backup methods. When the procedure is performed electively, preceding the approach for catheter placement with a 22-gauge needle attached to a 5- or 10-mL syringe filled with lidocaine facilitates local anesthesia and allows the operator to locate the vein.

In the *anterior approach* to the internal jugular vein, the needle should puncture the skin at the apex of a triangle formed by the tendinous and muscular heads of the sternocleidomastoid muscle. Held at a 60° angle with the plane of the skin, the needle is directed slightly lateral to the axis of the body. Blood return should be obtained within 3 cm, since the vein is very superficial here.

In the *lateral* or *posterior approach,* the head is turned slightly away from the selected side, and the needle is inserted at the posterior margin of the sternocleidomastoid muscle two to three fingerbreadths above the clavicle and directed toward the suprasternal notch. Blood should be aspirated within 4 to 5 cm.

For the *infraclavicular subclavian approach,* the needle is inserted beneath the clavicle medial to the midpoint and lateral to the medial third of the clavicle and directed toward the suprasternal notch. Inferomedial orientation of the needle bevel facilitates entry of the wire or catheter into the brachiocephalic vein. Vessel entry occurs at a depth of 3 to 4 cm.

For the *supraclavicular subclavian approach,* the patient's head is turned slightly away from the involved side. The needle enters just above the clavicle, 1 cm lateral to the insertion of the clavicular head of the sternocleidomastoid muscle and 1 cm posterior to the clavicle. It is then directed to bisect the angle formed between the sternocleidomastoid and the clavicle, at an angle of 10° above the horizontal, with the tip pointing just caudad to the contralateral nipple. Keeping the bevel up prevents trapping of the wire or catheter against the inferior wall of the vessel. Vessel puncture occurs at a depth of 2 to 3 cm.

Central Venous Pressure Measurement

Central venous pressure measurement is useful mainly in assessing volume status in the acutely ill or injured patient but may also assist in the diagnosis of specific disease processes and complications. It is the product of complex interactions among (1) circulating blood volume, (2) right ventricular function, (3) intrathoracic pressure, and (4) total systemic venous resistance. Absolute measurements of central venous pressure should be evaluated in light of the presence of right- or left-sided heart disease, which produces stable and chronic elevations. A low value in a patient with heart disease usually indicates volume depletion; however, hypovolemia should still be considered when the initial measurement is high and other signs are suggestive. A fluid challenge may be attempted, with a rising central venous pressure often indicating volume overload. Thus, (1) changes in central venous pressure over time are often more helpful than a single measurement, and (2) when heart disease is present it is especially important to evaluate central venous pressure in the context of other signs of volume status.

In patients who are healthy aside from acute trauma, a low value usually reflects hypovolemia, while a high value must be presumed to indicate a specific disease process or complication—such as pericardial tamponade or tension pneumothorax—or an error in measurement. Taking these considerations into account and keeping in mind that some controversy exists, the following may be referred to for use in clinical practice:

Low: <5 cm H_2O
Normal: 5–12 cm H_2O
High: >12 cm H_2O

In addition to heart failure, pericardial tamponade, and tension pneumothorax, abnormally high central venous pressure may also be caused by pulmonary embolism, superior vena cava obstruction, or MAST suit inflation. With an initial central venous pressure reading greater than 15 cm H_2O, fluid challenge is seldom warranted. Potentially confounding sources of high values include Valsalva's maneuver by the patient; positive-pressure ventilation; measurement in Trendelenburg's position; an external zero point reference too low on the chest wall; a catheter tip that is outside the thorax (e.g., in the internal jugular, axillary vein); a catheter that is kinked or partially occluded by the vein wall; a catheter that has crossed the tricuspid valve and is in the right ventricle; and a stopcock that is open to IV fluid rather than the patient.

A low central venous pressure is generally due to low circulating blood volume or decreased splanchnic venous tone (e.g., anaphylaxis, spinal shock, fear, or pain). Falsely positive low measurements are secondary to having the patient in a thorax-elevated position or having the external zero reference point too high on the chest wall.

Method of Measurement

To determine central venous pressure, the point of reference equivalent to the right atrium—the "zero point"—must be found and marked on the patient's chest wall. Although some disagreement exists on what landmark is ideal, the midaxillary line at the level of the fourth costochondral junction is frequently recommended. The manometer is filled to 20 to 25 cm with fluid by opening the three-way stopcock to the IV line leading to the source of IV solution. Then, with the patient level, supine, and breathing freely, the stopcock is opened to the patient so that fluid from the manometer runs into the patient until a steady state is reached. With the zero of the manometer at the zero reference point on the chest wall, the meniscus at end expiration gives the correct reading.

Complications

The three most common serious complications of central vein puncture are pneumothorax, arterial puncture, and local infection. With subclavian puncture the incidence of pneumothorax is 2 to 4 percent, significantly greater than with either internal jugular approach. The incidence of arterial puncture (3–7 percent) is similar for all approaches. Other, less common complications include hydrothorax, hydromediastinum, air or catheter embolisms, thrombosis, arrhythmias, nerve injuries, osteomyelitis of the clavicle, catheter tip perforation of the superior vena cava (causing hydromediastinum or hydrothorax) or right atrium (causing hydropericardium), knotting with other catheters, and puncture of endotracheal tube cuffs. Care in executing the procedure and in selection of patients who will benefit from central venous catheterization will minimize occurrence of complications.

VENOUS CUTDOWN

When percutaneous venous puncture is unsuccessful, cutdown is indicated. The basilic vein in the antecubital fossa and the saphenous vein in the leg are most commonly utilized. The basilic vein is located two fingerbreadths above and two fingerbreadths medial to the olecranon. The saphenous vein is just anterior to the malleolus at the ankle and is also accessible in the proximal thigh three fingerbreadths below the midpoint of the inguinal ligament.

Technique

Prep and anesthetize the skin. Make a transverse skin incision, and by blunt dissection separate the subcutaneous tissue until the vein is exposed. To avoid cannulating the artery, identify the artery and the vein before ligating or nicking a vessel. This is done by slipping a forceps or hemostat under the vessels and applying pressure; pulsatile flow will be evident in the artery. In patients with shock, this maneuver may be unsuccessful. After freeing the vein from the surrounding tissues, pass two separate sutures beneath the vein, one proximal and one distal. Leave the proximal suture untied. Tie the distal suture to occlude the vein, but keep the ends of the suture long so that they can be used for applying traction to the vein. Make a nick in the vein between the proximal and the distal suture. While applying traction on the vein, insert the catheter into the vein. Tie the proximal suture to secure the catheter in the vein. Suture the cutaneous incision. Care must be exercised throughout the procedure, since poor technique can result in tendon or nerve injury or extensive hemorrhage from soft tissue.

ARTERIAL CANNULATION

Arterial cannulation is indicated when arterial pressure monitoring or repeated arterial blood sampling is required, as in hypertensive crisis, cardiogenic shock treated with pressor and/or inotropic therapy, and respiratory failure. Although the radial artery is the most frequently employed site, the brachial, femoral, and dorsalis pedis arteries have also been employed in large series with little variation in occurrence of complications. While many operators are most familiar with the radial artery site, use of the femoral artery leaves the arm clear for other procedures and in the presence of shock is less difficult to cannulate percutaneously.

Assessment and Complications

Although catheterization of the radial artery is associated with up to a 20-percent incidence of temporary flow obstruction by Doppler study, permanent ischemic complications requiring surgical reanastomosis or amputation are quite rare. Confirmation of collateral flow through a patent ulnar artery can be obtained by performing Allen's test: while the patient clenches the wrist for 1 min, the examiner compresses the radial and ulnar vessels with thumb and forefinger. On release of ulnar compression, the patient partially extends the fingers, which are observed for rubor accentuated in comparison to the untested side. Patent ulnar circulation is indicated by return of rubor within 7 s, an equivocal result is 7 to 14 s, and greater than 14 s is considered definitely abnormal. If ulnar cannulation is contemplated, patency of the radial artery can be tested by the same test, with release of that vessel following compression.

Percutaneous cannulation of the brachial or femoral arteries may be possible when the radial pulse is absent in a hypotensive patient. The technique is similar to radial artery cannulation, although a careful groin prep, preceded by removal of hair at that site to minimize the risk of infection, is necessary. With profound hypotension, cutdown to the radial artery may be required to cannulate the artery. This is performed through a transverse incision, with the artery punctured utilizing a technique identical to the percutaneous approach, only under direct vision. The wound should be sutured, and the catheter affixed with a silk suture.

Serious complications—infection and occlusion—are most closely related to duration of cannulation and are much more common among critically ill patients than among those undergoing monitoring as an adjunct to a surgical procedure. During a typical intensive care unit stay, the incidence of local infection can be expected to approach 20 percent, while that of generalized sepsis from primary catheter infection is 4 percent, with little site-dependent variation. Other complications include hematoma formation and hemorrhage requiring transfusion.

Technique

The patient's nondominant extremity should be selected for radial artery cannulation. The wrist is placed in mild extension by placing a roll of gauze behind it and taping it to a splint. A sterile prep is applied and the operative area draped. Local infiltration should be performed with a small amount of lidocaine so that the pulse is not obscured. While a 20- or 22-gauge 1.25-in Teflon catheter over a needle is held in one hand, the radial pulse is palpated with the other. The skin over the radial aspect of the wrist is punctured with the needle pointing proximally and at a 45° angle with the plane of the skin. The needle is advanced into the artery until pulsations appear. The catheter is then slid off the needle into the artery. If pulsatile flow ceases, the catheter may be withdrawn until arterial flow again appears, and a second attempt may be made to advance the catheter. If this is unsuccessful, the procedure needs to be repeated. Once in the artery, the catheter is connected to the monitoring system and flushed through a three-way stopcock with a sterile cap. After each attempt, care should be taken to apply pressure to the site long enough to prevent hematoma formation.

BIBLIOGRAPHY

Allen EV: Thromboangiitis obliterans: Methods of diagnosis of chronic occlusive arterial lesions distal to the wrist with illustrative cases. *Am J Med Sci* 178:237, 1929.

Band JD, Maki DG: Infections caused by arterial catheters used for hemodynamic monitoring. *Am J Med* 67:735, 1979.

Conahan TJ III, Schwartz AJ, Geer RT: Percutaneous catheter introduction: The Seldinger technique. *JAMA* 237:446, 1977.

Dailey RH: Use of wire-guided catheters in the emergency department. *Ann Emerg Med* 12:489, 1983.

Dailey RH: External jugular vein cannulation and its use for CVP monitoring. *J Emerg Med* 6:133, 1988.

Dronen SC, Yee AS, Tomlanovich MC: Proximal saphenous vein cutdown. *Ann Emerg Med* 10:328, 1981.

Dula DJ, Muller HA, Donovan JW: Flow rate variance of commonly used IV infusion techniques. *J Trauma* 21:480, 1981.

Ersoz CJ, Hedden M, Lain L: Prolonged femoral arterial catheterization for intensive care. *Anesth Analg* 49:160, 1970.

Falchuk KH, Peterson L, McNeil BJ: Microparticulate-induced phlebitis: Its prevention by in-line filtration. *N Engl J Med* 312:78, 1985.

Getzen LC, Pollak EW: Short-term femoral vein catheterization: A safe alternative venous access. *Am J Surg* 138:875, 1979.

Gong V: Microwave warming of IV fluids in management of hypothermia. *Ann Emerg Med* 13:645, 1984.

Gurman GM, Kriemerman S: Cannulation of big arteries in critically ill patients. *Crit Care Med* 13:217, 1985.

Hedges JR, Barsan WB, Doan LA, et al: Central versus peripheral intravenous routes in cardiopulmonary resuscitation. *Am J Emerg Med* 2:385, 1984.

Iverson KV, Reeter AK, Criss E: Comparison of flow rates for standard and large-bore blood tubing. *West J Med* 143:183, 1985.

Iverson KV, Reeter A, Woods W, et al: Pressurization of IV bags: A new configuration and evaluation for use. *West J Med* 3:89, 1985.

Joyce SM, Barsan WG, Hedges JR, et al: Effect of a pneumatic antishock garment on drug delivery via distal venous access. *Ann Emerg Med* 13:885, 1984.

Knopp R, Dailey RH: Central venous cannulation and pressure monitoring. *J Am Coll Emerg Physicians* 6:358, 1977.

Kramer DA, Staten-McCormick M, Freeman SB: Percutaneous brachial vein catheterization: An alternate site for IV access (abst.). *Ann Emerg Med* 12:238, 1983.

Mandel MA, Dauchot PJ: Radial artery cannulation in 1,000 patients: Precautions and complications. *J Hand Surg* 6:482, 1977.

Mangiante EC, Hoots AV, Fabian TC: The percutaneous common femoral vein catheter for volume replacement in critically ill patients. *J Trauma* 28:1644, 1988.

Nadeau S, Tousignant M: Use of urologic set for improved fluid administration rates. *Can Anaesth Soc J* 32:283, 1985.

Posner MC, Moore EE, Greenholz SK: Natural history of untreated inferior vena cava injury and assessment of venous access. *J Trauma* 26:698, 1986.

Rosetti VA, Thompson BM, Miller J, et al: Intraosseous infusion: An alternative route of pediatric intravascular access. *Ann Emerg Med* 14:885, 1985.

Slogoff S, Keats AS, Arlund C: On the safety of radial artery cannulation. *Anesthesiology* 59:42, 1983.

Snazajder JI, Zveibil FR, Bitterman H, et al: Central vein catheterization: Failure and complication rates by three percutaneous approaches. *Arch Intern Med* 146:259, 1986.

Tucker JF, Danzl DF, Teague E, et al: Infusion of intravenous fluids distal to pneumatic antishock trousers. *J Emerg Med* 2:79, 1984.

Wilkins RG: Radial artery cannulation and ischaemic damage: A review. *Anaesthesia* 40:896, 1985.

Youngberg JA, Miller ED: Evaluation of percutaneous cannulations of the dorsalis pedis artery. *Anesthesiology* 44:80, 1976.

7
INVASIVE MONITORING AND PACING TECHNIQUES

Scott Syverud

Arterial pressure monitoring is gradually being introduced in emergency department resuscitation. Emergency physicians must have a familiarity with invasive pacing techniques in order to treat the unstable patient with bradycardia. In recent years the development of transcutaneous pacing has added a new pacing alternative. This chapter reviews the basics of these techniques as applied in emergency care.

INVASIVE MONITORING TECHNIQUES

General Considerations

Invasive pressure monitoring should never be the initial step in resuscitation. Airway assessment and stabilization and circulatory support clearly take priority. Early arterial line placement is appropriate when several physicians are available or when initial stabilization is completed. Continuous monitoring of arterial pressure is particularly helpful in prolonged emergency department resuscitations and in patients who require frequent adjustments in vasoactive infusions for circulatory support (i.e., hypertensive crisis, cardiogenic shock, hypothermic cardiac arrest). The arterial line also provides easy access for frequent sampling of blood gases to aid in ventilator management.

The placement of a pulmonary artery thermodilution catheter (PATC) is helpful in the diagnosis and management of a variety of critical illnesses. If possible, this procedure should be deferred until the patient reaches the more controlled and sterile environment of the intensive care unit. In many cases there may be a significant delay before a patient can be moved to intensive care or until a consultant reaches the hospital. When resuscitation management is critically dependent on hemodynamic monitoring, it may be helpful to place a PATC in the emergency department after initial resuscitation. Potential candidates include hypotensive patients with acute myocardial infarction and patients in shock, especially those with cardiopulmonary or renal disease. In such patients the information obtained with the PATC may significantly alter the physician's approach to fluid and pressor therapy.

The two essential components of any pressure monitoring system are a properly placed catheter and a functioning pressure transducer/monitor to connect it to. Failure of either of these components wastes valuable time during resuscitation. Ideally, the transducer and line for pressure monitoring should be set up and ready for use prior to the patient's arrival in the emergency department. Examples of transducer systems are illustrated in Fig. 7-1. The most common error made during the initiation of invasive monitoring is to focus on the procedure and forget about the patient until the procedure is completed. With an unstable patient, the physician must be constantly aware of the patient's status and be ready to discontinue efforts at line placement in favor of other procedures as circumstances dictate.

Arterial Cannulation

Arterial lines offer several advantages over monitoring of blood pressure with an arm cuff. The line provides continuous measurement of blood pressure and can be used for easy sequential sampling of blood gases. In the setting of marked vasoconstriction or hypotension, the arterial line usually gives more accurate pressure readings than a blood pressure cuff. The radial and femoral arteries are readily accessible to rapid cannulation. Percutaneous puncture is preferred. In hypotensive patients it may be easier to cannulate the femoral artery (larger vessel, constant landmarks) than the radial artery. Cutdown on the radial artery is an alternative in such patients. Allen's test for ulnar artery patency should always be performed prior to radial arterial line placement. If the ulnar artery is occluded, a different site should be used.

Landmarks for radial and femoral artery cannulation are shown in Fig. 7-2. The catheter (usually 20 gauge, 2 in long for radial cannulation and 18 gauge, 4 in long for femoral cannulation) can be introduced by direct puncture threaded over the needle or by Seldinger technique threaded over a guide wire. Free pulsatile flow of bright red blood indicates proper placement. With marked hypotension or hypoxia, correct placement may be mistaken for venous placement (nonpulsatile dark blood returned). In all cases, connection to the transducer should reveal an arterial waveform with proper arterial placement. Failure to visualize a waveform can be due to venous placement, air in the line, a closed stopcock, or a malfunction in the transducer or monitor.

Arterial line placement is a diagnostic aid, not a treatment modality. Therapeutic procedures or definitive care (i.e., airway management, transfer to the operating room) should not be delayed solely to allow arterial line placement. Local complications of line placement include local hematoma and hemorrhage; both can usually be controlled with a pressure dressing. Arterial occlusion, thrombosis, or embolization with distal ischemia may occur; they are associated with placement in smaller vessels or in atherosclerotic vessels, with prolonged catheterization, and with use of end arteries that supply areas with poor collateral circulation. These complications can be minimized by using the femoral or radial site, by checking for ulnar artery patency before using the radial artery , and by removing the line as soon as feasible after the patient is stabilized.

Sepsis may result from local infection at the insertion site. This complication can be avoided by proper attention to sterile technique and by frequent dressing changes with immediate removal of the catheter if evidence of site infection is detected. Early replacement of lines placed in the emergency department during resuscitation is also a rational intensive care unit policy to minimize these complications.

Pulmonary Artery Cannulation

Pulmonary artery cannulation offers several advantages over central venous pressure (CVP) monitoring (see Chapter 6, "Vascular Access"). When the balloon tip of a PATC is properly wedged in a branch of the pulmonary artery, the pressure sensed by the catheter tip is the same as that in the left atrium. Left atrial pressure (which equals left ventricular filling pressure) is an excellent indication of the adequacy of fluid resuscitation. If this pressure is low (less than 12 mmHg), additional fluid resuscitation is indicated. If this pressure is high (greater than 20 mmHg), additional fluids are unlikely to improve cardiac performance; vasopressors are probably indicated for circulatory support. Although the PATC can yield a vast amount of useful diagnostic information (Tables 7-1 and 7-2), this distinction between the need for more fluids or for more pressors is its most useful application during resuscitation. CVP monitoring is less reliable than PATC, especially in the presence of valvular or pulmonary disease.

The placement technique for PATCs is discussed at length in the chapter by Kaye in McIntyre's and Levis' text. Standard catheters have two lumens, a distal one which terminates at the tip of the catheter, and a proximal one which terminates 10 to 15 cm proximal to the tip (Fig. 7-3). A small balloon at the tip of the catheter helps float the catheter through the heart and also occludes a branch of the pulmonary artery to allow pulmonary artery occlusion (PAO) pressure measurement. It is the PAO pressure which best reflects the pressure in the pulmonary capillary bed and the left atrium.

In addition to the two lumens and the balloon, the PATC has a temperature sensor just proximal to the balloon. This sensor allows continuous central temperature monitoring, and measurement of car-

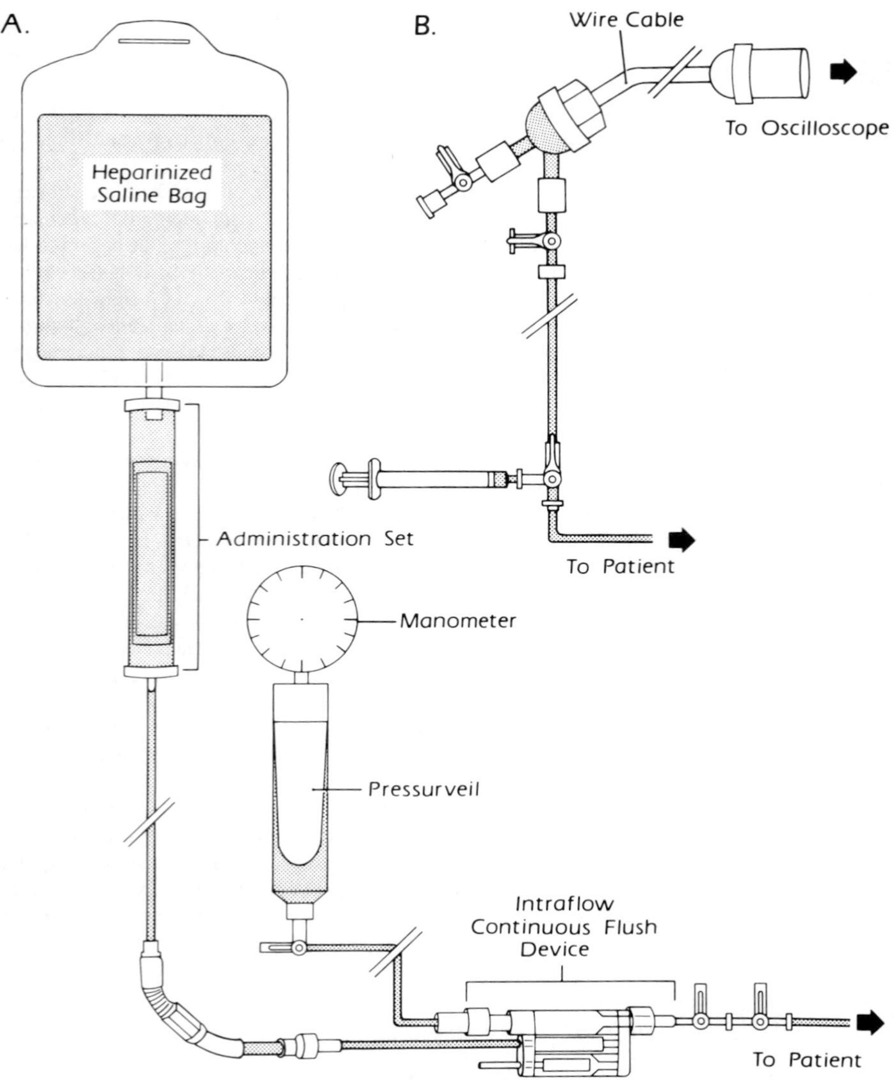

Fig. 7-1. Arterial pressure monitoring systems. **A.** System for continuous flush with heparinized saline connected to a mechanical pressure transducer. **B.** System for manual flush. Either system can be used with an electronic pressure transducer shown in **B.** The pressure dome should be maintained at the level of the patient's heart. (From Beal JM (ed): *Critical Care for Surgical Patients*. New York, Macmillan, 1982. Used by permission.)

Table 7-1. Hemodynamic Diagnosis of Shock States.

Type of Shock	CO	PAO	SVR
Cardiogenic	↓	↑	↑
Hypovolemic	↓	↓	↑
Septic	↓ *or* ↑	↓	↓
Neurogenic	↑	↓	↓
Anaphylactic	↓	↓	↓

CO = cardiac output; PAO = pulmonary artery occlusion pressure; SVR = systemic vascular resistance; (↑) increased; (↓) decreased; (−) unchanged from normal values.

Table 7-2. Hemodynamic Subsets in Acute Myocardial Infarction.

Cardiac Index (L/min/m^2)			
		I	II
	2.2		
		III	IV
		18	
		PAO (mmHg)	

Note: Initial therapy and prognosis can be determined by class. Mortality by class is 1%, 11%, 18% and 60% for classes I–IV, respectively. Patients in class I require supportive care only. Patients in class II require treatment for pulmonary edema to lower pulmonary artery occlusion pressure (PAO). Patients in class III may improve with fluid administration. Patients in class IV require maximal circulatory support for cardiogenic shock.

diac output, using the thermodilution technique. After central venous access is secured (see Chapter 6, "Vascular Access"), the catheter is advanced toward the heart through an introducer sheath. The pressure waveform sensed through the distal port changes as the catheter is advanced through the heart and is used to confirm proper placement in the pulmonary artery (Fig. 7-4). Fluoroscopy can also be used to place a PATC but is rarely available in the emergency setting.

Once a PATC is in position, the clinician can rapidly measure pulmonary artery pressure, PAO pressure, cardiac output (CO), and CVP. When combined with arterial pressure measurement, these parameters can be used to calculate systemic vascular resistance. These parameters are very useful in the diagnosis and treatment of various shock states and in determining therapy in acute myocardial infarction (Tables 7-1 and 7-2). With pericardial tamponade or tension pneumothorax, the right heart pressure waveforms flatten out until CVP, atrial, ventricular, and pulmonary artery pressures are almost the same.

As with arterial cannulation, therapeutic procedures or definitive care should not be delayed solely to allow PATC placement. Complications include all the complications of central venous line placement

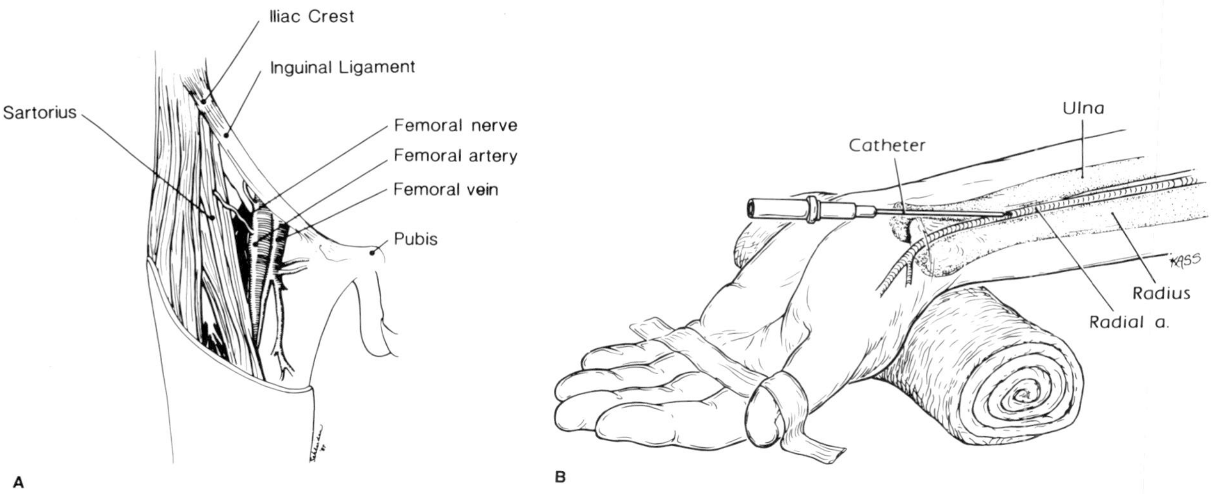

Fig. 7-2. Anatomic landmarks for arterial line placement. **A.** Femoral triangle. Note that the femoral artery lies lateral to the vein and midway between the pubis and the iliac crest. **B.** Radial aspect of the wrist. Note that mild extension of the wrist will aid successful placement. (From Beal JM (ed): *Critical Care for Surgical Patients*. New York, Macmillan, 1982. Used by permission.)

(Chapter 6). In addition, cardiac arrhythmias may occur as the catheter traverses the heart. Other potential complications include pulmonary embolism or infarction, knotting of the catheter, infection, and rupture of a small branch of the pulmonary artery.

EMERGENCY PACING TECHNIQUES

General Considerations

There is a distinct difference between *urgent* and *emergency* pacemaker placement. Urgent pacing is required in patients who are clinically stable yet may decompensate or become unstable in the near future. Provision of a standby pacer in these potentially unstable patients can be made in the emergency department using noninvasive techniques (transcutaneous pacing). If time and the clinical condition of the patient permit, all invasive cardiac pacing should be attempted in a controlled environment and should be performed by the most experienced physician available. Therefore, it is not advocated that urgent or prophylactic pacing be performed in the emergency department. Likewise, if the patient can be stabilized with drug therapy or is not in extremis, it is advised that the standard pattern of referral and consultation be used. Emergency pacing is required in those unstable patients with cardiac arrest, hemodynamically unstable bradyarrhythmia, or recurrent malignant escape rhythms who require pacing immediately. These patients cannot await the arrival of a consultant.

Since it can be instituted quickly and noninvasively, transcutaneous pacing is the technique of choice for emergent pacing. If transcutaneous pacing is not available or if it fails to produce electrical capture, transthoracic pacing should be used for emergent pacing. Transvenous pacing should be used for urgent pacing or after stabilization with drugs or another pacing technique. Electrodes and catheters for each of these techniques are illustrated in Fig. 7-5.

Transcutaneous Pacing

Transcutaneous pacing uses externally applied electrodes to deliver an electric impulse directly across the intact chest wall to stimulate the myocardium. Recent studies have demonstrated improved survival in bradyasystolic arrest patients who received pacing within 5 min of

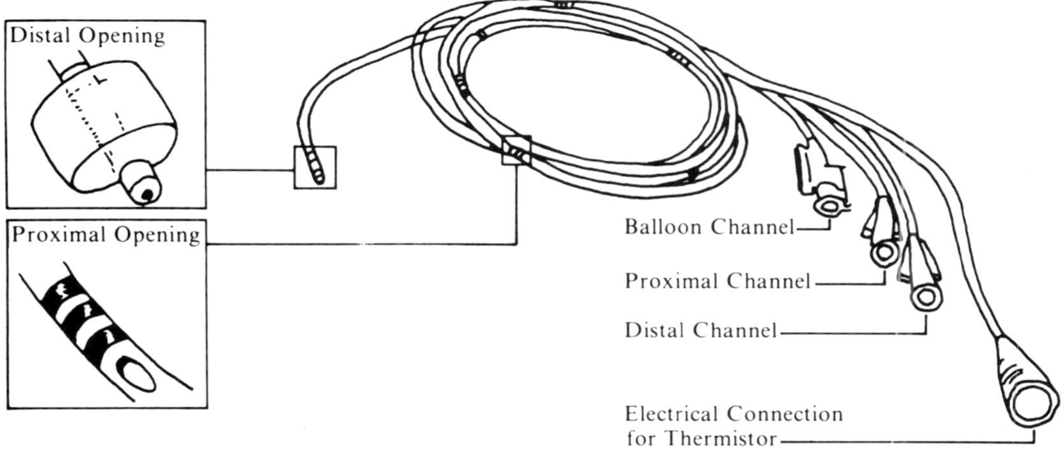

Fig. 7-3. Pulmonary artery thermodilution catheter (PATC). (From Beal JM (ed): *Critical Care for Surgical Patients*. New York, Macmillan, 1982. Used by permission.)

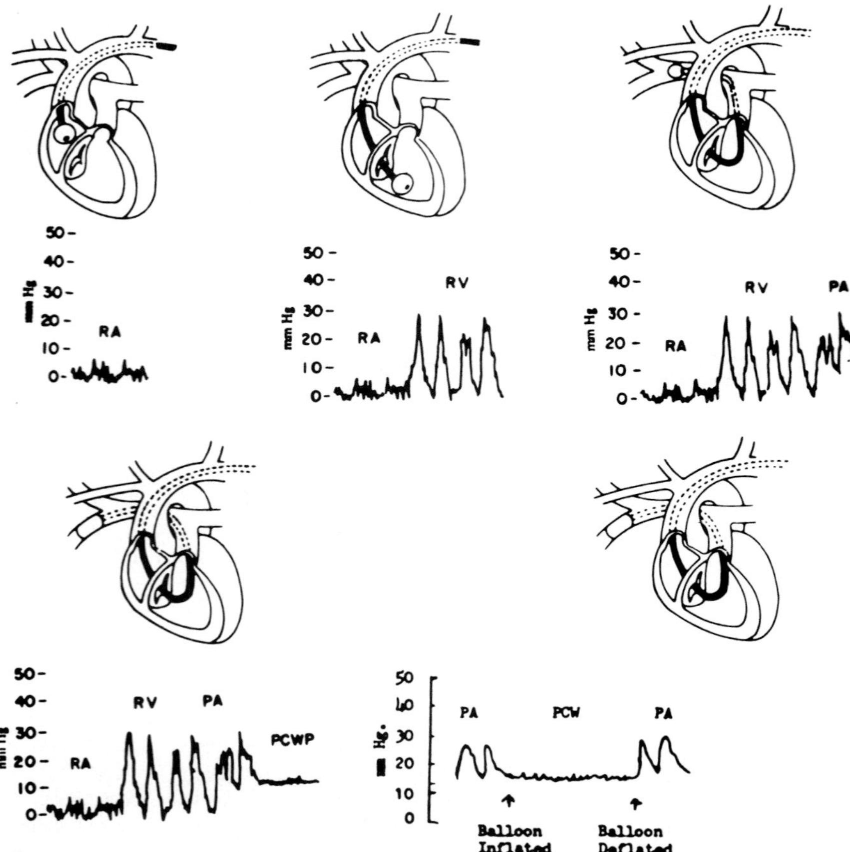

Fig. 7-4. Hemodynamic aspects of balloon catheter insertion into the pulmonary artery. (From Gottlieb AJ (ed): *The Whole Internist Catalog*. Philadelphia, Saunders, 1980. Used by permission.)

arrest onset. This observation combined with its relative ease of application has led to the application of transcutaneous pacing in prehospital settings. This technique is useful for initial stabilization of the patient in the emergency department who requires emergency pacing while arrangements for transvenous pacemaker insertion are being made.

Transcutaneous pacers differ from standard pacers in several important ways. The pulse duration of the simulating impulse is longer and the current output higher than for standard internal leads. Muscle contraction (usually the chest wall or diaphragm) is notable during pacing, especially at higher outputs. This results in a twitching or mild bucking activity that can make assessment of cardiac output by palpation of the radial, carotid, or femoral pulse unreliable during transcutaneous pacing. The higher current outputs used make cardiac monitoring with standard ECG monitors impossible due to interference from the large-amplitude pacing spike. Most transcutaneous pacing units come equipped with a monitor which automatically filters the pacing spike so that simultaneous monitoring is possible (Fig. 7-6).

The externally applied pacing electrodes are quickly and easily applied to the chest and back. There is little risk of electrical injury to health care providers during transcutaneous pacing. Chest compressions (CPR) can be administered directly over the insulated electrodes while pacing. Inadvertent contact with the active pacing surface results only in a mild shock. In the setting of bradyasystolic arrest, it is reasonable to turn the stimulating current to maximum output and then decrease the output if capture is achieved. In a patient with a hemodynamically compromising bradycardia (but not in cardiac arrest), the operator should slowly increase the output from the minimum setting until capture is achieved. Assessment of capture can be made by monitoring the electrocardiogram on the filtered monitor of the pacing unit. The hemodynamic response to pacing must also be assessed, either by blood pressure cuff or arterial catheter. Ideally, pacing should be continued at 1.25 times the threshold of initial electrical capture.

Failure to capture with transcutaneous pacing may be related to electrode placement or patient size. Patients who are conscious or who regain consciousness during transcutaneous pacing experience discomfort due to muscle contraction. Analgesia with incremental doses of morphine or sedation with a benzodiazepine makes this discomfort tolerable until transvenous pacing can be instituted. Transcutaneous pacing should be used for temporary stabilization only and should always be followed as soon as feasible by an internal pacing technique (usually transvenous).

An increasing number of defibrillators include a built-in transcutaneous pacemaker. This development insures that pacing will be available as soon as the defibrillator reaches the patient in cardiac arrest. Previous studies have clearly demonstrated that pacing will only improve survival if it is applied very early in the course of bradycardia or asystolic arrest. In the coming years, emergency physicians will treat more patients who have received pacing prior to hospital arrival by EMS providers who are equipped with combined defibrillator-pacers.

Transvenous Pacing

Transvenous pacing consists of endocardial stimulation of the right ventricle via an electrode introduced into a central vein. The major difficulties of transvenous pacing are venous access and proper placement of the stimulating electrode. Venous access routes most commonly used include the subclavian, internal or external jugular, femoral, and brachial. Transvenous pacing catheters can be inserted through a variety of venous introducers. A soft flexible semifloating bipolar catheter is preferred. This type of pacer is safest to use and takes advantage of any forward blood flow that may be present.

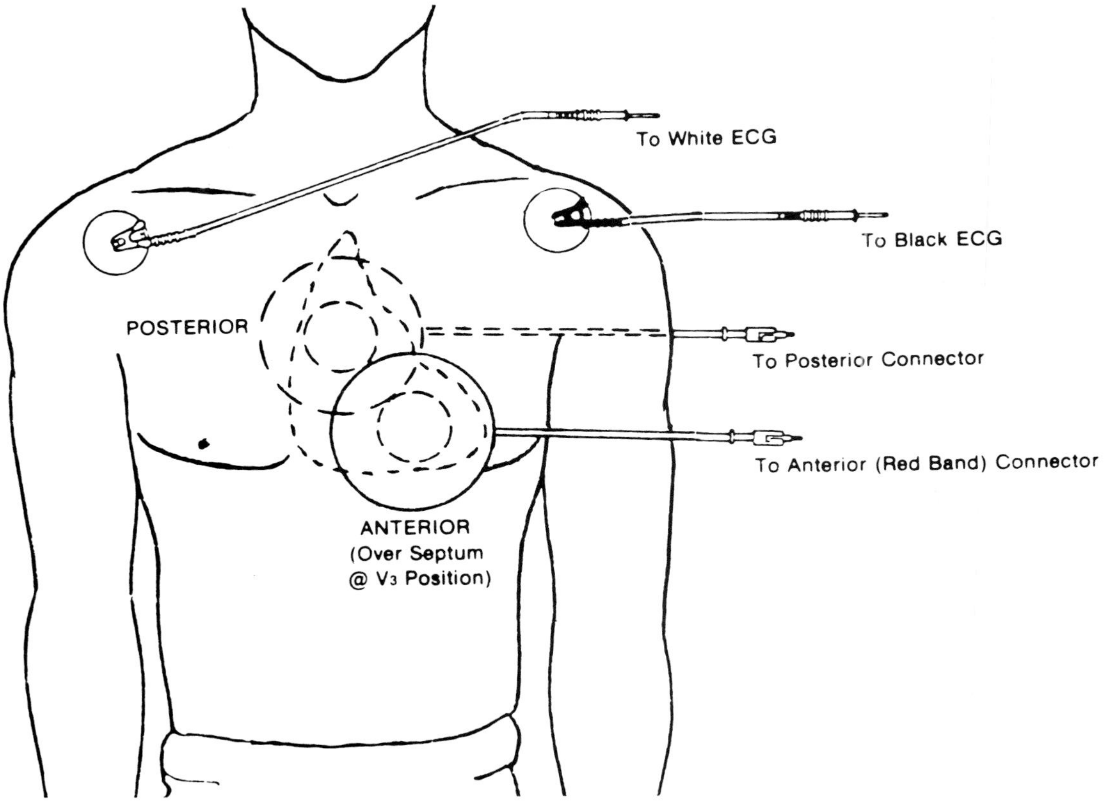

A

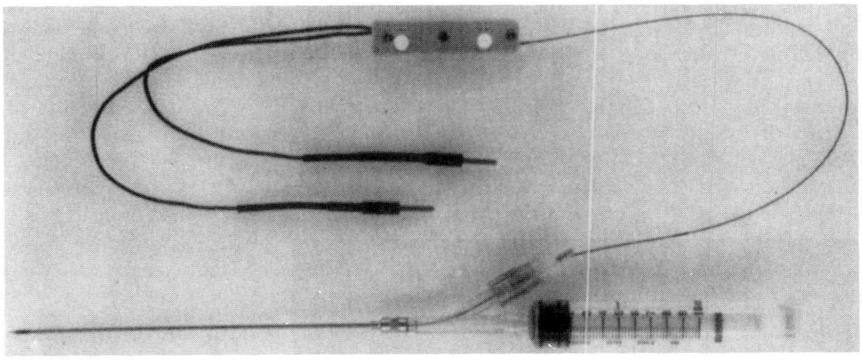

B

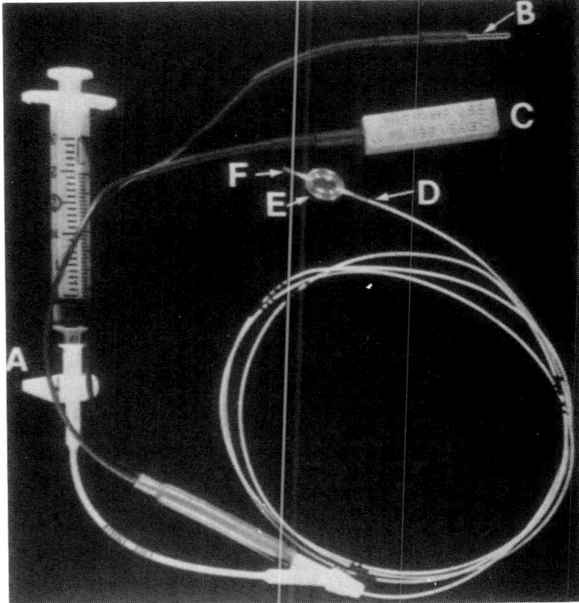

C

Fig. 7-5. Catheters and electrodes for emergency cardiac pacing. **A.** Transcutaneous. **B.** Transthoracic. **C.** Transvenous. [From Roberts JR (ed): *Clinical Procedures in Emergency Medicine*. Philadelphia, Saunders, 1985, and from Jastremski JS (ed): *The Whole Emergency Medicine Catalog*. Philadelphia, Saunders, 1985. Used by permission.]

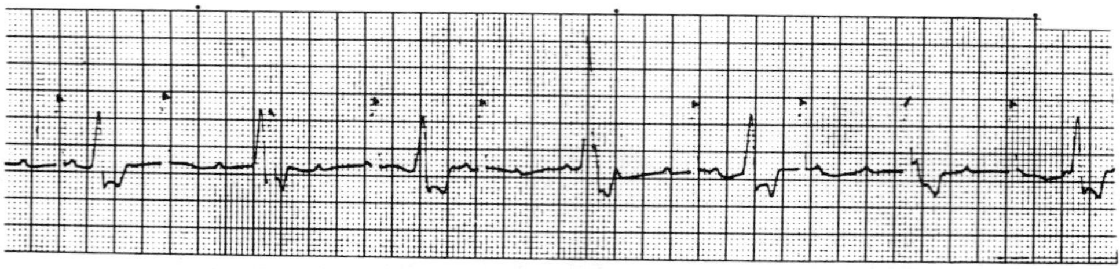

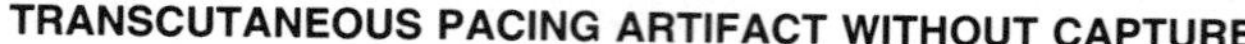

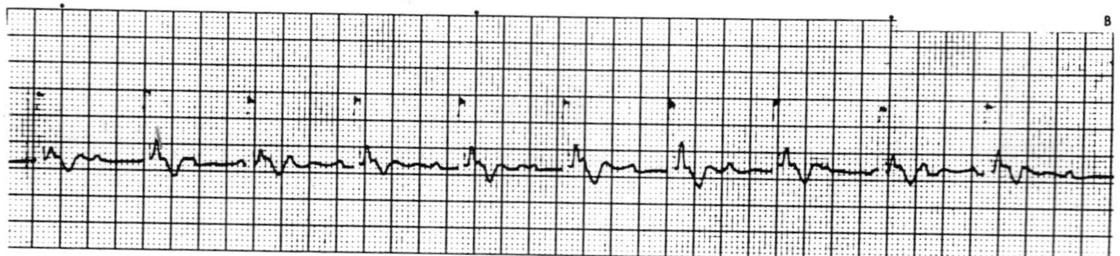

Fig. 7-6. ECG monitoring of the paced patient. Transcutaneous pacing without capture and with capture. Note the wide pacer artifact produced by the transcutaneous pacer. [From Roberts JR (ed): *Clinical Procedures in Emergency Medicine*. Philadelphia, Saunders, 1985. Used with permission.]

Placement of the catheter tip into the apex of the right ventricle is the key to successful transvenous pacing. Several techniques can aid successful placement. Fluoroscopic guidance is the surest method of right ventricular placement but is rarely available in the emergency department. Electrocardiographic guidance is useful in patients with narrow complexes and/or P waves when fluoroscopy is unavailable (see the chapter by Benjamin in Roberts' and Hedges' text for a description of this technique). Balloon-tipped "floating" catheters may aid placement when used in conjunction with ECG and fluoroscopic guidance or when used alone. The balloon is inflated after catheter insertion into a central vein. Forward blood flow then directs the catheter tip toward the ventricle as the operator slowly advances the catheter. As with all balloon-tipped catheters, the balloon should always be deflated prior to withdrawal; the catheter should never be pulled back with the balloon inflated.

When patients have decreased or no forward blood flow (including most circumstances in which transvenous pacing would be used in the emergency department) positioning of the pacer tip within the right ventricle is difficult. Balloon-tipped catheters are not much of an aid in placement during low- or no-flow states. In a true emergency the pacemaker electrodes are connected to the power source and the catheter advanced blindly in hopes that the tip will encounter the endocardium of the right ventricle and that capture will result. In this setting a *right internal jugular* venous access route should be used. From this approach, the catheter traverses a straight line into the right ventricle and rarely curls in the atrium or deflects into the inferior vena cava.

Pacer settings vary with the clinical situation. An initial rate of 80 to 100 per minute is appropriate in most patients. Asynchronous mode (sensitivity off) should be used initially in patients requiring emergency pacing for hemodynamically unstable bradycardias. The presence or absence of capture should be assessed by ECG (Fig. 7-7). Output should initially be set at maximum (usually 20 mA) and then decreased after capture is achieved. With optimal tip position, capture should occur at less than 2 mA. Pacing should be continued at 1.5 to 2 times the threshold output required for capture. Subsequent rate and sensitivity settings should be adjusted as clinically indicated by the patient's hemodynamic status and underlying rhythm disturbance.

Chest radiographs (anteroposterior and lateral) should be obtained after patient stabilization to ensure proper tip placement and to evaluate the possibility of pneumothorax from the preceding central venous line placement. Finally, care should be taken to firmly affix the pacing catheter to the insertion site prior to patient transfer. Transvenous pacing is a technique that can be easily mastered and rapidly performed in an emergency situation. Transvenous pacing is best used in urgent situations in which there is adequate time to utilize fluoroscopy. In the setting of cardiac arrest, transcutaneous or transthoracic pacing is preferred.

Transthoracic Pacing

Transthoracic pacing involves the percutaneous placement of a bipolar pacing wire directly into the right ventricular cavity via a trocar needle. The technique is quicker than transvenous pacer insertion. The intracardiac trocar needle can be properly positioned by an experienced physician, with only a brief interruption of CPR, in 30 to 45 s. Because of a significant incidence of serious complications associated with the procedure (pericardial tamponade, major vessel injury, pneumothorax), it should not be used indiscriminately. It is not indicated in the

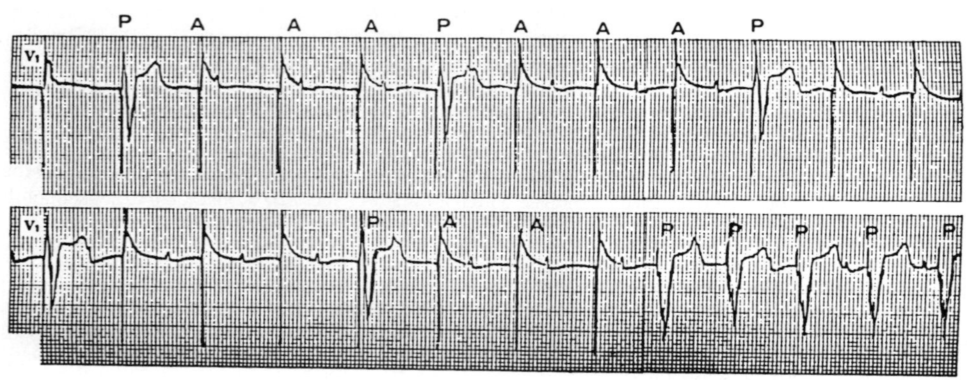

Fig. 7-7. Pacing with intermittent capture. "P" indicates paced beats. "A" indicates pacer artifact without capture.

stable patient, or in patients in which medication or transcutaneous pacing can buy time to pass a transvenous pacing catheter. Because of the risk of tamponade, transthoracic pacing should not be used in anticoagulated patients.

Because of its rapidity, transthoracic pacing may be preferable to transvenous pacing in unstable or arrested patients. If transcutaneous pacing is unavailable, or if it fails to produce electrical capture, transthoracic pacing can be attempted. In recent years, the widespread availability of transcutaneous pacing has markedly decreased the frequency with which transthoracic pacing is used. Many hospitals no longer stock transthoracic pacing kits with their resuscitation equipment.

If chest compressions are in progress, these should be interrupted until after intracardiac placement has been achieved to minimize the possibility of myocardial laceration by the sharp needle. The trocar needle is introduced into the left xyphocostal angle and directed at a 30 to 45° angle to the skin toward the sternal notch (Fig. 7-8). After the needle is advanced 8 to 12 cm, the trocar is removed. A free return of blood indicates intracardiac placement. Aspiration of blood with a syringe confirms position. After intracardiac position is confirmed, the pacing wire is inserted through the needle and connected to the pulse generator box.

After the pacing wire has been connected to the pulse generator, pacing is initiated with the same settings as were indicated for emergency transvenous pacing (asynchronous, maximum output, rate 80 to 100). The presence or absence of capture should then be assessed on the ECG rhythm strip or monitor (Fig. 7-7). If no pacer spikes are evident, the connection of the wire to the pulse generator should be checked. If pacer spikes are evident but no capture occurs, the wire should be gently manipulated to change its position within the ventricle. If capture is achieved and the patient's hemodynamic status is stabilized, the entire pacing apparatus should be securely taped to the chest while arrangements are made for placement of a transvenous pacing catheter. Chest radiographs (anteroposterior and lateral) should be obtained to confirm catheter position and assess for the possibility of pneumothorax induced during insertion. The transthoracic pacing catheter should be replaced by a transvenous pacemaker as soon as possible, although pacing may be accomplished with the transthoracic pacemaker for a number of days.

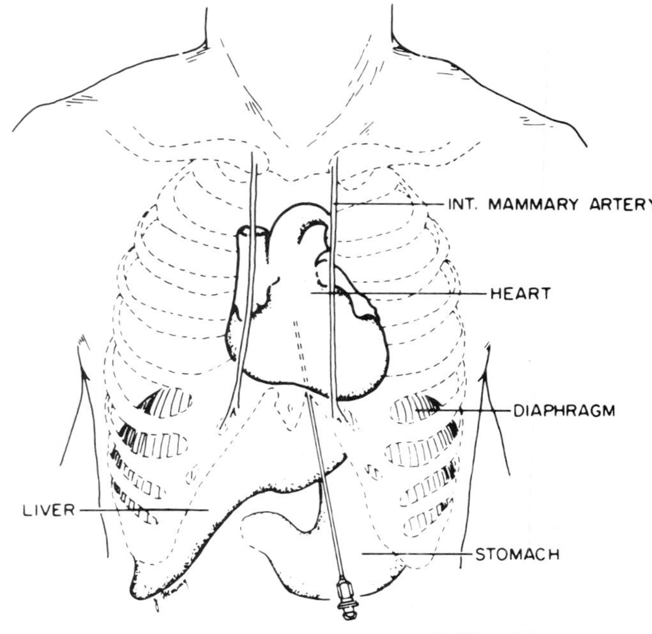

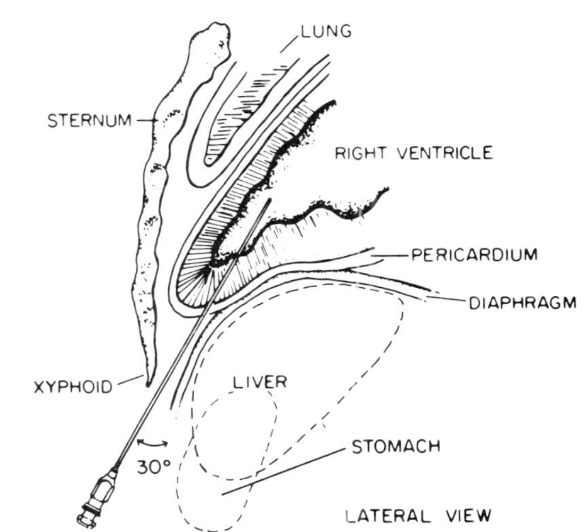

Fig. 7-8. Anatomic landmarks for transthoracic pacer placement. [From Roberts JR (ed): *Clinical Procedures in Emergency Medicine*. Philadelphia, Saunders, 1985. Used with permission.]

AUTOMATIC AND IMPLANTABLE DEFIBRILLATORS

In William Kouwenhoven's landmark 1957 report on the first DC defibrillator, he astutely observed:

> When ventricular fibrillation has been present for less than two minutes, application of this method results in survival in a high proportion of cases. . . . Effective use of closed chest defibrillation requires that the necessary equipment be available and rapidly applied.

Two recent technological developments have led to the more rapid application of defibrillation. Automatic external defibrillators allow first responders to institute defibrillation. In some cases even bystanders or family members can institute defibrillation with these devices. Implanted defibrillators allow patients with frequent malignant ventricular dysrhythmias to in effect carry their own defibrillators with them at all times. Emergency physicians need to be familiar with these devices and the special considerations associated with their use.

Automatic External Defibrillators

Automatic external defibrillators (AEDs) have relatively simple controls and can be applied by minimally trained providers to initiate defibrillation. AED use requires the operator to attach monitoring and defibrillation electrodes to the patient. Various models allow varying degrees of operator control. In most cases the device analyzes the cardiac rhythm and initiates defibrillation automatically after first warning the operator to stand clear prior to the actual delivery of the countershock. Some devices prompt the operator to initiate the countershock or rely on basic rhythm confirmation by the operator prior to defibrillating. As the rhythm recognition capability and reliability of these devices has improved, the need for time-consuming training of providers in rhythm recognition has decreased.

AEDs will shock patients in ventricular fibrillation several times sequentially until an organized cardiac rhythm results or until the maximum number of shocks allowed by the device's algorithm is reached. Many devices also provide a record of rhythms and events during their use which allows the emergency physician to subsequently reconstruct the sequence of events during resuscitation.

AEDs are most effective in tiered EMS systems where AED equipped first responders reach the patient rapidly and are backed up by the later arrival of paramedics with full advanced life-support capabilities. The failure of an AED to restore a perfusing rhythm is a poor prognostic sign often associated with long arrest times or arrest rhythms other than ventricular fibrillation. The emergency physician must be familiar with these devices. When an AED fails to resuscitate a patient in arrest, the cardiac rhythm should be identified and treated. If the rhythm is refractory ventricular fibrillation, drug therapy should be instituted simultaneously with instituting further defibrillation attempts.

Implantable Defibrillators

As of 1990, more than 3000 patients at high risk for ventricular fibrillation have had implanted defibrillators surgically attached to their myocardium. These devices continuously monitor cardiac rhythm. If a "treatable" rhythm is detected (ventricular tachycardia or ventricular fibrillation) and if it persists long enough (usually > 30 seconds), the device will attempt to restore a normal rhythm with a 20 to 40 joule countershock. Most devices will shock up to four times. If a normal rhythm is not restored after four shocks, no further pulses will be delivered. Conversion to a supraventricular rhythm at a rate less than 150 will usually reset the device so that it will initiate a series of shocks again if ventricular tachycardia or fibrillation recur.

Emergency providers need to be familiar with several key points about these devices. When a patient with an implanted defibrillator is found in cardiac arrest, it usually implies that the device did not work; e.g., a full set of shocks has been delivered without restoration of a normal rhythm. Normal resuscitation measures, as with any patient in cardiac arrest and including external defibrillation, are therefore indicated.

Emergency personnel may feel a small electrical shock if they are performing CPR when one of these devices delivers a countershock. No serious rescuer injuries have been reported, probably because the energy is delivered internally and is of a much lower magnitude (20–40 J) than that delivered in external defibrillation (200–400 J).

These devices can malfunction and inappropriately shock rhythms such as atrial fibrillation. In such cases, the implanted defibrillator can be deactivated by placing a donut magnet over the right upper quadrant of the pulse generator and holding it in place for 30 seconds. A detailed description of this technique is described in the article by Higgins (see bibliography).

BIBLIOGRAPHY

Invasive Monitoring

Barker WJ, Wyte SR: Arterial puncture and cannulation, in Roberts JR, Hedges JR (eds): *Clinical Procedures in Emergency Medicine*. Philadelphia, Saunders, 1985, pp 352–365.

Forrester JS, Diamond G, Chatterjee K, et al: Medical therapy of acute myocardial infarction by application of hemodynamic subsets. *N Engl J Med* 205:1356, 1976.

Kaye W: Invasive monitoring techniques, in McIntyre KM, Levis AJ (eds): *Textbook of Advanced Cardiac Life Support*. Dallas, American Heart Association, 1983, pp 165–196.

Shoemaker WC: Monitoring the critically ill patient, in Shoemaker WC (ed): *Textbook of Critical Care Medicine*. Philadelphia, Saunders, 1984, pp 105–121.

Pacing Techniques

Bing OH, McDowell JW, Hantman J, et al: Pacemaker placement by electrocardidographic monitoring. *N Engl J Med* 287:651, 1972.

Hazard PB, Benton C, Milnor P: Transvenous cardiac pacing in cardiopulmonary resuscitation. *Crit Care Med* 9:666, 1981.

Roberts JR, Syverud SA: Transthoracic and transcutaneous cardiac pacing; Benjamin GC: Emergency transvenous cardiac pacing, in Roberts JR, Hedges JR (eds): *Clinical Procedures in Emergency Medicine*. Philadelphia, Saunders, 1985, pp 170–207.

Syverud SA, Dalsey WC, Hedges JR: Transcutaneous and transvenous cardiac pacing for early bradyasystolic cardiac arrest. *Ann Emerg Med* 15:121, 1986.

Automatic and Implantable Defibrillators

Cummins RO: Review of the clinical experience with automatic external defibrillators. *Ann Emerg Med* 18:1269, 1989.

Higgins GL: The automatic implantable cardioverter-defibrillator: management issues relevant to the emergency care provider. *Am J Emerg Med* 8:342, 347, 1990.

Kouwenhoven WB: Closed chest defibrillation of the heart. *Surgery* 42:550, 1952.

8
ACID-BASE PROBLEMS

Robert F. Wilson

DEFINING TERMS

The acidity of any solution, whether blood, interstitial fluid, or cell water, is a measure of the hydrogen ion activity of that solution. Hydrogen ion activity is directly promotional to the concentration of hydrogen ions within the solution multiplied by an activity coefficient. Thus, an equation for hydrogen activity could be derived as

$$H^+ = K_A \frac{[HA]}{[A-]}$$

This equation assumes that the [A −] and [HA] are measurements of their activities, not of their concentrations. [HA] is any acid and [A −] is the conjugate base. The general equation for the acidity of any solution may now be written as

$$H^+ = K_A \frac{[\text{acid}]}{[\text{base}]}$$

The acidity of a solution is thus equal to the ratio of the activities of the acid to its corresponding base multiplied by its dissociation constant.

pH

The concentration of hydrogen ions, even in a very acid solution, is extremely low. In a so-called neutral solution, the number of hydrogen (H^+) ions equals the number of hydroxyl (OH −) ions; in water at 25°C (77°F) the number of hydrogen ions is 1/10,000,000, or 10^{-7} mol/L. The term *pH* refers to the negative logarithm of the hydrogen ion concentration. Thus, a solution with a pH of 1.0 has a hydrogen ion concentration of 1×10^{-1} and is extremely acidic, whereas a solution with a pH of 13.0 has a hydrogen ion concentration of 1×10^{-13} and is extremely alkaline.

Henderson-Hasselbach Equation

The Henderson-Hasselbach equation states that the pH is equal to the pK (the negative log of the dissociation constant or the pH at which half of the compound is ionized) plus the log of the ratio of the concentration of a base to its related acid.

$$pH = pK + \log \frac{\text{proton acceptor (base)}}{\text{proton donor (acid)}}$$

About 80 percent of the buffering for the extracellular fluid is the bicarbonate–carbonic acid system. The average normal concentration of bicarbonate is 24 mEq/L, and the average normal concentration of carbonic acid is 1.2 mEq/L. Thus, the ratio of bicarbonate to carbonic acid is normally 20:1. The log of 20 is 1.3, and adding 1.3 to 6.1 (the pK of the bicarbonate–carbonic acid system) results in 7.4, which is the normal arterial pH:

$$pH = 6.1 + \log \frac{HCO_3^-}{H_2CO_2} = 6.1 + \log \frac{24}{1.2}$$

$$= 6.1 + \log 20 = 6.1 + 1.3 = 7.4$$

If the ratio of bicarbonate to carbonic acid is doubled or reduced by half, the pH changes by 0.3. The normal ratio of HCO_3 to H_2CO_3 is 20:1 and the log of 20 is 1.3. Since the log of 10 is 1.0 and the log of 5 is 0.7, whenever the ratio of HCO_3 to H_2CO_3 is reduced by one-half, the pH falls by 0.3. On the other hand, if the HCO_3/H_2CO_3 ratio increases from 20:1 to 40:1, the pH rises from 7.40 to 7.70.

The H_2CO_3 can be calculated by multiplying the P_{CO_2} by 0.03. Thus, with a HCO_3^- of 12 and a P_{CO_2} of 40 mmHg, the H_2CO_3 would be 1.2, the ratio of HCO_3^- to H_2CO_3 would be 10 (log of 1.0), and the pH would be 7.1. If the HCO_3^- fell to 6 and the P_{CO_2} were still 40 mmHg, the ratio of HCO_3^- to H_2CO_3 would be 5 (log of 0.7) and the pH would be 6.8.

Hydrogen Ion Concentrations

Some investigators prefer to use hydrogen ion concentration, rather than pH, when discussing or calculating acidity (Table 8-1). At a pH of 7.40, the hydrogen ion activity is equivalent to 40 nmol/L. The clinical relationship between (H^+) (in nmol/L) and P_{CO_2} and HCO_3 can be expressed by the following formula:

$$H^+(\text{nmol/L}) = \frac{(24)\,(P_{CO_2})}{HCO_3}$$

If a table relating H^+ to pH is available, it is easy to calculate pH, P_{CO_2}, and HCO_3 if two of the three are known.

Thus, if the P_{CO_2} is 25 and the HCO_3 is 12,

$$H^+ = \frac{(24)\,(25)}{(12)} = \frac{600}{12} = 50 \text{ nmol/L}$$

A H^+ activity of 50 nmol/L is equivalent to a pH of 7.30 (Table 8-1).

Intracellular pH (pH_i)

There are many difficulties in measuring intracellular pH, especially in humans. Measurements from human quadriceps muscle by Sahlin in 1978 revealed a pH_i of 7.00 ± 0.06 in 13 studies. In 20 studies of human red blood cells by Warth and Desforges in 1978 the pH_i was found to range from 7.06 to 7.10. Thus, the pH_i is 0.30 to 0.40 units less than the arterial pH.

To maintain a chronic stable pH_i, acid must be extruded from the cell relatively soon after it is formed. However, the initial handling of acid in the cell is much more complex. When responding to an acute internal acid load, the cell first recruits several relatively rapid mechanisms that consume or bind H^+, thereby minimizing the magnitude of the pH_i decrease. Later, the pH_i slowly returns toward normal as acid is extruded from the cell.

The initial mechanisms for handling an acid load include (1) physicochemical buffering, (2) cellular consumption of nonvolatile acids, and (3) the transfer of acid or alkali between the cytosol and organelles. In the broadest sense, all three are buffering mechanisms, since they reversibly consume H^+. In combination they neutralize more than 99.99 percent of the acid or alkali introduced into a cell. For example, the addition of 10^{-3} mol of H^+ to 1 L of cell content might lower pH_i from 7.1 to 7.0, representing an increase of only about 2×10^{-8}

Table 8-1. Hydrogen Ion Activity and pH

H^+ (nmol/L)	pH
20	7.7
25	7.6
32	7.5
40	7.4
50	7.3
64	7.2
80	7.1
101	7.0
128	6.9
160	6.8

M in free [H^+]. All the rest of the H^+ is "consumed" or "buffered" by the three mechanisms described above.

The conversion of a weak acid (e.g., lactic acid) to a neutral product (e.g., glucose) or to one that can readily leave the cell (e.g., CO_2) results in the loss of intracellular H^+. Internal pH can also be influenced by other reactions, such as the hydrolysis of ATP (which releases H^+) or phosphocreatinine (which consumes H^+). Folbergrova et al. showed that intracellular acid loading (accomplished by increasing P_{CO_2}) leads to a reduction in the levels of several acidic metabolic intermediates (pyruvate, lactate, citrate, α-ketoglutarate, maleate, glutamate, and aspartate). Intracellular acid loading also causes an elevation of glucose and glucose-6-phosphate levels. This pattern suggests that reducing pH_i inhibits a step (possibly the phosphofructokinase reaction) in the glycolytic pathway. The maximum amount of H^+ that can be neutralized through these acidic intermediates is about 50 percent of that taken up by physicochemical buffers. Other evidence of metabolic consumption of acid comes from Cohen et al., who showed that increased lactate uptake by the isolated, perfused rat liver is associated with a rise in pH_i, as would be expected if lactate ions entered the cell and were converted to neutral products.

Intracellular alkalosis (produced by decreasing P_{CO_2}) leads to increased levels of pyruvate, lactate, and other acidic metabolic intermediates in rat brain, and these metabolic changes thereby partially neutralize the alkaline load.

Thus, physicochemical, biochemical, and organelle buffering mechanisms offer only partial and short-term solutions to acid loading. They can only minimize the decrease in pH_i and are of limited capacity. The restoration of a normal pH_i after an acute acid load requires the eventual extrusion of all added acid. As this extrusion proceeds, buffers release the H^+ which they previously consumed and are thereby restored to their initial state.

ACID PRODUCTION, TRANSPORT, AND EXCRETION

Carbon Dioxide (Volatile Acid)

With an average CO_2 production of 200 to 300 mL/min, the body's total CO_2 production is 288,000 to 432,000 mL/day. Since 22.4 mL CO_2 is equivalent to 1.0 mEq of acid, each day about 12,000 to 20,000 mEq of volatile acid is produced by the body's metabolism of carbohydrate, protein, and fat and is excreted by the lungs. Most carbon dioxide transport to the lungs from peripheral tissues is provided by plasma bicarbonate and red cell hemoglobin. Carbon dioxide present as carbonic acid in arterial blood averages about 1.2 (1.05 to 1.35) mEq/L, equivalent to a P_{CO_2} of 40 mmHg.

Nonvolatile Acid Excretion

Ordinarily the kidney excretes about 70 mEq of acid each day, but in acidotic patients, acid excretion may be increased more than tenfold. Renal tubular excretion of acid normally is accomplished by three mechanisms: (1) direct excretion of hydrogen, which accounts for only about 0.1 mEq of acid per day; (2) excretion with urine buffers, including the NaH_2PO_4 system, which accounts for about 20 mEq of acid per day; and (3) excretion with ammonia (produced in the distal tubal cells from glutamine and other precursors), which accounts for about 50 mEq of acid per day.

In the proximal tubule, sodium and bicarbonate are absorbed independent of the effects of aldosterone, and hydrogen is secreted into the tubular lumen in exchange for sodium ion. If the extracellular fluid volume is reduced or "contracted," increased amounts of sodium and bicarbonate are absorbed in the proximal tubule, and this may cause a "contraction metabolic alkalosis." If saline solution is given, expanding the extracellular fluid, proximal tubular absorption of sodium and bicarbonate is decreased. Sodium deficiency, increased aldosterone production, or decreased aldosterone metabolism by the liver also increase the absorption of sodium and bicarbonate in the proximal tubule.

In the distal tubule cells, H_2CO_3 is dissociated into H^+ and HCO_3^-. Here H^+ and K^+ are excreted into the urine in exchange for Na^+. The HCO_3^- which was formed in the cell and the Na^+ which is absorbed out of the tubule lumen move out the other side of the tubule cell into the bloodstream as $NaHCO_3$.

Anything that increases the intracellular concentration of hydrogen or potassium ions also increases the secretion of hydrogen and/or potassium ions into the distal tubular lumen and increases sodium reabsorption. When a potassium deficiency develops in the extracellular fluid, potassium ions leave tissue cells in exchange for hydrogen, resulting in an intracellular acidosis and an extracellular alkalosis. Increased potassium is also absorbed in the distal tubule in exchange for hydrogen ions, and increased hydrogen ions are then excreted in the urine. Thus, a hypokalemic alkalemic patient may put out a paradoxically acid urine.

Renal tubular acidosis may be classified as proximal or distal depending on the nephron segment primarily involved in the generation of this defect. In proximal tubular acidosis, urinary pH is increased at normal rates of bicarbonate filtration, denoting a failure of the proximal nephron to reabsorb the normal load of bicarbonate. However, when the filtered load of bicarbonate is decreased, urinary pH decreases to normal levels, indicating that the distal nephron is able to take care of the bicarbonate loads that are within the normal range.

When the distal nephron is predominately involved (distal tubular acidosis), the ability to create transepithelial pH gradients and thus to produce an acid urine is impaired at any filtered load of bicarbonate due to an intrinsic defect of the acidification capacity of the last tubule segments.

Acidification of urine by the distal nephron can be evaluated clinically by measuring urine and arterial P_{CO_2} after making the urine alkaline by bicarbonate loading. The urine-blood P_{CO_2} difference indicates the amount of urine CO_2 generation due to distal hydrogen ion secretion. When distal hydrogen ion secretion is impaired, as in distal tubular acidosis, urine P_{CO_2} falls, and urine-blood P_{CO_2} differences are reduced.

Buffers

A wide variety of metabolic and respiratory factors produce or take up hydrogen ions. These changes in hydrogen ion concentration could cause wide swings in the pH if it were not for a group of substances referred to as *buffers*, which are capable of partially neutralizing acids and bases. The acid-buffering capacity of any agent or solution is determined by the number of hydrogen ions that the agent can take up for each unit change in pH. In general, for each 1000 to 10,000 mEq of acid added to the body, only about 1 mEq remains unbuffered or free to produce a change in pH. Thus, about 99.99 percent of an acid load is buffered or combined with other compounds to prevent sudden pH changes.

The average adult male has a total buffer base, or buffering capacity, of about 1000 mEq. The chief buffers in blood are the hemoglobin in red blood cells and the bicarbonate and protein in plasma. Most of the total buffering against carbon dioxide is provided by hemoglobin, but moment-to-moment buffering of the blood and interstitial fluid is provided primarily by the bicarbonate–carbonic acid system. The most important intracellular buffers are phosphate and protein. Patients with anemia, low plasma protein levels, or decreased muscle mass have a reduced buffering capacity and are apt to have wide swings in pH when they become ill or injured. In such individuals, impaired tissue perfusion of relatively short duration may cause severe acidosis.

The body generally tolerates an acid load much better than a base excess. Most of the body's buffer systems are designed to neutralize acid. Mortality and morbidity tend to be much worse in patients with alkalosis than those with a corresponding amount of acidosis.

Buffer Base

To recognize and quantify nonrespiratory (metabolic) acidosis or alkalosis, changes in plasma bicarbonate concentrations are traditionally evaluated. However, since bicarbonate concentration in plasma is also affected by changes in P_{CO_2} (the respiratory disturbances), several P_{CO_2}-independent indexes of the nonrespiratory acid-base disturbance have been proposed, such as standard bicarbonate concentration or eucapnic pH (both standardized for P_{CO_2} of 40 mmHg), and buffer base, either in whole blood or in plasma; base excess or deficit is a measure of the deviation of buffer base from its normal value. Conceptually all the P_{CO_2}-independent indicators of the metabolic acid-base disturbances are meant to parallel the differences between the sums of all strong (i.e., completely dissociated) cations and anions in plasma.

Base Excess

An increase in the amount of buffer base present is referred to as a *base excess,* and a decrease may be referred to as a *base deficit* or a *negative base excess.*

The appropriate respiratory (ventilatory) component of the acid-base status of a patient is fairly predictable. A sudden increase of 10 mmHg in P_{CO_2} (with bicarbonate staying constant) causes the pH to decrease by about 0.10 unit; whereas a sudden decrease of 10 mmHg in P_{CO_2} (with bicarbonate staying constant) causes the pH to increase by about 0.13. Thus, the difference between the actual pH and the pH predicted from the P_{CO_2} represents a deviation from the normal buffer base status.

The metabolic component may also be estimated because a rise in HCO_3 of 5.0 mEq/L (with P_{CO_2} staying constant) raises the pH about 0.08, and a fall in HCO_3 of 5.0 mEq/L (again with P_{CO_2} staying constant) lowers the pH about 0.10.

As a general rule, the base deficit (negative base excess) represents the mEq/L of bicarbonate that is required to restore the total buffer base of the extracellular fluid to normal. There are a number of ways to determine the base deficit. One can estimate it by (1) subtracting the actual bicarbonate from 26 mEq/L at a pH of 7.30 to 7.34 or 28 mEq at a pH of 7.20 to 7.29; (2) using a nomogram, (3) using a table (Table 8-2); or (4) using a technique described by Shapiro (see below, steps 1 to 3).

Thus, if the pH is 7.04, according to Table 8-2, the sum of the HCO_3 and buffer base should be 32 mEq/L. Thus, if the HCO_3 is 19.9 mEq/L, the base deficit should be about 32 − 19.9 = 12.1 mEq/L.

If the pH is 7.47, according to Table 8-2, the sum of the HCO_3 and buffer base should be 23 mEq/L. Therefore, if the HCO_3 is 12.7 mEq/L, the base deficit should be 23 − 12.7 = 10 mEq/L.

Another method involves three steps for estimating the metabolic component (i.e., base deficit) of an acid-base abnormality.

1. Determine the P_{CO_2} variance, the difference between measured P_{CO_2} and 40. Move the decimal point two places to the left.
2. Determine the predicted pH from the P_{CO_2} variance: If the P_{CO_2} is over 40, subtract half of the P_{CO_2} variance from the 7.40. If the P_{CO_2} is under 40, add the P_{CO_2} variance to 7.40.
3. Estimate the base excess (or deficit) from the pH variance: Determine the difference between the measured and predicted pHs. Move the decimal point two places to the right, and multiply by two-thirds.

Example 1. pH 7.04, P_{CO_2} − 76 mmHg, HCO_3 19.9 mEq/L.

$$76 - 40 = 36$$
$$36 \times \tfrac{1}{2} = 18$$
$$7.40 - 0.18 = 7.22$$
$$7.22 - 7.04 = 18$$
$$\tfrac{2}{3} \times 18 = 12 \text{ mEq/L base deficit}$$

Example 2. pH 7.47, P_{CO_2} − 18 mmHg, HCO_3 12.7 mEq/L.

$$40 - 18 = 22$$
$$7.40 + 0.22 = 7.62$$
$$7.62 - 7.47 = 15$$
$$15 \times \tfrac{2}{3} = 10 \text{ mEq/L base deficit}$$

Nonvolatile Weak Acids

In addition to P_{CO_2} and plasma buffer base (BB), a third independent variable exists in body fluids, the total concentration of nonvolatile weak acids, designated as $[A_T]$. In plasma, the main constituent of $[A_T]$ is the protein (predominately albumin). The contribution of phosphate is less than one-tenth of the total $[A_T]$.

P_{CO_2} and buffer base are the controlled quantities in the biological regulation of acid-base balance. However, any abnormality in the amount of nonvolatile weak acids ($[A_T]$), especially plasma proteins, will produce an acid-base disturbance. Thus, hypoproteinemia tends to cause a nonrespiratory alkalosis, and abnormally high concentrations of plasma albumin can give rise to a nonrespiratory acidosis.

If the anion gap is normal in a hypoproteinemic patient, unidentified anions must be present. This increase in unidentified anions would be missed if the plasma protein level was not known.

Plasma proteins should be measured as part of the evaluation of acid-base status. Base excess or deficit does not distinguish strong acids (e.g., lactic, keto) from weak nonvolatile acids (plasma proteins, phosphate). The existing nomograms for the estimation of buffer base are based on data obtained in blood with normal concentrations of plasma proteins. Therefore, a deficit of novolatile weak acids appears as an apparent increase in plasma buffer base.

Carbon Dioxide Content

Carbon dioxide content refers to the total of all carbon dioxide present in the blood (normally 24 to 31 mEq/L). In the plasma, CO_2 content includes carbonic acid, bicarbonate, and carbamino compounds. The amount of carbonic acid present (averaging about 1.05 to 1.35 mEq/L) can be estimated by multiplying the P_{CO_2} by 0.03. The arterial bicarbonate concentration normally is 24 mEq/L. The concentration of the carbamino compounds, which consists of various forms of CO_2 combined with amino groups on proteins, averages about 0.5 to 1.0 mEq/L, depending on total CO_2 and protein concentrations.

Table 8-2. Estimating Base Deficit from the pH and Bicarbonate

pH	Sum of Base Deficit and Bicarbonate	Base Deficit if Bicarbonate is 24 mEq
7.00–7.09	32	8
7.10–7.19	30	6
7.20–7.29	28	4
7.30–7.34	26	2
7.35–7.45	24	0
7.45–7.49	23	−1
7.50–7.59	22	−2

EVALUATING ACID-BASE ABNORMALITIES

Checking the Consistency and Accuracy of Laboratory Reports

Correlating Carbon Dioxide Content and Bicarbonate

When obtaining blood for blood gas studies in patients with complicated acute problems, additional blood for electrolyte determinations should be drawn. The bicarbonate present can then be estimated from the CO_2 content as well as from the pH and P_{CO_2}.

Under ordinary circumstances, the arterial bicarbonate concentration is approximately 1.5 to 2.0 mEq/L less than the arterial CO_2 content reported as part of an electrolyte analysis. Since the venous P_{CO_2} is normally about 6 torr higher than the arterial P_{CO_2} and venous bicarbonate is 1.1 mEq/L higher than arterial bicarbonate, the venous CO_2 content is usually about 1.5 to 2.0 mEq/L higher than the arterial CO_2 content. Thus, if arterial blood is drawn for blood gas determinations and venous blood is drawn for electrolytes, the CO_2 content in venous blood should be about 3.0 to 4.0 mEq/L more than the arterial bicarbonate. One should not accept an arterial bicarbonate which is higher than a simultaneous venous CO_2 content.

Correlating pH and Electrolyte Values

Correlating pH with the potassium and other electrolyte values can also help estimate acid-base status. Patients with severe acidosis tend to have high serum potassium levels, and patients with severe alkalosis tend to have low serum potassium levels. In general, a rise or fall of 0.10 in pH is associated with a corresponding fall or rise of about 0.5 (0.3 to 0.8) mEq/L in serum potassium. Thus, if the pH of a patient with a pH of 7.30 and a plasma potassium of 4.8 mEq/L were raised to 7.50, the patient's plasma potassium level would fall to about 3.8. The potassium level in serum is slightly higher than that in plasma because the clotting process releases some potassium.

Correlating Chloride and Bicarbonate Levels

Plasma chloride and bicarbonate concentrations tend to move in opposite directions. Thus, patients who have a metabolic alkalosis (and high plasma bicarbonate levels) tend to have low plasma chloride levels, whereas those with metabolic acidosis (and low plasma bicarbonate levels) tend to have normal or elevated chloride levels. However, if there are increased amounts of unmeasured anions, such as lactate, present (causing an increased anion gap), bicarbonate may be very low and chloride may be normal or even low.

Effect of PCO_2 and HCO_3^- on pH

With mild to moderate acidosis (pH 7.25 to 7.35), a 1.0-mmHg rise in the P_{CO_2} produces a decrease of about 0.01 in pH, while a 1.0 mEq/L decrease in bicarbonate produces a pH decrease of about 0.02 (Table 8-3). Thus, a patient whose HCO_3 falls from 24.0 to 19.0 mEq/L and whose P_{CO_2} also falls from 40 to 30 mmHg will still have a pH of approximately 7.40. This "quick and dirty" way to estimate bicarbonate from the pH and P_{CO_2} can also be used as a check on the consistency and accuracy of the laboratory results, particularly if arterial bicarbonate is not 2.5 to 3.0 mEq/L less than the CO_2 content found on a venous electrolyte study.

Table 8-3. Acute pH and Bicarbonate Response to Changes in P_{CO_2}

P_{CO_2}, mmHg	pH	HCO_3, mEq/L
15	7.73	19
20	7.62	20
25	7.54	21
30	7.49	22
35	7.44	23
40	7.40	24
50	7.32	25
60	7.26	26
70	7.21	27
80	7.16	28

Categorizing the Abnormality

Single Disorders

Acid-base abnormalities can often be defined in terms of the pH and the relative amounts of arterial bicarbonate and carbonic acid. The normal average concentration of bicarbonate in arterial blood is 24 mEq/L, with a normal range of about 21 to 26 mEq/L. If the arterial bicarbonate is greater than 26 mEq/L and the pH is greater than 7.40, the patient is said to have a metabolic alkalosis. If the arterial bicarbonate is less than 21 mEq/L and the pH is less than 7.40, the patient is said to have a metabolic acidosis.

The P_{CO_2} is normally 35 to 45 mmHg. If the arterial P_{CO_2} is lower than 35 mmHg and the pH is greater than 7.40, the patient is said to have a respiratory alkalosis. In contrast, if the arterial P_{CO_2} is greater than 45 mmHg and the pH is less than 7.40, the patient is said to have a respiratory acidosis.

Mixed Disorders

In many instances, more than one acid-base problem is present at a time. For example, if a patient with chronic respiratory acidosis (pH, 7.35; P_{CO_2}, 50 mmHg; HCO_3, 26.7 mEq/L) develops pyloric stenosis and is vomiting large amounts of highly acidic fluid (which would ordinarily cause a metabolic alkalosis), the patient could develop a pH of 7.40 with a P_{CO_2} of 55 mmHg and a HCO_3 of 32 mEq/L. This might be confusing under many clinical circumstances. However, in general, if the arterial pH is relatively normal (7.36 to 7.44) and the P_{CO_2} and/or HCO_3 are abnormal, one can assume that a mixed abnormality is present. The mixed abnormality should also be detectable from the history and physical examination or other laboratory data. In this regard, the anion gap and buffer base may be helpful.

Compensatory Changes

Any abnormality that disturbs the normal ratio between arterial bicarbonate and carbonic acid tends to immediately stimulate a compensatory metabolic or respiratory response—to try to bring the ratio back to 7.35 if the primary problem is an acidosis or to 7.45 if the problem is an alkalosis.

Respiratory Compensation

Metabolic Acidosis

Respiratory compensation for a primary metabolic acidosis can occur very rapidly. For example, the patient who develops a metabolic acidosis with a bicarbonate of 14 mEq/L will tend to hyperventilate rather rapidly, producing a compensatory respiratory alkalosis. The P_{CO_2} would have to fall to 20 mmHg to produce complete compensation to a pH of 7.40; however, the acute compensation (within 1 to 2 h) may be only about 50 percent of that, and the compensation over 24 h may be only 75 percent complete (Table 8-4).

Table 8-4. Chronic pH and Bicarbonate Response to Changes in P_{CO_2}

P_{CO_2}, mmHg	pH	HCO_3, mEq/L
20	7.47	14
30	7.45	20
40	7.40	24
50	7.37	28
60	7.35	32
70	7.33	36
80	7.32	40

Metabolic Alkalosis

Compensation for an alkalosis is seldom as good as for an acidosis. Furthermore, the compensatory hypoventilation for a metabolic alkalosis is restricted by the hypoxemia that develops along with the hypoventilation. The P_{CO_2} seldom rises above 50 to 55 mmHg to compensate for a metabolic alkalosis unless oxygen is given.

If a patient develops a metabolic alkalosis with a HCO_3 of 36 mEq/L, the P_{CO_2} would have to rise to 60 mmHg for a complete compensation to a pH of 7.40. The acute compensation would only be about 25 to 40 percent, raising the P_{CO_2} to about 45 to 48 mmHg. Even after 48 h, the respiratory compensation is often only about 60 percent complete.

Metabolic Compensations

During acute and chronic hypocapnia and hypercapnia, the changes in HCO_3 are almost linear over the range of Pa_{CO_2} (20 to 100 mmHg) encountered in altered pathologic states (Tables 8-3 and 8-4). Thus, you can predict to some degree what the HCO_3 "should be" for any Pa_{CO_2}. This observation leads to certain rules of thumb to characterize various acid-base abnormalities:

1. During acute hypercapnia, HCO_3 increases 1 mmol/L for each 10-mmHg increase in Pa_{CO_2} above 40 mmHg.
2. During chronic hypercapnia, HCO_3 increases 4 mmol/L for each 10-mmHg increase in Pa_{CO_2} above 40 mmHg.
3. During acute hypocapnia, HCO_3 decreases 2 mmol/L for every 10-mmHg decrease in Pa_{CO_2} below 40 mmHg.
4. During chronic hypocapnia, HCO_3 decreases at least 5 mmol/L for every 10-mmHg decrease in Pa_{CO_2} below 40 mmHg.

Failure of Compensatory Mechanisms

Failure of compensatory mechanisms, or a combination of primary processes driving the pH in the same direction so that it rapidly falls and stays below 7.10 or rises above 7.60, is frequently lethal. Inability to compensate for an acid-base abnormality usually means a severe disturbance of ventilatory, renal, or general cellular function.

The Anion Gap

Definition

The concept of an anion gap in blood was described in 1939 by Gamble. It was felt that the law of electroneutrality required that the number of positive charges contributed by serum cations should equal the number of negative charges contributed by serum anions. Sodium (Na), chloride (Cl), and bicarbonate (HCO_3) are considered the measured ions. Potassium is ignored because its value changes so little. Thus, the concept of electroneutrality can be expressed by the simple equation:

$$Na + UC = Cl + HCO_3 + UA$$

where UC (unmeasured cations) indicates the sum of the charges of the cations other than sodium and UA (unmeasured anions) equals the sum of the charges of all of the anions other than chloride and bicarbonate.

The term *anion gap* was coined to indicate the difference between the measured sodium level and the measured chloride and bicarbonate (really CO_2 content) levels.

$$\text{Anion gap} = Na - (Cl + HCO_3)$$

The equation can also be written as

$$UA - UC = Na - (Cl + HCO_3) = \text{anion gap}$$

indicating that a rise in UA and/or a decrease in UC will cause an increase in the anion gap, independent of the presence or absence of an acid-base disorder. The reverse is also true. In other words, a decrease in UA and/or rise in UC will cause a decrease in the anion gap.

The "unmeasured cations" usually total about 11 mEq/L and include potassium (4 mEq/L), calcium (5 mEq/L), and magnesium (2 mEq/L).

The "unmeasured" serum anions include sulfates (1 mEq/L), phosphates (2 mEq/L), proteins (16 mEq/L), lactic acid (1 mEq/L), and other organic acids (3 mEq/L). Ordinarily, the sodium concentration is about 140 mEq/L, and the sum of the CO_2 content and chloride anions is about 128 mEq/L. Thus, the difference (or anion gap) between the sodium concentration and the sum of these two anions averages about 12 mEq/L. In patients with excessive acid production, the anion gap tends to be increased. On the other hand, in patients with metabolic acidosis due to loss of bicarbonate, the anion gap usually stays relatively normal.

Unmeasured Cations and Anions

Assigning numerical values for the charges of the serum constituents is accomplished easily for sodium, potassium, bicarbonate, and chloride, but is more difficult with phosphate and protein, which can have multiple charges. Although they are measured with relative ease, calcium and magnesium are also a problem (Table 8-5). The total concentration of serum calcium and magnesium, rather than just the ionized fraction, is used in the calculation of unmeasured cations because the nonionized portions of those cations are bound to protein (especially albumin, which is a polyanion) or are complexed with bicarbonate, phosphate, sulfate, lactate, or citrate. Thus, they "cover," or balance, an equivalent number of negative charges on these anions. In other words, protein-bound and complexed calcium and magnesium contribute to the charge balance in the serum.

The difficulty in establishing the precise charge contributions of sulfate and organic acid anions arises because clinical laboratories do not measure these serum constituents on a routine basis. At least 29 acid anions are detectable in plasma; however, in normal individuals the combined contribution to the serum anions by lactate, pyruvate, acetoacetate, 3-hydroxybutyrate, and citrate is only 1.8 to 2.6 mEq/L.

Although the concentration of serum phosphate is readily measured in the clinical laboratory, it is not a simple matter to derive its charge, which is a function not only of phosphate concentration but also serum pH. Serum phosphorus concentration in mg/dL is converted to mmol/L by multiplying by 10 and dividing by 31, the atomic weight of phosphorus. At a pH of 7.4, the ratio of $H_2PO_4^{2-}$ to $H_2PO_4^-$ is about 4 to 1. Thus, 80 percent of the phosphate contributes two negative charges as HPO_4^{2-}, and 20 percent contributes one charge as $H_2PO_4^-$; thus, the charge contribution of phosphate in mEq/L at pH 7.4 is equal to the mmol/L of phosphate multiplied by 1.8.

Normal serum proteins are polyanions. Although their net contribution to overall charge balance is difficult to assess exactly, a normal mixture of serum proteins is about 2.3 mEq/L per gram of protein at pH 7.40. This charge reflects three variables: the type of protein, the concentration of protein, and serum pH.

Albumin contributes about 2.6 mEq/L for each g/dL, and globulin provides approximately 1.7 mEq/L for each g/dL. Both Van Slyke and Van Leeuwen reported a 4 to 5 percent increase in the negative charge of protein for each 0.10 unit rise in pH.

Table 8-5. Conversion of Laboratory Values for Serum Constituents to mEq/L*

Ca^{2+} mg/dL × 10 ÷ 40 × 2
Mg^{2+} mg/dL × 10 ÷ 24 × 2
PO_4^- (mgP) mg/dL × 10 ÷ 31 × 1.8
SO_4^- (mmol) mmol/L × 2

* Conversion from mg/dL to mEq/L is done by multiplying by 10 to convert to mg/L, dividing by the molecular weight, and then multiplying by the valence.

Etiology of Increased Anion Gap

An increased anion gap may be caused by (1) artifacts; (2) an accumulation of organic acids, such as that seen in lactic acidosis, ketoacidosis, acute renal failure, and toxic ingestions; (3) exogenous anions; (4) reduced inorganic acid excretion, such as in chronic renal failure; (5) an increase in the anionic contribution of unmeasured weak acids; (6) a decrease in unmeasured cations; or (7) a combination of these factors.

Changes Due to Artifacts

A spurious increase in the anion gap (even in the presence of normal concentrations of the individual electrolytes) may result from excessive exposure of the serum to air. When serum placed in small measuring vessels for microautomated chemical analysis is not analyzed promptly, the percentage increases in Na, K, and Cl are similar, but HCO_3 decreases due to escape of CO_2. After 2 h, absolute increases in the concentrations of Na and Cl of 6.9 ± 1.9 and 4.2 ± 1.8 mEq/L, respectively, and a decrease in HCO_3 of 3.5 ± 1.2 mEq/L were observed. As a result, the anion gap increased 6.2 ± 2.3 mEq/L.

False elevations of serum Cl may result from the presence of other halide ions, as in patients intoxicated with bromide or iodide. These elevations occur because bromide and iodide interfere with both colorimetric and "ion-selective" techniques, resulting in reported values for Cl that exceed the sum of the true chloride concentration plus that of the other halide. Minimal interference with Cl measurement occurs with the use of chloridimetry, which should be used if halide poisoning is suspected.

Spurious hyperchloremia (with an equivalent apparent decrease in the anion gap) may also occur from the technical artifact caused by hypertriglyceridemia using colorimetric (but not titrimetric or potentiometric) techniques. In a prospective study by Graber et al., every patient with a triglyceride level exceeding 1000 mg/dL had a spurious elevation of Cl ranging from 9 to 93 mEq/L. This artifact would be independent of any change induced by displacement of the water phase of the plasma (i.e., pseudohyponatremia).

If there is excess heparin in the syringe in which arterial blood is drawn, the heparin will tend to cause an acidosis and lower the pH, P_{CO_2}, and bicarbonate, producing a picture of metabolic acidosis with partial respiratory compensation.

Increased Organic Acids

The organic acids most likely to increase the anion gap are lactic acid, keto acids, and a variety of other organic acids apt to increase in renal failure. Although an increase in unmeasured anions theoretically could result from increased phosphate, protein, sulfate, or organic anions, in practice, only increases in organic anions or major toxic ingestions account for large increases in the anion gap.

Patients with anion gaps greater than 35 mEq/L usually have ethylene glycol or methanol intoxication, hyperglycemic hyperosmolar coma, or lactic acidosis. In fact, such patients can have anion gaps greater than 50 mEq/L. Severe acidemia (pH < 7.00) occurs most commonly in such patients.

Lactic Acidosis

The causes of lactic acidosis have been divided into those due to inadequate tissue oxygenation (type A) and those due to other factors, such as diabetes mellitus, hypercarbia, tumors, etc. (type B) (Table 8-6). The presence of acidosis with an increased anion gap in a patient in severe shock most often is due to lactic acidosis.

Table 8-6. Classification of Lactic Acidosis (after Cohen and Woods)

Type A (tissue hypoxia)
Shock states
Profound anemia
Massive catecholamine excess
Type B (tissue oxygenation appears normal)
Diabetes mellitus
Liver failure
Renal failure
Carcinoma
Seizures
Alkaloses
Drugs or toxins
Inborn errors of metabolism
Hypoglycemia

Source: Cohen, Woods: *Diabetes* 32:181, 1983.

Ketoacidosis and Hyperglycemic Coma

A tendency to ketoacidosis will be less apparent in patients with a good urine output. In the presence of adequate hydration with a normal or increased urine output, ketoacidosis tends to be minimal because the increased ketones are rapidly excreted. However, if extracellular fluid volume is reduced, as is usually the case, the excretion of keto anions is retarded, producing a ketoacidosis with an increased anion gap. However, if the patient maintains an adequate salt intake and preserves normal or nearly normal extracellular fluid volume, renal perfusion, and glomerular filtration rate, keto anions are excreted almost as fast as they are produced. Under these circumstances, chloride is retained by the kidney in place of ketones, a rise in the serum chloride balances the fall in the serum bicarbonate concentration, and the serum anion gap remains or becomes normal. The increase in serum chlorides will be even greater if the patient is resuscitated with 0.9% saline rather than Ringer's lactate.

Although some ketonemia probably occurs in all spontaneously occurring instances of nonketotic hyperglycemic coma, increases in neither plasma β-hydroxybutyrate nor lactate are sufficient to explain the elevated anion gap levels, which some investigators have reported to average as high as 34 mEq/L.

Other Organic Acids

A wide variety of organic acids may be released into the blood in increased amounts in critically ill or injured patients. These may include fatty acids, amino acids, pyruvic acid, and a large number of other acid metabolites of incomplete cell metabolism.

Toxic Ingestions

Intoxications with salicylate, methanol, ethylene glycol, paraldehyde, toluene, sulfur, and formaldehyde lead to the formation of acid metabolites and/or organic acids that result in an increase in the anion gap. Some of these poisonings can be suspected clinically because of the presence of an increased osmolal gap (measured serum osmolality minus calculated serum osmolality). If the patient has a high anion gap metabolic acidosis without chronic renal failure, shock, or diabetic ketoacidosis, intoxication with methanol or ethylene glycol should be the first consideration, especially if the osmolal gap is increased.

Exogenous Anions

The influence of the poorly resorbable anion carbenicillin on the anion gap is a good example of the effect of the addition of unmeasured anion to the extracellular fluid. In addition to observing the renal tubular effects (a decrease in pH value and enhanced excretion of ammonium), Lipner et al. detected an increase in the anion gap from the control value of 11.2 to 18.3 mEq/L. In contrast, the administration of polymyxin B, a cationic antibiotic, has been reported to cause hyperchloremia and an apparently negative anion gap.

Reduced Inorganic Acid Excretions

In renal failure, increased quantities of sulfuric and phosphoric acid may accumulate in the bloodstream. With muscle damage a number of sulfur-containing compounds may greatly increase the anion gap.

Increased Unmeasured Weak Acids

In shock and sepsis, in particular, increased quantities of pyruvic acid, β-hydroxybutyric acid, fatty acids, citric acid, etc., may accumulate and add slightly to the anion gap. It is likely, however, that those known substances account for only a small increase in anion gap. Indeed, in sepsis, known compounds, including lactic acid, only account for 25 to 50 percent of the anion gap which develops.

Decreased Unmeasured Cations

The unmeasured cations are relatively constant in value. However, calcium could conceivably fall from 10 to 6 mg/dL (5 to 3 mEq/L). Potassium could fall from 5.0 to 3 mEq/L and magnesium could fall from 2.5 to 1.5 mEq/L without the patient becoming extremely ill. However, these changes combined would result in a decrease of only 5.0 mEq/L in the unmeasured cations.

Alkalemia

Alkalemia itself can induce an increase in organic acid production. However, an increased anion gap and alkalemia can coexist in the absence of a demonstrated increase in organic acids because (1) alkalemia tends to increase the net negative charge of serum proteins, and (2) certain exogenously administered anions (citrate, lactate, and acetate) can, via their metabolism, generate metabolic alkalosis and, by partial persistence in the circulation, elevate the anion gap. In Gabow's study of patients with an increased anion gap, 10 of the 42 subjects were alkalemic and 9 had a normal serum pH.

Alkalemia occurs in up to 50 percent of patients with alcoholic ketoacidosis or salicylate intoxication. Similarly, in one study 42 percent of patients with rhabdomyolysis and an increased anion gap were alkalemic. Four of seven normotensive patients with classic heat stroke had an increased anion gap. Alkalemia in alcoholic ketoacidosis, salicylate intoxication, rhabdomyolysis, and classic heat stroke is usually accounted for by enough respiratory and/or metabolic alkalosis to counteract the acidifying effect of organic acid overproduction.

Respiratory alkalosis frequently occurs in patients undergoing alcohol withdrawal. If one adds the increase in the anion gap to the actual serum bicarbonate concentration, a measure of the true extent of the metabolic alkalosis can be obtained. One can think of this value as the level of serum bicarbonate concentration that would have been present had the newly formed organic acids not titrated away a portion of the bicarbonate.

The interpretation of an increased anion gap in patients with alkalemia is complicated because alkalemia itself can increase the anion gap. Alkalemia can increase both organic acid generation and the negative charge on protein. In acute respiratory alkalosis, lactic acid production can increase modestly and thereby raise plasma lactate levels by 2 to 3 mEq/L. This increase in lactic acid production appears to result from an increased activity of phosphofructokinase, which enhances glycolysis via the Embden-Meyerhof pathway and thereby increases the conversion of glucose to lactate.

Two interrelated factors are responsible for alklemia increasing the net negative charge on serum proteins. First, alkalemic states are often associated with a reduced blood volume and hemoconcentration. Second, proteins surrender protons when titrated in an alkaline direction, thereby uncovering additional negative charges.

Utilizing Van Leeuwen's formula, one can anticipate that alkaline titration alone can increase the anion gap by about 0.6 mEq/L for every 0.10 rise in pH. Some investigators have reported that in humans, severe gastric alkalosis may increase the anion gap by 8 to 12 mEq/L. About 25 percent of the total increase results from increased organic acids and proteinate charge, and about 75 percent results from hemoconcentration. Before this phenomenon was emphasized in 1979, increases in the anion gap in hypotensive patients with severe gastric alkalosis were usually attributed (without confirmation) to lactic acidosis.

In summary, an anion gap greater than 30 mEq/L usually indicates the presence of an organic acidosis. Values between 23 and 30 mEq/L are also suggestive of an organic acidosis, but the nature of the retained anion frequently cannot be established. In acidotic patients with values between 16 and 22 mEq/L, uremia or mild organic acidosis may be present. If the patient is alkalemic, hemoconcentration or administration of an exogenous anion may be the cause of an increased anion gap.

Decreased Anion Gap

An anion gap of 7 or less is unusual. The main causes of a decreased anion gap are decreased unmeasured anions, increased unmeasured cations, and various analytical errors causing falsely low sodium levels or falsely high chloride levels (Table 8-7).

Decreased Unmeasured Anions

Hypoalbuminemia is probably the most common cause of a decreased anion gap in hospitalized patients. For each 1.0 gm/dL reduction in serum albumin the anion gap will fall approximately 2.5 to 3.0 mEq/L and the standard bicarbonate (the bicarbonate that would be present if the arterial P_{CO_2} were 40 mmHg) increases by an average of 3.4 mmol/L.

Rossing, based on his studies, presented somewhat different corrections in anion gap and bicarbonate related to changes in albumin.

$$[HCO_3] = [\text{albumin, g/dL}]\,(-2.63)$$

$$[AG] = [\text{albumin, g/dL}]\,(+4.20)$$

This mechanism is the most likely explanation for the decreased anion gap frequently observed in patients with nephrotic syndrome or advanced liver disease.

Some reduction in the anion gap occurs in hypoosmolar states, presumably as a result of dilution. This change is most apparent in the syndrome of inappropriate secretion of antidiuretic hormone (SIADH). Almost 25 percent of patients with SIADH have an anion gap of less than 6 mEq/L.

Increased Unmeasured Cations

The decreased anion gap in multiple myeloma is due to an increased serum concentration of cationic IgG paraproteins. Hypercalcemia and hypoalbuminemia can also contribute to a low plasma anion gap in patients with multiple myeloma.

Analytical Errors

One should never assume that all reported lab values are correct. Among the causes of nonrandom laboratory errors leading to artifactual reduction in the anion gap, hypernatremia and hyperviscosity are the most important. When the actual serum sodium concentration exceeds 170 mEq/L, certain flame photometers yield artifactually low values.

Table 8-7. Causes of a Decreased Anion Gap

Decreased unmeasured anions
Hypoalbuminemia
Dilution
Increased unmeasured cation
IgG multiple myeloma
Increased calcium, magnesium, or potassium
Acute lithium intoxication
Polymyxin B administration
Nonrandom analytical error
Hypernatremia (severe)
Hyperviscosity
Bromide intoxication
Iodide ingestion
Hyperlipidemia

Hyperviscosity can also lead to falsely low values for serum sodium and, hence, anion gap because the flame photometer apparatus may fail to aspirate a proper aliquot of hyperviscous serum.

Because bromide reacts very strongly with most reagents utilized to measure chloride, artifactually high values for serum chloride concentration are frequently seen in bromide-intoxicated patients. Indeed, this laboratory error may be sufficient to actually produce a negative anion gap.

Iodine, another halogen capable of accumulating in the serum, also can cause an artificial increase in serum chloride concentration and hence a decrease in the anion gap. Overestimation of serum chloride concentration also can occur in the presence of hyperlipidemia because lipids scatter light in such a way as to falsely elevate the concentration of chloride when determined by the colorimetric method.

Ratio of Change of Anion Gap to Change in Plasma Bicarbonate

In uncomplicated increased anion gap metabolic acidosis, the decrease (change) in plasma bicarbonate should be roughly equal to the increase (change) in the anion gap (that is, $dAG/dHCO_3 = 1.0$).

Whenever the anion gap changes much more or less than the bicarbonate, one should be suspicious of a coexisting or a mixed acid-base disorder. For example, in classical diabetic ketoacidosis (DKA) and lactic acidosis, the rise in anion gap is similar, quantitatively, to the decrease in HCO_3. The ratio of their changes, therefore, is close to 1.0. Since excretion of the keto anions tends to reduce the anion gap while not directly affecting the HCO_3, some patients with DKA, whose keto anion excretion is greater than usual, may have metabolic acidosis that is substantially or even entirely of the hyperchloremic variety. The hyperchloremic acidosis so frequently observed during the treatment of DKA is also believed to be largely explainable on the same basis. In a pure hyperchloremic metabolic acidosis, the ratio is close to 0. Ratios between 0.3 and 0.7 usually, but not always, indicate a mixed acid-base disorder or a preexisting low anion gap.

In renal failure, there is no cause-and-effect relationship between the rise in anion gap and fall in the HCO_3, since the latter is related largely to a failure of ammonia genesis, whereas the former is related to the reduction in the glomerular filtration rate (GRF), leading to anion retention. Thus, reciprocal stoichiometry between the anion gap and HCO_3 should not be expected. Even in end-stage chronic renal failure, the anion gap rarely exceeds 23 mEq/L. Indeed, in patients with mild to moderate chronic renal failure (serum creatinine concentration between 2 and 4 mg/dL), the anion gap is usually normal. In patients with more severe chronic renal failure, the anion gap averages about 16 mEq/L with an average $dAG/dHCO_3$ of only 0.4.

Thus, the $dAG/dHCO_3$ ratio is helpful in the diagnosis of mixed acid-base disorder because this ratio is usually close to 1.0 in typical organic acidoses. Values greater than 1.2 or less than 0.8 suggest the presence of a mixed acid-base disorder or an independent factor affecting the anion gap.

Urinary Anion Gap

Calculation of the urinary anion gap allows one to determine if NH_4 production is adequate or appropriate in patients with an acidemia. According to Hilton et al., the urinary anion gap (in mEq/L), which is determined by the difference between the UA and UC, equals Na + K − Cl. The value of potassium is included in the formula because, unlike the plasma potassium concentration, its concentration in urine is large and highly variable. The value for bicarbonate is not included because it is not easily measured in most clinical laboratories. At a urine pH of 6.8, the HCO_3 will generally be less than 10 mEq/L. Furthermore, if urine is more acidic (pH < 6.4), the HCO_3 concentration will be trivial.

The major ionic species in bicarbonate-free urine are

$$Na + K + Ca + Mg + NH_4 = H_2PO_4 + SO_4 + OA$$

Table 8-8. Average Daily Urinary Excretion of Cations and Anions in Four Normal Subjects on a Normal Diet*

Cations	mEq/day	Anion	mEq/day
Na	127 ± 6	Cl	135 ± 5
K	49 ± 2	SO_4	34 ± 1
Ca	4 ± 1	H_2PO_4	20 ± 1
Mg	11 ± 1	Organic anions	29 ± 1
NH_4	28 ± 2		
Total	219 ± 3		218 ± 6

* Values are shown as mean ± SE; modified by Goldstein et al.

$$\text{Urine AG} = (N + K) - Cl = (127 + 49) - 135 = 41$$

or

$$NH_4 = (N + K) - (Cl + 13) = (127 + 49) - (135 + 13) = 176 - 148 = 28 \text{ mEq}$$

where OA = organic anion. Excretion of phosphate, sulfate, and organic anions does not generally change importantly when acid-base status is modified. The normal mean anion gap in a 24-h collection of urine from a patient on a normal diet is approximately 40 mEq (Table 8-8).

In an acidemic patient with an acidic urine, a markedly negative anion gap (i.e., Cl much greater than the sum of Na + K) indicates a high (appropriate) level of ammonium ion (NH_4^+). On the other hand, finding a positive urine anion gap (Cl less than the sum of Na + K) in an acidemic patient suggests that NH_4 is inappropriately low.

Currently, it appears that the clinical use of urinary anion gap involves (1) the differential diagnosis (renal versus extrarenal origin) of hyperchloremic metabolic acidosis by providing an estimate of urinary ammonium levels and (2) assessment of the cause of renal potassium wasting by providing a clue to the excretion of large amounts of nonresorbable anion resulting in a kaliuresis (Table 8-8). Examples of nonresorable anions in an acid urine include carbenicillin, salicylate, and keto anions. Since most clinical laboratories cannot provide a measurement of urinary NH_4, the urinary anion gap can, in a sense, provide the clinician with a "poor man's" NH_4 measurement.

In general, when the cause of hyperchloremic metabolic acidosis is extrarenal, the normal kidney responds by markedly increasing the excretion of NH_4. In contrast, NH_4 excretion will be low (less than 40 to 80 mmol/day) in distal renal-tubular acidosis (RTA) or with decreased ammonia availability to the collecting tubule.

If the urinary anion gap is markedly negative (i.e., high NH_4 content), the differential diagnosis of a hyperchloremic metabolic acidosis includes (1) gastrointestinal alkali loss (e.g., secretory diarrhea), (2) proximal RTA with an acidic urine, (3) administration of extra chloride, and (4) high anion gap metabolic acidosis masquerading as hyperchloremic metabolic acidosis or renal origin (e.g., patients with hypoalbuminemia, halide poisoning, etc.) (Table 8-9).

If the urinary anion gap is positive or has a small negative value (e.g., representing a low rate of NH_4 excretion) in a patient with hyperchloremic metabolic acidosis, the different diagnosis includes

Table 8-9. Diagnostic Value of Urinary Anion Gap (Na + K − Cl) in an Acid urine (pH < 6.4)

Highly negative urine anion gap (high NH_4)
GI alkali loss
Proximal RTA
Increased Cl intake
Hypoalbuminemia
Halide ingestion
Positive or slightly negative urine anion gap (low NH_4)
Distal RTA
Decreased NH_4 production
Ketonuria
Highly positive urine anion gap (very low NH_4)
Organic aciduria

(1) distal RTA, (2) reduced NH_4 production, and (3) acid gain plus urinary excretion of the conjugate base (e.g., ketoanionuria). If ammonium excretion is very low, urinary pH may be low (i.e., high in free H^+) even if the rate of distal tubular H^+ secretion is subnormal.

If NH_4 is expressed per milligram of creatinine (and factored for an average creatinine excretion of 20 mg/kg per day), one can estimate the 24-h NH_4 excretion from data obtained from a random specimen.

Thus, the urinary anion gap appears to be helpful in the differential diagnosis of hyperchloremic metabolic acidosis by providing an estimation of urinary ammonium levels. Highly negative values for the urinary anion gap suggest exogenous or endogenous acid loads or an extrarenal loss of alkali. Positive values are seen in patients with impaired renal ammonium excretion.

Venous Studies

In critically ill patients with a puzzling acid-base picture or poor response to therapy, one should also analyze venous pH, P_{CO_2}, and bicarbonate. If, for some reason, it is difficult to obtain arterial blood or if a percutaneous sample is obtained and it is not clear whether the sample is arterial or venous, central venous blood from a subclavian or pulmonary artery catheter can be used to advantage. In patients with a normal cardiac output, arterial values can usually be obtained by adding 0.05 to the central venous pH, by subtracting 6 or 7 torr from the venous P_{CO_2}, and subtracting 1.1 mEq/L from the venous bicarbonate. However, during shock or severe heart failure, the differences between the arterial and mixed venous values may be much greater.

METABOLIC ACIDOSIS

Etiology

The causes of metabolic acidosis can be divided into two main groups: (1) those associated with increased production of organic acids (increased anion gap metabolic acidosis) and (2) those associated with a loss of bicarbonate or addition of chloride (normal anion gap metabolic acidosis).

Increased Anion Gap Metabolic Acidosis

The most frequent causes of increased production of organic acids and an increased anion gap metabolic acidosis are lactic acidosis, ketoacidosis, uremia, and drug intoxication (especially methanol, ethanol, ethylene glycol, and salicylates). Ketoacidosis may be diabetic, starvation, or alcoholic (nondiabetic) in origin (Table 8-10).

The most frequent cause of an organic acidosis in critically ill or injured patients, especially those with impaired blood flow or sepsis, is lactic acidosis. The causes of lactic acidosis in turn can be divided into those associated with poor tissue oxygenation (type A) and those with normal oxygenation (type B) (Table 8-6).

Table 8-10. Causes of High Anion Gap Metabolic Acidosis

Lactic acidosis
Type A—decrease in tissue oxygenation
Type B—no decrease in tissue oxygenation
Renal failure
Acute
Chronic
Ketoacidosis
Diabetes
Alcholism
Prolonged starvation (mild acidosis)
High-fat diet (mild acidosis)
Ingestion of Toxic Substances
Elevated osmolar gap
Methanol
Ethylene glycol
Normal osmolar gap
Salicylate
Paraldehyde

Table 8-11. Causes of Normal Anion Gap Metabolic Acidosis

With a tendency to hyperkalemia	With a tendency to hypokalemia
Subsiding DKA	Renal tubular acidosis—type I (classical distal acidosis)
Early uremic acidosis	Renal tubular acidosis—type II (proximal acidosis)
Early obstructive uropathy	Acetazolamide
Renal tubular acidosis—type IV	Acute diarrhea with losses of HCO_3 and K^+
Hypoaldosteronism (Addison's disease)	Ureterosigmoidostomy with increased resorption of H^+ and Cl^- and losses of HCO_3^- and K^+
Infusion or ingestion of HCl, NH_4Cl, lysine-HCl, or arginine-HCl	Obstruction of artificial ileal bladder
Potassium-sparing diuretics	Dilution acidosis

The immediate precursor of lactic acid is pyruvic acid. This 3-carbon acid may be transformed into fat or amino acids, or it may be transported into mitochrondria, where it is incorporated into the Krebs cycle after being oxidized to acetyl-CoA. Liver and kidney cortex contain enzymes that catalyze the conversion of pyruvate back to glucose (i.e., cause gluconeogenesis).

Lactate acid, in sharp contrast to its immediate precursor, pyruvic acid, represents a metabolic dead end. Its only means of metabolic transformation is via the lactate dehydrogenase (LDH) reaction, which regenerates pyruvate and converts nicotine adenine dinucleotide (NAD) to its reduced form (NADH).

An important cause of lactic acidosis is thiamine deficiency, particularly in patients with a heavy alcoholic intake. The severity of the lactic acidosis in some of these individuals, who have usually stopped drinking 1 to 5 days earlier, has caused this problem to be referred to as acute pernicious or fulminating beriberi. A similar problem can occur with TPN if inadequate thiamine is given with large amounts of glucose.

Normal Anion Gap (Hyperchloremic) Metabolic Acidosis

The most frequent causes of bicarbonate loss resulting in normal anion gap (hyperchloremic) metabolic acidosis include severe diarrhea, pancreatic fistulas, RTA, adrenal insufficiency, and therapy with carbonic anhydrase inhibitors, ammonium chloride, arginine hydrochloride, or amino acid hydrochlorides (as in TPN). The causes of normal anion gap metabolic acidosis can be further divided into those with normal or high serum potassium levels and those with hypokalemia (Table 8-11).

There are three main types of RTA: RTA I, RTA II, and RTA IV. RTA I involves failure of the distal renal tubules to excrete acid properly and RTA-II involves bicarbonate wasting in the proximal renal tubules. Both RTA I and RTA II tend to cause a normal anion gap metabolic acidosis with hypokalemia. RTA IV usually causes hyperkalemia.

Pathophysiology

Compensatory Changes

Any increase in the quantity of hydrogen ions in the bloodstream almost immediately results in an increase in alveolar ventilation. As a general rule, each mEq/L fall in bicarbonate tends to cause a relatively rapid 1.0- to 1.4-mmHg fall in the P_{CO_2}. Thus, if the bicarbonate falls to 14 mEq/L, the P_{CO_2} would be expected to fall to about 26 to 30 mmHg. If the fall in P_{CO_2} is less than 1.0 mmHg per mEq fall in bicarbonate, respiratory compensation is inadequate or abnormal. Further compensation is provided during the next several days by increased renal excretion of acid.

Muscle Function

In general, mild to moderate acidosis can increase the strength of muscular contraction. This is known as the *staircase phenomenon,* or *treppe,* in which a muscle which is rapidly and repetitively stimulated progressively increases its strength of contraction. However, a pH of less than 7.10 to 7.15 tends to impair muscular and cardiovascular function. Furthermore, if the bicarbonate is less than 5.0 mEq/L, any further reduction in bicarbonate can markedly reduce pH.

Catecholamines and Vascular Reactivity

Acidosis increases the secretion of catecholamines. However, if the acidosis is very severe (pH < 7.00 to 7.10), it decreases the end-organ response to the catecholamines. Severe acidosis tends to cause systemic arterial vasodilation and venous constriction, increasing the tendency to capillary stasis. Severe acidosis also tends to cause pulmonary vasoconstriction with increased strain on the right heart. β-Adrenergic receptors are particularly prone to develop rapid desensitization and uncoupling in the presence of severe lactic acidosis.

Oxygen Delivery and Availability

Oxygen delivery to tissues is affected differently by acute and chronic metabolic acidosis. Acute acidosis shifts the oxyhemoglobin dissociation curve to the right, thereby reducing the affinity of hemoglobin for oxygen and facilitating oxygen delivery to tissues. However, acidosis for more than 12 to 36 h results in impaired erythrocyte glycolysis, reducing the intraerythrocytic concentration of 2,3-diphosphoglyceric acid (2,3-DPG), which shifts the oxyhemoglobin dissociation curve to the left, reducing the release of oxygen from hemoglobin into plasma for use by the tissues. Chronic acidosis may also make red blood cells more rigid, thereby reducing their flow through nutrient capillaries. Consequently, one should not assume that a 90 to 95 percent arterial oxyhemoglobin saturation indicates that adequate oxygen is available to the tissues.

Diagnosis

The diagnosis of metabolic acidosis is usually based on a low pH with low bicarbonate levels. Calculation of the anion gap can help determine the cause of the metabolic acidosis. Severe metabolic acidosis, regardless of its origin, tends to cause nausea, vomiting, abdominal distress, and varying degrees of CNS dysfunction.

Increased Anion Gap Metabolic Acidosis

The mnemonic "muksleep" is used by some students to remember the first letters of some of the more common causes of increased anion gap metabolic acidosis: methanol, uremia, ketoacidosis, salicylates, lactate, ethanol, ethylene glycol, and paraldehyde. Patients being seen in the emergency department can have any one of these problems. However, if the problem develops in the hospital, toxic drug ingestions are much less likely. Another mnemonic used is "mudpiles," where "i" represents iron or isoniazid. Other causes of increased anion gap include toluene, carbon monoxide, and cyanide.

Lactic Acidosis

In type A lactic acidosis, there is poor tissue oxygenation and perfusion. In type B, however, there is no evidence of decreased tissue perfusion, and the mechanism of the acidosis is unknown.

Patients with lactic acidosis may present with nonspecific findings of nausea, vomiting, restlessness, Kussmaul respirations, and stupor or coma. The serum lactic acid level (as lactate) is elevated. Other laboratory abnormalities include hyperuricemia, hyperphosphatemia, and leukocytosis.

It is generally assumed that the development of metabolic acidosis during sepsis is secondary to lactic acidosis. However, Rackow et al. assessed the composition of the anion gap during severe sepsis induced by cecal perforation in rats. They found that the lactate concentration in the septic animals was 2.2 ± 0.3 mEq/L as compared to 0.9 ± 0.2 mEq/L in the controls ($P < .001$). Only 15 percent of the increase in the anion gap in septic animals could be accounted for by increases in lactate concentration. The other measured metabolic intermediates (such as pyruvate, citrate, β-hydroxybutyrate, acetoacetate, anionic amino acids, or albumin) also could not account for the anion gap metabolic acidosis.

An increase in unmeasured strong acids in sepsis could arise from several etiologies, including renal failure and ketoacidosis. Various organic and inorganic anions from skeletal muscle can be released as a result of septic proteolysis. Elevated purine nucleotide degradation products include uric acid and free fatty acids.

Ketoacidosis

Ketoacidosis can be caused by either an increase in the free fatty acid load to the liver or an increased conversion of free fatty acids to keto acids. The increased free fatty acid load may be due to increased catecholamine-induced lipolysis caused by stress or, occasionally, to a high-fat diet. Increased conversion of fatty acids to keto acids may occur in diabetic ketoacidosis, in alcoholism, and, to a lesser degree, in prolonged starvation or a high-fat diet.

The most common keto acid formed is β-hydroxybutyrate, followed by acetoacetate and hydroxybutyric acid. The nitroprusside test is commonly used to document the presence of ketones in serum and urine. This test is positive with increased levels of acetoacetate or acetone, but not with β-hydroxybutyric acid. The more acidotic the patient is, the more β-hydroxybutyric acid is formed from acetoacetate. Therefore, the test may reveal little or none of the ketoacidosis present in a severely acidotic patient.

Diabetic Ketoacidosis (DKA)

The patient with DKA is usually an insulin-dependent diabetic who is out of control and has developed polydipsia, polyuria, and polyphagia. On physical examination, the patient tends to be hyperventilating, with acetone breath and an altered mental status. The laboratory definition of DKA is a serum glucose level greater than 300 mg/dL (16.7 mmol/L), increased serum ketones, and a pH less than 7.30.

One should not assume that ketones are absent or only minimally present if the nitroprusside test is negative or only weakly positive in patients with severe acidosis. In ketoacidosis, the retained keto anions are β-hydroxybutyrate and acetoacetate and the usual ratio of β-hydroxybutyrate to acetoacetate is 3:1 to 4:1. With increasing acidosis, the amount of β-hydroxybutyrate increases and the amount of acetoacetate decreases. Since only acetoacetate reacts with nitroprusside (the key reagent to Acetest tablets and Ketostix), the severity of the ketosis may be underestimated. This occurs typically in patients suffering concomitantly from tissue hypoxia and/or lactic acidosis.

Other laboratory findings in DKA may include leukocytosis and an increased serum osmolality and osmolal gap. Serum sodium is often low secondary to hyperglycemia. Serum potassium is often elevated due to the acidosis, in spite of total body potassium deficits of up to 10 mEq/kg of body weight.

Although elevated glucose levels are considered characteristic of DKA, they can be deceptive. Modestly elevated serum glucose levels, 150 to 250 mg/dL, can occur in alcoholic ketoacidosis and salicylate intoxication. Conversely, hypoglycemia should suggest alcoholic ketoacidosis because serum glucose levels are lower than 50 mg/dL in about 13 percent of patients with this disorder. Ketonuria may also be helpful. It occurs in almost all cases of DKA, it is common in alcoholic ketoacidosis, and it occurs in approximately 25 percent of patients with salicylate intoxication.

Depending upon the amount of hydration and ability of the kidneys to excrete the increased keto acids in the blood, there may be a wide spectrum of acid-base patterns in DKA, ranging from pure high anion gap metabolic acidosis to pure normal anion gap (hyperchloremic) metabolic acidosis. Severe dehydration tends to result in increased retention of ketones and an increased anion gap. After 4 to 8 h of therapy with saline solution, many patients will develop a hyperchloremic acidosis because of retention of chloride in excess of sodium and because of excretion of ketones by the kidneys.

Alcoholic Ketoacidosis

Except for alcohol, the patient has generally fasted for at least 24 to 36 h. Patients tend to be dehydrated and malnourished, with epigastric pain, ethanol odor, and altered mental status. The increased anion gap is usually due to β-hydroxybutyrate. Laboratory studies usually reveal ketones, high normal or low glucose levels, elevated amylase levels, and hyperuricemia. A variable ethanol level may be present.

Starvation Ketosis

The patient has a history of starvation and is usually cachectic, hypoglycemic, and ketotic. There is accelerated gluconeogenesis with depletion of liver glycogen stores, hypoinsulinemia, and lipolysis. In prolonged starvation (4 to 6 weeks), ketogenesis serves to supply ketones for the brain.

High-Fat Diets

A diet with a high fat content may cause a mildly elevated anion gap due to ketosis from increased β oxidation of free fatty acids in the liver.

Renal Failure

In acute renal failure, the GFR is decreased. As a consequence, organic acids, phosphates, and sulfates (from endogenous metabolism) are retained, producing a metabolic acidosis with a high anion gap. In chronic renal failure, ammonia excretion is diminished, causing a further increase in anions. The anion gap in uremic acidosis is usually less than 24 mEq/L, and there is a poor correlation between the change in anion gap and the change in HCO_3.

Severe muscle damage may greatly increase the tendency to renal failure. The resulting myoglobinuric renal failure can produce a severe metabolic acidosis with a strikingly increased anion gap level. At least part of this acidosis is caused by the metabolism of large amounts of the sulfur-containing amino acids released from myoglobin.

Toxic Ingestions

Whenever one sees a patient with a metabolic acidosis of unknown etiology, the anion and osmolar gaps should be evaluated. Methanol ethylene glycol, salicylate, and paraldehyde poisoning can cause metabolic acidosis with a high anion gap. Ethylene glycol and methanol can also cause an increased osmolar gap.

Methanol

Methanol, also known as wood alcohol, is a clear liquid found in solvents, shellacs, and varnishes. It is sometimes ingested by alcoholics as a substitute for ethanol. The usual lethal dose is 30 mL of absolute methanol, but deaths have been reported after ingestion of as little as 6 mL. Peak methanol levels develop 30 to 60 min after ingestion, but there is usually a 12- to 24-h latent period before symptoms start. Classically, the patient describes cloudy, blurred, or misty vision. The person may see yellow spots or develop a central scotoma or blindness, which may or may not be reversible. These symptoms are caused by formaldehyde, a metabolite of methanol. Other symptoms include nausea, vomiting, weakness, epigastric pain, headache, dizziness, and CNS depression. Examination of the eyes may disclose optic disk hyperemia, edema, and decreased pupillary reaction to light.

Laboratory studies reveal metabolic acidosis with a high anion gap and an elevated osmolar gap. The high anion gap is caused mainly by formic acid, a metabolite of methanol.

Ethylene Glycol

This odorless substance is present in antifreeze, hydraulic brake fluid, cellophane softeners, and solvents for paints and plastics. The minimal lethal dose is 1.0 to 1.5 mL/kg. Peak ethylene glycol levels are reached after 1 to 4 h, but toxic manifestations are delayed 4 to 12 h. The three stages of toxicity are (1) CNS injury (during the first 12 h), (2) respiratory depression and cardiopulmonary failure (at 12 to 24 h), and (3) renal failure (at 24 to 72 h). The toxic effects of ethylene glycol poisoning are produced by metabolites of ethylene glycol, including glycoaldehydes, glycolic acid, glyoxylic acid, and oxalate. Glycolic acid and lactic acid are responsible for the high anion gap. Oxalate is the primary factor in renal toxicity.

The diagnosis of ethylene glycol poisoning is supported by a urine sediment with calcium oxalate crystals. The maximum production of oxalate occurs 8 h after ingestion, so there may be no crystalluria if the the patient presents earlier.

Other laboratory findings include hypocalcemia, leukocytosis, and an elevated osmolal gap that is caused by the serum concentration of ethylene glycol. The osmolal gap may be normal if it is measured many hours after ingestion when ethylene glycol is no longer present in the serum.

Salicylates

The usual toxic dose of salicylates is 200 to 300 mg/kg, with blood levels of 160 to 500 mg/dL reported as potentially lethal. Peak levels occur 2 to 4 h after ingestion of most preparations.

The first manifestations of salicylate poisoning include tinnitus and hearing impairment. These symptoms occur at an average adult dose of 4.5 g/day. In mild toxicity, there might also be vomiting 3 to 8 h after ingestion. In moderate toxicity, symptoms include severe hyperpnea and marked lethargy or excitability. Severe toxicity is frequently manifested by coma and seizures.

Salicylates directly stimulate the respiratory center, causing respiratory alkalosis. Later an increased metabolic rate with the production of more carbon dioxide may result in respiratory acidosis. Eventually the direct toxic effect on carbohydrate metabolism produces the classic high anion gap metabolic acidosis.

Paraldehyde

This sedative and antiseizure medication is rarely used now. The average minimal lethal blood level is approximately 500 μg/mL. Manifestations of toxicity include gastritis, renal failure, fatty changes in the liver, pulmonary hemorrhages, edema, and congestive failure. These patients have a characteristic offensive odor, mild to moderate dehydration, hypotension, and Kussmaul respirations.

The elevated anion gap is caused by acetic acid and chloracetic acid. Diagnosis is made by detection of paraldehyde in the serum and acetaldehyde in the urine and blood. When a nitroprusside reaction test is used, paralydehyde may cause a false-positive reaction for ketones, called "pseudoketosis."

Other Substances

Severe intoxication with lithium or magnesium reduces the anion gap by increasing unmeasured cations.

Rapid Laboratory Evaluation of Patients with High Anion Gap Metabolic Acidosis

A urine dipstick test that is positive for both ketones and glucose rapidly confirms DKA. If the test is negative for glucose, alcoholic or starvation ketoacidosis should be considered.

If there is a history of paraldehyde ingestion, and/or the urine contains acetaldehyde, paraldehyde poisoning is possible, and the finding of ketonuria may represent a false-positive reaction. A history of starvation and alcoholism suggests alcoholic ketoacidosis.

If the urine dipstick test is negative for ketones, the serum osmolality should be tested to determine whether there is an elevated osmolar gap. Causes of a high osmolar gap include ethylene glycol and methanol poisoning and DKA. If calcium oxalate crystals are found in the urine, ethylene glycol poisoning should be suspected. If there is a history of visual impairment or an abnormal funduscopic examination, methanol poisoning is the most likely cause.

When the osmolar gap is normal, the urine should be tested with ferric chloride. If a purple color develops, salicylate poisoning should be considered, although it is important to remember that the test is very sensitive. Renal failure is diagnosed when BUN and creatinine are elevated. Lactic acidosis is confirmed by an elevated lactic acid level.

If there is no renal failure or drug intoxication, an increased anion gap is usually due to ketoacidosis or lactate accumulation. In patients without uremia, drug intoxication, or DKA, an increased anion gap is usually due to lactate accumulation.

An anion gap of 30 mEq/L or more usually indicates an organic (lactic or keto) acidosis, even in the presence of uremia. With anion gaps of 20 to 29 mEq/L, 60 to 75 percent of patients will have an organic acidosis. Of those with no identified organic acidosis, changes in total proteins, phosphate, potassium, or calcium will account for about 50 percent of the increased anion gap. The etiology of the other 50 percent of the anion gap is usually apparent.

According to Gabow et al., if the anion gap exceeds 0.5 times the serum bicarbonate concentration plus 16.0, the diagnosis of an organic acidosis is justified. Thus, a patient with a HCO_3 of 6 mEq/L and an anion gap of 22 mEq/L probably has an organic acidosis, because the Gabow factor is 19 [$(HCO_3 \times 0.5) + 16 = (6 \times 0.5) + 16 = 3 + 16 = 19$], which is less than the anion gap of 22. On the other hand, if the HCO_3 is 18 mEq/L, the Gabow factor is $(18 \times 0.5) + 16 = 9 + 16 = 25$ and the cause of the anion gap is probably not an organic acidosis.

Normal Anion Gap Metabolic Acidosis

Normal anion gap metabolic acidosis is caused primarily by a loss of bicarbonate with little or no increase in organic acids. A mnemonic for the possible causes of normal anion gap metabolic acidosis is "used carp": *u*reteroenterostomy, *s*mall bowel fistulas, *e*xtra chloride (such as in NH_4Cl or amino acid hydrochlorides), *d*iarrhea, *c*arbonic anhydrase inhibitors (Diamox and Sulfamylon), *a*drenal insufficiency, *r*enal tubular acidosis, *p*ancreatic fistula. These and other causes of normal anion gap metabolic acidosis can be subdivided into those tending to cause hyperkalemia and those causing hypokalemia (Table 8-11).

In most of these problems, a careful history and routine laboratory studies should clarify the cause.

Treatment

The treatment of metabolic acidosis should be directed at (1) improvement of tissue perfusion and ventilation, (2) correction of the underlying problem, and (3) administration of sodium bicarbonate if needed.

Improved Tissue Perfusion and Ventilation

Almost every type of metabolic acidosis will be improved by restoration of an adequate or increased blood volume, cardiac output, and tissue oxygenation. If there is any problem with ventilation, so that the respiratory compensation is inadequate, early ventilatory assistance should be strongly considered.

Correction of the Primary Process

As the patient is being resuscitated, a strong effort should be made to determine the primary process causing the metabolic acidosis and correct it. An adequate resuscitation should correct any shock, but inotropic may occasionally be required. Sepsis may require eradication of the focus of infection plus antibiotics. For DKA, insulin and later glucose and potassium will be needed.

Treatment of toxic ingestions may require specific therapy. The treatment of severe methanol poisoning is administration of enteral or parenteral ethanol, because alcohol dehydrogenase (the enzyme that metabolizes ethanol, ethylene glycol, and methanol) has a significantly greater affinity for ethanol than for the other alcohols. Ethanol levels should be maintained at approximately 100 mg/dL. Hemodialysis is often required if the methanol blood concentration is greater than 50 mg/dL.

Ethylene glycol poisoning is treated with supportive measures (e.g., respiratory support) and administration of ethanol. If ethylene glycol levels exceed 50 mg/dL, or if renal failure is present, hemodialysis is indicated. Some authors also recommend thiamine, 100 mg IM, and pyridoxine, 100 mg IV or IM.

Therapy for salicylate poisoning consists initially of emesis with syrup of ipecac or, in a comatose patient, lavage coupled with activated charcoal. Salicylate excretion may be enhanced through alkalinization of the urine with or without concomitant diuresis. For severe poisoning (salicylate level greater than 100 mg/dL), hemodialysis is indicated.

Treatment of paraldehyde poisoning includes lavage, activated charcoal, and supportive measures. Emesis should not be promoted, since paralydehyde is locally corrosive to the gastrointestinal tract and is rapidly absorbed.

Bicarbonate Therapy

If a severe metabolic acidosis persists after maximal efforts to improve tissue perfusion with fluid, inotropes, and vasodilators as needed, sodium bicarbonate therapy to raise the pH from less than 7.10 to at least 7.25 should be considered. Sodium bicarbonate should probably also be given if the arterial bicarbonate falls below 5.0 mEq/L because any additional decrease in bicarbonate could cause a precipitous fall in pH.

The amount of bicarbonate given should not exceed 1.0 mEq/kg at a time so as to prevent alkaline overshoot. For each 0.1 rise in pH, oxygen availability to tissue drops by about 10 percent because of the shift of the oxyhemoglobin dissociation curve to the left. Giving bicarbonate to patients with hypoxemia due to a pulmonary or right-to-left heart shunt may rapidly lower the arterial P_{O_2} to dangerous levels. In patients with severe DKA, rapid bicarbonate administration can cause severe CNS changes.

Bicarbonate deficits are usually calculated using 30 to 50 percent of the body weight as the bicarbonate space. In patients with acute mild bicarbonate deficits of less than 10 mEq/L, calculations using 30 percent of the body weight as the bicarbonate space seem to provide adequate correction. For moderate bicarbonate deficits of 10 to 15 mEq/L, 40 percent of the body weight can be used as the bicarbonate space. However, in patients with severe acidosis with base deficits exceeding 15 mEq/L, the bicarbonate space involves almost the entire total body water and should be considered to be equal to 50 percent of the body weight.

Thus, in an acutely ill 80-kg man with a bicarbonate concentration of 10 mEq/L (i.e., a deficit of 14 mEq/L), one can assume a bicarbonate space of 40 percent, or 32 L. As a consequence, he would have a total bicarbonate deficit of $80 \text{ kg} \times 40) \times 14 = 448$ mEq. However, only about 1.0 mEq/kg is administered at a time, over 30 to 60 min. If the patient were hemodynamically unstable, more rapid infusion of bicarbonate might be desirable.

The American Heart Association now urges restraint in the use of sodium bicarbonate during cardiopulmonary resuscitation. Experimentally, HCO_3^- administered to correct severe hypoxic lactic acidosis actually increases lactate production. Part of the difficulty may be related to the fact that carbon dioxide (elaborated by the reaction of H^+ and HCO_3) diffuses rapidly across cell membranes, creating intracellular acidosis even while the extracellular acidosis is decreased.

Bicarbonate can also cause a paradoxical cerebral acidosis. The increased CO_2 generated by the bicarbonate readily crosses the blood-brain barrier while the bicarbonate crosses the blood-brain barrier very slowly. The increased cerebrospinal fluid CO_2 generates carbonic acid which causes cerebrospinal fluid acidosis in spite of an increasing alkalemia.

METABOLIC ALKALOSIS

Etiology

The two most frequent causes of metabolic alkalosis are excessive diuresis (with loss of potassium, hydrogen, and chloride) and excessive loss of gastric secretions (with loss of hydrogen and chloride).

Loss of Gastric Acid

Normally the stomach makes 2 to 5 mEq of free acid per hour. This may be increased two- to fourfold in patients with an active duodenal ulcer. Thus, a patient who is vomiting large amounts of acid due to pyloric stenosis from duodenal ulcer disease is particularly apt to develop a severe metabolic alkalosis. Removal of large amounts of gastric acid with a nasogastric tube may also produce the same effect.

Excessive Diuresis

Hypokalemia due to diuresis with excessive loss of potassium in the urine is probably the most common cause of metabolic alkalosis. Since potassium loss in urine averages 30 to 60 mEq/L, use of diuretics can easily produce a severe hypokalemia along with an excessive loss of chloride. Potassium will tend to come out of tissue cells to correct the hypokalemia, and hydrogen ions will tend to go back into the cells, causing an alkalemia. In addition, the kidney will tend to excrete hydrogen ions to conserve potassium. Diarrhea or excessive colostomy or ileostomy drainage may contain more than 25 to 50 mEq of potassium per liter and may also cause severe hypokalemia.

Mineralocorticoids

Mineralocorticoids tend to cause metabolic alkalosis by promoting the renal absorption of bicarbonate and sodium and by increasing the excretion of potassium, hydrogen, and chloride ions. Hypokalemia can produce a vicious cycle because the depletion of potassium causes even more excretion of hydrogen ions, aggravating the metabolic alkalosis. Reabsorption of potassium appears to be independent of aldosterone, but an aldosterone deficiency markedly reduces the ability of the distal tubule to secrete hydrogen ion and reabsorb bicarbonate.

Increased Intake of Citrate or Lactate

Patients receiving massive blood transfusions and large amounts of Ringer's lactate will tend to become alkalotic over the next 12 to 48 h. Massive transfusions of bank blood can greatly increase the quantity of citrate in the body (17 mEq from each unit of whole blood and 5 mEq from each unit of packed red blood cells). As this citrate is metabolized over the next 24 to 48 h, plasma bicarbonate levels rise proportionally, producing an increasing alkalosis. Ringer's lactate has a pH of about 5.5. However, after it is given, about half of it (L-lactate) is metabolized in the liver into bicarbonate, which tends to cause a metabolic alkalosis. The D-lactate is excreted in the urine.

Antacids

Clinicians often attempt to prevent stress gastric ulceration and bleeding in critically ill patients by maintaining a pH inside the stomach of 5.0 or higher with antacid and/or H_2-receptor antagonists, such as cimetidine. In some instances, large quantities of antacid are required. Absorption of these antacids and/or removal of the excess acid that they neutralize may significantly contribute to alkalosis.

Dehydration

One should not attempt to correct a severe metabolic alkalosis without first correcting any coexistent dehydration. Dehydration which it not severe enough to interfere with tissue perfusion may cause a "contraction alkalosis" because sodium and bicarbonate absorption in the kidney is increased. However, if the extracellular fluid is expanded, sodium and bicarbonate reabsorption in the kidney is reduced, and this may cause a "dilution acidosis."

Since the kidney is the organ responsible for excreting excess bicarbonate when the concentration is abnormally high, renal failure may make it very difficult to eliminate bicarbonate. However, if the renal failure is mild to moderate, the ability to excrete bicarbonate is still relatively well preserved.

Excretion of Nonresorbable Anions

The various penicillins when excreted into the tubular lumen have a negative charge and are not resorbed. This causes an increased loss of hydrogen ions in the urine. Increased excretion of phosphates may cause a similar problem.

Hypercapnia

After a period of respiratory acidosis, a compensatory rise in bicarbonate will tend to occur until the arterial pH is about 7.35. For example, with a chronic P_{CO_2} of 60 to 70 mmHg, the arterial bicarbonate will tend to rise to levels of 32 to 37 mEq/L, respectively. Even after the hypercapnia is corrected, bicarbonate levels may remain elevated for some time.

Severe Hypoproteinemia

To maintain electrical neutrality, a fall in serum proteins, especially albumin, will tend to cause a rise in bicarbonate. A fall in albumin levels from 4.5 to 1.5 g/dL can cause serum bicarbonate levels to rise by up to 9.6 mEq/L.

Other Problems

Other situations that tend to maintain high serum bicarbonate concentrations include hypokalemia and hypochloremia. Chloride deficiency is often listed as a cause of persistently high plasma bicarbonate levels, but chloride deficiency will only raise the renal bicarbonate threshold if it is accompanied by a reduced effective arterial volume. Resistant metabolic alkalosis may also be seen with secondary hypoparathyroidism (such as with milk alkali syndrome or malignancy-induced hypercalcemia).

Physiologic Effects

Although alkalosis tends to inhibit sympathetic nervous system activity and decrease adrenergic effects, it also tends to increase endogenous catecholamine release and accentuate adrenergic vasodilator effects.

Metabolic alkalosis reduces the amount of potassium in the blood by about 0.5 mEq/L for each 0.10 rise in pH. Ionized calcium and magnesium levels in the plasma also fall, about 4 to 8 percent for each 0.1 rise in pH. This tends to increase neuromuscular irritability and may impair cardiovascular function, particularly if the plasma ionized calcium levels fall below 1.6 to 1.7 mEq/L. The alkalosis also reduces oxygen availability by about 10 percent for each 0.1 rise in pH. Alkalosis may also cause tachyarrhythmias, probably due to potassium and/or calcium changes. The hypokalemia which develops secondary to an alkalosis may also interfere with muscle function, causing weakness and/or ileus.

Failure to compensate adequately for a metabolic alkalosis may be the first indication of an occult hypoxemia. The usual pulmonary compensation for a metabolic alkalosis is hypoventilation with slow, shallow breathing. As the P_{CO_2} rises because of hypoventilation, the

P_{O_2} falls, but the chemoreceptors will usually not allow the arterial P_{O_2} to fall much below 60 mmHg. Thus, the arterial P_{CO_2} will not usually rise above 50 to 55 mmHg unless the associated hypoxemia is prevented by giving oxygen.

One should probably not allow a patient to remain severely alkalotic, even if the patient appears to be doing well otherwise. With alkalosis, there is usually some degree of cerebral dysfunction. Blood ammonia levels tend to rise in metabolic alkalosis, and this may be part of the cause of the CNS changes.

If there is a combined metabolic and respiratory alkalosis, the arterial pH can rise rapidly to above 7.55. In a study at Detroit General Hospital, we found that the mortality rate of critically ill or injured patients was increased significantly if their arterial pH rose above 7.55. Almost all patients maintaining an arterial pH above 7.70 died.

Diagnosis

The diagnosis of metabolic alkalosis is made from laboratory studies revealing a bicarbonate level exceeding 26 mEq/L and a pH above 7.45. In most instances, there is also an associated hypokalemia and hypochloremia. Clinically, metabolic alkalosis is characterized by slow, shallow respiration (in contrast to the hyperventilation generally seen with metabolic acidosis). Determining the cause of the alkalosis can be facilitated by determining if urine chloride levels are above 20 mEq/L or below 10 mEq/L.

The causes of metabolic alkalosis are often divided into *chloride-responsive alkalosis* and *chloride-resistant alkalosis*. Chloride-responsive alkalosis is characterized by low urine chloride levels (< 10 mEq/L) and will usually respond well to saline. In chloride-resistant alkalosis urine chloride levels exceed 20 mEq/L and there is a poor response to saline alone. Chloride-resistant alkalosis is most frequently caused by increased endogenous or exogenous adrenal corticosteroids or severe hypokalemia. Bartter's syndrome (hypertrophy and hyperplasia of the cells of the juxtaglomerular apparatus) and Liddle's syndrome (pseudohyperaldosteronism with a clinical picture of hyperaldosteronism but normal aldosterone secretion) are interesting examples of chloride-resistant alkaloses.

Treatment

Chloride-responsive alkalosis, such as that caused by vomiting or excessive nasogastric suction, usually responds adequately to administration of fluid and chloride. If the patient is adequately hydrated, the chloride deficit can be calculated on the basis of 20 percent of the body weight. Thus, if the patient weighs 80 kg and has a serum chloride of 60 mEq/L, the chloride deficit can be calculated as (80 kg $\times$ 20 percent) $\times$ $(100 - 60) = 640$ mEq/L. If the patient is severely dehydrated, one can use 60 percent of the body weight to calculate the chloride deficit.

Half the chloride deficit is corrected over a period of 4 to 12 h. Approximately one-fourth of the chloride is given as potassium chloride and three-fourths as sodium chloride. Normally, the potassium is not given faster than 20 mEq/h and is not given if serum potassium levels exceed 5.0 mEq/L.

If the patient is hypokalemic, the kidneys tend to excrete H^+ and retain HCO_3^-, and this may result in a paradoxical aciduria (excretion of acid urine in the presence of an alkalemia). If adequate chloride is administered to patients with a chloride-responsive alkalosis, the increased chloride in the glomerular filtrate allows increased sodium absorption in the proximal tubule. As less sodium is presented to the distal tubule, less H^+ is excreted and less HCO_3^- is absorbed and the metabolic alkalosis begins to resolve.

Chloride-resistant alkalosis is usually not associated with hypovolemia. Consequently, relatively large quantities of Na^+ and Cl^- are filtered, and increased H^+ and K^+ are excreted as the Na^+ is resorbed in the distal tubule. These patients tend to require large quantities of potassium to correct the alkalosis.

If the alkalosis is severe (the CO_2 content exceeds 40 mEq/L, the pH exceeds 7.55, or the patient has tetany), one-half of the chloride deficit is given as sodium chloride, one-fourth as potassium chloride, and one-fourth as some type of hydrochloride (NH_4Cl, arginine hydrochloride, or 0.1 *N* hydrochloric acid). Ammonium chloride theoretically should be helpful, but many of these patients have renal or hepatic problems which increase the risk of giving ammonium compounds. Arginine hydrochloride may be helpful with hepatic insufficiency but is contraindicated in severe renal dysfunction. Interestingly, some investigators feel that these chlorides may acidify the ECF but not the cells.

If hydrochloric acid (0.10 *N*) is used, it must be given cautiously by slow infusion into a large vein at approximately 25 to 50 mL/h. The hydrochloric acid can be administered with amino acids to provide a higher pH and "gentler" solution than HCl alone.

In some instances, acetazolamide (Diamox), which inhibits carbonic anhydrase and thereby increases renal bicarbonate excretion, may be given by mouth or through a nasogastric tube to correct a mild to moderate metabolic alkalosis.

RESPIRATORY ALKALOSIS

Etiology

In stressful situations such as shock, sepsis, or trauma, there is a tendency to hyperventilate and develop respiratory alkalosis with a P_{CO_2} of 25 to 35 mmHg or less. If hypoxia or metabolic acidosis develops, the tendency to hyperventilation is increased even further.

Physiological Effects

Severe respiratory alkalosis tends to perpetuate itself. If the arterial P_{CO_2} falls, cerebral vasoconstriction occurs. In fact, each 1.0-mmHg drop in the arterial P_{CO_2} reduces cerebral blood flow by about 2 to 4 percent. Thus, a severe respiratory alkalosis, especially if the P_{CO_2} is less than 20 mmHg, can reduce cerebral blood flow enough to cause cerebral metabolic acidosis. This cerebral metabolic acidosis will then cause the respiratory center to increase ventilation even more, producing a progressively more severe respiratory alkalosis.

The initial response to hypocapnia is a shift of hydrogen chloride and lactate ions out of the cell. In severe respiratory alkalosis, lactic levels may increase by 2.0 to 3.0 mmol/L. This buffering is rapid and may be complete within 15 min of the initiation of the hypocapnia. The renal compensation will also begin to take effect within 2 to 4 h after the onset of hypocapnia.

Alkalosis shifts the oxyhemoglobin dissociation curve to the left, causing hemoglobin to hold oxygen more tightly. Each rise in pH of 0.10 lowers the P_{O_2} about 10 percent and reduces oxygen availability to tissues by about 10 percent.

Diagnosis

Respiratory alkalosis is diagnosed by a rise in pH above 7.40 and a decrease in Pa_{CO_2} below 35 mmHg. Occasionally, it may be difficult to differentiate hyperventilation of psychogenic origin from compensatory hyperventilation or hyperventilation due to sepsis or pulmonary emboli.

In such patients, careful continued observation of the patient and the blood gases is essential. It should be remembered that the arterial P_{O_2} may be 80 mmHg or higher in 15 percent of the patients who have pulmonary emboli demonstrated on pulmonary arteriogram. Although the P_{O_2} may be relatively normal initially, with continued sepsis, the P_{O_2} will eventually fall.

Treatment

The treatment of respiratory alkalosis is correction of the primary problem, and one must look particularly for underlying hypoxia, pulmonary embolism, and sepsis. If the problem is hysterical hyperventilation, treatment is best accomplished by having the patient rebreathe expired air, which has a P_{CO_2} about two-thirds that in arterial blood. Not infrequently, the most convenient rebreathing device is a paper bag. Once the P_{CO_2} begins to rise toward normal, the cerebral blood flow usually improves enough to correct the intracerebral acidosis and return the pattern of ventilation toward normal.

In critically ill patients who have severe respiratory alkalosis (P_{CO_2} less than 20 to 25 mmHg and pH more than 7.55 to 7.60) and are not on a ventilator, sedation may be given, but very cautiously. One must be sure that the patient does not reduce ventilation to the point of developing hypoxia.

A patient on a ventilator may be placed on intermittent mandatory ventilation (IMV) and the respirator rate progressively reduced as long as (1) the P_{CO_2} does not exceed 45 mmHg, (2) the pH is not below 7.35, and (3) the patient's respiratory rate is less than 30 per minute. In some instances, 60 to 300 mL of dead space may be added to the endotracheal tube or tracheostomy to increase the P_{CO_2}.

RESPIRATORY ACIDOSIS

Etiology

A P_{CO_2} elevated above 45 mmHg is usually due to inadequate minute ventilation and/or increased dead space. However, increased carbohydrate metabolism may contribute to hypercarbia if pulmonary function is marginal. This is most apt to occur in patients who are on a ventilator and are receiving three or more liters of 20 to 25% glucose IV per day.

Inadequate minute ventilation is most frequently due to head trauma, chest trauma, or disease or excess sedation. The chronic hypoventilation seen in extremely obese patients is often referred to as the *pickwickian syndrome,* after an obese character in Charles Dickens' *Pickwick Papers*. Patients with severe chronic obstructive pulmonary disease (COPD) have increased dead space and frequently also have a decreased minute ventilation.

In general, a rise in the P_{CO_2} stimulates the respiratory center to increase respiratory rate and minute ventilation. However, if the arterial P_{CO_2} chronically exceeds 60 to 70 mmHg, as may occur in 5 to 10 percent of patients with severe emphysema, the respiratory acidosis may depress the respiratory center. Under such circumstances, the stimulus for ventilation is provided primarily by hypoxemia acting on chemoreceptors in the carotid and aortic bodies. Giving oxygen could take away the main stimulus to breathe, causing the P_{CO_2} to rise abruptly to extremely dangerous levels. Consequently, one should not administer oxygen to patients with COPD without carefully watching for the development of apnea or hypoventilation.

Pathophysiology

With a sudden severe decrease in minute ventilation, the P_{CO_2} rises rapidly and the pH may fall abruptly because bicarbonate compensation by the kidney is very slow. In completely apneic patients, the arterial P_{CO_2} rises by about 2.0 to 3.0 mmHg/min. A rapid increase of the arterial P_{CO_2} to 60 mmHg can cause the pH to fall to about 7.22. However, over the next few hours or days, a rise in bicarbonate will gradually restore the pH to about 7.35. A high bicarbonate level in an ambulatory patient should make one suspicious of a chronic respiratory acidosis.

Acute, severe respiratory acidosis is usually accompanied by neurological signs or symptoms. The risk of brain acidemia is higher in respiratory acidosis than in metabolic acidosis. Carbon dioxide penetrates lipid structures, such as the blood-brain barrier, very readily and can markedly decrease the pH of the brain. Bicarbonate, which is water-soluble, penetrates much more slowly. Coma can occur at a P_{CO_2} exceeding 65 to 70 mmHg; however, if the respiratory acidosis develops very slowly, coma may not develop until the P_{CO_2} exceeds 100 to 110 mmHg.

Diagnosis

Respiratory acidosis, by definition, is present when the arterial P_{CO_2} exceeds 45 mmHg and the pH is 7.39 or less. If the pH is less than 7.30, the respiratory acidosis is usually acute or there is a superimposed metabolic acidosis. If the carbon dioxide content of an electrolyte study is high, one should suspect a chronic respiratory acidosis or a metabolic alkalosis. If the chloride and potassium levels are normal or high, the patient is likely to have respiratory acidosis. In contrast, metabolic alkalosis is usually associated with a hypokalemia and hypochloremia.

Treatment

Treatment of respiratory acidosis is primarily designed to improve alveolar ventilation. In general, if the minute ventilation is doubled, the P_{CO_2} will be reduced by 50 percent. In patients with COPD, bronchodilators such as aminophylline or various sympathomimetic agents such as isoproterenol or adrenalin, together with careful administration of small amounts of oxygen, may substantially improve ventilation. However, ventilating assistance may be required in some patients who do not respond adequately to lesser measures, particularly if the pH falls below 7.25 to 7.30. Unfortunately, it may be extremely difficult to extubate such patients later.

In patients with a chronic respiratory acidosis, reduction of the P_{CO_2} should generally proceed slowly. The minute ventilation for a 70-kg person is normally about 6 L/min, and in COPD patients it may be less than 4 L/min. In a patient with COPD and severe hypercarbia, it may be wise to start treatment with a minute ventilation of about 5 L/min and then gradually increase it according to the clinical response and changes in P_{CO_2}.

Rapid correction of a chronic respiratory acidosis can cause sudden development of a severe combined metabolic and respiratory alkalosis with resulting arrhythmias. A rapid rise in pH can cause an abrupt fall in ionized calcium. The resulting ionic hypocalcemia can then cause dangerous arrhythmias or seizures. In patients with a chronic respiratory acidosis, the arterial P_{CO_2} should not be reduced by more than 5.0 torr/hr.

More recently, the problems with ventilation in malnourished individuals has been explored in depth. Increased carbohydrate metabolism increases carbon dioxide production and may cause a respiratory acidosis. On the other hand, administration of adequate amounts of glucose may enable previously exhausted subjects to continue work. In malnourished individuals, increased protein intake can also gradually increase muscle mass and improve the maximal ventilatory response.

BIBLIOGRAPHY

Adrogue HJ, Wilson H, Boyd AE III: Plasma acid-base patterns in diabetic ketoacidosis, *N Engl J Med* 307:1603, 1982.

American Heart Association: Standards and guidelines for cardiopulmonary resuscitation and emergency cardiac care: III. Adult Advanced Cardiac Life Support. *JAMA* 255:2933, 1986.

Boysen PG, Kirby RR: Acid-base problem solving, in Civetta J, Taylor RW, Kirby RR (eds). Critical Care 1988. Philadelphia, JB Lippincott, pp. 337–339.

Brackett NC Jr, Cohen JJ, Schwartz WB: Carbon dioxide titration curve of normal man. *N Engl J Med* 272:6, 1965.

Brackett NC Jr, Wingo CF, Muren O, et al: Acid-base response to chronic hypercapnia in man. *N Engl J Med* 280:124, 1969.

Cohen RD, Woods H: Lactic acidosis revisited. *Diabetes* 32:181, 1983.

Folbergrova J, MacMillan V, Siesjo BK: The effect of moderate and marked hypercapnia upon the energy state and upon the NADH/NAD^+ ratio of the rat brain. *J Neurochem* 19:2497, 1972.

Foster DW, McGarry JD: The metabolic derangements and treatment of diabetic ketoacidosis. *N Engl J Med* 309:159–169, 1983.

Gabow PA: Disorders associated with altered anion gap (discussion). *Kidney Int* 27:472, 1985.

Gabow PA, Kaehny WD, Fennessey PV, et al: Diagnostic importance of an increased serum anion gap. *N Engl J Med* 303:854, 1980.

Goldstein MB, Bear R, Richardson RMA, et al: The urine anion gap: a clinically useful index of ammonium excretion. *Am J Med Sc* 292:198, 1986.

Graf H, Leach W, Arieff AI: Evidence for a detrimental effect of bicarbonate therapy in hypoxic lactic acidosis. *Science* 227:754, 1985.

Hilton JG, Vanderbroucke AC, Josse RG, et al: The urine anion gap: the critical clue to resolve a diagnostic dilemma in a patient with ketoacidosis. *Diabetes Care* 7:486, 1984.

Hood I, Campbell ENM: Is pK ok? *N Engl J Med* 306:864, 1982.

Krupp MA: Fluid and electrolyte disorders, in Schroeder SA (ed). *Current Medical Diagnosis and Treatment* 1988. Norwalk, Connecticut, Appleton and Lange, 1988, pp 34–45.

Moore SE, Good JT: Mixed venous and arterial pH: A comparison during hemorrhagic shock and hypothermia. *Ann Emerg Med* 11:300, 1982.

Ross A, Boron WF: Intracellular pH. *Physiol Rev* 61:296, 1981.

Sahlin K: Intracellular pH and energy metabolism in skeletal muscle of man. *Acta Physiol Scand Suppl* 455:1, 1978.

VanLeeuwen AM: Net cation equivalency (''base binding power'') of the plasma proteins: a study of ion-protein interaction in human plasma by means of in vivo ultrafiltration and equilibrium dialysis. *Acta Med Scand (suppl)* 422:1, 1964.

VanSlyke DD, Hastings AB, Hiller A, et al: Studies of gas and electrolyte equilibria in blood. XIV. The amounts of alkali bound by serum albumin and globulin. *J Biol Chem* 79:769, 1928.

Warth J, Desforges JF: Intraerythrocyte pH and physiochemical homogeneity. *Proc Soc Exp Biol Med* 159:136, 1978.

9
BLOOD GASES: PATHOPHYSIOLOGY AND INTERPRETATION

Robert F. Wilson

VENTILATION

Minute Ventilation

The minute ventilation, the total amount of new air moved in and out of the airways and lungs each minute, is equal to the tidal volume multiplied by the respiratory rate. The normal tidal volume (V_t) is about 500 mL, and the normal respiratory rate (*f*) is 12 breaths per minute. Therefore, the normal minute ventilatory volume averages about 6 L. A human being can live only for short periods with a 2-min ventilation as low as 1.5 L and with a respiratory rate as low as 2 to 4 breaths per minute unless the person's metabolism is severely depressed, such as in deep hypothermia.

The respiratory rate occasionally rises to as high as 40 to 50 breaths per minute, and the tidal volume can become almost as great as the forced vital capacity, which is about 4500 to 5000 mL or 65 to 70 mL/kg in a young adult male. However, at rapid rates a person usually cannot sustain a tidal volume greater than 40 percent of the vital capacity for more than several hours.

Alveolar Ventilation

The main function of the pulmonary ventilatory system is to continually renew the air in the alveoli, where it is brought in close proximity to the pulmonary capillary blood. The rate at which new air reaches these areas is called alveolar ventilation (V_A). During normal quiet ventilation, the tidal volume fills the respiratory passageways down as far as the terminal bronchioles, with only a portion of the inspired air actually flowing into the alveoli. The new air moves from the terminal bronchioles into the alveoli by diffusion. Diffusion is caused by the motion of molecules, with each gas molecule moving at high velocity among the other molecules. The velocity of the molecules in the respiratory air is so great and the distance from the terminal bronchioles to the alveoli so short that the gases move this remaining distance in only a fraction of a second.

Dead Space

Usually at least 30 percent of the air that a person breathes never reaches the alveoli. This portion of the upper and lower respiratory tract is called *dead space* (V_d) because it is not useful for the gas exchange process. The normal dead space in a young male adult with a tidal volume of 500 mL is about 150 mL (about 1 mL/lb of body weight), or about 30 percent of the tidal volume.

The volume of the airways to the gas exchange areas is called the *anatomic dead space*. Occasionally, some alveoli are not functional because of a lack of blood flow to their capillaries. From a functional point of view, these alveoli without capillary perfusion are considered to be pathologic dead space. When the alveolar (pathologic) dead space is included, the total dead space is called the physiologic dead space. In the normal person, the anatomic dead space is nearly equal to the physiologic dead space because all alveoli are functional. However, in those with poorly perfused alveoli, the total (physiologic) dead space may be greater than 60 percent of the tidal volume.

GAS PRESSURES

Pressure is caused by the constant impact of moving molecules against a surface. Therefore, the pressure of a gas acting on the surfaces of the respiratory passages and alveoli is proportional to the sum of the impaction forces of all the molecules striking the surface at any given instant.

In the lungs, one deals with mixtures of gases, particularly oxygen, nitrogen, and carbon dioxide. The rate of diffusion of each gas is directly proportional to its partial pressure.

The concentration of a gas in solution is determined not only by its pressure but also by the solubility coefficient of the gas. Some molecules, especially carbon dioxide, are physically or chemically attracted to water molecules while others are repelled. When molecules are attracted to water, more can become dissolved without building up excess pressure within the solution. On the other hand, those that are repelled develop excessive pressure with little solubility.

Henry's law states that both the partial pressure and the solubility coefficient determine the volume of gas dissolved in a volume of fluid. The solubility coefficients for the important respiratory gases at body temperature are oxygen, 0.024; carbon dioxide, 0.57; carbon monoxide, 0.018; nitrogen, 0.012; and helium, 0.008. Thus, carbon dioxide is more than 20 times as soluble as oxygen, and oxygen is more soluble than the other three major gases. These solubilities help determine the quantity of the gas that is dissolved in the fluids of the body, which in turn is a major factor in determining the rate at which the gas can diffuse through tissues.

When air enters the respiratory passageways, water immediately evaporates from the surfaces of these passages and humidifies the inhaled air. Water molecules, like other dissolved gas molecules, are continually escaping from the water surface into the gas phase. The pressure that the water molecules exert to escape through the surface is called the *vapor pressure* of water. At 37°C (98.6°F), this vapor pressure is 47 mmHg. Therefore, once the gas mixture is fully humidified, the partial pressure of the water vapor in the gas mixture is 47 mmHg. This partial pressure is designated P_{H_2O}.

Diffusion of Gases

Major factors that affect the rate of gas diffusion in a fluid include (1) the partial pressure of the gas, (2) the solubility of the gas in the fluid, (3) the area of the surface for diffusion, (4) the distance through which the gas must diffuse, (5) the molecular weight of the gas, and (6) the temperature of the fluid.

The greater the solubility of the gas and the greater the surface area for diffusion, the greater the number of molecules that are available to diffuse for any given pressure difference. On the other hand, the greater the distance that the molecules must diffuse, the longer it takes for the diffusion to occur. Finally, the greater the velocity of the molecules, which at any given temperature is inversely proportional to the square root of the molecular weight, the greater the rate of diffusion of the gas. All these factors can be expressed in a single formula:

$$D = \frac{PAS}{d\sqrt{\mathrm{MW}}}$$

where D = diffusion rate
P = pressure difference between the two ends of the diffusion pathway
A = cross-sectional area of the pathway
S = solubility of the gas
d = distance of diffusion
MW = molecular weight of the gas

The characteristics of the gas itself determine solubility and molecular weight, and these together are called the *diffusion coefficient* of the gas. The diffusion coefficient, which equals $S/\sqrt{MW}$, determines the relative rates at which different gases at the same pressure levels diffuse. If the diffusion coefficient of oxygen is 1.0, the relative diffusion coefficients of other gases of respiratory importance are carbon dioxide, 20.3; carbon monoxide, 0.81; nitrogen, 0.53; and helium, 0.95.

The gases that are of respiratory importance are highly soluble in lipids and, consequently, are also highly soluble in cell membranes, diffusing through them with very little impediment. The major limitation to the movement of gases in tissues is the rate at which the gases can diffuse through the tissue water.

The respiratory unit is composed of a respiratory bronchiole, alveolar ducts, atria, and alveoli. A respiratory bronchiole is the largest bronchiole that has any alveoli coming directly off of it. The alveolar walls are extremely thin and are closely applied to an almost solid network of interconnecting capillaries. Because of the extensiveness of the capillary plexus, the movement of blood past the alveoli has been described as a "sheet" of flowing blood. The membrane through which gaseous exchange between the alveolar air and the pulmonary blood occurs is known as the respiratory (pulmonary) membrane.

For oxygen to get from the alveolus into the pulmonary capillary bed, it must pass through four separate layers, referred to collectively as the *alveolar-capillary,* or *respiratory,* membrane. These include:

1. A layer of fluid lining the alveolus. Called alveolar fluid, it contains surfactant that reduces its surface tension.
2. The alveolar epithelium, composed of very thin epithelial cells and a basement membrane.
3. A very thin interstitial space between the alveolar epithelium and the capillary membrane.
4. The capillary endothelial membrane and its basement membrane, which fuses with the alveolar basement membrane in many places.

The overall thickness of the respiratory membranes averages 0.63 μm. The respiratory membrane in the normal adult is approximately 160 m^2. Although the lungs may contain about 700 mL of blood, the total quantity in the pulmonary capillaries at any given instant is only 60 to 140 mL.

The average diameter of the pulmonary capillaries is less than 8 μm, which means that red blood cells must actually squeeze through them. Therefore, at least part of the red blood cell membrane touches the capillary wall. Where this occurs, oxygen goes not have to pass through significant amounts of plasma as it diffuses from the alveolus to the red blood cell. This helps increase the rapidity of diffusion of gases between the alveolus and the hemoglobin molecules.

Gas Diffusion through the Respiratory Membrane

The factors that determine how rapidly a gas passes through the respiratory membrane are (1) the thickness of the membrane, (2) the surface area of the membrane, (3) the diffusion coefficient of the gas in the water of the membrane, and (4) the pressure difference between the two sides of the membrane.

The thickness of the respiratory membrane occasionally increases, usually as a result of fluid in the interstitial space. Also, some pulmonary diseases cause fibrosis of the lungs, which can further increase the thickness of some portions of the respiratory membrane. Because the rate of diffusion through the membrane is inversely proportional to its thickness, any factor that increases the thickness of the membrane to more than two to three times normal can interfere significantly with oxygenation of blood; however, diffusion is rarely a problem with carbon dioxide.

The surface area of the respiratory membrane may be greatly decreased by a variety of conditions, such as atelectasis or resection of lung tissue. In emphysema, many of the alveoli coalesce, with dissolution of alveolar walls. The new alveolar chambers are much larger than the original alveoli, but the total surface area of the respiratory membrane available for gas diffusion is considerably decreased, causing an increase in dead space. When the total surface area of the lung is decreased to approximately one-third to one-fourth normal, exchange of gases through the membrane is impeded significantly, even under resting conditions. During strenuous exercise, even the slightest increase in dead space in patients with severe emphysema can seriously interfere with the exchange of gases.

The pressure difference across the respiratory membrane is the difference between the partial pressure of the gas in the alveoli and the partial pressure of the gas in the blood. In room air, the normal alveolar-arterial oxygen difference ($PA_{O_2} - Pa_{O_2}$) or [$P(A - a)_{O_2}$] is 2 to 10 mmHg. The normal alveolar-arterial carbon dioxide difference ($PA_{CO_2} - Pa_{CO_2}$) or [$P(A - a)_{CO_2}$] is zero. An increase in the $P(A - a)_{CO_2}$ implies a significant increase in dead space.

Diffusing Capacity

The ability of the respiratory membrane to exchange gas between the alveoli and the pulmonary blood can be expressed in quantitative terms by what is known as *diffusing capacity,* defined as the volume of a gas that diffuses through the membrane each minute for a pressure difference of 1 mmHg. In the average young adult the diffusing capacity of oxygen under resting conditions averages 21 mL/min per mmHg. The mean oxygen pressure difference across the respiratory membrane during normal, quiet breathing is approximately 12 mmHg. Multiplication of this pressure by the diffusing capacity (21×12) gives a total of about 250 mL of oxygen diffusing through the respiratory membrane each minute; this is approximately equal to the rate at which an average adult uses oxygen under resting conditions.

During strenuous exercise, or during other conditions that greatly increase pulmonary blood flow and alveolar ventilation, the diffusing capacity of oxygen in young male adults can increase to a maximum of about 65 mL/min per mmHg, three times the diffusing capacity under resting conditions. This is caused both by opening up of previously dormant pulmonary capillaries, thereby increasing the surface area of the blood into which the oxygen can diffuse, and by dilation of pulmonary capillaries that were already open, further increasing the surface area available for diffusion.

The diffusing capacity of carbon dioxide has not been measured because carbon dioxide diffuses through the respiratory membrane so rapidly that the average difference between the P_{CO_2} in the pulmonary capillary blood and in alveoli is less than 1 mmHg. Since the diffusion coefficient of carbon dioxide is 20 times that of oxygen, one would expect the diffusing capacity of carbon dioxide under resting conditions to be about 400 to 450 mL/min per mmHg and during exercise to be about 1200 to 1300 mL/min per mmHg.

The oxygen diffusing capacity can be calculated from measurement of (1) the alveolar P_{O_2}, (2) the P_{O_2} in the pulmonary capillary blood, and (3) the rate of oxygen uptake by the blood. Because of the difficulties encountered in measuring oxygen diffusing capacity, carbon monoxide diffusing capacity is measured and then that value is used to calculate oxygen diffusing capacity. With the carbon monoxide method, a small amount of carbon monoxide is breathed into the alveoli, and the partial pressure of the carbon monoxide in the alveoli is measured from alveolar air samples. The carbon monoxide diffusing capacity can be determined by measuring the volume of carbon monoxide absorbed over time and dividing by the partial pressure of carbon monoxide in end-tidal gas.

The diffusion coefficient of oxygen is 1.23 times that of carbon monoxide. Thus, if the average diffusing capacity of carbon monoxide in young male adults is 17 mL/min per mmHg, the diffusing capacity of oxygen is 1.23×17, or about 21 mL/min per mmHg.

ALVEOLAR GASES

Inspired Gases

Air at sea level has an average barometric pressure of 760 mmHg and contains approximately 20.93 percent oxygen and 0.04 percent carbon dioxide, with nitrogen making up most of the remainder. Thus, the partial pressures of oxygen and carbon dioxide in the air at sea level are 159 and 0.3 mmHg, respectively (Table 9-1).

Alveolar air does not have the same concentration of gases as atmospheric air because (1) dry atmospheric air that enters the respiratory passages is humidified before it reaches the alveoli, (2) alveolar air is only partially replaced by atmospheric air with each breath, (3) oxygen is constantly being absorbed from the alveolar air, and (4) carbon dioxide is constantly diffusing from the pulmonary blood into the alveoli.

Humidification of Inspired Air

When air enters the upper airway, it is warmed and saturated with water, reducing the total partial pressure of the inhaled gases to about 713 mmHg. Thus, the inspired oxygen pressure (PI_{O_2}) in the trachea and bronchi falls to 713 × 0.2093, or 149 mmHg (Table 9-1). If the patient is breathing 60 percent oxygen (fraction of inspired oxygen FI_{O_2}) = 0.6, the PI_{O_2} in the trachea or bronchi is determined as follows:

$$\begin{aligned} PI_{O_2} &= (PB - P_{H_2O})\, FI_{O_2} \\ &= (760 - 47)\,(0.6) \\ &= 427.8 \text{ mmHg} \end{aligned}$$

Rate at Which Alveolar Air is Renewed by Atmospheric Air

The functional residual capacity of the lungs, which is the amount of air remaining in the lungs at the end of normal expiration, is approximately 2500 to 3000 mL (35 to 45 mL/kg). Only 350 mL of new air is brought into the alveoli with each new tidal volume, and the same amount of old alveolar air is expired. Therefore, the amount of alveolar air replaced by new atmospheric air with each breath is only 12 to 16 percent of the total gas present in the lungs. With normal alveolar ventilation, approximately half the old alveolar gas is exchanged in 17 s. When a person's rate of alveolar ventilation is only half normal, half the gas is exchanged in 34 s, and when the rate of ventilation is twice normal, half is exchanged in about 8 s.

The slow replacement of alveolar air helps prevent sudden changes in gas concentrations in the blood. This helps to prevent excessive changes in tissue oxygenation, tissue carbon dioxide concentration, and tissue pH when ventilation is temporarily interrupted.

Table 9-1. Partial Pressure of Gases While Breathing Room Air (mmHg)

	Air	Inspired Air in Trachea	Average Alveolar Gas	Average Expired Gas
P_{O_2}	159.0	149.3	104.0	120.0
P_{CO_2}	0.3	0.3	40.0	28.0
P_{N_2}	597.0	563.4	569.0	565.0
P_{H_2O}	3.7	47.0	47.0	47.0
Total	760.0	760.0	760.0	760.0

Oxygen Concentration and Partial Pressure in the Alveoli

Oxygen is continually being absorbed into the blood of the lungs, and new oxygen is continually entering the alveoli from the atmosphere. The more rapidly oxygen is absorbed, the lower its concentration in the alveoli. The more rapidly new oxygen is brought into the alveoli from the atmosphere, the higher its concentration becomes. Therefore, oxygen concentration in the alveoli is controlled by the rate of absorption of oxygen into the blood and the rate of entry of new oxygen into the lung.

Carbon Dioxide Concentration in the Alveoli

Carbon dioxide is continually formed and discharged into the alveoli and continually removed from the alveoli by ventilation. Therefore, the two factors that determine the partial pressure of carbon dioxide in the alveoli (PA_{CO_2}) are (1) the rate of excretion of carbon dioxide from the blood into the alveoli and (2) the rate at which carbon dioxide is removed form the alveoli by alveolar ventilation.

At a normal rate of alveolar ventilation of 4.2 L/min, the PA_{CO_2} is usually 40 mmHg. If alveolar ventilation is doubled, the PA_{CO_2} is reduced to 20 mmHg. If alveolar ventilation is decreased to 2.1 L/min, the PA_{CO_2} rises to 80 mmHg.

Alveolar Gas Equation

Inspired gas in the trachea has a P_{O_2} of about 149 mmHg and a P_{CO_2} of about 0.3 mmHg. As the water-saturated warmed air enters the alveoli, oxygen diffuses through the alveolar capillary membranes into the plasma and carbon dioxide diffuses from the blood into the alveoli. The mixed venous blood brought to the pulmonary capillaries normally has a P_{O_2} of about 40 mmHg and a P_{CO_2} of 46 mmHg. On the average, for each milliliter of oxygen that leaves the alveolus, 0.8 to 1.0 mL of carbon dioxide enters it. This relationship is defined as the respiratory quotient (RQ), which can be expressed as

$$RQ = \frac{\text{rate of } CO_2 \text{ output}}{\text{rate of } O_2 \text{ intake}}$$

To estimate alveolar P_{O_2} (PA_{O_2}) from the PI_{O_2} and PA_{CO_2} (which is assumed to be equal to the arterial P_{CO_2}), one needs a correction factor to determine how much oxygen is consumed for each 1.0 mmHg of P_{CO_2} resulting from carbon dioxide that enters the alveoli. If the RQ is 0.8, the correction factor is 1.2; if the RQ is 1.0, the correction factor is 1.0.

Thus, for the usual circumstances, in which the RQ is 0.8, the alveolar gas equation is

$$PA_{O_2} = (PB - P_{H_2O})(FI_{O_2})\,(Pa_{CO_2})(1.2)$$

In room air (FI_{O_2} = 0.21) at sea level with a Pa_{CO_2} of 40 mmHg, the $PA_{O_2}$is expected to be

$$PA_{O_2} = (760 - 47)(0.21) - (40)(1.2) = 150 - 48 = 102$$

Estimating the PA_{O_2}

In someone breathing room air, one can estimate the PA_{O_2} by just subtracting the Pa_{CO_2} from 145. Thus, if the Pa_{CO_2} is 45 mmHg, the PA_{O_2} should be about 100 mmHg.

If the patient is receiving supplemental oxygen, a quick way of estimating the PA_{O_2} is to multiply the percentage of inhaled oxygen by 6. Thus, a patient on 40 percent oxygen would be expected to have PA_{O_2} of about 240, and a patient on 60 percent oxygen would be expected to have a PA_{O_2} of about 360 mmHg.

Expired Air

Expired air is a combination of dead space air and alveolar air, and its overall composition is determined by the proportion of each in expired air. Dead space air is expired first. Then progessively more alveolar air becomes mixed with the dead space air until all the dead space air has finally been washed out. At the end of expiration nothing but alveolar air is expired. Therefore, to collect alveolar air for study, one simply collects end-tidal gas.

ARTERIAL BLOOD GASES

Arterial Pa_{CO_2}

Alveolar Ventilation

Carbon dioxide diffuses so rapidly that the Pa_{CO_2} usually provides an excellent index of the adequacy of overall ventilation of perfused alveoli. If the Pa_{CO_2} is greater than normal in a patient with a normal or low arterial pH, one can assume that ventilation is reduced. However, the patient may also have increased dead space due to emphysema, pulmonary emboli, or sepsis. An elevated Pa_{CO_2} in the presence of metabolic alkalosis usually reflects compensatory effort to restore arterial pH to normal. However, an elevated Pa_{CO_2} in a patient with metabolic acidosis generally indicates pulmonary insufficiency.

With adequate alveolar ventilation, the Pa_{CO_2} will be closely related to the aterial pHa. As a rough rule, the Pa_{CO_2} should fall by 5 to 10 mmHg for each 0.10 drop in pH. Thus, if the pH is 7.30, the Pa_{CO_2} should be 30 to 35 mmHg or less. If the arterial pH is 7.20 or less, the Pa_{CO_2} should be 25 to 35 mmHg or less.

As a rule, for each 5.0 mEq/L that the arterial bicarbonate concentration falls below 24.0 mEq/L, the Pa_{CO_2} should fall at least 5 mmHg. Otherwise one can assume that the patient has impaired minute ventilation, increased dead space, or increased carbohydrate metabolism.

Arterial pH is affected by both the bicarbonate level and the Pa_{CO_2}, and the Pa_{CO_2} can change 100 to 200 times faster than the bicarbonate level. Using this information, one can often gain some impression of the acuteness of various respiratory changes by noting the effects of the Pa_{CO_2} on the pH. For each 1 mmHg of acute rise or fall in the Pa_{CO_2} the pH decreases or increases by approximately 0.01, assuming the plasma bicarbonate level remains constant during that acute change.

Dead Space

When the ventilation of an alveolar-capillary unit is normal but perfusion of the alveolar capillary is absent, the ventilation of these alveoli and their associated airways is referred to as dead space. The volume of the dead space (V_d) and the tidal volume (V_t) are often expressed as a ratio (V_d/V_t). This is determined in the pulmonary function laboratory by measuring the Pa_{CO_2} in arterial blood, measuring the average expired gas (PE_{CO_2}), and using the following Bohr equation:

$$\frac{V_d}{V_t} = \frac{Pa_{CO_2} - PE_{CO_2}}{Pa_{CO_2}}$$

The normal values are

$$\frac{V_d}{V_t} = \frac{40 - 28}{40} = \frac{12}{40} = 0.3$$

When the physiologic dead space is increased, some of the work of ventilation is wasted because a greater fraction of ventilated air never reaches the blood.

Carbohydrate Metabolism

If the patient has to metabolize more than 450 g of carbohydrate per day, an increased alveolar ventilation may be required to excrete the increased carbon dioxide produced. This is most frequently a problem in patients with severe chronic obstructive pulmonary disease if they are receiving 2.5 to 3.0 L of 20 to 25% glucose per day.

Transport of Carbon Dioxide in the Blood

Under resting conditions, each 100 mL of blood transports an average of 4 mL of carbon dioxide from the tissues to the lungs. Transport of carbon dioxide is not as great a problem as transport of oxygen because, even in the most abnormal conditions, carbon dioxide can usually be transported in far greater quantities than oxygen. However, carbon dioxide in the blood does affect acid-base balance.

The carbon dioxide formed in cells diffuses out in the form of carbon dioxide rather than bicarbonate because the cell membrane is almost impermeable to bicarbonate ions. As the carbon dioxide enters the capillary, it initiates a number of almost instantaneous reactions essential for carbon dioxide transport.

A small portion of the carbon dioxide is transported to the lungs dissolved in plasma. The amount dissolved in plasma at 46 mmHg is about 2.76 mL/dL (vol%). The amount dissolved at 40 mmHg is about 2.4 mL/dL, or a difference of 0.36 mL/dL. Therefore, only about 0.36 mL of carbon dioxide is transported in the form of dissolved carbon dioxide by each 100 mL of blood. This is about 9 percent of all carbon dioxide transported.

Much of the dissolved carbon dioxide in the blood reacts with water to form carbonic acid. This reaction would occur too slowly to be of importance were it not for the fact that the enzyme carbonic anhydrase inside the red blood cells speeds up the reaction about 500-fold. The reaction occurs so rapidly that it reaches almost complete equilibrium within a fraction of a second. This allows tremendous amounts of carbon dioxide to react with red blood cell water even before the blood leaves the tissue capillaries.

In another fraction of a second, the carbonic acid formed in the red cells dissociates into hydrogen and bicarbonate ions. Most of the hydrogen ions then combine with the hemoglobin in the red blood cells because hemoglobin is a powerful acid-base buffer. At the same time, many of the bicarbonate ions diffuse into the plasma; to offset this ionic shift, chloride ions diffuse into the red blood cells. This is made possible by the presence of a special bicarbonate-chloride carrier protein in the red cell membrane that shuttles these two ions in opposite directions at rapid velocities. Thus, the chloride content of venous red blood cells is greater than that of arterial red blood cells. This phenomenon is called the *chloride shift.*

The reversible combination of carbon dioxide with water in the red blood cells under the influence of carbonic anhydrase accounts for at least 70 percent of all the carbon dioxide transported from the tissues. Indeed, when a carbonic anhydrase inhibitor (acetazolamide) is administered to an animal to block the action of carbonic anhydrase in the red blood cells, carbon dioxide transport from the tissues becomes very poor and the tissue P_{CO_2} rises abruptly.

Carbaminohemoglobin and Carbaminoproteins

Carbon dioxide also reacts directly with hemoglobin to form carbaminohemoglobin (Hb–CO_2). This reversible reaction occurs with a very loose bond, so the carbon dioxide is easily released into the alveoli, where the P_{CO_2} is lower than in the tissue capillaries. A small amount of carbon dioxide (usually equivalent to about 0.5 to 1.0 mEq of bicarbonate per liter) also reacts in this same way with the plasma proteins, but this is much less significant because the quantity of these proteins is only about one-fourth to one-half the quantity of hemoglobin.

The theoretical quantity of carbon dioxide that can be carried to the lungs in combination with hemoglobin and plasma proteins is approximately 30 percent of the total quantity transported—that is, about 1.5 mL of carbon dioxide in each 100 mL of blood. However, this reaction is much slower than the reaction of carbon dioxide with water, and it is doubtful that more than 15 to 25 percent of the total quantity of carbon dioxide is transported this way.

The Carbon Dioxide Dissociation Curve

Carbon dioxide can exist in the blood as free carbon dioxide and in chemical combinations with water, hemoglobin, and plasma proteins. The total quantity of carbon dioxide combined with the blood in all forms depends on the Pa_{CO_2}.

The normal blood Pa_{CO_2} averages about 40 mmHg in arterial blood and 46 mmHg in mixed venous blood. Although the normal total concentration of carbon dioxide in the blood is about 50 mL/dL (vol%), only 4 mL/dL of this is actually exchanged during normal transport of carbon dioxide. Thus, the concentration of carbon dioxide rises to about 52 mL/dL after the blood passes through the tissues, and falls to about 48 mL/dL after the blood passes through the lungs.

Effect of the Oxygen-Hemoglobin Reaction on Carbon Dioxide Transport—The Haldane Effect

An increase in the carbon dioxide level in the blood causes oxygen to be displaced from the hemoglobin, and this promotes oxygen release to tissues at the capillary level. The reverse is also true; binding of oxygen with hemoglobin tends to displace carbon dioxide as blood moves through the pulmonary capillaries. Indeed, this effect, called the Haldane effect, is quantitatively far more important in promoting carbon dioxide transport than the Bohr effect is in promoting oxygen transport.

The Haldane effect results because the combination of oxygen with hemoglobin causes hemoglobin to became a stronger acid. This displaces carbon dioxide from the blood in two ways: (1) the highly acidic oxyhemoglobin has less tendency to combine with carbon dioxide to form carbaminohemoglobin, thus releasing much of the carbon dioxide present in the red blood cell into the plasma; and (2) the increased acidity of oxyhemoglobin causes it to release hydrogen ions, and these in turn bind with bicarbonate ions to form carbonic acid. The carbonic acid then dissociates into water and carbon dioxide, and the carbon dioxide is released from the blood into the alveoli. Thus, in the presence of oxygen, much less carbon dioxide can bind with hemoglobin and conversely, in the absence of oxygen, considerably more carbon dioxide can be bound to the hemoglobin.

Therefore, in tissue capillaries, the Haldane effect causes increased pickup of carbon dioxide because oxygen has been removed from the hemoglobin, and in the lungs, it causes increased release of carbon dioxide because of oxygen pickup by the hemoglobin.

Change in Blood Acidity During Carbon Dioxide Transport

The carbonic acid formed when carbon dioxide enters the blood in the tissue decreases the pH. However, the buffers of the blood prevent the hydrogen ion concentration from rising greatly. Ordinarily, arterial blood has a pH of approximately 7.40, and as the blood acquires carbon dioxide in the tissue capillaries, the pH falls to approximately 7.35. The reverse occurs when carbon dioxide is released from the blood in the lungs. In conditions of high metabolic activity, or when blood flow through the tissues is extremely sluggish, the decrease in pH in the blood as it leaves the tissues can be 0.50 or more.

Changes in Respiratory Quotient

The value of the RQ changes under different metabolic conditions. When a person is metabolizing a mixed diet, the RQ averages about 0.8. If the patient were metabolizing only protein, the RQ would be 0.83. For carbohydrates, the RQ is 1.00, and if one is metabolizing only fats, the RQ falls to 0.7. When oxygen is metabolized with carbohydrates, one molecule of carbon dioxide is formed for each molecule of oxygen consumed. However, when oxygen reacts with fat, a large share of the oxygen combines with hydrogen atoms from the fats to form water instead of carbon dioxide. If the patient is eating enough carbohydrates to make fat, the RQ is greater than 1.0, and if the patient is making ketones but not metabolizing them, the RQ is less than 0.7.

Monitoring Oxygenation and Ventilation

The patient who is awake, alert, comfortable, and cooperative and has normal vital signs is generally oxygenating and ventilating adequately. However, if the patient is tachypneic and/or tachycardiac and appears to be anxious and/or confused, one should suspect a problem with the patient's ventilation or oxygenation and correct it as soon as possible. In comatose patients, it is sometimes very difficult to judge how well the patient is oxygenating or ventilating without serial blood gas determinations.

Cyanosis as a sign of inadequate oxygenation is almost worthless if the hemoglobin is less than 10 g/dL. Under such circumstances, the aterial oxygen saturation (Sa_{O_2}) must usually be less than 65 percent, corresponding to a Pa_{CO_2} of about 30 to 35 mmHg, before the patient looks cyanotic.

Arterial P_{O_2}

The arterial P_{O_2} (Pa_{O_2}) in normal, healthy young adults under ideal conditions is considered to be about 100 mmHg. However, many healthy young adults have a Pa_{O_2} of only 80 to 90 mmHg. The Pa_{O_2} is extremely important because it not only reflects the functional capabilities of the lungs but also determines the rate at which oxygen enters the tissue cells.

Factors that affect the Pa_{O_2} include the amount of alveolar ventilation; the concentration or fraction of oxygen in the inspired gases (FI_{O_2}); the functional capabilities of the lungs; and the oxyhemoglobin dissociation curve.

Alveolar Ventilation

If the patient hyperventilates, the Pa_{CO_2} tends to fall and the Pa_{O_2} tends to rise. If the Pa_{CO_2} falls by 1 mm Hg, the Pa_{O_2} rises by about 1.0 to 1.2 mmHg. The lungs can make up for some pulmonary dysfunction by hyperventilating.

Fraction of Inspired O_2

Unfortunately the FI_{O_2} is often not considered adequately in evaluating the Pa_{O_2}. If a patient is receiving oxygen by nasal cannula, the actual delivered FI_{O_2} is usually only 25 to 30 percent. With a properly fitting face mask, the inhaled FI_{O_2} is usually less than half that delivered to the mask. The approximate Pa_{O_2} values that might be expected in normal persons who are inhaling various concentration of oxygen are listed in Table 9-2.

The expected alveolar P_{O_2} when the patient is given oxygen can be estimated by multiplying the actual delivered percentage of oxygen by 6. Thus, a patient getting 60% oxygen would be expected to have a PA_{O_2} of about 60 × 6, or 360 mmHg.

Altitude

The Pa_{O_2} expected when a patient is breathing room air varies with height above sea level. The greater the altitude, the lower the P_{O_2} in

Table 9-2. Expected Pa_{O_2} in Patients Inhaling Various Concentrations of Oxygen

FI_{O_2} mmHg	0.21 (room air)	0.4	0.6	0.8	1.0
Expected Pa_{O_2}, mmHg*	100	227	370	512	655

* Assuming a $PA_{O_2} - Pa_{O_2}$ of 10 mmHg and a P_{CO_2} of 40 mmHg.

Table 9-3. Changes in P_{O_2} at Various Altitudes

Altitude, ft above Sea Level	Atmospheric Pressure, mmHg	P_{O_2} in Air, mmHg	$P_{A_{O_2}}$ in Alveoli, mmHg	Pa_{O_2} in Arterial Blood,* mmHg
0	760	159	105	100
2,000	707	148	97	92
4,000	656	137	90	85
6,000	609	127	84	79
8,000	564	118	79	74
10,000	523	109	74	69
20,000	349	73	40	35
30,000	226	47	21	19

* Assuming ideal circumstances with a $P_{A_{O_2}} - Pa_{O_2}$ of 5 mmHg or less.

the air and the greater the tendency for the patient to hyperventilate (Table 9-3).

The Pa_{O_2} drops about 3 to 4 mmHg for each 1000-foot rise above sea level. Up to an altitude of approximately 10,000 ft, the Sa_{O_2} remains about 90 percent. However, about 10,000 ft, the Sa_{O_2} progressively falls about 1 percent for each 1 mmHg drop in P_{O_2}, until at 20,000 ft altitude, the Pa_{O_2} is about 35 mmHg and the Sa_{O_2} is only about 65 percent.

When a person breathes air at 30,000 ft, where the barometric pressure is about 226 mmHg, the Pa_{O_2} is only 21 mmHg. At this height above sea level, almost three-fourths of the alveolar air is nitrogen. But if the person breathes pure oxygen instead of air, most of the space in the alveoli formerly occupied by nitrogen becomes occupied by oxygen. However, even if the person is breathing 100% oxygen at 30,000 ft, the Pa_{O_2} is only 139 mmHg (Table 9-4).

Age

Even in healthy individuals, pulmonary changes that cause a fall in the Pa_{O_2} occur with advancing age. On the average, the Pa_{O_2} falls about 3 to 4 mmHg per decade after the patient reaches 20 to 30 years of age. Thus, an otherwise normal 20-year-old patient with a Pa_{O_2} of about 90 to 100 mmHg (room air, at sea level) might be expected to have a Pa_{O_2} of only about 75 to 80 mmHg at 80 years of age.

Alveolar-Arterial Oxygen Differences

One method for determining the degree to which lung function is impaired is to determine the alveolar-arterial oxygen gradient [$P(A - a)_{O_2}$]. Arterial blood samples can be obtained easily. If there is a technique for trapping the end-expiratory gases (which generally represent average alveolar gases), the alveolar P_{O_2} ($P_{A_{O_2}}$) can be measured and the $P(A - a)_{O_2}$ calculated.

Table 9-4. Effects of Acute Exposure to Low Atmospheric Pressure on Alveolar Gas Concentrations and on Arterial Oxygen Saturation

		While Breathing Air		While Breathing 100% O_2	
Altitude, ft	Barometric Pressure, mmHg	Arterial P_{O_2} in Alveoli, mmHg	P_{CO_2} in Alveoli, mmHg	P_{O_2} in Alveoli, mmHg	Oxygen Saturation %
0	760	159	40	673	100
10,000	523	110	40	436	100
20,000	349	73	40	262	100
30,000	226	47	40	139	99
40,000	141	29	36	58	87
50,000	87	18	24	16	22

If alveolar gases are not directly measured, they can be estimated by the alveolar gas equation. One can also estimate alveolar oxygen in patients with a normal cardiac output breathing room air by subtracting the Pa_{CO_2} from 145. This is possible because $P_{A_{O_2}}$ and $P_{A_{CO_2}}$ add up to about 145 when a patient breathes room air at sea level. Since the $P_{A_{CO_2}}$ is usually the same as the Pa_{CO_2}, the $P_{A_{O_2}}$ can be estimated from the arterial gas pressure by the following formula:

$$P_{A_{O_2}} = 145 - Pa_{CO_2}$$

If the patient has a Pa_{CO_2} of 40 mmHg,

$$P_{A_{O_2}} = 145 - 40 = 105 \text{ mmHg}$$

This equation can be used to determine the $P(A - a)_{O_2}$. The $P_{A_{O_2}}$ is estimated from the above formula, and the Pa_{O_2} is determined from arterial blood-gases analysis. If the Pa_{O_2} were 90 mmHg, the $P(A - a)_{O_2}$ would be 15 mmHg, which is relatively normal. A $P(A - a)_{O_2}$ of 20 to 30 mmHg on room air usually indicates mild pulmonary dysfunction, and a $P(A - a)_{O_2}$ greater than 50 mmHg on room air usually indicates severe pulmonary dysfunction.

Oxyhemoglobin Saturation

Normal Relationships

It can be seen from oxygen-hemoglobin dissociation curves that even when the Pa_{O_2} is decreased to 59 mmHg, the arterial hemoglobin is still about 90 percent saturated with oxygen. Furthermore, if the hemoglobin level is 15.0 g/dL and the tissue removes 5.0 mL of oxygen from each 100 mL of blood, the P_{O_2} of the venous blood falls to about 36 mmHg, which is only 4 mmHg below the normal value. Thus, the tissue P_{O_2} often changes minimally despite a marked fall in Pa_{O_2}.

On the other hand, if the Pa_{O_2} rises far above the upper limit of normal (90 to 100 mmHg), the oxygen saturation of hemoglobin cannot rise above 100 percent. Therefore, even if the Pa_{O_2} should rise to 600 mmHg or more, the saturation of hemoglobin would increase only 1 to 2 percent because at Pa_{O_2} of 100 mmHg, the arterial oxygen saturation is only 98 to 99 percent.

Under circumstances of normal body temperature [37°C (98.6°F) and pH 7.40], certain standard relations exist between the oxygen-hemoglobin saturation and plasma P_{O_2} (Table 9-5).

Thus, the relation between Sa_{O_2} and plasma P_{O_2} is almost linear when the Sa_{O_2} is 60 to 90 percent. However, as the Sa_{O_2} rises above 90 percent, the P_{O_2} begins to rise much faster than the saturation.

Factors Affecting Oxyhemoglobin Dissociation

The best known of the factors affecting the oxyhemoglobin dissociation curve are pH, temperature, and the amount of 2,3-diphosphoglycerate (2,3-DPG) in the red blood cells.

pH

The more acidic the blood, the more readily hemoglobin gives up its oxygen and the higher the Pa_{O_2} is for a particular oxyhemoglobin saturation. In contrast, alkalosis makes hemoglobin hold onto its oxygen more tightly, lowering the Pa_{O_2} present at a particular oxygen-hemoglobin saturation. In general, a rise or fall in pH of 0.10 causes a fall or rise (i.e., an opposite change) in the Pa_{O_2} of about 10 percent (Table 9-6).

Table 9-5. Relation Between Oxygen-Hemoglobin Saturation and Plasma P_{O_2}

Oxygen saturation, %	100.0	98.4	95	90	80	73	60	50	40	35	30
P_{O_2}, mmHg	677	100	80	59	48	40	30	26	23	21	18

Table 9-6. Changes in P_{O_2} Produced by Changes in pH

pH	7.60	7.50	7.40	7.30	7.20	7.10	7.00
Pa_{O_2}, mmHg*	80	90	100	111	122	134	148

* Assuming a temperature of 37°C (98.6°F) and a hemoglobin saturation of 98.4%.

The P_{CO_2}

A shift of the oxygen-hemoglobin dissociation curve as a result of changes in the blood levels of carbon dioxide and hydrogen ions enhances oxygenation of the blood in the lungs and enhances release of oxygen from the blood in the tissues. This is called the *Bohr effect*. As the blood passes through the lungs, carbon dioxide diffuses from the blood into the alveoli. This reduces the blood P_{CO_2} and decreases the hydrogen ion concentration because of the resulting decrease in the blood carbonic acid level. Both changes shift the oxyhemoglobin dissociation curve to the left. With a shift to the left, the quantity of oxygen binding to hemoglobin at any given Pa_{O_2} is increased, allowing greater oxygen transport to the tissues. Then when the blood reaches the tissue capillaries, exactly the opposite effect occurs. Carbon dioxide entering the blood from the tissues shifts the curve to the right. This displaces oxygen from the hemoglobin and delivers oxygen to the tissues at a higher P_{O_2} than would otherwise occur.

Temperature

As blood temperature increases, hemoglobin gives up oxygen more readily, raising the P_{O_2} in the plasma. The opposite occurs during cooling. For each 1°C rise in temperature, the Pa_{O_2} rises about 5 percent (Table 9-7). With hypothermia, the P_{CO_2} falls by about the same amount.

Exercise

During strenuous exercise, several factors can shift the oxyhemoglobin dissociation curve to the right. Exercising muscles release large quantities of carbon dioxide and other acids, increasing the hydrogen ion concentration in muscle capillary blood. In addition, the temperature of the muscle often rises as much as 3 to 4° C, and phosphate compounds are also released. All these factors acting together shift the oxygen-hemoglobin dissociation curve of the blood in the muscle capillaries considerably to the right. Therefore, oxygen can sometime be released to the muscle at a P_{O_2} as high as 40 mmHg even though as much as 75 percent of the oxygen has been removed from the hemoglobin. In the lungs the shift occurs in the opposite direction, allowing pickup of extra amounts of oxygen from the alveoli.

2,3-DPG

Except for hemoglobin, the compound present in greatest quantity in red blood cells is 2,3-diphosphoglycerate (2,3-DPG). A normal concentration of 2,3-DPG in a red blood cell keeps the oxyhemoglobin dissociation curve shifted slightly to the right all the time. In addition, in hypoxic conditions that last longer than a few hours, the quantity of 2,3-DPG increases considerably, shifting the oxyhemoglobin dissociation curve even farther to the right. This can cause the P_{O_2} in the plasma to be as much as 10 mmHg higher than it would have been otherwise. However, the presence of increased 2,3-DPG makes it more difficult for the hemoglobin to combine with oxygen in the lungs.

If the concentration of 2,3-DPG falls, as it does in stored blood or during sepsis, the hemoglobin holds onto its oxygen more tightly and the Pa_{O_2} tends to fall.

Table 9-7. P_{O_2} Levels at Various Temperatures

Temperature, °F	104.0	102.2	100.4	98.6	95.0	86.6
Temperature, °C	40	39	38	37	35	32
Pa_{O_2}, mmHg*	117	111	105	100	90	76

* Assuming a pH of 7.40 and a hemoglobin saturation of 98.4%.

Other Methods for Evaluating Oxygenation

Pa_{O_2}/FI_{O_2} Ratio

A quick way to estimate the impairment of oxygenation is to calculate the Pa_{O_2}/FI_{O_2} ratio. Normally, the ratio is about 500 to 600, which usually correlates to a pulmonary shunt (Q_s/Q_t) of about 3 to 5 percent. However, if a patient has a Pa_{O_2} of 80 mmHg on 40% oxygen, the Pa_{O_2}/FI_{O_2} ratio is 80/0.4, or 200. A Pa_{O_2}/FI_{O_2} ratio of less than 200 corresponds with a Q_s/Q_t of about 20 percent and generally indicates a need for ventilatory support. The usual relationship between Pa_{O_2}/FI_{O_2} ratios and the Q_s/Q_t in patients with a normal cardiac output is tabulated as follows (Table 9-8).

Respiratory Index

Another method for evaluating the Pa_{O_2} in relation to the FI_{O_2} is to calculate the respiratory index (RI), which is the alveolar-arterial oxygen difference $[P(A - a)_{O_2}]$ divided by the Pa_{O_2}.

The PA_{O_2} can be calculated by the alveolar gas equation:

$$PA_{O_2} = PB - (P_{H_2O})(FI_{O_2}) - Pa_{CO_2}(CF)$$

where CF, the correction factor, is 1.2 if RQ = 0.8 and 1.0 if RQ = 1.0.

At sea level, one can assume $PB = 760$ and $P_{H_2O} = 47$. Thus, if the FI_{O_2} is 0.40, the Pa_{CO_2} is 40, and the RQ is 0.8, then

$$\begin{aligned} PA_{O_2} &= (760 - 47)(0.4) - (40)(1.2) \\ &= (713)(0.4) - 48 \\ &= 285 - 48 = 237 \text{ mmHg} \end{aligned}$$

One can also estimate the PA_{O_2} with an FI_{O_2} of 0.30 or higher by multiplying the percentage of oxygen inhaled by 6; for example, the PA_{O_2} on 40% O_2 is 40 × 6, or 240 mmHg.

Thus, if the patient has a Pa_{O_2} of 80 mmHg on 40% O_2, the $P(A - a)_{O_2}$ could be estimated as 240 − 80 = 160 mmHg.

A patient with an RI of 1.0 and a cardiac index of 3.0 L/min per meter has a Q_s/Q_t of about 15 percent. If the RI is 2.0 with a cardiac index of 2.0 L/min per square meter, the Q_s/Q_t is about 22 to 25 percent.

Physiologic Shunting in the Lung (Venous-Arterial Admixture) (Q_s/Q_t)

Although abnormal gas diffusion or distribution in the lungs can cause abnormal blood gases, the most important cause is usually ventilation-perfusion (V/Q) mismatching. When considering ventilation and perfusion, there can be four types of alveolar capillary units: (1) If ventilation and perfusion are normal, the unit is normal. (2) If there is ventilation without perfusion, the unit is considered to be dead space. (3) If there is perfusion without ventilation, the unit is considered to be a (right-to-left) shunt. (4) If there is neither ventilation nor perfusion, the unit is silent.

The amount of physiologic shunting in the lung (or venous-arterial admixture) (Q_s/Q_t) is probably the most sensitive guide to the onset and progression of acute respiratory failure. The *shunt* refers to that fraction of blood passing through the lungs without being oxygenated. Normally, the amount for venous-arterial admixture is about 3 to 5

Table 9-8. Interpretation of Pa_{O_2}/FI_{O_2} Ratio

Pa_{O_2}	FI_{O_2}	Ratio	Q_s/Q_t	Abnormality
240	0.4	600	5%	None
120	0.4	300	10%	Minimal
100	0.4	250	15%	Mild
80	0.4	200	20%	Moderate
60	0.4	150	30%	Severe*
40	0.4	100	40%	Very Severe*

* In trauma or septic patients, ventilatory assistance and PEEP to reduce the Q_s/Q_t to 15 percent should be considered. The higher the Q_s/Q_t, the greater the need for ventilatory assistance and PEEP.

percent of the cardiac output. This small amount of shunting is largely due to bronchial veins draining into pulmonary veins.

Physiologic shunting is harder to determine than alveolar-arterial oxygen differences because it requires drawing both arterial and mixed venous (pulmonary artery) blood samples and determining their oxygen contents. Mixed venous samples from the pulmonary artery are preferable to those obtained from central venous pressure catheters. However, central venous blood does give a reasonable estimate of the amount of shunting present if cardiac output is relatively normal.

Although an $F\text{I}_{O_2}$ of 1.0 was generally used in the past to determine the amount of physiologic shunting in the lung, the high $F\text{I}_{O_2}$ in itself may cause increased shunting. Now the shunt with an $F\text{I}_{O_2}$ of 0.4 is considered to be a better indicator of lung function.

The Q_s/Q_t can be calculated from a modification of Berggren's formula:

$$\frac{Q_s}{Q_t} = \frac{Cc_{O_2} - Ca_{O_2}}{Cc_{O_2} - Cv_{O_2}}$$

where Cc_{O_2} is the pulmonary capillary oxygen content, Ca_{O_2} is the arterial content, and Cv_{O_2} is the mixed venous oxygen content. Thus if Cc_{O_2} is 20 mL/dL, Ca_{O_2} is 19 mL/dL, and Cv_{O_2} is 14 mL/dL, the shunt is

$$\frac{Q_s}{Q_t} = \frac{20 - 19}{20 - 14} = \frac{1}{6} = 17\%$$

The amount of shunting in the lung can also be estimated from arterial blood alone, using an assumption that the arteriovenous oxygen difference is approximately 5 mL/dL.

In general, if cardiac output doubles, the amount of shunt associated with a particular $P(\text{A} - a)_{O_2}$ increases by about 50 percent (Table 9-9). This is partly related to the fact that if only a small amount of blood is going through the lung, the blood flow tends to go to well-ventilated alveoli. If cardiac output increases, there is increasing likelihood that some of the blood will go through less well-ventilated tissue.

Thus, if cardiac output is high, a relatively mild hypoxemia can result in a high shunt. For example, at a P_{O_2} of 300 mmHg, if the cardiac output is 2.5 L/min, the shunt might be 11 percent, but at a cardiac output of 10.0 L/min, the shunt would be 32 percent. To factor in the changes due to an increased or decreased cardiac output, we have utilized the concept of shunt index. The shunt index (SI) is the percent shunt divided by the cardiac index. For example, at a normal cardiac index of 3.5 L/min per square meter and a shunt of 5.0 percent, the SI is 5.0/3.5 = 1.4. If a patient has a shunt of 20 percent, with a cardiac index of 2.5 L/min per square meter, the SI is 8.0. Patients with an SI above 5.0 usually require ventilatory support.

If the cardiac index is not known, the critical Q_s/Q_t is about 20 to 25 percent. Above these values the patient usually has enough of a V/Q abnormality to warrant aggressive ventilatory support and positive end-expiratory pressure (PEEP).

Table 9-9. Relation between the Physiologic Shunt in the Lung (Q_s/Q_t) and $P(\text{A} - a)_{O_2}$ While Breathing 100% O_2

		Q_s/Q_t, %		
Pa_{O_2}	$P(\text{A} - a)_{O_2}$ on 100% O_2	CO = 2.5 L/min	CO = 5 L/min	CO = 10 L/min
600	70	2	4	8
500	170	5	10	17
400	270	8	16	25
300	370	11	19	32
200	470	13	24	38
150	520	14	26	42
100	570	18	31	47
90	580	20	34	50
80	590	22	36	53
70	600	24	39	56
60	610	28	44	61
50	620	33	50	67

Oxygen Availability

Oxygen availability is determined by the amount of oxygen brought to the capillaries, or oxygen delivery (D_{O_2}), and the dissociation of oxyhemoglobin at the tissues. To a certain extent, a good heart, which can increase cardiac output appropriately, can make up for bad lungs and a low hemoglobin level. The reverse is also true. However, a combination of poor oxygenation, low hemoglobin level, and low cardiac output may be rapidly fatal.

Oxygen Content

The oxygen content of blood is determined primarily by the hemoglobin level and the oxyhemoglobin saturation. Each gram of hemoglobin measured clinically, when fully saturated, can carry 1.34 mL of oxygen. "Pure" hemoglobin can carry 1.39 mL of oxygen per gram, but clinically measured hemoglobin includes about 4 percent other compounds not carrying oxygen. Thus, a patient with a hemoglobin concentration of 15.0 g/dL can carry about 20.1 mL of oxygen per 100 mL in the red blood cells when the hemoglobin is fully saturated. Although the Pa_{O_2} determines the rate at which oxygen enters the tissues, it contributes very little to the total oxygen content of blood. Each mmHg of Pa_{O_2} represents only 0.0031 mL of oxygen in 100 mL of blood. Thus, a patient with a normal Pa_{O_2} of 100 mmHg has only 0.31 mL of oxygen dissolved in the plasma.

The oxygen content of arterial blood (Ca_{O_2}) can be calculated from the following formula:

$$Ca_{O_2} = [\text{Hb}]\,(1.34)\,(Sa_{O_2}/100) + (Pa_{O_2})\,(0.003)$$

Thus, in a patient with a hemoglobin concentration of 15.0 g/dL, an Sa_{O_2} of 98 percent, and a Pa_{O_2} of 100 mmHg:

$$Ca_{O_2} = (15)\,(1.34)\,(98/100) + (100)\,(0.003)$$
$$= 20.0 \text{ mL of } O_2 \text{ per dL of blood}$$

If the hemoglobin concentration falls to 10.0 g/dL, even if Sa_{O_2} and Pa_{O_2} remain the same, Ca_{O_2} falls by about a third. For example,

$$Ca_{O_2} = (10)\,(1.34)\,(98/100) + (100)\,(0.003)$$
$$= 13.132 + 0.300$$
$$= 13.4 \text{ mL of } O_2 \text{ per dL of blood}$$

Even with only 10 g of hemoglobin, the red blood cells are carrying over 40 times as much oxygen as the plasma.

Cardiac Output

Oxygen content (in milliliters per liter of blood) multiplied by cardiac output (in liters per minute) is equal to oxygen delivery (D_{O_2}). Thus the D_{O_2} in a patient with 15.0 g of 98% saturated hemoglobin, a Pa_{O_2} of 100 mmHg, and a cardiac output of 5 L/min is

$$D_{O_2} = (Ca_{O_2} \text{ per dL})\,(10)\,(\text{cardiac output})$$
$$= \{[\text{HB}]\,(1.34)\,(Sa_{O_2}/100) + (Pa_{O_2})\,(0.003)\}(10)\,(\text{cardiac output})$$
$$= [(15)\,(1.34)\,(98/100) + (100)\,(0.003)](10)\,(5)$$
$$= [(19.698 + 0.3)](50)$$
$$= (19.998)\,(50) = (20)\,(50)$$
$$= 1000 \text{ mL/min}$$

The factor 10 is used to convert oxygen content from milliliters per 100 mL of blood to milliliters per liter of blood.

Since the normal oxygen consumption of an average resting adult male is about 250 to 300 mL/min, the tissue normally takes up about 25 percent of the oxygen brought to it. Thus, the oxyhemoglobin saturation (S_{O_2}) falls from about 98 percent in arterial blood to about 73 percent in mixed venous blood. If there is no change in oxygen consumption, but cardiac output doubles to 10 L/min, the amount of oxygen removed from each liter of blood is halved, and the venous oxyhemoglobin saturation will be about 85 percent. On the other hand, if cardiac output falls to 2.5 L/min, oxyhemoglobin saturation will fall to about 48 percent.

Oxygen Dissociation in the Tissues

The ability of blood to give up more oxygen (increasing the arteriovenous oxygen difference) as cardiac output falls is an important homeostatic defense mechanism sometimes referred to as oxygen reserve. Unfortunately, there is a limit to this so-called oxygen reserve because the P_{O_2} in most tissues seldom falls below 26 mmHg with an oxyhemoglobin saturation of about 50 percent.

The lowest value to which the P_{O_2} in capillaries can fall is about 18 to 20 mmHg because this is the usual capillary-mitochondrial gradient for oxygen. The saturation at a P_{O_2} of 20 is referred to as the S_{20}, and this is normally about 33 percent. The only place where the P_{O_2} in venous blood is normally as low as 20 mmHg is the coronary sinus and perhaps the jugular venous bulb at the base of the brain. A relatively mild degree of alkalosis can raise the S_{20} by 4 to 5 percent, thereby greatly reducing oxygen availability to the myocardium. Thus, alkalosis in low flow states can be deleterious.

Combination of Hemoglobin with Carbon Monoxide

Carbon monoxide combines with hemoglobin at the same point on the hemoglobin molecule that oxygen does. Furthermore, it binds about 230 times more strongly than oxygen does. Therefore, an alveolar carbon monoxide level of only 0.4 mmHg, which is only 1/230 that of the Pa_{O_2}, allows the carbon monoxide to compete equally with oxygen for combination with hemoglobin, causing half the hemoglobin in the blood to bind with carbon monoxide instead of with oxygen. An alveolar carbon monoxide level of 0.7 mmHg (about 0.1% in air) can be lethal.

Oxygen at high alveolar pressures displaces carbon monoxide from hemoglobin much more rapidly than atmospheric oxygen does. The patient can also benefit from simultaneous administration of 4 to 5% carbon dioxide which strongly stimulates the respiratory center, increasing alveolar ventilation, reducing the alveolar carbon monoxide concentration, and allowing increased carbon monoxide to be released from the blood. A 96% oxygen and 4% carbon dioxide therapy removes carbon monoxide from the blood 10 to 20 times more rapidly than would be removed by breathing room air. The half-life of Hb–CO in a patient breathing room air is 2 to 3 h; if the patient is breathing 100% O_2, the half-life is about 20 to 30 min.

OTHER METHODS FOR EVALUATING BLOOD GASES

Pulmonary Artery Catheters

A number of pulmonary artery catheters have been developed to continuously monitor mixed venouos oxygen saturation (Sv_{O_2}). The normal Sv_{O_2} is about 70 to 75%. Changes in the Sv_{O_2} can provide early warning of problems with function of the lungs or cardiovascular system. If the Sv_{O_2} rises to 80% or higher, either the catheter tip is wedged so that pulmonary capillary (oxygenated) blood is being analyzed or the cardiac output has risen. (Table 9-10).

A fall in Sv_{O_2} below 50 to 60% is usually due to a significant decrease in cardiac output or lung function and requires urgent investigation. A change in Sv_{O_2} indicates important physiologic changes, but there can be major changes in the patient's condition without corresponding changes in the Sv_{O_2}.

Table 9-10. Clinical Conditions Associated with Different Mixed Venous Oxygen Saturations

Sv_{O_2}, %	Cardiac Output* L/min/m²	Associated Condition
>79	>4.0 +	Sepsis, cirrhosis, left to right shunts wedged PA catheter†
70–75	3.0–3.5	Normal
60–65	2.5–3.0	Slight cardiac decompensation or increased V_{O_2}
50–60	2.0–2.5	Moderate to severe cardiac decompensation; increasing lactic acidosis
33–50	1.5–2.0	Increasingly severe shock, coma

* Estimated from Hb of 10.0 to 12.0 g/dL, V_{O_2} = 120 − 150 mL/min per m².
† Pulmonary venous rather than pulmonary arterial blood being analyzed.

Systemic Arterial Probes

A further development in the area of blood gas tension analysis is the intravascular probe. Although intravascular oxygen sensors have been available for some time, their usefulness has been limited by the loss of sensitivity if the electrode has protein deposits accumulated on the membrane. Recently, intravascular probes using fiberoptic light channels and specific fluorescent compounds to continuously measure pH, Pa_{O_2}, and Pa_{CO_2} have been developed. Some of the more recently developed probes are so small that they will pass through a 20-gauge catheter and still leave sufficient clearance for pressure measurements and blood sampling. Clinical experience with these intravascular fiberoptic "blood gas machines" is limited; however, these catheters should find wide acceptance as the technology is perfected.

Noninvasive Monitoring

Pulse Oximetry

The use of pulse oximetry for monitoring oxygen saturation and pulse amplitude in the fingers, nose, or toes can provide early warning of pulmonary or cardiovascular deterioration before it is clinically apparent. This technique employs a microprocessor that continuously measures pulse rate and oxyhemoglobin saturation. The photosensor is not heated and does not require calibration. Oxyhemoglobin (HbO_2) is red and reduced hemoglobin (Hb) is blue, and each has a different absorption of light at their given wavelengths. Because the ratio of transmittance at each of the two wavelengths (660 nm, red; 940 nm, infrared) varies according to the percentage of HbO_2, pulse oximeters can be programmed to calculate and display the percentage of oxyhemoglobin saturation at each pulse.

There is a predictable correlation between noninvasive Sa_{O_2} and arterial oxygen saturation over a wide range of Sa_{O_2} values. Pulse oximetry has many advantages which make it ideal for use in the intensive care unit (Table 9-11). However, a number of factors can limit the effectiveness and accuracy of pulse oximetry. These include impaired local perfusion, abnormal hemoglobin, and very high P_{O_2}. Carboxy hemoglobin and fetal hemoglobin falsely raise oxyhemoglobin saturation readings while methemoglobin lowers them.

Table 9-11. Advantages of Pulse Oximetry (Stasic)

1. Noninvasive
2. Continuous real-time information
3. No calibration
4. May be left in place for many hours
5. Rapid response time (5 to 7 s)
6. Minimal error (1 to 2 percent) over the range of 60 to 90 percent saturation
7. Unaffected by skin pigmentation

Pulse oximetry helps to reduce the number of arterial blood gas determinations needed and can provide rapid feedback on therapeutic interventions. In spite of its limitations, it is increasingly becoming the standard of care in neonatal, pediatric, and adult intensive care units.

Capnography

Capnography, by providing a real-time estimate of Pa_{CO_2}, is a useful and accurate means of assessing ventilatory adequacy, respiratory gas exchange, carbon dioxide production, and cardiovascular status (primarily cardiac output). Although the measurement of end-tidal carbon dioxide partial pressure (PET_{CO_2}) underestimates Pa_{CO_2} by about 1 to 2 mmHg normally, the difference is constant for a given patient provided that the dead space/tidal volume (V_d/V_t) ratio and airway resistance are not changing.

Mainstream and side stream infrared capnometers are commercially available. A mainstream capnometer connects directly to the endotracheal tube, thus providing real-time breath-by-breath analysis. The major disadvantage of this system is its size and bulk and the fact that it cannot be used in nonintubated patients. Side stream capnometers aspirate gas at the sample site. The principal advantages of this system are that it reduces mechanical dead space and can be used in nonintubated patients; however, there are many mechanical factors related to gas sampling which require much expert attention and time and which can affect the results.

Because carbon dioxide production is directly dependent on metabolic rate, there are a large number of conditions that can lower PET_{CO_2}. However, sudden decreases in PET_{CO_2} suggest mechanical problems in the airway, hypoventilation, or increased dead space. A gradual decrease in the PET_{CO_2} is usually due to changes in the lung itself. Increases in the PET_{CO_2} are generally due to hypermetabolic states.

If a simultaneous Pa_{CO_2} is available, one can estimate the $P(A - a)_{CO_2}$. Normally this is zero, and if it suddenly increases, one should suspect a pulmonary embolus or drastic reduction in cardiac output.

The most frequent use of PET_{CO_2} is to evaluate the adequacy of ventilation. Inadvertent esophageal intubation, tracheal extubation, and endotracheal tube obstruction can be readily detected. These monitors can reduce the number of arterial blood gas determinations obtained and be very useful in weaning patients from mechanical ventilatory support. They can also be useful in determining the adequacy of circulation during CPR. In general, capnographs are relatively inexpensive, and they are reliable in a wide variety of clinical settings.

Transcutaneous Monitoring of Oxygen and Carbon Dioxide

In 1951 Baumberger and Goodfriend discovered that a finger immersed in a 45°C (113°F) electrolyte solution had a P_{O_2} equal to the Pa_{O_2}. As a consequence, electrochemical sensors have been developed to detect the P_{O_2} and P_{CO_2} at the surface of the skin.

Transcutaneous oxygen and carbon dioxide tension (PTC_{O_2} and PTC_{CO_2}) are important variables for the early warning of disturbed pulmonary function or systemic circulation as well as for the evaluation of local tissue perfusion. Comparative studies indicate that PTC_{O_2} and PTC_{CO_2} are more sensitive indicators of circulatory changes than conventional monitoring variables such as arterial pressure, heart rate, CVP, ECG, and urine output. If tissue perfusion is severely reduced, PTC_{O_2} and PTC_{CO_2} values deviate from their relationship with arterial partial pressures and become flow-dependent, thereby providing only qualitative information on blood flow.

Oxygen

In adults, PTC_{O_2} is nearly always substantially lower than Pa_{O_2}, partly because the thicker skin layer acts as a barrier to oxygen diffusion. Rithalia has noted that heating of the skin produces three major effects: (1) vasodilation of the cutaneous blood vessels; (2) right shift of the oxyhemoglobin dissociation curve, increasing the P_{O_2}; and (3) altered lipid structure of the stratum corneum, allowing more rapid diffusion of oxygen. Oxygen molecules which diffuse from the "arterialized" capillary bed to the skin surface are consumed at the electrode in an electrochemical reaction which alters current flow between a cathode and anode, proportional to the oxygen tension present.

Carbon Dioxide

The transcutaneous CO_2 electrode is separated from skin by a thin hydrophobic membrane that is permeable to carbon dioxide. Carbon dioxide molecules diffuse through the membrane and form carbonic acid (H_2CO_3), which alters the pH across a conventional pH-sensitive glass electrode.

Carbon dioxide diffuses fairly rapidly through the skin. Heating the skin causes: (1) faster diffusion of carbon dioxide to the skin surface, (2) decreased solubility of carbon dioxide, and (3) increased local metabolism and carbon dioxide production. These three heating effects cause transcutaneous CO_2 readings to be 1.2 to 2 times greater than arterial values.

In critically ill adults, PTC_{O_2} responds rapidly to changes in Pa_{O_2} and cardiac output. Its 95 percent response time is less than 2 min, even in patients with low-flow circulatory shock. In a study of high-risk surgical patients monitored perioperatively with PTC_{O_2} sensors and pulmonary artery catheters, Nolan and Shoemaker found that decreases in cardiac output, oxygen delivery, oxygen consumption, and PTC_{O_2} were the earliest warning signs of impending circulatory deterioration.

Although transcutaneous monitoring is a noninvasive technique and can provide constant real-time monitoring, it has a number of disadvantages. If the electrode site is not changed every 2 to 6 h, there is a risk of burns from the heated electrode. There may also be skin irritation from the adhesive ring.

Conjunctival Oxygen and Carbon Dioxide Measurements

In 1971, Kawan and Fatt attached a Clark P_{O_2} electrode to the anterior surface of a scleral contact lens as a means of continuously monitoring conjunctival oxygen tension (PCJ_{O_2}). More recently, miniaturized fiberoptic electrodes have been developed for conjunctival PCJ_{CO_2} and pH monitoring.

If cardiac output is adequate, PCJ_{O_2} tracks Pa_{O_2} during variations in blood oxygenation. However, during hemorrhagic shock, PCJ_{O_2} tracks cardiac output. If PA_{O_2} is adequate, the PCJ_{O_2}, like the PTC_{O_2}, follows local oxygen delivery. PCJ_{O_2} does not require a heated electrode because the conjunctiva does not have a stratum corneum that impedes oxygen diffusion. Since the conjunctiva is supplied by the ophthalmic branch of the internal carotid artery, PCJ_{O_2} may also reflect carotid arterial oxygen transport.

PCJ_{O_2} monitoring has been used to manage patients on mechanical ventilation, during extubation, and during therapeutic interventions. Kram and Shoemaker found that abrupt alterations in PCJ_{O_2} may reflect changes in ventilator mode, FI_{O_2}, therapy with fluids, vasopressors and vasodilators, or endotracheal tube suctioning. A sudden drop in PCJ_{O_2} may also be due to hypoxemia, pneumothorax, reduced cardiac output, or altered local perfusion.

Mass Spectrometry

Mass spectrometry allows measurement of all respiratory gases (carbon dioxide, oxygen, and nitrogen) and anesthetic gases on a breath-by-breath basis. Analysis of inspired and expired respiratory gases by mass spectrometry is rapid and accurate to 0.1 percent of the measurement value.

A mass spectrometer can evaluate the P_{CO_2} curve in order to determine inspired and expired gas values. Sudden changes may indicate mechanical changes in the ventilatory system or airway. Slower changes may indicate important changes in cardiopulmonary function.

Mass spectrometry can be used to continuously monitor several patients at a time. However, as the number of monitored beds increase, so does the time between analysis and results. Data analyzed by the mass spectrometer are not real-time but are generally delayed by at least 9 to 22 s. This delay results from the aspirated sample having to traverse up 150 ft of the catheter tubing before reaching the mass spectrometer. In a system with more than 10 monitoring stations, sample determinations may be delayed by more than 2 min, which is not frequent enough to prevent serious injury to the patient. Unless sampling from each patient can occur at least once a minute, alarms for low oxygen levels and low ventilator pressures and flow should be included. Another disadvantage of mass spectrometers is their high cost (over $35,000).

BIBLIOGRAPHY

Kram HB, Shoemaker WC: Transcutaneous, conjunctival, and organ PO_2 and PCO_2 monitoring in the adult, in Shoemaker WC, Ayres S, Grenvik A, et al (eds): *Textbook in Critical Care*. Philadelphia, Saunders, 1989, pp 283–291.

Laghi F, Siegel JH, Rivkind AL, et al: Respiratory index/pulmonary shunt relationship: Quantification of severity and prognosis in the post-traumatic adult respiratory syndrome. *Crit Care Med* 17:1121, 1989.

Macklem PT: Respiratory mechanics. *Ann Rev Physiol* 40:157, 1978.

Plant JCD: Functional anatomy of the respiratory tract and lungs, in Wilson RF, Wilson JA (eds): *Pulmonary Function and Respiratory Failure in Critically Ill and Injured Patients*. Detroit, Wayne State University, 1974.

Pontopidan H, Geffin B, Lowenstein E: Acute respiratory failure in that adult. *N Engl J Med* 287:743, 1972.

Shapiro BA, Cane RD: Blood gas monitoring: Yesterday, today and tomorrow. *Crit Care Med* 17:966, 1989.

Stasis AF: Continuous evaluation of oxygenation and ventilation, in Civetta JM, Taylor RW, Kirby RR (eds): *Critical Care*. Philadelphia, Lippincott, 1988, pp 317–325.

Taylor MB, Whitman JG: The current status of pulse oximetry. *Anesthesia* 41:943, 1986.

Viale JP, Percival CJ, Annat G. et al: Arterial-alveolar oxygen partial pressure ratio: A theoretical reappraisal. *Crit Care Med* 14:153, 1986.

10 FLUID AND ELECTROLYTE PROBLEMS

Robert F. Wilson

Fluid and electrolyte and acid-base problems occur frequently in critically ill patients. A general approach to these problems is as follows.

1. One should never completely trust the laboratory. Some of the worst complications of fluid and electrolyte or acid-base management have occurred when aggressive therapy was based on an erroneous laboratory result. Errors may occur in obtaining the sample, labeling the sample, performing the test, or reporting the result. If the laboratory result does not seem to correlate properly with the patient's condition or other data, three things should be done: (a) The patient and the patient's record should be carefully reexamined. (b) If the laboratory result still does not seem to fit, the test should be repeated. (c) If there is still a question about the laboratory result, a sample from a normal individual should be analyzed.
2. Abnormalities should be treated at approximately the rate at which they developed since biologic systems react primarily to rate of change and not to absolute concentrations. For example, one should not rapidly correct a chronic asymptomatic abnormality. Even when an abnormality has developed rather rapidly, only half the calculated deficit should be corrected at a time. The patient is then reevaluated and the laboratory tests repeated to determine the rate and amount of correction still required.
3. The priorities for correcting multiple fluid, electrolyte, and acid-base abnormalities are as follows: first, fluid volume and perfusion deficits; second, pH; third, potassium, calcium, and magnesium abnormalities; and fourth sodium and chloride abnormalities. If blood volume and tissue perfusion are restored to normal, many electrolyte and acid-base abnormalities will correct themselves spontaneously.
4. One should not correct the pH without also evaluating potassium, calcium, and magnesium levels, and in no instance should one be corrected without considering the effect that it may have on the others. For example, acidosis is often associated with hyperkalemia and increased plasma levels of ionized calcium and magnesium. Alkalosis lowers plasma levels of potassium and ionized calcium and magnesium. If a severely acidotic patient has a low serum potassium level, one should suspect either laboratory error or severe potassium deficiency. As a general rule, if all the measured electrolyte levels are low, symptoms are apt to be less severe than if only one were decreased.

ATOMIC WEIGHTS

Proper correction of electrolyte abnormalities may be facilitated by some knowledge of the atomic weights of the elements most likely to be involved in fluid and electrolyte problems (Table 10-1). The equivalent weight is the atomic weight divided by its usual electrical charge or valence. For example, if the plasma level of ionized calcium, which has an atomic weight of 40 and an equivalent weight of 20, is 4.0 mg/dL, the concentration of ionized calcium can be expressed as 2.0 mEq/L or 1.0 mmol/L. Magnesium sulfate is usually stocked and given in terms of grams without indicating how many mEq of magnesium are present. Knowing the atomic weights, one can readily calculate the molecular weight of $MgSo_4 \cdot 7H_2O$ as 24 + 32 + (4)(16) + (7)(18) = 246. Thus, 1 g of $MgSO_4$ contains 4.06 mmol of Mg or 8.1 mEq Mg.

WATER

Normally about 55 to 60 percent of the body weight of an adult is water. In the newborn, there is relatively more water, usually equivalent to 70 to 80 percent of the body weight. Fat is relatively anhydrous, and muscle is about 77 percent water. Consequently, obese adult women may have less than 50 percent of their weight as water, and muscular men may have more than 60 to 65 percent of their weight as water.

Osmolarity and Osmolality

Alterations in the amount of water present in the various fluid spaces are primarily related to the *number* of particles present in a given volume of solution, or *colligative properties*. Osmotic pressure is one of the colligative properties with which we are most concerned. The osmotic pressure of serum is largely regulated by antidiuretic hormone (ADH), which increases water reabsorption in the collecting ducts of the kidney. The most important stimuli to ADH secretion, in descending order of potency, are nausea, pain, hypovolemia, and hyperosmolarity. Hypovolemia is a much stronger stimulus to ADH secretion than hypoosmolarity is an inhibitor. Consequently, increased ADH secretion tends to perpetuate hyponatremia in hypovolemic patients.

Serum osmolarity can be measured directly by determining the freezing point of the serum. Serum osmolarity can also be calculated from the sodium, glucose, and blood urea nitrogen (BUN) levels using the following formula:

$$\text{Osmolarity} = 2(\text{Na}) + \frac{\text{glucose}}{18} + \frac{\text{BUN}}{2.8}$$

where the glucose (mg/dL) and BUN (mg/dL) are divided by their respective molecular weights divided by 10 (because we are working with deciliters and not liters).

Thus, normal serum osmolarity, which is about 275 to 295 mOsm/L, can usually be calculated as

$$S_{\text{Osm}} = 2(140) + \frac{90}{18} + \frac{14}{2.8} = 280 + 5 + 5 = 290$$

The osmotic contributions from mannitol (mg/dL ÷ 18), glycerol (mg/dL ÷ 9), and ethanol (mg/dL ÷ 4.6) can also be included. This equation will not provide an accurate estimate of extracellular fluid (ECF) osmolality if other (unexpected or unknown) solutes are present in significant quantity. Thus, a difference or "gap" between measured and calculated osmolality of more than 10 mOsm/kg should suggest the presence of another solute, such as lactate, ethanol, methanol, etc. An osmolar gap of more than 50 mOsm/L is often fatal.

The terms osmolarity, osmolality, oncotic pressure, and tonicity are often confused. *Osmolarity* refers to the number of particles per liter of solution (e.g., plasma), whereas *osmolality* refers to the number of particles per liter of solvent (e.g., plasma water). Since plasma is

Table 10-1. Atomic and Equivalent Weights

Element	Symbol	Atomic Weight	Equivalent Weight
Calcium	Ca	40	20
Carbon	C	12	3
Chlorine	Cl	35.5	35.5
Hydrogen	H	1	1
Magnesium	Mg	24	12
Oxygen	O	16	8
Phosphorus	P	31	6.2
Potassium	K	39	39
Sodium	Na	23	23
Sulfur	S	32	5.3

about 91 to 93 percent water, osmolality reflects osmotic pressure better and is usually 7 to 9% higher than the osmolarity.

The plasma *oncotic pressure* is the difference in osmotic pressure created by the presence of protein or other relatively nonpermeable substances, assuming that the plasma is equilibrated against a solution having the same ionic composition as plasma but lacking protein. The concentration of diffusible ions is higher in the plasma by 0.43 mmol/L than in interstitial fluid. The sum of 0.43 mmol/L and the protein concentration, which is 0.8 mmol/L, determines the plasma oncotic pressure. Since each mmol/L generates 19.3 mmHg of oncotic pressure ($\Delta\pi$),

$$\Delta\pi = 1.23 \times 19.3 \text{ mmHg} = 23.7 \text{ mmHg}$$

When the extracellular osmolality is increased by solutes restricted to the extracellular fluid, the intracellular osmolality is increased by a shift of water from the cell to the extracellular fluid. The osmols which can cause a shift of water out of the cells are called "effective" osmols, and those that distribute across the cell membrane equally and therefore do not cause shift of water out of the cell may be termed "ineffective" osmols.

The osmolality produced by effective osmols is referred to as *tonicity* or *effective osmolality*. The principal extracellular electrolytes—sodium, chloride, and bicarbonate—are all effective osmols. Glucose is an effective osmol for most, but not all cells. For example, it easily enters red blood cells, hepatocytes, and osmoreceptor cells in the brain and hence does not draw water from them. Thus, when we consider a substance as an effective osmol, it is usually in reference to muscle, the organ that represents the greatest bulk of the body's tissues.

Some solutes (e.g., urea, ethanol, methanol, and ethylene glycol) pass freely across cell membranes and do not exert a force for water movement between the two major body fluid compartments. Such noneffective solutes contribute to body fluid osmolality but not to tonicity. Tonicity cannot be measured, but it can be estimated, under normal circumstances, as follows:

$$2 \times [Na^+] + \frac{[\text{glucose}]}{18} = (2 \times 140) + \frac{90}{18} = 285 \text{ mOsm/kg } H_2O$$

If mannitol, glycerol, and sorbitol are present in the ECF, they must be included in this calculation. Urea, ethanol, methanol, and ethylene glycol, no matter how severe the azotemia or the intoxication, need not be included.

Fluid Spaces

Total body water is normally divided into intracellular fluid (ICF) and extracellular fluid (ECF). Intracellular fluid is about 30 to 35 percent of the body weight, and ECF (which includes water in interstitial fluid, plasma, bone, connective tissue, and transcellular fluid) is about 25 to 30 percent of the body weight (Table 10-2).

Extracellular Fluid

Some of the fluid markers (such as sodium, chloride, and bromide) used to estimate the size of the ECF space also penetrate cells to varying degrees. Thus, they overestimate the ECF. Conversely, other ECF markers (such as insulin, mannitol, and sucrose) do not penetrate certain parts of the extracellular fluid space and therefore underestimate ECF. As a result, depending on the type of marker used, the calculated ECF may vary from 27 to 45 percent of the total body water.

Normally the intracellular water (ICW) is about 55 percent of the total body water (TBW), and the exchangeable potassium (K_e), which is primarily in ICW, is about 80 mEq/L in the TBW. In malnutrition, ICW falls, ECF increases, and K_e can fall to about 50 mEq/L in the TBW. In contrast, the total exchangeable Na (Na_e), which is normally about 75 mEq/L of TBW, can rise with malnutrition, trauma, or sepsis to about 95 mEq/L of TBW. Thus, the ratio of K_e to Na_e, which is normally about 1.05 to 1.10 (80/75), can fall to about 0.55 (50/95) in severe malnutrition. In sepsis, the K_e/Na_e can fall even lower.

Table 10-2. Size and Sodium and Potassium Content of Various Fluid Spaces

	% Body Weight	% Total Body Na	% Total Body K
Plasma	4.5	1.2	0.4
Interstitial fluid (lymph)	12.0	20.0	1.0
Dense connective tissue and cartilage	4.5	11.7	0.4
Bone	4.5	43.1	7.6
Transcellular	1.5	2.6	1.0
Total extracellular	27.0	97.6	10.4
Total intracellular	33.0	2.4	89.6
Total body	60.0	100.0	100.0

The electrolyte concentrations in the plasma and interstitial fluid are approximately the same except for protein-bound electrolytes, such as calcium and magnesium. Cellular fluid has much more potassium, magnesium, phosphate, and protein than ECF, but it has relatively little sodium and very little calcium or chloride (Table 10-3).

Interstitial Fluid (ISF)

Characteristics

The ISF space is not physiologically uniform. It consists of a small liquid and large gel phase invested by a fibrous meshwork, the latter made up largely of collagen fibers that hold the cells together. The ground substance between the collagen fibers consists largely of anionic polymers, referred to as glycosaminoglycans, which bind cations selectively and limit their mobility to varying degrees. Glycosaminoglycans also limit the mobility of water, holding some of the bound water in an icelike lattice.

Only a small part of the interstitial fluid is freely movable, and this portion is felt to have the following characteristics:

1. The ion concentrations are predictable by the Donnan equilibrium.
2. Interstitial protein is dissolved in this portion.
3. This portion exchanges water with the capillary fluid.
4. This is the route for water to move from capillaries to lymphatics.

The electrolyte concentrations of interstitial fluid, obtained primarily by the analysis of lymph fluid, probably reflect the average composition of the freely movable interstitial fluid fairly accurately.

Donnan Equilibrium

The concentrations of electrolytes in the interstitial fluid are different from those in the plasma because the concentration of proteins is much

Table 10-3. The Electrolyte Concentration of Body Fluids (mEq/L)

Solution	Seawater	Extracellular Fluid	Interstitial Fluid	Intracellular Fluid
Cations				
Sodium	425	142	144	10
Potassium	15	4.5	4.5	150
Magnesium	105	2	1.0	40
Calcium	35	4.5	2.5	
Total	580	153	152	200
Anions				
Chloride	500	102	113	—
Phosphates	10	2	2	120
Sulfates	45	1	1	30
Bicarbonate	25	27	30	10
Protein	—	16	1	40
Organic acids	—	5	5	
Total	580	153	152	200

lower in interstitial fluid. When two solutions are separated by a membrane permeable to water and small ions, and when one of the solutions contains more nonpermeable ions than the other, the distribution of permeable or diffusible ions occurs in a predictable manner which can be calculated from the products of the diffusible cations and anions in each solution according to the requirements of the Donnan equilibrium:

$$(C^+ \text{ plasma})(A^- \text{ plasma}) = (C^+ \text{ ISF})(A^- \text{ ISF})$$

On the average, the proteinate anion concentration in plasma is 16 mEq/L and in interstitial fluids the proteinate anion is 8 mEq/L. If the concentrations of diffusible cations and anions in the plasma are 156 and 140 mEq/L, respectively, the concentrations of diffusible cations and anions in the interstitial fluid can be calculated from the equation

$$156 \times 140 = c(c - 8)$$

where c is the diffusible cation concentration in the interstitial fluid and $c - 8$ is the concentration of diffusible anions. Thus, $c^2 - 8c - 21{,}840 = 0$, and $c = 152$ mEq/L. Thus, the concentration of diffusible anions is 144 mEq/L (Table 10-4).

Intracellular Fluid

Intracellular fluid has much more potassium, magnesium, phosphate, and protein than ECF, but it has relatively little sodium and almost no calcium or chloride. However, the electrolyte concentration of intracellular fluid varies greatly from tissue to tissue. For example, in muscle the concentration of chloride is 2 to 3 mEq/L, and the resting membrane potential of the cell membrane is about −90 mV. In contrast, in erythrocytes the concentration of chloride is about 70 mEq/L and the cell membrane potential is only about −7 mV.

The potassium concentration in muscle cells is about 160 mEq/L, whereas in platelets it is only 118 mEq/L. The concentration of sodium in muscle cells and in red blood cells is 12 to 17 mEq/L, but the sodium concentration in leukocytes is about 34 mEq/L. Because muscle represents the bulk of the body cell mass, it is customary to use the electrolyte concentration of muscle cells as representative of the total body's intracellular electrolyte concentration.

Daily Fluid Requirements

Daily fluid requirements include (1) basic needs for urine and insensible water loss; (2) current losses for gastrointestinal loss, sweat, or increased loss of insensible water; and (3) correction for any deficits or excesses.

Basic Needs

Basic needs include urine loss of about 600 to 1000 mL/m² per day and an insensible water loss of about 350 to 700 mL/m² per day. In a normal 70-kg adult man, this amounts to about 1000 to 1500 mL of urine and 1000 mL of insensible water loss per day. Insensible water loss includes about 300 mL from the skin and 700 mL from the lungs per day. It is pure water of evaporation and contains essentially no electrolytes. In contrast, sweat has an electrolyte content equivalent to about 0.2 to 0.3 N saline.

Table 10-4. Distribution of Electrolytes Across the Capilliary According to the Donnan Equilibrium (mEq/L)

	Plasma	Interstitial Fluid
Diffusible cations	156	152
Diffusible anions	140	144
Protein anions	16	8
Total	312	304

Table 10-5. Average Electrolyte Content of Various Body Fluids (mEq/L)

	Sodium	Potassium	Chloride	Bicarbonate	Volume/Day
Saliva	10–60	10–20	15–40	30–15	1000–2000
Stomach	40–100	5–15	15–20	—	1500–2500
Bile	130–140	4–6	95–105	30–40	50–1000
Pancreas	130–140	4–6	40–60	80–100	1000–2000
Small intestine	130–140	4–6	40–60	80–100	1000–2000
Colon	80–140	25–45	80–100	30–50	100–600
Sweat	40–50	5–10	45–60	—	200–1500

Current Losses

Current losses can include (1) about 500 mL of increased insensible water loss per 1°C fever, (2) 500 to 1500 mL extra for sweating, and (3) a mL for mL loss of gastrointestinal fluid. The electrolyte content of the various fluids that may be lost from the body vary greatly; some average values are given in Table 10-5.

Deficits

Water deficits can be estimated from weight loss, thirst, and physical signs. Severe thirst usually indicates a fluid deficit of at least 2 or 3 percent of the body weight. Soft eyes, tachycardia, severe oliguria, or organ dysfunction usually indicate severe dehydration. An adult patient who appears slightly, moderately, or severely dehydrated has lost fluid equal to 6, 8, or 10 percent of total body weight, respectively. Thus, a severely dehydrated 70-kg man has lost at least 7.0 L of fluid. An infant with mild, moderate, or severe dehydration has lost water equivalent to 5, 10, and 15 percent of total body weight, respectively.

Oliguria is generally due to hypovolemia and impaired renal perfusion causing a prerenal azotemia. Occasionally, however, oliguria may be due to renal disease or injury. Some of the tests used to differentiate these two entities are listed in Table 10-6.

In general, a urine output of 0.5 mL/kg per hour or more indicates adequate fluid repletion, except in the presence of high-output renal failure, glycosuria, or diuretics.

SODIUM

The total body sodium content is normally about 40 mEq/kg of body weight or about 2800 mEq in the normal 70-kg man. Almost 98 percent is present in ECF, where the concentration is about 140 mEq/L. About one-third is fixed in bone and the other two thirds is readily exchangeable in isotopic studies. However, intracellular sodium levels are usually less than 10 to 12 mEq/L.

Table 10-6. Tests Differentiating Oliguria due to Renal Failure from Oliguria Due to Prerenal Azotemia

Test	Prerenal Azotemia	Renal Failure
FeNa = $\dfrac{U_{Na}/P_{Na}}{U_{Cr}/P_{Cr}} \times 100\%$	$<1\%$	$>3\%$
BUN/Cr ratio ($S_{Cr} < 4.0$ mg/dL)	$>20:1$	$<10:1$
Urine osmolarity	>450	<300
Urine S.G.	>1.015	<1.010

Hyponatremia

Etiology

General Causes

Dilution

The total body sodium content tends to be kept rather constant by the kidneys, and consequently the most frequent cause of hyponatremia is too much TBW, producing a dilutional hypoatremia. The tendency to retain water can be greatly increased in patients with severe trauma, sepsis, cardiac failure, cirrhosis, renal failure, or chronic malnutrition.

Sodium Loss

Occasionally hyponatremia is due to sodium loss. Some of the more frequent causes of sodium loss include excessive vomiting, diarrhea, and sweating. If these losses are not corrected, the ECF and urine sodium concentration will fall. However, if these losses are treated with fluids that do not contain adequate sodium, a severe hyponatremia may develop. Increased urine sodium losses occur with diuretics, adrenal insufficiency, salt-losing nephritis, cystic disease of the renal medulla, the postoliguric phase of acute vasomotor nephropathy, and after renal transplantation or relief of urinary obstruction. Other less obvious causes of increased urine sodium loss include ketoacidosis and metabolic alkalosis with hypokalemia.

Factitious Hyponatremia

Factitious hyponatremia may be due to severe hyperglycemia, hyperlipidemia, or hyperproteinemia. Because glucose tends to stay in ECF, hyperglycemia tends to draw water out of cells into the ECF. Each 100 mg/dL increase in plasma glucose levels decreases the serum sodium concentration by about 1.6 to 1.8 mEq/L. Thus, if the blood glucose level of a previously normal patient rose to 1100 mg/dL, the patient's serum sodium concentration would fall to about 122 to 124 mEq/L.

In "true" hyponatremia, plasma osmolarity is reduced; in "factitious" hyponatremia, plasma osmolality is usually normal or increased. Mannitol, if present in excessive quantities, can produce factitious hyponatremia in a manner and quantity almost identical to that of glucose. If 100 g of mannitol is given rapidly and almost none is excreted, theoretically its concentration in the ECF of a 70-kg man could be as high as 7.0 g or 7000 mg/L (700 mg/dL). This could lower serum sodium levels by about 11.2 to 12.6 mEq/L, but plasma osmolarity would be normal.

Normally, plasma water occupies approximately 910 to 930 mL of each liter of plasma. High levels of plasma lipids or proteins increase plasma volume, decreasing the percentage that is water. This can be important if sodium determinations are performed with flame emission spectrophotometry (FES), which measures the mass of sodium in a given volume of serum. If the serum sodium concentration measured by FES is 140 mmol/L and if serum water occupies 93 percent of the serum volume, then the concentration of sodium in serum water will be 140 mmol/L divided by 0.93, which equals 150 mmol/L, which is normal. If the plasma contained only 86 percent water, then the serum sodium reported by FES would only be 129 mEq/L even though the concentration of sodium in the serum water would actually be 150 mEq/L.

In states of hyperproteinemia (e.g., multiple myeloma) or hyperlipidemia (familial, idiopathic, or secondary), there is an increased mass of the nonaqueous components of serum and a concomitant decrease in the proportion of serum composed of water. The serum water fraction can be estimated from the following equation adapted from Waugh:

$$S_W = 99.1 - 0.1(S_L) - 0.07(S_P)$$

where S_W is the percentage of serum volume occupied by water, S_L is the serum lipid concentration (g/L), and S_P is the serum protein concentration (g/L). Normally, the total serum lipids (triglicerides of 40 to 150 mg/dL and cholesterol of 140 to 220 mg/dL) are about 2 to 4 g/L and serum proteins are about 60 to 75 g/L. For example, in a patient with an abnormally high serum lipid concentration of 50 g/L and a normal protein concentration (74 g/L), only 88 percent of the serum volume will be occupied by water. If the concentration of sodium in serum water were normal (150 mmol/L), then the serum sodium concentration measured by the FES would be 150 mmol/L × 0.88 = 132 mmol/L, clearly below the normal range.

Ion selective electrodes measure sodium activity in serum water only. That activity is unaffected by the proportion of serum occupied by water. Thus, in the aforementioned case, the sodium activity in the undiluted specimen would be about 150 mmol/L, a normal value for the sodium concentration in serum water.

Hyperlipidemia is seen in 20 to 70 percent of persons with diabetes mellitus (DI) and in up to 50 percent of patients admitted to the hospital with diabetic ketoacidosis. Hyperlipidemia is more common and severe in patients with poor glucose control, and such patients are prone to ketoacidosis or hyperosomolar hyperglycemic nonketotic states. In one series, 38 percent of patients with severe diabetic ketoacidosis were found to be hyponatremic.

Classification by Functional ECF

The major causes of hyponatremia can be classified according to the functional ECF volume and urine sodium concentrations (Table 10-7). Once it is clear that the hyponatremia is "real" and plasma osmolality has been documented to be less than 280 mOsm/kg, one should make a clinical estimate of the ECF volume of the patient. This estimation can be assisted by looking for predisposing factors such as vomiting or diarrhea, diuretic use, and preexisting disease such as primary nephropathy, liver or heart disease, and CNS disorders. A careful review of the fluid intake and output as well as their composition over the past few days is important. The physical examination should emphasize findings that define the patient's state of hydration. Certain laboratory tests that may be useful include serum electrolytes, urea nitrogen, creatinine, glucose, and osmolality and urine electrolytes and osmolality. With these data, one can usually classify the patient's hyponatremia into one of three categories: (1) hypotonic hyponatremia associated with hypovolemia, (2) hypotonic hyponatremia associated with normal or only slightly increased ECF volume, and (3) hypotonic hyponatremia associated with hypervolemia or edema.

Table 10-7. Causes of Hyponatremia

- I. Hyponatremia with decreased ECF
  - A. Extrarenal losses; urinary Na < 20 mEq/L
    1. Sweating, vomiting, diarrhea
    2. Third-space sequestration (burns, peritonitis, pancreatitis)
  - B. Renal losses; urinary Na > 20 mEq/L
    1. Loop or osmotic diuretics
    2. Aldosterone deficiency (Addison's disease)
    3. Ketonuria
    4. Salt-losing nephropathies; renal tubular acidosis
- II. Hyponatremia with normal ECF; urinary Na > 20 mEq/L
  - A. Inappropriate ADH secretion
  - B. Sick-cell or "reset osmostat" syndromes
  - C. Physical and emotional stress or pain
  - D. Myxedema, Addison's disease, Sheehan's syndrome
- III. Hyponatremia with increased ECF
  - A. Urinary Na > 20 mEq/L
    1. Renal failure
  - B. Urinary Na < 20 mEq/L
    1. Cirrhosis
    2. Cardiac failure
    3. Renal failure
- IV. Pseudohyponatremia (hyperproteinemia, hyperlipidemia, hyperglycemia)

Hypovolemic Hyponatremia

These conditions are associated with loss of both water and sodium, with replacement with relatively more water than sodium. In hypovolemic patients with healthy kidneys not receiving diuretics, the urine sodium concentration is usually less than 20 mEq/L; however, in severe metabolic alkalosis secondary to vomiting, increased amounts of sodium are lost in the urine along with the increased urine bicarbonate.

By far the most common cause of hypovolemic hyponatremia in children is viral gastroenteritis causing vomiting and/or diarrhea. Fistulas and various types of gastrointestinal tubes occasionally cause this condition. Another cause is excessive sweating, especially in patients with cystic fibrosis and adrenal insufficiency. A similar disturbance occurs when isotonic body fluid is translocated within the body to a "third space." The unequal balance of electrolyte and water loss produces a contracted ECF and a hyponatremia that is maintained by the inability of the kidneys to excrete free water. The impairment of water excretion to defend ECF volume at the expense of tonicity is accomplished by (1) decreased glomerular filtration, (2) increased proximal tubular reabsorption of solute and water, (3) decreased delivery of fluid to the diluting segment of the nephron, and (4) the presence of ADH released by nonosmotic stimuli.

Excessive renal loss of sodium can be caused by a number of drugs, endogenous (osmotic) diuretics, mineralocorticoid deficiency, and certain primary kidney disorders. In these conditions the urine sodium concentration is greater than 20 mEq/L. Under the influence of loop diuretics, the kidneys cannot appropriately dilute or concentrate the urine. Loop diuretics can also cause volume depletion and hypokalemia. The hypokalemia, in turn, tends to cause an intracellular movement of sodium, further contributing to the hyponatremia.

Osmotic diuretics cause increased urinary losses of sodium and water, resulting in ECF volume depletion and hyponatremia. Other causes of increased urinary sodium losses in concentrations that are at least half isotonic are glucosuria associated with uncontrolled diabetes mellitus, urea diuresis after relief of urinary tract obstruction, and administration of mannitol for the treatment of cerebral edema. Hyperglycemia and mannitol also make hyponatremia worse by causing the movement of water from the intracellular space to the ECF compartment.

The combination of hyponatremia, ECF volume contraction, hyperkalemia, and renal sodium wasting without renal failure suggests the possibility of adrenal insufficiency. Decreased mineralocorticoid secretion impairs the reabsorption of sodium in exchange for potassium and hydrogen ions in the distal tubule.

Salt wasting sufficient to cause hyponatremia occurs in certain renal disorders, such as medullary cystic disease, polycystic kidney disease, and obstructive uropathy, even in the absence of any renal excretory impairment. Patients with advanced renal failure have an impaired ability to conserve sodium, but the defect is usually mild and does not cause hyponatremia unless the patient is severely sodium-restricted. Proximal renal tubular acidosis (type 2 RTA) may also cause sodium wasting, because the bicarbonate ion, which is lost in greatly increased quantities, obligates the excretion of sodium. Hyperkalemic renal tubular acidosis (type 4 RTA) is characterized by aldosterone insensitivity of the renal tubules, high aldosterone levels, hyperkalemia, metabolic acidosis, and hyponatremia. In all of these disorders the urinary sodium concentration is relatively high despite the presence of hypovolemia.

For the most part, extrarenal sodium losses are associated with a low urinary sodium concentration. Conversely, primary renal disorders and drug- and hormone-induced renal dysfunction are associated with renal salt wasting and a high urinary sodium concentration.

Euvolemic Hyponatremia

Patients described as having a combination of euvolemia and hyponatremia usually have a slightly increased ECF volume; however, these patients are not edematous and have a near-normal total body sodium content, despite the presence of hyponatremia. If symptoms are present, they are usually CNS manifestations of hypotonicity. Urinary sodium concentration is usually greater than 20 mEq/L and may be much higher in states of ADH excess, which is the most important factor in the initiation and perpetuation of most cases of euvolemic hyponatremia.

The syndrome of inappropriate (excess) secretion of ADH (SIADH) is the most common cause of euvolemic hyponatremia in children. The chronic hyponatremia of this syndrome is sustained by a constant or intermittent secretion of ADH, which is inappropriate in relation to both osmotic and volume stimuli. The diagnostic criteria are

1. Hypotonicity and hyponatremia (plasma osmolality $<$ 280 mOsm/kg H_2O)
2. Inappropriately concentrated urine (urine osmolality $>$ 100 mOsm/kg H_2O)
3. High urine sodium concentration (except during sodium restriction)
4. No clinical evidence of hypervolemia or hypovolemia
5. Normal renal, cardiac, hepatic, adrenal, and thyroid function
6. Correctable by severe water restriction

It should be noted that if serum osmolality exceeds 300 mOsm/L, urine osmolality should exceed 600 to 1200 mOsm/L. However, if serum osmolality is less than 270 to 280 mOsm/L, there should be almost no ADH secretion and urine osmolality should be 50 mOsm/L or less.

The diagnosis of SIADH is primarily one of exclusion. The diagnosis should be considered only in the absence of hypovolemia, hypervolemia (edema), endocrine dysfunction, renal failure, and drugs which may impair water excretion. Drugs which tend to cause hypotonic hyponatremia either stimulate the release of ADH centrally or potentiate its effect on the kidney, or both. The most frequent other causes of SIADH are malignancies, pulmonary disorders, and CNS infections or other CNS disorders (Table 10-8).

SIADH is most common in children with CNS infections, and the condition is worsened by the administration of usual volumes of parenteral fluids. Because the CNS symptoms and signs caused by hyponatremia may be obscured by primary CNS disease, hyponatremia itself may be the first clue to the diagnosis. It is important to remember that if the serum osmolality is less than 270 to 280 mOsm/kg, the urine osmolality should be less than 50 mOsm/kg. Furthermore, SIADH is a problem of water retention, not sodium depletion; therefore, aggressive sodium administration is appropriate only to relieve neurologic symptoms. Attempts to correct the hyponatremia of SIADH with sodium-rich solutions will cause an increase in urinary sodium excretion but little change in the serum sodium.

A variant of SIADH known as "reset osmostat" is not uncommon in chronically ill or malnourished individuals. This condition identifies

Table 10-8. Causes of SIADH

Central nervous system disorders	Drugs
Head trauma	Narcotics
Brain tumors, brain abscesses	Chlorpropamide
Meningitis, encephalitis	NSAIDs
Subarachnoid hemorrhage	Vincristine, vinblastine
Delirium tremens	Cyclophosphamide, phenothiazines
Tumors	Monoamine oxidase inhibitors
Lung cancer (especially small-cell), cancer of the pancreas, ovarian cancer	Tricyclic antidepressants
	Thiazide diuretics
Lymphoma	Endocrine disorders
Thymoma	Hypothyroidism
Pulmonary disorders	Glucocorticoid insufficiency
Tuberculosis	Miscellaneous
Pneumonia, empyema	Porphyria
Lung abscess	Pain, nausea
Cystic fibrosis, COPD	Idiopathic

a clinical state of hyponatremia which is characterized by a resetting downward of the plasma osmolality at which ADH is released. These patients have a chronic hyponatremia which is usually asymptomatic. They respond to water loading by decreasing ADH secretion and by diluting the urine. Likewise, sodium loading results in an increase in ADH secretion and hypertonic urine. Other than treatment of the underlying disease, no therapy is specifically indicated to correct the hyponatremia.

Endocrine disturbances that can cause hypotonic hyponatremia include glucocorticoid deficiency and hypothyroidism. Adrenal insufficiency allows increased ADH secretion and increased water reabsorption in the renal collecting ducts. The condition resembles SIADH except that these patients respond to exogenous glucocorticoid by abruptly increasing urine volume and decreasing urine osmolality. Severe hypothyroidism causes hyponatremia by promoting increased ADH secretion.

Acute water intoxication accounts for the diagnosis of hyponatremia in a few patients with impaired free water excretion. Since infants are unable to excrete a water load with the same efficiency as older children, they are at somewhat greater risk for developing hyponatremia from water loading. Postoperative patients are also at increased risk owing to their high ADH secretion secondary to pain and stress.

Other cases of acute water intoxication have been reported secondary to ingestion of low solute formula in infants, use of tap water enemas, and swallowing of swimming pool water. Chronic water intoxication or "psychogenic polydipsia" is rare except in mentally disturbed patients. The renal mechanisms resulting in hyponatremia in these patients include the "washing out" of the normal renal medullary concentrating gradient.

Hypervolemic Hyponatremia

These patients usually have TBW in great excess, often present with pulmonary or peripheral edema, and usually have impaired ability to excrete a water load. This allows water retention that is proportionately greater than sodium retention. These patients may be subcategorized into two groups: (1) generalized endematous states of congestive heart failure, cirrhosis of the liver, and the nephrotic syndrome; and (2) advanced acute or chronic renal insufficiency.

In the generalized edematous patients, hyponatremia is often the result of a decreased effective arterial blood volume. In heart failure, the decreased effective blood volume is caused by a low cardiac output, whereas in cirrhosis of the liver, the decreased effective arterial blood volume is related to decreased peripheral resistance with arteriovenous shunting and splanchnic venous pooling. The low blood volume found in the nephrotic syndrome is a result of low capillary oncotic pressure with resultant loss of fluid from the intravascular to the interstitial space. In each of these disorders, a decline in the effective arterial blood volume activates baroreceptors, leading to increased ADH release, renal water retention, dilution of ECF solutes, and hyponatremia. Furthermore, the edematous disorders are characterized by decreased glomerular filtration rate and enhanced proximal tubular reabsorption of fluid. The avid retention of sodium causes the urinary sodium concentration to be less than 20 mEq/L unless diuretics are being used.

Patients with oliguric acute or chronic renal failure may develop extreme salt and water overload through intravenous fluid administration. The decrease in glomerular filtration largely determines the extent of the impairment of water excretion. Urinary sodium concentration is variable but usually exceeds 40 mEq/L.

Pathophysiology

The pathophysiologic changes of hyponatremia are most obvious when serum sodium levels fall below 120 mEq/L in less than 12 to 24 h. The CNS effects are usually the most obvious, but cardiovascular and musculoskeletal dysfunction may also occur.

Central Nervous System

As serum sodium concentrations fall, the osmotic gradient that develops across the blood-brain barrier causes water to move into the brain, causing apathy, agitation, headache, altered consciousness, seizures, and even coma. The severity of symptoms is dependent not only on the rapidity, but also the magnitude, of the fall in the serum sodium concentration. Acute hyponatremia occurring in 24 h or less and resulting in a serum sodium concentration of less than 120 mEq/L, or a rate of fall of 0.5 mEq/L or more per hour, can cause muscular twitching, seizures, and coma. The mortality rate with acute severe hyponatremia with CNS changes has been reported to be as high as 50 percent in adults. In animals in which serum sodium is reduced to 110 mmol/L in 2 h, the mortality rate is 88 percent, and there is gross evidence of brain edema. When plasma sodium is lowered slowly during several days or weeks by a combination of sodium depletion and water ingestion, patients are usually less symptomatic, but even patients with chronic hyponatremia may experience focal weakness, hemiparesis, ataxia, and a positive Babinski sign.

As hyponatremia develops, the osmotic equilibrium between brain and plasma allows movement of increased amounts of water into the brain. However, brain swelling is less than would be predicted on the basis of the osmotic shifts alone. The brain's adaptation to hyponatremia is accomplished by two mechanisms: (1) movement of interstitial fluid into the cerebrospinal fluid and (2) loss of cellular potassium and organic osmolytes. With acute hyponatremia, water moves into the brain from the plasma, causing an increase in the hydrostatic pressure of the cerebral interstitial fluid. The increased interstitial pressure accelerates the clearance of interstitial fluid into the cerebrospinal fluid, which is returned to the systemic circulation via the arachnoid villi. The movement of sodium-rich interstitial fluid out of the brain reduces brain sodium, which in turn reduces the osmotic gradient for water moving into the brain.

The loss of sodium, potassium, and chloride from the brain provides most of the protection against cerebral edema in the first hours of hyponatremia; however, when hyponatremia is sustained, the brain slowly loses other intracellular osmolytes, mainly amino acids. Losses of organic osmolytes during prolonged or severe hyponatremia are especially important in defending the brain against swelling.

The adaptive changes that protect the brain from excessive swelling also render it susceptible to dehydration during correction of the fluid and electrolyte problem. Indeed, there is often more risk of brain damage during treatment than from the hyponatremia itself. The rate of rise of brain intracellular potassium and organic osmolytes during correction of the hyponatremia is much slower than the rate of loss of these substances during the development of the problem. If correction of hyponatremia occurs more rapidly than the brain can recover solute, the higher plasma osmolality may dehydrate and injure the brain, producing what is now called the *osmotic dymyelination syndrome*, or *central pontine myelinoysis*. (See section on "Complications of Therapy.")

Cardiovascular System

The cardiovascular response to hyponatremia depends primarily on the effective arterial blood volume, which may be increased, decreased, or normal depending on the underlying disorder. Intravascular volume is determined in part by the distribution of water between the ICF and ECF compartments. Thus, in the volume-depleted patient, hyponatremia can cause a further decrease in the intravascular volume by allowing movement of water out of the ECF compartment into the ICF space. Accordingly, shock occurs at lesser degrees of TBW depletion in hyponatremia than similar fluid deficits when the plasma is hypertonic or isotonic.

Antidiuretic hormone is one of the main factors opposing the hypovolemic effect of fluid shifts induced by hyponatremia. The ADH is released primarily as a response to the decreased effective arterial blood volume which often accompanies hyponatremic edematous disorders. Nonosmotic stimulation of ADH release overrides the hypoosmotic suppressive effect of hyponatremia, and increased ADH is present in almost all hyponatremic conditions. The function of ADH in this setting initially may seem paradoxical, because it potentiates the hyponatremic state by increasing water reabsorption by the renal tubules. ADH is also a potent vasocontrictor, however, and even at the low ADH concentrations which are characteristic of clinical hyponatremia, it increases peripheral vascular resistance, thereby increasing blood flow to the liver and kidneys at the expense of the skin and muscle.

Musculoskeletal System

Most patients with hyponatremia have normal muscle tone and function. However, muscle cramps and weakness can occur during strenuous exercise, especially if excess sweating is replaced with water. These symptoms usually resolve rapidly when the serum sodium concentration is corrected back toward normal.

Renal System

The usual renal response to hyponatremia is production of dilute urine; however, this process is abrogated to some extent by the presence of increased concentrations of ADH. The amount of ADH present depends on the primary disease process and the effective arterial blood volume.

A urine sodium concentration less than 10 mEq/L usually indicates that the renal handling of sodium is intact and that the effective arterial blood volume is contracted. In contrast, a urine sodium concentation greater than 20 mEq/L often indicates intrinsic renal tubular damage or a natriuretic response to hypervolemia. The urine sodium concentration will also vary somewhat according to the ongoing gains and losses of salt and water. Urine sodium will tend to increase if the underlying disease significantly impairs renal function.

Diagnosis

Most hyponatremia is due to dilution (a relative excess of TBW), which may be iatrogenic or due to disease (usually congestive heart failure, hepatic failure, or nephrotic syndrome). A decrease in the total body sodium due to excess diuresis, vomiting, diarrhea, or sweating is less common. The importance of each factor can usually be determined by careful review of the patient's history and intake and output of fluid.

Additional information can be obtained by comparing the sodium concentration and osmolarity of the serum and urine. A urine sodium less than 10 to 20 mEq/L in the presence of adequate renal perfusion suggests that either the ECF or the body content of sodium is low. If the urine sodium concentration is high, the patient usually has a water overload, is reacting to diuretics, or has renal disease. If the serum sodium is less than 120 to 125 mEq/L, there is often a decreased total body content of sodium as well as hemodilution. The patient may also have SIADH, but this is less common.

Treatment

Water Restriction

Since hyponatremia is usually due to hemodilution, fluid restriction is usually the best treatment in stable asymptomatic patients. One must, however, attempt to correct the underlying process and maintain an adequate tissue perfusion. If the effective ECF volume is depleted, too severe a water restriction program could cause complications.

Hypertonic Saline

If the hyponatremia is severe (less than 120 mEq/L) and develops rapidly (0.5 mEq/L decrease in serum sodium levels per hour) with CNS manifestations, administration of 3% saline solution is usually indicated. The 3% saline solution (which contains 513 mEq of sodium per liter) can be given at 25 to 100 mL/h, with careful observation for fluid overload and too rapid a rise in serum sodium levels. Attention should also be given to changes in urine sodium levels Unfortunately, hypertonic saline often only increases the serum sodium concentration transiently because much of the administered sodium is rapidly excreted in the urine. Consequently, in many patients it may be helpful to also give furosemide to reduce the amount of water present in the body.

Calculating Sodium Deficits

Methods of calculating sodium deficits are somewhat controversial. Most authors calculate sodium deficits using TBW (60 percent of body weight) as the sodium space because sodium tends to equilibrate with TBW even though most of the sodium is in the ECF. Thus, an 80-kg man with a serum sodium of 120 mEq/L would have a total sodium deficit of (80 kg × 60%) (140 − 120) = (48)(20) = 960 mEq. This calculation may be appropriate if the patient is normovolemic. However, most patients with hyponatremia are hypervolemic, and using 60 percent of the body weight in the calculations could result in administration of too much sodium. Accordingly, sodium deficits in hypervolemic patients are usually calculated using a sodium space equivalent to 20 percent of the body weight. Thus, a hypervolemic 80-kg man with a serum sodium of 120 mEq/L would be assumed to have a sodium deficit of (80 kg × 20%) (140 − 120) = (16) (20) = 320 mEq. Nevertheless, it must be stressed that unless there is a history or other evidence of sodium loss from the body, most patients with hyponatremia have a normal or even increased total body content of sodium, and fluid restriction is often the only treatment required.

Treatment of Pseudohyponatremia

Treatment of pseudohyponatrmia, such as that due to hyperglycemia, is directed at its cause. Once an adequate urine output is obtained and insulin becomes effective, glucose levels fall and serum sodium levels will usually correct spontaneously. No matter what type of hyponatremia is present, no treatment is usually necessary if serum osmolality is normal and the patient is asymptomatic.

Complications of Therapy

Complications with the treatment of acute hyponatremia, especially if there is no underlying CNS, hepatic, or renal disorder, are uncommon and occur in less than 2 percent of patients. In chronic hyponatremia, brain edema is usually not severe and little evidence exists that chronic hyponatremia itself causes brain damage. Nevertheless, these patients appear to be at greatest risk for brain injury during the correction process. The injury reportedly occurs after the hyponatremia has been corrected and progresses in a predictable manner that has been called the *osmotic demyelination syndrome* or *central pontine myelinolysis* (CPM). These neurologic changes are believed to be due to correction of the serum sodium at a rate faster than the brain can adapt to the higher osmolality. In patients with chronic hyponatremia, other factors contributing to the CPM may include alcoholism, malnutrition, toxins, and metabolic imbalance.

Brain histology in fatal cases shows myelinolysis and demyelination of central pontine and extrapontine myelin-bearing neurons. In typical cases the neurologic findings include fluctuating levels of consciousness, behavioral disturbances, dysarthria, dysphagia, or convulsions progressing to pseudobulbar palsy and quadriparesis. Improvement may occur after several weeks of severe debilitation, but some patients are permanently impaired.

In patients with chronic severe hyponatremia, the threshold for the production of CPM is a rate of correction of sodium levels faster than 0.5 mEq/L per hour (12 mEq/L per day). In patients with acute severe hyponatremia, correction at rates exceeding 0.5 to 1.0 mEq/L per hour, with or without diuretics, does not usually cause any problems.

Severe neurologic complications have occurred almost exclusively in clinically hypernatremic patients treated with hypertonic or isotonic saline without the addition of furosemide or an osmotic diuretic. Similar patients treated with the same fluids but with furosemide almost uniformly have done well. Patients with chronic hyponatremia corrected at a rate less than 0.5 mEq/L per hour have also done well.

Hypernatremia

Etiology

The most frequent cause of hypernatremia is a decrease in TBW because of reduced intake or excessive loss. The more common causes of hypotonic fluid losses are diarrhea, vomiting, hyperpyrexia, and excessive sweating. Less frequently, hypernatremia is due to oral lactulose, osmotic diuresis with mannitol or glycerol, or increased intake of salt (Table 10-9). The causes of hypernatremia can also be classified according to the status of the blood volume (Table 10-10).

Decreased Water Intake

Probably the main defense against hypernatremia is thirst. Although increased ADH secretion occurs before thirst, thirst generally is a far more important defense. However, patients who are in coma or who have a stroke and cannot move to get water will be unable to obtain adequate fluids.

Excess Water Excretion

Failure of ADH mechanisms is an important cause of hypernatremia, and it may be central or renal in origin. Neonates with immature kidney, and adults with certain types of renal disease, such as obstructive uropathy or renal dysplasia, may be unable to excrete sodium properly. Consequently, their urine osmolality may be fixed between 200 to 300 mOsm/kg with urine sodiums of 60 to 100 mEq/kg.

Increased Sodium Intake

The body tends to keep its total content of sodium remarkably constant, and if excessive sodium is given, the kidney will usually excrete it quite rapidly. However, if renal function is impaired, a dangerous expansion of the ECF may occur. One source of excessive sodium administration is the use of sodium-containing antibiotics, such as ticarcillin, which has an average of 5.2 mEq of sodium per gram.

Diabetic Insipidus

A particularly interesting cause of hypernatremia is DI, which results in excessive loss of hypotonic urine. Diabetes insipidus may be central in origin (due to a failure of secretion of ADH) or nephrogenic (due to renal unresponsiveness to ADH). About 30 percent of central DI is idiopathic and about 70 percent is secondary to neoplasms (25 percent), pituitary surgery (20 percent), or trauma (15 percent). Most of the remaining 10 percent is due to various granulomas (tuberculosis, sarcoidosis, eosinophilic granuloma) or local vascular problems (aneurysms, thrombosis, Sheehan's syndrome). Nephrogenic DI may be primary (familial) or secondary to a wide variety of causes including hypercalcemia, hypokalemia, renal disorders, various drugs (including lithium, demeclocycline, amphotericin B, aminoglycosides, cisplatin), hematologic disorders (sickle cell disease, myeloma), malnutrition, or amyloidosis.

Traumatic DI is typically triphasic. After an initial polyuria from insufficient ADH secretion by hypothalamic cells, there is a transient second phase lasting 1 to 7 days characterized by release of previously formed hormone from the posterior pituitary and resolution of the polyuria. In the third phase, central DI returns after the released hormone has been utilized. Regeneration of cells that secrete ADH may occur weeks to months after injury. The ADH-secreting cells have their cell bodies in the hypothalamus, and these are not usually completely destroyed by trauma.

Differentiation between central and nephrogenic DI is best achieved by noting (1) the response of serum and urine osmolarity to water deprivation (trying to reach a serum osmolarity greater than 295 mOsm/L) and (2) the response to 5 units of subcutaneous aqueous vasopressin. Patients with central DI show little or no response to dehydration, but respond well to vasopressin (urine osmolarity $\geq$ 800 mOsm/L). Nephrogenic DI shows little or no response to dehydration or vasopressin.

Pathophysiology

Because sodium does not freely penetrate tissue cell membranes, ECF and plasma volume tend to be maintained in hypernatremic dehydration until the water loss is greater than 10 percent of body weight. Although there may be rather profound dehydration in some patients with severe hypernatremia, shock is an infrequent occurrence. When the dehydration results in loss of 10 percent of body weight, skin turgor becomes reduced and the skin of the abdomen has a characteristic "doughy" feel when it is pinched between the fingers.

Acute symptomatology is seen in many patients once serum sodium concentrations exceed 158 mEq/L. Patients tend to become irritable, and infants may also have a high-pitched cry or wail alternating with periods of severe lethargy. As dehydration and hypernatremia become more severe, one may see increased muscle tone or even coma with eventual seizures. Fever can be both a contributing cause and a result of hypernatremic dehydration.

Restlessness and irritability occur when serum osmolality increases to between 350 and 375 mOsm/kg, while ataxia and tremulousness tend to occur when osmolality is between 375 and 400 mOsm/kg. When serum osmolality rises above 400 mOsm/kg, asynchronous jerks

Table 10-9. Causes of Hypernatremia

- I. Loss of water
  - A. Reduced water intake
    1. Defective thirst
    2. Unconsciousness
    3. Inability to drink water
    4. Lack of access to water
  - B. Increased water loss
    1. Vomiting, diarrhea
    2. Sweating, fever
    3. Hyperventilation
    4. Diabetes insipidus, osmotic diuresis
    5. Thyrotoxicosis
    6. Severe burns
- II. Gain of sodium
  - A. Increased intake
    1. Hypertonic saline ingestion or infusion
    2. Sodium bicarbonate administration
  - B. Renal salt retention (usually because of poor perfusion)

Table 10-10. Causes of Hypernatremia Related to Blood Volume

- I. Hypovolemia
  - A. Nonrenal H_2O losses ($U_{Na} < 10$ mEq/L, $U_{Osm} > 400$ mOsm/L) from skin or GI or respiratory tracts
  - B. Renal H_2O losses ($U_{Na} > 20$ mEq/L, $U_{Osm} < 300$ mOsm/L) from diuretics, renal disease, relief of urinary obstruction, adrenal failure, osmoreceptor failure
- II. Euvolemia
  - A. Impaired thirst (coma)
  - B. Nonrenal H_2O losses (GI, skin, respiratory)
  - C. Renal H_2O losses due to DI, reset osmostat, relief of urinary obstruction, renal disease, osmotic diuretics
- III. Hypervolemia
  - A. Iatrogenic (hypertonic saline therapy)
  - B. Mineralocorticoid excess ($U_{Na} > 20$ mE/L, $U_{Osm} > 300$ mOsm/L) due to hyperadosteronism, Cushing's disease, congenital adrenal hyperplasia, exogenous corticosteroids

and tonic spasms are apt to occur. Death usually occurs at an osmolality above 430 mOsm/kg.

Permanent sequelae are not uncommon in children when serum sodium concentrations exceed 160 to 165 mEq/L. Up to 16 percent of children with hypernatremia develop chronic neurologic deficits as a consequence. The overall mortality of hypernatremia is above 10 percent. If the plasma osmolality exceeds 350 mOsm/kg, the incidence of severe morbidity or mortality may exceed 25 to 50 percent.

Hypocalcemia, which is frequently seen in patients with hypernatremia, may contribute to the CNS symptomatology. However, the mechanism of the hypocalcemia is unclear.

Massive brain hemorrhage or multiple small hemorrhages and thromboses may occur when hypernatremia causes enough cellular dehydration and resultant brain shrinkage to cause tearing of cerebral blood vessels. This has been observed most frequently in neonates following acute administration of a large sodium load. As a consequence, the amount of sodium bicarbonate administered to acidotic infants must be limited.

If the hypernatremia persists for more than a few days, the brain dehydration may resolve, and brain water content may return to normal or near-normal levels due to accumulation in the brain cells of amino acids known as "idiogenic osmoles," particularly taurine. The formation of these idiogenic osmoles increases intracellular osmolality, attracts water back into the brain cells, and restores their cellular volume. If the hypertonicity develops gradually, this protective mechanism tends to prevent severe brain cell shrinkage.

Treatment

When dehydration is severe, plasma volume should first be restored with plasma-expanding fluids, such as normal saline or Ringer's lactate, which is administered until blood pressure and tissue perfusion are adequate. Once perfusion is reestablished, fluid containing 75 to 80 mEq/L of sodium (i.e., 0.45% saline) should be given until the urine output is at least 0.5 mL/kg per hour. Moderately hypotonic fluids can then be given with the aim of restoring normal hydration and bringing serum sodium concentrations down to normal in 48 to 72 h. The reduction of serum sodium concentration should not exceed 10 to 15 mEq/L per day.

The amount of water needed to correct hypernatremia can be estimated by the following equation:

$$\text{Water deficit (in liters)} = \text{TBW}\left(1 - \frac{\text{Na}_2}{\text{Na}_1}\right)$$

Where Na_1 is the current serum sodium and Na_2 is the desired serum sodium. TBW is normally expected to be about 60 percent of body weight. Thus for a 70-kg man, if Na_1 is 160 mEq/L and Na_2 is 145 mEq/L, the water deficit is

$$\text{Water deficit} = (60\% \times 70\text{ kg})\left(1 - \frac{145}{160}\right)$$

$$= (42)\left(\frac{15}{160}\right) = \frac{630}{160} = 3.9\text{ L}$$

As general rule, each liter of H_2O deficit results in a rise of serum sodium of 3 to 5 mEq/L or 8 to 15 mOsm/L. If there is any evidence of cardiac failure, rehydration must be done more slowly and with careful attention to changes in the central venous pressure (CVP) and/or pulmonary artery wedge pressure (PAWP). If the patient has significant ongoing fluid losses, these must be included in replacement therapy.

The sodium to be given can be calculated as 80 to 100 mEq per liter of estimated fluid deficit. Maintenance sodium needs can usually be disregarded. The sodium is given primarily as chloride, but sodium lactate or acetate can be given if the patient is acidotic. In hypernatremia with an excess total body sodium, the restoration of a normal ECF volume often initiates a substantial natriuresis. However, if this does not occur promptly, sodium should be removed with diuretics, such as furosemide, while 0.45% saline is administered.

Because of the predilection of children with hypernatremia to develop hyperglycemia, glucose should probably be given only as a 2.5% solution until glucose levels fall to relatively normal levels. Calcium gluconate may also be added, depending on serum calcium content. Once an adequate urine output is established, 20 to 40 mEq of potassium chloride should be added to each liter of fluid. Potassium aids water entry into cells.

Rapid correction of hypernatremia, especially if it is chronic, can cause seizures and severe neurologic sequelae. Unless the hypernatremia is of short duration, idiogenic osmoles are presumably present in brain cells. Consequently, too rapid rehydration and lowering of serum sodium concentration can cause brain cells to swell, resulting in cerebral edema and an increased likelihood of seizures, permanent neurologic sequelae, or even death. Serum electrolyte levels should be monitored frequently to ensure that the appropriate rate of decline of serum sodium concentration occurs.

In the case of acute hypernatremia, correction of serum sodium levels can be achieved rather rapidly with little fear of cerebral edema because idiogenic osmoles will not yet be present in brain cells. However, rapid fluid administration in patients with hypernatremia due to excessive sodium administration may result in hypervolemia and pulmonary edema.

In children with acute severe sodium excess and a serum sodium concentration of more than 180 to 200 mEq/L, peritoneal dialysis using a high-glucose (7.5%), low-sodium dialysate may be lifesaving, but must be done with frequent monitoring of serum electrolyte levels. Whenever the duration of the hypernatremia is unclear, rapid correction to a serum sodium of about 155 mEq/L is recommended followed by slower correction down to 145 mEq/L.

Hypercalcemia is a common, unexplained finding in hypernatremia, and the addition of calcium gluconate to rehydration fluids is often indicated. Hyperglycemia tends to accompany the hypernatremia. However, insulin treatment is not recommended because it may increase the idiogenic osmole content of the brain.

In the case of central DI, administration of either vasopressin or 1-deamino-8-D-arginine vasopressin (dDAVP) must be undertaken carefully, and fluid intake should be regulated so that the serum sodium concentrations do not drop too rapidly.

POTASSIUM

Elemental potassium is the major intracellular cation in the body. Total body potassium content is about 50 to 55 mEq/kg, or a total of about 3500 mEq in a young, healthy 70-kg man. However, "exchangeable potassium" measured with ^{42}K provides somewhat lower values, averaging about 45 mEq/kg. Over 70 to 75 percent of the total body potassium is in muscle. Thus, protein malnutrition may be associated with severe total body deficiencies in potassium. In women with severe muscle wasting, the total exchangeable body potassium content may be as low as 20 to 25 mEq/kg.

Almost 98 percent of the total body potassium is within cells where the concentration is 110 to 150 mEq/L. In contrast, the concentration of potassium in the ECF is normally only 3.5 to 5.0 mEq/L. This large K^+ gradient across cell membranes is critical for normal neuromuscular function.

The normal total daily potassium intake is about 50 to 150 mEq. Meat contains about 1 mEq of potassium for each gram of protein. Some of the fruits and vegetables with a high potassium content include oranges, grapefruit, tomatoes, bananas, avocados, and raisins. Of the average 100 mEq of potassium ingested daily, 5 to 10 mEq is lost in the feces and a similar amount in sweat, leaving 80 to 90 percent to be excreted by the kidneys.

Hypokalemia

Etiology

The most frequent causes of hypokalemia are intracellular shifts and increased losses, especially in urine (Table 10-11).

Intracellular Shifts

Increased Bicarbonate

Potassium tends to move inside cells and hydrogen ions tend to move out whenever the pH of the ECF rises, especially if the rise in pH is due to increased bicarbonate levels. A rise in the pH of 0.10 due to increased plasma bicarbonate levels generally causes a 0.5 (0.3 to 0.8) mEq/L fall in serum potassium levels. Thus, if a patient with a serum potassium level of 4.2 mEq/L and a pH of 7.40 is given bicarbonate and the pH is raised to 7.60, the serum potassium level will tend to fall to about 3.2 mEq/L. Interestingly, immediately after an elevation in the P_{CO_2}, plasma potassium levels rise transiently, but then return to baseline values fairly rapidly.

Loss of Gastric Acid

Hypokalemia seen with excessive vomiting is due primarily to the metabolic alkalosis which develops and not loss of the potassium present in the vomitus, even though the potassium content of highly acid gastric juice may exceed 10 mEq/L. The alkalosis in turn causes a shift of potassium ions into cells in exchange for hydrogen ions. The mild hypovolemia which also can develop with excess loss of gastric juice stimulates an increased secretion of aldosterone, which further contributes to the potassium loss and increased absorption of sodium and bicarbonate. Hypercalcemia can also cause increased potassium loss in the urine.

During the treatment of severe diabetic ketoacidosis, as insulin begins to become effective, potassium follows glucose into the cells, and a very dangerous hypokalemia may develop rapidly unless potassium is given as soon as glucose levels begin to fall. Although the glucose movement into cells brings potassium in with it, insulin also directly increases the cellular uptake of potassium. Furthermore, as the pH rises toward normal and urine volumes increase, serum potassium levels can fall even further because of increasing shift into the cells and loss in the urine. If potassium is not given as the hyperglycemia of diabetic ketoacidosis is corrected, severe hypokalemia may develop rapidly, causing dangerous arrhythmias.

Diuresis

Although normal kidneys conserve sodium well, potassium is much more difficult to preserve. Indeed, potassium losses in urine are almost "obligatory" and are usually directly proportional to the volume of urine. Urine potassium normally averages about 40 to 80 mEq/L. Even with severe acute potassium deficits, urine potassium losses will often exceed 30 mEq/L for at least several days.

Use of loop diuretics, such as furosemide (Lasix), may cause urine potassium losses to exceed 100 mEq/L. Indeed, loop diuretics are the most common cause of severe hypokalemia. Renal losses of potassium are also increased by alkalosis, hypochloremia, and hypomagnesemia. Renal tubular acidosis (type I), causes hypokalemia due to impaired hydrogen ion excretion in the distal tubule.

Hyperaldosteronism

Adrenal corticosteroids, especially aldosterone, cause the kidneys to excrete potassium and chloride and retain sodium and bicarbonate. This can cause a significant hypokalemic metabolic alkalosis. The combination of hypertension and hypokalemic metabolic alkalosis can be an important clue to hyperaldosteronism. Chronic or excessive ingestion of licorice can cause hypokalemia by a similar effect.

Bartter's syndrome, occurring mostly in children, is characterized by hypokalemic metabolic alkalosis, juxtaglomerular hyperplasia, hyperreninemia and hyperaldosteronism, kaliuresis, and sodium and bicarbonate retention, without hypertension or edema. Liddle's syndrome is a familial type of pseudohyperaldosteronism. The electrolyte changes are characteristic of hyperaldosteronism, but aldosterone levels are normal.

The normal colon conserves about 500 mL of water a day along with significant quantities of sodium, chloride, and bicarbonate (Table 10-12). Because of the high concentrations of potassium (up to 90 mEq/L) and bicarbonate (30 to 74 mEq/L) in stool, severe diarrhea can result in the loss of large quantities of these substances, producing a hypokalemic metabolic acidosis. Correction of only the metabolic acidosis will tend to cause an even worse hypokalemia. One should anticipate potassium deficits in patients with severe diarrhea and either prevent them or institute rapid correction.

Epinephrine Infusions

Another interesting cause of hypokalemia is infusions of epinephrine, which can cause serum potassium levels to fall by more than 0.5 mEq/L. This may be an important cause of arrhythmias in some patients with acute myocardial infarction. It is now known that β_2-adrenergic receptors are involved in the regulation of extrarenal potassium disposal. The generation of cyclic AMP activates Na^+, K^+-ATPase, which augments intracellular-extracellular exchange of K^+ for Na^+. This increases intracellular potassium levels, hyperpolarizing the cell membrane. Theophylline potentiates this tendency of epinephrine to increase potassium influx into cells.

Physiologic Effects

Severe hypokalemia with levels below 2.0 to 2.5 mEq/L may cause muscle weakness and increase the tendency to intestinal ileus. Indeed, respiratory paralysis has been seen with levels below 1.5 to 2.0 mEq/L.

It must be remembered that severe hypokalemia can cause nephrogenic DI and severe dehydration which must be considered when correcting the electrolyte abnormalities. Hypokalemia tends to cause

Table 10-11. Causes of Hypokalemia

I. Shift into the cell
   A. Raising the pH of blood
   B. Administration of insulin and glucose
II. Reduced intake
III. Increased loss
   A. Renal loss
      1. Primary hyperaldosteronism
      2. Secondary hyperaldosteronism associated with diuretics, malignant hypertension, Bartter's syndrome, renal artery stenosis
      3. Miscellaneous
         a. Hypercalcemia
         b. Liddle's syndrome
         c. Magnesium deficiency
         d. Renal tubular acidosis
         e. Acute myelocytic and monocytic leukemias
   B. Gastrointestinal loss (vomiting, diarrhea, fistulas)

Table 10-12. Daily Water and Electrolytes Delivered to and from the Normal Colon

	Delivered to Colon		Delivered to Stool	
Fluid or Electrolyte	**Amount**	**Concentration, mEq/L**	**Amount**	**Concentration, mEq/L**
Water	600 mL		100 mL	
Sodium	76 mEq	125	4 mEq	40
Potassium	5 mEq	9	6 mEq	60
Chloride	36 mEq	60	2 mEq	15
Bicarbonate	44 mEq	74	3 mEq	30

a metabolic alkalemia with increased acid excretion in the urine (paradoxical aciduria). It also increases the tendency to glycosuria.

The sensitivity of the heart to digitalis and the likelihood of digitalis toxicity with arrhythmias or an AV block is increased in the presence of hypokalemia. In patients treated with hydrochlorothiazide, there is a direct relationship between the severity of the hypokalemia, concomitant hypomagnesemia, and the incidence of ventricular ectopy. Administration of both potassium and magnesium are important parts of the treatment of arrhythmias due to digitalis toxicity.

Hypokalemia increases renal tubular production of ammonia, and this may aggravate hepatic encephalopathy in patients with advanced cirrhosis.

Diagnosis

The diagnosis of hypokalemia is made primarily on serum electrolyte studies. However, serum potassium levels should be interpreted relative to the arterial pH. A low serum potassium level may be expected in an alkalotic patient, but hypokalemia in an acidotic patient is either a laboratory error or evidence of a severe potassium deficit. In some instances, a patient with normal blood levels can seem to be hypokalemic, particularly after cardiopulmonary bypass and with metabolic alkalosis. In patients with metabolic alkalosis, paradoxical aciduria suggests a functional hypokalemia.

On ECG, hypokalemia less than 3.0 mEq/L may cause low-voltage QRS complexes, flattened T waves, depressed ST segments, prominent P and U waves, and prolonged QT and PR intervals. A U wave (between the T and P waves) can be seen in many normal individuals in the early precordial leads (V_1 to V_3), but it is somewhat more prominent with diastolic hypertension and coronary artery disease. The U wave may become especially prominent as potassium levels fall below 2.5 mEq/L. Potassium levels below 2.0 mEq/L also tend to widen the QRS complex.

Urine potassium levels can give some indication of the duration of hypokalemia and the severity of the total body deficit. Normal urine potassium levels (40 to 80 mEq/L) suggest that the potassium deficit is acute. However, if the hypokalemia is due to metabolic alkalosis from primary aldosteronism, urine potassium levels may be high despite severe chronic hypokalemia.

One should not attempt to correct hypokalemia rapidly if the urinary potassium is very low. Urine potassium levels less than 10 mEq/L suggest a chronic and severe potassium deficit that is not apt to respond well to attempts at rapid correction.

Treatment

Acute severe hypokalemia is treated by infusing 10 to 15 mEq of KCl per hour in 50 to 100 mL of 5% dextrose in water (D_5W) or 0.9 *N* saline by IV piggyback for 3 to 4 h. The ECG should be continuously monitored during potassium infusions. As a general rule, no more than 40 mEq of potassium should ever be put in a single liter of IV fluid (except by careful IV piggyback) and no more than 40 mEq should be given per hour.

Potassium equilibrates in the TBW, and it generally takes at least 40 to 50 mEq to raise the serum potassium level by 1.0 mEq/L. Chronic deficits usually require much larger amounts of potassium to maintain any increase in serum levels, and not infrequently, much of the infused potassium is promptly excreted in the urine.

Chronic hypokalemia may be associated with very severe potassium deficits, which often exceed 300 to 500 mEq. One way to estimate total body potassium deficits is from pH-corrected plasma potassium levels. The percentage by which serum levels (corrected for pH) are below 4.2 mEq/L is twice as large as the percentage of total body potassium deficit. Thus, a serum potassium level of 2.1 mEq/L at a pH of 7.4 indicates a 50 percent reduction in serum potassium and a 25 percent deficit in total body potassium. Total body potassium ranges between 20 mEq/kg in a markedly wasted woman to 45 mEq/kg in a normal muscular man. Thus, a serum potassium of 2.5 mEq/L at an arterial pH of 7.40 in a 50-kg woman with muscle wasting indicates a 40 percent pH-corrected potassium deficit in the plasma and a 20 percent deficit in total body potassium. The calculated total body potassium deficit would then be (20 percent)(50 kg)(20 mEq/kg) = 200 mEq.

Hyperkalemia

Etiology

There are many causes of hyperkalemia. It is easy to hemolyze blood as it is being drawn, producing a pseudohyperkalemia. Other causes of pseudohyperkalemia include leukocytosis, especially greater than $600{,}000/mm^3$, and thrombocytosis, especially greater than $10^6/mm^3$. These are particularly apt to cause hyperkalemia if the blood is not analyzed within 30 min of being drawn. Excessive opening and clenching of the fist while the tourniquet is on can raise potassium levels in veins below the tourniquet by 10 to 20 percent after several minutes. The more common causes of hyperkalemia are listed in Table 10-13.

Renal failure with oliguria is the most common cause of dangerous hyperkalemia. Normally, 90 to 95 percent of the potassium taken in is excreted in the urine. Thus, anuria can cause a severe progressive rise in serum potassium levels.

Since each kilogram of lean muscle tissue may contain over 100 mEq of potassium, breakdown of muscle from trauma or sepsis may release large quantities of potassium into the bloodstream. Occasionally, succinylcholine can raise serum potassium levels abruptly in patients with severe crush injuries or burns. A similar problem may develop with hemolysis due to transfusion reactions.

Excessive intake of potassium is an infrequent case of hyperkalemia, but can occur with IV administration of potassium-containing drugs. Aqueous (potassium) penicillin, for example, contains about 1.7 mEq of potassium per 1 million units.

Physiologic Effects

As potassium levels rise above 6.0 mEq/L, cardiac conductivity and contractility may be impaired. With severe hyperkalemia, above 6.5

Table 10-13. Common Causes of Hyperkalemia

Factitious
  Laboratory error
  Pseudohyperkalemia: hemolysis, thrombocytosis, leukocytosis
Metabolic acidemia (acute)
Increased intake into the plasma
  Exogenous: diet, salt substitutes, low-sodium diet, medications
  Endogenous: hemolysis, GI bleeding, catabolic states, crush injury
Inadequate distal delivery of sodium and decreased distal tubular flow
Oliguric renal failure
Impaired renin-aldosterone axis
  Addison's disease
  Primary hypoaldosteronism
  Other (heparin, β blockers, prostaglandin inhibitors, captopril)
Primary renal tubular potassium secretory defect
  Sickle cell disease
  Systemic lupus erythematosus
  Postrenal transplantation
  Obstructive uropathy
Inhibition of renal tubular secretion of potassium
  Spironolactone
  Digitalis
Abnormal potassium distribution
  Insulin deficiency
  Hypertonicity (hyperglycemia)
  β-Adrenergic blockers
  Exercise
  Succinylcholine
  Digitalis

to 7.0 mEq/L, an intracardiac block can be produced, first in the atria, then in the AV node, and finally in the ventricles, with the heart eventually stopping in diastole. Occasionally, hyperkalemia may cause such weakness that ventilatory failure may develop. The effects of hyperkalemia are increased if the patient has hyponatremia and hypocalcemia.

Diagnosis

One should suspect hyperkalemia in patients with oliguric renal failure, severe hemolysis, or excessive tissue breakdown. The potassium levels must also be correlated with the arterial pH. It is a bit unusual for a moderate to severe hyperkalemia to exist without acidosis.

Mild hyperkalemia brings the membrane potential closer to threshold, and conduction in the heart is initially improved. As the serum K^+ level rises above 5.6 to 6.0 mEq/L, the first ECG sign of hyperkalemia is usually the development of tall, peaked T waves, best seen in the precordial leads, as a result of speeded repolarization. With further increases in serum potassium levels to 6.0 to 6.5 mEq/L, impulse conduction decreases, often resulting in prolonged PR and QT intervals. At levels above 6.5 to 7.0 mEq/L, diminished P waves and depressed ST segments can occur. This finding is not specific for hyperkalemia, however, and may also be seen with massive cerebrovascular accidents and myocardial ischemia. Although ST segments are usually depressed with moderate to severe hyperkalemia, occasionally elevation resembling acute myocardial ischemia may be seen.

At serum potassium levels of 7.0 mEq/L or greater, impulses may still be conducted from the SA node to the ventricle because the intraatrial conduction fibers are less sensitive to hyperkalemia than are atrial muscle fibers. Since conduction may be delayed in the AV node, such conduction could result in an idioventricular rhythm. Delayed conduction in the interventricular conducting system can produce patterns resembling bundle branch block.

As the levels exceed 7.5 to 8.0 mEq/L, P waves disappear, the QRS complex widens, the S and T waves tend to merge, and the ventricular rhythm becomes irregular. At levels exceeding 10 to 12 mEq/L, a classic sine wave is usually seen.

Death from hyperkalemia is usually the result of a diastolic arrest caused by block of the distal Purkinje fibers or of ventricular fibrillation caused by reentrant circuits that develop because of prolonged ventricular conduction.

Treatment

If serum potassium levels rise above 5.0 to 5.5 mEq/L, one must begin to look for oliguric renal failure or increased red blood cell or other tissue breakdown. Whenever possible, all potassium-containing solutions and drugs should be discontinued. Diuresis is extremely helpful. Even when renal function is severely impaired, each liter of urine usually contains at least 30 to 40 mEq of potassium per liter.

If serum potassium levels rise above 5.5 to 6.0 mEq/L and diuresis is not possible or if there is extensive tissue damage, one should consider using an ion-exchange resin. Kayexalate (sodium polystyrene sulfonate) is an ion-exchange resin which may be administered by mouth or by retention enemas. Each gram of sodium resin exchanges with and eliminates about 1.0 mEq of potassium. When given orally, 15 to 25 g of Kayexalate are given with 50 mL of a 20% sorbitol solution every 4 to 6 h. Kayexalate tends to be constipating, and the sorbitol increases the speed of evacuation of bowel contents. Rectal administration is 20 g of Kayexalate in 200 mL of a 20% sorbitol solution every 4 h. The enema should be retained at least 30 min.

In patients with fluid overload or impaired cardiac function, the absorption of sodium from Kayexalate may precipitate acute heart failure. If serum potassium levels are less than 6.5 mEq/L and there are no ECG changes due to the hyperkalemia, treatment efforts may be slower. If serum potassium levels rise above 6.5 mEq/L, one should consider giving glucose and insulin and possibly also sodium bicarbonate. As glucose enters cells, it "pulls" potassium, magnesium, and phosphorus in with it. After an initial 50 mL of 50% IV glucose with 5 to 10 units of regular insulin, a liter of 20% glucose with 40 to 80 units of insulin may be given over the next 2 to 4 h.

Sodium bicarbonate causes an alkalosis which tends to reduce serum potassium levels. It also increases the serum concentration of sodium, which also helps oppose the potassium effects. Each ampule (50 mL of a 7.5% solution) should be given relatively slowly by continuous IV infusion over at least 10 to 20 min, depending on the urgency of the situation. Hypertonic (3%) sodium chloride in doses of 50 to 100 mEq IV over 30 to 60 min may also antagonize the effects of the high potassium levels.

Calcium gluconate or calcium chloride is usually only given for severe hyperkalemia with levels > 7.0 to 7.5 mEq/L. Ten mL of 10% calcium gluconate contains 4.6 mEq of calcium, while a similar ampule of $CaCl_2$ contains 13.4 mEq of calcium. The calcium is also more rapidly available from the chloride than from the gluconate. One ampule is given by slow IV infusion over at least 10 to 20 min. Additional calcium is given much more slowly as needed.

If calcium has to be given to patients on digitalis, it must be done with great caution, since hypercalcemia potentiates the toxic effects of digitalis on the heart. Therefore, if calcium must be given on an emergency basis to patients taking digitalis, an ampule should be added to 100 mL of D_5W and infused slowly over at least 20 to 30 min to permit a more even distribution throughout the extracellular space.

If a dangerous tachyarrhythmia develops in a hyperkalemic patient, all of the above steps may have to be done together and rapidly. Such emergency treatment must proceed rapidly according to a predetermined program (Table 10-14). If a patient is in acute oliguric renal

Table 10-14. Emergency Therapy of Hyperkalemia

Therapy	Mechanism	Dose	Onset of Action	Duration of Hypokalemic Effect
Ca gluconate (10%)	Antagonism	10–20 mL IV	1–3 min	30–50 min
Na bicarbonate	Antagonism and redistribution	50–100 mEq IV	5–10 min	1–2 h
Insulin plus glucose	Redistribution	20 U regular insulin with 50 g glucose IV over 1 h	30 min	4–6 h
Diuretics Furosemide Ethacrynic acid	Excretion	40 mg IV 50 mg IV	With diuresis	With diuresis
Cation-exchange resin (Kayexalate)	Excretion	15–50 g PO or rectally with sorbitol	1–2 h	4–6 h
Peritoneal dialysis or hemodialysis	Excretion		Within minutes	During dialysis

failure, hemodialysis and/or peritoneal dialysis should be set up while the above measures are being used.

CALCIUM

Calcium is the most abundant mineral in the human body. The total body calcium content is 15 to 20 g/kg body weight or about 1.0 to 1.5 kg in an adult of normal size. About 99 percent is in bone as the mineral apatite. The average daily calcium intake, about 800 to 1000 mg, is primarily from milk and milk products. About a third of this calcium is absorbed, primarily in the small bowel, by both active (vitamin D–dependent) and passive (concentration-dependent) absorption. Loss of calcium into the GI tract (150 to 200 mg/day) and urine (150 mg/day) usually balances the GI absorption quite closely.

Control of Calcium Levels

Calcium homeostasis is under the control of parathyroid hormone (PTH), calcitonin, and vitamin D metabolites, especially calcitrol (1α,25-dihydroxyvitamin D_3).

Parathormone

Parathormone (PTH) is secreted by the parathyroid gland, primarily in response to low ionized calcium or magnesium levels. Parathormone raises serum calcium levels primarily by stimulating osteoclasts to increase bone resorption. It has less activity in the intestine, where it works in combination with calcitrol. It also has an indirect action in the kidney through adenyl cyclase stimulation, whereby it increases calcium resorption and increases phosphorous excretion. PTH also stimulates conversion of 25-hydroxyvitamin D to the much more metabolically active 1α,25-dehydroxyvitamin D_3.

Calcitonin

Calcitonin is influenced by elevations in serum calcium, epinephrine, glucagon, and gastrin. It decreases the release of calcium from bone by inhibiting the activity of the osteoclasts. It also has a limited role in increasing calcium loss through the kidney.

Vitamin D

Vitamin D can be produced nonenzymatically by ultraviolet irradiation of skin or it can be absorbed directly from the GI tract, particularly from fortified milk products. Since it is a fat-soluble vitamin, its absorption requires bile salts and micelle formation. Vitamin D is hydroxylated in the liver to 25-hydroxycholecalciferol (25-(OH)-vitamin D) and in the kidney it is further hydroxylated to either 1α,25-$(OH)_2$-vitamin D or 24,25-$(OH)_2$-vitamin D. The synthesis of 1α,25-$(OH)_2$-vitamin D, which is much more potent metabolically, increases with hypocalcemia or hypophosphatemia. During hypercalcemia there is a reversal of the above sequence so that more 24,25-$(OH)_2$-vitamin D, which is much less active, is formed.

Functions

Calcium is vital to a wide variety of bodily functions, including neutrophil chemotaxis, lymphocyte activation, and membrane stability of a wide variety of cells. It is a required factor in the clotting cascade for activation or conversion of factors IX, VII, VIII, prothrombin, and fibrinogen, and it is necessary for platelet aggregation and granule release. However, very small amounts of calcium, probably less than 0.3 to 0.4 mEq/L, are needed for clotting. Calcium is also essential for the release of neurotransmitters in the central and peripheral nervous systems, and it plays a critical role in muscle depolarization.

Calcium ion influx into the depolarized myocardial cell prolongs depolarization. This is represented by the plateau or phase 2 portion of the cardiac action potential. Stimulation of skeletal muscle causes calcium ion to be released from the sarcoplasmic reticulum into the cytoplasm where it binds to and alters troponin. This alteration of troponin allows actin and myosin to interact, causing the muscle to contract.

Ionized and Protein-Bound Calcium

Total plasma calcium levels average 8.5 to 10.5 mg/dL. The calcium present in the plasma is in three forms: protein-bound calcium (normally 4.0 to 4.5 mg/dL), complexed (non-protein-bound, nonionized) calcium (normally 0.5 to 1.0 mg/dL), and ionized calcium (normally 4.2 to 4.8 mg/dL). Increasingly, calcium levels are being reported in milliequivalents per liter, which is half of the number expressed as milligrams per deciliter. Thus, 4.4 mg/dL of ionized calcium is the same as 2.2 mEq/L or 1.1 mmol/L. The ionized calcium fraction, which normally is 2.1 to 2.4 mEq/L or 1.05 to 1.3 mmol/L, is responsible for virtually all the physiologic effects of calcium, of which the neuromuscular changes are most obvious.

On an average, each gram of protein binds 0.8 mg of calcium. Thus, if the ionized calcium is 4.4 mg/dL and the total protein (TP) is 7.0 gm/dL, the total calcium is

$$\begin{aligned} Ca_{tot} &= 4.4 + (0.8)(TP) = 4.4 + (0.8)(7.0) \\ &= 4.4 + 5.6 = 10.0 \text{ mg/dL} \end{aligned}$$

If the albumin (alb) and globulin (glob) concentrations are unusual, one can estimate the normal total calcium (mg/dL) by the following formula:

$$Ca_{tot} = 4.4 + (1.1)(alb) + (0.2)(glob)$$

Thus, if the albumin is 3.0 g/dL and globulin is 4.0 g/dL,

$$\begin{aligned} Ca_{tot} &= 4.4 + (1.1)(3.0) + (0.2)(4.0) \\ &= 4.4 + 3.3 + 0.8 = 8.5 \text{ mg/dL} \end{aligned}$$

Because the relationships between total calcium, ionized calcium, and the plasma proteins vary so much, these formulas provide only a gross estimation of the relationship between ionized calcium and total calcium.

Hypocalcemia

Hypocalcemia is often defined as an ionized calcium below 2.0 mEq/L or 1.0 mmol/L. Total calcium levels, especially in the presence of hypoalbuminemia, may be very low and yet be associated with normal ionized calcium levels. Some of the more common causes of ionic hypocalcemia are shock, sepsis, renal failure, and pancreatitis (Table 10-15). Hypocalcemia is unusual in ambulatory patients except those

Table 10-15. Causes of Hypocalcemia

Shock or sepsis
Impaired production of 1α,25-dihydroxyvitamin D_3
- Malabsorption
- Severe hepatic failure
- Renal failure
- Anticonvulsant therapy

Pancreatitis
Hypomagnesemia
Alkalosis
Decreased serum albumin levels
Hypoparathyroidism
- Idiopathic
- Postsurgical
- Pseudohypoparathyroidism

Osteoblastic metastases
Fat embolism syndrome

with chronic hypoparathyroidism following surgery or in chronic renal disease.

Etiology

Movement into "Sick" Cells

The concentration of ionized calcium in the ECF is about 1.0 mmol/L or 10^{-3} *M*. The concentration of ionized calcium in the cytoplasm of most cells is about 10^{-7} *M*. This gradient of 10^4, or 10,000, to 1 is maintained by active metabolic processes. Any process which interferes with cell metabolism, such as shock or sepsis, will tend to reduce ionized calcium levels by allowing increased net movement of calcium across the cell membrane into the cytoplasm of the poorly functioning cells. Following trauma, serum calcium levels may be low, especially with the fat embolism syndrome, not only because of cell dysfunction and binding of calcium to free fatty acids, but also because of fatty acid inhibition of cell membrane calcium pumps.

Pancreatitis

Acute pancreatitis is an important cause of hypocalcemia. Pancreatic lipase breaks down fat into fatty acids and glycerol. The fatty acids combine with calcium to form insoluble calcium soaps and reduce serum calcium levels. The combination of necrotic fat cells plus calcium soaps makes up much of what is recognized as the fat necrosis of pancreatitis. In addition, as protein moves into the inflammatory exudate, the resultant hypoproteinemia may cause total calcium levels to fall. Pancreatitis can also reduce PTH secretion and the response of tissues to it. If total calcium levels fall below 7.0 or 8.0 mg/dL, there is an increased chance of severe complications from pancreatitis.

Drugs

A large number of drugs can cause hypocalcemia (Table 10-16). One of the most frequently used of these is cimetidine. This histamine receptor-blocking agent apparently lowers serum calcium levels by decreasing the synthesis or secretion of parathyroid hormone.

Postoperative Hypocalcemia

Hypoparathyroidism

Currently, more than 10 percent of postparathyroidectomy patients may have hypoparathyroidism as defined by a fasting calcium of less than 8.5 mg/dL and a simultaneous inorganic phosphorus of greater than 4.5 mg/dL. Postoperative hypocalcemia can be due to hypoparathyrodism from the permanent surgical removal of parathyroid tissue, from transient ischemia of the parathyroid glands in patients who have extensive bilateral neck surgery, or because of long-term hypercalcemic suppression of the nonadenomatous parathyroid glands.

Table 10-16. Drugs That Can Cause Hypocalcemia

Cimetidine
Phosphates (e.g., enemas, laxatives)
Dilantin, phenobarbital
Gentamicin, tobramycin
Cisplatin
Heparin
Theophylline
Protamine
Glucagon
Norepinephrine
Citrate (blood)
Loop diuretics
Glucocorticoids
Magnesium sulfate
Sodium nitroprusside

Hungry-Bone Syndrome

The term "hungry bone syndrome" was coined by Albright and now indicates postparathyroidectomy hypocalcemia due to rapid remineralization of the skeleton. During this accelerated remineralization, a persistent hypocalcemia and hypophosphatemia may be severe enough to cause tetany. These patients may require vigorous calcium and vitamin D supplementation for prolonged periods of time.

In a recent study, Brasier and Nussbaum found the hungry bone syndrome in 13 percent of their patients after parathyroid surgery. Patients were felt to have this problem if they had a fasting calcium level less than 8.5 mg/dL and a simultaneous inorganic serum phosphorus of less than 3.0 mg/dL on postoperative day 3 or later.

Renal Failure

Hypocalcemia is a frequent finding in renal failure. This may be partially due to the resulting hyperphosphatemia, but there is also decreased production of $1\alpha,25\text{-}(OH)_2$-vitamin D in the kidney, which, in turn, causes decreased intestinal absorption of calcium. Secondary hyperparathyroidism with increased PTH levels often results from the chronic hypocalcemia. If PTH levels remain elevated and hypercalcemia develops in spite of cure of the renal failure by renal transplantation, the patient is said to have tertiary hyperparathyroidism.

Phosphate Overload

Phosphate overload from nonrenal causes may also lead to hypocalcemia. This is the presumed mechanism in the acute rhabdomyolysis of hyperpyrexia and major trauma. Excessive use of phosphate cathartics and sodium phosphate enemas can cause significant hyperphosphatemia in patients with renal disease, in children with Hirschsprung's disease, and in small infants.

Hypomagnesemia

Hypomagnesemia as a cause of or association with hypocalcemia may be seen in alcoholism, diuretic use, epilepsy, and renal failure. Neonatal hypomagnesemia leads to low PTH secretion, decreased responsiveness of bone cells to PTH, and decreased calcium mobilization from bone.

Idiopathic Hypoparathyroidism

Idiopathic hypoparathyroidism is probably an autoimmune disorder in which pernicious anemia, exostoses, moniliasis, Hashimoto's disease, sterility, and Addison's disease may be seen. This syndrome may also be associated with cataracts, mental retardation, intracranial calcifications, and papilledema due to increased intracranial pressure.

Nonsurgical Primary Hypoparathyroidism

Hypocalcemia with primary hypoparathyroidism has been reported from parathyroid infarction, metastases to the parathyroids, and hemochromatosis of the parathyroids.

Pseudohypoparathyroidism

Pseudohypoparathyroidism is a familial disorder characterized by decreased end-organ responsiveness to PTH resulting in hypocalcemia, hyperphosphatemia, parathyroid hyperplasia, and excessive serum PTH concentrations. These patients usually have a very low urinary cyclic AMP excretion that only slightly increases with infusion of parathormone. This condition may be inherited as an X-linked dominant trait with variable penetrance; the male to female ratio is 2 to 1. Patients are short in stature and have round facies; brachycephaly; a short, thick neck; short, pudgy fingers and toes; and growth failure of the fourth and fifth metacarpals. Mental retardation, seizures, and subcutaneous soft tissue calcification may be seen. The skin can be dry and coarse, and the hair is often brittle.

Vitamin D Deficiency

Hypocalcemia due to vitamin D deficiency is rare in the United States. Infants born to vitamin D–deficient mothers who lack sunlight exposure and receive no vitamin D supplementation may have rickets. Breast milk has low vitamin D content, and breast milk feeding without sunshine exposure in unsupplemented infants may result in infantile rickets.

Physiologic Effects

Although normal ionized calcium levels are 2.1 to 2.6 mEq/L (1.05 to 1.3 mmol/L), serious physiologic changes do not usually occur until ionized levels in serum are less than 1.4 to 1.6 mEq/L (0.7 to 0.8 mmol/L). Below those levels, hypocalcemia can cause a wide variety of signs and symptoms (Table 10-17).

The severity of signs and symptoms depends greatly on the rapidity of the fall in calcium. The more acute the drop in the serum calcium, the more likely are significant pathophysiological changes. As serum calcium levels fall, neuronal membranes become increasingly more permeable to sodium, enhancing excitation. Potassium and magnesium have an antagonizing effect on this excitation.

Decreased ionized calcium levels reduce the strength of myocardial contraction primarily by inhibiting relaxation. They also decrease the sensitivity of the heart to digitalis. Hypocalcemia should be considered in patients with refractory heart failure.

Low ionized calcium levels increase PTH secretion, which mobilizes calcium from bone and decreases renal tubular absorption of phosphate and bicarbonate. This, in turn, may cause an increased absorption of chloride, producing a tendency to hyperchloremic hypophosphatemic renal tubular acidosis. A ratio of chloride to phosphate greater than 35 to 1 in mEq/mg in the plasma is sometimes considered to be highly suggestive of hyperparathyroidism.

Increased cytoplasmic calcium activates phospholipase, which increases prostaglandin production and alters cell lipids. Increased cytoplasmic calcium also interferes with cell metabolism. Efforts by mitochondria to pump the excess calcium from the cytoplasm into the mitochondrial matrix greatly reduce adenosine triphosphate (ATP) formation. Consequently, giving calcium during shock or sepsis may transiently improve hemodynamics, but if cell metabolism does not also improve, some of the additional calcium moves into the cytoplasm within 30 to 40 min and further impairs cell metabolism.

Movement of calcium into ischemic cerebrovascular smooth muscle cells may cause persistent cerebral vasoconstriction with resultant failure of cerebral reperfusion after strokes or cardiac arrest. This may be a major cause of the poor results in management of these problems. Consequently, there has been some interest in the use of calcium blockers for cerebral resuscitation.

Table 10-17. Symptoms and Signs of Hypocalcemia

General	Muscular
Weakness, fatigue	Spasms, cramps
Neurologic	Weakness
Tetany	Skeletal
Chvostek's sign, Trousseau's sign	Osteodystrophy
Circumoral and digital paresthesias	Rickets
Impaired memory, confusion	Osteomalacia
Hallucinations, dementia, seizures	Miscellaneous
Extrapyramidal disorders	Dental hypoplasia
Dermatologic	Cataracts
Hyperpigmentation	Decreased insulin secretion
Course, brittle hair	
Dry, scaly skin	
Cardiovascular	
Heart failure	
Vasoconstriction	

Diagnosis

Symptoms

The most characteristic initial symptom of hypocalcemia following thyroid or parathyroid surgery is parasthesias around the mouth or in the fingertips. Hypocalcemia should be suspected in any patient who is irritable and has hyperactive deep tendon reflexes following neck surgery. It should also be suspected in patients who have seizures, particularly if they have ever had thyroid surgery, even if many years previously.

Signs

A positive Chvostek's or Trousseau's sign is generally considered to be good clinical evidence of hypocalcemia. A positive Chvostek's sign is a twitch at the corner of the mouth when the examiner taps over the facial nerve just in front of the ear. However, it is present in about 10 to 30 percent of normal individuals. Nevertheless, eyelid muscle contraction with the Chvostek maneuver is said to be almost diagnostic of hypocalcemia.

Trousseau's sign, which is generally a more reliable indicator of hypocalcemia, is positive if carpal spasm is produced when the examiner applies a blood pressure cuff to the upper arm and maintains a pressure above systolic for 3 min. The fingers are spastically extended at the interphalangeal joints and flexed at the metacarophalangeal joints. The wrist is flexed and the forearm is pronated.

Laboratory Findings

Signs of hypocalcemia may be found with normal total serum calcium levels if the patient is very alkalotic. Each 0.1 rise in pH lowers ionized calcium levels by about 3 to 8 percent. Consequently, a very alkalotic patient may have normal total serum calcium levels with ionic hypocalcemia. Similar signs and symptoms may be caused by hypomagnesemia, strychnine, or tetanus toxin.

Decreased plasma levels of ionized calcium are diagnostic, but one should also suspect ionic hypocalcemia if the patient has decreased levels of total calcium in the presence of normal plasma proteins. Primary hypoparathyroidism is characterized by a low serum PTH concentration, hyperphosphatemia, and hypocalcemia.

ECG

The most characteristic ECG finding in hypocalcemia is prolonged QT intervals. However, the T wave is of normal width, and it is the ST segment which is really prolonged. This finding is usually seen with total serum calcium levels less than 6.0 mg/dL.

X-Rays

Radiologically, rickets is characterized by craniotabes, frontal skull bossing, rachitic rosary ribs, widened rib cage (Harrison's groove), bowed legs, and, often, fractures. Other radiographic changes include cupping and splaying of the metaphyseal ends of long bones, widening between the metaphyses and epiphysis, bone demineralization, and thinning of cortical bone.

Treatment

Treatment of hypocalcemia is tailored to the individual and directed toward the underlying cause. If the patient is asymptomatic, oral calcium therapy with or without vitamin D may be all that is required. Calcium lactate, calcium glubionate, calcium ascorbate, calcium carbonate, and calcium gluconate are available in oral preparations. Milk, because of the large amount of phosphate present, is not really a very good source of calcium, except in normal growing children who also need the phosphate.

Symptomatic patients following thyroid or parathyroid surgery are often treated with parenteral calcium (Table 10-18). With severe acute hypocalcemia, 10 mL of 10% $CaCl_2$ or calcium gluconate may be given IV over 10 to 20 min followed by a continuous IV drip providing 1 g of $CaCl_2$ over a period of 6 to 12 h. If the patient is not asymptomatic or if the hypocalcemia is not severe and prolonged for more than 10 to 14 days, treatment with calcium may not be required. One should not administer calcium rapidly IV to asymptomatic patients with mild to moderate hypocalcemia because it can cause severe unnecessary cardiovascular, neuromuscular, and renal complications. For chronic hypoparathyroidism, use of oral calcium salts and rather high doses of vitamin D may be required.

During massive transfusions, if the blood is being given faster than 1 unit every 5 min, 10 mL of 10% calcium chloride can be given after every 4 to 6 units of blood if the patient is in shock or heart failure in spite of adequate volume replacement therapy. Calcium is seldom required during transfusions for elective surgery.

Although, in the past, the use of calcium was advocated for the resuscitation of patients with asystole or electromechanical dissociation, it has now been shown that the chances of successful resuscitation are reduced by using calcium. On the other hand, patients with bradyasystolic arrest and chronic renal failure are apt to have hyperkalemia and hypocalcemia and may benefit from calcium administration.

For the prevention of rickets, 400 IU of vitamin D is the recommended daily allowance. Treatment of established rickets may involve a daily dose of vitamin D as high as 5000 to 10,000 IU until the electrolyte and bone changes are corrected.

Hypercalcemia

Etiology

Hypercalcemia may be defined as a total calcium level exceeding 10.5 mg/dL or an ionized calcium level exceeding 2.7 mEq/L. This abnormality has been found in 0.3 to 5.0 percent of patients studied in various biomedical profiles. A mnemonic used to remember some of the more common causes of hypercalcemia is "Pam P. Schmidt" for *p*arahormone, *A*ddison's disease, *m*ultiple myeloma, *P*aget's disease, *s*arcoidosis, *c*ancer, *h*yperthyroidism, *m*ilk-alkali syndrome, *i*mmobilization, excess vitamin *D*, and *t*hiazides.

Table 10-18. Treatment of Hypocalcemia

Parenteral			
Ca^{2+} gluconate (10%)	10-mL ampules	93 mg Ca^{2+} (4.6 mEq)	10–30mL in 100 mL D_5W over 10–15 min
Ca^{2+} chloride (10%)	10-mL ampules	272 mg Ca^{2+} (13.6 mEq)	2.5–10 mL in 100 mL D_5W over 10–15 min
Oral			
Ca^{2+} gluconate tablets	1000 mg (also 325-, 500-, and 600-mg tablets)	92 mg Ca^{2+} (4.5 mEq)	1–4 g/day in divided doses q 6 h
Ca^{2+} glubionate (Neo-calglucon)	5 mL syrup	23 mg Ca^{2+}/mL	1–4 g/day in divided doses q 6 h
Ca^{2+} lactate tablets	650 mg	79 mg Ca^{2+}	1–4 g/day in divided doses q 6 h
Ca^{2+} carbonate Titralac	5-mL solution, or 650-mg tablet	170, 400 mg Ca^{2+}	1–4 g/day in divided doses q 6 h
Os-Cal	Tablet	250 mg Ca^{2+} (125 U vitamin D)	

Malignancies

The most frequent cause of severe hypercalcemia is malignant neoplasms with either extensive metastases or PTH-like activity. Hypercalcemia is quite common in women with carcinoma of the breast being treated with estrogens. Hypercalcemia is also seen with increased frequency in lung cancer (especially of the squamous cell type) and renal carcinomas. Other malignancies associated with hypercalcemia but which are less frequent include multiple myeloma, pheochromocytoma, and some acute leukemias. In general, the higher the serum calcium level, especially above 14.0 mg/dL, the more likely the hypercalcemia is to be due to malignancy.

Primary Hyperparathyroidism

The next most common cause of hypercalcemia is primary hyperparathyroidism, which accounts for 25 to 50 percent of all hypercalcemia (Table 10-19). In ambulatory care settings, primary hyperparathyroidism is the most common cause of hypercalcemia. Primary hyperparathyroidism is caused by a parathyroid adenoma in 80 percent of cases and parathyroid hyperplasia in the remaining 20 percent. With very high calcium levels and no evidence of a malignancy, an enlarged parathyroid gland can sometimes be palpated in the neck. Parathyroid carcinoma is a rare cause of hyperparathyroidism.

Multiple Endocrine Adenomas

Parathyroid adenomas may be sporadic or familial. The familial type may be part of a multiglandular endocrinopathy, and one should look for associated pancreatic, pituitary, adrenal, and thyroid neoplasms in any patient with primary hyperparathyroidism. The combination of parathyroid, pituitary, and pancreatic islet adenomas is known as multiple endocrine neoplasia type I, or Wermer's syndrome. Multiple endocrine neoplasia type IIA (Sipple's syndrome) consists of hyperparathyroidism combined with pheochromocytoma and medullary cell carcinoma of the thyroid. In infants, parathyroid hyperplasia may be inherited as a familial autosomal dominant or recessive trait. It is sometimes seen in infants of hypoparathyroid mothers in response to chronic intrauterine hypocalcemia.

Immobilization

In patients who are immobilized, the parathyroid–vitamin D axis is suppressed, and calcium may leave bone rapidly, producing hypercalcemia, at least temporarily. Urinary excretion of calcium in such patients may exceed 200 to 300 mg/day, and there is an increased

Table 10-19. Causes of Hypercalcemia

Malignancy	Granulomatous disease
Lung (squamous cell cancer)	Sarcoid
Breast	Tuberculosis
Kidney	Histoplasmosis
Myeloma	Coccidiomycosis
Leukemia	Immobilization
Endocrinopathies	Miscellaneous
Primary hyperparathyroidism	Paget's disease of bone
Hyperthyroidism	Postrenal transplantation
Pheochromocytoma	Recovery from acute renal failure
Adrenal Insufficiency	Phosphate depletion syndrome
Acromegaly	
Drugs	
Hypervitaminosis D and A	
Thiazides	
Lithium	
Hormonal therapy for breast cancer	

tendency to nephrolithiasis. Patients with Paget's disease, especially if they are at bed rest because of their pain, may have severe hypercalcemia due to rapid bone turnover. Astronauts, due to their weightlessness, may rapidly lose large amounts of calcium from their bones and develop a severe prolonged negative calcium balance.

Hyperthyroidism

Although intestinal absorption of calcium is reduced in hyperthyroidism, up to one-third of patients with thyrotoxicosis will concurrently have hypercalcemia, which resolves with treatment of the thyroid disorder. The source of excess calcium is presumed to be bone, but the exact mechanism is not known.

Addison's Disease

Hypercalcemia has been seen in patients with Addison's disease and adrenal crisis perhaps because of a lack of the hypocalcemic effect of corticosteroids.

Hypervitaminosis

Hypervitaminosis A and D can cause hypercalcemia. In vitamin A toxicity, the patient will present with arthralgias, alopecia, a desquamating pruritus, and signs and symptoms of hypercalcemia. Vitamins A and D both cause increased osteoclastic resorption of bone, but vitamin D toxicity also causes increased intestinal absorption of calcium. Vitamin A toxicity usually subsides after discontinuation of vitamin A intake, but vitamin D toxicity may require treatment with corticosteroids.

Milk-Alkali Syndrome

Milk-alkali syndrome is an uncommon cause of hypercalcemia but has been reported in patients with peptic ulcer disease who drank excessive quantities of milk together with large amounts of antacids.

Granulomas

Many granulomatous diseases are associated with hypercalcemia. Hypercalcemia occurs in up to 17 percent of patients with sarcoidosis due to increased sensitivity to vitamin D in the intestine resulting in increased absorption of calcium. This hypercalcemia responds to corticosteroids or to vitamin D restriction. Hypersensitivity to vitamin D can also be seen in tuberculosis. There are a number of reports of hypercalcemia in patients with disseminated coccidioidomycosis, silicon granulomas, berylliosis, and histoplasmosis.

Thiazide Diuretics

Hypercalcemia may be seen with the use of thiazide diuretics, which increase the renal tubular reabsorption of calcium and decrease plasma volume. It is one of the more common causes of hypercalcemia in ambulatory patients. Other diuretics increase urinary calcium excretion and tend to cause hypocalcemia.

Syndromes in Infancy

Hypercalcemia may be seen in Williams syndrome, which is characterized by supravalvular aortic stenosis and elfin facies. Blue diaper syndrome, in which excessive amounts of indole derivatives cause blue urine because of an error in tryptophan metabolism, may also be associated with hypercalcemia.

Pathophysiologic Effects

The effects of hypercalcemia can be neuromuscular, cardiovascular, gastrointestinal, renal, and skeletal. Neuromuscular changes include decreased sensitivity, responsiveness, and strength of muscular contraction and nerve conduction. This causes increasing weakness and fatigue which may progress to ataxia and altered mental status.

In mild hypercalcemic states, the heart's conduction is slowed and automaticity is decreased with a shortening of the refractory period. There is also increased sensitivity to digitalis preparations. Gastrointestinal motility is impaired but there is increased acid secretion in response to gastrin.

Loss of renal concentrating ability, as might be expected with nephrogenic DI, is the most frequent renal effect of hypercalcemia. This is a reversible tubular defect, which results in polyuria and dehydration in spite of polydipsia. Sodium, potassium, and magnesium reabsorption are reduced in the proximal tubule. Potassium wasting results in hypokalemia in up to one-third of patients. Nephrocalcinosis and nephrolithiasis are caused by the hypercalcemia and aggravated by dehydration. As the hypercalcemia persists, increasing microscopic calcium deposits in the kidney may result in progressive renal insufficiency.

With serum concentrations greater than 16 mg/dL, calcium salts may deposit in the myocardium, kidneys, lungs, subcutaneous tissue, blood vessel walls, conjunctiva, and cornea. If phosphate is given, calcium phosphate can rapidly precipitate in tissues. Hypertension is seen with increased frequency in hypercalcemic patients, probably as a result of arteriolar vasoconstriction.

Diagnosis

Hypercalcemic patients with plasma total calcium levels below 12.0 mg/dL are usually asymptomatic, but higher levels can cause a wide variety of symptoms and signs (Table 10-20).

Patients with total calcium levels above 14 to 16 mg/dL are usually very weak, lethargic, and confused. Coma is uncommon, but calcium levels should probably be taken in any patient with coma of unknown etiology. Polyuria, in spite of polydipsia, tends to cause increasing dehydration. Weariness and weakness are common with hypercalcemia. Polyuria and polydipsia are due to impaired renal tubular reabsorption of water. Total calcium levels above 15.0 mg/dL may cause somnolence, stupor, and even coma.

A mnemonic sometimes used for the signs and symptoms of hypercalcemia is *stones* (renal calculi), *bones* (osteolysis), *psychic moans* (psychiatric disorders), and *abdominal groans* (peptic ulcer disease and pancreatitis). The most common gastrointestinal symptoms are anorexia and constipation, but these are very nonspecific.

Table 10-20. Symptoms and Signs of Hypercalcemia

General	Cardiovascular
Malaise, weakness	Hypertension
Polydipsia, dehydration	Arrhythmias
Neurologic	Vascular calcifications
Confusion	ECG abnormalities
Apathy, depression, stupor	QT shortening
Decreased memory	Coving of ST-T wave
Irritability	Widening of T wave
Hallucinations	Digitalis sensitivity
Headache	Gastrointestinal
Ataxia	Anorexia, weight loss
Hyporeflexia, hypotonia	Nausea, vomiting
Mental retardation (infants)	Constipation
Metastatic calcification	Abdominal pain
Band keratopathy	Peptic ulcer disease
Conjunctivitis	Pancreatitis
Pruritus	Urologic
Skeletal	Polyuria, nocturia
Fractures	Renal insufficiency
Bone pain	Nephrolithiasis
Deformities	

Hypercalcemia should be suspected in patients with extensive metastatic bone disease, particularly if the primary site involves the breast, lungs, or kidneys, and in individuals with combinations of clinical problems such as renal calculi, pancreatitis, or ulcer disease. As with hypocalcemia, ionized calcium levels should be measured and/or total calcium levels should be correlated with serum proteins. If the patient is hypoproteinemic, total calcium levels may be normal or low in spite of increased ionized calcium levels.

On ECG, hypercalcemia may be associated with depressed ST segments, widened T waves, and shortened ST segments and QT intervals. Bradyarrhythmias may occur, and bundle branch patterns may progress to second-degree block and then complete heart block. Levels above 20 mg/dL may cause cardiac arrest.

The diagnosis of primary hyperparathyroidism is primarily based on two laboratory findings: (1) elevated serum calcium levels on at least three different occasions and (2) a serum PTH level which is disproportionately high for a simultaneously measured serum calcium level. A serum chloride to phosphorus ratio exceeding 35 to 1 can help confirm the diagnosis.

Treatment

Treatment of hypercalcemia is particularly important for patients with (1) calcium levels greater than 12 mg/dL, (2) symptoms, (3) inability to maintain a good fluid intake, or (4) abnormal renal function. Treatment is aimed at correcting the dehydration, promoting urinary calcium excretion, and decreasing calcium influx into the ECF from the skeletal system and gastrointestinal tract.

Patients with hypercalcemia tend to be dehydrated because high calcium levels interfere with ADH and the ability of the kidney to concentrate urine. Consequently, the initial and safest treatment is restoration of the ECF with relatively large amounts of saline. More than 5 to 10 L of normal saline may be required in the first 24 h to correct the dehydration. Some authors attempt to achieve a urine output as high as 250 mL/m^2 per hour to facilitate calcium excretion and ensure continued adequate hydration. In patients with cardiac or renal disease, such fluid therapy may be dangerous, and peritoneal dialysis or hemodialysis may be required.

Once the ECF has been restored and a good urine output started, a wide variety of diuretics (but not thiazides) will further increase renal excretion of calcium. Furosemide in doses of 1 to 3 mg/kg has been advocated. Up to one-third of patients with hypercalcemia have hypokalemia, and in those with malignant disease, more than half the patients may have hypokalemia. Some patients will also have hypomagnesemia. The tendency to develop hypokalemia and hypomagnesemia will be aggravated by the diuresis and should be watched for carefully and promptly corrected.

A wide variety of modalities are available to treat hypercalcemia (Table 10-21). Mithramycin is a cytotoxic drug which suppresses bone resorption and calcium release from bone. It may be particularly helpful in patients with metastatic bone disease. Small daily doses of 15 to 25 μg/kg in 5% dextrose IV over a period of 3 h for 3 days can lower serum calcium levels within 24 to 48 h; however, the mithramycin often suppresses bone resorption for only 5 to 7 days. It must be used with caution in patients with bone marrow problems, thrombocytopenia, or renal or hepatic insufficiency.

Calcitonin (Calcimar) is also an osteoclast inhibitor and is less toxic than mithramycin. The dosage is usually 0.5 to 4 MRC units per kg given IM every 12 h. The dose may be increased to a maximum of 8 MRC units per kg every 6 h. Effects are usually seen within the first 12 h, but patients often become refractory to it within 2 days. When calcitonin is used in conjunction with corticosteroids, the action of calcitonin is more prolonged.

Glucocorticoids may reduce serum calcium levels in patients with sarcoidosis, vitamin A or D intoxication, multiple myeloma, leukemia, or breast cancer. Glucocorticoids work by inhibiting bone resorption and gastrointestinal absorption of calcium. Steroids may also cause calcium to shift inside cells where it may be bound to mitochondria. The dosage of hydrocortisone in adults is 25 to 100 mg IV every 6 to 8 h. The effect of this treatment may not be apparent until after the first 12 h. If no effect is seen after 7 to 10 days, the therapy may be discontinued.

Table 10-21. Treatment of Hypercalcemia

Drug	Dose	Cautions
Saline	Until ECF is restored	Watch for hypokalemia
Furosemide	40–100 mg IV q 2–4 h	Digitalis, renal failure
Decrease bone absorption		
Calcitonin	0.5–4 MRC units/kg IV over 24 h (or IM q 6 h in divided doses)	
Mithramycin	25 μg/kg IV	Bone marrow and renal toxicity
Hydrocortisone	3 mg/kg per day IV in divided doses q 6 h	May take 3 weeks to lower Ca^{2+}
Indomethacin	25 mg PO q 6 h	Peptic ulcer disease, GI bleeding

Intravenous phosphates and EDTA are rarely used now because of the rapid fall in calcium that may occur, along with tissue deposition of calcium phosphate, renal cortical necrosis, and even shock.

When possible, irradiation or resection of neoplasms producing PTH-like activity should be considered. If parathyroid hyperplasia or adenoma is suspected, it should be treated surgically as soon as possible.

MAGNESIUM

Magnesium is a vital element in all biologic systems and is the key element in chlorophyll, the first link in the world's food chain. The total body content of magnesium averages about 2000 mEq (24 g), with about 50 to 70 percent present in bone. The majority of the remaining magnesium is intracellular, with only 1 percent present in the ECF. The serum concentration of magnesium is about 1.8 to 2.4 mg/dL or 1.5 to 2.0 mEq/L. About 25 to 35 percent of the magnesium present in the blood is protein-bound, 10 to 15 percent is complexed, and 50 to 60 percent is ionized. The concentration of magnesium intracellularly is thought to be about 40 mEq/L, making it the second most abundant intracellular cation.

The usual daily requirement is about 24 to 28 mEq (288 to 336 mg), usually from vegetables and cereals. About 40 percent is excreted in the urine and 60 percent in feces. Renal excretion protects against hypermagnesemia, but not hypomagnesemia, which will develop if intake is consistently less than 3.0 mg/kg per day.

Hypomagnesemia

Etiology

A wide variety of problems can cause hypomagnesemia (Table 10-22). In adults, magnesium deficiencies are most frequently seen in alcoholics, in malnourished patients, and in patients with cirrhosis, pancreatitis, or excessive gastrointestinal fluid losses. Diarrhea is usually more of a problem (Mg^{2+} content of 10 to 14 mEq/L) then upper gastrointestinal loss (1 to 2 mEq/L). Chronic hyperparathyroidism increases urinary losses of magnesium and will eventually cause hypomagnesemia.

Table 10-22. Causes of Hypomagnesemia

Gastrointestinal	Drug-induced
Protein-calorie malnutrition	Diuretics
Hyperalimentation after malnutrition	Aminoglycosides
Malabsorption (diarrhea), fistulas	Cisplatin
Alcoholic cirrhosis	Vitamin D intoxication
Pancreatitis	Digoxin
Renal	Alcohol
Glomerulonephritis, pyelonephritis	Insulin
Diuretic phase of acute tubular necrosis	Citrate (blood)
Hypercalcemia	Miscellaneous
Endocrine	Lactation
Aldosteronism	Sweating
Hyperparathyroidism, hyperthyroidism	Hungry bone syndrome
	Burns
	Sepsis

Intravenous hyperalimentation or treatment of diabetic ketoacidosis without providing adequate magnesium, especially in a previously malnourished patient, can cause an abrupt fall in plasma magnesium levels. This is largely due to magnesium being "pulled" into cells with glucose or as new lean body mass is synthesized. Hypophosphatemia, which can also develop with IV hyperalimentation, can contribute to the hypomagnesemia.

Renal wasting of magnesium can be seen with loop diuretics, hypophosphatemia, ketoacidosis, aminoglycosides, and nephrotoxic chemotherapeutic agents.

The normal renal threshold for magnesium (1.5 to 2.0 mEq/L) is significantly decreased by cisplatin, diuretics, hypercalcemia, growth hormone, thyroid hormone, and calcitonin. Cisplatin causes dose-dependent, cumulative, reversible renal tubular injury. Even when the GFR is not diminished by cisplatin, renal magnesium wasting along with a secondary hypocalcemia and hypokalemia may develop. Potassium wasting is thought to occur as a result of impaired ATP production when magnesium is low. This in turn impairs the function of the membrane Na^+/K^+ transport system and causes loss of the normal Na^+/K^+ gradient. The accompanying hypocalcemia may be due to (1) impaired PTH release by the parathyroid gland, (2) decreased peripheral sensitivity to PTH, or (3) abnormal blood-bone calcium balance independent of PTH.

Physiologic Effects

Magnesium is essential to a large number of vital enzymes, including membrane-bound ATPase. Consequently hypomagnesemia may result in a wide variety of neuromuscular, gastrointestinal, and cardiovascular changes (Table 10-23).

Hypomagnesemia may cause increased muscular irritability similar to that seen with hypocalcemia. It can also cause many CNS signs and symptoms, including depression, vertigo, ataxia, and seizures. In severe chronic alcoholics, delirium tremens is often associated with moderate to severe magnesium deficiencies. Cardiac arrhythmias, particularly in patients on digitalis, is often due to both potassium and magnesium deficiencies.

Table 10-23. Symptoms and Signs of Hypomagnesemia

Neuromuscular	Gastrointestinal
Tetany	Dysphagia
Muscle weakness	Anorexia, nausea
Cerebellar (ataxia, nystagmus, vertigo)	Cardiovascular
Confusion, obtundation, coma	Heart failure
Seizures	Arrhythmias
Apathy, depression	Hypotension
Irritability	Miscellaneous
Paresthesias	Hypokalemia
	Hypocalcemia
	Anemia

Some metabolic manifestations of magnesium deficiency include difficulties in treating hypokalemia, impaired PTH secretion, decreased response to thiamine, and vitamin D–resistant hypocalcemia. Other manifestations include hypothermia, hypotension, nephropathy, incomplete distal renal tubular acidosis, dysphagia, and anemia due to shortened RBC survival.

It has been noted that patients with severe acute pancreatitis and hypocalcemia usually have normal serum magnesium levels; however, their mononuclear cell magnesium content may be significantly low and their retention of magnesium with a loading test may be significantly increased. This implies that, in spite of the normal serum magnesium levels, there is an intracellular and total body magnesium deficiency. This may contribute to the severity of the pancreatitis and the pathogenesis of the hypocalcemia.

Diagnosis

One cannot rely on plasma levels to diagnose magnesium deficiencies because it is not unusual to have total body magnesium fall rather severely before plasma levels are lowered. The diagnosis of hypomagnesemia in the presence of normal serum calcium levels is suggested by increased neuromuscular irritability (hyperreflexia, positive Chvostek's or Trousseau's signs, tremor, tetany, or even convulsions). Hypomagnesemia should be suspected in alcoholics, cirrhotics, and patients on IV fluids for prolonged periods. Hypomagnesemia may also develop rapidly during IV hyperalimentation, especially when anabolism begins.

The ECG changes seen with magnesium deficiencies include prolonged PR and QT intervals, widened QRS complexes, depression of ST segments, and inversion of T waves, especially in the precordial leads. The changes may be somewhat similar to those caused by hypokalemia and/or hypocalcemia, and many of these changes may be related to Mg^{2+} deficiency altering cardiac intracellular potassium content.

Treatment

Hypokalemia, hypocalcemia, and hypophosphatemia are often present with hypomagnesemia and must be monitored carefully. It must be emphasized that the physician treating a magnesium deficiency should look for and correct any associated potassium, calcium, or phosphate deficiencies.

Patients with magnesium deficiency may require more than 50 mEq or oral magnesium (6 g $MgSO_4$) per day. In chronic alcoholics with delirium tremens and in patients with severe proven hypomagnesemia, up to 8 to 12 g of $MgSO_4$ may be given intramuscularly or intravenously the first day. The first 10 to 15 mEq (1.5 to 2.0 g) of IV $MgSO_4$ can be given over 1 to 2 h. This may be followed by up to 4 to 6 g/day thereafter. If IV alimentation is being given to a hypomagnesemic patient, 12 to 16 mEq (1.5 to 2.0 g) should be added to each liter of total parenteral alimentation (TPN).

If magnesium is being given rapidly, as in the treatment of eclampsia, the deep tendon reflexes (which disappear at about 3 to 4 mEq/L) should be checked frequently, and blood levels should be measured once or twice daily. If deep tendon reflexes decrease or disappear, magnesium administration should stop, at least temporarily.

A variety of oral forms of magnesium are available for long-term treatment (Table 10-24).

Hypermagnesemia

Etiology

Hypermagnesemia occurs rather infrequently, except in patients with renal failure who are given magnesium-containing drugs, particularly

Table 10-24. Treatment of Hypomagnesemia

Drug	Size and Contents	Dose
Parenteral		
$MgSO_4$ (1 g = 98 mg of elemental Mg^{2+})	10% (20-mL ampules, 0.81 mEq/mL) or 50% (2-ml ampules), 4 mEq/mL)	1–2 g $MgSO_4$ or $MgCl_2$ by continuous IV every 4–6 h prn
$MgCl_2$ (1 g = 118 mg elemental Mg^{2+})	20% (30-mL bottle, 1.97 mEq/mL)	
Oral		
MgO	400-mg tablets (20 mEq)	1–4 per day
$Mg(OH)_2$ (milk of magnesia)	7.5% (2.9 mEq/5mL)	5–15 mL tid

antacids such as Maalox. Other less frequent causes include untreated diabetic acidosis and adrenal insufficiency. Hypermagnesemia may also be seen with tumor lysis, rhabdomyolysis, hyperparathyroidism, hypothyroidism, and ECF volume contraction, all of which lead to decreased magnesium clearance.

Physiologic Effects

Progressively increasing magnesium levels above 3.0 to 4.0 mEq/L can reduce neuromuscular irritability and cause deep tendon reflexes to disappear. Increasing muscular weakness is noted with levels above 4.0 mEq/L, and levels above 5.0 to 6.0 mEq/L may cause severe vasodilation and hypotension. Levels above 8.0 to 10.0 mEq/L can cause cardiac conduction abnormalities and neuromuscular paralysis with hypotension and/or ventilatory failure and death.

Diagnosis

Serum magnesium levels are usually diagnostic. The possibility of hypermagnesemia should be considered in patients with hyperkalemia or hypercalcemia. Hypermagnesemia should also be suspected in patients with renal failure, particularly in those who are on magnesium-containing antacids, such as Maalox.

Treatment

The initial treatment of hypermagnesemia is similar to that used for hypercalcemia and includes dilution by administering IV fluids and then using diuretics, especially furosemide, as needed. Any acidosis should be corrected and a slow infusion of calcium gluconate can also help to control symptoms. Peritoneal dialysis and hemodialysis are thought by some to be relatively ineffective with divalent cations, but removal of up to 700 mg of magnesium with one hemodialysis treatment has been reported.

PHOSPHORUS (PHOSPHATE)

The normal adult man contains about 700 g of phosphorus, of which about 80 percent is present in bones. Phosphorous is essential to a wide variety of reactions, especially energy metabolism in the form of high-energy phosphates and phosphocreatine. Serum phosphorus levels drop with age from a high of 4.0 to 7.0 mg/dL in the newborn to 3.0 to 5.0 mg/dL in adults. Serum calcium and phosphorus levels are inversely proportional, and the product of their two concentrations in milligrams per deciliter usually averages about 30 to 40. The normal oral intake is about 10 to 12 mmol, with urinary excretion largely regulated by PTH.

Hypophosphatemia

Etiology

Because phosphorus is available in so many foods and is so easily absorbed, hypophosphatemia is unusual unless (1) oral intake is reduced, (2) there is excess loss of phosphorus, or (3) there is excessive movement of PO_4 from the ECF into cells (Table 10-25).

One should look carefully for hypophosphatemia in patients on TPN, with low potassium or magnesium levels, or with hypercalcemia. Hypophosphatemia is being increasingly recognized, especially in patients with IV hyperalimentation, which increases phosphate movement into cells as anabolism occurs. Phosphorus is also consumed during phosphorylation of glucose as it moves into cells. Intracellular shifts also occur in the presence of respiratory alkalosis and with the adminstration of anabolic steroids, sodium bicarbonate, epinephrine, or glucagon.

Hypophosphatemia may be seen with metabolic alkalosis, especially after prolonged antacid therapy. Antacids with calcium and magnesium bind to phosphate and impair its intestinal absorption. Metabolic or respiratory alkalosis also increases phosphate loss in the urine. Respiratory alkalosis may also increase phosphate movement into cells. Hyperparathyroidism and alcoholism are additional causes of hypophosphatemia.

Other causes of hypophosphatemia include malignancy with hypercalcemia (due to phosphaturia), renal tubular defects, hypokalemia, hypomagnesemia, and use of phosphate-binding antacids. One should

Table 10-25. Conditions Associated with Hypophosphatemia

- Intake
  - Deficiency of dietary phosphate
  - Phosphate malabsorption in dialyzed patients, alcoholics
  - Overuse of phosphate-binding agents
  - TPN
- Redistribution
  - Glucose infusion
  - Treatment of diabetes mellitus
  - Respiratory alkalosis
  - β-Adrenergic agents
  - Increased skeletal uptake in healing phase of rickets
  - Osteoblastic metastases of cancer
  - Nutritional recovery syndrome
  - Androgens, estrogens
  - Diuretic phase of severe burns
- Renal Causation
  - Specific phosphate transport defect
    - X-linked dominant hypophosphatemia
    - Autosomal dominant hypophosphatemia
  - Multiple renal tubular transport defects
    - Idiopathic Fanconi syndrome
    - Cystinosis
    - Hereditary fructose intolerance
    - Galactosemia
    - Wilson's disease
    - Oculocerebrorenal (Lowe's) syndrome
  - Phosphaturia due to primary or secondary hyperparathyroidism
    - Primary hyperparathyroidism
    - Secondary hyperparathyroidism due to hereditary vitamin D dependency, types I and II
    - Hypocalcemia from any cause, provided parathyroid glands are intact
- Miscellaneous
  - Tumor-induced hypophosphatemia
  - Posttransplantation hypophosphatemia
  - Hypercalciuric nephrolithiasis

also look for and prevent or rapidly correct hypophosphatemia in patients during rapid healing or anabolism. During recovery from starvation or after severe burns, the body requirement for phosphate can greatly increase. The phosphate and potassium requirement of patients who undergo a partial hepatectomy may be particularly large, especially if more than 60 percent of the liver has been resected. In general, 5.0 mmol of phosphate is used to generate 1.0 g of protein; therefore, phosphate requirements may be as high as 30 to 60 mmol/day. Thus, extensive tissue repair or healing can quickly lead to severe phosphorous deficiency if there is inadequate intake.

Physiologic Effects

The most frequent consequences of hypophosphatemia are hematologic and neuromuscular. Hypophosphatemia may be associated with depletion of ATP in platelets, red blood cells, and white blood cells, reducing their survival time and function. Platelet membrane changes may result in a bleeding tendency due to impaired aggregation. Phosphate deficiency also causes tendency for red blood cells to become rigid spherocytes, thereby impairing capillary perfusion. In addition, decreased 2,3-diphosphoglycerate (2,3-DPG) increases the affinity of hemoglobin for oxygen, thereby reducing the arterial P_{O_2} and oxygen availability to tissues. Phosphate depletion in macrophages may impair chemotaxis, phagocytosis, and intracellular killing, resulting in decreased resistance to infection.

Progressive weakness and tremors may be noted as blood phosphate levels fall below 0.5 to 1.0 mg/dL. Circumoral and fingertip paresthesias may be present along with absent deep tendon reflexes. Mental obtundation, anorexia, and hyperventilation may also occur. Patients may become so weak that they cannot be weaned from a ventilator or ambulated. Myocardial function, as measured by left ventricular stroke work, may also be impaired.

Diagnosis

Patients with diabetic or alcoholic ketoacidosis or severe malnutrition are particularly prone to develop hypophosphatemia. This problem should be looked for with particular care within 12 to 48 h of beginning treatment of diabetic ketoacidosis, within 24 to 96 h of treating alcoholic ketoacidosis, and within 5 to 10 days of beginning IV hyperalimentation.

One should not rely completely on blood phosphorous levels to rule out phosphorous deficiency. The ratio of intracellular to extracellular phosphorus concentration is approximately 100 to 1. Since 80 percent of the total body phosphorus is in bone, serum phosphorus levels may not reflect total body stores, and the magnitude of the total body deficit cannot be estimated adequately from blood levels, particularly if there are acute changes.

Treatment

Treatment of hypophosphatemia should be primarily preventive and must be an integral part of any nutrition program. At least 7 to 9 mmol of phosphate, usually as a combination of KH_2PO_4 and K_2HPO_4 (dibasic and monobasic phosphates), should be given with each 1000 calories. In some instances, more than double that amount of phosphate may be required to bring phosphate levels up to normal. Because phosphate administration may cause a precipitous fall in serum calcium levels, calcium should also be given, usually as calcium gluconate in doses of 0.2 to 0.3 mEq/kg per day. The hazards of phosphate therapy include soft tissue calcification, hypotension, and hyperosmolality. If potassium phosphate is used, the therapy may also cause hyperkalemia.

For severe hypophosphatemia with blood levels less than 1.0 mg/dL (0.32 mmol/L) or symptoms, immediate IV replacement is required. Otherwise oral preparations can be often used.

If the hypophosphatemia is recent and uncomplicated, the initial recommended daily dose is 2.5 mg/kg. Prolonged or multifactorial hypophyosphatemia may require 5 mg/kg. Up to 25 to 50 percent more phosphorus is needed if the patient is symptomatic; however, less is required in the presence of hypercalcemia. Each dose is administered IV over 6 h, and serum phosphorus is checked after each dose. To minimize the risks of hyperphosphatemia, a total dose of no more than 7.5 mg/kg should be administered. Risks of phosphate therapy include hypocalcemia, metastatic calcification, hypotension, and hyperkalemia from the potassium salts. One should switch to oral therapy as soon as possible.

Hyperphosphatemia

Etiology

Hyperphosphatemia may be due to reduced renal excretion, increased phosphate movement out of cells into the ECF, or increased phosphorous or vitamin D intake (Table 10-26). Hyperphosphatemia is most apt to be seen with renal dysfunction. It may also be seen with hypoparathyroidism or any problem associated with hypocalcemia or hypomagnesemia.

Physiologic Effects

Problems due to hyperphosphatemia are usually those due to associated renal failure, hypocalcemia, or the hypomagnesemia which is usually present.

Therapy

Therapy is aimed at treating the underlying cause and restricting calcium phosphate intake to less than 200 mg/day. With normal renal function, PO_4 excretion can be increased with saline (1 to 2 L every 4 to 6 h) and acetazolamide (500 mg every 6 h). PO_4 absorption from the GI tract is decreased with oral PO_4 binders (i.e., aluminum carbonate or hydroxide 30 to 45 mL qid). These binders also absorb PO_4 secreted into the gut lumen and are of benefit even if no oral PO_4 is given. If clinically significant hypocalcemia exists, calcium should be cautiously administered. If renal failure is present, hemodialysis may be required.

CHLORIDE

Chloride is the major anion in the extracellular fluid. It fulfills several important physiologic functions. It is an important factor in maintaining (1) urine output and concentration in the renal countercurrent mechanisms, (2) ECF volume, (3) acid-base and potassium balance, and (4) a normal anion gap.

Chloride is readily absorbed in the large and small bowel by active and passive transport mechanisms which are either sodium or bicarbonate dependent. However, there is a $Cl–HCO_3$ exchange in the small

Table 10-26. Conditions Associated with Hyperphosphatemia

Intake	Renal Causation
Poisoning by phosphate-containing enema or laxative	Acute and chonic reduction in GFR
Redistribution	Hypoparathyroid State
Respiratory acidosis	Primary hypoparathyroidism
Lactic acidosis	Pseudohypoparathyroidism
Diphosphonate therapy	Suppression of PTH secretion from any hypercalemic condition
Chemotherapy for neoplasms	Miscellaneous Causes
Rhabdomyolysis	Hyperthyroidism
Septic shock	Vitamin D intoxication
	Acromegaly
	Cortical hyperostosis

bowel. Stomach parietal cells possess the unique capacity to secrete chloride plus hydrogen (H^+) ions into gastric fluid. About 90 percent of the chloride ingested is excreted in the urine and the remainder is lost in the stool and in sweat.

Chloride is almost entirely extracellular, and its concentration is usually about 70 to 75 percent that of sodium. There is little chloride in bone, and virtually all chloride in the body is diffusible and metabolically active.

The Role of Chloride in the Kidney

One should look for hypochloremia in patients who appear to be developing renal dysfunction. The activity of chloride in the kidney is extremely important in determining its ability to concentrate urine. In most of the tubule, chloride reabsorption occurs passively along with sodium transport. However, in the water-impermeable ascending thick limb of the loop of Henle, where about 20 to 30 percent of sodium and chloride is reabsorbed, chloride transport is active. This active transport of chloride apparently provides the crucial gradient needed for the "countercurrent" urine-concentrating mechanism to function properly. In the absence of ADH, this mechanism can also allow absorption of solute without water in the collecting ducts, allowing urine to be more dilute if needed.

Chloride is also significantly involved in plasma acid-base regulation. Although not directly responsible for regulation of H^+ ion concentration, reciprocal changes in plasma HCO_3 and Cl concentrations occur during renal adjustments of ECF pH, when hydrogen and chloride are secreted, and when HCO_3 is reabsorbed. Renal acid excretion and HCO_3 reabsorption can be greatly modified by insufficient quantity of readily reabsorbable anion, particularly chloride, in the glomerular filtrate.

Normal Levels

The range for normal serum chloride is 96 to 108 mEq/L. It can be measured in serum, plasma, urine, sweat, cerebrospinal fluid (CSF), stool, and other body fluids. Serum determinations are most commonly done, but heparinized (or EDTA) plasma may be used. Hemolysis can produce pseudohypochloremia secondary to a dilutional effect by RBC water; therefore, serum should be promptly separated from red cells. As with sodium, an increase in total serum protein may produce pseudohyperchloremia as a result of water displacement. Because all of the chemical methods for analyzing chloride also pickup the other halides, the presence of bromide and iodide can falsely elevate serum chloride levels.

Hypochloremia

Etiology

The most frequent causes of hypochloremia (< 95 mEq/L) are excessive diuresis, especially after administration of loop diuretics, and loss of highly acid gastric secretions through vomiting or nasogastric suction. Hypochloremia is usually associated with the presence of a metabolic alkalosis that can be divided into several types according to etiology. (Table 10-27).

Diuretic use promotes natriuresis, kaliuresis, and chloruresis. Vomiting and external gastric drainage lead to a complex series of events. Gastric parietal cells secrete hydrogen and chloride into gastric fluid while bicarbonate is generated into the circulation. Acid-base balance is maintained by hydrogen and chloride absorption in the more distal GI tract. Metabolic alkalosis results when this balance is upset by vomiting, or any other external loss of hydrochloric acid. This alkalosis is maintained by increased renal absorption of sodium and bicarbonate due to ECF volume depletion.

Because sodium conservation and volume maintenance take precedence over acid-base and potassium balance, the kidney is influenced by aldosterone to accelerate the exchange of sodium for potassium

Table 10-27. Types of Metabolic Alkalosis

Chloride-responsive (U_{Cl} < mEq/L)
GI losses
Vomiting, gastric drainage
Villous adenoma
Congenital chloride diarrhea
Diuretics
Cystic fibrosis
Rapid correction of chronic hypercapnia
Chloride-resistant (U_{Cl} >20 mEq/L)
Excess mineralcorticoid activity
Hyperaldosteronism
Cushing's syndrome
Bartter's syndrome
Excess licorice
Severe K^+ depletion
Unclassified (variable urine chloride)
Massive blood transfusion
Milk-alkali syndrome
Alkali administration
Nonparathyroid hypercalcemia
Large doses of carbenicillin or penicillin

and hydrogen ions. However, if abundant chloride is provided, the pattern is reversed, leading to bicarbonate diureses and correction of the alkalosis.

In contrast to gastric contents, stool is normally low in chloride and rich in potassium. Diarrheal diseases, unless vomiting is a prominent feature, are associated with metabolic acidosis rather than alkalosis. An exception is found with villous adenoma of the colon and in a rare congenital disorder known as chloride diarrhea that arises from a defect in the ileal and colonic C1–HCO_3 exchange mechanism. In both these situations, metabolic alkalosis is a consequence of loss of chloride augmented by ECF volume contraction.

Serious chloride depletion can occur from the skin secondary to severe sweating or severe burns. Patients with cystic fibrosis can develop metabolic alkalosis due to marked loss of chloride in sweat.

Physiologic Effects

The most frequent physiologic effects of hypochloremia are those due to the metabolic alkalosis and hypokalemia with which it is usually associated. Numerous studies have implicated chloride depletion in both the generation and maintenance of metabolic alkalosis. Because chloride is the only anion other than hydrochloric acid which is readily reabsorbed with sodium, chloride depletion accelerates Na–H exchange all along the tubule. Loss of H^+ in the urine results in alkalosis. In addition, because low blood chloride levels impair active chloride transport and the associated sodium reabsorption in the ascending limb, more sodium is delivered to the distal nephron for H^+ and potassium exchange. This exchange results in increased loss of H^+ and potassium in the urine, making the alkalosis more severe. Thus, urine chloride levels should be evaluated in all patients with hypochloremia.

Chloride-responsive alkalosis is established and maintained by ECF volume depletion and chloride deficits. Volume depletion supplies the stimulus for sodium retention, but chloride is not available in sufficient quantity to maintain electrical neutrality. Therefore, the exchange of sodium for hydrogen and potassium ions is accelerated. There is minimal urinary chloride excretion (less than 10 mmol/L), because there is nearly complete reabsorption of filtered chloride in the sodium-avid tubule.

Diagnosis

No signs or symptoms are specifically characteristic of hypochloremia. A history of vomiting, excessive nasogastric suction, or diuretic therapy, together with evidence of volume depletion, should signal the possible presence of hypochloremia and an associated metabolic alkalosis. Metabolic alkalosis may produce muscle weakness, neuromuscular irritability, and hypoventilation. This hypoventilation may be especially dangerous in patients already hypoxic secondary to chronic obstructive pulmonary disease (COPD).

If a patient has a metabolic alkalosis and the urinary chloride levels are low (less than 10 mEq/L), the patient is said to have a chloride-responsive alkalosis. Such patients usually have a relatively simple chloride deficit and will often respond to chloride administration alone. If urine chloride levels are 40 mEq/L or higher, the hypochloremia is probably due to dilution. If the patient is not overloaded with fluids, the hypochloremia is apt to be due to or associated with excessive corticosteroids and/or hypokalemia.

Hypochloremia with increased urine chloride can also be caused by excess mineralocorticoid activity which causes Na^+ and HCO_3^- retention and increased excretion of H^+, K^+, and Cl^- (Table 10-28). The ECF volume expansion results in diminished proximal tubule NaCl reabsorption and, therefore, an increased delivery of sodium to the distal tubule. The exchange of sodium for potassium and hydrogen ions is also enhanced, resulting in an even greater loss of H^+ and K^+.

It has been noted that metabolic alkalosis with severe potassium depletion may be resistant to correction with NaCl alone. Severe potassium depletion may directly alter the renal tubular handling of chloride, resulting in chloride wasting. To reverse this chloride-wasting nephropathy, at least a partial correction of the potassium deficit is required.

Treatment

Chloride-responsive metabolic alkalosis will usually respond to IV administration of sodium chloride alone. Chloride-resistant metabolic alkalosis usually also requires potassium and in severe cases may also require hydrogen ions. Hypochloremia due to dilution from excess total body water is usually best treated by cautious dehydration.

As a general rule, deficits in total body chloride are best treated by giving one-fourth of the calculated chloride deficit as KCl and three-fourths as NaCl. The total body chloride deficit can be estimated rapidly by multiplying 20 percent of the body weight by the serum chloride deficit. Thus, an 80-kg patient with a serum chloride of 60 mEq/L has a total deficit of (80 kg $\times$ 20%) (100 $-$ 60) = 16 $\times$ 40 or 640 mEq.

Table 10-28. Etiology of Hyperchloremia Associated with Primary Hypernatremic States

Administration of hypertonic or excess NaCl
Normal anion-gap metabolic acidosis
GI losses of HCO_3
Diarrhea
Small bowel
Biliary, pancreatic
Ureterosigmoidostomy, obstructed ileal loop conduit
$CaCl_2$, $MgCl_2$ ingestion
Cholestyramine ingestion
Renal losses of HCO_3
Renal tubular acidosis
Hypoaldosteronism
Hyperparathyroidism
Carbonic anhydrase inhibitors
Miscellaneous
Dilutional acidosis
Hyperalimentation acidosis
Sulfur ingestion
Compounds with Cl anion
Compensation of chronic respiratory alkalosis
Low anion-gap states
Hypoalbuminemia
Bromism (other halides)
Unmeasured non-Na cations

In attempting to correct chloride deficits, one should be aware that dehydration can greatly increase the total chloride deficit. If the patient is severely dehydrated, the total additional chloride deficit may be estimated by assuming that the mild, moderate, or severe dehydration involves a 6, 8, or 10 percent loss, respectively, of body weight as ECF containing 100 mEq of chloride per liter. Thus, if an 80-kg man is severely dehydrated, one can assume that he has lost at least 8 L of ECF containing 100 mEq of chloride per liter, or 800 mEq of chloride. Since he can be assumed to have only 8 L of ECF left, the deficit in the remaining ECF is 8 $\times$ 40, or 320 mEq. Thus, the total chloride deficit in a severely dehydrated 80-kg man with a serum chloride of 60 mEq/L would be 800 + 320 or 1120 mEq.

If the patient has renal dysfunction so that potassium cannot be given or if the metabolic alkalosis is very severe or does not respond to NaCl plus KCl, 0.1 *N* HCl or amino acid hydrochlorides may be useful. If 0.1 *N* HCl is used, it should be given slowly through a central IV line.

Hyperchloremia

Etiology

Hyperchloremia is usually due to dehydration, administration of excessive amounts of sodium chloride, or various problems which can cause a normal anion-gap metabolic acidosis (Table 10-28). The most frequent causes of normal anion-gap acidosis are gastrointestinal losses of bicarbonate (small bowel or pancreatic fistulas or diarrhea) or renal bicarbonate losses (Table 10-28). Excess administration of chloride as saline, KCl, and amino acid hydrochlorides can also cause hyperchloremia. All of these substances readily dissociate and consume HCO_3, resulting in hyperchloremic metabolic acidosis. The most frequent acid-base problem seen with IV hyperalimentation is a hyperchloremic metabolic acidosis because the amino acids are provided as chlorides or hydrochlorides.

Pathophysiology

The physiologic effects of hyperchloremia are due primarily to the underlying dehydration or metabolic acidosis. Clinically most changes in plasma chloride concentration parallel those of sodium. Primary hypernatremic states are, for the most part, predictably accompanied by hyperchloremia. In addition, changes in serum chloride accompany reciprocal changes in serum HCO_3. As a result, hypochloremia usually accompanies metabolic alkalosis, and hyperchloremia accompanies normal anion-gap metabolic acidosis.

The systemic effects of acute and severe metabolic acidosis are well known and include Kussmaul (slow, very deep) respirations, decreased myocardial contractility, and a drop in peripheral resistance. Bone disease associated with chronic acidosis, such as that seen in RTA, may manifest itself as stunted growth secondary to acidosis-induced bone mineral loss, as well as rickets and osteomalacia.

Diagnosis

Clinical features of hyperchloremia are difficult to list independently because the presentation is usually a manifestation of the primary underlying disorder and associated metabolic abnormalities. Elevated serum chloride and sodium levels usually indicate dehydration. Elevated chloride levels with normal or low serum sodium levels usually indicate either excess chloride administration as KCl or amino acid hydrochlorides or excess loss of bicarbonate from the body.

Anion gap and arterial pH can be extremely helpful in determining the cause and treatment of hyperchloremia. A low anion gap (less than 10 mEq/L) can be associated with hyperchloremia in several pathologic states. When reduced concentration of unmeasured anions exists, as in cirrhosis or nephrosis with hypoalbuminemia, the normally unmeasured anion albumin is partially replaced with the measured anions chloride and HCO_3 so that the anion gap will tend to fall. Unmeasured non-Na cations, such as cationic proteins in multiple myeloma or severe hypercalcemia, hypermagnesemia, and acute lithium overdose obligate an increased chloride or HCO_3 to counterbalance their positive charge.

An overestimation of serum chloride occurs when bromide (or other halide) is present because they interfere with all laboratory determinations of chloride. Bromism should be suspected when the anion gap is very small or negative.

Treatment

If there is excess administration of chloride or excessive losses of bicarbonate, this should be corrected. Hyperchloremia due to dehydration is best treated by slowly administering increased istonic fluids with little or no chloride. However, if too much hypotonic fluid is given too rapidly, seizures due to cerebral edema may develop.

BIBLIOGRAPHY

Arieff A, Llach F, Massry SG: Neurological manifestations and moridity of hyponatremia correlation with brain water and electrolytes. *Medicine (Baltimore)* 55:121, 1976.

Bartter FC, Schwartz WB: The syndrome of inappropriate secretion of antidiuretic hormone. *Am J Med* 42:790, 1967.

Berry PL: Hyponatremia. *Pediatr Clin North Am* 37:351, 1990.

Brem AS: Disorders of potassium homeostasis. *Pediatr Clin North Am* 37:419, 1990.

Chernow B, Smith J, Rainey TF, et al: Hypomagnesemia with implications for the critical care specialist. *Crit Care Med* 10:193, 1982.

Chernow B, Zaloga G, McFadden E, et al: Hypocalcemia in critically ill patients. *Crit Care Med* 10:848, 1982.

Cluitmans FHM, Meinders AE: Management of severe hyponatremia: Rapid or slow correction? *Am J Med* 88:161–166, 1990.

Conley SB: Hypernatremia. *Pediatr Clin North Am* 37:365, 1990.

DeCristofaro JD, Tsang RC: Calcium. *Emerg Med Clin North Am* 4:207, 1986.

Hartman F, Russier B, Zohlman R, et al: Rapid correction of hyponatremia in the syndrome of inappropriate secretion of antidiuretic hormone. *Ann Intern Med* 78:870, 1973.

Iseri LT, Freed J, Bures AR: Magnesium deficiency and cardiac disorders. *Am J Med* 58:837, 1975.

Martin ML, Hamilton R, West MF: Potassium. *Emerg Med Clin North Am* 4:131, 1986.

Podrid PJ: Potassium and ventricular arrhythmias. *Am J Cardiol* 65, 33E, 1990.

White BC, Winegar CD, Wilson RF, et al: The possible role of calcium blockers in cerebral resuscitation: A review of the literature and synthesis for future studies. *Crit Care Med* 11:202, 1983.

Zaloga G, Chernow B, Lake CR: *The Pharmacologic Approach to the Critically Ill Patient.* Baltimore, Williams and Wilkins, 1983, pp. 530–561.

11 DISTURBANCES OF CARDIAC RHYTHM AND CONDUCTION

J. Stephan Stapczynski

The interpretation and treatment of cardiac arrhythmias is basic to the practice of emergency medicine. This chapter reviews the important cardiac rhythm and conduction disturbances and their clinical significance and emergency treatment. Discussions of defibrillation, cardioversion, and artificial cardiac pacemakers are also included.

Although emphasis is appropriately placed on drug treatment of these arrhythmias, it is also important that underlying and reversible causes of rhythm and conduction disturbances—such as hypoxia, alkalosis, electrolyte abnormalities, or drug toxicity—be recognized and treated.

THE NORMAL CARDIAC CONDUCTING SYSTEM

The heart consists of three types of specialized tissue: (1) pacemaker cells that undergo spontaneous depolarization and can initiate an electric impulse, (2) conducting cells that form the specialized conducting system and rapidly propagate an electric impulse throughout the heart, and (3) contractile cells which contract when electrically depolarized.

The sinus node is normally the dominant cardiac pacemaker unless its activity is depressed by disease or drugs. The sinus node is located near the junction of the superior vena cava and right atrium. Blood supply is from the sinus node artery, which arises from either the proximal few centimeters of the right coronary artery in about 55 percent of individuals, or from the proximal few millimeters of the left circumflex artery in the other 45 percent. The sinus node is innervated by both sympathetic and parasympathetic nerve endings which can greatly modify the discharge rate. The intrinsic sinus node discharge rate is between 90 and 100 in middle-aged adults; the usual resting heart rate is lower, reflecting the predominance of parasympathetic activity at rest.

The electric impulse generated by the sinus node spreads like ripples throughout the right and then the left atrium, activating atrial contraction. Additionally, specialized atrial conduction tracts (anterior, middle, and posterior internodal tracts) serve to propagate the electric impulse through the atria and between the sinus node and the atrioventricular (AV) node.

The atria and ventricles are insulated electrically from each other by the fibrous connective tissue of the atrioventricular ring (annulus fibrosis). Normally, electric impulses from the atria can reach the ventricles only by passing through the AV node and infranodal conducting system.

The AV node is just beneath the right atrial endocardium and directly above the insertion of the septal leaflet of the tricuspid valve. The blood supply to the AV node in 90 percent of humans is by way of a branch off the right coronary artery as it turns to form the posterior descending artery, and in the other 10 percent, comes off the left circumflex artery. This accounts for the common occurrence of AV conduction disturbances with acute inferior myocardial infarctions. The AV node is innervated by both sympathetic and parasympathetic fibers. It has two important electrophysiological characteristics: a slow conduction velocity and a long refractory period. The slow conduction velocity through the AV node allows time for atrial contraction to give an extra boost to ventricular filling, which increases stroke volume according to the Frank-Starling principle. This "atrial kick" is most important in patients with ventricular failure. The long refractory period of the AV node protects the ventricles from excessively rapid stimulation; very rapid heart rates have a reduced cardiac output and may deteriorate into ventricular fibrillation. Cells around the AV node have pacemaker potential and can pace the heart should discharges from the sinus node fail or fall below a certain rate.

Electric impulses leave the inferior pole of the AV node along the bundle of His, which travels downward along the posterior margin of the membranous portion of the interventricular septum to reach the top of the muscular portion. The common bundle is only 1 to 2 cm in length before it divides at the crest of the muscular interventricular septum into the right and left bundle branches (RBB and LBB). The RBB is a compact group of fibers that travels down to the apex of the right ventricle before separating into smaller branches. The LBB travels 2 to 3 cm before fanning out into a virtual sheet of fibers to cover the left ventricle. There are two relatively distinct pathways to the base of the papillary muscles, the left anterior superior fascicle (LASF) and the left posterior inferior fascicle (LPIF).

The blood supply to the RBB and LASF is from the same sources: about half the time from both the AV nodal artery and branches from the left anterior descending coronary artery, and the other half from the left anterior descending artery alone. The LPIF is supplied about half the time from the AV nodal artery and the other half by both the AV nodal artery and left anterior descending artery. Infarction in the region supplied by the left anterior descending artery is capable of affecting the RBB and LASF but very rarely the LPIF.

Accessory tracts are embryologic remnants of myocardium found in the AV annulus that can transmit electric impulses between the atria and ventricles, bypassing all or part of the AV node and infranodal system. These bypass tracts are the anatomic basis for the preexcitation syndrome.

THE NORMAL ECG

The clinical surface ECG records the potential (voltage) differences between "neutral" ground and recording electrodes. The ECG is generated by the electrical activity of the heart and depicts the net sum of this activity recorded over time. By convention, a potential difference that points toward a recording electrode is assigned a positive deflection on the ECG, and a potential that points away from the recording electrode is assigned a negative deflection. Also by convention, routine ECG recordings are obtained with paper speed at 25 mm/s (2.5 cm/s) and signal calibration of 1.0 mV/10 mm (1.0 cm).

In Fig. 11-1, depolarization starts on the left side of the ventricular septum and initially proceeds to the right; this is recorded as a small negative deflection in the recording electrode. Subsequent depolarization involves the free walls of both ventricles, and since the left side has a much larger mass, the net sum of electrical activity is directed toward the recording electrode and a tall, positive deflection is recorded.

The P-QRS-T complex of the normal ECG represents electrical activity over one cardiac cycle (Fig. 11-2).

The P wave indicates atrial depolarization; atrial repolarization is usually obscured by the QRS complex. The normal P wave duration is less than 0.10 s (2.5 mm), and normal amplitude is less than 0.3 mV (3 mm). A P wave originating from the sinus node is directed inferiorly and to the left on the frontal plane.

The PR interval is the time between the onset of depolarization in the atria and ventricles and is commonly used as an estimation of AV nodal conduction time. For adults in sinus rhythm, the PR interval is 0.12 to 0.20 s (3 to 5 mm).

The QRS complex indicates ventricular depolarization. In general, depolarization starts on the endocardium and spreads outward to the epicardium. Despite the large amount of myocardium that must be depolarized, the specialized conducting system makes this a rapid process and the normal QRS duration is 0.06 to 0.10 s (1.5 to 2.5 mm). Any delay in conduction (such as bundle branch blocks) results in a wide QRS. Depolarizations which originate in the ventricles or

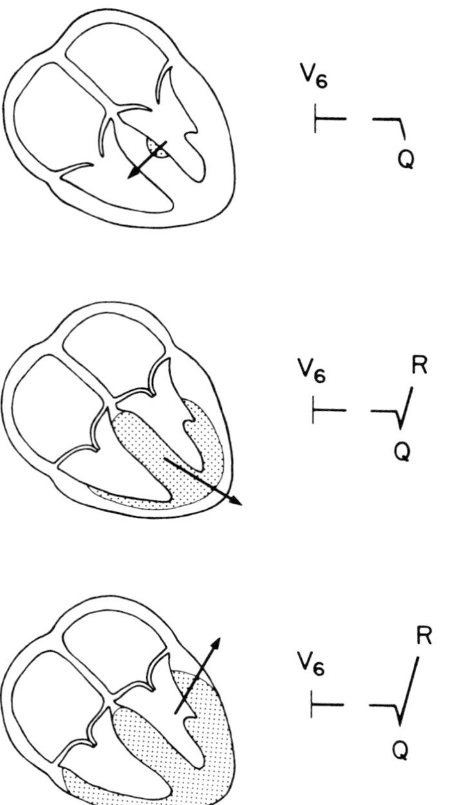

Fig. 11-1. Ventricular depolarization recorded in lead V_6

from a portion of the conducting system below the bifurcation of the bundle of His also have a wide QRS complex because of the slow cell-to-cell transmission (as opposed to propagation over the faster conduction system) of the electric impulse required to activate all the ventricular myocardium.

While small negative initial deflections (Q waves) are normal, large Q waves can be due to an electrically unexcitable area just under the recording electrode. An abnormal Q wave has a width of 0.04 s or greater and a height one-third that of the QRS complex.

The ST segment represents the plateau phase of ventricular depolarization. While the ST segment is usually isoelectric, small deviations, less than 0.1 mV (1 mm), are not always pathological.

The T wave indicates ventricular repolarization. Whereas depolarization is a rapid, near-simultaneous release of stored energy (like the release of a compressed spring), repolarization is a slow, asynchronous event where the metabolic machinery of each individual cell restores the transmembrane potential. Therefore, the T-wave duration is much longer and the amplitude much lower than those of the QRS complex. In general, repolarization starts on the epicardium and spreads to the endocardium. Many factors can influence this normal repolarization sequence: (1) metabolic (hypoxia, fever, drugs), (2) autonomic stimuli (abdominal pain, hyperventilation), (3) myocardial hypertrophy, (4) myocardial ischemia or inflammation, and (5) abnormal depolarization.

The QT interval represents the total duration of ventricular depolarization. While QT duration is commonly between 0.33 and 0.42 s, it does vary inversely with heart rate. The corrected interval is obtained by dividing the measured QT interval (in seconds) by the square root of the R-R interval (in seconds). The normal corrected QT interval is less than 0.47 s.

The U wave is produced by ventricular afterpotentials and can be seen as a normal component of the surface ECG, especially in leads V_1 and V_2. Afterpotentials that occur before full restoration of the transmembrane resting potential are considered early and are associated with disorders characterized by a prolonged QT interval. Early afterpotentials are exacerbated by slow heart rates. Delayed afterpotentials are seen after membrane potential is restored to the resting level and are associated with ischemia, electrolyte disorders, or sympathomimetic stimulation. Delayed afterpotentials are enhanced by faster heart rates.

CARDIAC ARRHYTHMIAS

Cardiac arrhythmias and conduction disturbances can be classified according to a number of methods: (1) heart rate; (2) site of origin, delay, or block; (3) mechanism; or (4) ratio of atrial to ventricular depolarizations (P waves to QRS complexes). For the cardiac arrhythmias, this chapter separates them into the site of origin.

Cardiac arrhythmias may decrease cardiac output if the ventricular rate is too fast or too slow. In the normal resting adult, heart rates between 40 and 160 are usually well tolerated as physiological adaptations are able to maintain an adequate cardiac output and blood

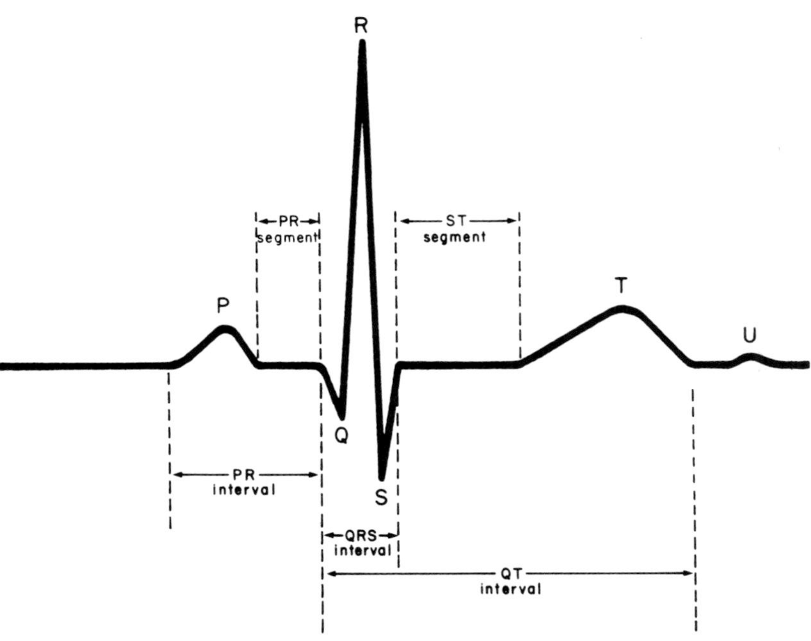

Fig. 11-2. Normal P-QRS-T ECG pattern.

pressure. However, in adults with significant heart or peripheral arterial disease, rates below 50 or above 120 may produce ischemia in susceptible organs.

Mechanisms of Tachyarrhythmias

Tachyarrhythmias are presumed to be caused by three mechanisms: ectopic focus, reentry, or triggered arrhythmias. While treatment would appear to be best directed by an understanding of the underlying process, uncertainty still exists over the precise mechanism of many arrhythmias, and therapy is still often empirical.

An ectopic focus is an area of the heart, away from the normal sinus node pacemaker, that acquires independent pacemaker activity and usurps the pacemaking role, resulting in single or multiple extra depolarizations. These ectopic pacemakers can be due to either (1) enhanced automaticity of subsidiary pacemaker cells (i.e., in the AV node or infranodal conducting system) or (2) abnormal automaticity of myocardial cells which seldom possess pacemaking activity (i.e., Purkinje cells). Arrhythmias due to an ectopic focus usually have a gradual onset (''warm-up period'') and offset, as opposed to the abrupt onset seen with reentry or triggered mechanisms.

Reentry occurs when a closed loop of conducting tissue transmits an electric impulse around the loop, either once or repeatedly, and stimulates an atrial and/or ventricular depolarization with each pass around the circuit. Electrophysiologically, reentry requires a temporary or permanent unidirectional block in one limb of the circuit and slower-than-normal conduction around the entire circuit. Both these conditions occur when cardiac conducting tissue is stimulated during the partial refractory period (before full repolarization).

For example, the inciting impulse traveling in the normal downward direction encounters the two limbs of the reentry circuit, finds limb a blocked, and travels down limb b (Fig. 11-3). Upon reaching the bottom portion of the circuit where the two limbs rejoin, the impulse can then travel retrograde up limb a and reach the upper connection of the circuit. Normally, conduction is so rapid that the impulse would encounter limb b still refractory to stimulation, and no further propagation would occur. However, if conduction around the circuit is slow enough, limb b would be able to conduct the impulse again in the antegrade direction. With the right size circuit and conduction velocity, an electric impulse can be maintained traveling around the circuit in a cyclical manner. Each time the impulse passes the upper and lower limb connections, a signal can be sent out stimulating atrial and ventricular depolarizations.

Reentry can occur around anatomically defined circuits, resulting in a regular rapid rhythm such as paroxysmal supraventricular tachycardia. Conversely, reentry can also occur in a disorganized and chaotic fashion through a syncytium of myocardial tissue, as seen, for example, in atrial or ventricular fibrillation.

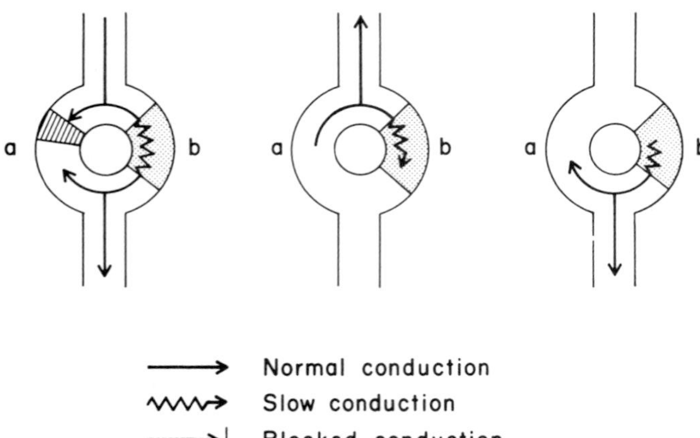

Fig. 11-3. Reentry circuit.

Triggered arrhythmias are due to the oscillations of the transmembrane potential during or after repolarization (afterpotentials), that may reach threshold and trigger a second complete depolarization. Once triggered, this process may be self-sustaining. Triggered arrhythmias associated with early afterpotentials are enhanced by slow heart rates and usually treated by accelerating the ventricular rate with positive chronotropic drugs or electrical pacing. Triggered arrhythmias associated with delayed afterpotentials are usually seen in states of myocardial ischemia and are enhanced by fast heart rates. Treatment is usually effective with agents that have a negative chronotropic action.

The urgency with which tachyarrhythmias require treatment is guided by two considerations: (1) evidence of hypoperfusion (shock, altered mental status, anginal chest pain, or pulmonary edema) and (2) the potential to degenerate into a more serious arrhythmia or cardiac arrest. The two treatment methods most commonly used are intravenous drugs for the clinically stable patient and synchronized cardioversion for the unstable patient. Occasional tachyarrhythmias may be treated with a short period of overdrive electrical pacing in selected patients.

Mechanisms of Bradyarrhythmias

Bradyarrhythmias can be caused by two mechanisms: depression of sinus nodal activity or conduction system blocks. In both situations, subsidiary pacemakers take over and pace the heart, and provided the pacemaker is located above the bifurcation of the bundle of His, the rate is generally adequate to maintain cardiac output.

The need for emergent treatment of bradycardias is guided by two considerations: (1) evidence of hypoperfusion and (2) the potential to degenerate into a more profound bradycardia or ventricular asystole. In general, emergent treatment is not required, unless: (1) the heart rate is below 50 and there is clinical evidence of hypoperfusion or (2) the bradycardia is due to structural disease of the infranodal conducting system (either transient or permanent) that has a risk of progressing to complete AV block. The first group of patients require immediate treatment during assessment of the etiology of the bradycardia and consideration as to whether internal cardiac pacing will be required. The second group of patients do not always require immediate treatment but should be monitored closely with therapy readily available while arrangements are made for further evaluation and possible internal cardiac pacing.

Three methods are currently available for emergent treatment of bradycardias: atropine, isoproterenol, and transcutaneous cardiac pacing.

Atropine should be the initial agent, at doses of 0.5 mg IV every 5 min until the desired response is achieved or a total vagolytic dose (about 0.05 mg/kg in humans) is given. Usually, if no response is seen by a dose of 2.0 mg, further doses are not effective. The vast majority of bradycardias due to problems of either the sinus or AV node respond to atropine. Even some patients with infranodal blocks may respond, so atropine deserves consideration in most bradycardias when emergent treatment is desired.

Isoproterenol can be used when atropine is ineffective, generally as a result of disease of the infranodal conducting system. Isoproterenol is given as a constant infusion, starting at a rate of around 0.5 μg/min and increasing as required to maintain a heart rate of 60. Isoproterenol increases myocardial oxygen demand, stimulates ventricular ectopy, and produces peripheral vasodilation, making it a less attractive agent than atropine. The reported response to isoproterenol is less than that observed with atropine, although isoproterenol is usually only used in patients who fail while receiving atropine; it is difficult to say how effective isoproterenol would be if used initially.

External cardiac pacing represents a reawareness of an old concept and should be available in every emergency facility. External pacing is most successful when the myocardium is still responsive to electrical stimuli (pulses with each depolarization) and must less successful when the myocardium is unresponsive (pulseless bradycardias or asystole). External pacing is discussed later in this chapter.

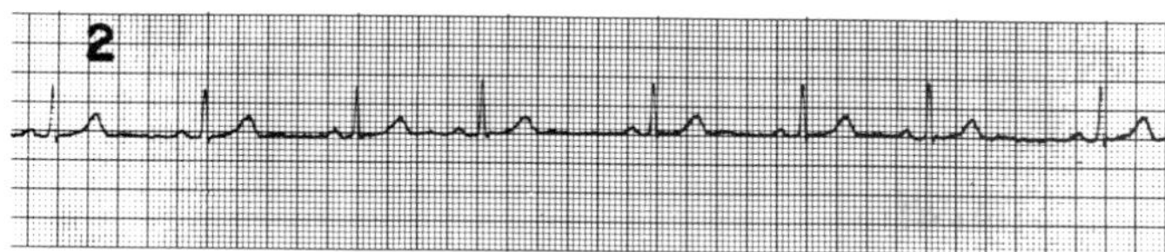

Fig. 11-4. Sinus arrhythmia.

Internal pacing is the definitive treatment for progressive or persistent bradycardias. Emergent internal pacing is possible with the use of balloon-tipped flotation catheters, although it is often technically difficult to achieve stable placement in a patient with low cardiac output without fluoroscopic guidance.

Supraventricular Arrhythmias

Sinus Arrhythmia

Some variation in the sinus node discharge rate is common, but if the variation exceeds 0.12 s between the longest and shortest intervals, sinus arrhythmia is present. The ECG characteristics of sinus arrhythmia are: (1) normal sinus P waves and PR intervals, (2) 1:1 AV conduction, and (3) variation of at least 0.12 s between the shortest and longest P-P interval (Fig. 11-4).

Clinical Significance

Sinus arrhythmias is most commonly found in children and young adults, disappearing with advancing age. Sinus arrhythmia varies in two manners: the more common phasic (respiratory) variety and the less common nonphasic variety. In the phasic variety, the sinus node rate accelerates during inspiration and decelerates during expiration due to changes in vagal tone occurring with respiration (Bainbridge reflex). The irregularity in either the phasic or nonphasic varieties can be exaggerated by conditions which increase vagal tone. During the long intervals of sinus arrhythmia, junctional escape beats may be seen.

Treatment

None is required.

Sinus Bradycardia

Sinus bradycardia occurs when the sinus node rate falls below 60. The ECG characteristics of sinus bradycardia are: (1) normal sinus P waves and PR intervals, (2) 1:1 AV conduction, and (3) atrial rate below 60 (Fig. 11-5).

Clinical Significance

Sinus bradycardia represents a suppression of the sinus node discharge rate, usually in response to three categories of stimuli: (1) physiological (well-conditioned athletes, during sleep, with vagal stimulation), (2) pharmacological (digoxin, narcotics, reserpine, β-adrenergic antagonists, calcium-channel blockers, quinidine), or (3) pathological (acute inferior myocardial infarction, increased intracranial pressure, carotid sinus hypersensitivity, hypothyroidism).

Treatment

1. Sinus bradycardia usually does not require specific treatment unless the heart rate is below 50 and there is evidence of hypoperfusion.
2. Initial therapy should begin with atropine as previously described. Most patients will respond to one or two doses.
3. Isoproterenol can be used if atropine is ineffective.
4. External cardiac pacing can be used in the patient refractory to atropine or isoproterenol.
5. Internal pacing is required in the patient with symptomatic recurrent or persistent sinus bradycardia.

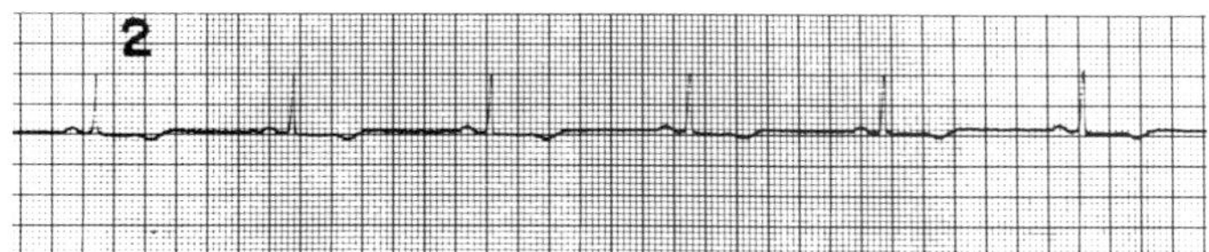

Fig. 11-5. Sinus bradycardia, rate 44.

Sinus Tachycardia

Sinus tachycardia originates from acceleration of the sinus node discharge rate. The ECG characteristics of sinus tachycardia are: (1) normal sinus P waves and PR intervals, (2) an atrial rate usually between 100 and 160, and (3) normally 1:1 conduction between the atria and ventricles (although rapid rates can occur with AV blocks) (Fig. 11-6).

Clinical Significance

Sinus tachycardia represents an acceleration of the sinus node discharge rate, usually in response to three categories of stimuli: (1) physiological (infants and children, exertion, anxiety, emotions), (2) pharmacological (atropine, epinephrine and other sympathomimetics, alcohol, nicotine, caffeine), or (3) pathological (fever, hypoxia, anemia, hypovolemia, pulmonary embolism). In many of these conditions, the increased heart rate is an effort to increase cardiac output to match increased circulatory needs.

Treatment

1. No specific treatment is usually required, but any underlying conditions should be investigated and treated.
2. Some patients with acute myocardial infarction have an "inappropriate" tachycardia and may benefit from slowing heart rate with β-adrenergic antagonists.

Premature Atrial Contractions (PACs)

PACs originate from ectopic pacemakers anywhere in the atrium other than the sinus node. The ECG characteristics of PACs are: (1) ectopic P′ wave appears sooner (premature) than the next expected sinus beat, (2) the ectopic P′ wave has a different shape and direction, and (3) the ectopic P′ wave may or may not be conducted through the AV node (Fig. 11-7). A PAC is not conducted through the AV node if it reaches the AV node during the absolute refractory period and is conducted with a delay (longer P′R interval) during the relative refractory period. Most PACs are conducted with typical QRS complexes, but some may be conducted aberrantly through the infranodal system. The sinus node is often depolarized and "reset" so that while the interval following the PAC is often slightly longer than the previous cycle length, the pause is less than fully compensatory.

Clinical Significance

PACs are common in all ages and often seen in the absence of heart disease. It is generally assumed, although remains unproven, that stress, fatigue, alcohol, tobacco, or coffee may precipitate PACs. Frequent PACs may also be seen in chronic lung disease, ischemic heart disease, or digitalis toxicity. PACs may trigger sustained atrial tachycardia, flutter, or fibrillation.

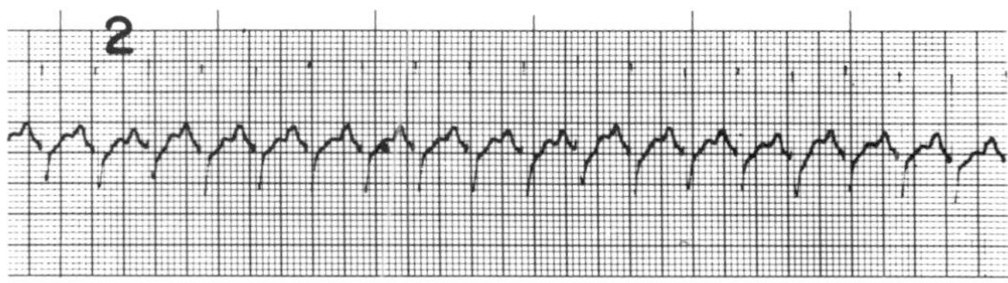

Fig. 11-6. Sinus tachycardia, rate 176.

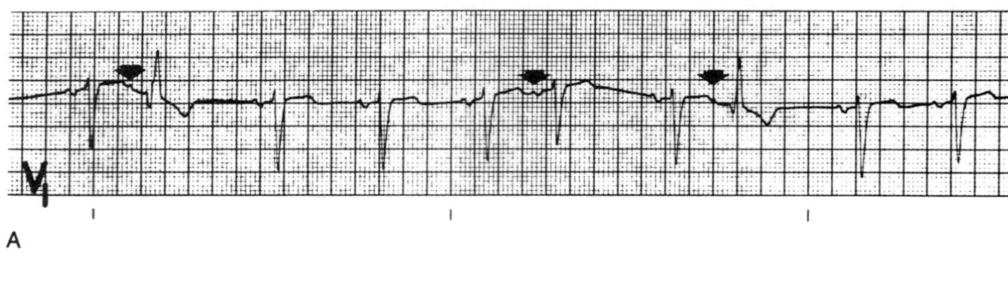

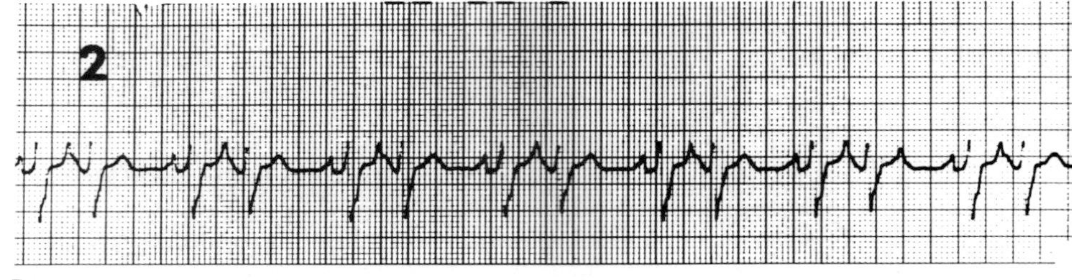

Fig. 11-7. Premature atrial contractions (PACs). Top: ectopic P′ waves (arrows). Bottom: atrial bigeminy.

Treatment

1. Any precipitating drugs or toxins should be discontinued.
2. Underlying disorders should be treated.
3. PACs that produce symptoms or initiate sustained tachycardias can be suppressed with quinidine, procainamide, or β-adrenergic antagonists.

Multifocal Atrial Tachycardia (MFAT)

Multifocal atrial tachycardia (MFAT, also known as "chaotic atrial rhythm" or "wandering atrial pacemaker") is an irregular rhythm caused by at least two different sites of atrial ectopy. The ECG characteristics of MFAT are: (1) three or more differently shaped P waves, (2) varying PP, PR, and RR intervals, and (3) atrial rhythm usually between 100 and 180 (Fig. 11-8). MFAT can be confused with atrial flutter or fibrillation.

Clinical Significance

MFAT is most often found in elderly patients with decompensated chronic lung disease, but also may complicate congestive heart failure, sepsis, or be caused by methylxanthine toxicity. Digoxin toxicity is an unlikely cause of MFAT.

Treatment

1. Treatment is directed toward the underlying disorder. With decompensated lung disease, oxygen and bronchodilators improve pulmonary function, arterial oxygenation, and decrease atrial ectopy.
2. Specific antiarrhythmic treatment is uncommonly indicated. Standard antiarrhythmics appear to be ineffective in suppressing these multiple sites of atrial ectopy, and toxic side effects from these agents have been reported. Likewise, attempts to slow the ventricular rate by depressing AV nodal conduction with digoxin is also difficult without producing toxic side effects. Recently, three modes of therapy have been described that may be helpful in some patients. Magnesium sulfate 2 g IV over 60 s followed by a constant infusion of 1 to 2 g/h has been shown to reduce atrial ectopy in these patients and sometimes is associated with conversion to sinus rhythm. The full antiarrhythmic effect of magnesium requires supplemental potassium to maintain serum potassium levels above 4 mEq/L. Intravenous verapamil (5 to 10 mg) slows the ventricular response in most patients, decreases atrial ectopy in some patients, and is associated with conversion to sinus rhythm in many patients. The β-adrenergic antagonists esmolol, acebutolol, and metoprolol all decrease the ventricular rate in MFAT, and metoprolol is associated with conversion to sinus rhythm in a majority of patients. However, the value of such specific antiarrhythmic treatment in MFAT is unproved.
3. Cardioversion has no effect on these multiple sites of atrial ectopy.

Atrial Flutter

Atrial flutter is a rhythm that originates from a small area within the atria. The exact mechanism—whether reentry, automatic focus, or triggered arrhythmia—is not yet known. As studied with intracardiac electrodes, electrical activity usually begins in the inferior right atrium and propagates upward and to the left. ECG characteristics of atrial flutter are: (1) regular atrial rate between 250 and 350 (most commonly 280 and 320); (2) sawtooth flutter waves directed superiorly and most visible in leads II, III, aV_F; and (3) AV block, usually 2:1, but occasionally greater or irregular (Fig. 11-9). One-to-one AV conduction may occur in patients with bypass tracts or when AV nodal conduction is enhanced by drugs such as quinidine. Aberrant conduction may occur and cause atrial flutter to resemble ventricular tachycardia. Carotid sinus massage is a useful technique to slow the ventricular response, increase the AV block, and unmask flutter waves.

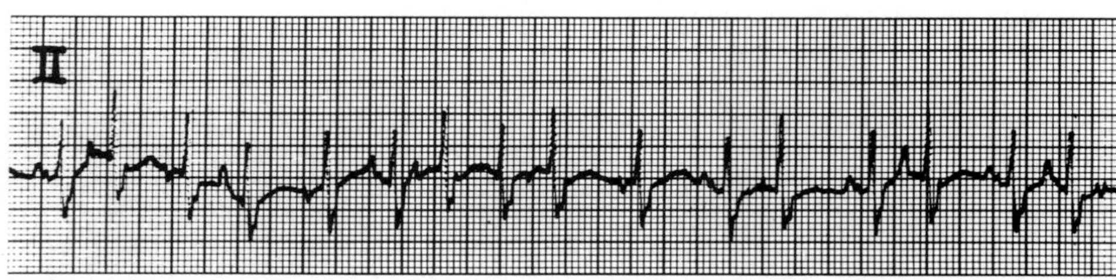

Fig. 11-8. Multifocal atrial tachycardia (MFAT).

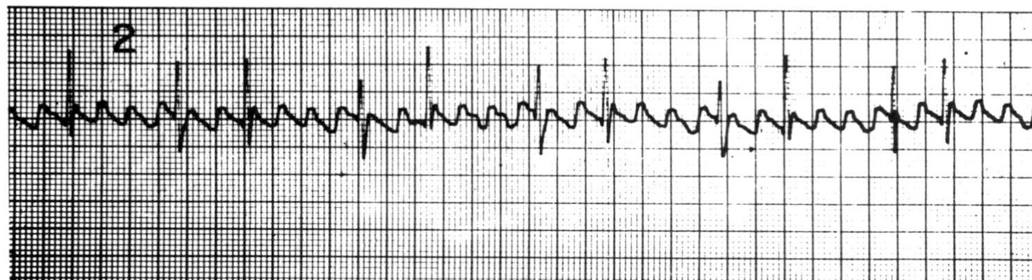

Fig. 11-9. Atrial flutter.

Clinical Significance

Atrial flutter rarely occurs in patients without heart disease. It is most commonly seen in patients with ischemic heart disease or acute myocardial infarction. Less common causes include congestive cardiomyopathy, pulmonary embolus, myocarditis, blunt chest trauma, and, rarely, digoxin toxicity. Atrial flutter may be a transitional arrhythmia between sinus rhythm and atrial fibrillation.

Treatment

1. Low-energy cardioversion (25 to 50 J) is very successful in converting more than 90 percent of cases of atrial flutter into sinus rhythm. Energies less than 10 J should be avoided as they are more likely to convert atrial flutter into atrial fibrillation than into sinus rhythm.
2. If cardioversion is contraindicated, ventricular rate control can be achieved with digoxin, verapamil, or β-adrenergic blockers.
3. Quinidine or procainamide can be used after ventricular rate control is achieved to chemically slow or convert atrial flutter or prevent recurrence of the arrhythmia.
4. Intravenous verapamil will occasionally convert atrial flutter into sinus rhythm (about 30 percent) or atrial fibrillation (about 20 percent).
5. Some of the newer antiarrhythmics may also have a role in the chemical conversion of atrial flutter. For example, early reports indicate that intravenous flecainide is associated with a conversion to sinus rhythm about 40 percent of the time.

Atrial Fibrillation

Atrial fibrillation occurs when there are multiple small areas of atrial myocardium continuously discharging and contracting. There is no uniform atrial depolarization and contraction, but instead, only a quivering of the atrial wall. While the atrial rate is usually above 400, the ventricular rate is limited by the refractory period of the AV node. The ECG characteristics of atrial fibrillation are: (1) fibrillatory waves of atrial activity, best seen in leads V_1, V_2, V_3, and aV_F; and (2) irregular ventricular response, usually around 170 to 180 in patients with a healthy AV node (Fig. 11-10). Disease or drugs (especially digoxin) may reduce AV node conduction and markedly slow ventricular response. A more rapid ventricular response may be seen in patients with bypass tracts; rates above 200 are possible. In this case, since ventricular activation occurs by way of the bypass tract, the QRS complex is usually wide. In addition, aberrancy—usually with a right bundle branch block configuration—is possible with rapid rates alone.

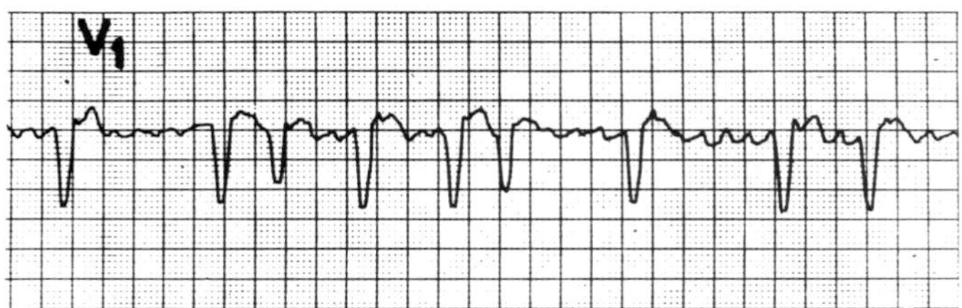

Fig. 11-10. Atrial fibrillation.

Clinical Significance

Atrial fibrillation can occur in a paroxysmal or sustained manner. Predisposing factors for atrial fibrillation are increased atrial size and mass, increased vagal tone, and variation in refractory periods between different parts of atrial myocardium. Atrial fibrillation is usually found in association with four disorders: rheumatic heart disease, hypertension, ischemic heart disease, and thyrotoxicosis. Less common causes are chronic lung disease, pericarditis, acute alcoholic intoxication, or atrial septal defect.

In patients with left ventricular failure, left atrial contraction makes an important contribution to cardiac output. The loss of effective atrial contraction, as in atrial fibrillation, may produce heart failure in these patients. Atrial fibrillation also predisposes to peripheral venous and atrial emboli, with the risk of pulmonary and systemic arterial embolism. Up to 30 percent of patients in chronic atrial fibrillation have at least one embolic episode. Conversion from chronic atrial fibrillation to sinus rhythm also carries up to a 1 to 2 percent risk of arterial embolism.

Treatment

1. Atrial fibrillation with a rapid ventricular response and acute hemodynamic deterioration should be treated with synchronized cardioversion. Over 60 percent can be converted with 100 J and over 80 percent with 200 J. Conversion to and retention in sinus rhythm is more likely when atrial fibrillation is of short duration and the atria are not greatly dilated. If initial cardioversion is unsuccessful, procainamide IV should be given to facilitate further cardioversion attempts.
2. In more stable patients, the first priority is to achieve ventricular rate control. Intravenous digoxin in an effective agent for this purpose, although the onset of action is slow. Verapamil 5 to 10 mg IV is effective in slowing the ventricular response in 60 to 70 percent of patients with atrial fibrillation and converts 10 to 15 percent into sinus rhythm. Intravenous β-adrenergic blockers (e.g., esmolol and propranolol) are effective, especially in patients with rheumatic mitral stenosis, but the depressive effects on myocardial contractility make them a poor agent to use in patients with ventricular failure.
3. Once ventricular rate control has been achieved, chemical conversion can be considered with procainamide, quinidine, or verapamil. Procainamide IV has also been used as a single agent to chemically convert atrial fibrillation of short duration into sinus rhythm. The intravenous administration of a number of the newer antiarrhythmias (disopyramide, pirmenol, flecainide, or amiodarone) is associated with a 40 to 70 percent conversion rate of acute atrial fibrillation to sinus rhythm. Because of the risk of intraatrial thrombi and arterial embolization, patients with atrial fibrillation of more than 3 days duration should be anticoagulated systemically for 1 to 3 weeks prior to attempts at either chemical or electrical conversion.

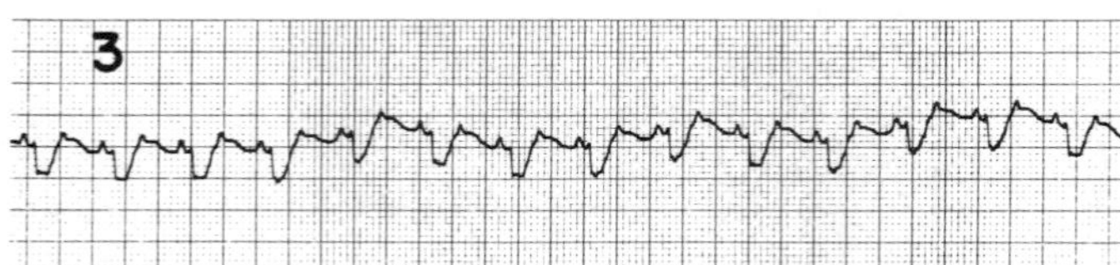

Fig. 11-11. Ectopic supraventricular, tachycardia (STV) with 2:1 AV conduction.

4. Patients with a slow ventricular response not due to digitalis have AV node disease and probably a more generalized disorder of cardiac conduction (sick sinus syndrome). These patients are at increased risk for profound bradycardias or asystole following cardioversion or antiarrhythmic drug therapy.

Supraventricular Tachycardia (STV)

Supraventricular tachycardia is a regular, rapid rhythm that arises from either reentry or an ectopic pacemaker in areas above the bifurcation of the bundle of His. The reentrant variety is clinically the most common. These patients often present with acute, symptomatic episodes termed *paroxysmal supraventricular tachycardia* (PSVT).

Ectopic SVT usually originates in the atria with an atrial rate of 100 to 250 (most commonly 140 to 200) (Fig. 11-11). The regular P waves can be mistaken for atrial flutter or, if there is a 2:1 AV block, sinus rhythm.

Reentrant SVT constitutes the majority of patients with SVT: about 60 percent of these patients have reentry within the AV node and 20 percent have reentry involving a bypass tract. The remainder have reentry in other sites. In the normal heart, reentrant SVT at the typical rates of 160 to 200 is often tolerated for hours or days. However, cardiac output is always depressed—regardless of the blood pressure—and rapid rates may produce heart failure.

Reentrant SVT within the AV node usually is initiated when an ectopic atrial impulse encounteres the AV node during the partially refractory period (Fig. 11-12). There are two functionally different parallel conducting limbs within the AV node that are connected above at the atrial end and below at the ventricular end of the node. This circuit is capable of sustained reentry when properly stimulated. In AV nodal reentry, the P wave is usually buried in the QRS complex and not visible, there is 1:1 conduction, and the QRS complex is normal.

In patients with bypass tracts, the two parallel limbs of the reentry circuit are the AV node and the bypass tract,with connections at the atrial and ventricular ends by myocardial cells. While reentry can occur in either direction, it usually occurs in a direction that goes down the AV node and up the bypass tract, producing a narrow QRS complex. In the Wolff-Parkinson-White syndrome, about 85 percent of the reentrant SVTs have narrow QRS complexes.

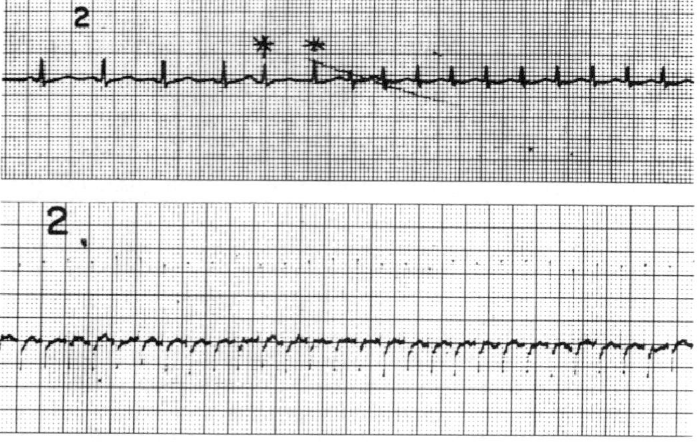

Fig. 11-12. Reentrant supraventricular tachycardia (STV). Top: 2d PAD (*) initiates run of PAT. Bottom: SVT, rate 286.

Clinical Significance

Ectopic SVT may be seen in patients with acute myocardial infarction, chronic lung disease, pneumonia, alcoholic intoxication, and digoxin toxicity [where it is often associated with AV block and termed *paroxysmal atrial tachycardia* (PAT) with block]. It is commonly held that a high percentage of SVT with block, as much as 75 percent, is due to digoxin toxicity. However, not all studies have found this to be the case. The common arrhythmias of digoxin toxicity are listed in Table 11-1.

Reentrant SVT can occur in a normal heart, or in association with rheumatic heart disease, acute pericarditis, myocardial infarction, mitral valve prolapse, or one of the preexcitation syndromes.

SVT often causes a sensation of palpitations and light-headedness. In patients with coronary artery disease, anginal chest pain and dyspnea may occur from the rapid heart rate. Frank heart failure and pulmonary edema may occur in patients with poor left ventricular function. The loss of atrial contribution to cardiac output is often poorly tolerated in patients with left ventricular failure.

Treatment

Ectopic SVT due to digoxin toxicity is treated by:

1. Discontinuing the digoxin.
2. As long as there is not a high-grade AV block, correcting any existing hypokalemia to bring serum potassium into the high-normal range in an effort to reduce atrial ectopy.
3. Digoxin-specific antibody fragments (Fab) should be considered for patients with hemodynamic deterioration or serious ventricular arrhythmias due to digoxin toxicity.
4. Atrial ectopy can be reduced by either phenytoin IV, lidocaine IV, or magnesium IV. Published reports are not adequate for determination of the response rate, risks, and benefits of each agent, so the choice is often guided by personal preference. Historically, phenytoin has been the most commonly used drug, but its response rate has not been impressive and toxic side effects are common with full loading doses (15 to 18 mg/kg IV). Lidocaine has not been considered a useful agent for this arrhythmia, but a recent report indicates some benefit. Recent studies indicate that magnesium sulfate 1 g IV impressively reduces atrial ectopy due to digoxin toxicity, and perhaps this agent has a greater effect than phenytoin or lidocaine.
5. Cardioversion is not effective and is potentially hazardous.

Ectopic SVT not due to digoxin toxicity is treated by:

1. Digoxin, verapamil, or β-adrenergic blockers to slow the ventricular rate.

Table 11-1. Common Arrhythmias of Digoxin Toxicity (Approximate Incidence)

PVCs (60%)
Unifocal, multifocal, bigeminy, or trigeminy
AV block (20%)
Second-degree
Mobitz I, Mobitz II
Third degree
Ectopic SVT (20–30%)
Rate 70–130
Gradual appearance and disappearance
AV dissociation and/or block
Junctional escape beats (10%)
Ventricular tachycardia (10%)
Bidirectional ventricular tachycardia associated with high mortality
Sinus bradycardia, SA block, and sinus pause (1–10%)

2. Antiarrhythmic therapy with either quinidine, procainamide, or magnesium.

Reentrant SVT can be converted by impeding conduction through one limb of the reentry circuit; sustained reentry is then impossible and extinguishes, allowing sinus rhythm to resume ventricular pacing.

1. Maneuvers which increase vagal tone have been shown to slow conduction and prolong the refractory period in the AV node. These maneuvers can be done by themselves or after administration of drugs.
   a. Carotid sinus massage attempts to massage the carotid sinus and its baroreceptors against the transverse process of C6. Massage should be done for 10 s at a time, first attempted on the side of the nondominant cerebral hemisphere, and should never be done simultaneously on both sides. Prolonged AV block during carotid massage may occur in patients with AV node disease or who are on digoxin. Patients with carotid artery stenosis may develop cerebral ischemia or infarction from overvigorous carotid massage.
   b. Facial immersion in cold water for 6 to 7 s with the nostrils held closed ("diving reflex"). This maneuver is particularly effective in infants.
   c. Gagging.
   d. The pneumatic antishock garment (PASG) increases arterial pressure, thereby stimulating the carotid sinus. One published report has described the effectiveness of the PASG in SVT, but many other physicians have not found it to be so useful.
   e. The Valsalva maneuver done in the supine position appears to be the most effective vagal maneuver for the conversion of reentrant SVT. For maximal effectiveness, the strain phase must be adequate (usually at least 10 s) with slowing or conversion seen during the release phase.
2. Verapamil is the drug of choice, 0.075 to 0.15 mg/kg (3 to 10 mg) IV over 15 to 60 s, with a repeat dose in 30 min if necessary. Studies have found that more than 90 percent of adults with reentrant SVT will respond within 1 to 2 min to verapamil. In patients with a normal blood pressure, intravenous verapamil is almost always associated with a decrease in blood pressure, even following successful conversion of SVT. The falls in systolic and mean arterial pressures are around 20 and 10 mmHg, respectively. There is good documentation that the drop in blood pressure due to verapamil can be prevented and/or treated with intravenous calcium without reducing the antiarrhythmic action of verapamil; the most commonly reported dose used is calcium chloride 1 g IV given over several minutes, but as little as 90 mg of calcium gluconate has been reported to be effective. Whenever verapamil is used intravenously, calcium should be readily available. Intravenous verapamil generally is considered to be contraindicated in the hypotensive patient. However, one small study of intravenous verapamil for the treatment of hypotensive patients with SVT reported that the conversion rate was about 80 percent, the ventricular rate almost always slowed, the systolic blood pressure usually increased, and only one patient out of 21 experienced a decrease in systolic blood pressure without a change in ventricular rate.
3. Adenosine is an ultrashort-acting (20 s) agent that produces AV block and has been observed to convert over 90 percent of reentrant SVT. The initial dose is 6 mg rapid IV bolus. If no effect is seen within 2 min, a second dose of 12 mg can be given. There is no proven benefit to repeated doses or administration of more than 20 mg. The majority of patients experience distressing, albeit transient, side effects. Because adenosine possesses no sustained antiarrhythmic effect, subsequent ectopic beats are able to initial the arrhythmia again, and early recurrences of SVT are seen in up to 25 percent of patients. The major advantage of adenosine is its ultrashort effect and its lack of hypotensive or myocardial depressive activity.
4. Parasympathetic tone can be increased with edrophonium. A standard treatment protocol is a 1 mg IV test dose, a wait of 3 to 5 min, followed by 5 to 10 mg IV over 60 s. Historically, edrophonium does not have the 90 percent response rate seen with verapamil.
5. Vagal tone can be enhanced by pharmacologically evaluating blood pressure with a pure peripheral vasoconstrictor; do not use agents with β-adrenergic activity. This method should be combined with carotid sinus massage. Blood pressure should be monitored frequently, and diastolic pressure should not be allowed to exceed 130 mmHg. This method should not be used if hypertension is already present.
   a. Metaraminol 200 mg/500 mL D_5W or norepinephrine 4 mg/500 mL D_5W can be infused at rates of 1 to 2 mL/min and titrated until the rhythm converts.
   b. Methoxamine or phenylephrine 0.5 to 1.0 mg IV over 2 to 3 min, with repeat doses as required.
6. Esmolol is an intravenous β-adrenergic blocker with an ultrashort duration of activity that can be titrated to effect. This agent can be used to control the ventricular rate in most tachycardias of supraventricular origin and is capable of converting about half of reentrant SVT. Esmolol is given as a bolus dose of 300 μg/kg over 60 s, followed by an infusion starting at 50 μg/kg per minute. If there is an inadequate response after 2 to 5 min, repeat bolus of 300 μg/kg and increases in the infusion rate in 50 μg/kg per minute increments should be done. The maximal recommended infusion rate is 300 μg/kg per minute, although most patients respond to rates of 200 μg/kg per minute or less. With aggressive dosing regimens, hypotension occurs in about half of patients but can be quickly reversed by halting the infusion.
7. Propranolol 0.5 to 1.0 mg IV slowly over 60 s, repeated every 5 min, until the rhythm converts or the total dose reaches 0.1 mg/kg. Overall, propranolol has about a 50 percent success rate in converting reentrant SVT: about 80 percent with AV nodal reentry and 15 to 20 percent with accessory tract retrograde reentry.
8. Digoxin 0.5 mg IV with repeat doses of 0.25 mg in 30 to 60 min until a response occurs or the total dose reaches 0.02 mg/kg. The chief drawback of digoxin has been its long onset of action and potential hazard in patients with accessory (bypass) tracts who develop either atrial fibrillation or flutter.
9. Synchronized cardioversion should be done in any unstable patient with hypotension, pulmonary edema, or severe chest pain. The dose required is usually small, less than 50 J.

Junctional Arrhythmias

Traditionally, a junctional impulse is considered to be one that arises from the AV node or bundle of His above the bifurcation. While pacemaker tissue cannot be found in the AV node itself in experimental animals, the matter is not settled in humans. From its source, the impulse spreads retrograde toward the atria and antegrade toward the ventricles. Depending on the site of origin, conduction velocity, and refractory periods, the atria may be activated before, during, or after ventricular depolarization. Atrial depolarization may not be visible if retrograde conduction is blocked or atrial activation occurs simultaneously with ventricular activation and the P waves are obscured by the QRS complex. AV dissociation may occur if the rate of discharge from the junctional pacemaker is faster than the sinus node rate and the junctional impulse is blocked from retrograde conduction toward the atria.

Junctional Premature Contractions (JPCs)

Junctional premature contractions are due to an ectopic pacemaker within the AV node or common AV bundle. The ECG characteristics of JPCs are: (1) the ectopic QRS complex is premature, (2) the ectopic P′ wave has a different shape and direction (usually inverted in leads II, III, and aV_F, (3) the ectopic P′ wave may occur before or after

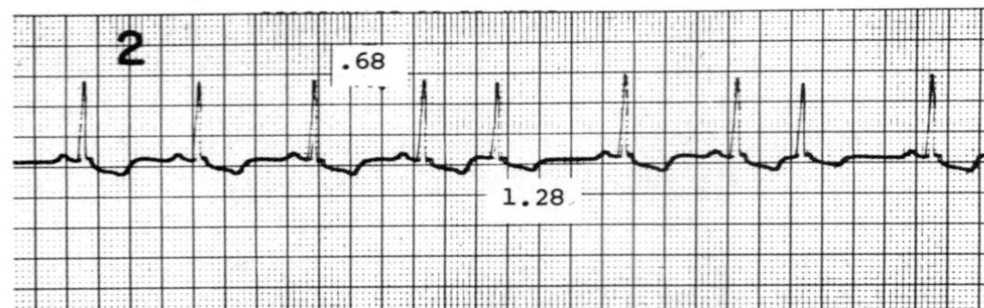

Fig. 11-13. Junctional premature contractions (JPCs).

the QRS complex, (4) the P′R interval of the ectopic beat is shorter than normal, (5) the QRS complex is usually of normal shape unless there is aberrant conduction, and (6) the sinus node is usually not affected and the postectopic pause is fully compensatory (Fig. 11-13). JPCs may be isolated, multiple (as in bigeminy or trigeminy), or multifocal.

Clinical Significance

JPCs are uncommon in healthy hearts. They occur in congestive heart failure, digoxin toxicity, ischemic heart disease, or acute myocardial infarctions (especially of the inferior wall).

Treatment

1. No specific treatment is usually required.
2. Treat the underlying disorder.
3. Antiarrhythmic therapy with quinidine or procainamide may be useful if JPCs are frequent, symptomatic, or initiate more serious arrhythmias.

Junctional Rhythms

Under normal circumstances, the sinus node discharges at a faster rate than the AV junction, so the pacemaker function of the AV junction is overridden. If sinus node discharges slow or fail to reach the AV junction, then junctional escape beats may occur, usually at a rate between 40 to 60, depending on the level of the pacemaker. Generally, junctional escape beats do not conduct retrograde into the atria so a QRS complex without a P′ wave is usually seen (Fig. 11-14).

Under other circumstances, enhanced junctional automaticity may override the sinus node and produce either an accelerated junctional rhythm (rate 60 to 100) or junctional tachycardia (rate greater than 100). Usually, both the atria and ventricles are captured by the enhanced junctional pacemaker (Fig. 11-15).

Clinical Significance

Junctional escape beats may occur whenever there is a long enough pause in the impulses reaching the AV junction: sinus bradycardia, slow phase of sinus arrhythmia, AV block, or during the pause following premature beats. Sustained junctional escape rhythms may be seen with congestive heart failure, myocarditis, hyperkalemia, or digoxin toxicity. If the ventricular rate is too slow, myocardial or cerebral ischemia may develop.

Accelerated junctional rhythm and junctional tachycardia may occur from digoxin toxicity, acute rheumatic fever, or inferior myocardial infarction. With digoxin toxicity, the rate is usually between 70 and 130. If this rhythm develops in a patient being treated with digoxin for atrial fibrillation, the ECG is characterized by regular QRS complexes superimposed on atrial fibrillatory waves. Regularization of ventricular response during digoxin therapy in a patient with atrial fibrillation should therefore raise the suspicion of digoxin toxicity.

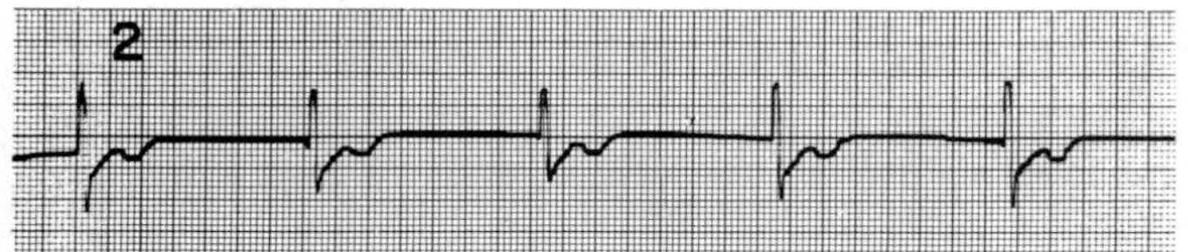

Fig. 11-14. Junctional escape rhythm, rate 42.

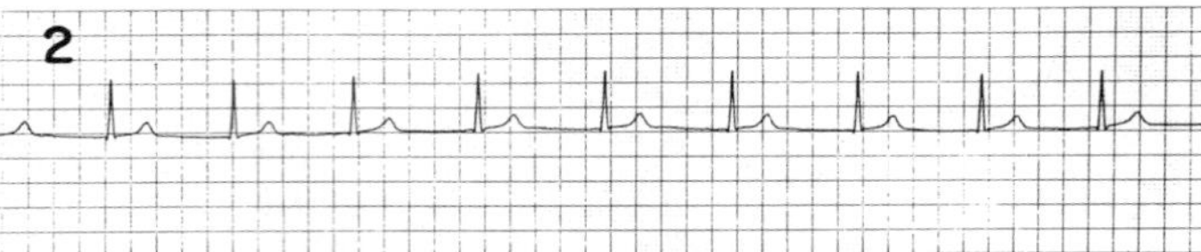

Fig. 11-15. Accelerated junctional rhythm, rate 61.

Treatment

1. Isolated, infrequent junctional escape beats usually do not require specific treatment.
2. If sustained junctional escape rhythms are producing symptoms, the underlying cause should be treated. Atropine can be used to accelerate temporarily the sinus node discharge rate and enhance AV nodal conduction.
3. Acccelerated junctional rhythm and junctional tachycardia usually do not produce significant symptoms. If the cause is digoxin toxicity, the drug should be discontinued. If the rate is fast and producing symptoms, it can be decreased by giving supplemental potassium to increase the serum level into the high-normal range.

Ventricular Arrhythmias

Premature Ventricular Contractions (PVCs)

Premature ventricular contractions are due to impulses originating from single or multiple areas in the ventricles. The ECG characteristics of PVCs are: (1) there is a premature and wide QRS complex; (2) there is no preceding P wave; (3) the ST segment and T wave of the PVC are directed opposite the major QRS deflection; (4) most PVCs do not affect the sinus node, so there is usually a fully compensatory postectopic pause or the PVC may be interpolated between two sinus beats; (5) many PVCs have a fixed coupling interval (within 0.04 s) from the preceding sinus beat; and (6) many PVCs are conducted into the atria, producing a retrograde P wave (Fig. 11-16).

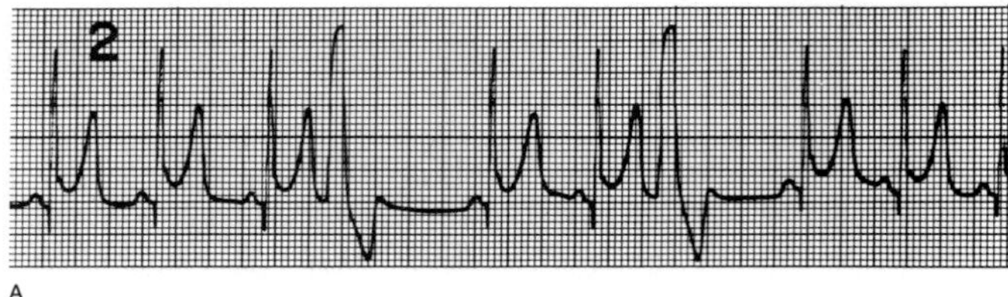

A

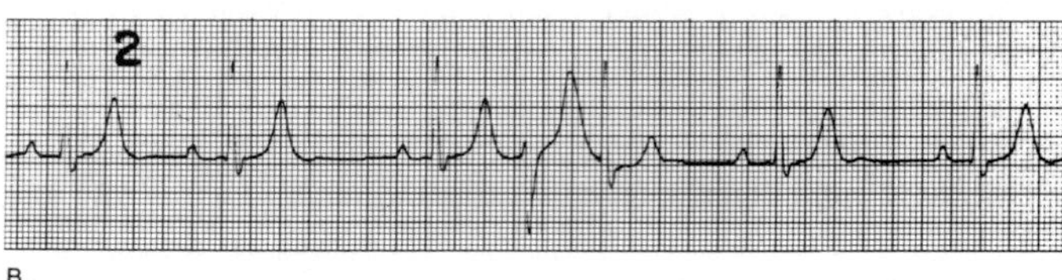

B

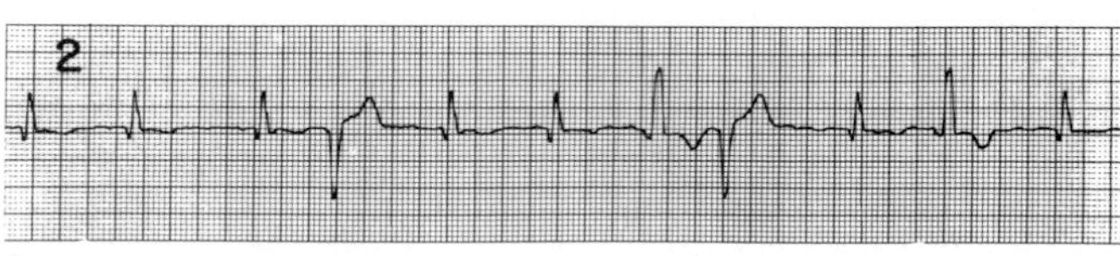

C

Fig. 11-16. Premature ventricular contractions (PVCs). Top: unifocal PVC. Center: interpolated PVC. Bottom: multifocal PVCs.

Occasionally, a ventricular fusion beat occurs when a supraventricular and ventricular impulse nearly simultaneously depolarize the ventricles. The QRS configuration of a fusion beat contains features of the individual components.

A PVC may be confused with an aberrantly conducted supraventricular beat. Several clinical and ECG criteria can be used to help differentiate between aberrantly conducted supraventricular beats and PVCs; this is discussed in a separate section.

Clinical Significance

PVCs are very common, even in patients without evidence of heart disease. They occur in most patients with ischemic heart disease and are universally found in patients with acute myocardial infarction. Other common causes of PVCs include digoxin toxicity, congestive heart failure, hypokalemia, alkalosis, hypoxia, and sympathomimetic drugs.

While there is a correlation between the severity of underlying coronary artery disease and the degree of ventricular ectopy, there is disagreement as to whether ventricular ectopy itself is an independent risk factor for future morbidity or mortality. Most studies indicate that repetitive PVCs (two or more in a row) do have some associated independent risk in patients with coronary artery disease, but the evidence for other forms of ventricular ectopy is less convincing. Lown has made an attempt with his classification to quantitate the risks associated with chronic ventricular ectopy, but his classification is not universally accepted (Table 11-2).

In the setting of an acute myocardial infarction, PVCs indicate the underlying electrical instability of the heart. The patients are at increased risk for the development of primary ventricular fibrillation. Current work indicates that various degrees of PVCs ("warning arrhythmias") are not reliable predictors of subsequent ventricular fibrillation.

Although it is experimentally established that electric impulses, such as PVCs, that occur during or soon after repolarization (the so-called vulnerable period) can initiate ventricular tachycardia or fibrillation, clinical studies have found that more paroxysms of ventricular tachycardia are initiated by late-coupled PVCs than early-coupled PVCs (R-on-T phenomenon).

Treatment

1. In the setting of possible or definite acute myocardial infarction, most physicians would treat frequent or multiform PVCs with intravenous lidocaine. In addition, some physicians would also treat the same group of patients prophylactically with lidocaine; this concept is discussed further in Chap. 17, "Myocardial Ischemia and Infarction." Most patients with PVCs respond to lidocaine, but occasional patients may require procainamide.
2. In patients with chronic ectopy, there is no current satisfactory method of identifying those who would benefit from oral antiarrhythmic therapy. The physician usually must consider several factors in deciding whether a patient with chronic PVCs should be treated: (a) the underlying heart disease, (b) the nature of the ectopy, (c) the presence or absence of symptoms, and (d) the potential side effects of oral antiarrhythmic therapy. There is little conclusive evidence that PVCs adversely affect survival and that treatment enhances survival. It would seem reasonable to treat those patients experiencing repetitive PVCs (two or more in a row). The case for treating other patients is much less conclusive. A wide variety of oral antiarrhythmics are available: quinidine, procainamide, disopyramide, tocainide, mexiletine, flecainide, encainide, propafenone, aminodarone, and β-adrenergic antagonists. All oral antiarrhythmics possess significant and occasionally severe or life-threatening side effects. For example, a recent multicenter study found that encainide and flecainide treatment of postinfarction patients with frequent PVCs was associated with a significantly increased risk of death within 1 year. It is possible that some of the increased mortality was due to the proarrhythmic activity of these drugs. Because of their relative safety and longer experience with their use, agents such as quinidine, disopyramide, procainamide, or propranolol usually are preferred as initial treatment for PVCs. Oral antiarrhythmic therapy should be carefully monitored.

Table 11-2. Lown Grading System for Ventricular Ectopy

Grade	
1	Uniform PVCs < 30/h
2	Uniform PVCs > 30/h
3	Multiform PVCs
4A	Couplets (2 consecutive PVCs)
4B	Triplets (3 or more consecutive PVCs)
5	R-on-T PVCs

Ventricular Parasystole

Parasystole occurs when an independent ectopic pacemaker is protected from the influence of outside impulses ("entrance block") and competes with the dominant pacemaker to produce myocardial depolarizations. A parasystolic pacemaker can arise anywhere in the heart, but is most often located in the ventricles where it produces a rhythm that operates alongside of and is independent of the sinus node.

The ECG characteristics of ventricular parasystole are: (1) variation in the coupling interval between the preceding sinus beat and the ectopic beat, (2) common relation between the interectopic beat intervals, and (3) occurrence of fusion beats (Fig. 11-17). Usually, long rhythm strips are necessary to establish that the interectopic intervals are multiples of a common parasystolic rate.

Clinical Significance

Ventricular parasystole is most often associated with severe ischemic heart disease, acute myocardial infarction, hypertensive heart disease, or electrolyte imbalance. Parasystole is often self-limited and benign, but infrequently, it may lead to ventricular tachycardia or fibrillation.

Treatment

1. The underlying disease should be treated.
2. Antiarrhythmics are indicated in patients with symptomatic episodes or beats which initiate ventricular tachycardia.

Accelerated Idioventricular Rhythm (AIVR)

Accelerated idioventricular rhythm is an ectopic rhythm of ventricular origin occurring at rates of 40 to 100. Even though AIVR is not a tachycardia, such terms as *idioventricular tachycardia*, *nonparoxysmal ventricular tachycardia*, or *slow ventricular tachycardia* are sometimes used to describe this rhythm.

The ECG characteristics of AIVR are: (1) wide and regular QRS complexes, (2) rate between 40 and 100 that is often close to the preceding sinus rate, (3) most runs of short duration (3 to 30 beats) and (4) an AIVR often beginning with a fusion beat (Fig. 11-18).

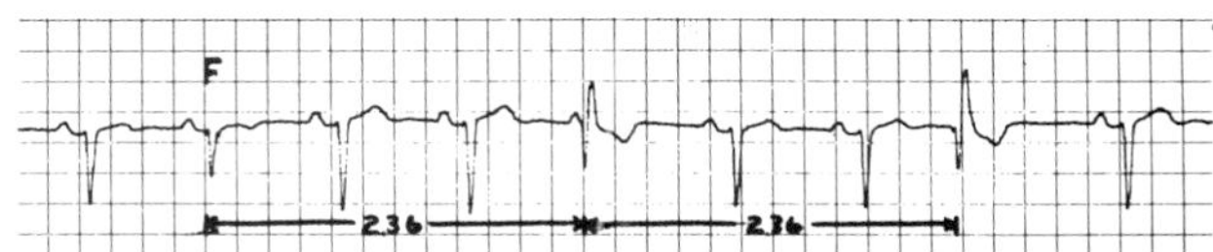

Fig. 11-17. The fifth and eighth ventricular complexes are premature and of similar morphology but have different coupling intervals. The second complex (marked "F") represents a fusion beat. The interectopic interval is 2.36 s. (From Heger JW, Niemann JT, Boman KG, et al: *Cardiology for the House Officer*. Baltimore, Williams & Wilkins, 1982. Used by permission.)

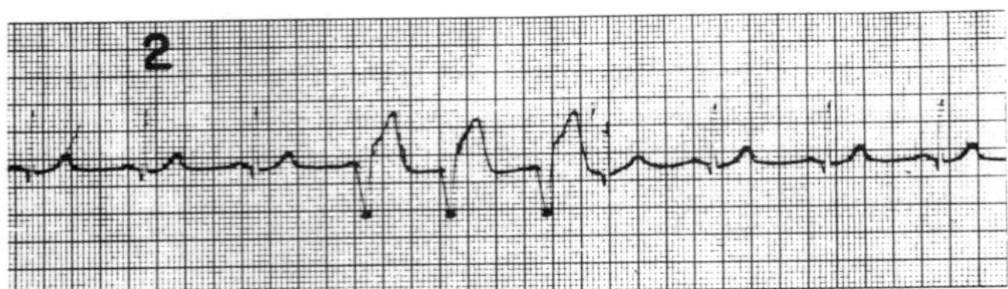

Fig. 11-18. Accelerated idioventricular rhythms (AIVR).

Clinical Significance

This condition is found most commonly in the setting of an acute myocardial infarction. Reports indicate that AIVR sometimes appears during successful thrombolysis of an occluded coronary. AIVR and other ventricular arrhythmias seen during this time are termed "reperfusion arrhythmias." AIVR may be seen infrequently in patients without organic heart disease. While there is some variable association with ventricular tachycardia, there is no apparent association with ventricular fibrillation. AIVR usually produces no symptoms itself. Sometimes the loss of atrial contraction and subsequent fall in cardiac output may produce hemodynamic deterioration.

Treatment

1. Treatment is not necessary. On occasion, AIVR may be the only functioning pacemaker and suppression with lidocaine can lead to cardiac asystole.
2. If sustained AIVR produces symptoms secondary to a decrease in cardiac output, treatment with atrial pacing may be required.

Ventricular Tachycardia

Ventricular tachycardia is the occurrence of three or more beats from a ventricular ectopic pacemaker at a rate greater than 100. The ECG characteristics of ventricular tachycardia are: (1) wide QRS complexes; (2) rate greater than 100 (most commonly 150 to 200); (3) rhythm usually regular, although there may be some beat-to-beat variation; and (4) QRS axis usually constant (Fig. 11-19). Ventricular tachycardia can occur in a nonsustained manner—usually short episodes, lasting seconds, with spontaneous termination—or occur in a sustained fashion—longer episodes that typically require treatment.

There are several variants of ventricular tachycardia. *Ventricular flutter* is the phrase used for a regular zigzag pattern without distinguishable QRS complexes or T waves. In *bidirectional ventricular tachycardia* the QRS complexes alternate polarity as recorded in a single lead. In *alternating ventricular tachycardia* the QRS complexes alternate in height (but not polarity) in a single lead. (Both bidirectional and alternating ventricular tachycardia indicate serious myocardial disease and are often due to digitalis toxicity.) In *polymorphous ventricular tachycardia* the QRS complexes have many different shapes in one lead. *Atypical ventricular tachycardia* (torsade de pointes, or "twisting of the points") is where the QRS axis swings from a positive to negative direction in a single lead (Fig. 11-20). Despite the appearance, this rhythm originates from a single focus and is considered to result from a triggered arrhythmic mechanism. Atypical ventricular tachycardia usually occurs in short runs of 5 to 15 s at a rate of 200 to 240. This form of ventricular tachycardia generally occurs in patients with serious myocardial disease who have a prolonged and uneven ventricular repolarization (prolonged QT interval) (Table 11-3).

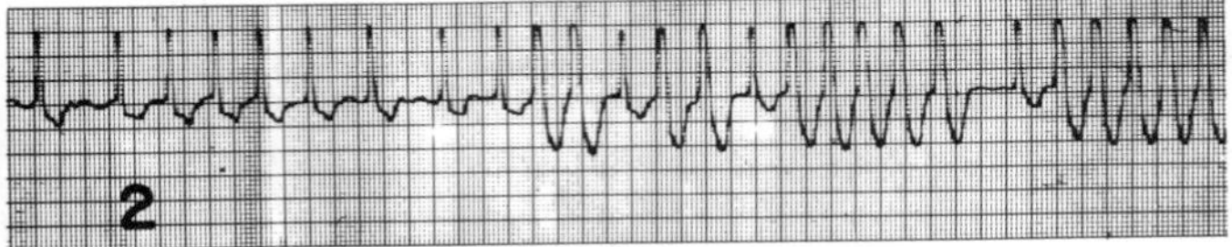

Fig. 11-19. Ventricular tachycardia.

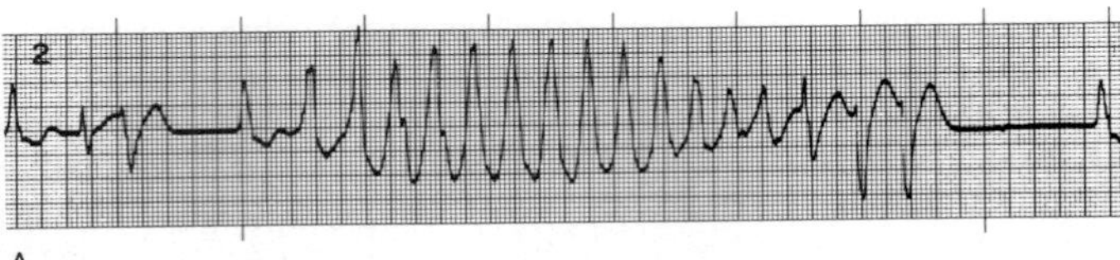

A

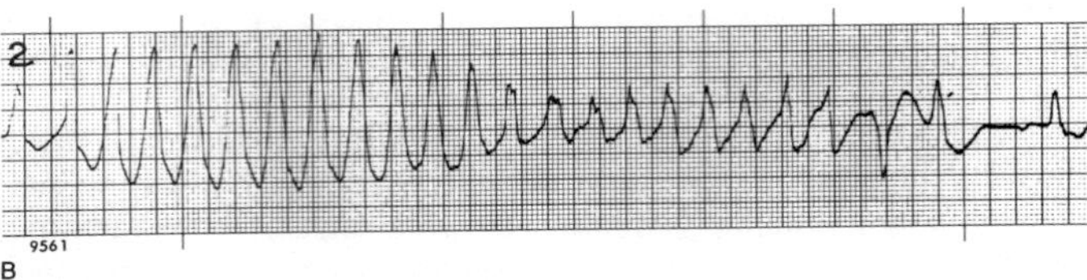

B

Fig. 11-20. Two examples of short runs of atypical ventricular tachycardia showing sinusoidal variation in amplitude and direction of the QRS complexes: "le torsade de pointes" (twisting of the points). Note that the top example is initiated by a late-occurring PVC (lead II).

Drugs which further prolong repolarization—quinidine, disopyramide, procainamide, phenothiazines, tricyclic antidepressants—exacerbate this arrhythmia. Conventional treatment with lidocaine often is ineffective. To date, treatment for torsade de pointes consisted of accelerating the heart rate (thereby shortening ventricular repolarization) with isoproterenol (2 to 8 μg/min) while making arrangements for a ventricular pacemaker to overdrive the heart at rates of 90 to 120. Temporary pacing is the most effective and safest method to treat torsades and prevent its recurrence. Recent reports have revealed that magnesium sulfate 1 to 2 g IV over 60 to 90 s followed by an infusion of 1 to 2 g/h is effective in abolishing these runs of torsade de pointes although recurrences are seen despite continued infusion. A wide variety of other agents and antiarrhythmics have reported anecdotal success, but overall efficacy has been inconsistent.

Clinical Significance

Ventricular tachycardia is very rare in patients without underlying heart disease. The most common causes of ventricular tachydardia are ischemic heart disease and acute myocardial infarction. Less common causes include hypertrophic cardiomyopathy, mitral valve prolapse, and toxicity from many drugs (digoxin, quinidine, procainamide, sympathomimetics). Hypoxia, alkalosis, and electrolyte abnormalities exacerbate the tendency toward ventricular ectopy and tachycardia.

Table 11-3. Etiologies and Associated Conditions in Torsades de Pointes

Familial	
	Jervell-Lange-Nielson syndrome (congenital deafness)
	Romano-Ward syndrome (without deafness)
Toxins and drugs	
	Antiarrhythmics: most common with classes IA, IC, and III
	Psychotropics: tricyclic antidepressants, some phenothiazines (thioridazine), tetracyclics (maprotiline)
	Organophosphate insecticides
	Liquid protein diets
Cerebrovascular disease	
	Cerebrovascular accidents, intracranial hemorrhage, carotid endarterectomy
Electrolyte disorders	
	Hypokalemia, hypomagnesemia, hypocalcemia
Endocrine disorders	
	Hypothyroidism
Cardiac disease	
	Acute rheumatic carditis, mitral valve prolapse syndrome, inflammatory myocarditis
Coronary artery disease	
	Myocardial ischemia or infarction, left ventricular failure
Pacemaker malfunction	
Postoperative complication	

It is a common misconception that patients with ventricular tachycardia appear clinically unstable; this is the basis for the mistaken assumption that patients who appear stable with a wide complex tachycardia have SVT with aberrancy rather than ventricular tachycardia. This is definitely wrong. Ventricular tachycardia cannot be differentiated from SVT with aberrancy on the basis of clinical symptoms, blood pressure, or heart rate. Patients who are unstable should be cardioverted; it is effective for both arrhythmias. In patients who are stable, a 12-lead ECG should be obtained first and examined for evidence which favors one arrhythmia over another; but even then, it is often difficult to decide. Therefore, in general, it is best to treat all wide complex tachycardias as ventricular tachycardia with lidocaine or procainamide. These drugs are obviously effective in ventricular tachycardia, often surprisingly effective in SVT with aberrancy and carry little risk of harming the patient. Conversely, verapamil is harmful in most patients with ventricular tachycardia, accelerating the heart rate and the decreasing blood pressure without converting the rhythm. Adenosine appears to have little harm in patients with ventricular tachycardia and has potential merit for the treatment for wide QRS complex tachycardias. However, until further experience is gained with this agent, it cannot be recommended for routine use in this setting.

Treatment

1. Unstable patients or those in cardiac arrest should be treated with synchronized cardioversion. Ventricular tachycardia can be converted with energies as low as 1 J and over 90 percent can be converted with less than 10 J. Rarely is more than 100 J needed. Current ACLS guidelines recommend that pulseless ventricular tachycardia be *defibrillated* (unsynchronized cardioversion) with 200 J.
2. Clinically stable patients should be treated with intravenous antiarrhythmics.
   a. Lidocaine 75 mg (1.0 to 1.5 mg/kg) IV over 60 to 90 s, followed by a constant infusion at 1 to 4 mg/min (10 to 40 μg/kg per minute). A repeat bolus dose of 50 mg lidocaine may be required during the first 20 min to avoid a subtherapeutic dip in serum level due to the early distribution phase.
   b. Bretylium 500 mg (5 to 10 mg/kg) IV over 10 min, followed by a constant infusion at 1 to 2 mg/min.
   c. Procainamide IV at a rate of less than 50 mg/min until the arrhythmia converts, the total dose reaches 15 to 17 mg/kg in normals (12 mg/kg in patients with congestive heart failure), or early signs of toxicity develop with hypotension or QRS prolongation. The loading dose should be followed by a maintenance infusion of 2.8 mg/kg per hour in normal subjects (1.4 mg/kg per hour in patients with renal insufficiency).
   d. A variety of other antiarrhythmics have been studied for the treatment of ventricular tachycardia. Most class I and III agents are effective for the acute termination of ventricular tachycardia when given intravenously. Recommendations concerning their routine use will have to await further studies.

Ventricular Fibrillation

Ventricular fibrillation is the totally disorganized depolarization and contraction of small areas of ventricular myocardium—there is no effective ventricular pumping activity. The ECG of ventricular fibrillation shows a fine to coarse zigzag pattern without discernible P waves or QRS complexes (Fig. 11-21).

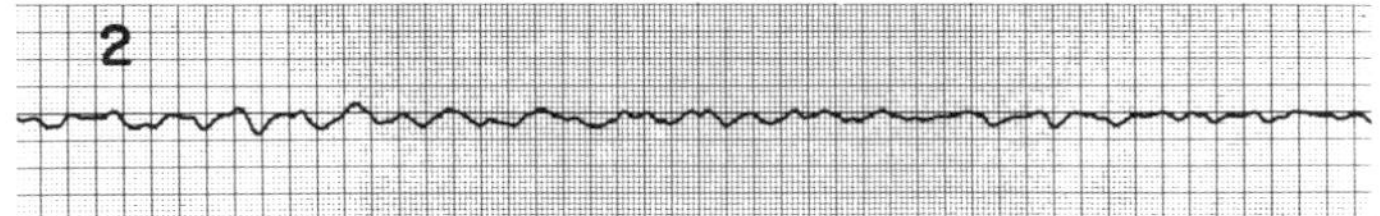

Fig. 11-21. Ventricular fibrillation.

Ventricular fibrillation is never accompanied by a pulse or blood pressure. In patients who are awake and responsive, the ECG pattern of ventricular fibrillation is caused by a loose lead artifact or electrical interference.

Clinical Significance

Ventricular fibrillation is most commonly seen in patients with severe ischemic heart disease, with or without an acute myocardial infarction. Primary ventricular fibrillation occurs suddenly, without preceding hemodynamic deterioration, while secondary ventricular fibrillation occurs after a prolonged period of left ventricular failure and/or circulatory shock. Ventricular fibrillation may also occur from digoxin toxicity, quinidine toxicity, hypothermia, blunt chest trauma, severe electrolyte abnormality, or myocardial irritation caused by an intracardiac catheter or pacemaker electrode.

Treatment

1. Current ACLS guidelines recommend immediate electrical defibrillation with 200 J. If ventricular fibrillation persists, defibrillation should be repeated immediately with 200 to 300 J for the second attempt and increased to 360 J for the third attempt.
2. If the initial three attempts at defibrillation are unsuccessful, CPR should be initiated and further electrical defibrillations done after the administration of various intravenous drugs according to ACLS guidelines.

ABERRANT VERSUS VENTRICULAR TACHYARRHYTHMIAS

Differentiation between ectopic beats of ventricular origin and those of supraventricular origin but conducted aberrantly can be difficult, especially in sustained tachycardias with wide QRS complexes (WCT). In general, the majority of patients with WCT have ventricular tachycardia and should be approached as ventricular tachycardia, until proved otherwise. Several guidelines might help in the distinction.

1. A preceding ectopic P′ wave is good evidence favoring aberrancy, although coincidental atrial and ventricular ectopic beats or retrograde conduction can occur. During a sustained run of tachycardia, AV dissociation greatly favors a ventricular origin of the arrhythmia.
2. Postectopic pause: A fully compensatory pause is more likely after a ventricular beat, but exceptions do occur.
3. Fusion beats are good evidence for ventricular origin, but again exceptions do occur.
4. A varying bundle branch block pattern suggests aberrancy.
5. Coupling intervals are usually constant with ventricular ectopic beats, unless parasystole is present. Varying coupling intervals suggest aberrancy.
6. Response to carotid sinus massage or other vagal maneuvers will slow conduction through the AV node and may abolish reentrant SVT and slow the ventricular response in other supraventricular tachyarrhythmias. These maneuvers have essentially no effect on ventricular arrhythmias.
7. A QRS duration of longer than 0.14 s is usually only found in ventricular ectopy or tachycardia.
8. QRS morphology: Wellens et al. have studied patients with both ventricular tachycardia and SVT with aberrancy using His bundle electrocardiography. Several morphologic ECG criteria were found useful in differentiating between the two (Table 11-4).
9. Historical criteria have also been found to be useful: age of the patient over 35 and/or history of myocardial infarction, congestive heart failure, or coronary artery bypass graft strongly suggest ventricular tachycardia in patients with WCT.

Table 11-4. Aberrancy versus Ventricular Ectopy

QRS Pattern in V_1	Favors	QRS Pattern in V_6	Favors
rSR′ (RBBB pattern) rR′	Aberrancy	qRS	Aberrancy
R qR RS Slurred downslope R	Ventricular	rS S qR or QR R qQ′	Ventricular
Slurred upstroke R	Either	RS Slurred R	Either

Source: Wellens HJJ, Frits WHMB, Lie KI: *Am J Med* 64:27, 1978. Used by permission.

CONDUCTION DISTURBANCES

Sinoatrial (SA) Block

The sinus node discharge must be conducted into the atria to pace the heart during sinus rhythm. If sinus node discharges are delayed or blocked in their outward propagation, then sinoatrial block is present. Sinoatrial block is divided into first-, second-, and third-degree varieties.

First-degree SA block means that the impulse is delayed in its conduction out of the sinus node into the atria—a condition that cannot be recognized on the clinical ECG.

Second-degree SA block means that some impulses get through and some are blocked. Second-degree SA block can be suspected whenever an expected P wave and the corresponding QRS complex are absent. In the variable (Wenckebach) type of second-degree SA block, the missing P wave would come after a period of progressive prolongation of the sinus node to atrium conduction time, again something undetectable on the clinical ECG. However, another ECG finding common to the Wenckebach phenomenon can be seen—progressive shortening of the P-P intervals prior to the missing P wave (Fig. 11-22). In the constant type of second-degree SA block, the sinoatrial conduction time remains constant before and after the blocked impulses. In this situation, the interval encompassing the missing beat is an exact or near-exact multiple of the cycle length (Fig. 11-23).

Third-degree SA block occurs when the sinus node discharge is completely blocked and no P wave originating from the sinus node is seen. There are three other causes of absent sinus P waves in addition to third-degree SA block: (1) sinus node failure, (2) a sinus node stimulus inadequate to activate the atria, and (3) atrial unresponsiveness.

Clinical Significance

Sinoatrial block usually arises from myocardial disease (acute rheumatic fever, acute inferior myocardial infarction, other causes of myocarditis) or drug toxicity (digoxin, quinidine, salicylates, β-adrenergic blockers, or calcium-channel blockers). In rare individuals, vagal stimulation can produce SA block.

Treatment

1. Treatment depends on the underlying cause, associated arrhythmias, and whether symptoms of hypoperfusion are present.

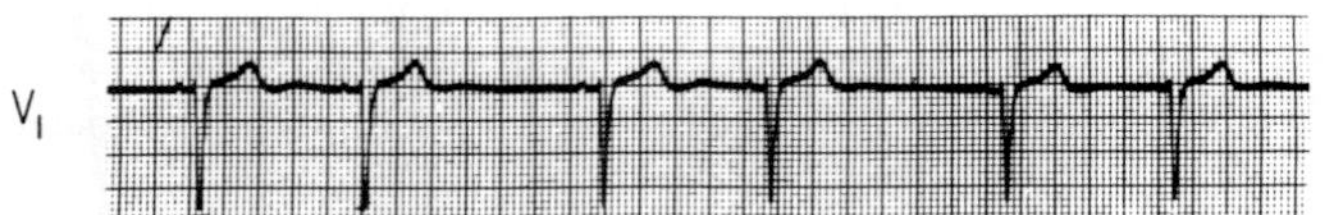

Fig. 11-22. Second-degree SA block type I (Wenckebach). (From Braunwald E: *Heart Disease. A Textbook of Cardiovascular Medicine.* Philadelphia, Saunders, 1980. Used by permission.)

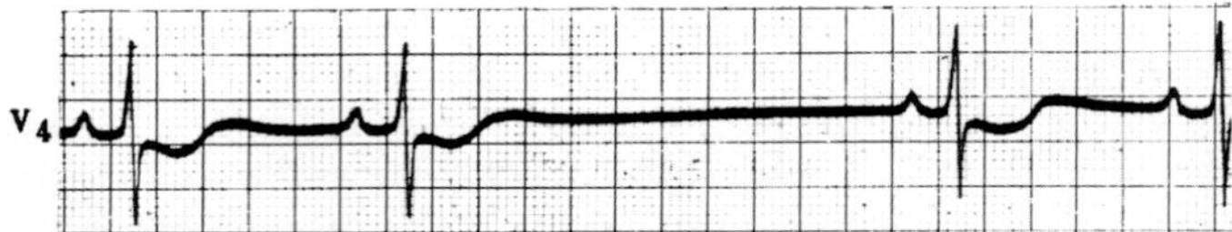

Fig. 11-23. Second-degree constant SA block type II (lead V_4)

2. Sinus node discharge rate and sinoatrial conduction can be facilitated by atropine or isoproterenol when clinically required.
3. Cardiac pacing is indicated for recurrent or persistent symptomatic bradycardia.

Sinus Arrest (Pause)

Sinus pause is a failure of impulse formation within the sinus node. In sinus arrest, the P-P interval has no mathematical relation to the basic sinus node discharge rate (Fig. 11-24).

Clinical Significance

The same conditions which produce SA block can also produce sinus arrest, especially digoxin toxicity. The combination of digoxin and carotid sinus massage is well known to be able to produce prolonged sinus arrest. Brief periods of sinus arrest may occur in healthy individuals from increased vagal tone. If sinus arrest is prolonged, AV junctional escape beats often occur.

Treatment

1. Treatment depends on the underlying cause, associated arrhythmias, and whether symptoms of hypoperfusion are present.
2. If sinus arrest is symptomatic, atropine will usually increase sinus node discharge rate.
3. Cardiac pacing is indicated for recurrent or persisent symptomatic bradycardia.

Atrioventricular (AV) Dissociation

Atrioventricular dissociation is a condition in which the atria and ventricles are driven by separate and independent pacemakers. It is not a primary rhythm disturbance, but is secondary to another conduction or rhythm abnormality. There are two varieties of AV dissociation: passive (default or "escape"), and active (usurpation).

Passive AV dissociation occurs when an impulse fails to reach the AV node due to sinus node failure or block. Usually an escape rhythm takes over and paces the ventricles. When the sinus node recovers, atrial activity resumes but there may be a period during which the ventricles are still driven by the escape pacemaker, and the P waves and QRS complexes occur independent of each other (Fig. 11-25).

Active AV dissociation occurs when a lower pacemaker accelerates

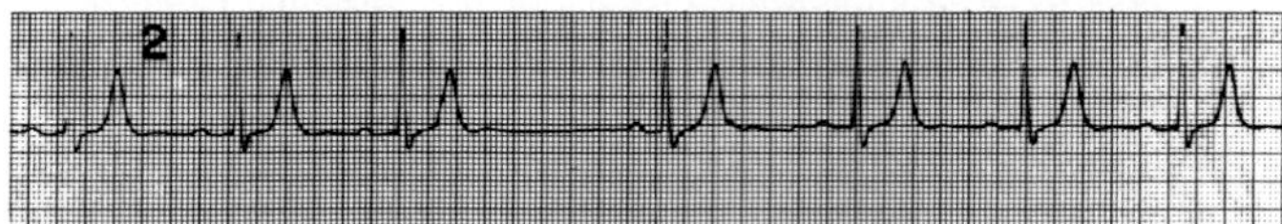

Fig. 11-24. Sinus pause.

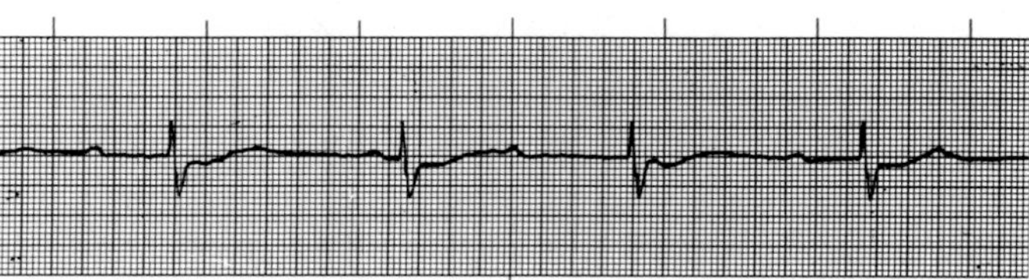

Fig. 11-25. Passive AV dissociation, secondary to third-degree AV block.

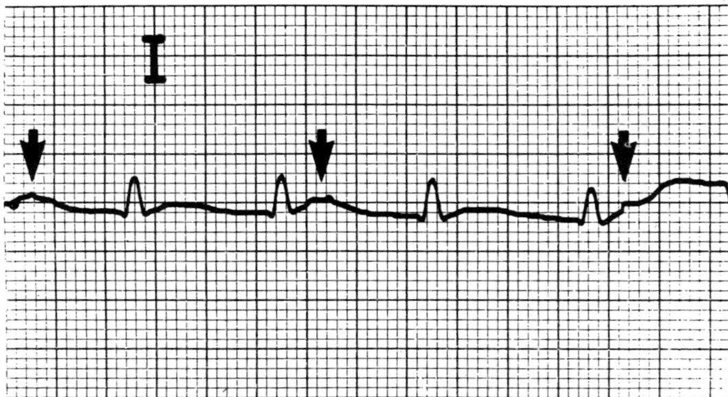

Fig. 11-26. Active AV dissociation. (Arrows indicate P waves.)

to usurp the sinus node and captures the ventricles, but the atria are still paced as before (Fig. 11-26).

In both varieties of AV dissociation, fusion beats are common. It is also common for the two pacemakers to operate with nearly identical rates, possibly as a result of mechanical or electrical influences which tend to keep them in phase with each other—a condition termed isorhythmic dissociation.

Clinical Significance

Passive AV dissociation occurs when the sinus node discharge rate is slowed by sinus bradycardia, sinus arrhythmia, SA block, or sinus pause. Common causes of this include: (1) ischemic heart disease (especially acute inferior myocardial infarction), (2) myocarditis (especially acute rheumatic fever), (3) drug toxicity (especially digoxin), and (4) vagal reflexes. It may also be seen in well-conditioned athletes.

Active AV dissociation occurs when the automaticity of lower pacemakers is enhanced. Common causes include myocardial ischemia and drug toxicity (especially digoxin).

Treatment

1. Most occurrences of AV dissociation have an acceptable heart rate and are well tolerated.
2. Therapy, if any, is directed toward the underlying cause.

Atrioventricular (AV) Block

Clincial classification of AV block was done before modern understanding of the sites and mechanisms involved in impairing conduction between the atria and ventricles. This is unfortunate because this classification is too simple to categorize all the problems that may occur with AV conduction. However, this system is almost universally used.

First-degree AV block is characterized by a delay in AV conduction, manifested by a prolonged PR interval. Second-degree AV block is characterized by intermittent AV conduction—some atrial impulses reach the ventricles and others are blocked. Third-degree AV block is characterized by complete interruption in AV conduction.

Precise localization of AV conduction blocks can be made with His bundle electrocardiography. Although this method is not available for us in the emergency department, correlations can be made between the clinical ECG, the approximate location of the block, and the risk of future progression.

AV blocks can also be divided into nodal and infranodal blocks, an important distinction because the clinical significance and prognosis vary with the site. AV nodal blocks are usually due to reversible depression of conduction, often self-limited, generally have a stable infranodal escape pacemaker pacing the ventricles, and therefore do not have a serious prognosis. Infranodal blocks are usually due to organic disease of the His bundle or bundle branches, often the damage is irreversible, they generally have a slow and unstable ventricular escape rhythm pacing the ventricles, and they may have a serious prognosis depending on the clinical circumstance.

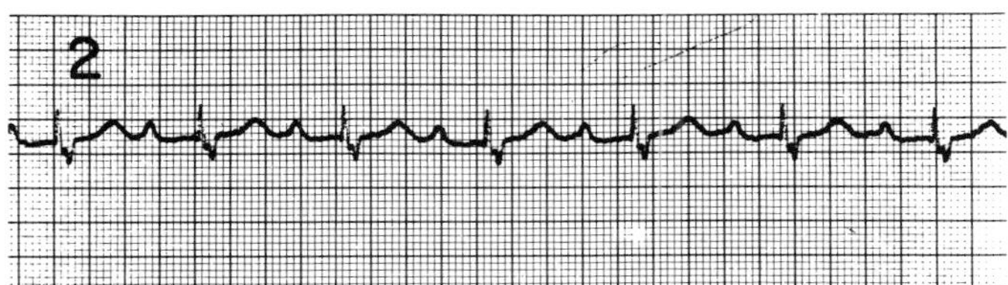

Fig. 11-27. First-degree AV block (PR interval = 0.3 s).

First-Degree AV Block

In first-degree AV block, each atrial impulse is conducted into the ventricles, but more slowly than normal. This is recognized by a PR interval of greater than 0.20 s (Fig. 11-27). The AV node is usually the site of conduction delay, although it may occur at any infranodal level.

Clinical Significance

First-degree AV block is occasionally found in normal hearts. Other common causes include increased vagal tone (whatever the cause), digoxin toxicity, acute inferior myocardial infarction, and myocarditis. Patients with first-degree AV block without evidence of organic heart disease appear to have no significant difference in mortality compared with matched controls.

Treatment

1. None is usually required.
2. Prophylactic pacing in acute myocardial infarction is not indicated unless more serious infranodal conduction disturbances are present.

Second-Degree Mobitz I (Wenckebach) AV Block

In this block there is progressive prolongation of AV conduction (and the PR interval) until an atrial impulse is completely blocked (Fig. 11-28). Conduction ratios are used to indicate the ratio of atrial to ventricular depolarizations: 3:2 indicates 2 out of 3 atrial impulses are conducted into the ventricles. Usually, only a single atrial impulse is blocked. After the dropped beat, the AV conduction returns to normal and the cycle usually repeats itself with either the same conduction ratio (fixed ratio) or a different conduction ratio (variable ratio). This type of block almost always occurs at the level of the AV node and is often due to reversible depression of AV nodal conduction.

The Wenckebach phenomenon has a seeming paradox. Even though the PR intervals progressively lengthen prior to the dropped beat, the increments by which they lengthen decrease with successive beats; this produces a progressive shortening of the R-R interval prior to the dropped beat (Fig. 11-28). This sign can be used to indicate that a Wenckebach phenomenon is occurring, even when the conduction delay cannot be seen, as in SA Wenckebach block.

Wenckebach block is believed to occur because each successive depolarization produces prolongation of the refractory period of the AV node. When the next atrial impulse comes upon the node, it is earlier in the relative refractory period and conduction occurs more slowly relative to the previous stimulus. This process is progressive until an atrial impulse reaches the AV node during the absolute re-

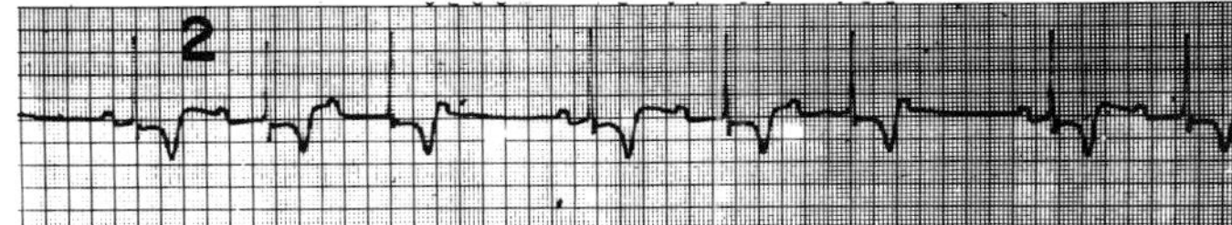

Fig. 11-28. Second-degree Mobiltz I (Wenckebach) AV block with 4:3 AV conduction.

fractory period and conduction is blocked altogether. The pause allows the AV node to recover and the process can resume.

Clinical Significance

This block is often transient and usually associated with an acute inferior myocardial infarction, digoxin toxicity, myocarditis, or is seen after cardiac surgery. Wenckebach block may also occur when a normal AV node is exposed to very rapid atrial rates.

Treatment

1. Specific treatment is not necessary unless slow ventricular rates produce signs of hypoperfusion.
2. 0.5 mg of atropine IV is given, repeated every 5 min as necessary, titrated to the desired effect, or until the total dose reaches 2.0 mg. Almost all cases will respond to atropine.
3. Isoproterenol is hazardous in the setting of acute myocardial infarction or digoxin toxicity and its use should be avoided.
4. Transvenous ventricular demand pacing should be initiated if atropine is unsuccessful.

Second-Degree Mobitz II AV Block

In this block, the PR interval remains constant before and after the nonconducted atrial beats (Fig. 11-29). One or more beats may be nonconducted at a single time.

Mobitz II blocks usually occur in the infranodal conducting system, often with coexistent fascicular or bundle branch blocks, and the QRS complexes are therefore usually wide. Even if the QRS complexes are narrow, the block is generally in the infranodal system.

When second-degree AV block occurs with a fixed conduction ratio of 2:1, it is not possible to differentiate between a Mobitz type I (Wenckebach) or Mobitz type II block. If the QRS complex is narrow, then the block is in the AV node or infranodal system with about equal incidence. If the QRS complex is wide, the block is more likely to be in the infranodal system.

Clinical Significance

Type II blocks imply structural damage to the infranodal conducting system, are usually permanent, and may progress suddenly to complete heart block—especially in the setting of an acute myocardial infarction.

Treatment

1. Emergent treatment is required when slow ventricular rates produce symptoms of hypoperfusion. Atropine should be the first drug used, and up to 60 percent of patients will respond. Isoproterenol is effective in up to 50 percent of cases but is potentially hazardous in the setting of acute myocardial infarction or digoxin toxicity, and its use should be avoided. Transcutaneous cardiac pacing is a useful modality in patients unresponsive to atropine.
2. Most cases, especially in the setting of acute myocardial infarction, will require permanent transvenous cardiac pacing.

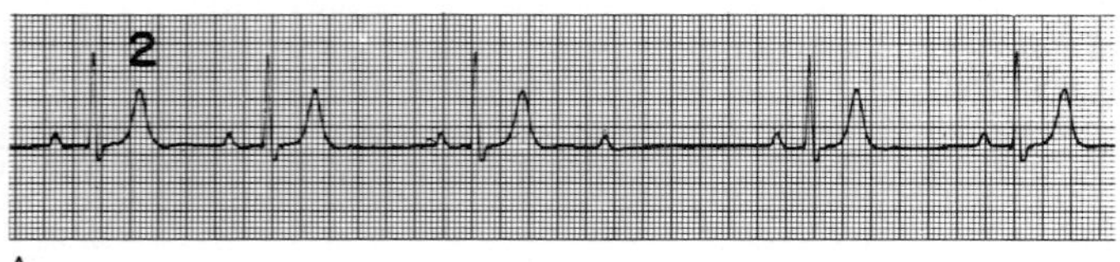

A

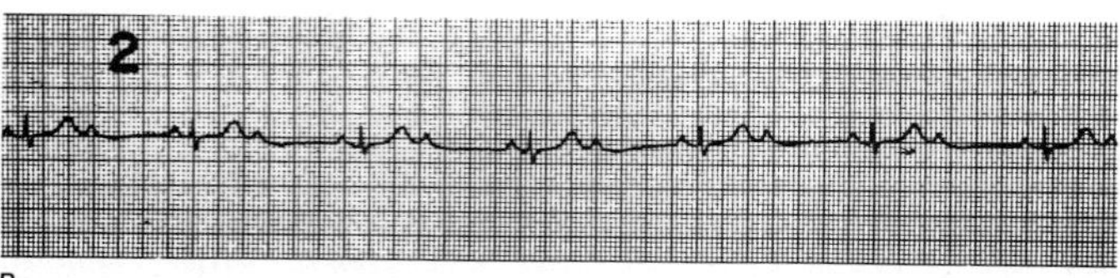

B

Fig. 11-29. Top: second-degree Mobitz II Av block. Bottom: second-degree AV block with 2:1 AV conduction.

Third-Degree (Complete) AV Block

In third-degree AV block, there is no atrioventricular conduction. The ventricles are paced by an escape pacemaker at a rate slower than the atrial rate (Fig. 11-30). Third-degree AV block can occur either at nodal or infranodal levels.

When third-degree AV block occurs at the AV node, a junctional escape pacemaker takes over with a ventricular rate of 40 to 60 and, since the rhythm originates above the bifurcation of the bundle of His, the QRS complexes are narrow.

When third-degree AV block occurs at the infranodal level, the ventricles are driven by a ventricular escape rhythm at a rate of less than 40. In third-degree AV block located at the His bundle level, the escape rhythm has narrow QRS complexes about half of the time. Presumably, in these cases, the escape pacemaker resides above the bifurcation of the conducting system into the separate bundle branches. Third-degree AV block located in the bundle branch or purkinje system invariably have escape rhythms with wide QRS complexes.

Clinical Significance

Nodal third-degree AV block may develop in up to 8 percent of acute inferior myocardial infarctions where it is usually transient, although it may last for several days.

Infranodal third-degree AV blocks indicate structural damage to the infranodal conducting system, as seen with an extensive acute anterior myocardial infarction. The ventricular escape pacemaker is usually inadequate to maintain cardiac output and is unstable with periods of ventricular asystole.

Treatment

1. Nodal third-degree AV blocks should be treated like second-degree Mobitz I AV blocks with atropine or ventricular demand pacemaker as required.
2. Infranodal third-degree AV blocks require a ventricular demand pacemaker. Isoproterenol can be used temporarily to accelerate the ventricular escape rhythm, or external cardiac pacing can be performed before transvenous pacemaker placement.

FASCICULAR BLOCKS

Unifascicular Block

Unifascicular block is a conduction block that affects one of the three major infranodal conduction pathways: right bundle branch (RBB), left anterior superior fascicle (LASF), and left posterior inferior fascicle (LPIF). A wide variety of disease processes can produce conduction block in the fascicles: ischemia, cardiomyopathies, valvular (especially aortic), myocarditis, cardiac surgery, congenital, and degenerative processes affecting the conduction tissue (Lenegre's or Lev's diseases).

In LASF block, left ventricular activation is by way of the LPIF and proceeds in an inferior-to-superior and right-to-left direction. The ECG characteristics of LASF block are: (1) normal QRS duration, (2) frontal plane mean QRS axis of less than $-45°$, (3) R wave in lead I greater than the R waves in leads II or III, (4) a qR complex in lead AVL, and (5) deep S wave in leads II, III, and AVF (Fig. 11-31). The LASF is small and easily affected by focal lesions. Other causes of left-axis deviation should be excluded—inferior myocardial infarction,

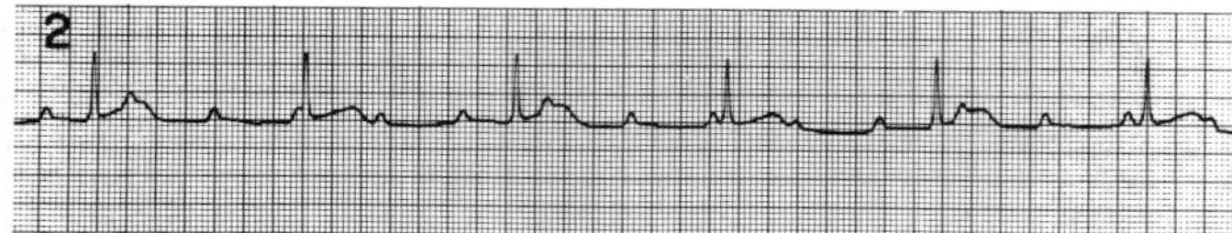

Fig. 11-30. Third-degree AV block.

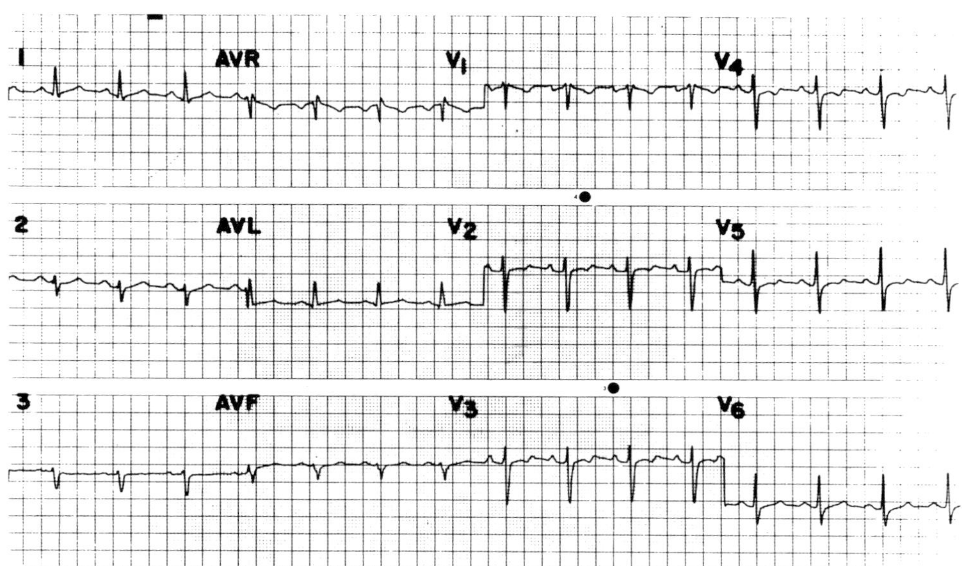

Fig. 11-31. Left anterior superior fascicular block (LASF block).

hyperkalemia, preexcitation syndromes, or body habitus. Left ventricular hypertrophy itself does not cause an extensive left-axis deviation as seen with LASF block.

In LPIF block, left ventricular activation is by way of the LASF and proceeds in a superior-to-inferior and left-to-right direction. The ECG characteristics of LPIF block are: (1) normal QRS duration, (2) frontal plane mean QRS axis greater than 110°, (3) small r and deep S wave in lead I, (4) an R wave in lead III larger than the R wave in lead II, and (5) a qR complex in lead III (Fig. 11-32). The LPIF is broad and not affected by focal lesions; its presence indicates widespread organic heart disease. Other causes of right-axis deviation are chronic cor pulmonale, right ventricular hypertrophy, and lateral myocardial infarction.

In RBB block, ventricular activation is by way of the left bundle branch, proceeding from the left to the right ventricle. The ECG characteristics of RBB block are: (1) prolonged QRS duration (greater than 0.12 s); (2) triphasic QRS complexes (RSR′) in lead V_1; (3) wide S waves in the lateral leads I, V_5, and V_6; and (4) normal onset of ventricular activation in lead V_6 (Fig. 11-33). The frontal plane mean QRS axis is usually not deviated to the right unless there is associated right ventricular hypertrophy or LPIF block.

Bifascicular Block

Bifascicular block refers to conduction blocks over two fascicles: (1) RBB and LASF, (2) RBB and LPIF, or (3) left bundle branch (LBB) block.

In LBB block, ventricular activation is by way of the RBB and proceeds from right to left and inferior to superior. The ECG characteristics of LBB block are: (1) prolonged QRS duration (greater than 0.12 s); (2) large and wide R waves in leads I, aV_L, V_5, and V_6; (3) small r wave followed by deep S wave in leads II, III, aV_F, and V_1 to V_3; and (4) no q waves in leads I, aV_F, V_5, and V_6 (Fig. 11-34).

Trifascicular Block

Trifascicular block refers to a combination of conduction blocks in all three fascicles, either permanent or transient: (1) RBB and LASF with first-degree AV block, (2) RBB and LPIF with first-degree AV block, (3) LBB with first-degree AV block, or (4) alternating RBB and LBB block.

While bi- and trifascicular conduction blocks indicate advanced organic heart disease, long-term follow-up studies of ambulatory patients indicate that the risk of sudden progression to complete heart

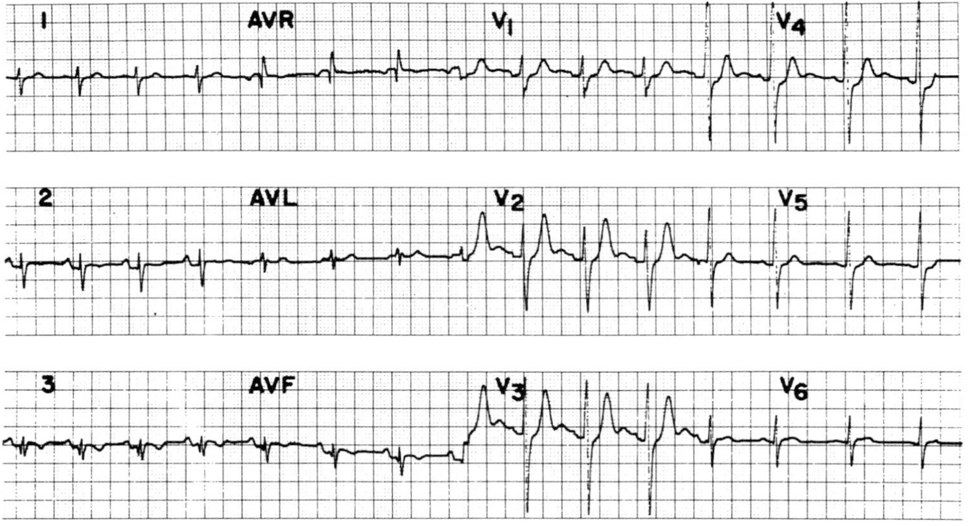

Fig. 11-32. Left posterior inferior fascicular block (LPIF block).

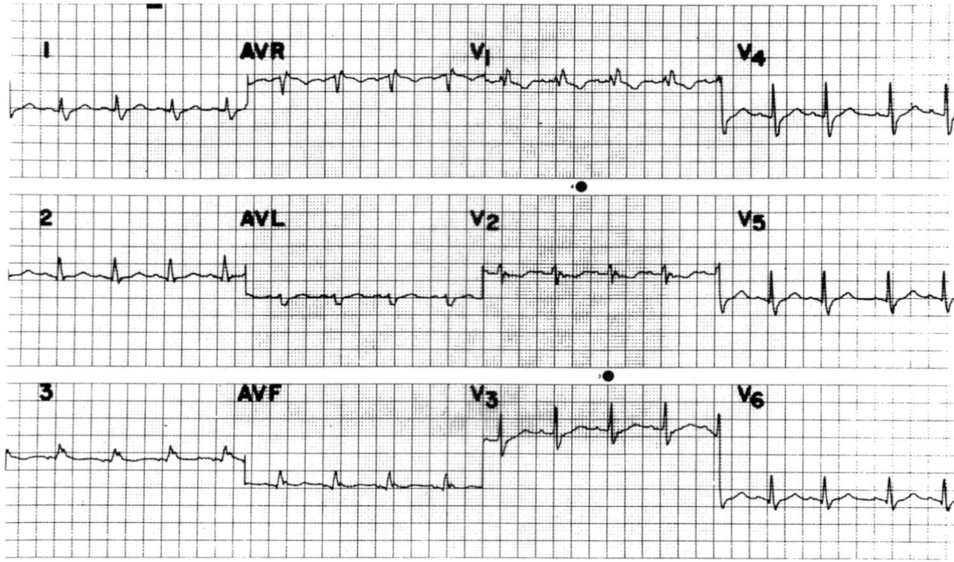

Fig. 11-33. Right bundle branch block (RBB block).

block and sudden death due to ventricular asystole is not high. Placement of a ventricular demand pacemaker is indicated only for symptoms due to documented bradyarrhythmias.

However, in the face of an acute myocardial infarction, the risks of complete heart block are much greater when new or preexistent bi- or trifascicular conduction blocks are present. In this setting, prophylactic placement of a ventricular demand pacemaker is indicated. This is further discussed in the chapter on acute myocardial infarction.

PRETERMINAL RHYTHMS

Several arrhythmias may be seen during cardiac resuscitation. Ventricular tachycardia and fibrillation potentially are treatable and resuscitation may result in a functional survivor. The four other arrhythmias included here have a low successful resuscitation rate and are much less likely to yield a functional survivor. Further discussion on this is included in the chapter on cardiac resuscitation.

Electromechanical Dissociation (EMD)

Electromechanical dissociation is the presence of electrical complexes without accompanying mechanical contraction of the heart (Fig. 11-35). In the setting of a cardiac arrest, EMD is due to a profound metabolic abnormality of the myocardium, rendering it noncontractile. At this time, there is no clearly beneficial therapy; the best that can be recommended currently is continued cardiopulmonary resuscitation and α-adrenergic agents. Although calcium has been advocated traditionally, most studies have found no consistent benefit, and there are serious biophysiologic reasons to question the use of calcium in the setting of cardiac arrest. Electrical pacing is, of course, not effective.

Other conditions which may mimic EMD are: (1) severe hypovolemia, (2) cardiac tamponade, (3) tension pneumothorax, (4) massive pulmonary embolus, and (5) rupture of the ventricular wall. The first three conditions are potentially treatable if recognized early.

Idioventricular Rhythm (IVR)

An IVR is an escape rhythm of ventricular origin with very wide QRS complexes (more than 0.16 s) and a rate less than 40 (Fig. 11-36). Effective cardiac contractions and pulses may or may not be present. Idioventricular rhythm may occur as the result of complete infranodal AV block, acute myocardial infarction, cardiac tamponade, or exsanguinating hemorrhage. Treatment consists of attempting to accelerate the heart rate and enhance mechanical contractility using cardiopulmonary resuscitation and α-adrenergic agents. There is no proven

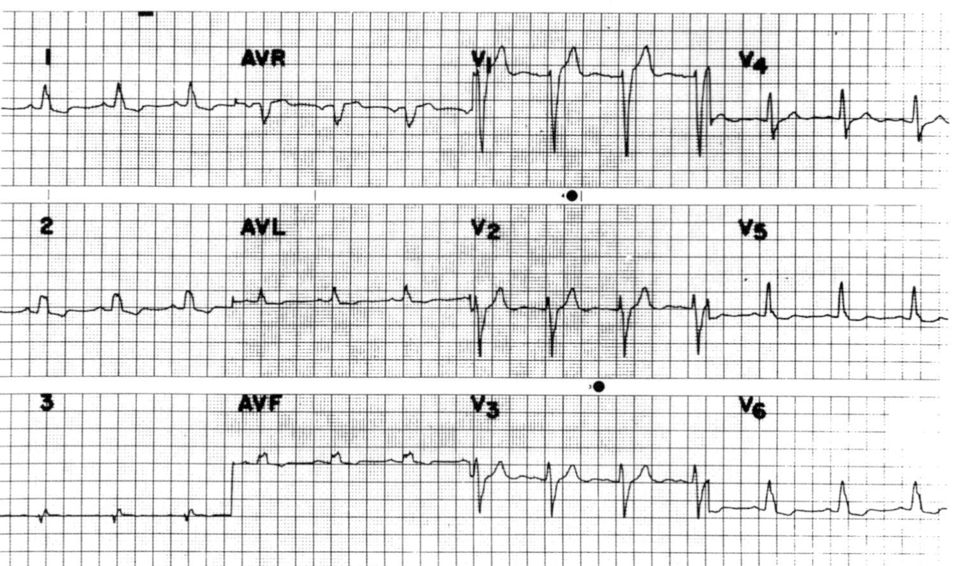

Fig. 11-34. Left bundle branch block (LBB block).

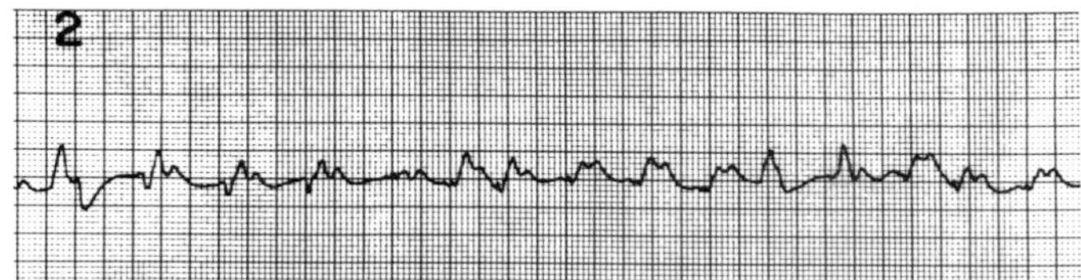

Fig. 11-35. Electromechanical dissociation (EMD).

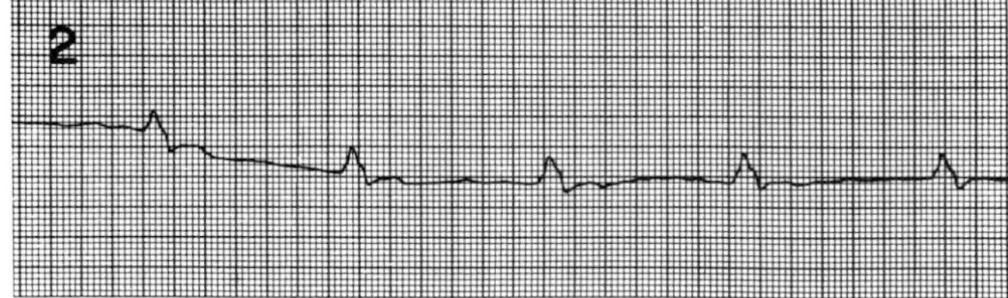

Fig. 11-36. Idioventricular rhythm (IVR).

benefit to the use of atropine or isoproterenol to treat IVR during cardiac resuscitation.

Agonal Ventricular Rhythm

Agonal rhythm is the occurrence of very broad and irregular ventricular complexes at a slow rate, usually without associated ventricular contractions (Fig. 11-37).

Cardiac Asystole (Cardiac Standstill)

Asystole is complete absence of any cardiac electrical activity. Treatment consists of attempting to stimulate electrical activity and mechanical contractions with continued cardiopulmonary resuscitation and α-adrenergic agents. Transthoracic or transvenous ventricular pacing occasionally may produce electrical capture but rarely yields effective pumping action if prior agents were unsuccessful.

TACHYCARDIA-BRADYCARDIA SYNDROME (SICK SINUS SYNDROME)

Sick sinus syndrome (SSS) is a heterogeneous disorder consisting of abnormalities of supraventricular impulse generation and conduction which produce a wide variety of intermittent supraventricular tachy- and bradyarrhythmias. The tachyarrhythmias are usually atrial fibrillation, junctional tachycardia, reentrant SVT, and atrial flutter. The bradyarrhythmias are marked sinus bradycardia, prolonged sinus arrest, and sinoatrial block usually associated with AV nodal conduction abnormalities and inadequate AV junctional escape rhythms.

Clinical Significance

Symptoms of SSS are due to the effects of either fast or slow heart rate. Common symptoms include syncope or near-syncope, palpitations, dyspnea, chest pain, and cerebrovascular accidents.

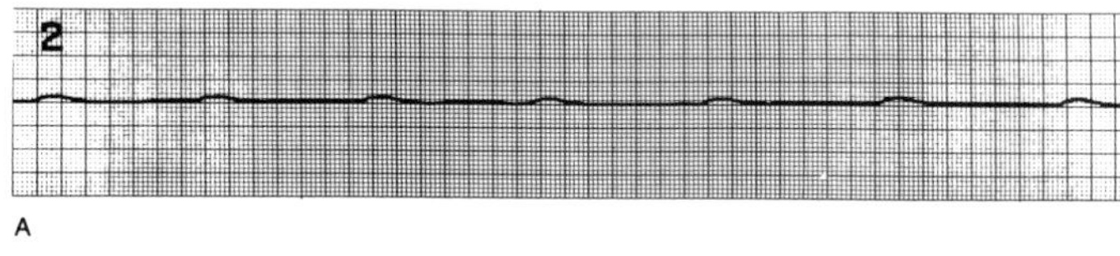

A

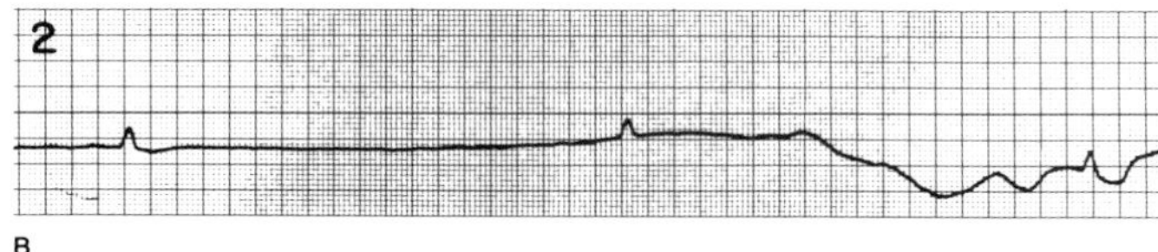

B

Fig. 11-37. Agonal ventricular rhythm. Top: regular. Bottom: irregular.

A wide variety of cardiac disease can affect the sinus and AV node, producing the arrhythmias of SSS: ischemic, rheumatic, myocarditis and pericarditis, rheumatologic disease, metastatic tumors, surgical damage, or cardiomyopathies.

Conditions such as abdominal pain, increased intracranial pressure, thyrotoxicosis, and hyperkalemia which increase vagal tone may exacerbate the abnormalities of SSS and cause increased symptoms. Drugs such as digoxin, quinidine, procainamide, disopyramide, nicotine, β-adrenergic antagonists, or calcium-channel blockers also cause increased symptoms.

Ambulatory ECG monitoring is usually necessary for the diagnosis of SSS since a routine ECG cannot be expected to show the intermittent arrhythmias common in this syndrome. The demonstration of increased sensitivity of the sinus node to carotid sinus massage, Valsalva's maneuver, or atropine suggests sinus node dysfunction but is not conclusive proof for the diagnosis of SSS.

Treatment

1. Symptomatic bradycardias require a permanent ventricular demand pacemaker. Because of the frequent association of AV conduction abnormalities, ventricular pacing is usually done, although atrial pacing is reasonable in selected patients.
2. Treatment of atrial tachyarrhythmias with digoxin, quinidine, disopyramide, procainamide, propranolol, or verapamil carries the risk of aggravating preexisting AV block or sinus arrest. Therefore, most patients should have pacemaker implantation before drug therapy is begun.

PREEXCITATION SYNDROMES

Preexcitation occurs when some portion of the ventricles are activated by an impulse from the atria sooner than would be expected if the impulse were transmitted down the normal conducting pathway. Several different forms of preexcitation have been described, based on anatomic, clinical, electrocardiographic, and electrophysiological abnormalities. All forms of preexcitation are felt to be due to accessory tracts that bypass all or part of the normal conducting system. These bypass tracts have specific names (Fig. 11-38).

James fibers are a continuation of the posterior internodal tract and connect the atrium and proximal His bundle. Atrial impulses can therefore completely bypass the AV node to activate the ventricles. On ECG, this appears as (1) a short PR interval because the usual delay in the AV node is bypassed and (2) a normal QRS because James fibers insert directly into the infranodal conducting system and the ventricles are activated normally. When this is associated with reentrant SVT, the clinical condition is termed the Lown-Ganong-Levine (LGL) syndrome.

Mahaim bundles are composed of myogenic tissue, originate from either the AV node, His bundle, or bundle branches, and insert into

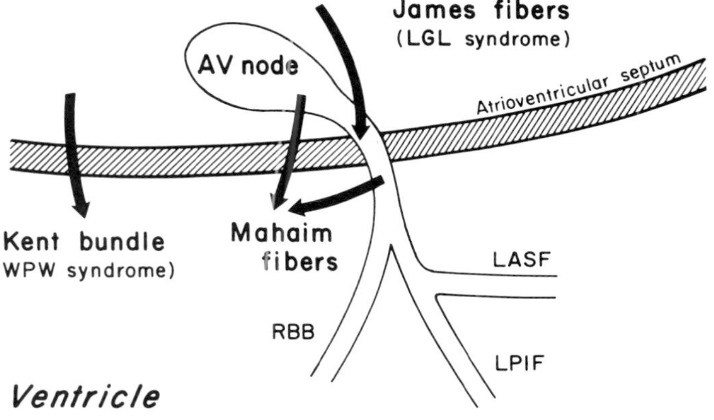

Fig. 11-38. Anatomic sites of bypass tracts.

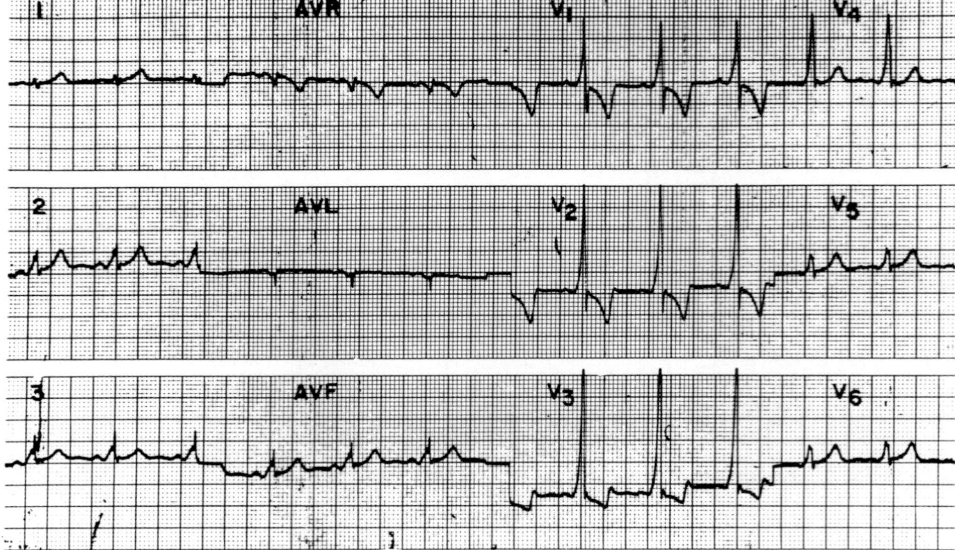

Fig. 11-39. Type A Wolff-Parkinson-White syndrome.

the ventricles in the septal region. Atrial impulses pass through the AV node but then bypass all or part of the infranodal conducting system to activate the ventricles. Ventricular activation then occurs from two sources, the bypass tract and the normal conducting system, and the QRS complex represents a fusion of the two. The initial depolarization starts at the ventricular insertion of the bypass tract and is spread slowly by cell-to-cell transmission of the impulse. Subsequent depolarization by way of the faster normal conducting system then overtakes the initial depolarization and activates the bulk of ventricular myocardium. The QRS complex is basically normal with a slurred and distorted initial portion termed a delta wave. On ECG, this appears as a normal PR interval, and an initial distortion of ventricular depolarization (delta wave).

Kent bundles are composed of myogenic tissue and directly link the atria to the ventricles, completely bypassing the AV node and infranodal system. This is the most common form of preexcitation and is the anatomic basis for the Wolff-Parkinson-White (WPW) syndrome. On ECG, this appears as a shortened PR interval and an initial distortion of ventricular activation (delta wave). Sometimes the bypass tract does not conduct an atrial impulse in the antegrade direction and the QRS complex is entirely normal. However, these concealed bypass tracts may conduct retrograde and be able to sustain reentrant SVT.

The WPW syndrome has been divided into types, depending on the direction of the initial delta wave on the surface ECG. This in turn is determined by where the bypass tract (bundle of Kent) inserts into the ventricles and which portion of the ventricles is activated first. In reality, accessory tracts can insert anywhere around the AV annulus; the three types are just the most common locations.

In type A WPW, ventricular activation first occurs in the inferior-posterior region of the left ventricle and the delta wave is directed anteriorly. A positive initial deflection with a dominant R wave is seen in lead V_1. Q waves in leads II, III, and aV_F are common (Fig. 11-39).

In type B WPW, ventricular activation first occurs in the inferior-posterior region of the right ventricle and the delta wave is directed posteriorly and to the left. A negative initial deflection and rS or QS pattern are seen in lead V_1 (Fig. 11-40).

In type C WPW, ventricular activation first occurs in the posterior-lateral region of the left ventricle and the delta wave is directed to the right, superiorly, and anteriorly. A positive delta wave is seen in lead V_1 with a negative or isoelectric delta wave in leads V_5 and V_6.

Because there is altered depolarization, repolarization is often abnormal with changes in the ST segments and T waves. The ECG changes of WPW may mimic changes seen with myocardial ischemia

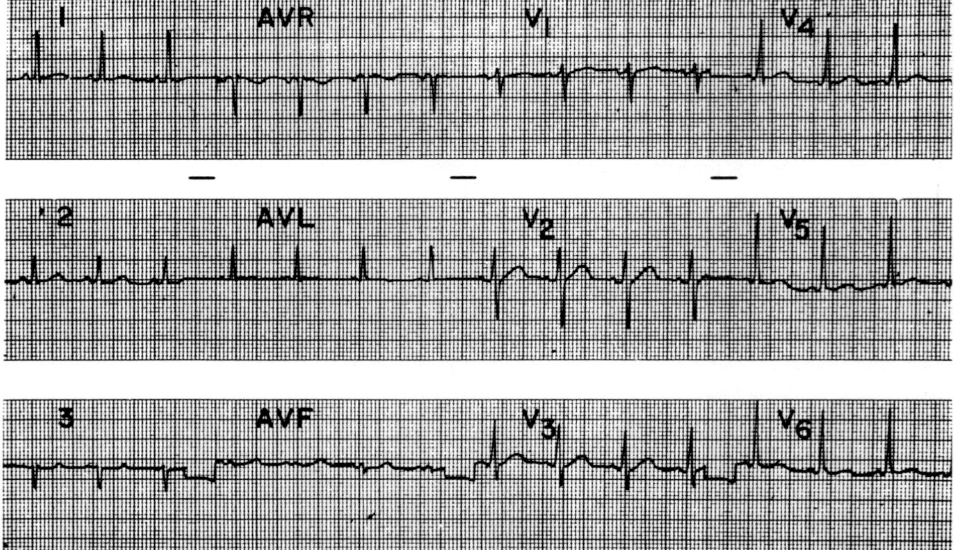

Fig. 11-40. Type B Wolff-Parkinson-White syndrome.

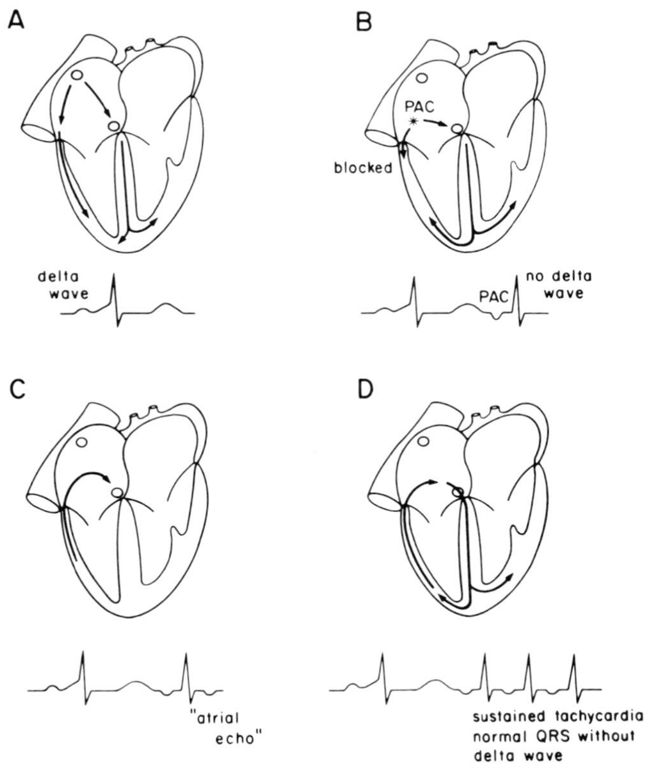

Fig. 11-41. Onset of reentrant SVT in Wolff-Parkinson-White syndrome.

or infarction. Type A WPW may appear as a posterior myocardial infarction, and type B WPW may appear as an inferior myocardial infarction.

Clinical Significance

There is a high incidence of tachyarrhythmias in patients with WPW—atrial flutter (about 5 percent), atrial fibrillation (10 to 20 percent), and paroxysmal reentrant SVT (40 to 80 percent).

Reentrant SVT occurs when an impulse is sustained around a loop composed of the bypass tract and the AV conducting system, the impulse traveling down one and up the other. Whether the QRS complex is wide or narrow depends on which limb of the circuit is used as the downward pathway to activate the ventricles. In about 80 to 90 percent of the time, reentrant SVT occurs with the impulse being conducted down the normal AV conducting system and up the bypass tract (orthodromic tachycardia). In this situation, ventricular activation occurs entirely over the normal system, the QRS complex is normal, and no delta wave is seen. Conversely, 10 to 20 percent of the time, the impulse is conducted down the bypass tract and retrograde up the AV node (antidromic tachycardia). In this case, the QRS complex is wide, and a delta wave may be visible. Reentry usually is initiated by a premature atrial contraction which encounters a bypass tract which still is refractory from the previous sinus beat, but the AV node has recovered partially and conducts the impulse more slowly than normal (Fig. 11-41). In some patients the bypass tract does not conduct antegrade during sinus rhythm and so no delta wave is seen, but it does conduct retrograde so reentrant SVT occurs. Patients with concealed bypass tracts account for about 20 percent of all patients with reentrant SVT.

If patients with WPW develop atrial flutter or fibrillation, impulses can reach the ventricles via the accessory tract, the normal conducting system, or both. Which pathway is used depends on the refractory periods of each. Most patients with WPW have longer refractory periods in their accessory tracts than in the AV node, but a minority have the opposite. In patients with short refractory periods in their accessory tracts, more atrial impulses can be conducted through the accessory tract than the AV node, so most of the QRS complexes will be wide. In atrial flutter, 1 : 1 AV conduction is possible with ventricular rates of 300 (Fig. 11-42). In atrial fibrillation, very rapid and irregular ventricular rates are possible. These rapid rhythms may resemble ventricular tachycardia, and excessive stimulation of the ventricles may precipitate ventricular fibrillation.

Treatment

1. Reentrant SVT (orthodromic, narrow QRS complex) in the WPW syndrome can be treated like other cases of reentrant SVT. Since the AV node is involved in the reentry circuit, any maneuver or drug that slows conduction through the AV node is usually effective. Verapamil or adenosine are very successful at terminating this arrhythmia in patients with WPW, but β-adrenergic blockers usually are ineffective.
2. Antidromic tachycardia (wide QRS complex) is usually associated with a short refractory period in the bypass tract, and such patients are at risk for rapid ventricular rates and degeneration into ventricular fibrillation. Stable patients should be treated with intra-

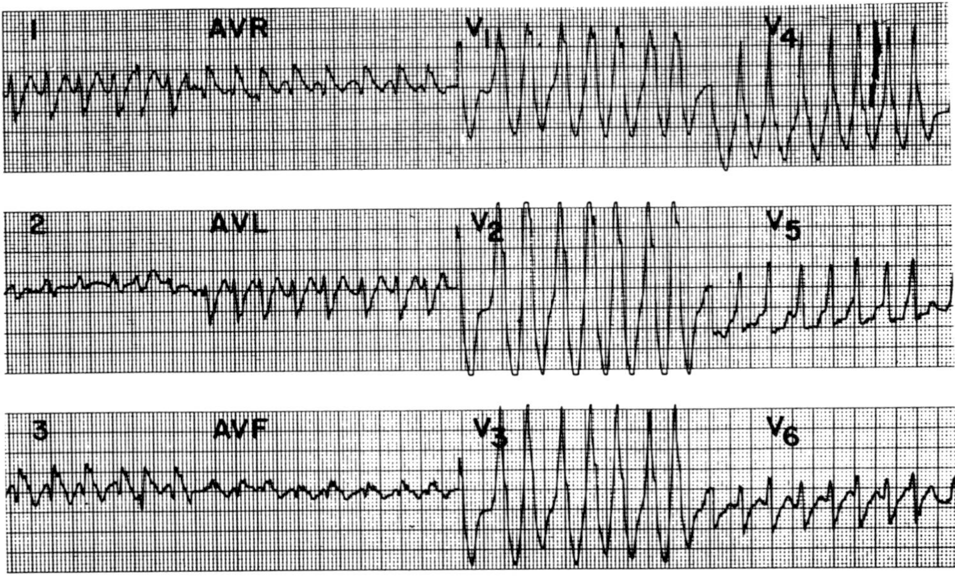

Fig. 11-42. Atrial fibrillation in Wolff-Parkinson-White syndrome.

venous procainamide and unstable patients should be cardioverted. β-adrenergic or calcium-channel blockers should be avoided.

3. Atrial flutter or fibrillation with a rapid ventricular response is best treated with cardioversion. As an alternative, agents which prolong the refractory period of the accessory tract—such as procainamide—can be used. Lidocaine may have some utility, and experimental studies with intravenous flecainide have shown promise. In general, phenytoin, esmolol, propranolol, or verapamil have a variable effect on accessory conduction and should not be used. Digoxin is contraindicated as it may shorten the refractory period and enhance conduction over the bypass tract.

DEFIBRILLATION AND SYNCHRONIZED CARDIOVERSION

Defibrillation and cardioversion is the technique of passing a short burst (about 5 ms) of direct electric current across the thorax to terminate tachyarrhythmias. The electric current simultaneously depolarizes all excitable cardiac tissue and terminates any areas of reentry by halting further propagation of the impulse around the reentry loop. This places all cardiac cells in the same depolarized state, and following repolarization a dominant pacemaker (usually the sinus node) paces the heart in a regular manner.

Defibrillation or cardioversion uses the same type of equipment. A device stores a known quantity of electrical energy in a storage capacitor and on command, discharges it through two paddles placed on the chest wall. Usually, a rhythm monitor and a synchronizer circuit are built into the device. Paddle placement can be either anterior-posterior or apex-right parasternal. While some authors found a lower energy requirement for conversion using anterior-posterior paddles, others have not. For emergency situations, paddle placement probably does not matter.

To reduce transthorax electrical impedance and increase the amount of current passing through the heart, certain techniques are important at the paddle-chest wall interface. Electrode paste, gel, or saline pads are applied to the surface of the paddles. Firm pressure of 10 to 12.5 kg/cm^2 (20 to 25 lb/in^2) is used to achieve good electrical contact. Larger paddles, within reason, have a reduced impedance, but this does not appear to significantly influence the energy required for conversion.

Older devices had significant internal energy losses and delivered as little as 40 percent of the stored energy to the patient. This is not a problem with modern defibrillators as they deliver very close to the stored amount.

Defibrillation should be done as soon as ventricular fibrillation is diagnosed. The longer ventricular fibrillation persists, the less likely resuscitation will be successful. Current ACLS guidelines recommend 200 J for the first attempt, 200 to 300 J for the second attempt, and 360 J for subsequent defibrillations. Several studies have found that most patients can be defibrillated with 160 to 200 J. Recommendations for children are 2 J/kg (1 J/lb) in the initial attempt and 4 J/kg on subsequent attempts.

Synchronized cardioversion applies the electric current at a time during the cardiac cycle well away from the vulnerable period when there is little chance of inducing ventricular fibrillation—usually about 10 ms after the peak of the R wave. On most machines, the synchronizer circuit must be turned on each time an impulse is desired. Many devices also display by the monitor screen or a flashing light that the synchronizer circuit is detecting properly the QRS complex. Cable leads, rather than the paddles, should be used to monitor the cardiac rhythm to avoid any movement artifact that could be misinterpreted by the synchronizer circuit as the QRS complex.

Complications include:

1. Direct myocardial damage: unusual unless there are repeated shocks at high energy (more than 325 J).
2. Ventricular fibrillation: incidence is less than 5 percent with a synchronized discharge but probably greater in the presence of digoxin or quinidine toxicity, hypokalemia, or acute myocardial infarction. However, patients on maintenance digoxin therapy can be safely cardioverted using low energies (less than 50 J).
3. Systemic emboli: about 1.2 to 1.5 percent in patients with chronic atrial fibrillation.
4. ST segment changes: transient elevations or depressions, usually resolving within 5 min.
5. Bradycardias: more common in patients with inferior myocardial infarctions and those requiring multiple defibrillations-cardioversions. Usually evident during the first 5 s after shock and may occasionally persist for longer than 20 s and require external or internal pacing.
6. Tachycardias: usually sinus tachycardia, occasionally atrial flutter or fibrillation, and usually resolving spontaneously within 5 min.
7. Atrial, junctional, or ventricular ectopy: usually transient and benign.
8. Pulmonary edema: uncommon but may occur in patients with mitral or aortic valvular disease or left ventricular failure.
9. Hypotension: rare, inexplicable, and may last for several hours before spontaneously resolving.
10. Muscle damage: elevated levels of creatine phosphokinase (CPK) and lactic dehydrogenase (LDH) are common but the myocardial fractions [CPK-MB, LDH1, LDH2, and α-hydroxybutyric dehydrogenase (HBD)] are rarely abnormal.

CARDIAC PACEMAKERS

Artifical cardiac pacemakers have two components: a power source (battery with pulse generator) and an electrode that delivers current to the heart (transvenous, epicardial, transthoracic, and transcutaneous). In permanent pacemaker placement, the power source is implanted subcutaneously, and the electrodes are run through the veins to inside the heart or through the subcutaneous tissue to the epicardial surface. In temporary pacemaker placement, the power source is external to the body and electrodes are placed in one of three ways: transvenous to an intracardiac location, transthoracic via a needle puncture through the skin into ventricular myocardium, or transcutaneous with electrodes placed on the thoracic skin.

The pulse generator can be designated to operate in either a fixed-rate mode (asynchronous or competitive) or a demand mode (synchronous or noncompetitive).

In the fixed-rate mode, the pulse generator produces an electrical signal at the preset rate regardless of the patient's own intrinsic cardiac rhythm. Serious arrhythmias or ventricular fibrillation may occur if the pacemaker discharges during the vulnerable period (T wave) and for this reason, fixed rate pacing is rarely done.

In the demand mode, the pulse generator has a sensing circuit which detects spontaneous cardiac activity and will discharge only if no cardiac depolarization is detected for a preset interval. Demand pacemakers may have two response modes, either inhibited or triggered. In the inhibited response mode (most commonly used), the pulse generator is inhibited by the sensed cardiac activity and does not generate an impulse. In the triggered response mode, the pacemaker detects the patient's intrinsic cardiac activity and then discharges during the absolute refractory period. On ECG, this appears as pacing spikes following each intrinsic QRS complex.

A five-letter code system is beginning to be used for pacemaker designation (see Table 11-5). The simplest type of pacemaker used—the ventricular demand inhibited response pacemaker—would be designated as VVI.

The modern permanent pacemaker is powered by a lithium battery which has an approximate lifetime of 8 to 12 years. Most units are preset for rates around 70 with a pacing interval of 0.84 s. The demand pacemaker has a built-in refractory period (0.2 to 0.4 s) during which

Table 11-5. Coding System for Permanent Pacemakers

First Letter Chamber Paced	Second Letter Chamber Sensed	Third Letter Mode or Response	Fourth Letter Programmable Functions	Fifth Letter Special Tachyarrhythmia Function
A = Atrium	A = Atrium	I = Inhibited	P = Programmable rate/output	B = Bursts
V = Ventricle	V = Ventricle	T = Triggered		N = Normal rate competition
D = Double (both)	D = Double (both)	D = Double	M = Multiprogrammable	
	O = None	R = Reverse	C = Communicating	S = Scanning
		O = None	O = None	E = External

it will not sense; this prevents it from being inhibited by its own stimulus. Most demand pacemakers have a magnetic switch which temporarily converts the pulse generator from the demand mode to the fixed-rate mode when a magnet is held over the unit. In this way the pacing rate can be quickly determined, but the magnet should be applied for only short periods to avoid initiating tachyarrhythmias. There are programmable pacemakers in which the rate and stimulus strength can be reset by noninvasive means. Since pacemaker complexity varies, the manufacturer supplies with each unit identification cards which patients should carry with them.

Temporary pacemakers are powered by 9-V radio-type batteries. On these pacemakers, there are settings for the mode (fixed or demand), rate (40 to 140), and stimulus strength (0.2 to 20 mA). During emergency pacing, initial settings should be in the demand mode with a rate around 70 and stimulus strength around 3.0 mA. The negative terminal should be connected to the distal electrode.

The transvenous intracardiac electrode may be either unipolar or bipolar. The unipolar setup has the negative electrode within the heart and the positive electrode in the chest wall. Permanent pacemakers using the unipolar setup have the positive electrode in their surface covering. Temporary pacemakers using the unipolar setup have their positive electrode connected to a needle implanted in the skin of the anterior thorax. With the bipolar setup, both electrodes are within a few millimeters of each other and both lie within the heart. Transvenous electrodes are placed most commonly into the apex of the right ventricle. Different catheters are used depending on the clinical situation. Right or semirigid catheters (No. 6 or No. 7 French) are inserted through a venous puncture or cutdown and usually require fluoroscopy for correct placement. Semifloating (No. 3 or No. 4 French) or flexible balloon-tipped catheters (No. 3 or No. 5 French) can be introduced and directed into the right ventricle without fluoroscopy using blood flow. Flexible catheters can become dislodged by patient or cardiac movement and usually are replaced with semirigid catheters within 24 h.

Transthoracic electrodes are inserted into the right ventricle through a left parasternal or subxiphoid intracardiac puncture. They are used in cardiac resuscitation when rapid placement is essential. The major disadvantage of transthoracic electrodes is that they can become dislodged with closed-chest compression. In addition, coronary artery laceration or pericardial tamponade is a hazard of percutaneous cardiac puncture. While electrical capture may be obtained in an occasional patient, it is rare to produce effective cardiac contractions with transthoracic pacing (Fig. 11-43).

Transcutaneous electrodes are self-adhesive pads which usually are placed with the negative electrode over the left anterior precordium and the positive electrode over the left infrascapular area. Transcutaneous pacing then is initiated by using the lowest current setting, which is increased until electrical capture is achieved. Most patients can be paced with 100 mA, but some may require up to 200 mA.

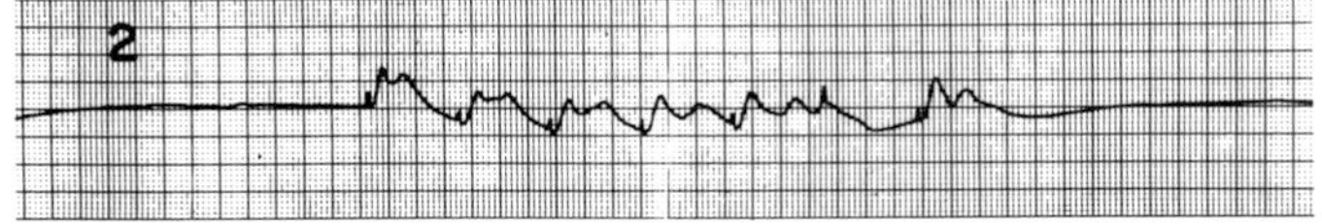

Fig. 11-43. Ventricular capture with transthoracic pacing.

Indications for Emergency Pacing

Emergency cardiac pacing is indicated either therapeutically (for symptomatic bradyarrhythmias) or prophylactically (for conduction defects which have a high risk of developing sudden complete heart block or asystole). (See Chapter 18.)

As noted before, symptomatic bradyarrhythmias should be treated with atropine and/or isoproterenol as a temporary measure to support cardiac rhythm prior to pacemaker placement. Some patients may respond adequately to atropine alone and do not require pacemaker insertion.

Most authors would recommend prophylactic placement of a pacemaker in any patient with acute myocardial infarction who has a new or age-indeterminant bi- or trifascicular block. In addition, second-degree Mobitz II and, of course, third-degree AV blocks are also indications for pacemaker insertion. Despite successful pacing, many patients with acute myocardial infarction and these serious conduction blocks have extensive left ventricular damage and a high mortality from pump failure.

Pacemaker Malfunction

Permanent pacemaker malfunction can be categorized as either (1) failure to sense, (2) failure to pace, (3) oversensing, or (4) combinations of the first three. With current lithium batteries and reliable circuitry, most pacemaker malfunctions are due to problems with the electrodes and not the result of battery exhaustion or pulse-generator failure.

Failure to sense may occur when the voltage of the patient's own intrinsic QRS complex is too low to be detected by the sensing circuit of the pacemaker. Changing from a bipolar to unipolar setup (if possible) may help the pacemaker sense the intrinsic cardiac activity. Failure to sense may cause the pacemaker to discharge during the T wave and trigger serious arrhythmias.

Failure to pace may occur when tissue reaction around the electrode makes the myocardium insensitive to the electric discharge generated by the pacemaker. It is common for the pacing threshold to increase during the first few weeks after insertion, but further rises are infrequent.

Failure to both sense and pace may be due to battery exhaustion, fracture of the wires in the catheter, or displacement of the electrodes. Battery exhaustion is indicated when the pacing rate slowly decreases. With lithium batteries, such decreases usually occur years before actual battery exhaustion. Greater than a 10 percent change from the initial rate is an urgent indication for replacement. Catheter wire fracture may cause either sustained or intermittent interruption in electrical conductivity. Sudden onset of symptoms and/or bradyarrhythmias suggests catheter fracture. Catheter fractures are rarely seen on routine chest radiographs. The transvenous electrode is usually positioned in the right ventricular apex, with a characteristic appearance on chest radiograph and ECG. Displacement can be suggested when changes on radiographs or ECG occur.

Oversensing is used to describe the situation where the pacemaker senses electrical activity not associated with atrial or ventricular depolarizations; it is thus inhibited, and pacemaker impulse generation is suppressed. Causes of oversensing include physiological electrical activity (T waves, muscle potentials), external electromagnetic interference, and signals generated by the interaction of different portions of the pacing system. Unipolar electrodes are more sensitive to physiological electrical activity and electromagnetic interference than bipolar electrodes.

Under certain conditions, pacemakers may initiate tachyarrhythmias despite functioning as designed; this usually results from an intrinsic depolarization occurring during the pacemaker refractory period, therefore not being sensed, and the pacemaker firing soon thereafter and initiating a reentrant tachycardia. In this setting, maintenance of the arrhythmia does not require further participation of the pacemaker. Dual-chamber pacemakers can also induce and sustain arrhythmias. In this situation, emergent treatment requires reprogramming the pacemaker, if possible, or converting to synchronous mode by placing a magnet over the pulse generator.

BIBLIOGRAPHY

Bar FW, Brugada P, Dassen WRM, et al: Differential diagnosis of tachycardia with narrow QRS complex (shorter than 0.12 second). *Am J Cardiol* 54:555, 1984.

DiMarco JP, Miles W, Akhtar M, et al: Adenosine for paroxysmal supraventricular tachycardia: Dose ranging and comparison with verapamil: Assessment in placebo-controlled, multicenter trials. *Ann Intern Med* 113:104, 1990.

Haft JI, Habbab MA: Treatment of atrial arrhythmias: Effectiveness of verapamil when preceded by calcium infusion. *Arch Intern Med* 146:1085, 1986.

Halperin BD, Kron K, Cutler JE, et al: Misdiagnosing ventricular tachycardia in patients with underlying conduction disease and similar sinus tachycardia morphologies. *West J Med* 152:677, 1990.

Haynes BE, Niemann JT, Haynes KS: Supraventricular tachyarrhythmias and rate-related hypotension: Cardiovascular effects and efficacy of intravenous verapamil. *Ann Emerg Med* 19:861, 1990.

Karlson BW, Herlitz J, Edvardsson N, et al: Prophylactic treatment after electroconversion of atrial fibrillation. *Clin Cardiol* 13:279, 1990.

Kastor JA: Multifocal atrial tachycardia. *N Engl J Med* 322:1713, 1990.

Ludmer PL, Goldschlager N: Cardiac pacing in the 1980s. *N Engl J Med* 311:1671, 1984.

Mehta D, Wafa S, Ward DE, et al: Relative efficacy of various physical maneuvers in the termination of junctional tachycardia. *Lancet* 1:1181, 1988.

Oronato JP, Hallagan LF, Reese WA, et al: Treatment of paroxysmal supraventricular tachycardia in the emergency department by clinical decision analysis. *Am J Emerg Med* 6:555, 1988.

Platia EV, Michelson EL, Porterfield JK, et al: Esmolol versus verapamil in the acute treatment of atrial fibrillation or atrial flutter. *Am J Cardiol* 63:925, 1989.

Rankin AC, Oldroyd KG, Chong E, et al: Value and limitations of adenosine in the diagnosis and treatment of narrow and broad complex tachycardias. *Br Heart J* 62:195, 1989.

Schweitzer P, Teichholz LE: Carotid sinus massage: Its diagnostic and therapeutic value in arrhythmias. *Am J Med* 78:645, 1985.

Steinman RT, Herrera C, Schuger CD, et al: Wide QRS tachycardia in the conscious adult: Ventricular tachycardia is the most frequent cause. *JAMA* 261:1013, 1989.

Stratmann HG, Kennedy HL: Torsades de pointes associated with drugs and toxins: Recognition and management. *Am Heart J* 113:1470, 1987.

Tzivoni D, Keren A: Suppression of ventricular arrhythmias by magnesium. *Am J Cardiol* 65:1397, 1990.

Viskin S, Belhassen B: Acute management of paroxysmal atrioventricular junctional reentrant supraventricular tachycardia: Pharmacologic strategies. *Am Heart J* 120:180, 1990.

Wellens HJJ, Brugada P: Mechanisms of supraventricular tachycardia. *Am J Cardiol* 62:10D, 1988.

Wellens HJJ, Frits WHMB, Lie KI: The value of the electrocardiogram in the differential diagnosis of a tachycardia with widened QRS complexes. *Am J Med* 64:27, 1978.

12 PHARMACOLOGY OF ANTIARRHYTHMIC AND VASOACTIVE MEDICATIONS

David B. Levy
Michael P. Peppers
Michael Ruffing

This chapter discusses the actions, pharmacokinetics, indications, dosing, and adverse effect profile of antiarrhythmic and vasoactive agents that are pertinent to emergency medicine practice. Specific antiarrhythmics include procainamide, quinidine, lidocaine, bretylium, and β blockers. In addition, calcium channel blockers, adenosine, and digoxin are discussed. Vasoactive medications include epinephrine, dopamine, norepinephrine, isoproterenol, dobutamine, amrinone, atropine, and nitroglycerin. Vasodilating agents such as phentolamine, hydralazine, and clonidine together with other drugs used in hypertension management are discussed in Chap. 23.

ANTIARRHYTHMIC AGENTS

Optimal therapy of arrhythmias requires knowledge of the mechanisms of action, pharmacokinetics, indications, appropriate dosing and administration, and types of adverse effects that may occur with each medication. Antiarrhythmic agents are divided into four classes based on their electrophysiological effects and properties. Class I agents are divided into three subgroups. (See Table 12-1.)

Class I Antiarrhythmic Agents

Procainamide

Actions

Procainamide shares the same basic mechanism of action as the other class IA antiarrhythmic agents in that it suppresses automaticity by decreasing the rate and amplitude of phase 4 diastolic depolarization, prolongs the action potential duration, and reduces the speed of impulse conduction. These effects directly depress myocardial conduction, suppress fibrillatory activity in the atria and ventricles, and prevent ectopic or reentrant arrhythmias.

Procainamide, like other class IA antiarrhythmic agents, possesses dose-dependent anticholinergic activity (less than disopyramide or quinidine) that may suppress automaticity in ectopic pacemakers. Large doses of procainamide provide extensive anticholinergic effects and may even increase automaticity.

Class IA antiarrhythmic agents may decrease the force of myocardial contraction by inhibiting calcium transport across the cell membrane. The negative inotropic effect is more pronounced in ischemic myocardial tissue. High doses of procainamide may cause hypotension from peripheral vasodilation.

Pharmacokinetics

The onset of action of procainamide is 5 to 10 min following intravenous (IV) administration and 15 to 60 min following intramuscular (IM) injection. Procainamide has an elimination half-life of 2.5 to 4.7 h (in normal renal function) and an apparent volume of distribution (Vd) of 2 L/kg. However, in patients with congestive heart failure (CHF) and renal dysfunction, the elimination half-life may increase and the Vd may decrease. Procainamide is metabolized to an active compound, *N*-acetyl procainamide (NAPA), in the liver via *N*-acetyltransferase. This active metabolite has an average half-life of 7 h in patients with normal renal function. Rapid acetylators convert greater amounts of procainamide to NAPA than do slow acetylators. Plasma procainamide levels of approximately 4 to 10 μg/mL are usually required to suppress ventricular arrhythmias. Refractory arrhythmias may require levels up to 20 μg/mL (usually 10–15 μg/mL). Adverse effects often appear with levels greater than 12 μg/mL.

Indications

Procainamide is generally used to treat and prevent recurrence of ventricular arrhythmias, specifically ventricular tachycardia and premature ventricular contractions (PVCs), which are resistant to lidocaine. It is infrequently used in ventricular fibrillation. Procainamide may also be used for slowing or converting supraventricular tachycardias (SVT) including atrial flutter and fibrillation [especially in Wolff-Parkinson-White (WPW) syndrome], paroxysmal supraventricular tachycardia (PSVT), paroxysmal atrial tachycardia, and paroxysmal AV junctional rhythm. Contraindications include complete AV heart block, second- or third-degree heart block (without an electrical pacemaker present), long QT intervals, and torsade de pointes. The drug should be used cautiously in patients with systemic lupus erythematosus (SLE), CHF, and hepatic or renal disease as well as those with allergies to procaine or amide-type drugs.

Dosing and Administration

The loading dose of procainamide for treating ventricular arrhythmias is 100 mg q 5 min at 20 mg/min until the arrhythmia is controlled, hypotension develops, the QRS complex widens greater than 50 percent, QT interval prolongation develops, or a total of 1 g has been given. Blood pressure and QRS complex must be monitored during IV administration. The rate of maintenance infusion is 1 to 4 mg/min. Lower doses may be necessary for patients with CHF or renal failure.

Adverse Effect Profile

The most serious adverse effects of procainamide are from myocardial depression. Electrocardiographic changes may include prolongation of the QRS and QT interval, impairment of AV conduction, ventricular fibrillation, torsade de pointes. High doses or rapid infusion can cause hypotension. Procainamide and NAPA levels should be monitored in the following patients: (1) those on procainamide longer than 24 h, (2) those on a maintenance infusion of 3 mg/min or higher, and (3) those with acute CHF or renal failure. SLE has been reported with chronic administration. Hypersensitivity reactions, characterized by angioedema, acute bronchoconstriction, vascular collapse, febrile episodes, and respiratory arrest, may occur. In addition, idiosyncratic reactions, including agranulocytosis, hepatitis, confusion, nausea, vomiting, urticaria, fever, maculopapular eruptions, and thrombocytopenia, can develop.

Quinidine (Gluconate or Sulfate)

Actions

Quinidine is a class IA antiarrhythmic agent with essentially the same mechanism of action as procainamide. However, anticholinergic effects are more pronounced with quinidine. These anticholinergic effects facilitate conduction across the AV node.

Pharmacokinetics

Onset of action following IV administration is within minutes, while the onset for the IM and oral routes usually occurs in 1 to 3 h. Therapeutic cardiovascular effects last for the half-life of the drug, 6 to 8 h. The oral sustained-release (SR) gluconate preparation, however, can last up to 12 h. Therapeutic serum levels range between 2 and 7 μg/mL. Quinidine has an average Vd of 2 L/kg in healthy adults. It is metabolized in the liver to two active metabolites. Approximately 10 to 20 percent of a dose is excreted as unchanged drug in the urine within 24 h.

Table 12-1. Electrophysiologic Actions of Antiarrhythmic Agents

Class, Sub-class		Generic Name	Trade Name	Electrophysiologic Actions
IA Fast channel blockers		quinidine disopyramide procainamide	— Norpace Pronestyl	↓ ↓ conduction velocity ↑ action potential duration 0/↓ automaticity (↓ ↓ automaticity in higher doses) ↑ ↑ effective refractory period 0/↑ PR, QRS, and QT intervals (drug- and dose-related)
	IB	lidocaine phenytoin mexiletine tocainide aprindine	Xylocaine Dilantin Mexitil Tonocard (investigat)	↓ ↓ phase 0 of action potential ↓ automaticity ↓ ↓ effective refractory period (in ischemic tissue) ↑ fibrillatory threshold ↓ repolarization period 0/↓ PR and QT intervals 0/↑ in AV nodal conduction
	IC	encainide flecainide propafenone indecainide moricizine	Enkaid Tambocor Rythmol Decabid Ethmozine	↓ ↓ phase 0 of action potential ↓ automaticity ↓ ↓ conduction velocity ↑ action potential duration ↑ effective refractory period ↑ PR and QRS intervals (drug and dose-related) 0/↑ QT intervals
II β Blockers		propranolol (also see Table 12–2)	Inderal	↓ conduction velocity ↑ automaticity ↑ effective refractory period ↓ ↓ AV nodal conduction 0/↑ PR interval 0/↓ QT interval
III		bretylium	Bretylol	↑ ↑ effective refractory period 0/↑ in automaticity 0/↑ in AV conduction
		amiodarone	Cordarone	↑ fibrillatory threshold ↑ action potential duration
		sotalol	Betapace	0/↑ PR, QRS, and QT intervals (amiodarone
IV Calcium channel blockers		verapamil diltiazem (also see Table 12-3)	Isoptin Calan Cardizem	0/↓ automaticity ↓/↓ ↓ AV nodal conduction ↑ AV node effective refractory period ↑ PR interval
Unclassified		digoxin adenosine (see text)	Lanoxin Adenocard	0/↓ automaticity; ↑ automaticity in high levels ↓ AV nodal conduction ↑ AV nodal refractory period ↓ refractory period in ventricle ↑ PR interval ↓ QT interval

Indications

Quinidine is effective in the treatment of atrial and ventricular arrhythmias and thus has the same indications as procainamide. Parenteral use of quinidine, however, is considerably more dangerous.

Dosing and Administration

The oral route is preferred when administering quinidine. Oral quinidine is available in three salts: sulfate (83% active drug), gluconate (62% active drug), and polygalacturonate (60% active drug). Only the gluconate and sulfate salts are available for parenteral use. IM administration is effective in acute, but not in critical, arrhythmias. IV administration should be reserved for acute symptomatic ventricular tachycardia. The dose for quinidine varies, depending on the indication and salt used. For example, the adult dose for suppressing atrial, AV junctional, and ventricular complexes is 324 to 660 mg of extended-release quinidine gluconate q 8 to 12 h, while the dose for quinidine sulfate to maintain sinus rhythm after conversion is 200 to 400 mg three or four times daily. The initial IM dose is 600 mg of quinidine gluconate, then 400 mg as often as q 2 h until desired effects are seen. Generally, the IV dosage required to abolish ventricular arrhythmias is 300 mg or less; however, 500 to 750 mg may be needed. The rate of infusion should not exceed 16 mg/min, and the ECG and blood pressure should be continuously monitored to gauge the efficacy and safety of treatment.

Adverse Effect Profile

The adverse effect profile of quinidine is similar to that of procainamide and includes torsade de pointes, SLE, and hypersensitivity reactions. High serum levels of quinidine may result in cinchonism. Symptoms of cinchonism include tinnitus, blurred vision, headache, nausea, and deafness. Severe cases may lead to delirium and psychosis.

Lidocaine

Actions

Lidocaine, a class IB antiarrhythmic agent, controls ventricular arrhythmias predominantly by blocking fast sodium channels. Lidocaine decreases the slope of phase 4 depolarization and suppresses automaticity in the His-Purkinje system. The action potential duration and effective refractory period (ERP) of Purkinje fibers and ventricular muscles are also decreased, while the ratio of ERP to action potential duration is increased. Lidocaine appears to act preferentially on ischemic myocardial tissue, causing little or no effect on AV nodal or His-Purkinje conduction velocity in normal heart tissue. Lidocaine has local anesthetic effects that stabilize membranes, elevate the ventricular fibrillation threshold, and suppress ventricular ectopy in tissues during acute myocardial ischemia. It has a negligible effect on the autonomic nervous system, myocardial contractility, and peripheral vascular tone.

Pharmacokinetics

The onset of action is 30 to 90 s following IV administration and 10 min following an IM dose. Subsequent bolus doses are generally required to attain therapeutic plasma levels early in treatment; maintenance infusions started without an initial bolus dose are unlikely to attain therapeutic levels for up to 30 to 60 min. Lidocaine has an approximate Vd of 1.3 L/kg in normal patients and 0.9 L/kg in those with liver disease or CHF. The drug is primarily metabolized in the liver, with less than 10 percent excreted unchanged in the urine. The major metabolites, monoethylglycinexylidide (MEGX) and glycinexylidide (GX), possess antiarrhythmic and neurotoxic actions and are excreted renally.

Lidocaine has a short distribution half-life of 7 to 8 min following an IV bolus and 12 to 28 min following IM administration. This short distribution half-life accounts for the short duration of action after a bolus injection. The elimination half-life in healthy patients ranges from 80 to 108 min but may increase up to 7 h in patients with CHF or liver disease and is also greatly prolonged in cardiac arrest. Therapeutic serum levels range from 1.5 to 6 μg/mL; serum levels greater than 5 μg/mL may cause CNS toxicity.

Indications

Lidocaine is the drug of choice for the suppression of and prophylaxis against ventricular arrhythmias and ventricular ectopy in the setting of acute myocardial ischemia. The drug is also indicated for ventricular tachycardia and ventricular fibrillation refractory to defibrillation. Lidocaine should be given prophylactically following successful conversion of ventricular tachyarrhythmias to normal sinus rhythm. Lidocaine can also be an adjunct to procainamide for the treatment of supraventricular arrhythmias in WPW syndrome.

Dosing and Administration

Lidocaine is given as an initial bolus dose of 1 mg/kg followed by additional bolus doses of 0.5 mg/kg q 5 to 10 min as needed up to a cumulative dose of 3 mg/kg. An alternative method is to give 1.5 mg/kg initially, followed by 50-mg bolus doses q 5 min up to a total dose of 225 mg or 3 mg/kg. Conscious patients should receive lidocaine at a rate not exceeding 50 mg/min to minimize adverse CNS effects. However, in pulseless ventricular tachycardia or ventricular fibrillation, lidocaine can be given by rapid IV push. IM injections are now facilitated by the availability of auto-injector devices that inject 300 mg of the 10% solution into the deltoid or the vastus lateralis muscles. An additional intramuscular dose can be given in 60 min if an IV line cannot be established. When IV lines are not available, the drug may be instilled endotracheally (ET); in doses less than 100 mg, however, the volume should be diluted with saline to at least 5 mL.

Ventricular fibrillation and pulseless ventricular tachycardia should be managed with bolus doses. Following a bolus dose, maintenance infusions should be started at 2 mg/min and titrated up to 4 mg/min as needed (30–50 μg/kg per min).

Patients greater than 70 years of age with CHF, liver disease, or impaired hepatic blood flow should have the loading dose and maintenance infusion rate lowered by 50 percent. Drug interactions that can prolong the half-life of lidocaine or increase toxicity include those that potentiate neurologic effects (e.g., procainamide and tubocurarine), drugs that also undergo metabolism in the liver and increase lidocaine levels (e.g., cimetidine and propranolol), and drugs that can produce excessive cardiac depression (e.g., phenytoin). Since the half-life of lidocaine can be increased after 24 to 48 h in any of the above, serum levels should be obtained and infusions adjusted accordingly if therapy is used for longer than 24 h. Lidocaine toxicity may also develop in patients with renal dysfunction due to accumulation of metabolites.

Adverse Effect Profile

Adverse effects from lidocaine usually occur when the drug is administered too rapidly in a conscious patient, when excessive doses are administered, or when a drug interaction potentiates toxicity. Symptoms of mild lidocaine toxicity that correlate with levels greater than 5 μg/mL include drowsiness, confusion, nausea, vertigo, ataxia, tinnitus, paresthesias, and muscle twitching. Serious symptoms occurring at plasma levels greater than 9 μg/mL may include psychosis, seizures, and respiratory depression. Lidocaine is contraindicated in patients with known sensitivities to amide-type local anesthetics and those with high-degree sinoatrial (SA) or AV block.

Class II Antiarrhythmics: β Blockers

General Information

Actions

Numerous β blockers have been introduced in the United States during the past several years. While these agents share the principal characteristic of blocking catecholamine effects on β receptors, they vary in other important properties, such as cardioselectivity, intrinsic sympathomimetic activity, α-adrenergic blocking activity, and pharmacokinetic properties (relative potency, route of elimination, distribution in fat and brain, and duration of action). See "Propranolol" for a basic discussion on the nonspecific β blocker (Table 12-2).

Cardioselective β blocking (specific for the β_1 receptor) drugs include acebutolol, atenolol, esmolol, and metoprolol. They may be better choices for use in patients with a history of asthma, congestive obstructive pulmonary disease (COPD), or diabetes, since the blockade of β_2 receptors may result in adverse outcomes. The hemodynamic effects of cardioselective β blockers are similar to those of propranolol, excluding the increase in vascular resistance. At high doses, some agents lose their cardioselectivity; the exact dose at which this occurs, however, has not been clearly established.

β blockers with intrinsic sympathomimetic activity, such as acebutolol or pindolol, occupy the β receptor and produce a low level of stimulation. Despite this stimulation, the receptor is functionally blocked to high sympathetic tone. Theoretically, these drugs would be safer to use in patients with low cardiac output states because of their intrinsic ability to stimulate the heart. This ability may prevent acute drug-induced heart failure, but this has not been demonstrated in clinical trials.

For information about β blockers with α blocking actions, see "Labetalol."

Pharmacokinetics

Refer to Table 12-3 for pharmacokinetic parameters of each of the β blockers.

Indications

Indications for each of the β blocking agents are similar to those for propranolol. The longer-acting agents are effective for the chronic treatment of hypertension. Cardioselective β blockers are used in patients with asthma or insulin-dependent diabetes, while drugs with intrinsic sympathomimetic activity may be better tolerated in some patients with underlying myodepression.

Table 12-2. Comparison Chart for β Blockers

Generic Name	Trade Name	Dosage Form	Receptor Selectivity	Elimination Half-life	Initial Dose	Maximum Dose	Approved Indications
acebutolol	Sectral	Oral	β_1	3–4 h (8–13 h for diacetolol)	400 mg/day	1.2 g/day	Hypertension, arrhythmias
atenolol	Tenormin	Injection	β_1	6–9 h	5 mg	10 mg	Acute myocardial infarction
		Oral		6–9 h	50 mg/day	200 mg/day	Hypertension
betaxolol	Kerlone	Oral	β_1	14–22 h	10–20 mg/day	20 mg/day	Hypertension
carteolol	Cartrol	Oral	β_1 β_2	6 h	2.5 mg/day	10 mg/day	Hypertension
esmolol	Brevibloc	Injection	β_1	9 min	25–50 μg/kg/min	300 μg/kg/min	Supraventricular tachycardia
labetalol	Normodyne Trandate	Injection	α_1 and β_1 β_2	5.5 h	20 mg IV push initially, then double the dose q 10 min	300 mg	Hypertension
		Oral	same	6–8 h	200 mg/day	2.4 g/day	Hypertension
metoprolol	Lopressor	Injection	β_1	3–7 h	5 mg IV push	15 mg	Acute myocardial infarction
		Oral		3–7 h	100 mg/day	450 mg/day	Hypertension, acute myocardial infarction
nadolol	Corgard	Oral	β_1 β_2	17–24 h	40 mg/day	320 mg/day	Hypertension, angina pectoris
oxprenolol	Trasicor	Oral	β_1 β_2	1–2 h	160 mg/day	320 mg/day	Hypertension, angina
penbutolol	Levatol	Oral	β_1 β_2	17–26 h	20 mg/day	80 mg/day	Hypertension
pindolol	Visken	Oral	β_1 β_2	3–4 h	20 mg/day	60 mg/day	Hypertension
propranolol	Inderal	Injection	β_1 β_2	3–6 h	1 mg IV	3 mg	Hypertension, arrhythmias, angina, post-myocardial infarction prophylaxis
		Oral		3–6 h	40–80 mg/day	480 mg/day	
sotalol	Betapace	Oral	β_1	7–15 h	80 mg/day	640 mg/day	Antiarrhythmic*
timolol	Blocadren	Oral	β_1 β_2	4–5 h	20 mg/day	60 mg/day	Hypertension, post-myocardial infarction prophylaxis

* Pending U.S. Food and Drug Administration approval.

Dosing and Administration

The dosing regimens for each β blocker vary according to its potency and pharmacologic half-life. Refer to Table 12-2 for initial and maximum daily dose information.

Adverse Effect Profile

Adverse effects include nausea, vomiting, lightheadedness, mental depression, bradycardia, hypotension, bronchospasm, hyperglycemia, and pulmonary edema. Cardioselective agents cause less bronchospasm and hyperglycemia than do nonselective agents. β blockers that are less lipophyllic have fewer CNS effects. These drugs are contraindicated in patients with second- or third-degree heart block, CHF, or cardiogenic shock.

Propranolol

Actions

In therapeutic doses, the major effect of propranolol is its β-adrenergic blocking activity. The drug blocks the effects of catecholamines on β receptors, inhibiting chronotropic, inotropic, and vasodilator responses to β-adrenergic stimulation. Propranolol slows the sinus rate, depresses AV conduction, decreases cardiac output, reduces blood pressure on exercise, and reduces both supine and standing blood pressures. In addition, propranolol decreases renin release and myocardial oxygen demand and protects against sudden cardiac death.

Pharmacokinetics

The onset of action of propranolol following IV administration is 1 min, with a half-life of elimination that varies with duration of therapy. In short-term treatment, the elimination half-life is 2 to 3 h, but in chronic treatment, the elimination half-life is 4 h. Propranolol is widely distributed throughout the body, undergoes extensive first-pass metabolism by the liver, and is also significantly bound to sites within the liver. For these reasons, propranolol has a low bioavailability when taken orally as compared to IV administration, making the IV dose approximately 10 times smaller than the oral dose. Several metabolites have been discovered, and they are primarily excreted in the urine and feces. In significant renal impairment, the proportion of metabolites excreted by the feces will increase. No dosage adjustments are required in these patients.

Indications

Propranolol is indicated for a wide variety of supraventricular arrhythmias. These include paroxysmal atrial tachycardia, particularly those induced by digoxin or catecholamines or associated with the

WPW syndrome; refractory sinus tachycardia; atrial flutter or fibrillation refractory to digoxin; persistent atrial extrasystoles that do not respond to conventional therapy; and tachyarrhythmias associated with thyrotoxicosis. Propranolol is less effective for ventricular than for supraventricular arrhythmias, but it can be used for ventricular tachycardia or ectopic beats due to digoxin or catecholamine toxicity.

Other indications for propranolol include the management of angina, and acute myocardial ischemia or infarction because it decreases myocardial oxygen demands; management of all chronic types of hypertension, either alone or in combination with other antihypertensive agents (propranolol is not indicated for hyptertensive emergencies); for the treatment of idiopathic hypertrophic subaortic stenosis; in prophylaxis for common migraine headaches; management of familial or hereditary essential tremor; and with α-adrenergic blockers for pheochromocytoma.

Dosing and Administration

For life-threatening arrhythmias, the IV dose of propranolol is 0.5 to 1 mg given as an IV bolus at a rate not exceeding 1 mg/min. The dose may be repeated in 2 to 5 min. Since significant myocardial depression can occur when doses greater than 3 mg are given, extreme caution should be used if additional doses are necessary.

Adverse Effect Profile

The adverse effect profile for propranolol is similar to that for other nonselective β blockers. The drug is generally not given to patients with asthma or allergic rhinitis and is contraindicated in those with sinus bradycardia or advanced SA or AV block. Propranolol should also not be used in CHF or cardiogenic shock, unless these conditions are due to tachyarrhythmias.

Esmolol

Actions

Esmolol possesses cardioselective β-adrenergic blocking properties, selectively blocking the β_1 receptor. As with other β blockers, this drug exhibits both negative inotropic and negative chronotropic effects. Esmolol prevents excessive adrenergic stimulation on the myocardium by blocking the β_1 receptors, thus producing an increase in sinus cycle length, prolongation of SA nodal recovery time, and a decrease in conduction through the AV node. Esmolol is effective for treating SVT and these also possesses antihypertensive effects. These may be due to its ability to decrease cardiac output, sympathetic outflow, and renin release from the kidneys, or perhaps from the direct vasodilatory action of the drug.

Pharmacokinetics

Within 1 to 4 min of IV loading with esmolol, both the heart rate and blood pressure decline, and the PR interval becomes prolonged on the ECG. Of all the available β blocking agents, esmolol has the shortest duration of action. The elimination half-life is approximately 9 min, and effects of the drug completely reverse within 30 min after cessation of IV therapy. This feature makes IV esmolol a promising agent for the treatment of acute and unstable SVT, since the adverse or toxic effects disappear quickly upon discontinuation of the drug. The short duration of action also allows the drug to be titrated to effect. Although 90 percent of an administered dose is excreted renally as metabolites, the metabolites possess minimal, if any, β blocking effects. Dosing adjustments are thus not required in hepatic or renal insufficiency.

Indications

Esmolol is currently indicated to control ventricular rate for the short-term when the termination of supraventricular tachyarrhythmias (SVT) is desired. It is effective to prevent or treat SVT resulting from increased sympathetic tone during or following surgical procedures. IV esmolol may also be used during surgery as replacement β blocker therapy to prevent rebound hypertension in patients who have been receiving long-term β blocker treatment. Esmolol is not indicated for long-term management of SVT.

Dosing and Administration

A loading dose of esmolol is given as an IV bolus of 500 μg/kg over 1 min, followed by IV infusion starting at 50 μg/kg per min infused over 4 min. Assess for therapeutic and adverse effects immediately following the infusion. If there is no response, give another loading dose over 1 min, and increase the infusion rate to 100 μg/kg per min for 4 min. If there is still no response, repeat this procedure, using the same bolus dose each time and increasing the infusion rate by 50-μg/kg per min increments until the rate of infusion reaches 200 μg/kg per min, the desired response is achieved, or adverse effects appear. The majority of patients will respond within this dose range. A dose-dependent action is noticed, however, and doses above 200 μg/kg per min are usually of no greater benefit. Once adequate therapeutic response is obtained, it is advisable to change infusion rates by no more than 25 μg/kg per min and not use a bolus dose. Also, avoid concentrations greater than 10 μg/mL.

Adverse Effect Profile

Esmolol shares the same toxic potential and adverse effect profile as the other β blocking agents. The most common adverse effect associated with esmolol use is hypotension, which occurs in approximately 20 to 50 percent of patients being treated for SVT. This usually occurs within 30 min of therapy initiation. Other common adverse effects include dizziness, somnolence, and nausea.

Labetolol

Actions

Labetalol possesses membrane-stabilizing effects and thus has some antiarrhythmic action; however, the drug is often used as an antihypertensive agent because it blocks both α- and β-adrenergic receptors. The β-adrenergic blocking effects are nonselective, while the α blocking effects are selective for the α_1 receptor. It appears that the β blocking effects of labetalol are much greater than its α blocking effects at a ratio between 3:1 for oral and 7:1 for IV. Additionally, studies have found labetalol to possess some ability to stimulate rather than block the β_2 receptors.

The mechanism by which labetalol elicits its antihypertensive effects may include any or all of the following: (1) synergistic effects resulting in hypotension when both α_1 and β_1 receptors are blocked; (2) β_2 receptor stimulation; and (3) direct vasodilatory action. Labetalol decreases heart rate, contractility, cardiac output, cardiac work, and total peripheral resistance.

Pharmacokinetics

Labetalol is primarily eliminated by the liver and undergoes extensive first-pass metabolism with approximately 30 percent of the drug reaching the circulation following oral administration. Geriatric patients and those with liver disease, however, may have greater bioavailability. The onset of action of IV labetalol is within 2 to 5 min, peaks in 10 to 15 min, and lasts 2 to 4 h. Oral labetalol acts within 20 min to 2 h, peaks within 1 to 4 h, and lasts 8 to 24 h. The elimination half-life is approximately 3 to 8 h in normal individuals. Only 5 percent of the drug is excreted as unchanged drug.

Indications

Labetalol is used in emergency medicine primarily for its antihypertensive actions. Intravenous labetalol rapidly and effectively reduces elevated pressures, causing only minimal alterations in heart rate and cardiac output. It is a good alternative for treating the hypertensive patient with myocardial ischemia. Oral labetalol may be substituted

Table 12-3. Cardiac Medications

Generic Name (Trade Name)	Main Uses	Therapeutic Effects	Routes of Administration	Usual Dosages	Side Effects	Contraindications	How Supplied	Comments
atropine	Hemodynamically unstable bradyarrhythmias (second- or third-degree heart blocks, bradycardias associated with hypotension or poor tissue perfusion); asystole; acute cholinergic poisoning (organophosphates, mushrooms)	Competes with acetylcholine at receptor sites at the synapse, blocking the parasympathetic (vagal) response on the heart; conduction is enhanced, and heart rate increases, improving cardiac output; decreases secretions (eyes, mouth, GI tract)	IV or ET rapid push (no dilution necessary for ET administration)	Bradycardia: 0.5 mg q 5 min up to 2.0 mg Asystole: 1.0 mg, repeat in 5 min up to 2.0 mg Cholinergic toxicity: 1.0–2.0 mg IV (additional doses of 2.0 mg can be given as needed to reverse toxic effects)	Tachycardia, palpitations, bradycardia (paradoxical reaction following low dose of atropine), seizures, hypertension, respiratory failure, anticholinergic symptoms, including blurred vision, dilated pupils, headache, flushing, dizziness, drowsiness, fever, confusion, delirium, hot, dry, flushed skin, decreased GI motility	None when used in emergency situations; *use caution* with tachycardia, myocardial infarction when a known sensitivity to anticholinergic drugs exists (narrow-angle glaucoma, GI obstructive disease, myasthenia gravis), and if an unstable cardiovascular condition exists during an acute hemorrhage	Preload syringes: 0.1 mg/mL, 5 and 10 mL 1 mg/mL, 10 mL 0.5 mg/mL, 5 mL Vials and ampoules: 0.4 mg/mL, 1 mL 0.4 mg/mL, 20 mL 0.5 mg/mL, 1 and 30 mL 0.8 mg/mL, 1 mL 1 mg/mL, 1 mL 1.2 mg/mL, 1 mL	If dose < 0.4 mg given or drug not administered rapid IV push, a paradoxical bradycardia may occur
bretylium (Bretylol)	Ventricular fibrillation or ventricular tachycardia that fail to respond to lidocaine and defibrillation treatments	Raises the fibrillation threshold and initially causes rapid depletion or release of norepinephrine; an adrenergic blockade occurs following this catecholamine release (this can result in a decrease in both heart rate and arterial blood pressure, but cardiac output and left ventricular filling pressure do not change)	IV bolus or IV infusion: 1 g/250 mL or 2 g/500 mL in D_5W (4 mg/mL); IM alternative route (maximum 5 mL per site, IM only when IV not possible)	Ventricular fibrillation: 5 mg/kg IV push rapid, undiluted; if fibrillation persists, second bolus of 5–10 mg/kg IV or 1–2 mg/min IV infusion Ventricular tachycardia: same as ventricular fibrillation but initial dose to be diluted and infused over 8–10 min	Hypotension and postural hypotension most frequent; bradycardia, PVCs, initial, hypertension, nausea and projectile vomiting after a rapid IV bolus in the conscious patient; vertigo, dizziness, lightheadedness, and syncope are symptoms of postural hypotension	No contraindications when used to treat ventricular fibrillation or life-threatening refractory ventricular arrhythmias; may aggravate digitalis toxicity	Vials and preload syringes: 50 mg/mL, 10 mL	Consider as initial drug for cocaine-induced ventricular fibrillation; keep conscious patients supine and monitor vital signs closely; smaller doses should be given in patients being treated with catecholamine sympathomimetics; also successful in reversing ventricular arrhythmias in hypothermic patients
calcium chloride, gluconate gluceptate	Acute hypocalcemic tetany from various etiologies; acute hyperkalemia; acute magnesium toxicity; acute symptoms of lead colic; to neutralize chemical burns; as an adjunct in therapy for insect and other venomous bites or stings (Portuguese man-o'-war, black widow spider, etc.); antidote for calcium channel blocker overdose; following multiple blood transfusions over a short period of time	Essential for normal function of the nervous and muscular systems in the body; functions as an important activator in many enzymatic reactions and is required for transmission of nerve impulses; contraction of cardiac, smooth, and skeletal muscles; renal function; blood coagulation; respirations; and many endocrine secretory effects	IV only for chloride and gluconate salts; IV or IM for gluceptate salt (IM only when IV not possible) SC injection used rarely for local infiltration for various stings, bites, or chemical burns (e.g., hydrofluoric acid)	Chloride: 250 mg–1 g slow IV push (2.5–10 mL) Gluconate: 250 mg–2 g IV push, IV infusion, or SC (2.5–10 mL) Gluceptate: 0.44–1.1 g IM (2–5 mL), 1.1–4.4 G (5–20 mL) IV or SC	Rapid IV administration: metallic or chalky taste, tingling or burning sensation, sense of "heat waves," peripheral vasodilation, hypotension, syncope, bradycardia, and cardiac arrest (effects are most prominent when using chloride salt). IM injection: mild-to-severe local reactions (never use chloride salt IM) such as burning, cellulitis, and necrosis	In ventricular fibrillation and in patients with the risk of existing digitalis toxicity (excluding ventricular fibrillation induced by hypocalcemia)	Chloride: 1 g/10 mL = 272 mg calcium (1.36 mEq calcium/mL) available in 10-mL ampoules, vials, and syringes Gluconate: 1 g/10 mL - 90 mg calcium (0.45 mEq calcium/mL) available in 10 and 20 mL Gluceptate: 1.1 g/5 mL = 90 mg calcium, 2–5 mL IM (0.44–1 g), 5–20 mL IV (1.1–4.4 g), available in 5 and 50 mL vials	IV incompatibility with sodium bicarbonate; flush line thoroughly before and after a dose is given

Various types of shock								
dopamine (Intropin)	Various types of shock, including cardiogenic, septic, anaphylactic, metabolic, and hypovolemic (after fluid resuscitation has failed to raise blood pressure)	Dopaminergic receptor: renal and mesenteric vasodilation improves blood flow to the kidney to increase urine output β_1 receptor; increases cardiac output and blood pressure via a direct inotropic effect on myocardium α receptor: peripheral vasoconstriction shifts blood to systemic circulation, thereby increasing blood pressure and organ perfusion	IV infusion: 800 mg/250 mL in D_5W or NS (3200 μg/mL) 800 mg/500 mL (1600 μg/mL) 400 mg/500 mL (800 μg/mL) 200 mg/500 mL (400 μg/mL)	Dopaminergic receptor: 1–5 μg/kg/min β_1 receptor: 2–10 μg/kg/min α receptor: $\geq$10 μg/kg/min	Low-dose effects: hypotension, tachycardia Moderate-dose effects: tachycardia, risk of angina, ectopic beats, ventricular arrhythmias and ectopy, dyspnea, nausea, vomiting, headache, palpitations High-dose effects: same as moderate plus decreased kidney function and hypertension	Hypovolemic patients prior to IV fluid resuscitation, patients with pheochromocytoma	Premade IV bags: 0.8 mg/mL, 100, 250, and 500-mL 1.6 mg/mL, 100, 250, and 500-mL 3.2 mg/mL, 100, 250, and 500-mL Ampoules, vials, and preload syringes: 40 mg/mL, 5 mL (200 mg) 80 mg/mL, 5 mL (400 mg) 160 mg/mL, 5 mL (800 mg)	Risk of extravasation if IV infiltrates; alkaline solutions will inactivate dopamine; flush IV line before and after if giving sodium bicarbonate; IV infusion should be titrated to desired effect and gradually tapered down when stopping infusion; monitor blood pressure, and ECG, and drip rate closely
epinephrine	Cardiac arrest with the following conditions: ventricular fibrillation, ventricular tachycardia with no pulse, electromechanical dissociation, asystole, idioventricular rhythm, or to maintain heart rate and/or arterial blood pressure	Increased contractile force of heart, SA, AV, and ventricular conduction, and heart rate (β_1 receptor agonist effects; increased systemic vascular resistance, perfusion pressure from external chest compress (α receptor agonist effects)	IV push or ET tube (no dilution necessary when 1:10,000 used) IV infusion: 1 mg in 250 mL in D_5W (4 μg/mL)	0.5–1 mg q 5 min during cardiac arrest resuscitation 1–4 μg/min to titrate good blood pressure	CNS stimulation, vomiting, nausea, headache, dizziness, tachycardia, palpitations, headache, hypertension, fatigue, muscle tremor, ventricular irritability, tachycardia, PVCs, PACs, stroke, acute MI	None when used in cardiac arrest; use caution in pregnant patients, in those with narrow-angle (congestive) glaucoma, and when used in conjunction with local anesthetics, since excessive vasoconstriction can cause sloughing of tissues	Preload syringes: 1:10,000, 0.1 mg/mL, 10 mL Ampoules, vials, and Tubex syringes: 1:1000, 1 mg/mL, 1 mL (not for bolus use)	Should be protected from light; can be deactivated if mixed with alkaline solutions; effects can be transient; monitor vital signs and ECG closely
isoproterenol (Isuprel)	Temporary adjunct therapy in hemodynamically unstable bradyarrhythmia (second- or third-degree heart blocks, bradycardias associated with hypotension or poor tissue perfusion) refractory to a vagolytic dose (2 mg) of atropine	Increased contractile force of heart, SA, AV, and ventricular conduction, and heart rate (β_1 receptor agonist effects); lower blood pressure and vasodilation due to lowered peripheral vascular resistance, bronchodilation (β_2 receptor agonist effects)	IV infusion only: 1 mg/250 mL in D_5W (4 μg/mL)	Maintenance: 2–10 μg/min titrating to desired heart rate (usually 60 beats/min) or until PVCs appear	Hypotension, palpitations, headache, dyspnea, angina, ventricular irritability, tachycardia, PVCs, PACs, ventricular fibrillation (most of these are from an increase in myocardial O_2 requirement)	Presence of tachyarrhythmias; should not be used to raise blood pressure in cardiogenic shock	Preload syringes, vials, and ampoules: 1:5000, 0.2 mg/mL, 5 and 10 mL	No longer recommended for asystole because of the vasodilation effect

Table 12-3. Cardiac Medications (*Continued*)

Generic Name (Trade Name)	Main Uses	Therapeutic Effects	Routes of Administration	Usual Dosages	Side Effects	Contraindications	How Supplied	Comments
lidocaine (Xylocaine)	Prophylactic use during myocardial infarction, to suppress multifocal PVCs, ventricular tachycardia, or ventricular fibrillation	Causes a membrane-stabilizing effect and raises fibrillatory threshold; also may decrease the velocity of an electrical impulse through the conduction system; has little to no effect on the autonomic nervous system	IV push, IM, or ET (ET dose <100 mg must be diluted to at least 5 mL) IV infusion: 1 g/250 mL or 2 g/500 mL in D_5W or NS (4 mg/mL)	Load: 1 mg/kg (≤50 mg/min for conscious patients), repeat load at 8–10-min intervals as needed, 0.5 mg/kg Maintenance: 1–4 mg/min, titrate to effect; for acute CHF or liver failure patients, reduce loading dose by 50 percent and start maintenance infusion at 1 mg/min	Rapid IV push in the conscious patient: euphoria; dizziness; ataxia; confusion; drowsiness; blurred or double vision; tinnitus; sensations of cold, heat, or numbness in peripheral extremities; shortness of breath; nausea or vomiting; slurred speech; and dyspnea. Other effects: muscle tremors, seizures, respiratory depression or arrest, widening of the QRS complex, bradycardia that can lead to cardiac arrest, or coma	Hypersensitivity to amide local anesthetics; WPW syndrome; Stokes-Adams syndrome; severe degrees of SA, AV, or intraventricular heart block in the absence of a cardiac pacemaker; idioventricular or escape rhythms	IM use, automatic injection: 300 mg/3 mL LidoPen Auto-Injector IM use, ampoules: 10% 100 mg/mL, 5 mL IV push, preload syringes, vials, and ampoules: 1% 10 mg/mL, 5 and 10 mL 2% 20 mg/mL, 5 mL IV infusion, preload syringes, vials, and ampoules: 4% 40 mg/mL, 25 and 50 mL 10% 100 mg/mL, 10-mL 20% 100 mg/mL, 5, and 10 mL Premade IV infusions: 0.2% mg/mL, 500 mL 0.4% 4 mg/mL, 250 mL, 500 mL, and 1L 0.8% 8 mg/mL, 250 and 500 mL	Do not administer faster than 50 mg/min in a conscious patient; can give rapid IV push in cardiac arrest; *use caution* for bradycardia with PVCs
procainamide (Pronestyl)	Treatment of ventricular tachycardia, ventricular fibrillation, or PVCs that are refractory to lidocaine and/or bretylium; to prevent recurrence of atrial fibrillation or flutter, PSVT, or ventricular tachycardia following conversion to normal sinus rhythm	Slows myocardial conduction velocity and decreases excitability (which may depress myocardial contractility); raises fibrillatory threshold, and suppresses ventricular ectopic activity	IV bolus injection IV infusion: 1 g/250 mL or 2 g/500 mL (4 μg/mL)	Loading dose: 50–100 mg given no faster than 20 mg/min q 5 min until rhythm is corrected, QRS complex begins to widen, hypotension develops, 1 g is administered Maintenance: 1–4 mg/min, titrate to effect	Precipitous hypotension may occur if IV dose excessive or administered faster than 20 mg/min; QRS complex widening and lengthening of the PR or QT interval possible warning signs of impending low blood pressure; AV conduction disturbances (heart block), PVCs, ventricular tachycardia, or fibrillation as asystole may follow; fever, nausea, vomiting, dizziness, giddiness, psychosis with hallucinations, seizures rare	Preexisting second- or third-degree heart block (without a pacemaker present) QT prolongation, or other severe conduction disturbances	For both IV push and IV infusion use vials: 100 mg/mL, 10 mL 500 mg/mL, 2 mL	Also used orally; is broken down in liver to form NAPA, which also has antiarrhythmic activity; accumulation of NAPA in patients with renal failure, increases potential for toxicity

verapamil (Isoptin, Calan)	PSVT, atrial fibrillation, or flutter with rapid ventricular response	Blocks influx and supply of calcium to cardiac muscle, exerting a negative inotropic effect, which lowers the myocardial oxygen demand, slows conduction, and prolongs the refractory period at the AV node, interrupting reentrant pathways during PSVT and helping to restore normal sinus rhythm; also, by inhibiting calcium influx, causes dilation of the main coronary, systemic, and peripheral arteries	IV push	Initial: 0.075–0.15 mg/kg (maximum dose not to exceed 10 mg) given no faster than 2.5 mg/min Repeated dose: not to exceed 10 mg, may be given 30 min after first dose if response not adequate	Symptomatic hypotension, abdominal cramps, nausea, vomiting, dizziness, or headache; prolongation of the PR interval correlating with verapamil plasma levels; PVCs, nodal escape rhythms, first-, second-, and third-degree AV blocks, bradycardia, and asystole rare; ventricular fibrillation in patients with WPW or Lown-Ganong-Levine syndromes	Hypersensitivity to verapamil, ventricular tachycardia, sick sinus syndrome without a functioning pacemaker, second- or third-degree AV blocks, severe hypotension or cardiogenic shock; do not administer verapamil and β-adrenergic blockers together (within a few hours), since both depress myocardial contractility and AV conduction	Ampoules, vials, and syringes: 5 mg/2 mL, 2 and 4 mL 5 mg/2 mL, 5-mL vials	Constant ECG and blood pressure monitoring essential; total dose not to exceed 15 mg (some physicians recommend 2.5-mg dose increments, as opposed to 5 or 10 mg); attempt to rule out WPW or Lown-Ganong-Levine syndromes prior to administration

once control of blood pressure has been established. Labetalol has been used safely in pregnant patients.

Dosing and Administration

Labetalol can be administered IV via multiple IV boluses or a continuous IV infusion. When initiating IV bolus, the clinician should start with 20 mg and repeat with 40 to 160 mg q 10 min until the desired effect is reached or until a total cumulative dose of 300 mg has been given. It is best to double the previous dose q 10 min, thus allowing gradual dosage increase. Alternatively, labetalol may be given via continuous infusion at a rate of 1 to 2 mg/min until desired response or a total cumulative dose of 300 mg has been reached. There are reports in which labetalol has been used as a continuous drip over a 24-h period in severe and refractory cases. Patients receiving labetalol via the IV route should be placed in a supine position and remain supine for approximately 3 h after receiving any IV doses, since symptomatic orthostatic hypotension may occur. Following patient stabilization, labetalol may be given orally up to 2400 mg/day in two to four divided doses.

Adverse Effect Profile

Labetalol has the same adverse effects profile as the other β blocking and α_1 blocking agents. The most common adverse effect associated with labetalol use is orthostatic hypotension, which occurs most frequently upon initial therapy. A loss of consciousness has occurred in some patients following both IV and oral administration. Symptomatic heart failure may also occur. Adverse CNS effects that may occur include lightheadedness, drowsiness, dizziness, fatigue, lethargy, and vivid nightmares. Tingling of the scalp and skin may occur with the initiation of therapy. Occasionally, reversible elevation of the hepatic enzymes may lead to jaundice and hepatitis. Other effects include lupus-like complaints, elevated renal function tests, blood dyscrasias, and allergic reactions.

Class III Antiarrhythmic Agents

Bretylium

Actions

Classified as a Class III antiarrhythmic, bretylium differs from lidocaine and procainamide in cardiovascular effects and electrophysiologic actions. The cardiovascular actions of bretylium are biphasic. Initially, bretylium releases norepinephrine from sympathetic ganglia and the terminal nerve endings of postganglionic nerves. This effect can cause a moderate increase in blood pressure, heart rate, and cardiac output lasting approximately 20 min, especially if the drug is infused too rapidly. At 45 to 60 min, bretylium blocks the release of norepinephrine in response to sympathetic nerve stimulation by depressing the excitability of adrenergic nerve terminals. This results in a sympatholytic effect that can cause orthostatic hypotension.

Bretylium affects phase 3 (repolarization) of the action potential and markedly prolongs refractoriness, action potential duration, and the QT interval.

Pharmacokinetics

The onset of action for IV bretylium in ventricular fibrillation is within minutes but may take from 20 min to 2 h when used for other ventricular arrhythmias. Peak effects occur in 1.5 to 6 h and last 6 to 12 h following a single dose. The drug is well absorbed following IM injection. Bretylium is eliminated primarily as unchanged drug via the kidney (70–85 percent) and thus may have a prolonged duration of action in patients with renal dysfunction. Dose adjustments may be necessary in patients with renal disease.

Indications

Bretylium is indicated for the treatment of both ventricular fibrillation and ventricular tachycardia refractory to other antiarrhythmic therapy and repeated countershocks. The drug is indicated as a first-line agent when lidocaine and procainamide are contraindicated (i.e., hypersensitivity reactions).

Dosing and Administration

The initial dose of bretylium for ventricular fibrillation is 5 mg/kg administered via rapid IV push. If ventricular fibrillation persists, the dose can be increased to 10 mg/kg and repeated at 15- to 30-min-intervals up to a maximum total dose of 30 mg/kg. For recurrent or refractory ventricular tachyarrhythmias, 5 to 10 mg/kg should be infused over a period of 8 to 10 min. If arrhythmias persist, repeated boluses of 5 to 10 mg/kg can be given q 1 to 2 h as necessary. If the IM route is used, no more than 5 mL should be injected at any one site, and injection sites should be rotated. Maintenance bolus injections with the same dosage can be given q 6 to 8 h. The standard dose for a bretylium infusion is 2 mg/min, with a dosing range of 1 to 4 mg/min.

Adverse Effect Profile

Postural hypotension is the most common adverse reaction and may occur within 15 to 30 min in as many as 60 percent of patients. If this occurs, the patient should be placed in a supine or Trendelenberg position and be resuscitated with crystalloid fluids. If hypotension persists, vasopressors may be employed. Nausea and vomiting, along with an increase in blood pressure and heart and ventricular irritability may also occur following a rapid IV injection in conscious patients. Bretylium should be avoided, if possible, in the setting of digoxin toxicity, since catecholamines are believed to exacerbate the toxic effects of digoxin.

Class IV Antiarrhythmic Agents: Calcium Channel Blockers

Verapamil

Actions

Verapamil, a calcium channel blocking agent, is classified as a class IV antiarrhythmic agent. In diseased tissue, verapamil decreases conduction velocity, prolongs the refractory period in the AV node, and decreases the discharge rate in the SA node. It interrupts the reentrant pathway associated with PSVT, thus causing the myocardium to return to NSR. In addition, verapamil can slow ventricular response in patients with atrial fibrillation and/or flutter by its action on the AV node. A decrease in heart rate and/or SA nodal block may occur in patients with SA nodal disease. Verapamil has minimal effects on normal conduction tissue.

Although verapamil has negative inotropic effects, they are often offset by the decrease in afterload. Those with severe heart failure, however, may experience a decrease in ejection fraction.

Most patients in PSVT and WPW demonstsrate narrow QRS complexes during tachycardia. This indicates antegrade conduction through the AV node, with retrograde conduction over the bypass tract completing the circuit. Verapamil is safe and effective in patients with narrow-complex PSVT, even in the presence of WPW, due to the pronounced negative dromotropic effects of verapamil on the AV node. If antegrade conduction occurs over the accessory pathway, the QRS complex is wide. Verapamil is contraindicated for atrial flutter or fibrillation due to WPW and in any type of wide-complex tachycardia, since it can increase rather than decrease the ventricular rate. In addition, wide-complex tachycardia could be ventricular tachycardia. In this case, verapamil could worsen hemodynamics because of vasodilation and negative inotropic effects.

By inhibiting the influx of calcium, verapamil impairs the contractile processes that calcium normally activates, thereby causing dilatation of coronary and systemic arteries. Dilatation of coronary arteries improves oxygen delivery, while dilatation of the systemic arteries decreases oxygen consumption by decreasing afterload. These effects provide the myocardium with a beneficial oxygen balance in patients with vasospastic, unstable, and chronic stable angina.

Pharmacokinetics

Verapamil elicits its hemodynamic effects in 5 min following IV administration, with effects lasting approximately 30 min. Effects on conduction begin within 2 min, peak in 10 to 15 min, and persist for 1 to 6 h. The Vd of verapamil is 4.5 to 7.1 L/kg. Verapamil undergoes first-pass metabolism in the liver and is metabolized to several metabolites. Norverapamil, an active metabolite, appears in the greatest amount. The elimination half-life of verapamil is 2 to 8 h, increasing to 4 to 12 h after 1 to 2 days of therapy.

Indications

Indications for verapamil include patients presenting with narrow complex PSVT from WPW syndrome. The drug may be used to control the ventricular rate in atrial fibrillation and/or flutter, but not if it is associated with an accessory bypass tract, since ventricular tachyarrhythmias may be precipiated. Diagnosis of PSVT should be confirmed by 12-lead ECG prior to administering verapamil whenever possible.

Oral verapamil is indicated for the management of vasospastic, chronic stable, and unstable angina and may also be used for the prophylaxis of PSVT.

Dosing and Administration

When managing patients with PSVT, the IV dose is 2.5 to 10 mg given initially over 2 to 3 min and repeated in 15 to 30 min if the response is inadequate. For the prevention of PSVT, oral administration of 240 to 480 mg daily should be given in three to four divided doses. Lower initial doses of verapamil should be considered in older patients and those with hepatic dysfunction. Calcium chloride, gluconate, or gluceptate (5–10 cm^3) can be given before or after verapamil infusion to prevent or reverse hypotension, although such reports have been largely anecdotal.

For the treatment of vasospastic, unstable, or chronic stable angina, oral doses of verapamil can be given (80 mg q 6–8 h), with doses titrated up or down to desired clinical response. In patients with hypertension, verapamil is initiated with 80 mg three times daily and titrated to blood pressure response. Although daily doses of 480 mg/day have been used, efficacy with doses greater than 360 mg/day has not been proven. The SR tablets, as an initial dose of 240 mg every morning, may be used for hypertension. Titration may be accomplished with 120-mg (one-half SR tablet) increments added in the evening. Breaking the SR tablet does not affect the therapeutic effect of verapamil SR.

Adverse Effect Profile

The majority of adverse effects secondary to verapamil are related to its pharmacologic action. The incidence is increased in patients with severe heart failure, hypertrophic cardiomyopathy, and conduction disturbances. Hypotension occurs in 5 to 10 percent with IV administration and may rarely require treatment with IV calcium salts or vasopressors. Conduction disturbances such as bradycardia, AV block, and bundle-branch block occur in approximately 2 percent of patients and usually respond to dosage reduction or discontinuation of the drug; rarely, use of atropine, isoproterenol, or cardiac pacing may be necessary. In addition, approximately 2 percent may develop acute or pulmonary edema secondary to the negative inotropic effects of verapamil.

Noncardiac side effects with verapamil include constipation, dizziness, headache, and nausea. Other side effects, reported to occur in less than 1 percent of patients, include sleep disturbances, blurred vision, shakiness, drowsiness, confusion, dry mouth, rash, urticaria, bruising, flushing, polyuria, sexual difficulties, dyspnea, and muscle cramps. Several cases of hepatocellular injury accompanied by clinical signs of hepatotoxicity have also been reported. Verapamil should be given with caution to patients receiving agents such as β blockers, digoxin, antihypertensives, and antiarrhythmics, since their effects may be additive. Cimetidine may decrease hepatic metabolism.

Nifedipine

Actions

Nifedipine (Procardia and Adalat) is a calcium channel blocker with actions similar to those of other agents in this class. The coronary artery dilatation results in improved oxygen delivery, benefitting patients with vasospastic angina. Systemic artery dilatation results in decreased afterload, leading to decreased oxygen consumption in patients with chronic stable angina. A reflex increase in heart rate and an increase in cardiac output may be seen with nifedipine. Unlike verapamil and diltiazem, nifedipine has little effect on the SA and AV node clinically. Nifedipine may, however, result in an increase in left ventricular and diastolic pressure (LVEDP) or left ventricular end diastolic volume (LVEDV) in patients with moderate to severely impaired LV function, thereby worsening their condition.

Pharmacokinetics

Nifedipine is 45 to 75 percent bioavailable as a result of significant first-pass liver metabolism. When taken orally (conventional capsules), the onset of action is 20 min and the duration of action is 4 to 6 h. Sublingual administration or capsules chewed and swallowed results in antihypertensive effects within 3 min, lasting 2 to 3 h. Extended-release capsules have a gradual onset of action which peaks at 6 h and persists for 24 h.

Nifedipine is metabolized in the liver to inactive metabolites. The elimination half-life of the parent drug is 2 to 5 h in patients with normal hepatic and renal function, increasing to 7 h in those with hepatic dysfunction

Indications

The primary use of nifedipine in emergency medicine is to rapidly lower the blood pressure in hypertensive crisis. The drug can be given sublingually or orally and is therefore particularly convenient when IV lines cannot be started and the blood pressure needs to lowered immediately.

Approved indications for nifedipine include management of vasospastic and chronic stable angina. It is considered to be as effective as β blockers or nitrates in the treatment of chronic stable angina. Nifedipine, either alone or in combination with other antihypertensives, is indicated for the management of essential hypertension. In comparison to other classes of antihypertensives (i.e., angiotensin-converting enzyme inhibitors and β blockers), nifedipine may benefit patients with low-renin hypertension, coexisting angina, or peripheral vascular disease.

Dosing and Administration

The initial dose of nifedipine for hypertensive crisis is 10 mg. The capsule contains liquid contents. To achieve rapid effects, the patient should chew and then swallow the capsule. If the patient is unconscious, several holes should be poked into the capsule using an 18-gauge needle, and the contents squirted below the tongue. A repeat dose can be administered 10 min later.

Adverse Effect Profile

The majority of side effects occurring with nifedipine are related to its vasodilatory activity on the smooth muscle and include lightheadedness, flushing, headache, and hypotension. Nifedipine may also cause a dose-related peripheral edema in 10 to 30 percent of patients. Other cardiovascular side effects associated with the use of nifedipine include myocardial infarction, CHF, and pulmonary edema. Since there have also been reported cases of reflex tachycardia, it should be used with caution in hypertensive crisis in patients who are already tachycardic.

Noncardiac-related adverse effects include nervousness, sleep disturbances, blurred vision, nausea, somnolence, insomnia, asthenia, diarrhea, dry mouth, rash, urticaria, dyspnea, polyuria, sweating, sexual difficulties, and joint pain. Rarely, thrombocytopenia, leukopenia, anemia, elevated liver function tests, and bruising have occurred in patients on nifedipine. Nifedipine should be used with caution in patients with aortic stenosis, CHF, and concomitant β blocker therapy, since CHF may be precipitated or exacerbated. Antihypertensive agents may enhance the hypotensive effects of nifedipine.

Nimodipine

Actions

Nimodine (Nimotop) is a calcium channel blocker structurally similar to nifedipine. Like other calcium channel blockers, it inhibits the influx of calcium across the transmembrane channels, thereby inhibiting the contractile activity in the cell. The inhibition of calcium influx is seen in myocardial, vascular smooth muscle, and neuronal cells. Nimodipine has a relative selectivity for vascular smooth muscle, as opposed to the myocardium, and therefore has minimal effects on the conduction and inotropy of the myocardium. Its greatest affinity is for the CNS vasculature. It increases cerebral blood flow and may shunt blood to ischemic areas. Although inhibition of cerebral vasospasm (which often occurs following SAH) was initially thought to be responsible for the beneficial effects of nimodipine in SAH, angiography has not supported this. Improved collateral blood flow and prevention of large calcium influxes into neurons (causing cell destruction) may be of greater importance.

Pharmacokinetics

Nimodipine is rapidly and well absorbed after oral administration; however, first-pass metabolism by the liver results in low and inconsistent bioavailability (3–30 percent). Peak concentrations occur in 30 to 60 min.

Nimodipine has a volume of distribution of 0.94 to 2.3 L/kg and is metabolized in the liver to several metabolites, most with little or no activity. The elimination half-life following oral administration is 1.7 to 9 h.

Indications

Nimodipine is indicated for the treatment of recent (within 96 h) SAH from ruptured congenital intracranial aneurysm in patients when postictal neurologic condition is good (e.g., Hunt and Hess grades I–III), where it can decrease morbidity and mortality. Patients with more severe disability (Hunt and Hess grades IV–V) do not seem to benefit and may worsen with nimodipine.

Dosing and Administration

The dose is 60 mg q 4 h for 21 days for managing patients with SAH. If oral administration is not possible, the capsules can be punctured, with the contents administered through a nasogastric tube, followed by a 30-mL saline flush.

Adverse Effect Profile

The most common adverse effect is hypotension, which is often dose-related. In addition, edema and headache have been reported in patients with SAH. Other, less frequent, dose-related adverse effects include tachycardia, bradycardia, palpitations, flushing, hypertension, rebound vasospasm, CHF, and pulmonary edema.

Other side effects reported include thrombocytopenia, anemia, disseminated intravascular coagulation, rash, pruritus, hematoma, abdominal discomfort, constipation, elevated liver test results, depression, lightheadedness, dizziness, drowsiness, hyponatremia, and hyperglycemia.

Other Calcium Channel Blockers: Diltiazem, Nitrendipine, and Nicardipine

Although other calcium channel blockers, such as diltiazem, nicardipine, and nitrendipine, are effective for chronic management of hypertension and angina, their use in the emergency department is minimal.

Actions

Nicardipine and nitrendipine are two calcium channel blockers structurally related to nifedipine. Like nifedipine, these agents inhibit the transmembrane flux of calcium into cardiac and vascular smooth muscle. The inhibition results in a decrease in the contractile activity within the myocardium and vascular smooth muscle. Unique to these agents is the selective activity on the vasculature as opposed to the myocardium. Nicardipine possesses both coronary and peripheral vasodilatation action, while nitrendipine exerts antihypertensive activity, primarily through a decrease in peripheral vascular resistance. Increases in cardiac output and cardiac index can be seen in a dose-dependent manner with nicardipine, whereas nitrendipine displays inconsistent effects on these values. Intravenous nicardipine, however, has been shown to produce a decrease in contractility in patients with severe heart failure.

Both nicardipine and nitrendipine have electrophysiologic actions similar to those seen with other calcium channels blockers, although reflex increases in heart rate may be seen with each. Neither agent has been shown to have demonstrable effects on renal blood flow or glomerular filtration rate; however, nitrendipine appears to have antihypertensive effects that are directly related to low renin activity.

Pharmacokinetics

Nicardipine and nitrendipine are well absorbed, with oral bioavailability being 35 and 23 percent, respectively. Both drugs are greater than 95-percent bound, have a Vd of 0.64 L/kg (nicardipine) and 6 L/kg (nitrendipine), and are metabolized to inactive metabolites. The onset of action of nicardipine following oral administration is approximately 20 min; it is 2 h for nitrendipine. The duration of action of nicardipine is approximately 3 h, while nitrendipine lasts between 8 and 24 h.

Indications

Nicardipine (Cardene) is indicated for chronic stable angina and essential hypertension. The drug can be used alone or in combination with other agents for both indications and appears to be equally effective as nifedipine in treating angina and hypertension. Nitrendipine (Baypress) is pending FDA approval for mild to moderate hypertension, particularly in patients with low baseline renin activity.

Dosing and Administration

The initial dose of nicardipine is 20 mg three times a day, titrating the dose to clinical response up to 40 mg three times a day. Nitrendipine is initiated at 10 mg/day and can be increased up to 40 mg/day in one or two divided doses. Dosage adjustments should be made for elderly patients or those with hepatic dysfunction: 20 mg twice a day for nitrendipine and 5 to 10 mg/day for nitrendipine.

Adverse Effect Profile

Adverse effects of these agents are similar to those of nifedipine and other calcium channel blockers.

Other Antiarrhythmic Agents

Adenosine

Actions

Adenosine is an endogenous adenine nucleoside produced by the dephosphorylation of adenosine monophosphate (AMP). Every cell of the body contains adenosine. This compound exerts negative chronotropic and negative dromotropic actions on SA and AV nodal tissue. Adenosine terminates PSVT primarily via blockage of the AV node without altering conduction through accessory pathways, as is seen with the WPW syndrome. Reentrant supraventricular tachyarrhythmias not involving the AV node are not terminated by adenosine. Adenosine is a potent vasodilator; however, there is no change in systemic blood pressure following administration because it is rapidly metabolized by circulating adenosine deaminase and undergoes rapid sequestration by vascular endothelial cells.

Pharmacokinetics

Onset of action is approximately 30 s with a duration of 60 to 90 s. The drug is rapidly metabolized in the liver, with a half-life of 1 to 7 s. The primary routes of elimination are cellular uptake and simple or facilitated diffusion by a nucleoside transport system, metabolism to various by-products, and renal excretion of these metabolic products. The predominant final metabolite of adenosine is uric acid. Specific pharmacokinetic parameters, such as Vd, therapeutic plasma concentrations, and clearance, are difficult to assess due to the extremely short half-life of the drug.

Indications

Adenosine (Adenocard) is approved as an antiarrhythmic drug for the emergency management of PSVT involving the AV node. The drug has also been used for distinguishing supraventricular from ventricular tachycardia as well as for diagnosing broad QRS complex tachycardias. Because adenosine shortens the action potential duration and slows the heart rate, it is contraindicated in second- and third-degree AV heart block, sick-sinus syndrome, atrial tachyarrhythmias (e.g., atrial fibrillation or flutter), and ventricular tachycardia.

Dosing and Administration

The initial dose for the treatment of acute PSVT is 6 mg given as a *rapid* IV bolus over 1 to 2 s, followed by a saline flush. If the heart rate does not decrease within 2 min, a second bolus injection of 12 mg should be given. A final third bolus dose of 12 mg may be given in 1 to 2 min if the arrhythmia persists. Adenosine has been shown to be at least as effective as verapamil in terminating PSVT and has the advantage of having a shorter half-life and fewer adverse effects.

Adverse Effect Profile

When adverse effects occur due to adenosine, they are minor and well tolerated because they last less than 1 min due to the drug's short half-life. The most common adverse effects are dyspnea, cough, syncope, vertigo, paresthesias, numbness, nausea, and metallic taste. Cardiovascular adverse effects may include facial flushing, headache, diaphoresis, palpitations, retrosternal chest pain, sinus bradydysrhythmias (i.e., bradycardia, sinus arrest, and AV block), atrial tachydysrhythmias (i.e., atrial fibrillation or flutter), premature ventricular contractions, and hypotension. These adverse effects rarely require specific management. Dipyridamole and carbamazepine have been shown to enhance the negative chronotropic and dromotropic effects of adenosine and may increase the degree of toxicity. Methylxanthines and caffeine, on the other hand, compete for adenosine receptors. Therefore, asthmatics or excessive coffee drinkers may require a higher dose of adenosine to achieve a therapeutic effect.

Digoxin

Actions

Digoxin has three basic actions: (1) it increases the force, strength, and velocity of cardiac contractions (positive inotropic effects); (2) it slows the heart rate (negative chronotropic effects); and (3) it slows conduction velocity through the AV node.

Digoxin exerts its direct inotropic and electrophysiologic effects by binding to and inhibiting the sodium and potassium ATPase pump in the cell membrane. This action results in higher intracellular levels of sodium and causes calcium to move intracellularly in exchange for sodium. The elevated intracellular calcium concentration allows more calcium to be available to increase the rate and force of cardiac contractions.

Digoxin increases the refractory period and decreases the conduction velocity of both the SA and AV nodes, but shortens the refractory period and increases conduction velocity in the atrial muscles (including atrial bypass tracts as present in WPW). The primary effect on SA and AV nodal conduction is secondary to direct enhancement of parasympathomimetic tone. ECG changes include PR interval prolongation and QT interval shortening. High doses of digoxin enhance ventricular automaticity.

Slowing of the heart results in a prolonged diastolic period, allowing a greater period for improving coronary blood and myocardial perfusion. A decrease in oxygen demand may also occur secondary to the decrease in heart rate.

Pharmacokinetics

The onset of action is about 30 min following IV administration and 30 to 120 min for oral tablets, while peak effects occur in 1 to 4 h and 2 to 6 h, respectively. The onset of action following parenteral therapy varies based upon the rate at which digoxin is administered. In oral dosing, however, patient variability is the primary cause for variation. The large variation in peak effect can be explained by the fact that digoxin has a large volume of distribution of 5.6 L/kg. Digoxin crosses the blood-brain barrier and the placenta, and high concentrations are found in the liver, heart, kidney, and intestines. Digoxin may also be given by oral tablets, elixir, and capsules, the bioavailability being approximately 70, 80, and 90 percent, respectively.

Digoxin is inactivated by hepatic degradation and is excreted unchanged in the urine. The half-life of digoxin in patients with normal renal function is 30 to 40 h and can extend to 4 to 6 days in anuric patients. Because digoxin concentrates in the tissues, serum levels of digoxin may not accurately reflect the amount of drug in the body, making procedures such as dialysis or exchange transfusion ineffective.

Indications

Digoxin is indicated to improve cardiac output in CHF and to control heart rate in atrial fibrillation, atrial flutter, and paroxysmal atrial tachycardia. Use of digoxin in the treatment of CHF should be considered only when diuretics and vasodilators fail to improve cardiac output. Digoxin may be particularly effective in providing beneficial hemodynamic and symptomatic improvement in heart failure patients presenting with an S_3 gallop or "low-output" heart failure associated with depressed ventricular function. Digoxin is less effective with "high-output" heart failure, which occurs in patients with bronchopulmonary insufficiency, anemia, infection, hyperthyroidism, or arteriovenous fistulas.

Dosing and Administration

Digoxin can be administered by oral or IV routes. The IV route is preferred when a more rapid onset of action and peak effect is desired. The IV dose is 20 to 30 percent less than an oral dose. Digoxin should not be administered by IM injection, since this route offers no advantages and can cause severe pain at the injection site.

For control of supraventricular tachycardias, digoxin should be administered IV in a dose of 10 to 15 μg/kg. This dose should be divided, with 0.25 to 0.5 mg given as the initial dose and 0.25 mg q 4 h as subsequent doses until the entire dose is administered or the heart rate is sufficiently lowered. The dose for patients with CHF without atrial fibrillation is generally lower (8 to 12 μg/kg) but can be given in a similar fashion (i.e., 0.25 to 0.5 mg initially, followed by 0.25 mg q 4 h until the complete dose is given) until the appropriate response has been achieved. Higher doses are often required to control the ventricular response to atrial fibrillation or flutter, but higher doses have more adverse effects. Cumulative doses should not exceed 1.0 mg. Loading doses should be calculated using lean body weight, since this method generally provides therapeutic effects with minimal risk of toxicity. Intravenous loading doses should be administered slowly over a 5-min period or longer, undiluted or diluted, to a fourfold or greater volume.

Maintenance therapy should be adjusted according to clinical response or to maintain a serum digoxin concentration between 0.8 and 2.0 ng/mL. Dosage adjustments are necessary in renal failure, dehydration, hypokalemia, hypercalcemia, hypomagnesemia, and hypothyroidism. Drugs that interact with digoxin to cause increases in serum digoxin levels include amiodarone, verapamil, nifedipine, nitrendipine, hydroxychloroquine, propafenone, quinidine, erythromycin, tetracycline, and anticholinergic agents. In contrast, cholestyramine, metoclopramide, kaolin-pectin, penicillamine, and dietary fiber have resulted in lower serum digoxin concentrations.

Adverse Effect Profile

When digoxin toxicity is suspected, the drug should be stopped and a serum level obtained. Digoxin serum levels do not always represent true toxicity. Toxicity may actually occur in some patients with low serum levels, since it is often myocardial tissue levels rather than serum levels that determine the degree of toxicity.

Symptoms of digoxin toxicity include mental depression, confusion, headache, drowsiness, anorexia, nausea, vomiting, weakness, visual disturbances (green or yellow vision and/or halo effects), delirium, EEG abnormalities, and seizures. Patients may also present with diarrhea and abdominal discomfort. Almost any type of arrhythmia may manifest in digoxin toxicity. The most common arrhythmias include an increased number of unifocal or premature ventricular contractions, ventricular tachycardia, junctional tachycardia, high-degree AV block, PSVT with block, and sinus arrest. Atrial fibrillation, bradycardia, and ventricular fibrillation may also occur. Other adverse effects may include gynecomastia, skin rash, eosinophilia, and thrombocytopenia.

While hypokalemia increases the risk of digoxin toxicity, significant digoxin toxicity itself may produce hyperkalemia due to paralysis of the transmembrane sodium-potassium pump. However, when hypokalemia develops in less severe cases of toxicity, potassium can be replaced by IV infusion, provided there is no evidence of high-degree AV conduction block. When digoxin toxicity is associated with hyperkalemia, a corresponding intracellular deficiency of potassium exists, which may be the causative factor of subsequent arrhythmias. Treatment in this circumstance is controversial. It is not clear whether methods should be taken to decrease the total body supply of potassium (at the risk of increasing intracellular hypokalemia), to increase the total body potassium in the face of extracellular hyperkalemia, or to use measures that would ordinarily encourage movement of potassium back into cells (e.g., use of bicarbonate, glucose, and insulin). These methods may all prove useless in the absence of a functioning transmembrane sodium-potassium pump.

Lidocaine and phenytoin are antiarrhythmics that have classically been used in digoxin toxicity, but their efficacy has not been proven. Atropine and electrical pacing have been tried in cases of bradyarrhythmias, but these methods too have had limited success. Hemodialysis and resin hemoperfusion have been attempted in some cases of severe digoxin poisoning but have generally been unsuccessful due to the large volume of distribution of digoxin. Digoxin antibody fragments, otherwise known as Digoxin Immune FAB (fragmented antibodies) or Digibind (Burroughs-Wellcome), have recently been approved for use in treating life-threatening digoxin toxicity. This antidote is indicated for life-threatening ventricular tachyarrhythmias, sinus bradyarrhythmias, severe AV blocks, resulting from overdose or accidental pediatric ingestion of digoxin and digitalis-like glycosides that is unresponsive to conventional therapy. An additional indication for FAB, by the manufacturer, is in patients experiencing severe digoxin toxicity who have serum potassium levels greater than 5 mEq/mL.

VASOACTIVE DRUGS

Vasoactive and Inotropic Agents

Epinephrine

Actions

Epinephrine is a nonselective α- and β-adrenergic agonist. The drug increases heart rate, ventricular contractility, and peripheral vascular resistance. Epinephrine increases mean arterial pressure by stimulating α_1-adrenergic receptors during cardiac arrest. This effect vasoconstricts arterioles in the skin, mucosa, and mesenteric vasculature, redistributing blood to the heart and brain. This effect results in improved cardiac and cerebral perfusion during resuscitation. Epinephrine also causes bronchodilation and antagonizes the effects of histamine.

Pharmacokinetics

Both the onset of action and the duration of action of epinephrine are relatively short: 1 to 2 min and 2 to 10 min, respectively. The drug quickly becomes fixed in the tissues and is rapidly inactivated via oxidation by monoamine oxidase (MAO) and via methylation by catechol-O-methyltransferase (COMT). Subsequent metabolites are excreted in the urine as sulfates and glucuronides.

Indications

Epinephrine is considered a first-line agent in the treatment of cardiac arrest and has been used as such in ventricular fibrillation, asystole, and electromechanical dissociation (EMD).

The drug has also been purported to "coarsen" fine ventricular fibrillation, but there is no documented evidence that this is true. Epinephrine does, however, increase the likelihood of continued hemodynamic stability in animals that have been successfully defibrillated. This result has been attributed to the effect of epinephrine on systemic vascular resistance. It is not clear whether this beneficial effect, seen in relatively healthy animals subjected to ventricular fibrillation, would be equally beneficial in unhealthy human hearts. Nevertheless, epinephrine remains a widely used and recommended agent following initially unsuccessful defibrillation attempts for ventricular fibrillation.

Epinephrine is also used as a vasopressor to increase blood pressure and as an antidote to reverse bronchospasm due to anaphylactic and hypersensitivity reactions.

Dosing and Administration

Current American Heart Association guidelines for dosing epinephrine state that 0.5 to 1 mg in 5 to 10 mL of a 1:10,000 solution may be used q 5 to 10 min, if required, to obtain return of spontaneous circulation (ROSC) in CPR. These dosing guidelines are being reevaluated as preliminary animal and human studies suggest larger doses may be more appropriate.

Epinephrine may be given via peripheral vein, via a central line, or endotracheally. Endotracheal administration is performed by placing 10 mL of a 1:10,000 solution down the ET tube and then performing several rapid ventilations to disperse the drug throughout the airways for maximal absorption.

Adverse Effect Profile

Adverse effects are of minimal importance in the setting of cardiac arrest. Epinephrine does increase myocardial oxygen consumption significantly and thus can exacerbate ventricular irritability in the setting of myocardial ischemia. The α-adrenergic activity of epinephrine produces increases in systemic vascular resistance, which could conceivably be detrimental to a failing myocardium, in that increased afterload can significantly decrease cardiac output. Also, should the patient survive cardiac arrest, hypertension, tachycardia and arrhythmias should be anticipated.

Dopamine

Actions

Dopamine, an endogenous catecholamine and the precursor of endogenous norepinephrine, acts on dopaminergic, β_1, and α receptors. In low doses (<5 μg/kg per min), dopamine acts on dopaminergic receptors, causing vasodilation of the renal, mesenteric, coronary, and intracerebral vascular beds. This effect improves organ perfusion and increases urine output. At moderate doses (2–10 μg/kg per min), dopamine exerts inotropic and chronotropic effects, increasing cardiac output by its actions on β_1-adrenergic receptors. Stimulation of α receptors increases peripheral resistance and decreases blood flow to the kidney. α Effects begin at 10 μg/kg per min and predominate above 15 μg/kg per min.

Pharmacokinetics

Dopamine has an onset of action within 2 to 4 min and a duration of action of less than 10 min. It is used only as an IV infusion. Renal response may take 20 to 30 min. Dopamine is metabolized primarily (75 percent) to homovanillic acid (HVA) and other metabolites (including norepinephrine) by MAO and COMT and subsequently excreted in the urine. Only a fraction of the dose eliminated by the kidneys is unchanged dopamine.

Indications

Dopamine is indicated for reversing hemodynamically significant hypertension due to myocardial infarction, trauma, sepsis, overt heart failure, renal failure, and chronic CHF when fluid resuscitation is not appropriate or unsuccessful. It is also used to improve renal blood flow to increase urine output.

Dosing and Administration

The range for low-dose dopamine is 1 to 5 μg/kg per min, while the moderate dose is 2 to 10 μg/kg per min. High dose begins at 10 μg/kg per min and should be titrated to adequate blood pressure response. As with all vasoactive infusions, dopamine should be discontinued by tapering the dosage. Most patients can be managed on 20 μg/kg per min or less.

Adverse Effect Profile

Dopamine may produce dose-dependent adverse effects, including hypotension at low infusion rates, hypertension at high infusion rates, ectopic beats, headache, nausea, vomiting, angina pectoris, and tachycardia. Necrosis may occur if the infusion extravasates. Gangrene of the extremities has occurred in patients with occlusive vascular disease or diabetes as well as in those who receive prolonged high-dose infusions. Monoamine oxidase inhibitors, halogen anesthetics, sympathomimetics, phenothiazines, and phosphodiesterase inhibitors will prolong and intensify the effects of dopamine, possibly causing hypertensive and arrhythmogenic activity. Phenytoin may interact with dopamine and cause hypotension, seizures, and bradycardia. Dopamine is contraindicated in cases of pheochromocytoma, tachycardia, or ventricular fibrillation.

Norepinephrine

Actions

Norepinephrine bitartrate (Levophed) is identical to the endogenous catecholamine synthesized in the adrenal medulla and sympathetic nervous tissue. Norepinephrine acts primarily on α receptors, inducing powerful vasoconstrictor actions on arterial and venous beds. The drug also has direct action on β_1 receptors, thus inducing inotropic and chronotropic effects. Paradoxical decreases in heart rate may result from reflex withdrawal of sympathetic tone. Norepinephrine differs from epinephrine in that norepinephrine has no effect on β_2 receptors.

Pharmacokinetics

Norepinephrine is administered only as an IV infusion. The pressor effect has an onset of action within 3 min and stops within 10 min of discontinuation of the infusion. The primary elimination of norepinephrine is via uptake by adrenergic neurons and metabolism in the liver and other tissues, mainly by COMT and to a lesser extent by MAO. Norepinephrine metabolites are excreted in the urine as sulfate and glucuronate conjugates.

Indications

Norepinephrine is primarily used as a second-line vasopressor for the treatment of severe hypotension refractory to fluids and other pressor agents, specifically dopamine. Norepinephrine may be particularly effective when endogenous norepinephrine stores are low. This scenario may arise in patients who have been on prolonged infusions of dopamine. To a certain degree, norepinephrine increases inotropic activity and may be indicated in severe hypotension occurring during an acute myocardial infarction or septic shock. Other specific uses for norepinephrine include controlling hypotension states during poliomyelitis, drug overdose (various phenothiazines and tricyclic antidepressants), spinal anesthesia, pheochromocytomectomy, and sympathectomy.

Dosing and Administration

As with any vasopressor, adequate fluid or blood replacement should be corrected before starting norepinephrine. Norepinephrine should only be used as an IV infusion. The initial adult dosage range is 8 to 12 μg/min (average dose, 2 to 4 μg/min), while the pediatric dose is 2 μg/min up to 6 μg/min (or 2 to 6 μg/m^2). An alternate pediatric dose is 0.1 μg/kg per min. Rates must be titrated carefully, increasing by 1 to 2 μ/min q 3 to 5 min until a systolic blood pressure of 80 to 100 mmHg is attained. The drug should be infused in the lowest effective dosage for the shortest period of time possible. Occasionally, high doses of norepinephrine may be necessary to reverse hypotension (e.g., 68 mg of norepinephrine daily). Usually, the maintenance dose is 2 to 4 μg/min. Adjust the rate of flow every 3 to 5 min to maintain blood pressure. Once the blood pressure is adequate, the infusion may be gradually titrated down. Abrupt withdrawal may result in acute hypotension.

Adverse Effect Profile

Large doses of norepinephrine may result in ventricular irritability, cardiac depression, decreased renal blood flow, and a reflex bradycardia. Acute hypertension may result in patients on MAO inhibitors or tricyclic antidepressants. Use norepinephrine with extreme caution in these patients. Use as large a vein as possible to minimize the risk of extravasation. If infiltration occurs, phentolamine may be used (see Chap.23). Check frequently for IV infiltration if a small vein is used. Norepinephrine is contraindicated in patients with hypotension resulting from cyclopropane or halogenated hydrocarbon anesthesia or uncorrected blood volume deficits as well as in mesenteric or peripheral vascular thrombosis.

Isoproterenol

Actions

Isoproterenol is a synthetic sympathomimetic with *strong* β_1 and β_2 adrenergic-agonist properties. β_1 actions increase the inotropic and chronotropic activity of cardiac muscle, resulting in increased cardiac output despite a reduction in the mean blood pressure. The drop in blood pressure can be attributed to the β_2-adrenergic relaxation of smooth muscle in the splanchnic vasculature bed and alimentary tract, the lungs, and skeletal muscle, which causes peripheral vasodilation and venous pooling.

Pharmacokinetics

After IV administration, isoproterenol has an onset of action within 1 to 5 min and a duration of action lasting 1 to 2 h. Fifty percent of the drug is eliminated unchanged in the urine, while 25 to 35 percent is metabolized primarily to 3-*O*-methylisoproterenol (which has been reported to have weak β-adrenergic blocking activity) by COMT in the lung, liver, and other body tissues and then excreted unchanged or as a sulfate conjugate.

Indications

Isoproterenol is indicated only for the temporary management of hemodynamically unstable bradyarrhythmias (i.e., bradycardia and heart block) refractory to atropine. The use of isoproterenol to increase the heart rate should be considered only when a pacemaker is not immediately available. Electronic pacing is the definitive treatment for this condition, since it provides better control and is a safer mode of therapy. The vasodilatory effects of isoproterenol have been shown to lower coronary perfusion pressure during cardiac arrest and to increase the mortality rate in experimental animals; the drug has not been shown to be efficacious in cardiac arrest.

Dosing and Administration

Isoproterenol should only be administered via IV infusion. The infusion rate, 2 to 10 μg/min, should be titrated to the desired heart rate.

Adverse Effect Profile

It must be emphasized that the β_1-agonist action of isoproterenol will cause an increase in chronotropic effect. This effect raises myocardial oxygen requirements and could possibly precipitate or exacerbate myocardial ischemia and induce serious arrhythmias (e.g., ventricular tachycardia and fibrillation). Other adverse effects include anxiety, mild tremors, and anginal pain in patients with previously reported angina pectoris. Therefore, the drug should be avoided in patients with preexisting ischemic heart disease. Isoproterenol may also induce tachyarrhythmias in hypokalemia and digoxin-toxic patients. The primary adverse effects from β_2-adrenergic actions are facial flushing, headache, and hypotension.

Dobutamine

Actions

Dobutamine (Dobutrex) is a synthetic sympathomimetic agent that exerts potent inotropic and mild chronotropic activity by directly stimulating β_1-adrenergic receptors. Dobutamine also has mild α_1-agonist activity, but the effects are balanced by the more potent β_2-agonist effects, cumulatively resulting in mild vasodilation. Doses of 2 to 15 μg/kg per min increase cardiac output and decrease peripheral resistance and pulmonary occlusive pressures, causing minimal increase in heart rate. However, higher doses of dobutamine will accelerate the heart rate and induce arrhythmogenic effects. An increased cardiac output usually results in increased renal and mesenteric blood flow.

Pharmacokinetics

Dobutamine has an onset of action of 1 to 2 min; however, peak plasma levels may not be reached for 10 min. Its duration of action is 10 to 15 min. The plasma half-life is 2 min. Dobutamine is metabolized in the liver and other tissues by COMT and glucuronic acid, and over two-thirds of a dose is excreted as metabolites in the urine within 48 h.

Indications

Dobutamine is used to increase inotropic activity in the short-term management of cardiac decompensation due to depressed contractility resulting either from organic heart disease or from cardiac surgical procedures. The drug should be used to increase cardiac output in the chronic CHF patient when standard therapy (diuretics, vasodilators, and digoxin) fail to improve symptoms and/or in the patient with pulmonary congestion and low cardiac output.

Dosing and Administration

Dobutamine is only administered via IV infusion. The dosage range is 2.5 to 20 μg/kg per min; however, most patients can be maintained on 10 μg/kg per min or less. In some cases, very low doses (0.5 μg/kg per min) may be effective. Conversely, infusions up to 40 μg/kg per min have been used, but doses greater than 20 μg/kg per min should be used with caution because of increased risks of tachyarrhythmias. To correctly assess the effectiveness of the drug, patients should be monitored with a Swan-Ganz catheter.

Adverse Effect Profile

The primary adverse effects of dobutamine are increased heart rate (increases greater than 5–15 beats/min are uncommon), blood pressure (increases greater than 10–20 mmHg are uncommon), and ectopic arrhythmias (escape beats, unifocal and multifocal ventricular ectopic beats, and ventricular bigeminy). Less common effects include headache, paresthesias, tremors, nausea, angina, and dyspnea. Heart rate increases greater than 10 percent may induce or exacerbate myocardial ischemia.

Amrinone

Actions

Amrinone (Inocor) is thought to be a positive inotropic agent not related to digitalis glycosides, catecholamines (e.g., dopamine and norepinephrine), or β_1-adrenergic agonists (e.g., dobutamine and isoproterenol), and possesses potent vasodilator activity. While its true mechanism is not known, amrinone is believed to act by inhibiting cyclic adenosine monophosphate (cAMP) phosphodiesterase activity, which results in increased levels of cellular cAMP. Increased levels of cAMP are thought to increase calcium availability to the myocardial contractile components. These actions increase myocardial contractility and force of contractions (i.e., positive inotropic effect). Some believe that the vasodilatory action is the primary mechanism responsible for increasing myocardial performance. Vasodilation resulting in conjunction with amrinone may be the result of direct action by the drug on the vessels or may be caused by a reflex withdrawal of sympathetic tone following the improvement of myocardial function. Nonetheless, the primary effect of amrinone is an increase in myocardial contractility and stroke volume with a reduction in preload and afterload.

Pharmacokinetics

Cardiovascular effects usually begin within 2 to 5 min and generally peak within 10 min at all doses. The duration of effect is dose-related. Following a 0.75-mg/kg bolus dose, the duration is about 30 min, while a 3-mg/kg dose will last approximately 2 h. Amrinone is metabolized in the liver and excreted in the urine and has a Vd of 1.2 L/kg. In patients with normal renal function, amrinone has an elimination half-life of 3.6 h. In patients with CHF and/or hepatic or renal dysfunction, amrinone has a prolonged elimination half-life (average, 5.8 h).

Indications

Amrinone is indicated for increasing myocardial performance in the short-term management of CHF. Due to its adverse effect profile, the drug should be used only when other therapies, such as diuretics, digoxin, and dobutamine, have failed. Amrinone has only been studied in classes III and IV CHF.

Dosing and Administration

The initial dose is 0.75 mg/kg, followed by a maintenance infusion at 5 to 10 μg/kg per min not to exceed to 10 mg/kg per day. A second

IV bolus injection may be given 30 min following the first dose if the desired effects have not been achieved. Adjustments in the maintenance infusion should be titrated to the clinical response. Amrinone can be administered as a slow direct IV injection (undiluted) over 2 to 3 min or as a continuous infusion diluted in 0.9% or 0.45% saline.

Adverse Effect Profile

The most common adverse effects are thrombocytopenia (<100,000/mm^3, 2.4 percent incidence), ventricular and supraventricular arrhythmias (3 percent), hypotension (1.3 percent), and nausea (1.7 percent). Other adverse effects, which occur in less than 1 percent of cases, include vomiting, anorexia, fever, chest pain, and burning at the site of injection. Although rare, hepatotoxicity has been reported. Acute marked elevations of hepatic enzymes along with clinical symptoms may suggest a hypersensitivity reaction, which would require prompt discontinuation of the drug.

Atropine

Actions

Atropine, an antimuscarinic agent, increases sinus node automaticity and AV conduction by blocking vagal activity and has thus been termed a parasympatholytic drug.

Pharmacokinetics

The onset of action of atropine following IV, IM, and ET administration is rapid, with peak increases in heart rate occurring within 5 min. The half-life of atropine is 2 to 3 h. Well absorbed and distributed throughout the body, atropine is metabolized in the liver and excreted in the urine.

Indications

Atropine is the treatment of choice for increasing heart rate in hemodynamically unstable bradycardias (e.g., decreased heart rate with hypotension, altered mental status, "escape beats," and chest pain). Higher doses have been used in cardiac arrest, specifically, asystole and/or pulseless idioventricular rhythm.

Dosing and Administration

The dose of atropine for hemodynamically unstable bradycardias is 0.5 mg *rapid* IV push and repeated as necessary q 5 min until a desired heart rate is achieved. Two milligrams is considered the maximum vagolytic dose in most patients. Bolus doses of 1 mg can be given for asystole and repeated once if necessary. Atropine can be administered IV push, IM, and via the ET tube. If given via the ET tube with a preload syringe (1 mg/10mL), no dilution is necessary. However, if the 1 mg/mL ampoules are used dilution with 5 to 10 mL normal saline is necessary.

Adverse Effect Profile

Atropine is not indicated for bradycardia in hemodynamically stable patients. If administered, marked increases in heart rate can increase myocardial oxygen consumption, possibly inducing ischemia and precipitating ventricular tachyarrhythmias or ventricular fibrillation. This is particularly true in doses greater than 0.5 mg. Doses less than 0.4 mg along with a therapeutic dose administered slowly can cause paradoxical bradycardia. Other effects that may occur include anticholinergic symptoms (e.g., blurred vision, dry mouth, CNS stimulation, hallucinations, mydriasis, tachycardia).

Vasodilator Agents

Nitroglycerin

Actions

Although the mechanism of action of nitroglycerin is not fully understood, its therapeutic benefit appears to be due to its actions on the peripheral circulation and the coronary blood flow. Nitroglycerin is a direct vasodilator that induces venodilation at low doses (<100 μg/min) and arteriolar vasodilation at high doses (>200 μg/min). Coronary artery dilation occurs throughout the dosage range.

Pharmacokinetics

Table 12-4 describes the onset and duration of various nitroglycerin products. Nitroglycerin has a plasma half-life of 1 to 4 min and is metabolized in the liver. Oral doses undergo an extensive first-pass metabolism.

Indications

Nitroglycerin is approved for the prophylaxis, treatment, and management of angina pectoris. Intravenous nitroglycerin is used to control hypertension associated with surgery and is also used in CHF associated with acute myocardial infarction.

Table 12-4. Nitroglycerin Chart

Dosage Forms	Onset (min)	Duration of Action	Dosing and Administration
Sublingual	1–3	1–3 min	Dissolve 1 tablet under tongue; repeat q 5 min if no relief up to 3 times in 15 min.
Translingual spray	2	30–60 min	Apply 1–2 metered dose sprays onto oral mucosa up to 3 times in 15 min if no relief.
Transmucosal tablets	1–2	3–5 h	Place 1-mg tablet between lip and gum above incisors or between cheek and gum.
Sustained-release tablet	20–45	4–8 h	Start at 2.5–2.6 mg tid–qid and titrate upward (swallow capsules whole).
Topical ointment	20–60	2–12 h	Apply 1–2 in to chest wall q 4–8 h.
Transdermal patch	30–60	Up to 24 h	2.5–15 mg patches are available; start with low dose and titrate upward; apply to hair-free area and rotate sites.
IV infusion	1–2	3–5 min	Start at 5–10 μg/min; titrate in increments of 5–10 μg/min q 3–5 min to desired response; most doses range between 50 and 200 μg/min.

Dosing and Administration

Nitroglycerin can be administered sublingually, lingually, intrabuccally, orally, topically, or by IV infusion. The sublingual and intrabuccal tablets should not be swallowed, and the extended-release buccal tablets (transmucosal) should not be chewed or swallowed. Patients should be in a sitting position immediately following sublingual, lingual, or intrabuccal administration.

An IV infusion of nitroglycerin should be administered via a controlled-infusion device. Since data on the incompatibility of nitroglycerin with other parenteral agents are unclear, a separate IV site for a nitroglycerin infusion should be used. Infusions should not be suddenly discontinued, since abrupt withdrawal reactions (including angina pectoris or myocardial infarction) may result. Attempts should be made to gradually wean patients off the infusion.

Specific dosing regimens are shown in Table 12-4. The dose of nitroglycerin for each patient should be titrated to the individual response, using the smallest effective dose.

Adverse Effect Profile

Most adverse effects are related to the cardiovascular actions induced by nitroglycerin. These effects include headache, dizziness, weakness, syncope, flushing, hypotension, reflex tachycardia, and occasionally bradycardia. Use in patients concomittantly using alcohol may result in hypotension; hypotension has been shown to decrease the anticoagulant effects of heparin. Also, rash has been reported with topical nitroglycerin use.

Caution is advised when using nitroglycerin in patients who are hemodynamically unstable (including those patients who are volume depleted) or who have increased intracranial pressure or severe anemia. The drug should also be used cautiously in cases of constrictive pericarditis, pericardial tamponade, and hypertrophic cardiomyopathy. Also, there have been reports of brief increases in intraocular pressure with angle-closure or open glaucoma. Extended-release preparations of nitroglycerin should be avoided in patients with GI hypermotility or malabsorption syndromes.

Transdermal patches and topical ointment must be removed prior to attempting defibrillation or synchronized cardioversion. Topical nitroglycerin products alter electrical conductivity and enhance the potential for electrical arcing to occur. To avoid excessive dosing, topical products should also be removed if additional nitroglycerin is given for acute symptoms.

BIBLIOGRAPHY

American Hospital Formulary Service Drug Information 90. Bethesda, Md., American Society of Hospital Pharmacists, 1990.

DiMarco JP, Miles W, Akhtar M, et al: Adenosine for paroxysmal supraventricular tachycardia: Dose ranging and comparison with verapamil. *Ann Intern Med* 113:104, 1990.

Drugdex. Micromedex, Inc., Denver, September–November 1990 update.

Drug Facts and Comparisons. St. Louis, Lippincott, 1990.

Gilman AG, Goodman LS, Gilman A: *The Pharmacological Basis of Therapeutics*, 7th ed. New York, Macmillan, 1990.

Gonzalez ER, Ornato JP, Garnett AR, et al: Dose-dependent vasopressor response to epinephrine during CPR in human beings. *Ann Emerg Med* 18:920, 1989.

Knoben JE, Anderson PO: *Handbook of Clinical Drug Data*, 6th ed. Hamilton, Ill. Drug Intelligence Publications, 1989.

Ornato JP, Gonzalez ER: *Drug Therapy in Emergency Medicine*. New York, Churchill Livingstone, 1990.

Parker RB, McCollam PL: Adenosine in the episode treatment of paroxysmal supraventricular tachycardia. *Clin Pharmacol* 9:261, 1990.

Textbook of Advanced Cardiac Life Support, 2nd ed. American Heart Association, 1987.

13
LIFE-THREATENING SIGNS AND SYMPTOMS IN ADULTS

A. CHEST PAIN

J. Stephan Stapczynski

Chest pain is a common presenting complaint in the emergency department and represents a diagnostic challenge for several reasons: (1) there is always the possibility of heart disease in every complaint of chest pain or upper abdominal pain; (2) pain from visceral organs can be referred to a variety of locations on the chest or abdominal wall; (3) accurate diagnosis requires interpretation of the patient's subjective perception of pain; (4) the diagnosis is based primarily on the history obtained, a process which is subject to the preconceptions and biases of the examiner; and (5) physical findings and ancillary tests are often not helpful in the emergency department. Protocols and algorithms have been devised for the evaluation of acute chest pain. However, their widespread clinical applicability is limited by several factors: (1) the studies have concentrated on the identification of patients with acute myocardial infarction, generally ignoring other diagnoses, many of which are potentially lethal and require urgent hospital admission; (2) on the basis of statistics, these algorithms assign a probability to a given diagnosis, but this probability is difficult to apply to an individual patient; (3) even if the probability of a serious problem, such as acute myocardial infarction, is low, local practice standards and potential liability often necessitate hospital admission; and (4) absolute sensitivity is not possible with any protocol. Nonetheless, these studies have been immeasurably helpful in quantifying and redefining the role of history, physical examination, and ancillary studies in the assessment of acute chest pain.

The emergency physician's immediate concerns are the potentially life-threatening causes of acute chest pain: unstable angina, acute myocardial infarction (AMI), aortic dissection, pulmonary embolus, spontaneous pneumothorax, and esophageal rupture (Boerhaave's syndrome). If serious or potentially life-threatening causes of chest pain can be excluded, the patient can usually be discharged with further outpatient evaluation as needed.

An understanding of the physiological basis of pain perception is helpful in evaluating pain symptoms. When peripheral nerve endings are stimulated, pain is perceived by the brain and its location interpreted by the parietal cortex. There are two categories of pain sensation: somatic and visceral. Somatic sensation results from irritation of fine pain fibers in the dermis. These nerves enter the spinal cord at a single level. Because of the high concentration of these fibers in the skin and their exact mapping onto the parietal cortex, somatic pain is usually perceived as sharp, piercing, and precisely located. Visceral pain results from stimulation of pain fibers located in internal organs. These nerves enter the spinal cord at multiple adjacent cord levels along with somatic pain nerves. There are connections between visceral and somatic fibers, which is why visceral pain is felt on some parts of the body surface. Visceral pain is perceived when impulses from the internal organs and the resting potential from the somatic nerves summate in the spinal cord to reach a pain perception threshold level. This threshold is not reached and pain is not felt if the impulses of the somatic resting potential are blocked by subcutaneous local anesthesia. Visceral pain is less distinct, usually dull or aching in quality, and less precisely located. Visceral pain nerves from the thorax and upper abdomen enter the spinal cord at the level of T1 to T6.

A useful classification of chest pain is based on this distinction between somatic and visceral pain. Superficial chest wall pain is a somatic type of pain. It is usually described as sharp or piercing, can be precisely localized, and is exacerbated by palpation. Respiratory (or pleuritic) pain is a somatic type of pain, but its main characteristic is a distinct accentuation by respiratory motion. It is important to remember that more than the pleura moves with respiration. Deep visceral pain is usually dull, aching, or pressurelike, but its distinguishing characteristic is its poor localization anywhere within the T1 to T6 dermatome range.

TREATMENT PRIORITY

Patients with acute chest pain should be given evaluation and treatment priority; certain steps should be done even before a complete history and physical examination. A principle developed from the First Hour program of the American Heart Association is to approach every patient with acute chest pain as a possible AMI. The American College of Emergency Physicians has developed a clinical policy for the management of adult patients with nontraumatic chest pain that can be used as a guide to evaluation. Because of the potential for sudden deterioration, any patient in obvious distress and with abnormal vital signs or deep visceral pain should have oxygen administered, a cardiac monitor applied, and an intravenous line established as soon as possible. Obviously, such generalizations should be applied with common sense, but it is better to err on the side of caution.

INITIAL EVALUATION

History

A careful, accurate history is the most important tool in the diagnosis of chest pain. However, recent work has pointed out the many pitfalls involved in relying on isolated factors in the history. No one part of the history can stand by itself; accurate diagnosis requires a composite picture. It is important to remember that a patient may have more than one cause of pain—coronary artery disease and hiatal hernia with reflux are very common in the middle-aged population.

Onset and Duration

Typical angina pectoris is episodic, usually lasts between 5 and 15 min, is induced by exertion, and is relieved within 3 to 5 min by rest or sublingual nitroglycerin. Unstable angina may occur at rest (angina decubitus), last longer, and not be relieved as readily. Variant (Prinzmetal's) angina occurs without provocation, often at rest or at night, but is usually relieved with nitroglycerin. Patients with variant angina can usually exercise to a moderate degree without difficulty. The pain of AMI generally lasts longer than 15 to 30 min. Pain from myocardial ischemia typically builds up to reach its maximum, whereas pain from aortic dissection or pulmonary embolus is usually severe at onset. Pain from the esophagus may be described as either heartburn, odynophagia (painful swallowing), and/or a "spasm"-like pain. Heartburn is a burning sensation located in the sternal region, often with an epigastric component. Heartburn generally occurs within 15 to 60 min after eating, more likely after large meals. Certain body positions, such as bending or lying supine or on the left side, may precipitate heartburn. Odynophagia is felt as the bolus of food passes through the esophagus and may be described either as a burning pain as the bolus contracts an inflamed esophagus or as a severe short-lived pain as the bolus encounters a narrowing. Esophageal spasm is described as a dull pain felt in the central chest, lasting for seconds to several minutes. Practically speaking, it is often impossible to distinguish esophageal pain from cardiac pain. Up to one-third of patients with AMI or unstable angina have "heartburn" as a chief complaint. Chest wall pain may last for only seconds or be prolonged over hours. The key elements of chest wall pain are a positional component and local chest wall tenderness. However, it is easy to be misled by the finding of chest wall tenderness; Lee found that patients whose pain was either fully or partially reproduced by palpation had acute myocardial ischemia with an incidence of 7 and 24 percent, respectively.

Quality

Sharp, piercing, stabbing pain is typical of pain of musculoskeletal chest wall origin. One large study of patients with documented pulmonary emboli found that 74 percent had pleuritic chest pain and an additional 14 percent had nonpleuritic pain. In differentiating between the various etiologies of visceral chest pain, the quality of the pain is not helpful; patients with AMI can have a burning type of pain and patients with esophageal reflux can have a pressure type of pain.

Location and Radiation

The specific location of deep visceral pain within the T1 to T6 dermatome range cannot be relied upon as diagnostic, but certain locations are classic. Angina almost always has a retrosternal component, as do most other causes of deep visceral pain. Ischemic pain often radiates to the neck, shoulders, and down the inside of the left or both arms. Up to 70 percent of patients with AMI report radiation to the arms, shoulders, and/or neck. Patients with aortic dissection typically have radiation of the pain to the back and upper abdomen as the dissection progresses over time. Patients with esophageal reflux almost always have both retrosternal and epigastric pain. Pain from reflux infrequently radiates; in about 20 percent of cases it radiates to the back. Less commonly, in severe episodes, it radiates into the arms.

Relief of Symptoms

A clear history of relieving factors is helpful, but diagnostic tests in the emergency department are neither sensitive nor specific. As with any cause of pain, a number of patients with chest pain will respond to the "placebo nature" of a therapeutic trial. Studies have found that about three-fourths of patients with coronary artery disease respond to sublingual nitroglycerin with complete relief within 3 min, although there is also a high false-positive rate. When a patient with prior stable angina presents to the emergency department with acute chest pain, less than half respond to nitroglycerin. Up to 90 percent of patients with diffuse esophageal spasm report relief with nitroglycerin; almost half within 5 min. While 70 percent of patients with a prior history of esophageal reflux give a history of moderate to good relief with antacids, only 25 percent respond while in the emergency department with acute chest pain. Pain caused by acid infusion of the lower esophagus (Bernstein test) is not relieved by local anesthetics, suggesting that a positive response to oral viscous lidocaine should not be considered significant.

Symptoms Other than Chest Pain

Symptoms of dyspnea, diaphoresis, nausea, or vomiting are more common in myocardial ischemia than in other causes of chest pain. Fatigue, lethargy, and confusion are infrequent symptoms reported in AMI, but their incidence increases with age. In fact, the presentation of the elderly patient with AMI may be dominated by symptoms other than chest pain. In addition, patients with AMI may report several days of prodromal symptoms before presenting to the hospital. The multicenter chest pain studies have found that failure to consider accompanying symptoms is a major factor in the misdiagnosis of AMI.

PHYSICAL EXAMINATION

Observation of the patient is important. General signs of tachypnea, diaphoresis, cyanosis, or pallor are significant. The vital signs should be obtained and recorded. Tachycardia is nonspecific but should never be disregarded entirely. Blood pressure should be checked in both arms, as a systolic pressure difference greater than 20 mmHg suggests arterial obstruction to the arm with the lower value.

The chest wall should be palpated and areas of point tenderness noted. The key point here is to note whether palpation fully or partially reproduces the pain. However, this finding does not exclude myocardial ischemia. The apical impulse is usually a small area (less than 2 cm or 2 fingerwidths) at or medial to the midclavicular line. Lateral displacement or enlargement of the apical impulse indicates cardiomegaly.

The heart should be ausculated carefully for heart sounds, murmurs, and rubs. The loudness of the first heart sound is due to the vigor of mitral valve closure and left ventricular contraction. A soft S_1 indicates preclosure of the mitral valve (severe aortic regurgitation) or weak left ventricular contraction. The second heart sound has two components, the first and second components due to aortic and pulmonary valve closure, respectively. Splitting normally increases during inspiration. With advancing age, splitting narrows and many patients over 50 have a single S_2. Wide splitting is most commonly caused by a right bundle branch block but is occasionally heard when an inferior myocardial infarction affects the right ventricle. Fixed splitting is usually due to an atrial septal defect and, occasionally, to severe heart failure. Paradoxical splitting is most commonly due to a left bundle branch block, and, rarely, aortic stenosis, aortic regurgitation, and AMI. The third heart sound is caused by the sudden deceleration of blood flow from the atria into the ventricle when the limits of ventricular distensibility are approached. The fourth heart sound is caused by atrial contractions strong enough to distend the left ventricle and produce vibrations. Physiological S_3s or S_4s can be heard in normal or hyperactive hearts in patients under 40. Pathological S_3s are accompanied by symptoms and signs of heart failure. Pathological S_4s are seen when left ventricular compliance is reduced, as occurs with acute ischemia. The key to classifying murmurs is their timing: systolic ejection, holosystolic, late systolic, diastolic decrescendo, or diastolic rumble. Most elderly patients have systolic ejection murmurs due to degenerative changes in the aortic valve leaflets (aortic sclerosis).

ANCILLARY STUDIES

An ECG is one of many tools used in patient assessment. Besides providing evidence of myocardial ischemia or infarction, the ECG is also helpful in deciding whether (1) to admit patients to intensive care units as opposed to monitored step-down beds, and (2) to urgently administer thrombolytic therapy. From the risk management viewpoint, ECG results, while not the sole factor used to make a decision, must be part of the body of evidence considered by the physician. Therefore, an ECG should be done on all patients with acute chest pain, except for those with trivial chest wall pain. An ECG characteristic of ischemic changes (new Q waves, ST segment elevation, ST segment depression, or symmetrical T wave inversions) is helpful, but a normal ECG does not exclude myocardial ischemia. Only about half of patients with spontaneous angina have ECG changes. Depending on the study and its criteria for electrocardiographic abnormality, between 60 and 90 percent of patients ultimately diagnosed as sustaining an AMI have abnormalities on the initial ECG obtained in the emergency department (Table 13A-1). If the criteria for electrocardiographic abnormalities are made purposefully broad (i.e., including minor ST segment and T-wave changes along with preexisting abnormalities), the sensitivity of the initial ECG will be high but the specificity will be low. If the criteria are more strict (i.e., new Q waves, ST segment elevation, or ST segment depression with deep, symmetrical T-wave inversions), sensitivity will be lower but specificity will be higher. Another way to view the value of the initial ECG is to look at the positive predictive value of the various ECG patterns, specifically, what percentage of patients displaying this pattern will ultimately be diagnosed as sustaining an AMI. The positive predictive value of new Q waves or ST segment elevation is obviously high, while that of minor ST-T changes is low. Conversely, emergency patients with an entirely normal ECG are at low risk for AMI, especially when the clinical impression does not suggest coronary disease (risk of AMI is

Table 13A-1. Value of Clinical Impression, ECG, and Serum Creatinine Kinase in the Emergency Department Diagnosis of Acute Myocardial Infarction

	Approximate Sensitivity, %	Approximate Specificity, %	Approximate Positive Predictive Value, %*
Clinical impression	95	60	20–30
Initial ECG			
New Q waves or ST segment elevation	65	90	70–80†
Above or subendocardial ischemia	75	80	20–30†
Above or prior changes of ischemia or infarction	85	75	5–10†
Above or nonspecific ST-T changes	90	65	<5†
Serum creatinine kinase (CK)			
Elevated total CK	45	70	25
Elevated CK-MB (electrophoresis)	35	90	50
Elevated CK-MB‡ (immunochemical)			
Upon presentation	50	90	75
3 h after presentation	90	95	85

* Since predictive value is dependent on the incidence of disease in the population under study, these values are for an emergency department population of adults over 30 with a 20 to 30 percent incidence of acute myocardial infarction.

† This is the predictive value for this ECG pattern alone.

‡ CK-MB level rising with each measurement obtained every hour for 3 h *or* one level above upper limits of normal for the specific assay method.

less than 1 percent). Patients with a clinical impression suggestive of myocardial ischemia and admitted to the hospital despite a normal initial ECG have a 6 to 21 percent incidence of AMI by the time of hospital discharge. Therefore, a normal ECG does not exclude myocardial ischemia. The electrocardiographic changes of pericarditis progress through evolutionary changes over several days, and depending on the stage of the process, the ECG may either be normal, show nonspecific changes, or appear similar to myocardial infarction. Electrocardiographic changes of pulmonary embolus are usually nonspecific and rarely diagnostic. Acute pain from the upper gastrointestinal tract or hyperventilation may cause ECG changes, typically ST segment depressions and T-wave inversions.

Measurement of serum enzymes is genereally considered not helpful in establishing the diagnosis of AMI in the emergency department. In patients with AMI, 4 to 8 h is required before total serum creatinine kinase (CK) exceeds the upper limits of normal (Table 13A-1). Depending on the amount of time between the onset of symptoms and the sampling of blood, only half or less of patients with AMI have elevated total serum CK levels in the emergency department. Specificity is also low, since many causes of skeletal muscle injury elevate serum CK. The MB isoenzyme of CK (CK-MB) is highly specific for the myocardium, but serum CK-MB contributes less than 3 to 6 percent of total serum CK activity normally. Small increases of CK-MB due to an AMI can be obscured by the larger quantities of the other CK isoenzymes. Consequently, CK-MB is less sensitive but much more specific than total CK for the diagnosis of AMI.

The electrophoretic method used to measure serum CK-MB is relatively insensitive and requires time for the serum level to rise sufficiently above the background concentration before it can be reliably detected. Thus, electrophoresis cannot detect the slight elevations in serum CK-MB found when patients first present to the emergency department. New immunochemical assays have been developed that can detect minimal elevations of serum CK-MB. There are at least four commercially available products that can measure serum CK-MB within 10 min to 2 h of processing time. A recent study of these four methods in adults with nontraumatic chest pain and ECGs without diagnostic ischemic changes found that all methods had a sensitivity of about 50 percent for AMI upon emergency department presentation. With serial sampling every hour for 3 h, the sensitivity increased to over 90 percent. The potential benefits of early AMI detection include correct in-hospital admission decisions, prevention of discharge of AMI patients with nondiagnostic ECGs, and possible early administration of thrombolytic or anti-ischemic therapy. The value of these early immunochemical methods to detect serum CK-MB is currently undergoing a larger multicenter study. At the time of this writing, such methods are not routinely available in most community hospitals.

Most patients with acute chest pain have a normal chest x-ray or one with only incidental findings. In acute pulmonary embolus, various combinations of infiltrates, atelectasis, pleural effusions, focal oligemia, and/or lung volume loss is found in most patients. In aortic dissection, a widened mediastinum is seen in about 40 to 50 percent of cases. A more specific sign of aortic dissection is separation of greater than 4 to 5 mm between the intimal calcium and edge of the aortic silhouette in the region of the aortic knob; unfortunately, however, this is found in less than 10 percent of cases. The chest x-ray is usually required to substantiate the diagnosis of pneumothorax or pneumomediastinum. The chest x-ray may also provide unexpected information: hiatal hernia, gallstones, or pleural or lung parenchymal disease.

Soon after the onset of myocardial ischemia, muscle contraction is impaired and can be detected by echocardiography as wall motion abnormalities. Experimentally, hypokinesis, akinesis, or dyskinesis can be seen within a few heartbeats after coronary occlusion. In selected CCU patients, echocardiography has a sensitivity of over 70 percent in AMI, but it has not been as well studied in emergency patients, where the prevalence of AMI is lower and the value of echocardiography would be less. Echocardiography has a low sensitivity for patients with unstable angina who are pain-free at the time of the study.

Thallium-201 scanning performed within 6 h after the onset of chest pain was found to have a high sensitivity for AMI in small studies. Unfortunately, thallium scans are less sensitive in small or non-Q-wave infarctions, detect less than 50 percent of patients with unstable angina, and have a low specificity (around 80 percent). It would be expected that in emergency department patients with chest pain, where the prevalence of AMI is low, thallium scanning would not be useful. The limited studies to date seem to indicate that is true.

The usefulness of both echocardiography and thallium scanning is further limited by their lack of ability to distinguish new abnormalities from old. In most facilities, the technical expertise required, the added cost, and the limited availability of these ancillary tests on an urgent basis restrict their routine use in the emergency department.

DIAGNOSTIC DECISION AIDS

As mentioned before, several large studies have devised protocols or algorithms to help organize the clinical decision-making process and quantify the risk of myocardial ischemia or infarction in adult patients with acute chest pain. The major benefit of these decision aids has been to preserve sensitivity at a level about equal to that of the physician's judgment, while improving, to a degree, specificity; i.e., decreased admissions to the CCU of patients without ischemia or infarction. The overall accuracy therefore increases and fewer patients are admitted to high-cost ICUs. It is not clear if any available algorithm indicates when a patient can or should be discharged from the emergency department. For example, some protocols have at their lowest a 1 to 4 percent risk of AMI despite answers pointing away from myocardial ischemia at all the decision points. For a practicing physician, it is difficult to feel comfortable discharging a patient when the decision aid yields a risk of 1 to 4 percent for AMI. Thus, until the decision aids become more accurate, these algorithms will not easily become an accepted part of emergency practice.

MAJOR CAUSES OF CHEST PAIN

There are several groups of patients who may present with chest pain where a knowledge of the most common diagnoses may be helpful. Chest pain in children and adolescents is very unlikely to be cardiac in origin and is most often due to chest wall, respiratory tract, anxiety, or idiopathic causes. Patients with multiple unexplained symptoms often have chest pain as a presenting complaint, but they can usually be recognized by their vast number of multiple symptoms without any coherent pattern, negative physical findings, or history of multiple medical encounters. Elderly patients who develop AMI are more likely to present with either nonretrosternal chest pain or no pain compared with younger individuals. In addition, the elderly who sustain an AMI are more likely to present with nonspecific symptoms such as syncope, stroke, weakness, mental confusion, or nausea.

Angina Pectoris

Typical angina is episodic, lasts 5 to 15 min (rarely, longer than 20), is provoked and reproducible by exertion, and is relieved by rest or sublingual nitroglycerin (NTG), usually within 3 min. In over 90 percent of patients, the location is retrosternal and about 70 percent have radiation, usually to the neck, shoulders, or arms. In individual patients, the character of each attack varies little with recurrent episodes. With angina, it is very unusual for a patient to feel better when recumbent, although some patients may lie down initially for the rest, but usually find that they feel better while sitting quietly. As noted before, only about half of patients with spontaneous angina have ECG changes during the acute painful episode. In addition, ambulatory ECG monitoring has found ST segment changes of ischemia without chest pain (termed ''silent ischemia'') occurring in most patients with coronary disease, and in only about half of ischemic episodes so detected does the patient report chest pain.

Variant (Prinzmetal's) Angina

This form of angina occurs without provocation, often while the patient is at rest or during a similar time each day. With acute attacks, there is ST segment elevation on the ECG representing transmural myocardial ischemia. Variant angina is thought to be caused by spasm of the epicardial coronary arteries, either in normal vessels (about one-third of these patients) or in vessels with atherosclerotic lesions (about two-thirds). Attacks may be complicated by tachyarrhythmias, bundle branch block, or atrioventricular nodal blocks. Variant angina is usually relieved by sublingual NTG.

Unstable (Crescendo or Preinfarction) Angina

Unstable angina is the clinical syndrome between angina and AMI. The natural history of untreated unstable angina is a high early infarction and death rate. Modern medical therapy greatly reduces this risk, so it is very important to recognize and hospitalize these patients. Three subgroups are recognized as unstable angina: (1) angina of recent onset—4 to 8 weeks; (2) angina of changing character—becoming more frequent, severe, or resistant to nitroglycerin; and (3) angina at rest—angina decubitus. The latter two subgroups are at higher risk for early infarction and death. In unstable angina, the ECG may show nondiagnostic ST segment or T-wave changes and the serum CK and CK-MB levels may also have minor nondiagnostic elevations.

Acute Myocardial Infarction

Anginal pain that lasts longer than 15 min, is not relieved by nitroglycerin, or is accompanied by diaphoresis, dyspnea, nausea, or vomiting suggests an AMI. Longitudinal population studies indicate about 20 percent of myocardial infarctions are clinically unrecognized. Although there is not universal agreement, diabetics are felt to be more susceptible to ''silent'' infarctions. Because of the potential liability of missing the diagnosis of myocardial infarction, most physicians are conservative and hospitalize patients who present with any episode suggestive of myocardial ischemia; this accounts for the reported 87 to 98 percent sensitivity of clinical impression in AMI (Table 13A-1), but it also means that specificity is low and generally less than a third of such patients admitted do, indeed, have an acute infarction. However, the value of admission cannot be gauged by these numbers alone because it does not include those patients with unstable angina who had their infarction prevented by hospitalization and aggressive treatment.

Multicenter studies have found that up to 5 percent of patients with AMI are discharged from emergency departments, even from the best of hospitals. Aware that patients discharged with AMI appear to have a worse outcome than those who are admitted, the emergency physician faces a serious responsibility. When discharging patients with chest pain, careful discharge instructions should be given and routine 24-h follow-up should be strongly encouraged.

Aortic Dissection

The incidence of aortic dissection is about 1000-fold less than myocardial infarction, so, unfortunately, the diagnosis is seldom initially considered when a patient presents with chest pain. About 80 percent of patients are hypertensive men between the ages of 50 and 70 years. Abrupt onset of tearing chest or interscapular back pain is the most common symptom of aortic dissection. About 30 percent will present with focal or general neurologic signs. The incidence of other symptoms and signs varies according to whether the ascending and/or descending aorta is affected (Table 13A-2). Acute treatment requires emergent blood pressure control to prevent further dissection and rupture. Once the blood pressure is controlled, angiography is recommended to make an accurate diagnosis and plan for possible surgery.

Pericarditis

The pain of pericarditis is often acute, steady, and severe with a retrosternal location and radiation to the back, neck, or jaw. Pain may

Table 13A-2. Signs and Symptoms of Aortic Dissection

	Aortic Involvement, %	
	Ascending	**Descending**
Location of pain:		
Anterior	45	17
Back	5	28
Both	38	45
None	12	10
Systolic BP > 160 mmHg	30	55
History of hypertension	50	70
Aortic regurgitation	65	7
Heart failure	20	3
Alteration of peripheral pulses	65	10

Source: Dalen JE, Pape LA, Cohn LH, et al: Dissection of the aorta: Pathogenesis, diagnosis, and treatment. *Prog Cardiovasc Dis* 23:237, 1980. Used by permission.

be pronounced with each cardiac systole, chest motion, or respiration and is relieved by sitting up and leaning forward. If there is associated pleuritis (pleuropericarditis), pain may be predominantly pleuritic. The diagnosis of pericarditis is confirmed by the presence of a pericardial friction rub, which can have one to three components: presystolic, systolic, and early diastolic. However, rubs may be only intermittently detectable clinically. The ECG can show ST segment elevation or T-wave inversion depending upon the stage of the disease process; serial ECGs best illustrate these changes. A small pericardial effusion is often present but can only be detected by echocardiogram.

Other Cardiac Conditions

Hypertrophic cardiomyopathy (idiopathic hypertrophic subaortic stenosis) and valvular aortic stenosis may cause anginal pain, presumably because of inadequate blood supply to the hypertrophied myocardium. Mitral valve prolapse and mitral stenosis also have occasional chest pain. Generally, these disorders are not responsive to nitroglycerin.

Pulmonary Embolism

Pleuritic chest pain, tachypnea, and tachycardia are the most common symptoms and signs in pulmonary embolism. Some patients have nonpleuritic chest pain, and a musculoskeletal component of pain is common. Most patients with documented pulmonary emboli have either (1) a history of predisposing factors for venous thrombosis (immobilization, cancer, massive obesity, pregnancy, oral contraceptives); (2) a previous history of congestive heart failure, venous thrombosis, or pulmonary embolism; or (3) physical findings of deep venous thrombosis. Arterial blood analysis is frequently used in the assessment of these patients because a normal arterial P_{O_2} while breathing room air is commonly thought to exclude pulmonary embolism. However, studies have found that up to 20 percent of patients with documented pulmonary emboli are not hypoxemic while breathing room air. Recent studies indicate that the combination of a normal alveolar-arterial oxygen gradient $P(\text{A-a})_{O_2}$ adjusted for age and a normal arterial P_{CO_2} is unusual in pulmonary embolism, suggesting this can be used as evidence against that diagnosis. The major distinction is between acute viral-idiopathic pleurisy and acute pulmonary embolism; the first condition is usually self-limiting and benign, while the second can be recurrent and fatal. While most patients with pulmonary embolism have some chest x-ray abnormality, patients with pleurisy usually have a normal chest x-ray and only 10 to 15 percent have a pleural effusion.

Mediastinitis

Mediastinitis usually follows spontaneous or traumatic esophageal perforation and is characterized by retrosternal pain, fever, and leukocytosis. A chest x-ray may show widening of the mediastinum or mediastinal emphysema due to infection with gas-producing organisms. Severe substernal pain and an audible mediastinal crunch suggest this diagnosis.

Other Pleuropulmonary Disorders

A wide variety of pleuritic or pulmonary disorders can produce chest pain. Spontaneous pneumothorax usually presents with sudden onset of sharp pleuritic chest pain and dyspnea, but small pneumothoraces may produce relatively few symptoms and signs. Spontaneous pneumomediastinum usually produces sharp precordial pain, dyspnea, dysphagia, neck pain, and subcutaneous crepitus. Pneumomediastinum may occur during asthmatic exacerbations or from forced insufflation as, for example, seen with nasal inhalation of cocaine and other drugs. The mediastinal crunching sound (Hamman's sign) is found in about half of the cases. Although both spontaneous pneumothorax and pneumomediastinum are often benign and self-limited, a liberal policy of obtaining chest radiographs is required to detect these conditions when the air collection is small. Pneumonia or respiratory infections usually present with productive cough, fever, dyspnea, and pleuritic or constant chest pain. Patients with obstructive airways disease may develop chest pain during an acute excacerbation, usually overshadowed by the symptom of dyspnea. Particularly in the older patient with COPD, such pain should be investigated with an ECG and chest x-ray to avoid missing myocardial ischemia or a pneumothorax.

Esophageal Disorders

A variety of esophageal disorders, occurring singly or in combination, may cause acute chest pain: gastroesophageal reflux, hiatal hernia, achalasia, diffuse esophageal spasm, "nutcracker" esophagus, hypertensive lower esophageal sphincter, and nonspecific esophageal motility disorders. The following factors are most helpful in identifying an esophageal origin of pain: (1) frequent heartburn, (2) symptoms of acid regurgitation, (3) odynophagia, (4) globus sensation, (5) easy satiety after eating, (6) pain beginning several minutes after stopping exercise, (7) pain that continues as a background ache for hours, and (8) absence of lateral radiation of pain. In addition, patients with peptic ulcer disease, biliary tract disease, or pancreatitis may present with chest pain, so an epigastric component to the pain should always be sought.

Musculoskeletal Chest Pain

Musculoskeletal causes of chest pain were first appreciated in the 1920s. Several specific syndromes have been defined, and a few are briefly discussed below.

The *costernal syndrome* is localized to the parasternal costochondral junctions, usually affecting multiple sites, most often between the second and fifth junctions. Diffuse tenderness without swelling is the major physical sign. Pain may occur at rest and is frequently exacerbated by exercise, changes in body position, or other stresses imposed on the chest wall. The pain is of variable duration, lasting seconds to hours. The specific cause is unknown. Tietze's syndrome is pain and swelling of the costochondral junctions. Usually only a single site is affected, most often the second or third. Both the costernal and Tietze's syndromes are self-limited and treated with heat, antiinflammatory medications, analgesics, and rest.

The *slipping rib syndrome* is pain at the inferior costal margins of the eighth to tenth ribs. The inferior rib slips upward and overrides the superior rib, producing pain and an audible click.

The *precordial catch syndrome* presents with episodes of sharp, short, stabbing precordial pain in the anterior chest wall. The pains are relieved within minutes by shallow respiration and rest.

The *thoracic outlet syndrome* can cause chest, neck, and shoulder pain. A careful history usually elicits occasional paresthesias of the upper extremities. Tenderness is common in the supraclavicular fossa. Hyperabduction and external rotation of the arms can reproduce symptoms and diminish radial pulses. Elevation and exercise of both arms cause paresthesias and weakness in both hands.

Radicular pain, caused by osteoarthritis or other spondyloarthropathies, may present as chest pain. Dorsal root pain is typically sharp and piercing in character with superficial paresthesias, whereas ventral root pain is deep, dull, and boring. Symptoms are usually bilateral and may occur over any area of the chest, axilla, shoulders, or arms. Pain may occur with movement, coughing or sneezing (Déjerine's sign), or after prolonged recumbency.

Hyperventilation

Hyperventilation can cause chest pain with many different qualities and locations. There is generally an inconsistent relationship to the onset or cessation of exercise. Pain may last for hours or days with episodes of sharp, stabbing pain superimposed upon a constant, dull ache. Hyperventilation may be obvious with increased rate and depth of respirations or may be subtle with frequent sighs interposed on a normal ventilatory pattern. The ECG may have nonspecific ST-T changes. There is a poor correlation between subjective symptoms and objective manifestations in the hyperventilation syndrome; measurement of arterial P_{CO_2}, will show it to be lower than 35 torr in about 50 percernt of cases. The most helpful maneuver is the provocation test: carefully have the patient breathe 30 to 40 times per minute for 5 min, provide ECG monitoring, have the patient recognize the symptoms, and realize relief with bag breathing. It is important to recognize that hyperventilation may occur in response to more serious conditions such as pneumothorax, pulmonary embolism, or any entity which causes severe pain or dyspnea.

SUMMARY

Certain patients with chest pain have an indefinable look or attitude that suggests serious illness and they deserve priority for evaluation and treatment. Others, sometimes despite loud and repeated outcry, can be relegated to waiting because the physician or triage nurse is certain that their chest pain is not life-threatening. Physicians must rely on their analytical and interrogative skills to arrive at the diagnosis. A careful history and physical examination are the physician's most important tools. Ancillary tests may support the diagnosis but cannot be expected to exclude it. The diagnosis of myocardial ischemia or infarction should never be discounted simply because the ECG is normal or unchanged from previous tracings.

BIBLIOGRAPHY

ACEP. *Clinical Policy for Management of Adult Patients Presenting with a Chief Complaint of Chest Pain, with No History of Trauma.* Dallas, American College of Emergency Physicians, 1990.

Bell WR, Simon TL, Menets DL: The clinical features of submassive and massive pulmonary emboli. *Am J Med* 62:355, 1977.

Bennett JR: Oesophageal symptoms. *Clin Gastroenterol* 14:591, 1985.

Branch WT, McNeil BJ: Analysis of the differential diagnosis and assessment of pleuritic pain in young adults. *Am J Med* 75:671, 1983.

Cvitanic O, Marino PL: Improved use of arterial blood gas analysis in suspected pulmonary embolism. *Chest* 95:48, 1989.

Dalen JE, Pape LA, Cohn LH, et al: Dissection of the aorta: Pathogenesis, diagnosis, and treatment. *Prog Cardiovasc Dis* 23:237, 1980.

Davies HA, Jones DB, Rhodes J, et al: Angina-like esophageal pain: Differentiation from cardiac pain by history. *J. Clin Gastroenterol* 7:477, 1985.

Fam AG, Smythe HA: Musculoskeletal chest wall pain. *Can Med Assoc J* 133:379, 1985.

Gibler WB, Lewis LM, Erb RE, et al: Early detection of acute myocardial infarction in patients presenting with chest pain and nondiagnostic ECGs: Serial CK-MB sampling in the emergency department. *Ann Emerg Med* 19:1359, 1990.

Lee TH, Cook EF, Weisberg M, et al: Acute chest pain in the emergency department: Identification and examination of low-risk patients. *Arch Intern Med* 145:65, 1985.

Lee TH, Goldman L: Serum enzyme assays in the diagnosis of acute myocardial infarction: Recommendations based on a quantitative analysis. *Ann Intern Med* 105:221, 1986.

Lee TH, Rouan GW, Weisberg MC, et al: Clinical characteristics and natural history of patients with acute myocardial infarction sent home from the emergency room. *Am J Cardiol* 60:219, 1987.

Lee TH, Short LW, Brand DA, et al: Patients with acute chest pain who leave emergency departments against medical advice: Prevalence, clinical characteristics, and natural history. *J Gen Intern Med* 3:21, 1988.

Malliani A, Lombardi F: Consideration of the fundamental mechanisms eliciting cardiac pain. *Am Heart J* 103:575, 1982.

McCarthy BD, Wong JB, Selker HP: Detecting acute cardiac ischemia in the emergency department: A review of the literature. *J Gen Intern Med* 5:365, 1990.

Pantell RH, Goodman BW: Adolescent chest pain: A prospective study. *Pediatrics* 71:881, 1983.

Russell NJ, Pantin CFA, Emerson PA, et al: The role of chest radiography in patients presenting with anterior chest pain to the accident and emergency department. *J Roy Soc Med* 81:626, 1988.

Selbest SM: Chest pain in children. *Pediatrics* 75:1068, 1985.

Travel ME: Hyperventilation syndrome: Hiding behind pseudonyms? *Chest* 97:1285, 1990.

B. SHOCK

Steven C. Dronen
Patrick Birrer

Shock is a state of inadequate tissue perfusion occurring secondary to circulatory failure. The causes of circulatory failure include (1) hypovolemia, which occurs with severe hemorrhage or dehydration; (2) pump failure, which occurs in cardiogenic shock; (3) loss of vascular tone, which occurs with septic or neurogenic shock; and (4) obstruction of cardiac filling, which occurs with such disorders as cardiac tamponade, tension pneumothorax, and pulmonary embolus. This chapter reviews the pathophysiology common to the various etiologies of shock and then discusses the individual disorders and their management.

Pathophysiology

Irrespective of etiology, all forms of shock are associated with inadequate perfusion and delivery of metabolic substrates at the tissue, and ultimately the cellular, level. The hypoperfusion state triggers a cascade of complex compensatory responses involving almost every organ system. In the early stages of shock, compensation is geared toward maximizing cardiac output and preserving critical organ perfusion. Catecholamine release causes an increase in heart rate and contractility as well as constriction of venous capacitance vessels and arteriolar pre- and postcapillary sphincters. The net effect of these responses is an increase in preload and cardiac output and redistribution of blood flow away from noncritical organs, such as the skin, mesentery, and skeletal muscle.

In the later stages of shock, compensatory measures begin to fail. Blood pressure and cardiac output drop, and flow to vital organs becomes compromised. Changes that occur in the microcirculation further impede oxygen delivery to cells. Precapillary sphincters relax, while postcapillary sphincters remain intact. The result is stagnation of flow and sludging. Rheologic abnormalities further contribute to sludging. The laminar flow, in part due to the driving pressure propelling the blood, is altered. Shear stress, which is normally able to bend red blood cells, thus enhancing their flow through capillaries, is lost. The result is rouleaux formation and further stagnation of flow in the microcirculation.

The cell, which has been the benefactor of all the body's efforts at compensation, begins to show signs of altered function as compensatory measures fail. The first effects of shock involve the cell membrane. There is a decrease in the membrane potential as sodium enters the cell while potassium leaves it. Stimulation of the ATPase-dependent Na-K pump then occurs. Adenosine triphosphate (ATP) is utilized, and mitochondria are stimulated. Cellular cyclic adenosine monophosphate (cAMP) decreases, and the ATP level further decreases. As the energy supply deteriorates, more sodium enters the cell, and swelling occurs in the cell, the mitochondria, and the endoplasmic reticulum. Eventually, lysosomes leak and autolysis occurs. Several stages, characterized by morphologic changes, occur in the cell subjected to shock. The observed alterations are reversible until stage 5 is reached, at which point resuscitation is of no benefit (Table 13B-1).

As the supply of oxygen and energy substrates diminishes, the cells revert to anaerobic metabolism to generate ATP. This grossly inefficient pathway also results in the formation of lactic acid. The net effect is an intracellular acid buildup and, ultimately, systemic aci-

Table 13B-1. Morphologic Changes in the Cell Subjected to Shock

Stage	Normal
Stages 1a and 2	Swelling of cytoplasm and endoplasmic reticulum
Stage 3	Mitochondria shrink, inner compartment gets smaller and more dense
Stage 4	Mitochondrial swelling
Stage 5	Continued swelling of mitochondria, clumps of flocculent, dense material appear
Stage 6	Interruptions of cell membrane; lysosomes disappear
Stage 7	Cell becomes a mass of debris

demia. The acidosis has a depressant effect on myocardial contractility and vascular smooth muscle.

There appears to be a point of no return for individual cells as well as for the overall organism in shock. Although this point is well defined for the cell, the clinician caring for patients in shock is less able to identify this landmark. It has been suggested that a sudden and substantial decrease in oxygen consumption may be the marker of irreversible shock. Animal studies support this hypothesis, but clinical verification is not yet available.

The sum of all the natural compensatory measures called into action in shock is designed to preserve cellular perfusion and thus prevent death. In addition to hemodynamic compensation, a number of neuroendocrine responses are aimed at optimizing blood flow and delivering adequate nutrients to the cells. The hormonal response to shock is mediated primarily through the hypothalamus, which is indirectly responsible for the release of glucocorticoids, growth hormone, and aldosterone. These hormones, along with insulin and glucagon, ensure adequate supply and utilization of glucose by cells. Likewise, catecholamines elevate serum glucose in addition to their hemodynamic effects. Antidiuretic hormone (ADH), renin, and angiotensin release are also stimulated by shock. They have a salutary effect on hemodynamics and blood volume.

The role of the physician in the management of shock is to supplement the body's response to shock by providing supportive care and eradicating the cause of the shock state. In carrying out this role, it is helpful to monitor a number of parameters that measure hemodynamic function and provide a means of gauging patient response. Such obvious clinical parameters as mentation and urine output are important bedside indicators of vital organ perfusion. Other routine measurements, such as blood pressure, pulse, and pulse pressure, are of obvious clinical benefit in treating shock. More sophisticated measurements requiring invasive procedures can also be obtained. Other than the central venous pressure (CVP), these parameters are not often followed in the emergency department. They do, however, provide important information diagnostically and therapeutically for critically ill patients. These determinations, along with their derivations and normal values, are listed in Table 13B-2.

Table 13B-2. Additional Indicators of Vital Organ Perfusion

Parameter	Derivation	Normal Values
CVP	Measured	5–12 cm H_2O
PAP	Measured	9–19 mmHg
PAEDP	Measured	4–13 mmHg
PCWP	Measured	4.5–13 mmHg
MAP	DP + ⅓(SP − DP)	80–90 mmHg
CO	SV × HR	4–8 L/min
CI	CO/BSA	2.8–3.8 L/(m^2 per minute)
LVSW	SV × (MAP − PCWP) × .0136	60–130 g/m per beat
LVSWI	LVSW/BSA	40–80 g/m per m^2/beat
SVR	$\frac{(MAP - CVP) \times 80}{CO}$	800–1400 dyn/(s · cm^5)
SVRI	SVR × BSA	1600–2200 dyn/(s · cm^5 m^2)
PVR	$\frac{(MPA - PCWP) \times 80}{CO}$	100–300 dyn/(s · cm^5)
PVRI	PVR × BSA	200–450 dyn/(s · cm^5 m^2)
O_2 consumption	(CaO_2 − CVO_2) × CO × 10	150–300 mL/min
O_2 delivery	CaO_2 × CO × 10	800–1200 mL/min

Abbreviations: CVP, central venous pressure; PAP, mean pulmonary artery pressure; PAEDP, pulmonary artery end-diastolic pressure; CO, cardiac output; CI, cardiac index; MAP, mean arterial pressure; DP, diastolic pressure; SP, systolic pressure; LVSW, left ventricular stroke work; MPA, mean pulmonary artery pressure; LVSWI, left ventricular stroke work index; SVR, systemic vascular resistance; SVRI, systemic vascular resistance index; PVR, pulmonary vascular resistance; PVRI, pulmonary vascular resistance index; O_2 consumption, oxygen consumption; O_2 delivery, oxygen delivery; BSA, body surface area; SV, stroke volume.

HEMORRHAGIC SHOCK

Pathophysiology

Hemorrhagic shock is defined as a state of impaired tissue perfusion occurring secondary to acute blood loss. Conditions causing hemorrhagic shock include blunt and penetrating trauma, ruptured or dissecting aneurysms, gastrointestinal hemorrhage, ruptured ectopic pregnancy or ovarian cyst, massive vaginal bleeding, and retroperitoneal hemorrhage. In victims of trauma it is important to distinguish hypotension secondary to blood loss from hypotension secondary to impaired cardiac filling or contractility, which may occur with tension pneumothorax and pericardial tamponade. Typically, the latter group will have an elevated CVP, demonstrated clinically by distended external jugular veins.

Clinical Presentation

The signs and symptoms of hemorrhagic shock vary with the degree of blood loss and the underlying physical condition of the patient. Although it is commonly taught that a blood volume loss of up to 25 percent may occur without symptoms, it is more likely that subtle symptoms of early shock frequently go undetected. Early symptoms are in large part caused by catecholamine release and reflect physiologic compensatory mechanisms. Blood is shunted away from the skin and distal extremities, causing cool, clammy skin and delayed capillary refill. Cardiovascular compensation includes an increased heart rate and constriction of the capacitance vessels, resulting in a narrowing of the pulse pressure. The respiratory rate increases, as does the depth of respiration.

As shock progresses beyond the initial compensatory phase, the clinical manifestations become much more apparent. Hypotension, marked tachycardia, diminished peripheral pulses, pallor, tachypnea, agitation, and decreased urine output are characteristic findings of this stage. Finally, when death is imminent, the patient becomes lethargic or comatose, respirations become irregular or absent, and the blood pressure is unmeasurable by standard techniques.

Management

Major goals in the early management of hemorrhagic shock are (1) control of hemorrhage, (2) restoration of circulating blood volume, and (3) maintenance of oxygen delivery. The first goal may be easily accomplished if the hemorrhage is superficial and accessible to manual compression. Generally this is not the case, and surgical intervention will be required. Thus, the emergency management usually is focused upon restoration of circulation and rapid preparation for surgery. Equally important, but sometimes neglected, is maintenance of oxygen delivery. The latter can be maximized by the use of supplemental oxygen, timely intervention with tracheal intubation if hypoventilation is suspected, and the early use of blood transfusions.

The treatment of the hemorrhagic shock victim often begins in the field. In recent years the concept of field stabilization of trauma victims has been popularized despite the fact that the primary pathophysiologic event—blood loss—generally cannot be controlled or corrected in the field. The value of such common prehospital interventions as the application of the MAST suit and the infusion of intravenous fluids remains controversial. Based on anecdotal reports of efficacy, use of the MAST suit has become standard prehospital therapy over the past 15 years. While there is no doubt that application of the MAST suit often raises blood pressure, there is no evidence suggesting that small and transient increases in blood pressure improve outcome. Only recently have large clinical trials been conducted directly comparing outcome with and without the MAST suit. These trials have failed to demonstrate a beneficial effect, and therefore enthusiasm for use of the MAST suit has begun to wane.

Intravenous fluid therapy is standard hospital treatment of hemorrhagic shock, yet its value in the field is uncertain. Proponents of prehospital fluid therapy argue that skilled paramedics can place lines with minimal or no delay in transport and can infuse large volumes of saline solution prior to arrival in the emergency department. Opponents claim that delays in transport occur commonly and that fluid infusion cannot keep pace with the bleed rate in severe hemorrhage. At the present time there is insufficient evidence for either position. It is likely that prehospital fluid therapy does not affect outcome in the vast majority of cases, but it may be valuable given a specific combination of hemorrhage severity and distance from the hospital. Until conclusive data for a particular position can be obtained, it is reasonable to place intravenous lines once en route to the hospital whenever possible. This practice avoids potentially lethal delays in the field and grants the patients the potential benefits of prehospital fluid therapy.

Emergency department management of the hemorrhagic shock victim begins with a rapid assessment of the adequacy of ventilation and circulation. Specific items to be assessed include patency of the airway, rate and depth of respirations, level of consciousness, skin color and temperature, pulse rate and amplitude, and blood pressure. During this brief examination, two or more large-bore intravenous lines should be started. As the lines are started, blood samples should be drawn for type and cross matching, a complete blood count (CBC), prothrombin time (PT), partial thromboplastin time (PTT), and a platelet count. Continuous monitoring of the hemorrhagic shock victim is essential. Although cardiac monitoring is commonly used, it provides relatively little useful information. It is far more valuable to monitor parameters that reflect adequacy of perfusion, oxygen delivery, and volume status, such as blood pressure, CVP, urine output, and noninvasive oximetry measurements.

The amount and type of volume expander used depends primarily on the clinical status of the patient and to a lesser extent on individual or institutional preference. In most hospitals, isotonic saline solutions (0.9% NaCl or Ringer's lactate) are the agents of choice for the initial management of acute hemorrhage. In the compensated shock patient, isotonic saline solution should be rapidly infused. If the patient continues to show signs of impaired perfusion after a total of 30 mL/kg, it is likely that blood loss exceeds 15 percent of the total blood volume. At this point, it is appropriate to begin red blood cell transfusions, particularly if blood loss has not been controlled. In this situation it is usually possible to wait for fully cross-matched blood, but that decision must be individualized based on the assessment of ongoing blood loss and the efficiency of the local blood bank in performing cross matches. When in doubt, it is advisable to use type-specific blood. Several studies have shown this to be a very safe practice, and delays in providing needed oxygen-carrying capacity are potentially more harmful to the patient.

More aggressive therapy is mandated in the uncompensated shock patient. These patients almost always require blood transfusions, and it is appropriate to begin type-specific blood early unless there is a prompt and steady improvement in perfusion with saline solution alone. Administration of large volumes of saline solution to patients who have sustained major blood loss has become a commonplace activity in recent years, as devices have been developed that facilitate rapid fluid infusion. The appropriateness of this therapy is unproven. Aggressive saline infusion may result in profound dilution of the remaining red blood cell mass as well as platelets and coagulation factors. Volume restored at the expense of oxygen-carrying capacity is of questionable therapeutic value, and therefore type-specific blood should be given in conjunction with asanguinous fluids.

The moribund patient requires even more prompt restoration of circulating red blood cell mass. In this case, type O blood should be used if it is available. Type O Rh negative blood should be given to females of childbearing age. In most other situations type O Rh positive blood is preferred because of its greater availability. A type and cross match should always be drawn before administration of type O blood. Autologous whole blood may also be given to these patients if the hemorrhage is intrathoracic or intraabdominal (without fecal contamination) and the capabilities for autotransfusion exist.

Although isotonic saline solution is most commonly used in the initial management of hemorrhagic shock, debate continues over the fluid of choice (crystalloid vs. colloid). Albumin has recently fallen into disfavor, but purified protein fraction (PPF) and fresh frozen plasma (FFP) continue to be recommended and used. Central to the issue are the effects of fluid resuscitation on the pulmonary interstitium. Proponents of protein replacement argue that saline resuscitation of hemorrhage results in a fall in intravascular oncotic pressure and a reversal of the normal gradient favoring intravascular fluid retention. Theoretically, this may lead to pulmonary edema and impaired tissue oxygenation. Colloid administration is advocated because it raises oncotic pressure in the pulmonary capillary bed. This argument ignores the fact that the pulmonary capillary endothelium permits considerable flow of fluids, including plasma proteins, between the capillaries and the interstitium. A fall in intravascular oncotic pressure is compensated for by a fall in pulmonary interstitial oncotic pressure, thereby minimizing changes in the pressure gradient. It appears likely that pulmonary capillary hydrostatic pressure (measured as pulmonary artery wedge pressure) is far more important than pulmonary capillary oncotic pressure in determining the amount of fluid flowing to the interstitium. Maintenance of the wedge pressure below 15 mmHg is probably the most important factor in preventing pulmonary edema. To date, there are few data to show that colloids are harmful, but the inability to convincingly demonstrate beneficial effects in scores of animal and clinical studies suggests that benefits are minimal. Clinicians inclined to use albumin, PPF, or FFP in the resuscitation of hemorrhagic shock should question whether the undocumented benefits of this therapy are worth the substantial increase in cost or, in the case of FFP, the risk of disease transmission.

Alternatives to the use of naturally occurring colloid preparations include synthetic colloid solutions such as hydroxyethyl starch (HES) and dextran 70. The volume-expanding properties of HES are equivalent to those of 5% albumin. HES differs significantly from albumin, however, in that it remains predominately in the intravascular space because of its high molecular weight. Interstitial edema is not a concern, as it is with albumin. Furthermore, the plasma-expanding effects of HES are more prolonged than those of albumin.

The volume-expanding properties of dextran 70 are slightly better than those of 5% albumin. Like HES, dextran remains predominately in the intravascular space because of its large, highly branched molecular structure. Interstitial edema is not a concern with dextran, as it is with albumin.

Another potential resuscitation agent that has shown considerable promise in animal studies is 7.5% hypertonic saline solution used in conjunction with dextran 70 (HTS/Dex). Numerous studies have demonstrated prompt and dramatic improvements in cardiac output and vital organ perfusion following the administration of a small bolus (3 to 5 mL/kg) of HTS/Dex during hemorrhagic shock. Clinically significantly hypernatremia is uncommon. If human studies demonstrate a comparable response, this agent is likely to become important for the prehospital resuscitation of severe shock.

CARDIOGENIC SHOCK

Pathophysiology

Cardiogenic shock is a clinical syndrome of hypotension with evidence of compromised perfusion in the presence of an acute myocardial infarction. Although the syndrome may develop on the basis of myocardial trauma, it is almost exclusively due to coronary atherosclerosis. Of all patients admitted with acute myocardial infarction, 10 to 15 percent develop cardiogenic shock. Autopsies of patients dying of cardiogenic shock demonstrate infarction of 35 to 75 percent of their left ventricle. It is generally agreed that 40 percent of the left ventricular myocardium must be damaged before shock develops. It has also been determined that all patients dying of the symptoms have apical involvement and that 84 percent have severe disease of the left anterior descending coronary artery. The majority of patients who develop cardiogenic shock have had a previous infarction, but some patients do present in shock with their first infarction. A small percentage of these patients do so as a result of mechanical complications of an infarction (papillary muscle dysfunction or rupture, intraventricular septum rupture, or rupture of the ventricular wall with tamponade). The majority of victims, however, develop cardiogenic shock as a result of massive myocardial necrosis. Additional uncommon causes of cardiogenic shock include right ventricular infarction, myocarditis, and cardiomyopathy. Despite aggressive therapy, cardiogenic shock still has a mortality rate in excess of 80 percent.

When 40 percent of the left ventricle is infarcted, its function is compromised to the extent that arterial pressure cannot be maintained. In this case, the normal compensatory measures mediated by the autonomic nervous system and circulating catecholamines can be deleterious. Increased peripheral vascular resistance increases afterload and thus the oxygen demand of the ventricle. Reflex tachycardia likewise increases oxygen demand. Venoconstriction results in an increased preload, further accentuating failure. A vicious cycle is thus established. Increased oxygen demand results in increased damage and less functioning myocardium. Blood pressure and cardiac output continue to fall. When mean arterial pressure falls below 70, coronary perfusion is inadequate, which further extends the area of infarction.

Clinical Presentation

The clinical presentation of cardiogenic shock depends on the degree to which the patient has decompensated. Patients may present with little evidence of compromise, only to deteriorate rapidly and expire while still in the emergency department. The clinical picture of cardiac decompensation includes hypotension (blood pressure less than 90 or a decrease of 80 mmHg in a normally hypertensive patient); cool, diaphoretic skin; cyanosis; dyspnea; clouded sensorium; and a decreased urine output. Pulmonary edema is usually evident on chest examination. Right ventricular infarction is suggested by hypotension with an elevated jugular venous pressure and electrocardiographic evidence of an inferior infarction in a patient who is not in congestive failure.

Management

The management of cardiogenic shock is aimed at myocardial preservation, supportive care, and acute interventions such as thrombolytic therapy and angioplasty.

A typical infarct consists of an area of necrosis intermingled with and surrounded by an ischemic zone. Treatment is directed to the ischemic area, which is functioning suboptimally and thereby contributing to the pump failure. Therapy is aimed at reducing myocardial oxygen use and improving its supply. Oxygen demand is minimized by preventing and correcting arrhythmias and by decreasing afterload and adjusting preload as needed. At this time, thrombolytic therapy is not generally used in the patient who is already in cardiogenic shock, even if the patient meets the other suggested criteria for its administration. Any additional interventions (e.g., use of a vasopressor) must be carefully chosen so as not to adversely affect this delicate balance of oxygen supply and demand.

The specifics of treatment depend on the severity of the patient's condition and the availability of invasive monitoring. Optimally, care should be guided by intraarterial blood pressure monitoring and Swan-Ganz catheter measurements. Without knowledge of left-sided heart pressures and cardiac output, treatment is empiric and may even be detrimental. Unfortunately, these monitoring lines are seldom inserted in the emergency department. Consequently, the emergency physician is often faced with choosing between transferring an unstable patient to an intensive care unit, taking the time to insert the lines, or treating empirically. The choice is dependent on physician experience, the availability of equipment, and to some extent institutional practice. Often the critical condition of the patient supervenes, mandating immediate intervention without benefit of sophisticated monitoring.

When it is necessary to treat empirically, the focus should be on airway maintenance and blood pressure support. High-flow oxygen should be supplied by a nonrebreather mask and the patient monitored by continuous pulse oximetry. An initial arterial blood gas determination should be obtained. Persistent cyanosis, fatigue, or deterioration in mental status are all indicators for intubation. Hypotension should be treated with small boluses of fluid, such as 150 to 200 mL of normal saline solution. About 20 percent of patients in cardiogenic shock have low or normal left ventricular end-diastolic pressure (LVEDP). A third of these respond to volume expansion, providing the rationale for a fluid bolus. If the blood pressure does not respond to fluid, a vasopressor should be started.

The best vasopressor for cardiogenic shock is somewhat controversial. Dopamine is a frequently used mixed inotrope and pressor agent that causes a prompt elevation of blood pressure and preserves renal and mesenteric blood flow. Its effects are primarily β adrenergic at low doses (5 to 10 μg/kg per min) and α adrenergic at high doses (10 to 15 μg/kg per min or greater). Although dopamine may cause a reflex tachycardia that increases myocardial oxygen consumption, prudent use can augment renal blood flow, perfusion, and cardiac output in shock states with low or normal peripheral vascular resistance.

Dobutamine is a β_1 agonist without α-adrenergic activity. It does not enhance sinus node automaticity as much as dopamine, and only modest increases in pulse rate are seen at doses less than 20 μg/kg per min. Dobutamine's primary effect is an augmentation of cardiac contractility and stroke volume. In addition, dobutamine causes a modest decrease in systemic vascular resistance. The net effect is a dose-related increase in cardiac output and a decreased pulmonary capillary wedge pressure. Because heart rate and afterload are not increased, there is little increase in myocardial oxygen demand. Enhanced emptying results in a decreased LVEDP and an improved gradient over the coronary vascular bed. When hypotension is severe, this effect may be a disadvantage in that coronary perfusion is not improved. Many authorities recommend dobutamine as the vasopressor of choice in cardiogenic shock. Dobutamine is a good drug to use in the setting of myocardial infarction with cardiogenic shock, particularly if the peripheral vascular resistance is high and the patient is tachycardic. The usual dose range of dobutamine is 2.5 to 15 μg/kg per min. The combined use of dopamine and dobutamine may be helpful, however, if the blood pressure is not improved by dobutamine alone.

Additional drugs that can be selectively applied include morphine, loop diuretics, and vasodilators. All of these drugs can produce adverse hemodynamic effects and should be used cautiously, preferably while monitoring left-sided heart pressures. Morphine's analgesic and anxiolytic effects reduce tachycardia, and its vascular effects decrease afterload and preload. Furosemide also decreases preload by causing venodilatation and initiating a diuresis. Potent vasodilators such as nitroprusside can be used in conjunction with a vasopressor to enhance cardiac output. Extreme caution and meticulous monitoring of all pressures are essential prerequisites to vasodilator therapy. Amrinone is an inotropic agent that increases cardiac contractility and promotes peripheral vasodilatation. It has been successfully used in patients with congestive heart failure refractory to other pharmacologic maneuvers. Amrinone is generally not available in most emergency departments, but as experience with the drug grows it may prove useful to the emergency physician. Esmolol is a short-acting β_1-adrenergic blocking agent that can be used to slow a noncompensatory sinus tachycardia in the setting of an acute myocardial infarction. Small doses of propranolol are equally appropriate in such a scenario.

If a Swan-Ganz catheter can be inserted, treatment can be more precisely tailored to the individual patient. A fluid bolus should be administered only if wedge pressures are low or normal. Optimal filling pressures in cardiogenic shock are 18 to 24 cm H_2O. The wedge pressure should be brought to this range through incremental infusion of crystalloid. Additional interventions are added as outlined above, depending on patient response and pressure measurements.

The Swan-Ganz measurements can also be used prognostically. Patients have been categorized on the basis of their cardiac index and indirect measurement of the pulmonary artery end-diastolic pressure (PAEDP; Table 13B-3). Four groups of patients, whose mortality ranges from 13 to 100 percent have been identified.

If pharmacologic therapy does not achieve satisfactory hemodynamic improvement, counterpulsation with an aortic balloon pump may prove beneficial. The balloon pump is particularly helpful as a temporizing measure in patients requiring surgical correction of an anatomic defect such as a ruptured papillary muscle. Its application in shock due to infarction is less clear-cut. A minority of authors feel that prolonged balloon support (up to 3 weeks) may be necessary and successful in allowing ischemic myocardium to heal. Most authorities argue that such an approach is unrewarding. The role of early angiography and coronary bypass of diseased vessels supplying ischemic myocardium is also unclear. Some surgeons report excellent short- and long-term survival if bypass is accomplished within 18 h of infarction. These good results are attributed to salvage of reversibly ischemic myocardial tissue. Therapeutic recommendations are further complicated by reports of successful management of cardiogenic shock by streptokinase with or without angioplasty.

In summary, the management of cardiogenic shock continues to evolve. The primary role of the emergency physician is prompt recognition of the syndrome, especially when it is caused by anatomic defects or right ventricular infarction. Diagnosis is followed by supportive measures aimed at enhancing myocardial salvage. Unless patient deterioration mandates it, specific treatment is best handled in an intensive care unit with invasive monitoring. Because of the high mortality of pharmacologic management alone, early surgical consultation should be obtained and therapy such as aortic balloon counterpulsation considered. The role and timing of surgical intervention (or thrombolysis and angioplasty) after angiography remains poorly defined.

Table 13B-3. Additional Parameters Providing Diagnostic and Prognostic Information

Group	PAEDP, mmHg	CI, L/m² per Minute	Mortality, %
I	>29		100
II	<29 + >15	<2	92
III	<15	<2	63
IV	<29	>2	13

Abbreviations: PAEDP, pulmonary artery end-diastolic pressure; CI, cardiac index.

SEPTIC SHOCK

Pathophysiology

Septic shock is a form of distributive shock in that blood volume is dispersed into a greatly dilated peripheral circulation. Other causes of such a maldistribution of circulating blood volume include anaphylaxis, spinal cord injury, and vasovagal reactions. This section will concentrate on the more common, and usually more serious, septic shock.

Septic shock is caused by bacteria and their products circulating in the blood. Although both gram-positive and gram-negative organisms are capable of producing shock, the gram-negative bacteria, and in particular gram-negative rods, are by far the most common etiologic agents. The bulk of this section will therefore deal with gram-negative rod bacteremia and the resultant shock that occurs in approximately 40 percent of cases.

Although the importance of gram-negative bacteremia has been appreciated since the early 1950s, it remains a very serious disease, with a mortality of 25 percent. If shock complicates the picture, the mortality is variously stated as 35 to 50 percent. Since the 1950s there has been a steady increase in the incidence of this syndrome, and it now has a prevalence of 12.75 cases per 1000 hospital admissions. This translates into an annual incidence of 330,000 cases. The syndrome occurs in all age groups but is more common in the elderly, with a peak incidence during the seventh decade of life. Several factors can predispose an individual to gram-negative bacteremia, including immunocompromise from chemotherapy or immunosuppressant drugs; underlying malignancy; autoimmune diseases; genitourinary tract manipulations; and respiratory tract manipulations, including tracheostomy and biopsy. Postsplenectomy patients are also at increased risk for gram-negative sepsis. The most common organism in postsplenectomy sepsis is *Streptococcus pneumoniae,* but the syndrome is also caused by a number of other organisms, including *Escherichia coli* and *Pseudomonas* species. The most common source of infection resulting in gram-negative bacteremia is the urinary tract, which accounts for 34 percent of cases. The next largest source of infection is the unknown category, which makes up 30 percent of all cases. Sources of bacteremia and their incidences are listed in Table 13B-4.

Infections arising in the biliary, genitourinary, and other sites result in a more benign course (mortality 15 percent). This figure contrasts with a mortality rate of 30 percent when the source of infection is in the respiratory or gastrointestinal tract or when the source is unknown. As mentioned, underlying disease predisposes one to bacteremia; it also results in a higher mortality resulting from bacteremia. Underlying diseases are categorized as rapidly fatal, ultimately fatal, or nonfatal. The mortality rates of gram-negative bacteremia in these three groups are 40, 31, and 15 percent, respectively.

The infecting organism in gram-negative bacteremia is most often *E. coli,* which causes 31 percent of all cases. Many other gram-negative organisms can result in bacteremia and shock. The more common of these are listed in Table 13B-5.

Most feel that the pathophysiologic effects of septic shock are due to endotoxin. Endotoxin is a lipopolysaccharide in the cell wall of gram-negative rods. Endotoxins have three component parts: oligo-

Table 13B-4. Sources and Incidence of Bacteremia

Source of Infection	Incidence, %
Urinary tract	34
Unknown	30
GI tract	14
Respiratory tract	9
Skin and soft tissue	7
Other	3
Biliary tract	2
Reproductive system	1

Table 13B-5. Organisms Causing Gram-Negative Bacteremia

Source	Percentage
E. coli	31
Klebsiella pneumoniae	12
Pseudomonas spp.	10
Enterobacter spp.	8
Proteus and *Providencia*	8
Bacteroides spp.	7
Other gram-negative bacilli	6
Serratia marcescens	2
More than one species	16

saccharide side chains; a core polysaccharide; and lipid A, which is responsible for the toxic effects of endotoxins. The side chains vary from species to species, whereas the core polysaccharide–lipid A complex is relatively constant regardless of bacterial species.

Experimental endotoxin shock may not be identical to gram-negative bacteremic shock, but striking similarities are present. Fever, shock, disseminated intravascular coagulation (DIC), complement activation, and transient leukopenia followed by leukocytosis are features of both entities. With such evidence, it is hard to refute an important if not a primary role of endotoxin in producing the symptoms of septic shock.

Precisely how the bacteria or their endotoxins result in the clinical picture of septic shock is not known. The complexity of the primary and secondary effects of bacteremia makes it difficult to arrive at a simple unifying theory. However, some of the pathophysiologic mechanisms have been demonstrated.

At the cellular level there is evidence of impaired energy utilization. Animal studies have documented a reduced transmembrane potential with concomitant increase in cellular Na, Cl, and water, presumably due to failure of the Na-K pump. A similar situation exists in severe hemorrhagic shock, in which these changes are due to an exhaustion of ATP supply. In endotoxic shock, even just prior to death, cellular ATP levels are normal. This finding suggests the possibility of inhibition of ATPase, the enzyme needed to utilize ATP for the Na-K pump.

In addition to impaired energy utilization, there is also evidence of faulty cellular ATP production via the Krebs cycle in septic shock. This suboptimal energy production is reflected in a decreased oxygen consumption, which is seen in the early phases of septic shock. In late septic shock, mitochondrial damage and ultimately cell autolysis are due to impaired oxygen delivery and subsequent cellular acidosis.

On a more macroscopic level, a pathophysiologic theory has been put forth based on simultaneous stimulation of fibrinolysis and activation of the intrinsic clotting system. The theory postulates complex alterations and interactions between the coagulation, fibrinolytic, kinin, and complement systems. The entire process starts with the activation of Hageman factor (factor XII) by endotoxin. Activated Hageman factor activates the intrinsic clotting system and converts plasminogen to plasmin. Plasmin stimulates fibrinolysis and also digests activated Hageman factor. Fragments of the Hageman factor then activate the kinin system, resulting in bradykinin release (a potent vasodilator). Finally, the complement system is activated both by gram-negative bacteria directly and by plasmin. Complement activation results in the production of anaphylatoxin, chemotactic factors, and histamine. The net result of complement activation is an increased capillary permeability.

Hence, many of the clinical findings of septic shock, including hypotension, vasodilation, transudation of fluid across capillary membranes, and DIC, can be explained by this theory. The theory is not without experimental support. Clinical studies have documented Hageman factor activation, bradykinin production and release, and depletion of the third component of complement in gram-negative bacteremia.

There is also evidence to suggest that endotoxin can alter the microcirculation, resulting in fluid loss across capillary membranes. Such studies have demonstrated endothelial cell thickening and red blood cell extravasation after infusion of endotoxin. It is postulated that capillary leak results from endothelial cell hydration and swelling, which produce gaps between cells.

Other factors that may contribute to the pathophysiology of septic shock include endorphins, vasopressin, prostaglandins, and myocardial depression. β Endorphins are endogenous opiates secreted by the same cells in the hypothalamus that secret ACTH. Hence, any stimulus, such as shock, that causes ACTH release will also cause β endorphin release. Opiates can cause hypotension through myocardial depression and lowered peripheral vascular resistance. The hypotensive effects of endogenous opiates may therefore contribute to the clinical picture of septic shock. The trend toward reversal of hypotension by naloxone, particularly in early septic shock, lends support to the theory that β endorphins may partially mediate the hypotension of septic shock.

Recent studies have documented very high levels of vasopressin during septic shock. Previous investigations have demonstrated that vasopressin causes intestinal smooth muscle constriction, vasoconstriction, reduced superior mesenteric artery flow, and myocardial depression. Again, some of these effects may contribute to the signs and symptoms of septic shock.

There is growing evidence that prostaglandins may play a role in the pathophysiology of septic shock. Thromboxane A_2 (TXA_2) is a potent vasoconstrictor and platelet aggregator, while prostacyclin (PGI_2) causes vasodilatation and prevents platelet aggregation. These combined effects may result in pulmonary hypertension, systemic hypotension, and DIC, all of which can be seen in septic shock.

Prostaglandins are formed from arachidonic acid by the enzyme cyclooxygenase. Several studies have shown that both TXA_2 and PGI_2 are elevated in septic shock. These studies have shown that administration of indomethacin, which inhibits cyclooxygenase, prevents these elevations. Likewise, those animals pretreated with indomethacin or given indomethacin after the onset of shock have less hypotension and an improved survival compared to controls. Other studies confirm the deleterious effect of thromboxane but show no increase in PGI_2 levels and, in fact, document a beneficial effect from administering PGI_2. Even though the data conflict, it is apparent that at least one prostaglandin contributes to the pathophysiology of septic shock. Future treatment of this disease may therefore include inhibition of prostaglandin formation.

The cardiovascular changes in septic shock include a hyperdynamic state with a depressed and dilated left ventricle. A myocardial depressant factor is thought to be at least partially responsible for the decreased myocardial contractility demonstrated during septic shock. This myocardial depressant factor is probably carried on the endotoxin.

Clinical Presentation

Typically, the clinical features of septic shock can be divided into two phases. In the early phase, vasodilatation predominates; patients are warm, flushed, and hyperdynamic, usually with a normal or elevated cardiac output. Agitation or confusion is frequently present, as is temperature elevation or lowering and hyperventilation. At this stage, hypotension may not be present, depending on the degree of compensation.

In the late phase of this syndrome, a more typical shock state prevails. Peripheral perfusion and vital organ perfusion are impaired. In its most severe form, patients are obtunded, urine output is reduced, cardiac output and blood pressure are diminished, and peripheral vasoconstriction is apparent. There may also be signs of severe DIC, including spontaneous ecchymosis or frank bleeding.

The foregoing description represents a typical presentation and course of septic shock. Unfortunately, when first seen, the patient may be anywhere in this course or may present in an atypical fashion. Less typical presentations of septic shock include fever alone, unexplained respiratory alkalosis, confusion, metabolic acidosis, or hypotension. The elderly or debilitated are more likely to have atypical presentations.

In addition to the history and physical examination, laboratory data are helpful in establishing the diagnosis of septic shock. Transient, initial leukopenia followed by leukocytosis with a leftward shift is the rule with bacteremia. The degree of leukocytosis is variable.

Arterial blood gases may reflect a respiratory alkalosis initially due to a central stimulation of the respiratory center. As shock develops, lactic acidosis ensues as a result of inadequate tissue perfusion and a reversion to anaerobic metabolism.

Coagulation defects are common in the setting of gram-negative bacteremia. In a retrospective review of 222 patients, some defect was observed in 64 percent of the patients. These defects can be divided into three groups: thrombocytopenia, DIC, and other defects with or without thrombocytopenia. Thrombocytopenia alone or with other defects occurred in 56 percent of the patients. The converse, other defects with or without thrombocytopenia, was seen in 31 percent of the patients. Although DIC was seen in 11 percent of patients, only 3 percent had clinical evidence of bleeding. Other studies have reported a 5-percent incidence of DIC in gram-negative bacteremia. The incidence of coagulation defects has been found to be higher in patients with rapidly fatal underlying disease. A higher incidence of shock and death has also been demonstrated in patients with coagulation defects compared to those with no defects. Likewise, patients with DIC more often had shock or a fatal outcome than did patients with other coagulation defects.

Blood cultures are the ultimate method by which bacteremia is confirmed. Unfortunately, blood cultures are not positive 100 percent of the time in bacteremia, suggesting that some cases may escape identification by blood culture. In one review, 69 percent of the 1258 cultures obtained from 404 patients were positive.

The technique of culture collection, especially the number of cultures taken, has a bearing on the percent of recovery of the organism. Except in neonates, multiple cultures should be obtained. One study found that the yield increased from 80 percent, to 89 percent, to 99 percent if one, two, or three sets of cultures were obtained, respectively. The timing of cultures in this study was over a 24-h period. Unfortunately, this is not possible in clinical practice, when the patient's condition requires prompt administration of antibiotics. An appropriate protocol for the emergency department is to obtain two sets of blood cultures from two separate sites at 30-min intervals. The first set could be obtained when initial screening samples are drawn. Most likely the diagnosis of sepsis has already been suggested by the patient's condition at this point in his or her presentation.

Management

The three primary goals in the management of septic shock are provision of cardiorespiratory support, administration of antibiotics, and drainage of pus. Cardiorespiratory support is geared to the severity of the patient's condition and may include fluid resuscitation, administration of vasopressors, and active airway management in the critically ill patient. The treatment of shock initially consists of giving adequate amounts of crystalloid. In less critical patients, fluid resuscitation can be gauged by the response in vital signs. More seriously ill patients and those patients needing vasopressors should undergo CVP monitoring or left atrial pressure monitoring. Patients whose blood pressure does not respond, despite restoration of adequate filling pressures, require vasopressor support. Dopamine is most commonly recommended as the agent of choice. Purely α-adrenergic drugs should be avoided, since they elevate blood pressure at the expense of peripheral perfusion. Dopamine has the advantages of being a positive inotropic agent at the lower dose range and of sparing renal perfusion. Patients unresponsive to volume infusion and dopamine may respond to norepinephrine. This potent vasoconstrictor is started at a rate of 8 to 36 μg/min and titrated to effect.

The second goal in the treatment of septic shock is the prompt and appropriate use of antibiotics. Antibiotics often rapidly inhibit or kill the causative organism, but the patient in septic shock may be unresponsive to antibiotic therapy as circulating toxins and mediators remain to be neutralized. It has been hypothesized that antibiotics may at times promote clinical deterioration secondary to release of endotoxins from gram-negative bacteria. Nevertheless, current practice mandates intravenous antibiotics; but the choice of antibiotics is often less than unanimous. One point of controversy is the use of multiple antibiotic regimens. Some feel that the synergistic effects of certain antibiotic combinations warrant their use, while others feel there is no advantage and potential detriment in such combinations. A logical approach to antibiotic choice is to establish the source of the infection, consider the organisms known to occur in a given instance, and employ the antibiotic(s) that provide specific coverage. Unfortunately, in 30 percent of cases, a specific source of infection is not apparent. In such a circumstance, broad-spectrum coverage with two or three antibiotics may be necessary, since both gram-positive and gram-negative coverage may be mandatory. Table 13B-6 lists various sites of infection, probable organisms, and at least one antibiotic regimen.

The final goal of therapy is the search for and surgical drainage of any pus collection that might exist. In most instances of abscess formation, recovery does not occur until the lesion is drained or excised. Potential pus collections include a perirectal abscess or a gangrenous gallbladder.

The use of steroids in the management of septic shock drew much attention in years past. Studies have not shown that steroids can reverse or prevent shock. In fact, steroids have been documented to cause superinfections in treated patients. Patients in septic shock should receive corticosteroid therapy only if they have suspected or documented adrenal insufficiency.

The lipid A core is thought to be the toxic portion of the endotoxin. The use of antiserum to endotoxin has been investigated in a prospective study of 212 patients with gram-negative sepsis. The antiserum utilized was developed against the J-5 mutant strain of *E. coli*, which contains only core determinants. Results indicate a beneficial effect of the antiserum. The mortality rate of the control group was 39 percent, compared to 22 percent in the antiserum group. In the critically ill patient with profound shock, the respective mortality rates were 77 percent compared to 44 percent. However, investigators were unable to demonstrate a similar beneficial effect using monoclonal antibodies against lipid A. Analogues of lipid A that may inhibit the toxic effects of endotoxin are currently being investigated. Though not presently available to practitioners, antiserum may play a significant role in the management of gram-negative bacteremia in the future.

NEUROGENIC SHOCK

Neurogenic shock has little in common with other forms of shock. It occurs when there is an interruption of vasomotor control affecting the balance between vasoconstrictor and vasodilator influences on both arterioles and venules. This form of shock may result from injury to the spinal cord or brain stem or from high spinal anesthesia. The hypotension that develops is due to generalized vasodilatation. The skin may be warm, dry, or even flushed. Despite a low blood pressure, the pulse rate is normal or perhaps slightly slow. Cardiac output is usually normal but made inadequate as the decreased arteriolar resistance and decreased venous tone serve to decrease venous return. Urinary retention and paralytic ileus frequently develop. The patient may become poikilothermic, with considerable heat losses from exposed skin surfaces with loss of autonomic control of cutaneous blood vessels. High spinal lesions may result in diaphragmatic paralysis and respiratory compromise. Reduced cerebral and renal blood flow which, manifest as decreased alertness and dwindling urine output, can occur in spinal shock, as are seen in classic hypovolemic shock.

Initial therapy of neurogenic shock requires crystalloid infusion through two large-bore catheters. Care must be taken to preserve patient warmth by using warmed blankets and avoiding cool or room-tem-

Table 13B-6. Antibiotic Regimens for Sepsis in Adults

Source of Infection	Probable Bacteria	Antibiotics
Biliary system	Enterobacteriaceae, *Enterococcus, Bacteroides, C. perfringens*	Mezlocillin + metronidazole; IMP; TC/CL; AM/SB
Peritonitis of GI origin	Enterobacteriaceae, *Enterococcus, Bacteroides*	Cefoxitin; ampicillin + APAG + metronidazole; IMP; TC/CL; AM/SB
Osteomyelitis (postoperative)	*S. aureus,* Enterobacteriaceae, *Pseudomonas*	Ciprofloxacin; TC/CL; vancomycin + P ceph 3 AP; IMP
Perirectal abscess	Enterobacteriaceae, *Bacteroides, Enterococcus*	Cefoxitin; TC/CL; AM/SB
Pelvic inflammatory disease (hospitalized)	*Gonococcus, Chlamydia, Bacteroides,* Enterobacteriaceae, *Streptococcus, Mycoplasma*	Cefoxitin + doxycycline; clindamycin + gentamicin
Pneumonia (CA without UD)	*Pneumococcus,* group A *Streptococcus*	Ceftriaxone; cefotaxime; cefuroxime; TMP/SMX
Pneumonia (CA with UD)	*M. pneumoniae, Legionella, Pneumococcus*	Erythromycin + (ceftriaxone, cefotaxime, cefuroxime, IMP, TC/CL, or AM/SB)
Pneumonia (HA)	*Pseudomonas, Klebsiella,* Enterobacteriaceae, *Serratia, Acinetobactor*	AP pen + APAG; P ceph 3 + APAG; IMP
Pneumonia (aspiration)	*Pneumococcus, Klebsiella,* Enterobacteriaceae, *Bacteroides*	Clindamycin + APAG; cefoxitin; IMP; TC/CL; AM/SB; P ceph 3; AP pen
Toxic shock	*S. aureus*	PRSP
Source unknown (uncompromised)	Enterobacteriaceae, group A or D *Streptococcus, Pneumococcus, Bacteroides, S. aureus*	Cefoxitin + APAG; ampicillin + APAG + clindamycin; TC/CL; AM/SB; IMP
Source unknown (splenectomized)	*Pneumococcus, H. influenzae, Meningococcus*	Cefotaxime; ceftriazone; or cefuroxime
Source unknown (neutropenic)	Enterobacteriaceae, *Pseudomonas, S. aureus* or *epidermidis, Streptococcus viridans*	Vancomycin + AP pen + APAG; vancomycin + P ceph 3 (ceftazidine) + APAG; or IMP
Pyelonephritis	Enterobacteriaceae (*E. coli* most common)	Ampicillin; cefazolin + APAG

Abbreviations: IMP, imipenem cilastatin; TC/CL, ticarcillin clavulanate; AM/SB, ampicillin sulbactam; APAG, antipseudomonal aminoglycoside; P ceph 3 AP, third-generation cephalosporin with increased antipseudomonal activity; TMP/SMX, trimethoprim/sulfoxazole; AP pen, antipseudomonal penicillin; P ceph 3, third-generation cephalosporin; PRSP, penicillinase-resistant synthetic penicillin; CA, community-acquired; HA, hospital-acquired; UD, underlying disease.

Source: Adapted from Sanford JP, 1990.

perature IV fluids. Correction of the fluid volume deficit generally will manifest as a prompt elevation of blood pressure. CVP should be normal or slightly low in uncomplicated neurogenic shock, while cardiac output is normal or slightly elevated. Monitoring CVP may be of aid when question arises as to whether the expanded vascular pool is filled.

A vasopressor such as ephedrine or phenylephrine can produce peripheral vasoconstriction and increase cardiac output to support blood pressure in spinal shock. Ephedrine can be given in 5-mg intravenous increments to increase blood pressure. Phenylephrine (10 mg in 250-mL intravenous solution) can be titrated to increase sympathetic tone and reverse hypotension. Phenylephrine can raise blood pressure rapidly at a dose of 100 to 180 μg/min. After hypotension is corrected, a maintenance infusion of 40 to 60 μg/min is used. Phenylephrine can also be given by intravenous injection of 0.1 to 0.5 mg for moderate hypotension and repeated as needed every 10 to 15 min. Neurogenic shock from spinal injury will abate in about 3 weeks, to be followed by return of reflex motor activity and permanent motor paralysis. Fluid administration and pressor support must be delicately balanced as vasopressors may compromise organ perfusion should intravascular volume be inadequate. Slight volume overload is less fraught with complications than overzealous pressor support.

SUMMARY

Although the clinical entity of shock has been known to physicians for centuries, there remain many unanswered questions concerning the pathophysiology and treatment of shock. Although different mechanisms are at work in the various forms of shock, all types of shock result in injury to a common target: the cell. Continued research regarding what happens to the cell in shock and what can be done to prevent such changes may provide the key to successful management of shock in the future. The material reviewed in this section touches on the macroscopic management of shock. In the future this therapy may be combined with measures directed at the cell itself. It is to be hoped that such measures will result in an improved outlook for an entity that currently exhibits a high morbidity and mortality.

BIBLIOGRAPHY

Baue AE, Chaudry I: Some clinical adventures and misadventures. *Adv Shock Res* 3:67, 1980.

Bolooki H: Emergency cardiac procedures in patients in cardiogenic shock due to complications of coronary artery disease. *Circulation* 79 (suppl 1):6, 1989.

Chaudry IH, Baue AE: The use of substrates and energy in the treatment of shock *Adv Shock Res* 3:27, 1980.

Chaudry IH, Clemens MG, Baue AE: Alterations in cell function with ischemia and shock and their correction. *Arch Surg* 116:1309, 1981.

Chudnofsky CR, Dronen SC, Syverud SA, et al: Early versus late fluid resuscitation: Lack of effect in porcine hemorrhagic shock. *Ann Emerg Med* 18:122, 1989.

Dewood MA, Notske RN, Hensley GR, et al: Intraaortic balloon counterpulsation with and without reperfusion for myocardial infarction shock. *Circulation* 6:1105, 1980.

Drucker WR, Chadwick CDJ, Gann DS: Transcapillary refill in hemorrhage and shock. *Arch Surg* 116:1344, 1981.

Geddes JS, Adgey AAJ, Pantridge JF: Prevention of cardiogenic shock. *Am Heart J* 99:244, 1980.

Gervin AS, Fischer RP: Resuscitation of trauma patients with type-specific uncrossmatched blood. *J Trauma* 24:327, 1984.

Keung EC, Ribner HS, Schwartz W, et al: Effects of combined dopamine and nitroprusside therapy in patients with severe pump failure and hypotension complicating acute myocardial infarction. *J Cardiovasc Pharmacol* 2:113, 1980.

Kleinman WM, Krause SM, Hess ML: Differential subendocardial perfusion and injury during the course of gram-negative endotoxemia. *Adv Shock Res* 4:139, 1980.

Kreger BE, Craven DE, Carling PC, et al: Gram-negative bacteremia: Reassessment of etiology, epidemiology and ecology in 612 patients. *Am J Med* 68:332, 1980.

Kreger BE, Craven DE, McCabe WR: Gram-negative bacteremia, reevaluation of clinical features and treatment in 612 patients. *Am J Med* 68:344, 1980.

Maddox KL, Bicknell WH, Pepe PE, et al: Prospective randomized evaluation of antishock MAST in postraumatic hypotension. *J Trauma* 26:779, 1986.

Monafo WW: Volume replacement in hemorrhagic shock and burns. *Adv Shock Res* 3:47, 1980.

Parrillo JE: The cardiovascular pathophysiology of sepsis. *Ann Rev Med* 40:469, 1989.

Parrillo JE et al: Septic shock in humans. *Ann Intern Med* 113:3, 1990.
Pennington DG: Emergency management of cardiogenic shock. *Circulation* 79 (suppl 1):6, 1989.
Perkins RM, Levin DL: Shock in the pediatric patient. *J Pediatr* 101:163, 1982.
Peters RM, Hargens AR: Protein vs. electrolytes and all of the Starling forces. *Arch Surg* 116:1293, 1981.
Putterman C: Modern approaches to the therapy of septic shock. *Am J Emerg Med* 8:2, 1990.
Rackely CE, Russell RO, Mantle JA, et al: Cardiogenic shock. *Cardiovasc Clin* 11:15, 1981.
Sanford JP: *Guide to Antimicrobial Therapy 1990*. San Antonio, Antimicrobial Therapy, Inc., 1990.
Schumer W: Modern concepts of treatment of septic shock. *Curr Surg* 1, 1982.
Schwab CW, Shayne JP, Turner J: Immediate trauma resuscitation with type O uncrossmatched blood: A two-year prospective experience. *J Trauma* 26:897, 1986.
Schwartz S, Frantz RA, Shoemaker WC: Sequential hemodynamic and oxygen transport responses in hypovolemia, anemia, and hypoxia. *Am J Physiol* 241:864, 1981.
Shawl FA et al: Emergency percutaneous cardiopulmonary bypass support in cardiogenic shock from acute myocardial infarction. *Am J Cardiol* 64:16, 1989.
Sheagren J: Septic shock and corticosteroids (editorial). *N Engl J Med* 305:456, 1980.
Trump BF: The role of cellular membranes in shock, in *The Cell in Shock: Proceedings of a Symposium on Recent Research Developments and Current Clinical Practice in Shock*. Scope Publ., 1974, pp 16–29.
Washington JA, Ilstrup DM: Blood cultures: Issues and controversies. *Rev Inf Dis* 8:792, 1986.

C. CYANOSIS

Ann L. Harwood-Nuss
Christina Drummond

DEFINITION

Cyanosis refers to that bluish color of the skin and mucous membranes which results from an increased amount of reduced hemoglobin or hemoglobin derivatives. The detection of cyanosis can be highly subjective and is not considered a sensitive indicator of the state of arterial oxygenation. In fact, cyanosis is determined by the absolute amount of reduced hemoglobin in the blood; the amount of oxygenated hemoglobin is of little influence. Cyanosis is usually present when there is 5 g or more of reduced hemoglobin in 100 mL of capillary blood. The increase in the amount of reduced hemoglobin in the cutaneous vessels can result from either an increase in the quantity of venous blood in the skin, dilatation of the venules, or a decrease in the oxygen saturation in the capillary blood. In some instances, cyanosis can be detected when the arterial saturation has fallen to 85 percent; in others, it may not be detected until saturation is 75 percent. The absolute rather than the relative amount of reduced hemoglobin produces cyanosis.

Factors which influence detection of cyanosis include the rate of blood flow through the capillaries, the light conditions under which the patient is examined, and the skill of the observer. The degree of cyanosis is modified by the quality of cutaneous pigment, the color of the blood plasma, thickness of skin, and state of the cutaneous capillaries. The tongue is considered one of the most sensitive sites for observing central cyanosis. The earlobes, conjuctivae, and nail beds are not reliable sites.

Additional factors which affect the detection of cyanosis include the complexities of the microcirculation. The amount of reduced hemoglobin in the capillaries will be affected by blood flow, oxygen content, tissue oxygen tension, oxygen extraction, and the hemoglobin dissociation curve. Accurate clinical detection of the presence and degree of cyanosis is often difficult.

Clinically, the presence of cyanosis must suggest the possibility of tissue hypoxia. However, the absence of cyanosis does not mean that there is no tissue hypoxia; severe states of tissue hypoxia are possible without the presence of cyanosis. Cyanosis demands a thorough clinical evaluation for possible tissue hypoxia. Additionally, unexplained cyanosis, particularly in association with normal arterial oxygen tension, should prompt a search for an abnormal hemoglobin.

CENTRAL AND PERIPHERAL CYANOSIS

Cyanosis can be divided into two categories, central and peripheral. The central type is seen under conditions where arterial blood is unsaturated or an abnormal hemoglobin derivative exists. The mucous membranes and skin are both affected. In contrast, peripheral cyanosis is due to the slowing of blood flow to an area and an abnormally great extraction of oxygen from normally saturated arterial blood. Congestive failure, peripheral vascular disease, shock states, and cold exposure all create states of vasoconstriction and decrease peripheral blood flow. The differentiation between central and peripheral cyanosis may not be possible in conditions where there may be an admixture of mechanisms (see Table 13C-1).

THE ROLE OF ARTERIAL BLOOD GAS DETERMINATION

To the clinician, the presence of cyanosis most often suggests the possibility of tissue hypoxia. Arterial blood gases are necessary for the further assessment of the cyanotic patient. Arterial oxygen saturation will be normal in peripheral cyanosis if cardiopulmonary function is normal. It will be decreased if cyanosis is due to hypoxia. An abnormal hemoglobin derivative is not detected by routine arterial blood gases. Spectrophotometry will be necessary to determine the presence of a hemoglobin derivative.

Few tests are as vulnerable to errors introduced by improper sampling, handling, and storage as are blood gas analyses. One study reports a 15.8 percent incidence of preanalytic error for arterial blood

Table 13C-1. Causes of Cyanosis

- Central cyanosis
  - Decreased arterial oxygen saturation
    - Decreased atmospheric pressure–high altitude
    - Impaired pulmonary function
      - Alveolar hypoventilation
      - Uneven relationships between pulmonary ventilation and perfusion
      - Impaired oxygen diffusion
    - Anatomic shunts
      - Certain types of congenital heart disease
      - Pulmonary arteriovenous fistulas
      - Multiple small intrapulmonary shunts
    - Hemoglobin with low affinity for oxygen
  - Hemoglobin abnormalities
    - Methemoglobinemia—hereditary, acquired
    - Sulfhemoglobinemia—acquired
    - Carboxyhemoglobinemia (not true cyanosis)
- Peripheral cyanosis
  - Reduced cardiac output
  - Cold exposure
  - Redistribution of blood flow from extremities
  - Arterial obstruction
  - Venous obstruction

Source: Braunwald E: Hypoxia, polycythemia, and cyanosis, in Wilson J, Braunwald E, Isselbacher KJ, et al (eds): *Harrison's Principles of Internal Medicine*, ed 12, New York, McGraw-Hill, 1991, pp 224–228. Used by permission.

gas samples from emergency departments. In contrast, a 0.1 percent incidence of error exists from samples obtained from an indwelling arterial catheter.

Special attention should be given to the following sources of preanalytic error for arterial blood gas samples:

1. Heparin is the anticoagulant of choice, but one must be cautious that the syringe be flushed with heparin and then emptied thoroughly. This will allow adequate anticoagulation of a 2- to 4-mL blood sample with assurance that the results will not be altered by the anticoagulant. Excessive heparin affects the pH, P_{CO_2} and P_{O_2}, as well as the hemoglobin determination.
2. Air bubbles that mix with the blood sample will result in gas equilibration, significantly lowering the P_{CO_2} values with an increase in pH and P_{O_2}. Any sample obtained with more than minor air bubbles should be discarded.
3. Reducing the temperature of the blood by placing the sample immediately in an ice slush will significantly deter changes in the P_{CO_2} and pH for a period of several hours. If the sample is not iced immediately, changes can be significant. As a general rule, arterial blood samples should be analyzed within 10 min or cooled immediately. A delay of up to 1 h for running a cool sample will have no significant effect on the results. Failure to properly cool the sample is a common source of preanalytic error.

DIFFERENTIAL DIAGNOSIS OF CYANOSIS

Hypoxia, anemia, and polycythemia can be diagnosed by means of hemoglobin, hematocrit, and arterial blood gas determination. The red cyanosis of polycythemia vera occurs because the increase in number of red blood cells and hemoglobin concentration results in sludging of blood flow in cutaneous capillaries and venules. Similarly, cyanosis is enhanced in chronic hypoxemia accompanied by polycythemia.

If arterial gases, hematocrit, and hemoglobin are normal, the cause of cyanosis may be due to abnormal skin pigmentation or an abnormal hemoglobin. The term "pseudocyanosis" is used to describe the blue, gray, or purple cutaneous discoloration which may mimic cyanosis. Pseudocyanosis can be caused by heavy metals (i.e., hemochromatosis, gold, silver, lead, arsenic) or drugs (i.e., phenothiazines, minocycline, amiodarone, chloroquine). Chrysiasis is a specific type of pseudocyanosis, characterized by a gray, blue, or purple pigmentation of areas exposed to light. It is a rare but dose-dependent complication of gold treatment that tends to cause permanent discoloration of the skin. Another example of pseudocyanosis is argyria, which is a slate blue to gray coloration of the skin resulting from either chronic ingestion or chronic local application of silver salts or colloidal silver. The color does not blanch with pressure, in contrast to true cyanotic skin, which will blanch. Skin biopsy confirms the diagnosis. Carboxyhemoglobinemia does not cause cyanosis. Occasionally, however, carboxyhemoglobinemia does produce a cherry-red flush of the skin, retina, or mucous membranes.

Cyanosis can be caused by methemoglobinemia and sulfhemoglobinemia. Most cases are due to acquired states secondary to chemicals or medications. Benzocaine, nitrates, and nitrites may produce methemoglobinemia. The sulfonamides, phenacetin, acetanilid, and aniline may produce sulfhemoglobinemia or methemoglobinemia. The incidence of acquired methemoglobinemia secondary to industrial exposure to aniline dyes and aromatic amino and nitro compounds has decreased with improvement in occupational health standards. Hereditary methemoglobinemia is a genetic disorder affecting the enzyme methemoglobin reductase, resulting in structural alterations of the hemoglobin molecule. Patients afflicted with this deficiency have cyanosis but are usually asymptomatic.

Although there exist a wide number of drugs that can produce methemoglobinemia, no currently used drug does so at therapeutic dose levels. Acetanilid and phenacetin are aniline derivatives and frequent causes of methemoglobinemia and sulfhemoglobinemia. Certain sulfonamides and local anesthetics may produce methemoglobinemia. Methemoglobinemia is manifest clinically by cyanosis with as little as 1.5 g of methemoglobin present in 100 mL of blood. Since methemoglobin is incapable of binding with oxygen, the symptoms of methemoglobinemia are secondary to hypoxia. The severity is related to the quantity of methemoglobin present, the rapidity of onset, and the patient's own cardiopulmonary system. Cyanotic patients without cardiovascular or pulmonary disease should be suspected of having methemoglobinemia, especially if cyanosis is not relieved by oxygen administration. Further, the venous blood will appear chocolate brown. Spectrophotometry is required for identification of the pigment and its quantity. In acquired methemoglobinemia, no treatment is necessary unless signs of hypoxia (i.e., angina, arrhythmias, hypotension, stupor, or coma) are present. Methylene blue in a dose of 1 to 2 mg per kilogram of body weight given intravenously over 5 min in a 1% solution is the agent of choice.

Sulfhemoglobinemia may result from one of the oxidizing drugs. Phenacetin (APC, Empirin compound) and acetanilid (Bromo Seltzer) are the most common causative agents. Sulfhemoglobin is inert as an oxygen carrier and when present can produce deep cyanosis at a level of less than 0.5 g of sulfhemoglobin per 100 mL of blood. Once formed, there is no way of converting sulfhemoglobin to hemoglobin and the treatment calls for the removal of the causative agent.

BIBLIOGRAPHY

Curry S: Methemoglobinemia. *Ann Emerg Med* 11:4, 1982.

Familton MJG, Armstrong RF: Pseudocyanosis: time to reclassify cyanosis? *Anaesthesia* 44:3, 1989.

Gold W: Cyanosis, in *MacBryde's Signs and Symptoms: Applied Pathologic Physiology and Clinical Interpretation*. Philadelphia, Lippincott, 1983.

Jaffe ER: Methemoglobinemia in the differential diagnosis of cyanosis. *Hosp Pract* 20:12, 1985.

Lees MH, King DH: Cyanosis in the newborn. *Pediatr Rev* 9:2, 1987.

Martin L, Khalil H: How much reduced hemoglobin is necessary to generate central cyanosis? *Chest* 97:1, 1990.

D. SYNCOPE

Andrew Wilson

Syncope and death are the same—except that in one you wake up.
Anonymous

The foregoing aphorism summarizes the clinical dilemma of syncope. Syncope is the final common pathway of a number of pathophysiological disturbances, some of which carry substantial morbidity and mortality, and most of which demonstrate few objective findings in the emergency department. The challenge, then, is to identify those patients who may not recover from a subsequent episode of syncope and who require admission to hospital.

DEFINITION

Syncope is a transient loss of consciousness, in most cases less than 5 min. Presyncope, a warning of syncope, shares, in most part, the pathophysiology and differential diagnosis for syncope.

INCIDENCE

The incidence of syncope in the general population is unknown but may be experienced at one time or another by as much as 50 percent of the population. Presyncope is nearly universal. Syncope accounts for about 3 percent of emergency department visits and may account for as many as 6 percent of hospital admissions.

Although older studies on syncope suggested that a definite etiologic diagnosis could be made in over 90 percent of cases, current works are much less optimistic. Probably because of more stringently defined criteria for diagnosis, current authors claim an eventual definitive diagnosis in about 50 percent of cases. These same authors suggest that of the patients who eventually have a diagnosis, about 50 percent can be diagnosed in the emergency department. While the emergency physician might be expected to arrive at a firm diagnosis in only about one quarter of the cases presenting to the emergency department, at least those patients at high risk for death or disability are more reliably identified.

PATHOPHYSIOLOGY AND CAUSES

Three basic pathophysiological mechanisms produce syncope: denial to the brain of oxygen, denial to the brain of glucose, and seizure activity. The latter two mechanisms are relatively straightforward. However, there are manifold mechanisms by which the brain may be denied oxygen, and more than one mechanism may be operational in an individual patient. In the elderly, in particular, multiple contributing factors may lead down the final common pathway of syncope. Such factors may include cerebral atherosclerosis, medications, and age-related blunting of the vascular reflexes required to maintain an upright position.

The differential diagnosis of syncope is listed in Table 13D-1. The first broad distinction to make in a patient with syncope is whether the interruption in consciousness was a seizure. If a seizure is unlikely, the manifold causes of fainting must be considered. These may be grouped, with a little artifice, into four categories: cardiac, peripheral vascular, cerebrovascular, and miscellaneous.

Seizure Disorders

A useful clue in the "fit versus faint" issue is the abrupt nature of the onset of most generalized seizures. An aura, if present, provides a valuable clue. While the onset of a seizure is abrupt, the clearing, the postictal phase, is slow. Injuries due to falling are also common with seizures. Usually the problem is not to ascertain whether the patient had seizure activity, for onlookers are very pleased to provide that information, but whether the seizure was the cause or an effect of syncope. Generalized clonic jerks often result from generalized cerebral anoxia. Likewise, tongue biting and incontinence of urine or feces may be found in syncope of any cause. If a history can be obtained of abrupt loss of consciousness with simultaneous tonic-clonic seizure activity and a slow recovery, seizure very likely is the cause of syncope.

Table 13D-1. Causes of Syncope

Seizure disorder
Cardiac
Arrhythmias
Obstructive lesions
Ischemia
Peripheral vascular
Vasovagal
Orthostatic
Carotid sinus hypersensitivity
Special situations
Cerebrovascular circulation
Transient ischemic attack
Subclavian steal
Miscellaneous
Hypoglycemia
Hyperventilation

Cardiac Causes

Cardiac causes of syncope fall into three groups: rhythm disturbances, ventricular outflow obstructive processes, and myocardial ischemia. Because cardiac causes of syncope are at once among the most lethal and the most remediable, identification of cardiac syncope can be crucial. Rhythm disturbances, when found in temporal proximity to syncope, should be suspected of causing syncope. Be aware, however, that proving a cause-and-effect relationship between an arrhythmia and syncope may be most difficult. The degree of arrhythmia tolerated in a given patient is dependent on many factors such as age, intravascular volume, position, and vagal tone. In general, to be considered as the cause of syncope, the heart rate should be over 150 or under 40 beats per minute. Any process causing acute or chronic obstruction to ventricular inflow or outflow may cause syncope. For the left ventricle, these processes include aortic stenosis (valvular or subvalvular), atrial myxoma, or mitral stenosis. For the right ventricle, pulmonary embolism and pulmonary hypertension are important considerations. Syncope in association with cardiac ischemia is usually secondary to arrhythmia or with-effort angina pectoris. Theories on the pathophysiology of the latter postulate an inability of the heart to increase output in response to demand, increased vagal tone, and hyperventilation. Cardiac syncope should be suspected in patients with underlying cardiopulmonary disease, especially with superimposed new cardiac symptoms. Cardiac syncope may occur with the patient in any position and usually has an abrupt onset and prompt (less than 1 min) resolution.

Peripheral Vascular Disorders

The peripheral vascular causes of syncope are the most diverse and include vasovagal syncope, orthostatic hypotension, carotid sinus hypersensitivity, and cerebrovascular circulation. The unifying concept is that, whatever the inciting phenomenon, a tendency to venous pooling of blood is increased. Pooling of blood in capacitance vessels decreases venous return, cardiac output, and, finally, cerebral perfusion, resulting in syncope. Factors such as drugs, peripheral neuropathy, and counterproductive reflexes can defeat the vascular responses needed to assume and maintain a standing position.

The most common cause of syncope is vasovagal syncope—the common faint. There are two contributory mechanisms: vasodepression causing venous pooling, and cardioinhibition resulting in bradycardia. Vasodepression is more important, as abolishing bradycardia with atropine still allows syncope. Clues to vasovagal syncope include the appropriate setting (fear, injury, sight of blood, illness); upright posture; and a warning period of progressive symptoms such as a feeling of warmth, light-headedness, nausea, roaring in the ears, and a dimming of vision, culminating in a loss of consciousness. After the syncopal episode, recovery should be prompt, that is, within seconds. The exception to this rule is when a well-intentioned bystander keeps the victim propped up, slowing resolution of symptoms. Although vasovagal syncope can occur at any age, be reluctant to make the diagnosis in a first episode occurring after age 40. Be reluctant, as well, to use the diagnosis as one of convenience; require the appropriate setting and warning symptoms as outlined. Because the symptoms of vasovagal syncope reflect nothing more than slowly progressive global cerebral ischemia, be wary of other conditions, such as cardiac arrhythmias, which can also occasionally have a slowly progressive onset.

Orthostatic syncope is syncope occurring when one assumes a more upright posture. An underlying disease, drugs affecting control of capacitance vessels, or both are responsible. Examples include diabetes mellitus, amyloid, pheochromocytoma, antihypertensives, phenothiazines, and nitrates. In addition, intravascular volume depletion through bleeding or dehydration may precipitate orthostatic syncope. The onset on changing position may be more abrupt than with vasovagal syncope, although the symptoms may linger prior to loss of consciousness. Criteria suggested for diagnosis are an orthostatic fall in systolic blood pressure of 25 mmHg, with symptoms, or a blood pressure of less than 90 mmHg systolic standing. The history and physical examination must also be directed to search for intravascular volume depletion, for example, by stool guaiac determination or evaluation for possible ectopic pregnancy.

Carotid sinus hypersensitivity is an uncommon cause of syncope. Three subtypes are described: peripheral, central, and cardioinhibitory. Carotid sinus stimulation causes capacitance vessel pooling of blood in the peripheral type, a bradycardia in the cardioinhibitory type, and direct loss of consciousness in the central type. Circumstances associated with syncope include tight collars, head turning, or shaving. Diagnosis can be made by carotid sinus massage. First, assure that there are no carotid bruits. Second, place the patient in a supine position with an intravenous infusion and cardiac monitor established, and atropine available. Third, monitor blood pressure and heart rate with gentle carotid massage of first one side and then the other. A positive result is considered to be asystole of 3 s or greater or a drop of systolic blood pressure of 50 mmHg or better. About 30 percent of normal asyncopal elderly people have a positive response to carotid sinus massage, so, again, correlation does not necessarily prove cause and effect.

The remaining causes of peripheral vascular syncope include syncope associated with special circumstances such as coughing, micturition, defecation, and swallowing. Causes include reflex-mediated changes in venous pressure, heart rate, and cardiac output.

Cerebrovascular Circulation

Syncope due to primary cerebral ischemia, or a transient ischemic attack, is rare. When present, it is referable to the vertebrobasilar circulation as the vertebrobasilar arteries supply the reticular activating system. Syncope due to anterior circulation transient ischemic attacks would require bilateral simultaneous compromise of circulation to the cerebral hemispheres and is only theoretically possible. If one entertains the diagnosis of a transient ischemic attack as the cause of syncope, focal neurological symptoms and signs should be reported by the patient. The brainstem is a compact structure with multiple functions, and other symptoms of brainstem ischemia should be present for syncope to be ascribed to this mechanism. Cerebrovascular disease may be a contributing factor, however, to other causes of syncope, especially in the elderly.

The subclavian steal syndrome should be sought if a blood pressure difference between the arms of at least 20 mmHg is noted, or if upper extremity exercise seems to be associated with syncope. In this entity, an obstruction of the brachiocephalic or subclavian artery causes shunting of blood through the vertebrobasilar system from the normal side past the obstruction, resulting, in effect, in a brainstem transient ischemic attack.

Miscellaneous

Two miscellaneous causes of syncope are worthy of mention. First is hypoglycemia, a frequent cause of coma but an unusual cause of syncope. The usual setting is that of a diabetic taking a hypoglycemic agent, usually insulin. The incidence of syncopal hypoglycemia in the absence of hypoglycemic agents is probably rare. Second is hyperventilation, a frequent cause of presyncope and sometimes a cause of syncope. Hypocarbia causes cerebral vasoconstriction and peripheral vasodilatation. Syncope, or at least presyncope, should be reproducible by a trial of hyperventilation in the emergency department. One should ascertain that hyperventilation in a given patient is psychogenic, and not secondary to an underlying cause such as pulmonary embolism.

EVALUATION

The goal in the emergency department evaluation of a patient with syncope is to establish the etiology so that the physician can best determine whether outpatient or inpatient management is appropriate. If the etiology cannot be established, then the physician must determine whether the patient is in a high-risk group and, if so, have the patient admitted for further evaluation.

The general history should attempt to establish whether the patient has underlying cardiopulmonary disease and should include a past history, gynecologic history (for female patients), and medication history. The history of the event may be considered in three phases: presyncope (environment, position, duration, symptoms), syncope (position and duration, from witnesses), and postsyncope (time to clear and injuries). Of these, the account of the presyncopal period is of most importance. The nature of the setting, the premonitory symptoms, and especially the duration are of great help in determining the potential morbidity or mortality associated with an episode of syncope. Description of events must be elicited from witnesses and emergency medical service personnel. The physical examination should include blood pressure and pulse in both arms, supine and upright, cardiovascular examination, and neurologic examination. A normal blood pressure with the legs dangling and the patient sitting should be followed with recordings taken with the patient standing, both immediately and after 2 min. Special maneuvers should be performed as indicated, for example, carotid sinus massage, rectal examination for occult blood, and a trial of hyperventilation. A careful history and physical examination will provide the diagnosis in about half the patients in whom a diagnosis can be made at all. The only other valuable emergency department test is the 12-lead electrocardiogram, which may provide an answer in about 10 percent of patients. Laboratory tests are usually unrewarding, except in selected cases, such as suspicion of bleeding. Cardiac monitoring, especially ambulatory monitoring, is quite useful and may be initiated in the emergency department in patients deemed safe for discharge.

The ultimate diagnoses depend on the patient population studied and stringency of the diagnostic criteria used. Patients who present to the emergency department after syncope are probably a selected group, in that many with benign disorders, such as vasovagal syncope, will not present to the emergency department. Since only about 50 percent of patients with syncope ever have an etiologic diagnosis, with only half of these diagnosed in the emergency department, those patients at risk for mortality or further morbidity should be identified. Several studies suggest that cardiac causes of syncope are associated with a 20 to 30 percent mortality in one year. However, patients with syncope of noncardiac and unknown causes experience morbidity and mortality similar to nonsyncopal patients matched for age and concomitant disease.

In the absence of an etiologic diagnosis, which patients should be admitted? A profile of a high-risk group is emerging and includes these characteristics: age over 55, a history of congestive heart failure and/or coronary artery disease and/or ventricular ectopy, an abrupt onset and clearing of the syncope, and an abnormal ECG (not necessarily specific for the etiology of the syncope). A low-risk profile is also emerging, with these characteristics: younger age group; absence of multiple diseases, especially renal disease and diabetes mellitus; absence of ventricular ectopy; and a normal ECG. Although these profiles may assist in determining disposition of patients, they remain guidelines only. If establishment of an etiology in a given patient is not possible, it is well to consider, in addition to the high-risk–low-risk assessment, the aphorism with which this chapter began.

BIBLIOGRAPHY

Eagle KA, Black HR, Cook EF: Evaluation of prognostic classifications for patients with syncope. *Am J Med* 79:455, 1985.

Kapoor WN, Karpf M, Wieand S: A prospective evaluation and follow-up of patients with syncope. *N Engl J Med* 309:197, 1983.

Kapoor W, Snustad D, Peterson J, et al: Syncope in the elderly. *Am J Med* 80:419, 1986.

Manolis AS, Linzer M, Salem D, et al: Syncope: Current diagnostic evaluation and management. *Ann Intern Med* 112:850, 1990.

Martin GJ, Adams SL, Martin HG: Prospective evaluation of syncope. *Ann Emerg Med* 13:499, 1984.
Wayne HH: Syncope: Physiological considerations. *Am J Med* 3:418, 1961.
Wright K, McIntosh HD: Syncope: A review of pathophysiological mechanisms. *Progr Cardiovasc Dis* 13:580, 1971.

E. ABDOMINAL PAIN

David T. Overton

IMMEDIATE LIFE THREATS

Abdominal aortic aneurysm
Splenic rupture
Ectopic pregnancy
Myocardial infarction

Abdominal pain is one of the most common presenting complaints in the emergency department. In up to 40 percent of patients, however, the etiology remains obscure. Further, misdiagnosis has been reported to occur in up to 30 percent. Studies suggest that microcomputer aids to clinical management may improve these sobering statistics.

TYPES OF ABDOMINAL PAIN

Three distinct types of pain response may be involved in the genesis of abdominal pain: visceral, somatic, and referred. A basic understanding of these pain responses aids the clinician in establishing a differential diagnosis.

Visceral Pain

Visceral (splanchnic) abdominal pain results from stretching of the autonomic nerve fibers surrounding a hollow or solid viscus. Obstruction is a common cause. The pain may be described as crampy, colicky, or gaseous and is often intermittent. Pure visceral pain is felt in the midline, the exact location depending on the embryologic origin of the intraabdominal organ involved. Foregut structures (stomach, duodenum, pancreatic-biliary tree) classically are referred in the epigastrium. Midgut structures (small bowel, ascending colon) are referred to the periumbilical area. Hindgut structures (descending colon) are referred to the suprapubic area or lower back.

Despite these typical patterns, visceral pain is usually ill defined and diffuse, and the patient may be surprised to find a disparity between the location of pain and the location of tenderness on examination. Visceral pain is an early manifestation of many disorders, including appendicitis, cholecystitis, bowel obstruction, and renal colic.

Somatic Pain

Somatic (parietal) pain occurs when pain fibers located in the parietal peritoneum are irritated by chemical or bacterial inflammation. Somatic pain is generally sharper, more constant, and more precisely localized to the area of disease. It represents the inflammation which often occurs subsequent to the obstruction of visceral pain. There is usually tenderness localized to the area of pathology, an important diagnostic feature.

Referred Pain

Referred pain is any pain felt at a distance from the diseased organ. Thus, in a strict sense, some kinds of visceral and somatic pain are types of referred pain. Referred pain generally follows certain classic patterns. For instance, diaphragmatic irritation, due to subphrenic collections of pus or blood, often radiates to the supraclavicular area. The pain of ureteral colic often radiates to the lower quadrants, genitalia, or inner thigh.

By thorough history taking and careful, often repeated, physical examination, the clinician may use this knowledge of pain classification to more accurately distinguish causes of pain. For instance, patients with appendicitis classically report an initial phase of ill-defined discomfort localized to the periumbilical or epigastric area, which is a visceral pain corresponding to obstruction and distention of the appendiceal lumen. Tenderness at this phase is generally vague and poorly localized. Later, as the appendix becomes progressively more inflamed and irritates the surrounding parietal peritoneum, the perceived area of pain migrates to the right lower quadrant. This somatic pain is accompanied by the development of tenderness localized to McBurney's point.

ORIGINS OF ABDOMINAL PAIN

Abdominal pain can arise from one of several origins: intraabdominal, extraabdominal, metabolic, or neurogenic.

Intraabdominal Origin

Pain arising from intraabdominal origins can be divided into three categories: peritoneal inflammation, obstruction of a hollow viscus, and vascular disorders.

Peritoneal Inflammation

Peritonitis is the somatic pain caused by inflammation of the peritoneum by an irritant. This irritant can be aseptic (e.g., gastric juice, bile, pancreatic juice, blood, or urine) or of bacterial origin. Peritoneal inflammation can be either primary or, more commonly, secondary. Primary ("spontaneous") peritonitis is a condition chiefly caused by *Pneumococcus, Streptococcus, Escherichia coli,* or *Mycobacterium tuberculosis.* It is most often seen in cirrhotic patients, or others with ascites. Secondary peritonitis is caused by disease or injury of the abdominal or pelvic viscera. Its microbiology parallels that of the gut flora and is often polymicrobial, involving both aerobes and anaerobes. Many causes of the acute abdomen, such as appendicitis, cholecystitis, and mesenteric infarction, eventually lead to peritoneal inflammation.

Obstruction of a Hollow Viscus

Obstruction of the intestine, ureter, or biliary tree produces the typical colicky sensation characteristic of visceral pain. Intestinal obstruction typically leads to colicky abdominal pain, nausea, and vomiting. Vomiting tends to be more pronounced the more proximal the obstruction. There may be a decrease in rectal gas. Abdominal distention may at first be discernible only on radiograph but eventually becomes clinically evident. The most common cause is adhesions from previous surgery, but other causes, such as hernias, neoplasm, and volvulus may also be involved.

Vascular Disorders

Bowel infarction and aortic dissection, leakage, or rupture represent the major vascular emergencies associated with acute abdominal pain. Bowel ischemia or infarction is a difficult and often delayed diagnosis. Classically, the early symptoms are severe, diffuse abdominal pain, with a paucity of physical findings. Systemic toxicity follows, with fever, acidosis, and shock. Hematemesis and loose, bloody stools tend to be late findings. Patients are often elderly, with underlying cardiovascular disease. Mortality is high.

An expanding or leaking abdominal aortic aneurysm is a true vascular emergency. It is characterized by abdominal pain, often radiating to the back, flank, or genitalia, and eventually, hypotension and cardiovascular collapse. It is easily mistaken for the pain of renal colic, so much so that when evaluating renal colic patients, the clinician should consciously keep the possibility of an aortic aneurysm in mind.

Extraabdominal Origin

A number of extraabdominal sources can lead to pain which is subjectively felt by the patient to arise in the abdomen. These include the abdominal wall, the pelvis, and the thorax.

Abdominal wall pain is usually traumatic in origin and may be caused by muscle strain, hematoma, or contusion. It is often accentuated by abdominal wall muscle contraction.

Intrathoracic disease, including pneumonia, pulmonary embolism, pneumothorax, and esophageal disease, may present as abdominal pain. Children with pneumonia commonly present with abdominal, rather than pulmonary, complaints. Acute myocardial ischemia may have many subtle presentations, particularly in the elderly and diabetics. Nausea, vomiting, diaphoresis, and vague abdominal distress may be the only clues to this life-threatening disorder. For this reason, clinicians should consider including an electrocardiogram in the evaluation of patients over the age of 40 with upper abdominal pain.

Pain from pelvic sources is usually reported as abdominal pain by the layperson. Disorders such as salpingitis, tuboovarian abscess, ovarian cyst torsion or rupture, or abortion commonly present with abdominal pain. Ectopic pregnancy is a common cause of acute abdominal pain in women and should be included in the differential diagnosis of these patients.

Metabolic Disorders

A number of metabolic disorders may cause pain in the abdomen. Perhaps the most common is diabetic ketoacidosis. In this instance, it is important to rule out true, intraabdominal pathology as a factor which exacerbated the diabetes. Porphyria, spider and scorpion bites, heavy-metal intoxication, systemic lupus erythematosus, periarteritis nodosa, and sickle cell crisis can all present with abdominal pain as the predominant symptom.

Neurogenic Causes

The preeruptive phase of herpes zoster can lead to confusing abdominal pain. Spinal disk disease and the now unusual crisis of tabes dorsalis may also present with abdominal pain.

CLINICAL APPROACH TO THE PATIENT WITH ACUTE ABDOMINAL PAIN

With virtually any chief complaint, but with abdominal pain in particular, the clinician should keep in mind a list of immediate life threats. The initial approach to the patient should bear these in mind, with the institution of immediate resuscitative and stabilization procedures, if necessary.

History

A detailed, careful history is the first step. The clinician should keep in mind the importance of individual patient variables (cultural, socioeconomic, educational, etc.), and confirmation of history with family or friends may be helpful.

The time of onset of pain, as well as severity at the onset, should be noted. Typically, the pain of aortic dissection, peptic ulcer perforation, and renal colic are abrupt in onset, while that of appendicitis is more gradual. The location of pain and its referral, both at the onset and subsequently, are important (see Fig. 13E-1). The character of the pain (colicky, steady, sharp, burning, tearing, gnawing, aching, etc.) and its severity are helpful.

The symptoms of anorexia, nausea, and vomiting so often accompany acute abdominal distress as to limit their usefulness in distinguishing etiologies. However, persistent vomiting may result in dehydration. Diarrhea and the presence of blood in either the diarrhea or vomitus should be noted. A chronic change in bowel habits may suggest an underlying malignancy. Dysuria, frequency, or hematuria suggest a urinary source. However, inflammatory conditions such as appendicitis can produce such symptoms if the inflamed appendix is in proximity to the ureter. A thorough gynecologic history is indicated in women with abdominal pain, including a pregnancy and menstrual history and a history of sexual activity and contraception. However, it is well recognized that patients may conceal such information, so a high index of suspicion is warranted.

Cardiorespiratory symptoms such as chest pain, shortness of breath, cough, sputum, hemoptysis, and orthopnea may suggest a thoracic source of pain. Any prior occurrence of similar symptoms should be sought. Other past medical history, including operations, diseases, and drug intake, especially steroids, antibiotics, or nonsteroidal anti-inflammatory agents should be elicited.

Physical Examination

The patient's general appearance should be noted, especially such signs as diaphoresis and pallor. Patients with visceral pain often are doubled over and tend to move about searching for a comfortable position. Patients with peritonitis, on the other hand, tend to lie still and resist movement. Jarring the bed or tapping on the heels may exacerbate their discomfort. The vital signs should be inspected. Tachycardia, hypotension, or orthostatic changes suggest volume depletion. Fever may present in many abdominal conditions, but its absence should not be given undue emphasis . Studies have shown a large percentage of patients with appendicitis to present with normal temperatures. High fever with shaking chills is typical of pyelonephritis and pneumonia.

The abdomen should be inspected for contour, scars, peristalsis, masses, distention, or pulsation. Cullen's sign (bluish umbilicus) and Grey Turner's sign (ecchymosis of the abdomen or flank) are unusual signs of internal hemorrhage. Auscultation should precede palpation. The diagnostic yield of abdominal auscultation is lower than that of palpation, especially in a noisy emergency environment. However, the presence and character of bowel sounds should be noted, as well as any bruits present.

Palpation is the most important physical examination modality available. It should be performed by the warmed hand in a comfortable environment. Placement of pillows under the head and knees, or having the supine patient bend the knees, may allow the abdominal musculature to relax. Palpation should be gentle, with only one or two fingers being necessary. It should begin at an area distal from the suspected location of pain. Tenderness is the patient's subjective feeling of pain exacerbated by the examiner's palpation. "Guarding" is muscular contraction in response to palpation. Involuntary guarding is the same as rigidity, which is reflex spasm of the abdominal musculature. Masses and organomegaly should be sought. Turning the patient on the right side may aid palpation of the left upper quadrant.

Certain physical signs may be of additional benefit. Murphy's sign (inspiratory arrest) is performed with the examining fingers held under the right costal margin while asking the patient to inspire. Painful midcycle arrest of inspiration occurs when an inflammed gallbladder comes into contact with the examining fingers. The iliopsoas sign is performed by asking the supine patient to keep the right knee extended and flex the thigh against the resistance of the examiner's hand. Pain in the pelvis indicates irritation of the iliopsoas muscle, as in appendicitis. The obturator sign is performed by having the supine patient flex the right knee to 90°. The examiner immobilizes the ankle and moves the knee laterally and medially, causing internal and external rotation. Pain in the pelvis also suggests appendicitis.

A genital examination is always indicated. It is important to check for hernias. Pain of testicular origin often radiates to the abdomen. All women with abdominal pain need a pelvic examination, as even

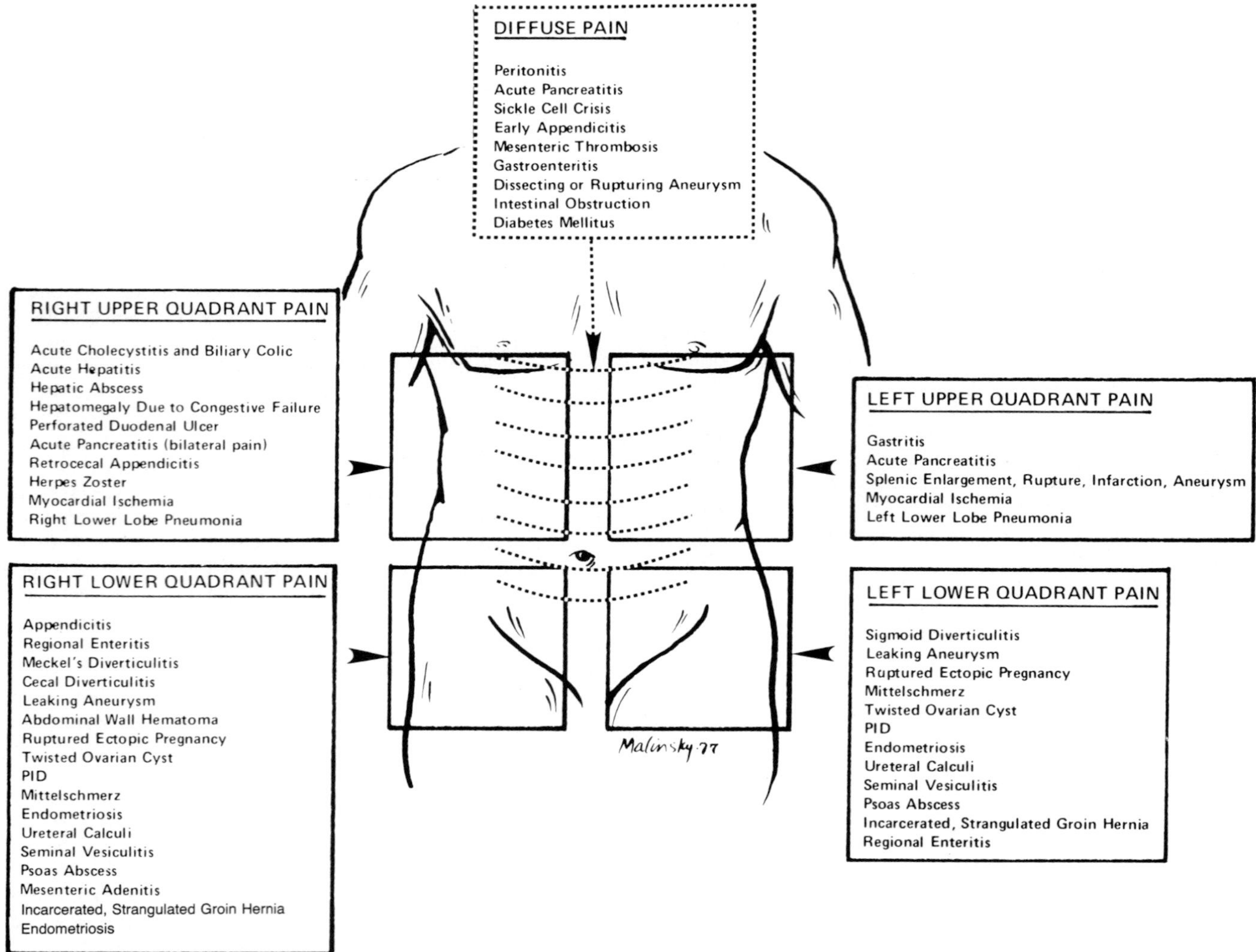

DIFFUSE PAIN
Peritonitis
Acute Pancreatitis
Sickle Cell Crisis
Early Appendicitis
Mesenteric Thrombosis
Gastroenteritis
Dissecting or Rupturing Aneurysm
Intestinal Obstruction
Diabetes Mellitus
RIGHT UPPER QUADRANT PAIN
Acute Cholecystitis and Biliary Colic
Acute Hepatitis
Hepatic Abscess
Hepatomegaly Due to Congestive Failure
Perforated Duodenal Ulcer
Acute Pancreatitis (bilateral pain)
Retrocecal Appendicitis
Herpes Zoster
Myocardial Ischemia
Right Lower Lobe Pneumonia
LEFT UPPER QUADRANT PAIN
Gastritis
Acute Pancreatitis
Splenic Enlargement, Rupture, Infarction, Aneurysm
Myocardial Ischemia
Left Lower Lobe Pneumonia
RIGHT LOWER QUADRANT PAIN
Appendicitis
Regional Enteritis
Meckel's Diverticulitis
Cecal Diverticulitis
Leaking Aneurysm
Abdominal Wall Hematoma
Ruptured Ectopic Pregnancy
Twisted Ovarian Cyst
PID
Mittelschmerz
Endometriosis
Ureteral Calculi
Seminal Vesiculitis
Psoas Abscess
Mesenteric Adenitis
Incarcerated, Strangulated Groin Hernia
Endometriosis
LEFT LOWER QUADRANT PAIN
Sigmoid Diverticulitis
Leaking Aneurysm
Ruptured Ectopic Pregnancy
Mittelschmerz
Twisted Ovarian Cyst
PID
Endometriosis
Ureteral Calculi
Seminal Vesiculitis
Psoas Abscess
Incarcerated, Strangulated Groin Hernia
Regional Enteritis
Malinsky 77

Fig. 13E-1. Differential diagnosis of acute abdominal pain by location. [*From* Wagner DK: Approaches to the patient with acute abdominal pain. *Current Topics* (a program of the Medical College of Pennsylvania). 1:3, 1978. Used by permission.]

upper abdominal pain may have a pelvic etiology. A classic example in the Fitz-Hugh–Curtis syndrome, in which periphepatitis occurs secondary to often unsuspected pelvic inflammatory disease. Similarly, the rectal examination is important to detect occult or gross blood in the stool, as well as areas of tenderness. A general physical examination is warranted, especially the cardiopulmonary and vascular examination.

Laboratory Evaluation

Laboratory evaluation, although helpful, cannot supplant a careful history and physical examination. The CBC is an integral part of the evaluation of the acute abdomen, but its limitations must be appreciated. Inflammatory conditions of surgical import such as appendicitis often have normal white blood cell counts. The hematocrit usually will not accurately reflect acute blood loss. However, serial values, together with careful clinical reevaluation, may be of value. The urinalysis may reveal hematuria, which is present in most, but not all, cases of renal colic. Pyuria suggests urinary tract infection but may be present when an inflammatory mass lies in close proximity to the urinary tract. The serum amylase level may be elevated in a number of conditions, including pancreatitis, biliary obstruction, cholecystitis, bowel obstruction, bowel infarction, salpingitis, ectopic pregnancy, or may be of salivary origin. A pregnancy test is valuable in women of childbearing age. Improvements in technology have made urinary tests more sensitive and specific. Serum measurements of the β subunit of human chorionic gonadotropin are very sensitive and a negative value virtually excludes the diagnosis of ectopic pregnancy.

An electrocardiogram should be considered in patients over 40, especially with upper abdominal or nonspecific symptomatology. Cardiac ischemia can and does present in atypical manners, and the presence of arrhythmias, such as atrial fibrillation, is associated with intestinal infarction.

Imaging Studies

The standard abdominal series, usually consisting of flat and upright views of the abdomen, as well as an upright view of the chest, have long been considered to be standard in the evaluation of abdominal pain. The flat plate may disclose biliary or renal calculi; air in the biliary tree; abnormal vascular calcifications, such as that of an aortic aneurysm; and abnormal gas patterns. An upright view may disclose air-fluid levels. The upright chest film may disclose free peritoneal air, or intrathoracic pathology related to abdominal pain. A right lateral decubitus view of the abdomen may also reveal free air.

A number of studies, however, have questioned the utility of standard radiographs. Several have recommended the use of the upright abdominal view only when obstruction or ileus are suspected clinically.

Still others have questioned the use of abdominal x-rays at all in patients with mild, nonspecific abdominal pain, uncomplicated gastrointestinal bleeding, or suspected ureteral colic.

Barium contrast studies have traditionally had limited usefulness and availability to the emergency physician. Recently, however, increasing use of these procedures in the emergency environment has occurred. The barium enema may prove helpful in the evaluation of suspected appendicitis in patients with equivocal findings. The barium enema is the diagnositic and therapeutic procedure of choice in intussusception. It may be of further value in patients with volvulus and other cases of suspected large bowel obstruction. Complications of barium enema are rare, but include perforation and barium extravasation.

Ultrasonography is a valuable diagnostic technique in a number of causes of the acute abdomen. It is a superior imaging procedure in patients with right upper quadrant pain. Cholelithiasis, choledocholithiasis, cholecystitis, and biliary duct dilatation can all be detected, as well as solid or cystic pancreatic masses. Hydroureter can be seen. It is of particular value in the evaluation of lower abdominal pain in women in childbearing age groups. Intrauterine and ectopic pregnancies, ovarian and tubal pathology, and free intraperitoneal fluid can be detected. Graded compression sonography has been shown to be useful in the evaluation of suspected appendicitis with equivocal findings. Ultrasonography is also very useful in evaluating abdominal aortic aneurysms. However, in the unstable patient with an acutely leaking or expanding aneurysm, the diagnosis is clinical and the treatment immediate.

Radioisotope studies using ^{99m}Tc-IDA have been found to be quite sensitive and specific for the cystic duct obstruction associated with acute cholecystitis. The procedure does take a number of hours to complete, making it somewhat less useful to the emergency physician.

Laparoscopy

Laparoscopy is reported to be a useful adjunct in the evaluation of selected cases of acute abdominal pain. The difficult distinction between appendicitis and gynecologic pathology can often be made, avoiding laparotomy in a number of patients.

ANALGESIA

Classic surgical teaching states that it is contraindicated to administer analgesics to patients with abdominal pain before a definitive diagnosis and plan of action is made. A vocal minority is now challenging this viewpoint, maintaining that judicious and careful use of analgesics in this situation is humane, does not obscure the diagnosis, and may even enhance patient evaluation. Further studies on this controversy are needed.

BIBLIOGRAPHY

Brewer RJ et al: Abdominal pain: An analysis of 1,000 consecutive cases in a university hospital emergency room. *Am J Surg* 131:219, 1976.

Doris PE, Strauss RW: The expanded role of the barium enema in the evaluation of patients presenting with acute abdominal pain. *J Emerg Med,* 3:93, 1985.

Eisenberg RL, Heineken P, Hedgcock MW, et al: Evaluation of plain abdominal radiographs of abdominal pain. *Ann Surg* 46:116, 1980.

Howie CR, Gunn AA: Temperature: A poor diagnostic indicator in abdominal pain. *J Roy Coll Surg Edinburgh* 29:249, 1984.

Irvin TT: Abdominal pain: A surgical audit of 1190 emergency admissions. *Br J Surg* 76:1121, 1989.

McAdam WA, Brock BM, Armitage T, et al: Twelve years' experience of computer-aided diagnosis in a district general hospital. *Ann R Coll Surg Engl* 72:140, 1990.

Mirvis SE, Young JWR, Keramati B, et al: Plain film evaluation of patients with abdominal pain: Are three radiographs necessary? *AJR* 147:501, 1986.

Reisertsen L, Rosseland AR, Hoivik B, et al: Laparoscopy in patients admitted for acute abdominal pain. *Acta Chir Scand* 151:521, 1985.

Simeone JF, Novelline RA, Ferrucci JT, et al: Comparison of sonography and plain films in evaluation of the acute abdomen. *AJR* 144:49, 1985.

Zoltie N, Cust MP: Analgesia in the acute abdomen. *Ann Roy Coll Surg Engl,* 68:210, 1986.

F. GASTROINTESTINAL BLEEDING

David T. Overton

Gastrointestinal bleeding should be considered potentially life-threatening until proved otherwise. Despite advances in medical care, the mortality for these patients has remained constant. While most patients will volunteer the chief complaints of hematemesis, hematochezia, or melena, gastrointestinal bleeding may have more subtle presentations. Patients with hypotension, tachycardia, angina, syncope, weakness, confusion, or even cardiac arrest may harbor occult gastrointestinal hemorrhage.

As with all true emergencies, the traditional triad of history, physical examination, and diagnosis often must be accomplished simultaneously with resuscitation and stabilization.

HISTORY

A carefully performed history can often point to the source of bleeding. The symptoms of hematemesis, coffee-ground emesis, melena, or hematochezia should be sought. Classically, hematemesis or coffee-ground emesis suggests a source proximal to the ligament of Treitz. Melena suggests a source at or proximal to the right colon, and hematochezia indicates a more distal colorectal lesion. The clinician, however, should remember that exceptions to these rules occur. Weight loss or changes in bowel habits are classic symptoms of malignancy. Vomiting and retching, followed by hematemesis, is suggestive of a Mallory-Weiss tear.

A history of drug ingestion should be carefully sought, particularly of salicylates, corticosteroids, nonsteroidal anti-inflammatory agents, and anticoagulants. Alcohol abuse is strongly associated with a number of causes of gastrointestinal bleeding, including peptic ulcer disease, erosive gastritis, and esophageal varices. Ingestion of iron or bismuth can simulate melena, and certain foods, such as beets, can simulate hematochezia. In such instances, stool guaiac testing will be negative.

A prior history of gastrointestinal bleeding should be noted. Although recurrent episodes of bleeding might appear to be from the same source, this is often not the case. A history of an aortic graft should suggest the possibility of an aortoenteric fistula.

PHYSICAL EXAMINATION

The vital signs may reveal obvious hypotension and tachycardia or more subtle manifestations such as a decreased pulse pressure or tachypnea. Orthostatic vital sign changes may unmask otherwise occult volume deficits. The clinician should remember that some patients can tolerate substantial volume losses with minimal or no changes in vital signs. Similarly, paradoxical bradycardia can occur in the face of profound hypovolemia.

Skin findings should be noted. Cool, clammy skin is an obvious sign of shock. Spider angiomata, palmar erythema, jaundice, and gynecomastia suggest underlying liver disease. Petechiae and purpura suggest an underlying coagulopathy. Skin findings may bring the Peutz-Jeghers, Rendu-Osler-Weber, or Gardner's syndrome to mind.

A careful ENT examination may occasionally reveal an occult bleeding source which has resulted in swallowed blood and subsequent coffee-ground emesis or melena. The abdominal examination may disclose tenderness, masses, ascites, or organomegaly. A rectal examination is mandatory, for detection of the presence of blood, its appearance (bright red, maroon, or frankly melanotic), and the presence of any masses.

LABORATORY DATA

In patients with significant gastrointestinal bleeding, the most important laboratory test is to type and cross-match blood. Other important laboratory data include CBC and coagulation studies. Additionally, BUN, creatinine, electrolytes, glucose, and liver function studies should be considered. The initial hematocrit level often will not reflect the actual amount of blood loss. Upper tract hemorrhage may elevate the BUN through digestion and absorption of hemoglobin. Coagulation studies, including prothrombin time, partial thromboplastin time, and platelet count are of obvious benefit in patients taking anticoagulants or those with underlying hepatic disease. Although coagulation studies are usually normal in other patients, they should be obtained nonetheless, as unsuspected abnormalities will lead to important changes in emergency management.

An ECG should be considered in patients in the coronary artery disease age group. Silent ischemia can and does occur secondary to the decreased oxygen delivery accompanying gastrointestinal bleeding.

RADIOGRAPHIC STUDIES

Routine abdominal radiographs are often obtained in patients with gastrointestinal bleeding. In the absence of specific indications, they are of limited value. Barium contrast studies are similarly of limited value in the emergency situation. Furthermore, barium limits the use of subsequent endoscopy or angiography.

Gastrointestinal angiography can sometimes detect the site of bleeding, particularly in cases of obscure lower gastrointestinal bleeding. However, it requires a relatively brisk bleeding rate (0.5 to 2.0 mL/min) to be diagnostic. Endoscopy is more accurate in most circumstances. Angiography, however, may allow intraarterial embolization, or the use of vasopressors.

MANAGEMENT

Primary

As with any emergency situation, immediate resuscitative measures take priority. Patients with profuse upper gastrointestinal hemorrhage may require definitive airway management in order to prevent aspiration of blood. Oxygen should be given to any patient with a significant gastrointestinal bleed, and cardiac monitoring is likewise indicated. Volume replacement should be initiated with crystalloids via large-bore intravenous lines. The decision to administer blood should be based on the clinical findings of volume depletion or continued bleeding more than on initial hematocrit values. Coagulation factors should be replaced as needed. A urinary catheter is indicated in patients with hypotension.

A nasogastric tube should be placed in all patients with significant gastrointestinal bleeding regardless of presumed source. Bright red blood per rectum often unexpectedly originates from massive upper gastrointestinal sources. A negative gastric aspirate does not conclusively rule out an upper gastrointestinal etiology and may result from intermittent bleeding or pyloric spasm or edema preventing reflux of duodenal blood. Standard guaiac paper may yield falsely negative results in the presence of low gastric pH.

If bright red blood or clots are found on nasogastric intubation, gastric lavage should be done. To be effective, a large-bore tube, usually oral, must be used. Room temperature saline is the preferred irrigant, as iced solutions have no proven benefit and have theoretical disadvantages. The addition of levarterenol to the lavage solution is similarly of unproven benefit. Overvigorous suction should be avoided, as it may produce gastric erosions which can confuse findings on subsequent endoscopy.

Secondary

Endoscopy

Upper gastrointestinal endoscopy is the most accurate technique for the identification of upper gastrointestinal bleeding sites. Traditional teaching has suggested that there is no reduction in mortality as a result of diagnostic endoscopy. However, this view is changing. Sclerotherapy of esophageal varices is rapidly becoming the treatment of choice of acute variceal bleeding, and can control acute hemorrhage in over 90 percent of patients. Sclerotherapy may decrease the duration of hospitalization and amount of blood transfused when compared with portal-caval shunting. It is less clear, however, if sclerotherapy is indicated in the prophylactic treatment of asymptomatic varices. Complications of sclerotherapy include perforation, sepsis, and portal and mesenteric venous thrombosis.

Endoscopic hemostasis has also been used successfully in nonvariceal etiologies of upper gastrointestinal bleeding, using technologies such as sclerotherapy, electrocoagulation, heater probes, and lasers.

Proctoscopy can often be diagnostic in patients with anorectal sources of bleeding. If an anorectal source such as hemorrhoids is suspected, the patient should be carefully evaluated for significant volume loss or more dangerous proximal sources of bleeding mimicking hemorrhoidal bleeding.

Sigmoidoscopy and colonoscopy can be diagnostic in other forms of lower gastrointestinal hemorrhage, such as diverticulosis or angiodysplasia. Attempted ablation of bleeding sites using the technologies noted above is being investigated.

Drug Therapy

Vasopressin has been used by both intravenous and intraarterial infusion to control gastrointestinal bleeding. Intravenous infusion has been shown to be as effective as intraarterial and is far easier to perform. Intravenous vasopressin infusion has been evaluated most extensively in the treatment of esophageal variceal bleeding. Infusion rates of 0.1 to 0.9 units/min are described, but adverse reactions are common. Hypertension, cardiac arrhythmias, myocardial and splanchnic ischemia, decreased cardiac output, and gangrene from local infiltration are all described. Thus, the use of vasopressin currently should be considered an adjunct to more definitive measures.

Histamine-2 antagonists are of unproven benefit in acute upper gastrointestinal hemorrhage. There is no conclusive evidence for reduction in the rates of rebleeding, surgery, or death.

Balloon Tamponade

Balloon tamponade with the Sengstaken-Blakemore tube or its variants can provide therapeutic benefit and presumptive diagnostic information. It can control documented variceal hemorrhage in 40 to 80 percent of patients. The device consists of gastric and esophageal balloons and, depending on the variation, often includes gastric and/or esophageal aspiration ports. The gastric balloon should be inflated first. If bleeding does not cease, the esophageal balloon should then be inflated, using a manometer to ensure that the pressure does not exceed 40 to 50 mmHg. Radiological confirmation of proper balloon placement is suggested. The balloon should be kept in place 24 h after bleeding has ceased. Some authors recommend deflating the esophageal balloon for 30 to 60 min every 8 h to prevent mucosal ulceration.

Like vasopressin therapy, balloon tamponade is frequently associated with adverse reactions, often severe. Mucosal ulceration, esophageal or gastric rupture, asphyxiation from dislodged balloons, tracheal compression secondary to balloon inflation, and aspiration pneumonia have been reported. Some authors recommend routine prophylactic endotracheal intubation to prevent pulmonary complications. Because of the incidence of adverse reactions, balloon tamponade should be considered an adjunctive or temporizing measure supplementing the more definitive modalities of sclerotherapy or surgical intervention.

Surgery

In patients who do not respond to medical therapy, and in whom endoscopic hemostasis, if available, fails, emergency surgical intervention is indicated. Surgical consultation on any patient admitted to the hospital for gastrointestinal bleeding is prudent, in case uncontrollable rebleeding occurs.

CAUSES OF UPPER GASTROINTESTINAL BLEEDING

Peptic Ulcer Disease

Peptic ulcer disease, including gastric, duodenal, and stomal ulcers, remains the most common etiology for upper gastrointestinal hemorrhage, encompassing approximately 50 percent of all cases. Duodenal ulcers, approximately 29 percent of the total, will rebleed in approximately 10 percent of cases, usually within 24 to 48 h. Gastric ulcers, approximately 16 percent of all cases, are more likely to rebleed. Stomal ulcers are uncommon (less than 5 percent of all upper gastrointestinal bleeds) and are present in only one-third of bleeding patients with a history of prior peptic ulcer surgery.

Erosive Gastritis and Esophagitis

Combined erosive gastritis, esophagitis, and duodenitis are responsible for approximately 20 percent of all cases of upper gastrointestinal hemorrhage. Irritative factors, such as alcohol, salicylates, or hiatal hernia, are predisposing factors.

Esophageal Varices

Esophageal or gastric varices result from portal hypertension, in the United States most often as a result of alcoholic liver disease. Although varices account for only about 10 percent of all cases of upper gastrointestinal hemorrhage, they are highly likely to rebleed and carry a high mortality rate. Despite this, it is interesting to note that many patients with end-stage cirrhosis never develop varices, many patients with documented varices never bleed, and many patients presenting with upper gastrointestinal bleeding and a documented history of varices will be bleeding from other sites.

Mallory-Weiss Syndrome

The Mallory-Weiss syndrome is upper gastrointestinal bleeding secondary to a longitudinal mucosal tear in the cardioesophageal region. The classic history is repeated retching followed by bright red hematemesis, but coughing and seizures have been reported as etiologic factors.

Other Etiologies

Stress ulcers (Cushing's or Curling's), arteriovenous malformations, and malignancies are other etiologies of upper gastrointestinal hemorrhage. ENT sources of bleeding can masquerade as gastrointestinal hemorrhage. An aortoenteric fistula secondary to an aortic graft is an unusual but important cause of bleeding to keep in mind. Classically, patients will present with a self-limited "herald" bleed prior to a subsequent massive hemorrhage.

CAUSES OF LOWER GASTROINTESTINAL BLEEDING

Upper Gastrointestinal Bleeding

The most common cause of apparent lower gastrointestinal bleeding remains upper gastrointestinal bleeding. Thus proximal etiologies should be sought.

Diverticulosis

Diverticulosis remains the most common cause of massive lower gastrointestinal bleeding. The bleeding is usually painless and results from erosion into the lumen of the penetrating artery of the diverticulum. Patients are often elderly with underlying medical illnesses which contribute to morbidity and mortality. If the hemorrhage does not cease spontaneously, arteriography with vasopressin infusion or injection of Gelfoam or autologous clot may be considered. Alternatively, colonoscopy with endoscopic hemostasis may be used. If these measures fail, emergency surgery may be necessary.

Angiodysplasia

Arteriovenous malformations or angiodysplasia, usually of the right colon, are a recognized etiology of obscure lower gastrointestinal bleeding, particularly in the elderly population. They are reputed to be more common in patients with hypertension and aortic stenosis.

Other Etiologies

Numerous other lesions may result in lower gastrointestinal hemorrhage. Carcinoma and hemorrhoids are common causes of bleeding, but massive hemorrhage is unusual. Similarly, inflammatory bowel disease, polyps, and infectious gastroenteritis rarely cause massive bleeding. Meckel's diverticulum is an unusual but important etiology to keep in mind.

BIBLIOGRAPHY

Collins R, Langman M: Treatment with histamine H_2 antagonists in acute upper gastrointestinal hemorrhage. *N Engl J Med* 313:660, 1985.

Fleischer D: Endoscopic therapy of upper gastrointestinal bleeding in humans. *Gastroenterology* 90:217, 1986.

Gogel HK, Tandberg D: Emergency management of upper gastrointestinal hemorrhage. *Am J Emerg Med* 4:150, 1986.

Jensen DM, Machilado GA, Taipa JI: Emergent colonoscopy in patients with severe hematochezia. *Gastrointest Endosc* 29:177, 1983.

Henderson JM, Kutner MH, Millikan WJ et al: Endoscopic variceal sclerosis compared with distal splenorenal shunt to prevent recurrent variceal bleeding in cirrhosis: A prospective, randomized trial. *Ann Intern Med* 112:262, 1990.

Lieberman D: Endoscopic therapy for bleeding from the upper gastrointestinal tract. *Postgrad Med* 87:75, 1990.

Long PC, Wilentz KV, Sudlow G, et al: Modification of the hemoccult slide test for occult blood in gastric juice. *Crit Care Med* 10:692, 1982.

Olsson R: The natural history of esophageal varices: A retrospective study of 224 cases with liver cirrhosis. *Digestion* 6:65, 1972.

Pitcher JL: Variceal hemorrhage among patients with varices and upper gastrointestinal hemorrhage. *S Med J* 70:1183, 1977.

Schuman BM, Beckman JW, Tedesco FJ, et al: Complications of endoscopic injection sclerotherapy: A review. *Am J Gastroenterol* 82:823, 1987.

Steele RJ: Endoscopic haemostasis for non-variceal upper gastrointestinal haemorrhage. *Br J Surg* 76:219, 1989.

Sugawa C: Endoscopic diagnosis and treatment of upper gastrointestinal bleeding. *Surg Clin North Am* 69:1167, 1989.

Terblanche J, Krige JE, Bornman PC: Endoscopic sclerotherapy. *Surg Clin North Am* 70:341, 1990.

Vellacott KD: Early endoscopy for acute lower gastrointestinal haemorrhage. *Ann R Coll Surg Engl* 68:243, 1986.

G. COMA AND ALTERED STATES OF CONSCIOUSNESS

Gregory L. Henry

Although coma is the most dramatic of the disorders of consciousness, it is only the endpoint in a continuum. Any disease process which can cause coma may initially present with mild alterations of, and progressively decreasing, mental status. It is often difficult or impossible to determine the direction and final outcome of a change in mental status until the most important test, time, has been applied.

In severe nervous system disease, a change in mental status is often the first sign of a severe pathological process. It is a well-recognized rule within the neurosciences that functional change is always greater and always precedes structural change in the brain and spinal cord. Of all the central nervous system functions, mental status is the most delicate and the most sensitive early bellwether of advancing disease.

It is important for any health professional dealing with altered mental status to realize that nothing replaces our standard approach to all emergency patients, namely, "A, B, C_3." *A*irway management and *b*reathing should be the first priorities of the evaluation of any patient in the emergency department. *C*ardiac status is next assessed and supported as necessary. The other two C's stand for *c*ervical spine immobilization and compression of obvious hemorrhage. It will be of little benefit to the patient or to society to have properly diagnosed a subdural hematoma if you have missed a fourth cervical vertebrae fracture and created a quadriplegic. The basic rule is that a comatose patient has suffered a cervical spine injury until proved otherwise.

The principal function of this chapter will be to review classification systems for patients with altered mental status and to provide a framework for evaluating such patients in the emergency setting. The immediate duty of the emergency department, with regard to patients with altered mental status, is to divide the potentially exhaustive list of disease entities into two major groups. The first and most common subset is that of diffuse metabolic and toxic disease. The second major group is that of structural, focal, central nervous system disease. Since the management of toxic and metabolic disease is principally medical and the management of focal disease is frequently surgical, it is important that these differentiations be made early so that correct treatment can be initiated. To delay making this important differential can mean severe disability and even death to the patient.

The determination of structural neurologic disease is based on a focal neurologic examination. Those patients who are developing discrete, isolated lesions of motor or sensory function or specific cortical defects will have structural or anatomic damage most of the time. This is the group of patients in whom immediate surgical therapy is most beneficial in salvaging meaningful life.

DEFINITIONS

A clear understanding of the terminology of altered mental status is necessary before classifying various diseases entities. The physician is better served by describing in the body of the chart exactly what he or she sees. Nonspecific terms are often misleading and not helpful for further examiners who must reassess the patient on an ongoing basis. It is much more useful to record in the chart objective findings such as the patient's ability to handle three-object retention and mathematical calculations as opposed to using terms such as "stuporous" or "lethargic." But since the following terminology has become universal in medical literature, some general understanding of the terms is needed. *Consciousness* is defined as an awareness of self and the environment. Disorders of consciousness can be divided into states where the patient appears asleep and states where the patient appears awake but is unresponsive.

Patients Who Appear Asleep

Sleep. A state of nonpathologic decreased mental status from which the patient can be easily aroused to full consciousness.

Lethargy. Depressed mental status in which the patient may appear wakeful but has depressed awareness of self and environment globally.

Stupor. Unresponsiveness from which the patient can be aroused with vigorous noxious stimuli constitutes stupor. The stuporous patient, however, does not return to a normal baseline of awareness of self or environment.

Coma. Coma is a state of unresponsiveness, from which the patient cannot be aroused by verbal and physical stimuli to produce any meaningful response.

Psychogenic coma. Psychogenic coma is a state of unresponsiveness, either voluntary or involuntary, from which the patient cannot be brought to reasonable cortical response by noxious verbal or physical stimuli. These patients do, however, have normal physiological testing and EEG responses.

Patients Who Appear Awake but Are Unresponsive

Abulic state. In the abulic state (also known as *akinetic mutism* or "coma vigil"), the patient is awake with eyes open but extremely slow to respond to questions asked. The patient's frontal lobe function is so depressed, from any number of processes, that meaningful response in a normal time frame is impossible. It should be noted that these patients often do have reasonable mental status, but because of the huge delays in their ability to process information and answer, they are often misdiagnosed in the emergency department. These patients may take several minutes to respond to any problem or question posed.

Locked-in syndrome. In the "locked-in" syndrome (also known as the "Count of Monte Cristo" syndrome) (M. Nortier de Villefort), patients appear absolutely motionless but their eyes are open. The lesion in the locked-in syndrome is the destruction of the ventral pontine motor tracts. The only function that these patients maintain is vertical eye movement. It is important, in all unresponsive patients who appear awake, that the examiner ask them to look up. In patients who can look up but cannot move their eyes from side to side, the diagnosis of locked-in syndrome is secured.

Psychogenic unresponsiveness. Also known as the *catatonic state*, psychogenic unresponsiveness is a level of unresponsiveness in which the patient appears awake and may maintain normal motor posturing and neurological testing, but who, for voluntary or involuntary reasons, is not able to communicate with the examiner.

Confusional States

This category covers a series of disorders in which mental status is not depressed, but in which the patient misinterprets external stimuli. These states may overlap with causes of depressed mental status and may be extremely difficult to differentiate in an emergency setting. The hallmarks of these conditions are global confusion. inability to appropriately process stimuli, or inability to make meaningful responses. Such findings are characteristic of a toxic ingestion, metabolic encephalopathy, or central nervous system infection.

THE PATHOPHYSIOLOGY OF ALTERED MENTAL STATUS

Although the specific causes of altered mental status are legion, the pathophysiology is either bilateral cerebral cortical disease or suppression of the brainstem reticular activating formation (RAF). Cellular disorders such as lipid storage disease or neuronal degeneration rarely present as acute changes in mental status.

Bilateral Cortical Disease

Focal lesions in one cerebral cortex cause neurological findings specific to that region but do not cause alteration of mental status. If the altered mental status is thought to be based on cortical disease, both cortices should be involved. For example, patients who have had large sections of the cerebral cortex removed by surgery can still be awake and alert. The most common causes of bilateral cortical disease altering mental status are toxins such as alcohol and illicit drugs and deficiencies of the metabolic substrates oxygen and glucose.

If the brain is deprived of its normal supply of oxygen by impairment of systemic oxygen uptake or distribution for more than about 10 s, loss of consciousness ensues. A marked decrease or increase of serum glucose can rapidly lead to changes in mental status.

Reticular Activating System Lesions

The other principal mechanism by which altered mental status is produced is through involvement of the reticular activating formation, a small grouping of fibers which traverses the brainstem and thalamus. Through continuous stimulation of the cortex, the RAF maintains the state of wakefulness. Any sudden interruption of RAF activity affects alertness. For example, it is postulated that the mechanism by which a boxer's blow to the chin causes sudden coma is not through damage to the cortical structures but rather through torque forces on the brainstem which interrupt RAF activity.

The reticular activating formation can be affected in three principal ways: by supratentorial pressure, by infratentorial pressure, and by intrinsic brainstem lesions.

Supratentorial pressure. The manner in which supratentorial lesions produce coma is by enlarging and displacing tissue. This causes compression of the opposite hemisphere, as well as deeper diencephalic and brainstem structures. By pressing on the brainstem through this remote mechanism, the RAF is also compressed. The skull is a limited area and the brain and its protective and supporting structures occupy the entire intracranial space. When additional volume accumulates in the skull, either as a discrete mass or from generalized edema, pressure is directed to the point of least resistance. The temporal lobes, which rest on the tentorium cerebelli, may be forced through the tentorial notch, compressing brainstem structures and cranial nerves. Therefore, the mechanism of coma in patients with acute supratentorial lesions such as epidural, subdural, or intraparenchymal bleeding is not due to destruction of specific cortex but rather from pressure directed toward deeper brainstem structures.

Infratentorial pressure. The brainstem lies below the tentorium cerebelli and is anatomically distinct from the great mass of cerebral tissue which lies above. The brainstem shares the posterior fossa with the ventricular aqueduct of Sylvius, the fourth ventricle, and the cerebellum. An increase in pressure in this area may be accompanied by movement of the posterior fossa contents upward through the tentorial notch or downward through the foramen magnum. For example, tumors involving the meninges, brainstem, and cerebellum, or acute cerebellar hemorrhage can increase pressure.This causes compression on the reticular activating formation and resultant coma.

Intrinsic brainstem lesion. Lesions intrinsic to the brainstem itself, such as traumatic or hypertensive pontine hemorrhage, may also compress the reticular activating formation directly.

In summary, severely depressed mental status is due to either bilateral cortical disease or involvement of the reticular activating formation. Bilateral cortical disease is almost always due to metabolic or toxic causes and generally shows no focal neurological findings. Reticular activating formation dysfunction, on the other hand, is more likely the result of structural disease and will most frequently have focal neurological findings.

GENERAL APPROACH TO THE PATIENT WITH ALTERED MENTAL STATUS

Initial Management

In the usual clinical approach to a patient, the examiner first obtains a history, then performs a physical examination and laboratory studies, and finally adminsters treatment. However, this sequence is not correct for patients in a coma. Coma is such a major variance from normal neurological functioning that immediate supportive efforts are required. The A, B, C_3 approach must be activated. For patients who do not have an active gag reflex, positive airway control is urgently needed to prevent aspiration. If cervical spinal fracture is suspected, or if the mechanism of coma is unknown, the neck must be stabilized while the airway is secured, and endotracheal intubation should be avoided. For patients in whom there is no obvious facial trauma and who are actively breathing, nasotracheal intubation is an excellent alternative. In patients who have had severe midfacial and oral trauma and in whom the standard approaches are contraindicated, a cricothyroidotomy may be necessary.

Once airway control is established, oxygenation and hyperventilation are necessary. Mild hyperventilation corrects acidosis, and lowering the P_{CO_2} reduces intracranial pressure. The P_{CO_2} should be lowered to approximately 25 torr. This level can usually be obtained by ventilating the patient approximately 20 to 25 times per minute.

Cardiac status should be assessed to make certain that the patient has reasonable cardiac output and that there is no reason to begin cardiac pulmonary resuscitation.

Immobilization of the cervical spine, as has been previously mentioned, is mandatory in patients in whom the cause of coma is unknown. Without a definite history, the possibility of trauma always exists. The mere smell of alcohol on the breath of the patient does not constitute a definite cause for that person's altered mental status. It is the general rule that all alcoholics fall and hit their heads. Encounters where the alcoholic is both intoxicated and suffering from an intracranial lesion *and* a cervical spine fracture are well within the experience of emergency physicians. Aggressive neck immobilization and restraints to the body so that the head and body function as a unit is the most effective way to anticipate cervical spine injury.

Finally, obvious hemorrhage should be stopped before detailed neurological examination is begun. One of the earliest signs of shock is apprehension and confusion. As shock worsens, mental status quickly deteriorates, and thus the patient in hemorrhagic shock may well be lethargic or comatose. Vital signs should be obtained and recorded at this point if not already done.

Initial Treatment

As an intravenous line is being inserted, blood should be removed for laboratory analysis. Generally, enough blood should be drawn to allow for CBC, glucose, BUN, creatinine, and electrolyte analyses. It is generally standard to administer intravenously thiamine, 100 mg; glucose, 25 to 50 g; and naloxone, 2 to 4 mg. Newer thiamine derivatives do not produce anaphylactoid reactions when given intravenously. Nutritionally deficient patients such as alcoholics or patients receiving cancer chemotherapy should receive thiamine prior to glucose administration. Thiamine is given to facilitate carbohydrate metabolism and to prevent the unwanted complication of Wernick's syndrome.

The standard dose of glucose is 25 to 50 g as a 50% solution. In the patient with an intracranial mass lesion glucose increases the osmotic load and is potentially beneficial in reducing intracranial pressure. In the patient who is comatose because of hyperglycemia, the recommended dose of glucose is inconsequential. Dextrostik determination of blood glucose may be done prior to glucose administration.

Generally, 2 mg of naloxone are given intravenously, and followed by two more mg if no response is seen. There are no dose-related adverse affects of naloxone reported, although the possibility of an acute opiate withdrawal syndrome increases along with the dose of naloxone. Unlike its predecessor, nalorphine, naloxone does not produce respiratory depression. Naloxone is an effective antagonist of opiates and synthetic narcotics such as propoxyphene and pentazocine. A very large dose of naloxone may be required to overcome the endorphin receptor effects of the synthetic narcotics. Any patient who can be aroused with naloxone may become combative and disoriented, so patients should be properly restrained before naloxone is given.

Obtaining the History

The patient may not be a reliable source of information, so other sources must be sought. One of the great mysteries in emergency medicine is the appearance of a comatose patient in the emergency department, without evident means of arrival. This defiance of the laws of physics is accomplished many times each week in any busy emergency department. Some data may be obtained from the patient's personal effects such as medical alert tags, wallet, purse, or pill containers.

Family and friends should be contacted to provide a history. They may be able to describe previous episodes or an event that led up to the current episode. Specific questions about abnormal motor movements, food or drug ingestions, trauma, and underlying diseases should be asked. It is important to provide reassurance that the medical history obtained will remain part of the medical record and will not be inappropriately given to law enforcement officials.

General Physical Examination

Vital signs should be regularly monitored. Arrhythmias should be monitored and treated as clinically indicated. Tachypnea should be considered a sign of inadequate oxygenation and not a sign of central nervous damage. Oxygenation and ventilation should be corrected and then mental status reevaluated. Both hypertension and hypotension should be considered to have a nonneurological cause in a patient with shock until proved otherwise. Although systemic hypertension can be caused by an elevation in intracranial pressure, systemic hypertension should not initially be ascribed to a primary neurological event. Constant cardiac monitoring of the comatose patient is useful to check for intermittent cardiac problems such as fluctuating bradycardias or ventricular arrhythmias. Although these are unusual causes of coma, they represent treatable entities from which a patient may have an excellent neurological recovery.

As the patient is examined, signs of trauma should be carefully sought. Blood behind the tympanic membranes as well as ecchymoses in the amstoid area should be particularly noted. Any patient with these findings should be considered to have a basilar skull fracture. Careful palpation of the head may reveal cephalohematomas which are not visible at first glance. Palpation of the neck, although often advocated is generally nonproductive in the comatose patient. It is best to assume that there is a cervical spine fracture, and immobilze the neck and perform necessary x-rays. Other general signs of trauma such as contusions, fractures, lacerations, and abrasions should also be noted.

Skin

Needle tracks suggest IV drug use. Cyanosis suggests hypoxemia, polycythemia, or an abnormal hemoglobin. Pallor likewise may be an early indication that the patient has inadequate oxygen-carrying capacity due to blood loss of anemia. Carbon monoxide poisoning may produce a cherry-red glow of the mucous membranes. Other more generalized skin findings such as multiple abscesses, cellulitis, uremic frost, or iceterus may point to underlying conditions which affect mental status.

Breath

One should never assume that coma is due to alcohol merely because the odor of alcohol is detectable. The fruity fragrance of acetone or the distinct odor of anaerobic infection should be noted. Fetor hepaticus indicates advanced liver disease. A feculent odor suggests bowel obstruction, while the distinctive odor of almonds indicates cyanide poisoning.

Cardiac Examination

Tachyarrhythmias or bradyarrhythmias can alter mental status because of decreased cardiac output. Endocarditis or arrhythmias which dislodge mural thrombi can produce cerebral emboli. Acute myocardial infarction may reduce cardiac output enough to depress consciousness. An intracranial lesion can result in static ECG changes, such as prolongation of the QT interval or ST-T changes, as well as arrhythmias. The mechanism is probably massive sympathetic outflow resulting in coronary spasm.

Abdominal Examination

Organomegaly, ascites, bruits, and pulsatile masses should be noted to detect conditions that are causative, or present but unassociated with a decrease in mental status. For example, hepatomegaly and ascites may be present in hepatic encephalopathy. The presence of an abdominal aortic aneurysm is consistent with advanced atherosclerotic disease. Grey Turner's or Cullen's signs suggest retroperitoneal hemorrhage. A pelvic/rectal examination should be performed in a comatose patient to detect bleeding, masses, infection, or foreign bodies.

Neurological Examination

The patient should be observed for involuntary movement of all four extremities and abnormal posturing. The patient who is agitated and yet has decreased mental status may have a toxic encephalopathy. Opisthotonic contractions may be due to tetanus, strychnine poisoning, dystonic reactions, or decerebration. Seizures should be observed to determine whether they are focal or generalized.

A simple system for classifying cancer patients is the Glasgow Coma Scale (see Table 13G-1). The Glasgow Coma Scale is useful for statistical analysis of EMS systems but cannot be used for decisions on an individual patient except to indicate in a basic way the severity of the injury and need for rapid intervention. The following more sophisticated evaluation is needed to understand actual brain and brainstem functioning.

Table 13G-1. The Glasgow Coma Scale

EYES		
Open:	Spontaneously	4
	To verbal command	3
	To pain	2
No response:		1
BEST VERBAL RESPONSE		
	Oriented and converses	5
	Disoriented and converses	4
	Inappropriate words	3
	Incomprehensible sounds	2
	No response	1
BEST MOTOR RESPONSE		
To verbal command:	Obeys	6
To painful stimulus:	Localizes pain	5
	Flexion-withdrawal	4
	Abnormal flexion (decorticate rigidity)	3
	Extension (decerebrate rigidity)	2
	No response	1
Total		3–15

Respiratory Pattern

The pattern and rate of respiration should be noted and recorded, as it may indicate the level of neurological injury in the patient.

An awake patient at rest generally breathes about 18 times per minute and has occasional sighing or deeper respirations as demanded by carbon dioxide levels. When the cortex is no longer functioning and the nervous system is relying on diencephalic control of breathing, *Cheyne-Stokes respirations* occur. This is a type of breathing characterized by periodic, regularly increasing breaths alternating with short periods of apnea. The breathing crescendoes to a peak and then ceases suddenly. The apneic phase is usually short. The most frequent causes for Cheyne-Stokes respirations are bilateral metabolic hemispheric disease or structural disease of the bilateral cerebral hemispheres and basal ganglia. The principal mechanism underlying Cheyne-Stokes respirations has to do with loss of forebrain control of ventilatory stimulation.

Hyperventilation in the stuporous or comatose patient may be from a variety of causes. Attempts to correct hypoxia, compensation for metabolic acidosis, and brain injury itself all cause hyperventilation. Central neurogenic hyperventilation is frequently seen with midbrain involvement with destruction of those areas which normally monitor ventilatory patterns. When hyperventilation is caused by central nervous system disease it indicates upper brainstem damage.

Apneustic breathing is characterized by a prolonged pause at the end of inspiration, much like breath-holding. It is seen with lesions about the fifth cranial nerve. *Cluster breathing* is breathing in short bursts and is almost always associated with lesions at the level of the pons. *Ataxic breathing*, irregular breathing without pattern or regularity, is a forerunner of agonal respirations and death.

Autisms are involuntary neurologic acts carried out for maintenance and protection of the body. Yawning, although its mechanism is not well understood, frequently accompanies expanding lesions of the posterior fossa.

The autisms of vomiting, hiccuping, and coughing have neurogenic centers involved in their control. In the face of altered mental status, hiccuping, coughing, and vomiting may be indications of lesions involving lower brainstem centers.

Mental Status

Mental status may be the most sensitive early indicator of nervous system disease and is the first function to be affected in a variety of lesions. The ability to respond to voice and follow commands should be recorded. If the patient cannot respond to voice, then response to firm but gentle touch must be assessed. Finally, response to noxious stimuli is recorded. There is no need to inflict pain on a patient suspected of feigning coma, since there are other more humane techniques for detecting functional disease.

Cranial Nerves

Visual threat is an unreliable test in unresponsive patients, since reactions can be checked voluntarily in certain awake patients. Lack of response to visual threat is not certain evidence for coma. Conversely, during visual threat, when air is moved toward the cornea in a comatose patient, a blink response can result.

Inspection of the ocular fundi gives the examiner the only opportunity to actually view the brain. Evidence of papilledema, hemorrhage, and spontaneous venous pulsations should be sought. Spontaneous venous pulsations in erect patients indicate normal intracranial pressure. This is often difficult to assess with comatose patients since they are recumbent. If spontaneous venous pulsations are seen when the patient is in the recumbent position, however, they clearly indicate that there is not increased intracranial pressure.

Pupils

The size, shape, and reactivity, both direct and consensual, of each pupil should be recorded. The pupillary pathways are relatively resistant to metabolic insult. They receive their parasympathetic supply from the thalamic pretectal region and their sympathetic supply from the superior cervical ganglion which courses along the carotid artery.

Pupillary findings must be interpreted along with the neurological examination. As a general rule, hemispheric disease has very little influence on pupillary function. Usually patients who are comatose from metabolic involvement of the cerebral hemispheres will have small to midrange pupils which are reactive to light. Structural lesions involving the diencephalon may cause small but reactive pupils.

Disparities in pupil size and reactivity can occur with eye trauma, ocular drugs, or previous eye surgery.

A unilateral fixed and dilated pupil should not necessarily be equated with an intracranial mass lesion. It may be the result of a cycloplegic agent instilled in one eye. An expanding aneurysm which compresses the third cranial nerve may cause an ipsilateral fixed and dilated pupil but not affect mental status. The general rule is that if a patient is alert, a dilated pupil is most likely not the result of increasing intracranial pressure. The mechanism for the fixed and dilated pupil seen with severe head injury is herniation of the uncus of the temporal lobe through the tentorial notch, which compresses the third cranial nerve. No patient with this degree of increased intracranial pressure will exhibit normal mental status.

Lesions which involve the midbrain tectal regions may cause midsized to large pupils which may respond poorly to light. Pontine lesions frequently cause fixed pinpoint pupils which are not affected by naloxone. Anoxia, atropine, and cycloplegics may all cause dilated pupils. Pinpoint pupils, which are reversible with naloxone, result from narcotics. Certain narcotics, however, such as propoxyphene, may leave the pupils intact and reactive. One cannot rule out a narcotic overdose strictly on the basis of pupillary size and reactivity.

Ocular Movements

In the awake patient, eye movements are directed by both anterior frontal lobe and posterior occipital lobe control centers which are connected to the pontine gaze centers. These gaze centers lie adjacent to the sixth cranial nerve and, in turn, direct eye movements by way of the medial longitudinal fasciculus (MLF). The MLF, which runs from the upper cervical spine through the area of the third cranial nerve, is the principal interconnection for all conjugate eye movements. Because it extends over a considerable length into the brainstem itself, testing of the MLF is the best single method for judging intactness of brainstem.

Without cortical control, most comatose patients will have roving eye movements, assuming that the brainstem is intact. Eye movements may be disconjugate or conjugate, but as long as both eyes cross the midline, there is no evidence of damage at the brainstem level.

The eyes may be abnormally deviated due to injury involving cortical gaze centers or pontine gaze centers. A general rule regarding cortical injuries is that the eyes will be directed toward a physiologically inactive lesion and away from an irritative or active focus. For example, during a seizure the eyes will be directed away from the side of the seizure focus.

To decide whether the cause of coma is a cortical or brainstem lesion, oculocephalic mechanisms must be tested. The presence of oculocephalic reflexes depends on the fact that the MLF receives constant information as to the position of the patient's head through the output of the semicircular canals. Without cortical influences, an intact brainstem maintains the eyes forward or upward when the patient is supine. This is the basis of the "doll's eye maneuver," the involuntary movement of the eyes upward and downward on passive flexion and

Table 13G-2. Oculovestibular Testing for Brainstem Integrity

Ice-Water Effect	Interpretation
Both eyes deviate and good nystagmus produced	Patient is not comatose
Both eyes deviate toward cold water—bilateral—no fast phase	Coma, but intact brainstem function
No eye movement despite cold stimuli to both sides—indirectly	Brainstem—complete dysfunction from structural, metabolic, or hypothermic causes
Movement of only eye ipsilateral to side stimulant but not opposite eye	Internuclear lesion

extension of the head. In a comatose patient in whom a cervical spine injury is suspected, the test is contraindicated.

Oculovestibular or cold caloric testing is a more sophisticated method to test the integrity of the brainstem (Table 13G-2). To perform the test, the examiner injects 50 mL of ice-cold water against the tympanic membrane. Countercurrent flow is set up in the semicircular canals, and information is transmitted to pontine gaze centers near the ipsilateral sixth nerve nucleus. The altered endolymphatic flow allows the centers to believe that the head has been rapidly turned in the opposite direction. Only four clinical responses are possible: (1) bilateral nystagmus, (2) bilateral conjugate deviation, (3) no response, and (4) unilateral eye deviation.

For the sake of the following discussion, we will assume that 50 mL of ice water has just been instilled in the right ear of a patient. If cold caloric stimulation of the right ear produces prominent nystagmus of both eyes, the cerebral cortex, MLF, and brainstem are intact. If both eyes move conjugately toward the side irrigated with cold water, and if they remain deviated in that direction, the midbrain and its brainstem reflexes are intact on that side. When cold water is instilled into the other ear, both eyes should again move conjugately toward the side of the cold-water irrigation. This assures that the entire brainstem reflex system is intact, that the pontine and midbrain structures are functioning normally.

If the eyes simply do not move in any direction despite bilateral testing, the brainstem is structurally or physiologically functionless. For example, severe hypothermia, drug overdose, or brainstem herniation can all result in absence of oculovestibular reflexes. Therefore, lack of response to cold caloric testing does not necessarily signify an irreversible process.

Finally, cold water stimulation may produce an ipsilateral ocular response only.

If the right ear is irrigated and the right eye moves but the left does not, an intranuclear ophthalmoplegia is present. That is, the sixth cranial nerve on the side tested is functioning, but it is not able to transmit information to the opposite side of the brainstem. The opposite third cranial nerve which would cause the conjugate medial movement of the left eye has not been stimulated. Such a situation almost always indicates structural damage of the brainstem. This finding necessitates a rapid evaluation to determine if there is a structural problem which can be surgically corrected.

Other Cranial Nerves

Other useful tests of the cranial nerves involve the corneal reflex and the facial muscles. The sensory portion of the corneal reflex is mediated through the fifth cranial nerve. Its efferent motor reaction is processed through the seventh cranial nerve. One must look for both the direct and consensual response to determine whether the reflex is working properly.

Facial asymmetry can only be judged in active motion. Particularly below the level of the nose, many normal people have mildly asymmetric faces. One cannot rule in or out a seventh-nerve lesion on the basis of a mild lower facial asymmetry at rest.

The eighth cranial nerve is of little localizing value in stuporous and comatose patients. Its fibers cross through the trapezoid body at the level of the lower pons and are therefore not strictly isolated to a particular side of the brainstem. Examination of the ninth, tenth, eleventh, and twelfth cranial nerves in comatose patients is likewise of little value in determining the level of functioning or underlying mechanism. Documentation of the gag response, however, is important to evaluate the risk of aspiration.

Motor Testing

The first part of the motor examination, observation, should have already been completed. Spontaneous motor movements are generally a good sign. The ability of the muscles to move without external stimuli indicates the patient is sending some cortical instructions down the motor pathway. Any patient who can follow a command or move a body part on command is showing high-level motor system function. Such a patient is not comatose.

Responses to stimuli help to isolate the level at which the nervous system is functioning. Abduction of the limbs or movements toward the site of noxious stimulation show motor system involvement, at least at diencephalic levels.

Decorticate posturing is hyperextension in the legs, and flexion at the arms and the elbows with the hands coming in toward the center of the body. Such posturing can occur with lesions of the internal capsule and upper midbrain which interfere with the corticospinal pathways.

Decerebrate rigidity, in which the teeth are clenched and the arms and legs extended, is seen in only a few situations. It usually is caused by severe disease involving the central midbrain, leaving the lower brainstem below the central midbrain regions intact. Posterior fossa lesions causing pressure against the brainstem may also cause this type of posturing. Decerebrate posturing can also accompany postanoxic cerebral demyelinization.

Total paralysis in the comatose patient with no posturing despite the application of noxious stimuli should be considered a grave finding. This indicates that no protective brainstem mechanisms are functioning. This can be seen in severe, deep, metabolic and toxic comas but is more likely in structural lesions which affect the brainstem nuclei. To be certain that no movement is possible, stimuli must be given both above and below the foramen magnum. Patients with cervical spinal injuries may only be able to grimace or move facial musculature if their motor tracts have been severed in the cervical cord region.

Sensory Examination

Sensory examination of the comatose patient essentially parallels the motor examination. Both the sensory or afferent fibers and the motor or efferent fibers should be tested. Hemisensory lesions as well as specific sensory levels should be sought.

Reflex Status

Reflexes in comatose patients may be sensitive but not terribly specific. An upgoing toe can indicate lesions along the cortical spinal tract all the way from the cerebral cortex down to the motor neuron. The importance of reflex testing in the comatose patient, as in the awake patient, lies in determining the general level of the lesion by comparing responses side to side and top to bottom. Abdominal reflexes are of extremely low value and not worth testing in comatose patients.

In summary, the neurological examination (see Table 13G-3) of the patient with altered mental status has only a few areas of vital importance. Correct assessment of the level of mental status is paramount. Examination of respiratory pattern, extraocular movements, pupils, and motor function all need to be simultaneously integrated to determine the level of neurological function. The principal goal of the

Table 13G-3. Rostrocaudal Brainstem Deterioration Secondary to Expanding Right Supratentorial Mass

Anatomic Level	Consciousness	Respiration	Pupils	Oculovestibular	Motor
Upper diencephalon	Drowsy (dull)	Eupnea with yawns and sighs	Small, reactive	Depression of ocular checking and fast component of nystagmus	Left hemiparesis, bilat. paratonia
Lower diencephalon	Coma	Cheyne-Stokes (CSR)	Small, reactive	Loss of above	Left hemiparesis, decorticate
Mesencephalon	Coma	CSR central neurogenic hyperventilation (CNH)	Midposition fixed (MPF)	Dysconjugate response (loss of medial rectus function on horizontal gaze)	Decerebrate
Upper pons	Coma	CNH: ataxic	MPF	As above	Weak decerebrate
Lower pons	Coma	Ataxic; eupnea	MFP	None	Flaccid; areflexic
Medulla	Coma	Apnea	MPF	None	Same

neurologic examination is to distinguish structural, localized lesions from diffuse metabolic disease.

LABORATORY AND X-RAY EVALUATION

The selection of laboratory and radiographic tests is guided by the history and initial evaluation. However, initial supportive therapy for the comatose patient must be done first, and an orderly approach to the laboratory can then follow.

A complete blood count is generally routine. Severe anemia or leukemias may be of diagnostic importance in coma.

Alterations in serum electrolytes, such as hyper- or hyponatremia or hypercalcemia, can cause altered mental status. Coma can result from sudden shifts in serum osmolality below 260 mOsm/L and above 330 mOsm/L. Glucose, sodium, and the alcohols are the most potent osmotically active substances generally encountered in clinical medicine. Hypoglycemia has been previously discussed.

Blood urea nitrogen (BUN), if it rises slowly, is usually not a cause of coma. Patients in whom there has been a sudden increase in BUN above 60 mg/100 mL may suffer significant alterations in mental status.

Arterial blood gases must be determined in all comatose patients. Hypoxia and hypercarbia can cause coma, and alkalosis and acidosis can change mental status.

Toxic drug screening should be ordered for those patients who have a nonfocal cause for coma and in whom no other discernible abnormal laboratory studies are found. However, toxic screens usually take several hours to complete and basic treatment decisions must be made before results are obtained.

The indication for emergency lumbar puncture is a strong suspicion of a nonfocal infection of the central nervous system. Lumbar puncture is contraindicated in the presence of a mass lesion. In all other circumstances lumbar puncture is at least relatively contraindicated until a CT scan is performed. In traumatic causes of coma the only immediate question of importance is the need for surgical intervention. Time is the critical factor in the salvage of brain function. Trauma Coma = CT Scan should be the rule. And the sooner this can practically be done the better. When there is a strong suspicion of an operable lesion—the neurosurgeon and surgical team should be mobilized even before the CT results are known.

The EEG evaluation should be reserved for in-hospital patients who have been properly stabilized and where the usual causes of coma are ruled out. Its basic function at that point is to document lack of cortical activity.

The most important radiological study is that of the cervical spine, to rule out fracture. A cross-table lateral view, followed by anteroposterior and odontoid views, are the minimum views needed. Even if the cervical spine films are found to be normal, if cervical cord injury is suspected, the neck must remain immobilized.

The CT scan has become the definitive test in the management of focal neurological disease. In coma patients, the CT scan can detect not only intracranial lesions but fractures of the skull as well. It can detect amounts of blood as minute as 5 mL. Cervical spine films must be done before a CT scan as it is impossible to position the patient in the scanner without flexing the neck. If an emergency department does not have access within its hospital to CT scanning, it should have transfer arrangements available to obtain the study when focal neurologic disease entities are suspected.

SPECIFIC CAUSES OF STUPOR AND COMA

There are literally hundreds of chemical agents and disease entities which can alter mental status. Before individual entities can be discussed it is necessary to review the most common general categories which cause coma. Two mnemonics can be useful: the word TIPS and the vowels A, E, I, O, and U (Table 13G-4). If these disease entities are considered, important causes of coma will not be overlooked.

From an operational standpoint, the neurological examination and laboratory studies divide the causes of altered mental status into toxic metaboic diseases and supratentorial and infratentorial structural lesions which affect the reticular activating formation. It is useful, therefore, to review some specific disease entities based on this categorization. The following etiologies of coma represent a review of the more common causes encountered in the emergency department.

Toxic and Metabolic Disorders

In most hospital emergency departments, metabolic causes dominate as the principal mechanism of coma. When toxic ingestions of drugs or other chemicals are included in this group, it is clearly the leading cause of coma in the United States. Intrinsic neurological diseases such as Schelder's leukodystrophy and other intrinsic nervous system diseases can cause coma but they develop over a long period of time, and will not usually be confused with acute decreases in mental status.

Glucose metabolism. In many series, the most common cause of altered mental status in the emergency department is hypoglycemia. Both hyper- and hypoglycemia may cause alterations of mental status. Diabetics are at high risk for altered mental status, not only because of abnormal glucose metabolism but also because of infection and

Table 13G-4. Mnemonic Aid for Coma Causes

TIPS	Vowels
T—Trauma; all types, temperature	A—Alcohol and ingested drugs and toxins
I—Infection—neurological and systemic	E—Endocrine—all types Exocrine—liver, electrolytes
P—Psychiatric and porphyria	I—Insulin—diabetes mellitus
S—Space-occupying lesions, stroke, subarachnoid hemorrhage, shock	O—Oxygen and opiates
	U—Uremia, renal causes including hypertensive problems

other metabolic derangements. Hypoglycemia is not seen only in diabetics. Patients with pancreatic tumors, retroperitoneal sarcomas, and chronic alcoholics with liver disease may also present in a hypoglycemic state. Severe hypoglycemia can be induced with oral hypoglycemic agents.

Liver disease. In advanced stages of cirrhosis and other degenerative liver diseases, cellular changes are seen in the brain. These abnormal cells probably contribute to decreased mentation but have an unknown affect on the actual level of consciousness. Rapid elevations of serum ammonia levels may contribute to depressed mental status. Patients with advanced liver disease frequently have decreased liver glycogen stores, predisposing to hypoglycemia.

Uremia. Uremic patients basically have no pathological changes in brain cells. The coma of uremia is related to changes in osmolality as the BUN rises. Cerebral water content will adjust to very gradual changes in the BUN, but coma may develop with a rapid rise in the BUN.

Oxygen. All portions of the cardiorespiratory system can be involved as causes of coma. Severe anemia decreases oxygen delivered to the brain. Low cardiac output due to arrhythmias or loss of myocardial contractility can cause decreased cerebral perfusion. Occasionally, older patients placed on antihypertensive medications will become lethargic. Blood pressure may have been reduced too rapidly, causing cerebral hypoperfusion. A rapid increase in P_{CO_2}, as with pulmonary disease, correlates closely with neurological symptoms. With chronic hypercarbia, however, mental status does not deteriorate because the brain can become adjusted to high levels of P_{CO_2}.

Endocrine disorders. Alterations in serum sodium affect the central nervous system by changing the serum osmolality and causing shifts in intracellular brain fluid. Extreme hypothyroidism can likewise cause metabolic shifts which result in depressed mental status or even coma. Hyperthyroidism, on the other hand, usually causes an agitated and tremulous state, and coma is not seen until the patient is in severe thyroid storm or suffers a cerebral vascular accident.

Carcinoma. Coma can be caused by the remote effects of cancer. Hyponatremia due to inappropriate antidiuretic hormone (ADH) secretion in carcinoma of the lung, pancreas, ovary, and prostate are well recognized. Metabolic alkalosis in association with Cushing's syndrome may become severe enough to alter mental status. The progressive multifocal leukoencephalopathies seen with lymphomas may first present with a depression of consciousness. Hyper- or hypocalcemia may also cause alterations in mental status.

Poisons and toxins. Alcohol is still the most widely used and most popular metabolic poison. Its effects are usually short-lived and it is metabolized within a matter of hours. Barbiturate comas, on the other hand, may be of extremely long duration, depending on the type of barbiturate ingested. Cases of barbiturate coma lasting several weeks followed by the return of normal mental status have been recorded. Severe metabolic acidosis from drugs such as methyl alcohol, ethylene glycol, and paraldehyde can be seen in patients who readily abuse the more traditional ethanol.

Central nervous system infections. Central nervous system infections and septicemia can be included in the toxic metabolic causes of coma. Meningitis can cause alterations in mental status. In bacterial meningitis, most notably tuberculous meningitis, the infecting organism can compete with the brain itself for glucose. Viral encephalitis may markedly alter consciousness and may at first present as an acute encephalopathy, followed by a rapid downhill course with depressed mental status. It should not be forgotten that severe infection anywhere in the body can produce little-understood substances which can cause depressed mental status.

Subarachnoid hemorrhage. Subarachnoid hemorrhage is the only intracranial hemorrhage which is not focal in nature. Bleeding into the subarachnoid space quickly spreads throughout the cerebral spinal fluid. The resultant vasospasm is an initial homeostatic attempt to stop subarachnoid bleeding. This vasospasm may be partially responsible for the rapid decrease in mental status. Subarachnoid hemorrhage should be considered high on the list of diagnostic possibilities in all patients who experience headache with decreasing mental status.

Epilepsy. A general rule is "all that seizes is not epilepsy." A patient who has had a seizure may present to the emergency department in postictal coma. If the underlying disease is truly idiopathic epilepsy, the patient usually has a rapid return to normal mental status without residual focal deficits. Seizures lasting for more than 15 min should be suspected to be structural in nature. It is always important to check for underlying causes of seizures such as encephalitis, meningitis, metabolic abnormalities, and trauma.

Disorders of temperature regulation. Hypothermia below the level of 32°C can in and of itself depress neurologic functioning enough to cause coma. Hypothermia may result from underlying diseases such as myxedema or hypopituitarism, or ingested toxins. Hyperthermia above the level of 42°C may also depress mental status to the point of coma. Patients with severe hyper- or hypothermia frequently have underlying neurovascular disease and are often left with severe neurologic residues.

Cofactor disease. Wernicke's encephalopathy due to carbohydrate overload and lack of thiamine can cause coma. Also, in rare instances of severe nutritional deprivation, altered mental status may be seen as the result of other minor cofactor deficiencies such as cobalt, manganese, or zinc.

Supratentorial Focal Lesions

These are localized anatomic lesions lying wholly or partially in the area above the tentorium cerebelli. They affect mental status principally by increased pressure, which compromises the reticular activating formation, and by bilateral cerebral hemisphere involvement. Such focal pressure may cause herniation of the temporal lobe (uncus) into the infratentorial space. This compresses the ipsilateral third cranial nerve, causing the uncal syndrome, with ataxic respirations, contralateral hemiparesis, and ipsilateral pupillary dilatation being the most common manifestations.

Subdural hematoma. In older patients, trauma victims, alcoholics, and those patients on anticoagulants, subdural hematoma is always a consideration. Even if focal neurologic findings are not present, if the patient belongs to one of these groups and has an acute change in mental status, subdural hematoma should still be considered. Subdural hematomas may compress supratentorial structures bilaterally and thus present much like dementia or progressive encephalopathy. A history of trauma, although helpful, is certainly not necessary to entertain the diagnosis of subdural hematoma. In chronic subdural hematomas, symptoms can fluctuate mildly from day to day. Laboratory tests, EEGs, and skull x-rays are of little value in diagnosis. The test of choice if the lesion is suspected in the enhanced CT scan.

Acute epidural hematoma. Acute epidural hematomas are almost always related to major trauma. The bleeding is usually the result of tearing of the middle meningeal artery due to skull fracture. Unlike subdural bleeding which is venous, epidural bleeding is arterial in nature and therefore progresses rapidly. The suspected epidural hematoma must be treated aggressively if the patient is to be salvaged.

Subdural empyema. This is a relatively rare cause of coma but must be considered in patients who have recently undergone otolaryngologic surgery, particularly related to acute sinusitis. It is occasionally seen in conjunction with acute meningitis when *Streptococcus* is the offending organism. Meningitis is not associated with focal neurologic signs. If a patient has symptoms of meningitis plus focal findings, a subdural empyema or brain abscess should be considered. Herpes simplex encephalitis, although a diffuse disease, tends to have a particular predilection for the temporal lobes. These patients thus present with temporal lobetype syndromes and may appear to have a focal neurological process.

Cerebral vascular accidents. The majority of thrombotic and embolic cerebral vascular accidents are not associated with coma or even significant decreased mental status. However, hemorrhagic cerebral vascular accidents are commonly associated with unconsciousness. Bleeding may be from a ruptured artery, aneurysm, or arterial venous malformation. When bleeding is the result of a hypertensive crisis, the exact site of the lesion is rarely found. If patients with severe hypertension become progressively obtunded, it is wise to stabilize the patient completely and reduce pressure to reasonable levels before attempting to localize the bleeding site.

Intraventricular hemorrhage is a particular subset of cerebral vascular accident. It is associated with an extremely poor prognosis, and death occurs within minutes to hours after pontine and medullary findings appear. The intraventricular hemorrhage does not, per se, harm brain tissue, but blood in the cerebrospinal fluid causes considerable increase in intracranial pressure. It is often very difficult to clinically differentiate intraventricular hemorrhage from pontine bleeding without the benefit of a CT scan. It is important to identify patients with acute cerebellar hemorrhage because this represents the most treatable of the intraparenchymal processes.

Cerebral neoplasms. It would be unusual for coma to be the first presenting sign of a cerebral neoplasm. More likely, the patient may present with a seizure followed by a prolonged postictal state. Bleeding into the tumor itself may cause symptoms indistinguishable from other types of cerebral vascular accidents. The slow enlargement of a supratentorial tumor produces brain swelling which can, over a period of time, dull mental status. Tumors in the lateral or third ventricles may obstruct outflow of cerebral fluid and cause acute downward pressure and displacement of the brainstem. In rare instances neoplasms directly infiltrate or destroy the cerebral connections of the reticular activating formation, causing irreversible coma. Almost all the findings in cerebral neoplasms, however, develop over an extended period of time.

Infratentorial Compressive Syndromes

The infratentorial compressive causes of coma are lesions which do not originate within the brainstem itself, but which by their proximity may compress the brainstem.

Basilar artery occlusion. The entire brainstem is supplied continuously by the vertebral basilar system. The reticular activating formation in particular receives paramedian branches off the basilar artery. Anything which interferes with the blood supply through the vertebral basilar system can cause alteration of consciousness. Posterior circulation transient ischemic episodes are often characterized as "drop-like" attacks in which they may be a total loss of muscular tone with or without a loss of consciousness. Problems involving the posterior circulation are extremely difficult to treat but need to be separated from other entities.

Traumatic posterior fossa hemorrhage. Severe trauma may result in bleeding below the tentorium cerebelli but without destruction of the brainstem itself. A hematoma in the posterior fossa can compress the brainstem and may be life-threatening. It is impossible to distinguish this type of hematoma from several other posterior fossa lesions on a physical examination basis alone. Since it represents a surgically correctable cause of coma it is imperative that it be diagnosed.

Acute cerebellar hemorrhage. Bleeding into the cerebellum is usually the result of a nontraumatic rupture of an arteriovenous malformation. Head pain and the onset of sudden vertigo with conjugate deviation of the eyes away to the opposite side of the cerebellar lesion are signs which strongly suggest acute cerebellar hemorrhage. This is the most treatable of the interparenchymal hemorrhages, and if relieved promptly, the possibility exists for good return of neurological function.

Pontine hemorrhage. Pontine hemorrhage is a devastating, acute brainstem parenchymal lesion which produces coma. It is often difficult to differentiate acute pontine hemorrhage from acute cerebellar hemorrhage. These two lesions are both associated with sudden decreases in consciousness and ataxic breathing, pinpoint pupils, absent or abnormal ocular vestibular responses, and meningismus. Although there are some reports of successful drainage of intrapontine hematomas, the prognosis remains grave. Rapid diagnosis is crucial to separate this problem from an acute cerebellar hemorrhage, which is a surgically treatable disease.

Brainstem tumors. Actual parenchymal lesions of the brainstem, including angiomas, gliomas, and ependymomas, can cause brainstem compression syndromes. Most of these, however, progress slowly over a period of time and present with other localized neurological findings before mental status is affected. Other posterior fossa tumors such as meningiomas and acoustic neuromas almost always present with cranial nerve findings before mental status is affected.

PRACTICAL ASSESSMENT AND MANAGEMENT GUIDELINES

Up to this point we have attempted to review the basic mechanisms and etiologies of decreased mental status. Translating this into action in the emergency department should now represent little problem. The following is a sample assessment checklist to be used for the patient with severely depressed mental status:

Airway established
Breathing checked (including auscultation to rule out pneumothorax)
Cardiac output assessed
Cervical spine immobilized
Obvious hemorrhage compressed
IV line started
Vital signs (full set)
Thiamine 100 mg IV
Glucose 50 mL 50% IV
Naloxone 2 ampoules IV, repeated if no response
The stable patient—historical features obtained including rate of onset, drugs, trauma, fever, prior episodes
General physical examination—signs of trauma; i.e., Battle's sign, hemotympanium, scalp hematomas and lacerations, subcutaneous emphysema of the chest
Obvious lesions of the abdomen, lesions of the pelvis, and long-bone injuries
Skin
- Needle marks, cyanosis, pallor, rashes, dehydration

Breath and odors
- Alcohol, acetone, fecal material, fetor hepaticus

Cardiac examination
- Rhythm, gallop, rub, murmurs

Abdominal findings
- Organomegaly, ascites, bruits, flank ecchymoses, rectal and pelvic examination

Neurological examination
Observation
Respiratory pattern
- Normal
- Cheyne-Stokes
- Hyperventilation
- Apneustic breathing
- Ataxic breathing
- Agonal breathing

Autisms
- Yawning
- Coughing
- Hiccuping
- Vomiting

Mental status
- Responds to voice
- Responds to touch
- Responds to noxious stimuli

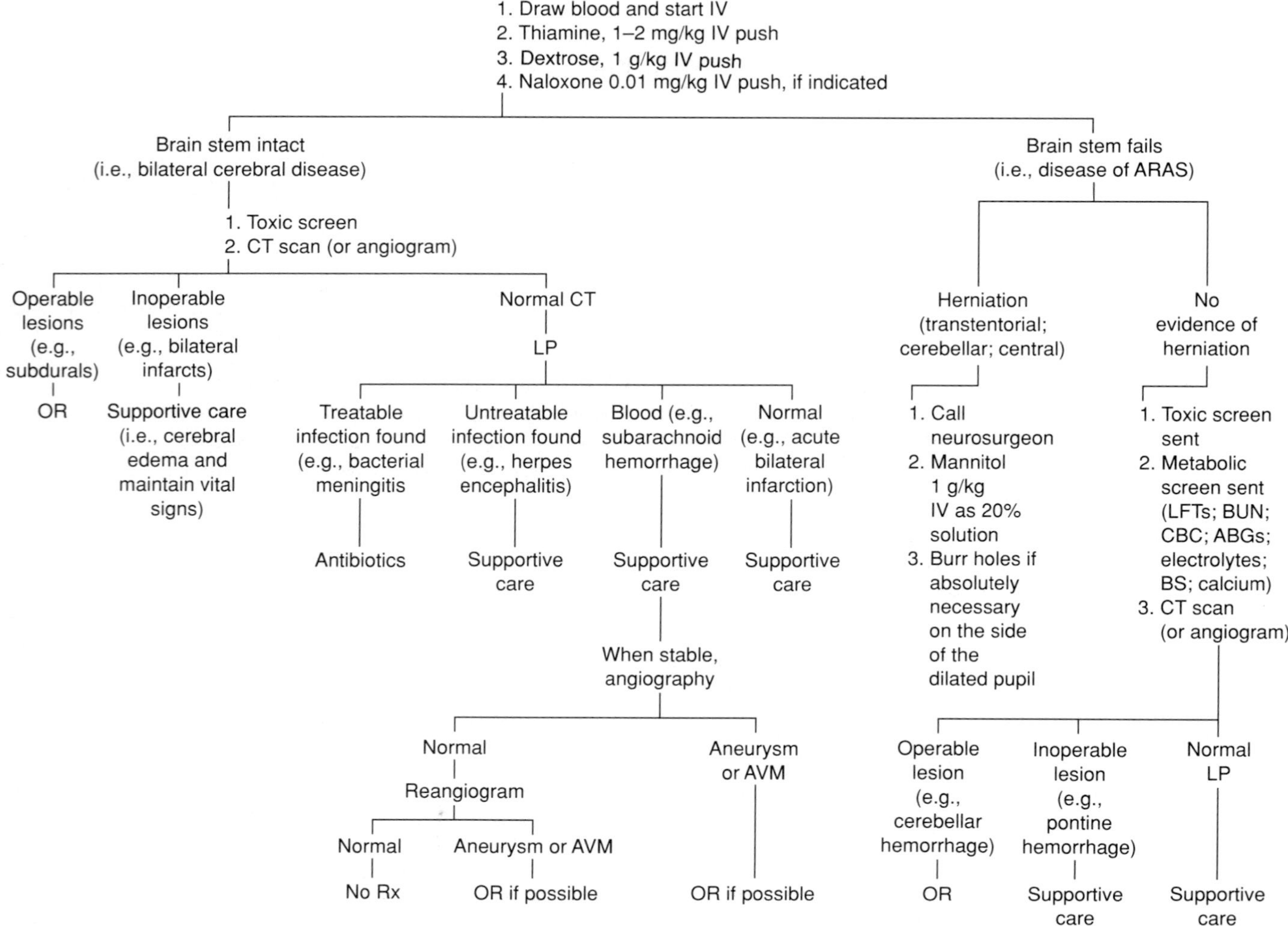

Fig. 13G-1. Diagnosis and treatment protocol in the comatose patient. (From Samuels MA: *Manual of Neurologic Therapeutics*. Boston, Little, Brown and Company, 1982, p. 13. Used by permission.)

Cranial nerves
  Visual threat
  Inspection of fundi for papilledema and hemorrhages
Pupils
  Size
  Reactions—direct and consensual
Extraocular movements
  Oculovestibular testing
  Oculocephalic testing (if appropriate)
Corneal reflex
Facial asymmetry
Motor system
  Posturing
  Ability of the limbs to move
  Stimuli
Decerebration, decortication, or true abduction by high-level centers
Pathlogical reflexes

X-rays and Laboratory Studies

The need for all x-ray and laboratory studies is relative. The need for the following tests will be guided by initial examination and patient's initial response to therapy:

CBC
BUN
Electrolytes
Glucose
Calcium
Toxic screen for drugs
Arterial blood gases
Cervical spine x-rays
Skull x-rays (rarely of use)
CT scan
Lumbar puncture

Treatment Algorithm

Figure 13G-1 illustrates an excellent decision tree algorithm for the management of the comatose patient.

BIBLIOGRAPHY

Barr M: *The Human System*, 2d ed. New York, Harper & Row, 1972.
De Jong R: *The Neurological Examination*, 4th ed. New York, Harper & Row, 1979.
Fisher CM: The neurological examination of the comatose patient. *Acta Neurol Scand* [*Suppl*] 45(36):56, 1969.
Plum F, Posner J: *Diagnosis of Stupor and Coma*, 4th ed. Philadelphia, Davis, 1984.

14
LIFE-THREATENING SIGNS AND SYMPTOMS IN CHILDREN

A. FEVER

Carol D. Berkowitz

Fever is the single most common chief complaint of children presenting to the emergency department, accounting for about 30 percent of pediatric outpatient visits. The physician evaluating the febrile child must differentiate the mildly ill from the seriously ill child, a challenge which may be compounded by the fact that no focus of infection is apparent. The extent of the diagnostic workup and the institution of appropriate management, including the use of antibiotics and the need for hospitalization, must be determined. Many factors, such as clinical assessment, physical findings, age of the patient, and height of the fever, influence the evaluation and management decisions.

PHYSIOLOGY OF FEVER

Fever is defined as a rise in deep body temperature associated with a resetting of the body's thermostat. This thermostat is located in the preoptic region of the anterior hypothalamus near the floor of the third ventricle. Exogenous fever-producing substances (pyrogens) such as bacteria, bacterial endotoxin, antigen-antibody complexes, yeast, viruses, and etiocholanolone, may stimulate the formation and release of endogenous pyrogens. Endogenous pyrogens are produced by neutrophils, monocytes, hepatic Kupffer's cells, splenic sinusoidal cells, alveolar macrophages, and peritoneal lining cells and are believed to induce the synthesis of prostaglandins in the hypothalamus. Endogenous pyrogens include interleukin-1, interleukin-6, and tumor necrosis factor. The body's thermostat is then reset at a higher setting,and the patient, whose own temperature is below that of the body's thermostat, experiences a chill. Peripheral vasoconstriction, shivering, central pooling, and behavioral activity (putting on a sweater, drinking hot tea) lead to an increase in body temperature.

FEVER AS A SYMPTOM

The possible beneficial effects of fever have been debated for many years. Aside from these considerations, it is important to recognize that fever represents a symptom of some underlying disease, and one must determine what this disease is.

An initial question is: "What degree of temperature elevation represents a fever?" One survey conducted among pediatric training programs revealed a wide variability in the temperature considered a "fever" in infants under 2 months of age. This figure has ranged from 38 to 39.4°C (100.4 to 103°F). It is important to recognize that oral temperatures are generally 0.6°C (1°F) lower than rectal temperatures and axillary temperatures are 0.6°C (1°F) lower than oral temperatures. Additionally, body temperature normally varies from morning to evening with the body's circadian rhythm. The degree of variation, which is greater in young women and small children, is about 1.1°C (2°F).

The relationship between height of fever and incidence of bacteremia is discussed below. In general, higher temperatures are associated with a higher incidence of bacteremia. A retrospective study of hyperpyrexia reported that the incidence of meningitis was twice as high in children with fever above 41.1°C (105.9°F), compared to children with fever between 40.5 and 41.0°C (104.9 and 105.8°F). The incidence of pneumonia and bacteremia was the same in the two groups.

AGE AS A FACTOR

The Infant Up To 3 Months

The age of the patient influences the extent of the workup. Early studies suggested that infants under the age of 3 months were at high risk for serious life-threatening infection. Recent studies based on outpatients show that the incidence of serious bacterial infection, including bacteremia and meningitis, is about 3 to 4 percent, although serious nonbacterial infections (e.g., aseptic meningitis) are a frequent cause of fever in this age group.

The history and physical examination may provide clues to the diagnosis. A history of lethargy, irritability, or poor feeding suggests a serious infection. A history of viral illnesses in other family members suggests a similar diagnosis in the infant. The physical examination may reveal a focus of infection such as an inflamed eardrum. Inconsolable crying, or increased irritability when handled, is frequently seen in infants with meningitis. Cough or tachypnea with a respiratory rate over 40 might suggest a lower respiratory infection and the need for a chest x-ray.

Clinical assessment of the severity of illness of a young, febrile infant is problematic. Young infants lack social skills, such as the social smile, and their ability to interact with the examiner is limited. There is a report in the literature of an infant with group B streptococcal bacteremia who was judged by house staff and faculty to be clinically well. The absence of any diagnostic abnormalities on history or physical examination suggests the need for extensive laboratory tests to detect occult infection. These tests would include a complete blood count and differential, ESR, blood culture, lumbar puncture, chest x-ray, urinalysis, and culture. Urinary tract infections may not produce symptoms other than fever, and so a urinalysis and culture should be included routinely in the workup. Antibiotic therapy and/or hospitalization should be instituted as suggested by the results of these studies.

The recognition of occult serious infection in the well-appearing young, febrile infant is problematic. Most investigators agree that no single variable can correctly identify these infants. Combinations of variables are more helpful in the differentiation process, and these variables include factors such as age under 1 month, ESR greater than 30 mm/h, white blood count at or over 15,000/mm^3, polymorphonuclear count of at least 10,000/mm^3, band count at or over 500/mm^3, evidence of soft tissue infection, pyuria (WBC $>$ 10/hpf), and leukocytes in the stool. The absence of these variables is usually (but not always) associated with the absence of serious illness.

The appropriate management of the young febrile infant presents another area of disagreement. There appears to be no "community standard of practice" regarding the need for hospitalization; some physicians hospitalize all febrile infants under 3 months, and others hospitalize only those under 1 month. Because the differentiation between sick and well infant is so difficult, all such febrile infants need extensive septic workups. The decision not to hospitalize the small febrile infant must be made after careful clinical and appropriate laboratory assessment and after assuring the reliability of follow-up.

Infants of 3 to 24 Months

Many of the considerations noted in the evaluation of the infant of less than 3 months apply for the older infant. Patients between 3 and 24 months have been the focus of considerable research because this group appears to be at higher risk for occult bacteremia. These studies have sought to identify clinical and laboratory characteristics of bacteremic patients.

Clinical judgment appears to be more reliable in the assessment of the older infant. Characteristics that the evaluating physician should note are willingness of the patient to make eye contact, playfulness and positive response to interactions, negative response to noxious stimuli, alertness, and consolability. The toxic infant will not respond appropriately.

Again, the history and physical examination will frequently reveal the source of infection. Viral illnesses, including respiratory infections and gastroenteritis, account for the majority of febrile illnesses and usually have system-specific symptoms. Bacterial infections of the respiratory tract include most notably otitis media, pharyngitis, and pneumonia. Otitis media is generally caused by *Streptococcus pneumoniae* or *Haemophilus influenzae*, and antibiotic therapy should be directed at these organisms. Although pneumonia is commonly of viral etiology, it is appropriate to institute antibiotic therapy to ensure coverage of *H. influenzae*. The physical signs of meningitis, such as nuchal rigidity and Kernig's and/or Brudzinski's signs, may be inapparent in the child under the age of 2 years. A bulging fontanelle, vomiting, irritability which increases when the infant is held, inconsolability, or a febrile seizure may be the only signs suggestive of meningitis. Infants with aseptic meningitis should generally be hospitalized and assured adequate long-term followup because they are at higher risk for subsequent neurological and learning disabilities. The presence of petechiae on physical examination should alert the physician to the potential presence of a serious underlying infection. About 20 percent of children will have bacteremia and/or meningitis most frequently with *Neisseria meningitidis* or *H. influenzae*. Petechiae in association with high fever (≥40°C), ESR at or above 30 mm/h, and white blood count of at least 15,000/mm^3 are most frequently correlated with bacteremia.

Bacteremic infants may or may not have an obvious focus of infection. The height of the fever is a clue to which infants are bacteremic. Although bacteremia may be seen at lower temperatures, a temperature of over 39.5°C (103.1°F) in infants 3 to 24 months is associated with a higher incidence of bacteremia. Certain laboratory tests have been recommended to assist in further identifying the bacteremic patient. White blood counts (WBC) over 15,000/mm^3, band count of at least 500/mm^3, total polymorphonuclear counts at or above 10,000/mm^3, and band plus polymorphonuclear counts equal to or greater than 10,500/mm^3 are associated with an increased incidence of bacteremia, although bacteremia also occurs in the absence of these findings. The incidence of bacteremia in children 3 to 24 months with a temperature of 39.5°C (103.1°F) or over is about 5 to 6 percent. The incidence increases to 12 to 15 percent in patients with WBCs of 15,000/mm^3 or over. An ESR at or above 30 mm/h has the same significance as a WBC of 15,000/mm^3 or greater. The organisms most commonly causing bacteremia in this age group are *S. pneumoniae* (65 percent) and *H. influenzae* (25 percent).

Is it important to perform a blood culture to detect occult bacteremia? Opinions vary on the answer to this question. It is apparent that bacteremic patients do better if they receive antibiotics early on. Many bacteremic children do have a focus of infection and so are treated anyway. Additionally, in a least 25 percent of bacteremic patients with no focus of infection the bacteremia is resolved without any antibiotics. Others develop soft tissue infections which are then appropriately managed. The ability of oral antibiotics to prevent the development of meningitis in the bacteremic child is still unclear. The blood culture appears to be useful for following a patient who may not be returning for periodic evaluations. Therefore, from a medical and epidemiological standpoint, blood cultures are indicated in the suspicious or high-risk infant.

Is there a role for the use of expectant antibiotics in children suspected of having occult bacteremia? Retrospective studies have all shown that early antibiotics diminished the incidence of persistent bacteremia. In a prospective randomized study comparing oral penicillin to no antibiotics, no improvement was reported in any bacteremic child who did not receive antibiotics. Other investigators report more equivocal results. Outpatient daily injections of ceftriaxone are being utilized by some physicians for children at increased risk of occult bacteremia. There are no controlled trials investigating the efficacy of this therapy. Parenteral ceftriaxone should never be initiated without appropriate antecedent diagnostic studies. Treatment should be discontinued if cultures are negative.

An additional dilemma surrounds the management of positive blood culture results. All patients with positive blood cultures should be recalled for repeat evaluation. If they are on the appropriate antibiotics, are clinically well, and have been afebrile, they should be instructed to complete the course of therapy. If they are afebrile and clinically well but have never been treated with antibiotics, opinions differ regarding the need for additional blood cultures and antibiotic therapy. Generally, neither is necessary unless the child has developed a specific focus of infection. However, any patient who remains febrile or does poorly even if on antibiotics should receive complete septic workup (CBC, blood culture, lumbar puncture, chest film, urine culture), be hospitalized, and receive parenteral antibiotics (see Fig. 14A-1).

Older Febrile Children

Children over the age of 2 are easier to evaluate. They can specify their complaints and have illnesses similar to younger children, particularly upper respiratory infections and gastroenteritis. The risk of bacteremia appears lower in this age group, but the incidence of streptococcal pharyngitis is higher, especially in children between the ages of 5 and 10. Infectious mononucleosis may present with fever, tonsillar hypertrophy, and exudate, like streptococcal pharyngitis. Marked lymphadenopathy or hepatosplenomegaly would confirm the diagnosis. Pneumonia in this age group may be caused by *Mycoplasma pneumoniae*. These children present with cough and fever. Rales may not be apparent early in the illness, although the chest film would show evidence of an infiltrate. Bedside cold agglutinins, if positive, provide clue to the correct diagnosis. Children with pneumonia secondary to mycoplasma should be treated with erythromycin, 30 to 40 mg/kg per day (maximum dose 1 g).

MANAGING THE FEVER

Once the issue of fever as a symptom has been addressed, it is appropriate to determine the need for fever-reducing measures.

Many parents are concerned about the harmful effects of the fever; many are aware of the risk of febrile seizures. Children who are prone to febrile seizures are not benefited by antipyretics alone. This is because the seizure frequently occurs early in the illness, often before the parents are aware that the child is ill. Aside from febrile seizures, fever is not known to produce any harmful effects in children. Many children, however, feel uncomfortable during the fever, and so it is appropriate to institute measures directed at symptomatically reducing the fever.

The body loses heat in four ways: (1) radiation (60 percent), heat loss from the body to the air in the surrounding environment; (2) evaporation (25 percent), heat loss through the evaporation of perspiration, water, or any liquid applied to the body surface; (3) convection (10 percent), heat lost when air currents blow over the skin; and (4) conduction (approximately 5 percent), heat loss through contact with solid surface. Heat loss through conduction is increased by the use of cooling blankets.

One can facilitate heat loss in a child using any combination of these measures. Unwrapping a bundled child increases heat loss through radiation, and rehydrating a dehydrated child will increase the heat loss through evaporation. Sponging also helps to reduce fever by evaporation. Sponging should be done slowly, using tepid water only. Very rapid cooling by sponging can result in peripheral vascular collapse, and death has been reported in the small critically ill infant. Sponging with ice water is uncomfortable and results in shivering, and sponging with alcohol carries the risk of intoxication, hypoglycemia, and coma. Vigorous rubbing of the skin induces vasodilatation and improves heat loss.

Studies have shown that sponging and antipyretics used together are more effective than either modality used alone. Acetaminophen and aspirin are equally effective, and both drugs appear to work centrally to block prostaglandin synthesis. Heat is lost through peripheral vasodilatation and sweating.

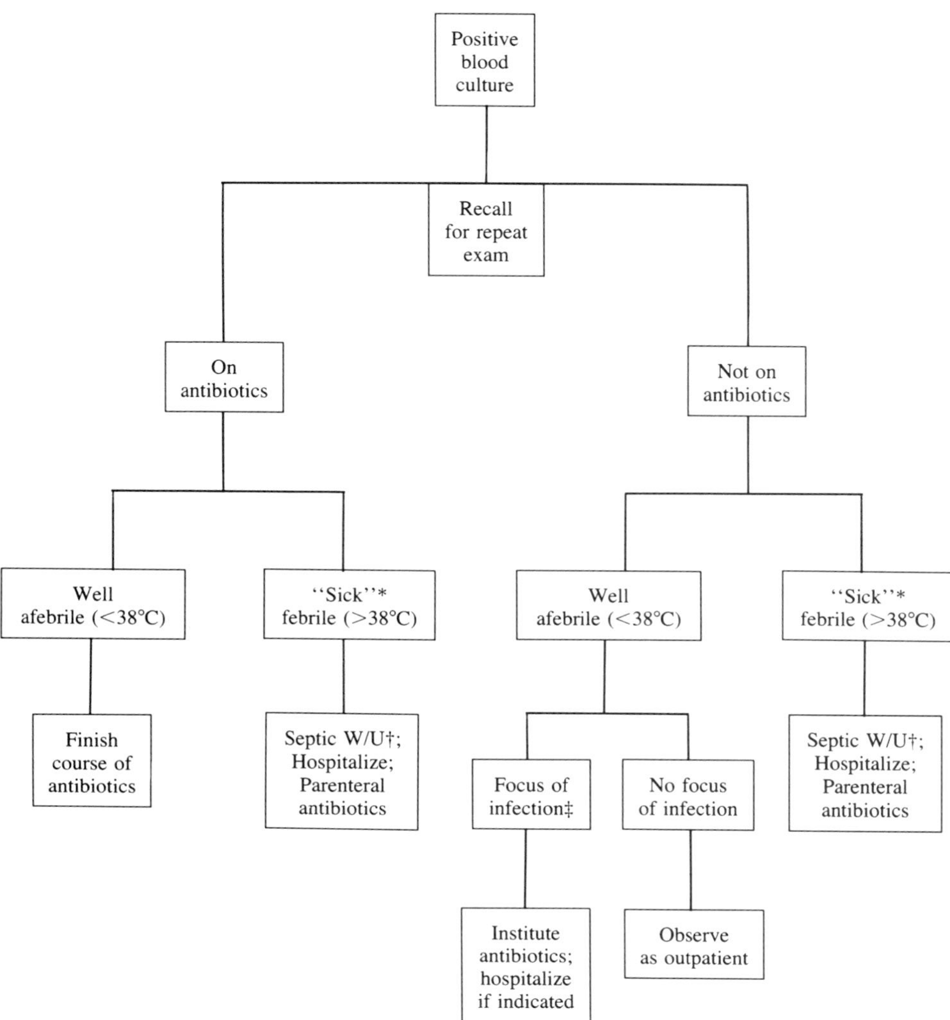

Fig. 14A-1. Management of the bacteremic child; (*"Sick"—irritable, lethargic, anorexic, vomiting; †septic W/U—blood culture, lumbar puncture, chest x-ray, CBC, differential, urinalysis, urine culture; ‡focus of infection—otitis media, pneumonia, cellulitis.)

Drug dosage is the same for either antipyretic and is 10 to 15 mg/kg per dose at 4-h intervals (maximum dose 600 mg). Increasing the dose does not result in a better or more sustained effect. Administration of the drug by rectal suppository results in a slight delay in absorption. There are no studies to evaluate the efficacy of alternating the two drugs at 2-h intervals, in an effort to avoid the recrudescence of fever. Administration of the drugs simultaneously at the usual dosage has been shown to produce a reduction in temperature that is sustained for 6 h rather than 2 to 4 h.

The use of aspirin has been curtailed following reports linking aspirin and Reye's syndrome. Aspirin should not be used in children with chickenpox or with influenzalike illnesses. The effects of aspirin are cumulative, and more than half of the reported overdoses involve therapeutic misuse. Other side effects of aspirin include gastrointestinal upset and hemorrhage and coagulation disturbances. Acetaminophen is also toxic if taken in inappropriate doses, but there is no cumulative effect, and children are less prone than adults to hepatotoxicity.

BIBLIOGRAPHY

Berkowitz CD, Uchiyama N, Tully SB, et al: Fever in infants less than two months of age: Spectrum of disease and predictors of outcome. *Pediatr Emerg Care* 1:128, 1985.

Carroll WL, Farrell MK, Singer JI, et al: Treatment of occult bacteremia. A prospective randomized clinical trial. *Pediatrics* 72:608, 1983.

Dagan R, Powell KR, Hall CB, et al: Identification of infants unlikely to have serious bacterial infection although hospitalized for sepsis, *J Pediatr* 107:855, 1985.

Dershewitz RA, Wigder HN, Wigder CM, et al: A comparative study of the prevalence, outcome, and prediction of bacteremia in children. *J Pediatr* 103:352, 1983.

Jaffe DW, Tanz RR, Davis AT, et al: Antibiotic administration to treat possible occult bacteremia in febrile children. *N Engl J Med* 317:1175, 1987.

Levi M: On managing the febrile child. *Emerg Med* 115, 1981.

McCarthy PL, Jekel JF, Stashwick CA, et al: History and observation variables in assessing febrile children. *Pediatrics* 65:1090, 1980.

Nguyen QV, Nguyen EA, Weiner LB: Incidence of invasive bacterial disease in children with fever and petechiae. *Pediatrics* 74:77, 1984.

Roberts KB (ed.): *The Febrile Infant and Occult Bacteremia.* Ross Roundtables on Critical Approaches to Common Pediatric Problems. 1988.

Soman M: Diagnostic work-up of febrile children under 24 months of age: A clinical review. *West J Med* 137:1, 1982.

B. FLUID AND ELECTROLYTE THERAPY

Deborah Lubitz
James Seidel

Important differences exist in fluid and electrolyte metabolism and homeostasis between young children and adults. The physiologic consequences of fluid and electrolyte disturbances are more pronounced in young children, who have a higher metabolic rate and turnover of fluid and solute per kilogram of body weight that is three times that of adults. The total body water (TBW) in normal newborns accounts for 70 to 75 percent of body weight, and in prepubertal children it is approximately 65 percent of body weight, significantly higher than that of adolescents and adults.

This chapter includes a discussion of normal maintenance fluid and electrolyte therapy in pediatric patients, assessment of deficits, treatment of deficits, special situations that will be encountered requiring modification of the basic guidelines of therapy, and a discussion of the use of oral rehydration for gastrointestinal (GI) losses due to diarrhea.

MAINTENANCE REQUIREMENTS

When maintenance intravenous therapy is needed for only a few days, the focus should be on maintaining water, sodium, potassium, chloride, and bicarbonate homeostasis and providing sufficient calories to prevent ketosis and minimize body protein catabolism. Normal maintenance requirements are the amounts of water and electrolytes lost through the usual routes: insensible water loss, urine, sweat (miniscule in the absence of visible sweating), and stool (usually minimal).

Maintenance requirements depend on the patient's rate of metabolism (caloric requirements), not body weight alone. An accurate estimate that includes basal metabolic expenditure plus an allowance for activity in bed can be made from body weight and is as follows:

From 0 to 10 kg, 100 cal/kg per 24 h;
From 10 to 20 kg, 50 cal/kg per 24 h;
From 20 to 70 kg, 20 cal/kg per 24 h.

Thus a child weighing 25 kg would have a daily maintenance caloric requirement of 1600 cal ($[10 \times 100] + [10 \times 50] + [5 \times 20] = 1600$). The caloric requirements (per unit of weight) decrease with increasing age and size because a greater percentage of weight is bones, muscles, and fat-tissues that are metabolically inactive at rest.

Normal maintenance water requirements equal 100 mL per 100 cal expended, with 40 to 45 percent as insensible water loss through the skin (two-thirds) and lungs (one-third), and 55 to 60 percent as urinary loss. Usually, stool and sweat losses can be ignored. Because of the 1:1 relationship, water requirements can be calculated directly from weight. Therefore, maintenance water requirements are 100 mL/kg for each kilogram from 0 to 10, +50 mL/kg for each kilogram from 10 to 20, and +20 mL/kg for each kilogram greater than 20. Normal maintenance requirements of sodium and potassium are 3 mEq/kg and 2 mEq/kg daily, respectively. All the anions can usually be given as chloride, with the kidney producing any needed bicarbonate. Potassium should be withheld from IV therapy if there is reason to suspect renal or adrenal insufficiency or if true hyperkalemia exists.

Replacement of approximately 20 percent of the total caloric expenditure is sufficient to prevent ketosis. This is accomplished by providing 5 g of glucose per 100 cal expended (or per 100 mL); 10 g/100 mL may be required for newborn infants. With this caloric intake, a daily weight loss of 1 to 2 percent of body weight can be expected.

Although rarely significant for our purposes here, it should be remembered that there are conditions that alter metabolic rates (e.g., fever, hyper- or hypometabolic states) or fluid losses (e.g., increased environmental humidity with artificial ventilation, sweating, oliguria or polyuria, and abnormal GI losses). Sometimes maintenance requirements need to be adjusted accordingly.

An intravenous solution that would provide these maintenance requirements can be calculated and would ideally contain 25 mEq Na/L, 25 mEq K/L, 50 mEq Cl/L, and 50 g dextrose/L. This is usually accomplished by using a solution of 5% dextrose in 0.2 or 0.25 normal saline ($D_5$0.2*N*S or $D_5$0.25*N*S) with 20 mEq KCl/L for infants and children.

DEFICITS

The most common causes of fluid deficits in pediatrics are abnormal gastrointestinal losses and environmental changes. Severe losses can occur very quickly. It is important to remember that this is not a static process but a combination of ongoing losses and gains. In the emergency setting, we need to compute and correct deficits of water and the electrolytes which are required to maintain extracellular volume or whose deficit might precipitate life-threatening problems. In the analysis of dehydration, four factors must be considered: (1) magnitude of dehydration, (2) type of dehydration, (3) total body potassium deficits, and (4) acid-base disturbances.

Magnitude of Dehydration

The *magnitude of dehydration* is an assessment of the amount of body water that has been lost in the course of an illness. This discussion concerns acute losses, which should be regarded as deficit primarily from extracellular fluids (ECF). Unless you have a recent previous weight (weight comparison is obviously the best method of estimating dehydration), the degree of dehydration must be estimated on clinical grounds. Important historical information includes the intake during the illness, with quantity and type of fluids; output, including site, type, and amount of loss; the patient's age; and other medical problems. Vital signs (weight, temperature, pulse rate, respiratory rate, and BP) are very important.

For estimating dehydration, we can divide the losses into mild (5 percent), moderate (10 percent), and severe (15 percent). Mild (5 percent or 50 mL water/kg body weight) dehydration may be present when it is suggested by the history and physical signs are minimal or absent. The skin may be pale but is moist with good turgor and capillary refill. Mucous membranes may be dry, tears may be absent, and urine output may be decreased. Pulse rate may be increased, but BP will be normal. In moderate (10 percent or 100 mL/kg) dehydration, skin may be dry with tenting and loss of turgor (in children less than 2 years), mucous membranes will be very dry, and fontanelle and eyeballs will be sunken. The patient will usually have an altered sensorium but may just be irritable. Oliguria, tachycardia, prolonged capillary refill (more than 2 s) and weak pulses may also be present, but the measured BP should be within normal limits. These patients are in the early stages of shock. In severe (15 percent or 150 mL/kg) dehydration, there is late shock or near circulatory collapse with skin that is clammy and mottled, poor capillary refill, weak or absent pulses, and an altered sensorium with or without a decrease in BP.

These signs and symptoms are for patients with isotonic dehydration and reflect changes in the ECF compartment as dehydration progresses. In older children and adults, whose ECF volume is relatively smaller, these estimates are 3 percent (mild), 6 percent (moderate), and 9 percent (severe). It takes a greater percentage of loss to cause shock in an infant, but dehydration of this magnitude will occur more readily than in adults.

Type of Dehydration

The *type of dehydration* refers to the relative degree of solute loss as reflected by the plasma sodium concentration. It is important to define the type of dehydration, since both hyponatremia and hypernatremia can be associated with special problems both prior to and during therapy.

Approximately 70 to 80 percent of pediatric patients will present with *isonatremic dehydration,* with a serum sodium of 130 to 150 mEq/L. This results from a proportionate loss of water and electrolytes. Estimation of the magnitude of water loss is as described above.

In *hyponatremic dehydration,* there is an abnormally low serum sodium of less than 130 mEq/L, indicating that the sodium deficit is greater than the water deficit. Practically, this usually occurs when sodium-poor fluids (e.g., tap water) are given to replace GI losses.

Because of the low serum sodium, there are water shifts from the ECF into cells, and plasma volume rapidly decreases. When this occurs, the child appears more seriously ill than would be expected by the actual weight loss, and shock occurs more rapidly. One may *over*-estimate total fluid losses using clinical signs. Specific signs and symptoms of hyponatremia are usually CNS related, and their presence depends on both the rate of fall of serum sodium and the absolute value. Seizures and coma seldom occur unless the serum sodium is less than 120 mEq/L, but intractable seizures are a common emergency department presentation of severe hyponatremia.

In *hypernatremic dehydration,* the serum sodium is greater than 150 mEq/L. This occurs when free water replacement is inadequate, as with incorrectly diluted formulas, or if sodium intake is abnormally high, as with the use of baking soda as a home remedy. This is a very important diagnosis to make, because hypernatremic dehydration is a prevalent cause of brain damage in infants and children. A relative cellular desiccation occurs as water moves into the ECF, and the magnitude of dehydration will tend to be *under*estimated. As a rule, if hypernatremia is present, there must be at least 10 percent dehydration. Rapid reinfusion of a hypotonic solution is not recommended, since it may lead to fluid and electrolyte shifts, brain swelling, and potentially serious complications. Historical factors that suggest hypertonic dehydration include massive GI losses, improperly mixed electrolyte solutions, and increased insensible losses (through fever, increased respiratory rate, and low environmental humidity). Specific signs and symptoms include dry, rubbery, or doughy skin; lethargy alternating with hyperirritability in response to stimuli; increased muscle tone and rigidity with hyperreflexia; and sometimes seizures, coma, and death.

Potassium Deficit

Potassium deficits occur in all conditions causing water and electrolyte deficits. Certain situations, including large diarrheal losses, increased renal losses (diuretics), or chloride loss with subsequent metabolic alkalosis, may result in an increased potassium deficit. With chronic dehydration, the extent of the intracellular potassium loss increases progressively, since renal losses increase in association with sodium retention.

It is important to remember that the change (or lack of change) in serum potassium concentration does not always reflect intracellular concentration. This is because serum potassium makes up only 2 percent of total body potassium, it is affected by acid-base status, and equilibration between intracellular fluid (ICF) and ECF potassium occurs more slowly than for free water.

Although a potassium deficit is present in all cases of dehydration, it seldom is significant initially. However, failure to repair the deficit during replacement therapy may produce the clinical effects of acute hypokalemia. Generally, potassium replacement should not begin until adequate urine output is assured, but *don't forget* to add it then.

Acid-Base Disturbances

Acid-base abnormalities may occur in patients with dehydration. In infancy, almost all hydration disturbances will produce some degree of metabolic acidosis. The mechanisms include bicarbonate losses in stool, ketone production secondary to carbohydrate starvation, and hypovolemia, which leads to both decreased tissue perfusion with lactic acid production and decreased GFR, which decreases acid excretion. Despite this, the most pressing problem is the *dehydration,* because as long as the kidneys function, the acidosis caused by other mechanisms can be compensated for. Therefore, acidosis is ameliorated mainly by the restoration of circulation and renal function. The administration of glucose decreases the production of ketones, and it may be necessary to provide intravenous bicarbonate for severe acidosis (see below).

Other clinical states which lead to metabolic acidosis include diabetes, starvation, salicylism, azotemia, hypoxia, organic acidosis (e.g., aminoacidemias), and renal disease leading to increased bicarbonate loss. When evaluating acidosis , it is important to look at the anion gap. The acidosis caused by dehydration has a normal anion gap (hyperchloremia). An increased anion gap can be caused by certain drugs and toxins (e.g., salicylates, methanol, propylene glycol), hyperglycemic nonketotic coma, ketoacidosis, lactic acidosis, and uremia.

Metabolic alkalosis can occur when there is fixed anion loss as in vomiting with a high intestinal obstruction. In this case, there is loss of hydrochloric acid without loss of intestinal bicarbonate. Therapy must be aimed at treating the underlying disease. Potassium losses are significant with alkalosis and must be replaced.

THERAPY

Replacement of the deficit is accomplished in three phases: (1) shock; (2) ECF volume; and (3) ICF volume and body potassium, protein, and fat stores. This discussion will be confined to the first two phases.

Shock

The treatment of shock is directed toward preventing circulatory failure. This phase should be instituted in any infant with estimated dehydration of 10 percent or greater (6 percent in older children) or with signs of shock: tachycardia, prolonged capillary refill (more than 2 s), pallor, weak peripheral pulses, and lethargy (hypotension is usually a very late and ominous sign of decompensated shock in infants and young children).

Unless the patient appears in imminent danger of cardiac arrest, a weight should be obtained. A peripheral intravenous line should be started and blood obtained for immediate chemical analysis (electrolytes, glucose, BUN, and creatinine), venous or arterial pH, and dextrostrip. If peripheral access cannot be obtained, percutaneous cannulation of the femoral or external jugular vein is an alternative. If skilled personnel is available, venous cutdown may be attempted. If the child is less than 3 years old and is hypotensive, an intraosseous infusion needle may be placed for initial volume expansion (since this is an extremely painful procedure, it should be reserved for critically ill patients). Patients in shock should also receive supplemental oxygen.

Regardless of the suspected type of dehydration, the patient should receive an initial fluid bolus of 20 mL/kg of isotonic crystalloid, either 0.9% NaCl (normal saline) or lactated Ringer's solution, over 5 to 20 min. Glucose-containing solutions should be avoided because repeated boluses can lead to hyperglycemia. Remember, 20 mL/kg of a 5% dextrose solution will give 1 g/kg of glucose! Rapid delivery can be achieved by attaching a three-way stopcock to the extension tubing of the intravenous line. A 20- to 50-mL syringe can then be used to push fluid aliquots. This method allows for rapid bolus infusion without disrupting fragile veins. Crystalloids are used because they are readily available, inexpensive, and free from reaction. Although large volumes must be used because only about one-fourth of the fluid remains in the plasma compartment, this quantity is well tolerated in infants and children unless they have underlying cardiac or pulmonary disease. If there is a concern regarding cardiac, pulmonary, or renal function, it may be preferable to use 10-mL/kg boluses of colloids such as salt-poor 5% albumin, fresh frozen plasma (FFP), or synthetic colloids. These solutions are more expensive and carry the risk of allergic reactions. If hypoglycemia is present, administer 0.5 to 1.0 g/kg of glucose (usually as 2 to 4 mL/kg of $D_{25}W$).

After the fluid bolus has been completed, the patient is reassessed (for heart rate, skin color, capillary refill, pulses, mental status, and urine output). If perfusion remains compromised, the fluid bolus should be repeated. If the shock state is attributable to dehydration alone, the only remedy is the restoration of vascular volume. In general, few patients require more than 60mL/kg of isotonic crystalloid in the first hour of therapy (circulating blood volume is 80 mL/kg). However, hypotensive children, those with severe third-spacing, and those with on-going volume losses may require more than 60 mL/kg of crystalloid infusion during the first hour or two of therapy. Patients receiving multiple fluid boluses should be monitored for signs of fluid overload (enlarged liver, pulmonary rales, or enlarged heart on chest radiograph) and serum electrolytes should also be reevaluated.

ECF Volume Restoration

The next phase of therapy is ECF volume restoration over 24 to 48 h. The aim of this phase is correction of the fluid deficit, restoring ECF volume, and partial ICF volume. To do this, one must determine the type of dehydration and make a precise assessment of the total fluid deficit on presentation.

Isonatremic Dehydration

For the patient with isotonic dehydration, calculate the deficit on the basis of the estimated percent dehydration. Once the deficit is calculated, subtract the initial fluids given as boluses. The net deficit is replaced over 24 h, with one-half given during the first 8 h and the remaining one-half over the subsequent 16 h, along with the calculated maintenance fluids.

For example, a 7-kg patient with an estimated 10 percent dehydration has a fluid deficit of 100 mL/kg or 700 mL. Initial fluids were 20 mL/kg of normal saline. The remaining deficit is therefore 700 − 140 = 560 mL. One-half, or 280 mL, should be given over the first 8 h (35 mL/h). This is added to the maintenance fluid rate of 29 mL/h (7 kg × 100 mL/kg = 700 mL/24 h = 29 mL/h), for a total of 64 mL/h. The rate for the next 16 h would be 46 mL/h.

In treatment of isonatremic dehydration in a patient with normal renal function, the IV solution used is flexible. Usually $D_5$0.25*NS* is used, but concentrations of up to $D_5$0.5*NS* can be used (theoretically, the deficit should be replaced with 0.5*NS* and the maintenance with 0.2*NS*). In addition, KCl should be added at 40 mEq/L.

Hyponatremic Dehydration

In hypotonic dehydration, the water deficit is calculated and replaced as above, but the sodium deficit will be different. Since most patients with hyponatremia will appear at least 10% dehydrated, relatively hypertonic saline (normal saline) will have been given initially. The remainder of the fluid deficit and the maintenance is given as calculated above, using $D_5$0.5*NS* or $D_5$0.33*NS*. Again, KCl is added at 40 mEq/L.

If the initial serum sodium is less than 120 mEq/L or the patient is symptomatic (e.g., seizures), an acute correction with 3% saline (0.5 mEq/mL), may be administered in addition to the normal saline bolus. This is done only to bring the sodium out of the "danger zone" according to the formula

(desired serum Na − present serum Na) (%ECF)(body weight)

(125 − serum Na) (0.2) (weight in kg)

This is given as a slow IV push while the patient is monitored. When symptoms are under control, proceed as above. Rapid correction has been associated with central pontine myelinolysis in alcoholic adults but has not been reported in children.

Hypernatremic Dehydration

In hypertonic dehydration, the critical factor is the high sodium and relative loss of intracellular water. The most important point to remember is that the serum sodium must be lowered *slowly*. Rapid rehydration (and, therefore, decrease in serum sodium) leads to rapid expansion of intracellular volume, especially in the CNS, which may cause serious complications. A large proportion of the mortality and neurologic sequelae that result from hypernatremic dehydration is secondary to the initial CNS cellular desiccation. Further complications from abrupt cellular swelling and cerebral edema can be avoided if careful attention is paid to *slow* rehydration. The goal should be to decrease the serum sodium by approximately 10 to 15 mEq/day, so that if the initial sodium is less than 170, rehydration is accomplished evenly over 2 days; if greater than 170, this is stretched to 3 days. If the sodium is greater than 200 mEq/L, the patient may require dialysis.

The first step is to estimate the patient's deficit. Clinically, these patients appear less dehydrated than they truly are because the ECF volume is preserved, and they may not appear to require therapy for shock. However, if there is any doubt regarding the adequacy of circulation, the use of a bolus of normal saline will not dilute the initially high sodium by more than 3 mEq/L. After the deficit is calculated, estimate the maintenance for the next 48 hours and add the two—this is the volume to be given evenly over 48 h.

For example, consider a 15-kg child with 10% dehydration and a serum sodium of 160. The deficit is 100 mL/kg or 1500 mL. Maintenance is 1250 mL/24 h (100 mL/kg × 10 + 50 mL/kg × 5). The total 48-h fluid need is 5500 mL or 115 mL/h. To bring the serum sodium down at the desired rate, use 0.25*NS*. As soon as urine output begins, add potassium to the solution to replace intracellular cation and draw water back into the cells. Hyperglycemia can aggravate hypertonicity and must be corrected slowly also, mainly by rehydration.

Acidosis

When acidosis accompanies dehydration or shock, inadequate perfusion is the primary problem. Mild to moderate acidosis is usually ameliorated by restoration of circulation to improve renal function and oxygen and substrate (glucose) delivery to the tissues, maintenance or restoration of ventilation, and the provision of sodium and potassium to alleviate the cation deficit.

If the blood pH is less than 7.10 or serum HCO_3 is less than 10, the administration of exogenous bicarbonate should be considered. Adequate treatment can usually be accomplished with a dose of 1 mEq/kg, added to the first hour of intravenous fluid. This dose may be repeated if necessary.

One must guard against an overly rapid correction of plasma bicarbonate concentration. Compensatory mechanisms do not abruptly cease when the blood pH reaches normal; this can result in an "overshoot," with resultant alkalemia. Additionally, changes in Pa_{CO_2} in the CSF alter the pH more rapidly and profoundly than do changes in arterial bicarbonate concentration (increased permeability to CO_2 relative to HCO_3). A rapid infusion of bicarbonate may correct the blood pH, but the P_{CO_2} in the CSF may rise, lowering the CSF pH and endangering neurological function.

SPECIAL SITUATIONS

Sepsis

Pediatric patients may be febrile (or even hypothermic) when they present with dehydration and/or shock. It may be difficult to ascertain after the initial assessment whether the patient is in shock from dehydration or sepsis or both. In sepsis, peripheral vasodilatation increases the size of the vascular compartment, leading to a relative hypovolemia. There is also an increase in capillary permeability, causing further third-space losses.

The treatment of septic shock is initially the same as outlined above (see "shock"). The patient must be supported and given intravenous fluids to expand the vascular volume. Unlike straightforward hypovolemia, there is a limit to the amount of crystalloid that should be administered. Sepsis frequently causes abnormalities of cardiac function, and increased capillary permeability in the lungs may result in the development of adult respiratory distress syndrome (ARDS). If a patient with suspected septic shock requires resuscitation with over 40 to 60 mL/kg of crystalloid, inotropic support should be instituted with an infusion of dopamine or epinephrine. In addition, appropriate cultures should be obtained and broad-spectrum antibiotics administered. Lumbar puncture should not be performed until the patient is hemodynamically stable.

Trauma

Pediatric patients will generally compensate for acute volume loss from hemorrhage up to 30 percent of their blood volume. Clinically, they may have tachycardia, decreased capillary refill, clammy skin, decreased pulse pressure, and altered sensorium. Hypotension is a late sign of impending circulatory failure in children. Treatment of the pediatric patient in compensated and uncompensated shock following trauma involves the administration of large volumes of fluids to replace continuing, as well as previous, losses. Normal saline or Ringer's lactate is given as 20 mL/kg boluses. The patient should be continually monitored and pulse, BP, perfusion, and urine output reassessed following each bolus. If the patient requires more than 40 mL/kg during the initial resuscitation, blood (10 mL/kg packed red blood cells) should be administered with further crystalloids, and possible sites of continuing losses investigated.

Diabetic Ketoacidosis

Diabetic ketoacidosis is a state characterized by (1) volume depletion, both intra- and extracellular, (2) osmotic imbalance between compartments, (3) metabolic acidosis, and (4) calorie deficiency.

In moderate or severe diabetic ketoacidosis, deficit therapy approximates that used for straightforward dehydration, but several important points must be emphasized. Rehydration and decreasing the serum glucose must be accomplished slowly to avoid complications of CNS edema. Bicarbonate should be used judiciously when the blood pH is less than 7.10 or when serum bicarbonate is less than 10, and should be given slowly over 1 h. Milder acidosis usually responds to adequate rehydration and insulin therapy. Dehydration should be corrected with normal saline initially (at least a 10 percent deficit in severe DKA). Since there is generally a large potassium deficit, potassium should be given early in therapy. Careful and frequent monitoring of glucose, pH, K, and PO_4 is essential.

Salicylate Intoxication

In salicylate poisoning, dehydration is due to large respiratory water losses, fasting, thirsting, sweating, and increased urinary losses.

Treatment is aimed at correction of the dehydration, hypokalemia, and metabolic acidosis. These guidelines may be followed: (1) first 2 h, give $D_5$0.33*NS* with 25 mEq/L $NaHCO_3$ at 10 to 15 mL/kg per hour, then (2) $D_5$0.25*NS* with 20 mEq/L $NaHCO_3$ and 40 mEq/L KCl at 5 to 10 mL/kg per hour. The goal is to achieve a diuresis of 3 to 6 mL/kg per hour. In cases of severe metabolic acidosis, an additional 1 to 2 mEq/kg of $NaHCO_3$ may be cautiously given every 1 to 2 h to titrate the plasma pH to 7.5.

Cystic Fibrosis

Cystic fibrosis is a hereditary disorder that occurs in 1 out of 2500 Americans. Patients with cystic fibrosis have increased sweat concentrations of Na and Cl. Most infant formulas have low salt content, and infants cannot increase their intake according to the body's need. Hyponatremic dehydration can occur in yet undiagnosed infants who are active and sweat profusely, secondary to either a hot environment or inappropriate bundling. This condition may be associated with a hypochloremic, hypokalemic metabolic alkalosis. Older children already diagnosed with cystic fibrosis may develop hyponatremic dehydration during prolonged exposure to hot environments or as a consequence of physical exertion. These patients must be distinguished from normal individuals with heat exhaustion, who have lost hypotonic sweat.

Pyloric Stenosis

Pyloric stenosis is a common condition that occurs in young infants, usually males. If this condition is diagnosed before there is significant dehydration, the acid-base abnormalities may be minimal. It is classic, however, for patients to have a hypochloremic, hypokalemic metabolic alkalosis.

Deficit therapy in these babies should be aimed at (1) restoring intravascular volume to restore perfusion and diminish renal factors that sustain the alkalosis and (2) replacing chloride and potassium to promote bicarbonate excretion. Use normal saline boluses if necessary (the use of Ringer's lactate may worsen the alkalosis), then $D_5$0.5*NS* with 40 mEq/L KCl. Dehydration and metabolic alkalosis should be corrected prior to surgical intervention.

Burns

In addition to airway and pulmonary management, fluid therapy is a cornerstone of the early care of the burned patient. Once the percent body surface area (BSA) burn has been determined, fluids may be given according to the following guidelines. Actual volumes should be titrated to clinical response, with the restoration of appropriate pulse, mental status, and a urine output greater than 0.5 mL/kg per hour as the goal of resuscitation:

1. Small burns (less than 25 percent BSA): Administer Ringer's lactate at 1.5 to 2.0 times normal maintenance.
2. Large burns (greater than 30 percent BSA) in older children (greater than 5 years): Use the Parkland formula and give Ringer's lactate at 4 mL/percent burn per kilogram body weight per 24 h, with one-half given over the first 8 h and the remainder over the next 16 h. Maintenance fluids and replacement for other third-space losses (intraabdominal, long-bone fractures, etc.) must be administered as well.
3. Children less than 5 years with large burns: With increased amounts of edema, colloid may be needed to maintain vascular volume. Administer colloid (5% albumin or FFP) at 1 mL/percent BSA per kilogram per 24 h, plus maintenance and third-space losses.

Syndrome of Inappropriate ADH

The syndrome of inappropriate antidiuretic hormone (SIADH) secretion results in excessive free water retention and plasma dilution. Any patient with hyponatremia who has an appreciable sodium excretion and is well hydrated may have SIADH. In pediatrics, this syndrome is often seen in patients with CNS infections, brain tumors, head injuries, and pulmonary disorders.

Treatment is directed at correcting the underlying cause while creating a negative water balance. Fluid intake is at least decreased to two-thirds maintenance with electrolytes and glucose given at normal rates (e.g., $D_5$0.33*NS* or 0.5*NS* with 20–30 mEq KCl/L)

ORAL REHYDRATION

While a great deal of attention over the past decade has been focused on the use of oral rehydration for the treatment of acute diarrheal illnesses and dehydration, appropriate oral therapy continues to be greatly underutilized. The advantages over IV therapy include lower cost, ease of administration (treatment can often be done at home by parents), decreased hospitalization, and less discomfort. Perhaps it is difficult to accept a simpler and less expensive therapy as an improvement over a still effective, but more complicated, solution.

A number of commercial formulas are available for use in oral therapy. The United Nations World Health Organization oral rehydration solution and Rehydralyte are intended for replacement therapy in patients who are dehydrated. Pedialyte, Infalyte, Lytren, Resol, and Ricelyte (in which rice syrup solids are used in place of glucose) are formulations appropriate for initial therapy to prevent dehydration and for maintenance therapy after rehydration has been accomplished. All of these solutions contain 2 to 2.5% glucose along with adequate concentrations of potassium, chloride, and base (either citrate or bicarbonate) to replace stool losses. The difference is that the maintenance solutions contain about 50 mEq Na/L, while the rehydrating solutions use 75 to 90 mEq Na/L. The higher ratio of sodium to glucose maximizes intestinal absorption of water and electrolytes. Starchy foods containing high concentrations of sugar polymers, such as rice, wheat, potatoes, and lentils, also appear to increase effective intestinal absorption. Such foods should probably be continued during the early treatment of patients with gastroenteritis and reintroduced early after rehydration is accomplished.

Oral rehydration therapy may be used for infants and children who are less than 10 percent dehydrated or after the initial IV volume resuscitation in patients with uncomplicated moderate to severe dehydration.

Therapy for an acute diarrheal illness should incorporate the use of one of the maintenance glucose-electrolyte formulas (the premixed formulations may be preferable for home use to avoid dilution errors) and continued feeding (breast milk and lactose-free, carbohydrate-rich foods are usually well tolerated). Fluid should be given ad lib, but intake should be at least 120 to 150 mL/kg per day to prevent dehydration. Smaller, more frequent glucose-electrolyte solution feedings are usually necessary if the patient is also vomiting (regular feedings must often be stopped for 24 h if there is significant vomiting). Infants should be closely followed to detect the development of dehydration.

Once the patient has become dehydrated, replacement is accomplished with one of the rehydrating solutions (75 to 90 mEq Na/L). The rehydration solution should be given ad lib hourly for the first 4 to 8 h. Once the signs of dehydration have resolved, the feeding schedule can be changed to every 3 h. During this maintenance period, give either a maintenance solution or the rehydration solution plus breast milk or low-carbohydrate juice. Again, the patient needs at least 120 to 150 mL/kg per day plus replacement for any ongoing losses. Feeding should be reintroduced during the first 24 h with breast milk or diluted formula for infants and rice cereal, bananas, potatoes, and bread for older patients.

Oral rehydration can be accomplished either at home or in the hospital but should be used only when there is confidence in the compliance with treatment instructions and the availability of appropriate follow-up evaluations.

BIBLIOGRAPHY

Avery ME, Snyder JD: Oral therapy for acute diarrhea. *N Engl J Med* 323:891, 1990.

Ellis D, Avner E: Fluid and electrolyte disorders in pediatric patients, in Puschett J (ed): *Disorders of Fluid and Electrolyte Balance*. New York, Churchill Livingstone, 1985.

Finberg L.: Oral electrolyte/glucose solutions: 1984. *J Pediatr* 105:939, 1984.

Finberg L, Kravath RE, Fleischman AR: *Water and Electrolytes in Pediatrics*. Philadelphia, Saunders, 1982.

Ichikawa, I: *Pediatric Textbook of Fluids and Electrolytes*. Baltimore, Williams & Wilkins, 1990.

Raphaely RC: Shock, in Fleisher G, Ludwig S (eds): *Textbook of Pediatric Emergency Medicine*, 2d ed. Baltimore, Williams & Wilkins, 1988, pp 42–51.

Winters RW: *Principles of Pediatric Fluid Therapy*. Boston, Little Brown, 1982.

C. VASCULAR ACCESS

William H. Spivey
Dee Hodge III

Vascular access in children, as in adults, is necessary for fluid and drug administration, monitoring blood pressure, and obtaining blood for diagnostic studies. However, children have fewer veins available for catheterization, their veins are smaller, and they have more adipose tissue overlying the veins.

Immobilization of the child and identification of a suitable vein are essential for venous access. To accomplish immobilization, the child may be placed in a commercial papoose or wrapped in a sheet with an assistant restraining the child's legs.

Sedation may be necessary for the insertion of central lines where movement could have disastrous consequences. A local anesthetic at the puncture site and a combination of morphine 0.1 mg/kg (maximum 8 mg) and pentobarbital 4 mg/kg (maximum 100 mg) IM will provide adequate sedation for most procedures. Other sedation regimens include: midazolam, 0.1 mg/kg IV: midazolam IV infusion at 0.4–1.2 μg/kg per minute; or chloral hydrate, 25–50 mg/kg PO or rectally.

PERIPHERAL VEINS

A suitable vein can usually be found in the antecubital fossa or on the dorsum of the hand between the third and fourth metacarpals. The feet and ankles are acceptable alternatives, especially the saphenous vein on the medial aspect of the ankle. Once a vein is located, immobilize the limb by taping it to a small armboard or, in the case of an infant, by splinting with two or three tongue depressors taped together.

A 21- to 27-gauge butterfly needle may be used for venous cannulation, or a 21- to 25-gauge plastic catheter-over-the-needle may be used to provide a more secure line. When using small-gauge needles, it is helpful to first puncture the skin with a larger needle and then insert the small-gauge butterfly or plastic catheter and needle through the skin puncture. This prevents the point of the small needle from puncturing both sides of the vessel as it overcomes skin resistance. After successful cannulation, the butterfly needle or catheter is taped into position. A piece of cotton may be placed underneath to provide a better needle angle for flow.

In infants and small children a microdrip fluid chamber should be used to accurately monitor the rate of infusion and to prevent large volumes from being accidentally infused. In trauma with hemorrhagic shock a microdrip chamber should not be used.

SCALP VEINS

Scalp veins are easily accessible in the infant under 1 year of age and provide a good route for maintenance fluid and drug administration. The infant should be immobilized and the head grasped by an assistant. Shave or clip the hair overlying the vein, large enough to accommodate the tape and the needle. The vein selected should be straight and long enough to accommodate the needle. It must also be differentiated from an artery. Arteries are generally more tortuous, pulsate, and fill from below, whereas veins fill from above.

Place a rubber band around the infant's head (Fig. 14C-1) to serve as a tourniquet. After the skin has been cleansed with povidone-iodine, grasp a butterfly needle (23- to 27-gauge) by the wings and insert it approximately 0.5 cm from the intended puncture site in the direction of blood flow. In order to prevent an air embolus, the butterfly tubing is filled with saline. When the vein is entered, blood will flow back into the tubing. The tourniquet is cut and 1 to 2 mL of fluid infused to establish the correct position of the needle. The needle is then taped in place with the plastic tubing, looped to prevent it from being accden-

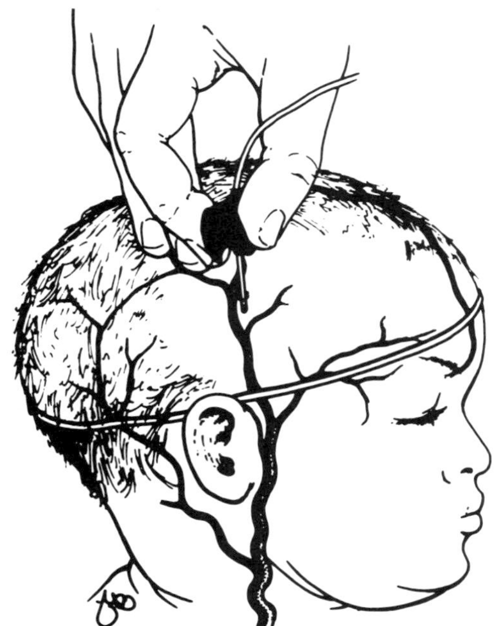

Fig. 14C-1. A tourniquet is placed around the infant's head and the needle inserted 0.5 cm from the intended puncture site in the direction of blood flow.

tally pulled. The needle and tubing may then be covered with a small medicine cup for protection.

Complications from this procedure include local hematoma, infiltration, infection, and inadvertent arterial puncture. This procedure should be carefully explained to parents since they often become upset when hair is cut or shaved off, for whatever reason.

VENOUS CUTDOWN

Venous cutdown catheterization is used when percutaneous attempts are not successful and rapid venous access is needed for treatment of shock or cardiac arrest.

The vein of choice for cutdown is the great saphenous vein, located between the medial malleolus and the anterior tibial tendon. Before exposing the vein, the child should be restrained and the site anesthetized with 1% lidocaine, cleansed with povidone-iodine, and draped with sterile towels. A tourniquet is not used since it increases bleeding. A 2-cm transverse incision is made between the medial malleolus and the anterior tibial tendon, and a curved hemostat is used to spread to subcutaneous tissue along the course of the vein (Fig. 14C-2). Anterior

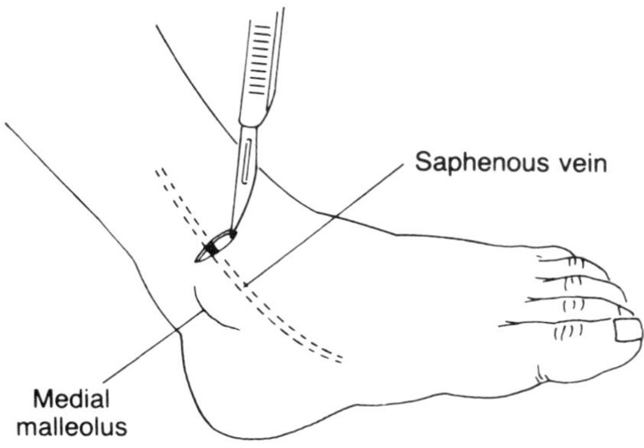

Fig. 14C-2. A 2-cm transverse incision is made between the medial malleolus and anterior tibial tendon. The incision should extend through the skin but not into the subcutaneous tissues.

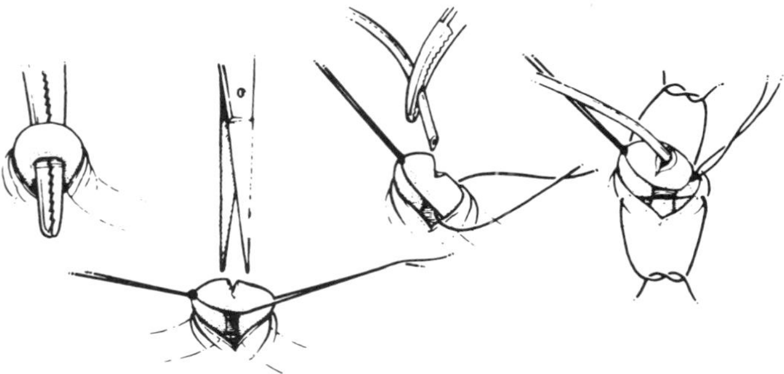

Fig. 14C-3. After the vein has been dissected from the subcutaneous tissues, it is elevated with a hemostat and retracted with ties. A V-shaped incision is made in the vessel and the cannula inserted. The ties may be tied or a pressure dressing applied to prevent bleeding.

to the vein is a sensory nerve that can be spared if the vein is carefully dissected. Once the vein is isolated, two 4–0 silk ties are placed under the vein, one distal and one proximal. The distal suture may be tied and used for stabilization during insertion of the catheter, since this will permanently occlude the vein; some prefer to avoid ligation to promote recannalization of the vein when the catheter is removed.

The vein is lifted with gentle traction using the two ties, and a V-shaped incision is made in the wall with a no. 11 scalpel or fine scissors. A beveled catheter previously filled with fluid and attached to a fluid-filled syringe may then be inserted as demonstrated in Fig. 14C-3. Patency is checked by aspirating blood and flushing the catheter. The proximal suture is then tied around the vein and catheter and the distal suture tied to the catheter. If the distal suture has not been tied, it may be removed.

An alternative method of cannulating the vessel, easier in the small infant, is to insert an over-the-needle plastic catheter directly into the vein once it is exposed. The vessel is elevated by holding traction on the sutures under the vessel as described above or by simply placing a hemostat under the distal end of the vessel and elevating it. The needle is then directly inserted into the vessel and the catheter advanced (Fig. 14C-4). Great care must be taken to avoid through-and-through puncture of the vein. This does not require that either end of the vessel be ligated. The incision is sutured and the catheter is taped or sewn in place.

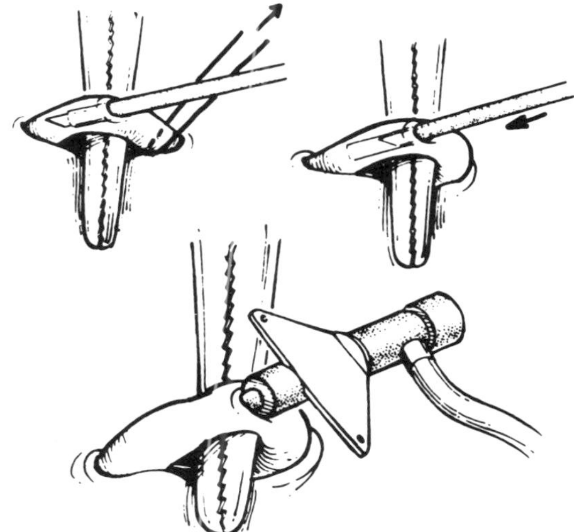

Fig. 14C-4. The vessel is elevated with a hemostat and occluded with gentle traction from a distal tie. The needle is inserted and the sheath is advanced into the vessel. The vessel should not be tied off with this technique.

Complications of a cutdown include infection, phlebitis, laceration of a nerve, and catheter loss into a vein.

INTERNAL JUGULAR CATHETERIZATION

Catheterization of the internal jugular vein for central venous access is preferable to using the subclavian vein in infants. The child is easier to immobilize for internal jugular catheterization, and the risk of pneumothorax is much less. Although there are several approaches to the internal jugular vein, the posterior approach and high central or anterior approach have a high success rate and fewer complications in infants and children.

In both techniques the infant is placed with head extended over the edge of the cart and rotated away from the intended puncture site. The neck is cleansed with povidone-iodine and the skin anesthetized. An 18- to 20-gauge needle and a J-shaped guidewire using the Seldinger technique is used to cannulate the vein.

In the high central approach the landmark is the apex of a triangle formed by the two heads of the sternocleidomastoid and clavicle (Fig. 14C-5). The needle is inserted pointing toward the ipsilateral nipple with the syringe elevated 45° above the plane of the table. Once the vein has been entered, the syringe is removed, a guidewire is inserted through the needle, the needle is removed, and a catheter is inserted over the wire. Care must be taken never to change direction of the needle while in the neck. The razor-sharp bevel of the needle can lacerate an artery or nerve.

In the posterior approach a needle attached to a syringe is inserted at the midpoint of the lateral border of the sternocleidomastoid muscle, and is directed toward the contralateral nipple. The syringe is elevated 10° and the needle advanced, maintaining negative pressure on the syringe. Cannulation of the vessel is accomplished as described for the high central approach.

Complications of internal jugular catheterization include carotid artery puncture with hematoma, pneumothorax, thoracic duct catheterization, and damage to the cranial and cervical sympathetic nerves. By using the right side of the neck, the incidence of complications may be reduced.

EXTERNAL JUGULAR VEIN

The external jugular vein is a good site for drawing blood when peripheral veins are not available and may be used for access to the central venous circulation. This route eliminates the danger of carotid artery puncture and pneumothorax, but the success rate of central venous catheter placement is only about 60 percent, as compared to about 80 percent for the internal jugular vein.

The child is immobilized with the head extended 15 to 20° over the edge of the bed and rotated away from the puncture site. In order to maximize the venous filling, the infant may be stimulated to cry and a finger placed over the base of the vein at the clavicle. After cleansing of the site, a 21- or 23-gauge butterfly needle attached to a syringe is inserted into the vein midway between the angle of the jaw and the shoulder (Fig. 14C-6). If central venous access is required, an 18- to 20-gauge needle attached to a syringe is likewise inserted and a J-tipped guidewire passed through it. The needle is removed and a Seldinger catheter passed over the wire. Complications of this procedure include hematoma and placement of central lines outside the thorax.

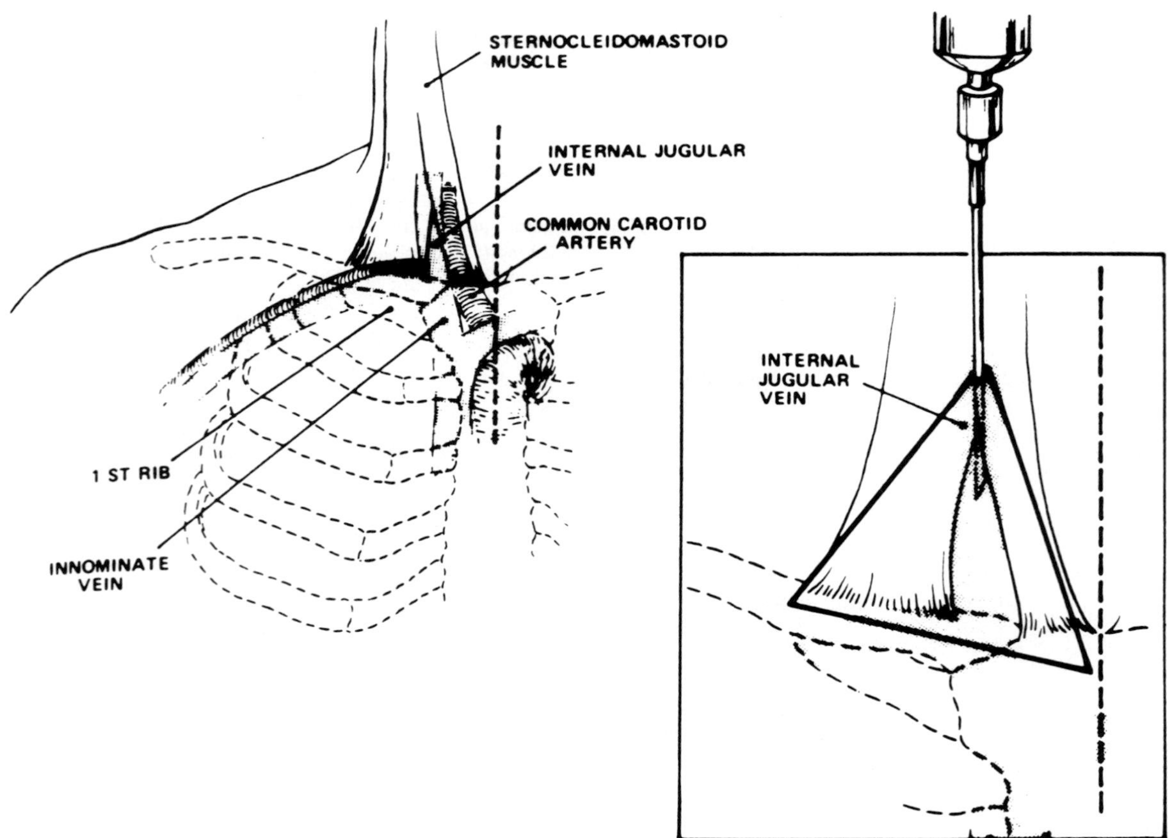

Fig. 14C-5. The position of the internal jugular vein is demonstrated on the left. It is cannulated by inserting a needle at the apex of the triangle formed by the two heads of the sternocleidomastoid muscle and pointing it at the ipsilateral nipple with 10° elevation of the syringe. Once the vessel has entered, a guide wire is inserted and the catheter inserted over the guide wire.

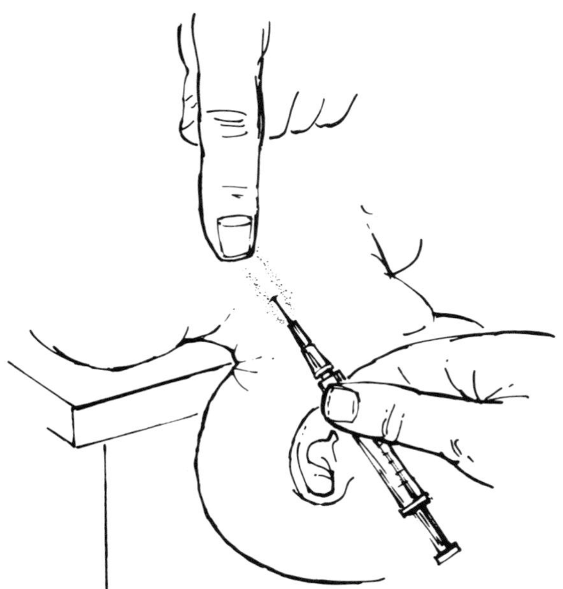

Fig. 14C-6. Venipuncture of the external jugular vein is accomplished by immobilizing the child and extending the head 15 to 20° over the edge of the bed, with the head rotated away from the puncture site. Venous return is occluded with light pressure over the vein above the clavicle and the vein punctured distally.

SUBCLAVIAN VEIN

This technique is indicated when emergency access to the venous circulation is required and percutaneous peripheral, femoral, or jugular access is not available. It is associated with pneumothorax, hemothorax, hydrothorax, and infection after emergency placement. It is also difficult to perform during closed-chest cardiac massage because of the motion of the chest and shoulders.

Adequate restraint is difficult unless the patient is heavily sedated. The child should be placed in the Trendelenburg position with a towel placed under the thoracic spine. The skin is cleansed and the puncture site anesthetized. A small nick is made in the skin over the medial portion of the clavicle with a scalpel. The needle is then inserted through this puncture site and advanced toward the junction of the clavicle and the first rib. When blood return occurs the catheter is then advanced into the vein (Fig. 14C-7). Blood is aspirated from the catheter and fluid infused. A catheter over the needle device such as the Intramedicut cannula is commonly used and ranges from 20-gauge in newborns to 14-gauge in children over 6 years. A Seldinger-type catheter may also be used. Care must be taken not to allow air to enter the catheter and produce an air embolus. An x-ray should be obtained to confirm the position of the catheter and to check for pneumothorax.

AXILLARY VEIN

The axillary vein may be used for central venous access when the femoral, subclavian, or internal jugular veins are not available. The incidence of pneumothorax is much lower than with the subclavian approach. Complications include infection, axillary artery puncture and nerve injury.

The child is immobilized and the arm is abducted to 45–90°. After cleansing the axillary region, the axillary artery is palpated and the needle inserted inferior and parallel to the artery. Once the vein is punctured, blood may be aspirated and catheter inserted.

Both Teflon coated over the needle catheters (18–24 gauge) and Seldinger-type catheters (3–8.5 French) may be used for this approach. If central venous pressure monitoring is desired, a catheter long enough to reach the superior vena cava should be used. Avoid introduction

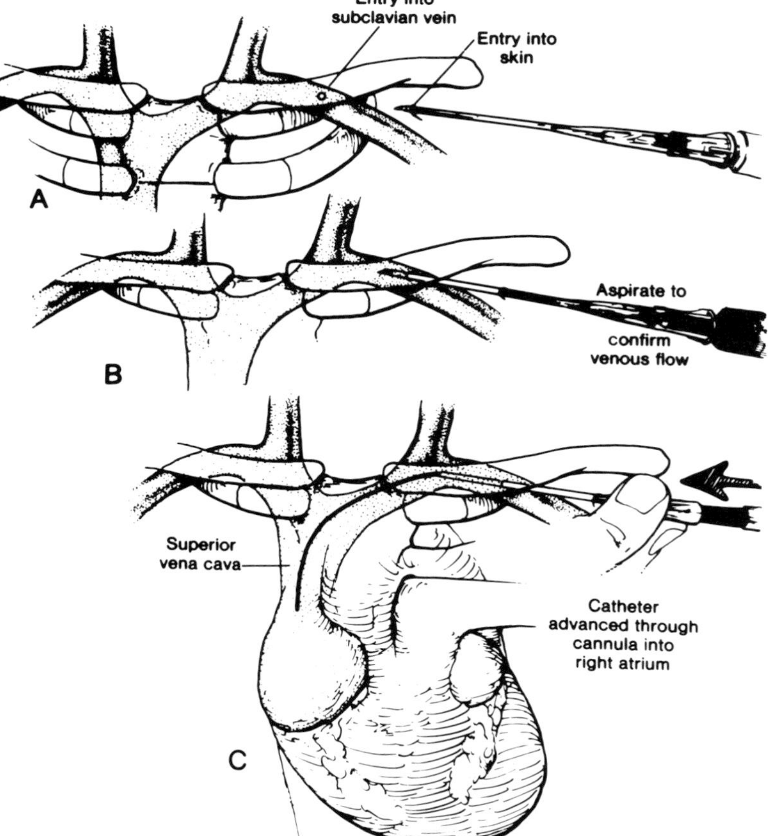

Fig. 14C-7. The anatomic position of the subclavian vein is demonstrated in *A*. A needle is inserted at the mid-portion of the clavicle and advanced until the vein is punctured, as demonstrated in *B*. Once venipuncture is successful a catheter may be inserted through the needle or a Seldinger-type catheter may be inserted (*C*).

of air through the cannula and check for catheter placement with an X-ray.

FEMORAL APPROACH

The femoral vein may be used for emergency central venous catheterization. It is more accessible than the external jugular vein during cardiac arrest and has a low incidence of short-term complications. The femoral vein may be cannulated percutaneously or by cutdown. The simplest method of percutaneous catheterization is to use the Seldinger technique. The leg is externally rotated and the artery palpated. The artery lies one-half the distance between the symphysis and anterior iliac spine and 1.5 cm below the inguinal ligament (Fig. 14C-8). The skin is cleansed and anesthetized and the needle inserted 0.5 cm medial to the artery into the femoral vein. When blood return is obtained, the guidewire is inserted through the needle, the needle removed, and the catheter inserted over the wire.

If the patient is in cardiac arrest, percutaneous cannulation is difficult. In this case, a 3-cm incision is made 1 to 2 cm below the inguinal ligament and the subcutaneous tissue dissected with a hemostat. When the vein is exposed, it may be cannulated under direct visualization or ligatures placed under it and cannulated as described for the great saphenous vein. Femoral cannulation may be complicated by thrombophlebitis or infection, but if it is used for only a short time, the incidence of infection is low.

INTRAOSSEOUS ROUTE

The intraosseous route was widely used for fluid and drug administration in the 1940s but was abandoned when venous catheters were perfected. Recently the intraosseous route has been demonstrated effective for the administration of sodium bicarbonate during cardiac arrest and for emergency fluid administration. Fluids and drugs that have been administered via this route include saline, glucose, epinephrine, dopamine, sodium bicarbonate, diazepam, glucose, and antibiotics. The technique is relatively simple and is indicated when emergency venous access is required and peripheral or central routes are not available.

The bone most commonly used is the proximal tibia. The anterior tibial tuberosity is palpated with the index finger and the medial aspect of the tibia grasped with the thumb. An imaginary line is drawn between the two, and the needle is inserted 1 cm distal to the midpoint of this line. An 18-gauge spinal needle is used in infants up to age 18 months, while other children require a bone marrow needle. Using strict sterile techniques, the needle is inserted in a perpendicular or caudal direction until the needle point is felt to puncture the cortex (Fig. 14C-9). The stylet is removed and blood or marrow contents aspirated to confirm position. Fluids or drugs may then be administered.

As soon as the child is resuscitated and conventional venous access obtained, the intraosseous needle should be removed and pressure applied to the puncture site. Complications include infection, fracture at the site of insertion and extravasation of drugs that may lead to sloughing of the skin. If sterile technique is used, the rate of infection is less than 1 percent.

UMBILICAL VEIN

Umbilical vein access is indicated for resuscitation and stabilization of the newborn. It may be performed up to seven days after delivery. The cord is cleansed, cut to a length of 2 cm and a purse string suture placed near the junction of the skin and cord. The single large vein and two smaller arteries are identified and a catheter filled with heparinized saline is inserted into vein. The catheter, 3.5 to 5.0 French, should only be advanced 4 to 5 cm in a term infant. Further advancement may damage the liver or result in improper placement. After the catheter is placed, the purse string is tightened and fluid is infused taking care not to introduce air through the catheter.

Fluids and drugs may be administered by this route for resuscitation and maintenance afterwards. Complications include infection, air embolus, hemorrhage, vessel perforation and hepatic sclerosis from injection of sclerosing substances into the liver.

ENDOTRACHEAL ROUTE

The endotracheal route is used when venous access cannot be obtained. It has been used for administration of epinephrine, atropine, naloxone, lidocaine, and diazepam in humans. Epinephrine and atropine have been administered most commonly, with no reports of adverse effects.

The drug is administered by injecting it directly into the endotracheal tube followed by several rapid insufflations with a bag-valve device to force the drug into the alveoli and terminal bronchioles. The optimum dose of drug has not been determined, but current dosages recommended are the same as intravenous doses. A recent study has demonstrated that much higher doses of endotracheal epinephrine are needed to produce similar cardiovascular changes in dogs when compared to intravenous epinephrine. Prolonged duration of action may result from a depot effect in the lungs.

Adverse effects include destruction of surfactant and the development of adult respiratory distress syndrome or pneumonia, although

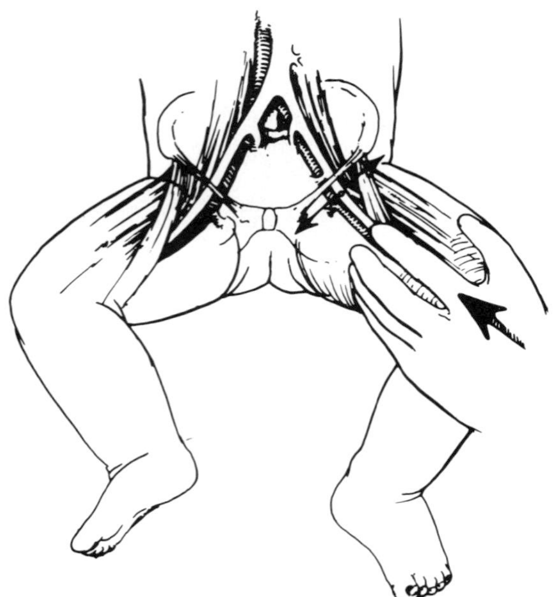

Fig. 14C-8. The femoral vein in children lies one-half the distance between the symphysis and anterior iliac spine and 1.5 cm below the inguinal ligament.

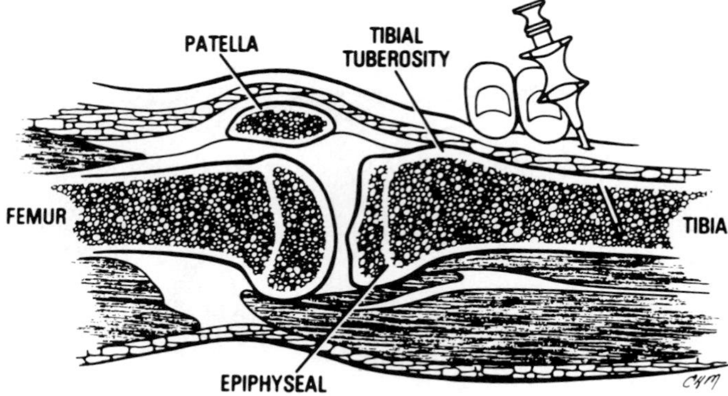

Fig. 14C-9. The needle is inserted 2-cm distal to the tibial tuberosity on the medial aspect of the tibia. It is inserted in a caudal direction, away from the joint space.

this has not been reported in humans. Sodium bicarbonate, calcium chloride, and bretylium tosylate should not be given via this route.

BIBLIOGRAPHY

Cote CJ, Jobes DR, Schwartz AJ, et al: Two approaches to cannulation of a child's internal jugular vein. *Anesthesiology* 50:371, 1979.

Hodge D, Delgado-Paredes C, Fleisher G: Intraosseous infusion flow rates in hypovolemic "pediatric" dogs (abstr). *Ann Emerg Med* 15:644, 1986.

Nicholson SC, Sweeney MF, Moore RA, et al: Comparison of internal and external jugular cannulation of the central circulation in the pediatric patient. *Crit Care Med* 13:747, 1985.

Prince SR, Sullivan RL, Hacket A: Percutaneous cannulation of the internal jugular vein in infants and children. *Anesthesiology* 44:170, 1976.

Ralston SH, Tacker WA, Showen L, et al: Endotracheal versus intravenous epinephrine during electromechanical dissociation with CPR in dogs. *Ann Emerg Med* 14:1044, 1985.

Rossetti VA, Thompson BM, Miller J, et al: Intraosseous infusion: An alternative route of pediatric intravascular access. *Ann Emerg Med* 14:885, 1985.

Spivey WH, Lathers CM, Malone D, et al: Comparison of intraosseous, central, and peripheral routes of sodium bicarbonate administration during CPR in pigs. *Ann Emerg Med* 14:1135, 1985.

D. NEONATAL RESUSCITATION AND EMERGENCIES

Seetha Shankaran
Eugene E. Cepeda

NEONATAL RESUSCITATION

Approximately 6 percent of all newborns require life support in the delivery room or nursery, and in those neonates whose birth weights are less than 1500 g, the need for resuscitation rises to 80 percent. Personnel skilled in neonatal resuscitation should be available at every delivery. It is important to anticipate the delivery of the high-risk neonate so that the delivery room personnel may be alerted to the possible need for resuscitation.

The following factors are associated with an increased risk for neonatal resuscitation.

Maternal factors
- Inadequate prenatal care
- Age <16 to >35 years
- History of previous perinatal morbidity or mortality
- Toxemia, hypertension
- Diabetes
- Chronic renal disease
- Anemia
- Drug therapy (e.g. reserpine, lithium carbonate, magnesium, adrenergic blocking agents)
- Substance abuse
- Infection or prolonged rupture of membranes
- Blood type or group isoimmunization
- Oligohydramnios

Intrapartum factors
- Abnormal presentation
- Caesarean section
- Prolonged labor or precipitous delivery
- Prolonged rupture of membranes
- Cephalopelvic disproportion
- Forceps delivery other than outlet or vacuum extraction
- Prolapsed cord
- Cord compression
- Maternal hypotension
- Analgesic or sedative drugs given within 2 h of delivery

Fetal factors
- Prematurity
- Postmaturity
- Intrauterine growth failure
- Multiple gestation
- Acidosis (fetal scalp capillary monitoring)
- Abnormal fetal heart rate per monitor
- Meconium-stained amniotic fluid
- Congenital infection
- Fetal malformation or edema diagnosed by ultrasound

The following conditions should alert nursery personnel to the possiblity of apnea: previous need for resuscitation, premature infants, sepsis and/or meningitis, congenital abnormalities, respiratory distress, or seizures.

Principles of Resuscitation

The Apgar Score (Table 14D-1) is assessed at 1 and 5 min of age for every newly delivered infant. Although the scoring system has been useful in evaluating the condition of the newborn, 1 min is too long to wait to make the decision to initiate resuscitation. If the 5-min score is less than 7, additional scores are obtained every 5 min for a total of 20 min.

In very low birth weight infants it should be noted that acidotic cord blood gases (cord pH $\leq$ 7.2) rather than low Apgar scores correlate with morbidity and mortality.

Equipment

The following is a list of the equipment necessary for resuscitation.

1. Bag and mask with manometer attached, connected to a source of 100% oxygen. Oxygen should be heated and humidified. The bag should be a rubber anesthesia bag, a rebreathing bag of 500-mL capacity, or a self-inflating bag designed for newborns.
2. Rubber face masks of varying sizes 1, 2, 3, and 4.
3. Wall suction, sterile catheters, and bulb syringes.
4. DeLee suction catheter with mucus trap
5. Laryngoscope with 0 and 1 blades.
6. Oral endotracheal tubes with stylet—size 2.5, 3.0, 3.5, and 4.0 mm
7. Radiant heater with servomechanism.
8. Sterile umbilical vessel catheterization tray.
9. Glucose oxidase blood test strips.
10. A heart rate monitor with easy applicable leads.
11. Intravenous infusion equipment.
12. Transcutaneous oxygen monitor or saturation pulse oximeter.
13. Appropriate light.
14. Infant stethoscope.
15. Nasogastric tubes 5- and 8-French size.
16. Clock with sweep second hand.

Table 14D-1. The Apgar Score

Sign	0	1	2
Heart rate	Absent	<100/min	>100/min
Respiratory effort	Absent	Weak cry	Strong cry
Muscle tone	Limp	Some flexion	Good flexion
Reflex irritability (when feet stimulated)	No response	Some motion	Cry
Color	blue: pale	Body pink; extremities blue	Pink

Steps to Follow During Resuscitation

Maintain Body Temperature

Maintain infant below the level of the placenta prior to clamping the cord. When the cord is clamped, blot the infant dry with a sterile towel and place the infant under a preheated radiant warmer on a sterile table. Neonates should be placed on either backs or the left side somewhat in Trendelenburg's position with the neck in a neutral position.

Clear the Airway

Gently suction the nose and mouth with a bulb syringe. DeLee trap, or mechanical suction apparatus with 8-French suction catheter. A 5- to 10-s examination should be performed to determine the need for resuscitation. This examination should include an assessment of heart rate, respiratory effort, color, and muscular activity. If the infant has a lusty cry, is pink, has spontaneous respirations, and a heart rate above 120/min (Apgar > 8), no further therapy is needed.

Initiate Breathing

If the infant is apneic or the heart rate is slow and irregular (<100 beats per minute) and the color is cyanotic (Apgar 4 to 7), administer positive-pressure ventilation with the mask over the infant's face and 100% oxygen. The respiratory rate should be maintained at 40 breaths/min with pressure applied to gently move the chest wall. In an infant who has not yet taken a breath, over 40 cm of H_2O pressure may be necessary to expand the lungs. In mildly depressed infants, this will produce a prompt increase in heart rate and the onset of regular spontaneous respirations. If no improvement is noted in 15 to 30 s and the condition deteriorates (Apgar ≤ 4), the trachea should be intubated and assisted ventilation continued.

Cardiac Massage

If the heart rate is below 50 beats per minute with assisted ventilation, cardiac massage should be initiated by placing both hands around the infant's chest with two thumbs over the midsternum so that the sternum will be depressed two-thirds of the distance to the vertebral column at 120 compressions per minute. Cardiac massage may be stopped periodically to assess improvement, and ventilation and cardiac massage should be synchronized (1:3 ratio). The chest should expand, bilateral breath sounds should be heard in the axilla, and heart rate should increase if the resuscitation is effective and the endotracheal tube is in good position. *In most instances* it is possible to obtain an adequate response with the use of external cardiac massage and assisted ventilation. If there is no response to these measures above, drug therapy should be considered. Any route of access to the circulatory system is acceptable, including a peripheral vein, the umbilical vein, or an umbilical artery.

Catheterize Umbilical Artery or Vein

The most expedient procedure for obtaining vascular access is to insert the venous catheter through the ductus venosus into the inferior vena cava (10 to 12 cm) or avoid the portal system by anchoring it superficially (4 to 5 cm). The first blood sample aspirated should be analyzed for blood gases. Either capillary gases, in the absence of shock, or arterial gases should be monitored. Obtain radiographs of chest and abdomen to rule out other abnormalities and evaluate the position of the catheters.

Drug Therapy in Resuscitation

There is a very minor role for drug therapy in resuscitation. Most resuscitative efforts in the delivery room respond to adequate support of ventilation and circulation without drug therapy.

Dextrose

To provide metabolic substrate and expansion of plasma volume, $D_{10}W$ at 100 mL/kg per day or 6 to 8 mg/kg per minute should be infused. If the Dextrostix is < 45 mg/dL, 5 mL/kg of 10 or 15% glucose solution should be infused; 25% dextrose infusions should be avoided because of the risk of rebound hypoglycemia.

Epinephrine

To stimulate heart rate if it is under 120/min, 0.1 mL/kg of a 1:10,000 solution may be given through the endotracheal tube or intravenously. Cardiac massage should continue following epinephrine administration.

Naloxone

To reverse narcotic depression, 0.01 mg/kg of a neonatal solution (0./2 mg/mL) may be administered intravenously, subcutaneously, or through the endotracheal tube. The time for peak concentration of transplacentally acquired narcotics in the fetus is 2 h, following administration of medication to the mother so that delivery of the fetus at that time would predispose the fetus to maximal depression.

Isoproterenol

If epinephrine has failed to raise the heart rate to at least 120 beats per minute, 1:10,000 solution or 0.05 to 0.1 μg/min may be infused.

A delay in onset of spontaneous regular respiration of more than 30 min following birth has been associated with a poor prognosis. Attempts at resuscitation after 30 min of no response do not appear to be warranted.

Certain neonatal conditions require specific measures during resuscitation besides those outlined above.

Neonatal Shock

The risk factors for shock and hypotension in the newborn infant are low birth weight, maternal sepsis, prolapsed cord, and acute onset of maternal vaginal bleeding. Clinical sign of hypovolemia in the neonate are pallor, tachycardia, grunting respirations in absence of pulmonary disease, mottling of skin, poor capillary filling, thready pulse and hypotension (systolic < 45 mmHg in a 1000-g premature neonate or < 60 mmHg in a term infant), and persistent metabolic acidosis. A hematocrit should be obtained, and if anemia (hematocrit < 45 vol %) or hypotension are diagnosed, immediate plasma expansion in the form of packed RBC 5 mL/kg or whole blood, fresh-frozen plasma, Plasmanate, or 5% salt-poor albumin 10 to 20 mL/kg should be given intravenously over 10 min.

Meconium Staining

Meconium staining of the amniotic fluid varies from 0.5 to 20 percent of all births. Aspiration of thick meconium carries a 20 to 50 percent mortality rate; however, with proper management it is almost entirely preventable. When gross meconium is noted at the time of delivery, the following procedure should be followed. After delivery of the infant's head (but before delivery of the shoulders), the nose, mouth, and pharynx should be thoroughly suctioned with a DeLee suction catheter. Repeat suctioning of the upper airway should be performed as the infant is placed under the radiant warmer. The trachea should then be visualized with a laryngoscope and meconium aspirated by direct suctioning through an endotracheal tube. Suctioning should be repeated until no more meconium is present in the trachea. The infant may then be ventilated with positive pressure as indicated. Failure to clear the trachea before assisted or spontaneous ventilation may result in dissemination of the meconium through the airways.

Complications of Asphyxia

Infants who were successfully resuscitated at birth should have continuous monitoring of vital signs, blood gases, hematocrit, dextrose, blood pressure, fluid status, and clinical condition. Complications associated with severe asphyxia are seizures, hypoxic-ischemic encephalopathy, intracranial hemorrhage, inappropriate ADH secretion, hypocalcemia, persistent pulmonary hypertension, ischemic cardiomyopathy, hypovolemia or shock, necrotizing enterocolitis, renal failure, and coagulopathy.

NEONATAL EMERGENCIES

Seizures

Seizures in neonates may represent primary central nervous system (CNS) disease or a systemic or metabolic disorder. Recent data suggests that seizure activity itself may adversely affect the growing brain.

Types of Seizures

Subtle

Subtle seizures occur in both preterm and term neonates. These consist of ocular movements, facial, oral, or lingual movements and respiratory manifestations, such as apnea or stertorous breathing.

Tonic

These are characteristic of premature infants. The seizures appear as decerebrate or decorticate posturing.

Multifocal Clonic

These seizures are seen in term infants. These are initially noted in one limb and migrate to another part of the body.

Focal Clonic

These are well localized and are accompanied by specific sharp activity on the EEG. These seizures occur more commonly in full-term infants.

Myoclonic

These seizures are expressed as single or multiple jerks of flexion of the upper or lower extremities. These seizures are rare and occur in both premature and full-term infants.

Differentiation of Seizures

It is important to distinguish seizures from tremors or jitteriness, which may be seen in infants who have hypocalcemia, hypoglycemia, drug withdrawal, or no identifiable morbidity. Tremors are uniform fine movements which respond to sensory stimuli, stop with manual stabilization, and do not occur spontaneously. They are not accompanied by eye, oral, or lingual movements.

Causes of Seizures

Hypoxic-Ischemic Encephalopathy

This is the most common cause of seizures. The seizures occur between 6 and 18 h of life. In full-term neonates the hypoxic injury may result in a cerebral hemorrhage, water-shed infarct, posterior fossa hematoma, or subarachnoid or subdural hemorrhage. In premature infants, hypoxic injury often results in periventricular-intraventricular hemorrhage. This type of seizure has a poor prognosis.

Metabolic Disturbances

The metabolic disturbances associated with neonatal seizures include hypoglycemia, hypocalcemia, hypomagnesemia, hyperammonemia, hypernatremia, and hyponatremia. Hypoglycemia, hypocalcemia, and hypomagnesemia are often found in premature infants with perinatal asphyxia. Hypernatremia occurs in neonates with dehydration secondary to excessive fluid losses or treatment with large doses of sodium bicarbonate. Hyponatremia may be seen secondary to inappropriate ADH secretion or acute volume overload. Inborn errors of amino acid metabolism also may present as seizures.

Meningitis or Encephalitis

These conditions include bacterial meningitis and encephalitis associated with TORCH complex (toxoplasmosis, rubella, cytomegalovirus infection, and herpes simplex infection) or Coxsackie B encephalitis.

Developmental Abnormalities

These include congenital hydrocephalus, microcephaly, and other congenital brain anomalies.

Drug Withdrawal

Drug withdrawal from maternal use of methadone, barbiturates, alcohol, pentazocine (Talwin) and tripelannamine (Pyribenzamine) rarely presents as seizures.

Pyridoxine Dependence

This condition occurs rarely but must be considered in neonatal seizures unresponsive to standard therapy.

Maternal Anesthesia

A rare cause of seizures is inadvertent fetal scalp injection of maternal local anesthetic agents.

Stroke

Neonatal stroke diagnosed by computed tomography (CT) has recently been described in term infants with focal motor seizures. Neonatal stroke may occur in the setting of diverse cerebrovascular disorders such as hypoxic-ischemic encephalopathy, polycythemia, acute severe hypertension, and cocaine use.

Diagnosis of Seizures

A careful history, including intrapartum monitoring data and physical examination, are essential when considering drug withdrawal, birth asphyxia, or metabolic disorders as a cause of the seizures. A lumbar puncture with analysis of cell count, culture and gram stain along with blood specimens for culture, sugar, calcium, magnesium, and BUN should be obtained. The skull x-ray, echoencephalogram, and EEG can be obtained after the seizures have been controlled. In a full-term infant a CT scan of the head to look for ischemic injury may be necessary as an echoencephalogram may not provide adequate visualization of the subarachnoid space or posterior fossa. Recently, positron emission tomography of the head has been utilized to evaluate the effects of asphyxia and seizures on cerebral blood flow.

Treatment of Seizures

Repeated seizures in neonates may be accompanied by hypoventilation and apnea, resulting in hypercapnia and hypoxemia. Increase in cerebral blood flow and arterial hypertension occur with neonatal seizures. Treatment of seizures should be initiated while awaiting results of laboratory data. An intravenous access route should be established immediately and the airway maintained; assisted ventilation should be initiated if apnea persists. Hypoglycemia and hypocalcemia should be treated as stated earlier in "Neonatal Resuscitation." Hypomagnesemia is often associated with hypocalcemia and should be treated by intravenous administration of 2 to 4 mL of a 2% magnesium sulfate solution.

The anticonvulsant drugs used most frequently include phenobarbital and diphenylhydantoin. The loading dosage of phenobarbital is 20 mg/kg IV given slowly over 10 min, and the maintenance dose is 5 mg/kg per day IM or PO in two divided doses. If the initial 20 mg/kg dose of phenobarbital is not effective in controlling the seizures, additional doses of 5 mg/kg may be administered every 5 min until the seizures have ceased or the total dose of 40 mg/kg has been reached. In unresponsive cases, diphenylhydantoin may be administered with a similar loading dose followed by maintenance dose of 3 to 5 mg/

kg per day by the IV route in only two divided doses 20 min apart to avoid disturbance of cardiac function. Diazepam (Valium) is recommended for status epilepticus, as long as ventilation and blood pressure are supported. The dose of diazepoam is 0.01 mg/kg administered intravenously. Infants with pyridoxine dependence respond immediately to an intravenous injection of 50 to 100 mg of pyridoxine.

Diaphragmatic Hernia

A failure of development of the posterolateral parts of the diaphragm at Bochdalek's foramen or retrosternally at Morgagni's foramen allows herniation of the gut into the chest cavity. Left-sided Bochdalek's hernias are more common than those on the right. The defect occurs in one out of 2200 births. Associated anomalies with diaphragmatic hernias include congenital heart disease, genitourinary anomalies, gastrointestinal anomalies, hydronephrosis, and cystic kidneys. Frequently the lungs are hypoplastic bilaterally and have abdominal pulmonary vasculature predisposing the infant to pulmonary hypertension.

Fifty percent of fetuses with diaphragmatic hernia have difficulty swallowing and the condition is therefore associated with polyhydramnios. The diagnosis can often be made by prenatal ultrasonography.

Clinical and Radiographic Findings

The clinical findings are localized to the respiratory and digestive tracts. The chest is large, while the abdomen is scaphoid. Bowel sounds are heard in the left chest, and the heart is displaced to the right. Dyspnea, cyanosis, retractions, and vomiting are proportional to the amount of abdominal viscera herniated into the thorax. Radiologic study will reveal air-filled loops of bowel in the chest cavity and an absent diaphragmatic margin. The heart is often displaced and the lungs are small in size.

Management

Immediate surgical repair is a method of treatment, and the neonate should be stabilized as much as possible prior to surgery. Alternatively, the neonate can be placed on extracorporeal membrane oxygenation (ECMO) prior to repair. The infant should be intubated immediately, and little or no attempt should be made to ventilate with a mask. The endotracheal tube should be positioned above the carina. Rapid ventilatory rates and low peak inspirator pressures are used to ventilate the infant and prevent reactive respiratory acidosis and hypercarbia, which are potentially conducive to the development of pulmonary hypertension. A large-caliber 10-French tube should be placed in the stomach with low continuous suction applied. An umbilical artery catheter is useful to monitor blood gases and pH. Any acidemia should be corrected and the pH maintained in the alkalotic range (pH > 7.45) if possible. Intravenous fluids should be given and the patient kept warm. Vasodilator therapy with tolazoline 2 mg/kg per hour infusion may need to be initiated (if pulmonary hypertension develops) prior to surgical repair.

The outcome of management of diaphragmatic hernia is dependent on pulmonary parenchymal and vascular hypoplasia, as well as the complex syndrome of persistent fetal circulation. The morbidity is higher when the symptoms present at birth and when the diaphragmatic hernia is detected prenatally. Morgagni hernias, if they do not affect cardiac output, generally have a better prognosis than do Bochadalek's hernias. Common complications that occur pre- and postoperatively are pneumothorax, persistent fetal circulation, overdistension of hypoplastic lungs, and chylothorax. The recent introduction of the use of ECMO for infants with persistent pulmonary hypertension after hernia repair has improved the prognosis.

Tracheoesophageal Fistula

A defect in the separation of the trachea from the esophagus results in a persistent channel connecting the trachea and the esophagus. There are five types of tracheoesophageal fistulas (TEF) which are descriptive of the malformation possible: (1) esophageal atresia with a distal communication between the trachea and the esophagus, the most common presentation (85 percent); (2) isolated esophageal atresia occurs, less common; (3) isolated TEF; (4) esophageal atresia with a proximal TEF; and (5) esophageal atresia with a double TEF.

Tracheoesophageal fistulas occur in one out of every 4500 births. One-third of the affected infants weigh less than 2500 g. The incidence of associated anomalies with TEF ranges from 40 to 55 percent. The smaller the infant with TEF, the greater the number of other associated anomalies. Congenital heart malformation, vertebral anomalies, imperforate anus, and radial aplasia are common associations.

Diagnosis

The inability to pass a catheter more than 20 cm through the gastrointestinal tract is the hallmark of esophageal atresia. An x-ray may show the air-filled proximal pouch, and if the catheter is left in place, it may coil in the proximal esophagus.

Management

It is important to provide respiratory support by assisted ventilation if needed to correct acidosis before any surgical repair can be undertaken. A plastic sump catheter should be left in the pouch and connected to constant, low-pressure suction. The patient should be maintained in the reverse Trendelenburg or semi-Fowler position to prevent further reflux of gastric secretions through the fistula into the trachea. Intravenous fluids and antibiotics are indicated. Other coexistent problems such as a heart defect should be evaluated. Primary anastomosis is done in cases of esophageal atresia with a distal tracheoesophageal fistula.

The majority (80 percent) of infants with TEF survive. Operative mortality is low. Complications of surgery are pneumonia, atelectasis, anastomotic leak, anastomotic strictures, and (rarely) recurrent fistulas.

Pulmonary Air Leaks

Pulmonary air leaks are a common occurrence in the neonatal intensive care unit. The air may present as a spectrum that includes pneumothorax, pulmonary interstitial emphysema, pneumomediastinum, pneumopericardium, and penumoperitoneum.

Spontaneous pneumothorax can occur in term and postterm infants following intrapartum asphyxia and meconium aspiration. Currently, however, pneumothorax has increased in incidence with the use of continuous positive airway pressure, positive end-expiratory pressure (PEEP), mechanical ventilation, and cardiopulmonary resuscitation. Uneven ventilation caused by aspirated blood, mucus, meconium, and amniotic fluid debris can also result in an air leak. Atelectasis, poor ventilation, and air trapping are common predisposing factors. The premature, low-birth-weight infant with surfactant deficiency has a high incidence of air leaks (30 percent) as does the newborn with meconium aspiration syndrome (40 percent).

Signs and Symptoms

The signs and symptoms of an air leak are those of respiratory distress and often present as an acute clinical deterioration. Grunting respirations and intercostal, sternal, and subcostal retractions may be seen. Cyanosis, elevated respiratory rate, and elevated heart rate are common. Auscultation of the chest will reveal decreased breath sounds on the affected side of a pneumothorax, distant heart sounds, and a shift of the mediastinum. Transillumination of the chest with a high-intensity lamp may aid in the diagnosis. A chest x-ray is diagnostic. The accuracy can be improved with a cross-table lateral film of the chest taken along with the anteroposterior and lateral views.

Treatment

An asymptomatic pneumothorax that is less than 20 percent of the volume of the affected side may be followed clinically with no therapy and with serial radiographic studies every 4 h. Any pneumothorax with severe respiratory distress and clinical deterioration will need emergency treatment. When there is mediastinal shift and cardiovascular collapse, rapid decompression at the fourth intercostal space with a 21-gauge needle attached to a three-way stopcock and a large syringe can be life-saving. A chest tube can be introduced by grasping the tube with a hemostat and passing it through a subcutaneous tunnel and hole in the intercostal space created by blunt surgical dissection. The chest tube is then connected to an underwater seal. This technique will prevent the occurrence of lung perforation, which may result when the chest tube is introduced with a steel trocar. The chest tube should remain as long as the neonate receives positive-pressure ventilation.

Gastroschisis and Omphalocele

An omphalocele is a defect in the umbilical ring which allows the intestines in a sac to protrude out of the abdominal cavity. A gastroschisis is a defect in the abdominal wall that allows the antenatal evisceration of abdominal structures, without a sac being present. There is some controversy as to the exact embryology of the two conditions.

Omphaloceles are found in one out of 6000 to 10,000 births, while gastroschisis occurs twice as frequently in the newborn population. Omphaloceles have a higher (37 percent) incidence of associated anomalies. Three specific syndromes are associated with omphalocele: the upper midline pentalogy of Cantrell, Haller, and Ravitch (sternal, ventral, diaphragmatic, pericardial, and cardiac defects); the lower midline syndrome (vesicointestinal fissure); and the Beckwith-Widemann syndrome (macroglossia, visceromegaly, and hypoglycemia).

Management

The emergency management of the two conditions is not different, especially when the sac in an omphalocele is ruptured. The eviscerated bowel should be wrapped in saline-soaked gauze and placed in a plastic bag to protect it from hypothermia and evaporative losses. A nasogastric tube should be inserted to decompress the intestines. Rapid infusion of 20 mL/kg of 5% Ringer's lactate may be necessary to restore vital signs, after which the infusion should be adjusted to maintain a urine output of at least 2 mL/kg per hour. Intravenous antibiotics should be administered.

Primary fascial closure is the treatment of choice and is often accomplished within hours after birth. When the defect is large, a Silastic silo may be used, but survival, nonetheless, correlates with rapid closure and removal of the prosthesis.

Complications include gastroesophageal reflux, malabsorption, diarrhea, dehydration, and failure to thrive. The mortality of omphalocele is 25 to 30 percent, largely as a result of congenital heart disease and sepsis, while death in patients with gastroschisis is associated with intestinal atresia.

Necrotizing Enterocolitis

Necrotizing enterocolitis is a disease entity that affects the asphyxiated or stressed premature infant of less than 2000-g weight. Full-term newborns with polycythemia or congenital heart disease and those who have had umbilical arterial or venous catheters in situ have been reported to also be at risk for necrotizing enterocolitis.

The exact cause of necrotizing enterocolitis remains unknown, and it is likely that there are multiple factors that ultimately lead to stasis, ischemia, and infection of the bowel wall. The risk factors include hypertonic feeding solutions producing damage to mucosal epithelium of the intestine, patent ductus arteriosus and episodes of apnea diverting blood flow away from the gastrointestinal tract, ischemia following exchange transfusions, and infections with *Escherichia coli, Klebsiella pseudomonas, Clostridium* species, coronavirus, rotavirus, and other enteroviruses.

Signs and Symptoms

The signs and symptoms seen in decreasing frequency are abdominal distension, gastric distension, retention of gastric feeds, apnea, gastrointestinal bleeding, and lethargy. Other signs are abdominal tenderness, redness of abdominal wall, and the presence of reducing substances in the stool.

Diagnosis

A supine anteroposterior and cross-table lateral and upright view will aid in the radiographic diagnosis. Nonspecific findings are distension, air-fluid levels, and separation of intestinal loops suggesting mural edema. Pneumatosis intestinalis is the radiographic hallmark, and its presence indicates gas in the bowel wall. Portal venous gas is an ominous sign, and pneumoperitoneum indicates perforation of the bowel.

Medical Management

The medical management consists of bowel rest, with the infant receiving nothing by mouth and gastric decompression with a nasogastric tube. Cultures of blood, urine, and CSF should be obtained and systemic antibiotics administered. The blood pressure and hydration status should be maintained with liberal use of crystalloids and Plasmanate. Fluid intake may have to be increased to 200 mL/kg per 24 h and inotropic agents used if needed. Thrombocytopenia, neutropenia, and disseminated intravascular coagulopathy are often seen in neonates who are deteriorating, and platelet transfusions should be administered if there is evidence of systemic or gastrointestinal bleeding. Respiratory support may be required, and any acidosis should be corrected. Patients with early necrotizing enterocolitis should have close clinical observations and serial x-rays to look for signs of gangrene or intestinal perforation. The medical treatment includes bowel rest for 2 weeks with nutritional support with parenteral alimentation. The complications of necrotizing enterocolitis are bowel stricture, fistula, abscess, malabsorption, and failure to thrive.

Surgical Management

Pneumoperitoneum related to signs of necrotizing enterocolitis is an absolute indication for surgical repair. Recent data indicate that paracentesis, indicative of intestinal gangrene prior to intestinal perforation, may be an indication for surgery. Persistent acidosis, oliguria, abdominal wall erythema, and portal vein air are associated with advanced disease. The surgical repair consists of removal of the segment of involved bowel and an enterostomy. Reanastomosis is usually performed after 4 to 6 weeks of bowel rest.

The Cyanotic Newborn

Cyanosis in the neonate may be central or peripheral. Central cyanosis is defined as cyanosis of the tongue, mucous membranes, and peripheral skin and indicates the presence of 5 g or more of reduced hemoglobin. Peripheral cyanosis is defined as blue discoloration confined to the skin of the extremities; the arterial saturation will be greater than 94 percent. Peripheral cyanosis is common in the neonate and may persist for 2 to 3 days. It is usually due to vasomotor instability secondary to a cold environment.

Causes of Central Cyanosis

Normal newborn infants have a P_{O_2} above 50 mmHg by 5 to 10 min of age; hence it is pathological for central cyanosis to persist beyond 20 min after birth.

Cyanotic Heart Disease

Congenital heart disease presenting with cyanosis secondary to intracardiac right-to-left shunt includes transposition of the great vessels, tricuspid atresia, truncus arteriosus, tetralogy of Fallot and total anomalous pulmonary venous return with obstruction, pulmonary atresia, and preductal coarctation.

Lung Disease Associated with Cyanosis

These lung disorders include hyaline membrane disease, pneumonia, meconium aspiration syndrome, and persistent fetal circulation due to pneumonia or asphyxia. Mechanical interference with lung function by air leaks (pneumothorax), diaphragmatic hernia, lobar emphysema, or mucous plugs also cause cyanosis.

Central Nervous System Disorders

Intracerebral hemorrhage, when severe, may be associated with shock and cyanosis.

Polycythemia

The increased viscosity and stagnation of blood may produce apparent cyanosis.

Shock and Sepsis

Shock and sepsis result in alveolar hypoventilation.

Methemoglobinemia

Methemoglobinemia is due to reduced oxygen carrying capacity of the blood because of abnormal hemoglobin.

Diagnostic Approach to Central Cyanosis

Physical Examination

Neonates with cyanosis secondary to cyanotic heart disease rarely have respiratory symptoms other than tachypnea. A murmur may be present. Neonates with lung disease producing cyanosis have respiratory distress, grunting, tachypnea, and sternal and intercostal retractions. The cyanotic infant with CNS disturbances or sepsis has apnea, bradycardia, lethargy, and seizures. Neonates with methemoglobinemia have minimal distress in spite of their cyanotic appearance.

Blood-Gas Profile and Response to 100% O_2 Breathing

The "hyperoxia test" (the response in Pa_{O_2} to 100 percent oxygen breathing) may be of use in distinguishing heart disease from other causes of cyanosis. The neonate with cyanotic heart disease will not demonstrate any increase in Pa_{O_2} over 20 mmHg because of the right-to-left shunting of the circulation. Most neonates with lung disease, however, will demonstrate an increase in Pa_{O_2} after breathing 100% oxygen for 20 min. The neonate with persistent fetal circulation, CNS disorders, polycythemia, sepsis, and shock also will demonstrate an increase in Pa_{O_2}. No response will also be elicited in the neonate with methemoglobinemia. When a blood specimen is exposed to air, it turns pink in all the conditions described above except in methemoglobinemia, where the blood remains chocolate-colored.

Radiographic Examination

The chest radiograph may demonstrate pulmonary oligemia with normal heart size in tetralogy of Fallot and pulmonary or tricuspid atresia while pulmonary vascularity is increased in transposition of great vessels, truncus arteriosus, anomalous pulmonary venous return, and hypoplastic left heart. The neonates with lung disease have radiographs that are characteristic of the underlying disease.

Electrocardiogram and Echocardiogram

These two studies will be useful in diagnosing cyanotic heart disease. Right ventricular hypertrophy may be seen in lung disease with associated pulmonary hypertension.

Management of Cyanotic Infants

Most of the cyanotic heart diseases are amenable to palliative or corrective surgery. Infants with severe or complete right ventricular outflow obstruction are dependent on the postnatal patency of the ductus arteriosus for maintenance of adequate pulmonary blood flow and systemic oxygenation. Short-term infusions of prostaglandin E_1 0.05 to 0.1 μg/kg per minute in these infants have allowed stabilization prior to surgery.

Congestive Cardiac Failure

Heart failure in the newborn infant is caused not only by structural heart disease but also by other systemic disorders.

Causes of Heart Failure

These include (1) structural heart disease (most commonly transposition of the great vessels and hypoplastic left heart syndromes), (2) heart disease without structural abnormalities (myocarditis, cardiac arrhythmias, glycogen storage disease, and endocardial fibroelastosis), (3) respiratory disease with patent ductus arteriosus with left-to-right shunt, (4) anemia (hemoglobin < 3.5 g/dL), (5) polycythemia, (6) cerebral or other arteriovenous malformation, and (7) sepsis.

Signs and Symptoms

The most frequent symptoms are feeding difficulties, tachypnea, increased sweating, tachycardia, rales and rhonchi, liver enlargement, and cardiomegaly. Less common signs and symptoms are ascites, gallop rhythm, pulsus alternans, and increase in central venous pressure. Peripheral edema is exceedingly rare. A clear distinction between right heart failure (characterized by liver enlargement, tachycardia, and dependent edema) and left heart failure (cardiomegaly, rales, tachypnea, and tachycardia) is not as obvious in the neonate as in the older child or adult.

Management

It is essential to monitor closely the heart and respiratory rates and blood pressure. Blood gases should be performed frequently to observe onset of hypoxemia or acidosis.

Fluid Intake

Fluid intake should be restricted to 100 mL/kg per day and adjusted according to the weight, liver size, and urine output. Electrolytes should be monitored closely. Anemia should be corrected with packed red cell transfusions.

Posture

The neonate should be on a 10 to 30° incline with the head elevated inside the incubator.

Digoxin

Infants with heart failure should receive digoxin unless the heart rate is below 100 beats per minute. The digitalizing dose of digoxin is 0.03 mg/kg PO for term neonates. For digitalization, half the calculated digitalizing dose should be given initially, a fourth in 8 h, and another fourth in 8 h, with maintenance started 12 h after the last digitalizing dose. The maintenance dose is one-fourth of the total digitalizing dose in two divided doses.

Diuretics

Furosemide (Lasix) is the drug of choice with rapid response and should be used intravenously (1 to 3 mg/kg). Maintenance therapy with hydrochlorothiazide (Diuril) and spironolactone (Aldactone) to help conserve potassium may be necessary.

β-Adrenergic Drugs

Neonates with severe heart failure from left-to-right shunts with cardiogenic shock and bradycardia may require β-adrenergic drugs for inotropic action. Isoproterenol (Isuprel) may be infused at 0.1 μg/kg per minute, increasing to 0.4 μg/kg per minute until the heart rate is 140 beats per minute. Dopamine is useful in hypotensive shock and should be infused at 5 to 15 μg/kg per minute. Both medications should be discontinued slowly while monitoring heart rate and blood pressure.

BIBLIOGRAPHY

American Heart Association: Standards and guidelines for cardiopulmonary resuscitation (CPR) and emergency cardiac care (ECC). Part VI: neonatal advanced life support. *JAMA* 255:2969, 1986.

Apgar V: A proposal for a new method of evaluation of the newborn infant. *Anesth Analg* 32:260, 1953.

Adsett DB, Fitz CR, Gill A: Hypoxic ischemic cerebral injury in the term newborn: Correlation of CT findings with neurological outcome. *Dev Med Child Neurol* 27:155, 1985.

Clancy R, Malin S, Laraque D, et al: Focal motor seizures heralding stroke in full term neonates. *Am J Dis Child* 139:601, 1985.

Donn SM, Grasela TH, Goldstein GW: Safety of a higher loading dose of phenobarbital in the term newborn. *Pediatrics* 75:1061, 1985.

Goldberg RN, Thomas DW, Sinatra FR: Necrotizing enterocolitis in the asphyxiated full term infant. *Am J Perinatol* 1:40, 1983.

Gregory GA, Gooding CA, Phibbs RH, et al: Meconium aspiration in infants. A prospective study. *J Pediatr* 85:807, 1974.

Grosfeld JL, Dawes L, Weber TR: Congenital abdominal wall defects: Current management and survival. *Surg Clin N Am* 61:1037, 1981.

Harrison MR, DeLorimer AA: Congenital diaphragmatic hernia. *Surg Clin N Am* 61:1023, 1981.

Heyman MA, Abraham MR: Ductus arteriosus dilatation by prostaglandin E1 in infants with pulmonary atresia. *Pediatrics* 59:325, 1977.

Koppe JG, Kleiverda G; Severe asphyxia and outcome of survivors. *Resuscitation* 12:193, 1984.

Kosloske AM: Pathogenesis and prevention of NEC: A hypothesis based on personal observation and a review of the literature. *Pediatrics* 74:1086, 1984.

Lindemann R: Resuscitation of the newborn. Endotracheal administration of epinephrine. *Acta Pediatr Scand* 73:210, 1984.

Perkins RP, Papile LA: The very low birth weight infant: Incidence and significance of low apgar scores, "asphyxia," and morbidity. Findings at delivery. *Am J Perinatol* 2:108, 1985.

Reynolds M, Luck SR, Lapper R: The "critical" neonate with diaphragmatic hernia. A 21 year perspective. *J Pediatr Surg* 19:364, 1984.

Sawyer SF, Falterman KW, Goldsmith JP, et al: Improving survival in the treatment of congenital diaphragmatic hernia. *Ann Thorac Surg* 4:75, 1986.

E. PEDIATRIC CARDIOPULMONARY RESUSCITATION

Robert Luten

The purpose of this chapter is to review cardiopulmonary resuscitation in children. Emphasis will be placed on pertinent differences between adults and children. Some subjects that are common to both groups have been reviewed elsewhere and will not be mentioned.

The most striking difference between adult and pediatric arrest is etiology. Adults tend to have primary cardiac arrest as a result of coronary artery disease. Adult advanced cardiac life support (ACLS) is based on this principle and heavily emphasizes recognition and management of cardiac disease. Children tend to have cardiac arrests secondary to respiratory arrest and shock syndromes.

Age-related differences must also be considered in pediatric resuscitation. What may be an appropriate drug dose for a 6-month-old is excessive for a 1-month-old and not enough for a 5-year-old. Other aspects of resuscitation, such as endotracheal tube size, tidal volume, cardiac compression rates, and respiratory rates, also vary with the child's age. Problems related to drug dosage and equipment selection are particular to the logistics of pediatric resuscitation and must be solved if one is to be able to effectively resuscitate infants and children. This problem is discussed below under "Drugs."

AIRWAY

A child's airway is much smaller than an adult's and varies in size, depending upon age. Functional differences are more pronounced in the infant or young child. The airway is higher and more anterior in the child's neck than in the adult's.

When the child is in the supine position, the prominent occiput causes flexion of the neck on the chest, occluding the airway. This can be corrected by mild extension of the head to the sniffing position. Overextension or hyperextension, as is recommended for adults, causes obstruction and may kink the trachea because the cartilaginous support is poor. The sniffing position can be maintained by placing a towel or other object beneath the occiput. Despite good head position the child's hypotonic mandibular tissues may still occlude the airway posteriorly. This can be relieved by a chin lift or jaw thrust which elevates the mandible anteriorly and separates the tongue from the posterior pharyngeal wall. If these maneuvers are unsuccessful, an oral airway or endotracheal tube should be considered.

Oral Airway

Oral airways are not widely used in pediatrics. However, they may be useful in the patient who does not respond to maneuvers to remove the mandibular tissues from the posterior pharyngeal wall. With the aid of a tongue blade they are inserted as in adults.

Intubation

Endotracheal intubation of infants and children is felt by many to be easier than the same procedure in adults. There are, however, some differences related to patient anatomy and equipment.

Hyperextension of the neck must be avoided and the sniffing position used for intubation.

The curved (MacIntosh) blade is rarely used in children less than 4 years old for two reasons. First, because of the high and anterior tracheal opening, the floppy mandibular mass of tissue may fill the field of vision when the blade is inserted in proper position. Second, an exact-sized blade must be used to fit the curvature of the tongue. For these reasons a straight (Miller) blade is preferred.

Tracheal tube sizes vary with the patient's age. A general rule is that the correct internal diameter tube size is approximately the same size as the end of the patient's little finger. Uncuffed tubes are used for children up to 7 or 8 years old, since the subglottic trachea usually narrows to form an adequate seal in this age group and cuffs are unnecessary. *One can almost always intubate with a laryngoscope blade that is too large and ventilate with a tube that is too small, but not vice versa.*

Once the child has been intubated, one person should be assigned to hold the endotracheal tube in place until it is securely fastened. Especially in small infants, minimum movements can easily displace the tube from the trachea into the esophagus.

Once intubated, if spontaneous ventilations are inadequate, mechanical ventilation should be instituted. For children weighing less than 10 kg, time-flow or pressure preset ventilators should be used. For time flow ventilators, inspiratory and expiratory times are selected. For pressure ventilators, inflating pressures are determined by checking pressures necessary to inflate the lungs and cause the chest to rise. Pressures usually range from 15 to 40 mm Hg. Excess pressures can cause barotrauma. For older children, volume ventilators can be used, using a volume of 10 mL/kg as for adults.

Foreign Body Management

Controversy exists as to the safest and most effective emergency maneuvers to use with the choking child. The American Heart Association specifically discourages two common maneuvers used with adult patients: (1) the Heimlich maneuver for patients less than 1 year of age because of the potential for injury to abdominal organs, and (2) blind finger sweeps, because of the possibility of pushing the foreign body further into the airway. Serious differences of opinion exist, but current recommendations rely on the back blow and chest thrust to clear the infant's airway.

The following sequence should be followed for emergency treatment of the choking infant less than 1 year of age who cannot cough, vocalize, or breathe. (1) With the infant's torso positioned prone and head down along the rescuer's arm, or the older child draped prone and head down across the rescuer's knees, four blows are delivered to the interscapular area. (2) If the airway is still obstructed, the infant is repositioned supinely along the rescuer's arm, or the older child is placed on the floor as for external cardiac compression, and four chest thrusts (cardiac compressions) are delivered. (3) The jaw thrust is used, the mouth is inspected, and a foreign body removed if seen. (4) If obstruction persists, mouth-to-mouth or mouth-to-mouth-and-nose ventilation is attempted. (5) If obstruction persists, the sequence is repeated. The back blow and chest thrust are thought by some to potentially worsen obstruction. Future investigation may well lead to revised recommendations. For children above 1 year of age, the Heimlich maneuver as described for adults is now recommended. This can be performed with the patient standing, sitting, or lying down.

The above recommendations are directed primarily at the first responder who has neither access to nor the skills to use airway management equipment. In the emergency department one would probably first attempt direct laryngoscopy, visualization, and removal of the foreign body with McGill forceps.

BREATHING

Mouth-to-Mouth

Whether to employ mouth-to-mouth or mouth-to-mouth-and-nose ventilation depends upon the size of the patient. The rate of ventilation is shown in Table 14E-1. Ventilations are done slowly to avoid the generation of high airway pressures which can overcome esophageal resistance and result in gastric distension.

Bag-Valve Mask

The self-inflating bag-valve-mask system is most commonly used for ventilation. A pop-off valve set near 40 cmH_2O is a feature of many bags. There is a common misconception that children are more susceptible to pneumothoraces at high inspiratory pressures than adults. In fact, pediatric lung compliance is very good, and children can tolerate high pressures. Pneumothoraces more commonly result from the administration of three to four times the required tidal volume. The tidal volume necessary to ventilate children is the same as that for adults, 10 to 15 mL/kg. It is impractical to calculate the tidal volume in emergency situations. One can start ventilating with minimal volumes and increase rapidly until adequate chest rise occurs. If a patient requires high pressures for ventilation, the pop-off valve may be occluded with a fingertip to produce adequate chest rise. 1987 AHA ACLS standards recommend pediatric bag-valve devices with either no pop-off valve or one that is easily occluded. Devices with manometers can also be used.

Table 14E-1. Rate of Ventilation

Age	Ventilation Rate, breaths/min
Infants	20 (every 3 s)
Children 1–8 years	15 (every 4 s)
Children over 8 years and adults	12 (every 5 s)

External Cardiac Compression

The brachial pulse is recommended for monitoring purposes for infants less than 1 year of age. Above this age, the carotid pulse is most easily accessible. Absence of pulses mandates external cardiac compression. Most patients should be placed on a hard surface, as are adults. With smaller infants, the wraparound technique is used.

Whether chest compressions produce blood flow by direct compression of the heart, by changes in thoracic pressure, or by both is unclear. New standards advocate compressions over the lower sternum as opposed to mid sternum since the infant heart has recently been shown to lie lower in the thoracic cage than previously believed. Whether to use two fingers, three fingers, or the heel of the hand depends upon the size of the child. Whichever method comfortably produces a compression depth of approximately one-fourth the anteroposterior diameter should be used. The rate of compressions is at least 100/min in infants and 80 to 100/min in older children. The ratio of ventilations to compressions is 1:5 for both one- and two-person CPR. A pause of 1 to 1.5 s between ventilations should be allowed for adequate exhalation.

VASCULAR ACCESS

Difficulty in obtaining rapid intravenous access is certainly one of the major differences between adult and pediatric resuscitation. Two important facts should be kept in mind. First, a significant portion of children respond to airway management alone, since most cardiac arrests in children are secondary to respiratory arrest. Time spent securing vascular access at the expense of adequate airway management is a common mistake in dealing with children, and nowhere is it more costly. Second, once a patient has been intubated, this route may be used to administer drugs such as epinephrine, atropine, and lidocaine.

Although central access would be ideal for administration of drugs during CPR, most studies demonstrating the safety and efficacy of virtually all central venous approaches in children were done under controlled situations and mostly by experienced personnel. Therefore, the most frequently used sites are peripheral: scalp, arm, hand, or antecubital veins; the external jugular vein; femoral vein; or distal saphenous vein via cutdown. Intraosseous infusion is a quick, safe route for resuscitation drugs as well as fluid administration. This is discussed in Chapter 14C, "Vascular Access."

FLUIDS

In the face of hypotension due to volume depletion, isotonic fluid boluses of 20 to 40 mL/kg should be given *as rapidly as possible* and repeated depending upon response. In neonates or small infants, a 20-mL syringe attached to a three-way stopcock and extension tubing can be used to deliver aliquots of fluid rapidly, until the entire bolus is administered. If volume depletion has been corrected and hypotension persists, a pressor agent should be strongly considered, preferably with the aid of a central venous pressure catheter. In the normotensive patient or when the IV line is being used for drug administration only, it should be maintained at the minimum rate that will keep the vein open (KVO). Fine fluid and electrolyte calculations and adjustments can be made after the emergency treatment has been completed. Overhydration, even when IV lines are set at KVO, is a common occurrence when adult equipment is used in pediatric resuscitations. A pediatric microdrip should always be used when resuscitating children.

DRUGS

The indications for the use of specific drugs are essentially the same for children as for adults. Particular to pediatrics, however, is the problem of drug dosage. Proper dosage in children requires knowledge of the patient's weight (Table 14E-2), knowledge of the dose (usually given in milligrams per kilogram), and error-free calculation and de-

Table 14E-2. Body Weight Estimation Guidelines

Age	Weight, kg	
Term infant	3.5	Birth weight (BW)
6 months	7	2 × BW
1 year	10	3 × BW
4 years	16	¼ adult weight of 70 kg
10 years	35	½ adult weight

livery. Problems may arise in remembering the correct dose, performing calculations in the crisis situation (the most common error involves the misplacement of a decimal point and results in 10 times or one-tenth the correct dosage), and delivery of the correct dosage (because of an error in drawing up the calculated amount). Use of a chart with precalculated drug dosages can help reduce dosage errors (Table 14E-3). However, estimating a child's weight accurately so that the proper dosage can be determined from the table is not easy, especially in a crisis situation. Choosing the proper size equipment for pediatric patients is similarly difficult. Valuable time can be lost in weight estimation, dosage calculations, and equipment selection.

Recently, systems based on a direct measurement of a patient's length have been developed for estimating dosages and selecting equipment in pediatric emergencies. In children, length has a direct correlation with weight. It has also been shown to be one of the most accurate predictors of correct equipment sizes for pediatric patients, especially endotracheal tube sizes. The Broselow Resuscitation Tape is one length-based system currently included in the American Heart Association's Pediatric Advanced Life Support Course (PALS). It is a two-sided tape; one side displays emergency resuscitation drug dosage and the other is for equipment selection (see Figs. 14E-1, 14E-2, and

Table 14E-3. Essential Drugs

Drug	Concentration	Dose	Adult Maximum Dose
Epinephrine	1:1000 *or* 1:10,000 (0.1 mg/mL)	0.01–.1 mg/kg	0.5–15.0 mg
Sodium bicarbonate	1 mEq/mL	1 mEq/kg	50–100 mEq
Atropine	1:10,000 (0.1 mg/mL)	0.02 mg/kg	0.5 mg
Calcium chloride	10% (100 mg/mL)	20.00 mg/kg	500 mg

PEDIATRIC DOSAGES

	1.0 kg		2.0 kg		3.0 kg	
	Dose	Vol	Dose	Vol	Dose	Vol
Epinephrine*	0.01 mg	0.1 mL	0.02 mg	0.20 mL	0.03 mg	0.30 mL
Sodium bicarbonate	1.00 mEq	1.0 mL	2.00 mEq	2.00 mL	3.00 mEq	3.00 mL
Atropine	0.15 mg	1.5 mL	0.15 mg	1.50 mL	0.15 mg	1.50 mL
Calcium chloride	20.00 mg	0.2 mL	40.00 mg	0.40 mL	60.00 mg	0.60 mL
	4.0 kg		**5.0 kg**		**6.0 kg**	
	Dose	Vol	Dose	Vol	Dose	Vol
Epinephrine*	0.04 mg	0.40 mL	0.05 mg	0.50 mL	0.06 mg	0.60 mL
Sodium bicarbonate	4.00 mEq	4.00 mL	5.00 mEq	5.00 mL	6.00 mEq	6.00 mL
Atropine	0.15 mg	1.50 mL	0.15 mg	1.50 mL	0.15 mg	1.50 mL
Calcium chloride	80.00 mg	0.80 mL	100.00 mg	1.00 mL	120.00 mg	1.20 mL
	7.0 kg		**8.0 kg**		**9.0 kg**	
	Dose	Vol	Dose	Vol	Dose	Vol
Epinephrine*	0.07 mg	0.70 mL	0.08 mg	0.80 mL	0.09 mg	0.90 mL
Sodium bicarbonate	7.00 mEq	7.00 mL	8.00 mEq	8.00 mL	9.00 mEq	9.00 mL
Atropine	0.15 mg	1.50 mL	0.16 mg	1.60 mL	0.18 mg	1.80 mL
Calcium chloride	140.00 mg	1.40 mL	160.00 mg	1.60 mL	180.00 mg	1.80 mL
	10.0 kg		**12.5 kg**		**15.0 kg**	
	Dose	Vol	Dose	Vol	Dose	Vol
Epinephrine*	0.10 mg	1.00 mL	0.13 mg	1.25 mL	0.15 mg	1.50 mL
Sodium bicarbonate	10.00 mEq	10.00 mL	12.50 mEq	12.50 mL	15.00 mEq	15.00 mL
Atropine	0.20 mg	2.00 mL	0.25 mg	2.50 mL	0.30 mg	3.00 mL
Calcium chloride	200.00 mg	2.00 mL	250.00 mg	2.50 mL	300.00 mg	3.00 mL
	17.5 kg		**20.0 kg**		**22.5 kg**	
	Dose	Vol	Dose	Vol	Dose	Vol
Epinephrine*	0.18 mg	1.75 mL	0.20 mg	2.00 mL	0.23 mg	2.25 mL
Sodium bicarbonate	17.50 mEq	17.50 mL	20.00 mEq	20.00 mL	22.500 mEq	22.50 mL
Atropine	0.35 mg	3.50 mL	0.40 mg	4.00 mL	0.45 mg	4.50 mL
Calcium chloride	350.00 mg	3.50 mL	400.00 mg	4.00 mL	450.00 mg	4.50 mL
	25.0 kg		**30.0 kg**		**35.0 kg**	
	Dose	Vol	Dose	Vol	Dose	Vol
Epinephrine*	0.25 mg	2.50 mL	0.30 mg	3.00 mL	0.35 mg	3.50 mL
Sodium bicarbonate	25.00 mEq	25.00 mL	30.00 mEq	30.00 mL	35.00 mEq	35.00 mL
Atropine	0.50 mg	5.00 mL	0.50 mg	5.00 mL	0.50 mg	5.00 mL
Calcium chloride	500.00 mg	5.00 mL	500.00 mg	5.00 mL	500.00 mg	5.00 mL

* Low dose epinephrine.

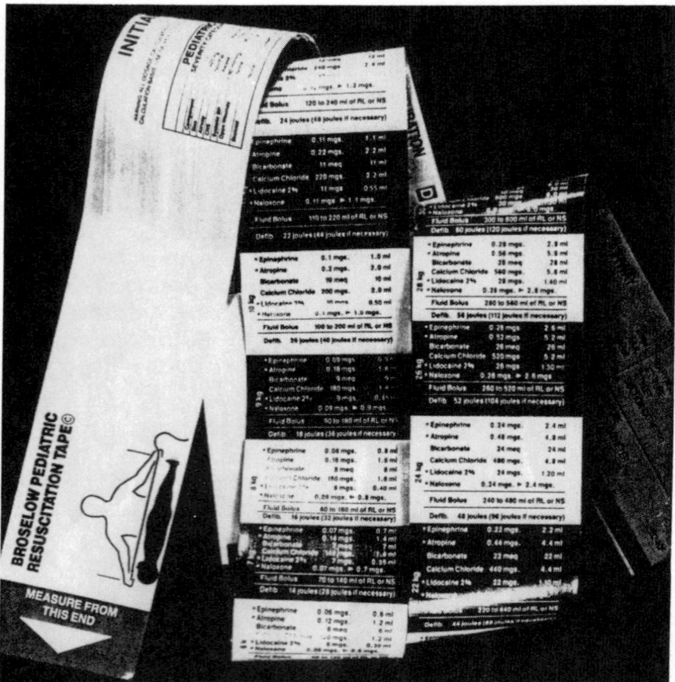

Fig. 14E-1. The Broselow Resuscitation Tape.

14E-3). Fluid volumes for resuscitation as well as appropriate basic life support techniques are also displayed on the Broselow tape. To make optimal use of these systems, emergency personnel must be able to find the proper equipment rapidly. Equipment can be stored in shelves or drawers labeled by age and weight, or a system of color codes can be used in which color-coded shelves, carts, or equipment organizers correspond to specific length categories.

Drugs delivered by constant infusion and the "rule of 6" used to calculate their dosage are listed in the accompanying box. The pharmacology of the drugs has been well described in other sections and will not be addressed here. A few peculiarities pertaining to pediatric drug use are discussed in the following paragraphs.

Atropine and epinephrine. Epinephrine is the one proven beneficial drug in cases of cardiac arrest. It is specifically indicated for hypoxia- or ischemia-induced *slow* rates that fail to respond to adequate oxygenation and ventilation, and full arrest *no pulse* situations (i.e., asystole, electromechanical dissociation, and ventricular fibrillation). In no pulse situations, if the initial dose of epinephrine is not effective, 2 to 10 times that dose should be given subsequently. As of this writing, the use of high dose (0.1 mg/kg) epinephrine for resuscitation in infants and children has not been clinically validated. Thus far, the lack of adverse effects associated with the use of high dose epinephrine in the clinical setting supports its use if there is no clinical response to a first low dose (0.01 mg/kg) of epinephrine. Primary cardiac causes of slow rates are rare and may be treated initially with atropine. The recommended dose is 0.01 mg/kg IV. Subsequent doses require at least twice the initial dose. When either atropine or epinephrine is given through an endotracheal tube, 2 to 3 times the IV dose should be used. If atropine is given in too small a dose, a paradoxical, centrally mediated bradycardia may result. This can be avoided by giving a minimum dose of 0.1 mg regardless of the size of the child.

Sodium bicarbonate. Sodium bicarbonate is no longer a first-line drug since its administration worsens acidosis when administered in the presence of inadequate ventilation *and* perfusion. It is administered

USEFUL DRUGS

RULE OF 6 FOR MEDICATIONS DELIVERED BY CONSTANT INFUSION

Dopamine	dose = 5–20 μg/kg per min
Lidocaine	dose = 20–50 μg/kg per min
Isoproterenol	dose = 0.1–1.0 μg/kg per min

Dosage of medications delivered by constant infusions is calculated in terms of micrograms per kilogram per minute. Actual calculation can be confusing and a source of lethal decimal errors. The *rule of 6* can be used for *dopamine* and *lidocaine* to simplify dosage calculation:

6 mg × wt (kg), *fill* to 100 mL with D_5W

The medication is mixed in an intravenous set with a measured chamber and a microdrip (1 drop/min = 1 mL/h). Rate of administration is best set by an electric pump.

Example: For a 10-kg infant requiring dopamine:

6 mg × 10 = 60 mg dopamine

In a measured chamber *fill* to 100 mL with D_5W. Weight is now factored in so that

1 mL/h = 1 μg/kg per min

5 mL/h = 5 μg/kg per min

10 mL/h = 10 μg/kg per min

For *isoproterenol* the rule of 6:

0.6 mg × wt (kg), *fill* to 100 mL with D_5W

1 mL/h = 0.1 μg/kg per min

5 mL/h = 0.5 μg/kg per min

Fig. 14E-2. Equipment side of the Broselow Resuscitation Tape. One of seven color equipment zones.

C **AIRWAY** | **INTUBATION** D

ORAL AIRWAY	Child	LARYNGOSCOPE	2 Straight or curved *
B.V.M.	Child		
O_2 MASK	Pediatric	E.T. TUBE	4.5 mm uncuffed
		STYLET	6F
		SUCTION CATHETER	8-10F
B.P. CUFF	Child	N.G. TUBE	10F
VASC. ACCESS	18-22 Catheter, 21-23 Butterfly, Intraosseus Needle	URINARY CATHETER	10F
		CHEST TUBE	20-24F
ARM BOARDS	8"		

* Most sources recommend a straight blade for this age child.

Left edge (partial): ...traight / ...cuffed / 6F / 8F / 8-10F / 8-10F / 16-20F

Right edge (partial): ORAL AIR... / B.V.M / O_2 MASK / B.P. CUFF / VASCULAR... / 21-23 Bu... / ARM BOA...

...SIONS RATE 80/min 5/1 BREATH DEPTH 1-1½" POSITION: HEEL OF HAND, 1 FINGER WI...

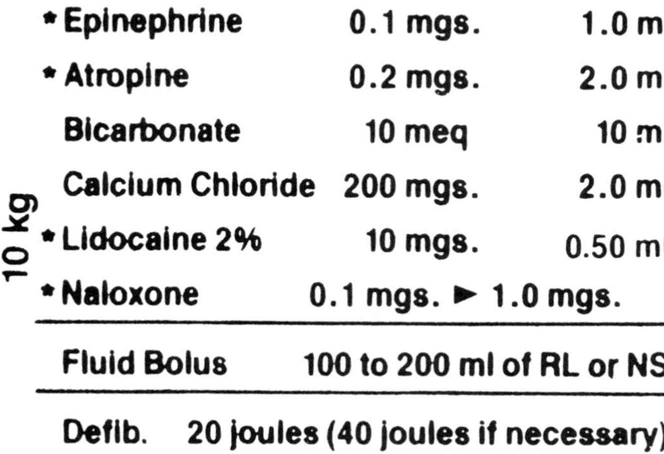

10 kg
• Epinephrine 0.1 mgs. 1.0 ml
• Atropine 0.2 mgs. 2.0 ml
Bicarbonate 10 meq 10 ml
Calcium Chloride 200 mgs. 2.0 ml
• Lidocaine 2% 10 mgs. 0.50 ml
• Naloxone 0.1 mgs. ► 1.0 mgs.
Fluid Bolus 100 to 200 ml of RL or NS
Defib. 20 joules (40 joules if necessary)

Fig. 14E-3. Drug side of the Broselow Resuscitation Tape. One of 25 precalculated weight zones for resuscitation drugs.

only after epinephrine administration has not improved the clinical situation. An initial dose of 1 mEq/kg IV is given only after the airway has been secured, the patient hyperventilated, and CPR initiated. Subsequent doses of 0.5 mEq/kg may be given at 10-min intervals. In the neonate or premature infant, sodium bicarbonate should be diluted 1 : 1 with sterile water, not saline.

Calcium. Because of lack of proven efficacy and possible deleterious effects, calcium has been removed from American Heart Association standards for resuscitation. It is indicated only for hyperkalemia, hypocalcemia, and calcium channel blocker overdose.

ARRHYTHMIAS

Arrhythmia management plays only a small role in the resuscitation of children. Since rhythm disturbances are usually secondary to respiratory arrest and not primary cardiac events, careful attention must be given to the correction of hypoxia, acidosis, and fluid balance. Ventilation and oxygenation must be accomplished first. Pulse oximetry, or arterial blood gas analysis if P_{CO_2} or pH abnormalities are suspected, should be obtained to assess oxygen and blood gas status. An IV of 0.9% NaCl or lactated Ringer's solution should be established and the child placed on a cardiac monitor.

A patient with an unstable cardiac rhythm or rate, coupled with evidence of poor end-organ perfusion (cyanosis, mottled skin, lethargy, etc.), requires immediate intervention. The parameters of clinical assessment and expression of instability vary with the child's age. In the neonate, blood pressure measurement is difficult, and a *heart rate* of 80 beats/min or less, coupled with evidence of poor end-organ perfusion, requires immediate intervention. In infants and children, variations in heart rate may be well tolerated clinically, and a *blood pressure* of 70 mmHg or less, coupled with evidence of poor end-organ perfusion is used to define instability. Table 14E-4 summarizes electrical and drug therapy of unstable cardiac rhythms.

The most common rhythms seen in pediatric arrest are the bradycardias, which lead to asystole if untreated. Outside of the code situation, by far the most common rhythm disturbance encountered is paroxysmal atrial tachycardia (SVT). It is most commonly seen in infants and usually presents as a narrow complex tachycardia with rates usually between 250 and 350 beats per minute. Treatment of the unstable patient has already been outlined. Treatment of the stable patient varies and is beyond the scope of this chapter. Verapamil is *not* recommended for infants less than 1 year of age as it has been associated with cardiovascular collapse.

Sometimes it is difficult to distinguish a secondary sinus tachycardia from a primary cardiac tachycardia. Although heart rates of 150 to 200 per minute in adults are usually cardiac in origin, it is not uncommon to have compensatory sinus tachycardia as fast as 200 to 220 per minute in small infants. Children can tolerate rapid primary cardiac heart rates for long periods of time before congestive heart failure (CHF) or lethal arrhythmias develop. Differentiating primary from secondary tachycardia is critical to patient management (see Table 14E-5). Note that an ECG is rarely helpful since at very fast rates, P waves are not usually distinguishable in either sinus tachycardia or SVT.

Table 14E-4. Summary of Therapy of Unstable Rhythms

Pulse Rate	Specific Common Diagnosis	Treatment
Slow	Secondary cardiac decompensation—sinus bradycardia, junctional or idioventricular rhythms, agonal rhythms, and heart blocks	Epinephrine q 5 min, atropine, epinephrine infusion, sodium bicarbonate, pacemaker
	Primary cardiac cause (rare); second- and third-degree blocks	Atropine, isoproterenol or epinephrine infusion, pacemaker
Fast	Narrow QRS SVT Atrial fibrillation Atrial flutter	Cardioversion [0.2–1.0 W·s/kg (low)]
	Wide QRS Ventricular tachycardia SVT with aberrancy	Cardioversion [0.2–1.0 W·s/kg (high)] Lidocaine 1 mg/kg
No pulse	Asystole and EMD	Epinephrine (give at least 2–10 times initial dose for continued arrest). Consider atropine, sodium bicarbonate
	Ventricular fibrillation	Defibrillate 2 W·s/kg; repeat if needed Epinephrine Defibrillate 4 W·s/kg Lidocaine Repeat defibrillation at 4 W·s/kg Bretylium tosylate

DEFIBRILLATION AND CARDIOVERSION

Electric conversion is used on an emergency basis to treat ventricular fibrillation and symptomatic tachyarrhythmias (Table 14E-6). Ventricular fibrillation as a cause of cardiac arrest is rare in children.

Paddle size. Paddle size is usually 4.5 cm for infants and 8 cm for children. The paddle should be in contact with the chest wall over its entire surface area.

Interface. Electrode cream, electrode paste, and saline-soaked

Table 14E-5. Sinus Tachycardia vs. SVT

Clinical Finding	Sinus Tachycardia	SVT
History	History usually compatible, e.g., vomiting, diarrhea, or bleeding.	In absence of known congenital heart disease, history is usually very nonspecific.
Physical examination	Clinical dehydration or pallor.	Patients may have rales and an enlarged liver if CHF is prolonged. The presence of a heart murmur is inconsistent.
Lab	Chest x-ray film shows small heart, clear lungs. Electrolytes and hematocrit usually consistent with underlying cause.	Chest x-ray film shows normal to large heart; patient may have pulmonary edema.

Table 14E-6. Defibrillation and Cardioversion—Pediatric

1. Blind defibrillation is not recommended. The incidence of ventricular fibrillation as a cause of arrest in children is very low.
2. Ventricular fibrillation:
   Children—2.0 W·s/kg
3. Tachyarrhythmias:
   Cardioversion (0.2–1.0 W·s/kg)
   Narrow QRS complex—lower dose ranges
   Wide QRS complex—higher dose ranges

gauze pads are all acceptable. Alcohol pads are to be discouraged as serious burns may be produced. Care must be taken so that the interface substance from one paddle does not come in contact with the substance from the other paddle. This creates a short circuit, and insufficient energy may be delivered to the heart.

Electrode position. One paddle is placed on the right of the sternum at the second intercostal space. The other is placed in the left midclavicular line at the level of the xyphoid. The AP approach can be used but is less desirable.

Defibrillation dose. Initially, 2 W·s/kg should be used; if that is unsuccessful, the amount should be doubled and attempted twice at the higher energy level if necessary. If the second attempt at the higher dose is unsuccessful, epinephrine should be given, and the oxygen and acid-base status should be assessed before repeating or increasing the energy dose.

Cardioversion. Tachyarrhythmias are generally very sensitive to electric conversion. There are no recent published standards for cardioversion. One can either use ¼ to ½ W·s/kg and double if unsuccessful, or initially place the defibrillator on the lowest possible energy setting and do the same. Of the two methods, the one that gives the lowest energy level is preferable.

SUMMARY OF MANAGEMENT GUIDELINES

It is the age-related differences that are difficult to remember and cause major problems in pediatric resuscitation. One should not have to memorize numbers such as drug doses, tube sizes, or cardiac compression ratios. The proper organization of equipment, the posting of pediatric CPR data and equipment sheets (Table 14E-7 and 14E-8), and use of a length-based system can eliminate the need to commit many variables to memory, thus reducing the possibility of errors. This eliminates much of the general anxiety connected with pediatric resuscitation and leaves the clinician free to apply the principles of resuscitation to the child as presented.

Table 14E-7. CPR

			Adult	
	Infant	Child	Rescuer 1	Rescuer 12
Compression/ventilation ratio	5:1	5:1	15:2	5:1
Cardiac compressions/minute	100	80–100	60–80	60–80

BIBLIOGRAPHY

Chameides L: *Textbook on Pediatric Advanced Life Support*. American Heart Association, 1988.

Chameides L: Guidelines for defibrillation in children. *Circulation* 56:502A, 1977.

Ehrlich R, Emmett S, Rodriquez-Torres R: Pediatric cardiac resuscitation team: A 6 year study. *J Pediatr* 84:152, 1974.

Eisenberg N: Epidemiology of cardiac arrest and resuscitation in children. *Ann Emerg Med* 12:672, 1983.

Friesen R, Duncan P, Tweet W, et al: Appraisal of pediatric CPR. *CMA Journal* 126:1055, 1982.

Greensher J: Emergency treatment of the choking child. *J Pediatr* 70:110, 1982.

Keep PJ, Manford ML: Endotracheal tube sizes for children. *Anesthesia* 29:181, 1974.

Kettrick L, Ludwig S: Resuscitation—Pediatric basic and advanced life support, in Fleisher B, Ludwig S (eds): *Pediatric Emergency Medicine*, Baltimore Williams & Wilkins, 1983, pp 1–29.

Lubitz A, et al: A rapid method of estimating weight and resuscitation drug dosages from length in the pediatric age group. *Ann Emerg Med* 17(6):576–81, June 1988.

Ludwig S, Fleisher G: Pediatric cardiopulmonary resuscitation: A review and a proposal. *Pediatr Emerg Care* 1:40, 1985.

Luten RC: Pediatric resuscitation chart and equipment shelf: Aids to mastery of age-related problems. *J Emerg Med* 4:9, 1986.

Melker R: CPR in neonates, infants and children. *Crit Care Q* 1:49, 1978.

Nichols DG, Kettrick RG, Swedlow DB, et al: Factors influencing outcome of cardiopulmonary resuscitation in children. *Pediatr Emerg Care* 2:1, 1986.

Oakley PA: Inaccuracy and delay in decision making in pediatric resuscitation and a proposed reference chart to reduce error. *Brit Med J* 297:817, 1988.

Orlowski JP: Pediatric cardiopulmonary resuscitation. *Emerg Med Clin North Am* 1:3, 1983.

Orlowski JP: Cardiopulmonary resuscitation in children. *Pediatr Clin North Am* 27:495, 1980.

Singer J: Cardiac arrests in children. *JACEP* 6:198, 1977.

Standards and guidelines for cardiopulmonary resuscitation (CPR) and emergency cardiac care (ECC). *JAMA* 255:2905, 1986.

Zaritsky A, Nadkarni V, Getson P, et al: CPR in children. *Ann Emerg Med* 16:1107, 1987.

Table 14E-8. Age- and Weight-Related Equipment Guidelines

	Premature, 3 kg	Newborn, 3.5 kg	6 Months, 7 kg	1–2 Years, 10–12 kg	5 Years, 16–18 kg	8–10 Years, 24–30 kg
C-collars	—	—	Small	Small	Small	Medium
Chest tubes	10–14 F	12–18 F	14–20 F	14–24 F	20–32 F	28–38 F
NG tubes	5 feeding	5–8 feeding	8 F	10 F	10–12 F	14–18 F
Foley	5 feeding	5–8 feeding	8 F	10 F	10–12 F	12 F
O_2 masks	Premature or newborn	Newborn	Pediatric	Pediatric	Pediatric	Adult
BVM	Infant	Infant	Pediatric	Pediatric	Pediatric	Pediatric or adult
Laryngoscopes	0	1	1	1	2	2–3
ET tubes/stylets	2.5–3.0/6F	3.0–3.5/6F	3.5–4.5/6F	4.0–4.5/6F	5.0–5.5/14F	5.5–6.5/14F
Suction catheters or stylets	6–8 F	8F	8–10F	10F	14F	14F
Oral airways	Infant	Infant or small	Small	Small	Medium	Medium or large
IV equipment	22–24 angio 25 scalp	22–24 angio 23–25 scalp	22–24 angio 23–25 scalp	20–22 angio 23 scalp	20–22 angio 19 scalp	20–22 angio 19 scalp
Arm boards	6 in	6 in	6–8 in	8 in	8–15 in	15 in
BP cuffs	Newborn	Newborn	Infant or child	Child	Child	Child or adult

F. UPPER RESPIRATORY EMERGENCIES

Nick Relich

The diseases which cause upper respiratory tract (URT) obstruction account for a significant percentage of pediatric emergency visits. Some are very common and, ordinarily, quite benign, while others are much less common, yet are true pediatric emergencies.

The physical examination sign common to all causes of URT obstruction is inspiratory stridor. This is a harsh, raspy noise produced by the flow of air through a partially obstructed airway. Stridor on inspiration is indicative of obstruction at or above the larynx. Biphasic stridor, heard during expiration as well as inspiration, places the obstruction in the trachea, while expiratory stridor usually means obstruction below the carina. According to the American Thoracic Society's definition of respiratory sounds, stridor is a type of wheezing, that is, a continuous sound originating from the airway. In common usage, though, only isolated expiratory stridor is referred to as *wheezing;* isolated inspiratory stridor is simply called *stridor*. Throughout this chapter, stridor and wheezing will refer, respectively, to inspiratory and expiratory sounds, usually associated with prolongation of inspiratory or expiratory phases of respiration. Many other physical examination signs are present in patients with URT obstruction. The significance of these, especially in patients under 6 months of age, will be discussed before the specific disease entities are presented.

PHYSICAL EXAMINATION

Cyanosis, while the most dramatic sign, has some inherent limitations as a diagnostic tool. It depends to a great extent on the amount of the hemoglobin in the blood and the status of the peripheral circulation. A child with severe anemia, for example, may have significant hypoxia without manifesting cyanosis. Conversely, a very young infant whose hemoglobin has not yet fallen from the normally high levels found at birth and whose peripheral circulation is normally somewhat sluggish may show varying degrees of peripheral cyanosis despite a normal P_{O_2}. Detection of cyanosis is sometimes quite difficult in black children. Finally, even when present, cyanosis is a late accompaniment of respiratory diseases. For all these reasons, cyanosis is of limited diagnostic value. However, when present, it is an extremely important and ominous sign.

Labored respirations consist of a triad of signs: tachypnea, chest retractions, and nasal flaring. Each of these has specific limitations that the physician must be aware of, especially in the infant less than 6 months old. As a group, however, these signs are the most valuable signs of respiratory distress. They appear early in the course of the disease and worsen as the disease worsens, thus serving as prognostic as well as diagnostic signs.

Tachypnea, an increased respiratory rate, is not specific for respiratory tract disease. It is also seen in cardiac problems, as well as diseases that cause metabolic acidosis, such as diabetic ketoacidosis and salicylate intoxication. Newborns *normally* breathe 40 to 50 times per minute. By 1 year of age, the respiratory rate is around 30 to 35, by 4 years 20 to 25, and by age 8 to 10 years it is at the usual adult rate of 12 to 15. Even with these limitations, tachypnea is an early sign of respiratory distress and correlates well with the severity of the disease.

Chest retractions and nasal flaring are much more specific for respiratory tract disorders than is tachypnea. They are both seen in respiratory tract obstruction and parenchymal lung disease. Both appear early in the course of the disease. They also correlate well with the severity of the disease, although semantically it may be difficult to distinguish "mild" from "moderate" or "moderate" from "severe" retractions or nasal flaring. Both the increased airway resistance of parenchymal lung disease and URT obstruction cause a greater than normal negative inspiratory pressure to be generated. This increased negative pressure causes the soft parts of the infant's chest, which is compliant and poorly ossified, to retract inward. Most commonly, retractions are seen in the intercostal, subdiaphragmatic, and supraclavicular spaces. If severe disease is present, the entire sternum may retract on inspiration. Nasal flaring, an outward and upward flaring of the nares on inspiration, is thought to be a primitive reflex seen in young infants, who are obligate nose breathers for the first 2 to 3 months of life. It probably is an attempt to decrease the airway resistance at the nares, which is quite high in the young infant.

Coughing is uncommon in the young infant less than 6 months old. This reflex is ordinarily not seen at this age, even in infants with large amounts of mucus in the airway. When a young infant does have a *persistent* cough, pertussis, *Chlamydia* pneumonia, or cystic fibrosis should be considered. Sneezing is more common in this age group and is much less significant. Because of the importance of nose breathing to young infants, sneezing can occur quite often, usually in the absence of any respiratory disease.

Grunting is an extremely valuable diagnostic sign. It occurs during expiration, when the glottis is partially closed, causing a delay and then a forceful, noisy expiration (the "grunt"). It seems to be the physiological counterpart of end-expiratory pressure in mechanically ventilated patients. In fact, it was through observations of neonates who grunted that continuous positive airway pressure (CPAP) and positive end-expiratory pressure (PEEP) first came to be used in the treatment of neonatal hyaline membrane disease. Grunting localizes the respiratory disease to the lower respiratory tract. That is, patients who grunt have pneumonia, asthma, or bronchiolitis. Patients with URT obstruction do not grunt. Therefore, grunting is not only specific to the airway, an early sign of disease which correlates with disease severity, but is also specific to a particular location in the respiratory tract.

Stridor is similar to grunting in its significance as a sign of respiratory distress. It appears early and correlates with the disease severity. It is specific not only for the airway but also for the URT; that is, patients with stridor have URT obstruction. Patients with pneumonia, asthma, or bronchiolitis do not have stridor. Stridor and grunting, then, are the most important signs of respiratory distress in the pediatric patient. When seeing a child who has either stridor or grunting, the physician can be confident that the disease is localized not only to the respiratory tract but to a specific part of the respiratory tract.

STRIDOR

The causes of stridor are listed in Table 14F-1. These diseases are occasionally referred to collectively as *croup syndrome*. This should not be confused with viral croup, which is a *cause* of stridor or of croup syndrome.

When confronted with a stridorous child, it is most helpful for the physician to ask two questions, the age of the patient and the duration of symptoms. The answers to these questions will narrow the differential diagnosis considerably. A child under 6 months old with a long duration of symptoms (weeks to months) characteristically has a *congenital* cause of stridor (see Table 14F-1). Most of these diseases present in the newborn nursery or in the pediatrician's office and are not emergency problems.

Laryngomalacia, the most common of these, is due to a developmentally weak larynx, which collapses with each inspiration. It is a self-limited disorder, resolving completely over 6 to 12 months, although there may be exacerbations with upper respiratory infections (URI). If asked, the parent will tell you, "My child has breathed that way since birth." It is usually an incidental finding and not the reason for the emergency visit. It is a benign problem requiring no therapy.

The patient over 6 months old with a relatively short duration of

Table 14F-1. Differential Diagnosis of Inspiratory Stridor

Congenital*
Laryngeal or tracheal webs, cysts, tumors
Laryngomalacia*
Vascular ring
Ectopic thyroid, thyroglossal duct cyst
Congenital vocal cord paralysis
Inflammatory
Viral croup†
Epiglottitis†
Retropharyngeal abscess
Diphtheria, tetanus
Noninflammatory
Aspiration of foreign body into airway†
Esophageal foreign body
Gastroesophageal reflux
Tetany, trauma, tumors

* Most common causes under 6 months of age.

† Most common causes over 6 months of age.

symptoms (hours to days) characteristically has an acquired cause of stridor. This may be inflammatory, such as viral croup or epiglottitis, or noninflammatory, such as foreign body aspiration. The remainder of the chapter deals with the most common acquired causes of stridor: epiglottitis, viral croup, foreign body aspiration, and retropharyngeal abscess.

EPIGLOTTITIS

Clinical

Epiglottitis is a life-threatening disease, a true pediatric emergency. The age range is 2 to 7 years old; the etiology is almost always *Haemophilus influenzae*. Classically, there is an *abrupt* onset over several *hours* of high fever, sore throat, stridor, dysphagia, and drooling. The parent can often tell you the exact time of day the child became ill. Physical examination reveals a toxic-appearing child with an ashen-gray color, very apprehensive and anxious looking, but with minimal movements. There is usually quiet breathing with little air exchange, no hoarseness, but a whispering voice. The characteristic position is sitting up with chin forward and neck slightly extended—the so-called sniffing position. Absence of a spontaneous cough can be a key historical point differentiating epiglottitis from viral croup.

Epiglottitis can also occur in teenagers and young adults, presenting with stridor, sore throat, fever, and drooling over several days, not hours. Epiglottitis should be considered at this age if the symptoms of sore throat, dysphagia, and drooling are out of proportion to the visible pharyngeal pathology. Although *H. influenzae* is the most common organism, gram-positive cocci are also common at this age. There are reports of rapid-onset URT obstruction due to traumatic epiglottitis, secondary to blind vigorous attempts, usually by the parents at home, at removal of a foreign body from the child's throat.

Diagnosis

The *ideal* approach is to take any patient with suspected epiglottitis to the operating room, administer anesthesia, and examine the airway with a laryngoscope while the patient is anesthetized. If the diagnosis of epiglottitis is made, the patient can be intubated. If it is ruled out, the patient can be returned to the ward or the emergency department to continue the workup, secure in the knowledge that epiglottitis is *not* present. However, most hospitals do not have the luxury of 24-h availability of an in-house anesthesiologist.

Therefore, a *less than ideal but perfectly acceptable approach* is the following. A portable lateral neck x-ray is done to establish the diagnosis. The physician *must* stay with the child at all times until the diagnosis is ruled out or the airway is secured. Do *not* send the patient to the x-ray department unattended. A *portable* lateral neck x-ray is quite adequate for diagnosing epiglottitis. Once the diagnosis is made, the patient can be treated accordingly. If total airway obstruction or apnea occurs before the airway has been secured, children with epiglottitis can be bagged effectively. A bag and mask should remain with the physician at the bedside until the diagnosis is ruled out or the airway is secured.

The patient with epiglottitis who is initially seen in the office, clinic, or nontertiary emergency department should be transported to a referral hospital by ambulance *with a physician in attendance*. Oxygen should be given en route, and equipment for airway stabilization, resuscitation, and ventilatory support should be available during the transport. The referring hospital should be alerted as soon as possible. If respiratory arrest occurs during transport, suction the patient, then ventilate with bag and mask.

Lateral neck x-rays must be taken with the neck extended, or the anatomy will be impossible to see. The x-ray should be taken during inspiration. The retropharyngeal space *normally* widens during expiration, and a film taken at that time may lead to a false diagnosis of retropharyngeal abscess. Fortunately, neither of these conditions is difficult to meet in the usual patient. The patient with epiglottitis is already in slight neck extension, and the audible stridor makes for easy timing of the film during inspiration.

A normal lateral neck x-ray is shown in Fig. 14F-1. There are four things to look for in any lateral neck x-ray performed for airway problems: the epiglottis, the retropharyngeal or prevertebral space, the tracheal air column, and the hypopharynx. The epiglottis is normally tall and thin, projecting up into the hypopharynx. In epiglottitis (Fig. 14F-2), it is very swollen and appears squat and flat, like a thumbprint at the base of the hypopharynx. The retropharyngeal space is normally 3 to 4 mm wide. The tracheal air column may need to be "bright-lighted" to be seen well. It should be of uniform width, without densities in the air column. Finally, the dimensions of the hypopharynx should be noted. Similarly to the gastrointestinal tract, although to a much lesser degree, the hypopharynx will distend proximal to a point of obstruction. This is illustrated by the different sizes of the hypopharynx in Figs. 14F-1 and 14F-2. While not specific for epiglottitis, this distension does indicate significant URT obstruction.

Until recently, attempted visualization of the epiglottis, with a tongue blade and flashlight, in the emergency department was considered a totally unacceptable approach to diagnosis. Accepted pediatric dogma was that you should *not* attempt direct visualization of the epiglottis unless the patient is sedated *and* you are ready and able to do endotracheal intubation at that moment. The swollen, cherry-red epiglottis of the patient with epiglottitis is not as mobile as normal and does not pop up into view easily when the patient gags with a tongue blade. Also, this forceful handling of the patient will cause increased anxiety and stridor, which may cause complete obstruction of the patient's airway. However, current pediatric literature argues that direct visu-

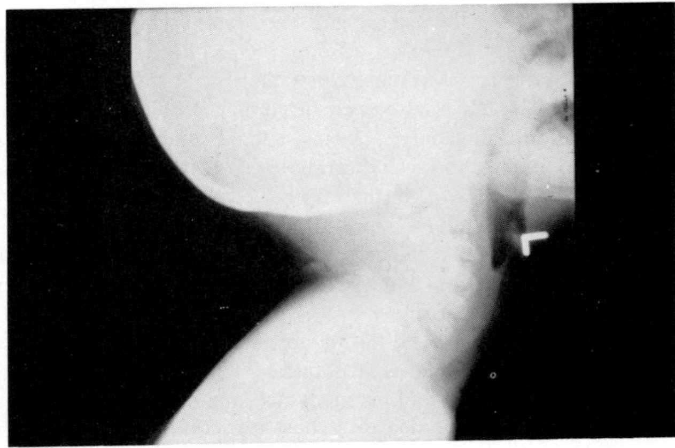

Fig. 14F-1. A normal lateral neck x-ray.

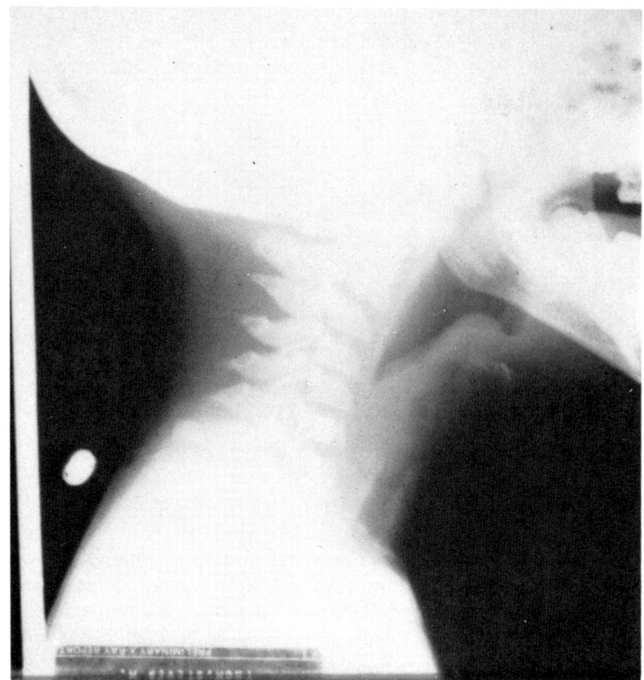

Fig. 14F-2. Lateral neck view of a child with epiglottitis.

alization is safe and accurate. Although this remains a controversial point, it seems prudent to ensure the availability of a person skilled in intubation before attempting direct visualization.

Airway Management

The airway may be secured either by immediate endotracheal intubation or immediate tracheostomy. The choice between these two depends on the particular institution and the 24-h availability of personnel trained in airway management. It is *mandatory* that each emergency department, along with pediatrics, anesthesia, and ENT departments, develop a protocol for managing the child with epiglottitis. Decisions concerning intubation or tracheostomy or transfer to a tertiary center must be made prior to the patient's arrival in the emergency department. It is totally unacceptable to "carefully" observe the patient in an intensive care setting for signs of deterioration. What will surely be observed is sudden and total obstruction of the patient's airway. The objective of airway management is to prevent this from occurring.

Most patients are treated with endotracheal intubation as soon as the diagnosis is made. This should be performed in the intensive care unit or operating room under controlled conditions in the sedated or anesthetized patient. We have had success using Valium (diazepam) and morphine as preintubation sedation, but some patients may require succinylcholine paralysis before intubation can be accomplished. If succinylcholine is used, the patient will have to be bagged using the endotracheal tube (ETT) until the drug effect is over, usually several minutes. Use an ETT that is one size smaller than ordinarily used for the patient's age to reduce the incidence of postintubation sequelae. Initial orotracheal intubation followed by nasotracheal intubation is the preferred method; however, orotracheal intubation alone is also well tolerated. If an oral ETT is used, an oral airway must also be inserted to prevent the patient from biting down on the ETT.

Tracheostomy has a higher morbidity in the patient with epiglottitis than does endotracheal intubation. However, in some hospitals, without adequate availability of intubation personnel, tracheostomy may be the treatment of choice. Again, these decisions should be agreed on ahead of time and made a part of the emergency department policy. Except for the patient who comes in in respiratory arrest and does not begin spontaneous ventilations after resuscitation (hypoxic brain damage) and the extremely rare patient with coexistent pulmonary edema, mechanical ventilation is not necessary. The duration of intubation is 36 to 48 h, after which time the patient can usually be extubated without visualizing the epiglottis. This should be done during day shift hours when adequate personnel are available. Once an ETT is in place, a lateral neck x-ray will not show the epiglottis. Occasionally, postextubation edema causes *mild* stridor which responds well to nebulized Vaponefrine (racemic epinephrine).

Supportive Therapy

Supportive therapy includes IV hydration, humidification of the air to the ETT, and administration of oxygen as necessary. Because of the possibility of ampicillin-resistant *H. influenzae,* most people use cefuroxime (100 to 150 mg/kg per day). Blood cultures are positive in 80 percent of the patients. Oral antibiotics should be continued after extubation for a total of 7 to 10 days. Steroids are *not* necessary. Sedation may be required for the duration of the intubation, although verbal reassurance is often adequate, especially in the older child.

VIRAL CROUP

This is usually a benign, self-limited disease. The age range is 6 months to 3 years; the etiology is almost always viral, usually parainfluenza virus. The male: female ratio is 1, although severe croup is more common in boys. The typical history is 2 to 3 days of a URI with a gradually worsening cough, especially at night. By the third or fourth day, there is a barking cough, stridor, and dyspnea, as well as varying degrees of anxiety. Physical examination reveals marked stridor, retractions, tachypnea, hoarseness, and mild cyanosis in room air. The patient may be fairly calm with little distress until the examination begins, at which time the patient's anxiety will increase markedly, causing a worsening of the stridor. The typical patient with croup can be differentiated from epiglottitis on clinical grounds, so x-rays are not necessary in every patient. In fact, in mild croup, x-rays are usually normal. In the more severely ill child, lateral neck x-rays will show a normal epiglottis, a distended hypopharynx, and a narrowed subglottic airway. A posteroanterior (PA) chest x-ray shows a narrowed tracheal air column in the form of a "steeple" rather than the normal "square shoulder."

Treatment is basically symptomatic: cool mist, oxygen when needed, and hydration either IV or PO. Antibiotics are not needed, unless there is an associated bacterial illness (otitis media or tonsillitis). Steroids are probably helpful, although controversy on this point continues. Mild sedation is often helpful, but codeine is *contraindicated* because of its cough suppressant effect.

Spasmodic croup, recurrent episodes of croup, usually without a preceding URI or fever, almost always occurring at night, is thought to be due to allergy. It is very sensitive to mist. Bacterial tracheitis, a more severe form of croup, has been increasing in the past few years. Also referred to as *membranous laryngotracheobronchitis,* it is usually caused by *Staphylococcus aureus.* The patient has significantly more respiratory distress because of the purulent secretions in the airway. The clinical presentation may be similar to epiglottitis; however, the x-ray shows the typical findings of croup, or the purulent secretions in the trachea may mimic a foreign body. The patient may need intubation as well as antibiotics.

In the severely ill patient, blood gases must be monitored and endotracheal intubation or tracheostomy considered. Vaponefrine can be administered by nebulized aerosol via a face mask [intermittent positive-pressure breathing (IPPB) is *not* necessary] for acute but sometimes temporary relief of obstructive symptoms. The dose is 0.5 mL in 3 mL of normal saline. It can be repeated as needed if a good response continues to occur and no cardiac toxicity, such as arrhythmias, is seen. Because of the possibility of rebound stridor, it is recommended that the patient sufficiently ill to require Vaponefrine be admitted or watched in the emergency department for 6 to 12 h.

FOREIGN BODY ASPIRATION

Clinical

Over 3000 people die from foreign body (FB) aspiration each year, and over half of these are children less than 4 years old. FB aspiration is the most common cause of in-home accidental death in children under 6 years old. It usually occurs in the 1- to 4-year-old but may occur as young as 6 months old. The most common FBs are peanuts and sunflower seeds, but almost any conceivable type of object (metal, plastic, food, grass) may be aspirated. Under 1 year, eggshell aspiration during feeding is a common cause.

The patient may present with a variety of signs depending on the location of the FB and the degree of obstruction: wheezing, persistent pneumonia, stridor, coughing, or apnea. Recurrent stridor and/or wheezing may indicate an FB which is changing position within the airway—stridor when it is proximal and wheezing when it moves more distally. Stridor from an FB implies a location in the larynx, trachea, or mainstem bronchus. The usual location is in a mainstem bronchus, often the right, producing cough, unilateral wheezing, or stridor, and classic x-ray signs. Laryngeal and tracheal FBs are less common but *not rare*, constituting 10 to 15 percent of all FBs. The patient with persistent stridor and croup who does not improve over 5 to 7 days may have an FB in the trachea.

Classically, symptoms will occur acutely (choking, coughing, gagging) but usually subside with passage of the FB into the smaller airways. This, in turn, may lead to pneumonia, atelectasis, or wheezing. This triphasic course of symptoms—acute, latent asymptomatic period, and delayed wheezing or stridor—is classic for mainstem bronchi FBs. As many as one-third of the aspirations may *not* be witnessed or remembered by the parent. Often, there is no history of the aspiration, or it is obtained only in retrospect. The physician must have a high index of suspicion of an FB.

Upper esophageal FBs can cause stridor. They may also cause dysphagia or failure to thrive, especially with a long-term radiolucent FB, such as an aluminum "pop-top." However, even in the absence of dysphagia, the possibility of an esophageal FB should be considered in the patient with stridor.

Diagnosis

If it is opaque, the FB can be easily seen on x-ray. However, most airway FBs are radiolucent and must be diagnosed by a change in airway appearance or dynamics. Laryngeal FBs can be outlined by air contrast on lateral neck x-rays. Tracheal FBs can also be outlined on x-rays, although this may require special techniques, such as xerograms or laminograms. Xerograms may also be useful in outlining small nonopaque FBs in the lower airway.

Mainstem bronchi FBs will cause air trapping in the involved lung on expiration because the bronchus constricts around the FB during expiration and obstructive emphysema occurs. This leads to hyperinflation of the obstructed lung and a shift of the mediastinum *during expiration away from the obstructed side* (Fig. 14F-3). This shift can be seen on inspiratory and expiratory PA chest x-rays or fluoroscopy. If necessary, the x-ray technician can apply pressure on the epigastrium during expiration, leading to a maximal exhalation and allowing for good timing of the films. In the young or uncooperative patient, it may be impossible to obtain accurately timed inspiratory and expiratory films.

This mediastinal shift may also be seen on bilateral decubitus x-rays of the chest. Normally, the "down" hemithorax is hypoinflated with an elevated hemidiaphragm and "splinted ribs." However, the reverse occurs on the side of the FB, where there is persistent hyperinflation and no loss of volume, even when the affected lung is

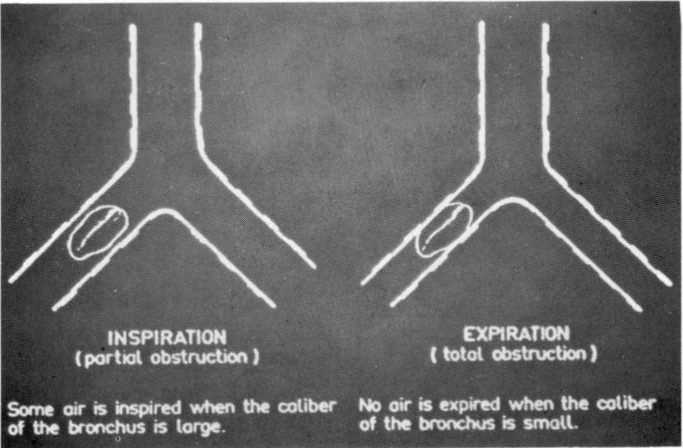

Fig. 14F-3. Inspiratory and expiratory films in foreign body aspiration.

"down" (Figs. 14F-4 and 14F-5). These films can be done even in young, uncooperative patients.

Most importantly, it takes some time for these findings to occur. A single negative x-ray examination does not rule out the presence of an FB. Computed tomographic scanning may be necessary for diagnosis in difficult cases. However, the most important rule is still to have a high index of suspicion. A preoperative diagnosis is made in only 60 percent of airway FBs. If you still suspect the diagnosis, even though x-rays are not confirmatory, you should probably proceed to bronchoscopy anyway.

Esophageal FBs are usually radiopaque and easy to detect on x-rays. Flat esophageal FBs, such as coins, are *almost* always oriented in the coronal plane, so that they are en face (facing forward) on a PA x-ray. Tracheal FBs are *almost* always oriented in the sagittal plane because of absent cartilage in the posterior tracheal wall. However, these "rules" do not always hold. PA *and* lateral x-rays will place the opaque FB without a doubt. Radiolucent esophageal FB may require barium swallow, xerograms, or tomograms to make the diagnosis.

Management

Treatment of airway FBs is laryngoscopy or bronchoscopy with removal of the object in the operating room under anesthesia. This may be a difficult procedure, especially in the very young patient with tiny

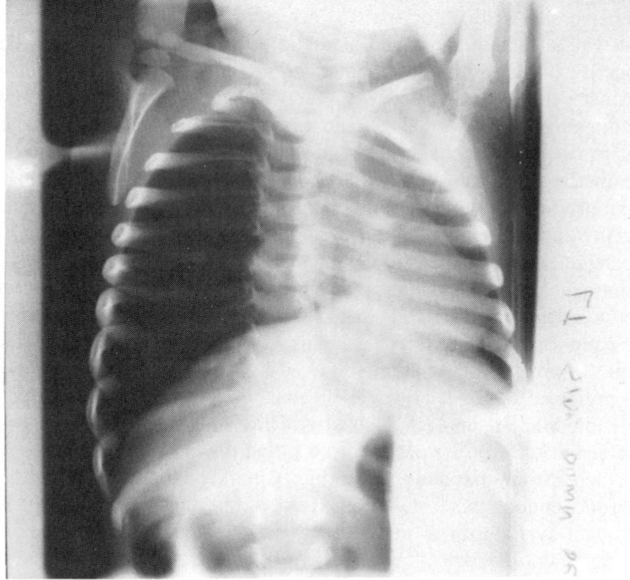

Fig. 14F-4. Normal decubitus film with left side down.

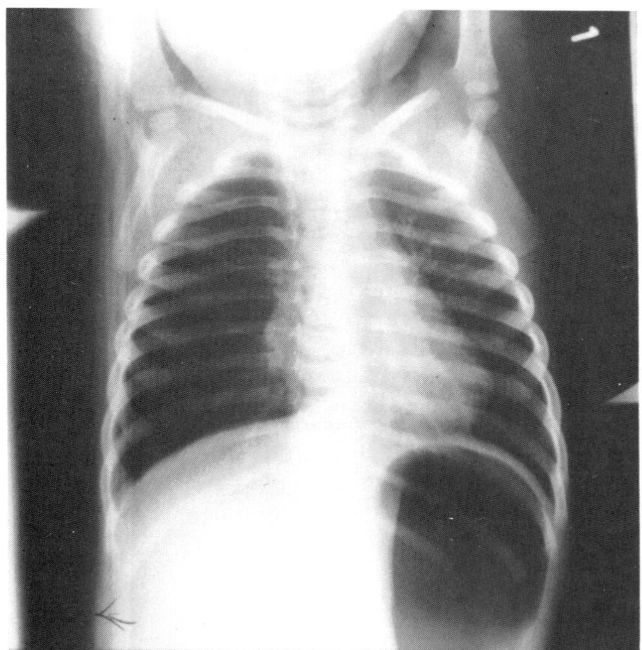

Fig. 14F-5. Decubitus film, right side down, in foreign body aspiration.

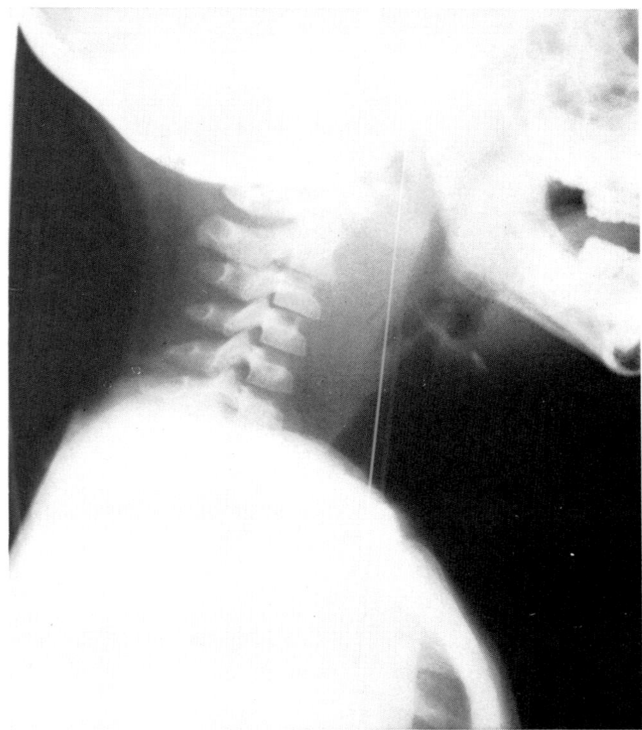

Fig. 14F-6. Lateral neck view of a child with retropharyngeal abscess.

airways. The FB may be too cumbersome to remove whole with the bronchoscope forceps, in which case a Fogarty catheter or urine stone basket may be needed for removal. Similarly, esophageal FBs can be removed by endoscopic forceps with or without a Foley catheter. However, if the latter is used, the FB must be smooth without sharp edges and in place for less than 2 weeks and there must be no underlying esophageal disease. It is *almost* never necessary to proceed immediately to bronchoscopy. One can usually wait and schedule it electively, especially if the patient has a full stomach.

Because of the edema of the airway from the FB itself and the instrumentation necessary for removal, as well as the chemical pneumonia in cases of food aspiration (especially peanuts), the patient with an airway FB will require respiratory care for 24 to 72 h after FB removal. Antibiotics, steroids, oxygen, mist, and chest physiotherapy may all be necessary. The patient with an FB is not dramatically improved after bronchoscopic removal as is the patient with epiglottitis after intubation.

RETROPHARYNGEAL ABSCESS

The usual age for retropharyngeal abscess formation is 6 months to 3 years. It is rare over the age of 3 because of a normal regression in the size of the retropharyngeal lymph nodes with age. It begins with a URI which localizes to the retropharyngeal lymph nodes over several days. Dysphagia and refusal to feed occur before significant respiratory distress. The child is usually toxic-appearing, febrile, and drooling and has inspiratory stridor and dysphagia. Characteristically, they assume an almost opisthotonic posture.

The diagnostic test is a lateral neck x-ray which shows a widened retropharyngeal space (Fig. 14F-6). This x-ray must be done in inspiration with the neck extended or a false-positive widening will be seen. Sometimes, lucencies or actual air-fluid levels can be seen within the widened retropharyngeal space. Physical examination of the pharynx shows a retropharyngeal mass which can often be seen with a tongue blade and a flashlight. Palpation of the mass is dangerous, as it may lead to rupture of the abscess.

Treatment is high-dose IV antibiotics, usually penicillin G in doses of 100,000 units/kg per day. The most common organism is β-hemolytic *streptococcus*. If fluctuation or severe respiratory distress occurs, an incision and drainage should be done in a controlled manner in the operating room by an experienced otolaryngologist. Complications include respiratory failure from obstruction, rupture of the abscess into the airway causing either asphyxia or bronchopneumonia, and spread of the abscess into the adjacent soft tissues of the neck.

BIBLIOGRAPHY

Black RE, Choi KJ, Syme WC, et al: Bronchoscopic removal of aspirated foreign bodies in children. *Am J Surg* 148:778, 1984.

Bottenfield GW, Arcinue EL, Sarnaik A, et al: Diagnosis and management of acute epiglottitis—report of 90 consecutive cases. *Laryngoscope* 90:822, 1980.

Fischer H: Oropharyngeal examination for suspected epiglottitis. *Am J Dis Child* 142:1261, 1988.

Gay BB Jr, Atkinson GO, Vanderzalm T, et al: Subglottic foreign bodies in pediatric patients. *Am J Dis Child* 140:165, 1986.

Hight DW, Philippart AI, Hertzler JH: The treatment of retained peripheral foreign bodies in the pediatric airway. *J Pediatr Surg* 16:694, 1981.

Liston SL, Gehrz RC, Jarvis CW: Bacterial tracheitis. *Arch Otolaryngol* 107:561, 1981.

Mauro RD, Poole SR, Lockhart CH: Differentiation of epiglottitis from laryngotracheitis in the child with stridor. *Am J Dis Child* 142:679, 1988.

O'Neill JA, Holcomb GW Jr, Neblett WW: Management of tracheobronchial and esophageal foreign bodies in childhood. *J Pediatr Surg* 18:475, 1983.

Schloss MD, Gold JA, Rosales JK, et al: Acute epiglottitis: Current management. *Laryngoscope* 93:489, 1983.

Vernon DD, Sarnaik AP: Acute epiglottitis in children: A conservative approach to diagnosis and management. *Crit Care Med* 14:23, 1986.

SECTION 2
Emergency Medical Services

15
EMERGENCY MEDICAL SERVICES

G. Patrick Lilja
Robert Swor

Emergency medical services (EMS) is the extension of emergency medical care into the community. Emergency physicians must be aware of and have input into the care provided to their patients prior to arrival in the emergency department. To be sure, many aspects of EMS are only indirectly under medical control, but strong medical leadership is absolutely essential for a safe and effective system.

The 1966 National Highway Safety Act authorized the U.S. Department of Transportation to fund ambulances, communications, and training programs for prehospital medical services. Coincidentally, Pantridge began using a mobile coronary care unit in Belfast, Northern Ireland, in 1967 to extend coronary care into the prehospital setting. In 1973 public law 93-154 defined a goal to improve emergency medical care and EMS on a national scale. This law identified 15 elements to be addressed in an EMS system as follows: (1) manpower, (2) training, (3) communications, (4) transportation, (5) facilities, (6) critical care units, (7) public safety agencies, (8) consumer participation, (9) access to care, (10) transfer of care, (11) standardization of patient records, (12) public information and education, (13) independent review and evaluation, (14) disaster linkage, and (15) mutual aid agreements.

STATE ROLE

The state legislatures provide laws that broadly outline what is safe and prudent for the public good. Such laws may define levels of ambulance service capability, training requirements, equipment requirements, and requirements for physician leadership and accountability. In addition, the state health department may be the lead agency in promoting and funding EMS activity.

LOCAL ROLE IN EMS

EMS systems must be planned, organized, and operated at the local level to be effective. Each community contemplating an EMS system must identify its resources and needs and how much service it is willing or able to afford. The 15 elements of an EMS system defined by public law 93-154 can provide very helpful guidance in this process.

Manpower

Who will provide prehospital medical care? In urban areas public safety personnel and ambulance personnel are obvious choices, but in rural or wilderness areas volunteers, park rangers, or ski patrols may be employed. The citizenry itself should not be overlooked. Public interest and participation are key ingredients in any EMS system.

Training

Training begins with education of the private citizen. Courses in EMS system access, CPR, and other forms of first aid are essential. Of course, the media can be utilized to reach large populations with the minimum information necessary to participate effectively. Some communities will opt to use a dual-response system consisting of first responders followed by ambulance personnel. First responders may be firefighters, police, park rangers, or citizen volunteers. Training for first responders may include advanced Red Cross first aid or the Department of Transportation's First Responder Course. The training for ambulance personnel is usually successful completion of an emergency medical technician (EMT) course. Although various levels of EMT training have evolved in different states, the three nationally recognized levels are emergency medical technician—ambulance (EMT-A), emergency medical technician—intermediate (EMT-I), and emergency medical technician—paramedic (EMT-P). EMT-As have the necessary first aid skills, including CPR, to take care of basic and immediately life-threatening prehospital emergency conditions. Other skills include safe extrication, immobilization, and transportation of emergency victims. EMT-I training adds the additional skills of IV access, pneumatic trouser use, and esophageal airway or endotracheal intubation. EMT-P training adds drug therapy for selected prehospital conditions, interpretation of ECG rhythms, and cardiac cardioversion and defibrillation. Recently, studies have demonstrated that EMT-As trained to operate defibrillators can markedly improve cardiac arrest survival. Obviously, physicians need to be deeply involved in all training efforts and must constantly be assured that skills and equipment are being used appropriately and safely.

Communications

The universal 911 emergency telephone number has greatly facilitated the citizen's access to emergency medical care. Physicians should promote this system and seek assurance that those answering the calls have the knowledge and training properly to dispatch rescue personnel and offer first aid information to the caller when appropriate. The public needs to be encouraged to use the 911 number rather than call the hospital or the physician when certain symptoms occur. Once a request for help is received, the system must assure a rapid dispatch of appropriate personnel. Ambulance personnel must be able directly or indirectly to communicate with the hospital of destination. Most importantly, ambulance personnel must be able to communicate with the physician approved to give them direction according to their standard operating procedure protocols. The overall goal of the communications system is to provide a means of early notification, prompt dispatch of the appropriate vehicles and personnel, hospital notification, and the provision of qualified medical control.

Transportation

Ambulances have evolved into sophisticated and efficient mobile patient care areas where life-saving maneuvers can be performed. Federal standards provide specifications for ambulance construction. The most important aspect of design is that the attendants must be able to provide airway and ventilatory support while safely transporting the patient. Basic life support (BLS) ambulances carry equipment appropriate for attendants trained to the EMT-A level. Advanced life support (ALS) ambulances are equipped for EMT-Ps or other health care personnel capable of drug therapy and other advanced medical procedures.

Air ambulances may be either airplane (fixed-wing) or helicopter ambulances. Both may be either BLS or ALS ambulances. Fixed-wing ambulances have faster air speed than do helicopters but are not as easily mobilized and, obviously, require landing strips. Fixed-wing ambulances are most practical for long transports when their greater speed can compensate for the associated delays. For transports over intermediate distances the helicopter ambulance is preeminent. Such transports may be from the scene of an accident to a hospital or from hospital to hospital. In addition to speed, the helicopter ambulance can reach victims in otherwise inaccessible locations. The helicopter also provides a smooth ride for patients who may be jeopardized by bumps and rolls and can also be used to deliver a skilled health care team to a locality where such is not available. The helicopter can provide an opportunity to concentrate the delivery of certain types of cases in specialized centers for economic and quality of care reasons. The delivery of major burn cases to burn centers is an example. Unfortunately, the dedication and the enthusiasm of medical personnel can influence decisions as to whether flights can be safely accomplished. It is obvious that strict safety operating rules must be followed and decisions regarding flight safety must take priority.

Physicians involved with air transport should be aware of some considerations unique to altitude physiology. As altitude increases, oxygen partial pressure decreases. At high altitude, hypoxia is made worse because of the resulting desaturation of circulating hemoglobin. Even pressurized aircraft maintain a cabin pressure equivalent to an altitude of 1500 to 4000 ft. Supplemental oxygen should be provided for any patient who may be compromised by a decrease in the partial pressure of oxygen. Another effect of decreased ambient atmospheric pressure is the expansion of balloons filled with air at ground level. In any catheter or endotracheal tube balloon filled with air, the air should be replaced with saline before ascent. Likewise, the pressure within pneumatic trousers and inflated blood pressure cuffs will increase with ascent and decrease with descent. Air within IV bottles and IV tubing will expand and contract similarly. Flow rates of IV solutions can be affected by this. Air embolism, of course, is the major concern. Plastic bags for IV solutions are preferred for these reasons.

Facilities

Emergency patients should be delivered to the hospital of their choice unless their condition can be better treated at another hospital that the system has identified as having overriding advantages under life-threatening conditions. Several systems of categorizing hospitals exist, and this process should either precede or coincide with the development of the EMS system. Prehospital personnel should not be pawns in a struggle between hospitals fighting for commercial advantage. In some areas there may be no hospital that meets system requirements for equipment and staffing. A well-functioning EMS system cannot always rely on interfacility transport to "bail out" its hospitals and medical personnel from the necessity of resuscitating critically ill or injured patients. Therefore, emergency departments capable of resuscitating and stabilizing these patients must be present or must be developed.

Critical Care Units

Tertiary care facilities should be identified either within the system or without. It is not feasible for every community to support a neonatal intensive care unit, burn unit, spinal cord injury unit, and so on.

Public Safety Agencies

It is obviously important that any EMS system have strong ties with police and fire departments. These public safety agencies may provide all or part of EMS care. Public safety officials must have input into EMS councils, and, conversely, EMS providers must have input into public safety decisions that impact on emergency medical care.

Consumer Participation

The public must have input into the governance of its EMS system. Lay participation on councils should be provided. The public must understand what a good EMS system offers, or support will dwindle. Involvement of the lay public in first aid training and in the implementation of a 911 system are important steps in constructing a successful system.

Access to Care

A successful EMS system assures that all individuals have access to emergency care regardless of ability to pay. A more difficult problem exists when population densities or terrain dictate longer response times for some citizens than others. EMS councils must be able to handle these inequities, which are both politically and economically difficult to adjust. EMS councils are typically advisory bodies to County Boards or other political entities. An informed, well-represented governing body will ultimately make the best decisions.

Transfer of Care

Patients must frequently be transferred from one medical care facility to another either within or without the system. These transfers must be made with maximum patient safety and convenience. Many problems can be avoided when a protocol is followed that has been previously agreed to by both of the involved medical centers. The referring physician should be assured of receiving follow-up information about the patient, and the receiving physician should be assured of receiving all the important information about the patient on arrival. Proper medical support en route should be assured by establishing radio contact with the receiving center as soon as possible and having appropriate medical personnel accompany the patient as needed.

Standard Patient Record

Patient care is dependent on good medical records, and prehospital records are no exception. Ambulance services within a specific region should all use a similar reporting form that can be quickly and easily interpreted by receiving nurses and physicians. It is more difficult to standardize emergency department records. However, flow sheets can be used which are easily interpretable by receiving physicians and nurses. It is also wise to design record systems that lend themselves to data extraction for trauma registries and severity scoring as well as cardiac arrest outcome studies.

Public Information and Education

As mentioned above, it is essential that the public be well informed. Consideration should be given to the following: (1) the public should understand how it stands to benefit by an excellent EMS system, (2) the public must be prepared to render first aid care, (3) the public must know how to access the system quickly, and (4) the public should understand that patients may be delivered to hospitals not of their choice under certain life-threatening conditions.

Independent Review and Evaluation

Governing agencies must be assured that ongoing review of the EMS system occurs. Monitoring radio communications, review of response times, and review of run sheets are relatively mechanical methods of quality control that are easily implemented. Outcome studies of such entities as cardiac arrest and multiple trauma require considerable physician input and cooperation. The system medical director should require that such studies be conducted periodically. System access to hospital charts should be a requirement for participating hospitals with due concern for patient privacy.

Disaster Linkage

Disaster care is discussed in the next chapter of this volume (Chapter 16, "Disaster Planning"). The EMS system is an integral part of disaster preparedness and should be involved in planning and practice drills along with the public safety agencies and others. Public safety agencies should keep the EMS system informed of potential disaster situations or hazards that may temporarily be present. Also, hospitals must be prepared to keep the EMS system informed of their capacity to receive certain kinds of patients under disaster conditions.

Mutual Aid Agreements

Communities should develop mutual aid agreements with their neighbors so that uninterrupted emergency care is available despite local exigencies.

MEDICAL CONTROL

A safe and effective EMS system requires considerable physician input and surveillance to provide the best possible patient care. Emergency physicians must be involved in providing this control. Medical control consists of immediate or "on line" and "off line" control (also called indirect medical control).

On line (immediate) medical control is the provision of direct medical orders to personnel in the field either in person or by radio or phone communication. The service medical director delegates this authority to other physicians, but must be assured that they understand the protocols under which the paramedics are allowed to administer care. Also, the medical director may allow ambulance personnel to carry out certain standing orders when contact with the controlling physician is not feasible in a timely fashion.

Off line (indirect) medical control is the responsibility of the service medical director. Three main components of the off line medical director are (1) development of protocols, (2) development of medical accountability (quality assurance) and (3) development of ongoing education. Protocol development describes those treatment procedures which prehospital personnel may perform under the medical license of the medical director. These protocols must be reviewed and rewritten on a regular basis to keep pace with current medical knowledge. Quality assurance requires ongoing surveillance and study of the system. It is mandatory that physicians be involved, both to review treatment and to suggest improvement in areas where deficiencies may be noted. Physicians must remember that they have the ultimate responsibility for the prehospital medical care provided. Lastly, the off line medical director is responsible for the ongoing educational needs of the prehospital care providers under his direction. This means that the quality and content of the training should be directed by the medical director.

MEDICAL BASIS FOR EMERGENCY MEDICINE SERVICES

Emergency Cardiac Care

It is clear that advanced life support (ALS) saves lives after sudden cardiac arrest. Early studies by groups in Seattle and King County, Washington, demonstrated that as many as 26 percent of patients may be resuscitated successfully from out of hospital cardiac arrest. Further work in Milwaukee demonstrated a 16 percent rate of survivors discharged home from the hospital. The overwhelming majority of survivors are from cardiac arrests that are witnessed and have an initial cardiac rhythm of ventricular fibrillation (VF). Survival clearly is related to the time from collapse of the patient to delivery of defibrillation by paramedics and declines dramatically with delays of a few minutes. Early literature documented 40 percent survival if treatment was within 4 min, but less than 10 percent if treatment was about 10 min. Few other systems have duplicated these impressive survival statistics, and many authors question the applicability of this work to EMS systems across the country.

The documentation that survival clearly is linked to rapid defibrillation led a number of authors to train basic EMTs, who arrive first at the scene of an emergency, to recognize and treat VF. Systems in King County and Iowa documented that this approach can improve survival from cardiac arrest if the interval between collapse and defibrillation is short. The development of the automatic external defibrillators (AEDs) has been the most significant contemporary change in EMS. AEDs have been shown to be clinically and cost effective and are rapidly becoming standard equipment for basic EMT units across the country. Effectiveness depends, in large part, on early application after cardiac arrest. For that reason, citizen awareness of the signs of cardiac arrest, quick access to the system, and rapid and appropriate dispatch of units are all critical links to maximize survival.

Despite the emphasis on treatment of cardiac arrest in the development of EMS systems, such cases make up less than 5 percent of an EMS system's volume. The most common clinical entities seen in EMS systems are the manifestations of cardiac disease. Paramedics frequently treat patients with ischemic chest pain and its complications. Common treatments include relief of ischemic chest pain with nitrates and narcotic analgesics, control of cardiac arrhythmias with antiarrhythmics, treatment of symptomatic bradyarrhythmias with external pacemakers, treatment of congestive failure with diuretics, and if necessary, endotracheal intubation. Most EMS authorities agree that prevention of cardiac arrest is the true benefit of an ALS system. There is a lack of research to document this assertion.

A new therapy that appears theoretically attractive for field use is early treatment of myocardial infarction with thrombolytic agents. Early administration can decrease ultimate mortality. Studies have also documented that delays may occur in the administration of thrombolytic agents once the patient arrives in the emergency department. Logistic obstacles to field therapy include the difficulty in diagnosing myocardial infarction in the field, identification of contraindications by paramedics, and management of complications by the limited resources available in the field. Diagnosis has been facilitated by the advent of cellular communications to transmit electrocardiograms to emergency departments. Studies to assess its feasibility are currently in progress.

Trauma Care

The care of the trauma patient is a more controversial role for EMS systems. There is widespread agreement that development of systems of trauma care, with delivery of the critically injured trauma patient to a trauma center, saves lives. Systems are then designed to bypass certain hospitals under predetermined protocols, based on the mechanism of injury or the patient's physiologic status.

There is less agreement on what therapy should be given by EMS providers at the time of a traumatic injury. Some early literature documented a decreased survival if a patient received ALS (intravenous lines and intubation) at the scene because of the delay of definitive care. A number of studies on ALS care have documented improvement in physiologic parameters and improved outcome from injury compared with historic controls. The most compelling literature has shown that paramedics may secure an airway, establish an intravenous line, and infuse significant volumes of fluid rapidly without delaying transport of the patient. New techniques such as administration of hypertonic fluid have been suggested as appropriate for field use, but are still being investigated. Emphasis on rapid transport of the trauma victim and provision of supportive measures en route are well accepted guidelines for EMS personnel.

Medical and Pediatric Care

While much of the initial research in EMS has centered on these topics, interest has evolved in the management of other emergencies by EMS providers. This interest has broadened the scope of practice of the EMS provider.

The management of respiratory distress is an important function of the EMS system. Provision of airway control via endotracheal and nasotracheal intubation has been shown to be performed readily by paramedics. This skill appears to be performed appropriately and with an acceptable complication rate. Early advanced airway measures for upper airway obstruction from burns, trauma, foreign body, or allergic causes may be lifesaving. Respiratory distress by patients with chronic obstructive pulmonary disease and asthma are common clinical entities. Most systems have utilized epinephrine and aminophylline for bronchodilators, but B_2 agonists have been shown to be safe and effective for field use. Some systems have also utilized pulse oximetry for evaluation of occult hypoxemia. While effective, oximetry is also costly and has not been widely utilized.

The management of altered mental status is an important paramedic function. Administration of glucose for hypoglycemia, naloxone for narcotic overdose, and control of seizures with diazepam or airway support for status epilepticus are similarly important functions.

Attention currently is focused on the care of the child in the EMS system. Up to 10 percent of a system's volume can be pediatrics. The most common entities treated are upper and lower respiratory emergencies, and pediatric trauma. Cardiac arrest in children is a rare event with poor outcome. The ability of paramedics to perform procedures to treat these entities are extremely variable and are patient-age dependent. For most age groups, rates of success for intubation are comparable to those for adults. As would be expected, endotracheal intubation and intravenous access are performed with poor levels of success in infants.

Aeromedical Transport

A critical function of an EMS system is the delivery of a critical patient to an appropriate facility as quickly as possible. One of the lessons learned in the Korean and Vietnam conflicts was the helicopter evacuation of such critically injured patients dramatically affected mortality. This concept now has been extrapolated to EMS care. Transfer of critical patients or transport from the scene of an injury have been shown positively to influence mortality of these patients, but some troubling issues persist. Initially all programs staffed helicopters with physicians, but little data exist regarding the need for this expensive arrangement. The costs and appropriateness of such programs have come under recent scrutiny as well. Most troubling is that during the initial decade of civilian experience, a number of health care providers died in helicopter crashes. Modifications in most programs have improved safety dramatically. While many questions remain regarding use of aeromedical care, it appears clear that it is here to stay and it needs to be integrated into existing EMS systems.

BIBLIOGRAPHY

National Academy of Sciences, National Research Council: *Accidental Death and Disability: The Neglected Disease of Modern Society*. Washington, DC, US Dept of Health, Education and Welfare, 1966.

Copass MK, Oreskovich MR, Bladergroen MR, et al: Prehospital cardiopulmonary resuscitation of the critically injured patient. *Am J Surg* 148: 20, 1984.

Eisenberg MS, Horwood BT, Cummins RO, et al: Cardiac arrest and resuscitation: A tale of 29 cities. *Ann Emerg Med* 19:179, 1990.

Gervin AS, Fischer RP: The importance of prompt transport in salvage of patients with penetrating heart wounds. *J Trauma* 22:443, 1982.

Pionkowski RS: Resusciation time in ventricular fibrillation: A prognostic indicator. *Ann Emerg Med* 12:733, 1983.

Seidel JS, Hornbein M, Yoshiyama K, et al: Emergency medical services and the pediatric patient: Are their needs being met? *Pediatrics* 73:769, 1984.

Stultz KR, Brown DD, Schug VL, et al: Prehospital defibrillation performed by emergency medical technicians in rural communities. *N Engl J Med* 310:219, 1984.

Weaver WD, Hill D, Fahrenbruch CE, et al: Use of the automatic external defibrillator in the management of out-of-hospital cardiac arrest. *N Engl J Med* 319:661, 1988.

West JG, Trunkey DD, Lim RC: Systems of trauma care: A study of two countries. *Arch Surg* 114:455, 1979.

16
DISASTER MEDICAL SERVICES

Brian D. Mahoney

Disasters may be natural, such as earthquakes, floods, or tornadoes. Or disasters may be of human origin, such as airplane or train crashes, fires, leaks of hazardous materials from industrial sites, or acts of terrorism. A disaster may involve the destruction of a great deal of property with few human victims. In this chapter the focus is on medical disaster planning. The American College of Emergency Physicians (ACEP) defines a *medical disaster* as an occurrence ''when the destructive effects of natural or manmade forces overwhelm the ability of a given area or community to meet the demand for health care.'' Emergency physicians play an integral role in the only civilian branch of medicine in the United States that considers disaster planning and management a primary field within its domain.

Medical disaster planning primarily involves preparations for managing multiple casualty incidents. In labeling a given multiple casualty incident as a medical disaster, the key issue is not the absolute number of victims. The key is the relation between the needs of the victims and the ability of a given health care system to meet those needs using normal operating procedures. For example, in one community a head-on collision involving two cars and eight severely injured victims may require implementation of the community's medical disaster response plan. In another community such a collision could easily be managed by the normal in-place medical resources. In the daily practice of emergency medicine, maximal care is provided to a limited number of patients. In a medical disaster with multiple casualties, changes in standard operating procedure are necessary. Instead of doing everything medically possible for one individual, field and hospital personnel strive to achieve the greatest good for the greatest number of potential survivors. For example: patients in cardiac arrest are pronounced dead, and precious resources are not spent on resuscitation attempts; patients are hospitalized only when absolutely necessary; laboratory and x-ray studies are used for critical information only; nurses have increased autonomy; and paramedics operate using standing orders, without the need for additional authorization from medical control.

Table 16-1. Disaster Management Team

Title	Role
Chief executive officer (e.g., mayor or designee)	Supervision of overall operation Communication with public Direction of requests for state or federal assistance
Fire chief	Overall scene command Supervision of victim rescue, extrication Hazard control
Police	Traffic management Scene security Overall scene command in some plans
Emergency medical services	Victim triage Stabilization Transportation
Public works	Support equipment such as heavy machinery for extrication Structural safety expertise
Emergency manager of civil defense	Communications Extra personnel Extra equipment
Red Cross	Food, shelter, clothing for displaced victims Disaster welfare inquiry system

Source: American College of Emergency Physicians: *Disaster Planning and Management for the Emergency Physician.* Emmitsburg, Md, Federal Emergency Management Agency, 1983. Used by permission.

A successful disaster response requires coordination of many governmental agencies and services (Table 16-1). The plan requires joint planning meetings, established lines of communication and authority, and regular coordinated multiagency drills. J. F. Waeckerle describes disasters as ''unexpected, chaotic, horrendous, catastrophes. . . . One is initially horrified, then bewildered and confused about what to do, where to start.'' Since a medical disaster will be a time of confusion under the best of circumstances, the plan must call for following normal operating procedures as much as possible. The fewer exceptions to the rules that stressed rescuers are expected to remember, the better. Mutual aid agreements between adjacent jurisdictions should be included in the plan and practiced regularly in drills.

PHASES OF A DISASTER RESPONSE

There are three phases to a disaster response (as taught in the ACEP course ''Disaster Planning and Management for the Emergency Physician''): activation, implementation, and recovery.

Activation

The first phase, the activation phase, has two components. The first component is notification and initial response. The first responder reports the nature of the incident, the extent of damage, the estimated number and types of injuries, the hazards for victims and rescuers, and the best access to the scene and or routes known to be blocked. It is crucial that the first responder take the time to ascertain and relay this information to medical control before attempting to render direct medical assistance. Early, accurate information leads to the appropriate mobilization of disaster response personnel and materials. The second component of the activation phase is the organization of an incident command post and further assessment of the scene. Typically the incident command post is set up by fire and rescue personnel, who locate it as close to the scene as safety allows, uphill and upwind of potential liquid and windborne hazards.

Implementation

The second phase, the implementation phase, has three components. The first is search and rescue. This is usually carried out by fire and rescue personnel because of the special expertise and equipment needed in a hazardous environment. Medical providers must remember that without this expertise and equipment they may themselves become victims. The second component involves triage, stabilization, and transport. The first arriving medical providers must assess medical needs, call to mobilize medical resources, establish contact with the overall incident commander (for example, the fire or police chief), and identify hazards and a safe casualty collection point, usually uphill and upwind from the scene. As more ambulances arrive, early treatment begins but it is limited to airway control, oxygen administration, hemorrhage control, and backboarding. Triage is begun: victims are grouped by priority within the casualty collection area. The third component of the implementation phase is definitive management of scene hazards and victims. Victims are transported to hospitals for definitive care according to the priorities identified by the triage officer.

Recovery

The first stage of the recovery phase is withdrawal from the scene, after making a systematic check for any missed victims. The second stage is the return to normal operations. Ambulances are restocked and standard operating procedures resumed. The Red Cross and the Salvation Army provide food, shelter, and clothing for displaced survivors. Concerned family members can use the Red Cross's disaster welfare inquiry system (DWIS) to locate victims.

The final stage of recovery is debriefing. A primary purpose of debriefing is to analyze the operation in order to improve future disaster responses. In addition, it plays a key part in the early identification and avoidance of potential psychological difficulties among the many rescuers.

TRIAGE

Triage is the process of sorting and classifying patients into categories according to priority of treatment. Its aim is to do the most good for the largest number of victims.

Multiple systems of triage exist. Many of them involve a tagging system. In all of them patients are classified according to priority of need. In a typical four-category system, a patient would be classified as severe, moderate, minor, or dead or expectant. In the severe category are patients who, given available care, have a reasonable chance of survival but without care have a markedly diminished chance of survival. This group gets the highest priority for care and transport. In the moderately injured group should be patients whose injuries will not lead to morbidity or mortality if they do not receive immediate care and transport. In the minor category are the "walking wounded," patients whose injuries will not lead to significant morbidity while they wait for treatment and transport of the two higher categories. In the fourth category are people in cardiac arrest, who are immediately pronounced dead and receive none of the scarce medical resources, and the "hopelessly wounded." Medical providers, who are accustomed to doing everything possible to save such patients on the chance that there will be a rare survivor, often have great difficulty limiting the care of patients in this category. These patients should receive supportive or palliative care until all higher-priority cases are managed. Which patients fall into which of these four categories depends on how large the medical disaster is and how thinly stretched the scarce medical resources have become. The rescuers must remember that the goal is to do the most good for the most potential survivors.

Triage is an ongoing, dynamic process. Patients' conditions are continually changing, and serial triage examinations must take place so that patients may be moved up or down in priority of treatment. Triage begins at first contact in the field. Rescuers check and correct, if possible, airway, breathing, and circulation on each victim and then rapidly move on to the next victim. Patients may or may not be tagged at this point. Only rapid life-saving maneuvers are carried out. For example, an oral airway may be placed, brief positive pressure ventilation done to see if a patient resumes spontaneous respiration, and a pressure dressing placed over a heavily bleeding wound. Cardiopulmonary resuscitation is not done.

Triage occurs again at the casualty collection point. This is usually the best time to apply triage tags. The victims are physically grouped according to priority of treatment to allow easy identification of those who should be transported first. The severe group should be collected at the location nearest to the ambulance loading area. More in-depth assessment and care may be provided according to the availability of resources. Serial examinations at the casualty collection point may lead to a change in the triage category. Triage influences the choice of a receiving hospital. Triage occurs again on arrival at the hospital. Each triage examination builds on and refines the sorting process that has already occurred.

There is some controversy over the value of triage tagging systems. Tags provide a record of critical medical interventions and prevent some redundancies in the triage survey by identifying those patients already checked. Vayer (1986) states that in many actual disasters tags are not used because they are such a marked departure from daily routine. He recommends using them as part of normal procedures, for a given period every year, in all accidents involving more than one victim. A disadvantage of tear-off tags is that they are unidirectional, allowing only for deterioration of the patient's condition. The author recommends sorting patients into physically separated groups according to degree of severity.

Each prehospital disaster plan should identify a medical response team consisting of a physician and paramedic group small enough to keep trained and up to date yet large enough that a nucleus can always be on call. The team responds to all disaster calls in a given geographic area, helping the other paramedic and medical providers to follow the philosophy and components of medical disaster management. Such medical response teams have proved valuable in actual medical disaster responses.

The members of the medical response team and their roles need to be identifiable at the scene: the best method is to use labeled vests. In reviewing the disaster response at the 1981 Hyatt Regency skywalk collapse, Orr and Robinson concluded that brightly colored overlay vests with large lettering are most effective. They reported that, initially, identification was less of a problem because rescuers recognized one another. Later, as more mutual aid providers arrived, identification became difficult. They also reported that police delayed some key personnel at the outer perimeter for lack of identification, and state that key personnel should carry some form of disaster identification card.

ORGANIZING THE MULTIPLE CASUALTY SCENE

The following discussion provides a framework for organizing a response to a multiple casualty incident confined to a single geographic location, for example, a fire or collapse in a single building, or an airplane crash. Modifications would be needed for larger, more diffuse multiple casualty incidents such as a tornado with multiple touchdowns, or an earthquake with multiple fires and collapses. In such cases, a response team would be required at each area of relative victim concentration.

Many systems have adapted the Incident Command System (ICS) to organize their disaster response. ICS was developed by the FIRESCOPE program in response to a series of wildfires in Southern California in 1970. It has since been taught and accepted nationally particularly by Fire services. There are seven key functions that the incident commander must manage. The ICS can be as small as one individual serving all seven functions or expand as needed by attaching divisions and task forces to each of four sections. If an incident commander is unwilling to delegate any of these seven functions, then he must assume them himself. The typical organization for the seven functions is as follows: an information officer, liaison officer, and safety officer all attached to the incident commander, and four section chiefs for finance, logistics, operations, and planning. EMS would typically fit in as a branch or division of the operations section.

Fire and rescue personnel usually provide overall incident command. They should establish an inner hazard perimeter within which emergency medical services (EMS) personnel are not allowed (Fig. 16-1). Fire and rescue personnel should conduct search, rescue, and extrication of victims, bringing them out of this hazardous area. Fire personnel should establish a scene command post uphill and upwind from any hazard.

EMS personnel should gather extricated victims at the casualty collection point, which should be close enough to the disaster for easy access yet far enough away, and far enough uphill and upwind, to be free of hazard. The collection site must afford easy access to direct transportation routes to hospitals.

EMS must provide several identifiable command personnel. The EMS branch director is in overall medical control and serves as liaison to the incident commander. This person should be a physician active in EMS and experienced in triage, resuscitation, stabilization, prehospital communications, and EMS capabilities. The EMS branch director must remember that EMS acts in support, not command, of the public safety agency in overall scene control. Ideally, a second physician, working under the EMS branch director, should have overall responsibility for triage operations. If there is only one physician, both these roles will be performed by one individual.

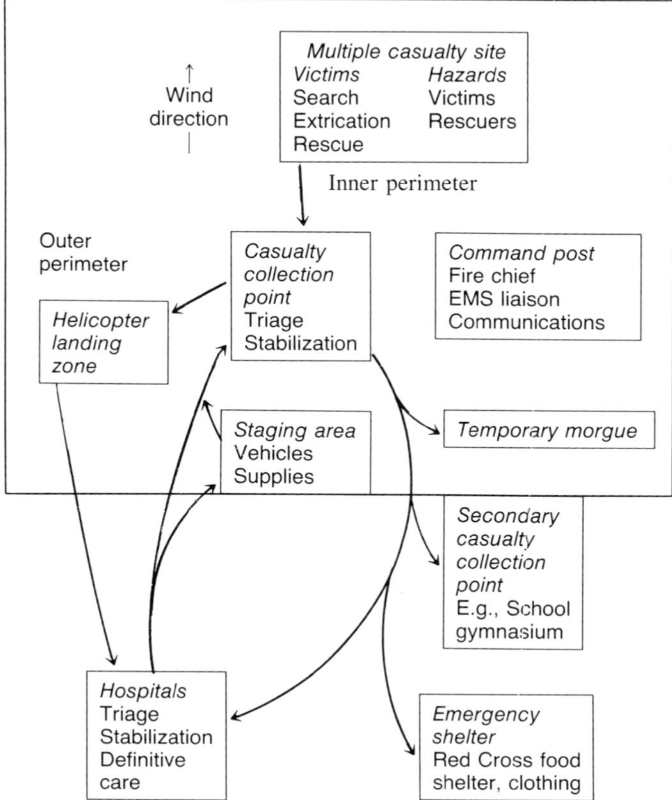

Fig. 16-1. Organization of a confined medical disaster site. (*Adapted from:* American College of Emergency Physicians: *Disaster Planning and Management for the Emergency Physician.* Emmitsburg, Md, Federal Emergency Management Agency, 1983. Used by permission.)

The EMS branch director should assign a paramedic to stay at the incident command post and act as communications liaison with the incident commander. The medical transportation officer, a paramedic supervisor, directs arriving crews in loading and transporting patients. The medical communications officer serves the transportation officer by relaying information to the regional medical control center and by relaying information back to the medical team at the scene regarding the ongoing capacity of various hospitals to handle patients.

In a large disaster extensive transport is needed. Resources to include in a regional disaster plan include metropolitan transit buses, school buses, and taxis. Many of the walking wounded will actually arrange their own transport to the nearest hospital. In general, the sicker patients are taken to the nearest capable hospital. However, the medical triage officer may elect to use helicopters and ambulances to take some patients to more distant hospitals, preserving some emergency capacity at the nearest hospital for patients who deteriorate or take longer to extricate. In smaller multiple casualty incidents, patient tracking is easier for families if all or most victims go to one or two hospitals. However, patient care must not be compromised by overloading a few hospitals.

Police need to establish an outer perimeter to ensure traffic control and deny scene access to unauthorized personnel. They must ensure crowd control and the safety of bystanders and the media, and in some cases prevent looting. Because a strong police presence is often necessary, in some systems the police chief, rather than the fire chief, is the incident commander.

Ambulance flow should be arranged in one direction. The ambulance exit route must not be blocked by other vehicles or fire hoses too large for ambulances to drive over. To avoid congestion, it is often necessary to designate a staging area where ambulances and supplies are collected and then directed to the casualty collection point as needed. Unfortunately, convergence is a common phenomenon in a disaster. Uninvited rescue agencies, and large numbers of civilians, will come from surprising distances, adding to the congestion and confusion at the scene. An obstruction-free helicopter landing zone should be established close enough to be usable but far enough away so that rotor wash and noise do not interfere with the rest of the operation. If there are many victims, or the weather is inclement, a secondary casualty collection point, e.g., a school gymnasium, should be established.

A temporary morgue may be needed. The medical examiner is in charge of removal, storage, and identification of bodies. Ice arenas and refrigerator trucks are possible resources.

COMMUNICATIONS

Communication problems are frequently identified in reviews of disaster responses. The multiple responding agencies typically do not have radios that operate on the same frequencies. Normal communications, principally the telephone, may be damaged or rapidly become overloaded. Alternatives to telephone systems include radio, cellular phones, messengers, and bullhorns. Orr and Robinson reported that in the Hyatt Regency skywalk collapse, bullhorns and messengers were necessary because of the noise of heavy extrication machinery Hand-held radios relying on outside repeaters proved unreliable.

To avoid overloading radio channels during a disaster, paramedic radio communications to their base hospital should be limited to key information. Paramedics should be authorized by their medical director to utilize all standard operating procedures without medical control.

The regional trauma center must rapidly obtain information from all hospitals in the region regarding emergency department capacity, operating room and critical care capabilities, and hospital bed availability. This information should be regularly updated and relayed to the incident medical director and transportation officer at the casualty collection point.

DISASTER MANAGEMENT TEAM

A disaster is a multifaceted event that requires expertise in many areas. So that personnel can adequately respond to a large, widely scattered, or prolonged disaster, a disaster management team is needed. Table 16-1 lists some key roles. In relatively small disasters, not all the personnel listed in the table may be needed, but they must be available. For large or prolonged disasters, an emergency operating center (EOC) should be provided for in the plan. Typically such a center is established in the city council offices in the nearest large city to the disaster site. The heads of each group involved in the disaster management team gather in the EOC to receive information, allocate resources, access additional supplies, and request outside assistance as needed.

HOSPITAL

The Joint Commission on Accreditation of Health Organizations requires every hospital to have a written disaster plan, covering every department and employee in the hospital, and to test that plan twice a year. To mobilize the disaster response without overloading hospital telephone lines, a chain call system can be established. Key hospital personnel should keep telephone lists at home or in their wallets. In massive disasters, community warning sirens can be sounded, alerting the public and the hospital staff to tune in to radio and television for announcements. Emergency physicians, who are needed in large numbers as soon as a disaster occurs, should have and carry their beepers at all times. On many beeper systems, dialing a single number can sound all the beepers at once.

Many steps must be completed in a short time to prepare for a large influx of patients. The decision to institute a hospital disaster response is usually a combined medical and administrative decision. It is better to call and mobilize early than to get caught behind. However, if information from a potential disaster scene is not sufficient to merit notifying all hospital personnel, an interim response plan may be effective, in which only emergency personnel are alerted. If the early disaster information suggests a prolonged event, then everyone should be notified. However, only half should come in at once so that the entire operation does not grind to a halt in 12 to 16 hours. The importance of writing the disaster plan so that it will be as close as possible to normal operating procedures, and of following the twice-a-year drill requirement, cannot be overemphasized. When a disaster occurs, all personnel need to be able to carry out their roles automatically. It is too late to read the manual.

Hospital administration must set up a control center with adequate telephone access. It should be near but not in the emergency department.

The emergency department must be rapidly cleared. Patients ready for discharge should be discharged and those needing admission admitted. Those without a disposition whose problem is not severe should be moved to a waiting area and told to expect a long wait. *The emergency department must be adequately stocked.* All stretchers must be returned from the wards immediately; extra oxygen and crystalloid infusion equipment must be prepared. The nursing supervisors need to obtain an accurate list of beds available. Dirty rooms need rapid cleaning, and inpatients ready for discharge should be discharged immediately.

Extra security officers should be in place as soon as possible. They must secure all doors to the hospital and keep driveways clear for ambulance access. They need to control patients, concerned family, the curious, and the media.

As patients arrive at the hospital, a medical triage officer should meet them at the door and reassess their treatment priorities. Categories similar to the four prehospital categories should be employed. The seriously injured must receive immediate stabilization. The moderate and minor groups need regular checks to be sure they do not deteriorate while waiting. The dead are moved to a temporary morgue, and the hopelessly injured continue to receive palliative care.

Documentation is limited to critical findings and treatments. Some plans call for the use of the prehospital disaster tag to record this limited information. Other plans include the preparation of kits containing the emergency department record, x-ray requests, laboratory slips and tubes, and wrist bands, all prelabeled with a discrete disaster number. Medical records and laboratory computers accept these numbers, which are used for patient identification until full normal registration is possible. At that point the computer will search previous medical records to match disaster numbers with the records of victims who have been patients previously. Such a prelabeled kit system can be used during normal operations, on unidentified critically ill or injured patients, so that all hospital departments are familiar with the concept. Admissions personnel are needed to log key information rapidly. Hours or days later they will be able to complete the registration process.

PUBLIC RELATIONS

The medical disaster plan should include a section on the proper relationship with the media. Representatives of the media are present at all medical disasters. They may be a valuable resource in announcing hazards or the need for evacuation. In addition, they may be used to make a general announcement that hospital or rescue personnel should report to work. The plan should include a means to provide the media with adequate information both at the site and in the hospital. At the disaster site, regular briefings help avoid the hazard of their becoming victims while in search of more information. At the hospital, regular briefings and a room with adequate telephone access will prevent the media from invading patient care areas. A hospital public relations officer should act as liaison with the media. His or her duties are to prepare the press room, hold regular briefings, and arrange appropriate photographic opportunities. These must be carried out while balancing the public's right to know against the individual victim's right to privacy.

In their review of managing the media during a disaster, Partington and Savage warned: "If an authoritative source does not provide this information reporters will talk to anyone and may receive unreliable information from which they, not surprisingly, make erroneous deductions. It is in the interest of the hospital, therefore, to release accurate information in a responsible way."

Designated waiting areas, away from treatment areas, must be available for family members. The public relations officer or other assigned personnel must regularly update these relatives on casualty lists and patient conditions. The hospital chaplain and volunteers should be present to provide support. These waiting areas should have adequate telephone lines as well as access to food, beverages, and bathrooms.

THE NATIONAL DISASTER MEDICAL SYSTEM

The National Disaster Medical System (NDMS) was created in 1984 to establish a mechanism to handle large numbers of casualties from a military or civilian disaster. It is a cooperative effort between the civilian hospital sector of the United States and the Department of Health and Human Services, the Department of Defense, the Federal Emergency Management Agency, the Veterans Administration, and state, regional, and local government agencies. In establishing the need for the NDMS, Mahoney et al. estimated that if the earthquake that destroyed Fort Tejon, California, in 1857 (Richter 8.3) occurred today it would cause 3000 to 14,000 deaths and from 12,000 to 55,000 injuries requiring hospitalization. No single metropolitan area or even a state could care for so many injuries. To meet the needs of an overwhelming medical disaster the NDMS is being developed to handle casualties of a magnitude of 100,000 victims arising from a massive peacetime disaster or an overseas conventional military conflict. This system builds on and replaces the Civilian Military Contingency Hospital System.

There are two component parts to the NDMS. The first part is the organization of the participating civilian hospitals and health care providers of 74 designated NDMS metropolitan areas. Each of these 74 areas is developing a system whereby large numbers of victims can be brought to that metropolitan area for definitive medical care provided by the many participating private hospitals. This system is a form of mutual aid agreement similar to that which many communities already have for local disasters. The NDMS is a mutual aid system on a national scale.

The second component of the NDMS is the development of disaster medical assistance teams (DMAT). These teams of volunteer health care providers will be provided with equipment and transportation to a site of a civilian disaster in the United States. There are two basic types of DMATs. The first is a 103-person clearing and staging team modeled after an Army medical clearing company. This type will provide medical care in field hospitals in the disaster area itself before evacuation of victims from the affected area to 1 or more of the 74 participating metropolitan areas. The second type of DMAT is a 215-person mobile surgical unit modeled after a mobile Army surgical unit. These civilian DMATs will not be used in military conflicts or outside the United States.

The NDMS does not replace state, regional, or local disaster plans. It will only be used for a massive disaster. The system can be deployed if a governor asks the Federal Emergency Management Agency for federal assistance and the request is approved by presidential declaration of a major disaster. It can be deployed by the Secretary of Defense in the event of a military conflict of sufficient magnitude. In both civilian and military scenarios, the patients are transported on military medical evacuation aircraft and distributed to participating areas under the direction of the Armed Services Medical Regulating Office.

MASS EVACUATION

The following is a summary of some key points in R. Leonard's review of mass evacuation. The first priority is the need to identify clearly who has the authority to order an evacuation. Often this authority rests with the fire chief. The overall disaster plan must specify the ordinance granting such authority. There are two types of evacuations—immediate, as in a toxic leak, and potential, as in a flood or hurricane. The news media can provide a valuable service in broadcasting announcements of potential mass evacuations.

There are four phases of a mass evacuation as developed by the Disaster Research Center of Ohio State University. The first phase is the warning. It is crucial that accurate, authoritative information be broadcast. The center found that people do not leave until they perceive a risk and do not evacuate if conflicting information causes doubt. Any announcements should explain the reason for evacuation, when it is to occur, and where people are to go. The second phase is withdrawal. The Disaster Research Center found that although persuading people to evacuate is often difficult, once they decide to go, they usually do so in an orderly fashion. An Environmental Protection Agency study of 500 evacuations involving 1.1 million people found that 99 percent of the people left by car. The difficult problem is in evacuating hospitals, jails, nursing homes, and mental institutions. The third phase is finding shelter. The center found that 72 percent of evacuees arrange their own shelter with friends, relatives, or motels. The other 28 percent go to public shelters (e.g., school gymnasiums, churches, and armories), where conflicts can be kept to a minimum by regular announcements on developments. The final phase is return. This is the most chaotic, as people make their own assessment of when it is safe to do so. Regular media broadcasts on continuing hazards help prevent premature return.

MENTAL HEALTH

An often overlooked but vital part of any medical disaster plan is attention to the mental health needs of the victims, their families, and the rescuers. Wilkinson studied the psychological sequelae of 102 victims, observers, and rescuers at the Hyatt Regency skywalk collapse in Kansas City. He reported that survivors in these groups suffered repeated recollections of the disaster (88 percent), sadness (83 percent), fatigue (57 percent), nightmares (52 percent), and guilt (44 percent). A debriefing should be organized as soon as possible after a disaster. This will help rescuers vent their feelings and help identify individuals in need of further counseling.

KEY POINTS

Following are the key points to remember when dealing with a disaster:

1. Do the most good for the most number of potential survivors.
2. Do not become a victim yourself.
3. Prioritize patient care, ensuring basic care for all potential survivors before organizing definitive care for lesser problems.
4. Remember that triage is an ongoing process requiring serial checks to record changes in treatment categories as patients improve or worsen.
5. Make your plan as close to day-to-day standard operating procedures as possible.
6. Remember that although limiting morbidity and mortality is the key goal in any disaster response, EMS is not in overall scene command.

TEN OF AUF DER HEIDE'S PRINCIPLES OF DISASTER RESPONSE*

1. Because of the limited resources available, disaster preparedness proposals need to take cost-effectiveness into consideration.
2. Interest in disaster preparedness is proportional to how recent and how extensive the last disaster was.
3. Base disaster plans on what people are likely to do, rather than what they should do.
4. For disaster planning to be effective, it must be interorganizational.
5. The process of planning is more important than the written document that results.
6. In disasters, what are thought to be "communications problems" are often coordination problems in disguise.
7. Panic is not a common problem in disasters; getting people to evacuate is.
8. Inquiries about loved ones thought to be in the impact zone are not likely to be discouraged, but can be reduced or channeled in less disruptive ways, if the needed information is provided at a location away from the disaster area.
9. Adequate disaster preparedness requires planning with the media rather than for the media.
10. Many of the questions that will be asked by reporters are predictable, and procedures can be established in advance for collecting the desired information.

* *Source:* Adapted from Auf der Heide, E., *Disaster Response: Principles of Preparation and Coordination,* Mosby, St. Louis, 1989.

BIBLIOGRAPHY

Auf der Heide, E: *Disaster Response: Principles of Preparation and Coordination.* St. Louis, Mosby, 1989.

American College of Emergency Physicians: Disaster medical services. *Ann Emerg Med* 14:1026, 1985.

American College of Emergency Physicians: *Disaster Planning and Management for the Emergency Physician.* Emmitsburg, Md, Federal Emergency Management Agency, 1983.

Feldstein BD, Gallery ME, Sanner PH, et al: Disaster training for emergency physicians in the United States: A systems approach. *Ann Emerg Med* 14:36, 1985.

Jacobs LM, Goody MM, Sinclair A: The role of a trauma center in disaster management. *J Trauma* 23:697, 1983.

Leonard R: Mass evacuation in disasters. *J Emerg Med* 2:279, 1985.

Mahoney BD, Ruiz E: Patient kits prelabeled with disaster numbers: Streamlining patient processing. University Association for Emergency Medicine, 11th Annual Meeting Abstracts, 1981, p 34.

Members of medical staff: Moorgate tube train disaster: Part I—Response of medical services. *Br Med J* 3:727, 1975.

Orr SM, Robinson WA: The Hyatt Regency skywalk collapse: An EMS-based disaster response. *Ann Emerg Med* 12:601, 1982.

Partington AJ, Savage PEA: Disaster planning: Managing the media. *Br Med J* 291:590, 1985.

Vayer JS, Ten Eyck RP, Cowan ML: New concepts in triage. *Ann Emerg Med* 15:927, 1986.

Waeckerle JF: The skywalk collapse: A personal response. *Ann Emerg Med* 12:651, 1983.

Wilkinson CB: Aftermath of a disaster: The collapse of the Hyatt Regency hotel skywalks. *Am J Psychiatry* 140:1134, 1983.

SECTION 3
Cardiovascular Diseases

17
MYOCARDIAL ISCHEMIA AND INFARCTION

J. Stephan Stapczynski

ISCHEMIC HEART DISEASE

Ischemic heart disease and its complications cause the greatest number of deaths in the United States, approximately 700,000 each year. Over 50 percent of these deaths occur prior to arrival at the hospital. While there are many processes which produce the imbalance between myocardial oxygen supply and demand that develops into ischemia, the most common cause by far is atherosclerosis of the epicardial coronary arteries; commonly termed *coronary artery disease* (CAD). CAD is a multifactorial disorder, and epidermiologic research has identified seven major risk factors for its development: age, male sex, family history, cigarette smoking, hypertension, hypercholesterolemia, and diabetes mellitus. Over the last 30 years, mortality due to CAD declined by about 40 percent in the United States. The decline is felt to be about half due to risk factor modification in the general population and half due to improvements in the medical care of symptomatic patients with CAD.

Pathophysiology of Myocardial Ischemia

Myocardial ischemia results from imbalance between myocardial oxygen supply and demand. Abnormalities in one or both of these factors may be present in the individual patient (Table 17-1). While the overwhelming majority of patients have fixed arterial obstruction due to atherosclerotic lesions, recent work has documented a greater incidence of coronary artery spasm than was previously appreciated. There are three major determinants of myocardial oxygen supply and three of myocardial oxygen demand (Table 17-2).

Ischemia produces major changes in two of the important functions of myocardial cells, electrical activity and contraction. The ischemic cell has a drastically altered transmembrane action potential. For example, the ischemic ventricular myocardial cell has an action potential in which the resting potential is elevated, the rate of rise is slower, and the plateau phase is shorter (Fig. 17-1). Between normal and ischemic myocardial tissues, an electrical potential difference exists which generates many of the arrhythmias seen with angina or acute myocardial infarction (AMI). Impaired myocardial contractility most importantly affects left ventricular function. Initially, there is a loss in normal diastolic relaxation, producing a decrease in ventricular distensibility and clinically manifested by an audible S_4. If ischemia becomes more profound, systolic contraction is lost and the affected area becomes hypokinetic or akinetic. If infarction develops, the area rapidly loses stiffness within minutes to hours and the area becomes dyskinetic, moving paradoxically with systolic contractions. All this results in a decreased ejection fraction. To maintain cardiac output, the cardiovascular system often compensates by increasing the filling pressure to maintain an adequate stroke volume, by the Frank-Starling principle.

Table 17-1. Etiology of Myocardial Ischemia

Decreased myocardial oxygen supply
Coronary artery obstruction
Fixed obstruction
Atherosclerosis
Miscellaneous causes
Arterial spasm
Systemic hypotension
Severe anemia
Increased myocardial oxygen demand
Myocardial hypertrophy
Tachycardia

Table 17-2. Major Determinants of Myocardial Oxygen Supply and Demand

Supply:
Aortic diastolic pressure
Coronary vascular resistance
Diastolic duration
Demand:
Heart rate
Wall tension:
Preload—left ventricular end diastolic pressure
Afterload—mean aortic pressure
Contractility

Natural History of Ischemic Heart Disease

The studies of the natural history of CAD done prior to 1970 cannot be applied to contemporary patients because of several limitations. Without coronary arteriography, there was no certainty about the specific diagnosis. There was no standard treatment protocol for all patients; some had no therapy, some had treatment with different medications, and some had surgery. In addition, more varieties of drugs and therapeutic agents are available now than in previous years. Studies have consistently shown that the natural history of CAD is primarily determined by two pathophysiologic factors: (1) the extent of arterial obstruction (one, two, or three vessels obstructed); and (2) the status of left ventricular function. The relation between symptoms, clinical observations, and the natural history of CAD can be accounted for by considering these two pathophysiologic factors. Some studies have found that complex ventricular ectopy (back-to-back ventricular ectopic beats or runs of ventricular tachycardia) is an independent factor in early mortality. During recent years, the mortality from CAD has

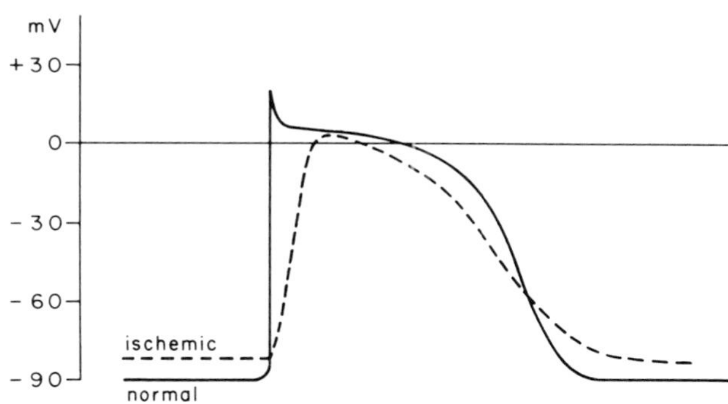

Fig. 17-1. Ventricular myocardial cell transmembrane action potential.

declined, primarily due to better application of medical treatment, and the previously grim prognoses given to certain subsets no longer apply. It has also been found that significant CAD can exist without clinical symptoms: such "silent" CAD has been found in 2.5 to 10 percent of various middle-aged population groups. These individuals appear to have a lower mortality than symptomatic individuals with CAD.

ANGINA PECTORIS

Clinical Features

Stable angina is characterized by episodic chest pain, lasting minutes (usually 5 to 15 min), provoked by exertion or stress, and relieved by rest or sublingual nitroglycerin. The pain almost always has a retrosternal component and commonly radiates to the neck, jaw, and shoulders, or down the inside of the left or both arms. Secondary symptoms—lightheadedness, palpitations, diaphoresis, dyspnea, nausea, or vomiting—may accompany the pain. Auscultation of the heart may find a transient S_4 or apical systolic murmur indicative of mitral regurgitation. An ECG taken during an acute attack shows changes about half the time, usually ST-segment depression or, less commonly, ST-segment elevation. Serum creatine kinase (CK) levels are not elevated.

Unstable (crescendo or preinfarction) angina represents a clinical state between stable angina and AMI. The subgroups included in the clinical definition of unstable angina are (1) exertional angina of recent onset, usually defined as within 4 to 8 weeks, (2) angina of worsening character, characterized by increasing severity, duration, or requirement for nitroglycerin, and (3) angina at rest (angina decubitus). Unstable angina is currently felt to be due to progression in the severity and extent of coronary atherosclerosis; coronary artery spasm; or hemorrhage into nonoccluding plaques with subsequent thrombotic occlusion developing over hours to days. The natural history of unstable angina can be partially assessed by analyzing five studies between 1956 and 1964 in which the only treatment was restriction of activities and sublingual nitroglycerin. Patients with either angina of worsening character or rest angina had a 40 percent incidence of acute infarction and a 17 percent incidence of death within a period of 3 months. A multicenter study from the 1970s found that intensive medical therapy reduces the risk of early infarction to 8 percent and the risk of early death to 3 percent. Therefore, it becomes important to recognize, hospitalize, and treat patients with unstable angina.

When obtaining a history of angina less responsive to nitroglycerin, it is important to inquire about the potency of the tablets, since nitroglycerin degrades over several months. If the patient has taken several tablets without the development of a local stinging or burning sensation under the tongue or a headache, the nitroglycerin is most likely old and ineffective. The sublingual spray retains its potency for more than 3 years. In unstable angina, ST-segment or T-wave changes may persist up to several hours after the pain episode, but there is no ECG evidence of new transmural infarction (new Q waves). Serum enzyme levels may show minor elevations without definite serial changes.

Variant (Prinzmetal's) angina occurs primarily at rest and without provocation. There is a tendency for attacks to recur at similar times of the day. Pain is associated with ST-segment elevation that represents transmural myocardial ischemia. Painless episodes may also occur with ST-segment elevation. Attacks may be associated with tachyarrhythmias, bundle branch blocks, or atrioventricular block. The current thought is that variant angina is due to spasm of the epicardial coronary arteries. When these patients are studied by coronary angiography, about one-third have no or insignificant atherosclerosis and about two-thirds have CAD in addition to spasm. The latter patients may have exertional angina in addition to variant angina. Spasm is not unique to variant angina; it has been found in patients with typical angina or AMI.

Treatment of Angina

For patients with ischemic heart disease, it is most important for the emergency physician to recognize and admit those patients with AMI and unstable angina. Occasionally a patient with stable angina may present with a typical acute attack. The most important concerns for the emergency physician are as follows: (1) Is there a new medical problem causing exacerbation of the angina? (2) Is this unstable angina? (3) Has the patient discontinued the prescribed medications? and (4) Are the medications ineffective? Many times, these patients can be managed by adjusting or refilling their medications. Ideally, this should be done with consultation of the patient's physician, and close follow-up should be arranged.

Treatment of angina should start with correction of modifiable risk factors: discontinuing smoking, controlling hypertension and diabetes, and lowering blood lipids by diet. Coexisting disorders that place stress upon the heart should be treated. Medications that increase myocardial oxygen demand, such as sympathomimetics and methylxanthine derivatives, should be discontinued if possible.

Drug treatment is usually started with nitrates (Table 17-3). Sublingual nitroglycerin is effective for most acute attacks; relief is usually felt within 3 min. Several long-acting forms are available to prevent anginal attacks: sublingual or oral long-acting nitrates, topical 2% nitroglycerin ointment, and prepackaged transdermal nitroglycerin delivery systems. However, there is evidence that tolerance to topical nitrates rapidly develops—sometimes within 24 h—suggesting that the continued treatment with long-acting nitrates is predominantly placebo in nature. It has been recommended that topical therapy be used for about half the day, allowing 10 to 12 h to recover nitrate responsiveness. Intravenous nitroglycerin is a potent vasodilator, with a quick onset of action, and can be rapidly titrated to the desired response; many physicians favor its use in patients with unstable rest angina.

β-adrenergic antagonists have been shown to be very useful in the treatment of angina but only moderately useful in patients with unstable angina or AMI. The theoretical risk of β-blockade therapy is unopposed α-adrenergic activity precipitating coronary vasoconstriction. Thus, while β blockers alone are useful in stable exertional angina, the combination of a β blocker and a vasodilator is logical for patients at risk for coronary artery spasm: those with variant angina, unstable rest angina, or AMI. Currently, 11 β blockers are available in the United States, four of which are FDA-approved for the treatment of angina (Table 17-4). Nonselective agents (e.g., propranolol) inhibit β receptors in the heart, lungs, and blood vessels. Selective agents (e.g., metoprolol) preferentially inhibit β_1 receptors of the heart at low and

Table 17-3. Nitrates

Agent	Dosage Size	Typical Dose	Duration of Action
Nitroglycerin (NTG)	Sublingual: 0.15, 0.3, 0.4, 0.6 mg	0.2–0.8 mg	Up to 30 min
	Buccal sustained release: 1.0, 2.0, 2.5, 3.0, 5.0 mg	1.0–3.0 mg	3–5 h
	Sublingual spray: 0.4 mg/puff	1–3 puffs	Up to 30 min
	Oral sustained release: 2.5, 2.6, 6.5, 9.0, 13.0 mg	2.5 mg	8–12 h
2% NTG ointment	20-, 30-, 60-g tubes; 1 in = 15 mg NTG	½–2 in	6–8 h
Transdermal NTG	0.1–0.6 mg/h	0.2–0.4 mg/h	12–24 h
Isosorbide dinitrate	Sublingual: 2.5, 5.0, 10.0 mg	2.5–5.0 mg	2–3 h
	Oral: 5.0, 10.0, 20.0, 30.0, 40.0 mg	5.0–20.0 mg	6 h
	Oral sustained release: 40 mg		8–12 h

Table 17-4. β-Adrenergic Antagonists

Agent	Brand Name	β_1 Selectivity	Tablet Size, mg	Typical Dose	Maximum Dose, mg
Acebutolol	Sectral	Yes	200, 300	200 mg bid	1200
Alprenolol	Aptin	Yes		200 mg qid	
	Betacard	Yes			
	Betapin	Yes			
Atenolol*	Tenormin	Yes	50, 100	50 mg qd	200
Betaxolol	Kerlone	Yes	10, 20	10 mg qd	40
Carteolol	Cartrol	No	2.5, 5.0	2.5 mg qd	10
Labetalol	Normodyne	No	100, 200, 300	100 mg bid	2400
	Trandate	No			
Metoprolol*	Lopressor	Yes	50, 100	50 mg bid	400
Nadolol*	Corgard	No	20, 40, 80, 120, 160	40 mg qd	240
Oxyprenolol	Transicor	No		40 mg qid	
Penbutolol	Levatol	No	20	20 mg qd	80
Pindolol	Visken	No	5, 10	5 mg bid	60
Practolol	Eraldin	Yes		25 mg tid	
Propranolol*	Inderal	No	10, 20, 40, 60, 80, 90	10–20 mg qid	320
	Inderal-LA	No	60, 80, 120, 160	80 mg qd	320
Timolol	Blocadren	No	5, 10, 20	10 mg bid	60
Sotalol	Betacordone	No		80 mg bid	
	Sotocor	No			

* FDA approved for treatment of angina pectoris.

intermediate doses. The β blockers are generally contraindicated in patients with congestive heart failure, atrioventricular block, variant angina, obstructive lung disease, or insulin-dependent diabetes mellitus. If given to patients with the last three diseases, selective β blockers instead of nonselective agents should be used whenever possible.

Calcium channel antagonists have been found effective for the treatment of stable angina and variant angina (Table 17-5). Several studies on the use of verapamil or nifedipine in the treatment of unstable rest angina or evolving AMI have shown no significant effect on the risk of progression to infarction, infarct size, or mortality. The three currently available calcium channel antagonists have different physiologic effects on the heart and blood vessels. Verapamil and diltiazem have major effects on the heart (decreased contractility and rate) and peripheral vessels (vasodilation). Nifedipine has predominant effects on the peripheral vessels (vasodilation) with only a small effect on the heart (decreased contractility).

ACUTE MYOCARDIAL INFARCTION

Pathogenesis of AMI

While the large majority of patients with AMI have CAD, there is no universal agreement about the exact process that precipitates the acute event. Current concepts concerning the immediate cause of AMI include the interaction of multiple factors: progression of the atherosclerotic process to the point of total occlusion, subintimal hemorrhage at the site of an existing narrowing, coronary artery embolism, coronary artery spasm, and thrombosis at the site of an intimal plaque. Recent studies strongly support the view that acute intracoronary thrombosis and, to a lesser extent, arterial spasm play frequent and important roles. These two processes are potentially reversible, and this has led to renewed interest in aggressive early intervention in AMI. The time period from the onset of symptoms to initiation of therapy is the key determinant of success. Emergency physicians commonly think of the "golden first hour" in determining the outcome of major trauma victims; it is time to consider the "first hour" in AMI as equally important. The previous approach to the treatment of AMI—resting the cardiovascular system while monitoring and treating only complications if they develop—is gradually being replaced by interventions which reverse the precipitating cause of infarction.

Pathophysiology of AMI

Like ischemia, infarction produces major changes in two important myocardial cell functions: electrical depolarization and contractility. The complications of AMI are caused by one or both of these events. During the first few hours, infarction is not a completed process; areas of infarction are interspersed with or surrounded by areas of ischemia or injury. The amount of infarcted tissue is a critical factor in determining prognosis, morbidity, and mortality. These ischemic areas are potentially salvageable through medical and surgical therapy.

Arrhythmias are frequent in AMI. Tachyarrhythmias and ventricular ectopy are usually caused by the electrical differences between adjacent areas of normal and ischemic myocardium. Bradyarrhythmias and atrioventricular blocks are due to either increased vagal tone or infarction directly affecting the conducting system.

Table 17-5. Calcium Channel Antagonists

Agent	Brand Name	Tablet Size, mg	Typical Dose	Maximum Dose, mg
Diltiazem	Cardizem	30, 60, 90, 120	30 mg qid	360
	SR*	60, 90, 120	60 mg bid	360
Nifedipine	Adalat	10, 20	10 mg tid	120
	Procardia	10, 20		
	SR	30, 60, 90	30 mg qd	120
Verapamil	Calan	40, 80, 120	80 mg tid	480
	Isoptin	40, 80, 120		
	SR	180, 240	180 mg qd	480
	Verelan SR	120, 240	120 mg qd	480

* SR = sustained release.

The major result of impaired contractility is left ventricular (LV) pump failure. If 25 percent of the LV myocardium is impaired, heart failure usually develops, and if 40 percent is affected, cardiogenic shock is common. Recent studies have also led to a greater appreciation of the effect of AMI on right ventricular (RV) pump function. If the papillary muscles of the mitral valve are impaired, acute mitral regurgitation may develop and cause acute pulmonary edema and hypotension.

The infarcted area can undergo autolysis, with distinct clinical syndromes resulting from rupture of the ventricular free wall, ventricular septum, or papillary muscle.

Stasis of the circulation can lead to venous thrombosis and pulmonary embolism. Stasis of blood within the ventricular cavity and exposure of collagen at the site of infarction can lead to development of mural thrombosis and systemic arterial embolism.

Clinical Features of AMI

The classic symptom is severe anginal pain lasting longer than 15 to 30 min, although severity and quality vary tremendously from individual to individual. As with angina, the pain may be accompanied by other symptoms such as lightheadedness, dyspnea, diaphoresis, palpitations, nausea, or vomiting. Elderly patients who develop an AMI are more likely to present with either nonretrosternal chest pain or no pain at all compared with younger patients. In addition, the elderly are more likely to present with the nonspecific symptoms. Longitudinal population studies indicate that up to 25 percent of myocardial infarctions are clinically unrecognized. Although there is disagreement, diabetic patients are felt by some physicians to be more susceptible to such "silent" infarctions.

The physical examination may be deceptively normal. Commonly, there is a mild to moderate increase in pulse rate although inferior infarctions frequently cause bradycardia. Depending on the degree of pain and sympathetic activation, blood pressure is elevated. Mild fever is common but rarely exceeds 39.5°C (103°F). Palpation of the apical pulse may show it to be diffuse or bulging. The loudness of S_1 may diminish as LV contraction is impaired. Uncommonly, the S_2 is paradoxically split owing to prolonged LV ejection. An S_4 is very common owing to decreased ventricular compliance, and a soft S_3 is occasionally heard. New systolic murmurs should be carefully examined. They may indicate (1) mitral regurgitation due to papillary muscle dysfunction or rupture, (2) ventricular septal rupture, or (3) friction rub of pericarditis.

Non-Q-wave versus Q-wave Infarction

The terms *Q-wave* and *non-Q-wave* infarction are often used to distinguish between a *transmural* and *nontransmural* (or *subendocardial*) infarction as determined by the presence or absence of Q waves. Autopsy studies have found very poor correlation between the development of a Q wave and the presence of transmural infarction seen on pathologic examination. Non-Q-wave infarction accounts for about 30 to 40 percent of AMIs. Such patients have a more frequent history of prior angina than do those with Q-wave infarcts. When studied with coronary angiography soon after the onset of pain, non-Q-wave infarctions have occlusion of the involved artery only about 20 percent of the time, as opposed to about an 80-percent occlusion rate for the involved artery in Q-wave infarcts. The incidence of complications and mortality in AMI depends on the extent of myocardial damage and not on the existence of a Q wave. On the whole, Q-wave infarctions tend to be larger (i.e., higher peak serum CK levels and lower radionuclide ejection fractions) and damage more myocardial tissue than non-Q-wave infarctions. As a group, non-Q-wave infarctions possess a lower in-hospital mortality but are more likely to be complicated by recurrent infarction or subsequent angina. As a result, the long-term mortalities of the two infarctions tend to equal out after about 3 years.

Ancillary Tests in AMI

Electrocardiography

The electrocardiographic diagnosis of AMI requires serial recordings. Depending on the electrocardiographic criteria for abnormality, between 60 and 90 percent of patients ultimately diagnosed as sustaining an AMI will have changes on their initial ECG in the emergency department (Table 17-6). However, a normal ECG does not exclude ischemia or negate the need for hospital admission; such decisions continue to be based on clinical assessment.

Acute ischemia may either be confined to the subendocardial area (manifested by ST-segment depression) or involve the complete transmural wall (manifested by ST-segment elevation). T waves often become inverted because ischemia or infarction reverses the sequence of repolarization, causing it to occur in the endocardial-to-epicardial rather than the normal epicardial-to-endocardial direction. Since many other conditions can cause ST-segment depression and T-wave inversion, "ischemic" subendocardial changes are considered to be (1) horizontal or downsloping ST segments of at least 1.0 mm and (2) deep, symmetrical T-wave inversions (Fig. 17–2). An important differentiating factor between ischemia and infarction is that the pain and ECG changes resolve as ischemia is relieved. Infarction eventually produces an electrically dead area of muscle, which may produce a Q wave in an overlying electrode. When they are observed in AMI, ST-segment changes occur rapidly, Q waves usually require several hours to become evident, and T-wave inversions are variable.

Table 17-6. ECG and Serum Creatine Kinase in the Emergency Department Diagnosis of Acute Myocardial Infarction

	Approximate Sensitivity, %	Approximate Specificity, %	Approximate Positive Predictive Value*, %
Initial ECG:			
A. New Q waves, or ST-segment elevation	65	90+	70–80†
B. As in A, or new subendocardial ischemia	75	80	20–30†
C. As in A, B, or prior changes of ischemia or infarction	85	75	5–10†
D. As in A, B, C, or nonspecific ST-T changes	90	65	<5†
Serum creatine kinase (CK) level:			
A. Elevated total CK	45	70	25
B. Elevated CK-MB (electrophoresis)	35	90	50
C. Elevated CK-MB (immunochemical)			
Upon presentation	50	90	75
3 h after presentation	90	95	85

* Since predictive value is dependent on the incidence of disease in the population under study, these values are for an emergency department population of adults (age >30) with a 20–30% incidence of acute myocardial infarction.

† The predictive value for this ECG pattern alone.

Source: From Gibler WB, et al: *Ann Emerg Med* 19:1359, 1990.

Fig. 17-2. Subendocardial ischemic ST-T changes.

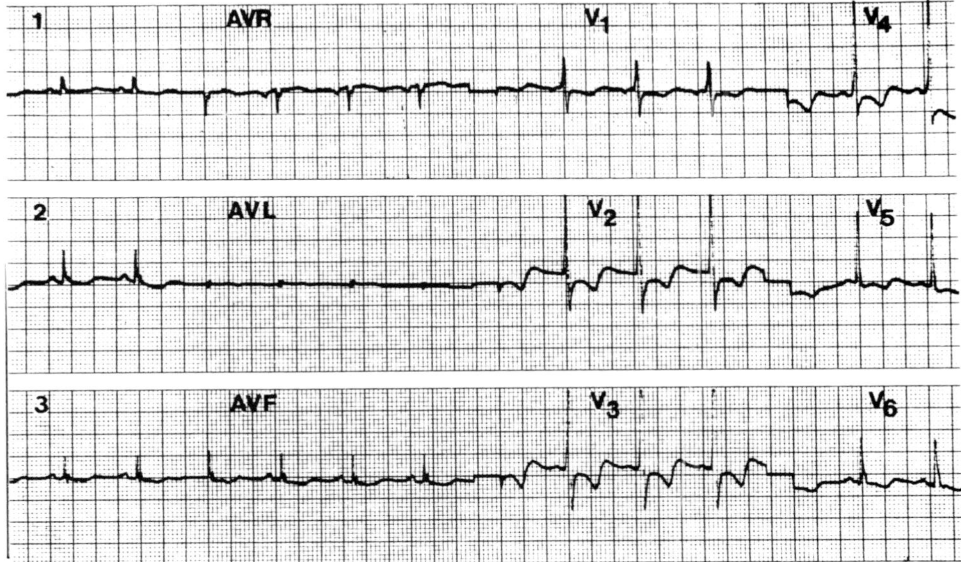

Using abnormal Q waves and ST-segment elevation on the ECG, one can localize the area of infarction (Fig. 17-3):

II, III, AVF inferior
V_1–V_3: anteroseptal
I, AVL, V_4–V_6: lateral
V_1–V_6: anterolateral

The one exception is a true posterior infarction, which produces a large R-wave and ST-segment depression in V_1 and V_2. Localization of AMI is important because the incidence and significance of complications vary with the site. For example, inferior wall infarctions may affect autonomic fibers in the atrial septum, resulting in increased vagal tone as manifested by sinus bradycardia or first-degree, or Mobitz I (Wenckebach), atrioventricular block (AVB). These blocks are generally benign and nonprogressive and respond readily to pharmacologic intervention if that becomes necessary. On the other hand, anterior wall infarction may directly damage the conducting system, producing Mobitz II second-degree or third-degree AVB. This is more grave and an indication for placement of a venticular pacemaker.

Cardiac Enzymes

When myocardial cells are irreversibly injured, they release enzymes into the serum. As discussed in Chapter 13A, "Chest Pain," the levels of commonly measured cardiac enzymes should not be used as criteria for hospitalization. The enzymes commonly measured in the coronary care unit are listed in Table 17-7.

CK is found in high concentrations in skeletal muscle, myocardial muscle, and brain tissue. Unfortunately, the total serum CK level is elevated by many disorders that affect skeletal muscle. The MB isoenzyme (CK-MB) is found primarily in myocardial cells, and elevated serum levels of this enzyme are more specific for myocardial injury. However, CK-MB normally contributes less than 3 to 6 percent of total serum CK activity, and small increases in CK-MB can be obscured by the larger amounts of other CK isoenzymes. The electophoretic method used to measure serum CK-MB is relatively insensitive and requires time for the serum level to rise sufficiently above background concentration before it can be reliably detected. Thus, electrophoresis cannot detect the slight elevations in serum CK-MB found when patients first present to the emergency department. New immunochemical assays have been developed that can detect minimal elevations of serum CK-MB. At least four commerically available products can measure serum CK-MB, requiring 10 min to 2 h of processing time. A recent study of these four methods in adults with nontraumatic chest pain and ECGs without diagnostic ischemic changes found that all methods had a sensitivity of about 50 percent for AMI upon emergency department presentation. With serial sampling every hour for 3 h, the sensitivity increased to over 90 percent. The potential benefits of early AMI detection include correct in-hospital admission decisions, prevention of discharge of AMI patients with nondiagnostic ECGs, and possible early administration of thrombolytic or anti-ischemic therapy. The value of these early immunochemical methods in detecting serum CK-MB is currently undergoing a larger multicenter study. At the time of this writing, such methods are not routinely available in most community hospitals.

Serum glutamic-oxaloacetic transaminase (SGOT) is found in many organs, and an elevated level is too nonspecific to be useful. Lactic dehydrogenase (LDH) is likewise found in many organs of the body, but two isoenzymes, LDH_1 and LDH_2, are confined primarily to the heart, and their serum concentration or ratio can be separately measured. These isoenzymes also have greater ability to dehydrogenate hydroxybutyric acid than other LDH isoenzymes. So while hydroxybutyrate dehydrogenase (HBD) is not a distinct enzyme, a measure of LDH_1 and LDH_2 concentration can be obtained by measuring serum HBD activity.

Table 17-7. Serum Enzymes in Diagnosis of Acute Myocardial Infarction

Enzyme	Earliest Rise, h	Peak, H	Normalize, Days
CK	6–8	24–30	3–4
CK-MB	3–4	18–24	2
AST (SGOT)	8–12	36–48	3–5
LDH	12–24	48–96	7–10
HBD	12	72	10–14

Echocardiography

Soon after the onset of myocardial ischemia, muscle contraction is impaired and can be detected by echocardiography as wall motion abnormalities. Experimentally, hypokinesis, akinesis, or dyskinesis can be seen within a few heartbeats after coronary occlusion. In selected critical care unit patients, echocardiography has a sensitivity of over 70 percent in AMI, but it has not been as well studied in emergency patients, where the prevalence of AMI is lower and the value of echocardiography would be less. Echocardiography has a low sensitivity for patients with unstable angina who are pain free at the time of the study.

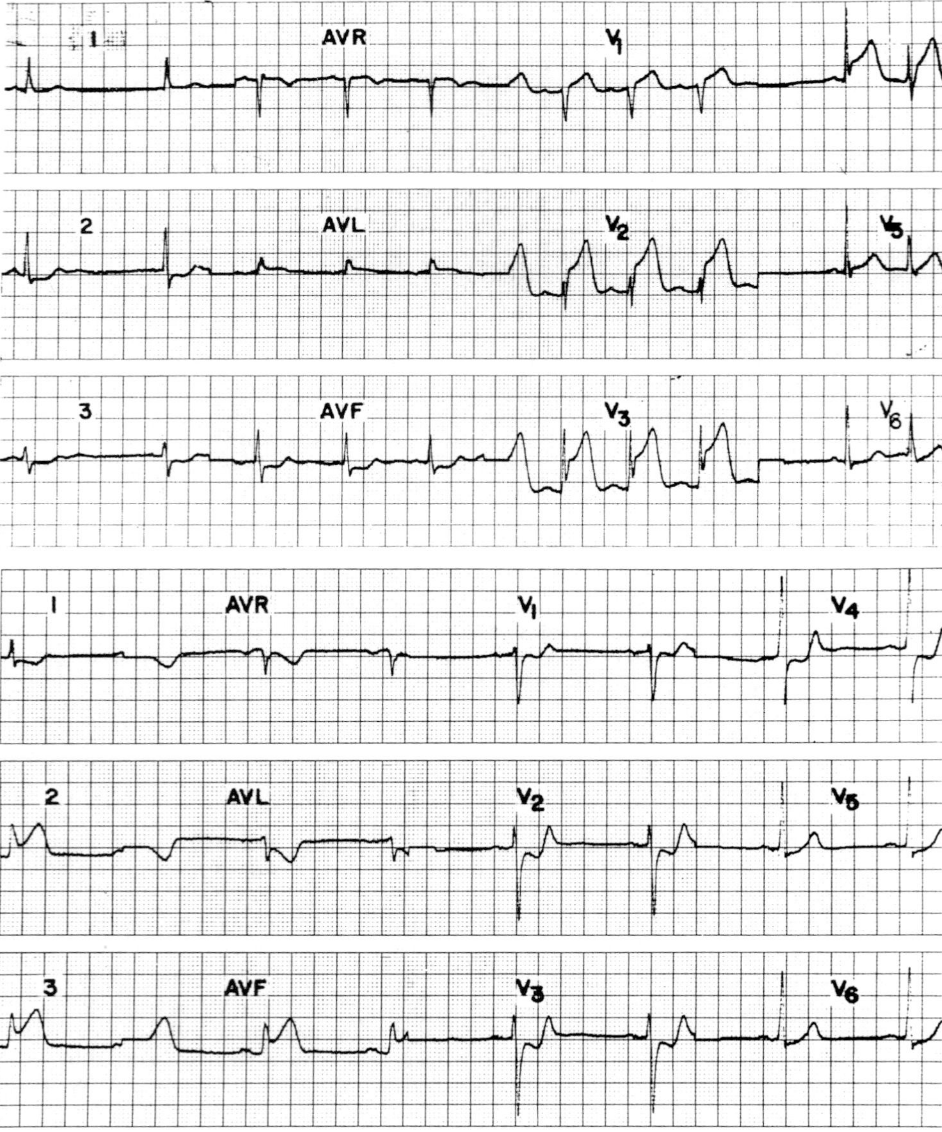

Fig. 17-3. Transmural ECG changes of acute myocardial infarction. Top: acute anterior MI; bottom: acute inferior MI.

Radionuclide Scans

Radionuclide scanning is not commonly available to evaluate patients in the emergency department nor should it be recommended at this time for use in the decision-making process. In certain situations, the radionuclide scan is helpful in evaluating inpatients. Two radionuclides, technetium 99 and thallium 201, are commonly used.

Technetium 99 pyrophosphate is deposited irreversibly in infarcted myocardial tissue, producing a "hot spot" on nuclear imaging. Scans first become positive within 10 to 12 h and become increasingly positive up to 24 to 72 h after onset of chest pain. Sensitivity is highest with Q-wave infarctions (about 85 percent) and less with non-Q-wave infarctions (about 50 percent).

Thallium 201 is reversibly taken up by normally perfused myocardial cells; the infarcted or ischemic area appears as a "cold spot" on nuclear imaging. Thallium 201 scanning performed within 6 h after the onset of chest pain was found to have a high sensitivity for AMI in small studies. Unfortunately, thallium scans are less sensitive in small or non-Q-wave infarctions, detect less than 50 percent of patients with unstable angina, and have a low specificity (around 80 percent). It would be expected that in emergency department patients with chest pain, where the prevalence of AMI is low, thallium scanning would not be useful. The studies to date seem to so indicate.

Both echocardiography and thallium scanning are hindered by the difficulty of separating new versus old abnormalities. In most facilities, the technical expertise required, the added cost, and the limited availability of these ancillary tests on an urgent basis restrict their routine use in the emergency department.

Complications of AMI

Arrhythmias

The out-of-hospital mortality in AMI is almost entirely due to arrhythmias; early assessment and treatment of these arrhythmias must first depend on their detection. All patients should be on continuous cardiac monitoring, and, equally important, the monitor must be watched by qualified personnel. The incidence of lethal arrhythmias is greatest in the prehospital phase. The site of infarction does not appear to influence the incidence of arrhythmias (Table 17-8).

Some studies have found a higher incidence of serious ventricular arrhythmias in patients experiencing an AMI who are initially hypokalemic or hypomagnesemic, especially if on prior diuretic therapy. Arrhythmias should be treated if the effect on the heart rate further exacerbates the myocardial oxygen supply and demand imbalance or has the potential to deteriorate into cardiac arrest. Experimental and

Table 17-8. Approximate Incidence of Arrhythmias in Acute Myocardial Infarction

	Incidence, %
Sinus tachycardia	40–60
Sinus bradycardia	3–10
Premature atrial contractions	15–40
Paroxysmal supraventricular tachycardia	2–7
Atrial fibrillation	10
Atrial flutter	5
Junctional tachycardia	5–10
Premature ventricular contractions	80–100
Ventricular tachycardia	10
Accelerated idioventricular rhythm	8–23
Primary ventricular fibrillation	5–10

clinical work indicate that the optimal heart rate is between 60 and 90 beats per minute in acute infarction.

Sinus tachycardia is potentially detrimental because of increased myocardial oxygen demand. Diagnosis and therapy should be directed toward the underlying cause: increased sympathetic activity, hypovolemia, hypoxia, etc.

Sinus bradycardia is usually due to increased vagal tone and is common with inferior AMIs. Treatment with atropine is usually not required unless the bradycardia is complicated by hypotension or premature ventricular contractions (PVCs). Premature atrial contractions (PACs) are common but generally are of no significance unless they initiate more serious arrhythmias, like paroxysmal supraventricular tachycardia (PSVT).

PSVT should be treated because the rapid rate increases oxygen demand and reduces cardiac output. The reentrant variety of PSVT should be treated with vagal maneuvers, adenosine, or cardioversion. Drugs that directly depress myocardial contractility (e.g., verapamil or β-adrenergic blockers) may have significant risk in the potentially unstable hemodynamics of AMI and should be used with caution.

Atrial fibrillation usually occurs within the first 48 h and often in association with pericarditis. The ventricular rate can be controlled with digoxin, verapamil, or propranolol. Cardioversion is effective if the patient is hemodynamically compromised. Recurrences are common and therapy with procainamide may be required. Atrial flutter responds readily to cardioversion, but digoxin, verapamil, or propranolol can also be used to control ventricular rate.

Junctional tachycardia is caused by enhanced automaticity of the junctional pacemaker due to infarction or digoxin toxicity. Treatment is not necessary unless the rapid rate produces hemodynamic deterioration.

PVCs occur in nearly all patients with AMI. The frequency or complexity of ventricular ectopy (so-called warning arrhythmias) is no longer felt to be a reliable predictor of subsequent ventricular tachycardia or fibrillation. However, some physicians consider the presence of PVCs an indicator of ventricular irritability and recommend treatment with lidocaine to prevent the occurrence of ventricular tachycardia or fibrillation (see below).

Ventricular tachycardia should be treated according to the hemodynamic status of the patient: if the patient is stable, intravenous lidocaine should be used, and if the patient is unstable, immediate synchronized cardioversion should be done.

Accelerated idioventricular rhythm (AIVR) is usually a transient arrhythmia, with wide QRS complexes, occurring at a rate of 60 to 90 per minute. It is thought to arise from a number of causes. While it is usually benign, there is some variable association with ventricular tachycardia but no apparent association with ventricular fibrillation (VF). Close monitoring is advised, but specific therapy is usually not indicated for AIVR.

Primary VF is the sudden development of VF in the absence of shock or LV failure. Primary VF occurs in about 5 to 10 percent of patients with AMI, usually early in the course; 60 percent with 4 h and 80 percent within 12 h after the onset of symptoms. In a monitored setting, primary VF should be rapidly detected and can nearly always be successfully defibrillated. Secondary VF occurs as a terminal event after a progressive course of LV pump failure. Treatment of secondary VF is unlikely to yield long-term success.

Prophylactic lidocaine therapy is recommended by some physicians to prevent primary VF in patients with definite or possible AMI during the first 24 to 48 h of hospitalization. Some studies have found prophylactic lidocaine partially effective in preventing primary VF while the patient with AMI is in the intensive care unit. However, meta-analysis of eight randomized in-hospital clinical trials showed a statistically significant increase in mortality during the treatment period in patients who received lidocaine. Similar meta-analysis of six prehospital clinical trials with prophylactic lidocaine showed no significant mortality difference. While the potential benefits of prophylactic lidocaine in the prehospital or emergency department setting are not proven, several points are worth noting. First, in untreated patients, the incidence of primary VF is low, about 5 to 10 percent in patients with AMI and less in patients with unstable angina. Second, primary VF should be easily detected and rapidly defibrillated in a monitored setting with a mortality of about 5 percent. Third, prophylactic lidocaine decreases the incidence of primary VF by about 90 percent. Fourth, the complications of lidocaine are minor, and the incidence is about 5 to 10 percent.

Conduction Disturbances

AMI may damage the conduction system and sometimes progress to complete (third-degree) AVB. The risk of complete AVB during an AMI depends on two major factors: (1) the site of the infarction, and (2) the occurrence of new conduction disturbances. While the site of infarction is usually known, many times the age of the conduction disturbance is not. This is reflected by the use of the term *new or age-indeterminant* conduction block in many studies. In addition, some studies use the term *high-grade AVB,* meaning that both third-degree AVB and forms of second-degree AVB are equally serious. This produces a wide variation in the reported rate of progression to AVB and yields divergent opinions as to what constitutes a high-risk situation in which prophylactic pacemaker insertion is warranted. With this in mind, data from six studies reported between 1973 and 1983 were pooled to yield the rates of progression to complete AVB with new or age-indeterminant conduction disturbances (Table 17-9). When the risk of complete AVB is above 10 to 15 percent, prophylactic pacemaker placement is probably indicated. In addition, two subgroups of patients are at particular risk. First, patients with some form of AV nodal conduction disturbance (first- or second-degree AVB) in addition to the infranodal conduction block (fasicular or bundle branch) are at increased risk for complete AVB. Second, patients with anterior infarctions are at risk for profound bradycardia if complete AVB develops because the escape ventricular pacemaker is often slow and unreliable.

First-degree AVBs and Mobitz I (Wenckebach) second-degree AVBs are usually due to increased vagal tone impairing AV nodal conduction and are generally seen in inferior ischemia or infarction. Progression to complete AVB is infrequent and rarely occurs suddenly, and if it does occur, a stable infranodal pacemaker with narrow QRS

Table 17-9. Approximate Incidence of Complete Atrioventricular Block in Acute Myocardial Infarction

New or Age-Indeterminant Conduction Defect	Incidence, %
No conduction abnormality	1–3
Left anterior superior fascicular block (LASFB)	2–4
Left posterior inferior fascicular block (LPIFB)	2–4
Right bundle branch block (RBBB)	6
Left bundle branch block (LBBB)	15
RBBB and either LASFB or LPIFB	30–40

Table 17-10. Killip-Kimball Classification

Class		Approximate Incidence, %	Approximate Mortality, %
I	No failure	30	5
II	Mild failure: bibasilar rales and S_3	40	15–20
III	Frank pulmonary edema	10	40
IV	Cardiogenic shock:	20	80
	Systolic BP < 90 mmHg		
	Peripheral vasoconstriction		
	Oliguria		
	Pulmonary vascular congestion		

complexes and a reasonable rate of about 50 is usually maintained. When treatment is necessary, these blocks usually respond to atropine.

Mobitz II second-degree AVBs are usually due to structural damage to the infranodal conduction tissue and are generally seen with anterior ischemia or infarction. Complete AVB may occur suddenly, with only a slow, unstable ventricular escape pacemaker available for cardiac activity. Mobitz II blocks are an indication for prophylactic pacemaker placement. Infarctions which cause Mobitz II blocks are usually large, and even with pacemaker treatment, many patients die of pump failure.

LV Pump Failure and Cardiogenic Shock

AMI nearly always produces impairment of LV pump function; whether this is clinically manifest depends on the extent of damage. Several classifications have been developed to correlate the extent of pump dysfunction with acute in-hospital mortality. The Killip classification is based on clinical criteria, and the Forrester-Diamond-Swan classification is based on hemodynamic measurements (Tables 17-10 and 17-11A and B). A rough, imprecise correlation exists between clinical and hemodynamic findings. Pulmonary vascular congestion occurs when pulmonary artery wedge pressure (PAWP) rises above 18 to 20 mmHg and is manifested by dyspnea and rales. Peripheral hypoperfusion occurs when the cardiac index falls below 2.2 to 2.5 L/min per square meter and is manifested by hypotension, oliguria, mental obtundation, peripheral vasoconstriction, and tachycardia. The terms *preload* and *afterload* are often used in discussions of LV dysfunction. Preload is the LV filling pressure during diastole. This filling pressure can be measured directly as LV end-diastolic pressure or, more commonly, indirectly measured as PAWP. Afterload is the pressure against which the left ventricle pumps and is usually measured as the mean aortic pressure.

Current management of LV pump dysfunction is based on the underlying hemodynamic derangement. Pulmonary vascular congestion is traditionally treated with vasodilators, morphine, or diuretics. Of these three modalities, vasodilators produce the most rapid and predictable decrease in PAWP. Because of the unstable hemodynamic situation, short-acting intravenous agents that can be titrated to effect are the most appropriate agents to use: nitroglycerin or nitroprusside. Sublingual, oral, and topical nitroglycerin act predominantly as venodilators, increasing venous capacitance and decreasing preload. Intravenous nitroglycerin is both a venous and an arterial dilator, but the greater effect is on the venous side. Intravenous nitroprusside is a "balanced" vasodilator, with about equal effects on systemic arterial resistance and venous capacitance. However, since nitroprusside sometimes causes a deterioration in myocardial oxygen supply and demand ratio, it is not routinely recommended as an afterload-reducing agent in AMI. Vasodilators reliably relieve pulmonary vascular congestion, but as PAWP falls, cardiac output may also fall if the filling pressure of the left ventricle decreases too much. Patients in heart failure usually have an elevated filling pressure, and vasodilator therapy generally improves cardiac output. Conversely, patients not in heart failure usually experience a fall in cardiac output with vasodilator therapy. Most of the clinical effect of morphine in LV pump failure is due to its general sedative actions rather than any direct effect on hemodynamics. So while morphine is still used for its sedative effect, vasodilators are more effective in reversing the abnormal pathophysiology. Intravenous furosemide is commonly thought to have a rapid venodilation action, although this has not been found in all studies, and there is evidence that intravenous furosemide acutely increases LV filling pressures for about 15 min after administration. To prevent this effect, vasodilators should be used simultaneously with intravenous furosemide. Regardless, the major effect of diuretics on pulmonary vascular congestion is to decrease the PAWP by producing a diuresis within an hour after intravenous administration of the potent loop diuretics (furosemide or bumetanide).

Table 17-11A. Forrester-Diamond-Swan Classification

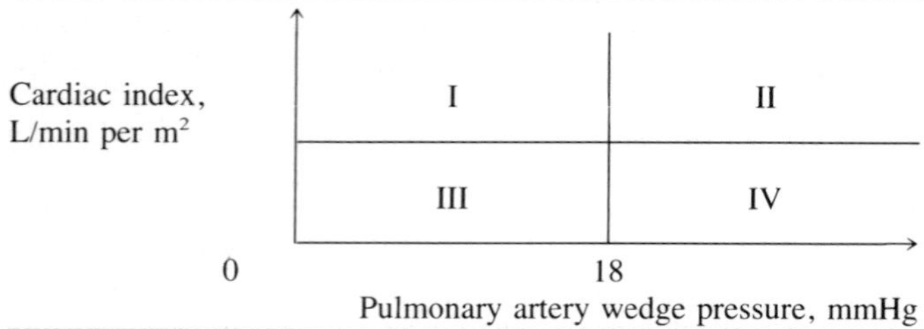

Table 17-11B. Approximate Mortality

Class	Approximate Mortality, %
I	3
II	9
III	23
IV	51

Depressed cardiac output should be treated by first optimizing preload, although most patients with cardiogenic shock already have an elevated PAWP. Patients without evidence of pulmonary vascular congestion can be given fluid challenges of saline or colloid, but once pulmonary edema develops, further therapy often requires measurement of the PAWP. Pharmacologic therapy to improve cardiac output is guided by the systolic blood pressure. If systolic blood pressure is above 100 mmHg, cardiac output can usually be increased with afterload reduction using intravenous nitroprusside. When systolic blood pressure is below 100 mmHg, vasodilator therapy should be undertaken cautiously. With mild hypotension (systolic blood pressure 75 to 90 mmHg), an inotropic agent such as dobutamine, dopamine, or amrinone is usually effective, although there are serious concerns about the short-term toxicity of amrinone in this setting. Experimental canine studies have found that dobutamine is a better agent in improving overall myocardial function in AMI, but unfortunately dobutamine is not a potent vasoconstrictor and does not adequately treat low blood pressure in frank shock. With severe hypotension (systolic blood pressure below 75 mmHg), a vasoconstrictor is generally required to maintain vital organ perfusion. Dopamine has both inotropic and vasoconstrictor properties (depending on the dose) and is a good agent to use in cardiogenic shock. If inotropic agents are ineffective or required for longer than a few hours, the intraaortic balloon pump or other LV-assisting devices can be used to mechanically support the circulation. Some patients require mechanical support for only a short time, allowing some myocardial recovery, and resumption of adequate LV function. However, if these devices are required for longer than 24 h, many or most patients do not recover adequate LV function for weaning and may need surgical intervention for survival.

Mechanical Defects

Cardiac rupture is a catastrophic event that presents with sudden recurrence of chest pain, hypotension, pericardial tamponade, cardiac arrest with electromechanical dissociation, and death. Patients at increased risk are those with first infarction, those with sustained hypertension after infarction, and the elderly; 50 percent of cardiac ruptures occur within the first 5 days and 90 percent within the first 14 days after infarction. Mortality is 95 percent; a few patients survive with volume replacement, pericardiocentesis for treatment of tamponade, and immediate surgery.

Ventricular septal rupture presents with sudden onset of pulmonary edema and a new harsh systolic murmur along the left sternal border. Septal rupture occurs about equally in anterior and inferior infarctions and is located in the muscular portion of the intraventricular septum. Clinical diagnosis may be difficult, often requiring the measurement of P_{O_2} in RV blood obtained via a Swan-Ganz catheter. Therapy should be initiated with afterload reduction by nitroprusside or, if this in ineffective, by the intraaortic balloon pump.

Papillary muscle dysfunction is common, especially with inferior infarctions. The clinical presentation is usually mild, with only a transient systolic murmur, but may become severe, with florid pulmonary edema. Treatment of the ischemia and afterload reduction is usually effective. Prognosis of mild dysfunction is very good.

Papillary muscle rupture is more serious, and the outcome depends on whether the whole muscle body is ruptured or only the head. Rupture of an entire muscle body is associated with a high mortality, up to 50 percent within 24 h. Rupture is usually associated with an inferior-posterior infarction and involves the posterior papillary muscle. Clinical diagnosis of papillary muscle dysfunction or rupture can be difficult and can require a Swan-Ganz catheter to measure large V waves in the PAWP.

Thromboembolism

Prolonged bed rest and generalized circulatory stasis predispose the patient with AMI to venous thrombosis and pulmonary embolism. Other predisposing factors include previous thromboembolism, atrial fibrillation, old age, and obesity. Early ambulation and low-dose subcutaneous heparin (5000 units bid) have reduced the incidence of deep venous thrombosis.

A mural thrombosis can develop at the site of infarction. Mural thrombi occur in less than 5 percent of patients with non-Q-wave or inferior infarction and in 30 to 40 percent of patients with anterior Q-wave infarction. Some patients form a thrombus within 48 h; these patients usually have large infarctions with hemodynamic complications and a high in-hospital mortality. Once formed, the LV thrombus may regress, remain asymptomatic, or embolize to the systemic circulation. Most large studies report an incidence of clinically evident systemic emboli of 1 to 6 percent of all patients with AMI, although the risk in patients with mural thrombi may be as high as 30 percent. Echocardiography is a good screening tool, and if a mural thrombus is detected, full-dose anticoagulation with intravenous heparin is initiated if there are no contraindications to its use.

Pericarditis

An acute form of pericarditis, manifested by pain and friction rub, can develop during the first 7 days postinfarction. The reported incidence is between 6 and 10 percent of all patients with AMI and is higher in patients with Q-wave infarctions. The cause is the inflammation associated with necrosis of the myocardium adjacent to the pericardium. The postmyocardial infarction (Dressler's) syndrome generally occurs later and is characterized by chest pain, fever, pleuropericarditis, and pleural effusion. The cause is an immunologic reaction to myocardial antigens exposed by AMI.

RV Infarction

RV infarction is now recognized as occurring in 19 to 43 percent of patients with inferior AMIs. RV infarction is due to right coronary artery obstruction, nearly always transmural, and almost always associated with LV damage. It was previously held that the right ventricle served as a volume conduit and that RV pump dysfunction is not clinically significant. However, severe RV pump failure does cause hypotension, usually with an elevated right atrial pressure and a normal or decreased left atrial pressure. Therefore, the clinical presentation is that of hypotension, jugular venous distension, and clear lungs. In addition, most patients with hemodynamically significant RV infarction have a rise in jugular venous pressure with quiet inspiration (Kussmaul's sign). RV pump dysfunction can be mimicked by occult LV failure, constrictive pericarditis, pericardial tamponade, and restrictive cardiomyopathy. Correct diagnosis of RV pump dysfunction may require simultaneous measurement of PAWP and right atrial pressure or visualization of poor RV contractions on radionuclide scanning. Patients with RV infarction are dependent on an elevated RV filling pressure to maintain cardiac output, and it is important to avoid or prevent decreases by the use of diuretics or nitrates. Volume infusions may produce a small improvement in cardiac output, but an inotropic agent like dobutamine is much more effective.

General Treatment of AMI

All patients with documented or suspected AMI should have an intravenous line established; a D_5W solution is generally used and saline solutions are avoided to prevent sodium overload and pulmonary congestion. The cardiac monitor should be applied and observed by qualified personnel. Supplemental oxygen should be administered to all patients. Patients with a history of oxygen sensitivity or chronic obstructive pulmonary disease should be given low concentrations (2 L/min or 24 percent) and all other patients given higher concentrations (4 to 6 L/min or 40 percent). Experimentally, supplemental oxygen at an FI_{O_2} of 40 percent reduces the degree of ST-segment elevation and size of the infarction. Severe hypoxia or hypercapnia often requires endotracheal intubation and mechanical ventilation, preferably with a volume-cycled respirator, since changes in lung compliance can make pressure-cycled ventilators unreliable. Underlying acid-base disorders, especially alkalosis, should be corrected since they contribute to arrhythmias.

With the potential liability for missing the diagnosis of an AMI, many physicians tend to overdiagnose myocardial ischemia and admit "soft" patients to the hospital as a precaution. Nationwide, this practice has led to over 1.5 million annual admissions to intensive care units for suspected ischemia, but less than 30 percent of these patients have acute infarctions. The policy in many hospitals is that all patients admitted because of chest pain (as "Rule out myocardial infarction") have to be admitted to the intensive care unit. Recent studies evaluating this process found that certain subgroups of these patients rarely, if ever, require intensive care unit interventions and have a very low in-hospital mortality. Patients with AMI or unstable angina who have either ongoing pain, ECG changes, arrhythmias, or hemodynamic complications often require intensive care unit interventions and rightly belong there. Patients with unstable angina who have a normal ECG and no arrhythmias or hemodynamic complications can appropriately be admitted to a step-down or telemetry unit without adversely affecting in-hospital mortality. Likewise, patients admitted as "Rule out myocardial infarction" and a normal ECG can be safely admitted to a step-down unit. Patients with unstable angina can be safely transferred out of the intensive care unit after they have remained hemodynamically stable and free of ischemic pain for 24 h. Likewise, patients who have sustained a relatively uncomplicated acute infarction can be safely transferred 24 h after their ischemic pain has resolved.

Arrhythmias should be treated as described above. The optimal heart rate during the early phase of AMI is believed to be between 60 and 90. Many physicians recommend prophylaxis with lidocaine for all suspected AMI patients during the prehospital and emergency department phases of treatment. However, the benefit of prophylactic lidocaine in these settings is not proven.

Pain relief is an important and humane goal. In addition, it reduces the circulatory load on the heart and decreases myocardial oxygen demand. The best treatment for pain is that which reduces or reverses ischemia: nitroglycerin, thrombolytics, anticoagulants, antiplatelet agents, or β-adrenergic blockers. Since such therapy takes time to provide relief, the early use of potent analgesics is often required. Intravenous morphine sulfate is the traditional treatment for the pain of AMI. Sequential small doses (4 to 6 mg) every 10 to 15 min should be used; however, complete pain relief may require up to a total dose of 15 to 20 mg of morphine. Morphine should be used with caution in patients with severe hypotension (systolic blood pressure < 80 mmHg) or chronic obstructive pulmonary disease. In the setting of AMI, the beneficial action of morphine is predominantly sedative and analgesic, which reduces oxygen demand. Morphine produces no consistent effect on preload and may actually decrease cardiac output. Meperidine hydrochloride has effects similar to those of morphine and can also be used. Pentazocine elevates preload and afterload, decreases contractility, and increases myocardial oxygen demand; it should not be used.

Nitroglycerin has traditionally been avoided in AMI for fear of inducing hypotension and tachycardia. However, recent studies have found that sublingual or intravenous nitroglycerin is both effective and safe in AMI. Additionally, nitroglycerin reduces the degree of ischemia and probably reduces infarct size and decreases in-hospital mortality in AMI. Repetitive small doses (0.4 to 1.6 mg) should be given sublingually at 3- to 5-min intervals as long as systolic blood pressure remains adequate (i.e., > 100 mmHg in most patients or > 120 mmHg in patients with a prior history of hypertension). The response of individual patients is quite variable and may require a total nitroglycerin dose of about 20 to 30 mg for complete pain control. Intravenous nitroglycerin can be initiated at an infusion rate of 10 μg/min and increased until pain is controlled or systolic blood pressure falls by about 10 percent; most patients require between 30 and 100 μg/min. Occasionally patients with AMI have what appears to be a vasovagal reaction marked by bradycardia and hypertension, to nitroglycerin. This is usually transient and responds to elevating the legs and, if required, atropine.

SUMMARY

Myocardial ischemia and infarction continue to present a diagnostic and therapeutic challenge to the emergency physician. There is no ideal method of excluding with certainty myocardial ischemia in the
ideal method of excluding with certainty myocardial ischemia in the
patient presenting with chest pain. Ischemia is even more difficult to diagnose in patients without chest pain or with atypical presentations. With these patients, the emergency physician's clinical judgment is the most important tool in diagnosis.

BIBLIOGRAPHY

Dell'Italia LJ, Starling MR, Blumhardt R, et al: Comparative effects of volume loading, dobutamine, and nitroprusside in patients with predominant right ventricular infarction. *Circulation* 72:1327, 1985.

deServi S, Ghio S, Ferrario M, et al: Clinical and angiographic findings in angina at rest. *Am Heart J* 111:6, 1986.

Forrester JS, Diamond G, Swan HJC: Correlative classification of clinical and hemodynamic functions after acute myocardial infarction. *Am J Cardiol* 39:137, 1977.

Gibler WB, Lewis LM, Erb RY, et al: Early detection of acute myocardial infarction in patients presenting with chest pain and nondiagnostic ECGs: Serial CK-MB sampling in the emergency department. *Ann Emerg Med* 19:1359, 1990.

Herlitz J, Hjalmarson A, Waagstein F: Treatment of pain in acute myocardial infarction. *Br Heart J* 61:9, 1989.

Hine LK, Laird N, Hewitt P, et al: Meta-analytic evidence against prophylactic use of lidocaine in acute myocardial infarction. *Arch Intern Med* 149:2649, 1989.

Hoekenga D, Abrams J: Rational medical therapy for stable angina pectoris. *Am J Med* 76:309, 1984.

Kim YI, Williams JF: Large dose sublingual nitroglycerin in acute myocardial infarction: Relief of chest pain and reduction of Q wave evolution. *Am J Cardiol* 49:842, 1982.

Lamas GA, Muller JE, Turi ZG, et al: A simplified method to predict occurrence of complete heart block during acute myocardial infarction. *Am J Cardiol* 57:1213, 1986.

Lavie CJ, Gersh BJ: Acute myocardial infarction: Initial manifestations, management, and prognosis. *May Clin Proc* 65:531, 1990.

Lee TH, Goldman L: The coronary care unit turns 25: Historical trends and future directions. *Ann Intern Med* 108:887, 1988.

Lee TH, Goldman L: Serum enzyme assays in the diagnosis of acute myocardial infarction. Recommendations based on a quantitative analysis. Ann Intern Med 105:221, 1986.

Maseri A: The changing face of angina pectoris: Practical implications. *Lancet* 1:746, 1983.

Rouan GW, Leee TH, Cook EF, et al: Clinical characteristics and outcome of acute myocardial infarction in patients with initially normal or nonspecific electrocardiograms: A report from the multicenter chest pain study. *Am J Cardiol* 64:1087, 1989.

18
ACUTE INTERVENTIONS IN MYOCARDIAL INFARCTION

Steven L. Almany
Cindy L. Grines
William W. O'Neill

Coronary artery disease is the leading cause of death in the United States. Despite major advancements in the treatment of acute myocardial infarction (AMI) during the last several years as well as an encouraging 47-percent reduction in age-adjusted coronary mortality rates over the past 25 years, coronary disease caused 514,000 deaths in 1987. More than 1,500,000 persons in the United States alone will suffer an AMI this year, with more than one person per minute succumbing to their disease. Sixty percent of the patients that die from AMI will die prior to hospital arrival. Over the past decade, with a greater understanding of pathophysiology, the diagnosis and treatment of these disorders has undergone significant change. It is now recognized that rapid diagnosis and treatment may have the greatest impact on mortality due to cardiovascular disease, and thus the emergency department physician's role is of utmost importance.

TRIAGE AND PREHOSPITAL TREATMENT

The complexity surrounding transportation of critically ill patients via the emergency medical system cannot be adequately addressed in this section. With the significant benefit associated with prompt administration of thrombolytic therapy, it would seem desirable to begin such treatment en route to the hospital. Several trials assessing such administration are currently under way. Preliminary data from the Nashville-Cincinnati prehospital tissue plasminogen activator (tPA) trials found that only 27 of 562 patients (4.8 percent) were candidates for prehospital thrombolysis. Trials have been plagued by numerous problems thus far, including difficulty transmitting acceptable electrocardiograms, misdiagnosis of acute infarctions, preparation and administration of the lytic agents, and adequate training of emergency medical services (EMS) personnel. Until such issues are resolved it would be prudent to pretreat suspected high-probability patients with aspirin, oxygen, sublingual nitroglycerin, heparin, and intravenous β blockers if indicated. These pharmacologic interventions are all associated with significant benefit-to-risk ratios.

The emergency physician needs to consider triage to centers capable of emergency revascularization (angioplasty or emergent coronary bypass surgery) in those patients who might not be candidates for thrombolytic therapy. As few as 9 to 38 percent of patients suffering from an AMI may actually qualify for intravenously administered thrombolytic therapy under strict inclusion guidelines established during the thrombolytic trials. Although the indications for thrombolytic therapy in the setting of AMI are likely to expand in the near future, nearly three-quarters of the excluded patients have been denied therapy on the basis of their age (over 75 years), delayed presentation (onset of symptoms greater than 4 h prior to admission), previous cerebrovascular accident or perceived inordinate bleeding risk, or nondiagnostic electrocardiogram. These patients should be considered for triage to hospitals with 24-h cardiology department availability where the risks of thrombolytic administration can be weighed against urgent diagnostic catheterization and potential revascularization. In patients who do receive thrombolytic therapy, transfer to revascularization centers should be considered if, after administration of the thrombolytic agent, the electrocardiogram fails to show evidence of improvement, the patient's symptoms have not improved, or hemodynamic compromise becomes evident. All patients in cardiogenic shock should be triaged to centers capable of revascularization. Patients in cardiogenic shock, who had an almost 90-percent mortality before development of urgent angioplasty, now survive in over 50 percent of the cases where urgent revascularization (angioplasty or bypass surgery) is performed. Thrombolytic therapy has had little impact on mortality in patients in cardiogenic shock.

NONLYTIC PHARMACOLOGIC THERAPY

Aspirin

Aspirin has been shown to be of definite benefit in the treatment of angina and AMI. The ISIS-2 study randomized approximately 18,000 patients to streptokinase or placebo as well as to low-dose aspirin (160 mg orally every day for 4 weeks) versus placebo. Mortality was reduced by 23 percent in the aspirin-treated group and nearly halved in those treated with aspirin and streptokinase. The effect of aspirin, unlike that of streptokinase, was independent of the delay from onset of symptoms to time of treatment. The combination of aspirin and streptokinase decreased the rate of early reinfarction and cerebrovascular events (cerebrovascular accidents and transient ischemic attacks).

The Antiplatelet Trialists' Collaborative Group reviewed all the long-term trials of antiplatelet agents in the secondary prevention of cardiovascular disease. The trials evaluated types of antiplatelet medications, dosages, and length of treatment required, with endpoints being cardiovascular events. With antiplatelet agents in the postinfarct setting, there was a 25-percent overall reduction in the risk of developing a major vascular event (AMI or stroke). There was no effect on noncardiac mortality.

There are no significant data to suggest that the use of aspirin plus dipyridamole of sulfinpyrazone is superior to the use of aspirin alone. The potential benefits of aspirin appear similar in doses between 160 and 1500 mg/day. There is, however, less gastrointestinal distress with the lower dosages. Enteric-coated aspirin may not be as effective as the noncoated variety in the treatment of ischemic syndromes. Because of the incidence of ileus in critically ill patients, the aspirin is probably best chewed to maximize bioavailability.

Aspirin is of definite benefit in the treatment of angina and AMI. In addition, it may be of benefit in the secondary prevention of cardiovascular disease in patients with known cardiac risk factors. It has been shown to decrease acute reocclusion after angioplasty and thus, in the absence of strict contraindications, should be given before a planned interventional procedure. In addition, it should be administered to all patients who present with unstable ischemic syndromes.

Heparin

There have been relatively few contemporary trials evaluating the independent effect of heparin therapy on mortality reduction in AMI. The pilot study performed prior to the ISIS-2 trial, in which about 600 patients were randomized to heparin or control, observed a trend toward less reinfarction among treated patients but found no difference in mortality. During the ISIS-2 trial there was a trend toward greater mortality reduction by streptokinase when more intense anticoagulation was attempted (risk reductions of 31 percent when streptokinase was used with intravenous heparin, 27 percent when used with subcutaneous heparin, and 12 percent with no heparin). Heparin resulted in a significant decrease in deep vein thrombosis, pulmonary embolism, reinfarction, and stroke. This trend toward improved mortality, however, was associated with a twofold increase in significant bleeding events. In addition, there are data suggesting that bolus intravenous heparin given early in the evolution of AMI may be a safe and effective alternative to thrombolytic therapy.

Studies involving postinfarction heparin have shown a more definite benefit. The use of heparin therapy during the periinfarction period has gained support recently because of its apparent effect on the genesis and embolization of left ventricular thrombus. Left ventricular mural thrombus formation usually occurs within the first 5 days after AMI and more commonly in anterior infarcts. Most systemic emboli occur within the first 3 months after AMI in patients with a mural thrombus, and the risk of embolization appears to be greater if the thrombus is mobile and protrudes into the left ventricular cavity. The SCATI group randomized 360 patients to 12,500 units of heparin subcutaneously twice daily and 351 patients to no heparin. None of the patients received aspirin; 433 patients received prior thrombolytic therapy. There was no difference in reinfarction, but mortality was significantly lower (21 of 360 vs. 35 of 351; $p < .03$).

In view of the consistent 10- to 20-percent reduction in mortality associated with the use of intravenous heparin during AMI, its use seems warranted despite the more than twofold increase in significant hemorrhagic events. Heparin in this setting is usually given as a 100-unit/kg bolus followed by a maintenance infusion of 10 units/kg per hour. Further therapy is guided by partial thromboplastin time (PTT) or activated clotting time (ACT) measurements. The use of heparin during the administration of thrombolytic therapy is not well studied, but current recommendations are to administer heparin concurrently with tPA and to delay therapy for 6 to 24 h in patients receiving streptokinase or APSAC (anisoylated plasminogen streptokinase activator complex). Patients are typically treated with intravenous heparin for 2 to 7 days.

Calcium Channel Blockers

Calcium channel antagonists have been used extensively in the treatment of chronic and unstable angina pectoris as well as in the treatment of hypertension. They have been shown to increase collateral flow, reduce the incidence of coronary spasm, lower blood pressure, lower vascular resistance, and decrease myocardial contractility. In addition, certain calcium channel antagonists may decrease heart rate and may be used in the treatment of supraventricular arrhythmias.

Despite these numerous beneficial cardiovascular properties, there is no clinical evidence to suggest that calcium antagonists are efficacious in the treatment of AMI.

The Diltiazem Reinfarction Study Group randomized patients to receive 90 mg every 6 h beginning 24 to 72 h after onset of infarction. They reported that diltiazem was effective in preventing early reinfarction and recurrent angina in patients with non-Q-wave (previously subendocardial) infarction. There was no statistically significant benefit in long-term diltiazem in either the Q-wave or the non-Q-wave infarction group. In fact, there was an increased incidence of adverse cardiac events in patients who received diltiazem who had evidence of left ventricular dysfunction. This may have negated any beneficial effect that would be seen in the long-term administration of diltiazem in patients with normal left ventricular function.

The Danish Verapamil Study randomized 3500 patients with suspected AMI to placebo or verapamil at a dose of 0.1 mg/kg intravenous push and oral therapy at 120 mg every 8 h. Fifteen hundred of these patients had documented AMI, with no difference in reinfarction or mortality at 6- or 12-month follow-up. Patients who had been randomized to verapamil therapy, however, had a twofold increase in the incidence of second- or third-degree heart block.

There have been numerous trials involving the use of nifedipine in AMI without conclusive evidence of any significant benefit. The Nifedipine Angina Myocardial Infarction Study consisted of 105 patients with threatened AMI and 66 patients with confirmed AMI. Patients were randomized to nifedipine, 120 mg/day orally or placebo, with randomization occurring a mean of 4.6 h from symptom onset. This study demonstrated that nifedipine was unable to prevent progression to AMI, which occurred in 75 percent in both groups, and unable to reduce infarct size. In addition, there was an alarming trend toward an increased mortality rate in the patients treated with nifedipine ($p < .02$).

In summary, there is no conclusive evidence that calcium channel blockers are of benefit in the treatment of AMI. Their use should be reserved for the treatment of hypertension, supraventricular arrhythmias, and angina; in postangioplasty patients (to prevent potential coronary vasospasm); and in patients with non-Q-wave infarctions without evidence of left ventricular dysfunction. Their benefit is less certain in patients with Q-wave infarctions and may be detrimental in any patient with impaired left ventricular function.

β Blockade

β blockers have convincingly been shown to reduce myocardial oxygen demand, limit infarct size, and reduce the incidence of recurrent ischemic events and nonfatal reinfarction. β blockers reduce myocardial oxygen demand by reducing heart rate and/or arterial pressure and have a favorable influence on myocardial blood flow distribution. In addition, the prolongation of diastole, resulting from a decrease in heart rate, allows for an increase in coronary blood flow. Almost 30 randomized trials have been reported in which intravenous β blockers were administered early in the course of AMI in the absence of thrombolytic therapy. In the largest of these trials, the ISIS-I study, more than 16,000 patients were enrolled within 12 h of onset of symptoms and administered intravenous β blockade (atenolol 5 to 10 mg) and then continued on 100 mg/day for 1 week. The 7-day mortality rate was reduced from 4.3 to 3.7 percent ($p < .02$). The 14-percent difference in mortality between the treated and nontreated groups was present by the end of day 1 and remained constant thereafter. Subsequent evaluations suggested that this early benefit may have been due to a decrease in the incidence of cardiac rupture. In the MIAMI trial, which enrolled over 5700 patients, the 15-day mortality was reduced from 4.9 to 4.3 percent, with the benefit again being evident on the first day. In this trial, metoprolol was given at doses of 5 mg intravenously every 2 min (up to 15 mg), followed by oral doses of 50 mg every 6 h. The TIMI-II trial showed in over 3200 patients that the early use of a β blocker in addition to tPA resulted in a 37-percent decrease in recurrent ischemic events and a 50-percent reduction of reinfarction compared to β-blocker therapy delayed for 6 days. Since several classes of β blockade (both cardioselective and nonselective) have been used in the studies, it appears as though the beneficial effects of these agents are not limited to particular subgroups of β blockers. However, it is generally felt that, given a choice, a β blocker without intrinsic sympathomimetic activity would be preferable.

With evidence of such profound benefit, the use of early intravenous β blockade should be considered in all AMI patients. Generally accepted guidelines for the use of early intravenous β blockade include:

Indicated/effective:

1. Patients, including those receiving thrombolytic therapy, with reflex tachycardia or systolic hypertension without signs of congestive heart failure or other contraindications to β blockade
2. Patients with continuing or recurrent ischemic pain, including those with tachyarrhythmias such as atrial fibrillation with a rapid ventricular response

Uncertain efficacy/probable benefit:

1. Patients presenting more than 6 h after symptom onset
2. Non-Q-wave AMIs

Generally accepted contraindications to early β-blocker therapy include:

Contraindications to β blockade:

1. Heart rate < 60 beats/min
2. Systolic blood pressure < 100 mmHg
3. Moderate to severe left ventricular dysfunction
4. Signs of peripheral hypoperfusion
5. Type I and II second-degree AV block
6. Third-degree (complete) AV block
7. Severe chronic obstructive pulmonary disease

Relative contraindications to β blockade:
1. History of asthma
2. Severe peripheral vascular disease
3. Concurrent use of calcium channel blockers (verapamil or diltiazem)
4. Difficult-to-control insulin-dependent diabetes
5. First-degree AV block

The benefit of long-term β blockade as it relates to reduction in reinfarction and mortality has been shown to extend at least 2 years postinfarct. These studies incorporated significant doses of β blockers, and this benefit must be weighed against the potential side effects that often accompany chronic β-blocker use.

Although significant benefit has been associated with the administration of early intravenous β blockers, as many as 51 percent of AMI patients in the TIMI-II trial were excluded from such therapy for relative contraindications such as bradycardia, hypotension, congestive heart failure, AV block, or a history of asthma. The introduction of short-acting intravenous β blockers, such as esmolol (half-life 9 min), may allow patients previously excluded from therapy more opportunities to benefit from β blockade.

INDICATIONS FOR TEMPORARY PACING

With the increasing use of thrombolytic therapy and its concomitant bleeding risk, the placement of inappropriate central cannulas needs to be closely monitored. In addition to the subsequent risk of bleeding, placement of a temporary pacing catheter has been associated with induction of arrhythmias, new right bundle branch block (7 to 25 percent), ventricular perforation, pneumothorax, hemothorax, and infection. The benefit of prophylactic temporary pacing in AMI has not been clearly defined, but the following are included as generally accepted guidelines:

Usually indicated and considered effective:
1. Complete heart block
2. Type 2 second-degree AV block
3. New left bundle branch block
4. Asystole
5. New right bundle branch block with left anterior or left posterior hemiblock
6. Symptomatic bradycardia not responsive to medications

Acceptable and probably of benefit:
1. Type 1 second-degree AV block with hypotension not responsive to atropine
2. Recurrent sinus pauses not responsive to atropine that result in bradycardia with hypotension
3. Atrial or ventricular overdrive pacing for incessant atrial flutter or ventricular tachycardia

Probably not harmful/benefit uncertain:
1. Left bundle branch block with first-degree heart block of uncertain duration
2. Bifascicular block of unknown duration

Not indicated/may be harmful:
1. First-degree heart block
2. Type 1 (Wenckebach) second-degree AV block with normal hemodynamics
3. Accelerated idioventricular rhythm causing AV dissociation
4. Bundle branch block known to exist prior to the AMI

In nonemergent situations, the use of external temporary pacing should be considered. It usually provides acceptable capture and allows the placement of a more stable system under controlled conditions. Temporary pacemakers (not external systems) can be used for overdrive pacing of ventricular tachycardia and some atrial arrhythmias (atrial flutter) as well as medically refractory torsade de pointes (polymorphic ventricular tachycardia). When ventricular function is severely compromised, particularly in the setting of a suspected right ventricular infarction, consideration should be given to placement of a temporary AV sequential pacemaker to preserve atrial augmentation.

REPERFUSION STRATEGIES IN AMI

Definitive reperfusion strategies in the treatment of AMI include nonlytic pharmacologic therapy (discussed above), thrombolytic therapy, emergency percutaneous coronary angioplasty (PTCA), and direct coronary artery bypass grafting (CABG).

CABG has received attention as a method of "controlled reperfusion" in the treatment of acute AMI. Additional support has been achieved through several uncontrolled studies that evaluated the efficacy of urgent bypass surgery in the setting of cardiogenic shock. Despite these apparent successes, the use of urgent CABG in the treatment of AMI has not become widespread, in part because of the success of other, less invasive modalities such as lytic therapy and emergent angioplasty. Elective or urgent CABG, however, remains a vital option in the management of patients with severe vessel disease that is not amenable to angioplasty.

PTCA has received considerable attention as a primary therapeutic option in the treatment of AMI. One study compared direct coronary angioplasty to intracoronary streptokinase and demonstrated that angioplasty improved ventricular function and reduced recurrent ischemic events. A recent review of 500 consecutive cases of AMI that were treated by direct coronary angioplasty without concomitant lytic therapy showed the procedure to be successful in over 94 percent of the patients. Reduction of infarct size and long-term mortality were similar to results obtained with lytic therapy. At this time, primary angioplasty has not gained widespread acceptance, probably in part because of the ease of administration of lytic agents and the logistics involved in urgent catheterization and angioplasty. At this time, only 12 percent of hospitals in the United States have sufficient facilities and trained personnel to perform urgent coronary angioplasty. However, approximately 60 percent of the United States population live within 30 min of such an institution, and as many as 80 percent live within 1 h. Studies are currently underway that directly compare the efficacy of thrombolytic agents to that of primary coronary angioplasty.

THROMBOLYTIC THERAPY FOR AMI

Studies involving the use of thrombolytic agents in the treatment of AMI have consistently shown that the timely administration of lytic therapy decreases infarction size and improves short- and long-term survival. Unfortunately, these drugs are not without serious, often life-threatening complications. Therefore, appropriate patient selection and drug administration are paramount to ensure that the maximum number of AMI patients can benefit from this therapeutic modality.

Patient Selection for Thrombolytic Therapy

The specific inclusion and exclusion criteria used by the major clinical trials have evolved as the currently accepted guidelines for thrombolytic therapy. Unfortunately, these exclusions allow as few as 9 to 38 percent of AMI patients to receive thrombolytic therapy. Conversely, for as many as 90 percent of AMI patients, the optimal reperfusion strategy has yet to be defined. It is important to recognize that many of these exclusion criteria evolved primarily as a result of historical recommendations in an attempt to reduce the risk of significant hemorrhage. Many of the criteria are based on little supporting scientific data.

Absolute contraindications:
1. Active internal bleeding
2. Suspected aortic dissection
3. History of hemorrhagic stroke or recent head trauma
4. Uncontrolled hypertension (systolic $>$ 220 or diastolic $>$ 110)
5. Menstruating or pregnant female

6. Previous allergic reaction to lytic agent
7. Recent trauma or surgery (2 weeks)
8. Known intracranial neoplasm

Relative contraindications:

1. Age over 76
2. History of cerebrovascular accident
3. Prior exposure to streptokinase of anisoylated plasminogen streptokinase activator complex (APSAC)
4. Delayed presentation (6 to 24 h after symptom onset)
5. Active peptic ulcer disease
6. Hemorrhagic retinopathy
7. Prior anticoagulation
8. Cardiopulmonary resuscitation

The most common reasons for exclusion from thrombolytic therapy in order of occurrence include delayed presentation, nondiagnostic ECG changes, age, and stroke or inordinate bleeding risk. Patients excluded from lytic therapy universally had a higher in-hospital mortality rate than did patients placed on the lytic protocols (11.8 vs. 3.9 percent).

Elderly patients have typically been excluded on the basis of a presumed increased risk of hemorrhage. This concern was probably fueled by the excessive rate of hemorrhagic complications (intracranial and retroperitoneal) that occurred in elderly patients following the use of intravenous streptokinase. The TIMI trials reported similar data, with significant bleeding occurring three times more frequently in patients over 70 years than in those under 60. In contrast, the ISIS-2 trial, which involved the largest cohort of elderly patients (1700 over age 70), showed a significant reduction in mortality (from 21.6 to 18.2 percent) without an increase in the rate of hemorrhagic complications.

With such conflicting data, other methods of reperfusion have been evaluated. Recent reports, including unpublished data from our institution, suggest that primary coronary angioplasty is associated with a high degree of technical success (94 percent) as well as a significant impact on mortality (reduced from 31 to 16 percent) when compared to age-matched controls.

At this time, with varied opinions regarding the potential complications associated with thrombolytic therapy in the elderly, it seems prudent to evaluate each case individually in regard to potential risk and benefit. The marked improvement in mortality associated with both methods of reperfusion (thrombolytic therapy and emergent angioplasty) suggests that the elderly cohort may have the most to gain from aggressive reperfusion strategies.

The exclusion of patients with delayed presentation (6 to 24 after symptom onset) was primarily based on canine models that showed evidence of irreversible cardiac damage after 4 h of coronary ischemia. Although the GISSI study did not show any significant benefit to late reperfusion, the ISIS-2 study, in which patients were treated with thrombolytics up to 24 h after onset of symptoms, revealed a significant mortality benefit. Studies from our institution have suggested that direct angioplasty is associated with a high rate of technical success (94 percent) and a significant impact on survival (4 vs. 13 percent).

Several trials under way at this time, including LATE, EMERAS, and TAMI-6, are designed to address the issue of delayed reperfusion. At this time, such therapy can only be recommended for those patients with evidence of continued ischemia or an uncertain time of symptom onset.

Patients with a history of cerebrovascular accident, recent head trauma or surgery, or known active bleeding diathesis are still routinely excluded from receiving thrombolytic therapy. A study of 154 patients with spontaneous intracranial hemorrhage following thrombolytic therapy found that these patients were frequently hypertensive (54 percent) at the time of presentation or had a history of a prior cerebral event or neoplasm (27 percent). It is alarming that over 40 percent had no predisposing condition identified. Currently, some cardiologists recommend avoiding thrombolytic therapy in all patients with any history of cerebrovascular disease, while some feel that lytic therapy is safe in patients with a remote history (>6 months) of ischemic stroke. This issue remains to be resolved, and at this time direct coronary artery angioplasty is probably the most universally accepted method of reperfusion in patients with a history of a cerebrovascular accident, bleeding diathesis, or recent trauma or surgery.

Patients entered into the thrombolytic trials have typically been required to show evidence of transmural infarction with ST elevation of more than 1 to 2 mm in two or more electrically contiguous leads. Although thrombolytic therapy has been shown to be of definitive benefit in this group, it has been shown to be of only minimal benefit in those patients without evidence of ST elevation. Both the ISIS-2 and GISSI-I trials showed that the mortality rate for patients with suspected myocardial infarction and ST depression was high (18 percent) and was only minimally improved with lytic agents. Several ongoing trials, including ISIS-3, TIMI-III, TIMIT, and the Multicenter Urokinase for Unstable Angina Trial, are currently evaluating reperfusion strategies in these patients. There are currently no convincing data to support the use of thrombolytic agents in unstable angina. At this time, optimal management includes the use of nonlytic pharmacologic methods with noninvasive (echocardiogram) assessment for new wall motion abnormalities. Those patients with refractory symptoms and/or new wall abnormalities should be triaged to more aggressive therapy (lytic therapy or catheterization/angioplasty).

Thrombolytic Agents

Complete thrombotic coronary occlusion is present in a majority of patients presenting with AMI. This process, which is multifactorial in nature, ultimately involves ruptured vascular endothelium at the site of an atherosclerotic plaque. In response to the vessel injury, platelets adhere to the damaged endothelium and activate coagulation factors, which results in fibrin formation. Although their precise mechanisms of action differ, all the current thrombolytic agents act by activation of plasminogen to the active enzyme plasmin, which dissolves the clot's fibrin component. The agents differ to some degree in their fibrin specificity, duration of action, potential allergic reactions, and cost.

Streptokinase

Streptokinase activates fibrin that is bound as well as circulating plasminogen and thus does not possess fibrin specificity. The product is derived from β-hemolytic streptococci and therefore elicits an antigenic response. Allergic responses, which can be especially pronounced in patients with a recent streptococcal infection, occur in approximately 5 percent of patients and consist of pruritus, rash, and low-grade fevers. This reaction is usually self-limited and responds to antihistamines and antipyretics. The incidence of anaphylaxis is less than 0.2 percent.

Streptokinase is given as a 1.5 million-unit dose over 60 to 90 min. This dose is usually sufficient to overcome the effect of any circulating neutralizing antibodies. At this dosage, most patients develop systemic fibrinolysis, which persists for up to 24 h. Antibodies develop approximately 5 days after the administration of streptokinase and persist for 6 months; therefore, retreatment with streptokinase (or the related compounds APSAC/Eminase) is not recommended. During administration of streptokinase, approximately 15 percent of patients develop hypotension, which improves with decreasing the infusion rate and volume expansion.

Streptokinase is perhaps the most well studied of the available thrombolytic agents. It has been shown to improve left ventricular function and decrease mortality in the setting of AMI. Its primary disadvantage is its potential for allergic reactions and hypotensive episodes during administration. It is the most inexpensive of the currently available agents.

Table 18-1. Characteristics of Currently Available Thrombolytic Agents

	Streptokinase	TPA	APSAC	Urokinase
IV dose and administration	1.5 million U: 1-h infusion	100 mg: 60 mg, 20 mg, and 20 mg over hours 1, 2, and 3	30 U: bolus 2–5 min	3 million U: 1.5-million U bolus, then 1.5-million U over 1 h
Systemic lysis or bleeding risk	High/high	Low/high	High/high	High/high
Antigenicity	Yes	No	Yes	No
Allergic reaction or hypotension	Yes	No	Yes	No
Acute patency rates	40–60%	60–80%	60–70%	50–70%
Cost*	~$200	$2100	$1700	$1700
Mortality reduction	Yes	Yes	Yes	?

* Pharmacy cost at William Beaumont Hospital, Royal Oak, Mich.

Tissue Plasminogen Activator (tPA, Activase)

Tissue plasminogen activator (tPA) is a naturally occurring human protein without antigenic properties, which makes readministration possible. It is derived from recombinant DNA technology, has a short half-life (5 min), and is fibrin-specific. This fibrin specificity allows for less depletion of circulating fibrinogen than occurs with streptokinase. In theory, this makes for fewer bleeding complications, although this has not yet been shown to be the case. The recommended dose of TPA is 100 mg over 3 h (60 mg over the first hour, 20 mg over the second, and 20 mg over the third). Newer dosing regimens have been developed in hope of limiting bleeding complications. Currently, in patients less than 65 kg, a total dose of 1.25 mg/kg is administered over 3 h, with 10 percent as a bolus, 50 percent over the first hour, and 40 percent over the last 2 h. Advantages of TPA include its lack of antigenicity and the possibility of subsequent allergic reactions. Although its reperfusion rates have been demonstrated to be higher than that of streptokinase, reocclusion rates may also be higher, thereby offsetting any potential benefit. tPA is the costliest thrombolytic agent.

Anisoylated Plasminogen (APSAC/Eminase) Streptokinase Activator Complex (APSAC)

APSAC/Eminase is a second-generation thrombolytic agent that was developed to overcome some of the limitations of streptokinase. The drug can be administered over 2 to 5 min as a bolus injection. This acylated derivative of streptokinase has several properties that differ from the parent compound. It has a longer duration of action (pharmacologic half-life 90 min), and the allergic effects may be fewer than those of streptokinase. The currently approved 30-mg dose has achieved coronary patency and mortality reduction similar to that of streptokinase administration. Potential advantages include easier administration, which might facilitate prehospital use. The cost is slightly below that of tPA.

Urokinase

Urokinase is a proteolytic enzyme produced from human fetal kidney tissue cultures. Although urokinase is approved for intracoronary use, the intravenous route of administration has yet to achieve FDA approval. The standard dose of 3 million units (over 1 h, with 1.5 million initially given as a bolus) usually causes systemic fibrinolysis. The incidences of coronary patency and reocclusion are comparable to those for streptokinase. In contrast to streptokinase, administration of urokinase is not usually accompanied by hypotension or allergic reactions. Severe shaking chills are occasionally noted and respond to intravenous meperidine and benadryl.

Comparison of Thrombolytic Agents

At this time there are no definitive data to advocate one thrombolytic agent over the others (Table 18-1). The GISSI-II trial showed no particular advantage between tPA and streptokinase. The ISIS-III trial, the first large-scale randomized trial to directly compare streptokinase, tPA, and APSAC, recently reported no difference in mortality between these agents. More cerebrovascular events, however, were noted in the tPA-treated patients.

PREPARATION FOR ANGIOGRAPHY

Although numerous trials have conclusively shown that intravenous thrombolytic therapy reduces mortality during AMI, not all patients are eligible for such therapy. In addition, a subset of patients who receive lytic therapy will fail to show evidence of successful reperfusion. Therefore, other reperfusion strategies have emerged, including emergent PTCA. This modality allows the cardiologist to determine arterial patency as well as to define subsets, such as left main or three-vessel disease, that might require urgent triage to angioplasty or CABG. In addition, it allows rapid diagnosis and treatment of patients who might exhibit evidence of mechanical complications of AMI, including ventricular septal rupture or acute mitral regurgitation.

Generally accepted risks of cardiac catheterization include death (<0.2 percent), other major adverse effects (<0.5 percent), such as cerebrovascular accident, cardiac perforation, arrhythmia, significant hemorrhage, nephrotoxicity, contrast allergy, or AMI. Complications at the vascular access site include hematoma, bleeding, infection, AV malformation, and pseudoaneurysm formation. Additional risks of PTCA include death (<1.3 percent), nonfatal AMI (<4 percent), and emergency CABG (3 percent). Certain subgroups of patients have been associated with an increased incidence of the above-mentioned complications.

Factors associated with increased risk of cardiovascular complications during cardiac catheterization/angioplasty:

1. Advanced age
2. Diabetes mellitus
3. Female sex
4. Congestive heart failure
5. Severe hypertension
6. Previous AMI or CABG
7. Peripheral vascular disease
8. Multiple PVCs

Factors associated with increased risk of contrast-mediated nephrotoxicity during cardiac catheterization/angioplasty:

1. Diabetes mellitus
2. Elevated serum creatinine
3. Dehydration

Factors associated with increased risk of contrast-mediated allergic reaction during cardiac catheterization/angioplasty:

1. Prior contrast media reaction
2. History of asthma or rhinitis
3. History of allergies (in particular to shellfish or iodine)

Transient renal impairment (defined as an increased creatinine) may occur in up to 20 percent of patients undergoing cardiac angiography. This impairment is usually self-limited, with less than 0.3 percent eventually developing overt renal failure. Certain subgroups, particularly diabetics, patients with preexisting renal disease, and patients with evidence of dehydration, are at increased risk of developing contrast-mediated nephrotoxicity. In addition, patients with poor left ventricular function or valvular disease (especially aortic stenosis) are more likely to experience hemodynamic compromise with contrast agents (particularly ionic compounds). Therefore, the emergency physician should attempt to identify these high-risk subgroups and pretreat them appropriately. Diabetics and patients with evidence of dehydration should be hydrated judiciously prior to the procedure. Patients with a history of marked left ventricular dysfunction or overt congestive heart failure would benefit most from pretreatment with diuretics and nitrates.

The estimated evidence of allergic reaction to contrast media is 1/100 for an intermediate reaction (i.e., itching, hives) to 1/2000 for a severe life-threatening anaphylactic reaction. Approximately 1/40,000 patients will expire because of a contrast-induced reaction. The generally accepted premedication (our institutional regimen) for known or suspected contrast allergy includes steroids (hydrocortisone 100 mg by intravenous push bolus q 6 h or prednisone 50 mg orally q 6 h), a histamine$_1$ receptor-blocker (benadryl 50 mg by intravenous push or orally q 6 h), and a histamine$_2$ receptor-blocker (cimetidine 300 mg orally or by intravenous push bolus q 6 h). Unfortunately, neither this combination nor any other currently in use has been shown to eliminate the risk of a potentially life-threatening reaction, and this risk should be weighed against the potential benefit of the proposed procedure.

BIBLIOGRAPHY

AIMS Trial Study Group: Effect of intravenous APSAC on mortality after acute myocardial infarction: Preliminary report of a placebo-controlled clinical trial. *Lancet* 1:545, 1988.

Almany SL, Cragg DR, O'Neill WW: Early and late results of delayed arterial recanalization in the treatment of acute myocardial infarction. 1991 (in press).

Antiplatelet Trialists' Collaboration: Secondary prevention of vascular disease by prolonged antiplatelet treatment. *Br Med J* 296:316, 1988.

Armstrong WF, West SR, Mueller TM, et al: Assessment of location and size of myocardial infarction with contrast enhanced echocardiography. *J Am Coll Cardiol* 2:63, 1983.

Austin JL, Preis LK, Crampton RS, et al: Analysis of pacemaker malfunction and complications of temporary pacing in the coronary care unit. *Am J Cardiol* 49:301, 1982.

Berman GO, Wolf NM, Schechter JA: Heparin induces coronary reperfusion in the very early myocardial infarction (abstr). *J Am Coll Cardiol* 7(suppl 2):17A, 1986.

Brott T, Thalinger K, Hertzberg V: Hypertension as a risk factor for spontaneous intracerebral hemorrhage. *Stroke* 17:1078, 1986.

Bussmann WD, Passek D, Seidel W, et al: Reduction of CK and CK-MB indexes of infarct size by intravenous nitroglycerin. *Circulation* 63:615, 1981.

Califf RM, Mark DB, Wagner GS: *Acute Coronary Care in the Thrombolytic Era*. Chicago, Yearbook Medical Publishers, 1988.

Chaitman BR, Thompson B, Wittry MD, et al: The use of tissue type plasminogen activator in the elderly: Results from the Thrombolysis in Myocardial Infarction Phase I, open-label studies and the Thrombolysis in Myocardial Infarction Phase II Pilot Study. *J Am Coll Cardiol* 14:1159, 1989.

Come PC, Pitt B: Nitroglycerin-induced severe hypotension and bradycardia in patients with acute myocardial infarction. *Circulation,* 1976.

Cragg DR, Almany SL, O'Neill WW: Early and late results of direct coronary angioplasty for acute myocardial infarction in patients over 76. 1991 (in press).

Cragg DR, Friedman HZ, Bonema JD, et al: Ineligibility for intravenous thrombolytic therapy predicts high mortality after acute myocardial infarction *Ann Int Med* 1991 (in press).

Danish Study Group on Verapamil in Myocardial Infarction: Verapamil in acute myocardial infarction. *Eur Heart J* 5:516, 1984.

Detre K, Holubkov R, Kelsey S: Percutaneous transluminal coronary angioplasty in 1985–86 and 1977–81. *N Engl J Med* 318:265, 1988.

DeWood MA, Spores J, Notske R, et al: Prevalence of total coronary occlusion during the early hours of transmural myocardial infarction. *N Engl J Med* 303:897, 1980.

Fillmore SJ, Shapiro M, Killip T: Arterial oxygen tension in acute myocardial infarction: Serial analysis of clinical state and blood gas changes. *Am Heart J* 79:620, 1970.

Fleckenstein A: History of calcium antagonists. *Circ Res* 52(suppl 1):111, 1983.

Forrester JS, Litvack F, Grundfest W, et al: A perspective of coronary disease seen through the arteries of a living man. *Circulation* 75:505, 1987.

Ganz W, Geft I, Shah PK, et al: Intravenous streptokinase in evolving acute myocardial infarction. *Am J Cardiol* 53:1209, 1984.

Graves EJ: 1989 National Hospital Discharge Survey: Annual Summary, 1987. *Vital Health Statistics* 13(99): 1987.

Grines CL, DeMaria AN: Optimal utilization of thrombolytic therapy for acute myocardial infarction: Concepts and controversies. *J Am Coll Cardiol* 16:223, 1990.

Gruppo Italiana per lo Studio della Streptochiinasi nell'Infarcto Miocardico (GISSI): Effectiveness of intravenous thrombolytic treatment in acute myocardial infarction. *Lancet* 1:349, 1986.

Gunnar RM: ACC/AHA Task Force Report on Acute Myocardial Infarction. *J Am Coll Cardiol* 16:247, 1990.

Gunnar RM, Lambrew CT, Abrams W, et al: Task force IV: Pharmacologic interventions. *Am J Cardiol* 50:393, 1982.

Hauser AM: The emerging role of echocardiography in the emergency department. *Emerg Med* 18:1298, 1989.

Hine LK, Laird N, Hewitt P, et al: Meta-analytic evidence against prophylactic use of lidocaine in acute myocardial infarction. *Arch Intern Med* 149:2694, 1989.

ISIS-I Collaborative Group: Mechanisms for the early mortality reduction produced by beta-blockade started early in acute myocardial infarction. *Lancet* 1:921, 1988.

ISIS-I (First International Study of Infarct Survival) Collaborative Group: Randomized trial of intravenous atenolol among 16,027 cases of suspected acute myocardial infarction: ISIS-I. *Lancet* 2:57, 1986.

ISIS Pilot Study Investigators: Randomized factorial trial of high-dose intravenous streptokinase, of oral aspirin and of intravenous heparin in acute myocardial infarction. *Eur Heart J* 8:634, 1987.

ISIS-2 (Second International Study of Infarct Survival) Collaborative Group: Randomized trial of intravenous streptokinase, oral aspirin, both, or neither among 17,187 cases of suspected acute myocardial infarction: ISIS-2. *Lancet* 2:349, 1988.

Jugdutt BI, Warnica JW: Intravenous nitroglycerin therapy to limit myocardial infarct size, expansion and complications: Effect of timing, dosing and infarct location. *Circulation* 78:906, 1988.

Kagen L, Scheidt S, Butt A: Serum myoglobin in myocardial infarction: The "staccato phenomenon." Is acute myocardial infarction in man an intermittent event? *Am J Med* 62:86, 1977.

Katus HA, Yasuda T, Gold HK, et al: Diagnosis of acute myocardial infarction by detection of circulating cardiac myosin light chains. *Am J Cardiol* 54:964, 1984.

Laks H, Rosenbranz E, Buckberg GD: Surgical treatment of cardiogenic shock after myocardial infarction. *Circulation* 74(suppl 3): 1, 1986.

Lester R: Achieving pain relief with physiologic management and analgesic agents during acute myocardial infarction, in Califf RM, Wagner GS (eds): *Acute Coronary Care: Principles and Practice,* Boston, Martinus Nijhoff, 1985, pp. 299–309.

Lown B, Vassaux C: Lidocaine in acute myocardial infarction. *Am Heart J,* 1968.

MacMahon S, Collins R, Knight C, et al: Reduction in major morbidity and mortality by heparin in acute myocardial infarction (abstr). *Circulation* 78:(suppl 2):98, 1988.

MacMahon S, Collins R, Peto R, et al: Effects of prophylactic lidocaine in suspected acute myocardial infarction: An overview of results from the randomized controlled trials. *JAMA* 260:1910, 1988.

May GS, Furberg CD, Eberlein KA, et al: Secondary prevention after myocardial infarction: A review of short-term acute-phase trials. *Prog Cardiovasc Dis* 25:335, 1983.

MIAMI Trial Research Group: Metoprolol in acute myocardial infarction (MIAMI). *Am J Cardiol* 56:1G, 1985.

Morris TW, Fischer HW: The pharmacology of radiocontrast media. *Ann Rev Pharmacol Toxicol* 26:143, 1986.

Muller JE, Morrison J, Stone PH: Nifedipine therapy for patients with threatened and acute myocardial infarction: A randomized, double blind, placebo-controlled comparison. *Circulation* 69:740, 1984.

Multicenter Diltiazem Postinfarction Trial Research Group: The effect of diltiazem on mortality and reinfarction after myocardial infarction. *N Engl J Med* 319:385, 1988.

National Center for Health Statistics: *Monthly Vital Statistics Report* 36(13): 1988.

O'Keefe JH, Rutherford BD, McConahay DR: Early and late results of coronary angioplasty without antecedent thrombolytic therapy for acute myocardial infarction. *Am J Cardiol* 64:1221, 1989.

O'Neill WW, Timmis GC, Bourdillion PD, et al: A prospective randomized trial of intracoronary streptokinase versus coronary angioplasty for acute myocardial infarction. *N Engl J Med* 314:812, 1986.

Reeder GS, Seward JB, Tajik AJ: The role of two-dimensional echocardiography in coronary artery disease: A critical appraisal. *Mayo Clin Proc* 57:247, 1982.

SCATI Group: Randomized controlled trial of subcutaneous calcium-heparin in acute myocardial infarction. *Lancet* 2:182, 1989.

Sobel BE, Braunwald E: The management of acute myocardial infarction, in Braunwald E. (ed): *Heart Disease: A Textbook of Cardiovascular Medicine,* 2d ed. Philadelphia, Saunders, 1984, pp. 1308–1309.

TIMI Study Group: Comparison of invasive and conservative strategies after treatment with intravenous tissue plasminogen activator in acute myocardial infarction: Results of the Thrombolysis in Myocardial Infarction (TIMI) Phase II trial. *N Engl J Med* 320:618, 1989.

Van de Werf F, Arnold AER, European Cooperative Study Group for Recombinant Tissue Type Plasminogen Activator (rt-PA): Intravenous tissue plasminogen activator and size of infarct, left ventricular function, and survival in acute myocardial infarction. *Br Med J* 297:2374, 1988.

Wilcox RG, Olsson CG, Skene AM, et al: Trial of tissue plasminogen activator for mortality reduction in acute myocardial infarction. *Lancet* 1:525, 1988.

Yusuf S: Interventions that potentially limit myocardial infarct size: Overview of clinical trials. *Am J Cardiol* 60:11A, 1987.

Yusuf S, Collins R, Peto R, et al: Intravenous and intracoronary fibrinolytic therapy in acute myocardial infarction: Overview of results on mortality, reinfarction and side-effects from 33 randomized controlled trials. *Eur Heart J* 6:556, 1985.

Yusuf S, Peto R, Lewis J, et al: Beta blockade during and after myocardial infarction: An overview of the randomized trials. *Prog Cardiovasc Dis* 27:335, 1985.

Zelis R, Mansour EJ, Capone RJ, et al: The cardiovascular effects of morphine: The peripheral capacitance and resistance vessels in human subjects. *J Clin Invest* 54:1247, 1974.

Zipes DP: Management of cardiac arrhythmias: Pharmacological, electrical and surgical techniques, in Braunwald E (ed): *Heart Disease: A Textbook of Cardiovascular Medicine,* 3d ed. Philadelphia, Saunders, 1988, pp. 625–627.

19 CONGESTIVE HEART FAILURE AND PULMONARY EDEMA

J. Stephan Stapczynski

CONGESTIVE HEART FAILURE

Heart failure is the clinical syndrome that occurs when cardiac pump function is inadequate—at normal filling pressures—to meet the circulatory demands of the body. Often, heart failure produces retention of fluid within many locations of the body (''congestion'' or edema), and the term *congestive heart failure* (CHF) is commonly used. Heart failure can be categorized in several respects: according to (1) rapidity of onset (acute or chronic), (2) which ventricle is predominantly impaired (right, left, or both), and (3) overall cardiac output (high, normal, or low). CHF occurs as the result of many different diseases, but often the clinical manifestations are exacerbated by coexistent diseases or other contributing factors. Therefore, appropriate therapy consists of treating both the primary process as well as any contributing factors.

Etiology

Right ventricular failure is most commonly caused by left ventricular failure. Isolated right-sided heart failure may occur as the result of pulmonary arterial hypertension, mitral or tricuspid valvular disease, restrictive or infiltrative cardiomyopathies, viral or idiopathic myocarditis, or some forms of congenital heart disease (CHD). Right-sided heart failure differs from left-sided failure in two important characteristics: (1) in right-sided failure, cardiac output and systemic blood pressure are usually decreased; and (2) in right-sided failure, fluid accumulation occurs primarily in dependent areas of the body and not the lungs. The common causes of left ventricular failure depress cardiac output: hypertension, coronary artery disease, aortic or mitral valvular disease, and dilated (congestive) cardiomyopathies. Less frequently, heart failure occurs with an elevated cardiac output, as the left ventricle is unable to meet the exceedingly high circulatory demands sometimes required in hyperthyroidism, septic shock, arteriovenous fistula, or Paget's disease.

As noted below, compensatory processes tend to preserve cardiac output and patients may remain asymptomatic with mild to moderate ventricular pump dysfunction, provided circulatory demands remain modest and stable. However, other factors may develop, demanding an increased cardiac output, and precipitating clinical symptoms and signs of heart failure. The most common precipitating factors of heart failure are (1) cardiac tachyarrhythmias, such as atrial fibrillation; (2) acute myocardial ischemia or infarction; (3) discontinuation of medications such as diuretics; (4) increased sodium intake; (5) administration of drugs which impair myocardial function, such as β-adrenergic or calcium channel antagonists; and (6) physical overexertion.

Acute left-sided heart failure usually produces pulmonary edema. However, pulmonary edema can also occur as the result of noncardiac causes. This process, termed *noncardiogenic pulmonary edema,* is discussed in Chapter 34.

Pathophysiology of Congestive Heart Failure

The fluid retention and peripheral edema of CHF are due to several factors. As right ventricular volume and pressure increase, the systemic venous and capillary pressure rise and fluid transudates from the vascular to interstitial space. As cardiac contractility and output decline, compensatory arteriolar vasoconstriction redistributes blood flow so that the brain and heart remain well perfused at the expense of flow to the bowel, kidneys, and muscle. The drop in renal blood flow activates the renin-angiotensin-aldosterone system, causing increased sodium retention. The hepatic metabolism of aldosterone is also impaired, so that the hormone remains active longer in the circulation.

Pulmonary vascular congestion and edema are due to a rise in left atrial pressure, which in turn elevates pulmonary capillary pressure. The major forces involved in the production of pulmonary edema are expressed in the Starling equation as the difference between pulmonary capillary hydrostatic pressure and plasma oncotic pressure. However, important roles are also played by interstitial-fluid hydrostatic and oncotic pressure, alveolar surface tension, and the pulmonary lymphatics. Pulmonary edema does not always occur when capillary hydrostatic pressure exceeds plasma oncotic pressure; the precise mechanisms involved in the production of pulmonary edema are still poorly understood.

As fluid transudates into the interstitial spaces of the lung, pulmonary arterial resistance rises and lung compliance falls. In an upright individual, this increase in pulmonary arterial resistance redistributes blood flow from the bases to the apices of the lung. The decrease in lung compliance produces the sensation of dyspnea. When the patient becomes supine for a period of time, fluid present in lower extremity edema can slowly be redistributed to other areas of the body, including the lungs, producing pulmonary vascular congestion and edema when the patient is supine; this symptom is termed *paroxysmal nocturnal dyspnea.* When heart failure is even more severe, the patient develops pulmonary vascular congestion as a result of the almost immediate slight rise in venous return seen in assuming the recumbent position; this symptom is termed *orthopnea.* Fluid is removed from the interstitial space by the pulmonary lymphatics, but when the system is overburdened, fluid spills over into the alveolar spaces. Severe pulmonary edema irritates the bronchioles and they often go into reflex spasm. Alveolar edema is clinically detected by rales and, when there is associated bronchospasm, by wheezes. There are regional differences in accumulation of fluid, so that ventilation perfusion inequality results, leading to variable degrees of arterial hypoxemia. In many patients respiratory stimulation produces alveolar hyperventilation and a lowered Pa_{CO_2}, while in others the alveolar edema is so severe that alveolar hypoventilation occurs with an elevated Pa_{CO_2}.

Preload and afterload are concepts used in discussions of left ventricular failure. *Preload* refers to the pressure which fills the left ventricle during diastole, measured either directly as the left ventricular end-diastolic pressure or indirectly as the pulmonary artery wedge pressure (PAWP). Afterload refers to the pressure against which the left ventricle pumps; measured as the mean aortic pressure.

As heart failure develops, three major compensatory mechanisms initially help maintain cardiac output, but they have effects that become deleterious in time.

The first compensation is through the Frank-Starling relation, a concept that states that a myocardial cell will contract with a greater force as its precontraction length is increased. The clinical correlate is that as the left ventricular filling pressure increases (increased preload), the left ventricle dilates, stretching individual myocardial cells which contract with greater vigor, and the sum of their individual efforts is an increased volume of blood ejected with systole. This relationship is often displayed showing how the left ventricular stroke volume or cardiac output varies with increases or decreases in PAWP. However, the Frank-Starling process has its limits: (1) myocardial cells can be stretched only so far before they reach their limits of contractility, beyond which they may even contract less; (2) increased left ventricular filling pressures are reflected back to the pulmonary veins, where such pressure may exceed plasma oncotic pressure and lead to pulmonary edema; and (3) this enhanced contractility increases myocardial oxygen demand—a potential harm in patients with ischemic heart disease. The second compensation is myocardial hypertrophy stimulated by pressure or volume overloads. Although hypertrophy (with its enhanced contractility) is potentially beneficial, it does entail the costs of increased oxygen demand, reduced ventricular compliance, and enhanced sus-

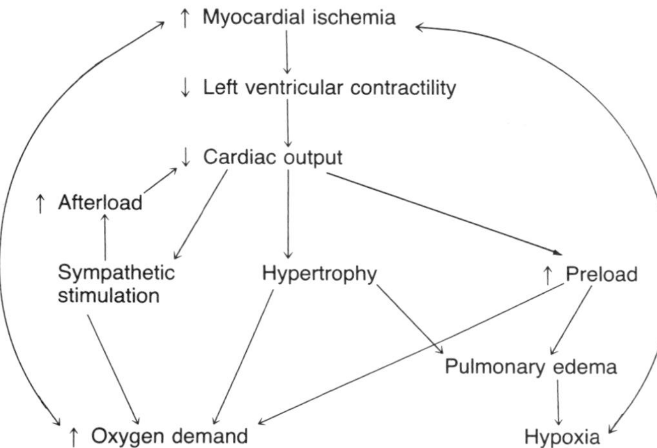

Fig. 19-1. Deleterious effect of sustained compensations in congestive heart failure.

ceptibility to pulmonary edema with small increases in left ventricular volume. The third compensation is stimulation of the sympathetic nervous system as the baroreceptors sense a declining cardiac output. Increased sympathetic activity produces peripheral vasoconstriction, increased heart rate, and increased myocardial contractility. Many patients with chronic CHF easily decompensate with β-adrenergic antagonists, appearing to require constant catecholamine stimulation to maintain cardiac output and perfusion pressure. However, there are some patients who improve with β-adrenergic antagonists, suggesting that constant sympathetic stimulation can be deleterious, perhaps because of the increased afterload due to peripheral vasoconstriction. All three compensatory mechanisms may eventually act to further depress cardiac output, an example of "positive" feedback, leading to the establishment of a vicious cycle of progressive cardiac deterioration (Fig. 19-1).

Clinical Features of Congestive Heart Failure

Edema, the classic sign of right-sided heart failure, generally occurs in dependent parts of the body such as the feet, ankles, and pretibial region. In bedridden patients sacral edema is prominent. Anasarca, or massive edema, may affect the genitalia, trunk, and upper extremities. If predominantly right-sided CHF is present, the patient can generally lie flat without dyspnea. Ascites is not common in right-sided CHF, although it is somewhat more prominent in patients with tricuspid valvular disease or constrictive pericarditis. Other causes of edema and ascites are cirrhosis, nephrotic syndrome, protein-losing enteropathy, inferior vena cava obstruction, and mesenteric or hepatic venous obstruction.

Transudative pleural effusion can occur in both right- and left-sided CHF because the pleura is perfused by both the systemic and pulmonic circulation. In CHF the pleural effusion is usually more prominent on the right side.

A positive hepatojugular reflux is an early sign of right-sided CHF and, if failure progresses, jugular venous distention will appear.

Hepatic tenderness and enlargement are generally present with moderate to severe right-sided CHF. The standard liver function tests usually indicate hepatocellular injury. The most common abnormality is a prolonged prothrombin time, while conversely, jaundice is unusual. In severe right-sided CHF or tricuspid regurgitation, the liver may be pulsatile. Nocturia is common and is due to mobilization and subsequent excretion of dependent edema while the patient is supine. Patients usually have an impaired ability to excrete sodium and water. Hyponatremia is common.

The first symptom of left-sided CHF is usually exertional dyspnea. As CHF progresses, paroxysmal nocturnal dyspnea followed by orthopnea develops. Interstitial edema often produces a dry cough, while alveolar edema causes coughing of frothy, pink sputum as fluid and red cells exude into the alveolar spaces. Some patients with pulmonary edema, especially the elderly, have Cheyne-Stokes respirations because the prolonged circulatory time between the lungs and brain slows the ventilatory response to alterations in Pa_{CO_2}.

On auscultation, moist pulmonary rales and an S_3 or S_4 are detectable. Pulsus alternans, or alternating weak and strong pulses, may be detected by palpation or sphygmomanometry.

There are nospecific electrocardiographic abnormalities due to CHF or pulmonary edema, but depending on the myocardial disease, the ECG will often show hypertrophy, chamber enlargement, subendocardial ischemia, or conduction disturbances.

Three progressive chest radiographic stages of CHF have been described; however there may be as much as a 12-h delay in visible radiographic changes after the onset of acute heart failure and up to a 4-day delay in resolution of radiographic changes after clinical improvement. The first stage occurs during chronic elevation in left atrial pressure, which causes reflex pulmonary vasoconstriction and redistribution of blood flow to the upper lung fields. This usually occurs when PAWP is elevated above 12 to 18 mmHg. The second stage occurs when further elevations in left atrial pressure produce interstitial edema, visible as blurred edges of blood vessels, and Kerley A and B lines. The PAWP is typically 18 to 25 mmHg. The third stage occurs when fluid exudes into the alveoli and is characterized by the classic bilateral hazy perihilar infiltrates ("butterfly"). The PAWP is usually above 25 mmHg.

Acid-base derangements in pulmonary edema cannot be predicted from the patient's clinical condition; therefore, arterial blood gases must be routinely obtained in pulmonary edema. The most common abnormalities are hypoxemia and acidosis. The acidosis is usually metabolic but may also be respiratory.

Treatment of Chronic Congestive Heart Failure

Treatment of chronic CHF consists of reducing circulatory demands, correcting precipitating factors, decreasing vascular congestion, increasing cardiac contractility, and treating the underlying myocardial disease if possible.

Vascular congestion can be reduced by restricting sodium intake and promoting diuresis with diuretics. Patients with advanced CHF are usually resistant to thiazide-type diuretics and generally require potent agents such as furosemide or bumetanide. In addition to relieving symptoms of vascular congestion, chronic diuretic therapy in CHF has been shown to lower systemic vascular resistance and increase cardiac output.

Digitalis has traditionally been used to improve cardiac contractility in CHF. Recent studies on the efficacy of long-term digitalis therapy for CHF have yielded variable results, but a reasonable consensus is that chronic digitalis therapy produces a sustained and measurable—albeit small—increase in cardiac output in CHF. Conversely, many or most stable patients with mild to moderate CHF can be maintained with diuretics alone. The most effective use of digitalis in CHF is to slow and control the ventricular rate when atrial fibrillation is present.

Nonglycoside inotropic agents are currently being investigated for use in CHF; some of them show promise for long-term oral therapy. The most recent development along these lines is the discovery of a new class of phosphodiesterase inhibitors which have both inotropic and vasodilatory effects, the bipyridine derivatives amrinone and milrinone. Intravenous amrinone is approved by the FDA for short-term treatment of severe CHF; however, some experts believe that amrinone may possess significant cardiac toxicity in this setting. Oral milrinone has been found in small studies to be safe and effective for periods as long as a year in the treatment of severe CHF. Milrinone is not currently released for general use in the United States.

As cardiac output falls in CHF, systemic vascular resistance rises, which has a further deleterious effect on the heart by increasing afterload and wall tension. Vasodilator therapy reverses this process, lowers systemic vascular resistance, and increases cardiac output. Several agents are currently used, some affecting predominantly the venous system and reducing preload, some affecting predominantly the arterioles and reducing afterload, and some exerting both actions. For example, sublingual or oral nitrates affect preload almost exclusively, oral hydralazine predominantly affects afterload, and oral prazosin, nifedipine, or captopril have more balanced effects on preload and afterload. Given acutely, vasodilators increase cardiac output in almost all patients with CHF, and most short-term studies have also revealed a relief in symptoms and improvement in exercise tolerance. However, with continued use, many patients do not maintain their initial improvement in left ventricular function, symptoms, or exercise tolerance, and the available evidence did not show any increase in survival. Recently, one large, multicenter study of men with moderate CHF did demonstrate a reduction in mortality over a 3-year period with the use of oral hydralazine and isosorbide dinitrate vasodilator therapy. Whether this observation applies to all patients with CHF and all classes of vasodilator agents remains to be determined.

β-Adrenergic antagonists are usually considered to be contraindicated in patients with chronic CHF for fear of further depressing left ventricular contractility. But some patients with CHF have excessive and harmful sympathetic activation where β-antagonist treatment is actually beneficial. At present, it is not possible—short of a therapeutic trial—to determine which patients will improve and which will not with β-blocker treatment. It is still uncertain whether such therapy will yield increased survival.

The long-term prognosis of chronic CHF is generally poor regardless of the etiology. In most studies, the 5-year mortality is usually around 50 percent or greater. Approximately half of the deaths appear to be sudden, suggesting that lethal ventricular arrhythmias play an important role and partially explains why vasodilators may not have a profound effect on long-term survival. It remains uncertain whether patients at risk for sudden death can be detected and treated.

Treatment of Acute Pulmonary Edema

Treatment of acute pulmonary edema consists of improving tissue oxygenation, reducing pulmonary congestion, and improving myocardial contractility.

Oxygen is the most important agent for treating acute pulmonary edema; it should be given at high concentrations by mask or nasal cannula. Large numbers of collapsed and fluid-filled alveoli make some patients unresponsive to supplemental oxygen. In this situation *positive end-expiratory pressure* (PEEP) can be used to prevent alveolar collapse and improve gas exchange. PEEP can be applied during spontaneous respirations with a tight-fitting mask or endotracheal tube, a method termed *continuous positive airway pressure*. If hypercapnea is present, then positive pressure ventilation, usually through an endotracheal tube, is required. Positive-pressure ventilation may adversely affect cardiac output, and it is important to use the lowest possible airway pressure.

Sodium bicarbonate may be considered for severe metabolic acidosis (pH $<$ 7.10) and *not* for respiratory acidosis. Sodium bicarbonate therapy of metabolic acidosis has several adverse effects, not the least of which is that it may actually decrease tissue oxygenation and exacerbate intracellular acidosis. Such treatment should be cautious and done only if respiratory acidosis is corrected and severe metabolic acidosis persists.

Pulmonary vascular congestion can be reduced by the use of vasodilators and diuretics. Preload can be decreased by the use of sublingual, oral, topical, or intravenous nitroglycerin. The dose of sublingual nitroglycerin used to reduce preload in pulmonary edema is larger than that normally used to treat angina (i.e., 0.8 to 2.4 mg as a single dose). Sublingual nifedipine has also been used to treat pulmonary edema with measured decreases in afterload, increases in cardiac output, and apparent clinical success. As opposed to sublingual nitroglycerin, it has been measured that sublingual nifedipine does not predictably decrease preload and some patients may experience a significant increase in LV filling pressures. Because of these occasionally unfavorable hemodynamic effects, sublingual nifedipine should be viewed with caution for the treatment of acute pulmonary edema. Intravenous nitroglycerin or nitroprusside are both effective in rapidly reducing preload and afterload but require close hemodynamic monitoring. The goal of intravenous vasodilator therapy is resolution of symptoms without undue systemic hypotension (i.e., systolic BP $<$ 100 mmHg). Intravenous furosemide is often considered to have an immediate venodilatory effect, although this has not been found in all studies, and there is evidence that intravenous furosemide acutely increases LV filling pressures for about 15 min after administration. To prevent this effect, vasodilators should be used simultaneously with intravenous furosemide. However, potent diuretics, such as furosemide, ultimately remain useful in the treatment of acute pulmonary edema because they induce a diuresis that promotes the resorption of lung water.

Many patients with acute pulmonary edema can be satisfactorily managed with oxygen, nitrates, and diuretics; a dramatic clinical response is usually seen within 20 min. However, some patients present with severe failure, sometimes in cardiogenic shock, and require more intensive treatment.

Myocardial contractility can be enhanced by the intravenous administration of various inotropic agents; the two most commonly used drugs are the β-adrenergic agonists dobutamine and dopamine. Dobutamine is predominantly an inotrope with few vasoconstrictor properties and is therefore most useful when heart failure is not accompanied by significant hypotension. Dopamine, a vasoconstrictor at moderate and high doses, is the preferred agent when shock is present. As previously mentioned, amrinone has been released for short-term intravenous use in severe CHF, but there is some suggestion of cardiac toxicity in this setting. Digitalis has no significant role as an inotrope in acute pulmonary edema.

Morphine has been a traditional agent in the treatment of acute pulmonary edema. Its major effect is sedative and analgesic; when carefully studied, preload and cardiac output remain unchanged. Available evidence indicates that morphine has no added benefit to oxygen, sublingual nitroglycerin, and intravenous furosemide in the treatment of acute pulmonary edema. Patients receiving intravenous morphine have a higher incidence of mental and respiratory depression.

Aminophylline is primarily a bronchodilator and is useful in treating the reflex bronchospasm of pulmonary edema (''cardiac asthma'').

Phlebotomy is a rapid method of reducing circulatory congestion and is worth remembering when treating pulmonary edema in the anuric patient.

Rotating tourniquets do not decrease preload, create potential complications due to venous stasis, and should, therefore, not be used.

The survival of patients following an episode of acute pulmonary edema remains poor; the acute in-hospital mortality is about 15 percent, and the 1-year mortality is about 40 percent.

BIBLIOGRAPHY

Applefeld MM: Contemporary issues in the management of chronic congestive heart failure. *Am J Med* 80:1, 1986.

Bertel O, Steiner A: Rotating tourniquets do not work in acute congestive heart failure and pulmonary edema. *Lancet* 1:762, 1980.

Bussman WD, Schupp D: Effect of sublingual nitroglycerin in emergency treatment of severe pulmonary edema. *Am J Cardiol* 41:931, 1978.

Clark LT, Garfein OB, Dwyer EM: Acute pulmonary edema due to ischemic heart disease without accompanying myocardial infarction. Natural history and clinical profile. *Am J Med* 75:332, 1983.

Cohn JN, Archibald DG, Ziesche S, et al: Effect of vasodilator therapy on mortality in chronic congestive heart failure. Results of a veterans administration cooperative study. *N Engl J Med* 314:1547, 1986.

Colucci WS, Wright RF, Braunwald E: New inotropic agents in the treatment of congestive heart failure. Mechanisms of action and recent clinical developments. *N Engl J Med* 314:290, 300, 1986 (two parts).

Engelmeier RS, O'Connell JB, Walsh R, et al: Improvement in symptoms and exercise tolerance by metoprolol in patients with dilated cardiomyopathy: A double-blind, randomized, placebo-controlled trial. *Circulation* 72:536, 1985.

Francis GS, Siegel RM, Goldsmith SR, et al: Acute vasoconstrictor response to intravenous furosemide in patients with chronic congestive heart failure. Activation of the neurohumoral axis. *Ann Intern Med* 103:1, 1985.

Goldberger JJ, Peled HB, Stroh JA, et al: Prognostic factors in acute pulmonary edema. *Arch Intern Med* 146:489, 1986.

Hoffman JR, Reynolds S: Comparison of nitroglycerin, morphine and furosemide in treatment of presumed prehospital pulmonary edema. *Chest* 92:586, 1987.

Kraus PA, Lipman J, Becker PJ: Acute preload effects of furosemide. *Chest* 98:124, 1990.

Lefkowitz CA, Moe GW, Armstrong PW: A comparative evaluation of hemodynamic and neurohumoral effects of nitroglycerin and nifedipine in congestive heart failure. *Am J Cardiol* 59:59B, 1987.

Mulrow CD, Feussner JR, Velez R: Reevaluation of digitalis efficacy. New light on old leaf. *Ann Intern Med* 101:113, 1984.

Packer M: Sudden unexplained death in patients with congestive heart failure: A second frontier. *Circulation* 72:681, 1985.

Roth A, Hochenberg M, Keren G, et al: Are rotating tourniquets useful for left ventricular preload reduction in patients with acute myocardial infarction and heart failure? *Ann Emerg Med* 16:764, 1987.

Timmis AD, Rothman MT, Henderson MA, et al:P Hemodynamic effects of intravenous morphine in patients with acute myocardial infarction complicated by severe left heart failure. *Br Med J* 1:980, 1980.

Wilson JR, Reichek N, Dunkman WB, et al: Effect of diuresis on the performance of the failing left ventricle in man. *Am J Med* 70:234, 1981.

20
VALVULAR HEART DISEASE

J. Stephan Stapczynski

The four heart valves function to force blood to flow in the forward direction only as the ventricles contract. Valvular heart disease may either be stenotic, causing obstruction to flow when the valve should be open, or incompetent, allowing backward regurgitation of blood when the valve should normally be closed. While cardiac catheterization and echocardiography have immensely increased our understanding of valvular heart disease, the emergency physician should remember that the ability to recognize and manage these disorders requires correlating clinical history and physical examination at the bedside. The ancillary tests of chest radiography and electrocardiography usually provide only confirmatory information.

The cardiovascular adaptations to valvular heart disease are complex and varied, depending on whether this disease is acute, subacute, or chronic. Most acute and subacute adaptations persist in the chronic state. The acute adaptations are primarily tachycardia, increased myocardial contractility, and arteriolar vasoconstriction—all in an attempt to maintain cardiac output and perfusion pressure to vital organs. A subacute adaptation is fluid retention producing an increase in venous volume and ventricular filling pressures. This attempts to maintain effective stroke volume by the Frank-Starling principle. Myocardial hypertrophy and cardiac dilatation develop in response to chronic pressure or volume overload. Ventricular hypertrophy and dilatation are seen when either the outflow valve is stenotic or incompetent or the inflow valve is incompetent. Atrial dilatation occurs when the atrioventricular valve is stenotic or incompetent.

Chronic adaptations are able to preserve cardiac output and prevent pulmonary congestion for many years. However, these processes cause myocardial injury that eventually becomes irreversible, and once clinical symptoms of heart failure develop, progressive clinical deterioration is common. Symptoms of aortic stenosis can develop rapidly, and sudden death is a well-recognized complication. Other chronic valvular lesions are better tolerated. Medical treatment is effective only for the side effects such as systemic and pulmonary venous congestion and does not affect the underlying mechanical problem. For this reason surgery is often recommended, even when symptoms are mild, to prevent irreversible myocardial injury.

The effects of aortic or mitral valvular disease on the pulmonary vascular bed are significant. As left ventricular diastolic pressure rises, pulmonary venous pressure also rises, causing interstitial pulmonary edema and reflex pulmonary arteriolar vasoconstriction. Initially the vasoconstriction and pulmonary artery hypertension are reversible, but persistence leads to irreversible pulmonary arteriolar changes and pulmonary artery hypertension becomes fixed. Pulmonary hypertension places a pressure overload on the right ventricle and may result in right-sided heart failure with venous engorgement and peripheral edema.

MITRAL STENOSIS

Valvular mitral stenosis is nearly always the result of rheumatic heart disease, usually requiring years of progressive damage to become clinically manifest. The murmur of rheumatic mitral stenosis is usually detected in the third or fourth decade of life, with symptoms developing 10 to 15 years later. The significant hemodynamic abnormality is an elevated diastolic pressure gradient across the mitral valve. The normal mitral valve area is 4 to 6 cm^2. A diastolic pressure gradient is usually found when the orifice size decreases below 2.5 cm^2; pulmonary congestion is seen below 1.5 cm^2; and right heart failure is found below 1.0 cm^2.

Clinical Features

The most common early symptom is dyspnea, which is precipitated by demands of increased cardiac output, such as exertion, tachycardia, anemia, pregnancy, or infection. Attempts to increase blood flow are resisted by the stenotic mitral valve, which produces an increase in left atrial pressure and pulmonary venous pressure. These patients need a slow heart rate and long diastole to allow for adequate left atrial emptying and keep left atrial pressure and pulmonary venous pressure as low as possible. Eventually, paroxysmal nocturnal dyspnea and orthopnea develop. The enlarged and irritable left atrium commonly produces premature atrial contractions, atrial fibrillation, and, rarely, atrial flutter.

Patients with mitral stenosis are susceptible to pulmonary infections because of sustained vascular congestion. Circulatory stasis predisposes to deep venous thrombosis, pulmonary embolism, and pulmonary infarction. Chronic interstitial edema and pulmonary hypertension can lead to pulmonary interstitial fibrosis and restrictive lung disease. Hemoptysis due to rupture of distended pulmonary-bronchial venous anastomoses is rare but potentially life-threatening. Thrombi may form in the atria or on the valve leaflets, especially in patients in atrial fibrillation, and may embolize to arteries supplying the brain, kidneys, spleen, or extremities.

There are several important physical signs of mitral stenosis. A prominent *a* wave in the jugular veins and an early-systolic left parasternal lift are signs of right ventricular pressure overload. The apical impulse is typically small and tapping in quality, indicating an underfilled left ventricle. The first heart sound is loud and snapping unless the valve is heavily scarred and immobile. An early-diastolic opening snap and a following low-pitched, middiastolic rumble that crescendos into S_1 is typical. The closer an opening snap occurs to S_2 and the longer the duration of the murmur during diastole, the greater is the severity of obstruction.

Pulmonary hypertension can be suspected from several possible physical signs: (1) an increase in the normal splitting of the two components of S_2 and an accentuation of the second component (pulmonic); (2) a pulmonary ejection click; (3) an early-diastolic blow along the left second or third intercostal spaces (Graham-Steell murmur), indicating pulmonary regurgitation; and (4) a holosystolic murmur of tricuspid regurgitation with severe pulmonary hypertension.

Two other conditions may also produce a middiastolic murmur. The Austin-Flint murmur is a middiastolic rumble associated with aortic regurgitation, but there is no accentuation of S_1 and no opening snap. A left atrial myxoma may obstruct flow across the mitral valve and produce a middiastolic murmur. Movement of the tumor may produce a loud sound ("tumor polyp"), and there are often signs of pulmonary hypertension. In atrial myxoma, systemic symptoms, such as fever, weight loss, anemia, embolic phenomena, and "pneumonia," are common.

The earliest radiographic change of mitral stenosis is straightening of the left heart border due to left atrial enlargement. Further left atrial enlargement can be recognized as a double density behind the heart. Pulmonary congestion is manifest by an increase in vascular markings, redistribution of flow to the upper lung fields, and Kerley B lines at the bases.

The ECG may show notched or diphasic P waves, indicating left atrial enlargement, and pulmonary hypertension may cause right axis deviation or right ventricular hypertrophy.

Treatment

The treatment of mitral stenosis as it relates to the emergency physician depends primarily on the recognition and initial management of acute complications. The development of fever in a patient with rheumatic heart disease should raise the suspicion of endocarditis. Sustained tachycardias are poorly tolerated by patients with mitral stenosis, particularly atrial fibrillation with a rapid ventricular response. Digoxin, propranolol, or verapamil should be used to control ventricular rate, although the latter two may impair myocardial contractility and precipitate heart failure. Occasionally, synchronized cardioversion may convert atrial fibrillation into sinus rhythm, but recurrences of the arrhythmia are common. Systemic arterial embolism may occur with electrical cardioversion, and a period of anticoagulation is necessary prior to treating chronic atrial fibrillation in this manner. Propranolol or verapamil is effective in preventing an exaggerated heart rate increase with exercise. Oral anticoagulation is indicated for patients in sustained atrial fibrillation to prevent systemic arterial emboli. Mild hemoptysis may occur secondary to a temporary rise in pulmonary venous pressure such as can be produced by exercise. Rarely, massive hemoptysis may require blood transfusion and emergency surgery. Pulmonary infarction should be considered in the differential diagnosis of hemoptysis. Bacterial endocarditis prophylaxis should be kept in mind for all procedures that may cause a bacteremia. Rheumatic fever prophylaxis is also recommended for children and young adults still at risk for acute rheumatic fever. Surgical treatment is advised for symptoms that interfere with the patient's pattern of living.

MITRAL REGURGITATION

The mitral valve may be incompetent from disease affecting any portion of the functional mitral valve apparatus: left atrial wall, mitral annulus, mitral valve leaflets, chordae tendineae, papillary muscles, and left ventricular wall. Mitral regurgitation may be acute, intermittent, or chronic, with corresponding clinical presentations.

Acute, severe mitral regurgitation is usually due to rupture of the chordae tendineae, rupture of the papillary muscles, or perforation of the valve leaflets, usually secondary to infective endocarditis or acute myocardial infarction. As blood attempts to regurgitate into the noncompliant left atrium, pressure rises to very high levels and acute pulmonary edema quickly develops. Reflex pulmonary vasoconstriction and signs of acute cor pulmonale may be present.

Intermittent mitral regurgitation is usually due to ischemia, which produces papillary muscle dysfunction or changes in left ventricular compliance. The anterior and inferior papillary muscles are sensitive to coronary artery disease because they are the last portion of the ventricle perfused by the coronary arteries. The inferior papillary muscle is more commonly affected by ischemia than the anterior papillary muscle.

There are many causes of chronic mitral regurgitation; redundant and "floppy" mitral valve leaflets, rheumatic heart disease, congenital heart disease, many connective tissue and rheumatologic disorders, hypertrophic and congestive cardiomyopathies, calcified mitral annulus, and complications of infective endocarditis or acute myocardial infarction. With chronic regurgitation, the left atrium dilates so that left atrial pressure rises little, even with large regurgitant flow. As an adaptation, the total stroke volume of the left ventricle increases so that effective forward flow into the aorta is maintained despite the large regurgitant volume across the mitral valve.

Clinical Features

Acute mitral regurgitation presents with dyspnea, tachypnea, and, eventually, pulmonary edema. The apical impulse is usually active, with prominent thrusts and a systolic thrill. Both an S_3 and an S_4 may be heard. The harsh, apical regurgitant murmur starts with S_1 and may end before S_2 because left ventricular and atrial pressures equalize before the end of systole. Acute right ventricular pressure overload may cause jugular venous distention, with a prominent a wave and a left parasternal lift.

Patients with intermittent mitral regurgitation usually present with acute episodes of respiratory distress due to pulmonary edema and are relatively asymptomatic between episodes. The predominant symptom of dyspnea may mask the anginal pain of ischemia. The murmur is usually a soft apical systolic murmur, which increases in intensity with acute episodes, often with S_3 and S_4 gallops. Ausculatory signs may also be obscured by the pulmonary edema signs.

Chronic mitral regurgitation is often well tolerated for years, the earliest signs being exertional dyspnea and fatigue, especially if atrial fibrillation develops. The jugular venous pressure is often normal. The large regurgitant flow into the left atrium may push the entire heart forward and produce a late systolic left parasternal lift. The high-pitched apical holosystolic murmur usually radiates to the axilla. The first heart sound is generally soft and obscured by the murmur. There is usually an S_3 followed by a short diastolic rumble indicating increased flow into the left ventricle. Chronic mitral regurgitation produces left ventricular and atrial enlargement, which is usually detected by chest radiography or electrocardiography.

Treatment

Patients with acute, severe mitral regurgitation need rapid treatment for cardiogenic pulmonary edema with oxygen, afterload reduction (even with normal blood pressure), diuretics, etc. The intraaortic balloon pump can be used to support the circulatory system prior to cardiac catheterization and surgery. Papillary muscle or chordae tendineae rupture often produces severe symptoms and entails a high mortality; emergent mitral valve replacement can be life-saving. Conversely, some patients may have only a small amount of regurgitation, experience mild symptoms, remain hemodynamically stable, and can be treated conservatively.

Intermittent mitral regurgitation usually responds to treatment for myocardial ischemia with nitrates. Diuretics are sometimes needed. Some patients achieve relief with the Valsalva maneuver.

Patients with chronic mitral regurgitation who develop congestive heart failure should be treated with digoxin and diuretics. If atrial fibrillation with a rapid ventricular response occurs, the ventricular rate should be controlled with digoxin. Afterload reduction can be used to decrease the percentage of regurgitation and increase forward cardiac output. Oral anticoagulation is occasionally needed to prevent development of atrial thrombi and systemic arterial embolism. Bacterial endocarditis and rheumatic fever prophylaxis are indicated for populations at risk.

MITRAL VALVE PROLAPSE

Mitral valve prolapse is due to a mismatch between the size of the left ventricular cavity and the mitral valve apparatus. Prolapse occurs when the "redundant" mitral valve prolapses into the left atrium as the left ventricle shrinks past the threshold volume for "mismatch" during systole. Prolapse most commonly involves a portion of the posterior mitral valve leaflet and occurs during mid to late systole. Often, the tricuspid valve may also prolapse, indicating a more generalized cardiac pathology.

Many disorders have a ventriculovalvular mismatch allowing mitral valve prolapse ("secondary" prolapse): connective tissue diseases (Marfan's syndrome), hypertrophic cardiomyopathy, atrial septal defect, Ebstein's anomaly, ischemic heart disease, rheumatic heart disease, trauma, etc. However, many patients have no discernible underlying cause ("primary" or idiopathic mitral valve prolapse). The incidence of auscultatory and/or echocardiographic evidence of primary mitral valve prolapse in studies of asymptomatic young adults has been found to be between 0.3 and 12 percent. The prevalence of mitral valve prolapse in the general population is estimated to be 6 to 8 percent. In studies from tertiary referral centers, many patients with mitral valve prolapse experience symptoms. However, epidemiological studies indicate that most patients with mitral valve prolapse are asymptomatic and many of the purported symptoms are just as common in a control population without mitral valve prolapse. This suggests to some investigators that mitral valve prolapse is more a variation in mitral anatomy rather than a specific syndrome. Even so, many clinicians still consider these reported symptoms to be related to mitral valve prolapse. Additionally, there are subgroups of patients (men older than 45 with systolic murmurs, individuals with thickened and redundant leaflets by echocardiography) who appear to be more susceptible to major complications (left ventricular failure, endocarditis, cerebral emboli, and sudden death) than the average patient with prolapse.

Most individuals with mitral valve prolapse have a benign course, with survival similar to a matched control population. However, patients with an enlarged left ventricle are more likely to eventually require mitral valve replacement for progressive mitral regurgitation. Additionally, patients with very redundant mitral valve leaflets have been reported to experience a higher incidence of sudden death, infective endocarditis, and cerebral embolism.

Clinical Features

Many patients are symptomatic and are diagnosed on the basis of incidental findings during routine physical examination. Some patients have chest pain (presumably due to tension on the papillary muscles) and palpitations (due to atrial or ventricular tachyarrhythmias). Patients may have syncope from tachyarrhythmias or orthostatic hypotension. Other symptoms, such as anxiety or fatigue, are poorly understood.

Patients with mitral valve prolapse are at increased risk for infective endocarditis, particularly if they have significant mitral regurgitation and redundant valve leaflets. Thrombi may form on the redundant leaflets and embolize to the ophthalmic or cerebral circulation, presenting as amaurosis, transient ischemic attacks, or strokes. Sudden death, perhaps due to ventricular fibrillation or other lethal arrhythmia, is the least understood complication of mitral valve prolapse.

The classic auscultatory findings are a mid- to late-systolic click followed by a late-systolic murmur. The click is caused by the sudden tensing of the loose chordae tendineae as the leaflet reaches the maximal prolapsed position. At this point the valve is often slightly incompetent, allowing for a small amount of mitral regurgitation. The timing of the click and murmur is established by when the threshold ventricular volume for ventriculovalvular mismatch is reached during systole. Maneuvers which decrease left ventricular volume (strain phase of the Valsalva maneuver, tachycardia, sudden standing, or use of amyl nitrate) allow prolapse to occur sooner in systole and the click-murmur moves closer to S_1. Maneuvers which increase left ventricular volume (squatting, maximal isometric handgrip, bradycardia, passive leg raising, or β-adrenergic blockers) prevent prolapse until late in systole and the click-murmur moves away from S_1. Clicks and murmurs commonly vary in intensity and may not be heard all the time.

The ECG may have nonspecific flattened or inverted T waves, especially in leads II, III, aV_f, and V_4 to V_6. The QT interval may be prolonged. Certain arrhythmias are common: marked sinus arrhythmia, premature atrial contractions, premature ventricular contractions, paroxysmal supraventricular tachycardia, and, in older patients, atrial fibrillation. Some patients with these arrhythmias have no auscultatory findings but do have echocardiographic evidence of mitral valve prolapse.

Heart size and shape are usually normal on chest radiograph. Rare cases with severe mitral regurgitation will show left ventricular and atrial enlargement.

Diagnosis of mitral valve prolapse is generally confirmed by echocardiography or, if necessary, cardiac catheterization.

Treatment

β-Adrenergic antagonists are effective in suppressing arrhythmias and, to some extent, chest pain, presumably by increasing left ventricular size, reducing the ventriculovalvular mismatch, and lessening tension on the papillary muscles. Some patients may require additional antiarrhythmic therapy. Prophylaxis against bacterial endocarditis during dental and other procedures associated with bacteria is commonly recommended, although the risk of endocarditis is very small. Patients with a history of systemic embolism should receive antiplatelet or anticoagulant therapy. Since emboli are uncommon, preventive therapy is not recommended in all patients.

VALVULAR AORTIC STENOSIS

Valvular aortic stenosis develops primarily from either rheumatic heart disease, a congenitally bicuspid aortic valve, or, rarely, idiopathic sclerosis. Rheumatic inflammation of the aortic valve leaflets causes fusion at the commissures, which may be followed by progressive fibrosis and varying degrees of calcification, producing a valve that is usually both stenotic and incompetent. A bicuspid aortic valve is a common congenital abnormality (found in up to 2 percent of the general population) that may, but does not invariably, undergo fibrosis and calcification from a lifetime of hemodynamic stress. Patients with rheumatic or bicuspid aortic stenosis usually present with symptoms at ages between 40 and 60 years. Idiopathic sclerosis of the aortic valve leaflets is common in the elderly and often produces a hemodynamically insignificant systolic ejection murmur. Rarely, calcification of aortic valve sclerosis produces significant stenosis.

The principal hemodynamic abnormality in aortic stenosis is obstruction to left ventricular outflow. The normal aortic valve area is 3 to 4 cm^2, and usually stenosis does not produce significant impairment to forward flow until the orifice has become narrowed to between 1.0 and 1.5 cm^2, in which case the systolic pressure gradient across the valve usually exceeds 50 mmHg. Cardiac output can be maintained for many years by hypertrophy of left ventricular myocardium. With severe obstruction, stroke volume is partially dependent on adequate filling pressure, which is augmented by an effective left atrial contraction just before ventricular systole (''left atrial kick''). Conversion from sinus rhythm to atrial fibrillation can markedly reduce stroke volume and exacerbate left heart failure.

Clinical Features

The patient with aortic stenosis may remain asymptomatic for many years, but once symptoms occur, average life expectancy is less than 5 years if the disease remains untreated. The characteristic symptoms of aortic stenosis are angina pectoris, syncope, and left heart failure. Exertional dyspnea and other symptoms of left heart failure result from an elevated left ventricular end-diastolic pressure that is transmitted to the pulmonary venous bed and causes pulmonary congestion. Angina pectoris occurs because of the markedly increased oxygen demand of the hypertrophied myocardium and, to some extent, decreased blood flow to the subendocardium due to increased wall tension compressing small arterioles. However, coronary artery disease is also common in these middle-aged patients. Exertional syncope may result when a stenotic valve prevents cardiac output from increasing during exercise, or may be due to inhibition of vasoconstrictor reflexes during exercise. Sudden death has been related to syncopal attacks and seems to occur primarily in adults with acquired aortic stenosis. Congestive heart failure indicates advanced disease, with average survival estimated to be less than 2 years after its onset. Atrial fibrillation or sustained tachycardias are poorly tolerated and often produce symptoms.

Initially blood pressure is normal, but as disease progresses, systolic blood pressure falls and pulse pressure narrows. However, elderly patients have a loss in aortic compliance and may have systolic hypertension despite significant aortic stenosis. The carotid pulse has a slow upstroke (often with a ''shuttering'' feeling), diminished amplitude, and slow downstroke. The apical impulse is enlarged, sustained, and laterally displaced owing to left ventricular hypertrophy and dilatation. An S_4 is usually prominent. Aortic stenosis produces a coarse, low-pitched systolic ejection murmur, loudest at the right second intercostal space, with radiation to the carotids and to some extent the apex. The later the murmur peaks in systole, the more severe the obstruction. As stenosis increases in severity, the splitting of S_2 becomes narrowed, often producing a single S_2. Aortic valve leaflets that are still mobile may have an early systolic ejection click, but increasing age, fibrosis, and calcification usually reduce this finding. The ECG usually shows left ventricular hypertrophy and secondary repolarization changes (''strain pattern'').

Aortic stenosis usually produces left ventricular hypertrophy, which causes little cardiac enlargement on chest radiography. Poststenotic dilatation of the ascending aorta is common. Calcification of the aortic valve leaflets indicates severe aortic stenosis.

Treatment

Strenuous physical exertion should be avoided. Prophylaxis for bacterial endocarditis is indicated. Symptoms of congestive heart failure can be treated with salt restriction, diuretics, and digoxin. However, these patients are partially dependent on an adequate left ventricular filling pressure to maintain cardiac output, and hypovolemia may be life-threatening. Nitrates may be cautiously tried for treatment of chest pain, although they may exacerbate syncope and orthostatic hypotension. Prosthetic replacement of the aortic valve is strongly advised in most patients who develop symptoms of angina, syncope, or heart failure.

AORTIC REGURGITATION

Aortic regurgitation may be acute or chronic, with correspondingly different pathophysiology, clinical features, and treatment.

Acute aortic regurgitation may result from destruction of valve leaflets (due to infective endocarditis, acute rheumatic fever, trauma, or spontaneous rupture) or from sudden dilatation of the aortic root (due to aortic dissection). With acute aortic regurgitation, left ventricular diastolic pressure rises rapidly to very high levels as blood regurgitates into the noncompliant left ventricle, producing acute left ventricular failure and pulmonary edema. Effective stroke volume and cardiac output fall and heart rate increases. The systolic blood pressure does not increase, and the diastolic blood pressure cannot fall below the very high left ventricular end-diastolic pressure so that pulse pressure does not increase substantially.

Chronic aortic regurgitation can occur from processes which slowly destroy the valve leaflets (rheumatic heart disease or myxomatous degeneration) or dilate the aortic root (cystic medionecrosis of the aorta, Marfan's syndrome, tertiary syphilis, ankylosing spondylitis, or Reiter's syndrome). With chronic aortic regurgitation, the left ventricle dilates and hypertrophies so that end-diastolic volume markedly increases with little change in end-diastolic pressure. The ejection fraction increases so that effective stroke volume and cardiac output are maintained despite a large regurgitant volume. Heart rate remains unchanged and systolic blood pressure rises while diastolic blood pressure falls, producing an increased pulse pressure. If unchecked, chronic aortic regurgitation will ultimately result in heart failure.

Clinical Features

Acute Aortic Regurgitation

Acute aortic regurgitation is characterized by the sudden onset of dyspnea, tachypnea, tachycardia, and chest pain. Signs of specific causes, such as bacterial endocarditis, aortic dissection, or trauma, may be present. Low cardiac output and vasoconstriction produce pale extremities and sometimes peripheral cyanosis. Heart rate is increased. Systolic and diastolic blood pressures are normal or decreased and pulse pressure widens little. Pulse signs of chronic aortic regurgitation are absent.

The apical impulse is usually normal in position and quality. Auscultation may be difficult because of marked tachycardia and respiratory distress. An important diagnostic feature is a diminished S_1 because the rapidly rising left ventricular diastolic pressure closes the mitral valve before the onset of systole. If the aortic valve leaflets are also destroyed, the aortic component of S_2 is soft. An S_3 is common. The murmur of acute aortic regurgitation is medium-pitched, soft, and of short duration because the early equalization of pressures in the aorta and left ventricle diminishes regurgitant flow. There may be a soft systolic ejection murmur due to increased flow across the aortic valve during systole.

The ECG is generally characterized by nonspecific ST-T changes without evidence of left ventricular hypertrophy. Infectious endocarditis may cause various conduction disturbances as the infection spreads to the nodal and infranodal conducting system.

The chest radiograph will show a normal cardiac size with pulmonary venous congestion and edema. Special attention should be directed to aortic and mediastinal contours in a search for evidence of aortic dissection.

Chronic Aortic Regurgitation

A patient with chronic aortic regurgitation may relate a history of specific causes: rheumatic fever, syphilis, infective endocarditis, different varieties of arthritis, or Marfanoid habitus.

Compensatory mechanisms enable the patient with chronic aortic regurgitation to remain asymptomatic for many years. Characteristic symptoms include dyspnea on exertion, paroxysmal nocturnal dyspnea, and palpitations. Chest wall pain may also occur, presumably owing to excessive force of cardiac contractions against the thorax. Patients with severe chronic aortic regurgitation may exhibit bobbing of the head with each systole. Severe aortic regurgitation may cause neck and abdominal pain, presumably due to stretching of the carotid artery or aorta from the large stroke volume. Postural dizziness may occur from a low diastolic pressure inadequate to maintain cerebral circulation.

The carotid pulse is pounding, rapidly rising and falling (water-hammer or Corrigan's pulse). A pistol shot sound or a to-and-fro murmur (Duroziez's sign) may be heard over the femoral artery. Capillary pulsations (Quincke's sign) can be seen in the nailbeds. The pulse pressure is usually widened, and a rough guide to the severity of regurgitation can be obtained from the ratio of pulse pressure to systolic pressure, which in mild disease is usually < 0.5, in moderate disease between 0.5 and 0.7, and in severe disease > 0.7. These pressure ratios are not pathognomonic for aortic regurgitation as they may be seen in other hyperdynamic states, such as fever, sepsis, or thyrotoxicosis.

Significant aortic regurgitation will displace the apical impulse laterally owing to left ventricular dilatation. A diastolic thrill may be palpable along the left sternal border and, rarely, a systolic thrill may be felt in the second right intercostal space. The first heart sound is preserved. The aortic component of S_2 is usually normal but may be diminished or absent. A third heart sound is occasionally present. With advanced scarring of the valve leaflets, a systolic ejection sound may be heard, which is presumably due to sudden aortic dilatation at the onset of systole.

The classic murmur of rheumatic aortic regurgitation is a high-pitched, blowing, decrescendo diastolic murmur best heard along the left sternal border. If the murmur is more audible along the right sternal border, a nonrheumatic cause is more likely. The regurgitant stream may cause posterior displacement of the anterior mitral valve leaflet, partially narrow the mitral valve orifice during diastole, and cause a middiastolic to presystolic rumble (Austin-Flint murmur).

Mild aortic regurgitation may cause no ECG abnormalities, but severe disease produces left ventricular hypertrophy and secondary repolarization changes (''strain pattern''). The chief radiographic feature of chronic aortic regurgitation is left ventricular enlargement.

Dilatation of the ascending aorta is typical in Marfan's syndrome and tertiary syphilis.

Treatment

Acute aortic regurgitation is a medical emergency which causes rapid clinical deterioration and has a high mortality without surgical treatment. Prompt diagnosis is essential. Medical stabilization should be initiated with oxygen, diuretics, and antibiotics, if endocarditis is present. Some patients may also require afterload reduction with vasodilators and/or the intraaortic balloon pump. Cardiac catheterization and surgery are recommended as soon as practical.

The heart failure of chronic aortic regurgitation is treated with sodium restriction, diuretics, and digoxin. Cardiac arrhythmias and infections may exacerbate the left heart failure. Prophylaxis for bacterial endocarditis is indicated. Afterload reduction is effective on a short-term basis for increasing effective stroke volume, especially if hypertension, pulmonary venous congestion, and left ventricular failure are present. Currently, there is little information concerning the long-term benefits of vasodilator therapy, but it is reasonable to assume that such therapy will not halt or slow the progression of left ventricular failure. Aortic valve replacement in patients with symptomatic chronic aortic regurgitation almost always results in symptomatic improvement, and most studies indicate better survival than with medical therapy. It is generally recommended that asymptomatic patients also undergo aortic valve replacement when evidence of left ventricular dysfunction develops. Repeat evaluations with serial echocardiographic studies is advised to detect developing myocardial failure.

TRICUSPID STENOSIS

Tricuspid stenosis is an uncommon valvular disease which is most often due to rheumatic heart disease and associated with some tricuspid regurgitation, mitral stenosis, and, occasionally, aortic stenosis. In patients with rheumatic tricuspid stenosis, the symptoms are primarily due to left heart valvular damage and/or the resulting pulmonary hypertension. Rare causes of tricuspid stenosis include the carcinoid syndrome, endomyocardial fibroelastosis, endomyocardial fibrosis, and systemic lupus erythematosus. The most significant hemodynamic abnormality is an increased diastolic gradient across the tricuspid valve. The normal tricuspid valve has a diastolic area about 7 cm^2, and significant obstruction occurs when the orifice size narrows below 1.5 cm^2.

Clinical Features

While dyspnea and fatigue are common symptoms of rheumatic tricuspid and mitral stenosis, signfiicant obstruction at the tricuspid level prevents the development of pulmonary congestion with exertion. Severe tricuspid stenosis is characterized by signs of increased systemic venous pressure such as hepatomegaly, splenomegaly, ascites, and peripheral edema. Pulmonary congestion is absent and cardiac output is usually diminished, especially with exertion.

The jugular venous pressure is elevated, with a prominent *a* wave and decreased *y* descent. The first heart sound is accentuated and often split; both findings are enhanced by inspiration. A tricuspid opening snap is rarely audible at the bedside. The rumbling diastolic murmur is best heard along the lower left sternal border or over the xyphoid process. The murmur usually increases in intensity as a result of right atrial contraction and then declines as the right atrium relaxes and the right ventricle begins to contract. This is heard as a crescendo-decrescendo murmur just prior to S_1. The murmur characteristically increases in intensity with inspiration and decreases with expiration; this is Carvallo's sign, a useful sign in detecting a tricuspid murmur.

Characteristic ECG changes are tall, peaked P waves in lead II, indicating right atrial enlargement. The chest radiograph demonstrates an enlarged right atrium and dilated superior vena cava without pulmonary artery enlargement or signs of pulmonary hypertension.

Treatment

Medical therapy is directed toward relief of systemic venous congestion. Appropriate prophylaxis for bacterial endocarditis and rheumatic fever is indicated. Severe cases may require valve replacement.

TRICUSPID REGURGITATION

Right ventricular failure and dilatation constitute the most common cause of tricuspid regurgitation. Combined tricuspid stenosis and regurgitation may result from rheumatic heart disease. Less common causes of isolated tricuspid regurgitation include infective endocarditis, congenital abnormalities of the valve leaflets, endocardial cushion defects, Ebstein's anomaly, prolapsed leaflet syndrome, blunt chest trauma, and papillary muscle damage.

Clinical Features

Since tricuspid regurgitation is most often caused by right ventricular failure secondary to left-sided failure or mitral stenosis, the common symptoms are dyspnea, orthopnea, and peripheral edema. However, tricuspid regurgitation may protect the patient against symptoms of augmented venous return, and paroxysmal nocturnal dyspnea is uncommon. The clinical features of isolated tricuspid regurgitation are the result of increased systemic venous pressure and decreased cardiac output. Patients with advanced cases have peripheral edema, pulsatile hepatomegaly, splenomegaly, and ascites. The jugular veins are distended, with a large *v* wave and rapid *y* descent. The murmur is soft, blowing, holosystolic, and best heard over the lower sternal border of xyphoid. The murmur often increases in intensity with inspiration (Carvallo's sign).

The ECG findings include tall, peaked P waves of right atrial enlargement, but these may be masked by the common occurrence of atrial fibrillation. The chest radiograph usually shows enlargement of both the right atrium and ventricle.

Treatment

Treatment for the systemic venous congestion and right-sided heart failure consists of salt restriction, diuretics, and digoxin. Functional tricuspid regurgitation due to pulmonary hypertension will often improve with attempts to lower pulmonary artery pressure. If right ventricular failure is due to mitral stenosis, prosthetic replacement of the mitral valve is indicated.

PULMONARY STENOSIS

Right ventricular outflow obstruction may result from infundibular, valvular, or supravalvular stenosis. The most common cause of valvular pulmonary stenosis is congenital and the most common cause of infundibular obstruction is the tetralogy of Fallot. The significant hemodynamic abnormality is a systolic pressure gradient across the pulmonary valve. Stenosis can be graded by the peak right ventricular systolic pressure: mild, < 65 mmHg; moderate, between 65 to 120 mmHg; and severe, > 120 mmHg.

Clinical Features

Many patients remain asymptomatic for years. Severe pulmonary stenosis causes external dyspnea and signs of right heart failure. Syncope and sudden death can occur. The jugular veins have a prominent *a* wave. An early right parasternal lift is usually present and a systolic thrill may be felt in the second left intercostal space or suprasternal notch. The second heart sound is widely split. A systolic ejection click followed by a harsh systolic ejection murmur, which increases with inspiration, is usually heard in the left second intercostal space and radiates to the left clavicle.

The ECG findings of severe pulmonary stenosis are right atrial enlargement, right-axis deviation, and right ventricular hypertrophy with secondary repolarization changes ("strain pattern"). The chest radiograph usually shows poststenotic dilatation of the main pulmonary artery and evidence of right ventricular enlargement. Pulmonary blood flow is normal in the absence of a right-to-left shunt.

Treatment

Medical management consists of treating the symptoms of venous congestion. Prophylaxis for bacterial endocarditis is indicated. Pulmonary valve surgery is recommended when the peak right ventricular systolic pressure is over 70 mmHg or the peak systolic gradient across the pulmonary valve is over 50 mmHg.

PULMONARY REGURGITATION

Pulmonary regurgitation may be secondary to pulmonary hypertension, producing dilatation of the valve ring and resultant valvular incompetence. Symptoms are more likely to be due to the pulmonary hypertension than to the regurgitation itself. Isolated pulmonary regurgitation may result from a congenital lesion, acute rheumatic fever, or infective endocarditis.

Clinical Features

Isolated pulmonary regurgitation is tolerated for many years. The characteristic symptoms of severe pulmonary hypertension are dyspnea, fatigue, and syncope. The classic murmur of pulmonary regurgitation is a high-pitched, blowing, diastolic murmur at the second left intercostal space. The murmur starts with the pulmonic component of S_2 and has a brief crescendo, followed by a longer decrescendo. A brief midsystolic ejection murmur, reflecting increased flow across the pulmonary valve, is typical.

Treatment

Treatment of pulmonary hypertension, if present, with diuretics, digoxin, vasodilating agents, and mitral valve replacement is the first step. Isolated pulmonary regurgitation is often well tolerated and valve replacement is indicated in only severe cases.

PROSTHETIC VALVE COMPLICATIONS

Complications of prosthetic valves may occur early after surgery or be delayed for years after implantation. The type and incidence of the different complications depend on such factors as (1) the underlying heart disease, (2) the specific valve replaced, (3) the type of prosthetic valve, and (4) the need for anticoagulation.

Prosthetic valves can be divided into four main types (Table 20-1). The valves themselves can be covered with a variety of materials, such as cloth, Silastic, or Teflon.

Table 20-1. Four Varieties of Prosthetic Valves

Caged-ball
Starr-Edwards (aortic and mitral)
Smeloff-Cutter (aortic and mitral)
Braunwald-Cutter (mitral and tricuspid)
Magovern-Cromie (aortic only)
DeBakey-Surgitool (aortic only)
Disk
Central occluder disk
Beall-Surgitool (mitral and tricuspid)
Kay-Shiley (mitral and tricuspid)
Starr-Edwards (mitral and tricuspid)
Cooley-Cutter
Tilting Disk
Bjork-Shiley
Lillihei-Kaster
Medtronic Hall (Hall-Kaster)
Bioprosthesis
Hancock porcine
Carpentier-Edwards porcine
Ionescu-Shiley pericardial
Bileaflet
St. Jude Medical

A normally functioning prosthetic valve can have distinctive auscultatory features: (1) audible opening and closing sounds, (2) a murmur during normal forward flow of blood through the prosthesis, and (3) a murmur caused by turbulence of blood around the metal portions of the prosthesis. Most prosthetic valves produce systolic ejection murmurs in both the mitral and aortic position. Disk and porcine valves produce diastolic murmurs in the mitral position. Opening sounds in the aortic position are common with ball and bileaflet valves. Opening sounds in the mitral position are common with ball and porcine valves.

Thromboembolism is a major problem with the completely artificial valves, its prevention usually requiring lifelong anticoagulation. Although less of a problem, thrombosis may also occur on the porcine heterograft, especially in the mitral position. Most patients who have an aortic porcine heterograft or a mitral porcine heterograft and stay in sinus rhythm do not need chronic anticoagulation. The presentation of aortic or mitral prosthetic valve thrombosis is usually acute, with obvious development of left heart failure. The presentation of tricuspid prosthetic valve thrombosis is much more insidious.

Mechanical hemolysis of red cells by the prosthetic valve can occur from either a normally functioning or an incompetent valve. Mechanical hemolysis sufficient to produce anemia generally indicates perivalvular incompetence. Bacterial endocarditis soon after implementation is most commonly caused by staphylococci or gram-negative rods. Delayed endocarditis is most often due to viridans streptococci or *Staphylococcus epidermidis*.

Valvular incompetence can develop from leakage around the valve or, in the case of a porcine heterograft, from cusp rupture. Symptoms suggestive of prosthetic valve dysfunction are increased angina, heart failure, and syncope.

A change in murmurs or muffled valve sounds suggest prosthetic valve dysfunction. Chest radiographs should be done to confirm correct position of the prosthesis. Blurring of the prosthetic valve margins may be secondary to normal valve motion or respiration as well as dysfunction. Cinefluoroscopy, angiography, or echocardiography is necessary to confirm the diagnosis of dysfunction.

Sudden cardiovascular collapse may occur as a result of sticking of the valve in one position or, rarely, catastrophic embolization of the ball portion of a ball-in-cage valve.

BIBLIOGRAPHY

Barnett HJM, Boughner DR, Taylor DW, et al: Further evidence relating mitral-valve prolapse to cerebral ischemic events. *N Engl J Med* 302:139, 1980.

Bor DH, Himmelstein DU: Endocarditis prophylaxis for patients with mitral valve prolapse. A quantitative analysis. *Am J Med* 76:711, 1984.

Cha SD, Desai RS, Gooch AS, et al: Diagnosis of severe tricuspid regurgitation. *Chest* 82:726, 1982.

DePace NL, Nestico PF, Morganroth J: Acute severe mitral regurgitation. Pathophysiology, clinical recognition, and management. *Am J Med* 78:293, 1985.

Grayburn PA, Smith MD, Handshoe R, et al: Detection of aortic insufficiency by standard echocardiography, pulsed doppler echocardiography, and auscultation. A comparison of accuracies. *Ann Intern Med* 104:599, 1986.

Harrison EC, Rashtian MY, Allen DT, et al: An emergency department physician's guide to prosthetic heart valves: Identification and hemodynamic function. *Ann Emerg Med* 17:194, 1988.

Harrison EC, Rashtian MY, Allen DT, et al: An emergency physician's guide to prosthetic heart valves: Valve-related complications. *Ann Emerg Med* 17:704, 1988.

Jeresaty RM: Mitral valve prolapse. An update. *JAMA* 254:793, 1985.

Marks AR, Choong CY, Sanfilippo AJ, et al: Identification of high-risk and low-risk subgroups of patients with mitral-valve prolapse. *N Engl J Med* 320:1031, 1989.

Morganroth J, Perloff JK, Zeldis SM, et al: Acute severe aortic regurgitation. Pathophysiology, clinical recognition, and management. *Ann Intern Med* 87:223, 1977.

Retchin SM, Fletcher RH, Earp J, et al: Mitral valve prolapse. Disease or illness? *Arch Intern Med* 146:1081, 1986.

Selzer A: Changing aspects of the natural history of valvular aortic stenosis. *N Engl J Med* 317:91, 1987.

Smith ND, Raizada V, Abrams J: Auscultation of the normally functioning prosthetic valve. *Ann Intern Med* 95:594, 1981.

Stein PD, Sabbah ND: Aortic origin of innocent murmurs. *Am J Cardiol* 39:665, 1977.

Wooley CF, Fontana ME, Kilman JW, et al: Tricuspid stenosis. Atrial systolic murmur, tricuspid opening snap, and right atrial pressure pulse. *Am J Med* 78:375, 1985.

21
THE CARDIOMYOPATHIES, MYOCARDITIS, AND PERICARDIAL DISEASE

James T. Niemann

THE CARDIOMYOPATHIES

Classification and Definition

The term *cardiomyopathy* is broadly used to describe a group of diseases that directly impair myocardial function and cardiac structure. Primary cardiomyopathies are those diseases which originate in the myocardium itself. By current definition, a primary cardiomyopathy is of unknown origin (idiopathic). Secondary cardiomyopathies are those which result from a systemic disease that involves the heart as part of a recognized disease process or from a variety of toxins which alter cardiac structure and function.

Three types of cardiomyopathies are recognized: (1) dilated, (2) hypertrophic, and (3) restrictive. Some secondary cardiomyopathies may present with restrictive or dilated characteristics. The cardiomyopathies, as a group, are the third most common form of cardiac disease encountered in the United States, and follow coronary (ischemic) heart disease and hypertensive heart disease in prevalence.

Dilated Cardiomyopathy

This subgroup is characterized hemodynamically by depressed myocardial systolic function or *systolic pump failure*. Left ventricular (LV) contractile force is diminished, resulting in a low cardiac output and increased end-systolic and end-diastolic ventricular volumes and intracavitary pressures. Cardiomegaly results from both dilatation and hypertrophy. Systemic diseases that may involve the heart and produce a dilated cardiomyopathy as part of a recognized disease process are shown in Table 21-1. However, a specific etiology or associated disease will be found in fewer than 15 percent of patients. Most cases are idiopathic. With increasing use of percutaneous endomyocardial biopsy as a diagnostic tool, many patients with the presumptive diagnosis of idiopathic cardiomyopathy have been found to have active lymphocytic myocarditis presumably of viral origin.

Clinical Profile

As a result of systolic pump failure, the patient presents with signs and symptoms of congestive heart failure: dyspnea on exertion, orthopnea, and paroxysmal nocturnal dyspnea. Depressed ventricular contractile function and dilatation may result in the formation of mural thrombi, and the patient may present with manifestations of peripheral embolization, e.g., an acute neurological deficit, flank pain and hematuria, or a pulseless, cyanotic extremity.

Murmurs are frequently heard during cardiac auscultation and are not necessarily indicative of primary valvular disease. Ventricular dilatation and the resultant annular dilatation and displacement of the papillary muscles of the atrioventricular valves inhibit leaflet coaptation and complete valve closure. Holosystolic regurgitant murmurs of mitral and tricuspid valve origin are frequently heard at the apex or lower left sternal border in the patient with biventricular failure. On occasion an apical "diastolic rumble" may be heard and is due either to accentuated, early-diastolic atrial-to-ventricular flow (the result of mitral regurgitation and left atrial overload) or to a loud summation gallop. An enlarged, pulsatile liver may be found if tricuspid insufficiency is present. Bibasilar rales and dependent edema are common additional findings.

The chest x-ray invariably shows an enlarged cardiac silhouette and increased cardiothoracic ratio; biventricular enlargement is common. Evidence of pulmonary venous hypertension ("cephalization" of flow, enlarged hila) is also frequent and may serve to differentiate cardiac enlargement due to myocardial failure from that due to a large pericardial effusion.

The electrocardiogram is almost always abnormal. Left ventricular hypertrophy and left atrial enlargement are the most common findings. Q or QS waves and poor R-wave progression across the anterior precordium may produce a pseudoinfarction pattern.

Echocardiography in the symptomatic patient demonstrates a decreased ejection fraction, increased systolic and diastolic volumes, and ventricular and atrial enlargement.

Table 21-1. Dilated Cardiomyopathy: Known Cause or Association

Infectious	*Associated with neuromuscular disorders (the muscular dystrophies)*
Viral	*Associated with collagen vascular diseases*
Protozoal (Chagas's disease)	*Sarcoidosis*
Metabolic	*Myocardial toxins*
Thyrotoxicosis	Ethanol
Myxedema	Heavy metals
Acromegaly	Emetine
Hemachromatosis	Adriamycin
Glycogen storage disease	Cobalt
Thiamine deficiency (beriberi)	
Hypophosphatemia	
Peripartum	
Amyloidosis	

Therapy

Management of the patient with dilated cardiomyopathy is symptom-directed, and the prescribed therapeutic regimen almost always employs the digitalis glycosides and diuretics. Patients unresponsive to these agents may respond to preload and afterload reduction with nitrates and hydralazine or angiotensin-converting enzyme inhibitors (captopril, enalapril). A thorough diagnostic evaluation should be undertaken for all patients with unexplained heart failure or cardiomegaly. Such an evaluation may reveal an underlying disease which is amenable to specific therapy in patients with secondary forms of dilated cardiomyopathy.

Hypertrophic Cardiomyopathy

Hypertrophic cardiomyopathy (HCM) is a familiar (autosomal dominant) or sporadic cardiac muscle disorder characterized by increased left ventricular muscle mass without associated ventricular dilatation. The diagnostic hallmarks of the disease are echocardiographic asymmetrical septal hypertrophy and histologic myocardial fiber disarray.

Hemodynamically HCM is characterized by abnormal left ventricle (LV) diastolic function due to reduced compliance of the hypertrophied left ventricle. This decreased compliance is reflected by an increase in LV filling pressure. Cardiac output, ejection fraction, and end-systolic and diastolic volumes are usually normal. A systolic pressure gradient between the body of the left ventricle and the subvalvular outflow tract can be recorded in some patients at rest or after provocation (exercise, isoproterenol infusion). The majority of clinical symptoms in this heart muscle disease are the result of impaired diastolic relaxation and restricted LV filling.

Clinical Profile

Severity of symptoms in most instances is related to patient age; the older the patient, the more severe the symptoms. Dyspnea on exertion is the most frequent initial complaint and is due to elevated LV diastolic pressure accentuated by exercise. Additional symptoms include chest pain, palpitations, and syncope. A family history of death due to cardiac disease, frequently described as ''massive heart attack'' or ''heart failure,'' is not uncommon. Complaints of paroxysmal nocturnal dyspnea and pedal edema are uncommon.

Chest pain in HCM patients is due to an imbalance between the oxygen demand of the hypertrophied left ventricle and the available myocardial blood flow. In older patients, associated atherosclerotic coronary artery disease may further limit myocardial perfusion. Precordial or retrosternal chest discomfort in HCM may mimic angina pectoris or may be ''atypical.'' Response to nitroglycerin administration is poor and highly variable.

The HCM patient may be aware of forceful ventricular contraction and complain of an abnormal heartbeat or ''palpitations.'' Atrial and ventricular arrhythmias are not uncommon in these patients; rapid atrial arrhythmias, especially atrial fibrillation, are particularly poorly tolerated because of the increased importance of the atrial contribution to LV filling in the poorly compliant heart.

Jugular venous pressure is usually not elevated; however, a prominent *a* wave may be noted on close inspection of the neck veins. The upstroke of the carotid arterial pulse is rapid and frequently biphasic or bifid (pulsus bisferiens). The apical impulse is sustained and hyperdynamic and a presystolic lift is common.

The first and second heart sounds are usually normal, and a fourth sound (S_4) will be heard in most patients. The characteristic systolic ejection-type murmur of HCM is heard best at the lower left sternal border or at the apex and rarely radiates to the carotid arteries. Easily performed bedside maneuvers can be used to increase the intensity and duration of the murmur (Table 21-2). Interventions that decrease LV filling and the distending pressure in the LV outflow tract or that increase the force of myocardial contraction accentuate the murmur of HCM. Such interventions include standing, the Valsalva maneuver, amyl nitrate inhalation, and isoproterenol infusion. The murmur will also be louder with the first sinus beat following a premature ventricular contraction. Maneuvers that increase LV filling (squatting, passive leg elevation, handgrip) have an opposite effect on murmur characteristics.

ECG findings of LV hypertrophy and left atrial enlargement are found in 30 percent and 25 to 50 percent, respectively, of HCM patients. Evidence of chamber enlargement is most common in patients with large gradients across the LV outflow tract. Q waves of considerable amplitude (> 0.3 mV), termed *septal Q waves,* are seen in about 25 percent of patients and may be encountered in the anterior, lateral, or inferior leads. These Q waves may mimic those seen following myocardial infarction (*pseudoinfarction pattern*). The polarity of the T wave serves as a diagnostic clue in the separation of HCM septal Q waves from Q waves due to myocardial infarction. Upright T waves in those leads with QS or QR complexes are usually found in HCM; T-wave inversion in such leads is highly suggestive of ischemic heart disease.

The chest x-ray is frequently normal, and identifiable abnormalities are largely nonspecific. Many patients do not show radiographic evidence of LV or left atrial enlargement. Evidence of pulmonary venous congestion is unusual but has been reported.

Echocardiography has played a substantial role in the diagnosis of HCM, in the correlation of the auscultatory and hemodynamic events with LV anatomic changes, and in defining inheritance patterns. The characteristic echocardiographic finding is disproportionate septal hypertrophy. Additional described echocardiographic abnormalities include normal or reduced LV end-diastolic dimensions, systolic anterior motion of the mitral valve, and midsystolic closure of the aortic valve.

Therapy

The mainstay of medical therapy for the symptomatic patient, specifically the patient with chest pain, has been the liberal use of β blockers (propranolol, usual dose 120 to 320 mg/day in divided doses). Studies have demonstrated that calcium blocking agents may be of value in a carefully defined population of HCM patients who do not respond to β blockade. Surgical therapy (septal muscle excision or mitral valve replacement) has not been conclusively shown to offer advantages over medical therapy. Antibiotic prophylaxis is recommended for dental procedures and potentially unsterile surgery. Several authorities discourage competitive athletics of any type, since sudden death following vigorous exertion is not infrequent in patients with HCM.

Restrictive Cardiomyopathy

This is the least common of the clinically recognized and described cardiomyopathies. The hemodynamic characteristics of a restrictive cardiomyopathy include (1) elevated left and right ventricular end-diastolic pressures, (2) normal LV systolic function (ejection fraction > 50 percent), and (3) an abrupt and rapid rise in early-diastolic ventricular pressure following a marked decline at the onset of diastole. The rapid rise and abrupt plateau in the early-diastolic ventricular pressure tracing results in a characteristic (but not diagnostic) ''square-root sign'' or ''dip-and-plateau'' filling pattern. Simultaneously recorded left and right ventricular diastolic pressures are frequently mirror images, varying by only a few millimeters of mercury. These hemodynamic findings are similar to those reported in constrictive pericarditis, and differentiation at times may require surgical biopsy. Causes of restrictive cardiomyopathy are listed in Table 21-3. In the vast majority of cases, no specific etiology can be defined.

Clinical Profile

In patients with advanced cardiac disease of known etiology, clinical symptoms are similar to those noted in patients with a dilated cardiomyopathy, namely, pedal edema and decreased exercise tolerance or other evidence of pulmonary venous hypertension. Chest pain, either typical for angina or atypical, is also a frequent presenting complaint, and its cause is unknown.

Findings on physical examination depend on the stage or severity of myocardial involvement. An S_3 and/or S_4 is commonly heard in the asymptomatic or minimally symptomatic patient. Gallop rhythms and systolic murmurs (due to mitral regurgitation) are usually heard in advanced cases, as are pulmonary rales, and pedal edema is present.

The routine chest x-ray may be normal and, combined with symptoms and physical findings, may suggest constrictive pericarditis. In advanced cases, enlargement of the cardiac silhouette and pulmonary vascular redistribution are seen.

The ECG is frequently abnormal, but ''diagnostic'' changes have not been described. The most frequently reported ECG changes include chamber enlargement (ventricular and atrial) and repolarization abnormalities (nonspecific ST-T-wave changes). Low-voltage QRS complexes (< 0.7 mV) have been frequently reported in patients with

Table 21.2 Effect of Bedside Interventions on Murmur Intensity and Duration in HCM

Increase	Decrease
Valsalva maneuver	Passive leg elevation in the supine patient
Standing	Handgrip
Amyl nitrate inhalation	Squatting
β Agonists (isoproterenol infusion)	α Agonists (phenylephrine infusion)

Table 21-3. Causes of Restrictive Cardiomyopathy

Idiopathic (includes endomyocardial fibrosis and Loeffler's eosinophilic endomyocardial disease)
Secondary (associated with systemic disease)
Hemachromatosis
Amyloidosis
Sarcoidosis
Progressive systemic sclerosis (scleroderma)

restrictive cardiomyopathy secondary to amyloidosis and hemochromatosis.

Therapy

With the exception of hemachromatosis (variably responsive to chelation therapy with desferroxamine), therapy for restrictive cardiomyopathy is symptom-directed and consists mainly of diuretics, digoxin, vasodilators, and class I antiarrhythmic agents for complicating rhythm disturbances. However, patients with amyloid cardiomyopathy may be "sensitive to digoxin" (prone to toxicity) because of amyloid fibril binding of digoxin, and this medication should be used with caution in such patients.

MYOCARDITIS

Definition

Myocarditis is broadly but nonspecifically defined as inflammation of the heart muscle and is most frequently characterized pathologically by focal infiltration of the myocardium by lymphocytes, plasma cells, and histiocytes. Varying amounts of myocytolysis and destruction of the interstitial reticulin network are also seen. The pathologic changes have been ascribed to a number of disease entities (Table 21-4), some of which involve the myocardium secondarily as part of a systemic disease process. Myocarditis is frequently accompanied by pericarditis.

Clinical Profile

Fever is common, as is sinus tachycardia, usually "out of proportion" with respect to the extent of temperature elevation. Signs and symptoms depend on the extent of myocardial involvement and resultant depression of myocardial systolic function. In severe cases, progressive heart failure with its associated symptoms may be seen. With less extensive myocardial involvement, pericarditis and the clinical manifestations of systemic illness (fever, myalgias, headache, rigors) may overshadow clinical signs of myocardial dysfunction. Retrosternal or precordial chest pain is a frequent presenting complaint and is most commonly secondary to associated pericardial inflammation (myopericarditis). This chest pain may mimic angina in its character. A pericardial friction rub is commonly heard in patients with myopericarditis.

The chest roentgenogram is usually normal, and reported abnormalities (cardiomegaly and pulmonary venous hypertension and/or pulmonary edema) vary with disease severity and are nondiagnostic. Reported ECG changes include nonspecific ST-T-wave changes, ST segment elevation (due to associated pericarditis), atrioventricular block, and prolonged QRS duration. Echocardiography may reveal depressed systolic function in severe cases.

Treatment

Current therapy in cases of idiopathic or viral myocarditis is largely supportive and symptom-directed. Myocarditis in rheumatic fever and complicating diphtheria or meningococcemia necessitates directed antibiotic therapy.

Table 21-4. Common Infectious Causes of Myocarditis

Viral agents	Bacteria
Coxsackie B virus	*Corynebacterium diphtheriae*
Echovirus	*Neisseria meningitidis*
Influenza virus	*Mycoplasma pneumoniae*
Parainfluenza virus	β-Hemolytic streptococci (rheumatic fever)
Epstein-Barr virus	
Hepatitis B virus	

UNEXPLAINED HEART FAILURE OR CARDIOMEGALY: DIFFERENTIAL DIAGNOSIS AND EVALUATION

Symptoms of congestive heart failure and associated cardiomegaly or evidence of cardiomegaly in the asymptomatic patient necessitates a directed evaluation. In the vast majority of instances, one of the following seven disease entities will eventually be diagnosed. Where appropriate, recognized diagnostic clues are noted.

1. *Hypertensive Heart Disease.* Systemic arterial hypertension affects 10 to 20 percent of the adult population. This is a disease with a high prevalence which may be diagnosed at a number of stages. The patient with a dilated cardiomyopathy and untreated cardiac failure will frequently present with an elevated blood pressure due to autonomically mediated compensatory reflexes. Isolated involvement of the myocardium as the major manifestation of systemic arterial hypertension is rare. A careful search for evidence of other end-organ damage due to arterial hypertension should be undertaken (examination of fundi, assessment of renal function, evaluation for focal neurological changes, or history of such).
2. *Ischemic Heart Disease (Ischemic Cardiomyopathy).* Most patients with clinical signs of biventricular heart failure and cardiomegaly due to obstructive coronary arterial disease will relate a history of typical anginal pain or documented myocardial infarction(s). A few will not, and clinical presentation and physical findings in these cases will mimic those of an idiopathic dilated cardiomyopathy.
3. *Valvular Heart Disease.* Although the incidence of rheumatic heart disease in the United States is low, it remains a prevalent disease in underdeveloped countries and is frequently first diagnosed in recent immigrants. The growing "geriatric" population is prone to calcific aortic stenosis and mitral annular calcification. In addition, bicuspid or unicuspid aortic valve abnormalities remain as the most common congenital heart disease. All may present with congestive heart failure or incidental cardiac enlargement, and systolic and diastolic murmurs may be noted. Echocardiography is the diagnostic test of choice in the patient with suspected valvular heart disease. Hemodynamic and angiographic studies may be confirmatory.
4. *Constrictive Pericardial Disease.* Constrictive pericarditis frequently presents with clinical manifestations that mimic right-sided failure. A past history of pericarditis and minimal cardiac enlargement, clear lung fields, and pericardial calcification on chest x-ray are diagnostic clues.
5. *Myocarditis.* The patient with severe myocarditis may present with signs and symptoms of cardiac insufficiency. Such patients are usually young, have no significant past cardiac history, have few risk factors for atherosclerotic coronary arterial disease, and present with a recent, abrupt onset of symptoms during or immediately following a systemic or viral illness.
6. *Hypertrophic Cardiomyopathy.* The patient with hypertrophic cardiomyopathy may present with a history of shortness of breath or decreased exercise tolerance. Symptoms thus mimic left heart failure. Echocardiography and, if necessary, left heart catheterization are critical diagnostic aids.
7. *Idiopathic Cardiomyopathy.* This diagnosis should be considered only if the first six entities have been excluded. A careful search for potential etiologic causes should then be undertaken.

PERICARDIAL DISEASE

The pericardium consists of a serous or loose fibrous membrane (visceral pericardium) overlying the epicardium and a dense collagenous sac (parietal pericardium) which surrounds the heart. The space between the visceral and parietal pericardium may contain up to 50 mL of fluid under normal conditions, and intrapericardial pressure is normally subatmospheric. Because its layers are serosal surfaces and

Table 21-5. Common Causes of Acute Pericarditis

Idiopathic
Infectious
Viral (especially Coxsackie virus and echovirus)
Bacterial [especially staphylococcus, *Streptococcus pneumoniae*, β-hemolytic streptococci (acute rheumatic fever), *Mycobacterium tuberculosis*]
Fungal (especially *Histoplasma capsulatum*)
Malignancy (leukemia, lymphoma, metastatic breast and lung carcinoma, melanoma)
Drug-induced (procainamide, hydralazine)
Connective tissue disease
Radiation-induced
Postmyocardial infarction (Dressler's syndrome)
Uremia
Myxedema

because of its proximity and attachments to other structures, the pericardium may be involved in a number of systemic or localized disease processes (Table 21-5). The clinical presentation of pericardial heart disease is variable and dependent on the pericardium's response to injury and how this response affects cardiac function. In this section the clinical manifestations and evaluation of acute and constrictive pericarditis are discussed.

Acute Pericarditis

Symptoms and Signs

The most common symptom is precordial or retrosternal chest pain, which is most frequently described as sharp or stabbing. It may be of sudden or gradual onset and radiate to the back, neck, left shoulder, or arm; referral to the left trapezial ridge (due to inflammation of the adjoining diaphragmatic pleura) is a particular distinguishing feature. Chest pain due to acute pericarditis may be aggravated by inspiration or movement. It may be most severe when the patient is supine and is often relieved when the patient sits up and leans forward. In most instances, these characteristics allow the pain of acute pericarditis to be distinguished from the ischemic pain of angina or acute myocardial infarction.

Associated symptoms include (1) low-grade, intermittent fever, particularly if pericarditis is infectious in origin or of the idiopathic type; (2) dyspnea, due to accentuated pain with inspiration; and (3) dysphagia, ascribed to irritation of the esophagus by the posterior pericardium.

A pericardial friction rub is the most common and important physical finding in pericarditis. A pericardial rub most closely resembles a superficial grating or scratching sound. It is best heard with the diaphragm of the stethoscope at the lower left sternal border or apex when the patient is sitting and leaning forward or in the hands-and-knees position. It may be audible only during a certain phase of respiration and characteristically is transient, i.e., heard one hour and not the next. No inference as to the amount of pericardial fluid should be drawn from the presence or absence of a pericardial friction rub.

A pericardial rub is most often triphasic in character, consisting of a systolic component, an early diastolic component occurring during the early phase of ventricular filling, and a presystolic component synchronous with atrial systole. It is less commonly biphasic, i.e., a systolic component with either an early diastolic or presystolic component. A monophasic rub is unusual (18 percent of cases) but is most often systolic.

Other common associated physical findings include fever and resting sinus tachycardia. Additional signs (paradoxical pulse, venous distention, Kussmaul's sign) may result from the effects of an expanding pericardial effusion on ventricular filling.

Diagnostic Findings

Electrocardiogram

Serial ECGs recorded over a number of days may be diagnostic in acute pericarditis. The evolutionary ECG changes during acute pericarditis and convalescence have been divided into four stages. During stage 1 or the acute phase, ST segment elevation (reflecting associated subepicardial inflammation and/or injury) is prominent in the precordial leads, especially V_5 and V_6, and in standard lead I. PR segment depression may be noted in leads II, aV_F, and V_4 to V_6 (Fig. 21-1). In stage 2, the ST segment begins returning to the isoelectric line and T-wave amplitude decreases. T-wave inversion is rarely seen until stage 3. Stage 3 is characterized by an isoelectric ST segment and T-wave inversion in those leads previously showing ST segment elevation. Resolution of repolarization abnormalities is the hallmark of stage 4.

If a large pericardial effusion develops during the course of acute pericarditis, additional ECG abnormalities may be noted and include low-voltage QRS complexes and electrical alternans. These phenomena are due to the "insulating" effect of pericardial fluid, which attenuates electrical signals of myocardial origin, and the pendular motion of the heart within the fluid-filled pericardial space.

Although serial ECG tracings are of diagnostic value in acute pericarditis, sequential ECG assessment is not a diagnostic luxury afforded the emergency physician. Differentiating pericarditis from the normal variant with "early repolarization" is a common problem and can be difficult when only a single 12-lead ECG is available. Acute pericarditis is a common cause of chest pain and abnormal ECGs in young adults. The ST-T-wave changes present in the early repolarization or normal variant ECG mimic those of pericarditis and have been reported in 2 percent of healthy young adults. Investigations attempting to distinguish these two conditions have yielded conflicting results. However, a simple criterion offers considerable diagnostic utility, namely, the ST segment/T-wave amplitude ratio in leads V_5, V_6, or I. Using the end of the PR segment as baseline, or 0 mV, the amplitude or height of the ST segment at its onset is measured in one of the above leads and recorded in millivolts. The height of the T wave in the same lead is measured from the baseline to the T-wave peak. If the ratio of ST amplitude (in millivolts) to T-wave amplitude (in millivolts) is below 0.25, a normal variant or early repolarization is most probable. If the ratio is above 0.25, acute pericarditis is likely. This criterion may allow differentiation of acute pericarditis (stage 1) from early repolarization during emergency department evaluation (Fig. 21-1).

Radiographic Assessment

Conventional PA and lateral chest x-rays are of limited value. The cardiac silhouette may be of normal size and contour in acute pericarditis and, in some instances, the setting of cardiac tamponade. If previous chest x-rays are available for comparison, a recent increase in the size of the cardiac silhouette or an increase in the cardiothoracic ratio without radiographic evidence of pulmonary venous hypertension aids in distinguishing an expanding pericardial effusion from left heart failure. The epicardial "fat pad sign" is rarely seen on the lateral chest x-ray and has been reported in only 15 percent of cases of acute pericarditis during fluoroscopy with image intensification. If acute pericarditis is suspected on the basis of history, physical examination, or ECG, PA and lateral chest x-rays, which may demonstrate a pleuropulmonary or mediastinal abnormality, may assist in establishing an etiology, e.g., neoplastic or infectious.

Echocardiography

Echocardiography has become the procedure of choice for the detection, confirmation, and serial follow-up of patients with acute pericarditis and a pericardial effusion.

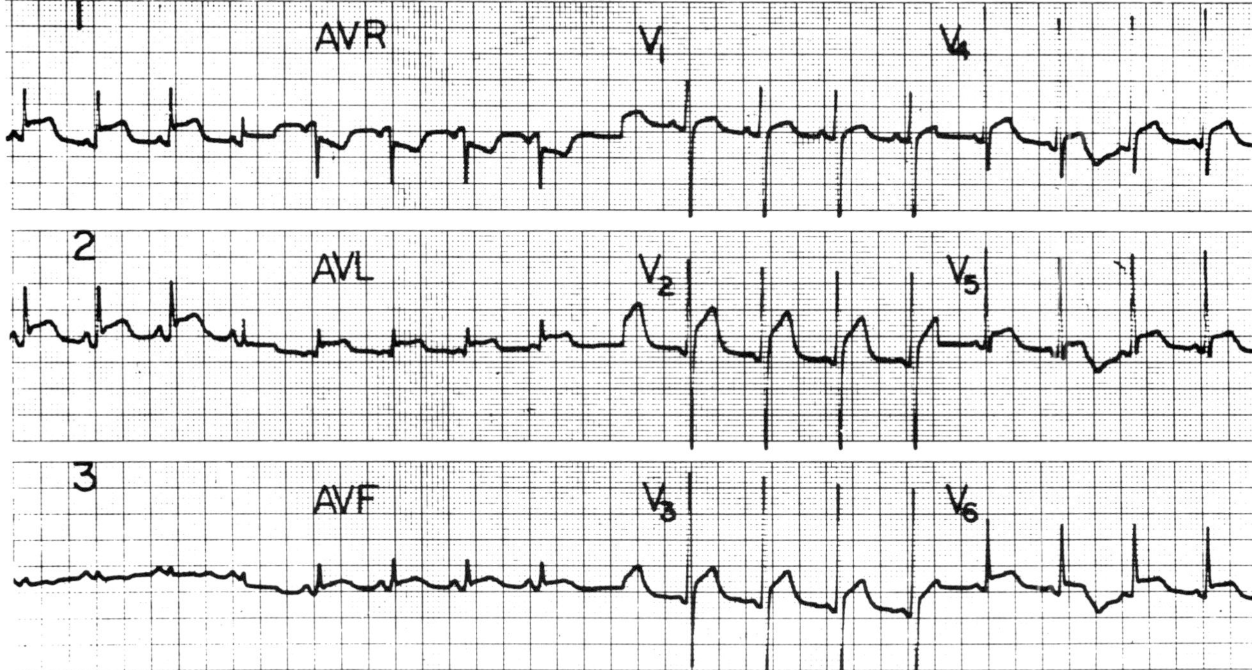

Fig. 21-1. This ECG was obtained from a 24-year-old male complaining of retrosternal pleuritic chest pain. A three-component pericardial friction rub was heard on examination. ECG abnormalities consistent with pericarditis are present. There is diffuse ST segment elevation, and PR interval depression is evident in the standard limb leads (PR interval below the isoelectric TP segment). The ST segment/T-wave amplitude ratio in V_6 is approximately 0.75. (*From* Ginzton LE, Laks MM: The differential diagnosis of acute pericarditis from the normal variant: New electrocardiographic criteria. *Circulation* 65:1004, 1982. Used by permission.)

Normally, the pericardial sac is only a "potential" space and the myocardium is echocardiographically in direct contact with surrounding thoracic structures. The anterior right ventricular wall is in contact with the chest wall and the posterior LV wall is in contact with the posterior pericardium and adjacent pleura. When a pericardial effusion is present, the pericardial space fills with echo-free fluid. Echocardiographically, a separation is seen between the right ventricle and the chest wall and between the left ventricle and the posterior pericardium. Quantitation of the size of the effusion is arbitrary and is determined by where the echo-free space is seen (anterior or posterior) and when in the cardiac cycle it occurs. For example, when an echo-free space is seen only posteriorly and only during systole, a "small" effusion is said to present.

Ancillary Laboratory Evaluation

The laboratory studies listed in Table 21-6 may be of value in establishing an etiologic diagnosis. Creatine kinase (CK) and CK-MB may be elevated in acute pericarditis due to associated myocarditis.

Table 21-6. Ancillary Diagnostic Studies in Acute Pericarditis

CBC and differential WBC count: may suggest infection or leukemia
BUN/creatinine: may suggest a diagnosis of uremic pericarditis
Streptococcal serology (antistreptolysin O, anti-DNAse, antihyaluronidase): of particular value in the patient with an antecedent history of rheumatic heart disease or history of pharyngitis
Blood cultures (if bacterial infection suspected)
Acute and convalescent viral titers
Serological studies: antinuclear antibodies, anti-DNA titers, or RA latex fixation in the patient with systemic symptoms
Thyroid function studies
Erythrocyte sedimentation rate: will not facilitate an etiologic diagnosis but can be followed serially to assess response to therapy.

Constrictive Pericarditis

Pathology

Constrictive pericarditis is pathologically distinct from acute pericarditis. Following pericardial injury and the resultant inflammatory and reparative process, fibrous thickening of the layers of the pericardium may occur. This fibrous reparative process is most commonly encountered after cardiac trauma with intrapericardial hemorrhage, after pericardiotomy (open-heart surgery, including coronary revascularization), in fungal or tuberculous pericarditis, and in chronic renal failure (uremic pericarditis). When the fibrous and/or collagenous response prevents passive diastolic filling of the normally distensible cardiac chambers, constriction is said to be present. Intrapericardial fluid is not required to produce such a hemodynamic effect. By its nature, constrictive pericarditis is most commonly a clinically chronic process. However, clinical manifestations may occur early if fluid also accumulates within the thickened, noncompliant pericardial sac (so-called effusive constrictive pericarditis). In the vast majority of cases of constrictive pericarditis, proved by hemodynamic assessment (see below), a specific etiology is never determined.

Symptoms and Signs

The symptoms of constrictive pericarditis usually develop gradually and may mimic those of congestive heart failure (CHF). If symptoms develop within months of a pericardial injury, a combination of pericardial effusion and constriction should be suspected. Exertional dyspnea and decreased exercise tolerance are common patient complaints; however, orthopnea, paroxysmal nocturnal dyspnea, and chest pain are unusual. Lower extremity swelling (pedal edema) and increasing abdominal girth (ascites) are also common complaints and are the result of decreased right ventricular diastolic compliance and resultant increase in systemic venous pressure.

In most instances, physical findings and their correct interpretation will lead the clinician to suspect constrictive pericarditis. Examination of the neck veins with the torso of the patient at a 45° angle from the horizontal will reveal jugular venous distension and a rapid *y* descent of the cervical venous pulse. Elevated venous pressure is also seen in CHF but a rapid *y* descent is infrequently encountered. Kussmaul's sign (inspiratory neck vein distension) is frequently but not invariably noted in constrictive pericarditis but rarely noted in uncompensated CHF. A paradoxical pulse is found in a minority of patients, and thus its absence does not exclude a diagnosis of constrictive pericarditis. On cardiac auscultation, an early diastolic sound, a pericardial "knock," may be heard at the apex 60 to 120 ms after the second heart sound. The pericardial knock sounds like a ventricular gallop but occurs earlier than the S_3 of CHF, which it may mimic. The knock is due to accelerated right ventricular inflow in early diastole and early myocardial distension, followed by an abrupt slowing of further ventricular expansion. There is usually no pericardial friction rub.

Hepatomegaly, ascites, and dependent edema of varying severities are usually found.

Diagnostic Findings

Electrocardiogram

Diagnostic ECG changes have not been described in constrictive pericarditis. However, low-voltage QRS complexes and inverted T waves are common.

Radiographic Assessment

Conventional PA and lateral chest x-rays most commonly demonstrate a normal or slightly enlarged cardiac silhouette, clear lung fields, and little or no evidence of pulmonary venous congestion. Pericardial calcification, which may be evident in up to 50 percent of patients with constrictive pericarditis, is seen best on the lateral chest x-ray but is not diagnostic of constrictive pericarditis.

Echocardiography

On occasion, echocardiography may demonstrate pericardial thickening and abnormal ventricular septal motion in the patient with suspected constrictive pericarditis. However, its diagnostic utility is much less than in the patient with acute pericarditis.

BIBLIOGRAPHY

Agner RC, Gallis HA: Pericarditis: Differential diagnostic considerations. *Arch Intern Med* 139:407, 1979.

Benotti JR, Grossman W, Cohn PF: Clinical profile of restrictive cardiomyopathy. *Circulation* 61:1206, 1980.

Cameron J, Oesterle SN, Baldwin JC, et al: The etiologic spectrum of constrictive pericarditis. *Am Heart J* 113:354, 1987.

Dec GW, Jr, Palacios IF, Fallon JT, et al: Active myocarditis in the spectrum of acute dilated cardiomyopathies: Clinical features, histologic correlates, and clinical outcome. *N Engl J Med* 312:885, 1985.

Ginzton LE, Laks MM: The differential diagnosis of acute pericarditis from the normal variant: New electrocardiographic criteria. *Circulation* 65:1004, 1982.

Guberman BA, Fowler NO, Engel PJ, et al: Cardiac tamponade in medical patients. *Circulation* 64:633, 1981.

Johnson RA, Palacios I: Dilated cardiomyopathies of the adult. *N Engl J Med* 1982; 307:1051, 1119.

Maron BJ, Bonow RO, Cannon RO, et al: Hypertrophic cardiomyopathy: Interrelations of clinical manifestations, pathophysiology, and therapy. *N Engl J Med* 1987; 316:780, 844.

Montague TJ, Marrie TJ, Bewick DJ, et al: Cardiac effects of common viral illnesses. *Chest* 94:919, 1988.

Spodick DH: Differential characteristics of the electrocardiogram in early repolarization and acute pericarditis. *N Engl J Med* 295:523, 1976.

Spodick DH: The normal and diseased pericardium: Current concepts of pericardial physiology, diagnosis, and treatment. *J Am Coll Cardiol* 1:240, 1983.

22
PULMONARY EMBOLISM

Robert S. Hockberger

Pulmonary embolism (PE) is the third most common cause of death in the United States, with an estimated incidence of approximately 650,000 cases annually. There are no historical, physical, or laboratory findings which are specific for the disease, and it may mimic clinically many other serious and benign medical disorders. If the diagnosis of this disease is missed in the emergency department, the overall mortality of 8 percent increases four- to fivefold.

PREDISPOSING FACTORS

Injury to the vascular endothelium, venous stasis, and alterations in the coagulating system may predispose an individual to significant thromboembolic phenomenon. Table 22-1 lists the most commonly recognized predisposing factors. Less than 6 percent of all PEs occur in the absence of any predisposing factor.

Pulmonary emboli may arise from pelvic vein thrombosis secondary to pelvic trauma or pelvic surgery (including abortion attempts) or occurring during the postpartum period. In 70 to 90 percent of cases, however, PEs arise from the deep venous system of the lower extremities. Venous thromboses confined to veins of the calf rarely embolize. The incidence of embolism from popliteal thrombosis is 50 percent, and when the thrombosis extends to involve the femoral vein, it approaches 70 percent. Unfortunately, the clinical diagnosis of deep venous thrombosis of the lower extremities, particularly when isolated in the calf, is difficult and may be missed in up to 50 percent of cases.

CLINICAL FEATURES

A "classic" picture is infrequently seen. PE may mimic many serious and benign medical disorders (see Table 22-2) and must be considered in any patient at risk who experiences any acute nonspecific cardiopulmonary complaint.

The frequencies of various symptoms and signs reported in one of the largest series of patients with angiographically documented PE are shown in Table 22-3. Chest pain is the most common symptom, occurring in approximately 90 percent of patients. While the pain is usually pleuritic in nature, it may mimic the pressurelike pain of myocardial ischemia as well as the vague discomfort of nonspecific chest wall pain. Chest pain is often noted for 3 to 4 days prior to diagnosis. Over 80 percent of patients experience dyspnea at some point but it may occur only briefly and, therefore, may not be a symptom at the time of presentation. Anxiety or apprehension, probably caused by hypoxemia, occurs in approximately 60 percent of cases, and 10 to 20 percent of patients may present following a syncopal episode.

Table 22-1. Factors Predisposing to Thromboembolism

Heart disease, especially	Alterations in coagulation
Congestive heart failure	Oral contraceptive use
Myocardiopathy	Neoplastic disease
Atrial fibrillation	Polycythemia
Myocardial infarction	Trauma
Stasis of blood flow	Postoperative states
Pregnancy and parturition	Leg or pelvic trauma
Obesity	
Varicose veins	
Prolonged immobilization (e.g., long-distance travel)	
Prolonged bed rest (with burns or fractures)	

Once a thromboembolism migrates to the lungs and lodges in the pulmonary vasculature, platelets degranulate and release a wide variety of biologically active substances, including histamine, catecholamines, serotonin, and prostaglandins. These act to cause smooth muscle constriction of the bronchi and pulmonary arteries. The increased airway resistance and decreased total lung volume with uneven ventilation contribute to the dyspnea and tachypnea found in the majority of patients with pulmonary embolism. Tachypnea (respiratory rate more than 16 per minute) is found in over 90 percent of patients. Localized rales, rhonchi, wheezes, or a pleural friction rub are often, but not invariably, seen.

The hemodynamic reaction to PE depends on the extent of vascular occlusion as well as on the patient's prior cardiovascular status. The previously healthy patient does not develop clinical signs of significant pulmonary hypertension (distended neck veins, a right ventricular heave, and a loud pulmonary component of the second heart sound) unless total pulmonary vascular obstruction approaches 40 to 50 percent. Patients with preexisting cardiopulmonary disease, however, may experience life-threatening changes in hemodynamic status with only minor insult. Some degree of hypotension is present in up to 25 percent of pulmonary emboli, but frank shock occurs in less than 10 percent.

Fever [over 38°C (100.4°F)], tachycardia (more than 100 beats per minute), and clinical evidence of deep venous thrombosis (DVT) of a lower extremity are each present in less than one-third of cases.

LABORATORY INVESTIGATION

Arterial Blood Gases

Most patients with PE will experience some degree of hypoxia. This is due to underperfusion of well-aerated segments of lung secondary to the emboli themselves, decrease in total lung volume secondary to diffuse bronchial constriction, inadequate respirations secondary to pain and splinting, and occasionally some degree of cardiac decompensation. The mean P_{O_2} values among patients with documented PE in two large series were 62 and 72 mmHg, respectively, but 10 to 15 percent of patients with PE have a P_{O_2} greater than 80 mmHg, and up to 5 percent have a P_{O_2} greater than 90 mmHg. The presence of an increased alveolar-arterial (A-a) gradient of oxygen is more sensitive although nonspecific. It can be calculated using the following simplified formula: $140 - (P_{O_2} + P_{CO_2})$. A normal value is less than 10 mmHg for a healthy person without cardiopulmonary disease.

Table 22-2. Diseases in the Differential Diagnosis of PE

Skin	Pericardium
Herpes zoster	Acute pericarditis
Muscle	Myocardium
Mytosis	Myocardial infarction
Muscle strain	Intraabdominal disorders
Bone	Splenic flexure syndrome
Rib fracture	Renal colic
Thoracic vertebral compression fracture	Acute pancreatitis
Costochondritis	Acute cholelithiasis
Pleura	Subdiaphragmatic abscess
Pleurisy	Hepatitis
Lung	Psychiatric
Emphysema	Hyperventilation syndrome
Bronchitis	
Asthma	
Carcinoma	
Tuberculosis	
Spontaneous pneumothorax	
Pneumonia	

Table 22-3. Incidence of Symptoms and Signs in 327 Patients with Angiographically Proven Pulmonary Emboli

Symptoms and Signs	Total Series, %
Symptoms	
Chest pain	88
Pleuritic	74
Nonpleuritic	14
Dyspnea	84
Apprehension	59
Cough	53
Hemoptysis	30
Sweats	27
Syncope	13
Signs	
Respirations > 16/min	92
Rales	58
$P_2 > S_2$	53
Pulse > 100/min	44
Temperature > 37.8°C (100.04°F)	43
Phlebitis	32
Gallop	34
Diaphoresis	36
Edema	24
Murmur	23
Cyanosis	19
Predisposing condition	
Current venous disease	49
Immobilization	55
Congestive heart failure and chronic lung disease	38
Malignant neoplasm	6

Source: Bell WR, Simon TL, DeMets DL: The clinical features of submassive and massive pulmonary emboli. *Am J Med* 62:358, 1977. Used by permission.

Electrocardiogram

The ECG is usually abnormal in pulmonary embolism. The ECG changes seen in pulmonary embolism are listed in Table 22-4.

In the clinical setting of suspected pulmonary embolism, the sudden appearance of ECG findings of acute right heart strain correlates very highly with the presence of pulmonary embolism. In the clinical setting of suspected myocardial infarction, an ECG indicating multiple areas of infarction is highly suggestive of PE. The most common ECG finding in pulmonary embolism is nonspecific ST-T-wave changes that are transient (lasting for hours to days). Comparison with previously obtained ECGs or sequential ECGs obtained in the emergency department may be helpful in raising an initial suspicion of PE. A normal ECG argues against, but does not rule out, acute PE.

Chest X-Ray

When the chest x-ray is normal in a patient with severe dyspnea, PE should be strongly suspected. Roentgenograms of the chest are, however, most often abnormal in pulmonary embolism. The chest x-ray in nearly half of all patients with acute PE will show an elevated dome of one hemidiaphragm secondary to the decrease in lung volume. Other common but nonspecific radiographic findings include pleural effusions, atelectasis, and transient pulmonary infiltrates (particularly when ''wedge-shaped'').

Two radiographic features that are uncommon but relatively specific for pulmonary embolism are Hampton's hump and Westermark's sign. *Hampton's hump* is an area of density or lung consolidation with a rounded border pointing toward the hilus. *Westermark's sign* refers to the presence of a dilated pulmonary outflow tract on the side of embolization with an area of decreased perfusion distal to it.

Chest x-rays are often diagnostic in conditions that mimic acute PE such as acute pulmonary edema, cardiac tamponade, and tension pneumothorax. Even when these conditions are absent, chest x-rays are essential for the correct interpretation of radionuclide studies and can be helpful for pulmonary angiography.

Ventilation-Perfusion Lung Scan

When the diagnosis of PE cannot be excluded, a radionuclide perfusion lung scan should be employed. This measures blood flow in pulmonary vessels as small as 50 μm in diameter and is therefore extremely sensitive. A normal perfusion lung scan excludes the diagnosis of PE.

Abnormal perfusion scans are not only caused by PE but also by a large number of pulmonary disorders, including asthma, emphysema, bronchitis, bronchiectasis, pneumonia, pleural effusions, atelectasis, congestive heart failure, pulmonary carcinoma, and congenital cysts. In the clinical setting of suspected PE, an abnormal perfusion scan should be followed by a ventilation scan. Normal ventilation in an area of diminished perfusion is suggestive of PE. The larger the area of ventilation-perfusion ''mismatch'' on lung scan, the greater the correlation with PE as documented by pulmonary angiography. High-probability lung scans (lobar or multiple segmental mismatches) correlate highly (in a recent study, 88 percent) with documented PE. This finding can be used to justify anticoagulation therapy for most patients. Further investigative testing is indicated for otherwise healthy young adults who possess no predisposing factors for PE and for patients at high risk for complications of anticoagulation.

In addition, recent evidence has shown that no other findings on ventilation-perfusion lung scans are either sensitive or specific enough to establish or exclude a diagnosis of PE. The study mentioned above, involving over 900 patients, found that medium- and low-probability scans were associated with angiographically documented PE in 33 and 12 percent of patients, respectively. All perfusion abnormalities, therefore, with the exclusion of the high-probability scan, should be further evaluated.

Table 22-4. Electrocardiographic Manifestation: 90 Patients with Massive or Submassive Pulmonary Embolism without Prior Cardiac or Pulmonary Disease*

Manifestation	% of Series
Normal electrocardiogram	13
Rhythm disturbances	
Premature atrial beats	2
Premature ventricular beats	3
Atrioventricular conduction disturbances	
First-degree AV block	1
P pulmonale	6
QRS abnormalities	
Right-axis deviation	7
Left-axis deviation	7
Clockwise rotation (V_5)	7
Incomplete right bundle branch block	6
Complete right bundle branch block	9
Right ventricular hypertrophy	6
$S_1S_2S_3$ pattern	7
$S_1Q_3T_3$ pattern	12
Pseudoinfarction	11
Low voltage (frontal plane)	6
Primary RST segment and T-wave abnormalities	
RST segment depression (not reciprocal)	26
RST segment elevation (not reciprocal)	16
T-wave inversion	42

* Some patients had more than one abnormality. The prevalence of none of the various electrocardiographic abnormalities differed significantly between patients with massive or submassive pulmonary embolism ($\chi^2 > .05$).

Source: Adapted from Stein PD, Dalen JE, McIntyre KM, et al: The electrocardiogram in acute pulmonary embolism. *Progr Cardiovasc Dis* 17:247, 1975. Used by permission.

Venography or Impedance Plethysmography (IPG)

Since 70 to 90 percent of PEs arise from proximal DVT of the lower extremities, a search for DVT with venography or IPG will often preclude the need for pulmonary angiography in patients suspect for PE having medium- or low-probability ventilation-perfusion lung scans. A positive venogram or IPG examination should be followed by anticoagulation. Since up to 30 percent of angiographically documented cases of PE have no evidence of DVT on venogram or IPG examination, negative test results should be followed by pulmonary angiography to rule out PE that might have originated in the deep pelvic veins, renal veins, inferior vena cava, or right atrium.

Pulmonary Angiography

Pulmonary angiography is the "gold standard" for diagnosing PE. Pulmonary vessels as small as 0.5 mm in diameter are visualized. In one study of over 800 pulmonary angiograms performed for suspected PE, the morbidity of the test was less than 1 percent and the mortality was less than 0.01 percent. Complications occur almost exclusively in elderly patients with ventricular aneurysms, cardiomyopathies, severe congestive heart failure, or chronic obstructive pulmonary disease.

The following are indications for performing pulmonary angiography for suspected PE: (1) when patients have medium- or low-probability lung scans and negative tests for DVT; (2) when patients are at high risk for bleeding complications during anticoagulation because of severe uncontrolled hypertension, actively bleeding gastrointestinal or genitourinary lesions, a craniotomy or cerebrovascular accident within the previous month, recent intraocular surgery, or evidence of lesions known to be associated with intracranial hemorrhage; (3) in unstable patients thought to be suffering from massive PE prior to the use of expensive and potentially hazardous fibrinolytic therapy or surgical embolectomy; (4) in patients with suspected recurrent PE despite appropriate anticoagulation who are also candidates for surgical procedures; (5) *perhaps* in otherwise healthy young adults without predisposing factors for PE even in the presence of high-probability lung scans, since the test may be inaccurate in up to 12 percent of cases.

TREATMENT

Stabilization

Most patients with PE suffer from some degree of hypoxia secondary to ventilation-perfusion imbalance. The administration of oxygen at 4 to 10 L/min by nasal cannula relieves or diminishes the symptoms of hypoxia in many patients. Early initiation of adequate oxygen therapy may well prevent hypoxia-induced cardiac arrhythmias and should, therefore, not be withheld in the dyspneic patient prior to obtaining blood gases.

The patient with PE is at greatest risk for succumbing to shock or cardiac arrhythmias during the first few hours. Early initiation of vigilant monitoring of vital signs and cardiac rhythm is essential. Hypotension may be caused by low cardiac output secondary to right ventricular outflow obstruction or by myocardial dysfunction due to ischemia. Initial therapy should include the aggressive administration of crystalloid fluids if the central venous pressure is low or the use of a vasopressor such as dopamine if it is normal to high. The persistently hypotensive patient with suspected PE should be managed with Swan-Ganz catheter placement, immediate pulmonary arteriography, and early consideration of either fibrinolytic therapy or surgical pulmonary embolectomy.

Anticoagulation

Anticoagulation with heparin has been the cornerstone of therapy for venous thrombosis and PE for over 30 years. Heparin acts through inhibition of certain steps of the coagulation system by combining with antithrombin III, a naturally occurring circulating heparin cofactor. Heparin acts to prevent the extension of an existing thrombus. One study of 516 patients revealed survival after diagnosis of pulmonary embolism in 92 percent of anticoagulated patients versus 42 percent in cases where anticoagulants were withheld because of medical contraindications. In addition, pulmonary emboli recurred in only 16 percent of anticoagulated patients but in 55 percent of nonanticoagulated patients.

The continuous intravenous infusion of heparin appears to result in fewer bleeding complications but requires special equipment, experienced and competent nursing care, and frequent laboratory monitoring. When these requirements are met, therapy should be initiated with a 10,000-unit IV bolus of heparin followed by approximately 25 units/kg per hour by continuous infusion. The partial thromboplastin time is the most commonly used test for assessing control of anticoagulation. It should be checked prior to anticoagulation as a baseline, after several hours of therapy, and then as often as necessary to achieve a value of 1½ to 2 times the control value, although rigid control may not be necessary.

Heparin does not cross the placenta and can, therefore, be used safely in pregnant women with PE. Peripartum bleeding remains a problem, however, requiring that heparin be discontinued just prior to delivery and resumed only after proper postpartum hemostasis has been obtained. All cases of abnormal bleeding caused by heparin may be reversed through administration of protamine sulfate. Each milligram of protamine sulfate neutralizes approximately 100 units of heparin activity.

Thrombolytic Therapy

The thrombolytic agents streptokinase, urokinase, and recombinant tissue plasminogen activator activate the body's own fibrinolytic system by converting the normally present proenzyme plasminogen to the proteolytic enzyme plasmin. Potential advantages of thrombolytic therapy include rapid dissolution of the thrombus with subsequent hemodynamic improvement, reduction in the frequency of recurrent PE, and prevention of the long-term sequelae of chronic pulmonary hypertension. Studies have documented accelerated lysis of thrombi in patients treated with heparin and thrombolytics, as compared to patients treated with heparin alone; however, no overall difference in mortality or morbidity has yet been proved in large controlled clinical trials. Presently, the major indication for the use of fibrinolytic therapy is in hemodynamically unstable patients, that is, those with acute massive embolization accompanied by shock. Emergency physicians should consider the utilization of thrombolytic therapy for acute PE only when all the following criteria have been fulfilled: (1) the patient with suspected PE is hemodynamically compromised and has not responded to initial stabilization procedures; (2) pulmonary angiography has documented massive pulmonary embolization; and (3) consultation with a pulmonary specialist has been sought.

Vena Cava Interruption

Surgical techniques for vena cava interruption include ligation, clips, intraluminal devices such as umbrella filters, and transvenous balloon occlusion. Interruption of the inferior vena cava should be considered in the following instances: (1) when there is a contraindication to heparin therapy; (2) when pulmonary emboli recur despite adequate anticoagulation; (3) in the presence of multiple small pulmonary emboli that are thought to be causing chronic pulmonary hypertension; (4) following pulmonary embolectomy; and (5) in cases of septic pelvic thrombophlebitis with recurrent PEs.

Pulmonary Embolectomy

The treatment of massive life-threatening PE by directly removing a potentially fatal embolus has been used with some success in patients on cardiopulmonary bypass. However, since such patients are a poor risk for the added stresses of general anesthesia and surgery, fibrinolytic therapy is rapidly supplanting pulmonary embolectomy in such patients; it has been shown that massive embolization with shock can usually be managed with greater success medically. In the case of severe PE accompanied by cardiopulmonary arrest, however, transvenous pulmonary embolectomy, support with the membrane lung, and induced hypothermia should be considered.

PROGNOSIS

Approximately 10 percent of patients with PE die within 1 h of the event. When the diagnosis of PE is made and approriate therapy instituted, initial survivors have a mortality of approximately 8 percent. Death after 24 h occurs almost exclusively in chronically ill patients, particularly those with congestive heart failure. The recurrence rate of PE in appropriately treated patients has been reported to be 6 to 25 percent. Most experts agree that the prognosis for PE patients ultimately depends on the outlook for any underlying disease present, as well as on the rapidity and care with which treatment is initiated.

BIBLIOGRAPHY

Bell WR, Simon TL: Current status of pulmonary thromboembolic disease. *Am Heart J* 103:239, 1982.

Benotti JR, Dalen JE: The natural history of pulmonary embolism. *Clin Chest Med* 5:403, 1984.

Branch WT, McNeil BJ: Analysis of the differential diagnosis and assessment of pleuritic chest pain in young adults. *Am J Med* 75:671, 1983.

Caracci BF, Rumbolo PM, Mainini S: How accurate are ventilation-perfusion scans for pulmonary embolism? *Am J Surg* 156:477, 1988.

Goldhaber SZ, Savage DD, Garrison RJ, et al: Risk factors for pulmonary embolism. *Am J Med* 74:1023, 1983.

Goodman PC: Pulmonary angiography. *Clin Chest Med* 5:465, 1984.

Greenfield LJ: Vena caval interruption and pulmonary embolectomy. *Clin Chest Med* 5:495, 1984.

Hirsh J, Hull RD: Treatment of venous thromboembolism. *Chest* 89:427S, 1986.

Hull RD, Hirsch J: Pulmonary angiography, ventilation lung scanning and venography for clinically suspected pulmonary embolism with abnormal perfusion lung scan. *Ann Intern Med* 98:891, 1983.

Hull RD, Raskob CE, Hirsch J: The diagnosis of clinically suspected pulmonary embolism: Practical approaches. *Chest* 89:417S, 1986.

Mohr DN, Ryu JH, Litin SC: Recent advances in the management of venous thromboembolism. *Mayo Clin Proc* 63:281, 1988

PIOPED Investigators: Value of the ventilation-perfusion scan in acute pulmonary embolism. *JAMA* 263:2753, 1990

Stein PD, Willis PW, Demets DL: History and physical examination in acute pulmonary embolism in patients without preexisting cardiac or pulmonary disease. *Am J Cardiol* 47:218, 1981.

23 HYPERTENSIVE EMERGENCIES

Raymond Jackson

This chapter outlines the approach to the diagnosis and management of hypertension in the emergency department. Hypertensive syndromes are defined and specific treatments recommended. The most useful antihypertensive medications are discussed, as well as management of complications of acute and chronic treatment.

DEGREE OF HYPERTENSION

There are four general categories based on presentation and the level of aggression required for treatment: (1) emergencies; (2) urgencies; (3) mild, uncomplicated hypertension; and (4) transient hypertension. An understanding of the differences in the pathophysiology of these syndromes is essential to the successful and safe management of these patients.

Hypertensive Emergencies

A *hypertensive emergency* is an increased blood pressure with evidence of end-organ damage or dysfunction. The organs which are at risk for injury during a hypertensive emergency are the brain, the heart, and the kidneys. This now uncommon condition is experienced in 1 percent of all hypertensives. There are no predetermined criteria for the level of blood pressure necessary to induce a hypertensive emergency. Evidence of altered organ function, not the level of blood pressure, is the basis for this diagnosis. The most striking example of minimally elevated blood pressure inducing a hypertensive emergency is eclampsia, where hypertensive encephalopathy may occur with a blood pressure of 160/90 mmHg.

Signs and symptoms of organ dysfunction can develop progressively over hours to days. After the recognition of a hypertensive emergency, the treatment goal is to lower the blood pressure to a level which is "normal" for that patient within 30 to 60 min in a controlled, graded manner. A 30 percent reduction in 30 min is a good initial guideline. The resolution of the signs and symptoms should be used as a guide in control of pressure, although in elderly patients improvements in the signs and symptoms may lag behind the drop in pressure.

Hypertensive Urgencies

A *hypertensive urgency* is an elevation of blood pressure to a level which may be potentially harmful, usually sustained at greater than 115 mmHg diastolic, without signs, symptoms, or other evidence of end-organ dysfunction. This condition is most often due to noncompliance with medications. The treatment goal is to reduce the pressure gradually within 24 to 48 h to a level appropriate for the patient. Rapid reductions in blood pressure are potentially harmful and should be avoided. Recent evidence suggests that prescribing an antihypertensive medication, whether or not emergency department blood pressure reduction has been achieved, results in control of the hypertension on follow-up exams.

Mild, Uncomplicated Hypertension

Mild, uncomplicated hypertension is a blood pressure less than 115 mmHg diastolic without symptoms of end-organ damage. It should not be treated acutely, but requires follow-up care. New-onset, mild hypertension should not be diagnosed on the basis of emergency department pressure alone.

Transient Hypertension

Transient hypertension can be seen in many conditions, such as anxiety, pancreatitis, thrombotic stroke, early dehydration, alcohol withdrawal syndromes, epistaxis, and some overdoses (pentachlorophenol, clonidine). Treatment of the underlying condition, rather than administration of antihypertensive medication, is the rule.

To summarize, the level of blood pressure should not be the guide to treatment; rather, the golden rule of hypertension is *treat the patient, not the blood pressure.*

APPROACH TO THE HYPERTENSIVE PATIENT

The initial approach to the hypertensive patient in the emergency department is the systematic exclusion of a hypertensive emergency. This is accomplished with a thorough history and physical examination directed at uncovering signs and symptoms of organ dysfunction. With the exclusion of an emergency, nonhypertensive reasons for the blood pressure elevation are sought and, if negative, the diagnosis of an urgency is made by exclusion. The blood pressure must be taken in both arms and repeated prior to the initiation of therapy. Often the pressure will fall with rest and recumbency, making it unnecessary to use powerful antihypertensive medications.

History

Any past history of hypertension, hypertensive complications, cardiac disease, or renal disease should be elicited. Medication history, especially of antihypertensives and monoamine oxidase inhibitors, and the history of recent compliance, is important. Special attention is paid to CNS symptoms such as blurred vision, diplopia, hemiparesis, and seizures. Symptoms such as headache and dizziness are nonspecific unless they occur with grade 3 or 4 fundoscopic changes or other signs of CNS dysfunction. Symptoms of ischemic chest pain or acute congestive heart failure establish the diagnosis of an acute hypertensive cardiovascular emergency. A history of renal insufficiency may alter the diagnosis and treatment of the elevated blood pressure. Most of the above symptoms have a history of gradual onset followed by rapid progression. If the patient is pregnant, previous history of hypertension or renal disease is important as well as previous blood pressures during the pregnancy.

Physical Examination

The blood pressure should be determined by the physician in both arms with palpation of pulses in all extremities. The "tilt test" should be done on elderly patients with no signs of organ dysfunction and a history compatible with dehydration. The physical examination focuses on the neurological, cardiac, and pulmonary evaluation, searching for signs of organ dysfunction. The abdomen should be auscultated for bruits. A fundoscopic examination is mandatory.

Laboratory and Other Studies

A complete blood count, serum glucose, and blood urea nitrogen (BUN), creatinine, electrolytes, and urinalysis should be obtained in cases of suspected hypertensive emergencies. Microangiopathic hemolytic anemia is a result of ongoing medial necrosis which exposes the red cell to subendothelial collagen and fibrin. This shears the red cells as they pass by. On the peripheral smear, this results in histocytes and target cells. Hypokalemia may be observed with high-renin forms of hypertension and in patients on diuretic therapy and increases the risk of malignant arrhythmias. The BUN and creatinine determine the renal function and aid in the determination of the severity of the hypertensive episode and the choice of antihypertensive medications. The urinalysis in an emergency may show proteinuria, red cells, and red cell casts.

Evidence of cardiac ischemia and left ventricular hypertrophy is

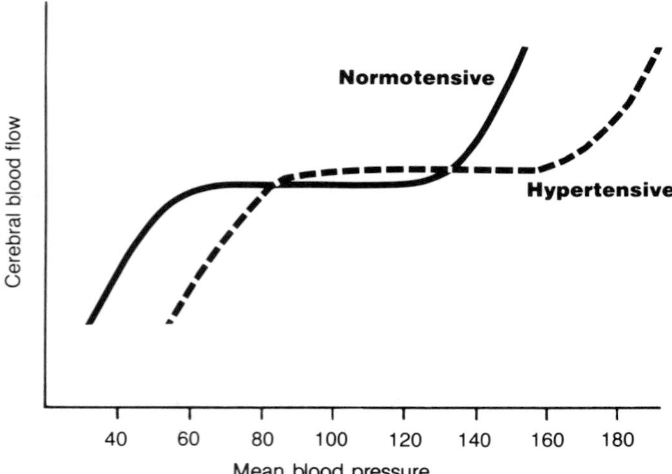

Fig. 23-1. Cerebral autoregulation of blood flow: changes seen with chronic hypertension.

determined by ECG. Signs of pulmonary edema, aortic dissection, or coarctation of the aorta may be seen on the chest x-ray. Patients with a suspected emergency should be placed on a cardiac monitor and given oxygen. A head CT scan should be obtained when the physical findings indicate cerebral ischemia or hemorrhage and in the presence of focal neurological signs of coma.

HYPERTENSIVE EMERGENCIES INVOLVING THE CENTRAL NERVOUS SYSTEM

Hypertensive Encephalopathy

The most devastating complication of hypertension is hypertensive encephalopathy. Signs and symptoms include severe headache, nausea and vomiting, and altered mental status ranging from lethargy or confusion to coma. Focal findings include cranial nerve palsies, blindness, aphasia, and hemiparesis. Twitching and myoclonus indicate neuromuscular hyperirritability. Retinal findings include hemorrhage, exudates, cotton wool spots, papilledema, and sausage linking. These signs and symptoms often progress over hours and can lead to coma and death in that time span.

Encephalopathy is secondary to cerebral hyperperfusion with loss of the integrity of the blood-brain barrier. The autoregulation of cerebral blood flow maintains a constant cerebral perfusion over a large range of mean blood systemic pressures. In normotensive patients, this range is from 60 to 125 mmHg. Flow increases with excessively high mean arterial pressures, whereas flow decreases with low mean pressures. This is demonstrated schematically in Fig. 23-1 as the cerebral-autoregulation curve.

For poorly controlled hypertensive patients, partially because of changes in the structure of the cerebral arteriole, this curve shifts to the right, so that adequate cerebral blood flow is not maintained during periods of low arterial pressure that normotensive patients easily tolerate. This shift in the autoregulation curve can occur over a period of weeks to months and may be reversible with proper control of the blood pressure in younger patients.

When high blood pressure exceeds the limits of autoregulation, excessive blood flow develops and there is loss of the integrity of the blood-brain barrier at the arteriole and the glial venules. Alterations of the endothelial membrane transport mechanisms and the opening of tight junctions result in an exudation of fluid into the brain. Experimentally, symptoms of hypertensive encephalopathy seem to correlate with an increase in permeability of the blood-brain barrier. Disruption of the blood-brain barrier occurs prior to the decrease in blood flow seen late in hypertensive encephalopathy. With persistent elevation in pressure, vascular necrosis occurs. This progression of pathologic findings can be witnessed in the retina with the finding of alternating areas of arteriolar constriction and dilation (sausage linking) and exudates. Late findings include generalized vasodilation, decreased blood flow, cerebral edema, and papilledema.

However, this is an oversimplified view of the dynamics of the cerebral vasculature occurring during hypertensive encephalopathy. The intracellular mechanism for the vasodilation seen has been hypothesized to be secondary to abnormal arachidonic acid metabolism and the development of oxygen-free radicals. This affects the smooth muscle cells of a media by preventing the sustained contraction needed in the face of elevated pressure. It has been noted that this functional impairment persists hours after the reduction of pressure and can be partially prevented with free-radical scavengers and prostaglandin inhibitors. Without lowering the pressure, this intracellular process continues, resulting in necrosis of the media layer. Exposure of the passing blood to these necrotic structures shears the red cells, causing further disruption to flow and resulting in micrangiopathic hemolytic anemia.

The treatment goal of hypertensive encephalopathy is to lower the mean arterial pressure so that the cerebral blood flow becomes normal and the stimulus for the vascular pathology ends in a controlled fashion over 30 to 60 min. Care is taken not to lower the pressure beyond the lower limits of autoregulation, which in a chronic hypertensive is a mean arterial pressure of approximately 120 mmHg.

The best agent for use in the setting of hypertensive encephalopathy is sodium nitroprusside. Intravenous labetalol is also an excellent choice. Avoid clonidine and pure beta blockers.

Hypertension and Other CNS Disorders

Differentiation of the cause-and-effect relationship between hypertension and CNS dysfunction is often very difficult. All other forms of CNS dysfunction (thrombotic stroke, intracranial hemorrhage, subarachnoid hemorrhage) are more common than hypertensive encephalopathy. The neurological event may be the etiology of the elevation in pressure (Cushing's effect), or the event may be related to the hypertension. History is often the principal means of differentiating these syndromes (see Table 23-1). The coma due to hypertensive encephalopathy is often not as dense as that with intracranial hemorrhage and may wax and wane.

In cases where the cause-and-effect relationship of the CNS dysfunction to the blood pressure is uncertain, severe elevations of pressure (BP > 220/130 mmHg) should be decreased in a controlled, graded manner with an initial decrease in mean blood pressure of 20 to 30 percent. The final pressure is modified according to the previous history of hypertension and medication compliance of the patient. Treatment should also be modified when the hypertension is secondary to stroke or the stroke is a complication of aortic dissection of myocadial infarction. A too rapid and vigorous reduction in pressure with a thrombotic stroke may lead to further ischemia from decreased blood flow to the watershed areas. The natural course of blood pressure levels after an acute stroke is mild hypertension with a gradual decrease to prestroke levels without treatment.

Treatment of hypertension in acute stroke syndromes must be executed in a controlled manner with an agent without CNS effects. The best agents are sodium nitroprusside and labetalol.

PREGNANCY-INDUCED HYPERTENSION

The upper limit of normal blood pressure in the third trimester of pregnancy is 125/75 mmHg, and pressures higher than 140/90 mmHg with signs and symptoms of hyperreflexia, confusion, headache, epigastric pain, seizures, or coma should be considered an emergency. Eclampsia occurs most commonly in young primagravidas and in multigravidas over the age of 35, especially those with a prior history of renal or hypertensive disease. Pregnancy-induced hypertension usu-

Table 23-1. Differential Diagnosis of Hypertensive Cerebrovascular Events

	Hypertensive Encephalopathy	Cerebral Thrombosis	Intracerebral Hemorrhage	Subarachnoid Hemorrhage	Transient Ischemia
Onset	Gradual, over 24–48 h	Acute, over 1–2 h	Rapid	Rapid	Rapid, may be recurrent
Neurological progression	Yes, over 24–48 h	May occur over several hours	Over minutes to hours	Rapid, in minutes	No
Impaired consciousness	Late	Not unless bilateral or brainstem	Usual	Usual and predominant	No
Other symptoms	Progressive headache, lethargy, seizures	Possible prior TIA* may occur during sleep	Sudden headache and vomiting initially		No
Focal signs	Transient and migratory	Present and fixed	Present and fixed	Frequently absent	Present but brief
CSF findings	Pressure may be elevated	Normal unless severe edema	Frequently blood, increased pressure	Blood, increased pressure	Normal

* Transient ischemic attack.

ally appears in the third trimester unless a molar pregnancy is present or there is a prior history of hypertensive or renal disease.

During eclampsia, uterine blood flow decreases, necessitating monitoring of fetal heart tones. The initial emergency treatment is to lower the blood pressure with magnesium sulfate and hydralazine. Magnesium sulfate has both antihypertensive and antiepileptic properties. It is given as a 4- to 6-g bolus intravenously, followed by a 1 to 2 g/h infusion. Therapeutic levels are 6 to 8 mEq/L. Excessive magnesium sulfate administration can lead to loss of reflexes (>8 mEq/L), hypotension, and eventual respiratory arrest (>12 mEq/L). Thus reflexes must be monitored, and when they disappear, the infusion must be stopped. Hydralazine 10 to 20 mg IV is also given. Diazoxide decreases uterine motility, requiring the use of oxytocin, and can, rarely, cause fetal hyperglycemia and hyperbilirubinemia. Sodium nitroprusside has also been used but infusions should not be prolonged and thiocyanate levels monitored. Labetalol has been shown to be safe and efficacious in this setting. The definitive treatment is evacuation of the uterus. Postpartum eclampsia can manifest itself for up to 2 weeks postpartum and may be treated as above or with any other appropriate antihypertensive medication. Diuretics are contraindicated in pregnancy-induced hypertension.

HYPERTENSIVE CARDIOVASCULAR EMERGENCIES

Left Ventricular Failure and Coronary Insufficiency

Alterations in left ventricular performance secondary to increased afterload is the primary mechanism by which an acute rise in pressure affects the cardiovascular system. This increases oxygen demand and may decrease coronary blood flow, which may result in angina, myocardial infarction, or acute left ventricular dysfunction with pulmonary edema.

Treatment of these syndromes is with agents which decrease both preload and afterload, thereby decreasing myocardial work and oxygen demand. Sodium nitroprusside and intravenous nitroglycerin are excellent agents, although the degree of blood pressure reduction is not as great with nitroglycerin. Oral nifedipine has been used successfully in these situations but is not approved for this use in the United States. Agents to avoid are diazoxide, hydralazine, minoxidil, and labetalol in patients with a history of congestive heart failure. Oxygen and morphine sulfate are adjuvant therapy in this setting. Furosemide or bumetanide may be used if there is evidence of volume overload.

Thoracic Aortic Dissection

Hypertension is the etiology for aortic dissection in about 90 percent of cases. Symptoms of chest or back pain usually begin abruptly and are severe. The location of pain varies depending on the site of dissection. The dissecting segment may involve the carotid arteries, leading to signs of acute cerebral infarction. Proximal dissection of the ascending aorta may occlude the coronary arteries, resulting in myocardial infarction, or can cause aortic insufficiency or tamponade.

The blood pressure is generally elevated but may also be normal or low. There may be discrepancies in the pulse character and blood pressure in different extremities. Any patient with acute chest pain and neurological deficit should be evaluated for possible aortic dissection.

The agents of choice for blood pressure reduction are a β-adrenergic antagonist, such as propranolol, and sodium nitroprusside. Trimethaphan may also be used. The goal of the pharmacologic therapy is to reduce the blood pressure and decrease the aortic pressure wave (dP/dt). Surgery is indicated with dissections involving the ascending aorta and in cases of inadequate control of the blood pressure.

ACUTE RENAL COMPLICATIONS OF HYPERTENSION

Deterioration of renal function in the face of an elevated pressure is considered a hypertensive emergency. Previous levels of the creatinine and BUN aid in the diagnosis. Proteinuria and the presence of red cells and red cell casts in the urine with elevation of the BUN and creatinine are diagnostic.

CATECHOLAMINE-INDUCED HYPERTENSIVE EMERGENCY

Acute elevations of circulating catecholamines with or without hypersensitivity of adrenergic receptors can lead to acute symptomatic hypertension. Pheochromocytoma presents as episodic elevations of blood pressure, headache, flushing, and diarrhea. Use of MAO inhibitors prevents the metabolism of adrenergic agents and can cause hypertension if sympathomimetics are used concurrently. Tyramine is the precursor to the adrenergic compounds, and patients on MAO inhibitors who ingest tyramine-containing foods (Chianti wine, aged cheese, beer, pickled herring) develop hyperstimulation of the adrenergic receptors resulting in acute symptomatic hypertension. Hypertension may also be precipitated in these patients with over-the-counter cold preparations and diet pills. Clonidine withdrawal, especially when withdrawn concurrently with a β blocker, leads to a severe hypertensive condition. These hyperadrenergic states are best treated with an α and β blocker, such as labetalol.

MEDICATION OPTIONS

Overview

The ideal antihypertensive agent for a hypertensive emergency would act rapidly, in a controllable and predictable manner, with few side effects; would be safe in combination with other medications and have few contraindications; and would not have adverse effects on cardiac output or myocardial, cerebral, and renal blood flows. The final com-

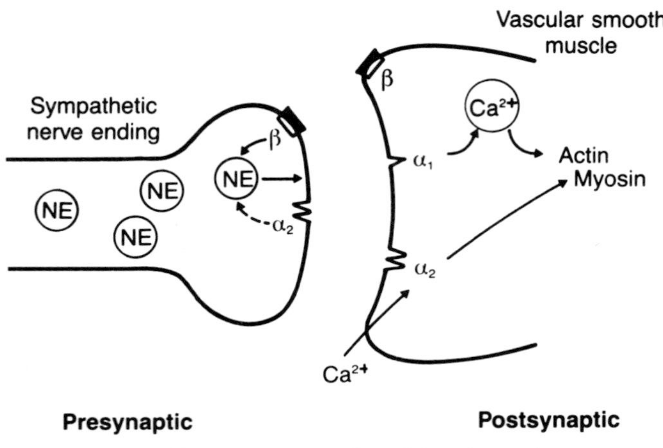

Fig. 23-2. Diagrammatic representation of the adrenergic receptors at the smooth-muscle synapse. ⟶, Stimulates; ----→ inhibits.

mon pathway in the acute setting is vasodilation by alteration of the membrane receptors or intracellular messengers.

Cellular Physiology

Postsynaptic α_1 receptors are stimulated by synaptically released norepinephrine, causing a release of intracellular calcium stores, resulting in smooth muscle contraction. Alpha-2 receptors are found both pre- and postsynaptically. The postsynaptic α_2 receptor is stimulated by circulating norepinephrine, causing an influx of calcium and resulting in smooth muscle contraction. Stimulation of the presynaptic α_2 receptor by norepinephrine prevents further release of norepinephrine (negative-feedback loop) (see Fig. 23-2). Agents which are nonspecific blockers of α receptors can lower pressure by smooth-muscle dilation but do not prevent the further release of norepinephrine from the nerve terminal. Agents which selectively block α_1 receptors cause a similar decrease in pressure but allow the negative-feedback cycle to operate by not blocking the presynaptic α_2 receptors.

Stimulation of CNS α_2 receptors decreases sympathetic outflow, resulting in bradycardia, hypotension, and somnolence.

Calcium entry into cells follows a strong concentration gradient. Once in the smooth-muscle cells, calcium binds with calmodulin, which then allows myosin and actin to bond, resulting in contraction. Small changes in intracellular calcium cause large changes in vascular tone.

Calcium channel blockers vary in effect on different vessels. In general, they prevent the calcium influx seen with depolarization of the cell membrane by blocking entry through the slow channel, resulting in decreased peripheral vascular resistance.

PRIMARY AGENTS FOR USE IN HYPERTENSIVE EMERGENCIES

The medications most commonly used for hypertensive emergencies are listed in Tables 23-2 and 23-3.

Sodium Nitroprusside (Nipride)

Actions and Pharmacology

Sodium nitroprusside, a rapidly acting arteriolar dilator and venodilator, can be used for all hypertensive emergencies, although it is not the agent of choice in pregnancy-induced hypertension. It acts by reacting with cysteine to form nitrosocysteine, which is a potent activator of guanylate cyclase. Guanylate cyclase stimulates the formation of cyclic GMP, which relaxes smooth muscle. Both arterial and venous smooth muscle dilate, decreasing preload and afterload, resulting in decreased myocardial oxygen demand. Despite the lack of a direct chronotropic effect, the heart rate increases slightly secondary to a baroreceptor-mediated reflex. There is no change in cardiac output or myocardial blood flow. The dilation of small-resistance coronary vessels may lead to a "steal" syndrome in face of coronary insufficiency. Cerebral blood flow may decrease in a dose-dependent manner. There is no change in renal blood flow with treatment, and plasma renin activity is increased. Pulmonary shunting may be induced, aggravating hypoxia.

The onset of action is almost immediate, with a duration of action of 1 to 2 min, and the plasma half-life is 3 to 4 min. Nitroprusside is metabolized initially to cyanide by sulfhydryl groups in the blood and then converted to thiocyanate in the liver by rhodanase. Thiocyanate is excreted by the kidney.

Indications

Sodium nitroprusside is the first drug of choice for all hypertensive emergencies except eclampsia prior to delivery. It may be used in predelivery eclampsia if other treatments have failed and in postpartum eclampsia. It is safe for use in children.

Use

A reasonable initial goal is a 30 percent reduction of the diastolic pressure in 30 to 60 min. Assessment of the patient's signs and symptoms are the ultimate guide for treatment.

Mix 50 mg of Nipride in 500 mL of D_5W (10 μg/mL) and start the infusion at 0.5 μg/kg per min and then titrate rapidly until the desired blood pressure has been achieved. The average effective dose needed is 3 μg/kg per min, with a range of 0.5 to 10 μg/kg per min. Maintenance antihypertensive medication should be started concurrently with the infusion of nitroprusside. The blood pressure should be monitored every few minutes during the initial titration. An arterial line is not necessary for the institution of therapy, but with long-term use it is necessary. The infusion fluid should not be used for simultaneous infusion of other medications. The infusion bottle should be covered with aluminum foil and not used for more than 24 h.

Table 23-2. Selection of Medications for Various Hypertensive Emergencies

Type of Hypertensive Emergency	First-Line Medication	Second-Line Medication	Medications to Avoid
Hypertensive encephalopathy	Nitroprusside, labetalol	Trimethaphan, diazoxide	Methyldopa, clonidine, propranolol
Acute pulmonary edema	Nitroprusside, nitroglycerin	Trimethaphan, furosemide, bumetanide	Labetalol, diazoxide, hydralazine, minoxidil
Myocardial ischemia	Nitroglycerin, nitroprusside	Nifedipine, labetalol	Diazoxide, hydralazine, minoxidil
Dissecting aortic aneurysm	Nitroprusside + propranolol	Trimethaphan	Diazoxide, hydralazine, minoxidil
Catecholamine crisis	Labetalol, phentolamine + propranolol	Nitroprusside + propranolol	Minoxidil
Pregnancy-iduced hypertension	Magnesium sulfate + hydralazine, labetalol	Diazoxide, nitroprusside	Trimethaphan, furosemide, bumetanide

Table 23-3. Medication Characteristics

Medication	Mode of Action	Route	Onset of Action	Duration of Action
Nitroprusside	Direct arterial & venous dilator	IV	Seconds	1–2 min
Labetalol	α_1, β_1, β_2 Blocker	IV	5 min	8 h
	Direct arteriolar dilator	PO	2 h	8 h
Nitroglycerin	Direct arterial &	IV	Seconds	4 min
	venous dilator	SL	Minutes	15–20 min
Diazoxide	Direct arteriolar dilator	IV	2 min	Varies: 8–24 h
Nifedipine	Calcium channel blocker	PO SL	5 min	2–4 h
Hydralazine	Direct arteriolar dilator	IV	10 min	3–8 h
		IM	20 min	3–8 h
		PO	30 min	3–8 h
Minoxidil	Blocks calcium uptake	PO	2 h	12 h
Prazosin	Postsynaptic α_1 blocker	PO	2 hr	>4 h
Phentolamine	α blocker	IV	Rapid	?
Clonidine	Central α_2 agonist	PO	30 min	2–4 hr

Side Effects and Contraindications

Hypotension is the most common complication. Cyanide toxicity is rare but may occur with prolonged infusions, in infusion rates greater than 10 μg/kg per min, or in hepatic dysfunction. Thiocyanate toxicity, manifesting as tinnitus, blurred vision, muscle weakness, changes in mental status, and seizures, is more common and seen after prolonged infusions and in patients with renal failure. Close monitoring of the infusion is required, which can present a staffing problem in many emergency departments. Nitroprusside inhibits hypoxia-induced vasoconstriction in the pulmonary vasculature and therefore may increase perfusion to nonventilated areas of the lung. Concomitant use with clonidine has caused myocardial infarction. It is inappropriate for use in prehospital situations.

Labetalol (Normodyne, Trandate)

Labetalol is a competitive, selective α_1 blocker and a competitive, nonselective β blocker ($\beta_1 = \beta_2$). The β-blocking action is approximately 4 to 8 times the α-blocking action. Labetalol is 6 to 10 times less potent than phentolamine as an α blocker. Propranolol is 1.5 to 4 times more potent as a β blocker. The hypotensive response is a result of the α- and β-blocking actions and a direct vasodilatory effect.

Labetalol is rapidly absorbed when taken orally, with an absorption half-life of 0.23 h for the tablets and peak plasma concentrations at 0.82 h. There exists significant first-pass hepatic metabolism, and care should be taken in oral dosing in the presence of hepatic disease. Bioavailability is only 25 percent after an oral dose, but increases if taken with food or with cimetidine, and in the elderly. Elimination half-life after an oral dose is approximately 8 h.

After an intravenous dose, the distribution to peripheral tissues is rapid, with a large volume of distribution of 15.7 L/kg. Elimination half-life is 5.5 h. Onset of action after an intravenous injection is 5 to 10 min, with a duration action of 8 h.

There is extensive hepatic metabolism, with less than 5 percent of the active compound excreted in the urine. It is safe for use with severe renal insufficiency without alteration of dosages.

The major hemodynamic effects are reduction of systolic arterial pressure and total peripheral vascular resistance. The reflex tachycardia associated with nonselective α blockade is avoided by the selective postsynaptic α_1 blockade and the β_1 blocking action. Cardiac output may not change or may slightly decrease after an intravenous dose. Pulmonary artery and wedge pressures decrease. Labetalol does not reduce cerebral blood flow despite significant reduction in blood pressure. There is no change in renal blood flow or glomerular filtration rates, and angiotensin II activity is decreased with use of labetalol. Fluid retention may occur with chronic use.

Because of its nonselective β-blocking activity, labetalol decreases the forced expiratory volume FEV_1 in patients with asthma and chronic obstructive pulmonary disease (COPD). It may blunt the β-agonist response in the treatment of bronchospastic disease.

Indications

Labetalol is a good intravenous medication for use in hypertensive emergencies and may be used in cases of treatment failure with sodium nitroprusside. It may be used orally for urgencies. It provides a steady, consistent drop in blood pressure and can be used in patients with cerebral vascular disease because there is no change in cerebral blood flow. Since it does not produce a reflex tachycardia, it is safe for use in the presence of coronary artery disease. It is an ideal choice for states of excessive catecholamine stimulation such as pheochromocytoma, MAO inhibitor–induced emergencies and abrupt clonidine withdrawal. It has been used in pregnancy-induced hypertension. Use in prehospital care has not been reported.

With an intravenous bolus, blood pressure falls in 5 min, with a maximum response in 10 min, and may last for up to 6 h. The rate of fall of the blood pressure is related to the rapidity of the injection. Labetalol can be given with repeated, incremental boluses starting with 20 to 40 mg IV. If the antipressor response is inadequate, repeat with double the dose every 30 to 60 min until adequate response is obtained or a total of 300 mg has been given. Labetalol may also be given as a continuous infusion, mixing 200 mg in 200-mL of D_5W to run at 2 mg/min (2 mL/min). When the goal pressure is achieved, the infusion should be stopped. The initial oral dose for labetalol in hypertensive urgencies is 200 mg.

Side Effects and Contraindications

Because of its large volume of distribution and long elimination half-life, labetalol has a prolonged action. Orthostatic hypotension occurs in 5 percent of patients. The nonselective β-blocking action of labetalol can exacerbate heart failure and induce bronchospasm. Tingling of the scalp has been noted. A paradoxical hypertensive effect can be seen when the drug is used in low doses in catecholamine-induced crisis because of the predominance of the β-blocking effect, leaving the α-receptors unblocked for the circulating catecholamines.

Intravenous Nitroglycerin

Actions and Pharmacology

Nitroglycerin causes arteriolar dilation and venodilation and dilates large coronary arteries with a greater effect on capacitance vessels. Onset is almost immediate when nitroglycerin is given intravenously, with a half-life of 4 min. The mechanism of action is postulated to be formation of disulfide bonds from reduced sulfhydryl groups at a smooth-muscle nitrate receptor, resulting in an increase in cyclic GMP. Metabolism in the liver occurs by denitration by a glutathione-reductase system. The cardiac output may decrease slightly or remain unchanged.

Indications

Intravenous nitroglycerin is the drug of choice for moderate hypertension complicating unstable angina, myocardial infarction, or pulmonary edema. It has a less deleterious effect on pulmonary gas exchange and collateral coronary blood flow than sodium nitroprusside in patients with ischemic heart disease.

Use

Start infusions at 10 μg/min, then augment by 5 to 10 μg every 3 to 5 min until symptoms are resolved or adverse effects become predominant.

Side Effects and Contraindications

The most common side effects are headache, tachycardia, nausea, vomiting, hypoxia, and hypotension.

SECONDARY AGENTS FOR USE IN HYPERTENSIVE EMERGENCIES

These agents have been used extensively in the past for hypertensive emergencies, but their role has diminished with the introduction of newer, safer, and equally efficacious medications. However, these agents still have a limited but significant role in the treatment of hypertensive emergencies.

Trimethaphan Camsylate (Arfonad)

Actions and Pharmacology

Trimethaphan produces its antihypertensive effects by ganglionic blockade, affecting both adrenergic and cholinergic ganglia with an additional direct vasodilatory effect. Reflex tachycardia develops, and cardiac output and renal and uterine blood flow decrease. The decrease in the aortic pressure wave *dP/dt* make this agent ideal for aortic dissections.

Indications

Trimethaphan camsylate is used in thoracic aortic dissection of the descending type if nitroprusside and propranolol fail to control the blood pressure. It is also useful in acute pulmonary edema secondary to hypertension.

Use

Mix 500 mg in 500 mL of D_5W (1 mg/mL), begin the infusion at 1 to 4 mg/min, and titrate the dose to the desired response. Because of loss of the vasomotor reflexes, the blood pressure can be modified by postural changes.

Side Effects and Contraindications

Tachycardia, paralytic ileus, urinary retention, mydriasis, and cycloplegia are very common. Tachyphylaxis develops within 24 h. This drug is contraindicated in pregnancy because it decreases uterine motility. It should be used with caution in patients with cardiac disease, adrenal insufficiency, and diabetes; in patients with an allergic history (because of histamine release); and in those on steroids.

Diazoxide (Hyperstat)

Actions and Pharmacology

Diazoxide is a direct arteriolar dilator. Reflex tachycardia results, and increased myocardial contractility, cardiac output, and myocardial oxygen demand are ramifications of the use of diazoxide. It has no sedative effects. Blood flow to the brain, kidneys, and coronary arteries is maintained.

The onset of hypotensive effect is 1 to 2 min after an intravenous dose, with a peak effect in 5 to 10 min. The initial distribution half-life is 48 h. The hypotensive action may last for up to 12 to 24 h. Diazoxide is metabolized in the liver and excreted in the urine.

Indications

The major indication for use of diazoxide is in hypertensive emergencies in which nitroprusside may be impractical, such as in prehospital care, but its use should be avoided with cardiovascular disease. The introduction of other equipotent agents which cause fewer complications has limited its usefulness.

Use

A 50-mg bolus every 5 to 10 min is given until the desired blood response is achieved. Alternatively, a constant infusion may be used, with a rate of 15 to 30 mg/min until a loading dose of 5 to 8 mg/kg has been given or an adequate hypotensive response is achieved. Furosemide may be given to counteract the sodium and water retention. Propranolol may be needed if symptomatic tachycardia develops. Propranolol may also significantly potentiate the hypotensive effects of diazoxide.

Side Effects and Contraindications

This agent does not allow for a controlled reduction in blood pressure. With more than a 150-mg bolus, hypotension may be severe and prolonged. Reflex tachycardia has induced angina and myocardial infarction in some cases. Sodium and water retention may occur as well as hyperglycemia. Renal disease seems to potentiate the hypotensive response. The potential use for diazoxide for eclampsia is complicated by fetal hyperglycemia, hyperbilirubinemia, and decreased uterine contractility, which can be reversed with oxytocin.

Diazoxide is contraindicated in coronary artery disease, angina, myocardial infarction, aortic dissection, coarctation of the aorta, intracerebral hemorrhage, and pulmonary edema. It should not be used with thiazide diuretics or aminophylline, hydralazine, reserpine, clonidine, or α-methyldopa. It can potentiate the effect of warfarin.

Hypotension secondary to the use of diazoxide may be reversed with volume infusion or sympathomimetic agents.

AGENTS FOR USE IN HYPERTENSIVE URGENCIES

Calcium Channel Blockers

Nifedipine (Procardia)

Actions and Pharmacology

Nifedipine is a coronary and peripheral arterial dilator with no direct chronotropic effect and a mild negative inotropic effect. This results in a slight increase in heart rate but does not often cause postural hypotension. This agent undergoes extensive hepatic metabolism, and no adjustment is needed in renal insufficiency. With oral administration, the plasma level correlates to the size of the dose, but the clearance half-life of 2 to 4 h and the time to the peak level remain constant with all doses. Plasma levels of nifedipine correlate with hypotensive action. Oral administration causes a rapid surge in sympathetic activity, with an increase in plasma norepinephrine, cortisol, renin, and angiotensin I and II. There are no long-term effects on the renin-angiotensin system.

The maximal hypotensive response is observed in 30 min after an oral dose. There is a slight increase or no change in glomerular filtration rate and renal blood flow and some diuretic natriuric, and uricosuric effects. It is effective in control of pressure with renovascular hypertension. Tachycardia has been noted for 1 to 2 h after an oral dose, but in most cases it is mild.

With an oral dose, peripheral vascular resistance falls, cardiac output increases, and pulmonary capillary wedge pressures decrease in patients without congestive heart failure. Maximal dP/*dt* remains unchanged or slightly decreases. Nifedipine may improve cardiac performance with impaired ventricular function. With severe congestive heart failure, the beneficial effects seen are balanced by the small but significant negative inotropic effect, and this agent should be used with caution in these patients.

Indications

Nifedipine is an excellent agent for use in hypertensive urgencies.

Use

Nifedipine is primarily absorbed by the gastric mucosa. To achieve the most rapid onset of action, the patient is instructed to bite, chew, and then swallow a capsule which has been punctured. Alternatively, 10 to 20 mg may be given orally. After a 20-mg oral dose, the onset of hypotensive effect occurs in 5 min, with a maximal effect in 20 to 30 min that persists for up to 4 to 5 h.

Side Effects and Contraindications

Headache, a burning sensation, flushing, and pedal and periorbital edema are observed. Postural hypotension may result if nifedipine is used concomitantly with diuretics. The effect on the cardiac index with left ventricular dysfunction is variable, and heart failure may develop. There is a negligible effect on the conduction system with therapeutic doses. There have been reports of reversible renal deterioration after a short course with nifedipine. Rebound hypertension has been described, as well as worsening of myocardial ischemia with rapid withdrawal. These symptoms can begin within 24 h of the last dose and are reversed by giving a calcium channel blocker. Nifedipine should not be used in dissection of the aorta unless a β-blocker is also given.

Direct Arteriolar Dilators

Hydralazine (Apresoline)

Actions and Pharmacology

One of the first antihypertensive agents available, hydralazine acts as a direct arteriolar dilator, with onset of action within 10 min after an intravenous dose and a duration of action of 3 to 8 h. The onset of action is 20 min when hydralazine is given intramuscularly and 30 min when given orally. Hydralazine causes reflex tachycardia and increases cardiac output. It causes sodium and water retention and increases plasma renin and catecholamines.

The plasma half-life is 2 to 4 h, but the antihypertensive effect lasts much longer than the plasma levels would indicate. Hydralazine has been detectable in the vascular walls long after being cleared from the plasma. It is metabolized by acetylation in the liver and gut walls. Approximately 50 percent of the population in the United States are "slow acetylators," and these patients have a higher incidence of hypotension and toxic complications. Hydralazine is also metabolized by ring hydroxylation and conjugation. Eighty percent of hydralazine and its metabolites are excreted within 24 h. Renal insufficiency prolongs the elimination half-life, and doses should be decreased in renal patients.

Indications

Pregnancy-induced hypertension is now the major indication for parenteral use. It is now used principally orally as an adjunct to other drugs.

Use

During eclampsia, 10 to 20 mg of hydralazine is given intravenously or 10 to 50 mg intramuscularly. The dose can be repeated in 30 min.

Side Effects and Contraindications

Undesirable cardiac effects prevent use of hydralazine when there is a history of coronary artery disease and in aortic dissection. This agent causes sodium and water retention and frequently causes headache, nausea, tachycardia, lethargy, and postural hypotension. Chronic oral administration can result in a lupuslike syndrome.

Minoxidil (Loniten)

Actions and Pharmacology

Minoxidil is a potent oral arteriolar dilator. It acts by blocking calcium uptake through the cell membrane. The onset of action is in 2 h, with a maximal effect in 4 h and a duration of action of 12 h. Ninety percent of the drug is absorbed orally, with peak plasma levels in 1 h. Minoxidil is conjugated in the liver, and no accumulation of action is seen in renal insufficiency. It causes fluid retention and should be used with a diuretic. Reflex tachycardia is a common finding.

Indications

Minoxidil can be used for the rapid oral control of pressure during a hypertensive urgency when other medications have failed. It is safe for use in the azotemic patient.

Use

Ten to twenty mg should be given orally and the dose repeated in 4 h if needed. A β blocker may be needed to control symptomatic tachycardia, but an excessive hypotensive effect may result. Sodium and water retention necessitates the use of diuretics.

Side Effects and Contraindications

Minoxidil is contraindicated with recent myocardial infarction, pheochromocytoma, congestive heart failure, and known hypersensitivity. Hirsutism may result from chronic use.

Adrenergic Blocking Agents

Prazosin (Minipress)

Actions and Pharmacology

Prazosin acts by α_1 (postsynaptic) blockade without blocking the presynaptic α_2 receptor, allowing for prevention of further release of norepinephrine into the synapse. It has an equipotent effect on the arterial and venous vessels. Acute use results in no reflex tachycardia, no change in cardiac index, and myocardial and cerebral perfusion. Renal blood flow and glomerular filtration rates remain the same.

Indications

Prazosin may be used for hypertensive urgencies.

Use

A 1-mg oral dose is given initially. Doses greater than 1 mg are not intended for initial therapy. The onset of hypotensive action in 30 min, peaking in 2 to 4 h.

Side Effects and Contraindications

Orthostatic hypotension, usually seen only with the first dose, is exacerbated by mild dehydration and with doses greater than 2 mg. β Blockers increase hypotensive effects. Overdose causes drowsiness and depressed reflexes.

Phentolamine (Regitine)

Actions and Pharmacology

Phentolamine competitively blocks postsynaptic and presynaptic α-adrenergic receptors and vasodilates both arterial and venous beds, resulting in a reduction of total peripheral vascular resistance. The drug also has directed, but less marked, positive inotropic and chronotropic effects on the heart, causing an increase in cardiac output. Onset of action following an IV dose of phentolamine is within 5 min, and the duration of action is 30 to 60 min. The average half-life is 19 min and approximately 13 percent is recovered unchanged in the urine.

Indications

Phentolamine is indicated for the prevention and treatment of hypertension associated with pheochromocytoma as a result of stress or manipulation during preoperative preparation and surgical excision. Phentolamine is approved for prevention and treatment of dermal necrosis, sloughing, or extravasation following IV administration of α-adrenergic agents.

Dose

The adult dose for phentolamine for control of hypertension in a patient with pheochromocytoma is 5 mg IV or IM. For prevention of extravasation, 10 mg can be added to each liter of norepinephrine. Phentolamine at this dose does not affect the pressor effect of norepinephrine. When treating an extravasation, dilute 5 to 10 mg of phentolamine in 10 mL of 0.9% saline and inject it intradermally into the affected area. This therapy is most effective when given with 12 h of extravasation.

Adverse Effects

Intravenous phentolamine has been noted to cause acute and prolonged hypotensive episodes, myocardial infarction, stroke, reflex tachycardia, cardiac arrhythmias, and death. Less severe effects that are also reported include weakness, dizziness, flushing, orthostatic hypotension, nausea, vomiting, diarrhea, and nasal congestion.

Adrenergic Agonists

Clonidine (Catapres)

Actions and Pharmacology

Clonidine, at doses used for hypertension, has potent central α_2-agonist effects. Stimulation of the postsynaptic receptors in the central nervous system results in a marked decrease in sympathetic system activity, lowering plasma catecholamine levels. While clonidine decreases basal sympathetic tone, vasomotor reflexes are not altered; thus there is no postural hypotension seen with therapeutic doses. Clonidine decreases renin secretion by a central mechanism. The net effect is a lowering of the blood pressure, bradycardia, and sedation. There is no change in renal blood flow or glomerular filtration rates. Cardiac output is decreased at rest but responds normally to exercise.

The onset of action is 30 to 60 min with oral loading, with a peak effect in 2 to 4 h. The duration of action of a single dose is 6 to 8 h. Clonidine readily passes the blood-brain barrier. Approximately 50 percent is excreted unchanged in the urine in the first 24 h. In renal failure, it is excreted in the feces. Very little is removed with dialysis.

Indications

Clonidine is an excellent agent for use in hypertensive urgencies. It can be used in the elderly and in renal failure. There are several unapproved uses of clonidine, including for migraine, and opiate and nicotine withdrawals.

Use

Oral loading is accomplished by giving 0.2 mg. Additional doses of 0.1 mg may be given hourly until the diastolic pressure is below 115 mmHg or a maximum of 0.7 mg has been given. The typical dose needed for adequate reduction of blood pressure is 0.3 to 0.4 mg. with an average time for reduction of pressure of 2¾ h. It is not necessary to discharge the patient on clonidine after its use.

Side Effects and Contraindications

Sedation and dry mouth are the most common side effects. Occasional bradycardia, especially in patients with sick sinus syndrome, has been reported. Orthostatic hypotension is not expected with therapeutic doses but may occur if used with diuretics. Rebound and "overshoot" hypertension may be seen with rapid withdrawal from high doses of clonidine. Caution should also be used with patients on the following drugs: cyclic antidepressants, where the antihypertensive effects of clonidine may be blocked; alcohol, which enhances the sedative effects of clonidine; β blockers, may worsen clonidine withdrawal; negative inotropic agents, which may cause bradyarrhythmias and disturbances when used with clonidine. Clonidine may inhibit the antiparkinsonism effect of levodopa.

Modifiers of the Renin-Angiotensin System

Captopril (Capoten)

Actions and Pharmacology

This angiotensin-converting enzyme inhibitor is a potent oral antihypertensive agent. It is rapidly absorbed after an oral dose, with an onset of action in 30 min. The peak effect is in 50 to 90 min, lasting for 4 to 6 h. Captopril is effective in congestive heart failure. No change in cardiac output or in heart rate has been observed. Captopril is not a reliable agent in patients with low renin activity. Cerebral blood flow is unchanged. The drug is metabolized rapidly and excreted in the urine. With renal insufficiency, plasma levels rise and the dose must be decreased when used chronically. Baroreceptor reflexes remain intact, and postural hypotension is rare.

Indications

Indications are limited to use in hypertension urgencies with known renovascular hypertension such as hypertension associated with scleroderma.

Use

Captopril should be administered in 25-mg doses orally three times a day.

Side Effects and Contraindications

Leukopenia and proteinuria may appear after chronic use. Skin rash, coughing, and loss of taste (ageusia) are not uncommon. This drug should not be used with potassium-sparing diuretics or with potassium supplements because hyperkalemia can develop.

ADJUVANT AGENTS IN HYPERTENSIVE TREATMENT

Loop Diuretics: Furosemide (Lasix) and Bumetanide (Buminex)

Actions and Pharmacology

Hypotensive effects are due to increased venous capacitance and decreased plasma volume. The diuretic effect begins within 5 min, peaks in 30 min, and lasts for 2 h. The drugs may decrease cardiac output but dilate renal arteries. They are usually excreted unchanged renally, but with renal impairment are cleared by biliary excretion. With renal and hepatic impairment, furosemide should be used with caution.

Indications

The primary use of furosemide and bumetanide is with antihypertensive agents which cause sodium and water retention. They should not be used as primary therapy of hypertensive urgencies or emergencies because volume depletion will stimulate the renin system and increase vasoconstriction.

Use

The initial dose of furosemide is 40 mg intravenously. This may be repeated with double the dose in 30 to 60 min. The initial dose of bumetanide is 1 to 2 mg.

Side Effects and Contraindications

Hypokalemia, hypovolemia, and orthostatic hypotension are the most common acute side effects. Ototoxicity may occur with very high doses and with rapid intravenous injections of furosemide. These drugs are contraindicated in pregnancy-induced hypertension.

Propranolol (Inderal)

Actions and Pharmacology

Propranolol is a nonselective β blocker, and the postulated mechanisms for its blood pressure reduction action includes reduced cardiac output, a readjustment to blood flow, readjustment of the baroreceptors, altered high pressure reflexes from the heart, reduced plasma renin activity, altered catecholamine synthesis, inhibited presynaptic β receptors, and a central action of an active metabolite of the agent.

Indications

Propranolol is used primarily as adjuvant therapy with other medications. In catecholamine overdrive states (pheochromocytoma, clonidine withdrawal, and MAO inhibitor reaction), propranolol may be used in conjunction with phentolamine or sodium nitroprusside. Along with sodium nitroprusside, it is the treatment of choice for thoracic aortic dissection. It may be needed to counteract reflex tachycardia induced by many vasodilatory agents.

Side Effects and Contraindications

The nonselective β blockade may induce bronchospasm in susceptible individuals. Left ventricular decompensation may be seen. Acute heart blocks and bradycardia have been observed. Sudden withdrawal of β blockers can precipitate angina or infarction. Because of the impaired adrenergic response seen with hypoglycemia, propranolol should be used with caution in insulin-dependent diabetics. It should not be used with clonidine, since simultaneous withdrawal from both medications may precipitate a hypertensive emergency. When used concurrently or within 1 h of verapamil or diltiazem, significant bradycardias or heart blocks may result.

COMPLICATIONS OF HYPERTENSIVE THERAPY

Unique complications of antihypertensive therapy include symptoms caused by abrupt withdrawal from antihypertensive medications or from overdose.

Rapid Withdrawal

Withdrawal from antihypertensive medications which affect the adrenergic system may lead to one of five responses in the patient: (1) a small percent remain normotensive, possibly because of resetting of the "baroreceptors"; (2) the blood pressure returns to pretreatment levels over a few weeks; (3) the majority of patients have an asymptomatic return to pretreatment levels; (4) the blood pressure may "rebound" rapidly to pretreatment levels and may show signs of sympathetic overactivity; and (5) the blood pressure may "overshoot" to exceed the pretreatment levels, with evidence of excessive sympathetic activity and end-organ dysfunction. It is the overshoot in pressure that may lead to a hypertensive emergency. Medications which can place the patient at risk for complications include clonidine, β blockers, and calcium channel blockers.

The mechanism of withdrawal overshoot with clonidine involves increased sympathetic discharge, increased plasma renin activity, and enhanced responsiveness of the adrenergic receptors to norepinephrine. These actions are enhanced when a β blocker is withdrawn simultaneously with clonidine, and with high daily doses of clonidine. Chronic use of β blockers leads to sensitization of the β receptors, which, along with the sympathetic surge seen with clonidine withdrawal, may lead to a hypertensive emergency.

Treatment depends on the symptoms. If the patient presents with sympathetic hyperactivity, the first drug of choice is labetalol. Care must be taken with the use of labetalol since low doses may exacerbate the elevation of pressure because of the predominance of the β-blocking effect. Use of phentolamine with propranolol is an adequate second choice. Sodium nitroprusside is also an excellent option. Symptoms of angina or myocardial infarction should be treated with labetalol, propranolol, or intravenous nitroglycerin.

Rapid withdrawal of β blockers and calcium channel blockers has been reported to precipitate arrhythmias, angina, and myocardial infarction.

BIBLIOGRAPHY

Alpert M, Bauer J: Rapid control of severe hypertension with minoxidil. *Arch Intern Med* 142:2009, 1982.

Anderson R, Hart G, Crumpler C, et. al: Oral clonidine loading in hypertensive urgencies. *JAMA* 246:848, 1981.

Baumbach G, Heistad D: Heterogenicity of brain blood flow and permeability during acute hypertension. *Am J Physiol* 249:H629, 1985

Beer N, Gallegos I, Cohen A, et al: Efficacy of sublingual nifedipine in the acute treatment of systemic hypertension. *Chest* 79:571, 1981

Bertel O, Conen D, Radu E, et al: Nifedipine in hypertensive emergencies. *Br Med J* 286:19, 1983.

Calhoun D, Oparil S: Treatment of hypertensive crisis. *N Engl J Med* 323:1177, 1990.

Cohn J, Burke L: Nitroprusside. *Ann Intern Med* 91:752, 1979.

Cressman M, Vidt D, Gifford R, et al: Intravenous labetalol in the management of severe hypertension and hypertensive emergencies. *Am Heart J* 107:980, 1984.

Elkayam U, Weber L, McKay C, et al: Spectrum of acute hemodynamic effects of nifedipine in severe congestive heart failure. *Am J Cardiol* 56:560, 1985.

Fagan T: Acute reduction of blood pressure in asymptomatic patients with severe hypertension: An idea whose time has come—and gone. *Arch Intern Med* 149:2169, 1989.

Ferguson R, Vlasses P: Hypertensive emergencies and urgencies. *JAMA* 255:1607, 1986.

Ferguson R, Vlasses P: How urgent is 'Urgent' hypertension? *Arch Intern Med* 149:257, 1989.

Finnerty F: Slowing the return of hypertension after stopping medication. *JAMA* 254:503, 1985

Frohlich E: Antihypertensive therapy: Newer concepts and agents. *Cardiology* 73:349, 1985.

Garrett B, Kaplan N: Efficacy of slow infusion of diazoxide in the treatment of severe hypertension without organ hypoperfusion. *Am Heart J* 103:390, 1982.

Given B, Lee T, Stone P, et al: Nifedipine in severely hypertensive patients with congestive heart failure and preserved ventricular systolic function. *Arch Intern Med* 145:281, 1985.

Hachinski V: Hypertension in acute ischemic strokes. *Arch Neurol* 42:1002, 1985.

Haft J, Litterer W: Chewing nifedipine to rapidly treat hypertension. *Arch Intern Med* 144:2357, 1984.

Halpern A, Cubeddu L: The role of calcium channel blockers in the treatment of hypertension. *Am Heart J* 104:363, 1986.

Hass D, Anderson G, Streeten D: Role of angiotensin in lethal cerebral hypoperfusion during treatment of acute hypertension. *Arch Intern Med* 145:1922, 1985.

Hill N, Antman E, Green L, et al: Intravenous nitroglycerin: A review of pharmacology, indications, therapeutic effects and complications. *Chest* 79:69, 1981.

Houston M: Treatment of hypertensive emergencies and urgencies with oral clonidine loading and titration. *Arch Intern Med* 146:586, 1986.

Jaker M, Atkin S, Soto M, et al: Oral nifedipine vs. oral clonidine in the treatment of urgent hypertension. *Arch Intern Med* 149:260, 1989.

Lavin P: Management of hypertension in patients with acute stroke. *Arch Intern Med* 146:66, 1986.

Lebel M, Langlois S, Belleau L, et al: Labetalol infusion in hypertensive emergencies. *Clin Pharmacol Ther* 37:615, 1985.

MacCarthy E, Bloomfield S: Labetalol: A review of its pharmacology, pharmokinetics, clinical use and adverse effects. *Pharmacotherapy* 3:193, 1983.

McLain L: Therapy of acute severe hypertension in children. *JAMA* 239:755, 1978.

Mayhan W, Heisted D: Disruption in the blood-brain barrier in veins. *Stroke* 16:137, 1985.

Panzer R, Feibel J, Barker W, et al: Predicting the likelihood of hemorrhage in patients with stroke. *Arch Intern Med* 145:1800, 1985.

Reid I: The renin-angiotensin system and body function. *Arch Intern Med* 145:1475, 1985.

Reid J: Alpha-adrenergic receptors and blood pressure control. *Am J Cardiol* 57:6E, 1986.

Smith W, Clifton G, O'Neill W, et al: Antihypertensive effectiveness of intravenous labetalol in accelerated hypertension. *Hypertension* 5:579, 1983.

Strandgaard S: Autoregulation of cerebral blood flow in hypertensive patients: The modifying influence of prolonged antihypertensive treatment on the tolerance to acute, drug induced hypotension. *Circulation* 53:720, 1976.

Strandgaard S: Cerebral blood flow in hypertension. *Acta Med Scand* 678(suppl):11, 1983

Strandgaard S: Cerebral autoregulation. *Stroke* 15:413, 1984.

Strandgaard S, Olesen J, Skinhoj E, et al: Autoregulation of brain circulation in severe hypertension. *Br J Med* 1:507, 1973.

Strauss F, Franklin S, Lewin A, et al: Withdrawal of antihypertensive therapy. *JAMA* 238:1734, 1977.

Van Zwieten P: Overview of alpha 2-adrenergic agonists with a central action. *Am J Cardiol* 57:3E, 1986.

Van Zwieten P, Timmermans P, Thoolen M, et al: Inhibitory effect of calcium antagonist drugs on vasoconstriction induced by vascular alpha 2 adrenergic stimulation. *Am J Cardiol* 57:12D, 1986.

Vidt D, Bravo E, Fouad F: Drug therapy: Captopril. *N Engl J Med* 306:214, 1982.

Yatsu FM, Zivin J: Hypertension in acute stroke: Not to treat. *Arch Neurol* 4:999, 1984.

Zeller K, Von Kuhnert L, Matthews C: Rapid reduction of severe asymptomatic hypertension: A prospective, controlled trial. *Arch Intern Med* 149:2186, 1989

24
THORACIC AND ABDOMINAL AORTIC ANEURYSMS

A. Joel Feldman

Any portion of the aorta may be involved with aneurysmal disease. Although the asymptomatic patient is not a problem for the emergency physician, the symptomatic patient requires prompt, accurate diagnosis and expeditious therapy. Delay, incorrect diagnosis, or improper therapy will frequently cost these patients their lives.

ACUTE DISSECTING ANEURYSM OF THE AORTA

Acute dissection is the most common catastrophe involving the aorta. It affects 5 to 10 patients per million population each year and is two to three times more common than an acutely ruptured abdominal aortic aneurysm. Untreated, it is lethal. The mortality rate is 28 percent at 24 h, 50 percent at 48 h, 70 percent in 1 week, and 90 percent in 3 months. Men are much more commonly affected than women. The vast majority of patients are hypertensive.

Etiology

The final common pathway leading to this entity is necrosis of the medial layer of the aortic wall, usually due to atherosclerosis. However, approximately 10 percent have cystic medial necrosis associated with Marfan's syndrome. Medial necrosis also occurs during pregnancy, with coarctation, with congenital abnormalities of the great vessels, and with various hormonal abnormalities. Half of the dissections occurring in young women occur during pregnancy.

Classifications

Dissecting thoracic aortic aneurysms are classified according to the location of the dissecting process and not the site of origin of the tear. In Debakey's classification, type I involves the ascending aorta as well as varying lengths of the distal aorta; type II is limited to the ascending aorta only and does not involve the arch or the more distal portions of the aorta; and type III is a dissection of the descending aorta, usually starting just distal to the origin of the left subclavian artery and most commonly involving the entire descending aorta down to the iliac arteries. In the Stanford classification, types I and II are grouped together, as type A, because the principles of treatment and the prognosis are the same. A Stanford type B dissection is the same as a Debakey type III. In the Stanford experience two-thirds of the patients presented with ascending aortic dissections and one-third with descending aortic dissections.

Presentation

In acute dissection, 70 to 90 percent of patients present with severe pain that is more intense than they have ever experienced. The pain may be located in the back, the anterior chest, the epigastrium, the flanks, and/or the extremities. The most important characteristic of the pain is its severity and short duration of onset.

Patients may present with an acute stroke (approximately 3 percent due to occlusion of a cerebral vessel), with acute paraplegia because of spinal ischemia (2 to 4 percent), acute loss of pulse in an extremity (approximately 16 percent), and/or renal or visceral ischemia (60 percent). Congestive heart failure and pulmonary edema are present in 22 percent of patients. Less commonly, the initial presentation is acute ischemia of the lower extremities without other associated symptoms.

The blood pressure may be elevated, normal, or low. It should be measured in both upper extremities and one of the lower extremities. Significant differences in extremity blood pressure should suggest the diagnosis in the proper clinical setting. Likewise, the patient who presents with both acute chest pain and an acute neurologic deficit (uncommon in acute myocardial infarction), or with acute chest pain and an acutely ischemic leg should be suspected of having an acute aortic dissection.

Diagnosis

The most important differential diagnosis is acute myocardial infarction. Less commonly, stroke, acute surgical abdomen, pulmonary embolism, or an acutely ischemic extremity due to thrombosis or embolus may be confused with an acute aortic dissection.

In addition to extremity blood pressure differences, physical examination may reveal the murmur of aortic insufficiency, signs of cardiac tamponade, or murmurs at the base of the neck, in the abdomen, or over the femoral arteries that have not been previously present.

The electrocardiogram is abnormal in 90 percent of these patients; however, changes compatible with acute myocardial infarction are rare.

A chest x-ray should be obtained immediately. A normal chest x-ray is rare. Roentgenographic findings suggestive of an acute aortic dissection are (1) mediastinal widening, (2) a change in the configuration of the thoracic aorta as compared with old films, (3) extension of the aortic shadow beyond a calcified aortic wall, (4) a localized hump on the aortic arch, and (5) pleural effusion, most commonly on the left.

The diagnostic gold standard remains the thoracic arteriogram. However, rapid-sequence CT scanning with intravenous contrast injection can accurately diagnose acute dissecting aneurysm. The false lumen and its hematoma can usually be visualized and the extent of the aneurysm defined. In our institution, we use the CT scan to evaluate patients in whom we have a low suspicion of an aortic dissection. However, the CT scan may be more readily available in many institutions and can accurately diagnose an aortic dissection. Patients requiring surgery will ultimately require an arteriogram. Transesophageal echocardiography can also be used to make the diagnosis.

Management

The most important contribution of the emergency physician is to suspect the diagnosis and initiate proper diagnostic maneuvers. In institutions not equipped to definitely diagnose or treat this problem, arrangements should be made for immediate transfer. Hypertensive patients are treated by continuous intravenous infusion of nitroprusside, and intravenous β blockers such as propranolol, metoprolol, labetalol, or esmolol. Frequent monitoring of blood pressure (preferably by an indwelling arterial line) is necessary. Hypotensive patients can usually be resuscitated with small quantities of a crystalloid solution or blood.

All patients with acute type A (ascending) aortic dissections should be treated with emergency surgical repair. The appropriate long-term therapy for those with descending aortic dissections (type B) is more controversial. Long-term results for surgical therapy as compared with medical therapy are approximately the same. This may in large part be due to the fact that the indications for acute surgical repair of a descending aortic dissection are themselves independent indicators of increased operative mortality. Nonetheless, patients with persistent pain, lower extremity ischemia, visceral or renal ischemia, or rupture are candidates for surgical repair.

THORACIC AORTIC ANEURYSMS

Thoracic aortic aneurysms are most commonly located in the descending aorta but may occur in the ascending aorta.

Etiology

Atherosclerosis has replaced syphilis as the most common cause of thoracic aortic aneurysms. These aneurysms can occur in patients with Marfan's syndrome and cystic medial necrosis. Trauma is also a common cause of thoracic aortic aneurysms, but strictly speaking, these are pseudoaneurysms and will not be discussed here.

Presentation

In approximately half the patients the diagnosis is an incidental finding on chest x-ray. Forty-two percent of patients had back or chest pain when first seen. Symptoms are usually due to compression or erosion of surrounding structures or to frank rupture. Large aneurysms (uncommon) may erode into the vertebral column or ribs. Dysphagia from compression of the esophagus, hoarseness from traction on the laryngeal nerve, cough because of bronchial compression, or hemoptysis because of compression of the left lung can occur. Hemoptysis from erosion into the esophagus or a bronchus also occurs.

Prognosis

The prognosis is poor if the condition is left untreated. Exact data are difficult to obtain because most series are old and contain large percentages of syphilitic aneurysms. Nonetheless, a mean survival time of 2.4 years for untreated descending thoracic aneurysms and a 20 percent 5-year survival has been established. In most series the average survival time after onset of symptoms is less than 1 year.

Diagnosis

Diagnosis is accomplished by chest x-ray and aortography. The widened mediastinal or aortic silhouette is suggestive. Serial chest x-rays showing enlargement of the thoracic aorta indicate aneurysm formation. A CT scan is useful in nonemergency situations, but ultimately an aortogram must be performed to diagnose the size and extent of the aneurysm.

Management

The asymptomatic patient is not a problem for the emergency physician. Nonetheless, such patients should be assured of adequate follow-up. Patients with symptomatic aneurysms that have not ruptured should be admitted for close observation and an expedient workup.

The treatment of this entity is surgical. All patients with a symptomatic aneurysm or documented enlargement of their aneurysm should undergo surgery. Patients with asymptomatic aneurysms should undergo surgery if their overall condition permits.

EXPANDING AND RUPTURED ABDOMINAL AORTIC ANEURYSMS

Abdominal aortic aneurysms affect approximately 2 percent of the population. Of these 98 percent are infrarenal, which facilitates both diagnosis and surgical management. Approximately 90 percent are atherosclerotic in nature; a small percentage are syphilitic or myotic in origin.

Over 80 percent of abdominal aortic aneurysms are asymptomatic when first diagnosed and are not emergency management problems. However, a symptomatic or ruptured aneurysm presents both diagnostic and management dilemmas. This entity is uncommon, and a diagnosis may not be considered unless one consciously searches for it and is aware of the many ways in which it may present. If inordinate delays are to be avoided and a reasonable salvage rate achieved, treatment must be initiated on the basis of clinical suspicion only.

An expanding aneurysm is one in which the aneurysmal wall is intact but symptoms are caused by compression and inflammation of surrounding structures. Rupture is imminent in such cases. The ruptured aneurysm has lost continuity of the aneurysm wall at some point. If the bleeding is tamponaded by the retroperitoneal tissues, the patient may be normotensive when initially seen.

Presentation

Patients almost always present with the sudden-onset pain. However, there is a rare entity of so-called chronic ruptured aneurysm in which the pain may be present for weeks or months. Typically, the pain is severe and constant (however, it may be mild) and cannot be relieved by changing position. It may be located in the low back, flanks, periumbilical area, or pelvis. There is no clearly characteristic pattern, and the diagnosis should be considered in any patient over the age of 50 with a sudden onset of abdominal or low back pain. The pain is usually somatic rather than visceral in nature, due to compression of the somatic sensory nerves in the retroperitoneum by the expanding aneurysm sac or hematoma. This may give rise to unusual presentations. There may be a neurologic deficit caused by compression of the femoral or sciatic nerve from a ruptured aortic and/or iliac artery aneurysm. The patient may present with thigh, testicular, or peroneal pain. Ecchymoses may be present along the groins, scrotal sac, or perineum as a result of dissection of retroperitoneal blood into the pelvis or inguinal canals. In the elderly patient, unless there is an obvious explanation for these symptoms or signs, one should think of the diagnosis of a ruptured aortic or iliac artery aneurysm.

A pulsatile abdominal mass is usually present on abdominal examination. However, this may be obscured by the presence of a retroperitoneal hematoma, low blood and pulse pressure, or obesity. Seventy percent of patients are normotensive when first seen, so that the hemodynamic stability of a patient should not dissuade the physician from making this diagnosis.

Any older patient presenting with the sudden onset of abdominal pain associated with an abdominal mass (whether pulsatile or not) or who is hypotensive with an abdominal mass (whether pulsatile or not) is presumed to have an expanding or ruptured abdominal aortic aneurysm. Similarly, any patient with a known history of an aortic aneurysm and the sudden onset of severe low back pain and/or hypotension is presumed to have a ruptured abdominal aortic aneurysm. These are emergency situations, and the patients should be taken quickly to the operating room. No laboratory studies—including ultrasonography, plain films of the abdomen, CT scan of the aorta, or arteriography—are of diagnostic value. The patient may well die during the delay caused by these studies.

In other situations, however, additional diagnostic studies may help avoid unnecessary emergency surgery or allow for elective repair of a nonruptured aneurysm. The cross table lateral x-ray of the abdomen is not particularly useful, since only 60 percent of abdominal aortic aneurysms are calcified. Moreover, the study cannot determine whether the aneurysm is ruptured or not. Ultrasonography of the abdominal aorta will determine the presence or absence of an aneurysm, but it cannot reliably differentiate a ruptured from unruptured aneurysm. A CT scan of the abdominal aorta can accurately define the presence or absence of an aneurysm, its extent, and whether it is ruptured or not. If a previous CT scan or ultrasound study exists, an emergency CT scan will reveal whether enlargement of the aneurysm has occurred in the interim.

In the hemodynamically stable patient with a known history of abdominal aortic aneurysm in whom there is a low suspicion of rupture, we obtain an emergency CT scan. The CT scan is also used in the older patient without any background or evidence on physical examination of an abdominal aortic aneurysm who presents with back or abdominal pain of unknown etiology or hypotension thought secondary to intraabdominal bleeding. If an emergency CT scan is not possible, then emergency ultrasound of the aorta can at least determine if an aneurysm is present.

Management

The definitive treatment of an expanding or ruptured abdominal aortic aneurysm is surgical. The goal of the emergency physician is to get the patient into an operating room as soon as possible.

If transfer is necessary, two large-bore intravenous catheters and a Foley catheter should be placed. Transfer should not await the availability of laboratory results, blood products, or x-rays. If the patient is stable when first seen, intravenous fluid should be given at a rate adequate to maintain urine output but not to elevate the patient's blood pressure. Patients who become unstable or who are hypotensive on arrival in the emergency department should be resuscitated with fluids up to a systolic pressure of 90 to 100 mmHg. Military antishock trousers (MAST) may be applied to the hypotensive patient in whom transfer is necessary. There is no wide experience with this particular mode of therapy, but it seems a rational adjunctive measure to support the patient's blood pressure.

At an institution prepared to treat the problem definitively, the stable patient is taken to the operating room as soon as possible. The remainder of the evaluation and preparation of the patient for surgery can be done there. Two large-bore intravenous catheters should be placed in the unstable patient on arrival in the emergency department and the patient should then be transferred directly to the operating room. Control of the suprarenal aorta is required in severely hypotensive patients who do not respond to fluid resuscitation and vasopressors, and in patients in full cardiac arrest who do not respond to closed-chest cardiac massage, fluids, and vasopressors. This is best performed in the operating room. If an operating room is not available, then anterolateral thoracotomy and occlusion of the thoracic aorta performed in the emergency room may be life-saving. The patient's survival is then dependent on restoring flow to the renal and mesenteric vasculature within 30 to 45 min.

Prognosis

The overall mortality rate for this disease is approximately 45 percent in most centers. The patient who is stable on admission has a better prognosis, with some centers achieving mortality rates as low as 15 percent but more commonly 30 to 35 percent. The patient who is unstable on presentation has a poor prognosis, with mortality rates ranging from 60 to 80 percent. Salvage in this particular group of patients is contingent on quick diagnosis and treatment.

BIBLIOGRAPHY

Debakey M, McCollum CH, Crawford ES, et al: Dissection and dissecting aneurysms of the aortic: Twenty-year followup of five hundred twenty-seven patients treated surgically. *Surgery* 92:1118, 1982.

Lawrie GM, Morris GC, Crawford EJ, et al: Improved results of operation for ruptured abdominal aortic aneurysms. *Surgery* 85:483, 1979.

Miller DC, Stinson EB, Shumway NE: Realistic expectations of surgical treatment of aortic dissection: the Stanford experience, *World J Surg* 4:571, 1980.

Sarris GE, Miller DC: Peripheral vascular manifestations of acute aortic dissection, in Rutherford RB (ed): *Vascular Surgery*. Philadelphia, Saunders, 1989, p 942.

Szilagyi DE: Clinical diagnosis of intact and ruptured abdominal aortic aneurysms, in Bergan JJ, Tao JST (eds): *Aneurysms: Diagnosis and Treatment*. New York, Grune & Stratton, 1982, p 205.

25 MESENTERIC ISCHEMIA

John L. Glover
Geoffrey B. Blossom

Mesenteric ischemia is a relatively rare condition, but the incidence may be increasing in association with the advancing age of the population. It may present as an acute abdominal catastrophe or as a cause of chronic weight loss. In both circumstances, the diagnosis is usually not considered until the patient is critically ill. Consequently, morbidity and mortality are high (at least 70 percent mortality for laparotomy done for dead bowel), even though there is reasonably good understanding of the pathophysiology and the appropriate treatment. Therefore, early diagnosis is the key to improving results; and early diagnosis can be facilitated by instituting appropriate tests based on prodromal symptoms.

ANATOMY AND PATHOPHYSIOLOGY

Knowledge of the anatomy of the intestinal blood supply is necessary to understand the pathophysiology of ischemia, especially since ischemia may be acute or chronic, and may affect either the arterial or the venous supply.

Abdominal viscera are supplied with blood by three major arterial branches which arise from the anterior aspect of the abdominal aorta. The celiac trunk originates at the diaphragmatic crura. Its three main branches, the splenic, left gastric, and common hepatic arteries, supply the upper abdominal viscera and small bowel to the ligament of Treitz. The remainder of the mesenteric circulation comes from the superior and inferior mesenteric arteries. These two vessels supply a portion of the pancreatic circulation as well as the small bowel and colon. Together, the three splanchnic vessels receive 25 percent of the cardiac output at rest and contain up to one-third of the total blood volume.

The venous drainage of the intestines is by the superior and inferior mesenteric veins. These vessels join the splenic vein beneath the pancreas and form the portal vein. Each drains the area supplied by its corresponding artery.

Mesenteric ischemia may be caused by (1) arterial embolism, nearly always to the superior mesenteric artery; (2) arterial thrombosis, usually due to arteriosclerotic plaques; (3) venous thrombosis, often associated with a coagulopathy; or (4) insufficient arterial flow due to poor cardiac performance, the so-called low-output ischemia.

Arterial embolism accounts for 40 to 50 percent of all episodes of acute mesenteric ischemia, and the source of the embolus is nearly always the heart. In most cases, the clot is from a mural thrombus associated with a myocardial infarction; but in some cases it comes from the left atrium and is associated with acute or chronic atrial fibrillation. In the past, atrial thrombus associated with mitral valvular stenosis due to rheumatic fever was the most common source of embolism; but the decrease in rheumatic fever and the aging of the population have made mural thrombus overlying an infarcted segment of left ventricular wall or septum more common. In most cases, patients have no preexisting significant obstruction of their mesenteric vessels, and consequently there is no development of collateral circulation. When embolism occurs, therefore, it causes acute cessation of distal arterial flow. In most cases, the point of obstruction is the main trunk of the superior mesenteric artery, just beyond its right colic branch. As a result, the entire small bowel except for the most proximal jejunum becomes acutely ischemic.

Arterial thrombosis, on the other hand, is usually preceded by long periods (months at least) of relative ischemia caused by progressive stenosis at the origins of the celiac and superior mesenteric arteries. In most patients, the narrowing is due to progressive buildup of arteriosclerotic plaque, but in some cases it is due to fibromuscular hyperplasia. As stenosis increases, collateral circulation develops. For example, when there is plaque at the origins of both the celiac and the superior mesenteric artery, the inferior mesenteric artery becomes very large, supplying blood through connections with the superior mesenteric, including the marginal artery which courses along the mesenteric aspect of the colon. The gradual nature of this process and the rich collateral connections make it possible to supply enough arterial flow to maintain viability under resting, basal conditions. When more blood is required, however, as when a large meal is ingested, flow becomes inadequate. The patient feels cramping abdominal pain, and may vomit, expelling the source of "stress" from the intestine and possibly relieving the pain. The intermittent nature of this phenomenon and the analogy with pain related to myocardial stress generated the term "intestinal angina." This chronic situation may become acute if complete occlusion occurs or if the metabolic requirements of the intestine exceed the ability of the collateral circulation to supply adequate blood flow.

In view of the excellent arterial perfusion of the intestinal tract, it is not surprising that most instances of venous occlusion are associated with factors affecting coagulation. Some of these are hereditary disorders, such as deficiencies of antithrombin III or protein C. Others are more general, for example, dehydration, relative polycythemia, and hypercoagulable states associated with medications such as birth control pills (less common with present oral contraceptives). Venous occlusion in the presence of normal arterial flow results in massive congestion, and by the time infarction occurs, a large proportion of the blood volume is sequestered in the intestine. Consequently, large volumes of fluid are required to replenish intravascular volume, and anticoagulation is necessary to prevent further clotting.

Since the mucosa has a higher metabolic rate than the other layers of the intestine, it is the first area affected by ischemia, and may be the only area affected if there is enough remaining blood flow to support the muscular layer. This situation occurs commonly in chronic intestinal ischemia, and the resulting sloughing of mucosa accounts for the presence of occult blood in the stool. Mucosal sloughing occurs in the first stages of acute ischemia from all causes. As long as the loss is patchy, or of only partial thickness, there will be no abdominal tenderness because there is no stimulation of the somatic nerve fibers which lie outside the bowel wall. When more mucosa sloughs, the combination of bacterial invasion of the muscular layer and the damaging effects of toxic products of breakdown of intestinal cells stimulates the visceral nerve endings which lie within the muscular layers of the intestine. The result is poorly localized, intermittent abdominal discomfort which makes the patient feel restless and change positions frequently. When the inflammatory process involves the full thickness of the bowel wall, the somatic nerve endings are irritated and the patient experiences constant, severe abdominal pain which is associated with abdominal tenderness. This stage usually corresponds with infarction of the full thickness of the bowel wall, and the patient must be assumed to have peritonitis whether or not perforation has occurred.

CLINICAL PRESENTATION

The mortality rate for patients with gangrenous bowel is extremely high, and the most important factor in improving the chances for survival is to make the diagnosis before infarction occurs. This, in turn, means suspecting the diagnosis in patients with vague symptoms of abdominal distress and few, if any, clinical signs. The key to early diagnosis is to think of mesenteric ischemia in patients with abdominal pain and no obvious related problem such as previous abdominal surgery, an incarcerated hernia, or symptoms of biliary disease or ulcer. The initial presentation always involves abdominal discomfort but varies with the mechanism of mesenteric ischemia.

In acute ischemia due to embolism to the superior mesenteric artery or due to arterial thrombosis, the onset of abdominal discomfort is sudden and dramatic. With either etiology, there is pain "out of proportion to the physical findings" before peritonitis is present. The patients are nearly always over 50 and have some general evidence of cardiovascular disease. With acute ischemia due to embolism there is often atrial fibrillation or evidence of a myocardial infarction in the relatively recent past. In some cases, however, the infarction has been silent or subendocardial and the abdominal catastrophe is its first manifestation. Patients who have recently discontinued anticoagulant therapy for controlled chronic atrial fibrillation are at an increased risk for recurrent atrial thrombosis and subsequent embolization.

In patients with arterial thrombosis occurring due to progressive occlusion of the celiac and superior mesenteric arteries, one can nearly always elicit a history of unexplained weight loss over the preceding several months. It is rare, however, to elicit the classical history of intestinal angina: abdominal pain after a large meal, relieved by vomiting. More often the history is one of weight loss and "fear of food." These patients have gradually become accustomed to eating smaller and smaller meals in order to avoid abdominal pain, and this is the characteristic history for chronic mesenteric ischemia without infarction.

"Nonocclusive" intestinal ischemia usually occurs in patients hospitalized for cardiac failure, and it was much more frequent before interventional cardiology became common and measurement of cardiac output became so easy. It may still be seen in an emergency department setting in patients who are being given outpatient intensive diuretic therapy for cardiac failure and who have concurrent hypokalemia and digitalis toxicity or near toxicity.

Finally, venous thrombosis tends to occur in younger patients because venous thrombi are associated with disorders of coagulation instead of complications of arteriosclerosis. In these patients, the onset of pain is more insidious because the occlusion is on the venous side of the circulation, and a thorough history is especially important in raising a suspicion for this diagnosis. For example, a previous spontaneous episode of venous thrombosis *either in the patient or a relative* may be a clue to protein C or antithrombin III deficiency. Other factors in the history include concurrent use of birth control pills, a history of malignancy, evidence of polycythemia (either "true" polycythemia or polycythemia secondary to other diseases), and evidence of portal hypertension.

Other important aspects of the history and general physical examination include any evidence of cardiac or peripheral vascular disease, such as a history of symptoms of cerebrovascular disease or claudication or a history of myocardial infarction or angina pectoris. Auscultation for bruits in the neck and abdomen should be done, and the status of all peripheral pulses should be recorded. Physical evidence of chronic weight loss may be important, especially in elderly patients unable to give a good history.

Patients are usually afebrile unless infarction has been present long enough to cause peritonitis. Blood pressure is stable until sequestration of a large percentage of the blood volume causes hypovolemia, or until bacteremia occurs. These findings are not present as a rule until the patient has obvious abdominal tenderness and rigidity. The lack of abnormal vital signs except for mild tachycardia in the preinfarction stage of the disease is one of the reasons that physicians may dismiss prodromal symptoms of mesenteric ischemia as gastroenteritis.

The abdominal examination varies depending on the stage of ischemia and on whether or not infarction has occurred. Distension is not present initially, but develops when ileus occurs secondary to peritonitis or to impaired motility before peritonitis occurs. If the visceral component of pain is predominant, the patient may writhe and will have difficulty localizing the pain. When the somatic component develops, patients lie still and have diffuse abdominal tenderness and rigidity. As long as some bowel is viable, bowel sounds will be active until peritonitis becomes generalized. The presence of rebound tenderness, of course, is dependent on the presence of peritoneal irritation caused by transmural inflammation of the intestine.

DIAGNOSTIC STUDIES

A leukocytosis is present in most patients, frequently in excess of 15,000, and about half of the patients will exhibit a metabolic acidosis. Hemoglobin and hematocrit reveal hemoconcentration, and occasionally serum amylase and phosphate may be elevated, although these are nonspecific findings.

Abdominal radiographs should be obtained, primarily to look for other conditions which can have similar prodromes, such as an early bowel obstruction or gallstone ileus. Although one looks for thickening of the bowel wall, or air in it, these findings are rare, and are never clear enough to make a definitive diagnosis. Air in the portal vein is a late finding indicative of dead bowel and a grim prognosis.

Duplex ultrasound may be used to diagnose chronic mesenteric ischemia, but at the current stage of development it requires expert interpretation. Furthermore, a successful examination depends on a relative paucity of gas in the abdomen, and therefore is best done after an overnight fast. However, since abdominal duplex techniques are developing rapidly, duplex ultrasound may become a useful technique even in emergency situations. The same can be said for laparoscopy, but the necessity of a general anesthetic limits its use as an early method for diagnosis in a condition with such vague and varied initial symptoms.

Arteriography, which is the mainstay of diagnosis and early treatment, should be obtained promptly in all patients who are hemodynamically stable if there is a strong suspicion of mesenteric ischemia. Embolic occlusion of the superior mesenteric artery is usually manifested by a sharp cutoff of the column of dye several centimeters from its origin, below the takeoff of the middle colic artery. Thrombosis is represented by occlusion at the origin, and nonocclusive ischemia manifests as segmental narrowing of arterial arcades. Findings in venous thrombosis are more subtle and may not be diagnostic.

If there is strong enough suspicion of the diagnosis of mesenteric ischemia to believe that angiography should be obtained, surgical consultation should be requested because the study may indicate need for an emergency operation. In addition, it may be desirable to leave a catheter in place for intraarterial infusion of vasodilating agents.

TREATMENT

As stated previously, the challenge is to make the diagnosis of ischemia before infarction occurs. Emboli can be removed relatively easily; and the results of celiac and superior mesenteric revascularization are quite good, but cannot be done safely in the presence of generalized peritonitis. Venous infarction nearly always requires resection, but usually enough bowel can be spared to allow survival and normal nutrition if the hypercoagulability is reversed. It is crucial *to avoid laparotomy* in patients with "nonocclusive" ischemia because the anesthetic exacerbates the cause of the problem (the low cardiac output) and operative manipulation increases vasospasm and can cause ischemia to progress to necrosis. The marked differences in treatment for different varieties of ischemia point out the importance of early angiography. There is also substantial evidence that infusion of vasodilating drugs through angiographic catheters increases the amount of bowel which can be saved in cases of embolism and thrombosis, and may be therapeutic in low output ischemia.

Other adjunctive therapies are anticoagulation with heparin, decompression of dilated bowel, and use of broad-spectrum antibiotics. Heparin, which should be started as soon as feasible after angiography, prevents propagation of thrombus in conditions of decreased arterial flow and reverses the hypercoagulability associated with venous thrombosis. Bowel decompression and antibiotics have been shown to prolong the period between ischemia and necrosis when there is marginally adequate intestinal blood supply.

Other measures include replacement of plasma volume and adequate monitoring of hemodynamic parameters. These are best accomplished in the perioperative period by placing an arterial line, a Swan-Ganz catheter, and a Foley catheter while giving appropriate fluid and electrolyte therapy.

Since all forms of intestinal ischemia may cause loss of so much intestine that life cannot be sustained, bowel with marginal viability is often left in place at the initial procedure. In such cases, a "second look" operation is done after 12 to 24 h.

Adopting an aggressive attitude toward arteriography in patients with early and vague symptoms suggestive of ischemia will undoubtedly lead to some unnecessary arteriograms, but the risk of morbidity from angiography is negligible compared to the risk of mortality from bowel which has become necrotic while physicians waited for symptoms to become clearer.

BIBLIOGRAPHY

Bergan JJ: Diagnosis of acute intestinal ischemia, in *Seminars in Vascular Surgery*. Philadelphia, Saunders, 1990.

Bergan JJ, Pearce WH: *The Management of Visceral Ischemic Syndrome*, ed 3. Philadelphia, Saunders, 1989.

Boley SJ, Spraynagan S: Initial results from an aggressive roentgenological and surgical approach to acute mesenteric ischemia. *Surgery* 82:848, 1977.

Clavien PA, Muller C: Treatment of mesenteric infarction. *Br J Surg* 74:500, 1987.

Fry WJ: *Mesenteric Ischemia in Current Surgical Therapy*-3, Toronto, Decker, 1989.

Kaleya RN, Boley SJ: Mesenteric ischemic disorders, in *Maingot's Abdominal Operations*, ed 9. Connecticut, Appleton and Lange, 1989.

Serreyn RF, Schoofs PR: Laparoscopic diagnosis of mesenteric venous thrombosis. *Endoscopy* 18:249, 1986.

Sitges-Serra A, Mas X, Roquenta F, et al: Mesenteric infarction: An analysis of 83 patients with prognostic studies in 44 cases undergoing massive small bowel resection. *Br J Surg* 75:544, 1988.

26 PERIPHERAL VASCULAR DISEASE AND THROMBOPHLEBITIS

A. Joel Feldman

PERIPHERAL VASCULAR DISEASE

The emergency physician is frequently the first contact for patients with acute vascular emergencies. To intelligently assess and initiate treatment, it is important to understand the several etiologies of acute vascular disease and their underlying pathophysiology.

Acute Ischemia of the Extremities

Acute extremity ischemia is most commonly due to embolism, thrombosis in situ of a preexisting atherosclerotic lesion, or trauma. The latter diagnosis is obvious from the history and physical examination. The lower extremities are more frequently involved by both embolism and thrombosis in situ. Ninety percent of emboli originate in the heart, although infrequently the source is a proximally located arterial lesion (arterioarterial embolus). Thrombosis occurs at a site of a severe stenosis of the vessel (usually due to severe atherosclerosis) because of low flow through the stenotic area and abnormal intima. Because atherosclerosis is a systemic disease, the patient will frequently have evidence of chronic arterial occlusive disease on both history and physical examination. Both lower extremities may show diminished pulses, absent hair on toes, thinning of the skin, and thickening of the nails.

There are a number of conditions that may present as acute ischemia of the extremities. The false lumen of an acute dissecting thoracic aortic aneurysm involving the abdominal aorta may occlude the blood flow to one or both legs.

Patients with low cardiac output (either cardiogenic or hypovolemic) may present with acutely ischemic limbs due not to acute mechanical obstruction of a major artery but rather to decreased delivery of blood. These patients are usually easily diagnosed because of the clinical setting of an acute myocardial infarction, blood loss, intravascular volume depletion (e.g., sepsis, dehydration), or treatment with intravenous vasopressors. Patients with severe atherosclerotic occlusive disease are at a much higher risk to develop ischemia or tissue loss in situations of low flow.

Intraarterial injection of illegal drug substances is an increasingly common problem. In our experience intraarterial injection into the femoral arteries rarely results in acute ischemia and tissue loss. Injection into the arteries of the wrist, hand, or fingers results in intense burning pain, frequently followed over a period of days by extensive swelling of the hand and digital gangrene of varying degree. Vasospasm, the presence of particulate matter used to cut the drug, crystallization of the injected substance on injection, and arterial necrosis have all been implicated as causes of this injury. Rarely, massive iliofemoral thrombosis may be confused with acute ischemia. This is discussed elsewhere.

Emboli most commonly lodge at the bifurcation of arteries and are more common in the lower extremities. In a recent series, 46 percent of emboli lodged at the bifurcation of the femoral artery, 18 percent at the iliac arteries, 13 percent in the terminal aorta, and 10 percent in the popliteal arteries. The most common site of an upper extremity embolus was the distal brachial artery. Approximately 8 percent of emboli lodged in the visceral circulation, in either the renal or the superior mesenteric arteries. Emboli may be multiple, and the patient should be carefully examined for evidence of embolization to other extremities or to visceral arteries.

Microemboli are small collections of platelets and fibrin (platelet-fibrin emboli) and/or atheromatous debris that originate from atherosclerotic ulcers, stenoses, or aneurysms in the aorta or the iliac, femoral, or popliteal arteries. These are so-called arterioarterial emboli. These small emboli do not occlude major vessels but become lodged in smaller digital, muscular, and skin vessels, causing ischemia in the small amount of tissue supplied by the occluded vessel. Clinically, this is manifest by painful, cyanotic toes (or portion of a toe), petechialike skin lesions, or muscle infarcts with associated muscle tenderness and pain. These lesions may be present despite palpable pulses. Occasional massive showers of microemboli may occur. Both lower extremities can be affected. The patient's extremity may be mottled, with areas of muscle tenderness and pain, and cyanosis and pain of several toes may be present.

Upper extremity microemboli do occur but are less common, just as atherosclerosis is less common in the upper extremities. Patients with upper extremity microemboli should be evaluated for atherosclerotic lesions of the proximal subclavian vessels and poststenotic aneurysm of the subclavian artery due to compression at the thoracic outlet.

Pathophysiology

The severity of the ischemic episode depends on the site of occlusion and the quality of collateral circulation around this point. Progressive thrombosis occurs in the stagnant column of blood both proximal and distal to the acutely occluded site. As thrombosis progresses, sources of collateral blood supply are occluded, causing progression of ischemia. Anticoagulation prevents this propagation and helps to limit the ischemic insult.

Pain is the most common symptom of an acutely ischemic extremity. Loss of sensory nerve function (resulting in hypesthesia-anesthesia) and of motor nerve function (resulting in paresis or paralysis) occurs within minutes of severe ischemia. If the severe ischemic insult persists, muscle necrosis occurs. Much later, necrosis of skin, bone, and fat intervenes. The time sequence in which these events occur is dependent on the severity of ischemia. In general, patients presenting with sensorimotor deficits have a severe ischemic insult, and if flow cannot be restored within 3 to 4 h, permanent loss of function and possible gangrene may ensue.

Initial Evaluation

The history and physical examination are the most important parts of the initial evaluation of the acutely ischemic extremity. Both the normal and the symptomatic extremity are carefully examined because the former provides evidence of the patient's baseline condition. A careful sensorimotor examination is performed. The temperature and color of the skin of both extremities are noted. The presence of gangrene is important. The consistency of the limb musculature to palpation is evaluated. Of course, pulses are examined.

This initial assessment not only determines the severity of the ischemic insult but also provides a reference point for evaluating progression of ischemia and response to treatment.

Differential Diagnosis

The most common problem in acute ischemia of the lower extremities is differentiating embolus from thrombosis. The signs and symptoms of ischemia are the same regardless of the etiology. Nonetheless, various aspects of history and physical examination tend to favor one diagnosis or the other. A history of cardiac disease (arrhythmia, myocardial infarction, valvular heart disease, etc.), an asymptomatic opposite extremity with normal pulses, and the absence of the skin changes of chronic arterial insufficiency favor embolism. Conversely, if the patient's history reveals no source for an embolus (no clinically significant heart disease), if the opposite extremity shows evidence of chronic arterial occlusive disease, and if there is a history of symptoms compatible with chronic peripheral vascular disease (claudication or rest pain), thrombosis in situ is favored. Unfortunately, the patient with underlying chronic occlusive disease as well as cardiac disease who has thrown an embolus is quite common. Patients with emboli almost always have a known history of cardiac disease. Examination of the involved extremity may reveal an absent pulse when one is palpable at the same level on the opposite extremity. An arteriogram is usually needed to differentiate the two entities.

Petechial areas of cyanosis or necrosis; cyanotic, painful toes; muscle tenderness; and pain suggest microemboli. The rest of the limb seldom is ischemic, and pulses may be intact.

Management

The management of these patients is outlined in Figure 26-1. After the history and physical examination, patients with salvageable limbs are anticoagulated with approximately 100 units/kg of heparin IV.

Patients suspected of having an acute aortic dissecting aneurysm are not anticoagulated. Patients whose history and physical examination clearly indicate an embolus undergo embolectomy. All others undergo emergency arteriography with visualization of both lower limbs. The radiographic appearance of the uninvolved limb will provide a clue as to the cause of ischemia in the symptomatic limb. A patient with a sharp cutoff on arteriogram most likely has had an embolic episode. On the other hand, thrombosis in situ frequently presents in the setting of diffuse atherosclerotic disease and commonly shows a tapering lumen. Patients thought to have emboli undergo immediate embolectomy if their condition permits. Those who have thrombosis undergo emergency revascularization if they have sensory or motor deficits or tissue loss. Patients with rest pain but without neurologic deficits or tissue loss are treated with anticoagulation and observation. They undergo elective reconstruction. A number of these patients will experience improvement in symptoms and may not require reconstruction as collateral flow improves with time.

Patients with microemboli are anticoagulated for 3 to 5 days if seen acutely (although the benefit of this has not been proved). An arteriogram is performed to identify the source of the emboli. An abdominal aortic ultrasonograph is obtained to detect the presence of an aortic aneurysm.

Some success has been reported in the treatment of acute lower extremity ischemia with fibrinolytic agents. These are infused in low doses through an intraarterial catheter placed in the clot for periods of 24 to 72 h. Such therapy is contraindicated if the patient has neurologic deficits or early tissue necrosis because flow must be restored within a few hours to salvage the extremity.

ARTERIAL TRAUMA

Arterial injury is due to either blunt or penetrating trauma. Although penetrating trauma is more common, blunt trauma is potentially more dangerous since it is not so obviously associated with vascular injury. Severe soft tissue and bone injuries may obscure a vascular injury. The blunt trauma may appear so mild that an accompanying arterial injury may be missed unless it is searched for. In blunt or penetrating extremity trauma, for any injury potentially involving the vasculature, further vascular evaluation is necessary.

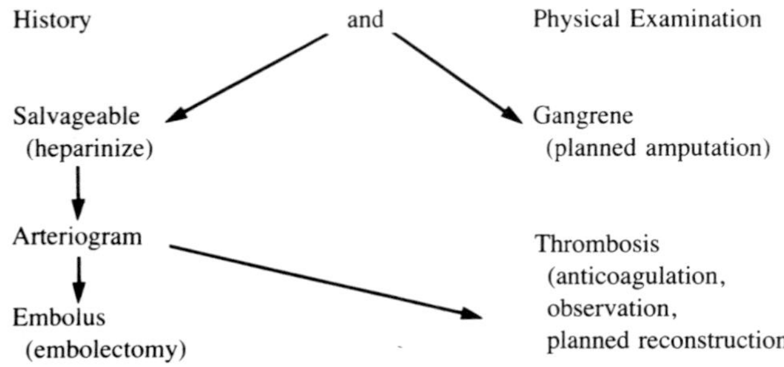

Fig. 26-1. Management of acute ischemia of the extremities.

Diagnosis

The signs and symptoms of acute ischemia, the five P's, should be sought in patients suspected of having an arterial injury. Patients with severe ischemia frequently complain of *pain*. The patient may note *paresthesias* or *paralysis* due to direct nerve injury, ischemia distal to the injury, or nerve compression due to hematoma within the neurovascular sheath. Of course, a *pulseless* extremity and/or one with *pallor* distal to an injury indicates an arterial injury. Patients with any of these signs or symptoms should undergo arteriography. A biplane arteriogram obtained using transfemoral or transaxillary catheterization is preferred. If this is not possible, the emergency physician may elect to obtain an arteriogram of the involved extremity by placing a small intravenous catheter in the artery proximally and injecting the dye by hand. This provides less accurate information.

If the trajectory of a penetrating injury is thought to have passed in proximity to a neurovascular bundle, arteriography is indicated. This is true even in the absence of any obvious physical signs or symptoms of arterial injury. Under these circumstances, if good-quality biplane angiography is normal, surgical exploration is not needed. This has been questioned recently by several authors. The incidence of abnormal arteriograms in patients without physical findings suggestive of arterial injury is low. Moreover, the injuries that are identified in the asymptomatic patient tend to be "minor" (e.g., intimal tears, intimal flaps, disruption of small branch vessels, etc.). Patients with such injuries have been safely observed and surgery reserved for those who become symptomatic at a later date. This approach is not yet universally accepted. We believe that arteriographic examination of asymptomatic patients with proximity injuries (or blunt trauma) and surgical repair of so-called minor injuries is indicated.

Patients with knee dislocations have a high incidence of accompanying popliteal arterial and venous injuries, and arteriography should be performed in these patients.

A venogram of the injured extremity should be obtained, and popliteal venous injuries should be repaired if found. Injuries of more proximally located major veins are repaired if the patient's condition is stable and the repair does not unduly prolong surgery.

Emergency arteriography is contraindicated in any unstable patient. Obviously, the patient's life takes priority over salvage of an extremity. Bleeding injuries are controlled by direct pressure and taken to the operating room, where the injury is explored and repaired. Other potentially life-threatening injuries take precedence over peripheral vascular injuries.

SYMPTOMATIC POPLITEAL ANEURYSMS

Any patient with acute ischemia of the lower leg may have a symptomatic popliteal aneurysm. Such aneurysms are among the most common of peripheral arterial aneurysms and present with either thrombosis of the aneurysmal sac or embolization of an intramural thrombus into the distal vasculature. Rupture is uncommon. These aneurysms are generally due to atherosclerosis and are more common in older males; 47 percent are bilateral, and there is a high incidence (78 percent) of associated aortic, iliac, or femoral artery aneurysms.

A popliteal mass (whether pulsatile or not) in the symptomatic leg or a pulsatile mass in the asymptomatic extremity indicates a possible symptomatic aneurysm. An arteriogram is obtained to document the diagnosis and to plan operative treatment.

THROMBOPHLEBITIS

In patients with acute venous disease, thrombosis occurs because of mechanical injury to the vein, a hypercoagulable state, and/or venous stasis. The signs and symptoms of acute venous disease vary and are related to the patient's underlying disease and the location and extent of the thrombosis.

Superficial Thrombophlebitis

In the lower extremities, superficial thrombophlebitis involves the greater or lesser saphenous veins or varicosities. Redness, tenderness, and induration are present along the course of the involved vein. If the greater saphenous vein is involved, it is clinically not possible to distinguish phlebitis from lymphangitis, as the major lymphatic drainage of the leg runs along the vein.

The diagnosis is confirmed by Doppler examination (with a reported 94 percent accuracy rate) or by obtaining a venogram. The Doppler examination, although easy to do, requires an experienced examiner. Superficial thrombophlebitis of varicosities or the lesser saphenous system is treated conservatively with bed rest, elevation, local heat, and analgesics as needed. Nonsteroidal anti-inflammatory drugs are useful in treating the inflammatory process and pain associated with this disease. Involvement of the greater saphenous vein below the knee is treated similarly. Thrombophlebitis of the saphenous vein in the thigh may also be treated conservatively unless there is some question of the involvement of the saphenofemoral junction. A venogram is then obtained. If the thrombotic process involves the iliofemoral system, anticoagulation as for deep-vein thrombosis is performed.

Acute Deep-Vein Thrombosis

The signs and symptoms of acute deep-vein thrombosis are quite unreliable, and confirmatory testing is necessary. Again, the lower extremities are most commonly involved. The classical findings of edema, warmth, erythema, pain, and tenderness are present in 23 to 50 percent of patients. Unfortunately, massive iliofemoral thrombosis can be present with minimal physical findings. Homan's sign is unreliable. The common femoral vein and popliteal vein are superficially located in the groin and popliteal fossa; tenderness, induration, or erythema in these areas is highly suggestive of acute thrombosis of the underlying vein.

A previous history of thrombotic disease, recent lower extremity trauma, treatment with estrogen, use of birth control pills, recent surgery (especially urologic, orthopedic, or gynecologic surgery), advanced age, recent myocardial infarction, congestive heart failure, carcinoma, and obesity are all associated with an increased risk of deep-vein thrombosis. Patients with one or more of these factors should be evaluated by additional testing even if the physical examination is negative.

A variety of tests are available for diagnosis of deep-vein thrombosis. The venogram remains the accepted standard. However, duplex evaluation of the venous system using real-time ultrasound Doppler imaging and simultaneous Doppler flow evaluation of the venous system with color flow has proved to be an accurate noninvasive diagnostic modality. A large number of series have reported accuracy ranging from 90 to 100 percent. The venous duplex examination eliminates the need for x-ray exposure as well as the risk of allergy to the intravenous contrast medium. It can differentiate acute from chronic disease and characterize the age of the thrombus. In some hospitals, it has replaced the venogram as the standard diagnostic test for acute deep-vein thrombosis.

Impedance plethysmography is readily and easily performed in the emergency department setting. Accuracies of 80 to 90 percent have been reported. It is insensitive to infrapopliteal thrombus. Accuracy may be decreased in patients with chronic venous disease and venous collaterals, in patients with elevated central venous pressure, in patients with severe peripheral vascular disease, and in patients with mechanical compression or obstruction of the venous system. In our institution both duplex color-flow imaging of the deep venous system and impedance plethysmography are readily available and both are performed by experienced technicians. We have found the duplex scan to be more accurate and useful in the diagnosis of acute deep-vein thrombosis, and it is our diagnostic test of choice in this setting.

Management of Acute Deep-Vein Thrombosis of the Lower Extremities

Patients who are at high risk for deep-vein thrombosis based on history and/or physical examination should be heparinized immediately pending the results of confirmatory tests. We prefer the color-flow venous duplex examination or venogram to establish the diagnosis. The patient is then treated with continuous intravenous infusion of heparin for 7 to 10 days. The patient is kept in bed with strict elevation of the legs for the first 4 days after the diagnosis is established. Local heat and analgesia are used as needed. Patients with significant pain secondary to a marked inflammatory response to the thrombotic process may obtain relief with the addition of nonsteroidal anti-inflammatory agents to the regimen. However, we have generally avoided this because of the fear that the antiplatelet effect of these agents may increase the incidence of bleeding complications in the fully anticoagulated patient. Long-term anticoagulation with oral anticoagulants may be begun soon after the patient's admission.

Massive Deep-Vein Thrombosis

Phlegmasia alba dolens (milk leg) is caused by extensive iliofemoral thrombosis with swelling of the entire leg to the groin. The leg frequently has a doughy consistency but is not tensely swollen. Arterial inflow is not compromised. The leg is treated as above.

Phlegmasia cerulea dolens is due to extensive iliofemoral thrombosis involving most of the venous collateral circulation as well. The leg is tensely swollen and cyanotic. Skin bullae may be present. Swelling within the muscular compartments of the leg may cause arterial insufficiency. If all venous outflow is occluded, stasis occurs in the capillary and arteriolar beds and retrograde thrombosis of the arterial system will occur. Venous gangrene occurs in this setting.

The treatment consists of strict bed rest with maximum elevation of the affected extremity. Anticoagulation with heparin is instituted immediately. Treatment with fibrinolytic therapy should be considered in these patients if no contraindication exists. These patients may have intravascular volume depletion because of fluid sequestration within the affected extremity. Fasciotomy should be performed if indicated. Finally, amputation of gangrenous tissue may be necessary.

Deep-Vein Thrombosis of the Upper Extremity

This most commonly involves the axillary and subclavian veins and is usually iatrogenic following catheterization. Effort thrombosis of the axillary or subclavian vein is seen in young persons following strenuous activity and may be more common in people who have some narrowing of the thoracic outlet.

The patient with axillary or subclavian vein thrombosis usually presents with mild swelling involving the forearm or occasionally the entire extremity. Edema is pitting and not tense. The color of the extremity is normal. Arterial flow is well preserved, and pulses are present.

The risk of pulmonary embolism in this setting is between 12 and 15 percent. Accordingly, the patient should be treated with elevation of the extremity, application of local heat, analgesia as needed, and anticoagulation, if not contraindicated by the patient's overall condition. Postphlebitic sequelae are common in these patients.

Thrombolytic Therapy

Thrombolytic therapy can be used to treat patients with acute deep venous thrombosis. Streptokinase combines with plasminogen to form a plasminogen-streptokinase activator complex. This, in turn, can combine with a plasminogen-fibrin complex in the thrombus to cause lysis. The activator complex may also combine with circulating plasminogen, forming plasmin and causing fibrinolysis. Urokinase, which is derived from human embryonic kidney cells, is a direct plasminogen activator. It is not antigenic and has a low pyrogenicity.

This is a useful treatment in experienced hands for appropriately selected patients. It should be considered in patients with proven venous thrombosis of the iliofemoral or above-knee venous segments of less than 4 days' duration. Some consider this the treatment of choice for phlegmasia cerulea dolens. There are a number of contraindications to its use. Patients with a history of peptic ulcer disease, severe hypertension, recent stroke, liver disease, blood dyscrasia, recent surgery, recent arterial punctures, or intracranial neoplasms are not candidates for this treatment. In addition, it is still controversial as to whether this treatment method results in a lower incidence of postphlebitic sequelae. It does result in a higher incidence of bleeding complications than standard heparin therapy.

BIBLIOGRAPHY

Adams JT, DeWees JA: Effort thrombosis of the axillary and subclavian veins. *Trauma* 11:923, 1971.

Astedt B, Robertson B, Haeger K: Experience with standardized streptokinase therapy of deep venous thrombosis. *Surg Gynecol Obstet* 139:387, 1974.

Dale WA: The swollen leg. *Curr Concepts Surg* 1973.

Elliott JP, Hageman JH, Belanger AC, et al: Phleborrheography: A correlative study with venography. *Henry Ford Hosp Med J* 28:189, 1980.

Quinones-Baldrich WJ, Gomez AS: Thrombolytic therapy, in Rutherford RB (ed): *Vascular Surgery*. Philadelphia Saunders, 1989, p 313.

Salzman EW, Dykin D, Shapiro RM, et al: Management of heparin therapy, *N Engl J Med* 292:1046, 1975.

Silver D: Non-operative management of acute venous thromboembolism, in Rutherford RB (ed): *Vascular Surgery*. Philadelphia, Saunders, 1989, p 1561.

Summer DS: Diagnosis of deep venous thrombosis, in Rutherford RB (ed): *Vascular Surgery*. Philadelphia, Saunders, 1989, p 1520.

27
CARDIOVASCULAR PHYSIOLOGY OF AGING

Michael Maddens

Because of the marked reduction in childhood and early adult mortality over the last 100 years in the United States, there has been a rapid increase in the elderly population. Between 1900 and 1980 life expectancy from birth increased 23 years. However, over the same period life expectancy in persons reaching the age of 65 increased by only 3 years. The growth in the elderly population has had a major impact on the economics of health care in this country. People over 65 years of age make up less than 15 percent of the general population in the United States, yet consume 25 percent of all prescription drugs and account for nearly 50 percent of all hospital days and one-third of all health care expenditures. The elderly account for 22 to 25 percent of EMS runs and a comparable number of emergency department visits.

The prevalence of cardiovascular disease increases so much with advancing age that it may be the norm rather than the exception. However, in order to make accurate assessments and optimize therapy for elderly patients, it is important to distinguish between the physiologic changes of normal aging and the pathophysiologic changes of common diseases in the elderly. The morphologic changes of the cardiovascular system that occur as a result of normal aging have been reviewed by Wei and Gersh and are presented in Table 27-1. A slight increase in the cardiothoracic ratio on chest radiographs has also been demonstrated. However, in the absence of major chest deformities it does not exceed 0.51, thus maintaining the specificity of a cardiothoracic ratio of > 50 percent for detecting cardiac pathology. Age-related physiologic changes can be divided into changes in cardiac function (summarized in Table 27-2), changes in blood vessel function, and changes in baroreceptor and endocrine homeostatic mechanisms. Particular note should be made of the increased dependence on the "atrial kick" to complete ventricular diastolic filling. This causes elderly patients to be more prone to congestive heart failure in the setting of atrial fibrillation or supraventricular tachycardia.

Changes in blood vessel function include decreased β-adrenergic-mediated vasodilatation and impaired α_1-adrenergic responsiveness. Animal data suggest that although vascular smooth-muscle relaxation in response to nitrovasodilators remains intact, age-related alteration in endothelial-cell modulation of this response leads to decreased relaxation. The previously noted morphologic changes of the blood vessels are associated with increased peripheral vascular resistance and impedance, both of which contribute to an increased left ventricular workload. The nonpulsatile component of the left ventricular load, peripheral resistance, increases by 37 percent from the second to the sixth decade, while the pulsatile component, characteristic impedance (an index of aortic elasticity), increases by 137 percent over the same time span.

Table 27-1. Morphologic Changes Associated with Normal Aging

Histologic changes
Myocardium
Lipofuscin accumulation
Amyloid deposition
Increases in cell size
Decrease in number of pacemaker cells
Blood vessels
Intimal cells become heterogeneous in size and spatial orientation
Medial thickening and calcification
Macroscopic changes
Heart
No change in chamber size
Slight increase in left ventricular wall thickness
Decreased number of conducting fascicles between the main bundle and the left bundle
Thickening of the atrial surface and atrioventricular valves
Blood vessels
Increased diameter and thickness of the aorta
Increased tortuosity

Table 27-2. Physiologic Changes in Cardiac Function with Normal Aging

Diminished early (passive) left ventricular filling with increased dependence on the "atrial kick" to fill the ventricle (considered secondary to an age-related decrease in left ventricular compliance)
Preserved contractility of the left ventricle
No change in resting cardiac output
Increase in end diastolic volume
Operating further up the Frank-Starling curve
Relatively greater dependence on increases in end diastolic volume relative to increases in heart rate to increase cardiac output during exercise
Decreased inotropic and chronotropic responses to catecholamines
No change or small decrease in peripheral vascular resistance
No change in ejection fraction

A wide variety of baroreceptor- and endocrine-mediated homeostatic responses have been shown to decline with advancing age. These are summarized in Table 27-3. Of particular clinical relevance is the smaller increase in heart rate with standing or tilting in the elderly. Shannon et al. reported that the heart rate of young patients increased by 15 beats per minute after 3 min of 60-degree head-up tilt while that of older patients (average age, 75) increased by only 6 beats per minute. Neither group experienced significant changes in blood pressure. In the face of a modest diuretic-induced sodium depletion young patients increased their heart rates even more and were able to maintain blood pressure. In contrast, elderly patients were unable to mount further heart rate increases despite significant drops in blood pressure. Thus the sensitivity of a 20-beat-per-minute heart rate increase as a clinical indicator of volume depletion declines with advancing age. The specificity of a 20-mmHg drop in blood pressure as an indicator of volume depletion also declines, partially because of the physiologic alteration in the baroreceptors but to a greater extent because of the high prevalence of other conditions which produce orthostatic hypotension (drugs, varicose veins, Parkinson's disease, diabetes mellitus, and vitamin deficiency). Nonetheless, a 20-mmHg drop in systolic blood pressure within 3 min of standing has been shown to be a significant risk factor for falls and syncope.

CARDIOVASCULAR DISEASES

Hypertension

Hypertension is the most common cardiovascular disease in the elderly, affecting up to 50 percent of people over the age of 70. The Joint National Committee (JNC) on Detection, Evaluation and Treatment of High Blood Pressure defines this condition as a systolic blood pressure greater than 159 mmHg and/or a diastolic blood pressure greater than 89 mmHg. Isolated elevation of systolic blood pressure accounts for up to half of the cases of hypertension in the elderly; it

Table 27-3. Age-Related Changes in Baroceptor- and Endocrine-Mediated Blood Pressure Homeostatic Mechanisms

Decreased chronotropic response to standing, tilt, cough, valsalva
Decreased carotid baroreceptor response
Little or no change in cardiopulmonary baroreceptor responses
Decreased aldosterone and renin responses to hypovolemia
Decreased antidiuretic hormone response to hypovolemia
Decreased thirst after water deprivation
Impaired natriuretic capability

is especially prominent in the African-American population and in females. Not only does the prevalence of hypertension increase with age, but the Framingham Study has shown that the importance of a given systolic blood pressure elevation also increases with age, producing a morbidity 2 to 5 times higher than that observed in the nonhypertensive elderly and a mortality 30 to 100 percent higher. Additionally, isolated systolic hypertension in this population is associated with a high incidence of carotid bruits (20 to 40 percent) and lower-extremity peripheral arterial disease. Despite its proven morbidity, studies suggest that 40 to 70 percent of elderly patients with isolated systolic hypertension are either unaware of it or not taking medication for it. Given the increased variability of blood pressure readings in the elderly and the stress of the usual emergency department visit, it is important to remember that the JNC guidelines call for multiple measurements in the seated position, with a cuff of appropriate size, after at least 5 min of quiet rest, confirmed on at least two subsequent visits, before diagnosing hypertension. Patient evaluation should seek to exclude the relatively rare secondary causes of elevated blood pressure, such as hyperthyroidism, severe bradycardia, Paget's disease, and aortic regurgitation. Evidence of end-organ damage such as retinopathy, papilledema, peripheral vascular disease, aortic aneurysms, carotid bruits, congestive heart failure, or sequelae of stroke should be documented. In the absence of such evidence and the absence of other risk factors, such as diabetes or smoking, the Canada Consensus Conference on Hypertension proposes treatment of isolated systolic hypertension only for systolic pressures greater than 200 mmHg (SBP > 200 mmHg). When target-organ damage or associated medical conditions are present, they recommend treating SBP > 180 mmHg. They suggest no treatment for SBP < 160 mmHg, and the physician's discretion for SBP 160 to 179 mmHg. In any case, in the absence of acute end-organ damage (papilledema, angina, congestive heart failure) or aneurysm, there is rarely any need for immediate reductions in blood pressure. Given the previously noted baroreceptor impairments, and the high prevalence of orthostatic hypotension, most elderly hypertensive patients are best served by referral to a primary care physician rather than by institution of antihypertensive therapy in the emergency department. When urgent therapy is indicated, the choice of agent is dictated by the concomitant illnesses and the side-effect profile most likely to be tolerated. It should be noted that β blockers may be less effective in older hypertensives due to the high prevalence of low-renin hypertension, and to the diminished sensitivity to β blockade, observed in the elderly.

Coronary Artery Disease

Coronary atherosclerotic heart disease is the most common cause of death in persons over 65 years, and the elderly account for over 50 percent of admissions to the hospital for acute myocardial infarction. Despite the high prevalence of coronary disease, only about 10 percent of the elderly population have angina pectoris. Evidence from the Honolulu Heart Study shows no difference between the elderly population and the general population in the percentage (approximately 33 percent) of clinically unrecognized myocardial infarctions ascertained by ECG changes at repeated examinations. However, with advancing age the presenting symptoms of a myocardial infarction tend to change. Beyond the age of 80, fewer than 50 percent experience chest pain, and less than 20 percent experience diaphoresis. Syncope, acute confusion, and stroke become increasingly more common presenting symptoms of myocardial infarction in the elderly, while the prevalence of weakness, giddiness, and vomiting are unchanged. Among elderly patients whose heart attack includes syncope as a presenting symptom, less than one-third have associated chest pain, but the prevalence of truly silent infarctions probably does not increase dramatically.

Risk factors for myocardial infarction and coronary heart disease mortality are similar to those seen in younger adults, though their relative importance changes. With advancing age the relative risk of hypertension increases dramatically. The relative risk of elevated total cholesterol levels declines dramatically, but high-density lipoprotein (HDL) remains significantly inversely related to coronary mortality. Smoking remains a significant risk factor in the elderly, and is associated with a 50 percent increase in coronary mortality. Diabetes mellitus remains an extremely potent risk factor, especially in older women. Electrocardiographic abnormalities associated with left ventricular hypertrophy and nonspecific ST-T changes both confer added risk for coronary artery disease. Obesity remains a powerful risk factor in elderly men and to a much smaller degree in elderly women. Physical activity, even at modest levels, has been shown to reduce mortality (both cardiac-specific and total mortality) in the elderly. Left ventricular hypertrophy is also an independent risk factor in the elderly, conferring a 1.6- to 1.67-fold increased risk for every 50 g/m in the left ventricular mass to height index. Use of estrogens is associated with a significant reduction in coronary mortality rates in elderly women, and there is some evidence that aspirin may reduce the risk of myocardial infarction in elderly men.

Treatment of unstable angina or acute infarction is similar to treatment in younger patients, with a few caveats. Infarctions associated with elevated CK-MB isoenzymes but a normal total CK level occur twice as often in the elderly as in younger patients. The elderly also have a higher frequency of complications, including arrhythmias, heart failure, and cardiac rupture. Although increasing age is associated with higher complication rates from most invasive treatments for myocardial infarction, surgical repair of remediable postinfarction cardiogenic shock should not be excluded on the basis of age alone. The role of thrombolytic therapy remains uncertain. Initial studies showed no reduction in mortality in elderly patients and an increased rate of hemorrhagic complications, but pooled analysis of several recent studies suggests that the elderly do derive significant benefit. Additionally, primary angioplasty has been reported as an effective treatment in patients over age 75. Nitrates and sodium nitroprusside must be used with additional caution in the elderly due to the age-related impairments in baroreceptor responses. It is prudent to start with an infusion rate of 5 μg/min and increase the rate by 5 μg/min every 5 min in elderly patients requiring intravenous nitroglycerin. Beta-blocker therapy in the acute phase of infarction can be undertaken cautiously, but it should be recalled that elderly patients may have a higher incidence of CNS side effects and are more likely to have contraindications to β blockade than younger patients. Lidocaine prophylaxis has recently been called into question both for prehospital and in-hospital use. Lidocaine toxicity is twice as common in patients over 70 years as it is in patients under 50. This may be due to an increased drug sensitivity as well as to the twofold increase in lidocaine half-life observed in the elderly. Wei suggests reducing the loading dose by one-third to one-half and keeping the maintenance dose under 25 μg/kg per min as a way of avoiding toxicity.

Elderly postmyocardial infarction patients demonstrated reductions in subsequent mortality when treated with metoprolol, propanalol, or timolol, without a significant increase in side effects. The value of aspirin for secondary prevention of coronary events remains unproven. Elderly patients have up to a fourfold increase in 1-year mortality compared to younger adults, and those with non-Q-wave infarctions have been reported to have a 12 percent annual mortality rate from the third year on.

Treatment of chronic coronary artery disease is also similar to treatment in younger patients. Indications for surgical therapy remain essentially the same, but the prevalence of contraindications increases. Perioperative mortality increases progressively with advancing age (under age 65: 1.9 percent; age 65 to 69: 4.6 percent; age 70 to 74: 6.6 percent; and age 75 and over: 9.5 percent). However, in elderly patients surviving surgery, 5-year survival is 87 percent (77 percent in those 75 and older), and recurrence of angina is less common than in younger patients. Survival results after angioplasty are equally favorable.

SYNCOPE

Syncope is defined as a sudden, transient loss of consciousness characterized by unresponsiveness and loss of postural tone; recovery is spontaneous, not requiring resuscitative procedures. Among the very elderly, the 10-year prevalance of syncope is 23 percent. The yearly incidence is 6 percent, with 30 percent of patients experiencing recurrences and up to 6 percent experiencing seven or more episodes during a 2-year follow-up. Among late middle-aged adults with syncope, subsequent mortality may depend on the etiology of the episode (for example, higher mortality in cases where a cardiovascular cause is identified). However, among the elderly, no significant differences in 2-year mortality rates exist between those with cardiovascular, noncardiovascular, and unknown causes. Syncope in the elderly is associated with functional decline, as well as a substantial morbidity rate (37 percent). Morbidity includes a 10 percent incidence of major complications such as fractures, subdural hematomas, or injuries resulting from car accidents, and the iatrogenic morbidity resulting from hospitalization and diagnostic evaluation.

Any factor or combination of factors which results in a transient insufficiency in oxygen or nutrient delivery to the brain can produce syncope. Since oxygen transport capacity is directly proportional to hemoglobin content, even modest degrees of anemia may be a major contributory factor in elderly patients who have age-related physiologic declines in baroreceptor and endocrine homeostatic responses. Likewise, modest reductions in cardiac output secondary to congestive heart failure, volume depletion, or drug-induced orthostatic hypotension may also contribute. Finally, postprandial drops in blood pressure are common among the elderly and may contribute to the incidence of syncope.

Carotid sinus hypersensitivity is frequently overlooked as a cause of syncope in the elderly, and should be sought by means of carotid massage during ECG monitoring. Ventricular asystole greater than 2.5 to 3 s constitutes a positive cardioinhibitory response. A systolic blood pressure decline of more than 40 to 50 mmHg or a systolic blood pressure drop below 90 mmHg is considered a positive vasodepressor response. Cardioinhibitory response is the most common (51 to 84 percent), followed by mixed response (11 to 33 percent), with pure vasodepressor response being the least common (5 to 12 percent). Digitalis, propanalol, and α-methyldopa have all been reported to be associated with carotid sinus hypersensitivity. Patients with a known history of stroke or intracranial arterial disease, or who present with carotid bruits on physical examination, should be excluded.

Vasovagal syncope accounts for only 1 to 5 percent of syncopal episodes in the elderly. In most cases it probably results from initial sympathetic overstimulation of ventricular sensory receptors, resulting in a dramatic reflex reduction in peripheral vascular tone and increased parasympathetic tone which causes bradycardia and decreased mesenteric vascular resistance.

Evaluation and Treatment

History and Physical Examination

Twenty-five percent of elderly syncope patients can be diagnosed by history and physical examination alone, accounting for nearly half of all cases where a cause is eventually established. History taking in the elderly patient with syncope should first establish the cognitive ability of the patient, with corroboration by family or friends whenever possible. Next, explicit details regarding the circumstances preceding the syncopal episode should be determined. These include the time of the last meal; postural changes before the episode; sensation of pain, nausea, or strong emotions before the episode; or an urge to void or defecate. Any correlation with activities that may precipitate syncope, such as exercise, coughing, swallowing, voiding, or defecating, should be sought. Simple activities such as shaving or turning the head may occasionally precipitate syncope in patients with carotid sinus hypersensitivity. A list of the patient's medications and the time of the last few doses should be noted.

The patient's description of sensations immediately preceding or during the episode, as well as eye-witness accounts, should be obtained if possible. The presence of nausea and vague abdominal distress accompanied by a flushed sensation suggests the presence of vasovagal syncope. The feeling of a prodrome or aura suggests the presence of epilepsy.

Clonic jerks may occur in the presence of cerebral hypoperfusion and do not necessarily indicate the presence of a seizure. The presence of urinary incontinence, a prolonged recovery period, or Todd's paralysis suggest the diagnosis of a seizure. Rapid onset, especially in the seated or supine position, suggests the presence of arrhythmia. A jugular venous pulse rate greater than the peripheral pulse rate, or a pulse of 20 to 40 beats per minute that is unaffected by atropine, are both suggestive of a Stokes-Adams attack. Careful note should be made of the patient's rhythm, blood pressure (including response to orthostatic stress and any concomitant symptoms), and respiratory rate. Detection of a prolonged, harsh, loud (IV, V, or VI) systolic murmur associated with a diminished second heart sound is strong evidence for significant aortic stenosis. However, many elderly patients with significant lesions have atypical murmurs and may have fairly well-preserved carotid upstrokes secondary to diminished arterial compliance. By age 50, 50 percent of people have audible ejection murmurs; by age 90, 70 percent. Due to the high prevalence of aortic ejection murmurs from hemodynamically insignificant aortic sclerosis, an echocardiogram is often required to ascertain with certainty whether sclerosis or stenosis is the cause of the murmur. The extremities should be examined for pallor, distal perfusion, clubbing, or cyanosis. After a careful neurologic examination and auscultation of the neck to determine that there are no bruits, patients without a previous history or evidence of cerebrovascular disease should have carotid sinus massage performed.

Laboratory Evaluation

Due to the high prevalence of disease and the nonspecific presentation of many diseases in the elderly, a number of screening tests are usually performed. These include a complete blood count, creatinine and blood urea nitrogen, and a blood glucose. Some authors have questioned the diagnostic value of such tests for syncope, stating that positive findings relevant to syncope are found in less than 4 percent of patients.

Creatine kinase levels may be helpful in diagnosing myocardial infarction. However, 10 percent of elderly patients with syncope but without myocardial infarction and 10 percent of age-matched controls also have mildly elevated isoenzymes. The survival rate for patients with syncope and mildly elevated isoenzymes who have no other evidence of myocardial infarction is no different from the survival rate for those with syncope and normal isoenzyme levels.

An ECG should be obtained as the first laboratory test in ruling out myocardial infarction or significant arrhythmia. In over 30 percent of elderly patients with syncope caused by arrhythmia, the arrhythmia can be diagnosed on the admission ECG. Although there is a significantly increased risk of sudden death associated with frequent or complex premature ventricular complexes (PVCs), the relative risk is lower in men older than 49 compared to those 49 and younger.

Despite the relative frequency of EEG abnormalities, several series have reported the yield of new seizure diagnoses as a result of routine electroencephalography to be from 0 to 1.5 percent. Similarly, CT scanning of the brain in the absence of focal neurologic signs is generally not contributory.

Echocardiography can distinguish hemodynamically significant aortic stenosis from the more common systolic murmur produced by hemodynamically insignificant aortic sclerosis. Additionally, the echocardiogram may diagnose hypertrophic obstructive cardiomyopathy, a condition which is often missed on clinical evaluation in the elderly, even when moderate to severe.

Ambulatory Electrocardiographic Monitoring

In elderly syncope patients, electrocardiographic monitoring for at least 24 h is the single most useful study after the history and physical examination, establishing a diagnosis in over 25 percent of patients in whom an etiology was eventually determined. However, a number of authors have reported low rates of temporal association (8 percent) of arrhythmias with symptoms of syncope or presyncope as documented by ambulatory monitoring. In 1512 adult (not exclusively elderly) patients with syncope, 15 patients (1 percent) experienced syncope during ambulatory monitoring, and 241 experienced presyncope. Among those with syncope, only half the episodes were related to an arrhythmia (most commonly ventricular tachycardia); among those with presyncope, only 10 percent were related to an arrhythmia. In total, only 2 percent of studies led to a definitive diagnosis of arrhythmia. Clark et al. have reported that although 42 percent of their patients monitored for symptoms of syncope or dizziness had symptoms during monitoring, only 23 out of 41 symptomatic patients had major arrhythmia, and in only three of these cases was the arrhythmia temporally related to the symptoms reported. There was no significant difference in the incidence or type of arrhythmia between symptomatic and asymptomatic patients. Similarly, Kala et al. have reported low rates of symptoms during monitoring. Fifteen percent of their subjects experienced symptoms, with 50 percent demonstrating a simultaneous causative arrhythmia. They also found a sizable number of ''significant arrhythmias'' among the asymptomatic group.

The significance of asymptomatic arrhythmias remains a subject of much debate. In Kapoor's study of prolonged ECG monitoring in syncope patients, mean age 56.6 ± 19.5 years, 25 percent of patients reported symptoms with corresponding arrhythmias. However, they found that frequent PVCs (more than nine per hour), or repetitive PVCs, and sinus pauses of greater than 2 s were both independent predictors of mortality. Likewise, Abdon et al. reported that 15 of 21 patients with a significant arrhythmia during an asymptomatic 24-h recording later had the same arrhythmia during symptoms. However, the likelihood of most arrhythmias increases with advancing age, increasing the chances of finding a coincidental arrhythmia with ambulatory monitoring. In a study of 13 asymptomatic active individuals 67 to 84 years old, all had at least some supraventricular and some ventricular arrhythmia; five demonstrated complex ventricular arrhythmia; and seven had complex atrial arrhythmia. In another study, major arrhythmias occurred in 13 percent of active asymptomatic elderly subjects. In a group of healthy people 60 to 85 years old screened with maximal treadmill exercise testing, 80 percent had ventricular arrhythmia, 35 percent had multiform PVCs, 11 percent had couplets, and 4 percent had ventricular tachycardia. Although 88 percent had supraventricular arrhythmia and 13 percent had paroxysmal atrial tachycardia, marked sinus bradycardia (less than 40 beats per minute) and prolonged sinus pauses (longer than 1.5 s) were each present in only 2 percent.

Transtelephonic Monitoring

A continuous-loop ECG recorder may be a useful alternative to traditional ambulatory monitoring. The device continually records and erases cardiac rhythm. Activation of the ''record'' button stores in memory the preceding 64 s and the ensuing 32 s. The preserved rhythm can then be transmitted over the telephone. In this manner, patients can record rhythms accompanying their symptoms. One month of continual use is reported to cost the same as one 24-h holter recording.

Signal-Averaged Electrocardiography

A newer noninvasive electrocardiographic technique available to evaluate patients with syncope is signal-averaged ECG. This technique uses high-gain amplification and passband filtering of the surface ECG. Late potentials (low-amplitude potentials at the terminal portion of the QRS complex) are correlated with the likelihood of sustaining ventricular tachyarrhythmia. Kuchar et al found that late potentials were present in 11 of 13 patients (85 percent) with ventricular tachycardia, and absent in 94 percent of patients with other causes for their syncope. In patients with recurrent syncope, late potentials had a 73 percent sensitivity and 89 percent specificity, but only a 55 percent positive predictive value for serious ventricular arrhythmia as a cause of syncope. Gang et al. reported an 89 percent sensitivity and 100 percent specificity in predicting inducible ventricular tachycardia on electrophysiologic studies in patients with unexplained syncope. Winters et al. reported that an abnormally low root mean square of the terminal 40 ms had an 82 percent sensitivity and a 91 percent specificity in distinguishing individuals with syncope of unknown origin who had inducible ventricular tachycardia.

Head-Up Tilt Test

The use of the head-up tilt test to provoke syncope may be useful in the evaluation of syncope of unknown origin. This maneuver produces syncope in 37 to 67 percent of patients, usually of the vasovagal type. The administration of isoproterenol before tilting may increase the sensitivity of the maneuver. However, the number of controls studied has not been large enough to establish the significance of a positive test. In studies with Lipsitz, the author has observed only one tilt-induced episode of syncope or near syncope in a group of elderly subjects (average age 85 years old) with unexplained syncope; a recent study by Hackel et al. reported that 4/5 controls experienced syncopal symptoms during prolonged tilt.

VALVULAR HEART DISEASE

Significant aortic stenosis (AS) may be present in elderly patients in the absence of the classic *pulsus parvus et tardus* because of the increased transmission of the pulse secondary to decreased elasticity. The cause of AS in older patients is usually degenerative rather than congenital or rheumatic, as in younger patients. The male predominance seen in younger patients disappears, and the ejection click is usually absent. Severe symptomatic AS is associated with a 40 to 70 percent reduction in life expectancy among the elderly, with a 3-year survival of about 25 percent. Valve replacement is associated with a 16 percent operative mortality, but survivors usually achieve functional improvement and improved subsequent survival. Balloon angioplasty has also shown promise as a palliative treatment for elderly patients with AS. However, although symptoms improve in the majority of patients, restenosis is common.

Mitral annular calcification is almost exclusively a disease of the elderly. Over 30 percent of women and 12 percent of men over the age of 70 are affected. Fifty to seventy-five percent of patients have a systolic murmur which is usually holosystolic, crescendo-decrescendo, and radiates to the axilla, and thus can be confused with either aortic stenosis or mitral regurgitation. Although conduction abnormalities are often present, only right bundle branch block is more common than in age-matched controls. Although mitral annular calcification is associated with a higher incidence of cerebral embolic events and infective endocarditis, preventive treatment for either remains controversial.

CONGESTIVE HEART FAILURE

Congestive heart failure increases exponentially with advancing age after the fifth decade. Special note should be made of the high prevalence of impaired diastolic function in the elderly, since 50 to 60 percent of old persons with congestive heart failure have normal or only slightly reduced ejection fractions. Treatment in these cases should be directed at improving diastolic relaxation (for example, with calcium channel blockers) rather than augmenting contractility or decreasing afterload, which may aggravate the condition.

For elderly patients with impaired systolic function (diminished ejection fraction), digoxin may improve the ejection fraction even in patients who are in sinus rhythm; however, maximum improvement is frequently seen with serum levels of 0.4 to 1.0 μg/mL. Given the increased prevalence of digoxin toxicity in the elderly, close monitoring of levels is indicated, and physicians should have a high index of suspicion for toxicity when patients on digoxin present with nonspecific complaints.

DRUG THERAPY

A final note of caution regarding treatment of elderly individuals is warranted. The emergency physician must keep in mind that many drugs in the usual arsenal have longer half-lives or more pronounced effects in elderly patients. As a group, the elderly have decreased renal function and are less able to metabolize drugs that require hepatic oxidation or deamination. However, although mean responses change with age, the variability of responses also increases. Thus one 80-year-old may require a fraction of the usual adult dose while another requires a full dose. Where there is uncertainty, it is usually safest to start with small doses and titrate up to the desired effect or level.

BIBLIOGRAPHY

Abdon NJ, Johansson BW, Lessem J: Predictive use of routine 24 hour electrocardiography in suspected Adams-Stokes syndrome. Comparison with cardiac rhythm during symptoms. *Br Heart J* 47:553, 1987.

Agarwol AK. Aortic stenosis: Diagnosis and treatment in the elderly patient. *Geriatrics* 40(2):105, 1985.

Aranow WS, Starling L, Etienne F, et al: Risk factors for coronary artery disease in persons older than 62 years in a long-term health care facility. *Am J Cardiol* 57:518, 1986.

Bayer AJ, Chadha JS, Faray RR, et al: Changing presentation of myocardial infarction with increasing old age. *J Am Geriatr Soc* 34:263, 1986.

Bush TL, Barrett-Connor E, Cowan E, et al: Cardiovascular mortality and noncontraceptive use of estrogen in women: Results from the lipid research clinics program follow-up study. *Circulation* 75:1102, 1987.

Clark PI, Glasser SP, Spoto E: Arrhythmias detected by ambulatory monitoring. *Chest* 77:722, 1980.

Fleg JL: Alterations in cardiovascular structure and function with advancing age. *Am J Cardiol* 57:33C, 1988.

Gang ES et al: Detection of late potentials on the surface electrocardiogram in unexplained syncope. *Am J Cardiol* 58:1014, 1986.

Gerson LW, Skvarch L: Emergency medical services utilization by the elderly. *Ann Emerg Med* 11:610, 1982.

Gribbin B, Pickering TG, Sleight P, et al: Effect of age and high blood pressure on baroreflex sensitivity in man. *Circ Res* 29:424, 1971.

Hackel A et al: Cardioversion and catecholamine responses to head-up tilt in the diagnosis of recurrent unexplained syncope ion elderly patients. *J Am Geriatr Soc* 39:663, 1991.

Jajich CL, Ostfeld AM, Freeman DH: Smoking and coronary heart disease mortality in the elderly. *JAMA* 252:2831, 1984.

Kala E, Vitasola MT, Toivonen L, et al: Ambulatory ECG recording in patients referred because of syncope or dizziness. *Acta Med Scand (Supp)* 668:13, 1982.

Kannel WB, Vokonas PS: Primary risk factors for coronary heart disease in the elderly: The Framingham study, in Wenger NK, Furkberg CD (eds): *Coronary Heart Disease in the Elderly.* New York, Elsevier, 1986, pp 60–95.

Kapoor, et al: Syncope in the elderly. *Am J Med* 80:419, 1986.

Kapoor WN et al: Prolonged electrocardiographic monitoring in patients with syncope. Importance of frequent or repetitive ventricular ectopy. *Am J Med* 82:20. 1987.

Kuchar DL, Thorburn CS, and Sammel NL: Signal-averaged electrocardiogram for evaluation of recurrent syncope. *Am J Cardiol* 58:949, 1986.

Lew AS, Hod H, Cercek B, et al: Mortality and morbidity rates of patients older and younger than 75 years with acute myocardial infarction treated with intravenous streptokinase. *Am J Cardiol* 59:1, 1987.

Lipsitz LA: Orthostatic hypotension in the elderly. *N Engl J Med* 321:952, 1989.

Lipsitz LA: Syncope in the elderly patient. *Hosp Pract* 21(10):33, 1986.

Lipsitz, LA: Syncope in the elderly. *Ann Intern Med* 99:92, 1983.

Lipsitz LA, Wei JY, Rowe JW: Syncope in an elderly, institutionalized population: Prevalence, incidence and associated risk. *Q J Med* 54:45, 1985.

Maddens ME: Isolated systolic hypertension: The rationale for treating elderly patients. *Consultant* 29:125, 1989.

Maddens ME, Lipsitz LA, We JY, et al: Impaired heart rate responses to cough and deep breathing in elderly patients with unexplained syncope. *Am J Cardiol* 60:1368, 1987.

O'Brien IAD, O'Hare P, Corrall RJM: Heart rate variability in healthy subjects: Effect of age and the derivation of normal ranges for tests of autonomic function. *Br Heart J* 55:348, 1986.

Rajala SA, Geiger UKM, Haavisto MV, et al: Electrocardiogram, clinical findings and chest X ray in persons aged 85 years or older. *Am J Cardiol* 55:1175, 1985.

Rowe JW: Clinical consequences of age-related impairments in vascular compliance. *Am J Cardiol* 60:686, 1987.

Rowe JW, Troen BR: Sympathetic nervous system and aging in man. *Endocr Rev* 1(2):167, 1980.

Schaff HV, Gersh BJ: Feasibility of coronary artery bypass surgery in elderly patients. *Geriatr Med Today* 3(3):81, 1984.

Shannon RP, Wei JY, Rosa RM, et al: The effect of age and sodium depletion on cardiovascular response to orthostasis. *Hypertension* 8:438, 1986.

Tsumoda K, et al: Effect of age on the renin-angiotensin-aldosterone system in normal subjects: Simultaneous measurement of active and inactive renin, renin substrate, and aldosterone in plasma. *J Clin Endocrinol Metab* 62:384, 1986.

Wei JY, Gersh BJ: Heart disease in the elderly. *Curr Probl Cardiol* 12(1):1, 1987.

Weintraub RM, Wei JY, Thurer RL: Surgical repair of remediable post-infarction cardiogenic shock in the elderly: Early and long term results. *J Am Geriatr Soc* 34:389, 1986.

SECTION 4
Pulmonary Emergencies

28
BACTERIAL PNEUMONIA

Georges C. Benjamin

Bacterial pneumonia remains a leading cause of death and is responsible for as many as 10 percent of hospital admissions in the United States. The pneumococcus accounts for up to 90 percent of all bacterial pneumonias, with *Escherichia coli, Pseudomonas aeruginosa, Klebsiella pneumoniae, Staphylococcus aureus, Hemophilus influenzae,* and group A streptococci accounting for most of the rest. Other bacteria, such as *Legionella pneumophila* and the anaerobes, are discussed in later sections. The frequency with which each of these organisms causes disease varies from study to study.

Patients with chronic diseases such as congestive heart failure, diabetes, cancer, bronchiectasis, sickle-cell anemia, and hypogammaglobulinemia are at greater risk for pneumonia, as are smokers and postsplenectomy patients. Essentially all bacterial pneumonia is the result of aspiration of oropharyngeal contents. Therefore, patients with seizures, obtundation, suppressed cough reflex, and increased secretions are also predisposed to it. These and other predisposing factors are shown in Table 28-1.

Sterility of the lower airways and alveoli is due to a very effective system utilizing the cough reflex, mucociliary clearance, phagocytosis, and in situ bacterial killing. Cilia located in the tracheal bronchial tree are responsible for removing most infected particles greater than 5.0 μm.

Particles smaller than this are removed by alveolar macrophages and local factors (surfactant, complement, IgG, IgA) which limit bacterial growth. Because of a variance in the susceptibilities of different bacterial species to these clearance mechanisms, most pneumonias are ultimately the result of a single species. This is of interest in light of the multiplicity of organisms in oropharyngeal secretions.

LABORATORY TESTS

Laboratory tests useful in the emergency department diagnosis of bacterial pneumonia include the white cell count, chest x-ray, arterial blood gas, sputum examination, blood cultures, and pleural fluid examination.

Table 28-1. Factors Predisposing to Bacterial Pneumonia

Debilitation	Chest wall disorders
Alcoholism	Myopathies and neuropathies
The extremes of life	Chest wall trauma
Neoplasia	Postoperative pain
Immunosuppression	Syncope
Chronic diseases	Seizures
Diabetes	Bronchial obstruction (tumor or foreign body aspiration)
COPD	Pulmonary embolism
Valvular heart disease	Iatrogenic invasion
Congestive heart failure	Bronchoscopy
Leukemia	Intubation, respiratory support
Lymphoma	Transthoracic procedures
Hemoglobinopathies	Stroke
Viral infections	

The white cell count remains a useful way to document the presence of the inflammatory response from pneumonia. In healthy young patients, marked elevation usually occurs. This elevation is not diagnostic, however, and the presence of a normal count does not rule out pneumonia or suggest a viral etiology. Also, in the elderly or debilitated patient, a normal or low white cell count may represent overwhelming sepsis. In these cases the presence of a left shift may be the only clue to bacterial infection.

Radiographically, bacterial pneumonias are frequently characterized as in Table 28-2. Note that these classic patterns frequently are the exception and serve only as a guide in radiographic diagnosis. Another reason to obtain a chest x-ray is to look for evidence of effusion, abscess formation, or pneumothorax. Special views such as the lateral decubitus and apical lordotic are frequently of value to further define the nature of pulmonary abnormalities. Patients with marked leukopenia or dehydration may not initially demonstrate an infiltrate. A diagnosis of pneumonia in these patients rests with a strong clinical suspicion on serial chest x-rays.

Pulmonary infarction, atelectasis, neoplasia, pulmonary edema, parenchymal scarring, and pleural thickening may all simulate pneumonitis radiographically. In these patients, clinical examination, history, and comparison with prior radiographs may aid in proper diagnosis.

Ventilation-perfusion abnormality is the most common functional disorder in acute pneumonias. This is the result of sustained perfusion of poorly ventilated areas of the lung. Measurement of the oxygen content of arterial blood in patients with respiratory compromise is useful to document hypoxia and to ensure adequate oxygenation in patients on oxygen therapy. Arterial blood gases are especially important in patients with chronic lung disease because the acute hypoxia will be superimposed on an underlying ventilation-perfusion mismatch.

Sputum examination and culture remain the most important guides to proper antibiotic therapy. Frequently the patient is unable to generate an adequate specimen because of dehydration, obtundation, or a weak cough. Occasionally postural drainage or heated saline nebulization may be helpful to induce sputum.

Although not usually an emergency department procedure, transtracheal aspiration is frequently of value in patients who are unable to produce adequate sputum. Complications from this procedure include subcutaneous or mediastinal emphysema, cardiac arrhythmias, esophageal perforation, bleeding, and infection. This procedure should be done by physicians thoroughly familiar with the technique and its complications. It is contraindicated in the patient who requires restraint, has uncorrected hypoxia, or has a coagulopathy.

Gross examination of the sputum is done first and may reveal the bloody or rusty sputum of pneumococcal pneumonia (not diagnostic, as other bacterial pneumonias may involve rusty sputum); the thick "currant jelly" sputum produced by both type 3 pneumonococcus and *K. pneumoniae;* the green sputum caused by *P. aeruginosa, H. influenzae,* and *Streptococcus pneumoniae;* or the foul-smelling sputum of an anaerobic infection. The sputum is then Gram-stained and viewed under the low-power objective (100 ×) to determine whether the sputum is suitable for examination and culture. If more than 10 squamous epithelial cells are present per low-power field, the specimen is contaminated and of low diagnostic value. An adequate specimen should demonstrate more than 25 polymorphonuclear leukocytes and less than

Table 28-2. Characteristics of Bacterial Pneumonia

Organism	Sputum	Chest X-ray	Therapy	Complications
Streptococcus pneumoniae	Rusty, gram-positive encapsulated diplocci (type III, thick)	Usually lobar in LLL, RLL, RML; occasionally patchy, small pleural effusion, 10%	Phenoxymethyl penicillin 500 mg PO q 6 h for 10 days; erythromycin 500 mg PO q 6 h for 10 days *or* Aqueous penicillin G 20 million units/day q 4–6 h *or* Procaine penicillin G 1.2 million units IM followed by phenoxymethyl penicillin 500 mg PO q 6 h for 10 days *or* Vancomycin 1 g q 12 h IV (penicillin-resistant)	Sepsis, abscess, congestive heart failure, meningitis, peritonitis, herpes labialis, septic arthritis, endocarditis, pericarditis
Group A streptococci	Purulent, bloody, gram-positive cocci in chains, pairs	Often lower lobes, patchy, multilobar large pleural effusion	See above	Sepsis, pleural effusion, hemoptysis
Hemophilus influenzae	Short, tiny, gram-negative, encapsulated cocci-bacilli	Patchy, frequently basilar, occasional pleural effusion	Cefamandole 6–12 g/day IV q 4–6 h *or* Cefuroxime 0.75–1.5 g IV q 8 h *or* Ampicillin 500 mg PO q 6 h for 10 days *or* Tetracycline 500 mg q 6 h for 10 days *or* Chloramphenicol 50–100 mg/kg per day IV q 6 h and ampicillin 9–12 g/day IV q 6 h	Septic arthritis, sepsis, meningitis, empyema
Klebsiella pneumoniae	Brown jelly, thick; short plump, gram-negative, encapsulated paired cocci-bacilli	Upper lobes, lobular bulging fissure sign, abscess formation	Cefazolin 0.25–1.0 gm q 8 h IV *or* Aminoglycoside (gentamicin, tobramycin, or amikacin)	Sepsis, empyema, pneumothorax, effusion, necrotizing pneumonia, hemoptysis, thick sputum
Staphylococcus aureus	Purulent; gram-positive cocci in pairs and clumps	Patchy, multicenter with early abscess formation, empyema, pneumothorax	Oxacillin 8–12 g/day IV *or* Nafcillin 40 mg/kg per day IV 10–14 days* *or* Vancomycin 500 mg q 6 h IV	Sepsis, endocarditis, empyema, necrotizing pneumonia, hemoptysis
Escherichia coli	Gram-negative cocci-bacilli	Patchy, bilateral, lower lobes	Ampicillin 6–8 g/day IV q 6 h *or* Cephalosporin 9–12 g/day plus gentamicin 3–5 mg/kg per day IV q 8 h (tobramycin or amikacin as needed)	Sepsis, empyema
Pseudomonas	Gram-negative cocci-bacilli	Patchy, mid- and lower lung, with abscesses	Tobramycin 3–5 mg/kg per day IV *or* Gentamicin 3–5 mg/kg per day IV q 8 h plus carbenicillin 5–6 g q 4 h IV	Sepsis, empyema

* May require 4 weeks of therapy.

10 squamous epithelial cells per low-power field. In addition, a predominant bacterial form should be evident, as a mixture of morphological forms suggests oropharyngeal contamination. Such contamination frequently makes interpretation difficult. Enteric organisms are uncommon habitants in the pharynx of healthy people. However, recent viral infections, chronic obstructive pulmonary disease (COPD), chronic bronchitis, recent hospitalizations, and debilitating diseases favor colonization with gram-negative bacteria.

Blood cultures are frequently of diagnostic value in patients who have presumed bacteremia, immunosuppression, or rigors, or who are seriously ill. Two to three cultures from separate sites are done when indicated.

Examination of the pleural fluid by thoracentesis, although generally not an emergency department procedure, is useful in ruling out empyema. Patients who may require a pleural biopsy should have only a diagnostic tap (10 to 20 mL) done by the emergency physician. Patients with respiratory compromise may require more extensive therapeutic drainage.

Streptococcus pneumoniae

Pneumonococcal pneumonia is caused by *S. pneumoniae,* a gram-positive lancet-shaped, encapsulated bacterium. On the basis of its capsular antigens it has been divided into at least 83 serotypes. Disease is usually caused by types 1, 3, 4, 6, 7, 8, 12, 14, 18, and 19 in adults and types 1, 6, 14, and 19 in children.

This organism is the most common cause of community-acquired bacterial pneumonia. Its peak incidence is winter and early spring, but it does occur year round. Mortality from this disease is less than 5 percent.

Clinical disease presents as an acute shaking chill, tachypnea, and tachycardia. A single rigor lasting several minutes is so common that recurrent rigors should suggest another etiology. Sharp chest pain which causes marked splinting on the affected side occurs in 70 percent of patients. Cough may be absent in the early phases but rapidly becomes a prominent symptom. In 75 percent of patients a rust-colored sputum develops. With type 3 pneumococcus a thick, jellylike sputum may be present and must be differentiated from that caused by *K. pneumoniae*. Additional symptoms include malaise, anorexia, myalgias, flank or back pain, and vomiting.

On physical examination, the classic signs of consolidation, including bronchial breath sounds, egophony, and increased tactile and vocal fremitus are present. Pleural friction rubs, cyanosis, and jaundice are occasionally found. Abdominal distention from acute gastric dilatation or paralytic ileus may also develop.

The white blood cell count generally ranges from 12,000 to 25,000 cells per cubic millimeter but may reach 40,000 per cubic millimeter. Normal or decreased white cell counts are seen and suggest overwhelming infection. The chest x-ray usually demonstrates a singular infiltrate in the right middle lobe, right lower lobe, or left lower lobe. The infiltrate frequently has a lobar or segmental pattern but patchy involvement is frequent in infants and the elderly. Occasionally bulging fissures similar to those seen with *K. pneumoniae* are noted. In 10 percent of patients a small, sterile pleural effusion is seen. Sputum culture is positive in only approximately 50 percent of cases and blood cultures in only 30 percent. This illustrates the difficulties in establishing a definitive diagnosis.

Untreated, this disease frequently resolves in 7 to 10 days by a clinical syndrome known as the "crisis" (prompt defervescence with diaphoresis and a rapid increase in well-being). Treated patients are often afebrile within 24 to 72 h, but in some the fever gradually decreases over 4 to 7 days. Physical signs take from 14 to 21 days to resolve, with radiographic signs resolving over another 21 days. Delayed resolution may be noted in some patients and is seen most frequently in the debilitated and the aged.

Complications include sepsis, lung abscess, congestive heart failure, meningitis, peritonitis, herpes labialis, septic arthritis, endocarditis, and pericarditis. In less than 20 percent of patients, empyema develops.

A poor prognosis is associated with type 2 and type 3 disease, multilobar involvement, leukopenia, bacteremia, jaundice, splenectomized states (including sickle hemoglobinopathies), congestive heart failure, COPD, alcoholism, and diabetes.

Penicillin is still the drug of choice for pneumococcal pneumonia despite recently recognized resistant strains. The current recommendations for therapy are listed in Table 28-2. In penicillin-allergic patients, erythromycin may be used. Tetracycline is not effective because of increased resistance.

Hemophilus influenzae

Hemophilus influenzae is a gram-negative pleomorphic rod, which exists in both encapsulated and unencapsulated forms. The capsular forms are divided into six serotypes (a through f) based on their capsular antigens. Of these, type b is found to cause 95 percent of all human infections. Both forms are able to cause pneumonia, but only the encapsulated form consistently causes bacteremia. The peak incidence of this disease occurs in winter to early spring and tends to occur in debilitated or immunocompromised patients.

The clinical presentation is one of fever, shortness of breath, and occasionally pleuritic chest pain. Lung examination may reveal rales without clear signs of consolidation. The white blood count is frequently normal but may be as high as 30,000. The chest x-ray usually demonstrates patchy alveolar infiltrates, generally without effusion. Lobar consolidation does occur, but abscess formation is rare. This organism is frequently overlooked on Gram stains and diligence is required to find it and to recognize its small coccobacillary form.

Outpatient management consists of oral ampicillin or tetracycline (Table 28-2). For those patients requiring intravenous therapy, a third generation cephalosporin is now generally used.

Complications include septic arthritis, sepsis, meningitis, and, rarely, empyema. As with other serious pneumonias, the morbidity and mortality are highest in the young or compromised patient.

Klebsiella PNEUMONIA

Klebsiella pneumonia is found most frequently in patients with alcoholism, diabetes, or COPD. It is a necrotizing lobar pneumonia, which is most frequently seen in the right upper lobe. In approximately 20 percent of cases empyema occurs within 24 to 48 h, along with intrapulmonary abscess formation in 4 to 5 days.

Klebsiella pneumonia presents as a sudden cough with rigors, shortness of breath, malaise, and often cyanosis; 80 percent of patients develop pleuritic chest pain. Pulmonary examination frequently reveals signs of consolidation and cyanosis. The white cell count is elevated in 75 percent of cases. Chest x-ray frequently reveals a necrotizing lobar pneumonia in the right upper lobe. In 35 percent of cases a bulging minor fissure is seen. Occasionally, perihilar and patchy infiltrates are also seen. Sputum examination reveals a dark brown tenacious sputum, occasionally blood-stained. Gram stain reveals short, plump, encapsulated gram-negative bacilli in pairs, which in poorly decolorized Gram stains can be easily confused with pneumococci. Sepsis, empyema, and pneumothorax are complications of this disease.

Initial therapy usually consists of an aminoglycoside and a cephalosporin intravenously. Attention to airway management is a must, as frequently the sputum is so thick that clearance is difficult.

OTHER GRAM-NEGATIVE PNEUMONIAS

Othe gram-negative organisms, including *E. coli, Pseudomonas, Enterobacter,* and *Serratia,* are rare causes of pneumonia. Their presence should be considered in the recently hospitalized, debilitated, or immunosuppressed patient. Therapy usually consists of intravenous carbenicillin or ticarcillin, and an aminoglycoside.

STAPHYLOCOCCAL PNEUMONIA

Staphylococci cause 1 percent of bacterial pneumonias. Although this pneumonia occurs sporadically, it has its peak incidence during influenza and measles epidemics. Patients presenting after a viral illness with the abrupt onset of productive cough, pleurisy, multiple chills, and hectic fever are suspect for this disease. Lung examination may show fine to coarse rhonchi and rales; however, signs of consolidation are rare. The chest x-ray reveals a patchy infiltrate, which rapidly progresses to abscess formation and lobar consolidation. Empyema is common, white blood counts are usually above 15,000 per cubic millimeter, and blood cultures are usually negative unless the pulmonary involvement is metastatic. Gram stain of the sputum reveals large gram-positive cocci in pairs and clumps.

Patients at particular risk include intravenous drug abusers, hospitalized patients, and the debilitated. Therapy includes intravenous oxacillin or nafcillin unless penicillin resistance or allergy is suspected. In these patients vancomycin can be used.

STREPTOCOCCAL PNEUMONIA (GROUP A)

Although a rare cause of pulmonary infection, group A streptococci can cause rapidly progressive pneumonitis. The clinical syndrome is characterized by the sudden onset of fever, chills, and productive cough. In most patients pleuritic pain is a prominent symptom. Pulmonary examination usually reveals fine rales without signs of consolidation. The chest x-ray is usually consistent with a multilobar bronchopneumonia, often with a large pleural effusion. The sputum is frequently bloody and purulent. Gram stain reveals gram-positive cocci in pairs and chains. Penicillin is the drug of choice.

EMPIRIC THERAPEUTIC GUIDELINES

In general, initial therapy is based on clinical presentation, sputum Gram stain, or culture results. The emergency physician is often faced with a nonspecific clinical presentation or nondiagnostic Gram stain with which to initiate outpatient therapy. In this situation, an excellent choice is erythromycin 500 mg every 6 h for 10 to 14 days with close clinical follow-up. *Hemophilus influenzae* is not covered by this approach and must be considered in patients who do not respond to therapy.

ADMISSION GUIDELINES

Pregnant patients and those with serious underlying diseases, volume depletion, toxicity, or severe hypoxia require hospital admission. Social admissions include all patients who cannot care for themselves at home. Patients who, after an appropriate evaluation, are felt to be well enough for outpatient therapy should be followed up in 3 to 5 days. A chest x-ray is frequently done after 1 month to document resolution of the infiltrate.

BIBLIOGRAPHY

Biggs DD: Pulmonary infections. *Med Clin North Am* 61:163, 1977.

Burmeister RW, Overholt EL: Pneumonia caused by hemolytic streptococcus. *Arch Intern Med* 111:367, 1963.

Chodosh S: Examination of sputum cells. *N Engl J Med* 282:854, 1970.

Everett D, Rahn A, Adaniya R, et al: *Hemophilus influenzae* pneumonia in adults. *JAMA* 238:319, 1977.

George LW, Finegold SM: Bacterial infections of the lung. *Chest* 81:501, 1982.

Johanson WG, Gould KG: Lung defense mechanisms. *Basics Respir Dis* 6:66, 1977.

Johanson WG, Pierce AK, Sanford JP: Changing pharyngeal bacterial flora of hospital patients. *N Engl J Med* 281:1137, 1969.

Kalinske RW, Parker RH, Brandt D, et al: Diagnostic usefulness and safety of transtracheal aspiration. *N Engl J Med* 276:604, 1967.

Klein RS, Steigbigel NH: Bacterial pneumonia, in Edlich RF, Spyker DA (eds): *Current Emergency Therapy,* 3d ed. Rockville, MD, Aspen Pub. 1986, p 519.

Manfredi F, Daly WJ, Beinke RH: Clinical observation of acute Friedländer pneumonia. *Ann Intern Med* 58:642, 1963.

Musher DM, McKenzie SO: Infections due to *Staphylococcus aureus. Medicine* 56:383, 1977.

Norden CW: *Hemophilus influenzae* infections in adults. *Med Clin North Am* 62:1037, 1978.

Ramirez-Ronda CH, Fuxeuch-Lopez Z, Nevarez M: Increased pharyngeal bacterial colonization during viral illness. *Arch Intern Med* 141:1599, 1981.

Reyes MP: The aerobic gram-negative bacillary pneumonias. *Med Clin North Am* 64:363, 1980.

Scanlon GT, Unger JD: The radiology of bacterial and viral pneumonias. *Radiol Clin North Am* 11:317, 1973.

Tuazon CU: Gram-positive pneumonias. *Med Clin North Am* 64:343, 1980.

29
VIRAL AND *Mycoplasma* PNEUMONIAS IN ADULTS

K. P. Ravikrishnan

INTRODUCTION

Respiratory viruses and *Mycoplasma* infections have a tremendous impact on society. Over half of the acute disabling illnesses in the United States is caused by respiratory viruses. The spectrum of disease caused by these agents ranges from the common cold to life-threatening pneumonia. Predominantly two common types of lower respiratory infections are caused by viruses and *Mycoplasma:* tracheobronchitis and pneumonia. Without localizing clinical and radiographic findings, it is not easy to separate severe tracheobronchitis from pneumonia. Classic pneumonia is characterized by chills followed by high fever, cough, pleuritic chest pain, and dyspnea. Depending upon the host response, the intensity of clinical manifestations and complications varies.

Viral and *Mycoplasma* pneumonia contribute to more than a third of community-acquired pneumonias, and an understanding of the disease is helpful in planning management strategies. Though most often these nonbacterial infections are seasonal minor illnesses, their potential for causing overwhelming pneumonia and respiratory failure is well known. Epidemics should be anticipated so that the effect on the normal population and the highly vulnerable elderly, debilitated, cardiac, and pulmonary patients can be minimized. Since there is no specific treatment for most of these pneumonias, the emphasis is placed on identification of the responsible agent and supportive treatment.

INCIDENCE AND ETIOLOGY

The spectrum of acute respiratory illnesses caused by viruses and *Mycoplasma* include pharyngitis, laryngitis, tracheobronchitis, and bronchitis. Nonbacterial agents account for over 90 percent of infectious respiratory ailments. Common complications from these infections are listed in Table 29-1. In hospitalized patients, bacteria predominate as the causative agents of pneumonia. Viral agents and *Mycoplasma* account for 10 to 25 percent of community-acquired pneumonia.

Increased airway reactivity from viral and *Mycoplasma* infections is well known. The inflammatory reaction and hyperreactivity to cholinergic stimulation occur during both the infectious and postinfectious phase. The mechanism of airway hyperreactivity is not clear, but patients with preexisting pulmonary diseases such as bronchiectasis and chronic obstructive pulmonary disease are prone to deterioration of pulmonary function during and after episodes of infection. This underscores the importance of prophylaxis and early management during each episode of respiratory infection.

VIRAL PNEUMONIA

Viral infections of the respiratory tract occur commonly as epidemics in the general population or in small groups such as school children or army recruits. However, sporadic cases do occur both in healthy and immunocompromised hosts. Children and debilitated older patients, especially those with underlying cardiopulmonary disorders, can become the victims of viral pneumonia or the associated secondary bacterial infections.

Table 29-1. Complications of Viral and *Mycoplasma* Pneumonia

1. Secondary bacterial infections
2. Recurrent pneumonia
3. Altered pulmonary function
4. Respiratory failure due to overwhelming infection
5. Bronchial hyperactivity
6. Chronic bronchitis
7. Bronchiolitis obliterans

Influenza and Parainfluenza Viruses

Of all the viruses, influenza and parainfluenza viruses cause the most serious respiratory infections. Influenza causes significant morbidity and mortality, either directly or secondary to bacterial superinfection. The major effect of the parainfluenza virus is in causing severe upper respiratory infections in children.

Influenza viruses are classified by their antigenic variation and are denoted by the initial place of isolation. They belong to the Orthomyxo viruses. Surface projections possess hemagglutinin and neuraminidase activity and are the antigenic determinants. Antigenic variability causes the perpetuation of infection. Horses, pigs, and birds serve as reservoirs.

Other Viral Infections

Respiratory syncytial viruses generally cause lower respiratory infections, again usually in children. Rhinovirus (the virus of the common cold), adenovirus, Coxsackie A and B, and echoviruses cause predominantly upper respiratory infections. It is important to differentiate these infections from pneumonia, and the potential for secondary bacterial infection should be recognized. Herpesvirus and lymphocytic choriomeningitis virus also cause pneumonia in healthy and in compromised hosts. The measles virus causes predominantly mucosal inflammation leading to bronchitis and bronchiolitis. An overwhelming interstitial pneumonia from this infection can occur. Secondary bacterial infections are common following epidemics of measles, usually in debilitated infants and children.

Varicella-zoster infection causes pneumonia. Adults with chickenpox can develop an interstitial pneumonia as a complication. Although varicella pneumonia is often self-limiting, at times it is associated with severe systemic disorders, such as encephalitis and myelitis, and adult respiratory distress syndrome (ARDS) requiring ventilatory management.

Pathology and Pathogenesis

Influenza and viruses in general are known for their potential to cause respiratory infection rapidly after exposure, often spreading like a brush fire in the susceptible population. Droplet particles containing the virus are carried as aerosols and are deposited in the airways. Within 24 to 48 h, symptomatic disease develops. Mucosal and interstitial inflammation and impaired mucociliary clearance predispose to secondary bacterial infection. Interstitial pneumonia, either due to infection or an antigen-antibody response, occurs in a small group of patients. If pneumonia is diffuse and progressive, acute hypoxemic respiratory failure results.

Diagnosis

Viral pneumonia is diagnosed in a patient presenting with chest pain, cough, fever, and dyspnea during the flu season. Patients usually complain of a prodrome comprised of malaise, upper respiratory symptoms, and, often, gastrointestinal symptoms. Clinical findings are minimal and variable. Chest examination may reveal wheezing. Fine rales, if heard, are indicative of interstitial involvement. Chest x-ray may show patchy densities or interstitial involvement. In cases complicated by respiratory failure, there is diffuse radiographic involvement indistinguishable from other causes of ARDS.

Leukocytosis is mild (the white blood cell count is 10,000 to 15,000). Gram stain of the sputum will not demonstrate bacteria in substantial quantities. Confirmation of the diagnosis is based on the identification of viral particles and serologic studies. Secretions from the respiratory tract during this phase of pneumonia can be used for isolation of the virus. The immunofluorescent staining technique is an excellent aid in the rapid diagnosis of influenza infections. Serologic tests, though not helpful in the acute setting, are extremely useful in epidemiological studies. If secondary bacterial infection is suspected, appropriate studies should be undertaken. Fiberoptic bronchoscopy is useful in isolating the agents from the lower respiratory tract and excluding other forms of pneumonia. On occasion, a lung biopsy is necessary for definitive diagnosis.

Management and Prophylaxis

Supportive treatment of viral pneumonia is aimed at decreasing the severity of symptoms. General management should include bed rest, analgesics, decongestants, antihistaminics, and expectorants. Older patients must guard against dehydration and some may require parenteral fluid therapy. Patients with significant wheezing should be treated with bronchodilators, including theophylline and aerosolized β_2 agonists. Associated bacterial infections like the secondary staphylococcal infection should be treated with appropriate antibiotics.

Severity of respiratory functional impairment should be assessed with pulmonary function studies, arterial blood gas analysis, and close assessment of the patient's clinical status. In case of progressive respiratory difficulty, supportive respiratory care should include oxygen supplementation and, if necessary, ventilatory assistance.

Amantadine (1-adamantanamine hydrochloride) has been shown to have in vitro action against influenza A virus. This drug is useful for specific treatment and in prophylaxis. If started following exposure or within the first 48 h of infection, treatment results in reduction of clinical symptoms. This drug is advised in high-risk patients who could not be vaccinated prior to the flu season. Amantadine is given in doses of 100 to 200 mg daily. For prophylaxis amantadine should be used throughout the flu season. Side effects have been noted in 5 to 7 percent of patients taking the drug and are due to its CNS effects. Insomnia, jitteriness, difficulty in concentrating, dizziness, and rarely syncopal episodes have been described. The drug and its metabolites are excreted by the kidneys and should be used with caution in patients with renal disease.

Aerosolized ribavirin has been found to be useful against upper and lower respiratory infections, caused by respiratory syncytial virus. Acyclovir is useful in the treatment of herpes viral infections.

Influenza Vaccine

High attack rates have been noted in recent epidemics of influenza. An increase in the size of the elderly population and in the survival rates of patients with chronic pulmonary diseases such as cystic fibrosis has compelled us to be more vigorous in preventing influenza. Influenza vaccine is effective against influenza A and B viruses. Attenuated whole or split viruses are used in vaccine manufacture. The formulation of vaccine is determined by the World Health Organization (WHO) and the Centers for Disease Control (CDC). Emphasis is on effective vaccination of the majority of the high-risk groups (Table 29-2). Current vaccines cause minimal side effects and have not been associated with Guillain-Barré syndrome.

Table 29-2. High-Risk Patients and Groups Targeted for Influenza Vaccination

1. Adults and children with chronic cardiopulmonary disorders
2. Residents of nursing homes and other institutions
3. Healthy individuals over the age of 65 years
4. Adults and children with chronic metabolic disorders: diabetes mellitus, renal failure, anemia, immunosuppression, asthma
5. Medical personnel who have contact with high-risk patients

Mycoplasma PNEUMONIA

Introduction

Mycoplasma pneumoniae, traditionally known to cause mild upper respiratory infection, is an important agent capable of causing pneumonia in otherwise healthy individuals. *M. pneumoniae* lacks a cell wall and this feature makes it resistant to common antibiotics which act on the cell wall. This agent is dispersed widely in the environment and accounts for nearly 25 percent of community-acquired pneumonia. It can cause extrapulmonary manifestations such as meningitis, encephalitis, pericarditis, hepatitis, and hemolytic anemia.

Pathology and Pathogenesis

The cell structure of *Mycoplasma* is conducive to receptor attachment to host cell membranes, causing an inflammatory response in host cells. The predominant direct effect is hyperemia and polymorphonuclear leukocyte response. Host response is the production of IgG and IgM antibodies. An aggressive host response rather than the direct infection may result in predominant clinical manifestations. Hence, pneumonia caused by this agent is probably a postinfectious hypersensitivity phenomenon mediated by T lymphocytes. The delay in manifestation of pneumonia, lack of *Mycoplasma* antigen in fulminant cases, and the difficulty in identifying the agent in body fluids other than sputum, support this theory. Hence, it is likely that *Mycoplasma* infection results usually in bronchitis with the capability of an aggressive hypersensitivity pneumonia mediated by humoral and cellular mechanisms.

Clinical Manifestations

Manifestations include upper and lower respiratory symptoms with varying severity, often associated with headache, malaise, and fever. The spectrum of disease, which is widespread, extends from a "trivial cold," pharyngitis, and bronchitis to an acute interstitial pneumonia culminating in respiratory failure.

Patients with pneumonia (less than 10 percent of cases) have initial upper respiratory symptoms followed by fever, chills, cough, headache, and malaise. The cough is nonproductive and often annoying, and is due to bronchitis, airway obstruction, and an interstitial form of pneumonia. In some patients the cough may become chronic and may last for 4 to 6 weeks, representing a postbronchitic hyperreactivity phenomenon associated with significant airway obstruction. Earache is helpful in the diagnosis of *Mycoplasma* pneumonia, especially if bullous myringitis can be identified. In patients with chronic obstructive lung diseases, as with any other associated infections, there is exacerbation of airway obstruction. Manifestations of extrapulmonary involvement include musculoskeletal and gastrointestinal symptoms. Pleural involvement is rare and is manifested by pleuritic pain and in a minority of cases, pleural effusion. Splenomegaly and lymphadenopathy are rare. Central nervous system involvement could lead to aseptic meningitis and encephalitis. In uncomplicated disease, symptoms abate within a week to 10 days. Treatment reduces the duration and intensity of both respiratory and systemic symptoms.

Complications and Extrapulmonary Manifestations

Most patients have self-limited disease and respond well to antibacterial treatment with erythromycin. Acute complications are due to hypoxemic respiratory failure leading to adult respiratory distress syndrome. Secondary bacterial infection in a small number of cases increases the morbidity. Other complications include increased airway reactivity, atelectasis, mediastinal adenopathy, pneumothorax, pleural effusion, and lung abscess.

Extrapulmonary manifestations are not necessarily complications. They may precede the pneumonia or occur during the pneumonia. Headache is often associated with pneumonia and is mild. Aseptic meningitis and (rarely) encephalitis with pleocytosis in the CSF have been described. Guillain-Barré syndrome can occur, though this is uncommon. Serologic changes are often a manifestation of infection, yet an interesting complication, the presence of IgM antibodies, results from the hemolytic potential of the cold agglutinins. Significant hemolysis is rare, and if it occurs it usually develops during the recovery phase. On rare occasions hemolysis leads to renal failure, thromboembolism and disseminated intravascular coagulopathy. Cardiac complications result from pericarditis and myocarditis with the clinical manifestations of chest pain, congestive cardiac failure, pericardial effusion, and cardiac arrhythmia, including heart block.

Laboratory Findings

Moderate leukocytosis (>10,000/mm^3) is the rule and leukopenia is rare. Exceptionally high counts over 25,000/mm^3 are seen rarely. A negative tuberculin skin test, due to a transient suppression of delayed hypersensitivity, and a false positive VDRL have been reported.

ECG changes are seen in patients with myocardial and pericardial involvement. Findings of pericarditis, myocarditis, and nonspecific ST and T wave changes along with cardiac arrhythmias are seen occasionally.

Sputum studies help to distinguish this disease from acute bacterial infections by the lack of identifiable organisms. Specific diagnosis is dependent on isolation of the organism in the phase of acute infection or the demonstration of rise in antibody titers. These tests do not serve as an immediate tool at the time of initial presentation, yet they are very helpful in confirmation of the diagnosis. Culture and identification take 7 to 10 days. Enriched media which enhance the rapidity of growth are promising and should be available for rapid diagnosis of this infection in the near future.

Serology

Complement-fixing antibody titers are diagnostic if there is a fourfold increase in the titers. If the initial titer is $>1/64$ it is highly suggestive of the infection. This IgM antibody rises at about the tenth day, peaks at 4 to 6 weeks, and could last as long as 6 months.

Cold Agglutinins

This IgM antibody capable of fixing complement is also directed against the I antigens of the red blood cells. Titers $>1/64$ in the acute phase and a fourfold rise during the convalescent period are diagnostic. The hemagglutination property can be used as a bedside test, but it cannot be overemphasized that cold agglutinins are nonspecific and rise in both infectious and noninfectious disorders (Table 29-3).

Radiology

Patchy densities to dense consolidation involving a whole lobe may be seen. An acute interstitial pneumonia, characterized by a reticulonodular pattern, is usually accompanied by significant pulmonary functional impairment, at times leading to respiratory failure, in which case the findings are indistinguishable from other causes of ARDS. Cavities, pneumatoceles, abscesses, significant pleural effusions, mediastinal adenopathy, and atelectasis have been described with clinically suspected *Mycoplasma* infection. However, these manifestations are rare and every attempt should be made to exclude an associated bacterial infection or other diagnosis if such features are present.

Table 29-3. Some Conditions Associated with Elevated Cold Agglutinin Titers

1. *Mycoplasma* pneumonia
2. Other viral pneumonias
3. Tuberculosis
4. Collagen vascular disorders
5. Malignancy
6. Lymphoma

Management

Erythromycin is the drug of choice in *Mycoplasma* infections. Penicillin, which acts by destroying the cell wall of organisms, is ineffective due to the lack of a defined cell wall in these organisms. Tetracycline is also effective against *Mycoplasma* infection. However, since erythromycin is effective against the common bacterium, *Streptococcus pneumoniae*, it is the favored antibiotic for the initial treatment of community-acquired pneumonia. The drug treatment reduces the duration of illness and decreases the severity of clinical symptoms during the period of illness. Treatment should be continued for 10 to 14 days, and the possibility of recurrence should be considered because *Mycoplasma* organisms can be isolated up to 12 weeks after drug treatment.

Supportive treatment should include bronchodilators, expectorants, analgesics, and antipyretics. Cough is often bothersome and may last weeks after the acute infection. Codeine-containing cough suppressants are useful in management. Patients with marked respiratory symptoms will require hospitalization.

Chlamydial Pneumonia

The chlamydia group of organisms consists of *Chlamydia psittaci, C. trachomatis,* and the newly described TWAR strain. They are a well-known cause of urogenital tract infection and are also capable of causing an atypical pneumonia. Pneumonia occurs as a sporadic case or in small epidemics. *C. psittaci* causes infections in patients who have had contact with infected birds harboring these organisms. Clinical features are indistinguishable from other forms of atypical pneumonia. TWAR pneumonia outbreaks have been known to occur in young adults. They are characterized by a prodrome of upper respiratory infection. Pulmonary symptoms include cough, chest pain, mucoid-to-greenish sputum production, and findings of diffuse or localized parenchymal involvement. In some studies, TWAR strain accounted for pneumonia in up to 6% of cases. Serological studies and special cultures are useful in confirming the diagnosis due to this group of organisms. Treatment consists of the use of erythromycin, 1 g/day for 5–10 days. This regimen has been inadequate in some patients with TWAR infection. They require treatment with tetracycline, 2 g/day for 7–10 days.

COMPARATIVE ANALYSIS OF COMMUNITY-ACQUIRED PNEUMONIA

This chapter would be incomplete without describing the differential features of common pneumonias, both typical and atypical. Table 29-4 gives a list of agents capable of causing atypical pneumonia in normal and debilitated hosts. The emergency physician is faced with the task of separating various forms of pneumonia with limited data. Initial analysis has to be thorough and complete in laying the groundwork for a definitive diagnosis, which may be possible at a later time. Separating a normal from an immune-compromised host becomes very important in the diagnosis and management. Underlying cardiopulmonary or other disorders which predispose to certain forms of bacterial pneumonia should be diagnosed appropriately. Separating pneumonia from severe laryngotracheal bronchitis is difficult at times. Once the diagnosis of pneumonia is established, the next step is the identification of an etiological agent and a logical approach to management.

Table 29-4. Atypical Pneumonias

1. *Mycoplasma* pneumonia
2. *Legionella* pneumonia
3. Viral pneumonia
4. *Chlamydia* pneumonia
5. Rickettsial pneumonia
6. Atypical presentation of a bacterial pneumonia

The spectrum of pneumonia extends from a simple, uncomplicated *Mycoplasma* pneumonia in a previously healthy individual to a complicated gram-negative pneumonia with sepsis in a debilitated elderly nursing home patient. Differentiating features are extremely helpful in distinguishing various forms of pneumonia. Physical and radiographic findings usually portray the severity of infection and do not help in defining an etiology.

Following are some of the common features which help to distinguish different forms of pneumonia:

1. Mixed bacterial infections are common in patients with chronic bronchitis.
2. Anaerobic and gram-negative infections occur commonly in alcoholics and in patients prone to develop aspiration pneumonia.
3. Staphylococcal infection occurs following viral pneumonia.
4. *Legionella* pneumonia occurs in elderly patients, and in the summer months as opposed to the winter months.
5. A patchy, consolidative pattern with a diffuse finding of rales are the features of nonbacterial pneumonia.
6. Predominant upper airway symptoms preceding the development of pneumonia are indicative of a viral or *Mycoplasma* pneumonia.
7. Earache with bullous myringitis is a feature of *Mycoplasma* pneumonia.
8. Dense consolidation with a bulging fissure in a chest x-ray is indicative of *Klebsiella* pneumonia, especially in an alcoholic patient.
9. Elderly patients with severe constitutional and gastrointestinal symptoms, and with relative bradycardia should be suspected of having *Legionella* pneumonia.

Combined features of bacterial and viral infections are indicative of concurrent bacterial infection. Travel, occupation, animal exposures, and environmental factors are helpful in diagnosing chlamydial infections, tularemia, Q fever, and especially noninfectious forms of hypersensitivity pneumonias which share the manifestations of community-acquired pneumonia. High leukocyte counts with polymorphonuclear leukocytosis suggest a bacterial etiology. Elevated liver enzymes with hypophosphatemias have been reported with *Legionella* infections. Multilobar involvement, especially the superior segments of lower lobes, with early findings of cavitation, should be diagnostic of anaerobic infections following an episode of aspiration. Multiple patchy lesions with a cavity or pneumatocele suggest the crucial possibility of septic pulmonary embolism, and the importance of this distinction cannot be overemphasized because of the radical difference in management. In the patient with risk factors for acquired immunodeficiency syndrome (AIDS) (i.e., homosexuals, intravenous drug addicts, patients requiring repeated transfusions) pulmonary infections with opportunistic organisms such as *Pneumocystis carinii,* cytomegalovirus, and *Mycobacterium avium-intracellulare,* should be suspected. Lastly, this chapter is incomplete without emphasizing the need to rule out tuberculosis, both for epidemiologic reasons and proper patient management. A disease so common in the past still could be confusing to a young physician, since the manifestations are varied.

BIBLIOGRAPHY

Bogart DB, Liu C, Ruth WE, et al: Rapid diagnosis of primary influenzal pneumonia. *Chest* 68:513, 1975.

Dolin R, Reichman RC, Madore HP, et al: A controlled trial of amantadine and rimantadine in the prophylaxis of influenza A infection. *N Engl J Med* 307:580, 1982.

Empey DW, Laitinen LA, Jacobs L, et al: Mechanisms of bronchial hyperreactivity in normal subjects after respiratory tract infection. *Am Rev Respir Dis* 113:131, 1976.

Fine NL, Smith LR, Sheedy PF: Frequency of pleural effusion in mycoplasma and viral pneumonias. *N Engl J Med* 283:790, 1970.

Glezen WP: Viral pneumonia as a cause and result of hospitalization. *J Infect Dis* 147:765, 1983.

Hall CB, McBride JT, Gala CL, et al: Ribavirin treatment of respiratory syncytial viral infection in infants with underlying cardiopulmonary disease. *JAMA* 254:3047, 1985.

Helmes CM, Viner JP, Strum RH, et al: Comparative features of pneumococcal, mycoplasmal and Legionnaires' disease pneumonias. *Ann Intern Med* 90:543, 1979.

Knight V, Gilbert BE: Chemotherapy of respiratory viruses, in Stollerman GH, et al (eds): *Advances in Internal Medicine,* vol. 31. Chicago, Year Book Medical Publishers, pp 95–118, 1986.

Linz DH, Tolle SW, Elliot DL: *Mycoplasma pneumoniae* pneumonia—experience at a referral center. *West J Med* 140:895, 1984.

Marrie TJ, Grayston JT, Wang SP, et al: Pneumonia associated with the TWAR strain of chlamydia. *Ann Intern Med* 106:507, 1987.

Murray HW, Masur H, Senterfilt LB, et al: The protein manifestations of mycoplasma pneumonia infections in adults. *Am J Med* 58:229, 1975.

Noriega ER, Simbercoff MS, Gilroy FJ, et al: Life threatening *Mycoplasma pneumoniae* pneumonia. *JAMA* 229:1471, 1974.

Prevention and control of influenza. *MMWR* 33:253, 1984.

Yu VL, Krubotn FK, Shonnard J, et al: New clinical perspective from a prospective pneumonia study. *Am J Med* 73:357, 1982.

30
LEGIONNAIRES' DISEASE AND *Pneumocystis* PNEUMONIA

Mark Zwanger

LEGIONNAIRES' DISEASE

In 1976 an outbreak of an unknown illness in 200 people at an American Legion Convention in Philadelphia heralded the birth of Legionnaires' disease. A few months later the etiologic agent, a fastidious gram-negative bacillus, *Legionella pneumophila,* was isolated. Evidence of the involvement of *Legionella* in previous outbreaks of disease has been shown by serologic testing. It appears that the *Legionella* organism was involved in an outbreak of pneumonia in Washington, D.C., in 1965 and was the likely cause of "Pontiac fever" in Pontiac, Michigan, in 1968. *Legionella* bacterium have now been recovered in clinical specimens from as early as 1943. The majority of *Legionella* infections are caused by *L. pneumophila,* with approximately 15 percent caused by other *Legionella* species.

Transmission and Incubation

L. pneumophila is ubiquitous in nature. It has been found in natural and synthetic water systems and has been cultured from mud. One study isolated the *Legionella* bacterium from 32 percent of the households in a Chicago neighborhood. It is estimated that 25,000 to 50,000 cases of *Legionella* occur yearly in the United States, but the actual incidence is unknown. The *Legionella* bacterium is estimated to be responsible for 6 to 30 percent of bacterial pneumonias. Recent studies of patients hospitalized with pneumonia suggest that *Legionella* is an important cause of both hospital- and community-acquired pneumonias. Outbreaks of Legionnaires' disease are more common than sporadic cases, with most epidemics occurring in summer and fall months.

The usual incubation period is from 2 to 10 days, although the incubation period in the Pontiac fever outbreak was much shorter, in the range of 24 to 48 h. The presumed mechanism of infection is airborne transmission of *L. pneumophila* with inhalation of contaminated aerosols, but the exact mode of transmission is still in debate. Domestic water systems are a potentially important source of transmission, as are cooling towers, heat-exchange systems, respiratory therapy devices, shower stalls, and whirlpool spas. Direct person-to-person transmission does not appear to occur. Most cases are in middle-aged males, with a 2.6:1 male-female preponderance. The age range of people who have contracted the disease has been from 5 months to 90 years.

Risk factors include smoking, diabetes, surgery (trauma), chronic lung disease, alcohol use, and living or working near construction or excavation sites. At greatest risk are immunocompromised individuals, such as kidney transplant recipients and individuals with underlying cardiorespiratory, renal, or neoplastic disorders.

Clinical Presentation

Legionnaires' disease can progress rapidly from mild, nonspecific symptoms to a severe respiratory illness with the classical features of a bacterial pneumonia. After an initial low-grade fever, the temperature rises rapidly, reaching 39.5 to 40.0°C (103.1 to 104°F).

The patient develops symptoms of anorexia, weakness, malaise, cough (95 percent), shaking chills (77 percent), and watery diarrhea (47 percent). Weakness is frequently the only presenting complaint. Headache (75 percent), drenching sweats, nausea (40 percent), vomiting, myalgia (75 percent), and arthralgias may all be present. Dyspnea, pleuritic chest pain, and hemoptysis are seen in about one-third of the patients. The cough is typically nonproductive and not bothersome to the patient. Eventually, small amounts of watery or bloody sputum may be produced. Disorientation and confusion may be seen in up to one-third of the patients during the initial days of high fever. Coma occurs in 15 to 20 percent of the patients.

Physical examination reveals an acutely ill toxic-appearing individual who is diaphoretic and tachypneic. Auscultation of the chest reveals fine inspiratory rales in multiple areas. As the infection continues, classical findings of pneumonic consolidation and sepsis are found.

Laboratory Studies

Leukocytosis in the range of 10,000 to 20,000 with a left shift is common. Sputum Gram stain findings that demonstrate few polymorphonuclear leukocytes and no predominant bacterial species should suggest *Legionella* as a possible agent causing pneumonia. An elevated sedimentation rate and mild elevation of liver function tests (SGOT, LDH, alkaline phosphatase, and bilirubin) are frequently seen. Microscopic hematuria is noted in up to 10 percent of the patients, but its significance is unclear. It is not unusual to find hyponatremia (less than 130 mEq/L) or hypophosphatemia. No cerebrospinal fluid abnormalities have been reported.

Radiographs

Radiographic patterns are very variable. The chest film may initially indicate only a small unilateral alveolar infiltrate (70 percent), which can rapidly progress to multiple bilateral patchy, nonsegmental pulmonary infiltrates in about two-thirds of the patients. As the disease continues, pulmonary consolidation is commonly seen around the tenth day of the illness, with radiographic findings easily mimicking the appearance of pneumococcal pneumonia. Pleural effusions occur in from 9 to 16 percent of patients and can be present in the absence of lung field infiltrates. Pulmonary cavitary lesions can also be seen on chest roentgenograms. Serial radiographic findings may not correlate with the patient's clinical course. Serial chest radiographs frequently show progression of infiltrates despite the patient's being on appropriate antibiotics, since resolution of roentgenographic changes lags far behind clinical improvement. Infiltrates have been noted to persist on radiographs for as long as 6 to 12 months after clinical resolution.

Differential Diagnosis

The diagnosis of Legionnaires' disease is suggested by the clinical picture. A constellation of fever, respiratory symptoms, severe toxicity, extrapulmonic complaints, and a chest radiograph with infiltrates suggest the diagnosis. A sputum Gram stain of one predominant pathogen should suggest another infectious agent. Patients who have failed on a trial of antibiotics such as penicillin or ampicillin are more likely to have *Legionella.*

Mycoplasma pneumonia, pneumococcal pneumonia, psittacosis, Q fever, influenza, viral pneumonia, and tularemia all must be considered in the differential diagnosis, since *Legionella's* presenting signs and symptoms can be similar to these diseases. Current diagnosis involves culture, which has a sensitivity of from 50 to 80 percent and a specificity of 100 percent. At least 2 days are necessary for positive cultures, with colonies frequently not present for up to 2 weeks.

Tests that use direct immunofluorescence testing of respiratory specimens have a high specificity but low sensitivity (25 to 50 percent), which can be improved by obtaining multiple specimens. Investigators are studying radioimmunoassay and enzyme-linked immunosorbent assays for the detection of *L. pneumophila* antigen in urine samples. Initial results suggest a very high specificity and sensitivity, which may allow diagnosis as early as 24 h after the onset of symptoms. However, since the antigen is excreted for a long period of time, a positive test result may reflect a prior, rather than a current, infection.

Elevation of antibody titers from acute to convalescent phase sera of at least 1:128 is necessary for serologic diagnosis of *Legionella* infection using indirect immunofluorescence tests. Convalescent titers of greater than 1:256 are suggestive of recent infection with *L. pneumophila*. Although titers may be positive within 1 week, it usually takes 3 to 6 weeks for titers to increase and thereby confirm the diagnosis. This delay makes the results of serologic titer testing of limited value clinically.

Therapy

Early aggressive antibiotic therapy is essential. The drug of choice is 750 to 1000 mg of erythromycin IV every 6 h. Patients who have failed to respond have been shown to have inadequate erythromycin blood levels. This mandates the initial need for intravenous therapy. Oral therapy should be continued for 3 weeks, since shorter courses are associated with relapse. Delay in treatment affects prognosis; therefore, erythromycin must be started as early as possible in pneumonias where a definite diagnosis is not known and Legionnaires' disease is suspected. Tetracycline is not as efficacious as erythromycin. Rifampin may be an alternative drug to use.

Course and Prognosis

Legionnaires' disease varies in severity and duration from mild pneumonitis to severe respiratory failure. Symptoms frequently last for several weeks after diagnosis. Spiking fevers may continue even after specific therapy has been instituted. Respiratory failure is common, and ventilatory support is required in 11 to 49 percent of hospitalized patients. Shock occurs in 10 percent of patients and almost universally indicates a very unfavorable prognosis. The pneumonia may resolve spontaneously, but the mortality rate in untreated patients is significant. Mortality from Legionnaires' disease can be as high as 75 percent in patients who do not receive appropriate therapy but is only about 5 percent with the use of erythromycin and aggressive ventilatory support. Extrapulmonary manifestations of Legionnaires' disease disappear much more rapidly than the fever or pneumonia.

Extrapulmonic Manifestations

L. pneumophila can cause extrapulmonic manifestations without evidence of simultaneous pneumonia. In the summer of 1968, workers in Pontiac, Michigan, experienced an outbreak of a febrile illness that was proved to be due to *L. pneumophila*. It was an acute, short-lived illness with chills, fever, headache, and myalgias. There were no documented cases of pneumonia or death. The incubation period was only 24 to 48 h. There was a very high infectivity rate, with 95 percent of the visitors and employees of the building experiencing complaints. The incidence of Pontiac fever is not known, but this fever closely resembles that of viral respiratory infections and might easily be attributed to the flu rather than to the *Legionella* bacterium.

L. pneumophila has also been documented as the cause of myocarditis in children without evidence of pneumonia. Similar cases of *Legionella* pericarditis and endocarditis in adults have been reported.

PNEUMOCYSTIS CARINII PNEUMONIA

In 1981, researchers in New York and California reported that *Pneumocystis carinii*, an opportunistic infection rarely seen other than in immunocompromised individuals, was occurring in homosexual men and intravenous drug abusers. It was subsequently proven that a human retrovirus, HIV-1, was responsible for this new acquired immune deficiency syndrome (AIDS). By 1992, over 200,000 AIDS cases will be diagnosed in the United States, with over 1 million Americans presumed to be currently infected with the virus and more than 100,000 individuals already dead from AIDS. The highest incidence of infection has continued to be in the traditional high-risk groups of gay men and intravenous drug abusers. Transfusion-related AIDS is estimated at 2 percent of all cases and is diminishing with screening of the blood supply for antibodies to the virus. Hemophiliacs represent 1 percent of AIDS cases. The largest rate of increase is in heterosexual women who are sexual partners of infected members of high-risk groups and through maternal spread of disease by the perinatal route.

HIV-infected patients have both reduced functional and quantitative numbers of T-helper lymphocytes, which increases patient susceptibility to opportunistic infections and neoplastic processes. *P. carinii* is the most common opportunistic infection in HIV patients and has the potential for severe morbidity and mortality. Approximately 60 to 85 percent of HIV-infected individuals not receiving chemoprophylaxis therapy against *P. carinii* will develop *P. carinii* pneumonia (PCP) as their first opportunistic infection.

Prior to the AIDS epidemic, PCP was relatively uncommon, with approximately 100 cases reported per year. Since the start of the AIDS epidemic in 1981, more than 100,000 cases of PCP have occurred. The annual incidence of PCP in AIDS patients is approximately 30 percent, with a case fatality rate of 20 percent per episode.

Transmission and Incubation

P. carinii is ubiquitous in nature, although the natural habitat and mode of acquisition are unclear. It is commonly found in asymptomatic individuals and rarely causes disease except in immunosuppressive states. The infection is most likely transmitted by the airborne route. Most children have antibodies to the organism by the age of 4 years, which suggests a high incidence of exposure and subclinical infection by an early age. A slight seasonal variation, with more infections in summer than in winter, has been noted.

The organism was noted in guinea pig lungs in 1909. The first human reports of infection were described in the United States in the 1950s. The organism develops from a trophozoite into a cystic structure containing sporozoites. *P. carinii's* life cycle is similar to those of both protozoa and fungi, and therefore its classification has been confusing, with the organism being described by some as fungus and by others as protozoan. *P. carinii* causes disease as a result of defects in cellular immunity. Patients with primary immunodeficiency disorders, malignant tumors, lymphomas, leukemias, collagen vascular diseases, organ transplants, or patients on immunosuppressive medications are at highest risk of developing pneumocystis pulmonary disease. The development of the disease may occur from a new primary infection, reactivation, or reinfection. The annual attack rate for PCP in transplant, leukemic, and lymphoma patients is approximately 0.01 to 1 percent.

Clinical Presentation

Clinical manifestations of PCP are nonspecific, range from mild to severe, and can be similar to those of other pneumonias. Patients typically present with a slow and insidious onset of disease and are frequently symptomatic for weeks prior to diagnosis. The triad of fever, dyspnea, and cough in an HIV-infected individual should suggest PCP. Exertional dyspnea is noted by 30 to 95 percent of patients with *P. carinii* infection. Cough is present in 60 to 91 percent of these patients. The cough is typically nonproductive, although one-third of the patients report the production of sputum. Weight loss (32 to 100 percent), chest pain (14 to 23 percent), night sweats (12 to 26 percent), chills (12 to 26 percent), and fatigue (12 to 100 percent) can be present.

Fever is noted in 80 to 100 percent of patients, with a 2- to 3-week prodrome of fever of 39 to 40°C common. Clinical signs include tachypnea (55 to 62 percent), with a respiratory rate greater than 30 suggesting a worse prognosis. Rales or rhonchi are heard in 30 to 46 percent of the patients. Since in the majority of patients no unusual lung sounds are auscultated, the absence of abnormal chest findings does not rule out the diagnosis of PCP.

Other clinical manifestations of immune suppression may be noted, such as oral candidiasis, hairy leukoplakia, seborrheic dermatitis, Kaposi's sarcoma, or generalized lymphadenopathy. When seen in HIV patients, these findings are specific for the potential development of other opportunistic infections, including PCP.

Extrapulmonary Infections

It is uncommon to see *P. carinii* infection outside of the lung. However, *P. carinii* has been found as ear masses and retinal cotton-wool spots and in the thyroid, heart, lungs, gastroinestinal tract, kidney, adrenal glands, bone marrow, and pleural effusions.

Laboratory Studies

White blood cell counts are variable, with normal values reported most often, followed by leukopenia (32 percent) and leukocytosis (9 percent). Lymphopenia, anemia, and thrombocytopenia are common and suggest more advanced disease. The T helper-T suppressor cell ratio is inverted, with the total number of T helper cells (CD4 lymphocyte count) markedly reduced. A CD4 lymphocyte count less than 200 cells/mL correlates with marked immunosuppression and greatly increases the patient's risk of developing opportunistic pulmonary infections such as PCP. Mean serum LDH levels are elevated in 90 percent of the patients with *Pneumocystis* pulmonary disease. A rising LDH level or a value greater than 450 IU is suggestive of PCP. LDH levels decrease as the infection is controlled. A low serum albumin level is common and indicates a worse prognosis. An erythrocyte sedimentation rate (ESR) above 50 mm/h may be useful in helping to diagnose PCP. For a symptomatic HIV-infected patient with a normal chest radiograph, an elevated ESR, and an LDH level above 220 IU/L, the probability that the patient has PCP is 47-percent.

While arterial blood gas abnormalities are common, a normal blood gas does not exclude the diagnosis of PCP. Arterial blood gas abnormalities include hypoxemia, hypocarbia, respiratory alkalosis, and an increased arterial-alveolar (A-a) oxygen gradient. Hypoxia is almost uniformly present (80 percent), with a low Pa_{O_2} (less than 70 mmHg) suggesting a worse prognosis. Sixty-four percent of patients with PCP have an abnormal $P(\text{A-a})_{O_2}$ gradient (greater than 20 mmHg) at rest. The $P(\text{A-a})_{O_2}$ gradient can frequently be accentuated with exercise and can be useful in helping to diagnose pulmonary infection in the symptomatic HIV-infected patient who has a normal chest radiograph. During exercise, an increase of more than 10 mmHg in the $P(\text{A-a})_{O_2}$ gradient from rest is suggestive of PCP. This simple test has a 91-percent sensitivity but only an 11-percent specificity for PCP.

Pulmonary function tests can be abnormal in HIV-infected patients, with the diffusing capacity for carbon monoxide (DLCO) frequently decreased. Although the DLCO is not specific for PCP, a diffusion capacity of less than 80 percent of the predicted value has a sensitivity of near 100 percent for *P. carinii* infection.

Gallium scans of the lung have sensitivities of 90 to 98 percent in patients with PCP but have a specificity of from 20 to 82 percent. Gallium scans can be useful in diagnosing PCP in the symptomatic patient who has both a normal chest radiograph and arterial blood gas. In these patients, a normal gallium lung scan has a positive predictive value of 96 percent that the patient does not have PCP. A combination of a negative gallium lung scan and a diffusion capacity greater than 80 percent virtually rules out the diagnosis of pulmonary infection by *P. carinii*.

Radiographs

The chest roentgenogram will be abnormal in 90 to 95 percent of patients. The most common radiographic finding (56 to 94 percent) is diffuse bilateral interstitial or alveolar infiltrates. The classic radiograph shows a perihilar distribution that extends in a "bat-wing" pattern. As the infection progresses, infiltrates may involve all lung fields or produce consolidation. One-third of the patients present with an atypical appearance of asymmetric infiltrates, unilateral infiltrates, or infiltrates near the periphery of the lungs. The lung periphery and apices are frequently spared, except in patients on prophylactic aerosolized antibiotics who are likely to have disease predominantly in the upper lobes of the lungs. This pattern is thought to result from less of the aerosolized antibiotic reaching the upper lobes.

Radiographically, PCP can also simulate tuberculosis, a solitary pulmonary nodule, and occasionally even pulmonary edema. Approximately 7 percent of patients have cystic-appearing radiographic abnormalities, and 6 percent develop spontaneous unilateral or bilateral pneumothoraces. Bronchopleural fistulas, lymphadenopathy, pulmonary cavitation, and pleural effusions can occur but are not common and should suggest other pulmonary disease processes. Approximately 10 percent of patients with PCP infection have a completely normal chest radiograph.

Differential Diagnosis

The differential diagnosis for pneumonia in the HIV-positive patient includes *P. carinii, Mycobacterium tuberculosis*, bacterial pneumonia, cryptococcus, histoplasmosis, coccidioidomycosis, nocardia, cytomegalovirus, lymphocytic interstitial pneumonitis, *Mycobacterium avium-intracellulare*, and *Mycobacterium kansasii*. Concurrent pulmonary infections occur in 10 to 20 percent of patients, and the physician should be alert for these coinfections.

Diagnosis

Cytologic evaluation of induced sputum yields positive results for PCP in 15 to 90 percent of patients. The negative predictive value of sputum, however, is only about 50 percent. Current research is focusing on the development of direct fluorescence assays using monoclonal antibodies to screen for the detection of *P. carinii* in sputum specimens. Reports indicate these assays have sensitivities of near 90 percent. Sputum should also be Gram-stained and examined for acid-fast bacilli and fungal causes of infection. Routine bacterial, fungal, and tuberculosis cultures must be done.

If sputum examination is unsuccessful for identification of the organism, fiberoptic bronchoscopy is the method of choice for the rapid diagnosis of *P. carinii*. The combination of transbronchial biopsy, bronchial brushings and washings, and bronchoalveolar lavage have a diagnostic yield for *P. carinii* of near 100 percent. Bronchoalveolar lavage alone has a sensitivity of 79 to 98 percent. For solitary lesions or cavitary lesions that might represent associated infections, fine-needle aspiration using computerized tomography guidance assists in diagnosis. Open lung biopsy offers the greatest diagnostic yield but is expensive and time-consuming and entails the risks of anesthesia and the complications of thoracotomy.

For the HIV-positive symptomatic patient with a normal chest radiograph and a satisfactory blood gas, it is necessary to pursue further evaluation and workup with gallium scans or exercise testing to rule out the diagnosis of PCP.

Therapy

Treatment of immunocompromised patients suspected of having PCP includes aggressive respiratory management and support, mechanical ventilation, antibiotics, and corticosteroids. Patients need to be admitted for treatment because they can acutely decompensate, and there is a very high incidence of adverse drug reactions. Oxygen therapy should be guided by arterial blood gases and the results of pulse oximetry. If oxygen therapy with a nasal cannula or simple face mask does not rapidly improve hypoxia, continuous positive airway pressure with a mask is useful but has the potential complications of developing pneumothoraces or aspirating stomach contents.

Antibiotics

The initial drug of choice is currently either trimethoprim-sulfamethoxazole (TMP-SMZ) or pentamidine isethionate, with most studies suggesting similar efficacy and no clear preference for one drug over the other. Because of the high incidence of adverse drug reactions with these medications, it is not uncommon for the patient to be started on one antibiotic and because of side effects have to be switched to the other drug during therapy. Combination therapy with both TMP-SMX and pentamidine is not more advantageous than using a single antibiotic and increases the risk of side effects.

Many clinicians begin with TMP-SMZ, which also provides antimicrobial coverage for some bacterial pneumonias and allows the patient to eventually be switched to oral medication. The dosage of TMP-SMX is 15 to 20 mg/kg per day of TMP and 75 to 100 mg/kg per day of SMX intravenously divided into four doses for 14 to 21 days. Estimates of side effects from TMP-SMX in AIDS patients ranges from 50 to 90 percent. Adverse reactions include fever, nausea, vomiting, bone marrow suppression, rash, increased liver enzymes, renal insufficiency, and electrolyte abnormalities. In the patient with a history of prior allergic reactions to sulfa drugs, renal failure, or blood cell dyscrasias (neutropenia, anemia, or thrombocytopenia), TMP-SMX should be avoided and pentamidine used.

The dose of pentamidine is 4 mg/kg given as a single daily intravenous infusion over 1 to 2 h for 14 to 21 days. The drug is infused over a period of 1 to 3 h with frequent monitoring for hypotension. Up to 50 percent of patients on pentamidine develop adverse reactions, including hypotension, tachycardia, facial flushing, pruritis, syncope, renal toxicity, elevated liver enzymes, taste disturbances, hallucinations, thrombocytopenia, rash, nausea, hypoglycemia, and pancreatitis.

Aerosolized pentamidine or oral TMP-SMX may also be used judiciously as initial therapy in patients with mild PCP. Some authors report success rates of from 60 to 80 percent in the treatment of PCP by giving 300 or 600 mg of aerosolized pentamidine daily.

Recent studies suggest that giving dapsone (100 mg/day) and trimethoprim (15 to 20 mg/kg per day in four divided doses) together is as effective as the traditional therapies. The benefits of this combination include less toxicity and the option of giving the drugs orally, which allows for continuation of therapy on an outpatient basis. Trimetrexate gluconate, eflornithine hydrochloride, and a combination of clindamycin and primaquine phosphate are all being evaluated as possible drugs for treatment of PCP and can be used if the patient cannot tolerate the established treatment therapies for PCP.

Corticosteroid Therapy

Patients with PCP can be stratified into mild or severe disease based on their arterial oxygen pressure or A-a oxygen gradient. This distinction is important, since it aids in differentiating who should receive steroids. A P_{O_2} greater than 70 mmHg or arterial $P(\text{A-a})_{O_2}$ gradient less than 35 mmHg suggests a mild infection and has a more favorable prognosis than patients with a P_{O_2} less than 70 mmHg or a $P(\text{A-a})_{O_2}$ gradient greater than 35 mmHg who have severe pulmonary dysfunction are more likely to have a grave prognosis.

Patients who have severe disease should be given corticosteroid therapy as early as possible. Corticosteroids as an adjunct in the therapy of severe PCP are clearly beneficial, since they substantially reduce mortality, decrease respiratory failure, limit oxygen deterioration, and accelerate recovery. It is postulated that steroids act by reducing the lung's inflammatory response to *P. carinii* infection. Since prolonged steroid administration has been associated with the development of PCP in a variety of patients, the finding that steroids decrease mortality in AIDS patients with PCP is surprising. Concerns about the possibility of increasing other life-threatening opportunistic infections or augmenting the spread of Kaposi's sarcoma by using steroids have not been supported. The following regimen is based on the consensus recommendations of the National Institutes of Health. In patients with severe pulmonary disease, oral prednisone in the dose of 40 mg twice a day is given for days 1 through 5, 40 mg daily for days 6 through 10, and 20 mg daily for days 11 through 21. Intravenous methylprednisolone can be alternatively given at 75 percent of these dosages. There is currently no compelling information to suggest that steroids are beneficial in mild *Pneumocystis* pulmonary disease.

Prophylaxis

Patients with a CD4 count below 200 cells/mL are at very high risk for developing PCP, while patients who are not on suppressive therapy and have had a prior infection with *P. carinii* have a 60-percent probability of developing a recurrent episode of PCP. The Centers for Disease Control recommend that HIV-infected patients with a CD4 count less than 200 cells/mL or patients who have had a prior episode of PCP be given 300 mg of aerosolized pentamidine every 4 weeks via nebulizer for prophylaxis against *P. carinii*. This prophylactic regimen has reduced the rate of relapse by 50 to 80 percent to a recurrence rate of 6 to 16 percent. In patients not receiving prophylactic treatment, the fatality rate is 20 percent, compared with 9 percent for those on prophylactic therapy.

Local side effects include cough and upper airway irritation (10 to 20 percent) and bronchospasm (1 to 2 percent). Systemic side effects are infrequent (1 percent) but can include hypoglycemia and pancreatitis. When on prophylaxis, these patients can develop atypical apical pneumonias and are more likely to present with disseminated *P. carinii* infection.

Other prophylaxis regimens include the oral administration of 160 mg of trimethoprim and 800 mg of sulfamethoxazole with 5 mg of lecovorin calcium twice a day.

Clinical Course and Prognosis

Compared to other patients with PCP, AIDS patients take longer to respond clinically and show slower radiographic improvement when treated. These patients can be unstable and decompensate quickly, which mandates initial in-hospital treatment of *Pneumocystis* infection. Initial survival rates for PCP were approximately 57 percent. With more aggressive treatment, a wider spectrum of antibiotics available, and the use of steroids, recent studies suggest survival rates of 80 to 95 percent for the first PCP admission. AIDS patients may need a change in therapy if there is no clinical improvement in 4 to 5 days or if there is no radiographic improvement after 7 to 10 days. Patients necessitating a change in therapy usually do worse and have a higher mortality.

Respiratory failure can occur in as many as 5 to 30 percent of hospitalized patients. Although initial reports suggested mortality rates of 90 to 100 percent with patients who need mechanical ventilatory support, new studies suggest that the mortality rate with severe respiratory failure has declined to 58 to 64 percent.

Failure to respond to therapy indicates the need for reevaluation and a search for other infectious agents that may coexist. Patients who have mixed pulmonary infections have a worse prognosis, with mortality rates as high as 92 percent, compared to 18 percent for patients with only PCP. Recurrent bouts of pneumonia also have a worse prognosis.

Some authors have suggested empirically treating patients who have clinical and radiographic features consistent with PCP and forgoing further diagnostic studies. This approach is unwise and is not in the patient's best interest. It is necessary to make a diagnosis, since current recommendations include using steroids that are life-saving in PCP but potentially catastrophic in patients who have bacterial or other fungal pulmonary infections. Without a diagnosis, the treating physician will have difficulty identifying those patients who should receive steroids.

BIBLIOGRAPHY

Legionnaires' Disease

Fraser DW, Tsai TR, Orenstein W, et al: Legionnaires' disease: Description of an epidemic of pneumonia. *N Engl J Med* 297:1189, 1977.

Glick TH, Gregg MB, Berman B, et al: Pontiac fever. *Am J Epidemiol* 107:149, 1978.

Helms CM, Viner JP, Strum RD, et al: Comparative features of pneumococcal, mycoplasmal, and Legionnaires' disease pneumonias. *Ann Intern Med* 90:543, 1979.

Kirby BD: Community-acquired pneumonia. *Emerg Med Clin North Am* 3:179, 1985.

Kohler RB: Antigen detection for the rapid diagnosis of mycoplasma and *Legionella* pneumonia. *Diag Microbiol Infect Dis* 4(suppl 3):47S, 1986.

Miller AC: Early clinical differentiation between Legionnaires' disease and other sporadic pneumonias. *Ann Intern Med* 90:526, 1979.

Nelson DP, Rensimer ER, Raffin TA: *Legionella pneumophila* pericarditis without pneumonia. *Arch Intern Med* 145:926, 1985.

Pastoris MC, Nigro G, Midulla M: Arrhythmia or myocarditis: A novel clinical form of *Legionella pneumophila* infection in children without pneumonia. *Eur J Pediatr* 144:157, 1985.

Ruf B, Schurmann D, Horbach I, et al: The incidence of *Legionella* pneumonia: A 1-year prospective study in a large community hospital. *Lung* 167:11, 1989.

Winn WC: Legionnaires disease: Historical perspective. *Clin Microbiol Rev* 1:60, 1989.

Pneumocystis Pneumonia

Bozette S, Sattler F, Chiu J, et al: A controlled trial of early adjunctive treatment with corticosteroids for *Pneumocystis carinii* pneumonia in the acquired immunodeficiency syndrome. *N Engl J Med* 323:1451, 1990.

Friedman Y, Franklin C, Rackow EC, et al: Improved survival in patients with AIDS, *Pneumocystis carinii* pneumonia, and severe respiratory failure. *Chest* 96:862, 1989.

Gagnon S, Boota A, Fischl M, et al: Corticosteroids as adjunctive therapy for severe *Pneumocystis carinii* pneumonia in the acquired immunodeficiency syndrome. *N Engl J Med* 323:1444, 1990.

Garay SM, Greene J: Prognostic indicators in the initial presentation of *Pneumocystis carinii* pneumonia. *Chest* 95:769, 1989.

Guidelines for prophylaxis against *Pneumocystis carinii* pneumonia for persons infected with human immunodeficiency virus. *MMWR* (suppl 5):1, 1989.

Katz MH, Baron RB, Grady D: Risk stratification of ambulatory patients suspected of *Pneumocystis* pneumonia. *Arch Intern Med* 151:105, 1991.

Kramer EL, Sanger JH, Garay SM, et al: Diagnostic implications of Ga-67 chest-scan patterns in human immunodeficiency virus-seropositive patients. *Radiology* 170:671, 1989.

Levine SJ, White DA: *Pneumocystis carinii*. *Clin Chest Med* 9:395, 1988.

Medina I, Mills J, Leonug G, et al: Oral therapy for *Pneumocystis carinii* pneumonia in the acquired immunodeficiency syndrome: A controlled trial of trimethoprim-sulfamethoxazole versus trimethoprim-dapsone. *N Engl J Med* 323:776, 1990.

Miller RF, Millar AB, Weller IVD, et al: Empirical treatment without bronchoscopy for *Pneumocystis carinii* pneumonia in the acquired immunodeficiency syndrome. *Thorax* 44:559, 1989.

National Institutes of Health: Consensus statement on the use of corticosteroids as adjunctive therapy for *Pneumocystis carinii* in the acquired immunodeficiency syndrome. *N Engl J Med* 323:1500, 1990.

Stover DE, Greeno RA, Fagliardi AJ: The use of a simple exercise test for the diagnosis of *Pneumocystis carinii* pneumonia in patients with AIDS. *Am Rev Respir Dis* 139:1343, 1989.

31
ASPIRATION PNEUMONIA, EMPYEMA, AND LUNG ABSCESS

Georges C. Benjamin

Aspiration pneumonia is an inflammation of the lung parenchyma resulting from the entrance of foreign material into the tracheobronchial tree. The clinical consequences of pulmonary aspiration of gastric contents were described in 1946 by Mendelson, who observed this complication in obstetrical patients undergoing anesthesia. Predisposing risk are depression of the cough or gag reflex, alterations in the normal physiologic handling of secretions or gastric contents, and structural alterations of the normal physiologic protective mechanisms.

PATHOPHYSIOLOGY

The clinical and pathologic results of pulmonary aspiration depend on the pH of the aspirated material, the volume of the aspirate, the presence in the aspirate of particulate matter such as food, and bacterial contamination.

Aspiration of large particles of food or other objects that can cause upper airway obstruction is an important and easily reversible cause of mortality. This complication must be quickly recognized and treated.

Neutral Fluids

It is generally accepted that serious injury results if the pH of the aspirate is 2.5 or less. However, many of the early pathologic changes are nonspecific and occur regardless of the pH of the aspirate. These include collapse and expansion of individual alveoli, reflex airway closure, and interstitial edema. These changes occur within seconds, producing significant ventilation-perfusion mismatch and marked hypoxia. If material with a pH greater than 2.5 is aspirated, the severity of injury depends additionally on the composition of the aspirate and the volume. The aspiration of lipid materials results in a chronic granulomatous reaction resulting in lipoid pneumonia. The consequences of aspiration of neutral, clear liquids are more easily reversible with supportive therapy; however, large-volume aspiration results in high mortality and morbidity.

Neutral Fluids with Food Particles

Neutral fluids with food particles produce a persistent inflammatory reaction resulting in a hemorrhagic pneumonitis within 6 h after aspiration. As the pneumonitis progresses, a chronic granulomatous reaction develops which resembles the granuloma of pulmonary tuberculosis and may be visible on roentgenography.

Acid Aspiration

The aspiration of fluids with a pH of less than 2.5 results in severe pulmonary changes analogous to those produced by a chemical burn. Volumes as low as 1 mL/kg have been shown to result in pathologic changes throughout the pulmonary parenchyma within seconds. These changes include reflex airway closure, destruction of surfactant-producing alveoli, alveolar collapse, and pulmonary capillary destruction. In the first few hours after aspiration, intrapulmonary mucosal hemorrhage, bronchial epithelial degeneration, and pulmonary edema occur. Shunting may be massive and pulmonary compliance decreases. The loss of integrity of the alveolocapillary bed results in large fluid losses that can be severe enough to require volume repletion. Secondary bacterial infection results. In community-acquired aspiration, anaerobes comprise the most common bacterial isolates. In a patient who develops aspiration following hospitalization, gram-negative aerobes, including *Pseudomonas, Proteus,* and *Escherichia coli* in addition to anaerobes, are frequent isolates.

Foreign Body Aspiration

Foreign body aspiration may represent an acute threat to life and is responsible for approximately 3000 deaths each year. Eighty percent of these cases occur in children, especially those under the age of 6. Running with food or other objects in the mouth, seizures, and forced feeding are common risk factors for this problem in children. In adults, it can result from dental or nasal surgery, unconsciousness, or poorly chewed food. Sixty percent of foreign bodies are found in the right bronchus, 19 percent in the left, and 21 percent at the larynx or cords. When complete obstruction occurs, death from asphyxiation occurs within minutes unless the condition is relieved. In these cases the patient usually is aphonic, cyanotic, and may be grabbing his or her throat. Prompt therapy with a chest or abdominal thrust is required for relief. Patients without complete obstruction present with spasmodic cough, choking, and wheezing. Physical examination may reveal fever, wheezing on the involved side, decreased breath sounds, hyperresonance on percussion, and asymmetric chest movement. Chest radiography will reveal the object if radiopaque. However, atelectasis, air trapping, or mediastinal shift on inspiratory and expiratory chest films are more commonly seen.

Therapy consists of prompt bronchoscopic removal. In some cases, tracheotomy or open thoracotomy and bronchotomy are required for removal. Patients who aspirate massive amounts of particulate matter such as dirt or sand have an increased risk for obstruction from impacted material. Bronchoscopy is indicated in severe cases; however, postural drainage with percussion has been demonstrated to be of benefit when used in a controlled setting.

Long-term complications from foreign body aspiration include bronchiectasis, hemoptysis, spontaneous perforation of the chest wall, abscess, emphysema, and pneumonia.

CLINICAL FEATURES

Aspiration of fluid and oropharyngeal bacteria can occur in healthy persons during sleep. Pathologic aspiration also can be silent and a high index of suspicion must be maintained in order to detect this problem. Signs of hypoxemia such as tachypnea, tachycardia, and cyanosis may develop immediately or may not be present for a number of hours. Auscultation of the chest may disclose wheezing, rales, or rhonchi, and the patient may produce large amounts of frothy, bloody sputum.

Blood gas abnormalities include marked hypoxia with respiratory alkalosis. Severe aspiration may result in respiratory failure with a combined respiratory and metabolic acidosis.

Hypotension and hypovolemic shock may develop rapidly owing to the outpouring of fluid into the alveolar spaces. Although the clinical picture may resemble pulmonary edema, left ventricular function remains normal and hemodynamic monitoring usually reveals a high cardiac index with normal to low right-sided pressures.

The chest roentgenogram may show a diffuse alveolar and interstitial infiltrate or a segmental or lobar infiltrate. The lower lobe of the right lung is most frequently involved because the right mainstem bronchus courses more directly toward the right lower lobe. If the patient is in the Trendelenburg position, the infiltrates tend to involve the axillary segment of the right upper lobe and the apical segment of the right lower lobe.

Patients with chronic aspiration may have repeated bouts of pneumonia, especially involving the right lower lobe or the axillary segment of the right upper lobe.

COMPLICATIONS

While acute respiratory failure is the most serious complication of acute pulmonary aspiration, chronic sequelae include pulmonary fibrosis, lung abscess, and empyema. The mortality due to this problem ranges from 40 to 70 percent for aspiration of fluids with a pH less than 2.5 and is higher for fluids with a pH less than 1.8. Patients who aspirate material which is grossly contaminated, as in bowel obstruction, have a mortality approaching 100 percent.

Lung Abscess

A lung abscess is a cavitation in the pulmonary parenchyma that develops as a result of local suppuration with central necrosis, usually after the aspiration of oropharyngeal secretions. As with other forms of pneumonitis, factors that suppress the cough or gag reflexes, such as anesthesia, tooth extraction, esophageal motility disorders, strictures, or carcinoma, predispose to aspiration. Other pulmonary disorders that may lead to lung abscess formation include pneumonia, pulmonary embolism with cystic infarction, septic emboli, vasculitis, and infected cysts. The presence of peridontal disease plays an important role in the formation of anaerobic lung abscess by increasing the inoculum of organisms available for aspiration. Lung abscess is rare in edentulous people.

The flora in a lung abscess secondary to aspiration are usually polymicrobial, with as many as 60 percent exclusively anaerobes and the rest a mixture of both aerobes and anaerobes. The anaerobes include microaerophilic and anaerobic streptococci, *Fusobacterium*, and *Bacteroides*. Aerobic organisms such as *Staphylococcus aureus, Pseudomonas,* alpha streptococci, *Streptococcus pneumoniae, Proteus, Escherichia coli,* and *Klebsiella pneumoniae* can cause a severe necrotic pneumonitis with abscess formation. *Mycobacterium, Histoplasma, Coccidioides,* lung flukes, and *Entamoeba* can also present with abscess formation.

In patients with pulmonary aspiration, cavitation usually develops 1 or 2 weeks after the aspiration. Clinical illness is usually insidious but may present as an acute pneumonitis. Presenting signs and symptoms include a cough productive of a fetid and bloody sputum, fever, chest pain, shortness of breath, weakness, and weight loss. Oral examination usually reveals gingivitis and poor dentition. Signs of localized consolidation or cavitation may be present on pulmonary auscultation. Clubbing is rarely seen. Complete blood count usually reveals a leukocytosis with a left shift and anemia.

Diagnosis is confirmed by chest roentgenogram that demonstrates the cavity (Fig. 31-1). An air-fluid level is generally present. The most common sites for aspiration-induced abscesses are the posterior segment of the right upper lobe and the superior segments of the right and left lower lobes. A lung abscess that develops secondary to pulmonary parenchymal disease, carcinoma, opportunistic infection, or septicemia may occur anywhere in the lung.

Occasionally it may be difficult to distinguish a lung abscess from empyema on the chest roentgenogram. Schachter et al. suggest several signs that favor the diagnosis of empyema over lung abscess. These include (1) the development of an air-fluid level at the site of a previous pleural effusion, (2) a cavity with an air-fluid level that tapers at the pleural border, (3) an air-fluid level that crosses a fissure, and (4) an air-fluid level that extends to the lateral chest wall.

Sputum Gram stains are of some value in the diagnosis of aerobic infection. However, only transtracheal or transthoracic aspiration are reliable for anaerobic culture, since expectorated sputum is always contaminated with oral anaerobes. Pleural effusions are occasionally a source of positive cultures and should be cultured both aerobically and anaerobically. In patients with septic emboli, blood cultures are frequently positive.

Hemoptysis

Hemoptysis, although usually not life-threatening, may be of concern because of the risk of airway obstruction, which initially is more life-threatening than hemorrhagic shock. Mattox defines massive hemoptysis as the expectoration of 200 mL of blood per cough, 400 mL of blood per 24 h, or hemoptysis requiring transfusion to maintain a stable hematocrit. Certain radiologic signs described by Thoms et al. are useful in identifying actual or impending hemoptysis: (1) emptying and refilling of the abscess cavity on serial firms, (2) variations in the lucency and height of the air-fluid level, and (3) variable parenchymal densities representing blood clots within the cavity. Other complications include chronic lung abscess, empyema, brain abscess, and bronchopleural fistula.

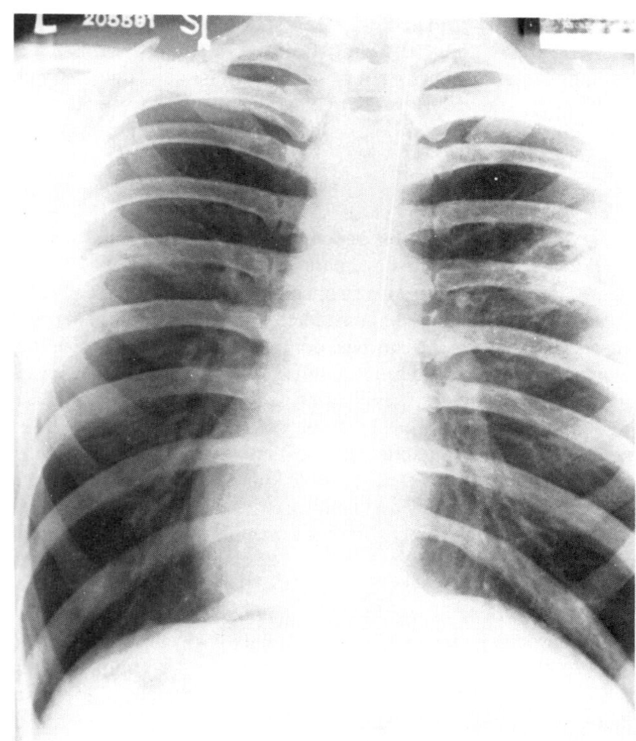

Fig. 31-1. Lung abscess in the superior segment of the right lower lobe.

Empyema

Empyema is the collection of purulent material in the pleural space or its loculation between fissures. It generally develops secondary to hematogenous or lymphatic spread from pneumonia, or by direct extension or rupture of a lung abscess into the pleural space. Other causes of empyema include esophageal perforation and mediastinitis; rupture of a mediastinal lymph node; direct extension from vertebral osteomyelitis, retropharyngeal or subdiaphragmatic abscesses; or infection as a complication of needle aspiration, thoracostomy tubes, or thoracotomy. The common causative organisms are *Staphylococcus,* gram-negative, and anaerobic organisms.

Presenting signs and symptoms are fever and chills, pleuritic chest pain, and shortness of breath. Weight loss, fatigue, and clubbing of fingers may be present with chronic disease. On examination, dullness to percussion, decreased breath sounds, and diminished excursion of the affected hemothorax are evident.

The chest roentgenogram demonstrates an air-fluid level in the pleural space, or evidence of loculated fluid. The radiologic distinctions between empyema and lung abscess were discussed earlier. Diagnosis is made by thoracentesis with aspiration of purulent material.

Complications of empyema include empyema necessitans, bronchopleural fistula, or permanent loss of parenchyma. Empyema necessitans is an encapsulated empyema that dissects into the subcutaneous tissues or through the chest wall.

An empyema may rupture into the bronchus, spreading infections throughout the tracheobronchial tree or causing airway obstruction. In chronic empyema or fibrothorax, restrictive lung disease may result.

TREATMENT

The prevention of aspiration pneumonia is the most important consideration in the management of patients at risk. This is accomplished by particular attention to airway management. Nasotracheal or orotracheal intubation should be considered in any patient with depressed or absent gag reflexes. This is best done in adults with a high-volume, low-pressure cuffed endotracheal tube. In children and newborns, a noncuffed tube provides adequate protection in most cases. Gastric lavage is performed cautiously in the comatose or obtunded patient. Preventive measures include placing patients in the Trendelenburg position on their left sides if possible, with endotracheal intubation before lavage. The presence of a nasogastric tube does not ensure that a patient's stomach is empty. The tube may not be positioned properly to completely evacuate the stomach, or large particles may be present that cannot be removed by the nasogastric tube. Patients with an esophageal obturator airway in place must always have their airway protected prior to removal as vomiting usually occurs in this setting.

The use of nonparticulate antacids such as 0.3M sodium citrate has been shown to reduce morbidity and mortality if the pH of the gastric contents is reduced to below 2.5 and the gastric volume to below 0.4 mL/kg before aspiration occurs. Recently, H_2 receptor blockers such as cimetidine have been demonstrated to raise the pH of gastric contents acutely in trauma patients and may play a role in the prevention of pulmonary injury. Drugs which hasten gastric emptying such as metoclopramide may also be of value.

If pulmonary aspiration is observed, the trachea should be immediately suctioned and a sample of the aspirate checked for pH. Even in the best of circumstances, however, endotracheal suctioning cannot be expected to remove all of the aspirate.

Bronchoscopy is indicated for removal of large particles and for further clearing of the large airways. Irrigation of the tracheobronchial tree with large volumes of neutral or alkaline solution appears to have no beneficial effect and is harmful, since it may force the aspirate deeper into the terminal airways, increasing the extent of injury. Small amounts of saline may be used to clear the airway, but large volumes should be avoided.

Oxygen should always be administered. Endotracheal intubation and mechanical ventilation are indicated for hypercarbia or in the management of severe hypoxemia that cannot be corrected with oxygen by nasal cannula or face mask. Continuous positive airway pressure or positive end-expiratory pressure (PEEP) is indicated if adequate oxygenation cannot be accomplished by the above means. Both increase functional residual capacity and diminish atelectasis and interstitial edema, resulting in a reduction of ventilation and perfusion inequality. In addition, Cameron and others have shown that PEEP decreases mortality if it is begun within 6 h after aspiration.

Fluid loss into the interstitium and alveoli should be compensated for by adequate volume replacement, generally with crystalloid solution. Despite the clinical finding of wet pulmonary rales, cardiogenic pulmonary edema is usually not present in uncomplicated aspiration pneumonia. Fluid replacement should be guided by changes in central venous pressure, by urine output, and by frequent monitoring of the pulse and blood pressure. If cardiac failure is suspected, it may be necessary to monitor the pulmonary capillary wedge pressure in order to administer fluids safely and effectively.

Steroids and prophylactic antibiotics are of no value and should not be used. The patient should be monitored closely and antibiotics instituted when there is clinical evidence of infection. An antibiotic is chosen that is effective against the most likely organisms, namely selected aerobes and anaerobes. This selection is further guided by sputum culture when possible.

Follow-up supportive care includes appropriate chest physical therapy, humidification and oxygenation, and bronchodilators to treat bronchospasm.

Penicillin remains the drug of choice for uncomplicated lung abscess. Generally, aqueous penicillin G is given 6–12 million units/day until clinical improvement occurs, followed by oral penicillin V-K 500–750 mg every 6 h for up to 6 weeks. Metronidazole 500 mg every 6 h PO may be added to penicillin to cover penicillin-resistant organisms. In patients with penicillin allergy, clindamycin (600 mg q 6 h IV then 300 mg every 6 h) or chloramphenicol 500 mg every 4 h (IV or PO) or cefoxitin 1–2 gm every 4 h IV are suitable alternatives. Antibiotic therapy for hospital-acquired lung abscess is guided by culture results or gram stain. Elective bronchoscopy is valuable to evaluate the presence of a tumor or foreign body, to obtain material for culture, and to facilitate drainage. Surgery is indicated for life-threatening hemoptysis, tumor, and, rarely, a residual cavity.

Patients with life-threatening hemoptysis should be placed in Trendelenburg's position, vigorously suctioned, and oxygenated. If the side of the bleeding is known, the patient should be placed with that side down. Fluid and blood must be rapidly replaced as well, and immediate consultation for bronchoscopy must be obtained, generally from a thoracic surgeon. Bronchoscopy can aid in localizing the bleeding site, can provide a route for suctioning, and the rigid bronchoscope can be used to maintain the airway. By use of a bronchoscope, the patient can be intubated with a double-lumen endobronchial tube (Carlens, Robert Shaw, or White), or selective endobronchial intubation can be done. The bleeding mainstem bronchus can then be occluded, which ensures a patent airway through the other mainstem bronchus. Both bronchoscopy and endobronchial intubation should be attempted only by trained, experienced individuals.

Empyema requires appropriate intravenous antibiotic therapy combined with tube thoracostomy with closed drainage, or by open drainage and decortication for resolution.

BIBLIOGRAPHY

Bartlett JG, Finegold SM: Anaerobic infections of the lung and pleural space. *Am Rev Respir Dis* 110:56, 1974.

Bynum LJ, Pierce AK: Pulmonary aspiration of gastric contents. *Am Rev Respir Dis* 114:1129, 1976.

Cameron JL, Mitchell WH, Zuidema GD: Aspiration penumonia: Clinical outcome following documented aspiration. *Arch Surg* 106:49, 1973.

Goitein KJ, Rein AJ-JT, Gornstein A: Incidence of aspiration in endotracheally intubated infants and children. *Crit Care Med* 12,1:19, 1984.

Gregory GA, Gooding CA, Phibbs RH, et al: Meconium aspiration in infants: A prospective study. *J Pediatr* 85:848, 1974.

Johanson WG, Harris GD: Aspiration pneumonia, anaerobic infections, and lung abscess. *Med Clin North Am* 64,3:385, 1980.

Katz S: Primary lung abscess, in *Conn's current therapy*, Rakel RE (ed). WB Saunders, p 163, 1990.

Lorber B, Swenson RM: Bacteriology of aspiration pneumonia: A prospective study of community and hospital acquired cases. *Ann Intern Med* 81:329, 1974.

Mattox KL: Hemoptysis, in Schwartz G: *Principles and Practice of Emergency Medicine*, Safar P et al (eds). Philadelphia, WB Saunders, p 547, 1978.

Mendelson CL: The aspiration of stomach contents into the lungs during obstetric anesthesia. *Am J Obstet Gynecol* 52:191, 1946.

Robertson C: A review of the use of corticosteroids in the management of pulmonary injuries and insults. *Arch Emerg Med* 2,2:59, 1985.

Schachter EN, Kreisman H, Putman C: Diagnostic problems in suppurative lung disease. *Arch Intern Med* 136:167, 1976.

Solanki DR, Suresh M, Ethridge HC: The effects of intravenous cimetidine and metoclopramide on gastric volume and pH. *Anesth Analg* 63:599, 1984.

Strain JD, Moore EE, Markovchick VJ: Cimetidine for the prophylaxis of potential gastric acid aspiration pneumonitis in trauma patients. *J Trauma* 21,1:49, 1981.

Thoms NW, Puro HE, Arbula A: The significance of hemoptysis in lung abscess. *J Thorac Cardiovasc Surg* 59:617, 1970.

32 TUBERCULOSIS

K. P. Ravikrishnan

Despite the great strides in the treatment of tuberculosis with successful drug regimens since the 1950s, it still looms as a major worldwide health problem. The goal of completely stamping out tuberculosis by the turn of this century now appears to be a formidable task. Even in the developed countries, the increase in the incidence of tuberculosis is real and is likely to continue throughout the 1990s. Due to the impact of acquired immunodeficiency syndrome (AIDS), tuberculosis has become a major problem in many third world countries. A significant increase in international travel and the influx of new cases to developed countries has resulted in a new twist in the epidemiology of tuberculosis in the United States. In some cities, up to 30 to 40 percent of cases occur among the immigrant population.

In the United States, increased awareness of tuberculosis is a prerequisite for effective case finding and management. Emergency physicians and emergency department staff should be familiar with the incidence of tuberculosis in their communities and with the AIDS population. They must also know the typical clinical presentations of tuberculosis, as well as emergency department and local health department policies and procedures for isolation, treatment, and follow-up care. Early isolation of cases is helped by maintaining a high index of suspicion for patients in one of the six population subsets that have a disproportionately high prevalence of tuberculosis (Table 32-1).

PATHOPHYSIOLOGY

Tuberculosis, which has infected both humans and animals since antiquity, is the clinical illness caused by species of *Mycobacterium* and characterized by the formation of *tubercles*. Known by many other names historically, such as phthisis, galloping consumption, and white plague, tuberculosis was rampant in the late nineteenth and early twentieth centuries.

Mycobacteria are a family of widely distributed organisms characterized by acid-fast staining properties and slow growth. They are aerobic, non-spore-forming, nonmotile bacilli which commonly cause a granulomatous infection. Members of the mycobacteria family with varying in vitro properties cause a spectrum of clinical illness in the susceptible host (Table 32-2). In immunocompromised patients, tubercle bacilli cause a massive systemic infection. With the increasing incidence of HIV infection and AIDS, there has been an alteration in the rate of infection and in the postinfectious manifestation of tuberculosis. A classic example of this new phenomenon is the rampant infection and bacteremia caused by *Mycobacterium avium-intracellulare* (*M. avium*) in AIDS patients.

Table 32-1. Population Subsets with a High Prevalence of Tuberculosis

1. Homeless
2. Alcoholics
3. AIDS and HIV-positive patients
4. Drug addicts
5. Immigrants
6. Elderly and nursing home population

PATHOGENESIS

Tuberculosis is transmitted from person to person by an aerosol of organisms suspended in tiny droplets. The thin, watery spray may contain millions of bacteria. The number of organisms inhaled by a susceptible host is the determining factor in transmission of the disease. Cavitary and laryngeal tuberculosis, with their high number of organisms, are extremely infectious forms. Members of the same household as an index case, schoolmates, fellow employees, and anyone who has recurrent contact with an infected person are susceptible to the droplet infection of tuberculosis.

Initial Infection

A sizable number of airborne organisms are required to cause the initial infection. Upper airway defense mechanisms intercept many of these droplets. Once settled in the peripheral airways, tuberculosis bacilli multiply slowly over a period of 2 to 3 weeks. A mild inflammatory reaction with an asymptomatic infection occurs in a majority of patients. Regional lymphatic spread and concomitant hematogenous spread are part of the initial infection. Hematogenous spread takes the organisms to places of high vascularity. Because the tubercle bacillus requires high oxygen tension for survival, lung zones with high oxygen tension, especially the apical and posterior segments of the upper lobes, and the superior segments of the lower lobes, are sites of initial spread. Other favored locations are the renal cortex, the meninges, the pericardium, the vertebral column, and the epiphysis of long bones. As the infection spreads, immunologic events with T-cell participation result in granuloma formation. Organisms are surrounded by a tubercle consisting of macrophages, histiocytes, and giant cells. The resulting granulomatous fibrous scar kills many of the organisms. Initial infection is thwarted and the prevailing host immunity prevents subsequent tuberculous disease.

Host immunity is manifested by a hypersensitivity to the tuberculin skin test [purified protein derivative (PPD) test], which is the marker of initial infection. The host immunity lasts as long as the number and quality of sensitized T-cells are preserved. Eventually, all that remains from the original infection is a calcific focus in the lung with a calcified regional lymph node. This is known as the Ghon complex. At times,

Table 32-2. Tuberculosis and Common Mycobacteria

Organisms	In Vitro Characteristics	Comments
Mycobacterium tuberculosis	Niacin positive, nonpigmented, 3–6 weeks' growth in culture	Cause of pulmonary and extrapulmonary TB
M. bovis	Niacin negative, nonpigmented	Cause of intestinal TB; from use of nonpasteurized milk
Bacillus Calmette-Guérin (BCG)	Niacin negative, nonpigmented	Used for BCG vaccination; at times, virulent in immunocompromised host
M. avium	Niacin negative, nonpigmented, 3 weeks' growth	Common with HIV infection; can cause chronic illness in elderly patients
M. kansasii	Niacin negative, pigmented colonies	Cause of pulmonary cavitary disease in patients with chronic pulmonary illness
Rapid growers *M. gordonae* *M. fortuitum*	Niacin negative, nonpigmented, 1 week growth	Not usually pathogenic; at times capable of causing massive infection in immunocompromised patients

minimal apical calcification and small calcified foci in all the hematogenously seeded areas, called Simon foci, also result.

CLINICAL MANIFESTATIONS

The majority of infected patients do not develop any sequelae. Reactivation of tuberculosis results from an imbalance between the host immunity and the pathogen. Areas with a large bacterial population, like the lungs, are sites of reactivation resulting in intense inflammatory process, cavitation, and necrosis. The host immunity continues to participate with systemic reactions of fever, weight loss, and an accelerated local inflammatory process. The hallmark of tuberculous infection, the *tubercle,* is characterized by a caseating granuloma surrounded by histiocytes and giant cells containing the engulfed tubercle bacillus.

Primary Tuberculosis

Primary tuberculosis occurs following the initial infection. In over 90 percent of cases it is not associated with a clinical illness. The primary lesion is subpleural and is associated with regional hilar lymph node involvement. The PPD skin test is positive. In a few patients with primary tuberculosis, the disease is characterized by a consolidative process in the lung, similar to common pneumonia. Associated pleural effusion and hilar and mediastinal adenopathy may be seen (Figs. 32-1 and 32-2).

Reactivation Tuberculosis

This is the most common form of tuberculosis seen clinically. In over 90 percent of patients, pulmonary involvement is noted. The disease manifests as a chronic illness with symptoms of fever, malaise, and weight loss, associated with pulmonary symptoms of cough, sputum production, and at times hemoptysis. Chest x-ray shows the characteristic involvement of the apical and posterior segments of the upper lobes (Fig. 32-3). Atypical x-ray presentations are seen in 5 to 7 percent

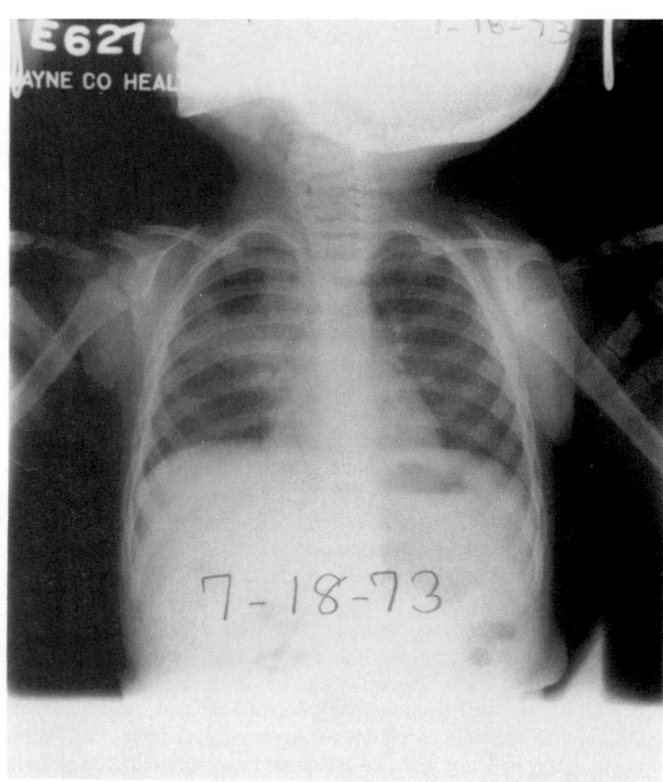

Fig. 32-2. Right upper lobe consolidation with hilar and paratracheal adenopathy due to primary tuberculosis.

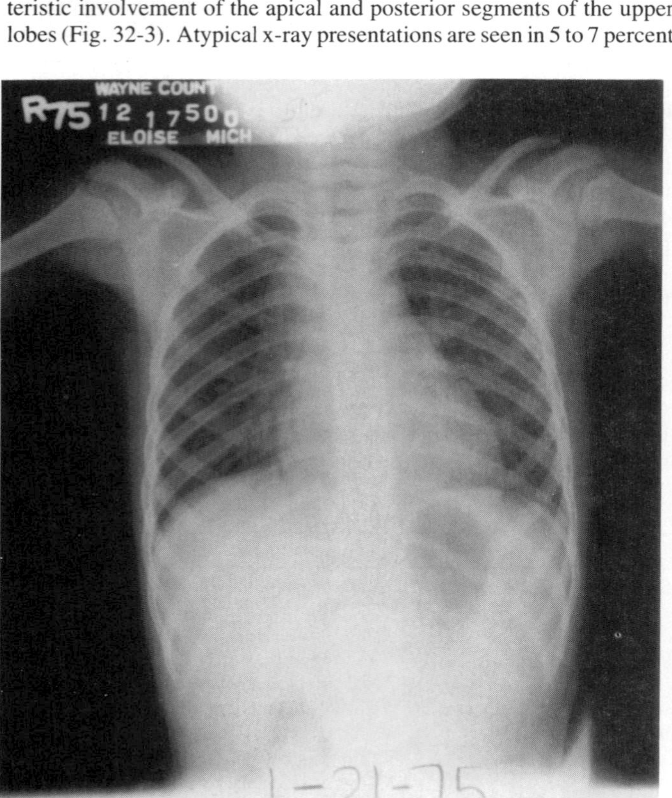

Fig. 32-1. Right paratracheal adenopathy due to primary tuberculous infection in a child.

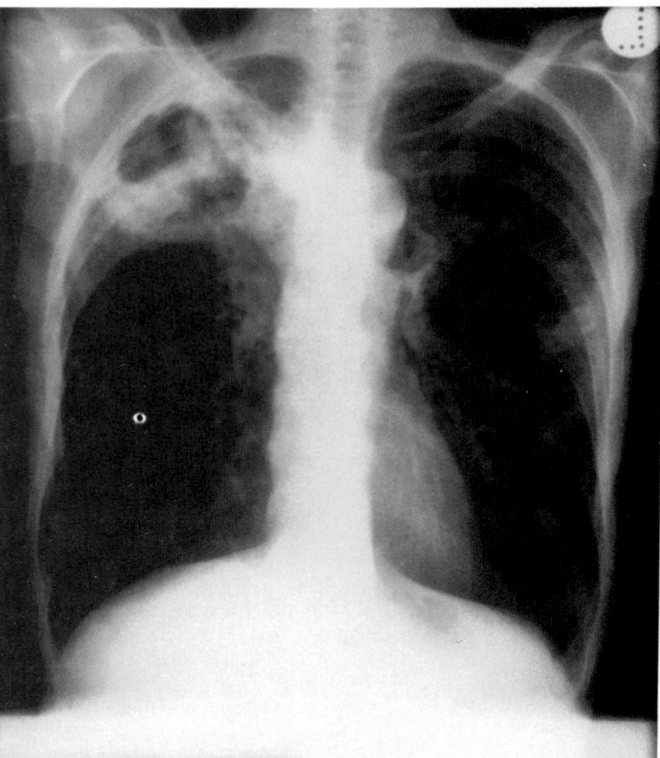

Fig. 32-3. Classic cavitary disease in the upper lobe due to reactivated tuberculosis. Left mid-lung abnormality due to endobronchial spread.

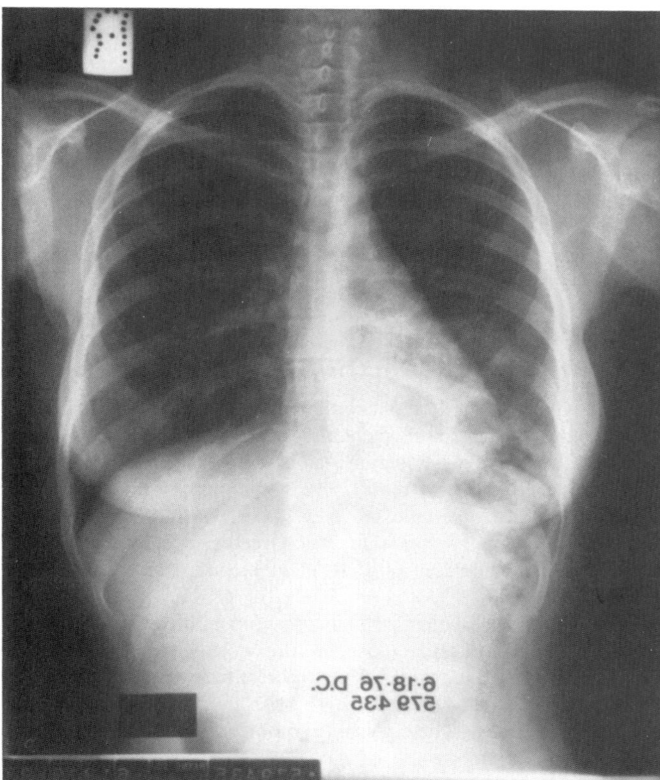

Fig. 32-4. Cavitary disease in the left lower lobe—an atypical manifestation of reactivated tuberculosis.

of cases (Fig. 32-4). In 80 percent of cases, the PPD skin test is positive. Anergy is a manifestation of advanced disease in debilitated and malnourished patients. Culture of acid-fast bacilli with the characteristics of M. tuberculosis from the respiratory secretions is the gold standard for diagnosis. Specimens from gastric fluid, bronchial washings, bronchoalveolar lavage, and bronchial and lung biopsy are sometimes necessary for definitive diagnosis. Fluorescent staining and Ziehl-Neelsen acid-fast staining remain the standard techniques for early identification of tubercle bacillus in the sputum.

Excellent response to combination chemotherapy is the rule. In advanced cases, pulmonary and systemic complications occur as initial manifestations or during the course of the disease. Pulmonary complications result in morbidity and mortality in 10 to 15 percent of cases (Table 32-3).

Tuberculous Pleural Effusion

Tuberculous pleurisy is usually a manifestation of primary tuberculosis. In massive fibrocaseous tuberculosis and in the presence of a bronchopleural fistula, pleural effusion is also seen in the reactivated form of tuberculosis. Tuberculous pleurisy is thought to be a hypersensitivity phenomenon, and the majority of patients (80 to 90 percent) exhibit a positive reaction to the PPD skin test. It should be assumed that a lymphocytic pleural exudate in a patient with a positive tuberculin skin test is due to tuberculosis, unless proved otherwise.

Table 32-3. Complications of Tuberculosis

1. Massive infection
2. Acute respiratory failure
3. Chronic respiratory failure
4. Miliary TB
5. Bronchopleural fistula
6. Hemoptysis
7. Extrapulmonary TB
   a. TB meningitis
   b. TB pericarditis
   c. TB peritonitis
   d. TB arthritis

Patients with tuberculous pleural effusion present with pleuritic chest pain, cough with minimal sputum production, and low-grade fever. The chest radiograph will show a varying amount of pleural fluid. The pleural fluid is characteristically exudative in nature, with absolute elevation of protein and LDH, and elevation of the pleural-fluid-to-serum ratio of protein and LDH. A low glucose level and a decrease in pleural fluid pH are also characteristics of tuberculous pleurisy. Early pleural effusions are characterized by polymorphonuclear leukocytosis, while more chronic effusions are predominantly lymphocytic. Acid-fast smears are often negative because of the hypersensitive nature of the effusion and the small number of organisms present. A pleural biopsy will often show the characteristic tubercle.

Cases of tuberculous pleural effusion should be treated for 6 to 9 months with two antituberculous medications (see Table 32-6). Response to drug therapy is excellent.

Extrapulmonary Tuberculosis

Extrapulmonary tuberculosis is due to a disseminated form of the infection which results in tuberculous meningitis, pericarditis, peritonitis, or skeletal tuberculosis and is associated with high morbidity and mortality.

Despite the overall decrease in cases of tuberculosis, the incidence of extrapulmonary tuberculosis remains very high. Nonpulmonary manifestations, alone or in combinations with pulmonary involvement, occur in 10 to 20 percent of patients. Common extrapulmonary sites of involvement are pleura, lymph nodes, bones (Fig. 32-5), GI tract,

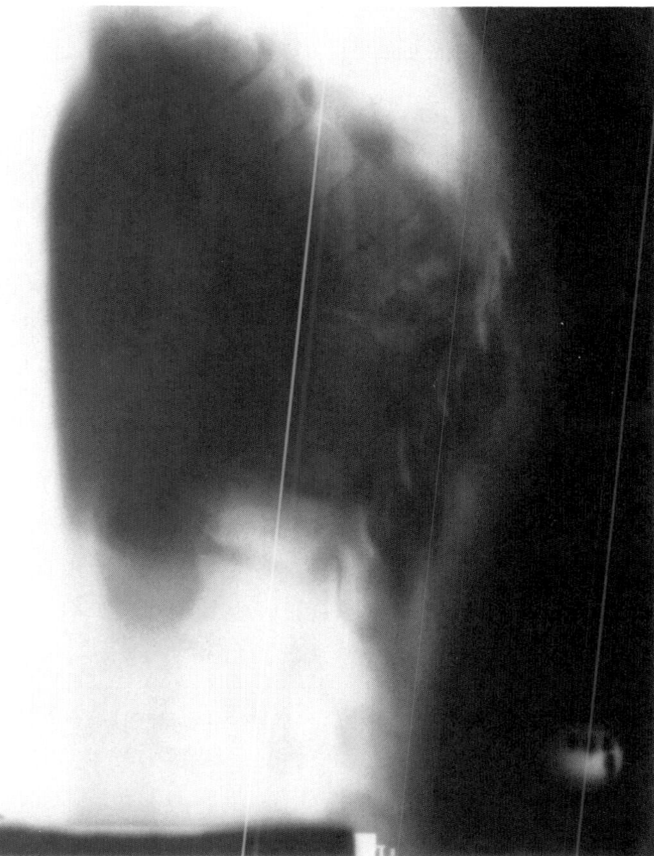

Fig. 32-5. Extensive spinal involvement from extrapulmonary tuberculosis.

GU tract, meninges, and pericardium. Nonspecific, nonpulmonary manifestations in cases of extrapulmonary tuberculosis often lead to misdiagnosis and delay in treatment.

Miliary Tuberculosis

Once common, this acute hematogenous form of tuberculosis, with its high morbidity and mortality, is now rare. The characteristic clinical and radiographic picture has given miliary tuberculosis a special place in the annals of clinical medicine. Manifestations of multisystem involvement, with meningitis, pericarditis, and peritonitis, in the presence of fever and acute and chronic illness should alert the clinician to the likelihood of miliary tuberculosis. Hepatomegaly, splenomegaly, pleuropericardial rub, arthralgia, arthritis, and generalized lymphadenopathy may be present. Anemia, thrombocytopenia, hypoxemia, hyponatremia, and, at times, a leukemoid reaction, with a chest x-ray showing miliary nodules 1 to 3 mm in size, are seen in classic cases (Fig. 32-6). Diagnostic confirmation may require bronchoscopy with biopsy, BAL, bone marrow aspiration, liver biopsy, or lymph node biopsy. Bronchoscopy with biopsy is successful in up to 70 percent of cases in establishing the diagnosis. Upon clinical diagnosis, a two-drug treatment regimen should be initiated promptly.

Tuberculosis in the Elderly

Thirty percent of all cases of tuberculosis occur in patients over the age of 65. Elderly patients are likely to develop a chronic, indolent form of tuberculosis with extrapulmonary, atypical manifestations that can delay diagnosis. Many epidemics resulting from unrecognized sporadic cases in the debilitated and elderly nursing home population have been reported. To prevent such epidemics, the health practitioner should maintain a high index of suspicion of tuberculosis when treating elderly patients with pneumonia and other chronic systemic illnesses.

Better epidemiologic studies, a diligent search for index cases, early diagnosis and treatment, and constant surveillance are necessary if the incidence of tuberculosis in the elderly and nursing home population is to be decreased.

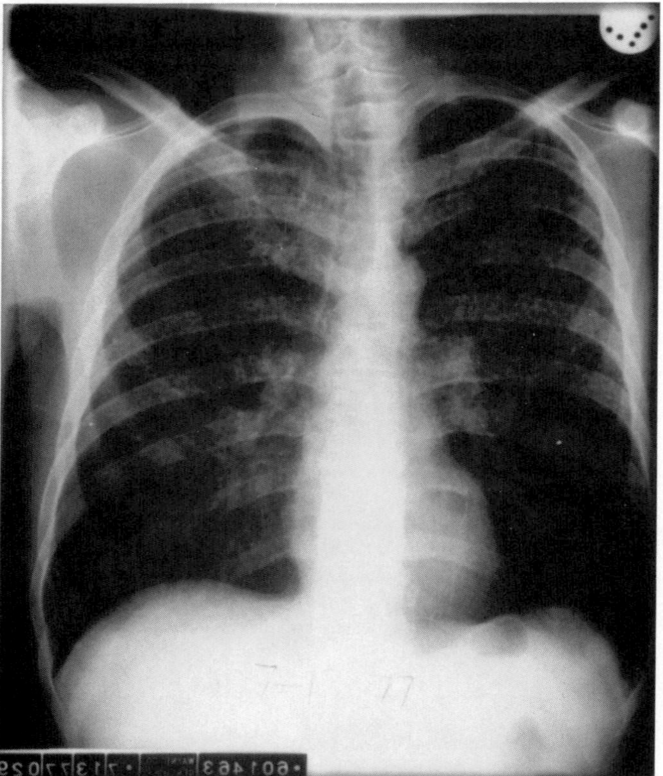

Fig. 32-6. Diffuse, fine, nodular pattern of miliary tuberculosis.

RADIOGRAPHIC FEATURES

Right upper lobe cavitation with parenchymal involvement is a classic finding for tuberculosis. In the reactivated form of tuberculosis, apical and posterior segments of the upper lobes of the lung are often involved. Common radiographic features of tuberculosis are listed in Table 32-4. The chest x-ray is useful in the initial diagnosis and in assessing response to treatment.

TUBERCULOSIS AND ACQUIRED IMMUNODEFICIENCY SYNDROME (AIDS)

With the advent of modern chemotherapy there came a steady 5 to 7 percent annual decline in the incidence of tuberculosis. In 1986, however, there was no decline, and in 1987 and 1988 there was an increase in the incidence. Most of these increases could be attributed to the impact of AIDS on tuberculosis. Over 10 percent of AIDS patients in the United States have concomitant tuberculosis, and Haitians with AIDS have a greater than 60 percent incidence of concomitant tuberculosis.

AIDS-related tuberculosis is a major epidemiologic problem impacting the control of tuberculosis in third-world countries and in the inner cities of the United States. The 36 percent increase in tuberculosis in New York City in 1986, the highest in the nation, was directly correlated with AIDS. The disturbing combination of tuberculosis and AIDS was noted among the Hispanic, Asian, and non-Asian black populations, and in intravenous drug abusers. HIV infection is also strongly correlated with tuberculosis. In Dade County, Florida, 31 percent of tuberculosis patients (71 patients) were HIV-positive.

Several factors account for the high incidence of tuberculosis in patients who are HIV-positive or have AIDS:

1. There is an increase in susceptibility to the initial infection in patients with AIDS and HIV infection.
2. The compromised immune systems of AIDS and HIV patients favor the rapid reactivation of tuberculosis.
3. Decreased T-cell function favors widespread dissemination of tuberculosis, leading to the development of extrapulmonary and miliary forms of tuberculosis.

Some of the differences between the usual features of tuberculosis and those found in AIDS-related tuberculosis are listed in Table 32-5. Tuberculosis in AIDS patients has responded to drug therapy in the usual fashion. However, there are no good control studies, and short-course chemotherapy, which is the state-of-the-art treatment for tuberculosis, has not been reliably tested in AIDS patients. The American Thoracic Society recommends the use of isoniazid, rifampin, and pyrazinamide for 2 months to be followed by isoniazid and rifampin for 9 months, or for 6 months after sputum conversion, whichever is longer. There is an increase in the incidence of drug reactions and drug intolerance in patients with AIDS-related tuberculosis.

Table 32-4. Radiographic Manifestations of Tuberculosis

1. Cavitation
2. Diffuse, patchy densities
3. Pleural effusion
4. Lymphadenopathy
5. Calcific or noncalcific granulomatous nodules
6. Miliary (1 to 3-mm) nodules
7. Pleuropulmonary changes due to:
   a. Thoracoplasty
   b. Plombage
   c. Pneumothorax treatment
8. Lower lobe cavity

Table 32-5. Characteristics of Tuberculosis and Aids-Related Tuberculosis

Features	Tuberculosis	Aids-Related TB
PPD skin test	Positive in up to 80% of cases	Variable
Location of infection	Upper lobes of lung; superior segments of lower lobe	Any segment of lung or diffuse lung involvement; extrapulmonary TB > 60% of the time
Treatment	Predictable good response to short-term treatment in over 90%	Good response early; unpredictable in massive late infection
Drug reaction	3–5%	Over 5%
Other mycobacterial infection	Rare	Combined infections common, e.g., *M. avium* infection

DRUG TREATMENT FOR TUBERCULOSIS

Combination chemotherapy has been extremely successful in treating tuberculosis. Table 32-6 lists commonly used drugs, dosages, and side effects. Two basic principles of treatment are

1. Effective treatment requires the initial concomitant administration of at least two drugs to which the patient's organisms are susceptible.
2. Cure of tuberculosis requires that treatment be continued for the full course beyond the time of sputum conversion and amelioration of symptoms.

National Consensus of Chemotherapy for Tuberculosis

1. A 9-month regimen of isoniazid and rifampin, at times supplemented during the initial phase by ethambutol, streptomycin, or pyrazinamide, should be standard therapy for tuberculosis in the United States and Canada.
2. Infants, children, and adolescents with tuberculosis should be treated with a 9-month regimen of isoniazid and rifampin.
3. When drug resistance is suspected, the initial use of at least three drugs is mandatory.
4. A 6-month regimen of therapy is acceptable if four drugs (isoniazid, rifampin, pyrazinamide, and streptomycin or ethambutol) are given for 2 months, followed by an additional 4 months of isoniazid and rifampin, with all drugs given under close supervision.
5. Immunosuppressed patients with tuberculosis should be treated with 9 to 12 months of isoniazid and rifampin, supplemented during the initial phase by ethambutol, streptomycin, or pyrazinamide.
6. Extrapulmonary tuberculosis should be treated as outlined above.

PREVENTION

Preventive therapy with isoniazid given for 6 to 12 months is effective in decreasing the risk of future tuberculosis. Persons for whom preventive therapy is indicated include:

Table 32-6. Common Drugs Used in the Treatment of Tuberculosis

Drugs	Daily Dosage	Side Effects
Isoniazid	5–10 mg/kg up to 300 mg PO or IM	Peripheral neuritis, hepatitis
Ethambutol	15–25 mg/kg PO	Optic neuritis
Rifampin	10–20 mg/kg up to 600 mg PO	Hepatitis, febrile reaction, purpura (rare)
Streptomycin	15–20 mg/kg up to 1 g IM	8th nerve damage, nephrotoxicity
Pyrazinamide	15–30 mg/kg up to 2 g PO	Hepatotoxicity, hyperuricemia

1. Household members and other close contacts of potentially infectious persons
2. Newly infected persons (recent conversion of tuberculin skin test within 2 years)
3. Persons in whom active tuberculosis has been excluded but who have a history of tuberculosis or a positive tuberculin reaction and an abnormal chest film
4. Persons with a positive PPD test in the following situations:
   - Silicosis
   - Diabetes mellitus
   - Corticosteroid therapy
   - Other immunosuppressive therapy
   - AIDS or positive tests for antibodies to HIV
   - Hematologic and reticuloendothelial malignancies
   - End-stage renal disease
   - Conditions associated with rapid weight loss or chronic malnutrition
5. People younger than 35 years with a positive tuberculin skin test

In persons younger than 35 years, routine monitoring for adverse effects of isoniazid should consist of a monthly clinical evaluation. For persons 35 and older, in addition to monthly evaluation, hepatic enzymes should be measured prior to starting isoniazid and periodically throughout treatment. As with treatment of tuberculosis, the key to success of preventive therapy is patient compliance.

BIBLIOGRAPHY

Alvarez S, McCabe WR: Extrapulmonary tuberculosis revisited: A review of experience at Boston City and other hospitals. *Medicine* 63:25, 1984.

American Thoracic Society. Treatment of tuberculosis (TB) and tuberculosis infection in adults and children. *Am Rev Respir Dis* 134:355, 1986.

Centers for Disease Control. Epidemiologic notes and reports: Tuberculosis, final data—United States, 1986. *MMWR* 36:817, 1988.

Centers for Disease Control. Perspectives in disease prevention and health promotion: A strategic plan for the elimination of tuberculosis in the United States. *MMWR* 38:269, 1989.

Centers for Disease Control. TB and AIDS—New York City. *MMWR* 36:785, 1987.

Dutt AK, Stead WW: Present chemotherapy for tuberculosis. *J Infect Dis* 146:698, 1982.

Dyer RA, Chappel WA, Potgieter PO: Adult respiratory distress syndrome associated with miliary tuberculosis. *Crit Care Med* 13:12, 1985.

Murray JF; The white plague: Down and out, or up and coming? J. Burns Amberson Lecture. *Am Rev Respir Dis* 140:1788, 1989.

Rieder HL, Snider DE Jr: Tuberculosis and the acquired immunodeficiency syndrome. *Chest* 90:469, 1986.

Welty C, Burstin S, Muspratt S, et al: Epidemiology of tuberculous infection in a chronic care population. *Am Rev Respir Dis* 132:133, 1985.

33
SPONTANEOUS AND IATROGENIC PNEUMOTHORAX

Kimberlydawn Wisdom

PNEUMOTHORAX

Collection of air in the pleural space causes malfunction of the thoracic pump, resulting in pulmonary and hemodynamic complications. Accumulation of air in the pleural space—*pneumothorax*—occurs in patients with or without underlying pulmonary disorders. The term *spontaneous pneumothorax* refers to the collection of air in the pleural space without any local trauma. Pneumothorax occurring spontaneously in young adults is due to the rupture of a subpleural bleb. Chest trauma or diagnostic or therapeutic procedures can also lead to pneumothorax or hemopneumothorax with resultant complications. The term *pulmonary barotrauma* is used to describe the complications resulting from increased airway pressures generated during ventilatory assistance, such as mediastinal and subcutaneous emphysema, and tension pneumothorax. Pneumothorax causes hypoxia, especially in the setting of obstructive airway disorders; immediate complications are due to the hemodynamic impact of a tension pneumothorax. Emergency thoracostomy is needed to correct the hemodynamic compromise of tension pneumothorax.

Spontaneous Pneumothorax

Spontaneous pneumothorax is more common in males than in females. The characteristic male is tall and 20 to 40 years old. Pneumothorax is generally due to the rupture of a pulmonary or subpleural bleb into the pleural space but may develop when excessive mechanical stress is placed upon a segment of weakened pleura. Leakage of air from the alveoli into the pleural space causes a rise in the intrapleural pressure, leading to pulmonary collapse. Spontaneous pneumothorax may occur in conjunction with pulmonary infection, such as staphylococcal pneumonia or tuberculosis, asthma or emphysema, pulmonary carcinoma, "honeycomb" lung disorders such as tuberous sclerosis or histiocytosis X, occupational pulmonary disease, sarcoidosis, postpulmonary irradiation, and Marfan's and Ehlers-Danlos syndromes. Rarely, cyclical pneumothorax may occur in young or middle-aged females. In such cases the development of "catamenial" pneumothorax is coincident with menstruation and may be related to the presence of pelvic, pleural, or diaphragmatic endometriosis. In 40 percent of patients no underlying pathology can be determined. Some patients may have recurrent episodes of spontaneous pneumothorax. In some cases there is a history of deep inspiration or hyperventilation, followed by the generation of excessive intrathoracic pressures such as can be induced by screaming, coughing, or the Valsalva maneuver (when smoking marijuana).

Clinical Features

The most common symptom of spontaneous pneumothorax is sudden sharp chest pain, which is often pleuritic in character. The pain is generally anterior but it may radiate to the neck or back. Dyspnea, tachycardia, and tachypnea may be present if the degree of pneumothorax compromises pulmonary function. There may be a cough, occasionally productive of blood-streaked sputum. Subcutaneous emphysema involving the neck and chest wall may be present if air has dissected through mediastinal structures. On physical examination there may be decreased breath sounds, hyperresonance to percussion on the side of the pneumothorax, and decreased tactile fremitus. However, in some patients, especially those with emphysema, the clinical findings may be subtle. In addition, the development of pneumothorax in this group is serious and can lead to respiratory failure. In every individual with chronic obstructive pulmonary disease, pneumothorax should always be suspected as a cause for clinical deterioration.

A chest roentgenogram is necessary to confirm the diagnosis. Pneumothorax is characterized by hyperlucency and a lack of lung markings at the periphery of the lung and by the appearance of a fine line that represents the retraction of the visceral from the parietal pleura.

If a suspected pneumothorax is not visible on an inspiratory film, it may be seen on an expiratory film, since the constant volume of the pneumothorax is more evident when the size of the hemithorax decreases with expiration. A lateral decubitus film with the patient lying on the affected side may be helpful for the same reason. Tomograms are also useful in assessing emphysematous lesions.

A small amount of pleural fluid, usually represented by blunting of the costophrenic angle, is generally present. Bullae or emphysematous blebs or pulmonary infiltration may be seen on the x-ray film.

Visual estimates of pneumothorax size are inaccurate. A technique for more accurate estimation of pneumothorax size based upon measurement of interpleural distances has been described, but has not found wide acceptance of application.

Pneumothorax must be differentiated from skin folds, outlines of tubing, artifacts on the chest wall such as clothing, and bullae or cysts. Bullae and cysts have concave inner margins and rounded edges.

Hypotension, cyanosis, and marked respiratory distress may develop if the degree of pneumothorax is large, if underlying pulmonary function is poor, or if tension pneumothorax has developed (Fig. 33-1). Tension pneumothorax is characterized by severe dyspnea, cyanosis, and hypotension. The chest will be hyperresonant on the side of the pneumothorax and the trachea and mediastinal structures will deviate to the opposite side. Deviation of the mediastinal structures results in kinking of the inferior vena cava and a marked decrease in venous return. Uncorrected tension pneumothorax rapidly leads to cardiorespiratory collapse. Chest x-ray is generally not necessary to make this diagnosis. Emergency thoracostomy is necessary, and procrastination to obtain a confirmatory chest x-ray can result in cardiac arrest in the patient.

Iatrogenic Pneumothorax

Iatrogenic pneumothorax can occur secondary to procedures such as cannulation of the subclavian vein, lung inflation at high pressures, intercostal nerve block, thoracentesis, percutaneous lung biopsy, and bronchoscopy. It is the most commonly described complication of subclavian vein catheterization and generally occurs if the angle of introduction of the needle is too sharp or if the tip of the needle is directed too deeply, nicking the parietal pleura and allowing air to accumulate in the pleural cavity. It can also occur if catheterization is attempted while the patient is moving or during chest compression in CPR. It may be more common in apical procedures, as opposed to procedures generally performed at the lung bases such as thoracentesis, because airflow is greater in the apices than the bases. Consequently, subclavian vein catheterization should be approached cautiously in patients with hyperventilation or Kussmaul respirations. Simple pneumothorax can lead to tension pneumothorax rapidly in such circumstances. Chest x-ray is routinely performed immediately after subclavian vein catheterization to detect immediate pneumothorax, but delayed pneumothorax could also develop.

Lung inflation at high pressures can also lead to pneumothorax. Mouth-to-mouth or bag-mask ventilation in infants and children or even in adults can lead to pneumothorax or pneumomediastinum if excess airway pressures are generated. Pneumothorax has resulted when an oxygen cannula is inserted directly into an endotracheal tube. Oxygen is delivered at high flow rates through the cannula into the tube, but because the cannula itself nearly fills the tube lumen, adequate expiration is not possible. Lung pressures build up until pneumothorax

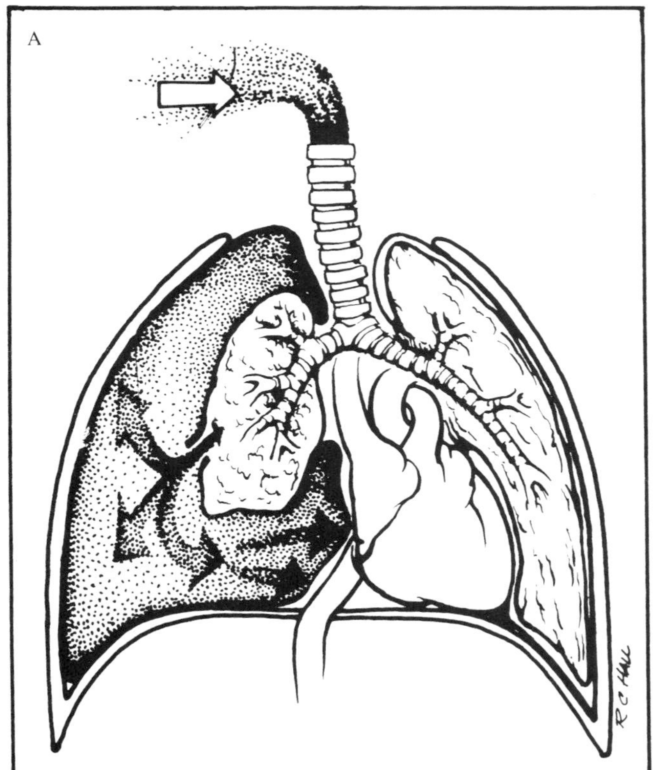

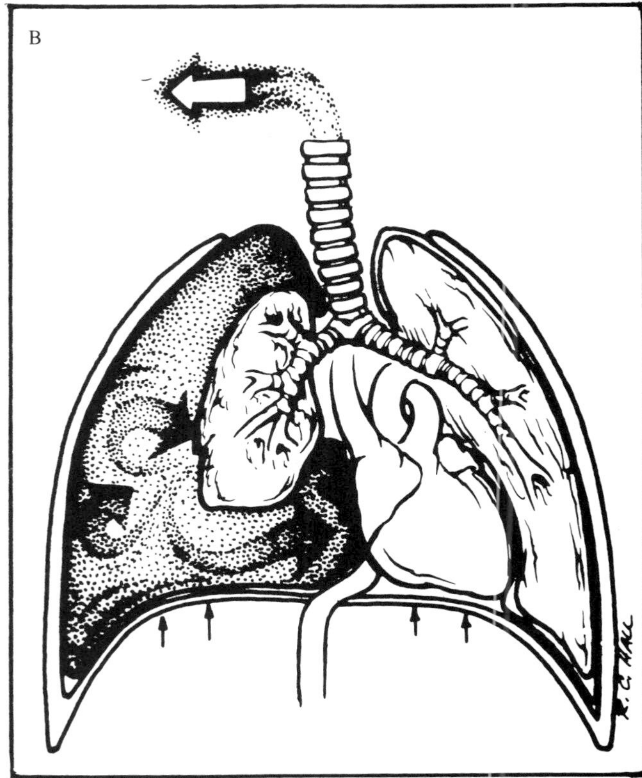

Fig. 33-1. A. Tension pneumothorax (inspiration). **B.** Tension pneumothorax (expiration).

results. The institution of mechanical ventilation or positive end-expiratory pressure can cause pneumothorax in patients with previous lung disease or can quickly lead to tension pneumothorax if there has been prior simple pneumothorax. In the latter case a thoracostomy tube is necessary before mechanical ventilation is begun.

In patients with recent subclavian vein catheterization or in those on mechanical ventilation, pneumothorax should be considered as a cause of cardiopulmonary deterioration. Intercostal nerve block for relief of pain from rib fractures or severe costochondritis should be followed by a chest x-ray to rule out iatrogenic pneumothorax.

Treatment

If the pneumothorax involves 20 percent or more of the hemithorax, tube thoracostomy with water-seal or vacuum drainage is generally performed. The technique of tube thoracostomy is discussed in Chapter 174, "Thoracic Trauma."

If the pneumothorax is under 20 percent, the decision for tube thoracostomy varies with the clinical situation, the patient's pulmonary reserve, and the treatment philosophy of the institution.

Simple catheter aspiration in pneumothorax has been described as an alternative method to tube thoracostomy in selected patients (Fig. 33-2). Two methods have been described: the nonsequential and the sequential.

In the *nonsequential* method a 14- to 16-gauge catheter is introduced into the pleural space at the level of the second or third interspace at the midclavicular line, and air is aspirated with a syringe using a three-way stopcock. Chest x-ray is repeated immediately after aspiration, and 6 h later is used to confirm success of the technique. Patients without evidence of pneumothorax after 6 h can be discharged with a follow-up scheduled at 24 or 48 h. Recurrence of pneumothorax at 6 h is variable, but tends to be more frequent with large pneumothoraces or with trauma.

The *sequential* method involves several steps. If the pneumothorax has not been successfully reexpanded after aspiration, a Heimlich flutter valve is attached to the catheter. If after 1 h reexpansion has been unsuccessful, then the catheter is connected to wall suction for 1 h. If a pneumothorax persists, tube thoracostomy is performed.

The catheter aspiration technique has been used successfully in patients with spontaneous pneumothorax who have no underlying pulmonary disease, have not been subject to trauma, have no hemo- or hydrothorax, who are not in any respiratory distress, and who have normal vital signs. Catheter aspiration can also be used in patients with recurrent spontaneous pneumothoraces in whom it is desirable to avoid tube thoracostomy. Admission is the practice for this latter group, especially if there is underlying pulmonary disease.

If tube thoracostomy or catheter aspiration is deferred, the patient must be frequently and carefully examined and serial chest x-ray films taken to detect the development of an increasing or tension pneumothorax. If the pneumothorax is increasing, if the patient is on mechanical ventilation, or if general anesthesia is contemplated, tube thoracostomy should be performed. If tension pneumothorax is evident, the pressure should be immediately relieved by insertion of a large-bore needle into the pleural space, followed by tube thoracostomy.

On occasion, rapid expansion of pneumothorax with excessive negative pressure may result in the development of unilateral or even bilateral pulmonary edema. This is more likely to occur if there is bronchial obstruction. It is postulated that the increase in pulmonary blood flow with rapid lung reexpansion can cause transudation of capillary fluid into the alveoli. With judicious fluid management and respiratory care this condition is self-limited.

Spontaneous Pneumothorax and AIDS

Spontaneous pneumothorax as a complication of pneumonia is rare, but when it occurs it is usually due to organisms such as *Staphylococcus aureus, Mycobacterium tuberculosis,* or *Klebsiella,* which cause necrotizing infections. Although pneumothorax associated with *Pneumocystis carinii* pneumonia (PCP) was described over 20 years ago in malnourished and immunosuppressed infants and more recently in

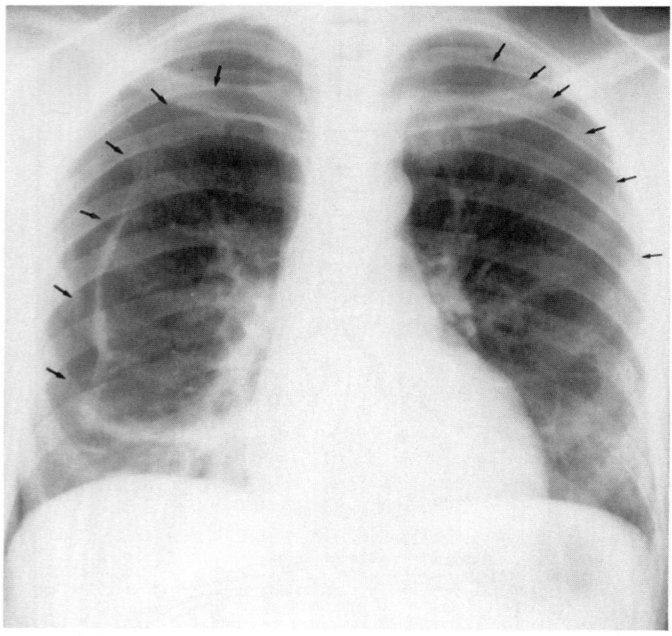

A

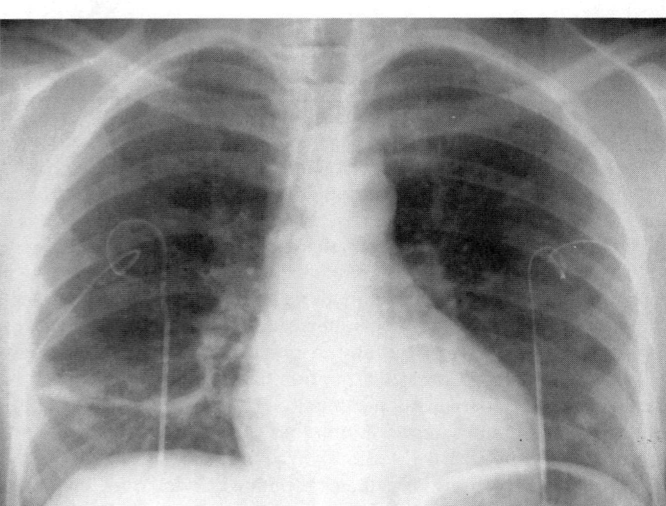

B

Fig. 33-2. Bilateral pneumothorax in an intravenous drug abuser. **A.** The catheter aspiration of the simple pneumothorax (CASP) technique was used. **B.** As shown, the catheters were successful in complete reexpansion of the lungs. (Courtesy Henry Ford Hospital.)

leukemics, it has been reported with increased frequency in the AIDS population.

The pathophysiology is not well understood. The literature reports the etiology of the pneumothorax as lymphocytic alveolar exudate, interstitial inflammation and subpleural necrosis, and cavitation with subsequent development of a bronchopleural fistula. These pathologic findings may progress to fibrosis, which predisposes the patient to pneumothorax. Usually, pneumothorax occurs with concurrent infection.

Recurrence is characteristic of pneumothorax associated with PCP. Eng and associates reported one patient who had seven separate episodes. Patients with bilateral pneumothorax have also been reported.

Management of the small asymptomatic pneumothorax is observation. The symptomatic patient should be managed with tube thoracostomy unless there are persistent or large air leaks, in which case thoracotomy, stapling of blebs, and pleurodesis may be indicated. Decisions regarding surgical intervention should be made on an individual basis.

Pneumothorax must be ruled out in an AIDS patient with prior or active PCP who presents with respiratory deterioration, and an AIDS patient who presents with a pneumothorax should be evaluated for active PCP.

BIBLIOGRAPHY

Beers MF, Sohn M, Swartz M: Recurrent pneumothorax in AIDS patients with pneumocystis pneumonia: A clinicopathologic report of three cases and review of the literature. *Chest* 98:266, 1990.

Childress ME, May G, Mottram M: Unilateral pulmonary edema resulting from treatment of spontaneous pneumothorax. *Am Rev Respir Dis* 104:119, 1974.

Eng RH, Bishburg E, Smith SM. Evidence for destruction of lung tissues during pneumocystis carinii infection. *Arch Intern Med* 147:746, 1987.

Greene RG, McCloud TC, Stark P: Pneumothorax. *Semin Roentgenol* 12:313, 1977.

Jones JS: A place for aspiration in the treatment of spontaneous pneumothorax. *Thorax* 40:66, 1985.

Obeid FN, Shapiro MJ, Richardson HH, et al: Catheter aspiration for simple pneumothorax (CASP) in the outpatient management of simple traumatic pneumothorax. *J Trauma* 25:882, 1985.

Rhea JT, DeLuca SA, Greene RE: Determining the size of pneumothorax in the upright patient. *Radiology* 144:733, 1982.

Vallee P, Sullivan M, Richardson HH, Bivins B, Tomlanovich M: Sequential treatment of a simple pneumothorax. *Ann Emerg Med* 17:936, 1988.

Wisdom K, Nowak RM, Richardson HR, Martin GB, Obeid FN, Tomlanovich MC: Alternate therapy for traumatic pneumothorax in ''pocket shooters.'' *Ann Emerg Med* 15:428, 1986.

34 PERMEABILITY PULMONARY EDEMA AND THE ADULT RESPIRATORY DISTRESS SYNDROME

Marilyn T. Haupt
Richard W. Carlson

INTRODUCTION

Permeability pulmonary edema is a distinct form of edema which is frequently fulminant and leads to severe hypoxemia, intrapulmonary shunting, reduced lung compliance, and, in some cases, irreversible parenchymal lung damage. When these features develop, they are usually termed the "adult respiratory distress syndrome" (ARDS). This syndrome may be associated with a variety of diseases and injuries and it is not clear if the mechanisms of lung injury are similar for each disorder.

Permeability edema differs from the more commonly encountered "cardiac," "high-pressure," or "hemodynamic" edema with respect to the characteristics of the volume and the composition of the fluid which escapes the pulmonary microcirculation, as well as a rapidly expanding list of the associated conditions that precipitate edema (Table 34-1). In turn, the therapeutic approach for permeability edema differs from the approach for high-pressure edema.

PATHOPHYSIOLOGY

The Starling equation quantitates fluid movement across the pulmonary microvascular (capillary) membrane in relation to the microvascular and perimicrovascular hydrostatic and oncotic forces:

$$\dot{Q}_f = K_f\,[(P_{mv} - P_{pmv}) - \delta(\pi_{mv} - \pi_{pmv})]$$

in which $\dot{Q}_f$ = fluid flow across pulmonary microvascular membrane

K_f = hydraulic filtration coefficient

P_{mv}, P_{pmv} = hydrostatic pressures on microvascular and perimicrovascular sides of the microvascular membrane, respectively

π_{mv}, π_{pmv} = corresponding oncotic pressures

δ = reflection coefficient and represents the degree to which the microvascular membrane presents a physical barrier to protein molecules

It is the factor δ that can be used to distinguish high-pressure from permeability edema. In high-pressure edema, the membrane remains an effective barrier to protein equilibrium and δ approaches 1. Therefore, in high-pressure edema the primary forces which lead to an increase in fluid flux are the hydrostatic and oncotic pressure differences and the filtration coefficient K_f. In permeability edema, the microvascular membrane is no longer an effective barrier to protein. In this condition δ approaches zero and the oncotic pressure difference ($\pi_{mv} - \pi_{pmv}$) therefore influences fluid flux minimally. Hydrostatic pressure thus assumes an even greater importance in edema formation, and an increase in hydrostatic pressure will accelerate fluid flux into the lung to a far greater extent than in hemodynamic edema. Assessment or estimation of pulmonary hydrostatic pressure therefore has major therapeutic implications in the management of permeability pulmonary edema.

A variety of biochemical mediators produce the inflammatory response of permeability pulmonary edema. Some mediators are the result of a series of reactions facilitated by enzyme systems. Therefore, in many of the disorders associated with permeability edema, activation of these enzyme cascades can be demonstrated. One of these is the complement system, which may be triggered by a variety of substances (Fig. 34-1), including antibody antigen complexes (classical pathway), endotoxin, exposure to cell surfaces (bacteria, fungi), and to complex polysaccharides. The intermediate products C3a and C5a lead to neutrophil aggregation and the release of proteases and superoxide radicals which damage the pulmonary vascular endothelium. In addition, metabolism of membrane-bound phospholipid on leukocyte membranes leads to the formation of arachidonic acid. In turn, this compound is the parent for a host of leukotrienes and prostaglandins (Fig. 34-2), which contribute to further endothelial and alveolar injury.

Permeability pulmonary edema may also develop in the neutropenic host. Injury to the pulmonary endothelium in neutropenic patients may be secondary to the direct effects of bacterial endotoxin and complement, to oxygen toxicity, or to the release of prostaglandins and leukotrienes from alveolar macrophages.

Another enzyme cascade involves the coagulation pathways. Collagen in exposed subendothelial basement membrane will activate Hageman factor (factor XII) when exposed to plasma. The components of the coagulation system, the fibrinolytic system, and kinin system are activated and result in additional mediator release and endothelial damage (Fig. 34-3).

To complicate this process, the mechanical properties of the lung are adversely affected. Surfactant is inactivated or reduced with consequent destabilization of lung units. The lung becomes stiffer, and greater pressure is required to inflate it to a given volume; that is, pulmonary compliance decreases. When pulmonary edema is observed in a critically ill or injured patient with reduced lung compliance and severe hypoxemia refractory to supplemental oxygen, the criteria for the diagnosis of ARDS are met. A vicious cycle of ongoing pulmonary destruction and continued interaction of the enzymatic and biochemical

Table 34-1. Conditions Associated with Clinical Pulmonary Edema

Hemodynamic edema
Left ventricular failure
Acute myocardial infarction
Cardiomyopathies
Valvular heart disease
Volume overload
Crystalloid
Colloid
Blood or blood products
Permeability edema
Bacterial and other types of shock
Drug use and overdose—heroin, methadone, aspirin, paraquat, ethchlorvynol
Liquid aspiration—gastric contents, fresh water, salt water
Toxin inhalation—smoke, corrosive chemicals (Cl_2, NH_3, SO_2, NO_2, phosgene)
Bacterial and viral pneumonia
Pulmonary thromboembolism, fat embolism, amniotic fluid embolism, air embolism
Thermal injury
Hematologic disorders—disseminated intravascular coagulation, thrombotic thrombocytopenic purpura
Multiple trauma
Pulmonary contusion
Multiple transfusions
Eclampsia (pregnancy-induced hypertension)
Reexpansion of collapsed lung
High-altitude pulmonary edema
Acute neurologic crises
Tumor lysis
Radiation

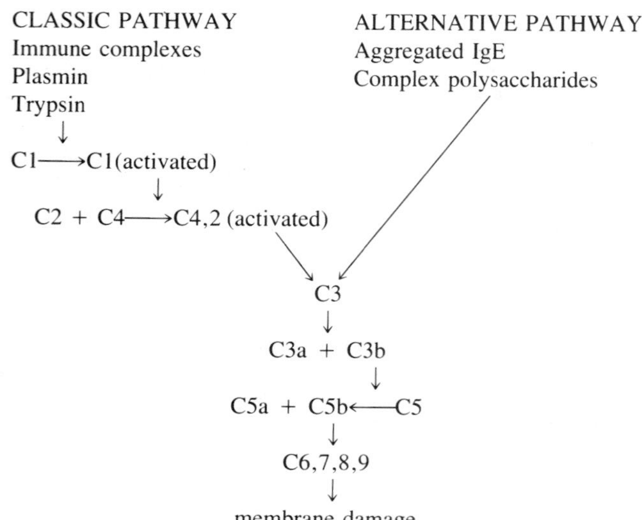

Fig. 34-1. The complement system is activated in many of the conditions associated with ARDS. C3a and C5a have a variety of physiologic actions including membrane damage and chemotaxis of neutrophils. Additional membrane damage is produced by activation of the C6–C9 components.

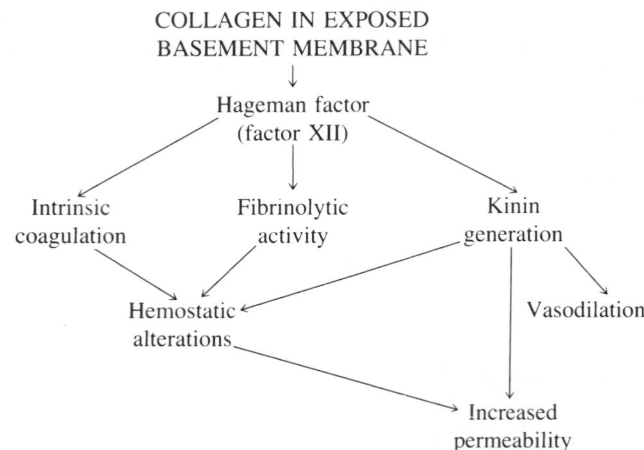

Fig. 34-3. Activation of Hageman factor can be triggered by subendothelial collagen, leading to involvement of the coagulation system, the fibrinolytic system, and the kinin system. Thus, cascading secondary reactions amplify membrane damage and increase vascular permeability.

cascading reactions develops. This process is often irreversible (approximately 50 percent of cases are fatal) unless the inciting event is controlled.

DIAGNOSIS

The clinical features of ARDS usually develop 12 to 72 h after the initial injury or medical crisis. Tachypnea, labored breathing, and impaired gas exchange (arterial P_{O_2} less than 50 torr with an FI_{O_2} of more than 0.5) are characteristic of this stage of the syndrome. Serial chest radiographs demonstrate progressive, bilateral alveolar infiltrates. Pulmonary compliance is reduced. Accordingly, airway pressures are high when the patient is placed on mechanical ventilation.

The diagnosis may be facilitated by sampling and analysis of pulmonary edema fluid. Sampling may be performed by suctioning fluid from the endotracheal tube with a soft plastic catheter and collecting the fluid in a Lukens trap. The fluid should be rejected if it is contaminated with mucus, sputum, or other debris. Colloid osmotic pressure and total protein are measured on edema fluid and simultaneously collected plasma. In permeability edema, the edema fluid-to-plasma ratio or colloid osmotic pressure ratio exceeds 60 percent. For high-pressure edema, the ratio is less than 60 percent. Substances such as collagenase, elastinase, and angiotensin-converting enzyme may be detected in increased quantities in edema fluid. Some recent studies have suggested that fluid obtained from the lower airways of patients with ARDS contains large numbers of neutrophils, and that the number of neutrophils correlates with the magnitude of impaired gas exchange.

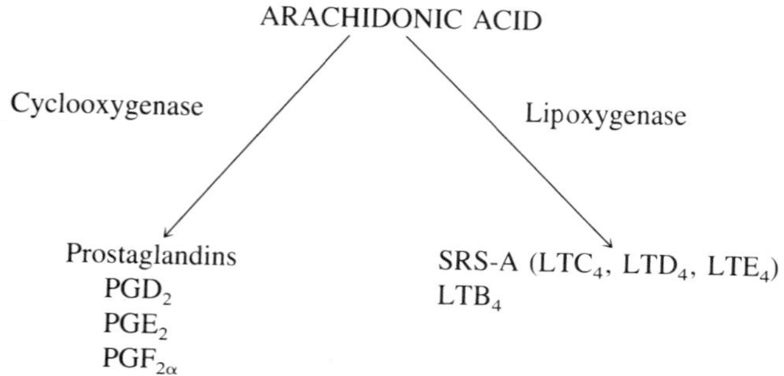

Fig. 34-2. Metabolism of arachidonic acid through major biochemical pathways leads to a variety of physiologically active mediators.

MANAGEMENT

Since most instances of permeability pulmonary edema are associated with other disorders (e.g., bacterial infection, gastric aspiration, trauma, drug intoxication), therapy should be directed primarily to treating the underlying insult. However, supportive therapy to maintain oxygenation and hemodynamic function must be assured.

Mechanical ventilatory support will be required for most patients with moderate to severe edema. Oxygen supplementation to increase arterial P_{O_2} is of limited effectiveness in ARDS, even with the use of mechanical ventilation. Accordingly, the physician must use other techniques to improve oxygenation. The use of positive end-expiratory pressure (PEEP) has virtually revolutionized the treatment of oxygenation deficits. PEEP recruits and helps stabilize lung units that may be filled with fluid and susceptible to collapse. Therefore, an increased number of lung units participate in gas exchange when PEEP is used. Because elevated inspired oxygen fractions (FI_{O_2}) may contribute to additional lung injury, the use of PEEP allows the reduction of FI_{O_2} to safer levels. As the level of PEEP increases, venous return, cardiac output, and oxygen delivery can decrease. PEEP may also cause pneumothorax or pneumomediastinum. Pressure control inverse ratio ventilation may also be useful, especially when pulmonary compliance is reduced.

Invasive hemodynamic monitoring allows the measurement of cardiac output, arterial and mixed venous oxygen tensions, and pulmonary artery pressures, including the wedge or occluded pressure (PAWP). This serves as a clinical index of pulmonary microvascular hydrostatic pressure (P_{mv}) as well as left ventricular volume and compliance. Because P_{mv} plays a major role in transcapillary fluid flux in permeability pulmonary edema, PAWP should be maintained at levels as low as possible—provided that peripheral perfusion is maintained. Diuretics or vasodilators may be required when PAWP is elevated, or if pulmonary edema or gas exchange worsen.

Adequacy of peripheral perfusion can be assessed by bedside guides (blood pressure, sensorium, urine output, etc.) as well as by the determination of cardiac output, systemic oxygen delivery, and oxygen consumption. These values are dependent upon cardiac output and hemoglobin, as well as arterial and mixed venous oxygen tensions and saturations. The level of blood lactic acid will reflect the adequacy of oxygen transport and utilization.

Fluid infusion may be required to maintain satisfactory cardiac output and peripheral perfusion, particularly in the face of the decreased venous return that may be produced by sudden increases of PEEP. The choice of fluid in this setting remains controversial (crystalloid or colloid), but the goal of fluid therapy should be to augment intravascular and intracardiac volumes with improvement of cardiac output and consequently oxygen transport to the system tissues. Careful hemodynamic assessment before and after a fluid challenge is necessary to interpret the response.

Current experimental studies are directed to analyzing the role of anticoagulants, antihistamines, and cyclooxygenase and oxygen radical inhibitors, as well as corticosteroids, in reducing permeability damage. Other novel experimental approaches to therapy include the administration of anticomplement and antiendotoxin antibodies, chelating agents, and protease inhibitors. To date, however, the effectiveness of these agents in humans is unproven. Some authorities have stated that it is likely that the simultaneous administration of several drugs or agents will be required to combat ARDS since multiple mediators and enzymatic pathways contribute to the pathophysiology of this condition.

SUMMARY

Permeability edema may be distinguished from the more common cardiogenic or hemodynamic edema on the basis of associated clinical conditions, pathophysiology, and, if available, analysis of pulmonary edema fluid. This distinction has important therapeutic implications. The goals of successful management of permeability edema and ARDS include treatment of the underlying condition and maintenance of adequate pulmonary oxygen loading with mechanical ventilation and PEEP, while assuring adequate circulatory function and tissue oxygen delivery.

BIBLIOGRAPHY

Biondi JW, Hines RL, Barash PG, et al: The adult respiratory distress syndrome. *Yale J Biol Med* 59:575, 1986.

Carlson RW, Schaeffer RC, Michaels SG, et al: Pulmonary edema fluid. Spectrum of features in 37 patients. *Circulation* 60:1161, 1979.

Lain PC, DiBenedetto R, Morris SL, et al: Pressure control inverse ratio ventilation as a method to reduce peak inspiratory pressure and provide adequate ventilation and oxygenation. *Chest* 95:1081, 1989.

Ognibene FP, Martin SE, Parker MM, et al: Adult respiratory distress syndrome in patients with severe neutropenia. *N Engl J Med* 313:547, 1986.

35
ACUTE ASTHMA IN ADULTS

Stanley Sherman

DESCRIPTION AND DEFINITION

Asthma is a common chronic disease. While it is more common in children and young adults, onset of symptoms can occur in any decade of life. Childhood asthma often dissipates with age, but adult-onset disease is usually persistent. Despite this chronicity, the clinical course is quite variable, and only a minority suffer serious debilitation. However, despite optimal medical management, asthma *can* be a fatal disease.

While asthma is difficult to define succinctly, several concepts are central to the definition and understanding of this disease. Asthma, in contrast to other obstructive lung diseases, is defined mainly in physiologic rather than anatomic or clinical terms. *Asthma* is reversible airflow obstruction, associated with a state of increased responsiveness of the tracheobronchial tree to many different stimuli (which do not affect normal individuals). This state of increased responsiveness, manifest by widespread bronchospasm, reflects the condition of *bronchial hyperreactivity,* a concept which will be discussed later. The bronchospasm characteristic of the acute asthmatic attack is typically reversible; it improves spontaneously or within minutes or hours of treatment.

Within the spectrum of chronic obstructive lung disease, asthma may either exist as a relatively ''pure'' entity or coexist with chronic bronchitis, emphysema, or bronchiectasis in various combinations. In either case, patients experience dypsnea, cough, and wheezing as the major complaints. The patterns of airflow obstruction vary greatly, depending on the frequency of the acute episodes and the state of the airways between episodes. Asthma may occur sporadically or manifest as chronic airflow obstruction with episodic exacerbations.

CLASSIFICATION

Traditionally, asthma has been classified as extrinsic or intrinsic. *Extrinsic asthma* is said to be ''allergic'' or immunologic in origin, occurring in atopic individuals. *Atopy* refers to the genetic predisposition to manifest immediate wheal and flare reactions to skin tests with multiple antigens, to which normal individuals do not respond. Atopic patients are usually younger and often have a history of allergic rhinitis and elevated serum levels of IgE. *Intrinsic asthma* exists when no obvious extrinsic causes are identified. Patients are typically older, nonatopic, and more likely to have a chronic course.

This timeworn division is less valuable today because understanding of the disease has evolved. A greater understanding of the complex mechanisms of bronchospasm has enabled us to view asthma as a state of bronchial hyperreactivity with many potential ''triggers'' (Table 35-1). An immunologic response (type I allergic reaction or immediate hypersensitivity) mediated by IgE is but one trigger, which may occur in atopic individuals (as in classic ''extrinsic'' asthma) as well as in nonatopic patients.

Table 35-1. Provocation of the Asthmatic Response (Triggers)

Immunologic reaction (exposure to antigen with mediator release)
Viral respiratory infections (upper and lower respiratory tract)
Changes in temperature and humidity (especially cold air)
Strong odors (perfume, etc.)
Pollutants, dusts, fumes, and other irritants (including occupational exposures)
Certain drugs and chemicals: aspirin, nonsteroidal antiinflammatory drugs, tartrazine dye (yellow dye no. 5), sulfiting agents, β-adrenergic blocking drugs
Sinus infections
Exercise
Strong emotions, laughing, coughing
Deep inspiration or forceful expiration
Gastroesophageal reflux

In addition, research and experience in recent years have revealed an increasing number of agents that cause asthma, either through immunologic mechanisms or by direct irritant effects. Occupational asthma has emerged as an important entity. In fact, it is estimated that as many as 5 to 10 percent of asthmatic patients (atopic and nonatopic) may have a significant trigger in the work environment. Because of the varying patterns of occupational asthma, it is difficult to correctly diagnose. Responses can be immediate, delayed 4 to 6 h following exposure, or repetitive at 24-h intervals (often in the morning).

PATHOPHYSIOLOGY

The rapidly reversible airflow obstruction that characterizes asthma is due mainly to bronchial smooth muscle contraction. However, in addition to abnormalities in the control of airway smooth muscle, the asthmatic attack is frequently associated with mucus hypersecretion and inflammatory changes in the bronchial walls, resulting in mucosal edema. Thus, the increased airway resistance seen in the asthmatic patient usually implies a three-component response. While the focus of therapy usually centers around pharmacologic manipulation of airway smooth muscle, it is important to recognize the physiologic impairment caused by mucus production and mucosal edema. Bronchospasm can be reversed within minutes, but the airflow obstruction due to mucous plugging and inflammatory changes in bronchial walls does not resolve for days or weeks. Failure to rapidly reverse an acute asthmatic attack strongly suggests that all three mechanisms are operative.

In addition to contributing to airflow obstruction, mucous plugging may lead to atelectasis, infectious bronchitis, and pneumonitis, with consequent impairment in gas exchange efficiency. The syndromes of allergic bronchopulmonary aspergillosis and mucoid impaction of the bronchus attest to the potential complications of mucus hypersecretion and impaired mucociliary clearance seen in some asthmatic patients.

Bronchial Hyperreactivity

The hallmark of asthma is bronchial hyperreactivity—an extreme sensitivity of the airways to physiologic, chemical, and pharmacologic stimuli. This results in a greater degree of bronchoconstriction than seen in normal individuals. Bronchial hyperreactivity in asthmatics is, thus, an exaggerated response—an extreme irritability of airway smooth muscle to stimuli such as exercise, cold air, dust, irritants (smoke, atmospheric pollutants), inhaled antigens, histamine, serotonin, bradykinin, and various cholinergic agonists.

While the cause of bronchial hyperreactivity is not fully understood, many theories have been proposed (Table 35-2). In any case, it is important to understand the role of the autonomic nervous system in the control of airway smooth muscle, since these relationships provide the rationale for certain pharmacologic interventions in acute asthma.

The parasympathetic nervous system (PSNS) has an abundance of vagal efferent fibers ending in airway smooth muscle. Vagus nerve stimulation releases acetylcoholine at postganglionic nerve endings, causing bronchospasm. Under normal conditions, a minor degree of PSNS predominance is observed, mainly in large, central airways (the main resistance airways). This tonic cholinergic activity produces a baseline bronchial smooth muscle tone, which, when abolished, produces bronchodilation. Strong emotions may lead to significant neural output from the central nervous system to airway smooth muscle (traveling through vagal efferent pathways), resulting in bronchospasm. In addition, the PSNS functions in the efferent limb of reflexive bron-

Table 35-2. Postulated Mechanisms of Bronchial Hyperreactivity in Asthma

Decrease in baseline airway caliber
Alterations in bronchial smooth muscle (hypertrophy, hyperplasia)
Increased number of mast cells
Increased synthesis of mediators
Lowered receptor threshold
Damage to airway epithelial cells (greater exposure to subepithelial irritant receptors)
Alterations or imbalance in autonomic nervous system regulation:
Increased parasympathetic activity
Decreased β-adrenergic responsiveness
Increased α-adrenergic responsiveness
Decreased responsiveness of the nonadrenergic (purinergic) inhibitory system

choconstriction, following afferent stimulation arising from the nasopharynx, larynx, trachea, and airways. The subepithelial irritant receptors in these locations may be stimulated by mechanical pressure, dust, chemical irritants, and certain drugs. Damage to airway epithelium disrupts the tight intercellular junctions, increases the exposure of the subepithelial irritant receptors and mast cells, and sensitizes the subepithelial irritant receptors. This increased airway permeability has been cited as a possible mechanism of bronchial hyperreactivity.

Compared to the PSNS, the sympathetic nervous system (SNS) innervation of airway smooth muscle is not as abundant and is limited to smaller airways. The role of the SNS in baseline airway smooth muscle tone appears small. Direct effects are less significant than those of circulating catecholamines. β-Adrenergic stimulation promotes bronchodilation of peripheral airways more than of central airways, while α-adrenergic stimulation may produce bronchoconstriction.

A third component of the autonomic nervous system consists of fibers which appear to travel with the vagus nerves to the airways. The transmitter(s) have not yet been identified. This nonadrenergic (purinergic) inhibitory system prevents bronchial smooth muscle contraction, possibly serving as the major opposition to the parasympathetic nervous system.

Mechanisms of Bronchospasm

Physiologic reactions in the asthmatic target cells (bronchial smooth muscle cells, mast cells, mucous gland secretory cells, vagus nerve cells, and inflammatory cells) are calcium-dependent processes—i.e., activation of these cells requires mobilization of free calcium ions with a transmembranous movement to the intracellular cytoplasmic matrix. Regardless of the inciting stimulus, it appears that calcium flux represents the final common pathway for cellular response.

While the factors capable of triggering an asthmatic reaction are numerous (Table 35-1), the known mechanisms of bronchospasm are relatively few. The best known (but not necessarily the most prevalent) is the immunologic reaction. Immediate hypersensitivity (type I allergic reaction) involves IgE antibody attached to the abundant airway mast cells (scattered throughout smooth muscle bundles, in the submucosa of airways, and adjacent to submucous glands). Exposure to a specific antigen establishes a bivalent cross-linking and results in mast cell degranulation. Preformed mediators are released (histamine, eosinophil chemotactic factors of anaphylaxis, neutrophil chemotactic factors, serotonin, and others) and other mediators are rapidly synthesized and then released (leukotrienes, prostaglandins, thromboxanes, platelet-activating factor). Mediators act directly on airway smooth muscle to produce bronchoconstriction. In addition, by inciting inflammation and increasing vascular permeability, mediators may produce mucosal edema and greater airflow obstruction. They may also elicit bronchospasm indirectly, by stimulating subepithelial irritant receptors and creating a vagal-mediated reflexive response.

The autonomic nervous system may function directly in the contraction of bronchial smooth muscle. Cholinergic neural output, from the central nervous system or as part of an irritant receptor reflex, produces bronchoconstriction. Imbalance in autonomic control—reduced β-adrenergic stimulation, increased α-adrenergic stimulation, or reduced purinergic stimulation—can also result in bronchospasm.

In exercise-induced bronchospasm hyperventilation with large volumes of cold, dry air promotes a cooling of the airways, which triggers a bronchospastic response. This exercise-induced respiratory mucosal heat loss appears to involve mediator release, because the response is most consistently blocked by the prior administration of disodium cromoglycate, an inhibitor of mast cell degranulation.

In some asthmatics, bronchoconstriction may be caused by drugs which inhibit cyclooxygenase (e.g., aspirin and nonsteroidal anti-inflammatory agents). The mechanism is believed to involve an alteration in the metabolism of arachidonic acid toward the lipoxygenase pathway, with production of greater amounts of leukotrienes. Leukotrienes (formerly known as the *slow-reacting substance of anaphylaxis*) comprise a family of related compounds which are potent bronchoconstrictors.

Consequences of Airflow Obstruction

The physiologic consequences of airflow obstruction are outlined in Table 35-3. The initial abnormality is increased airway resistance, stemming from a combination of bronchoconstriction, mucosal edema, and mucus hypersecretion. These conditions result in a reduction in maximum expiratory flow rates, best determined by objective measurements of pulmonary function.

As impairment of the expiratory phase of ventilation progresses, the complete tidal volume is not exhaled, and air trapping ensues. This process, reflected in elevation of the residual volume and functional residual capacity of the lungs, has both beneficial and adverse effects on lung mechanics. Air trapping tends to maintain airway patency through a tethering effect on the airways, thus reducing airway resistance. However, an elevated residual volume places the diaphragms in a mechanically disadvantageous position and, for all the inspiratory muscles, increases the elastic work of breathing.

Increased airway resistance and air trapping combine to produce increased airway pressures, which may result in barotrauma (subcutaneous emphysema, pneumomediastinum, or pneumothorax) and may impair cardiac performance through several mechanisms.

The acute asthmatic attack also results in an uneven distribution of ventilation, which in turn results in ventilation-perfusion imbalance. While hypercarbia may be seen in extreme cases, hypoxemia is more commonly observed. Worsening of hypoxemia has been demonstrated during the early treatment of acute asthma, an effect attributed to the vasoactive nature of β-adrenergic bronchodilators (which promote increased perfusion to poorly ventilated lung zones). Since most asthmatics receive oxygen supplementation during the initial phase of treatment, this sequence is not clinically significant.

During an acute asthmatic attack, the combination of increased airway resistance, increased respiratory drive, and air trapping creates

Table 35-3. Physiologic Consequences of Airflow Obstruction

Increased airway resistance
Decreased maximum expiratory flow rates
Air trapping
Increased airway pressure
Barotrauma
Adverse hemodynamic effects
Ventilation-perfusion imbalance
Hypoxemia
Hypercarbia
Increased work of breathing
Pulsus paradoxus
Respiratory muscle fatigue with ventilatory failure

greater demands on the muscle of inspiration. Excessive contractions of these muscles (during inspiration and, for unknown reasons, during expiration also) and an increased workload contribute to the patient's sensation of dyspnea. Respiratory muscles can fatigue. When the energy supply to these muscles fails to match energy requirements, lactic acidosis ensues, followed by overt ventilatory failure. When the major muscles of inspiration, the diaphragms, begin to tire, accessory inspiratory muscles assume a greater proportion of the ventilatory work. Retraction of the sternocleidomastoids (accessory neck muscles) closely correlates with severe asthma and is not usually observed until the FEV_1 falls below 1.0 L.

An abnormal pulsus paradoxus (> 20 mmHg) is associated with severe asthma. A dual mechanism has been proposed, relating to excessive negative intrathoracic pressure swings. During labored breathing, the generation of excessive negative intrathoracic pressure increases left ventricular afterload and accelerates venous return to the right heart, shifting the interventricular septum and further impairing left ventricular output. The net effect is transient reduction in cardiac output and systolic blood pressure.

PATHOLOGY

Precise pathologic descriptions of the asthmatic lung are hampered by difficulty in determining what constitutes pure asthma. Mucous plugging of the airways is a common finding, almost universally present in fatal asthma. Within the mucus, one finds abundant eosinophils and sloughed mucosal epithelial cells. In addition, mucus may contain other characteristic elements: Charcot-Leyden crystals (crystalline structures representing coalescence of free eosinophilic granules), Creola bodies (large compact clusters of sloughed mucosal epithelial cells), and Curschmann's spirals (bronchiolar casts of sputum components). Bronchial walls demonstrate mucosal edema, thickening of the basement membranes, submucosal eosinophilic inflammatory infiltrate, smooth muscle hypertrophy, and hyperplasia of mucous glands and goblet cells. The lung parenchyma may demonstrate areas of atelectasis, secondary to mucous plugging, but destructive changes are not observed.

CLINICAL PRESENTATION

Even though it may be difficult to define asthma precisely, and to appreciate the great variability in clinical patterns, the emergency physician easily recognizes the severe asthmatic attack. The diagnosis of asthma is secure when the key elements of the database are identified and the other conditions that may mimic acute asthma are excluded (Table 35-4). In practical terms, it is not essential to distinguish between the various obstructive lung diseases, since acute management is the same, focusing on reversible components.

History

While most patients relate a history of asthma at the onset, many will not. The patient complains of progressive dyspnea, chest tightness, wheezing, and cough. Persistent cough is often the major complaint, overshadowing the airflow obstruction and delaying recognition of the asthmatic state. The duration of acute symptomatology is important because episodes lasting more than several days are likely to be associated with significant mucosal edema and mucous plugging, factors which reduce the likelihood of successful emergency treatment and which necessitate hospitalization.

Table 35-4. Asthma Mimickers

Congestive heart failure ("cardiac asthma")
Upper airway obstruction
Aspiration of foreign body or gastric acid
Bronchogenic carcinoma with endobronchial obstruction
Metastatic carcinoma with lymphangitic metastasis
Sarcoidosis with endobronchial obstruction
Vocal-cord dysfunction
Multiple pulmonary emboli (rare)

Physical Examination

The patient presenting with a severe asthmatic attack is in obvious respiratory distress, with rapid, loud breathing. At times, wheezing may be audible without a stethoscope. The use of accessory muscles of inspiration (neck muscles are most prominent) indicates diaphragmatic fatigue, while the appearance of paradoxical respirations (inward movement of the upper abdominal wall due to inspiratory ascent of the diaphragms) reflect impending ventilatory failure. Alteration in the mental status—e.g., lethargy, exhaustion, agitation, or confusion—also heralds respiratory arrest.

Direct physical examination reveals hyperresonance to percussion, decreased intensity of breath sounds, and prolongation of the expiratory phase, usually with wheezing. Although wheezing results from the movement of air through narrowed airways, the intensity of the wheeze may not correlate with the severity of the airflow obstruction. The "quiet chest" reflects very severe airflow obstruction with air movement insufficient to promote a wheeze. A pulsus paradoxus above 20 mmHg is also indicative of severe asthma.

Pulmonary Function Testing

The objective demonstration of reversible airflow obstruction is central to the diagnosis. Characteristic changes in pulmonary function during acute asthma include a reduction in expiratory flow rates, such as the peak expiratory flow rate (PEFR) and forced expiratory volume in 1 s (FEV_1), a slight reduction in the forced vital capacity (FVC), and a ratio of FEV_1/FVC of less than 75 percent (defining a state of airflow obstruction). The residual volume, functional residual capacity, and total lung capacity are increased, although the latter elevation is less pronounced. Diffusing capacity is normal. In response to bronchodilator treatment, asthmatics typically demonstrate a greater than 15 percent improvement in FEV_1, FVC, and PEFR.

Chest Radiograph

Despite a low diagnostic yield in the setting of acute asthma, the chest radiograph is essential in excluding other conditions which may mimic asthma (Table 35-4) and in monitoring for associated complications. Abnormalities directly related to the asthmatic attack include pneumomediastinum, pneumothorax, atelectasis, and pneumonia. The difficulty of diagnosing pneumothorax by physical examination in the patient with acute asthma should be emphasized; the consequences of missing such a diagnosis are obvious. In the uncomplicated asthmatic, chest radiographic findings may include hyperinflation (flattening of the diaphragms, increased retrosternal air space) and increased bronchial markings, which are due to thickening of bronchial walls and which reflect an associated chronic bronchitic state.

Additional Laboratory Investigations

With the exception of arterial blood gases (see below), other studies are not diagnostically useful. The electrocardiogram may demonstrate many nonspecific findings, such as sinus tachycardia, right ventricular strain (right-axis deviation, clockwise rotation of the heart, right atrial enlargement, right bundle branch block), and atrial or ventricular arrhythmias. Blood and sputum eosinophilia may be present, reflecting the asthmatic condition. The total white blood cell count is frequently elevated, even without overt infection.

ASTHMA AND PREGNANCY

When asthma and pregnancy coexist (about 1 percent of all pregnancies), appropriate management is based on an understanding of the changes in respiratory physiology that accompany pregnancy, and a recognition of the hazards that the acute asthmatic attack poses for the mother and fetus.

The gradual increase in circulating progesterone during pregnancy increases central chemoreceptor sensitivity, resulting in an increase in minute ventilation (mainly tidal volume, not rate). This effect explains the frequent complaint of dyspnea during pregnancy. As a result of the increased minute ventilation, a moderate respiratory alkalosis (with appropriate renal compensation) is observed. In addition, oxygen consumption is increased during pregnancy. Pulmonary mechanics, however, are not affected by the enlarging uterus until the later half of the pregnancy, when the functional residual capacity is reduced. Vital capacity, total lung capacity, and large airway function are unchanged.

The effect of pregnancy on the course of the asthma varies and is unpredictable. Most reports describe worsening of asthmatic symptoms in about 25 percent of cases, improvement in another 25 percent, and no change in the remaining half. Patients tend to repeat the same pattern established during preceding pregnancies.

The effect of asthma on pregnancy is also unpredictable. However, maternal complications are slightly increased. In addition, there is a greater likelihood of premature births, and the rate of perinatal mortality is twice as high. These risks correlate with the severity of the asthma. Fetal complications are due to impaired fetal oxygenation resulting from maternal hypoxemia and from the adverse effects of alkalosis on the oxyhemoglobin dissociation curve.

Management of Asthma during Pregnancy

With few exceptions, the treatment of the pregnant asthmatic patient is no different from that of the nonpregnant asthmatic. Management should emphasize prompt and aggressive measures aimed at avoiding uncontrolled asthma and preventing hypoxemia. Most drugs used to treat asthma are safe for use during pregnancy and for nursing mothers. These include theophylline, β-adrenergic agents, corticosteroids, atropine, and most antibiotics. Caution should be exercised with the use of parenteral β-adrenergic agents near term, since these drugs may inhibit uterine contractility and occasionally produce maternal pulmonary edema. If essential for the treatment of asthma near term, β-adrenergic agonists should be administered using the aerosolized route, to minimize systemic absorption.

The use of parenteral epinephrine during the early months of pregnancy has been associated with a significant increase in fetal malformations; accordingly, this medication should be avoided. Other medications to avoid include iodides (which may cause fetal goiter and hypothyroidism), tetracycline (damage to fetal teeth, bone, and liver), and sulfonamides (interference with folic acid metabolism). Because erythromycin may interfere with theophylline metabolism (resulting in increased serum concentrations), close monitoring of serum theophylline levels is necessary when the two drugs are administered simultaneously.

ASSESSING THE SEVERITY OF THE ASTHMATIC ATTACK

When patients present with acute asthma, the physician must assess the severity of the attack, not only to rapidly determine which patients will require hospital admission, but also to identify those at risk of respiratory failure. It is fortunate that asthmatics rarely require intubation and mechanical ventilation. However, when necessary, these measures may be lifesaving because asthmatic patients can deteriorate rapidly.

What is "severe" asthma? In the past, the term *status asthmaticus* was used to indicate the severest condition experienced by the asthmatic, short of respiratory failure. However, the term lacks precision and offers no additional insight to the treating physician. Because the meaning of status asthmaticus is likely to differ among physicians, it is best to avoid the phrase and use instead the more accurate term "severe" asthma. *Severe asthma* is a high-risk, refractory condition requiring immediate and intensive treatment to avoid respiratory failure. The patient with severe asthma has not responded with objective improvement in airflow obstruction to initial emergency treatment consisting of nebulized β-adrenergic drugs, intravenous theophylline and corticosteroids, and even nebulized anticholinergics. In terms of the mechanism of airflow obstruction, failure to rapidly improve with bronchodilator therapy indicates significant mucous plugging and mucosal edema—conditions that require many days or even weeks for complete resolution.

Profile of the High-Risk Asthmatic

Certain characteristics of the patient and distinctive features of the acute episode enable the physician to predict a high-risk situation. Steroid-dependent patients with a labile clinical pattern (marked, rapid fluctuations in severity of bronchospasm) and a prior history of respiratory failure requiring intubation and mechanical ventilation are at greater risk of a poor outcome. Asthmatic patients who do not respond to emergency treatment are more likely to have ignored escalating symptoms for several days prior to seeking medical attention, thus allowing mucous plugging and mucosal edema to proceed unchecked. In this respect, severe asthma is often viewed as a "crisis of neglect" on the part of the patient. However, the physician often contributes to the poor outcome through inadequate assessment of the severity of the attack, delayed and suboptimal use of corticosteroids, and, during initial treatment, the use of sedation, which may lead to respiratory arrest.

Subjective versus Objective Assessment

Both the patient and the physician often underestimate the severity of the airflow obstruction. In fact, in acute asthma, the degree of physiologic impairment correlates poorly with most signs and symptoms. While studies using objective measurements, such as the peak expiratory flow rate (PEFR), have shown that many experienced patients are more accurate than their physicians in predicting their degree of airflow obstruction, not all patients are capable of such an analysis. The perception of dyspnea is often related more to changes in inspiratory resistance and the work of breathing than to the degree of expiratory airflow limitation. Patients often have difficulty in determining when their baseline function has returned, usually underestimating the functional impairment. Nevertheless, physicians are well advised to take note of the asthmatic patient's subjective complaints.

The physician's assessment relies on physical examination findings such as increased respiratory rate, contraction of the sternocleidomastoid muscles, paradoxical respirations, the presence of pulsus paradoxus, and reduced intensity of the breath sounds with prolongation of the expiratory phase. Despite the emphasis placed on "wheezing," this sign does not correlate with the severity of the obstructive process.

Numerous studies have demonstrated that successful emergency treatment of acute asthma depends on the degree of objective improvement in pulmonary function. Measurements of the FEV_1 and PEFR are useful in predicting which patients are likely to require hospital admission. Physicians using objective criteria can more confidently determine who is likely to do well following discharge and who is likely to relapse.

Warning Signs of Severe Asthma

Certain objective findings during the emergency evaluation should alert the physician to a potentially adverse outcome (Table 35-5). The performance of spirometry and measurement of PEFR have greatly enhanced the physician's ability to recognize a severe asthmatic attack. However, some asthmatics have difficulty in performing spirometry because forced expiratory maneuvers produce bronchospasm. In such cases, measurement of the PEFR may be tolerated since it does not

Table 35-5. Warning Signs of Severe Asthma

Impaired pulmonary function:
FEV_1 < 1.0 L
PEFR < 80 L/min
Hypoxemia (Pa_{O_2} < 60 mmHg)
Hypercarbia (Pa_{CO_2} > 45 mmHg) and acidosis (pH < 7.35)
Change in mental status: agitation, confusion, lethargy, exhaustion
Atrial or ventricular arrhythmias
Pulsus paradoxus > 20 mmHg
Pneumothorax

require the forced expiration of the entire vital capacity. The correlation between these two objective measurements of airflow obstruction is good. Severe asthma is characterized by an FEV_1 of less than 1.0 L and a PEFR of less than 80 L/min, while a moderate impairment is associated with an FEV_1 of 1.0 to 1.5 L and a PEFR of 80 to 200 L/min.

Deterioration in arterial blood gases (ABGs) is a grave sign in the acutely ill asthmatic; hypoxemia (Pa_{O_2} less than 60 mmHg on room air) and hypercarbia (Pa_{CO_2} greater than 45 mmHg) portend respiratory failure (Table 35-6). While ABGs are usually drawn early in the emergency management of the acute asthmatic, this diagnostic study is clearly overused. Assessment of oxygenation status does not require ABGs. Because mild or moderate hypoxemia is nearly universal during the acute attack, one could argue that empiric oxygen supplementation be initially administered. Adequate arterial oxygen saturation (≥ 90 percent) can be confirmed with pulse oximetry. The true purpose of drawing ABGs is to measure the Pa_{CO_2}. In this regard, ABGs do not inform the physician "how well" the patient is doing; rather, they serve to relate "how poorly" he or she is doing. Accordingly, measurement of ABGs should be reserved for the patient who presents with obvious exhaustion and signs of mental deterioration or who does not improve or appears worse following initial emergency treatment. The use of ABGs outside of this framework rarely serves to alter management decisions. Arterial blood gases must be interpreted in light of the total clinical picture. For example, the physician must note whether the patient is clinically improved or worse; normocarbia is an ominous finding only if the patient is doing poorly. In the heavy smoker or the obese patient, hypercarbia may occur prematurely and not imply the same degree of risk. Fortunately, only a minority of hypercarbic episodes in acute asthmatics require mechanical ventilation; with good medical management, rapid reversibility is the rule.

Changes in mental status suggest severe physiologic impairment and, unless promptly reversed, indicate a need for intubation and mechanical ventilation. Atrial and ventricular arrhythmias may reflect multiple stresses such as hypoxemia, acidosis, and elevated levels of circulating catecholamines. A pulsus paradoxus greater than 20 mmHg indicates severely impaired pulmonary status, usually correlating with an FEV_1 of less than 1.25 L. A pneumothorax in the midst of an acute asthmatic attack is a potentially fatal complication that must be managed promptly. In most instances, tube thoracostomy is desirable to prevent respiratory failure or circulatory compromise due to a tension pneumothorax. Other frequently mentioned "warning" signs such as hypertension, tachycardia, and even the "quiet" chest do not provide additional insight beyond the findings already discussed.

Table 35-6. Clinical Stages of Asthma According to Arterial Blood Gases*

Clinical Stage†	Pa_{O_2}, mmHg	Pa_{O_2} mmHg	pH
1	Normal (> 80)	< 35	> 7.45
2	Reduced (60–80)	< 35	> 7.45
3	Low (< 60)	35–40	7.35–7.45
4	Low (< 60)	35–40	< 7.35‡
5	Low (< 60)	> 45	< 7.35

* Clinical correlation is advised.

† Clinical stages 1 and 2 reflect "mild" disease, stage 3 is "moderate," and stages 4 and 5 indicate "severe" asthma.

‡ Reflects lactic (metabolic) acidosis related to increased work of breathing.

TREATMENT OF ACUTE ASTHMA

The goals are simple: Improve airway function rapidly, avoid hypoxemia, and prevent respiratory failure and death. In addition, it is desirable to quickly identify those patients who require hospital admission, and avoid discharging patients who will return within hours or days. In most cases, disposition of the acute asthmatic patient can be made within 1 h.

Indications for Hospital Admission

Criteria for hospital admission are detailed in Table 35-7. Admission decisions can and should be made early. Because bronchoconstriction is rapidly reversible with appropriate treatment, an asthmatic attack of recent onset due mainly to bronchial smooth muscle contraction can be distinguished from the slowly responding episodes associated with mucous plugging and significant mucosal edema. Thus, asthmatics who do not demonstrate significant subjective and objective improvement within 30 to 60 min are likely to require many days of further intensive treatment to resolve the complex airflow obstruction. Objective assessment (FEV_1 or PEFR) is crucial to proper management of acute asthma.

Basic Approach to Management

While many accepted treatment measures have a secure foundation in pulmonary physiology, few have been rigidly assessed with well-controlled double-blind studies. Nevertheless, a rational approach to the therapy of acute asthma can be constructed on the basis of current concepts of the disease process, the principles of pharmacology, and clinical experience.

Oxygen should be administered immediately to all acute asthmatics, using nasal cannula at 2 to 3 L/min. Empiric treatment is justified because most patients will manifest some degree of hypoxemia and the potential for rapid fluctuation is great. Furthermore, in the "pure" asthmatic, the risk of oxygen-induced respiratory depression is insignificant. The adequacy of supplemental oxygen should be determined—preferably by pulse oximetry.

Because mucous plugging is prominent in patients hospitalized with acute asthma, intravenous fluids are essential for proper liquefaction and clearance of secretions. Generous fluid therapy will also benefit the many asthmatics who are dehydrated due to excessive respiratory water loss and reduced oral intake. Percussion and postural drainage may also assist in the removal of secretions, but because they are difficult to perform in the acutely dyspneic patient and can produce reflex bronchospasm, they are best avoided during early treatment.

Several measures must always be avoided in the treatment of acute asthma. Sedatives and tranquilizers are absolutely contraindicated, regardless of how "nervous" the patient appears; respiratory arrest often follows such ill-advised treatment. Mucolytic agents (acetyl-

Table 35-7. Criteria for Hospital Admission in Acute Asthma*

Emergency visit within the preceding 3 days
Failure of subjective improvement following treatment
Failure of posttreatment FEV_1 to increase by > 500 mL, or absolute value < 1.6 L
Failure of posttreatment PEFR to increase more than 15% above initial value, or absolute value < 200 L/min
Change in mental status (lethargy, agitation, exhaustion, confusion)
Failure of hypercarbia to resolve after treatment
Presence of pneumothorax

* Presence of any of these conditions warrants admission to the hospital.

cysteine) are similarly contraindicated during the acute episode because they may provoke further bronchospasm. Since the benefits of iodides and glyceryl guaicolate are uncertain, these drugs should also be avoided. β-Adrenergic blocking agents (even "selective" agents) should not be used to treat arrhythmias, hypertension, or angina in the face of acute asthma. Many asthmatics respond poorly to ultrasonic nebulization and treatments with an intermittent positive pressure breathing machine (IPPB). Hydration can be achieved through the intravenous route, and airway medications can be delivered using a compressor-driven nebulizer.

β-Adrenergic Agonists

β-Adrenergic agonists are preferred as the initial medication for the treatment of acute bronchospasm and for the stable ambulatory patient. These drugs produce greater and more rapid improvement in pulmonary function than parenteral theophylline. The addition of theophylline to β-adrenergic therapy is reserved for the more difficult cases.

Description

β-Adrenergic receptors are divided into two types: β_1 and β_2. Stimulation of β_1 receptors in the heart increases rate and force of contraction, while in the small intestine motility and tone are decreased. β_2-Adrenergic stimulation promotes bronchodilation (in airways) vasodilation (in blood vessels), uterine relaxation, and skeletal muscle tremor.

The mechanism of bronchodilator action of β-adrenergic drugs involves stimulation of the enzyme adenylcyclase, which converts intracellular adenosine triphosphate (ATP) to cyclic adenosine monophosphate (cAMP). This action enhances the binding of intracellular calcium to cell membranes, reducing the myoplasmic calcium concentration, and results in relaxation of bronchial smooth muscle. In addition to bronchodilation, β-adrenergic drugs inhibit mediator release and promote mucociliary clearance.

The issue of tachyphylaxis with β-adrenergic agents is frequently raised. The consensus view is that if this does occur in asthmatics, the effects are not clinically significant. These drugs are metabolized by monoamine oxidase (MAO) and catechol-*O*-methyltransferase (COMT) to inactive compounds. In the intestine, sulfatases also inactivate these agents.

The most common side effect of β-adrenergic drugs is skeletal muscle tremor. Patients may also experience nervousness, anxiety, insomnia, headache, hyperglycemia, palpitations, tachycardia, and hypertension. Despite earlier concerns over potential cardiotoxicity, especially when these drugs are used in combination with theophylline, clinical experience has not revealed significant problems. Arrhythmias and evidence of myocardial ischemia are rare, especially in patients without prior history of coronary artery disease.

The Aerosol Route

Aerosol therapy with β-adrenergic drugs produces superior bronchodilation and is favored over both oral and parenteral routes. The aerosol route achieves topical administration of a relatively small dose of drug, producing local effects with minimum systemic absorption and fewer side effects. Optimum deposition and retention of appropriately sized particles (1 to 5 μ in diameter) containing a bronchodilator drug is enhanced by slow inspiratory flow rates followed by prolonged (10 s or more) breath-holding. Aerosol delivery may be achieved with a metered-dose inhaler, a compressor-driven nebulizer, or an IPPB. Treatment with an IPPB device offers no advantage over compressor-driven nebulizers and may be irritating to some asthmatics. While nebulizers and inhalers are equally effective in the stable patient, the nebulizer may offer certain advantages in the acute asthmatic since the metered-dose inhaler is less effective when the respiratory pattern is rapid and shallow and the patient has difficulty coordinating actuation of the inhaler with inspiration. A spacer device attached to the inhaler can improve drug deposition when patient technique is inadequate. Even with optimum technique, however, a maximum of 15 percent of the drug dose is retained in the lungs, regardless of the aerosol method used.

β_2-Adrenergic Drugs

The β-adrenergic agonists used today are analogs of naturally occurring sympathomimetics. The ideal bronchodilator in this class of drugs would possess pure β_2-receptor activity—bronchodilation without cardiac effects. The older catecholamine bronchodilators (isoproterenol and epinephrine) are not β_2-specific and have a short duration of action. Isoetharine is more β_2-selective, but still has a short duration of action. These drugs have nearly been replaced by newer agents produced by chemical modification of the parent compound. There are two new classes of β-adrenergic drugs which share greater β_2 specificity (relative, not absolute), as well as longer duration of action (due to resistance to COMT and MAO) and effectiveness through the oral route (due to resistance to gut sulfatases). These include the resorcinol bronchodilators (metaproterenol, terbutaline, and fenoterol) and the saligenin bronchodilators (albuterol and carbuterol). Bitolterol represents an even newer concept in β-adrenergic therapy. This "prodrug" is inactive until hydrolyzed by esterases to the active β_2-specific catecholamine, colterol. Because the concentration of necessary esterases is higher in the lungs than in the heart, β_2 selectivity is maintained. Currently, bitolterol is available only in a metered-dose inhaler.

Table 35-8 lists the β-adrenergic bronchodilators approved for emergency use. Terbutaline, albuterol, and bitolterol are not available in solutions for use with compressor-driven nebulizers, although metered-dose inhalers are available. Fenoterol and carbuterol are not commercially available. Although subcutaneous injections of epinephrine and terbutaline are widely used, this mode of treatment is no more effective and is associated with more systemic side effects. The parenteral route should probably be avoided in patients over 40 years of age. Similarly, the use of continuous intravenous isoproterenol should be discouraged.

Theophylline

Until recently, intravenous theophylline has been the first-line drug for treatment of acute asthma. But this approach has been challenged by studies showing that, in acute asthma, theophylline produces less bronchodilation than β-adrenergic agents. Furthermore, theophylline in combination with inhaled β-adrenergic drugs appears to increase the toxicity but not the efficacy of treatment. Although the issue remains controversial, it is clear that nebulized β_2-adrenergic agents are the favored initial treatment for acute asthma. This is not to say that theophylline should be eliminated from the treatment program. In fact, since many severe asthmatics will require hospitalization and multidrug therapy, the addition of theophylline is rational. Theoretically, the addition of theophylline to may be beneficial by providing a more sustained bronchodilator effect, contributing to small airway bron-

Table 35-8. β-Adrenergic Bronchodilators for Acute Asthma

	Dose, mg	Duration, h	Dosing Interval
Subcutaneous route*			
Epinephrine	0.3	4	20 min × 3
Terbutaline sulfate	0.25	4–6	20 min × 3
Nebulized route			
Isoetharine mesylate	2.5–5.0	3–4	3 h
Metaproterenol sulfate	10–15	3–5	3 h
Albuterol	2.5–5.0	3–4	1–2 h

* Not the preferred route—should be restricted to children and young adults. Avoid in patients over 40 years old or with history of hypertension or coronary artery disease.

chodilation (especially when mucous plugging prevents uniform distribution of the nebulized drug) and improving respiratory muscle endurance and resistance to fatigue.

Pharmacology

For many years, bronchodilation with theophylline was viewed as a consequence of phosphodiesterase inhibition (preventing degradation of cyclic AMP). Several lines of reasoning have demonstrated that this is not the case, and the mechanism of action of theophylline remains unknown. The majority of theophylline metabolism (90 percent) is by the liver, by two separate oxidases. The remainder is excreted unchanged through the kidneys. Theophylline has numerous beneficial effects on pulmonary physiology. Bronchodilation, proportional to the serum concentration, is well recognized. In addition, theophylline increases the contractility and endurance of the diaphragm (and possibly other inspiratory muscles), improving mechanical efficiency and delaying the onset of muscle fatigue. Other actions include stimulation of mucociliary clearance, increased respiratory drive, inhibition of mediator release, increased myocardial contractility, increased gastric acid secretion, and promotion of diuresis.

The toxicity of theophylline is well described. The most common side effect is gastrointestinal disturbance (nausea, cramps, diarrhea). Also common are headache, nervousness, insomnia, and sinus tachycardia. The more serious adverse effects such as confusion, agitation, seizures, and arrhythmias are uncommon and usually associated with serum theophylline concentrations greater than 40 μg/mL. Symptomatic theophylline toxicity with a serum concentration greater than 30 μg/mL should be treated with oral charcoal (30 g every 2 h for four doses). The use of charcoal hemoperfusion should be determined on an individual basis.

Serum Theophylline Levels

As with the beneficial effect of bronchodilation, the side effects of theophylline are related to the serum concentration. Because metabolism (hepatic clearance) of theophylline varies, the relationship between dose and serum level is unpredictable. The prudent physician will carefully monitor the serum theophylline concentration until a steady-state condition exists and also whenever events develop which are likely to alter theophylline disposition. Theophylline has a narrow therapeutic range, with a therapeutic serum concentration defined as 10 to 20 μg/mL. Some patients may benefit at levels less than 10 μg/mL. Toxicity increases in frequency at levels above 20 μg/mL but is still observed at lower levels, occasionally below the therapeutic range. In the acute setting, maintaining serum levels between 10 and 15 μg/mL is the safest approach.

Numerous factors alter theophylline metabolism by affecting hepatic oxidases. Reduced theophylline clearance (increased serum levels) is associated with liver disease, congestive heart failure, cor pulmonale, febrile viral respiratory infections, advanced age, cimetidine, erythromycin, oral contraceptives, and allopurinol. Increased theophylline clearance (decreased serum levels) is seen with cigarette smoking, phenobarbital, phenytoin, significant consumption of charcoal-broiled beef, and elimination of the factors which reduce clearance.

Theophylline Dosing

Extensive insight into the pharmacokinetics of theophylline has provided rational dosing recommendations. Because the beneficial effects are directly related to the serum concentration, it is desirable to maintain a constant therapeutic concentration of theophylline. This requires administration of a loading dose (to establish blood levels) immediately followed by a constant infusion (Table 35-9). Of course, proper utilization of theophylline requires a knowledge of prior drug administration, as well as clinical assessment of the factors likely to alter theophylline metabolism.

Table 35-9. Guidelines for Intravenous Theophylline in Adults

	Dose
LOADING DOSE*	
No previous theophylline	5 mg/kg IBW
Short-acting theophylline taken < 12 h, or long-acting theophylline taken < 24 h, *and* serum levels therapeutic	None
Oral theophylline as above *and* serum levels subtherapeutic	3 mg/kg *or* ½ (desired level − observed level) mg/kg
MAINTENANCE INFUSION†	
Patients taking oral theophylline *and* serum levels therapeutic	Same dose‡
Patients taking oral theophylline *and* serum levels subtherapeutic	Increase by 25%
Patients not taking oral theophylline:	
Smoking adult	0.8 mg/kg/h
Nonsmoking adult, seriously ill patient	0.5 mg/kg/h
Congestive heart failure, liver disease	0.2 mg/kg/h

* Loading dose should be administered in 50 mL of 5% dextrose in water over 20 to 30 min, *never as a bolus,* and *never through a central venous catheter.*

† Serum theophylline level should be monitored 24–36 h after infusion.

‡ Divide daily dose (mg) by 24 to determine the hourly infusion rate.

Corticosteroids

Corticosteroids are highly effective drugs in asthma; in fact, they form the cornerstone of treatment of the severe episode. While the mechanism of action is unknown, many believe that steroids produce beneficial effects by restoring β-adrenergic responsiveness and reducing inflammation. It is generally accepted that the onset of steroid action is delayed at least 6 to 8 h following intravenous administration, but recent studies suggest that improvement may be observed within 1 h, possibly as a result of improved β-adrenergic responsiveness. Many controversies remain concerning steroid use, including the basic issue of efficacy. The following recommendations represent one of many approaches, and should by no means be construed as the single standard of care.

Corticosteroids should be used immediately in all asthmatics who are currently taking, or have recently taken, these drugs. They should also be administered to patients who demonstrate any of the warning signs of severe asthma (Table 35-5) and to those who do not show objective improvement in pulmonary function (Table 35-7) after the first nebulized bronchodilator treatment. While there is considerable disagreement over what constitutes the optimum dose of corticosteroid (ranging from 100 to 4000 mg of hydrocortisone equivalent during the first 24 h), this author favors low-dose treatment with an initial intravenous bolus of 60 to 80 mg of methylprednisolone. The bolus is followed by 15 to 20 mg every 6 h until the patient's airway function is restored to near-baseline levels. Subsequent tapering to a single morning dose of oral corticosteroid depends on the patient's condition and past history. Because aerosolized corticosteroids may be irritating during the acute episode, they should be avoided.

Anticholinergics

Plants containing anticholinergic alkaloids have been smoked for hundreds, if not thousands, of years to treat respiratory disorders. In recent years, anticholinergics have been rediscovered as potent bronchodilators in patients with asthma and other forms of obstructive lung disease. Although comparisons of bronchodilator response between anticholinergics and β-adrenergic agonists have produced conflicting results, when the drugs are used in combination, the effects are additive. This is probably true because the sites of action of both drugs are different: Anticholinergics affect large, central airways while β-adrenergic drugs bronchodilate smaller airways.

Anticholinergic drugs competitively antagonize acetylcholine at the postganglionic, parasympathetic effector-cell junction. This process effectively blocks the bronchoconstriction induced by vagal (cholinergic-mediated) innervation to the larger central airways. In addition, concentrations of cyclic GMP in airway smooth muscle are reduced, further promoting bronchodilation.

Earlier concerns with potential adverse effects of anticholinergics, such as mucous plugging and systemic toxicity, have not proved clinically significant, probably due to the use of the aerosol route of administration and the tendency to use small doses. Potential side effects with nebulized anticholinergics include drying of the mouth (most common), thirst, and difficulty swallowing. Less commonly, one observes tachycardia, change in mental status (restlessness, irritability, confusion), difficulty in micturition, ileus, blurring of vision, or an increase in intraocular pressure.

The major anticholinergic nebulized in the United States is atropine sulfate. Unfortunately, this is not the ideal agent because significant systemic absorption can occur. However, newer synthetic atropine derivatives such as ipratroprium bromide, atropine methonitrate and glycopyrrolate methylbromide are more potent, longer acting, and produce fewer systemic side effects.

A nebulized dose of atropine sulfate [between 0.4 and 2.0 mg (0.025 mg/kg maximum)] appears to produce maximum effect with minimum toxicity. Atropine sulfate and metaproterenol or albuterol can be nebulized together. The onset of action is slower than that of the β-adrenergic drugs, with peak effects not observed for 60 to 90 min in many cases. The duration of action is in the range of 4 h.

Other Medications

The empiric use of a single broad-spectrum antibiotic during the treatment of acute asthma is acceptable, because secondary bacterial bronchitis is seen in many instances. Disodium cromoglycate and inhaled corticosteroids should be avoided during the acute asthmatic attack, since they are only minimally beneficial and may cause further airway irritation. Antihistamines are not beneficial in asthma.

Calcium channel blockers can inhibit the calcium-dependent reactions that lead to bronchial smooth muscle contraction, mucus secretion, mediator release, and nerve impulse conduction. These agents have been shown to prevent bronchospasm in response to exercise, hyperventilation, cold air, histamine, and various additional antigens. While the prophylactic value of calcium channel blockers has been demonstrated, these drugs have not proved to be significant or consistent bronchodilators. Neither has magnesium sulfate. At the present time, they have no role in the acute treatment of asthma.

Mechanical Ventilation

When all efforts to relieve the severe airflow obstruction fail and the patient manifests progressive hypercarbia and acidosis or becomes exhausted or confused, intubation and mechanical ventilation are necessary to prevent respiratory arrest. Mechanical ventilation does not relieve the airflow obstruction; it merely eliminates the work of breathing and allows the patient to rest while the airflow obstruction is resolved. Fortunately, only a small percentage of asthmatics (less than 1 percent) ever require mechanical ventilation. Direct oral intubation is preferred over the nasotracheal route.

The potential complications of mechanical ventilation in the asthmatic patient are numerous. Increased airway resistance may lead to extremely high peak airway pressures (potentially resulting in frequent high-pressure alarming of the ventilator), barotrauma, and hemodynamic impairment. Due to the severity of airflow obstruction, during the early phases of treatment, the tidal volume may be larger than the returned volume; this condition leads to air trapping and increased residual volume. These effects may be partially avoided by utilizing rapid flow rates at a reduced respiratory frequency (12 to 14 per minute), allowing adequate time for the expiratory phase. In this manner, one can achieve the major goal of ventilatory support—maintenance of an adequate arterial oxygen saturation (90 percent), without concern for "normalizing" the hypercarbic acidosis (an undesirable initial strategy). This approach is referred to as *controlled mechanical hypoventilation*. Mucous plugging is frequent, often leading to increased airway resistance, atelectasis, and pulmonary infection. Finally, an endotracheal tube may cause some asthmatics to become even more "twitchy," resulting in further bronchospasm.

BIBLIOGRAPHY

Edelson JD, Rebuck AS: The clinical assessment of severe asthma. *Arch Intern Med* 145:321, 1985.

Fanta CH, Rossing TH, McFadden ER: Emergency room treatment of asthma: Relationships among therapeutic combinations, severity of obstruction and time course of response. *Am J Med* 72:416, 1982.

Hendeles L, Weinberger M: Theophylline: A "state of the art" review. *Pharmacotherapy* 3:2, 1983.

Kelsen SG, Kelsen DP, Fleegler BF, et al: Emergency room assessment and treatment of patients with acute asthma: Adequacy of the conventional approach. *Am J Med* 64:622, 1978.

Newhouse MT, Dolovich MB: Control of asthma by aerosols. *N Engl J Med* 315:870, 1986.

Pak CCF, Kradjan WA, Lakshminarayan S, et al: Inhaled atropine sulfate: Dose-response characteristics in adult patients with chronic airflow obstruction. *Am Rev Respir Dis* 125:331, 1982.

Raimondi AC, Figueroa-Casas JC, Roncoroni AJ: Comparison between high and moderate doses of hydrocortisone in the treatment of status asthmaticus. *Chest* 89:832, 1986.

Rebuck AS, Read J: Assessment and management of severe asthma. *Am J Med* 51:788, 1971.

Turner ES, Greenberger PA, Patterson R: Management of the pregnant asthmatic patient. *Ann Intern Med* 6:905, 1980.

Westerman DE, Benatar SR, Potgieter PD, et al: Identification of the high-risk asthmatic patient: Experience with 39 patients undergoing ventilation for status asthmaticus. *Am J Med* 66:565, 1979.

36
CHRONIC OBSTRUCTIVE PULMONARY DISEASE

Joel C. Seidman

Individuals with chronic obstructive pulmonary disease frequently present to emergency departments in severe respiratory distress, and are among the most frustrating, frightening, and challenging patients encountered there. In a fearful state of mixed anxiety, intense physical effort, and disoriented fatigue, such people face a constant battle against asphyxiation. At other times, presentation is prompted by otherwise uncomplicated medical or surgical disease, which becomes more serious or catastrophic as the impact of chronic respiratory disease is unmasked.

CAUSES AND PREDISPOSING FACTORS

The most important predisposing factor to chronic airflow obstruction is cigarette smoking. Other less well understood environmental exposures, genetic aberrations, and, probably, sustained bronchospastic airflow obstruction can cause disease in nonsmokers as well as smokers. Less is known about the roles of environmental and industrial air pollution and passive smoking than about active cigarette smoking. Some forms of industrial asthma such as byssinosis and diisocyanate-induced bronchospasm can cause irreversible airflow obstruction. Recent public communications by the Surgeon General highlight medical evidence of the serious irreversible impact of passive smoking on some individuals. Genetic disorders such as α_1-antitrypsin deficiency and cystic fibrosis account for only a small fraction of disease. Recognition of heritable markers is of academic interest, facilitates genetic counselling, and may alter long-term clinical management (e.g, intravenous α_1-proteinase inhibitor repletion therapy). Asthma alone, if sufficiently sustained and punctuated by repetitive endobronchial infections, may progress to chronic obstructive pulmonary disease, even in the absence of other known risk factors.

PATHOPHYSIOLOGY

Almost three decades ago, the American Thoracic Society defined the dominant clinical forms of chronic obstructive pulmonary disease as follows: (1) *pulmonary emphysema* (defined pathologically) as a condition of the lung characterized by abnormal, permanent enlargement of the air spaces distal to the terminal bronchiole, accompanied by destruction of their walls; and (2) *chronic bronchitis* (defined clinically) as a condition of excess mucus secretion in the bronchial tree, occurring on most days for at least three months in the year for at least two consecutive years. Although not included in the above definition, increased airways resistance is also a fundamental feature of either condition.

The earliest objective changes in the evolution of chronic obstructive pulmonary disease are clinically imperceptible and are measured as small increases in peripheral airways resistance or lung compliance. The slow, insidious appearance of dyspnea and hypersecretion often require several decades of disease; the sedentary life habits of many cigarette smokers result in failure to unmask exertional dyspnea; and the frequent use of denial in smokers results in suppression of symptoms or attribution of symptoms to aging, poor conditioning, obesity, or allergies. Further, the respiratory consequences of cigarette smoking are a continuum of slowly evolving and latent effects, unique to each individual, in a complex dose-response relationship. Early in disease evolution, abstinence from smoking may eliminate symptoms and result in physiologic improvement. Once well developed, however, abnormalities persist and may still progress despite abstinence.

Pathologic specimens from patients with early disease demonstrate minor metaplasia of bronchial epithelium and an increase in bronchial gland number and size. As disease evolves, such findings are exaggerated, acute and chronic inflammatory changes in the epithelium are more notable, and acinar expansion, destruction, and coalescence are seen. Elements of emphysematous disease are invariably present in concert with those of bronchitic disease, though one often predominates.

Despite recognition of causative factors, what determines the clinical onset and rate of progression of chronic airflow obstruction, and the direction toward either emphysematous or bronchitic patterns, is uncertain. Clearly, there is a great deal of variability in disease pattern and severity among individuals with seemingly similar predispositions to disease.

The central element in the pathophysiology of chronic airflow obstruction is impedance to airflow, especially expiratory airflow, due to increased resistance or decreased caliber throughout the small bronchi and bronchioles. This results from obstruction due to secretions and mucosal edema, bronchospasm, and bronchoconstriction from impaired elastance. Impedance to airflow alone accounts substantially for the abnormal physiology of the disease. Exaggerated airway resistance either reduces total minute ventilation, or increases respiratory work. To the degree that alveolar hypoventilation occurs, hypoxemia and hypercarbia result. Ventilation-perfusion mismatching occurs, so that regional relative overperfusion widens the alveolar-arterial oxygen difference, promoting hypoxemia. Increased physiologic dead space ventilation leads to alveolar hypoventilation, hypercarbia, and further hypoxemia. Even if all challenges to increased respiratory work are met, hypoxemia resulting from regional low ventilation-perfusion relationships or true physiologic right-to-left shunts cannot be overcome.

In addition to obstruction of the peripheral airways, all forms of advanced chronic airflow obstruction involve other pathophysiologic elements to complete the overall picture. Particularly in dominantly emphysematous disease, destruction and coalescence of alveolar architecture results in reduction of total "matched" alveolar-capillary surface area for diffusion of gas, while vascular destruction results in "unmatched" regions where ventilation is wasted.

Neurochemical and proprioceptive ventilatory responses in chronic airflow obstruction may be aberrant. For example, ventilatory response to hypercarbia may be blunted during sleep, and ventilatory drive and dyspnea may be exaggerated in spite of normal pulmonary inflation. The composition of muscle fiber types, breathing pattern, and resistance to fatigue of respiratory muscles are also altered in advanced chronic airflow obstruction. Finally, pulmonary arterial hypertension supervenes as chronic airflow obstruction progresses. The right ventricle transiently hypertrophies, and then dilates with the evolution of overt cor pulmonale. A low-output state in the pulmonary circulation translates into low left ventricular output. Arterial hypoxemia increases as the effects of right-to-left shunt on poorly oxygenated mixed venous blood are exaggerated. Right ventricular pressure overload is clinically poorly tolerated and associated with atrial and ventricular arrhythmias.

COMPENSATED CHRONIC AIRFLOW OBSTRUCTION

Clinical Features

Despite the pathophysiologic segregation of chronic airflow obstruction into categories of pulmonary emphysema, chronic bronchitis, and bronchiectasis, none of these exists as pure entities in clinical medicine. Most patients demonstrate a mixture of symptoms and signs. The hallmark symptom is exertional dyspnea. Chronic, productive cough is common, and minor hemoptysis is frequent, especially in chronic bronchitis and bronchiectasis. Physical findings include tachypnea, accessory respiratory muscle use, and pursed-lip exhalation. Airflow obstruction causes wheezing during exhalation, especially maximum forced exhalation, and prolongation of the expiratory time. In dominantly bronchitic disease, coarse crackles are heard as uncleared secretions move about the central airways. In dominantly emphysematous disease, there is hyperexpansion of the thorax, impeded diaphragmatic motion, and global diminution of breath sounds. Weight loss is frequent due to poor dietary intake and excessive caloric expenditure for the work of breathing. Plethora due to secondary polycythemia, cyanosis, and tremor, somnolence, and confusion due to hypercarbia may be seen in advanced disease. Findings of secondary pulmonary hypertension with or without cor pulmonale may be present. The physical signs of left ventricular dysfunction are often disguised or underestimated by the seemingly more overwhelming signs of respiratory disease, or because pulmonary hyperinflation prohibits adequate auscultation.

Roentgenographic examination is often misleading. Mild chronic airflow obstruction is likely to be roentgenographically inapparent. Dominantly bronchitic disease may be associated with subtle or absent x-ray findings. On the other hand, dominantly emphysematous disease may be associated with remarkable signs of hyperaeration such as increased anteroposterior diameter, flattened diaphragms, increased parenchymal lucency, and attenuation of pulmonary arterial vascular shadows, despite only mild-to-moderate physiologic alterations. Right or left ventricular enlargement may not produce relative enlargement of the cardiac silhouette. Certainly, roentgenography is of unquestionable value in diagnosing complications such as pneumothorax, pneumonia, pleural effusion, or pulmonary neoplasia.

The most valuable tool in characterizing disease severity is pulmonary physiologic testing, including examination of lung mechanics, analysis of arterial blood gases, description of ventilatory response patterns, tests of respiratory muscle performance, metabolic assessment, and survey of hemodynamic reserve. In clinically apparent chronic airflow obstruction, the FEV_1 (forced expiratory volume in 1 s) as a fraction of the FVC (forced vital capacity), also called $FEV_{1\%}$, correlates remarkably well with day-to-day functional performance, morbidity incidents, and mortality. Reduction of the FVC in the absence of restrictive ventilatory disease favors the emphysematous pattern, while improvement in the $FEV_{1\%}$ in response to bronchodilator inhalation is more commonly seen in bronchitic patients. All such studies are adaptable for use in the emergency department.

Arterial blood gas analysis can show exaggeration of the predicted normal alveolar-arterial oxygen difference as disease progresses; an increase in hypoxemia during exercise in emphysematous disease; resting hypercarbia in advanced bronchitic disease; and chronic, resting hypoxemia in all forms of advanced disease, especially with secondary pulmonary hypertension and cor pulmonale.

When ventricular function is clinically unclear, echocardiography or gated nuclear scans to estimate ejection fractions may prove invaluable. ECGs are useful to identify arrhythmias or ischemic injury, but do not assess the severity of pulmonary hypertension or right ventricular dysfunction.

Other laboratory analyses may indicate advanced disease: polycythemia, with or without elevation of packed red blood cell 2,3-diphosphoglycerate (2,3-DPG) concentration, as a feature of chronic hypoxemia; elevated serum bicarbonate reflecting chronic hypercarbia and respiratory acidemia; and elevated hepatic enzymes and albuminuria indicative of high central venous pressure in cor pulmonale.

Therapy

The appropriate and optimal management of decompensated chronic airflow obstruction in an emergency department setting requires an appreciation of chronic day-to-day therapy. Specific management limits further insults to the respiratory system, treats reversible bronchospasm, and prevents or treats complications. Seven actions comprise the core of strategy: (1) elimination of extrinsic irritants, (2) bronchodilator and glucocorticoid therapy, (3) antibiotics, (4) mobilization of secretions, (5) "respiratory" vaccines, (6) oxygen, and (7) treatment of complicating systemic disease. Cigarette smoking and other aggravating environmental factors must be limited or thoroughly eliminated.

Some combination of regular as well as symptom-guided nonsteroidal bronchodilator therapy is chronically prescribed. This may include oral theophylline or aminophylline in immediate- or sustained-release forms, oral or inhaled selective β-adrenergics, and oral or inhaled glucocorticoids. The use of these agents varies with disease severity and lability, physician preference, the patient's subjective response, compliance, drug cost, and availability of facilities to monitor serum concentrations of theophylline or toxicities of systemic glucocorticoid therapy.

Knowledge of certain features of the maintenance regimen are essential to the emergency physician: (1) If theophylline or aminophylline is taken, the formulation prescribed, last dose time, and total daily dose must be determined. (2) If systemic glucocorticoid is taken, the product prescribed and total daily dose, or dose as otherwise prescribed, must be known. (3) The dose and frequency of use of oxygen therapy should be identified, if only to assure continuity of therapy.

Broad-spectrum antimicrobials are frequently prescribed, and sometimes initiated independently by the patient, to treat acute mucopurulent tracheobronchitis. In mild-to-moderate bronchitis uncomplicated by pneumonia, antibiotic selection need not concur with in vitro sensitivities to assure clinical efficacy. Most commonly, tetracyclines, ampicillin or amoxicillin, sulfamethoxazole/trimethoprim, erythromycin, ciprofloxacin, or first-generation cephalosporins are given; infrequently used agents include chloramphenicol and clindamycin.

Various actions are taken to mobilize respiratory secretions: assurance of generous oral fluid intake and atmospheric humidification, avoidance of antihistamine/decongestant/anticholinergic agents, and limitation of antitussive use. The efficacy of specific expectorant products is dubious.

Preventive respiratory vaccines are recommended: polyvalent (23) pneumococcal vaccine and annual trivalent influenza vaccine.

Chronic intermittent or continuous oxygen therapy is indicated if the oxygen saturation is less than 90 percent while at rest and breathing room air.

Complications of chronic airflow obstruction include those in direct consequence to respiratory disease (secondary pulmonary hypertension and cor pulmonale) or nonrelated diseases with an adverse physiologic impact upon underlying respiratory disease (left-sided) heart failure, anemia, hyperthyroidism). Such problems are sometimes managed with difficulty as their treatments may aggravate bronchospasm, and vice versa.

DECOMPENSATED CHRONIC AIRFLOW OBSTRUCTION

Clinical Features

Tissue oxygen delivery is decreased as a result of ventilation-perfusion mismatching and alveolar hypoventilation. The former reflects intensification of bronchospastic airflow obstruction, and the latter, increased work of breathing. The end result is increasing hypoxemia and hypercarbia.

Progressive hypoxia is characterized by tachypnea, cyanosis, agitation and apprehension, tachycardia, and systemic hypertension. Signs of hypercarbia are confusion, tremor, plethora, stupor, and, finally, apnea. The patient complains primarily of dyspnea and orthopnea. The intensified effort to ventilate is further dramatized by sitting-up-and-forward posturing, pursed-lip exhalation, accessory muscle use, and diaphoresis. Pulsus paradoxus may be noted during blood pressure recording. Complications such as pneumonia, pneumothorax, or an acute abdomen may be neglected or minimized by the patient's generalized respiratory distress, tachypnea, or global diminution of breath sounds.

Clearly the most life-threatening feature of decompensation is critical hypoxemia where arterial saturation falls below 90 percent under ambient conditions. Correction is mandatory, even if oxygen supplementation sufficiently suppresses hypoxemic drive to require mechanical ventilation. Cyanosis alone has poor clinical correlation with hypoxia, and arterial blood gases are necessary to evaluate oxygenation and carbon dioxide retention. While pulse oximetry may identify hypoxemia, it cannot identify hypercarbia or acid-base disturbances. The finding of an arterial pH below that consistent with renal compensation for chronic respiratory acidosis implies either acute exaggeration of hypercarbia or acute metabolic acidosis.

Decompensation is usually due to worsening of airflow obstruction resulting from increased bronchospasm, superimposed respiratory infection, interference with respiratory drive, cardiovascular deterioration, smoking, noncompliance with medication, noxious environmental exposures, use of medications that prohibit bronchorrhea, and adverse responses to medication (e.g., anaphylactoid responses or institution of β-adrenergic blockade). Other respiratory pathophysiology, often with a restrictive pattern, may add to the impact of chronic airflow obstruction: pneumonia, pneumothorax, pulmonary embolism, pulmonary edema, blunt chest injury, or abdominal pain are considerations. Disordered ventilatory drive most commonly arises from misuse of oxygen therapy, hypnotics, or tranquilizers. Metabolic disturbances such as diabetic ketoacidosis, uremia, or hepatic encephalopathy may also impair ventilatory drive. Inadequate tissue oxygen delivery independent of respiratory function results from left ventricular failure, anemia, hyperthyroidism, or hyperthermia.

Therapy

The primary goal of emergency therapy in decompensated chronic airflow obstruction is to correct tissue oxygenation. This requires the restoration of the lungs as gas exchange organs, assurance of hemodynamic efficiency, repletion of red blood cell mass where deficient, and limitation of excessive oxygen demands and carbon dioxide production.

Certain medical historical details are critical to appropriate therapy. These include the patient's current medical regimen (medications, doses, and schedule of administration), with special attention to use of theophylline, glucocorticoids, and oxygen; medication allergies; duration of symptomatic decompensation (recognizing that slow, protracted deterioration will often be slowly responsive and comparatively refractory to immediate interventions); and recent "upgrading" of therapy (recognizing that a failure to provide continued therapy of at least similar intensity will represent a "downgrading" of intervention).

The membrane gas transport capabilities of the alveolar-capillary interface in chronic airflow disease are little affected by therapies. However, the gas exchange process is facilitated by increasing the inspired partial pressure of oxygen. Oxygen is a drug with a therapeutic-toxic range. The need to increase P_{O_2} must be balanced against the possibility of suppression of hypoxic ventilatory drive. If hypercarbia is present, a fixed-concentration mask with 24 to 35 percent FI_{O_2} should be used, with frequent reassessment of clinical response. Arterial saturation should be corrected to above 90 percent.

The application of assisted ventilation increases alveolar ventilation by accelerating the rate and depth of total ventilation, augments mean alveolar oxygen partial pressure by more effectively matching the distribution of pulmonary blood flow and alveolar ventilation, and minimizes the patient's work of ventilation. Pharmacologic bronchodilatation accomplishes similar ends by minimizing the impedance to bronchial airflow and facilitating mobilization of excessive airway secretions.

Assisted mechanical ventilation is indicated for inability to maintain oxygen saturation at 90 percent, or severe hypercarbia associated with stupor, narcosis, or acidosis. Other parameters which reflect respiratory muscle effort, extent of dead space ventilation, and the work of breathing have prognostic bearing, but none can be used to determine the need for ventilator therapy. A volume-cycled ventilator should always be used. Security of the airway should be accomplished with a cuffed endotracheal tube of generous diameter inserted orally whenever possible. Small tubes or nasotracheal tubes provide impedance to suctioning, make fiberoptic bronchoscopy more difficult, and make spontaneous ventilation with the tube in situ intolerable (because of upper airway resistive impedance). The endotracheal tube must be maintained above the carina. Excessive tidal volumes (over 15 mL/kg ideal body weight) can cause barotrauma and hypotension due to reduction of venous return and can produce a severe combined metabolic and respiratory alkalosis. Initially, high inspired oxygen concentrations should be used. In an emergency department setting, there is no clear role for the application of intermittent mandatory ventilation (IMV) or positive end-expiratory pressure (PEEP); the mode of ventilation should be assist/control (A/C).

The use of assisted mechanical ventilation in chronic airflow obstruction is a two-edged sword. Placement of an endotracheal tube, with or without assisted ventilation, impairs normal mucociliary clearance, initiates or exaggerates microbial colonization of the tracheobronchial tree, obstructs the cough mechanism, allows catheter suctioning of predominantly the right bronchial system, and injures the laryngeal and proximal tracheal supporting structures, to say nothing of the psychological impact upon the patient. It should be avoided if at all possible.

Pharmacologic intervention is the most essential and least traumatic method to treat decompensated chronic airflow obstruction. Three groups of agents are used: (1) parenteral methylxanthines, (2) β-adrenergic agonists, and (3) systemic glucocorticoids.

Methylxanthines

The methylxanthines, aminophylline (theophylline ethylenediamine) and theophylline, are most effective for emergency treatment when given intravenously. Drug concentration should be maintained at 10 to 20 μg/mL (10 to 20 mg/L). Incremental benefit is often observed at the upper region of this range. Many schemes of dosing have been described, each dependent upon estimations of the patient's volume of distribution (usually approximately 0.5 times ideal body weight expressed in liters) and probable clearance rate.

The loading dose (of theophylline) to obtain an initial serum concentration of 10 μg/mL (10 mg/L) is 5 to 6 mg/kg ideal body weight in a patient currently receiving no drug. In a patient previously medicated orally with theophylline already present in serum, a mini-loading dose may be alternatively selected as: (target concentration − currently assayed concentration) × volume of distribution (i.e., 0.5 × ideal body weight in liters). With the mini-load method, the target concentration should be between 10 μg/mL (10 mg/L) and 15 μg/mL (mg/L).

The maintenance dose is 0.2 to 0.8 mg/kg ideal body weight per hour. Lower maintenance rates are given to patients with congestive cardiac failure or hepatic insufficiency with low clearance rates, while higher rates are given to smokers with rapid clearance. Unfortunately, no regimen suits a given patient, and the above are only guidelines. Relatively rapid determination of dosage can be obtained from the Chiou approximation of total body theophylline clearance measured during continuous, uninterrupted intravenous infusion, while two serum assays are drawn approximately 8 h apart:

$$CL = 2K_0/(C_1 + C_2) + 2VD(C_1 - C_2)/[(C_1 + C_2)(T_2 - T_1)]$$

where CL = total body clearance (L/h)
K_0 = current infusion rate (mg/h)
C_1 = first serum theophylline concentration (mg/L)
C_2 = second serum theophylline concentration (mg/L)
VD = volume of distribution (assumed to be 0.5 × ideal body weight in liters) (L)
$T_2 - T_1$ = actual time interval between blood draws (h)

Further derivation concludes:

$$K_1 = CL \times C_3$$

where K_1 = new infusion rate (mg/h)
C_3 = desired target serum theophylline concentration (mg/L)

The accuracy of this methodology assumes that theophylline clearance is constant over the short term (e.g., there has been no activated charcoal administered for toxicity), and enteric absorption of theophylline is negligible.

Maintenance theophylline infusion in a patient on chronic oral therapy is complex (whether or not a mini-loading dose has been given), particularly in attempting to account for enteric drug yet to be absorbed. A single serum assay upon arrival in the emergency department is of little value in calculating dose requirements, unless the measurement is in the toxic range. Alternatively, the already established daily dose can be administered as an intravenous infusion over 24 h. If the optimal daily dose is unknown, then the above guidelines should be used. In addition, the hourly infusion rate selected (in miligrams per hour) should be reduced for $(6 - t)$ hours by $D/6$, for rapid-release formulations; and for $(12 - t)$ hours by $D/12$, for sustained-release preparations (including 24-h release forms), where t is the time in hours since the last oral dose taken, and D is the usual oral dose. This guideline will likely minimize the risk of "summation toxicity" due to continued enteric absorption. Theophylline and aminophylline should not be given orally (unless decompensation is not severe, alimentary motility is assured, and forthcoming ambulatory care is imminent), and certainly not by rectal suppository, in an emergency setting.

β-Adrenergic Agonists

β-Adrenergic agonists produce the promptest of responses and are available in oral, parenteral, and aerosolized dosage forms. In critical settings, reliance should be placed upon parenteral or aerosolized forms of epinephrine or, preferably, relatively selective β_2 agonists. Epinephrine 1:1000 (0.1 to 0.3 mL) or terbutaline sulfate (0.25 to 0.50 mL) may be given subcutaneously. Aerosol therapy minimizes systemic toxicity and is a favored delivery route. Isoetharine 1% 2.5 to 5.0 mg (0.25 to 0.50 mL), metaproterenol 5% 10 to 15 mg (0.2 to 0.3 mL), or albuterol sulfate 0.6% (0.5% as albuterol base) 1.25 to 2.50 mg (0.25 to 0.50 mL) can be delivered by compressed-gas-driven nebulizer. Acceptable dose intervals for adrenergic therapies range from 1 to 4 h, depending on clinical response and signs of drug toxicity. Both parenteral and aerosol routes should not be used concurrently. Occasionally, dramatic benefit can be obtained by continuous, closely monitored, intravenous infusion of isoproterenol (0.25 to 4.0 μg/min). Continuous infusion of isoproterenol should not begin until all other adrenergic therapy (regardless of administration route) has ceased. Cardiac arrhythmias are the major hazard. Self-contained, fluorocarbon-pressurized adrenergic inhalation devices are unreliable in severe, decompensated chronic airflow obstruction and are not recommended.

Systemic Glucocorticoids

Systemic glucocorticoids elicit delayed bronchodilatory responses and undoubtedly attribute part of their effect to facilitation of concurrently given methylxanthine or β adrenergics and to anti-inflammatory effects. Because of a delay of hours in onset of response, corticosteroids should be given early. Optimally effective daily doses range between one and three times the maximal physiologic adrenal secretion rate (i.e., the equivalent of 60 to 180 mg prednisone daily). Higher doses have demonstrated dubious additional efficacy and excessive toxicity. The choice of steroid is generally not critical, though hydrocortisone should probably be avoided because of excess mineralocorticoid effect, unless primary adrenal insufficiency is concurrently present. There is no role for inhaled glucocorticoids in acute treatment.

Other Agents

Although unpredictable in efficacy, inhaled anticholinergic agents may sometimes be useful adjuvants superimposed upon other therapies. Atropine sulfate, 1.0 to 3.5 mg, or glycopyrrolate, 0.2 to 1.0 mg, is usually administered. Doses may be repeated as often as every 3 to 4 h. Alternatively iprotroprium bromide may be administered by metered dose inhaler (preferably with a spacing device), pending approval of the inhalant solution for use in the United States.

Further Considerations

Aggravating events other than simple "decompensation" should be identified quickly: Pneumonia, pneumothorax, pleural effusion, lobar atelectasis, pulmonary thromboembolism, and acute myocardial infarction should all be considered in the differential diagnosis.

From another perspective, the possibility of previously recognized or unrecognized chronic airflow obstruction should be considered in *any* patient over 40 years of age presenting to an emergency department with a catastrophic medical or surgical problem—and treated appropriately.

Tissue oxygen delivery must be maximized by correcting left ventricular failure or arrhythmia to improve cardiac output, replacing red blood cell mass and intravascular fluid to increase arterial oxygen content, and suppressing fever to decrease oxygen consumption. In mathematical terms, attempts should be made to optimize the mixed venous oxygen content ($c_{\bar{v}}$) derived from algebraic rearrangement of Fick's equation for cardiac output.

$$c_{\bar{v}} = c_a - \dot{V}_{O_2}/\dot{Q}_t$$

where c_a = arterial oxygen content (mL O_2/100 mL blood)
$\dot{V}_{O_2}$ = minute oxygen consumption (or delivery) (mL O_2/min)
$\dot{Q}_t$ = cardiac output (mL blood/min)

Common errors encountered in emergency department care of decompensated chronic airflow obstruction include:

1. Use of parenteral or aerosolized sympathomimetics alone for sustained decompensation
2. Inadequate theophylline dosage or failure to deliver by parenteral route
3. Failure to discontinue sodium cromolyn or inhaled glucocorticoid altogether, or failure to discontinue metered-dose inhalers in patients receiving concurrent adrenergic aerosols by other means
4. Denial of systemic glucocorticoid therapy to patients already so medicated or with established "steroid-dependent" disease
5. Indiscriminate use of sedation, antihistamine/decongestants, or anticholinergics
6. Misuse of an intermittent positive pressure breathing machine (IPPB) to deliver adrenergic aerosols
7. Misuse of ultrasonic aerosols
8. Uncontrolled use of supplemental oxygen (including pressurized, high-concentration sources to drive aerosol equipment)
9. Use of pressure-cycled ventilators rather than volume-cycled machines

10. Inadvertent mechanical hyperventilation following prolonged hypercarbia (resulting in unchallenged extreme metabolic alkalosis, hypotension, arrhythmias, and seizures)
11. Failure to recognize respiratory failure or need for hospital admission.

BIBLIOGRAPHY

American Thoracic Society: Definitions and classifications of bronchitis, asthma and pulmonary emphysema. *Am Rev Respir Dis* 85:762, 1962.

Chiou WL, Gadalla AF, Peng GW: Method for the rapid estimation of the total body drug clearance and adjustment of dosage regimens in patients during a constant-rate intravenous infusion. *J Pharmacokinet Biopharm* 6:135, 1978.

Dantzker DR (ed): *Cardiopulmonary Critical Care*. Orlando, Grune & Stratton, 1986.

Diener CF, Burrows B: Further observations on the course and prognosis of chronic obstructive lung disease. *Am Rev Respir Dis* 111:719, 1975.

Fishman AP: Chronic cor pulmonale. *Am Rev Respir Dis* 114:775, 1976.

Hendeles L, Weinberger M: Theophylline: A ''state of the art'' review. *Pharmacotherapy* 3:2, 1983.

Nocturnal Oxygen Therapy Trial Group: Continuous or nocturnal oxygen therapy in hypoxemic chronic obstructive lung disease. *Ann Intern Med* 93:391, 1980.

Piafsky KM, Ogilvie RI: Dosage of theophylline in bronchial asthma. *N Engl J Med* 292:1218, 1975.

Sahn S: Corticosteroids in chronic bronchitis and pulmonary emphysema. *Chest* 73:389, 1978.

Snyder JV, Pinsky, MR: *Oxygen Transport in the Critically Ill*. Chicago, Year Book Medical Publishers, Inc, 1987.

SECTION 5
The Digestive System

37
ESOPHAGEAL EMERGENCIES

Richard E. Burney
James R. Mackenzie

INTRODUCTION

Esophageal disease is a relatively infrequent source of emergency problems, but one that must be considered with respect to a number of more common emergency complaints, including chest pain, gastrointestinal hemorrhage, and dysphagia. While most esophageal conditions are benign, both esophageal hemorrhage and perforation carry a high morbidity and mortality if not recognized and treated promptly. Specific knowledge of the anatomy, physiology, and history of esophageal diseases, and familiarity with the diagnostic methods of identifying esophageal problems, all assist in the identification of emergency problems of esophageal origin.

ANATOMY AND PHYSIOLOGY

The esophagus begins at the hypopharynx opposite the sixth cervical vertebra and the lower border of the cricoid cartilage; passes through three visceral compartments, the neck (cervical esophagus), the mediastinum, and the upper abdomen; and ends at the cardia of the stomach opposite the body of the eleventh thoracic vertebra. The anatomic relations of the esophagus are shown in Fig. 37-1.

The pharynx and esophagus lie immediately in front of the prevertebral fascia and are surrounded by a layer of fascia which fuses with cellular tissue of the superior mediastinum. A layer of this tissue separates laterally in the neck to unite with the prevertebral fascia, forming the retropharyngeal space of Henke. The retropharyngeal and retroesophageal space is in direct communication with the superior mediastinum, and bleeding, perforations, or abscesses in this space have a direct conduit to the superior mediastinum.

The esophagus is composed of an inner mucosal layer covering a tough, fibrous submucosal layer. There are two muscle layers surrounding the mucosal and submucosal layers. The innermost is spiral to circular while the outer is longitudinal. There is no serosa, and as a result, once the submucosa is perforated or destroyed, the perforation tends to extend into the surrounding mediastinal structures, leading to a diffuse, malignant, and often rapidly progressive and fatal mediastinitis. The striated muscle of the upper esophagus gradually gives way to the smooth muscle which forms the rest of the esophagus and the gastrointestinal tract.

The mucosa and submucosa are the layers usually involved in peptic esophagitis, which, when severe and prolonged, may result in scarring and stricture formation. However, it is only when the esophageal muscle layer is split beyond the submucosal scar in bouginage or by repeated dilatations that the muscle layer becomes involved in the scarring process. When the muscle becomes scarred, stricture formation continuously recurs after instrumentation. On the other hand, when the muscle is not involved, elimination of the cause for esophagitis, and one or two dilatations, eliminate the stricture. Ingestion of lye and some other corrosives destroys the muscular layer to a greater or lesser degree, and dilatation of the scar formation in this layer tends to cause tearing and further scarring and stricture.

The Venous System

The submucosal plexus of veins drains to an intercommunicating plexus which surrounds the esophagus. This network anastomoses with the inferior thyroid vein in the neck, the azygous system in the thorax, and the coronary and short gastric veins (part of the portal venous system) in the abdomen. Obstruction of the portal system from such diseases as cirrhosis of the liver causes submucosal esophageal varices (Fig. 37-2).

Deglutition and Propulsion of the Food Bolus: Physiology

A food bolus is passed from the anterior part of the tongue backward by a sequential contraction of the tongue upward against the roof of the mouth and backward against the hard and soft palate and posterior pharyngeal wall. At the same time there is a sequential contraction of the esophageal constrictor muscles from above downward. The pressure of the tongue and the contraction of the muscles of the soft palate and the superior constrictor cause an airtight closure of the nasal pharynx to the food bolus. The resulting high-pressure wave which is created by the sequential contraction of the aforementioned muscles propels food toward the esophagus.

Laryngeal muscles contract involuntarily as the bolus is passed from the front of the tongue to the middle pharynx, causing the larynx to rise and be sealed from the pharynx by the epiglottis. The cricopharyngeal muscle forms the UES and is in tonic contraction at all times, except when it relaxes as the food bolus approaches.

The bolus is then propelled caudad by a peristaltic wave which starts at the UES and is controlled by the reflex arcs of Meissner's and Auerbach's plexuses located between the inner and outer muscle layers. When the bolus reaches the distal 1 to 2 cm of the esophagus, it meets another high-pressure area, the LES, which relaxes to allow food to enter the stomach. A secondary peristaltic contraction wave starts at the level of the aortic arch, which is another area of raised pressure, and propels any leftover liquid caudad. Finally, a tertiary contraction wave may be initiated at the level of the lower one-third of the esophagus, usually by reflux of gastric contents. This may be an important mechanism for keeping the lower esophageal mucosa clear of gastric contents.

PRESENTING SYMPTOMS

Dysphagia

Definition

Dysphagia is an awareness of something wrong with the smooth pattern of swallowing, i.e., the patient mentions that food sticks, hesitates, or pauses, or that it just won't go down right. The presence of dysphagia almost always signifies esophageal pathology. It is different from "globus hystericus"—the sensation of "something always stuck in the throat"—but is akin to transfer dysphagia, which is the inability to initiate the act of swallowing and is usually due to pharyngeal muscular weakness or central nervous system disease.

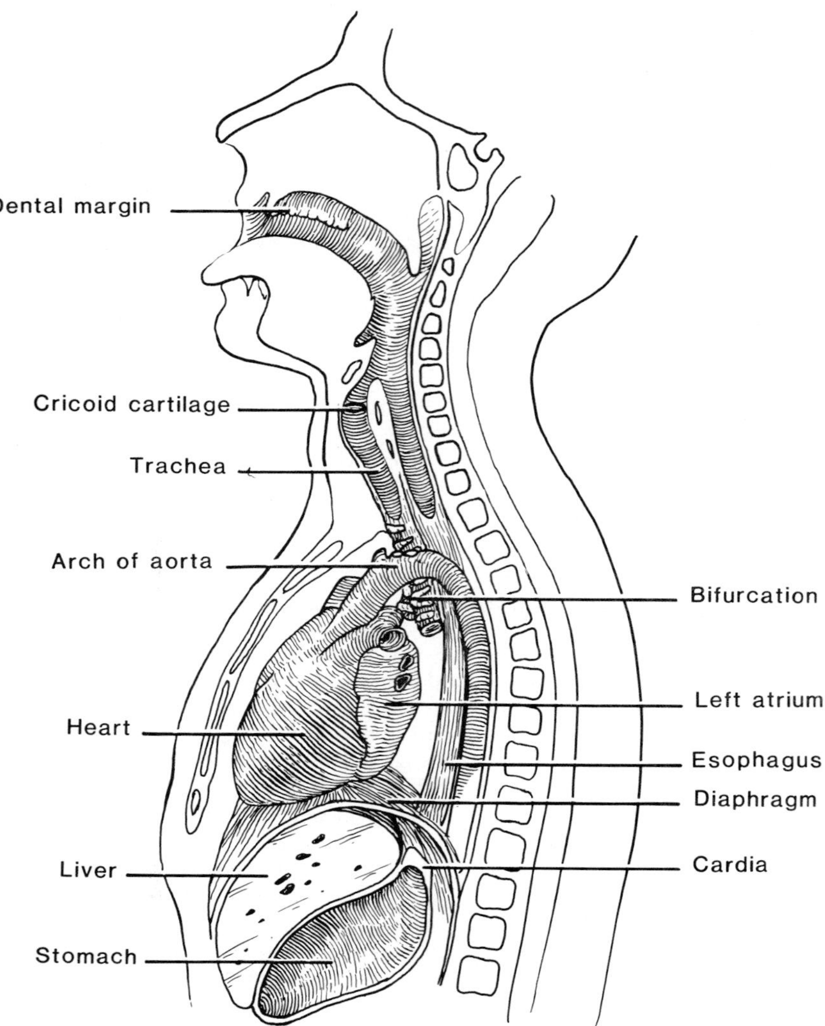

Fig. 37-1. Anatomic relations of the esophagus (seen from the left side). The esophagus is about 25 cm (10 in) long. The distance from the upper incisor teeth to the beginning of the esophagus (cricoid cartilage) is about 15 cm (6 in); from the upper incisors to the level of the bronchi, 22 to 23 cm (9 in); to the cardia, 40 cm (16 in). Structures contiguous to the esophagus that affect esophageal function are demonstrated.

Cause

There are two basic causes for dysphagia, either mechanical narrowing or obstruction of the lumen, or motor disorders (Table 37-1). Mechanical problems stem from abnormality in the lumen (e.g., foreign body), in the wall (peptic stricture of the submucosa, or esophageal cancer), or extrinsic to the esophagus from encroachment by surrounding structures (goiter, enlarged subcarinal lymph nodes). Motor disorders include those due to intrinsic muscular or nervous disorders of the esophagus or pharynx, and those due to central nervous lesions.

Characteristics

Dysphagia can be characterized by (1) the onset, that is, the caliber, character, and temperature of food causing it, (2) the location of the dysphagia, and (3) how it is relieved (Table 37-2).

Mechanical problems cause solid foods to stick in the esophagus. The caliber of spongy-type foods which can be swallowed decreases relentlessly over a short period of time if dysphagia is due to esophageal cancer, and more slowly if it is due to benign stricture. Fluids can usually be swallowed until the stricture is far advanced or the narrowing is suddenly blocked by a solid bolus of food or another foreign body (e.g., enteric-coated pills). Peptic stricture can produce the same symptoms, but usually the dysphagia is mild, and accompanied by heartburn due to the esophagitis. Difficulty in swallowing liquids, especially if they are cold, is a symptom of a motor disorder.

Specific Types of Dysphagia

Transfer Dysphagia

Transfer dysphagia is the inability of to initiate the act of swallowing (deglutition). Inflammatory lesions which are painful or cause mechanical obstruction, and neuromuscular disorders, are the usual causes for this disorder. Failure of the muscles of mastication and salivary lubrication also cause this problem, but less frequently.

Painful lesions of the tongue, oropharynx, and larynx can cause transfer dysphagia, along with odynophagia. Examples include pharyngitis of bacterial (streptococcal), viral (herpetic), and fungal (monilial) origin. The latter two occur especially in the immunocompromised patient. Parapharyngeal abscesses and tonsillitis may cause mechanical obstruction as well as odynophagia with dysphagia. Foreign bodies stuck in the throat, especially in the young and the old, and epiglottitis in the young also can lead to this symptom. Finally, cancers of the head and neck which invade the tongue and throat, and operations to cure the lesions, are an increasing cause of transfer dysphagia.

Patients with mechanical causes of transfer dysphagia tend to drool because of mechanical obstruction or pain. They are often hoarse and have a bad cough because of the laryngeal involvement. The diagnosis is made by direct laryngoscopy, except in the child with possible epiglottitis, who must be intubated in the operating room under anesthesia.

Neuromuscular causes of transfer dysphagia include cerebrovascular accidents, polio and bulbar palsies, dermatomyositis, and poly-

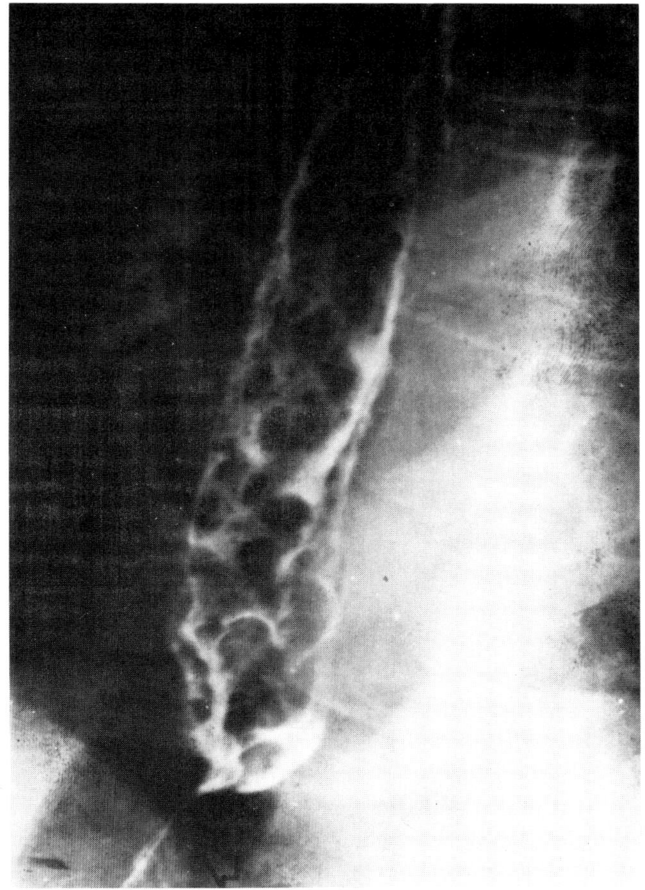

Fig. 37-2. Esophageal varices. Current therapy includes a vasopressin drip followed by esophagoscopy and an attempt at sclerotherapy to stop the bleeding.

myositis. The symptoms most associated with neuromuscular weakness are nasopharyngeal regurgitation, and cough and hoarseness due to laryngeal aspirations. A Zenker's diverticulum may also be found associated with these diseases (Tables 37-1 and 37-2).

Rare but curable, causes of transfer dysphagia in younger age groups include myasthenia gravis, thyrotoxic myopathy and lead poisoning.

Table 37-2. Characteristics of Dysphagia

	Mechanical Narrowing (Tumors, Strictures)	Motor Disorder (Achalasia, Scleroderma)
Onset	Gradual or sudden	Usually gradual
Progressive	Often	Usually not
Type of bolus	Solids (unless high-grade obstruction)	Solids and/or liquids
Temperature-dependent	No	Worse with cold liquids; may improve with warm liquids
Response to bolus impaction	Often must be regurgitated	Can usually be passed by repeated swallowing or by washing it down with fluids

Esophageal Body Dysphagia

Mechanical causes of esophageal body dysphagia in the young include congenital stricture, swallowed foreign bodies, and vascular ring anomalies of the aortic arch. In the older patient the most common causes include reflux esophagitis, webs, rings, and cancer of the esophagus (Table 37-1). Increasingly, infections caused by herpesvirus, cytomegalovirus, and *Candida albicans* are the cause of dysphagia in the immunocompromised or immunosuppressed patient.

The most important neuromuscular causes of dysphagia include achalasia, diffuse spasm, and scleroderma; achalasia-caused dysphagia is associated with esophageal retention and regurgitation of retained food. X-ray films show a dilated esophagus with a distal beak. The diagnosis is confirmed by manometry of the LES, where the pressure remains high even during swallowing.

Diffuse spasm causes dysphagia associated with esophageal colic (see ''Esophageal Colic'' below). Segmental contractions are seen on barium swallow, and some peristaltic waves interspersed with simultaneous prolonged high-amplitude contractions are seen on manometric studies. Many patients are admitted to the coronary care unit on several occasions before a barium swallow, esophageal manometry, and coronary arteriography prove the esophageal rather than the myocardial origin of the pain.

Dysphagia associated with scleroderma usually is associated with symptoms of reflux. Aperistalsis seen on a simple barium swallow is diagnostic, but often single or multiple contractions are seen, and in such cases the barium swallow is not diagnostic.

If a patient has dysphagia, odynophagia, or esophageal colic, an emergency barium swallow, when positive, will lead to a diagnosis

Table 37-1. Causes of Dysphagia

	Extrinsic	Intrinsic
Acquired, infectious		Poliomyelitis, diphtheria, botulism, rabies, tetanus, *Candida*, herpes, cytomegalovirus
Congenital	Vascular abnormalities, webs	
Immunologic		Dermatomyositis, polymyositis scleroderma, multiple sclerosis, myasthenia gravis
Neurologic		Stroke, Parkinson's, chorea, pseudobulbar palsy
Physical, inflammatory	Cervical spurs, stricture (caustic, reflux), Schatzki's ring	Esophagitis
Mechanical	Foreign body, food, pills	
Cardiovascular	Aortic aneurysm, left atrial enlargement	
Endocrine, metabolic	Goiter	Lead poisoning, magnesium deficiency, thyrotoxicosis
Neoplastic	Benign and malignant tumors of esophagus, larynx, lung, pericardium, tracheobronchial tree, thyroid; metastatic disease in mediastinal lymph nodes	
Others	Zenker's diverticulum, paraesophageal hernia	Achalasia, spontaneous intramural hemorrhage

of mechanical or neuromuscular esophageal disease, and appropriate referral. Unfortunately, motor diseases of the esophagus, except for achalasia, may not be evident at the time of the initial barium swallow, especially diffuse esophageal spasm.

Odynophagia (Pain on Swallowing)

Odynophagia is defined as pain upon swallowing. It can be associated with bolus arrest (dysphagia) but may be experienced without arrest of the bolus. Odynophagia and dysphagia are the cardinal symptoms of esophageal disease.

The pain is associated with inflammation of the esophageal mucosal surface commonly seen in such conditions as gastroesophageal reflux, radiation, viral esophagitis, or trauma causing laceration or perforation.

Odynophagia appears at the time of bolus transmission and disappears when the material has left the esophagus. Therefore, unlike pain of cardiac origin, it comes with swallowing and disappears within 10 s. It may be mild or so intense that the patient refuses to swallow solids, liquids, or saliva.

Esophageal Colic

Esophageal colic is an acute, agonizing, spasmodic, or crescendo-like pain that can mimic myocardial ischemia. Like all colic, it is due to an acute stretching or distension of a hollow muscular tube when the forward propulsion of the contents is blocked; or it is due to the acute vigorous contraction or spasm of the esophageal musculature secondary to stimulation. The spasm may be a direct consequence of odynophagia or reflux but is not relieved by antacids. Colic may therefore occur both in conditions that cause mechanical narrowing of the lumen and in motor disorders that cause esophageal spasm. Both distension and spasm may be caused by the same disease.

The acute and crescendo-like pain is experienced substernally and radiates directly through to the back into the interscapular area. It may also radiate into the neck, jaw, or arms. It lasts from 5 to 10 s to hours and usually is indistinguishable from angina pectoris in terms of intensity, radiation, and relation to exercise or relief with nitroglycerin, except that it usually takes 7 to 10 min for relief instead of 2 to 3 min. It is often an associated symptom in patients with dysphagia.

Heartburn (Pyrosis)

Heartburn is the most common symptom of esophageal disease. Unlike the first three symptoms, it is not associated with the swallowing of solids or fluids but rather with reflux of acid or alkaline contents of the stomach into the esophagus, altering the pH and causing inflammation and/or ulceration.

The inflammatory response depends upon the frequency and amount of acid or alkali refluxed and the rate at which it is cleared from the mucosal surface. Biopsy changes show thickening of the basal layer of the esophageal mucosa with extension of the dermal pegs to the free surface in the mildest cases of reflux esophagitis. In more severe cases the epithelial layer is obviously inflamed at esophagoscopy, and microscopically the mucosa is covered with microulcers and the lamina propria has the classic pathologic signs of inflammation.

Heartburn is perceived as a burning discomfort in the substernal area. It appears after meals, especially large ones containing fat, is worse in recumbency or with exercise, and is relieved by antacids, if only temporarily.

Regurgitation

Regurgitation is the retrograde propulsion of fluid into the mouth. It is different from rumination, in which recently eaten food is propelled back into the mouth by a strong contraction of the abdominal wall musculature.

Regurgitation is usually due to the stomach or duodenal contents leaking through an incompetent LES. It is, therefore, associated with reflux esophagitis and heartburn. It can also be associated with the emptying of a diverticulum or with regurgitation of the retained portion of fluid in achalasia.

Regurgitation causes a bitter or acid taste in the mouth, and is usually associated with increased intraabdominal pressure resulting from bending over, lying down, or lifting heavy objects.

Regurgitation of diverticular contents or from achalasia, on the other hand, usually produces undigested, foul-tasting food, with an odor from the mouth due to the presence of putrid food. Both types of regurgitation may produce aspiration, recurrent pneumonia, and failure to thrive.

The Bleeding Esophagus

Patients with bleeding from the esophagus may present in a variety of ways, including acute, life-threatening hematemesis, coffee-ground emesis or gastric aspirate, melena, hematest-positive stools, or anemia of chronic, occult loss, depending upon the rate and duration of bleeding. Bleeding from the esophagus, like bleeding from other parts of the gastrointestinal tract, may be classified according to the amount, source, and symptoms produced by the bleeding at presentation.

Amount

Bleeding from the esophagus can be classified according to the amount of blood replacement needed to restore blood volume while the patient is in the emergency department. There are four degrees: mild, moderate, major, and life-threatening.

Mild Blood Loss

Mild blood loss (less than 10 percent of blood volume) is due to capillary bleeding or to sudden, nonrecurring aterial bleeding. Volume replacement is unnecessary. The cause may be inflammation, infection (especially in immunosuppressed persons), or injury.

Moderate Blood Loss

Moderate blood loss (10 to 20 percent) is due to laceration of an artery or nondistended vein. Bleeding may not stop during treatment in the emergency department. Infusion of 1 L of crystalloid, and possibly 1 to 2 units of blood, is needed to restore blood volume. The patient may be sent to a regular hospital bed if there is no need to continue intravenous replacement (signifying the bleeding has stopped) or to a critical care unit if continued volume replacement indicates continued bleeding.

Major Blood Loss

Major blood loss (20 to 40 percent) is due to a lacerated varix or an artery that has been eroded by a peptic ulcer but cannot retract because it is bound down by scar tissue. The measure of major bleeding in the emergency department is that the patient needs at least 1 L of saline and 2 to 4 units of blood to restore blood volume. These patients must be sent to a critical care unit. Fiberoptic endoscopy should be carried out promptly to establish the diagnosis.

Life-Threatening or Massive Blood Loss

Massive blood loss (more than 40 percent) can be due to a perforated artery at the base of a peptic ulcer, but is more likely due to a ruptured varix. The patient needs more than 4 units of blood in addition to the initial crystalloid replacement, and the source tends to continue bleeding. The source of bleeding should be confirmed by endoscopy in the emergency department. Coagulation abnormalities should be sought and corrected. If esophageal varices are the cause, a vasopressin drip using 20 units in 200 mL of saline at 0.25 to 0.5 unit per minute is given. If bleeding continues, sclerotherapy or Gelfoam embolization of the left gastric vein or use of a Blakemore or similar type tube should be considered. Other methods to control esophageal bleeding are inpatient decisions.

Source

Gastrointestinal bleeding originates from three sources:

1. *Capillary bleeding* is usually due to esophagitis. Capillary bleeding is mild, but it also tends to cause anemia, which may be profound because of its chronic and undetected nature. If bleeding from esophagitis produces emesis, it is a coffee-ground color rather than bright red because the blood drips into the stomach and is changed before regurgitation. Capillary bleeding is rarely the cause of melena or vomiting of red blood.
2. *Arterial bleeding* is usually due to an artery which has been perforated by a penetrating peptic esophageal ulcer or to a laceration of the esophagus due to instrumentation, foreign body ingestion, or violent vomiting (Mallory-Weiss tear).

   Arterial bleeding is usually mild or moderate, and presents with vomiting of bright-red blood and/or melena. The bleeding is episodic, and the episode has usually stopped by the time the patient reaches the emergency department, although he or she may be in hypovolemic shock.
3. *Venous bleeding* from lacerations of the submucosal plexus of veins in a patient without portal hypertension may produce mild to moderate bleeding. However, the most common form of venous bleeding is from varices. It is usually massive and life-threatening, associated with portal pressure in excess of 15 mmHg, and usually with a liver-derived coagulopathy.

EXTRAESOPHAGEAL MANIFESTATIONS OF ESOPHAGEAL DISEASE

Many patients with esophageal disease present with symptoms that do not directly relate to the esophagus but which are extraesophageal manifestations (EEM) of esophageal disease.

The common EEM in the adult include pulmonary symptoms, weight loss due to starvation, and iron deficiency anemia. The EEM in infants and retarded children include pulmonary symptoms and failure to thrive.

Chest Pain of Esophageal Origin

Pain arising from the esophagus is the most alarming esophageal symptom since it often mimics chest pain due to mediastinitis or cardiac ischemia. Pain due to esophageal abnormality tends to be associated with dysphagia, odynophagia, pyrosis, epigastric bloating, belching, and reflux. If a careful search for these symptoms is made, many patients with esophageal causes for their chest pain can be separated from those who have myocardial infarction. Relief of chest pain by antacids or repeated swallowing, especially of warm liquids, and liberal use of a barium swallow can identify most of the leftover group.

Unfortunately, precipitation of pain by exercise and relief by rest, mimicking angina pectoris, are found in patients with atypical esophageal colic due to reflux esophagitis or diffuse spasm. Moreover, Nitroglycerin relieves pain of both esophageal and cardiac origin. Pain relief in the esophageal group, however, usually takes 7 to 10 min, while pain from angina responds in 2 to 3 min and pain due to a myocardial infarction does not respond at all. Both types of patients may also have ST abnormalities on an ECG.

Pulmonary Manifestations

Material regurgitated or refluxed into the larynx and the tracheobronchial tree can cause asthmatic-like symptoms in adults, nocturnal or early morning cough, nocturnal wheezing, hoarseness especially on arising, the need to repeatedly clear the throat, and a feeling of constant pressure deep in the neck. Patients may have recurrent bouts of pneumonia with radiographic changes in the right middle lobe and superior segments of both lower lobes. Infants, retarded children and adults, and debilitated people who have suffered strokes are especially prone to aspiration pneumonia.

Aspiration may be caused by transfer dysphagia while awake, reflux from an incompetent LES, or reflux from retained food in achalasia or diverticula while asleep.

Starvation and Failure to Thrive

Starvation and failure to thrive is seen in infants, children, and adults. In adults it is seen with increasing obstruction of the esophagus due to stricture, achalasia, or cancer, or with reflux esophagitis, especially if esophageal colic is present or the patient is mentally retarded or debilitated by a stroke.

MANUAL SKILLS

Nasogastric Intubation

Indications

A nasogastric tube should be passed for diagnostic purposes in all cases of gastrointestinal bleeding and multisystem trauma, most cases of potential esophageal injuries due to ingestion, and intestinal obstruction (Fig. 37-3). Exceptions include actual or suspected laceration or perforation of the esophagus (usual sites are at the upper weak point between the inferior constrictor and the crycothyroid muscle or at the level of LES), near-complete obstruction of the esophagus due to benign or malignant stricture, and the presence of an esophageal foreign body. The nasogastric tube must be placed orally in patients with severe midfacial trauma or rhinorrhea associated with head trauma.

A relative contraindication for placement of a nasogastric tube is a lacerated posterior larynx from whatever cause. In this case the tube should be placed under the direct visualization of a laryngoscope (after the larynx has been anesthetized with a suitable local anesthetic).

Anatomic Considerations

The following points should be recognized when passing a nasogastric tube (see Fig. 37-3).

1. One naris may be blocked. If so, the other naris or the mouth should be used.
2. The tip of the nose should be directed cephalad while the tip of the nasogastric tube is directed horizontally and slightly downward toward the floor of the posterior nares (rather than toward the roof of the anterior nares). Improper direction of the tube is the commonest cause of damage to the nasopharynx (Fig. 37-3).
3. The resistance caused by the spasmodic closure of the soft palate pressing against the superior constrictor can be overcome by having the patient swallow. Swallowing always facilitates tube passage.
4. The next level of resistance is the inferior constrictor approximately 15 to 20 cm from the ala of the nares. The tip of the nasogastric tube will catch, either on the lip formed by the cephalad surface of the cricothyroid muscle posteriorly, the pyriform fossa on either side of the larynx, or the vallecula anterior to the vocal cords or Killian's mouth. These recesses disappear with a conscious swallow with or without the use of water.

   By spasm of the constrictors, the tip may be directed anteriorly through the vocal cords into the trachea. This problem can be alleviated by two maneuvers: first by advancing the tube past this area only during the swallowing motion when the larynx rises to and is covered by the epiglottis, thus making the curve from the posterior tongue continuous with the epiglottis and the anterior lip of the esophagus (Fig. 37-3); and second by flexing the neck so that the chin is on the chest, thus directing the tip of the nasogastric tube posteriorly. Oral intubation with the patient sucking on the tube before swallowing often overcomes the problem when other maneuvers fail.

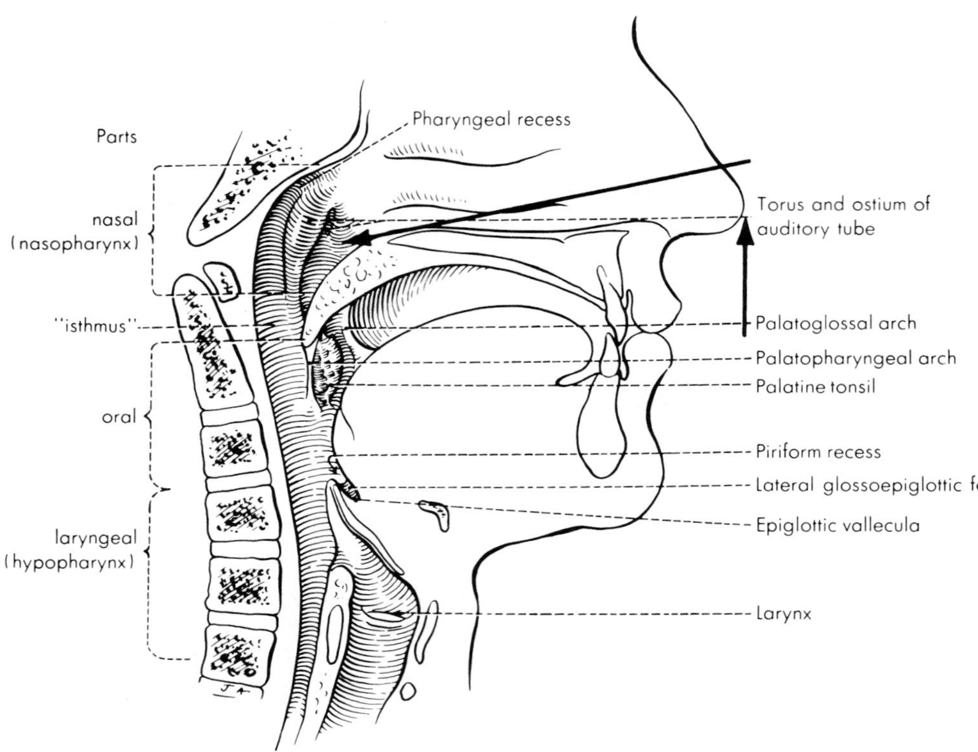

Fig. 37-3. Functional anatomy regarding the passage of tubes into the esophagus. The arrows indicate that the tip of the nose needs to be elevated and the tip of the tube directed along the floor of the naris in order to make the curve at the isthmus.

5. Insertion of the tube by way of the nasal or oral route directly into the esophagus using the Magill forceps and direct laryngoscopy may be used in the patient with an absent swallowing reflex or when it is dangerous to flex the neck, as in the unconscious trauma patient.
6. An alternative method for overcoming misdirection of the nasogastric tube is to place the second and third fingers over the tongue and direct the tips to touch the posterior pharyngeal wall. The tip of the tube is then directed over the dorsal groove formed by the approximation of the fingers.
7. The final resistance to the passage of the tube is at the proximal end of the gastroesophageal junction. This usually is overcome by slow, gentle pressure or, if this fails, by gently injecting 15 to 20 mL of water to relax the lower esophageal sphincter. Occasionally the tip may fail to pass because of a large hiatus hernia, esophageal dilation from achalasia or epiphrenic hernia, or stricture, but this is rare.

Polyethylene nasogastric tubes need not be iced before placing them. Gentle pressure should be sufficient in every case. Resistance to gentle passage indicates misdirection or obstruction. Tube placement should be confirmed by aspiration of gastric contents. If there is any question as to proper location, a radiograph should be taken.

Endoscopy

Endoscopy using a laryngoscope is indicated for removal of foreign bodies from the hypopharynx and those lodged in the constrictor muscle and to aid direction of the tips of esophageal tubes into the esophagus. Local anesthesia must be used in the awake patient, the neck is not extended as in endotracheal intubation, the cervical vertebrae must be known to be intact, and a straight blade is more useful than a curved blade.

Flexible, fiberoptic esophagoscopy should be used for removal of foreign bodies from the esophagus. It is also used to diagnose the site of gastrointestinal bleeding before introduction of a Blakemore tube or to confirm the absence of esophageal bleeding and varices in a patient going directly to surgery for massive bleeding from a suspected gastroduodenal site.

Both topical pharyngeal anesthesia and intravenous sedation are usually required for esophagoscopy.

Blakemore Intubation

Indications

Blakemore intubation is indicated for massive or uncontrolled bleeding which is suspected to arise from the lower 10 cm of the esophagus or from the cardia of the stomach and which is not controlled by vasopressin (see discussion on the bleeding esophagus) or other measures.

Contraindications include bleeding from complete or incomplete lacerations of the esophagus; or peptic ulceration with stricture.

Anatomic Considerations and Procedure

A complete description of how to place the Blakemore tube can be found in the package with the tube. There are, however, some precautions:

1. The tube can be placed through either the nose or the mouth.
2. The same points of obstruction found in placing nasogastric tubes obstruct passage of the Blakemore tube.
3. The oropharynx should be anesthetized prior to placement unless the patient is unconscious or lacks a gag reflex.
4. The site of bleeding must be identified by endoscopy prior to placement unless the rate of bleeding precludes it.
5. The airway must be protected by endotracheal intubation prior to placement.
6. The tip of the tube is best directed over a dorsal groove formed by the second and third fingers, which are in turn pressed loosely against the midposterior pharyngeal wall.

Endotracheal intubation should precede placing a Blakemore tube in any patient, and should be considered with any type of esophageal tube in the unconscious patient. It is necessary to release the cuff pressure while passing the tip of the esophageal tube past the level of the balloon cuff of the endotracheal tube.

ESOPHAGEAL TRAUMA

Etiology

Esophageal injury results from a variety of causes and agents. Because the esophagus is well protected deep in the thoracic cavity, external forces or agents are relatively infrequent causes of esophageal injury, and iatrogenic and self-induced problems predominate.

Pathogenesis and Clinical Presentation

Esophageal injury may be partial- or full-thickness. Partial-thickness tears occur as a result of swallowed foreign bodies or sharp objects (including tortilla chips) and heal spontaneously. They may be associated with dysphagia, odynophagia, esophageal colic, and mild upper gastrointestinal bleeding. Full-thickness injury without perforation results from ingestion of caustic substances or after injection of sclerosing agents in patients with esophageal varices. Perforation of the esophagus from penetrating trauma, foreign bodies, or instrumentation leads to mediastinitis. Early diagnosis is critical to successful treatment. If surgical repair of the perforation is made in less than 24 h, mortality is 5 percent, but if surgical treatment is delayed, mortality is as high as 75 percent.

Laceration of the mucosa and submucosa (Mallory-Weiss syndrome) and perforation of the full thickness of the thoracic and abdominal esophageal wall (Boerhaave's syndrome) are associated with a sudden, violent, and usually repeated increase in the intraabdominal pressure against a weakened esophageal wall. The cause of the sudden increase in abdominal pressure is a Valsalva movement, which usually implies a closed glottis during hiccuping, defecation, labor, epileptic attack, or lifting a heavy weight. Other causes include striking the steering wheel or compression during external heart massage. The most common cause of increased intraabdominal pressure is violent and repeated emesis.

Predisposing causes for a weakened esophageal wall include emesis in which the mucosa at the gastroesophageal junction prolapses into the esophageal lumen through the narrow hiatus and gastroesophageal junction. The mucosa becomes edematous and even bruised and inflamed after such an event. The mucosa can also be weakened by the prolonged presence of a nasogastric tube; reflux esophagitis; epiphrenic hernias; or hemorrhage into the esophageal wall.

Mallory-Weiss lacerations, are thought to occur in weakened mucosa, usually on the right posterolateral side, but Boerhaave's perforations tend to rupture on the left posterolateral side of the unsupported part of the abdominal esophageal wall. The lacerations or perforations tend to extend cephalad into the thoracic esophagus. The second most common site for both syndromes is on the right side just below the level of the azygos vein. Laceration or perforation of the cervical esophagus from flexion-hyperextension injury has also been reported as a cause of mediastinitis.

Lacerations cause usually moderate and self-limiting bleeding of the submucosal plexus of veins and arteries. They may also produce dysphagia and odynophagia and be associated with symptoms of reflux esophagitis (predisposing factor).

Perforations of the esophagus associated with Boerhaave's syndrome cause the most malignant type of mediastinitis. The force of expulsion of fluid through the perforation spreads it rapidly through the mediastinum, causing an acid burn to the mediastinal tissues and rapid spread of very virulent bacteria. The patient complains of severe abdominal pain and chest pain which often radiates into the neck. Patients rapidly develop shock and septicemia, leading to death within 48 h. There is often an associated peritonitis with air under the diaphragm, as well as air-fluid levels in the mediastinum and pyopneumothorax.

Symptoms of Laceration and Perforation

Bleeding and dysphagia following at least one episode of previous emesis are the common signs of laceration (see the discussion of the bleeding esophagus, above). Severe and unrelenting chest and neck pain secondary to chemical and then bacterial mediastinitis, followed by shock and collapse, are the most outstanding symptoms related to perforation. The clinical and radiologic signs of perforation are related to the level of the perforation, and include pleural effusion pneumothorax and pneumomediastinum.

Diagnosis

The most important clue to the diagnosis of esophageal injury is to suspect if from the history. All patients who swallow foreign bodies that obstruct the esophagus are at risk for laceration and perforation. This is especially true of the infant or young child who swallows small alkaline batteries which lodge for an extended time in the hypopharynx or at the level of the aortic arch. Patients who vomit blood or develop chest or abdominal pain after emesis are especially suspect. All unconscious patients who have had instrumentation of the pharynx, larynx, or esophagus, cardiopulmonary resuscitation in the field, or instrumentation or cardiopulmonary resuscitation in the emergency department (with the exception of very routine procedures) should be suspected of having esophageal perforation.

Patients with penetrating wounds of the neck or chest and with crushing wounds to the chest must be suspected of having a ruptured esophagus. In addition, patients who have suspected splenic rupture treated nonoperatively should be observed for a late Boerhaave's rupture, since a predisposing factor to this syndrome is intramural rupture of a short gastric artery that may lead to esophageal intramural hemorrhage.

Patients with chest pain or a history outlined in the previous two paragraphs must have a chest x-ray examination for evidence of a foreign body, perforation, mediastinal fluid, or cardiac and pleural effusions.

If there is radiologic evidence of perforation on posteroanterior and lateral chest x-ray films, a water-soluble contrast study should be done to confirm the diagnosis. Esophagoscopy is only performed if a perforation is suspected but cannot be confirmed by contrast studies, or if there is upper gastrointestinal bleeding associated with a partial-thickness laceration, or if the patient with chest trauma is unconscious and a contrast study cannot be done. Anyone suspected of having a perforation should be given intravenous antibiotics immediately (e.g., cefoxitin and clindamycin), and surgical consultation obtained. Survival is inversely proportional to the length of time between perforation and operative repair.

BIBLIOGRAPHY

Ach RD: Abdominal pain, in Blacklow RS (ed): *MacBryde's Signs and Symptoms, Applied Pathologic Physiology and Clinical Interpretation*, ed 6. Philadelphia, Lippincott, 1983, pp 165–179.

Castell DO: Esophageal chest pain. *Am J Gastroenterol* 79:969, 1984.

Cello JP, Grass RA, Grendell JH, et al: Management of the patient with hemorrhaging esophageal varices. *JAMA* 256:1480, 1986.

Cotton PB, Williams CB: *Practical Gastrointestinal Endoscopy*, ed 2. Oxford, Blackwell Scientific, 1982.

Edwards DAW: Discriminating information in the diagnosis of dysphagia. *J R Coll Physicians Lond* 9:257, 1975.

Fiddian-Green RG, Turcotte JG (eds): Evaluation of the bleeding patient, *and* Variceal bleeding in *Gastrointestinal Hemorrhage*. New York, Grune & Stratton, 1980, pp 3–80 and 233—328.

Han SY, McElvein RB Aldrete JS: Perforation of the esophagus: Correlation of site and cause with plain film findings. *AJR* 145:537, 1985.

Henderson RD, et al: Atypical chest pain of cardiac and esophageal origin. *Chest* 73:24, 1978.

Rostein OD, Rhame FS, Molina E, et al: Mediastinitis after whiplash injury. *Can J Surg* 29:54, 1986.

Shackelford RT: *Surgery of the Alimentary Tract*, vol. 1, ed 3. Philadelphia, Saunders, 1990.

Temple DM, McNeese MC: Hazards of battery ingestion. *Pediatrics* 71:100, 1983.

38
SWALLOWED FOREIGN BODIES

Wade R. Gaasch
Robert A. Barish

INTRODUCTION

The problem of swallowed foreign bodies is common, and can range from innocuous to life-threatening. In the United States, approximately 1500 people die yearly as a result of ingesting foreign bodies. Often thought to be confined to the pediatric population, foreign-body ingestion occurs in all age groups. The pediatric age group accounts for approximately 80 percent of all cases, followed by edentulous adults, prisoners, and psychiatric patients. The presence of dentures eliminates the tactile sensitivity of the palatal surface vital to the identification of small items. A correlation exists between age groups and specific types of ingested material. Children most often ingest coins, toys, crayons, and ballpoint pen caps; adults tend to have problems with meat and bones. In addition, psychiatric patients and prison inmates may ingest such unlikely objects as spoons and razor blades.

PATHOPHYSIOLOGY

The majority of objects pass spontaneously; 10 to 20 percent require some intervention, and only 1 percent require surgical treatment. Ingested foreign bodies may be found anywhere throughout the digestive tract, but there are several physiologic "narrow spaces" where the majority of articles tend to lodge. In the pediatric esophagus, there are five areas of constriction where coins and other objects may become trapped: cricopharyngeal narrowing (C6), the most common site; thoracic inlet (T1); aortic arch (T4); tracheal bifurcation (T6); and hiatal narrowing (T10-T11).

Once an object has traversed the pylorus, it usually continues to the rectum and is passed in the stool. If, however, the object has irregular or sharp edges, it may become lodged anywhere in the GI tract. Objects that lodge in the esophagus (not necessarily limited to sharp or irregular contour) can result in airway obstruction, stricture, or perforation with resultant mediastinitis, cardiac tamponade, paraesophageal abscess, or aortotracheoesophageal fistula.

Perforation may be the result of direct mechanical erosion, as with bones, or chemical corrosion, as with button batteries. Button batteries may cause burn damage in addition to chemical damage. The chemical composition of the battery may also play a role in the degree of mucosal injury. Batteries with mercury and alkaline manganese cells have been reported to result in more significant damage than batteries with silver and lithium cells and therefore may require more expeditious evaluation and treatment. Esophageal damage can occur within a short period of time after a button battery becomes lodged in the esophagus. Once the battery has traversed the esophagus, it is unlikely to lodge at any other location. The theoretical threat of heavy metal poisoning from button batteries has not been supported by clinical experience. Most ingested objects pass through to the rectum in 48 to 72 h, although it may take up to 6 days in some cases. It has been reported to take as long as 14 days to pass a button battery.

CLINICAL PRESENTATION

Objects lodged in the esophagus generally produce anxiety and discomfort. Adult patients often complain of retrosternal pain. Patients are likely to retch or vomit, and there may be dysphagia resulting in choking, coughing, or aspiration when the patient attempts to wash down the object. Eventually, the patient may be unable to swallow his or her own secretions. In the adult, the history often provides all the pertinent information necessary for diagnosis and treatment. However, this is often not true with foreign-body ingestion in the pediatric population. In the 16-and-under age group, symptoms include refusal to eat, vomiting (with or without hematemesis), gagging, choking, stridor ("pseudo-asthma"), neck or throat pain, inability to swallow, increased salivation, and foreign-body sensation in the chest.

Physical examination must include the careful evaluation of the nasopharynx, oropharynx, neck, and subcutaneous tissues for air resulting from perforation of a hollow viscus. Laryngoscopy, either direct or indirect, should be done, especially when the patient complains of a sticking sensation or has ingested a bone. Although physical signs are not always present, findings consistent with foreign-body ingestion in the 16-and-under age group consist of red throat, dysphagia, palatal abrasion, temperature elevation, anxiety and distress, and peritoneal signs.

EMERGENCY DEPARTMENT MANAGEMENT

General Care

Since the great majority of ingested foreign bodies traverse the entire GI tract without any problem, treatment can be expectant once the object has passed through the pylorus. If, however, a foreign body obstructs the esophagus, prevention of aspiration is paramount. This can be accomplished by inserting a nasogastric tube above the obstructing body to remove unswallowed fluids above the impaction.

The offending object can be located in several ways. If radiopaque, the object will be demonstrated on standard x-rays of the neck and/or abdomen. If the foreign body is not visible on x-ray, the physician must use indirect methods, such as an esophagram, or direct visualization utilizing fiberoptic endoscopy. The use of endoscopy may enable the physician to remove the object at the time of visualization, making surgical intervention unnecessary. Progress of the object through the GI tract must be monitored with repeat abdominal x-rays, usually 2 to 4 h apart. Repeated abdominal examinations should be done to detect early signs of developing peritonitis should perforation occur. Virtually all symptomatic patients will require observation and esophagoscopy. If a nonfood object becomes lodged in the esophagus or is unable to pass through the pylorus, it must be removed as soon as possible, utilizing esophagogastroscopy. Fatal lead encephalopathy has been reported in a child who had ingested a lead curtain weight which theoretically had been in the stomach for an extended period of time.

Food Impaction

Meat impaction may be treated expectantly providing the patient can manage his or her own secretions. Time and sedation will often allow the meat to pass into the stomach. The bolus should not be allowed to remain impacted longer than 12 h. Endoscopy is the preferred method for removal. Alternatives have been suggested if endoscopy is not available.

The use of proteolytic enzymes, such as an aqueous solution of papain (e.g., Adolph's meat tenderizer), to dissolve a meat bolus has been advocated by some. There have been several reports in the literature, however, of esophageal perforation secondary to the enzymatic action of the solution. Mucosal ischemia resulting from distension of the esophageal wall renders the esophagus more susceptible to enzymatic degradation. Hemorrhagic pulmonary edema has also been reported with aspiration of Adolph's meat tenderizer. Because of this increased incidence of reported complications, and the increasing expertise in the use of endoscopy, proteolytic enzyme therapy is not recommended.

The use of intravenous glucagon to relax esophageal smooth muscle has also been suggested as a method of treating food impaction. The recommended dose is 1 mg, following a test dose to ensure that hypersensitivity does not exist. If the food bolus is not passed in 20 min, an additional 2 mg is given intravenously. An esophagogram must be performed following treatment to ensure passage.

Bell reports the successful use of nifedipine. Nifedipine reduces lower esophageal sphincter (LES) pressure and the amplitude of LES contractions, without changing the amplitude of contractions in the body of the esophagus. By this mechanism a bolus of food lodged in the vicinity of the GE junction may pass. The recommended dose is 10 mg administered sublingually.

Some authors have suggested the use of gas-forming agents in patients with esophageal food impactions, causing the bolus either to be forced into the stomach or regurgitated into the oropharynx where it can easily be retrieved. Pathology of the esophagus is present in 97 percent of adults presenting with meat impaction, and barium swallow must be performed to confirm foreign-body clearance and to evaluate possible underlying pathology.

Coin Ingestion

Up to 35 percent of children with a coin lodged in the esophagus will be asymptomatic, and some authors recommend that all children who swallow coins have radiographs performed to determine the location of the coin. Coins in the esophagus lie in the frontal plane; coins in the trachea lie in the sagittal plane. The coin in the esophagus will show on routine films, but a coin in the trachea will be viewed on end and may not be visible. The use of a Foley catheter, initially reported in the late 1960s, has been promoted as a safe and effective technique for removal when the coin has been impacted for less than 24 h. The catheter is passed down the esophagus beyond the object, and the balloon inflated. As the catheter is slowly withdrawn, the object is withdrawn along with it. Retrieval of a coin by this technique is less effective after 24 h. Although most prefer using the Foley catheter under fluoroscopy, Foster notes his preference to perform the procedure in the emergency department, where the necessary experienced personnel, equipment, and supplies are available to perform pediatric resuscitation. Foley catheter retrieval of foreign bodies may be complicated by aspiration.

Button Battery Ingestion

A button battery lodged in the esophagus is a true emergency because of the extremely rapid action of the alkaline substance on the mucosa. Once the battery is in the stomach, it usually passes without difficulty; however, daily radiographs should be taken to confirm movement through the GI tract. Kuhns and Dire have developed a flowchart for the management of ingested button batteries (see Fig. 38-1).

Miscellaneous Ingestion

Management of sharp and pointed foreign bodies is controversial. Objects longer than 5 cm and wider than 2 cm will rarely pass the stomach. These and objects with extremely pointed edges such as open safety pins or razor blades, must be removed by endoscopy. In general, all sharp and pointed foreign bodies should be removed before they pass from the stomach because 15 to 35 percent will cause intestinal perforation, usually in the ileocecal valve.

Paul recommends the following management for *children* who have swallowed sharp objects. All patients should have an initial x-ray and physical examination. If the patient is symptomatic, or has ingested a sewing needle, surgical consultation for possible endoscopy and laparotomy is indicated. Management of asymptomatic sharp object ingestion other than sewing needles may be on an expectant basis. Progression of sharp object ingestion should be documented with serial radiographs. If progression past the stomach is not seen, a water-soluble contrast x-ray may document GI perforation. At the first sign of perforation the object should be removed even if the patient remains asymptomatic. If the object does not progress through the GI tract, surgical retrieval is indicated.

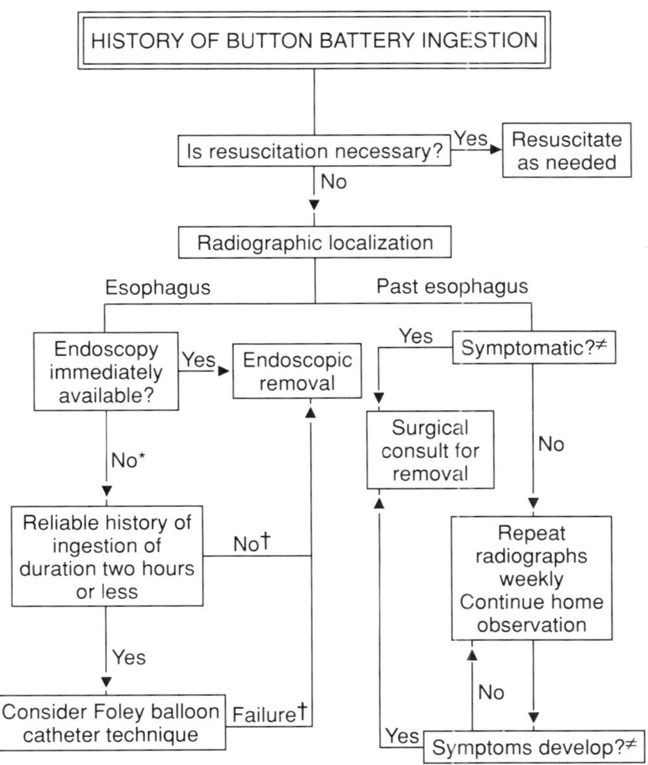

* Button batteries in the esophagus must be removed. Endoscopy should be used if available. The balloon catheter technique can be used if the ingestion is less than two hours old, but should not be used after this since it may increase the amount of damage to the weakened esophagus.

† When the Foley technique fails or is contraindicated due to a greater than two-hour elapsed time period, the button battery should be removed endoscopically. This may require transfer of the patient.

≠ Acute abdomen, tarry or bloody stools, fever, persistent vomiting

Fig. 38-1. Algorithm for management of button battery ingestion. (*Adapted from* Kuhns DW, Dire DJ: Button battery ingestions. *Ann Emerg Med* 18:293, 1989.)

Cocaine ingestion is an increasingly widespread problem. Carriers will ingest multiple small packets of cocaine in the attempt to conceal the drug. A favored packet is the condom, which may hold up to 5 g of cocaine. Rupture of even one such packet may be fatal. Webb recommends surgery as the safest method of recovery to lessen the likelihood of packet rupture during endoscopic retrieval. If the packet appears to be passing intact through the intestinal tract, one may choose to observe and wait for it to be spontaneously delivered through the rectum.

CONCLUSION

Most cases of foreign-body ingestion require nothing more than observation. Clear exceptions to this are nonfood items lodged in the esophagus and sharp or pointed items that have not yet passed the pylorus. Those foreign bodies which are sharp or pointed and have passed the pylorus present an ongoing risk of perforation or obstruction and mandate endoscopic or surgical consultation.

Endscopy remains the most effective nonsurgical interventional method of foreign-body management. There are three indications for surgical removal of a foreign body: (1) GI obstruction or perforation,

(2) the existence of toxic constituents, and (3) a length, size, and/or shape that will likely prevent the object from passing safely. Management of asymptomatic patients with prolonged passage should be approached on an individual basis.

Following removal of a foreign body from the esophagus, the patient should have a complete evaluation of esophageal function to ensure that underlying pathology did not lead to the obstruction.

BIBLIOGRAPHY

Bell AF, Eibling DE: Nifedipine in the treatment of distal esophageal food impaction. *Arch Otolaryngol Head Neck Surg* 114:682, 1988.

Binder L, Anderson WA: Pediatric gastrointestinal foreign body ingestions. *Ann Emerg Med* 13:112, 1984.

Caravati EM, Bennett DL, McElwee NE: Pediatric coin ingestion: A prospective study on the utility of routine roentgenograms. *Am J Dis Child* 143:549, 1989.

Dunlap LB: Removal of an esophageal foreign body using a Foley catheter. *Ann Emerg Med* 10:101, 1981.

Durback LF, Wedin GP, Seidler DE: Management of lead foreign body ingestion. *J Toxicol Clin Toxicol* 27:173, 1989.

Fernandes ET, Hollabaugh RS, Boulden T: Mediastinal mass and radiolucent esophageal foreign body. *J Pediatr Surg* 24:1135, 1989.

Friedman EM: Caustic ingestions and foreign bodies in the aerodigestive tract of children. *Pediatr Clin North Am* 36:1403, 1989.

Glauser J, Lilja GP, Greenfield B, et al: Intravenous glucagon in the management of esophageal food obstruction. *JACEP* 8:228, 1979.

Gracia C, Frey CF, Bodai BI: Diagnosis and management of ingested foreign bodies: A ten-year experience. *Ann Emerg Med* 13:30, 1984.

Green GG, Durham TM, King TA: Management of patients with swallowed dental objects. *Am J Dent* 1:147–150, 1988.

Hall ML, Huseby JS: Hemorrhagic pulmonary edema associated with meat tenderizer treatment for esophageal meat impaction. *Chest* 94:640, 1988.

Hugelmeyer CD, Moorhead JC, Horenblas L, Bayer MJ: Fatal lead encephalopathy following foreign body ingestion: Case report. *J Emerg Med* 6:397, 1988.

Krome RL: Swallowed foreign bodies, in Tintinalli JE, Krome RL, Ruiz E (eds): *Emergency Medicine: A Comprehensive Study Guide*, 2/e. New York, McGraw-Hill, 1988, pp 307–308.

Kuhns DW, Dire DJ: Button battery ingestions. *Ann Emerg Med* 18:293, 1989.

Kuzon WM, McFadyen CA, Moffat FL: Unusual gastric foreign body: A case report. *Can J Surg* 31:413, 1988.

Paul RI, Jaffe DM: Sharp object ingestions in children: Illustrative cases and literature review. *Pediatr Emerg Care* 4:245, 1988.

Phillipps JJ, Patel P: Swallowed foreign bodies. *J Laryngol Otol* 102:235, 1988.

Savitt DL, Wason S: Delayed diagnosis of coin ingestion in children. *Am J Emerg Med* 6:378, 1988.

Schunk JE, Corneli H, Bolte R: Pediatric coin ingestions: A prospective study of coin location and symptoms. *Am J Dis Child* 143:546–8, 1989.

Sigalet D, Lees G: Tracheoesophageal injury secondary to disc battery ingestion. *J Pediatr Surg* 23:996, 1988.

Suita S, Ohgami H, Nagasaki A, et al: Management of pediatric patients who have swallowed foreign objects. *Am Surg* 55:585, 1989.

Webb WA: Management of foreign bodies of the upper gastrointestinal tract. *Gastroenterology* 94:204, 1988.

Winkler AR, McClenathan DT, Borger JA, et al: Retrograde esophagoscopy for foreign body removal. *J Pediatr Gastroenterol Nutr* 8:536, 1889.

Yasui T: Hazardous effects due to alkaline button battery ingestion: An experimental study. *Ann Emerg Med* 15:901, 1986.

Young TL, Lubitz RM: Cylindrical battery ingestion: A case of endoscopic retrieval. *J Tenn Med Assoc* 82:415, 1989.

Zimmers TE, Chan SB, Kouchoukos PL, et al: Use of gas-forming agents in esophageal food impactions. *Ann Emerg Med* 17:693, 1988.

39 PEPTIC ULCER DISEASE

Ronald L. Krome

Although considered a chronic disease characterized by long asymptomatic periods interspersed with symptomatic episodes, peptic ulcer disease can run a rapidly fulminant course.

A peptic ulcer is a mucosal defect extending beyond the muscularis mucosae and occurring in acid-secreting epithelium. Most peptic ulcers occur along the lesser curvature of the stomach or in the first portion of the duodenum. Less common sites include the distal esophagus, ectopic gastric mucosa in a Meckel's diverticulum, or margins of surgical anastomoses. Factors that predispose to ulcer formation include cigarette smoking and coffee, cola, or alcohol ingestion. Ulcer symptoms tend to become more severe in the spring and in the fall.

Duodenal ulcer is more common in emphysematous patients and in those with chronic pancreatitis. Gastric ulceration and erosive gastritis are associated with cirrhosis and/or heavy, chronic alcohol ingestion.

Endocrine abnormalities associated with an increased frequency of peptic ulceration are the Zollinger-Ellison syndrome and hyperparathyroidism. Ulcers associated with the Zollinger-Ellison syndrome tend to occur, or reoccur, in unusual locations and are very resistant to antacid therapy. Ulcers also occur in children. Most often they are duodenal or prepyloric in location.

Although the incidence of peptic ulcer and its complications appears to be decreasing, this is not the case in the elderly, where the incidence seems to be increasing, perhaps as a result of the increased use of NSAIDs or other physiologic changes in the mucosal barrier. In one study, there was a 35-percent recurrence rate within 1 year of demonstrated healing.

PATHOPHYSIOLOGY

Normally, the epithelium of the stomach and duodenum are protected from the effects of acid and pepsin by mucosal resistance. When an imbalance occurs, peptic ulceration results. Mucosal resistance may be disrupted by the depletion of endogenous prostaglandins.

Although clinically it may be difficult to distinguish gastric and duodenal ulcers, there are substantial differences in development. Gastric ulcers are associated with prolonged gastric emptying times and low, or normal, gastric acid secretions. Duodenal ulcers are associated with hypersecretion, and there is no delay in gastric emptying except as a complication of the ulcer. Duodenal ulcers are more common than gastric ulcers. The development of gastric ulcers may be related to an impairment of the resistance of the gastric mucosa to hydrogen ions. The back diffusion of hydrogen ions into the gastric mucosa is thought to cause bleeding and ulceration. Some agents that alter the mucosal barrier in the stomach are bile salts, aspirin, alcohol, NSAIDs, and indomethacin.

Several factors appear important in the development of duodenal ulcers, but not everyone with a duodenal ulcer demonstrates these characteristics. These include an increased number of parietal cells and an increased sensitivity of the parietal cells to stimulation, impaired inhibition of gastrin release when the antrum is acidified, and faster gastric emptying with the rapid loss of the buffering capacity of food. Factors concerned with mucosal defense are probably more important than acid and pepsin activity, and may be related to the depletion of endogenous prostaglandins.

CLINICAL FEATURES

The primary manifestation of peptic ulcer disease is burning epigastric distress. The burning pain may extend across the upper abdomen, or, if the ulcer is located posteriorly and penetrates into the pancreas, the pain may go straight through to the back. The pain of a gastric ulcer tends to occur immediately after eating, while that of a duodenal ulcer tends to occur between meals, typically 2 h after eating. The burning pain of a duodenal ulcer also tends to wake the patient during the night.

Pain relief may result from a wide variety of over-the-counter medications, and the patient often gives a history of trying several different kinds before seeking medical attention. Even though almost one-third of patients with complications from their ulcers give no history of diagnosed ulcer disease, the majority describe the use, sometime in the past, of over-the-counter medication.

Characteristically, then, the pain is burning, located in the epigastric region, occasionally radiating into the back (straight back), and may be worse at times when the stomach is empty—at night and between meals. Symptoms are usually periodic and recurrent. Definitive diagnosis is made with endoscopy and/or barium studies.

TREATMENT

Mild pain is generally treated with medical therapy: frequent feeding; avoidance of alcohol, coffee, tea, and smoking; antacids; perhaps mild sedatives or tranquilizers; and possibly anticholinergics, except when there is suspicion of pyloric obstruction or if bladder outlet obstruction may be present. If the patient is taking NSAIDs, they should be discontinued. About 50 percent of patients experience recurrence within a year of termination of antiulcer medication.

More severe pain requires more stringent treatment, which may acutely include nasogastric suction, bed rest, sedation, H_2-receptor antagonists, and antacids. For a duodenal ulcer, 30 mL of antacid should be given 1 and 3 h after eating with an additional 30 mL at bedtime. If the patient is on nasogastric suction, no antacids are required, since the tube keeps the stomach empty and prevents the accumulation of acids. The buffering effect of antacids is prolonged if they are taken with food. Without food, the buffering effect lasts about 45 to 60 min.

The nasogastric tube not only removes acid-containing gastric fluid but also decreases gastric retention, distension, and stasis. Gastric distension acts as a stimulus to the antrum, increasing gastrin secretion and then acid secretion.

Cimetidine, a member of a class of drugs that are histamine (H_2 receptor) antagonists and inhibit gastric acid secretion, may be useful in the treatment of duodenal ulcer disease. It has been shown to decrease gastric acid secretion by about 70 percent.

The use of cimetidine and other H_2 receptor antagonists has made a significant impact on the treatment of peptic ulcer disease. The necessity for elective surgery for peptic ulcer problems has greatly diminished, although the incidence of perforation and rebleeding has not been significantly reduced. The use of H_2-receptor antagonists in bleeding has reduced the mortality from the initial bleeding episode. Both cimetidine and ranitidine have been shown to produce healing in about 70 percent of cases for 1 year. However, they are palliative, not curative, and neither has been shown to be any better, overall, than antacids. Carafate has produced healing in 75 percent of uncomplicated peptic ulcers for 1 year.

When cimetidine has been used at a dosage of 400 mg twice a day, short-term healing of gastric and duodenal ulcers has been impressive, with a healing rate of 68 to 95 percent. Complications of therapy do occur, including interaction with other medications dependent on hepatic degradation. H_2-receptor antagonists decrease hepatic blood flow, and consequently, blood levels of drugs that are metabolized by the liver will be higher than anticipated. These drugs include warfarin-type anticoagulants, phenytoin, propranolol, diazepam, lidocaine, and theophylline. In addition, care must be taken in administering H_2-receptor antagonists in patients with diminished renal function. Adverse reactions to cimetidine itself do not appear to be significantly different from those in patients taking placebo. Use of H_2-receptor antagonists in children has also been successful, and complications have been minimal.

COMPLICATIONS

In addition to intractable pain, i.e., pain that does not respond to conventional medical therapy, or pain that repeatedly incapacitates the patient for a prolonged period of time, the other major complications are bleeding, pyloric obstruction, and perforation.

Hemorrhage

Peptic ulcer disease, despite the advent of cimetidine, remains one of the major causes of massive upper gastrointestinal (GI) bleeding in the United States. Massive bleeding is generally defined as a loss of 1500 or 2000 mL of blood in an adult, or the need to replace 30 percent of a patient's blood volume over 12 h in order to maintain vital signs.

Initial management should consist of rapid fluid replacement using either Ringer's lactate or normal saline with transfusions of blood as indicated to maintain the patient's vital signs. Two large-bore intravenous lines should be inserted; one of them should be a central line to monitor central venous pressure (CVP). The rapidity of fluid replacement should be assessed by monitoring the patient's vital signs, CVP, and hourly urinary output. Transfusion of blood, or blood components, should be based on the patient's response to fluid administration. In addition, if the patient has angina or an earlier history of a myocardial infarction, transfusion may be indicated to maintain the patient's oxygen-carrying capacity. When chest pain consistent with angina occurs in these patients it should be interpreted as an indication for transfusion. Oxygen should be administered at a flow rate of 6 to 8 L/min, depending on the presence of any intercurrent disease.

Nasogastric suction should be instituted to confirm the presence of acute and current bleeding and to begin lavage of the stomach. Constant nasogastric suction is indicated, with lavage to slow or stop the bleeding. Antacids may be given through the nasogastric tube, even as a constant drip. Saline lavage is not universally successful, but it should be done in every patient. All clot should be removed because the presence of clot in the stomach may produce gastric distension and increase gastric acid secretion. When transfusion becomes mandatory to maintain vital signs, some would consider surgical exploration.

Perforated ulcers are rarely the cause of massive upper GI bleeding, although they are often associated with some bleeding.

Diagnosis should be established as quickly as feasible, since definitive therapy depends on the cause of the bleeding. Endoscopic examination of the esophagus, stomach, and duodenum is becoming the new standard of diagnosis. Upper GI bleeding is probably an indication for emergency and immediate endoscopic examination. If necessary, once stabilized, the patient may have to be transferred to a center where endoscopy can be done. Other diagnostic tools include angiography and barium studies. To be diagnostic, angiography must be done while the patient is actively bleeding.

The chances of the patient's survival with minimum morbidity improve if the patient's bleeding can be controlled without emergency surgical intervention and surgery can be done on an elective basis. Some people consider that one episode of massive bleeding from an ulcer is an indication for surgery, even if done on an elective basis. Cimetidine therapy (300 mg IV every 6 h) may modify this position. However, if massive bleeding occurs, or active bleeding continues despite adequate fluid therapy and blood replacement, prolonged medical management is associated with a greater risk, and emergency surgical intervention is indicated.

Little is known about the factors predisposing to recurrent hemorrhage from peptic ulcers. Patients with chronic ulcers seem to have an increased risk. According to Northfield, patients without any evidence of bleeding for 48 h are unlikely to rebleed in the near future. Patients with a large blood loss in the first episode are more likely to rebleed. Elderly patients with generalized arteriosclerosis have a greater propensity to continue to bleed because the vessels are not soft enough to contract.

Obstruction

Since most ulcers heal by scar formation, when the ulcer is in the pyloric channel or in the antrum, there is a chance for pyloric obstruction to develop, or for antral narrowing to occur and produce gastric outlet obstruction. Obstruction can result in severe gastric distension with intractable vomiting, producing dehydration and metabolic alkalosis. Bile in the vomitus of a patient with peptic ulcer disease rules out, in essence, gastric outlet obstruction.

Treatment consists of constant nasogastric suction for a prolonged period of time. Fluid replacement and correction of electrolyte abnormalities are mandatory. Anticholinergic agents are contraindicated because they may aggravate the distension by decreasing gastric motility. Many surgeons consider that persistent gastric outlet obstruction after several days of nasogastric suction is an indication for surgical intervention.

Perforation

Despite the impact of cimetidine on the treatment of peptic ulcer disease and some complications, the incidence of perforation does not appear to have been significantly reduced. Perforation is characterized by the sudden onset of severe epigastric pain. Often the patient can give the exact time that the pain began. If the gastric contents run down the colonic gutter, right lower quadrant pain may also occur. In this case, the picture may resemble that of acute appendicitis. The abdomen may be rigid. Percussion may reveal a lack of liver dullness in the right upper quadrant because of the presence of free air in the peritoneum. An upright view of the chest may show free air under the diaphragm, but this is not a universal finding. Free air under the diaphragm on an upright abdominal film is more difficult to detect. If free air is not demonstrated on the upright film of the chest, a lateral decubitus film of the abdomen may be helpful. If a further attempt to demonstrate free air is needed, the stomach can be filled with air (300 to 500 mL) using the nasogastric tube. Clamping the tube and allowing the patient to sit up for 5 to 15 min may make the air demonstrable. Both ports of the Salem sump tube must be clamped when air is inserted. Free air is present in only 51 percent of patients with perforations. Shock results from primary chemical and secondary bacterial peritonitis; generalized sepsis will follow if aggressive treatment is not instituted. Posterior penetration may result in pancreatitis.

Treatment consists of constant nasogastric suction, fluid and electrolyte replacement, and appropriate antibiotic therapy. In the United States, surgery remains the definitive therapy for perforations. Histamine H_2 antagonists may reduce the incidence of rebleeding (10 percent), surgery (20 percent), and death (30 percent), although data are still not definitive.

STRESS EROSIONS AND HEMORRHAGIC GASTRITIS

The term *acute mucosal lesions* refers to a variety of lesions involving the gastric mucosa that include Curling's and Cushing's ulcers, stress ulcers, and acute erosive gastritis.

Stress erosions are superficial lesions that do not extend through the muscularis mucosae. They may be multiple and discrete, or diffuse and extensive, and most often they involve the body and fundus of the stomach. They are a common cause of gastric bleeding. Multiple factors involved in the development of stress erosions include an increase in gastric secretion, an alteration in the mucosal barrier to hydrogen ions, and local ischemia.

Stress erosions or acute mucosal lesions can occur after a variety of systemic insults and can develop within hours in conditions such as CNS tumors, head trauma, fractures, burns, sepsis, or shock. Steroids, aspirin, and alcohol all predispose to the development of erosions. In a large series collected by Josen, acute hemorrhagic gastritis accounted for the bleeding in more than half of the patients.

The diagnosis is best made by endoscopic examination. Barium studies are of little help. Since surgery is rarely indicated in these patients, it is imperative that the diagnosis be established as quickly as possible in patients with upper GI bleeding.

Because the gastric mucosa renews itself in 48 to 72 h, medical management is often effective. Cimetidine appears to be of questionable use. In one study of intensive care unit patients, there was a lack of statistical benefit associated with the routine, prophylactic use of cimetidine. Nasogastric suction with saline lavage and the use of antacids may also be effective.

If bleeding is massive and cannot be controlled with the methods described, surgery may be indicated. Because the lesions are generally extensive, the surgery must also be extensive.

BIBLIOGRAPHY

Brooks RP: The pathophysiology of peptic ulcer disease. *Dig Dis Sci* 30:155, 1985.

Collins R, Langman M: Treatment with histamine H_2 antagonists in acute upper gastrointestinal hemorrhage. *N Engl J Med* 313:660, 1985.

Freston MS, Freston JW: Peptic ulcers in the elderly: Unique features and management. *Geriatrics* 45:39, 1990.

Lucas CE, Sugawa C, Riddle J, et al: Natural history and surgical dilemma of stress gastric bleeding. *Arch Surg* 102:266, 1971.

Mouawad E, Deloof T, Genette F, et al: Open trial of cimetidine in the prevention of upper gastrointestinal hemorrhage in patients with severe intracranial injury. *Acta Neurochir* 67:239, 1983.

Northfield TC: Factors predisposing to recurrent hemorrhage after acute gastrointestinal bleeding. *Br Med J* 2:26, 1971.

Paterson WL: Pathogenesis and therapy of peptic ulcer disease. *J Clin Gastroenterol* 12 (suppl 2):1, 1990.

Richter JM, Colditz GA, Huse DM, et al: Cimetidine and adverse reactions: A meta-analysis of randomized clinical trials of short-term therapy. *Am J Med* 87:278, 1989.

Tam PK, Saing H: The use of H_2-receptor antagonists in the treatment of peptic ulcer disease in children. *J Pediatr Gastroenterol Nutr* 8:41, 1989.

Tsang TM, Saing H, Yeung CK: Pediatric ulcer in children. *J Pediatr Surg* 25:744, 1990.

Zuckerman G, Welch R, Douglas A, et al: Controlled trial of medical therapy for active upper gastrointestinal bleeding and prevention of rebleeding. *Am J Med* 76:361, 1984.

40
PERFORATED VISCUS

W. Kendall McNabney

INTRODUCTION

In most cases, perforated viscus leads to such a profound set of symptoms and clear physical findings that recognition and subsequent treatment are straightforward when the patient presents for care. However, there are variables which contribute to a more subtle presentation either because of altered host response to inflammation or because the perforation may be walled off or not involving the free peritoneum.

Nontraumatic perforation of the gastrointestinal (GI) tract is rare if the wall of the viscus is normal. Diligent search will reveal an etiologic factor either involving the wall or leading to rapid, marked increase in intraluminal pressures secondary to distal obstruction. The underlying process may be inflammatory, neoplastic, or iatrogenic, or the result of stone formation. The presence of a self-ingested foreign body must be considered if no other obvious cause is present. Whatever organ is involved, the signs and symptoms of perforation are due first to chemical irritation of the peritoneum and then to infection or sepsis. Therefore, the chemical composition of the contents of the viscus has a significant effect on the development of chemical peritonitis, including the onset and severity.

Patients receiving glucocorticosteroids do not demonstrate the classic signs of perforation. Because symptoms and signs are minimal, such patients have a significant delay in treatment, and mortality approaches 80 percent. Other immunocompromised patients, such as those receiving chemotherapy, AIDS patients, and patients who have received allografts, are subject to both increased risk of perforated viscus as well as delayed recognition.

Sometimes the signs and symptoms of perforation are the first evidence of underlying disease. At other times, there is a symptomatic period relating to the disease process before signs or symptoms of perforation appear. Although most perforations of the GI tract are free into the peritoneum, they may be localized, walled off by the surrounding viscera or omentum, or occur into a limited or restricted space, such as the lesser sac. Perforations may also occur into the retroperitoneal space. Symptoms and signs, then, are generally determined by (1) the viscus involved, (2) the location of the perforation, (3) the volume and chemical composition of the leaking fluids, (4) the underlying disease, and (5) the host response mechanism.

Unless the patient has some significant contraindication, surgical intervention is indicated at the time of diagnosis. Ideally, intervention should occur before any significant contamination or sepsis has occurred, since the amount of contamination is a significant factor in survival. Emergency treatment in all suspected perforations includes (1) nasogastric suction, (2) volume replacement, (3) antibiotics consistent with local protocols, and (4) rapid surgical consultation. Use of analgesia prior to surgical consultation must be guided by the need to provide relief without masking signs or symptoms.

PATHOPHYSIOLOGY

The combined surface area of the peritoneum (visceral and parietal) constitutes about 50 percent of the area of the exterior body surface. Contact of intestinal contents with the peritoneum produces a sudden increase in capillary permeability, with the subsequent exudation of large volumes of plasma into the peritoneal cavity, the bowel lumen, and the bowel wall and mesentery. As much as 4 to 12 L can be shifted into this "third space" within 24 h.

Inflammation of the visceral peritoneum produces a brief period of bowel irritability and hypermotility followed by bowel atony with paralytic (adynamic) ileus and distension. The inflamed bowel no longer absorbs fluid and secretes increased salt and water into the lumen. When distension becomes sufficient to compress capillaries and prevent or compromise circulation to the inflamed area, exudation ceases. The ultimate clinical picture is one of severe hypovolemia and shock.

Fluid loss into this third space causes hypovolemia. Hypovolemia, in turn, results in inadequate cardiac output, compensatory vasoconstriction, and inadequate tissue perfusion. Oliguria, severe metabolic acidosis, and respiratory insufficiency follow if hypovolemia is not rapidly corrected. Peritonitis and septicemia may evolve into septic shock. Correction of hypovolemia is therefore mandatory.

The local response to bacterial invasion from intestinal perforation is complex. Bacterial contamination is generally necessary to produce fatal peritonitis. Endotoxins and exotoxins increase cell permeability and compound the already significant fluid losses into the third space.

Distal obstruction, the amount of contamination, the elapsed time prior to the institution of treatment, and the host response to infection account for the variations in the clinical response to perforation.

Perforated Ulcer

Gastric or duodenal perforations develop more commonly in benign than in malignant ulcers, although malignant gastric ulcers may also perforate. Chemical peritonitis develops in the first 6 to 8 h and is due to the effect of the gastric acid and pepsin on the peritoneum.

In general, posterior duodenal ulcers penetrate into the pancreas rather than freely perforate into the peritoneum, and produce pancreatitis. Free perforation is prevented because of the adherence of the pancreas to the posterior duodenum. Posterior gastric or duodenal ulcers may perforate into the lesser sac, resulting in abscess formation, but this is relatively rare. Anterior ulcers generally perforate into the peritoneal cavity, although the omentum or adjacent structures such as liver or gallbladder may be adherent to the ulcer bed and limit signs and symptoms. An antecedent history of ulcer disease is not always present, and perforation may be the first manifestation. If carefully sought, though, a history of antacid use, mostly of over-the-counter preparations, will usually be found.

The pain of ulcer perforation is usually sudden and severe. The patient may even be able to give the exact time of onset. The pain is usually localized to the epigastric region, although if penetrating or posterior, it may radiate straight through to the back (not around to the back).

Significant upper GI bleeding does not accompany perforation. Whatever bleeding occurs is minimal. Chronic blood loss may occur if the ulcer has been present for a time. As a rule of thumb, massive upper GI bleeding rules out the presence of a perforated ulcer; however, a second penetrating ulcer should be considered.

Gallbladder Perforation

Perforation of the gallbladder is associated with a high mortality, although it has decreased from 20 to 7 percent in the past 25 years. Early surgical intervention improves mortality. The highest mortalities are associated with nonoperative management. Peritonitis is the result of chemical irritation of the peritoneum as well as bacterial contamination.

Because sterile bile may cause only well-tolerated ascites, bacteria must be present to produce clinical peritonitis.

Obstruction of the cystic or common bile duct by stones produces distension of the gallbladder with eventual compromise of the vascular supply and gangrene of the wall with perforation. The stones can erode through the wall of the gallbladder, cystic duct, or common duct. Such erosions more commonly produce fistulas between the gallbladder and another portion of the GI tract than free perforation into the peritoneal cavity. Large gallstones have been found to produce obstruction of the small bowel after such fistula formation, resulting in a syndrome known as *gallstone ileus*.

Gangrene can occur in the gallbladder free of stones, and perforations have been reported in acalculous cholecystitis, especially in diabetics. In one recent study, perforation occurred in the absence of stones in 40 percent of patients. Acalculous cholecystitis most commonly occurs in postoperative, posttrauma, or burn patients secondary to dehydration; with hemolysis from blood transfusions; or with use of narcotics.

Those most at risk are the elderly, the diabetic, and those with a history of stones or repeated cholecystitis. Perforations have also been reported in patients with sickle cell disease or hemolytic anemias. Infection is often associated with cystic or common bile duct obstruction and stone formation. There is a male predominance of 2 or 3 to 1.

The diagnosis is difficult. In Stevens's series of 35 patients, none were diagnosed preoperatively. Although not always present, antecedent signs and symptoms of biliary disease should be sought. Gallbladder perforation should be suspected in an elderly patient with a tender right upper quadrant mass, fever, and leukocytosis who is deteriorating clinically or who develops signs of peritonitis. The bilirubin level may be elevated, and slight elevation of the amylase level is not unusual. Nonalcoholics may give a past history of episodes of jaundice or pancreatitis, which should suggest the presence of common duct stones. Subhepatic or subphrenic abscesses may form as a result of perforation of the gallbladder. On routine x-ray, a stone may be seen free in the abdomen.

Ultrasonography should be performed in all patients suspected of having stones.

Perforation of the Small Bowel

Nontraumatic perforations of the mid-GI tract are very uncommon. Jejunal rupture may result from certain drugs such as enteric-coated potassium tablets which produce ulcerations of the small bowel; infections, such as typhoid or tuberculosis; tumors; strangulated hernia, either internal or external; and, rarely, regional enteritis.

In general, jejunal perforation produces a more severe chemical peritonitis than ileal rupture since the pancreatic juice that leaks out of the upper jejunum has a pH of about 8 and is rich in enzymes such as trypsin, lipase, and amylase. Fluid that leaks from lower jejunal and ileal perforations has less enzymatic activity, and the pH may also be lower. Perforations of the ileum have significant bacterial contamination. If, however, perforation is the result of obstruction, as in appendicitis followed by perforation, the clinical course is likely to be serious regardless of the level of perforation. This is because of the effect of the duration of the obstruction and the underlying inflammatory disease process. Mortality is directly proportional to degree of contamination and delay in diagnosis, and treatment.

Perforations of the jejunum and ileum, especially if due to regional enteritis, may become quickly walled off, and signs of generalized peritonitis may be delayed. Free air may be detected on radiologic examination, or air may be seen in a retroperitoneal location or in the wall of the bowel. There is an elevated white blood count and a shift to the left, and the serum amylase level may also be elevated. Metabolic acidosis may be present. Tachycardia and fever are common. The abdomen may be distended. Hypoactive bowel sounds are present. Tenderness, rebound, guarding, and rigidity, usually associated with peritonitis, may all be absent, especially in the elderly. Perforations of the appendix are more likely in the extremes of age and if symptoms are prolonged prior to exploration. Suprapubic peritoneal paracentesis may help in diagnosis.

Perforation of the Large Bowel

Nontraumatic perforations of the lower GI tract are most commonly the result of diverticulitis, carcinoma, colitis, and foreign bodies. They may result from barium enemas, colonoscopy, and sigmoidoscopy as well. Perforations of the colon produce signs and symptoms predominantly due to sepsis as opposed to chemical irritation, and therefore the abdominal symptoms are more subtle in onset.

Carcinoma of the large bowel detected by a perforation has a higher mortality than carcinoma detected because of obstruction, changes in bowel habits, or bleeding. If there is no obstruction, the more proximal the perforation, the more serious the clinical picture, probably because the fecal stream is more liquid and disseminates rapidly. An antecedent history of partial or complete obstruction, change in bowel habits, and other findings consistent with carcinoma should be sought.

Perforation secondary to obstruction, as in carcinoma of the colon or acute diverticulitis with abscess formation, may be associated with a temporary amelioration of abdominal pain because the local distension has been relieved, although this is not common. Perforation in diverticulitis is usually the result of abscess formation, so that signs and symptoms of the abscess, and a mass, may predominate. Perforation resulting from carcinoma is the result of erosion of the carcinoma and not rupture of a normal bowel wall. This is quickly followed, however, by evidence of peritonitis, hypovolemia, and sepsis.

CLINICAL FEATURES

The hallmark of perforated viscus is abdominal pain. The severity, location, and suddenness of onset are a reflection of where the perforation has occurred. Patients presenting in the emergency department may be in acute distress and want to stay in a sitting or rocking position. Patients at later stages of peritonitis want to maintain immobility, lying on one side with hips flexed.

Usually vomiting is present. Bile in the vomitus indicates that the pylorus is open and that gastric outlet obstruction is not present. Coffee-ground vomitus may be present in patients with duodenal or gastric ulcer, or even in patients in whom common duct or cystic duct stones erode into the duodenum or stomach. A feculent drainage from the nasogastric tube, or vomiting of that sort of material, may indicate the presence of a long-standing small bowel obstruction or the presence of dead bowel. Abdominal distension, the inability to pass gas, and constipation are all signs and symptoms of the accompanying ileus or bowel obstruction.

Fever, tachycardia, a narrowed pulse pressure, oliguria, and tachypnea are signs of hypovolemia and sepsis. A fall in blood pressure usually indicates the presence of the full-blown shock state. Aggressive fluid therapy should occur before shock develops, while the patient's vital signs, including urinary output, are monitored. Fluid correction and aggressive treatment of sepsis are a part of the resuscitation process in the emergency department, but often resuscitation cannot be completed until surgical intervention has occurred.

Marked tenderness is frequently detected on abdominal examination, usually accompanied by rebound tenderness over the area of inflammation. Rigidity is also present if generalized peritonitis has developed. Pain is aggravated by any motion of the patient, including sneezing and coughing. The patient frequently lies in the fetal position to reduce the pain by minimizing the tension in the peritoneum.

Considerable effort should be made to obtain an accurate physical examination in patients already in distress. Use of percussion tenderness as opposed to rebound tenderness gives the examiner the same indication of peritonitis but without the patient discomfort. Gentle palpation with warm hands while the patient is in a comfortable position will help measure objectivity of changes detected by repeated examinations. Bowel sounds are absent if adynamic ileus has developed as a result of the inflammation. If early obstruction is present, the bowel sounds may be hyperactive. When the obstruction is long-standing, the bowel sounds disappear. If free air has accumulated, there may be a loss of liver dullness to percussion. Subcutaneous emphysema of the lower abdominal wall or thighs may result from perforation of the colon or rectum. The intraluminal gas spreads along neurovascular bundles and other planes to reach the subcutaneous tissues.

When a great deal of fluid is present in the peritoneum, shifting dullness may be found. Rectal and pelvic examinations are essential to determine if any pelvic or lower abdominal masses are present, or if tenderness can be elicited.

Laboratory studies may be of little help. Leukocytosis with a shift to the left is common. The blood urea nitrogen (BUN) level may be elevated if the degree of dehydration is significant. Electrolyte imbalance is frequent. Respiratory alkalosis is present early on in sepsis. Metabolic acidosis follows if the hypovolemia and sepsis are uncorrected. A mild elevation of the amylase level does not necessarily reflect pancreatitis since such elevations frequently accompany perforation, especially of the small bowel.

The elderly senile patient with multiple chronic complaints, vague history, equivocal physical findings, and no confirming laboratory findings is at high risk for delayed diagnosis and treatment. Hoffmann has reported on the utility of diagnostic peritoneal lavage (DPL) in this setting.

The open technique of DPL seems to offer the greatest degree of safety, especially when the patient has distension or has had prior abdominal operations. Lavage technique is identical to post-trauma DPL. If gas, food, bowel content, bile, or turbid or bloody fluid is detected on initial aspiration, lavage need not be done. Pus, bile, or bowel content are most consistent with free perforation. Although proven safe, this relatively simple but invasive diagnostic procedure has not achieved the same acceptable status for nontrauma as it has for abdominal trauma.

An upright chest x-ray is necessary to rule out the presence of thoracic disease, and to detect free air under the diaphragm (Fig. 40–1). The leaves of the diaphragm are much more clearly demonstrated on this view. The left lateral decubitus film of the abdomen may also be helpful in detecting free air. In either case, the patient should be left in position for 10 min before obtaining the films.

Abdominal x-rays may show air-fluid levels in a stepladder pattern indicating the presence of mechanical obstruction, or simply dilated loops of bowel indicating adynamic ileus (Fig. 40-2). Air along the biliary tract may be present if a gallstone has eroded into the small or large bowel. Neighboring loops of bowel may be widely separated if the intestinal walls are edematous. Free stones may be seen.

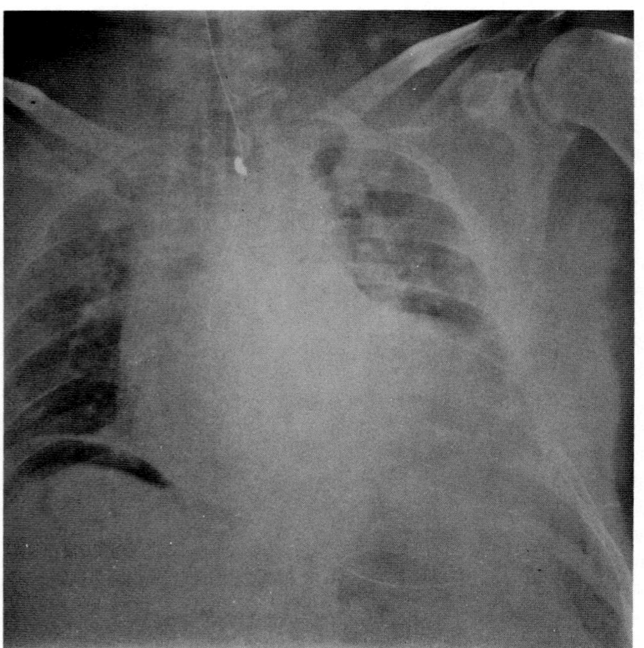

Fig. 40-1. Perforated viscus as shown in upright chest film. (Courtesy of Detroit General Hospital.)

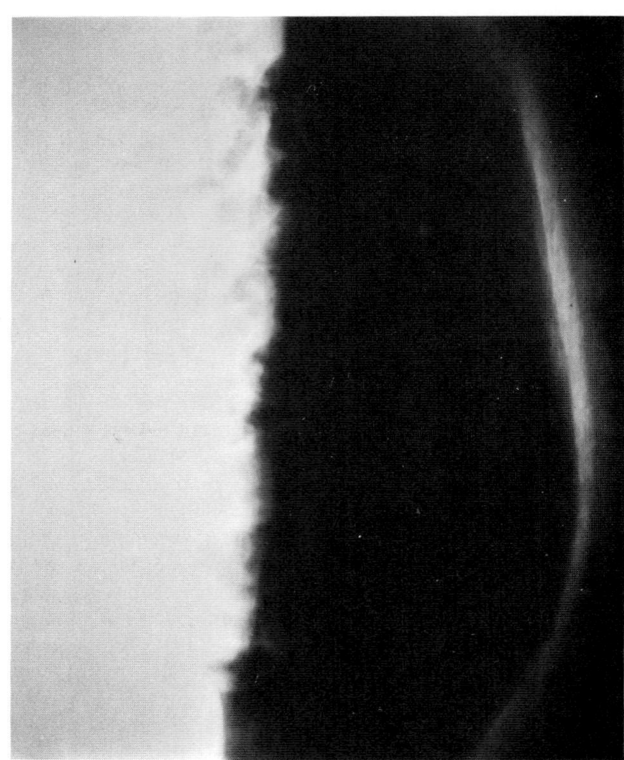

Fig. 40-2. Perforated viscus as shown in cross-table lateral film of abdomen. (Courtesy of Detroit General Hospital.)

Unquestionably, pneumoperitoneum, when present, expedites the diagnosis and treatment of perforated viscus. Since only 60 to 70 percent of perforated ulcer patients have this finding, one-third of patients with perforated viscus have potential for harmful delay of diagnosis. Most such patients will have clinical findings suggesting the diagnosis, but some will be equivocal. Insufflation of 400 to 500 mL of air into the nasogastric tube (pneumogastrography) followed by an upright chest x-ray has been used for equivocal cases. In Maull's series, perforated viscus patients who were diagnosed using air insufflation were operated on within 6 h of diagnosis and had an overall mortality of 9.7 percent. Failure to use insufflation led to average operative delays of 27 h and a 28 percent mortality.

The psoas shadows may be obscured by the presence of fluid in the abdomen or in the retroperitoneal space. If there is a distinct lack of gas in the intestine, dead bowel may be present.

Ultrasonography may be necessary to rule out the presence of cystic or common duct stones. There is some suggestion that CT scanning may also be helpful in identifying perforation and abscess formation by detecting masses in the mesentery or adjacent to organs. While radionuclide hepatobiliary scans can demonstrate gallbladder perforation, they are not universally available.

TREATMENT

Vigorous fluid resuscitation, as quickly as possible, is mandatory. In general, a balanced electrolyte solution should be used. Central venous pressure (CVP) and hourly urinary output should be monitored, in addition to the pulse and blood pressure, in continuous assessment of the patient's volume status. In the presence of significant blood loss, transfusions are necessary. Nasogastric tube insertion should be done early, even if the diagnosis is only suspected. Broad-spectrum antibiotics are indicated intravenously when the diagnosis of perforation is suspected. The particular antibiotics used should be discussed with the surgical consultant. Operative intervention is indicated as soon as volume replacement and urine output have been established, unless the risk of surgery exceeds the risk of death from perforation.

BIBLIOGRAPHY

Ackerman NB, Sillin LF, Suresh K: Consequences of intraperitoneal bile: Bile ascites versus bile peritonitis. *Am J Surg* 149:244, 1985.

Felice PR, Trowbridge PE, Ferrara JJ: Evolving changes in the pathogenesis and treatment of the perforated gallbladder. *Am J Surg* 149:466, 1985.

Gately JF, Thomas EF: Acute cholecystitis occurring as a complication of other diseases. *Arch Surg* 118: 1137, 1983.

Hinchey EJ, Schaal PGH, Richards GK: Treatment of perforated diverticular disease of the colon. *Adv Surg* 12:85, 1978.

Hoffmann, J: Peritoneal lavage in the diagnosis of the acute abdomen of non-traumatic origin. *Acta Chir Scand* 153:561, 1987.

Howe HJ: Acute perforation of the sigmoid colon secondary to diverticulitis. *Am J Surg* 137:184, 1979.

Koepsell, TD, Inui TS, Farewell VT: Factors affecting perforation in acute appendicitis. *Surg Gynecol Obstet* 153:508, 1981.

Larmi TK, Kairaluoma MI, Junila J, et al: Perforation of the gallbladder: A retrospective comparative study of cases from 1946–1956 and 1969–1980. *Acta Chir Scand* 150:557, 1984.

Lee H, Vibhakar SD, Bellon EM: Gastrointestinal perforation: Early diagnosis by computed tomography. *J Comput Assist Tomogr* 7:226, 1983.

Leijonmarck CE, Raf L: Ulceration of the small intestine due to slow-release potassium chloride tablets. *Acta Chir Scand* 151:273, 1985.

Massie JD, Austin HM, Kuvula M, et al: HIDA scanning and ultrasonography in expeditious diagnosis of acute cholecystitis. *South Med J* 75:164, 1982.

Maull KI, Reath DB: Pneumogastrography in the diagnosis of perforated peptic ulcer. *Am J Surg* 148:340, 1984.

Nadkarni KM, Shetty SD, Kagzi RS, et al: Small bowel perforations: A study of 32 cases. *Arch Surg* 116:53, 1981.

Nylander WA: The acute abdomen in the immunocompromised host. *Surg Clin North Am* 68(2): 457, 1988.

ReMines SG, McIlrath DC: Bowel perforation in steroid-treated patients. *Ann Surg* 192:581, 1980.

Sievert W, Vakil NB; Emergencies at the biliary tract. *Gastroenterol Clin North Am* 17(2): 245, 1988.

Silen W: *Cope's Early Diagnosis of the Acute Abdomen*, ed. 17. New York, Oxford, 1987.

Stephen M, Loewenthal J: Generalized infective peritonitis. *Surg Gynecol Obstet* 147:231, 1978.

Taylor R, Weakley FL, Sullivan BH Jr: Nonoperatrive management of colonoscopic perforation with pneumoperitoneum. *Gastrointest Endosc* 24:124, 1978.

Wilson DG, Lieberman LM: Perforation of the gallbladder diagnosed pre-operatively. *Eur J Nucl Med* 8:135, 1983.

41 ACUTE APPENDICITIS

James A. Catto

Appendicitis is a common cause of emergency surgery. Approximately 6 percent of the population will experience appendicitis in their lifetimes. While classically a disease of persons 10 to 30 years of age, it affects all ages. Appendicitis is most difficult to diagnose in the young, the elderly, the pregnant, and those afflicted with other diseases, such as acquired immunodeficiency syndrome or diabetes. However, it may also be difficult to diagnose in other patients, even for the most capable practitioner.

Seventy to eighty percent of appendicitis specimens reveal a nonruptured appendix; 20 to 30 percent are perforated. Of the total group, 1 percent of cases will be associated with delay of presentation, delay of recognition, error in diagnosis, and increased morbidity and mortality.

Mortality is low (0.1 to 0.2 percent) for unruptured appendicitis, but higher (3 to 5 percent) for ruptured appendicitis. There is a direct relationship between the morbidity and mortality rates associated with acute appendicitis and delay between onset of symptoms and definitive treatment. The more common immediate morbidities include soft tissue wound infection, intraabdominal abscess, ileus, and prolonged hospitalization. Delayed morbidities may include subsequent small bowel adhesive obstruction. In women with perforation and peritonitis, infertility can result.

Other pathologic processes involving the appendix are relatively rare. They include Crohn's disease of the appendix, diverticulitis of the appendix, pinworms, inspissated barium, foreign bodies, neoplastic diseases, and mechanical complications such as intussusception and torsion. Disease entities afflicting adjacent organs are a more frequent cause of misdiagnosis. Mesenteric lymphadenitis, pelvic inflammatory disease, mittelschmerz, acute gastroenteritis, and Crohn's disease are the most common of the multitude of conditions which simulate appendicitis. Despite the newer diagnostic tests available to the clinician, no single evaluation can substitute for the diagnostic accuracy of the experienced physician.

A complete knowledge of the development of the appendix and embryologic rotation of the colon (or incomplete rotation) is essential to develop an awareness that the appendix may be anywhere within the coelomic cavity. A healthy skepticism regarding the location of the appendix is essential to diagnosing the atypical presentations of appendicitis as seen in situs inversus viscerum, malrotation, hypermobile cecum, and the extremely long pelvic appendix.

The fact that the occurrence of appendicitis parallels the development of lymphoid tissues within the gastrointestinal tract has given rise to theories that appendicitis is caused by luminal obstruction secondary to lymphoid hyperplasia. Such theories gain credence from the fact that appendicitis often follows a flulike syndrome, an upper respiratory infection, mononucleosis, measles, bacterial enterocolitis, or some other inflammatory illness which produces generalized lymphoid hyperplasia. Other causes of luminal obstruction known to be associated with appendicitis include fecaliths, inspissated barium, seeds, pinworms, strictures, and carcinoma. Some patients present with recurrent bouts of a nonobstructive variant of appendicitis. This condition, while uncommon, is known to most clinicians.

CLINICAL PRESENTATION

The classic presentation of (1) anorexia, (2) periumbilical pain associated with nausea or modest emesis, and (3) the development of steady pain in the right lower quadrant developing over a 24-h period is present in approximately 60 percent of cases. Anorexia and pain are the more frequent symptoms. Nausea, modest emesis, and/or diarrhea are usually described. Localized tenderness within the abdomen or pelvis is usually present. Rebound tenderness supports a diagnosis that appendicitis or some significant intraperitoneal disease is present, but need not be obvious. Rebound is muted in the obese and the elderly.

Less common is a severe, crampy, colicky presentation associated with acute appendiceal luminal obstruction secondary to a fecalith. Recurrent diarrhea associated with the pelvic location of the inflamed appendix is often misdiagnosed as acute gastroenteritis. A rectal exam may clarify the issue when localizing pain is demonstrated within the pelvis.

A high index of suspicion that all abdominal pain presentations may reflect an atypical appendicitis is necessary in evaluating the acute abdomen. Rectal and pelvic exams are essential and may demonstrate localizing tenderness within the pelvis. The results of one study of the symptoms of 53 patients over 40 years of age are listed in Table 41-1. In another study of 305 patients with appendicitis, another order of signs, symptoms, and laboratory findings, based on predicted value, was determined (Table 41-2). Other physical signs associated with appendicitis have been described. Left lower quadrant abdominal palpation may produce pain in the right lower quadrant; this is known as Rovsing's sign. Cutaneous hyperesthesia in T10, T11, and T12 dermatomes may be present. The psoas sign is characterized by right lower quadrant pain on thigh extension while lying in the left lateral decubitus position. Internal rotation of the flexed right thigh, while supine, may produce right lower quadrant pain and is known as the obturator sign. These signs are often helpful when dealing with inflamed appendices in a more posterior position.

Appendicitis in the young taxes a physician's clinical skills in obtaining a reliable history and conducting comprehensive examination. In the less than 2 year age group, appendicitis is associated with a high degree of perforation and associated mortality. The diagnosis is evasive and must be suspected even in the absence of the classic presentation of adulthood. Irritability, emesis, and distension, while commonly present, are not very specific. The clinical presentation in young children tends to parallel that in adults. However, in children the incidence of mesenteric adenitis and acute gastroenteritis is higher than in adults.

Appendicitis in the elderly is associated with an even higher percentage of rupture than that seen in childhood, and leukocytosis is less pronounced. Diagnosis is difficult, and delay from admission to surgery tends to be longer than in other age groups.

Appendicitis occurs frequently during pregnancy (1 per 2200 pregnancies). It is associated with pain at a higher location than normally seen, but consistent with migration of the cecum from the right lower quadrant to the subcostal position during the evolution of the pregnancy. Perforating appendicitis during pregnancy carries an increased risk to the fetus and mother from septic complications. Appendectomy for nonruptured appendicitis during pregnancy seems to be well tolerated. However, the failure to identify intraabdominal pathology at appendectomy during pregnancy seems to be associated with an increased risk of abortion as the clinical presentation usually reflects some undiagnosed complication of the pregnancy.

LABORATORY EVALUATION

In 98 to 99 percent of appendicitis cases an elevated total leukocyte count (with a mean value of 16,000) or a left shift is present. In only 1 percent of cases is a normal leukocyte count and the absence of band forms found. However, the magnitude of leukocytosis does not correlate with the histologic severity of the appendicitis. If the inflammatory process lies close to the ureter, urinalysis will often reveal microscopic hematuria.

Table 41-1. Symptoms in Acute Appendicitis in Patients Over 40

Symptom	No.	%
Right lower quadrant (RLQ) pain	31	58
Nausea	26	49
Vomiting	24	45
Anorexia	19	36
Crampy abdominal pain	10	18
General pain—RLQ	9	17
Umbilical pain—RLQ	6	11
Diarrhea	6	11
Constipation	5	9
Fever	3	6

Source: Adapted from Stair T, Corlette MB: Appendicitis over forty. *Ann Emerg Med* 9:77, 1980.

Radiography

Plain abdominal radiologic investigation of the abdomen thought to possess appendicitis has neither the sensitivity nor the specificity to make it a useful test. While a fecalith of the appendix, gas in the appendix, or an air fluid level in the distal small bowel may suggest appendicitis, these signs are frequently absent.

Barium enema may be useful when the results are considered along with the rest of the clinical evaluation, but is not needed if the diagnosis is already reasonably certain. Use of the test is based on the premise that the lumen of the appendix is obstructed in appendicitis. While this is usually the case, it is not necessarily true. Barium enema is available in most hospitals, is safe, and does not require special radiologic equipment or personnel. In addition, results can be interpreted by the clinician. Nonfilling of the appendix associated with spasm, thickening, or cecal indentation is suggestive, but not pathognomonic, of appendicitis. Simple nonfilling of the appendix may reflect appendicitis or luminal fibrous obliteration seen with advancing age. Visualization of the appendix with a gas collection at the tip, loculated extraluminal gas in an abscess, extravasation of barium into an abscess, or a sharp cutoff sign in a shortened appendix suggests appendicitis. Visualization of a "normal" appendix suggests the absence of appendicitis but does not exclude it. Furthermore, partial filling of the appendix may be misconstrued as complete filling. If barium enema demonstrates an abnormal location of the appendix, such as a cecum beneath the liver (incomplete rotation of the colon) or deep within the pelvis, atypical presentations of appendicitis are more likely. Diseases often confused with appendicitis, such as terminal ileitis, diverticulitis, and neoplasia of the colon, may be diagnosed by the unprepared barium enema.

Table 41-2. Predictive Factors in the Diagnosis of Appendicitis

Localized tenderness—right lower quadrant
Leukocytosis
Migration of pain
Left shift
Temperature elevation
Nausea/vomiting
Anorexia/acetone
Rebound tenderness

Source: Adapted from Alvarado A: A practical score for the early diagnosis of acute appendicitis. *Ann Emerg Med* 15:557, 1986.

Other Diagnostic Studies

In a few selective studies, ultrasound examination was shown to have a 75 to 90 percent sensitivity and an 86 to 100 percent specificity. Visualization of the appendix as an immobile, tender, noncompressible structure is suggestive of appendicitis. Ultrasound examination is a noninvasive procedure possessing no radiation hazards and can be used in pregnancy. However, it requires special equipment, trained technicians, and physicians skilled in interpretation.

Computed tomography is not effective in detecting early appendicitis but is useful in the differential diagnosis of a right lower quadrant abdominal mass. It can differentiate between appendicitis, appendicitis with perforation and abscess, carcinoma of the cecum or appendix, appendiceal mucocele, or pseudomyxoma peritonei.

Diagnostic laparoscopy is an invasive study requiring special equipment, special surgical skills, and general anesthesia. It is relatively contraindicated in patients with obesity or abdominal distension, pregnant patients, and patients with previous laparotomies. Visualization of an inflamed appendix is not always diagnostic of appendicitis, and identification of another cause of intraabdominal pathology does not exclude appendicitis. However, studies report high sensitivity and specificity using diagnostic laparoscopy, and the advent of therapeutic endoscopic appendectomy techniques may enhance the use of this approach for diagnosis.

Diagnostic peritoneal tap or peritoneal lavage has been studied in moderation, but has not gained wide popularity. A leukocyte-rich effusion reflects intraabdominal pathology which may include appendicitis, mesenteric adenitis, or pelvic inflammatory disease. A leukocyte-sparse effusion may be found in early appendicitis, late well-established appendicitis with chronic abscess, or early closed-loop intestinal obstructions.

Other diagnostic aids, including clinical scoring systems, computer assisted programs, radioactive isotope imaging, and barium swallow, have been evaluated. No single test exceeds the diagnostic accuracy of the experienced physician, aided when necessary by hospital admission, serial examination of the patient, and, if appropriate, surgical consultation. An experienced surgeon may then choose to utilize ultrasound examination, barium enema, or diagnostic laparoscopy to enhance diagnostic accuracy.

TREATMENT

In the United States, surgical intervention is the treatment of choice for acute appendicitis. The patient suspected of having appendicitis should be instructed to refrain from oral consumption. Intravenous fluids should be administered to maintain current needs and to correct any deficits that may be present. A nasogastric tube may be inserted to diminish gastric distension. Antibiotics are indicated after commitment to surgical intervention has been made. The incidence of wound infection has been shown to decrease with the use of prophylactic antibiotics. Delay in operation is associated with a higher percentage of perforation and increased morbidity and mortality.

BIBLIOGRAPHY

Alvarado A: A practical score for the early diagnosis of acute appendicitis. *Ann Emerg Med* 15:557, 1986.

Fitz RH: Perforating inflammation of the vermiform appendix, with special reference to its early diagnosis and treatment. *Trans Assoc Am Physicians* 1:107, 1886.

Stair T, Corbette, MB: Appendicitis over forty. *Ann Emerg Med* 9:76, 1980.

42
INTESTINAL OBSTRUCTION
John L. Glover

Intestinal obstruction occurs when anything interferes with the normal peristaltic progression of intestinal contents. In the past, the term *ileus* was used as a synonym for intestinal obstruction, and ileus was either *paralytic* or *dynamic*. Paralytic ileus is intestinal obstruction caused by inadequate muscular contraction of the intestine and, therefore, failure of intestinal contents to progress through the intestinal tract. The most common cause is abdominal surgery, which normally causes a temporary cessation of intestinal motility. By common usage in recent years, the term *paralytic ileus* has been shortened to *ileus;* and dynamic ileus is usually referred to as *intestinal obstruction*. In some situations it can be difficult to distinguish between these two.

Mechanical intestinal obstruction can be subdivided into obstruction due to lesions (1) extrinsic to the bowel wall, (2) intrinsic to the bowel wall, and (3) within the lumen of the bowel. From a clinical standpoint, however, obstruction of the small intestine and obstruction of the large intestine should be considered as different entities because they have different causes, different clinical presentations, and different kinds of treatment.

Small intestinal obstruction is usually caused by postoperative adhesions. Adhesions follow all intraabdominal procedures, and they usually cause no symptoms. Some people and some disease processes, however, are associated with greater numbers and apparently greater density of adhesions. In most cases, intestinal obstruction does not occur until long after the surgery that caused the adhesions, sometimes many years. On the other hand, it can occur during the first two postoperative weeks.

The second most common cause of small intestinal obstruction is incarceration of a groin hernia. In most cases the hernia is a small one, and the patient is usually aware that the "knot" or lump in the groin became constant (and tender) when the symptoms of bowel obstruction began. In infants, or obtunded patients, however, this history is lacking. In infants, the hernia may present as a painful testicle and, therefore, be confused with acute torsion of the testis. In adults, a femoral hernia may be confused with inflamed inguinal lymph nodes. Small umbilical hernias may not be readily apparent, and large umbilical hernias in obese patients occasionally become incarcerated. Finally, there are two kinds of hernias which cause obstruction but are not apparent on examination. The first is a hernia through the obturator foramen, an *obturator hernia*. This rare lesion is nearly always seen in elderly women, and the diagnosis may be established presumptively by the presence of mechanical small bowel obstruction in a patient who has not had surgery in the past and who also complains of pain in one knee or along the medial aspect of one thigh (in the distribution of the obturator nerve). The other occult hernia is an internal hernia, which occurs through defects in the mesentery.

Causes of small bowel obstruction other than adhesions and hernias are quite rare. An important one is a primary tumor of the small bowel, such as an adenocarcinoma or a polypoid lymphoma, both examples of lesions intrinsic to the wall causing obstruction. Finally, the most common lesions within the bowel lumen which cause obstruction are gallstones and bezoars. The former usually occur in older patients and cause obstruction which waxes and wanes as the gallstone (or gallstones) progresses toward the ileocecal valve, where it stops. Since such stones have eroded through the gallbladder into the intestinal tract, there will usually be air in the biliary tree, a subtle finding which can be easily missed. Bezoars obstructing the small intestine are usually composed of vegetable fiber, such as orange or persimmon pulp; they are more likely to be found in patients who have lost the function of the pylorus, as by pyloroplasty or pyloric resection with gastric surgery.

Inflammatory bowel disease can present as low small bowel obstruction, but there is usually a history of preexisting disease. The same is true for radiation enteritis, which causes stricture and may even be associated with development of enteroliths. Finally, intraabdominal abscesses can cause small bowel obstruction, and, while these usually occur in postoperative patients, they can be the initial manifestation of a perforated retrocecal appendix.

Colonic obstruction is almost never caused by adhesions or by a hernia. Except for fecal impaction, which should be apparent, the most common cause is carcinoma of the colon or rectum. Since carcinoma begins in the mucosa, it tends to obstruct the part of the colon where the lumen is relatively narrow and the fecal stream solid—the left colon. The next most common cause of colonic obstruction in adults is diverticulitis. In acute diverticulitis, there is obstruction due to the swelling at the site of perforation of a diverticulum, usually sealed by the mesentery. Chronic scarring from this same process can cause colonic obstruction which presents in a manner identical to that of carcinoma.

After cancer and diverticulitis, the next most common cause of large bowel obstruction is *volvulus,* which is an obstruction of a loop of bowel by twisting on itself. The most common form is volvulus of the sigmoid colon; it is usually seen in older patients with chronic constipation, often from nursing homes. The radiographic appearance is characteristic (Fig. 42-1). Cecal volvulus occurs also but less commonly.*

PATHOPHYSIOLOGY

In the initial phase of obstruction, the bowel immediately proximal to the obstruction becomes distended with fluid and electrolytes, as well as with gas which is mostly from swallowed air. The amount of fluid increases even if the patient is not eating, since gastric, pancreatic, and biliary secretion continue. Furthermore, as obstruction persists, the bowel loses its ability to absorb fluid and electrolyte, and the resulting dehydration is a major systemic manifestation of intestinal obstruction. Additional fluid and electrolyte loss occurs into the bowel wall and, if there is venous congestion, from the serosal surface into the peritoneal cavity. Finally, the buildup of fluid and gas is associated with vomiting, and the body's extracellular fluid may be rapidly depleted from all these routes, resulting in hemoconcentration, hypovolemia, and hypotension. If not corrected rapidly, renal insufficiency, shock, and death will occur.

When mechanical obstruction occurs, intestinal peristalsis increases initially, as if it were attempting to overcome the blockage. As a result, bowel sounds are initially hyperactive and then assume a pattern of intermittent vigorous "rushes" of peristalsis and quiescent periods. These rushes are associated with severe, cramping pain. The bowel distal to the obstruction becomes inactive by reflex, and when obstruction persists, the proximal bowel loses its ability to contract vigorously. When this occurs, the bowel sounds become infrequent and very high pitched.

When the bowel becomes very distended, there may be venous congestion, and other mechanical factors, such as pressure from an adhesive band, may contribute to impairment of the circulation. At this stage, bacteria may pass into the lymphatics or the bloodstream, and the bowel wall may become gangrenous—strangulation obstruction is now present. This condition is usually associated with shock, and mortality may be as high as 70 percent. These changes occur early if there is a *closed-loop obstruction,* one in which a segment of intestine is blocked proximally and distally. Examples of closed-loop obstruction include a loop of small intestine herniated through a defect in the

**Volvulus* is a general term referring to twisting of the intestine. A loop of small intestine, for example, may twist behind an adhesion and therefore undergo volvulus. The entire small intestine in an infant may undergo volvulus if the mesentery is not attached normally to the posterior abdominal wall.

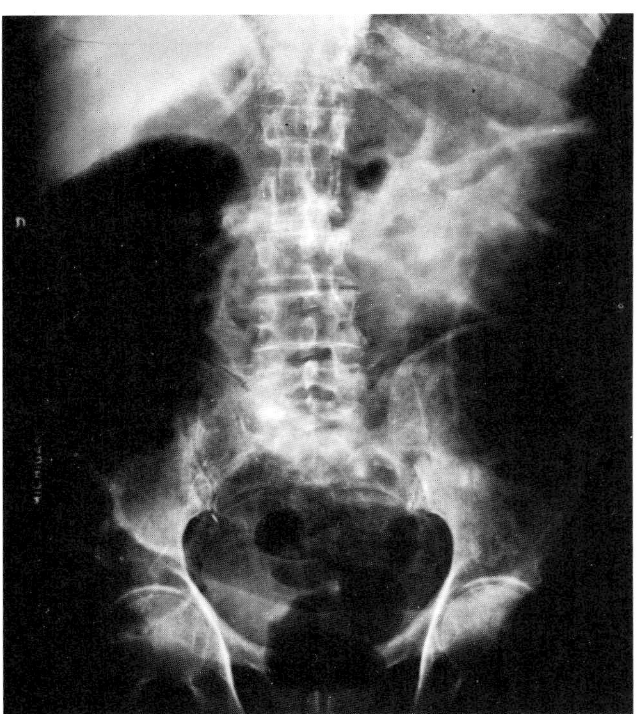

Fig. 42-1. Sigmoid volvulus. (Courtesy of Detroit General Hospital.)

omentum or mesentery, a loop of intestine caught in a hernia sack, and all cases of complete colonic obstruction as long as the ileocecal valve is closed.

CLINICAL FEATURES

The first manifestation of intestinal obstruction is abdominal pain which is poorly localized but generally felt in the midline. The pain fluctuates and gives the patient a feeling of restlessness and sometimes nausea. This initial visceral pain is due to the abdominal distention and contraction in the early phases of obstruction. When peristaltic rushes begin, there is associated severe cramping pain which causes the patient to double over; coincident with this pain, peristaltic rushes can be heard with a stethoscope. As the bowel loses the ability to contract because of prolonged obstruction, the pain becomes more constant but remains dull and generalized. In small bowel obstruction, the pain begins earlier and is more severe, whereas it is vague and less severe in colonic obstruction. In contrast, distention is often absent in small bowel obstruction but pronounced in colonic obstruction. This latter difference is partially explained by differences in the pattern of vomiting, which occurs early in small bowel obstruction and is usually bilious. In colonic obstruction, vomiting is less frequent and occurs later; the contents look and smell feculent. Feculent vomiting can occur in low small bowel obstruction, of course, but usually after a period of early bilious vomiting.

Most patients with intestinal obstruction stop having stools soon after obstruction. Also, there is decreased passage of flatus. Failure to pass any flatus generally means that a complete obstruction is present.

Decreased passage of stool and flatus are present, of course, in anyone who becomes constipated, and constipation can occur in a variety of situations. Some people have chronic constipation due to chronic use of laxatives because of irregular bowel habits. Constipation may occur in people with normal bowel habits because of decreased bowel motility resulting from use of narcotics. Oral pain medications containing codeine are a very common cause. Since regular defecation is due to the gastrocolic reflex and usually follows a routine, so that the urge to defecate occurs soon after a meal, travel across several time zones can interfere with the routine and cause constipation. Dehydration aggravates any of these situations because absorption of fluid from the bowel hardens the feces and decreases its bulk. These changes can result in fecal impaction, which causes a clinical picture identical with large bowel obstruction due to cancer. Furthermore, this kind of picture also occurs most commonly in patients of the same age as those with large bowel cancer.

Differentiating between colonic obstruction due to cancer and that due to impaction can be especially confusing in patients sent from nursing homes for evaluation of abdominal distention and vomiting. They often have irregular bowel habits related to immobility and poor dietary habits. In addition, they may be unable to give an accurate medical history. The biggest danger in these patients is to delay the diagnosis of cancer by attributing the symptoms to constipation and impaction because digital exam shows hard stool in the rectum.

Patients with relatively normal bowel habits who get fecal impaction normally have tenesmus, the constant feeling of needing to defecate but passing little or no stool. Tenesmus is also a symptom of bulky rectal cancers, but such lesions are usually associated with a history of changing bowel habits for several weeks.

The abdominal examination may be misleadingly nondescript in small bowel obstruction because of lack of distention and tenderness. If *cardiac sounds* are clearly heard in the midabdomen, fluid-filled loops of intestine are undoubtedly present all the way to the diaphragm (since sound is transmitted readily through fluid and poorly through air), and this is an early sign of obstruction. When localized tenderness or rebound tenderness occurs, there is transmural inflammation of the bowel, and strangulation obstruction is imminent or present, thus requiring urgent surgical consultation. In colonic obstruction, distention will be impressive and bowel sounds will be distant because of the massive amount of air.

Rectal and pelvic examinations must always be done in suspected bowel obstruction because of the importance of colorectal tumors and pelvic abscesses in the pathogenesis of obstruction.

LABORATORY FINDINGS

Generally, laboratory findings reflect the degree of fluid loss and the associated electrolyte disturbances and acid-base imbalances. Leukocytosis ($>20,000/mm^3$) with a shift to the left is, of course, indicative of the presence of an inflammatory process and can occur with gangrene of the bowel, perforation, vascular occlusion, or abscess. The serum amylase level is frequently mildly elevated in the presence of obstructed bowel, primarily as a result of systemic absorption of pancreatic enzymes from the bowel wall, although obstruction of pancreatic secretions may be related in some cases.

Elevation of the blood urea nitrogen (BUN) level correlates with the degree of dehydration or the presence of blood in the bowel lumen. The more complete and long-standing the obstruction, the more severe the dehydration.

Leukocytosis, elevation of the BUN, tachycardia, tachypnea, and elevated temperature, with or without a decrease in the blood pressure, are signs of toxicity and require vigorous fluid resuscitation. Decreased urinary output, monitored as part of the continuing evaluation of the patient, is an additional clue to the development of toxicity and sepsis. Broad-spectrum antibiotics, in keeping with local practice, are indicated.

Initial radiographic studies should include flat and upright views of the abdomen and radiographs of the chest. When possible, an upright radiograph of the chest should be obtained to rule out the presence of free air. The presence of air-fluid levels, with a stepladder pattern on the upright film, is considered diagnostic of mechanical obstruction (Fig. 42-2). The presence of dilated loops of bowel without air-fluid levels is not diagnostic. The presence of air in the rectum and/or the sigmoid colon after a rectal examination does not help in deciding whether a complete obstruction is present. There are times when dilated

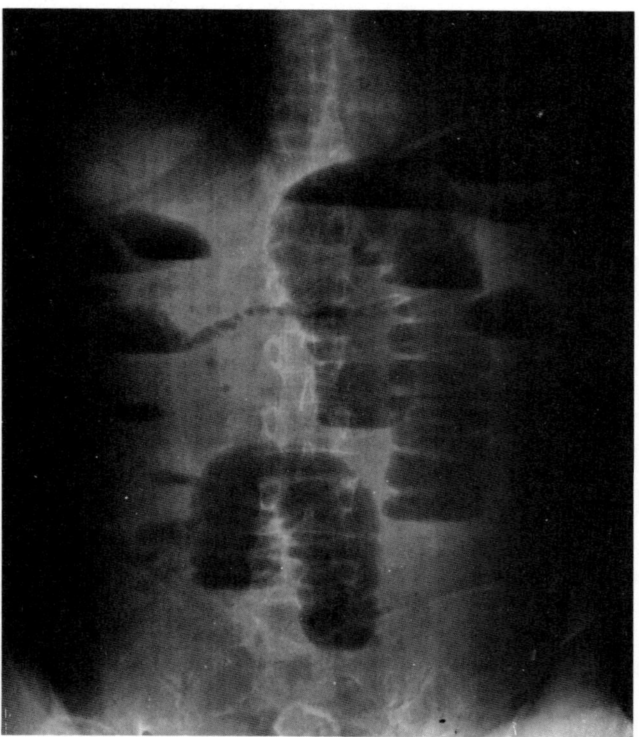

Fig. 42-2. The presence of steplike air-fluid levels suggests a mechanical intestinal obstruction. (Courtesy of Detroit General Hospital.)

loops of bowel are present and terminate at the point of an obstruction, and this should be used as a clue to the diagnosis.

Sigmoidoscopic examination is a part of the diagnostic evaluation of patients with suspected obstruction, especially when the diagnosis is obscure. In general, sigmoidoscopic examination should be done before barium examination, so that the radiologist is aware of the results. If completely occluding lesions are seen, a barium enema examination is not necessary, and biopsy may be done if barium enema examination is to be deferred.

During sigmoidoscopic examination, the examiner should look not only for masses but also at the mucosa. Friable, erythematous mucosa, with or without a granular appearance, may be indicative of an underlying inflammatory disease. Dark blue or frankly gangrenous mucosa is present when dead bowel, or bowel with compromised vascular supply, is entered with the sigmoidoscope.

Barium enema examination is helpful in determining not only the presence of large bowel obstruction but also its cause; sooner or later every patient suspected of having mechanical large bowel obstruction requires such a study. The hazards of a barium enema examination include perforation, especially of already damaged bowel or if a biopsy has been done, and the theoretical possibility of converting a partial bowel obstruction to a complete one with inspissated barium. Introduction of barium into the small bowel by a tube passed through the stomach and into the duodenum—enteroclysis—is useful if a mechanical small bowel obstruction is suspected but plain films are not diagnostic. Although barium administered above a partial or a complete obstruction may theoretically increase morbidity and mortality, one study of 172 patients with mechanical small bowel obstruction revealed that orally administered barium produced no untoward side effects.

Tachycardia, tachypnea, and a fever, even in the presence of a normal blood pressure, may be indicative of significant hypovolemia, with or without sepsis. In the elderly, the only signs of dead bowel may be the presence of deteriorating vital signs. Inflammatory lesions, of course, are commonly associated with tachycardia, tachypnea, and fever. Intraabdominal abscesses, like abscesses elsewhere, may be associated with spiking temperatures, so that the patient may be afebrile when initially seen. When the mechanical obstruction is of recent onset, vital signs may be within normal limits.

Mechanical obstruction and paralytic ileus are sometimes difficult to distinguish. Repeated radiographic examination, laboratory studies, and physical examinations, while correcting any electrolyte and fluid imbalances, may provide the only means of differentiation between these two disorders. If possible, the same physician should repeat the examinations.

TREATMENT

Insertion of a nasogastric tube should be done at the first suspicion of intestinal obstruction because it prevents additional distention from swallowed air and gastric secretions and may provide partial decompression, especially in relatively high small bowel obstruction.

Long intestinal tubes (Baker, Cantor, or Miller-Abbott tubes) are available also, but their use is generally restricted to the early obstruction that occurs in some patients within 2 weeks of abdominal surgery. Such obstructions are frequently relieved by passage of a long intestinal tube. Attempts to pass them preoperatively, however, in other cases of mechanical obstruction usually delay operative treatment because of the time required to ascertain that the tube is beyond the ligament of Treitz. Furthermore, further passage depends on peristalsis, which may be impaired as a result of the obstruction. When a long tube is used, it does not supplant the need for a nasogastric tube to evacuate gas and secretions from the stomach.

Mechanical bowel obstruction should be treated surgically as soon as appropriate fluid resuscitation has been done, as shown by adequate urine output and correction of hypotension. In small bowel obstruction, the obstruction and its cause are usually treated simultaneously, by lysis of adhesions, resection of any gangrenous bowel, and primary anastomosis. In obstruction of the colon, however, the obstruction is often treated separately, as by a decompressing colostomy. An obstructing cancer may be removed, but primary anastomosis of unprepared colon is rarely done.

In all cases of bowel obstruction, preoperative administration of broad-spectrum antibiotics is indicated because of bacterial invasion of the bowel wall and because the bowel may be opened. It is useful to establish protocols for this type of treatment because sepsis is a major hazard of intestinal obstruction.

Fecal impaction requires digital evacuation of the hard stool in the distal rectum. Gentle, slow dilatation of the anal canal so that the index and middle finger can be inserted into the rectum allows one to manually extract most of the hard, impacted feces. To insure complete relief, an oil retention enema is administered as high as possible, and followed in a half an hour by a cleaning enema. Patients often have a small amount of bleeding from mucosal tears after "disimpaction," and they may have some fecal soiling for a few days afterwards because the dilatation decreases sphincter tone.

PSEUDOOBSTRUCTION

Intestinal pseudoobstruction is a clinical entity in which signs and symptoms of obstruction are present but no mechanical obstruction can be demonstrated. Although it may affect any segment of the bowel, its most common clinical presentation is that of low colonic obstruction, with large amounts of gas in the colon and some gas in the small intestine. It is associated with use of anti-Parkinson drugs and tricyclic antidepressants, as well as many other possible contributing factors. Its significance is that, since it mimics colon obstruction, a barium enema may be done and result in obstruction due to inability to evacuate barium. Furthermore, the distention of the cecum may be so great as to warrant consideration of surgery because of fear of perforation. In such cases, the first examination (after digital rectal exam) should be colonoscopy, which can both rule out the presence of tumor and treat the pseudoobstruction by decompression. This entity is being recognized more frequently; surgery is not helpful and can, in fact, be harmful.

BIBLIOGRAPHY

Anderson A, Bergdahl L, Van der Linden W: Volvulus of the cecum. *Ann Surg* 181:876, 1975.

Golladay ES, Byrne WJ: Intestinal pseudo-obstruction. *Surg Gynecol Obstet* 153:257, 1981.

Grodsinsky C, Ponka JL: Volvulus of the colon. *Dis Colon Rectum* 20:314, 1977.

Khoury GA, Pickard R, Knight M: Volvulus of the sigmoid colon. *Br J Surg* 64:587, 1977.

Laws HL, Aldrete JS: Small-bowel obstruction: A view of 465 cases. *S Med J* 69:733, 1976.

Stewardson RH, Bombeck CT, Nyhus LM: Critical operative management of small bowel obstruction. *Ann Surg* 187:189, 1978.

Wolmark N, Wieand HS, Rockette HE, et al: The prognostic significance of tumor location and bowel obstruction in Dukes B and C colorectal cancer. *Ann Surg* 198:743, 1983.

43
HERNIA
Ronald L. Krome

A *hernia* is classically defined as the protrusion of any viscus which is enclosed in a peritoneal sac from its normal position through a congenital or acquired opening into another area. This classic description does not include all hernias. It does not, for example, include internal hernias, herniation of omentum, herniation of preperitoneal fat, or traumatic herniation of a variety of organs.

An *external hernia* is one that protrudes through to the outside and can be seen or palpated. External hernias include femoral, inguinal, umbilical, obturator, and incisional hernias.

An *internal hernia* is one in which the herniated organ and the herniation itself occur within the confines of a body cavity. Examples of this are diaphragmatic hernias, both acquired and congenital; hernias through the foramen of Winslow into the lesser sac; or hernias through a tear in the omentum or mesentery.

An *incisional hernia* is one that results as a postoperative complication and occurs through a previous incision site. It is an acquired hernia.

A *reducible hernia* is any hernia in which the herniated organ can be returned to its normal anatomic position without surgical intervention, simply by manipulation.

An *incarcerated hernia*, or irreducible hernia, is one which cannot be returned to its normal anatomic position by manipulation, and therefore surgical intervention may be necessary to replace the contents. Incarceration may be either *acute* or *chronic*. The incidence of incarceration is increased when the hernia occurs in association with a disease which causes increased intraabdominal pressure, for example, asthma, chronic obstructive pulmonary disease, benign prostatic hypertrophy, prostatism, and colon or rectal tumors producing obstruction and constipation. All these conditions may result in increased intraabdominal pressure because of the strain necessary to breathe, urinate, or defecate.

Incarceration is more likely to occur when the defect is small and the contents are large. This holds true wherever the hernia is; the incidence of incarceration decreases as the size of the defect increases. Once edema develops, and as it progresses, the hernia becomes increasingly difficult to reduce. Impingement of the vascular supply may result.

When the hernia is associated with vascular compromise, either venous or arterial, then it is said to be *strangulated*. As the vascular compromise progresses or if it is not relieved, gangrene develops. Although all strangulated hernias are by definition incarcerated, not all incarcerated hernias are strangulated. Strangulated hernias require surgical intervention. Not all incarcerated hernias require intervention. Chronic incarcerations will most likely not strangulate, and therefore emergency surgery is not generally necessary.

Strangulation and incarceration may occur in both external and internal hernias.

PATHOPHYSIOLOGY

Direct inguinal hernia. A *direct inguinal hernia* is one that protrudes through Hesselbach's triangle, which is bounded by the inguinal ligament, the inferior epigastric vessels, and the lateral border of the rectus abdominis muscle. Direct hernias rarely, if ever, incarcerate (Fig. 43-1).

Indirect inguinal hernia. An *indirect inguinal hernia* is one that comes down the inguinal canal and occurs lateral to the inferior epigastric vessels. Incarceration of these hernias is not uncommon. Although indirect hernias are much more common in men because of the embryological descent of the testes, they do occur in women.

Femoral hernia. A *femoral hernia* is one that protrudes below the inguinal ligament into the femoral canal. They are much more common in women, most likely because of the different structure of the pelvis. Femoral hernias are often associated with ipsilateral inguinal hernia. Nevertheless, by far the most common hernia in the population as a whole is the inguinal hernia. Femoral hernias are frequently misdiagnosed in children because they are uncommon in this age group.

A hernia that occurs above the epigastric vessels in the linea semilunaris is called a *Spigelian hernia*.

Bilateral inguinal hernias are referred to as a *double hernia;* a *pantaloon hernia* is an inguinal hernia with both direct and indirect components occurring on the same side. When one wall of the hernia sac is made up by the viscus involved, regardless of the anatomic location of the hernia, it is called a *sliding hernia*. There are therefore sliding inguinal hernias and sliding hiatal hernias. When an incarceration or a strangulation contains only one wall of a viscus, it is a *Richter's hernia*.

Although a number of factors play an etiologic role in the development of groin hernias, most often multiple factors are involved. Congenital development defects and heredity play roles in the indirect hernias present at birth. There is a failure to develop a portion of the abdominal wall. Persistence of the processus vaginalis peritonei in the inguinal canal, with an inguinal ring large enough to permit a hernia to occur, may be hereditary. Similarly, generalized connective tissue weakness may be hereditary.

Direct inguinal hernias have an increasing frequency as age increases and are uncommon in children. Indirect hernias, on the other hand, are more common in the younger age groups.

A slow, chronic increase in intraabdominal pressure is a major factor in the development of acquired hernias and is the precipitating factor in indirect hernias, in spite of the existence of a congenital sac.

Obturator hernias. Protrusion of abdominal contents through the obturator foramen, located between the superior and inferior rami, into the medial thigh is known as an obturator hernia. This is a rare hernia, occurring more frequently in elderly women for some unknown reason.

Umbilical hernias. Although an umbilical defect is common in newborns, in the majority of cases the defect is closed by the second year of age. Obese patients, especially those in the older age groups, have an increased incidence of umbilical hernias, perhaps because of increasing intraabdominal pressure. Such hernias also develop with some frequency in persons with chronic and severe ascites. Pregnancy plays a significant role in their development. Umbilical hernias can incarcerate and strangulate, especially if small and the hernial contents are large.

CLINICAL FEATURES

The majority of hernias are asymptomatic and are detected either on routine physical examination or inadvertently by the patient. Mild symptoms, such as a sensation of "dragging" or a lump in the groin, may be the only manifestations. If incarceration is acute, pain may develop suddenly. When strangulation occurs, the patient may be toxic, with signs and symptoms of bowel obstruction or perforation. The most common complaint is a tender swelling or a sense of bulging. Patients with obturator hernias have intermittent bouts of partial small bowel obstructions over years.

Patients with incarceration frequently give a history of having a hernia. The patient can no longer return the hernia to its normal position and thus seeks help. Acute incarcerations are painful and tender; they may be accompanied by nausea and vomiting if partial or complete obstruction has occurred. The tenderness is due to inflammation of the bowel wall or omentum and the surrounding tissues. Incarcerated hernias are a leading cause of bowel obstruction in the United States, second only to postoperative adhesions.

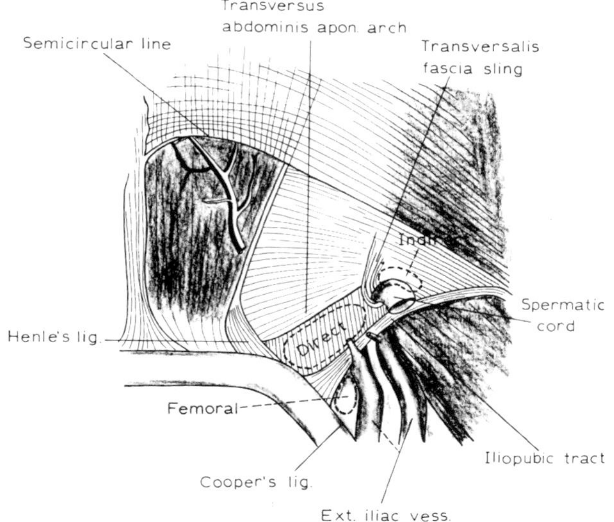

Fig. 43-1. The posterior inguinal wall viewed from the preperitoneal side. The peritoneum and all preperitoneal fat and lymphoid tissue have been excised, exposing the transversalis fascia. The areas through which the three common groin hernias occur are indicated, as are the transversalis fascia analogues, which are utilized in the iliopubic tract repair. [From Nyhus LM: Preperitoneal approach in the repair of inguinal hernia in adults, in Ellison EH, Friesen SR, Mulholland JH (eds): *Current Surgical Management III*. Philadelphia, Saunders, 1965, p. 465. Used with permission.]

Initial symptoms, produced by traction on a portion of the small bowel or omentum, may be located in the epigastrium. If only a portion of the bowel wall is caught in the defect (Richter's hernia), strangulation may occur without signs and symptoms of intestinal obstruction.

Pain along the medial aspect of the thigh to the knee and hypesthesia in the same area is associated with obturator hernias.

On physical examination, an abnormal swelling may be noted. If incarceration is present, the swelling is tender. The consistency of this mass varies depending on the contents of the hernia sac.

Tachycardia and mild temperature elevation frequently are present if incarceration is also present. Unrelieved incarceration or strangulation may result in bowel obstruction, perforation, abscess formation, or peritonitis and septic shock.

Groin hernias can be confused with tender lymph nodes and hydroceles. Lymph nodes are generally movable, firm, and multiple. Hydroceles may transilluminate and are not tender. Incarcerated hernias will not transilluminate and are tender. If bowel is contained in the hernia sac, bowel sounds may be heard and peristalsis may be seen. Testicular torsion may be confused with incarcerated hernias.

When incarceration is acute, the white blood cell count is slightly elevated with a shift to the left. Electrolyte abnormalities and elevation of the blood urea nitrogen (BUN) level occur as a reflection of both the patient's state of hydration and the toxic state. In the elderly, laboratory studies may not be reliable indicators of the patient's state. There are times when a barium enema is obtained as part of a diagnostic evaluation for abdominal pain that a hernia is detected.

Upright chest films should be obtained to rule out free air under the diaphragm, which may result from perforation or dead bowel. Flat and upright films of the abdomen, including the groin, should be obtained to assess the possible presence of bowel obstruction. Loops of bowel may be seen entering a hernial sac.

TREATMENT

If there is a good history that the incarceration is of very recent onset, an attempt can be made to reduce the hernia. If there is any question of the duration of the incarceration, no attempt should be made so that no dead bowel is reintroduced into the abdomen. Before an attempt is made to reduce the hernia, the patient should be placed in Trendelenburg's position and given some mild sedation. A warm compress over the area may make the task easier by reducing the swelling and relaxing the abdominal musculature. Only gentle compression of the hernia should be used, and nothing should be forced back. Attempts at reduction should be limited in time and force.

If the incarceration is tender, if it cannot be reduced, or if strangulation is suspected, the patient should not be fed by mouth, and a nasogastric tube should be inserted. Intravenous fluid should be started with the thought of correcting the patient's volume and electrolyte problems.

The treatment of choice for an incarceration which cannot be reduced, or for a strangulation, is surgical. Broad-spectrum antibiotics and vigorous fluid resuscitation may be necessary, but only as a prelude to operation. Mortality is higher in the elderly when emergency surgery is required.

BIBLIOGRAPHY

Bjork KJ, Mucha P Jr, and Cahill DR: Obturator hernia. *SGO* 167:217, 1988.
Glassow F: Femoral hernia. *Am J Surg* 150:353, 1985.
Nehme AE: Groin hernias in elderly patients. *Am J Surg* 146:257, 1983.
Norton J: Abdominal wall hernias, in *Principles of Surgery*, 5th ed. Schwartz SI et al (eds). McGraw-Hill, 1989.
Rozk TA, Deshmukh N: Obturator hernia: a difficult diagnosis. *South Med J* 6:709, 1990.
Tam PK, Lister J: Femoral hernia in children. *Arch Surg* 119:1161, 1984.

44 ILEITIS AND COLITIS

Howard A. Werman
Hagop S. Mekhjian
Douglas A. Rund

CROHN'S DISEASE

Crohn's disease is a chronic inflammatory disease of the gastrointestinal (GI) tract of unknown etiology. The disease was first described by Crohn, Ginzberg, and Oppenheimer in 1932 and was thought to involve only the distal ileum. We now know that it can involve any part of the GI tract from the mouth to the anus. Characteristically, there is a segmental involvement of the intestinal tract by a nonspecific granulomatous inflammatory process. The ileum is involved in the majority of cases. In 20 percent, the disease is confined to the colon, making differentiation from ulcerative colitis, at times, a difficult clinical problem. The terms *regional enteritis, terminal ileitis, granulomatous ileocolitis,* and *Crohn's disease* are used to describe the same disease process.

Etiology and Pathogenesis

Environmental, genetic, and host factors have all been implicated as a cause. Atypical mycobacteria have also been considered as a possible cause of Crohn's disease. There are few data to support the causative role of psychogenic factors. Immunologic factors have received great attention recently. There is considerable similarity between bacterial and gut mucosal cell antigens. It is postulated that T lymphocytes are sensitized by external antigens from enterobacteria, and in the presence of antibodies the T lymphocytes produce a cytotoxic response. The presence of T and B lymphocytic infiltrates in involved tissues, increased circulating plasma cells, and decreased antibody and cell-mediated response further suggest an immunologic mechanism in Crohn's disease. Whether immune factors play a primary or secondary role in the pathogenesis is not known. Some extraintestinal manifestations suggest a role for immune complexes or an autoantibody response at various involved sites.

Epidemiology

The peak incidence of Crohn's disease occurs in patients between 15 and 22 years of age with a suggestion of a secondary peak at age 55 to 60 years. The prevalence varies from 10 to 100 cases, and the incidence from 1 to 7 cases per year per 100,000 population in the United States. The incidence has been increasing over the past 20 years. The disease has a worldwide distribution but is more frequent in people of European extraction. It is four times more common in Jews than non-Jews and is more common in whites than blacks. Family history of inflammatory bowel disease is present in 10 to 15 percent of patients. Ulcerative colitis, as well as Crohn's disease, may be present in other family members, and siblings are more frequently affected with Crohn's disease.

Pathology

The most important feature of the pathology of Crohn's disease is the involvement of all the layers of the bowel as well as the mesenteric lymph nodes. In addition, the disease is discontinuous, with normal areas of bowel ("skip areas") between one or more involved areas. On gross inspection, the bowel wall is thickened; the lumen narrowing results in stenosis and obstruction of the intestine. The mesenteric fat often extends over the bowel wall ("creeping" fat). The appearance of the mucosa varies with the extent and severity of the disease. Longitudinal deep ulcerations are characteristic. These often penetrate the bowel wall, resulting in fissures, fistulas, and abscesses. Late in the disease, a "cobblestone" appearance of the mucosa results from the crisscrossing of these ulcers with intervening normal mucosa.

Microscopically, there is an inflammatory reaction that extends through all layers of the intestine, but which is most marked in the submucosa. This inflammatory response consists of infiltration by mononuclear cells, lymphocytes, plasma cells, and histiocytes. Fissure ulcers frequently penetrate the muscle layer. Unlike the situation in ulcerative colitis, crypt abscesses are infrequent. Discrete granulomas consisting of epithelioid cells, giant cells, and lymphocytes are seen in 50 to 75 percent of the specimens. Although the finding of granulomas is helpful, it is not essential for the diagnosis of Crohn's disease.

Clinical Features and Course

The clinical course of Crohn's disease varies and in the individual patient is unpredictable. Abdominal pain, anorexia, diarrhea, and weight loss are present in 75 to 80 percent. Occasionally, a patient with Crohn's disease may present with acute right lower quadrant abdominal pain and fever and on examination be found to have a mass in the right lower quadrant. The more common course is an insidious onset of recurrent abdominal pain, fever, and diarrhea for several years before the definitive diagnosis is made. Approximately 90 percent of patients develop perianal fissures or fistulas, abscesses, or rectal prolapse. In 10 to 20 percent of patients the extraintestinal manifestation of arthritis, uveitis, or liver disease could be presenting symptoms. Crohn's disease should also be considered in the differential diagnosis of fever of unknown etiology.

The clinical manifestations, as well as the course, of the disease seem related, in part, to its anatomic distribution. This has been classified as disease involving only the small bowel (33 percent), the colon only (20 percent), or both, as in ileocolitis (45 percent). The latter is the most frequent pattern and is characterized by the highest recurrence rate following surgery. The incidence of hematochezia and perianal disease is higher when the colon is involved, as in ileocolitis or Crohn's colitis. A slight increase in the incidence of arthritis may be associated with Crohn's colitis. With the exception of growth retardation, childhood-onset Crohn's disease seems to have a course similar to that of adult-onset disease.

Extraintestinal manifestations of inflammatory bowel disease may precede bowel symptoms, and this may be the patient's presenting complaint. These complications are seen in 25 to 36 percent of patients with Crohn's disease, and the incidence of these complications does not differ between patients with Crohn's disease and those with ulcerative colitis. Extraintestinal manifestations are divided among arthritic (19 percent), dermatologic (4 percent), hepatobiliary (4 percent), ocular (3.5 percent), and vascular (1.3 percent) complications. Dermatologic complications include erythema nodosum and pyoderma gangrenosum. Ocular manifestations include episcleritis and uveitis. Peripheral arthropathies are commonly seen in both ulcerative colitis and Crohn's disease and tend to manifest during exacerbations of the underlying disease process. Ankylosing spondylitis can be detected in up to 20 percent of patients with inflammatory bowel disease. Symptoms may occur before, during, and after bouts of Crohn's disease or ulcerative colitis. Eight percent of these patients with ankylosing spondylitis will have the antigen HLA-B27. Conversely, 18 percent with ankylosing spondylitis have inflammatory bowel disease.

Hepatobiliary disease is common in patients with inflammatory bowel disease and includes pericholangitis, chronic active hepatitis, primary sclerosing cholangitis, and cholangiocarcinoma. Gallstones are detected in up to 33 percent of patients with Crohn's disease. Vascular complications include thromboembolic disease, vasculitis, and arteritis. Patients with thromboembolic complications have a mortality rate of approximately 25 percent. Growth retardation can be seen in children. Hyperoxaluria is a common and potentially treatable occurrence in patients with ileal disease and steatorrhea. This results from the colonic hyperabsorption of dietary oxalate and accounts for the occurrence of nephrolithiasis in 20 to 25 percent of patients with ileal disease.

Complications

More than 78 percent of patients with Crohn's disease will require surgery within the first 20 years from the onset of initial symptoms. Abscess and fissure formation are seen in approximately 30 percent of patients with Crohn's disease. Abscesses can be characterized as intraperitoneal, retroperitoneal, interloop, or intramesenteric. Patients may present with abdominal pain and tenderness typical of their underlying disease but may also have a palpable mass. Patients with retroperitoneal abscesses may present with hip or back pain and difficulty ambulating. Liver abscesses are also found in patients with Crohn's disease.

Fistulas are the result of extension of intestinal fissures noted in patients with Crohn's disease. The most common sites are between the ileum and the sigmoid colon, the cecum, another ileal segment, or the skin. Internal fistulas should be suspected when there is a change in the patient's symptom complex including bowel frequency, amount of pain, or weight loss. Enterovesical fistulas are rare complications of Crohn's disease.

Obstruction is the result of both stricture formation due to the inflammatory process and of edema of the bowel wall. The distal small bowel is the most common site. Symptoms include crampy abdominal pain, distension, nausea, and bloating.

Perianal complications are seen in 90 percent of patients and include perianal or ischiorectal abscesses, fissures, fistulas, rectovaginal fistulas, and rectal prolapse. These are more commonly seen in patients with colonic involvement of Crohn's disease.

While gastrointestinal bleeding is common in patients with Crohn's disease, only 2.5 percent of patients develop life-threatening hemorrhage. In patients with Crohn's disease, bleeding is the result of erosion into a vessel in the bowel wall. Toxic megacolon occurs in 6 percent of all cases of Crohn's disease and is associated with massive gastrointestinal bleeding in over half the cases. Fifty percent of all cases of toxic megacolon occur in patients with Crohn's disease. Free perforation is rarely seen in patients with this disease.

When bowel symptoms are present, malnutrition, malabsorption, hypocalcemia, and vitamin deficiency can be severe. Added to the complications of the disease itself are complications associated with the treatment of the disease.

The incidence of malignant neoplasms of the GI tract is three times higher in patients with Crohn's disease than the incidence in the general population.

Diagnosis

In the majority of patients, the definitive diagnosis of Crohn's disease is made months or years after the onset of symptoms. Occasionally the initial presenting complaint is an extraintestinal manifestation such as arthritis or iritis. A provisional diagnosis of appendicitis or pelvic inflammatory disease may change to Crohn's disease at the time of surgery. A careful and detailed history for bowel symptoms before the onset of acute right lower quadrant pain may provide clues to the correct diagnosis before surgery.

Diagnosis is confirmed by UGI, an air contrast barium enema, and colonoscopy, performed in conjunction with consultation from a gastroenterologist. Oral barium studies with fluoroscopy are the most sensitive and specific for detecting ileal involvement. The classic radiographic findings in the small intestine include segmental narrowing, destruction of the normal mucosal pattern, and fistulas. The segmental involvement of the colon with rectal sparing is the most characteristic feature.

Colonoscopy is the most sensitive technique for examining patients with Crohn's colitis. This technique is useful in detecting early mucosal lesions, in defining the extent of colonic involvement, and in surveillance for the occurrence of colon cancer. Air contrast enemas are also useful in defining mucosal detail.

Intraabdominal abscesses and fistulas are best diagnosed using either CT scan or ultrasound.

Diseases that should be considered in the differential diagnosis include lymphoma, ileocecal amebiasis, tuberculosis, other deep chronic mycotic infections involving the GI tract, gastrointestinal tuberculosis, Kaposi's sarcoma, and yersinial ileocolitis. Fortunately, most of these are uncommon and can be differentiated by appropriate laboratory tests. Yersinial ileocolitis is an acute problem that can be diagnosed by stool culture. Acute ileitis should not be confused with Crohn's disease. Patients with acute ileitis usually recover without sequelae and should not be operated upon. When the disease is confined to the colon, ischemic bowel disease and pseudomembranous enterocolitis as well as ulcerative colitis have to be included in the differential diagnosis of Crohn's colitis.

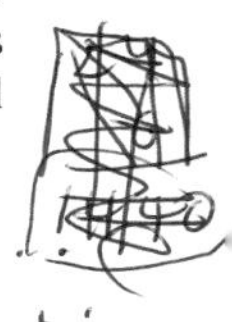

Treatment

The aim of therapy includes relief of symptoms, suppression of the inflammatory disease, treatment of complications, and maintenance of nutrition. In a disease that is virtually incurable, the emphasis should be on relief of symptoms and avoidance of complications.

Prednisone, 40 to 60 mg/day, and sulfasalazine (Azulfidine), 3 to 4 g/day, have both been demonstrated to be effective in treating patients with mild to moderately active Crohn's disease. Patients with severe disease should be hospitalized and receive intravenous steroids. Patients who have not previously been treated with steroids respond best to ACTH, 120 U/day, whereas those on steroids should receive hydrocortisone, 300 mg/day. Supportive measures include intravenous fluids, nasogastric drainage, and correction of nutritional and electrolyte abnormalities.

The presumed mechanism of action of sulfasalazine is the breakdown of the drug to 5-aminosalicylic acid, which appears to be the active component in suppression of the disease. Sulfapyridine is also a byproduct of this breakdown. This drug appears to be responsible for side effects noted in 20 to 45 percent of patients taking sulfasalazine, which include nausea, vomiting, anorexia, epigastric distress, headache, diarrhea, and male infertility. As a result, oral and topical preparations of 5-aminosalicylic acid are being used in patients with inflammatory bowel disease.

Immunosuppressive drugs such as 6-mercaptopurine (1.5 mg/kg per day) or azothioprine (2 mg/kg per day) are useful as a steroid sparing agent and in patients with refractory disease in whom surgery is contraindicated. Additionally, these agents have proved useful in patients with enterocutaneous fistulas, producing a closure rate of up to 75 percent. Both agents have been associated with leukopenia, fever, and pancreatitis. Metronidazole (20 mg/kg per day) has been shown to be useful in treatment of patients with perianal complications of Crohn's disease.

Unlike the situation with ulcerative colitis, there is no conclusive evidence that any drug is useful in maintaining remission in patients with Crohn's disease. The addition of sulfasalazine to prednisone does not improve the response rate and increases the risk of side effects.

Diarrhea can be controlled by the use of loperamide (Imodium), 4 to 16 mg/day, diphenoxylate (Lomotil), 5 to 20 mg/day, and, in some cases, cholestyramine (Questran), 9 g one to six times daily. The latter is particularly useful in patients who have limited ileal disease, no obstruction, and mild steatorrhea. Cholestyramine acts by binding bile acids and eliminating their cathartic action. The primary aim of dietary therapy is the maintenance of nutrition and the alleviation of diarrhea. Lactose intolerance is quite common in these patients and may be a major contributing factor to the diarrhea. When such intolerance is present, elimination of lactose from the diet should be of therapeutic benefit. Reduction in dietary oxalate should be considered in every patient. In addition, supplementation of trace metals, fat-soluble vitamins, and medium-chain triglycerides should be considered in selected patients.

Surgical intervention is indicated in those patients with certain complications of the disease, including intestinal obstruction of hemorrhage, perforation, abscess or fistula formation, toxic megacolon, and perianal disease. In addition, a patient may need surgery because of the failure of medical therapy. The recurrence rate after surgery approaches 100 percent.

ULCERATIVE COLITIS

Ulcerative colitis is a chronic inflammatory and ulcerative disease of the colon and rectum characterized most often clinically by bloody diarrhea. The etiology, like that of Crohn's disease, remains unknown even though extensive investigations into the cause continue. Epidemiological considerations are similar to those of Crohn's disease: the disease is more prevalent in the United States and northern Europe, and peak incidence occurs in the second and the third decades of life. The incidence of ulcerative colitis is about 5 to 8 per 100,000 and has not risen significantly in the last few years, even though the incidence of new cases of Crohn's disease has increased during this period. First-degree relatives of patients with ulcerative colitis have a 15-fold risk of developing ulcerative colitis and a 3.5-fold risk of developing Crohn's disease.

Pathology

Ulcerative colitis involves primarily the mucosa and submucosa. Microscopically, the disease is characterized by mucosal inflammation with the formation of crypt abscesses, epithelial necrosis, and mucosal ulceration. The muscular layer and serosa are often spared. In the usual case the disease increases in severity more distally, the rectosigmoid being involved in 95 percent of cases. In the early stages of the disease, the mucous membranes appear finely granular and friable. In more severe cases, the mucosa appears as a red spongy surface dotted with small ulcerations oozing blood and purulent exudate. In very advanced disease, one sees large oozing ulcerations and pseudopolyps (areas of hyperplastic overgrowth surrounded by inflamed mucosa).

Clinical Features and Course

The clinical features and course of ulcerative colitis vary but are somewhat dependent on the anatomic distribution of the disease in the colon. The disease is classified as mild, moderate, or severe depending on the clinical manifestations. Patients with mild disease have fewer than four bowel movements per day, no systemic symptoms, and few extraintestinal manifestations. Of all patients, 60 percent present with mild disease; in 80 percent of cases the disease is limited to the rectum. Occasionally, constipation and rectal bleeding are the presenting complaint. Progression to pancolitis occurs in 10 to 15 percent.

Patients with severe disease constitute 15 percent of those with ulcerative colitis. Severe disease is associated with more than six bowel movements per day, anemia, fever, weight loss, tachycardia, and more frequently extraintestinal manifestations. Severe disease accounts for 90 percent of the mortality from ulcerative colitis. Virtually all severely affected patients have pancolitis.

Moderate disease accounts for 25 percent of patients. The clinical manifestations are less severe and demonstrate a good response to therapy. These patients usually have colitis extending to the splenic flexure (left-sided colitis) but may develop pancolitis.

The most frequent clinical course of ulcerative colitis is characterized by intermittent attacks with complete remission between attacks. This occurs in the majority of patients. In other patients, the first attack is followed by a prolonged period of inactivity. Least commonly, patients run a chronically active course. The factors associated with an unfavorable prognosis and increased mortality include the severity and extent of disease, a short history before the first attack, and onset of the disease after 60 years of age.

Extraintestinal complications of ulcerative colitis include peripheral arthritis, ankylosing spondylitis, episcleritis, posterior uveitis, pyoderma gangrenosum, and erythema nodosum.

Complications

Although blood loss from sustained hemorrhage may be the most common complication of the illness, toxic megacolon is a complication that must not be missed.

Toxic megacolon develops in advanced colitis when the disease process begins to extend through all layers of the colon. The result is a loss of muscular tone within the colon and localized peritonitis. The colon begins to dilate as muscular tone is lost. If the colon continues to dilate without treatment, signs of toxicity will develop. Plain radiography of the abdomen demonstrates a long, continuous segment of air-filled colon greater than 6 cm in diameter. The distended portion of the atonic colon can perforate, causing peritonitis and septicemia. Mortality from this complication is approximately 50 percent if perforation occurs but less than 10 percent if surgery is undertaken prior to perforation.

A patient with toxic megacolon appears severely ill; the abdomen is distended, tender, and tympanitic. Severe diarrhea (more than 10 bowel movements per day) is often seen. Fever, tachycardia, and signs of hypovolemia are typically part of the portrait. Leukocytosis, anemia, electrolyte disturbances, and hypoalbuminemia are the supporting laboratory data.

Some of the more toxic aspects of ulcerative colitis such as leukocytosis and peritonitis can be masked in the patient taking corticosteroids. When such therapy is being administered, greater suspicion is required to make the diagnosis. Antidiarrheal agents, hypokalemia, narcotics, cathartics, and enemas have been implicated as precipitants of toxic megacolon. Medical therapy with nasogastric suction, intravenous prednisolone, 60 g/day, or hydrocortisone, 300 mg/day, parenteral antibiotics active against coliforms and anaerobes (ampicillin and clindamycin) and intravenous fluids should be attempted as initial therapy and in preparing the patient for possible surgery. However, prolonged medical treatment of these patients increases mortality; therefore, early surgical consultation must be sought with the aim of performing a colectomy if clinical improvement is not noted in 24 to 48 h with medical treatment.

Local complications such as small rectovaginal fistulas occur infrequently in cases of ulcerative colitis. Perirectal fistulas and abscesses are much more common in patients with Crohn's disease but occur in approximately 20 percent of patients with ulcerative colitis. Massive gastrointestinal hemorrhage, obstruction secondary to stricture formation, and acute perforation are other complications of the disease.

Clinically apparent liver disease may occur in 5 to 10 percent of patients. The liver disease may be any of the following: pericholangitis, chronic active hepatitis, fatty liver or cirrhosis, cholelithiasis, sclerosing cholangitis, and bile duct carcinoma.

There is a 10- to 30-fold increase in the development of carcinoma of the colon in patients with ulcerative colitis. Carcinoma of the colon is the cause of 5 to 15 percent of the deaths attributed to ulcerative colitis. The major risk factors for the development of carcinoma of the colon are the extent and the duration of the disease. The cumulative risk of cancer after 15, 20, and 25 years is 8, 12, and 25 percent, respectively. Additional factors that increase the risk of cancer in patients with ulcerative colitis include early onset of the disease and a family history of colon cancer. Carcinoma developing in patients with ulcerative colitis is more evenly distributed in the colon and is often multicentric and virulent in clinical behavior. The availability of fiberoptic colonoscopy allows one to perform periodic colonoscopies and biopsies to detect metaplastic change thought to predict the development of colon cancer. In patients with pancolitis such surveillance should start 7 to 10 years after the onset of the disease.

Diagnosis

Laboratory findings in patients with ulcerative colitis are nonspecific; they may include leukocytosis, anemia, thrombocytosis, decreased serum albumin, and abnormal liver function studies. Therefore, the diagnosis of ulcerative colitis rests on the following: a history of abdominal cramps and diarrhea, mucoid stools, stool examination negative for ova and parasites, stool cultures negative for enteric pathogens, and confirmation by sigmoidoscopic examination. The results of the latter examination are abnormal in 95 percent of the patients with ulcerative colitis. The observed pathologic changes vary depending on the severity and duration of the disease. Granularity, friability, ulceration of the mucosa, and, in more advanced cases, pseudopolyposis are quite characteristic.

Rectal biopsy is helpful in very early cases and in excluding amebiasis and metaplasia (see under "Pathology," above). Barium enema examination is useful in confirming the diagnosis and defining the extent of involvement of the colon. It is usually done before biopsy as it is used to differentiate ulcerative colitis from other conditions. Colonoscopy is the most sensitive method for making the diagnosis and defining the extent and severity of the disease. In addition, in the evaluation of the patient for the development of metaplasia or colon cancer, colonoscopy is extremely useful. Barium enema examination and colonoscopy should not be performed in moderately or severely sick patients. One should not shy away from performing a rigid or fiberoptic proctosigmoidoscopy, however, even in the severely ill patient, provided it is done gently and without the administration of any enemas or laxatives.

The major diseases that should be considered in the differential diagnosis of ulcerative colitis include infectious colitis, Crohn's colitis, ischemic colitis, irradiation colitis, and pseudomembranous colitis. When the disease is limited to the rectum, particular attention should be paid to sexually acquired diseases that are seen frequently in the male homosexual population ("gay bowel disease"). Some of the more common diseases in this category include rectal syphilis, gonococcal proctitis, lymphogranuloma venereum, and inflammations caused by herpes simplex virus, *Entamoeba histolytica, Shigella,* and *Campylobacter.*

Treatment

The majority of patients with mild and moderate disease can be treated as outpatients. Corticosteroids are effective in inducing a remission in the majority of cases and constitute the mainstay of therapy in an acute attack. Long-term steroid therapy should be initiated in conjunction with a referral to a gastroenterologist. Daily doses of 40 to 60 mg of prednisone are usually sufficient and can be adjusted depending on the severity of the disease. 5-Aminosalacylic acid enemas have been used with great success to treat patients with active proctitis, proctosigmoiditis, and left-sided colitis (less than 60 cm of active disease). This therapy has also been used to maintain remission in these patients. Once clinical remission is achieved, steroids should be slowly tapered and discontinued. There is no evidence that maintenance dosages of steroids reduce the incidence of relapses. Sulfasalazine has been used in the treatment of acute attacks but is probably inferior to steroids, especially in the more severe cases. Its primary usefulness is in the form of adjunctive therapy and in the maintenance of a remission. Maintenance dosages of 1.5 to 2 g/day significantly reduce the recurrence rate of the disease.

Supportive measures in the treatment of mild to moderately sick patients include the replenishment of iron stores, a nutritious diet with the elimination of lactose, and adequate physical and psychological rest. Hydrophilic bulk agents such as psyllium (Metamucil) can be used in some patients to improve stool consistency. Antidiarrheal agents should be avoided because they may precipitate toxic megacolon and because they are generally ineffective.

Patients with severe ulcerative colitis should be treated in the hospital. Intravenous steroids or ACTH, replacement of fluids, correction of electrolyte abnormalities, broad-spectrum antibiotics active against coliforms and anaerobes (ampicillin and clindamycin or metronidazole), and hyperalimentation may be considered for the individual patient. When toxic megacolon is suspected, nasogastric suction and a surgical consultation should be obtained, and the patient should be observed by frequent examinations and flat films of the abdomen. When the diagnosis of toxic megacolon is established and the patient fails to show dramatic clinical improvement within 24 to 48 h, emergency surgery should be considered. In addition to toxic megacolon, the indications for surgery are colonic perforation, massive lower GI bleeding, suspicion of colon cancer, and disease that is refractory to medical therapy (large doses of steroids required for the control of the disease). The surgical treatment of choice is total proctocolectomy with ileostomy. Because this is not well accepted by most patients, subtotal colectomy with ileorectal anastomosis is being performed in a greater number of cases. Unlike the effects of surgery in Crohn's disease, in ulcerative colitis surgical intervention is curative.

PSEUDOMEMBRANOUS ENTEROCOLITIS

Pseudomembranous enterocolitis is an inflammatory bowel disorder in which membranelike yellowish plaques of exudate overlay and replace necrotic intestinal mucosa. Three different syndromes have been described: neonatal pseudomembranous enterocolitis, postoperative pseudomembranous enterocolitis, and antibiotic-associated pseudomembranous colitis. In the latter, it is presumed that broad-spectrum antibiotics, most notably clindamycin, cephalosporins, and ampicillin, alter the gut flora in such a way that toxin-producing *Clostridium difficile* can flourish in the colon. The result is a clinical picture of mucoid watery diarrhea that may progress to a full-blown ulcerative colitis. Rarely, toxic megacolon or colonic perforation may occur in patients with pseudomembranous colitis. The disease typically begins 7 to 10 days after the institution of antibiotic therapy, although in some cases symptoms may be noted up to 2 to 4 weeks after the antibiotic is discontinued.

The diagnosis is made by a history of antibiotic use and the observation of the characteristic yellowish plaques on sigmoidoscopy. Lesions may be seen throughout the entire alimentary tract although they are typically limited to the right colon. For this reason colonoscopy may be needed in some cases. The diagnosis is confirmed by the demonstration of the presence of *Clostridium difficile* toxin in stool filtrates.

The treatment of pseudomembranous colitis includes discontinuing antibiotic therapy and instituting supportive measures such as the administration of fluids and the correction of electrolyte abnormalities. Severely ill persons may be hospitalized. Oral vancomycin, 125 mg four times a day for 7 to 10 days, is effective in the majority of patients. The symptoms resolve in a few days. Relapses occur in 10 to 20 percent of patients, necessitating a second course of treatment with vancomycin. Other agents that are useful in the treatment of pseudomembranous colitis include metronidazole, 500 mg four times a day, or bacitracin, 1 g per day, both administered for 7 to 10 days orally. The use of antidiarrheal agents may prolong or worsen symptoms in patients with pseudomembranous colitis and should be avoided. Steroids and surgical intervention are rarely needed for patients with pseudomembranous colitis.

BIBLIOGRAPHY

Crohn's disease

Bozdech JM, Farmer RG: Diagnosis of Crohn's disease. *Hepatogastroenterology* 37:8, 1990.

Danzi M: Extraintestinal manifestations of idiopathic inflammatory bowel disease. *Arch Intern Med* 148:297, 1988.

Meyers S, Sachar DB: Medical management of Crohn's disease. *Hepatogastroenterology* 37:42, 1990.

Reddy SB, Jeejeebhoy KN: Acute complications of Crohn's disease. *Crit Care Med* 16:557, 1988.

Ruderman WB: Newer pharmacologic agents for the therapy of inflammatory bowel disease. *Med Clin North Am* 74:133, 1990.

Zenilman ME, Becker JM: Emergencies in inflammatory bowel disease. *Gastroent Clin North Am* 17:387, 1988.

Ulcerative Colitis

Hawkey CJ, Hawthorne AB: Medical treatment of ulcerative colitis: scoring the advances. *Gut* 29:1298, 1988.

Sutherland SR: Topical treatment of ulcerative colitis. *Med Clin North Am* 74:119, 1990.

Pseudomembranous Colitis

Burden DW: Treatment of pseudomembranous colitis and antibiotic-associated diarrhea. *J Antimicro Chemother* 14 (Suppl D):103, 1984.

Fortson WC, Tedesco FJ: Drug-induced colitis: A review. *Am J Gastroenterol* 79:878, 1984.

Gross MH: Management of antibiotic-associated pseudomembranous colitis. *Clin Pharm* 4:304, 1985.

Trnka YM, Lamont JT: *Clostridium difficile* colitis. *Adv Intern Med* 29:85, 1984.

45
COLONIC DIVERTICULAR DISEASE

Stephen G. Priest
Steven N. Klein

Acquired diverticular disease of the colon has become an increasingly common disorder of industrialized nations. Diverticulosis coli was first described in the early 1700s by Littre but was not identified as a pathologic entity until the mid-nineteenth century by Cruveilhier. Radiologic studies have suggested that one-third of the population will have acquired the disease by age 45 and two-thirds by age 85. Diverticula of the colon are rare in individuals under age 20.

Inflammation resulting in clinical diverticulitis has been estimated to occur in 10 to 25 percent of patients with known diverticulosis, and the incidence increases with age. Diverticulitis in the younger age group tends to be a more virulent form of the disease, with frequent complications requiring earlier surgical intervention.

Early literature indicated that the frequency of the disease was higher in men. Recent reports have shown an increased incidence in women.

PATHOPHYSIOLOGY

Colonic diverticula are, by definition, false diverticula because they do not include all the layers of the bowel wall. They consist of mucosa and submucosa with the peritoneal covering that has herniated through a defect in the circular muscle layer of the wall. The sites of herniation are located between the mesenteric and antimesenteric taenia where intramural blood vessels penetrate the muscularis.

A pathophysiologic mechanism to explain the development of diverticular disease is not apparent. It is still unresolved whether diverticular disease is a disorder of colonic motility, a colonic muscle abnormality, a connective tissue disorder, or a normal concomitant of aging. The most common hypothesis is that acquired diverticula arise because of high intraluminal pressures in areas of relative weakness of the colonic wall. This is based upon observations that the majority of patients have diverticula located within the sigmoid colon. Laplace's law states that the tension on the wall of a hollow cylinder is proportional to the radius of the cylinder multiplied by the pressure within the cylinder. This suggests that the intraluminal pressure in the colon is greatest where the lumen is narrowest. The diameter of the colon is smallest in the sigmoid region, and thus this region of the colon is the most likely location for the development of diverticula.

The complications of diverticular disease that bring the patient to the emergency department can be divided into two broad categories: (1) inflammation and its associated complications and (2) bleeding.

Diverticulitis, or inflammation, is the most common complication of diverticular disease. It results when fecal material becomes inspissated in the neck of an acquired diverticulum, resulting in subsequent bacterial proliferation and adjacent peridiverticulitis. Fortunately, fecal contamination of the peritoneum is usually limited because perforation of a diverticulum is into the leaves of the mesentary, or because the contamination is walled off by the mobile loops of the sigmoid colon or small bowel and adjacent pelvic structures. Free perforation may occur with generalized peritonitis, but fortunately it is uncommon.

DIAGNOSIS

The most common symptom of diverticulitis is pain. This is most commonly described as a steady, deep discomfort in the left lower quadrant. Rarely, the clinical presentation may be indistinguishable from that of acute appendicitis. This may occur when the patient has a redundant sigmoid colon lying on the right side of the abdomen which becomes inflamed. Cases of diverticulitis in the cecum or ascending colon have also been reported. In patients 50 years or older, the possibility of diverticulitis should always be considered in the patient with right lower quadrant abdominal pain.

Often, patients will complain of a change in their bowel habits, either in the form of diarrhea or increasing constipation. Tenesmus is another common symptom. The involved diverticulum may irritate the bladder or ureter, causing the patient to have urinary frequency, dysuria, or pyuria. If a fistula develops between the colon and the bladder, the patient may present with recurrent urinary tract infections or pneumaturia. Paralytic ileus with abdominal distension, nausea, and vomiting may develop secondary to intraabdominal irritation and peritonitis. Small bowel obstruction may also occur if an adjacent loop of small bowel becomes kinked or narrowed in the inflammatory mass.

The patient with free perforation will often present with a history of sudden onset of abdominal pain usually beginning in the lower abdomen and then progressing to generalized abdominal involvement. The patient appears quite toxic with signs of diffuse peritonitis.

PHYSICAL EXAMINATION

Physical examination frequently demonstrates a low-grade fever around 38°C (100.4°F). The temperature may, however, be more elevated in patients with generalized peritonitis or in those who have formed an abscess. The abdominal examination then reveals localized tenderness often with voluntary guarding and localized rebound tenderness. With careful palpation, one may be able to appreciate a fullness or a mass over the involved segment of the colon. Rectal examination will often reveal tenderness on the left side. In the female patient, a pelvic examination should always be carried out to eliminate a gynecologic source of symptoms.

LABORATORY STUDIES

Laboratory studies should include routine screening blood tests, urinalysis, and an acute abdominal series. Unfortunately, in many cases laboratory studies are not helpful in the diagnosis. Leukocytosis was seen in only 36 percent of 130 patients treated at the Lahey Clinic for acute complications of diverticular disease. The acute abdominal series may be normal or may demonstrate associated ileus, partial small bowel obstruction, colonic obstruction, free air indicating bowel perforation, or extraluminal collections of air that might indicate a walled-off abscess. Additional noninvasive studies which may be useful include abdominal and pelvic ultrasonography or a CT scan of the abdomen and pelvis. These studies may show bowel wall thickening, mesenteric inflammation, or abdominal fluid collections indicating abscess formation.

Controversy exists regarding the use of sigmoidoscopy or contrast radiographic studies in the acute inflammatory state. The general opinion is that these studies should be performed after the acute inflammatory process has subsided following conservative medical management.

DIFFERENTIAL DIAGNOSIS

In patients over the age of 40 presenting with complaints of abdominal pain, a change in bowel habits, and urinary symptoms, a diagnosis of colonic diverticulitis should be entertained. These symptoms, however, are nonspecific, and a number of pathologic entities may present with similar signs and symptoms (Table 45–1).

Irritable Bowel Syndrome

One-third of the patients surgically treated for diverticulitis lack microscopic inflammatory changes in the resected specimen. These patients are said to have had "painful diverticular disease," or irritable bowel syndrome. Their symptoms included diffuse crampy or colicky abdominal pain, brought on by meals or emotional upset. The passage

Table 45-1. Differential Diagnosis for Diverticulitis

1. Irritable bowel syndrome
2. Carcinoma of the colon
3. Acute appendicitis
4. Ulcerative colitis
5. Crohn's disease
6. Pelvic inflammatory disease
7. Ischemic colitis
8. Leaking aortic aneurysm
9. Renal calculus
10. Other colonic diseases
    a. Amebiasis
    b. Lymphogranuloma venereum
    c. Gonorrheal proctitis
    d. Fecal impaction
    e. Foreign-body granuloma
    f. Endometriosis
    g. Collagen disease
    h. Postirradiation proctosigmoiditis
    i. Hyperplastic tuberculosis
    j. Syphilis
    k. Actinomycosis

of flatus or a bowel movement may bring relief of symptoms. Bowel habits can include alternating bouts of constipation and diarrhea. On physical examination, these patients may have a cordlike mass in the left lower quadrant corresponding to the sigmoid colon but lack signs of localized or generalized peritonitis. Laboratory studies are normal and the patient is afebrile.

Carcinoma of the Colon

The differentiation of diverticulitis from colon carcinoma is usually not difficult. If a cancer has progressed in size to cause luminal narrowing, then a patient may present with a change in bowel habits, with either diarrhea or constipation, and/or abdominal pain which can mimic symptoms of acute diverticulitis. There may be blood mixed with the patient's stools, and weight loss. Physical examination may reveal a palpable mass, usually nontender. Fever and chills are less common, and laboratory studies may demonstrate anemia without evidence of leukocytosis.

If a patient with colonic obstruction but without symptoms of acute diverticulitis has evidence of diverticular disease on barium enema, the diagnosis could be either obstruction due to an inflamed diverticuloma or colon carcinoma with underlying diverticulosis. X-ray changes which may be helpful in differentiating between the two include the length of the segment involved and whether or not the mucosa is intact. Adenocarcinoma of the colon is a mucosal disorder that results in mucosal destruction, a short segment of involvement, and overhanging edges. Diverticular disease originates outside the lumen of the colon so that the bowel mucosa remains intact, and the segments of bowel involvement tend to be longer. If there are no signs of acute inflammation, then fiberoptic colonoscopy can be used to differentiate between diverticular disease and carcinoma.

Acute Appendicitis

A redundant loop of inflamed sigmoid colon or inflamed diverticula of the right side of the colon may mimic acute appendicitis. Therefore, in patients over the age of 50, diverticulitis should always be considered in the differential diagnosis of acute appendicitis.

Ulcerative Colitis

Inflammatory bowel disease is commonly seen in individuals under the age of 30. There does, however, exist a secondary peak in the incidence of newly diagnosed ulcerative colitis and Crohn's disease in individuals in their sixth decade. Patients with ulcerative colitis may present with frequent loose bowel movements and rectal bleeding. On physical examination, abdominal tenderness is usually absent and no masses are palpable. Difficulty again arises in the individual who has diverticulosis and concomitant ulcerative colitis. In these individuals, radiographic and endoscopic studies are most helpful.

Crohn's Disease

Crohn's disease is a transmural disease which can cause fistulae and abscesses. Patients may present with symptoms indistinguishable from those of acute diverticulitis, and a careful history should be taken. Patients with Crohn's disease will often present with diarrhea, mucous discharge, and rectal complaints. The association of perianal disease, such as unusual fissures, fistulas, or large skin tags, is suggestive of Crohn's disease. Sigmoidoscopy and biopsy can establish the diagnosis.

Pelvic Inflammatory Disease

Pelvic inflammatory disease may present with abdominal pain, fever, and leukocytosis, and it usually occurs in young women. A careful pelvic examination should be carried out in all female patients. A history of irregular menses, and the finding of vaginal discharge, should aid in the diagnosis.

Ischemic Colitis

Ischemic colitis can present with a broad range of clinical manifestations. Mild transient ischemia may result in mucosal sloughing and painless rectal bleeding. If the disease progresses to gangrene, the patient develops severe abdominal pain and peritonitis. Pain may be out of proportion to physical findings. A plain film of the abdomen may reveal thumb printing in the region of the involved colonic segment. In more advanced cases, there may be gas within the bowel wall, or, if perforation has occurred, free air in the abdomen. Cautious endoscopic evaluation and contrast x-ray studies are helpful in distinguishing ischemic colitis from diverticulitis.

MEDICAL TREATMENT

Patients who have localized pain without signs and symptoms of local peritonitis or systemic infection may be treated on an outpatient basis. Treatment consists of bowel rest and broad-spectrum oral antibiotic therapy. Patients are instructed to limit activity and to maintain a liquid diet for 48 h. If symptoms improve, low-residue foods are added to the diet. Broad-spectrum antibiotics covering both aerobic and anaerobic bacteria are given. Predominant colonic aerobes include *Escherichia coli, Klebsiella,* and *Enterobacter,* while *Bacteroides fragilis, Peptostreptococcus,* and *Clostridium* are the predominant colonic anaerobes. Common oral antibiotic agents effective against aerobic organisms include ampicillin (500 mg) or a cephalosporin such as Keflex (500 mg), in combination with metronidazole (Flagyl, 500 mg), which is utilized to treat the anaerobic organisms. These drugs are taken orally every 6 h for 7 to 10 days. If the patient has an allergy to penicillin, then tetracycline, 500 mg qid, can be substituted. Patients are instructed to contact their physicians if increasing abdominal pain, fever, or malaise occurs. Once the patient has improved, elective evaluation with contrast barium enema is performed.

If a patient has systemic signs and symptoms of infection, or localized peritonitis, then hospitalization is necessary. Again, the patient is placed on bowel rest, but in this case, nothing by mouth is given and intravenous fluids are administered. Nasogastric suction is necessary only if the patient manifests signs of bowel obstruction or an adynamic ileus. Surgical consultation should be obtained at the time of hospitalization. Intravenous antibiotics, usually ampicillin and an aminoglycoside, and clindamycin or metronidazole, are given for aerobic and anaerobic coverage.

LOWER GASTROINTESTINAL BLEEDING AS A COMPLICATION OF DIVERTICULOSIS

In the past, most cases of massive lower gastrointestinal bleeding were attributed to diverticular disease. Over the last 20 years, however, with the development of selective mesenteric angiography and endoscopy, it has been shown that arteriovenous malformations are as common a cause of lower gastrointestinal bleeding as diverticulosis.

Nevertheless, bleeding occurs in 5 to 15 percent of the patients with diverticulosis. Diverticular bleeding is generally massive, but, fortunately, in 75 to 95 percent of the cases, bleedings stops spontaneously and can be managed with supportive therapy.

Although the majority of cases of massive lower gastrointestinal bleeding are caused by colonic diverticula or arteriovenous malformations, other etiologic factors should be considered. These include colonic tumors, inflammatory bowel disease, ischemic colitis, Meckel's diverticulum, and radiation enteritis.

Pathogenesis

Diverticula form in areas of relative weakness created by the penetrating vasa recta. As the colonic mucosa herniates, the vasa recta are stretched and displaced over the fundus of the herinated pouch. Bleeding results when the vasa recta rupture into the diverticulum.

Management

Lower gastrointestinal bleeding may originate from anywhere within the gastrointestinal tract. Upper gastrointestinal tract sources of bleeding must always be considered. The most common sites of upper gastrointestinal bleeding include duodenal ulcers, gastric erosions, gastric ulcers, esophageal varices, and Mallory-Weiss tears.

A careful history must be obtained, with particular attention to previous gastric or duodenal ulceration and associated abdominal, rectal, or anal symptoms. One should inquire about the onset and duration of bleeding, and whether the stools are bright red in nature and forming clots, or melanotic. Since diverticular bleeding is usually painless, the presence of abdominal pain suggests another disease process. Certain medications, and alcohol abuse, also predispose to bleeding.

Physical examination is often unremarkable. Abdominal examination may reveal a mass or tenderness suggesting causes of bleeding other than diverticula. Careful anorectal examination is necessary to ensure that fissures or hemorrhoids are not the source of bleeding. Normally, the latter do not cause serious gastrointestinal hemorrhage; however, severe hemorrhage can occur if portal hypertension is present. Proctosigmoidoscopy is necessary to identify lesions within the rectum or lower sigmoid colon that might cause bleeding, and also to ensure that no significant abnormalities within the distal bowel are present if emergent total abdominal colectomy becomes necessary. In this situation, the rectum can be saved and used for a primary anastomosis.

If anorectal causes of major lower gastrointestinal bleeding have been excluded, then a nasogastric tube should be inserted and the gastric contents aspirated to detect blood. Bilious return should be identified to be sure that an adequate sampling has been taken. Even if the nasogastric aspirate does contain bile but no gross blood, bleeding from an upper gastrointestinal source cannot be completely excluded. If there is evidence of bleeding, then an urgent esophagogastroduodenoscopy should be carried out.

At the time of resuscitation, blood should be drawn for type and crossmatch, CBC, coagulation profiles including bleeding time, and screening evaluations including serum electrolyte and liver function studies. Two large-bore IVs should be initiated in all patients with significant blood loss.

Once the patient is stabilized, and no obvious source of bleeding has been identified, then further studies are necessary. The next diagnostic test is a ^{99m}Tc-labeled red blood cell scan, which can identify bleeding rates as low as 0.12 mL/min. If an area of active bleeding is identified, then selective mesenteric arteriography should be carried out. However, in order for an arteriogram to identify bleeding, the rate of blood loss must be rapid, greater than 0.5 mL/min.

If arteriography positively identifies a bleeding site, then selective perfusion of vasopressin may be used in an attempt to control bleeding. If bleeding remains uncontrolled, a segmental resection of the involved colon should be carried out.

If the ^{99m}Tc-labeled red blood cell scan is negative and bleeding stops, total colonoscopy is necessary in an attempt to identify the bleeding source. If no bleeding source is identified, but hemorrhage continues, requiring transfusions of more than 6 units of blood within 24 h, then emergency surgery should be considered. Total abdominal colectomy with ileorectal anastomosis or a temporary ileostomy is usually performed.

Fortunately, most diverticular bleeding stops spontaneously with supportive therapy. Twenty-five percent of patients will require subsequent hospitalization for recurrent bleeding. After a second bleeding episode, the risk of a third hemorrhage approaches 50 percent.

BIBLIOGRAPHY

Almy TP, Howell DA: Diverticular disease of the colon. *N Engl J Med* 302:324, 1980.

Connell AM: Applied physiology of the colon: Factors relevant to diverticular disease. *Clin Gastroenterol* 4:23, 1975.

Hackford AW, Veidenheimer MC: Diverticular disease of the colon: Current concepts and management. *Surg Clin North Am* 65:347, 1985.

Meyers MA, Volberg F, et al: The angioarchitecture of colonic diverticula, significance and bleeding diverticulosis. *Radiology* 108:249, 1973.

Milsom JW, Singh G.: Diverticulitis in young patients. *Semin colon* and *rectal surg* 1:103, 1990.

Opelka FG, Timmcke AE: Management of Bleeding Diverticulosis: Colonic diverticulitis. *Semin Colon Rectal Surg* 1, 1990.

Parks TG: Natural history of diverticular disease of the colon. *Clin Gastroenterol* 4:53, 1975.

Potter GD, Sellin JH: Lower gastrointestinal bleeding. *Gastroenterol Clin North Am* 17:341, 1988.

Roth JL: Diagnosis and differential diagnosis of colonic diverticulitis. *Postgrad Med* 60:85, 1976.

Schoetz DJ Jr, Murray JJ: Diverticular Disease: Post Graduate Advances in Colon and Rectal Surgery, II-I, Forum Medicum, Inc. 1989.

46
ANORECTAL DISORDERS

James K. Bouzoukis

Anorectal disorders are varied and multiple and may also be complex, manifesting signs and symptoms of underlying serious local or systemic disorders that could be life-threatening. The symptoms with which these patients invariably present include one or more of the following:

Bleeding

Constipation

Diarrhea

Discharge

Incomplete evacuation

Incontinence

Pain

Protrusion or palpable mass

Pruritus

ANATOMY

The anorectum is an anatomical structure in which the entodermal intestine unites with and opens into an orifice of ectodermal origin: the anal canal. The junction of these two embryonic structures (the anorectal line) is the dentate line, which marks the anatomical beginning of the anal canal (2 to 3 cm long) and is in continuity with the perianal skin at its distal anal verge. The mucosa of the anal canal consists of stratified squamous epithelium but contains no hair follicles or sweat glands. At the anal verge (perianal region), the anoderm thickens and includes in its structure hair follicles and other cutaneous appendages. Proximal to the dentate line the rectal ampulla narrows to conform to the opening of the anal canal, and in doing so its mucosa takes on a pleated appearance, forming 8 to 14 convoluted longitudinal folds: the columns of Morgagni. Each adjacent column is connected at the dentate line by a flap of mucosa that forms a small anal crypt, normally 1 to 3 mm in longitudinal depth.

At the base of approximately one-half of these crypts is a small rudimentary anal gland that may extend centrifugally through the internal sphincter as far as the intersphincteric plane (an extension of the rectum's longitudinal muscle layer) but does not penetrate into the external sphincter. Infection and inflammation of these crypts and glands become the source of anal sepsis as characterized by the development of cryptitis, fissures, abscesses, and fistulas.

The inner structure (wall) from the mucosal lining to the intersphincteric plane that separates the internal from the external sphincters is a continuation of the usual layers of the wall of the colon and rectum. The innermost lining, mucosa, continues to the anal verge, undergoing a transition, just proximal to the dentate line, from rectal columnar to cuboidal to squamous epithelium. The submucosa, which normally contains the bulk of the bowel's blood vessels (and autonomic nerves), thickens considerably proximal to the dentate line, and its dilated veins in this area are referred to as the internal hemorrhoidal plexus. Likewise, the inner circular muscle layer of the rectum thickens considerably as it terminates distally in the anorectum to form the internal sphincter muscles, while the more attenuated longitudinal muscles of the rectum extend caudally, blending with fibers of voluntary skeletal muscles from the levator ani and external sphincter groups to form the intersphincteric plane (Fig. 46-1).

Additional sphincteric support is provided by an outer layer of voluntary skeletal muscles, the external sphincters, that are divided into three parts: deep, superficial, and subcutaneous. The external sphincters are actually a caudal extension of the puborectalis muscle, which interacts with the levator ani muscle that forms the pelvic floor. The puborectalis, the proximal external sphincters, and the internal sphincters form the ring of muscles that one palpates when performing a digital examination of the anorectum.

Lateral to the external sphincters and superior to the levator ani are the ischiorectal and pelvirectal spaces, where deep, life-threatening infections can occur.

EXAMINATION OF THE PATIENT

No matter how much historical information is obtained, no definitive diagnosis can be made without a careful examination of the anus and rectum, including anoscopy and, if necessary, proctoscopy.

The patient should be placed in any one of three positions (Fig. 46-2). The lateral, or Sim's, position, performed with the patient lying on his or her left side with the left leg extended and the right knee and hip flexed, is probably the most commonly used approach for performing a routine digital rectal examination and is the preferred position for elderly or pregnant patients who would not otherwise tolerate the knee-chest position. In debilitated patients, one may have to perform the examination with the patient in a supine, lithotomy position. From the Sim's position, one should elevate the upper right buttock to provide better exposure of the perianal area, and, if needed, endoscopic examination of the anus and distal rectum can be performed with the patient in this position.

Examining a patient placed in the knee-chest position requires a cooperative patient who is not too ill or in too much distress. This provides for a thorough inspection of the perianal area and is convenient for anoscopy and proctoscopy. Thighs should be at right angles to the table with the feet extended over the end of the table.

The optimal position for examining and treating anorectal lesions is with the patient prone on a proctoscopic table that is tilted to place the anus in an uppermost position (Fig. 46-2C).

A digital examination should always be performed before doing any endoscopic procedure. No bowel preparation is needed to perform an anoscopic examination. After performing a digital examination and determining that the patient will tolerate passage of an anoscope, introduce a well-lubricated, lighted anoscope (Fig. 46-3); remove the obturator; and gently rotate it 360° to view the anorectum circumferentially.

It is usually difficult to perform a proper sigmoidoscopic examination in an emergency department setting. Ordinarily, the lower bowel has to be prepped; a natural bowel movement, spontaneous or induced, 1 to 2 h before examination is usually sufficient preparation. In some acute situations, such as trying to determine the source of lower GI bleeding or obtaining cultures in a case of suppurative proctitis, emergency proctoscopy may be performed. A rigid sigmoidoscope should be utilized, with the patient placed in a proctoscopic or Sim's position, depending on how hemodynamically stable the patient is. An inexperienced endoscopist should not attempt to pass the sigmoidoscope beyond the rectosigmoid junction, where the lumen is greatly angulated, because of the risk of perforation.

HEMORRHOIDS

The anorectal area is drained by the internal and external hemorrhoidal venous system. The internal hemorrhoidal veins, which in essence are submucosal vascular cushions that may contribute to anal continence, are located proximal to the dentate line and drain into the portal system through the superior rectals and the inferior mesenteric vein. They

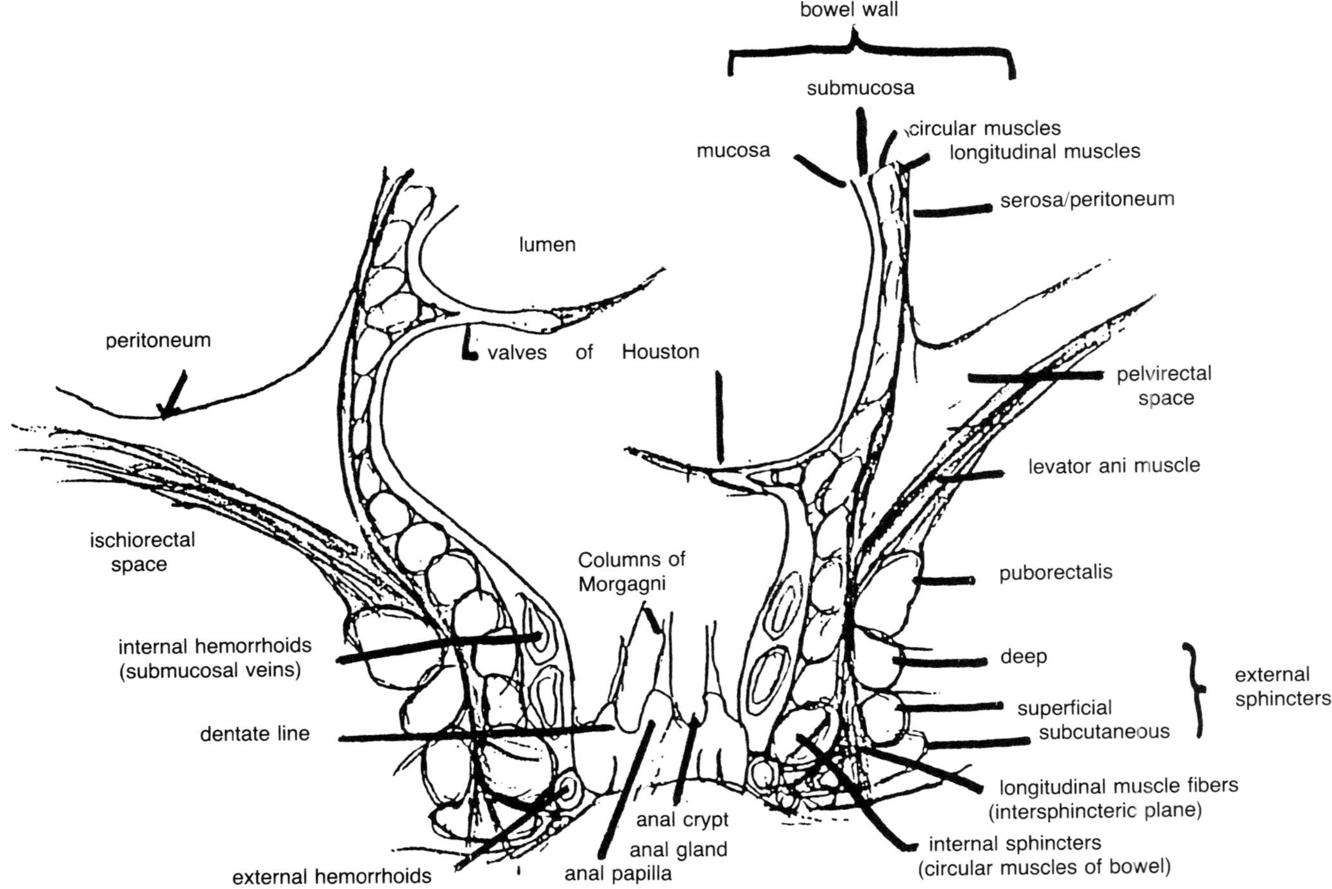

Fig. 46-1. Coronal section of the anorectum.

also communicate freely with the external hemorrhoidal veins, which are subcutaneous to the anoderm and which drain primarily through the pudendal and iliac venous systems. When these hemorrhoidal plexuses become excessively engorged, prolapsed, or thrombosed, they are referred to as hemorrhoids—one of the most common problems afflicting human beings.

Internal hemorrhoids, which course along the terminal branches of the superior rectal artery, are constant in their location, coursing longitudinally at the right posterolateral, right anterolateral, and left lateral positions (at the 2-, 5- and 9-o'clock positions when the patient is viewed prone). Internal hemorrhoids are not palpable and can best be visualized through an anoscope. External hemorrhoids are seen as dilatation of veins at the anal verge and can be seen at external inspection.

Although the cause of hemorrhoids is not always known, there is an association with constipation and straining at stool. They are very common during pregnancy and may be the result of sustained increased pressure on the venous drainage of the rectum. One of the physiologic shunts of the portal system involves the hemorrhoidal veins. Consequently, increased portal pressure, occurring as a result of chronic liver disease, may produce marked dilatation and varix formation of the hemorrhoids. The bleeding that can result is extremely difficult to control.

Tumors of the rectum and sigmoid colon, often associated with constipation, tenesmus, and incomplete evacuation, may cause hemorrhoids and must be ruled out in all cases of rectal bleeding in patients over the age of 40.

Clinical Features

Uncomplicated internal hemorrhoids are usually painless, and the chief complaint is painless, bright-red rectal bleeding with defecation. Bleeding is usually slight, with the blood being found on the surface of the stool, on the toilet tissue, or dripping into the toilet bowl. Although the most common cause of rectal bleeding is hemorrhoids, other, more serious causes should be sought in all patients who present with bleeding as the chief complaint. Chronic, slow blood loss may go unnoticed but can result in a significant anemia. Pain, when present, is most severe at the time of defecation and subsides with time. Pain is usually associated with thrombosed external hemorrhoids.

As they increase in size, hemorrhoids may prolapse, requiring periodic reduction by the patient (Table 46-1). When prolapse occurs, the patient may develop a mucous discharge and pruritus ani.

If the prolapse cannot be reduced, strangulation can result. Other complications include severe bleeding and thrombosis. Both strangulation and thrombosis are extremely painful and are accompanied by significant edema that must be treated before surgical intervention. Ulceration of the overlying mucosa may also occur.

Treatment

Most treatment is local and nonsurgical unless a complication is present. Hot sitz baths for at least 15 min three times a day and after each bowel movement are the most effective way to relieve pain and edema. Following the bath, the anus must be dried gently but thoroughly to avoid maceration of the perianal skin. Use of topical antibiotics, an-

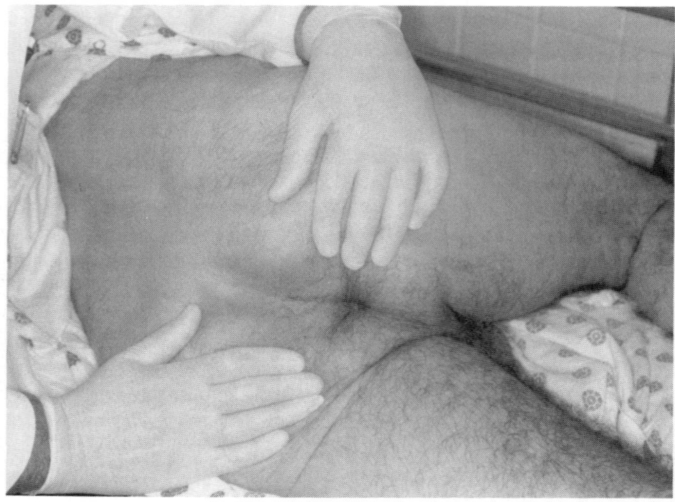

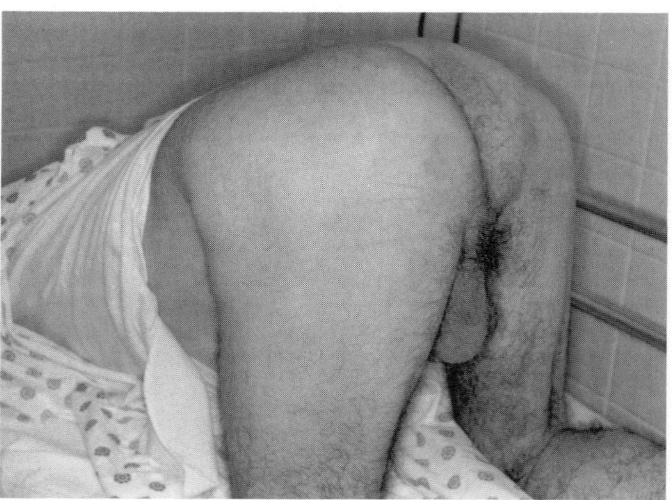

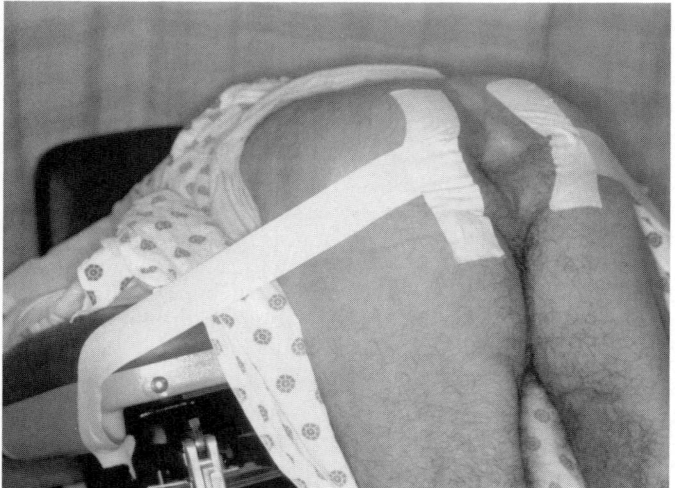

Fig. 46-2. Positioning the patient for anorectal examination. **A.** Lateral, or Sims' position. **B.** The knee-chest position. **C.** Position on the proctoscopic table. See the text for detailed descriptions.

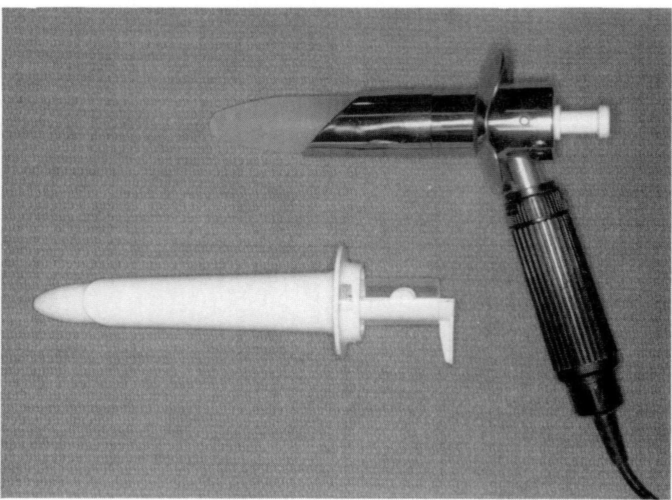

Fig. 46-3. Two types of anoscope. *Top:* Lighted anoscope with power source attached to handle. *Bottom:* Disposable anoscope. An extrinsic light source is required.

esthetics, or steroidal creams are of limited value and may cause more harm. The patient should not sit for a prolonged period on the commode. Bulk laxatives, such as psyllium seed compounds, or stool softeners should be used after the acute phase is treated. Laxatives causing liquid stool must be avoided; this can result in cryptitis and anal sepsis. The addition of bran or other forms of roughage to the patient's diet should help ameliorate future problems.

As a rule, internal hemorrhoids bleed and, if not prolapsed, are not palpable. External hemorrhoids thrombose. Selection of therapy for thrombosed external hemorrhoids depends on the severity of symptoms: if the thrombosis has been present more than 48 h, the swelling is not tense, and the pain is tolerable, the patient may be treated with sitz baths and bulk laxatives. Suppositories, which are placed proximal to the anorectal ring, are of no help. If, on the other hand, thrombosis is acute and recent in origin, significant relief can be provided by excising the clots. With the patient in prone position, the area of the overlying skin to be incised is infiltrated with a local anesthetic using a 30-gauge needle. While applying gentle traction to the skin adjacent to the thrombosed hemorrhoid, an elliptical incision is made in the overlying skin, exposing the thrombosed vein, which is locally excised with the elliptical flap of skin. Because of the multiloculated clots that are invariably present, the technique of unroofing a thrombosed hemorrhoid with an elliptical incision gives far better results than the simple incision and evacuation of a clot. Bleeding is controlled by tucking the corner of a small piece of gauze into the wound and leaving it in place for a few hours. A small pressure dressing may be applied external to the gauze and removed when the patient takes the first sitz bath 6 to 12 h after the drainage procedure. Narcotics may be prescribed, but only judiciously, since they produce constipation and may produce more problems.

Surgical referral and intervention for hemorrhoids is indicated for continued bleeding; incarceration and/or strangulation; severe, unrelenting pruritus; and intractable pain. Surgical treatment can consist

Table 46-1. Classification of Internal Hemorrhoids

Degree	Symptoms
First	Bleeding; local, compressible swelling
Second	Protrude with defecation, reduce spontaneously; ± bleeding
Third	Protrude with defecation; must be reduced manually; ± bleeding
Fourth	Incarcerated

of sclerosing injections, the use of rubber band ligation (the current, most common form of surgical treatment), or excision. Up to 5 percent of patients undergoing rubber band ligation may develop acute thrombosis of external hemorrhoids, and immunocompromised patients treated with band ligation may develop pelvic sepsis.

CRYPTITIS

Anal crypts are the superficial mucosal pockets that lie between the columns of Morgagni. They are formed by the puckering action of the sphincter muscles and normally flatten out during the passage of a stool. Sphincter spasm and superficial trauma caused by repeated bouts of diarrhea or trauma produced by evacuation of large, hard stools associated with constipation cause breakdown in the mucosal lining of the crypts. This permits infecting organisms to enter pockets and inflammation to extend into the lymphoid tissue of both the crypts and anal glands. Cryptitis could well be the common denominator for the development of such anal infections as fissure in ano, perianal and rectal abscesses, and fistula in ano.

Associated with cryptitis is the development of hypertrophied anal papillae, which lie between adjacent crypts. When hypertrophy occurs, the papillae may be palpated as small, hard nodules along the wall of the anal canal. Rarely, papillae may hypertrophy and present as a prolapsing polypoid tumor. The crypts most commonly involved are in the posterior half of the anal ring and, in most cases, in the posterior midline, the same location where anal fissures occur.

Clinical Features

Initially, the locally inflamed crypts produce no symptoms, but as the trauma from recurrent diarrhea or passage of large, hard stools continues, the inflammation of the crypts extends to the adjacent papillae, producing an edematous swelling of the sensitive anoderm that lines this part of the canal. At this stage, the patient will experience pain with bowel movements, and if there is an associated papillitis or fissure in ano, there will also be a small amount of bleeding. Anal pain, spasm, and itching with or without bleeding are the cardinal signs and symptoms of cryptitis.

Treatment

Treatment of anal cryptitis, which should be conservative, is based on establishing a definitive diagnosis and ruling out the possibility of more serious anorectal problems. The diagnosis can be suspected clinically from the history and the palpation of the tender, swollen crypt and its associated hypertrophied papillae. Definitive diagnosis of cryptitis is made by anoscopic examination. Gentle insertion of a hooked probe into the crypts brought into view through the anoscope will reveal the involved crypt(s) to be deeper than normal and definitely more tender.

The goal of treatment is to control the trauma of abnormal bowel movements and thus enable the inflammation to subside. Bulk laxatives and additional roughage to the diet to produce formed, soft stools combined with hot sitz baths and/or warm rectal irrigations greatly enhance healing by keeping the anus clean and the crypts empty.

Surgical intervention is indicated when the infection has progressed and there is a deep, redundant crypt that will not drain adequately on its own. In these cases, the roof (mucosal surface), as outlined by the passage of a hooked probe, should be infiltrated with local anesthetic and excised. Thus, what had been a deep pocket is converted into an open wound that should heal with proper control of bowel movements and frequent sitz baths.

FISSURE IN ANO (ANAL FISSURE)

This disorder is the result of a linear tear of the anal canal beginning at or just below the dentate line and extending distally along the anal canal. The epithelium in this area consists of anoderm, which has a rich supply of somatic sensory nerve fibers. Consequently, anal fissures are the most common cause of painful rectal bleeding.

Anal fissures are often associated with swelling of the surrounding tissues, producing hypertrophic papillae proximally and the characteristic sentinel pile distally. The latter is frequently misdiagnosed as an external hemorrhoid when in actuality it is the result of edema and fibrosis secondary to the ulcerating fissure. In more than 90 percent of cases, anal fissures occur in the midline posteriorly. In 10 percent of women but in only 1 percent of men, it may be in the midline anteriorly. This almost constant location of anal fissures may be because of the posterior angulation of the rectum on the anus where the posterior midline of the proximal anal canal becomes the "lesser curvative" for the passage of stool. A fissure not located in the midline should arouse suspicion that another, potentially life-threatening cause may be involved. Such diagnostic possibilities include Crohn's disease, chronic ulcerative colitis, squamous cell carcinoma of the anus, adenocarcinoma of the rectum invading the anal canal, localized anal cancers such as Bowen's disease and extramammary Paget's disease, leukemia, lymphoma, syphilitc fissures, and tuberculous ulcer. Such patients must be referred for a diagnostic biopsy of the ulcer edge, culture of the anal canal, and a systemic evaluation.

Most often, the traditional midline anal fissure is caused by the trauma produced by the passage of a particularly hard and large fecal mass, but it is also seen after acute episodes of diarrhea. Fissures persist because of the severe, chronic internal sphincter spasm that occurs along with the secondary infection of its base.

Clinical Features

Pain of the sharp, cutting variety is the most common symptom. Typically, the pain is most severe during and immediately after a bowel movement. The pain may persist for a few hours after each bowel movement, but invariably it subsides between movements, which is a distinguishing feature of fissures from other forms of painful anorectal disease. The bleeding is bright and small in quantity, usually being noticed only on the toilet paper. In infants, the presence of small amounts of bright blood on the stool or toilet paper is usually the presenting complaint for an anal fissure. Sphincter spasm and pain may be severe enough to make the patient retain stool and avoid defecation.

Diagnosis of anal fissure is usually suggested by the history; however, the anal area must be examined in all cases. With proper exposure, the sentinel pile, if present, and frequently the distal end of the fissure itself, may be seen. The mere retraction of the buttocks and the anal skin may cause considerable discomfort; sphincter spasm may be so severe that the patient will not permit digital examination. Application of a topical anesthetic may provide some relief. If the fissure can be visualized and is present in the posterior midline, rectal examination can be deferred until the patient is having less spasm and pain.

Treatment

Treatment is aimed at providing symptomatic relief, relieving the anal sphincter spasm, and preventing stricture formation. Hot sitz baths for at least 15 min three to four times a day and after each bowel movement will relax the sphincter and provide symptomatic relief. The addition of bran to the diet will serve to prevent stricture formation by providing a bulky stool. Use of local analgesic ointments, although providing symptomatic relief, is not associated with rapid healing. Indeed, there is a risk of hypersensitivity reaction. The use of hydrocortisone-containing ointments does little to help and may even retard healing. There is one study that demonstrates that most rapid healing of the fissure occurs with sitz baths and a diet rich in bran and that healing was not aided by either an analgesic ointment or a hydrocortisone-containing ointment. Meticulous anal hygiene is imperative; following defecation, the anus must be cleaned thoroughly. Healing is by the development of granulation tissue and the reepithelialization of the ulcerated area. If healing does not occur in a reasonable amount of time, operative treatment consisting of partial sphincterotomy and excision of the fissure may be required.

ANORECTAL ABSCESSES

Abscesses are common in the perianal and perirectal regions, as are fistulas, which are common sequelae. Almost all begin with involvement of an anal crypt and its gland. From there, the infection can progress to involve any of the potential spaces that are normally filled with fatty areolar tissue and have little inherent resistance to the progression of infection. These spaces, which can become infected alone or in combination with each other, are as follows: the perianal space, the intersphincteric space, the ischiorectal space, the deep postanal space (connecting the ischiorectal space on each side posteriorly), and the supralevator space (Fig. 46-4).

The perianal abscess is the most common anorectal abscess and occurs when pus spreads caudally between the internal and external sphincters to form a painful, tender, erythematous swelling at the anal verge, most often at the midline posteriorly. When it presents as a localized, superficial, fluctuant mass that is not associated with any other form of perirectal infection, it is only this type of abscess that can be adequately treated under local anesthesia in an emergency department setting.

Ischiorectal and other deep abscesses pose a different problem. The ischiorectal fossa forms a large potential space on either side of the rectum, communicating behind it through the deep postanal space, and, in males, has extensions anteriorly above the perineal membrane to the prostate. Infections in this area are insidious and extensive and can point in an area some distance from the anal verge. These abscesses can be large, and yet only a diffuse, nonfluctuant, tender ''mass'' is palpable either through the rectal wall or the overlying perineal skin.

Most abscesses in the anorectal area are the result of obstruction of an anal gland that opens in the base of an anal crypt and normally drains into the anal canal. When obstruction occurs, the gland orifice is blocked, resulting in infection and abscess formation. An element of cryptitis can frequently be identified by anoscopic examination. A variety of diseases are associated with the development of fistulous abscesses, including Crohn's disease, carcinoma of adjacent organs, Hodgkin's disease, tuberculosis, and gonococcal proctitis.

Clinical Features

Initially, the patient notices a dull, aching, or throbbing pain that becomes worse immediately before defecation, is lessened after defecation, but persists between bowel movements. The pain is increased by the increased pressure in the rectum that occurs just before defecation.

As the abscess spreads, increases in size, and comes nearer the surface, the associated pain becomes more intense. Pain will be aggravated by straining, coughing, or sneezing, which cause motion of the region. As the abscess progresses, pain and tenderness interfere with walking or sitting.

The patient appears markedly uncomfortable and may be febrile. A tender mass may be present, or there may be a tender, erythematous area with or without fluctuance. On rectal examination, a tender mass or induration is detected. Leukocytosis may be present.

Treatment

Treatment is surgical and should be performed as soon as the diagnosis is made, before the abscesses become fluctuant. Drainage should be both early and extensive. All these abscesses should be drained in the operating room. A recent publication revealed that 32 percent of patients who had undergone a simple incision and drainage under local anesthesia were required to have a second operation because of inadequate drainage and recurrence of disease.

Isolated, simple, fluctuant perianal abscesses that are not associated with the presence of any deeper abscesses may be drained using local anesthetics in an emergency department setting. The local anesthetic should be administered with the finest-gauge needle available (30-gauge) and should be complemented with the administration of systemic analgesia, including the use of nitronox. To ensure adequate drainage, a cruciate incision should be made over the fluctuant part of the abscess, and the ''dog ears'' resulting from the cruciate incision should be excised so as to prevent premature closure of the cutaneous wall of the abscess. No packing is required; sitz baths should be started the next day.

As a rule, antibiotics are not necessary after an abscess has been adequately drained. On the other hand, patients whose immune system may be compromised by diabetes mellitus, AIDS, malignancies, and chemotherapy and/or those patients who have extensive cellulitis should be started on a regimen of broad-spectrum antibiotics.

FISTULA IN ANO

An anal fistula is an abnormal tract that connects the anal canal with the skin and is lined with epithelium and granulation tissue. A fistula in ano most commonly results from a perianal or ischiorectal abscess (Fig. 46-4). It may, however, be associated with ulcerative colitis, Crohn's disease, or tuberculosis. Although anterior-opening fistulas tend to follow a simple, direct course to the anal canal (Goodsall's rule), posterior-opening fistulas may follow a devious, curving path, including some that are horseshoe-shaped.

Clinical Features

As long as the tract remains open, there is a persistent, blood-stained, malodorous discharge. More commonly, the tract becomes blocked periodically, producing bouts of inflammation and even local, recurrent abscess formation that is relieved by spontaneous rupture. An abscess may be the only sign of fistula in ano.

Treatment

The only definitive treatment is surgical excision. Improperly excised fistulas may result in permanent fecal incontinence.

VENEREAL PROCTITIS

Sexually transmitted diseases (STDs) of the anorectum are not uncommon among patients who practice anal sex. The infecting organisms, for the most part, are the same ones that are transmitted with vaginal coitus; infection is transmitted and perpetuated almost entirely by men who fail to use condoms (Table 46-2). Exceptions to this occur with women whose lymphogranuloma venereum (LGV) variety of chlamydia infection extends directly to the rectum from the vagina and on occasions when there is a contamination of the anus with gonococcal-laden discharge emanating from the urethra or cervix.

As a rule, if the patient has an anorectal infection caused by one of the STDs, the assumption must be made that another STD may be present; appropriate blood tests must be obtained, and patients should be anoscoped or proctoscoped in order to obtain specimens for Gram's stain as well as for viral and bacterial cultures.

Clinical Features

Most venereal diseases involving the anorectal area manifest themselves initially with itching, seepage, and mild pain or irritation. Indeed, these mild early symptoms may heighten the sexual desire of certain patients, which could result in the rapid dissemination of the disease to other unwary and unprotected partners. Some infections may persist with mild to minimal symptoms, rendering the patient a carrier of the disease who will be detected only by epidemiologic surveys, if they are ever conducted. Most venereal infections, however,

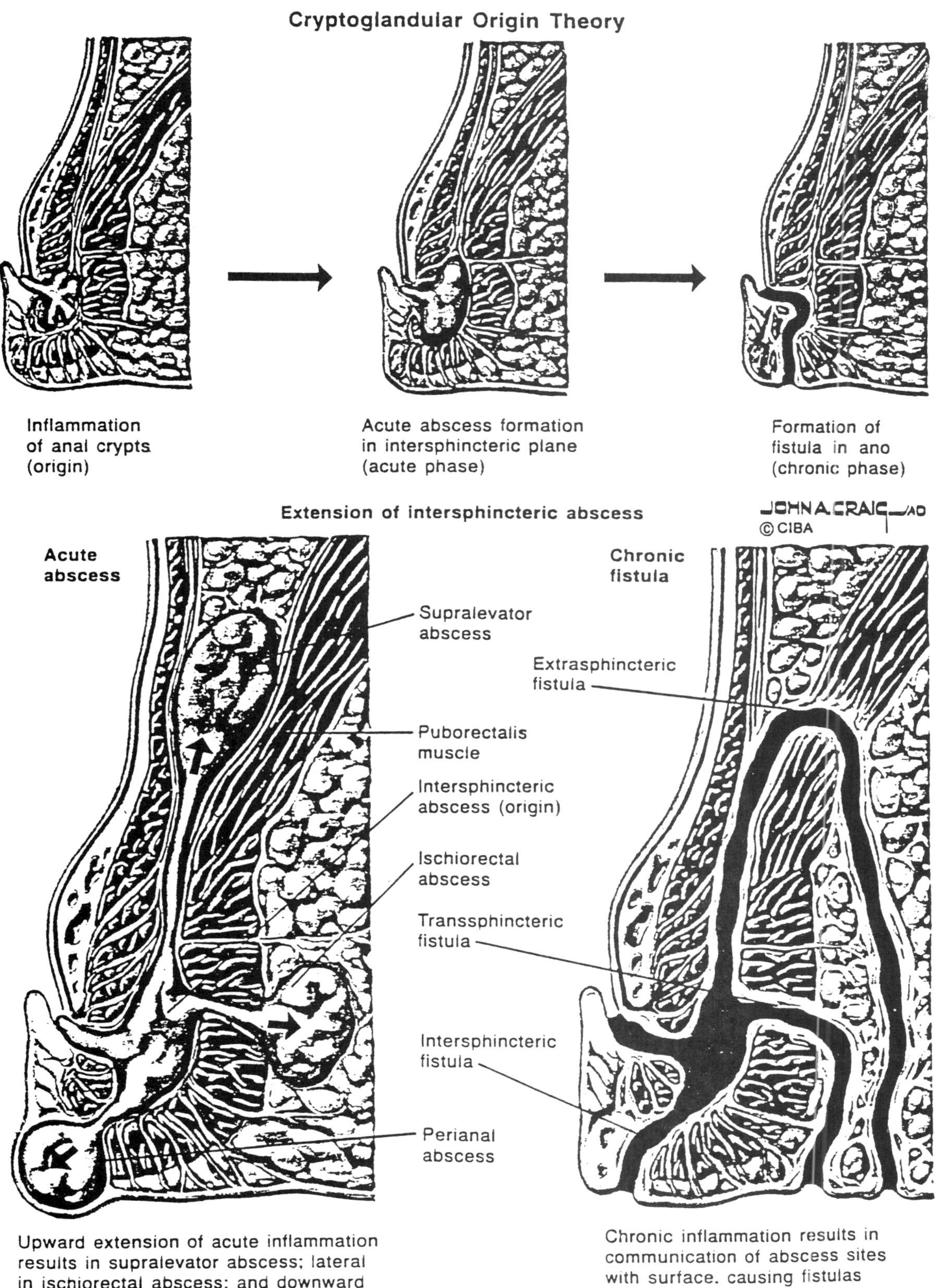

Fig. 46-4. Illustration of mechanism for anorectal abscess and fistula formation. (From Fry RD, Kodner IJ: *Clinical symposia: Anorectal disorders,* Vol. 37, No. 6. West Caldwell, NJ: CIBA Pharmaceutical Co., 1985. Used by permission.)

Table 46-2. Anorectal Sexually Transmitted Diseases

Bacteria
Neisseria gonorrheae
Chlamydia trachomatis, lymphogranulomatous
C. trachomatis, nonlymphogranulomatous
Spirochete
Treponema pallidum
Virus
Herpes simplex type 2
Human immunodeficiency virus
Papilloma virus

will produce significant symptoms of pain, bleeding, and discharge in addition to a bothersome pruritus that will force them to seek medical attention.

Condylomata Acuminata

Condylomata acuminata, commonly known as anal warts, are caused by a papilloma virus and are probably sexually transmitted in more than 90 percent of cases. They begin as discreet, soft fleshy growths on the skin of the perianal area as well as on the squamous epithelium of the anal canal. Occasionally, the mucosa of the lower rectum becomes involved. Patients usually first notice the presence of a growth in the perianal areas as well as associated pruritus and varying degrees of anal pain. With time, bleeding and anal discharge become part of the symptom complex. Evaluation of a patient with condyloma acuminata must include ruling out the presence of other STDs. Because cases of squamous cell carcinoma arising in association with condyloma acuminata have been reported, multiple biopsies must be taken.

Gonorrhea

Gonococcal proctitis occurs most commonly among homosexual men, although it may also be found among others who have had anal sex. Symptoms vary, ranging from none to severe rectal pain with profuse yellow discharge. Patients in the acute phase generally have mild anal burning and/or pruritus with some purulent seepage. Proctoscopic examination during this phase of the disease reveals marked hyperemia and edema of the rectal mucosa and diffuse inflammation with purulent discharge from the anal crypts. Unlike nonvenereal cryptitis, infection is not confined to the posterior crypt. Diagnosis is made by Gram's stain and cultures on appropriate media.

Chlamydial Infections

Chlamydia trachomatis is an obligate human intracellular parasite that causes, among other conditions, both urogenital and anorectal infections. The lymphogranulomatous (LGV) variety occurs mainly in tropical and subtropical climates. Infection can involve the rectum by perirectal lymphatic invasion from vaginal seeding or from direct anorectal mucosal infections. The non-LGV chlamydial organisms may infect the rectal mucosa, although they do not cause the extensive rectal scarring and stricturing that its lymph gland–invading cousin from the tropics does. A patient with chlamydial proctitis may be asymptomatic or may present with nonspecific symptoms, including anal pruritus, pain, and purulent discharge. Bleeding may also be present.

The more severe form of proctitis occurring with this infection is usually due to the LGV type of chlamydia. In addition to rectal scarring, which is a late sequel, infection of the perirectal tissue results in perirectal abscesses and chronic fistulas.

Chlamydia may be identified by culture. The LGV forms may be distinguished from the non-LGV variety by the Frei intradermal test or the LGV complement fixation test. Treatment for LGV chlamydial infections should be maintained for at least 21 days.

Syphilis

Chancres, the characteristic lesion of primary syphilis, usually manifest themselves at the anal verge or in the anal canal. Rarely will a chancre involve the rectal mucosa, although proctitis due to syphilis can occur in the absence of a chancre. Anal chancres are usually very painful. If they are not identified and treated, they will resolve and the patient will proceed to develop secondary and tertiary syphilis. Condylomata lata, which are flatter and firmer than the condylomata acuminata, appear in the perianal region as a manifestation of the secondary stage of syphilis.

Herpes

Anorectal herpes is almost always caused by the type II herpes simplex virus (HSV-2). Infection is initially manifested with itching and soreness in the perianal area; this soon progresses to severe anorectal pain. Initially, the virus manifests itself as small, discreet groups of vesicles superimposed on an erythematous base. These vesicles enlarge, coalesce, and rupture, forming exquisitely tender aphthous ulcers that appear on the perianal skin, the anoderm, and even the rectal mucosa. The pain and tenesmus from these lesions may be so intense that the patient is reluctant to have a bowel movement, resulting in constipation and possibly fecal impaction.

AIDS-Related Infections

Ironically, infection of the rectum by the human immunodeficiency virus (HIV) per se does not cause any local reaction or symptoms, but its affect on the patient inoculated with this virus is invariably devastating. Patients who have been rendered immunodeficient by the HIV virus are subject to a variety of opportunistic infections that affect the intestinal, anorectal, and other body systems. Chronic perianal infections with herpes simplex type I as well as type II are commonly seen in AIDS patients. Table 46-3 lists other, more common enteric organisms that infect AIDS patients who continue to practice anal intercourse. Severe rectal pain, diarrhea, and hematochezia are common presenting symptoms.

Treatment

Success in the management of patients with acute venereal proctitis depends on suspecting the diagnosis, obtaining specimens to confirm the diagnosis, and initiating therapy as expeditiously as possible. Patients presenting with symptoms of anorectal pain, rectal discharge, and/or tenesmus should be considered to have proctitis until proven otherwise. These patients should have an anoscopy or proctoscopy, and a Gram's stain should be performed to document the presence of acute proctitis. In addition to the appropriate culture specimens, blood should be drawn to check for syphilis.

Antibiotic therapy should not be delayed, pending the results of cultures. Empirical therapy aimed at eradicating gonorrhea, non-LGV chlamydia, and incubating syphilis should be initiated for any patient presenting with symptoms and physical signs suggestive of acute proctitis. This therapy should be administered to all patients with acute proctitis even if there are concomitant lesions suggestive of herpetic or papilloma virus infections.

Table 46-3. Anorectal AIDS-Related Infections

Herpes simplex type 1
Mycobactrium avium intracellulare
Cytomegalovirus
Salmonella enterocolitis
Shigella
Campylobacter
Entamoeba
Giardia

Although treatment for certain causes of venereal proctitis may be initiated in the emergency department, all patients must be referred to appropriate specialists for continued therapy and follow-up.

RECTAL PROLAPSE

Rectal prolapse, known as procidentia, is the circumferential protrusion of part or all layers of the rectum through the anal sphincters. There are three classes of rectal prolapse: (1) prolapse involving the rectal mucosa only, (2) prolapse involving all layers of the rectum, and (3) intussusception of the upper rectum into and through the lower rectum so that the apex of the intussusception protrudes through the anus.

In the first group, seen primarily in children under the age of 2, the prolapse occurs because of the loose attachment of the mucosa to the submucosal layers, and there is an associated weakness of the anal sphincter. In the second and third groups, prolapse occurs because of the laxity of the pelvic fascia and muscles in addition to a generalized weakening of the anal sphincters. In all cases, the rectum does not conform with, but lies anterior to, the sacral concavity, thus obliterating the angulation that normally occurs between rectum and anus. The prolapsing mucosa of a partial prolapse rarely protrudes more than 4 cm beyond the anal verge; the mucosal folds emanate in a radial fashion from the central lumen of the prolapsed mucosa. Mucosal prolapse is frequently associated with third- and fourth-degree hemorrhoids (see Table 46-1).

Complete rectal prolapse occurs at the extremes of life, most commonly in elderly women. Multiparity is not a contributing factor to rectal prolapse; there appears to be a higher incidence of prolapse in women who have had a hysterectomy.

Clinical Features

Most patients are able to detect the presence of a mass, especially following defecation or strenuous activity. In more advanced cases, this may be present when they stand or walk. Irritation to the rectal mucosa caused by recurrent prolapse results in a mucous discharge with some associated bleeding. Some patients may present because of blood-stained mucus on their undergarments, others because of fecal incontinence caused by associated anal sphincter weakness. In pediatric patients, parents often mistakenly believe that the prolapsed mucosa is hemorrhoids.

Treatment

In young children, after appropriate analgesia and sedation, prolapse can be reduced manually by replacing the protruding mucosa proximal to the anorectal ring of sphincter muscles. Every effort should be made to prevent the child from becoming constipated, and the child should be referred for further evaluation.

Surgical intervention is generally indicated in all other age groups unless the prolapse is minimal. A variety of effective surgical procedures is available and may be used depending on the degree of prolapse and the general health of the patient. All adults should have or be referred to have a proctosigmoidoscopic examination to rule out the presence of a tumor that could have caused the intussusception. In addition, one should check for the possibility of an anterior rectal wall ulcer that may occur in patients with recurrent prolapse.

If vascular compromise appears to have occurred, reduction may be necessary on an emergency basis. Because of the risk of having reduced ischemic bowel that could perforate, these patients must be hospitalized.

ANORECTAL TUMORS

Carcinoma of the anal area represents less than 5 percent of all large bowel malignancy. At the level of the dentate line and extending approximately 1 cm proximal is a transitional zone of epithelium connecting the squamous cell epithelium of the anoderm with the columnar epithelium of the rectum. This transition zone includes columnar, cuboidal, transitional, and squamous epithelial cells that represent the source for a variety of malignancies that arise in the anal canal (Table 46-4). For the purpose of grading malignancies, the United Nations World Health Organization has divided the anal canal into two regions: (1) malignancies of the portion proximal to the dentate line and including the transitional zone are referred to as anal canal neoplasms and (2) tumors arising in the anoderm distal to the dentate line are referred to as anal margin neoplasms.

Anal margin neoplasms have a low-grade malignant potential and are slow to metastasize. Anal gland neoplasms, on the other hand, are far more virulent, metastasize early, and have a poor prognosis. Squamous cell carcinoma of the anal canal has a much poorer prognosis than its anal margin counterpart. Anal canal malignancies metastasize not only to mesenteric lymph nodes and the portal circulation but also to the regional inguinal nodes and via the systemic circulation.

Included among the anal canal neoplasms is Kaposi's sarcoma, the most common AIDS-related malignancy. The anal canal is the third most common site for malignant melanoma (after the skin and the eye), which, when it occurs there, is usually not pigmented and frequently overlooked.

Clinical Features

Early anal canal malignancies usually cause nonspecific symptoms such as pruritus, pain, and bleeding admixed with stool. The sensation and presence of a lump in the anal canal may be erroneously diagnosed as a hemorrhoid. As the neoplasms progress, the patient experiences anorexia, weight loss, constipation, narrowing of the caliber of the stool, and eventually tenesmus with or without bowel movement. Complete obstruction may also occur.

Anal canal tumors may produce partial rectal prolapse; hemorrhoidal dilatation and prolapse may also occur. More advanced malignancies may present as perirectal abscesses or fistulas.

Villous adenomas, which arise from the rectal columnar epithelium, frequently produce diarrhea and a profuse rectal discharge, with secondary excoriation of skin and pruritus. These patients may suffer a significant loss of electrolytes, resulting in a clinically significant hypokalemia and/or hyponatremia.

Treatment

The anal margin neoplasms may present as persistent ulcers or as chronic dermatologic conditions such as eczema or mycotic infections. Any ulcer that fails to heal within 30 days or any discrete skin lesion that fails to improve with appropriate therapy must be biopsied to rule out the presence of malignancy.

Virtually all anorectal tumors can be detected by careful visual examination of the perianal area, digital palpation of the distal rectum and anal canal, and procto- or sigmoidoscopic examination. In one review of anal malignancies, 80 percent were in the canal and 20

Table 46-4. Neoplasms of the Anal Region

Anal canal neoplasms (proximal to dentate line)
Adenocarcinoma of the rectum
Adenocarcinoma of anal glands and ducts
Mucoepidermoid carcinoma
Transitional cloacogenic (basaloid) carcinoma
Squamous cell carcinoma of the anal canal
Malignant melanoma
Kaposi's sarcoma
Anal margin neoplasms (distal to dentate line)
Bowen's disease
Squamous cell carcinoma of anal margin
Extramammary Paget's disease
Basal cell carcinoma
Giant solitary trichoepithelioma

percent at the anal margin. Failure to look, feel, and think would be the only reason not to suspect the presence of these curable but life-threatening lesions.

RECTAL FOREIGN BODIES

The medical literature is replete with the variety of foreign bodies that have been reported to have been inserted into the rectum (Fig. 46-5). Most foreign bodies are "low-lying," that is, in the rectal ampulla and therefore palpable through digital examination and detectable on proctoscopic examination. Any patient presenting with an intrarectal foreign body must have multiple x-rays of the abdomen taken to demonstrate not only the position, shapes, and number of foreign bodies but also the possible presence of free air. Perforation of the rectum or colon is the most frequent and most serious complication. Perforation may be either extraperitoneal or intraperitoneal; both can result in life-threatening sepsis.

Treatment

Although many foreign bodies can be removed in the emergency department, some require surgical intervention. If the foreign body is removed in the emergency department and is of a size or shape that could cause perforation, a follow-up sigmoidoscopic examination and x-ray studies must be performed. In questionable cases, observations for at least 12 h should be done to ensure that perforation has not occurred. Rectal and anal lacerations may be present and require repair.

Sphincter relaxation is mandatory for removal of foreign bodies. If the patient's sphincters are taut or otherwise not sufficiently relaxed, local infiltrative anesthesia must be administered to achieve proper relaxation. After the patient has been sedated and placed on the proctoscopic table (condition permitting), local anesthetic is injected through a fine, 30-gauge needle to raise an intradermal wheal at the 6- and 12-o'clock positions. The index finger of the physician's non-dominant hand is then inserted into the anal canal to act as a guide for a $1\frac{1}{2}$-in, larger-gauge needle through which anesthetic is injected circumferentially along the course of the external sphincter muscles as they course along the anal canal. Five milliliters of anesthetic should suffice for each quadrant of infiltration. Large bulbar objects create a vacuumlike effect in the rectal ampulla, making it difficult to retrieve the object by simple traction. The vacuum can be overcome by passing a catheter beyond the object and injecting air. A modification of this technique is to insert Foley catheters around the foreign body and, after the vacuum is relieved by injecting air, inflate the balloons of the Foley catheters and use the catheters as traction devices to deliver the foreign body or manipulate it into a more accessible position.

If there is a risk of perforation, either by the foreign body itself or by local attempts to remove the foreign body, the patient should be prepared for emergency surgery, which includes obtaining appropriate laboratory studies, initiating intravenous therapy with crystalloid solution, passing a nasogastric tube, and administering a loading dose of broad-spectrum (second-generation cephalosporin) antibiotics.

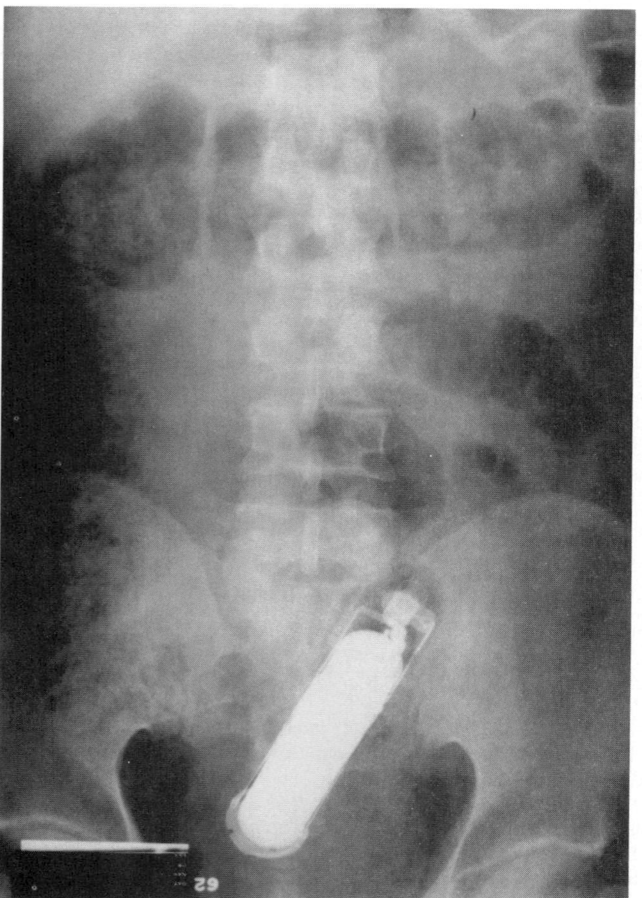

Fig. 46-5. Vibrator device lodged in rectum. (Courtesy of Medical Center of Delaware, Inc.)

PILONIDAL SINUS

Pilonidal sinus has nothing to do with the anorectum, anatomically or embryologically. Pilonidal sinuses or cysts occur in the midline in the upper part of the natal cleft overlying the lower sacrum. Because of their proximity to the anus, infected pilonidal cysts (abscesses) are sometimes mistakenly diagnosed as perirectal abscesses. An abscessed pilonidal sinus is always located in the midline (although there may be secondary fistulous openings on either side of the midline) and does not communicate with the anorectum. On the other hand, long, horse-shoe-type fistulas emanating from a perirectal abscess may drain close to the location of a pilonidal sinus but not in the midline.

Although once thought to be congenital in nature, pilonidal sinus is now considered an acquired problem. The sinus is formed by the penetration of the skin by ingrowing hair, which causes a foreign body granuloma reaction. The sinus is perpetuated by the presence of the hair and repeated bouts of infection. Although pilonidal sinuses or infected pilonidal cysts occur most commonly before the third decade of life, a small portion of patients may develop this problem in their fourth decade. Pilonidal sinus and abscess formation should be considered a chronic and recurring disease.

Carcinoma is a rare complication of chronic, recurring pilonidal sinus disease. It is more frequent in men and is usually a well-differentiated squamous cell carcinoma.

Clinical Features

Depending on whether the disease presents as a cyst or a sinus, the patient generally complains of swelling, pain, or a persistent discharge. When abscess formation occurs, the patient complains of a tender mass. Although there may be more than one sinus with several tiny openings in the midline of the intergluteal cleft, the most common finding is that of a single opening from which hair is protruding. Patients usually present to the emergency department when an abscess has formed that can no longer drain.

Treatment

Surgery is the treatment of choice. Ideally, a patient should undergo elective excision of the entire pilonidal sinus system and primary closure of skin when there is no infection present in any of the sinuses. Recent literature that suggests minimal excision, marsupialization, and packing using a local anesthetic in the emergency department is, in effect, advocating inadequate surgery that has proven to have a high failure and recurrence rate. Patients presenting with acute inflammation should have their abscess drained in the emergency department. Their wounds should be allowed to heal, and then, at least 6 weeks later, if there is no evidence of active infection, they should undergo definitive surgical excision and closure as described above.

The technique for incising and draining a pilonidal abscess is as follows: Place the patient prone on the proctoscopic table with the buttocks retracted laterally (see Fig. 46-2C). The patient should be sedated or have the option of self-administering nitronox analgesia. Tuck an ABD pad between the lower gluteal cleft to prevent the prep solution from pooling at the anus or genitals. After having prepped the skin, infiltrate the area to be incised with an intradermal injection of anesthetic solution, using a fine-gauge needle. A suction apparatus should be available to aspirate the unusually foul-smelling pus that has accumulated within the abscess. Following drainage, gently break down any loculations that may be present and loosely pack the wound with iodoform gauze. Bulk dressing should then be applied and secured with tape to the patient's buttocks. The patient should be given a prescription for a strong oral analgesic and advised to begin hot sitz baths the following day. Before the sitz bath, the patient should remove the outer dressing but should not attempt to remove the packing until after having soaked in hot water for a few minutes. Ideally, one should allow the hot water current to flush the packing out of the wound. The patient should be seen in 48 to 72 h for evaluation and further advice concerning wound management.

Unless the patient is immunocompromised or there is extensive cellulitis, there is no need to obtain cultures or prescribe antibiotics for an abscess that has been adequately drained.

PRURITUS ANI

Pruritus ani is a symptom complex that occurs secondary to a variety of anal and systemic problems. It is not in itself a specific disease process. It effects men far more often than women, and it occurs most commonly during the fifth and sixth decades of life.

There is an entity of primary or idiopathic pruritus ani, the etiology of which is unknown. To make such a diagnosis, one has to rule out the many specific, known causes of secondary pruritus ani. Even so, idiopathic pruritus ani may occur in association with or be precipitated by secondary pruritus ani. Table 46-5 lists the major categories of the various likely causes of secondary pruritus ani.

In Table 46-5, "anorectal disease" includes the various categories that have been discussed in this chapter. The pruritus that accompanies such conditions as fissures, fistulas, hemorrhoids, and prolapses occurs as a result of the perianal skin's being exposed to and macerated by constant mucous and purulent discharge. It is probably the increased perianal moisture caused by these conditions that results in itching. The itching triggers a vicious cycle of scratching, excoriation, and more itching.

Numerous dietary factors have been implicated and are associated with secondary pruritus ani, although proof of cause is lacking for most of them. Those dietary factors most commonly listed include excessive consumption of caffeine-containing liquids, such as coffee, tea, or colas, and beer, although one recent study failed to demonstrate any correlation between pruritus ani and alcohol consumption. Milk, chocolate, tomatoes, and citrus fruits are other food products that allegedly contribute to pruritus ani. Likewise, certain drugs, such as colchicine and mineral oil, have been associated with pruritus ani. Ingestion of these products can result in increased liquidity and seepage of fecal material, which in itself is a probable cause of pruritus ani.

Table 46-5. Pruritus Ani

Anorectal disease
Dietary factors
Local infection
Local irritants
Dermatologic conditions
Systemic illness
Psychogenic factors

Infectious agents that have to be considered as causes of pruritus ani include bacteria, viruses, fungi, spirochetes, and parasites. More common bacterial infections, such as staphylococci and streptococci, in addition to all sexually transmitted organisms, will cause pruritus, if not actual pain. Pinworms (*Enterobius vermicularis*) are the most common cause of anal pruritus in children. *Candida albicans* is commonly found on the perianal skin but is not usually associated with pruritus; the *Trichophyton* species, on the other hand, are always associated with pruritus.

Local irritants, if not the initial cause, commonly contribute to the incidence of pruritus. Fecal contamination, resulting from poor anal hygiene, is by far the most common irritant to the perianal skin. Lysozyme from intestinal mucous secretions, acting together with bacterial exotoxins to raise the stool and skin pH, will cause pruritus. Ironically, patients who compulsively clean their anus, particularly if they use perfumed toilet tissue, soaps, or detergents or hygiene sprays, cause pruritic reactions. Also, wearing of synthetic, tight-fitting underwear retains moisture that normally occurs in the perianal area, another leading cause of pruritus.

Dermatologic conditions contributing to this symptom complex include atopic dermatitis, lichen planus, psoriasis, and seborrheic dermatitis. Any of the anal margin neoplasms, particularly Bowen's disease and extramammary Paget's disease, may initially manifest themselves as pruritus.

Finally, certain systemic conditions, such as diabetes mellitus, lymphoma, and certain vitamin deficiencies (vitamins A and D and niacin), because of their secondary effect on the perianal skin, will cause pruritus.

Clinical Features

Appearance of the perianal skin will depend on the severity and chronicity of the underlying conditions that are causing the pruritus. The skin will appear normal with early, mild cases. With acute, more severe exacerbations, the perianal skin will appear reddened, edematous, and moist; frequently, there are excoriations caused by scratching. In chronic cases, the perianal skin takes on a thickened, almost leathery, depigmented appearance. The normal radiating folds of skin thicken into rugae and may include superficial fissures factitiously induced.

Treatment

Pruritus, like any other symptom, suggests the presence of an underlying cause that should be diagnosed and treated appropriately. Thus, excision of malignancies or surgical correction of fistulas, prolapses, or hemorrhoids would be the definitive treatment for patients with those conditions.

In most cases, specific anorectal lesions are not apparent, and the patient must be referred to a proctologist or dermatologist for probable long-term management.

In the meantime, the patient should be advised to make certain dietary changes, if appropriate, and should be instructed about proper anal hygiene. Scratching of the area must be avoided; if necessary, the patient should be advised to wear gloves at bedtime, when most of the scratching is likely to occur. Patients with maceration of perianal skin should use moist cotton rather than toilet paper. Soaps should be avoided, and the patient should take sitz baths for at least 15 min two to three times a day. The skin should then be thoroughly dried either with a hair dryer or by gently blotting the area with a soft cloth. Zinc oxide ointment can provide a protective covering for the perianal skin and may enhance the healing. Fungicidal creams should be prescribed for patients with secondary fungal infections. One percent hydrocortisone cream is effective for the allergic component of the inflammation.

Finally, as an adjunct to providing symptomatic relief, consider prescribing hydroxyzine hydrochloride (Atarax) as an effective bedtime sedative.

BIBLIOGRAPHY

Abcarian H: Rectal trauma, *Gastroenterol Clin North Am 16:1, 1987.*

Aucoin EJ: Pruritus ani, *Postgrad Med* 82:7, 1987.

Barone JE, Yee J, Nealon TF Jr: Management of foreign bodies and trauma of the rectum. *Surg Gynecol Obstet* 156:453, 1983.

Brenner BE, Simon RR: Anorectal emergencies. *Ann Emerg Med* 12:367, 1983.

Connolly SM: Nonvenereal perianal conditions. *Dermatol Clin* 5:4, 1987.

Fry RD, Kodner IJ: Anorectal disorders. *Ciba Clin Sym* 37:6, 1985.

Goldstein SD: Anal fissures and fistulas. *Postgrad Med* 82:7, 1987.

Gordon PH: The anorectum. *Gastroenterol Clin North Am* 16:1, 1987.

Hanno R, Murphy P: Pruritus ani: Classification and management. *Dermatol Clin* 5:4, 1987.

Jensen SL: Treatment of first episodes of acute anal fissure: Prospective randomized study of lignocaine ointment versus hydrocortisone ointment or warm sitz bath plus bran. *Br Med J* 292: 1167, 1986.

Meban S, Hunter E: Outpatient treatment of pilonidal disease. *Can Med Assoc J* 126:941, 1982.

Nehme-Kingsley A, Arcarian R: Colorectal foreign bodies: Management Update. *Dis Colon Rectum* 28:941, 1985.

Roberts JW: Rectal prolapse. *Clin Geriatr Med* 1:445, 1985.

Rompalo AM, Roberts P, Johnson K et al: Empirical therapy for the management of acute proctitis in homosexual men. *JAMA* 260:3, 1988.

Smith LE: Hemorrhoids: A review of current techniques and management. *Gastroenterol Clin North Am* 16:1, 1987.

Sohn N, Weinstein MA, Robbins RD: Anorectal disorders. *Cur Probl Surg* vol 20, January 1983.

47
DIARRHEA AND FOOD POISONING

James S. Seidel

Vomiting, diarrhea, and gastrointestinal (GI) upset are common complaints. The cause is usually food poisoning or an acute infectious illness. Diarrhea occurs in 3 to 5 billion persons worldwide and is responsible for 5 to 10 million fatalities in people of all age groups in Asia, Africa, and Latin America. In the industrialized nations, diarrheal disease is responsible for the death of more than 700 preschool children each year. It is the third most common reason for hospitalization of children in the United States. Traveler's diarrhea occurs frequently in visitors in developing nations and, if not managed properly, may persist when they return home.

The causes of diarrheal illness include infection by viruses, bacteria, parasites, and fungi; entercolitis induced by antibiotics and other drugs; inflammatory bowel disease; cystic fibrosis; endocrinopathies; acrodermatitis enteropathica; lactose intolerance; milk allergy; malignancy; obstruction (as seen in Hirschsprung's disease); and extraintestinal infections such as otitis media or urinary tract infection.

Food poisoning may be caused by:

1. Toxic contaminants of food and water
   a. Heavy metals (zinc, copper, cadmium)
   b. Organic chemicals: polyvinylchlorides
   c. Pesticides
   d. Radioactive substances
   e. Alkyl mercury
2. Bacterial, fungal, viral, and parasitic contaminants of food
   a. Invasive organisms
   b. Chemical metabolites of the microorganisms
3. Toxic substances naturally present in the food: akee fruit, mushrooms, thallophytes, fish (ciguatera, scombroid poisoning), dinoflagellates, shellfish
4. Altered host response to a food substance, e.g., foods containing tyramine, monosodium glutamate, tryptamines, etc.
5. Food intolerance: shellfish, moray eel, chili pepper

We will only consider ciguatera fish poisoning and the infectious causes of food poisoning and diarrhea.

PATHOPHYSIOLOGY

Organisms that cause diarrhea may produce (1) a noninflammatory, or secretory diarrhea usually due to enterotoxin production, (2) an inflammatory diarrhea or dysentery due to mucosal invasion and/or (3) enteric fever due to penetration of the mucosa and intracellular infection. The type of diarrheal syndrome found in the patient depends on the organism and the host defenses.

A watery, profuse noninflammatory diarrheal syndrome may be produced by the loss of the absorptive surface of the small intestine or the actions of enterotoxin on the intestine. The diarrhea is watery and not associated with fecal leukocytes (Table 47-1). The classic example of this type of infection is cholera in which organisms colonize the small intestine and produce an enterotoxin that causes an adenyl cyclase–mediated secretory diarrhea. Large amounts of isotonic solution are lost through the bowel. Similar problems may be caused by enterotoxin-producing *E. coli.* A profuse, watery diarrhea may also be produced by direct damage to the intestinal epithelium by such organisms as *Giardia lamblia, Cryptosporidium, Isospora,* Rotavirus, and Norwalk agent. Diarrhea produced by enterotoxins is not usually associated with fecal leukocytes.

Invasion of the epithelium of the distal small bowel and colon may lead to an inflammatory diarrhea with the clinical findings of fever, diarrhea (often dysentery), and abdominal pain. The stool may contain blood, mucus, and sheets of fecal leukocytes. The severity of the clinical findings is dependent on the severity of damage to the intestinal lining, the extent of tissue invasion, and the presence or absence of bacteremia. Invasive organisms include *Shigella, Campylobacter, Salmonella, Yersinia,* and *E. coli.* Diarrhea caused by invasive organisms frequently has fecal leukocytes.

Enteric fever is usually caused by invasive organisms such as *Salmonella typhi* and *Yersinia enterocolitica,* which pass through the mucosa of the intestinal tract, invade lymphatic structures and phagocytic cells, and cause systemic disease. Although the patient may be constipated at first, diarrhea is often present and the stool may contain fecal monocytes rather than polymorphonuclear cells.

Factors which may protect the host from diarrheal disease include (1) gastric acidity; (2) the normal flora of the intestinal tract, which may be altered by systemic broad-spectrum antibiotics; (3) the normal motility of the intestine, which serves to mix and help in the absorption of fluids, electrolytes, and nutrients and to maintain the distribution of the indigenous microflora of the gut; (4) the gastrointestinal mucus, which protects the lining from damage and invasion of organisms; and (5) the presence of secretory immunoglobulin and phagocytic cells which are immune barriers. Iatrogenic alterations of immune barriers may make the host more susceptible to severe diarrheal disease.

Diarrhea is an increase in both the volume and frequency of stool. There may be a large increase in the volume of water lost. In most cases, the intestinal tract is changed from a site of absorption of water and electrolytes to one of secretion or loss of water and electrolytes. Leukocytes and blood may be present in the stool. Dehydration and electrolyte imbalance are seen frequently, and are responsible for the high morbidity and mortality, particularly in the very young and very old. Interventions such as the use of broad-spectrum antibiotics and agents that inhibit motility, such as loperamide and diphenoxylate, may add to the disease process. In more chronic diarrheal illness, loss of nutrients, essential minerals, and vitamins may further compromise the patient.

ETIOLOGY OF DIARRHEAL DISEASE (Tables 47-2 and 47-3)

Viral Infections

Most cases of acute diarrheal disease are caused by viral infections. The best-understood and probably the most common viruses are Rotavirus and Norwalk agent. Other viral organisms include enteroviruses, enteric adenovirus (serotypes 40 and 41), and calicivirus. Clinical manifestations include watery diarrhea, nausea, and vomiting and are usually self-limiting. Infection occurs primarily in the winter and spring months and is more frequent in children.

Rotavirus has been studied most extensively and a number of serotypes are responsible for endemic infantile gastroenteritis. It is spread

Table 47-1. Fecal Leukocytes in Diarrheal Illness

Present	Sometimes Present	Absent
Shigella	*Salmonella*	*Vibrio cholerae*
Campylobacter	*Yersinia*	Toxigenic *E. coli*
Invasive *E. coli*	*Vibrio parahaemolyticus*	Enteropathogens:
	Clostridium difficile	*E. coli*
	Aeromonas (20%)	*Bacillus cereus*
		Clostridium perfringens
		Rotavirus
		Norwalk agent
		Giardia lamblia
		E. histolytica
		Cryptosporidium

Table 47-2. Viral Causes of Acute Diarrhea

Agent	Clinical Syndrome	Symptoms: Diarrhea	Vomiting	Fever	URI	Pneumonia
Rotavirus	Endemic infantile gastroenteritis	+ + +	+ +	+ +	+	±
Norwalk agent	Endemic gastroenteritis Family outbreaks	+ + +	+ + +	+	−	−
Enteric type adenovirus	Intestinal "flu"	+ +	+ +	+	+	±
Enterovirus	Variety of syndromes associated with mild GI upset	+	±	+ +	+	±
Calicivirus	"Flu" in children under 2	+ +	+	±	−	−

from person to person through the fecal-oral route, and contamination may be associated with diaper changing. Nosocomial spread has occurred among hospitalized pediatric patients and medical personnel. Infection is sporadic and occurs primarily in infants less than 1 year of age. The incubation period is 1 to 3 days, and the typical patient has fever, vomiting, and diarrhea, but may also have an upper respiratory infection or pneumonia. The diarrhea generally lasts for 3 to 10 days, but may be protracted.

Norwalk virus occurs in school-aged children and adults. Community outbreaks and epidemics are common. The illness is generally self-limiting and resolves in several days.

Enteroviruses, adenoviruses, and calicivirus have also been implicated in outbreaks of acute gastroenteritis. These viruses, the clinical syndromes, and typical clinical course are shown in Table 47-2.

Bacterial Infections

Bacterial infections are responsible for approximately 20 percent of acute infectious diarrheal illnesses. Bacterial diarrhea is divided into two classes—disease caused by direct invasion and disease caused by enterotoxins.

Escherichia coli

Toxogenic and invasive *E. coli* are primary agents of traveler's diarrhea. Infection is acquired by ingestion of contaminated food and water. Typically, the patient experiences mild abdominal pain and watery diarrhea 2 to 4 days after infection. Infection may be fulminant and resemble clinical cholera, but is usually self-limited and rarely associated with systemic symptoms.

The organism can cause diarrhea by three mechanisms. Enterotoxigenic strains produce heat-labile toxin, stable toxin, or both. The genes for toxin production are carried on a plasmid; thus, any serotype of *E. coli* may elaborate the toxins. The enterotoxins produced act at the cellular level, stimulating an increased production of cyclic AMP that leads to the loss of electrolytes and water into the lumen of the bowel. The enteropathogenic strains colonize the small and large intestines. They are associated with epidemics of acute diarrhea in hospital nurseries. The exact mechanism of disease is not fully understood but is thought to involve toxin production. *Escherichia coli* may also produce invasive disease and a clinical picture described below for *Shigella*.

Treatment with an antibiotic (doxycycline or trimethoprim with sulfamethoxazole) may be required in cases which are moderate to severe, but most patients will require only supportive therapy. Identification of enterotoxigenic organisms in the laboratory requires special techniques not widely available.

Table 47-3. Infectious organisms Associated with Diarrheal Syndromes

Noninflammatory	Inflammatory	Enteric Fever
Vibrio cholerae	*Shigella*	*Salmonella*
Aeromonas hydrophila	*Campylobacter*	*Yersinia enterocolitica*
Vibrio parahaemolyticus	*E. coli*—Invasive	*Campylobacter fetus intestinalis*
Rotavirus	*Salmonella*	
Norwalk agent	*Clostridium difficile*	
Cryptosporidium	*Yersinia enterocolitica*	
Isospora	*Aeromonas* (20%)	
E. coli	*Entamoeba histolytica*	
Staph. aureus		

Shigella

Shigella infections are common in all parts of the world and are associated with food-borne, nosocomial transmission and fecal and oral contamination. The organism is highly infectious, and ingestion of only 100 organisms may cause disease. The spectrum of illness may vary from mild—an asymptomatic carrier—to severe—a fulminant disease resulting in severe dehydration and death in the very young and old. The patient may become symptomatic 36 to 72 h after exposure. Infection is associated with abdominal pain and fever which may reach 40° or 41°C (104° or 105.8°F) in children. Bowel movements may be explosive and associated with blood and mucus in 50 to 75 percent of these patients. Young children may present with high fever and a febrile convulsion without a history of diarrhea; the diarrhea may begin in the emergency department, often when the child is being held for lumbar puncture.

A stool specimen should be sent to the microbiology laboratory in holding media as soon as possible. Even under the best circumstances, cultures may be negative in 30 percent of the cases and should be repeated. *Shigella,* like *E. coli,* generally causes a self-limited disease. The largest number of bowel movements are usually within the first 24 h, and dehydration may occur in young children. Deaths have been reported in infants within 8 h after the onset of symptoms. Although rare, bacteremia can occur with *Shigella* infections.

A complete blood cell count may be helpful in differentiating *Shigella* enteritis. The white blood cell count may be low, high, or normal, and a marked left shift is common. Fecal leucocytes are usually present.

Antibiotics promptly alter the course of *Shigella* infections but are only recommended in cases of *Shigella* dysentery or institutional outbreaks of *Shigella flexneri*. Although many strains are sensitive to ampicillin, trimethoprim with sulfamethoxazole or ciprofloxacin is considered the treatment of choice by some. Without specific therapy the majority of patients have an uneventful recovery in 5 to 7 days. Complications of shigellosis include diarrhea and dehydration, Reiter's syndrome, arthralgias, and the hemolytic uremic syndrome.

Salmonella

Salmonella is responsible for wide range of diseases, which, however, may be divided into five clinical syndromes: (1) self-limiting enteritis, (2) enteric fever, (3) bacteremia without metastatic disease, (4) gastroenteritis, and (5) the asymptomatic carrier.

This organism is ubiquitous and is found in many animals as well as humans. Most human infections occur as a result of contamination of food and water. Eggs, egg products, chicken, and turkey are often implicated as a source of infection. Pet turtles have also been known to carry the organism.

The clinical presentation is often a self-limiting enteritis with watery diarrhea associated with abdominal pain and cramping. Infection may produce septicemia with systemic symptoms including fever, cough, and meningismus (enteric fever). There may be a relative bradycardia associated with high fever; this is most often seen with infection of *Salmonella typhi*. Typhoid fever may present as an unremitting fever with abdominal pain, cramps, rose spots (10 to 20 percent), and meningismus. Diarrhea may be absent. Drug addicts, and persons with AIDS, splenectomies, or sickle cell disease, are particularly susceptible to *Salmonella* infections. The diagnosis is based on recovery of the organism from blood, urine, and stool cultures. Febrile agglutinins may be positive, but generally this test lacks sensitivity and specificity.

Therapy depends on the clinical syndrome. Gastroenteritis is treated with replacement of fluid losses and control of nausea and vomiting. Drugs which reduce bowel motility should not be used as they may prolong the illness. Enteric fever and bacteremia should be treated in the hospital with chloramphenicol and ampicillin or trimethoprim with sulfamethoxazole. The carrier state may require prolonged treatment with antibiotics and, when accompanied by biliary disease, cholecystectomy may be necessary.

Yersinia Enterocolitis

Domestic animals including household pets have been implicated in the transmission of *Yersinia* to humans. Food, water, and fecal-oral transmission have also been shown to occur. Infection is associated with acute enteritis, dysentery, and fever. Mesenteric adenitis, terminal ileitis, and pseudoappendicitis may also occur. Blood is found in the stool in 25 percent of the cases and erythema nodosum may be present, particularly in women.

Yersinia is difficult to isolate in the laboratory, and when infection is suspected, one should specifically request the laboratory to isolate the organism. This may take days to accomplish, and often the symptoms have subsided when the report is returned from the laboratory. Symptomatic cases may be treated with chloramphenicol, tetracycline, trimethoprim with sulfamethoxazole, or a third-generation cephalosporin, although there is no agreement about a precise treatment protocol.

Campylobacter fetus spp. *jejuni*

Campylobacter fetus spp. *jejuni* was first described in 1977 as a frequent cause of diarrhea. Isolation of the organism requires special laboratory techniques, and when such isolation has been performed routinely, the organism has been shown to be more common than *Salmonella* and *Shigella* as a cause of bacterial diarrhea. The majority of patients present with fever and bloody diarrhea; two-thirds have abdominal pain, and one-third have vomiting. *Campylobacter* gastroenteritis is most frequently reported in children. Waterborne infections have been reported. Erythromycin is the treatment of choice in children, and tetracycline in adults. Parenteral treatment with gentamicin may be required to treat serious infections.

Clostridium perfringens

Clostridium perfringens is a common cause of food poisoning. The organism is part of the normal flora of the colon of humans and other animals, but only heat-resistant strains have been associated with enteritis. Human intestinal carriage of heat-resistant strains is in the range of 2 to 9 percent. The incubation period is 6 to 24 h, with an average of 12 h to the onset of symptoms. These include abdominal cramps and diarrhea. Constitutional symptoms such as headache, chills, and fever may occur, although they are not prominent features of clostridial food poisoning. Nausea and vomiting are not common. Meat and meat products are usually implicated in the transmission. Clostridial food poisoning is generally self-limited and requires no therapy. Antitoxin to the β toxin has been considered useful in the treatment of necrotizing enteritis of type C *C. perfringens*.

Clostridium difficile

An overgrowth of this organism has been associated with pseudomembranous enterocolitis, which may develop after the administration of antibiotics. The organism releases cytotoxins that produce a profuse diarrhea that may be indistinguishable from that of severe shigellosis. If untreated, the disease is associated with high mortality. Treatment includes vancomycin, the binding of the toxin with cholestyramine, and the administration of supportive fluids.

Staphylococcus aureus

Infections with *Staphylococcus* may occur after antibiotic therapy, with an overgrowth of the organism in the bowel and resultant enterocolitis. The enterotoxins may also contaminate food such as ham, poultry, meats, and dairy products. The organism and the enterotoxins it produces are the most common cause of food-borne disease. Vomiting and diarrhea are the most common symptoms, but abdominal cramps, headache, and prostration may occur when large amounts of toxin are ingested. The incubation period is 2 to 24 h with symptoms appearing most often 6 to 12 h after ingestion of the toxin. The disease is generally self-limited, and supportive therapy is all that is required.

Bacillus cereus

Bacillus cereus enterotoxins cause two clinical syndromes. It has been associated with a predominantly upper GI tract illness with vomiting that may develop 1 to 6 h after ingestion of contaminated food, particularly fried rice. A lower intestinal tract illness that resembles *C. perfringens* enteritis may also develop 6 to 24 h after ingesting a contaminated meal; *B. cereus* should be suspected if more than 10^5 organisms are isolated from the stool. Treatment is symptomatic.

Aeromonas hydrophila

Aeromonas hydrophila is a vibrio, found in soil and water, which can cause a choleralike GI disorder when contaminated food or water is ingested. There is generally no fever or other constitutional symptoms. The disease is mediated by an enterotoxin. Treatment is symptomatic, but serious infections can be treated with chloramphenicol or aminoglycosides.

Vibrio cholerae

Cholera is an acute infectious diarrhea caused by *Vibrio cholerae*. The disease is transmitted by contaminated water or food. A large inoculum of the organism is required to produce disease because of the acid sensitivity of the bacteria. The illness may begin with vomiting, but production of copious watery diarrhea is the hallmark of clinical cholera. Large volumes of "rice water" stool may lead to (1) severe dehydration due to loss of isotonic fluid from the bowel, (2) acidosis due to loss of bicarbonate in the stool, and (3) hypokalemia due to potassium loss in the stool. The disease may be complicated by renal failure and hypovolemic shock. Therapy is aimed at oral or parenteral replacement of fluids. Antibiotics may shorten the clinical course; tetracycline and trimethoprim with sulfamethoxazole are the drugs of choice.

Vibrio parahaemolyticus

This organism has been associated with the ingestion of raw or improperly prepared seafood, particularly oysters, clams, and crabs. The spectrum of disease varies from mild gastroenteritis to explosive diarrhea associated with cramps, vomiting, and dysentery. The average incubation period is 12 h but may vary from 2 to 24 h. As is the case with cholera, symptomatic treatment is important. It is unclear if oral antibiotics are beneficial. In severe infections, however, tetracycline and chloramphenicol have been used.

Bacteria may be transmitted venereally in persons engaging in anal intercourse. Those associated with enteritis include *Shigella* and *Campylobacter*. Others may cause enteritis and/or proctitis such as *Chlamydia, Campylobacter, Neisseria gonorrhea,* and *Treponema pallidum*.

Parasites

A variety of parasitic protozoa and helminths may produce diarrhea during the course of infection. Only several, however, are important in the United States as a cause of acute diarrheal disease. (See Table 47-3.)

Entamoeba histolytica

Entamoeba histolytica is found in 10 percent of the world's population, with 35 to 50 million individuals developing clinical symptoms each year. The prevalence of *E. histolytica* infection in the United States is probably between 1 and 5 percent. The majority of those infected are asymptomatic. Asymptomatic cyst passers may transmit the disease through the fecal-oral route as well as by contaminating the environment with infected cysts. The disease may also be venereally transmitted through anal intercourse.

Infection may cause colitis with abdominal cramps and diarrhea, or acute amebic dysentery with profuse bloody diarrhea. Vomiting is usually absent. Approximately 5 percent of the patients with dysentery develop extraintestinal amebiasis. The liver is the most common site of amebic abscesses, but they can also develop in the lung, heart, kidney, or brain. Treatment includes the use of metronidazole, tetracycline, or, for severe infections, emetine hydrochloride or dehydroemetine plus chloroquine. Iodoquinol should also be given to eradicate the cyst stage.

Giardia lamblia

Giardia is the most common intestinal parasite in the United States. Infection may be asymptomatic. Transmission is through fecal or oral contamination with infective cysts or through other contamination of water and food. Beavers have been shown to play a role in transmission through infection of mountain streams in Colorado and the northwest. Patients most often complain of abdominal pain, distension, postprandial urgency to defecate, and feeling bloated and gaseous. They may have profuse foul-smelling diarrhea. Classically the stools are floating, frothy, and foul-smelling. Diagnosis may be difficult as the cysts are only passed sporadically. At least three stools should be submitted for examination for ova and parasites. If these are negative and there is a high index of suspicion, an Enterotest (string test) or duodenal aspiration may be performed to look for trophozoites.

Although metronidazole has been used effectively for the treatment of giardiasis, it is not approved for use in this infection. Quinacrine hydrochloride is the drug of choice. Furazolidone may be used as an alternative to other drugs and is preferred by some for children as it comes in a liquid preparation.

Cryptosporidium

Cryptosporidium is an intestinal protozoan that was described in mice in 1907. It was subsequently found to be responsible for diarrhea in a variety of animals. The first case in humans was reported in 1976 and it is now recognized as a significant pathogen in immunosuppressed patients. The organism has been implicated in diarrheal disease in preschoolers and travelers. The prevalence in cases of acute diarrhea varies from 1 to 8 percent.

The organism is acquired by the ingestion of infective cysts from fecal-oral contamination of food and water from human or animal sources. The infective stage is extremely resistant to various agents and may also be transmitted on fomites or contaminated environmental surfaces.

Cryptosporidiosis usually presents as a profuse, watery diarrhea without gross blood. Other symptoms may include nausea, vomiting, anorexia, abdominal pain, and cramping. Diagnosis may be made by an acid-fast stain of the stool. The severity and duration of the illness depend on the immunologic status of the patient. It is usually self-limiting but may cause severe dehydration. There is no effective therapy. In patients with AIDS, cryptosporidiosis may cause a chronic diarrheal syndrome with hepatobiliary disease and is associated with significant morbidity and mortality.

Isospora belli

Like *Cryptosporidium, I. belli* is a sporozoan parasite which is probably transmitted from person to person. In normal individuals it produces a self-limited disease consisting of mild fever, headache, diarrhea, and colicky abdominal pain. In the immunocompromised host, it produces profuse diarrhea which may occur cyclically and is associated with significant weight loss. Diagnosis is difficult and must be made by examination of the stool by an experienced technician. Treatment with trimethoprim with sulfamethoxazole is usually successful, but relapses in AIDS patients are common.

Dientamoeba fragilis

Dientamoeba fragilis is an ameboflagellate that is probably transmitted by fecal-oral contamination, although the exact mechanism is not known. Transmission in the ova of the pinworm has been suggested as a likely mode of infection. The prevalence of diarrheal disease is probably about 1 percent. The organism is not invasive and generally produces abdominal pain, anorexia, and intermittent diarrhea. Diagnosis is by examination of the stool by an experienced technician. Treatment with iodoquinole or tetracycline has been successful.

Ciguatera Fish Poisoning

Although many exogenous toxins may cause GI upset, they are too numerous to discuss in this chapter. Ciguatera fish poisoning is worth mentioning, as its prevalence is increasing in the southeastern United States. Fish whose ingestion can cause the disease are found in tropical and subtropical waters. These fish, particularly grouper, snapper, and kingfish, become sporadically poisonous when a particular dinoflagellate is present in the food chain in the late spring and summer months. The incubation period varies from 2 to 30 h after ingestion of the toxin (median 6 h). The illness may begin with vomiting and diarrhea, which are present in 78 percent of the patients. Neuromuscular and neurosensory manifestations may be particularly severe and lead to prolonged discomfort. These include myalgia of the legs and thighs, weakness, and dysesthesia and paresthesia of the perioral region and distal extremities. Occasionally patients describe a "burning" sensation of their feet or hands. Itching of various parts of the body is common and may be a late manifestation on day 2 or 3 of the illness. The disease is self-limited, and there is no specific therapy. Symptoms generally subside in several days, but some patients have reported having sensory problems for months after the ingestion of affected fish.

GENERAL MANAGEMENT

A complete history, including the time and onset of symptoms, travel, and the relation of symptoms to ingestion of a particular food, is important in determining the cause of the GI illness. The presence and frequency of fever may be helpful as well as the consistency, frequency, and odor of the stool. The presence of mucus or blood in the stool should also be determined. Physical examination should include all systems, as extraintestinal disease may cause GI upset and diarrhea. Particular attention should be paid to the signs of dehydration,

Table 47-4. Drug Therapy for Diarrhea

Organism	Drug	How Supplied	Dosage
Campylobacter jejuni	Erythromycin	Ethyl succinate: 200-, 400-mg/5 mL, 400-mg tabs	50 mg/kg (maximum 2 g) divided qid for 7–10 days
	or	Estolate: 125 mg/5 mL, 125-, 250-mg tabs	
		Salt: 125-, 250-mg tabs	
		Stearate: 125-. 250-, 500-mg tabs	
	Tetracycline (older children and adults)	250-, 500-mg tabs Syrup: 25 mg/mL Drops: 100 mg/mL	25–50 mg/kg divided qid (maximum 500 mg qid) 7–10 days
Clostridium difficile	Vancomycin	Oral solution: Mix to make 250 mg/5 mL or 500 mg/5 mL Injectable 1-g vials	20–40 mg/kg PO divided qid (maximum 500 mg qid) 7–10 days
Entamoeba histolytica			
Asymptomatic cyst passers	Iodoquinol		13 mg/kg tid × 21 days (maximum 650 mg tid)
	or		
	Paramomycin	250-mg capsules	7–10 mg/kg tid × 10 days
Passers of cysts and trophozoites	Metronidazole	250-mg tabs	12–17 mg/kg tid × 10 days (maximum 750 mg tid)
	plus		
	Iodoquinol		13 mg/kg tid × 21 days
	or		
	Tetracycline	250-, 500-mg tabs Syrup: 25 mg/mL Drops: 100 mg/mL	2.5–5 mg/kg qid × 7 days (maximum 2g/day)
	plus		*plus*
	Iodoquinol	650-mg tabs	Iodoquinol as above
Amebic dysentery	Metronidazole		12–17 mg/kg tid × 10 days
	plus		*plus*
	Iodoquinol		13 mg/kg tid × 21 days
	or		
	Dehydroemitine		1.5 mg/kg IM × 5 days (maximum 90 mg/day)
	plus		
	Chloroquine phosphate	125-, 250-mg tabs	5 mg/kg/d × 14–21 days
	or		
	Tetracycline, iodoquinol, and chloroquine		Doses as listed above
Escherichia coli (Only persistent infections)	Trimethoprim with sulfamethoxazole	Suspension: 40 mg TMP/200 mg SMZ/5 mL 80/400-mg or 160/800-mg tabs	8–10 mg TMP/kg 40–50 mg/kg SMZ divided bid (maximum 160/800 mg PO bid) 5–7 days
Giardia lamblia	Quinacrine HCl	100-mg tabs	7 mg/kg divided tid × 7 days (maximum 100 mg tid)
	or		
	Metronidazole	250-mg tabs	10–15 mg/kg divided tid × 7 days (maximum 250 mg tid)
	Furazolidone	100-mg tabs Suspension: 50 mg/15 mL	1.5 mg/kg divided qid × 7 days (maximum 100 mg qid)
Salmonella sp. (Only persistent symptomatic infections)	Ampicillin	Suspension: 125, 250 mg/5 mL Capsules: 250, 500 mg Drops: 100 mg/mL Chewable tabs: 125 mg	50–100 mg/kg divided qid × 7–14 days (maximum 500 mg qid)
	or		
	Trimethoprim with sulfamethoxazole	As above	As above
	or		
	Chloramphenicol	Suspension: 150 mg/5 mL 100-, 250-mg capsules	50 mg/kg divided qid for 7–14 days (maximum 500 mg qid)
Shigella sp.	Trimethoprim with sulfamethoxazole	Suspension: 40 mg TMP/200 mg SMZ/5 mL, 80/400 or 160/800 tabs	8–10 mg TMP/40–50 mg SMZ/kg divided bid (max 160/800 mg bid × 7–14 days)
Shigella sp. (resistant cases)	Ciprofloxacin HCl	250-mg tabs	250 mg bid × 5–7 days
Yersinia enterocolitica	Trimethoprim with sulfamethoxazole	As above	As above
	or		
	Tetracycline	250-, 500-mg capsules	20–50 mg/kg divided qid × 7–10 days (maximum 500 mg qid)
	or		
	Third-generation cephalosporin		As directed

mucous membrane, skin turgor, postural changes in blood pressure, level of consciousness, and the fontanel in young infants. Many patients with acute diarrheal disease will have abdominal tenderness, but if this is severe or persistent, the patient should be observed for a process that may require surgical intervention.

Laboratory studies are not generally helpful in the acute management of food poisoning and infectious diarrhea. A high white blood cell count with a left shift may suggest a bacterial cause; however, this condition is not always present. In typhoid fever one may see a relatively low white blood cell count, neutropenia, or a marked shift to left. Electrolytes are indicated when dehydration is suspected, and urine specific gravity should be obtained. If a stool sample is available, a wet mount may be made by mixing a small amount of feces with normal saline or methylene blue on a slide. Microscopic examination of this preparation may show white and red blood cells, mucous strands, and trophozoites or cysts of parasitic protozoa. A Hemoccult test of the stool may also reveal the presence of blood. Cultures should be sent to the laboratory in transport media when *Salmonella, Shigella, Campylobacter,* or *Vibrio* infections are suspected, because of the public health importance of these infections. An acid-fast stain of the stool may show Cryptosporidium. Ova and parasite examinations may reveal *Entamoeba histolytica, Giardia, Cryptosporidium, Isospora,* or *Dientamoeba fragilis.*

Many prescription and over-the-counter preparations are available for the treatment of diarrhea, vomiting, and GI upset. Few have been shown to be effective in altering the course of the illness. Most infectious and noninfectious GI illnesses are self-limited and do not require specific therapy.

Antibiotics should be reserved for patients who are febrile and toxic, and only for diseases for which they have been shown to be effective. Contraindications to antibiotic therapy may exist in some uncomplicated infections, such as salmonellosis, as they prolong the carrier state.

Other medications such as diphenoxylate hydrochloride with atropine (Lomotil) or loperamide (Immodium) may provide temporary symptomatic relief and may be efficacious if the patient has uncontrollable diarrhea. These preparations and others that slow peristalsis and delay intestinal emptying may prolong the illness, as infective organisms and toxins have continued contact with the bowel. The mainstay of therapy is putting the intestinal tract at rest and maintaining hydration. Most patients can be managed with a clear liquid diet. Liquids may include clear fruit juices, sodas, gelatin dessert water, rice water, etc. The diet may be advanced to include rice, applesauce, bananas, and toast when the diarrhea has subsided. Small sips of clear liquids should be recommended when vomiting is prominent. Using Popsicles is also recommended.

Phenothiazine preparations may be used with severe vomiting but are not recommended in children because of a higher incidence of dystonic reactions. Hospitalization should be considered in the very young and old when there is evidence of dehydration.

Table 47-4 lists some of the organisms responsible for diarrhea and the drugs commonly used in treatment.

BIBLIOGRAPHY

Black RE, Jackson RJ, Tsia T, et al: Epidemic *Yersinia enterocolitica* infection due to contaminated chocolate milk. *N Engl J Med* 298:76, 1978.

Communicable Disease Surveillance Center, PHLS: Surveillance of food poisoning and *Salmonella* infections in England and Wales 1170–9. *Br Med J* 281:817, 1980.

Gorbach SL (ed): Infectious diarrhea. *Infect Dis Clin North Am* 2: 1988.

Harris JC, Dupont HL, Hornck RB: Fecal leukocytes in diarrheal illness. *Ann Intern Med* 76:697, 1972.

Kimmey M: Infectious diarrhea. *Emerg Clin N Amer* 3:127, 1985.

Lawrence DN, Enriquez MB, Lumish RM, et al: Ciguatera fish poisoning in Miami. *JAMA* 244:254, 1980.

Lowenstein MS: Epidemiology of *Clostridium perfringens* food poisoning. *N Engl J Med* 286:1026, 1972.

Markell EK, Voge M, John DT: *Medical Parasitology,* 6th ed. Philadelphia, Saunders, 1986.

Rodriquez WJ, Kim HW, Arrobio JO, et al: Clinical features of acute gastroenteritis associated with human reovirus-like agent in infants and young children. *J Pediatr* 91:188, 1977.

Soave R, Johnson WD: *Cryptosporidium* and *Isospora belli* infections. *J Infect Dis* 157:225, 1988.

48 CHOLECYSTITIS

John L. Glover

Cholecystitis is an acute inflammation of the gallbladder, usually associated with gallstones. It is significantly more common in women than in men; most cases occur in the third through the fifth decade of life, though it can occur in the very young or the very old. It is characterized by recurring episodes of symptoms, many of which are relatively minor. It is an extremely common problem; in 1985, nearly 500,000 cholecystectomies were done in the United States.

A less frequent form of cholecystitis not associated with gallstones, and known, therefore, as *acute acalculous cholecystitis,* occurs as a complication of burns, sepsis, major trauma, and any major illness or operation. This form of cholecystitis usually occurs in hospitalized patients. Diagnosis may be difficult; gangrene and perforation are relatively frequent, in contrast to acute calculous cholecystitis.

Cholecystitis is the most frequent cause of acute pancreatitis, the mechanism being passage of a gallstone into the common bile duct and occlusion of the pancreatic duct at the sphincter of Oddi.

Passage of stones into the common bile duct can also cause *ascending cholangitis,* purulent infection of the bile ducts extending into the liver. This condition, characterized by shaking chills, high fever, and jaundice (Charcot's triad), is a surgical emergency and is associated with a high mortality rate.

Finally, cholecystitis can occur from gallstones resulting from hemolytic processes, since the increased breakdown of hemoglobin can cause gallstones composed exclusively of bile pigment. Such conditions include congenital spherocytosis, acquired hemolytic anemias, and sickle cell disease.

PATHOGENESIS

In most cases, acute cholecystitis is associated with an obstruction of the neck of the gallbladder or the cystic duct due to gallstones. About 20 million people in the United States have gallstones; the incidence increases with age, and the majority of women in their eighties probably have gallstones, Above certain concentrations of cholesterol, lecithin, and bile salts, bile is either a supersaturated liquid or a two-phase system of liquid bile and solid crystalline cholesterol. When the crystals achieve macroscopic size, while bile is stored in the gallbladder, gallstones are formed. A number of factors, including stasis, presence of bacteria, and reflux of intestinal contents or pancreatic juice, may contribute to the precipitation of cholesterol.

Obstruction of the cystic duct is followed by increased pressure in the gallbladder. If unrelieved, there is damage to the mucosa, followed by intramural inflammation. The extent of this process depends on the duration of obstruction. If it is relieved promptly, as by the stone becoming spontaneously dislodged, there is relief of pain and resolution of the inflammation. Repeated episodes of this sort are the rule rather than the exception, and the result is chronic fibrosis in the wall of the gallbladder. This fibrosis limits the degree to which the gallbladder can distend and probably protects against perforation. It also explains why a palpable distended gallbladder in a jaundiced patient is usually a sign of malignant obstruction of the bile duct instead of obstruction due to stones. In some cases, however, there is relatively rapid necrosis of the wall, resulting in perforation. Elderly patients and diabetics are more prone to this complication than others. When perforation occurs, the omentum tends to wall off this de facto subhepatic abscess initially; but bile peritonitis is present by definition and must be treated on an emergency basis.

In some instances gallstones will erode into an adjacent viscus, most commonly the duodenum or the colon. If large stones erode into the duodenum, they can cause intestinal obstruction because they rarely pass the ileocecal valve. Stones that erode into the colon are usually passed unnoticed in the feces, but these patients usually have persistent cholecystitis.

Empyema of the gallbladder is an advanced stage of cholecystitis in which there is bacterial invasion of the gallbladder wall and gross suppuration associated with it. Emphysematous cholecystitis is a rare form of cholecystitis in which there is infection with gas-forming bacteria. The gallbladder fills with gas due to *Escherichia coli, Clostridium perfringens,* anaerobic streptococci, or some combination of these organisms.

Because of recent improvements in diagnostic techniques, more young women, often in their early twenties or younger, are found to have cholecystitis but no gallstones. Examination of the excised gallbladder shows chronic cholesterolosis, which is an early stage of calculous cholecystitis. It might be termed *precalculous cholecystitis* to differentiate it from the *acalculous cholecystitis* which occurs as a complication of major illness or trauma and which probably has a different etiology.

CLINICAL FEATURES

Patients with gallbladder disease may present with a variety of symptoms, usually on an urgent basis, due to different pathophysiologic conditions: pain from intermittent obstruction of the cystic duct, pain from an acute exacerbation of chronic cholecystitis, severe pain and tenderness due to gangrene of the gallbladder wall with adjacent abscess formation, ''biliary colic'' due to stones passing into the common duct, pancreatitis due to gallstones obstructing the pancreatic duct, and any combinations of these. In addition, a patient with prior cholecystectomy may have recurrences of right upper quadrant pain several months after surgery, symptoms called *biliary dyskinesia* or *postcholecystectomy syndrome.* A review of the mechanisms of visceral and somatic pain helps sort out these different presentations of biliary tract disease.

Visceral pain arising from the gallbladder wall comes from stimulation of the nerve endings in the muscular layer of the gallbladder wall by strong distension or contraction of the gallbladder. The distension or contraction is caused by obstruction of the cystic duct, either by a gallstone or by inflammation. This visceral pain, like that from other abdominal viscera, is felt *in the midline,* not in the right upper quadrant. Furthermore, it may not be construed as pain at all, but as a vague, intermittent discomfort in the epigastrium associated with varying degrees of nausea. The patient may be restless, and frequently walks around, or tosses and turns at night, to get relief, which is another characteristic of visceral pain. Symptoms of this type are associated with intermittent cystic duct obstruction or early cholecystitis. It is a clinical challenge to differentiate such symptoms from gastroenteritis and initiate a proper evaluation so that later, more serious stages of cholecystitis may be avoided.

If obstruction of the cystic duct persists, pressure in the gallbladder rises enough to cause necrosis of some of the mucosal cells. As a result, there is a chemical inflammation of the gallbladder wall; and if bacteria are present (as they usually are when gallstones are present), infection is initiated. These changes result in a full-thickness inflammation of the gallbladder wall which, in turn, stimulates the somatic nerve endings adjacent to the gallbladder wall. At this stage, the pain becomes constant and is localized to the right upper quadrant. (Somatic pain is characteristically localized to the area in which the nerve endings are being stimulated by the inflammatory process.) Any movement of the peritoneal covering exacerbates the pain—coughing, taking a deep breath, or having an examiner percuss the abdominal wall over the gallbladder. At this stage, the patient usually has fever due to the inflammation, which may vary in severity from mild cholecystitis to gangrene of the wall and pericholecystic abscess.

Complicating these clinical features is the possibility of passing a stone into the common bile duct. This occurs in 20 percent or more of patients with acute cholecystitis, although one might suppose that obstruction of the cystic duct from cholecystitis would prevent the phenomenon. When a stone reaches the common duct, it may cause severe colicky pain, or the patient may be asymptomatic. Some patients develop jaundice, while others, even those with a large number of stones, have no jaundice or other symptoms. Furthermore, some patients pass stones into the duodenum without symptoms, while others with transient obstruction of the pancreatic duct develop severe pain due to pancreatitis. Undoubtedly, these variations are in some instances related to differences in the motility of the bile duct and to the amount of muscular contraction in the biliary and pancreatic sphincters, factors which are probably also related to two other poorly understood clinical manifestations of bilary tract disease: postcholecystectomy syndrome and formation of "primary" stones in the common bile duct. The former usually occurs within the first 2 years after cholecystectomy, and the latter, many years later. Although the specific pathophysiologic events are not thoroughly understood, "emptying" of the biliary tree into the intestinal tract is thought to be the fundamental cause.

Important features in the history of patients presenting with pain possibly due to cholecystitis include a family history of gallbladder disease and a history of intolerance to certain foods, often fatty or greasy foods. Nausea is a prominent feature of acute cholecystitis. Vomiting is variable; and in spite of the theoretical consideration that the obstruction of the cystic duct should block the flow of gallbladder bile, the vomitus is bile-stained and described as bitter. In cholecystitis alone, jaundice is usually absent; if present, the situation becomes more urgent because of the possibility of ascending cholangitis due to obstruction of the common bile duct.

In most cases the temperature is mildly elevated, 38.3° to 38.8°C (100.9° to 101.8°F); and there is mild tachycardia. Tachypnea may be present, and the breathing may be shallow. A good way to elicit the characteristic localized tenderness is to have the patient take a slow, deep breath while the examiner holds gentle, steady pressure against the abdominal wall, just below the costal margin in the midclavicular line. At the height of the patient's inspiration, when the liver and gallbladder have descended to the costal margin, an increase in pressure of the examining hand will cause the patient to wince with pain due to direct pressure on the inflamed gallbladder. In some patients, an ill-defined mass is palpable due to the omentum being adherent to the gallbladder. Abdominal distension is usually mild or absent, and bowel sounds may be normal unless there is significant peritonitis.

Generally there is mild leukocytosis with a left shift. Bilirubin and alkaline phosphatase may be slightly elevated due to cholecystitis alone, but higher values usually mean that a common duct stone is present also. If there is a significant elevation of serum amylase, one can make the diagnosis of pancreatitis on the basis of a common duct stone.

Plain films of the abdomen will be nonspecific except when the gallstones are radiopaque (about 10 percent of cases) and when there is air in the biliary tree due to a biliary enteric fistula. In classical emphysematous cholecystitis, the gallbladder is either filled with air or has an air-fluid level. There may be localized ileus in the right upper abdomen, manifest by loops of air-filled intestine adherent to the inflamed gallbladder.

Ultrasonography has become the first diagnostic test because of ease of performance and high accuracy, both in detecting the presence of gallstones and measuring the thickness of the gallbladder wall (5 mm or greater being diagnostic of cholecystitis). In addition, ultrasound can detect stones in the common duct and the presence of a dilated common duct. Finally, it can identify a pericholecystic abscess caused by localized (and walled-off) perforation of the gallbladder.

If ultrasonography shows no stones and equivocal thickness of the gallbladder wall, biliary scintiscanning (HIDA, PIPIDA) may be done. The isotope normally is concentrated in the liver and excreted in bile; the course of the common bile duct is easily outlined by the radioactivity, as is passage into the duodenum. If there is no passage of isotope into the gallbladder, the cystic duct is presumed to be obstructed, therefore providing evidence in favor of cholecystitis.

Although CT scanning may be done, it rarely offers any advantage over ultrasound for the diagnosis of cholecystitis. Endoscopic retrograde cholangiography is not often indicated to diagnose cholecystitis, but it may be considered for rapid decompression of ascending cholangitis, though its role is yet unproven.

TREATMENT

When the diagnosis of cholecystitis has been confirmed, cholecystectomy is indicated; but the timing of admission to the hospital and the scheduling of surgery may vary. In some instances, patients are obviously not sick; they have experienced transient cystic duct obstruction and have no significant inflammatory process, as shown by the lack of fever, leukocytosis, and significant abdominal tenderness. Such patients may be discharged, with instructions to limit diet to liquids initially and to avoid fats, which stimulate contraction of the gallbladder. They may be given antinauseants, but any need for pain medication at this stage suggests the need to reevaluate the patient. Diabetic patients with these "early" symptoms should not be sent home until specific arrangements for care are made, and diabetics with definite cholecystitis should be admitted to the hospital and given antibiotics (cefotetan 1g every 12 h IV or cefoxitan 1g every 8 h). The need for surgical consultation is urgent. Other patients with persistent vomiting, significant abdominal tenderness, fever, and leukocytosis should be admitted and treated with nasogastric suction and intravenous fluids (nothing by mouth should be given). Parenteral antibiotics are generally given also.

Timing of surgery is slightly controversial. In the past, the usual practice was to allow the acute episode to subside and perform cholecystectomy electively 6 weeks later. A significant number of patients, however, had recurrent or persistent cholecystitis and required surgery sooner. This common recurrence of symptoms, the lack of specific nonoperative therapy, and the increased costs of a second hospitalization have led to a trend to operate as soon as "convenient" after the diagnosis is established. One may, for example, admit the patient one evening and operate the following day, or wait an additional day if a complicated preoperative cardiac evaluation is required. The surgery is considered urgent, but need not be done within the first few hours of diagnosis unless empyema of the gallbladder or impending perforation is suspected. If pancreatitis is present, operation is usually delayed until the serum amylase falls to normal. On rare occasions, for example, when a patient has acute cholecystitis during convalescence from a myocardial infarction, cholecystostomy, under local anesthesia, may be done instead of cholecystectomy, which requires a general or spinal anesthesia.

Treatment of the different stages of biliary disease is changing due to newer medical and surgical techniques. Some patients are being treated with agents designed to dissolve pure cholesterol stones, but the treatment has several drawbacks. It is expensive, has significant side effects, and must be continued for the rest of the patient's life. Another method is fragmentation of gallstones by extracorporeal shock wave lithotripsy. This treatment is limited at present to patients with a few relatively small stones, and it may require endoscopic papillotomy to allow the stone fragments to pass into the duodenum.

More recently, it has been shown that cholecystectomy can be done laparoscopically. The advantage of this technique, which requires general anesthesia, is that it may be done on an outpatient basis, and that patients return to full preoperative function within 1 week (in contrast to 4 to 6 weeks after standard cholecystectomy). At present, laparoscopic surgery is not done if acute or extensive inflammation is present. Thus the importance of making the diagnosis of gallbladder disease when the symptoms are relatively mild cannot be overemphasized, as early diagnosis allows for definitive therapy with a minimum of incapacitation.

Finally, even in severe cholecystitis in high-risk patients, less invasive techniques are being used. Percutaneous drainage, for example, has been used to provide palliative treatment while other serious medical conditions, such as cardiac failure, are treated.

BIBLIOGRAPHY

Carroll BA: Preferred imaging techniques for the diagnosis of cholecystitis and cholelithiasis. *Ann Surg* 210:1, 1989.

Cheung LY, Maxwell JG: Jaundice in patients with acute cholecystitis: Its validity as an indication for common bile duct exploration. *Am J Surg* 130:746, 1975.

Cornwell EE III, Rodriguez A, Mirvis SE, et al: Acute acalculous cholecystitis in critically injured patients. *Ann Surg* 210:52, 1989.

Cucchiaro G, Watters CR, Rossitch JC, et al: Deaths from gallstones: Incidence and associated clinical factors. *Ann Surg* 209:149, 1989.

Diettrich NA, Cacioppo JC, Davis RP: The vanishing elective cholecystectomy. *Arch Surg* 123:810, 1988.

DuBois F, Icard P, Berthelot G, Levard H: Coelioscopic cholecystectomy. *Ann Surg* 211:60, 1990.

Escallon A Jr, Rosales W, Aldrete JS: Reliability of pre- and intraoperative tests for biliary lithiasis. *Ann Surg* 210:640, 1985.

Glenn F: Acute acalculous cholecystitis. *Ann Surg* 189:458, 1979.

Glenn F, Becker CG: Acute acalculous cholecystitis: An increasing entity. *Ann Surg* 195:131, 1982.

Heberer G, Paumgartner G, Sauerbruch T, et al: A retrospective analysis of 3 years' experience of an interdisciplinary approach to gallstone disease including shock waves. *Ann Surg* 208:274, 1988.

Hickman MS, Schwesinger W, Page CP: Acute cholecystitis in the diabetic. *Arch Surg* 123:409, 1990.

Jarvinen HJ, Hastbacka J: Early cholecystectomy for acute cholecystitis. *Ann Surg* 191:501, 1980.

McAvoy JM, Roth J, Rees WV, et al: Role of ultrasonography in the primary diagnosis of cholelithiasis: An analysis of fifty cases. *Am J Surg* 136:309, 1978.

McGahan JP, Lindfors KK: Acute cholecystitis: Diagnostic accuracy of percutaneous aspiration of the gallbladder. *Radiology* 167:669, 1988.

Misra DC Jr, Blossom G, Fink-Bennett, D, Glover JL: Results of surgical therapy for biliary dyskinesia. *Arch Surg* 126:(*in press*), 1991.

Pinto DJ, Burke M, Wilkins A, et al: Infusion cholecystography in the diagnosis of acute cholecystitis. *Br J Surg* 66:173, 1979.

Pitluk HC, Beal JM: Choledocholithiasis associated with acute cholecystitis. *Arch Surg* 114:887, 1979.

Saltzstein EC, Peacock JB, Mercer LC: Early operation for acute biliary tract stone disease. *Surgery* 94:704, 1983.

Savoca PE, Longo WE, Zucker KA, et al: The increasing prevalence of acalculous cholecystitis in outpatients. *Ann Surg* 211:433, 1990.

Zwemer FL, Coffin-Kwart VE, Conway MJ: Biliary enteric fistulas: Management of 47 cases in native Americans. *Am J Surg* 138:310, 1979.

49 ACUTE JAUNDICE AND HEPATITIS

Richard Owen Shields, Jr.

ACUTE JAUNDICE

Jaundice is the yellowish discoloration of the sclera, skin, and mucous membranes by bilirubin. The presence of carotene or long-standing hemochromatosis may also cause yellow-orange discoloration of the skin, but the sclera is not affected.

Bilirubin, a breakdown product of hemoglobin from injured or senescent red blood cells and other heme-containing proteins, is produced in the reticuloendothelial system and transported on albumin to the liver. There it is conjugated mostly as the diglucuronide and excreted through the bile channels into the small intestine. An increase in the production of bilirubin or a defect in the elimination pathway may produce clinical jaundice and hyperbilirubinemia.

Hyperbilirubinemia can be divided into two subtypes: unconjugated and conjugated. *Unconjugated* hyperbilirubinemia results from an increased bilirubin load or a defect in the ability of the hepatocyte to take up and conjugate bilirubin. *Conjugated* hyperbilirubinemia results from a decrease in the ability of the liver to excrete conjugated bilirubin (cholestasis). The site of cholestasis may be either intrahepatic or extrahepatic in origin. *Intrahepatic cholestasis* is caused by decreased excretion of conjugated bilirubin, hepatocellular damage, and damage to the biliary endothelium. Obstruction of biliary outflow by a congenital defect, inflammation, a mass lesion, or gallstones produces *extrahepatic cholestasis* (see Table 49-1).

Emergency Department Evaluation

A careful history and physical examination coupled with judicious use of the clinical laboratory frequently enable the emergency physician to make a reasonable diagnosis and decide if hospitalization is indicated. Often, more extensive diagnostic procedures are needed before the cause can be determined.

History

Jaundice without other complaints and with a positive family history of jaundice suggests a hereditary cause. Viral hepatitis should be suspected in male homosexuals, patients on hemodialysis, and intravenous drug abusers, and when the history reveals raw seafood ingestion, recent blood transfusion, ear piercing, tattoos, needle puncture, foreign travel, or close contact with someone with hepatitis. Toxic hepatitis must be considered if there is a history of exposure to toxic chemicals or the use of hepatoxic drugs. Older patients with right upper quadrant abdominal pain, vomiting, and fever probably have extrahepatic biliary obstruction. Heavy ethanol abusers with fever and abdominal pain are likely to have alcoholic hepatitis or cirrhosis.

Physical Examination

Jaundice can most easily be detected in the mucous membranes of the mouth and in the conjunctiva using natural light. The presence of ascites, edema, and spider angiomata suggests cirrhosis. Right upper quadrant tenderness, a positive Murphy's sign, or a palpable gallbladder might indicate biliary disease. Cachexia and an epigastric mass suggest a neoplastic process, while a hard, nodular liver may represent hepatic metastases. Hepatomegaly with pedal edema, jugular venous distension, and a gallop rhythm make congestive cardiac failure the likely cause of jaundice. Needle tracks should raise the likelihood of viral hepatitis.

Laboratory

The total bilirubin level is elevated if clinical jaundice is present. With unconjugated hyperbilirubinemia, 85 percent or more of the total bilirubin is of the indirect fraction. A direct-reacting fraction of at least 30 percent (and usually higher) is present with conjugated hyperbilirubinemia. A bedside test to determine if bilirubin is conjugated is to test the urine for bilirubin. Conjugated bilirubin is water-soluble and appears in the urine at very low serum concentrations. Unconjugated bilirubin is bound to albumin and is not present in urine.

Some cholestasis is present if the serum alkaline phosphatase level is elevated to greater than three times normal. Anemia with reticulocytosis and an abnormal peripheral smear are characteristic of hemolysis. Markedly elevated aminotransferase levels are most compatible with a viral hepatitis. A prolonged prothrombin time, a low serum albumin level, and anemia suggest alcoholic hepatitis or decompensated cirrhosis.

VIRAL HEPATITIS

Viral hepatitis produces inflammation of the liver and necrosis of hepatic parenchymal cells. The severity of illness ranges from inapparent, subclinical infections to fulminant hepatic failure. Viral hepatitis is a significant public health problem, not only because of the associated morbidity and mortality, but also because of its sequelae: chronic hepatitis, cirrhosis, and hepatocellular carcinoma.

The initial prodromal symptoms are usually constitutional, may be variable, and may be abrupt or insidious in onset. Nausea, vomiting, fatigue, malaise, and alterations in taste are common. Low-grade fever with pharyngitis, coryza, and headache may lead to an early misdiagnosis of upper respiratory infection or "flulike" syndrome. The majority of cases do not develop jaundice and recover uneventfully.

In icteric cases, jaundice develops 1 to 2 weeks following the onset

Table 49-1. Causes of Jaundice

I. Unconjugated
  A. Hemolytic anemia
  B. Hemoglobinopathy
  C. Transfusion reaction
  D. Gilbert's disease
  E. Crigler-Najjar syndrome
  F. Prematurity in neonates
  G. Congestive heart failure
II. Conjugated
  A. Intrahepatic
    1. Infectious
      a. Viral hepatitis
      b. Leptospirosis
      c. Infectious mononucleosis
    2. Toxic
      a. Drugs
      b. Chemicals
    3. Familial
      a. Rotor syndrome
      b. Dubin-Johnson syndrome
    4. Alcoholic liver disease
    5. Other
      a. Sarcoidosis
      b. Lymphoma
      c. Liver metastases
      d. Amyloidosis
      e. Cirrhosis
      f. Biliary cirrhosis
  B. Extrahepatic
    1. Gallstones
    2. Pancreatic tumors or cysts
    3. Cholangiocarcinoma
    4. Bile duct stricture
    5. Sclerosing cholangitis

Table 49-2. Distinguishing Features of the Hepatitis Viruses

Feature	Hepatitis A	Hepatitis B	Hepatitis C
Size	27 nm	42 nm	?
Nucleic acid	RNA	DNA	RNA
Incubation	15–49 days	45–160 days	15–160 days
Mean	30 days	120 days	55 days
Oral-fecal	Yes	No	?
Percutaneous	Rare	Yes	Yes
Carrier state	No	Yes	Yes
Severity	Mild	Often severe	Moderate
Mortality	0.1–0.2%	1%	?

of the prodrome and may be preceded by a few days of pruritus and dark urine. Other prodromal symptoms usually disappear during the icteric phase, but malaise and gastrointestinal symptoms frequently persist. Right upper quadrant abdominal pain may develop because of hepatic enlargement. Physical examination during the icteric phase may reveal hepatomegaly or splenomegaly. In the recovery phase, the symptoms disappear, and complete clinical and biochemical recovery is the rule in 3 to 4 months. (See Table 49-2)

The first biochemical abnormality is an elevation of serum transaminase levels before the onset of the prodromal phase. The levels peak during the phase of clinical hepatitis and return to normal during recovery; the magnitude of elevation is not a good indicator of the disease's severity. Prolongation of the prothrombin time by more than a few seconds indicates extensive hepatic necrosis and a poorer prognosis, as does a persistent bilirubin level elevation to greater than 20 mg/dL. An early transient neutropenia is often followed by a relative lymphocytosis with many atypical lymphocytes. Blood glucose levels may be depressed because of poor intake, depleted glycogen stores, and decreased hepatic gluconeogenesis.

Hepatitis A

Hepatitis A, formerly known as infectious hepatitis, is caused by a small RNA picornavirus (HAV) which is spread primarily by the fecal-oral route and has a peak seasonal incidence in the fall and winter. Victims are usually children or adolescents. Adult victims of HAV hepatitis tend to have more severe and prolonged disease. Common-source outbreaks among people exposed to contaminated food or water are common. About 30,000 cases are reported yearly in the United States, but this represents only a small fraction of actual cases. Most cases of HAV hepatitis are mild, anicteric, and undiagnosed, as suggested by the fact that, although more than 50 percent of adults in the United States have serologic evidence of past HAV infection, fewer than 10 percent can recall an episode of hepatitis or jaundice.

The incubation period is 15 to 50 days with viral shedding in the stool for 1 to 2 weeks prior to and up to a week after the onset of symptoms. Symptom onset is often more abrupt than with other types of viral hepatitis. If jaundice develops, it appears several days later and is usually mild. No carrier state or chronic liver disease has been described following HAV infection. IgM and anti-HAV appears in the serum during the phase of clinical hepatitis but is soon replaced by IgG anti-HAV, which persists indefinitely and confers immunity.

Hepatitis B

Hepatitis B, formerly known as serum hepatitis, is caused by a double-stranded DNA hepadnavirus (HBV) with an inner core and an outer coat, both of which are antigenic. It is spread primarily by the percutaneous route, although in as many as 50 percent of acute cases there is no clear history of exposure. Infective particles are present in semen, saliva, and other bodily fluids as well as in blood, which accounts for at least some of the nonpercutaneous transmission of the disease. HBV is maintained in humans in a large reservoir of chronic carriers; the carrier rate in the United States is 0.1 to 0.5 percent. Certain subpopulations such as intravenous drug abusers, male homosexuals, and patients on chronic hemodialysis have a much higher carrier rate.

The incubation period of hepatitis B is 70 to 160 days with a mean of 70 to 80 days. Most cases are inapparent and anicteric. The onset of symptoms is usually insidious and preceded, in 5 to 10 percent, by a "serum-sickness-like" illness with polyarthritis, proteinuria, and angioneurotic edema thought to be caused by circulating antigen-antibody complexes. The symptoms tend to be more prolonged and severe than with hepatitis A, but complete recovery is expected in 90 percent.

Fulminant hepatic failure develops in about 1 percent, and is characterized by encephalopathy, rapidly rising bilirubin levels, and a significant coagulopathy. Complete recovery is possible, but 80 percent of those developing coma will die. About 5 to 10 percent of victims of hepatitis B develop chronic hepatitis or a chronic carrier state. Patients developing chronic HBV hepatitis frequently have a relatively mild acute illness.

The identification of three distinct HBV antigens and the capability to detect viral DNA in the serum (HBV-DNA) have provided serologic methods with which to diagnose and monitor patients with HBV infection. Hepatitis B surface antigen (HBsAg) represents the outer protein coat of the viral particle. It appears in the serum of more than 90 percent of patients before the appearance of transaminase elevations and clinical symptoms and persists until 1 to 2 months following the icteric phase, with total antigenemia lasting about 6 months.

Antibody to HBsAg (anti-HBs) appears in the serum from 2 to 6 months following the disappearance of HBsAg. The presence of anti-HBs implies prior HBV infection or vaccination, and confers immunity to subsequent infection. Anti-HBs is present in 5 to 10 percent of healthy, volunteer blood donors in the United States. Chronic carriers of HBV usually have persistence of HBsAg in the serum and do not develop anti-HBs.

The core of the HBV particle, called *hepatitis B core antigen* (*HBcAg*), does not appear in the serum. Anti-HBc antibody appears in the serum about 2 weeks after the appearance of HBsAg, and during the "window" between the disappearance of HBsAg and the appearance of anti-HBs, it may be the only serologic marker of recent infection. IgM anti-HBc in high titer indicates the presence of acute HBV hepatitis with high infectivity, while its persistence at low levels is found in chronic HBV hepatitis. IgG anti-HBc is also found along with HBsAg in chronic hepatitis, but its presence along with anti-HBs implies remote HBV infection.

Hepatitis B e antigen (*HBeAg*) is a soluble antigen found in serum containing HBsAg. Its presence implies ongoing viral replication and high infectivity. This antigen disappears in those who recover from HBV hepatitis but persists in those who develop chronic hepatitis. Antibody to the e antigen (anti-HBe) appears in the acute phase or illness and usually signifies reduced infectivity. This antibody persists for some months after HBeAg disappearance.

The presence of HBV-DNA in the serum is the most sensitive indicator of ongoing viral replication and, therefore, of infectivity. In the typical acute HBV hepatitis, HBV-DNA is detectable in the serum in the incubation period and peaks about the time that symptoms appear. HBV-DNA is rapidly cleared from the serum in those with acute HBV hepatitis and is already undetectable in more than half of patients first seeking medical attention for the disease.

Hepatitis Non-A, Non-B

The term *hepatitis non-A, non-B* (*HNANB*) is used to denote typical viral hepatitis that is not caused by HAV, HBV, or other known viral agents (e.g., cytomegalovirus or Epstein-Barr). As new hepatitis viruses are identified and characterized, this term will become outmoded, but it is now a useful shorthand notation.

Evidence currently suggests the existence of two categories of HNANB: enterically transmitted and parenterally transmitted. The parenterally transmitted form accounts for from 20 to 40 percent of all reported cases of acute viral hepatitis in the United States, and 80 to 95 percent of all transfusion-related viral hepatitis. Posttransfusion HNANB has an incubation period of 2 to 26 weeks with a mean of 7 weeks. The clinical course is similar to HBV hepatitis although usually milder. Incubation periods of HNANB associated with clotting factor transfusions may be considerably shorter and probably represent infection with a different agent.

In the early 1980s, about 10 percent of transfusion recipients developed HNANB. About 50 percent of those developed a chronic hepatitis, and as many as 5 to 10 percent developed cirrhosis. The screening of potential blood donors for "surrogate" markers of HNANB had helped to reduce this incidence by the late 1980s.

In 1989, both radioimmune and enzyme-linked assays were developed to detect antibodies to a protein produced by a viral agent now referred to as the hepatitis C virus (HCV). HCV is a linear, single-stranded RNA virus with characteristics similar to the flaviviruses. Retrospective serologic studies of chronic transfusion-related HNANB strongly suggest that HCV is the predominant etiologic agent of this disease. By early 1990, blood banks in the United States were screening all donor units for the presence of anti-HCV. This policy should significantly reduce the incidence of transfusion-related viral hepatitis.

Other HNANB agents exist, as suggested by patients with typical posttransfusion HNANB who fail to develop serologic markers for infection with HCV, and by patients with multiple episodes of HNANB. The majority of reported cases of HNANB are not transfusion-related, and show modes of transmission similar to that of HBV.

Enterically transmitted HNANB, resembling HAV in route of transmission, has been identified sporadically and in waterborne epidemics in Africa, Asia, and Mexico. A causative agent has been identified and is referred to as hepatitis E (HEV). Hepatitis E is a single-stranded RNA virus of the Calicivirus family. This type of HNANB carries a higher incidence of fulminant liver failure and mortality than does HAV and has an especially high mortality rate among pregnant women. It does not appear to progress to a chronic hepatitis.

Hepatitis D

The hepatitis D virus (HDV) is an important cause of both acute and chronic viral hepatitis. This virus consists of the HDV antigen (HDV Ag) and a small, circular piece of single-stranded RNA enclosed by a coat of HBsAg. HDV is considered a "defective" virus because it can replicate only in the presence of acute or chronic HBV infection. Thus, the mode of transmission of HDV is inextricably linked to the transmission of HBV.

Acute HDV infection can occur as a coinfection with acute HBV hepatitis, or as a superinfection in HBsAg carriers. Acute coinfection is usually self-limited, with HDV being cleared as the HBV infection clears. Superinfection, however, produces a mortality rate much higher than acute infection with HBV, and chronic hepatitis develops in as many as 80 percent of cases. Chronic HDV hepatitis results in cirrhosis in 70 to 80 percent of cases, and often progresses quite rapidly. Fulminant liver failure is seen more often in high-risk groups such as intravenous drug users.

Diagnosis of HDV infection is made by the demonstration of anti-HDV in the serum by radioimmunoassay. This antiboidy appears late and in low titer in acute infections, but is persistent in high titer in chronic infections.

No specific treatment exists for HDV infection, nor does a vaccine currently exist. Prevention of HDV infection is best achieved by immunization against HBV and by the avoidance of high-risk behaviors.

Emergency Department Management and Evaluation

When faced with a patient with suspected viral hepatitis, the emergency physician must utilize the history and physical examination as well as readily available laboratory testing to determine if hospital admission is required. Outpatient management with emphasis on rest, adequate diet, good personal hygiene, and the avoidance of hepatotoxins (e.g., ethanol) is sufficient for the majority. Discharged patients must have adequate follow-up care. Patients meeting any one of the criteria listed in Table 49-3 should be admitted for further evaluation, monitoring, and supportive care.

Every patient should have serologic testing done to confirm the diagnosis of viral hepatitis and to identify, if possible, the etiologic agent. At a minimum, assays for HBsAg, IgM anti-HBc, and IgM anti-HAV should be done, with other studies ordered based on the history and clinical situation. Baseline coagulation studies and bilirubin and transaminase levels should also be obtained.

Documented cases of viral hepatitis should be reported to the appropriate public health agency, and close personal contacts of the patient should be advised of the potential risks and offered prophylaxis if indicated (see Table 49-4).

Prevention and Prophylaxis

At this time, no vaccines are available for the prevention of hepatitis caused by HAV, HDV, HCV, HEV, or HNANB. In 1982, a vaccine for the prevention of HBV hepatitis was introduced and has proved to be both highly effective and free of significant adverse effects. This vaccine consists of HBsAg prepared from the pooled plasma of chronic carriers of HBV. The deltoid muscle is the preferred site of vaccine injection, producing consistently better responses than other sites. Despite some early concern about a possible risk of contamination of the HBV vaccine with the then-unknown infectious agent causing acquired immunodeficiency syndrome (AIDS), no evidence exists linking the vaccine to AIDS. The sequential inactivation treatment used in purifying the vaccine has been shown to totally inactivate the human immunodeficiency virus (HIV). Vaccines consisting of HBsAg produced by genetically engineered yeast are now available and should be used instead of the plasma-derived vaccine, except in special situations (yeast allergy).

The currently recommended series of three doses of vaccine produces adequate anti-HBs response in greater than 90 percent of adults. This response provides virtually complete protection against HBV infection. The need for booster doses of vaccine has not been established.

Vaccination against HBV has been recommended for high-risk groups such as intravenous drug abusers, homosexual men, patients on chronic hemodialysis, household and sexual contacts of HBV carriers, infants of HBV carriers, and selected groups of health-care providers. The risk to health-care providers is proportional to the degree of exposure to blood products and to patients with HBV infection and to the degree of preventive measures practiced. No serious adverse effects of vaccination have yet been reported. Because of the nature of emergency medicine, it seems prudent to suggest that emergency personnel be immunized against HBV hepatitis.

Immune globulin (formerly known as gamma globulin or serum immune globulin) is a solution of antibodies obtained by cold ethanol extraction of pooled human plasma. It contains anti-HAV and low-titer anti-HBs. Hepatitis B immune globulin (HBIG) is obtained from the plasma of donors known to have high titers of anti-HBs. Serious adverse effects from the use of immune globulin or HBIG are very

Table 49-3. Indications for Admission with Viral Hepatitis

1. Encephalopathy
2. Prothrombin time prolonged > 3s
3. Dehydration
4. Hypoglycemia
5. Bilirubin > 20 mg/dL
6. Age > 45 years
7. Immunosuppression
8. Diagnosis uncertain

Table 49-4 Postexposure Immunoprophylaxis for Viral Hepatitis

Source	Treatment
HEPATITIS A	
1. Household and sexual contacts of known cases	IG, 0.02 mL/kg IM
2. Day-care center, school, and custodial institution contacts of known cases if evidence of transmission.	Same
3. Exposure to contaminated water or food before cases begin to appear	Same
4. All staff and attendees of day-care centers caring for children in diapers with any known case among children or staff	Same
HEPATITIS B WITH PERCUTANEOUS OR PERMUCOSAL EXPOSURE	
1. Known HBsAg-positive	Unvaccinated: single dose HBIG ASAP, initiate vaccine series.* Vaccinated: Known responder: test for anti-HBs. If adequate (> 10 mIU), no treatment. If inadequate, vaccine booster.† Known nonresponder: two doses HBIG, one ASAP, one in 30 days. Response unknown: test for anti-HBs. If adequate (> 10 mIU), no treatment. If inadequate, single dose HBIG STAT and vaccine booster.†
2. Known HBsAg-negative	Unvaccinated: initiate vaccine series.* Vaccinated: no treatment.
3. Source untested or unknown	Unvaccinated: initiate vaccine series.* Vaccinated: Known responder: no treatment. Known nonresponder: two doses HBIG, one ASAP, one in 30 days if high-risk source. Response unknown: test for anti-HBs. If adequate (> 10 mIU), no treatment. If inadequate, vaccine booster.†
4. Known HNANB infection	Consider single dose IG 0.06 mL/kg IM (clinical studies inconclusive).
HEPATITIS B SEXUAL EXPOSURE	
1. Acute and chronic hepatitis B	Unvaccinated: single-dose HBIG STAT; consider vaccination.* Vaccinated: test for anti-HBs. If adequate (> 10 mIU), no treatment. If inadequate, single dose HBIG ASAP and vaccine booster.†
HEPATITIS C D AND E	
No Recommendations	

* Hepatitis B vaccine is given in a three-injection series; the second injection is given 1 month after the first, and the third six months after the first. Each dose is 1.0 mL (20 μg). For children under 11 years old, the dose is 0.5 mL (10 μg).

† Vaccine booster is a single injection of vaccine.

IG = immune globulin; HBIG = hepatitis B immune globulin 0.06 mL/kg given IM; HBsAg = hepatitis B surface antigen; ASAP = as soon as possible.

Source: Centers for Disease Control: Protection against viral hepatitis: Recommendations of the Immunization Practices Advisory Committee (ACIP). *MMWR* 39(RR-2):4, 1990.

rare and no contraindications to their use exist except for previous hypersensitivity reaction. Immune globulin (IG) is 80 to 90 percent effective in preventing HAV hepatitis when given within 14 days of exposure. A regimen of two doses of HBIG (each dose 0.06 mL/kg IM) following percutaneous exposure to HBsAg-positive blood is about 75 percent effective in preventing the development of HBV hepatitis, but the first dose must be given within 7 days of exposure or the HBIG becomes much less effective. An alternative regimen combines a single dose of HBIG, given as soon as possible after exposure, with the initial dose of the HBV vaccine. This regimen is at least as effective, and less expensive, than the two-dose HBIG regimen and has the added advantage of providing permanent immunity to HBV infection.

Recommendations for postexposure prophylaxis of HAV hepatitis are based on the nature and timing of the exposure, and assume that the patient being considered for prophylaxis has not developed clinical hepatitis. IG should be given to all household and sexual contacts of persons with confirmed HAV hepatitis. IG should also be given to employees and children of day-care facilities caring for children in diapers if one or more cases develop among the children or staff. In centers not enrolling children in diapers only the classroom contacts of the index case need receive IG. School contacts of index cases in elementary or secondary schools need not be treated unless a classroom-centered outbreak is identified. Prophylaxis for hospital staff caring for a patient with HAV hepatitis is not necessary. Prophylaxis in the situation of a common-source outbreak is not indicated unless the exposure is discovered before cases begin to appear. When indicated, IG should be given in a single IM dose of 0.02 mL/kg.

Decision making regarding postexposure prophylaxis for hepatitis B is more complex and must take into account the immunity status of the exposed person and the relative risk that the source of exposure was HBsAg-positive. Prophylaxis should be given to newborns of HBsAg-positive mothers, sexual contacts of an HBsAg-positive partner, and percutaneous or permucosal contacts to HBsAg-positive blood.

Persons with percutaneous exposure to blood from a patient known to have HNANB should receive a single dose of IG at 0.06 mL/kg as soon as possible after exposure, although such prophylaxis is of unproven benefit.

Measures to prevent infection with hepatitis B are sufficient to prevent HDV infection in a person susceptible to HBV infection. There is no known prophylaxis against HDV in persons with chronic HBV infection.

The current recommendations of the Immunization Practices Advisory Committee of the Centers for Disease Control, Department of Health and Human Services, for the postexposure prophylaxis of viral hepatitis are shown in Table 49-4. These recommendations are reviewed periodically and have undergone changes over the past few years.

TOXIC HEPATITIS

A large number of industrial chemicals and pharmaceutical agents are capable of producing hepatic injury. Although hepatic injury accounts for only a small percentage of all adverse drug effects, this etiology accounts for a significant number of hospitalizations for jaundice, especially among the elderly. Acute liver injury may be primarily cytotoxic (e.g., halothane), may be primarily cholestatic (e.g., anabolic steroids), or may present as a mixed form (e.g., amrinone).

Intrinsic hepatotoxins cause rapid, predictable, dose-related injury through a direct toxic effect of the agent or its metabolites on the liver. Other agents cause damage sporadically and unpredictably as a result of hypersensitivity or idiosyncratic reactions. This type of hepatic injury is not dose-related, may be delayed in onset, and may be accompanied by systemic signs and symptoms such as arthralgias, rash, fever, and eosinophilia.

Halothane, methyldopa, isoniazid, and other drugs may produce morphologic changes in the liver resembling those of acute viral hepatitis. Other drugs such as anabolic steroids, oral contraceptives, chlorpropamide, chlorpromazine, and erythromycin estolate may produce cholestatic changes. Massive hepatic necrosis may be produced by carbon tetrachloride, phosphorus, acetaminophen, and mushroom poisoning (e.g., *Amanita phalloides*).

Some drugs and toxins, including methyldopa, vinyl chloride, arsenic, and isoniazid, have been implicated in the development of chronic active hepatitis and cirrhosis.

Halothane

Halothane hepatitis is an idiosyncratic reaction to a metabolite, resulting in a combination of toxic and immunologic injury that may be mediated by genetic factors. It appears much more often in patients with multiple prior exposures to halothane and is more common in adults, especially women, and the obese. In about 25 percent, rash, fever, and eosinophilia are present. Severe icteric cases have a 20 to 40 percent mortality; even mild reactions to halothane must be recognized so that susceptible patients are not reexposed.

Acetaminophen

Acetaminophen has become a very popular nonprescription analgesic and antipyretic, as well as an increasingly common cause of hepatic injury and death when taken in accidental or intentional overdose. A toxic metabolite produces hepatic necrosis when the liver's capacity to conjugate and excrete the metabolite is overwhelmed. Liver injury may be minimized or avoided when overdosage is recognized and treated as described in Chapter 101.

Methyldopa

Methyldopa causes mild, usually transient elevation of transaminase levels in about 5 percent of those treated with this popular antihypertensive. In fewer than 1 percent of those treated, acute hepatitis (occasionally with cholestasis) develops, usually within the first month of therapy. A prodrome of rash, arthralgias, and lymphadenopathy may precede the onset of jaundice. Clinical improvement occurs with discontinuation of the drug, but cases of chronic hepatitis and cirrhosis have been reported. The mechanism of hepatic injury is unclear but may be a combination of immunologic and direct toxic injury.

Chlorpromazine

Chlorpromazine induces intrahepatic cholestasis in 1 to 4 percent of those taking it, usually within 1 to 4 weeks of exposure. A prodrome of anorexia, nausea, vomiting, malaise, and pruritus may precede the onset of jaundice. Clinical recovery occurs within 4 to 6 weeks after withdrawal of the drug, with only a rare fatality reported. Chlorpromazine-induced liver injury is not dose-related and appears to be immunologically mediated.

Treatment

During the evaluation of the patient with acute liver injury, the emergency physician must obtain a detailed history of current and recent medications as well as possible occupational and recreational exposure to drugs and chemicals. Stopping the exposure to the offending agent is vital, other treatment being nonspecific and supportive in most cases. In cases of exposure to toxic chemicals, possible injury to other organs should be suspected as well.

ALCOHOLIC LIVER DISEASE

More than 10 million people in the United States are alcohol abusers, and alcohol-related injuries and illnesses are major causes of death and disability. Alcohol adversely affects all the organ systems of the body, but it is the liver that bears the brunt of its deleterious effects. Three syndromes of alcoholic liver injury—hepatic steatosis (fatty liver), alcoholic hepatitis, and alcoholic cirrhosis—have been described based on clinical and histologic criteria.

Hepatic Steatosis

Most people who regularly consume even moderate amounts of alcohol develop some degree of hepatic steatosis. It is usually a benign, asymptomatic condition in which fat is deposited in the hepatocytes because of alterations in cell oxidation-reduction potentials caused by the oxidation of ethanol to acetaldehyde. This change reduces the rate of oxidation of fatty acids and favors the synthesis of triglycerides. The most common clinical finding is nontender hepatomegaly with laboratory evidence of minimal hepatic injury. Less commonly, patients with fatty liver develop a syndrome of jaundice, malaise, anorexia, and a tender, enlarged liver. Rarely, severe cholestasis or portal hypertension develops. When the patient abstains from alcohol and receives adequate nutrition, steatosis resolves in 4 to 6 weeks without residual scarring or necrosis.

Alcoholic Hepatitis

Alcoholic hepatitis (also known as alcoholic steatonecrosis) is a syndrome characterized histologically by hepatocellular necrosis and intrahepatic inflammation. It develops in only a small percentage of chronic alcohol abusers. The clinical severity ranges from very mild illness to acute liver failure. Typically, the patient reports the gradual onset of anorexia, nausea, abdominal pain, weight loss, and weakness. Fever, dark urine, and jaundice are frequently reported.

On examination, tender hepatomegaly, low-grade fever, and jaundice are commonly noted. Laboratory evaluation usually shows elevation of the levels of serum amino transaminases in the range of 2 to 10 times normal, with an AST (aspartate aminotransferase) to ALT (alanine aminotransferase) ratio greater than 1.5. Alkaline phosphatase and bilirubin levels are usually mildly elevated, although marked elevations may occur and imply more severe disease. Anemia, leukopenia, and thrombocytopenia are common and may be caused by the toxic effects of alcohol on bone marrow or by nutritional deficits. The prothrombin time is frequently prolonged a few seconds, but prolongation greater than 8 s is a poor prognostic sign. The presence of fever and leukocytosis in the alcoholic patient mandates a thorough search for concurrent pneumonia, peritonitis, urinary tract infection, sepsis, and meningitis.

Treatment

In-hospital treatment is mainly supportive with correction of electrolyte abnormalities, good nutrition with correction of specific deficits (e.g., folate, thiamine), rest, and abstinence from alcohol. Treatment is frequently complicated by the development of alcohol withdrawal symptoms. Symptoms of hepatic failure must be closely watched for and aggressively treated. A number of specific therapies have been advocated to speed recovery from alcoholic hepatitis or to halt the progression to cirrhosis, but at this time none is considered established. These include the use of corticosteroids, anabolic androgenic steroids, colchicine, penicillamine, propylthiouracil, and insulin-glucagon combinations.

The histologic, biochemical, and clinical abnormalities of alcoholic hepatitis do not rapidly resolve with abstinence from drinking. Instead, from 15 to 50 percent deteriorate during the first weeks of hospitalization despite abstinence and nutritional support. The overall mortality is 10 to 15 percent, and death results from hepatic failure with encephalopathy, gastrointestinal bleeding, and infections. Survivors face a convalescence lasting weeks to months, with a significant number developing cirrhosis.

Emergency Department Management

Because of the difficulty of ruling out concurrent infection, the tendency toward clinical deterioration, and the significant mortality, all but the mildest cases of alcoholic hepatitis should be hospitalized. A complete blood count, prothrombin time, and levels of transaminases, alkaline phosphatase, bilirubin, albumin, blood urea nitrogen, creatinine, glucose, magnesium, and phosphorus should be obtained as indicated. In the febrile patient, a chest radiograph and cultures of blood, urine, and ascitic fluid are needed. If the patient has an altered mental status, occult head trauma, meningitis, hepatic encephalopathy, and hypoglycemia must be considered and aggressively treated when present.

Alcoholic Cirrhosis

Alcoholic (Laennec's) cirrhosis is the irreversible stage of alcoholic liver disease. The liver is usually a golden yellow and may be shrunken or enlarged. Nodules of regenerating hepatocytes are separated by bands of fibrous tissue which represent scarring from previous necrosis. The normal pattern of hepatic blood circulation is disrupted, with a resultant decrease in the total blood flow through the liver as well as the shunting of blood away from the remaining functioning hepatocytes and into the systemic circulation. This portosystemic shunting and concomitant portal hypertension result in many of the clinical findings of cirrhosis as well as the associated complications.

Cirrhosis develops in only about 10 percent of chronic alcoholics and may remain unrecognized in a significant number. Genetic, nutritional, and other factors probably determine which heavy drinkers will develop cirrhosis.

Clinical Features

A characteristic clinical feature of symptomatic cirrhosis is a general, gradual deterioration in health. Weight loss (sometimes masked by edema and ascites), weakness, peripheral muscle wasting, easy fatigability, and anorexia are the rule. Nausea, vomiting, and diarrhea are commonly reported. Fever, usually low-grade and continuous, is much more common in alcoholic than in other types of cirrhosis and often develops in decompensated disease. Hypothermia may develop in the terminal stages. Jaundice, spider angiomata, palmar erythema, pedal edema, ascites, hepatosplenomegaly, and gynecomastia are common.

Laboratory abnormalities include elevated bilirubin and alkaline phosphatase levels, a prolonged prothrombin time, decreased albumin, anemia (from chronic disease, nutritional factors, or blood loss), leukopenia, and thrombocytopenia. Hyponatremia may be dilutional secondary to increased antidiuretic hormone activity or the result of total body sodium deficit, frequently aggravated by the injudicious use of diuretics. Hypokalemia is almost always present as a result of GI losses, secondary hyperaldosteronism, and diuretic use. Arterial hypoxemia is common in decompensated cirrhosis and may be caused by abnormal alveolar-capillary diffusion or restricted respiratory expansion secondary to massive ascites.

Management

The clinical course of cirrhosis is marked by periods of relative stability interspersed with episodes of decompensation. No therapy has been shown effective in reversing the histologic changes of cirrhosis. The mainstay of outpatient management is total abstinence from alcohol, which has been shown to significantly improve 5-year survival. Other measures include salt and water restriction, the cautious use of diuretics (especially those that spare potassium), and a nutritious diet with protein restriction as needed. Emergency management may involve making alterations in diuretic dosage, correcting symptomatic anemia or fluid and electrolyte abnormalities, and recognizing and initiating treatment of the life-threatening emergencies seen in decompensated cirrhosis.

COMPLICATIONS OF ALCOHOLIC LIVER DISEASE

Bleeding Esophageal Varices

Bleeding esophageal varices are the most dramatic and immediately life-threatening complications of alcoholic liver disease. The mortality rate from variceal hemorrhage is high and rebleeding is common. As many as 30 percent of all cirrhotic patients die from this complication alone. The patient usually arrives in the emergency department in hemorrhagic shock with massive hematemesis complicated by underlying coagulation and electrolyte derangements. A significant number of patients with documented varices who develop hematemesis, however, are bleeding from other lesions, including gastric erosions, gastric or duodenal ulcers, or a diffuse gastritis. Since definitive therapy varies, emergency endoscopy should be done as soon as possible to confirm the diagnosis.

Management

Initial management includes securing a stable airway and restoring intravascular volume. Fresh whole blood or packed red cells augmented by fresh frozen plasma should be rapidly infused through large-bore intravenous lines to maintain adequate tissue perfusion and replace depleted clotting factors. Transfusion of platelet concentrates may be necessary if thrombocytopenia is severe (see Table 49-5). Monitoring of central venous or pulmonary wedge pressure may be needed to aid fluid resuscitation.

Control of bleeding can be attempted using IV vasopressin, endoscopic sclerotherapy, tamponade with a Sengstaken-Blakemore tube, or emergency portal decompression. All these methods have significant morbidity even in experienced hands. More detailed discussion of emergency management of variceal bleeding is described in Chapter 37, "Esophageal Emergencies."

Particular attention must be paid during emergency treatment to the evacuation of blood from the GI tract with gastric lavage, vigorous catharsis, and enemas. Otherwise, some patients in whom bleeding is controlled will die in hepatic coma.

Portosystemic Encephalopathy

Portosystemic encepalopathy (PSE), also referred to as *hepatic encephalopathy* and *hepatic coma*, is a complex neuropsychiatric syndrome of altered consciousness and impaired intellectual functioning seen in cirrhotics with extensive spontaneous or surgical portosystemic shunting. It results from an accumulation in the blood of substances which the damaged liver is unable to detoxify. The severity ranges from subtle changes in personality and performance to coma.

Elevated blood ammonia apparently plays a role in the pathogenesis of PSE, but the precise role has not yet been clearly defined. Elevated levels of some amino acids, short-chain fatty acids, biogenic amines, mercaptans, and false neurotransmitters have also been implicated, and it may be a synergistic effect of combinations of these substances that produces encephalopathy.

The finding of elevated levels of plasma gamma-aminobutyric acid (GABA) in PSE appears to implicate this inhibitory neurotransmitter system. Increased GABA-ergic tone can cause alterations in con-

Table 49-5. Management of Variceal Bleeding

1. Secure the airway
2. Large-bore IV lines
3. Volume replacement with blood and plasma
4. Evacuate blood from GI tract
5. Endoscopic sclerotherapy (if readily available)
6. IV vasopressin
7. Esophageal tamponade
8. Portal decompression

sciousness and motor control similar to that seen in PSE. These changes are mediated through the GABA-benzodiazepine (GABA–BZ) complex on postsynaptic neurons by an endogenous diazepamlike substance.

This finding led to the experimental use of the BZ receptor blocker flumazenil in PSE. Single doses of flumazenil have produced temporary improvement in consciousness in patients with PSE, but its future role in treating PSE is far from established.

PSE can be precipitated or exacerbated in susceptible patients by a variety of factors. Azotemia, either renal or prerenal, provides more urea to urease-producing intestinal bacteria, thereby increasing ammonia production in the gut. Gastrointestinal bleeding and high-protein diets provide large amounts of nitrogenous substrates. The careless use of analgesics, sedatives, and tranquilizers is an occasional cause of PSE in hospitalized patients. Diuretic-induced hypokalemic metabolic alkalosis results in a pH gradient favoring the passage of ammonia into cells. Other metabolic derangements, such as hypoglycemia, anemia, with hypoxia, as well as infection and hypotension, may also contribute.

Clinical Features

The patient with PSE has the stigmata of chronic liver disease including edema, ascites, spider angiomata, and hepatosplenomegaly. Fetor hepaticus, a musty odor on the breath attributed to elevated blood mercaptan levels, is often noted. Asterixis (''liver flap'') is characteristic of, but not specific for, PSE. It is demonstrated most readily in the dorsiflexed wrist, but may be noted in other muscles as well. Neurologic examination may reveal a level of consciousness ranging from lethargy to coma with variable appearance of hyperreflexia, generalized seizures, and spasticity. Occult head injury should be suspected if focal or lateralizing signs are present.

Laboratory studies reflect the underlying liver failure with jaundice, coagulopathy, and decreased albumin levels. The acid-base status and serum electrolytes must be closely monitored. Arterial ammonia levels correlate more closely with the severity of PSE than venous levels, but there is a 24- to 72-h lag between the rise in ammonia levels and the onset of symptoms. Serial changes in ammonia levels rather than absolute levels are more useful in monitoring the course of PSE and evaluating the effectiveness of treatment.

Treatment

The initial treatment in the comatose patient is to maintain oxygenation and perfusion. Precipitating factors such as GI bleeding should be treated aggressively. Efforts to cleanse the gut of bacterial flora and nitrogenous substances include cathartics, enemas, and the use of poorly absorbed broad-spectrum antibiotics such as neomycin. Lactulose is a nondigestible disaccharide which produces an acidic diarrhea that may trap nitrogenous substances in the colon and eliminate them in the stool. Lactulose may be given orally, through a nasogastric tube, or by enema.

Many other therapies have been suggested, but clinical studies have been inconclusive. With meticulous supportive care and the aggressive treatment of complications, PSE is potentially reversible, although the mortality remains very high.

Hepatorenal Syndrome

Hepatorenal syndrome is a syndrome of acquired renal failure without other obvious cause in patients with decompensated cirrhosis. It almost always occurs in the presence of ascites, jaundice, and portal hypertension in the hospitalized patient. This implies that iatrogenic factors may play a significant role in the pathogenesis. The mortality of HRS approaches 100 percent.

HRS probably represents a functional disturbance in the control of renal vascular tone with a decreased glomerular filtration rate due to intense vasoconstriction and shunting of blood away from the renal cortex. This results in the production of small volumes of concentrated urine with very low sodium content, and a progressive azotemia unresponsive to attempts to expand intravascular volume. No significant histologic changes are evident in the kidneys of patients dying with HRS. In fact, kidneys from HRS donors function normally if transplanted into recipients with normal hepatic function.

Spontaneous Bacterial Peritonitis

Spontaneous bacterial peritonitis (SBP) is now recognized as a common complication of severe liver disease complicated by ascites. Using diagnostic paracentesis, up to one-third of admitted patients with ascites have been demonstrated to have the disease. The pathogenesis of SBP is felt to be the result of spontaneous bacteremia with seeding of ascitic fluid. Defects in patient defenses which allow seeding include complement deficiency, abnormal neutrophil function, and deficient reticuloendothelial system function. A precondition for SBP is low ascitic fluid protein concentration, which correlates directly with low opsonic activity. Ascitic fluid with a high protein content, such as in peritoneal carcinomatosis or heart failure, is relatively resistant to SBP.

SBP should be suspected in all patients with increasing ascites, worsening hepatic function, fever, or abdominal tenderness. The major consideration in differential diagnosis is secondary peritonitis resulting from viscus perforation or an intraabdominal or hepatic abscess. The diagnosis of SBP is established by evaluation of ascitic fluid obtained by paracentesis, and the procedure should be accomplished as part of the emergency department evaluation. Although absolute guidelines have not been determined, a neutrophil count greater than $250/mm^3$ is used to clinically establish the diagnosis. At least 10 mL of ascitic fluid should be cultured, using blood culture bottles. The demonstration of ascitic fluid leukocytosis is an indication for intravenous antibiotic administration, usually with a third-generation cephalosporin. Additional treatment includes the use of diuretics, which increase ascitic fluid protein and opsonic activity. Underlying hepatic disease and associated complications should also be treated. Even with early detection and appropriate treatment of SBP, mortality is high, varying from 30 to 100 percent. Reoccurrence of SBP is common and carries an even higher morality than the first episode.

BIBLIOGRAPHY

Bansky G, Meier PJ, Riederer E, et al: Effects of the benzodiazepine receptor antagonist flumazenil in hepatic encephalopathy in humans. *Gastroenterology* 97:744, 1989.

Burnett DA, Rikkers LF: Nonoperative emergency treatment of variceal hemorrhage. *Surg Clin North Am* 70:291, 1990.

Cuthbert JA: Southwestern Internal Medicine Conference: Hepatitis C. *Am J Med Sci* 299:346, 1990.

Epstein M: The hepatorenal syndrome. *Hosp Prac* 24:65, 1989.

Frank BB: Clinical evaluation of jaundice: A guideline of the patient care committee of the American Gastroenterological Association. *JAMA* 262:3031, 1989.

Hoofnagle JH: Type D (delta) hepatitis. *JAMA* 261:1321, 1989.

Jones EA, Skolnick P, Gammal SH, et al: NIH Conference: The gamma-aminobutyric acid A (GABA A) receptor complex and hepatic encephalopathy: Some recent advances. *Ann Intern Med* 110:532, 1989.

Lewis JH, Zimmerman HJ: Drug-induced liver disease. *Med Clin North Am* 73:775, 1989.

Lieber CS, Guadagnini KS: The spectrum of alcoholic liver disease. *Hosp Prac* 25(2A):51, 1990.

Runyon, BA: Spontaneous bacterial peritonitis: An explosion of information. *Hepatology* 8:171, 1988.

Terblanche J, Burroughs AK, Hobbs, KEF: Controversies in the management of bleeding esophageal varices. *N Engl J Med* 320:1393, 1989.

Tito L, Rimola A, Gines P, et al: Recurrence of spontaneous bacterial peritonitis in cirrhosis: Frequency and predictive factors. *Hepatology* 8:27, 1988.

50
ACUTE PANCREATITIS

Donald Weaver

The diagnosis of acute pancreatitis rests primarily on clinical grounds. The severity of the disease may range from mild pancreatic edema to frank necrosis and hemorrhage. No clinical findings are pathognomonic, and the symptoms depend largely on the amount of glandular destruction. In the mildest form, patients present with epigastric pain, abdominal distension, nausea, vomiting, and hyperamylasemia. Refractory hypotensive shock, blood loss, and respiratory failure may accompany the most severe forms. In 1977 Ransom and Posterbach proposed a schema to grade the severity of acute pancreatitis (Table 50-1). They found that the rate of serious morbidity and mortality was 14 percent in patients with fewer than three positive findings, and 95 percent in patients with three or more positive findings.

Etiology

Acute pancreatitis is most often due to alcohol abuse or gallstones (Table 50-2). The incidence with which each is associated with pancreatitis depends largely on the age of the population and the reporting institution. Patients over the age of 50 who present in a community hospital setting most often have "biliary pancreatitis," while younger patients presenting to large inner-city emergency departments almost always have alcoholic pancreatitis.

Pathophysiology

A complete understanding of the pathophysiology of acute pancreatitis is lacking. The common-channel concept of Opie dominated the literature for years, but anatomic studies of cadavers have shown that only a fraction of patients with pancreatitis have a true common channel. Moreover, in fatal cases, careful dissection at postmortem examinations rarely discloses an impacted stone in the ampulla of Vater. In animal experiments, neither the anastomosis of bile ducts to the pancreatic duct nor the injection of bile into the pancreatic duct without pressure produces pancreatitis. Only when trypsin or bacteria are added to bile and the mixture is injected under pressure can consistent experimental pancreatitis be produced.

A vascular insult is important either as a cause or perpetuator of acute pancreatitis. The hyperlipemic serum sometimes seen in patients following a drinking binge may be responsible for peripancreatic vascular sludging and relative pancreatic ischemia. Small-microsphere injections (8 to 20 U) result in profound pancreatitis because of plugging of the terminal arterioles. The acinar and ductal injury which then results leads to extravasation of proteolytic enzymes, and this may be responsible for the progression of the inflammatory state. Alcohol increases pancreatic ductal permeability, and this may result in a similar escape of proteolytic enzymes.

Table 50-1. Criteria for Projecting the Outcome from Acute Pancreatitis

On Admission	48 H Later
Age over 55	Change in HCT (falling) decreased more than 10 percent
Blood sugar > 200 mg/dL	Rise in BUN over 5 mg/dL
WCB > 16,000/mm^3	↓ CA^{2+} below 8 mg/dL
SGOT > 250 Sigma-Fankel units/L	↓ Arterial P_{o2} below 60 mmHg
	Rapid fluid sequestration over 6 L
LDH > 700 IU/L	Base deficit over 4 mEq/L

Alcoholic pancreatitis may result from duodenal inflammation that produces some degree of pancreatic duct obstruction, with increased ductal pressure. The latter may occur secondary to sphincter of Oddi spasm or pancreatic hypersecretion.

Hyperparathyroidism has been associated with an increased incidence of pancreatitis, but the mechanism by which this occurs is unknown.

Patients with primary hyperlipemias (Frederickson types I, IV, and V) are susceptible to acute pancreatitis, but patients with pancreatitis may develop transient secondary hyperlipemia because of the release of an inhibitor of lipoprotein lipase during the attack of pancreatitis.

Various drugs, such as methyl alcohol, thiazide diuretics, and phenformin, can produce pancreatitis (Table 50-3). Inflammation and infection, such as mumps or hepatitis, can also result in pancreatitis. Penetrating posterior duodenal and gastric ulcers may involve the head of the pancreas, producing a local pancreatitis. Once the pancreas becomes edematous and swollen, especially if there is significant involvement of the head, partial obstruction of the common bile duct or even gastric outlet may occur. For these reasons elevation of the bilirubin level, and even clinical jaundice, may occur. Pancreatitis may also produce adynamic ileus secondary to the peritoneal irritation.

DIAGNOSIS

Laboratory

Since no clinical features are pathognomonic for acute pancreatitis, the diagnosis must often rest on the presence of abnormal results from laboratory tests, most often the serum amylase level in combination with the clinical findings. Amylase is a product of two genes located on chromosome 1, known as AMY_1 and AMY_2. Each organ that makes

Table 50-2. Etiologic or Contributing Factors in Acute Pancreatitis

Ethanol ingestion
Biliary tract disease
Trauma, penetrating or blunt
Penetrating peptic ulcer
Postoperative
Obstruction secondary to neoplasms, diverticula, roundworms, benign polyps
Perisphincteric fibrosis
Metabolic disturbances
- Hyperlipemia (Frederickson types I, IV, and V)
- Hypercalcemia
- Diabetes mellitus, diabetic ketoacidosis
- Uremia
- Hemochromatosis
- Hereditary pancreatitis

Viral infections
- Mumps
- Viral hepatitis
- Infectious mononucleosis
- Coxsackie group B
- Pregnancy—any trimester, postpartum

Collagen vascular disease
- Systemic lupus erythematosus
- Polyarteritis nodosa

Liver disease
Generalized infections
- Typhoid fever
- *Salmonella typhimurium* infection
- Scarlet fever
- Streptococcal food poisoning
- Dysentery
- Scorpion sting
- Other causes

Source: Adapted from Kowlessar OD: Pathogenesis of pancreatitis, in Clearfield HR, Dinoso VP (eds): *Gastrointestinal Emergencies*. New York, Grune & Stratton, 1976, p 226.

Table 50-3. Drugs Reported to be Associated with the Occurrence of Acute Pancreatitis

Oral contraceptives	Donidine
Estrogens	Salicylates
Phenformin	Indomethacin
Azathioprine	Dextropropoxyphene
Corticosteroids	Calcium
Rifampin	Warfarin
Tetracyclines	L-Asparaginase
Isoniazid	Acetaminophen
Thiazides	Ethacrynic acid
Furosemide	

amylase expresses either one or the other, and no organ has been found that expresses both genes. The only known site to express the AMY_2 gene is the pancreas. All other organs, such as the fallopian tubes, ovaries, lungs, salivary glands, lacrimal glands, and endocrine glands, express the AMY_1 locus. Pancreatic (AMY_2) amylase can be separated from nonpancreatic (AMY_1) amylase by a variety of electrophoretic techniques. Normally there is a nearly even distribution in the serum between AMY_1 and AMY_2 amylase. Many other isoamylases can occur but result from posttranslational modifications of the major isoenzymes.

During the last decade, recognition of the multiple organ sources of amylase has resulted in less reliance on the simple measurement of the serum amylase level as an indicator of pancreatic disease. In one study, 32 percent of the patients admitted with the clinical diagnosis of acute pancreatitis made on the basis of upper abdominal pain, nausea, vomiting, and an elevated amylase level were found to have nonpancreatic hyperamylasemia. This suggests that the clinical criteria used to make the diagnosis of acute pancreatitis may be too variable.

Since the electrophoresis of serum to differentiate isoamylases is time-consuming (approximately 2.5 h), other laboratory tests have been proposed to improve the accuracy of pancreatitis diagnosis. Observations that the amylase-creatinine clearance ratio is high in patients with acute pancreatitis suggests this might be a valuable diagnostic test. The ratio is determined using the following formula:

$$\frac{\text{Amylase clearance}}{\text{Creatinine clearance}}\ \% = \frac{\text{urine amy.}}{\text{serum amy.}} \times \frac{\text{serum creat.}}{\text{urine creat.}} \times 100$$

The normal clearance ratio is about 3 percent, and levels of 5 percent or greater are consistent with the diagnosis of acute pancreatitis. The mechanism for the increased renal clearance of amylase may be a tubular defect in the reabsorption of amylase. Unfortunately, elevated ratios have been found with other diseases, and not every patient with acute pancreatitis has an elevated ratio.

The level of lipase, another enzyme liberated by pancreatic disease, is nearly always elevated in acute pancreatitis. Although the lipase level is a more sensitive sign of acute pancreatitis than the serum amylase level, it too lacks specificity and immediate availability. Reports that the lipase level rises later and remains elevated longer than the serum amylase level have not been confirmed, but the course of the lipase level elevation more closely follows the clinical course than does the serum amylase level.

When pancreatic hemorrhage occurs, hemoglobin may be split by the action of pancreatic enzymes, and methemalbumin is formed. The presence of this pigment in patients with acute pancreatitis indicates hemorrhagic pancreatitis. Unfortunately, the finding of methemalbumin in the serum is not pathognomonic, since it may be elevated in any condition in which there is intraabdominal or retroperitoneal bleeding.

The finding of a wheat germ protein that inhibits the activity of salivary amylase nearly 100 times more than the activity of pancreatic amylase has led to a rapid test for approximating the levels of the serum isoamylases. Analysis of serum amylase levels before and after reaction with the inhibitor allows an estimation of what portion of the amylase comes from pancreatic sources. This test holds promise as a simple way to improve the accuracy of serum amylase interpretations. Patients with severe edema of the pancreatic head from pancreatitis may have elevation of the bilirubin and alkaline phosphatase levels.

As with most inflammatory conditions, leukocytosis is usually present but rarely exceeds 20,000/mL in uncomplicated pancreatitis.

Low calcium levels may be detected on laboratory analysis. Persistent hypocalcemia, less than 7 mg/100 mL, is associated with a poor prognosis. Hypocalcemia may result when calcium reacts with free fatty acids and precipitates as calcium soap, but a complete explanation for this phenomenon is lacking.

Radiography

Plain radiographs of the abdomen have little role in the diagnosis of acute pancreatitis, although calcification, when present, suggests preexisting pancreatic disease. More often their importance is to exclude other diseases which may be confused with pancreatitis. Patients with acute pancreatitis who show evidence of ileus, and air trapped in the small bowel near the inflamed pancreas, have been described as having a sentinel loop. Gaseous distension of the colon with a distally collapsed colon suggests colonic ileus (colon-cutoff sign). None of these signs is truly diagnostic. Contrast studies of the upper GI tract occasionally show narrowing or edema of the duodenum, but the routine use of this procedure or barium enema examination to confirm the diagnosis is not helpful.

Evidence of pancreatic edema or lesser sac fluid on ultrasound or CT may be indicative of acute pancreatic inflammation. Reports indicate that CT scanning may not only aid in the diagnosis of acute pancreatitis but also provide important prognostic information. The routine use of this test, however, seems unnecessary. It should be employed only for the most severe cases or when late complications are suspected.

The injection of contrast material under pressure into the duct of an inflamed pancreas is unwise. Although cases of severe pancreatitis following endoscopic retrograde cholangiopancreatography (ERCP) have been reported, these are rare, most likely because of prudence on the part of endoscopists. Nearly all patients undergoing ERCP have a mild elevation of pancreatic amylase levels following the procedure.

TREATMENT

The mainstay of treatment for acute pancreatitis is fluid resuscitation. Recognition that profound shock may result from high-volume fluid sequestration in the retroperitoneum has lowered morbidity as resuscitation efforts have improved. Although some controversy exists about the optimum regimen of fluid replacement, most agree that the use of a balanced electrolyte solution is essential. The observation that albumin reduces the amount of pancreatic edema in a whole perfused pancreatitis model has suggested to some that colloid solution may be of benefit. Although an uncontrolled clinical trial of fresh frozen plasma given in large amounts to patients with acute pancreatitis seemed beneficial, most believe that these measures add little if anything to standard fluid regimens except cost. Fluids should be given in volumes adequate to ensure renal perfusion. When the pancreatitis is severe, admission to an intensive care unit with maximum hemodynamic monitoring is needed. A falling hematocrit should suggest hemorrhagic pancreatitis, and in this case blood replacement is mandatory.

Although the use of the nasogastric tube is widely accepted, no controlled clinical trial has shown its value in altering the course of the disease. The theoretical advantage of reducing pancreatic stimulation and its established value in preventing vomiting, however, make the nasogastric tube a standard part of therapy. Since acute pancreatitis is a self-limiting disease under most circumstances, attention to fluid needs, treatment of pain, and the prevention of vomiting are often sufficient treatment. A small number of patients may develop a severe systemic illness, complicated by acidosis, renal failure, severe hypocalcemia, and respiratory failure.

Acute pancreatitis is not a bacterial disease in its early stages, and the initial use of antibiotics is unwarranted. Sepsis, when it occurs results from secondary infections and is usually encountered late in the course of the disease. The exception to this is when pancreatitis is complicated by biliary tract infection in the presence of choledocholithiasis. In this case, ampicillin and third-generation cephalosporins are indicated.

The use of a variety of medications, such as anticholinergic drugs, apoprotein, and cimetidine, has been proposed to hasten the usual recovery from pancreatitis; however, none has been shown in controlled clinical trials to alter the course of the disease.

Peritoneal lavage should be considered for patients who fail to respond to initial supportive measures. The rationale for this approach is that the dilution or removal of "toxic" shock factors released by pancreatic necrosis may be beneficial to the patient. Although the precise mechanism by which peritoneal lavage benefits patients with acute pancreatitis is speculative, more than anecdotal observations by a number of clinicians have validated its usefulness in severe cases.

The role of surgery in the treatment of acute pancreatitis is limited. Patients whose clinical course deteriorates despite maximum supportive efforts should undergo laparotomy to ensure that another more treatable condition has not been missed and to debride and drain devitalized pancreatic tissue. Patients with gallstone pancreatitis and choledocholithiasis may benefit from early biliary tract decompression.

Acute pancreatitis can be considered to be a disease of limited duration. Failure to show significant improvement by the end of a week should lead the physician to suspect a complication such as pancreatic abscess, pseudocyst, or pancreatic ascites.

Pancreatic abscess or pseudocyst should be considered in any patient with an abdominal mass, an elevated serum amylase level, an elevated serum bilirubin level, and leukocytosis.

Pseudocysts may rupture spontaneously while the patient is under observation in the emergency department with catastrophic results. Erosion into the upper gastrointestinal tract or an adjacent vessel with massive bleeding has occurred.

Pancreatitis may be a difficult diagnosis to establish. It presents as an acute surgical abdomen, and repeated observation and surgical consultation are often necessary to determine the indicated treatment.

BIBLIOGRAPHY

DeBernardinis M, Violi V, Roncoroni L, et al: Automated selection of high-risk patients with acute pancreatitis. *Crit Care Med* 17:318, 1989.

Block P, Kelly TR: Management of gallstone pancreatitis during pregnancy and the postpartum period. *Surg Gynecol Obstet* 168:426, 1989.

Nordestgaard AG, Wilson SE, Williams RA: Early computerized tomography as a prediction of outcome in acute pancreatitis. *Am J Surg* 152:127, 1986.

Weaver DW, Bouwman DL, Walt AJ, et al: A correlation between clinical pancreatitis and isoenzyme patterns of amylase. *Surgery* 92:576, 1982.

Wilson C, Imrie CW, Carter, DC: Fatal acute pancreatitis. *Gut* 29:782, 1988.

51
COMPLICATIONS OF GENERAL SURGICAL PROCEDURES

Geoffrey B. Blossom
John L. Glover

The role of outpatient surgery, and the early discharge of hospitalized postoperative patients, has led to an increase in the numbers of these patients presenting to emergency centers with surgical complications. Currently, 30 percent of all surgical procedures are performed on an outpatient basis and that number is expected to rise to 60 percent in the next decade. Eleven of the 24 most common general surgical procedures now are performed routinely on an outpatient basis including inguinal herniorrhaphy, breast biopsy, wound debridements, hemorrhoidectomy, anal fissures and fistulas, and gastrostomy. In addition, recent advances in laparoscopic surgery are likely to make cholecystectomy an outpatient or same-day surgical procedure. Many patients undergoing more complex surgical procedures are being discharged early from the hospital to be followed by home health care workers or extended-care facilities. All these patients may present to emergency centers with a variety of postoperative complications.

GENERAL CONSIDERATIONS

Wound Complications

The majority of wound complications are the result of infection; however, hematoma, seroma, and wound dehiscence also are seen occasionally.

The incidence of wound infection varies with the type of procedure performed. Atraumatic wounds not involving the respiratory, gastrointestinal, or genitourinary tracts are associated with a 3 percent incidence of infection, while old traumatic wounds or those involving perforation of a viscus may be associated with a 30 percent incidence of infection. Additionally, elderly, diabetic, obese, or immunocompromised patients are at a higher risk.

Most wound infections are manifest between the 5th and 9th postoperative days, but symptoms may be delayed if patients have been receiving antibiotic therapy. Excessive tenderness at the incision site is the most common presenting complaint. Patients may describe an intermittent low-grade fever and malaise. The wound appears edematous and erythematous and may be fluctuant on palpation. Seropurulent discharge may be noted from a portion of the wound. If the diagnosis is not obvious, a 16- or 18-gauge needle may be introduced into the incision site and the wound aspirated for pus. Definitive treatment of infected wounds requires drainage by removing skin sutures or staples, thorough irrigation with saline, and loosely packing the wound with gauze. Cultures should be taken at the time of drainage. In general, wound infections do not require treatment with antibiotics. Exceptions include wounds infected by hemolytic streptococci, wounds of the central face where intracranial extension is possible, and those associated with spreading cellulitis.

A wound hematoma results from inadequate hemostasis at the time of the procedure. The incidence is higher in patients with coagulation defects or in those receiving anticoagulant therapy. Wounds appear edematous and discolored, and drainage of serosanguineous fluid may be appreciated. A wound hematoma should be drained because blood affords an excellent culture medium and delays healing. After drainage, the wound should be left open if infection is suspected or may be loosely reapproximated if clean.

Wound seromas commonly are encountered after procedures in which lymphatics have been disrupted. Large skin flaps such as those used in mastectomy and procedures that involve the axilla or groin are usual sites of seroma formation. Typically, a seroma will present as a fluctuant, nontender, fluid collection in proximity to a surgical wound. Initial treatment involves sterile needle aspiration of the fluid to appose tissue planes and facilitate healing.

Wound dehiscence is separation of the fascial layer of an abdominal wound. If the overlying skin remains intact, an abdominal-wall hernia results. If the entire wound separates, intraperitoneal contents may be exposed and result in evisceration. The overall incidence of this after abdominal surgery is 2 to 3 percent with advancing age, poor nutritional status, obesity, and carcinoma all increasing the incidence. Wound dehiscence may not be readily apparent but is seen most commonly on the 5th postoperative day. Drainage of serosanguineous fluid from the wound more than 24 h postoperatively is pathognomonic. If the skin remains intact, it may be possible to palpate fascial edges and the resulting ventral hernia. Treatment normally involves secondary operative closure if the dehiscence occurs in the immediate postoperative period. If the skin is intact, however, an abdominal binder may be placed, and the wound repaired on an elective basis. If evisceration should occur, the bowel or omentum should be covered with sterile saline-moistened towels, and the patient transported to the operating room.

Respiratory Complications

Atelectasis accounts for 90 percent of all postoperative respiratory complications and is commonly seen after upper abdominal and thoracic surgery. It results from bronchial obstruction with distal gas absorption and ineffective respiration. Clinical findings include basilar rales, diminished breath sounds, mild tachycardia, and fever. It generally occurs within 24 h postoperatively and rarely after 48 h. Chest radiographs usually demonstrate small areas of consolidation and arterial blood gases may reveal a decreased P_{O_2} and normal P_{CO_2}. Treatment involves nasotracheal aspiration and encouraging patients to cough and deep breathe.

Persistent atelectasis may result in pneumonia. Collapsed, poorly drained areas of the lung are especially vulnerable to infection from aspirated material or nosocomial infection. This generally occurs 3 to 4 days postoperatively and is manifest by fever, tachycardia, and dyspnea.

Pneumothorax is a rare complication after general surgical procedures, but it has been noted following excision of chest wall lesions, breast biopsy, mastectomy, and insertion of long-term intravenous-access catheters. Patients present with shortness of breath, dyspnea, and occasionally, with pleuritic chest and shoulder pain. Chest radiography should be obtained and will reveal the extent of the pneumothorax.

A pneumothorax of 25 percent or less in an otherwise healthy individual may be treated conservatively by observation for 24 h as long as serial chest radiographs and clinical evaluations are done to identify an increasing pneumothorax. Some advocate aspiration of small pneumothoraces using a 16- or 18-gauge angiocatheter connected to a three-way stopcock and underwater-seal vacuum. Larger pneumothoraces require hospitalization, tube thoracostomy, and underwater-seal vacuum. Healthy young patients may be managed on an outpatient basis if flutter valves are used instead of standard tube thoracostomy drainage.

Vascular Complications

Superficial thrombophlebitis is a relatively common complication after catheterization of upper extremity peripheral veins. In the lower extremity, phlebitis is most commonly associated with varicose veins. Pain, induration, erythema, and tenderness are noted along the course of the involved vein, and a palpable cord is sometimes appreciated. Swelling of the extremity should not be observed, and its presence suggests deep venous thrombosis. Treatment is the application of local moist heat and analgesics. Bed rest and anticoagulation are not indicated in superficial phlebitis because the chance of pulmonary embolism is remote. Suppurative thrombophlebitis (high fever, chills, and presence of pus) should be treated with antibiotics and excision of the involved vein.

Deep venous thrombosis has been seen after a variety of general surgical procedures, but it is most common after abdominal or pelvic surgery. Venous stasis, endothelial damage, and hypercoagulability, the three risk factors associated with this entity, are common in postoperative patients. Most lower-extremity deep venous thrombosis begins as small clots in the valveless venous sinuses in the soleus muscle, and patients are asymptomatic until the clot propagates and causes significant obstruction. Consequently, patients may be discharged before symptoms are evident clinically. Patients often present to the emergency center with a swollen extremity and frequently describe a stiff leg and aching in the calf region, with discomfort aggravated by muscular activity. Swelling varies with a variety of factors, including the level of obstruction and whether or not there is complete occlusion of major veins. Infrapopliteal thrombosis produces edema in the ankle and calf tenderness, while iliofemoral involvement causes a diffusely swollen lower extremity.

The following risk factors make the physician more suspicious of venous thrombosis: age older than 45, upper abdominal surgery, diagnosis of malignancy, obesity, previous venous disease, cardiac disease, and prolonged immobility. Evidence of previous venous disease includes varicose veins, hyperpigmentation of the skin at the ankles, and a history of fractured hip or femur and joint replacement. The most common cause of postoperative ankle swelling, however, is simple edema related to the bed rest and inactivity associated with major surgery. Consequently, a simple and repeatable test is needed to differentiate deep venous thrombosis, superficial phlebitis, and simple edema.

In the past, venography was considered the most definitive diagnostic test. It has a 90 percent sensitivity and still is used. It has the disadvantages of being invasive and painful, is associated with reactions to dye, and rarely, can induce venous thrombosis.

Doppler ultrasonography may be utilized at inguinal and popliteal sites, and a lack of flow augmentation with inspiration or compression suggests venous obstruction. Correct interpretations depend, however, on the experience of the examiner, and it will not detect nonocclusive thrombi. Plethysmography also is used as a screening test for occlusive thrombi. Radiolabeled fibrinogen scans primarily are used for research, since results depend on changes over several days. Duplex ultrasonography is rapidly becoming the method of choice for diagnosis because it is noninvasive, can be repeated at will, and has excellent overall accuracy.

Goals of treatment include minimizing the risk of pulmonary embolus, preventing further propagation of thrombi, and potentiating the resolution of the existing thrombus. Anticoagulation should be initiated with heparin, 100 to 150 units/kg by intravenous bolus, followed by 10 to 15 units/kg per hour by continuous infusion. Effectiveness of therapy should be monitored by the activated clotting time or partial thromboplastin time. Patients should be placed at absolute bed rest, with the foot of the bed elevated 10 to 15 in. Warfarin therapy is initiated also and may be used as the sole agent after about 5 days.

Pulmonary embolism accounts for significant postoperative morbidity and mortality and is the most serious complication of deep venous thrombosis. It has been estimated to account for 90,000 deaths per year in the United States and is responsible for 5 percent of postoperative deaths. Clinical manifestations depend on the size of the embolus and the cardiopulmonary status of the patient. Dyspnea, anxiety, pleuritic chest pain, cough, and hemoptysis are the most frequently described symptoms. Tachypnea and tachycardia usually are seen, with an accentuated second heart sound, cyanosis, prominent neck veins, and wheezing occasionally noted. Clinical evidence of deep vein thrombosis is present in one-third of cases. Differential diagnosis should include myocardial infarction, pneumonia, esophageal perforation, dissecting thoracic aneurysm, or pneumothorax. ECG, arterial blood gases, and chest radiograph should be obtained quickly. Ventilation-perfusion lung scan may be utilized to exclude or suggest the diagnosis, but pulmonary angiography is the most definitively diagnostic procedure. Anticoagulation is initiated with heparin, and more recently thrombolytic therapy has been advocated. Patients refractory to medical management may require pulmonary embolectomy.

Genitourinary Complications

Urinary retention is a common postoperative complication after a variety of surgical procedures. Inguinal hernia repair, gynecologic surgery, anorectal surgery, and spinal anesthesia are common offenders. An elderly man with a benign prostatic hypertrophy may first manifest symptoms following surgical procedures. The bladder should be drained promptly by Foley catheterization with continued drainage dependent on the etiology of the retention. Generally, with urine volumes less than 500 mL in an otherwise healthy patient, a single decompression will suffice. In the presence of chronic retention (volume greater than 500 mL) and concurrent disease, persistent drainage should be instituted.

Urinary tract infections are the most frequent nosocomial infection in postoperative surgical patients. Existing urinary tract contamination and urinary retention in combination with instrumentation of the bladder are etiologic factors. Symptoms may include dysuria, elevated leukocyte count, and fever. Progression to pyelonephritis with high fever and flank pain occasionally may be seen. Treatment involves Foley catheter drainage, hydration, and appropriate antibiotics.

Postoperative Fever

The etiology of postoperative fever generally can be determined by the chronologic nature of the fever. Onset of fever within 24 h of a procedure is most commonly the result of atelectasis and should not be of undue concern as long as prompt treatment is instituted. Fever as a result of infection from environmental sources normally will manifest on days 2 to 5 postoperatively. This includes, most commonly, Foley catheterization or intravenous access cannulas. Fever on days 5 to 9 is likely to be associated with wound infections and should be investigated accordingly. Intraabdominal abscesses are associated with intermittent spiking fevers. Deep venous thrombosis also must be considered in patients who present with fever later in the postoperative course.

COMPLICATIONS OF GASTROINTESTINAL SURGERY

General Considerations

Intestinal Obstruction

Functional bowel obstruction due to adynamic ileus is common immediately after abdominal surgical procedures. It results from the excitation of sympathetic splanchnic nerves during manipulation of abdominal viscera. The small bowel normally recovers function within 24 h postoperatively, the stomach within 48 h postoperatively, and the colon in 3 to 5 days. Prolonged ileus is likely the result of continued splanchnic stimulation from peritonitis, hemoperitoneum, retroperitoneal hematoma, basal pneumonia, or electrolyte imbalance. Manifestations include abdominal distension, anorexia, hypoactive bowel sounds, and failure to pass flatus or stool. Evaluation should include appropriate laboratory and radiologic studies. A flat-plate and upright abdominal x-ray will reveal diffuse gas throughout the large and small bowel and in some cases air-fluid levels. Treatment involves correction of the underlying pathologic condition, placement of a nasogastric tube to prevent further distension, and correction of electrolyte abnormalities. Discontinuing or decreasing narcotic-containing pain medication also may be helpful.

At times, it is very difficult to distinguish postoperative ileus from mechanical bowel obstruction, which involves a physical barrier to passage of intestinal contents, especially between postoperative days 7 and 14. In that period, bowel distension may be due to prolongation of adynamic ileus, to ileus secondary to intraabdominal infection, or to early mechanical intestinal obstruction. The most common cause of postoperative mechanical obstruction is fibrinous adhesions, although internal hernias occasionally are seen. Initial symptoms include crampy abdominal pin, nausea and vomiting, failure to pass stool, and abdominal distension. Flat-plate and upright abdominal x-rays are the most important diagnostic modalities. In the presence of mechanical obstruction, they will reveal multiple air-fluid levels, with a stair-step appearance, and a paucity of gas in the distal bowel. As opposed to other forms of mechanical intestinal obstruction, early postoperative bowel obstruction initially should be treated conservatively. Aggressive fluid and electrolyte replacement should be instituted and a nasogastric tube placed. Some advocate a decompressive "long tube" in the early postoperative period. Serial abdominal x-rays then should be obtained, and if symptoms of obstruction persist, a contrast radiologic study should be obtained. Reoperation may then be necessary.

Intraabdominal Abscess

An intraabdominal abscess in the postoperative period may be due to a variety of processes. Spillage of enteric contents during the operative procedure, contamination of a hematoma, or anastomotic leaks are all likely etiologies. Also, overwhelming preoperative contamination from peritonitis may be a factor. Abscesses commonly are located in the dependent portions of the abdomen, such as the subdiaphragmatic spaces, paracolic gutters, or pelvis. They also may occur between loops of bowel. Clinical manifestations include intermittent fever, and occasionally, chills, anorexia, abdominal distension, paralytic ileus, and abdominal tenderness. Diagnosis is established by CT scan or ultrasonography, and treatment includes antibiotics and drainage either by radiologically guided catheter placement or through surgical intervention.

Fistulas

Postoperative enterocutaneous fistulas are connections between the bowel or an abscess cavity and the skin. They may complicate gastric, small intestinal, or colonic operations and result from inadvertent enterotomy during the surgical procedure or from anastomotic leaks. Fistulas are defined by the amount of fluid discharged (high or low output) and their location. In general, the more proximal the fistula, the more serious the problem. Proximal fistulas involve large-volume fluid and electrolyte losses and may result in severe malnutrition. Since fistulas commonly track to the incision, diagnosis usually is made when an infected-appearing wound is opened and the initial bloody or purulent discharge is followed shortly by obvious bowel contents. If in doubt, the diagnosis is established by administering charcoal by mouth and noting its appearance at the fistula site. Treatment involves control of sepsis, protection of surrounding skin, preventing fluid and electrolyte imbalance, and provision of adequate nutrition. Many fistulae close spontaneously with conservative management. Those involving cancer, inflammatory bowel disease, distal obstruction, foreign body, or output greater than 500 mL/day are unlikely to close and eventually should be treated surgically.

Complications of Stomas

Ileostomies may be done as part of operations on the large and small bowel for inflammatory disease, ischemia, or neoplasia, and they may be loop or end in stomas. The normal high-volume liquid content from an ileostomy will quickly excoriate the peristomal skin unless it is protected by careful fitting of the stomal appliance. Complications involving either retraction or recurrent stomal prolapse require surgical revision. Because of the inability of the small bowel to absorb large volumes of fluid, simple insults such as infectious diarrhea or viral gastroenteritis may cause devastating dehydration in the patient with an ileostomy.

Colostomies also are constructed in either a loop or end fashion following a variety of surgical procedures. Loop-type colostomies usually are temporary and may be associated with several distinct complications. The bowel loop is held outside the abdomen by a bridge of skin, fascia, or plastic tubing. If an opened loop retracts back into the abdomen, laparotomy to retrieve it is indicated. Evisceration of small bowel around a loop colostomy also is seen occasionally and this generally requires operative reduction. Prolapse of proximal or distal colon through the stoma may occur in up to 25 percent of all loop colostomies. Treatment involves manual reduction. Recurrence is likely, however; and the problem is well tolerated.

The majority of complications after end colostomy relate to skin irritation, minor bleeding, or the appliance itself. More serious complications of end colostomy include necrosis, retraction, stenosis, and parastomal hernias. A fresh stoma should be checked daily for pink, viable mucosa; in the presence of ischemia or necrosis, the ostomy should be revised. Retraction of a stoma below the skin occasionally is seen, especially in obese individuals, and treatment is operative revision. Stomal necrosis or retraction eventually may result in stenosis of the colostomy site and subsequent fecal impaction. Initial treatment involves gentle digital dilation and irrigation with a rectal tube or Foley catheter. A parastomal hernia may be seen in 25 percent of end colostomies. It involves herniation of small bowel or adjacent colon through the fascial opening of a colostomy. The herniated bowel usually is contained within the rectus sheath or subcutaneous tissue. Most do not require treatment, but in the presence of pain or irreducibility, the colostomy should be relocated.

Specific Considerations

Gastric Surgery

Complications of gastric surgery can be divided into those occurring within the first postoperative week and those that occur weeks to months after surgery. Early complications may include gastric bleeding, delayed gastric emptying, postoperative pancreatitis, and leakage from the divided end of the duodenum in certain types of gastric reconstruction. Later complications are more likely to be seen in the emergency center. Patients who have had a Billroth II-type reconstruction after gastric surgery may experience partial obstruction of the jejunal limb arising from the duodenum (afferent loop syndrome). These patients complain of severe pain several hours after eating and may vomit bile without food. The food has passed down the efferent limb while bile and pancreatic juice remain obstructed in the afferent. Diagnosis is by endoscopy. Patients with persistent peptic ulcer disease after surgery may develop stenosis of the gastrointestinal stoma. These patients present with gastric-outlet obstruction and need to be evaluated to ascertain the reason for persistent acid peptic disease. Bile gastritis and dumping syndromes are also occasional late complications of gastric surgery.

Gastrostomy tubes may be placed surgically or endoscopically. Most complications involve inadvertent removal of the tube or excoriation and infection around the gastrostomy site. Tubes which are removed from gastrostomies more than 7 days old normally can be replaced without difficulty. The stomach should be reintubated within 3 to 4 h to prevent stomal stenosis. If a gastrostomy is removed in the immediate postoperative period, intubation should be attempted gently and confirmation of placement obtained by contrast radiography if doubt exists. Inflammation of the skin commonly is noted around gastrostomy sites due to the acidity of gastric contents. Treatment involves adequate daily cleansing of the ostomy site and properly securing the gastrostomy tube. Evidence of induration and cellulitis should be treated with antibiotics.

Biliary and Pancreatic Surgery

The majority of complications arising from surgery of the biliary tract result from leakage of bile, ductal obstruction, infection, or iatrogenic injury. Bile leaks may become evident as early as 4 or 5 days postoperatively or may be delayed several weeks. Symptoms are normally insidious in onset and include abdominal pain of variable intensity, nausea, and vomiting. Pain usually is located in the right upper quadrant or epigastrium and may radiate to the right shoulder. Large bile leaks may result in acholic stools and bilious ascites. Patients normally exhibit a low-grade fever, abdominal tenderness, tachycardia, and mild jaundice. Bile leaks are well demonstrated using biliary scanning and fluid collections best appreciated by CT scan or ultrasonography. Treatment involves radiologically guided percutaneous drainage of symptomatic bile collections followed by surgical correction of persistent leaks.

Postoperative biliary obstruction may result from iatrogenic bile duct injury, retained common bile duct stones, bile duct stricture, or an obstructing T-tube. The most common clinical manifestation is jaundice. Patients most often complain of upper abdominal pain, nausea, and occasional vomiting. They may present with acute cholangitis, exhibiting fever, chills, jaundice, and abdominal pain. This syndrome requires prompt institution of intravenous antibiotics with decompression and drainage of the biliary system. Other forms of biliary obstruction normally are not surgical emergencies. Definitive diagnosis involves cholangiography with a T-tube, percutaneous transhepatic cholangiogram, or endoscopic retrograde cholangiopancreatography (ERCP). Retained common bile duct stones may be removed through a mature T-tube tract or by endoscopic sphincterotomy. Iatrogenic bile duct injuries resulting in obstruction require operative intervention.

The sudden absence of bile drainage from a T-tube should alert the physician to the possibility of obstruction or malposition of the tube. A T-tube cholangiogram should be performed promptly, and displaced or obstructing tubes require surgical replacement. Tubes removed inadvertently within 5 days of a surgical procedure need to be replaced operatively. After this period, a patient may be observed for signs and symptoms of bile leak or peritonitis, then treated accordingly.

Laparoscopic cholecystectomy is commonly performed today and has led to a new spectrum of postoperative complications. Many complications are related to the initial pneumoperitoneum and result from perforation of a viscus, injury to a solid organ, or vascular injuries. Patients normally are discharged within 24 h of the procedure. Complications likely to be seen in the emergency room are similar to those seen with open cholecystectomy and include intraabdominal bleeding, bile duct injury and leak, and retained common bile duct stones.

Postoperative pancreatitis may follow any type of intraabdominal surgery and may account for up to 9 percent of all cases of pancreatitis. It also may occur after ERCP. Clinical diagnosis is established in the presence of abdominal pain and hyperamylasemia. CT scan generally will demonstrate acute pancreatitis, although 20 percent of patients will not show any changes. Treatment involves bowel rest and pain control. Pancreatic pseudocysts, pancreatic fistulas, and abscesses are all complications of pancreatic surgery.

Appendectomy

Complications following appendectomy are related to the disease state preoperatively. Complications are unusual after straightforward appendicitis but may be seen frequently following operations for perforated appendicitis involving peritonitis or abscess formation. Wound infection is the most common postoperative complication, occurring in 7 percent of cases of nonperforated appendicitis and in 35 percent of cases where peritonitis was present.

Intrabdominal or pelvic abscesses may follow complicated appendectomy. Patients normally exhibit fever, localized tenderness, and a mass on abdominal or rectal examination. The pelvis and right paracolic gutter are the most likely locations for the abscess. Diagnosis is usually established by ultrasonography or CT.

Fever, jaundice, and shaking chills are manifestations of pylephlebitis and disseminated intrahepatic abscess following appendectomy. This rare but serious complication should be treated with high-dose antibiotics and surgical drainage.

Anorectal Surgery

Many of the surgical procedures involving the anus and rectum are done on an outpatient basis, and complications may be seen occasionally in the emergency center. These include benign conditions such as hemorrhoids, anal fissures, anorectal abscesses, and fistulas, and malignant conditions such as anal or rectal carcinoma.

Hemorrhage following anorectal surgery is unusual generally but occurs in up to 2 percent of patients following hemorrhoidectomy. Bleeding normally occurs within several hours of the procedure or between 7 to 10 days when sutures dissolve. A surprising amount of blood may be sequestered within the rectum, and patients may present with hypotension. Treatment involves examination under anesthesia and ligation of bleeding vessels. In the event of exsanguinating hemorrhage, a temporary pack or Foley catheter with a large balloon inflated should be placed in the rectum.

Urinary retention after anorectal surgery has been reported to occur in up to 10 percent of cases. Urethral sphincter spasm, overdistension of the bladder from intraoperative fluid, and spinal anesthesia are contributing factors. Men are affected much more often than women. Treatment involves catheterization as mentioned previously.

Constipation and fecal impaction may also be seen following anorectal surgery. Patients generally complain of increasing anorectal pain or pressure or experience diarrhea on the 3rd or 4th postoperative day. A gentle rectal examination may reveal the fecal impaction. If firm stool is encountered, a tap water or Fleet's enema may be given to relieve discomfort.

Infection after anorectal surgery surprisingly is uncommon, unless a patient is immunosuppressed or diabetic. Patients normally complain of increasing perianal pain and fever postoperatively. There may be swelling, induration, and redness of the perianal area. An adequate anal examination is necessary to confirm the possibility of an abscess; however, this may need to be done under anesthesia. A particularly virulent form of necrotizing perineal infection, Fournier's gangrene, may follow anorectal surgery. Perineal pain and swelling are present, and evidence of suppuration or gangrene of overlying skin may be noted. Numerous aerobic and anaerobic organisms have been cultured from these patients. Intravenous clindamycin or metronidazole should be started immediately in suspected cases, and thorough operative debridement is required.

Inguinal Hernia

Inguinal hernia repair is one of the most common general surgical procedures, and almost all patients are discharged within 24 h postoperatively. Serious complications are rare, but occasionally, minor complications may be seen in the emergency center. Urinary retention occurs in up to one-third of patients undergoing hernia repair. Older men and young healthy men are the two most commonly affected groups, the former due to prostatic hypertrophy and the latter due to sphincter spasm. Treatment requires catheter decompression as discussed earlier.

Scrotal ecchymosis may be noted on the 1st or 2nd postoperative day and, unless massive, requires only patient reassurance. A swollen testicle may result from a tight repair, and the impaired venous and lymphatic drainage should be treated by scrotal elevation and inactivity. Symptoms normally resolve.

Wound infection rates after repair of groin hernias are approximately 1 percent, slightly higher in a recurrent hernia. Local care should be instituted as described previously. If infection seems to extend below external oblique fascia, repair may be compromised, and the risk of recurrence is high. Antibiotic treatment is only necessary if evidence of spreading cellulitis exists or if the repair involved foreign material.

Chronic pain in proximity to a repaired hernia may be the result of a neuroma, from division of a nerve during the procedure, or entrapment of a nerve within a suture. Symptoms most often resolve spontaneously, but persistence may require reexploration.

Vascular complications after hernia repair are rare but are more serious in nature. Both the femoral artery and the femoral vein are close to the site of hernia repair and may be injured during the procedure. Unrecognized arterial injury may result in retroperitoneal hematoma and hemodynamically significant blood volume loss. Arterial thrombosis or distal embolus also may occur resulting in an ischemic extremity which demands prompt treatment, but this is very rare. Venous injury is a little more common and usually results in thrombosis. When it occurs, it is usually a complication of direct hernia repair using Cooper's ligament. If recognized immediately, surgical treatment can prevent venous insufficiency if the vein is obstructed by extrinsic compression or if extensive thrombosis has not occurred.

BREAST SURGERY

Since breast cancer will affect one in 10 women in the United States during their lifetime, operations to diagnose and treat breast cancer are very common. Complications may arise as a consequence of both breast biopsy and mastectomy. The breast is a very vascular organ, and postoperative hemorrhage is not uncommon. A tense, bulging, and discolored biopsy site are signs of postoperative hematoma, and patients need to be taken back to the operating room for evacuation and hemostasis. A seroma may develop postoperatively in the axilla or chest wall after drains have been removed. This is not a serious problem and will resolve with frequent aspiration.

Infection after breast surgery is a serious complication because it may lead to necrosis of skin flaps and lymphedema of the arm. Antibiotics should be initiated when erythema, induration, or excessive tenderness are noted at the biopsy site or mastectomy wound. Purulent drainage requires opening of the wound.

BIBLIOGRAPHY

Condon RE, Nyhus LM: Complications of groin hernia, in, *Hernia,* 3d ed. Philadelphia, Lippincott, 1989.

Corman ML: *Colon and Rectal Surgery,* 2d ed. Philadelphia, Lippincott, 1989.

Doherty VC, O'Donovan TR, Hill GJ: Current status of ambulatory surgery in the United States, in *Outpatient Surgery,* 3d ed., Hill, GJ (ed.). Philadelphia, Saunders, 1988.

Goldberg SM, Gordon HP, Nivatvongs S: *Essentials of Anorectal Surgery.* Philadelphia, Lippincott, 1980.

Greenfield LJ: *Complications in Surgery and Trauma.* Philadelphia, Lippincott, 1990.

Hardy JD: *Complications in Surgery and Their Management.* Philadelphia, Saunders, 1981.

Leand P: Pneumothorax, in *Current Surgical Therapy,* 3d ed. Cameron, JL (ed.): Toronto, Decker, 1989.

Ponsky JL: Complications of laparoscopic cholecystectomy. *Am J Surg* 161: 493, 1991.

Schwartz SI: Complications, in Schwartz SI (ed): *Principles of Surgery,* 5th ed. New York, McGraw-Hill, 1989.

SECTION 6
Renal and Genitourinary Disorders

52
EMERGENCY RENAL PROBLEMS

K. Venkateswara Rao

Discussion in this chapter is limited to acute renal failure, rapidly progressive glomerulonephritis, kidney stones, and emergency medical problems associated with chronic renal failure.

ACUTE RENAL FAILURE

Acute renal failure is a constellation of clinical findings associated with sudden impairment in renal function leading to excessive accumulation of nitrogenous waste products in the serum. Depending on the amount of urine produced in a 24-h period, acute renal failure is classified as (1) oliguric form (< 500 mL) and (2) nonoliguric form (> 500 mL).

Etiology

The causes of acute renal failure can be broadly divided into (1) prerenal, (2) renal, and (3) postrenal. Table 52-1 lists some of the causes of acute renal failure under the three categories.

Differential Diagnosis

The history and physical examination may provide important clues as to the etiology of acute renal failure. A history of acute abdominal pain with nausea and vomiting may point toward a prerenal cause, while oliguria associated with suprapubic discomfort and increased area of dullness to percussion over the bladder suggests obstructive uropathy.

The diagnostic studies listed in Table 52-2 can be completed within an hour or two of the patient's arrival in the emergency department and require only a small amount of urine for analysis. They are innocuous and pose no danger to the patient's health. An intravenous pyelogram, renal angiography, and kidney biopsy may provide additional diagnostic information, but they are invasive and can cause significant morbidity, and are therefore not used routinely in the evaluation of acute renal failure. They should be reserved for specific situations only.

Management

Postrenal Failure

In patients with a postrenal cause of acute renal failure, an appropriate channel for urinary drainage should be established. The exact procedure employed may vary depending on the level of obstruction. For example, a Foley catheter may be adequate for obstruction arising from a benign prostatic hypertrophy, whereas a percutaneous nephrostomy tube is required for a ureteral occlusion. Once the patient's medical status is optimized, definitive surgery for the correction of the obstructive lesion should be considered.

For the patient with acute anuria, obstruction is the major consideration. If no urine is obtained after proper urethral catheterization, ultrasonography and urologic consultation should be obtained on an emergency basis.

Prerenal Failure

In those patients where a prerenal cause is suspected, every effort should be made to restore the effective intravascular volume. In states of volume depletion, isotonic fluids (normal saline, plasma, or Ringer's solution) should be administered at a rapid rate. When cardiac failure is contributing to prerenal azotemia, the intravascular volume should be reduced to enhance cardiac performance. Surgical correction of the underlying problem (e.g., segmental bowel resection for infarction, peritoneovenous shunt for massive ascites, valve replacement for left ventricular outflow tract obstruction, pericardiectomy for con-

Table 52-1. Causes of Acute Renal Failure

Prerenal	Renal	Postrenal
Reduction in cardiac output	Vascular	Lower urinary tract
Congestive heart failure	Thrombosis of renal vasculature	Phimosis
Acute pulmonary edema	Systemic vascular disorders [thrombotic thrombocytopenic purpura (TTP), disseminated intravascular coagulation (DIC), scleroderma, malignant hypertension, etc.]	Meatal stenosis
Valvular heart disease	Preferential reduction in renal cortical blood flow (e.g., nonsteroidal anti-inflammatory drugs)	Urethral stricture
Myocardial dysfunction	Glomerular	Blood clots
Pericardial tamponade	Primary glomerular diseases (e.g., rapidly progressive glomerulonephritis, poststreptococcal nephritis)	Stones
Hypovolemia	Glomerular involvement in systemic disease (e.g., lupus erythematosus, bacterial endocarditis, systemic vasculitis)	Bladder tumors
Fluid loss from skin, kidney, GI tract, or hemorrhage	Tubulointerstitial	Prostatic hypertrophy
Redistribution of intravascular fluids, as in peritonitis, pancreatitis, hepatic failure, anaphylaxis, and septic shock	Ischemic acute tubular necrosis	Cancer of prostate
	Toxic tubular damage from antibiotics, pigments, radiographic dyes, anesthetics, and other chemicals	Neurogenic bladder
	Drug-induced allergic interstitial nephritis (e.g., sulfonamides, penicillin, allopurinol)	Upper urinary tract (usually requires bilateral involvement)
	Intraparenchymal obstructive lesions (e.g., myeloma kidney, acute uric acid nephropathy, ethylene glycol poisoning)	Papillary necrosis
		Calculi
		Tumors (intrinsic or extrinsic)
		Retroperitoneal fibrosis

Table 52-2. Laboratory Studies Aiding in the Differential Diagnosis of Acute Renal Failure

Test Employed	Prerenal	Renal	Postrenal
Urine sodium (mEq/L)	<20	>40	>40
FE_{Na}(%)*	<1	>2	>2
Renal failure index†	<1	>2	>2
Urine osmolality (mosm/L)	>500	<300	<400
Urine/serum creatinine ratio	>40:1	<20:1	<20:1
Serum urea nitrogen/creatinine ratio	>20:1	≈10:1	≈10:1
Kidney size by ultrasonic exam	Normal	Normal	May be increased
Radionuclide scan	Poor uptake, delayed excretion	Good uptake but marked delay in excretion	Good uptake but minimal or no excretion

$$* \text{ Fractional excretion of sodium (\%)} = \frac{\text{urine sodium/serum sodium}}{\text{urine creatinine/serum creatinine}} \times 100$$

$$† \text{ Renal failure index} = \frac{\text{urine sodium}}{\text{urine creatinine/serum creatinine}} \times 100$$

strictive pericarditis) is recommended when the patient's medical status is stable.

Renal Failure

Acute tubular necrosis (ATN) resulting from an ischemic injury or a nephrotoxic agent is the most common cause of intrinsic renal failure. Other parenchymal diseases such as acute glomerulonephritis or allergic interstitial nephritis are less frequent causes. The history, physical examination, and simple laboratory tests may provide useful clues in distinguishing one form of intrinsic renal disease from the other. The acute onset of oliguria, hypertension, pulmonary edema, and a telescopic urine sediment (red cells, white cells, protein, red blood cell casts) would suggest acute glomerulonephritis as the primary cause of acute renal failure. In these situations, the physician should avoid the use of drugs such as nephrotoxic antibiotics or nonsteroidal anti-inflammatory agents, which are potentially toxic. Renal function can be supported with dialysis until recovery.

The general principles followed in the management of patients with established intrinsic acute renal failure are discussed in the following paragraphs.

Diet

The diet should be high in calories (3000 to 4000), low in protein (40 to 60 g), low in sodium (2 to 3 g), and low in potassium (60 to 80 mEq). Fluids should be restricted (500 mL + urine output). In patients who cannot eat, sufficient caloric intake should be ensured with tube feeding. If the gastrointestinal tract is not functioning, intravenous hyperalimentation is preferred. Provision of adequate calories will prevent further tissue breakdown and minimize the daily rise in serum urea nitrogen level.

Diuretics

The role of diuretics in the management of established acute renal failure is limited, although in a rare instance they may augment diuresis and thus convert an oliguric form of renal failure into a nonoliguric form. Hyperoncotic solutions, such as mannitol, may cause acute blood volume expansion in an oliguric patient and lead to massive pulmonary edema. Rapid infusion of large doses of furosemide may cause ototoxicity. These drugs should be used with extreme caution in patients with intrinsic renal failure.

Dialysis

Both hemodialysis and peritoneal dialysis are effective methods of supporting the patient until the kidneys recover. The choice of hemodialysis or peritoneal dialysis is made on an individual basis, considering the facilities available, the patient's hemodynamic stability, and the status of the patient's abdomen. In recent years, slow, continuous hemofiltration has been used in patients with hemodynamic instability resulting from cardiogenic or septic shock.

Intermittent dialysis facilitates the removal of not only the nitrogenous waste products but also excess fluid volume and thus may improve the patient's blood pressure. It also helps to correct metabolic acidosis and hyperkalemia, which, if untreated, could lead to cardiac instability and death. Most patients with acute renal failure require 4 h of hemodialysis every other day.

Drugs

Dopamine in low concentrations (1 to 3 μg/kg per min) may improve renal cortical blood flow and is frequently used in the early phase of acute renal failure. At 4 to 6 μg/kg per min, dopamine begins to exert a β-adrenergic effect, increasing the heart rate and contractility. Other drugs which are renally excreted (e.g., digoxin, magnesium compounds, sedatives) should be used with caution. The usual therapeutic doses may cause serious side effects as the drugs accumulate in excess concentration.

Other Measures

Whenever possible, procedures that disrupt the host defense barriers (skin and mucosa) should be avoided to prevent the risk of microbial infection. When prolonged urinary drainage or intravenous infusion is required, changing the catheters and infusion devices every fifth day may help to reduce the risk of infection. Other common extrarenal complications developing in the setting of acute renal failure, such as sepsis, GI bleeding, and pericardial tamponade, should be anticipated and promptly treated.

Prognosis

Prognosis depends on the cause. Recovery can be expected in most cases of prerenal and postrenal acute renal failure. Among the patients with intrinsic renal failure, a majority of those with toxin-induced acute renal failure (aminoglycosides, radiographic contrast agents, myoglobinuria) regain renal function. The prognosis is poor in patients with posttraumatic and postsurgical acute tubular necrosis. Elderly patients with involvement of multiple organ systems have a poor outcome compared to young individuals who have been healthy before the onset of acute renal failure. Most patients regain renal function within 2 to 3 weeks following the acute insult, although rare cases have been reported in which patients regained renal function after 6 months.

Prevention

Even at the present time, 60 to 70 percent of patients with established acute renal failure die during the course of the illness. Therefore, every effort should be made to prevent the onset of renal failure. Such measures would include identification of high-risk patients, avoidance of nephrotoxic agents, and adequate hydration with intravenous fluids prior to angiographic studies. High-risk patients are those 60 years old and above, those undergoing cardiovascular or gastrointestinal surgical procedures, and those developing renal failure in association with multiorgan dysfunction or a systemic disease such as diabetes, lupus, or scleroderma. The use of crystalloid or colloidal solutions before, during, and after major surgical procedures has reduced the incidence of ischemic ATN in the perioperative period.

RAPIDLY PROGRESSIVE GLOMERULONEPHRITIS

Rapidly progressive glomerulonephritis (RPGN) is a clinical syndrome with the following features: (1) evidence of inflammation of the glomeruli, usually manifest by hematuria with or without red cell casts in the urine; (2) rapid decline in renal function leading to azotemia; (3) oliguria or anuria, which is a frequent finding; and (4) hypertension, edema, and massive proteinuria, which may or may not be found. Histologically, this entity is characterized by circumferential crescents involving more than 50 percent of the glomeruli in the renal biopsy specimen. The exact etiology of the parietal epithelial cell proliferation of Bowman's capsule leading to crescent formation is unclear, although an immunologic basis [due to the presence of antiglomerular basement membrane (GBM) antibodies and circulating immune complexes] has been implicated in the pathogenesis of this disorder. The term *Goodpasture's syndrome* is used when the rapidly progressive anti-GBM glomerulonephritis is preceded by pulmonary hemorrhage and clinical hemoptysis. On occasion, acute poststreptococcal glomerulonephritis, IgA nephropathy, mesangiocapillary glomerulonephritis, and systemic vasculitis may present with clinical and histologic features similar to those of idiopathic RPGN.

The differential diagnosis of RPGN with glomerular inflammation includes (1) lupus nephritis, (2) polyarteritis nodosa, (3) hypersensitivity angiitis, (4) Wegener's granulomatosis, (5) anaphylactoid purpura, (6) scleroderma renal disease, (7) thrombotic thrombocytopenic purpura, (8) hemolytic uremic syndrome, and (9) malignant hypertension. Most of these can be diagnosed on the basis of the patient's history, physical findings, other routine laboratory studies (peripheral blood smear, platelet count, chest x-ray, etc.), and finally the renal biopsy.

The principles of therapy are similar to those for acute renal failure. Once the patient's clinical status is stable, a renal biopsy has to be performed. The specific therapy is directed at the histologic diagnosis. Most patients with crescentic poststreptococcal glomerulonephritis recover renal function spontaneously within a few weeks. Plasmapheresis in conjunction with immunosuppressive drugs has been found beneficial in the setting of anti-GBM nephritis and Goodpasture's syndrome. Isolated case reports have appeared in the literature, showing successful treatment of idiopathic RPGN using massive doses of intravenous steroids.

In idiopathic RPGN, despite the currently available treatment modalities, the prognosis for survival and recovery of renal function remains poor. Sepsis is the leading cause of death in patients receiving aggressive therapy with plasmapheresis and cytotoxic agents. Despite an initial improvement in the clinical course and the findings on chest x-ray, approximately 50 percent of patients receiving cytotoxic drug therapy die from a septic complication during the second or third week after the initiation of treatment. Those who have survived but lost renal function have tolerated intermittent dialysis quite well, and many of them have received successful renal transplants. Recurrence of RPGN in the renal allografts is extremely rare.

URINARY CALCULI

Stones in the urinary tract, or nephrolithiasis, should be distinguished from nephrocalcinosis. In nephrocalcinosis calcium is deposited within the renal tubules, and on plain x-ray of the abdomen, it appears as multiple small radiopaque shadows distributed uniformly over both kidneys. Patients with urinary calculi develop acute renal colic. In contrast, patients with nephrocalcinosis are often asymptomatic and the diagnosis is made as an incidental finding on x-ray. The stones formed in the collecting system, i.e., the renal calyces and the pelvis, travel along the ureter and are passed in the urine. When they lodge along the urinary tract, obstructive uropathy and secondary infection may occur. Stones less than 5 mm in diameter are generally passed spontaneously.

Pathogenesis

Supersaturation of urine with a particular mineral such as calcium, phosphate, oxalate, cystine, or urate is the principal reason for the formation of renal stones. Other mechanisms include reduced urinary concentration of natural inhibitors such as magnesium, citrate, and pyrophosphate. Infection with urea-splitting organisms often contributes to the growth of "struvite" stones or triple phosphate (calcium, magnesium, and ammonium phosphate) stones. Decreased urine volume from reduced intake or excess losses can augment the risk in patients predisposed to nephrolithiasis. Most stones consist of calcium oxalate or mixed calcium oxalate and phosphate. About 40 percent of stone formers never have a second episode. In the remaining patients, management should be directed at the potential etiologic factors to prevent recurrence.

Clinical Features

Patients with urinary calculi develop severe, acute abdominal or flank pain. The typical history is of intermittent colicky pain which radiates from the loin to the groin and scrotum or labia. The patient often curls up in bed to find a comfortable position, and may exhibit anxiety or apprehension. Associated signs and symptoms include anorexia, nausea, vomiting, and gross or microscopic hematuria. Physical examination may reveal signs of dehydration, hypotension, costovertebral angle (CVA) tenderness, and diminished bowel sounds secondary to ileus.

The urinanalysis often (but not always) shows red cells, but the presence of casts or protein is rare. Urinalysis is necessary to detect infection, which, if present, alters disposition and management. Bacteriuria may occur if there is superimposed infection, and the urine pH may be alkaline. The serum chemistry profile may suggest an underlying metabolic abnormality such as hypercalcemia, hypophosphatemia, hyperuricemia, or hypokalemia. Hyperchloremic metabolic acidosis together with hypokalemia is characteristic of distal renal tubular acidosis in which nephrocalcinosis and nephrolithiasis are common findings.

Radiologic Examination

Most stones are radiopaque and if a plain x-ray (kidney and upper bladder, KUB) is done can be visualized along the renal pelvis, calyces, or bladder. The KUB abdominal film may be normal if the principal component of the stone is a nonopaque material such as cystine, xanthine, or uric acid. Radiolucent stones are best diagnosed by intravenous pyelogram (IVP). However, a filling defect in the IVP can be due to a radiolucent calculus, thrombus, or tumor. In follow-up studies, a filling defect caused by tumor is persistent, whereas it disappears when the thrombus lyses or the stone passes. The IVP is useful in diagnosing renal calculi, in estimating the size of the stone, in identifying extravasation of the dye, and in evaluating renal function. The test should be avoided in patients with a history of allergy to radio contrast materials, iodinated compounds, or seafood. It is contraindicated in patients with concurrent or preexisting renal failure.

Before ordering the IVP, the patient should be asked about a history of renal disease, diabetes, or hypertension. If there is a possibility of renal disease, the physician should obtain renal function studies. Blood urea nitrogen greater than 50 mg/dL, or a serum creatinine level of 3 mg/dL or above, are generally considered contraindications for infusion of the contrast material. However, any elevation of BUN or creatinine should prompt reevaluation of the need for the study.

There is no satisfactory test that will predict which patients will develop an allergic reaction following the infusion of radio contrast material. Minor allergic reactions such as pruritus or skin rash can be treated effectively with cessation of infusion and administration of antihistimines (25 to 50 mg Benadryl IM or IV) and corticosteroids (100 to 200 mg Solu-Cortef IV). More severe reactions require treatment with epinephrine and crystalloids.

Under such conditions, ultrasonography is a useful alternative. It can identify the stone and its location, demonstrate proximal obstruction such as hydroureter or a dilated pelvis, and also the size and configuration of each kidney. Rarely, ultrasonography may be inconclusive, and CT scanning (with or without radio contrast) may be required.

Adequate analgesia, 1 to 2 mg/kg meperidine IV or IM, or the equivalent, should be given based on the clinical diagnosis and before subjecting the patient to confirmatory but time-consuming studies.

Differential Diagnosis

Although the pain of renal colic is quite classic, the physician should consider and exclude other acute intraabdominal and retroperitoneal problems such as acute pancreatitis, perforated peptic ulcer or diverticulum, acute appendicitis, bowel obstruction, acute cholecystitis, acute pyelonephritis, thrombosis of renal vein, renal infarction, aneurysmal dilatation and rupture of the abdominal aorta, acute cholecystitis, and acute biliary calculus. Abdominal pain referred from the thorax (pleurisy, pericarditis, or coronary ischemia) should be differentiated from renal colic. Most of these conditions can be distinguished on the basis of the background history, signs and symptoms, physical examination, and confirmatory laboratory or radiographic studies.

Complications

The major complications associated with renal stones are obstruction, infection, and intractable pain. If obstruction and infection are untreated, they may lead to acute oliguria, renal failure, and septic shock. Emergency urologic consultation, adequate analgesia, and intravenous antibiotics, including aminoglycosides, are necessary.

Management

The management of a patient with kidney stones is divided into (1) emergency therapy, (2) elective procedures to remove the stone, and (3) prevention of recurrence.

Emergency Therapy

Since 90 percent of stones are passed spontaneously, the management is directed at relief of pain and providing adequate hydration. Morphine or meperidine intramuscularly or intravenously provides adequate analgesia and relieves anxiety, allowing the patient to pass the stone with ease. In the emergency department, intravenous saline should be administered to ensure a urine volume of 100 to 200 mL/h. Most patients with renal colic can be discharged to urologic follow-up. They should be instructed to urinate through a sieve and capture the stone for chemical analysis. Indications for admission are (1) persistent pain requiring continued parenteral narcotics, (2) urinary tract infection, (3) stone greater than 5 mm in diameter, (4) deteriorating renal function, (5) failure to visualize the obstructed kidney on IVP, and (6) extravasation of dye. Note that extravasation of dye on IVP is not commonly observed in patients with urinary calculi unless the calculus erodes through the renal pelvis or ureter.

Surgical removal is recommended if the stone is not passed within 2 to 3 days of hospitalization and the patient continues to have renal colic; the stone is obstructing the urine flow, causing hydronephrosis; or the stone is a large staghorn calculus. Lithotripsy is available in major medical centers. This form of therapy will minimize the hospital stay and prevent the surgical complications associated with exploration of the kidney and urinary tract.

EMERGENCIES IN CHRONIC RENAL FAILURE

Patients with chronic renal failure are initially managed with conservative medical therapy and subsequently by intermittent dialysis (hemodialysis or peritoneal dialysis). The accepted indications for initiation of chronic dialysis are (1) uremic symptoms (e.g., nausea, vomiting, mucosal erosions, increased fatigue, pruritus, and insomnia), even in the absence of high serum urea nitrogen level; (2) uncontrolled hypertension secondary to volume overload; (3) hyperkalemia, requiring repeated use of ion-exchange resins; (4) fluid overload and congestive heart failure; (5) uremic pericarditis; (6) rapidly progressing uremic peripheral neuropathy; and (7) uremic encephalopathy. Emergencies occurring in uremic patients either before or after initiation of dialytic therapy are discussed in this section.

Uremic Pericarditis

The classic symptom is chest pain, which is partially relieved by sitting up and leaning forward. A pericardial friction rub may not be heard in all instances, or it may be heard intermittently. Low-grade fever and atrial arrhythmias (paroxysmal atrial tachycardia, atrial flutter–atrial fibrillation) are common accompaniments. Echocardiography may reveal a pericardial effusion. The pericardial fluid may impede venous return into the right atrium, leading to low output congestive heart failure and hypotension. The tamponade is relieved by pericardiocentesis. The instillation of corticosteroids into the pericardial sac after the pericardiocentesis has been recommended to prevent relapses. Regular dialysis at frequent intervals (utilizing minimal doses of heparin) also reduces the incidence of recurrence and is the preferred form of therapy at many dialysis centers. The definitive treatment is the creation of a pericardial window or an anterior pericardiectomy.

Cardiac Arrhythmias and Cardiac Arrest

The etiology of cardiac arrhythmias in uremic patients is multifactorial and includes such diverse causes as hyperkalemia, hypocalcemia, hypokalemia, hypermagnesemia, coronary ischemia, metastatic calcification involving the cardiac conduction system, and the effect of drugs such as digitalis and quinidine. The most frequent arrhythmia encountered during dialysis is hypokalemia-induced ventricular irritability manifest by premature beats and ventricular fibrillation. This problem can be prevented by frequent monitoring of the serum potassium level and adjusting the potassium concentration in the dialysate solution.

The most common cause of cardiac arrest in uremic patients presenting to the emergency department is hyperkalemia. Resuscitation should therefore include immediate administration of calcium gluconate, followed by infusion of 50 mL of 50% glucose along with 20 units of regular insulin and 50 to 100 mEq sodium bicarbonate IV.

Alterations in Blood Pressure

Hypertension

In about 90 percent of hypertensive uremic patients the hypertension is related to excess intravascular volume secondary to salt and water retention. Only a minority of patients have renin-dependent hypertension. When patients present with hypertensive emergencies such as encephalopathy or pulmonary edema, blood pressure should be lowered immediately with an intravenous infusion of sodium nitroprusside and removal of excess volume with ultrafiltration dialysis. The usual methods of management of acute pulmonary edema, such as phlebotomy or administration of larger doses of intravenous diuretics, are not practical in patients with renal failure. Other agents employed in lowering the blood pressure acutely are intravenous labetalol, captopril, diazoxide, hydralazine, and α-methyldopa.

Hypotension

A sudden drop in blood pressure is a common complication during dialysis and, if not promptly treated, can lead to cardiac arrest. Subjective symptoms such as muscle cramps, nausea, yawning, and mental confusion may precede actual hypotension in most patients but not in all. The treatment is rapid infusion of isotonic saline or hypertonic solutions such as 3% saline, plasma, or albumin. In rare instances the use of vasopressors may be required.

Neurologic Problems

Dialysis Disequilibrium

Symptoms of increased intracranial pressure, manifest by nausea, vomiting, headache, and mental confusion, can be experienced soon after or within a few hours of a dialysis treatment. This is extremely common after the first dialysis but can also occur with chronic dialysis. Intracranial pressure increases because of the osmotic shift of water from the bloodstream into cerebrospinal fluid (CSF) as a result of a higher urea content in the CSF relative to plasma. During dialysis, the concentration of urea in plasma is lowered quickly but the concentration of urea in the CSF remains high because of the blood-brain barrier. After a few hours the osmotic gradient between plasma and CSF becomes equilibrated and the patient's symptoms gradually resolve.

Diagnosis is based on the history and evaluation of BUN levels before and after dialysis. It should be differentiated from other causes of raised intracranial pressure such as subdural hematoma, cerebrovascular accident, or brain tumor. Therapy of dialysis disequilibrium is purely symptomatic. Reassurance, bed rest, and administration of analgesics and antiemetics will alleviate the symptom within a few hours. Patients usually return to their normal state of health the next day following dialysis. Dialysis disequilibrium does not occur following peritoneal dialysis treatment because of the slower pace at which the urea is removed from plasma.

Subdural Hematoma

Both spontaneous and posttraumatic subdural hematomas occur in patients receiving chronic hemodialysis. A history of trauma may or may not be elicited as patients tend to ignore simple events such as a fall from bed or tripping over an object. The risk is increased in uremic patients as a result of defective platelet function and heparinization during dialysis.

Diagnosis is based on the history, alteration in mental status, and computed tomographic (CT) scanner confirmation of a subdural hematoma. Focal neurologic signs, such as dilated pupils, hemiplegia, or monoplegia, may not be present in all cases. Therapy is directed at evacuation of hematoma and relieving the pressure on the vital structures. Preventive measures are cautious heparinization and avoidance of falls.

Other Neurologic Problems

Uremic patients may present with seizures, coma, or mental obtundation. The evaluation should include a complete review of the medications; physical examination; measurement of plasma levels of calcium, magnesium, electrolytes, BUN, and blood glucose; and an emergency head CT scan. Therapy is directed at the cause. Most patients require in-hospital management unless the problem is a simple one such as a seizure from severe hypoglycemia.

Gastrointestinal Disorders

Upper gastrointestinal bleeding may result from uremic gastritis, peptic ulcer disease, or excess anticoagulation in patients with chronic renal failure. The management does not differ from that employed in nonuremic patients. However, caution should be exercised in using large doses of magnesium-containing antacids. Since magnesium is normally excreted by the kidney, abnormal levels could accumulate in the plasma, leading to mental obtundation and respiratory depression.

Bowel obstruction symptoms are not uncommon in uremic patients receiving phosphate-binding antacids. The plain abdominal x-ray may demonstrate a nonspecific bowel gas pattern with a large amount of stool in the colon. Therapeutic measures should include fecal disimpaction, tap water enemas, and laxatives such as sorbitol or mineral oil. Phosphate-containing enemas such as Fleet's Phospho-soda (Na biphosphate) should be avoided. Since most of the phosphate-binding antacids [Amphojel, Basaljel (Al carbonate), ALternaGEL (Al hydroxide)] induce bowel constipation, it is a good practice to prescribe a stool softener such as 200 mg of docusate sodium (Colace or Pericolace) daily.

Diverticulitis and bowel perforation are commonly observed in patients with renal failure from polycystic kidney disease. They also have a higher incidence of spontaneous intracerebral bleeding due to rupture of congenital berry aneurysms.

Peritonitis is a frequent problem in patients receiving chronic peritoneal dialysis. The symptoms are abdominal discomfort, pain during dialysate inflow, and fever. Physical examination may reveal abdominal tenderness, particularly around the catheter site, and decreased bowel sounds. Laboratory evaluation should include CBC, analysis of peritoneal fluid for cell count, protein, culture, and sensitivity. A variety of microorganisms (bacterial, fungal, and parasitic) have been found in the cultures from the peritoneal fluid. Treatment is with an appropriate antimicrobial agent which is infused into the peritoneal cavity. In patients with associated bacteremia, intravenous antibiotics are recommended. The incidence of peritonitis can be reduced by educating the patient about the use of sterile technique in connecting and disconnecting the dialysate tube with the peritoneal catheter and daily cleaning of the catheter exit site with an antiseptic solution. In patients with recurrent bouts of peritonitis, tunnel infection, or intraabdominal abscess, the catheter may need to be changed. Appropriate surgical drainage may also be required.

Problems Related to Vascular Access

A variety of vascular access devices have been developed to facilitate blood flow between the patient and dialyzer during the dialysis process. They are of two basic types: (1) external shunts and (2) internal shunts. The former category includes (1) a Scribner shunt (two plastic tubes, one in the radial artery and the other in the cephalic vein, connected together on the outside with a Teflon piece); (2) a Thomas shunt (a device similar to the Scribner shunt, but usually placed in the groin, connecting the femoral artery and saphenous vein segments); and (3) Hemasite, a small button-shaped titanium body with a puncturable rubber septum which allows the entry of dialysis needles during the treatment and seals off when the needles are removed. Hemasite access devices are placed either in the upper arm or in the anterior thigh near the groin.

The best of the internal access shunts is the Brescia-Cimino fistula, in which the radial artery is anastomosed to an adjacent vein. In patients with inadequate veins in the forearm, alternative methods of internal access include using a bovine heterograft (a specially treated carotid artery segment from a cow) or a Gore-Tex graft made from a synthetic material. These grafts are interposed between the patient's artery and the vein in the forearm. Occasionally they are placed in the upper arm.

The most frequent complications associated with external shunts are clotting and infection. When the shunt is acutely clotted, the vascular surgeon must be notified immediately. Irrigation of the cannula with heparinized saline should be avoided as it may cause the clot to spread, increasing the risk of pulmonary or peripheral embolization. Declotting procedures are generally accomplished by the surgeon in the operating suite.

Infection of the cannula site is another common complication in dialysis patients. Coagulase-positive staphylococci and *S. epidermidis* are the bacteria which are frequently cultured from the cannula tips. Physical examination reveals local inflammation, tenderness over the cannula tips, and purulent drainage at the exit sites. As soon as blood cultures and cannula tip cultures are obtained, antibiotic therapy should be initiated with a drug which is effective against penicillinase-resistant organisms (e.g., oxacillin, vancomycin, or cephalosporins). The most dreaded complications associated with cannula infection are septic pulmonary embolism and brisk hemorrhage resulting from dislodgment of the cannula tip. An alternative site for dialysis (such as peritoneal dialysis or subclavian venous catheter dialysis) should be considered while the patient is being treated for cannula infection.

Clotting and infection are rare with the Brescia-Cimino fistula, but they occur with bovine and Gore-Tex fistulas. Other problems are (1) stricture of the arterial or venous segment, causing poor blood flow and inefficient dialysis; (2) aneurysmal dilatation with the threat of rupture; (3) vascular ischemia of the fingertips secondary to a steal syndrome; and (4) prolonged bleeding at the puncture sites. To control the bleeding at the puncture sites, one should apply firm pressure. If pressure is unsuccessful, other measures, such as topical thrombin or neutralization of excess anticoagulation with protamine sulfate or aqueous vitamin K, should be considered. Aneurysms and strictures require surgical intervention by an experienced vascular surgeon. When a bovine or Gore-Tex fistula is clotted, the declotting procedure should be left to the surgeons in the operating room.

To prevent some of these complications, patients should be advised to (1) practice good cannula care [instructed how to clean the cannula tips with povidone-iodine (Betadine) and apply a sterile dressing], (2) avoid drawing blood from the fistula site, and (3) avoid taking blood pressure measurements on the arm containing the vascular access device. Patients should also be educated to seek emergency care as soon as these problems arise, since life-sustaining dialysis treatment cannot be provided without a functioning vascular access shunt.

Resuscitation of the Potential Organ Donor

With the adoption of brain-death laws in most states, organs are now removed from brain-dead donors while the heart is still beating and the kidneys are perfused and oxygenated by the donor's own blood. Brain death can be determined only after resuscitation, stabilization, and admission to the hospital. Emergency physicians should, of course, aggressively resuscitate all brain-injured patients without regard to this potential.

The following measures are undertaken by the transplant team after consent for organ donation is obtained by the attending physician: (1) the blood pressure in the donor is maintained within normal range by means of plasma expanders or vasopressors depending on the individual circumstance, (2) adequate diuresis is established with a urine output of 100 mL/h, (3) α-adrenergic blockers such as phentolamine are administered to reduce agonal vasospasm, (4) large doses of corticosteroids are administered prior to nephrectomy, and (5) tissue hypoxia is minimized with proper ventilation.

After the kidneys are removed, they are preserved and transported by means of either the surface cooling method or a hypothermic pulsatile perfusion machine. The use of these preservation techniques has allowed the transplant team to find the best possible recipient for the available kidneys on the basis of tissue typing and crossmatching. Engraftment has been successful even after 72 h of cold perfusion. A nationwide computer system has facilitated the use of nearly all donated kidneys in the United States and abroad.

Because of the large number of patients waiting for a transplant and the relative scarcity of donor kidneys, an effort should be made to obtain consent for organ donation from all brain-dead victims. However, the donor is considered unsuitable under the following circumstances: (1) age greater than 60 years, (2) hypertension or other significant vascular disease, (3) evidence of septicemia or renal infection, (4) a history of malignancy with primary or metastatic involvement of the kidneys, or (5) serum creatinine concentration greater than 3.0 mg/dL at the time of death or history of prior renal disease.

BIBLIOGRAPHY

Comty CM, Shapiro FL: Cardiac complications of regular dialysis therapy, in Drukker W, Parsons FM, Maher JF (eds): *Replacement of Renal Function by Dialysis.* The Hague, Martinus Nijhoff, 1983, pp 595–610.

Corwin HL, Bonventre JV: Acute renal failure. *Med Clin North Am* 70:1037, 1986.

Giacchino JL, Geis WP, Buckingham JM, et al: Vascular access: Long term results, new techniques. *Arch Surg* 114:403, 1979.

Miller TR, Anderson RJ, Linas SL, et al: Urinary diagnostic indices in acute renal failure. A prospective study. *Ann Intern Med* 89:47, 1978.

Nolph KD, Boen FST, Farrell PC, et al: Continuous ambulatory peritoneal dialysis in Australia, Europe and the United States. *Kidney Internatl* 23:3, 1983.

Preminger GM, Peterson R, Peters PC, et al: The current role of medical treatment of nephrolithiasis: The impact of improved techniques of stone removal. *J Urol* 134:6, 1985.

Rao KV: Status of renal transplantation. A clinical perspective. *Med Clin North Am* 68:427, 1984.

Rao KV: Mechanism, pathophysiology, diagnosis and management of renal transplant rejection. *Med Clin North Am* 74:1039, 1990.

Stevens ME, McConnell M, Bone JM: Aggressive treatment with pulse methyl prednisolone or plasma exchange is justified in rapidly progressive glomerulonephritis. *Proc Eur Dialysis Transplant Assoc* 19:724, 1982.

Vaziri ND: Topical thrombin and control of bleeding from the fistula puncture sites in dialyzed patients. *Nephron* 24:254, 1979.

53
URINARY TRACT INFECTIONS

David S. Howes

Urinary tract infection is defined as significant bacteriuria in the presence of symptoms. It affects an estimated 20 percent of women at some point during their lifetime and accounts for a significant number of emergency department visits. Controversial aspects of the diagnosis and management of apparent lower urinary tract infection in adult women will be discussed. In the elderly, urinary tract infection is a major cause of nosocomial gram-negative sepsis, and 1 to 3 percent of all patients with pyelonephritis die.

NATURAL HISTORY

The natural history of urinary tract infection varies with age and sex (Fig. 53-1). In neonates a urinary tract infection is part of the syndrome of overwhelming gram-negative sepsis. The incidence of urinary tract infection in preschool children is approximately 2 percent, with the incidence in girls at least ten times greater than in boys. In school-age children the incidence rises to 5 percent, almost exclusively girls.

Bacteriuria is rare in males under the age of 50 and symptoms of dysuria or urinary frequency are usually due to infection of the urethra or prostate. However, in men older than 50 years the incidence of urinary tract infection rises because of prostatic obstruction or subsequent instrumentation.

Dysuria in females is a common clinical problem and symptoms increase with age and sexual activity. Most urinary tract infections occur in otherwise normal females possibly due to sexual contact and attendant local trauma.

The infecting organisms are generally those found colonizing the perineum, and in women with a traditional "positive" culture of 10^5 colony forming units (CFU) per mL, *Escherichia coli* is responsible for approximately 90 percent of infections. However, one-third to one-half of cases of dysuria are characterized by sterile or low bacterial colony count culture results. This formerly was termed the "acute urethral syndrome" and was not felt to represent true urinary tract infection. In fact, further study revealed that many of these patients had low-grade or early *E. coli*, *Staphylococcus saprophyticus*, or *Chlamydia trachomatis* infections. Therefore, the definition of urinary tract infection based on early studies that reported only upper tract disease may be inappropriate. Such studies established that a colony count of at least 10^5/mL is necessary to indicate the presence of "significant bacteriuria." Current research suggests that with regard to lower urinary tract infection, in the presence of symptoms, a colony count of $\geq 10^3$/mL may represent significant bacteriuria which merits treatment.

The majority of urinary tract infections in women recur either because of relapse or reinfection. Relapse is caused by the same organism; when symptoms recur in less than 1 month this represents treatment failure. When symptoms recur in 1 to 6 months it is generally due to reinfection. Reinfection is usually from a different enteric organism or a different serotype of the same organism and may represent a defect in the defense mechanisms of the host. If a patient has a cluster of infections of more than three recurrences in 1 year, a more complete workup may be warranted to look for the presence of tumor, tuberculosis, renal calculi, structural abnormalities, or associated systemic illness such as diabetes mellitus.

A urinary tract infection during pregnancy poses special problems. If untreated, asymptomatic bacteriuria (ABU) may progress to symptomatic urinary tract infection. Urinary tract infection and pyelonephritis have a high incidence in the third trimester and may lead to preeclampsia, sepsis, or miscarriage. This is the single area in which treatment of ABU is definitely indicated.

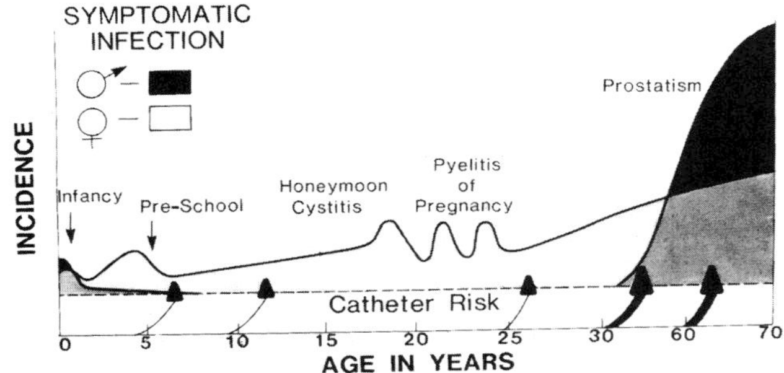

Fig. 53-1. Natural history of urinary tract infections.

BACTERIOLOGY

Urinary tract infection should be thought of as either complicated, that is, occurring in patients with underlying renal or neurologic disease; or uncomplicated, occurring in patients in which no defect can be demonstrated. Most uncomplicated urinary tract infections are caused by gram-negative aerobic bacilli from the gut, the vast majority due to *E. coli* (Table 53-1). As we will discuss in the management section, these coliform bacteria respond to a wide variety of antimicrobial agents. Anaerobic organisms do not grow well in urine and are rarely pathogenic. Complicated urinary tract infections are more often caused by unusual pathogens that may be resistant to multiple antibiotics. These infections will ultimately require management by a urologist or nephrologist.

NORMAL HOST DEFENSE MECHANISMS

Urine is generally a good culture medium depending on its pH and chemical constituents. Factors unfavorable to bacterial growth are a low pH (5.5 or less); a high concentration of urea; and the presence of organic acids derived from a diet including fruit juice and methionine, a breakdown of protein food, which enhances acidification of the urine. A thin film of urine remains in the bladder after voiding. An intact bladder mucosa removes organisms from the film, probably by the production of organic acids by the mucosal cells and not by antibody formation or phagocytosis. Incomplete bladder emptying renders this mechanism ineffective.

Frequent and complete voiding has been associated with the reduction of recurrence of urinary tract infection. Investigators have shown that the concentration of bacteria in the bladder may increase tenfold after sexual intercourse due to a "milking action" of the female urethra during intercourse. It is suggested that prompt voiding after intercourse may lessen the frequency of urinary tract infection. A large urinary flow also dilutes the bacterial inoculum that occasionally occurs; several authors suggest that urinary hydrodynamics may be the most important host defense mechanism.

Table 53-1. Etiologic Agents in Uncomplicated Urinary Tract Infection

Organism	Incidence
E. coli	>80%
Klebsiella *Proteus* sp. *Enterobacter* *Pseudomonas*	5–20%
Group D streptococci *Chlamydia trachomatis** *Staphylococcus saprophyticus**	<5%

* Much more common in the "dysuria-pyuria" syndrome where sterile or low colony count culture results are obtained.

If the mechanisms of the lower urinary tract fail and ascending infection of the urinary tract occurs, renal defense mechanisms are called into play. Local antibodies are produced in the kidney and kill bacteria in the presence of complement. Local leukocytosis and phagocytosis also help eradicate bacteria.

CLINICAL FEATURES

The clinical symptoms of urinary tract infection in an adult are dysuria, frequency, and lower abdominal pain. In females, a history of vaginal discharge should be sought and a pelvic examination must be performed to rule out vaginitis, cervicitis, or pelvic inflammatory disease as the cause of dysuria. Fever, chills, and malaise may also be present.

Flank pain and costovertebral angle tenderness can be associated with cystitis because of referred pain. However, when these are found clinically, one should assume that pyelonephritis is present.

In the male, dysuria with discharge indicates urethritis, and a Gram stain of the discharge is necessary to establish the diagnosis. If gram-negative intracellular diplococci are present, the patient must be treated for gonococcal urethritis. If the Gram stain is inconclusive, the diagnosis is most likely nonspecific urethritis, which is mainly chlamydial infection. In either case, a VDRL test and a culture for gonorrhea should be obtained. It should be emphasized to the emergency department triage personnel that urinary tract infection in young adult males is extremely rare; therefore, a urine specimen should be obtained after examination by the physician. This will enhance the likelihood of a positive urethral swab in the male patient with minimal discharge. If bacteriuria is present and is not clinically associated with urethritis or prostatitis, then treatment, followed by a complete urologic workup, is indicated.

DIAGNOSIS

If urinary tract infection is suspected, the first step in establishing the diagnosis is the careful collection of urine for a urinalysis and potentially for culture. The midstream voiding specimen is as accurate as urine obtained by catheterization if the patient is given and follows careful instructions. Instruct the woman to remove her underwear, sit facing the back of the toilet, spread the labia with one hand, cleanse from front to back with povidone-iodine swabs or liquid soap, pass a small amount of urine into the toilet, and then urinate into a sterile cup. Instruct the man to carefully cleanse the urethral meatus, retracting the foreskin if uncircumcised, and obtain a midsteam specimen as described above.

If the sample is properly collected, it should contain no or few epithelial cells. The many sources of contamination include material in the collection bottle, menses, vaginal discharge, urethral or periurethral tissue, and organisms multiplying in the urine after collection. Bacteria in urine double each hour at room temperature; therefore urine should be refrigerated if not sent directly to the laboratory. In addition to special care in cleansing, the use of a tampon also helps women to obtain a clean-cup specimen if menstruation or profuse discharge is present.

Catheterization is indicated if the patient cannot void spontaneously, is too ill or immobilized, or is extremely obese. It may also be performed as part of a urologic evaluation, and to relieve obstruction. However, routine catheterization should be avoided, as 1 to 2 percent of patients develop urinary tract infection after a single catheter insertion, according to Kunin. This seems to be a problem especially if done just prior to delivery.

Though blood or bile may be detected by gross examination of the urine, visual inspection or the smell of the urine is generally not helpful in determining infection. Cloudiness is usually not due to white blood cells or bacteria but large amounts of protein or crystals. Malodorous urine may be caused by diet or medication ingestion and is not a reliable sign of infection.

Current emphasis is on the detection of pyuria and bacteriuria in the initial examination of the urine. The assessment of pyuria is imperfect. Variables include the method of centrifuging the specimen, the amount of supernatant in which the sediment is resuspended, and the final volume of urine under the cover slip that is examined. Laboratories which use a white-cell counting chamber diminish some of this variability and increase accuracy in assessing both centrifuged and uncentrifuged urine. Stamm has used the latter technique and defined pyuria as the presence of ≥ 8 leukocytes per mL of uncentrifuged urine. This figure roughly corresponds to 2 to 5 leukocytes per high-power field (HPF) in a centrifuged specimen.

Both Komaroff and Stamm feel that this low-level pyuria is clinically important. Other authors have suggested that, in women, pyuria is significant only if there are more than 10 white blood cells (WBC) per HPF, and only if bacteria are present on the microscopic examination. Though this is more likely to be true with typical coliform infection, lower degrees of pyuria with or without bacteriuria may be significant, especially with regard to infection with *Chlamydia*.

As knowledge of urinary tract infection in adult women evolves, it is clear that women with symptoms and low-grade pyuria (fewer than 10 WBC/HPF) do have significant bacteriuria which will symptomatically and bacteriologically respond to antimicrobial therapy. In the past, these women were not treated initially and their cultures often did not establish $> 10^5$CFU/mL. Sensitivity to causes of lower urinary tract infection other than typical coliforms has brought the designation of the "dysuria-pyuria syndrome" which almost always benefits from treatment. It is in this subgroup of women that the urinalysis may well be more useful than the urine culture, which is often misleading, especially as reported in standard microbiological laboratories. In addition, a positive urinalysis would dictate more immediate management interventions than would awaiting a urine culture.

In men, more than 1 to 2 WBC/HPF can be significant in the presence of bacteria. Again it must be remembered that urethritis or prostatitis are far more likely causes of pyuria in young males.

Bacteriuria is also felt to be a sensitive tool for detection of urinary tract infection in the symptomatic patient. The presence of any bacteria on a Gram stain of uncentrifuged urine is significant. In a clean specimen this correlated to a high degree with culture results. This statement is also true if more than 15 bacteria per HPF are found in a centrifuged specimen. Both of these methods will fail to detect low colony count urinary tract infection or infection caused by *Chlamydia*. False positives occur when vaginal or fecal contamination is present.

Several authors have advocated the use of the nitrate urine test. Although a positive nitrate reaction has a very high specificity, its sensitivity is very low, rendering it much less useful as a screening examination.

More recently, the presence of leukocyte esterase in the urine has been evaluated as an indicator of the presence of pyuria. Initial reports of high sensitivity supported use of this test as a screening tool for pyuria. However, Propp found an unacceptable rate of false-negative results for low-level pyuria (6 to 20 WBC/HPF) in an emergency department setting.

When the clinical presentation suggests pyuria, a positive leukocyte esterase test supports the diagnosis, and treatment should be initiated. If the test is negative, a microscopic examination should be performed to detect lower levels of clinically significant pyuria.

Unfortunately, we are still left with women who complain of dysuria, have no pyuria or demonstrable pathogen on culture, and who do not respond to antimicrobial treatment. The absence of pyuria in these patients is useful because it indicates that antimicrobial treatment is probably unnecessary. Presuming that vulvovaginitis has been excluded, causes of this dysuria may include inflammation of the urethra from physical trauma or due to the use of chemical agents, e.g., spermicides, cleansing douches, or other feminine hygiene products.

In a symptomatic patient who has less than 2 to 5 WBC/HPF, other causes of false-negative pyuria should be considered. These include ingestion of large amounts of fluids which wash out the bladder and produce a dilute urine, and, more likely, old or leftover medication, or a drug belonging to another person, being taken by the patient on a self-directed basis. It should be remembered that, in the case of an obstructed kidney, pyuria may be intermittent or absent.

The classical definition for diagnosis of urinary tract infection has been a count of > 10^5/mL from a midstream catch. If the patient is symptomatic, a single positive culture is significant. For asymptomatic bacteriuria two or three positive cultures are necessary before treatment is undertaken, with the rejoinder that treatment is always indicated in pregnancy. Lastly, the classical definition of urinary tract infection as based on culture results is changing, and current emphasis is on detection of pyuria. Most authors agree that a urine culture must be obtained in the following settings: acute pyelonephritis; subclinical pyelonephritis (which should be especially suspected in those patients with underlying urinary tract disease, diabetes mellitus, immunocompromised state, recent instrumentation, prolonged symptoms before seeking care, three or more infections in the past year, or a history of acute pyelonephritis in the recent past); any patient who needs to be hospitalized; those patients who have a chronic indwelling catheter; and all children and adult males.

TREATMENT

The selection of antibiotics depends upon the suspected bacteriology of the infection, the patient's compliance, potential drug toxicity, and cost. In uncomplicated urinary tract infection *E. coli* is the offending microorganism in the vast majority of cases. This and other typical coliform pathogens are susceptible to a wide variety of agents: sulfonamides, trimethoprim, co-trimoxazole, extended-spectrum penicillins (e.g., amoxicillin), nitrofurantoin macrocrystals, cephalosporins, and the quinolones (Table 53-2).

Most authorities have, until recently, recommended treating the first episode of urinary tract infection with a 10- or 14-day antibiotic regimen. A sulfonamide, trimethoprim or the combination (co-trimoxazole), is generally recommended as these are cheap and effective (Table 53-3). Alternatives include cephalosporins and amoxicillin. In cases of treatment failure or in the host with a structural or immunologic defect, use of amoxicillin with clavulanic acid, nitrofurantoin macrocrystals, or one of the quinolones may be considered. Concern about the emergence of resistant organisms and expense preclude indiscriminate use of the latter agents. The urine should be bacteria-free in 24 to 48 h with substantial relief of symptoms within the same time period. The offer of 1 to 2 days of an oral bladder analgesic, e.g., phenazopyridine (Pyridium), is considerate when urination is painful for the patient.

Recently, multiple investigational reports of shorter treatment regimens for uncomplicated infections in nonpregnant adult women have been published. Single-dose treatment appears to offer a number of advantages: Cost and side effects are substantially reduced, compliance

Table 53-3. Cost Comparison of Urinary Antimicrobial Agents

Generic name	Cost of 10-Day Course, $*	Brand Name	Cost, $*
Trimethoprim	12.91	Proloprim	23.19
Sulfamethoxazole	9.16	Gantanol	25.19
Co-trimoxazole	9.29	Bactrim or Septra	24.59
Amoxicillin	10.99	Amoxil	NA
Doxycycline	12.19	Vibramycin	62.69
Amoxicillin with clavulanic acid	NA	Augmentin	54.19
Nalidixic acid	NA	NegGram	44.09
Ciprofloxacin or norfloxacin	NA	Cipro or Noroxin	53.72
Nitrofurantoin macrocrystals	NA	Macrodantin	25.79

* The prices given are retail prices in the Chicago metropolitan area in January 1991 obtained by telephone survey by the author.

Table 53-2. Guidelines to Outpatient Management of Uncomplicated Urinary Tract Infection

Type of Patient	Presumed Type of Infection	Clinical Characteristics	Antimicrobial Regimens	Comments
Adult female	Lower	Few prior episodes with brief duration of symptoms and no risk factors for subclinical pyelonephritis	1. Co-trimoxazole, 2 double-strength tablets *or* 2. Co-trimoxazole, 1 double-strength tablet bid × 3 days	Singe-dose or brief-duration regimen Good follow-up available No culture needed.
Adult female	Lower/upper	Risk of subclinical pyelonephritis: prolonged symptoms, relapse or recurrent UTI, diabetes mellitus, urinary tract abnormalities, recent pyelonephritis, indigent patients	1. Sulfamethoxazole, 2 g initially then 1 g bid 2. Co-trimoxazole, 1 double-strength tablet bid 3. Cefadroxil, 500–1000 mg bid 4. Amoxicillin, 250–500 mg tid 5. Nitrofurantoin macrocrystals, 50–100 mg qid *or* Amoxicillin with clavulanic acid, 250–500 mg tid *or* Norfloxacin or ciprofloxacin, 250–500 mg bid (if resistant organism suspected)	10–14 day course advised Consider culture Coliforms typical
Adult male	Lower/upper	Suspect underlying anatomic abnormality; R/O urethritis, prostatitis	Same as above	Same as above
Adult female	Lower	Stuttering symptoms, new sexual partner or partner with urethritis, signs and symptoms of cervicitis, pyuria without bacteriuria	1. Doxycycline, 100 mg bid 2. Co-trimoxazole, 1 double-strength tablet bid 3. Sulfamethoxazole, 1 g bid 4. Erythromycin, 500 mg qid (in allergy or pregnancy-related cases and will only eradicate *Chlamydia*)	10–14 day course Culture for GC advisable

improves, and the development of resistant strains of bacteria is less likely.

These reports have also generated concern. The entity of subclinical pyelonephritis has become increasingly apparent during studies of what was felt to be uncomplicated lower urinary tract infection. Detection of this entity requires sophisticated differentiation based on analysis of immunofluorescent antibody results or analysis for β-glucuronidase and lactate dehydrogenase isoenzymes. At this time these tests are principally useful as research tools and are not helpful in the routine clinical arena.

Because of this, single-dose or short-term (e.g., 3-day) regimens have limitations. In several series, a disturbing number of patients with apparent simple cystitis exhibited tissue invasion as demonstrated by the presence of antibody coated bacteria (ACB), i.e., unsuspected or subclinical pyelonephritis. This group had a poor response to short-term therapy when compared to patients who received traditional 10- or 14-day treatment and had positive ACB. Since ACB testing is justifiable only in research settings, this raises questions about the efficacy of short-term therapy in episodic care settings.

On the other hand, several authors suggest that single-dose treatment may as reliably identify patients with subclinical pyelonephritis as available diagnostic tests. This is because a single-dose or a short course of antibiotics is less likely to eradicate bacteriuria in the patient with tissue invasion. In practice, they suggest that all women with urethrocystitis symptoms be given a single dose or brief course of co-trimoxazole with the expectation of cure in the vast majority. The few patients with recurrence of symptoms, pyuria, and bacteriuria will be promptly identified as having complicated infection necessitating more prolonged therapy.

In certain emergency department settings, especially those serving indigent populations where there is delay in seeking care, the incidence of subclinical pyelonephritis may approach 70 percent of patients. In this circumstance, single-dose therapy is difficult to justify. This is especially important because acute pyelonephritis following single-dose therapy has been reported. Therefore, before an emergency physician decides to utilize a single-dose treatment, the patient's ability to follow up within 1 week must be ensured. If follow-up compliance is not expected, or the epidemiologic risk of subclinical pyelonephritis is great, then the patient should be placed on a conventional regimen. Three-day regimens are as effective as 10-day regimens in those patients who do not demonstrate ACB, but the efficacy in patients with possible tissue invasion is likely to be lower than a conventional prolonged course of therapy.

One should be suspicious that *Chlamydia* is responsible for symptoms in the following settings: a woman with a recent, new sexual partner; a partner with urethritis; examination findings of cervicitis; or when there is low-grade pyuria with no bacteria seen on urinalysis. A 10-day course of sulfonamides or doxycycline is the preferred treatment. Though erythromycin is very effective for chlamydial infections, it is ineffective against coliform bacteria. Therefore, it cannot be recommended as empiric therapy.

For recurrent infection, culture and sensitivity tests are essential. The infection is often due to a new serotype of *E. coli,* or it may be due to newly resistant organisms which develop as a result of antibiotics excreted into the gastrointestinal tract. Empiric therapy for recurrent infections includes co-trimoxazole, nitrofurantoin macrocrystals, or the quinolones. However, successful management depends on sensitivity testing. Again, it must be emphasized that these patients need referral in the setting of chronic, recurrent infection. The institution of chronic, suppressive therapy should be left to a specialist.

Aggressive therapy is warranted for pregnant women with pyuria or bacteriuria, whether or not associated symptoms are present. Most authors suggest ampicillin or a cephalosporin as the outpatient treatment of choice. A sulfa drug can also be used, except near term and in those with G6PD deficiency. All regimens should be continued for 14 days. Inpatient management is stressed for suspected pyelonephritis as the incidence is higher in pregnancy, and maternal and fetal morbidity is substantial. Urine culture is mandatory.

Adjunctive therapy should include plenty of fluids to enhance diuresis, fruit juices containing vitamin C to acidify the urine, a proper diet, and frequent voiding (at least every two hours) to diminish tissue contact with bacteria. Women should be reminded that postintercourse voiding may be helpful in reducing recurrent infection.

Once the infection is eradicated management should be directed toward prevention of reinfection. This is designed to prevent ascending kidney infection. Up to 80 percent of women who have had a urinary tract infection develop recurrence. Since many factors are involved in reinfection and some of these are correctable, continuity of care is essential.

PYELONEPHRITIS

On occasion, it may be difficult to distinguish lower from upper urinary tract infection. Classically, acute pyelonephritis is characterized by shaking chills and fever, flank pain, and costovertebral angle tenderness following several days of dysuria and frequency. The urine will often demonstrate white blood cell casts and clumps as well as bacteria.

Factors associated with pyelonephritis include pregnancy, prolonged symptoms prior to seeking care, three or more infections in the past year, immunocompromised state, and diabetes mellitus. Less often one may find congenital or acquired anatomic urinary tract abnormality, neurogenic problems that result in incomplete bladder emptying, recent urinary tract instrumentation, renal calculi and nephrocalcinosis, prostatic hypertrophy, or prostatitis present.

Young, otherwise healthy females with uncomplicated acute pyelonephritis may be candidates for outpatient management. A popular regimen at our institution is referred to as "treatment by [the rule of] twos." While in the emergency department, the patient is given 2 L of IV fluid, 2 Tylenol #3 capsules, and 2 g of ceftriaxone. If the fever drops by 2 degrees and the patient is able to hold down 2 glasses of water, an outpatient prescription for co-trimoxazole DS, 2 times per day for 2 weeks, is given. The patient is to follow up in 2 days, for a progress check. A recent study showed that outpatient therapy for selected patients was as safe and effective and considerably less expensive than in a comparable group of patients treated on an inpatient basis.

The decision to admit a patient with acute pyelonephritis is based on age, host factors, and response to initial emergency department interventions. Fluid replacement and parenteral antibiotics are necessary if the patient is vomiting or dehydrated. Unremitting fever and loss of vasomotor tone mandate inpatient therapy. For initial management in an otherwise healthy host with no prior or recent history of urinary tract infection, the typical offending bacteria would include *E. coli* as well as other coliform bacteria. Recent recommendations favor a single intravenous agent such as trimethoprim-sulfamethoxazole, 160 and 800 mg, q 12 h; a third-generation cephalosporin, e.g., ceftriaxone, 1 g q 12 h; or an aminoglycoside, e.g., gentamicin, 1.5 mg/kg, q 8 h. The selection of which drugs to use depends on cost considerations and on local sensitivity patterns.

Younger patients without complicating factors have the least morbidity or mortality. Despite appropriate intervention, 1 to 3 percent of patients with acute pyelonephritis die. Factors associated with an unfavorable prognosis are old age and general debility, renal calculi or obstruction, a recent history of hospitalization or instrumentation, diabetes mellitus, evidence of chronic nephropathy, sickle cell anemia, underlying carcinoma, or intercurrent cancer chemotherapy. In this type of patient it is imperative that broad-spectrum antibiotic coverage to include *Pseudomonas* spp. be provided. A urologic or infectious disease consultation should be considered as part of the initial management of such patients.

Complications of acute pyelonephritis include acute papillary necrosis with possible ureteric obstruction, septic shock, and perinephric abscesses. Adequate fluid hydration must be emphasized in these settings.

BIBLIOGRAPHY

Carlson KJ, Mulley AG: Management of acute dysuria: A decision-analysis model of alternative strategies. *Ann Intern Med* 102:244, 1985.

Fihn SD, Johnson C, Roberts PL, et al: Trimethoprim-sulfamethoxazole for acute dysuria in women: A single-dose or 10-day course. *Ann Intern Med* 108:350, 1988.

Hankins GDV, Whalley PJ: Acute urinary tract infections in pregnancy. *Clin Obstet Gynecol* 28:266, 1985.

Hooton TM, Running K, Stamm WE: Single-dose therapy for cystitis in women: A comparison of trimethoprim-sulfamethoxazole, amoxicillin, and cyclacillin. *JAMA* 253:387, 1985.

Johnson JR, Stamm WE: Urinary tract infection in women: Diagnosis and treatment. *Ann Intern Med* 111:906, 1989.

Komaroff AL: Acute dysuria in women. *N Engl J Med* 310:368, 1984.

Komaroff AL: Urinalysis and urine culture in women with dysuria. *Ann Intern Med* 104:212, 1986.

Lipsky BA: Urinary tract infections in men: Epidemiology, pathophysiology, diagnosis, and treatment. *Ann Intern Med* 110:138, 1989.

McCabe JB, Hamilton GC: Single-dose antibiotic therapy of urinary tract infection: Is it appropriate in the emergency department? *Ann Emerg Med* 13:432, 1984.

Propp DA, Weber D, Ciesla ML: Reliability of a urine dipstick in emergency department patients. *Ann Emerg Med* 18:560, 1989.

Sanders LL, Harrison HR, Washington AE: Treatment of sexually transmitted chlamydial infections. *JAMA* 255:1750, 1986.

Safrin S, Siegel D, Black D: Pyelonephritis in adult women: inpatient versus outpatient therapy. *Am J Med* 85:793, 1988.

Schulta HJ, McCaffrey LA, Keys TF, et al: Acute cystitis: A prospective study of laboratory tests and duration of therapy. *Mayo Clin Proc* 59:391, 1984.

Shaw ST, Poon SY, Wong ET: "Routine urinalysis": Is the dipstick enough? *JAMA* 53:1596, 1985.

Stamm WE, Running K, McKevitt M, et al: Treatment of the acute urethral syndrome. *N Engl J Med* 304:956, 1981.

Strom BL, Collins M, West SL, et al: Sexual activity, contraceptive use, and other risk factors for symptomatic and asymptomatic bacteriuria: A case control study. *Ann Intern Med* 107:816, 1987.

54
MALE GENITAL PROBLEMS
Robert E. Schneider

One of the most anxiety-provoking problems presenting to an emergency department is the male with acute genital pain. The extensive sensory innervation of this area produces severe symptoms, and the close relationships of the abdominal and genital sensory afferent pathways in the male account for the common association of abdominal pain with some acute genitourinary disorders.

ANATOMY

Penis

The penis is composed of three cylindrical bodies: the two corpora cavernosa, which form the main bulk of the penis, and the corpus spongiosum, which surrounds the urethra (Fig. 54-1). The corpora cavernosa are the major erectile bodies, extending distally from the pubic rami and capped by the glans penis. These two cylindical structures are encased in a thick tunic of dense connective tissue, the tunica albuginea. All three cylinders are collectively covered by a thinner Buck's fascia, which fuses with Colles' fascia at the level of the urogenital diaphragm.

The blood supply is primarily from the internal pudendal artery, which branches to form the deep and superficial penile arteries. Lymphatic drainage is into the deep and superficial inguinal nodes.

Scrotum

The prepubertal scrotal skin is thin and thickens with subsequent hormonal stimulation. Immediately beneath the skin are the smooth muscle and elastic tissue layers of dartos fascia, the continuous conjoined Camper's and Scarpa's fascial layers of the abdominal wall (Fig. 54-2). This fused layer extends into the perineum as Colles' fascia. The blood supply is primarily derived from branches of the femoral and internal pudendal arteries. Lymphatics from the scrotum drain into the inguinal and femoral nodes.

Testes

The testes usually lie in an upright position with the superior portion tipped slightly forward and outward. The average size is between 4 and 5 cm in length and approximately 3 cm in width and depth. The overall volume is about 25 mL. Each testis is encased in a thick fibrous

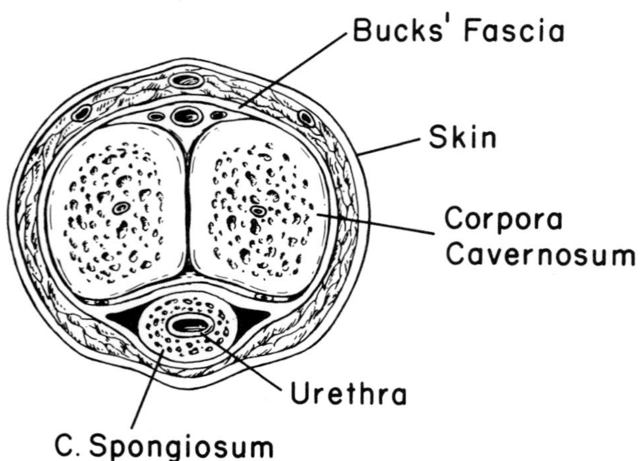

Fig. 54-1. Cross section of the penis.

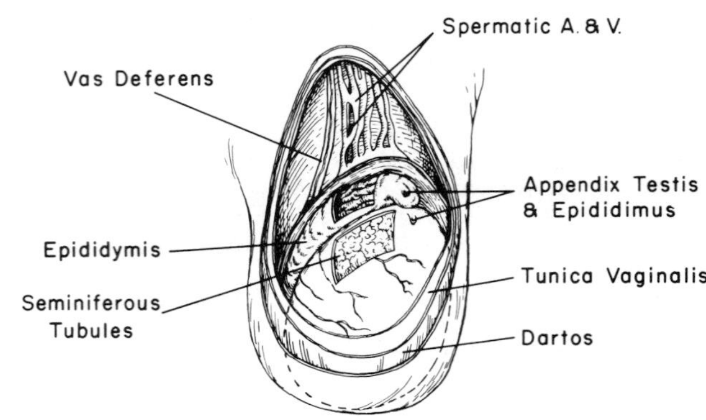

Fig. 54-2. Anatomy of the scrotum and the testis.

tunica albuginea except posterolaterally, where it is in tight apposition with the epididymis. The enveloping tunica vaginalis anchors each testis and epididymis to the posterior scrotal wall. Inferiorly, the testis is anchored to the scrotum by the scrotal ligament (gubernaculum). A lack of proper fixation leaves both structures at risk for torsion. The posterior (visceral) leaf of tunica vaginalis is contiguous with the tunica albuginea testis. A potential space exists between this visceral leaf and the anterior (parietal) tunica vaginalis. Any traumatic or inflammatory event will impede the normal parietal tunica vaginalis from absorbing viscerally secreted fluid, resulting in a hydrocele (Fig. 54-3).

The blood supply is by the internal spermatic, differential, and external spermatic arteries, which travel together in the spermatic cord. Venous return is primarily by the internal spermatic, epigastric, internal circumflex, and scrotal veins. The lymphatics drain toward the external, common iliac, and periaortic nodes.

The epididymis is a single, fine, tubular structure approximately 4 to 5 m long compressed into an area of about 5 cm. The function of the epididymis is to promote sperm maturation and motility. Vestigial embryonic structures, the appendix epididymis and the appendix testis, which have no known physiologic function, are often associated with the testes and epididymis. The appendix epididymis, a remnant of the epigenitales, is found attached to the head of the epididymis, or globus major. The appendix testis, a pear-shaped structure of müllerian duct origin, is usually situated on the uppermost portion of the testis at the junction of the testis and the globus major.

The vas deferens, a prominent part of the adnexa of the scrotal contents, is a distinct muscular tube that is easily palpable within the scrotal sac. It extends cephalad in the spermatic cord from the tail of the epididymis (globus minor), traveling the inguinal canal and crossing medially behind the bladder over the ureters to form the ampullae of the vas, where it joins with the seminal vesicles to form the paired ejaculatory ducts in the prostatic urethra.

Prostate

The prostate originates from the urogenital sinus at approximately the third month of embryonic life. It is continually enlarging and in the young male is approximately 10 to 15 g, often not definable on rectal examination. As a man matures, the prostate may enlarge dramatically, resulting in significant outlet obstruction. The hyperplastic adenoma envelops the urethra between the bladder neck and the urogenital diaphragm. Positioned just anterior to the rectal ampulla, its posterior surface is readily palpable on rectal examination.

PHYSICAL EXAMINATION

Physical examination should be carried out with the patient in both the supine and upright positions in a well-illuminated, warm room. If the scrotum is contracted despite proper room temperature, a warm

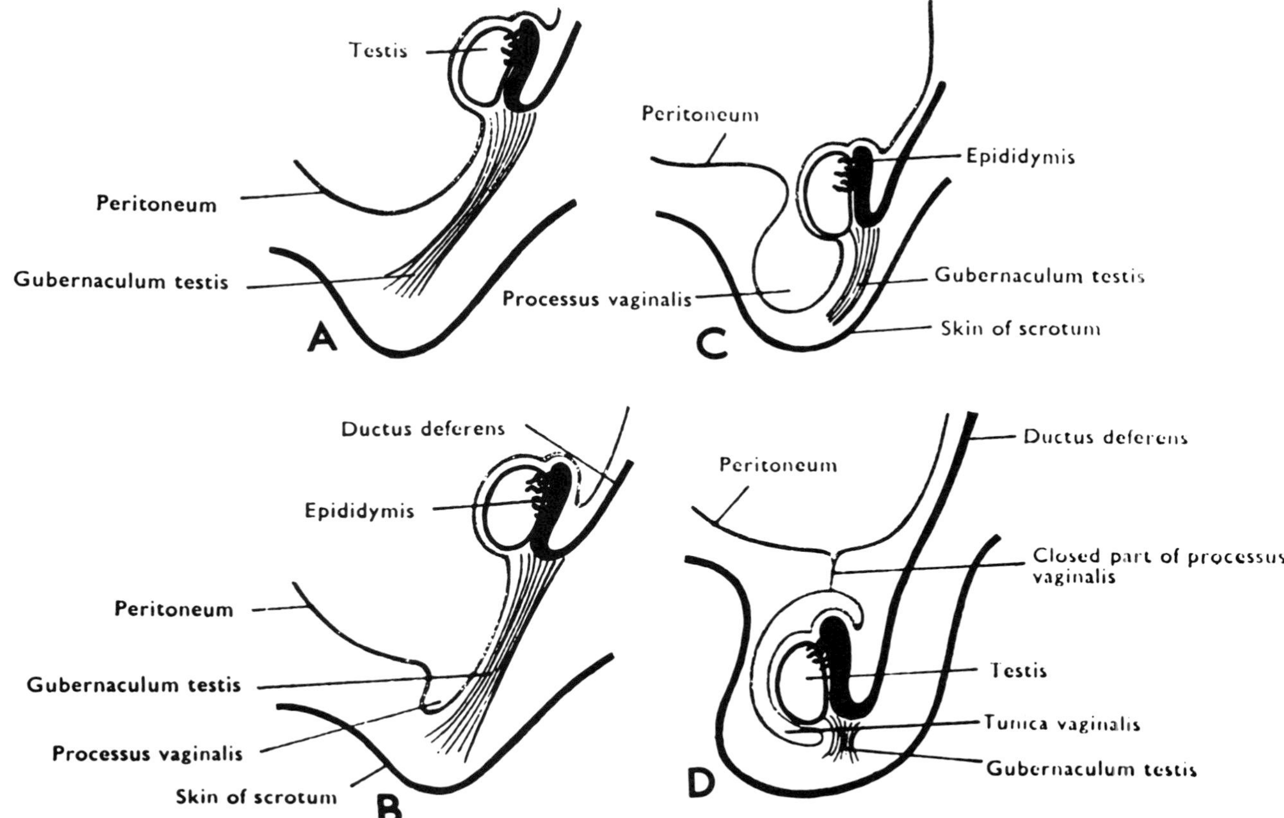

Fig. 54-3. Embryonic retroperitoneal testis descends into the scrotum and invaginates into the tunica vaginalis which anchors it to the posterior scrotal wall. Note the potential space in the tunica vaginalis for development of a hydrocele.

towel placed over the genitalia permits the scrotum and testes to descend and be comfortably examined.

Examination should always begin with visual inspection. In uncircumcised males, the foreskin should be fully retracted to inspect the glans, coronal sulcus, and preputial areas. The location of the urethral meatus and presence of discharge should be noted. The penile shaft should be carefully palpated for plaques, cysts, or early abscesses.

Examination of the inguinal canals for hernias and the scrotal spermatic cords for varicoceles is best done in the upright position, with the patient straining at the appropriate time. When the patient is upright, it should be determined whether the testes are aligned along a vertical or horizontal axis. Horizontally aligned testes are at risk of torsion. Actual testicular examination, with palpation of the testes and epididymis, should be performed in the supine position to prevent an infrequent vasovagal response. Testicular nodularity or firmness should be considered carcinoma until proven otherwise. The epididymis usually lies on the posterolateral aspect of the testis and, if not inflamed or involved with other pathological entities, has a soft, fleshy feel similar to that of the earlobe. Many males experience pain and tenderness with palpation of a normal globus major (head), body, and globus minor (tail) of the epididymis.

The supine or modified lithotomy position seems to be more comfortable for both the examiner and the patient and allows a more thorough examination of the prostate, seminal vesicles, and rectal ampulla.

When the prostate is palpated, it normally has a heart-shaped contour with its apex located more distally, abutting the urogenital diaphragm (anatomic soft spot). The posterior lobe is small and thin, allowing palpation of the median raphe that distinguishes the two lateral lobes. A common analogy used to describe the consistency of the prostate is that normal tissue has the same resiliency as the cartilaginous tip of the nose, while suspicious carcinogenic areas feel more like the bony prominence of the chin. A normal rectal examination does not exclude outlet obstruction secondary to an obstructing median bar or large intravesical prostate. The seminal vesicles, lying just superior to the prostate, cannot normally be distinguished unless there is inflammation, induration, or enlargement.

The uncircumcised male patient should retract his foreskin and wash the glans penis with plain tap water before collecting a midstream specimen. Failure to do so will result in preputial contamination. The often described three-cup specimen used to localize male lower urinary tract infections is time-consuming and requires patient compliance, both factors that tend to limit its usefulness in the emergency department. The differential diagnosis of hematuria or pyuria in a properly collected urine specimen is listed in Table 54-1.

COMMON GENITOURINARY DISORDERS

Scrotum

Because the scrotal skin is loose and elastic, dramatic enlargement of the scrotum may occur secondary to either scrotal or testicular pathological conditions.

Scrotal Edema

Simple isolated scrotal edema is uncommon and usually occurs secondary to insect or human bites or in young boys secondary to idiopathic scrotal edema. Contiguous scrotal and penile edema occurs in older men in conjunction with lower extremity edema in fluid overload states (congestive heart failure), hypoalbuminemia, and generalized anasarca.

Table 54-1. Etiology of Hematuria and Pyuria

Genitourinary trauma
Blunt or penetrating
Urethral instrumentation
Tumor
Stones
Sloughed papillae
Sickle cell anemia
Non-steroidal anti-inflammatory drugs (NSAIDs)
Diabetes mellitus
Infection
Pyogenic
Tuberculous

Fournier's Gangrene

An acutely swollen, edematous, necrotic scrotum with no demonstrable urinary problem is often a presenting sign of Fournier's gangrene, or idiopathic scrotal gangrene (Fig. 54-4). In its later stages, gangrene, subcutaneous emphysema, and crepitance develop. A roentgenogram or sonogram of the genitalia will identify gas or an abscess. The etiology may be a traumatic abrasion or scratch that allows the entrance of anaerobic streptococci beneath the skin, or invasions of gram-negative rods and anaerobes from perirectal disease. A mean of 3.4 organisms has been isolated in most studies, more commonly in men who are immunocompromised, whether from self-induced immunosuppression from chronic alcoholism or drug addiction or from iatrogenic steroid therapy or diabetes mellitus.

Fournier's gangrene is a life-threatening surgical emergency. Aggressive fluid resuscitation and the administration of antibiotics such as penicillin, clindamycin, or flagyl and an aminoglycoside, and hyperbaric oxygenation are immediately necessary. Urologic consultation is mandatory for debridement and suprapubic urinary drainage.

Phlegmon

The physical findings for an intraurethral or periurethral phlegmon are similar to those for Fournier's gangrene, but the patient also complains of marked urinary symptoms, usually urinary retention or overflow incontinence. Urethral extravasation of infected urine due to either a stricture or trauma causes acute necrosis of the skin with subsequent infection. Infection characteristically does not extend below the inguinal folds of the thigh but can extend cephalad as far as the chest.

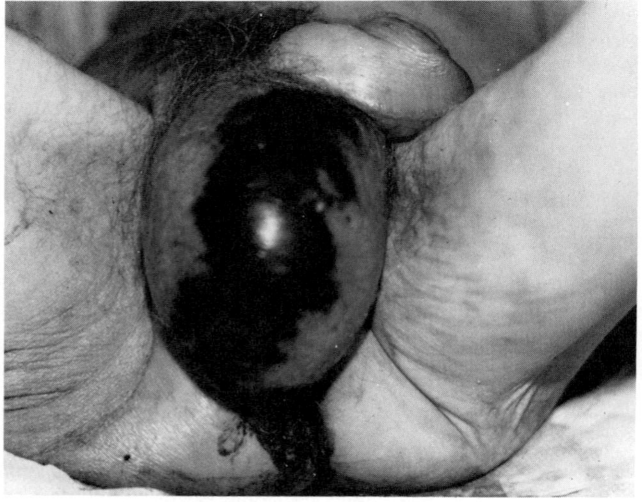

Fig. 54-4. A patient with idiopathic gangrene of the scrotum. Note the sharp demarcation of gangrenous changes and the marked edema of the scrotum and the penis.

Treatment includes antibiotic administration, incision and drainage, and suprapubic urinary diversion.

Other Problems

Simple hair folliculitis, more common in diabetic men, should be treated as a superficial abscess. Careful examination before incision and drainage is necessary to confirm that the abscess involves only the scrotal skin and is not contiguous with the intrascrotal contents. Intrascrotal extension may require surgery, including orchiectomy.

Penis

Balanoposthitis

Balanitis is inflammation of the glans penis. Posthitis is inflammation of the foreskin. Balanoposthitis is inflammation of both the glans and foreskin. When foreskin retraction is attempted, the glans and apposing prepuce appear purulent, excoriated, malodorous, and tender. When recurrent, it can be the sole presenting sign of diabetes. Treatment consists of cleansing the area with mild soap, assuring adequate dryness, application of antifungal creams (nystatin and Lotrimin) and possibly circumcision. If secondary bacterial infection is present, a broad-spectrum antibiotic, usually a cephalosporin, should be given.

Phimosis

Phimosis is the inability to retract the foreskin proximally and posterior to the glans penis. Causes include infection, poor hygiene, or previous preputial injury with scarring. Scarring at the tip of the foreskin can occlude the meatus, causing urinary retention. Hemostatic dilation of the preputial ostium relieves the urinary retention until definitive dorsal slit or circumcision can be done.

Paraphimosis

Paraphimosis is the inability to reduce the proximally existing edematous foreskin over the distal glans penis into its naturally occurring position (Fig. 54-5). The resulting glans edema and venous engorgement can progress to arterial compromise and gangrene.

Paraphimosis is a true urologic emergency. If the surrounding tissue edema can be successfully compressed, the foreskin may be reduced, as demonstrated in Figure 54-5. If arterial compromise is suspected or has occurred, urologic consultation is necessary. Local infiltration of the constricting band with 1% plain lidocaine followed by superficial vertical incision of the band will decompress the glans and allow foreskin reduction.

Entrapment Injuries

Various objects can be placed around the penis, initially occluding the venous, and subsequently the arterial, blood supply. String, metal rings, and wire have been wrapped around the penis for sexual, experimental, or accidental reasons. One of the most insidious objects that can become entrapped behind the coronal ridge is human hair, usually found in young circumcised boys aged 2 to 5 years (Fig. 54-6). The child presents with swelling of the glans. The offending hair may be invisible within the edematous coronal sulcus. If the hair has been chronically occluding, the urethra and dorsal nerve supply of the penis may be partially or completely involved. Removal of the offending object requires ingenuity and care. Urethral integrity (retrograde urethrogram) and distal penile arterial blood supply (Doppler) must be assured prior to emergency department discharge.

Fracture of the Penis

An acute tear or rupture of the penile tunica albuginea is rare but easily diagnosed. The penis is acutely swollen, discolored, and tender. The

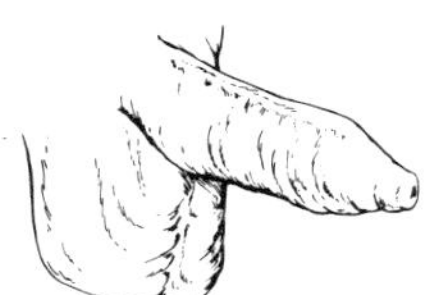

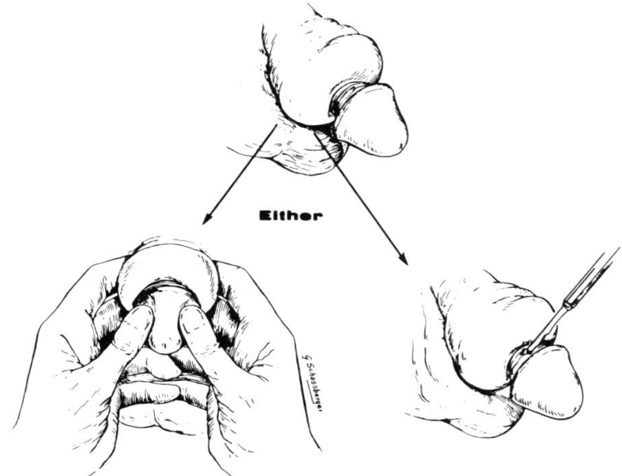

Fig. 54-5. Phimosis and paraphimosis. (The lower figure depicts the method of reduction.)

history is of trauma during intercourse or other sexual activity, when a sudden "snapping sound" occurs. Even though the urethra is infrequently injured, a retrograde urethrogram is necessary to assure urethral integrity. Surgical treatment consists of hematoma evacuation and suture apposition of the disrupted tunica albuginea.

Peyronie's Disease

The patient complains of either gradual or sudden onset of dorsal penile curvature with erections. Examination of the dorsal penile shaft will disclose a thickened plaque involving the tunica albuginea of the corpora bodies without urethral involvement. Reassurance and urologic referral are warranted. Peyronie's disease of the penis has been noted in association with Dupuytren's contracture of the hand.

Carcinoma

Carcinoma of the penis is a rare disease occurring in about 1 out of every 100,000 malignancies reported, usually appearing in the fifth or sixth decade in an uncircumcised male. Carcinoma may appear as a nontender ulcer or warty growth beneath the foreskin in the area of the coronal sulcus or glans penis. It is often hidden by an inflamed phimotic foreskin.

Priapism

Priapism is a painful, hard, tender, pathological erection in which both corpora cavernosa are engorged with stagnant blood. Even though the glans penis and the corpus spongiosum urethra are characteristically soft and uninvolved, urinary retention may occur. Infection and impotence are other common complications.

Priapism is commonly called reversible or nonreversible depending upon etiology and the response to medical treatment. Reversible priapism may respond to medical treatment, while nonreversible priapism usually does not respond to medical treatment and requires shunt surgery. Urologic consultation is necessary for both reversible or nonreversible forms.

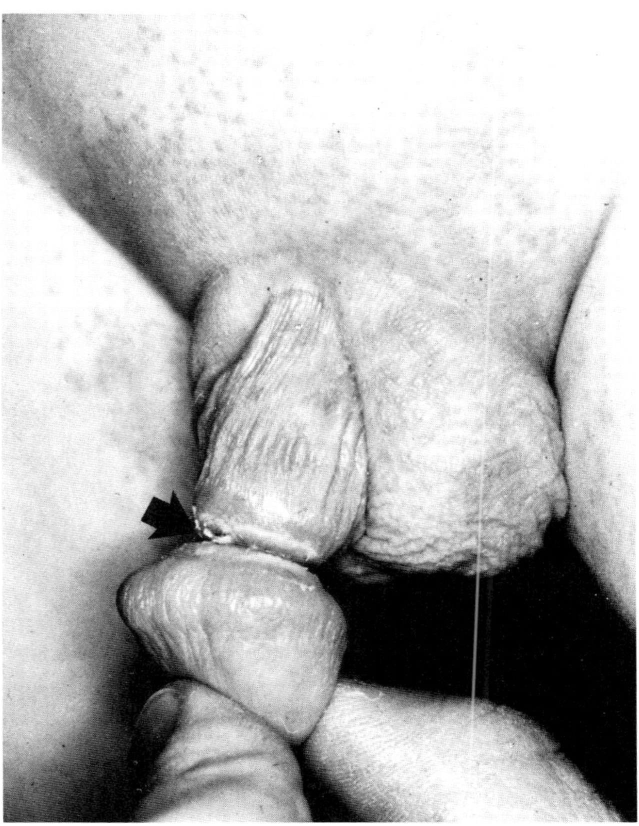

Fig. 54-6. Hair is entrapped behind the corona (arrow), constricting and progressively amputating the glans.

Table 54-2 lists the etiology and treatment of priapism. Regardless of etiology, initial therapy is terbutaline, 0.25 to 0.5 mg subcutaneously every 4 to 6 h. Neither sedation nor ice water enemas are effective.

Testes and Epididymis

Testicular Torsion

The differential diagnosis of acute scrotal pain includes testicular torsion, torsion of the appendix testis, and epididymitis, but testicular torsion must be the primary consideration (Fig. 54-7). While the peak incidence of intravaginal torsion occurs at puberty in conjunction with maximal hormonal stimulation, it may occur at any age.

Table 54-2. Causes and Treatment of Priapism

Reversible Causes
1. Sickle cell anemia
   Treatment: Terbutaline, 0.25–0.5 mg subcutaneously every 4 to 6 h; packed red blood cell transfusion; hyperbaric oxygenation
2. Iatrogenic injection (of PGE1, papaverine, or phentolamine) for impotence
   Treatment: Terbutaline, 0.25–0.5 mg sc q 4 to 6 h; aspirate 30–90 mL corporal blood, then inject 30–90 mL of 10 mg neosynephrine in 500 mL NS
3. Leukemic infiltration
   Treatment: Terbutaline, 0.25–0.5 mg sc q 4 to 6 h; specific chemotherapy

Nonreversible Causes
1. Idiopathic
2. High spinal cord lesion
3. Medication (phenothiazines, desyrel)
   Treatment of all nonreversible causes: Terbutaline, 0.25 to 0.5 mg sc q 4 to 6 h; pseudoephedrine instillation; corporal aspiration and heparin irrigation; shunt surgery

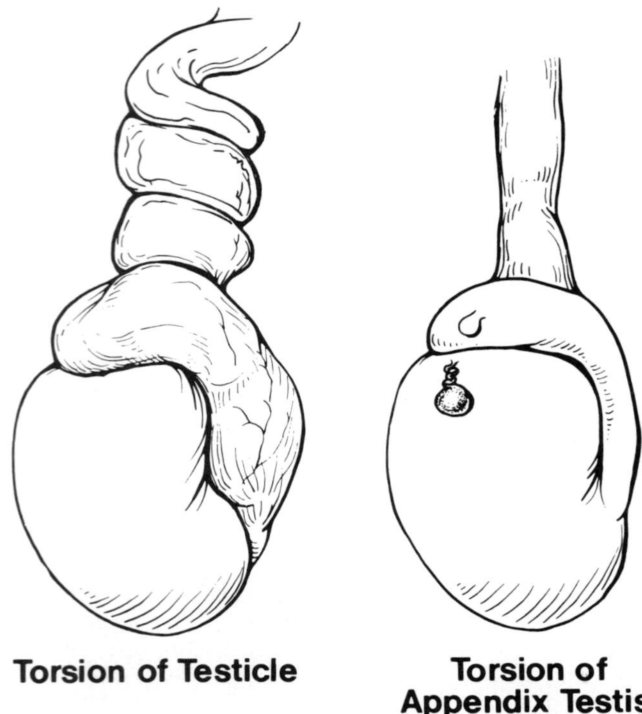

Fig. 54-7. Diagrams of testicular torsion and torsion of the appendix testis.

Torsion of the testis or spermatic cord results from bilateral maldevelopment of fixation between the enveloping tunica vaginalis and the posterior scrotal wall. Characteristically, the at-risk testis is aligned along a horizontal rather than a vertical axis. The axis of alignment can only be determined with the patient in an upright position, and even then the determination may be difficult.

Frequently there is a history of an athletic event or strenuous physical activity just prior to the onset of scrotal pain. However, a fair number occur during sleep. Unilateral cremaster muscle contraction results in testicular torsion. The pain usually occurs suddenly, is severe, and is felt in either lower abdominal quadrant, the inguinal canal, or the testis. The pain may be constant or intermittent.

Once the diagnosis is considered, urologic consultation is necessary. Radionuclide imaging can be a helpful diagnostic study, but availability and reader sensitivity make this a time-intensive procedure in a very time-dependent condition. The often quoted 4-h warm ischemia time for testicular salvage comes from controlled animal studies and cannot be extrapolated to clinical medicine. There are no readily available clinical or laboratory parameters to judge either the degree or the duration of testicular ischemia. Therefore, no matter how long the patient has been symptomatic and no matter what the presenting physical examination suggests, if testicular torsion cannot be excluded, emergency scrotal exploration is the definitive diagnostic test and procedure of choice.

Torsion of the Appendages

The appendages of the epididymis and testis have no known physiologic function. These pedunculated structures are, however, capable of torsion and in prepubertal boys probably torse more often than the testes. If the patient is seen early, the pain is more intense near the head of the epididymis or testis, and an isolated tender nodule can often be palpated. When the involved appendage is brought close to the thin, prepubertal scrotal skin, a blue reflection may be seen when light shines upon it. This "blue dot sign" is pathognomonic of torsion of the appendix testis or epididymis. If the diagnosis can be absolutely assured and confirmed by radionuclide scan showing normal blood flow to the involved testis, immediate surgery is not necessary, since most appendages will calcify or degenerate over 10 to 14 days and cause no harm. If testicular swelling is present, urologic consultation and surgical exploration may be necessary to exclude testicular torsion.

Epididymitis

The onset of pain in epididymitis or epididymo-orchitis is usually more gradual than that of testicular torsion. Bacterial infection is the most common cause and tends to be age-dependent. In patients less than 40 years of age, epididymitis is due to sexually transmitted diseases (STDs) or their complications, i.e., urethral stricture. In patients over 40 years of age, epididymitis is caused by common urinary pathogens such as *Escherichia coli* and *Klebsiella*. These patients will most often have pyuria on urinalysis, but the absence of white cells or bacteria does not exclude the diagnosis. Occasionally, young patients may present with chemical epididymitis secondary to retrograde reflux of sterile urine into the globus minor (tail of the epididymis) and may well have a normal screening urinalysis.

Epididymitis causes lower abdominal, inguinal canal, scrotal, or testicular pain alone or in combination. The retrograde progression of infection from the prostatic urethra to the epididymis explains the location of pain. Patients with epididymitis are more prone to lower urinary tract irritative voiding symptoms and may note transient relief of pain in the recumbent position with scrotal elevation. Initially, isolated firmness and nodularity of the affected globus minor is noted on examination. As the disease progresses, the sulcus between the epididymis and testis becomes obliterated, and the inflammatory epididymal mass becomes contiguous with the testis, producing a large, tender scrotal mass (epididymo-orchitis) that cannot be differentiated from testicular torsion or carcinoma. At this stage the patient may appear toxic and require admission for IV antibiotic therapy (see Table 54.3). Adjunctive diagnostic modalities such as radionuclide imaging are no more helpful here than with testicular torsion.

Admission criteria for epididymitis include fever, elevated white blood cell count, and subjective toxicity, all of which can be indicative of epididymal or testicular abscess formation. Patient management includes: (1) absolute bed rest for the first 24 to 48 h, with scrotal elevation and ice application (10 to 15 min every 4 to 6 h) to the involved testis/epididymis; (2) nonsteroidal anti-inflammatory drugs; (3) intravenous antibiotic based on etiology (Table 54-3); and (4) narcotics for pain control, with concomitant stool softeners. These measures will prevent further progression of the inflammatory process. Once the bedridden patient is pain-free, he should begin ambulation with a scrotal supporter, being careful not to lift heavy objects or strain when having a bowel movement, both of which will increase intra-abdominal pressure and exacerbate the inflammation. Urologic follow-up should begin 5 to 7 days after initial presentation. Any significant deviation from this plan will prolong the recovery period.

Table 54-3. Etiology and Treatment of Epididymitis and Epididymo-orchitis

Etiology	Treatment
Chemical	Tetracycline, NSAID
Gonococcal	Ceftriaxone, tetracycline, NSAID
Chlamydia	Ceftriaxone, tetracycline, NSAID
E. coli	Trimethoprim/sulfamethoxazole, NSAID
Klebsiella	Trimethoprim/sulfamethoxazole, NSAID

DOSAGES

Tetracycline 500 mg q.i.d. × 10 days or doxycycline 100 mg b.i.d. × 10 days
Ceftriaxone 125–250 mg IM
Trimethoprim/sulfamethoxazole DS 1 tablet bid × 10 days

Orchitis

Isolated orchitis, or inflammation of the testicle, is quite rare. It usually occurs in conjunction with other systemic diseases, such as mumps, other viral illnesses, or syphilis. Orchitis usually presents as bilateral testicular tenderness and swelling over a few days' duration. Treatment is symptomatic and disease-specific with urologic follow-up.

Testicular Malignancy

Any asymptomatic testicular mass, firmness, or induration is the hallmark of testicular carcinoma. Ten percent of tumors will present with pain secondary to acute hemorrhage within the tumor. Metastatic testicular tumors can be insidious and must be suspected in any male with unexplained supraclavicular lymphadenopathy, abdominal mass, or chronic nonproductive cough that appears resistant to antibiotic or other supportive therapy. Testicular examination may be diagnostic. While not a urologic emergency, any unexplained testicular mass must be approached as a tumor, with urgent urologic referral.

Urethra

Urethral Stricture

Urethral strictures are becoming more prevalent secondary to the rising incidence of STDs. Increasingly, in teenagers and young adults, gonococcal and chlamydial infections have resulted in bulbous urethral obstruction (Figs. 54-8), while trauma and urethral instrumentation are less common and tend to be localized to areas where a traumatic event has occurred. In the older population, postendoscopy meatal stenosis or localized urethral strictures are more common.

If a patient is in urinary retention and a 14- or 16-French Foley catheter or coudé catheter cannot be easily placed into the bladder, the differential diagnostic possibilities include urethral stricture, voluntary external sphincter spasm, bladder neck contracture, or benign prostatic hypertrophy (BPH). If time permits, retrograde urethrography can be done and will define the location and extent of urethral stricture. Only endoscopy can confirm a bladder neck contracture or the extent of an obstructing prostate gland. Suspected voluntary external sphincter spasm can be overcome when the patient relaxes his perineum and breathes slowly during the procedure.

When a urethral stricture is encountered, copious anesthetic lubrication (Anestacon) is placed intraurethrally. A 12- or 14-French coudé catheter may negotiate the strictured area, since this catheter has an angled bend near its tip. If there are previous false passages from attempts at dilation or unsuccessful instrumentation, passage of the coudé catheter may be difficult. Further urethral manipulation may create new false passages, leading to unnecessary hemorrhage and possible gram-negative sepsis. If two or three gentle attempts to pass the catheter fail, urologic consultation is indicated.

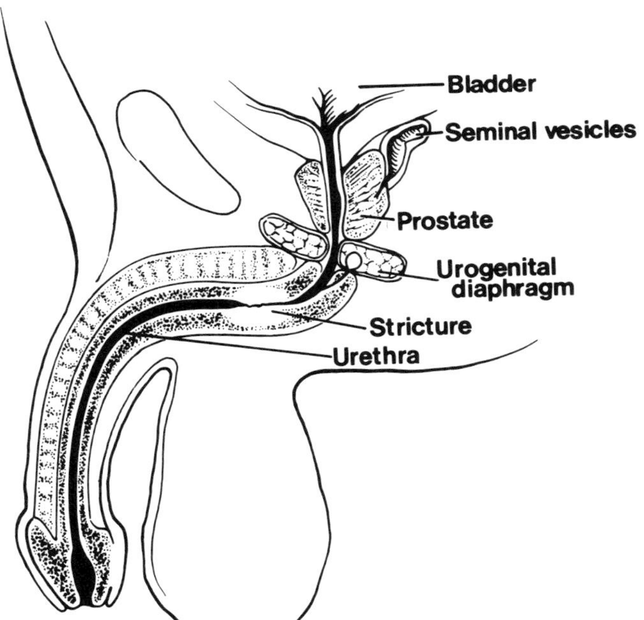

Fig. 54-8. Stricture of the bulbous urethra.

In an emergency situation, suprapubic trocar cystotomy can be performed with the least amount of morbidity. The infraumbilical and suprapubic area is prepped with povidone-iodine (Betadine) solution. A 25- to 27-gauge spinal needle is used to locate the bladder. This step is important in cases of previous lower abdominal surgery where normal anatomic relationships may be distorted. Suprapubic trocar cystotomy kits utilizing a catheter-inside-the-needle technique or Stamey suprapubic catheters utilizing a catheter-over-a-needle obturator are readily available and allow easy access to the bladder for temporary drainage. Once temporary suprapubic drainage has been achieved, appropriate urologic follow-up is necessary.

Urethral Foreign Bodies

Patients of all ages, but especially young children, may be victims of innocent urethral exploration or attempts to heighten sexual experiences utilizing a variety of foreign bodies such as bobby pins; long, thin paint brushes; or ball point pens. Bloody urine combined with infection and slow, painful urination should suggest a possible foreign body in the lower urinary tract. An x-ray of the bladder and urethral areas may disclose the presence of a foreign body.

Foreign bodies often require endoscopic removal or even open cystotomy. Occasionally a gentle milking action of the proximal end of the urethral foreign body by an experienced examiner will allow its retrieval from the distal urethral meatus. Even then, retrograde urethrography or endoscopic confirmation of an intact, nontraumatized urethra is indicated.

Urinary Retention

Obstructive uropathy causes a wide expanse of signs and symptoms. Overt urinary retention represents one end of the spectrum, while symptoms of insidious overflow incontinence will often fool an unsuspecting examiner. Prior to acquiring a detailed genitourinary history, questions regarding chronic systemic medical illnesses that have as sequelae sensory or motor neurogenic side effects or complications must be addressed. A detailed medication history, including over-the-counter medications, will often reveal a sympathomimetic agonist that has secondarily caused outlet obstruction due to its muscle-constricting effect on the abundant α fibers in the bladder neck. Inconvenient, and therefore infrequent, voiding during a prolonged car trip by a vacationing patient with borderline obstructive symptoms may be just enough to result in urinary retention.

A thorough voiding history begins with questions regarding problems holding or initiating the urinary stream, voiding completely with one continuous stream rather than starting and stopping of the stream, a feeling of complete bladder emptying as opposed to incomplete emptying and postvoid residual, and the relative frequency of nocturia. Most men do not void as well or completely empty their bladders when sitting down to urinate, which happens most often during the night. Infrequent ejaculation may lead to secondary prostatic congestion and subsequent spurious symptoms of irritation and outlet obstruction. Unless specific questions are asked about the latter circumstances, these easily treatable causes of obstructive symptoms can be missed.

The most difficult evaluation involves the patient with silent prostatism. Historically, voiding symptoms have gradually worsened over the years, but at such a pace that the patient often makes adjustments and then perceives each worsening state as "normal" for him. The ultimate result is retention, with a large palpable bladder and often

Table 54-4. Etiology of Outlet Obstruction

Meatal stenosis
Urethral stricture
Bladder neck contracture
Benign prostatic hyperplasia

1600 to 2000 mL residual urine. An intact sensory examination, anal sphincter, and bulbocavernosus reflex differentiate chronic outlet obstruction from the sensory or motor neurogenic bladder.

Intraurethral causes of urinary retention are the same as those of outlet obstruction (Table 54-4). Appropriate physical examination requires inspection of the meatus for stenosis, palpation of the entire urethral length for masses or fistulas consistent with urethral stricture disease or abscess formation, lower abdominal examination for palpation of a suprapubic mass, and rectal examination to evaluate anal sphincter tone and the size and consistency of the prostate. Outlet obstruction due to a large intravesical prostate can result in a palpably normal prostate on rectal examination. Similarly, rectal examination in a patient in urinary retention may initially reveal a spuriously enlarged, nodular prostate that will shrink considerably once bladder decompression is achieved.

Most patients with bladder outlet obstruction are in distress, and passage of a urethral catheter alleviates both their pain and their urinary retention. Copious intraurethral lubrication must be used, and if attempts at passage of a straight 16-French Foley catheter fails, a 16-French coudé catheter should be passed. Be certain to pass either catheter used to its fullest extent, obtaining a free flow of urine, and only then inflate the catheter balloon. This will prevent balloon inflation in the prostatic urethra. If the catheter drainage holes become obstructed with lubricating jelly, gentle irrigation with sterile saline or water will quickly establish urinary drainage. Spontaneous, complete drainage of a distended bladder can be accomplished rapidly without the need for repeated clamping of the catheter. Occasionally, when a bladder has been chronically distended, bladder mucosal edema develops. Rapid decompression following catheter placement may result in transient gross hematuria. The transient hematuria is usually self-limited, of little consequence, and responds to orally induced diuresis. Postmicturitional or bladder decompression syncope is rare and should be treated symptomatically.

The catheter should be left indwelling and connected to a portable leg drainage bag. The patient or his family must be instructed in the care and drainage of this simple device. Belladonna and opium (B and O) suppositories, one every 4 to 6 h, can be prescribed to alleviate the constant urge to urinate secondary to bladder spasm that frequently accompanies an indwelling catheter. The initiation of antibiotic therapy depends on the presence or absence of infected urine and on how long the catheter will be left indwelling. Since infection tends to be universal after 5 to 7 days of permanent drainage, appropriate antibiotic therapy should be started when the catheter is inserted. Trimethoprim alone without sulfa (Trimpex or Proloprim) is a good choice, 100-mg tabs once or twice daily. The patient or a family member should be instructed on Foley balloon deflation, should it become necessary to remove the catheter.

If urinary retention has been chronic or insidious, postobstructive diuresis may occur secondary to osmotic diuresis or interstitial tubular dysfunction. Postobstructive diuresis may occur in the presence of a normal BUN and creatinine and may become an emergency if the patient suddenly becomes hypovolemic or hypotensive without warning. Thus, close monitoring of urine output is essential, with appropriate fluid replacement. For these reasons, all patients with chronic or insidious obstructive voiding symptoms and urinary retention should either be observed for 4 to 6 h or be admitted, with particular attention paid to hourly intake, urinary output, vital signs, and urine and serum electrolytes. Osmotic diuresis will dissipate or the dysfunctional tubules will recover within 24 to 48 h. In all cases of urinary retention, consultation and follow-up with a urologist for a complete genitourinary evaluation are necessary.

BIBLIOGRAPHY

Bertram RA, Webster GD, Carson CC: Priapism: Etiology, treatment and results in series of 35 presentations. *Urology* 26:229, 1985.

Caldamone AA, Valvo JR, Altebarmakian VA, et al: Acute scrotal swelling in children. *J Pediatr Surg* 19:581, 1984.

Cattolica EV: Preoperative manual detorsion of the torsed spermatic cord. *J Urol* 133:803, 1985.

Chen DCP, Holder LE, Kaplan GN: Correlation of radionuclide imaging and diagnostic ultrasound in scrotal diseases. *J Nucl Med* 24:735, 1983.

Clayton MD, Fowler JE, Sharifi R, et al: Causes, presentation and survival of fifty-seven patients with necrotizing fasciitis of the male genitalia. *Surg Gynecol Obstet* 170:49, 1990.

Coldiron B, Jacobson C: Common penile lesions. *Urol Clin North Am* 15(4):671, 1988.

Ganti SU, Sayegh N, Addonizio JC: Simple method for reduction of paraphimosis. *Urology Urotech* 26, 1986.

Joo R, Peters WJ: Fournier's gangrene. *Can J Surg* 28:180, 1985.

Likitnukul S, McCraken GH, Nelson JD, et al: Epididymitis in children and adolescents. *Am J Dis Child* 141:41, 1987.

Lindsey D, Stanisic TH: Diagnosis and management of testicular torsion: Pitfalls and perils. *Am J Emerg Med* 6:42, 1988.

Melekos MD, Hans WA, Markou SA: Etiology of acute scrotum in 100 boys with regard to age distribution. *J Urol* 139:1023, 1988.

Muschat M: The pathological anatomy of testicular torsion: An explanation of its mechanism. *Surg Gynecol Obstet* 54(5):758, 1932.

O'Brien WM, O'Connor KP, Lynch JH: Priapism: Current concepts. *Ann Emerg Med* 18:980, 1989.

Orvis BR, McAninch JW: Penile rupture. *Urol Clin North Am* 16(2):369, 1989.

Pfaf G, Balkenius M: Hands off the prepuce. *Lancet* 2:874, 1984.

Rabinowitz R: The importance of the cremasteric reflex in acute scrotal swelling in children. *J Urol* 132:89, 1984.

Shantha TR, Finnerty DP, Rodriquez AP: Treatment of persistent penile erection and priapism using terbutaline. *J Urol* 141:1427, 1989.

Sidi AA, Lange PH: Recent advances in the diagnosis and management of impotence. *Urol Clin North Am* 13:489, 1986.

Son KA, Koff SA: Evaluation and management of the acute scrotum. *Primary Care* 12(4):637, 1985.

Yeates WK: Pain in the scrotum. *Br J Hosp Med* 33(2):101, 1985.

SECTION 7
Gynecology and Obstetrics

55
GYNECOLOGIC EMERGENCIES
John R. Musich

In evaluation of gynecologic emergencies in women, particularly those of reproductive age, a delay in or improper management of the patient may compromise care and jeopardize future reproductive capabilities. Although there are several gynecologic "urgencies" that warrant expeditious management, there are only three life-threatening gynecologic "emergencies": (1) ruptured ectopic pregnancy, (2) ruptured hemorrhagic ovarian cyst, and (3) ruptured tuboovarian abscess. If these are kept constantly in mind, diagnostic failures should not occur and proper management of the similar-presenting but less concerning gynecologic urgencies will be enhanced.

The possibility of pregnancy in every reproductive-age female must always be excluded before radiological procedures or treatment plans are initiated, regardless of the chief complaint. The presence of a pregnancy could alter the decision to obtain x-rays, or could change a choice of antibiotics.

The objective of this chapter is to provide a suggested approach to the evaluation and management of the more common and important urgent and emergency gynecologic problems occurring in women of reproductive age. After a brief discussion of nongynecologic causes of abdominal and pelvic pain, the chapter will focus on early pregnancy-related problems, adnexal accidents, endometriosis, abnormal genital bleeding conditions, and pelvic inflammatory disease (PID).

NONGYNECOLOGIC CAUSES OF ABDOMINAL OR PELVIC PAIN

In the initial evaluation of a woman with lower abdominal or pelvic pain, there is a tendency for physicians to quickly assume a gynecologic etiology for the presenting symptoms. The prudent physician, however, should first always approach each such patient with the thought of ruling out nongynecologic conditions as the source of the problem. The causes of abdominal pain are numerous and may involve gastrointestinal, musculoskeletal, urologic, or reproductive tract organs either independently or in combination. Since the somatic distribution of pain due to noxious stimuli or tissue damage will be influenced by pain referral patterns, one cannot always depend on finding a precise location for the pain as the sole means of making a diagnosis. This is particularly true when a considerable amount of time has elapsed between the onset and emergency presentation of the problem.

A detailed description of the presentation and management of the many nongynecologic causes of lower abdominal pain and pelvic pain is beyond the scope of this chapter. The following common causes of pain may, with varying degrees of likelihood, falsely suggest a gynecologic problem: (1) lower lobe pneumonia, (2) cholecystitis, (3) pancreatitis, (4) gastric or duodenal ulcers, (5) gastroenteritis, (6) colitis, (7) ileitis, (8) diverticulitis, and most commonly (9) appendicitis. A few moments of initial history-taking will usually correctly rule out these causes or at least minimize their priority in an eventual differential diagnosis. Having done so, one can then proceed with confidence to the consideration of specific gynecologic problems.

EARLY PREGNANCY COMPLICATIONS AS CAUSES OF GYNECOLOGIC PAIN AND BLEEDING

A most useful dictum is that, until proved otherwise, amenorrhea is a normal result of pregnancy and abnormal uterine bleeding is a complication of pregnancy. The possibility of an ectopic pregnancy must be considered in every patient who presents with a clinical scenario that includes lower abdominal or pelvic pain or abnormal uterine bleeding. A spontaneous abortion, infected abortion, hemorrhagic corpus luteum of pregnancy, and uterine incarceration are additional early pregnancy complications that frequently present to the emergency department (ED).

To firmly establish the possibility of a pregnancy in the woman with pelvic pain and/or bleeding, a brief but accurate gynecologic and menstrual history that provides the following information must be obtained:

Last menstrual period (LMP). Not only the LMP, but also the timing of two or more immediate past periods should be ascertained to determine the intervals between "normal" menses. Any regularly menstruating woman whose LMP is greater than 4 weeks prior to the current date is very likely to be pregnant. After being given an LMP date by the patient, the physician must determine that the LMP was, in fact, a normal menses. If normal, the described LMP will have the same characteristics of menstrual flow length, volume, and symptoms as *several prior menses.* Volume is best assessed by determining the number of pads used per day. A soaked pad suggests 20 to 30 mL of blood loss. If the LMP is determined to be normal and the patient is less than 4 weeks past that date, the possibility of a pregnancy complication is highly unlikely, as spontaneous abortion and ectopic pregnancies do not present clinically before the first missed menses. If the LMP was normal and occurred more than 4 weeks prior to the onset of the current problem, the patient is by definition amenorrheic and is, therefore, pregnant until proved otherwise. An interval of amenorrhea, regardless of length, followed by abnormal uterine bleeding or pelvic pain must be considered as a pregnancy complication. Similarly, if the stated LMP was lighter and shorter than normal, pregnancy must also be considered since many women, rather than "missing" their menses after blastocyst implantation, instead will have such an abnormal menstrual flow.

Past pregnancy history. Acquiring information about prior pregnancies, especially prior ectopic pregnancy, is important because the patient, if prompted, (1) will likely suggest the possibility of a pregnancy if she is experiencing symptoms similar to those in previous pregnancies, and (2) may also suggest the possibility of a specific pregnancy complication if she has experienced one in the past. Spontaneous abortions and ectopic pregnancies have a minimum 15 and 12 percent recurrence risk, respectively, and it is common for a recurrent episode to be clinically similar to previous episodes.

Sexual activity. One must historically confirm that vaginal intercourse has occurred once or several times since the LMP. The denial of sexual activity must be viewed with skepticism if all other historical and physical examination features are compatible with a pregnancy-related concern.

Contraception. Although contraceptive practices minimize the possibility of pregnancy, they do not completely eliminate it. All popular methods of contraception, including tubal sterilization and vasectomy, have failure rates ranging from less than 1 percent for oral contraception use and sterilization to 30 to 40 percent for methods such as rhythm, withdrawal, and postcoital douching. It is important, therefore, to determine whether sexual activities were associated with the use of effective and reliable means of contraception.

Pregnancy signs and symptoms. Commonly beginning shortly after the first missed menses, the findings of breast engorgement and tenderness, polyuria, easy fatigability, and occasional nausea and vomiting should make one very suspicious of pregnancy in the presence of a compatible menstrual history. Occasional pregnant patients do not experience such signs and symptoms.

Once the possibility of a pregnancy has been quickly established through historical means, vital signs, including blood pressure sitting *and* standing, are necessary to determine the presence of hypovolemia. If orthostatic signs are present, crystalloid infusion must be begun and blood sent for typing and cross-matching. A pelvic examination, and pregnancy testing confirm the diagnosis.

All currently-used qualitative and quantitative pregnancy tests are dependent on the ability to detect in serum or urine human chorionic gonadotropin (HCG), a glycoprotein hormone produced by the pregnancy trophoblast (placenta). Advances in immunochemistry, radioimmunoassay, and monoclonal antibody technology in the past decade have resulted in the modern-day ability to detect HCG within 2 to 3 days after implantation of the blastocyst into the uterine endometrium. Accordingly, it is now possible to readily make the laboratory diagnosis of pregnancy before the first missed menses, if need be, and certainly within the first few days after a missed menstrual period. Qualitative serum radioimmunoassays specific for the β-HCG fragment can detect as little as 10 mIU β-HCG/mL with a test time of 30 to 60 minutes while the quantitative application of such tests takes 3 hours to perform and can detect as little as 2.5 mIU β-HCG/mL. Detection of as little as 50 mIU of HCG/mL within 20 min is possible with current immunoenzymatic tests. In normal pregnancies, blood levels of β-HCG double approximately every 2 days for the first 6 to 8 weeks of pregnancy. Therefore, knowledge of the absolute HCG values when obtained serially may also be helpful in monitoring and predicting early pregnancy status. The degradation half-life of HCG in serum following abortions, ectopic pregnancies, or term deliveries is also approximately 2 days.

Ectopic Pregnancy

Most life-threatening of the several early pregnancy complications is an ectopic pregnancy. Ectopic pregnancies occur in the fallopian tubes in 95 percent of cases and rarely in the ovaries, cervix, pelvic interstitia, or elsewhere in the abdomen. The frequency of tubal ectopic pregnancies has tripled over the past decade to account for nearly 1.5 percent of all pregnancies. Ruptured ectopic pregnancies now account for nearly 13 percent of all maternal deaths and are the leading cause of maternal deaths in the first trimester.

Although ectopic pregnancies may occur in apparently normal fallopian tubes, predispositions to the development of an ectopic pregnancy are pelvic-inflammatory disease (PID), prior ectopic pregnancy, previous pelvic surgery (particularly tubal reconstructive surgery), tubal sterilization, induced abortions, and intrauterine contraceptive device (IUCD) use.

Most tubal ectopic pregnancies present between the fifth and eighth weeks after the LMP. Accordingly, the usual history will include that of a short interval of amenorrhea (80 percent of patients), followed by pain (95 percent) and abnormal bleeding (75 percent).

Tubal pregnancy-related pelvic pain is usually localized and unilateral initially and is of an intermittent and crampy nature as a result of tubal distention and minimal bleeding at the implantation site. *The pain usually develops before bleeding, unlike spontaneous abortion, where the reverse often occurs.* After further growth of the pregnancy, the tube will either rupture or abort the pregnancy out its fimbriated end, either of which may cause severe unilateral pain. By the time the patient is seen in the ED, the pain is usually diffused across the entire lower abdomen and pelvis, making its source indistinguishable from other pain etiologies. The location of the pain at its onset must be determined to help arrive at the diagnosis.

The abnormal bleeding associated with an ectopic pregnancy usually follows the event (rupture or abortion) that disrupts the tubal implantation site. The decidual tissue and the uterine endometrium, hormonally stimulated and supported by HCG from the intact tubal trophoblast and progesterone from the ovarian corpus luteum of pregnancy, will, as a consequence of tubal disruption, lose their endocrine support and be sloughed from the uterine cavity. Although scanty irregular shedding of decidual tissue may occur prior to tubal rupture, most bleeding will occur afterward. The amount of bleeding is usually minimal, unlike that associated with the spontaneous abortion of an intrauterine pregnancy, and may be accompanied by the passage of a decidual cast which should be examined histologically in all cases.

Abdominal examination findings may be entirely normal in a patient with an ectopic pregnancy, although unilateral lower-quadrant tenderness is common in the patient with an evolving tubal rupture or abortion. If frank rupture and hemoperitoneum have occurred, there is abdominal distention, severe pain to deep palpation, and rebound tenderness throughout the lower abdomen. The complaint of shoulder pain (due to irritation of the diaphragm) during examination in the supine position strongly suggests the presence of a significant hemoperitoneum.

Pelvic examination findings vary and are often nonspecific. Inspection of the vagina and cervix may reveal a minimal reddish-brown discharge due to sloughing of the decidua, but it is common for this portion of the examination to be entirely normal. Extremely heavy uterine bleeding and tissue passage through the cervix will more likely be seen with spontaneous abortions. In most patients with ectopic pregnancy the uterus will be normal in size but, when enlarged, will usually be smaller than expected for gestational dates. Unilateral adnexal tenderness is the most consistent pelvic examination finding and when accompanied by the finding of a mass, an ectopic pregnancy is very likely. An adnexal mass may also represent the corpus luteum of an intrauterine pregnancy, particularly if the uterine size is more compatible with gestational dates. If significant intraperitoneal hemorrhage has occurred, cervical motion tenderness may be present and cul-de-sac fullness or bulging may be palpated. With or without such a finding, however, culdocentesis must be considered in all patients with a suspected ectopic pregnancy. The positive finding of clotting or nonclotting blood by culdocentesis in a patient with a positive pregnancy test and clinical presentation suggestive of an ectopic pregnancy mandates surgical exploration either laparoscopically or by laparotomy. A negative culdocentesis, while ruling out a hemoperitoneum, does not eliminate the possibility of an ectopic pregnancy. In such a situation, greater reliance on laboratory studies may be necessary to make the proper diagnosis.

Although one may make a tentative diagnosis of an ectopic or any other pregnancy complication on the basis of the clinical history and examination, laboratory confirmation of a pregnancy must always be obtained unless the patient is so unstable that immediate surgical intervention is required.

A positive pregnancy test, regardless of the absolute HCG value, confirms the diagnosis of a pregnancy in either the uterus or an ectopic location. The HCG value does not differentiate ectopic from intrauterine pregnancy. Further localization of the pregnancy can then be attempted with a real-time ultrasound examination of the pelvis, the findings on which will be greatly dependent on the gestational age and the type of sonographic approach used. In general, real-time sonography using an abdominal transducer can find an intrauterine gestational sac by the fifth week, a sac with an embryonic or fetal pole by the sixth week, and an embryonic mass with cardiac motion by the seventh week. Using an intravaginal transducer, the same intrauterine pregnancy parameters may be found nearly one week earlier. It is uncommon for a tubal ectopic pregnancy, even if unruptured, to demonstrate such unequivocal localizing sonographic findings. Therefore, the sonographic diagnosis of a tubal ectopic pregnancy is suggested, but not absolutely confirmed, by excluding the presence of an intrauterine pregnancy. A final and accurate diagnosis will be provided by laparoscopy.

When confronted with a patient with abdominal pain and vaginal bleeding, the first and foremost diagnosis is an ectopic pregnancy. A detailed gynecologic and menstrual history, complete abdominal and pelvic examination, and pregnancy testing are the next steps. An intravenous line of 5% dextrose in Ringer's lactate (D_5RL) or normal saline (D_5NS) should be established, volume replaced to correct orthostatic signs, and type and cross matching for 2 to 6 units of blood should be obtained. Emergency gynecologic consultation is required.

Spontaneous Abortion

The most common early pregnancy complication, a spontaneous abortion, occurs in 15 percent of pregnancies. It can cause significant abnormal uterine bleeding resulting in acute anemia and hypotension. There are several postulated causes of abortions, but most are due to genetic defects in the early embryo, uterine anomalies, or ovulatory endocrine deficiencies. Repetitive abortions occur in 5 percent of women, who are usually quite accurate in diagnosing their own pregnancy complications on the basis of personal past history.

The differences between the clinical presentation of an ectopic pregnancy and a spontaneous abortion are several. Most spontaneous abortions also occur prior to 8 or 9 weeks of gestation, but unlike ectopic pregnancies, it is common for abortions to present in the 8- to 13-week interval. The aborting patient initially experiences minimal intermittent or continuous spotting that progresses to very heavy bleeding with the passage of clots and gestational tissue. The pain associated with the abortive process usually occurs after bleeding has commenced and is very characteristically midline and cramping in nature, as opposed to the acute, severe, and unilaterally localized pain of an ectopic pregnancy or ruptured ovarian cyst.

The abdominal examination of the aborting patient is usually very unremarkable, with the possible finding of midline suprapubic tenderness to deep palpation. On pelvic examination, a patient with a threatened abortion will be found to have a closed cervical os and minimal bleeding. In a woman with an actively progressing abortion, however, the bleeding will be profuse and accompanied by the passage of blood clots and products of conception through an obviously dilated cervical opening. The uterus will usually be enlarged to a size compatible with gestational dates unless significant tissue sloughage has occurred. In the case of a complete abortion, the uterus may be found to be small and firm shortly after all tissue has been passed. The adnexal examination is unlikely to be abnormal, although slight tenderness and palpation of a fullness on the side of the corpus luteum of pregnancy is common.

In a full-blown abortive situation, the proper diagnosis is easy to determine. However, in earlier stages of the abortion process, a definitive diagnosis can be difficult and is easily confused with an ectopic pregnancy. An ultrasound examination can help to rule out an ectopic pregnancy if an intrauterine gestational sac is seen and may even be predictive of a possible abortion if absent heart tones or irregular margins of the sac are seen. However, the rare case of a twin intrauterine and ectopic pregnancy should also be considered. When the diagnosis of an intrauterine pregnancy is uncertain, intrauterine instrumentation must be avoided until an accurate diagnosis can be made. Most patients with early pregnancy bleeding problems have normal pregnancy outcomes. If the diagnosis of a threatened abortion is made, the patient may be sent home for continued expectant management and close follow-up by her obstetrician. Discharge instructions should include bed rest, no intercourse, and no tampon use. The patient should be instructed to return to the ED if bleeding or cramping intensify, if orthostatic symptoms develop, or if there is fever or chills. Incomplete abortions require immediate evacuation of the uterine contents to prevent excess bleeding and postabortal endometritis. Occasionally, a patient will present with massive vaginal bleeding when the fetal tissue is in the cervical canal. The fetal contents should be gently withdrawn and bleeding will abate. All tissue obtained either from spontaneous passage or at the time of a dilatation and curettage must be histologically evaluated to confirm the presence of normal trophoblastic tissue, chorionic villi, or fetal tissue, thereby ruling out an ectopic pregnancy or hydatidiform molar pregnancy.

Infected Abortion

Endometritis following a spontaneous abortion is uncommon, even if instrumentation of the uterine cavity with a dilatation and curettage (D&C) is necessary. Postabortal endometritis following an induced abortion is more likely to occur, particularly if unsterile catheters or other foreign objects are used to stimulate the abortion.

Retained gestational tissue following a spontaneous or induced abortion can serve as a nidus for an infection that is usually polymicrobial in etiology. Continued bleeding, cramping pain, fever, nausea, and generalized malaise usually accompany a postabortal endometritis. On examination, a purulent, hemorrhagic cervical discharge is seen associated with a boggy, tender, and enlarged uterus. Significant adnexal tenderness may also be elicited if the myometrium, parametrium, and fallopian tubes are followed in the process. In severe cases where uterine perforation has occurred, an infected tender mass compatible with an abscess may be palpated in the adnexae or in the cul-de-sac. Patients with postabortal endometritis require hospitalization, intensive parenteral antibiotic therapy, and possible repeat dilatation and curettage in an effort to prevent abscess formation and development of septic pelvic thrombophlebitis.

Hemorrhagic Corpus Luteum

The corpus luteum of pregnancy usually persists until the eighth week or so of gestation and frequently is palpable as a 3- to 4-cm adnexalovarian mass associated with a normal intrauterine pregnancy. Rupture of the luteal cyst or hemorrhage into the corpus luteum may occur in early pregnancy and cause a clinical picture indistinguishable from that of a ruptured ectopic pregnancy, in terms of the patient's menstrual history and physical examination. An ultrasound examination demonstrating an intrauterine pregnancy will clearly distinguish between the two entities.

More common than a ruptured corpus luteum of pregnancy, however, is the rupture of a persistent corpus luteum in a nonception menstrual cycle. In normal circumstances, the corpus luteum of an ovulatory cycle undergoes spontaneous luteolysis 2 weeks after ovulation. Resultant decreases in estrogen and progesterone blood levels initiate a series of endometrial events that culminate in a menstrual flow. For reasons poorly understood, the corpus luteum may persist for an interval greater than 2 weeks and continue to support endometrial growth past the time of the expected menses. In such a case, the patient usually will experience amenorrhea for an additional 1 to 3 weeks, after which luteolysis occurs and a heavy menstrual flow results. If the corpus luteum persists and the cyst ruptures, the clinical presentation again could be very similar to that of an ectopic pregnancy or spontaneous abortion. HCG determinations and ultrasonography will be required for differentiation between the possible diagnoses.

Acute rupture of a corpus luteum cyst with consequent hemoperitoneum, in either a pregnant or nonpregnant state, usually requires surgical intervention and an ovarian cystectomy. Outpatient management in suspected cases is contraindicated, although expectant management on an inpatient basis may be feasible if, in the judgment of the consultant gynecologist, the clinical picture warrants close observation only.

Uterine Incarceration

An uncommon complication of a late first-trimester pregnancy, but one that can be associated with pelvic pain and other signs and symptoms of a threatened abortion, is an incarceration of a pregnant uterus. Incarceration occurs only in patients who have a retroverted and retroflexed uterus as a normal anatomic variant or as a result of endometriosis or retrouterine adhesions. Normally the uterus rises out of the pelvis as it enlarges as a result of a pregnancy and is safely beyond the bony confines of the pelvic walls by 12 to 13 weeks of gestation. However, if anteversion of such a uterus does not occur during the expansion process, the uterus may become trapped within the bony pelvis. Clinically, the patient will note progressively severe pelvic and rectal pressure, and because of marked upward anterior displacement of the cervix to a position behind the pubic symphysis, urinary retention may also be noted. The diagnosis is easily made by noting the cervical displacement and by an inability to mobilize the uterus on a combined abdominal-vaginal examination.

Treatment of this condition must be fairly immediate, to both alleviate urinary retention and prevent a certain spontaneous abortion. Placing the patient in a knee-chest position may spontaneously, or with appropriate pressure applied through the rectum, correct the problem. If needed, repositioning can be accomplished under a general or regional anesthetic.

ADNEXAL ACCIDENTS (NONPREGNANCY-ASSOCIATED) AS CAUSES OF PELVIC PAIN

Once nongynecologic and pregnancy-related causes have been eliminated, one should next consider the possibility of torsion or rupture of a cyst or a solid ovarian, tubal, or uterine mass. With the exception of rupture of a persistent corpus luteum cyst, all such adnexal accidents occur in patients whose menstrual cycles have been normal, and except for the pain itself, any other associated localizing or systemic symptoms are unlikely.

Most such problems occur in reproductive-age women who commonly have ovarian endometriomas, benign cystic teratomas (''dermoid''), dysfunctional follicular cysts, or serous or mucinous cystadenomas. Ovarian enlargement due to cystic or neoplastic processes is usually asymptomatic as a result of poor afferent innervation of ovarian tissue. The patient may experience pelvic and abdominal discomfort due to ovarian pressure on adjacent visceral organs. When ovarian rupture occurs, acute pain is caused by the irritation of pelvic peritoneum, richly endowed with sensory innervation, by the spillage of ovarian contents.

Ovarian torsion is an uncommon event and will not occur unless limited enlargement has developed. In such a circumstance the enlarging ovarian mass may stretch the mesovarium to the point where the ovary effectively becomes a pedunculated structure that may acutely twist on its pedicle. When torsion occurs, the ovarian blood supply is compromised, causing painful progressive anoxic degeneration of the ovary and eventual gangrenous necrosis. Torsion of tubal masses (hydrosalpinx, pyosalpinx) and pedunculated uterine leiomyomata (''fibroids'') may also cause acute pelvic pain.

Adnexal pain in the reproductive-age patient may be due to *mittelschmerz* (''middle pain'') which is unique to ovulatory cycles. The key to the diagnosis of mittelschmerz is the relationship of the timing of the pain to the menstrual cycle. In a woman with typically regular 28- to 30-day cycles, the pain associated with ovulation will usually occur between cycle days 14 to 16, be unilateral in location, be mild to moderate in severity, and last for less than a day. The pain may also be accompanied by light midcycle endometrial spotting. Although the source of the pain has not exactly been determined, it is thought to be due to follicular fluid irritation of the periovarian visceral peritoneum associated with release of the ovum at the time of ovulation. No diagnostic studies are helpful in evaluating the possibility of mittelschmerz, and treatment is symptomatic, with analgesics or nonsteroidal antiinflammatory agents.

Confronted with such an acute pelvic problem, there are few specific diagnostic modalities that will be helpful to the ED physician. Most importantly, a complication of pregnancy or an infectious process (to be discussed) must be ruled out. Aside from pregnancy testing, other laboratory and routine radiologic studies are of no value. An emergent ultrasound evaluation of the pelvis may be revealing if an adnexal mass cannot be palpated on pelvic examination. In nearly all cases, however, laparoscopic evaluation is needed to make a definitive diagnosis and direct further management.

ENDOMETRIOSIS

Although one of the most common diagnostic entities in gynecology, endometriosis continues to be an enigmatic disease of the menstruating female. When the tissue that characterizes the normal epithelial lining of the uterine cavity, the endometrium, is found in ectopic locations, it is called endometriosis. Most commonly, endometriosis is found on or in the ovaries. All pelvic tissues, however, are subject to endometriosis growth, including the uterine serosal surface, fallopian tubes, ovarian fossae, uterosacral ligaments, cul-de-sac peritoneum, and the utero-vesical peritoneal fold.

Much of the difficulty in making a diagnosis of endometriosis is due to the fact that there is no consistent symptom complex that characterizes affected women and that there is no direct relationship between the location and extent of the disease to the severity of symptoms. The diagnosis of endometriosis should be considered in any reproductive-aged woman complaining of any one or combination of the following signs and symptoms: acute adnexal pain, premenstrual pelvic pain, worsening dysmenorrhea, and deep dyspareunia. The most serious complication is rupture of an ovarian endometrioma. The approach is that directed at acute adnexal accidents.

The diagnosis of endometriosis of any extent or variety cannot be made by any combination of historical, examination, laboratory, or radiographic studies. Visual inspection of the disease either at laparoscopy or laparotomy is necessary to confirm the clinical suspicion. Therefore, unless the clinical circumstances warrant immediate operative diagnostic or therapeutic intervention by the gynecology team, the emergency physician should offer the patient analgesia and refer her to a gynecologist for definitive diagnosis and management.

ABNORMAL GENITAL BLEEDING (NONPREGNANCY)

When abnormal bleeding occurs, pregnancy complications such as an ectopic pregnancy, an abortion, or a ruptured corpus luteum cyst will probably be the first considerations. Once these have been ruled out, it is then necessary to systematically consider pathologic and traumatic causes of lower genital tract and uterine bleeding. Except for trauma, the bleeding is usually painless.

Trauma to the vulva and vagina from a variety of causes may result in profuse bleeding and hypotension. Patient stabilization with intravenous fluids is the first priority, and a thorough pelvic examination will easily indicate the bleeding source. In most cases, hemostasis and other indicated surgical procedures will require an anesthetic and the assistance of a gynecologist.

If the bleeding is determined not to be of vulvar, vaginal, rectal, or bladder origin, attention must then be given to the following pathologic causes of uterine cervix or corpus bleeding: (1) erosion of the cervical vasculature by an invasive cervical carcinoma, (2) endometrial carcinoma, (3) endometrial polyps, and (4) submucosal leiomyomata. A detailed description of the management of each of these entities is beyond the scope of this chapter. In all cases, it is the ED physician's responsibility to locate the bleeding source, stabilize the patient, and quickly refer the patient for gynecologic care.

If pathologic and pregnancy-related causes of uterine bleeding have been eliminated, it is then possible to ascribe the cause of uterine bleeding to that of anovulatory dysfunctional uterine bleeding (DUB). The gynecologist must eventually determine the hypothalamic-pituitary-ovarian axis disturbance that underlies the DUB, but in severe cases, the ED physician must immediately initiate management. Fortunately, most DUB problems do not require emergency treatment and are comfortably dealt with in an office or clinic setting. Virtually all severe cases of DUB occur in adolescent girls shortly after the onset of menstruation. Bleeding is occasionally severe enough to cause hemorrhagic shock. The ED management of such a patient should follow these suggested steps in an expeditious and overlapping manner:

1. Ascertain the adolescent perimenarcheal status of the patient and historically rule out a pregnancy. A lack of pain, and profuse, tissue-free blood loss dramatically reduces the possibility of a ruptured ectopic pregnancy or spontaneous abortion.
2. Localize the bleeding source to the uterine cavity and assure normal uterine and adnexal anatomy with a pelvic examination.
3. Stabilize the patient with intravenous fluids, or blood or blood-component transfusions as needed. Obtain the following minimum laboratory studies: (*a*) complete blood count including platelet count; (*b*) blood type and Rh factor for a transfusion cross match; (*c*) pregnancy test; and (*d*) coagulation profile. Coagulopathies, particularly platelet function disorders, may first manifest as severe perimenarcheal bleeding.
4. Administer 20 mg of conjugated estrogen intravenously slowly over 10 to 15 min. Acute intravenous estrogen therapy causes vasospasm of the uterine arterial vasculature and initiates several coagulation-related functions that often dramatically decrease the uterine bleeding.
5. Seek emergency gynecologic consultation for continuing hormonal or surgical management.

PELVIC INFLAMMATORY DISEASE

Pelvic inflammatory disease (PID) is the most common serious infection among reproductive-age women in the United States. An estimated 2.5 million physician visits occur annually for acute salpingitis, resulting in 250,000 hospitalizations and 150,000 surgical procedures for complications of this disease. Long-term sequelae of salpingo-oophoritis may include chronic pelvic pain, dyspareunia, infertility due to tubal occlusion or pelvic adhesions, tuboovarian abscess, and an increased risk of tubal ectopic pregnancies. The seriousness of the acute and chronic problems associated with PID makes it mandatory to recognize the diagnosis as early as possible in order to institute early, appropriate, and intensive antibiotic therapy.

Salpingitis is a polymicrobial disease whose commonly found pathogens may include *Neisseria gonorrhoeae;* anaerobic bacteria such as *Peptococcus, Peptostreptococcus,* and *Bacteroides* species; *Escherichia coli;* and *Chlamydia.* Antibiotic selection must take into consideration the polymicrobial nature of the disease and make special note of the increasing frequency with which *Chlamydia trachomatis* is being found to play a role in PID and its sequelae.

Risk factors for the development of PID include (1) a history of previous gonococcal salpingitis, (2) frequent sexual activity with multiple partners, (3) adolescence, and (4) use of an intrauterine contraceptive device. In addition to those cases related to sexual transmission, it must be determined whether recent instrumentation of the uterine cervix or cavity has occurred. Dilatation and curettage, endometrial biopsy, hysterosalpingography, tubal insufflation, and cautery or cryotherapy of the cervix may also predispose to the development of endometritis and salpingitis.

Acute salpingitis may present with a variety of clinical manifestations. Swelling and edema of infected tubes and parametrial tissues cause lower abdominal pain, adnexal and cervical motion tenderness, fever, and generalized malaise. The discharge of pus from the tubes onto adjacent peritoneal surfaces or around the liver may cause a more localized pain of pelvic peritonitis (Fitz-Hugh–Curtis syndrome). Gastrointestinal symptoms of nausea and anorexia are not uncommon and may suggest appendicitis or viral gastroenteritis. Onset frequently occurs shortly after a menstrual flow, but uterine bleeding abnormalities are uncommon. In general, the lack of an amenorrhea history and bleeding abnormalities and the usual presence of fever and malaise should strongly detract from diagnoses such as ectopic pregnancy, spontaneous abortion, and adnexal accidents.

Few physical examination findings are specific for salpingitis but include lower abdominal tenderness with possible rebound, cervical motion tenderness (''chandelier sign''), and adnexal tenderness. A purulent or mucopurulent cervical discharge is commonly found and should always be Gram-stained. The finding of unilateral or bilateral adnexal or cul-de-sac masses strongly suggests the presence of a tuboovarian or pelvic abscess. Only one-third of patients with PID will be febrile with temperatures over 38°C (100.4°F).

A Gram stain of cervical secretions should be done on all patients with suspected salpingitis to detect gram-negative intracellular diplococci (*N. gonorrhoeae*). Bacteriologic studies of the cervix should be limited to gonococcal and chlamydial cultures only. A complete blood count should be obtained, although not all patients with PID will have the expected increase in white blood cell count. An HCG assay should be ordered if there is any possibility of a pregnancy. Pelvic sonography should be obtained if the pelvic examination is inadequate as a result of severe pelvic tenderness or if there is a lack of response to antibiotic therapy in the initial 48 to 72 h of treatment.

Because of its variable presentation, the diagnosis of acute salpingitis may be difficult to make. In addition, the clinical criteria on which a diagnosis is based are multiple in number and variously defined and have not been standardized. Adding to the potential diagnostic confusion is the fact that there is no correlation between the extent of the disease and the severity of symptoms. Table 55-1 lists the diagnostic criteria that have been proposed for the clinical diagnosis of acute salpingitis. In all situations in which diagnostic doubt exists, a laparoscopic evaluation of the pelvis is indicated.

Treatment must take into consideration the polymicrobial nature of the disease process and, because of the seriousness of PID sequelae, should usually be offered on an inpatient basis. Inpatient parenteral (intravenous) antibiotic therapy should be utilized for patients who exhibit any of the following criteria: (1) diagnosed or suspected pyosalpinx or tuboovarian abscess, (2) temperature greater than 38°C (100.4°F), (3) pregnancy, (4) nausea and vomiting that prevent the use of oral antibiotics, (5) upper peritoneal signs, (6) presence of an IUCD, (7) failure to respond to oral antibiotics within 48 h, and (8) uncertain diagnosis.

The CDC's (Table 55-2) most current treatment schedules should be used. Ambulatory treatment should be reserved for patients with suspected gonorrheal cervicitis, chlamydial cervicitis, or the mildest forms of salpingitis. In all such cases, the treatment regimen must include a 10- to 14-day course of a tetracycline derivative and the

Table 55-1. Criteria for Clinical Diagnosis of Acute PID

All three of these conditions must be present:
- Abdominal direct tenderness with or without rebound tenderness
- Tenderness with motion of cervix and uterus
- Adnexal tenderness

One of these conditions must be present:
- Gram stain of endocervix—positive for gram-negative, intracellular diplococci
- Temperature greater than 38°C (100.4°F)
- Leukocytosis greater than 10,000/mm^3
- White blood cells and bacteria in peritoneal fluid collected by culdocentesis or laparoscopy
- Inflammatory mass documented by pelvic examination and/or sonogram

Source: Adapted from Hager WD et al: Criteria for diagnosis and grading of salpingitis. *Obstet Gynecol* 61:113, 1983. Used by permission.

Table 55-2. Centers for Disease Control Recommended Treatment for Acute PID—1989

Outpatients
Cefoxitin 2 g IM plus probenecid, 1 g orally *or*
ceftriaxone 250 mg IM *or*
equivalent cephalosporin
followed by
Doxycycline 100 mg orally 2 times a day for 10–14 days *or*
Tetracycline HCl 500 mg orally 4 times a day for 10–14 days
Inpatients
Recommended regimen A
Cefoxitin 2 g IV every 6 hrs *or*
Cefotetan 2 gm IV every 12 hours
plus
Doxycycline 100 mg every 12 hrs orally or IV for at least 48 hours
After hospital discharge, doxycycline 100 mg orally 2 times a day for 10–14 days
Recommended regimen B
Clindamycin 900 mg IV every 8 hrs
plus
Gentamicin loading dose IV or IM (2 mg/kg) followed by a maintenance dose (1.5 mg/kg) every 8 hours
for at least 48 hours
After hospital discharge, doxycycline 100 mg orally 2 times a day for 10–14 days. Continuation of clindamycin, 450 mg orally, 4 times a day for 10–14 days may be considered

Source: Adapted from MMWR (Suppl) 38, 1989.

patient must be reevaluated after 2 days of such therapy. Failure to respond to oral outpatient therapy mandates hospitalization and parenteral antimicrobial therapy.

BIBLIOGRAPHY

CDC: Ectopic pregnancy in the United States, 1970–1983. *MMWR* 35:2955, 1986.

DeVore GR, Owens O, Kase N: Use of intravenous Premarin in the treatment of dysfunctional uterine bleeding—a double-blind randomized control study. *Obstet Gynecol* 59:285, 1982.

Jones OG, Saida AA, St. John RK: Frequency and distribution of salpingitis and pelvic inflammatory disease in short stay hospitals in the United States. *Am J Obstet Gynecol* 138:905, 1980.

Landers DV, Sweet RL: Current trends in the diagnosis and treatment of tuboovarian abscess. *Am J Obstet Gynecol* 151:1098, 1985.

Ory SJ: Ectopic pregnancy: current evaluation and treatment. *Mayo Clin Proc* 64:874, 1989.

Reyniak JV: Pelvic endometriosis. *Sem Reprod Endocrinol* 3:303, 1985.

Sweet RL, Gibbs RS: *Infectious Diseases of the Female Genital Tract.* Baltimore, Williams & Wilkins, 1985, pp 53–77.

Washington AE, Cates W, Zadi AA: Hospitalization for pelvic inflammatory disease. Epidemiology and trends in the United States, 1975 to 1981. *JAMA* 251:2529, 1984.

Weckstein LN: Current perspectives on ectopic pregnancy. *Obstet Gynecol Surv* 40:259, 1985.

56 VULVOVAGINITIS

Gloria Kuhn

The commonest causes of acute vulvovaginitis include (1) infections with *Candida albicans*, *Trichomonas*, *Gardnerella*, and herpes simplex virus type 2, (2) contact vulvovaginitis, (3) local response to a vaginal foreign body, and (4) atrophic vaginitis.

Candidal and atrophic vaginitis may occur in virgins and after menopause, but other forms of vulvovaginitis are generally found only in sexually active women. A detailed gynecologic history, pelvic examination, and routine use of both normal saline and potassium hydroxide slide preparations for microscopic evaluation of vaginal secretions will, in most instances, provide a diagnosis. Secretions should be checked for pH with nitrazine paper, as this is a clue to the type of infection present.

NORMAL

In the female of child-bearing age estrogen causes the development of a thick vaginal epithelium with a large number of superficial cells serving a protective function and containing large stores of glycogen. This glycogen is used by the normal flora consisting of lactobacilli and acidogenic corynebacteria to form lactic and acetic acid. The resulting acidic environment favors the normal flora and discourages growth of pathogenic bacteria. Lack of estrogen or a dominance of progesterone results in an atrophic condition with loss of the protective superficial cells and their contained glycogen and loss of the acidic environment. Normal vaginal secretions may vary in consistency from a thin, watery material to one which is thick, white, and opaque. The quantity may also vary from scant to a rather copious amount. This material is odorless and produces no symptoms. The normal vaginal pH varies between 3.5 and 4.1. Alkaline secretions from the cervix before and during menstruation or semen, which is alkaline, reduce acidity, predisposing to infection. Before menarche and after menopause, the vaginal pH varies between 6 and 7. Because of scant nerve endings in the vagina, the patient usually does not have symptoms until both the vagina and vulva are involved in a disease process.

CANDIDA VAGINITIS

Candida species are the commonest cause of vaginitis. *Candida albicans* is present as part of the normal vaginal flora in up to 50 percent of healthy, asymptomatic women, and therefore this infection is not considered a sexually transmitted disease. The growth of this organism is held in check by the normal vaginal flora, and infection usually occurs only when the normal balance is upset. Conditions which inhibit growth of normal vaginal flora (systemic antibiotics), diminish the glycogen stores in vaginal epithelial cells (diabetes mellitus, pregnancy, the use of birth control pills, and the postmenopausal state), or increase the pH of vaginal secretions (menstrual blood or semen) may cause colonization by *Candida*, which is an opportunistic organism, and subsequent symptomatic infection.

Clinical symptoms include leukorrhea, vaginal pruritus, and, occasionally, dysuria and/or dyspareunia. Gynecologic examination may reveal vulvar erythema and edema, vaginal erythema (20 percent), and an occasional thick "cottage cheese" discharge seen most often in pregnant patients. Often the onset of symptoms will coincide with menses or coitus.

The diagnosis of *Candida* vaginitis is made by microscopically examining a sample of vaginal secretions on a potassium hydroxide slide preparation. Two drops of 10% potassium hydroxide are applied to dissolve vaginal epithelial cells, leaving yeast buds and pseudohyphae intact.

A number of treatment regimes are effective, but 3- and 7-day regimens are superior to single-dose therapy. Creams, tablets, and vaginal suppositories are all available. Creams rather than suppositories should be used for ease of application when there is extensive involvement of the vulvar area. All of the following treatment courses are effective: miconazole nitrate, 200 mg vaginal suppositories intravaginally at bedtime for 3 days, clotrimazole 200 mg vaginal tablets intravaginally at bedtime for 3 days, and butoconazole 2% cream intravaginally at bedtime for 3 days.

Patients with recurrent infections should have documentation of infection by culture and should be evaluated for predisposing causes, especially diabetes mellitus, use of antibiotics, pregnancy, and human immunodeficiency virus (HIV) infection. Treatment of sexual partners is not necessary unless candidal balanitis is present.

Trichomonas VAGINITIS

Trichomoniasis is almost always a sexually transmitted disease. The causative organisms is a flagellated protozoa that may live quiescently in the paraurethral glands and from this nidus of infestation cause overt infection in the susceptible vagina. *Trichomonas vaginalis* may survive up to 24 h in tap water, in hot tubs, in urine, on toilet seats, and in swimming pools, but the usual sequence of events begins with the deposit of a large inoculum of organisms contained in the alkaline semen at time of intercourse. Up to 50 percent of women harboring the organisms are asymptomatic, and only about 10 percent of men infested with the organisms will have any symptoms at all.

The discharge may vary from the classic gray to yellow to green, is malodorous, and is described as frothy in character. The pH is greater than 4.5. Pruritus, pain, dyspareunia, dysuria, and a sense of vulvovaginal fullness may be intense or mild. Intermenstrual or postcoital spotting may occur. Symptoms may be more severe before, during, or after the menstrual period when the vaginal pH is more alkaline. The infection may cause changes on the Pap smear which are inflammatory but not premalignant.

Gynecologic examination reveals the classic "strawberry cervix" secondary to diffuse punctate hemorrhages in only 20 percent of patients, but diffuse erythema of the vaginal vault is seen in 80 percent of cases.

The diagnosis of *Trichomonas* vaginitis is made through use of the "hanging drop" slide test: A cotton swab is used to obtain a specimen of secretions from the vaginal vault (not the endocervix) and is placed within a drop of normal saline on a glass slide. Microscopic examination reveals many polymorphonuclear leukocytes and motile, pear-shaped, flagellated trichomonads which are slightly larger than the leukocytes.

Treatment in the nonpregnant patient is best accomplished with a single 2-g oral dose of metronidazole (Flagyl). Metronidazole, 500 mg, bid for 7 days, is recommended for treatment failures. Since metronidazole is an acetaldehyde dehydrogenase inhibitor, concomitant alcohol ingestion may precipitate an Antabuse-like reaction. Thus, alcohol should be avoided for 24 h following ingestion of the drug. Up to 90 percent of infected males are asymptomatic; thus, all male consorts should be referred for therapy. Failure of the asymptomatic male partner to seek treatment is probably responsible for the high recurrence rate of this infection. Metronidazole is a folic acid inhibitor and, therefore, is not recommended for use in the first trimester of pregnancy.

For patients with severe symptoms after the first trimester, treatment with 2 g of metronidazole may be considered, after gynecologic consultation, as the safety of metronidazole after the first trimester has not been established.

BACTERIAL VAGINOSIS

Symptomatic bacterial vaginosis (BV), also known as *Gardnerella* vaginitis, *Haemophilus* vaginitis, *Corynebacterium* vaginitis, and nonspecific vaginitis, is the clinical result of alterations in the vaginal microflora that promote the synergistic activity of aerobic *G. vaginalis* and vaginal anaerobes. Presence of the gram-negative rod designated *G. vaginalis* is not necessarily indicative of disease. The Centers for Disease Control (CDC) states that in order for the disease to be diagnosed, three or four of the following criteria should be present: (1) homogeneous discharge, (2) pH of discharge greater than 4.5, (3) positive amine odor test, or (4) presence of clue cells.

The gram-negative rod is found in 40 percent of asymptomatic women and in children with no prior sexual contact. Males can harbor the organism in the urethra and serve as a potential source of infection.

When symptomatic, patients have mild pruritus and a copious vaginal discharge which has a disagreeable fishy odor. Gynecologic examination is usually normal except for occasional mild vaginal erythema and the presence of a thin, frothy gray-white vaginal discharge.

The diagnosis of *Gardnerella* vaginitis is often made from the wet-mount saline preparation, which shows pathognomonic *clue cells* (clusters of bacilli clinging to the surface of desquamated epithelial cells). Often, the diagnosis must be suspected from the typical presentation accompanied by the absence of *Candida* and *Trichomonas* on microscopic examination.

Treatment for asymptomatic infection is not recommended by the CDC. Symptomatic patients may be treated with metronidazole 500 mg orally bid for 7 days. Alternatively, clindamycin 300 mg orally bid for 7 days may be used. Treatment of the male sex partner has not been shown to be beneficial.

In pregnancy, recent studies have suggested that BV may be a factor in premature rupture of membranes and premature delivery. Until this is confirmed, routine treatment of the pregnant patient is not recommended. If it is necessary to treat the patient, clindamycin, 300 mg orally bid for 7 days is used, as metronidazole is contraindicated in the first trimester of pregnancy.

GENITAL HERPES

Genital herpes is a sexually transmitted infection caused by a DNA-containing virus specific to humans. There are two antigenic groups (HSV-1 and HSV-2). Initially, HSV-1 caused oral lesions and HSV-2 genital lesions, but that is no longer true, as up to 30 percent of genital lesions have been found to be due to HSV-1 in some studies. Generally it is felt that 85 to 90 percent of genital infections are caused by HSV-2. Symptomatic genital herpes is the most frequent cause of painful lesions of the lower genital tract in American women. It has been associated with cervical cancer, although a causative role has not been proven. Neonatal infection with high mortality and morbidity after passage through an infected birth canal has been seen. While the actual prevalence is not known, it may be one of the most frequent sexually transmitted diseases. It is a recurrent disease with no cure at this time.

Initial presentation occurs 1 to 45 days (mean 5.8 days) after exposure. Usually initial infection is more severe and lasts longer than subsequent recurrences. There may be both local and systemic manifestations. The lesions begin as painful fluid-filled vesicles or papules which progress to well-circumscribed, occasionally coalescent, shallow-based ulcers. They then heal by reepithelialization of mucous membranes or by crusting by the epidermal surface. Symptoms peak in 8 to 10 days and decrease over the next week. Ulcers last 4 to 15 days with total healing in 21 days. Lymphadenopathy is usually present, and when the deep inguinal nodes are involved, severe pelvic pain may result. Urethritis is usually present, causing severe dysuria which may cause urinary retention. Initial disease involves the cervix in over 80 percent of cases. Pharyngitis and secondary spread of lesions to other body sites, usually below the waist, have been reported in up to two-thirds of patients. Systemic symptoms such as fever, malaise, headache, and myalgias are common. Hepatitis, aseptic meningitis, and autonomic nervous system dysfunction can occur. Aseptic meningitis has been seen more frequently with HSV-2 than with HSV-1 infection and has been reported in about 30 percent of patients. Sacral autonomic nervous dysfunction is rare but can result in decreased cutaneous sensation and bladder and bowel dysfunction. After the attack is over, the inactive virus resides in the dorsal root of the sacral ganglia. Under various stimuli both exogenous and endogenous, the virus travels down the sensory nerve root to the lower genital area where it replicates and becomes symptomatic.

Recurrent episodes are usually milder than the initial disease, and the patient usually does not have systemic symptoms. A recurrence may be heralded by genital tingling. Genital lesions are fewer, smaller, and more often unilateral. Lesions may be ulcerations or resemble a fissure or excoriations. Recurrences tend to occur in the same location and have the same appearance from episode to episode. Symptoms last 4 to 8 days, and the lesions have usually disappeared by 10 days. Frequency of attacks and intervals between attacks are highly variable. The average number of symptomatic recurrences is 5 to 8 per year. Asymptomatic infections, defined as culture positive viral shedding in the absence of symptoms or lesions, have been documented.

Approximately 25 percent of initial presentations occur in women with preexisting antibody to HSV. These initial episodes tend to be less severe and resemble recurrent infections. These may, in fact, represent recurrent infections in patients who had previous asymptomatic infections. Clinically it is impossible to distinguish between HSV-1 and HSV-2 infections, but HSV-1 usually causes milder initial disease, results in recurrence less frequently, and the recurrent episodes are milder and less frequent.

Diagnosis is suspected by clinical presentation and confirmed by culture. The virus can be isolated from vesicle fluid and the base of a wet ulcer. Intact vesicles, if present, should be unroofed and the fluid cultured directly. These cultures will be positive in 85 to 95 percent of cases. Scrapings of an ulcer may be taken for a Pap smear or Tzanck preparation. A Tzanck smear stained with either Wright's or Giemsa stain is positive if multinucleated giant cells are present, as they are in up to 50 percent of cases. Antibody testing is usually of no value, as even if the test is positive, it does not denote active disease.

Treatment is not curative. Systemic acyclovir provides partial control of the signs and symptoms and accelerates healing of lesions, but does not affect the frequency or severity of recurrences. Topical treatment with acyclovir is less effective. For first infections, the dose of acyclovir is 200 mg orally, five times a day for 7 to 10 days or until clinical resolution. For patients with severe disease or complications necessitating hospitalization, acyclovir, 5 mg/kg IV every 8 h for 5 to 7 days or until clinical resolution occurs, may be used. Most patients with recurrent disease do not benefit from acyclovir. In severe recurrent cases, some patients may benefit if therapy with the drug is begun within 2 days and 200 mg of acyclovir is given five times a day for 5 days. Efficacy has not been proven. Daily suppression therapy may be indicated in those patients with more than six recurrences per year. Recurrences are decreased by 75 percent when acyclovir 200 mg orally two to five times a day or 400 mg bid is taken. While acyclovir-resistant strains have been isolated, they have not been associated with treatment failures among immunocompetent patients. After 1 year, suppressive therapy should be discontinued to reassess recurrence rates. In pregnant patients with life-threatening disease such as encephalitis, pneumonitis, or hepatitis, intravenous acyclovir may be used. It should not be used for recurrent episodes or as suppressive therapy in pregnant patients. HIV-positive patients should initially be treated with the same dose of acyclovir as immunocompetent patients. If failure of this regimen occurs, an infectious disease expert, or one familiar with HIV disease, should be consulted.

CONTACT VULVOVAGINITIS

Contact dermatitis results from the exposure of vulvar epithelium and vaginal mucosa to either a primary chemical irritant or an allergen. In either case, characteristic local erythema and edema occur. Severe reactions may progress to ulceration and secondary infection. Common irritants and/or allergens include chemically scented douches; soaps; bubble baths; deodorants; perfumes; dyes and scents in toilet paper, tampons, and pads; feminine hygiene products; topical vaginal antibiotics; tight slacks panty hose; and tight elastic underwear.

Clinically, patients report local swelling and itching or a burning sensation. The gynecologic examination reveals a vulvovaginal area which is erythematous and edematous. Local vesiculation and ulceration are seen more commonly with allergens or when primary irritants are used in strong concentrations. Vaginal pH changes may promote colonization and infection with *Candida albicans*, thus obscuring the primary cause.

The diagnosis of contact vulvovaginitis is made by ruling out an infectious cause and by identifying the offending agent. Most cases of mild vulvovaginal contact dermatitis resolve spontaneously when the causative agent is withdrawn. For patients with severe painful reactions, cool sitz baths and wet compresses of dilute boric acid or Burrow's solution may afford relief. Topical corticosteroids such as hydrocortisone acetate (Cortef), fluocinolone acetonide (Synalar), or triamcinolone acetonide (Aristocort) relieve symptoms and promote healing. Oral antihistamines should be avoided since they may actually dry the vaginal mucosal membrane and result in further irritation and discomfort.

VAGINAL FOREIGN BODIES

Children and adolescent females may insert objects intravaginally during periods of genital exploration or sexual stimulation. In young girls the most commonly inserted foreign bodies are rolled up pieces of toilet paper, toys, and small household objects. In adolescents it is often a forgotten tampon or diaphragm. Foreign objects left in place for more than 48 h can cause severe localized infections due to *Escherichia coli,* anaerobes, or overgrowth of other vaginal flora. Patients present with a foul-smelling and/or bloody vaginal discharge. The only treatment necessary for vaginitis secondary to foreign bodies is removal of the object. In most cases, the patient's associated vaginal discharge and odor will disappear without further therapy within several days.

PINWORMS

Pinworms (Enterobius vermicularis) may migrate from the anus to the vagina in children and cause intense pruritus. Cellophane tape can be used to obtain material for a slide that can be looked at microscopically for presence of ova, which are large and double-walled in appearance. The child and family members may all need treatment with an antiparasitic agent.

ATROPHIC VAGINITIS

During menarche, pregnancy, lactation, and after menopause, the vaginal epithelium lacks the stimulation of estrogen. As a result, squamous cells proliferate at a lower rate, they do not mature into glycogen-containing forms, acidogenic flora are not present, and the pH rises to 6.5 to 7.5. Lactobacilli and corynebacteria are diminished, while coliforms, gut anaerobes, and pyogenic cocci are frequent isolates. Unless estrogenic replacement therapy is used, *Candida* and *Trichomonas* infections are rare. Because of the thin, friable epithelium, inflammatory denudation causes rupture of surface blood vessels, and a pinkish or blood-tinged discharge results. The vagina will be pale and pasty in appearance with adhesions which bleed easily. The discharge is thin, scant, and yellowish with an alkaline pH. A Pap smear of the cervix and vagina is mandatory to rule out carcinoma. A wet preparation will show RBCs, WBCs, and round or oval parabasal cells. Specific topical therapy consists of a sulfa-containing cream and estrogen cream. The patient should be referred for follow-up to monitor therapy and for results of the Pap smear.

BIBLIOGRAPHY

Crane JK, Bump RC: Vulvovaginal infections, in Rayburn WF, Zuspan FP (eds): *Drug Therapy in Obstetrics and Gynecology*. East Norwalk, CT, Appleton Lang, 1986, pp 371–390.

Friedrich EG Jr: *Vaginitis in Vulvar Disease*, 2d ed, Major Problems in Obstetrics and Gynecology Series, vol 9). Philadelphia, Saunders, 1983, pp 9–33.

Gibbs RS: Sexually transmitted diseases in the female. *Med Clin North Am* 67:221, 1983.

Kistner RW: *Gynecology Principles and Practice*, 4th ed. Chicago, London, Year Book Medical, 1986, pp 677–695.

Lossick JG: Single-dose metronidazole treatment for vaginal trichomoniasis. *Obstet Gynecol* 56:508, 1980.

Morbidity and Mortality Weekly Report: *1989 Sexually Transmitted Disease Treatment Guidelines*. U.S. Dept. of Health and Human Services, Public Health Service, 1989.

Robertson WH: A concentrated therapeutic regimen for vulvovaginal candidiasis. *JAMA* 244:2549, 1980.

57 SEXUAL ASSAULT

Marion Hoelzer

Rape is the carnal knowledge, to a lesser or greater degree, of a victim without consent and by compulsion, through fear, force, or fraud, singly or in combination. Thus there are three elements of rape: (1) carnal knowledge, (2) nonconsensual coitus, and (3) compulsion. Carnal knowledge can consist of anything from complete coitus to slight penile penetration of female genitalia irrespective of seminal emission. Nonconsent must be an integral part of coitus unless the victim is a minor (under statutory age of consent), intoxicated, drugged, asleep, or mentally incompetent. Finally, there should be compulsion or fear of great harm, threats with a real or alleged weapon, or use or threat of brute force. Any use of intimidation invalidates any consent on the victim's part. Rape has also been further subdivided into four degrees of criminal sexual conduct: first to fourth degree. The first and third degrees require penetration, which is defined as protrusion into genital or anal openings by an object or any part of an assailant's body. The second and fourth degrees include intentional touching or fondling of intimate parts of the victim or coercing the victim to fondle the assailant's intimate parts.

EPIDEMIOLOGY

Most rape victims feel that there is a stigma attached to being a victim of sexual assault. As a result, authorities believe that only one in four cases is reported.

The vast majority of information and statistics relates to female rape victims. Only recently has male sexual assault been recognized and reported. The median age range of victims is 15 to 26 years, and about 80 percent are single, divorced, or separated. About half of the assailants are known to their victims. Many victims are threatened with a weapon, the majority of women suffer minor injuries, and only 1 to 2 percent require hospitalization. When injuries are encountered, they are usually facial or extremity injuries, and seldom genital.

THE FEMALE RAPE EXAMINATION

History

The purpose of the history is to tactfully obtain data about pertinent events and personal information for proper medical care without having the rape victim relive in minute detail the events of the attack.

1. *Who.* Was the assailant known to the victim? Was it a single attacker? If more than one, how many?
2. *What happened.* Was the victim physically assaulted? If so, with what (i.e., heavy object, gun, bat), and where? This information will determine whether x-rays are necessary to rule out a fracture.
3. *When.* When approximately did the assault take place? This will determine the probability of detecting sperm or acid phosphatase.
4. *Where.* Where did penetration occur—vaginally, orally, or rectally? This will direct the physical examination to areas of potential injury.
5. *Last menstrual period.* This will help to determine pregnancy risk.
6. *Birth control method.* This will also help to determine pregnancy risk.
7. *Last intercourse.* If the patient had recent intercourse (less than 3 days) prior to the attack, it may confuse laboratory analysis of sperm and acid phosphatase.
8. *Douche, shower, change clothes.* Any of these activities performed prior to seeking medical attention may decrease the probability of sperm or acid phosphatase recovery.
9. *Allergies and medical history.* This information is necessary before giving antibiotics or postcoital contraception.
10. *Prior sexual assault.* This is necessary when considering postcoital contraception and counseling referral.

Physical Examination

Document bruises, lacerations, or other visible signs of trauma. Predrawn diagrams aid in an accurate representation of injuries. A pelvic examination should be done, taking note of any vaginal discharge or genital lacerations or abrasions. Most hospitals have a prepackaged rape kit with equipment and directions on sample collection. If no kit is available, smears of material from the vagina and cervix are made, labeled, and air-dried. The swabs are placed in tubes, labeled, and air-dried. A wet mount of cervix and vagina is prepared for the examining physician to be microscopically inspected for sperm and documented on the emergency chart. A plastic-tip catheter on a syringe is filled with 5 to 10 mL of sterile saline, injected into the vaginal canal, and aspirated. This is labeled "vagina aspirate" and tested for acid phosphatase. A culture for gonorrhea and chlamydia may be obtained, but many physicians prefer to treat patients prophylactically and consider cultures irrelevant. A Wood's lamp will cause semen to fluoresce. When indicated by a history of extravaginal ejaculation, a cotton-tip applicator moistened with saline is used to retrieve semen. If indicated by history, premoistened rectal or buccal swabs for sperm may be collected. If sodomy is involved, a routine rectal examination is performed with attention to perianal fissures or lacerations. If blood is present, anoscopy or sigmoidoscopy should be done to detect any internal injuries. Any film or photographs taken as well as all specimens collected should be labeled with the patient's name and the date and given to the police.

MALE RAPE EXAMINATION

History-taking is similar to that in the female rape examination. The physical examination must be tailored to the particulars of the assault. For example, since the anus is penetrated and the victim is lying prone in the majority of cases, one should search for abrasions on the thorax or abdomen. The male victim may be subdued by blows to the jaw, face, or abdomen. Male children are often less apt to be harmed because fear and intimidation by adult authority may compel them to be passive.

Swabs should be taken of buccal and gingival areas even if the patient has brushed, rinsed, or eaten. Gonorrhea and chlamydia cultures of the pharynx can be taken.

Inspect the anus externally for signs of trauma such as abrasions, lacerations, or fissures. Injuries are the result of friction or disproportion between the diameter of the anus and the erect penis. If no injuries are seen, either the anus was not penetrated or the victim is a homosexual. Other signs of chronic sodomy include decreased sphincter tone, hemorrhoids, and chronic fissures. Rectal swabs should be taken and slides made, labeled, and air-dried. If there is evidence of bleeding, the source should be located and documented. Then 10 mL of sterile saline is injected into the rectum, allowed to equilibrate for a few minutes, and aspirated. The fluid is then examined for sperm. The acid phosphatase determination has little value in sodomy.

CHILD SEXUAL ABUSE

The term *sexual misuse* has replaced the term *sexual abuse* in reference to children to alter the misconception that physical injury is an integral part of the diagnosis. Sexual misuse refers to "any situation where a child is exposed to sexual stimulation inappropriate for that child's age or psychosocial development." The emphasis in this explanation is on the broad range of sexual experiences that may occur, often repeatedly (see Table 57-1).

The spectrum of sexual misuse includes rape, molestation, and incest. Rape has been described previously and usually involves vi-

Table 57-1. Spectrum of Sexual Abuse

Verbal sexual abuse
Inappropriate disrobing and nudity
Genital exposure
Inappropriate observation of the child
Viewing and/or participating in the production of pornographic materials
Inappropriate kissing
Fondling of breasts and genitals
Masturbation—mutual or single
Penetration of mouth by penis (fellatio)
Female genitalia manipulated by another's mouth (cunnilingus)
Penetration of penis in rectum (sodomy)
Digital or object penetration of anus
Digital or object penetration of vagina
Rubbing penis or ejaculating between child's legs or against child's body
Penile penetration of vagina

Source: Blythe MJ, Orr DP: Childhood sexual abuse: Guidelines for evaluation. *Indiana Med* 78:11, 1985. (Used by permisssion.)

olence or the threat of violence. It is usually a single act, and victims often present for help after the incident. Children who are raped know the assailants in most cases. Child molestation is any illegal act performed on or with the body of a child where there is lewd intent. The median age is 11 years; most victims are premenarcheal, and most know their assailant. Most assailants are neighbors, friends, or "shirttail relatives." Because the assailant is known to the victim, most episodes of molestation are nonviolent and recur for weeks to years before being reported. Incest is a sexual offense involving related victim and assailant who could not legally be married. Usually a parent or guardian is involved. Father-daughter incest accounts for most cases, while mother-son incest is considered the most pathological pairing. The long-term impact of incest on children is not encouraging. Many exhibit regressive or antisocial behavior (see Table 57-2) when first evaluated, and even with therapy, adjustment is difficult.

The Physical Examination

The interview of the child and family members should be done individually. Often the use of dolls and play acting encourages the young child to talk about the event. The details of the assault sought are similar to those for the rape victim. However, in cases of incest or repetitive molestation, the physician needs to know when the last episode occurred. If 3 or more days have elapsed since the sexual encounter, recovery of sperm or acid phosphatase will be negligible.

For victims of rape or single-episode molestation there are signs of minor physical or genital trauma observed in 80 percent of all victims examined. A complete extragenital physical examination should be done. Most injuries are external and involve the posterior fourchette labia or hymen. Genital injuries are often noted in the absence of semen or sperm. Bruises should be sought and carefully noted, especially in the perineal and thigh areas. Diagrammatic representation of injuries is the easiest and most accurate method of recording. Chronic molestation or incest presents with subtle signs of previous intercourse rather than actual signs of trauma. The physician will find well-healed circumferential transections of the hymen, healed hymenal tears at 6 o'clock extending into the posterior fourchette, a spacious introitus, and possibly a vaginal discharge. Woodling and Kossoris explain in detail the genital injuries sustained in acute and chronic sexual abuse of children and is a good reference for those who wish to know more.

Most important in the exam is an assessment of female sexual development with description of breast development and presence of axillary or pubic hair, since this may change by the time of trial. An easy method of classification is the Tanner scale (see Table 57-3). The genital examination must be tailored to the age of the patient and circumstances of the assault. The physician should concentrate on signs of forced vaginal or rectal entry. Once again, bruises, abrasions, or lacerations should be diagrammed and the presence of blood or discharge in the vagina or rectum noted and the discharge cultured. Any vaginal discharge in a premenarcheal child should be presumed secondary to sexual abuse until proved otherwise. Since the prepubertal vagina is short and lined with epithelium conducive to bacteria growth, gonorrhea and chlamydia cultures may be obtained from the vagina instead of the cervix. Suspicious lesions or vesicles should be cultured for herpes. The presence of blood should prompt the physician to visually inspect the vagina and rectum, which in a small child may be accomplished easily with the use of a nasal speculum instead of a vaginal speculum. The sodomized infant may be evaluated for lacerations or fissures by using the rounded end of a 5-mL glass test tube inserted into the anus and illuminated with an otoscope or penlight. Rectal sphincter tone should be noted when a digital examination is done since frequent sodomy causes reflex relaxation following perianal stimulation. Sometimes, however, because of the child's emotional state, the vaginal or rectal examination must be done under general anesthesia.

Specimens and washings for forensic purposes should be collected and handled in the same way as outlined in the section on female rape examination. In the child, vaginal washings may be atraumatically obtained with the catheter portion of an IV angiocatheter attached to a syringe. The specimens must be labeled and handled to maintain the chain of evidence.

If possible, siblings of the victim should be examined for signs of physical or sexual abuse. The victim should be protected from further abuse either by admission to the hospital or immediate referral to the appropriate child protective service agency. The family should be referred as a group for counseling, and individual counseling should be provided for the victim.

Physical injuries are treated as indicated by the specific injury, such as lacerations repaired and fractures casted or surgically set. Some patients may need to be hospitalized for such injuries as skull fractures and subdural hematomas. Venereal disease prophylaxis should be given according to Centers for Disease Control (Atlanta, GA) (CDC) guidelines (see "Treatment of the Victim"). Postmenarcheal girls at risk for pregnancy should be given pregnancy prophylaxis after obtaining a pregnancy test.

Table 57-2. Behaviors Suggestive of Sexual Abuse

Infants–toddlers
Irritability
Sleep disturbances
Feeding difficulties
Altered leveling activity
Toddlers–preschoolers
Regressive behavior (thumb-sucking, eneuresis, encopresis)
Age-inappropriate understanding of sexual behavior
Persistent and inappropriate sexual play with peers, toys, or themselves
Acting out, aggressive behavior
Preschoolers–school-age children
Excessive fears, phobias
Sudden changes in behavior such as withdrawal, depression
Sleep disturbances such as night terrors, nightmares
Hints of sexual activity with age-inappropriate understanding of sexual behavior
School-age children–adolescents
Sudden drop in school performance or inability to concentrate in school
Arriving early at school, leaving late with few absences
Poor peer relationships or inability to make friends
Nonparticipation in school and social activities
Adolescents
Extremely seductive with precocious sexual behavior
Running away from home
Prostitution
Suicide attempts

Source: Blythe MJ, Orr DP: Childhood sexual abuse: Guidelines for evaluation. *Indiana Med* 78:11, 1985. (Used by permission.)

Table 57-3. The Tanner Classification

		AGE IN YEARS				AGE IN YEARS			
Stage	**Pubic Hair**	**−2 SD**	**Mean**	**+2 SD**	**Breasts**	**−2 SD**	**Mean**	**+2 SD**	**Comments**
1	None; prepubertal				Prepubertal; elevation papilla only				
2	Long, lightly pigmented, downy; along labia	9.27	11.69	14.11	Breast bud stage; elevation breast and papilla as small mound and enlargement of areolar diameter	8.95	11.15	13.25	Onset of breast and pubic hair development more or less simultaneous; initiation of height spurt will soon follow
3	Increased in amount and pigmentation; curly; still limited to labia	10.16	11.69	14.56	Breast and areola show further enlargement with no separation of contours	9.97	12.15	14.33	Menarche usually occurs about this time or 1½ years after onset of breast development; axillary hair first appears here or in stage 5
4	Adult in type; covers mons and extends about half-way out to inguinal regions	10.83	12.95	15.07	Areola and papilla project to form a secondary mound above the level of the breast itself (variable; not always present)	10.81	13.11	15.31	Height spurt begins to decelerate
5	Adult in type, quantity, and lateral distribution; extending out to thighs	12.17	14.41	16.65	Mature with projection of papilla only due to recession of general contour of entire breast	11.85	15.33	18.81	Growth almost complete and most epiphyses closed; may grow 1–2 cm more

Source: From Fleisher G, Ludwig S: *Textbook of Pediatric Emergency Medicine,* Baltimore, Williams & Wilkins, 1983, Chapter 71. (Used by permission.)

PREGNANCY PROPHYLAXIS

When treating postmenarcheal female rape victims, the physician must consider whether pregnancy prophylaxis is indicated. One must first consider the risk of pregnancy after an isolated sexual encounter. Several studies have found the risk of pregnancy after a single act of intercourse to be rare. In a prospective study of 4000 rapes in Minnesota no pregnancies were found. In another prospective study of 117 rapes, no pregnancies were detected among 17 victims treated with diethylstilbestrol (DES) and 100 given no pregnancy prophylaxis. In a 9-year, retrospective study no pregnancies were found.

Despite the very low probability of pregnancy, women rape victims should be offered the informed choice of pregnancy prophylaxis. Women who were not using any form of contraception at the time of assault and are midcycle in the menses (days 10 to 16) are at greatest risk of pregnancy. Prophylaxis must be initiated within 72 h of the sexual assault to be effective in preventing pregnancy.

DES has lost favor for pregnancy prophylaxis because of the risk of carcinogenesis. Currently accepted therapy is the birth control pill, Ovral (norgestrel + ethinyl estradiol), two tablets orally initially and two tablets 12 h later. This regimen replaces the older 5-day DES regimen, which had more side effects and lower compliance, and seems effective.

TREATMENT OF THE VICTIM

Treat abrasions, lacerations, and other physical injuries according to the standards of care; for instance, lacerations should be sutured and fractures casted. Tetanus prophylaxis should be given when indicated.

A pregnancy test should be obtained in postmenarcheal women and should always be documented as negative before providing postcoital contraception. Many authors recommend also drawing a Venereal Disease Research Laboratories VD test (VDRL). At the discretion of the physician, a drug screen or alcohol level may be indicated.

Most of the literature demonstrates poor compliance with followup in sexual assault victims. Therefore, VD prophylaxis should be given according to CDC guidelines to all sexual assault victims irrespective of their age. (See Table 57-4 for current CDC guidelines on antibiotic and age-related doses.)

The possibility of pregnancy should be discussed with the victim; postcoital contraception should also be discussed and the patient's acceptance or refusal documented on the chart. Postcoital contraception should not be offered if there are medical contraindications to its use, such as the possibility of preexisting pregnancy.

Ideally, counseling for sexual assault victims should be available 24 h a day in the emergency department. If this is not available, the physician should provide information on local mental health or rape counseling centers where patients may seek further help.

Table 57-4. CDC Treatment Guidelines for Gonococcal Infections

Adults and children weighing > 100 lb (45 kg)
- Ceftriaxone 250 mg IM; *or*
- Amoxicillin 3.0 g PO; *or*
- Ampicillin 3.5 g PO; *or*
- Procaine penicillin G 4.8 million units IM
- (Each of these regimens except ceftriaxone is accompanied by probenecid 1.0 g PO)

Followed by
- Tetracycline 500 mg PO qid for 7 days; *or*
- Doxycycline 100 mg PO bid for 7 days

Penicillin allergy
- Spectinomycin 2 g IM *plus*
- Erythromycin stearate 500 mg PO qid for 7 days; *or*
- Ciprofloxacin 500 mg PO once

Children weighing < 100 lb (45 kg)
- Ceftriaxone 125 mg IM; *or*
- Amoxicillin 50 mg/kg (accompanied by probenecid 25 mg/kg PO); *or*
- Procaine penicillin G 100,000 units/kg IM *plus*
- Probenecid 25 mg/kg PO

Penicillin allergy
- Spectinomycin 40 mg/kg IM; *or*
- Tetracycline 40 mg/kg PO qid for 5 days (for children > 8 years old)

Source: 1989 STD Treatment. *MMWR* 38 (number 5-8) Sept, 1, 1989.

The physician should provide for follow-up medical care to ensure that injuries have healed properly. A follow-up appointment with a gynecologist in 7 to 14 days is necessary to ensure adequate pregnancy prophylaxis and venereal disease treatment. For male rape victims a follow-up urologic appointment would be appropriate. Young children should be referred to a pediatrician for reevaluation.

SPERM SURVIVABILITY

The presence of sperm or seminal constituents in the vagina is evidence of recent sexual intercourse. The detection of sperm is dependent on several factors, including time lapse between the rape and the physical examination, whether the assailant is azoospermic, whether the patient douched prior to examination, and whether the assailant ejaculated. The recovery rate of sperm has been variably reported in the literature to span from 20 to 75 percent depending on the method employed to detect sperm.

Because of the difficulties in sperm detection, several researchers attempted to determine, in controlled settings, how long sperm persisted in the vagina and cervix. In one study of Papanicolaou smears of the cervix of 980 patients, 64 percent of the Pap smears prepared on the first day after intercourse were found to contain sperm. As the interval between intercourse and smear preparation increased, the percentage of smears with sperm decreased. Sperm were irregularly detected to nonexistent after the seventh postcoital day. In another study 15 volunteer couples were enlisted to investigate the rate of decay of sperm and prostatic acid phosphatase after a single act of intercourse (see Fig. 57-1). Only 50% of the women had motile sperm after 3 h, and their presence in the vagina decreased rapidly thereafter. Nonmotile sperm were present in all subjects for up to 18 h, and at 72 h 50 percent had persistent sperm. The level of acid phosphatase enzyme decreased more rapidly than sperm after intercourse. Fifty percent of the subjects had significant levels after 9 h, but by 36 h there were no positive findings. The investigators also found no correlation betweens sperm and acid phosphatase decay, which implies that seminal fluid with a high sperm count may not necessarily indicate a high acid phosphatase level.

There is general agreement in the literature that 2 to 3 h is the average time for loss of sperm motility in 50 percent of controls. Most rape examinations do not take place within this time frame. The normal range of decay for sperm in the cervix or vagina varies widely from study to study, from 14 h to 19 days. This discrepancy may be explained by the methods of specimen collection ranging from Pap smears of the cervix to wet mounts of the vaginal fluid, as well as the criteria used for reporting positive sperm.

There is very little published data on sperm persistence in the anus or rectum. In one study, sperm were observed to be present up to 24 h after intercourse; however, it was rare to find tails on sperm from rectal swabs, especially after 6 h.

RECENT ADVANCES IN LABORATORY EVALUATION

Historically, courts and the legal profession have placed a high significance on sperm detection as confirmatory evidence of rape. It is well documented how elusive sperm detection during a rape examination may be. Several factors influencing sperm detection include long delay in seeking medical attention, azoospermia, vasectomy, sexual dysfunction during rape, and alcohol in the assailant. Researchers have investigated other laboratory tests that, in the absence of sperm, would still be sensitive indicators of recent intercourse.

Acid phosphatase detection in vaginal washings is helpful in cases of azoospermic ejaculation. The time period for detection of this enzyme is variably reported in the literature as 2 to 9 h. Acid phosphatase is also present in erythrocytes, thrombocytes, leukocytes, and bone but may be differentiated from seminal acid phosphatase by various chemical means. However, one must be careful in comparing acid phosphatase levels from different laboratories, for they are reported in different units on the basis of the assay employed. An acid phosphatase level greater than 20 to 25 King-Armstrong units is generally considered indicative of recent intercourse.

Comparisons of gamma glutamyl transferase activity (GGT) and acid phosphatase have shown that GTT is not sensitive or specific enough to be used as a substitute test for acid phosphatase.

A male-specific semen protein, p30, is derived from the prostate gland and is isolated in seminal plasma and prostate tissue. It is an ideal marker because it (1) is found in high concentration in semen, (2) is male-specific, (3) follows a regular pattern of postcoital decline, and (4) is reliably detected by a sensitive and specific enzyme-linked immunoabsorbent assay (ELISA). The shortest postcoital interval at which p30 is no longer detected is 13 h. The ELISA assay for p30 confirmed the presence of semen in 7 out of 27 alleged rape cases where acid phosphatase was negative.

A sperm coating antigen from human seminal vesicles, MHS-5, is present in normal and vasectomized males but absent in all human tissues or fluids other than semen. It is localized to the surface of

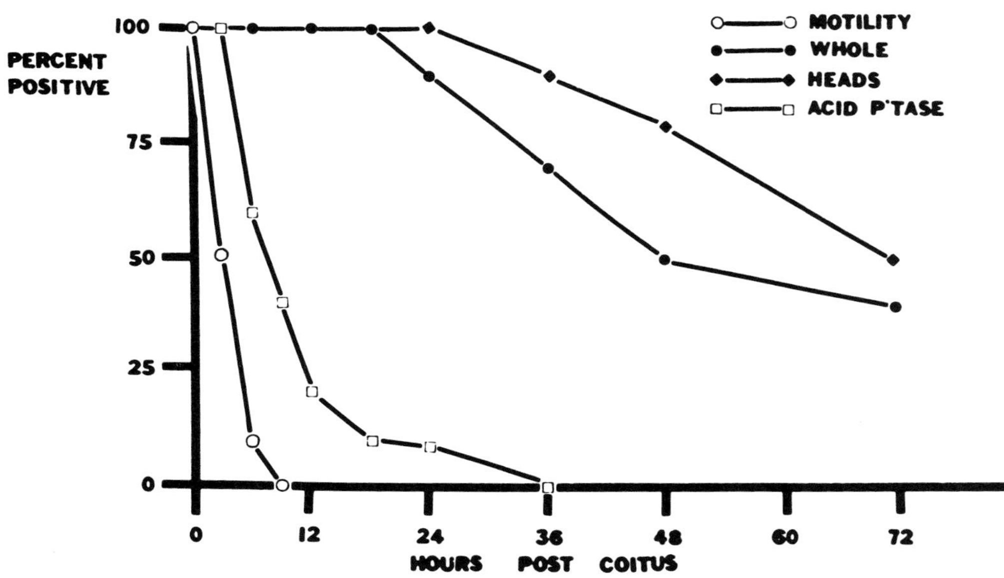

Fig. 57-1. Survival of motile and nonmotile sperm and seminal acid phosphatase in the vagina. Percent positive = percent of subjects in whom each constituent was still present at each time interval after coitus (n = 10). (From Soules MR, Pollard AA: The forensic laboratory evaluation of evidence in alleged rape. *Am J Obstet Gynecol* 130:142, 1978. (Used by permission.)

ejaculated sperm. There is an ELISA assay sufficiently sensitive to detect MHS-5 in 1 ng of seminal protein. It is biochemically distinct from p30.

Until more sensitive and specific tests are available, determination of the presence of sperm or acid phosphatase is the most widely used and widely available marker. The absence of sperm or acid phosphatase, however, does not mean that sexual penetration has not occurred.

BIBLIOGRAPHY

Blythe MJ, Orr DP: Childhood sexual abuse: Guidelines for evaluation. *Indiana Med* 78:11, 1985.

Braen GR, Martin CA: Rape and the rape trauma syndrome. *South Med J* 78:1230, 1985.

Dixon GW, Schlesselman JJ: Ethinyl estradiol and conjugated estrogens as postcoital contraceptives. *JAMA* 244:1336, 1980.

Goldenring JM: Estrogen treatment for victims of rape (letter). *N Engl J Med* 312(15):989, 1985.

Jenny C, Hooton TM, Bowers A: Sexually transmitted diseases in victims of rape. *N Engl J Med* 322:713, 1990.

1989 STD Treatment Guidelines. *MMWR* vol. 38, No. 5-8, Sept. 2, 1989.

Schiff AF: Examination and treatment of the male rape victim. *S Med J* 73:1498, 1980.

Silverman EM, Silverman AG: Persistence of spermatozoa in the lower genital tracts of women. *JAMA* 240:1875, 1978.

Soules MR, Pollard AA: The forensic laboratory evaluation of evidence in alleged rape. *Am J Obstet Gynecol* 130:142, 1978.

Tintinalli J, Hoelzer M: Clinical findings and legal resolutions in sexual assault. *Ann Emerg Med* 14:447, 1985.

Woodling BA, Evans JR, Bradbury MD: Sexual assault: Rape and molestation. *Clin Obstet Gynecol* 20:509, 1977.

Woodling BA, Kossoris PD: Sexual misuse: Rape, molestation, and incest. *Pediatr Clin N Am* 28:481, 1981.

58
TOXIC SHOCK SYNDROME

Ann L. Harwood-Nuss
Christina Drummond

Toxic shock syndrome (TSS), first described in 1978 by J. Todd in seven children with *Staphylococcus aureus* infections, is an acute febrile syndrome characterized by diffuse, desquamating erythroderma, mucous membrane hyperemia, vomiting, diarrhea, pharyngitis, and myalgias. It may progress rapidly to hypotension and multisystem dysfunction. There is a convalescent peeling of digits, palms, and soles.

In 1980, TSS was noted in menstruating women, and by 1981, an epidemic associated with continuous tampon use was widely recognized. In Table 58-1 a TSS case definition is given. This case definition was formulated in 1980 by the Centers for Disease Control (CDC) to ensure that cases included in various surveillance studies were the same clinical entity of TSS. In the absence of a definitive laboratory marker, the strict application of the case definition undoubtedly excludes the less severe (subclinical) cases.

Since 1980, there have been significant advances in the understanding of the clinical and epidemiologic aspects of TSS. Since 1984, the incidence of reported cases has declined. In addition, the case fatality ratio has fallen and the proportion of cases associated with menstruation has decreased.

ETIOLOGY AND PATHOGENESIS

Most cases of TSS have been directly associated with *S. aureus* infection or colonization. Approximately 67 percent of the organisms are phage type I, while 25 percent are nontypable. Recent reports have demonstrated a disease clinically indistinguishable from TSS caused by group A streptococci, *Streptococcus pneumoniae,* and *Pseudomonas aeruginosa.*

The most impressive aspect of the pathophysiology is the massive vasodilation and rapid movement of serum proteins and fluids from the intravascular to the extravascular space. This results in the rapid onset of oliguria, hypotension, edema, and low central venous pressure, and the requirements for large amounts of fluid to restore and maintain blood pressure. The multisystem involvement seen in TSS may be a reflection of the rapid onset of hypotension and decreased perfusion, or there may be direct effects of a toxin or toxins on the parenchymal cells of different organs. Current evidence indicates that pyrogenic toxin C and enterotoxin F are the same protein, called *toxic shock syndrome toxin-1* (TSST-1). TSST-1 mediates the disease, although the mechanism remains unclear. TSST-1 enhances susceptibility to normal or sublethal amounts of endotoxin while directly damaging cell membranes, activating coagulation, kinin, and prostaglandin cascades. While TSST-1–producing strains of *S. aureus* have been found in 95 percent of cases of menstrual-related TSS, approximately 40 percent of isolates from non-menstrual-related TSS do not produce the toxin. This suggests that while TSST-1 plays an important role in the pathogenesis of TSS produced by some strains of *S. aureus,* other bacterial products may be capable of inducing the syndrome.

Furthermore, the immunologic status of the individual may play a role in the pathogenesis of the disease. Anti-TSST-1 antibody titers of 1:100 were seen in approximately 80 percent of control patients, whereas only 17 percent of patients with TSS had such titers.

The means by which *S. aureus* enters the host in TSS are numerous. Although an exogenous source of *S. aureus* has been suggested for nonmenstrual cases, no such source has been identified for menstrual cases. It is presumed that women who develop menstrual TSS were colonized with *S. aureus* before the onset of menstruation.

Table 58-1. Criteria for Diagnosis (Must Have All)

1. Temperature > 38.9°C (102°F)
2. Systolic BP < 90 mmHg, orthostatic decrease of systolic BP by 15 mmHg, or syncope
3. Rash (diffuse, macular erythroderma) with subsequent desquamation, especially on palms or soles of feet
4. Involvement of three of the following organ systems clinically or by abnormal laboratory tests:
   a. Gastrointestinal: Vomiting, profuse diarrhea
   b. Musculoskeletal: Severe myalgias or twofold increase in CPK
   c. Renal: Increase in BUN and creatinine two times normal; pyuria without evidence of infection
   d. Mucosal inflammation: Vaginal, conjunctival, or pharyngeal hyperemia
   e. Hepatic involvement: Hepatitis (twofold elevation of: bilirubin, SGOT, SGPT)
   f. Hematologic: Thrombocytopenia < 100,000 platelets/mm^3
   g. CNS: Disorientation without focal neurologic signs
5. Negative serologic tests for Rocky Mountain spotted fever, leptospirosis, measles, hepatitis B surface antigen, fluorescent antinuclear antibody, VDRL, and monospot; and negative blood, urine, and throat cultures

EPIDEMIOLOGY

The CDC reports a decrease from 900 cases in 1980 to 351 cases in 1988, presumably due to the general public's increased awareness of risk factors from tampon use.

TSS is most often seen in menstruating women between the ages of 15 and 24 years. Although the proportion of cases associated with menstruation has decreased since 1980, 50 percent of TSS cases reported by the CDC in 1986 and 1987 were found in menstruating women. *S. aureus* has been isolated from the vaginas of 98 percent of women with TSS, versus an 8 to 10 percent carrier rate in the control group.

The proportion of cases not associated with menstruation has increased since 1980 primarily because of the decrease in the number of menstruation-related cases. The nonmenstrual cases occur in a variety of clinical settings. Nearly 25 percent are associated with postpartum and *S. aureus* vaginal infections. Other cases of TSS have been reported in association with cutaneous and subcutaneous *S. aureus* infections (burns, abrasions, abscesses, etc.). Nasal packing (nasal tampons) is also associated with TSS, with 20 to 40 percent of the adult population carrying *S. aureus* in the nasal vestibule.

Prior to 1980, the case fatality rate was 10 percent. Since 1980, there has been a marked decline in TSS mortality.

DIFFERENTIAL DIAGNOSIS

There are other systemic illnesses that are characterized by fever, rash, diarrhea, myalgias, and multisystem involvement and resemble TSS (Table 58-2). Kawasaki disease (mucocutaneous lymph node syndrome) is characterized by fever, conjunctival hyperemia, and erythema of the mucous membranes with desquamation.
Although the exanthems may be quite similar, Kawasaki disease may

Table 58-2. Differential Diagnosis of Toxic Shock Syndrome

Acute pyelonephritis	Acute viral syndrome
Septic shock	Leptospirosis
Acute rheumatic fever	Systemic lupus erythematosus
Streptococcal scarlet fever	Rocky Mountain spotted fever
Staphylococcal scarlet fever	Tick typhus
Staphylococcal scalded skin syndrome	Gastroenteritis
Legionnaires' disease	Kawasaki disease
Pelvic inflammatory disease	Reye's syndrome
Hemolytic uremic syndrome	

present with target lesions resembling erythema multiforme, and the bright-red appearance of the vermillion border is not common in TSS.

Further differentiation of Kawasaki disease from TSS lies in the facts that more than 99 percent of those afflicted with Kawasaki disease are under 10 years of age and that Kawasaki disease is not characterized by hypotension, renal failure, or thrombocytopenia.

The clinical picture of staphylococcal scarlet fever is so similar to TSS that only pathology specimens or serologic evidence of the exfoliatin toxin will differentiate the two entities. However, streptococcal scarlet fever is rare after 10 years of age. Further, the "sandpaper" rash of scarlet fever is distinct from the macular rash of TSS.

Septic shock must always be considered in the differential diagnosis of TSS. In general, the appearance of a rash and the laboratory abnormalities associated with TSS will aid in distinguishing these two entities. Scalded skin syndrome may be distinguished from TSS primarily by the lack of serious multisystem involvement and by rapid, superficial peeling in contrast to the full-thickness desquamation of TSS. In addition, the scalded skin syndrome usually occurs in children less than 5 years old.

CLINICAL PRESENTATION

TSS should be considered in any unexplained febrile illness associated with erythroderma, hypotension, and diffuse organ pathology, especially in menstruating women. The clinical criteria for the diagnosis of TSS are listed in Table 58-1. Patients with menstruation-associated TSS usually present between the third and fifth day of menses. The median time to onset of illness in postsurgical toxic shock is two postoperative days.

The CDC case definition may exclude mild cases of TSS, so one must keep in mind the spectrum of the disease in diagnosis. A milder form of TSS may occur in any patient. It is generally characterized by fever and chills, myalgias, abdominal pain, sore throat, nausea, vomiting, and diarrhea. Hypotension does not occur, and the illness is self-limited.

Severe TSS is an acute-onset, multisystem disease with symptoms, signs, and laboratory abnormalities reflecting multiple-organ involvement. Some patients may experience a prodrome consisting of malaise, myalgias, headache, and nausea. Most patients, however, will present with the sudden onset of fever and chills, headache, nausea, vomiting, and diarrhea. Sudden onset of fever and chills occurs approximately 1 to 4 days prior to presentation. Diffuse myalgias, particularly in the proximal aspects of the extremities, abdomen, and back are reported by virtually all patients; arthralgias are also common. Profuse, watery diarrhea and repeated vomiting are reported by 90 to 98 percent of patients. Patients also complain of sore throat, headache, paresthesias, and photophobia, as well as orthostatic dizziness or syncope. The patient may additionally complain of abdominal pain, cough, or sore throat.

Physical examination reveals hypotension or an orthostatic decrease in systolic pressure by 15 mmHg in 100 percent of cases since this is an inclusion criterion of the disease. Milder forms of the disease may not present with hypotension, however.

Patients may show edema of the face and extremities. Orthostatic light-headedness or syncope may be present. In general, victims of TSS appear acutely ill. In the acute state, which usually lasts about 24 to 48 h, the patient may be obtunded, disoriented, oliguric, and hypotensive. Dermatologic manifestations include erythema of the skin and mucous membranes.

The rash is classically a diffuse blanching erythroderma which fades within 3 days of its appearance and is followed by full-thickness desquamation, especially of the palms and soles. Variations include patchy erythroderma and localized maculopustular eruptions. Between the fifth and tenth hospital days, a generalized pruritic maculopapular rash develops in about 25 percent of patients. In all cases, a fine generalized desquamation of the skin, with peeling over the soles, fingers, toes, and palms, occurs between 6 and 14 days after the onset of illness. More than 50 percent of severely ill patients experience loss of hair and nails 2 to 3 months later. Other prominent signs and symptoms may include profound muscle weakness and tenderness and/or abdominal pain and tenderness; vomiting and diarrhea persist. The diarrhea is usually watery and profuse. One-half to three-quarters of patients have pharyngitis with a strawberry-red tongue; conjunctival hyperemia and vaginitis are also seen. Tender, edematous external genitalia, diffuse vaginal hyperemia, scant purulent cervical discharge, and bilateral adnexal tenderness are seen in 25 to 35 percent of patients with menstruation-related TSS.

Specific focal neurologic findings rarely occur, but altered states of consciousness are common. Approximately 75 percent of patients have nonfocal neurologic abnormalities without signs of meningeal irritation. Confusion, disorientation, agitation, hysteria, somnolence, and seizures have been reported, consistent with a toxic encephalopathy.

Figure 58-1 illustrates the temporal relationships of the major manifestations.

Abnormal laboratory values reflect the multisystem involvement in TSS. Leukocytosis with an increase in immature forms is frequently seen; lymphocytopenia has also been reported. Azotemia and abnormal urinary sediment (sterile pyuria and red blood cell casts) are seen with the development of acute renal failure. Liver function abnormalities and hyperbilirubinemia are seen in approximately half the patients. Despite increases in the prothrombin time, partial thromboplastin time, and fibrin split products in association with thrombocytopenia, only 3 percent of patients have clinical evidence of a coagulopathy. Electrolyte abnormalities including hypocalcemia, hypophosphatemia, hyponatremia, and hypokalemia are common. Metabolic acidosis secondary to hypotension is also seen.

Acute renal failure secondary to acute tubular necrosis is a complication of TSS. Ventricular arrhythmias, adult respiratory distress syndrome (ARDS), and refractory hypotension represent the ultimate end organ damage secondary to TSS.

MANAGEMENT

Management of TSS depends on its severity. The most important aspect of initial management is the aggressive volume replacement. Continuous monitoring of heart rate, respiratory rate, arterial blood pressure, urinary output, central venous pressure, and pulmonary capillary wedge pressure is necessary. During the first 24 h, patients may require 4 to 5 L of crystalloids and fresh-frozen plasma. There have been reports of patients requiring up to 20 L of fluid in the first 24 h of hospitalization. A dopamine infusion beginning at 5 to 10 μg/kg per minute may be used if volume correction fails to restore normal arterial pressure. Chest radiographic findings, blood gases, and serum electrolytes should be monitored.

Patients with abnormal coagulation profiles and evidence of bleeding require colloid replacement and replacement of fresh-frozen plasma, or transfusions; thrombocytopenia may require platelet transfusions. If ARDS occurs, both mechanical ventilation and positive end-expiratory pressure will likely be necessary.

A focus of infection should be sought and promptly treated. Women with tampon-related TSS should have the tampon removed; some authors recommend irrigation of the vagina with saline or povidone-iodine solution. Cultures of all potentially infected sites should be obtained, including blood cultures, prior to initiating antibiotic therapy.

Although antimicrobial agents have not been shown to affect the outcome of the acute illness, they are recommended and have been given to most patients to eradicate the focus of toxin-producing staphylococci as well as to decrease the recurrence rate.

Antibiotic selection should include an antistaphylococcal penicillin or cephalosporin with β-lactamase stability. Nafcillin or oxacillin in doses of 1 to 2 g every 4 h provides adequate antimicrobial coverage. Cefazolin, 2 g every 6 h, also provides adequate coverage, but the

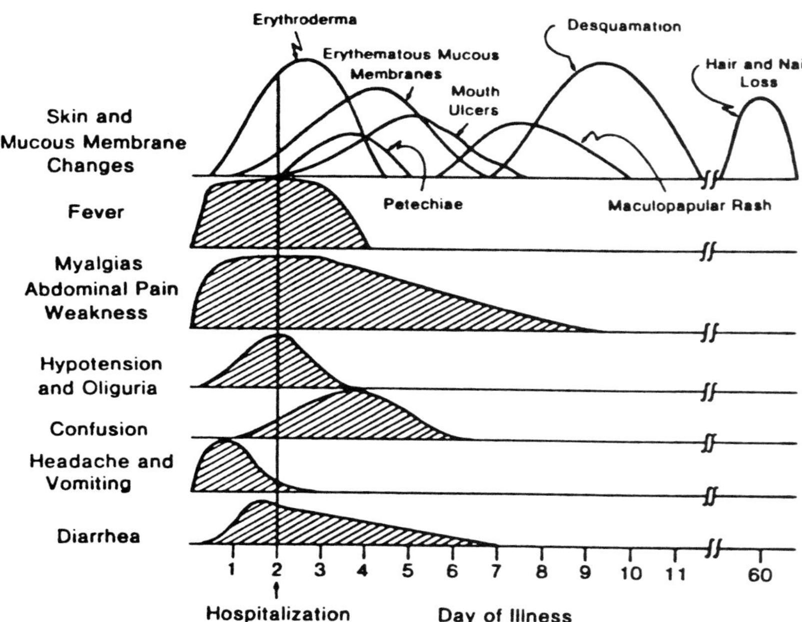

Fig. 58.1. Composite drawing of major systemic, skin, and mucous membrane manifestations of toxic shock syndrome. (*From* Chesney PJ, David JP, Purdy WK, et al: Clinical manifestations of toxic shock syndrome. *JAMA* 246:741, 1981.)

first-generation cephalosporins are less β-lactamase stable than the antistaphylococcal penicillins. Vancomycin, trimethoprim-sulfamethoxazole, or rifampin may be used if methicillin-resistant strains are encountered. Although data on the optimum duration of antimicrobial therapy are not available, it seems prudent to administer parenteral antibiotics for at least 3 days or until the patient clinically improves. Oral antistaphylococcal antibiotics should then be administered for an additional 10 days. Although prospective studies are lacking, the addition of rifampin to the oral regimen is suggested because of the ability of this drug to eradicate the carrier state.

There is clinical evidence that methylprednisolone, 30 mg/kg, may reduce the severity of the illness if administered within the first 2 to 3 days of illness.

The majority of patients become afebrile and normotensive within 48 h of hospitalization. The laboratory abnormalities seen initially resolve within 1 to 2 weeks. Full anemia correction occurs in 4 to 6 weeks.

SEQUELAE

Numerous sequelae of TSS have been reported and include late onset of maculopapular rash, decreased renal function, reversible loss of hair and nails, prolonged neuromuscular abnormalities, and cyanotic extremities. Neurologic sequelae have been documented. Memory deficits, reflexia, and diffuse electroencephalographic abnormalities are consistently seen in those patients with neurologic sequelae.

Table 58-3. Clinical Settings Associated with Variant Toxic Shock Syndrome

Childbirth (vaginal or cesarean section)
Septic abortion
Mastitis
Nasal surgery with packing
Fasciitis
Osteomyelitis
Peritonsillar abscess
Subcutaneous abscess or lesion (furuncles, hydradenitis, insect bites, burns, abrasions)
Staphylococcal colonization of mucous membranes
Sinusitis
Postoperative
Burns
Diaphragm use
Bronchitis (influenza)

The exact mechanism associated with the appearance of these sequelae is not yet clear. Possible explanations may include a delayed effect of the toxin, the presence of circulating immune complexes, or drug-mediated reactions.

RECURRENCES

Up to 60 percent of patients not treated with β-lactamase-stable antimicrobial drugs had recurrences. Most recurrent episodes occur by the second month following the initial episode, on the same day of menses as the prior attack, although some have recurred in less than 1 month, and some more than 1 year later. In the majority of patients having a recurrence, the initial episode was the most severe, although deaths have occurred from recurrences of initially mild cases of TSS.

NONMENSTRUAL TOXIC SHOCK SYNDROME

The proportion of reported cases not associated with menstruation has been increasing, accounting for 29 percent of cases of TSS in 1983. These are either associated with *S. aureus* infections or follow childbirth by vaginal delivery or cesarean section (see Table 58-3). Cases of TSS associated with subcutaneous and cutaneous lesions and with surgical wound infections show that life-threatening illness can result from infections with *S. aureus* at these sites. TSS has also been reported following nasal surgery and nasal packs. Staphylococcal infections at diverse sites can be responsible for producing TSS. Finally, TSS can occur in patients with no apparent source of infection.

Patients with TSS not associated with menstruation differ in age and racial distribution from those with menstruation-associated TSS, one-third of them being male. TSS can occur in many clinical settings in patients of both sexes and of all ages and racial groups.

BIBLIOGRAPHY

Broome CV: Epidemiology of toxic shock syndrome in the United States: Overview. *Rev Infect Dis* 2(suppl 1):S14, 1989.

Centers for Disease Control: Summary of notifiable diseases—United States. *Morbid Mortal Week Rep* 37:51, 1989.

Resnick ST: Toxic shock syndrome: Recent developments in pathogenesis. *J Pediatr* 116:3, 1990.

Todd JK: Toxic shock syndrome. *Clin Microbiol Rev* 1:4, 1988.

59 OBSTETRIC EMERGENCIES

Robert P. Lorenz

Pregnancy requires major physiologic adaptations of all organ systems to allow normal fetal growth and development and finally birth and maternal recovery. These physiologic changes should be understood by the emergency department physician because (1) appropriate management of nonobstetric emergencies in a pregnant patient should reflect an appreciation of pregnancy-related symptoms, adaptive physiologic alterations, and altered physical examination and laboratory findings; and (2) appropriate management of obstetric emergencies should be based on an understanding of altered physiology of the mother and fetus.

This chapter deals with the following topics: (1) the diagnosis of pregnancy; (2) decision making regarding diagnostic radiologic procedures and therapeutic drug selection in pregnancy; (3) selected medical complications of pregnancy; and (4) surgical complications including ectopic pregnancy, disorders causing bleeding during pregnancy, and postmortem cesarean section.

DIAGNOSIS OF PREGNANCY

All female patients of childbearing age are assumed to be pregnant until proven otherwise. This maxim is useful in the emergency department because (1) pregnancy may explain the presence of mild symptoms such as breast pain, nausea, urinary frequency, or fatigue; (2) the complications of pregnancy must be considered in any woman of childbearing age with abdominal pain or vaginal bleeding; (3) the complications of pregnancy must be considered in the differential diagnosis of women of childbearing age with hypertension, seizures, thromboembolic disease, or jaundice; (4) radiation exposure and drug therapy must take into account a possible pregnancy; and (5) many common problems (e.g., herpes, rubella, diabetes mellitus) may adversely affect normal fetal development and survival and require genetic counseling or specialized obstetric care later in pregnancy.

The pregnant woman usually has a history of mistimed, light, or absent menses. By 4 weeks from the last normal menstrual period (LMP), she may notice mild breast pain and/or nipple sensitivity. Fatigue, nausea, and urinary frequency often appear in the next few weeks. However, these signs are merely presumptive and not totally reliable in the diagnosis. Often, even in the absence of particular symptoms, multiparous women state that they "feel pregnant."

At approximately 4 weeks from the LMP, there may be slight breast swelling and tenderness. A pelvic examination by an experienced gynecologist usually can identify a pregnancy by 6 to 8 weeks of amenorrhea by findings of softening and bluish discoloration of the cervix (in a woman not on oral contraceptives), and softening and enlargement of the uterus (in the nonobese patient). The uterus becomes an abdominal organ after 12 weeks gestation. A pelvic examination should be considered whenever the differential diagnosis includes pregnancy.

All pregnancy tests are based on the determination of the level of human chorionic gonadotropin (HCG), which is produced after implantation of the fertilized ovum (about 9 days after conception). HCG levels peak at 50 to 75 days of amenorrhea but are still detected until 14 days (median) after a term delivery. The latest generation of HCG assays offers improved sensitivity, rapid turnaround time, and only rare false-positive results. Assays with multiple monoclonal antibodies provide improved specificity. Clinicians are cautioned that assays (and clinical correlation) vary with the reference standard, the most recent being the World Health Organization Third International Standard. The clinician should learn which test the laboratory employs, the sensitivity, specificity, reference standard, and whether intact HCG, or "total" (intact plus free β subunit) is measured.

Examples of pregnancy tests are listed in Table 59-1. Any pregnancy test results should be integrated into overall clinical assessment of the patient.

Transabdominal real-time pelvic ultrasonography can identify a normal intrauterine pregnancy by 6 weeks of gestation. Transvaginal sonography if available can detect the same about 1 week earlier.

DRUG AND RADIATION EXPOSURE IN PREGNANCY

An important principle of teratogenesis is that one cannot prove any individual exposure is safe. One may be able to prove an increased risk of teratogenic effects if sufficient human data are available. Most clinical exposures are associated with risks that fall between these extremes. Although most adverse outcomes are not due to drug or radiation exposure, the list of adverse pregnancy outcomes each pregnancy faces is formidable; spontaneous abortion 15 to 20 percent, preterm birth 8 percent, stillbirth 1 percent, congenital anomalies 3 to 5 percent, cerebral palsy 0.25 percent, mental retardation 0.25 percent, learning or behavioral disorders 8 percent. Patients are often unaware that Mother Nature has more adverse impact than most medical exposures.

Drugs

Only 2 percent of congenital malformations are attributable to a drug. Nevertheless, the institution and selection of medication during pregnancy should reflect consideration of benefits and risks to mother and fetus. Resources available include helpful texts and on-line computer databases. It is important to consider whether human or only animal data are provided and whether proven adverse effects have been found.

Antibiotics

The penicillins, cephalosporins, and erythromycin have been used extensively in pregnancy without proven adverse effects. The estolate form of erythromycin, however, should not be used because of an increased risk of cholestatic hepatitis in the mother. Sulfonamides compete with bilirubin for albumin binding sites and can cause kernicterus when used late in pregnancy. In severe infections, one may

Table 59-1. Examples of Laboratory Methods For Pregnancy Testing*

Method	Specimen	Endpoint	Sensitivity,† mIU/mL	Earliest Detection Days From LMP	Assay Time
ELISA (qualitative)	Urine	2 monoclonal antibodies with colorimetric assay	50	25	5 min
Immunoradiometric (quantative)	Blood	3 monoclonal antibodies, one with I^{125}	5	23	60 min

* Commercial labs vary considerably. See text.

† World Health Organization Third International Standard.

have to use aminoglycosides, but the potential fetal ototoxicity and nephrotoxicity make them relatively contraindicated. Tetracyclines may cause maternal hepatocellular necrosis and fetal hypoplasia of bones and teeth. The gray syndrome observed in newborns following maternal chloramphenicol therapy provides a relative contraindication to its use late in pregnancy. Oxidant drugs such as the nitrofurantoins should be avoided in pregnant patients who are potentially deficient in glucose-6-phosphate dehydrogenase (G6PD). Because of animal studies demonstrating mutagenicity, metronidazole (Flagyl) is relatively contraindicated, especially in the first trimester. However no adverse effects in humans have been proved.

Analgesics

Salicylates, with potent effects on prostaglandin metabolism and platelet function, are associated with a slight increase in stillbirths, prolonged pregnancy, and fetal intraventricular hemorrhage. Potent analgesics, such as morphine and meperidine (Demerol) may have transient CNS depressant effects on the newborn after short-term exposure, or cause a life-threatening neonatal withdrawal syndrome with chronic use. Single use of nitrous oxide, enflurane, or halothane early in pregnancy has not been shown to be teratogenic. However chronic occupational exposure may increase risk of spontaneous abortion.

Anticoagulants

Warfarin (Coumadin) crosses the placenta and is associated with adverse pregnancy outcome in 35 percent of first trimester exposures, including a specific fetal warfarin syndrome (8 percent). Fetal hemorrhagic complications can result from third trimester exposure. Heparin, on the other hand, does not cross the placenta and has no described adverse fetal effects. Chronic (>6 months) therapeutic doses in pregnancy may predispose to reversible osteoporosis and fractures. Heparin is the anticoagulant of choice in pregnancy. The safety of thrombolytic agents such as streptokinase and tissue plasminogen activator has not been demonstrated.

Anticonvulsants

Offspring of epileptic patients have an increased risk of congenital anomalies, regardless of therapy. In addition, phenytoin (Dilantin) increases the risk of a specific syndrome (craniofacial anomalies, limb deformities, deficient growth, and mental retardation). Trimethadione (Tridione) has been linked to multiple malformations, as well as increased risk of spontaneous abortion. There is no current evidence to contraindicate the rapid intravenous use of standard drugs to control status epilepticus. Epileptic women in the reproductive years should undergo preconception counseling and evaluation of possible medication change in anticipation of pregnancy.

Psychotropic Drugs

Lithium may cause fetal cardiac and other defects and should be avoided if possible during pregnancy. Conflicting reports concerning all other psychotropic medications (minor tranquilizers, phenothiazines, tricyclics, etc.) have led to the recommendation that they not be used, particularly in the first trimester, unless absolutely necessary.

Asthma Medications

Exacerbations of asthma may occur at any time during pregnancy. Therapy is directed at maintaining optimal maternal and fetal oxygenation. Upright positioning of the patient with administration of supplemental oxygen and the maintenance of adequate hydration are essential. β-Adrenergic drugs have been used extensively in pregnancy for treatment of preterm labor. Treatment of asthma in pregnancy with them is not contraindicated.

There are no proven adverse effects of currently used medications for acute asthma, including steroids and cromolyn sodium. The inhalation may be as effective as other routes for many drugs, with a lower fetal dose resulting.

Antinauseants

Changes in eating patterns and dietary constituents may alleviate symptoms in many cases of nausea associated with pregnancy. If such changes are unsuccessful, the use of both prochlorperazine (Compazine) and trimethobenzamide (Tigan) is preferable to the development of dehydration and electrolyte imbalance.

Radiation Exposure

High doses of radiation (>100 rad, therapeutic radiation) increase risks of mental retardation and pregnancy loss. Exposure >10 rad increases risk of fetal growth retardation. Fetal exposure <10 rad does not carry a proven increase in risk. Radiographic studies such as skull series, cervical spine series, chest x-ray films, and extremity films result in less than 1 to 10 mrad of fetal radiation exposure if the uterus is shielded during the procedure. Larger doses (100 to 350 mrad) of radiation are delivered to the fetus during abdominal, pelvic, and lumbosacral spine x-ray examination. When considering obtaining x-ray films in women of childbearing age, (1) always take a menstrual history and a contraceptive history and consider obtaining a pregnancy test if indicated; (2) never withhold necessary x-ray studies; (3) obtain informed consent if possible; (4) shield the uterus if possible; (5) if the patient is pregnant, arrange for radiation dosimetry calculations for use in further (usually reassuring) counseling.

MEDICAL COMPLICATIONS

Nausea of Pregnancy and Hyperemesis Gravidarum

Approximately 50 percent of pregnancies result in nausea, usually worst in the first trimester. Symptoms beyond that stage should be an indication for a further evaluation for other causes, such as cholecystitis, hepatitis, gastroenteritis, or pyelonephritis.

When the presence of other medical or surgical disease has been eliminated, the nausea of pregnancy may be treated with frequent small meals of dry food such as crackers, toast, and cereal during periods when the patient is symptomatic. Trimethobenzamide or prochlorperazine may be used if this fails. Starvation, dehydration, and acidosis may result from unremitting nausea and vomiting, a condition referred to as hyperemesis gravidarum. Hospitalization, intravenous rehydration, emotional support, and gradual reinstitution of oral nourishment usually are effective. While ketonuria is not a direct fetal risk, it may reflect a severity of illness warranting hospitalization. Occasionally, parenteral alimentation is necessary.

Preterm Labor

Preterm birth is defined as birth between 20 and 37 completed weeks of gestation, and occurs in 8 percent of births in the United States. It is the cause of 75 percent of perinatal mortality and most long-term morbidity in newborns. Prevention of preterm birth is the most significant problem facing obstetrics, and all physicians seeing pregnant women should be sensitized to early sign of preterm labor. Early identification of signs of preterm birth may increase the success of treatment of preterm labor with prolongation of the pregnancy.

Patients at increased risk of preterm birth include those with multiple gestations, diethylstilbesterol (DES) exposure in utero, uterine anomalies, previous cervical conization, previous preterm birth, a cerclage, and cocaine use.

Pregnant patients in early preterm labor usually don't describe "contractions," but may complain of any of the following: change in vaginal discharge; new pain in the back, thighs, pelvis, or abdomen; pressure in the pelvis, bladder, or rectum; abdominal tightenings; menstrual-like cramps; or vaginal pain. Although many of these symptoms may be due to a normal pregnancy, patients with new complaints should receive obstetric evaluation for possible preterm labor. If frequent contractions are identified on external tocodynamometry and cervical change is noted, then treatment with intravenous fluids, bed rest, and tocolytics (e.g., β mimetics or magnesium sulfate) may be indicated. If advanced dilation is found (>4 cm), treatment is ineffective and delivery should be anticipated.

Premature Rupture of Membranes

Premature rupture of membranes (PROM) is defined as spontaneous rupture of fetal membranes before the onset of labor, regardless of gestational age. At term, 70 percent of patients are in labor within 12 h of PROM, 80–90 percent are in labor within 24 h. In preterm gestations labor begins within 24 hours in only 35–50 percent of patients and within 72 hours in 70 percent of patients.

Diagnosis

A history of a trickle or a sudden gush of fluid from the vagina should be evaluated with a perineal preparation and a careful sterile speculum examination. Sterile swabs of the posterior vaginal vault (not the cervix, which can give false-positive results) should be evaluated by nitrazine paper (amniotic fluid is alkaline) and microscopic examination of a dried slide for ferning. Blood can give a false-positive nitrazine test. Either blood or inflammatory secretions can lead to a false-negative ferning test. Because amniotic fluid leakage may be intermittent, one cannot prove intact membranes by a negative nitrazine and ferning examination. If clinical suspicion for PROM is high, admission, observation, and serial speculum examination is warranted. Remote from term, cervical cultures for beta streptococcus, gonococcus, and *Chlamydia* may guide perinatal antibiotic therapy. A bimanual examination should be deferred until active labor ensues.

Treatment

In a term patient with a dilated and effaced cervix, induction of labor is usually undertaken. With an unfavorable cervix at term, bed rest in the hospital usually is followed by spontaneous labor and is associated with a lower operative delivery rate than induction. In the preterm patient, there is considerable controversy regarding ideal management. Because prematurity is a more common cause of perinatal loss than infection, conservative inpatient observation is frequently undertaken, depending on gestational age. Amniocentesis to asses fetal pulmonary maturity and identify early chorioamnionitis can often be done, and the results can guide therapy. If chorioamnionitis develops, delivery is indicated. Spontaneous labor is usually managed by allowing delivery, preferably in a tertiary center if significant prematurity is present.

Hypertensive Disorders In Pregnancy

Hypertensive disorders complicate approximately 8 percent of pregnancies and are a leading cause of maternal mortality. They are the leading cause of preventable perinatal mortality in the U.S. Fetal growth retardation, abruptio placentae, and stillbirth are more common in hypertensive pregnancy.

Hypertension in pregnancy is classified into five categories: (1) chronic hypertension, (2) preeclampsia-eclampsia, (3) preeclampsia superimposed on chronic hypertension, (4) transient hypertension, and (5) unclassified.

Chronic Hypertension

Because of the above risks, patients with chronic hypertension may benefit from antihypertensive therapy preconceptually and throughout pregnancy. Treatment may reduce the risk of superimposed preeclampsia. Because diuretics in pregnancy adversely affect the normal maternal plasma volume expansion, they are not the first choice of treatment. Methyldopa, β blockade, or hydralazine (Apresoline), in that order, are frequently used, with diuretics as an adjunct if necessary.

Preeclampsia

Preeclampsia occurs in approximately 5 percent of pregnancies and is defined as acute hypertension after 20 weeks of gestation with either (1) proteinuria (>300 mg/24 h) or (2) generalized edema. This clinical syndrome is unique to humans, usually occurs in primagravidas, and has an unknown cause. Its pathophysiology is characterized by diffuse vasospasm, reduced intravascular volume, and decreased colloid osmotic pressure, and is not reversed until after delivery.

Like syphilis, it has been labeled the "great imitator" because of its varied presentation with cardiopulmonary, hepatic, hematologic, renal, and CNS involvement. Although the blood pressure elevation may be slight, any pregnant woman with any of the following should undergo obstetric consultation: persistent headache, visual disturbance, change in mentation, epigastric pain, hepatic dysfunction, thrombocytopenia, or proteinuria. The difficulty for the emergency department physician is the common absence of information about previous blood pressure measurements in pregnancy, and mild elevations, especially in a young woman, may be significant in comparison with previous measurements. Criteria for diagnosis are shown in Table 59-2.

Treatment

Definitive therapy is delivery. However, cases of mild preeclampsia remote from term can often be managed conservatively with bed rest and observation, with resultant extended prolongation of pregnancy, allowing fetal growth and development.

All patients presenting with preeclampsia should be evaluated for hospital admission, management that has been shown to have significant benefit. Antepartum fetal heart rate assessment and intrapartum electronic fetal monitoring should be used in all patients.

If severe preeclampsia (see Table 59-2) or eclampsia develops at any gestational age, the treatment is stabilization and delivery. Such patients should be transferred from the emergency department to an obstetric unit experienced in management of this disorder as soon as possible.

Prophylactic anticonvulsant treatment with magnesium sulfate should be considered in all preeclamptic patients during risk periods (in labor, in delivery, and at least 24 h postpartum) (see Table 59-3). Magnesium sulfate is also effective as acute therapy in eclampsia.

Table 59-2. Criteria for Diagnosis of Preeclampsia and Eclampsia

I. Preeclampsia (A *and* B criteria necessary)
  A. Acute elevation measured twice at least 6 h apart, of either
    1. SBP ≥140 torr or rise ≥30 torr above baseline or
    2. DBP ≥90 torr or rise ≥15 torr above baseline, *and*
  B. Either
    1. Proteinuria >300 mg/24 h or
    2. Generalized edema
II. Indication for delivery regardless of gestational age (i.e., severe preeclampsia)
  A. SBP persistently ≥160 torr
  B. DBP persistently ≥110 torr
  C. Proteinuria ≥5 g/24 h
  D. Oliguria <500 mL/24 h
  E. Persistent headache or visual disturbances
  F. Epigastric pain
  G. Pulmonary edema or cyanosis
  H. Thrombocytopenia
  I. Liver dysfunction
III. Eclampsia
  The occurrence of grand mal seizures or coma in a patient with preeclampsia

Note: BP = blood pressure; SBP = systolic blood pressure; DBP = diastolic blood pressure.

Table 59-3. Preeclampsia Treatment: Anticonvulsant Prophylaxis and Control

Dosage
Loading dose 6 g ($MgSO_4 \cdot 7H_2O$) IV. Infuse slowly over 5–10 min (30 mL of a 10% solution or 4mL of a 50% solution = 4 g)
Maintenance dose 1–2 g/h IV; continuous calibration infusion
Precautions
Obstetrician should be notified immediately
Patient should be transferred to obstetric unit
Respirations must be normal
Serial examination of deep tendon reflexes is required
Monitor urine output hourly with a Foley catheter and discontinue $MgSO_4$ (which is excreted solely by the kidney) if urine output is less than 25 mL/h
Discontinue $MgSO_4$ if deep tendon reflexes disappear or serum Mg^{2+} exceeds 10 mg/dL
Antidote
1 g calcium gluconate IV slowly, if patient is not digitalis toxic (calcium chloride may be used if gluconate not available)
Adverse effects
Depression of reflexes
Respiratory depression
Bradyarrhythmias, heart block, cardiac standstill
Laboratory studies
Hemoglobin, hematocrit, platelet count, BUN, creatinine, glucose, sodium, potassium, chloride, bicarbonate, transaminases, urinalysis

Most preeclamptic patients do not require antihypertensive drugs, and there is no convincing evidence that fetal outcome is improved with such therapy. Acute lowering of blood pressure may actually jeopardize the fetus by lowering uterine blood flow. Antihypertensive therapy is instituted if the blood pressure reaches levels of acute maternal risk of cerebrovascular accident or myocardial infarction (e.g., systolic blood pressure >170 torr; diastolic, >110 torr). A target for such therapy would be approximately 140/100. In the presence of thrombocytopenia, many obstetricians begin antihypertensive therapy at somewhat lower levels. Hydralazine in small intravenous doses (10 mg) followed by a continuous infusion is usually effective and is preferred over diazoxide or nitroprusside before delivery, due to the risks of fetal hypoperfusion with hypotension and the fetal accumulation of cyanide.

Urinary Tract Infection

Mechanical occlusion of the ureters by the enlarging uterus, flaccidity of the ureters due to progesterone, and the increased volume of the urinary tract during pregnancy are factors in the increased incidence of asymptomatic bacteriuria and pyelonephritis in pregnancy. Asymptomatic bacteriuria (5 to 7 percent of all pregnancies) if untreated carries a 30 to 40 percent risk of development of subsequent pyelonephritis in pregnancy. Ampicillin or a cephalothin is a frequent choice for treatment.

In pregnancy, pyelonephritis carries an increased risk of sepsis and preterm labor and is an indication for intravenous antibiotics and fluid therapy.

Diabetes Mellitus

Gestational (first diagnosis or onset during pregnancy) diabetes mellitus occurs in 2 to 3 percent of all pregnancies, and carries an increase in fetal macrosomia, birth trauma, preeclampsia, multiple neonatal metabolic problems, and, possibly, stillbirth. Preexisting (types I and II) diabetes mellitus occurs in an additional 0.4 percent of pregnancies. These patients are at high risk for the above problems and spontaneous abortion, congenital anomalies, fetal growth impairment, and urinary tract infection. Human placental lactogen (hPL) antagonizes the effects of insulin. Also, placental insulinase may contribute to this process by accelerating insulin degradation. The nausea of pregnancy and the predisposition of hyperglycemic patients to develop infections make management of diabetes during pregnancy difficult. When pregnant, even in the absence of diabetes, a woman is more prone to develop metabolic acidosis than when nonpregnant. This is most likely due to the carbohydrate sparing and lipolytic action of hPL. When diabetic ketoacidosis occurs in the pregnant patient, it is often severe. Diabetic ketoacidosis can also cause acute fetal death. The emergency physician treating any hyperglycemic woman of child-bearing age should be aware that most pregnancy complications can be reduced by aggressive long-term diabetic management utilizing multiple insulin injections every day and multiple self-measurements of glucose every day with the feasible goal of normalization of blood sugar levels. Preconception normalization of blood sugar levels may reduce congenital anomaly risk from 23 to 3 percent in types I and II diabetic patients. All diabetic patients should be on effective contraceptive therapy during preconception normalization of blood sugar levels, and any pregnant patient with hyperglycemia should be treated aggressively acutely, counseled, and referred for intensive long-term management. Oral hypoglycemic agents are contraindicated in pregnancy. During pregnancy, hypoglycemia has no proven adverse effects but should be treated if CNS symptoms develop. The goal should be normalization of blood sugar while minimizing hyperglycemia when possible.

Persistent hyperglycemia (e.g., >200 mg %) warrants admission due to risks of pregnancy loss.

In healthy women, the fasting plasma glucose concentration falls somewhat during pregnancy because of the metabolic needs of the developing fetus. The placenta is known to synthesize and secrete a growth hormone–like substance, hPL, which promotes lipolysis and increases the level of plasma free fatty acids, thereby providing alternative fuel substrates for the mother. If dietary intake is insufficient or if metabolic needs are increased (as with marked physical activity or systemic infections), overt symptomatic hypoglycemia may occur.

Thromboembolism

The risk of thromboembolism is increased five to six times in a pregnant woman, and the time of greatest risk is the early postpartum period. This is because of increased levels of clotting factors; increased venous distensibility; and compression of the vena cava by the enlarged uterus.

Iodinated radiodiagnostic agents should not be used during pregnancy because of concentration in the fetal thyroid and subsequent permanent ablation of thyroid function. Nuclear medicine studies (ventilation/perfusion scans) should be considered, and an estimate of pelvic radiation dosimetry may assist in selecting a diagnostic test. Pulmonary angiography with pelvic shielding is an alternative. It has the advantage of being definitive. In many cases, nuclear medicine study results are inconclusive, requiring another test with additional radiation exposure in pregnancy. Impedance plethysmography is noninvasive, useful in evaluating possible proximal venous thrombosis, and predictive if normal. This study must be done with the patient in the lateral supine position to avoid pregnancy artifact from the enlarged uterus.

Treatment of both deep venous thrombosis and embolism is heparin (see above) and should be maintained throughout the risk period.

Viral or Protozoal Infection in Pregnancy

Primary infections with cytomegalovirus, herpes genitalis, rubella, varicella, or *Toxoplasma gondii* may be teratogenic. Pregnant patients presenting with these possible diagnoses should undergo aggressive diagnostic workups (cultures, acute and convalescent titers, virus-specific IgM titers) and follow-up to reinforce the diagnosis for further management. If a primary infection with any of these agents is identified, especially in the first trimester, genetic counseling should be sought. If a newborn contracts herpes during birth, there is a 50 percent mortality and a high rate of neurologic sequelae in surviving infected infants. If at the time of labor or shortly after rupture of membranes, active infection in the birth canal is proved or likely, cesarean section is indicated.

Acute maternal varicella (chickenpox) may be life-threatening if pneumonia develops. For this reason, some offer varicella zoster immune globulin to nonimmune pregnant women after exposure. Varicella infection in a newborn can be severe if delivery occurs at the time of acute maternal infection (approximately one week before to one week after outbreak of maternal rash).

One of the leading causes of acquired immunodeficiency syndrome (AIDS) in young children is congenital transplacental infection. Women with AIDS should avoid pregnancy; those who are at risk for AIDS and who are pregnant should be screened for AIDS very early in pregnancy and referred for counseling.

Liver Disease in Pregnancy

Jaundice in pregnancy may be unrelated to the pregnancy (hepatitis, choledocolithiasis, etc.). Pregnancy-related causes of liver disease include preeclampsia with hepatic involvement, acute fatty liver of pregnancy, and cholestatic jaundice of pregnancy. Preeclampsia complicated by hepatic involvement usually reflects a process that is only reversed by delivery, and delivery is frequently necessary. Acute fatty liver of pregnancy is a dreaded complication that often presents as jaundice, coma, or altered mentation, and has a high maternal and fetal mortality. The cause is unknown, although it may also be related to preeclampsia. Treatment is delivery and supportive care. Cholestatic jaundice of pregnancy is more common and less serious, although for unknown reasons there is risk of preterm birth and fetal compromise. It has a genetic predisposition: familial patterns are seen, and it is more common among Scandinavians and Chileans. It tends to recur in subsequent pregnancies and with oral contraception. It usually presents as pruritus, followed by mild jaundice. The conjugated bilirubin level is increased but seldom above 5 mg/dL. Transaminase levels are also elevated but below levels seen with hepatitis. Characteristically serum bile acid levels are markedly elevated. Cholestyramine resin (10 to 12 g/day) relieves pruritus but does not address the fetal risk, and appropriate surveillance for the remainder of pregnancy is indicated.

Cholecystitis

Pregnancy appears to increase the risk of cholelithiasis and cholecystitis. Following the first trimester, a doubling of gallbladder volume, combined with incomplete gallbladder emptying following meals, predisposes to the formation of cholesterol gallstones. Acute attacks of gallbladder disease during pregnancy are managed in the same way as in nonpregnant patients with the following exceptions. (1) Radionuclide scanning of the gallbladder should be avoided during pregnancy, and ultrasonography should be used to confirm a clinical suspicion of cholelithiasis. (2) Ideally, cholecystectomy should be delayed until following delivery. If this is not possible, the second trimester is the optimal time for surgery since the risk of spontaneous abortion or delivery of an immature fetus during surgery is reduced and the uterus is not yet large enough to impinge on the field of operation. Emergent cholecystectomy should be considered regardless of gestational age in patients who present "toxic" and fail attempts at aggressive medical management. Delaying surgery in such instances only places the woman and her fetus in greater jeopardy.

Appendicitis in Pregnancy

Appendicitis occurs in approximately 1 in 850 pregnancies. Although it is not more common in pregnancy, the outcome is worse. In pregnancy, perforation is found more frequently, peritonitis is more frequent and more severe, delay in diagnosis is more frequent, and historically mortality has been higher. Babler said in 1908, "The mortality of appendicitis in pregnancy is the mortality of delay." Difficulty in diagnosis and fetal mortality increase with increasing gestational age. Cunningham found delay in diagnosis in 75 percent of patients in the third trimester, 18 percent in the second trimester, and 0 percent in the first trimester. Symptoms are more nonspecific in pregnancy: pain may be diffuse, anorexia and fever are often absent, and nausea and vomiting are variable. Baer's barium studies in 70 pregnancies of varying gestational age demonstrated the anatomic changes as pregnancy advances: by term the appendix has migrated to near the right subcostal margin and rotated counterclockwise, with the distal end pointed toward the diaphragm. This anatomic change explains the frequently different presentation in pregnancy, with pain and tenderness being more diffuse or located in the right upper quadrant. Laboratory studies are equally uninformative. Often the white blood cell count does not exceed the usual pregnancy values of 12,000 to 15,000. Fever may be low-grade or absent. Diagnosis must begin with a high index of suspicion. Treatment is surgical, with postoperative observation for preterm labor.

Acute appendicitis presenting late in pregnancy is most commonly misdiagnosed as acute pyelonephritis. Several points may be of help in differentiating these two disease entities. (1) The absence of gastrointestinal distress does not diminish the likelihood of acute appendicitis in pregnancy. (2) Pyuria without bacteriuria in the gravid patient should strongly suggest the diagnosis of acute appendicitis. (3) Pyelonephritis usually causes a fever greater than 38°C (100.4°F), which is often accompanied by chills, while appendicitis rarely causes these findings unless perforation has occurred.

Substance Abuse

The emergency department is often the site of initial identification or treatment of abuse of narcotics, alcohol, cocaine, or other substances. Substance abuse during pregnancy carries a major risk to the fetus, and early identification and appropriate referral may reduce the risks. Narcotic abuse increases risk of fetal growth retardation, stillbirth, preterm labor, neonatal withdrawal and death, and long-term neurodevelopmental problems. Initiation of methadone therapy, rather than substance withdrawal, is the ideal mangement. Heavy alcohol use is a leading cause of mental retardation in this country and also causes growth retardation and other neurodevelopmental problems. The adverse effects of cocaine use on pregnancy include increased risk of abruptio placentae, preterm birth, and fetal loss. Specific interventions are available at experienced centers but are dependent on accurate and early identification and referral. Management should be directed at treatment and support to maximize pregnancy outcome and subsequent care. Attempts at criminal prosecution of pregnant substance abusers may only force such patients out of the health care system with worse results.

Postpartum Fever

Fever in the postpartum period is common, and evaluation is similar to that of any febrile patient. The process of delivery can result in trauma and devitalization of the structures of the pelvis and urinary tract, creating an environment conducive to infection. In any postpartum patient, careful pelvic examination is necessary. The frequency of surgical infection following cesarean section varies between 5 to 45 percent in different populations. Episiotomy infections are uncommon, but when they occur they can be severe (e.g., necrotizing fasciitis). Urinary tract infection should be considered in any postpartum febrile patient.

Endometritis is characterized by the development of a boggy, tender uterus 1 to 3 days postpartum and is more common after abdominal delivery. Diagnosis is based on physical examination and exclusion of other causes of fever. A foul lochia is often found.

Hospitalization and intravenous therapy with broad-spectrum antibiotics with anaerobic coverage is recommended.

Persistent fever despite aggressive antibiotic therapy and without evidence of infection elsewhere may indicate pelvic thrombophlebitis, an occasional sequela of pelvic infection. It may present with pulmonary embolus. If endometritis does not respond within a few days, heparinization should be considered.

Mastitis

Women who choose bottlefeeding initially or who later stop breastfeeding will develop transient bilateral breast engorgement (pain, fullness, tenderness, and often a low-grade fever). These can be treated with mild analgesia, breast binding, and ice, and they will resolve in a few days.

Mastitis presents differently: usually the symptoms and findings are unilateral, located in one quadrant, and occur in a breastfeeding patient. Milk from that quadrant should be cultured and gram-stained. The responsible organism is frequently staphylococcus. Treatment is antibiotics, analgesia, continuing breastfeeding, and emptying the affected quadrant. The pediatrician should be alerted to the use of medication.

Rh Immunoprophylaxis

An Rh-negative woman with an Rh-positive fetus may develop antibodies that can cause fetal anemia, hydrops, and fetal loss in that or subsequent pregnancies. All Rh-negative women with vaginal bleeding in pregnancy, an ectopic pregnancy, spontaneous or induced abortion, or trauma, should undergo antibody screening, and if there are no Rh antibodies, receive Rh immunoglobulin. After delivery of an Rh-positive infant, management should be similar. Ideally, therapy should occur within 72 h of the event. In addition all Rh-negative women are offered Rh immunoglobulin at approximately 28 weeks of gestation.

SURGICAL COMPLICATIONS

Ectopic Pregnancy

Ectopic pregnancy is defined as the implantation of the fertilized ovum in any location other than the endometrium. It remains a leading cause of maternal mortality in the United States. A high index of suspicion is necessary in the emergency department, in that iatrogenic delay in diagnosis has been a common problem. Early intervention reduces blood loss and transfusion requirements, and frequently allows conservative surgery that may help subsequent fertility. Risk factors for ectopic pregnancy include a history of previous salpingo-oophoritis, previous ectopic pregnancy, previous tubal ligation, and use of an intrauterine device.

Symptoms

Bleeding and pain is an ectopic pregnancy until proved otherwise. A clear history of amenorrhea is often absent. If rupture has occurred, the pain may be severe, colicky, or referred to the shoulder due to diaphragmatic irritation from intraabdominal blood.

Physical Examination

Appearance and vital signs may be normal in the supine young patient, despite significant intraabdominal bleeding. Orthostatic vital signs are a useful guide to occult blood loss. With progressive loss in circulating blood volume, tachycardia followed by hypotension is observed when the patient is in the upright position. The uterus may be enlarged. An adenexal mass is an inconsistent finding and often if present actually represents a corpus luteum, not infrequently on the contralateral side from the ectopic pregnancy.

Culdocentesis

Culdocentesis offers valuable information in patients with pelvic abnormality and should be used liberally. In a normal patient, a few milliliters of straw-colored fluid is obtained (negative culdocentesis). If an ectopic pregnancy is present, or there is intraabdominal bleeding, nonclotting blood is obtained (positive culdocentesis). A pelvic infection produces purulent fluid; a ruptured ovarian cyst, free-flowing straw-colored fluid. If clotted blood or no fluid results, improper placement has occurred and the test is nondiagnostic.

Pregnancy Test

Modern quantitative HCG tests (see above) are very useful in excluding an ectopic pregnancy if the test is negative. Significant elevation of HCG levels (e.g., >6500 mIU/mL) coupled with an ultrasound examination showing an empty uterus (see below) is predictive of an ectopic pregnancy.

Pelvic Ultrasonography

Abdominal real-time ultrasound examination should detect a gestational sac at 6 weeks of gestation when a pregnancy is intrauterine. Transvaginal sonography can identify a sac approximately 1 week earlier. Ultrasound examination is less useful in visualizing an ectopic gestation. Abdominal pain in a patient with a positive pregnancy test, especially with quantitative HCG >6500 mIU/mL and an empty uterus on ultrasound examination, is an indication for emergent gynecologic consultation.

Differential Diagnosis

The most commonly encountered misdiagnoses in ectopic pregnancy include salpingo-oophoritis, ovarian cyst, dysfunctional uterine bleeding, spontaneous abortion, and acute appendicitis. Adhering to a standardized approach similar to that shown in Fig. 59-1 may decrease the incidence of misdiagnoses.

Treatment

Once the diagnosis is made or suspected, the treatment is surgical. In hypotensive patients, placement of a military antishock trousers (MAST) suit, administration of crystalloid fluids through two large-bore intravenous lines, and early administration of blood are potentially lifesaving. Rh immunoglobulin should be administered to all Rh-negative patients.

Vaginal Bleeding in Pregnancy

Abortion

Abortion is defined as termination of pregnancy, spontaneous or induced, before 20 weeks of gestation.

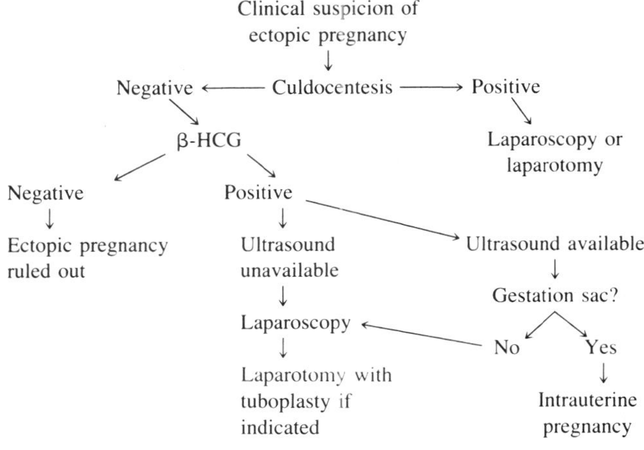

Fig. 59-1. Differential diagnosis for ectopic pregnancy.

First Trimester Bleeding

Approximately 30 percent of first trimester pregnancies have some bleeding. It may be from any lesion in the genital tract, from hematuria, or rectal in origin. If it is uterine in origin, then the diagnosis is either ectopic pregnancy, molar pregnancy, or some type of abortion.

Threatened Abortion

If uterine bleeding in pregnancy occurs with a closed cervix, no tissue has been passed, and ectopic pregnancy is eliminated; the diagnosis is threatened abortion. Approximately one-half of such patients subsequently spontaneously abort. Management is expectant, with instructions to avoid intercourse and douching. Patients should return if bleeding or cramping increases, there are symptoms of excess blood loss, or tissue is passed. The tissue should be brought in.

Inevitable, Complete, and Incomplete Abortion

If the cervix is open to a ring forceps, or if tissue has been passed, inevitable abortion is diagnosed. If all tissue has been passed and there is minimal bleeding, a complete abortion is identified. This diagnosis is difficult at times, and many patients require a dilatation and curettage to ensure that the products of conception are removed.

Molar Pregnancy

Hydatidiform mole is a rare cause of late first trimester bleeding. Classically, there is excessive uterine growth, nausea, and vomiting, and/or the development of preeclampsia before 24 weeks of gestation. In addition, the patient has abdominal pain, is anemic, and has passed grapelike clusters of tissue characteristic of a mole. The uterus may also be smaller than the expected gestational age.

Although a presumptive diagnosis may be made from the history and physical examination, the definitive diagnosis is made by ultrasound examination or by the identification of molar tissue in the vagina.

Treatment

A careful suction dilatation and curettage is performed, with intravenous oxytocin. Although the coexistence of a hydatidiform mole and a fetus is rare, it has been reported; consequently the unsensitized Rh-negative woman should receive Rh immunoglobulin. All such patients should be followed closely subsequently by serial HCG titers to identify the occasional choriocarcinoma.

Third Trimester Bleeding

Third trimester vaginal bleeding is bleeding that occurs after 27 weeks of gestation; it occurs in 3.8 percent of pregnancies. The causes are placenta previa 22 percent, abruptio placentae 31 percent, and assorted other causes (cervical effacement, cervicitis, vaginitis, neoplasia in the birth canal, trauma to the birth canal) in 47 percent.

All patients with third trimester bleeding should be evaluated for admission to the hospital. Because a bimanual examination of a placenta previa may result in profuse bleeding, pelvic examination should be deferred until placenta previa is excluded by ultrasonography.

Placenta previa

Placenta previa is defined as implantation of the placenta in the lower uterine segment in advance of the fetal presenting part after 24 weeks gestation. At 16 weeks of gestation, 10 percent of all pregnancies have sonographic evidence of the placenta over the cervix: at delivery the incidence is approximately 0.4 percent. Differential growth of the uterus throughout pregnancy accounts for this changing relationship of the placenta and the lower uterine segment. Late in pregnancy, patients often present with bleeding resulting from disruption of the implantation site from progressive uterine activity and thinning of the lower uterine segment. Bleeding tends to be recurrent and often progressively worse with each episode, the basis for the British description "inevitable hemorrhage." Risk factors for placenta previa are previous cesarean section, multiparity, previous placenta previa, multiple gestation, and multiple induced abortions. All patients with third trimester bleeding should be considered for admission to the hospital, and pelvic examination should be deferred. If stable, such patients can undergo real-time ultrasonography for placental localization. Because bleeding is recurrent and progressively worse, long-term hospitalization is necessary for most. D'Angelo found a better outcome with inpatient versus outpatient management in a nonrandomized study, although Cotton found no difference. Outpatient care after initial hospitalization requires complete bed rest, immediate and close access to transportation to a hospital, and a compliant patient. Delivery is recommended if sustained hemorrhage occurs, or if fetal compromise or active labor develops. Elective delivery is used if fetal maturity can be determined. As an alternative, Cotton used temporization with transfusions and tocolytics, and this procedure had a favorable outcome, but intensive surveillance is required in this population. Pelvic examination in the operating room ("double setup") at the time of planned delivery may identify the minority of patients with a low-lying placenta that does not obstruct the birth canal, allowing rupture of membranes, internal fetal monitoring, and possible vaginal delivery.

Abruptio Placentae

Abruptio placentae (accidental hemorrhage) is separation of the normally located placenta before delivery of the fetus. It occurs in approximately 1 percent of births. Risk factors are hypertension, smoking, previous abruptio placentae, multiparity, and trauma.

In its severe form, it may present as painful vaginal bleeding, active labor with a hypertonic, tender uterus, fetal compromise or fetal death, shock, and disseminated intravascular coagulation. Most patients, however, do not present this dramatic picture, and any third trimester uterine bleeding for which placenta previa has been excluded should be considered possible abruptio placentae. Hospitalization and close surveillance of maternal and fetal status are indicated. If maternal vital signs are stable, electronic fetal monitoring is reassuring, the uterus is soft and nontender between contractions, uterine contractions are normal in frequency and intensity, coagulation studies are normal, and bleeding is minimal or moderate, observation may continue. A large-bore intravenous line and ready availability of blood replacement and an operating team are required. If any of the above conditions deteriorate, intervention by delivery is indicated. If vaginal delivery is not imminent, cesarean section is necessary. Surveillance for and aggressive management of hemorrhagic shock are similar to those of the nonpregnant patient, except that shock may result from intrauterine bleeding without obvious vaginal bleeding. The coagulation disorder of abruptio placentae responds rapidly to delivery, and component therapy is often not required beyond red blood cell replacement.

Out-of-Hospital Delivery

When birth occurs before arrival at the hospital, the emergency department must respond to two patients simultaneously, and adequate resources should be mobilized. The newborn should be quickly assessed for color, respiration, heart rate, muscle tone, and reflex response (Apgar score). A healthy term baby needs to be dried and kept warm. Preterm or depressed newborns often respond to oxygen administration and positive-pressure ventilation by mask while emergent consultation is sought. If these measures don't work, then endotracheal intubation and cardiopulmonary resuscitation by experienced personnel are necessary. In a healthy mother, the average blood loss of delivery, 500 mL, is well-tolerated. All patients should undergo a thorough inspection of the perineum, cervix, and vagina for lacerations that may require closure. The uterus should be firm and below the umbilicus unless uterine atony is present. Uterine massage, breast feeding, and intravenous oxytocin (10 units in 1000 mL of crystalloid run rapidly) resolve most uterine atony, although surgical therapy is sometimes necessary. If the placenta does not deliver within 30 min, surgical removal should be considered.

In approximately 5 percent of births, postpartum hemorrhage, or significant blood loss beyond average, occurs. It usually appears in the first few hours after birth and remains a major cause of maternal mortality. The causes are uterine atony, lacerations, or retained placenta. Management begins with an accurate identification of the cause and prompt treatment along with aggressive supportive measures for the patient with impending or actual hemorrhagic shock.

Postpartum Hemorrhage

Most postpartum hemorrhage occurs within a few hours of birth. Rarely a patient may return a few days to weeks after delivery with a complaint of bleeding. If bleeding is less than menstrual flow, there is no evidence of infection or hypovolemia, and the pelvic exam is normal, nothing further need be done. More significant bleeding usually is related to retained placental fragments and/or endometritis and warrants consultation. Note that uterine atony, a common cause for hemorrhage in the first postpartum day, is not a cause for later hemorrhage.

Postmortem Cesarean Section

Emergency cesarean section is justified if the fetus has reached 26 weeks of gestation and the interval from maternal death to delivery is short. If the interval is more than 20 min, the fetal outcome is poor. If an attempt at postmortem cesarean section is to be made, personnel must be immediately available for vigorous resuscitation of the newborn.

This area is fraught with medical, legal, and ethical considerations, and extreme care must be taken in exercising this option.

BIBLIOGRAPHY

Pregnancy Tests

Huber R: Human Chorionic Gonadotrophin: Chemical Review Core Chemistry V.5 #6 1989 p 1–8.

Rattle SJ, Purnell DR, Williams P, et al: New separation method for monoclonal immunoradiometric assays and its application to assays for thyrotropin and human choriogonadotropin. *Clin Chem* 30:1457, 1984.

Drugs

Briggs GG, Freeman RK, Yaffe SJ: *Drugs in Pregnancy and Lactation,* 3rd ed. Williams & Wilkins, Baltimore, 1990.

Koren G: *Maternal Fetal Toxicology—A Clinicians Guide.* Marcel Dekker, New York, 1990.

Reproductive Toxicology Center Colombia Hospital for Women Medical Center, 2440 M Street, N.W., Suite 217, Washington, D.C., 20037-1404.

Shepard TH: *Catalog of Teratogenic Agents,* 6th ed. Johns Hopkins University Press, Baltimore, 1989.

Medical Complications

Babler EA: Perforative appendicitis complicating pregnancy. *JAMA* 51:1310, 1908.

Baer JL, Reis RA, Arens RA: Appendicitis in pregnancy with changes in position and axis of the normal appendix in pregnancy. *JAMA* 98:1359, 1932.

Creasy RK, Resnick R: *Maternal Fetal Medicine,* 2d ed. Philadelphia, Saunders, 1989.

Duff P, Huff RW, Gibbs RS: Management of premature rupture of membranes and unfavorable cervix in term pregnancy. *Obstet Gynecol* 63:697, 1984.

Gilstrap LC, Cunningham FG, Whalley PJ: Management of pregnancy-induced hypertension in the nulliparous patient remote from term. *Semin Perinatol* 2:73, 1978.

Hughes EC (ed): *Obstetric & Gynecologic Terminology.* Philadelphia, Davis, 1972.

Miller E, Hare JW, Cloherty JP, et al: Elevated maternal hemoglobin A1 in early pregnancy and major congenital anomalies in infants of diabetic mothers. *N Engl J Med* 304:1331, 1981.

Nicholas G, Lorenz RP, Botti JJ, et al: The frequent occurrence of false positive results in phleborheography during pregnancy. *Surg Gynecol Obstet* 161:133, 1985.

Pritchard JA, Cunningham FG, Pritchard SA: The Parkland Memorial Hospital protocol for treatment of eclampsia: Evaluation of 245 cases. *Am J Obstet Gynecol* 148:951, 1984.

Surgical Complications

Brenner WE, Edelman DA, Hendricks CH: Characteristics of patients with placenta previa and results of expectant management. *Am J Obstet Gynecol* 132:180, 1978.

Crosby WM: Trauma during pregnancy—Maternal and fetal injury. *Obstet Gynecol Surg* 29:683, 1974.

Cunningham FG, McCubbin JH: Appendicitis complicating pregnancy. *Obstet Gynecol* 45:415, 1975.

D'Angelo LJ, Irwin LF: Conservative management of placenta previa: A cost benefit analysis. *Am J Obstet Gynecol* 149:320, 1984.

Hurd WW, Miodovich M, Hertzberg V, et al: Selective management of abruptio placentae: A prospective study. *Obstet Gynecol* 61:467, 1983.

Rothenberger D: Blunt maternal trauma—A review of 103 cases. *J Trauma* 18:173, 1978.

Weber CE: Postmortem cesarean section: Review of the literature and case reports. *Am J Obstet Gynecol* 110:158, 1974.

60
BLUNT ABDOMINAL TRAUMA DURING PREGNANCY

Mark D. Pearlman

Trauma during pregnancy is the most frequent cause of nonobstetrical maternal death. The three major causes of maternal injury are vehicular accidents, falls, and penetrating objects. Diagnosis and treatment of the injured gravida follows the same general guidelines as management of the nonpregnant trauma victim, but several critical differences exist. Marked changes occur in almost every organ system of the gravida's body, and a basic understanding of these changes is a prerequisite to initiating treatment and interpreting diagnostic tests. This chapter will review those aspects of trauma care which are peculiar to the gravid trauma patient.

ANATOMIC AND PHYSIOLOGICAL CHANGES ASSOCIATED WITH PREGNANCY

Treatment priorities require an understanding of the anatomic and physiological changes of pregnancy. In addition, pathological states which are unique to pregnancy such as abruptio placentae or amniotic fluid embolism may be initiated by injury and must be considered both diagnostically and therapeutically. After initial maternal stabilization, diagnosis and treatment of the second patient (fetus) must be considered.

Cardiovascular Changes

Cardiac output increases during the first 10 weeks of pregnancy (up to 1.0 to 1.5 L/min) and then maintains this increased level throughout pregnancy. In the supine position late in pregnancy, the inferior vena cava can be occluded by the enlarging uterus and cardiac output falls dramatically as a result of decreased preload. By displacement of the gravid uterus off the inferior vena cava, cardiac output can increase by 25 percent late in pregnancy. This can be accomplished by either placing the patient in the left atrial decubitus position, placing a 6-in. wedge under the right hip, or manual displacement of the uterus to the left.

Heart rate normally increases during pregnancy. This physiological tachycardia reaches a maximum of 15 to 20 beats above baseline late in the third trimester. Tachycardia as a sign of hypovolemia must be interpreted with caution in the pregnant trauma victim.

Both *systolic and diastolic blood pressure* in normal pregnancy fall by 10 to 15 mmHg in the second trimester, with a gradual increase to prepregnancy levels toward the end of pregnancy.

Electrocardiographic changes are influenced by displacement of the heart by the enlarging uterus. This is demonstrated by a left-axis deviation of 15° as well as flattened or inverted T waves in lead III. Supraventricular ectopy is also more frequent during pregnancy.

Hematologic Changes

Blood volume expands by a maximum of 45 percent at term. Red blood cell mass does not increase to the same degree as does plasma volume; therefore, *dilutional "anemia"* is a normal physiological finding in pregnancy. This increase in plasma volume allows a greater red blood cell loss to take place without the usual signs of hypovolemia. Fluid replacement estimates may need to be increased when considering the pregnant trauma patient.

A moderate *leukocytosis* is seen during normal pregnancy, as high as 18,000 in the second and third trimester, and as high as 25,000 during labor.

Coagulation factors are affected by pregnancy: fibrinogen and factors VII, VIII, IX, and X are all increased. However, bleeding time, clotting time, prothrombin time, and partial thromboplastin time are unchanged. These coagulation alterations (a result in part of elevated estrogen levels) increase the risk of formation of venous thrombosis. In addition, the release of thromboplastic materials from traumatic abruptio placentae can initiate a fulminant coagulopathy (DIC).

Erythrocyte sedimentation rate is elevated in normal pregnancy (average ESR = 78 mm/h).

Pulmonary Changes

Tidal volume increases by approximately 40 percent, and *residual volume* decreases by approximately 25 percent. *Respiratory rate* changes little.

Arterial blood gases are affected by the increased tidal volume and decreased residual volume resulting in a reduced alveolar and arterial P_{CO_2}; P_{CO_2} averages 30 torr. Normal pH is maintained by increased bicarbonate excretion by the kidney.

Gastrointestinal Changes

Decreased gastric motility and *decreased gastric emptying time* both predispose to an increased risk for aspiration, especially in those patients requiring general anesthesia or with an altered sensorium.

Cephalad displacement of the intraabdominal contents by the gravid uterus seems to have a protective effect on these organs in blunt abdominal trauma. However, in penetrating trauma of the upper abdomen, intestinal injury is almost assured.

Signs of peritoneal irritation are less reliable in the gravida in comparison to those of the nonpregnant trauma victim. Rebound tenderness and rigidity are often diminished, delayed, or absent in pregnant women. This is presumably due to the gradual stretching of the peritoneum and abdominal musculature by the gravid uterus.

The placental component of *alkaline phosphatase* results in levels which are increased two to three times those of nongravid levels near term.

Urinary System Changes

Dilatation of the renal pelves and ureters (right > left) occurs from 10 weeks' gestation to 6 weeks' postpartum.

The *bladder* is displaced both superiorly and anteriorly, becoming an abdominal organ around the twelfth week of gestation and rendering it more susceptible to injury.

Decreased serum creatinine and BUN (0.5 and <10 mg/dL, respectively, in late pregnancy) occur as a result of increased renal blood flow and increased glomerular filtration rate.

Reproductive Organ Changes

The *uterus* increases in size from a 7-cm, 70-g organ to a 36-cm, 1000-g organ at term.

Blood flow to the uterus increases from 60 to 600 mL/min at term, predisposing to massive blood loss if the uterine vasculature is disrupted.

MATERNAL INJURIES

In a prospective series by Crosby of 411 pregnant victims of serious automobile accidents, there were 16 fatalities (3.4 percent). Of these fatalities, 7 died of head injuries, 6 died of exsanguination from internal injuries, and 3 died of pelvic fractures associated with retro- or intraperitoneal hemorrhage. In addition, 7 other women suffered life-threatening injuries, including 5 pelvic fractures and 2 liver or spleen ruptures. The pattern and severity of injury depend on several factors, including speed, restraint system, direction of impact, and the victim's position in the vehicle.

Seat Belt Injuries

In 1971 Crosby and Costiloe published a series of severely injured pregnant women and focused specifically on whether two-point restraint systems were protective or deleterious to the pregnancies. In this study, seat belts protected against death of the mother, and death of the mother was the leading cause of fetal death. In addition, abruptio placentae was not increased as a result of seat belt use. However, in a separate animal study of trauma during pregnancy, it appeared that decelerative-type injuries where the pregnant subject is in two-point restraint are at increased risk for abruptio placentae compared to three-point restraint.

Pelvic Fracture

Fracture of the maternal pelvis may be associated with life-threatening hemorrhage; bladder, urethral, or ureteral laceration; fat embolism; vaginal lacerations; lumbar plexus injury; fetal skull fracture; and maternal death. Retroperitoneal hemorrhage is common following major trauma to the pelvis. Hypovolemic shock is frequently associated with injuries of this type as the retroperitoneum has a volume capacity of at least 4 L.

Pelvic deformity following pelvic fractures may interfere with normal passage of the fetus through the pelvic inlet during labor and delivery. However, cesarean section is necessary only 5 to 10 percent of the time as a result of pelvic fracture. Recent pelvic fracture is not a contraindication to vaginal delivery.

Intraabdominal Injuries

The enlarged gravid uterus and the contained amniotic fluid together act as a hydraulic shock absorber and has a protective affect on intraabdominal organs during blunt abdominal trauma. Life threatening hemorrhage as a result of trauma is most often found in the retroperitoneum during pregnancy, however, intraperitoneal hemorrhage should *always* be considered in the gravid victim of abdominal trauma. Splenic rupture, injury to the kidney, and liver laceration remain the three most common intra-abdominal injuries.

Uterine Rupture

Up to the twelfth week, the uterus is protected by the bony pelvis. After the twelfth week, it becomes an abdominal organ and is more vulnerable to injury. Crosby (1968) noted tremendous increases in intrauterine pressure (up to 550 mmHg) in restrained pregnant baboons subjected to experimental impacts. This is 10 times the pressure observed during normal labor. During abrupt deceleration, the uterus is thrown against the anterior abdominal wall, causing it to flatten and elongate. Rapid deceleration may cause an increase in intrauterine pressure great enough to produce uterine rupture. Traumatic uterine rupture is uncommon. Asymmetry of the uterus, signs of peritoneal irritation, the presence of maternal shock, and ultrasound visualization of the fetus free in the abdominal cavity all suggest the diagnosis.

Abruptio Placentae

Abruptio placentae occurs when the placenta prematurely separates from the uterine wall. The common presenting signs and symptoms include vaginal bleeding (78 percent), abdominal pain (66 percent), uterine irritability (17 percent), tetanic uterine contractions (17 percent), and fetal death (15 percent). Crosby and Costilloe found the incidence of placental abruption in severely traumatized pregnant victims to be about 5 percent. The mechanism of abruptio placentae in this type of injury is due to compression of the elastic uterus around the relatively inelastic placenta, causing a shearing of the placenta away from the underlying decidua basalis. A simultaneous increase in the intraamniotic pressure propagates this shearing effect. In a decelerative-type injury, hyperflexion of the torso over the pregnant uterus is prevented to a great degree by a shoulder harness. In addition to the bleeding from the separated uteroplacental site, release of thromboplastic materials into the maternal circulation predisposes to the development of DIC. In the presence of vaginal bleeding, uterine tenderness, or tetanic uterine contractions following trauma, fibrinogen levels, PT, PTT, and a platelet count should be obtained. A peripheral smear should also be examined for the presence of schistocytes.

Fetomaternal Hemorrhage

The human placenta is a hemochorial system, that is, the fetal and maternal blood circulations are normally separate. Fetomaternal hemorrhage (FMH) is a condition where fetal blood is found in the maternal circulation, and some degree of FMH frequently occurs following delivery, amniocentesis, and spontaneous vaginal bleeding. Fetomaternal hemorrhage following trauma was first described in a case report by Bickers and Wennberg. Since that initial report, Rose, Pearlman, and Goodwin have studied the incidence, volume, and significance of FMH following trauma. All three studies identified a four- to fivefold increase in incidence of FMH in pregnant trauma victims compared to uninjured controls regardless of severity of injury. In addition, the volume of FMH was several-fold higher in the injured group.

The most important unfavorable consequence of FMH is isoimmunization, the development of maternal antibodies against the $Rh_o(D)$ antigen on the surface of the Rh-positive fetal cells. These maternal IgG antibodies can cross the placenta and may cause fetal red blood cell hemolysis in the current or future pregnancies. $Rh_o(D)$ immune globulin (Rhogam) has been utilized for the last two decades to protect $Rh_o(D)$-negative gravidas against the possible exposure to $Rh_o(D)$-positive blood and the development of anti-$Rh_o(D)$ antibodies. Events which increase the risk of FMH (e.g., bleeding during pregnancy, amniocentesis, chorionic villus sampling, and delivery) are generally followed by prophylaxis with Rh immune globulin in $Rh_o(D)$-negative women. Based on the available data, trauma which occurs during pregnancy should be added to this list of events.

Calculating the volume of the FMH following trauma is important because a standard dose of $Rh_o(D)$ immune globulin (300 μg) will only protect against FMH $\leq$ 30 mL of whole blood. Administration of this standard dose of $Rh_o(D)$ immune globulin in the face of a larger bleed may not adequately protect the gravida against Rh isoimmunization. The Kleihauer-Betke assay is a test to identify and quantitate FMH. In this test a phosphate acid buffer is added to a peripheral smear of a pregnant (or recently pregnant) woman's blood. The phosphate buffer elutes adult hemoglobin from red blood cells (RBC), whereas the fetal hemoglobin is resistant to elution and remains within the RBC. A hemoglobin counterstain is then applied to the smear, and the ratio of maternal (ghost) RBCs to fetal (stained) RBCs is counted. By multiplying this ratio by the estimated maternal blood volume, an estimate of the volume of FMH can be made. For example, if 1000 maternal cells are counted and 3 fetal cells are seen, and if the estimated maternal blood volume is 5 L, the calculated FMH is $^3/_{1000} \times 5000 = 15$-mL bleed. Fetal blood volume does not reach 30 mL until approximately 16 weeks, so the use of Kleihauer-Betke or similar quantitative assays would be unnecessary in these early gestations if 300 μg of Rh immune globulins is administered empirically to Rh-negative women following trauma.

A second reason to quantitate the volume of FMH (rather than just treating Rh-negative women empirically) is to identify those occasional pregnancies in which large FMH occur, which may compromise the fetus. In Rose's study, 33 percent of fetuses who suffered a FMH developed some adverse outcome (neonatal anemia, supraventricular tachycardia, and fetal death) related to that event.

In summary, FMH occurs frequently following trauma during pregnancy (8 to 30 percent), and the Rh_o(D)-negative gravida should be protected against isoimmunization by the administration of Rh immune globulin. Beyond 16 weeks' gestation, a Kleibauer-Betke assay should be considered to quantitate the volume of the transfusion so that the appropriate dose of Rh immune globulin is administered and so that the rare episode of massive FMH is recognized, allowing appropriate intervention.

EVALUATION AND MANAGEMENT

Because fetal survival depends wholly on maternal integrity, maternal stabilization is of primary importance. Maternal shock is associated with fetal mortality approaching 80 percent. During the initial stage of evaluation, concentration should be entirely directed toward maternal status. The steps in the initial examination of a seriously injured trauma victim should be no different than in a nonpregnant trauma victim with the following exceptions: (1) in positioning the injured gravida of greater than 20 weeks' gestation, the left lateral tilt position is preferred as the uterus lies directly over the inferior vena cava, subsequently decreasing venous return; and (2) the physiological hypervolemia of pregnancy often allows 30 to 35 percent blood loss before the usual signs of hypovolemia develop, and aggressive fluid replacement, 50 percent above nonpregnant needs, is necessary. Maternal vital signs and fetal heart tones must be obtained at intervals. There are no specific studies regarding the use of MAST in pregnancy.

Maternal and fetal resuscitation are best accomplished by restoring the circulating blood volume.

Vasopressors decrease uterine blood flow and therefore decrease fetal oxygen delivery. Where vasopressors are required to maintain maternal vital signs, ephedrine is the drug of choice in our institution. However, no drug should be withheld if needed to save the life of the mother regardless of the known or unknown fetal risk. If excessive bleeding is occurring from an already emptied uterus (i.e., postpartum or postabortal), dilute intravenous oxytocin or intramuscular ergonovine are both useful.

Once the patient is adequately oxygenated and her circulating volume has been restored, maternal evaluation and assessment of fetal condition should follow. The obstetric portion of the abdominal examination must be included in the general physical examination. Uterine tenderness or irritability, tetanic contractions, and vaginal bleeding are all suggestive of abruptio placentae. Uterine size should be assessed by measuring the fundal height (pubic symphysis to the top of the fundus). The fundal height is a rough estimate of gestational age (centimeters = gestational age in weeks), which allows some indication of fetal viability if delivery is necessary. Fetal heart tones should be auscultated with a Doppler instrument (after 10 weeks' gestation) or with a fetoscope (after 18 weeks' gestation). A pelvic examination is mandatory to assess trauma to the genital tract, dilatation and effacement of the cervix, the presenting fetal part, and the station of the presenting part (relationship of the presenting part to the ischial spines). The presence of amniotic fluid must be sought. Nitrazine paper (turns blue with amniotic fluid, pH >7) and "ferning" (dried amniotic fluid under a microscope reveals a fern pattern) are both highly reliable for diagnosing ruptured membranes.

Radiographs that are clinically necessary should be obtained. CT scanning of the pregnant abdomen has been used without fetal complication. Open diagnostic peritoneal lavage, using a supraumbilical approach, can also be used. Appropriate laboratory studies, including clotting studies, should be obtained when evaluating severe maternal trauma.

Cardiotocodynamometry

In a prospective study, Pearlman et al. evaluated the sensitivity and specificity of a 4-h cardiotocodynamometry monitoring period for predicting immediate adverse outcomes following trauma during pregnancy beyond the twentieth week of gestation. Adverse outcomes in this study included abruptio placentae, fetal death, preterm delivery, or rupture of the amniotic membranes. When eight or more uterine contractions per hour at any time during the first 4 h of monitoring was used as threshold criterion, over 10 percent of pregnancies suffered immediate adverse outcomes. More importantly, when this frequency of contractions was *not* found in the first 4 h of monitoring, no episodes of immediate adverse outcomes were identified. A 4-h monitoring period appears to be a highly sensitive test for predicting immediate adverse outcome. In addition, monitoring appears to be more sensitive than ultrasound for predicting abruptio placentae in this setting (100 percent vs. 50 percent). Subjects who did not suffer immediate adverse outcomes and who were discharged after the monitoring period had pregnancy outcomes comparable to noninjured controls.

Based on the results of this and other studies, all pregnant women beyond 20 weeks' gestation with direct or indirect abdominal trauma should undergo at least 4 h of cardiotocographic monitoring. Monitoring should begin as soon as the gravida's vital signs are stable. The presence of uterine contractions, fetal brady- or tachycardia, or loss of fetal beat-to-beat variability requires immediate obstetrical consultation.

Additional indications for emergent obstetrical consultation include vaginal bleeding; abdominal tenderness, pain, or cramping; evidence of maternal hypovolemia; absence of fetal heart tones; suspected leakage of amniotic fluid; and sonographic evidence of fetal injury or suspicious retroplacental structure.

CARDIAC ARREST AND POSTMORTEM CESAREAN SECTION

Nearly 200 cases of successful postmortem cesarean section have been reported in the literature. Several factors have been suggested to be important in predicting the chance of fetal survival:

1. Gestational age >28 weeks (or fetal weight >1000 g).
2. Interval between maternal death and delivery
   a. <5 min—excellent
   b. 5–10 min—good
   c. 10–15 min—fair
   d. 15–20 min–poor
   e. >20 min—unlikely
3. Maternal cause of death—if unrelated to *chronic* hypoxia, fetal chances are improved.
4. Fetal status prior to maternal death.
5. Quality of maternal resuscitation.

When postmortem cesarean section is performed, the abdomen should be opened as rapidly as possible, and the infant delivered through a "classical" (vertical) uterine incision. Neonatology consultation and attendance during the procedure should be attempted. Informed consent from the next of kin should be obtained if possible, but implied consent can be assumed if the next of kin is not available.

Cardiac arrest during pregnancy presents a difficult clinical and ethical challenge. The lives of two patients are at stake, and decisions made for one patient may adversely affect the other. There is evidence that early thoracotomy and open-chest massage may improve both maternal and fetal outcome. In addition, timely emergency cesarean section has been shown to improve both maternal venous return and cardiac output during cardiopulmonary resuscitation and to increase the likelihood of intact neonatal survival. On the basis of this, it is suggested that if there is no response to Advanced Cardiac Life Support efforts in several minutes following maternal cardiac arrest, both of these methods should be seriously considered.

BIBLIOGRAPHY

Buchsbaum HJ: *Trauma in Pregnancy*. Philadelphia, Saunders, 1979.

Crosby WM, Costilloe JP: Safety of lap belt restraint for pregnant victims of automobile collisions. *N Engl J Med* 284:632, 1971.

Crosby WM, Snyder RG, Snow CC, et al: Impact injuries in pregnancy. 1: Experimental studies. *Am J Obstet Gynecol* 101:100, 1968.

Goodwin TM, Breen MT. Pregnancy outcome and fetomaternal hemorrhage after noncatastrophic trauma. *Am J Obstet Gynecol* 162:665, 1990.

Hayashi RH: Hemorrhage shock in obstetrics. *Clin Perinatol* 13:755, 1986.

Avin JP, Polsky SS: Abdominal trauma during pregnancy. *Clin Perinatol* 10:423, 1983.

Pearlman MD, Tintinalli JE, Lorenz RP. A progressive controlled study of outcome after trauma during pregnancy. *Am J Obstet Gynecol* 162:1502, 1990.

Pearlman MD, Tintinalli JE, Lorenz RP. Blunt trauma during pregnancy. *N Engl J Med* 323:1609, 1990.

Rolbin SH, Levinson G, Shinder SM, et al: Dopamine treatment of spinal hypotension decreases uterine blood flow in pregnant ewes. *Anesthesiology* 51:36, 1979.

Rose PG, Strohm PL, Zuspan FP: Fetomaternal hemorrhage following trauma. *Am J Obstet Gynecol* 153:844, 1985.

Rothenberger D, Quattlebaum FW, Zabel J, et al: Diagnostic peritoneal lavage for blunt trauma in pregnant women. *Am J Obstet Gynecol* 129:479, 1977.

Rothenberger D, Quattlebaum FW, Perry JF, et al: Blunt maternal trauma: A review of 103 cases. *J Trauma* 18:173, 1978.

61
EMERGENCY DELIVERY

Paul T. von Oeyen

The necessity for emergency delivery outside a hospital obstetric unit is relatively uncommon (1 in 695, or 0.14 percent in Weir's large series) but is an event met with extreme anxiety by medical personnel as well as parents. Despite careful planning, precipitous labor can result in the need for delivery either at home, in transit, or in the emergency department of a hospital without an obstetric unit. Precipitous labor is often unpredictable and can occur in nulliparous teenagers, who may not recognize periodic lower abdominal cramping as labor, as well as in experienced multiparas. Other reasons for emergency delivery include inadequate preparations (including inability to make arrangements for sudden care of other children), lack of transportation, remote geographic location, fear of arriving at the hospital too early or in false labor, fear of delivery in transit, and premature labor. The issue of purposeful out-of-hospital delivery is the source of continuing heated controversy, although such delivery is fortunately still statistically quite rare, and will not be dealt with here.

TRANSPORT OF MATERNAL PATIENTS

The current emphasis on maternal transport of high-risk pregnancies to tertiary perinatal centers rather than transport of newborns increases the importance of proper preparedness for emergency delivery in transit. The regionalization of obstetric and newborn care, and especially the establishment of neonatal intensive care centers in the 1960s and 1970s resulted in a marked decline in neonatal mortality. Although regional centers at first operated largely for neonates, several studies have now established the desirability of maternal over neonatal transports. This is especially true for the premature neonate weighing less than 1500 g and born prior to 34 weeks gestation. Maternal transports can result in improved neonatal mortality and neonatal morbidity when measured in terms of lower hospitalization costs and length of stay. Maternal transports in general are faster and less expensive than neonatal transports. Clearly, the human uterus is the best transport incubator.

Reasons for maternal transport include placental bleeding, pregnancy-induced hypertension, fetal abnormalities, multiple gestation, diabetes mellitus, and other maternal medical problems, but by far the most common indications for transfer to tertiary perinatal centers are preterm labor and premature rupture of membranes. This creates the necessity to be prepared for emergency delivery and resuscitation of premature infants in transit. Delivery while en route by air or ground transportation should be relatively rare if adequate communication and proper consultation are performed. Clearly, in-utero transport should not be attempted if there is maternal or fetal cardiovascular instability or if cervical dilatation has not been arrested by tocolytic agents.

Maternal-transport vehicles should carry sterile delivery packs, intravenous solutions and tubing, medications for both maternal and neonatal use, neonatal-resuscitation equipment, and monitoring equipment for both mother and baby (see Tables 61-1 and 61-2). The transport team should be familiar with the use and side effects of the β-adrenergic drugs terbutaline and ritodrine, used for treatment of preterm labor, as well as magnesium sulfate, used for treatment of pregnancy-induced hypertension and sometimes also for preterm labor.

In general, ground ambulance appears to be the most efficient means of transportation up to a 50- or 60-mile radius. However, helicopter transport has been advocated in some densely populated urban areas even for short distances because of concern over emergency-transport delays caused by traffic congestion. Fixed-wing aircraft are most useful for transports in rural settings with transport distances greater than 100 miles where the additional speed more than adequately makes up for the time lost between hospital and airport.

Air transport, however, also brings up the issue of potential additional hazards to the fetus because of the altitude during fights as well as safety issues for emergency flights occurring in stressful conditions and sometimes hazardous weather. The small ambulance types of aircraft utilized for maternal transport are pressurized to an altitude equivalent of 5000 to 8000 ft, but accidental decompression may expose the fetus to hypoxia during transport. This could be especially deleterious to the fetus already partially compromised by pregnancy-induced hypertension, or by placental infarction or abruption. Adequate oxygen supplies for face mask or nasal administration should be available for use during high-altitude transports as well as for emergency resuscitation.

PREPARATION FOR EMERGENCY DELIVERY

The same basic equipment as that needed for maternal transports should be available in the emergency department for emergency delivery (see Tables 61-1 and 61-2).

Any pregnant woman arriving in an emergency ward who is beyond 20 weeks gestation and appears to be actively contracting should be rapidly evaluated with a bimanual pelvic examination to assess cervical dilatation, and maternal vital signs and fetal heart rate should also be checked. An exception to this is the gravida with active vaginal bleeding, who should be evaluated with ultrasound to rule out placenta previa before pelvic examination is attempted. Also, the pregnant woman with suspicion of ruptured membranes should be evaluated with sterile speculum, with Nitrazine paper and ferning tests done to confirm ruptured membranes unless delivery appears imminent. The speculum examination should afford a view of the cervix to estimate the dilatation of the cervix and allow collection of specimens for culture (in particular for group B streptococcus and *Neisseria gonorrhoeae,* if the history is unknown or there has been no prenatal care). Occasionally a pregnant woman who denies knowledge of the pregnancy will present to the emergency department. This is seen most often in the teenage years, but any woman between 12 and 45 who presents to the emergency ward with vaginal bleeding or abdominal pain should be evaluated for possible pregnancy whether or not she exhibits an obviously enlarged abdomen. A Doppler fetoscope should be available for conformation of fetal life, although the inability to detect fetal heart tones does not rule out the possibility of a viable pregnancy.

Bimanual examination should be performed with sterile gloves and lubricant with the patient in the dorsal lithotomy position. Stirrups are not necessary as an adequate examination can be made with the mother's feet drawn close to her perineum on the examining table with her knees flexed and abducted. The cervix should be checked for dilatation and effacement and the presenting part (i.e., vertex or breech) identified. Prolapse of the cord should be excluded. The pregnant woman should not be left lying flat on her back for long, however, as the weight of the pregnant uterus can compress the major vessels, resulting in supine hypotension syndrome and decreased uterine perfusion.

Prenatal records should be quickly perused, if available. Gestational age can be determined from the last normal menstrual period (LMP), if this is known, and the due date (estimated date of confinement, or EDC) can be calculated by using Naegele's rule (add 9 months and 7 days to the date of the LMP). If ultrasound examination is readily available, it may be useful for making a reasonable estimate of potential fetal viability in a premature pregnancy of uncertain dates, but third trimester ultrasound measurements are unreliable for accurate dating (± 3 to 4 weeks). Between 20 and 35 weeks, there is a rough correlation between the gestational age and the height of the uterine fundus measured in centimeters from the pubic symphysis.

If the cervix is 6 cm or more dilated in a woman experiencing active contractions, further transport even for short distances is impossible

Table 61-1. Medications for Emergency Delivery

Oxytocin, 10 units/mL	Epinephrine, 1:1000
Methylergonovine (Methergine), 0.2 mg/mL	Diazepam, 10 mg
Magnesium sulfate, 50% (5 g/10 mL)	Lidocaine (Xylocaine), 1%
Magnesium sulfate, 10% (2 g/20 mL)	Sodium bicarbonate, 50 mEq
Calcium gluconate, 10 mL	Prochlorperazine (Compazine), 10 mg/2 mL
Hydralazine, 20 mg/mL	Diphenhydramine (Benadryl) 50 mg/mL
Ephedrine sulfate, 0.05 g	Naloxone (Narcan), 0.4 mg/mL
Sodium amytal, 250 mg	Dimenhydrinate (Dramamine), 50 mg
Terbutaline sulfate, 1 mg/mL	Sterile water for injection

and preparations should be made for emergency delivery. An intravenous line should be established with lactated Ringer's solution, if there is time before delivery, in order to be prepared for the administration of medications, fluids, or blood products immediately post partum if this becomes necessary. Minimal blood testing should include hemoglobin or hematocrit measurement (or a complete blood cell count), hepatitis B surface antigen (HB_sAg), blood typing (if unknown), and a clotted tube of blood to be available for emergency cross matching if necessary. If possible, urine should be tested for protein and glucose.

Maternal temperature, blood pressure (between contractions), and heart rate should be evaluated at least every 1 to 2 h. In the absence of continuous electronic monitoring, the fetal heart rate should be evaluated by Doppler fetoscope or a fetal stethoscope every 15 min prior to complete cervical dilatation (10 cm) and every 5 min during the second stage of labor (complete dilatation to delivery). The normal fetal heart rate is between 120 and 160 beats per minute and can be differentiated from the maternal heart rate if necessary by simultaneous manual assessment of the radial pulse. The fetal heart rate should be counted for at least a 30-s period following a contraction. If bradycardia is detected, the mother should be given oxygen and an intravenous fluid bolus and positioned on her side. This will maximize uterine blood flow and fetal oxygenation as well as possibly relieve cord compression. If bradycardia is associated with tetanic contractions, and delivery is not imminent, consideration should be given for the administration of tocolytic agents to relax the uterus, such as terbutaline 0.25 mg subcutaneously or magnesium sulfate 4 to 6 g intravenously over 15 to 20 min. If uterine tenderness, severe back pain, or excessive vaginal bleeding is also present, the possibility of placental abruption should be considered.

If membranes are intact, there is generally no reason to rupture them artificially until actual delivery. Amniotomy may result in prolapse of the umbilical cord if the baby's head is not well-engaged in the pelvis. Bladder distension should be avoided, and if it occurs and the mother is unable to spontaneously void, straight catheterization is indicated.

Around the time the cervix has become fully dilated, the gravida will feel a nearly uncontrollable urge to bear down with a Valsalva maneuver to expel the baby. The cervix should be checked to ensure full dilatation before allowing the mother to "push." If the cervix can still be palpated, serious laceration may occur from her uncontrolled expulsive efforts. Although important throughout labor, constant reassurance and emotional support are especially crucial at this point. Suggesting an alternative behavior, such as focusing on breathing and panting through the contractions, may help the mother to follow instructions and stay in control of expulsive efforts. A lateral position may also be helpful.

Once full dilatation has been established, expulsive efforts will most likely occur spontaneously. However, the inexperienced mother may need to be coached with instructions to take a deep breath at the start of each contraction, and with breath held, exert downward pressure as if having a bowel movement. Indeed, expulsion of feces during the second stage of labor is quite common, and the perineum should be frequently cleansed with a mild soap solution. The mother should not, however, be encouraged to push beyond the duration of each uterine contraction, which can be judged by direct palpation.

Table 61-2. Equipment and Supplies for Emergency Delivery

Sterile gloves	Plasma
Doptone stethoscope	IV tubing
Ultrasound gel	Alcohol sponges
Blood pressure cuff with stethoscope	Adhesive tape
Surgical scissors	Adhesive bandages
Rubber bulb syringe	Ambu bag
Plastic airway	Towels
Padded tongue blade	Hemostats
Reflex hammer	Cord clamps
Elastic tourniquet	Gauze sponges, 4 × 4
Syringes	Umbilical tape
Needles	Neonatal laryngoscope
Angiocaths	Neonatal endotracheal tubes
Lactated Ringer's solution, 1000 mL	Neonatal Ambu bag
Dextrose, 5% in 1000 mL of water	

EMERGENCY DELIVERY PROCEDURE

As the baby's head descends, imminent delivery can be anticipated by bulging of the perineum and the appearance of the fetal scalp at the introitus. At this point, no attempt should be made to delay delivery, but a controlled delivery is important in preventing both fetal and maternal injury. Either a traditional dorsal lithotomy or lateral Sims's position may be used for the actual delivery. The lateral Sims's position has the advantage of slower descent and lessening tension in the perineal tissues, and this may allow easier delivery without an episiotomy. On the other hand, with the dorsal lithotomy position the less-experienced attendant may be better able to visualize and manually control the delivery process and perform episiotomy as necessary. If the dorsal lithotomy position is chosen, the mother should be tilted slightly to one side to lessen vena caval compression and brought to the edge of the bed or stretcher, or the buttocks raised on pillows, to allow room for delivery of the baby's head and shoulders. The mother's legs should be widely separated and supported with her knees flexed.

With each contraction the vaginal outlet bulges to accommodate a greater portion of the fetal head, and this process may be aided by gentle digital stretching of the perineum. Episiotomy may be performed at this time if necessary to allow delivery without spontaneous lacerations. A local anesthetic should be injected just prior to episiotomy with 5 to 10 mL of 1 percent lidocaine (Xylocaine) in a syringe with a small-gauge needle. If a local anesthetic is unavailable, an episiotomy may be cut with minimal pain when the perineum is most stretched, taking care to protect the infant's head with gloved fingers. A midline perineal incision should be made, taking care not to extend into the rectum.

As the head emerges, the palm of one hand should be placed over the head to assist with the normal extension of the head and at the same time prevent the head from suddenly popping out of the vagina. At this point the mother is asked not to push in order to minimize the trauma associated with uncontrolled expulsive efforts. The best method to inhibit the overwhelmingly strong desire to bear down when the fetal head is distending the perineum is generally reassurance and asking the mother to pant or breathe through her nose.

With expulsive efforts under control, and one hand on the infant's crowning head, the second hand draped with a sterile cloth can be used to gently lift the infant's chin posterior to the maternal anus. This facilitates further extension and a slow, controlled emergence of the baby's head (modified Ritgen's maneuver; see Fig. 61-1). As the head is delivered, usually with the face down, it tends to restitute to one or the other lateral positions.

The baby's neck region should be palpated immediately after delivery of the head to check for a nuchal cord, which may be found

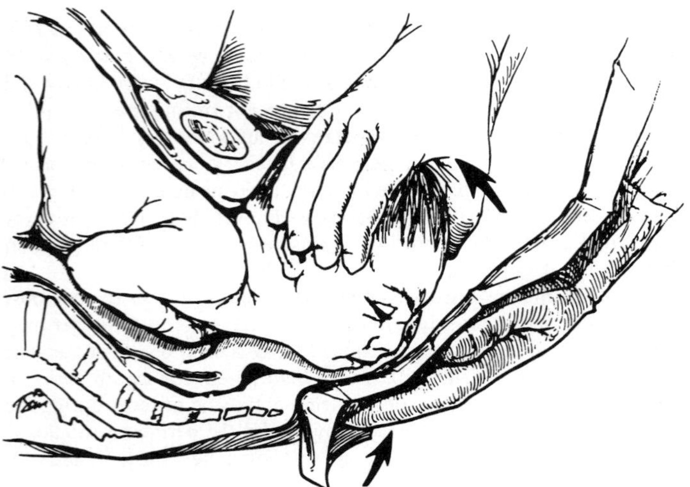

Fig. 61-1. Modified Ritgen's maneuver. Palm of hand on infant's head while second hand draped with sterile cloth gently lifts the infant's chin. (*From* Pritchard JA, McDonald PC, Gant NF (eds): *Williams Obstetrics*, ed 17. Norwalk, Conn, Appleton-Century Crofts, 1985, p 341. Used by permission.)

about 25 percent of the time. If the cord is relatively loose, it can be slipped out of the way over the baby's head. If the cord is tight, two clamps should be placed close together on the most accessible portion of the cord (usually anteriorly) and the cord cut in between. The cord can then be unwound if there are multiple loops.

Before the delivery of the shoulders and thorax is continued, the baby's face should be wiped off and the mouth and nose aspirated with a soft rubber bulb syringe to clear the airway. This is especially important to prevent meconium aspiration if there has been meconium staining of the amniotic fluid. If no bulb syringe is available, the mouth should be scooped out with the finger as well as possible. Squeezing the nose between the fingers and stroking the upper neck from the larynx toward the mandible may also be helpful.

Attention should now be turned toward delivery of the shoulders. This can be facilitated by placing both hands on either side of the body's head, and a gentle downward traction will ease the anterior shoulder under the pubic symphysis (see Fig. 61-2). Care should be taken not to use undue force, as this may result in brachial plexus injury. If there is resistance, an assistant should be asked to employ suprapubic pressure (not fundal pressure) to avoid impaction of the shoulder behind the symphysis. When the anterior shoulder is visible, gentle upward traction will deliver the posterior shoulder. Care should be taken not to let the posterior shoulder pop out uncontrolled, as this may result in a laceration of the anal sphincter and into the rectum (third-degree perineal laceration).

The baby will be very slippery, especially if there is thick vernix (white, cheesy desquamated skin). The posterior hand should slide down onto the posterior shoulder as it is delivered and then behind the back of the neck to support the baby's head. The anterior hand should then be brought along the baby's back as the body delivers spontaneously. Placing the index finger between the lower legs, and the third finger and thumb around each leg, ensures a safe grip. The baby should not, however, be held by its heels upside down. The body can easily be cradled in the same arm that is gripping the legs, and the other hand can be used to further wipe the body off and suction out the mouth and pharynx as needed.

If the baby is breathing spontaneously and is close to term, there is no need to rush cutting the cord. The baby can be dried off, wrapped in a warm blanket, and placed on the mother's abdomen to help minimize heat loss. The cord should be doubly clamped before cutting

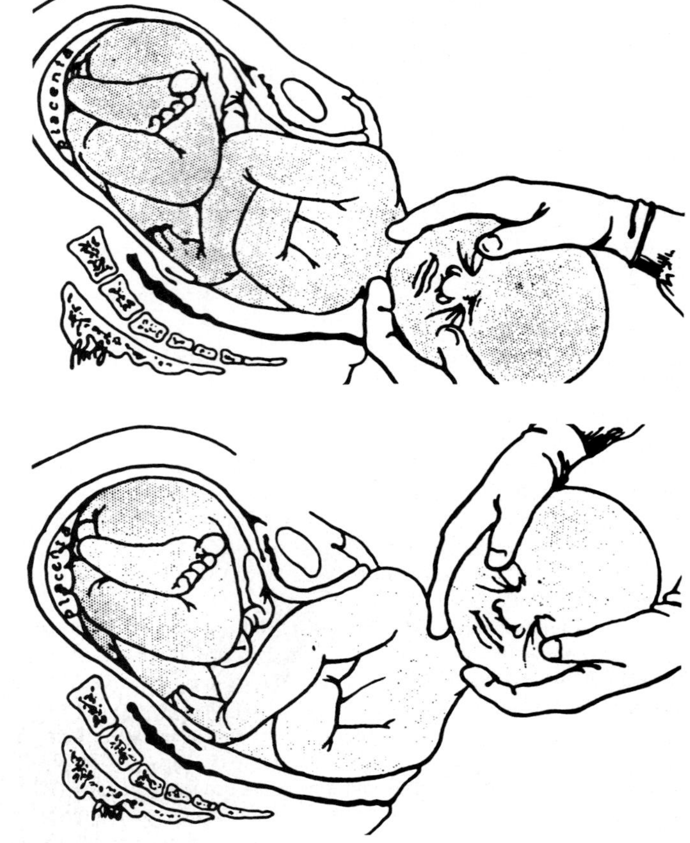

Fig. 61-2. Delivery of shoulders. **Top.** Gentle downward traction to ease anterior shoulder under pubic symphysis. **Bottom.** Delivery of anterior shoulder completed; gentle upward traction to deliver posterior shoulder. (From Pritchard JA, McDonald PC, Gant NF (eds): *Williams Obstetrics*, ed 17. Norwalk, Conn, Appleton-Century-Crofts, 1985, p 343. Used by permission.)

with a sterile scissors. If sterile scissors are unavailable, it is better to leave the cord uncut until sterile instruments can be found.

An immediate assessment of the baby with Apgar scoring should be done to determine the need for resuscitation. See Chapter 14D for details of neonatal resuscitation.

PRETERM DELIVERY

Since preterm labor is a common cause for unexpected childbirth, emergency deliveries frequently involve premature infants. It is very important to deliver a premature infant in a slow, controlled fashion, because the premature baby has greater fragility and may be more susceptible to rupture of intracranial blood vessels as well as superficial bruising. For this reason, it may be best to avoid artificial rupture of the membranes with preterm delivery and to allow delivery to occur *en cul* or with the membranes intact. In spite of the premature infant's smaller head size, an episiotomy should be liberally performed to prevent prolonged pounding of the infant's head against a resistant perineum as well as sudden popping of the head out of the introitus. Premature infants should be dried off quickly to reduce their rapid heat loss. The cord should be rapidly clamped and cut so the infant can be quickly assessed for resuscitation. Any ventilation assistance that may be required should be performed with a small Ambu bag, taking care to avoid higher pressures that would result in pneumothorax.

Premature babies are more often in breech presentation than term infants are. Although the procedure of choice for premature breech delivery is by cesarean section, this may not be possible in an emergency situation. As much as possible, the breech infant should be allowed to deliver spontaneously, at least until the level of the umbilicus has been reached. A warm towel should be placed on the baby's lower back and buttocks, and with gentle handling of the baby's pelvic bones and back (not abdomen!) one shoulder should be rotated anteriorly and delivered by raising the infant's entire body. Reversing the movement, the remaining shoulder should be rotated anteriorly and delivered. An assistant should apply pressure suprapubicly to help maintain flexion of the baby's head. As the neck appears, a finger can be placed over the baby's maxilla or, if done gently, into the baby's mouth, to flex the head for delivery and avoid entrapment in the cervix. The breech infant is more likely to require resuscitation.

MANAGEMENT IMMEDIATELY POSTPARTUM

The placenta should be allowed to separate spontaneously, unless there is considerable active bleeding. Pulling on the cord risks cord rupture, or the possible catastrophe of inversion of the uterus. The usual signs of placental separation are a gush of blood and lengthening of the cord. As the placenta is expelled, the membranes may be teased out by rotating the placenta and twisting the membranes.

After the placenta is out, the uterus should be massaged to help it to contract and remain firm. Oxytocin, 10 units, may be given slowly intravenously (or mixed in the intravenous bag), or by intramuscular injection if no intravenous line is available, to help maintain uterine contraction. Excessive bleeding calls for vigorous uterine massage, an increased amount of intravenous crystalloid solutions, and additional oxytocin or methylergonovine (Methergine). Bleeding sites for lacerations should also be identified and controlled with clamps or direct pressure. Episiotomy or laceration repair should await the availability of an experienced practitioner or obstetrician.

It should be emphasized that the infant should be thoroughly dried and wrapped in warm towels or blankets to minimize heat loss. Meconium should be suctioned out immediately after delivery of the head and before the infant takes its first breath. If personnel skilled in neonatal intubation are present, the infant with thick meconium should be intubated and suctioned under direct laryngoscopy. If a warm isolette is not available, the infant can be kept in close contact with the mother to conserve heat.

The goal of every delivery, including in the emergency situation, is a safe delivery with minimal trauma to the mother and without injury to the infant. Usually this can be accomplished even with minimal equipment if the attending individual(s) have the basic knowledge and skills for the mechanics of delivery and can give emotional support to the mother during the process. If need be, the basic points of delivery can be reviewed with a consultant by telephone in order to accomplish a safe outcome to both mother and baby.

BIBLIOGRAPHY

American Academy of Pediatrics Committee on Fetus and Newborn, American College of Obstetricians and Gynecology Committee on Obstetrics: Maternal and Fetal Medicine, Guidelines for Perinatal Care, 1983.

Anderson CL, Aladjem S, Ofelia A, et al: An analysis of maternal transport within a suburban metropolitan region. *Am J Obstet Gynecol* 140:499, 1981.

Bowes WA: Delivery of the very low birth weight infant. *Clin Perinatal* 8:183, 1981.

Crenshaw C, Payne P, Blackmon L, et al: Prematurity and the obstetrician: A regional neonatal intensive care unit is not enough. *Am J Obstet Gynecol* 147:125, 1983.

Elliot JD, O'Keeffe DF, Freeman RK: helicopter transportation of patients with obstetric emergencies in an urban area. *Am J Obstet Gynecol* 143:157, 1982.

Harris BA, Wirtshafter DD, Muddleston JF, et al: In utero versus neonatal transportation of high-risk perinates: A comparison. *Obstet Gynecol* 57:496, 1981.

Knox GE, Korliss AS: In-utero transport. *Clin Obstet Gynecol* 27:11, 1984.

Parer JT: Effects of hypoxia on the mother and fetus with emphasis on maternal air transport. *Am J Obstet Gynecol* 142:957, 1982.

Pritchard JA, MacDonald PC, Gant NF (eds): *Williams Obstetrics*, ed 17. Norwalk, Conn, Appleton-Century-Crofts, 1985.

62 COMMON COMPLICATIONS OF GYNECOLOGIC PROCEDURES

Veronica T. Mallett

With the advent of same-day surgery, and the increasing necessity to discharge patients within 3 days of a major procedure, postsurgical gynecologic patients are presenting to emergency departments with increasing frequency. The objective of this chapter is to provide an overview of the common complications of gynecologic procedures likely to lead to an emergency department visit and the diagnostic and therapeutic approach to these patients.

COMMON COMPLICATIONS OF ENDOSCOPIC PROCEDURES

Laparoscopy

Gynecologic laparoscopy, both diagnostic and therapeutic, involves the use of a rigid endoscope which is inserted usually through a small subumbilical incision bluntly into the abdominal cavity. Prior to the insertion of the laparoscope, the abdomen is insufflated with nitrous oxide or carbon dioxide gas administered through a small-diameter verres needle.

Laparoscopy can be used to diagnose existing pelvic disease and to perform simple and complex gynecologic surgeries. The most common surgical procedure in the United States today is female sterilization. Greater than 50 percent of sterilizations are performed through the laparoscope, making laparoscopy the most common surgical procedure today. With advanced technology and increased operator skill, use of the laparoscope is growing. In addition to sterilization, the laparoscope is used for laser ablation of endometriosis and pelvic adhesions, sharp lysis of adhesions, linear salpingostomy, and salpingectomy for the treatment of ectopic pregnancy, laser ablation of small myomata, and even uncommonly oophorectomy and hysterectomy.

All of these procedures, although varied in complexity, have the same range of complications. The major complications associated with the use of the laparoscope are (1) thermal injuries to the bowel, (2) bleeding at the site of tubal interruption or sharp dissection, and (3) infection.

Of these complications the most serious and dreaded is that of thermal injury to the bowel. This injury most commonly occurs in the terminal ileum, although injuries to the rectosigmoid and colon have been reported. Various series have reported the incidence of electrothermal injuries to be in the range of 0.5 to 3.2 per 1000 cases. The injury that goes unrecognized presents the most serious problem. These patients generally appear 3 to 7 days postoperatively, depending upon the degree of necrosis, with signs and symptoms of peritonitis, including bilateral lower abdominal pain, fever, elevated white count, and direct and rebound tenderness, X-rays may show an ileus or free air under the diaphragm. Although gas has been used to insufflate the abdomen, it should be absorbed totally within 3 postoperative days. If thermal injury is a serious consideration and cannot be distinguished from other causes of peritonitis, it is best to err on the side of early laparotomy.

Traumatic bowel injury is less problematic than thermal injury. This is because it is usually caused by the very small diameter verres needle and is recognized when the needle is withdrawn. Peritonitis rarely develops following this complication and hospital revisits are uncommon.

Bleeding may occur with any laparoscopic procedure, but due to direct visualization, it is usually arrested during the original procedure.

Infection has not been a frequent or particularly serious complication of laparoscopy. Excluding minor incisional infection, pelvic infection is reported in less than 1 per 1000 cases. When pelvic infection does occur, it is probably secondary to a subacute coexisting infection present prior to the procedure or secondary to the introduction of skin contaminants. Its presentation is not unique and broad-spectrum antibiotic treatment provides a rapid response.

Infection, dehiscence, and herniations of the laparoscopic abdominal incision are rare but have been reported. Infection is usually treated with drainage. Dehiscence usually involves protrusion of the omentum and, in rare cases, the small bowel through the opening. Immediate wound reclosure is usually sufficient, provided no bowel injury has occurred, and there is no evidence of infection.

Hysteroscopy

Hysteroscopy involves the direct investigation of the interior of the uterine cavity using a rigid fiberoptic instrument. It can be carried out as an office procedure using the contact hysteroscope or under IV sedation or general anesthesia using the panoramic hysteroscope. It is used for both diagnostic and therapeutic purposes. Indications for use include investigation of any intrauterine pathology, i.e., endometrial polyps, submucous myomata, and foreign bodies. Therapeutic applications include directed biopsies, removal of small myomata, endometrial ablation using laser for menorrhagia, and division of small uterine septae.

Complication of hysteroscopy fortunately are rare. They include: (1) reaction to the distending media, (2) uterine perforation, (3) cervical laceration, (4) anesthesia reaction, (5) intraabdominal organ injury, (6) infection, and (7) postoperative bleeding.

Postoperative bleeding will be the most likely cause of hospital revisit. Surgical procedures that could result in postopertive uterine bleeding include lysis of adhesions, resection of myomata, and YAG laser obliteration of the endometrium. After hemodynamic stabilization of the patient, an intrauterine tampon such as a pediatric foley generally can control this problem. Occasionally reexploration to cauterize a bleeding area is necessary. Rarely, abdominal control of the bleeding is required.

Infection as a result of the hysteroscopic procedure is uncommon, considering the number of cases done, and has rarely been reported.

Damage to intraabdominal contents has been reported. The seriousness of these complications ranges from the inconsequential rupture of a hydrosalpinx to damage to the bowel at the time of electrical sterilization, intrauterine biopsy, uterine perforation, or laser ablation. These are not common and generally are eliminated by the concomitant use of laparoscopy, the current standard of care. Should injury go unrecognized, it would present as described.

Uterine perforations are mentioned only because they are a relatively common complication associated with the procedure but seldom require more than observation.

COMPLICATIONS RELATED TO MAJOR ABDOMINAL PROCEDURES

Those complications which would lead to an emergency department visit would, by their nature, present greater than 3 days postoperatively. Late-onset complications include, but are not confined to, wound infection and related morbidity, phlebitis (superficial and deep), urinary tract infection, and ureteral or bladder injury.

Wound Infection

Wound infection may occur as late as several months following surgery, but more than 90 percent of the cases present within the first 2 weeks. The first sign is usually fever followed by tachycardia and varying degrees of increased tenderness. As the infection progresses, the wound may be fluctuant or firm. The incision is swollen, erythematous, edematous, and tender. There may be spontaneous purulent drainage from the wound. Initial management consists of opening the wound and probing with a cotton-tipped swab to ensure the fascia is intact, then allowing the wound to drain. If the patient has been discharged with staples in place, the wound opens easily after staple removal. If the staples have been removed, gentle probing will open the wound. Aerobic and anaerobic wound cultures should be obtained for use if the patient does not respond rapidly. Once a wound infection has been opened and drained, care is directed toward debridement and packing with saline-soaked gauze or half-strength peroxide. Rarely are antibiotics required unless there is an underlying cellulitis. Readmission is common practice, at least for observation and patient teaching.

Wound Hematoma

Hematomas are a common complication of wound closure that are more frequent in transverse than vertical incisions. The wound itself may swell and be painful, but in general, the smaller hematoma can and should be managed expectantly. If there are any signs of infection, the wound should be managed accordingly. The patient should be instructed to return if signs of infection develop.

Wound Seroma

Wound seromas are relatively uncommon in the gynecologic incision, with the exception of groin dissection. It is, by definition, a collection of serous fluid, which may drain spontaneously. In general, it is the presence of drainage, not fever or pain, which brings the patient to the emergency department. If the wound remains intact after gentle probing, the seroma can be watched and usually will disappear. Wound infection precautions should be given.

Dehiscence and Evisceration

Dehiscence is a failure of normal healing and literally means disruption of any layers of a surgical incision. Clinically dehiscence connotes disruption of all layers including fascia, but not peritoneum. Evisceration is a complete breakdown of the healing processes through all levels of the abdominal wall, with the omentum or bowel presenting through the incision. The classic sign and symptom of impending wound disruption is the sudden outpouring of serosanguinous fluid from the abdominal incision. Most often this occurs between postoperative days 5 and 8. The patient may describe a pop or tearing sensation. About one-third of the cases of wound dehiscence will be associated with evisceration. When evisceration has occurred, the abdomen should be covered with moist sterile towels and supported with tape to prevent further extrusion of the gut. The patient should be taken directly to the operating room for closure. In those cases in which there is a sudden appearance of fluid but no bowel, it is best to follow the same procedure because evisceration usually is imminent.

Ureteral Injury

Operative injury to the ureter results from one of three types of trauma: crushing, transection, and ligation. Each type of injury may be either partial or complete. This complication occurs more often during the performance of abdominal hysterectomy than any other pelvic surgery. Unilateal ureteral injury usually is discovered within 48 to 72 h postoperatively but may go undiscovered for up to 2 to 3 weeks. Occasionally permanent and complete occlusion will lead to renal atrophy without symptoms. In most instances, ureteral injury produces symptoms of fever flank pain, and costovertebral angle tenderness. These symptoms may indicate pyelitis, but if the patient has unexplained or persistent fever, persistent abdominal distention, unexplained hematuria, or especially escape of a watery discharge, an intravenous pyelogram (IVP) should be obtained. Further indications for an IVP include oliguria or the appearance of a lower abdominal or pelvic mass following pelvic surgery. If the diagnosis is made 2 to 3 weeks postoperatively, percutaneous nephrostomy with delayed repair is the treatment of choice.

MISCELLANEOUS COMPLICATIONS OF MAJOR GYNECOLOGIC PROCEDURES

Cuff Cellulitis

Cuff cellulitis refers to infections of the contiguous retroperitoneal space immediately above the vaginal apex and including the surrounding soft tissue. It is a common complication following both abdominal and vaginal hysterectomy. It usually produces a fever between the postoperative days 3 to 5 and thus, generally will, delay discharge of the postabdominal hysterectomy patient. The postvaginal hysterectomy patient conceivably will have been discharged and present with a complaint of fever and lower quadrant pain. Pelvic tenderness and induration are prominent during the bimanual examination. A vaginal cuff abscess may be palpable. Readmission drainage and intravenous antibiotics is the treatment of choice.

Urinary Retention

Voiding difficulties in the healthy female are uncommon. However, many women experience an inability to void or incomplete emptying of the bladder during the postoperative period. Inability to void is more frequent after operations that involve the urethra and bladder neck, i.e., anterior repair or any modification of the retropubic urethropexy. Most problems with voiding following any of these procedures resolve without medication with time. If mechanical obstruction is not suspected to be a factor, intermittent straight catheterization is the treatment of choice. The patient should be instructed to attempt to void on a timed schedule with an interval of less than 3 h. She should be discharged with instruction on self-catherization should she be unable to void and reassured voiding function will return in time.

Postconization Bleeding

Laser vaporization and laser excision conization currently are popular for the treatment of cervical intraepithelial neoplasia. The most common complication associated with these procedures is bleeding. If delayed hemorrhage occurs, it usually occurs 7 days postoperatively. Bleeding following this procedure can be rapid and excessive. Visualization of the cervix is the key to controlling it. Application of Monsel's solution is a reasonable first step if it easily available. Usually, however, suturing of the bleeding arteriole is necessary. Quite often, the patient must be taken to the operating room for repair secondary to poor visualization. Cold-knife conization also remains popular and is association with the same complication. Treatment for both types of hemorrhage is identical.

Induced Abortion

There are three major methods for termination of pregnancy: instrumental evacuation by the vaginal route, stimulation of uterine contraction, and major surgical procedures. Vacuum evacuation of the uterus has known immediate and delayed complications. Immediate complications include uterine perforation, hemorrhage, and cervical laceration. Delayed complications of all methods of abortions include retention of products of conception causing bleeding, infection, and possibly thrombophlebitis.

The majority of immediate complications will be arrested at the time of the abortion; however, uterine perforation, if unrecognized, could be complicated further by injury of intraabdominal contents with the suction. If this should occur and go unrecognized, the patient will present with the appropriate signs of organ injury. The organ most commonly injured is the bowel; however, the ureter has been injured as a consequence of this mishap. Management of these complications was discussed previously.

Retained products of conception and a resulting endometritis is a far more common complication. The patient usually will present 3 to 5 days posttermination with complaints of excessive bleeding, fever, and abdominal pain. She may not present for up to 2 weeks. Pelvic examination reveals a subinvoluted tender uterus with foul-smelling blood vaginally. An elevated white blood count is common. Treatment must include evacuation of intrauterine contents and intravenous antibiotic therapy. Triple antibiotic therapy is the standard; however, there is increasing evidence that ampicillin with salbactum (Unasyn) is equally as effective. If the patient has pain, bleeding, or both, unaccompanied by fever, ectopic pregnancy must be ruled out. The presence of villi on the pathology report (if available) confirms the presence of an intrauterine gestation but cannot rule out the rare occurrence of both ectopic and intrauterine gestations.

BIBLIOGRAPHY

Baggish MS, Lee WK: Abdominal wound disruption. *Obstet Gynecol* 46:530, 1975.

Burke L: The use of the carbon dioxide laser in the therapy of cervical intraepithelial neoplasia. *Am J Obstet Gynecol* 144:337, 1982.

Daly JW: Dehiscence, eviseration and other complications. *Clin Obstet Gynecol* 31:754, 1988.

Loffer FD, Pent D: Indications, contraindications and complications of laparoscopy. *Obstet Gynecol* 30:407, 1975.

Masterson BJ, Krantz K, Calkins JW, et al: The carbon dioxide laser in cervical intraepithelial neoplasia, a five year experience in treating 230 patients. *Am J Obstet Gynecol* 139:565, 1981.

SECTION 8
Pediatrics

63
COMMON NEONATAL PROBLEMS

Niranjan Kissoon

The assessment of the neonate in the emergency department is more difficult than that of the older child or the adult. Symptoms are usually vague and nonspecific. Signs are usually subtle and even when recognized may not be helpful in pinpointing the exact diagnosis. For example, respiratory distress may be due to primary respiratory or cardiac disease, generalized sepsis, abdominal pathology, or metabolic derangements. Examination of the neonate is time-consuming and requires special skills in the approach to the infant as well as to the anxious parent.

The prerequisites for the proper evaluation of neonates are a great deal of patience as well as an appreciation for the marked variations in normal vegetative functions in this population. Many visits are initiated because of parental concerns relating to feeding patterns, weight gain, stool frequency, color, and consistency, and breathing patterns.

NORMAL VEGETATIVE FUNCTIONS

Feeding Patterns

During the first few weeks of life, feeding is usually dictated by the infant, with a specific pattern established by 1 month in 90 percent. Most bottle-fed infants will want six to nine feedings per 24 h by the first week of life, while breast-fed infants may require feeding every 2 to 4 h. Parents usually need reassurance that their infant is obtaining adequate nutrition because of the wide variation in the intakes of normal infants compared to one another.

Weight Gain

While it is difficult to judge the exact caloric intake of breast-fed infants and feeding frequency varies widely, intake is adequate if the neonate is gaining weight appropriately and appears content between feeds. Intake is satisfactory if infants are no longer losing weight by 5 to 7 days and gaining 10 to 30 g/kg per day by 12 to 14 days of age.

Stool Patterns

The number, color, and consistency of bowel movements vary greatly in the same infant and between infants regardless of diet or environment. Stool frequency may vary from one to seven times per day, with loose stools frequent in breast-fed infants. Infrequent bowel movements do not necessarily mean constipation, since breast-fed infants may occasionally go 5 to 7 days without a bowel movement. Stool color is of no significance unless blood is present.

Breathing Patterns

In the first month of life breathing patterns vary widely. Normal full-term infants have episodes during sleep when periodic breathing occurs, manifested as an interruption of respiration two or more times within a 20-s period. It is, however, not associated with heart rate or color changes and has no prognostic significance.

REASONS FOR EMERGENCY DEPARTMENT VISITS

A review of presenting complaints in our pediatric emergency department, a tertiary care referral center, over a 6-month period indicates the spectrum most likely to be seen by the emergency physician (Table 63-1). Complaints in neonates are usually not single but can more correctly be referred to as "symptom complexes." These reflect the nonspecific nature of signs and symptoms in the neonate and the similar presentation of many commonly seen diseases of diverse etiology.

CRYING/IRRITABILITY/LETHARGY

This group of symptoms is fairly common yet difficult to treat even in the presence of an identifiable cause. Most neonates will exhibit varying degrees and periods of crying during a 24-h period. However, those infants who present with an episode of acute inconsolable crying should be observed closely for an underlying cause (Table 63-2).

Intestinal Colic

The most common cause of crying is intestinal colic. This usually occurs in normal, healthy, thriving babies in the second or third week of life and persists until 3 months of age. Episodes commonly occur in the late afternoon or evening and begin with screaming episodes with drawing up of knees, as if the infant is in pain, and usually passage of flatus. Intestinal colic is not known to have any grave clinical significance or long-term effects.

The diagnosis is usually made when there is no evidence of physical illness (normal growth and development) and if the bouts of crying are episodic in nature. However, a careful history, physical examination, and appropriate laboratory investigations will enable the emergency physician to diagnose colic and exclude the serious conditions listed in Table 63-2. In doubtful situations, admission for observation or return for reassessment is reasonable. More often than not, parents have visited several physicians and are angry, frustrated, or dissatisfied

Table 63-1. Common Presenting Complaints

1. Crying/irritability/lethargy
   (See Table 63-2)
2. Gastrointestinal tract symptoms
   a. Feeding difficulties
   b. Regurgitation
   c. Vomiting
   d. Diarrhea
   e. Abdominal distension
   f. Constipation
3. Cardiorespiratory symptoms
   a. Rapid breathing
   b. Cough and nasal congestion
   c. Noisy breathing and stridor
   d. Apnea/periodic breathing
   e. Blue spells/cyanosis
4. Jaundice
5. Eye discharge/redness
6. Diaper rash/oral thrush
7. Fever and sepsis
8. Sudden infant death

Table 63-2. Conditions Associated with Uncontrollable Crying and/or Irritability and/or Lethargy in Neonates

1. Intestinal Colic
2. Traumatic conditions
   a. Battered child syndrome (fractures, burns, etc.)
   b. Falls (skull or extremity fractures)
   c. Open diaper pin
   d. Strangulation of digit or penis
   e. Corneal abrasion or foreign body
3. Infections
   a. Meningitis
   b. Generalized sepsis
   c. Otitis media
   d. Urinary tract infection
   e. Gastroenteritis
4. Surgical
   a. Incarcerated hernia (umbilical or inguinal)
   b. Testicular torsion
   c. Anal fissure
5. Improper feeding practices

with the advice and care given. While colic cannot be treated or cured in the emergency department, reassurance that all is well and follow-up are essential in all cases.

Abuse and Trauma

Traumatic conditions, though less common, are frequently overlooked in the neonate. A careful history (inconsistent or implausible history) may lead the physician to strongly suspect the diagnosis of child abuse, while physical examination may reveal unexplained injuries (bruises of varying ages, skull fractures, extremity fractures, cigarette burns, etc.). If the diagnosis is suspected, the child should be admitted for protection and further investigations. An examination of the eye, though difficult, is essential since the presence of retinal hemorrhage especially in the absence of external signs of trauma suggests a whiplash injury due to severe shaking. The examination of the eye is also useful to rule out an eyelash in the eye or a corneal abrasion as reasons for the infant's symptoms. Congenital glaucoma, though rare, may also present with irritability and crying. The piercing of the skin with an open diaper pin as well as strangulation of integuments with hair are not uncommon reasons for distress in the neonate.

Infections

Infections in the neonate will manifest as a variety of symptoms and signs such as feeding difficulties, fever, jaundice, or respiratory distress. Neck rigidity and Kernig's and Brudzinski's signs are usually absent in the neonate with meningitis. A septic neonate may present with a normal or subnormal temperature rather than fever. Urinary tract infections in neonates are often associated with nonspecific signs such as irritability, diarrhea, or poor feeding, and diagnosis is established by urine culture rather than urinalysis.

Surgical Lesions

Surgical lesions such as incarcerated hernia (umbilical or inguinal) as well as testicular torsion require prompt diagnosis and surgical referral. The most common signs are irritability and crying, followed by poor feeding, vomiting, constipation, and abdominal distension. Physical examination may reveal a red, edematous, tender lump at the site of the hernia or testicular torsion. These findings are very easy to overlook when irritability is the only symptom and the neonate has not been undressed fully for examination. Anal fissures may also present at this age and may be difficult to diagnose. Most can easily be seen if the bottom of a small test tube is inserted into the anal verge and the fissure is examined through the bottom glass surface.

Improper Feeding Practices

Improper feeding practices may result in an irritable infant with periods of inconsolable crying. This usually results from overfeeding with inadequate burping during feeds. The infant subsequently swallows large amounts of air resulting in bowel distension and occasionally respiratory distress. Instruction in proper feeding practices usually alleviates the problem.

GASTROINTESTINAL TRACT SYMPTOMS

Feeding Difficulties

Most visits for feeding difficulties are due to parental perception that the infant's food intake is inadequate. The neonate's pattern of intake is not fully established until about 1 month of age. If weight gain is satisfactory and the infant is satisfied after feeds, intake is adequate. Parents can usually provide accurate information of the intake of the bottle-fed infant. The weighing of the breast-fed infant before and after feeds is not advised, since weights may be inaccurate. In addition, weighing may have adverse psychological effects on the mother whose infant is doing poorly.

Rarely, anatomic abnormalities can cause difficulty in feeding and swallowing. A careful history usually pinpoints these difficulties as occurring from birth. Infants appear malnourished and dehydrated. The most likely causes are esophageal obstruction (stenoses, strictures, laryngeal clefts, cleft palate) and double aortic arch compressing the esophagus or trachea. Infants with a recent decrease in intake, who were feeding normally previously, have an acute disease, usually an infection.

Regurgitation

Regurgitation of small amounts is common in the neonate and is due to reduced lower-esophageal sphincter pressure and relatively increased intragastric pressure. Parents may confuse regurgitation with vomiting. Vomiting results from forceful contraction of the diaphragm and abdominal muscles, whereas regurgitation is independent of any effort. If the neonate is thriving, parents can be reassured that regurgitation is of no clinical significance and will decrease as the infant grows. Infants who are not thriving or having respiratory symptoms should be investigated for anatomical causes of regurgitation or chronic aspiration.

Regurgitation rarely results from pathological processes such as intrinsic compression of the esophagus or occasionally compression of the trachea in which case it is usually accompanied by stridor and cough. Dysphagia, irritability, anemia due to chronic blood loss, and malnutrition are sequelae of chronic regurgitation with esophagitis, but this condition is rare.

Vomiting

Vomiting usually results from a variety of causes and rarely presents as an isolated symptom. During the first few weeks of life, vomiting is uncommon and often is confused with regurgitation. Vomiting from birth is most likely due to an anatomic abnormality such as a tracheoesophageal fistula, upper gastrointestinal obstruction, or midgut rotation. More commonly, acute vomiting may be part of the symptom complex of some diseases (Table 63-2), especially increased intracranial pressure, and infections (sepsis, urinary tract infections, gastroenteritis).

Projectile vomiting is usually seen in infants with pyloric stenosis and usually assumes its characteristic pattern after the second and third week of life. This condition usually occurs in firstborn males and is characterized by projectile vomiting at the end of feeding or shortly thereafter. The vomitus does not contain bile or blood. Examination of these infants should be done with the infant relaxed and the stomach empty. Prominent gastric waves may be seen going from left to right as well as a firm olive mass felt by palpating up and down under the liver edge. Malnutrition and dehydration may be evident. Hospitalization is necessary for rehydration and surgical referral.

Diarrhea

Diarrhea is associated with the excessive loss of fluid and electrolytes in stools. The complaint of diarrhea in the neonate in many cases reflects ignorance of the marked normal variation in stool frequency and consistency. Where the infant is feeling well and gaining weight appropriately, the only treatment necessary is to reassure parents that all is well.

Diarrhea may be associated with systemic diseases such as generalized sepsis, otitis media, and urinary tract infections. This entity, termed *parenteral diarrhea,* is nonspecific and does not contain blood or mucus. Infectious diarrhea, on the other hand, is usually associated with fever and is mostly of viral etiology, with rota and enteroviruses being most common. Bacterial causes (*Escherichia coli, Salmonella, Shigella*) and parasitic causes (*Giardia, Entamoeba histolytica*) are rare in neonates. Causes of bloody diarrhea in the neonate include necrotizing enterocolitis, bacterial enteritis, antibiotic-associated diarrhea, milk allergy, and rarely, intussusception. In the absence of other signs of infection, a bleeding diathesis should also be suspected. Close attention to hydration and nutritional status as well as fluid and electrolytes is mandatory. Infants who are moderately or severely dehydrated should be admitted for treatment, while those with mild dehydration can be followed closely as outpatients if parents are reliable and follow-up ensured.

Necrotizing enterocolitis usually presents with other signs of sepsis (jaundice, lethargy, fever, poor feeding, abdominal distension, and discoloration). Abdominal radiography may demonstrate pneumatosis intestinalis. True milk allergy presents with abdominal distension, explosive bloody diarrhea, and, in severe cases, shock. Intussusception usually occurs in the older infant and toddler but can also occur in the neonate, with abdominal distension, feeding difficulty, and a mass in the right upper quadrant.

Abdominal Distension

Abdominal distension is normal in the neonate and is usually due to lax abdominal musculature and relatively large intraabdominal organs. It may also be accentuated by excessive gas within the bowel. In the majority of cases, if the infant is comfortable and feeding well and the abdomen is soft, there is no need for concern. Abdominal distension may also occur in association with bowel obstruction, constipation, or as a result of ileus due to sepsis or gastroenteritis. Congenital organomegaly (hepatomegaly, splenomegaly, renal enlargement) undetected in the perinatal period may also present as abdominal distension.

Constipation

Infrequent bowel movements in neonates do not necessarily mean constipation. The breast-fed infant may on occasion go without a bowel movement for 5 to 7 days and then pass a normal stool. However, if the infant has never passed stools, the possibility of intestinal stenosis or atresia, Hirschsprung's disease, and meconium ileus or plug should be considered.

Constipation occurring after birth but within the first month of life suggests Hirschsprung's disease, hypothyroidism, or anal stenosis. The diagnosis of Hirschsprung's disease is supported by absence of feces on rectal examination and abrupt change in bowel luminal size on barium enema, and is confirmed by rectal biopsy demonstrating absence of ganglion cells. Hypothyroidism is manifested as feeding problems, a weak, hoarse cry, hypothermia, hypotonia, and peripheral edema.

CARDIORESPIRATORY SYMPTOMS

The neonate is prone to respiratory problems (Table 63-1) for a variety of reasons. Anatomic reasons that are disadvantageous are the barrel-shaped chest, flattened diaphragm, limitation of diaphragmatic movement by abdominal compression, smaller airway diameter, and higher closing volumes. In addition, the high compliance of the chest wall, low compliance of the infant lung, and less fatigue-resistant fibers in the diaphragm and intercostal muscles are also significant contributory factors. Cardiorespiratory symptoms are also more common in this age group, since structural and functional abnormalities of the airway and heart are more likely to present at this time.

Cardiorespiratory symptoms in neonates are nonspecific and may be due to primary organ failure (cardiovascular or respiratory) or secondary to a variety of systemic diseases such as sepsis and metabolic acidosis, abdominal pathology, and severe meningitis. Regardless of etiology, the concern is, first, the assessment and stabilization of airway, breathing, and circulation; and second, establishing the diagnosis.

Rapid Breathing

Rapid breathing can be due to minor problems such as abdominal distension or life-threatening illnesses such as sepsis. Rapid breathing or grunting should always be considered a medical emergency. Admission for investigations, monitoring, and therapy should be considered in all but the mildest cases. When a cause cannot be identified on initial presentation, a full sepsis workup (full blood count, blood culture, urinalysis, chest x-ray, and cerebrospinal fluid examination) should be done and broad-spectrum antibiotic therapy instituted (Table 63-3).

Pneumonia

Bacterial pneumonias (pneumococcal, streptococcal, staphylococcal) as well as viral pneumonias may present as a period of fussiness, stuffy nose, and decreased appetite followed by an abrupt onset of high fever (<39°C), nasal flaring, grunting, retractions, tachypnea, and tachycardia. *Chlamydia* pneumonia usually occurs after 3 weeks of age and is accompanied by conjunctivitis in 50 percent of cases. The infants are tachypneic, afebrile, and have a prominent cough. Chest examination reveals rales but few wheezes. Chest x-ray shows hyperinflation with diffuse patchy infiltrates. Aspiration pneumonia is more likely

Table 63-3. Causes of Rapid Breathing in the Neonate

1. Pneumonia
   a. Bacterial
   b. Viral
   c. *Chlamydia*
   d. Aspiration
2. Bronchiolitis
3. Illness to other organ systems
   a. Septicemia
   b. Central nervous system, e.g., meningitis
   c. Abdomen, e.g., distension, gastroenteritis
   d. Metabolic acidosis
4. Congenital diseases:
   a. Respiratory disease
      (1) Delayed presentation of diaphragmatic hernia
      (2) Tracheoesophageal fistula
      (3) Lobar emphysema
      (4) Tracheal stenosis, webs
   b. Heart disease
      (1) Cardiac failure, e.g., hypoplastic left heart, critical coarctation of aorta, aortic stenosis, patent ductus arteriosus
      (2) Cyanotic disease, e.g., transposition of great arteries
      (3) Vascular ring
   c. Neuromuscular disease
      (1) Infantile botulism
      (2) Muscle weakness

Table 63-4. Antibiotic Therapy for Infections

Indications	Drugs*
Pneumonia (bacterial) Generalized sepsis Necrotizing enterocolitis Bacterial meningitis Gonococcal infections Urinary tract infections	Ampicillin (100 mg/kg per day q 6 h) and Gentamicin (7.5 mg/kg per day q 8 h) or Cefotaxime (200 mg/kg per day q 6 h) Length of therapy depends on infection being treated.
Bronchiolitis (RSV)	Ribavirin (nebulized) 20 mg/mL water for 12–18 h/day for 3–7 days.
Conjunctivitis (bacterial)	Sodium sulamyd 10% or topical erythromycin, 2 drops to each eye, q 4 h for 5–7 days. Erythromycin 40 mg/kg per day q 6 h for 14 days.
Pneumonia (chlamydial)	Erythromycin 40 mg/kg per day q 6 h for 14 days.
Oral thrush	Oral nystatin suspension 100,000 units q 4–6 h after feeds for 7–14 days.
Candida dermatitis	Nystatin/amphotericin cream to affected area q 4–6 h for 7–14 days.

to occur in infants with a tracheoesophageal fistula, swallowing dysfunction, and debilitated infants. Following aspiration, symptoms such as tachypnea and cough usually occur within 1 h and are seen within 2 h in almost all cases. Infants with pneumonia should be admitted for monitoring and institution of antibacterial therapy (Table 63-4) as indicated.

Bronchiolitis

Acute bronchiolitis usually presents in infancy as a serous nasal discharge accompanied by sneezing. These symptoms are followed by fever (38.5 to 39°C), diminished appetite, cough, dyspnea, irritability, and, commonly, periods of apnea. Physical examination reveals a rapid respiratory rate (<60 breaths per minute), cyanosis, air hunger, hyperinflation, intercostal and subcostal retractions, and palpable liver and spleen due to hyperinflation of the lungs. Prolonged expiration, wheezes, and fine rales are present. Chest x-rays usually reveal hyperinflation with atelectasis. Admission for monitoring and therapy is required (Table 63-4).

Illness Involving Other Organ Systems

The search for pathology in other organ systems is mandatory since the presence of respiratory symptoms may divert attention from the underlying significant problem. For example, generalized sepsis, meningitis, gastroenteritis, and metabolic acidosis may present with respiratory distress as the predominant symptom.

Congenital Diseases

Respiratory Disease

Occasionally, H-type tracheoesophageal fistula may present in the first month of life or later with recurrent pneumonia, respiratory distress after feeds, and problems handling mucus. Tracheal stenosis may present initially with noisy breathing or high-pitched cry and tremendous respiratory difficulty even after mild upper respiratory infections. Similarly, neonates with chronic respiratory insufficiency, e.g., bronchopulmonary dysplasia, may present in respiratory failure even after mild upper respiratory infections.

Heart Disease

Rapid breathing due to cardiac disease is usually not associated with significant retractions and use of accessory muscles. As a general rule, the well-developed neonate who presents with unexplained cyanosis and tachypnea should be suspected of having congenital cardiac disease. In neonates with transposition of the great arteries and ventricular septal defect or critical coarctation of the aorta, congestive cardiac failure may be the presenting feature. Signs of heart failure may be very subtle but are life-threatening and require emergent referral. Dyspnea, hepatomegaly, cyanosis, and cardiomegaly are present, and peripheral pulses are weak.

Neuromuscular Disease

Any form of muscle weakness may be associated with shallow breathing and an increase in respiratory rate as a compensatory mechanism.

Cough and Nasal Congestion

Cough may be a prominent feature of most of the primary respiratory conditions listed in Table 63-3. It may also be the initial presentation of a variety of congenital anomalies including cleft palate, laryngotracheomalacia, laryngotracheal cleft, tracheal webs, tracheoesophageal fistula, tracheal hemangiomas, and vascular rings. Although congenital malformations resulting in cough and nasal congestion are more likely to occur in the neonate, in the majority of instances, cough is due to a viral upper respiratory infection and may be associated with sneezing and nasal congestion. It may also be a prominent feature of bronchiolitis, and *Chlamydia* and *Pertussis* infections. Treatment of the underlying condition is the therapy of choice. Cough suppressants should be used with extreme caution in neonates. Nasal congestion is best treated with instillation of saline drops when necessary.

Noisy Breathing and Stridor

Noisy breathing is a common presenting complaint in the neonate and is usually benign. Stridor is usually due to congenital anomalies (webs, cysts, atresia, stenosis, clefts, hemangiomas) extending anywhere from the nose to the trachea and bronchi. Infants who were intubated in the neonatal period are prone to develop subglottic stenosis. Infection (croup, epiglottitis, abscess) as a cause of stridor in the neonate is rare. Stridor worsening with cry suggests laryngomalacia or subglottic hemangioma; stridor and feeding difficulties suggest vascular ring, laryngeal cleft, or tracheoesophageal fistula; stridor with hoarseness suggests vocal cord paralysis. Laryngomalacia is the most common cause of stridor in the neonate. It is characterized by noisy, crowing inspiratory sounds which usually improve during the first year of life.

Apnea and Periodic Breathing

Periodic breathing, which may occur in normal neonates, should be differentiated from apnea. However, periodic breathing may precede apnea and both may occur in the same patient. *Apnea* is defined as a cessation of respiration for 10 to 20 s with or without bradycardia and cyanosis. It signifies critical illness and warrants prompt investigation and admission.

Apnea may be precipitated by any of the disease conditions listed in Table 63-3 and usually indicates respiratory muscle fatigue and impending respiratory arrest. Resuscitation including airway support and ventilation should be followed by a thorough search for the inciting condition. If no obvious cause is found, the neonate should be assumed to be septic. Cultures should be obtained and broad-spectrum antibiotics started.

Cyanosis and Blue Spells

The infant with cyanosis and blue spells usually presents a diagnostic challenge since these findings may be due to a variety of disorders. If breathing is rapid but not labored, the most likely cause is cyanotic congenital heart disease with right-to-left shunting. Methemoglobinemia, though rare, may present similarly. Irregular or shallow breathing may be associated with sepsis, meningitis, cerebral edema, or intracranial hemorrhage and may also be accompanied by cyanosis.

If breathing is labored (grunting, indrawing), pulmonary disease (pneumonia, bronchiolitis) is likely. Infants with cyanosis should be admitted for monitoring and further investigation.

JAUNDICE

Jaundice (Table 63-5) is a yellowish-green pigmentation of the skin and sclera due to excess bilirubin. It may appear at varying times during the neonatal period and requires a complete diagnostic evaluation. Jaundice during the first 24 h rarely presents to the emergency department (ED). The commonest causes of jaundice seen in the ED are physiologic, secondary to sepsis, breast-milk jaundice, and, occasionally, hemolysis due to autoimmune congenital causes.

Physiologic jaundice is due to the breakdown of fetal red blood cells, and bilirubin rises at a rate of <5 mg/dL per 24 h with a peak of 5 to 6 mg/dL during the second to the fourth day of life, returning to <2 mg/dL by 5 to 7 days. The septic infant with hyperbilirubinemia will also have other features of sepsis, i.e., vomiting, abdominal distension, respiratory distress, and poor feeding. Jaundice associated with breast-feeding may start as early as the third to fourth day and reaches a peak of 10 to 27 mg/dL by week three. Cessation of breast-feeding causes rapid decline in 2 to 3 days. This is thought to be due to the presence of substances which inhibit glucorinyl transferase in breast milk.

A proper history and physical examination will provide a clue to the causes of jaundice. The well-looking child who is gaining weight and feeding well is unlikely to be septic. Laboratory evaluation should include full blood count for anemia, smear for hemolysis, direct and total bilirubin, a reticulocyte count, and Coombs' test. In addition, admission, appropriate cultures, and antibiotics are appropriate for neonates who are unwell and have any of the signs or symptoms listed in Table 63-6. In all cases, arrangements should be made for monitoring of bilirubin and hemoglobin levels. While most well infants can be monitored out of hospital, infants who are anemic or those with bilirubin levels approaching transfusion levels (approximately 20 mg/dL) should be admitted.

EYE DISCHARGE AND REDNESS

Most commonly, the neonate with red eye will be suffering from conjunctivitis. While the commonest cause of conjunctivitis in the neonate is chemical, due to silver nitrate, this rarely presents to the emergency department. For the first 2 weeks of life, the commonest causes of conjunctivitis are chlamydial infection, *Neisseria gonorrhoeae*, and gram-negative bacilli (*Escherichia coli* and *Pseudomonas*). In neonates older than 2 weeks of age, these infections along with other viral infections (herpes) and staphylococcal and streptococcal species should be considered.

Gonococcal conjunctivitis begins after an incubation period of 2 to 5 days with a mild inflammation accompanied by a serosanguinous discharge which becomes purulent within 24 h. *Chlamydia* trachomatis has an incubation period of 5 to 14 days and is associated with a thick, purulent discharge in an afebrile and alert infant. It may also accompany pneumonia in the neonate greater than 3 weeks of age.

The neonate with a red eye and irritability may also be suffering from a corneal irritation or abrasion usually due to an eyelash. Acute glaucoma, though rare, will present as a red, teary eye. In these instances, the cornea may be stained or cloudy, the anterior chamber shallow and intraocular pressure increased. Prompt ophthalmological referral of all suspected cases of glaucoma is essential. Infectious causes should also be treated (Table 63-4).

Table 63-5. Causes of Jaundice in Neonates

<24 h	ABO, Rh incompatibility Sepsis Congenital infections (rubella, toxoplasmosis, cytomegalic inclusion disease) Secondary to bruising
2–3 days	Physiologic
3 days–1 week	Septicemia Syphilis, toxoplasmosis, cytomegalic inclusion disease
>1 week	Septicemia, congenital atresia of bile ducts, serum hepatitis Congenital hemolytic anemias (sickle cell anemia, spherocytosis) Hemolytic anemia due to drugs (e.g., in glucose-6-phosphate dehydrogenase deficiency) Rubella, herpetic hepatitis Hypothyroidism Breast-milk jaundice

Table 63-6. Signs and Symptoms of Neonatal Sepsis

Temperature instability	Fever, hypothermia
CNS dysfunction	Lethargy, irritability, seizures
Respiratory distress	Apnea, tachypnea, grunting
Feeding disturbance	Vomiting, poor feeding, gastric distension, diarrhea
Jaundice	
Rashes	

DIAPER RASH AND ORAL THRUSH

Candida diaper dermatitis is an erythematous plaque with a scalloped border, sharply demarcated edge, and studded by satellite lesions. It usually occurs in the moist, occluded diaper area and intertriginous zones. It usually results from the action of organisms harbored in the gastrointestinal tract. Treatment consists of an anticandidal agent with each diaper change or four times daily. Protection of the area with zinc oxide paste overlying the cream will prevent friction. In addition, an oral course of treatment is usually warranted to prevent colonization of the gut (Table 63-4).

Oral lesions are white, flaky plaques covering the tongue, lips, gingiva, and mucous membranes. These lesions are common in debilitated infants and in those on antibiotics. Oral lesions may affect oral intake because of pain and discomfort. Treatment of ill infants consists of treating the underlying pathology, oral antifungal therapy, and an anesthetic gel prior to feeding. Cool liquids may prevent discomfort and pain.

FEVER AND SEPSIS

Fever (Table 63-6) is most commonly due to infectious causes. Most infections occurring in the first 5 days of life are acquired by vertical transmission from the mother. Bacterial infections are usually caused by group B streptococci (30 percent), *E. coli* (30 to 40 percent), other gram-negative enteric organisms (15 to 20 percent), and gram-positive cocci (10 percent). Viral infections are also common and are most likely due to enteroviruses (Coxsackie and echovirus) acquired at the time of delivery or respiratory syncytial viruses acquired postnatally. Neonates with presumed sepsis should be admitted and started on broad spectrum antibiotics after a full sepsis workup.

SUDDEN INFANT DEATH

Neonates may occasionally develop cardiorespiratory arrest. Although sudden infant death syndrome should be considered, catastrophic deterioration is more likely to be due to infectious causes (septicemia, meningitis), trauma (intracranial bleed, child abuse), and inborn errors of metabolism (medium-chain acyl dehydrogenase deficiency).

In most cases, cardiopulmonary resuscitation is unsuccessful since the myocardium has suffered severe hypoxic ischemic damage. The physician's role in these cases is to provide supportive care for the family. In most cases, this entails reassurance that all appropriate efforts were made to save their child's life and that the infant has been treated with dignity. Other personnel (chaplain, social worker, family physician, etc.) may also be required to provide support.

When the cause of death is not known, physicians should obtain appropriate samples (blood, urine, skin biopsy, etc.) and obtain permission for an autopsy. This is very important because of the genetic implications of metabolic disease. A postmortem protocol for sudden neonatal deaths should be available in all EDs.

BIBLIOGRAPHY

Behrman RE, Vaughan VC: *Nelson, Textbook of Pediatrics.* Philadelphia, Saunders, 1983.

Fleisher G, Ludwig S: *Textbook of Pediatric Emergency Medicine,* 2d ed. Baltimore, Williams & Wilkins, 1988.

Jaffe D, Torrey S: Diagnostic approach to febrile illness, in Ludwig S (ed): *Clinics in Emergency Medicine, Pediatric Emergencies.* New York, Churchill Livingstone, 1988.

McBride JT: Infantile apnea. *Ped Rev* 5:275, 1984.

Report of the Committee on Infectious Diseases, American Academy of Pediatrics, 1988; 141 Northwest Point Boulevard, P.O. Box 927, Elk Grove Village, Illinois 60009-0927.

64 THE NICU GRADUATE

Daniel G. Batton

The graduate of the neonatal intensive care unit (NICU) may be a frequent visitor to the emergency department and often requires rehospitalization during the first few months following discharge. Most NICU graduates are low-birthweight infants who may have a variety of complications related to prematurity. These infants should be evaluated based upon *postconceptional* age, not chronologic age. For example a 32-week-gestation premature infant with an 8-week chronologic age since birth is evaluated as a term infant.

Premature infants are usually discharged from the hospital at a postconceptional age of 35 to 40 weeks, although a few infants will be much older. The normal respiratory rate at this age is 30 to 40 per minute, although an infant with bronchopulmonary dysplasia may breathe 60 to 70 times per minute. The heart rate ranges from 120 to 160 beats per minute but can be considerably lower during quiet sleep. Most laboratory values will be similar to adult values although the hematocrit can be as low as 20 to 25 percent because of physiologic anemia. Neurodevelopmental milestones most appropriate for a given infant are those corresponding to the postconceptional age. When caring for the NICU graduate, attention must be paid not only to the presenting signs and symptoms but also to general problems related to prematurity.

GENERAL CONSIDERATIONS

Cold Stress

Following hospital discharge, premature infants remain susceptible to cold stress when exposed to lower environmental temperatures primarily because of decreased subcutaneous tissue. Infants who are cold-stressed are not capable of responding by shivering but rather attempt to maintain body temperature by increasing their metabolism of brown fat, which results in heat production. However, this increases oxygen consumption and can lead to hypoglycemia. If this compensatory increase in metabolic rate is insufficient to overcome the low environmental temperature, then body temperature will fall. A normal body temperature, however, does not eliminate the possibility of cold stress since body temperature may be maintained at a considerable metabolic expense. The best way to avoid cold stress is to provide an adequate environmental temperature for the infant who is being evaluated in the emergency department. If the room temperature cannot be adjusted appropriately, a heat lamp should be available. Commercial heat lamps are available which have automatic timers and can be adjusted to provide varying amounts of heat. These should be standard equipment in emergency departments which treat infants and children.

Hypoglycemia

Premature infants are at risk of developing hypoglycemia with an acute illness. This may be due in part to increased glucose consumption, cold stress, poor enteral intake during the illness, or suboptimal glycogen stores. Since hypoglycemia can have severe consequences, glucose testing is necessary for all premature infants presenting with an acute illness. If the blood sugar is less than 45 mg percent, intravenous glucose (2 mL/kg of D10/W) should be administered.

Hypertension

Longitudinal studies of convalescing premature infants have demonstrated that systemic hypertension may develop in as many as 9 percent. The possible causes include thromboembolic renal artery occlusion following umbilical artery catheterization and bronchopulmonary dysplasia. Although the normal range is age-dependent, a systolic blood pressure greater than 120 mmHg or a diastolic pressure greater than 75 mmHg warrants consideration of systemic hypertension.

Fractures

Because of decreased bone mineralization (osteopenia) related to prematurity, fractures of the long bones and ribs are not uncommon in premature infants during their initial hospitalization. Usually by the time of hospital discharge, bone mineralization has improved to such an extent that new fractures are uncommon, but there may be evidence of healing fractures on x-ray examination. This should be kept in mind if fractures are incidentally noted on an x-ray because of the confusion this may create with child abuse. Comparison of current x-rays with previous films may help to clarify the issue.

Failure to Thrive

The establishment of consistent weight gain with oral feedings is a standard criterion for discharge from the hospital for most premature infants. However, this does not ensure that the pattern of weight gain will continue following discharge. Failure to thrive may occur either because of an ongoing chronic disease (i.e., bronchopulmonary dysplasia, malabsorption, or central nervous system disease) or because of dysfunctional parenting. NICU graduates should be consuming approximately 150 mL/kg per day of a standard formula if not breast feeding and should be consistently gaining approximately 20 g/day. A comparison of the current weight with the discharge weight (which parents usually remember) allows for a quick evaluation of this problem. Any infant with failure to thrive requires a thorough diagnostic evaluation and often hospitalization for accurate documentation of caloric intake.

Immunizations

The recommendation by the American Academy of Pediatrics is to immunize premature infants on the same schedule as normal full-term infants. However, because of a prolonged hospitalization and complicated follow-up, it is possible immunizations might be missed. Inquiry about the immunization status may uncover such a situation. Although it may not be desirable to immunize an infant during an acute illness, appropriate recommendations for follow-up should be made.

ACUTE RESPIRATORY DETERIORATION IN INFANTS WITH BRONCHOPULMONARY DYSPLASIA

Many infants are discharged from the NICU with ongoing pulmonary disease, most commonly bronchopulmonary dysplasia (BPD). BPD is usually a sequela of prematurity, hyaline membrane disease, and mechanical ventilation, although it may be associated with other conditions. Features of BPD include tachypnea, hypercarbia, suboptimal oxygenation, and sometimes reactive airway disease. In some cases, pulmonary hypertension, pulmonary edema, and cor pulmonale are prominent. The cornerstones of therapy for bronchopulmonary dysplasia are oxygen and nutrition. Chronic diuretic or bronchodilator therapy have a role in selected patients although their value remains poorly defined.

Acute deterioration in patients with BPD is usually manifested by an increase in respiratory rate, an increase in respiratory effort, a decrease in oxygenation, and poor feeding. The most common causes of an acute respiratory deterioration in infants with BPD are listed in Table 64-1. A careful history can usually delineate the likely etiology. For example, infants with infectious causes usually have a history of an upper respiratory infection for a few days preceding the development of respiratory distress and may have fever. Sudden respiratory dete-

Table 64-1. Causes of Acute Respiratory Deterioration in Infants with Bronchopulmonary Dysplasia

Respiratory infection
Aspiration
Gastroesophageal reflux
Incoordinate suck/swallow
Bronchospasm
Pulmonary edema
Dehydration
Gastroenteritis
Diuretic therapy
Anemia
Cor pulmonale

Table 64-2. Most Common Causes of Apnea and Bradycardia at Home in NICU Graduates

Respiratory infection
Respiratory Syncytial Virus or Pertussis
Gastroesophageal reflux and aspiration
Aspiration with feedings
Anemia
Hypoglycemia
Seizures
Cardiac arrhythmias
Posthemorrhagic hydrocephalus

rioration is usually due to aspiration, either from gastroesophageal reflux or to a poorly coordinated suck/swallow reflex. Exposure to cigarette smoke or some other environmental pollutant may precipitate acute bronchospasm. An increase in pulmonary edema is usually accompanied by the development of peripheral edema and excessive weight gain.

Dehydration is an important cause of acute respiratory deterioration since many infants possess an altered myocardial compliance (Starling curve shifted to the right) making cardiac output more dependent on end-diastolic filling. Therefore, if an infant becomes dehydrated secondary to either vomiting and diarrhea or to aggressive diuretic therapy, cardiac output will decrease and secondary respiratory deterioration will follow. When evaluating and treating an infant with BPD with respiratory distress, there is often a temptation to use diuretics. However, one must be sure the infant is not already hypovolemic since in that case diuretics make the infant worse.

Anemia may also exacerbate respiratory distress in an infant with BPD and is suggested by the presence of pallor on examination. Acute cor pulmonale can develop secondary to hypoxemia from any of the above mentioned causes, and deterioration can be very rapid. The only effective way to treat acute cor pulmonale in infants with BPD is to treat hypoxemia and its underlying cause.

The usual evaluation of an infant with acute respiratory deterioration includes a complete blood count, arterial blood gas determination, and a chest x-ray. However, the chest x-ray can be difficult to interpret because of the presence of chronic abnormalities. Therefore, it is essential to compare the current x-ray with previous films to identify acute changes. Therapy should be directed toward the specific cause of deterioration, but oxygenation is the cornerstone of treatment. Although BPD infants often have chronic CO_2 retention, there is no evidence that respiratory drive is decreased with oxygen administration. Therefore, oxygen should be used liberally while definitive diagnosis and treatment are debated.

APNEA AND HOME APNEA MONITORS

Most infants resolve the apnea of prematurity before discharge and do not require apnea monitoring at home. However, home monitoring is sometimes utilized for premature infants with severe apnea or if apnea persists beyond 38 weeks' postconceptional age. Infants may be brought to the emergency department because of an actual apneic episode or because the parents were not sure of the significance of an alarm. Studies have demonstrated that the majority of alarms at home are not associated with a change in cardiorespiratory status and probably represent monitor dysfunction, such as loose leads. However, caution must be exercised before attributing an alarm to a mechanical problem with the monitor.

All episodes associated with cyanosis or bradycardia; directly observed episodes of apnea; and any episode requiring intervention, such as stimulation or mouth-to-mouth resuscitation, should be thoroughly evaluated and require admission. A recurrence of apnea in a premature infant who was discharged home apnea-free warrants admission and a thorough search for the cause. The differential diagnosis (Table 64-2) includes respiratory infection (especially respiratory syncytial virus or pertussis), gastroesophageal reflux and aspiration, aspiration with feedings, anemia, and metabolic problems such as hypoglycemia. Other more unusual causes include seizures, cardiac arrhythmias, and posthemorrhagic hydrocephalus. Therapy is directed to the specific cause.

POSTHEMORRHAGIC HYDROCEPHALUS

Premature infants who have had an intraventricular hemorrhage may develop posthemorrhagic hydrocephalus in the newborn period. This can progress during the initial hospitalization, in which case the infant will usually be discharged with a ventriculoperitoneal (VP) shunt in place, or the hydrocephalus may develop gradually following discharge. Such infants can present to the emergency department because of progressive hydrocephalus, if unshunted, or shunt obstruction or infection. Infants presenting with infection usually have nonspecific signs such as poor feeding, lethargy, irritability, fever, and vomiting similar to those of any other child presenting with central nervous system infection. Infants with obstructed shunts most often present with a tense fontanelle and a history of vomiting although the infant usually does not appear particularly ill. A comparison of the current head circumference with the head circumference at discharge (if available) is helpful in evaluating for progressive hydrocephalus. Cranial ultrasound can also rapidly determine the size of the ventricles if the anterior fontanelle remains open. Shunt infections usually require removal of the foreign body, although successful treatment without removal has been reported for *Staphylococcus epidermidis* infections. For both shunt infections and hydrocephalus neurosurgical consultation is required.

THE EXPECTED HOME DEATH

Some infants are discharged from the NICU with lethal conditions for which further medical intervention is futile, and the parents are expecting the child to die at home. In many cases the parents are instructed to take the infant to the emergency department to be pronounced dead by a physician. The parents should be given a letter at the time of the original hospital discharge by their physicians delineating the infant's problems to provide guidance to the emergency physician facing such a situation.

This is a very traumatic time for the parents, and a futile resuscitation effort is not indicated and can prolong the parents' agony. However, it is very important to try to request autopsy permission to completely delineate the infant's problems and to provide optimal counseling for future pregnancies.

BIBLIOGRAPHY

Abman SH, Bradley AW, Lum GM: Systemic hypertension in infants with bronchopulmonary dysplasia. *J Ped* 104:928, 1984.

Anas N, Boettrich C, Hall CB, Brooks JG: Clinical and laboratory observations:

The association of apnea and respiratory syncytial virus infection in infants. *J Ped* 101:65, 1982.
Ballard RA: *Pediatric Care of the ICN Graduate*. Philadelphia, Saunders, 1988.
Berger LR, Schaefer AR: The premature infant goes home. *Am J Dis Child* 139:200, 1985
Consensus Statement: National Institutes of Health Consensus Development Conference on Infantile Apnea and Home Monitoring, Sept 29 to Oct 1, 1986. *Pediatrics* 79:292, 1987.
Groothuis JR, Gutierrez KM, Lauer BA: Respiratory syncytial virus infection in children with bronchopulmonary dysplasia. *Pediatrics* 82:199, 1988.
Klaus MH, Fanaroff AA: *Care of the High-Risk Neonate*, 3d ed. Philadelphia, Saunders, 1986.
Martin RJ, Miller MJ, Waldemar AC: Pathogenesis of apnea in preterm infants. *J Pediatr* 109:733, 1986.
Mutch L, Newdick M, Lodwick A, Chalmers L: Secular changes in rehospitalization of very low birth weight infants. *Pediatrics* 78:164, 1986.
Sauve RS, Singhal, N: Long-term morbidity of infants with bronchopulmonary dysplasia. *Pediatrics* 76:725, 1985.
Sheftel DN, Husted V, Friedman A: Hypertension screening in the follow-up of premature infants. *Pediatrics* 71:763, 1983.

65
SUDDEN INFANT DEATH SYNDROME

Carol D. Berkowitz

SUDDEN INFANT DEATH SYNDROME

Sudden death may affect persons of any age, but it is especially devastating when it affects previously healthy individuals. Nearly 10,000 infants (2 per 1000 live births) succumb yearly to sudden infant death syndrome (SIDS), also known as "crib death."

The term SIDS was officially designated in 1963 to describe a syndrome of unexpected death in infants under 1 year of age for which no pathologic cause could be determined by a thorough postmortem examination. The syndrome is the leading cause of death of infants between 1 month and 1 year.

An understanding of SIDS is essential for the emergency physician so that he or she can recognize the syndrome, initiate resuscitation, manage the infant who has experienced an apparent life threatening event (ALTE or "near miss" SIDS), and counsel the family of the victim.

PATHOPHYSIOLOGY

Over 70 different theories for SIDS have been proposed, including suffocation from sleeping with the parent, milk allergy, and thymic enlargement (status thymicolymphaticus). The main disturbance appears to be with the infant's ventilatory response, and SIDS and infantile apnea appear related, although the exact nature of this relation is uncertain. Death is due to respiratory rather than cardiac arrest, and some potential SIDS victims may be successfully resuscitated with ventilation alone. Arrhythmias probably occur only as a terminal event, and syndromes such as prolonged QT interval or Wolff-Parkinson-White syndrome are very rare associations. Prospective studies monitoring normal infants showed no antecedent arrhythmias in infants who eventually succumbed to SIDS. Conversely, approximately 2 percent of premature and low-birth-weight infants experienced bradycardia (<50 beats per minute) without apnea 1 week after discharge.

Information implicating ventilation and hypoxemia has been obtained from two sources: autopsies of infants who succumbed to SIDS, and studies of those who experienced an ALTE but survived. This latter group represents infants who were found limp, cyanotic, pale, and lifeless, without any respiratory effort, but who were successfully resuscitated.

Autopsies of SIDS victims reveal pathologic changes initially felt to be indicative of long-standing hypoxemia. These changes include smooth muscle thickening in small pulmonary arteries, right ventricular hypertrophy, hematopoiesis in the liver, increase in periadrenal brown fat, adrenal medullary hyperplasia, and abnormalities of the carotid body. The only marker now reported with regularity is brain stem gliosis.

SIDS AND APNEA

Four groups of infants who appear at increased risk of SIDS have been identified: (1) term infants who have had a life-threatening episode of apnea, or ALTE; (2) premature infants of low birthweight; (3) siblings of infants who have succumbed to SIDS, and (4) infants of substance-abusing mothers.

Studies of infants with ALTE may reveal (1) hypoventilation (P_{CO_2}>45 torr) and chronic hypoxemia, (2) a depressed ventilatory response to CO_2 breathing, (3) prolonged sleep apnea (>15 s, associated with cyanosis or pallor), (4) bouts of frequent short apnea, (5) increased periodic breathing (characterized by repeated 3-s pauses in breathing followed by normal breathing for less than 20 s with bradycardia), (6) obstructive apnea, (7) mixed obstructive and central apnea.

Recently, Southall described three separate components associated with respiratory abnormalities in infants.

First, there is central apnea, in which immaturity, tumor, lead injury, infection, or congenital malformation leads to primary failure of respiratory center control. In addition, peripheral chemoreceptors act in an abnormal manner, particularly in response to hypercarbia and hypoxia. The dive reflex may contribute to apnea on a central basis. Young monkeys receiving a cold or wet stimulus to the face in the area of the trigeminal nerve stop breathing. This situation may be analogous to the young infant lying in a regurgitated feeding.

Airway obstruction is the second component. Obstructive apnea may occur in response to nasal occlusion, as with an upper respiratory infection, and is noted with tonsillar enlargement, hypotonia of the hypopharynx, or glossoptosis. It is a contributing factor in about 5 percent of ALTE episodes. It is detected by the presence of increased chestwall movement, with bradycardia and decreased P_{O_2} (by surface oximeter). It is a contributing component to SIDS in infants with upper respiratory infection.

The third and most significant component is expiratory apnea. Prolonged expiratory apnea is associated with sudden atelectasis. Ventilation perfusion inequalities, hypoxia, and sudden cyanosis within 5 to 10 s occur. There is a rapid loss of consciousness. These episodes may occur even in the face of nasotracheal intubation. In older children, they may occur with crying, as cyanotic breath-holding spells.

Acute hypoxic episodes are felt to occur in 80 percent of SIDS cases.

EPIDEMIOLOGIC FACTORS

The diagnosis of SIDS is confirmed by autopsy, but there are many clinical and epidemiologic features which characterize the syndrome. Although the overall incidence is 2 per 1000 live births, there is variation among different ethnic groups, with an incidence of 0.51 per 1000 among Asian Americans and 5.93 per 1000 among Native Americans. Victims range in age from 1 month to 1 year, with peaks at 2½ months and at 4 months. The infant frequently has been premature or small for gestational age, and there is a higher incidence of SIDS among infants with residual bronchopulmonary dysplasia. One study reported that 11 percent of premature infants with bronchopulmonary dysplasia subsequently died of SIDS.

The syndrome is rare in the first month of life, probably because the neonate has a better anaerobic capacity for survival, and with a gasp may be able to raise his or her arterial P_{O_2} over 20 torr and continue breathing. Of the infants who are otherwise healthy, 30 to 50 percent have some acute infection, usually of the upper respiratory tract, at the time of the event. Infection with respiratory syncytial virus has been associated with apnea, particularly in premature infants and those with an antecedent history of apnea. Otitis media and gastroenteritis have also been associated with SIDS. Infected infants tend to be older than noninfected infants, and males outnumber females in the infected group by 2:1. The sex ratio is equal in the noninfected group. There is a disproportionate number of babies from the lower socioeconomic group, although this is true for deaths in infancy from all causes. Mothers frequently are under 20 years and unwed, smoke, use drugs, and have made few prenatal and postpartum visits. SIDS is more likely to occur during the winter months and when the infant is asleep.

CLINICAL PICTURE

A number of scenarios may confront the physician in the emergency department. These scenarios mirror the range of problems which may be broadly categorized under the heading "Rule out SIDS."

Some infants are completely well appearing at the time they are examined, and the parents relate a history of cessation of respiration. The physician must then determine if the event represented an episode of apnea, was severe enough to be life-threatening, or represents a different disorder.

The sequence of events prior to the episode may be a clue to the cause. If the infant stiffened or exhibited clonic movements, the cessation of respiration may have been postictal apnea following a seizure. With a seizure, an infant is frequently awake before becoming apneic. Gastroesophageal reflux may lead to apnea and also may occur in the awake infant following a feeding. A history of an upper respiratory infection followed by paraoxysmal cough with an apneic episode would be suggestive of pertussis. Hypoglycemia may also be associated with apnea, with or without a seizure. The differential diagnosis also includes infection (sepsis or meningitis) and cardiomyopathy. Infantile botulism may be the cause in 5 to 10 percent of SIDS victims.

The evaluation of the healthy-appearing infant with a history of apnea is problematic. Occasionally parents may have misinterpreted acrocyanosis, postprandial regurgitation, or color changes with stooling as an episode of apnea. The parents should be carefully questioned about what they did to revive the baby, for example, stimulation or mouth-to-mouth resuscitation. No resuscitative efforts suggest a benign event. Conversely, the need for mouth-to-mouth resuscitation bespeaks a more serious event. The finding of irregular respiration or poor muscle tone on physical examination would assist in the diagnosis of an ALTE.

Some infants who appear in the emergency department have not been fully resuscitated in the field. They should receive the benefit of vigorous cardiopulmonary resuscitation, unless signs of irreversible death (livedo reticularis, blood pH of 6, box-car venous pooling in the fundi) are apparent. Frequently the heart will resume beating after prolonged arrest. The infant heart is a remarkably resistant organ and may be revived after irreversible brain damage.

EVALUATION

In general, all ALTE victims and infants with a history of apnea and/or cyanosis should be admitted to the hospital. The evaluation of these infants is designed to rule out treatable causes of apnea and to determine if, in the absence of these other causes, the infant is at risk for recurrences of SIDS, an event reported in from 20 to 100 percent of infants with an ALTE.

The evaluation of the infant should include a complete history, particularly of the event itself, and take into account the perinatal and epidemiologic factors associated with SIDS. A history of other infant deaths in the family should be obtained because of the familial incidence of SIDS. Initial reports suggested that siblings of SIDS victims are at increased risk (about 10-fold) for subsequent SIDS. More recent studies show at most a twofold increase in the incidence of SIDS among SIDS siblings.

Familial cases of SIDS also raise the possibility of child abuse. Although it is an infrequent cause of SIDS, there are case reports of ALTE and SIDS attributed to child abuse. Some of these children with ALTE have been purposefully asphyxiated, a problem referred to as Munchausen by proxy. Child abuse is the diagnosed cause of death in 2000 cases a year. The presence of bruises, long bone fractures, internal hemorrhages, evidence of physical neglect, or trauma around the nares suggest abuse. A history inconsistent with the usual events surrounding a SIDS death may also raise the suspicion of abuse. An interesting report on death-scene investigations revealed that in 23 of 26 infants studied, circumstantial evidence of accidental death was present. It is beyond the scope of the emergency department physician to conduct such investigations. It is important, however, to be aware of the possible role of accidental or intentional trauma in some SIDS victims.

The physical examination should be complete with special emphasis on the neurologic evaluation and the presence of any injuries. The initial laboratory assessment should include a complete blood cell count; determination of levels of serum electrolytes, blood sugar, calcium, phosphate, and magnesium; and a 12-lead ECG. A septic workup including blood culture, cerebrospinal fluid analysis, urine culture, and chest x-ray is indicated in most cases. In the infant with ALTE, stool should be sent for clostridial culture and botulinum toxin testing. Other studies should be obtained if suggested by the history and physical examination; these include determination of serum and urine levels of amino acids; sleep and awake EEGs; skull x-rays; barium swallow; and CT scan.

Apnea monitoring should be carried out in the hospital. Most hospitals are able to obtain pneumograms which give evidence of abnormalities related to periodic breathing or episodes of apnea. Polysomnography measures the amount of air flowing in at the mouth and nose and can detect obstructive apnea; the test is complicated and is generally done in a sleep laboratory. Certain tertiary care centers are equipped to evaluate responses to CO_2 breathing and diminished FI_{O_2}.

HOME MONITORING

Two major treatment modalities are recommended for infants who have experienced an ALTE or are at risk for SIDS. Xanthine derivatives such as caffeine and theophylline are used frequently in treating apnea of prematurity because of their central excitatory effect. Their use is associated with the normalization of the respiratory pattern in over 80 percent of such children. Their efficacy in the prevention of SIDS is unclear. A pragmatic approach to the use of theophylline would be to limit it to infants with abnormal pneumograms. Reversal of these abnormalities with theophylline would be an indication for its use. Theophylline is given at 6 mg/kg per day, and a serum level of 5 to 15 mg/mL should be maintained.

Home apnea monitoring is the second modality which can be offered. Three groups have been defined in a National Institutes of Health Consensus Statement in 1986 as being candidates for home monitoring. Group 1 consists of term infants with unexplained apnea of infancy, usually manifested by a life-threatening episode and/or abnormal pneumogram. The absence of an abnormal pneumogram does not preclude home monitoring. The second group consists of preterm infants who have continued to manifest apnea beyond term (i.e., after 40 weeks postconception). The third group consists of subsequent siblings of two or more SIDS victims, but not of one SIDS victim. Twins of SIDS victims were reported in the past to have a 20-fold increase in their risk for SIDS. More recent studies suggest their chance is the same as for nontwin siblings. Additional candidates for home monitoring include infants with bronchopulmonary dysplasia, especially if oxygen-dependent, and infants who require tracheostomy for airway support.

Home-monitoring devices usually measure chest-wall movement and heart rate. The detection of bradycardia is particularly important in infants with an obstructive component because chest-wall movement is not diminished with obstructive apnea. Parents must be instructed in equipment maintenance, interpretation of the alarm, and cardiopulmonary resuscitation. Home monitoring does not mean simply supplying a family with a mechanical device. It involves the development of a medical team to support the family, interpret any episodes of apnea, and decide when home monitoring can be discontinued. Technicians who are available 24 h a day to maintain the equipment are also required.

Emergency physicians are frequently consulted about monitor

alarms. Infants are brought to the emergency department because of alarm triggering. The physician must be able to differentiate the false alarm from a true episode. The need for vigorous stimulation or mouth-to-mouth resuscitation again suggests a serious episode. If there is concern about equipment malfunction, technical assistance should be obtained from the monitoring company.

The use of home monitors has increased dramatically in recent years. The estimated cost of monitoring (including initial assessment) is about $3000 per infant, with monthly rental and maintenance costs ranging from $150 to $300. Although parental anxiety is frequently reduced, the reduction in the incidence of subsequent SIDS in monitored infants is questioned. Recent reports have shown a mortality as high as 50 percent in infants on home monitoring. In many cases, technical errors and parental noncompliance contributed to the infant's demise. There were, however, some infants who simply failed to respond to aggressive cardiopulmonary resuscitation.

The decision to discontinue monitoring is usually made by the infant's primary physician. In general, most infants remain on a monitor for 6 to 8 months. Criteria for discontinuing the monitor include 2 to 3 months with no episodes requiring stimulation or resuscitation, 3 months without apnea of 20 s or more, no apnea associated with an upper respiratory infection or immunization, and an improvement in any neurologic problem for which the monitoring was instituted (e.g., apnea associated with seizures.)

THE SIDS VICTIM

The management of the nonresuscitatable SIDS infant and his or her family is equally challenging for the physician. The emergency department physician is confronted by the distraught mother who had fed her infant several hours earlier, went to check the sleeping infant, and found the baby cold, blue, and lifeless. Frequently, valiant though unsuccessful efforts are carried out in the emergency department, or the infant is revived briefly, only to succumb after several hours in the intensive care unit.

The major responsibility of the physician is then to notify, counsel, and educate the family. In most jurisdictions, victims of sudden and unexplained deaths must be referred to the coroner's office, where an autopsy is performed at the coroner's discretion. If the physician believes the infant is a victim of SIDS, the family should be so advised but told that the final confirmation awaits the autopsy report. The emergency physician should assure the family about their lack of responsibility for the infant's death and assuage their feelings of guilt. He or she should then serve as a facilitator maintaining contact with the family to advise them of the autopsy results. The hospital chaplain or social worker may provide additional support, but the physician's empathy is especially supportive to the family. Most communities have organizations for parents of SIDS victims, and information about these organizations can be obtained from the National Foundation for Sudden Infant Death, 101 Broadway, New York, New York 10036. Parents should be referred to these organizations.

BIBLIOGRAPHY

Bass M, Kravath RE, Glass L: Death-scene investigation in sudden infant death. *N Engl J Med* 315:100, 1986.

Church NR, Anas NG, Hall CB, et al: Respiratory syncytial virus-related apnea in infants. *Am J Dis Child* 138:247, 1984.

Goyco PG, Beckerman RC: Sudden infant death syndrome. *Curr Prob Pediatr* XX:299, 1990.

Kelly DH, Shannon DC: Sudden infant death syndrome and near sudden infant death syndrome: A review of the literature, 1964–1982. *Pediatr Clin North Am* 29:1241, 1982.

Merritt TA, Bauer WI, Hasselmeyer EG: Sudden infant death syndrome: The role of the emergency room physician. *Clin Pediatr* 14:1095, 1975.

Oren J, Kelly D, Shannon DC: Identification of a high-risk group for sudden infant death syndrome among infants who were resuscitated for sleep apnea. *Pediatrics* 77:495, 1986.

Peterson DR, Sabotta EE, Dalind JR: Infant mortality among subsequent siblings of infants who died of sudden infant death syndrome. *J Pediatr* 108:911, 1986.

Rosen CL, Frost JD Jr, Glaze DG: Child abuse and recurrent infant apnea. *J Pediatr* 109:1065, 1986.

Shannon DC, Kelly DH: SIDS and near-SIDS. *N Engl J Med* 306:959, 1022, 1982.

Southall DP: Role of apnea in the sudden infant death syndrome: A personal view. *Pediatrics* 80:73, 1988.

66
HEART DISEASE

James H. McCrory

The incidence of congenital heart disease is only 8 per 1000 live births. The incidence of acquired pediatric heart disease is also relatively rare. This low incidence rate contrasts sharply with the prevalence of cardiovascular disease in the adult population.

Congenital heart disease is usually classified on the basis of presence or absence of cyanosis or according to the nature of the anatomic defect (shunt, obstruction, transposition, or complex). The common acquired conditions include complications secondary to rheumatic fever and to severe chronic anemias, as well as myocarditis, pericarditis, endocarditis, and supraventricular tachycardia.

Because of the low incidence and the age-related differences in presentation, recognition of heart disease in infants and children remains a challenge for the primary care physician. This chapter is written with a view toward pediatric heart disease as it presents in the emergency department or outpatient setting, as opposed to the nursery or inpatient setting. Emphasis is placed on the recognition of pediatric heart disease, the evaluation of life-threatening physiologic instability if present, the planning of emergent interventions, and the timing of referral to a pediatric cardiologist.

INITIAL EVALUATION

There are eight common clinical presentations of pediatric heart disease: cyanosis, pathological murmur in an asymptomatic patient, abnormal pulses, hypertension, syncope, congestive heart failure, cardiogenic shock, and tachyarrhythmias. Table 66-1 lists the most common lesions in each category.

All eight of these presentations are discoverable by a routine history and physical examination. Pertinent points of focus in the history include growth, cyanosis, syncope, feeding difficulty, tachypnea, and sweating on feeding. The physical examination includes determination of vital signs, inspection of skin color and perfusion, palpation of pulses and liver, and auscultation of the heart and breath sounds.

Chest x-ray, arterial blood gases, and electrocardiogram can next be helpful in establishing the working diagnosis in the primary setting, but definitive diagnosis often requires referral to a pediatric cardiologist for echocardiography, catheterization, and other procedures.

Table 66-1. Clinical Presentation of Pediatric Heart Disease

Cyanosis	TGA, TOF, TA, TAt, TAVR
Murmur, asymptomatic patient	Shunts: VSD, PDA, ASD
	Obstructions
	Valvular incompetence
Abnormal pulses	
Bounding	PDA, AI, AVM
Decreased	Coarctation, HPLV
Hypertension	Coarctation
Syncope	
Cyanotic	TOF
Acyanotic	Critical AS
Congestive heart failure	See Table 61-3
Cardiogenic shock	HPLV, coarctation, myocarditis
Tachyarrhythmias	ST, SVT

Abbreviations: AI = aortic insufficiency, AS = aortic stenosis, ASD = atrial septal defect, AVM = arteriovenous malformation, HPLV = hypoplastic left ventricle, SVT = supraventricular tachycardia, PDA = patent ductus arteriosus, ST = sinus tachycardia, TA = truncus arteriosus, TAt = tricuspid atresia, TAVR = total anomalous venous return, TGA = transposition of the great arteries, TOF = tetralogy of Fallot, VSD = ventricular septal defect.

Cyanosis

Cyanosis is a classical presenting sign of congenital heart disease. It is produced by right-to-left intracardiac shunting. Cyanosis is noticeable when the amount of desaturated hemoglobin is 5 g or greater. It can sometimes be quite difficult to detect clinically, especially in dark-skinned infants in a resting state. It may become apparent only when the infant is active or crying. Chronic cyanosis can produce polycythemia, digital clubbing, squatting, and hypercyanotic fainting spells.

When suspected, the presence of cyanosis should be confirmed by measurement of arterial blood gases on room air. If present ($P_{O_2} <$ 55), a second blood gas is performed on an increased FI_{O_2} (0.80 to 1.00). Failure of improvement of P_{O_2} and arterial saturation on an increased FI_{O_2} points to intracardiac shunting, as opposed to pulmonary disease.

Table 66-1 lists the most common lesions which produce cyanosis. Since these problems usually present in the first few days of life in the newborn nursery, the reader is referred to standard pediatric textbooks for further details.

Tetralogy of Fallot, however, deserves special consideration in this chapter for three reasons: it is a common lesion, it often escapes detection in the nursery, and it can present in the emergency department with life-threatening hypercyanotic spells (see "Syncope" below).

Murmurs

Murmurs are extra heart sounds produced by turbulent blood flow and are detected by routine auscultation of the heart. Murmurs are common in infants and children and are usually innocent, that is, not associated with heart disease. Pathological murmurs are produced by shunts, obstructions, or valvular incompetence. The left-to-right shunts [ventricular septal defect (VSD), atrial septal defect (ASD), and patent ductus arteriosus (PDA)] often fall into this category. VSD and PDA can also present in congestive heart failure (see below). The murmurs associated with ASD are not produced directly by the shunt. Rather, they are produced by a relative pulmonary stenosis and/or tricuspid stenosis due to the increased right-sided blood flow.

A complete discussion of murmurs is beyond the scope of this chapter. In general, further evaluation is indicated in all murmurs which produce a thrill or are holosystolic or diastolic. The initial approach consists of a chest x-ray and an electrocardiogram. Since murmurs are usually discovered in physiologically stable patients with no other cardiac signs or symptoms, referral to a pediatric cardiologist can be made electively rather than emergently.

Abnormal Pulses

Peripheral pulses should be palpated in both the upper and lower extremities. Vascular lesions which produce bounding pulses include PDA, aortic insufficiency, and arteriovenous malformations.

Temperature instability and shock are the most common causes of diminished peripheral pulses in infants and children. A hypoplastic left ventricle may present with diminished pulses in all four extremities. Usually, this occurs in the first week of life and is accompanied by cyanosis, congestive heart failure, or cardiogenic shock. Coarctation of the aorta produces diminished pulses in the lower extremities after closure of the patent ductus. Patency of the ductus is usually maintained until the second week of life in this lesion. Until closure occurs, right ventricular stroke volume produces pulses below the coarctation.

Hypertension

The normal blood pressure in a term newborn is 60 mmHg. In toddlers and children, the following formula can be helpful in estimating normal blood pressure:

$$\text{Systolic pressure} = 90 + (2 \times \text{age in years})$$

The size of the blood pressure cuff should be sufficient to cover one half to two-thirds of the infant's forearm.

Essential hypertension is rare below 2 years of age; thus etiology should be carefully determined to guide specific therapy. Coarctation of the aorta can be readily diagnosed on initial physical examination. The diagnosis of renal artery stenosis, on the other hand, requires invasive studies, which are deferred until after other renal and metabolic causes have been excluded.

Syncope

Transient loss of consciousness in the pediatric age group is usually due to seizures, breath holding spells, or vagal stimulation. Cardiac syncope is rare, but in many cases portends sudden death from arrhythmias. Cardiac syncope can be cyanotic as a result of tetralogy of Fallot or acyanotic due to critical aortic stenosis. Both require prompt recognition and immediate referral to a pediatric cardiologist.

Tetralogy of Fallot

Ventricular septal defect, pulmonary stenosis, overriding aorta, and right ventricular hypertrophy are the four components of tetralogy of Fallot. The degree of cyanosis from right-to-left shunting is determined by the degree of pulmonary stenosis. If the pulmonary stenosis is severe, the cyanosis is obvious at birth. If the pulmonary stenosis is mild, the right-to-left shunting may be minimal and the patient may be acyanotic.

The other cardinal features on physical examination are the holosystolic VSD murmur in the third intercostal space at the left sternal border and the diamond-shaped, systolic murmur of pulmonary stenosis in the second intercostal space at the left sternal border. The history may reveal exercise intolerance relieved by squatting. The main radiographic findings are a boot-shaped heart with decreased pulmonary vascular markings. A right-sided aortic arch is present in 25 percent of tetralogies. Right ventrical hypertrophy with right axis deviation are the primary ECG abnormalities.

Dynamic obstruction below the pulmonary valve can lead to an acute increase in the right-to-left shunt and produce a hypercyanotic spell or syncope with cyanosis. Prolonged or recurrent syncope due to tetralogy of Fallot can be a life-threatening emergency; therefore, referral after initial stabilization is indicated for further diagnostic evaluation and possible urgent surgical intervention.

The initial medical management of a hypercyanotic spell includes placing the infant in the knee-chest position, maximizing the FI_{O_2} and administering intravenous morphine. The infant should be made comfortable and kept quiet. The knee-chest position can be maintained while the infant is held upright in the parent's arms and the parent is seated. If the infant is aggravated by a face mask after consciousness has returned, the parent can administer oxygen blown by the infant's face at a high flow rate. Direct manipulation of the infant is limited to establishing an IV line for medications. Morphine in the dosage of 0.1 mg/kg can relieve the hyperdynamic spell. If the syncope does not respond to this therapy, the dose of morphine can be repeated before considering usage of propranolol.

Because of the high rates of mortality and CNS morbidity associated with hypercyanotic spells, surgical intervention is indicated. The two options are total repair, which requires heart-lung bypass, or a palliative shunt between the aorta and the pulmonary artery. Since the use of propranolol is considered a contraindication to bypass surgery, initiation of this form of therapy should be done in coordination with the pediatric cardiologist and the cardiovascular surgeon.

Critical Aortic Stenosis

Critical aortic stenosis is a noncyanotic lesion which can be life-threatening and present at any age. In an older child, exercise intolerance with easy fatigability and chest pain can be present in the history. Prominent physical findings are a systolic ejection click and a diamond-shaped murmur which radiates to the neck and can be accompanied by a suprasternal thrill. Left ventricular hypertrophy with strain can be present on ECG and the chest x-ray may show poststenotic dilitation of the aorta, although neither of these signs are consistently present.

Syncope without cyanosis due to critical aortic stenosis can signal an imminent fatal arrhythmia. The patient should be kept strictly at rest, using sedation if necessary. Immediate referral for further diagnosis and possible urgent surgical repair is indicated.

Congestive Heart Failure

The first task confronting the physician in the emergency department is to recognize congestive heart failure and to differentiate it from more common conditions, such as pneumonia or sepsis. The distinction between pneumonia and congestive heart failure in infants requires a high index of clinical suspicion and is difficult. Pneumonia can cause a previously stable cardiac condition to decompensate, so that both problems can present simultaneously. The common symptoms and signs of an infant presenting in congestive heart failure are outlined in Table 66-2.

Auscultation of the heart may be normal or reveal a gallop rhythm. Depending on the etiology of the failure, a murmur characteristic of PDA, VSD, coarctation, or valvular disease secondary to rheumatic fever may be present. Severe anemias can produce systolic flow murmurs. The electrocardiogram may also be normal. The diagnosis is clinical and depends mainly on signs of fluid accumulation in the lungs, liver, and other areas.

Although hepatomegaly appears long before ascites, anasarca, or peripheral edema in right-sided failure in infants, it is usually a late sign. Hepatomegaly exists when the liver is situated more than 2 cm below the right costal margin in the absence of downward displacement of the diaphragm by hyperexpanded lungs. In hepatomegaly, the liver border is rounded rather than sharp.

Tachycardias

Sinus Tachycardia

The normal newborn heart rate ranges from 120 to 160 beats per minute. Heart rates of 180 to 210 are not uncommon in a variety of stress situations under age 5. Serious causes of tachycardia such as hypovolemic shock, acidosis, hypoxia, and hypercapnia must be ruled out before the tachycardia can be attributed to a more benign disorder such as fever, fear, or agitation.

Supraventricular Tachycardia

With the exception of supraventricular tachycardia (SVT), primary arrhythmias are uncommon in the pediatric age group. In infants, SVT presents with a 4- to 24-h history of poor feeding, tachypnea, pallor, and lethargy. In the older child, palpitations and chest pain can be prominent in the symptomatology. Physical examination reveals thready pulses and a tachycardia which can be too rapid to be counted accurately. Depending on the time since onset of SVT, other physical

Table 66-2. Recognition of Congestive Heart Failure in Infants

	Right-sided Failure	**Left-Sided Failure**	**Both**
Cardinal signs	Hepatomegaly	Tachypnea; dyspnea and sweating on feeding	Cardiomegaly, failure to thrive, tachycardia
Unusual signs	Jugular venous distention, peripheral edema	Rales	

signs can vary from congestive heart failure to cardiogenic shock with pending arrest. Low cardiac output is secondary to inadequate ventricular diastolic filling time.

An ECG rhythm strip shows a ventricular rate of 220 to 360, as opposed to a range of 150 to 200 in adults with SVT. The QRS complexes are narrow and regular. P waves are absent or abnormal.

Digoxin remains the standard medical management of SVT in infants in most pediatric referral centers. Its main disadvantage is that it usually requires 4 to 6 h before the rhythm converts to a normal sinus rhythm. In the previously undigitalized patient, the initial intravenous dose is 0.02 mg/kg. Care must be taken in calculation and administration of the proper dosage, since an error can be fatal. Other forms of medical management include verapamil, Tensilon (edrophonium chloride), and Neo-Synephrine (phenylephrine). Intravenous verapamil rapidly converts SVT but is contraindicated under 2 years of age because of a number of deaths reported in infants. As of January 1991, adenosine has emerged as the drug of choice for rapid conversion. Rapid administration of 0.1 mg/kg is given by intravenous push. Conversion occurs within one minute and metabolism of the compound within 4 minutes. The dosage can be repeated if necessary.

Vagal maneuvers to convert SVT can be attempted but are usually not successful until after the first dose of digoxin. The diver's reflex, which is elicited by submersing the face in ice water, usually produces the greatest vagal tone. An alternative to submersion is to place the ice water in a plastic bag which can be lowered briefly on the infant's face.

Cardioversion with 0.25 to 1 W/s per kilogram is indicated in infants and children presenting in profound cardiogenic shock with pending arrest.

BIBLIOGRAPHY

Artman M, Graham TP: Congestive heart failure in infancy: Recognition and management. *Am Heart J* 103:1040, 1982.

Lees MH: Heart failure in the newborn. *J Pediatr* 75:139, 1969.

Rankin AC, Oldroyd KG: Adenosine or adenosine triphosphate for treatment of supraventricular tachycardia? *Am Heart J* 119:316, 1990.

Talner NS: Congestive heart failure in the infant: A functional approach. *Pediatr Clin N Am* 18:1011, 1971.

67
OTITIS AND PHARYNGITIS

David M. Jaffe
Susan Fuchs

OTITIS

Otitis Media

Otitis media, defined as inflammation of the middle ear, is one of the most common diagnoses made by pediatricians. Acute otitis media (AOM) (acute suppurative, purulent, bacterial) is associated with signs and symptoms of inflammation of the middle ear, such as otalgia, otorrhea, fever, or recent onset of irritability. Otitis media with effusion (OME) (secretory, nonsuppurative, serous, mucoid) is a relatively asymptomatic collection of fluid in the middle ear. The duration (not the severity) of OME can be divided into acute (<3 weeks), subacute (3 weeks to 3 months), and chronic (>3 months). The most important distinction between OME and AOM is that the signs and symptoms of acute infection (otalgia, otorrhea, and fever) are lacking in OME, but hearing loss may be present in both conditions.

Infants and young children are at greatest risk for the development of otitis media with the peak incidence occurring between 6 and 13 months. By 3 years, more than two-thirds of children have had at least one episode of AOM and one-third have had three or more episodes. The incidence is higher in males, Native Americans, Alaskan and Canadian Eskimos, and children with cleft palate or other craniofacial anomalies (e.g., Down's syndrome). The incidence is lower in breast-fed infants.

Middle ear effusion may persist for weeks to months after an episode of AOM. Antibiotic therapy generally sterilizes the effusion but does not clear it from the middle ear space. After the first episode of AOM, 70 percent of children still have a middle ear effusion at 2 weeks, 40 percent at 1 month, 20 percent at 2 months, and 10 percent at 3 months.

Etiology

Bacteria are the most common cause of AOM and can be isolated in a pure culture from the middle ear exudate in 60 to 75 percent of cases. These organisms colonize the nasopharynx and enter the middle ear via the eustachian tube. *Streptococcus pneumoniae* and *Haemophilus influenzae* are still the most common agents, accounting for approximately two-thirds of bacterial isolates (*S. pneumoniae* 25 to 50 percent, *H. influenzae*—primarily nontypable strains—15 to 25 percent). *Branhamella catarrhalis* has been replacing *Streptococcus pyogenes* (group A) as the third most common organism in many areas. *Staphylococcus aureus* is found in approximately 2 percent of cultures, and the remaining 5 to 10 percent are mixed. However, in infants 6 weeks or less, gram-negative enteric bacilli and *S. aureus* account for 10 to 20 percent of isolates. Although viruses are rarely recovered from middle ear effusions, recent studies have shown an increased risk of OME following an upper respiratory tract infection due to respiratory syncytial virus, adenovirus, and influenza virus A or B.

Pathophysiology

Abnormal function of the eustachian tube appears to be the dominant factor in the pathogenesis of middle ear disease. Two types of tube dysfunction may result in otitis media: obstruction and abnormal patency. Obstruction can result from persistent collapse of the eustachian tube due to increased tubal compliance, an inadequate active opening mechanism, or both. Infants and younger children are prone to eustachian tube obstruction because the cartilage which supports the eustachian tube is less stiff than in adults. In addition, an upper respiratory tract infection or allergies can obstruct the eustachian tube and decrease its function. The obstructed eustachian tube prevents equilibration of air pressure between the middle ear and the atmosphere and creates conditions favorable to the development of purulent or sterile effusions. The other type of dysfunction is abnormal patency, which may allow reflux of nasopharyngeal secretions.

Clinical Findings

Classic signs and symptoms of AOM include ear pain (otalgia), otorrhea, and fever; however, ear pulling and irritability may be the only clues in an infant. The most important diagnostic tool is the pneumatic otoscopic examination. Before adequate visualization of the external canal and tympanic membrane (TM) can be obtained, cerumen must be removed from the canal by blunt curettage, or by irrigation with warm water. The presence or absence of discharge; and position, color, degree of translucency and mobility of the TM must be assessed. The light reflex is of no diagnostic value. The normal eardrum is translucent and pearly gray but may become reddened with crying. The eardrum should be freely mobile in response to positive and negative pressure by the pneumatoscope; however, retracted TMs have reduced mobility. The TM of AOM is usually opaque, hyperemic, and sometimes bulging, and bony landmarks (long and short process of the malleus) are not easily discernible. However the most significant sign is the loss or decrease in mobility of the TM.

Tympanometry is a noninvasive diagnostic technique which is used to determine the compliance of the TM and the middle ear. A fixed tone at a given intensity is delivered through a probe snugly placed in the external ear canal, as the air pressure in the canal is varied from positive to negative. The tympanogram is a recording of the acoustic compliance of the middle ear, and patterns obtained are useful in distinguishing a normal ear from one with an effusion. Acoustic reflectometry is a technique that in the uncooperative infant or child is easier to perform than tympanometry and provides similar information about the presence of middle ear fluid.

Aspiration of the middle ear is the most definitive method of verifying the presence and type of middle ear effusion and infecting organism; however, its use for this purpose in the emergency department setting is rarely practical. It may be beneficial in (1) children with overwhelming sepsis, (2) immunologically deficient children, (3) neonates, or (4) children with persistent symptoms of AOM after more than 48 to 72 h on antimicrobial therapy, or (5) otitis media with confirmed or potential suppurative complications. Diagnostic tympanocentesis may be performed by inserting an 18-gauge spinal needle or catheter over a needle, attached to a syringe, through the inferior portion of the TM. When therapeutic drainage is required, a myringotomy should be performed. The incision should be made in the lower half of the TM and should be large enough to allow adequate drainage and aeration of the middle ear. Myringotomy may relieve unusually severe otalgia, either at initial examination or at any time during the course of the disease. In addition, it should be performed when a suppurative complication (meningitis, facial paralysis, mastoiditis) is present.

Treatment

Selection of the appropriate antibiotic is based on several factors: (1) knowledge of the likely etiologic agent or recovery of a specific pathogen from middle ear fluid, (2) the efficacy of certain antibiotics against the organism responsible for AOM, (3) antibiotic penetration into middle ear fluid, and (4) a history of drug allergy. Amoxicillin (30 to 40 mg/kg per day tid) [or ampicillin (50 to 100 mg/kg per day qid] for 10 days is still the drug of choice for the treatment of AOM, because of its in vitro and in vivo activity against *S. pneumoniae* and most strains of *H. influenzae*. However, if β-lactamase-producing *H. influenzae* or *B. catarrhalis* are suspected or documented, appropriate antibiotics include trimethoprim-sulfamethoxazole (TMP-SMZ) (Bactrim, Septra) (8 and 40 mg/kg per day, respectively, given bid), erythromycin and sulfisoxazole in combination (Pediazole) (40 and 100 to

120 mg/kg per day, respectively, qid); cefaclor (40 mg/kg per day tid), or amoxicillin/clavulanate potassium (Augmentin) (40 mg/kg per day tid). In children in whom the aforementioned medications have failed, cefuroxime axetil (Ceftin—30 mg/kg per day bid) or cefixime (Suprax—8 mg/kg per day once daily or 4 mg/kg per day bid) can be used, as both are active against β-lactamase producing organisms. In infants 6 weeks of age or less, cefaclor (30 to 40 mg/kg per day bid or tid) is preferred because of the potential presence of gram-negative enteric bacilli or *S. aureus* as pathogens. If the child is allergic to penicillin, erythromycin and sulfisoxazole in combination, or TMP-SMZ are recommended.

In the numerous trials of antibiotics in the treatment of otitis media, adverse reactions requiring the discontinuation of the drug have occurred in less than 5 percent of patients. With ampicillin and amoxicillin, diarrhea is the most common side effect, followed by rash. TMP-SMZ can also cause diarrhea and skin rash (including Stevens-Johnson syndrome), but the major concern is the development of neutropenia and thrombocytopenia. In addition, a patient with glucose 6-phosphate dehydrogenase deficiency should not receive sulfonamides. Erythromycin often causes gastrointestinal symptoms including abdominal cramps, nausea, vomiting, and diarrhea. Cefaclor, besides the possible cross-sensitivity in patients with pencillin allergy, can cause a serum sickness-like reaction consisting of a rash, arthralgia or arthritis, and fever.

Additional therapy including antipyretics and analgesics may be helpful in alleviating some of the acute symptoms. A topical analgesic (Auralgan) instilled into the external ear canal often provides some relief from otalgia, but it should not be used when a TM perforation is present. Decongestants, antihistamines, or corticosteroids have no demonstrable role in the treatment of AOM. With appropriate antimicrobial therapy, most children with AOM are significantly improved within 48 to 72 h. Persistent or recurrent pain or fever or both indicate a need for reexamination of the child and the possible selection of another antimicrobial agent. Reasons for response failure include a resistant organism, noncompliance, and host-related structural or immunologic abnormalities.

Children should be reexamined within 10 to 14 days of the completion of antibiotic therapy. At this time, some children have a persistent (but asymptomatic) middle ear effusion. Two further treatment options exist: (1) ''watchful waiting'' (no treatment) in children who have asymptomatic OME, with reexamination 6 weeks later, or (2) treatment for 10 days with another antimicrobial agent that is effective against possible resistant bacteria; then reexamination.

Recurrent AOM

Many children have repeated episodes of AOM (recurrent AOM). Some develop symptoms and a new ear effusion after a previous effusion has resolved, while others develop symptoms with no documentation of resolution of a previous effusion. If these attacks are frequent and close together, prevention of further episodes is desirable. A more thorough physical examination or laboratory or x-ray studies should be performed to rule out submucous cleft palate, a tumor of the nasopharynx, sinusitis, allergies, and immune deficiencies (C3 and C5 deficiency). If none of these are present, several methods of prevention are available. These include (1) prophylaxis with antibiotics: amoxicillin (20 mg/kg per day qhs), sulfisoxazole (50 mg/kg per day qhs), or (2) myringotomy with tympanostomy tubes.

Complications and Sequelae of Otitis Media

The complications and sequelae of otitis media predominantly involve the middle ear and adjacent structures within the temporal bone, but in rare instances, intracranial complications may occur. The aural or intratemporal complications and sequelae include hearing loss, perforation or retraction pocket of the TM, tympanosclerosis, adhesive otitis media, ossicular discontinuity and fixation, chronic suppurative otitis media, cholesteatoma, mastoiditis, labyrinthitis, and facial paralysis. Suppuration in the middle ear or mastoid, or both, may extend into the intracranial cavity producing the following intracranial complications: meningitis, extradural abscess, subdural empyema, focal encephalitis, brain abscess, and lateral (sigmoid) sinus thrombosis. These complications are uncommon except in neglected cases.

OME

OME is the (relatively asymptomatic) collection of fluid in the middle ear, which often follows an episode of AOM. Hearing loss is by far the most prevalent complication and morbid outcome of OME. The extent of hearing loss is dependent on the volume of the effusion rather than the physical properties of the effusion. Audiometry is of limited value as a diagnostic method for the identification of OME, but it can be helpful in the evaluation of the effect of middle ear disease on hearing. The relation between persistent or episodic conductive hearing loss and impairment in the cognitive linguistic and speech development of children has been reported. However, the degree and duration of the hearing loss required to produce such deficits have not been defined.

Other factors that should be considered in addition to hearing loss when deciding whether to treat OME include (1) occurrence in young infants, as they are unable to communicate their symptoms and may have suppurative disease, (2) an associated acute purulent upper respiratory infection, (3) permanent conductive/sensorineural hearing loss, (4) vertigo, (5) alterations in the tympanic membrane: severe atelectasis and/or a deep retraction pocket in the posterosuperior quadrant or the pars flaccida, (6) middle ear changes such as adhesive otitis or ossicular involvement, (7) persistence of the effusion for more than 3 months (chronic OME), or (8) occurrence of the episodes so close together that the child has OME for 6 out of 12 months. A thorough search for an underlying cause (sinusitis, allergy, submucous cleft, tumor) should be attempted before treatment is begun. If an antimicrobial treatment has not been tried recently, since bacteria that cause OME are similar to those found in AOM, the antibiotics used are the same. Amoxicillin is the drug of choice except in chronic OME, in which cefaclor, erythromycin-sulfisoxazole; trimethoprim-sulfamethoxazole, amoxicillin/clavulanate potassium, or cefuroxime axetil should be used. The other nonsurgical methods available, including oral combinations of decongestants and antihistamine, topical intranasal or systemic corticosteroids, and immunotherapy, have not been shown to be effective in clinical trials. If antibiotic therapy fails, the situation warrants referral to a pediatric otolaryngologist for evaluation for surgical therapy such as myringotomy alone or myringotomy with the insertion of tympanostomy tubes. Myringotomy alone improves the conductive hearing loss, but the effusions may recur. Tympanostomy tube placement improves the conductive hearing loss for longer periods of time than myringotomy alone. Tympanostomy tubes remain in place for a few weeks to several years, with an average of 6 months. Possible complications of myringotomy tubes are scarring (tympanosclerosis), localized atrophy, persistent perforation, and the rare development of a cholesteatoma. For children who have recurrent chronic otitis media with effusion and who have had one or more myringotomy and tympanostomy tube operations in the past, adenoidectomy is a reasonable option. The presence of upper airway obstruction, recurrent acute/chronic adenoiditis or both would be another indication to consider adenoidectomy.

Otitis Externa

External otitis (OE) is any inflammatory condition of the auricle, external ear canal, or outer surface of the tympanic membrane. It can be caused by infection, inflammatory dermatoses, trauma, or combinations of the three.

Etiology and Pathophysiology

The flora of the ear canal are the same as those of normal skin. They include *Staphylococcus epidermidis,* diphtheroids, β-hemolytic streptococcus, *Staphylococcus aureus,* anaerobes, and fungi. Compromise of any of the protective features of the ear canal (shape and cerumen) can lead to OE due to colonization and invasion by pathogenic organisms, especially gram-negative enteric bacteria, pseudomonads, and fungi. Causes include (1) high environmental temperature and humidity, (2) hyperhydration and maceration of epithelial tissue in the canal, (3) absorption of moisture by the stratum corneum, (4) lack of cerumen through blocked gland ducts and/or mechanical removal (scratching); (5) obstruction of gland ducts by edema and keratin debris, (6) invasion by exogenous or endogenous organisms through breaks in the damaged epithelial surface, and (7) trauma.

Clinical Findings

The mildest form of OE is characterized by itching or a sense of fullness in the ear. As it progresses, increasing pain, itching, redness, swelling, tenderness of the canal, and cheesy discharge occur. Inward pressure on the tragus, or pulling the auricle up and back, usually results in discomfort. If the TM can be visualized, it is often red, thick, and covered with the flat vesicles or areas of desquamating epithelium. In some cases, the pain is intense and constant, aggravated by any motion of the jaw or external ear. The regional lymph nodes may be enlarged and tender. When otomycosis is present (either as primary or secondary cause), intense itching is usually more prominent than pain.

Differential Diagnosis

The hardest part of the diagnosis is to distinguish between OE and OM. Ideally, clinical inspection of the TM with a pneumatic otoscope will help establish the diagnosis; however, the TM of a child with OE may be as red and distorted as one with OM, although mobility of the TM is normal or slightly decreased in OE. In addition, visualization of the TM may be difficult because of edema of the canal in OE. Tympanometry can be helpful if the canal is clear and a tight seal for the earpiece can be formed without too much discomfort. Parotitis, periauricular adenitis, mastoiditis, dental pain, and temporomandibular joint dysfunction should be considered when the discomfort is poorly localized and the ear canal and TM appear normal. In addition, pain can be referred from pharyngitis or tonsillitis, but this pain is often made worse by swallowing or eating. Foreign bodies in the ear can also cause OE.

Treatment

Cleansing of the ear canal is the most important part of therapy. For mild infections, dry mopping using a small tuft of cotton attached to a wire applicator is sufficient and may be curative. If the canal is inflamed, edematous, and occluded by debris, cleansing can be done with gentle suctioning, a soft plastic infant feeding tube (with an opening at the tip) attached to a DeLee trap can be used. If there is no perforation of the TM, irrigation with warm hypertonic (3%) saline or 2% acetic acid in Burow's solution (Otic Domeboro) is helpful. Acidified isopropyl alcohol (equal parts vinegar and alcohol) can also be used, followed by drying with suction, compressed air, or a hair dryer. The use of cotton swabs to clean the ears should be strongly discouraged.

Acetic acid ear drops are the easiest and least expensive way to eliminate the infecting agent. A 2% solution is effective and available commercially in aqueous (Otic Domeboro) or propylene glycol (Vosol, Orlex) solutions. These drops should be used 3 to 4 times a day for at least 1 week. However, when OE is accompanied by a TM perforation, burning or stinging will occur with the use of acid or alcohol-containing medication, so an antibiotic preparation containing neomycin, polymyxin B, and hydrocortisone (Cortisporin Otic suspension) is less irritating. Another option is the use of Cortisporin ophthalmic suspension, which is free of both acid and alcohol. Ophthalmic gentamicin or tobramycin are alternative drugs; however, they have ototoxic properties, although hearing loss due to their topical use has not been documented. Otic chloramphenicol should be avoided because of the risk of aplastic anemia. Swimming should be prohibited during the course of treatment. After brief showers (with infrequent hair washing), drops should be instilled into the ear.

The basic treatment of otomycosis is similar to that for acute bacterial OE, with cleansing followed by 2% acetic acid or M-cresyl acetate (25%) preparations. Patients who do not respond can be treated with topical ophthalmic suspensions of miconazole, nystatin, or amphotericin B. Corticosteroids are present in many topical otic preparations, but their value is unproven. Topical benzocaine and lidocaine may be useful to reduce the itching, but they are inadequate for the relief of moderate to severe pain, for which oral analgesics may be required.

Children who fail to respond to treatment within 48 h must be reevaluated. Examination should confirm the presence of a clear, dry, and patent canal, free of foreign bodies, and an intact TM. Evidence of other conditions, including cellulitis, abscess formation, or underlying dermatoses requires specific treatment, depending on the condition.

Patients with progressive, unresponsive, or severe infection may require parenteral (IV) therapy. Cultures of canal secretions should be taken and a combination of an aminoglycoside (gentamicin or tobramycin) and an antipseudomonal penicillin (ticarcillin or piperacillin) started. If the clinical findings and course of the illness suggest an infection due to *S. aureus,* a penicillinase-resistant penicillin (nafcillin) should also be given.

PHARYNGITIS

Pharyngitis, infection of the pharynx and the tonsils, is a very common pediatric problem which accounts for as many as 5 percent of visits to pediatric offices in the United States. It is estimated that $300 million are spent annually in its diagnosis and treatment. Despite physicians' long-standing familiarity with pharyngitis, there remains wide variability in approach. Controversies and new developments pertain to (1) selection of patients for throat culture and antibiotic treatment, and (2) use of new rapid diagnostic tests for group A β-hemolytic streptococcus (GABHS).

Etiology

Many organisms—viral, bacterial, fungal, and even protozoal—have been associated with pharyngitis; however, only a relatively few are of practical significance to the emergency evaluation of pharyngitis in the immune competent child. Common viral isolates include adenovirus, Epstein-Barr virus (see below), influenza virus, parainfluenza virus, and enteroviruses. In one series, viral isolates were obtained from 37 percent of children with nonstreptococcal pharyngitis. *Chlamydia* and *Mycoplasma* have been implicated as common pharyngeal pathogens in adults. While only 3 percent of children and adolescents with pharyngitis as the major manifestation of illness were found to have *Mycoplasma pneumoniae,* pharyngitis was present in 32 percent of children with pneumonia caused by *M. pneumoniae.* A recent study of *Chlamydia trachomatis* in adolescents with and without pharyngitis found a prevalence of only 2 percent among symptomatic adolescents, and 0 percent among those asymptomatic. Among bacterial pathogens, GABHS is clearly the most important, accounting for nearly half of all pharyngeal infections in patients between the ages of 5 and 15 years. GABHS pharyngitis is unusual in children under 3 years of age, and rheumatic fever is vanishingly rare in this age group.

Differential Diagnosis

The few non-GABHS organisms that occasionally require specific diagnosis are *Corynebacterium diphtheriae, Neisseria gonorrhoeae,* and Epstein-Barr virus. Despite the many etiologic possibilities, in school-age children the diagnostic task is most often reduced to distinguishing GABHS, which requires specific antibiotic therapy, from nonstreptococcal pharyngitis.

Diphtheria is a rare but serious cause of pharyngitis in developed countries. Immunization in infancy with an alum-precipitated toxoid combined with pertussis antigen and tetanus antigen (DPT) has been effective in nearly eliminating diphtheria in childhood, but it can occur in crowded conditions in which there are socioeconomic barriers to immunization. Morbidity occurs because of both infectious and toxic reactions. Infectious invasion and spread occurs with enough tissue necrosis to produce a pseudomembrane which can progress to cause airway obstruction. The *C. diphtheriae* bacteria also produce an exotoxin which can cause widespread organ damage, including myocarditis and cardiac arrhythmia, neuritis with both bulbar and peripheral paralysis, nephritis, and hepatitis. Diagnosis must be clinical in order to expedite effective therapy; however, the bacteria can be grown on Loeffler's media. Treatment is directed both at killing the bacteria and neutralizing the exotoxin. Therefore, both antibiotic (penicillin or erythromycin) and horse-serum antitoxin must be given.

Neisseria gonorrhoeae is an important cause for pharyngitis in sexually active adolescents. Gonococcal pharyngitis in younger children strongly suggests child sexual abuse. Gonococcal pharyngitis may be either asymptomatic or cause very mild symptoms with occasional exudative tonsillitis and/or cervical lymphadenopathy. Pharyngeal throat swabs should be plated on Thayer-Martin medium to recover the organism. Rectal and vaginal or urethral cultures as well as serum to test for syphilis should be obtained whenever gonorrhea is suspected or documented. Gonoccocal pharyngitis in children should be treated with ceftriaxone (125 mg IM once). Children who cannot tolerate ceftriaxone may be treated with spectinomycin (40 mg/kg IM once). Children 8 years or older should also receive oral doxycycline (100 mg BID for 7 days). Children $\geq$ 45 kg should be treated with adult regimens. (Ceftriaxone 250 mg IM once or ciprofloxacin 500 mg in a single oral dose with repeat culture in 4 to 7 days.)

Epstein-Barr virus (EBV) is a herpesvirus that is a common cause of infection in childhood and adolescence. While EBV has been associated with a variety of clinical syndromes, most children infected with EBV are asymptomatic or have only mild nonspecific symptoms. EBV can cause isolated tonsillopharyngitis, and pharyngitis as a manifestation of infectious mononucleosis (IM). Clinically, the classic IM syndrome begins with malaise, fatigue, and sore throat. Fever and adenopathy are the most common signs. Splenomegaly and hepatomegaly are also present in the majority of infected children, while skin rash, enanthem, eyelid edema, and jaundice occur much less commonly. Pharyngitis occurs in nearly all children with IM. The appearance of the throat can resemble that of bacterial GABHS disease. Dual infection with EBV and GABHS has also been documented. Classic IM is much less common in children under the age of 2 years, when EBV tends to cause a nonspecific febrile illness. However, recently IM has been reported to occur in toddlers more commonly than was once thought. These younger children most often have a syndrome characterized by fever, tonsillitis, lymphadenopathy, and hepatosplenomegaly.

The laboratory can be helpful in establishing the diagnosis of IM. There is an increase in both the proportion and the absolute number of atypical lymphocytes in the peripheral blood smear (generally $\geq$50 percent lymphocytes and $\geq$10 percent atypical lymphocytes). Liver transaminase levels show moderate elevation (generally SGOT is $<$600 U/dL). The heterophil antibody is present (and can be demonstrated by rapid slide test methods) in over 90 percent of children over the age of 5 with IM, but in only 75 percent between the ages of 2 and 4, and in fewer than 30 percent under the age of 2. While not yet routinely available in most centers, EBV-specific serologic testing can provide information as to the likelihood of acute, post-acute, old quiescent, and reactivation-type infection. These determinations are made on the basis of the presence of specific patterns of IgM and IgG antibodies to viral capsid antigen, and IgG responses to EBV early antigen, and to the Epstein-Barr nuclear antigen.

IM is generally a benign, self-limited, though somewhat prolonged, illness. In general, treatment involves nonspecific supportive modalities (fluids, acetaminophen, and rest). Fatal complications are rare. Mortality can be caused by neurologic complications (meningoencephalitis, Guillain-Barré syndrome), splenic rupture and hemorrhage, and bacterial and fungal sepsis. Children with the X-linked lymphoproliferative syndrome have unusual susceptibility to fulminant EBV infection. Airway obstruction secondary to tonsillar hypertrophy can also occur. This complication responds rapidly to corticosteroid administration (dexamethasone 1 mg/kg to 10 mg maximum; then 0.5 mg/kg every 6 h) and rarely requires insertion of an artificial airway. Airway obstruction is the only complication for which the use of steroids is widely accepted.

Streptococcal Pharyngitis

GABHS pharyngitis is the most common treatable cause of pharyngitis in children. The peak months of infection are January to May, but because of the high frequency of occurrence in school-age children, the beginning of school in the fall is also associated with GABHS pharyngitis in many areas. The peak ages are 4 to 11 years, with GABHS infection being uncommon under the age of 3 years.

Diagnosis

No set of symptoms or signs is completely specific for GABHS. Nonetheless, there are findings which are typically, but not exclusively, associated with GABHS. Generally, the infected child experiences sudden onset of sore throat and fever. The tonsils and pharynx appear markedly red and have a moderate to large amount of exudate. The soft palate and uvula are also red and may have petechiae. The anterior cervical lymph nodes are enlarged and tender. The presence of a scarlatiniform rash and pharyngitis is virtually diagnostic of GABHS. Headache, vomiting, abdominal pain, meningismus, and torticollis can occur as well. These are of little diagnostic importance but must be recognized as possibly attributable to GABHS. The presence of significant coughing and/or rhinorrhea suggests an alternative diagnosis. Diagnostic accuracy on the basis of clinical findings alone is reported at about 50 to 75 percent for children thought to have GABHS and 75 to 85 percent for children thought not to have GABHS. There is general agreement that clinical diagnosis alone would result in an unacceptably high rate of misdiagnosis.

The mainstay of laboratory diagnosis is still the throat culture, although rapid antigen-detection techniques are gaining popularity in pediatric offices and emergency departments. The tonsil or posterior pharyngeal wall should be swabbed vigorously. In many centers, the swab is sent to the laboratory in appropriate culture medium for further handling. The sample is plated on a blood agar culture medium with neomycin and nalidixic acid added. Colonies which show β-hemolysis are identified as group A by bacitracin disk tests, fluorescent antibody staining, or latex agglutination. The rate of false-negative results from single throat culture is about 10 percent. Recovery rates are maximized by good swabbing technique, multiple cultures (rarely actually performed), and incubation in a carbon dioxide-enriched environment. Positive cultures may indicate either an acute GABHS infection or the carrier state. Rates of GABHS carriage vary with season but have been reported as high as 15 percent. There is imperfect correlation between the amount of growth (generally reported on a scale of 1+ to 4+) and the likelihood of true infection. Chronic carriers of GABHS are not at increased risk for developing true GABHS pharyngitis or suppurative and nonsuppurative (rheumatic fever and nephritis) sequelae, nor do they pose an increased risk for disease transmission.

Incubation of throat cultures takes 24 to 48 h, during which time management must occur with uncertainty as to the diagnosis. Recently, antigen-detection procedures have become available for commercial use. The tests involve extraction of group A carbohydrate antigen from a throat swab and then combining the antigen with a latex agglutination, coagglutination, or enzyme-linked immunosorbent assay. The tests take 10 to 30 min to perform and are generally more expensive per test than direct plate culturing. Sensitivity under controlled laboratory conditions using the culture as the "gold standard" ranges from 85 to 90 percent, and specificity ranges from 98 to 100 percent. Unfortunately, when measured in the field under less well-controlled circumstances, sensitivity has been as low as 50 percent. In other words, the false-positive rate is low, but the false-negative rate may be unacceptably high. Any emergency department or office planning to use a rapid diagnostic test must assess the performance of the test on site. A safe and commonly used approach is to obtain swabs for both throat culture and rapid test simultaneously. Children with positive rapid tests are treated for GABHS. If the test is negative, the throat culture is processed and the children are managed according to an acceptable strategy while awaiting throat culture results.

Management

The objectives of treatment for GABHS are (1) to prevent rheumatic fever, (2) to prevent suppurative complications (peritonsillar abscess and cellulitis, suppurative cervical lymphadenitis, and retropharyngeal abscess), and (3) to hasten clinical recovery. GABHS is highly sensitive to penicillin, and there has been no evidence of development of resistance despite decades of use. A single dose of intramuscular penicillin G benzathine—600,000 units if the patient is ≤27 kg (60 lb) and 1.2 million units if >27 kg—is effective but causes significant local discomfort in over 50 percent of recipients. A preparation containing 900,000 units of penicillin G benzathine and 300,000 units of penicillin G procaine (CR Bicillin 900/300, introduced in 1976) is effective for children at all ages and significantly reduces the magnitude and frequency of local reactions. Oral penicillin V is a popular alternative. A regimen of 250 mg three times daily for 10 days effectively eradicates infection and prevents rheumatic fever. Variable levels of compliance have been reported. Improvements in compliance can be achieved with careful parent education at the time of discharge. If compliance or follow-up are problematic, the intramuscular route should be used. Alternatives to penicillin for children with penicillin allergy include erythromycin, first-generation cephalosporins, and clindamycin.

The overall incidence of rheumatic fever has been declining in the developed countries and is now approximately 0.6 per 100,000 in the continental United States, although it has recently been reported to be much higher in Hawaii. A number of scattered outbreaks of acute rheumatic fever have been reported in the United States during the latter part of the 1980s. There is ample justification for adherence to the American Heart Association's recommendations that one of the above antibiotic regimens for documented GABHS pharyngitis must be provided. Antibiotic treatment begun within 9 days of the onset of infection is effective in preventing rheumatic fever.

Poststreptococcal glomerulonephritis is a nonsuppurative complication of GABHS disease that is not preventable with antibiotic therapy. Its occurrence is related to infection with nephritogenic strains of streptococci.

Recent research has also clearly demonstrated the beneficial effects of early antibiotic therapy on reduction of signs and symptoms of GABHS pharyngitis. In addition, because it is recommended that children with GABHS receive antibiotics for 24 h prior to returning to school or day care, early treatment benefits both the children and their parents, especially parents who work outside the home. Based on these considerations, many strategies for testing and treatment have been proposed ranging from treating all children with pharyngitis with antibiotics to withholding antibiotics from all pending culture results. Cost-effectiveness studies employing decision-analysis methods have been performed to compare some of these strategies. The best strategy for a given institution depends on the local prevalence of GABHS, the availability and accuracy of rapid antigen testing, and the ability to follow up successfully on untreated children found to have positive cultures. A widely accepted strategy that incorporates the latest technology is to perform rapid antigen testing on all children with pharyngitis and to treat all positives. In addition, children with classic clinical findings or a scarlatiniform rash should be treated regardless of the result of rapid testing. Those with a negative rapid test and equivocal or atypical clinical features for GABHS should have a throat culture sent, but treatment may be withheld pending culture results. Positive culture results indicate the need for treatment. It is not necessary to reculture to test for eradication of GABHS in asymptomatic children. Children with recurrent or persistent symptoms and those with previously documented rheumatic fever do require reculturing. Children with persistent positive cultures in this context can be treated with a different antibiotic. Although the asymptomatic carrier state need not be treated, a combination of penicillin and rifampin has been shown to be effective in eradicating GABHS in carriers.

Indications for tonsillectomy remain uncertain and controversial. Paradise and his colleagues have shown that for children with many recurrent episodes of pharyngitis (seven or more episodes in 1 year, five or more annually for 2 years, or three or more annually for 3 years) tonsillectomy reduces the incidence of pharyngitis for the subsequent 2 years compared with nonsurgical management. However, 5 of 6 children in the nonsurgical groups experience significant improvement as well. Decision as to tonsillectomy for such children should be individualized to account for various considerations of risks, benefits, and quality of life, including the quality of available anesthetic and surgical services, impact of recurrent illness vs. surgery on the child and parents, school performance, and comparative costs to the family.

Symptomatic therapy for both GABHS and nonstreptococcal pharyngitis includes acetaminophen for analgesia. A throat spray (e.g., Chloraseptic) can be used before meals and bedtime if further analgesia is required. Lozenges should be avoided in children under 5 years because of the possibility of aspiration. Recent outbreaks of pharyngitis caused by group G streptococci have been reported. Although the acute clinical syndromes associated with these organisms are identical to that of GABHS pharyngitis, they are not known to cause preventable non-suppurative sequelae. Nonetheless, by analogy to GABHS, treatment of children with pharyngitis caused by group G streptococci with the same penicillin regimens as in GABHS is recommended to hasten clinical recovery. Indications for treatment of group C-associated pharyngitis have not been established.

BIBLIOGRAPHY

Otitis

Bluestone CD: Otitis media in children: To treat or not to treat. *N Engl J Med* 306:1399, 1982.

Bluestone CD: Modern management of otitis media. *Pediatr Clin North Am* 36:1371, 1989.

Bluestone CD, Klein JO: Epidemiology, in Bluestone CD, Klein JO: *Otitis Media in Infants and Children*. Philadelphia: Saunders, 1988, pp. 31–43.

Bluestone CD, Klein JO, Paradise JL, et al: Workshop on effects of otitis media on the child. *Pediatrics* 71:639, 1983.

Marcy SM: Infections of the external ear. *Pediatr Infect Dis* 4:192, 1985.

McCracken GH: Management of acute otitis media with effusion. *Pediatr Infect Dis* 7:442, 1988.

Nelson JD: Changing trends in the microbiology and management of acute otitis media and sinusitis. *Pediatr Infect Dis* 5:749, 1986.

Paradise JL: Otitis media in infants and children. *Pediatrics* 65:917, 1980.
Paradise JL, Bluestone CD, Rogers KD, et al: Efficacy of adenoidectomy for recurrent otitis media in children previously treated with tympanostomy-tube placement. Results of parallel randomized and nonrandomized trials. *JAMA* 263:2066, 1990.

Pharyngitis

1989 STD Treatment Guidelines. *MMWR* 38(suppl):58, 1989.
Bass JW: Treatment of streptococcal pharyngitis revisited. *JAMA* 256:740, 1986.
Bisno AL: Acute rheumatic fever: Forgotten but not gone. *N Engl J Med* 316:476, 1987.
Bisno AL: The diagnosis of streptococcal pharyngitis. *Ann Intern Med* 90:426, 1979.
Breese BB: A simple scorecard for the tentative diagnosis of streptococcal pharyngitis. *Am J Dis Child* 131:514, 1977.
Breese BB, Denny FW, Dillon HC, et al: Consensus: Difficult management problems in children with streptococcal pharyngitis. *Pediatr Infect Dis* 4:10, 1985.
Brien JH, Bass JW: Streptococcal pharyngitis: Optimal site for throat culture. *Clin Lab Observ* 106:781, 1985.
Broughton RA: Infections due to *Mycoplasma pneumoniae* in childhood. *Pediatr Infect Dis* 5:71, 1986.
Brunell PA: Non-streptococcal pharyngitis. *Pediatr Infect Dis* 4:S44, 1985.
Colcher IS, Bass JW: Penicillin treatment of streptococcal pharyntitis. *JAMA* 222:657, 1972.
Denny FW: Effect of treatment on streptococcal pharyngitis: Is the issue really settled? *Pediatr Infect Dis* 4:352, 1985.
DuBois D, Ray VG, Nelson B, et al: Rapid diagnosis of group A strep pharyngitis in the emergency department. *Ann Emerg Med* 15:157, 1986.
Fleisher G, Lennette ET, Henle G, et al: Incidence of heterophil antibody responses in children with infectious mononucleosis. *J Pediatr* 94:723, 1979.
Gerber MA: Critical appraisal of the clinical relevance of rapid diagnosis in pediatrics. *Diagn Microbiol Infect Dis* 3:39S, 1985.
Gerber MA: Culturing of throat swabs: End of an era? *J Pediatr* 107:85, 1985.
Gerber MA, Markowitz M: Management of streptococcal pharyngitis reconsidered. *Pediatr Infect Dis* 4:518, 1985.
Gerber MA, Randolph MF, Chanatry J, et al: Antigen detection test for streptococcal pharyngitis: Evaluation of sensitivity with respect to true infections. *J Pediatr* 5:654, 1986.
Gerber MA, Randolph MF, Martin NF, et al: Community wide outbreak of group G streptococcal pharyngitis. *Pediatrics* 87:598, 1991.
Gerber MA, Spadaccini LJ, Wright LL, et al: Twice-daily penicillin in the treatment of streptococcal pharyngitis. *Am J Dis Child* 139:1145, 1985.
Grose C: The many faces of infectious mononucleosis: The spectrum of Epstein-Barr virus infection in children. *Pediatr Rev* 7:35, 1985.
Haggerty RJ: Sore throats and tonsillectomy. *N Engl J Med* 298:453, 1978.
Howie JGR, Foggo BA: Antibiotics, sore throats and rheumatic fever. *J R Coll Gen Pract* 35:223, 1985.
Huss H, Jungkind D, Amadio P, et al: Frequency of *Chlamydia trachomatis* as the cause of pharyngitis. *J Clin Microbiol* 22:858, 1985.
Kaplan EL: The group A streptococcal upper respiratory tract carrier state: An enigma. *J Pediatr* 97:337, 1980.
Kaplan EL: Benzathine penicillin G for treatment of group A streptococcal pharyngitis: A reappraisal in 1985. *Pediatr Infect Dis* 4:592, 1985.
Kaplan EL, Top FH Jr, Dudding BA, et al: Diagnosis of streptococcal pharyngitis: Differentiation of active infection from the carrier state in the symptomatic child. J Infect Dis 123:490, 1971.
Levin RM, Grossman M, Jordan C, et al: Group A streptococcal infection in children younger than three years of age. *Pediatr Infect Dis* 7:581, 1988.
Lieu TA, Fleisher GR, Schwartz JS: Clinical performance and effect on treatment rates of latex agglutination testing for streptococcal pharyngitis in an emergency department. *Pediatr Infect Dis* 5:655, 1986.
Meier FA, Centor RM, Graham L, et al: Clinical and microbiological evidence for endemic pharyngitis among adults due to group C streptococci. *Ann Int Med* 150:825, 1990.
Neinstein LS, Inderlied C: Low prevalence of *Chlamydia trachomatis* in the oropharynx of adolescents. *Pediatr Infect Dis* 5:660, 1986.
Paradise JL, Bluestone CD, Bachman RZ: Efficacy of tonsillectomy for recurrent throat infection in severely affected children. *N Engl J Med* 310:674, 1984.
Poses RM, Cebul RD, Collins M, et al: The accuracy of experienced physicians' probability estimates for patients with sore throats. *JAMA* 254:925, 1985.
Randolph MF, Gerber MA, DeMeo KK, et al: Effect of antibiotic therapy on the clinical course of streptococcal pharyngitis. *J Pediatr* 106:870, 1985.
Schwartz RH, Hayden GF, Wientzen R: Children less than three-years-old with pharyngitis. *Clin Pediatr* 25:185, 1986.
Shulman ST: The decline of rheumatic fever. *Am J Dis Child* 138:426, 1984.
Sumaya CV: Epstein-Barr virus serologic testing: Diagnostic indications and interpretations. *Pediatr Infect Dis* 5:337, 1986.
Sumaya CV, Ench Y: Epstein-Barr virus infectious mononucleosis in children. I. Clinical and general laboratory findings. *Pediatrics* 75:1003, 1985.
Sumaya CV, Ench Y: Epstein-Barr virus infectious mononucleosis in children. II. Heterophil antibody and viral-specific responses. *Pediatrics* 75:1011, 1985.
Tanz RR, Shulman ST, Barthel MJ, et al: Penicillin plus rifampin eradicates pharyngeal carriage of group A streptococci. *J Pediatr* 106:876, 1985.
Veasy LG, Wiedmeier SE, Orsmond GS, et al: Resurgence of acute rheumatic fever in the intermountain area of the United States. *N Engl J Med* 316:423, 1987.

68
SKIN AND SOFT TISSUE INFECTIONS

Gary R. Fleisher

This chapter will discuss several of the more common skin and soft tissue infections of childhood. The diseases will include conjunctivitis, impetigo, sinusitis, and cellulitis. Because of its particular severity, orbital/periorbital cellulitis will be highlighted in a section separate from the general discussion of cellulitis; however, the pathophysiology and clinical manifestations which are shared will not be repeated.

CONJUNCTIVITIS

Definition

Conjunctivitis is an inflammation of the conjunctivae, the membranes that line the surface of the eye. This inflammation may be the result of infection, allergy, or mechanical or chemical irritation. Keratoconjunctivitis involves the cornea as well as the conjunctivae.

Etiology

The etiology of infectious conjunctivitis differs between the newborn and the older child (Table 68-1). In the newborn, pathogens that reside in the birth canal play a major role in ocular infections. *Chlamydia trachomatis* is the most frequent, but *Neisseria gonorrhoeae* poses the greatest threat to the integrity of the eye. Later in childhood, the respiratory tract pathogens predominate, particularly *Haemophilus* species. Trachoma, a recurrent chlamydial conjunctivitis seen in tropical regions, will not be discussed.

Epidemiology

Conjunctivitis is the most common ocular infection of childhood. It may occur at any age. Neonates acquire most infections during passage through colonized birth canals; in older children, respiratory tract pathogens spread from person to person. Conjunctivitis is usually a sporadic disease, but epidemics of viral illness may occur.

Pathophysiology

Pathogens introduced into the conjunctival sac may proliferate and produce hyperemia and an inflammatory exudate. This exudate may be purulent, fibrinous, or serosanguinous. With certain organisms, corneal involvement (keratitis) may also occur.

Table 68-1. Etiology of Infectious Conjunctivitis

Frequency	Neonate	Child
Very frequent	*Chlamydia trachomatis*	Adenoviruses *Haemophilus* species
Moderately frequent	*Streptococcus pneumoniae* *Streptococcus fecalis* (enterococcus) *Neisseria gonorrhoeae*	*Streptococcus pneumoniae*
Infrequent	*Haemophilus influenzae* Herpes simplex *Staphylococcus aureus*	*Neisseria gonorrhoeae* *Neisseria meningitidis* *Chlamydia trachomatis* Herpes simplex *Staphylococcus aureus* *Corynebacterium diphtheriae*

Clinical Findings

Older children with conjunctivitis may complain of photophobia, ocular pain or pruritus, a sensation of a foreign body in the eye, crusting of the eyelids, or conjunctival erythema. Infants and young children are usually brought by their parents for "pink eye" or crusting. The duration of symptoms with infectious conjunctivitis is most often 2 to 4 days but may be longer in cases which are untreated or resistant to therapy.

As with any ocular complaint, the physician should perform a thorough examination of the structure and function of both eyes including, when age appropriate, examination of visual acuity, visual fields by confrontation, extraocular muscle function, periorbital area, eyelids (with eversion), conjunctivae, cornea with fluorescein staining, pupillary reflex, anterior chamber, and fundus. Erythema and increased secretions characterize conjunctivitis. Chemosis may be seen. Intense erythema and purulent discharge are more common with an infectious rather than an allergic cause. The cornea does not stain with fluorescein in children with conjunctivitis unless an associated keratitis has developed, as with herpes simplex or adenoviruses. Most importantly, visual acuity is normal.

Fever and/or other systemic symptoms do not occur with isolated conjunctivitis. However, conjunctivitis may be only one manifestation of a viral upper respiratory tract infection, in which case the temperature may be elevated.

Diagnosis

The diagnosis of infectious conjunctivitis rests primarily on the clinical examination. A Gram stain, which should be performed in neonates or in confusing cases, usually shows more than five white blood cells per oil immersion field and, in many cases, bacteria. The finding of gram-negative intracellular diplococci presumptively identifies *N. gonorrhoeae* in the first few weeks of life. Conjunctival scrapings and/or cultures may be performed in selected circumstances to diagnose *C. trachomatis* or specific viral and bacterial pathogens.

Differential Diagnosis

The differential diagnosis of the "red (or pink) eye" includes conjunctivitis, orbital/periorbital infection, foreign body, corneal abrasion, uveitis, and glaucoma. Periorbital and orbital infections cause obvious swelling and tenderness around the eye and/or loss of ocular mobility. Foreign bodies should be visible on direct examination, often only following eversion of the upper eyelid. Thus, the differential diagnosis usually revolves around four conditions: conjunctivitis, corneal abrasion, uveitis, and glaucoma (Table 68-2). Both uveitis and glaucoma are uncommon. The erythema in these conditions is concentrated around the limbus, and the discharge consists primarily of tears. Additionally, the vision is decreased in glaucoma, and the cornea may be cloudy. A corneal abrasion is easily identified by the uptake of fluorescein.

The physician must keep in mind that conjunctivitis may be only one manifestation of a systemic disorder. Examples include measles and Kawasaki disease.

Complications

Conjunctivitis is generally self-limited, with the notable exceptions of herpes simplex and *N. gonorrhoeae*. The potential complications are corneal ulceration and scar formation leading to visual impairment.

Management

Bacterial and viral conjunctivitides are far and away the most common cause for the complaint of a red eye in childhood. Once the diagnosis of conjunctivitis is established on the basis of diffuse injection, purulent discharge, and normal vision (Table 68-2), infectious and noninfectious

Table 68-2. Differential Diagnosis of the "Red Eye"

	Conjunctivitis	Corneal Abrasion	Uveitis	Glaucoma
History	URI	Trauma, contact lens	JRA, sarcoid, trauma	Prematurity, Marfan's syndrome, homocystinuria
Visual acuity	Normal	Normal or decreased	Normal or decreased	Decreased
Ocular exam				
External	Watery or purulent discharge	Watery discharge	Watery discharge	Watery discharge
Cornea	Usually normal; staining if keratitis	Staining	Normal or band keratopathy	Cloudy, staining
Anterior chamber	Normal	Normal	Cells, hypopyon, hyphema	Normal or shallow
Pupil	Normal	Normal	Small	Fixed
Intraocular pressure	Normal	Normal	Variable	Increased

Note: URI = upper respiratory infection; JRA = juvenile rheumatoid arthritis.

causes are next separated. Allergic conjunctivitis is usually distinguished by chronicity, seasonality, pruritus, and associated symptoms of allergic rhinitis; if the physician is uncertain, a Gram stain can be done (Table 68-3).

In approaching infectious conjunctivitis (Fig. 68-1), the physician must decide whether the ocular disorder is one manifestation of a systemic illness such as measles or is occurring in relative isolation. Isolated conjunctivitis may be due to various viruses and bacteria, of which herpes simplex and *N. gonorrhoeae* are particularly severe, or to *C. trachomatis,* especially in the first 3 months of life.

Fluorescein staining should always be performed in an effort to identify the dendritic corneal ulcerations characteristic of herpetic disease. If they are identified, treatment is with acyclovir or other antiviral agents under the supervision of an ophthalmologist. Because *N. gonorrhoeae* is usually acquired during passage through the birth canal, infants under 1 month of age must always be tested for this pathogen with a Gram stain and culture. The visualization of gram-negative intracellular diplococci on smear mandates admission to the hospital for intravenous penicillin therapy, although a definite diagnosis must await the results of culture. Recent data pointing to the efficacy of a single dose of intramuscular ceftriaxone await wider confirmation.

Infants beyond 1 month of age and older children with an obvious clinical diagnosis of conjunctivitis do not routinely require smears or cultures. In patients under 3 months of age, treatment is instituted with erythromycin (50 mg/kg per day) orally for *C. trachomatis* (Table 68-4). Older children require only topical antibiotic instillation into the conjunctival sac. A child who has unusually severe disease or who fails to respond to therapy within 48 h may benefit from a laboratory investigation. Appropriate studies in the infant under 1 month of age would include a Gram stain and bacterial culture and either a scraping or culture for *C. trachomatis.* Older children require only a Gram stain and bacterial culture. Diagnostic tests for herpes simplex are not usually rewarding in the absence of corneal ulceration; culture for adenoviruses may be helpful in persistent or severe hemorrhagic infections to avoid unnecessary additional testing, but there is no specific treatment.

Table 68-3. Differential Diagnosis of Allergic and Infectious Conjunctivitis

	Allergic	Infectious
History		
Pruritus	Yes	No
Chronic	Yes	No
Recurrent	Yes	No
Seasonal	Yes	No
Associated sneezing, rhinorrhea	Yes	Variable
Exam		
Discharge	Watery	Watery or purulent
Chemosis	Present	Usually absent
Fluorescein	Negative	Negative, except keratitis
Lab		
Gram stain	Negative	White cells, bacteria

All children with conjunctivitis should be reevaluated within 48 h. Failure to improve warrants further investigation and continued, careful follow-up.

IMPETIGO

Definition

Impetigo is a superficial bacterial infection of the skin confined to the epidermis. Deeper spread to the dermis leads to ecthyma. There are two varieties of impetigo: impetigo contagiosa and bullous impetigo.

Etiology

Group A β-hemolytic streptococcus (GABHS) is the major pathogen in impetigo contagiosa. Any strain of GABHS, including nephritogenic varieties, may infect the skin. *Staphylococcus aureus* has been recovered in an increasing proportion of cases in recent years. In bullous impetigo, the primary pathogen in *S. aureus.*

Epidemiology

Impetigo is the most common skin infection seen in the emergency department. The prevalence is greatest in young children, particularly those under the age of 6 years. Impetigo may occur sporadically or, occasionally, in epidemics. Conditions favoring epidemic spread include warm weather, overcrowding, and poor hygiene. Bullous impetigo is less common than impetigo contagiosa.

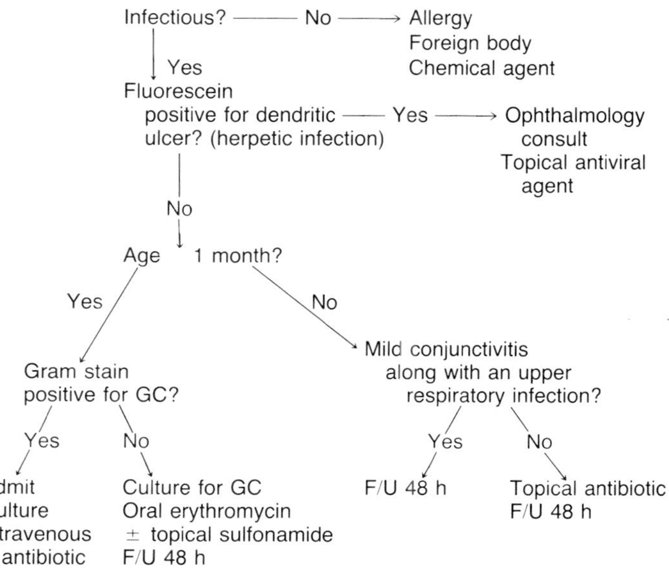

Fig. 68-1. Approach to the child with an isolated, infectious conjunctivitis. F/U: follow-up; GC: gonorrhea culture.

Table 68-4. Treatment of Conjunctivitis by Pathogen

Viruses	
Herpes simplex	Trifluridine, vidarabine, or acyclovir, topically (neonate may also have systemic infection)
Other	Supportive
Chlamydia	
Chlamydia trachomatis	Erythromycin, 50 mg/kg per day orally, for 14 days
Bacteria	
Neisseria gonorrhoeae or *meningitidis*	Child: penicillin, 50,000 units/kg per day, intravenously, for 7 days Adult: penicillin, 10 million units/day, intravenously, for 5 days Penicillinase-producing strains: cefotaxime, 75–100 mg/kg per day
Haemophilus influenzae, Streptococcus pneumoniae, and others	Topical antibiotic ointments: sulfonamide, erythromycin, etc.

Pathophysiology

The intact epidermis forms a relatively impervious barrier to bacteria. The development of impetigo follows a breach in the integument; this may be an obvious abrasion or an inconspicuous insect bite. Bacteria then invade the skin and elaborate toxins, such as streptolysins, which promote local spread.

Clinical Findings

The chief complaint of children with impetigo is most often that of sores on the body. There are no associated systemic manifestations such as fever or malaise. Regional lymph nodes may be minimally enlarged.

The typical lesion of impetigo contagiosa begins as an erythematous papule. Small vesicles may follow transiently, but rapid progression to crusted lesions occurs. These crusts, which are initially honey-colored and fine in consistency, may appear on any area of the body; between the upper lip and the nose is a very characteristic site. The lesions enlarge over days to weeks, and the crusts become thicker. Erythema is mild. No induration is present.

In bullous impetigo, the characteristic skin lesions are superficial bullae filled with purulent material. The bullae range in size from 0.5 to 3 cm and have minimal, if any, surrounding erythema.

Diagnosis

The diagnosis of impetigo rests with the visual appearance of the lesions. Rarely are laboratory tests needed.

In cases where the diagnosis of impetigo is uncertain, Gram stain of the lesions is helpful, showing abundant polymorphonuclear leukocytes and gram-positive bacteria. Local culture may be obtained from patients whose disease does not respond to standard therapy. If performed, the peripheral white blood cell count is normal.

Differential Diagnosis

Several dermatologic disorders may resemble either impetigo contagiosa or bullous impetigo. These include tinea corporis, nummular eczema, small burns or abrasions, allergic contact dermatitis, eczema herpeticum (with underlying atopic dermatitis), and scalded skin syndrome.

Complications

Impetigo may spread locally or, in the case of streptococcal infections, lead to remote, nonsuppurative sequelae. Occasionally, impetigo may progress to cellulitis or lead to lymphadenitis in the regional nodes. The attack rate for acute poststreptococcal glomerulonephritis has been as high as 1 percent in certain epidemics; however, the disease is unusual following sporadic skin infections.

Management

The treatment of impetigo is oral antibiotic therapy or an appropriate topical antibiotic for limited eruptions. Erythromycin, 50 mg/kg/day, provides an effective oral therapy. Alternative oral agents include dicloxacillin (50 mg/kg/day) or cephalexin (50 mg/kg/day). Mupirocin is the only topical agent with proven efficacy. Combination topical and systemic therapy in unnecessary. Vigorous scrubbing, in addition to topical or systemic antibiotic agents, offers no advantage; routine cleanliness is sufficient.

Antibiotic therapy hastens the resolution of impetigo and limits suppurative complications. Although the incidence of glomerulonephritis may be reduced, it has not been possible to demonstrate this effect with certainty in clinical studies due to the low incidence of this disease.

SINUSITIS

Definition

Sinusitis is an inflammation of the paranasal sinuses: maxillary, ethmoid, frontal, or sphenoid. This inflammation may be on the basis of infection or allergy; it may be acute, subacute, or chronic.

Etiology

The major pathogens in acute bacterial sinusitis in childhood are *Streptococcus pneumoniae* and *Haemophilus influenzae.* Wald and colleagues studied the etiology of infectious sinusitis using culture of material obtained by aspiration. Bacteria were recovered from 79 aspirates performed on 50 children as follows: 22 *S. pneumoniae,* 15 *Branhamella catarrhalis,* 15 *H. influenzae* (nontypable), 1 group A streptococcus, 1 group C streptococcus, 1 α-hemolytic streptococcus, 1 *Eikenella corrodens,* 1 *Peptostreptococcus,* and 1 *Moraxella.* Similar clinical investigations in adults have been in general agreement, finding nontypable *H. influenzae* and *S. pneumoniae* in 60 to 70 percent of the cases. Although *Staphylococcus aureus* and anaerobic organisms are isolated occasionally, they rarely play a role in acute infections in childhood.

Epidemiology

Severe sinusitis is not a common illness in children. However, the incidence of mild or subacute disease is less certain. Among 2613 patients seen in an office practice, Breese made this diagnosis in only 6 (0.23 percent). Investigators in Cleveland reported that 1 in 200 viral upper respiratory infections led to sinusitis in children.

Pathophysiology

The ethmoid and maxillary sinuses are present at birth, but the frontal and sphenoid sinuses do not become aerated until 6 or 7 years of age. The sinuses are lined primarily by ciliated columnar epithelium and connect with the nasopharynx via narrow ostia. Normally, the epithelium is coated by a double layer of mucus: a viscid gel layer superficially and a more fluid layer underneath. Resistance to infection depends on the patency of the ostia, the function of the ciliary mechanism, and the quality of the secretions.

Obstruction of the ostia results either from mucosal swelling or, less commonly, mechanical obstruction. By far the most frequent offenders are viral upper respiratory infection and allergic inflammation. Less common causes include cystic fibrosis, trauma, choanal atresia, deviated septum, polyps, foreign body, and tumor.

Factors that impair normal mucociliary function include viral infections, cold or dry air, certain chemicals or drugs, and, rarely, inborn

Table 68-5. Signs and Symptoms in Children with Sinusitis

	Acute, Severe Disease	Mild, Subacute Disease
Headache	+ + +	+ +
Fever	+ + +	+
Facial tenderness	+ +	—
Facial swelling	+ +	—
Nasal discharge	+ + +	+ + + +

errors of motility. Alterations of the mucus occur in asthma and cystic fibrosis.

The bacteria that cause sinusitis often colonize the nasopharynx of healthy children. Disruptions in one or more of the barriers described above allow these organisms to ascend through the ostia and multiply within the sinuses.

Clinical Findings

The spectrum of sinusitis has not been completely defined as it relates to clinical manifestations. However, there are two major types of infection which can usually be distinguished on clinical grounds: acute, severe sinusitis, and mild, subacute sinusitis (Table 68-5).

Acute, severe infections of the sinuses are infrequent during childhood. Such patients often have a history of headache and an elevated temperature. Findings include fever, localized swelling and/or erythema, and facial tenderness. A mucopurulent discharge usually accompanies severe sinusitis but may also indicate a nasal foreign body when unilateral.

Mild, subacute sinusitis is encountered more commonly than the severe form during childhood. This type of infection usually manifests as a protracted "cold." Rather than improving in 3 to 7 days, these children persist with the symptoms of an upper respiratory infection beyond 2 weeks. They have a nasal discharge, which may be serous or mucopurulent. Fever is infrequent.

Bacterial infection of the sinuses must be contrasted with congestion of brief duration found in association with some viral upper respiratory infections. Such congestion per se does not constitute a purulent infection.

Diagnosis

The diagnosis of sinusitis is usually made on clinical grounds without any laboratory or radiographic studies. In older children and adolescents, transillumination of the maxillary or frontal sinuses may provide assistance. Absence of light transmission has been shown to correlate with the recovery of pathogens on aspiration.

Standard radiographs, including anteroposterior, lateral, and occipitomental views should be obtained in patients with an uncertain clinical diagnosis and in cases of severe sinusitis. The most diagnostic findings for purulence are an air-fluid level or complete opacification. Mucosal thickening greater than 4 mm is usually indicative of infection but may accompany viral upper respiratory disease, particularly in the first year of life. A normal radiograph suggests, but does not prove, that a sinus is free of disease.

Several studies have shown that ultrasonography may be useful for the diagnosis of sinusitis, but there is not sufficient experience to recommend this modality for routine use. The anatomy of the paranasal sinuses is superbly defined by computed tomography (CT).However, the cost of CT does not justify its substitution for plain radiography, except in cases where complications are suspected.

Ultimate confirmation of infection within the paranasal sinuses rests with demonstration of organisms by Gram stain and quantitative culture of aspirated secretions. Aspiration is not routinely indicated but can easily be performed in selected cases of maxillary sinusitis in the outpatient setting via the intranasal route. The presence of organisms on Gram stain and a count of at least 10^4 colony-forming units point to bacterial infection. Appropriate circumstances for aspiration include (1) life-threatening complications, (2) immunosuppressive conditions, (3) clinical unresponsiveness, and (4) unusually severe disease.

Differential Diagnosis

Sinusitis may cause local swelling, facial pain, or nasal discharge. Other causes of swelling include superficial infection (cellulitis), trauma, cold injury, and allergic edema. Facial pain may be neurogenic, odontogenic, or related to the temporomandibular joint. Nasal discharge, particularly unilateral, should lead to a suspicion of a foreign body within the nares.

Complications

The proximity of the paranasal sinuses to the brain sets the scene for the occurrence of life-threatening complications from sinusitis; however, the use of antibiotics has reduced their incidence in recent times. Infection may spread from the sinuses to surrounding structures through the diploic veins, which have no valves, or by erosion through bone.

The most commonly encountered complications are periorbital cellulitis and orbital cellulitis/abscess. Periorbital infection causes swelling around the eye, while intraorbital accumulation of pus may be recognized on the basis of proptosis and decreased ocular motion. Infection may also produce osteomyelitis of the surrounding bone; in the frontal region this is referred to as Pott's puffy tumor. Less commonly, complications follow intracranial extension and may include epidural, subdural, or brain abscess; meningitis; and cavernous sinus thrombosis. Meningitis rarely follows sinusitis; it more commonly occurs after bacteremia. Focal intracranial involvement can be demonstrated by CT.

Management

In deciding upon appropriate therapy, the first step is to differentiate bacterial sinusitis from nasal congestion accompanying viral upper respiratory tract disease. Although the latter resolves spontaneously or may be treated with decongestants, sinusitis requires therapy with antibiotics (Table 68-6). Mild, subacute infections respond well to oral therapy for 10 to 14 days; as for otitis media, amoxicillin (40 mg/kg per day) remains the first-choice antimicrobial (Fig. 68-2). Failure to improve with amoxicillin therapy suggests infection with pathogens that are often resistant to this drug, such as *B. catarrhalis* or *H. influenzae*. A second course of treatment with cefixime, erythromycin/sulfisoxazole, or amoxicillin/clavulanic acid should then be instituted; aspiration for culture is necessary to select specific antimicrobial therapy for those patients in whom the infection still persists after a second course of therapy.

Table 68-6. Antibiotic Therapy for Sinusitis

	Acute, Severe Sinusitis	Mild, Subacute Sinusitis
Initial	Cefuroxime, 100 mg/kg per day IV *or* Ceftriaxone, 75 mg/kg per day IV *or* Oxacillin, 150 mg/kg per day IV, and chloramphenicol, 100 mg/kg per day IV	Amoxicillin, 40 mg/kg per day PO
Persistent	Antibiotics as above plus surgical drainage	Cefixime, 8 mg/kg per day PO *or* Erythromycin/sulfisoxazole; 40 mg/kg per day of erythromycin PO
Penicillin allergic	Cefuroxime, 100 mg/kg per day IV	As for persistent cases

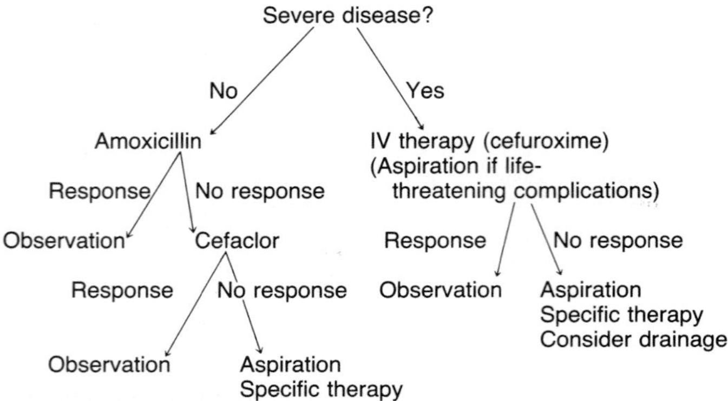

Fig. 68-2. Approach to sinusitis in the immunocompetent child.

Acute, severe sinusitis may result in life-threatening complications and requires intravenous antibiotic therapy directed at *S. pneumoniae*, amoxicillin-resistant *H. influenzae*, and less commonly *S. aureus*. Cefuroxime (100 mg/kg per day) or ceftriaxone (75 mg/kg per day) represent single-drug regimens effective for this disease; the combination of oxacillin (150 mg/kg per day) and chloramphenicol (100 mg/kg per day) is an alternative. Failure of severe disease to respond promptly to antibiotic therapy and/or the occurrence of complications indicates the need for surgical consultation in regard to drainage procedures.

CELLULITIS

Definition

Cellulitis is an infection of the skin and subcutaneous tissues. It extends below the dermis, differentiating it from impetigo, but does not involve muscle (pyogenic myositis) or bone (osteomyelitis). Any region of the body may be involved, but two divisions are important in regard to predicting the most likely pathogens: (1) the trunk and extremities and (2) the face (buccal and periorbital cellulitis).

Etiology

The organisms that play an important role in the immunocompetent host under normal circumstances include *Staphylococcus aureus*, *Streptococcus pyogenes* (group A β-hemolytic streptococcus), and *Haemophilus influenzae* (Table 68-7). In general, *S. aureus* is the most common and *H. influenzae* the least, among the three major pathogens. However, in certain anatomic locations and under differing clinical conditions, the likelihood may vary among these three pathogens. Additionally, unusual organisms may cause cellulitis in immunocompromised hosts or following their introduction in special types of wounds (Table 68-7).

Table 68-7. Etiology of Cellulitis

	Most Likely	Less Likely
IMMUNOCOMPETENT HOST		
Trunk/extremity	*Staphylococcus aureus* *Streptococcus pyogenes*	*Haemophilus influenzae*
Face (periorbital/buccal)	*H. influenzae*	*S. aureus* *S. pneumoniae*
Any site/animal bite	*S. aureus*	*Pasteurella multocida*
Any site/human bite	Anaerobic organisms	*S. aureus*
IMMUNOCOMPROMISED HOST		
Any site	*S. aureus*, gram-negative rods	Anaerobic organisms

Epidemiology

Cellulitis is a frequent infection, particularly in the warm weather. The precise incidence is unknown; however, in a study at an urban children's hospital, this infection accounted for 1 of every 500 visits. Children of any age may develop cellulitis, but disease due to *H. influenzae* occurs most often in the first 3 years of life.

Pathophysiology

Cellulitis may occur either when a pathogen is directly inoculated into the subcutaneous tissue or following an episode of bacteremia. The majority of infections involve local invasion after a breach in the integument. The organisms responsible are usually *S. aureus* and *S. pyogenes*. In contradistinction, *H. influenzae* disseminates hematogenously.

Clinical Findings

The child with cellulitis manifests a local inflammatory response at the site of the infection, including erythema, edema, warmth, and tenderness. There may be a history of a preceding wound or a complaint related to loss of function, such as limp with an infection of a lower extremity. Fever is unusual except in infections due to *H. influenzae* (Table 68-8).

Inspection of the area of cellulitis usually shows intense erythema. A violaceous hue suggests *H. influenzae* but has been reported with other pathogens including *Streptococcus pneumoniae*. Red streaks may radiate proximally along the course of the lymphatic drainage, and the regional nodes may enlarge.

Diagnosis

The diagnosis of cellulitis is made by inspection. Laboratory studies including a WBC count, blood culture, and aspirate culture are obtained for specific indications: immunocompromise, fever, severe local infection, facial involvement, and failure to respond to therapy.

The WBC count is normal in most cases of infection due to *S. aureus* or *S. pyogenes*, which are locally invasive. On the other hand, cellulitis due to *H. influenzae* results from bacteremia and is usually accompanied by a polymorphonuclear leukocytosis. In one study of children with cellulitis, the WBC count was over 15,000/mm^3 in 3 of 4 children infected with *H. influenzae*, and 0 of 19 infected with *S. aureus* or *S. pyogenes*. Among 194 patients with *H. influenzae* cellulitis reported in the literature as reviewed in 1983, the WBC count was greater than 15,000/mm^3 in 84 percent, with a mean of 20,850/mm^3.

The blood culture is usually negative in infections due to *S. aureus* and *S. pyogenes*. On the other hand, *H. influenzae* as a rule causes a bacteremic infection.

Aspirate cultures are best obtained close to the center of an infected lesion, as the periphery may consist primarily of edema fluid devoid of organisms. The needle should be sufficiently large to permit the evacuation of purulent material—22 gauge for the face and 19 gauge for the trunk and extremities. Using a 5- or 10-mL syringe prefilled

Table 68-8. Usual Clinical and Laboratory Features of Children with Cellulitis

Characteristic	*H. influenzae*	*S. aureus*
Age	<3 yrs	Any
Fever	Yes	No
Color of lesion	Violaceous	Erythematous
Location	Cheek, periorbital	Trunk, extremity
Preceding wound	No	Yes
WBC count	>15,000/mm^3	<15,000/mm^3
Bacteremia	Yes	No

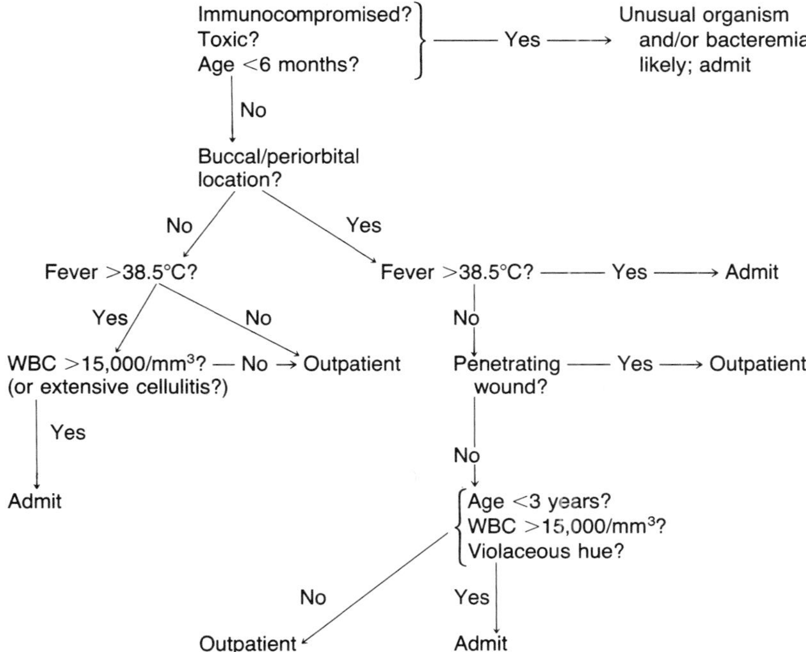

Fig. 68-3. Approach to the child with cellulitis.

with 1 mL of sterile, nonbacteriostatic saline, the needle is directed into the subcutaneous tissue to a depth of approximately 0.5 to 1.0 cm, and aspiration is attempted. If there is no return, the saline is injected and reaspirated. The material obtained is used for culture and Gram stain.

Differential Diagnosis

Cellulitis must be differentiated from other causes of erythema and edema, including trauma and allergic reaction. Allergic edema is not tender and usually only mildly erythematous. Traumatic lesions may be easily distinguished when there is a history of injury and absence of fever. Cold injury, especially on the cheeks (''popsicle panniculitis''), may be confused with cellulitis.

Complications

Cellulitis due to *S. aureus* and *S. pyogenes* may at times spread locally or involve the regional lymph nodes; distant foci occur only rarely. Bacteremic *H. influenzae* infections are more likely to spread hematogenously, involving the central nervous system, epiglottis, joints, or pericardium.

Management

The treatment of cellulitis is the administration of systemic antibiotic therapy. Although most patients respond rapidly to oral antistaphylococcal agents, the clinician must identify those individuals who require broad-spectrum or intravenously administered drugs (Fig. 68-3).

Obviously, signs of sepsis are indicative of hematogenous dissemination and demand treatment as an inpatient. Additionally, children under 6 months of age and those with impaired immunity are unable to contain local bacterial infections and will benefit from intravenous therapy. All patients admitted to the hospital should have WBC counts and cultures of blood.

Among otherwise healthy children over 6 months of age, only those with bacteremic disease, usually from *H. influenzae* or severe infections, need to be admitted to the hospital. Those patients with *H. influenzae* can be identified fairly reliably on the basis of clinical risk factors including buccal/periorbital location, fever, and a WBC count greater then 15,000/mm^3. Although most physicians are well aware of the association of *H. influenzae* with facial cellulitis, it is important to remember that the young, febrile child with extremity involvement stands a reasonable chance of being infected with this organism.

The usual therapy for patients discharged from the emergency department is an antistaphylococcal antibiotic, such as dicloxacillin or cephalexin. Broad-spectrum therapy is recommended presumptively for patients who are immunocompromised or suspected to have bacteremia, pending a definitive isolate (Table 68-9).

PERIORBITAL/ORBITAL CELLULITIS

Definition

Cellulitis as previously defined may involve the tissues anterior to the orbital septum (periorbital cellulitis) or within the orbit (orbital cellulitis).

Etiology

Periorbital disease is usually due to *H. influenzae;* orbital infections are more often caused by *S. aureus.*

Epidemiology

Children under the age of 3 years are more likely to become bacteremic than those who are older; thus, they experience the highest incidence of periorbital disease. Orbital cellulitis may occur at any age.

Pathophysiology

Organisms reach the periorbital area either hematogenously or by direct extension from the ethmoid sinus. In the case of orbital disease, contiguous spread is most common.

Clinical Findings

Orbital and periorbital cellulitis cause the periorbital area to appear red and swollen. The periorbital edema is usually more prominent with preseptal infections. Proptosis or limitation of extraocular muscle function indicates orbital involvement. Fever is more common with periorbital cellulitis.

Table 68-9. Initial Antibiotic Therapy for Cellulitis

	Drug(s)	Dose	Route
I. Presumptive			
Immunocompetent			
1. Extremity			
a. Afebrile	Dicloxacillin	50–100 mg/kg per day	PO
	or		
	Cephalexin	50–100 mg/kg per day	PO
b. Febrile/leukocytosis	Oxacillin	150 mg/kg per day	IV
	and		
	Chloramphenicol	100 mg/kg per day	IV
	or		
	Cefuroxime	100 mg/kg per day	IV
	or		
	Ceftriaxone	75 mg/kg per day	IV
2. Buccal/periorbital	As above	As above	As above
Immunocompromised			
Any site	Oxacillin	150 mg/kg per day	IV
	or		
	Cefazolin	100 mg/kg per day	IV
	and		
	Gentamicin	5–7.5 mg/kg per day	IV
	or		
	Tobramycin	5–7.5 mg/kg per day	IV
II. Specific organism			
Streptococcus pyogenes	Penicillin	100,000 units/kg per day	PO *or* IV
Staphylococcus aureus	Dicloxacillin	50–100 mg/kg per day	PO
	or		
	Oxacillin	150 mg/kg per day	IV
Haemophilus influenzae			
Ampicillin-sensitive	Ampicillin	200 mg/kg per day	IV
Ampicillin-resistant	Cefuroxime	100 mg/kg per day	IV
	or		
	Ceftriaxone	75 mg/kg per day	IV

Diagnosis

Periorbital and orbital cellulitis are distinguished from noninfectious disorders on the basis of the clinical findings and the WBC count. Leukocytosis occurs frequently with cellulitis, more often with bacteremic preseptal infections. A blood culture is often positive.

Computed tomography is performed when orbital involvement is likely. An inflammatory mass is easily demonstrated when present using this modality.

Differential Diagnosis

As for cellulitis in other regions, allergic and traumatic causes for edema must be considered. Additionally, tumors and metabolic disease may cause swelling, discoloration, and/or proptosis. Thyrotoxicosis usually occurs in adolescents. The most likely tumor is metastatic neuroblastoma. Pseudotumor occurs rarely.

Complications

Periorbital cellulitis may serve as a focus for metastatic bacterial disease; of particular concern is the occurrence of meningitis. Orbital cellulitis may evolve into a subperiosteal abscess; this condition threatens the integrity of the eye and should be considered a surgical emergency. Intracranial extension may occur rarely.

Management

Admission and treatment with intravenous antibiotics is the rule. Blood cultures should always be done, and an aspirate culture is indicated for any ill child. Presumptive therapy of periorbital or orbital cellulitis is directed against *S. aureus* and *H. influenzae* (Table 68-9). Surgical drainage may be necessary with abscess formation or sinusitis.

BIBLIOGRAPHY

Conjunctivitis

Gigliotti F, Hendley JO, Morgan J, et al: Efficacy of topical antibiotic therapy in acute conjunctivitis in children. *J Pediatr* 104:623, 1984.

Gigliotti F, Williams WT, Hayden FG, et al: Etiology of acute conjunctivitis in children. *J Pediatr* 98:531, 1981.

Hammerschlag MR: Conjunctivitis in infancy and childhood. *Pediatr Rev* 5:285, 1984.

Sandstrom KI, Bell TA, Chandler SW, et al: Microbial causes of neonatal conjunctivitis. *J Pediatr* 105:706, 1984.

Vichgamond P, Brown Q, Jackson D: Acute bacterial conjunctivitis: Bacteriology and clinical implications. *Clin Pediatr* 25:506, 1986.

Impetigo

Barton LL, Friedman AD, Sharbey AM, et al: Impetigo contagiosa VII: Comparative efficacy of oral erythromycin and topical mupirocin. *Pediatr Dermatol* 6:134, 1989.

Barton LL, Friedman AD: Impetigo: A reassessment of etiology and therapy. *Pediatr Permatol* 4:185, 1987.

Fleisher, GR, Wilmott CM, Campos JM: Amoxicillin combined with clavulanic acid for the treatment of soft tissue infections in children. *Antimicrob Agents Chemother* 24:679, 1983.

Sinusitis

Hamory BH, Sande MA, Sydnor A Jr., et al: Etiology and anti-microbial therapy of acute sinusitis. *J. Infect Dis* 132:197, 1979.

Lew D, Southwick FS, Montgomery WW, et al: Sphenoid sinusitis: A review of 30 cases. *N Engl J Med* 309:1119, 1983.

Wald ER, Milmoe GJ, Bowen A, et al: Acute maxillary sinusitis in children. *N Engl J Med* 304:749, 1981.

Wald ER, Reilly JS, Casselbrant M, et al: Treatment of acute maxillary sinusitis in childhood: A comparative study of amoxicillin and cefaclor. *J Pediatr* 104:297, 1984.

Wald ER, Byers C, Guerra N, et al: Subacute sinusitis in children. *J Pediatr* 115: 28, 1989.

Cellulitis

Barkin RM, Todd JR, Amer J: Periorbital cellulitis in children. *Pediatrics* 62:390, 1978.

Fleisher GR, Heger P, Topf P: *Hemophilus influenzae* cellulitis. *Am J Emerg Med* 3:274, 1983.

Fleisher GR, Ludwig S, Campos J: Cellulitis: Bacterial etiology, clinical features, and laboratory findings. *J. Pediatr* 97:591, 1980.

Gellady AM, Shulman ST, Ayoub EM: Periorbital and orbital cellulitis in children. *Pediatrics* 61:272, 1978.

Goldberg F, Berne AS, Oski FA: Differentiation of orbital cellulitis from preceptal cellulitis by computed tomography. *Pediatrics* 62:1000, 1978.

Teele DW: Management of the child with a red and swollen eye. *Pediatr Infect Dis* 2:258, 1983.

69
BACTEREMIA, SEPSIS, AND MENINGITIS

Joseph A. Zeccardi

Bacteremia, sepsis, and meningitis in children may be considered different points on a spectrum of bacterial invasion. Although all bacteremia does not progress through sepsis and meningitis, it is helpful to consider the three entities simultaneously.

BACTEREMIA

Positive blood cultures with symptomatology confined to fever constitute the definition of bacteremia. Most bacteremias are caused by *Streptococcus pneumoniae* and *Hemophilus influenzae* with *Salmonella, Neisseria meningitidis,* and group A streptococci causing a significant minority. The incidence of various pathogens varies from study to study. However, the major cause is *S. pneumoniae,* which accounts for 60 to 80 percent, whereas *H. influenzae* accounts for 10 to 30 percent. The preponderance of bacteremias is identified in the 6- to 24-month-old population, with many fewer occurring before or after that age. Bacteremia may progress to a focal infection such as meningitis, abscess, or sepsis, or the condition may spontaneously improve. Since factors influencing susceptibility have not been well defined, it is not possible to identify the child at risk for progression to sepsis or meningitis.

Diagnosis and Treatment

A number of studies have shown that the strongest evidence for bacteremia is in children under 24 months of age who have white blood cell (WBC) counts of 15,000 or more and a fever of 39.4°C (102.9°F) or higher. Therefore, a WBC count should be obtained in children in the following circumstances: (1) those 3 to 24 months old with a temperature of 39.4°C or more without a demonstrable focus of infection and (2) all patients 3 to 24 months old who appear toxic and have a fever less than 39.4°C. Those children with a WBC count of 15,000 or a polymorphonuclear count over 9000 should have blood cultures done. Antibiotic therapy may be administered on an ambulatory basis, on the presumption that therapy may reduce the incidence of progression to serious infection. Amoxicillin, 50 to 100 mg/kg per day; Amoxicillin/clavulanate, 50 mg/kg per day; or cefuroxime, 125 to 250 mg orally q 12 h, is appropriate, considering the likely bacterial causes. All discharged patients should be reevaluated in 24 h or less if the clinical condition warrants.

On reevaluation, the patient whose blood cultures are positive for *S. pneumoniae* and who is now asymptomatic and afebrile may be treated with oral penicillin, 50,000 units/kg per day, for the next 10 days. All children with blood cultures positive for *H. influenzae* should be admitted to the hospital. Children who continue to have symptoms or who develop a focus of infection should be admitted to the hospital for parenteral antibiotic therapy.

Children under 3 months of age with fever or who appear toxic should be admitted because of the possibility of sepsis, since neither the WBC count nor the physical assessment is reliable enough to distinguish those with sepsis from those with a more benign condition.

SEPSIS

Sepsis is bacteremia with focal findings in addition to fever. The commonest organisms causing sepsis in the neonate are group B streptococcus and *Escherichia coli*. After the newborn period, *H. influenzae, N. meningitidis,* and *S. pneumoniae* become the most frequently isolated pathogens, with streptococcus A, *Staphylococcus aureus,* and *Salmonella* reported much less commonly. Increased risks for sepsis include exposure to communicable pathogens such as meningococcus; suppressed immune competence from conditions such as primary immunodeficiency disease or chemotherapy; hyposplenism due to surgical removal for hemoglobin disorders; and sickle cell disease or trait, which is associated with sepsis and bacteremia from *S. pneumoniae* and *Salmonella*.

Clinical Presentation

The patient's illness may range from hours, in the case of meningococcemia, to several days of mild to moderate symptoms, such as listlessness or poor feeding. Hypothermia is more likely than fever in those under the age of 3 months. Any child under the age of 3 months with hypothermia or fever should be admitted for treatment and evaluation of sepsis. Symptoms may progress through tachycardia, hypotension, cold and clammy skin, lethargy, and coma. Occasionally, hemorrhagic skin lesions may be noted.

Focal findings can be varied and include urinary tract infections or otitis, but the clinician should suspect sepsis when more than one focus is identified. Skin lesions indicative of embolic phenomena should also be sought.

Laboratory studies should include a complete blood count (CBC) with platelets; determination of prothrombin time and partial thromboplastin time; determination of fibrin split product, aterial blood gas, glucose, electrolyte, blood urea nitrogen (BUN), serum glutamic oxaloacetic transaminase (SGOT), and serum glutamic pyruvic transaminase (SGPT) levels; blood culture; and a lumbar puncture with cultures. Pupuric skin lesions should be opened with a lancet and smeared, and a Gram stain obtained. Laboratory studies usually reveal a normal hemoglobin and hematocrit. The WBC count is almost always elevated, but neutropenia may accompany an overwhelming infection. The differential should show a shift to the left with immature forms. If there are hemorrhagic skin lesions, the platelets may be decreased on the smear, and the platelet count will be lowered. Clotting studies may also be abnormal in the presence of disseminated intravascular coagulation. Measurement of blood gases usually demonstrates a metabolic acidosis. Sodium may be lowered because of inappropriate antidiuretic hormone secretion. The BUN is usually normal. A lowered glucose level may be noted in infants.

Treatment

If the patient is in shock, an infusion of 20 mL/kg per hour of normal saline solution with 5% dextrose should be given following determination of the central venous pressure. Urinary output should be monitored with a catheter and maintained at 1 mL/kg per hour. Antibiotics of choice are ampicillin, 200 mg/kg per day, and gentamycin, 7.5 mg/kg per day. In the older child, because of the increased frequency of infection with *H. influenzae,* chloramphenicol, 100 mg/kg per day, should be used instead of gentamycin. Chloramphenicol in the same doses is indicated in the infant with bloody diarrhea because of the possibility of *Salmonella* infection. Steroid therapy is still controversial, but pharmacologic doses in severely ill patients are commonly used by some physicians. Hypoglycemia should be treated with glucose infusion. Further stabilization may require infusion of packed red blood cells to correct blood loss or anemia, and of platelet concentrates and fresh frozen plasma for bleeding disorders.

MENINGITIS

In children, *H. influenzae, S. pneumoniae, N. meningitidis, E. coli,* and group B streptococci are the commonest causes of meningitis. In the first month of life, group B streptococci and *E. coli* are usually the causative agents. After this period, *H. influenzae* becomes the most frequent cause of meningitis, with *S. pneumoniae* and *N. meningitidis* following in incidence. Unusual pathogens such as *Salmonella* should be considered in patients with sickle cell disease or a history of gastroenteritis. Bacterial invasion of the meninges occurs either directly from contiguous infections such as otitis or by seeding from sepsis. The mode of entry in the newborn can be from the maternal vaginal tract into the bowel or respiratory tract, whereas in the older child the nasopharynx is more frequently the site of entry for the organism. Splenectomized patients and patients with sickle cell disease or immunodeficiency are at higher risk for meningitis following showers of bacteria. The clinician should look carefully for infections in the middle ear and sinuses and for associated fractures of these structures in addition to searching for midline defects such as meningomyelocele. Direct extension of infection from these sites may be associated with unusual organisms.

Clinical Presentation

The presentation varies significantly, depending on the age of the child. In the first 3 months of life, the degree of symptoms is low, and the clinician needs to be especially alert to subtle findings. Increased or decreased activity level, vomiting, or decreased appetite, as evidenced by poor sucking or rooting, should alert the physician to infection in the infant. Increased irritability, as opposed to being soothed, when held is a useful symptom. The cuddling that would normally reduce crying may cause movement of the inflamed meninges and, therefore, more crying. A bulging fontanelle is a significantly late but important and reliable sign of increased intracranial pressure in meningitis.

Other late symptoms include a high-pitched cry and reduced consciousness. In the first few months of life, patients frequently do not have fever and may even be hypothermic. In the presence of fever over 38.5°C (101.3°F) or hypothermia below 36.8°C (98°F), meningitis must be ruled out by lumbar puncture.

Symptoms become more reliable as the child develops beyond 3 months. Irritability and a significant change in sleep and wake patterns become much more noticeable. The child's level of activity is usually significantly decreased. As maturation continues, meningitis presents more frequently with nuchal rigidity and headache. Presenting complaints may also include back pain, petechial rash, and focal neurologic signs.

In a child older than 3 months, a febrile response is a more common finding. Seizures as an initial manifestation are rare in meningitis. However, in children under the age of 6 months with a fever and seizure, meningitis must be ruled out. Over the age of 6 months, controversy exists in management because the likelihood of a febrile seizure is greater. However, in general, a lumbar puncture is indicated in every case of a first febrile seizure or seizure with fever. If there is a definite history of febrile seizures, a lumbar puncture need not be done unless there are other findings indicating the need for investigation. The patient with meningitis may also present in shock initially. The clinician should search for skin lesions and nuchal rigidity in the febrile child with no history of blood or fluid losses. Signs of meningitis should be sought in febrile children with non-CNS problems such as vomiting, dehydration, or respiratory infections if the child appears to be more toxic than is usually expected from apparent primary problems.

Laboratory Findings

Accurate diagnosis is crucial, and prompt therapy must be instituted in order to reduce mortality. The critical diagnostic procedure is the lumbar puncture. If the child appears stable, however, it is wise to obtain blood for a CBC; determination of electrolyte and glucose levels and osmolarity; clotting studies; blood culture; and blood typing and cross matching. Then a lumbar puncture may be performed. The blood should be tested with a glucose oxidase tape. Immunoelectrophoresis may aid in the identification of the pathogen. Blood, urine, and cerebrospinal fluid may be submitted for this study. Cultures should be obtained from the most likely sites of entry, including the throat, nasopharynx, stool, urine, and skin. The accuracy of cultures is low from the nasopharynx and higher from blood, urine, and skin. A lumbar puncture is necessary before antibiotic treatment is begun, unless the patient is too unstable. In this case, oxygenation, fluid resuscitation, and antibiotics are first necessary. Cerebrospinal fluid should be sent for a cell count, differential blood count, Gram stain, and determination of protein and glucose levels. Culture of and sensitivity to aerobes and mycobacteria should be done only if there is clinical indication.

Rapid interpretation of cerebrospinal fluid results is important. A cloudy spinal fluid that is not blood-tinged indicates a need for immediate antibiotic treatment while awaiting the analysis. If (1) the WBC count is over 1000 cells/mL and is primarily polymorphonuclear, (2) the glucose is less than one-half the blood sugar, and (3) the Gram stain demonstrates bacteria, the patient obviously has bacterial meningitis. Patients with less clear-cut findings should be admitted and repunctured in 6 h. Antibiotics are generally withheld for repuncturing in order to avoid committing the patient to a prolonged and unnecessary course of parenteral antibiotic therapy. A completely clear tap in an infant with signs and symptoms of meningitis should be repeated within 6 to 8 h and the child admitted for close observation without antibiotics during this time. It is not unusual for symptoms to begin prior to the demonstration of bacteria in the cerebrospinal fluid. There is a lag period between the showers of bacteria and a positive Gram stain (especially in pneumococcal meningitis), and the onset of cerebrospinal pleocytosis. Therefore, the Gram stain becomes an essential part of the evaluation despite the absence of any abnormal cells, protein, or glucose. Other tests that are helpful but not universally available are immunoelectrophoresis; determination of cerebrospinal fluid, lactic acid dehydrogenase, and lactic acid concentrations; and the quelling reaction.

A urine sample should be sent for analysis, including osmolality measurement and culture. If counterimmunoelectrophoresis is available, it should be obtained. Blood gas values should be obtained initially. Skin lesions may be incised with a lancet and a Gram stain obtained; the material should be cultured in an attempt to identify the pathogen. In addition, Gram stains of the buffy coat may be useful in identifying the pathogen.

Treatment

After the lumbar puncture, an intravenous infusion should be started at a maintenance rate to avoid increasing intracranial pressure. A Foley catheter is appropriate in all cases. Seizures should be managed in the usual manner with Valium, 0.3 mg/kg, to terminate seizure activity, followed by loading with phenytoin or phenobarbital. Therapy for seizures should be specific and not prophylactic. Shock should be treated with volume infusion consisting of normal saline solution with 5% dextrose at 20 mL/kg. The patient's urinary output should be monitored and maintained at 1 mL/kg per hour. Methylprednisolone at 30 mg/kg is used by some. As of this writing, some support the routine administration of steroids prior to administration of antibiotics. Positive inotropic or pressor agents may be necessary if the volume loading is unsuccessful. Cerebral edema or subdural effusions may lead to signs of increased intracranial pressure. Treatment for signs of impending herniation should be instituted immediately using mannitol, 1 mg/kg, and dexamethasone, 0.15 mg/kg. Collections of fluid may be relieved by subdural taps. Fluid recovered should be treated as spinal fluid for laboratory purposes. The presence of cerebral edema is a significant risk, and it should preclude a lumbar puncture. Cultures can be obtained from another site, such as skin lesions, the pharynx, urine, blood, or any obvious infected site. A lumbar puncture may be attempted after a trial of therapy to reduce intracranial pressure. Then, a small needle, with the stylet held in the opening so the immediate control of leakage is possible, should be utilized, and the smallest sample of cerebrospinal fluid necessary for culture and Gram stain should be obtained.

Antibiotic Therapy

Although 3 months of age has been used as a dividing line for decisions because of the paucity of symptoms and increased risk, when considering antibiotic choice, 2 months of age becomes a significant milestone because during the second month *E. coli* and group B streptococci diminish in frequency, while *H. influenzae* is isolated more frequently. *H. influenzae* becomes the major organism by the third month, with *S. pneumoniae* and *N. meningitidis* following in incidence. Therefore, in the patient under 1 month of age, antibiotic therapy should include ampicillin and an aminoglycoside. The choice of aminoglycoside should be hospital-specific, depending on the sensitivity of the pathogens in the particular nursery. A common choice is gentamycin. The doses are gentamycin, 5 mg/kg per day q 12 h for children under 7 days of age and 7.5 mg/kg per day q 8 h for children over 7 days of age; ampicillin, 100 mg/kg per day q 12 h for children under 7 days of age and 200 mg/kg per day q 4 h for children over 7 days of age.

In children in their second month and beyond, antibiotic choice changes to ampicillin and chloramphenicol because of the resistance of some strains of *H. influenzae*. Ampicillin is given in a dose of 300 mg/kg per day and chloramphenicol at 100 mg/kg per day given as a rapid IV infusion q 4 h. The patient must be monitored closely for signs of increasing intracranial pressure or focal neurologic signs.

Prehospital and hospital professionals and family who have had contact with the child will be concerned with prophylaxis. Family members should have cultures of the pharynx, and prophylaxis with rifampin for meningococcemia should be considered. Prophylactic rifampin is given in a dose of 600 mg po qd for 4 days to adults. For children under one month of age, the dose is 10 mg/kg qd for 4 days, and for children over 1 month, 20 mg/kg qd for 4 days. Prehospital and hospital professionals who transported and cared for the child do not need prophylaxis, but if mouth-to-mouth resuscitation has occurred, prophylaxis should be offered.

BIBLIOGRAPHY

Alpert G, Hibbert E, Fleisher G: Case-control study of hyperpyrexia in children. *Pediatr Infect Dis J* 9:161, 1990.

Baker MD, Avner JR, Bell LM: Failure of infant observation scales in detecting serious illness in febrile, 4- to 8-week-old infants. *Pediatrics* 85:1040, 1990.

Baron MA, Fink HD, Cicchetti DV: Blood cultures in private pediatric practice: An eleven-year experience. *Pediatr Infect Dis J* 8:2, 1989.

Crocker PJ, Quick G, McCombs W: Occult bacteremia in the emergency department: Diagnostic criteria for the young febrile child. *Ann Emerg Med* 14:1172, 1985.

Fleisher GR: Infectious disease emergencies, in Fleisher G, Ludwig S (eds): *Textbook of Pediatric Emergency Medicine,* 2d ed. Baltimore, Williams & Wilkins, 1988, pp 416–425.

Geiseler RJ, Nelso KE: Bacterial meningitis without clinical signs of meningeal irritation. *South Med J* 75:448, 450, 1982.

Jaffe DM, Tanz RR, Davis AT, et al: Antibiotic administration to treat possible occult bacteremia in febrile children. *N Engl J Med* 317:1175, 1987.

Lembo RM, Marchant CD: Acute phase reactants and risk of bacterial meningitis among febrile infants and children. *Ann Emerg Med* 20:36, 1991.

Mazur LJ, Jones TM, Kozinetz CA: Temperature response to acetaminophen and risk of occult bacteremia: A case-control study. *J Pediatr* 115:888, 1989.

McCarthy PL, Lembo RM, Baron MA, et al: Predictive value of abnormal physical examination findings in ill-appearing and well-appearing febrile children. *Pediatr* 76:167, 1985.

70 VIRAL AND BACTERIAL PNEUMONIAS

Duane D. Harrison

Infections of the lung remain a leading cause of serious morbidity in infancy and childhood. Infections range from mild to life-threatening and from gradually progressive to fulminant. The multiplicity of agents which can cause pneumonia as well as limitations of diagnostic testing often make precise etiologic diagnosis difficult. However, consideration of clinical data, epidemiologic factors, roentgenographic findings, and common laboratory tests provides a basis for a reasonable approach to most children.

CLINICAL HISTORY

Pneumonia often presents in a school-age child or adolescent with cough, fever, pleuritic chest pain, dyspnea, increased sputum production, or tachypnea. These typical symptoms may be absent in the young child or infant, who may present with nonspecific symptoms not readily attributable to pneumonia. Such symptoms include apneic spells, fever without other localizing signs, poor feeding, decreased physical activity, vomiting or diarrhea, hypothermia, grunting, bradycardic episodes, abdominal pain, shock, or lethargy. Because of the diverse clinical presentations of pneumonia in young children and infants, heightened suspicion for this diagnosis should be maintained.

Fever may be the sole manifestation of pneumonia. Although there is much overlap between bacterial and viral pneumonia, very high fever [above 40°C (104°F)] increases the likelihood of a bacterial etiology. A history of prodromal coryza followed by sudden onset of high fever suggests bacterial pneumonia complicating a viral illness. Insidious onset of fever with gradual worsening of symptoms is more characteristic of viral or *Mycoplasma* pneumonia.

The presence of associated symptoms should be considered. Viruses causing pneumonia often infect the upper respiratory tract first, with rhinorrhea initially, followed sequentially by sore throat, coughing, croup, hoarse voice, or wheezing. Pleuritic chest pain is found most often in acute bacterial pneumonia. Exanthemata are associated with mycoplasma or viral infections. Conjunctivitis frequently precedes chlamydial pneumonia in young infants. Fulminant septicemia suggests a bacterial etiology.

The feeding history aids assessment of the severity of illness, particularly in young infants. Infants who feed slowly, taking extra time to breathe, or who refuse feedings entirely are more severely affected than infants who are able to maintain their usual feeding patterns. Vomiting may follow severe coughing spells and lead to dehydration.

The presence of underlying diseases should also be noted. Children with preexisting cardiac or pulmonary disease are likely to be most severely compromised by pulmonary infections. A history of frequent infections, previous episodes of pneumonia, immunosuppressive therapy, or primary immune deficiency raises concern about both the potential severity of infection and the possibility of infection with opportunistic organisms. Acute pulmonary infections may exacerbate the course of children with chronic disease outside of the respiratory tract, such as chronic liver disease, metabolic diseases, or chronic renal failure.

CLINICAL EXAMINATION

In a child with a history suggestive of pneumonia, an examination should begin with observation of the child's breathing pattern. The respiratory rate should be measured; tachypnea is the most frequent sign of pneumonia in children. The amount of extra effort used for breathing can be assessed from the child's use of accessory muscles of respiration, or retraction of the sternum, intercostal spaces, or suprasternal spaces during inspiration. Flaring of the nares also indicates increased respiratory effort. A prolonged expiratory phase suggests outflow obstruction, as in foreign-body obstruction, asthma, or bronchiolitis. Very rapid respirations suggest parenchymal pulmonary disease. Pleuritic chest pain may be evident in the child who splints the involved area by lying on the affected side or holding support over the area. Irregular or gasping respirations in a young infant are an ominous sign portending respiratory failure.

Auscultatory findings in infants are less consistent than in older children. Transmission of sounds throughout the chest makes precise localization of sounds difficult. End-inspiratory crackling rales, so typical of pneumonia in older children, are seldom noted in young children who ventilate involved lung areas poorly. Rales can occasionally be elicited by requesting the older child to inspire deeply. For children too young to cooperate, careful "back and forth" comparison of sounds in the left and right chest may reveal areas of diminished breath sounds. Very noisy large airway sounds heard during both inspiration and expiration may be noted, especially in pneumonia caused by respiratory viruses. These viruses seldom cause pneumonia without antecedent or concurrent involvement of higher levels of the respiratory tract. Dullness to percussion over the lung suggests the possibility of pleural fluid or consolidation.

EPIDEMIOLOGIC FACTORS

Cases of pneumonia caused by communicable agents often occur in clusters. Awareness of outbreaks in a particular locale may therefore facilitate diagnosis of pneumonia in individual children (Table 70-1).

In the neonatal period, major bacterial pathogens include group B streptococci, *Listeria monocytogenes*, and enteric gram-negative bacilli. Chlamydial pneumonia has been diagnosed with increasing frequency. Viruses responsible for early neonatal pneumonia include rubella virus, cytomegalovirus, or herpesvirus.

Infants who are exposed postnatally to a respiratory viruses may also develop pneumonia. In early infancy (1 to 6 months), these commonly include respiratory syncytial virus, parainfluenza viruses, and adenovirus. Other viruses incriminated less frequently include the influenza viruses and enteroviruses. Beyond about 4 weeks of age, *Streptococcus pneumoniae* and *Haemophilus influenzae* assume their roles as the dominant bacterial pathogens. Pneumonia due to *Bordetella pertussis*, *Staphylococcus aureus*, *Streptococcus pyogenes*, gram-negative bacilli, or *Pneumocystis carinii* is recognized rarely.

After 6 months of age, respiratory syncytial virus is found less frequently as a cause of pneumonia. Important viral causes of pneumonia in young children 6 to 48 months old include the parainfluenza viruses, adenovirus, and Epstein-Barr virus. *Streptococcus pneumoniae* remains the predominant cause of bacterial pneumonia in this age group. *Haemophilus influenzae* is the next most frequent bacterial pathogen and occurs less frequently with advancing age. It is only occasionally found after 4 or 5 years of age. *Mycobacterium tuber-*

Table 70-1. Principal Causes of Pneumonia in Children

Newborn to 3 months	Young Children 1 month-5 years	School-Age Children
Group B streptococci	Respiratory syncytial virus	*M. pneumoniae*
Coliforms	Parainfluenza virus	*S. pneumoniae*
L. monocytogenes	*S. pneumoniae*	Influenza virus
Herpes simplex	*H. influenzae*	
Rubella	Adenovirus	
Cytomegalovirus	Epstein-Barr virus	
	Influenza virus	

culosis is now an uncommon pathogen but should be considered in any child with progressive or unresponsive pneumonia.

Viral agents seldom cause primary pneumonia in children older than 4 years. However, viral infections, particularly influenza viruses, predispose children to develop secondary bacterial pneumonia. *Streptococcus pneumoniae* remains an important bacterial pathogen, and *Mycoplasma pneumoniae* assumes a major role in school-age children. Rarely, pneumonia due to fungi, *Legionella*, or parasites may be seen.

In temperate climates, infections due to respiratory syncytial virus and influenza virus follow distinct seasonal patterns, with widespread wintertime outbreaks. Enteroviral infections characteristically occur in late summer. The parainfluenza viruses, adenoviruses, and Epstein-Barr virus cause infections throughout the year; local seasonal outbreaks of illness may occur. *Mycoplasma pneumoniae* infections increase in frequency during late fall, with fewer infections occurring during other seasons. Pneumococcal and *Haemophilus* infections occur predominantly in late fall to early spring but can be found at any time of year. Simultaneous illness in several members of a household suggests viral or *Mycoplasma* disease.

ROENTGENOGRAPHIC FINDINGS

Chest x-rays are frequently used to supplement information gained from the history and physical examination and may reveal unsuspected pulmonary infiltrates. The pattern of pulmonary infiltrates suggests the etiology of pneumonia. Widespread, patchy involvement of both lungs with perihilar densities is characteristic of respiratory viruses or *Mycoplasma*. A diffuse, homogeneous pattern is seen with neonatal group B streptococcal disease, *Pneumocystis*, cytomegalovirus, varicella-zoster virus, or *Chlamydia*. Segmental or lobar patterns, restricted to one lung, are noted with bacterial pneumonia, *Mycoplasma pneumoniae*, or airway obstruction.

Pulmonary effusions may be evident. They suggest bacterial infection, although occasionally such effusions are caused by *Mycoplasma*. Pleural fluid collections are most commonly due to *S. pneumoniae*; however, *H. influenzae*, *S. pyogenes*, and *S. aureus* should also be considered. Diagnostic thoracentesis may yield the offending organism by culture or by detection of bacterial antigen. Effusions complicate up to 10 percent of bacterial pneumonia and usually resolve with appropriate antibiotic therapy. Thick purulent fluid may indicate the need for continuous drainage via closed-chest tube suction.

Pulmonary hyperinflation is particularly characteristic of respiratory syncytial virus infections in infants. Involvement of smaller bronchioles results in air trapping; expiratory wheezing may be heard by auscultation of the chest. Hyperinflation may also be seen in foreign body aspiration. Partial obstruction of an airway creates a "ball-valve" effect, preventing release of trapped air. Left and right decubitus views or inspiratory-expiratory films reveal persistent hyperinflation of the obstructed area compared to normal areas of lung. Atelectasis of a portion of lung may lead to relative hyperinflation of other areas of lung.

Hilar lymphadenopathy suggests consideration of tuberculosis, fungal pneumonia, or malignancy. Enlarged hilar lymph nodes have also been described in *Mycoplasma* infections. Pneumatoceles or abscesses raise suspicion for staphylococcal or anerobic pneumonia.

Serial chest x-rays are of use in following the course of a clinically worsening or unresolving pneumonia. For children whose pneumonia is clinically improving with therapy, routine follow-up chest x-rays are not needed. Up to 25 percent of pulmonary infiltrates require longer than 1 month for radiologic resolution.

LABORATORY TESTS IN PNEUMONIA

For each child, individual consideration should guide the selection of laboratory studies. Commonly performed tests include a peripheral white cell count and differential, erythrocyte sedimentation rate, blood culture, sputum Gram stain and culture, cold agglutinins, and tests for detection of viral antigen (as for respiratory syncytial virus).

Very high peripheral white cell counts (above 18,000 cells/mm^3) with a left shift are suggestive of bacterial infection. Pneumococcal pneumonia, lung abscesses, and pneumonia with effusion classically produce the highest white cell counts. It is essential to note that infants normally have higher peripheral white cell counts than do adults. Normal or low white cell counts are sometimes found in overwhelming bacterial infections in infants and young children. A high white cell count with lymphocytosis may be seen in viral infections or in pertussis. Eosinophilia suggests chlamydial or parasitic infection.

The erythrocyte sedimentation rate frequently parallels the white cell count and is highest in bacterial infections. Use of both tests together increases the sensitivity for detecting bacterial infection. The sedimentation rate is frequently elevated in *M. pneumoniae*, infection, even though the peripheral white cell count is normal.

Blood cultures grow pathogens in only a minority—up to one-third—of cases of bacterial pneumonia. Yet, when positive, they provide helpful identification of the specific bacteria responsible. Such cultures should be considered when bacterial pneumonia is suspected.

Cultures of expectorated sputum may also identify a specific bacterial pathogen. A Gram-stained smear of sputum can be examined in suspected bacterial pneumonia and provide immediately useful information. Cultures are most reliable if the sputum sample contains polymorphonuclear white blood cells. Sputum can seldom be obtained satisfactorily from children younger than 6 to 8 years.

Cold agglutinins develop in response to a variety of infectious agents but are present in highest titer in mycoplasmal infections. They are positive in up to 90 percent of *M. pneumoniae* in adolescents but are less consistently positive in younger children. A rough but rapid qualitative test may be done at the bedside by placing several drops of anticoagulated blood in a tube, placing the tube in ice water until cold, and visually observing agglutinated blood. These cold agglutinins should disappear on warming of the tube and reappear when the blood is cooled again. Cold agglutinins are present in low titer early in the course of infection and increase rapidly. When *M. pneumoniae* is strongly suspected but cold agglutinins are absent, repeated measurements may demonstrate their development. More specific *M. pneumoniae* antibodies can be measured on paired sera obtained several weeks apart.

Rapid specific diagnosis of viral pneumonia is made possible by detection of viral antigen in respiratory secretions. Such tests are ordinarily reserved for children requiring hospitalization and facilitate antiviral chemotherapy. Usual methods employed include enzyme immunoassays or indirect fluorescent staining of antigen.

Other laboratory tests are useful in specific situations. Efforts at diagnosis should be more rigorous in children with severe disease, unusual courses, or immune deficiencies. Tests for common bacterial antigens may be performed on pleural fluid, urine, blood, or pulmonary secretions. Serologic tests can be performed for viral infections, fungal infections, and parasitic infections and on an experimental basis for tuberculosis. Total IgM antibody may be elevated in congenital viral infections or in chlamydial pneumonia. Skin testing should be performed if tuberculosis is possible. The proliferative response of sensitized lymphocytes has also been measured to detect previous exposure to tuberculosis. Material obtained directly from the lungs via bronchial washings, from endotrachael tubes, or by lung biopsy may permit precise diagnosis in severely affected children. Transtracheal aspiration of bronchial secretions is rarely performed because of hazardous, even fatal, complications which might occur.

SPECIFIC CAUSES OF PNEUMONIA

Group B Streptococci

Group B streptococcal pneumonia is primarily a disease of the newborn who is colonized with the organism at birth. Disease may be apparent at birth in infants infected in utero or may appear in the first few weeks of life. The incidence of group B streptococcal septicemia in recent years varied from 0.5 to 4 per 1000 live births; the incidence of pneumonia is lower. Very young infants with pneumonia due to streptococci or other bacteria are frequently bacteremic and may present with signs not readily attributable to the respiratory tract. Affected infants may have apneic episodes, diminished activity, poor feeding, or hypothermia or may exhibit tachypnea, grunting respirations, tachycardia, bradycardia, or cyanosis.

Chest x-rays in affected infants show evidence of diffuse pulmonary disease simulating hyaline membrane disease. All group B streptococci are susceptible to penicillin G, which is recommended for culture-proven infections. Some strains of streptococci are killed only by relatively high concentrations of penicillin G. In the laboratory, addition of aminoglycosides to penicillin provides a synergistic effect for such "tolerant" strains. Because bacterial pneumonia in young infants may be caused by other bacteria, such as coliforms or *Listeria,* a combination of ampicillin and gentamicin has been used for initial therapy of neonatal bacterial pneumonia before results of cultures are available. In the rare circumstances where staphylococci are particularly likely (empyema, pneumothorax, pneumatoceles), a penicillinase-resistant penicillin may be substituted for ampicillin.

Chlamydia

Pneumonia due to *C. trachomatis* typically presents between 4 and 11 weeks of age following colonization of the infant at birth. A history of conjunctivitis during the first few weeks of birth is noted in nearly half of affected infants. Such infants are afebrile and develop frequent "staccato" coughing followed by tachypnea increasing over several days. More than three-fourths have a prodrome extending back over 1 week at the time of presentation.

In contrast to infants with bacterial pneumonia, infants with chlamydial pneumonitis rarely appear systemically ill and may not have fever. Symptoms are related to the degree of respiratory involvement and resulting hypoxia. Infants seem quite alert and responsive, although remarkably tachypneic. On examination, infants have tachypnea, with respiratory rates up to 100 per minute. Auscultation reveals fine crepitant end-inspiratory rales diffusely. Such infants do not typically have the nasal congestion or large-airway sounds seen with respiratory viral pneumonia.

Infants with chlamydial pneumonia have modest eosinophilia and elevated levels of immunoglobulins compared with age-specific normal values. Diagnosis is confirmed by culture of *Chlamydia* in cell culture or by direct stains from nasopharyngeal swab specimens. Treatment with erythromycin usually results in clinical improvement. Other causes of afebrile pneumonia in young infants include cytomegalovirus, *Pneumocystis,* and respiratory viruses.

Respiratory Syncytial Virus

Respiratory syncytial virus (RSV) is unique in causing widespread outbreaks of serious disease yearly. The disease occurs in discrete sudden outbreaks. In temperate zones it occurs in 9- to 13-month intervals, usually during winter. Up to one-half of all infants are infected during the first year of life: about 1 out of each 100 infants so infected are admitted to hospital. The usual age of presentation is between 1 and 6 months. RSV is the single most important agent of bronchiolitis, causing over half of cases. RSV is also a major pathogen in pediatric viral pneumonia.

RSV in infants is often acquired from older household contacts who may have common cold symptoms. Following an incubation period of 4 to 6 days, infants develop nasal congestion. In the smallest infants, who are obligate nasal breathers, obstructed nares can occasionally lead to poor feeding, respiratory distress, or frank apnea. Over the succeeding 2 or 3 days, the virus spreads to involve the lower respiratory tract. Coughing develops, followed by audible wheezing, respiratory distress, or tachypnea. Fever is present, particularly in pneumonia, but is low-grade.

Some degree of bronchiolitis usually accompanies pneumonia, although either may occur alone. Examination of such infants reveals variable degrees of respiratory distress, tachypnea, or retractions. The infant is usually quite alert, unless fatigued by increased effort of breathing. Observation also reveals a prolonged expiratory phase of respiration and chest hyperexpansion. The liver is pushed down by the flattened diaphragm and is readily palpable. Auscultation demonstrates noisy large-airway sounds, variable degrees of expiratory wheezing, and inspiratory rales. Chest x-rays demonstrate hyperexpansion, with flattened diaphragms and patchy infiltrates throughout both lungs.

Morbidity due to respiratory syncytial virus infection is related to the presence of underlying diseases and is highest in the youngest infants. Infants with preexisting cardiac disease, particularly with pulmonary hypertension, are at highest risk of fatal disease. Infants with bronchopulmonary dysplasia or immune deficiency are also at high risk of serious disease.

Apnea is a frequent (up to 20 percent) complication of RSV in hospitalized infants with RSV infections. Infants in the first month or two of life and infants born prematurely are at highest risk of developing apnea. Otitis media has also been associated with RSV infection.

During an outbreak of RSV, the infection is readily identifiable by its presenting signs and symptoms. In young infants, parainfluenza viruses may also cause bronchiolitis and viral pneumonia. In those infants with minimal upper- and large-airway disease, bacterial pneumonia may be simulated. Congenital heart disease may be suspected and should be ruled out. Treatment of severely affected infants includes maintenance of hydration, monitoring of respiratory status, and provision of oxygen or ventilation if needed. Ribavirin, an antiviral compound effective against RSV, may be given in a small-particle aerosol to hospitalized children. Ribavirin may shorten the hospital course or lessen disease severity in some children. Indications for use of this costly drug are evolving at this time. Ribavirin aerosol should particularly be considered for severely ill infants and for infants with preexisting cardiorespiratory disease or immune deficiency. Inhaled β sympathomimetics, given as aerosols, have been beneficial for some infants with bronchiolitis.

Haemophilus influenzae

Haemophilus influenzae is the second most frequent bacterial cause of pneumonia in childhood, behind the pneumococcus. It is a disease of early childhood. Approximately half of cases occur during the first year of life and another one-fourth during the second year. Mild prodromal upper respiratory symptoms are followed by the sudden onset of higher fever, toxicity, cough, and prostration. Otitis media is found concomitantly in up to half of cases. Decreased breath sounds over the affected area are appreciated on auscultation of the chest. Consolidation is evident in three-fourths of cases; disease is bilateral in one-fouth. Pleural effusions are common. Peripheral white cell counts are variable. Leukocytosis above 18,000/mm^3 is found in half of children. White cell counts may be low in some children, particularly infants with septicemia.

A specific diagnosis of *Haemophilus* pneumonia is most frequently made when blood cultures yield the organism. Other foci of infection may also be found, including meningitis, epiglottitis, septic arthritis, or soft tissue infections. The diagnosis may be suspected by detection of *Haemophilus* bacterial antigen in urine or throat cultures growing abundant type B *Haemophilus.* Children with bacteremia should initially be treated parenterally in hospital. Up to 20 percent of *H. influenzae* type B are resistant to ampicillin. For this reason, children with bacteremic disease should be treated with antibiotics effective against both ampicillin-sensitive and ampicillin-resistant *Haemophilus* until results of sensitivity testing are available. These antibiotics include cefuroxime, cefotaxime, ceftriaxone, and chloramphenicol. Doses sufficiently high to attain bactericidal levels in cerebrospinal fluid should be used. Rifampin prophylaxis should be given to each member of the household if there are young household contacts exposed to invasive *Haemophilus* disease.

Streptococcus pneumoniae

The pneumococcus is the most common cause of bacterial pneumonia in all children beyond the first month of life. Onset of disease is characteristically abrupt, with high fever and cough, followed by tachypnea. Pleuritic chest pain and pleural effusion are observed in up to 10 percent of cases. Unilateral involvement of the lungs is the rule; lobar or segmental consolidations are seen. Pneumococcal pneumonia may be diagnosed during evaluation of otherwise asymptomatic children with fever. The peripheral white cell count is very high.

Penicillin is the drug of choice for known pneumococcal pneumonia. Dramatic resolution of fever can be expected. Persistent fever should raise suspicion of pleural fluid collections or alternative diagnoses.

Mycoplasma pneumoniae

Mycoplasma pneumoniae competes with *S. pneumoniae* as the most frequent cause of pneumonia in school-age and adolescent children. *Mycoplasma* is uncommon as a cause of pneumonia in children under 2 years.

These infections begin insidiously, without the abrupt, sudden onset characteristic of pneumococcal pneumonia. Many patients have prodromal symptoms of fever, cough, malaise, headache, and other nonspecific complaints for several days before seeking medical attention. Upper respiratory tract symptoms are unusual. Illness is frequently found in other family members, which helps to distinguish mycoplasmal infections from pneumococcal infections. Multiple-organ involvement is also noted frequently. Exanthemata are noted in 9 to 17 percent of patients. Arthritis, hematologic abnormalities, gastrointestinal complaints, and neurologic disease have also been associated with mycoplasmal infections.

Inspiratory rales are noted on auscultation of the chest. Expiratory wheezes are frequently heard. Involvement of the lung is protean and includes lobar or segmental consolidations, diffuse interstitial patterns, or patchy bronchopneumonia. Pleural effusions develop rarely. The peripheral white cell count is usually normal, but modest elevations may occur. The erythrocyte sedimentation rate is characteristically markedly elevated. The normal white count and elevated sedimentation rate distinguishes mycoplasmal infections from other bacterial pneumonia (in which the white cell count is elevated) and from viral pneumonia (in which the sedimentation rate is usually normal). Serum cold agglutinins develop in up to 90 percent of adolescents with pneumonia but are infrequently found in younger children.

Mycoplasma pneumoniae infections may be treated with erythromycin or tetracycline. Tetracyclines are not recommended for school-age or younger children because of adverse effects on teeth.

Pertussis

Pertussis (whooping cough) occurs following infection of susceptible individuals by *Bordetella pertussis*. Incompletely immunized infants and children are most frequently affected.

Following an incubation period of 6 to 20 days, symptoms begin with rhinorrhea, mild cough, low-grade fever, and mild conjunctivitis. Symptoms during this stage, the *catarrhal stage*, simulate the common cold. After a week of nonspecific upper respiratory tract symptoms, the *paroxysmal stage* begins. This stage, which lasts 2 to 6 weeks, is heralded by sudden paroxysms of unrelenting coughing. At the end of a prolonged coughing spell, one may hear the characteristic "whoop" caused by sudden, forceful inspiration. However, the whoop is often absent in infants. During severe paroxysms, children may develop signs of increased venous pressure (engorgement of neck veins, subconjunctival hemorrhage, intracranial hemorrhage) or pulmonary pressure (subcutaneous emphysema, pneumothorax). Respiratory distress during this stage may also be caused by mucus plugging, atelectasis, or pneumonia. Coughing paroxysms interfere with feeding, and dehydration is also a major presenting sign. During the *convalescent stage,* the severity and frequency of coughing paroxysms gradually diminish.

Pertussis may be suspected in the presence of typical clinical symptoms, and by a marked lymphocytosis (20,000 to 50,000/mm^3) which appears during the catarrhal stage in many, but not all, children. It may be confirmed by culture of nasal wash specimens on Bordet-Gengou media, or by detection of pertussis antigen on dried specimens.

Pneumonia is the most frequent complication of pertussis, and the most frequent cause of death. Pneumonia can be caused by *B. pertussis* itself, but is more commonly caused by other invasive bacteria. Erythromycin (50 mg/kg per day) should be given to children suspected of having pertussis. Household contacts less than 7 years of age should be immunized. All household contacts should also be given erythromycin prophylaxis (40 to 50 mg/kg per day up to 2 g/day for 14 days). Corticosteroids given during the paroxysmal stage improved symptoms in one study. If pneumonia is present, antibiotics (ampicillin, cefotaxime, ceftriaxone) to provide coverage for other bacteria should also be given.

PNEUMONIA IN IMMUNOCOMPROMISED CHILDREN

Children who have deficient immune mechanisms are susceptible to severe or fulminant pneumonia from opportunistic organisms as well as from the more usual childhood respiratory pathogens. Extra effort at precise etiologic diagnosis is warranted in such children. Invasive procedures, such as open lung biopsy, are sometimes required. Opportunistic pathogens responsible for pneumonia in immunodeficient children include cytomegalovirus, *P. carinii,* and *Candida* species, although a long list of opportunistic bacteria, fungi, parasites, and common viruses can cause severe pneumonia in such hosts. Neutropenic children with pneumonia should be hospitalized. While the patient is awaiting diagnostic testing, antibiotic combinations active against a broad spectrum of gram-positive cocci and gram-negative bacilli should be started. Examples of such combinations include ticarcillin-tobramycin or the combination of nafcillin or vancomycin plus ceftazidime.

Children with cystic fibrosis may have acute exacerbations of disease due to staphylococci or, more commonly, to *Pseudomonas aeruginosa*. Children with hypogammaglobulinemia often develop severe infections due to common pathogenic bacteria such as pneumococci or *Haemophilus*. Provision of exogenous immune globulin intravenously may be of benefit.

MANAGEMENT OF CHILDREN WITH PNEUMONIA

Decisions regarding admission to hospital should be individualized and based on the seventy and progression of disease, age of the child, presence of underlying disease, ability of caregivers to monitor the child's course, and presence of associated symptoms. In general, infants under 3 months of age, children with tachypnea above 40 to 50 breaths per minute, and "toxic" appearing children should be hospitalized.

Adequate hydration should be maintained with parenteral fluids if necessary. Parenteral nutrition may be required in some children with severe disease. Excessive levels of antidiuretic hormone are secreted by some children with pneumonia and may result in hyponatremia.

Appropriate specimens for culture should be obtained before antimicrobial therapy is instituted. Results from these cultures may be used to guide subsequent therapy.

For hospitalized children, monitoring and management of the respiratory status rivals antimicrobial therapy in importance. Oxygen should be provided to hypoxic children. Oxygen saturation can be monitored continuously by oximetry. In young infants, transcutaneous monitors can continuously monitor oxygen pressures. Blood-gas measurements should be performed in hypoxic children to assess acid-base status and measure carbon dioxide levels. Development of hypercarbia requires consideration of intubation and artificial ventilation. In infants, respiratory failure, acidosis, and apnea can develop precipitously. Those who fail to clear secretions or who are evidently in severe and increasing respiratory distress should be intubated on clinical grounds alone, without waiting for development of hypercarbia. Young infants with respiratory syncytial virus infections should be observed for development of apnea.

Antimicrobial therapy should be started on the basis of age and likely pathogens. In newborns, ampicillin plus gentamicin should be started. Infants between 1 and 3 months of age may develop pneumonia due to neonatal pathogens or due to bacteria found in childhood. A combination of ampicillin plus cefotaxime provides broad coverage against likely pathogens in this age group.

Children with bacterial pneumonia between 3 months and 5 or 6 years of age should be treated with antimicrobial agents effective against the two most frequent pathogens; *S. pneumoniae* and *H. influenzae*. Appropriate oral agents for children with mild disease include ampicillin or amoxicillin. Up to 20 percent of *Haemophilus* strains are resistant to ampicillin. Nonetheless, the much lower frequency of *Haemophilus* pneumonia as compared to pneumococcal pneumonia still permits amoxicillin therapy initially in most circumstances. Other considerations for outpatient therapy include amoxicillin-clavulanate, cefaclor, cefixime, cefuroxime, or erythromycin-sulfa. More seriously ill children should be treated parenterally in hospital. Ampicillin given intravenously remains a first choice. Dosages sufficiently high to attain protective levels in cerebrospinal fluid should be given initially. Other parenteral antimicrobial agents active against both *Haemophilus* and pneumococci include cefuroxime, cefotaxime, ceftriaxone, ampicillin-chloramphenicol, and ampicillin-sulbactam.

Erythromycin is preferred for initial therapy of mild to moderate pneumonia in school-age and adolescent children, particularly when the white cell count is normal. This agent is active against both pneumococci and *Mycoplasma*. Erythromycin is not active against *Haemophilus*, but such infections are uncommon in this age group. In all age groups, added coverage for staphylococcal pneumonia should be considered if disease is fulminant.

BIBLIOGRAPHY

Boyer KM, Cherry JD: Nonbacterial pneumonia, in Feigin RD, Cherry JD (eds): *Textbook of Pediatric Infectious Diseases*. 2d ed. Philadelphia, Saunders, 1987.

Bruhn FW, Mokrohisky ST, McIntosh K: Apnea associated with respiratory syncytial virus infection in young infants. *J Pediatr* 90:382, 1977.

Cherry JD: Mycoplasma and ureaplasma infections, in Feigin RD, Cherry JD (eds): *Textbook of Pediatric Infectious Diseases*, 2d ed. Philadelphia, Saunders, 1987.

Cherry JD, Hurwitz ES, Welliver RD: Mycoplasma pneumoniae infections and exantherns. *J Pediatr* 87:369, 1975.

Cohen GJ: Management of infections of the lower respiratory tract in children. *Ped Infect Dis J* 6:317, 1987.

Ginsburg CM, Howard JB, Nelson JD: Report of 65 cases of Haemophilus influenzae pneumonia. *Pediatrics* 64:283, 1979.

Hail CB: Respiratory syncytial virus, in Feigin RD. Cherry JD (eds): *Textbook of Pediatric Infectious Diseases*. 2d ed, Philadelphia, Saunders, 1987.

Hall CB, McBride JT, Walsh EE, et al: Aerosolized ribavirin treatment of infants with respiratory syncytial viral infection. *N Engl J Med* 308:143, 1983.

Klein JO: Bacterial pneumonias, in Feigin RD, Cherry JD (eds): *Textbook of Pediatric Infectious Diseases*. 2d ed. Philadelphia, Saunders, 1987.

Peter G, Lepow ML, McGacken GH Jr, et al (eds): Report of the Committee on Infectious Diseases, 22d ed. American Academy of Pediatrics, Elk Grove Village, Ill, 1991.

Stagno S, Brasfield DM, Brown MB, et al: Infant pneumonitis associated with cytomegalovirus. Chlamydia, Pneumocystis, and Ureaplasma: A prospective study. *Pediatrics* 68:322, 1981.

Stagno SS, Pifer LL, Hughes WT, et al: Pneumocystis carinii pneumonitis in young immunocompetent infants. *Pediatrics* 66:56, 1980.

Taber LH, Knight V, Gilbert BE, et al: Ribavirin aerosol treatment of bronchiolitis associated with respiratory syncytial virus infection in infants. *Pediatrics* 72:613, 1983.

Tipple MA, Beem MO, Saxon EM: Clinical characteristics of the afebrile pneumonia associated with Chlamydia trachomatis infection in infants less than 6 months of age. *Pediatrics* 63:192, 1979.

Turner RB, Hayden FG, Hendley JO: Counterimmunoelectrophoresis of urine for diagnosis of bacterial pneumonia in pediatric outpatients. *Pediatrics* 71:780, 1983.

71 URINARY TRACT INFECTIONS AND VULVOVAGINITIS

Denise J. Fligner

URINARY TRACT INFECTIONS IN CHILDREN

Urinary tract infection (UTI) is an important problem in pediatrics. UTI in young children is associated with significant later morbidity, including renal insufficiency and hypertension; the majority of damage occurs before 5 years of age. The goals of diagnosis are to provide relief for acute symptoms, to prevent damage to the upper urinary tract, and to identify those children at risk for late complications.

Incidence

The incidence of UTI varies with age and sex. In infants younger than 3 months, the rate of bacteriuria is 1 percent. In febrile infants (temperature >38.1°C) the rate increases tenfold and ranges from 7 to 17 percent. Infection is two to three times more common in boys than in girls, and 80 to 90 percent of male infant UTIs occur in uncircumcised boys. Sepsis associated with UTI is reported in 10 to 35 percent of infants.

Past 3 months of age, girls are at many times greater risk of both bacteriuria and symptomatic infection, and this risk persists in adults. School-age girls have a 1- to 2-percent prevalence of bacteriuria, compared to less than 0.1-percent prevalence in boys. The cumulative risk of UTI in girls is 3 to 5 percent.

Microbiology

Bacteria usually enter the urinary tract system following colonization of the urethral meatus with perineal flora. Gram-negative enteric bacteria are thus the most common organisms found in UTI. *Escherichia coli* accounts for 90 percent of acute, uncomplicated infections. Other pathogens include *Klebsiella* and *Enterobacter* species. *Staphylococcus saprophyticus* is common in adolescent girls. Enterococci, *Proteus* species, and *Pseudomonas* are more likely with recurrent infections and in children receiving antibiotic prophylaxis for chronic infections.

Clinical Findings

Infants and young children present with nonspecific complaints including unexplained fever, irritability, vomiting, diarrhea, feeding problems, and failure to thrive. Older children may complain of abdominal pain. Toilet-trained children may develop enuresis or urge incontinence (dribbling) and complain of dysuria and frequency. Constipation is frequently present.

Findings on physical examination are usually minimal. There may be suprapubic or abdominal tenderness; flank pain suggests upper urinary tract infection but is not specific for pyelonephritis. The external genitals of all children who present with dysuria or other symptoms of UTI should be specifically examined for vulvovaginitis in girls and urethritis in boys.

Diagnosis

The diagnosis of UTI requires urine culture. Presumptive diagnosis based on clinical symptoms or urinalysis is unreliable. Confirmation of UTI by culture has critical importance in children under 5 years of age because of the prognostic implications of UTI in this age group.

Bacteriuria

Microscopic examination of fresh, unspun urine provides a rapid, reliable estimate of probable culture results. One bacterium per high-power field (hpf) seen in unspun urine correlates well with growth of greater than 10^5 colonies on urine culture.

Pyuria

The presence of leukocytes in spun urine is suggestive of UTI but not diagnostic. Pyuria (>10 leukocytes/hpf of spun urine) can be found in gastroenteritis, vulvovaginitis, appendicitis, and other acute abdominal conditions. Pyuria is also common in the sexually transmitted diseases (STDs). Of greater concern, pyuria is often absent in culture-positive bacteriuria; in infants with culture-proven UTI, less than half have pyuria.

Specimen Collection

Specimen collection for culture in infants and young children is problematic. Bag specimens are easily contaminated by fecal and skin flora even following proper cleansing of the perineum. In addition, the specimen usually remains in contact with the perineum for an undetermined length of time, allowing for overgrowth of bacteria. A negative culture from bag urine reliably excludes UTI. Positive bag urine cultures (and indeterminant results) are unreliable in the diagnosis of UTI and must be confirmed by a suprapubic or catheterized specimen. In young children, if antibiotics are to be started pending culture results, it is crucial that urine for culture first be obtained by bladder catheterization or suprapubic aspiration. In older children, a midstream clean-catch specimen obtained following careful cleansing of the genitals is adequate. The specimen should be plated immediately or refrigerated at 4°C (39.2°F) to prevent bacterial overgrowth.

Culture Results

The definition of a positive culture depends on the method of collection. In fresh urine obtained from a midstream clean-catch specimen, the presence of 10^5 colonies of a single organism per milliliter of urine is diagnostic. The probability of infection with one positive culture is 80 percent; with two separately collected positive cultures it is 90 percent. Colony counts between 10^4 and 10^5 are uninterpretable and should be repeated. Colony counts less than 10^4 or the presence of two or more organisms indicates contamination. Several factors may lower the colony count in the presence of significant infection. These factors include dilution, low urine pH and specific gravity, recent antibiotic therapy, fastidious organisms, inappropriate culture techniques, bacteriostatic agents in the urine, and complete obstruction of the ureter.

The presence of greater than 10^3 colonies per milliliter of urine in a catheterized specimen or any bacteria in a suprapubic specimen indicates infection.

Differential Diagnosis

Dysuria can be the presenting complaint in urethral, vulvar, and vaginal inflammation. Vulvovaginitis is a far more common cause of dysuria than is UTI. Dysuria due to vulvar inflammation can often be distinguished by older adolescents and adults as being external, in contrast to the deeper discomfort that occurs with UTI. Dysuria from UTI is usually associated with urinary frequency.

Pyuria and dysuria with negative urine cultures is frequently seen with *Neisseria gonorrhoea, Chlamydia trachomatis,* and *Trichomonas* in both sexes. In adolescent boys, sterile pyuria is strongly suggestive of sexually transmitted urethritis.

Complications

Reflux nephropathy, previously termed chronic pyelonephritis, is the major preventable cause of renal insufficiency in childhood. The main determinants of renal scarring in children are vesicoureteral reflux (VUR), obstruction, UTI during the first year of life, and delay in diagnosis and treatment. Almost half of children less than 1 year of age with UTI have vesicoureteral reflux or other significant abnormalities. In boys, this is usually a structural abnormality. In girls with a first UTI, 25 to 30 percent have significant reflux. Vesicoureteral reflux (VUR) predisposes the child with UTI to renal scarring, which progresses with each subsequent infection. After 5 years of age, the likelihood of progressive damage from reflux decreases.

Management

Following proper collection of a specimen for culture, treatment of the symptomatic patient may be started pending culture results. In the afebrile, nontoxic patient, outpatient therapy can be instituted with oral antibiotics. Amoxicillin (50 mg/kg per day in three doses), sulfisoxazole (150 mg/kg per day), or trimethoprim/sulfamethoxazole (TMP/SMX; 6 to 8 mg/kg per day TMP, 30 to 40 mg/kg per day SMX in two doses) are reasonable choices. Since resistance develops rapidly to amoxicillin and sulfonamides, TMP/SMX or TMP alone is preferred for suspicion of pyelonephritis, recurrences, and prophylaxis. The new fluoroquinolones are neither approved by the U.S. Food and Drug Administration nor recommended for routine therapy in childhood UTI because of possible toxicity to cartilage of weight-bearing joints.

Duration of Therapy

Treatment for 5 to 7 days in uncomplicated UTI is adequate, while longer courses promote candidiasis and diarrhea. Upper tract infection should be treated for 10 days. Single-dose therapy is not recommended in children because, although the cure rate at 48 h is comparable to that for conventional therapy, the recurrence rate at 10 days is unacceptably high.

Hospitalization and parenteral therapy are preferred for infants under 3 months of age; for children who appear toxic, febrile, or unable to tolerate oral therapy; and when pyelonephritis is suspected. Parenteral ampicillin alone or in combination with an aminoglycoside is used initially. Antibiotic therapy should be adjusted once culture results and sensitivities are known.

Prophylaxis

Prophylaxis is recommended in children with recurrent UTI, children under 5 to 7 years of age with vesicoureteral reflux, and children awaiting radiologic evaluation following a first UTI. A single nightly dose of TMP/SMX (1 to 2 mg/kg TMP, 5 to 10 mg/kg SMX) is effective.

Asymptomatic Bacteriuria

In the child with a radiologically normal urinary tract, asymptomatic bacteriuria does not require treatment.

Follow-up

Children with UTI should be seen within 48 h to assess the clinical response and obtain repeat cultures. Additional cultures should be done following cessation of therapy to exclude persistent bacteriuria or recurrence. The risk of recurrence after the first infection is 30 percent and increases to 75 percent in children with three or more previous infections. Children with a documented UTI need periodic examination and culture of the urine.

Radiologic Evaluation

The majority of children should have radiologic evaluation of the urinary tract system within 2 to 4 weeks following the first documented UTI. The goals of radiographic evaluation are to diagnose structural abnormalities of the urinary tract system, to determine the presence and severity of vesicoureteral reflux, and to assess the renal parenchyma for scarring.

Voiding cystourethrography is done initially to evaluate vesicoureteral reflux and to delineate structural abnormalities of the lower urinary tract. Intravenous pyelography has been the standard test for evaluation of the upper urinary tract and to detect renal scars; it is still preferred by some when severe reflux is present. Ultrasonography may substitute for intravenous pyelography in some centers. It is most commonly recommended for renal imaging in infants and for screening the upper urinary tract in children without reflux. Nuclear renal scanning has been used in the evaluation and follow-up of documented reflux and scarring.

PEDIATRIC VULVOVAGINITIS

Vulvovaginitis is a common problem in females of all ages. Estrogen effects are a major determinant of susceptibility to vulvovaginitis; therefore, the likely causes vary with physiologic age and stage of pubertal development. The neonate shows the effects of intrauterine maternal estrogen stimulation. In the prepubertal girl, unestrogenized vulvar skin is thin, easily inflamed, and unprotected by the adult labial fat pads and pubic hair. The vulva is vulnerable to trauma, contact irritants, and bacterial contamination from both proximity to the anus and typical childhood hygiene. Puberty moves the spectrum of vulvovaginitis toward infections that prefer estrogenized vaginal epithelium. The causes of vulvovaginitis in adolescent girls are similar to those in adult women and are likewise effected by sexual experience. This section focuses on vulvovaginitis in prepubertal and peripubertal girls; the diagnosis and treatment of adult vulvovaginitis (Chapter 56) and sexually transmitted disease (Chapter 81) apply to sexually active adolescents and are not reviewed here. Table 71-1 lists the causes of pediatric vulvovaginitis.

Clinical Findings

Vulvar inflammation can cause redness, itching, and burning. Squirming and an awkward walk may be seen in younger children. Dysuria

Table 71-1. Causes of Pediatric Vulvovaginitis

Vulvitis and nonspecific inflammation
Nonspecific vulvovaginitis: poor hygiene, local irritants
Enterobius vermicularis (pinworms)
Candida albicans and other yeasts
Vaginal infections
Respiratory: group A and B streptococci, *Streptococcus pneumoniae, Neisseria meningitidis, Hemophilus influenzae**
Skin: *Staphylococcus aureus**
Enteric: *Shigella, Yersinia, Escherichia coli**
Sexually transmitted infections
Vaginitis: *Neisseria gonorrhoea, Chlamydia trachomatis, Trichomonas vaginalis, Gardnerella vaginalis**
Vulvitis: condyloma acuminata, herpes simplex
Vulvar skin disease and systemic illness
Childhood exanthems: measles, chicken pox, scarlet fever
Generalized skin disorders: seborrheic and atopic dermatitis
Infestations: scabies, pediculosis, molluscum contagiosum
Noninfectious causes
Trauma
Sexual misuse
Foreign body: toilet paper wads, tampons
Structural anomalies of the genitourinary tract

* Can be found as normal vaginal flora (in asymptomatic children).

is a common symptom and more often caused by vulvovaginitis than by UTI. A complaint of vaginal discharge suggests a specific infectious etiology, although a persistent, foul, or bloody discharge also occurs with retained foreign bodies. On examination, inflammation of the vulva and distal vagina should be distinguished from a primary vaginitis without prominent vulvar symptoms.

Etiology by Age and Pubertal Status

The Infant

A physiologic vaginal discharge commonly occurs in newborn girls during the first 2 weeks of life due to intrauterine estrogen stimulation. The discharge may become slightly bloody secondary to maternal estrogen withdrawal. During this time, the infant's estrogenized vagina is also susceptible to candidiasis and, less commonly, to trichomoniasis, which are acquired from the mother during vaginal delivery. Maternally transmitted condyloma may appear up to 1 year of age.

The Prepubertal Girl

Approach to the Child

The general appearance, hygiene, and pubertal stage according to Tanner classification should be noted and the child examined for signs of systemic illness and dermatologic disorders. Thorough inspection of the perineum and external genitals provides sufficient examination for most children with symptoms of vulvovaginitis. Young girls may be more comfortably examined while sitting on their parent's lap with their legs placed outside the parent's legs. The child's perineum is then easily exposed by having the parent recline slightly and spread his or her own legs. The perineal skin, perianal area, labia majora, labia minora, and periurethral area are observed for signs of inflammation and trauma. The hymen and distal vagina are inspected by outward traction on the posterior labia majora. Signs of sexual abuse should be specifically looked for and the shape, width, and any irregularities of the hymen noted. If sexual misuse is suspected or vaginal discharge is present, specimens should be collected for microscopic examination and cultures; however, a discharge is found in only half the children with this complaint. Specimens are collected by gentle swabbing with a moistened applicator or by aspiration following saline irrigation. The cooperative child should be further examined in a prone knee-chest position, which allows visualization of the upper vagina and often the cervix. Vaginoscopy is indicated acutely for vaginal bleeding, suspicion of foreign body, and trauma. Vaginoscopy for persistent symptoms following treatment may be deferred to the pediatric gynecologist. Bimanual rectal examination is helpful to assess for masses and foreign bodies and to milk any discharge from the vagina.

Vulvitis

Nonspecific Vulvovaginitis

The most common condition in this age group, nonspecific vulvovaginitis is defined by lack of any identifiable pathogen or etiology. On examination, the vulva is erythematous and swollen, with secondary inflammation of the distal vagina. Discharge is usually scanty. Excoriations and, in severe cases, ulcerations may be present. Cultures, when done, grow mixed vaginal and enteric flora. Multiple factors contribute to inflammation of the vulva. Management consists of eliminating local and chemical irritants and improving hygiene by the use of absorbent cotton underpants, loose clothing, bland soaps, front-to-rear wiping after bowel movements, and frequent handwashing. For severe inflammation, cool sitz baths or wet compresses will provide relief within 2 to 3 days. Amoxicillin may be tried for cases resistent to conservative therapy.

Enterobius vermicularis

Enterobius vermicularis should be routinely tested for, since 20 percent of infestations have an associated vulvovaginitis characterized by prominent nocturnal itching.

Candidiasis

Candidiasis is far less common than nonspecific vulvovaginitis in prepubertal girls, and topical antifungal treatment should be based only on microscopic diagnosis. Factors associated with candidiasis include recent antibiotic therapy, diabetes mellitus, underlying skin disorders, and exogenous estrogen exposure.

Specific Vaginal Infections

Respiratory and Enteric Pathogens

Respiratory and enteric pathogens develop primarily or concurrently with infection at another site. Transmission occurs through autoinoculation, and handwashing should be stressed for treatment and prevention. A bloody discharge suggests *Shigella* or group A streptococcus; both can occur without signs of infection at another site. Diagnosis is by culture, and treatment is an antibiotic appropriate to the organism.

Foreign Bodies

Foreign bodies, most commonly wads of toilet paper, cause a persistent, foul, or bloody discharge and are found in 4 percent of symptomatic children. Vaginoscopy is required for diagnosis and to assure complete removal.

Candida, Trichomonas,* and *Gardnerella vaginalis

The three primary causes of vaginitis in adults, *Candida, Trichomonas,* and *Gardnerella vaginalis,* are all unusual in prepubertal girls because the unestrogenized vaginal epithelium is relatively resistant to these organisms. Typical clinical and microscopic features are usually adequate for diagnosis; unclear or persistent cases may require culture.

Sexually Transmitted Infections

Prepubertal Gonorrhea

Prepubertal gonorrhea presents as a vaginitis rather than the endocervicitis typical past puberty. The primary symptoms are dysuria; purulent vaginal discharge; and, less commonly, abdominal pain. Culture is mandatory for diagnosis and documentation, since nongonococcal *Neisseria* can also cause infection. Asymptomatic infection is usual and has been found in one-third of children residing in the household of an infected child. In culture-proven gonorrhea, all household members should have cultures of the vagina (urethra in boys), rectum, and pharynx.

Other STDs

Gonorrhea, *Chlamydia, Trichomonas,* genital herpes, and condylomata acuminata usually indicate sexual contact. *Gardnerella* can be cultured from asymptomatic girls, but symptomatic infection is found more commonly in girls who report sexual misuse. Although nonsexual transmission of most sexually transmitted pathogens has been suggested, their presence should prompt a thorough investigation into possible sexual misuse of the child.

The Pubertal Girl

Pubertal girls and adolescents are more likely than younger girls to have an infectious cause for vulvovaginitis, although nonspecific cases and retained foreign bodies also occur in this age group. The onset of sexual activity increases the incidence of sexually transmitted infections and the occurrence of pelvic inflammatory disease. A speculum examination should be performed in most adolescents; it may be omitted in the young virginal girl with physiologic discharge or candidiasis. Bimanual examination is necessary to assess for pelvic tenderness. The examination offers a good opportunity to discuss proper hygiene, the virtues of safe sexual practices, and contraception.

Physiologic Vaginal Discharge

The onset of pubertal estrogenic influence precedes menarche by up to a year; the timing corresponds roughly to breast bud development. Estrogen results in a physiologic discharge, often termed leukorrhea, which is composed of mucus and normal vaginal epithelial cells without leukocytes. The discharge is mucoid or gray-white, odorless, and generally nonirritating. The amount increases prior to menarche, and minor irritation can result from copious discharge, especially if nonabsorbent underpants are worn. Yellow staining of the underpants, a common complaint, is due to the protein content, which discolors when heated during washing. No treatment is necessary other than reassurance that this is a healthy sign of puberty and advising absorbent cotton underpants if the discharge is copious or irritating.

Vaginitis and STD

Candidiasis occurs in the pubertal girl both before and after menarche and is the most common cause of pruritic vulvovaginitis in premenarchal pubertal girls. *G. vaginalis* deserves mention because it is found in normal vaginal flora of asymptomatic girls. A diagnosis of bacterial vaginosis associated with *G. vaginalis* is reserved for symptomatic patients and requires a gray-white vaginal discharge with a characteristic fishy odor (positive ''whiff'' test when KOH is added) in addition to clue cells on microscopic examination. Asymptomatic patients do not require treatment. Since both bacterial vaginosis and *Trichomonas* are suggestive of sexual activity, any adolescent with *Trichomonas* or bacterial vaginosis should also have cultures for gonorrhea and *Chlamydia*.

BIBLIOGRAPHY

Vulvovaginitis

Altchek A: Pediatric vulvovaginitis. *J Reprod Med* 29:359, 1984.

Emans SJ: Vulvovaginitis in the child and adolescent. *Pediatr Rev* 8:12, 1986.

Farmer MY, Hook EW, Heald FP: Laboratory evaluation of sexually transmitted diseases. *Pediatr Ann* 15:715, 1986.

Rosenfeld WD, Clark J: Vulvovaginitis and cervicitis. *Pediatr Clin North Am* 36:489, 1989.

Williams TS, Callen JP, Owen LG: Vulvar disorders in the prepubertal female. *Pediatr Ann* 15:588, 1986.

Urinary Tract Infections

Alon U, Berant M, Pery M: Intravenous pyelography in children with urinary tract infection and vesicoureteral reflux. *Pediatrics* 83:332, 1989.

Burns MW, Burns JL, Krieger JN: Pediatric urinary tract infection. *Pediatr Clin North Am* 34:1111, 1987.

Crain EF, Gershel JC: Urinary tract infections in febrile infants younger than 8 weeks of age. *Pediatrics* 86:363, 1990.

Magill HL, Riggs W, Boulden TF, et al: Diagnostic imaging in children with urinary tract infection: Review of current concepts and suggested guidelines. *South Med J* 80:1557, 1987.

McCracken GH: Diagnosis and management of acute urinary tract infections in infants and children. *Pediatr Infect Dis J* 6:107, 1987.

McCracken GH: Options in antimicrobial management of urinary tract infections in infants and children. *Pediatr Infect Dis J* 8:552, 1989.

72
ASTHMA AND BRONCHIOLITIS

Stanley H. Inkelis

Asthma is a disorder of the tracheobronchial tree characterized by bronchial hyperirritability and subsequent obstruction to airflow after exposure to any one of many stimuli. Examples of these stimuli include extrinsic allergens, viral respiratory infections, vigorous exercise, cold air, cigarette smoke, and air pollutants. Narrowing of the airways is dynamic and improves either spontaneously or as a result of therapy. The symptom which is most characteristic of asthma is wheezing. However, the often-quoted statement, "all that wheezes is not asthma" is certainly true, and emphasizes the importance of the differential diagnosis which will be addressed later in this chapter. Asthma may occur, on the other hand, without evidence of overt wheezing and is often missed in children who are diagnosed as having recurrent pneumonia, recurrent or chronic bronchitis, or recurrent colds with chest congestion. Because misdiagnosis and undertreatment occur frequently, some authors feel that a more appropriate statement may be, "most things that wheeze, plus some things that do not, are asthma."

Asthma is one of the leading causes of chronic illness in children, with a prevalence rate of 5 to 12 percent. About 80 to 90 percent of children with asthma have their first symptoms before 4 to 5 years of age. One review of children admitted with status asthmaticus to a children's hospital found a doubling of admissions for asthma between 1973 and 1987. In a group of 100 patients admitted between February and June 1988, demographic data indicated that these patients tended more often to be young, male, and black than did other patients admitted to the same hospital. Forty-five percent of these patients also had sinusitis, otitis, or pneumonitis. Although there was not an increase in mortality in asthmatic patients in this study, many others have reported an increase in the number of deaths from asthma over similar time periods. Children at risk of dying from asthma are those who (1) have been intubated for asthma; (2) have had two or more hospitalizations for asthma in the past year; (3) have had three or more emergency department visits for asthma in the past year; (4) have had an emergency department visit or hospitalization for asthma in the past month; and/or (5) use systemic steroids.

In children dying of asthma, the assessment of the severity of their illness by both patient and physician is often inadequate. In addition, compliance with medication schedules is poor in these patients, and there is frequently a delay in the initiation of therapy for progressively worsening illness.

Although there has been an increase in morbidity and mortality in recent years, the prognosis for asthmatic children in general is very good. About half of these children will be free of symptoms by the time they are adults.

Bronchiolitis is the term used to describe a clinical syndrome in infancy characterized by rapid respiration, chest retractions, and wheezing. It typically occurs during the winter and spring months, more often in male than female infants less than 2 years of age, with the greatest frequency between the ages of 2 and 6 months.

ETIOLOGY

The etiology of asthma is multifactorial. Immunologic, infectious, endocrine, and psychological factors play a role in the development of asthma in different individuals. Rather than being one disease, asthma may, in fact, be a number of diseases that have in common the physiological finding of reversible obstructive airway changes.

Asthma is usually categorized as extrinsic (atopic or IgE-mediated), intrinsic (nonatopic, usually triggered by infection), mixed, and exercise-induced. In extrinsic asthma, the most common type of asthma seen in children, environmental factors such as dust, pollens, dander, molds, tobacco smoke, and foods are the cause of bronchial hyperirritability. Antibodies (IgE) are produced in response to allergens and bind to receptors of mast cells. Interaction with the antigens causes the release of mediators of inflammation such as histamine and leukotrienes. In children with intrinsic asthma, no evidence of IgE involvement is found. There is little correlation with skin tests and known allergens. This type of asthma is seen most frequently in the first 2 years of life and in adults. The precipitant of asthma in these individuals is usually viral respiratory infection, most commonly caused by the respiratory syncytial and parainfluenza viruses. In mixed asthma, symptoms are worsened by both extrinsic and intrinsic factors.

Exercise-induced asthma (EIA) is seen in patients with asthma of all types but may also be the only manifestation of asthma such as in the child with allergic rhinitis. There is no relationship between the degree of EIA and the severity of asthma. The type of exercise influences the extent of the airway obstruction. For example, running causes more severe symptoms than bicycling, whereas swimming rarely causes bronchial hyperactivity. As ventilation increases with exercise, airways are cooled by the loss of water to the relatively dry air. It is postulated that mast cells respond to this cooling by releasing mediators which induce bronchoconstriction.

The most common cause of bronchiolitis is the respiratory syncytial virus (RSV). It is the etiologic agent in approximately 75 percent of infants admitted to the hospital with this disorder. Other organisms which cause bronchiolitis are parainfluenza virus, influenza virus, mumps virus, adenovirus, echovirus, rhinovirus, *Mycoplasma pneumoniae*, and *Chlamydia trachomatis*. Adenovirus, particularly types 3, 7, and 21, may cause a more destructive form of bronchiolitis, known as bronchiolitis obliterans, a chronic, obstructive lung disease.

PATHOPHYSIOLOGY

Most of the information available regarding the pathology of asthma comes from postmortem examination. The lungs are hyperinflated and pale and are difficult to collapse with pressure. Numerous tenacious mucous plugs exude from the larger and middle-sized bronchi. On microscopic examination, sloughing of mucosal cells, edema of the bronchial mucosa, and hyperplasia and hypertrophy of bronchial and bronchiolar smooth muscle are seen. Often, there is infiltration of the submucosa by eosinophils.

In the past, bronchial smooth muscle hyperreactivity has been considered the main reason for the pathological findings associated with asthma. Hyperreactive airways play a major role in the pathology of the asthmatic patient, particularly in the new-onset asthmatic or in the early phase of an asthmatic attack. In patients with chronic asthma, inflammation of the airways plays an equal or greater role in the pathological changes. Biopsies of bronchial tissue as well as bronchoalveolar lavage have demonstrated an increased proportion of inflammatory cells, particularly eosinophils and lymphocytes.

Bronchial smooth muscle hyperreactivity is characteristic of asthma. The smooth muscle lining the respiratory tract is under autonomic control, with sympathetic fibers causing bronchodilation (β_2 receptors) and parasympathetic fibers causing bronchoconstriction.

The eosinophil is the inflammatory cell most characteristic of asthma. These cells release proteins that are toxic to airway epithelial cells. In one study, the number of peripheral blood eosinophils and levels of eosinophils and eosinophil cationic protein in bronchoalveolar lavage fluid correlated with the severity of asthma. In addition, intraepithelial eosinophils were present only in patients with asthma.

Neutrophil infiltration is not commonly found in asthmatic patients. T lymphocytes are commonly found in the airways of asthmatic patients, but their role is uncertain. Mediators released from T lymphocytes may affect the eosinophils and their function in airway inflammation.

Numerous inflammatory mediators contribute to pathological findings in the asthmatic patient. IgE-sensitized mast cells, which are antigenically stimulated, begin a reaction that results in the release of preformed mediators, including histamine, chemotactic factors, proteases, and platelet-activation factor (PAF). Metabolism of membrane phospholipids is also activated to release arachidonic acid, which is metabolized to form the generated mediators, leukotrienes, thromboxanes, and prostaglandins. These mediators are responsible for bronchial hyperreactivity, edema, and mucus formation as well as chemotaxis for other inflammatory cells, which release more mediators and continue the inflammatory process.

The early phase of an asthmatic attack is characterized by bronchoconstriction secondary to release of histamines and leukotrienes. Chemotactic factors, PAF, and other mediators bring on inflammatory cells, which cause the late phase of an asthmatic attack. This phase begins 2 to 8 h later and is characterized by airway hyperreactivity lasting for days to weeks.

The combination of mucosal edema, bronchospasm, and mucous plugging results in airway obstruction which leads to increased airway resistance and gas trapping. Varying degrees of obstruction, atelectasis, and decreased compliance cause ventilation-perfusion mismatch. Hypoxia occurs because of perfusion of inadequately ventilated portions of the lung. Early in severe asthma, carbon dioxide tensions are usually below normal because of compensatory hyperventilation. As the obstruction increases, the number of alveoli being adequately ventilated and perfused decreases, giving rise to CO_2 retention. A "normal" P_{CO_2} of 40 mmHg in the setting of asthma may be an indication of respiratory muscle fatigue and impending respiratory failure.

Acidosis results from both hypoxia and hypercapnia. Along with hypoxia, acidosis leads to pulmonary vasoconstriction, pulmonary hypertension, right heart strain, and, occasionally, cardiac failure.

Infants with asthma have more severe respiratory symptoms and are more vulnerable to respiratory failure. The anatomic and physiological reasons for this are (1) increased peripheral airway resistance, (2) decreased elastic recoil pressure and early airway closure, (3) deficient collateral channels of ventilation, and (4) an unstable rib cage and mechanically disadvantaged diaphragm.

The most important pulmonary lesion associated with bronchiolitis is bronchiolar obstruction characterized by submucosal edema, peribronchiolar cellular infiltrate, mucous plugging, and intraluminal debris. These pathological changes lead to narrowing of the lumens of small bronchi and bronchioles, increasing airway resistance, and concomitant wheezing. The obstruction is not uniform throughout the lungs, so that some of the small bronchi and bronchioles are affected while others are not. However, normal exchange of gases in the lung is impaired. Hypoxia is the major result of abnormal gas exchange in which alveoli are poorly ventilated but remain well perfused (ventilation-perfusion imbalance). Compensation for the hypoxia results in hyperventilation, which is a more sensitive indicator of reduced oxygen tension than is cyanosis. Carbon dioxide retention does not occur in mild cases of bronchiolitis, but in more severe cases where larger numbers of alveoli are obstructed, hypercapnia and respiratory acidosis ensue. Carbon dioxide retention is associated with respiratory rates of greater than 60 and increases in proportion to the increasing rate.

Clinical Findings

Wheezing is the hallmark of asthma and is present in almost every child presenting to the emergency department with this disorder. The notable exceptions to this are (1) the child who is in extreme respiratory distress and is so "tight" that there is not enough movement of air to produce audible wheezing and (2) the child who has a persistent nonproductive cough or who coughs and becomes short of breath with exercise. In the latter case, many of the patients will have findings characteristic of asthma on pulmonary function testing and will respond to bronchodilator therapy.

Attacks of asthma may be acute or may be of gradual onset. Exposure to allergens or bronchial irritants causes the acute attack of asthma which is due to spasm and inflammation of the small and medium airways. Viral upper respiratory infections usually cause attacks of slower onset with a gradual increase in frequency and severity of cough and wheezing over a few days.

Other signs and symptoms in addition to wheezing and cough associated with asthma include tachypnea, shortness of breath with prolonged expiration and use of accessory muscles of respiration, cyanosis, hyperinflation of the chest, tachycardia, abdominal pain, and feeling of "tight chest," poor exercise tolerance, "recurrent chest colds," "recurrent" or "chronic" bronchitis, or "recurrent pneumonia."

On physical examination the chest is hyperinflated and hyperresonant to percussion. A barrel chest deformity suggests chronic, severe asthma. Expiratory wheezes are prominent; occasionally inspiratory wheezes will be heard as well. Musical rales may be present. The child usually is restless with tachypnea and tachycardia and may, if severely obstructed, use accessory muscles. If the child is in extreme respiratory distress, wheezing may be absent, as noted above. To make breathing easier, the child may assume a hunched-over, tripod-like sitting position. Cyanosis may be apparent. Pulsus paradoxus may be present and will increase as airway obstruction increases. However, it is often difficult to assess because of the rapid heart rate in children. The liver and spleen may be palpable because of hyperinflation of the lungs and downward movement of the diaphragm. Successful treatment will produce color improvement and wheezing as air begins to move through the lungs.

Bronchiolitis usually occurs in children in contact with family members who have an upper respiratory infection. The infant is first noted to have signs of upper respiratory infection, such as runny nose and sneezing, accompanied by a low-grade fever, 38 to 39°C (100 to 102°F), and decreased appetite. Lower respiratory symptoms develop over a few days and include dyspnea, tachypnea, intercostal retractions, wheezing, and cyanosis. In more severely affected patients, the symptoms may develop more rapidly, within a few hours.

On examination of the patient with bronchiolitis, one will typically see a tachypneic infant in mild to severe respiratory distress, with respirations ranging from 60 to 80 per minute, flaring of the alae nasi, and using the accessory muscles of respiration with intercostal and subcostal retractions. Cyanosis may not be present, but significant abnormalities of gas exchange may develop in the absence of cyanosis. Respirations are shallow because of the persistent distention of the lungs by trapped air. Diffuse, fine sibilant and/or muscial rales are often present and the expiratory phase of breathing may be prolonged with audible wheezing. Barely audible breath sounds are a sign of impending respiratory failure. The liver and spleen may be palpated below the costal margins, suggesting hepatosplenomegaly; however, their position is secondary to downward displacement of the diaphragm from pulmonary hyperinflation. Signs of dehydration are often present, usually caused by inadequate oral fluid intake secondary to respiratory distress.

It is during the first 48 to 72 h after the onset of cough and dyspnea that the infant is most critically ill. Improvement occurs quickly after this time and the infant is usually fully recovered within a few days.

Laboratory and X-ray Findings

Most asthmatic children have normal blood counts; however, an elevated white blood cell count does not necessarily indicate infection. Both the "stress" of an acute asthma attack and the injection of epinephrine may cause leukocytosis. Blood eosinophilia above 250 to 400 cells/mm^3 is common in asthmatic children with the total eosinophil count being preferred to estimation from differential white counts. Eosinophils in the sputum and nasal secretions are usually present, as well. Sputum cultures are not very helpful in children. Polymorphonuclear leukocytes and bacteria on a nasal smear in an allergic child are suggestive of sinusitis.

A chest x-ray should be taken on every child under 1 year of age with the first episode of wheezing or a history of persistent symptoms of asthma, such as "chronic cough" or "chronic bronchitis" (if no x-ray was taken previously) to rule out foreign body aspiration, heart disease, parenchymal disease, and congenital anomaly.

The need for an x-ray in children over 1 year of age with first episodes of wheezing is controversial. The results of one study of 371 children over 1 year of age presenting with their first episode of wheezing suggest that routine chest x-rays in children of this age are not necessary since evaluation of vital signs [respiratory rate ≥60, pulse ≥160, and/or temperature ≥38.3°C (100.9°F)] and pretreatment auscultation (localized rales and/or localized decreased breath sounds) provides sufficient information to reveal which patients will have abnormal radiographic findings that might influence therapeutic decisions. One should consider obtaining an x-ray on any child admitted to the hospital. Vital signs and auscultatory findings noted above are helpful in determining which of these children need x-rays. Although the chest x-ray may be normal in an acute attack of asthma, the lungs are usually hyperinflated with flattening of the diaphragms and increased bronchial markings. The AP diameter is increased on lateral view. In addition, there may be patchy areas of infiltrate or atelectasis and, less commonly, pneumomediastinum and pneumothorax. Routine chest x-ray is not necessary, however, for the known asthmatic with an uncomplicated attack.

Pulmonary function tests are useful determinants of response to therapy in the asthmatic child. The forced expiratory volume (FEV_1) or peak expiratory flow rate (PEFR) are the most reliable measurements of the degree of airway obstruction. The spirometer measures FEV_1 and is useful in older children. The hand-held mini-Wright peak flow meter measures PEFR and may be used for children 5 years of age or older. Because the FEV_1 correlates well with PEFR, many physicians have chosen to use the mini-Wright peak flow meter for adults as well as children. These measurements are helpful in conjunction with clinical evaluation in identifying patients needing admission or close outpatient follow-up. If the initial PEFR is less than 25 percent of the predicted level, hypercarbia is likely. Rapid and aggressive treatment is indicated, and admission is warranted. If the PEFR is less than 60 percent of the predicted level after aggressive emergency department therapy, admission is indicated. Selected patients may be treated as outpatients if close, frequent follow-up can be arranged or if a holding area is available.

Arterial blood gases should be obtained from the radial or brachial artery in the severely ill asthmatic child to monitor for respiratory failure. Measurement of a PEFR less than 25 percent of the predicted level is helpful in determining which children are hypercarbic and therefore need arterial blood gas monitoring. Unfortunately, the PEFR is difficult to obtain in small children, and the need for a blood gas must be based on the clinical severity. The P_{CO_2}, which is usually low during the early part of an asthmatic attack, begins to rise as the obstruction increases. When the P_{CO_2} is >35 mmHg, it is an indication for concern, and blood gases should be monitored frequently. The blood pH usually remains normal until the buffering capacity of the blood is superseded.

Hypoxia commonly occurs in patients with PEFRs of 25 percent or higher. Because of this, all patients with moderate or severe asthma should have their oxygen saturation measured with a pulse oximeter. An initial O_2 saturation of 91 percent or less has been found to differentiate between an unfavorable and a favorable outcome. A rise in O_2 saturation after treatment with bronchodilators was *not* a determinant of outcome. Another study found that PEFR and initial O_2 saturation were useful in determining the severity of an acute asthmatic attack but that the initial O_2 saturation was a better predictor of outcome in those not initially admitted to the hospital.

The chest x-ray in bronchiolitis shows hyperinflation of the lungs and an increased AP diameter on lateral view. There are sometimes small areas of atelectasis which may mimic pneumonitis. The white blood cell count and hemoglobin level are usually within the normal range. Viral cultures are positive in the majority of infants with bronchiolitis, with respiratory syncytial virus (RSV) being by far the most frequently identified. Pulse oximetry and blood gases almost always reveal hypoxia, which correlates with the respiratory rate. Carbon dioxide retention occurs infrequently in children with bronchiolitis, but is present in those infants in severe respiratory distress. Infants with moderate to severe bronchiolitis should have their O_2 saturation monitored with a pulse oximeter. Arterial blood gases should be obtained in those children with severe bronchiolitis.

DIFFERENTIAL DIAGNOSIS

Bronchiolitis and infantile asthma are very similar in their clinical presentation and their differentiation provides a challenge for even the best of clinicians. In fact, in some situations, it may be impossible to clinically differentiate between the two. The most important differential clue to infantile asthma is a history of recurrent episodes of wheezing and/or coughing in an infant, regardless of age. Other clinical features suggesting asthma are a positive family history of asthma or allergy, physical evidence of atopic disease in the patient, sudden onset of wheezing without preceding infection, markedly prolonged expiration, and rapid reversibility of bronchospasm with sympathomimetic therapy.

Acute bronchiolitis usually occurs in children between 2 and 6 months of age (but may occur until age 2 years) in the winter and spring months. There are often other family members with an upper respiratory infection (URI) and the infant's illness begins with signs of a URI. There is usually no history of associated atopic disease in the patient or family.

Some physicians are reluctant to diagnose asthma in a child less than 1 year of age and label children who have recurrent episodes of coughing and wheezing with diagnoses such as asthmatic bronchitis, wheezy bronchitis, and recurrent bronchiolitis. There is good evidence, however, that approximately 30 percent of children with asthma are symptomatic in their first year of life.

The relationship between bronchiolitis and the subsequent development of asthma is very intriguing. Considering that 25 to 50 percent of children with bronchiolitis develop asthma later in life, bronchiolitis may constitute the first attack of asthma in these children. It is not clear whether the airways of some children are genetically hyperactive, thus predisposing them to bronchiolitis, or the first viral infection and resultant epithelial damage sensitize irritant receptors and lead to hyperactive airways.

It is known that RSV and other viruses are potent stimulants of wheezing in the individual prone to asthma. This suggests that bronchiolitis may be the first attack of asthma in the atopic child and that these children may be more likely to wheeze if infected with RSV or other viruses. A recent study determined that infants with diminished lung function before the age of 6 months and prior to any lower respiratory illness were more likely to have a wheezing lower respiratory illness in their first year of life than those infants with normal lung function.

In most patients with RSV infection of any kind, IgE is bound to exfoliated nasopharyngeal epithelial cells. The persistence of cell-bound IgE in patients with RSV-induced bronchiolitis or asthma, in contrast to those patients with mild upper respiratory tract infection or pneumonia from RSV, may explain the recurrent episodes of wheezing that occur in infants after RSV-induced bronchiolitis. Other studies have demonstrated pulmonary function abnormalities in symptom-free children years after their episode of bronchiolitis, indicating that these children are left with residual parenchymal or airway lesions which may predispose them to chronic obstructive lung disease. Mild bronchiolitis, on the other hand, does not seem to be associated with abnormal pulmonary function. It is probable that environment, genetic predisposition, and lung injury, either individually or in combination, play roles in the development of wheezing in children.

A helpful way to differentiate between bronchiolitis and asthma is by giving a trial of a β-adrenergic drug such as albuterol by nebulizer. Those infants responding to the β-adrenergic medication are more likely asthmatic. Since acute viral bronchiolitis is rarely a recurrent condition, infants with recurrent attacks (three or more episodes) of "bronchiolitis" should be considered asthmatic and treated as such.

Infants with bronchopulmonary dysplasia often have hyperreactive airways and are more likely to have a positive family history of asthma. They are predisposed to developing bronchiolitis or asthma with respiratory infections. Infants with bronchopulmonary dysplasia may be identified by a previous history of prematurity complicated by the respiratory distress syndrome for which they required mechanical ventilation. Their chest x-rays show evidence of chronic lung disease not seen in the infant with wheezing due to bronchiolitis or asthma alone. These children often present with mild illness that rapidly progresses to severe respiratory distress with tachypnea and cyanosis. Occasionally, the cause of the wheezing and respiratory embarrassment in these children is from pulmonary edema and may present a confusing clinical picture.

Other disease processes associated with wheezing which can be confused with bronchiolitis and asthma may be excluded by a careful history and physical and radiographic examination (Table 72-1). Recurrent food aspiration from gastroesophageal reflux or tracheoesophageal fistula usually presents with a history of frequent vomiting after feeding and associated coughing and choking. Foreign bodies in the trachea, bronchus, or esophagus may be differentiated from bronchiolitis in that severe coughing, cyanosis, and respiratory distress usually develop suddenly in a well child who has recently being eating peanuts, popcorn, coins, seeds, etc. Often, the wheezing will be unilateral. A chest x-ray may identify the foreign body if it is radiopaque. If it is not, one may see hyperinflation on the affected side of an expiratory film. Since expiratory films are difficult to obtain in small children, bilateral, lateral decubitus films are very helpful. Normally, the dependent lung against the table will have less volume than the other lung because of its immobility. However, if a foreign body is present on the side closest to the table, air trapping persists and hyperinflation is evident.

Bronchial stenosis is commonly manifest by wheezing and recurrent lower respiratory infection. This disorder can be diagnosed by bronchoscopy.

Children with cystic fibrosis on initial presentation may be difficult to differentiate from those with bronchiolitis or asthma. If there is a history of recurrent wheezing, pneumonitis, and respiratory distress in an infant who is failing to thrive, one must strongly consider this diagnosis.

Congestive heart failure from congenital heart disease or viral myocarditis may present in a fashion similar to bronchiolitis or asthma, especially with a palpable liver and spleen confusing the issue. A history of normal growth and development and the absence of a heart murmur makes the diagnosis of bronchiolitis or asthma more likely. The chest x-ray in congestive heart failure will usually demonstrate a large heart. Infants with heart disease sometimes go into congestive heart failure with viral infections, and may present with both conditions at once.

Vascular rings, mediastinal cysts, and tumors may compress the trachea or a bronchus. If one suspects a vascular ring but cannot see compression of the trachea on chest x-ray, a barium swallow may demonstrate constriction of the esophagus at the site of the ring. A mediastinal cyst or tumor will be apparent as a mass on chest x-ray.

Salicylate intoxication or other metabolic disorders may mimic bronchiolitis clinically because of the rapid respiratory rate. These disorders may be diagnosed by asking specifically about salicylate ingestion from aspirin or from other salicylate-containing products such as Pepto-Bismol, and by obtaining measurements of arterial blood gas, salicylate levels, and serum electrolytes, especially if no wheezing is present.

Table 72-1. Differential Diagnosis of Wheezing

Asthma
Bronchiolitis
Bronchopulmonary dysplasia
Foreign body aspiration
Viral pneumonitis
Cystic fibrosis
Heart disease
Vascular rings
Gastroesophageal reflux
Stenosis: tracheal and bronchial
α_1-Antitrypsin deficiency
Neoplasms
Adenomas
Papillomas
Bronchogenic cysts
Lymph gland enlargement
Hypersensitivity pneumonitis

Croup, epiglottitis, and other causes of upper airway obstruction usually present with inspiratory wheezing (stridor) but rarely with expiratory wheezing. If there is doubt about the diagnosis, chest and lateral neck x-rays may be helpful. If one is seriously considering the diagnosis of epiglottitis, however, one should follow the hospital protocol for this disease and, above all, never leave the patient unattended by a physician, especially if the child is going for an x-ray.

TREATMENT OF ASTHMA

Theory

The treatment of asthma is aimed at decreasing smooth-muscle spasm (early phase) and airway inflammation (late phase). Smooth muscle spasm or bronchial hyperreactivity is assisted by increasing levels of cyclic AMP (cylic adenosine 3′5′monophosphate) and is opposed by cyclic GMP (cyclic guanosine monophosphate). Elevation of cyclic AMP causes smooth muscle relaxation (bronchodilation) and may inhibit the release of mediators from airway mast cells, while elevation of cyclic GMP causes constriction of smooth muscle (bronchoconstriction). Sympathomimetics increase levels of cyclic AMP by activating the enzyme adenyl cyclase, which catalyzes ATP to cyclic AMP. Methylxanthines were originally thought to increase cyclic AMP by inhibiting the enzyme phosphodiesterase, which degrades cyclic AMP. Although there are a number of proposed theories, currently the mechanism of action of theophylline is unknown.

Sympathomimetic (adrenergic) agents, which are often the first-line medication used in the treatment of asthma, exert their activity by combining with receptors on cell surfaces. The two types of adrenergic receptors are α and β. Usually, drugs affecting α-adrenergic receptors are associated with excitatory functions while drugs affecting β-adrenergic receptors are associated with inhibitory functions (e.g., muscle relaxation). Stimulation of α-adrenergic receptors by agents such as norepinephrine decreases the amount of available cyclic AMP, and stimulation of β-adrenergic receptors increases the amount of available cyclic AMP. Consequently, adrenergic drugs which stimulate β receptors are useful in treating the asthmatic patient. The β-adrenergic system has two groups of receptors: the β_1 receptors, which control heart rate, myocardial contractility, and lipolysis; and the β_2 receptors, which control bronchiolar and arteriolar dilatation. Therefore, adrenergic drugs with more β_2-selective activity, such as albuterol and terbutaline, affect bronchodilation without affecting an increase in heart rate and myocardial contractility that occur with epinephrine and isoproterenol, which stimulate both β_1 and β_2 receptors.

Levels of cyclic GMP are controlled by the parasympathetic nervous system. Vagal stimulation or cholinergic drugs increase production of the enzyme guanylate cyclase, which increases the concentration of cyclic GMP. Atropine and other anticholinergic drugs block cholinergic (muscarinic) receptors. This prevents the binding of acetylcholine and decreases the availability of cyclic GMP. The side effects associated with atropine limit its use. Ipratropium bromide, a derivative of atropine, has minimal side effects and is becoming a much more used medication in the treatment of asthma.

Corticosteroids and cromolyn sodium are agents used to treat the airway inflammation. The mechanism of action of corticosteroids is not entirely understood, but it is known that they inhibit the release of mediators from macrophages and eosinophils. In addition, they reduce microvascular leakage, decrease the number of inflammatory cells coming to the lung by effecting the chemotactic response, reduce eosinophilia in the peripheral blood, and increase the number of β-adrenergic receptors available for response to β-agonists. Cromolyn sodium appears to stabilize mast cells and prevent release of mediators.

Treatment of Acute Attacks of Asthma

Most children presenting to the emergency room with asthma have an acute episode of airway obstruction that can be reversed relatively easily with bronchodilators. Epinephrine by injection had been the preferred treatment for acute asthma for many years, but bronchodilator aerosols, especially those with more selective β_2 activity, are now the treatment of choice. Several studies have demonstrated that, because of their selectivity, β_2 agonists delivered by inhalation provide equal or better bronchodilation and fewer systemic side effects than parenteral therapy. Moreover, providing bronchodilation by inhalation rather than injection is not painful, and children with frequent asthmatic attacks are less likely to be frightened when they come to the emergency department.

The nebulized β_2 agonist most commonly used is albuterol because it has the most β_2 selectivity with the longest duration of action. In children with severe asthma, high-dose albuterol (0.15 mg/kg per dose) nebulized and given frequently provides significantly greater improvement in pulmonary function than low-dose albuterol (0.05 mg/kg per dose) with no significant increase in side effects. Thus, albuterol (0.5% solution) should be given at 0.15 mg/kg (0.03 mL/kg) to a maximum dose of 5 mg diluted in 3.0 mL of saline solution and administered every 20 min by nebulization for up to six doses. If there is little or no improvement after six doses, consider continuous nebulized albuterol using 0.5 mg/kg per h (maximum 15 mg per h). Hospitalization is likely at this point unless marked improvement is evident. Albuterol should be delivered with an oxygen flow of 6 to 7 L/min, and the pulse should be monitored to keep it less than 180.

In children with moderately severe asthma, 0.15 mg/kg of albuterol to a maximum of 5 mg/dose may be administered and repeated twice at 60-min intervals. A recent study indicates that hourly use of 0.30 mg/kg for three doses to a maximum of 10 mg provides greater improvement in the FEV_1 than three doses of 0.15 mg/kg over the same time period and is equally safe. The authors suggest that the higher dose should be considered in some children with moderately severe asthma, particularly those who relapse between lower hourly doses.

The use of albuterol by metered-dose inhaler (MDI) with a spacer has been advocated by some authors because of the familiarity of patients with this method, ease of use, and decrease in therapist time. Two puffs of albuterol are given every 2 min and titrated until improvement stops to a maximum of 20 puffs.

If albuterol is not available, terbutaline may be used as an alternative. Presently, terbutaline is available in the United States only as an injectable solution (1 mg/1 mL). It may be used in a nebulizer at 0.03 mg/kg up to 0.5 mg in 2 mL of normal saline every 1 to 2 h or more often as tolerated, or by continuous nebulization at 2 to 4 mg/h. Terbutaline in this form is not generally recommended because it offers no advantage over albuterol and is not FDA approved for nebulizer use.

It should be remembered, however, that nebulized and MDI medications are dependent on patient cooperation and inspiratory effort. In administration of nebulized drugs to the very young child, the drug must be delivered properly so that the patient's airways are receiving it. Also, in very severe asthma, the nebulized drug may not get to as much of the bronchial tree as will the systemic medication which will reach it through the bloodstream. In such cases, particularly if the patient is unable to generate a PEFR or has decreased consciousness, parenteral adrenergics are indicated. Aqueous epinephrine, 1:1000, may be administered subcutaneously at a dose of 0.01 mL/kg up to a maximum dose of 0.3 mL. This dose may be repeated twice at 20-min intervals with monitoring of respiratory status and heart rate. Terbutaline (1 mg/mL), which is more β_2-specific, may be given subcutaneously in place of epinephrine at a dose of 0.01 mL/kg (up to 0.25 mL). The dose may be repeated in 20 min if no adverse effects occur. If there is improvement in airway obstruction in the very severe asthmatic with the use of parenteral adrenergics, nebulized β_2 agonists should be started.

Close monitoring of the pulse, respiratory rate, auscultatory findings in the chest, use of accessory muscles, oxygen saturation, and PEFR should be done before and after each treatment with adrenergic agents and should be recorded in the chart. The decision to repeat or withhold these agents should be based on the above clinical findings rather than rigidly following a protocol.

Anticholinergics are effective bronchodilators but until recently have been associated with many undesirable side effects. With the introduction of ipratropium bromide (Atrovent), a derivative of atropine, side effects are negligible. In several studies of patients treated with nebulized ipratropium bromide in combination with nebulized β_2 agonists, the two drugs provide more bronchodilation than a β_2 agonist alone. Unfortunately, nebulized ipratropium bromide is not available for commercial use in the United States at this time, although it is available in Canada and Europe. Physicians who have access to nebulized ipratropium bromide should combine it with albuterol in patients 5 years of age or older who do not respond satisfactorily to albuterol alone at 40 and 80 min after the first dose. If the child is severely ill, ipratropium bromide may be added to the first dose of albuterol and repeated at 40 and 80 min. The dosage of ipratropium bromide is 250 mg (1.0 mL). Its use in children less than 5 years of age has not been established, but it may be beneficial.

Ipratropium bromide is available as a metered-dose inhaler in the United States. The safety and effectiveness in children below the age of 12 have not been established. However, since metered-dose inhalers with spacers have been shown to deliver inhaled bronchodilators to the lungs as effectively as nebulizers, the administration of ipratropium bromide and a β_2 agonist in this manner may prove beneficial.

Theophylline does not increase bronchodilation in patients optimally treated with β agonists. Therefore, theophylline is no longer recommended in the management of the acutely ill asthmatic child in the emergency department. In the hospital setting, however, theophylline therapy over time may improve outcome, and its use is recommended. Consequently, children who are admitted to the hospital for status asthmaticus may have theophylline therapy started in the emergency department (see "Treatment of Status Asthmaticus").

Corticosteroids are potent anti-inflammatory medications that are particularly useful in the inflammatory or late phase of asthma (2 to 8 h into the attack). Their benefit in the acute asthmatic attack is controversial, but most studies indicate that recovery time is decreased and there is less need for hospitalization in those patients treated with corticosteroids. Moreover, corticosteroids have been shown to improve oxygenation, decrease airway obstruction, and work synergistically with β agonists to improve bronchodilation in acute asthmatic attacks. Therefore, the question of when to start corticosteroids rather than who deserves corticosteroids is now more the issue. Clearly, however, not every child with a mild attack of asthma needs corticosteroids to reverse the attack.

If a child presents to the emergency department with an infrequent acute attack of asthma and responds quickly to β_2 agonists (within 1 h) corticosteroids are probably not necessary. Corticosteroids should be given early to children with an acute attack of asthma in the following cases: (1) a child with an infrequent acute attack of asthma who does not respond to inhaled β_2 agonists after 1 h of treatment, (2) a child with a severe attack of asthma, (3) a child who is well known to the treating physician or the hospital or has a history of frequent emergency department visits or hospitalizations, (4) a child who is known to respond for a short period of time to bronchodilators but who subsequently develops wheezing again and returns to the emergency department for further therapy or to be admitted for status asthmaticus, (5) a child who has a second attack of asthma requiring an emergency department visit within a period of 1 week while on bronchodilators at home and who has responded on both emergency department visits to β_2 agonists, (6) a child with a viral upper respiratory infection who may or may not have symptoms of asthma when presenting to the emergency department but who is known to have rapid progression of symptoms once an attack begins, and (7) a child who is chronically on corticosteroids or who has needed frequent short-term bursts in the past.

With the exception of the first and sixth situation described above, corticosteroids should be administered very soon after β_2 agonists are started. Prednisone at 1 to 2 mg/kg per day, given in two divided doses, is not associated with toxicity and does not cause adrenal suppression. Liquid preparations have made administration to small children easier. Steroid bursts for 5 days or less, if done no more than four times per year, do not require tapering, since there is no adrenal suppression. Occasionally, after a viral illness, steroids may be required for 7 to 10 days. If they are needed for longer than 5 days or if the child has had four or more bursts per year, they should be tapered over 10 to 14 days. If a child is receiving chronic steroid treatment he or she should be given high doses of prednisone for acute exacerbations and returned to a maintenance dose when the acute exacerbation is resolved. Steroids may be given orally, except in the severely ill child, since intravenous administration does not offer additional benefit.

After an acute attack of asthma, all children should be sent home with an inhaled β_2 agonist, an oral β_2 agonist, or theophylline for 1 to 2 weeks to prevent further exacerbation of their symptoms (for dosages see "Treatment of Chronic Asthma").

Treatment of Status Asthmaticus

Status asthmaticus may be defined as severe, persistent wheezing and dyspnea that fail to respond to usually effective outpatient therapy. Respiratory failure may occur in patients with status asthmaticus; this makes this disorder a true medical emergency. Hospitalization is mandatory for these patients.

All patients with status asthmaticus are hypoxic and some are hypercapneic. Consequently, all patients should be monitored with a pulse oximeter. Arterial blood gas levels should be obtained to determine baseline P_{O_2}, P_{CO_2}, and pH, particularly in patients whose PEFR is less than 25 percent of predicted. These should be repeated frequently if one does not have an available pulse oximeter or if the P_{CO_2} is high until the patient's clinical condition improves. Humidified oxygen should be administered to every child with status asthmaticus immediately. The pulse oximeter should be maintained above 90-percent saturation and/or the P_{O_2} should be maintained between 70 and 90 mmHg. Mist tents are not indicated, both because water does not reach the lower airway in any significant way, and because mist irritates the airways of many asthmatics.

Many children with status asthmaticus become dehydrated. This is the result of several factors, including decreased fluid intake, excessive work of breathing, pulmonary insensible water loss, and the diuretic effect of theophylline. When hydrating children with status asthmaticus, it must be taken into account that they have increased secretion of antidiuretic hormone, and there is danger of overhydration and subsequent pulmonary edema. Consequently, fluid administration must be carefully monitored. Hydration in excess of maintenance is usually unnecessary and may be harmful.

In the patient who has metabolic acidosis, i.e., a pH of less than 7.2 and a base deficit greater than 5 mEq/L, intravenous sodium bicarbonate should be administered because acidosis may blunt the effect of bronchodilator therapy. The following calculation may be helpful in correcting metabolic acidosis:

$$\text{Bicarbonate (mEq)} = 0.3 \times \text{body weight (kg)} \times \text{base deficit (mEq)}$$

Give one-half of the calculated dose initially over 20 min and the other half after repeating the blood gas measurements. Adequate ventilation is necessary to prevent a rise in P_{CO_2} from bicarbonate breakdown. Respiratory acidosis should be treated with appropriate medication and with assisted ventilation in those who fail to respond.

Nebulized albuterol or other β_2 agonist should be administered every 20 min or continuously if necessary (see "Treatment of Acute Attacks of Asthma").

Although theophylline has not proven to be of benefit in the emergency department treatment of asthma, it does appear to improve outcome in severely ill patients in an intensive care unit setting. In addition to its bronchodilator properties, it can stimulate respiration centrally and can increase contractility of respiratory muscle. Consequently, if a child is going to be admitted to the hospital, aminophylline (85% theophylline) should be administered as a loading dose of 7 mg/kg (lean body weight) diluted in 25 to 50 mL of saline given intravenously over a period of 20 min. If the child is a known asthmatic who has taken a dose of oral theophylline at home within 4 to 6 h prior to arriving at the hospital, the loading dosage of aminophylline should be adjusted by deducting the amount given in the past 4 to 6 h from the ordinary bolus of 7 mg/kg of aminophylline. Canavan, et al., suggested that even if the child has taken theophylline within 6 h of arriving at the hospital, a loading dose of 6 mg/kg may be given with few side effects. In this study, time zero theophylline levels ranged from 0 to 24.0 μg/mL (mean 6.7 μg/mL) and peak theophylline levels ranged from 8.1 to 35.2 μg/mL (mean 15.2 μg/mL). There was no consistent relationship, in the immediate period after the bolus was given, between side effects and peak levels even if the peak level was >20 μg/mL. If a recent theophylline level is known, one may calculate the loading dose with the knowledge that, as a general rule, 1 mg/kg of theophylline will raise the serum concentration by approximately 2 μg/mL. The loading dose can thus be calculated with the following formula:

$$\text{Loading dose (mg)} = \frac{\text{desired level} - \text{measured level}}{2} \times \text{kg}$$

Another approach, advocated by some physicians, is to give 7 mg/kg of aminophylline to patients who have not taken a recent dose of theophylline and 5 mg/kg to patients who have taken a recent dose.

A theophylline level should be obtained prior to the administration of aminophylline if the child has been on an oral theophylline preparation. The loading dose should be followed by a constant maintenance infusion of aminophylline of 1.0 to 1.2 mg/kg per hour for children 1 to 9 years old, 0.8 to 1.0 mg/kg per hour for children 10 to 16 years, and 0.6 to 0.8 mg/kg per hour for children over 16 years. This will usually maintain serum concentrations of approximately 10 μg/mL. If there is significant fever, liver disease, or heart failure, the maintenance infusion should be reduced by 50 percent. Because infants, particularly those under 6 months of age, are erratic in their clearance rate of theophylline, a formula for infants less than 1 year of age is useful.

$$\text{Dose (mg/kg per day)} = 0.3 \times \text{age in weeks} + 8$$

It is extremely important to measure serum theophylline levels because of the variable clearance rates from one patient to the next. If, after the initial theophylline level is obtained, the patient continues to have significant wheezing, the dose of aminophylline can be increased until a theophylline level of 15 μg/mL is reached. Levels should also be measured whenever toxicity is suspected on the basis of symptoms such as gastrointestinal upset, CNS irritability, and headaches. Theophylline should be delivered by a constant infusion pump. If constant infusion cannot be delivered safely, boluses of aminophylline at 5 mg/kg every 6 h (or an amount which will give a serum concentration of 10 to 15 μg/mL) should be administered over a period of 30 min.

Intravenous corticosteroids should be started in the child with status asthmaticus. The beneficial effects of corticosteroid therapy, i.e., decreasing inflammation, facilitating recovery from hypoxia, increasing cyclic AMP, and possibly restoring β-adrenergic responsiveness to adrenergic drugs in patients who have become unresponsive to these drugs, outweigh the remote possibility of adverse effects from short-term corticosteroid use. Hydrocortisone (Solu-Cortef) or methylprednisolone (Solu-Medrol) may be administered. The dosage of hydrocortisone is 4 to 6 mg/kg every 6 h for 48 to 72 h. Methylprednisolone may be administered at 1 to 2 mg/kg every 6 h for 48 to 72 h. When intravenous corticosteroids are discontinued, the patient should be maintained on oral prednisone at 1 to 2 mg/kg per day in two divided doses for a total of 5 days or more if clinically indicated.

Sedation is contraindicated in patients with status asthmaticus. Antibiotics should not be used routinely. If bacterial infection is suspected, attempts should be made to identify the causative organism; the patient should be started on a broad-spectrum antibiotic while the culture results are pending.

Occasionally, the patient with status asthmaticus develops respiratory failure. Clinical signs and symptoms of respiratory failure are decreased or absent breath sounds, severe retractions and use of accessory muscles, cyanosis on 40% oxygen, depressed level of consciousness, decreased response to pain, and poor skeletal muscle tone. Arterial blood gas levels are the final determinant of respiratory failure and must be monitored frequently in the distressed child. Respiratory failure may be defined as a P_{O_2} <50 mmHg on 100% inhaled O_2, or P_{CO_2} >50 mmHg. The child with a rapidly rising P_{CO_2} (e.g., from 35 to 40 mmHg in 1 h) who is receiving optimal therapy and is tiring, should be considered to be in respiratory failure and treated as such.

In a child whose arterial P_{CO_2} is rising rapidly but is less than 55 mmHg and whose arterial P_{O_2} is more than 60 mmHg on oxygen, continuously nebulized albuterol should be administered in an attempt to avert the need for mechanical ventilation. The dosage of albuterol is 0.5 mg/kg per hour. An alternative to albuterol is continuously nebulized terbutaline at 4 mg/kg per hour.

Some studies advocate the use of intravenous albuterol to avert the need for mechanical ventilation. At the present, albuterol is not available for intravenous use in the United States, but it is available in Canada and Europe. If intravenous albuterol is used, the dosage is 10 μg/kg over 10 min, followed by 0.2 μg/kg per minute. This should be increased by 0.1-μg/kg increments every 15 min as needed and titrated according to response. Potassium levels should be obtained, since hypokalemia occurs frequently in patients receiving intravenous albuterol. Supplementary potassium is often needed with this treatment. If albuterol is not available, terbutaline may be used instead. The dose is 10 μg/kg over 10 min, followed by 0.2-μg/kg per minute increments titrated according to clinical response. The pulse with all of these medications should not be higher than 180. Continuous delivery of an intravenous β_2 agonist will ordinarily be administered in a properly equipped intensive care unit. If admission to the intensive care unit is delayed, initial therapy may be undertaken in the emergency department, but only with continuous cardiac monitoring and a constant infusion pump.

Intravenous isoproterenol was used in the recent past to avert mechanical ventilation. It is no longer recommended because β_2 agonists are more specific, they decrease P_{CO_2} more rapidly, and they have fewer side effects than intravenous isoproterenol.

If medical therapy fails to control respiratory failure, mechanical ventilation is required. Any child with a P_{CO_2} rising at 5 to 10 mmHg/h during aggressive therapy, a P_{CO_2} greater than 55 mmHg after 1 to 2 h of aggressive therapy, or a P_{O_2} less than 50 mmHg on 100% inspired oxygen should be started on assisted ventilation. If a child has a P_{CO_2} of more than 65 mmHg initially, immediate intubation should be strongly considered. Rapidly changing lung compliances make the use of a volume respirator preferable. An initial tidal volume of 10 mL/kg should be used with a short inspiratory time and an expiratory time as long as possible. A Swan-Ganz catheter should be placed if there is right heart strain, low pulse pressure, or low urine output. The patient may be given diazepam for sedation and pancuronium bromide for muscle relaxation. These medications will help with synchronization of respiration with the ventilator. Parenteral and inhaled medication should be continued throughout the period of ventilation.

Management of Complications

Atelectasis occurs in 10 percent and pneumomediastinum occurs in 5 percent of children hospitalized with asthma. Treatment of atelectasis and pneumomediastinum should be conservative; they will usually resolve with drug therapy. Percussion and postural drainage are helpful for the resolution of atelectasis. Pneumomediastinal air is absorbed over 7 to 10 days.

Pneumothorax occurs rarely in children with asthma. When it does occur, a pneumothorax may be small and cause minimal respiratory compromise or it may be large or under tension, causing significant respiratory distress. A small pneumothorax may be managed conservatively and will often respond to the treatment of asthma. A large pneumothorax or tension pneumothorax will require placement of a chest tube.

Treatment of Chronic Asthma

An attempt should be made to determine the environmental factors which may trigger an attack of asthma. Some of these factors include allergens such as animal dander, pollen, house dust, molds, and foods; irritants such as smoke, perfumes, and aerosol spray products; and climate. If these environmental stimuli are identified, their removal may "cure" the child's asthma.

More often than not, the physician is unable to identify a precipitating environmental factor and must resort to medication to control a child's asthma. Mild or intermittent asthma may be controlled with inhaled β_2 agonists such as albuterol or terbutaline. The use of one of these medications three or four times a day may be the only treatment necessary to control symptoms. Aerosolized adrenergics are particularly recommended for children with exercise-induced bronchospasm. Two inhalations may provide more bronchodilation and fewer side effects than the oral preparations of these medications. Since metered-dose inhalers are often used improperly, it is important to instruct patients in their use. Even after instruction, some older children have difficulty with metered-dose inhalers. In these children and especially those who are 3 to 4 years of age, spacers or holding chambers have provided an easy way to take advantage of aerosolized β_2 agonists. The addition of a sustained-release theophylline to the β_2 agonist may prove beneficial if symptom control is not maximally achieved, particularly at night when the bronchodilator effect of the β_2 agonist may wear off. Because metered-dose inhalers are occasionally abused, parents and patients must be warned about this tendency.

Several medications can be used alone or in combination to control symptoms in children with moderate chronic asthma. These children have many asthmatic episodes per year either requiring more than one medication for several days or requiring emergency department therapy or hospitalization. This group of patients should be on daily medication.

Cromolyn sodium, because of its anti-inflammatory properties and an effectiveness equal to that of theophylline in controlling symptoms with fewer associated side effects, may be used alone. Theophylline, however, continues to be favored by many allergists as the first-line medication for these children. Because of its side effects, particularly behavioral ones, it should be considered an alternative to cromolyn sodium. Other medications to be considered are inhaled β_2 agonists and oral β_2 agonists. Often these medications work well in combination with cromolyn sodium, particularly after an acute attack of asthma in a child who needs the bronchodilating effect of β_2 agonists or theophylline and the anti-inflammatory effect of cromolyn sodium. Inhaled steroids are often useful with inhaled β_2 agonists in a child who has more of an inflammatory component or cannot tolerate oral medication. Short-burst oral steroids are sometimes needed to control symptoms (See "Treatment of Acute Attacks of Asthma").

Cromolyn sodium stabilizes mast cells and prevents the release of mediators and thus decreases inflammation. It is useful in all forms of asthma (extrinsic, intrinsic, mixed, and exercise-induced). Since it is a prophylactic antiasthmatic medication and has no bronchodilating effect, it should not be used to treat acute attacks of asthma. Cromolyn sodium is available in three preparations: 20-mg powder capsules, 20-mg solution for nebulizer use, and a metered-dose inhaler at 1 mg/puff to be administered at 2 mg (2 puffs) per dose. Each preparation should be administered four times per day.

As noted above, theophylline is considered by many the oral bronchodilator of choice in the outpatient management of chronic asthma. Theophylline comes in many forms. Depending on the specific theophylline preparation chosen and individual patient clearance, it may be given every 6 h, every 8 h, or every 12 h. Sustained-release preparations, those given every 8 or 12 h, are preferred because they decrease fluctuations in serum concentrations and increase compliance. In children who clear theophylline rapidly, sustained-release theophylline should be given every 8 h.

The initial dose for most children is 20 mg/kg per day. Depending on individual differences in metabolism, smaller or larger doses may be needed to maintain serum concentration between 5 and 15 μg/mL. In many cases, children do very well at levels of 5 to 10 μg/mL. Levels greater than 15 μg/mL rarely have to be exceeded to gain good control. Children less than 6 months and over 9 years of age should be started on doses of 12 to 16 mg/kg per day because of their slower clearance rate of theophylline. Infants less than 6 months of age have erratic clearance rates of theophylline, and their serum theophylline levels should be checked in 24 h and then monitored accordingly (see formula in "Treatment of Status Asthmaticus" section). Any child receiving theophylline should always be observed for signs of toxicity such as nausea, vomiting, restlessness, irritability, and seizures. If any of these signs appear, theophylline levels should be obtained and the medication stopped.

Oral β agonists (albuterol, terbutaline, and metaproterenol) may be used alone or in combination with other bronchodilators or anti-inflammatory medications, particularly if the child continues to be symptomatic on only one medication. Albuterol is the most commonly used oral β agonist in children. It is available as a liquid (2 mg/5 mL), with a starting dose of 0.1 to 0.2 mg/kg per dose three times a day not to exceed 6 mg, or as a tablet (2 mg and 4 mg), with starting doses for children 6 to 12 years of 2 mg three or four times a day; for children over 12 the dose is 2 or 4 mg three or four times a day. Albuterol is also available in a longer-acting form known as a Repetab, which may be used in children older than 12 years of age at a dose of 4 to 8 mg every 12 h. Metaproterenol is available as a liquid (10 mg/5 mL) or as a tablet (10 mg and 20 mg). The dose is 10 mg for children from 6 to 9 years of age or who weigh less than 27 kg (60 lb), and 20 mg in children who are over 9 years of age or over 27 kg (60 lb), given 3 to 4 times a day. The dose for children under 6 has not been clearly established, but dosages of 1.3 to 2.6 mg/kg per day are well tolerated. Terbutaline is available as 2.5- and 5-mg tablets. The dose for children from 12 to 15 years of age is 2.5 mg three times a day. For adolescents over age 15, the dose is 5 mg three times a day. Terbutaline tablets are not currently recommended for children less than 12. If tachycardia, nervousness, tremors, palpitations, or nausea develop in patients taking β_2-adrenergic drugs, the dose should be reduced.

Corticosteroids are rarely needed in the patient with chronic asthma. However, if the patient has severe chronic asthma with intractable symptoms, continuous use of oral (prednisone) or aerosolized (beclomethasone, triamcinolone, and flunisolide) corticosteroids is indicated in combination with inhaled or oral bronchodilators. Treatment should begin with beclomethasone since fewer side effects are associated with it than with oral preparations. The latter should be reserved for the more intractable symptoms and should preferably be given as alternate-day doses. In any case of difficult-to-manage asthma, especially in a child in whom chronic steroids may be indicated, consultation with an allergist should be obtained.

Small infants who respond well to nebulized therapy but not as well to oral medication may benefit from a home nebulizer.

Other Therapeutic Modalities

A number of medications are being tested for their effectiveness in the treatment of asthma. Calcium channel blockers have been studied but have not up to now demonstrated proven benefit. Magnesium sulfate causes bronchodilation and is considered an adjunct to β_2-agonist therapy by some, but its effects have not been studied in children. Ketotifen is used in a manner similar to cromolyn sodium, but some studies of its effectiveness have not shown it to be any better than placebo. Azelastine, an inhibitor of mediators, is a bronchodilator that has shown some effectiveness in the treatment of asthma. Troleandomycin potentiates the anti-inflammatory effects of steroids and may prove useful in chronic asthmatic patients on high-dose corticosteroid therapy.

Treatment of Bronchiolitis

Treatment of bronchiolitis is primarily supportive and should be based on the child's clinical condition. The infant with mild bronchiolitis (alert, playful, feeding well with good hydration, respiratory rate <50, and no subcostal retractions) and no significant associated illness such as BPD or congenital heart disease, may be managed conservatively as an outpatient with careful observation and small frequent feedings. Almost all other children with bronchiolitis are hypoxic, especially when they are asleep.

Consequently, the most important therapy for bronchiolitis is humidified oxygen at an FI_{O_2} of 28 to 40%. This should be delivered by mask, hood, or tent, since nasal prongs may produce reflex bronchoconstriction. Pulse oximetry and arterial blood gases are useful in monitoring those patients in moderate to severe respiratory distress (respiratory rate >60). Mist has not proved helpful since almost no moisture reaches the lower respiratory tract to liquefy secretions.

Many children with bronchiolitis become dehydrated because of decreased fluid intake secondary to the excessive work of breathing and pulmonary insensible water loss. Intravenous fluids (D_5 one-fourth normal saline solution with added KCl) must be administered to these children, but should be given with some caution as pulmonary edema may occur with overaggressive fluid therapy. Hydration in excess of replacement and maintenance is unnecessary.

Routine administration of antibiotics has not proved beneficial in bronchiolitis. If the child is desperately ill, or if the infant's clinical condition suddenly deteriorates, one should consider bacterial infection superimposed on viral infection. In this case, a broad-spectrum antibiotic such as cefuroxime may be useful. Prior to administering the antibiotic, tracheal secretions should be examined by Gram stain and by culture, and blood cultures should be obtained. Recently, two forms of inpatient therapy have been used to alter the course of the very ill child with bronchiolitis. Ribavirin, an antiviral agent, administered by aerosolization, has been shown to decrease mortality and morbidity due to RSV infections, and extracorporeal membrane oxygenation (ECMO) has been used successfully in children with bronchiolitis whose condition deteriorates despite maximal ventilator management.

Corticosteroids have been studied extensively in bronchiolitis and have not been shown to alter the course of this disease.

Sedation should be avoided because of its effect on suppression of the respiratory drive. In very agitated infants, who are closely monitored, one may consider using chloral hydrate, 10 to 20 mg/kg per dose every 6 to 8 h.

Bronchodilator therapy in infants with bronchiolitis is controversial. Since many children with bronchiolitis go on to develop asthma, it is beneficial to give a trial of nebulized albuterol at 0.15 mg/kg per dose for three doses at 1-h intervals. If the child responds, it suggests that he or she has reversible bronchospasm and should be followed closely for future wheezing episodes. A trial of oral albuterol (or other β agonists) should be considered in the child who responds to nebulized albuterol. The dose is 0.1 to 0.2 mg/kg per dose three times a day.

One may consider managing a child with bronchiolitis as an outpatient if the child is well hydrated, drinking fluids well, is not cyanotic, appears comfortable, and is not in visible respiratory distress (respiratory rate <60). Since hypoxia is a common finding in bronchiolitic children, pulse oximetry and/or arterial blood gases should be obtained in most instances. Children who are not drinking fluids well, are having apneic episodes or have a history of apnea, and/or appear to be in respiratory distress should be admitted. Occasionally, children with severe bronchiolitis develop respiratory failure. These infants and those with frequent episodes of apnea may need endotracheal or nasotracheal intubation for ventilatory support. Infants with a past history of respiratory distress syndrome resulting in bronchopulmonary dysplasia who develop bronchiolitis need close observation and should, in almost all cases, be hospitalized.

If the social situation is such that following instructions and giving adequate home care seem unlikely, or if parental anxiety is so great that the parents are having trouble coping with their child's illness, the child should be admitted. If one chooses to discharge a patient with mild bronchiolitis, parents should be given detailed instructions regarding hydration and increasing respiratory distress. All these children should be seen again 12 to 24 h after their presentation to the emergency department.

SUMMARY

Pediatric asthma is characterized by tachypnea, wheezing, and cough. It is caused by multiple factors, the most common of which is exposure to environmental stimuli such as allergens, air pollutants, etc. Since there are many diseases which are associated with wheezing in children, it is important to differentiate them from asthma. Once the diagnosis of asthma has been established, control of the environment is an important adjunct to therapy. Pharmacologic therapy is aimed at decreasing smooth-muscle spasm and reducing bronchial mucosal edema and mucus secretion. This is usually achieved with the use of sympathomimetics and corticosteroids. A child who is refractory to conventional outpatient management of asthma has status asthmaticus and must be admitted to the hospital for more intensive therapy. Once discharged from the hospital, the child must be followed closely and treated as necessary for long-term control of the asthma.

Bronchiolitis is characterized by rapid respiration, chest retractions, and wheezing in the infant. It is most often caused by the respiratory syncytial virus and usually occurs in the winter and spring. Bronchiolitis is commonly confused with infantile asthma and attempts should be made to differentiate the two. Treatment is supportive. Bronchiolitis is usually a mild disease but may cause significant respiratory distress and necessitate admission to the hospital.

BIBLIOGRAPHY

Asthma

Barnes PJ: A new approach to the treatment of asthma. *N Engl J Med* 321:1517, 1989.

Canny GJ, Reisman J, Healy R, et al: Acute asthma: Observations regarding the management of a pediatric emergency room. *Pediatrics* 83:507, 1989.

Ellis EF: Asthma: Current therapeutic approach. *Pediatr Clin North Am* 35:1041, 1988.

Goldenhersh MJ, Rachelefsky GS: Childhood asthma: Management. *Pediatr Rev* 10:259, 1989.

Harris JB, Weinberger MM, Nassif E, et al: Early intervention with short courses of prednisone to prevent progression of asthma in ambulatory patients incompletely responsive to bronchodilators. *J Pediatr* 110:627, 1987.

McWilliams B, Kelly HW, Murphy S: Management of acute severe asthma. *Pediatr Ann* 18:774, 1989.

Neddenriep D, Schumacher MJ, Lemen, RJ: Asthma in childhood. *Curr Prob Pediatr* 19:329, July 1989.

Reisman J, Galdes-Sebalt M, Kazim F, et al: Frequent administration by inhalation of salbutamol and ipratropium bromide in the initial management of severe acute asthma in children. *J Allerg Clin Immunol* 81:16, 1988.

Schuh S, Reider MJ, Canny G, et al: Nebulized albuterol in acute childhood asthma: Comparison of two doses. *Pediatrics* 86:509, 1990.

Stein R, Canny GJ, Bohn DJ, et al: Severe acute asthma in a pediatric intensive care unit: Six year's experience. *Pediatrics* 83:1023, 1989.

Bronchiolitis

Schuh S, Canny G, Reisman JJ, et al: Nebulized albuterol in acute bronchiolitis. *J Pediatr* 117:633, 1990.

Wright PF: Bronchiolitis. *Pediatr Rev* 7:219, 1986.

73
REYE'S SYNDROME

Carol D. Berkowitz

Reye's syndrome is the most common neurological complication of a viral illness in children. Early recognition and prompt management may be life-saving and may significantly reduce the long-term morbidity.

The disorder was first reported by Reye, Morgan, and Basal in 1963. They described 21 children seen between 1951 and 1962 at the Royal Alexander Hospital for Children in Australia. These children had "encephalopathy and fatty degeneration of the viscera." Other authors in earlier reports had also noted encephalopathies of unknown cause associated with fatty accumulation in the liver, but it was only after the report by Reye and colleagues that the disorder became a recognized clinical entity. The Centers for Disease Control defines Reye's syndrome as follows:

1. Acute non-inflammatory encephalopathy documented by the clinical picture of alteration in the level of consciousness and, if available, a record of cerebrospinal fluid containing eight leukocytes or less per mm, or histologic sections of the brain demonstrating cerebral edema without perivascular or meningeal inflammation.
2. Fatty metamorphosis of the liver diagnosed by either biopsy or autopsy or threefold or greater rise in the levels of either the SGOT [AST], SGPT [ALT] or serum ammonia.
3. No known more reasonable explanation for the cerebral or hepatic abnormalities. The incidence is reported to be between 0.58 and 2.7 cases per 100,000 per year in children under 18 years of age.

ETIOLOGY

The primary insult in Reye's syndrome is a disruption of mitochondrial function, primarily in the brain and liver. Other organs, such as the heart, kidneys, pancreas, and skeletal muscle are also affected. Electron microscopy demonstrates swelling and pleomorphism of the mitochondria, with disruption of the outer membrane and deformation of the cristae.

The agent responsible for initiating the mitochondrial dysfunction has not been identified. A heat-stable factor which affects mitochondrial function in vitro has been found in the serum of some patients with Reye's syndrome. Viruses, virus neutralization, genetic predisposition (e.g., heterozygotes for urea cycle disorders), exposure to toxins or drugs, and a synergistic interaction among these factors have also been implicated.

Influenza B and chickenpox are the viruses usually antedating Reye's syndrome. However, live-virus immunization and multiple other viruses have also been associated with the disorder; these include Coxsackie, influenza A, herpes (including simplex and zoster), Epstein-Barr, parainfluenza, rubella, rubeola, and vaccinia virus; reovirus, adenovirus, poliovirus 1, and echovirus.

Numerous toxins have also been studied. Two disorders which clinically resemble Reye's syndrome are associated with the ingestion of specific toxins. Jamaican vomiting sickness follows the consumption of the unripe fruit of the akee tree, which contains hypoglycin A. Udorn encephalopathy, seen in southeast Asia, follows the ingestion of grains and nuts which contain aflatoxin B, a toxic metabolite of *Aspergillus flavus*.

The drug most recently implicated in Reye's syndrome is aspirin. In 1980, a report from the Centers for Disease Control showed a statistical association between the use of aspirin and the development of Reye's syndrome following an outbreak of influenza A in a group of schoolchildren. Those who developed Reye's syndrome had fever more often than controls, and among those who had fever, patients who developed Reye's syndrome used aspirin more frequently than those who did not. In addition, the investigators found increasing severity of Reye's syndrome with increasing aspirin dosage. Others have corroborated these findings. Additionally, decreasing occurrence of Reye's syndrome has been reported following the decreasing use of aspirin. The data are sufficiently convincing to recommend that children with chickenpox or influenza-like illnesses avoid aspirin. Older children who may self-medicate should also be warned to avoid aspirin under these circumstances.

Of theoretical interest is that salicylate diminishes mitochondrial function and uncouples oxidative phosphorylation, the phenomena seen in Reye's syndrome. Glycogen stores are diminished in the liver and muscle in both Reye's syndrome and salicylate ingestion.

Reports also link pesticide exposure to Reye's syndrome.

CLINICAL PICTURE

Classically the disorder presents in a biphasic manner. There is generally an antecedent viral illness, usually influenza B (most common in "epidemic" Reye's syndrome) or chickenpox (20 percent). Reye's syndrome occurs in 1 case per 1700 children afflicted with influenza B and in 1 case per 15,000 children with chickenpox. The clustering of cases of Reye's syndrome in late winter and early spring follows the seasonal nature of these viruses. The child is recovering from the viral illness when he or she develops new symptoms, particularly intractable vomiting. There is a subsequent alteration in mental status with either lethargy or combative behavior, which may progress to coma, the encephalopathic phase. The mean duration between the two phases of the illness is 3 days but may range between 0.5 and 7 days, or may be as long as 2 to 3 weeks. Nonsurvivors have been noted to have a longer interval between the antecedent illness and the onset of Reye's syndrome.

The clinical features of Reye's syndrome are influenced by the age of the patient. The syndrome has been reported in patients from early infancy to adulthood. Most children are between 6 and 11 years. The median age of children afflicted following chickenpox is 6 years as opposed to 11 years following influenza.

Infants under 1 year may present with seizures. These may be secondary to hypoglycemia or central nervous system (CNS) insult. Respiratory disturbances such as apnea or hyperventilation are also noted, but the hallmark of Reye's syndrome, vomiting, may be minimal in the infant. Diarrhea, however, is more frequent. The child over the age of 1 year may also manifest respiratory disturbances, particularly hyperventilation. Breathing may be shallow, irregular, or rapid, or may mimic that seen with ketoacidosis or salicylate intoxication. Changes in mental status, such as lethargy, irritability, disorientation, delirium, hallucinations, and combativeness occur. Seizures may also be seen in older children. Adults with Reye's syndrome present with similar symptoms.

DIAGNOSIS

The diagnosis of Reye's syndrome should be suspected clinically in any one of the following classes of patients:

1. Any child showing an alteration of mental status, such as lethargy, irritability, or combativeness.
2. A child with right upper quadrant tenderness. Fifty percent of children with Reye's syndrome have hepatomegaly, with the liver being either soft or firm.
3. A child with antecedent chickenpox or influenza who presents with new complaints.
4. A child with abnormal neurologic examination. Fundoscopic examination should be included because the finding of papilledema, although unusual, is associated with a higher mortality. More fre-

quent neurologic findings include increased muscle tone and deep tendon reflexes, and dilated, sluggishly reactive pupils.
5. All infants with unexplained hypoglycemia and seizures.

It is crucial that the emergency physician maintain a high index of suspicion for this disorder, obtain the appropriate tests, and initiate early treatment.

LABORATORY

The detection of abnormalities is confirmatory evidence of Reye's syndrome. The following laboratory studies are suggested.

1. *Liver function tests* The liver panel should include tests for prothrombin time, partial thromboplastin time (prolonged), serum glutamic oxaloacetic transaminase, serum glutamic pyruvic transaminase (elevated 2 to 20 times normal), serum ammonia (2 to 20 times normal), and bilirubin (usually normal). It would be difficult to entertain the diagnosis of Reye's syndrome in the absence of abnormal liver function tests, or in the presence of an elevated bilirubin level (total greater than 5 mg/dL).
   Elevation of the blood ammonia level is the sine qua non of Reye's syndrome. The ultimate outcome does not correlate completely with the ammonia level, although levels greater than 350 mg/dL (venous) are associated with a poor prognosis. The elevated ammonia level reflects a disturbance of the urea cycle. Carbamoylphosphate synthetase and ornithine carbamoyltransferase, urea cycle enzymes, are located within the mitochondrial matrix.
   Transient elevations of liver function tests may occur with varicella hepatitis even in the absence of Reye's syndrome.
   Liver function studies return to normal in 3 to 5 days in Reye's syndrome. This rapid recovery helps differentiate Reye's syndrome from acute yellow atrophy due to hepatitis or poisoning.
2. *Creatine phosphokinase* The creatine phosphokinase (CPK) level is also elevated. This includes MM (skeletal), MB (cardiac), but not BB (brain) fractions. The elevation of the CPK level may correlate with the ultimate outcome; patients with the highest levels of CPK have the highest mortality.
3. *Blood glucose levels* Hypoglycemia was initially considered a hallmark of Reye's syndrome. It is now felt to occur in 40 percent of affected children, usually those less than 5 years old and especially those under 1 year. A low blood glucose level is correlated with a poor outcome. It is related to diminished glycogen stores and increased sugar utilization often seen with elevated ammonia levels.
4. *Serum electrolyte and blood urea nitrogen levels* These levels are either normal or reflect a degree of dehydration secondary to anorexia and vomiting. Baseline values must be present before further fluid restriction and diuretic therapy are instituted.
5. *Complete blood count and differential blood count with platelet count* These values are usually normal. The white blood cell count may be elevated secondary to stress or metabolic acidosis. Platelet counts are rarely decreased.
6. *Amylase levels* Amylase levels are elevated in about 4 percent of children with Reye's syndrome secondary to pancreatic involvement.
7. *Urinalysis* This is obtained as a baseline assessment prior to fluid restriction and diuretic therapy.
8. *Lumbar puncture* A lumbar puncture is recommended to exclude CNS infection. Some controversy exists about the risk of a spinal tap in a child with suspected elevation of intracranial pressure. The results of cerebrospinal fluid (CSF) examination are usually normal and may show a slightly low glucose level or mild monocytosis.
9. *CT scan* The CT scan shows diffuse cerebral edema with slitlike ventricles.
10. *ECG* The ECG may show arrhythmia or evidence of myocarditis, although neither is usually severe enough to require treatment.
11. *Other laboratory studies* Other laboratory results include abnormal amino acid patterns, increased free fatty acid (serum dicarboxylic acids) levels but diminished lipid levels, respiratory alkalosis and metabolic acidosis, and ketonuria.

PATHOLOGIC CONFIRMATION

The diagnosis of Reye's syndrome, while suspected clinically, may be confirmed by liver biopsy. The biopsy is characteristic and shows microvesicular fat droplets in the hepatocytes without inflammatory cell response. Electron microscopy reveals dilatation of the endoplasmic reticulum and the mitochondria. There is also an absence of glycogen stores.

The National Institutes of Health Consensus Development Conference on the Diagnosis and Treatment of Reye Syndrome concluded that the clinical and laboratory findings are diagnostic in children over the age of 1 year and liver biopsy is not necessary in all cases. Liver biopsy is recommended in infants under 1 year, children who have recurrences or atypical presentations (no prodromal illness, no vomiting), familial cases, or when unproven therapeutic interventions are planned. Some investigators have reported pathognomonic changes in the mitochondria with muscle biopsy and suggest that this may be an alternative tissue for disease confirmation.

DIFFERENTIAL DIAGNOSIS

The differential diagnosis includes other disorders producing hepatic and CNS dysfunction. These include:

1. *Fulminant hepatic failure* This may occur in association with infection (viral hepatitis), or drug or toxin ingestion. Salicylates, acetaminophen, isopropyl alcohol, and valproate may produce drug-induced hepatitis resembling Reye's syndrome. The absence of jaundice and the unique liver biopsy in Reye's syndrome help differentiate the two disorders.
2. *Pancreatic encephalopathy* This is a very rare disorder associated with a confusional state during a bout of acute pancreatitis.
3. *Infections of the CNS* Viral and bacterial meningitis or encephalitis may present with vomiting and lethargy. Varicella encephalitis may be confused with Reye's syndrome, but the absence of hepatic involvement leads to the diagnosis of encephalitis.
4. *Inborn errors of metabolism* Inborn errors of metabolism should be considered in young infants with Reye's syndrome, in familial cases, and in recurrent cases. Metabolic defects include urea cycle disturbances (ornithine carbamoyltransferase and carbamoylphosphate synthetase deficiencies), organic acid disorders (glutaric aciduria and isovaleric acidemia), and systemic carnitine deficiency.

The liver biopsy usually helps to differentiate these disorders when differentiation on clinical or laboratory grounds is uncertain.

STAGING

Once the diagnosis is suspected and supported by the laboratory data, one should assign the patient to a clinical stage. Lovejoy and coworkers have delineated stages helpful in determining the aggressiveness of the intervention.

Stage 0
Biochemical dysfunction without clinical syndromes. Patients demonstrate abnormalities on liver biopsy.

Stage I
Vomiting, lethargy, sleepiness, liver dysfunction. Mortality is less than 5 percent.

Stage II

Disorientation, delirium, combativeness, hyperventilation, increased deep tendon reflexes, liver dysfunction. Patients appear hyperexcitable with tachycardia, fever, sweating, and pupillary dilatation.

Stage III

Coma, increased respiratory rate, decorticate rigidity, intact pupils and oculovestibular reflexes, liver dysfunction. The mortality is 50 to 60 percent.

Stage IV

Deepening coma, decerebrate rigidity, no oculovestibular reflexes, loss of corneal reflexes, minimal liver dysfunction.

Stage V

Seizures, loss of deep tendon reflexes, respiratory arrest, flaccidity. Liver dysfunction is absent. The mortality is 95 percent in this group.

Staging based on the EEG is nonspecific and does not facilitate diagnosis but may have some predictive value. The neurologic symptoms as reflected in the staging move in a rostral to caudal manner. Seizures are associated with brainstem dysfunction. Poor prognostic signs include

1. Rapid passage through the first three clinical stages
2. The onset of seizures while in stage III
3. Initial ammonia levels greater than 300 μg/mL
4. Prothrombin time that is 13 to 14 s greater than that of the control
5. An increased CSF pressure in stage III
6. Type 3 EEG

MANAGEMENT

The management of the noncomatose patient with stage I or II Reye's syndrome is supportive, with intravenous fluids (10% dextrose), and observation in the hospital. The management of the comatose patient is directed toward preventing and reversing the potentially lethal complications, particularly increased intracranial pressure. Few cases of herniation have been seen with Reye's syndrome in spite of massive swelling and flattening of gyri. Additionally, neuronal damage appears to be reversible, and neuronal necrosis is not extensive at the time of autopsy.

Elevated intracranial pressure is suggested by the presence of slit-like ventricles on CT scan and is documented with the use of an intracranial pressure monitor (subarachnoid or epidural bolt, or intraventricular catheter). The catheter transmits pressure via a transducer to a recorder and also permits instant removal of CSF. It is preferred by many centers but is difficult to insert because of the small size of the ventricles. It also carries an increased risk of bleeding and infection.

The main goal of management is to maintain the intracranial pressure at less than 15 torr. Cerebral blood flow is often compromised when the cerebral perfusion pressure falls to less than 50 torr. The cerebral perfusion pressure equals the mean arterial pressure [diastolic + ⅓ (systolic minus diastolic)] minus the intracranial pressure.

The following are measures to manage increased intracranial pressure and to ensure adequate cerebral perfusion:

1. The head should be elevated to 30° in a midline position. This ensures adequate cerebral venous return and helps reduce vasogenic swelling.
2. Intubation and controlled ventilation with a respirator may be used to maintain a P_{CO_2} of 20 to 25 torr. This achieves optimum vasoconstriction and decreases the intracranial volume by decreasing the blood proportion. Further reduction of the P_{CO_2} to less than 20 torr may reduce flow too much and result in cerebral anoxia.
3. The patient may be paralyzed with pancuronium bromide, 0.1 to 0.2 mg/kg, to facilitate mechanical respiration and prevent an increase in intracranial pressure associated with movement.
4. Furosemide may be given orally in a dosage of 1 to 2 mg/kg per day divided every 6 to 8 h, or intramuscularly or intravenously 0.5 to 1.0 mg/kg per day in divided doses every 2 h; the maximum dose is 80 mg. The exact method by which furosemide works is unclear. It has been noted to produce an immediate effect with a reduction in pupillary size minutes after the dose is given. This occurs before the diuretic effect can occur.
5. Mannitol may be given as a bolus of 1 to 2 g/kg intravenously over 30 to 60 min. A continuous infusion may also be given using 1 to 2 g/kg per hour or alternately 13 g/h per 1.73 m^2. The goal of continuous mannitol infusion is to maintain the serum osmolality at 310 mOsm. Glycerol is an alternative to mannitol and may be given at 1 to 2 g/kg per dose every 4 to 6 h orally. It may produce gastrointestinal irritation. Glycerol is a smaller molecule than mannitol and may recouple oxidative phosphorylation.
6. Dexamethasone is usually given as 0.25 to 0.5 mg/per day in divided doses every 4 to 6 h. The dosage may be increased to 1 mg/kg per day. Theoretically, the mechanism of action of dexamethasone is to stabilize vascular membranes and prevent leakage. Since cerebral edema in Reye's syndrome is on a cytotoxic rather than a vasogenic basis, it is unclear why dexamethasone should be effective. It is thought that intracellular membrane stabilization or decreased CSF production may be the mode of action.
7. Pentobarbital coma may be induced with an initial intravenous bolus, 3 to 5 mg/kg, followed by 2.5 mg/kg every 2 h. The serum should be monitored to maintain a level of 3.5 mg/dL. Pentobarbital is thought to decrease cerebral blood flow and metabolic rate. Its use should be reserved for children whose elevated intracranial pressure is not responsive to other measures.
8. If positive end-expiratory pressure (PEEP) must be used for ventilation, pressure should be kept at a minimum, so as not to impede cerebral venous return. Vigorous chest physiotherapy should not be given since this increases intracranial pressure. Gentle vibration and suctioning remove mucus plugs and facilitate ventilation.

In addition to the control of the elevated intracranial pressure, there are other considerations in the management of the child with Reye's syndrome.

1. *Fluid management* There is controversy about the appropriate fluid management. Some maintain the child should be on full maintenance, while others state that the patient should receive between ⅔ and ¾ maintenance fluids. Regardless of the regimen chosen, it is important to maintain the urine output at a minimum of 0.5 mL/kg per hour to avoid renal failure.
2. *Use of hypertonic glucose* Hypertonic glucose (10 to 15%) is recommended to provide substrate for metabolism. Insulin may be given at 1 unit per 5 g of glucose, but most patients seem to be in a hyperinsulinemic state and do not need exogenous insulin. Insulin may help reduce free fatty acid levels by stimulating the activity of lipoprotein lipase.
3. *Coagulation problems* Coagulopathy should be managed with the use of vitamin K, 5 mg intravenously or intramuscularly every 12 h. Fresh-frozen plasma at a dose of 5 mL/kg per dose may be given especially if one is contemplating any invasive procedures such as liver biopsy or the placement of a subarachnoid bolt.
4. *CVP line* A central venous pressure (CVP) line is useful to monitor pressure in a patient who is being fluid-restricted. The CVP should be maintained at 4 to 6 cmH_2O to avoid renal complications secondary to dehydration.
5. *Ulcer prevention* Patients with Reye's syndrome are at risk for gastrointestinal hemorrhage and ulcer. Gastrointestinal hemorrhage is exacerbated by the coexistent coagulopathy. Antacids may be

given via nasogastric tube, or the patient may be managed with cimetidine.

6. *Bowel sterilization* Neomycin, 500 mg by nasogastric tube every 6 h, or lactulose may be used to decrease bowel flora and ammonia production.

Additional features which have been tried with variable results include total body washout (removal of the blood and replacement with normal saline for a brief period of time), peritoneal dialysis (60 percent mortality), and exchange transfusion using fresh heparinized blood. None of these measures have any proven advantage.

COMPLICATIONS

Renal failure and pancreatitis are two additional complications that may occur with Reye's syndrome. Although the kidneys frequently show pathologic changes, renal failure is an unusual complication. Changes are confined to the tubules and are reversible, and the kidneys of children who have died with Reye's syndrome have been used for renal transplantation. In the three cases of renal failure with Reye's syndrome described in the literature, the children also exhibited coagulopathy, and the renal failure was felt to resemble hemolytic-uremic syndrome.

Pancreatitis occurs in about 1 out of every 25 cases of Reye's syndrome and may progress to acute hemorrhagic pancreatitis. Hypertension, hypercalcemia, and glucose lability may herald the onset of acute pancreatitis in these patients. The role of steroids in precipitating the pancreatitis is unclear. There may be an inherent predisposition to the development of pancreatitis in some patients with Reye's syndrome.

The lungs may also show some abnormalities with alveolar wall thickening and alveolar capillary block, but this does not appear to produce symptoms.

RECOVERY PHASE

The duration of coma is variable, but typically persists for 24 to 96 h. Some children, however, remain unconscious for several weeks.

Withdrawal of measures regulating intracranial pressure may begin after the intracranial pressure has been maintained at 15 to 20 torr for 24 h. If the intracranial pressure increases, the support must be reinstituted.

1. Ventilation may be decreased to allow Pco_2 to increase by 5 mmHg every 4 to 6 h until it is a normal range.
2. Once this has been achieved, pancuronium bromide may be discontinued.
3. The mannitol bolus may be decreased in frequency from every 8 h to every 12 h to every 24 h.
4. Steroids should be decreased by 50 percent per day.
5. Mechanical ventilation may be discontinued.
6. The bolt or catheter may be discontinued.
7. Sedation may be discontinued.
8. Extra glucose and oxygen may be discontinued.

PROGNOSIS

The prognosis for Reye's syndrome has improved significantly, with the Centers for Disease Control reporting a decline in overall mortality from 40 percent in 1973 to 25 percent in 1981. Infants under the age of 1 year and children admitted in stage V Reye's syndrome continue to do poorly. In others, the prognosis for survival and normal neurologic functioning are excellent in spite of severe abnormalities at the time of initial evaluation.

Early recognition of Reye's syndrome and institution of appropriate management are the keys to successful outcome for these children.

BIBLIOGRAPHY

Consensus conference. Diagnosis and treatment of Reye's syndrome. *JAMA* 246:2441, 1981.

DeVivo DC: Reye syndrome. *Neurol Clin North Am* 3:95, 1985.

Haller J: Intracranial pressure monitoring in Reye's syndrome. *Hosp Practice* 15:101, 1980.

Herebi JE, Partin JC, Partin JS, Schubert WK: Reye's syndrome: Current concepts. *Hepatology* 7:155, 1987.

Hurwitz ES, Nelson DB, Davis C, et al. National surveillance for Reye syndrome: a five-year review. *Pediatrics* 70:895, 1982.

Lichenstein PK, Heubi JE, Daugherty CC, et al: Grade I Reye's syndrome. A frequent cause of vomiting and liver dysfunction alter varicella and upper-respiratory-tract infection. *N Engl J Med* 309:133, 1983.

Orlowski JP, Gillis J, Kilham HA: A catch in the Reye. *Pediatrics* 80:638, 1987.

Remington PL, Rowley D, McGee H, et al: Decreasing trends in Reye syndrome and aspirin use in Michigan. *Pediatrics* 77:93, 1986.

Reye RDK, Morgan G, Baral J: Encephalopathy and fatty degeneration of the viscera: A disease entity in childhood. *Lancet* 2:749, 1963.

Trauner DA: Reye's syndrome. *Curr Probl Pediatr* 12:1, 1982.

74
SEIZURES AND STATUS EPILEPTICUS IN CHILDREN

Michael A. Nigro

Approximately 2 percent of the United States population has some form of epilepsy. Many more experience seizures in association with febrile illnesses or other acute problems. In children aged 0 to 9 years, the prevalence is 4.4 cases per 1000, and in those 10 to 19 years, the prevalence is 6.6 cases per 1000. Simple febrile convulsions constitute a separate category, with an incidence of 3 to 4 percent in children.

These numbers alone do not reveal the most important features of the seizure phenomenon—the increased morbidity and mortality that are a direct result of seizures, their cause, or their treatment. Epidemiologic studies indicate an overall mortality two to three times higher in epileptic patients than in nonepileptics. The earlier the onset of seizures and the more deprived the social environment, the higher the morbidity and the mortality.

Typically a patient with seizures arrives at the emergency department with one of the following:

1. The initial or a recurrent seizure
2. Status epilepticus
3. Complications of medication
4. A history of seizures with an acute, underlying disease—e.g., sickle cell anemia, metabolic disease, or febrile illness—that needs treatment

Emergency care should include (1) safely stopping the seizure, (2) identifying and correcting immediately treatable or reversible causes, and (3) initiating appropriate diagnostic studies and arranging follow-up. If management is difficult, the patient should be admitted. There are significant enough differences in the treatment of children that unless the physician is experienced in pediatric management or able to readily obtain pediatric consultation, the child should be transferred to a pediatric facility. When the treatment or the diagnostic studies promise to be complex, time is important in reducing morbidity.

DEFINITION

A *seizure* is an episodic, involuntary alteration in motor activity, behavior, sensation, or autonomic function. It represents an abrupt change in brain function. The term *epilepsy* indicates recurring seizures without a simple discernible and reversible cause. Physiologically, a seizure is an abnormal, sudden, and excessive electric discharge of neurons (gray matter) which propagates down the neuronal processes (white matter) to affect end organs in a clinically measurable fashion.

The International Classification of Epileptic Seizures is accepted as the contemporary standard (see Table 74-1).

THE FIRST SEIZURE

The first seizure in a child usually causes some degree of panic in the parents, and an accurate account of seizure and preseizure events may not be obtainable. If it lasts seconds to minutes, and if others in the family have experienced seizures, an emergency visit may not be made. Unless the child is in status epilepticus, or seizures recur in the emergency department, the physician can defer immediate anticonvulsant treatment and concentrate on defining the cause and the risk of recurrence.

Hauser and co-workers categorized seizure recurrence for all ages according to the presumed cause. Of their patients, 73 percent were categorized as having idiopathic seizures, and 27 percent as having remote symptomatic seizures. Idiopathic seizures recurred in 17 percent of the patients by 20 months after the initial seizure, and in 26 percent of the patients by 36 months after the first seizure, but the recurrence rate was greater in patients with generalized spike-wave EEGs, and in patients with siblings who had had seizures. In patients with prior neurologic insult (cerebrovascular accident, meningitis, etc.) the recurrence rate was 34 percent by 20 months after the initial seizure.

Immediate diagnostic evaluation (see Table 74-2) can be initiated in the emergency situation, and if the seizure was brief and appears to be idiopathic, the decision to initiate anticonvulsant therapy can be deferred until the appropriate neurologic assessment is completed. The causes of the first seizure vary, but idiopathic seizures account for 26.3 to 47 percent of the children with seizures seen, depending on the study cited. Secondary seizures occur for a variety of reasons (e.g., inflammatory, structural, metabolic, or secondary to general illness).

In any group of seizure patients, there is a subgroup in whom the seizure is a symptom of an underlying disorder, and in such cases correction of the primary problem makes seizure recurrence unlikely. Thus, the primary goal must be to uncover disorders that are readily identifiable and reversible. Symptomatic seizures of hypoglycemia, hypocalcemia, and electrolyte imbalance can be treated immediately; there is little risk of recurrence, and they usually do not require anticonvulsant use. Seizures occurring as a result of intracranial infections and craniocerebral trauma may require only immediate or short-term anticonvulsant use. Symptomatic seizures of systemic lupus erythematosus (SLE), sickle cell anemia, leukemia, arteriovenous malformations, and neoplasms may be the heralding symptoms of a complex, yet treatable, underlying disease.

If the initial seizure is prolonged or classified as status epilepticus, appropriate therapy and diagnostic workup must be initiated (Tables 72-2, 72-3, or 72-6). If several seizures occur, or if the initial seizure is prolonged or occurs in a patient at higher risk for recurrence (such as one with prior neurologic insult), anticonvulsant therapy can be initiated (Table 72-3). For tonic, tonic-clonic, clonic, or partial seizures, pheonobarbital is used most often, and the initial doses need not be the higher, loading doses required in status epilepticus (Table 72-6). Phenytoin is the second most commonly used drug in this

Table 74-1. International Classification of Epileptic Seizures

I. Partial seizures (seizures beginning locally)
   A. Partial seizures with elementary symptomatology (generally without impairment of consciousness)
      1. With motor symptoms (includes Jacksonian seizures)
      2. With special sensory or somatosensory symptoms
      3. With autonomic symptoms
      4. Compound forms
   B. Partial seizures with complex symptomatology (generally with impairment of consciousness)
      1. With impairment of consciousness only
      2. With cognitive symptomatology
      3. With affective symptomatology
      4. With "psychosensory" symptomatology
      5. With "psychomotor" symptomatology
      6. Compound forms
   C. Partial seizures secondarily generalized
II. Generalized seizures (bilaterally symmetric without local onset)
   A. Absences (petit mal)
   B. Bilateral massive epileptic myoclonus
   C. Infantile spasms
   D. Clonic seizures
   E. Tonic seizures
   F. Tonic-clonic seizures (grand mal)
   G. Atonic seizures
   H. Akinetic seizures
III. Unclassified epileptic seizures

Source: Gastaut, H. Clinical and electroencephalographical classification of epileptic seizures. *Epilepsia* 11:102, 1970. Used by permission.

Table 74-2. Diagnostic Studies in Seizure Patients*

Study	Neonatal Seizure	First Seizure in Children	Status Epilepticus	Recurring Breakthrough (nonstable)
CBC with differential	X	X	X	—
Random blood sugar	X	X	X	X
Electrolytes	X	X	X	X
Creatinine	X	—	X	—
Magnesium	X	X	X	—
Calcium	X	X	X	X
BUN	X	X	X	—
Blood gases	X	—	X	—
Serum ammonia	X†	—	—	—
Urine and serum amino acid screen	X†	—	—	—
TORCH titers	X†	—	—	—
Lumbar puncture	X†	X†	X§	—
Anticonvulsant levels	—	—	X	X
EEG	X	X	X§	—
Echoencephalogram (real-time)	X†	—	—	—
CT scan	X†	X‡	X§	X†
MRI scan	X§	X§	X§	X§
Chest x-ray	X§	X§	X§	X§
Skeletal (x-ray) survey	X†	—	—	—
Cardiac/pulmonary evaluation	X†	—	X	—
Evaluation for superimposedmedical problems	—	—	X§	X
Infectious disease workup	X	X	X§	X

* X = diagnostic studies to be performed; — = studies need not be performed.

† When history or physical examination warrants it.

‡ If there is evidence of structural lesion or hereditary disorder.

§ If indicated.

situation. Carbamazepine is considered equal to phenytoin in anticonvulsant properties but has a different spectrum of potential side effects.

Absence (petit mal) seizures rarely require emergency care, and an EEG should be obtained for confirmation before one starts drugs that are more specific, namely, ethosuximide, valproate, and acetazolamide.

FEBRILE SEIZURE

Febrile seizure is a unique and common form of seizure in childhood. Although various types occur (tonic, tonic-clonic, clonic), the characteristics of a simple febrile seizure separate it from other symptomatic and idiopathic seizure disorders. The National Institutes of Health Consensus Development Conference of Febrile Seizure defined it as "an event in infancy or childhood usually occurring between three months and five years of age, associated with fever but without evidence of intracranial infection or defined cause." Typically, these seizures are generalized and last less than 10 min (some physicians say 15 to 20 min is more typical), and there is no postictal neurologic deficit. The EEG usually does not reveal paroxysmal (epileptic) activity, and there often is a family history of similar seizures. Typically a rapid rise in temperature, usually above 38.8°C (101.8°F), occurs at the onset of the illness and, on occasion, recurs several times in the course of the illness. Three to four percent of young children experience febrile seizures, and of these, 30 to 40 percent have recurrences, especially when the first seizure occurs under 1 year of age. The mortality from simple febrile seizures is extremely low.

Evaluation

The first febrile seizure warrants the most concern, because the benign nature of the illness has not been established. More concern regarding intracranial infection is justified with the febrile-seizuring child before the propensity for recurring simple febrile seizures has been established. The initial evaluation concentrates on serious causes, such as meningitis, encephalitis, and sepsis or bacteremia. Lumbar puncture is warranted with the first febrile seizure or whenever intracranial sepsis appears likely. If a cause it not found and the child is ill, admission, workup, and therapy are warranted. Underlying diseases should be

Table 74-3. Initial and Maintenance Doses in the First Seizure (*Nonstatus* Partial and Tonic, Clonic, and Tonic-Clonic Seizures of Childhood)

Drug	Initial Dose, mg/kg	Maintenance Dose, mg/kg per 24 h	Doses/Day	Therapeutic Level, μg/mL	Half-Life, h
Phenytoin (Dilantin)	8	4–8	2–3	10–20	24 ± 12
Phenobarbital	6	3–8	1–2	15–20	60 ± 20
Carbamazepine (Tegretol)	5	10–20	2–4	6–12	20 ± 5
Primidone (Mysoline)	5	10–20	2–4	5–12	12
Valproic acid (Depakene/Depakote)	10	20–60	2–4	50–100*	6–12
Ethosuximide (Zarontin)	20	20–30	2–3	50–100	30
Clonazepam (Clonopin)	0.05	0.1–0.3	2–4	NA	18–50
Acetazolamide (Diamox)	10	10	1–2	NA	24–42

* Supratherapeutic levels (up to 130 μg/mL) have been tolerated.

Note: NA = not applicable.

diagnosed. Toxic encephalopathy with fever as a symptom should be identified and treated. An EEG can be done electively, and, although its benefits are arguable, it can be helpful in identifying the child who is at greater risk of recurrent seizure.

Treatment

Therapy for the cause of the fever is the main goal. If a child appears well after experiencing a single febrile seizure, anticonvulsant therapy can be deferred, the child can be evaluated electively, and the family and attending physicians can decide whether anticonvulsants will be used. Phenobarbital at therapeutic levels (15 to 30 μg/mL) may reduce febrile seizure frequency. A recent study indicated no significant benefit from phenobarbital prophylaxis and a 6-point loss in full-scale I.Q. in lower functioning children. At this time, prophylaxis for febrile seizures remains an unresolved issue. If the child is ill, has had recurring seizures with this febrile illness, or has had several seizures with prior febrile illnesses, administration of phenobarbital can be initiated and maintained until the child improves and a decision is reached regarding the use of long-term anticonvulsants. There are subgroups of febrile seizure patients who warrant long-term anticonvulsant (phenobarbital) use, including the child (1) with a preexisting neurologic deficit, such as mental retardation or cerebral palsy, (2) with repeated seizures in the same febrile illness, (3) under 1 year of age, (4) with prior nonfebrile seizures and siblings or parents with epilepsy, or (5) with more than three febrile seizures in 6 months. When parents request phenobarbital prophylaxis, having been informed of the risks and benefits, it is reasonable to treat the child.

The protocol to follow when treating a child with febrile seizure is as follows:

1. Administer a loading dose of phenobarbital (15 mg/kg) orally, intravenously, or intramuscularly, followed by 4 to 6 mg/kg per day to attain therapeutic levels of 15 to 30 μg/mL.
2. Interrupt the fever gradually with tepid baths (use no alcohol) and acetaminophen.
3. Identify the source of infection and do a lumbar puncture if meningitis or encephalitis is suspected, or if unexplained febrile seizure occurs for the first time.
4. Arrange for follow-up studies with the child's family physician.
5. Admit the ill child without an easily treatable problem or one in whom recurrent seizures have occurred within several hours or 1 day.
6. Obtain an EEG when appropriate. An EEG may be helpful (if definitely abnormal) as a further indication of a convulsive disorder.

Phenobarbital is the most effective medication for febrile seizures. Phenytoin is less effective. Rectally administered diazepam has been used in Europe and Great Britain, but it is not in standard use in the United States. Respiratory depression associated with rectal diazepam is a potential problem when administered at home. Valproic acid has been effective, but its relative toxicity increases its risk, which contraindicates its use in the prevention of febrile seizure.

NEONATAL SEIZURES

Seizures in the neonate are difficult to identify and often require aggressive therapy. All neonates experiencing seizures should be considered to be at serious risk from the underlying disorder and also to be at increased risk of epilepsy. Electroconvulsive activity should be of as much concern as the outward clinical signs of seizure. Prompt, effective anticonvulsant therapy and other specific therapies lessen the impact of short-term detrimental effect on long-term neurologic functioning. In many instances, the seizure itself is less important for its immediate effects than it is as an indicator of significant underlying disease (e.g., galactosemia, meningitis) that will ultimately have more effect on the morbidity and mortality.

The difference in seizure presentation is due to the predominantly inhibitory brain of newborns and the particular illnesses to which they are subject. Multifocal or fragmentary seizures occur more commonly at this age, and clonic or tonic movements independently affect the limbs simultaneously or fleetingly. Progressive migratory partial seizures (jacksonian) are rarely seen at this age. Autonomic seizures manifest as variable changes in respiration (tachypnea, depression, or apnea), temperature, and color (cyanosis), and also as cardiac arrhythmias and pupillary changes. Myoclonic seizures usually have hypoxic or metabolic causes and indicate a poor prognosis unless the cause is easily identifiable and readily reversible (e.g., hypocalcemia, hypoglycemia). Myoclonic seizures can, however, be refractory in metabolic disorders such as urea cycle defects and nonketotic hyperglycinemia. Unilateral (partial or focal) seizures may be associated with structural lesions, and permanent neurologic deficit may be associated with them. The causes of neonatal seizures are diverse, but the majority of the seizures are attributable to a few well-defined causes.

Evaluation

Common neurologic nonepileptic problems encountered in the newborn are hyperexcitability in the tremulous infant, and nonepileptic cerebral manifestations of sepsis, cardiac disease, and hypoxia. Benign myoclonus is also seen. Respiratory immaturity with apnea is a particularly difficult problem at this age.

The workup includes early assessment for treatable causes. Sepsis and metabolic derangements are frequent causes of neonatal seizures. The highest incidence of neonatal seizures is in infants with hypoxia/ischemia, sepsis, or hypoglycemia.

Complex hereditary metabolic disorders—e.g., urea cycle defects with hyperammonemia; maple syrup urine disease; and methylmalonic acidemia—usually become evident days or weeks after feedings with protein are initiated. Others may appear symptomatic in utero or soon after delivery, e.g., nonketotic hyperglycinemia, in which the mother reports fetal hiccoughs, and soon after birth the infant is flaccid, exhibiting myoclonic seizures. Seizures in these metabolic disorders are a signal that significant CNS impairment may be present.

Some of these disorders may be completely controlled or the effects may be reversed with appropriate dietary manipulation (galactosemia) or coenzyme replacement (pyridoxine dependency, subtypes of methylmalonic acidemia).

In evaluating the infant, the cause of the seizures may be readily apparent. The dysmorphic newborn could have a chromosomal defect (trisomy, deletion) or be identifiable only by the combination of unusual features (Cornelia de Lange's syndrome). Neurocutaneous diseases infrequently cause seizures in the newborn but are readily identifiable by certain signs, e.g., encephalotrigeminal hemangiomatosis in Sturge-Weber syndrome, or achromic patches in tuberous sclerosis. Cutaneous herpes with seizures may be an indication that herpes simplex encephalitis is present. Chorioretinitis is a clear sign of an intrauterine infection which could cause seizures (e.g., herpes, toxoplasmosis, cytomegalovirus, rubella). The laboratory assessment may require real-time ultrasound or a CT scan to diagnose cerebral hemorrhage or malformation.

Treatment

There are several factors influencing treatment in the neonate: (1) variations in the metabolic half-lives of drugs; (2) associated etiologic conditions (e.g., hypoxia prolongs the half-life of many drugs and may affect the renal or gastrointestinal clearance rate); and (3) greater difficulty in identifying the end point of seizure control in neonates.

Effective seizure control is obtained by rapidly achieving therapeutic blood levels of the anticonvulsant chosen. Newborns have different rates of metabolism and excretion of anticonvulsants from older infants and children. In infants less than 7 days old, the half-life of pheno-

Table 74-4. Drug Regimen for Neonatal Seizures

1. Vitamin B_6 (pyridoxine), 50 mg IV—used in the absence of an obvious cause of seizures
2. Glucose, 2 mL/kg (25% solution) bolus—given to infants stressed with proven hypoglycemia or when merely suspect
3. Calcium gluconate, 4 mL/kg IV
4. Magnesium—magnesium sulfate, 50%, 0.2 mL/kg IM—given to infants with a proven deficiency
5. Phenobarbital loading
   Premature infant 10–20 mg/kg IV
   Full-term infant 10–15 mg/kg IV
6. Phenytoin (Dilantin), loading dose, 10–15 mg/kg IV
7. Diazepam (Valium) for continuous seizures, 0.2 mg/kg IV, repeat twice if necessary (see text)
8. Lorazepam, 0.05 mg/kg IV (may repeat twice if necessary)
9. Clonazepam (Klonopin), 0.1 mg/kg NG if high therapeutic levels of phenobarbital and phenytoin (Dilantin) are ineffective

barbital, the drug of first choice, is 100 h, and after 28 days of continuous therapy, the half-life of the drug is reduced to 60 to 70 h.

In the presence of hypoxia with tissue acidosis and renal and hepatic compromise, anticonvulsant half-lives may be increased, with toxic levels reached more readily.

Blood levels of phenobarbital above 16 μg/mL are necessary to achieve seizure control, but levels of above 40 μg/mL are of no proven benefit. Dosages of phenobarbital of 3 to 4 mg/kg per day maintain mid to high therapeutic levels and prevent toxicity.

Phenytoin is the second drug of choice in treating neonatal seizures and has the disadvantage of requiring intravenous use to obtain and maintain therapeutic levels. Loading doses vary from 10 to 20 mg/kg, and maintenance dosages of 3 to 4 mg/kg per day (similar to those of phenobarbital) are satisfactory and not likely to produce toxicity. Pyridoxine (vitamin B_6) is empirically used when no reasonable cause of the seizure is found. The only reasonable determinant of its effectiveness is a cessation of seizure activity. The electroencephalogram does not immediately improve with intravenous pyridoxine use.

In status epilepticus of the neonate, diazepam or lorazepam must be used with caution since its half-life may be prolonged, and respiratory depression superimposed on an immature and possibly compromised respiratory apparatus should be anticipated. Diazepam may exaggerate hyperbilirubinemia by uncoupling the bilirubin-albumin complex and should be used with caution in jaundiced babies.

Treatment principles in the management of neonatal seizures are as follows:

1. Identify and correct treatable causes (hypocalcemia, hypoglycemia, electrolyte imbalance).
2. Identify and treat associated problems such as sepsis, hyperbilirubinemia, acidosis, etc.
3. Initiate anticonvulsant therapy with appropriate loading doses, and carefully observe blood levels to adjust the maintenance dosage (see Table 74-4).

INFANTILE SPASMS

Infantile spasms are a unique form of seizures. The onset is typically between 3 and 9 months of age and may begin as late as 18 months. Concurrently, the child exhibits a regression in development. The spasms are very brief, lasting a split second, often with flexion or extension of the head and trunk. They occur singly or repeatedly in bursts of 5 to 20 spasms at a time, usually occurring several times per day and more often upon arousal from sleep or with sudden auditory or physical stimulation. The EEG is abnormal in most cases (hypsarrhythmic in 50 percent). Mental retardation is as high as 85 percent of patients with this disorder. Parents are often frustrated because medical professionals fail to diagnose these spasms as seizures.

There are many causes of infantile spasm (secondary type) including trauma, vitamin B_6 deficiency, infection, and metabolic disorders. The idiopathic type is the most alarming because it most often affects children with no prior neurologic disorder.

Early diagnosis and aggressive management with adrenocorticotropic hormone (ACTH) within a month of onset result in an optimum response. Since this is a neurologic emergency, hospitalization, neurologic referral, appropriate diagnostic workup, and initiation of treatment must be rapidly conducted. Aggressive management with steroids or anticonvulsants, careful monitoring of the EEG, and identification of side effects make this therapeutic problem beyond the scope of emergency care with one exception: recognizing the problem.

HEAD TRAUMA AND SEIZURES

Head trauma can result in seizures of three types: immediate seizures, early posttraumatic seizures, and late posttraumatic seizures. Immediate seizures result from impact and presumably are due to traumatic depolarization of neurons. The risk of recurring seizures in these patients is minimal unless there are more serious prognostic factors such as prolonged coma and penetrating head injury. Anticonvulsants are sometimes used because of the unknown potential for immediate recurring seizures. In the patient who recovers rapidly, chronic anticonvulsant use is usually not indicated. An exception would be a patient with a prior seizure history or a family history of epilepsy.

Early posttraumatic seizures occur within the first week after trauma, and epilepsy results in 20 to 25 percent of these patients. These early seizures are presumed to result from the focal effects of contusions or lacerations and the associated hypoperfusion, which causes ischemia and related metabolic changes.

Treatment of immediate and early posttraumatic seizures requires the correction of neurologic problems (depressed fracture, hematoma), the reduction of cerebral edema, proper oxygenation (airway maintenance, correction of shock), and the careful administration of anticonvulsants. With immediate and early posttraumatic seizures when impaired consciousness already prevails, it is important to avoid the use of significant sedative medication (barbiturates or diazepam) if possible. Phenytoin may be used successfully with relative safety (see Table 74-3). The dosage is determined by the clinical presentation; rapid loading is warranted to obtain immediate therapeutic levels in the patient in whom repeated seizures are occurring or likely to recur, especially when a seizure may further aggravate associated medical or surgical conditions.

Immediate posttraumatic seizures warrant anticonvulsant therapy for initial control, while long-term management of immediate seizures remains controversial.

Late posttraumatic seizures occur after 1 week and may be seen as late as 10 years after the trauma. Structural changes such as atrophy with cicatrix and permanent local vascular changes, altered dendrite branching, and presumably modified neurotransmitter function account for the development and permanence of these seizures. Of these seizures, 40 percent are focal or partial seizures and 50 percent are temporal lobe seizures, indicating the predilection for traumatic injury and known epileptogenic properties of this structure. The risk of recurring seizures in this group is reported to be as high as 70 percent.

Early and late posttraumatic seizures warrant long-term anticonvulsant therapy in view of the risk of immediate and later recurrence. Late-onset posttraumatic seizures are most likely to recur, and long-term anticonvulsant therapy is necessary. Patients at greater risk for chronic posttraumatic seizures include those with depressed skull fractures, posttraumatic amnesia more than 24 h after the trauma, dural penetration, acute intracranial hemorrhage, early posttraumatic epilepsy, and a foreign body in a cerebral wound. The more severe the seizure and the later the onset, the less likely remission will occur.

Emergency management of seizures related to trauma should emphasize neurosurgical assessment, the rapid, careful administration of nonsedative anticonvulsants, the interruption of the seizures, and the stabilization of the general medical condition.

BREAKTHROUGH SEIZURES IN THE KNOWN EPILEPTIC

When seizures recur in a known epileptic, something has occurred to alter the balance of the excitation-inhibition complex, and the seizure threshold has been lowered. Complete seizure control is not always possible. The child with mental retardation, cerebral palsy, and generalized (most often myoclonic) seizures is most likely to have recurring seizures. Tonic-clonic (grand mal) seizures are the most dramatic and often lead to emergency treatment. The usual causes of seizure breakthrough can be summarized as follows:

1. Lowered anticonvulsant blood levels.
   a. Due to noncompliance. This is a common cause, most often in the preteen or teen who has been given the responsibility for self-medication.
   b. Related to intercurrent infection. Anticonvulsant levels fall during acute infections (viral or bacterial) with or without fever. Quite often the child's seizure recurrence is an indication of the infection before the acute problem is evident, e.g., with varicella or otitis media.
   c. The interaction of different drugs. An example is the reduction of the phenytoin level by the induction of parahydroxylators when barbiturates are used concomitantly (see "Problems of Anticonvulsant Use").
2. Change in habits.
   a. Altered sleep patterns because of trips, holidays, or parties.
   b. A job, exams, or an emotional stress. In the active teen, this may lead to seizures. If a pattern develops, knowledge of the pattern is quite helpful in defining treatment.
   c. Alcohol use. This can lower the seizure threshold and can also increase noncompliance.
   d. The use of illicit drugs or prescription drugs that lower the threshold. Examples are phenothiazine, lindane (Kwell), theophylline, PCP, LSD, and anesthetic agents (e.g., ethrane).
3. Complicating factors of epilepsy management.
   a. Toxic levels of drugs. An example is phenytoin intoxication, which can increase seizure frequency. Carbamazepine in therapeutic dosage has been found to infrequently increase seizures.
   b. The use of phenytoin in some myoclonic epilepsies.
   c. Valproic acid. Its use in complex partial seizures with secondary generalization has been reported to increase the partial (focal) seizure.
   d. Anticonvulsant-induced osteomalacia with hypocalcemia (ricketts). This uncommon problem may increase the seizure frequency and typically occurs after 5 to 7 years' use.
4. The progression of the underlying cause. Examples are subacute focal (Rasmussen's) encephalitis, neoplasm, arteriovenous malformation, and degenerative disease (ceroid lipofuscinosis). Blume and co-workers reported that 16 of 38 children undergoing cerebral resection for intractable seizures were found unexpectedly to have a cerebral tumor.
5. The vagaries of epilepsy. An unprovoked episode of seizures may occur in a well child with adequate therapeutic levels of anticonvulsants.
6. Superimposed head trauma may precipitate seizures.

When a child known to have epilepsy presents with recurring seizures, several steps may minimize the treatment time and disclose the reason for the breakthrough. The physician should first assess the obvious factors: the airway and the vital signs. Next, if the patient is having seizures at the time, the physician should test for the levels of anticonvulsants, electrolytes, calcium, and glucose and should obtain a complete blood cell count with differential. An intravenous catheter should be inserted if the child is not alert, so that medication can be administered if necessary. If the patient if febrile, a source of infection should be sought.

Once these procedures have been completed, anticonvulsant management is initiated. Assume the anticonvulsant levels are low and give a partial loading dose. If the patient is compliant, give the daily dose of phenobarbital or phenytoin orally if the patient is able to swallow, or intravenously if not. If the patient is known to be noncompliant or if the levels of the anticonvulsant are found on testing to be significantly below the therapeutic range, give the daily dose twice (e.g., in the child on 60 mg of phenobarbital, give 60 mg initially and repeat the dose if the seizures recur despite levels in the low therapeutic range).

If the anticonvulsant levels are within a high therapeutic range and the child is well without an obvious source of infection or other cause of breakthrough, then one can decide if another anticonvulsant is necessary. One may decide to wait and see if there is a trend toward increased seizure frequency, warranting additional medication, or if this is a solitary episode, warranting observation, monitoring of drug levels, and follow-up. If the levels are within the high therapeutic range and seizures recur, additional anticonvulsants are warranted in appropriate loading doses (Table 74-3).

Recurring or frequent tonic, tonic-clonic, and clonic seizures warrant loading doses that produce therapeutic levels rapidly. Phenobarbital and phenytoin can be given orally or intravenously to achieve therapeutic levels. Primidone (Mysoline) and carbamazepine (Tegretol) and not typically used as emergency drugs or given in large loading doses because of their side effects. Valproic acid (Depakene) or its enteric-coated form, divalproic acid (Depakote) is usually given orally; the enteric-coated form may be used with less likelihood of abdominal discomfort and nausea. Liquid valproate (60 mg/kg with equal amounts of saline) has been used rectally to achieve therapeutic levels rapidly in patients in status epilepticus. It can be given this way in patients temporarily unable to swallow.

Seizures which begin with focal features, partial or complex partial (temporal lobe, psychomotor), may appear less dramatic and typically warrant a slower modification of drug therapy unless the seizures are prolonged or postictal Todd's paralysis occurs. If the patient requires additional drugs, phenobarbital, phenytoin, and carbamazepine can be used interchangeably, although the last cannot be loaded rapidly without producing uncomfortable side effects. Patients with petit mal (generalized absence) epilepsy rarely are brought to the emergency room, since the seizures are not alarming to the parents. If some injury occurs because of the absence spells, or if the parent is unusually concerned and brings the child for emergency treatment, determining the blood levels of anticonvulsants is most useful. Addition of another anticonvulsant can be initiated, for example, ethosuximide (Zarontin), valproate, clonazepam (Klonopin), or acetazolamide (Diamox).

Most often the epileptic patient can be sent home and modification of the drug regimen can be carried out by the attending physician. Following the initial evaluations, modification of drug therapy, and treatment for any superimposed problems, the emergency physician should (1) arrange for follow-up evaluations by the attending physician, (2) emphasize the need for compliance, and (3) provide continued treatment for infections.

STATUS EPILEPTICUS

Status epilepticus represents a state of "epileptic seizure that is so frequently repeated or so prolonged as to create a fixed and lasting epileptic condition." This definition applies to continuous seizures lasting at least 30 min. More specific classification is listed in Table 74-5.

About 5 to 10 percent of children with epilepsy and 60,000 to 100,000 total epileptics experience one bout of status grand mal (SGM). This condition is a neurologic emergency which could be fatal. The

Table 74-5. Classification of Status Seizures

I. Primary generalized convulsive status grand mal (continuous and noncontinuous)
  A. Tonic-clonic status
  B. Myoclonic status
  C. Clonic-tonic status
II. Secondary generalized convulsive status (continuous and noncontinuous)
  A. Tonic-clonic status with partial onset
  B. Tonic status
III. Simple partial status
  A. Partial motor status including EPC*
  B. Partial sensory status
  C. Partial status with vegetative or autonomic symptoms
  D. Partial status with cognitive symptoms
  E. Partial status with affective symptoms
IV. Complex partial status
V. Absence (petit mal) status

* Epilepsia partialis continua.

Source: Modified from Delgado-Escueta AV, Bajorek JG: Status epilepticus: Mechanisms of brain damage and rational management. *Epilepsia* 23(suppl 1):S29, 1982. Used by permission.

longer the SGM persists, the greater the morbidity and the mortality and the more difficult it is to control the seizures. In patients with no neurologic sequelae, the mean duration of SGM is 1½ h. Neurologic sequelae result when SGM lasts an average of 10 h. The mean duration of SGM in patients who die is 13 h.

Effects of SGM

Experimental models in animals provide evidence of the neurologic effects of SGM. Selective permanent cell damage in the hippocampus, amygdala, cerebellum, thalamus, and middle cerebral cortical layers develops after 60 min of seizure activity. Even with artificial ventilation and correction of existing metabolic derangements, most changes still occur. This cell death results from the increased metabolic demands and the exhaustion of the continuously firing neurons. In addition, there are secondary effects which probably exaggerate the adverse effects of SGM. After unremitting SGM, the cerebral P_{O_2} and amounts of cytochrome *A* and cytochrome A_3 reductase decrease, enhancing the risk of cell damage. Increases in calcium, arachidonic acid, arachidonal diglycerol, prostaglandin, and leukotriene levels in the neurons exaggerate or cause cerebral edema and cell death. Increased levels of cyclic AMP and increased release of prolactin, growth hormone, ACTH, cortisol, insulin, glycogen, epinephrine, and norepinephrine may contribute to the progression of cell damage with the loss of physiologic responsiveness.

Late secondary effects include lactic acidosis, elevated cerebrospinal fluid pressure, hyperglycemia (followed later by hypoglycemia), dysautonomia with hyperthermia, diaphoresis, dehydration, hypertension followed by hypotension, and eventually shock. In addition, excessive muscle activity leads to myolysis, myoglobinuria, and renal failure. Neuropathologic studies indicate nucleovacuolation and ischemic nerve cell damage leading to neuronal dissolution.

Treatment

Treatment is best initiated when the type of seizure is identified. To obtain the most effective and rapid cessation of status epilepticus, the following specific therapeutic goals must be reached.

1. Specific delineation of the type and subtype of status epilepticus so that appropriate treatment can be chosen. For example, tonic-clonic generalized status epilepticus is very responsive to diazepam or phenytoin; noncontinuous clonic or tonic-clonic seizures may be refractory to diazepam.
2. Identification and treatment of the reversible precipitating cause of status epilepticus, e.g., cerebral infection, trauma, electrolyte disturbance, brain abscess, hypoglycemia.
3. Rapid cessation of status epilepticus to prevent secondary effects that both prolong the seizures and cause irreversible neuronal damage.
4. Full support of medical systems to prevent unwarranted complications of the seizures or the treatment, e.g., respiratory depression, arrhythmia, aspiration pneumonia, shock, myoglobulinuria.

In treating the patient with continuous grand mal or tonic-clonic seizures, the end point is clear: the cessation of seizures. The amount of diazepam necessary to stop the seizures has been derived from studies that confirm one significant point—complications usually occur in markedly ill patients with complex disorders or with prior use of high dosages of other hypnotic drugs. The safety of diazepam to a maximum dose of 2.6 mg/kg over the course of treatment has been substantiated. Smith and co-workers described an effective dose of diazepam as 0.08 to 2.72 mg/kg in infants and young children with an average effective dose of 0.68 mg/kg. Many authors recommend initial doses of 1 mg per year of age with a maximum total dose of 5 mg in infants and 10 mg in children. Eckert reported maximum doses in adolescents as 35 mg in brief periods and 100 mg in 24 h.

A starting diazepam dose of 0.2 to 0.5 mg/kg, given at a rate of 1 mg/min and repeated as needed to a maximum of 2.6 mg/kg, is recommended to stop continuous tonic-clonic and clonic seizures. This higher dose is rarely used since most patients stop seizing at lower doses and additional drugs such as phenytoin may be employed. Care must be taken to ensure adequate ventilation.

The drug of choice in continuous SGM is diazepam, with 80 percent success within 5 min reported. To maintain the seizure-free state, one must use a long-term anticonvulsant. Therefore, after diazepam causes the seizures to cease, a phenytoin loading dose of 15 mg/kg is administered with maintenance dosages of 5 to 8 mg/kg per day to maintain therapeutic blood levels of 10 to 20 μg/mL. Phenobarbital may be necessary if phenytoin is ineffective.

Lorazepam is an alternative benzodiazepam, useful in the treatment of SGM. Theoretically, lorazepam is better than diazepam because of its pharmacokinetic properties, exhibiting a slower onset of action (latency) but a longer duration of action, allowing for a more prolonged seizure-free interval following initial infusion. In an open study by Lacey and co-workers, lorazepam was administered to 31 children exhibiting status epilepticus. The initial dose was 0.05 mg/kg, with 20 patients receiving two injections and 1 receiving three injections. The median dose was 0.05 mg/kg, with a total median accumulative dose of 2.0 mg. The median latency was 10 min; control lasted at least 3 to 6 h in 83 percent of the patients and 24 h in nearly 50 percent of the patients. In a double-blind randomized trial by Leppik and co-workers, 78 adult patients were treated with either lorazepam (4 mg) or diazepam (10 mg). Latency (2 to 3 min), efficacy (76 to 89 percent), and adverse effects (12 to 13 percent) did not differ significantly in both groups. At this time, lorazepam may be used interchangeably with diazepam in the treatment of status epilepticus. Whether it will be superior to diazepam will probably depend on whether or not the duration of action is significantly longer and whether or not respiratory depression is as prominent.

The following 10 steps should be followed when treating continuous SGM (tonic-clonic status epilepticus) (Table 74-6):

1. Assess basic functions immediately and maintain blood pressure, airway, and pulse.
2. Obtain blood to be tested for levels of anticonvulsants, electrolytes, BUN, calcium, and glucose, and for a complete blood cell count with differential while inserting an IV catheter for fluid administration.
3. Administer IV a bolus of 25% glucose, 2 mL/kg.

Table 74-6. Doses for Status Epilepticus in Children

Drug	Recommended Loading Dose	Route	Repeat	Rate	Maximum Dose
Diazepam (Valium)	0.2 mg/kg	IV	3 times	1 mg/min	5 mg 0–2 years 10 mg 2 years and older
Lorazepam	0.05 mg/kg	IV	2 times	over 2 min	0.2 mg/kg
Phenobarbital	15.0 mg/kg	IV	0		400 mg
Phenytoin (Dilantin)	15.0 mg/kg	IV	0	1 mg/kg per min	1000 mg
Paraldehyde*	0.3 mL/Kg	Rectal	q 4 h		15 mL
Clonazepam (Klonopin)	0.3 mg/kg	NG	q 6 h		10 mg
Valproic acid (Depakene*)	60.0 mg/kg	Rectal	0		
Lidocaine	2.0 mg/kg	IV		5–10 mg/kg per h	

* See text.

4. Administer IV diazepam, 0.2 mg/kg, and repeat up to a total dose of 2.6 mg/kg or early signs of respiratory depression. Alternatively, administer IV lorazepam, 0.05 mg/kg over 2 min, repeating in 15 min and 30 min if necessary.
5. Administer IV phenytoin, 15 mg/kg, after diazepam is infused, at a rate of 25 mg/min.
6. Administer IV phenobarbital, 10 to 15 mg/kg, if phenytoin is ineffective. When the patient requires step 6, transfer to the intensive care unit is warranted.
7. Administer rectally paraldehyde, 0.3 mL/kg, mixed with an equal amount of mineral oil, if step 6 is ineffective.
8. Administer IV a bolus of lidocaine, 2 mg/kg, if step 7 is ineffective.
9. In noncontinuous SGM, administer clonazepam (Klonopin) through nasogastric tube in a single dose of 0.2 to 0.6 mg/kg initially followed by 0.1 to 0.4 mg/kg per day maintenance.
10. General anesthesia.

Noncontinuous status epilepticus can be more difficult to treat since the end point is more elusive. Rapidly acting drugs such as diazepam are less effective, and a more sustained effect is necessary. Often noncontinuous status epilepticus is not responsive to appropriate therapeutic levels of phenytoin and phenobarbital. Large doses (0.2 to 0.6 mg/kg) of clonazepam via nasogastric tube may be used to produce the desired effect of rapid cessation of noncontinuous seizures, and the anticonvulsant effect maintained by additional drugs (phenytoin, phenobarbital) and clonazepam (0.1 to 0.3 mg/kg per day).

Paraldehyde administered rectally can be very effective in noncontinuous status epilepticus. Paraldehyde should be administered only with glass syringes and rubber tubing in view of its degradation to toxic forms in the presence of certain plastics.

Absence (petit mal) status is a much simpler form of status epilepticus to deal with since it is exquisitely responsive to diazepam given intravenously. It rarely happens that a patient requires emergency care for this form of epilepsy.

Epilepsia partialis continua is a serious neurologic condition, although it does not appear threatening at first glance. The patient exhibits repeated continuous or minimally interrupted clonic jerking of one side of the body and usually one part of an extremity for days, weeks, or months. It is typically due to encephalitis or cerebrovascular accident and indicates a relatively poor prognosis. Its management is similar to that of noncontinuous SGM.

DIFFERENTIAL DIAGNOSIS OF SEIZURES

It is necessary to identify nonepileptic paroxysmal disorders to prevent confusion with epilepsy. The differential diagnosis of seizures must take into account many disorders that can produce loss of consciousness, unusual movements, impaired awareness, or bizarre behavior. Many of these disorders depend on age.

In the newborn, the problems partly reflect the intrauterine experience. Jitteriness or hyperexcitability appears as high-amplitude tremulousness easily brought out by passive movement of the extremities or jarring of the crib. The drug-withdrawn infant is irritable and tremulous and may have diaphoresis, vomiting, and diarrhea; in addition, seizures may occur. Sepsis, hypoglycemia, and hypocalcemia may produce nonepileptic paroxysmal activity in addition to seizures. Near-miss sudden death syndrome (SIDS) remains a multifactorial condition in which seizures are part of the differential diagnosis and might be considered part of the cause.

In the older infant it is more common to see cyanotic and pallid breath-holding spells, which typically occur following an abrupt trauma (fall, minor spanking) or a verbal reprimand. The infant gives a sudden cry followed by prolonged inhalation or exhalation, resulting in no air exchange, and a Valsalva maneuver, often with bradycardia. A brief tonic nonepileptic seizure often occurs. Drug intoxication manifested by hyperkinesis, impaired awareness, or altered behavior (hallucinations) is usually accidental at this age. Later in childhood, phencyclidine (PCP) intoxication mimics complex partial seizures and may result in seizures with more severe overdoses.

Congenital heart disease can produce paroxysmal events at all ages. Abrupt mental-status changes may occur in patients with pulmonary hypertension, aortic stenosis, tetralogy of Fallot, atresia of the ventricles, cardiac rhabdomyomas, etc. Acquired cardiomyopathy may result in decreased cardiac output (Adams-Stokes disease) or cerebrovascular accident.

Hyperkinetic movement disorders can be difficult to differentiate from complex partial seizures. Sydenham's chorea is infrequently seen today, and drug-induced chorea (ethosuximide, carbamazepine, diphenhydramine hydrochloride) and lupus-induced chorea are likewise very uncommon. Tourette's syndrome is more frequently seen, but rarely does the child appear acutely ill.

Immediate posttraumatic migraine may recur after relatively minor injury and cause confusional states mimicking concussion or complex partial seizures.

In the adolescent, syncope due to stretching and yawning or following hair combing (vasovagal) is more common. Many children experience syncope when standing in church.

Pseudoseizures represent a particular problem for the treating physician because the "seizures" appear to represent a significant threat to the patient's safety, and vigorous anticonvulsant therapy is often initiated. Unfortunately, pseudoseizures often occur in patients with documented epilepsy. Secondary gain should become evident in these cases. The "seizures" are atypical in that the patient may waken fully in the interictal phase and require repeated large doses of anticonvulsants even to the point of protracted drug-induced depression. Another form of pseudoseizures consists of those described by the parent and never observed by other witnesses.

To distinguish pseudoseizures from true epileptic spells, a bedside technique may be dramatic and diagnostic, and prevent overtreatment. One method is to gently insert a nasopharyngeal tube and observe the patient's response. The pseudoseizure patient will become responsive immediately. Experience dictates referral for patients with a diagnosis of pseudoseizure, or even hospitalization, to prevent recurrences, provide family education, and lessen the likelihood of inappropriate treatment.

Simple sleep myoclonus and night terrors are of concern to parents. They are, however, easily distinguished from nocturnal seizures.

Preventing misdiagnosis and mistreatment is an essential part of the emergency management of seizures and related disorders.

PROBLEMS OF ANTICONVULSANT USE

Unwanted features of anticonvulsants may be seen soon after the drug is initiated or may develop weeks, months, or years later. These problems may turn up during evaluation for other illnesses (e.g., macrocytic anemia) or be the basis for emergency treatment.

Immediate side effects often subside in time. Lethargy occurs more often with barbiturates, is usually dose-related, and subsides with chronic use and half-life stabilization. Irritability and changes in cognition can persist and be so significant that a nonbarbiturate anticonvulsant must be substituted. Rashes may occur within days or weeks of initiation of therapy but must be differentiated from concurrent viral exanthem. Pruritic and/or morbilliform rashes usually require cessation of medication. Stevens-Johnson syndrome, with bullous skin lesions affecting mucous membranes, is a serious potential reaction. There is a risk of serious sequelae—blindness, esophageal stenosis, or loss of life.

With valproic acid use, hepatic failure may occur within days or up to 2 years after first use. The drug reaction results in alteration of behavior, increasing lethargy, and vomiting. Levels of liver enzymes may be minimally to markedly elevated, and hyperammonemia with or without symptoms of hepatic failure may be found. Immediate cessation of valproate, hospitalization, and observation are necessary if symptomatic hepatic reaction is evident. In the asymptomatic patient with enzyme-level elevations, a reduction of the dosage and careful observation are warranted. Gastrointestinal side effects are common with initial use of valproic acid and may be so severe that more serious hepatic problems are considered. These side effects can be avoided by a more frequent dosage schedule, by taking the drug with meals, and by avoiding carbonated beverages and citric juices, or alternatively by using the enteric-coated form. Pancreatitis secondary to valproate use also has been reported.

Toxicity due to overdosage at any time can produce some readily identifiable symptoms and signs. Phenytoin toxicity occurs when serum levels exceed 25 μg/mL in most patients (above 20 μg/mL in some). Nausea, dysarthria, diplopia, and ataxia are seen early, with progression to impaired levels of consciousness and decerebrate posturing. Virtually all anticonvulsants produce ataxia and lethargy with significant overdosage. Cardiopulmonary monitoring during high-dose drug use in status epilepticus should be employed since cardiac collapse or respiratory depression can occur. Burning in the limb used for the infusion of phenytoin has also been reported. Using a free-flowing, well-positioned needle and a short tubing distance and infusing at a rate of 50 mg/min or less lessens the likelihood of phenytoin side effects. Chronic phenytoin use can result in folate deficiency with macrocytic anemia, acquired osteomalacia (increased vitamin D turnover), neutropenia (often transient), peripheral neuropathy, lupus-like syndromes, and myasthenic weakness.

Valproate-induced thrombocytopenia is a significant side effect warranting lowering or discontinuation of the drug. Lower carnitine levels due to valproate metabolism may be a contributing factor of valproate hepatotoxicity.

Drug interactions may be quite dramatic. Valproate and aspirin can result in a bleeding diathesis. Antihistamines used in conjunction with barbiturates can be very sedating, warranting smaller doses of the antihistamine. When erythromycin is used, particular care must be exercised since the carbamazepine levels may rise to toxic levels rapidly. Toxicity is greater when carbamazepine and lithium are used together, and blood levels may be in the therapeutic range. Total phenytoin levels are typically reduced when valproic acid is also used, but free phenytoin usually remains therapeutic. It is essential to measure free phenytoin when valproate is used concurrently. When barbiturates are used concomitantly with phenytoin, increased parahydroxylation can cause enhanced metabolism of phenytoin so that therapeutic levels fall, resulting in seizure breakthrough. Hyperbilirubinemia and hypoalbuminemia can affect anticonvulsant binding and blood levels.

Movement disorders (e.g., chorea) can result after several weeks' or months' use of ethosuximide and rarely with carbamazepine. The movements may be profound and usually respond promptly to the cessation of use of the drug and the use of diphenhydramine (Benadryl), 12.5 to 25 mg given intravenously. Clonazepam and diazepam can cause acute bladder dysfunction with urinary retention.

Many problems of dose-related toxicity can be avoided by maintaining therapeutic blood levels. Blood level determinations should be done randomly to determine compliance and at times of increased seizure frequency or when signs of toxicity develop. In some patients, side effects develop at therapeutic levels. Idiosyncratic effects cannot be predicted, but families must be made aware that significant side effects can develop with little warning, and evaluation by a physician is recommended before a drug is dismissed. Obtaining the patient's history, consulting with the primary physician or consultant, and reviewing readily available drug information in the package insert or *Physicians' Desk Reference* make emergency evaluation and treatment of anticonvulsant drug reactions simpler.

PITFALLS OF EMERGENCY MANAGEMENT OF SEIZURES

After the patient arrives for treatment, the initial assessment may be incomplete, resulting in inappropriate or inadequate therapy. Not identifying treatable infections, electrolyte imbalance, child abuse, and accidental trauma can lead to rapidly progressive deterioration and demise, or may make seizure control difficult. By not ascertaining anticonvulsant levels in the patient with epilepsy, the physician loses an opportunity to determine if the anticonvulsant is ineffective or simply at too low a level.

If the emergency physician communicates with the primary physician, unnecessary studies, and drugs which either were ineffective or produced some side effects, can be avoided. Additionally, it is important to consult with the patient's physician when prescribing nonanticonvulsants which might interfere with anticonvulsants or produce unwanted side effects.

In the aggressive treatment of seizures (status epilepticus and recurring breakthrough seizures), inadequate loading doses or improper drug selection may prolong the seizures and worsen the prognosis. Excessive dosage can result in respiratory depression or hypotension and, in rare instances, can exacerbate the seizures. If nonepileptic paroxysmal disorders are not recognized, the patient is put at the additional risk of unnecessary medication and inadequate treatment of the real disorder.

The emergency physician cannot deal with all the problems facing the patient with epilepsy. Follow-up care by the primary physicians or appropriate consultants ensures better compliance and, one hopes, lessens emergency situations in the future.

BIBLIOGRAPHY

Commission on Classification and Terminology of the International League Against Epilepsy: Proposal for revised clinical and electroencephalographic classification of epileptic seizures. *Epilepsia* 22:489, 1981.

Delgado-Escueta AV, Treiman DM, Walsh GO: The treatable epilepsies (first of two parts). *N Engl J Med* 308:1508, 1983.

Delgado-Escueta AV, Treiman DM, Walsh GO: The treatable epilepsies (second of two parts). *N Engl J Med* 308:1576, 1983.

Farwell, JR, Lee YJ, Hertz DG, et al: Phenobarbital for febrile seizures—effects on intelligence and on seizure recurrence. *N Engl J Med* 322:364, 1990.

Gal P, Toback J, Boer HR, et al: Efficacy of phenobarbital monotherapy in treatment of neonatal seizures—Relationship to blood levels. *Neurology* 32:1301, 1982.

Gross M, Hureta E: Functional convulsions masked as epileptic disorders. *J Pediatr Psychol* 5:71, 1980.

Juul-Jensen P, Denny-Brown D: Epilepsia partialis continua. *Arch Neurol* 25:97, 1971.

Lacey DJ, Singer WD, Horwitz SJ, et al: Lorazepam therapy of status epilepticus in children and adolescents. *J Pediatr* 108:771, 1986.

Leppik IE, Derivan AT, Homan RW, et al: A double blind study of lorazepam and diazepam in status epilepticus. *JAMA* 249:1452, 1983.

Lombroso CT: A perspective study of infantile spasm: Clinical and therapeutic correlations. *Epilepsia* 24:135, 1983.

National Institutes of Health: Consensus Development Conference on Febrile Seizures, May 1980, *Epilepsia* 22:377, 1981.

Nelson KB, Eleenberg JH: Prognosis in children who have experienced febrile seizure. *Pediatrics* 61:720, 1978.

Painter MJ: General principles of treatment: Status epilepticus in neonates. *Adv Neurol* 34:385, 1983.

Pippenger CE: An overview of antiepileptic drug interactions. *Epilepsia* 23(suppl 1):581, 1982.

Riikonen R: A long term follow up study of 214 children with the syndrome of infantile spasms. *Neuropediatrics* 13:14, 1982.

Staudt F, Scholl ML, Coen RW, et al: Phenobarbital therapy in neonatal seizures and the prognostic value of the EEG. *Neuropediatrics* 13:24, 1982.

Tassinari CA, Daniele O, Michelucci R, et al: Benzodiazepines: Efficacy in status epilepticus. *Adv Neurol* 34:465, 1983.

Thurston JH, Thurston DL, Hixon BB, et al: Prognosis in childhood epilepsy—Additional follow up of 148 children 15–23 years after withdrawal of anticonvulsant therapy. *N Engl J Med* 306:831, 1982.

75
GASTROENTERITIS

Ronald D. Holmes
William M. Belknap

Gastroenteritis is a major public health problem; up to one-fifth of all acute-care outpatient visits to hospitals are by families with infants or children affected by acute gastroenteritis. Acute diarrhea is the most prominent symptom of gastroenteritis in infants and children. Most enteric infections are self-limited, but excessive loss of water and electrolytes, resulting in clinical dehydration, may occur in 10 percent and is life-threatening in 1 percent. Pathogenic viruses, bacteria, or parasites may be isolated from nearly 50 percent of children with diarrhea. Viral or nonbacterial gastroenteritis is the most common cause of acute infectious diarrhea and accounts for the vast majority of cases. Bacterial pathogens may be isolated in 1 to 4 percent of cases. Parasitic infestations are the least common but may be pervasive in certain day-care settings.

ETIOLOGY

Enteric infections causing diarrhea are spread by the fecal-oral route, with contaminated food, water, fomites, or direct inoculation as the vehicles of transmission. Rotaviruses, Norwalk-like agents, the enteric adenoviruses, calicivirus, and astroviruses are the most commonly recognized viral pathogens in children. Of these, rotavirus is the most common, typically occurring in the cooler months of the year (October through April), and infects every child in the United States by age 4 years. This virus causes potentially lethal dehydration in 0.75 percent of children under 2 years of age. Older children and adults have acquired immunity against the rotaviruses and are less likely to develop the severe dehydrating syndrome. Norwalk-like agents are implicated in causing epidemic gastroenteritis. In addition to developing nausea, vomiting, diarrhea, and abdominal cramps, affected children and adults may have headache, fever and chills, and myalgias. Vomiting is more prevalent in children, while diarrhea is more common in adults. Symptomatic enteric adenovirus infection, with serotypes 40 and 41, causes diarrhea that is associated with concurrent respiratory symptoms. Infections occur throughout the year with no clear peaks and may be responsible for 5 to 20 percent of hospitalizations for childhood diarrhea.

The major bacterial enteropathogens in the United States are *Campylobacter jejuni, Shigella* species, *Salmonella* species, *Yersinia enterocolitica, Clostridium difficile,* and *Aeromonas. Escherichia coli* is the most common bacterial organism causing diarrhea in children around the world but is not common in the United States.

Giardia lamblia is responsible for causing diarrhea in infants and young children in day-care centers. Asymptomatic infestations may be present in as many as 50 percent of these children. *Cryptosporidium* infestations occur in a similar epidemiologic pattern. Although *Cryptosporidium* was first recognized as an opportunistic pathogen in immunocompromised children, it is now recognized as a cause of protracted watery diarrhea in otherwise healthy children. *Entamoeba histolytica* causes diarrhea, proctitis, dysentery, or hematochezia; symptomatic infection in children results from exposure by travel to a geographic locale endemic for the organism or in adolescents through sexual transmissions.

Infants and children who attend day-care centers that care for infants in diapers are at risk of acquiring a variety of enteric infections. In some areas, *G. lamblia* is the most common cause of diarrhea, but outbreaks of *Shigella, Campylobacter, C. difficile, Salmonella,* and *Cryptosporidium* are frequently reported. The attack rate during outbreaks may range from 30 to 100 percent; shigellosis is particularly contagious.

PATHOPHYSIOLOGY

Viral pathogens cause acute gastroenteritis by tissue invasion and a directly cytopathic effect to small intestinal villous cells. As a consequence, there is villous damage and decreased intestinal absorption of electrolytes and water, resulting in watery diarrhea in volumes that may exceed 50 mL/kg body weight per day (normal less than 5 mL). The villous injury reduces the total cell population of mature, villous-tip absorptive enterocytes, which are replaced by immature crypt secretory cells; total mucosal glucose-coupled sodium transport is diminished and abolishes the major route of intestinal water absorption by osmotic effect. The volume of fluid delivered from the lumen of the damaged small intestine exceeds the colon's limited ability for fluid absorption, and the net result is secretory diarrhea. Giardiasis causes a similar pathologic effect but is probably not invasive.

The pathogenic mechanisms causing bacterial diarrhea are complex and incompletely understood but can be divided into the following basic processes: mucosal adherence, production of enterotoxins, production of cytotoxins, and the ability to survive phagocytosis. Enteric infections with *E. coli* are prototypic for understanding several of these pathogenic processes. Enterotoxigenic *E. coli* (ETEC) and enteropathogenic *E. coli* (EPEC) adhere to the mucosa and produce enterotoxins or damage the microvilli, respectively. Certain strains of enteroinvasive *E. coli* (EIEC) invade the colonic mucosa, resulting in inflammation and an illness similar to shigellosis. Enterohemorrhagic *E. coli* (EHEC) has emerged as a cause of outbreaks of bloody diarrhea in the United States. EHEC (*E. coli* 0157.H7) typically produces a hemorrhagic colitis with little inflammation and may produce verotoxins that have been implicated in causing hemolytic-uremic syndrome in children. *Vibrio cholerae* and ETEC are the classic bacterial organisms that produce an enterotoxin causing watery diarrhea. The toxin of *V. cholerae* activates adenylate cyclase, resulting in increased intracellular levels of cyclic adenosine 3′, 5′-monophosphate (cAMP). Increased intracellular cAMP levels cause electrolyte secretion by crypt cells and impaired intestinal water absorption; the net result is secretory diarrhea. ETEC species elaborate a heat-labile toxin (LT) and/or a heat-stable toxin (ST), which increases enterocyte cAMP levels and enterocyte cyclic guanosine 3′,5′-monophosphate (cGMP) levels, respectively, resulting in secretory diarrhea.

Inflammatory diarrhea occurs when organisms invade the bowel wall and produce colitis or dysentery, resulting in bloody and mucousy diarrhea. *Shigella, Campylobacter, Salmonella,* and enteroinvasive *E. coli* cause this type of diarrhea. Antibiotic-associated diarrhea and colitis due to cytotoxigenic *C. difficile* causes a similar pattern of diarrhea.

DIAGNOSIS

The approach to diagnosis and successful treatment involves careful history and selective laboratory testing (Fig. 75-1). Various cultures and immunoassays of stool for the presence of the enteric pathogens are now well established in most hospital laboratories. Routine stool culture for bacterial pathogens now include *C. jejuni* and *Y. enterocolitica* in addition to *Salmonella* and *Shigella;* subculturing for *E. coli* serotypes or stool assays for *C. difficile* toxin activity are available. Many enzyme-linked immunosorbent assays (ELISA) are available to test stool for the presence of rotavirus; although electron microscopy is a reference method of defining the presence of a virus, it is rarely utilized.

Most children present with a nonspecific gastroenteritis and not dysentery. In these cases the clinician must assess the likelihood of defining a treatable etiology and, as a consequence, the indication for doing a stool culture. If the patient is febrile, has abrupt onset of diarrhea occurring more than four times per day, or blood in the stool,

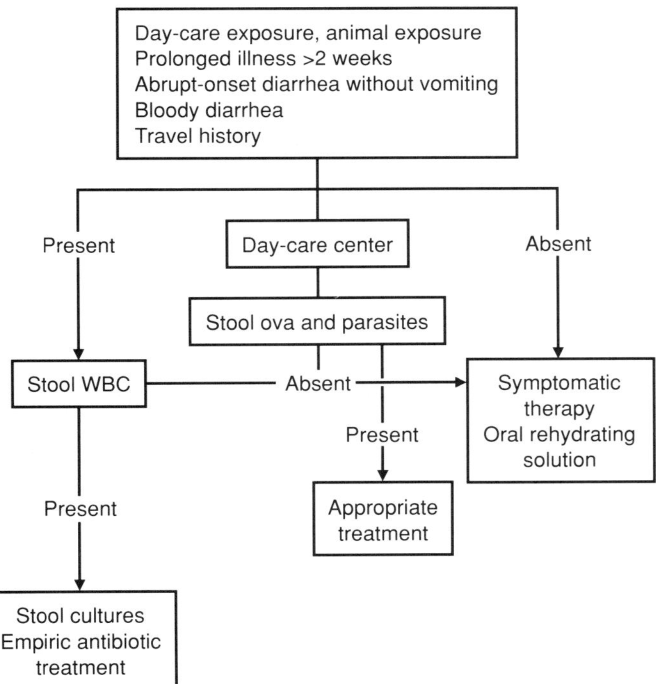

Fig. 75-1. Approach to diagnosis and treatment. Empiric antibiotic treatment may occasionally be justified for inflammatory diarrhea (see text).

the illness is more likely to have been caused by a bacterial pathogen. Stool cultures are indicated. The likelihood of identifying bacterial pathogens is increased if the patient's stool or accompanying exudate contains polymorphonuclear leukocytes (PMNs). A fresh stool sample must be collected to be stained for fecal leukocytes by methylene blue stain. A loopful of mucus or bloody exudate from the stool specimen is mixed with a drop of nonbacteriostatic saline or methylene blue stain on a clean slide, placed under a cover slip, and examined under high-dry magnification. More than five PMNs seen in several high-dry fields is postive. The stool should also be tested for occult blood using a modified guaiac test (Hemoccult). The positive test for fecal leukocytes correlates 90 percent of the time with the presence of bacterial enterocolitis if there are no anal fissures or perianal skin lesions that could provide a source of blood and a falsely positive test.

Stool cultures should also be obtained if there is a history of seafood ingestion, prior antibiotic treatment, or day-care center exposure even if fecal leukocytes or blood is not seen. If there has been a history of unexplained fever or abdominal pain, exposure to a sick pet with diarrhea, or signs and symptoms suggesting appendicitis or mesenteric adenitis, then a culture for *Y. enterocolitica* and other pathogens should be obtained. Any child presenting with a dysentery-like illness should have stool sent for culture and, if indicated, examination for ova and parasites regardless of the results of fecal leukocyte smear. A swab of mucus or bloody exudate from the stool, which has been collected in a cup, should be placed in transport medium, such as Culturette II, and sent to the laboratory. *Shigella* is a fastidious pathogen and is more likely to be recovered from a swab than from a fresh stool specimen. In cases of persistent or recurrent diarrhea, especially with weight loss or day-care center exposure or in immunocompromised children, a fresh stool sample should be collected in fixative, such as Fekal, and examined for *G. lamblia*, *E. histolytica*, and *Cryptosporidium*. Infants and children who present with bloody or mucousy diarrhea after having received antibiotics may have antibiotic-associated pseudomembranous colitis due to infection with cytotoxigenic *C. difficile*, and anaerobic stool cultures and assay of stool for toxin activity should be obtained. Finally, serologic testing or sigmoidoscopy for confirming *Entamoeba histolytica* infection may be necessary.

Watery diarrhea is usually a sign of viral gastroenteritis but may also be caused by infections with enterotoxigenic bacteria such as *V. cholerae* and *E. coli*. Bacterial toxins may also be ingested directly in food. *Staphylococcus aureus* produces five distinct heat-stable toxins in improperly stored meats, poultry, and dairy products. *Bacillus cereus* also produces a heat-stable toxin typically ingested with boiled or fried rice. Although *Shigella* is considered a prototype organism causing dysentery, it can also produce a toxin that causes watery diarrhea, encephalopathy, and/or convulsions.

Table 75-1 lists the causes of enteric infections in children presenting with symptoms of watery diarrhea, bloody diarrhea, or enteric fever.

TREATMENT

Most cases of acute diarrhea are self-limited, and little more than oral rehydration therapy is required. Certain infections require antibiotics to reduce morbidity and reduce the risk of contagion. The use of antimotility agents is contraindicated in acute infectious diarrhea.

The most important part of the treatment of acute gastroenteritis begins with the evaluation of the child's state of hydration (Table 75-2). Kussmaul's respiration secondary to systemic metabolic acidosis, decreased peripheral perfusion visualized as poor capillary refill, decreased skin turgor, and blood urea nitrogen greater than 6.5 mmol/L with blood pH less than 7.35 constitute the best combination of clinical and laboratory findings defining severe dehydration in infants and young children. Severely dehydrated infants should be hospitalized for parenteral rehydration. However, the majority of children with diarrhea and dehydration can be treated with oral rehydrating solutions, even if they are vomiting. Oral rehydration therapy capitalizes on the fact that glucose-coupled sodium and water absorption remain sufficiently intact during most infections, and the oral glucose-electrolyte solutions utilized are remarkably effective. Two types of glucose-electrolyte solutions are commercially available. Rehydration solutions contain 75 to 90 mEq of sodium per liter, and maintenance fluids contain 40 to 60 mEq of sodium per liter; the glucose concentration of both these solutions is 2.0 to 2.5% and does not exceed the sodium concentration in millimolar units by more than 2:1.

The osmolality of the commercial rehydration solution is 310 mOsm/L. Other clear fluids such as soft drinks, juices, and sherbet are largely carbohydrate-based and have osmolalities ranging from 510 to 1225! The routine use of such highly osmolar sugar-based solutions to treat acute diarrhea will predictably amplify net small intestinal fluid secretion and increase diarrhea.

Rehydration solutions should be used for rapid rehydration of dehydrated infants, regardless of initial serum osmolality. The estimated fluid deficit should be replaced over 4 to 6 h. After the calculated deficit has been replaced, the maintenance solution is given to replace ongoing gastrointestinal losses. The daily volume should not exceed 150 mL/kg per day. Water, breast milk, or infant formula should be

Table 75-1. Diagnosis of Enteric Infection

Watery diarrhea	Bloody diarrhea (dysentery)
Vibrio cholerae	*Shigella*
Escherichia coli (toxigenic)	*Salmonella*
Staphylococcal food poisoning	*E. coli* (enteroinvasive)
Bacillus cereus	*Campylobacter jejuni*
Rotavirus	*Yersinia*
Norwalk-like viruses	*Clostridium difficile*
Adenovirus (enteric)	*Aeromonas*
Giardia	*Entamoeba histolytica*
Cryptosporidium	Enteric fever
	Salmonella
	Yersinia
	Campylobacter fetus

Table 75-2. Clinical Criteria for Estimating Extent of Dehydration

	Estimated Body Weight Loss (%)		
Parameter	**5**	**5–10**	**>10**
Skin turgor	Slight decrease	Decreased	Very decreased
Oral mucosa	Dry	Very dry	Parched
Tears	± Decreased	Absent	Absent
Fontanelle	Normal	Depressed	Sunken
Heart rate	± Increased	Increased	Marked tachycardia
Blood pressure	Normal	± Decreased	Decreased
Urine output	Mild oliguria	Oliguria	Oliguria-anuria
Level of consciousness	Irritable	Lethargic	Unresponsive

Source: From Bonadio et al., with permission.

used if additional fluid is needed to satisfy thirst. In general, reintroduction of food may begin after the 4 to 6 h of rehydration and never be delayed more than 24 h. These guidelines are for patients of all ages; however, children weighing more than 10 kg have lower maintenance water requirements. The recommendations for use of oral glucose-electrolyte solutions are outlined in Table 75-3.

Breastfeeding should be routinely continued in infants with acute gastroenteritis. Infants who have been receiving formula feedings and who are well nourished and not dehydrated may rapidly return to their feeding. Formula should rapidly be reintroduced into the diet and never delayed beyond 24 h of treatment with oral rehydration solution.

If the child has had diarrhea lasting longer than 10 to 14 days, has a significant fever or systemic complaints, or has inflammatory cells in the stool, then empiric antimicrobial treatment may be indicated after obtaining a stool sample for bacterial culture. Therapy should provide coverage for the usual dysenteric agents (*Shigella* and *Salmonella*), and either ampicillin or trimethoprim-sulfamethoxazole are reasonable choices. Erythromycin is usually given for *Campylobacter*.

Antibiotic therapy does not affect the clinical course in most cases of acute gastroenteritis and is contraindicated in some infections. Patients with uncomplicated *Salmonella* gastroenteritis should not be given antibiotics unless they appear septic or are bacteremic, have a hemoglobinopathy, or have an underlying chronic gastrointestinal disease. However, infants less than 6 months of age are generally treated with antibiotics because of their overall risk of bacteremia or suppurative disease. In these cases ampicillin, chloramphenicol, or trimethoprim-sulfamethoxazole may be used. *Shigella* dysentery responds to treatment with trimethoprim-sulfamethoxazole (8 to 10 mg/kg trimethoprim plus 40 to 50 mg/kg sulfamethoxazole per day divided every 12 h) or ampicillin (50 to 100 mg/kg per day divided every 6 h to a maximum of 2 to 4 g/day). The usual clinical course of shigellosis with antibiotic therapy is shortened, and the period of fecal shedding may be reduced. Most cases of *C. jejuni* will spontaneously resolve without antibiotics, but early administration of erythromycin ethyl succinate (50 mg/kg per day in four equal doses) may reduce the duration of diarrhea and fecal excretion of the organism. Mild to moderate cases of *Y. enterocolitica* enteritis resolve spontaneously, but infants less than 3 months of age and children with severe diarrhea may be treated with chloramphenicol or trimethoprim-sulfamethoxazole. The efficacy of antibiotics in altering the course of this infection has not been proved.

Most cases of antibiotic-associated colitis caused by *C. difficile* resolve spontaneously if antibiotics are discontinued. Infants and children with protracted diarrhea that has not improved after discontinuing antibiotics may benefit from receiving cholestyramine (240 mg/kg per day divided into three equal doses). Cholestyramine is an anion exchange resin which absorbs *C. difficile* cytotoxin. Debilitated patients, children with underlying gastrointestinal disorders, immunocompromised children, and children with severe bloody diarrhea should be treated orally with vancomycin (10 to 40 mg/kg per day divided every 6 h) or metronidazole (15 to 40 mg/kg per day in three divided doses).

Any infant or child with infectious diarrhea who appears toxic should receive intravenous fluids and should be hospitalized. Patients with severe dehydration and vascular compromise should be given a rapid infusion of normal saline solution or Ringer's lactate, 20 mL/kg, regardless of the serum osmolality. This rapid infusion should be followed by a more gradual replacement of estimated fluid and sodium deficit over 24 to 72 h. Hypernatremic dehydration requires gradual total body water repletion over 48 to 72 h.

Table 75-3. Recommendations for Using Oral Glucose-Electrolyte Solutions

Treatment of Acute Dehydration

Rehydration solution:

1. Give volume equal to estimated fluid deficit (e.g., 5% dehydration = 50-mL/kg deficit).
2. Usually 40–50 mL/kg is given over 4 h.
3. Reevaluate clinical status and therapy after 3–4 h.

Prevention of Dehydration or Maintenance of Hydration after Rehydration

Maintenance solution:

1. Daily volume should not exceed 150 mL/kg per day.
2. Supplement with water, breast milk, or lactose-free formula to satisfy thirst.
3. Do not delay refeeding more than 24 h.

BIBLIOGRAPHY

American Academy of Pediatrics Committee on Nutrition: Use of oral fluid therapy and posttreatment following enteritis in children in a developed country. *Pediatrics* 75:358, 1985.

Bonadio WA, Hennes HH, Machi J, et al: Efficacy of measuring BUN in assessing children with dehydration due to gastroenteritis. *Ann Emerg Med* 18:755, 1989.

Conway S, Ireson A: Acute gastroenteritis in well-nourished infants: Comparison of four feeding regimens. *Arch Dis Child* 64:87, 1989.

Finberg L: Water and solute imbalance in oral rehydration. *J Pediatr Gastroenterol Nutr* 5:4, 1986.

Guerrant R, Lohr J, Williams E: Acute infectious diarrhea. I. Epidemiology, etiology and pathogenesis. *Pediatr Infect Dis* 5:353, 1986.

Kim K, DuPont H, Pickering L: Outbreaks of diarrhea associated with *Clostridium difficile* and its toxin in day-care centers: Evidence of person-to-person spread. *J Pediatr* 102:376, 1983.

Lebaron CW, Furutan NP, Lew JF, et al: Viral agents of gastroenteritis: Public health importance and outbreak management. *MMWR* 39:1, 1990.

MacKenzie A, Barnes G, Shann F: Clinical signs of dehydration in children. *Lancet* 2:605, 1989.

Radetsky M: Laboratory evaluation of acute diarrhea. *Pediatr Infect Dis* 5:230, 1986.

Rodriguez W, Kim H, Brandt C, et al: Fecal adenoviruses from a longitudinal study of families in metropolitan Washington, D.C.: Laboratory, clinical, and epidemiologic observations. *J Pediatr* 107:514, 1985.

Walker WA: Acute infectious diarrhea. *Semin Ped Gastro Nutr* 1:1, 1990.

Williams E, Lohr J, Guerrant R: Acute infectious diarrhea: II. Diagnosis, treatment and prevention. *Pediatr Infect Dis* 5:458, 1986.

Zwiener RJ, Quan R, Belknap WM: Severe pseudomembranous enterocolitis in a child: Case report and literature review. *Pediatr Infect Dis* 8:876, 1989.

76
ABDOMINAL EMERGENCIES
Robert W. Schafermeyer

Evaluation of abdominal emergencies in childhood presents a diagnostic challenge to the emergency physician. Some diseases are common to adults and children and others are age-specific, such as congenital anomalies, volvulus, and Hirschsprung's disease. One must understand the differential diagnoses of the presenting symptoms, recognize the clinical manifestations of the more common and life-threatening diseases, and be sensitive in approaching the infant and child.

One can classify these disease processes in several ways. Is the child febrile or afebrile? Does the disease appear to be obstructive or nonobstructive, abdominal or extraabdominal in nature? Is it due to a local process, or is it a systemic process? Does the child appear healthy and happy or sick and/or septic?

Implicit in the elucidation of the problem presented by a gastrointestinal (GI) emergency in childhood is the recognition of the importance of age. The spectrum of pathologic GI conditions of a 2-day-old infant is vastly different from that of a 2-week-old, and both are quite different from that of a 2-year-old.

EVALUATION

History

The infant or young child cannot give a complete history, but if the child is verbal, one should try to get historical information from him or her and then obtain and listen carefully to what the parent or caretaker says. Find out an accurate chronology of events, whether fever has been a part of the illness, the quality and location of pain, feeding and bowel habits, and the quality and quantity of vomiting and bowel losses. Inquire whether bleeding has been present in vomitus or stools. It is very important to ask about weight changes.

A history of prematurity, necrotizing enterocolitis, congenital anomalies, inborn errors of metabolism, cystic fibrosis, intussusception, or sickle cell anemia are all associated with abdominal complications. The important symptoms referable to the GI tract are pain, vomiting, diarrhea, bleeding, jaundice, and masses. These symptoms are very important and must be explored thoroughly.

Unfortunately, because a child either is too young or too frightened to speak for him- or herself or has not been under continuous observation, trauma as a factor in the development of a GI emergency may be missed—particularly a form of trauma peculiar to children: that of the battered or abused child. In this situation, there may be a purposeful attempt by the parent or care giver to hide the background of the problem and confuse the physician by evasion and lies. Trauma must always be considered by the physician evaluating the pediatric patient presenting with what appears to be an abdominal emergency.

EXAMINATION

Children vary greatly in their ability to cooperate with a physical examination. One should take a few moments to gain the confidence of the child before any painful examination or procedures occur. Allowing the child to rest or be on the care giver's lap may help. Clothing must be removed to avoid missing an incarcerated hernia, petechiae, visible masses, or peristalsis. Look first, then feel. Consider some nontouch maneuvers and observations such as the child's responses during coughing, walking, climbing onto the table, or jumping up and down.

The child can also be invited to self-palpate or palpate with the physician. Start in the least painful areas. Also evaluate extraabdominal areas such as the pharynx, mucous membranes, neck, lung fields, inguinal regions, femoral triangles, testes, and scrotum. Failure to do so may result in delayed or missed diagnoses. Never omit the rectal examination and guaiac test. The diagnosis of Hirschsprung's disease or intussusception will be missed without them.

Laboratory Studies

The most important studies include a urinalysis, a complete blood count and differential, and a test of the stool for occult blood. Other tests and x-ray evaluation should be guided by history, physical examination, how ill the child appears, and the differential diagnoses. Electrolyte and amylase studies, a pregnancy test, and chest and abdominal x-rays may be useful in certain cases.

Assessment and Therapy

Once the history, physical examination, and laboratory studies have been performed, one should have a good idea of the causes. If the child is critically ill, he or she should receive active resuscitation during the whole process of evaluation and not wait for an exact diagnosis. Early consultation must be part of the child's care. If the child is ill but stable and the findings are worrisome and equivocal, then the patient should be admitted for observation and reassessment.

KEY SYMPTOMS

Pain

Abdominal pain is a manifestation of a variety of disease states not necessarily related to the intestinal tract. The origin of the pain may be abdominal or extraabdominal, such as one might see in the 3- to 6-year old with tonsillitis and pneumonia. Pain (subjective) as opposed to tenderness (objective) tends to be periumbilical in this age group. One ought to distinguish between two types of pain, peritonitic and obstructive:

1. Peritonitic pain tends to be exacerbated by motion and thus keeps the patient relatively immobile, as, for example, in appendicitis.
2. Obstructive pain is usually spasmodic and associated with restlessness and motion, as, for example, with intussusception.

In the very young (up to 2 years of age), pain is usually described by the care giver in general terms, such as fussiness, irritability, and inconsolableness. With severe peritonitic pain, the care giver may state that the child is very irritable or lethargic or seems to be grunting as if in pain. Peritonitis or pain from intussusception may present as lethargy or an altered level of consciousness. Between 2 and 6 years of age, pain of GI origin is usually referred to the periumbilical region, and diagnosis requires correlation of the patient's observations and the physician's visual and tactile evaluation. The youngster with pain of peritonitic origin walks with obvious discomfort and prefers to lie still. In contrast, the youngster with obstructive pain may be unable to remain immobile on the examining table. The etiologies of pain vary significantly with age (Table 76-1). Every emergency physician must be familiar with and recognize the life-threatening causes of pain (Table 76-2).

Vomiting

Vomiting is a common childhood problem and may be a specific or nonspecific manifestation of a benign process or a serious, life-threatening illness or injury. Vomiting or regurgitation may be a manifestation of a relatively minor problem (e.g., a nervous parent, poor feeding habits, or gastroesophageal reflux) or it may be a sign of a more serious illness.

Bilious vomiting is always a serious manifestation in an infant or a child, and it must be evaluated quickly and completely. Vomiting may be a sign of obstructive or nonobstructive diseases of abdominal or nonabdominal processes, or, of infectious or abnormal metabolic

Table 76-1. Etiology of Pain

Under 2 Years	2–5 Years
Appendicitis	Appendicitis
Colic	Diabetic ketoacidosis
Congenital anomalies	Gastroenteritis
Gastroenteritis	Hemolytic uremic syndrome
Incarcerated hernia	Henoch-Schönlein purpura
Intussusception	Incarcerated hernia
Malabsorption	Intussusception
Malrotation	Malabsorption
Metabolic acidosis	Metabolic acidosis
Obstruction	Obstruction
Sickle cell pain crises	Pneumonia
Toxins	Sickle cell pain crises
Urinary tract infection	Toxins
Volvulus	Urinary tract infection
	Volvulus
6–11 Years	**Over 11 Years**
Appendicitis	Appendicitis
Diabetic ketoacidosis	Cholecystitis
Gastroenteritis	Diabetic ketoacidosis
Henoch-Schönlein purpura	Dysmenorrhea
Incarcerated hernia	Ectopic pregnancy
Inflammatory bowel disease	Gastroenteritis
Obstruction	Incarcerated hernia
Peptic ulcer disease	Inflammatory bowel disease
Pneumonia	Obstruction
Renal stones	Pancreatitis
Sickle cell syndrome	Peptic ulcer disease
Streptococcal pharyngitis	Pneumonia
Torsion of ovary or testicle	Pregnancy
Toxins	Renal stones
Urinary tract infection	Sickle cell syndrome
	Torsion of ovary or testicle
	Toxins
	Urinary tract infection

Table 76-2. Life-Threatening Causes of Pain

Appendicitis	Metabolic acidosis
Congenital anomalies	Peptic ulcer disease: complications
Diabetic ketoacidosis	Pneumonia
Ectopic pregnancy	Sepsis
Hemolytic-uremic syndrome	Toxins
Incarcerated hernia	Trauma
Intussusception	Volvulus

processes (Table 76-3). Vomiting (bilious or not) is a classic symptom of mechanical intestinal obstruction in the child. In the early phases of the condition, before the child has developed electrolyte abnormalities (e.g., in the child with pyloric stenosis) or before the child has reached the stage of harboring gangrenous bowel (e.g., internal volvulus), the child's general condition may appear to be good. In the early phases of such a process, it is not unusual for the youngster to be hungry immediately after vomiting and even wanting to feed vigorously. One must therefore not ignore the possibility of a serious underlying intraabdominal pathologic condition merely because the vomiting child appears to be systemically well.

Diarrhea

When the presenting symptom is diarrhea, one must quantitate the number and volume of stools, consistency, and the presence of blood. Ascertain the norm for the child, since there is great individual variability in frequency and type of stools. Associated symptoms or the presence of diarrheal illness in other members of the family helps in establishing the diagnosis. Dehydration and electrolyte imbalance should be assessed and treated. Diarrhea may represent fluid expelled

Table 76-3. Causes of Vomiting

Newborn (0–3 Months)	Under 2 Years
Congenital anomalies	Appendicitis
Congenital adrenal hyperplasia	Congenital adrenal hyperplasia
Gastroesophageal reflux	Diabetic ketoacidosis
Gastroenteritis	Foreign body
Hirschsprung's disesease	Gastroenteritis
Hydrocephalus	Head trauma
Inborn errors of metabolism	Hirschsprung's disease
Incarcerated hernia	Hydrocephalus
Kernicterus	Incarcerated hernia
Malrotation	Intussusception
Meconium ileus	Malrotation
Meningitis	Meningitis
Necrotizing enterocolitis	Metabolic acidosis
Obstruction: anatomic causes	Neurologic diseases
Obstruction: renal system	Obstruction
Pneumonia	Pneumonia
Pyloric stenosis	Pyloric stenosis
Sepsis	Sepsis
Toxins	Toxins
Urinary tract infection	Urinary tract infection
Volvulus	Volvulus
Over 2 and Adolescents	
Appendicitis	Neurologic diseases
Diabetic ketoacidosis	Pancreatitis
Foreign body	Peritonitis
Gastroenteritis	Pneumonia
Head trauma	Pregnancy
Hirschsprung's disease	Sepsis
Incarcerated hernia	Toxins
Meningitis	Urinary tract infection
Metabolic acidosis	

around an obstructive mass such as an impaction or as one might see in Hirschsprung's disease (absence of parasympathetic ganglia cells in the muscle layers of the colon). Bloody diarrhea may be infectious or a manifestation of a systemic disease (e.g., hemolytic-uremic syndrome; Table 76-4).

Bleeding

Bleeding may be a sign of GI inflammation, duplication, foreign body infection, or systemic illness, or it may be nothing more than an anal fissure or milk allergy. Apparent major GI bleeding in the newborn, whether blood is vomited or evaluated per rectum, may be the result of the child's having swallowed maternal blood. The laboratory can differentiate between maternal and fetal blood by the Kleihauer-Bedke test or hemoglobin electrophoresis. Rarely do hemorrhagic states cause GI bleeding in the newborn. Small amounts of blood in the stool of an infant, if fresh, may be a manifestation of anal fissures, which are easily identified. In children 2 to 10 years of age, painless bleeding of small to moderate amounts of fresh blood usually mixed through the stool might well be an indication of benign GI polyps or infection giving rise to bloody diarrhea.

The presence of small to moderate amounts of blood in the stool of an infant (particularly associated with vomiting) must lead the physician to consider the malrotation of the midgut. This is an urgent,

Table 76-4. Causes of Diarrhea

Anatomic: Hirschsprung's disease
Dietary: allergy, malabsorption, overfeeding
Infectious: bacterial, parasitic, toxic, viral
Inflammatory: Crohn's disease, hemolytic-uremic syndrome, ulcerative colitis
Malabsorption: cystic fibrosis, enzyme deficiencies
Systemic: endocrinopathy, immunodeficiencies

Table 76-5. Causes of GI Bleeding

Under 2 Months	Under 2 Years	Over 2 Years
	UPPER	
Bleeding diathesis	Bleeding diathesis	Esophageal varices
Swallowed maternal blood	Foreign body	Foreign body
Vascular malformation	Gastroenteritis	Gastroenteritis
	Traumatic hemobilia	Traumatic hemobilia
	Vascular malformation	Mallory-Weiss tear
		Peptic ulcer disease
		Vascular malformation
	LOWER	
Congenital duplications	Anal fissure	Allergy
Intussusception	Congenital duplication	Colitis
Meckel's diverticulum	Gastroenteritis	Gastroenteritis
Necrotizing enterocolitis	Hemolytic-uremic syndrome	Hemolytic-uremic syndrome
Swallowed maternal blood	Henoch-Schönlein purpura	Henoch-Schönlein purpura
Vascular malformation	Inflammatory bowel disease	Inflammatory bowel disease
Volvulus	Intussusception	Meckel's diverticulum
	Meckel's diverticulum	Polyps
	Milk allergy	
	Polyps: benign, familial	

life-threatening disease process that requires immediate investigation and surgical consultation because of volvulus of the midgut and the possibility of midgut gangrene if the problem is not identified and corrected early in its course.

Major painless upper GI bleeding in the infant or child is most commonly the result of bleeding varices secondary to portal hypertension. Major painless lower GI bleeding in the infant or child is frequently ascribable to a Meckel's diverticulum.

Frequently, the cause of minimal to moderate amounts of blood in the stool of an infant or a child may never be identified. Repeated episodes of bleeding require GI x-ray, endoscopic evaluation, and Meckel's isotope scanning (Table 76-5).

Jaundice

Jaundice is an ominous sign, since it represents hepatic dysfunction. It might represent sepsis, congenital infection (TORCHS), or postnatal viral hepatitis. It might represent a minor ABO incompatibility or a major ABO or Rh factor incompatibility, with the possibility of kernicterus or death. It may represent the first signs of cystic fibrosis, galactosemia, or other hepatic enzyme deficiencies, or it could be the harbinger of an anatomic problem such as biliary atresia, a choledochal cyst, or even pyloric stenosis. All jaundiced patients must be admitted and evaluated promptly (Table 76-6).

Table 76-6. Causes of Bilirubin Abnormalities

Unconjugated	Conjugated
ABO or Rh incompatibility	Anatomic defect: biliary, hepatic
Autoimmune hemolytic anemia	Hemolytic-uremic syndrome
Hepatic: Crigler-Najjar syndrome, Gilbert's disease	Hepatic abscess
Hypothyroidism	Hepatitis: congenital, acquired
Sepsis	Hepatitis: TORCHS
Sickle cell anemia	Inflammatory bowel disease
G-6-PD	Metabolic: cystic fibrosis, galactosemia, etc.
	Sepsis
	Sickle cell anemia
	Toxins
	Urinary tract infections
	Wilson's disease

Masses

The presence of a mass could be the first sign of a congenital anomaly or a tumor (e.g., Wilms' tumor or neuroblastoma). It could be a pyloric "olive" or the intussusception mass if associated with vomiting or a guaiac-positive stool. If the child has an acute surgical or obstructive abdomen, resuscitation and prompt surgical consultation are necessary. Otherwise, admission and pediatric consultation should be started along with appropriate laboratory studies.

DIAGNOSES AND MANAGEMENT OF SELECTED EMERGENCIES

GI Emergencies in Infants in the First Year of Life

Malrotation with and without Volvulus

Volvulus is a major life-threatening complication of malrotation. The complications of malrotation occur most commonly in the first year of life, although malrotation can give rise to symptoms at any time in a person's life. It is the most urgent of GI emergencies in infants and children because of consequent gangrene of the total midgut. The process from the first symptoms to the development of total midgut gangrene may occur within a few hours.

The presenting symptoms are usually vomiting (ultimately becoming bilious), with or without abdominal distension, and streaks of blood in the stool. Pain is usually constant, not colicky. This symptom complex usually occurs in a previously healthy child. However, there may have been minor episodes in the past of vomiting or abdominal discomfort. The child suspected of harboring a malrotation with possible midgut volvulus should have a flat and upright abdominal x-ray. The presence of a loop of bowel overriding the liver is suggestive of the diagnosis. An upper GI examination may reveal an abnormal location of the ligament of Treitz.

An infant with symptoms of obstruction or bilious vomiting must receive prompt surgical consultation and active resuscitation. Intravenous fluids should be started, a nasogastric tube placed, and blood typed and crossmatched. Any child with vomiting or bloody stools who is identified as having an incompletely rotated bowel warrants urgent laparotomy to prevent the development of midgut volvulus and total midgut gangrene.

Incarcerated Hernia

An incarcerated hernia will not be detected unless the infant or child is totally undressed at the time of examination. The symptoms include irritability, poor feeding, vomiting, and an inguinal or scrotal mass. the differential diagnosis of an inguinal or scrotal mass most frequently includes hydrocele of the cord or the scrotum, undescended testicle, torsion of the testicle, torsion of the appendix testis, inguinal lymphadenopathy, inguinal node abscess, orchitis, and inguinal or scrotal trauma. The incidence of incarceration of inguinal hernias is highest in the first year of life. In both boys and girls, the incarcerated sac may contain small or large bowel. In girls there is a high incidence of cases in which ovary is present in the sac.

In most instances, provided the child is examined gently and his or her confidence obtained, it is possible to achieve manual reduction of the incarcerated hernia (if it has been present for only a short period of time) without the use of sedation. When this maneuver is unsuccessful, most cases can be successfully reduced following the administration of intramuscular meperidine (up to 2 mg/kg of body weight in the first year of life). After an hour, only minimal disturbance is necessary to examine the child and observe the status of the incarcerated hernia. Quite often, as a result of the relaxation induced by the meperidine, spontaneous reduction of the hernia is apparent. In the absence of spontaneous reduction, one should attempt to reduce the hernia. The few patients that do not respond to these maneuvers must undergo surgical reduction.

Intestinal Obstruction

Intestinal obstruction presents in infants and young children in the classic manner, with symptoms of pain (manifested by irritability); vomiting; abdominal distension; and, later, absence or diminution of bowel movements. The differential diagnosis of intestinal obstruction in the newborn and infant includes intestinal atresia or stenosis, meconium ileus (newborn only), incarcerated inguinal hernia, malrotation, malrotation with volvulus, volvulus around a congenital intraabdominal band, duplication cysts of the intestinal tract, imperforate anus, and Hirschsprung's disease.

Diagnosis necessitates immediate flat and upright films of the abdomen, which show dilated loops of bowel with air-fluid levels (Fig. 76-1). Such an appearance on the plain x-ray film warrants a barium enema examination with a Hirschsprung's catheter, which helps to differentiate between Hirschsprung's disease, malrotation, and colonic stenosis and also separates lower large bowel obstruction from upper small bowel obstruction.

Once intestinal obstruction has been diagnosed, the patient should be prepared for surgical intervention by having an intravenous line and a nasogastric tube placed.

Pyloric Stenosis

The child presenting in the emergency department with a history of nonbilious projectile vomiting must be considered to have pyloric stenosis. This is a familial disease, and one parent (usually the father) or relative has usually been treated for pyloric stenosis. The classic patient is a healthy 3- to 6-week-old infant with projectile nonbilious vomiting after feeding who is hungry enough after vomiting to take another feeding. Initially, the vomiting may not be forceful, but over a period of days it becomes projectile. As time passes and vomiting becomes more prolonged, dehydration and electrolyte imbalance develop. Examination of the patient may reveal the presence of gastric peristaltic waves traveling from the left quadrant to the midline across the abdominal wall. On palpation with care and gentleness, after emptying the stomach with a nasogastric tube, the classic olivelike pyloric tumor may be identified in the right upper quadrant. The differential diagnosis of pyloric stenosis includes gastroesophageal reflux, pylorospasm, and gastroenteritis. The diagnosis can be confirmed by obtaining an ultrasound examination to locate the "olive." Alternatively, an upper GI examination can be completed to rule out the other diseases. The barium should be removed after the x-ray to prevent aspiration of barium. After rehydration and reestablishment of electrolyte balance, definitive treatment involves pyloromyotomy.

Intussusception

Intussusception presents with recurring attacks of cramping abdominal pain. The classic patient is a robust 6- to 18-month-old infant without prior difficulty. Suddenly, the child appears to be in pain. The youngster may be playing quietly in the playpen and suddenly stop playing, begin to cry, and even roll around in discomfort. Just as suddenly, the pain ceases, and the child appears to be as happy and content as before the onset of the pain and returns to playing with toys. This process is repeated at decreasing intervals, with the duration of the painful attacks increasing. Some children become very still, listless, and pale, and appear to be in a shocklike state due to the visceral pain. Vomiting is rare in the first few hours but usually develops after 6 to 12 h. The classic "currant-jelly" stool associated with intussusception is a later manifestation of the disease complex, resulting from interference with mucosal circulation, and is present in only 50 percent of the cases. Its absence should not delay evaluation for intussusception in the patient. However, a positive stool guaiac test is present in almost every case.

Examination between attacks may reveal the oft-described sausage-shaped tumor mass of intussuscepted bowel in the right abdomen. The absence of this finding, however, should not delay further investigation.

The presumptive diagnosis of intussusception is made on the basis of the history and may be seriously considered as a result of a telephone description of the child's problem by the care giver. The apparent well-being of the child and the absence of clinical findings should not mislead the physician. X-ray films of the abdomen may show a mass

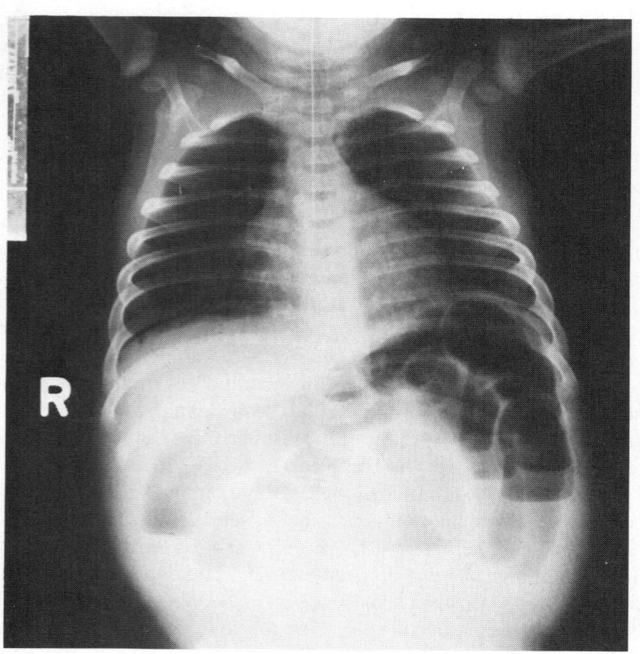

A

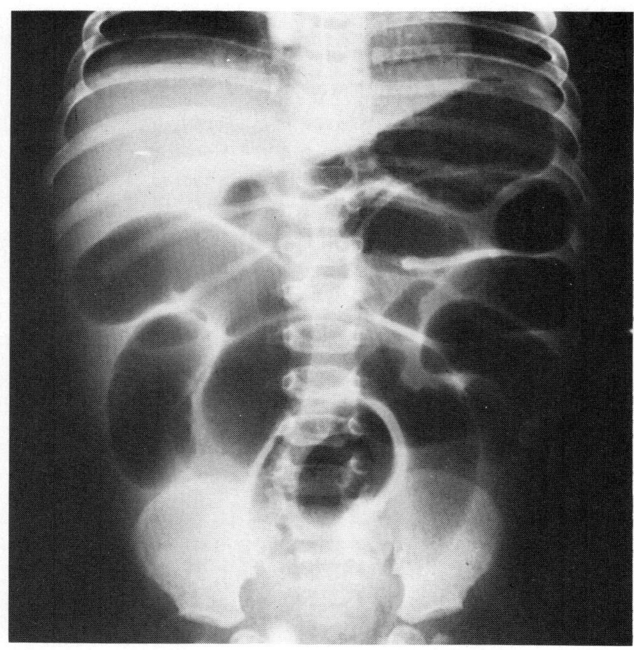

B

Fig. 76-1. Mechanical intestinal obstruction. **A.** Upright film. **B.** Flat film.

or filling defect in the right upper quadrant of the abdomen (Fig. 76-2A). Even in the presence of normal plain x-ray films, the history described demands a barium enema examination, which demonstrates the classic "coiled spring" (Fig. 76-2B). The barium enema examination is not only a diagnostic tool in the management of this disease but is also frequently curative. If it is obtained in the first 12 to 24 h of the developing intussusception, up to 80 percent of cases can be corrected by barium enema alone. When barium enema does not resolve the intussusception, surgical intervention is indicated. If barium enema reduces the intussusception, the parents should be warned of the 5- to 10-percent chance of recurrence of the same process. Recurrence usually takes place within the first 24 to 48 h following the barium enema reduction.

GI Emergencies in Children 2 Years and Older

Appendicitis

While appendicitis can occur under age 2, the presentation is usually one of peritonitis or sepsis because of the delay in diagnosis. Over age 2, appendicitis becomes a more important part of the differential diagnoses of abdominal pain. The classic progression of symptoms associated with appendicitis applies equally to children and adults. The events involve early anorexia followed by the development of mild to moderate periumbilical pain and then vomiting and the movement of the pain to the right lower quadrant of the abdomen. The youngster should be observed walking into the examining room; in most instances the child appears to be in discomfort as he or she moves along. This discomfort associated with motion can be exacerbated by asking the youngster to jump up and down before he or she lies down on the examining table. On inspection of the patient, the physician may find limited motion of the lower abdomen due to inflammation of the peritoneum, and depending on the duration of the symptoms, there may be abdominal distention. Palpation may reveal the presence of tenderness in the right lower abdominal quadrant. The position of the appendix may vary greatly, and thus tenderness on examination may vary. Guarding and rebound tenderness may or may not be present in this area. The longer the duration of the symptoms, the greater the possibility of finding a right lower quadrant mass representing localized perforation with the development of an appendiceal abscess. A rectal examination should be performed in order to detect the presence of a low-lying, intrapelvic, acutely inflamed appendix or to palpate a mass. The child may have a mild fever and an elevated white blood cell count in the range of 11,000 to 20,000. When there is doubt in the overall symptom complex, an x-ray may reveal the presence of an appendicolith (Fig. 76-3). Symptoms consistent with appendicitis together with the presence of an appendicolith warrant the clinical diagnosis of appendicitis and laparotomy. Intravenous fluids should be given and surgical consultation obtained.

The following signs and symptoms may be misleading:

1. The temperature may be normal.
2. The white blood cell count may be normal.
3. The child may not be anorexic and may actually request food.
4. A heavily built child may manifest minimal right lower quadrant tenderness and minimal tenderness on rectal examination.
5. Gastroenteritis is not infrequently associated with appendicitis. Thus, a child presenting with a several-day history of vomiting and diarrhea, perhaps even with siblings suffering from the same problem, should not have the diagnosis of appendicitis discounted on this basis. Intensification of pain in the presence of a history of gastroenteritis should suggest an acutely inflamed appendix secondary to gastroenteritis.
6. Appendicitis has been identified in children under 1 year of age and is not uncommon in the second year. The incidence of per-

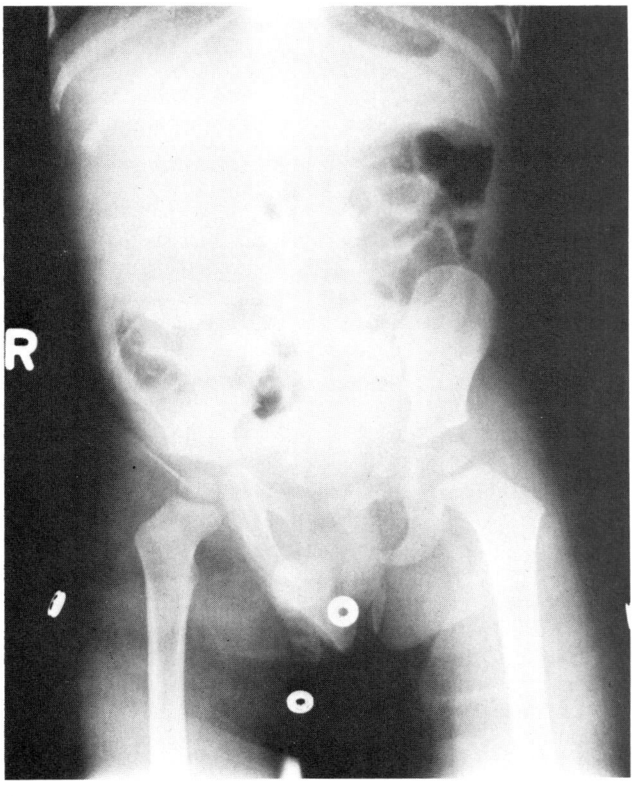

A

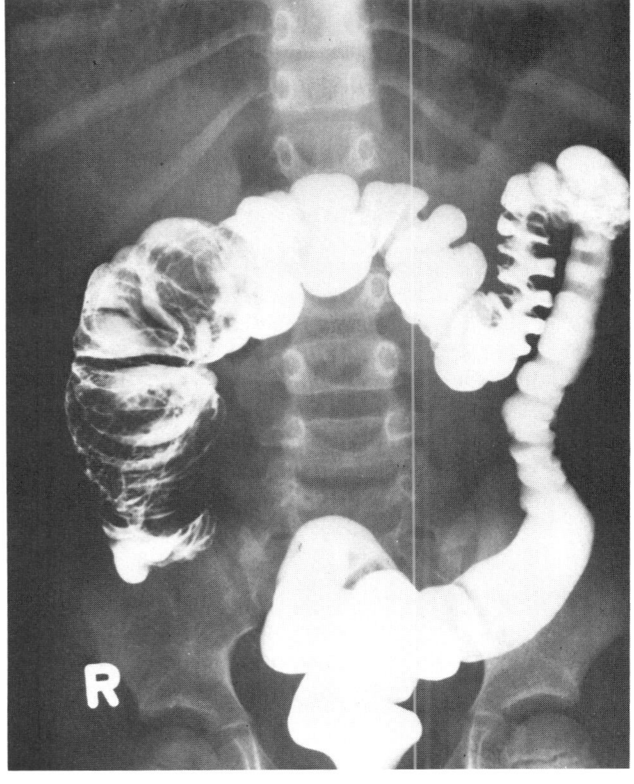

B

Fig. 76-2. Intussusception. **A.** Plain film showing a filling defect in the right upper quadrant. **B.** With barium enema, showing a "coiled spring" in the ascending colon.

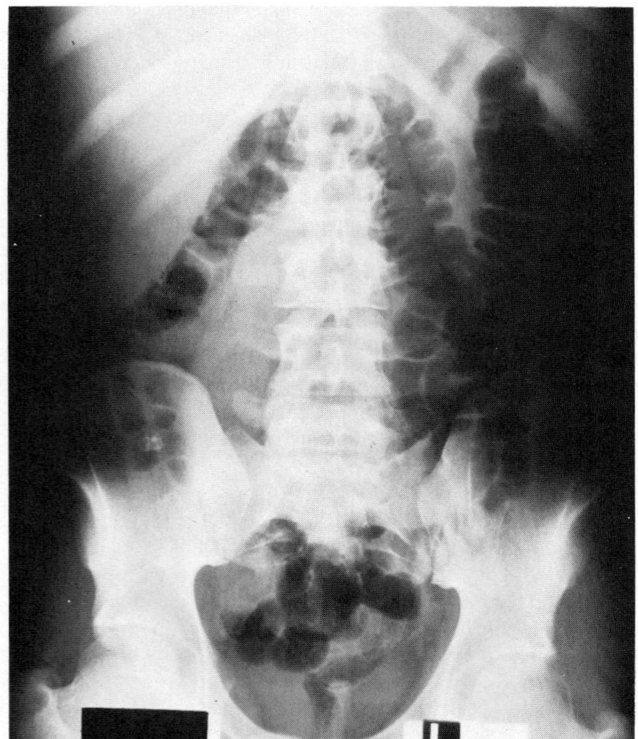

Fig. 76-3. Appendicitis; appendicolith in the right lower quadrant.

foration in this age group is much higher because of the difficulty of making the diagnosis and the confusion with gastroenteritis.

Meckel's Diverticulum

A Meckel's diverticulum can cause a variety of signs and symptoms, such as bleeding, peritonitis, intussusception, and intestinal obstruction. The presence of gastric mucosa in the diverticulum may give rise to an ulcer in the adjacent ileum, which may cause symptoms such as painless rectal bleeding or perforation with attendant peritonitis. Isotope scanning reveals the presence of a Meckel's diverticulum containing gastric mucosa in up to 50 percent of the cases. A negative scan does not eliminate the diagnosis.

Acute inflammation in a Meckel's diverticulum may simulate acute appendicitis or may initiate intussusception. Finally, the vitellointestinal remnant attaching the apex of a Meckel's diverticulum to the intraabdominal umbilical region may be the focus around which volvulus of the small bowel or an internal hernia develops, each of these giving rise to intestinal obstruction.

Colon Polyps

Single polyps or multiple or classic familial polyposis may give rise to painless bright-red lower intestinal bleeding. Most commonly the polyp is single, or perhaps there are two or three. Single polyps are usually benign (juvenile), with no propensity for malignant degeneration. Frequently, the parent describes what is obviously a prolapsed polyp, easily palpated on rectal examination. It is rare for bleeding originating from a polyp to be life-threatening. Familial polyposis is rare and is a premalignant syndrome. The child should be referred to a pediatric surgeon for care of these conditions.

Other Causes of GI Bleeding

Blood represents local irritation or erosion in the majority of children. What appear to be small amounts of blood on the stool or diaper of a healthy child are probably due to an anal fissure or could be related to food substances that have a red or melanotic coloration. A stool test for occult blood and a gentle rectal examination may be all that is needed in the healthy child

On the other hand, if the child is sick- or ill-appearing or shocklike or has petechiae, one must consider vascular malformation, Meckel's diverticulum, or intestinal duplication. In adolescents, one must consider stress ulceration, peptic ulcer disease, and inflammatory bowel disease (chronic and ulcerative colitis). Sepsis, severe gastroenteritis, Henoch-Schönlein purpura, and hemolytic-uremic syndrome should be part of the differential diagnoses.

In the infant, a coagulation survey should be included in the evaluation if the child is ill or shocklike or has a family history of a clotting disorder. Also remember that this could be the presentation of intussusception or volvulus.

Intraabdominal Masses

Every child should have a careful abdominal examination because intraabdominal masses grow silently at first until they cause obstruction, bleeding, or hemorrhage into the tumor or until a parent sees a mass protruding in the abdomen. The child should be supine with his or her head turned toward the parent and one should carefully palpate all quadrants of the abdomen. If a mass is palpated, the child should be referred to a pediatric surgeon and diagnostic imaging studies obtained. A careful rectal examination, especially if the child has constipation or a gait abnormality, must be done to check for a presacral teratoma and for ovarian masses; both of these tumors can show calcifications on plain film x-rays in approximately 50 percent of cases.

Neuroblastomas can arise from adrenal glands or along the sympathetic chain. They often cross to the midline, and the best cure rate is obtained in the child under 1 year of age. CT scan is the best way to evaluate this tumor. Wilms' tumor is an intrarenal tumor initially and should be considered in the child with hematuria. Ultrasound and CT scan help define this tumor. Bone scan is also needed. Rhabdomyosarcoma occurs in the pelvis or anywhere there is striated muscle, and it is highly malignant.

In girls over the age of menarche, one must consider pregnancy, and if there is lower quadrant pain, one must consider ectopic pregnancy. One should obtain a serum pregnancy test and consider the use of pelvic, intravaginal ultrasound.

Foreign Bodies in the GI Tract

It is safe to generalize that anything that reaches the stomach will eventually traverse the GI tract and be spontaneously evacuated per rectum. Nails, open safety pins, pieces of glass, and coins are examples of objects that have traveled the complete journey. It may take weeks for a coin, for example, to complete the trip to the anus. Any foreign body caught in the esophagus must be removed by esophagoscopy. (See Chap. 38.) Very rarely is surgical removal of a foreign body in the stomach or distal to the stomach warranted. Occasionally, a long, thin foreign body may not traverse the duodenum and may need to be removed surgically. Round objects almost always pass spontaneously.

Portal Hypertension

Portal hypertension is rare in children but is one of the common causes of major upper GI hemorrhage. Extrahepatic portal thrombosis, parenchymal liver disease associated with fibrocystic disease, and biliary cirrhosis in the youngster with congenital biliary atresia surviving as a result of portal enterostomy are examples of conditions that can result in portal hypertension and esophagogastric varices.

BIBLIOGRAPHY

Altman RP, Krug J: Portal hypertension. *J Pediatr Surg* 17:567, 1982.

Andrassy RJ, Mahour GH: Malrotation of the midgut in infants and children. *Arch Surg* 116: 158, 1981.

Benson CD, Lloyd JR: Infantile pyloric stenosis. *Am J Surg* 107:429, 1964.

Boyle JJ: Gastrointestinal bleeding, in Ludwig S, Fleisher GR (eds): *Textbook of Pediatric Emergency Medicine,* 2d ed. Baltimore, Williams & Wilkins, 1988, pp 171–179.

Cloud DT: Appendicitis. *J Pediatr Surg* 925:498, 1980.

Eichelberger MR, Randolph JG: Pediatric trauma: An algorithm for diagnosis and therapy. *J Trauma* 23:91, 1983.

Ein SH, Stephens CA: Intussusception: 354 cases in 10 years. *J Pediatr Surg* 6:16, 1971.

Fleisher GR: Diarrhea, in Ludwig S, Fleisher GR (eds): *Textbook of Pediatric Emergency Medicine,* 2d ed. Baltimore, Williams & Wilkins, 1988, pp 133–137.

Fuchs S, Jaffe D: Vomiting. *Pediatr Emerg Care* 6:164, 1990.

Puri P, O'Donnell B: Appendicitis in infancy. *J Pediatr Surg* 13:173, 1978.

Raffensperger JG, Luck SR: Gastrointestinal bleeding in children. *Surg Clin North Am* 56:413, 1976.

Rowe MJ, Marchildon MB: Inguinal hernia and hydrocele in infants and children. *Surg Clin North Am* 61:1137, 1981.

Ruddy RM: Abdominal pain, in Ludwig S, Fleisher GR (eds): *Textbook of Pediatric Emergency Medicine,* 2d ed. Baltimore, Williams & Wilkins, 1988, pp 70–77.

Schnaufer L, Mahboubi S: Abdominal emergencies, in Ludwig S, Fleisher GR (eds): *Textbook of Pediatric Emergency Medicine,* 2d ed. Baltimore, Williams & Wilkins, 1988, pp 936–965.

Seagram CGF, Louch RE, Stephens CA, et al: Meckel's diverticulum: A 10-year review of 218 cases. *Can J Surg* 11:369, 1968.

Singer J: Jaundice: Conjugated hyperbilirubinemia, in Ludwig S, Fleisher GR (eds): *Textbook of Pediatric Emergency Medicine,* 2d ed. Baltimore, 1988, pp 205–209.

Ward JA Jr, Otherson HB: The juvenile polyp of the colon. *Am J Surg* 34:566, 1968.

Watkins JB: Jaundice: Unconjugated hyperbilirubinemia, in Ludwig S, Fleisher GR (eds): *Textbook of Pediatric Emergency Medicine,* 2d ed. Baltimore, Williams & Wilkins, 1988, pp 201–204.

77 CHILD ABUSE

Carol D. Berkowitz

Child abuse and neglect are problems which have been recognized with increasing frequency in recent years. Over 1 million cases of child abuse and neglect are reported annually in the United States. It is estimated that approximately 6 infants per 1000 live births are physically abused during childhood. The prevalence of physical abuse is about 500 cases per 1 million population per year. In spite of improved physician awareness and reporting, these figures are probably gross underestimates. The extent of sexual abuse has been recognized increasingly. It is estimated that one-fourth of all girls and one-sixth of all boys are sexually abused before adulthood.

The physician in the emergency department is often the first, and frequently the only, person to evaluate a child who is a victim of child abuse or neglect. Approximately 10 percent of all injuries in children under 5 years of age being evaluated in the emergency department result from inflicted, nonaccidental trauma. Failure to recognize this fact carries a high morbidity and mortality. Approximately 5 percent of these children will die from future inflicted trauma, and another 35 percent will be seriously injured again.

This chapter discusses the spectrum of the syndrome of child abuse and neglect, focuses on the features of the history and physical examination which assist the physician with the diagnosis, and describes the legal obligations for reporting suspected cases.

SPECTRUM OF CHILD ABUSE AND NEGLECT

The concept of child maltreatment, defined as harm to a child because of abnormal child-rearing practices, is a broadening of the initial description of the battered child syndrome. Child maltreatment is an all-inclusive term covering physical abuse; sexual abuse; emotional abuse; parental substance abuse; physical, nutritional, and emotional neglect; supervisional neglect; and Munchausen by proxy.

The ease with which the physician is able to recognize these disorders in part depends on his or her knowledge of normal children and normal development. The physical stigmata of maltreatment are characteristic, although the findings of neglect and sexual abuse are more subtle than those of gross physical trauma.

CHILD NEGLECT

Child neglect can result in an array of physical and emotional problems. Child neglect from early infancy results in the syndrome of failure to thrive (FTT). This syndrome usually affects children under the age of 3 years, although older children who remain in a non-nurturing environment show similar manifestations.

The patient is often brought to the emergency department because of other medical problems, such as intercurrent infections; skin rashes, particularly severe monilial diaper dermatitis; or acute gastroenteritis.

The history of the acute illness may not alert the physician to the chronic nature of the underlying problem. The physical examination provides the clue to the diagnosis of long-standing malnutrition. Overall physical care and hygiene are frequently poor. The infant has very little subcutaneous tissue. The ribs protrude prominently through the skin, and the skin of the buttocks hangs in loose folds. There may be alopecia over a flattened occiput, reflecting the fact that the baby has been allowed to lie on his or her back all day. Muscle tone is usually increased (although sometimes these babies are hypotonic). This increased tone is most notable in the lower extremities, and infants may manifest scissoring, similar to infants with cerebral palsy.

FTT infants also show distinct behavioral characteristics. They are wide-eyed and wary. If brought in close proximity to the examiner's face, they may purposely turn away to avoid eye contact. They become irritable if interpersonal interaction is pursued. They are difficult to console and are not cuddly. They prefer inanimate over animate objects and spend much time with their hands in their mouths. When left alone, they assume a "straphanger's position" with their arms flexed at the elbows and extended over their shoulders.

Weights and lengths should be plotted on the appropriate growth curves. In general, weight is more adversely affected than length, although this depends on the duration of the neglect. Likewise, long-standing neglect results in a diminution in the rate of growth of the head.

In addition to observing for these physical signs, the physician should obtain certain historical information. This includes the birth weight (to assess the rate of growth); any maternal use of cigarettes, alcohol, and/or drugs during pregnancy; previous hospitalizations; and the parental stature. A full social service assessment should also be obtained, although this is usually done by a medical social worker.

Infants suspected of suffering from significant environmental FTT should be admitted to the hospital. Weight gain in the hospital is felt to be the sine qua non of environmental FTT. Most infants gain weight within 1 to 2 weeks following admission; in addition the hositalization allows a more extensive social service assessment while the infant is in a protected environment. A skeletal survey of the long bones should be carried out to detect any evidence of physical abuse.

Children over the age of 2 to 3 years with environmental neglect are termed psychosocial dwarfs. Their short stature is a more prominent finding than their low weight. These children manifest a classic triad of short stature, bizarre voracious appetite (eating from trash cans), and a disturbed home situation. They are frequently hyperactive and have delayed or unintelligible speech. Psychosocial dwarfs have been studied endocrinologically and have been found to have a low to normal level of growth hormone which fails to increase with stimulation with insulin or arginine. These children should also be admitted for evaluation and initiation of appropriate social intervention. The endocrinologic disturbances rapidly reverse following hospitalization or placement in a foster home.

SEXUAL ABUSE

Victims of sexual abuse are frequently difficult for the inexperienced physician to assess because of an unfamiliarity with the normal prepubertal genital examination. Children who have been sexually abused are brought to the emergency department because of a disclosure about the abuse or because of other symptoms such as those referrable to the genitourinary tract, including vaginal discharge, vaginal bleeding, dysuria, urinary tract infections, or urethral discharge; behavior disturbances, including excessive masturbation, genital fondling, or other sexually oriented or provocative behavior; encopresis; regression; nightmares; and unrelated complaints. Approximately 15 percent of children diagnosed as victims of sexual abuse in one report had unrelated complaints such as abdominal pain, asthma, and sore throat.

Children who are sexually abused rarely disclose their abuse until time has elapsed from the acute episode. Children who are seen immediately after an assault should be evaluated for evidence of acute injuries and for the presence of forensic material, such as semen.

More often, several years have elapsed since the abuse was initiated, although it may be ongoing. Children 8 to 11 years of age frequently disclose that they have been victims of sexual abuse for a significant period of time. The assailant is known to the child in over 90 percent of cases.

A medical history should be obtained from all children being evaluated for sexual abuse. Because evidence of the abuse may not be apparent until the child is examined, the physician may have to obtain additional historic information after the physical assessment. The medical history should include pertinent statements about whether the child has any underlying condition or has undergone any previous procedures that might account for changes in the anogenital area. Genitourinary surgery or trauma would be particularly important to note.

The child should be questioned directly about what happened. The child's name for genitalia and other body parts should be recorded, and all statements that the child makes concerning the abuse should be recorded verbatim. The demands of a busy emergency department may make it difficult for the physician to conduct a detailed and sensitive interview. In such cases, the hospital social worker should be consulted.

The examining physician must maintain a high index of suspicion of sexual abuse when evaluating children presenting with anogenital or behavioral complaints. The physical assessment should include an evaluation of the child's overall well-being and a general physical examination. The skin should be examined for bruises. Nongenital physical injuries are unusual, even following acute abuse. Rarely, there may be grip marks on the forearms or puncture wounds on the inner aspects of the lips resulting from a slap to the face. The age of the child and the degree of sexual development should be noted.

The genital examination should be confined to a careful inspection of the genitalia and perianal area. Generally, there is no need for a speculum examination unless the victim is an older adolescent or unless perforating vaginal trauma is suspected. Likewise, sedation is rarely needed, and most children can be reassured verbally if they are at all apprehensive. Careful inspection of the external genitalia is sufficient to establish physical evidence of genital injury. The examination is sometimes augmented by the use of a colposcope, an instrument used primarily by gynecologists to magnify, allowing detection of minor changes in the cervical mucosa. The colposcope also facilitates photographing the external genital area. However, most emergency departments are not equipped with a colposcope, and this instrument is, in fact, not critical to an adequate assessment of the anogenital area. Magnification can easily be achieved with the use of hand-held lenses. Toluidine blue dye applied to the genital area may also detect subtle acute injuries.

A number of different positions have been used to facilitate the examination. Infants may be seated on their parents' laps. Children are easily examined supine on the examining table with their legs in a frog-leg position. Some physicians also place all children in a prone knee-chest position to help fully assess the contour and homogeneity of the hymen. Placing a child in "stirrups" is usually unnecessary unless she is obese or has achieved adult stature.

The normal prepubescent girl has full labia majora and small thin labia minora. The vaginal opening is covered by the hymen, a fine reddish-orange, thin-edged membrane. The thickness and color of the hymen varies as a function of age. It is normally thick during infancy and again with the onset of puberty. In between, it is thinner, most often annular or crescentric, and smooth-edged. The hymenal orifice should be measured, although there is a range of variation depending on the child's age, position, and degree of relaxation. Trauma may result in changes such as hymenal notches or indentations. Indentations at the 6:00 position are associated with prior penetrating trauma. Attenuation or reduction in the amount of hymenal tissue may lead to a gaping opening. Irregularities in the contour, particularly deep notches, are also associated with prior injury. Scarring, as evidenced by marked alteration in the vascular pattern (white areas or swirling vascularity), is an additional sign of healed injury. Erythema, on the other hand, may be secondary to irritation, inflammation, and/or chronic manipulation and is not specific for abuse.

Physical findings indicative of a sexually transmitted disease should also be noted, including a vaginal discharge, warts consistent with condylomata acuminata or condylomata lata, and vesicles or ulcers consistent with herpes genitalia.

It is critically important for the emergency physician to be aware that the absence of physical findings does not preclude abuse. There are many sexually abusive activities (such as orogenital contact) that would not be expected to produce scarring trauma. In addition, as is true elsewhere in the body, injuries can heal without residual scarring.

The genital examination in the sexually victimized young boy is less revealing. Rarely, there may be bite marks on the penis or scrotum. There may be a urethral discharge; the penis may become erect without tactile stimulation and remain erect.

The perianal examination is often more revealing, although it too may be completely normal in the case of either acute or chronic sodomy. Acute penetration may produce no changes or may be associated with fissures; abrasions; hematomas; and changes in tone, including both dilatation and anal spasm. In the young female patient, anal penetration is easier than vaginal penetration, and changes in this area may be seen. Anal fissures or tags may be noted. The perianal folds, or rugae, may be thickened in some areas, thinned out in others, and distorted. The perianal skin may be lichenified and thickened secondary to frictional rubbing. Anal tone may be reduced when there has been repeated prior anal penetration. However, stool in the rectal ampulla may lead to similar dilatation, and one should be careful to note the presence or absence of stool.

The laboratory evaluation of the sexually abused child should include cultures of the throat, vagina (or urethra), and rectum for gonorrhea; and a culture from the vagina (or urethra) for *Chlamydia*. A serologic test for syphilis is indicated if there is clinical evidence of syphilis, a history of syphilis in the assailant, or the presence of another sexually transmitted disease. HIV testing should only be done after appropriate counseling and if there is reason to suspect infection.

A suspicion of child sexual abuse mandates that a report be filed with child protective services or law enforcement agencies. These agencies will pursue an investigation and attempt to ensure that the child is placed in a protected environment.

Although there is the likelihood that the child may be removed from the home, a return appointment for follow-up of cultures for sexually transmitted diseases and a referral for psychologic counseling should be given.

PHYSICAL ABUSE

The spectrum of injuries in the child who has been intentionally traumatized is wide. Familiarity with this spectrum enables the physician in the emergency department to arrive at the correct diagnosis in a timely manner. Two-thirds of the victims of physical abuse are under the age of 3 years, and one-third are under 6 months. The physical vulnerabilty of such small children is easy to understand.

Historical data may raise suspicions of inflicted trauma. A history which is inconsistent with the nature or the extent of the injuries (e.g., a fractured femur in an infant from a fall off a bed), a history which keeps changing as to the circumstances surrounding the injury, a discrepancy between the story the child gives and the story the caretaker gives, a history of previous trauma in the patient or siblings, or a delay in seeking medical attention should raise one's index of suspicion of physical abuse. Knowledge of normal motor development assists the physician in determining the likelihood that the injury happened in the stated manner. Children under the age of 6 months are incapable of inducing accidents or accidentally ingesting any drugs or poisons. The evaluating physician should record the developmental milestones the child has achieved, e.g., the age of sitting unsupported, walking, etc. Parental behavior in the emergency department should be observed, and it should be noted if the parents appear intoxicated or under the influence of drugs. The level of parental concern about the injury should also be noted.

Toddlers and older children should be questioned about the circumstances of the injury, and the comments should be recorded verbatim on the medical record. These statements are frequently admissible in court under exceptions to the hearsay rule and may help establish the diagnosis of child abuse.

The physical examination should note the child's overall hygiene and well-being. Normal children, especially toddlers who are just learning how to walk, may have multiple ecchymoses over the anterior shins, the forehead, and other bony prominences. Most falls result in bruises on only one body surface. Bruises over multiple areas, especially the low back, buttocks, thighs, cheeks, ear pinnae, neck, ankles, wrists, corners of the mouth, and lips suggest physical abuse. Handprints may be observed, or there may be uniform but bizarre bruise marks caused by belts, buckles, cords, or blunt instruments. Bite marks produce bruising in a characteristic oval pattern, with teeth indentations along the periphery. Lacerations of the frenulum or oral mucosa may be present, especially in an infant who has been force-fed. Lacerations and abrasions in the genital area are seen in toddlers who are "punished" because of toilet-training accidents.

The duration of a bruise can be estimated by the color of the lesion. No discoloration is noted initially, although the bruised area may be swollen and tender. Within a day or two the lesion becomes reddish-blue, and this lasts for about 5 days. This changes to green (days 5 to 7), then to yellow (days 7 to 10), and finally to brown (days 10 to 14) before resolving. For instance, reddish-blue lesions are inconsistent with a 2-week-old injury.

Children with multiple bruises should be evaluated with a complete blood cell count, a differential blood count, and coagulation studies including a platelet count, a prothrombin time, and a partial thromboplastin time. Rarely, a child with leukemia, aplastic anemia, or thrombocytopenia is brought for evaluation because of multiple bruises.

Burns constitute another form of inflicted injuries. These may be scald burns caused by immersion in hot water. Such burns do not conform to a splash configuration; rather, an entire hand or foot ("glove-and-stocking" pattern) may be involved. There is sharp demarcation of the burn margin. The buttocks may be burned during toilet training "punishment" by immersion in a bathtub filled with hot water. Knees, anterior thighs, feet, and portions of the abdomen are spared, and the buttocks and genitalia are scalded. Cigarette burns leave small (approximately 5 mm) circumferential scab-covered injuries. These lesions may resemble impetigo, as do scald injuries, which may resemble bullous impetigo. A culture of material from these lesions differentiates the burn from the infection. Other inflicted burns can result from forced contact with metal objects such as an iron, curling iron, or heater grid.

Skeletal injuries may be detected when a child presents with unexplained swelling of an extremity or refusal to walk or to use an extremity. These fractures may take any form, but spiral fractures caused by torsion (twisting) of a long bone, and metaphyseal chip fractures, suggest inflicted injury, especially when present in infants under 6 months of age. Skeletal surveys referred to as a trauma series (or trauma x) should be obtained. These include films of all long bones, the ribs, the clavicles, the fingers, the toes, the pelvis, and the skull. They may reveal periosteal elevation secondary to new bone formation at sites of previous microfractures or periosteal injury; multiple fractures at different stages of healing; fractures at unusual sites such as the ribs, the lateral clavicle, the sternum, or the scapula; or repeated fractures to the same site. Such x-ray findings are supportive of the diagnosis of child abuse.

Head injuries are a serious and potentially lethal form of child abuse. In addition to having bruises around the ears, eyes, and cheeks, these children may exhibit swelling of the scalp secondary to subgaleal hematomas or underlying skull fractures. Fundoscopic examination may reveal retinal hemorrhages, which are usually associated with subdural hematomas. Such hemorrhages may result from direct trauma to the skull or severe shaking of the child. These children should be evaluated with a CT scan, and coagulation studies should be performed to rule out underlying coagulopathies. MRI studies are also being used to help differentiate recent from older intracranial bleeding episodes. Additional eye injuries caused by trauma may include hyphema, lens dislocation, and retinal detachment.

Injuries to the abdomen are equally serious and are a common cause of death from child abuse. Symtoms include recurrent vomiting, abdominal pain and tenderness, diminished bowel sounds, and/or abdominal distension. A history of injury as well as bruising of the overlying skin may be absent. Abdominal x-ray films may reveal a distended stomach with a "double-bubble sign" secondary to a duodenal hematoma. Diffuse distension may also be noted. Laboratory studies may reveal anemia, an elevated amylase level from traumatic pancreatitis, or hematuria from kidney trauma. Other abdominal injuries caused by trauma may include hepatic or splenic rupture, intestinal perforation, or rupture of intraabdominal blood vessels.

Any serious injury in a child under the age of 5 years should be viewed with suspicion. Other injuries which may be viewed as suggestive of child abuse include those which the child states were inflicted by another, were self-inflicted, or were inflicted by an unknown assailant.

The behavioral interaction between the child, the parent, and the physician may provide supportive evidence of the diagnosis of abuse. These children are often very compliant and submissive. They do not resist the medical examiner and readily submit to painful procedures such as blood drawing. They are overly affectionate to the medical staff, frequently preferring the nurse or the physician over the parent. Sometimes they are protective of the abusing parent, try to foster to his or her needs, and lie to cover up the true nature of the injury.

Parental behavior is less uniform, but certain distinct characteristics may be noted. The parents may not interact with the child in a comforting or supportive manner during the examination. They may become angry at the physician early in the course of the evaluation and may refuse diagnostic studies. They may appear to be intoxicated or under the influence of drugs. They may have brought the child in for seemingly minor complaints and ignored the major injuries or lesions. They may insist on hospital admission of the child for these minor problems and may readily confess they can no longer cope with the child. They may express fears of losing control.

The social service assessment may reveal an unstable home situation with frequent moves, poor parental-support systems, low parental self-esteem (often caused by battering during their own childhood), and/or domestic violence. This adds further supportive evidence of a high-risk situation.

MANAGEMENT

Once the medical assessment has been completed, the physician must initiate the appropriate treatment. The medical management should be guided by the physical findings. Frequently these children require hospitalization.

Although the specifics of the laws surrounding child abuse and neglect vary from state to state, every state does require that suspected cases be reported. A verbal report is made initially to the police department and/or the child protection agency of the locality in which the abuse occurred. Law enforcement officers often appear in the emergency department, especially if the child does not require hospitalization. The child may be removed from the home and placed in protective custody, taken to a juvenile facility, placed temporarily with other relatives, or placed in a foster shelter home. The final disposition is dependent on a court hearing. The physician is also required to complete an official report detailing the specifics of the evaluation and giving his or her diagnostic opinion as to why the injuries or neglect are nonaccidental. The report should use nontechnical terms, e.g., *bruise* instead of *ecchymosis*, so that law enforcement and social service workers can understand the extent of the injuries.

Physicians are sometimes hesitant to report suspected cases. They are not "100 percent" certain. They are fearful of the parental response to the report. They are concerned about removing a child from the natural home. It is important to remember that the physician is required by law to report all suspected cases of abuse and neglect. Failure to report suspected cases can result in misdemeanor charges and lead to a fine or imprisonment. Additionally, the physician is protected by the law from legal retaliation by the parents.

Parental anger is a natural response to the filing of a report of suspected child abuse. The physician should refrain from being accusatory. Instead, the physician should note his or her concern about the child's well-being and advise the family that a physician is required by law to report any suspicions. The physician should verbally acknowledge the anger but persist in the role of child advocate. This job is facilitated in hospitals which have child abuse teams available to assist the physician in the emergency department.

BIBLIOGRAPHY

Child Neglect

Berkowitz CD, Sklaren B: Environmental failure to thrive—The need for intervention. *Am Fam Physician* 29:191, 1984.

Cupoli JM, Hallock JA, Barness LA: Failure to thrive. *Curr Probl Pediatr* 10:5, 1980.

Helfer RE: The neglect of our children. *Pediatr Clin North Am* 37:923, 1990.

Sexual Abuse

Berkowitz CD: Sexual abuse of children and adolescents. *Adv Pediatr* 34:275, 1987.

Chadwick DL, Berkowitz CD, Kerns D, et al: *Color Atlas of Child Sexual Abuse*. Chicago, Year Book Medical Publishers, 1989.

DeJong AR, Finkel MA: Sexual abuse of children. *Curr Probl Pediatr* 20:491, 1990.

Seidel JS, Elvik SL, Berkowitz CD, et al: Presentation and evaluation of sexual misuse in the emergency department. *Pediatr Emerg Care* 2:157, 1986.

Woodling BA, Kossoris PD: Sexual misuse: Rape, molestation, and incest. *Pediatr Clin North Am* 28:481, 1981.

78
THE DIABETIC CHILD

David A. Poleski

INTRODUCTION

Type I, or insulin-dependent, diabetes mellitus (IDDM) is an increasingly common disease in childhood. Diabetic ketoacidosis (DKA) remains the leading cause of death in pediatric diabetes. Life expectancy for patients developing the disease under age 20 is reduced by one-third. Morbidity from the complications of retinopathy, nepropathy, neuropathy, premature coronary and peripheral vascular disease, and stroke significantly impairs patients' life-styles. Meticulous attention to the diagnosis and treatment of IDDM on the part of emergency physicians is important in the effort to reduce the morbidity and mortality of IDDM.

INCIDENCE

IDDM affects 1 in 300 children, making it the most common endocrine disorder of childhood. Males and females are equally affected, with a mean age of onset of 12½ for males and 11 for females. New cases are more common in winter and summer months, although this seasonal variation is not noted in patients presenting under 5 years of age. Socioeconomic factors do not appear to play a role in the incidence of IDDM.

ETIOLOGY

Type I diabetes is probably an autoimmune disease. Its onset is associated with the appearance of circulating islet-cell antibodies and autoreactive T lymphocytes. Factors involved in triggering the autoimmune destruction of pancreatic insulin-secreting β cells remain to be delineated. Viruses, particularly rubella, CMV, Epstein-Barr, mumps and coxsackie have all been implicated as triggering agents. In addition a genetic predisposition for acquiring IDDM exists. Ninety percent of patients diagnosed with IDDM carry the HLA antigens HLA-DR3, HLA-DR4, or both. In addition, individuals with the HLA-B7 or HLA-DR2 antigens seem to be protected from IDDM. Other etiologic factors may be involved, but all the puzzle pieces are not yet in place.

DIAGNOSIS

The diagnosis of IDDM is relatively easy. The triad of polyuria, polydipsia, and polyphagia is the classic presentation. In children and particularly infants, (DKA) and coma are frequent presenting findings. Symptoms which occur prior to the onset of polyuria, polydipsia, polyphagia, and DKA include anorexia, weight loss, malaise, nocturia, erratic behavior, and changes in school performance. These are nonspecific, and usually only serendipity allows the diagnosis of IDDM to be made early in the development of the disease. Glycosuria associated with elevated serum blood glucose values will establish the diagnosis. Glucose tolerance tests in children are of little value and may be detrimental, particularly if elevated serum glucose levels are already present.

DIABETIC KETOACIDOSIS

DKA is a common complication of childhood diabetes, accounting for 14 to 31 percent of hospitalizations related to diabetes. Mortality is reported to be as high as 15.4 percent, although the actual incidence is probably lower. Treating DKA costs over $1 billion annually and accounts for 160,000 hospital admissions. Emergency physicians must be prepared to recognize and treat DKA effectively and expeditiously.

The details of the physiology of DKA are reviewed comprehensively elsewhere. A brief summary is necessary to understand treatment and to avoid pitfalls in management.

DKA develops because of a relative lack of insulin and because of increased activity of the counterregulatory hormones glucagon, cortisol, growth hormone, and epinephrine. Glycogen is mobilized, contributing to the rise in glucose levels; proteolysis and muscle breakdown result in increased amino acid levels; and lipolysis results in increased free fatty acids. Ketone bodies (acetoacetate and β-hydroxybutarate) increase, resulting in ketosis and metabolic acidosis. The hallmarks of DKA are thus hyperglycemia, metabolic acidosis, and ketosis.

Hyperglycemia leads to increased serum osmolality and a subsequent osmotic diuresis. Depending on the duration and extent of the hyperglycemia significant dehydration and possibly shock can result from the diuresis. Infants, whose fluid intake is dependent on their parents, are more apt to develop dehydration and shock than older children, who can compensate by increasing their oral intake at least for a period of time. In addition to volume contraction induced by the osmotic diuresis other important metabolic disturbances are the increased loss of sodium, potassium, and phosphate. Potassium loss may impair cardiovascular function if severe, and phosphate depletion may result in reduced oxygen transport by red blood cells due to diminished levels of 2,3-diphosphoglycerate. Hyperglycemia also may play a role in the development of cerebral edema by leading to the increased production of "idiogenic osmoles." Renal function is impaired as GFR drops due to the osmotically induced hypovolemia.

Ketoacidosis results from increased production in the liver of acetoacetate and β-hydroxybutarate, both of which are strong organic acids. β-hydroxybutarate predominates in the serum (by a 3 : 1 ratio), but acetoacetate is the one measured by commonly available techniques. Measurement of serum ketones during the management of DKA is thus misleading and of little clinical value. The metabolic acidosis produced by increased ketone body production (and by hypoperfusion if fluid loss is advanced) results in a compensatory respiratory alkalosis manifested clinically in advanced stages by Kussmaul respirations. In addition, severe acidosis depresses myocardial function and may contribute to arrhythmias or cardiovascular collapse. Acidosis also can cause paralytic ileus and gastric distension and may account for the abdominal pain and vomting which frequently accompany DKA.

The diagnosis of DKA should be suspected in any patient with polyuria, polydipsia, hyperventilation, acetone-smelling breath, and lethargy. Abdominal pain and vomiting can also be presenting complaints. In young children the diagnosis can be more difficult, and in particular in children under 2 years of age DKA can mimic bacterial sepsis. The diagnosis should be apparent, however, once laboratory results are available. Infection is frequently the stress precipitating DKA, and a thorough search for sources of infection must be performed.

Treatment of DKA

Volume replacement is the mainstay of treatment for DKA. The average deficit is 100 to 150 mL/kg. If possible the fluid deficit should be calculated by comparing the patient's weight on presentation to the emergency department with a known recent weight. If such an estimate is not possible, assume a deficit of 10 percent unless the patient is in shock. Given the importance of fluid replacement in DKA therapy, it is better to overestimate rather than underestimate the amount of fluid loss.

In most cases initial replacement should be a 20 mL/kg bolus of normal saline given over 1 h. If shock is present (rapid pulse, capillary refill greater than 2 sec, obtundation, orthostatic blood pressure changes in the older child, and in the extreme case a falling blood pressure), modify initial therapy by repeating 20 mL/kg boluses until the shock state is corrected. Reevaluate the patient's hydration state and clinical condition frequently, preferably every 30 min. After the initial resuscitation is completed, the calculated remaining deficit should be replaced over 24 to 36 h and will average a rate of infusion approximately 1.5 times maintenance needs per hour. Use 0.45% NaCl as the maintenance and replacement fluid. Once the blood glucose is 250 mg/dL D_5 0.45% NaCl should be substituted. Urinary output during the first 6 h should be measured and replaced with 0.45% NaCl. Oral fluids can be started as soon as nausea and vomiting are no longer clinical problems.

The net effect of adequate fluid resuscitation includes improved renal perfusion with a subsequent increased urinary excretion of glucose and drop in serum glucose levels. In addition peripheral perfusion is improved with partial correction of the metabolic acidosis.

Fluid resuscitation and correction of metabolic derangements in DKA should not be carried out too rapidly in order to avoid the complication of cerebral edema (see "cerebral edema," below).

Once fluid resuscitation has commenced and hyperglycemia (greater than 250 mg/dL on a Dextrostix) has been verified, insulin therapy should be started. Low-dose continuously infused short-acting (regular) insulin is now the method commonly used, although frequent IM injections will also work. The dose recommended is 0.1 unit/kg per hour. Continuously infused insulin has the advantage of smoother and more predictable correction of the metabolic abnormalities associated with DKA. The insulin should be mixed in normal saline (NS) with a concentration of 1 unit per 5 mL of saline. Infusions must be made with an IV infusion pump to avoid inadvertent administration of excess insulin. An initial bolus of 0.1 unit/kg IV can be given but is not necessary. Before administering the insulin infusion, approximately 50 mL of the solution should be run through the intravenous tubing in order to saturate the insulin binding sites of the tubing. With the infusion running, glucose determinations should be made hourly and once levels have declined to 250 mg/dL, 5% glucose should be added to the maintenance and replacement fluid (D_5 0.45 NS). If the glucose level has fallen below 250 mg/dL before the patient's pH has reached 7.30, continue both the insulin infusion and 5% glucose until the acidosis has resolved. This may require titrating the amount of insulin versus the amount of infused dextrose to maintain a glucose level between 200 and 250 mg/dL. Once a pH of 7.30 is reached and the glucose is below 250, subcutaneous short-acting insulin can be started. This should be given about 1 h prior to discontinuing the insulin infusion. Ideally this should be done by the physicians who will be providing the child's long-term follow-up care since meticulous monitoring is needed and is unfortunately difficult to provide in a busy emergency department.

As important, if not more important, as insulin therapy in DKA is the monitoring and correction of electrolyte imbalances. Na^+ and K^+ are both lost in the urine with the osmotic diuresis induced by hyperglycemia, which results in total body depletion of these electrolytes. The loss of Na^+ is not as clinically significant as that of K^+. Sodium levels should be monitored, but fluid resuscitation with normal saline or 0.45% NS will ordinarily prevent problems with rapid osmolar shifts due to hypo- or hypernatremia. The management of potassium disturbances with DKA is much more critical. Serum K^+ does not reflect total body potassium levels since most potassium is intracellar. The acidosis of DKA exacerbates the problem by causing additional shifting of K^+ from the intracellar to extracellular space. This results in high serum K^+ levels even in the face of total body deletion. Patients with DKA should have cardiac monitoring to detect hypo- or hyperkalemia pending the results of serum potassium levels. Once the serum level is known, decisions regarding the amount and rate of replacement can be made. If the pH is 7.10 or less and the K^+ normal or reduced, replacement should begin immediately since hypokalemia will be exacerbated as the pH improves and can cause life-threatening cardiac dysfunction. If the K^+ level is high (greater than 6.0), however, replacement should be withheld so that iatrogenic hyperkalemia is not induced with its potential for cardiac complications as well. Once the K^+ level is normal and the pH is improving, therapy can begin. Forty mEq of KCL added to each liter of maintenance fluid given at the calculated maintenance replacement rate on an infusion pump is sufficient. Some clinicians recommend replacing potassium with potassium phosphate (20 mEq/L) and potassium chloride (20 mEq/L). This approach has the theoretical but as yet unsubstantiated clinical advantages of maintaining the level of 2,3-diphosphoglycerate which is important in the transfer of oxygen to the tissues. Phosphate and calcium levels should be measured at some point in the management of DKA but are seldom of concern to the emergency physician.

Finally, the issue of bicarbonate therapy in the treatment of DKA needs to be addressed. As yet no convincing evidence exists that bicarbonate therapy affects the outcome of DKA. Classically, arguments favoring bicarbonate use have pointed out that myocardial function and ventilatory effort are impaired when the pH falls below 7.1. At least in children these considerations do not appear to be clinically significant. On the other hand, use of bicarbonate may contribute to the complications of DKA treatment, although again the clinical relevance of these problems is still unclear. Bicarbonate therapy can result in a paradoxical CNS acidosis which may alter CNS function; a shift of the oxyhemoglobin dissociation curve to the left with impaired tissue oxygentation, worsening hypokalemia; and possibly in hypernatremia contributing to rapid osmolar shifts which may play a role in the development of cerebral edema. Since there is no convincing evidence of the benefit of bicarbonate therapy, it is probably best avoided except in life-threatening situations. These would include cardiac arrhythmias due to hyperkalemia or cardiac dysfunction due to severe acidosis.

Laboratory tests necessary in the management of DKA are glucose, electrolytes, urinalysis, venous pH (which accurately correlates which arterial pH and is easier to obtain in children), BUN, and creatinine. Serum acetone can be obtained but is usually unnecessary. The degree of ketosis can be estimated by calculating the anion gap which will be due primarily to the ketone bodies and lactate. It is advisable to check glucose, electrolytes (particularly potassium), and venous pH on an hourly basis and adjust therapy accordingly. Cardiac monitoring until the dangers of potassium-induced cardiac problems are passed is recommended. If the stress inducing DKA is not apparent from the history and physical examination, a CXR, blood cultures, lumbar puncture, and complete blood count should be considered to look for occult sources of infection. If serious infection is suspected, antibiotics should be started pending the results.

Cerebral Edema

Although rare, cerebral edema can be a fatal complication of DKA in children. Increasing evidence suggests that subclinical cerebral edema exists in most children with DKA. For reasons that are not clear some patients develop malignant edema, which will lead to death in over 90 percent of cases. The etiology of this complication is not well understood. Overly aggressive fluid resuscitation with its attendant rapid osmotic shifts has been implicated, but cerebral edema has occurred without such therapy. Hyponatremia, bicarbonate therapy resulting in paradoxical CSF acidosis, cerebral hypoxia, and elevated intracellar potassium levels due to insulin therapy have also been implicated. The complication usually occurs when the child appears to be improving, about 6 to 10 h after treatment has started. Typical symptoms are abrupt mental status changes with progression to coma. Treatment attempts have been discouraging. Intubation with hyperventilation to reduce intracranial pressure should be performed. Mannitol 1 to 2 g/kg may help. Fluid restriction should be instituted. Until more is understood about this complication, the slowest correction of fluid deficits and metabolic derangements associated with DKA consistent with patient well-being is the prudent course to follow.

HYPOGLYCEMIA

In children the initial treatment of a hypoglycemia episode depends on the clinical presentation. In those with mild symptoms, such as dizziness, diaphoresis, or weakness, oral supplements including candy, table sugar, or commerically prepared glucose supplements are adequate. When hypoglycemia leads to significant mental status changes such as unconsciousness or seizures, treatment consists of administering 0.5 mL/kg of $D_{50}W$ or 1.0 mL/kg of $D_{25}W$ intravenously. If IV access cannot be obtained, glucagon 0.5 mg IM can be given to children under 6 years of age or 1 mg IM to those 6 years old or older. In children with already depleted glycogen stores, glucagon may not work; in all cases, efforts to establish IV access should continue. In children under 3 years of age, intraosseous infusions may be used for glucose infusions if IV access cannot be obtained and glucagon is unsuccessful. Once normal mental status is regained, oral glucose supplements or a regular meal can be given.

Important to note is the growing concern for overtreatment of hypoglycemia. If serious symptoms such as coma or seizures are not present, treatment with a maintenance infusion of $D_{10}W$ is preferable to repeated boluses of $D_{25}W$ or $D_{50}W$ to avoid unnecessary hyperglycemia. Overtreatment can also occur if one doesn't recall that approximately 10 min will elapse between initial glucose therapy and the time the patient begins to feel better. It is during this time frame that excessive amounts of glucose are frequently administered.

Finally, whenever possible, hypoglycemia should be verified by Dextrostix or serum glucose determinations prior to treatment. Treating presumed hypoglycemia can delay the diagnosis of other entities in diabetic children with altered mental status, such as sepsis, meningitis, toxic overdoses, and head injuries.

OTHER CONSIDERATIONS

With the increasing realization that IDDM is an autoimmune disease, interest is growing in starting treatment with immunosuppressive drugs, particularly cyclosporine, as soon as the diagnosis of new-onset IDDM has been made. As tempting as this idea is, the treatment is still experimental and is not currently recommended in newly diagnosed emergency department cases.

The treatment of childhood diabetes in the emergency department is primarily concerned with the acute management of hypoglycemia and DKA. Long-term day-to-day management of childhood diabetes is complicated and requires a good long-term physician-patient relationship. Emergency department physicians are not in a position to provide this and should make efforts to coordinate any decisions about care with the patient's primary physician. Follow-up with the patient's primary doctor should always be assured prior to emergency department discharge.

BIBLIOGRAPHY

Ainslee MB, Spencer ML: New approaches to diabetes in the young. *Compr Ther* 14:65, 1988.

Bach JF, Feutren G, Boitard C: The prospects of immunosuppression in type-I diabetes. *Adv Nephrol* 17:321, 1988.

Chase HP, Garg SK, Jelley DH: Diabetic ketoacidosis in children and the role of outpatient management. *Pediatr Rev* 11:297, 1990.

Drash AL: The epidemiology of diabetes mellitus in children and adolescents. *Pediatr Ann* 12:629, 1983.

Duck SC, Wyatt D: Factors associated with brain herniation in the treatment of diabetic ketoacidosis. *J Pediatr* 113:10, 1988.

Edwards GA, Kohaut EC, Wehring B, et al: Effectiveness of low-dose continuous intravenous insulin infusion in diabetic ketoacidosis. *J Pediatr* 91:701, 1977.

Eisenbarth GS: Type I diabetes mellitus: A chronic autoimmune disease. *N Engl J Med* 314:1360, 1986.

Fisher JN, Kitabchi AE: A randomized study of phosphate therapy in the treatment of diabetic ketoacidosis. *J Clin Endocrinol Metab* 57:177, 1983.

Franklin B. Liu J, Ginsberg-Fellner F: Cerebral edema and opthalmoplegia reversed by mannitol in a new case of insulin-dependent diabetes mellitus. *Pediatrics* 69:87, 1982.

Ginsberg-Fellner F: Insulin-dependent diabetes mellitus. *Pediatr Rev* 11:239, 1990.

Krane EJ: Diabetic ketoacidosis. *Pediatr Clin North Am* 34:935, 1987.

Krane EJ, Rockoff MA, Wallman JK, et al: Subclinical brain swelling in children during treatment of diabetic ketoacidosis. *N Engl J Med* 312:1147, 1985.

Lever EL, Jaspan JB: Sodium bicarbonate therapy in severe diabetic ketoacidosis. *Am J Med* 75:263, 1983.

Morris LR, Murphy MB, Kitabchi AE: Bicarbonate therpay in severe diabetic ketoacidosis. *Ann Intern Med* 105:836, 1986.

Rayfield EJ, Seto Y: Viruses and the pathogenesis of diabetes mellitus. *Diabetes* 27:1126, 1978.

Rosenbloom AL, Riley WJ, Weber FT, et al: Cerebral edea complicating diabetic ketoacidosis in childhood. *J Pediatr* 96:357, 1980.

Scibilia J, Finegold D, Dorman J: Why do children with diabetes die? *Acta Endocrinol* 113(suppl):326, 1986.

Skyler JS: Why control blood glucose? *Pediatr Ann* 16:713, 1987.

Stiller CR, Dupre J, Gent M, et al: Effects of cyclosporine immunosuppression in insulin-dependent diabetes mellitus of recent onset. *Science* 223:1362, 1984.

79
PEDIATRIC EXANTHEMS

Michael S. Weinstock
Michael S. Catapano

Rashes with diverse etiologies can look alike. The emergency physician's task is to obtain an accurate history regarding prior immunizations, potential human or animal contacts, and recent environmental exposure. This, along with the signs and symptoms either preceding or presenting with the exanthem, helps to determine the diagnosis. The various etiologic agents and associated exanthems are noted in Table 79-1.

BACTERIAL

Bullous Impetigo

Bullous impetigo, or staphylococcal impetigo, is a local skin infection caused by phage group II staphylococci. The staphylococci produce an epidermolytic toxin that acts locally to cause separation of the skin at the granular layer, giving rise to bullae. The infection occurs primarily in newborn infants and young children. The characteristic skin lesions of bullous impetigo are superficial, flaccid, thin-walled bullae that occur most often on the extremities but can occur anywhere. They range in size from 0.5 to 3 cm. They can arise from normal skin or may have a thin, red halo. The bullae are filled with a clear, pale-to-yellow fluid and rupture easily, leaving a moist, denuded base that dries rapidly with a shiny coating. Extensive areas of skin may be involved if untreated.

The clinical appearance of the lesions usually makes diagnosis easy. However, single lesions or extensive involvement may not be as typical. Staphylococci cultured from fluid from aspirated bullae will establish the diagnosis.

Systemic antistaphylococcal antibiotics, usually oral, along with local wound cleansing and topical antibiotics (such as neosporin) are effective in eradicating the infection. Prognosis for complete recovery is good.

Impetigo Contagiosum

Impetigo is a superficial pyoderma caused by infection with group A, β-hemolytic streptococci, although staphylococci may also be cultured. It is a common skin infection, primarily affecting young children, especially in warm, humid conditions. Impetigo can arise at the site of insect bites or superficial cutaneous trauma; sometimes there is no apparent predisposing skin lesion. Fever and systemic signs are uncommon.

The skin lesions start as small erythematous macules and papules. These develop into discrete, thin-walled vesicles which become pustular and quickly rupture (see Fig. 79-1). As the vesicles rupture, a yellow fluid forms an exudate, which dries to form a stratified golden, yellow crust that accumulates. The crusts can be readily removed, leaving a smooth, red surface. The crusts can spread the infection to other parts of the body. Initially, the lesions are discrete, but they may enlarge and become confluent. Local adenopathy may be present. The infection occurs most frequently on the face, neck, and extremities.

The diagnosis of impetigo can be readily made on the basis of the typical clinical appearance. Cultures are generally not necessary. Systemic antibiotic therapy must be combined with wound scrubbing and cleansing and application of neosporin or mupirocin ointment for optimal results. Effective antibiotics include benzathine penicillin and oral antibiotics such as penicillin V, erythromycin, cephalosporin, and dicloxacillin.

Erysipelas

Erysipelas, or St. Anthony's fire, is cellulitis and lymphangitis of the skin caused by group A, β-hemolytic streptococci. It is frequently accompanied by fever, chills, malaise, headache, and vomiting.

The rash is characterized by local redness, heat, swelling, and a raised, indurated border. There is marked involvement of the superficial dermal lymphatics. The rash starts as an erythematous plaque that rapidly enlarges by peripheral extension. At first, it is scarlet, hot, brawny, swollen, and tender. The edge is raised and sharply demarcated. The rash can vary in appearance from a transient hyperemia to intense inflammation, vesiculation, and bullae. The face is the most frequent site. A skin wound, fissure, or ulcer may act as a portal of entry.

Diagnosis is made on clinical grounds, although aspiration of the leading edge of the lesion will frequently demonstrate streptococci. A brief course of parenteral penicillin is usually warranted because of the rapid advancement of the infection, the acutely toxic state of the patient, and the possibility of suppurative complications. Rapid clinical response is usually obtained. Erythromycin may be used in patients unable to take penicillin.

Mycoplasma Infections

Mycoplasma pneumoniae infections are a common cause of pneumonia, upper respiratory infections, and bronchitis in children between 5 and 19 years of age. The most frequent presenting clinical findings in children and adults are fever, cough, sore throat, malaise, headache, chills, and rash. An erythematous maculopapular rash, the most fre-

Table 79-1. Differential Diagnosis of Exanthems

Vesiculopustules	Maculopapules	Urticaria	Petechiae
Drug eruption	Drug eruption	Varicella (urticaria around vesicle)	Drug eruption
Herpes simplex	Secondary lues	Coxsackie A5, A9	Bacterial endocarditis
Variola	Scarlet fever	Infectious hepatitis	Echovirus
Vaccinia	Echovirus 9, 16	Mononucleosis	Coxsackie A5, A9
Varicella	Coxsackie A5, A9, A16, B5	*Mycoplasma pneumoniae*	Mononucleosis
Generalized zoster	Reovirus 2	Hepatitis	Rubella
Rickettsialpox	Erythema infectiosum		Thrombocytopenia with many acute infections
Coxsackie A and B	Gianotti-Crosti syndrome		
Reovirus 2	Rubella		
Mycoplasma pneumoniae	Rubeola		
Echovirus 4	Hepatitis		
Contagious ecthyma (orf)	Infectious mononucleosis		
	Arbovirus (dengue)		
	Rickettsioses		

Source: From Burnett JW, Crutcher WA: Viral and rickettsial infections in Moschella SL, Hurley, HJ: *Dermatology*, Philadelphia, Saunders, 1985, vol 1, chap 12, pp 673–738.

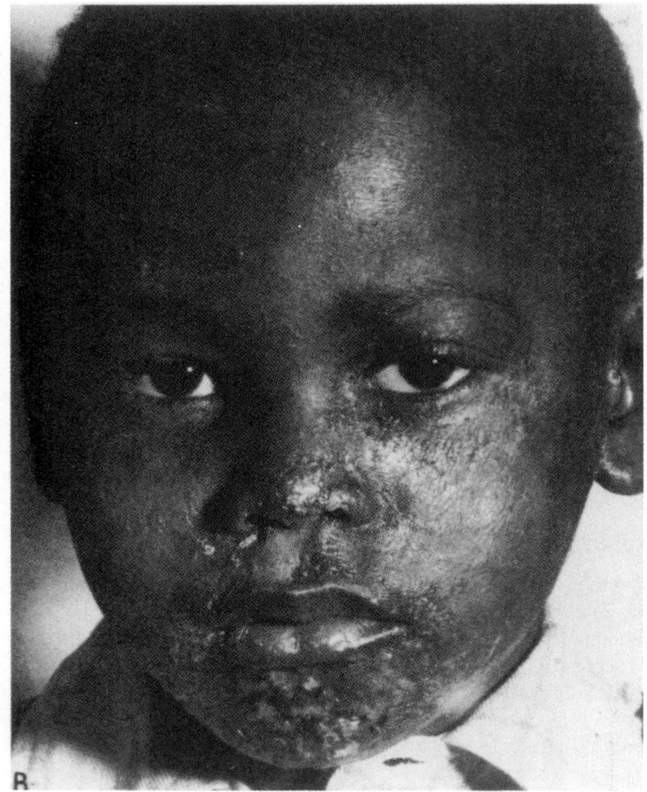

Fig. 79-1. Impetigo contagiosum. (*From* Marples RR, Leyden JL: Bacterial infections, section I, Fundamental cutaneous microbiology in Moschella SL, Hurley HJ (eds): *Dermatology*, Philadelphia, Saunders, 1985, vol I, chap 11, pp. 590–642, with permission.)

quent presentation, is located on the trunk and may be discrete or confluent. However, the most frequently reported exanthem is consistent with *Erythema multiforme* and Stevens-Johnson syndrome, with lesions occurring primarily on the trunk, legs, and arms. The rash occurs most commonly during the febrile period. An enanthem of generalized ulcerative stomatitis or pharyngitis-tonsillitis associated with the exanthem is common. The diagnosis can be confirmed by the use of either serum cold agglutinins or several specific antibody tests.

Mycoplasma responds to several antimicrobials, including erythromycin, tetracycline, chloramphenicol, and aminoglycosides. Infection with *M. pneumoniae* should be suspected in patients with pneumonia and a rash.

Scarlet Fever

Scarlet fever is an acute febrile illness, primarily affecting young children, caused by group A, β-hemolytic streptococci. Recently group C streptococci have been implicated as well. Clinical manifestations include acute onset with fever, sore throat, headache, vomiting, and abdominal pain followed by a distinctive exanthem in 1 to 2 days.

There are both an exanthem and an enanthem associated with scarlet fever. They are caused by an erythrogenic toxin elaborated by the streptococcal organism. The tonsils and pharynx are red and covered with exudate, although occasionally pharyngeal findings are minimal. The tongue has a white coating through which red and hypertrophied papillae project, creating the appearance of a "white strawberry tongue." The white coating disappears by day 4 or 5, and the tongue acquires a bright-red appearance, the "red strawberry tongue." Bright-red or hemorrhagic spots may be seen on the soft palate or anterior pillars of the tonsillar fossae.

The exanthem of scarlet fever begins 1 or 2 days after the onset of the illness. It starts on the neck, axillae, and groin, spreading to the trunk and extremities. The rash is red and finely punctate, consisting of 1- to 2-mm papules giving the rash a characteristic rough, sandpaper feel. It is sometimes easier to identify the rash by palpation. The rash blanches with pressure. Linear petechial eruptions, Pastia's lines, are often present in the antecubital and axillary folds. There is facial flushing with circumoral pallor. A branny desquamation occurs at 2 weeks, yielding fine flakes of dry skin.

The diagnosis of scarlet fever is readily made on clinical grounds. Throat swabs usually culture group A, β-hemolytic streptococci, although group C may be cultured as well. Treatment with antibiotics is necessary to reduce the incidence of rheumatic fever and nephritis and will probably ameliorate the course of the disease. Penicillin is the antibiotic of choice with erythromycin also being effective for those who are penicillin-allergic.

Staphylococcal Scalded-Skin Syndrome

The staphylococcal scalded-skin syndrome (SSSS) is a febrile illness of neonates and young children characterized by a generalized, confluent superficial exfoliation of skin. It is also called Ritter's disease or dermatitis exfoliativa neonatorum. SSSS is caused by the action of an epidermolytic toxin, exfoliatin, elaborated by phage group II *Staphylococcus aureus*. The staphylococci do not occur in the involved skin but rather in a distant, separate focus such as the pharynx, nose, conjunctiva, skin wounds, or even septicemia. Exfoliation causes the skin to separate at the granular layer, resulting in a superficial exfoliation.

The illness starts with fever, malaise, irritability, and skin tenderness. There is a diffuse macular erythroderma of the face, neck, axillae, and groin with rapid extension. The palms, soles, and mucous membranes are spared. Within 1 to 3 days there is wrinkling of the skin or separation in response to gentle stroking, a positive Nikolsky's sign. Large, flaccid, thin-walled bullae appear which rupture spontaneously. The epidermis separates in large sheets leaving moist, glistening denuded areas, which quickly dry and undergo a flaky desquamation. Healing occurs without scarring unless secondary infection occurs.

The diagnosis of SSSS can usually be made clinically. Cultures are not necessary. SSSS can be distinguished from toxic epidermal necrolysis (TEN) by biopsy of exfoliated skin. In SSSS the cleavage plane is at the granular layer, while in TEN the skin separates at the dermal-epidermal junction or within the dermis.

Therapy for SSSS includes parenteral antistaphylococcal antibiotics, fluid resuscitation, temperature regulation, and wound care. Topical antibiotics are of no benefit, and steroids should not be used. Staphylococci should be eliminated from the focus of infection, ending toxin production. Prognosis for complete recovery is good.

RICKETTSIAL

Rocky Mountain Spotted Fever

Rocky Mountain spotted fever (RMSF) is an infectious disease caused by *Rickettsia rickettsii* which is transmitted by ticks. The prominent clinical manifestations of RMSF can be directly related to the primary pathologic lesion in the endothelial cells lining small blood vessels where the rickettsia multiply. Rash, headache, mental confusion, terminal heart failure, and shock are manifestations of the generalized vasculitis.

The incubation period is from 2 to 12 days with either a sudden or gradual onset of symptoms. Peak severity usually occurs within 1 to 2 weeks. Headache, fever, toxicity, rash, and myalgia are the major clinical features. The rash (Fig. 79-2), a pathognomonic feature of the disease, usually appears on the second or third day. The initial lesions first appear on the wrist and ankles spreading rapidly to the extremities and trunk. These lesions also are found on the palms and

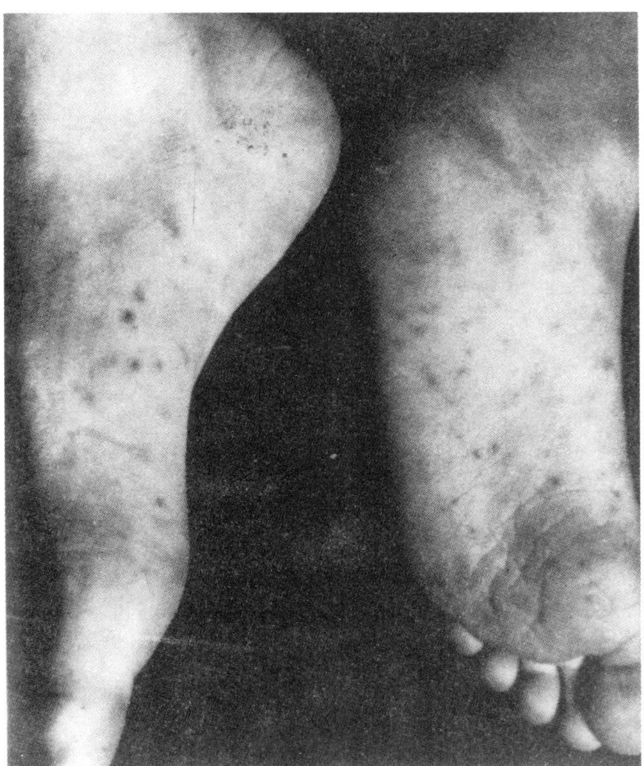

Fig. 79-2. Rocky Mountain spotted fever. (*From* Burnett JW, Crutcher WA: *Viral and rickettsial infections,* in Moschella SL, Hurley HJ (eds), *Dermatology,* Philadelphia, Saunders, 1985, vol 1, chap 12, pp. 673–738, with permission.)

soles of the patient. Initially, lesions are small, erythematous macules which blanch on pressure. They rapidly become maculopapular and petechial.

Laboratory diagnostic confirmation is difficult during the early phase of the disease, frequently mandating treatment based on clinical criteria. Serologic tests are mainly used to confirm the diagnosis of RMSF. Some laboratory data may be helpful in establishing the presumptive diagnosis early, such as leukopenia and thrombocytopenia.

Specific therapy consists of tetracyclines or chloramphenicols. In seriously ill children 100 mg/kg per 24 h of chloramphenicol up to 3 g total dose is advised. As improvement is noted, therapy can be changed to 50 mg/kg per 24 h in four divided doses orally. Treatment can be terminated 2 or 3 days after fever returns to normal for 24 h. The mortality of RMSF in the United States has held steady for a decade at 3 to 6 percent of identified cases despite treatment.

VIRUSES

Enteroviruses

Enteroviruses are an exceedingly common cause of illness and exanthem in young children. Enteroviruses are small, single-stranded RNA viruses belonging to the picornavirus group and consist of polioviruses and nonpolioviruses (coxsackievirus and echovirus). There are many types of coxsackieviruses and echoviruses that have been associated with illnesses. They usually occur in epidemics and are most prevalent in the summer and early fall. Transmission usually occurs by fecal-oral route and possibly by the respiratory route.

The clinical manifestations of infection with coxsackieviruses and echoviruses are extensive. The spectrum of disease includes nonspecific febrile illness, upper respiratory infection, parotitis, croup, bronchitis, pneumonia, bronchiolitis, vomiting, diarrhea, abdominal pain, hepatitis, pancreatitis, conjunctivitis, pericarditis, myocarditis, orchitis, nephritis, arthritis, meningitis, and encephalitis.

Similarly, the associated skin manifestations include an array of exanthems. Diffuse macular eruptions, morbilliform erythema, vesicular lesions, petechial and purpural eruptions, rubelliform rash, roseola-like rash, and scarlatiniform eruptions have been reported.

Strict clinical-virologic associations have been difficult to demonstrate. A single clinical syndrome can be associated with many types of coxsackieviruses and echoviruses. On the other hand, some types of coxsackieviruses and echoviruses have been associated with multiple illnesses and exanthems.

Hand, foot, and mouth disease is an acute infectious illness that primarily affects children. Initial manifestations include fever, anorexia, malaise, and sore mouth. Oral lesions appear 1 to 2 days later and cutaneous lesions shortly thereafter. The oral lesions begin as vesicles on an erythematous base which ulcerate. The vesicles are usually 4 to 8 mm in size, and are very painful. They are located on the buccal mucosa, tongue, soft palate, and gingiva. The exanthem starts as red papules which change to gray vesicles about 3 to 7 mm in size. They are found on the palms and soles but may occur on the dorsum of the feet and hands and on the buttocks, as well. They may be oval, linear, or crescentic and may run parallel to skin lines. They heal in 7 to 10 days.

Herpangina is a febrile disease of children associated with many types of coxsackieviruses and echoviruses. The onset is acute with fever to 40°C, headache, sore throat, dysphagia, anorexia, and, occasionally, stiff neck. In the pharynx, there are one or more yellowish-white 2-mm vesicles with hyperemic borders. They are located in the posterior pharynx on the tonsils, uvula, soft palate, and anterior faucial pillars. The vesicles will usually ulcerate, leaving a shallow, gray-yellow crater 2 to 4 mm in size. The lesions persist for 5 to 10 days.

Boston exanthem is caused by echovirus 16. It is an acute illness with fever, anorexia, pharyngitis, and lymphadenopathy. An enanthem similar to herpangina may be present. The exanthem begins as small, discrete, pink macules that develop into papules. It appears on the face and chest, spreads centrifugally, and may involve the palms and soles. As in roseola, the rash may appear with defervescence of the fever.

Infection due to echovirus 9 is prevalent and produces a typical enteroviral illness. Clinical manifestations include fever, headache, nausea, vomiting, abdominal pain, cough, coryza, pharyngitis, and nuchal rigidity. The exanthem is rubelliform, a maculopapular rash beginning on the face and neck or extending to the trunk and feet and sometimes the palms and soles. Occasionally, there are lesions on the buccal mucosa and soft palate that resemble Koplik's spots. Petechiae may occur. The appearance of this rash and the presence of nuchal rigidity makes this illness occasionally mimic meningococcemia. The exanthem persists for about 5 days.

Infection with coxsackievirus A9 is a common cause of exanthem. It is an acute febrile illness with a discrete erythematous maculopapular rash that begins on the face and neck and extends to the trunk and extremities. Aseptic meningitis may occur. The rash may also be vesicular or urticarial.

The clinical differentiation of enteroviral disease is difficult. Since there is no specific therapy for enteroviral infection, it is more important to consider bacterial diseases in the differential diagnosis in order to exclude treatable causes of sepsis, meningitis, myocarditis, and pneumonia. Symptomatic therapy for enteroviral infections includes adequate hydration, antipyretics, and viscous lidocaine gel for painful oral lesions.

Erythema Infectiosum

Erythema infectiosum (fifth disease) is an acute, febrile illness with a unique exanthem. Outbreaks of erythema infectiosum occur primarily in the spring. During epidemics, the attack rate is highest in children

5 to 15 years of age, but all age groups can be affected. The illness is caused by infection with human parvovirus, a single-stranded DNA virus.

The abrupt appearance of the rash is frequently the first manifestation of erythema infectiosum. It begins with a characteristic fiery red rash on the cheeks. The rash is a diffuse erythema or closely grouped tiny papules on an erythematous base. The edges are slightly raised. The erythema is most intense below the eyes and extends over the cheeks in a pattern reminiscent of butterfly wings; it is sometimes referred to as a *slapped-cheek appearance*. There is circumoral pallor as well as sparing of the eyelids and chin. The facial rash fades after 4 to 5 days. Approximately 1 to 2 days after the appearance of the facial rash, a nonpruritic macular erythema or erythematous maculopapular rash occurs on the trunk and limbs. It is at first localized to the deltoid areas, trunk, and forearms but usually extends to involve a large area. This stage of the exanthem may last 1 week. A distinctive aspect of the rash is that it fades with central clearing, giving a reticulated or lacy appearance. The palms and soles are rarely affected.

The exanthem may recur in the ensuing 3 weeks, sometimes briefly. The intensity of the recurrent exanthem varies and may be related to exposure to environmental factors such as sunlight, hot baths, and, perhaps, physical exertion or emotional upset. Associated symptoms frequently occur and may include fever, malaise, headache, sore throat, cough, coryza, nausea, vomiting, diarrhea, and myalgia. Arthralgias and arthritis can occur, but usually only in adults. These symptoms may occur before or after the onset of the rash.

There is no specific treatment for human parvovirus infection. Symptomatic therapy is all that is required. Recovery is usually complete.

Measles

Prior to a nationwide immunization program in 1965 measles was an expected disease of childhood. It is a highly contagious, endemic myxovirus infection. It is a winter-spring disease in temperate climates, but it occurs throughout the world.

After exposure, the incubation period for the disease is about 10 days. The prodromal period lasts approximately 3 days and is characterized by upper respiratory symptoms. The onset of clinical measles is characterized by general malaise, systemic toxicity, fever, coryza, conjunctivitis, photophobia, and cough.

The exanthem develops about the fourteenth day following exposure. The rash first appears behind the ears and at the hairline of the forehead. It spreads in a centrifugal pattern from the head to the feet. It is initially erythematous and maculopapular but rapidly progresses to confluence, especially on the face. Initially the rash is red and blanches on pressure. As it fades, it takes on a copper-to-brownish hue. With healing there may be some fine desquamation. The rash generally lasts 7 days.

Koplik's spots are an associated pathognomonic enanthem. The lesions are white, 1-mm discrete spots which first appear on the buccal mucosa opposite the lower molars and then spread to involve the entire buccal mucosa. The treatment of measles is supportive.

Infectious Mononucleosis

The diagnosis of infectious mononucleosis can be entertained in those children, adolescents and young adults who present with fever, sore throat, malaise, and fatigue accompanied by tonsillopharyngitis and lymphadenopathy.

There is strong evidence for Epstein-Barr virus (EBV) as the etiologic agent of the "mononucleosis syndrome." The age of initial (primary) infection varies and appears to depend upon socioeconomic status. The mononucleosis symptom complex is associated with the primary infection. A 2- to 5-day prodromal period of malaise and fatigue with or without fever may precede the full onset of the syndrome. The adenopathy is usually confined to the anterior and posterior cervical chain but may be generalized. There is a 5 percent incidence of a generalized erythematous maculopapular rash associated with an enanthem consisting of petechiae on the soft palate. The incidence of the rash increases to almost 100 percent in those patients taking ampicillin or its congeners. The treatment for infectious mononucleosis is supportive.

Rubella

Rubella (German measles) is a common childhood disease with its highest incidence during the spring. The incubation period is 12 to 25 days following exposure with a 1- to 5-day prodrome of fever, malaise, headache, and sore throat.

The exanthem varies and is sometimes difficult to identify. It may present as a short-lived blush, or it may have the more common 2- to 3-day course. The exanthem begins as irregular pink macules and papules on the face spreading to the neck, trunk, and arms in a centrifugal distribution. It coalesces on the face as the eruption reaches the lower extremities and then clears in the same fashion. An exanthem of pinpoint petechiae involving the soft palate (Forschheimer's spots) may accompany the rash but is nonspecific.

Lymphadenopathy is a clinical manifestation of rubella, with the enlargement characteristically in the suboccipital and posterior auricular nodes. The clinical diagnosis of the individual case is often difficult, but the epidemic nature of the illness, along with the seasonal variation and high expression rate of the exanthem, help in establishing the diagnosis. A history of inadequate immunizations may assist in the diagnosis. There is no specific therapy.

Varicella

Varicella, or chickenpox, is a result of infection with varicella-zoster virus, a herpes virus. In normal children it is characterized by a pruritic generalized vesicular exanthem with mild systemic manifestations. Cases generally occur in late winter and early spring. It is highly contagious in the prodromal and vesicular stage. Varicella most frequently occurs in children less than 10 years old, but it may occur at any age.

The exanthem starts on the trunk or scalp and first appears as faint, red macules. Within 24 h, the rash acquires the typical vesicular appearance of varicella. The rash consists of teardrop vesicles on an erythematous base, which then dry and crust over (see Fig. 79-3). Successive fresh crops may appear for a few days. The extent of the rash may be minimal but usually will spread centrifugally and become widespread. Palms and soles are spared. Vesicles may occur on mucous membranes and proceed to rupture and form shallow ulcers. Low-grade fever, malaise, and headache are frequently present but are usually mild. The diagnosis of varicella is usually made clinically on the basis of its distinctive rash. A Tzanck smear of the vesicle contents will demonstrate varicella giant cells with inclusion bodies.

Complications of varicella can occur, including encephalitis, pneumonia, nephritis, and infection of the vesicles with staphylococci or streptococci. Neonates born to mothers with perinatal varicella infection may develop serious illness.

Uncomplicated varicella requires no specific therapy. Acetaminophen may be used as needed, but aspirin should be avoided as it may predispose to the development of Reye's syndrome. Oral antihistamines may be useful to reduce itching. Most importantly, lesions should be cleansed regularly to prevent secondary infection. In the absence of central nervous sytem complications, the prognosis is excellent.

Immunocompromised patients with varicella require aggressive treatment with antiviral drugs such as acyclovir. Administration of varicella-zoster immune globulin (VZIG) should be considered for immunocompromised patients exposed to individuals with varicella.

ETIOLOGY UNCLEAR

Erythema Nodosum

Erythema nodosum is an inflammatory exanthem of unknown etiology. It is probably an inflammatory reaction to a stimulus. In the past,

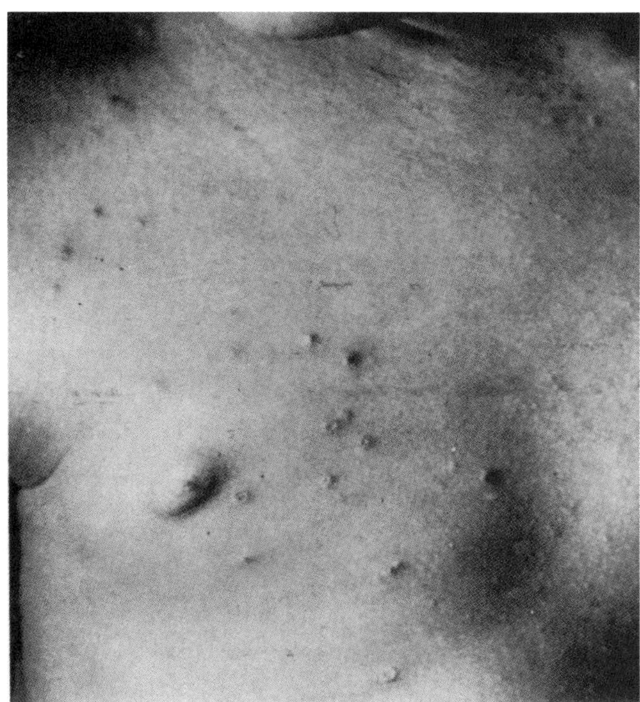

Fig. 79-3. Varicella. (*From* Burnett JW, Crutcher WA: *Viral and rickettsial infections*, in Moschella SL, Hurley HJ: *Dermatology*, Philadelphia, Saunders, 1985, vol 1, chap 12, pp. 673–738, with permission.)

erythema nodosum was associated with streptococcal infections, tuberculosis, sarcoid, fungal infections, *Yersinia* infections, vasculitis, inflammatory bowel disease, and leukemia. Now it is more commonly associated with drugs, especially oral contraceptives. Any age can be affected. Constitutional symptoms may be present at the onset, including fever, malaise, myalgias, and arthralgias.

Erythema nodosum presents a distinctive clinical appearance. Bilateral, very tender nodules develop symmetrically. They usually occur on the shins but can occur on the arms, thighs, calves, and buttocks. The nodules are 1 to 5 cm in diameter, and individual lesions may coalesce to form sizable areas of induration. The skin over the nodules is red, smooth, and shiny. No ulceration occurs. After a week or two, the color of the lesions changes from red to blue and may achieve a dull, purple, bruised appearance. The eruption lasts several weeks.

The diagnosis of erythema nodosum is usually readily made on clinical grounds. A thorough history and physical, and perhaps laboratory evaluation, must be performed to exclude an underlying cause. There is no known therapy to alter the course of the disease. Nonsteroidal anti-inflammatory drugs may provide relief from the sometimes significant pain associated with these lesions.

Kawasaki Disease (Mucocutaneous Lymph Node Syndrome)

Kawasaki disease, or mucocutaneous lymph node syndrome (MLNS), is a disease of unclear etiology found predominantly in children under 9 years of age.

The diagnosis of this disorder is based on a constellation of clinical findings. The patient must exhibit a prolonged fever associated with at least four of the following: (1) conjunctivitis, (2) rash, (3) lymphadenopathy, (4) changes in the oropharynx consisting of injection of the pharynx and lips with prominent papillae of the tongue (strawberry tongue), and (5) extremity erythema and edema.

The rash has been described as erythematous, morbilliform, urticarial, scarlatiniform, or erythema multiforme-like. It has a predilection for the perineum. Additional supportive evidence which may help in the presumptive diagnosis are leukocytosis, elevation of acute-phase reactants, elevated liver function tests, arthritis, arthralgia, and irritability.

In the second phase, there is usually a sharp rise in the platelet count, desquamation of the fingers and or toes, and the most serious complication, the development of coronary artery aneurysm. A small percentage (1 to 2 percent) of patients with coronary artery anuerysm develop sudden cardiac failure, resulting in death from myocardial infarction with coronary artery thrombosis.

The differential diagnosis includes drug allergy, toxic epidermal necrolysis, staphylococcal toxin–mediated syndromes, erythema multiforme, and scarlet fever. The etiologic speculations are a hyperimmune response to a variety of infections, a viral syndrome, allergic or toxic response to pollutants, drugs, toxic agents, and a possibility of a rickettsial disease.

Treatment of Kawasaki disease is controversial and includes various antibiotics, salicylates, and steroids. Intravenous gamma globulin is now routinely recommended. Aspirin may be the most promising therapy. Bed rest, supportive therapy, and frequent monitoring are mainstays of treatment.

Pityriasis Rosea

Pityriasis rosea is a mild inflammatory exanthem of unknown cause. The available evidence suggests a viral etiology. Pityriasis rosea affects all age groups but occurs most commonly in patients 10 to 35 years old. It tends to occur in spring and fall but not in epidemics. Pityriasis rosea is not contagious. A pityriasis rosea–like eruption has been associated with some drugs and viruses. Occasionally there are prodromal symptoms including malaise, headache, sore throat, fatigue, and arthralgia.

The rash of pityriasis rosea evolves over a period of several weeks. It begins with a "herald patch," a solitary, erythematous lesion with a raised edematous border most frequently occurring on the chest or back. It is 2 to 6 cm in diameter. About 1 or 2 weeks later, there is a widespread, symmetrical eruption of pink- or salmon-colored maculopapular lesions. The patches are oval to circinate and are covered with dry epidermis which desquamates to form a collarette of scale at the periphery. The lesions are 0.5 to 1.5 cm in diameter and are at first discrete, but can become confluent. The long axes of the patches frequently run parallel to lines of skin tension, giving rise to the Christmas tree pattern seen on the back. The eruption is generalized and chiefly affects the trunk, although it can occur anywhere. The lesions can be localized. Mucous membranes can be involved with plaques, hemorrhagic punctate spots, or ulcers. Successive crops of skin lesions can occur, and the entire illness can last 3 to 8 weeks. Healing is complete, without sequelae or evidence of organ involvement.

The diagnosis of pityriasis rosea is made by the clinical appearance. It can be confused with viral exanthem, drug eruptions, and seborrheic dermatitis. Potassium hydroxide preparation of skin scrapings will serve to distinguish pityriasis rosea from tinea corporis. A serologic test for syphilis must be done to exclude that diagnosis.

Therapy is directed at alleviating symptoms. No treatment has been shown to shorten the duration of the rash. The rash is sometimes very itchy. Oatmeal baths and oral antihistamines will provide temporary relief. Emollients will help dryness and irritation. Secondary infection must be prevented with thorough cleansing.

Roseola Infantum

Roseola infantum, or exanthem subitum, is a common acute febrile illness of childhood. There appears to be no seasonal preponderance to its occurrence. Roseola has long been considered to be an infectious disease, probably viral in origin. It has been associated with human herpesvirus 6 infection.

Roseola is characterized by a febrile period of 3 to 5 days, defervescence, and the appearance of a rash for 1 to 2 days. Primarily, young children are affected, with most patients being between 6 months and 3 years. The illness beings abruptly with high fever, sometimes as high as 40.6°C. The child is usually alert and active but may be irritable, especially with very high fever. Associated symptoms are usually mild and may include cough, coryza, anorexia, and abdominal discomfort. Lymphadenopathy may be present. Febrile convulsions may occur. The fever persists for 3 to 5 days, and most often returns to normal by crisis. The child rapidly becomes well.

The exanthem in roseola usually coincides with defervescence of the fever, but it may follow a short afebrile interlude. The rash is an erythematous macular or maculopapular eruption that consists of discrete, rose or pale-pink lesions 2 to 5 mm in size. It is most prominent on the neck, trunk, and buttocks, but the face and proximal extremities may also be involved. The lesions blanch with pressure. There is no mucous membrane involvement. The rash lasts 1 to 2 days but may fade rapidly, usually without desquamation.

There is no specific treatment for roseola. Acetaminophen is useful for fever control and convulsions should be treated vigorously. Recovery is usually complete.

BIBLIOGRAPHY

Anderson MJ, Lewis E, Kidd IM, et al: An outbreak of erythema infectiosum associated with human parvovirus infection. J Hyg, 93:85093, 1984.

Burnett JW, Crutcher WA: Vial and rickittsial infections, in Moschella SL, Hurley HJ(eds): *Dermatology*. Philadelphia, Saunders, 1985.

Cherry JD, Hurwitz ES, Williver RC: *Mycoplasma pneumonia* infections and exanthems. *J Pediatr* 87:3, 1975.

Cherry JD: Mycoplasma and ureaplasma infections, in Feigin RD, Cherry JD (eds): *Textbook of Pediatric Infectious Diseases*. Philadelphia, Saunders, 1987.

Corkey RJ et al: Diagnosis and treatment of impetigo. *J Am Acad Dermatol* 17:62, 1987.

Hurwitz S: Kawasaki disease, in Hurwitz S (ed): *Clinical Pediatric Dermatology: A Textbook of Skin Disorders of Childhood and Adolescence*. Philadelphia, Saunders, 1981, pp. 397–401.

Melish ME, Hlsdhoe LD: The staphylococcal scalded skin syndrome. *N Engl J Med* 282:1114, 1970.

Miller GD, Tindall JP: Hand, foot, and mouth disease. *JAMA* 203:827, 1968.

Nihill MR, Feign RD, Gruber R, Morens D: Kawasaki disease in Feigin RD and Cherry JD (eds): *Pediatric Infectious Disease*, 2d ed. Philadelphia, Saunders, 1987.

Odom RB, Olson E6: Mucocutaneous lymph node syndrome. *Arch Dermatol* 113:339, 1977.

Parrono JM: Pityriasis rosea update. *J Am Acad Dermatol* 15:159, 1986.

Teisch JA, Shapiro L, Walzer RA: Vesiculopustular eruption and *Mycoplasma* infection. *JAMA* 211:10, 1970.

Urbach AH, McGregor RS, Malatack JJ, et al: Kawasaki disease and perineal rash. *Am J Dis Child* 142:1174, 1988.

Yamanishi K, Okuno T, Shiraki K et al: Identification of human herpesvirus-6 as a casual agent for exanthem subitum. *Lancet* 11:1065, 1988.

80
PEDIATRIC ANALGESIA AND SEDATION

Roy M. Kulick
Elaine S. Pomeranz

Analgesia and sedation for children in the emergency department is fraught with misconceptions and controversy. Although some of the discussion and guidelines that follow are extrapolated from studies done either in a preoperative setting or in adults, there is growing interest and investigation in the area of analgesia and sedation for acutely sick and injured children.

It is crucial to distinguish between analgesics and sedatives. Although decreasing anxiety with sedatives may increase the pain threshold to some extent, no amount of sedation will allow a child to comfortably undergo a painful procedure. On the other hand, analgesics are not ideal for sedation. In reality, the emergency setting frequently calls for both.

The underuse of analgesics and sedatives has been well documented. There are several reasons for this underuse. The expression of pain in infants and young children is nonspecific and easily overlooked. Children are often perceived as being fragile and more vulnerable than adults to the respiratory depressant effects of many of these agents. Yet pharmacokinetic studies show that infants and young children are actually more tolerant of some of these medications. Nevertheless, the risk of respiratory depression must be anticipated when using systemic agents. To complicate matters, there is an approximately 15-percent failure rate with any of these agents, and the risk of untoward side effects increases with the dose and the number of different agents used. In addition, many drugs can occasionally cause paradoxical excitement instead of the desired effect. However, when used correctly and with adequate monitoring, these agents can be safely utilized to make the emergency department encounter more humane for the child, parent, and physician.

ASSESSMENT OF PAIN IN CHILDREN

The presence or absence of pain in infants must be inferred from physiologic and behavioral responses. Physiologic responses include increases in heart rate, blood pressure, and respiratory rate. Behavioral clues include facial expression, cry, posture, and vocalization.

Preschool children understand and can begin to describe their experience of pain. Creative self-report scales have recently been developed to help young children indicate their degree of pain. These scales include, for example, line drawings of faces or a photographic scale of facial expressions (''Oucher!''). The child selects the facial expression on the analogue scale that best represents the intensity of pain. Physiologic and behavioral parameters remain important in this age group.

Older children and adolescents are better able to directly express their perception of pain intensity, although self-report scales such as the Linear Analogue Scale may still be useful.

NONPHARMACOLOGIC APPROACHES

The emergency department is a frightening place for any sick or injured child, particularly for those in pain. The child's level of anxiety and discomfort can greatly influence the ability to perform an adequate physical examination or successfully complete a procedure. There are several simple, easily applied nonpharmacologic interventions that can decrease patients' anxiety and even alter their perception of pain. However, few children will be completely anesthetized by purely behavioral techniques for a truly painful procedure. These techniques should be considered an adjunct to the appropriate use of analgesics and sedatives.

It is a challenge to establish rapport and earn a child's trust in the short time generally available in an emergency department encounter. One must take a developmentally appropriate approach to communicating with a child, considering issues such as language development, pain, separation, body image, fear of death, and autonomy. A gentle, unhurried approach is helpful. Preparation for a procedure should always include an honest, clear explanation of what is to be expected and an opportunity for questions to be addressed. To the extent that it is practical in the emergency setting, the child may be allowed to handle the equipment and practice the procedure on a doll. If, however, there is no time for this more extensive preparation, it is probably best to minimize the time the child must anticipate a painful procedure by saving the explanation until just prior to its execution.

Environmental alterations such as dimmed lights, a quiet room, or stereo headphones may relieve anxiety. Specific relaxation techniques such as deep breathing exercises may be beneficial. Some children may respond to distractions such as storytelling or singing. Another technique that takes advantage of a child's unique ability to daydream or pretend is guided imagery. During guided imagery, children as young as 3 to 4 years old are encouraged to imagine they are in a favorite place or participating in their favorite activity and to describe their fantasies in great detail.

Hypnosis combines distraction, imagery, and progressive muscle relaxation. It has been used successfully to treat pain in children in many different settings, including the emergency department. Formal application requires trained personnel and often some practice on the part of the patient.

To complete a procedure safely and efficiently, many children will require restraint despite all of the above efforts as well as the addition of sedation and analgesia. Manual restraint may be sufficient for quick, simple procedures such as venipuncture. Sheets or ''papoose'' boards are more appropriate for longer procedures and are usually well tolerated after an initial protest. Parents should be relieved of the responsibility of restraining a child and allowed instead to provide comfort.

LOCAL ANALGESIA

Infiltrative

With any local anesthetic, it is important to remember to infiltrate slowly, with frequent aspiration to avoid injecting into an artery. Slower infiltration and small needles also decrease the pain of infiltration. Jet injection devices are useful in minimizing the pain of injection for such procedures as lumbar puncture.

Lidocaine

Although lidocaine is the local anesthetic most frequently used in the emergency department setting, it is often argued that the pain upon infiltrating the skin with this drug is worse than the pain of ''one quick stick'' for obtaining cerebrospinal fluid or an arterial sample. The truth of this belief is debatable, as is the myth in pediatrics of ''one quick stick.''

Neutralizing lidocaine's acidity by adding 8.4 % sodium bicarbonate greatly diminishes the pain of infiltration. This can be accomplished by adding sodium bicarbonate to lidocaine in a ratio of 1:10. This should be done just prior to use, as it reduces the shelf life.

Lidocaine is available in 1 or 2% solutions with or without epinephrine. Epinephrine's vasoconstricting effect makes it a helpful addition when bleeding would otherwise obscure the field and prolongs the half-life of the lidocaine by slowing absorption. However, preparations containing epinephrine should not be used on a distal extremity, nose, penis, or pinna of the ear.

The maximum recommended dose of lidocaine is 5 mg/kg for preparations without epinephrine and 7 mg/kg for preparations with epinephrine.

Bupivicaine

Bupivicaine is four times as potent as lidocaine and has a duration of action of up to 7 h. Although it is frequently used for both children and adults in the postoperative setting, its use in children has not been well studied. Commercial preparations of bupivicaine are even more acidic than lidocaine, but they too can be buffered with sodium bicarbonate. They are available in 0.25 and 0.5% solutions with and without epinephrine. The maximum recommended dose is 2 to 3 mg/kg with or without epinephrine.

Topical

TAC

TAC is a topical anesthetic that has gained increasing acceptance for children with superficial dermal lacerations. but its use remains controversial. Although the original formulation arbitrarily consisted of tetracaine 0.5%, adrenaline 1:2000, and cocaine 11.8%, one-half strength TAC appears to be equally effective and presumably has a wider margin of safety.

TAC has been shown to provide anesthesia equivalent to infiltrated lidocaine for superficial lacerations on the face and scalp and has several advantages. The application of TAC is painless and therefore decreases psychic trauma and encourages trust and cooperation. In addition, there is no distortion of the wound margins. However, TAC is not as effective on less vascular areas, such as the extremities, where supplemental infiltrated lidocaine is often required. Since the epinephrine component causes vasoconstriction, the same restrictions for lidocaine with epinephrine apply to the use of TAC.

Although rare, the potential adverse effects associated with the misuse of TAC include disorientation, hallucinations, seizures, and death, which are related to the excess systemic absorption of cocaine and tetracaine. These events have been associated with the inappropriate application of TAC on the mucous membranes of the eyes, nose, and mouth or the use of repeated applications. TAC should therefore never be used on or near a mucosal surface. Similarly, the inadvertent dripping of TAC onto a mucosal surface must be prevented. Its use on burns, abraded areas, or a child with a history of seizures or cardiac arrhythmias should also be avoided.

The maximal allowable dose of TAC has not been determined. However, 3 mL of one-half strength TAC appears to be safe and provides adequate anesthesia for the great majority of wounds. Supplemental lidocaine can generally be comfortably infiltrated into those wounds not adequately anesthetized for suturing. The use of repeated applications of TAC is strongly discouraged. Adherence to these precautions will ensure the safe use of TAC.

TAC may be applied in the following manner:

1. Gently cleanse the wound.
2. Place the wound in a gravity-dependent position, instill TAC into the wound cavity, and allow to stand for 3 min.
3. Saturate a 2 × 2 gauze pad, cotton ball, or swab with additional TAC and hold or tape in place over the wound for 10 to 15 min prior to irrigation and suturing. The child's caretaker should apply gentle pressure to promote the even distribution of TAC throughout the wound cavity and margins.

Regional Nerve Blocks

Regional nerve blocks are described in Chap. 189 and are appropriate for children as long as the physician adheres to the recommendations for the maximum allowable doses for the local anesthetics.

SYSTEMIC ANALGESIA

"The American Academy of Pediatrics defines conscious sedation as a minimally depressed level of consciousness that retains a patient's ability to maintain a patent airway . . . and respond appropriately to physical stimulation and/or verbal commands." Conscious sedation is distinguished from deep sedation and general anesthesia, for which separate guidelines for patient monitoring are suggested. However, the difference between conscious and deep sedation is sometimes only a matter of quantity rather than quality of drug and of individual variations in response.

Whenever a systemic analgesic or sedative is used, it is ideal to have the patient continuously monitored and under the constant observation of a physician or nurse trained in airway management. A busy emergency department offers the advantage of having such personnel and airway equipment nearby at all times but rarely has the staffing capability to allow the physician or nurse to remain at the bedside constantly. Since the major risk of these agents is respiratory depression, a more practical approach would be to have such a skilled individual at the bedside whenever possible and to have the patient monitored continuously with at least a pulse oximeter. Oxygen, suction equipment, oral airways, bag and mask, and intubation equipment should be readily accessible. When narcotics are used, it is wise to have the appropriate naloxone dose (5 to 10 μg/kg per kilogram) precalculated and available.

When choosing a pharmacologic agent for a pediatric patient, important considerations include the nature of the procedure (painful or nonpainful), the desired onset and duration of action, and the route of administration most appropriate for the clinical situation. Therefore, the following discussion of individual agents is structured according to the nature and duration of the planned procedure (see Table 80-1).

Suggested initial and supplemental dosages, routes of administration, timing of onset, duration of action, and risks are summarized in Table 80-2.

Analgesia for Brief, Painful Procedures

Fentanyl

The synthetic narcotic fentanyl is well suited for use in the emergency department. It is 100 times more potent than morphine and has an almost immediate onset and a brief duration of action (approximately 30 min) when administered intravenously. Respiratory depression can be minimized by administering it slowly over 3 to 5 min. Because it

Table 80-1. Suggested Strategy for Analgesia and Sedation in Children

Analgesia for brief, painful procedures (30–45 min)
Fentanyl (Sublimize) IV*
Nitrous oxide inhalation
Ketamine IV, IM†
Analgesia for painful procedures (1 h or longer)
Morphine IV§
Meperidine (Demerol) PO, IV, IM§
"DPT cocktail"
Sedation for brief nonpainful procedures (30–45 min)
Midazolam (Versed) PO, PR, intranasally, IV, IM
Methohexital (Brevital) PR, IM
Sedation for nonpainful procedures (1 h or longer)
Diazepam (Valium) PO, IV
Pentobarbital (Nembutal) IV, IM
Chloral hydrate PO, PR

* May be supplemented with midazolam for synergistic sedative/analgesic effect.

† Ketamine has both sedative and analgesic properties.

§ May be supplemental with hydroxyzine for synergistic sedative/analgesic effect.

Table 80-2. Guidelines for Usage of Analgesics and Sedatives in Children

	Initial Dose	Onset	Effective Duration	Supplemental/ Maximum Dose	Precautions/ Comments
Analgesics					
Pentanyl	2–3 μg/kg IV	2 min	30 min	Titrate to effect in 0.5 μg/kg increments	Respiratory depression (especially with rapid IV push); bradycardia; muscle rigidity; have naloxone available
Nitrous oxide	30–50% mixture with O_2	1–2 min	———	———	Fail-safe system to avoid hypoxia; scavenger system; contraindications: previous sedative, altered mental status, dyspnea, pneumothorax, eye injury, obstructed viscus
Ketamine	1.0 mg/kg IV 4.0 mg/kg IM	Rapid IV 3–5 min	10 min 20 min	Titrate IV dose to effect; 2 mg/kg IM supplementation	Laryngospasm; hypertension (not recommended for closed head injury patients); hypersalivation (can be controlled with atropine 0.01 mg/kg); hallucinations (can be avoided with midazolam or diazepam)
Morphine	0.1 mg/kg IV	5–10 min	3–4 h	0.05 mg/kg supplementation, titrate to effect	Respiratory depression (especially with rapid IV push); hypotension; have naloxone available
Meperidine	1.0 mg/kg IV, IM 1–2 mg/kg PO	Rapid IV 10–15 min IM 15–30 min PO	2–3 h	0.5 mg/kg supplementation; maximum 100 mg IV, IM; maximum 150 mg PO	Precautions as with other narcotics above; can be combined with hydroxyzine, 0.5 mg/kg IM or PO; have naloxone available
Sedatives					
Midazolam	0.15 mg/kg IV, IM 0.2–0.3 mg/kg PR, intranasally 0.5 mg/kg PO	2 min IV 10–15 min IM, PR, intransally, or PO	30 min IV 45 min IM, PR, intransally, or PO	Titrate IV dose to effect in 0.02-mg/kg increments; 0.1 mg/kg IM supplementation; 12 mg/kg maximum dose PO	Respiratory depression, apnea, hypotension (especially when combined with fentanyl); anterograde amnesia for 1–2 h
Methohexital	20 mg/kg PR	15 min PR	20 min	Maximum PR dose 25 mg/kg	Adverse effects similar to those of pentobarbital
Diazepam	0.1 mg/kg IV 0.2 mg/kg PO, PR	Rapid IV 30–60 min PO, PR	1–2 h	Maximum IV dose 0.6 mg/kg over 8 h; maximum PO dose 10 mg over 6–8 h	Adverse effects similar to those of midazolam
Pentobarbital	4–5 mg/kg IV, IM	Rapid IV 15 min IM	30 min IV 2 h IM	1 mg/kg slow IV push supplementation, titrate to effect; 100–200 maximum IM dose	Hiccups, respiratory depression, apnea, hypotension, cardiac depression
Chloral hydrate	75 mg/kg PO, PR	30 min	3–4 h	2 g maximum dose	GI irritation, cardiac arrhythmias (rare), increased hyperbilirubinemia in premature infants

is so concentrated, care should be taken not to flush any small amount that might be left over in heparin lock tubing, since this could represent a significant overdose in a small child. Fentanyl was used safely and successfully in a series of 2000 children undergoing facial laceration repairs in the emergency department with the use of a pulse oximeter as a monitor for respiratory depression.

Pharmacokinetic studies suggest that fentanyl may be less likely than morphine to cause respiratory depression in young infants.

Nitrous Oxide

Although nitrous oxide has been used in emergency departments for over 20 years, experience with children in this setting is somewhat limited. Delivered as a 30 to 50% mixture with oxygen, it is an effective analgesic and induces a state of conscious sedation with feelings of euphoria and dissociation. Nitrous oxide is used alone or, more commonly, as an adjunct to local anesthesia for orthopedic procedures, lacerations, burns, and abrasions.

Nitrous oxide must be administered through a system that has a fail-safe against delivery of a hypoxic mixture. It is generally recommended that a self-administered demand valve system be used such that the patient must deliberately inhale through a mask or mouthpiece to receive the analgesic mixture. When oversedated, the mask or mouthpiece falls and the patient breathes room air, leading to rapid arousal. The system should also include an oxygen analyzer and a scavenger device. The patient should be continuously monitored with a pulse oximeter and by maintaining verbal communication.

The advantages of nitrous oxide include its rapid uptake and excretion. Peak effects are reached in 1 to 2 min, and the patient is fully aroused within minutes after cessation of delivery. It has minimal respiratory or cardiovascular effects when administered in the 30 to 50% range.

A limitation to the use of nitrous oxide is that young children often have difficulty accepting or understanding the self-administered system, making it more practical for school-aged patients. Risk of aspiration is minimal. Use of nitrous oxide in the emergency setting also requires specially designed equipment and appropriately trained personnel.

Nitrous oxide is contraindicated for children who have recently received another sedative and those with an altered mental status, dyspnea, pneumothorax, eye injuries, or suspicion of an obstructed viscus.

Ketamine

Ketamine is considered a dissociative analgesic that also has sedative properties. Although ansthesiologists have much experience with ketamine, it has only recently become popular for children in the emergency department. It can be administered by a variety of routes, including orally. Although airway reflexes are usually protected, ketamine can cause laryngospasm. Atropine is often used as an adjunct to control associated hypersalivation, and the addition of midazolam is helpful in older children, who may otherwise be prone to unpleasant hallucinations. Since ketamine raises blood pressure and intracranial pressure, it should not be used under circumstances in which this is a concern (e.g., head trauma). Moreover, it may be unsatisfactory for CT scanning due to random movements that can occur despite full sedation.

Analgesia for Longer, Painful Procedures

Morphine

Morphine is still the gold standard. There is substantial experience using it, and it is easily reversed with naloxone. Unfortunately, its bioavailability is poor in oral form. Infants less than 3 months of age may be particularly susceptible to its respiratory depressant effects.

Opioids in general have analgesic effects at lower doses than those required for sedation. If both effects are desired, it is wise to combine fentanyl with midazolam (see below) or morphine or meperidine with hydroxyzine. In fact, hydroxyzine (0.5 mg/kg orally or intramuscularly) appears to have significant analgesic effects on its own and is clearly synergistic with narcotics.

"DPT Cocktail" (Meperidine, Promethazine, and Chlorpromazine)

This combination of drugs is extremely popular and was the most commonly cited "sedative" in a recent survey of pediatric emergency departments. The reason for this may be that it has been available for a long time and that familiarity with it has led to the false belief that it is completely safe. However, it was developed for inpatient cardiac catheterization and has several drawbacks that, in the opinion of these authors, make it less suitable for use in the emergency department. The most serious problem is the risk of respiratory depression, which was as high as 13 percent in one series. The rationale behind this combination has been questioned. Moreover, DPT can only be given intramuscularly, and the majority of patients sleep for more than 7 h.

Adding to the confusion surrounding the use of DPT is the wide range of doses used, with meperidine ranging from 1.0 to 3.0 mg/kg and promethazine and chlorpromazine ranging from 0.06 to 1.0 mg/kg in a recent survey. The most common combination seems to be 2 mg/kg of meperidine and 1 mg/kg each of promethazine and chlorpromazine.

Meperidine

Meperidine is a synthetic derivative of morphine that is about one-tenth as potent an analgesic when used alone and has a briefer duration of action. It is less effective in its oral form than when given parenterally, but the difference between the two routes is less than with morphine. As with other narcotics, nausea and vomiting are possible side effects, although the addition of hydroxyzine as described above decreases the frequency. Meperidine appears less likely to cause respiratory depression in neonates than does morphine.

Nonsteroidal Anti-inflammatory Drugs (NSAIDs)

Ibuprofen and naprosyn are generally used for less severe pain than are narcotics. However, a more potent formulation, ketorolac, has recently become available. It shows promise as a relatively safe analgesic that is purported to rival narcotics but has a longer duration of action. It can be given orally, intravenously, or intramuscularly. Although data are not yet available regarding use in children, most common adverse effects appear to be gastrointestinal irritation and other problems typical of NSAIDs.

SEDATION

For Brief, Nonpainful Procedures

Midazolam

Midazolam is a drug well suited for use in pediatric outpatients. It is a short-acting benzodiazepine that offers great versatility in routes of administration. Although it is only supplied in vials for intravenous use, it has been given successfully via oral, rectal, intramuscular, subcutaneous, and intranasal routes.

Midazolam is a potent sedative and has a duration of action of 30 to 40 min. As with the narcotics, the oral dose needed for effects equivalent to the intravenous route is much higher. Regardless of the route chosen, children require higher doses than do adults. Children given midazolam are generally awake but drowsy and disinhibited. Therefore, it is useful in rendering children cooperative for such procedures as suspected sexual abuse examinations or as a prelude to administering local anesthesia for suturing, lumbar puncture, bone marrow aspiration, and the like. Midazolam is also an excellent amnestic agent and makes, for instance, the return visit for suture removal easier. It is less suitable for procedures such as CT scanning, which requires the patient to lie motionless.

Flumazenil is a benzodiazepine antagonist that has been used effectively in Europe as a reversal agent in much the same way that naloxone is used for narcotic overdoses. It will soon be available in the United States, which should allow practitioners to feel more comfortable using benzodiazepines.

Methohexital

Methohexital is frequently given per rectum to children under the age of 5 prior to general anesthesia. Experience using it in the pediatric emergency department is more limited, but it does have properties that make it an attractive choice in this setting. It takes effect in 10 to 15 min and can be given without an injection. Its intramuscular use has been reported but is felt by some to be unduly painful. It is available in a variety of concentrations, but the more concentrated solutions are suggested for intramuscular and parenteral routes.

For Longer, Nonpainful Procedures

Diazepam

Diazepam has been widely used in children as an effective anxiolytic, amnestic, and anticonvulsant agent. It has not been specifically studied as a sedative for emergency department procedures.

Pentobarbital

Pentobarbital is a longer-acting barbiturate that has been used to sedate children in the emergency department. However, it was administered intravenously in the only published report of its use in pediatric outpatients, which is a distinct disadvantage for those children who do not require an intravenous line for other purposes. There are anecdotal reports of its safety and efficacy when administered intramuscularly, but our experience with this route is limited.

Chloral Hydrate

Chloral hydrate has been used for a century. There is much experience using it both orally and rectally, and it is unlikely to cause respiratory depression. It can cause gastric or mucosal irritation. Reported success rates range from 70 to 85 percent with a wide range of doses (30 to 80 mg/kg). The disadvantages of its use in the emergency department include its relatively slow onset of action (30 to 60 min) and its prolonged sedative effect (up to several hours).

BIBLIOGRAPHY

Beyer JE, Wells N: The assessment of pain in children. *Pediatr Clin North Am* 36:837, 1989.

Billmire DA, Neale HW, Gregory RO: Use of IV fentanyl in the outpatient treatment of pediatric facial trauma. *J Trauma* 25:1079, 1985.

Bonadio WA: TAC: A review. *Pediatr Emerg Care* 5:128, 1989.

Bonadio WA, Wagner V: Half-strength TAC topical anesthetic. *Clin Pediatr* 27:495, 1988.

Christoph RA, Buchanan L, Begalla K, et al: Pain reduction in local anesthetic administration through pH buffering. *Ann Emerg Med* 17:117, 1988.

Committee on Drugs, Section on Anesthesiology: Guidelines for the elective use of conscious sedation, deep sedation, and general anesthesia in pediatric patients. *Pediatrics* 76:317, 1985.

Gamis AS, Knapp JF, Glenski JA: Nitrous oxide analgesia in the pediatric emergency department. *Ann Emerg Med* 18:177, 1989.

Green SM, Nakamura R, Johnson NE: Ketamine sedation for pediatric procedures: I. A prospective series. *Ann Emerg Med* 19:1024, 1990.

Hawk W, Crockett K, Ochsenschlager DW, et al: Conscious sedation for the pediatric patient for suturing: A survey. *Pediatr Emerg Care* 6:84, 1990.

Kohen DP: Applications of relaxation/mental imagery (self-hypnosis) in pediatric emergencies. *Int J Clin Exp Hypn* 34:283, 1986.

Mitchell AA, Louik C, Lacouture P, et al: Risks to children from computed tomographic scan premedication. *JAMA* 247:2385, 1982.

Paris PM: Pain management in the child. *Emerg Med Clin North Am* 5:699, 1987.

Selbst SM, Henretig FM: The treatment of pain in the emergency department. *Pediatr Clin North Am* 36:965, 1989.

SECTION 9
Infectious Diseases

81
SEXUALLY TRANSMITTED DISEASES

David Nolan

Venereal, or sexually transmitted, diseases (STDs), are commonly encountered in nearly all fields of medical practice. Recorded numbers of STDs may be misleading due to underreporting. Former favorable trends in occurrence have reversed, and STDs that had become uncommon are again being found. The picture is worsening in some localities and some population groups. STDs that cause genital ulcers may contribute to the acquisition of AIDS. The issue of concurrent AIDS is addressed in Chapter 82.

It must be remembered that the STDs considered here are only part of the picture. Venereal exposure can facilitate transfer of virtually any disease normally transmitted by skin-to-skin, fecal-oral, or fluid exchange routes. These include hepatitis B, scabies, fungi, parasites, AIDS, and others.

Further, the agents of STDs may infect tissue distant from the portal of entry and present in extremely varied fashion. It is necessary to maintain a high index of suspicion to reduce missed diagnoses not only for the welfare of the patient but also for the patient's contacts. Groups known to represent high risk of STDs (substance abusers, prostitutes, the previously infected) are not the only ones at risk, and history taking for all patients must include sexual habits.

Beyond establishing the diagnosis and starting treatment, several other steps are in order. Cases should be reported to the public health department as required by local regulations. Patients should be encouraged to report contacts to the appropriate facility; educated in how to prevent repeat infections and avoid new STDs; and directed, when appropriate, to return to the hospital or clinic to make sure the cure has been effective. When children are involved, it may also be necessary to report possible abuse.

Because epidemiology and/or resistance patterns change rapidly in given locations, effective communication should be established with local public health authorities. The information exchange should be two-way. Other sources of current information include the Centers for Disease Control publications *Morbidity and Mortality Weekly Report*, *Medical Letter*, and *Infectious Disease Newsletter*.

GONORRHEA (GC)

Historically the most common STD, GC usually presents in males as a purulent urethral discharge associated with dysuria. Symptoms in women are similar but more likely to be overlooked. It may be asymptomatic in either sex. Pharyngeal and anal infections, and dissemination with resultant infection of joints, heart, or meninges, may occur in either sex. The latter may be destructive of tissue and life-threatening. Pelvic inflammatory disease (PID) is described in Chapter 55.

Diagnosis is made by smear of discharge or lesion revealing gram-negative intracellular diplococci and culture of *Neisseria gonorrhea*. False-negative smear and culture are common. Repeated cultures including anal and pharyngeal specimens may be needed. Treatment should be started based upon adequate suspicion or history of exposure.

The disease is usually acquired by genital contact with an infected person, but contamination of fingers or fomites can transmit it to another body site (e.g., eyes) of the same or another person. Sexual practices may result in infections of the pharynx or anus. GC can be acquired at birth in the vaginal canal.

The incubation period is a few days to about a week. The communicable period varies, possibly being very prolonged. The communicability ceases with appropriate treatment. It may be self-limiting.

Treatment choices must be influenced by likelihood of resistance to commonly used drugs and the probability of concurrent and undiagnosed chlamydia and/or syphilis.

Present treatment calls for ceftriaxone, 250 mg as a single IM dose. Doxycycline, 100 mg orally bid for 7 days, should be given concurrently for *Chlamydia,* which is present in about half of cases but is often difficult to detect. This should also suffice for incubating syphilis.

If the patient is unable to take ceftriaxone, spectinomycin, 2 g as a single IM dose, should be given, with doxycycline for *Chlamydia,* as above. Syphiliis is not treated by this regimen. If appropriate, treat it as noted below.

For children, drugs must be adjusted for age and weight.

SYPHILIS

Syphilis, although most often transmitted by genital contact, can be acquired congenitally and by blood transfusion (if the donor was in a very early stage of the disease and the blood was transfused fresh). Modern handling of blood and serologic screening of donors protects the U.S. blood supply from this risk.

The infectious agent *Treponema pallidum* is a spirochete. It may be found in lesions, infected mucous membranes, saliva, semen, and blood. It is thought to be able to enter through defects of skin or mucous membranes, even those too small to be easily noted.

The disease occurs in recognizable phases, all requiring treatment:

Primary. Occurs with or without an ulcerated, usually genital, lesion approximately 3 weeks after exposure.

Secondary. Occurs with constitutional signs and symptoms, and skin eruptions, within weeks to months.

Tertiary. Involves cardiovascular and/or neurological system(s) years after original infection.

Diagnosis in early phases may be made by examination of material from lesions by dark-field or phase contrast microscopy. Serologic studies may reveal evidence of prior exposure without indicating the time since first infection. Biologic false positives occur. The decision to treat may be made in seropositive cases if prior effective treatment is not known to have been administered.

Treatment of known or suspected cases of primary disease through the first year of infection is as follows:

1. For those who can tolerate penicillin, benzathine penicillin G, 2.4 million units IM as a single dose.
2. If unable to use penicillin, tetracycline HCl 500 mg qid orally for 15 days *or* erythromycin 500 mg qid orally for 15 days

Initiation of treatment for later stages of the disease is not urgent, and appropriate studies, including cerebrospinal fluid examination, should be undertaken.

CHLAMYDIA INFECTIONS

The incidence and scope of *Chlamydia* infections have increased in recent years. It mimics or coexists with GC, and patients may present with PID or perihepatitis. The frequency of concurrence and difficulty of culture have led to recommendations to treat for *Chlamydia* in all cases of GC. *Chlamydia* infection may also present as lymphogranuloma venereum with skin lesions and lymphadenopathy.

The usually painless skin lesions associative with *Chlamydia* infections may wax and wane, taking the form of shallow ulcerations, papular or nodular lesions, or herpetiform vesicles. They are noted most often in genital tissues. Lymphadenopathy in the inguinal region follows. These latter lesions may become fluctuant, bind down overlying skin, and develop sinus tracts. In women, sinus formation may be extensive and involve the vagina and rectum. Constitutional signs of chills, fever, headache, and general malaise may be present. Infection of joints and meninges, while uncommon, has been noted. If the infection is untreated, the course may be very long, but death is unusual.

Chlamydia is communicable while active lesions are present. The incubation period is 1 to 3 weeks or longer. The culture and serologic tests currently available may still result in false-negative results.

Treatment is with doxycycline, 100 mg orally bid for 7 days, or tetracycline HCl, 500 mg orally qid for 7 days. For pregnant women, erythromycin base, 500 mg orally qid for 7 days, should be used. Erythromycin estolate should not be used in pregnant women. Incision and drainage of fluctuant lesions may be indicated.

Late complications, including elephantiasis and rectal stricture, do not respond to drug treatment.

CHANCROID

This disease is caused by *Haemophiolus ducreyi* in discharges from ulcerated or suppurating genital or lymphatic tissue. Lesions may heal within weeks but are infectious during that time. The incubation period varies from 3 to 14 days.

Presentation is usually with one or more painful necrotic lesion(s) or suppurating inguinal lymphadenopathy. Lesions can also be located elsewhere, depending upon site of inoculation.

Diagnosis is suspected on basis of clinical presentation. Proof is sought by smear and culture. Histologic characteristics are also regarded as diagnostic.

The treatment of choice is erythromycin, 500 mg orally qid for 7 to 10 days or longer, until lesions are healed. Alternatively, a single dose of ceftriaxone, 250 mg IM, or erythromycin, 500 mg orally qid for 7 days, may be used. Incision and drainage of fluctuant lesions may be indicated. Failure to respond may indicate resistance and call for sensitivity testing.

GRANULOMA INGUINALE

Caused by *Calymmatobacterium granulomatis*, this disease is thought to be an STD; however, sexual partners of infected persons rarely develop the disease. It is uncommon in the United States.

The incubation period may be as long as 3 months.

Presentation depends upon the stage of disease. It begins with small papular, nodular, or vesicular lesions that develop slowly into extensive granulomatous or ulcerative lesions. These are found in the skin and mucous membranes of genital, inguinal, and anal areas. The lesions are generally painless, but, if untreated, extensive destruction of local tissue ensues.

Diagnosis depends upon staining and histologic appearance of granulomatous tissue.

Treatment with tetracycline HCl, 2 g orally daily for 15 days, should result in resolution of the lesions. Streptomycin and chloramphenicol have also been used.

TRICHOMONIASIS

Trichomoniasis is caused by the protozoan *Trichomonas vaginalis*. It is contracted by contact, usually genital, with infected secretions of genital and urinary tracts. It is communicable for the duration of the infection. The incubation period is from 4 to 20 days, usually 1 week. In women, vaginitis and copious, foamy yellow discharge having a foul odor are symptomatic. Diagnosis is made by microscopic identification of the motile parasites on a wet slide. Treatment is with metronidazole, 250 mg orally, tid for 7 days. Other dosage schedules are sometimes used. Metronidazole should not be used in pregnant women.

HERPES PROGENITALIS

This rather common disease is caused by Herpesvirus hominis, type II. It usually presents as recurring genital lesions of typical clustered vesicles, which can be painful. Ulceration and crusting precede healing. In women cervical and vulvar sites are most common; in men, glans and prepuce. Lesions may be seen at any site. Newborns may acquire the virus at birth with devastating results. In women, the initial episode may be associated with a self-limiting meningitis. Herpesvirus hominis type I may also cause lesions in genital tissue.

The virus is usually acquired by sexual contact. With or without visible lesions, the infected individual may be shedding virus and is contagious at such times. The incubation period is 2 to 12 days.

Diagnosis is usually made by clinical findings but can be confirmed by virus culture or other studies depending upon the level of laboratory support available.

Curative treatment is not available, and treatment which may hasten resolution of symptoms does not prevent recurrences. The initial episodes may be treated with acyclovir, 200 mg orally five times a day for 7 to 10 days, or less if clinical improvement occurs. For proctitis the dosage should be doubled. Severe symptoms may require hospital admission for intravenous treatment.

If recurrences are frequent or severe, daily long-term treatment with acyclovir may be undertaken.

GENITAL WARTS

Human papillomavirus are associated with warts which may occur in anal and genital tissue. The condition is contagious and no known treatment eradicates the virus. When symptoms warrant, the lesions are removed using podophyllin or by physical means, such as surgical excision or laser treatment.

BIBLIOGRAPHY

Benenson, AS: *Control of Communicable Diseases in Man: An Official Report of the APHA*, ed 15. American Public Health Association, 1990.

Centers for Disease Control: *MMWR* 38:6, 1989.

Year Book of Infectious Diseases: Chicago, Yearbook, 1990.

82
HIV INFECTION AND AIDS

Catherine A. Marco

INTRODUCTION

The spectrum of disease caused by human immunodeficiency virus (HIV) infection is commonly encountered in the practice of emergency medicine. Its presentation may vary from asymptomatic HIV infection in a patient who has an unrelated complaint to life-threatening complications of AIDS. The acquired immunodeficiency syndrome (AIDS) has been recognized since 1981, when several cases of *Pneumocystis carinii* pneumonia (PCP) and Kaposi's sarcoma were described. AIDS was initially defined by the Centers for Disease Control in 1982. Since that time, recognition of the disease has improved as modes of transmission and identification of risk factors have been studied and as serologic testing has become readily available. The Centers for Disease Control published an updated definition of AIDS for surveillance purposes in 1987. The diagnosis of AIDS is most commonly made with laboratory evidence of HIV infection and the presence of one or more indicator diseases. Table 82-1 lists some of the conditions that, together with laboratory results, are diagnostic of AIDS.

The number of patients infected with HIV is growing dramatically worldwide. Actual seroprevalence is not known, as HIV seropositivity is currently not a reportable disease. As of May 1991, over 174,000 cases of AIDS had been reported in the United States. Reported cases are thought to greatly underestimate the number of actual cases. In the United States alone, 800,000 to 1.2 million people are thought to be infected with the HIV virus. Reports of the rate of HIV infection in inner-city emergency department patients range from 4.2 to 8.9 percent. The majority of these patients have unrecognized HIV infection. Studies in suburban hospitals have shown significantly lower rates. Risk factors which are commonly associated with HIV infection include homosexuality or bisexuality, intravenous drug use, heterosexual exposure, blood recipients prior to 1985, and maternal-neonatal transmission.

Infection with HIV may be diagnosed by several methods: detection of antibodies to HIV, detection of viral-specific antigens, isolation of the virus by culture, and assays for HIV nucleic acid. At this time, because of difficulties in assuring confidentiality and providing adequate counseling, HIV testing is rarely indiçated in the emergency department. However, recognition of risk factors and referral for counseling and testing may be appropriately initiated in the emergency department.

Table 82-1. AIDS Defining Conditions

Esophageal candidiasis
Cryptococcosis
Cryptosporidiosis
Cytomegalovirus retinitis
Herpes simplex virus
Kaposi's sarcoma
Brain lymphoma
Mycobacterium avium complex
P. carinii pneumonia
Progressive multifocal leukoencephalopathy
Brain toxoplasmosis
HIV encephalopathy
HIV wasting syndrome
Disseminated histoplasmosis
Isosporiasis
Disseminated *M. tuberculosis* disease
Recurrent *Salmonella* septicemia

PATHOPHYSIOLOGY

The human immunodeficiency virus is a cytopathic retrovirus which kills infected cells. It appears to selectively attack cells involved in immune function, primarily T4 helper cells. The viral genes are carried as single-stranded RNA within the viral particle. Within the host cell, the RNA template is reverse-transcribed into DNA, which becomes permanently integrated into the host's DNA. As a result of infection, immunologic abnormalities ensue, including lymphopenia, qualitative T4 lymphocytic function defect, autoimmune phenomena, and circulating immune complexes. The profound defect in cellular immunity is typically manifest as a variety of opportunistic infections and neoplasms.

Transmission of HIV has been shown to occur via semen, vaginal secretions, blood or blood products, and by transplacental transmission in utero. HIV has also been isolated from saliva, urine, cerebrospinal fluid, brain, tears, breast milk, alveolar fluid, synovial fluid, and amniotic fluid. Transmission has not been documented by casual contact. The HIV is a very labile virus and is easily neutralized by heat or common disinfecting agents, such as Lysol, a 1:10 solution of household bleach, 0.3% hydrogen peroxide, 35% isopropyl alcohol, or 50% ethanol.

Progression of disease after infection varies among individuals. Antibodies may be detected within several weeks to months after exposure. A study of homosexual males showed that 5 to 10 percent of patients will develop symptoms within 3 years of seroconversion. Predictors of high rates of progression include high serum B2-microglobulin level, low T4 count, presence of p24 antigen, and hematocrit less than 40. The mean incubation time from the time of exposure to the development of AIDS is estimated at 8.23 years for adults and 1.97 years for children under age 5. The average survival time following a diagnosis of AIDS is approximately 9 months, although newer treatments under evaluation may alter this prognosis.

CLINICAL PRESENTATIONS AND MANAGEMENT

The spectrum of disease caused by HIV infection varies greatly. Many patients with asymptomatic HIV infection may be encountered for complaints unrelated to HIV disease. Other patients may be seen with involvement of virtually any organ system, commonly with more than one concurrent problem. Because of the complexity of HIV infection, and related opportunistic infection or malignancy, many specific diagnoses cannot be made in the emergency department. Diagnostic and therapeutic maneuvers are directed toward recognition of organ system involvement, assessment of the severity of disease, and, when appropriate, institution of specific therapy. Table 82-2 lists some of the common causative conditions of organ system involvement in HIV-infected patients. Table 82-3 contains a summary of common infections and current recommendations for therapy.

Systemic Symptoms

HIV infection has been increasingly recognized as a spectrum of disease rather than a series of discrete disease phases. As a result, the term ARC (AIDS-related complex), which was once commonly used to describe early symptoms of HIV infection such as lymphadenopathy, fever, malaise, weight loss, and fatigue, is less often found in the literature.

Within a few weeks of infection with HIV, a period of malaise, fever, arthralgias, myalgias, lymphadenopathy, and weight loss may occur, followed by a long asymptomatic period. Once the first symptoms appear, others may occur at any time. In such cases, systemic infection and malignancy must be ruled out. In addition to a complete history and physical examination, appropriate laboratory investigation may include electrolytes, complete blood count, blood cultures (aerobic, anaerobic, and fungal), urinalysis and culture, liver function tests, chest radiograph, serologic testing for syphilis, and blood tests for cryptococcal antigen and *Toxoplasma* and *Coccidioides* serologies.

Table 82-2. Common Conditions Causing Organ System Involvement in AIDS Patients

	Systemic	Pulmonary	GI	Neurologic
BACTERIA				
Staphylococcus aureus	X	X		
Streptococcus pneumoniae	X	X		
Clostridium perfringens	X			
Hemophilus influenzae	X	X		
Shigella species	X		X	
Salmonella species	X		X	
Listeria monocytogenes	X			
Treponema pallidum	X			X
Neisseria gonorrhea			X	
Campylobacter jejuni			X	
Nocardia asteroides	X	X		
Chlamydia species	X		X	
Legionella species	X	X		
M. avium complex	X	X		
M. tuberculosis	X	X		
Anaerobic species	X			
VIRUSES				
Human immunodeficiency virus	X		X	X
Hepatitis viruses	X			
Epstein-Barr virus	X			
Herpes simplex virus	X	X	X	X
Cytomegalovirus	X	X	X	X
Herpes zoster virus	X			X
Adenoviruses	X	X	X	
FUNGI				
Aspergillus species	X			
Histoplasma capsulatum	X	X		
Cryptococcus neoformans	X	X		X
Coccidioides	X	X		
Candida species	X	X	X	
PROTOZOA				
Cryptosporidium species	X		X	
Toxoplasma gondii	X	X		X
Pneumocystis carinii	X	X		
Isospora species	X		X	
Entamoeba species	X		X	
Giardia lamblia			X	
Strongyloides			X	
MALIGNANCY				
Kaposi's sarcoma	X	X	X	
Lymphoma	X	X	X	X
Hodgkin's disease	X			

Lumbar puncture may also be considered if no source of fever is identified.

Although fever may indicate any of a variety of infections, including bacterial, fungal, viral, and protozoal pathogens, the most common etiologies of fever include HIV-related fever, systemic infections such as *Mycobacterium avium-intracellulare* (MAI), cytomegalovirus (CMV), Hodgkin's disease, and non-Hodgkin's lymphoma.

MAI causes disseminated disease in up to 50 percent of AIDS patients. It is usually associated with weight loss, diarrhea, fever, malaise, and anorexia. It may also cause pulmonary involvement. Anemia and liver function test abnormalities may be seen. Diagnosis may be made by acid-fast stain of stool or other body fluids, or by blood culture. Treatment is often ineffective, especially for disseminated disease, due to wide resistance to isoniazid and rifampin.

CMV also commonly causes disseminated disease in HIV-infected individuals. It is often associated with PCP. It is the most common cause of retinitis in such patients. Gastrointestinal involvement is also common. Although still under investigation, DHPG (ganciclovir), a drug similar to acyclovir, is commonly used in an attempt to combat infection with CMV. It is thought to be especially effective for patients with retinitis and colitis.

Many HIV-infected patients with fever may be managed as outpatients. Outpatient management may be attempted if the source of the fever does not dictate admission, appropriate laboratory studies have been initiated, the patient is able to function adequately at home (e.g., ambulation and sufficient oral intake), and appropriate medical follow-up can be arranged.

Cutaneous Manifestations

Cutaneous manifestations of HIV infection are commonly encountered in the emergency department. Generalized cutaneous complaints such as xerosis (dry skin) and pruritus are common, and may be manifest prior to development of opportunistic infections. Treatment of these conditions is identical to traditional therapy. Xerosis may be treated with emollients, and if necessary, with mild topical steroids. Pruritus may respond to oatmeal baths, and if necessary, antihistamines. Exacerbation of any underlying dermatologic condition is common.

Table 82-3. Treatment Recommendations for Common HIV-Related Infections

Organ System	Infection	Therapy
Systemic	MAI	No known effective therapy
	CMV	Ganciclovir, 7.5–15 mg/kg/d; maintenance therapy required
Pulmonary	*P. carinii*	TMP-SMX, 15–20 mg TMP/kg/d and 75–100 mg SMX/kg/d, PO or IV, for 3 weeks *or* Pentamidine, 4 mg/kg/d, IV or IM, for 3 weeks
	M. tuberculosis	Isoniazid, 5–10 mg/kg/d PO *plus* Rifampin, 9 mg/kg/d *plus* Pyrazinamide, 25 mg/kg/d PO *or* streptomycin, 0.75–1.0 mg/kg/d IM
CNS	Toxoplasmosis	Pyrimethamine, 25–50 mg/d PO *plus* Sulfadiazine, 100 mg/kg/d, for 3–6 months
	Cryptococcosis	Amphotericin B, 0.4–0.6 mg/kg/d; maintenance therapy required
Ophthalmologic	CMV	Ganciclovir, 5 mg/kg/d for 2 weeks; maintenance therapy required
GI	Candidiasis	Clotrimazole, 30–50 mg/d *or* Ketoconazole, 200–400 mg/d; maintenance therapy required
	Salmonellosis	TMP-SMX, 10 mg TMP/kg/d and 50 mg SMX/kg/d, IV or PO *or* Ampicillin, 12 g/d IV; maintenance therapy required
	Cryptosporidiosis	No known effective therapy
Cutaneous	Herpes simplex	Acyclovir, 1000 mg/d PO *or* Acyclovir, 15 mg/kg/d IV
	Herpes zoster	Acycolovir, 25–30 mg/kg/d IV
	Candida, tricophyton	Clotrimazole, miconazole, or ketoconazole, topical therapy bid-tid for 3 weeks

Infections including *Staphylococcus aureus* (manifest as bullous impetigo, ecthyma, or folliculitis), *Pseudomonas aeruginosa* (which may present with chronic ulcerations and macerations), herpes simplex, herpes zoster, syphilis, and scabies are commonly seen and should be treated with standard therapies.

Kaposi's sarcoma is the second most common manifestation of AIDS (second to PCP). It is usually widely disseminated, and may involve mucous membranes. Since Kaposi's sarcoma is not generally associated with significant morbidity or mortality, therapy is only indicated for extensive, painful, or cosmetically disfiguring lesions. Chemotherapy with vincristine, vinblastine, or doxyrubicin, or radiation therapy may be used.

Varicella zoster eruptions are commonly seen. In the HIV-positive patient, outpatient management may be sufficient. However, in the AIDS patient, or with disseminated disease, admission is frequently indicated for therapy with intravenous acyclovir (30 mg/kg per day). Varicella immune globulin (VZIG) may be useful in patients with primary infection and visceral involvement.

Herpes simplex infections are common among AIDS patients. Both HSV-1 and HSV-2 are seen, and may present as either local infection or systemic involvement. Herpes simplex infections respond well to standard therapy with oral acyclovir (200 mg five times daily for 10 days). Intravenous therapy (15 to 30 mg/kg per day) may be required in extensive disease.

Molluscum contagiosum presents with small flesh-colored papules with a white core and is commonly seen in HIV-infected individuals. Since cure is difficult, treatment is recommended for symptomatic lesions only. Treatment may be instituted by a dermatologist with cryotherapy or curettage.

Intertriginous infections with either *Candida* or *Tricophyton* are common, and may be diagnosed on microscopic examination of potassium hydroxide preparation of lesion scrapings. Treatment may include topical imidazole creams (such as clotrimazole, miconazole, or ketoconazole).

Seborrheic dermatitis is a common eruption, and may present with erythematous, hyperkeratotic, scaling plaques involving the scalp, face (typically in a malar distribution), ears, chest, and genitalia. Treatment with topical steroids is effective in most patients.

Human papillomavirus infections occur with increased frequency in immunocompromised patients. Treatment is cosmetic or symptomatic, and may include cryotherapy, topical therapy, or in extreme cases, laser therapy.

Other dermatologic conditions which occur with increased frequency among HIV-infected patients include psoriasis, atopic dermatitis, and alopecia. Referral for dermatologic consultation is generally indicated.

Neurologic Complications

Central nervous system disease occurs in 75 to 90 percent of patients with AIDS, and 10 to 20 percent of AIDS patients initially present with CNS symptoms. The most common symptoms are seizures or altered mental status, but headache, meningismus, and neuropathy also commonly occur. Emergency department evaluation should include a complete neurologic examination, and when appropriate, computed tomography and lumbar puncture. Specific CSF studies which may be of value include opening and closing pressures, cell count, glucose, protein, gram stain, India ink stain, bacterial culture, viral culture, fungal culture, *Toxoplasma* and *Cryptococcus* antigen, and coccidiomycosis titer. The most common etiologies of neurologic symptoms include AIDS dementia, *T. gondii, C. neoformans, M. tuberculosis,* and herpes simplex.

AIDS dementia complex (also referred to as HIV encephalopathy, or subacute encephalitis) is a progressive dementia, commonly heralded by impairment of recent memory, caused by direct HIV infection. It occurs in over one-third of AIDS patients. Zidovudine (AZT) is the recommended therapy.

Toxoplasmosis is the most common cause of focal encephalitis in patients with AIDS. Symptoms may include headache, fever, focal neurologic deficits, altered mental status, or seizures. Diagnosis may be made by a contrast-enhanced CT scan showing ring-enhancing lesions. However, because of possible false-negative CT scans, MRI or a delayed CT scan may be necessary to establish the diagnosis. Other etiologies in the differential diagnosis of ring-enhancing lesions include lymphoma, fungal infection, cerebral tuberculosis, CMV, Kaposi's sarcoma, and hemorrhage. Often the diagnosis may be definitively established only with brain biopsy. Treatment for toxoplasmosis should be instituted with oral sulfadiazine (100 mg/kg per day) and pyrimethamine (25 to 50 mg/d), with folinic acid added to reduce the incidence of hematologic toxicity. Short courses of steroids may be employed. Chronic suppressive therapy is usually indicated after acute treatment.

Cryptococcal CNS infection may be seen in up to 10 percent of AIDS patients and may cause either focal cerebral lesions or diffuse meningoencephalitis. Presenting symptoms may include headache, lightheadedness, depression, seizures, or cranial nerve palsies. Diagnosis is made by India ink preparation or fungal culture, or by the presence of cryptococcal antigen in the CSF. Treatment should include intravenous amphotericin B (0.4 to 0.6 mg/kg per day). Flucytosine

(75 to 100 mg/kg per day) may be added to this therapy. Sixty percent of patients may be expected to respond to therapy. Initial therapy should continue for 6 weeks, and chronic suppressive therapy is often indicated.

Tuberculous meningitis is common, with symptoms of headache, fever, meningismus, seizures, altered mental status, or focal neurologic deficits. CSF studies may reveal low glucose, high protein, and lymphocytic pleocytosis.

Patients with HSV encephalitis may present with headache, seizures, or altered mental status. CT scanning may reveal enhanced cortical uptake in the temporal area, but biopsy is usually required to establish the diagnosis.

Disposition may be considered after appropriate evaluation is undertaken in the emergency department. Most patients with new or changed neurologic involvement should be admitted.

Psychiatric Disorders

AIDS and its associated disease states may manifest as physiologic, neurologic, or psychiatric abnormalities, and may also involve complex psychological and social issues. Interactions with family and friends may be altered, and issues of confronting chronic illness and death may prove devastating. The most common psychiatric presentations include delirium, dementia, depression, and psychosis.

Delirium or dementia suggest the presence of a primary physiologic disease state and should be thoroughly investigated as discussed above.

Depression is common among AIDS patients, and may be initially manifested as a primary complaint or as a suicide attempt. Patients with a previous history of depression are at increased risk. Depression is often responsive to hospitalization and psychosocial intervention. Antidepressant therapy may be considered if symptoms of depression continue longer than 2 weeks.

AIDS psychosis is poorly understood; and the patient may present with psychiatric symptoms such as hallucinations, delusions, or other abnormal behavioral changes. The etiology is unclear at this time, and treatment is identical to that for psychoses of other etiologies.

Ophthalmologic Manifestations

Eye complaints such as change in visual acuity, photophobia, redness, or pain are common among AIDS patients and may represent retinitis or malignant invasion of the eye or periorbital tissues.

The most common eye finding in AIDS patients is cotton-wool spots. The etiology is uncertain, but is thought to perhaps occur in conjunction with PCP.

Cytomegalovirus retinitis occurs in 10 to 15 percent of patients. It accounts for the majority of retinitis among AIDS patients. It may be asymptomatic or may present with photophobia, scotoma, redness, pain, or change in visual acuity. It has a characteristic appearance of fluffy white retinal lesions, often perivascular. Treatment should be initiated with ganciclovir (5 mg/kg per day) for 2 weeks, followed by long-term maintenance therapy.

Pulmonary Complications

Pulmonary manifestations of HIV infection are one of the most common reasons for emergency department visits among AIDS patients. Common presenting complaints may include cough, hemoptysis, shortness of breath, or chest pain. Evaluation in the emergency department may include history, lung examination, arterial blood gas, sputum culture, gram stain, acid-fast stain, blood cultures, and chest radiograph. Leukocytosis, productive cough, and presence of a focal infiltrate are suggestive of bacterial pneumonia. The most common etiologies of pulmonary abnormalities include PCP, *Mycobacterium tuberculosis* pneumonia (MTB), CMV, *Cryptococcus neoformans, Histoplasma capsulatum,* and neoplasm. Nonproductive cough and the presence of a diffuse infiltrative process on chest radiography suggest PCP, CMV, or pulmonary involvement of Kaposi's sarcoma. Hilar adenopathy with a diffuse pulmonary infiltrate may be associated with cryptococcosis, histoplasmosis, mycobacterial pneumonia, or neoplasm. Table 82-4 summarizes common radiographic findings in the AIDS patient.

Emergency department management may include supplemental oxygen, volume repletion if indicated, and, when appropriate, initiation of antibiotic therapy. Admission should be considered for patients with new-onset pulmonary symptoms and for those with a change in respiratory status.

PCP is the most common opportunistic infection among AIDS patients. More than 80 percent of patients will acquire PCP at some time during their illness. It is often the initial opportunistic infection which establishes the diagnosis of AIDS. Common presenting symptoms may include cough, typically nonproductive, and shortness of breath. Chest radiography may show a diffuse interstitial infiltrate, but may be falsely negative. Gallium scanning of the chest is more sensitive but may result in more false positives. Other diagnostic tests include bronchoscopy with lavage, biopsy, and culture or examination of induced sputum by indirect immunofluorescence using monoclonal antibodies. Initial therapy for PCP should be instituted with TMP-SMX (trimethoprim, 20 mg/kg per day, and sulfamethoxazole, 100 mg/kg per day), either PO or IV for 2 to 3 weeks. Pentamidine isothionate (4 mg/kg per day) may be used as an effective alternate therapy. A majority of patients respond to therapy. Relapses are common; 65 percent of patients will have a reinfection within 18 months. Repeat infections may be less responsive to therapy. Prophylactic therapy with an agent such as TMP-SMX, inhaled pentamidine, or dapsone may be used.

The incidence of MTB among AIDS patients is increasing. Reactivation of prior infection due to immunosuppression is common. Chest radiography may be nondiagnostic, since the typical pulmonary upper lobe involvement is less common among AIDS patients. Negative PPD tests are frequent among AIDS patients due to immunosuppression. Diagnosis may be made by sputum stain and culture or by bronchoscopy with biopsy. Triple therapy with isoniazid, rifampin, and ethambutal should be initiated. This regimen may be supplemented with pyrazinamide or streptomycin. It is currently recommended that all HIV-

Table 82-4. Chest Radiographic Abnormalities: Differential Diagnosis in the AIDS Patient

Finding	Etiologies
Diffuse interstitial infiltration	*P. carinii* CMV *M. tuberculosis* *M. avium* complex Histoplasmosis Coccidioidomycosis Lymphoid interstitial pneumonitis
Focal consolidation	Bacterial pneumonia *M. pneumoniae* *P. carinii* *M. tuberculosis* *M. avium* complex
Nodular lesions	Kaposi's sarcoma *M. tuberculosis* *M. avium* complex Fungal lesions Toxoplasmosis
Cavitary lesions	*P. carinii* *M. tuberculosis* Bacterial infection Fungal infection
Adenopathy	Kaposi's sarcoma Lymphoma *M. tuberculosis* Cryptococcosis

infected patients with positive PPD should receive isoniazid prophylaxis.

Gastrointestinal Complications

Gastrointestinal manifestations of HIV infection are common. Approximately 50 percent of AIDS patients will present with GI complaints at some time during their illness. The most common presenting symptoms include abdominal pain, bleeding, and diarrhea. Common causes include *Candida,* Kaposi's sarcoma, MAI, HSV-1 and HSV-2, CMV, *Campylobacter jejuni, Shigella, Salmonella, Giardia, Entamoeba histolytica, Cryptosporidium,* and *Isospora* species. Emergency department evaluation should focus on identification and severity of symptoms and on obtaining appropriate initial diagnostic studies. Therapy should include rehydration and initiation of antibiotic therapy when appropriate.

Oral candidiasis affects more than 80 percent of AIDS patients. The tongue and buccal mucosa are commonly involved. Differentiation from hairy leukoplakia, also common in this patient population, may be difficult, but microscopic examination on potassium hydroxide smear can confirm the diagnosis. The development of oral candidiasis is a poor prognostic sign and is predictive of progression to AIDS. Most oral lesions can be managed symptomatically on an outpatient basis. Clotrimazole troches (five times daily) are the preferred treatment. Oral ketoconazole may be used if clotrimazole is ineffective. Nystatin suspension is not recommended due to limited duration of application in the oropharynx.

Oral involvement with HSV, MAI, and Kaposi's sarcoma are also common and may usually be managed on an outpatient basis with symptomatic therapy.

Esophageal involvement may occur with *Candida,* HSV,and CMV. Esophagitis may present with complaints of dysphagia or odynophagia. Endoscopy, fungal stains, viral cultures, or biopsy may be necessary to establish the diagnosis. An air-contrast barium swallow may be obtained in the emergency department as a means to establish the diagnosis of *Candida* esophagitis. A pattern of ulceration with plaques is typically seen. Treatment should be initiated with oral ketoconazole (400 mg/d). Relapses are common and intravenous amphotericin B may occasionally be required. Herpes esophagitis may produce punched-out ulcerations without associated heaped-up plaques. Treatment with acyclovir should be initiated.

Hepatomegaly occurs in perhaps 50 percent of AIDS patients. Elevation of alkaline phosphatase is commonly seen. Jaundice is uncommon. Coinfection with hepatitis B and hepatitis C is common, especially among IV drug users. Opportunistic infection with CMV, MAI, and MTB may produce a clinical picture similar to that of hepatitis.

Diarrhea is the most common gastrointestinal complaint, and is estimated to occur in 50 to 90 percent of AIDS patients. Emergency department evaluation may include microscopic examination of stool for leukocytes, acid-fast stain, and examination for ova and parasites, as well as bacterial culture of stool and blood. Management should be directed toward repletion of fluid and electrolytes. *Cryptosporidium* and *Isospora* infection in particular are common etiologies and are associated with prolonged watery diarrhea. Salmonella also occurs commonly among AIDS patients, and may cause bacteremia. Long-term management of diarrhea not requiring specific therapy may be established with attapulgite (Kaopectate), psyllium (Metamucil), and if necessary, diphenoxylate hydrochloride with atropine (Lomotil).

Cardiovascular Manifestations

Clinically significant cardiac disease among AIDS patients is uncommon. Findings such as pericardial effusion, cardiomyopathy, and congestive heart failure have been reported but are often clinically silent.

Renal Manifestations

Renal insufficiency among AIDS patients may be secondary to prerenal azotemia, drug nephrotoxicity, or HIV nephropathy, which may cause chronic renal insufficiency due to focal and segmental glomerulosclerosis. Dialysis may be considered for the usual clinical criterion, and may be done either by peritoneal dialysis or hemodialysis. This decision should be made in conjunction with a nephrologist.

IMMUNIZATIONS OF HIV-INFECTED PATIENTS

According to the U.S. Public Health Service Immunizations Practices Advisory Committee (ACIP), routine immunizations of DPT, Td, and MMR are unchanged among HIV-infected patients. Other vaccinations are generally not indicated in the emergency department. Response to vaccination may be variable among individuals. Table 82-5 summarizes the Centers for Disease Control recommendations for common immunizations.

DRUG REACTIONS

Reactions to pharmacologic therapy are common among HIV-infected patients and must always be considered as a possible etiology of new symptomatology. In a recent series, 5 percent of emergency department visits by symptomatic HIV-positive patients were related to complications of pharmacologic therapy. Table 82-6 illustrates common side effects of medications used in AIDS patients.

ETHICAL CONSIDERATIONS

Many ethical considerations are involved in testing and treatment of HIV-infected patients. Testing for HIV in the emergency department is at this time generally not indicated. Many departments have adopted strict policies against such testing, due to the difficulties of ensuring adequate confidentiality and counseling. This may change as the need for early identification and treatment of patients is demonstrated. Initiation of counseling and referral for testing are recommended for patients at high risk.

Resuscitation in patients with advanced AIDS is a controversial subject. Since emergency department physicians may have limited information about individual patients, their wishes, and the state of their disease, it is recommended that appropriate therapy and resuscitative measures be undertaken, unless specifically requested otherwise by the patient.

Confidentiality regarding HIV-related diagnoses is paramount in providing appropriate patient care. Treatment without discrimination, as with all disease states, should be initiated in all patients unless they specifically request otherwise.

PRECAUTIONS FOR HEALTH CARE WORKERS

Health care workers are often exposed to HIV-infected patients and their body fluids. Precautions in handling potentially infectious fluids

Table 82-5. Immunization Recommendations for HIV-Infected Patients

Vaccine	Asymptomatic	Symptomatic
DPT (to age 7)	Yes	Yes
Td	Yes	Yes
OPV	No	No
IPV (inactivated polio vaccine)	Yes	Yes
MMR	Yes	Consider vaccine
H. flu (HbCV)	Yes	Yes
Pneumococcal	Yes	Yes
Influenza (inactivated)	No (although not contraindicated)	Yes

Source: Adapted from Centers for Disease Control, *MMWR* 38:205, 1989.

Table 82-6. Common Drug Reactions Seen in the HIV-Infected Patient

	Symptoms									Laboratory Abnormalities							
Medication	**Fever**	**Rash**	**Nausea and Vomiting**	**Diarrhea**	**Constipation**	**Headache**	**Mental Status Change**	**Phlebitis**	**Neuropathy**	**↑ LFT**	**↑ Glucose**	**↓ Glucose**	**↓ K**	**↓ Mg**	**↓ WBC**	**↓ Plt**	**↓ Hct**
Antimicrobials																	
TMP-SMX	X	X	X							X					X	X	
Pentamidine		X									X	X			X		X
Isoniazid	X	X	X						X	X					X	X	X
Clindamycin		X															
Dapsone	X	X	X			X			X	X					X		X
Antifungal agents																	
Amphotericin	X		X			X		X					X	X			X
5-FU			X	X						X					X		
Ganciclovir			X	X				X							X		
Clotrimazole			X	X													
Nystatin			X	X													
Ketoconazole			X	X						X							
Antiviral agents																	
Zidovudine			X			X	X								X		X
Acyclovir			X	X		X											
Pain medications																	
Ibuprofen		X	X	X	X					X					X		X
Narcotics			X		X												

are crucial to protect against occupational acquisition of HIV infection. Since HIV infection is often undiagnosed at the time of the emergency department encounter, the use of universal precautions is strongly recommended. Departments should educate employees regarding specific precautions regarding needle handling, cleaning of patient areas and equipment, and the use of gloves, gown, glasses, and masks. However, it should also be noted that the risk of acquiring HIV through occupational exposure is low. The risk of contracting AIDS after such exposure has been estimated at 0.5 percent. Approximately 80 percent of cases of documented occupational exposure have been due to needlestick injuries. If a significant occupational exposure to a patient occurs, HIV testing of the patient, with the patient's consent, is recommended. If the patient tests positive for HIV, HIV testing of the employee is recommended at 6 weeks, 3 months, and 6 months following exposure. Some centers currently advocate the immediate oral administration of AZT following exposure, although its clinical efficacy is to date unproven.

DISPOSITION

Consultation with an infectious disease specialist, neurologist, psychiatrist, or gastroenterologist is often necessary to provide proper disposition.

Disposition decisions, as for all patients, are based on determination of the patient's ability to function as an outpatient, with special consideration regarding oral intake and ambulation; availability of adequate outpatient therapy for the specific condition; and the availability of appropriate medical follow-up. Admission is generally indicated for patients with abnormal vital signs, unexplained neurologic findings or seizures, hypoxia worse than baseline, significant volume depletion, bone marrow suppression, or any other condition causing extreme debilitation or requiring intravenous therapy.

BIBLIOGRAPHY

Centers for Disease Control: AIDS and human immunodeficiency virus infection in the United States: 1988 update. *MMWR* 37, 1988.

Centers for Disease Control: Guidelines for prevention of transmission of human immunodeficiency virus and Hepatitis B virus to health-care and public safety workers. *MMWR* 38(suppl no. S-6), 1989.

Centers for Disease Control: *HIV/AIDS Surveillance Report*. May 1991.

Centers for Disease Control: Public Health Service statement of management of occupational exposure to human immunodeficiency virus, including considerations regarding zidovudine postexposure use. *MMWR* 39(RR-1), 1990.

Centers for Disease Control: Revision of the CDC surveillance case definition of acquired immunodeficiency syndrome. *MMWR* 36(suppl 1), 1987.

Cohen PT, Sande MA, Volberding PA (eds): *The AIDS Knowledge Base*. Waltham, Massachusetts, Massachusetts Medical Society, 1990.

Fischl MA, Richman DD, Grieco MH, et al: The efficacy of azidothymidine (AZT) in the treatment of patients with AIDS and AIDS-related complex: A double-blind, placebo-controlled trial. *N Engl J Med* 317:185, 1987.

Glatt AE, Chirgwin K, Landesman S: Treatment of infections associated with human immunodeficiency virus. *N Engl J Med* 318:1439, 1988.

Henderson DK: HIV in the health care setting, in Mandell GL, Douglas RG, Bennett JE, eds: Principles and practice of infectious diseases, ed 3. New York, Churchill Livingstone, 1990.

Kelen GD, DiGiovanna T, Bisson K, et al: Human immunodeficiency virus infection in emergency department patients: Epidemiology, clinical presentations and risk to health care workers: The Johns Hopkins experience. *JAMA* 262:516, 1989.

Kelen GD, Fritz S, Qaqish B, et al: Unrecognized human immunodeficiency virus (HIV) infection in general emergency patients. *N Engl J Med* 318:1645, 1988.

Murray JF, Garay SM, Hopewell PC, et al: Pulmonary complications of the acquired immunodeficiency syndrome: Report of the second National Heart, Lung and Blood Institute workshop. *Am Rev Respir Dis* 135:504, 1987.

83 TETANUS

Donna L. Carden

Tetanus is an acute, frequently fatal disease which results from a wound infected with the organism *Clostridium tetani*. The clinical manifestations of tetanus are all secondary to an exotoxin, tetanospasmin, elaborated at the wound site by the clostridial organism and consist of generalized muscular rigidity and violent muscular contractions.

MICROBIOLOGY

Clostridium tetani is an anaerobic gram-positive rod which exists in either a vegetative or sporulated form. The spores formed by the organism are extremely resistant to destruction and can survive in soil and on environmental surfaces for years. *Clostridium tetani* is usually introduced into a wound in the sporulated form where it may later germinate into the tetanospasmin-producing vegetative form if tissue oxygen tension is sufficiently low. Any factor which lowers the local oxidation-reduction potential, such as the presence of crushed, devitalized tissue or a foreign body, or the development of suppuration, favors the development of the vegetative form of *C. tetani*.

The infection caused by *C. tetani* remains localized at the site of injury, but the exotoxin produced is transported to the central nervous system where it is responsible for all of the clinical manifestations of tetanus. Tetanospasmin acts on the motor end plates of skeletal muscle, in the spinal cord, in the brain, and in the sympathetic nervous system. This extremely potent exotoxin prevents transmission at inhibitory interneurons in the CNS resulting in disinhibition of the motor system and the clinical manifestations of the disease. The toxin probably also disinhibits the sympathetic nervous system, resulting in autonomic dysfunction.

EPIDEMIOLOGY

Although safe and effective immunization exists for the prevention of tetanus, the disease is still a major health problem worldwide and is an important cause of infant mortality in developing countries. In the United States, approximately 60 cases of tetanus are reported each year, the majority of cases occurring in patients over 50 years of age who are inadequately immunized. In fact, the majority of Americans over 60 years of age lack adequate immunity to tetanus. The overall case fatality rate in the United States for the disease in 1987 and 1988 was 21 percent.

Tetanus occurs most frequently following an acute, unreported injury, most commonly a puncture wound to an extremity. However, tetanus can also develop after minor trauma, surgical procedures, otitis media, and abortion, and can develop in neonates through infection of the umbilical cord. Although the majority of tetanus in the United States occurs in the rural southern states, the disease has been reported with surprising frequency in urban areas in drug addicts.

CLINICAL MANIFESTATIONS

The incubation period of tetanus, that is, the period from infection to the first appearance of symptoms, can range from less than 24 h to over 1 month. The shorter the incubation period, the more severe the disease and the worse the prognosis for recovery.

Clinical tetanus can be categorized into four forms: local, generalized, cephalic, and neonatal. *Local tetanus* is manifested by persistent rigidity of the muscles in close proximity to the site of injury and usually resolves after weeks to months without residue. Local tetanus may progress to the generalized form of the disease.

Generalized tetanus is the most common form of the disease and usually follows minor trauma. The most frequent presenting complaints are pain and stiffness in the jaw and trunk muscles. The transition from muscle stiffness to rigidity leads to the development of trismus and the resultant characteristic facial expression, risus sardonicus (sardonic smile). Reflex convulsive spasms and tonic contractions of muscle groups are responsible for the development of dysphasia, opisthotonos, flexing of the arms, clenching of the fists, and extension of the lower extremities. Patients are completely conscious and alert unless laryngospasm and tonic contraction of the respiratory muscles result in respiratory compromise.

Disturbances of the autonomic nervous system, generally a hypersympathetic state, occur during the second week of clinical tetanus and present as tachycardia, labile hypertension, profuse sweating, hyperpyrexia, and increased urinary excretion of catecholamines. The autonomic complications of generalized tetanus are particularly difficult to manage and contribute significantly to the morbidity and mortality of the disease.

Cephalic tetanus follows injuries to the head or occasionally otitis media and results in dysfunction of the cranial nerves, most commonly the seventh. This form of tetanus has a particularly poor prognosis. *Neonatal tetanus* is an important cause of infant mortality in developing countries and carries an extremely high mortality rate.

The differential diagnosis of tetanus is presented in Table 83-1. Strychnine poisoning most closely mimics the clinical picture of generalized tetanus.

MANAGEMENT

The patient with tetanus is best managed in the intensive care unit. Respiratory compromise may require immediate neuromuscular blockade (succinylcholine) and orotracheal intubation, but tracheostomy provides the best method of prolonged ventilatory control. Environmental stimuli must be minimized in order to prevent the precipitation of reflex convulsive spasms.

Identification and debridement of the wound through which the clostridial spores were introduced are necessary to minimize further toxin production and to improve the oxidation-reduction potential of the infected tissue. A wound may not be identified in approximately 20 percent of patients.

Tetanus Immune Globulin

Human tetanus immune globulin (TIG) neutralizes circulating tetanospasmin and toxin in the wound but not toxin that is already fixed in the nervous system. Despite the fact that TIG does not ameliorate the clinical symptoms of tetanus, there is evidence that its administration significantly reduces mortality. The recommended single intramuscular dose of TIG is 3000 to 5000 units. Although there are theoretical advantages to administering TIG intrathecally, this route is not currently licensed in the United States.

Antibiotics

Clostridium tetani is sensitive to a number of antibiotics (e.g., penicillins, cephalosporins, tetracycline, erythromycin) but parenterally

Table 83-1. Differential Diagnosis of Tetanus

Strychnine poisoning
Dystonic reaction (phenothiazines)
Hypocalcemic tetany
Peritonsillar abscess
Peritonitis
Meningeal irritation (bacterial meningitis, subarachnoid hemorrhage)
Rabies
Temporomandibular joint disease

administered penicillin G is most frequently recommended. Metronidazole has been shown to be superior to penicillin in some studies.

Muscle Relaxants

As noted above, tetanospasmin prevents transmission at inhibitory interneurons, and consequently therapy of tetanus is aimed at restoring inhibition. The benzodiazepines are centrally acting inhibitory agents which have been used for this purpose. Diazepam has been extensively utilized and results in a desirable degree of sedation. Methocarbamol, baclofen, and long-acting benzodiazepines have been suggested as alternative modalities for restoring central inhibition and providing muscle relaxation. Dantrolene is a peripherally acting muscle relaxant which has been successfully employed in a limited number of cases.

Neuromuscular Blockade

Neuromuscular blockade may be required in the treatment of tetanus for control of ventilation and muscular spasms as well as for prevention of fractures and rhabdomyolysis. Concomitant sedation with barbiturates or benzodiazepines is mandatory.

Treatment of Autonomic Dysfunction

The combined α- and β-adrenergic blocking agent labetolol has been successfully used to treat the manifestations of sympathetic hyperactivity in tetanus. However, several investigators have reported fatal cardiovascular complications in patients treated with β-adrenergic blocking agents alone. Adrenergic blocking drugs, although effective in the treatment of the autonomic dysfunction of tetanus, may precipitate dangerous myocardial depression if sympathetic activity transiently diminishes.

Magnesium sulfate, because of its ability to inhibit catecholamine release, has been advocated as a means of treating the autonomic dysfunction of tetanus. Continuous epidural block with bupivacine has been employed recently to provide sympathetic blockade, muscle relaxation, and analgesia in the treatment of the generalized form of the disease. Morphine sulfate provides control of the sympathetic hyperactivity of tetanus without compromising cardiac output. The central α-receptor agonist clonidine has met with initial success in managing the cardiovascular instability seen in tetanus, presumably by decreasing sympathetic tone and causing peripheral vasodilation.

Active Immunization

Patients who have recovered from tetanus must undergo active immunization since the disease does not confer immunity. Tetanus toxoid 0.5 mL should be administered intramuscularly at 1 and 6 weeks and at 6 months after injury.

A summary of the treatment used in the management of tetanus is presented in Table 83-2.

Table 83-2. Treatment of Tetanus

Respiratory management	Succinylcholine, 80 mg for emergency oral intubation; tracheostomy except in localized or mild tetanus
Immunotherapy	TIG 3000–5000 units IM as a single dose *and* Tetanus toxoid, 0.5 mL IM at 1 and 6 weeks and at 6 months
Antibiotic therapy	Penicillin G, 10,000,000 units IV every 24 h *or* Metronidazole, 500 mg every 6 h *or* Erythromycin, 2 g/day
Muscle relaxation	Diazepam, 10 mg IV every 1–3 h prn *or* Dantrolene, 1–2 mg/kg IV every 4 hours
Neuromuscular blockade	Pancuronium bromide, 2 mg IV to paralysis
Management of autonomic dysfunction	Labetolol, 0.25–1.0 mg/min continuous IV infusion *or* Magnesium sulfate, 70 mg/kg IV loading, then 1–4 g/h continuous infusion to maintain blood level of 2.5–4 mmol/L Morphine sulfate, 5–30 mg IV infusion every 2–8 h Clonidine, 300 μg every 8 h per nasogastric tube

SUMMARY

Despite the fact that tetanus is a completely preventable disease, it remains a source of significant morbidity and mortality in the rural southern states and in urban intravenous drug abusers. The sporulated form of *C. tetani* survives in soil and on environmental surfaces indefinitely and often gains access to the host through a minor, unreported wound. Once introduced into tissue, the spores of *C. tetani* may germinate and result in the production of tetanospasmin, the exotoxin responsible for all of the clinical manifestations of tetanus. Human tetanus immune globulin (TIG) neutralizes circulating exotoxin but not tetanospasmin fixed within nervous tissue. Nevertheless, administration of TIG lowers the case fatality rate of tetanus and is an important therapeutic intervention. Because of the extreme potency of tetanospasmin, the quantity of the exotoxin necessary to produce clinical disease is insufficient to confer immunity and therefore all patients recovering from tetanus require active immunization.

BIBLIOGRAPHY

Blake PA, Feldman RA, Buchanan TM, et al: Serologic therapy of tetanus in the United States, 1965–1971. *JAMA* 235:42, 1976.

Bleck, TP: Pharmacology of tetanus. *Clin Neuropharmacol* 9:103, 1986.

Centers for Disease Control. Tetanus—United States: 1987 and 1988. *JAMA* 263:1192, 1990.

Heurich AE, Burst JC, Richter RW: Management of urban tetanus. *Med Clin North Am* 57:1373, 1973.

James MFM, Manson EDM: The use of magnesium sulfate infusions in the management of very severe tetanus. *Intensive Care Med* 11:5, 1985.

Shibuya M, Sugimoto H, Sugimoto T, et al: *J Trauma* 29:1423, 1989.

Stoll BJ: Tetanus. *Pediatr Clin North Am* 26:415, 1979.

Sutton DN, Tremlett MR, Woodcock TE, et al: Management of autonomic dysfunction in severe tetanus: The use of magnesium sulfate and clonidine. *Intensive Care Med* 16:75, 1990.

Weinstein, L: Tetanus. *N Engl J Med* 289:1293, 1973.

Wright DK, Lallo UG, Nayiager S, et al: Autonomic nervous system dysfunction in severe tetanus: Current perspectives. *Crit Care Med* 17:371, 1989.

84 RABIES

Louis S. Binder

Rabies is a near uniformly fatal disease and represents the most serious potential complication of an animal bite. The disease is caused by an RNA-containing rhabdovirus and is transmitted by inoculation with infectious saliva from a carnivore or bat bite, or by salivary contact with a break in the skin or mucous membrane. The disease exists primarily in wildlife, which serves as the viral reservoir in endemic areas and which represents the most important source of infection for humans and domestic animals in the United States. The prevalence of rabies in wild carnivores varies in different geographic areas, which accounts for differences in prevalence of rabies in domestic animal population (as the virus is transferred from wild to domestic animals and subsequently to humans).

Worldwide, rabies is endemic throughout Latin America, Asia, Africa, South American, Europe, the Middle East, India, and Southeast Asia. A few island countries are free of rabies: England, Australia, Japan, and parts of the Caribbean.

In the United States, the rabies virus is most prevalent in the mid-Atlantic and southern Atlantic states (New York to Florida), the south central states (Arkansas; Louisiana; Oklahoma; and Texas, especially the U.S.-Mexico Border), and the midwest (the Dakotas, Minnesota, Iowa, Missouri, and Kansas). It is rare in New England, the Ohio Valley, and the Rocky Mountain states. Skunks are the most commonly identified species in California and the midwest, while raccoons are commonly infected in the Atlantic states.

Approximately 2400 cases of animal rabies were reported to the Centers for Disease Control (CDC) in 1989, a decrease of approximately 25 percent from 1978; early 1990 animal figures suggest a further 30-percent decrease from 1989. Ten cases of human rabies were reported in the United States in the 1980s (three since 1985); four of these were related to exposure to rabid dogs outside the United States, while the other six had no definite history of animal bites or other exposure. Twenty-eight percent of cases since 1960 have had no history of bite exposure. This is greatly decreased from an average animal rate of 8000 cases of dog rabies and 22 cases of human rabies reported in 1946, reflecting the implementation and effectiveness of immunization programs for domestic animals. Inactivated animal rabies vaccination induces adequate rabies antibody titers for at least 1 year and prevents canine and feline infections during this period.

In developing countries where rabies is endemic and animal immunizations are uncommon, dogs are the primary (but not only) reservoir of disease and the principle source of human exposure. In developed countries, such as the United States, dog and cat bites are the most common reason for implementation of postexposure prophylaxis, but the most important source of active rabies transmission is wildlife transmission (85% of reported animal rabies since 1970). Animal bites contracted outside the United States in an undeveloped country should be considered at high risk for rabies transmission.

Rabid wildlife species reported to the CDC in 1980 include skunks (60 percent), bats (15 percent), raccoons (10 percent), cows (4 percent), dogs (4 percent), foxes (3 percent), and cats (3 percent). Rodents (squirrels, chipmunks, rats, mice, etc.) and lagomorphs (rabbits, hares, etc.) have never been implicated as carriers, and bites by these animals are not at risk for transmission.

Rabid animals are agitated and labile, may indiscriminately attack anything that moves, and may otherwise wander aimlessly. Feeble bark, drooling, stupor, and convulsions mark more advanced disease preceding death of the animal.

Transmission through inhalation without bite exposure or from laboratory accidents is rare but has been reported. Human-to-human transmission by tissue transplantation (corneal transplants) has been reported in six cases.

PATHOPHYSIOLOGY

Once introduced, the initial infection and multiplication occurs within local myocytes for the first 48 to 96 h. Subsequently, the virus spreads across the motor endplate and ascends and replicates along peripheral nervous axoplasm to the dorsal root ganglia, the spinal cord, and the central nervous system (CNS). Following CNS replication in the gray matter, the virus spreads outward by peripheral nerves to virtually all tissues and organ systems. Viral infection of the salivary glands, kidneys, and intestine engenders infectivity of saliva, urine, and feces.

Histologically, rabies manifests the same findings as seen in other forms of encephalitis: monocellular infiltration with focal hemorrhage and demyelination, predominantly in perivascular areas in the gray matter of the CNS, basal ganglia, and the spinal cord. Negri bodies are the characteristic histologic finding for rabies, which is the site of CNS viral replication. They are eosinophilic intracellular lesions found within cerebral neurons and are highly specific for rabies. Negri bodies are encountered in only 75 percent of proven animal rabies cases; thus, although their presence is pathognomonic for rabies, their absence does not exclude rabies as a diagnostic possibility.

CLINICAL PRESENTATION

As human rabies has decreased in the United States, the proportion of rabies patients without animal bite exposure has increased. In 60 percent of the cases in the 1980s, a source of infection was not identified. Rabies is often overlooked diagnostically in persons without such exposure. In untreated rabid bites, the risk of contracting rabies ranges from 5 to 80 percent. Rabid hand and foot bites carry a 15- to 20-percent mortality; rabid head and neck bites, a 50-percent mortality.

Incubation periods average 35 to 64 days; periods as short as 12 days and as long as 700 days have been reported. Variations in incubation period are dependent on the size of the viral inoculum, host immunity, and bite location: the more rostral the bite, the shorter both the travel distance and the incubation time for the virus.

The initial symptoms of human rabies are nonspecific: fever, malaise, headache, anorexia, and nausea, sore throat, cough, and pain or paresthesias at the bite site (80 percent). This initial phase may last for 1 to 4 days. Subsequently, evidence of CNS involvement becomes apparent, with restlessness and agitation, altered mental status, painful bulbar and peripheral muscular spasms, opisthotonos, and bulbar or focal motor paresis. Alternatively, in 20 percent an ascending, symmetric, flaccid, and areflexic paralysis, comparable to the Landry-Guillain-Barré syndrome, may be seen. Hypersensitivity to sensory stimuli (light, noise, and touch) and hydrophobia may occur at this stage, the latter resulting from the sight, sound, swallowing, or even mention of water. Progressively, lucid and confused intervals may become interspersed, cholinergic nervous abnormalities may manifest (hyperpyrexia, mydriasis, and increased lacrimation and salivation), and brainstem dysfunction (dysphagia, optic neuritis, and facial palsies) with hyperreflexia and extensor plantar responses may occur. Coma, convulsions, and apnea are the final manifestations of rabid death.

Death universally occurs in 4 to 7 days in untreated patients, which may be prolonged to 25 days if supportive care is instituted. There are three reported cases of neurologically intact survivors of rabies, who received rabies vaccine before onset of symptoms and intensive supportive care. In these patients, supportive care maintained vital functions while the patient's stimulated immune response eradicated the infection. Such recoveries, however, are exceedingly rare.

DIAGNOSIS

The diagnosis of rabies in animals and humans is made by analysis of brain tissue from biopsy. Analysis for Negri bodies is highly specific, but carries a 25-percent false-negative rate. Fluorescent antibody testing (FAT) has become the procedure of choice due to low cost, speed, and reliability when performed in a competent laboratory. Mouse inoculation tests and tissue culture tests are used for confirmation or as the primary test in less sophisticated laboratories. More recently, enzyme-linked immunosorbent assay techniques have been employed, with satisfactory results comparable to those with FAT and tissue culture. Serum antibody titers in unimmunized patients become positive between days 6 and 12, and a fourfold increase in these patients in antibody titers is considered diagnostic. In vaccinated patients, cerebrospinal fluid (CSF) analysis for rabies antibodies suggests the diagnosis, as immunizations alone rarely produce detectable antibodies in the CSF. CSF titers for rabies antibodies become positive between days 8 and 16, with titers of 1:200 or higher being diagnostic. Elevated CSF protein and a mononuclear pleocytosis are also seen.

The differential diagnosis includes viral or other infectious encephalitis, polio, tetanus, viral process, meningitis, brain abscess, septic cavernous sinus thrombosis, cholinergic poisoning, and Landry-Guillain-Barré syndrome. The diagnosis is especially difficult without history of exposure but should be considered in patients with a picture of progressive and unexplained encephalitis.

Common complications include adult respiratory distress syndrome, diabetes insipidus, syndrome of inappropriate antidiuretic hormone, volume depletion, fluid and electrolyte complications, pneumonia, and cardiogenic hypotension and arrhythmia from rabies myocarditis.

Management consists of institution of postexposure immunoprophylaxis as early as possible (preferably before the onset of symptoms) and institution of intensive supportive care to maintain vital functions, with hope that the stimulated immune system can overcome the infection.

POSTEXPOSURE PROPHYLAXIS

On 6th July, 1885, Louis Pasteur attempted to protect, for the first time in the history of medicine, a child bitten by a rabid dog. He prepared a modified rabies virus (''virus fixe'') which he inoculated intracerebrally into a rabbit, and subsequently prepared a suspension of rabbit spinal cord. The nervous tissue suspension was used to inoculate the boy during eleven days with thirteen doses containing increasing amounts of active virus. The boy survived.

Thus was reported the first (and most dramatic) antirabies vaccine ever produced and employed to induce immunity and protection against rabies in man. It has been subsequently shown that the use of hyperimmune serum (conferring passive immunity) or interferon inducer together with a vaccination regimen (conferring active immunity) yielded complete survival from rabies. Both the passive antibodies and interferon perform a critical biological function in controlling local propagation and spread of the virus until the patient can develop active immunity from the vaccine.

Following inoculation, the rabies virus often remains latent for a period in myocytes prior to spreading to nervous tissue. Employment of local cleansing (to eliminate the virus from the infection site) and local infiltration of hyperimmune serum may successfully control the spread of infection. Postexposure immunization of an infected individual can induce active antibody production and prevent CNS infection if the propagation and spread of local rabies infection can be initially controlled. Postexposure treatment must be instituted promptly, since effectiveness decreases proportionately to the delay in institution of treatment.

Currently indicated pharmaceuticals for rabies prophylaxis are rabies immune globin (RIG) for passive immunization and human diploid cell vaccine (HDCV) for active immunization. RIG is antirabies gammaglobulin concentrated by cold ethanol fractionation of the plasma of hyperimmunized human donors. Neutralizing antibody content is standardized to contain 150 IU/mL. HDCV is an inactivated virus vaccine grown in human diploid cell tissue culture, is rich in rabies antigen, and engenders a universally excellent antibody response in recipients. HDCV induces IgM rabies-specific antibodies on day 3, IgG rabies-specific antibodies on day 7, early IgM/IgG conversion, and a 99- to 100-percent incidence of adequate titers at 42 and 90 days, respectively.

Figure 84-1 presents a clinical algorithm for the evaluation of animal exposures for rabies postexposure prophylaxis. Critical factors in the process of deciding whether to institute prophylaxis are the animal species, the nature of the exposure (whether salivary contact with wounds or mucous membrane did or did not occur), and whether the animal is available for observation or rabies testing.

Dogs and cats with normal behavior when captured may be quarantined for 10 days, which is sufficient time in these species for the disease to manifest if the animal is infected. If no signs become apparent, the animal can be considered nonrabid. The principle indication in clinical practice for the initiation of postexposure prophylaxis is a bite wound by an uncaptured dog or cat in an endemic area or a bite wound by an uncaptured bat or appropriate species of carnivore. State or local health officials should be consulted regarding the possibility of rabies in local dog, cat, rodent, and lagomorph populations before decisions on initiating postexposure rabies prophylaxis are made.

Pre-exposure prophylaxis should be considered for persons involved in rabies animal diagnosis and control, wildlife trapping, rabies vaccine production, animal handlers, hunters, veterinarians, and travelers to areas where rabies is endemic. Seroconversion for antirabies antibody titers is 100 percent for a three-dose regimen (see below), and titers remain adequate for 2 years. Prophylaxis should be completed at least 30 days prior to anticipated exposure. Either booster doses or antibody titer determinations have been recommended every 2 years for persons with continuing risk of exposure and every 6 months for persons working with live rabies virus in research laboratories or vaccine production facilities.

TREATMENT GUIDELINES

Prompt debridement and cleansing of wounds to remove rabies virus is important in reducing the viral inoculum. Scrubbing and cleansing the wound with soap, derbridement of devitalized tissue, and thorough irrigation with sterile saline solution or water should be undertaken, along with tetanus prophylaxis and prophylactic antibiotic coverage as indicated. If there is strong concern for rabies virus contamination of the wound, it should not be sutured, as this promotes rabies virus replication.

RIG is administered only once at the onset of therapy. The dose is 20 IU/kg, with half the dose (if possible, based on volume constraints) infiltrated locally at the exposure site and the remainder administered intramuscularly. RIG can be given up to 8 days after the first dose of HDCV; beyond this time, RIG is unnecessary due to the developing active immunity from HDCV. Each vial of RIG contains 2 mL (300 IU); hence, a 70-kg man will require 1400 IU, or five vials. HDCV should be administered in five 1-mL doses intramuscularly as soon as possible following exposure, on days 0, 3, 7, 14, and 28. The World Health Organization also recommends a sixth dose on day 90.

Rabies antibody titers are not recommended following the fifth dose on day 28 for healthy individuals but are recommended for an incomplete immunization course or immunocompromised patients (particularly those on corticosteroids). Both RIG and HDCV should be administered in the deltoid muscle rather than in the gluteal area. A reduced rabies antibody response has been shown with gluteal administration, presumably due to interference of HDCV immunogenicity by subcutaneous fat, and gluteal injection has been implicated as the chief factor in vaccine failure.

Preexposure prophylaxis for susceptible individuals consists of HDCV 1 mL intramuscularly on days 0, 7, and 21. Patients who have been previously immunized with rabies vaccine (either preexposure or postexposure prophylaxis with HDCV or other vaccine), who have a documented adequate rabies titer, and who have sustained another exposure or potential exposure to rabies virus should receive two doses of HDCV at days 0 and 3. Rabies antibody titers are subsequently

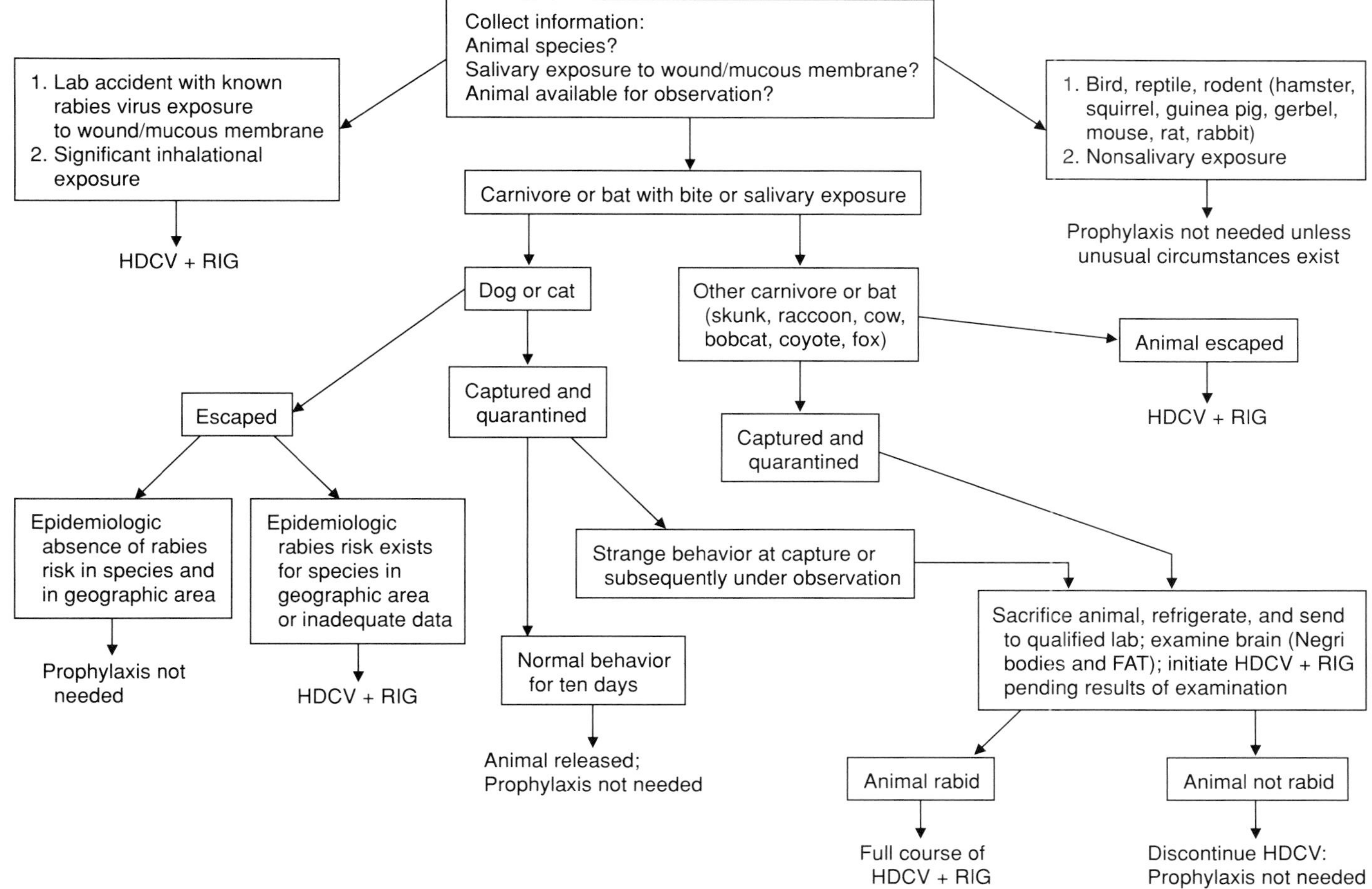

Figure 84-1. Clinical guidelines for administration of rabies postexposure prophylaxis. (Adapted from Mann, JM: Rabies risk: Systematic evaluation and management of animal bites. *Comp Ther* 7:53, 1981. Used by permission.)

recommended to determine the adequacy of the immune response. An HDCV booster followed by repeat titers in 2 to 3 weeks is indicated for inadequate rabies antibody titers.

Adverse reactions following the use of RIG have been limited to local pain and low-grade fever, which are transient and can be treated with salicylates or nonsteroidal anti-inflammatory medication. HDCV can precipitate similar local reactions in 25 percent of recipients. Up to 20 percent of HDCV recipients may manifest mild headache, nausea, dizziness, and myalgias, and 6 percent of booster recipients have experienced an immune complex-like reaction. Rare cases of anaphylaxis and transient neuroparalytic reactions similar to Landry-Guillain-Barré syndrome have also been reported with HDCV use. Rabies prophylaxis should not be stopped due to mild reactions, but serious neuroparalysis or anaphylaxis during treatment poses a therapeutic dilemma. Postexposure assessment of the clinical risk of rabies must be weighed against the risks of treatment, with possible choices consisting of continuation of therapy, switching to an alternative vaccine, pretreatment with antihistamine for hypersensitive patients, or discontinuation of treatment. Both the CDC and state or county health departments can provide assistance in the management of complications.

Since no fetal abnormalities have been reported and because of the possibility of rabies infection without passive and active treatment, pregnant patients may receive passive and active immunization for rabies prophylaxis.

Both animal bites and rabies are reportable entities in all states. Physicians should notify the county or state public health department of cases of rabid animals or humans. Animal bites should be reported to the local animal control unit (usually associated with public health or police departments) so that appropriate animals are captured and quarantined for observation in a timely fashion.

BIBLIOGRAPHY

Anderson LJ, Nicholson KG, Tauxe RV, et al: Human rabies in the United States, 1960 to 1979: Epidemiology, diagnosis, and prevention. *Ann Intern Med* 100:728, 1984.

Anderson LJ, Sikes RK, Langkop CW, et al: Postexposure trial of a human diploid cell strain rabies vaccine. *J Infect Dis* 142:133, 1980.

Anderson LJ, Winkler WG, Hofkin B, et al: Clinical experiences with a human diploid cell rabies vaccine. *JAMA* 244:781, 1980.

Bahmanyar M: Benefit versus risk factors in prophylactic vaccination against rabies. *Dev Biol Stand* 43:305, 1979.

Bourhy H, Rollin PE, Vincent J, et al: Comparative field evaluation of the fluorescent antibody test, virus isolation from tissue culture, and enzyme immunodiagnosis for rapid laboratory diagnosis of rabies. *J Clin Microbiol* 27:519, 1989.

Fishbein DB, Baer GH: Animal rabies: Implications for diagnosis and human treatment. *Ann Intern Med* 109:935, 1988.

Mann, JM: Rabies risk: Systematic evaluation and management of animal bites. *Comp Ther* 7:58, 1981.

National Association of State Public Health Veterinarians, Inc.: Compendium of animal rabies control, 1990. *Morbid Mortal Weekly Rep* 39:1, 1990.

Recommendation of the immunization practices advisory committee (ACIP): Rabies prevention. *Morbid Mortal Weekly Rep* 29:265, 1980.

Shill M, Baynes RD, Miller SD: Fetal rabies encephalitis despite appropriate post-exposure prophylaxis. *N Engl J Med* 316:1257, 1987.

Udwadia ZF, Udwadia FE, Katrak SM, et al: Human rabies: Clinical features, diagnosis, complications, and management. *Crit Care Med* 17:834, 1989.

85
MALARIA

Jeffrey D. Band

With the increase in international travel and the continued shift of travel to tropical locales, it is not surprising that physicians are seeing more patients with infectious diseases acquired in the tropics. Malaria, a protozoan disease transmitted by the bite of the *Anopheles* mosquito, remains one of the most significant of these. Annually, over 200 million persons develop malaria and more than 1.5 million persons die. The incidence of malaria has been increasing in recent years despite worldwide aggressive attempts at control. Not only is the mosquito vector becoming less susceptible to a variety of insecticides, but *Plasmodium falciparum*—the parasite responsible for the most deadly form of malaria—is becoming increasingly resistant to antimalarial medications.

Malaria, especially disease due to *P. falciparum*, represents a medical emergency in any nonimmune host. Its early manifestations are largely nonspecific and can mimic other infectious diseases. Failure to rapidly diagnose infection can be disastrous. Likewise, failure to use specific antimalarial agents to which the individual strain is susceptible can result in early death. A diagnosis of malaria must be considered in any person returning from the tropics with an unexplained febrile illness. Questions regarding recent travel should become routine in emergency departments.

ETIOLOGY

Four species of the genus *Plasmodium* infect humans; *P. vivax, P. ovale, P. malariae* and *P. falciparum*. The organism is transmitted primarily by the bite of an infected female anopheline mosquito. This vector is most frequently found in tropical and subtropical regions below 8200 ft (2500 m) above sea level. Plasmodial sporozoites are injected into the host's bloodstream during the mosquito's blood meal and are carried directly to the liver. The hepatic parenchymal cells are invaded, and asexual reproduction of the parasite begins (preerythrocytic schizogony or exoerythrocytic stage). As thousands of daughter merozoites are formed, the parenchymal liver cell ruptures, releasing daughter merozoites back into the circulation where they rapidly invade erythrocytes (erythrocytic stage). In *P. vivax* and *P. ovale* infection, a portion of the intrahepatic forms are not released and remain dormant for months. These forms can later activate and cause clinical relapses.

The clinical manifestations of malaria first appear during the erythrocytic stage. Once merozoites enter this stage, they never reinvade the liver. Merozoites mature within the erythrocyte and take on various morphologic forms including the early ring forms, trophozoites, and schizonts (which represent a mass of new merozoites). Eventually, the target erythrocyte lyses and new merozoites invade uninfected red blood cells, continuing the infection and causing clinical manifestations. Lysogeny may become regular, occurring at 2- to 3-day intervals in established and untreated infections, producing the classic periodicity of symptoms.

After several cycles, a proportion of the merozoites develop into sexual forms (gametocytes). Upon ingestion by another feeding anopheline mosquito, male and female gametocytes undergo sexual reproduction and become infective sporozoites ready for their next host.

Each species of plasmodium has specific characteristics, including typical morphologic forms and selective red blood cell tropism (Table 85-1). Many of these characteristics are responsible for important pathophysiologic consequences.

Malaria may also be transmitted by direct transfusion of infected blood or passed transplacentally from mother to fetus. In these cases an exoerythrocytic phase is absent.

EPIDEMIOLOGY

Malaria transmission occurs in large areas of Central and South America, the Caribbean, sub-Saharan Africa, the Indian subcontinent, Southeast Asia, the Middle East, and Oceania. Certain species may predominate in a given geographic area. For example, *P. vivax* is more common in the Indian subcontinent and in Central America, while *P. falciparum* is the most prevalent form in Africa, Haiti, and New Guinea.

The risk of malaria varies considerably between regions. It is largely dependent upon the intensity of transmission in both urban and rural areas, and, for travelers, upon the itinerary and time and type of travel. From 1980 to 1988 the Centers for Disease Control reported 3436 cases of malaria among U.S. civilians. Of the 546 cases which occurred in 1988, 358 (65 percent) were acquired in sub-Saharan Africa; 82 (15 percent) in Asia; 68 (13 percent) in the Caribbean and Central America; and only 5 (1 percent) in South America. *Plasmodium falciparum* accounted for 46 percent of all cases, and *P. vivax* for another 43 percent. Mixed infections were uncommon, representing less than 1 percent of all cases. Thus, nearly two-thirds of all cases of malaria, including the majority of cases due to *P. falciparum*, are acquired from travels in sub-Saharan Africa. Yet for every traveler to sub-Saharan Africa, at least 10 travelers visit potential malarious areas of Asia and South America each year. Clearly, the intensity of exposure appears to be much higher in sub-Saharan Africa.

Resistance of *P. falciparum* to chloroquine continues to spread (Table 85-2). In addition, strains exist of *P. falciparum* that are resistant to other chemotherapeutic agents, including pyrimethamine-sulfadoxine, quinine, mefloquine, and possibly doxycycline. Recently, strains of *P. vivax* have been isolated from patients who have failed chloroquine therapy. Prior to 1990, no strains of *P. vivax, P. ovale,* or *P. malariae* were resistant to chloroquine.

Table 85-1. Characteristics of Malaria-Causing *Plasmodium* Species

	P. falciparum	*P. vivax*	*P. ovale*	*P. malariae*
Incubation period (mean)	8–25 days (12)	8–27 days (14)	9–17 days (15)	15–30 days
Asexual erythrocytic cycle	48 h	48 h	48 h	72 h
Relapse	No	Yes	Yes	No
Red blood cell preference	Reticulocytes (but can infect RBCs of all ages)	Reticulocytes	Reticulocytes	Older cells
Morphologic characteristics				
Degree of parasitemia	High (multiple rings per RBC)	Low	Low	Low
Ring forms and early trophozoites	Ring forms predominate; threadlike cytoplasm with double chromatic dots	Amoeboid cytoplasm	Compact cytoplasm	Compact cytoplasm
Mature trophozoites	Rarely seen	Observed	Observed	Observed
Schizonts	Rarely seen	Observed	Observed	Observed
Gametocytes	Banana-shaped	Round	Round	Round

Table 85-2. Geographic Distribution of Malaria Including Resistant Strains

Geographic Region	Areas with Malaria	Countries with Chloroquine-Resistant *P. falciparum*	Countries with Fansidar-Resistant *P. falciparum*
Central America	All countries	None	None
Caribbean	Dominican Republic and Haiti		
South America			
Temperate	Argentina	None	None
Tropical	All countries	All countries except Paraguay	Interior Amazon Basin
East Asia	China	China	South China
Eastern South Asia	All countries except Brunei and Singapore	All infected areas	Infected areas except Malaysia and Philippines
Middle South Asia	All countries	All countries except Iran	Afghanistan and Bhutan
Western South Asia and Middle East	Iraq, Oman, Saudi Arabia, Syria, Turkey, and UAE	None	None
Northern Africa	All countries except Tunisia	Algeria	None
Sub-Saharan Africa	All countries except Cape Verde, Réunion, São Tomé/Príncipe, and Seychelles	Widespread	Widespread
Southern Africa	All countries except Lesotho and St. Helena	Widespread	None
Oceania	Limited to Papua New Guinea, Solomon Islands, and Vanuatu (small foci elsewhere)	Widespread	Papua New Guinea and Vanuatu

PATHOGENESIS

After an incubation period ranging from 8 days in the nonimmune and unprotected host to several weeks or more, disease ensues. Both incomplete suppression by partially active chemoprophylaxis and incomplete immunity can markedly prolong the incubation period to months or even years. Only the asexual intraerythrocytic parasite is responsible for the symptoms and pathophysiologic consequences. The hallmark of malaria is the recurring febrile paroxysm which corresponds to hemolysis of infected erythrocytes and release of antigenic products with activation of macrophages and production of cytokines.

Hemolysis can be high with *P. falciparum* infection since parasitemia can be overwhelming and erythrocytes of all ages are susceptible. Parasitized erythrocytes lose flexibility and are removed in the microcirculation with resultant obstruction and tissue anoxia of the lungs, kidneys, brain, and other vital organs. Noncardiac pulmonary edema, renal failure, and cerebral malaria may result. Sequestration accounts for the paucity of observed mature parasites in the peripheral smear of patients infected with *P. falciparum*.

In addition to prolonged high fever, hemolysis, and, in the case of infection with *P. falciparum,* obstruction to capillary flow, immunologic sequela may also occur, resulting in glomerulonephritis, nephrotic syndrome, thrombocytopenia, and polyclonal antibody stimulation.

Lastly, hypersplenism with resultant pancytopenia may occur, especially in cases of prolonged, untreated malaria.

CLINICAL MANIFESTATIONS

Typically, patients develop a prodrome of malaise, myalgia, headache, and low-grade fevers often accompanied by chills. In some patients, headache, chest pains, cough, abdominal pain, arthralgias, or diarrhea may be prominent. The early manifestations are quite nonspecific and can easily become confused with a viral syndrome, influenza, hepatitis, and other less severe self-limited clinical entities. Illness usually progresses to severe chills followed by high-grade fevers accompanied by tachycardia, nausea, orthostatic dizziness, and extreme weakness. After several hours the fever abates and the patient becomes diaphoretic and exhausted. Over time, the paroxysms of malaria—chills and fever followed by diaphoresis—may occur at nearly regular intervals which correspond to the length of the asexual erythrocytic cycles (Table 85-1). The classic paroxysms of malaria are often lacking in malaria due to *P. falciparum*.

The findings on physical examination are also not specific for malaria. Most patients appear acutely ill with high fevers, tachycardia, and tachypnea. Splenomegaly and tender abdomen are commonly present in advanced infection. The liver may or may not be enlarged. Features quite atypical for malaria include lymphadenopathy and a maculopapular skin rash.

Laboratory features include normochromic normocytic anemia with findings suggestive of hemolysis, a normal or mildly depressed total leukocyte count, thrombocytopenia, an elevated erythrocyte sedimentation rate, and mild abnormalities in liver and renal functions. Other laboratory abnormalities include hyponatremia, hypoglycemia, and a biologic false-positive VDRL.

Complications of malaria can occur rapidly in untreated infection, especially when the agent is *P. falciparum*. Infections caused by any species of plasmodium can result in hemolysis, splenic enlargement, and occasionally splenic rupture. An immune-mediated glomerulonephritis is also common to all forms but tend to occur most often in *P. malariae* infection. With the ability to cause high parasitemia levels and sequestration with capillary sludging, *P. falciparum* infection can be fatal. Cerebral malaria—characterized by somnolence, coma, delirium, and seizures—is associated with mortality rates in excess of 20 percent. Reversible causes of encephalopathy must be excluded. The cerebrospinal fluid is usually normal with the exception of a slightly elevated opening pressure and protein concentration. A mild pleocytosis might also be present. Other life-threatening complications associated with *P. falciparum* infection include respiratory failure due to noncardiogenic acute pulmonary edema (similar to adult respiratory distress syndrome), renal failure (acute tubular necrosis), and severe metabolic abnormalities including lactic acidosis and profound hypoglycemia. Any target organ is susceptible to the effects of severe tissue hypoxia from the cytoadherence between the parasitized erythrocyte and the vascular endothelium of the host.

Persons at greatest risk for complications due to *P. falciparum* include the very young, the elderly, and pregnant women.

DIAGNOSIS

Certain clinical and epidemiologic clues provide supportive evidence for a presumptive diagnosis. The definitive diagnosis is established by the visualization of parasites on Giemsa-stained thick and thin blood smears. In early infection, especially infection due to *P. falciparum*, in which parasitized erythrocytes are sequestered from the bloodstream,

Table 85-3. Guidelines for Preparing Malaria Smears

1. Use scrupulously clean slides; manufacturers' precleaned slides may have residual debris.
2. Obtain a large drop of blood from the patient's finger using a blood lancet.
3. Place the cleaned surface of the slide against the drop of blood; with a quick circular motion, make a film the size of a dime. Do not mix excessively or distortion will result. The thick smear should be of such depth that newsprint would be barely legible. (Let the smear air-dry for 30 to 60 min.)
4. Obtain a small drop of blood from the patient's finger, and with a second clean slide, spread the blood gently over the slide. Air-dry the thin film, fix it with methyl alcohol, and stain it with Giemsa stain.
5. If the thin smear is negative, examine the thick smear. Once air-dried, the thick film should not be fixed prior to staining with Giemsa.

parasitemia may be undetectable. Also, parasitemia fluctuates over time. It generally is highest during chills and as the fever is on the rise. High fevers are schizonticidal.

In highly suspicious cases, failure to detect parasitemia is not an indication to withhold therapy. Delay in the diagnosis and treatment of malaria can have disastrous results. If parasitemia is not seen in the stained thin smear, a thick smear which concentrates blood cells may provide the diagnosis. Extreme care in the preparation of slides is important, since debris may result in false-positive smears. If parasites are not visualized, repeated smears should be obtained at least twice daily for 3 days to fully exclude malaria (Table 85-3). The two major questions to be answered by the blood smear are the degree of parasitemia present (correlates with prognosis) and whether or not *P. falciparum* is responsible for infection. Most patients with *P. falciparum* infection should be managed in the hospital setting as should any patient with at least 1 to 2 percent parasitemia. Clues to the diagnosis of *P. falciparum* infection include the presence of small ring forms with double chromatin knobs within the erythrocyte, multiply infected rings in individual red blood cells, a paucity of trophozoites and schizonts on smear, the pathognomonic crescent-shaped (banana-shaped) gametocyte, and parasitemia exceeding 4 percent. Repeated smears should be obtained twice daily to assess the efficacy of drug treatment .

Serologic measurement of antibodies against *Plasmodium* is of limited value.

THERAPY

Therapeutic decisions are based upon the severity of the illness, the agent, and whether the patient may be infected with chloroquine-resistant *P. falciparum.* If *P. falciparum* infection can be excluded, most persons can be managed in the ambulatory setting. Close follow-up, including repeated smears, is necessary. Patients with significant hemolysis or who have underlying severe chronic medical problems which can be aggravated by high fevers or hemolysis are best hospitalized. Infected infants and pregnant women are also best managed in the hospital.

The drug of choice for treatment of infection due to *P. vivax, P. ovale,* and *P. malariae* is chloroquine. Table 85-4 summarizes the treatment regimens for malaria. With treatment, the parasite load

Table 85-4. Treatment Regimens for Malaria

		Dosage Guidelines	
Clinical Setting	**Drug**	**Adults**	**Children**
Uncomplicated infection with *P. vivax, P. ovale, P. malariae,* and chloroquine-sensitive *P. falciparum*	Chloroquine phosphate	1-g load (600-mg base), then 500 mg (300-mg base) in 6 h, then 500 mg (300-mg base) per day for 2 days (total dose 2.5 g)	10 mg/kg base to maximum of 600 mg load, then 5 mg/kg base in 6 h and 5 mg/kg base per day for 2 days
	plus		
	Primaquine phosphate [a]	26.3 mg load (15-mg base) per day for 14 days upon completion of chloroquine therapy	0.3 mg/kg base for 14 days upon completion of chloroquine therapy
Uncomplicated infection with chloroquine-resistant *P. falciparum*	Quinine sulfate	650 mg PO tid for 5–7 days	8.3 mg/kg PO tid for 5–7 days [b]
	plus		
	Pyrimethamine-sulfadoxine (Fansidar)[c]	3 tablets (75 mg/1500 mg) PO × 1 dose	Over 2 months old:
	plus		>50 kg 3 tabs
			30–50 2 tabs
			15–29 1 tab
			10–14 ½ tab
			4–9 ¼ tab
	Doxycycline	100 mg PO bid for 10 days	Contraindicated in children <8 years of age
	or		
	Mefloquine	1250 mg PO × 1	1 tablet/10 kg PO × 1[d]
	plus		
	Doxycycline[e]	See above	See above
Complicated infection with chloroquine-resistant *P. falciparum*	Quinidine gluconate	24 mg/kg load (15-mg base) over 4 h, then 7.5 mg base/kg over 4 h q 8 h until patient stabilizes and is able to tolerate PO therapy (see above)	6.2 mg base/kg load over 2 h, then continuous infusion at rate of 0.0125 mg base/kg per min[f]
	plus		
	Doxycycline	100 mg IV q 12 h until tolerating PO therapy (see above)	Contraindicated in children <8 years of age

[a] Terminal treatment of *P. vivax* and *P. ovale* only.
[b] If unable to administer with doxycycline due to patient's age, extend treatment to full 10 days.
[c] Optional; of unlikely value if acquisition in area with Fansidar resistance.
[d] Not formally approved yet by FDA in this setting.
[e] Optional; many experts feel comfortable with mefloquine alone.
[f] Consult an expert in pediatric infectious disease immediately for guidance.

should decrease significantly within the first 24 to 48 h. No asexual forms of the parasite should be detectable 3 to 4 days after treatment is completed. Gametocytes, the sexual forms, may persist for several weeks after treatment and are not an indicator of treatment failure. Gametocytes do not cause disease in the human host. Chloroquine has no effect on the exoerythrocytic parasites which may be dormant in the liver with infection due to *P. vivax* and *P. ovale*. Unless terminal treatment is administered with primaquine, clinical relapses commonly occur. Primaquine should not be used in patients with G6PD deficiency because it may induce massive hemolysis of erythrocytes. Table 85-5 summarizes the commonly described adverse effects and precautions or contraindications of the antimalarial medications. Despite treatment with both chloroquine and primaquine, persistence of infection or relapse may occur.

Treatment of *P. falciparum* infection is generally best managed in a hospital setting, particularly if the level of parasitemia exceeds 1 to 2 percent. Unless one is certain that the patient could not have chloroquine-resistant *falciparum* infection (based upon geographic exposure, Table 85-2), it is best to assume the infecting strain is resistant to chloroquine and to initiate treatment with a combination of quinine and pyrimethamine-sulfadoxine and/or doxycycline. Mefloquine, a newly approved antimalarial compound, is also an effective therapy for chloroquine-resistant *P. falciparum* (and the asexual erythrocyte stages of the other plasmodium species).

Persons presenting with complications due to *P. falciparum* or with high parasitemia but unable to tolerate oral medications due to vomiting should receive intravenous medications. Supportive care is critical in these patients and includes close hemodynamic monitoring, use of judicious fluid replacement, correction of significant metabolic abnormalities, and additional support as needed (dialysis, mechanical ventilation, etc.). Exchange transfusions have been lifesaving in some patients with parasitemia in excess of 10 percent. Corticosteroids have not been shown to be of benefit in the treatment of cerebral malaria and should not be used. Quinidine is probably the intravenous drug of choice due not only to its widespread availability but also to its enhanced activity against *P. falciparum*. Parenteral quinine is only available from the Centers for Disease Control.

Quinine and quinidine are potent inducers of insulin release and may cause severe hypoglycemia. Sudden changes in orientation, sweating, tremor, tachycardia, or anxiety should prompt measure of plasma glucose concentration. Cinchona alkaloids are myocardial depressants, so cardiac monitoring is needed during administration. Terminal treatment with primaquine is not needed in patients with falciparum malaria due to the absence of dormant asexual forms in the liver.

PREVENTION

Malaria is largely preventable through use of personal protection measures and appropriate chemoprophylaxis. A recent study confirmed that travelers to malarious areas frequently do not use antimosquito measures or take antimalarial drugs. Between dusk and dawn, travelers should remain in well-screened areas, use mosquito nets if needed, and wear long-sleeved clothing. A pyrethrum-containing insect spray should be used during evening hours and before retiring to bed. Permethrin can be sprayed on clothing for additional protection and an insect repellent containing *N,N-diethylmetatoluamide (DEET)* applied to exposed skin.

Appropriate chemoprophylaxis depends upon where one will be traveling. If potential exposure to infected mosquitos is likely, prophylaxis is warranted even if such exposure will be brief. Table 85-6 summarizes the chemotherapeutic agents of choice. The Centers for Disease Control maintains a 24-h malaria hotline [(404) 332-4555], which provides up-to-date information on resistance patterns in countries. Chemoprophylaxis should generally be taken for 4 weeks following the exposure.

Lastly, even with the religious use of antimosquito measures and chemoprophylaxis, malaria can be contracted or can recur. For reasons discussed earlier, malaria must be considered whenever fever occurs

Table 85-5. Adverse Effects, Precautions, and Contraindications of Antimalarial Drugs

Drug	Minor Toxicity	Major Toxicity	Precaution or Contraindication
Chloroquine	Nausea and vomiting, diarrhea, pruritus, postural hypotension, rash, fever, headache, dizziness	Rare; hypotension and shock after parenteral therapy; retinopathy after prolonged use	Avoid in patients with severe psoriasis and some types of porphyria
Mefloquine	Nausea and vomiting, cramps, diarrhea, anorexia, dizziness, headaches, bradycardia	Rare unless there is underlying heart disease with bradycardia or the patient is on selected cardiotoxic medications (arrhythmias, arrest); acute toxic confusional states may also occur on occasion	Contraindicated during pregnancy and in infants; avoid if receiving quinine, quinidine, calcium-channel blockers or β blockers.
Fansidar	GI disturbances, phototoxicity, headaches, dizziness, skin rash	Fatal cutaneous eruptions reported, agranulocytosis.	Contraindicated during pregnancy and in infants or if allergic to sulfonamides or pyrimethamine
Tetracycline	GI disturbances, phototoxicity, vaginal candidiasis	Rare	Contraindicated during pregnancy, in children <8 years of age; may depress prothrombin time in patients receiving anticoagulants
Proguanil*	Generally well tolerated; may have oral sores, dizziness	Rare; anemia after prolonged use	Contraindicated in allergy to proguanil
Quinine or quinidine	Cinchonism (nausea and vomiting, headache, tinnitus, dizziness, visual disturbance), skin reactions	Hypotension, cardiac arrhythmias, hypoglycemia, Coombs'-positive hemolysis, abortions, neuromuscular paralysis (myasthenia)	Contraindicated in cardiac disease; cautiously in pregnancy, myasthenia gravis
Primaquine†	Nausea and vomiting, diarrhea, cramps, methemoglobulinemia	Massive hemolysis in patients with G6PD deficiency, exacerbation of SLE or RA	Contraindicated in G6PD deficiency, pregnancy

* Not used for acute therapy.

† Terminal treatment for *P. vivax* and *P. ovale* infections only.

Table 85-6. Recommended Chemoprophylactic Regimens for Prevention of Malaria[a]

Drug	Adult Dose	Pediatric Dose
TRAVEL TO AREA WHERE CRPF HAS NOT BEEN REPORTED		
Primary drug		
Chloroquine phosphate	300-mg base (500 mg salt) PO, 1/week	5 mg/kg base (8.3 mg/kg salt) PO, 1/week, up to adult dose
Second-line drugs		
Doxycycline	100 mg PO, qd	>8 years of age: 2 mg/kg PO qd up to adult dose
TRAVEL TO AREAS WHERE CRPF HAS BEEN REPORTED		
Primary drug		
Mefloquine	228-mg base (250 mg salt) PO, 1/week	>45 kg: 1 tab/week 31–45 kg: ¾ tab/week 20–30 kg: ½ tab/week 15–19 kg: ¼ tab/week
Second-line drugs		
Chloroquine	See above	See above
plus		
Fansidar[b]	See Table 85-5	See Table 85-5
plus		
Proguanil[c]	200 mg PO qd	> 10 years: adult dose 7–10 years: 150 mg/day 2–6 years 100 mg/day <2 years: 50 mg/day
or		
Doxycycline[d]	See above	See above

[a] For prolonged exposure in areas with *P. vivax* or *P. ovale*, primaquine (Table 85-5) should be added at completion of prophylaxis.

[b] Fansidar may be used for unexplained febrile illnesses if medical assistance is not readily available. See a physician as soon as possible.

[c] Some experts add proguanil to chloroquine prophylaxis for alternate prophylaxis in selected sub-Saharan countries (Angola, Burundi, Kenya, Malawi, Mozambique, Rwanda, Tanzania, Uganda, Zaire, Zambia).

[d] Doxycycline is the preferred second-line agent for travels where Fansidar resistance is prevalent such as the Amazon-basin area; the sub-Saharan countries listed above; and Southeast Asia, Burma, and Papua New Guinea.

in someone who has traveled to a malarious area or who has received "successful" therapy in the past.

BIBLIOGRAPHY

Bygbjeig IC, Schapira A, Flachs H, et al: Mefloquine resistance of falciparum malaria from Tanzania enhanced by treatment. *Lancet* 1:774, 1983.

Centers for Disease Control: *Health Information for International Travel 1990*. HHS Publication No. (CDC)90–8280, 1990

Centers for Disease Control. Intravenous quinidine gluconate in the treatment of severe *Plasmodium falciparum* infections. *MMWR* 34:371, 1986.

Centers for Disease Control: *Malaria Surveillance Annual Summary 1988*. U.S. Government Printing Office 90–731–011(09187), 1990.

Hoffman SL, Rustama D, Punjabi NH, et al: High-dose dexamethasone in quinine-treated patients with cerebral malaria: A double-blind, placebo-controlled trial. *J Infect Dis* 158:325, 1988.

Krogstad DJ, Herwaldt BL, Schlesinger PH. Antimalarial Agents: Specific treatment regimens. *Antimicrob Agents Chemother* 32:957, 1988.

Lobel HO: Malaria and use of prevention measures among United States travelers, in Steffen R, Lobel HO, Waworth J, et al (eds): *Travel Medicine*. Berlin, Springer-Verlag, 1989.

Okitolonda W, Dellacollette C, Mallengrean M, et al: High incidence of hypoglycemia in African patients treated with intravenous quinine for severe malaria. *Br J Med* 295:716, 1987.

Peterson C, Leech JH. Diagnosis, treatment and prevention of malaria due to *Plasmodium falciparum*, in Leech JH, Sande MA, Root RK (eds): *Parasitic Infections*. New York, Churchill Livingstone, 1988.

Phillips RE, Warrell DA, White NJ, et al: Intravenous quinidine for the treatment of severe falciparum malaria. *N Engl J Med* 312:1273, 1985.

Rieckmann KH, Davis DR, Hutton DC. *Plasmodium vivax* resistance to chloroquine? *Lancet* 2:1183, 1989.

Scuderi P, Sterling KE, Lam KS, et al: Raised serum levels of tumour necrosis factor in parasitic infection. *Lancet* 2:1364, 1986.

White NJ, Looareesuwan S, Warrell DA, et al: Quinine loading dose in cerebral malaria. *Am J Trop Med Hyg* 32:1, 1983.

White NJ, Plorde JJ: Malaria, in Wilson JD, Braunwald E, Isselbacher KJ, et al (eds): *Harrison's Principles of Internal Medicine*, ed 12. New York, McGraw-Hill, 1991.

World Health Organization: *International Travel and Health—Vaccination Requirements and Health Advice*. Geneva, Switzerland, 1991.

86
COMMON PARASITIC INFECTIONS
Harold Osborn

INTRODUCTION

Despite significant advances in medical knowledge and technology over the last half century, parasitic disease remains prevalent worldwide. It is estimated that 200 million people, living mostly in the rural tropics, suffer from schistosomiasis and that hookworm infects approximately a quarter of the world's population. Parasites such as *Ascaris* and *Enterobius* each infect 1 billion people.

In the United States parasitic disease is becoming increasingly recognized. In addition to the persistence of endemic parasites in this country, three factors account for this trend: (1) immigration to the United States of infected individuals from countries such as Asia, Africa, and Latin America; (2) increased travel by Americans, particularly to the underdeveloped parts of the world; and (3) the rise of parasitic infections among immunosuppressed patients, especially those afflicted with the human immunodeficiency virus (HIV-1).

Arcaris is said to infect 3 million people in North America, while *Enterobius* infection rates among United States children vary from 10 to 45 percent. Serologic surveys in the United States have demonstrated that 20 to 70 percent of the population have antibodies to *Toxoplasma* and over 90 percent have antibodies to *Pneumocystis carinii*. These two parasites can cause significant morbidity and mortality when they reactivate in immunosuppressed individuals and create opportunistic infections.

The agents that cause parasitic diseases belong to three major groups: helminths (worms), protozoa, and arthropods. The multicellular helminths include nematodes (roundworms), cestodes (flatworms), and trematodes (flukes). The protozoa are single-celled organisms which cause a variety of diseases ranging from malaria to amoebiasis. Arthropods are classified as ectoparasites and are medically important as obligatory intermediate hosts and as mechanical vectors in many diseases. This chapter will review diseases caused by helminths and protozoa. Malaria is discussed in Chapter 85.

HISTORY

The recognition of parasitic disease begins with the elicitation of a careful history. Specifically, the clinician should inquire about travel to or immigration from high-risk areas. Parasites flourish in warm, moist climates where sanitation is poor and where many of the people share a low socioeconomic status and have inadequate nutrition. Children are infected with parasites more frequently than adults because of their oral behavior, poor hygiene, and inability to ward off arthropod vectors.

Parasitic disease should be considered in any patient with unexplained fever, abdominal pain, diarrhea, skin ulcers, rash, or eosinophilia. The history should include dates of travel or immigration, destination or country of origin, living conditions and activities. Certain specific areas of the world may implicate particular parasitic agents. Hmong tribesmen, who came to this country from Indochina in large numbers in 1979 and 1980, often harbor *Paragonimus westermani* (lung fluke), while visitors to Leningrad or the Rockies may return with *Giardia*. The history should also include questions about sexual orientation and contacts, drug use, past illnesses, and a complete review of systems. The use of pretravel medications, including antimalarial and antidiarrheal agents, should be elicited.

The presence of risk factors can provide a clue to specific parasitic diseases (see Table 86-1). Recently cases of acute Chagas' disease (trypanosomiasis) and babesiosis following blood transfusions have been described in the United States and Canada. Institutionalized patients may suffer from amoebiasis and can become infected with *Hymenolepis nana* (the most common tapeworm in the United States) or *Giardia*. Immunocompromised hosts, most notably those with AIDS, are susceptible to inflection by *Strongyloides, Toxoplasma, Cryptosporidium*, and *Pneumocystis carinii*. Finally, the consumption of raw food has been associated with a variety of parasitic diseases including fish, pork, and beef tapeworm.

SYMPTOMS

Unfortunately symptoms may be nonspecific and the latency period between exposure and symptom appearance may be years. Symptoms can be acute or chronic, specific or vague. Parasitic disease can present with relatively common complaints such as headache, fever, cough, and malaise or with acute, life-threatening complications such as seizures, hemoptysis, melena, and intestinal obstruction. A differential diagnosis can be made on the basis of the history and knowledge of typical symptoms associated with different parasitic agents (see Table 86-2).

Parasites differ in their pathogenicity and in their capacity to produce invasive or systemic disease. The subclass Coccidia, for example, incudes both *Toxoplasma* and *Isospora*. However, *Isospora* is unable to invade the intestinal mucosa and thus produces only an enterocolitis, while *Toxoplasma* crosses the intestine and produces severe systemic illness.

Sometimes different forms of the same parasite differ in their ability to cause illness. The adult form of *Trichinella spiralis* remains in the intestine, while the larval form crosses and migrates to striated and cardiac muscle. Amoebiasis can result in both intestinal and visceral infections. Pathogenicity may vary among different strains within a genus. Infection with *Entamoeba* can result in an asymptomatic cyst carrier state or hepatic abscesses, depending on the strain involved. Table 86-3 shows the most commonly used antiparasitic drugs.

HELMINTHS

Nematodes (Roundworms)

Nematodes are cylindrical, unsegmented, elongated white worms. Their mode of entry into the human host varies from ingestion of eggs (*Ascaris* and *Enterobius*), to penetration of the skin (*Necator, Ancylostoma*, and *Strongyloides*), to inoculation by insect bite (*Wucheria*).

Ascaris

Ascaris lumbricoides has a worldwide distribution with an estimated 3 million Americans infected each year. Its life span untreated is 2 to 7 years. Larval invasion follows the ingestion of *Ascaris* eggs, and during this stage the parasite migrates through the lungs. Patients can present with fever, cough, dyspnea, hemoptysis, and eosinophilia. The diagnosis is made by finding eggs or occasionally the adult worm in the stool. Serological tests including bentonite flocculation, ELISA,

Table 86-1. Risk Factors for Parasitic Disease

Blood transfusion: *Plasmodium* species, *Trypanosoma, Babesia, Toxoplasma*
IV drug use: *Plasmodium species*
Homosexuality: *Entamoeba* (often seen after colonic irrigation therapy), *Giardia*
Immunocompromised host: *Toxoplasma, Cryptosporidium, Pneumocystis, Strongyloides*
Institutionalization: *H. nana, E. histolytica, Giardia*
Pica: *Toxocara* (visceral larva migrans), hookworm (*N. Americanus*)
Consumption of raw food:
  Sushi, sashimi, gefilte fish—*Diphyllobothrium*
  Pork—*T. solium, Trichinella, Sarcocystis*
  Beef—*T. saginata, Toxoplasma, Sarcocystis*

Table 86-2. Symptoms of Parasitic Disease

Symptom	Possible Cause
Hemoptysis	*Ascaris, Paragonimus, Echinococcus*
Meningitis	*Trichinella, Toxocara, Nageleria, Acanthamoeba, Trypanosoma, Malaria*
Malaria	(*P. falciparum*), primary amebic meningoencephalitis
Urticaria	*Ascaris, Strongyloides, Dracunculus, Trichinella, Fasciola*
Diarrhea	*Hookworm, Strongyloides, Trichuris, Trichinella, Schistosoma, Fasciola, Fasciolopsis, Taenia, Hymenolepis, Entamoeba, Giardia, Dientamoeba, Palantidium, Leishmania donovani*
Abdominal pain	*Ascaris,* hookworm, *Trichuris, Schistosoma, Entamoeba, Clonorchis, Fasciola, Taenia, Hymenolepis, Diphyllobothrium, Giardia*
Pruritus	*Enterobius, Trichuris, filariae (Onchocerca volvulus), Dientamoeba, Leishmania*
Nausea and vomiting	*Ascaris, Trichuris, Trichinella, Taenia, Entamoeba, Giardia, Leishmania*
Seizures	*Hymenolepis, Trichinella, Paragonimus,* tapeworm (*Echinococcus, Cysticercus*)
Anemia	*Plasmodium* species, *Babesia,* hookworm (*N. americanus, Ancylostoma duodenale*), Trichuris, *Diphyllobothrium, Leishmania donovani*
Pneumonia	*Ascaris, Strongyloides, Trichinella,* filariae (*Wuchereria bancrofti, Brugia malayi*), fluke (*Paragonimus westermani*)
Myocardial disease	*Trichinella, Taenia, Trypanosoma (T. cruzi)*
Conjunctivitis and keratitis	*Trichinella,* filariae (*O. volvulus*) Taenia, Trypanosoma
Jaundice	*Toxoplasma, fluke (Clonorchis sinensis, Opisthorchis viverrini), Plasmodium* species
Asthma	*Ascaris*
Skin ulcers	*Dracunculus,* hookworm (Ancylostoma duodenale), Leishmania donovani, Trypanosoma
Splenomegaly	*Babesia, Toxoplasma, Plasmodium* species
Intestinal obstruction	*Arcaris, Strongyloides,* fluke (*Fasciolopsis buski*), *Taenia, Diphyllobothrium*
Eosinophilia	*Srongyloides,* hookworm, *Trichuris, Dracunculus, Fasciola, Toxocara, Ascaris, Trichinella,* filariae (*Wuchereria bancrofti, Brugia malayi*) *Hymnenolepis, Schistosoma,* fluke (*Paragonimus westermani, Clonorchis sinesis, Fasciolopsis leuski*), *Taenia*
Fever	*Ascaris, Toxocara,* hookworm, *Trichuris, Trichinella,* filariae (*Wuchereria bancrofti*), *Schistosoma,* fluke (*Clonorchis sinensis*), *Fasciola, Entamoeba, Giardia, Trypanosoma, Leishmania donovani, Babesia, Plasmodium* species
Hepatomegaly	*Trypanosoma, Leishmania donovani, Toxocara, Schistosoma,* fluke (*Clonorchis sinensis, Opisthorchis viverrini, Fasciola*), tapeworm (*Echinococcus*), *Plasmodium* species
Edema	*Trichinella,* filariae (*Wuchereria bancrofti*) *Fasciolopsis, Trypanosoma*

and indirect hemagglutination may be helpful. Treatment is with mebendazole or pyrantel pamonate. Intestinal obstruction may necessitate surgery, especially in children.

Enterobius (Pinworm)

Adult *Enterobius* (pinworm) resides in the cecum, appendix, ileum, and ascending colon after its eggs are ingested. The gravid female migrates to the anus especially at night where it causes intense pruritus. Autoinfection with hand-to-mouth transmission is possible after scratching. Whether or not *Enterobius* can cause appendicitis has not yet been settled. A host of problems from vaginitis to enuresis have been attributed to infection with *Enterobius* but none too convincingly. Pinworm infection is most prevalent in temperate climates during the winter and fall. The diagnosis is confirmed with cellophane tape swab of the anus. All family members should be examined. Treatment is with pyrantel pamoate or mebendazole and should be repeated after 2 weeks. All those living in close contact with the patient should be treated.

Hookworm

Necator americanus (American hookworm) prevails in the southern United States and is often seen in immigrants from warmer climates. Infection is associated with the use of human fertilizer and the lack of shoes and latrines. Since each worm can withdraw 0.03 to 0.2 mL of blood a day, infection often leads to chronic anemia. Pica and geophagy are often seen in infected children. Patients may present with cough, low-grade fever, abdominal pain, diarrhea, weakness, weight loss, guaiac-positive stools, and eosinophilia. The diagnosis is made by finding ova in the stool. In mild infections multiple stool specimens or concentration techniques may be necessary. The parasite burden can be estimated using Beaver's stool or Kato's slide smear method. Infections with less then 2100 eggs per gram of feces (< 50 adult worms) are usually not hemalotogically important, while infections with over 11,000 eggs per gram result in a significant anemia. Hookworm is best treated with mebendazole or pyrantel pamoate.

Strongyloides (Threadworms)

Adult threadworms reside in the mucosa of the small intestine. Since entry of the parasite is through the skin, penetration can lead to allergic manifestations, pruritus, and an erythematous rash. Migration throughout the lungs can produce cough, dyspnea, and pneumonia, while the intestinal phase is manifested by abdominal pain, diarrhea with mucus and blood, and eosinophilia. Larval migration in the skin produces cutaneous larva migrans. Fatalities may occur in the elderly and the immunocompromised (those with AIDS, leprosy, nephrotic syndrome, hepatic disease, and lymphoproliferative disorders, and those on steroids). *Strongyloides* is probably a hyperinfection rather than an opportunistic infection. The diagnosis is confirmed by finding larvae in the stool. Occasionally a formol-ether concentration method or duodenal aspiration may be necessary. Various stages of the parasite may be found in the sputum. An upper GI series may reveal a deformed duodenal bulb, and *Strongyloides* may be confused with ulcer disease. Treatment is with thiabendazole.

Trichuris trichiura

Trichuris trichiura, like *Ascaris,* is found in rural communities in the southern United States. The infection is most often acquired in childhood because the ova are deposited in the soil where children play and defecate freely. The adult worm resides in the cecum. Patients complain of anorexia, insomnia, abdominal pain (including pain in the right upper quadrant), fever, flatulence, diarrhea, weight loss, and pruritus, and may have eosinophilia and a microcytic hypochromic anemia. *Trichuris* can result in colitis or rectal prolapse in children. The diagnosis is made with the finding of ova in the stool. Mebendazole is the treatment of choice.

Trichinella Spiralis

Trichinosis is common in Mexico and the United States and results from the consumption of infected pork and, less commonly, bear and walrus meat. Autopsy studies have revealed an infection rate in human diaphragms of 4 to 5 percent. In the early stages of infection with *Trichinella spiralis,* the patient may present with acute myocarditis, nonsuppurative meningitis, bronchopneumonia, or catarrhal enteritis. The primary lesions are in striated muscle. Clinical symptoms depend on the number of worms ingested, the number of larvae produced, and the site of invasion. Patients may present with nausea and vomiting, diarrhea, fever, urticaria, periorbital edema, splinter hemorrhages,

Table 86-3. Commonly Used Antiparasitic Drugs

Drug	First-Line Agent	Alternative Agent	Side Effects
Albendazole	Tapeworm (*E. granulosus, Cysticecus*)	*Capillaria*	Diarrhea, abdominal pain
Amphotericin B	Amebic meningoencephalitis (*Nageleria*)	Leishmania (*L. braziliensis, L. mexicana*)	Fever, headache, anorexia, nausea, diarrhea, muscle and joint pain, azotemia, anemia, RTA, leukopenia
Cholorquine	Plasmodium species (except resistant *P. falciparum*)		Pruritis, vomiting, headache, confusion, skin eruptions, myalgias, EOM palsies
Iodoquinol	*Entamoeba* (*E. histolytica*)	*Balantidium*	Rash, acne, enlarged thyroid, nausea, diarrhea, anal pruritis, rarely: optic atrophy, peripheral neuropathy
Ivermectin	Filariae (*O. volvulus*)		Fever, pruritis, tender nodes, bone and joint pain, headache
Lindane		Lice, scabies	Eczema, conjunctivitis, aplastic anemia
Mebendazole	*Angiostrongylus, Ascaria, Capillaria, Enterobius,* filariae (*Mansonella Perstans*), *Gnathosoma, Trichuris*	*Leishmania*	Diarrhea, abdominal pain, agranulocytosis
Metronidazole	Entamoeba (*E. histolytica, E. polecki*), *Dracunculus, Trichomonas*	*Balantidium, Giardia*	Nausea, headache, dry mouth, reaction with alcohol, rarely: seizures, ataxia, leukopenia, pancreatitis
Nicosamide	Fluke (*F. buski*), tapeworm (*Diphyllobothrium, Taenia, Dipylidium*)	Tapeworm (*Hymenolepis*)	Nausea, abdominal pain
Paromomycin	*Dientamoeba*	*E. histolytica*	GI disturbance, rarely: eighth nerve and renal damage, GI damage
Pentamidine isethionate	*Leishmania* (*L. donovani*)	*Pneumocystis, Trypanosoma* (*T. brucei*)	Hypotension, hypoglycemia, vomiting, blood dyscrasias, renal damage, GI disturbance
Piperazine			
Praziquantel	Fluke, *Schistosoma*, tapeworm (*Hymenolepsis, Cysticecus*)		Malaise, headache, dizziness, abdominal upset, fever, eosinophilia
Primaquine phosphate	*P. vivax, P. orale* (prevention of relapses only)		G6PD hemolysis, neutropenia, GI disturbance
Pryantel pamoate	*Ascaria, Enterobius,* hookworm, *Trichostrongylus*		GI disturbances, headache, dizziness, rash, fever
Pyrimethamine	Chloroquine-resistant *P. falciparum, Toxoplasma*		Blood dyscrasias, folate deficiency, rarely: rash, vomiting, seizures, shock
Quinacrine	*Giardia*		Dizziness, headache, vomiting, diarrhea, yellow skin, toxic psychosis, insomnia, rash, blood dyscrasias
Quinine sulfate	*Babesia*, chloroquine-resistent *P. falciparum*		Cinchonism, hemolytic anemia, blood dyscrasias, photosensitivity, hypoglycemia, arrhythmias, hypotension
Stibogluconate sodium	*Leishmania*		Muscle pain, joint stiffness, nausea, diarrhea, rash, pruritus, liver and heart damage, bradycardia, rarely: hemolytic anemia, sudden death
Thiabendazole	*Angiostrongylus, Strongyloides,* visceral larva migrans, cutaneous larva migrans	*Capillaria, Dracunculus, Trichostrongylus*	Nausea, vertigo, rash, leukopenia, hallucinations, erythema multiforme, Stevens-Johnson syndrome, rarely: shock, seizures
Trimethoprim-sulfamethoxazole	*Isospora, Pneumocystis*		Nausea, anorexia, urticaria, agranulocytosis, Stevens-Johnson syndrome, hepatitis

Source: Adapted from Drugs for parasitic infections. *Med. Lett.* 32:23, 1990.

myalgia, muscle spasm, stiff neck, headache, and psychiatric disturbances. The periorbital edema is pathognomonic.

Laboratory manifestations of trichinosis include leucocytosis, eosinophilia, elevated CPK, and ECG changes. The diagnosis can be confirmed with latex agglutination, skin test, and a complement fixation or bentonite flocculation test available from the Centers for Disease Control. A new ELISA test is very specific and sensitive after the third week of infection. Biopsy of tender muscle may be helpful after the fourth week. Since *T. spiralis* encysts in striated muscle, stool examination is not helpful after the initial gastrointestinal phase in making the diagnosis. The differential diagnosis includes staphyococcal and salmonella food poisoning, shigellosis, and amoebiasis. Mebendazole is indicated for treatment of the intestinal phase but may be ineffective after encystment. Steroids are indicated for CNS disease and myocarditis but are not advocated routinely since their use can increase the number of circulating larvae. Most cases are mild and never come to medical attention.

Trematodes (Flukes)

Trematodes are leaflike, symmetical flatworms lacking a body cavity but possessing a ventral sucker to hold their position. They live in intermediate hosts like snails, crabs, and fish and shed their eggs from the human host in the feces (*Schistosoma, Clonorchis, Fasciola*), urine (*S. haematobium*) or sputum (*Paragonimus*).

Schistosoma

Schistosomes penetrate the skin, creating a papular pruritic rash. The adult form resides in the venous system. Symptoms of acute disease—fever, lymphadenopathy, and hepatosplenomegaly (so-called "Katayama fever")—are rarely seen. More typically patients present in the chronic stage with granulomas in the liver (portal hypertension) and bladder (obstructive hydroureter). Patients may present with diarrhea, abdominal pain, melena, hepatospenomegaly, hematemesis, and in the late stages, ascites and liver failure. With *S. haematobium* dysuria and hematuria may be found. The diagnosis can be confirmed by finding eggs in the feces or on rectal biopsy. Treatment is with praziquantel.

Cestoda (Flatworms)

The cestodes are flatworms commonly referred to as tapeworms. They have a scolex or head equipped with suckers or hooks. Cestodes grow by segmentation, extending proglottids from the neck.

Taenia

Taenia solium (pork tapeworm) is occasionally encountered in the United States today in immigrants or visitors from Central America and the Middle East. *Taenia saginata* (beef tapeworm) is seen more often, especially in those who consume raw beef (e.g., steak tartare). Adult worms live in the small intestine. Infected patients can be asymptomatic or present with nausea and vomiting, headache, abdominal pain, pruritus, constipation, diarrhea, and intestinal obstruction. The larval stage of *T. solium* can cause clinical disease (cysticercosis) which can be serious and sometimes fatal. *Taenia* cysts may be found in subcutaneous tissue, the eye, the brain, and the heart. Radiographs of the soft tissues may reveal curvilinear calcifications indicative of cysts, and cysts can be seen in the meninges and brain parenchyma on CT scanning. The diagnosis is made by finding gravid proglottids in the stool. An ELISA or hemagglutination reaction may be helpful, but both can be falsely negative if the cysts are calcified. Treatment is with niclosamide or praziquantel.

Diphyllobothrium

Diphyllobothrium (fish tapeworm) has been reported in the Pacific Northwest, Minnesota, Michigan, and other areas where raw fish (e.g., sushi and sashimi) and gefilte fish are consumed. *Diphyllobothrium* can compete with the host for vitamin B_{12}, and thus patients can present with pernicious anemia. Treatment is the same as for *Taenia*.

PROTOZOA

Amebas

Amebiasis, which is caused by *Entamoeba histolytica,* occurs worldwide and is associated with poor sanitation. Outbreaks have been reported in institutions for the mentally retarded and in the homosexual community. Amoebae inhabit the cecum and large intestine, where they cause ulcers and diffuse inflammation which can mimic ulcerative colitis. An ameboma can rarely develop in the liver and present as a liver abscess. Approximately half of all infected patients are asymptomatic. Symptoms include nausea and vomiting, anorexia, diarrhea, fever, abdominal pain, and leucocytosis. Protozoan infections, amebiasis included, do not produce eosinophilia. The diagnosis is established with stool testing including postcathartic stools and concentration and staining techniques. Stool specimens should be fixed in polyvinyl alcohol, formalin, or merthiolate-iodine-formalin. Serological tests (ELISA and indirect hemagglutination reaction) can be helpful in the presence of extraintestinal disease. Treatment is with metronidazole followed by iodoquinol.

Giardia

Giardia is probably the most common intestinal parasite in the United States. It inhabits the duodenum and upper jejunum where the alkaline pH creates a favorable milieu. Cysts are ingested in fecally contaminated water or are passed by hand-to-mouth transmission. Symptoms depend on the duration of infection at the time of presentation. Patients may complain of explosive, foul-smelling diarrhea, flatus, abdominal distension, fatigue, fever, and weight loss or general debilitation. Stools should be examined with routine and concentration techniques. Occasionally duodenal aspiration or small-bowel biopsy is necessary to make the diagnosis. The drug of choice for treatment is quinacrine.

Trypanosoma

American *Trypanosoma* (*T. cruzi*) causes Chagas' disease, while three strains of African *Trypanosoma* cause sleeping sickness. Chagas' disease is usually transmitted by the reduvid (kissing) bug, but infection can also follow breast-feeding and blood transfusion, as has occurred in the United States. A nodular swelling or chagoma develops at the site of inoculation following a bite. The acute phase of the disease can last 2 to 3 months, and patients present with fever, headache, anorexia, conjunctivitis, and myocarditis. Infants can develop a meningocephalitis, and heart involvement can lead to CHF and ventricular aneurysms. The organism can attack the myenteric plexus of the GI tract resulting in megacolon. Laboratory abnormalities include anemia, leucocytosis, an elevated sedimentation rate, and ECG changes (PR interval, T-wave changes, heart block, and arrhythmias). During the acute phase serological tests are helpful and *trypomastigotes* can be seen on a peripheral smear. In the chronic phase the diagnosis is made with a complement fixation test or biopsy of the liver, spleen, or bone marrow. Treatment is with nifurtimox.

Babesia

Babesia is a protozoan which, like *Plasmodium* species, possesses an erythrocytic phase. It is transmitted by *Ixodes* ticks and occasionally by blood transfusion. Babesiosis has been reported in Europe and in the northeastern United States (especially Nantucket, Massachusetts, and Long Island). Babesiosis in the northeastern United States is invariably caused by the murine species, *B. microti,* and is transmitted by the deer tick, *Ixodes dammini,* which also serves as a vector for Lyme disease. Patients may present with intermittent fever, splenomegaly, hemolysis, and jaundice. Infection can be fatal in splenectomized patients but is apparently not increased in incidence in immunocompromised patients. Diagnosis can be made on a Giemsa-stained peripheral smear, but occasionally *Babesia* smear can be confused for the ring forms of *P. falciparum* malaria. Babesiosis can simulate rickettsial diseases like Rocky Mountain spotted fever and Lyme disease. Treatment is with clindamycin and quinine.

Protozoan Infections in the Immunocompromised Host

Respiratory Tract

Pneumonia occurs commonly in immunocompromised patients and is often due to *Pneumocystis carinii*. Since most normal children have antibodies to *P. carinii, P. carinii* pneumonia probably represents a reactivation of a latent infection. The natural habitat and mode of transmission of *P. carinii* are poorly understood. Patients present acutely with fever, dyspnea, a nonproductive cough and scant rales. Arterial blood gases may reveal hypoxia or an increased alveolar-arterial gradient. Early, the chest x-ray may be normal. Later, the classical appearance is of symmetrical interstitial infiltrates in the mid and lower lung zones. *Pneumocystis carinii* occurs in premature and debilitated infants, AIDS patients, those receiving organ transplants, and those with inherited immune deficiencies. Diagnosis is usually made by obtaining tissue from lung biopsy. The specimen should be stained with methenamine–silver nitrate or toluidine blue. Serological tests are of limited value, since so many normal individuals have antibodies to *P. carinii.* Treatment is with trimethoprim-sulfamethoxazole or pentamidine isethionate.

Gastrointestinal Tract

Gastrointestinal disease in the immunocompromised host is often due to *Cryptosporidium,* a small intestinal parasite belonging to the subclass Coccidia, which includes *Toxoplasma, Isospora,* and *Plasmodium.* The recently available ELISA assay indicates a high rate of subclinical infection in the general population. In the person with an uncompromised immune system, following a 14-day incubation period, one can see watery diarrhea, abdominal pain, flatulence, and fever. GI disease due to *Cryptosporiduim,* which forms part of the spectrum of traveler's diarrhea, is usually self-limited. In contrast, immunocompromised patients experience prolonged, intractable diarrhea with fever, malabsorption, and severe weight loss. The diagnosis is now more easily made with a modified Ziehl-Neelsen acid-fast stain or Kinyoun stain. An ELISA assay is also available for the detection of antibodies to *Cryptosporidium.* A vast array of antimicrobial and antidiarrheal agents have been tried without much success in the treatment of cryptosporidiosis. Spiramycin has a limited effect in some patients. Recently octreotide has been used to control the diarrhea but not the infection. The high rate of recurrence and relapse in this disease is probably related more to the underlying immunodeficiency. *Isospora belli* is another protozoan which can cause significant gastrointestinal disease. As with *Cryptosporidium,* infection with *Isospora* occurs after ingestion of oocysts in contaminated food or water and following sexual contact. Symptoms may vary from acute gastroenteritis in the immunointact individual to severe, protracted diarrhea in the immunocompromised. Characteristic oocysts can be detected in the stool with acid-fast stains. Treatment is with trimethoprim-sulfamethoxazole.

Central Nervous System

Toxoplasma is an intracellular parasite carried by cats and other intermediate hosts which can cause significant disease in the immunocompromised patient. Infection can come from the ingestion of oocysts or undercooked meat, by placental transfer, following organ transplant, or during a blood transfusion. Acquired toxoplasmosis is usually asymptomatic. During acute infection, transient lymphadenopathy and splenomegaly may be present. Reactivation can result in encephalitis, chorioretinitis, myocarditis, and pneumonia. Symptoms of cerebral toxoplasmosis can include severe headache, seizures, confusion, and lethargy. Focal deficits may appear, and cerebellar, brain stem, and cranial nerve lesions may be seen. Making the diagnosis may be difficult. Ventricular fluid, brain tissue, or the buffy coat from a blood sample may be inoculated into test animals. The Sabin-Feldman dye test is fairly specific. An ELISA test is now available but is less reliable in AIDS patients due to low antibody titers. CT scanning may reveal characteristic intracerebral lesions with ring enhancement following the use of contrast. Treatment is with pyrimethamine plus trisulfapyrimidine or sulfadiazine.

BIBLIOGRAPHY

Cook GC: Opportunistic parasitic infections associated with AIDS: Parasitology, clinical presentation, diagnosis and management. *Q J Med* 65:967, 1987.

Drugs for parasitic infections. *Med Lett* 32:23, 1990.

Gibler WB: Parasitology: The emergent presentation, in Rosen P, Baker FJ, Barkin RM, et al (eds): *Emergency Medicine.* St. Louis, Mosby, 1988, pp 1013–1031.

Grant IH, Gold JWM, Wittner M, et al: Transfusion-associated acute Chagas disease acquired in the United States. *Ann Int Med* 111:849, 1989.

Mandell WF, Neu HC: Parasitic Infections: Therapeutic considerations. *Med Clin North Am* 72:669, 1988.

Most H: Treatment of parasitic infections of travelers and immigrants. *N Engl J Med* 310:298, 1984.

Tanowitz HB, Weiss LM, Wittner M: Diagnosis and treatment of protozoan diarrheas. *Am J Gastroenterol* 83:339, 1988.

Thomson RB, Haas RA, Thompson JH: Intestinal parasites: The necessity of examining multiple stool specimens. *Mayo Clin Proc* 59:641, 1984.

Wittner M, Otteren EA, Mahmoud A, et al: Parasitic diseases in Rudolph AM (ed.): *Pediatrics,* ed 18. Norwalk, Connecticut, Appleton and Lange, 1987, pp 637–693.

87
TICK-BORNE DISEASE

Bruce S. Auerbach

Ticks (phylum Arthropoda, class Arachnida, order Acarina) are hematophagous parasites found almost worldwide in wilderness areas. Their requirement for several blood meals during their lifetime tends to make them particularly prevalent where there are large congregations of warmblooded animals.

Ticks are particularly well adapted for obtaining blood. In addition to the body proper, there is a head (capitulum) whose barbed mouthparts are capable of burrowing into and imbedding themselves under the skin, allowing its hypostome (the needlelike structure through which the tick obtains its blood meal and can infect its host) to penetrate the source of blood. Once implanted, these barbed parts are quite difficult to remove.

There are three families of ticks; two of these, the Ixodidae (hard ticks) and Argasidae (soft ticks), are known to cause human and animal disease. Starting as an egg, all ticks go through three stages during their growth: larva, nymph, and adult. Ticks generally feed (take a blood meal) between each stage and can, therefore, be infectious at any stage. Depending upon the tick, feeding may occur over several hours to several days. In addition, it may take some ticks up to 24 h to find a preferred site of implantation. These facts are of significance when looking at ways to prevent tick-borne disease.

Ticks can transmit a great number of diseases, including Lyme disease, Rocky Mountain spotted fever (RMSF), tick paralysis, tularemia, relapsing fever, and babesiosis and are, in fact, second only to mosquitoes as vectors of human disease. The diseases they cause can be secondary to the transmission of viral or bacterial agents or the result of envenomation.

Lyme Disease

Currently the most frequently transmitted tick-borne disease, Lyme disease was first described in 1977 after an epidemic of oligoarticular arthritis broke out in three Connecticut communities surrounding the town whose name it bears. Its causative agent, the spirochete *Borrelia burgdorferi,* was discovered in 1982, in conjunction with *Ixodes dammini* (the deer tick), which is endemic to the Lyme, Connecticut, area. Subsequently, this spirochete was isolated from the blood, CSF, and skin lesions of patients with the clinical syndrome, confirming it as the etiologic agent. While the *I. dammini* tick appears to be the most common vector, other ixodid ticks have been implicated (e.g., *I. pacificus, Amblyomma americanum,* and *Dermacentor variabilis*). The ticks feed on the deer mouse, deer rabbits, and domesticated animals. Females may transmit the spirochete transovarially to their offspring.

Although initially thought to be a disease isolated to the northeastern United States, Lyme disease has now been reported in 33 of the 50 states (with the highest frequency in the five northeastern states of Connecticut, Massachusetts, New Jersey, New York, and Rhode Island and the two upper midwestern states of Minnesota and Wisconsin), as well as on every continent except Antarctica.

The large majority of cases occur between late spring and late summer, with the peak incidence in July. Less than a third of patients recall having had a tick bite, probably because the adult *I. dammini* tick is only the size of a sesame seed, and the nymph stage (responsible for as many as 50 percent of the cases) is only the size of a poppy seed. The number of reported cases has increased dramatically from approximately 500 cases in 1982 to almost 7997 in 1990.

Clinical Presentation

Lyme disease is a multisystemic disorder which is generally divided into three stages, although there may be remissions between any stage.

Stage I

Stage I is most characteristically identified by the presence of erythema chronicum migrans (ECM), an annular, erythematous lesion with central clearing which expands from the tick bite lesion site. This occurs 3 to 32 days (median 7) after the bite. It may be accompanied by generalized malaise and fatigue (80 percent of patients), headache (64 percent), fever and chills (59 percent), stiff neck and arthralgias (48 percent), and a multitude of other generalized constitutional symptoms. The ECM fades an average of 4 weeks after its appearance.

Stage II

Stage II begins approximately 4 weeks after the onset of ECM and may last for several months. Approximately 10 percent of untreated patients develop neurologic manifestations, including headache, meningoencephalitis, or unilateral or bilateral facial nerve palsy. Other findings of this stage may be radiculoneuropathy, ophthalmitis, and first-, second-, or third-degree cardiac atrioventricular block.

Stage III

Approximately 60 percent of untreated ECM patients develop arthritis several weeks to years after onset of skin lesions (median 4 weeks). This presents as brief, recurrent episodes of migratory oligoarthritis with periods of remission longer than the exacerbations. The joints affected in decreasing order of frequency are the knee, shoulder, elbow, temporomandibular, ankle, wrist, hip, and the small joints of the hands and feet. Pain is the most common symptom and it is unusual for any joint other than the knee to swell.

Diagnosis

Diagnosis of Lyme disease may be difficult. Careful search for the tick is mandatory, with removal immediately upon discovery. The tick is best removed by using a fine-nosed forceps to grasp the imbedded head and applying gentle, constant traction to dislodge the mouthparts and force the tick to release its grip. The clinician should be careful not to squeeze or otherwise injure the body proper, which may cause the remaining contents to be "injected."

Laboratory evaluation adds little in the early phases. The erythrocyte sedimentation rate may be mildly elevated, and the lymphocyte count may be slightly decreased (very nonspecific findings). Serologic studies are usually negative early on and patients may not show a rise in specific antibody titer until stage II or stage III disease is present. Both immunofluorescent and immunoadsorbent assays accurately diagnose antibodies to the *B. burgdorferi* spirochete. Diagnosis is best made by careful history and physical examination keeping in mind the clinical and epidemiologic information. It is important to keep in mind that most patients do not recall being bitten.

Treatment

Treatment is with doxycycline, 100 mg PO bid, or tetracycline, 250 mg PO qid, for 10 to 21 days in nonpregnant, nonlactating adults and children over 8 years of age. Amoxicillin, 250 to 500 mg PO tid (20 to 40 mg/kg per day in three divided doses for children for 30 days), is recommended for pregnant or lactating women and children under 8. However, the unknown risk of transplacental infection in pregnant women has caused some experts to recommend intravenous penicillin 5 million units qid for 10 to 14 days. Penicillin V, 250 to 500 mg PO qid, is recommended for doxycycline and tetracycline failures. Erythromycin, 250 mg PO qid, can be used in patients who cannot tolerate penicillin or tetracycline.

Stages II and III disease can be treated with the above mentioned oral regimens for 30 days or with intravenous penicillin or ceftriaxone depending upon the severity of symptoms.

Rocky Mountain Spotted Fever (RMSF)

Now the second most commonly acquired tick-borne disease, RMSF has been recognized in the northwestern United States since the late 1700s. Recently a shift in the geographic distribution of reported cases to the southern and eastern portions of the United States has been noted, making the name something of a misnomer.

The etiologic agent for this disease, *Rickettsia rickettsii,* is transmitted by the bite of ixodid ticks, most notably *Dermacentor andersonii* (the wood tick) in the west and *D. variabilis* (the American dog tick) in the southeast. Both are significantly larger than *I. dammini.* Only the female tick becomes infected, and the female may transmit the disease transovarially to offspring.

Peak incidence, as for Lyme disease, is from late spring to early fall. With RMSF, approximately two-thirds of patients remember having a tick bite.

Between 500 and 1000 cases of RMSF are reported annually, with peak rates in the south Atlantic region (32 percent) and the west south central region (24 percent).

Clinical Presentation

RMSF has a wide clinical spectrum, probably related to the fact that the tick invades small blood vessels throughout the body, leading to vascular damage and a vasculitis secondary to an immunologic response. This response gives way to the varied manifestations of the disease: rash, fever, edema and other manifestations of third spacing, disseminated intravascular coagulation (DIC), encephalitis, myocardial necrosis, pulmonary interstitial disorders, and adult respiratory distress syndrome.

Symptoms begin in 2 to 14 days (average 5) after exposure. The incubation period is seemingly inversely proportional to the ultimate severity of disease. Initial symptoms are fever, usually high [up to 40°C (104°F)], followed by a rash. The rash, which is initially erythematous, macular, and blanching, rapidly progresses to a deep red, dusky more papular one, and ultimately becomes petechial. Rash is present in 75 to 80 percent of patients. It begins on the flexor surfaces of the wrist and ankles and spreads centripetally and centrifugally. Other common symptoms are headache (75 to 85 percent), nausea and vomiting (66 percent), myalgias (85 percent), cough (33 percent), and other signs of meningoencephalitic involvement (20 to 25 percent). A triad symptom complex of fever, headache, and rash has been seen in up to 55 to 65 percent of patients. In severe cases every organ system can be involved and the disease may progress on to DIC, shock, and death.

Diagnosis

Diagnosis may be difficult. Clinicians must rely on clinical and epidemiologic criteria, i.e., tick exposure or presence of patient, pet, or family member in an endemic area.

Laboratory evaluation is almost always nonspecific. The WBC count may be increased or decreased. Other laboratory abnormalities will be related to the organ systems involved in the primary vascular damage or to secondary vasculitis, for example, decreased serum sodium levels in patients with SIADH, kidney or liver function test abnormalities, and elevations in cardiac enzyme levels in those with myocarditis. Essentially any organ system can be involved.

More specific testing relates to the microbiologic and/or serologic search for *R. rickettsii.* Immunofluorescent antibody staining can be performed on a skin biopsy specimen obtained from an area of rash. This test is very specific (100 percent) and quite sensitive (70 percent), and is currently the best rapid diagnostic tool available.

Serologic tests are less helpful because they are most often negative in the early phases (first few days) of the illness. As a result antibiotic therapy should not be withheld while awaiting serologic confirmation. Of the three serologic tests available—complement fixation, Weil-Felix reaction, and fluorescent antibody titer—only the fluorescent antibody titer is still recommended because the complement fixation and Weil-Felix reaction require both acute and convalescent sera). A titer of greater than 1:64 or a fourfold rise in paired sera is diagnostic.

Treatment

Treatment of suspected RMSF should not await laboratory confirmation of the disease. Patients from an endemic area presenting with fever and any one or more of the other symptoms (rash, headache, myalgias, vomiting), with or without a history of tick exposure, should receive prompt antibiotic therapy. Tetracycline and chloramphenicol are the drugs of choice; they are equally effective in eradicating RMSF. Severely ill or vomiting patients should be treated intravenously.

For adults and children over 8 years old, tetracycline is given as follows: 10 to 20 mg/kg per day IV in two divided doses (up to a maximum of 500 mg per dose) or 25 to 50 mg/kg per day PO in four divided daily doses (up to a maximum of 500 mg per dose). For children under 8 years of age, chloramphenicol, 50 mg/kg per day IV or PO, is given in four divided daily doses.

Both treatment regimens should be followed for no less than 10 days and continued for 2 to 3 days after defervescence. Prophylactic therapy is not recommended.

Other treatment modalities will be focused on the specific organ system dysfunction, for example, fluid resuscitation for those suffering from dehydration secondary to the fever and vomiting, fresh frozen plasma for those with DIC, etc.

Prompt tick removal is necessary. The use of various hydrocarbon products or heat (a lighted match) is not recommended. The former may not be effective and the latter may cause the tick to burst or regurgitate, increasing the likelihood of exposure to infected body fluids. The site should be disinfected before the tick is manually removed, as described in the section on Lyme disease.

All patients should be hospitalized for at least the early course of treatment.

Tick Paralysis

Tick paralysis is a relatively uncommon tick-borne disease resulting in an ascending paralysis. The disease is of clinical importance because with prompt recognition and treatment (*which consist solely of tick removal*), it is curative, but mortality in untreated cases may be as high as 12 percent. It is caused by a venom secreted from the female tick salivary glands during feeding. The venom is most likely a neurotoxin which produces a conduction block at the peripheral motor nerve branches, resulting in a failure of acetylcholine release at the neuromuscular junction.

Cases in North America are usually caused by *D. andersonii,* but up to 43 tick species, from both Ixodidae and Argasidae families, have been implicated as causative agents.

Tick paralysis occurs during the months of heavy tick feeding (late spring to late summer) and seems to affect children more commonly than adults. The incidence is higher in girls than in boys.

Clinical Presentation

Symptoms develop within 4 to 7 days (median 5) after attachment by the female tick. Irritability, restlessness, and hand and feet paresthesias may initially be reported. Within 1 to 2 days the presenting symptoms are followed by a symmetric, ascending, flaccid paralysis accompanied by loss of deep tendon reflexes. In severe untreated cases death results from bulbar and respiratory paralysis. Loss of coordination and ataxia may indicate cerebellar involvement.

Diagnosis and Treatment

Tick discovery and removal are both diagnostic and therapeutic for this disease. Careful search must be made, with particular attention paid to the scalp. Most patients begin showing signs of recovery within hours after tick removal. Complete resolution within 48 to 72 h is the rule.

Other treatment modalities should be directed at the complications of the disease which may have occurred before tick removal, most notably respiratory support.

Relapsing Fever

Relapsing fever is a relatively uncommon acute disease whose endemic form is caused by a spirochete of the *Borrelia* species. Its vector is argasid ticks of the genus *Ornithodoros,* which tend to inhabit caves and burrows and feed on various rodents. An epidemic variety exists, transmitted by body lice, although it has not been reported in the United States in some time. Transmission is transovarial, so ticks at all stages of development can be infective.

The disease distribution is isolated to the western and southwestern United States, with peak incidence in summer months.

Clinical Presentation

After an incubation period of 5 to 9 days (median 7), infected individuals may experience an acute febrile episode. This lasts approximately 3 days (range 1 to 17) followed by an afebrile period and then a return of fever (relapse). Fever may be high [up to 39°C (102.2°F)]. The fever is generally accompanied by chills, malaise, vomiting, headache, lethargy, and myalgias. Approximately 40 percent of patients develop splenomegaly, and almost 20 percent develop hepatomegaly. Neurologic involvement occurs in less than 10 percent of patients. A pruritic eschar frequently appears at the bite site but is usually not seen, having resolved prior to onset of the other clinical symptoms. Petechia or erythema multiforme develops in up to 30 percent of patients [25].

Diagnosis

Because most laboratory analysis reveals nonspecific findings only, diagnosis is usually made using epidemiologic and clinical criteria. However, peripheral blood smear demonstrates spirochetes in up to 70 percent of patients. There are, as yet, no helpful serologic tests.

Treatment

Tetracycline, 500 mg PO qid, or erythromycin, 250 mg PO qid, are equally effective. Both should be continued for a 5- to 10-day course. Penicillin appears to result in some treatment failures. The spirochete also appears to be sensitive to chloramphenicol.

The first dose of any of these agents commonly results in what is known as the Jarsch-Herxheimer reaction. This reaction can be quite severe. Patients' clinical condition may worsen, and profound vasodilatation and drop in blood pressure may develop. No pretreatment regimens appear to be effective in preventing this reaction, although an isotonic saline infusion may reduce the severity of the hypotension.

Q Fever

Q fever is a flulike illness caused by *Coxiella burnetii*. Fever, myalgias, headache, and cough are common. Diagnosis is based on two complement-fixing antibody titers.

Q fever normally resolves spontaneously in 2 to 4 weeks. *Coxiella burnetii* appears to be sensitive to tetracycline, and treatment with 500 mg PO qid for 10 days may speed resolution. The chronic form of the disease may require as much as 12 months of tetracycline therapy.

Tularemia

The bacteria *Francisella tularensis* is the causative organism for tularemia. *Dermacentor variabilis* and *A. americanum* are the main tick vectors in the United States. Tick transmission is transovarial, so ticks at all stages of development can be infective. Although it was initially thought that tularemia was primarily transmitted through rabbits and rabbit meat, it is now recognized that ticks are the most frequent vectors.

The peak occurrence of the tick-borne variety of tularemia is in the summer months. Most cases in the United States are reported from the southern and midwestern states.

Clinical Presentation

The clinical presentations of tularemia have been classically typed into six groups: ulceroglandular, glandular, oculoglandular, typhoidal, pneumonic, and oropharyngeal. More recently, a simpler classification, using only the ulceroglandular and typhoidal groups, has been suggested. The ulceroglandular type appears to be the most common, with an overall incidence of approximately 50 percent reported by Jacobs et al. (using the six-group classification). Glandular, pneumonic, and typhoidal types are the next most common, with overall incidences of approximately 18, 16, and 10 percent, respectively). Evans et al., using the two-group classification, reported an approximate 80 percent incidence of the ulceroglandular group.

Lymphadenopathy is the most frequent sign, and is present in 65 to 96 percent of patients (with the greater frequency in children). In children it is most commonly cervical adenopathy (82 percent), whereas in adults the location is more often inguinal (54 percent). In children, fever is the next most frequent sign (87 percent), and in adults, ulceration (51 percent). Ulcerations are, however, also common in children (45 percent). The ulcerations usually begin as reddened nodules which indurate and then ulcerate. They sometimes originate at the initial tick bite site.

The typhoidal form typically presents with fever, chills, debility, abdominal pain, diarrhea, anorexia, and weight loss. It is more commonly contracted by the ingestion of improperly cooked, infected rabbit meat than by tick bite.

Diagnosis

Clinicians practicing in or caring for patients from endemic areas must maintain a high index of suspicion. Serologic tests are helpful. A presumptive diagnosis can be made if an acute specific agglutination titer is greater than 1:160; a fourfold increase is confirmatory.

Treatment

Streptomycin is the drug of choice. It should be given as a dose of 30 to 40 mg/kg per day in two divided doses (q 12 h) IM for 3 days and then 20 mg/kg per day in two divided doses IM for an additional 4 to 7 days. For streptomycin-sensitive patients, an alternative is tetracycline, 50 to 60 mg/kg per day in four divided doses PO for 14 days. There is an incidence of relapse after tetracycline therapy which can usually be overcome by repeating the 14-day course.

Babesiosis

Babesiosis is caused by members of the genus *Babesia,* a malarialike, intrarythrocytic protozoan parasite. The first human case was described in 1957, and approximately 100 cases were documented in the United States through 1984.

Babesiosis was initially reported only in splenectomized individuals, with only scattered cases reported throughout the world literature. Since 1969, however, there has been a dramatic rise in reported cases, seemingly related to an outbreak of infection with the species *B. microti,* which can cause disease in those with intact spleens.

The major tick vector is *I. dammini,* the main vector for Lyme disease, and both diseases have been seen in the same patient. Additionally, the distribution of babesiosis appears to be similar to that of Lyme disease. Cases from the area of southern New England are still the most common, but a few cases from the upper Midwest have been reported.

Clinical Presentation

The clinical spectrum is broad, ranging from subclinical infection (mild febrile illness) to severe disease with hemolytic anemia, hemoglobinuria, and death. More severe disease appears to occur in splenectomized patients.

Fever, malaise, anorexia, and fatigue are almost universally present, and headache and mild to moderate hemolytic anemia are common. There appears to be a correlation between age and disease severity, with younger patients having a milder form.

Physical examination is generally nondiagnostic. Mild splenomegaly may be seen in approximately 40 percent of patients.

Diagnosis

Thick or thin Giemsa-stained blood smears will usually reveal intraerythrocytic organisms. The *Borrelia microti* organism has a ring form which resembles *Plasmodium falciparum.* In the appropriate clinical setting a presumptive diagnosis may be made by using indirect immunofluorescent testing for antibody if the titer is >1:256. Diagnosis can be confirmed by inoculating splenectomized hamsters with the patient's blood.

Treatment

Use of chloroquine and other antimalarial agents has shown only limited efficacy. Combined therapy with clindamycin, 600 mg bid, and quinine, 650 mg bid, has been shown to be effective at eliminating parasites from the blood. Exchange transfusion has been effective in severe cases.

Colorado Tick Fever

A multitude of viruses may be transmitted by the tick vector; however, a member of the genus *Orbivirus* of the family Reoviridae, which causes Colorado tick fever, is the only one to present with any frequency in North America. This virus is mainly transmitted by the tick *D. andersoni,* which becomes infective by feeding on a viremic rodent host. Peak incidence is from late spring to early fall. Approximately 90 percent of patients remember the tick bite or exposure. Only about 200 cases are reported annually.

Clinical Presentation

Approximately 3 to 6 days (range 0 to 14) after exposure patients may develop sudden-onset fever, headache, lethargy, myalgias, anorexia, and nausea and vomiting. The headache is retroorbital, and photophobia is common. In approximately 50 percent of cases, the patient experiences 2 to 3 days of fever, followed by 1 to 2 afebrile days and then an additional 2 to 3 days of fever.

Other clinical findings occur rarely, but may be severe. In children meningoencephalitis and death resulting from blood loss associated with a coagulopathy have been reported.

Treatment

Since the disease is self-limited, treatment is supportive. Recovery usually takes about 3 weeks. Some patients, particularly those over 30, may suffer from a prolonged period of generalized weakness not dissimilar to that seen in the postinfectious stages of patients with Epstein-Barr virus.

Prevention of Tick-Borne Disease

Adherence to the following practices will reduce the likelihood of contracting a tick-borne disease:

1. Wear protective clothing when traveling in endemic areas, especially where there is long grass.
2. Use insect repellents of limited benefit.
3. When travelling in known endemic areas, examine yourself and your pets for ticks at least twice daily.
4. Once discovered, remove ticks *promptly*. The longer the exposure, the greater the likelihood of infection.

BIBLIOGRAPHY

Abbott KH: Tick paralysis: A review. *Proc Mayo Clin* 18:39, 1943.

Butler T: Relapsing fever: new lessons about antibiotic action. *Ann Intern Med* 102:397, 1985.

Butler T, et al: Borrelia recurrentis infection: Single dose regimens and management of the Jarisch-Herxheimer reaction. *J Infect Dis* 137:573, 1978.

Burgdorferer W, et al: Lyme disease: A tick-borne spirochetosis? *Science* 216:317, 1982.

Centers for Disease Control: Lyme disease surveillance 1989–1990. *MMWR* 40:418, 1991

Centers for Disease Control: Rocky mountain spotted fever—United States, 1988. *MMWR* 38:513, 1989.

Centers for Disease Control: Rocky mountain spotted fever—United States 1987. *MMWR* 37:388–9, 1988.

Centers for Disease Control: Rocky mountain spotted fever—United States 1985. *MMWR* 35:247, 1986.

Centers for Disease Control: Rocky mountain spotted fever—United States, 1983. *MMWR* 33:188, 1984.

Centers for Disease Control: Tick paralysis—Wisconsin. *MMWR* 30:217, 1981.

Centers for Disease Control: Update: Lyme disease and cases occurring during pregnancy—United States. *MMWR* 34:376, 1985.

Evans ME, et al: Tularemia: A 30 year experience with 88 cases. *Medicine* 64:251, 1985

Gombert ME, et al: Human Babesiosis—Clinical and therapeutic considerations. *JAMA* 248:3005, 1982.

Goodpasture HC, et al: Colorado tick fever: Clinical, epidemiologic and laboratory aspects of 228 cases in Colorado in 1973–1974. *Ann Intern Med* 88:303, 1978.

Gorman RJ and Snead C: Tick paralysis in three children: the diversity of neurologic presentations. *Clin Pediatr* 17:249, 1978.

Hoogstaal H: Argasid and nuttallielid ticks as parasites and vectors. *Adv Parasitol* 24:135, 1985.

Jacobs RF, et al: Tularemia in adults and children: A changing presentation. *Pediatrics* 76:818, 1985.

Jacoby GA, et al: Treatment of transfusion-transmitted babesiosis by exchange transfusion. *N Engl J Med* 303:1098, 1980.

Linneman CC: Rapid recognition and specific intervention in Rocky mountain spotted fever. *Emerg Med Rep* 8:105, 1987.

Linnemann CC and Janson PJ: The clinical presentations of Rocky mountain spotted fever. *Clin Pediatr* 17:673, 1978.

Needham GR: Evaluation of five popular methods for tick removal. *Pediatrics* 75:997, 1985.

Pachner AR and Steere AC: The triad of neurologic manifestations of Lyme disease: meningitis, cranial neuritis and radiculoneuritis. *Neurology* 35:57, 1985.

Riley HD: Rocky mountain spotted fever. *Hosp Pract* 12:51, 1977.

Rosner F, et al: Babesiosis in splenectomized adults. *Am J Med* 76:696, 1984.

Ruebush TK, et al: Human Babesiosis on Nantucket Island. *Ann Intern Med* 86:6, 1977.

Ruebush TK, et al: Human Babesiosis on Nantucket Island. *N Engl J Med* 297:825, 1977.

Schmitt N, et al: Tick paralysis in British Columbia. *Can Med Assoc J* 100:417, 1969.

Southern PA, Sanford JP: Relapsing fever: A clinical and microbiological review. *Medicine* 48:129, 1969.

Spruance SL, and Bailey A: Colorado tick fever: A review of 115 laboratory confirmed cases. *Arch Intern Med* 131:288, 1973.

Steere AC, et al: The early clinical manifestations of Lyme disease. *Ann Intern Med* 99:76–82, 1983.

Steere AC, et al: Erythema chronicum migrans and Lyme arthritis: the enlarging clinical spectrum. *Ann Intern Med* 86:685, 1977.

Steere AC, et al: Erythema chronicum migrans and Lyme arthritis: Epidemiologic evidence for a tick vector. *Am J Epidemiol* 108:312, 1978.

Steere AC, et al: Lyme arthritis: An epidemic of oligoarticular arthritis in children and adults in three Connecticut communities. *Arthritis Rheum* 20:7, 1977.

Steere AC, et al: The spirochetal etiology of Lyme disease. *N Engl J Med* 308:733, 1983.

Steketee RW, et al: Babesiosis in Wisconsin. *JAMA* 253:2675, 1985.

Walker DH, et al: Laboratory Diagnosis of Rocky mountain spotted fever. *South Med J* 73:1443–1446, 1980.

Williamson PK, et al: Lyme disease: A review of the literature. *Semin Arthritis Rheum* 13:229, 1984.

Woodward TE, et al: Prompt confirmation of Rocky mountain spotted fever: Identification of rickettsiae in skin tissues. *J Infect Dis* 134:297, 1976.

SECTION 10
Toxicology

88
GENERAL MANAGEMENT OF THE POISONED PATIENT

Michael V. Vance

INCIDENCE OF POISONING

The American Association of Poison Control Centers (AAPCC) reported, through its national network of certified regional poison control centers, a total of over 1.5 million poison exposures during 1989. Estimates of the total number of actual poisonings in the United States may be more than twice that number, placing the incidence of poisoning in the same category as injury due to motor vehicle accidents.

CHARACTERISTICS OF POISONING

Pediatric Poisoning

Well over half of poisonings reported to the AAPCC by participating poison centers occur in young children (1 to 5 years). Exposures in this age group are generally "accidental" (implying no harmful intent) and relatively mild. Although they represent a large number of exposures, pediatric patients account for only about 10 percent of all hospital admissions due to poisoning. Despite the almost universally accidental nature of pediatric poisoning, the emergency physician should be aware of other reasons for a child to present with a toxic exposure, including child abuse through intentional poisoning by parents, other caretakers, and even siblings. More common reasons for exposure in older children (including the preteen age group) include intentional drug experimentation/abuse and adolescent and preadolescent suicide attempts. A good rule of thumb is to consider a toxic exposure in any child over the age of 5 with normal intellectual development to be suspicious.

Adult Poisoning

While adult poisoning is responsible for less than half of calls to poison centers, these result in 80 to 90 percent of hospital admissions due to toxic exposures. Although an increasing number of adult poisonings are accidental, due to chemical exposures in the workplace or at home, most are intentional. Although the motives for these intentional exposures may be very different—recreational drug abuse, suicide "gestures," or bona fide suicide attempt—the emergency physician must recognize and be prepared to deal with the associated psychological factors in these patients. Above all, a firm but nonjudgmental approach may avoid violent verbal and even physical confrontations and may well pave the way for appropriate psychiatric intervention.

EVALUATION OF THE POISONED PATIENT

History

A thorough, accurate history provides a working diagnosis and assists with management decisions for most patients in the emergency department. Unfortunately, the history in a poisoning is notoriously unreliable (pediatric patients, drug abuse, suicide attempts), whether it is obtained from the patient, friends, and family members or EMS personnel. Despite the possible inaccuracies, the important historical factors include *what* poison was involved, *how much* was taken, *how* it was taken, *when* it was taken, *why* it was taken, and especially *what else* was taken (a significant number of intentional ingestions involve more than one substance).

Physical Examination

A complete head-to-toe physical examination may offer supportive evidence and credence to the history, may indicate the presence of additional or entirely different substances, or may provide an exact diagnosis. The approach to the physical examination of the poisoned patient includes (1) vital signs, (2) identification of toxic syndromes, (3) evaluation for complications, and (4) evaluation for underlying disease states.

Vital Signs

As in any emergency department patient, physical assessment of the poisoned patient starts with the ABCs. *Airway* evaluation should include not only the usual factors indicating gross airway compromise (stridor, snoring, vomitus, etc.), but also specific evaluation of the gag reflex. If there is any question about the integrity of the airway, active airway management should be initiated as soon as possible to protect against further compromise or aspiration. *Breathing* evaluation includes not only a baseline respiratory rate but also evaluation of the quality of respirations: shallow respirations suggest the need for early ventilatory support; deep respirations suggest the presence of an underlying hypoxemia or metabolic acidosis. *Circulation* evaluation includes a baseline pulse rate and blood pressure, and any suggestion of serious poisoning should dictate continuous ECG monitoring and serial blood pressure determinations.

Temperature

In addition to the usual vital signs discussed above, a baseline temperature should be obtained. This is given special emphasis because an oral or rectal temperature is frequently not obtained early—if at all—in the poisoned patient for a variety of reasons. The patient may be uncooperative, combative, or require a number of other important diagnostic or therapeutic measures on arrival in the emergency department. However, the emergency physician must recognize that environmental exposure (hot or cold) or direct toxic effects may produce a wide range of thermoregulatory and core temperature abnormalities. Hyperthermia and hypothermia frequently accompany toxic exposures and may well interfere with treatment if they are not identified and managed appropriately. Thus, despite the possible difficulty of obtaining an oral or rectal temperature in a cursing/spitting/vomiting/seizing/dying patient, its importance should not be forgotten.

Toxic Syndromes

Numerous toxic syndromes may be identified virtually at first glance with certain poisonings. Many, including the anticholinergic syndrome, the cholinergic syndrome, and the sympathomimetic syndrome, are described in detail in later chapters in this section. Table 88-1 lists some basic elements of the more common toxic syndromes, and the rapid identification of such presentations saves considerable time and frustration in the evaluation and management of the poisoned patient.

Table 88-1. Toxic Syndromes (Multiple-Cause Symptom Complexes)

Syndrome	Causes	Manifestations
Anticholinergic	Belladonna alkaloids: Atropine (hyoscyamine) Belladonna alkaloid mixtures: belladonna leaf, fluid extract, tincture Stramonium Homatropine Methscopolamine Methylatropine nitrate Plants: *Atropa belladonna, Datura stramonium, Hyoscyamus niger, Amanita muscaria or pantherina* Scopolamine (I-hyoscine) Synthetic anticholinergics: Adiphenine Anisotropine Cyclopentolate Dicyclomine Diphemanil Eucatropine Glycopyrrolate Hexocyclium Isopropamide Mepenzolate Methantheline Methixene Oxyphenonium Oxyphencyclimine Pentapiperide Pipenzolate Piperidolate Poldine Propantheline Thiphenamil Tridihexethyl Tropicamide Incidental anticholinergics: Antihistamines Tricyclic antidepressants Benactyzine Phenothiazines	Peripheral antimuscarinic: Dry skin and mucous membranes Thirst Dysphagia Vision blurred for near objects Fixed dilated pupils Tachycardia Sometimes hypertension Rash, scarlatiniform Hyperthermia, flushing Abdominal distension Urinary urgency and retention Central: Lethargy Confusion to restlessness, excitement Delirium, hallucinations Ataxia Seizures Respiratory failure Cardiovascular collapse
Acetylcholinesterase inhibition	Organophosphates: TEPP OMPA Dipterex Chlorthion Di-Syston Co-ral Phosdrin Parathion Methylparathion Malathion Systox EPN Diazinon Guthion Trithion	Muscarinic effects: Sweating, constricted pupils, lacrimation, excessive salivation, wheezing, cramps, vomiting, diarrhea, tenesmus, bradycardia *or* tachycardia, hypotension *or* hypertension, blurred vision, urinary incontinence Nicotinic effects: Striated muscle: fasciculations, cramps, weakness, twitching, paralysis, respiratory failure, cyanosis, arrest Sympathetic ganglia: tachycardia, elevated blood pressure CNS effects: Anxiety, restlessness, ataxia, seizures, insomnia, coma, absent reflexes, Cheyne-Stokes respirations, respiratory and circulation depression
Cholinergic	Acetylcholine *Areca catechu* Betel nut Bethanechol Carbachol *Clitocybe dealbata* Methacholine Muscarine Pilocarpine *Pilocarpus* species	Same as Muscarinic under Anticholinesterases, also Nicotinic
Extrapyramidal	Acetophenazine Butaperazine Carphenazine Chlorpromazine Haloperidol Mesoridazine Perphenazine Piperacetazine Promazine Thioridazine Thiothixene Trifluoperazine Triflupromazine	Parkinsonian: Dysphonia, dysphagia, oculogyric crises, rigidity, tremor, torticollis, opisthotonos, shrieking, trismus, laryngospasm
Hemoglobinopathies	Carboxyhemoglobin Carbon monoxide Methemoglobin	Headache, nausea, vomiting, dizziness, dyspnea, seizures, coma, death Cutaneous bullae, gastroenteritis Epidemic occurrence with carbon monoxide Cyanosis, chocolate blood with methemoglobin
Metal fume fever	Fumes of oxides of Brass Cadmium Copper Iron Magnesium Mercury Nickel Titanium Tungsten Zinc	Chills, fever, nausea, vomiting, muscular pain, throat dryness, headache, fatigue, weakness, leukocytosis, respiratory distress

Table 88-1. Toxic Syndromes (Multiple-Cause Symptom Complexes) (*Continued*)

Syndrome	Causes			Manifestations
Narcotic	Alphaprodine Anileridine Codeine Cyclazocine Dextromethorphan Dextromoramide Diacetylmorphine Dihydrocodeine Dihydrocodeinone Dipaone	Diphenoxylate (Lomotil) Ethohepatazine Ethylmorphine Fentanyl Heroin Hydromorphone Levorphanol Meperidine Methadone	Metopon Morphine Opium Oxycodone Oxymorphone Pentazocine Phenazocine Piminodine Propoxyphene Racemorphan	CNS depression Pinpoint pupils Slowed respirations Hypotension Response to naloxone Pupils may be dilated and excitement may predominate
Sympathomimetic	Aminophylline Amphetamines Caffeine Cocaine Dopamine Ephedrine	Epinephrine Fenfluramine Levarterenol Metaraminol Methylphenidate (Ritalin)	Pemoline Phencyclidine Phenmetrazine Phentermine	CNS excitation Seizures Hypertension Hypotension with caffeine Tachycardia
Withdrawal	Alcohol Barbiturates Benzodiazepines Chloral hydrate Cocaine	Ethchlorvynol Glutethimide Meprobamate Methaqualone	Methyprylon Narcotics Opioids Paraldehyde	Diarrhea, mydriasis, piloerection, hypertension, tachycardia, insomnia, lacrimation, muscle cramps, restlessness, yawning, hallucinosis Depression with cocaine

Source: Adapted from Done AK: *Poisoning—A Systematic Approach for the Emergency Department Physician.* Presented Aug. 6–9, 1979, at Snowmass Village, CO, Symposium sponsored by Rocky Mountain Poison Center. Used by permission.

Complications of Poisoning

Whether a toxic syndrome is readily identified or not, the primary goal of physical assessment of the poisoned patient is to identify any effects on the three vital organ systems most likely to produce immediate morbidity and mortality: the respiratory system, the cardiovascular system, and the central nervous system.

Respiratory Complications

Airway compromise in the patient with an altered level of consciousness is as common in the poisoned patient as in patients with any other serious illness or injury. Ventilatory insufficiency frequently accompanies airway problems, as does the risk of aspiration. Other respiratory complications include the early development of noncardiogenic pulmonary edema or the later development of adult respiratory distress syndrome (ARDS); bronchospasm due to direct or indirect toxic effects may also be present.

Cardiovascular Complications

The most common cardiovascular complication of poisoning is rhythm disturbance. *Tachyarrhythmias* are fairly common but are usually not associated with serious perfusion problems unless the patient has underlying cardiovascular disease. *Bradyarrhythmias* are relatively uncommon and usually are associated with more serious underlying metabolic problems, such as hypoxia or acidosis. *Hypotension* is frequently seen and is almost always associated with decreased vascular tone. *Hypertension* is occasionally seen and may be accompanied by serious sequelae, such as cerebrovascular hemorrhage.

Neurologic Complications

Altered level of consciousness is a frequent complication of poisoning and may range from mild drowsiness to agitation, hallucinations, coma, medullary depression, cardiopulmonary depression, and death. In addition, advanced levels of central nervous system depression are typically associated with many of the primary respiratory and cardiovascular complications listed above. *Seizures* are one of the most serious complications seen in the poisoned patient and may be due to underlying perfusion or metabolic problems, or due to primary drug effect. *Behavioral abnormalities,* while not as lethal as other central nervous system complications, are nonetheless among the greatest problems for emergency department personnel. Confused, combative patients create additional difficulties in the treatment of patients with potentially severe toxic effects of poisoning.

Underlying Disease States

The final emphasis on physical assessment of the poisoned patient is to evaluate for the presence of underlying disease states which may increase the likelihood of complications. Patients with asthma or chronic obstructive pulmonary disease are obviously at increased risk for the respiratory complications, while patients with underlying cardiovascular disease are more likely to develop severe arrhythmias. As is the usual case, the very young and very old are also more susceptible to toxic effects of poisoning.

EMERGENCY DEPARTMENT MANAGEMENT

Management of the poisoned patient in the emergency department is directed toward a number of goals: *Decontamination* limits absorption and minimizes the extent of toxicity; *supportive care* limits the effects of the serious complications of poisoning on the primary organ system at risk; and *definitive care* limits the severity or duration of toxicity through the use of pharmacologic antagonists (*antidotes*) or the enhanced *elimination* of the toxin itself.

Decontamination

The vast majority of serious poisonings are due to ingestion of toxic substances. Thus, *gastrointestinal decontamination* is a common consideration in the management of the poisoned patient. As the stomach is the first recipient of a bolus of ingested material, this organ has long received the most attention for recovery of toxic material and prevention of absorption.

For decades, *syrup of ipecac* has been the most commonly accepted method of accomplishing gastric emptying, although the routine use of ipecac has come under increased scrutiny and criticism in recent years. While ipecac has the advantages of widespread acceptance and active promotion by poison centers for use in home management, its utility in the context of serious poisoning in the emergency department is virtually nonexistent. Studies consistently show that ipecac-induced emesis only reduces absorption by about 30 percent (leaving 70 percent to be absorbed to produce toxic effects) and actually interferes with the efficacy of other methods of decontamination (such as administration of activated charcoal). In addition, the vomiting produced by ipecac may interfere with other diagnostic and therapeutic measures necessary for the well-being of the patient. In the 1990s, ipecac appears to be nothing more than an interesting historical footnote in the management of poisoning in the emergency department.

Gastric lavage is one alternative to the use of ipecac as a method of gastrointestinal decontamination. The proper technique requires the use of a large-bore (36 to 40 French in an adult) *orogastric hose* connected to appropriate irrigation and drainage tubing, with infusion and recovery of 250- to 300-mL aliquots of fluid until the return is clear. Gastric lavage has the advantages of providing immediate recovery of gastric contents (compared with a 15- to 30-min delay with ipecac-induced emesis), control of lavage duration, and direct access for instillation of activated charcoal. Disadvantages include the invasive nature of the procedure and the technical difficulties of having a relatively alert patient accept a tube somewhat larger than his or her trachea. In experienced hands, recovery of gastric contents is at least as good as ipecac-induced emesis. However, the efficacy of gastric lavage after the first 1–2 h post-ingestion in all but the most serious presentations is questionable.

Activated charcoal is the agent of choice for gastrointestinal decontamination in acute poisoning. Activated charcoal acts by adsorbing molecules of chemicals on its surface, thereby inhibiting their absorption and preventing systemic toxicity. In addition, technologic advances have produced a superactivated charcoal, which boasts an adsorptive surface area of 3000 m^2/g, approximately three times the older preparations. While ipecac or lavage may recover 30 percent of an ingested dose, studies suggest that the use of activated charcoal alone, given in timely fashion, may reduce absorption by as much as 50 percent. The dose is 1 g/kg. Disadvantages of activated charcoal include poor patient acceptance and the messy result if the patient happens to regurgitate stomach contents.

Cathartics are another method of gastrointestinal decontamination with a long history of endorsement by poison centers and medical personnel. In theory, cathartics (sorbitol, magnesium sulfate, magnesium citrate) speed up gastrointestinal motility, thereby shortening absorption time for chemicals in the gut. However, studies do not show that cathartics positively affect patient outcome, and the osmotically increased gastrointestinal fluid load may even *increase* systemic absorption and toxicity of some substances. Their major disadvantage is frequent liquid stools, which may become distracting to nursing and other personnel responsible for continuing care of the patient and may interfere with more appropriate evaluation and monitoring needs. In young children, dehydration and electrolyte dehydration and electrolyte imbalance can occur.

Future directions in gastrointestinal decontamination will most likely see the increased use of activated charcoal in both prehospital and emergency department settings. Administration of activated charcoal prior to gastric lavage (20 to 30 min) has been shown to double the effectiveness of lavage, and the use of activated charcoal immediately following lavage, or as a primary method of decontamination, and even as a tool to enhance elimination of already absorbed toxin, continues to gain acceptance and popularity, although much of the previous literature on multiple-dose charcoal has not been based on controlled studies.

Other decontamination concerns include removal of toxic substances from the *skin*, primarily through complete removal of clothing followed by thorough soap and water wash; *eye* decontamination, using 15 to 30 min of constant irrigation for chemical exposures until a conjunctival pH of 7 is attained (perhaps even longer for alkalis) (see Chapter 154, "Ocular Emergencies"), and decontamination of *special areas*, which may produce increased or prolonged absorption, such as hair, skin folds, mucous membranes, and damaged skin.

Supportive Care

Supportive care of the poisoned patient is directed toward the prevention or limitation of respiratory, cardiovascular, and neurologic complications. The initiation of standard diagnostic and therapeutic measures including administration of oxygen, establishing intravenous access, and placing the patient on a cardiac monitor should be routine in any serious poisoning.

Management of Respiratory Complications

Airway protection is an essential step in the treatment of a poisoned patient. If any airway compromise (vomitus, stridor, diminished gag reflex) is present in a patient with altered level of consciousness, orotracheal or nasotracheal intubation should be accomplished as soon as possible. Correction of airway problems frequently resolves associated *ventilatory insufficiency*, but if any doubt remains, assisted ventilation should be instituted until ventilatory status may be further evaluated. *Bronchospasm* may cause significant problems in patients with underlying pulmonary disease but usually responds to standard bronchodilator therapy. *Noncardiogenic pulmonary edema* may be seen early and is due to increased alveolocapillary permeability, requiring treatment with high-flow oxygen, positive-pressure ventilation, and consideration of positive end-expiratory pressure (PEEP). In contrast, true ARDS is rarely seen as an emergency department complication, but early anticipation may allow early, aggressive treatment and limit its consequences. *Aspiration* is best treated by prevention through early airway control, but if it has already occurred, it requires only simple ventilatory support. Although antibiotics and steroids are frequently used, studies do not support their efficacy and neither is recommended.

Management of Cardiovascular Complications

Tachyarrhythmias are, as previously mentioned, rarely associated with serious perfusion problems and usually require nothing more than cardiac monitoring. However, ventricular irritability should be aggressively managed with appropriate antiarrhythmic agents. Bradyarrhythmias are best treated with atropine but may require chronotropic agents or even pacing. *Hypotension* usually reflects decreased peripheral vascular resistance and should be treated with fluid administration; only rarely are vasopressors required. *Hypertension* which is complicated by pulmonary edema, cardiac ischemia, or encephalopathy should be controlled with direct arterial vasodilators (nitroprusside, calcium channel antagonists, etc.).

Management of Neurologic Complications

Coma, or altered level of consciousness, represents no significant problems except as it relates to the respiratory and cardiovascular complications previously discussed. *Seizures,* on the other hand, are one of the most dangerous complications encountered in the poisoned patient, requiring treatment early and often. Standard anticonvulsant therapy with short-acting benzodiazepines and barbiturates (diazepam, pentobarbital) in concert with phenytoin controls most seizure activity, although repeated or prolonged seizures should be controlled with paralyzing agents (pancuronium) to avoid progressive metabolic acidosis, hyperthermia, and rhabdomyolysis. *Behavioral abnormalities,* including hallucinations, combativeness, and agitation, are most often due to early stages of central nervous system depression (the excitation stage of anesthesia). Therefore, the use of "chemical restraints" only compounds the intoxication and may on occasion precipitate catastrophic cardiopulmonary complications. Therefore, physical restraints should be used as much as possible, although patients who continue to be unmanageable to the extent that essential diagnostic or therapeutic measures are unable to be carried out may require sedation. Short-acting benzodiazepines (diazepam, etc.) may be used for rapid control of patients, while haloperidol is very effective for longer-term control.

Diagnostic Studies

As information is being obtained via history and physical examination and supportive care is being initiated, ancillary studies may be important to confirm the presence of suspected or unsuspected toxins, to confirm the clinical status or chronic effects on organ systems, or to obtain baseline information for future comparison.

Drug screens rarely alter the basic management of patients, because of delayed turnaround times or a limited scope of the assays. However, specific management of some toxins, such as acetaminophen, will be directly determined by blood levels; the emergency physician should be acquainted with time-dependent laboratory studies and the interpretation of blood levels relative to the time since ingestion. Generally, comprehensive drug screens or isolated blood levels are still controversial, and the emergency physician must weigh the poor return against the possibility of "missing" the presence of a significant toxin. In all cases, drug levels should be guided to the extent possible by history and physical findings. It is essential that emergency physicians be familiar with their own laboratories' capabilities and limitations in providing rapid, accurate drug screens. Other laboratory studies may include the usual baseline determinations, including a complete blood cell count, electrolyte levels, glucose levels, arterial blood gas levels, osmolality, and organ function (renal, hepatic, etc.). However, these studies also rarely alter the emergency department management of the poisoned patient. *Arterial blood gases* may be important in the evaluation of the oxygenation, ventilation, and metabolic status of seriously poisoned patients. However, laboratory studies should be ordered on an individual basis depending on the exposure, the presence or absence of complications, and the overall clinical status of the patient. Similarly, ancillary studies (electrocardiograms, x-ray studies, etc.) should also be ordered based on specific indications.

Definitive Care

In most instances, "definitive" care of the poisoned patient is accomplished by decontamination and supportive care. However, there are a number of conditions in which the use of an *antagonist* is indicated. Any patient presenting with an altered level of consciousness deserves a trial of two essential cellular substrates, oxygen and glucose,

Table 88-2. Emergency Antidotes

Poison	Antidote	Adult dosage*	Comments
Acetaminophen	*N*-Acetylcysteine	Initial dose: 140 mg/kg	Most effective within 16 h
Arsenic	*See* Mercury		
Atropine	Physostigmine	Initial dose: 0.5–2 mg (IV)	Can produce convulsions, bradycardia
Carbon monoxide	Oxygen		
Cyanide	Amyl nitrite;	Inhale contents of crushed pearl for 30 s; breathe oxygen for 30 s	Methemoglobin-cyanide complex
	then Sodium nitrite	10 mL of 3% solution over 3 min (IV) in adults 0.33 mL (10 mg 3% sol.)/kg initially in children	Causes hypotension. Dosage assumes normal level hemoglobin
	Sodium thiosulfate	25% solution—50mL (IV) over 10 min in adults; 1.65 mL/kg in children	Forms harmless sodium thiocyanate
Ethylene glycol	See Methyl alcohol		
Gold	See Mercury		
Iron	Deferoxamine	Initial dose: 10–15 mg/kg/per hour (IV)	Deferoxamine mesylate—forms excretable ferrioxamine complex
Lead	Calcium disodium edetate *or* Dimercaptosuccinic acid	1 ampoule/250 mL D_5W over 1 h 250 mg (PO)	5-mL ampoule (IV) 20% solution. Dilute to less than 3% solution. Calcium displaced by lead
Mercury (arsenic, gold)	BAL (British anti-Lewisite)	5 mg/kg (IM) as soon as possible	Each mL BAL in oil has dimercaprol, 100 mg, in 210 mg (21%) benzyl benzoate and 680 mg peanut oil. Forms stable nontoxic excretable cyclic compound
	Dimercaptosuccinic acid (DMSA)	250 mg (PO)	Oral, water soluble preparation of BAL
Methyl alcohol (ethylene glycol)	Ethyl alcohol in conjunction with dialysis	1 mL/kg of 100% ethanol initially in glucose solution; maintain blood level of 100 mg/100 mL	Competes for alcohol dehydrogenase; prevents formation of toxic metabolites
Nitrites	Methylene blue	0.2 mL/kg of 1% solution (IV) over 5 min	Exchange transfusion may be needed for severe methemoglobinemia
Opiates	Naloxone	0.4–0.8 mg (IV) in adults; up to 8–22 mg 0.01 mg/kg (IV) in children	Higher doses may be required for certain high-affinity substances such as propoxyphene (Darvon) and diphenoxylate (Lomoil)
Organophosphates	Atropine	Initial dose: 2–5 mg (IV) in adults; 0.05 mg/kg (IV) in children	Physiologic: blocks acetylcholine (at muscarinic receptor sites). Up to 5 mg (IV) every 15 min (or more) may be necessary in the critical adult patient
	Pralidoxime (2-PAM chloride) (Protopam)	Initial dose: 1 g (IV) in adults; 25–30 mg/kg (IV) in children	Specific: breaks alkyl phosphate-cholinesterase bond, regenerating acetylcholinesterase activity

* Dosages listed may require modification according to specific clinical conditions.

Source: Adapted from the American College of Emergency Physicians poster on poisoning, Dallas, TX, 1980.

and the opiate antagonist naloxone. Additional antagonists used in the treatment of poisoning are listed in Table 88-2.

The other technique considered a part of definitive care is the enhancement of *elimination* of toxic substances already absorbed into the system. Previously, such efforts concentrated on increasing renal excretion by manipulating urinary pH. And while alkalinization is still an important technique in increasing the elimination of many drugs (salicylates, barbiturates, etc.), acidification is unlikely to remove any significant amount of total body drug burden and may contribute to renal complications from some of the chemicals supposedly undergoing "ion-trapping" by acidification (amphetamine, phencyclidine, etc.). Some studies have demonstrated the marked efficacy of activated charcoal in enhancing the elimination of certain toxins, including parent compounds and active metabolites. Repeated doses may be given every 2 to 4 h, although decreased gastrointestinal motility (anticholinergics, etc.) may require that the dosage interval be much longer. It appears that the administration of activated charcoal is as important in removing some substances such as theophylline and phenobarbital from the system as it is in preventing absorption in the first place but the routine use of multi-dose charcoal in all poisonings is not recommended at present. Finally, enhancement of elimination may include extracorporeal methods. However, hemodialysis and hemoperfusion are only effective in removing chemicals found in high concentration in the vascular space. In addition, the use of these techniques is generally limited to cases involving very specific chemicals (methanol, ethylene glycol), progressive deterioration despite adequate supportive care, or the presence of renal failure.

Disposition

While the continued care of victims of accidental poisoning is straightforward and depends on clinical condition (ambulatory discharge versus emergency department observation versus admission), the disposition of the patient with intentional exposure is frequently difficult. If the patient shows no significant toxicity, psychiatric evaluation should be a prerequisite for discharge. Above all, emergency physicians must avoid the temptation to accept the demands of an excited, angry, combative, and potentially intoxicated patient who states "You can't keep me here against my will!" A patient who is under extreme emotional distress and perhaps unable to make a rational decision because of a drug or alcohol intoxication requires attention to his or her psychiatric needs.

BIBLIOGRAPHY

Gastrointestinal Decontamination

Albertson TE, Derlet RW, Foulke GE, et al: Superiority of activated charcoal alone compared with ipecac and activated charcoal in the treatment of acute toxic ingestions. *Ann Emerg Med* 18:56, 1989.

Burton BT, Bayer MJ, Barron L, et al: Comparison of activated charcoal and gastric lavage in the prevention of aspirin absorption. *J Em Med* 1:411, 1984.

Krenzelok EP, Keller R, Stewart RD: Gastrointestinal transit times of cathartics combined with charcoal. *Ann Emerg Med* 14:1152, 1985.

Kulig K, Bar-Or D, Rosen P, et al: Management of acutely poisoned patients without gastric emptying. *Ann Emerg Med* 14:562, 1985.

McNamara RM, Aaron CK, Gemborys M, et al: Sorbitol catharsis does not enhance efficacy of charcoal in a simulated acetaminophen overdose. *Ann Emerg Med* 17:243, 1988.

McNamara RM, Aaron CK, Gemborys M, et al: Efficacy of charcoal cathartic versus ipecac in reducing serum acetaminophen in a simulated overdose. *Ann Emerg Med* 18:934, 1989.

Merigian KS: Prospective evaluation of gastric emptying in the self-poisoned patient. *Am J Emerg Med* 8:479, 1990.

Tandberg D, Diven BG, McLeod JW: Ipecac-induced emesis versus gastric lavage: a controlled study in normal adults. *Am J Emerg Med* 4:205, 1986.

Tenenbein M, Cohen S, Sitar DS: Efficacy of ipecac-induced emesis, orogastric lavage, and activated charcoal for acute drug overdose. *Ann Emerg Med* 16:838, 1987.

Additional Textbooks

Ellenhorn MJ, Barceloux DG: *Medical Toxicology: Diagnosis and Treatment of Human Poisoning*. New York: Elsevier Science Publishing Company, 1988.

Goldfrank LR, Flomenbaum NE, Lewin NA, Weisman RS, Howland MA: *Goldfrank's Toxicologic Emergencies,* 4th ed. East Norwalk, Conn, Appleton & Lange, 1990.

Haddad LM, Winchester JF (eds): *Clinical Management of Poisoning and Drug Overdose,* 2nd ed. Philadelphia, WB Saunders Co., 1990.

89
CYCLIC ANTIDEPRESSANT OVERDOSE

Michael Callaham

The cyclic antidepressants (CAs), chiefly the tricyclic antidepressants, are the most popular therapy for the treatment of major depression and were the third most common cause of drug-related death in the United States throughout the 1980s. This, combined with their unpredictable clinical course and their cardiovascular toxicity, make them major management problems for the emergency physician.

PHARMACOLOGY

The CAs are a group of closely related cyclic compounds that share to different degrees the anticholinergic and amine pump blocking properties of the phenothiazines. The CAs also have adrenergic stimulating effects, block the uptake of norepinephrine at the synapse, and block the sodium channel in cell membranes. Classically, the original agents in this group were all tricyclic, but newer agents are also unicyclic, bicyclic, and tetracyclic.

In overdose, CAs are absorbed slowly because they are ionized in the acid stomach and they slow peristalsis dramatically. The drug may remain in the gut for 12 h or more; pills may dissolve very slowly. Once absorbed, the CAs enter the plasma, where they are 85 to 98 percent bound to plasma proteins. From plasma, the CAs are rapidly taken up at the tissue level and bound to various cellular sites, including endoplasmic reticulum and mitochondria. Tissue entry is dependent on two factors: the CAs' lipid solubility, which is high when ionized, and their ionic dissociation at various pH levels (pK_a), which favors ionization (and thus decreased tissue entry) at a low pH. Tissue affinity for CAs is great, and levels in tissue such as the heart are often much greater than plasma levels. Due to the great affinity for tissue, the volume of distribution is very high (about 20 L/kg).

Metabolism occurs by demethylation, hydroxylation, and glucuronidization in the liver. The liver microsomal systems that metabolize CAs are enhanced by barbiturates, tobacco smoking, and alcohol, but at toxic levels this pathway is saturated. After hepatic metabolism the CAs are excreted in the bile and enter an enterohepatic cycle. Another 5 to 16 percent is excreted in gastric juices, since CAs have a pK_a of 9.5 and are highly ionized (and thus unable to cross cell membranes) at acid pH, favoring concentration in an acid medium.

The CAs have a half-life in the α (distribution between body compartment) stage of only a few minutes, but the half-life of the β (elimination) stage is measured in days, and rebound effects can occur as the drug redistributes from tissue compartments into the plasma. Genetic differences in individual metabolism produce differences in overdose half-life of from 25 to 81 h.

The CAs block the neuronal amine pump in the central nervous system, blocking the reuptake of norepinephrine and serotonin and thus reversing depression. Unfortunately, these same actions also block norepinephrine reuptake at the adrenergic synapse outside the central nervous system and lead to adrenergic blockade of the cardiovascular system. In addition, the CAs possess α-adrenergic blocking properties, anticholinergic effects, membrane stabilizing effects (similar to those of quinidine or local anesthetics), and even some calcium channel blocking properties. Of these activities, the membrane stabilizing properties are probably most important in producing major complications. The cardiac toxicities are induced by CA blocking of the fast sodium channel, responsible for depolarization of conduction tissue; CAs also slow repolarization (prolonging the QT interval) and depress automaticity. In addition, CAs have some α-adrenergic blocking activities, adding to their pharmacologic complexity.

All these pharmacologic actions produce significant side effects and toxicities in both therapy and overdose. These effects are discussed in more detail under the respective complications with which they are associated. However, it should be emphasized that our understanding of the pharmacologic pathophysiology of CA overdose is poor, and the relative importance of these effects is a matter of debate. Similarly, treatments based on these pharmacologic mechanisms (such as the use of physostigmine or β blockers) have been neither successful nor safe.

Since no major differences have been shown to exist among the older cyclic antidepressants in terms of toxicity, the treatment is the same for all. New cyclic antidepressants are being continually developed, with claims of decreased toxicity in overdose that often are not substantiated. For example, maprotiline (Ludiomil) is a tetracyclic antidepressant that demonstrates more seizures in overdose. Amoxapine (Asendin) is a metabolite of loxapine that has few cardiovascular side effects in overdose but a dramatically higher incidence of seizures (36 percent) and death (15 percent), compared to 5 to 10 percent and less than 1 percent, respectively, for all tricyclic antidepressants combined.

Two new compounds seem to be genuinely safer and are already reducing the incidence of CA overdose deaths. Trazadone (Desyrel) is a triazolopyridine compound unrelated to the tricyclic antidepressants that has equal clinical efficacy and virtually no cardiac and few CNS effects in overdose. The few overdose cases reported so far had a benign course comparable to benzodiazepine overdose. Fluoxetine (Prozac), a pure serotonin blocker with little adrenergic activity, is as effective as previous drugs, but of the 38 overdoses reported so far, none has had significant cardiovascular effects, and major CNS effects were rare.

SIGNS AND SYMPTOMS

The symptoms and signs of CA overdose are those of CNS depression, anticholinergic toxicity, and depression of cardiac conduction and contractility. CNS signs include disorientation, coma, myoclonus, clonus, and seizures; other signs include tachycardia, mydriasis, decreased bowel sounds, and respiratory depression. Generally, tachycardia, slurred speech, and lethargy are the earliest signs of toxicity, but life-threatening complications can develop in their absence. Coma is seen in about 35 percent. Twitching, jerking myoclonic movements are seen in 40 percent, are commonly confused with seizures, and do not respond to phenytoin. Grand mal seizures are seen in 10 to 20 percent of cases.

ECG changes are common and include ST- and T-wave changes, prolonged QT and QRS interval, rightward deviation of the QRS axis, bundle branch blocks, AV conduction blocks, aberrant conduction, ventricular arrhythmias, and eventually idioventricular rhythm and electromechanical dissociation (EMD). Arrhythmias such as ventricular tachycardia and frequent aberrant beats occur after there is significant intraventricular conduction block (with a widened QRS) and before bradycardia. By the time these arrhythmias occur, cardiac contractility is severely depressed. Although much human literature has focused on these ventricular arrhythmias, in the laboratory they do not seem to be an important mechanism of mortality. Myocardial depression is much more significant. Most patients who die suffer from hypotension, conduction blocks, and supraventricular tachycardia, not ventricular arrhythmias.

TREATMENT

There is little effective prehospital treatment for the major toxicity of CA overdose, and rapid transport should be instituted. In 25 percent of fatal cases, patients were alert and awake at first prehospital contact. All patients with a history of possible CA ingestion should be placed on a monitor, have an intravenous (IV) line and oxygen started, and be under constant observation while being transported to an emergency department. Ipecac is not recommended, since the level of consciousness may rapidly decrease, leading to aspiration. Activated charcoal, 50 to 100 g, should be given prehospital if the patient has an active gag reflex. Obtunded patients should have assisted ventilation and oxygen supplementation. Stabilization of a toxic patient is unlikely under field conditions.

The mainstays of treatment in CA overdose are prevention of absorption of the drug and respiratory support. Once absorbed, the drug is highly tissue bound; thus, even efficient methods of removal, such as charcoal hemoperfusion, have little impact.

Mandatory Preventive Care for All Patients

Fatal cases can present with only trivial signs of poisoning and develop major toxicity and life-threatening complications in a very short time. Therefore, every patient who presents to medical care with any history of ingestion of CAs must be immediately placed on a cardiac monitor, have an IV line established, and receive gastric lavage. Gastric lavage is preferred over ipecac, although the relative risks and benefits of these two approaches have never been specifically studied in CA overdose. Ipecac may produce vomiting just as the patient loses his or her gag reflex, and it delays administration of activated charcoal by at least an hour. Instilling charcoal down the lavage tube before lavage may further limit the amount of drug absorbed. If this is done, lavage should not be delayed, and a repeat dose of charcoal must be administered after lavage. The patient should be lavaged with large quantities of water, but recent study has demonstrated that further lavage is not necessary if return is clear after 5 L.

Activated charcoal effectively binds CAs, and multiple doses of charcoal every 2 h are even more effective. Such multiple doses reduce the drug half-life from 36 h to 4 h. Cathartics such as sodium and magnesium sulfate (250 mg/kg) are routinely recommended to speed drug removal from the gastrointestinal tract, although their clinical effectiveness has not been demonstrated. There may be no cathartic effect or passage of stool until the patient begins to awaken, since CAs have anticholinergic properties that inhibit peristalsis.

Ventilatory support and careful monitoring of acid-base status is even more important than for most other overdoses, because many cardiovascular complications of CAs are directly pH-dependent and worsened by acidosis. Any CA-overdosed patient with even a minimal decrease in level of consciousness should have arterial blood gases drawn and a chest x-ray (30 percent of patients with serious overdose develop either pulmonary edema or aspiration pneumonitis). Arterial pH should be maintained at or above 7.40 (see alkalinization under "Cardiac Complications"), and a high normal Pa_{O_2} should be maintained with oxygen administration.

An electrocardiogram should be obtained as soon as the patient arrives to evaluate QRS duration, QRS axis, and cardiac rhythm and rate. Toxicity is not closely related to the QRS duration. Although an early study claimed that a QRS duration of 100 ms or less put the patient at relatively low risk for complications, those findings have been contradicted. A QRS of $>$ 100 ms has a sensitivity for major complications of only 59 percent and a specificity of 76 percent. Another variable studied is a rightward deviation of the vector of the terminal 4 ms of the QRS complex of between 130 and 270° (i.e., negative in lead I and positive in aV_R). This deviation of the vector identifies CA overdose with a positive predictive value of 49 percent and a negative predictive value of 90 percent, making it useful only when absent. Consequently, a normal ECG does not rule out serious overdose.

In patients with serious overdose, serum sodium and potassium should be checked, because the former antagonizes CAs and the latter increases toxic effects. Significant hyponatremia or hyperkalemia should be corrected.

Drug removal from the body cannnot be achieved by peritoneal dialysis or forced diuresis. Hemoperfusion with activated charcoal removes only very small quantities, but this technique may be attempted in the critically ill patient in whom simpler, safer, and better-proven measures, such as alkalinization, fluid loading, and pressors, have been unsuccessful.

Prognosis

Accurate plasma CA levels are measurable by gas chromatography and are clinically important for monitoring therapy but are not predictive in individuals in overdose because of the large volume of distribution, the long half-life, and the extremely variable individual metabolism.

Just as plasma levels are not sensitive predictors of outcome, neither are ingested doses, even when they are accurately known. There are huge individual differences in sensitivity and metabolism. Due to the unpredictable variation in response, it is wise to anticipate complications in all patients and treat on the basis of the clinical condition, not the amount or type of drug ingested.

A Glasgow Coma Scale (GCS) of 8 or less predicts serious complications with a sensitivity of 86 percent and a specificity of 89 percent, which is better than the QRS duration. However, since cases of alertness shortly before sudden deterioration and death have been reported, a high GCS does not rule out significant ingestion.

TREATMENT OF SPECIFIC COMPLICATIONS

Despite an enormous literature, specific and effective treatment for CA complications does not exist. The preventive measures listed above are far more important. Currently recommended therapy is summarized in Table 89-1, and a few key points are emphasized in the text below. Despite the tidy explanations in review articles, the relative importance of the various pharmacologic effects is a matter of debate. Similarly, treatments based on these pharmacologic mechanisms (such as the use of physostigmine or β blockers) have not been successful or safe. Life-threatening complications generally fall into the category of seizures or cardiac depression (resulting in conduction blocks and hypotension).

Seizures

Seizures are seen in 10 percent of CA overdoses, and patients who seize have a mortality of 10 percent. Most patients' seizures are brief (less than 2 min) and few; 80 percent terminate spontaneously before any treatment can be given. Unfortunately, neither the duration nor the frequency of seizures predicts which patients will have cardiovascular complications. Since most seizures induced by CAs are brief and benign, it is not clear that treatment has any benefit, and most patients probably do not need treatment.

Nonetheless, many authors have recommended many different anticonvulsants, none of which has been proved both effective and safe. In the case of repeated or protracted seizures (most likely to be seen with amoxapine and maprotiline), one of the treatments below will have to be attempted.

Physostigmine is a specific and very effective antidote. However, it is short-acting and itself causes seizures, which usually occur within 20 min of administration. Physostigmine increased both seizures and mortality in experimental CA overdose in mice. For this reason, it is not recommended.

Diazepam (5 to 10 mg IV) has anecdotally been a successful initial treatment for seizures. Diazepam causes CNS and respiratory depression, but, as most of these patients are already comatose and intubated, this is a minor drawback. However, since most CA-induced seizures are brief and since diazepam does not protect long against subsequent seizures, its usefulness is questionable.

Phenobarbital and phenytoin have been reported only rarely and anecdotally, although the use of the latter is probably widespread.

Table 89-1. Summary of Treatment of Specific CA Complications (in Order of Preference and Effectiveness)

Coma
- Arterial blood gas monitoring and respiratory support

Seizures
- Respiratory support and alkalinization for all patients
- No drug treatment unless repeated or prolonged seizures
- Diazepam
- Phenytoin (not effective for myoclonic jerks)
- Phenobarbital
- General anesthesia
- Paralysis plus anticonvulsants

Tachycardia
- Alkalinization by ventilation
- No other treatment unless hypotensive

Conduction blocks and ventricular arrhythmias
- Alkalinization by hyperventilation
- Sodium loading with isotonic saline or sodium bicarbonate
- Phenytoin (unproven and may increase ventricular tachycardia)
- Only if hypotensive and the above fail:
  - Lidocaine (unstudied)
  - All other antiarrhythmics significantly worsen myocardial depression

Hypotension
- Alkalinization by hyperventilation
- Cautious fluid loading (high incidence of pulmonary edema)
- Pulmonary artery catheter monitoring for persistent hypotension
- Sodium loading with hypertonic saline or sodium bicarbonate
- Pressors with predominant α-adrenergic effect:
  - Epinephrine
  - Norepinephrine
  - High-dose dopamine
  - Phenylephrine
- Digitalis (unstudied)
- Physostigmine (in extremis only)
- Charcoal or resin hemoperfusion
- Cardiopulmonary bypass

Contraindicated drugs
- Absolute: Procaineamide
  - Quinidine
  - Disopyramide
  - Other type Ia antiarrhythmics
  - β Blockers
- Relative: Corticosteroids
  - Metaraminol
  - Mephentermine
  - Isoproterenol, dobutamine, low-dose dopamine (may worsen hypotension and arrhythmias)
  - Type Ia and type III antiarrhythmics: bretyllium, amiodarone (may promote torsade de pointes)
  - Type Ic antiarrhythmics: flecainide, encainide

Phenytoin given rapidly IV can cause hypotension and bradycardia, especially in patients with already depressed cardiac function. Therapeutic phenytoin caused significant hypotension in amitriptyline overdose in dogs and can worsen ventricular arrhythmias; one study found it to be ineffective in 188 human cases. Phenytoin is definitely ineffective against the typical frequent myoclonic jerks of CA overdose. Despite this lack of convincing therapeutic effectiveness, phenytoin has become widely used in CA overdose to treat both seizures and conduction defects, with no ill effects reported to date.

Occasionally, patients—especially those ingesting amoxapine, maprotiline, or desipramine—develop status epilepticus (often complicated by hyperthermia) that only appears to respond to general anesthesia or paralysis. When using the latter, it should be remembered that paralysis ends muscle activity but not electrical seizure activity in the brain, which still requires treatment. Since depolarizing agents such as succinylcholine may have potent vagal effects, a nondepolarizing agent such as vecuronium is theoretically safer.

Cardiac Complications

Treatment of the cardiac complications of CA overdose is equally complex and equally poorly studied. Physostigmine (given 2 mg IV over 2 min and repeated every 20 to 30 min, or 2 mg IM every 2 h) has enjoyed periodic popularity. Physostigmine is a very short-acting cholinergic drug that reverses the anticholinergic effects of cyclic antidepressants. Unfortunately, physostigmine is also a nonspecific analeptic and will waken patients obtunded due to a wide variety of causes. It has a very narrow therapeutic/toxic ratio and can produce cholinergic crisis, cause seizures, worsen conduction blocks, and produce cardiac arrest and asystole. The use of physostigmine should be avoided.

Alkalinization of the blood to a pH of 7.5 is probably the best treatment available for most forms of cardiovascular CA toxicity; this can narrow the QRS complex duration, abolish arrhythmias, and improve perfusion in minutes. Alkalinization can be accomplished by either hyperventilation or administration of IV sodium bicarbonate (1 to 5 mEq/kg over several minutes or titrated to pH). Hyperventilation can be implemented instantly (via bag-valve-mask or bag-valve-endotracheal tube) and is completely reversible. Sodium bicarbonate can cause hypernatremia and paradoxical intracellular acidosis, lower oxygen-carrying capacity, and worsen myocardial ischemia. However, in CA overdose bicarbonate seems to be more effective than hyperventilation alone. Hyperventilation is a safe and reversible initial choice; it can be followed with bicarbonate if not effective.

Part of the reason sodium bicarbonate is effective is that the sodium ion reverses the CA-induced block of the cell membrane sodium channel; in some animal studies hypertonic saline solution has been as effective as bicarbonate. Isotonic saline solutions should be used to correct hypovolemia, and any hyponatremia should be promptly corrected. Whether hypertonic saline solution has a role in treating CA toxicity in humans is unknown.

Phenytoin is a theoretically logical treatment that also has its advocates. Early studies mistakenly concluded that phenytoin improved cardiac conduction and produced no myocardial depression; both of these conclusions are false. However, phenytoin has never been studied in any large series of human CA-overdose patients and was ineffective in several animal studies. Its widespread use for "prophylaxis" in CA overdose is not defensible, particularly since a recent animal study in our laboratory has shown that it dramatically increases ventricular tachycardia.

Hypotension is present in 14 percent of CA overdoses, but significant depression of cardiac contractility is present long before hypotension develops. Usually accompanied by conduction blocks, apparent ventricular arrhythmias, and often pulmonary edema, it progresses to cardiac arrest and death in about 2 percent. Since the healthy myocardium of the younger patient will recover fully once the drug toxicity is past, markedly prolonged cardiopulmonary resuscitation (CPR) (for hours) or cardiopulmonary bypass may be successful in cases not responding to other measures.

Hypotension can be treated with isotonic saline solutions or alkalinization with bicarbonate. Presumably this is due both to the fact that increased vascular volume corrects for vasodilatation and to the fact that sodium loading helps reverse the sodium channel block. Due to the risk of pulmonary edema, fluid volume should be limited to the minimum necessary to maintain adequate perfusion; consequently, persistent hypotension requires pulmonary artery catheter monitoring. If isotonic saline solution and alkalinization with bicarbonate fail, catecholamine pressors are a rational choice. Agents with potent vasoconstricting properties, such as epinephrine, norepinephrine, and phenylephrine, are desirable, since CAs produce α-adrenergic blockade. Cases have been reported in which patients unresponsive to dopamine regained normal pressure with norepinephrine. Use of isoproterenol may worsen hypotension and cardiac irritability through an unopposed β-adrenergic effect. All vasopressors may increase the risk

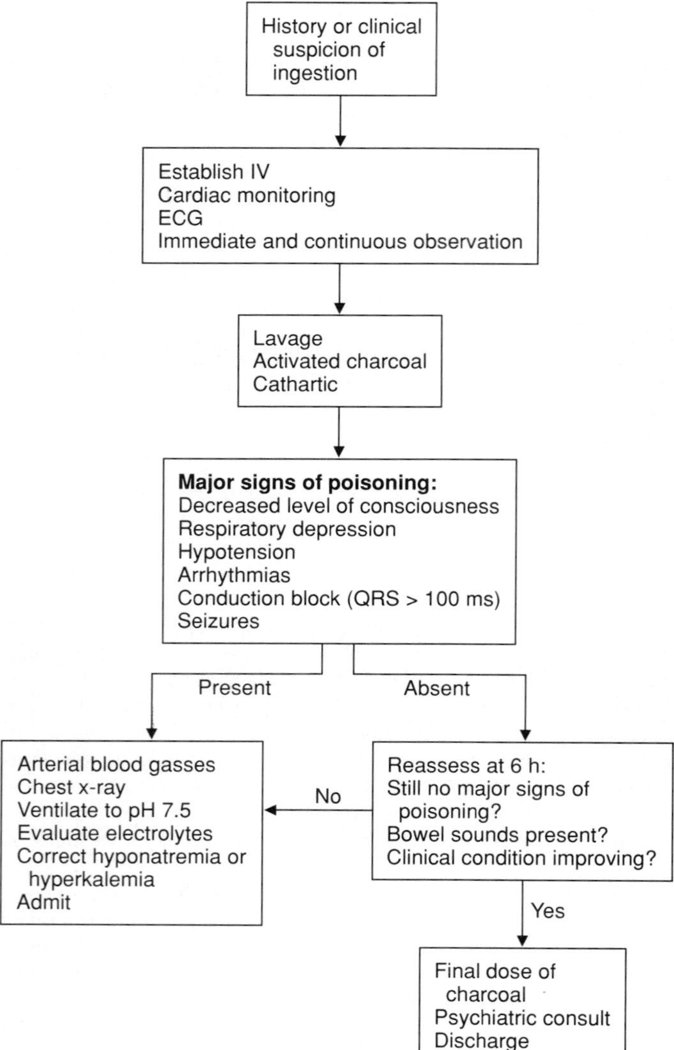

Fig. 89-1. Management of CA ingestion. [Modified with permission from Callaham M: Cyclic antidepressant overdose, in Callaham M (ed): *Current Practice in Emergency Medicine,* 2nd ed., B.C. Decker, Philadelphia, Pa., 1991.]

of arrhythmias. Dopamine has not been studied in humans; its use would be logical at high doses (although some patients fail to respond), but at low doses it carries the same risk as isoproterenol. Dobutamine, a predominantly β-adrenergic drug, is contraindicated. Indirect-acting sympathomimetics, such as metaraminol and mephentermine, are not logical choices, since CAs block their uptake into the adrenergic neuron and they act by releasing endogenous norepinephrine, which may already be depleted.

The list of noncatechol inotropic agents is short. Digitalis has been used clinically with and without conduction blocks with good results. In dogs there was no effect on the already increased PR and QRS duration. The literature suggests that digitalis must be used with caution in patients with significant block or ectopy but may be useful as a last resort. Glucagon has never been studied.

Physostigmine has been recommended for hypotension, but it can worsen hypotension and block and cause asystole. Many of the anecdotal beneficial effects of physostigmine may have been due to its CNS and respiratory analeptic properties. It should be avoided.

Hemoperfusion with activated charcoal or resin is highly efficient, but so much of the drug is bound to body tissues that this procedure can remove only a few milligrams of drug. Although its impact appears minor, it occasionally seems to be effective and should be considered in severe overdoses when simpler methods are failing.

Other experimental modalities include α-1-acid glycoprotein, which affects drug binding but has not proven useful in experimental studies. Fragments of CA-specific antibodies (analogous to digoxin antibodies) have been studied, but such large quantities are required (1 kg in an adult) that this method has not yet found clinical usefulness.

Disposition and Admission Criteria

Patients should receive cardiac monitoring, an IV line, gastric lavage, activated charcoal, and cathartics and should be observed for at least 6 h. If at any time during this period patients develop signs or symptoms of poisoning (decreased level of consciousness, respiratory depression, seizures, hypotension, arrhythmia, conduction block, or rightward terminal QRS vector), they should be admitted to a monitored bed. If after 6 h of observation the patient is free of these signs and symptoms, he or she should receive a final dose of charcoal and may be discharged to psychiatric evaluation. Patients who after 6 h demonstrate only minor signs, such as tachycardia less than 120 or minimally slurred speech, may be discharged if the presence of active bowel sounds suggests that both the ingested CA and the administered charcoal and cathartic are progressing on their way out of the GI tract and if their signs of poisoning are decreasing rather than increasing. If bowel sounds are absent or markedly decreased, peristalsis may be inhibited by the anticholinergic effects of CAs, and delayed absorption is more likely. In this case, admission for further monitoring and observation is prudent.

Management by this algorithm (Fig. 89-1) will allow proper identification and treatment of seriously poisoned patients. At the same time, the high rate of hospitalization and unnecessary cost for trivial ingestions will be lowered, while an adequate margin of safety for borderline cases will still be provided.

Delayed Complications

Virtually all major complications and deaths occur in the first 24 h when patients are treated according to the algorithm in Fig. 89-1. Most major complications and deaths occur in the first few hours, and most complications are present at the time of emergency department admission. After the first 24 h, continued monitoring is needed only for those patients manifesting major signs of toxicity, which should be very few. Monitoring inpatients for 6 h after all cardiovascular toxicity (including any ECG abnormalities other than sinus tachycardia less than 120) disappears is safe and effective.

BIBLIOGRAPHY

Bajaj K, Woosley R, Roden D: Acute electrophysiologic effects of sodium administration in dogs treated with *0*-desmethyl encainide. *Circulation* 80:994, 1989.

Callaham M: Cyclic antidepressant toxicity in Rosen P, Baker F, Braen R, et al. (eds): *Emergency Medicine: Concepts and Clinical Practice,* 2d ed. St. Louis, Mosby, 1987, pp 2087–2098.

Callaham M, Kassel D: Epidemiology of fatal tricyclic antidepressant overdose: Implications for management. *Ann Emerg Med* 14:1, 1985.

Callaham M, Schumaker H, Pentel P: Phenytoin prophylaxis of cardiotoxicity in experimental amitriptyline poisoning. *J Pharmacol Exp Ther* 245:216, 1988.

Emerman C, Connors A, Burma G: Level of consciousness as a predictor of complications following tricyclic overdose. *Ann Emerg Med* 16:326, 1987.

Foulke G, Albertson T: QRS interval in tricyclic antidepressant overdosage: Inaccuracy as a toxicity indicator in emergency settings. *Ann Emerg Med* 16:160, 1987.

Wolfe T, Caravati E, Rollins D: Terminal 40-ms frontal plane QRS axis as a marker for TCA overdose. *Ann Emerg Med* 18:348, 1989.

90 NEUROLEPTICS

William P. Kerns, II

INTRODUCTION

The term *neuroleptics* is now used to refer to a diverse group of antipsychotics and major tranquilizers utilized in the treatment of schizophrenia and other functional psychoses. Patients for whom neuroleptics are prescribed present a risk for therapeutic misadventure and intentional ingestion because of their behavioral unpredictability. Thus the emergency physician needs a firm understanding of the pharmacology of the neuroleptic agents, potential adverse reactions, and the effects of acute ingestion.

PHARMACOLOGY

Neuroleptics comprise a group of five classes of drugs (Table 90-1) which share a basic three-ring structure. While all five classes share the same general therapeutic and adverse effects, modifications of the base structure alter the potency of the drug and prevalence of the various side effects.

Neuroleptics act by blocking dopaminergic (D_1 and D_2), adrenergic (α_1 and α_2), muscarinic, and histaminic (H_1 and H_2) neurotransmission receptors. The D_2-dopaminergic receptor blockade provides the beneficial effects of behavior modification but is also responsible for the extrapyramidal symptoms which may occur. Blockage of α-adrenergic receptors results in vasodilation with orthostatic hypotension. Since muscarinic receptors are integral in the parasympathetic nervous system, their blockade results in anticholinergic effects including mydriasis, tachycardia, hyperthermia, flushing, dry mouth, urinary retention, and constipation. Histamine blockade may produce either CNS stimulation or sedation.

PHARMACOKINETICS

Chlorpromazine, an aliphatic phenothiazine, is the best-studied neuroleptic. Chlorpromazine may be administered orally or parenterally with peak serum levels attained in 2 to 3 h via the oral route. Oral bioavailability is approximately one-third of a given dose. Once absorbed, the drug binds greater than 95 percent to plasma protein. Chlorpromazine has a large volume of distribution (V_D = 20 L/kg). The high degree of protein binding and large volume of distribution preclude the use of hemodialysis in therapy of overdoses. The hepatic microsomal enzymes metabolize the drug via oxidation and glucuronidation to many metabolites, several of which are active and undergo enterohepatic circulation. This permits the use of multidose activated charcoal in cases of acute ingestion. The elimination half-life is biphasic and difficult to evaluate, but averages approximately 20 h. A negligible amount of the drug is cleared via the kidneys.

Haloperidol, a frequently used neuroleptic in the emergency department, has kinetics similar to those of chlorpromazine. Peak action occurs within 30 to 45 min after IM injection. Plasma proteins bind 92 percent of the drug. Metabolism occurs in the liver, via oxidation and reduction, and by the kidneys with 40 percent of an oral dose eliminated renally.

The above data are obtained from individuals taking therapeutic doses under well-controlled conditions. The kinetics may be altered in overdose situations due to the effects of large amounts of ingested drug, delays in gastric emptying, the effects of coingestants, or the premorbid condition of the patient.

THERAPEUTIC INDICATIONS

Psychiatric indications for neuroleptics include schizophrenia, schizoaffective disorders, mania, major depression with psychotic features, paranoid disorders, and atypical psychoses.

Neuroleptics are also used for nonpsychiatric conditions. Patients suffering with involuntary motor movements from Gilles de la Tourette syndrome, Huntington's chorea, chorea in rheumatic fever, and Meige syndrome will often experience relief of symptoms when treated with neuroleptic agents. Hiccoughs may be controlled with chlorpromazine, although the mechanism is unknown. Recent reports have shown beneficial effects of chlorpromazine in relief of vascular and tension headaches.

The most common nonpsychiatric use of neuroleptics (especially the phenothiazine class) is to control nausea and emesis. The antiemetic action results from dopaminergic blockade in the chemoreceptor trigger zone of the medulla, the area which controls vomiting stimulus. Prochlorperazine and promethazine are both class C fetal risk agents and should not be given to pregnant patients unless the potential benefit justifies the risk to the fetus.

Neuroleptics should not be used as sedating agents for drug-induced agitation in patients who have taken an overdose, for alcohol-intoxicated patients, for patients with delerium tremens or sedative-hypnotic withdrawal, or for pediatric patients. Neuroleptics lower the seizure threshold, have a prolonged duration of action, and form active metabolites. The central nervous system effects of abused drugs such as amphetamines, cocaine, and phencyclidine include seizure activity. The use of neuroleptics may theoretically increase the risk of seizures in the stimulant-intoxicated patient.

ADVERSE EFFECTS

The adverse effects of neuroleptic therapy are based on the types of neurotransmitter receptors each drug antagonizes. The lower-potency agents such as chlorpromazine and mesoridazine have more anticholinergic, antiadrenergic, and antihistaminic adverse reactions. The higher-potency agents such as thiothixene and haloperidol have predominantly antidopaminergic side effects. The antimuscarinic, antihistaminic, and antiadrenergic effects are common adverse reactions of many medications and will not be considered further. Dopamine antagonism results in a variety of abnormal motor movement disorders which may be classified by time of presentation during therapy. Early reactions develop in the first few days to weeks of therapy, while late complications occur after several months of treatment (see Table 90-2).

Dystonias are idiosyncratic drug reactions which consist of acute involuntary muscle movement and spasm. Unless a medication history is sought, the reactions may be confused with tetanus, strychnine toxicity, atypical seizures, or hysteria. Relief of symptoms can be achieved with parenteral administration of 50 mg diphenhydramine or 2 mg benztropine. Resolution should occur within 5 to 15 min. Oral therapy with either agent should be maintained for 2 to 3 days because of the prolonged action of the neuroleptic medication and subsequent risk of recurrence of the dystonic reaction. Because dystonias are idiosyncratic and not dose-dependent, prophylactic therapy is not indicated when using neuroleptics unless there is a prior history of a dystonic reaction.

Akathisia is a condition of motor restlessness. The symptoms may be subtle and falsely ascribed to worsening psychosis. As a result, the patient is often given increased doses of medication which result in worsening symptoms. Dosage decrease or change to a less potent neuroleptic will relieve akathisia and should occur in consultation with the patient's psychiatrist. Treatment of akathisia has also included amantadine, benztropine, and propranolol therapy.

Drug-induced parkinsonism may occur due to dopamine blockade in the nigrostriatal brain pathway. Parkinsonian symptoms are re-

Table 90-1. The Five Neuroleptic Classes

Class	Dose Range, mg/day	Potency* Equivalent, mg	Dopaminergic Effects	Anticholinergic Effects	Adrenergic Effects
Phenothiazines					
aliphatics					
Chlorpromazine	25–2000	100	Low	High	High
Promethazine	50–150	—	Low	High	Moderate
piperidines					
Mesoridazine	75–400	50	Low	High	High
Thioridazine	50–800	100	Low	High	Moderate
piperazines					
Prochlorperazine	15–150	15	Moderate	Moderate	Low
Fluphenazine	1–25	2	High	Moderate	Moderate
Thioxanthenes					
Thiothixene	6–60	4	High	Low	Moderate
Dibenzoxazepines					
Loxapine	10–300	10	Low	Moderate	Low
Butyrophenone					
Haloperidol	1–30	2	High	Low	Moderate
Dihydroindolone					
Molindone	15–225	10	Low	Low	Low

* Compared to 100 mg of chlorpromazine.

Table 90-2. Adverse Reactions to Neuroleptics

Type of Disorder	Presentation	Incidence, %	Treatment
Dystonic reaction Torticollis, facial grimacing, opisthotonos, oculogyric crisis, laryngeal spasm	Early	12 > males	Diphenhydramine 50 mg IM or benztropine 2 mg IM
Akathisia Restlessness, jittery feeling, insomnia	Early	20 > females	Lower dose or change to less potent drug. Benztropine, amantadine, or propranolol
Parkinsonism Resting tremor, rigidity, masked facies, shuffling gait	Early	13 > females	Lower dose or change to less potent agent. Benztropine or amantadine
Tardive dyskinesia Lip smacking, tongue protrusion, grimacing, chewing motion	Late	30 > females	No proven treatment
NMS Hyperthermia, rigidity, altered mental status, autonomic instability	Variable	<1 > males	A,B,C's, muscle relaxation, rehydration

versible with reduction in dosage, change to a less potent neuroleptic, or treatment with either benztropine or amantadine.

Tardive dyskinesia is a movement disorder in which the patient experiences repetitive, rhythmic motions of facial muscles and limbs. It is secondary to increased dopaminergic effects on the nigrostriatal pathway. Postulated mechanisms include the development of supersensitivity to dopamine at the receptor site or an increased number of dopamine receptors which occur in response to the dopaminergic blockade by the neuroleptic medication. Tardive dyskinesia is a disfiguring and debilitating adverse effect which is not readily reversible. One follow-up study showed no change in symptoms in two-thirds of the patients 2 years after diagnosis. There is no proven beneficial treatment.

Neuroleptic Malignant Syndrome

Neuroleptic malignant syndrome (NMS) is a dramatic, life-threatening reaction to neuroleptic medication which may occur at any time during therapy. The cardinal features of the syndrome include hyperthermia, muscular rigidity, altered level of consciousness, and ANS instability. The incidence is approximately 0.05 to 1 percent in patients treated with neuroleptic drugs, especially haloperidol. The differential diagnosis includes meningitis, encephalitis, tetanus, strychnine poisoning, vascular CNS events, malignant hyperthermia, heat stroke, and fatal catatonia.

Several mechanisms for NMS have been proposed, but the antidopaminergic theory is favored. Support for this theory is derived from the fact that muscular rigidity may result from dopamine antagonism in the nigrostriatal pathway and hyperthermia may occur from blockade of hypothalamic thermoregulation. NMS has also been reported following withdrawal of dopamine agonists in parkinsonian patients. Still others suggest that endorphins may have a role via modulation of dopaminergic neurotransmission.

The typical picture at presentation is that of a young male who is brought to the hospital because of high fever and altered mental status. Temperatures may be as high as 41°C (106°F). Other signs are tachycardia and a labile blood pressure. The muscular hypertonicity has been likened to lead-pipe rigidity. The mental status ranges from slight confusion to coma, but coma is more common.

Predominant laboratory findings include leukocytosis, elevated CPK and elevated hepatic transaminases. Electrolyte and renal function tests reflect the patient's degree of dehydration. Cerebrospinal fluid is normal. Blood, sputum, urine, and spinal fluid cultures are negative unless a secondary infection ensues. Myoglobinuria may occur secondary to rhabdomyolysis.

Successful management of NMS hinges on considering and making the diagnosis followed by meticulous intensive care aimed at providing adequate ventilation, rehydration, relief of muscle rigidity, reversal

Table 90-3. Initial Care of NMS

1. Airway, breathing, IV access, and cardiac monitor; ABG.
2. Immediate skeletal muscle relaxation with repeated doses of intravenous diazepam and, if necessary, rapid-sequence intubation followed by paralysis with pancuronium.
3. Reverse hyperthermia using mist and fan technique or packing in ice.
4. Rehydrate with IV crystalloid.
5. Obtain blood samples for WBC, Hgb, Hct, glucose, electrolytes, BUN, creatinine, CPK, hepatic enzymes, PT, PTT. Send urine for myoglobin.

of hyperthermia, and recognition of complications. Neuroleptics should be discontinued. (See Table 90-3.)

The use of specific drug agents in NMS is controversial and, unfortunately, the rarity of this disease makes controlled clinical trials of therapeutic modalities difficult. Intravenous benzodiazepines and, if necessary, neuromuscular paralytic agents are the first-line agents for muscular relaxation. Their onsets of action are rapid and predictable. Large doses of diazepam may be required to achieve the desired effect. If muscular rigidity remains after 10 to 15 min of diazepam therapy, the patient should undergo rapid-sequence intubation followed by treatment with a paralytic agent such as pancuronium. Bromocriptine, a dopamine agonist, and dantrolene, a direct skeletal muscle relaxant, have been reported effective. However, their lack of rapid effect precludes their use in the immediate therapy of NMS and their roles as delayed therapeutic agents have yet to be evaluated in clinical trials.

Mortality ranges from 5 to 20 percent. Complications of NMS occur in one-third of affected patients. Pulmonary complications predominate and include aspiration pneumonia, pulmonary embolism, pulmonary edema, and acute respiratory failure secondary to restricted chest wall motion. Other reported complications include rhabdomyolysis, cardiac arrhythmias, disseminated intravascular coagulation, and seizures.

ACUTE OVERDOSE

Clinical Findings

Central nervous system depression, from mild sedation to coma, typically occurs. Both coma and respiratory depression are less common with isolated neuroleptic ingestion; however, their incidence increases with the coingestion of other central nervous system depressants. Dysfunction of hypothalamic thermal regulation may occur, resulting in either hyperthermia or, more commonly, hypothermia. Pinpoint pupils have been associated with phenothiazine ingestion. Any of the previously described abnormal motor movement reactions may occur. Seizures have been reported.

Anticholinergic symptoms (flushing, dry mouth, hyperthermia, tachycardia, urinary retention, and constipation) are seen with ingestion of lower-potency agents such as chlorpromazine, thioridazine, or mesoridazine.

Hypotension and reflex tachycardia due to α-adrenergic blockade occur frequently. Thioridazine and mesoridazine (aliphatic phenothiazines) exert a quinidine-like action on myocardial tissue and can produce prolongation of the PR or QT interval and widening of the QRS complex. Ventricular arrhythmias, including torsades de pointes, have occurred in patients on therapeutic doses of thioridazine and mesoridazine as well as in overdose patients. Supraventricular tachycardia and atrioventricular dissociation have been reported.

Management

Supportive care and gastrointestinal decontamination are the main components of successful management. (See Table 90-4.) Initial attention should be focused on providing a patent airway and assuring adequate ventilation. Any patient with altered mental status should be given naloxone, dextrose, and thiamine. Assure adequate tissue perfusion by administering crystalloid. If crystalloid therapy fails and hypotension persists, vasopressor therapy with a predominant α-agonist agent should be initiated.

Table 90-4. Care of Acute Ingestion

1. Airway, breathing, IV access, cardiac monitor
2. Naloxone, dextrose, thiamine
3. Hypotension
   a. Crystalloid therapy
   b. Norepinephrine or phenylephrine
4. Ventricular arrhythmias
   a. Bicarbonate, 1–2 mEq/kg IV bolus, followed by continuous bicarbonate infusion to keep serum pH between 7.45 and 7.50
   b. Lidocaine or phenytoin
5. Torsades de pointes
   a. Isoproterenol
   b. Magnesium
   c. Overdrive pacing
6. Gastrointestinal decontamination:
   a. Activated charcoal 1 gm/kg initially, then 0.5 gm/kg q4h in all patients
   b. If patient is intubated, orogastric lavage using > 34 FR tube, followed by activated charcoal
7. Warming or cooling techniques for hypo- or hyperthermia
8. Seizures
   a. Benzodiazepines
   b. Phenobarbital
   c. Phenytoin

Continuous cardiac monitoring and a 12-lead ECG are essential. Ventricular arrhythmias should be managed with class IB antiarrhythmics or bicarbonate therapy. Bicarbonate is felt to restore the activity of sodium channels responsible for the phase 0 depolarization of myocardial conducting tissue. Avoid class IA antiarrhythmics (disopyramide, quinidine, and procainamide) as they may exacerbate the cardiac toxicity. Ventricular tachycardia with torsades de pointes is amenable to isoproterenol, overdrive pacing, or magnesium.

Appropriate diagnostic studies should be obtained to identify any reversible effects of neuroleptics and other coingestants. Laboratory tests should include glucose, electrolytes, and renal function. Toxicology analysis should include a drug screen and ethanol, salicylate, and acetaminophen levels. A flat plate radiograph of the abdomen may demonstrate radiopaque phenothiazine pills.

Gastrointestinal decontamination is an integral part of treatment in cases of acute ingestion. All patients need activated charcoal (1 g/kg with cathartic) initially. Multidose charcoal (0.5 g/kg q4h) may be helpful in removing the drug from the enterohepatic circulation, thus reducing drug bioavailability and accelerating the elimination half-life. Whether or not the symptomatic patient will benefit from a gastric emptying procedure should be weighed on a case-by-case basis. The mildly symptomatic patient may do well with charcoal therapy alone. The severely obtunded patient who requires intubation should have a large-bore orogastric tube placed and lavaged until clear, prior to the instillation of charcoal. The abdominal radiograph may assist in determining the need for gastric lavage and judge its efficacy. A patient found to have radiopaque pills in the GI tract might benefit from lavage. Attempts at enhancing elimination via hemodialysis are futile as the neuroleptics are highly protein-bound and have large volumes of distribution. Forced diuresis will not be of benefit as most of these drugs have minimal renal clearance.

Once the patient's condition is stabilized and gut decontamination initiated, therapy is directed to other complications. Temperature abnormalities should be corrected. Abnormal motor reactions should be treated as previously described. Seizures should be treated with intravenous benzodiazepines, phenobarbital, or phenytoin. Physostigmine has no role in acute neuroleptic ingestion.

With strong supportive care and adequate gut decontamination, the acutely intoxicated patient should experience little morbidity or mortality. Data from the *1989 AAPCC Report* revealed that only 21 deaths occurred in 9139 isolated phenothiazine ingestions.

BIBLIOGRAPHY

Bell J, Bass GE, Escobar JI: Management of neuroleptic overdoses. *Clin Toxicol Consult* 2:21, 1980.

Black JL, Richelson E, Richardson JW: Antipsychotic agents: A clinical update. *Mayo Clin Proc* 60:777, 1985.

Briggs GG, Freeman RK, Yaffe SJ: *Drugs in Pregnancy and Lactation*, 2d ed. Baltimore, Williams and Wilkins, 1986.

Danlon PT, Tupin JP: Successful Suicides with thioridazine and mesoridazine: A result of probable cardiotoxicity. *Arch Gen Psychiatry* 34:955, 1977.

Dubin WR, Feld JA: Rapid tranquilization of the violent patient. *Am J Emerg Med* 7:313, 1989.

Ellenhorn MJ, Barceloux DG: *Medical Toxicology: Diagnosis and Treatment of Human Poisoning*. New York, Elsevier, 1988.

Goldfrank LR, Flomenbaum NE, Lewin NA, et al: *Goldfranks Toxicologic Emergencies*, ed 4. Norwalk, Connecticut, Appleton and Lange, 1990.

Guze BH, Baxter LR: Neuroleptic malignant syndrome. *N Engl J Med* 313:163, 1985.

Maars-Simon PA, Zell-Kanter M, Kendzierski DL, et al: Cardiotoxic manifestations of mesoridazine overdose. *Ann Emerg Med* 17:1074, 1988.

Richelson, E: Neuroleptic affinities for human brain receptors and their use in predicting adverse effects. *J Clin Psychiatry* 45:331, 1984.

Rosenberg MR, Green M: Neuroleptic malignant syndrome: Review of response to therapy. *Arch Intern Med* 149:1927, 1989.

91
LITHIUM
P. J. Ryan

Since 1970 in the United States, the use of lithium carbonate has been an accepted treatment for bipolar (manic-depressive) affective disorders. Because of its narrow therapeutic index, the range between adequate dosage and drug toxicity is very close. Acute toxicity may result from greater than 40 mg/kg overdose, and toxicity may develop from a change in drug kinetics during chronic lithium therapy. Both are potentially life-threatening.

PHARMACOLOGIC PROPERTIES

Lithium, a monovalent cation, in the carbonate salt form is 99 percent absorbed following an oral dose. Peak absorption is in 1 to 4 h; complete absorption occurs in 8 h. During a 12- to 18-h distribution phase, it circulates unbound to plasma proteins, with an equilibrium volume of distribution approximating total body water, 0.6 to 0.8 L/kg. Lithium moves into and out of tissues slowly due to its property of delayed cellular membrane transfer. A blood-brain equilibrium (therapeutic state) may take 8 to 10 days. The average plasma half-life of lithium is 20 to 24 h, increasing with age and renal dysfunction.

Excretion is primarily renal and occurs in two phases. Two-thirds of a single dose is cleared in the urine by 6 to 12 h. The remainder is completely cleared over 10 to 14 days. Lithium has complete glomerular filtration; the proximal tubule reabsorbs 60 to 80 percent. No absorption occurs in the distal tubule. Renal clearance of lithium is 15 to 30 mL/min. An increased clearance is found with an alkaline urine and a decreased clearance results with hyponatremia and renal insufficiency.

Therapeutic serum levels are 0.6 to 1.2 mEq/L. Levels should be obtained 10 to 15 h post dosage to make sure absorption and distribution are complete. A 300-mg dose of lithium carbonate equals 8.1 mEq and may increase serum levels by 0.2 to 0.4 mEq/L. Both therapeutic action and toxic effects of lithium are mediated intracellularly. Thus lithium serum levels may not be a true reflection of the biologically active tissue portion. Lithium levels are considered toxic above 2.0 mEq/L; however, the significance of laboratory levels must always be closely correlated with the patient's clinical presentation.

PATHOPHYSIOLOGY

The exact mechanism and site at which lithium exerts its therapeutic effect remains uncertain. Lithium is known to compete with other cations, sodium, potassium, and calcium, and interferes with cyclic adenosine 3′,5′-monophosphate (cAMP) mediated processes that are regulated by polypeptide hormones. Many organ systems are affected by lithium which may be manifested as tolerable side effects or changes with chronic lithium therapy. These are outlined in Table 91-1.

Table 91-1. Potential Effects of Lithium Therapy

Initial side effects	Endocrine
Polydipsia	Nontoxic goiter
Polyuria	Hyperparathyroidism
Dry mouth	Teratogenesis (lithium crosses placenta and is excreted in breast milk)
Nausea	Ebstein's anomaly or other heart defects
Fine tremor of hands	Neonatal diabetes insipidus
Chronic effects	Dermatologic
Ophthalmologic	Acne
Tearing	Localized edema
Blurring of vision	Cutaneous ulcers
Scotomatas	Hematologic
Exophthalmos	Neutrophilia
Papilledema (pseudotumor cerebri)	Aplastic anemia (rare)
Renal	
Lowered urine osmolarity	
Nephrogenic diabetes insipidus	
Nephrotic syndrome	
Structural damage (+/−)	

ACUTE LITHIUM TOXICITY

Clinical Presentation

The most prominent symptoms of acute lithium toxicity are central nervous system and neuromuscular changes. Lethargy, confusion, muscle jerking, and tremor are early signs. Progression to stupor, seizures, and coma are evidence of severe lithium toxicity. Gastrointestinal reactions of nausea, vomiting, and diarrhea are frequent. Cardiovascular events are varied and are usually seen when the toxicity is severe. Conduction defects, bradycardia, and ST-T-wave changes may occur. Severe hypertension has been reported, but is rare. Hypotension is usually secondary to volume depletion. Laboratory studies will show a reduced anion gap. Blood lithium levels are not strictly predictive of the severity of toxicity. An acute overdose in a patient who has not previously received lithium may produce less severe toxicity than in a patient who has had maintenance lithium therapy. Careful clinical correlation is required in the interpretation of lithium levels. Signs and symptoms of acute lithium toxicity are outlined in Table 91-2. When a patient on chronic lithium therapy presents with a clinical picture of lithium toxicity, there should be an effort to discover anything which may have caused the lithium level to rise other than extra drug. Such factors could be decreased salt intake, a disturbance of the sodium balance, dehydration, or impaired renal function. There have been reports of drug interactions which might increase the serum lithium level, for example, ibuprofen, indomethacin, methyldopa, thiazides, chlorthalidone, triamterene, spironolactone, and acetylcholinesterase inhibitors.

Treatment

The treatment of lithium toxicity includes gastrointestinal decontamination, replacement of sodium depletion, supportive care, and occasionally hemodialysis. There are no effective antidotes.

Gastric lavage. In the overdose state, gastric lavage may be helpful even several hours after ingestion, especially if sustained-release tablets were taken. Repeated gastric lavage in 2 to 4 h may remove additional lithium. The use of charcoal is not effective in binding lithium, but should be used if there is any question of multiple drug ingestion. Cathartics are not helpful.

Intravenous normal saline. Sodium administration assures a good supply of sodium ions to the proximal renal tubules, producing an increase in lithium excretion.

Table 91-2. Signs and Symptoms of Acute Lithium Toxicity

CNS/Neuromuscular:	
Tremor	Gastrointestinal
Neuromuscular irritability: muscle twitching, hyperreflexia, clonus, fasciculations	Nausea and vomiting
	Diarrhea
	Cardiovascular:
Ataxia	ST-T-wave changes
Transient neurologic asymmetries	Sinus bradycardia
Lethargy	Conduction defects
Dysarthria	Ventricular arrhythmias
Confusion	Hypertension (rare)
Stupor	
Convulsions	
Coma	

Alkalinization of urine and osmotic diuresis. If renal function is adequate, these measures may increase lithium excretion. Sodium bicarbonate and carbonic anhydrase inhibitors have been advised by some but should be used with caution in the absence of good clinical studies. Aminophylline and osmotic diuretics (mannitol or urea) have been used to increase urinary output and lithium excretion.

Good supportive care. Supportive care should include cardiac monitoring. Careful electrolyte and renal function monitoring is required. Fluid balance needs attention. Intensive care may be required for severely toxic patients.

Hemodialysis. Dialysis is an effective means for removing lithium ions from the serum. The goal of hemodialysis is a lithium level of 1 mEq/L 6 to 8 h after dialysis. This will allow for redistribution of lithium from tissue stores. Repeat dialysis may be necessary based on clinical response and resultant serum lithium levels. Indications for hemodialysis are as follows:

1. Clinical signs of severe poisoning
2. Deteriorating clinical condition: seizures, coma, or ventricular arrhythmias
3. Decreasing urine output, or renal failure
4. Lack of expected drop in serum lithium level (20 percent in 6 h)

BIBLIOGRAPHY

Amdisen A: Lithium and drug interactions. *Drugs* 24:133, 1982.

Clendeninn NJ, Pond SM, Kaysen G, et al: Potential pitfalls in the evaluation of the usefulness of hemodialysis for the removal of lithium. *J Toxicol Clin Toxicol* 19:341, 1982.

DePaulo JR, Folstein MF, Correa EI: The course of delirium due to lithium intoxication. *J Clin Psychiatry* 43:11, 1982.

El-Mallakh RS: Treatment of acute lithium toxicity. *Vet Hum Toxicol* 26:31, 1984.

Jaeger A, Kopferschmitt SJ: Toxicokinetics of lithium intoxication treated by hemodialysis. *Clin Toxicol* 23:501, 1986.

Kondziela JR: Extreme lithium intoxication without severe symptoms. *Hosp Community Psychiatry* 35(7):727, July 1984.

Clinical Toxicology Review 2(5), 1980.

Mateer JR, Clark MR: Lithium toxicity with rarely reported ECG manifestations. *Ann Emerg Med* 11(4):208, April 1982.

Ramsey TA, Cox M: Lithium and the kidney: A review. *Am J Psychiatry* 139:4, 1982.

Simard M, Gumbiner B, Lee A, et al: Lithium carbonate intoxication. *Arch Intern Med* 149:36, 1989.

Singer I, Rotenberg D: Mechanisms of lithium action. *N Engl J Med* 289:254, 1973.

Thomsen K: Renal handling of lithium at non-toxic and toxic serum lithium levels. *Dan Med Bull* 25(3):106, April 1978.

92
BARBITURATES

P. J. Ryan

Barbiturates were first introduced as a sedative in 1903. Current use has increased to include treatment of seizure disorders, induction of anesthesia, and management of increased intracranial pressure. Barbiturate poisoning is not as frequently seen now that there are numerous other tranquilizers and sedatives, but is still remains a very serious, potentially lethal problem.

PHARMACOLOGY

The basic structure common to all barbiturates, barbituric acid, has no central nervous system activity. Only when its C-5 position is substituted with an alkyl, alkenyl, or aryl group does the resulting compound have a central nervous system effect. Four categories are classified by the duration of hypnotic activity, ranging from 0.3 h for the ultrashort-acting thiobarbiturates to 6 to 12 h for long-acting phenobarbital. The duration of action of barbiturates is dependent on lipid solubility, which is determined by the side chain structure at C-2 and secondarily by pH gradients. Thiobarbiturates, which have the oxygen at C-2 replaced by sulfur, are more lipid-soluble than oxybarbiturates.

Barbiturates with lipid solubility readily diffuse into body tissues and rapidly cross the blood-brain barrier. They are mainly metabolized by the liver. The mean half-life varies from 3 h for the ultrashort-acting drugs up to 37 h for intermediate-acting drugs.

Long-acting barbiturates such as phenobarbital are 80 percent absorbed by oral dosage. The volume of distribution is 0.8 L/kg, and 50 percent of the drug becomes protein-bound in the serum. Hepatic metabolism occurs, but approximately 25 percent of phenobarbital is excreted unchanged in the urine. Urinary pH varies the rate of renal clearance. The elimination half-life of phenobarbital varies from 48 to 200 h. In children, the elimination half-life is ½ times greater than in adults, but in infants the elimination half-life is 2 to 5 times greater than in adults. The elderly and those with hepatic disease have an increased elimination half-life. Phenobarbital readily crosses the placenta to the fetus and enters breast milk. Therapeutic levels are 10 to 40 mg/L.

Repeated use of hepatic metabolized barbiturates can lead to their shortened elimination half-life by induction of metabolizing enzymes (cytochrome P_{450}). Chronic use of phenobarbital can accelerate metabolism of oral anticoagulants, digoxin, corticosteroids, quinidine, phenytoin, tricyclic antidepressants, tetracycline, and phenothiazines.

The major site of action of barbiturates is in the central nervous system, where they enhance the action of the inhibitory neurotransmitter γ-aminobutyric acid (GABA). They may also inhibit noradrenergic excitation at neuronal junctions. Barbiturates are general depressants to nerve and muscle tissues. Tolerance develops after chronic use of all barbiturates; as much as six times the usual dose may be required for the same effect.

CLINICAL PRESENTATION

Mild to moderate barbiturate intoxication closely mimics the presentation of alcohol intoxication. Lethargy, emotional lability, and impaired thinking occur. General incoordination, slurred speech, and nystagmus may be seen.

Severe acute barbiturate toxicity results in progressive central nervous system depression ranging from lethargy to profound coma. Respiratory depression develops and may progress to respiratory arrest. Cardiovascular functions are altered, resulting in hypotension, vasodilatation, and shock. Hypothermia is common. Pupillary size may vary, either constricted or dilated. Flaccid muscle tone is present, and deep tendon reflexes are depressed or absent. Gastrointestinal activity is slowed. Skin bullae occur in about 6 percent of patients, and sweat gland necrosis has been reported. A severe overdose may show a flat line EEG.

The lethal dose of barbiturates varies considerably, but as a rule of thumb, 10 times the hypnotic dose is capable of producing severe toxicity. Short-acting, lipid-soluble barbiturates induce toxicity more rapidly and at a lower dose than the longer-acting agents. Neither drug dose nor the blood levels should be exclusively relied upon to predict the severity of an overdose or to correlate it to potential mortality. Measured plasma concentrations of barbiturates may not reflect the actual level in the brain. The laboratory should report the specific type of barbiturate ingested, which is important in understanding its duration of action and its route of excretion. Chronic barbiturate use and the patient's tolerance need to be considered.

The clinical presentation, such as the depth of coma, respiratory depression, or cardiovascular depression, must be the primary consideration in determining the severity of a barbiturate overdose. Early deaths are generally cardiovascular-related (shock or arrest) while late deaths most commonly are due to secondary pulmonary complications (aspiration pneumonitis or pulmonary edema). Less often, deaths are related to cerebral edema or renal failure. Fatalities usually have developed multiple system catastrophes.

Table 92-1. Barbiturate Classification

General Formula and Substituted Derivatives

```
        R3    O
        |    //
        N—C
        3         R1
                 /
*O=C2         5C
                 \
                  R2
        N—C
        |   \\
        H     O
```

Barbiturate	Duration of Action, h	R_1	R_2	R_3
Ultrashort-acting:				
Thiopental*	0.3	Ethyl	1-Methyl butyl	—H
Thiamylal*	0.3	Allyl	1-Methyl butyl	—H
Methohexital	0.3	Allyl	1-Methyl-2-pentynyl	$—CH_3$
Short-acting:				
Hexobarbital	3	Methyl	1-Cyclohexen-1-yl	$—CH_3$
Pentobarbital	3	Ethyl	1-Methyl butyl	—H
Secobarbital	3	Allyl	1-Methyl butyl	—H
Intermediate-acting:				
Amobarbital	3–6	Ethyl	Isopentyl	—H
Aprobarbital	3–6	Allyl	Isopropyl	—H
Butabarbital	3–6	Ethyl	*sec*-Butyl	—H
Long-acting:				
Barbital†	6–12	Ethyl	Ethyl	—H
Mephobarbital†	6–12	Ethyl	Phenyl	$—CH_3$
Phenobarbital†	6–12	Ethyl	Phenyl	—H
Primidone*	6–12	Ethyl	Phenyl	—H

* Has S substitution for O, except in thiamylal and thiopental which is replaced by S, and 2H substitution for primidone.

† Only drugs responsive to alkaline diuresis.

TREATMENT

The key to eventual recovery is the careful and skillful management of multiple depressed organ systems until the patient metabolizes and clears the drug. Because of this type of attention to critical care, most patients with serious barbiturate overdose now survive; only a few years ago such patients were frequently fatalities.

Airway management in the patient with severe overdose frequently requires intubation. Blood gas levels and chest x-ray films should be obtained periodically. Protection of the airway before gastric lavage cannot be overemphasized.

Gastric lavage is the method most commonly used for gastric emptying. Induction of emesis is dangerous in any patient with potential central nervous system depression.

Activated charcoal is instilled at the completion of an adequate lavage. In the management of patients with phenobarbital overdoses, good results occur with the use of multiple doses of charcoal. Thirty-gram doses have been used every 6 h via a nasogastric tube for a total of six doses. Results have shown a decrease in the elimination half-life of phenobarbital with use of repeated doses of charcoal.

Intravenous fluids are necessary for supportive or maintenance balance. A fluid challenge is the first treatment which should be given if hypotension develops. Low doses of dopamine may be used if an adequate fluid load is ineffective. Total parenteral nutrition should be considered if the coma duration is greater than 2 to 3 days.

Forced diuresis and alkalinization of the urine are helpful for the management of long-acting phenobarbital intoxication. Sodium bicarbonate used in 1 to 2 mEq/kg doses every 4 to 6 h to maintain urine pH at 7.5 or greater may significantly (5- to 10-fold) increase the phenobarbital excretion rate. This is not effective for intermediate- or short-acting barbiturates. Care should be taken that fluid overload does not result from too vigorous attempt of diuresis.

Hemodialysis can remove significant amounts of phenobarbital and is six to nine times more effective than forced diuresis and alkalinization. Charcoal hemoperfusion is even more efficacious, but is not without potential complications. Hemodialysis and hemoperfusion should only be used in the most critical overdose cases, or if the patient has underlying hepatic or renal insufficiency.

BARBITURATE WITHDRAWAL SYNDROME

If an abrupt discontinuation of barbiturates occurs after a state of physical dependence has been established by their chronic use, withdrawal symptoms occur. Minor symptoms generally develop within 24 h after cessation of the drug. These include restlessness, anxiety, insomnia, depression, nausea, vomiting, abdominal cramps, sweating, and tremor. Such symptoms subside within 3 to 7 days. Occasionally there is progression to more severe withdrawal symptoms.

Following 2 to 3 days of abstinence, major withdrawal symptoms may appear. Increased muscular tone and jerking may progress to grand mal seizures. Auditory hallucinations and delirium could result. Hyperpyrexia, cardiovascular collapse, and death are possible.

Treatment of seizures is first the administration of diazepam and then, if this is ineffective, administration of a barbiturate. Gradual withdrawal of the addicting agent is the safest way to prevent major withdrawal symptoms.

BIBLIOGRAPHY

Baltarowich LL: Barbiturates. *Topics in Emergency Medicine*. October 1985, pp 46–54.

Costello JB, Poklis A: Treatment of massive phenobarbital overdose with dopamine diuresis. *Arch Intern Med* 141:938, 1981.

Gaudreault P: Barbiturates. *Clinical Toxicology Review* 3:1, 1981.

Goldberg MJ, Berlinger WG: Treatment of phenobarbital overdose with activated charcoal. *JAMA* 247:2400, 1982.

Ho IK: Mechanism of action of barbiturates. *Annu Rev Pharmacol Toxicol* 21:83, 1981.

McCarron MM, Schulze BW, Walbert CB, et al: Short-acting barbiturate overdosage. *JAMA* 248:55, 1982.

Pond SM, Olson KR, Osterloh JD, et al: Randomized study of the treatment of phenobarbital overdose with repeated doses of activated charcoal. *JAMA* 251:3104, 1984.

Preskorn SH, Schwin RL, McKnelly WV: Analgesic abuse and the barbiturate abstinence syndrome. *JAMA* 244:369, 1980.

Rosenbaum JL, Kramer MS, Raja R: Resin hemoperfusion for acute drug intoxication. *Arch Intern Med* 136:263, 1976.

Zawada ET, Nappi J, Done G, et al: Advances in the hemodialysis management of phenobarbital overdose. *South Med J* 76:6, 1983.

93 PHENYTOIN TOXICITY

Brad S. Selden

Death or severe morbidity is unusual following intentional phenytoin overdose, and an intact outcome is typical if good supportive care is provided. Most deaths have not been overdose-related. Instead, they have almost always been iatrogenic in nature, and due to hypersensitivity reactions, rapid IV administration in critically ill or digoxin-intoxicated patients, coingested drugs, or complications of extravasated infusions. The infrequently seen life- and limb-threatening manifestations of phenytoin intoxication (Table 93-1) may be readily treated using conventional therapies immediately available to any acute care facility (Table 93-2).

TOXIC MECHANISM AND PATHOPHYSIOLOGY

The Brain

Phenytoin exerts its antiepileptic and antiarrhythmic actions by a stabilizing effect on all excitable membranes, through sodium and calcium channel blocking effects, and through facilitation of potassium and chloride conductance. Phenytoin also enhances activity at the receptor site of γ-aminobutyric acid, which functions as an inhibitory neurotransmitter in the cerebral cortex to limit repetitive firing and propagation of seizure activity. Conversely, γ-aminobutyric acid has an excitatory effect on the cerebellum. This acts to suppress cortical seizure formation at therapeutic phenytoin levels via stimulation of inhibitory cerebellar pathways, but gives rise to the cerebellar-vestibular signs seen at toxic phenytoin concentrations.

Cardiovascular System

The membrane-stabilizing effect of phenytoin on the heart is similar to that of lidocaine and other class IB antiarrhythmics. Although phenytoi has been used to enhance atrioventricular conduction in treatment of digitalis toxicity, impaired cardiac conduction with prolonged PR and QRS intervals and increasing degrees of AV block occurs with phenytoin toxicity. Similarly, therapeutic effects of depressed pacemaker and ventricular Purkinje cell automaticity are increased and accompanied by a direct negative inotropic effect on myocardium at toxic levels. Peripheral vasodilation may also contribute to hypotension. This effect, as well as negative inotrophy, has been attributed to rapid intravenous administration. However, clinically significant hypotension, bradycardia, and even cardiac arrest have occurred at much lower drug infusion rates than the recommended 50 mg/min.

Effects of Propylene Glycol and Ethanol Diluents

The acute cardiovascular toxicity seen with intravenous phenytoin infusion has frequently been ascribed to its diluent. The vehicle for the most widely used parenteral formulation of phenytoin (Dilantin) is 40% propylene glycol and 10% ethanol, adjusted to a pH of 12 with sodium hydroxide. The glycol component has been shown to cause coma, seizures, circulatory collapse, ventricular arrhythmias, cardiac nodal depression, and hypotension in humans and animals. Propylene glycol is a strong myocardial depressant and vasodilator and increases vagal tone. Other toxic effects of propylene glycol include hyperosmolality, hemolysis, and lactate-associated metabolic acidosis. Louis et al. compared the acute toxicities of intravenous phenytoin and propylene glycol both alone and in combination. In a feline model, phenytoin alone did not cause significant cardiovascular effects, and instead partially reversed the toxic effects that occurred when propylene glycol was given. Acute toxic effects of propylene glycol are also strongly related to rate of infusion. This is further evidence for its etiologic role in intravenous phenytoin toxicity, a phenomenon which is almost always related to infusion rate. The ethanol intravenous diluent fraction may precipitate a reaction in patients taking disulfuram.

Table 93-1. Life-Threatening Manifestations of Acute Phenytoin Toxicity

Coma with loss of protective airway reflexes
Seizures
Bradyarrhythmias and heart block
Hypotension
Extravasation of intravenous phenytoin (limb-threatening)

PHARMACOKINETICS

Absorption

Bioavailability differs markedly between phenytoin formulations, so a patient may become toxic with a change in product brand at the same dose, or when tablets or suspension are substituted for capsules.

Peak levels are seen within 10 min of intravenous infusion and approximately 8 h (range 3 to 10 h) after an oral therapeutic dose. Because of phenytoin's poor gastrointestinal (acidic) solubility, which further decreases at higher doses, the absorption phase will be markedly extended after large oral overdose. Peak levels are delayed until 31.5 h after a 1600-mg oral dose and have been shown to increase for up to 6 days after overdose, remaining in the toxic range for over 2 weeks.

Distribution

Phenytoin is highly protein-bound with a free drug fraction of approximately 0.1 and a relatively low volume of distribution of 0.6 L/kg. Brain tissue concentrations equal those in plasma within about 10 min of intravenous infusion and correlate with therapeutic effects, while cerebrospinal fluid and myocardium equilibrate within 30 to 60 min. This slower distribution into tissue is further evidence that hypotension and arrhythmias occurring during phenytoin infusion are due to propylene glycol toxicity.

Free Phenytoin Fractions

Toxic signs appear to be more closely related to free phenytoin fractions in plasma than total drug levels, and, indeed, the *proportion* of active free drug to bound drug increases as serum levels rise into the toxic range. Clinically significant increases in free drug fraction have been associated with hypoalbuminemia, uremia, severe hyperbilirubinemia from viral hepatitis or other liver disease, acidosis, therapeutic use of (or toxic hepatitis from) valproic acid, and use in elderly patients.

Metabolism

Phenytoin is metabolized by hepatic microsomal enzymes that transform almost all of the drug to inactive metabolites; only 1 to 4 percent

Table 93-2. Emergency Treatment of Life-Threatening Phenytoin Toxicity

Airway management with endotracheal intubation and mechanical ventilation as needed
Treatment of seizures with phenobarbital, 20 mg/kg IV; repeat as needed and manage airway as above
Atropine and temporary pacemaker as required for symptomatic bradyarrhythmias and heart block, *avoiding other membrane-stabilizing antiarrhythmic drugs*
Intravenous crystalloid boluses followed by pressor therapy as needed for hypotension
Urgent consultation with orthopedic or plastic surgeon if extravasation injury or other damage in extremity is observed

is excreted unchanged in the urine. The rate of metabolism and elimination is proportional to the serum phenytoin concentration (first-order kinetics) only at low drug levels. As phenytoin levels increase, metabolism changes to fixed-rate (zero-order or saturation) kinetics. This change from first-order to zero-order metabolism occurs even at low therapeutic levels in some patients. As a result, plasma drug concentrations increase disproportionately as dosage is increased, which can result in intoxication shortly after a patient's daily dose is changed. This effect also serves to markedly prolong elimination in overdose.

Drugs that inhibit microsomal enzyme activity will also cause phenytoin levels to increase. Clinically significant increases in phenytoin levels or toxicity have been documented with chloramphenicol, disulfuram, isoniazid (but only in slow acetylators), cimetidine, miconazole, valproic acid, dicoumarol, and high daily doses of propoxyphene.

SERUM LEVELS AND RANGE OF TOXICITY

Therapeutic phenytoin levels for seizures and arrhythmias are described as being 10 to 20 μg/mL (40 to 80 μmol/L),* although 50 percent of seizure patients achieve reduction of seizure frequency below these levels.

Individual variation in toxicity is a function of baseline mental status, neurologic status, individual response to the drug, and free drug fraction. Patients with underlying brain disease are predisposed to toxicity and may become toxic at much lower levels than usual. Historically, nystagmus has been held to be the initial sign of toxicity at phenytoin levels of approximately 20 μg/mL, but it may occur at much lower levels or not appear until much higher levels are attained. Ataxia usually begins at about 30 μg/mL, and lethargy at 40 μg/mL. Altered mental status and other motor signs may occur at levels well below 20 μg/mL and are not necessarily preceded by nystagmus . Conversely, some patients may tolerate levels of ≥ 40 μg/mL and only demonstrate mild impairment on neuropsychologic testing. Almost all patients with phenytoin-induced seizures will have levels ≥ 30 μg/mL, but serum concentrations are usually much higher. Similarly, deaths have occurred at levels >50 μg/mL, but most have been at levels >90 μg/mL. However, survival in children is also reported with levels of >100 μg/mL. Signs of toxicity occur at serum free phenytoin levels of 1.5 to 3.5 μg/mL and are consistently severe over 5 μg/mL.

CLINICAL PRESENTATIONS

Central Nervous System Toxicity

As toxic phenytoin levels are reached, both inhibitory cortical and excitatory cerebellar-vestibular effects begin to occur. The usual initial excitatory sign of toxicity is nystagmus, which is seen first on forced lateral gaze and then becomes spontaneous. Upward-beating, bidirectional, or alternating nystagmus may occur with severe intoxication.

Decreased level of consciousness is routine, with initial sedation, lethargy, ataxic gait, and dysarthria progressing to confusion, coma, and even apnea in large overdose. Chronically impaired cognitive function or acute encephalopathy may occur without other common signs of ataxia and nystagmus. This is usually seen at toxic levels but again may occur in the therapeutic range. Nystagmus will commonly disappear at levels sufficient to cause coma (above 35 to 55 μg/mL), and complete ophthalmoplegia and loss of corneal reflexes may occur. Therefore, absence of nystagmus does not exclude severe phenytoin toxicity. Nystagmus then returns as serum drug levels decrease and coma lightens. This depression of oculovestibular reflexes persists as mental status recovers, demonstrating the relatively greater effect of phenytoin on the vestibulo-oculomotor system.

Phenytoin-induced seizures are usually brief, and may be partial or generalized. They are almost always preceded by other signs of toxicity, especially in acute overdose. However, some patients will develop seizures first.

Cerebellar stimulation and alteration in dopaminergic and serotonergic activity may be responsible for acute dystonias and movement disorders seen in overdose, including opisthotonos and choreoathetosis. Either depressed or hyperative deep tendon reflexes, clonus, and extensor toe responses may also be elicited. Some signs of neurologic toxicity may outlast the presence of drug by months, especially mild peripheral neuropathy or acute reversible cerebellar degeneration with ataxia.

Psychosis, toxic delirium, visual and auditory hallucinations, euphoria, irritability, agitation, and combativeness have all been reported with toxicity.

Cardiovascular Toxicity

Cardiac toxicity after oral phenytoin overdose in an otherwise healthy patient has never been reported and, if observed, should mandate a rapid assessment for other causes (e.g., hypoxia, other drugs). Cardiovascular complications have been almost entirely limited to cases of intravenous administration in otherwise extremely ill or digitalis toxic patients. These include hypotension with decreased peripheral vascular resistance, bradycardia, conduction delays progressing to complete AV nodal block, ventricular tachycardia, primary ventricular fibrillation, and asystole. Electrocardiographic changes include increased PR interval, widened QRS interval, and altered S-T and T-wave segments. However, bradycardia, hypotension, and syncope in healthy volunteers have been reported even after small intravenous doses. Slowly administered (<25 mg/min) intravenous phenytoin has also been reported to cause precipitous, refractory hypotension and cardiac arrest in critically ill patients receiving dopamine infusions to support blood pressure. Again, most of these complications can be attributed to rapid intravenous administration of the propylene glycol diluent fraction and cannot be demonstrated at infusion rates of less than 30 mg/min of phenytoin in otherwise stable patients.

Vascular, Extravasation, and Soft Tissue Toxicity

An important but infrequently considered toxic effect is local vascular and tissue injury after injection. Although still recommended by the manufacturer, intramuscular injection results in localized crystallization of the drug, with erratic and unpredictable absorption, hematomas, sterile abscess, and myonecrosis at the injection site. Complications after intravenous infusion have included skin and soft tissue necrosis requiring skin grafting, compartment syndrome with multiple fasciotomies, gangrene, amputation, and death (at a fatality rate exceeding that from oral overdose). A syndrome of delayed bluish discoloration of the affected extremity, followed by erythema, edema, vesicles, bullae, and local tissue ischemia, has also been described. This has been reported after intravenous push administration of undiluted phenytoin *even in the absence of extravasation,* and has eventually necessitated amputation in some cases. The propylene glycol diluent, strong alkalinity of the intravenous solution, and crystallization of the drug contribute.

Hypersensitivity Reactions and Other Side Effects

Hypersensitivity reactions usually occur within 1 to 6 weeks of beginning phenytoin therapy and can include fever, systemic lupus erythematosus, erythema multiforme, toxic epidermal necrolysis, Stevens-Johnson syndrome, hepatitis, rhabdomyolysis, acute interstitial pneumonitis, lymphadenopathy, leukopenia, disseminated intravascular coagulation, and renal failure. An erythematous morbilliform rash is extremely common (up to 50 percent of cases) after initiation of phenytoin, occurring more frequently in the summer. Another clin-

* Multiply traditional units of μg/mL or mg/L by 3.964 to convert to SI units μmol/L).

ically significant effect in some is hyperglycemia, felt to be secondary to inhibition of insulin release. This can lead to diabetic ketoacidosis or nonketotic hyperosmolar coma. The teratogenic fetal hydantoin syndrome is well described, so oral phenytoin therapy in a pregnant patient should never be initiated or continued by the emergency physician without consultation and close follow-up from the attending neurologist and obstetrician.

DIFFERENTIAL DIAGNOSIS

Intoxication with almost any CNS-active or sedative-hypnotic drug may mimic early phenytoin intoxication, especially ethanol, carbamazepine, benzodiazepines, and lithium. Disease states resembling phenytoin toxicity include hypoglycemia, Wernicke's encephalopathy, and posterior fossa hemorrhage or tumor. Although seizures may be caused by phenytoin at toxic levels, other epileptogenic medication overdoses and seizures due to withdrawal from ethanol or other sedative-hypnotics must be considered in adults.

LABORATORY DIAGNOSIS AND ANCILLARY STUDIES

In oral overdose, the prolonged absorption phase mandates serial assessment to determine peak serum phenytoin levels. Phenytoin concentrations are most commonly measured by an enzyme-mediated immunoassay (EMIT) technique, which is specific and sensitive to ≤ 1 μg/mL. If available, free phenytoin concentrations are more useful to predict toxicity. Corrected serum phenytoin levels can be calculated in hypoproteinemia patients with a known serum albumin level. To calculate the phenytoin concentration (C_{normal}) that would be present if the patient's serum albumin were normal, the following equation is used:

$$C_{\text{normal}} = \frac{C_{\text{measured}} \times 4.4}{\text{albumin concentration}}$$

where phenytoin concentrations are in micrograms per milliliter and albumin concentration is in grams per deciliter.

Similarly, the free phenytoin fraction (FPF) (normally about 0.1) may be corrected for hypoalbuminemia with this equation:

$$\text{FPF} = \frac{1}{1 + (2.1 \times \text{albumin})}$$

where phenytoin concentrations are in micrograms per milliliter and albumin concentration is in grams per deciliter.

TREATMENT

Initial treatment of oral phenytoin overdose, including airway management and cardiac monitoring, is similar to that for other ingested drugs. Respiratory acidosis due to ventilatory insufficiency or metabolic acidosis should be corrected to decrease the active free phenytoin fraction. Two or three additional 1g/kg doses of oral activated charcoal in the first 24 h may be of benefit, given the known poor solubility and resultant extended absorptive phase of oral phenytoin in overdose. However, this therapy remains clinically unproven and should not be given to a patient with concomitant anticholinergic drug ingestion or absent bowel sounds for other reasons. Hemodialysis and hemoperfusion are of no clinical benefit in phenytoin poisoning. Cathartics are not recommended.

Seizures may be treated with intravenous benzodiazepines or phenobarbital, again with the caution that seizures are not common in phenytoin overdose and other etiologies must be ruled out. *Cardiovascular toxicity* is extremely rare in oral overdose and requires no specific therapy. Hypoxia and coingested drugs are possible causes. Atropine and temporary cardiac pacing may be used as usual for *symptomatic bradyarrhythmias,* and the additive negative inotropic effects of membrane-stabilizing antiarrhythmics should be avoided, especially after intravenous poisoning. Hospital admission and appropriate orthopedic or plastic surgery consultation should be obtained for patients with any significant *extravasation of intravenous phenytoin* or other signs of local vascular or tissue toxicity after infusion.

To minimize complications due to infusion, intravenous phenytoin should be administered only under close observation with constant cardiac and blood pressure monitoring. The infused solution should be given slowly ($\leq$ 30 mg/min) through a large, well-positioned catheter.

DISPOSITION

All acute overdose patients should be admitted to an intensive care unit setting for monitoring. *Given the long and erratic absorption phase of phenytoin after oral overdose, the decision to discharge or medically clear a patient for psychiatric evaluation cannot be based on a single serum level.* Patients with symptomatic chronic intoxication should be admitted for observation unless signs are minimal, adequate care can be obtained at home, and they are 8 to 12 h from their last therapeutic dose. Phenytoin therapy should be stopped in all cases and if toxicity continues to decrease, a serum level may be reassessed in 2 to 3 days to guide resumption of therapy.

BIBLIOGRAPHY

Booker HE: Serum concentrations of free diphenylhydantoin and their relationship to clinical intoxication. *Epilepsia* 14:177, 1973.

Demey HE, Daelmans RA, Verpooten GA, et al; Propylene glycol-induced side-effects during intravenous nitroglycerin therapy. *Intensive Care Med* 14:221, 1988.

Hansten PD, Horn JR: Phenyton (Dilantin) interactions, in Hansten PD, Horn JR (eds): *Drug Interactions.* Philadelphia, Lea and Febiger, 1989, pp 129–150.

Haruda F: Phenytoin hypersensitivity: 38 cases. *Neurology* 29:1480, 1979.

Louis S, Kutt H, McDowell F: The cardiocirculatory changes caused by intravenous Dilantin and its solvent. *Am Heart J* 74:523, 1967.

Mellick LB, Morgan JA, Mellick GA: Presentations of acute phenytoin overdose. *Am J Emerg Med* 7:61, 1989.

Rao VK, Feldman PD, Dibbell DG: Extravasation injury to the hand by intravenous phenytoin. *J Neurosurg* 68:967, 1988.

Spengler RF, Arrowsmith JB, Kilarski DJ, et al: Severe soft-tissue injury following intravenous infusion of phenytoin. *Arch Intern Med* 148:1329, 1988.

Stilman N, Masdeu JC: Incidence of seizures with phenytoin toxicity. *Neurology* 35:1769, 1985.

Winter ME, Tozer TN: Phenytoin, in Evans WE, Schentag JJ, Juski WJ, et al (eds): *Applied Pharmacokinetics,* ed. Spokane, Washington, Applied Therapeutics, Inc., 1986.

York RC, Coleridge ST: Cardiopulmonary arrest following intravenous phenytoin loading. *Am J Emerg Med* 6:255, 1988.

94 NARCOTICS

George L. Sternbach

The narcotic of most frequent illicit use is heroin, which is produced by the acetylation of morphine. Other narcotics include methadone, morphine, codeine, meperidine, hydromorphone (Dilaudid) and oxycodone (Percodan). Street heroin is adulterated, usually in a 20 to 200:1 ratio, with a number of agents such as quinine, lactose, sucrose, mannitol, magnesium silicate (talc), procaine, or baking soda. Quinine is most commonly used, and in itself can produce auditory, ophthalmic, muscular, gastrointestinal, and renal toxicity.

CLINICAL FEATURES OF NARCOTIC USE

Intoxication

Acute narcotic intoxication is characterized by drowsiness, euphoria, miosis, conjunctival injection, and slowed respirations. Decreased sensitivity of the CNS respiratory center to carbon dioxide causes a decrease in minute and tidal volume. Nausea, vomiting, and pruritus can also occur.

Withdrawal

The classic picture of narcotic withdrawal includes piloerection, lacrimation, yawning, rhinorrhea, sweating, nasal stuffiness, myalgia, vomiting, abdominal cramping, and diarrhea. The patient may be irritable, hyperactive, or confused.

Heroin withdrawal symptoms are generally seen 12 to 14 h after the last dose, whereas symptoms of methadone withdrawal occur in 24 to 36 h. On occasion, the treatment of an overdose patient with naloxone may precipitate a withdrawal syndrome. Though discomforting, acute narcotic withdrawal in the adult is in itself not life-threatening. Many of the symptoms resemble those of a febrile illness, however, and the physician must be alert to the possibility of sepsis in a patient who appears to be undergoing withdrawal. Treatment of withdrawal is symptomatic.

The most common long-term treatment of narcotic withdrawal syndrome is through the substitution and gradual withdrawal of methadone. The antihypertensive agent clonidine has also been utilized to effect narcotic detoxification. Clonidine has been shown to alleviate the symptoms of withdrawal, especially chills, lacrimation, rhinorrhea, abdominal cramping, sweating, myalgia, and arthralgia. Although the severity of symptoms is ameliorated, their presence is not entirely eliminated by clonidine. The mechanism by which the drug acts to reduce the symptoms of opiate withdrawal appears to be by inhibiting adrenergic activity at α_2-adrenergic receptors. Side effects of clonidine include hypotension, dizziness, drowsiness, and dry mouth. Dosage must be adjusted to individual reaction.

Narcotic Overdose

The cardinal physical findings of narcotic overdose are pinpoint pupils and hypoventilation. However, the pupils may be midrange or dilated if CNS hypoxia has occurred. Hypertension may be present secondary to hypoxia. An injection site may be visible or absent, depending on whether the patient injected, inhaled, or ingested the drug.

Street methods of overdose "resuscitation" include packing the victim in ice, pouring milk down the throat, and injecting milk or saline intramuscularly or intravenously. Complications of such actions include hypothermia, aspiration pneumonia, and cellulitis.

TREATMENT

The treatment of coma due to narcotic overdose is the administration of naloxone, 0.4 to 2.0 mg in an adult, 0.01 mg/kg in a child or neonate. The drug may be given subcutaneously, intratracheally, intramuscularly, or intravenously. When administered intravenously, it is effective in 1 to 2 min. The dose may be repeated as needed. Naloxone can also be given as a continuous intravenous infusion, with the dose titrated to clinical response; 2 mg of naloxone in 500 mL of normal saline or 5% dextrose produces a concentration of 0.004 mg/mL, or 0.4 mg/100 mL. The usual dose is 400 μg (0.4 mg) per hour.

Through antagonism at opiate receptor sites in the CNS, naloxone rapidly reverses coma and respiratory depression caused by narcotics. Pentazocine has been shown to occupy receptor sites other than those of the opiates, and although naloxone can reverse the CNS depressant effects of this drug, larger doses are generally required. High-dose administration of naloxone has also been shown to reverse respiratory depression produced by propoxyphene.

Many heroin addicts also use other drugs or alcohol, so that overdose may be of a mixed type. Coma due to the action of other drugs will not be antagonized by naloxone.

The serum half-life of naloxone is about 1 h, with a duration of action of 2 to 3 h. Close observation and repeated injection or continuous intravenous infusion may be necessary, since the action of the narcotic is likely to be significantly longer than that of the antagonist. This is especially true of methadone, whose duration of action may be as long as 72 h.

Naloxone is virtually without adverse effect, even when given chronically and in large doses. Its action is purely narcotic-antagonistic, and the drug displays no intrinsic agonistic effects. In the truly addicted patient, however, its administration may precipitate a withdrawal syndrome of sudden and alarming proportions.

COMPLICATIONS OF NARCOTIC ABUSE

Skin

The tracks of repeated venous injection may be accompanied by the hallmark of subcutaneous use: small, oval, punctate, or depressed ulcers, or hyperpigmented atrophic lesions. Nonpitting edema of the extremities is often seen in addicts of long standing. This is the result of occlusive thrombophlebitis, lymphatic obstruction, and lymphedema.

Infections

Among the most common sequelae of heroin addiction are infections. Narcotics cause inhibition of leukocyte motility and phagocytosis, and both humoral and cellular immune function abnormalities have been described in heroin addicts. Intravenous drug use is a known risk factor for acquired immunodeficiency syndrome (AIDS). In addition, the notorious lack of sterile technique among users contributes to the high incidence of infection.

Abscesses, Cellulitis, Thrombophlebitis

Abscesses and cellulitis, especially of the hands and forearms, are common to subcutaneous injectors. These abscesses most often contain staphylococci, but may harbor other flora, including anaerobic bacteria. Small abscesses with no surrounding cellulitis can be treated with drainage and soaks. More extensive lesions require antibiotic therapy, usually with an agent effective against penicillinase-producing staphylococci. Since septicemia and endocarditis cannot be ruled out with certainty in most patients with fever, hospitalization is often necessary. Blood cultures should be obtained before antibiotic therapy is begun.

Infections of the hand or fingers often require surgical drainage, as progression to gangrene can be rapid. Abscesses in the neck or groin are generally drained in the surgical suite because of their proximity to major vessels. Mycotic aneurysm should be considered in differential diagnosis of abscesses in these areas.

Septic thrombophlebitis, most often involving the legs or thighs, is a common result of intravenous heroin use. It is characterized by painful swelling and warmth of the affected extremity. Unlike uncomplicated deep venous thrombosis, septic thrombophlebitis requires treatment with antibiotics, not heparin alone.

Mycotic aneurysm of the brain, neck, or groin can result in life-threatening hemorrhage. Masses in the neck or groin of a drug user should be carefully evaluated for pulsation or bruits, to rule out the presence of mycotic aneurysm. Ultrasonography or angiography may be necessary to establish the diagnosis.

Endocarditis

Endocarditis is a serious complication among addicts, with a high mortality reported in some series. The left or right side of the heart may be affected; the relative incidence varies widely in different reports.

Right-sided infections are the most common in addicts. These usually spare the pulmonic valve, attacking a previously normal tricuspid valve in almost all cases. Murmurs may be absent, faintly heard, or audible in atypical locations. Indeed, there may be no physical findings of tricuspid valvular disease per se, the diagnosis being made on the basis of multiple or repeated septic pulmonary emboli. The infecting organism is most often *Staphylococcus aureus*. The clinical picture of septic pulmonary emboli in the these cases is often that of pneumonia with staphylococcal septicemia. The radiologic appearance may be one of pulmonary consolidation. Alternatively, round or wedge-shaped lesions may appear successively in the periphery of the lungs. On the other hand, initial chest roentgenograms may be unremarkable or display only minor abnormality, with typical findings appearing only as the disease progresses. Pulmonary infarcts may progress to cavitation, abscess, or empyema formation. Following treatment, the chest film may revert to normal or may display residual atelectasis or pleural thickening.

Left-sided cardiac valves may be affected in the presence or absence of previous aortic or mitral abnormality. The aortic valve in particular is susceptible even without preexisting disease. Classic physical findings of bacterial endocarditis are frequently present in left-sided disease. Organisms may be cultured from sites of extravascular embolization, such as Osler's nodes and Janeway lesions. *Escherichia coli, Streptococcus, Klebsiella,* and *Pseudomonas* species, as well as *Candida albicans* are the most frequent pathogens involved in left-sided heroin-related endocarditis. *C. albicans* never affects previously normal valves.

Complications of infective endocarditis include systemic embolization to the viscera, extremities, and brain; and acute valvular insufficiency. Focal CNS signs and progressive renal failure may develop. Embolization to a coronary vessel can result in acute myocardial infarction. Acute aortic insufficiency can lead to death within hours, and may be difficult to diagnose because the classic hallmarks of chronic aortic insufficiency (such as widened pulse pressure and prominent diastolic murmur) are often absent. The clinical picture is most often one of unexplained dyspnea, tachycardia, and hypotension, followed by cardiovascular collapse. Acute mitral valve rupture is characterized by sudden, severe pulmonary edema. A loud mitral insufficiency murmur is usually present.

Malaria

Malaria was first described as a complication of narcotic use in 1929. During the following decade, the disease was considered endemic among addicts in New York City. Although the incidence has greatly diminished since that time, sporadic cases of syringe-transmitted malaria continue to be reported in the addict. Due to the rarity of the disease in this country, it is seldom considered in the differential diagnosis of the febrile addict, and patients experiencing the symptoms of chills, fever, and malaise may be mistakenly diagnosed as undergoing withdrawal.

Tetanus

Tetanus was first described in addicts in 1876 and has been a relatively frequent observation among them ever since. An inordinately high mortality follows tetanus infection in the heroin user. It is a disease predominantly of the older, long-standing addict, especially the female. Some have speculated that adolescents and males are more likely to be protected by childhood or military immunization. Tetanus is more frequently seen in subcutaneous injectors, and many of these tend to be women, perhaps because the less prominent veins in many females preclude regular intravenous use. Emergency patients should be routinely questioned on the status of tetanus immunizations.

Pulmonary Complications

The occurrence of pulmonary complications in addicts is related to the duration of heroin use, but not to the amount used or to overdose. Pneumonia is frequently seen. The bacterial agent is usually *Streptococcus pneumoniae, Haemophilus, Klebsiella,* or *Staphylococcus aureus*. Factors predisposing the drug user to pneumonia include direct drug effects: slowing of the epiglottic, cough, and sighing reflexes; alveolar hypoventilation; aspiration of gastric contents; and alterations of humoral and cellular immunity.

Lung abscess may complicate bacterial pneumonia, aspiration pneumonitis, or pulmonary infarction. Pathogens may be either aerobic or anaerobic. Heroin addicts also contract tuberculosis more frequently than nonusers. Pneumothorax may result from attempted subclavian or internal jugular vein injection.

Pulmonary edema following use of heroin is a serious complication. Although the onset of symptoms usually immediately follows injection, it may also be delayed 24 to 48 h. The mechanism is unclear, but heroin-induced pulmonary edema is characterized by an increase in capillary permeability with exudation of fluid into the alveoli. Whether the edema is due to hypoxia, allergic reaction, or the direct toxic effects of heroin is unclear. Pulmonary edema is usually bilateral, though it may appear in one or only a part of one lung.

Physical signs include cyanosis, diffuse rales, tachypnea, tachycardia, and the presence of foamy sputum. Extensive rales may be absent if pulmonary edema is perihilar or localized. Arterial blood gases reveal a profound hypoxemia and there may be hypercarbia as well.

The chest roentgenogram displays unilateral or bilateral fluffy, ill-defined densities in an alveolar pattern, radiating centrally to peripherally. The heart is usually normal in size, but may be slightly enlarged. The differential diagnosis should include head trauma, subarachnoid hemorrhage, near-drowning, noxious gas inhalation, and allergic reaction.

The treatment of heroin-induced pulmonary edema consists of ventilatory support and the administration of naloxone. Other components of cardiogenic pulmonary edema therapy—digitalis, diuretics, and rotating tourniquets—are neither effective nor necessary. Response is usually dramatic, with physical findings clearing within 1 day and radiologic changes reverting to normal within 72 to 96 h.

Angiothrombotic pulmonary hypertension, a syndrome of pulmonary hypertension and cor pulmonale, results from recurrent embolization of injected material to the pulmonary vasculature. This is most frequently seen in those injecting oral preparations intravenously, but also affects heroin users because of the talc and starch adulterants of street heroin and the cotton through which the narcotic may be filtered prior to its use. Clinical presentation of the syndrome includes dyspnea, a pulmonic ejection murmur, and signs of right ventricular hypertrophy. Roentgenographic findings include a nodular, irregular perihilar shadow pattern that is symmetrical.

Pulmonary function studies in chronic intravenous narcotic users have shown that diffusing capacity and vital capacity are decreased. It is uncertain whether these effects are due to a direct toxic action of heroin or represent sequelae of repeated episodes of the pulmonary diseases to which these patients are prone. Pulmonary infarction has been previously mentioned as a complication of right-sided endocarditis.

Hepatic Complications

The most common side effect of parenteral drug use is acute or chronic hepatic dysfunction. Liver function tests consistent with acute hepatitis may be seen in 10 to 15 percent of addicts sampled, and approximately another 60 percent display less dramatic abnormalities. The latter are usually attributed to chronic hepatitis and, indeed, chronic hepatitis has been found in a substantial number of addicts who died suddenly and came to autopsy. This has commonly been assumed to represent type B, or serum hepatitis. However, a significant proportion of drug users with acute hepatitis test negative for hepatitis B surface antigen.

Experimental morphine addiction in animals has not been found to induce hepatitis or to exacerbate preexisting liver disease, so a toxic or allergic narcotic effect cannot be invoked to explain this extremely common association. Some heroin addicts are heavy alcohol users as well, so liver disease in addicts may in actuality be alcohol-induced. Treatment of addicts with hepatitis is essentially the same as treatment for liver impairment of any other origin. Progression from acute to chronic disease or a fatal outcome is best correlated with greatly elevated transaminase levels in the acute state.

Gastrointestinal Complications

Intestinal hypomotility, a direct narcotic effect, may give rise to ileus. Abdominal distension and dilated loops of bowel seen on radiologic examination can be associated with this condition and may mimic intestinal obstruction. Termed "intestinal pseudoobstruction," this must be differentiated from a surgical abdomen.

Because of constipation due to hypomotility, there is a significantly increased incidence of symptomatic hemorrhoids and fecal impaction in narcotic addicts.

CNS Complications

The neurologic complications of heroin injection are many and varied. Some have clear etiologies and others are less readily explained. Traumatic mononeuritis is easily diagnosed because there is immediate postinjection pain and paresthesia in a definite nerve distribution. The loss of function sustained in this manner is usually permanent.

Heroin and meperidine overdose have been reported to cause seizures, although this is uncommon. These are usually grand mal and of short duration. The result may be a typical postictal stupor. Seizures induced by narcotis may also be focal, even in the absence of focal lesions. However, focal CNS lesions resulting in altered states of consciousness may have grave implications in view of the addict's increased propensity for meningitis and intracerebral abscess. Focal neurologic signs are not a feature of uncomplicated addiction per se. Subarachnoid hemorrhage is a less common, though well-recognized complication of heroin addiction. This is thought to be due to vascular weakness caused by necrotizing angiitis or mycotic aneurysm.

The most frequent neurologic complication of narcotic abuse is nontraumatic mononeuropathy. This appears as a painless weakness 2 to 3 h after injection, with no history suggestive of pressure neuropathy. An entire brachial or lumbosacral plexitis may be seen, unrelated either to direct injection or pressure effect. This often occurs in association with other neurologic complications.

The narcotic user is susceptible to the development of spinal epidural abscess, most commonly on the basis of hematogenous dissemination of bacteria to the epidural space, but occasionally via direct extension of infection from vertebral osteomyelitis. *Staphylococcus aureus* is the most common infecting organism, though gram-negative bacilli may be the cause.

The progression of signs and symptoms proceeds through phases involving spinal ache, nerve root pain, muscular weakness and, ultimately, paralysis. Fever, leukocytosis, and focal lumbar or thoracic spinal tenderness may be present in the early stage of the process, but the diagnosis may be difficult to make on early clinical grounds. Plain spinal radiographs may reveal vertebral osteomyelitis, compression fracture, or evidence of a paravertebral mass, but radiographs are often negative. Contrast-enhanced computed tomography or magnetic resonance imaging are required to make the diagnosis.

Transverse myelitis involving thoracic segments of the spinal cord is seen particularly in patients reinstituting heroin injections after a 1 to 6 month abstinence. The cause is unclear, but it has been speculated to be toxic or hypersensitive mechanisms or vascular insufficiency to a portion of the thoracic cord. Horner's syndrome can occur as a result of neck injection.

Polyneuritis indistinguishable from Guillain-Barré syndrome has been reported. This may progress to respiratory failure.

The heroin user who presents with pain in an extremity may be the victim of a number of phenomena. Intraarterial injection, like neural trauma, results in immediate pain—in this instance in the distribution of the affected artery. Initial physical signs may be subtle and easily overlooked. The eventual outcome may include ischemic necrosis of the extremity. This is more likely if the lower extremities are involved, less so if there is involvement of the arms.

The pathophysiology of this ischemic necrosis has been postulated to include several factors. Certainly, distal embolization of particulate matter poses a threat to the circulation via occlusion. Damage caused by the needle to the intimal layer of the vessel may also result in occlusion. Arteries may release catecholamines upon such an insult, and although vasospasm has long been assumed to be a major factor in this process, recent work casts doubt upon this particular theory. Various therapeutic modalities have been employed, including sympathectomy and infusion of heparin or dextran, but the eventual outcome may not be greatly affected by such actions.

Muscular Complications

Fascial compartment syndrome may be produced by compression of the limbs during drug-induced stupor. A vicious cycle is established in which ischemic injury produces edema, which raises pressure in fascial compartments, which in turn aggravates ischemia. This "crush" syndrome creates a situation in which open fasciotomy may be necessary to save the involved extremity. The patient complains of increasing pain and progressive weakness as intrafascial pressure mounts, but external signs may be few. The physician may be forced to exercise clinical judgment upon hearing this history, with no more than a firm, wooden feeling to the extremity as a guide.

Signs of generalized sepsis along with raised pressure in the fascial compartment pose an even more ominous situation, these being the hallmarks of necrotizing fasciitis. This constitutes a spreading septic necrosis resulting from subfascial injection. The extremity is frequently dusky, edematous, and tender, and systemic signs of fever, tachycardia, chills, and leukocytosis are present. The bacterial agent is most likely to be streptococcal, staphylococcal or a gram-negative organism. The entity produces a mortality rate as high as 30 percent. Treatment includes antibiotic therapy and surgical debridement.

Generalized necrosis of skeletal muscle unrelated to muscle compression sometimes occurs acutely in addicts. The rhabdomyolysis syndrome may occur in a variety of clinical situations, but if there is a mechanism peculiar to narcotic use, this is unknown. Muscles over much of the body may be tender and edematous, and the extremities weak. The hallmark of this syndrome is myoglobin in the urine. Prompt treatment is in order to prevent renal damage.

A syndrome of fever, paraspinal myalgia, and periarthritis has been reported in association with the use of brown heroin. Although this clinical picture frequently mimics an acute febrile illness, no infectious organism has been implicated, and antibiotics do not affect the outcome of this self-limited illness.

Bone and Joint Pain

Bone or joint pain in the addict must call to mind at least two potential complications: septic arthritis and osteomyelitis. When injecting veins in the antecubital fossa or in the hand, the addict may inadvertently enter joint spaces at the elbow or wrist introducing foreign material and bacteria. More frequently, however, organisms are spread hematogenously to infect sites distant from their site of introduction. There is a curious predilection for the axial skeleton in such hematogenous metastases, particulary the sternoclavicular joint. Organisms infrequently seen in septic arthritis of nonaddicts, including *Pseudomonas aeruginosa* and *Serratia marcescens,* are frequently the cause.

Hematogenous osteomyelitis, although rare, is a recognized complication of heroin addiction. There is a predilection for the spine, but other bones may be involved. *Pseudomonas* is a frequent pathogen. Osteomyelitis should come to mind whenever back pain is a presenting symptom in a patient with evidence of self-injection. Indeed, the presentation of osteomyelitis may include little more than acute localized pain, as fever is rarely present, and the white blood count and x-ray films are normal early in the course. Spinal epidural abscess should also be considered in the differential diagnosis.

Abnormalities of Pregnancy and Menstruation

Secondary amenorrhea is common in female heroin users. In several studies, one-third of adolescent girls using narcotics ceased menstruating. An additional group displayed oligomenorrhea and hypomenorrhea. Normal menses resumed after discontinuation of the drug, but amenorrhea sometimes persisted for several months to a year.

Complications of pregnancy are frequent, and include a high incidence of toxemia, as well as delivery of premature or growth-retarded babies. Up to 70 percent of babies born to drug-using mothers experience neonatal withdrawal, a potentially fatal condition.

BIBLIOGRAPHY

Blanck RR, Ream NW, Deleese JS: Infectious complications of illicit drug use. *Int J Addict* 19:221, 1984.

DeGans J, Stam J, van Wijngaarden GK: Rhabdomyolysis and concomitant neurological lesions after intravenous heroin abuse. *J Neurol Neurosurg Psychiatry* 48:1057, 1985.

Ford M, Hoffman RS, Goldfrank LR: Opioids and designer drugs. *Emerg Med Clin North Am* 8:495, 1990.

Frand UI, Shim CS, Williams MH Jr: Heroin-induced pulmonary edema. *Ann Intern Med* 77:29, 1972.

Gifford DB, Patzakis M, Ivler D, et al: Septic arthritis due to *Pseudomonas* in heroin addicts. *J Bone Joint Surg* 57A:631, 1975.

Gilroy J, Adaya L, Thomas VJ: Intracranial mycotic aneurysms and subacute bacterial endocarditis in heroin addiction. *Neurology* 23:1193, 1973.

Kleber HD, Riordan CE: The treatment of narcotic withdrawal: A historical review. *J Clin Psychol* 43:30, 1982.

Stern WZ, Subbarao K: Pulmonary complications of drug addiction. *Semin Roentgenol* 18:183, 1983.

Washton AM, Resnick RB: Outpatient detoxification with clonidine. *J Clin Psychol* 43:39, 1982.

95
CLONIDINE

E. Martin Caravati

INTRODUCTION

Clonidine hydrochloride, a synthetic imidazoline derivative, was initially investigated as an α-adrenergic agonist for use as a nasal decongestant. It was discovered to have a potent blood pressure lowering effect and is now commonly used as an antihypertensive agent. Clonidine has also been used to ameliorate withdrawal symptoms from opiates, nicotine, and alcohol. It is of particular interest because of a recent increase in therapeutic usage; the manifestations of toxicity, which resemble those in cases of opiate overdose; and controversy regarding each of a proven antidote for clonidine poisoning.

PHARMACOLOGY AND PATHOPHYSIOLOGY

Formulations

Clonidine is available in 0.1-, 0.2-, and 0.3-mg tablets, alone (Catapres) or in combination with chlorthalidone (Combipres). Also available are transdermal patches (Catapres-TTS), which supply 0.1-, 0.2-, or 0.3-mg/day for 7 days. These patches contain 2.5, 5.0, and 7.5 mg total drug, respectively, and the amount of active drug remaining in a patch after 7 days of use has been reported as high as 75 percent of the total content. Therefore, the patch designed to deliver only 0.1 mg/day of clonidine may still contain up to 1.9 mg of active drug after it has been used and discarded.

Pharmacokinetics

Clonidine is rapidly and almost completely absorbed from the gastrointestinal tract. Antihypertensive effects are noted within 30 to 60 min and peak between 2 and 4 h after ingestion. It is lipid-soluble and 20 to 40 percent protein-bound in the plasma. It has a large volume of distribution (3 to 6 L/kg). The serum half-life is approximately 12 h, with a range of 6 to 24 h. Approximately 50 percent of a therapeutic dose is excreted unchanged in the urine while the remainder is metabolized in the liver; none of the metabolites are pharmacologically active.

Mechanism of Action

The mechanism by which clonidine lowers blood pressure is not fully understood. The primary site of action appears to be in the medulla oblongata where it is a presynaptic α_2-adrenergic agonist. This results in decreased sympathetic outflow from the central nervous system with a subsequent decrease in heart rate, cardiac output, and peripheral vascular resistance. At high doses, it may act as a peripheral α adrenoreceptor agonist at vascular smooth-muscle sites and cause vasoconstriction.

Clonidine also depresses the central nervous system as reflected by decreased levels of norepinephrine and metabolites in the cerebrospinal fluid after a therapeutic dose.

Toxic Dose

The minimum toxic dose of clonidine has not been established. Significant toxicity has been reported in a 24-month-old child (11 kg) who ingested a single 0.1-mg tablet, and in a 9-month-old boy (11 kg) found sucking on a used transdermal patch. Adults have survived ingestions of up to 100 mg. The amount ingested does not always correlate with the severity of symptoms. There has been only one reported fatality from clonidine overdose: a 37-year-old who ingested an unknown amount and suffered a cardiac arrest shortly after administration of tolazoline.

Clonidine does not appear to be teratogenic in animals, and no human congenital defects have been associated with its use. It has been administered therapeutically in the second and third trimesters of pregnancy without adverse fetal effects.

CLINICAL PRESENTATION

Manifestations of acute toxicity vary and reflect both the central and peripheral effects of the drug. Symptoms are usually present within 2 h of ingestion and recovery is generally complete within 72 h.

Infants and children are particularly sensitive to the drug and may manifest toxicity after ingestion of a single tablet. In a report of 42 pediatric ingestions by Wiley, 76 percent of patients had symptoms within 1 h and 100 percent within 4 h. None of these patients demonstrated clinical deterioration more than 4 h after presentation. Therefore, if a patient is asymptomatic 4 h after ingestion, it is unlikely that significant toxicity will occur. Renal insufficiency may predispose a patient to delayed or prolonged toxic effects, however.

The common signs and symptoms of clonidine poisoning are illustrated in Table 95-1. After clonidine poisoning children tend to have a higher incidence of hypothermia and respiratory depression, particularly recurrent apnea, than adults. Hypertension may be present initially due to the peripheral α-adrenergic agonist effect of clonidine in high doses. It is usually transient and may be followed by significant hypotension. The effects of clonidine are additive with the CNS depressant effects of other sedative-hypnotics. Irritability, pallor, mydriasis, seizures, atrioventricular block (first-, second-, and third-degree), extensor plantar reflex, and diarrhea have also been reported.

Table 95-1. Common Signs and Symptoms of Clonidine Poisoning

Central nervous system	Cardiovascular
Lethargy or coma	Sinus bradycardia
Respiratory depression	Hypotension
Apnea	Hypertension
Miosis	Other
Hyporeflexia	Hypothermia
Hypotonia	Pallor

Toxicity may mimic narcotic overdose with the classic triad of coma, miosis, and respiratory depression. Other agents which may cause a clinical presentation similar to clonidine include β-blocking drugs (bradycardia, hypotension, coma), phenobarbital and chloral hydrate (miosis, coma, respiratory depression), phenothiazines (miosis, coma, hypotension), and pesticides (miosis, coma, bradycardia).

LABORATORY

No laboratory tests are specific for clonidine poisoning. It can be measured in the plasma by high-pressure liquid chromatography (HPLC). Clonidine is not detected by usual hospital toxicology screening methods, but toxicology screening may help by detecting coingestants or excluding other possible agents responsible for the clinical presentation.

An ECG may reveal sinus bradycardia or heart block. An arterial blood gas can help in assessing the patient's oxygenation and ventilatory status.

TREATMENT

Stabilization. All patients suspected of clonidine overdose should have intravenous access established and continuous respiratory and cardiac monitoring for at least 4 h. Symptomatic patients should be admitted and observed for at least 12 h. The patient's vital signs, mental status, and pupil size should be checked frequently. An adequate airway and ventilation must be maintained.

Decontamination. After the patient has been stabilized, measures to decontaminate the gut should be initiated. Gastric emptying may be of benefit in cases of recent ingestion (within 1 h) consisting of more than one or two tablets. Gastric lavage with a large-bore orogastric tube is the procedure of choice. Because of the possibility of rapid deterioration in the patient's mental status and subsequent inability to protect the airway when vomiting, it is inadvisable to use ipecac to induce emesis. Activated charcoal probably binds clonidine and should be administered to all patients after gastric lavage.

Elimination Enhancement. Forced diuresis is not recommended. It does not hasten renal elimination of clonidine and may complicate management of the patient's hemodynamic status. Urinary pH manipulation, dialysis, and hemoperfusion are unlikely to add any benefit to supportive care.

Supportive Care. The mainstay of treatment for clonidine toxicity is supportive care. Respiratory compromise may require endotracheal intubation and assisted ventilation. Apnea in the child should be closely monitored. It usually responds to tactile stimulation, but if it is recurrent, elective intubation should be considered. Hypothermia is generally mild and resolves with passive rewarming. Bradycardia should be treated only in association with hemodynamic compromise and is responsive to standard doses of atropine. Hypertension is usually transient, and aggressive treatment should be undertaken only when end-organ damage is evident. An appropriate agent is sodium nitroprusside, which is short-acting and easily titratable. The hypotensive patient often responds to being placed in the Trendelenburg position and given a bolus of intravenous fluids. Dopamine is indicated for hypotension not alleviated by volume expansion. Seizures, a rare complication, respond to diazepam and phenytoin, but potential underlying causes such as hypoxia or hypoglycemia must be excluded.

Antidotes. Although there are no proven antidotes for clonidine poisoning, agents purported to have antagonistic effects on clonidine toxicity include naloxone, tolazoline, yohimbine, and idazoxan.

Since clonidine overdose has manifestations similar to opiate intoxication, naloxone has been recommended as a potential antidote. There are conflicting reports as to its efficacy in reversing the cardiovascular and opioid effects of clonidine. There is no evidence for a consistent or predictable clinical response and naloxone cannot be relied upon to replace supportive care. It is possible, however, that there exists a subset of patients in whom naloxone is beneficial. Naloxone should be administered to patients with significant symptoms in order to reverse potential narcotic toxicity and possibly alleviate some signs of clonidine toxicity. The dose is similar to that used for narcotic overdose. No complications of naloxone therapy for adult clonidine toxicity have been reported, but hypertension has been reported as a complication of naloxone treatment in a few children.

Tolazoline is a relatively nonselective α-adrenoreceptor blocker. Two case reports have suggested that it reverses the cardiovascular toxicity of clonidine, but in the majority of reported cases it had no effect. Significant complications such as seizures, hypotension, gastrointestinal hemorrhage, and death have been reported with its use in other settings. In addition, the only reported fatality from clonidine overdose occurred shortly after the administration of tolazoline. It is not recommended as an antidote for clonidine toxicity.

Yohimbine, a selective α-adrenoreceptor blocker, readily penetrates the CNS and causes an increase in blood pressure, heart rate, and motor activity. It is available in tablet form only and has not been specifically studied as an antidote. Idazoxan, also a specific α_2-adrenoreceptor antagonist, has been shown to reverse clonidine-induced miosis in healthy adults. It is currently an investigational drug.

CLONIDINE WITHDRAWAL SYNDROME

Abrupt cessation of chronic clonidine therapy may result in symptoms of adrenergic hyperactivity as early as 12 h after the last dose. The symptoms last approximately 5 to 7 days and consist of anxiety, diaphoresis, headache, nausea and abdominal pain, tachycardia, and hypertension. Ventricular arrhythmias, hypertensive encephalopathy, and death have been reported. Tapering the dose of clonidine over 3 to 5 days usually prevents development of withdrawal symptoms. The syndrome is most effectively treated by restarting the clonidine. Severe hypertension may require nitroprusside therapy. Theoretically, treatment with β blockers alone may exacerbate rebound hypertension due to unopposed α-adrenergic stimulation. Clonidine withdrawal has not been reported after an acute overdose.

BIBLIOGRAPHY

Bamshad MJ, Wasserman GS: Pediatric clonidine intoxications. *Vet Hum Toxicol* 30:220, 1990.

Banner W Jr, Lund ME, Clawson L: Failure of naloxone to reverse clonidine toxic effect. *Am J Dis Child* 137:1170, 1983.

Caravati EM, Bennett DL: Clonidine transdermal patch poisoning. *Ann Emerg Med* 17:175, 1988.

Geyskes GG, Boer P, Mees EJD: Clonidine Withdrawal: Mechanism and frequency of rebound hypertension. *Br J Clin Pharmacol* 7:55, 1979.

Gremse DA, Artman M, Boerth RC: Hypertension associated with naloxone treatment for clonidine poisoning. *J Pediatr* 108: 776, 1986.

Olsson JM, Pruitt AW: Management of clonidine ingestion in children. *J Pediatr* 103:646, 1983.

Niemann JT, Getzug T, Murphy W: Reversal of clonidine toxicity by naloxone. *Ann Emerg Med* 15:1229, 1986.

Stein B, Volans GN: Dixarit overdose: The problem of attractive tablets. *Br Med J* 2:667, 1978.

Wiley JF, Wiley CC, Torrey SB, et al: Clonidine poisoning in young children. *J Pediatr* 116:654, 1990.

Williams PL, Drafcik JM, Potter BP, et al: Cardiac toxicity of clonidine. *Chest* 72:784, 1977.

96
ALCOHOLS
William K. Chiang

METHANOL

Methanol (wood alcohol) is obtained from destructive distillation of wood and is synthesized from carbon oxides and hydrogen. Methanol is an important solvent in the manufacturing industry and is present in a variety of substances found at home and in the workplace, such as antifreeze, paint solvent, duplicating fluids, canned fuels (Sterno), gasoline additives, and home heating fuels. Life-threatening poisoning can occur even if a small amount of methanol is ingested. Historical epidemics of methanol toxicity have resulted from ingesting methanol-contaminated spirits.

Pathophysiology

Most cases of methanol toxicity result from intentional or accidental oral ingestion. Toxicity can also occur if methanol is absorbed via dermal and pulmonary routes. Accidental inhalation has been reported when windshield solvent was applied to interior windows in a closed space, such as an automobile. The volume of distribution (V_d) of methanol is similar to other alcohols at 0.6 L/kg. The potential maximal serum concentration of methanol can be estimated by the following formula if the amount of methanol ingested is known (see Table 96-1):

$$C = \frac{\text{dose}}{V_d}$$

The toxic dose of methanol is variable. Doses as small as 15 mL of 40% methanol have been reported as lethal, while ingestions as large as 500 mL of 40% methanol have been reported without toxicity. Generally, a dose of 30 mL of 100% methanol in an adult should be regarded as lethal and any amount ingested as toxic or potentially lethal. Toxicity may be modified by concomitant ethanol consumption, folate deficiency, and the total dose per body weight of methanol absorbed.

Methanol is converted in the liver, by alcohol dehydrogenase to formaldehyde, and formaldehyde by aldehyde dehydrogenase to formate. These two metabolites are responsible for the toxicity of methanol. However, formate appears to be most important, since formaldehyde is rapidly metabolized to formate and does not accumulate in the serum. Formate inhibits cytochrome oxidase and mitochondrial respiration leading to diffuse cellular hypoxia. Formate accounts for the majority of the anion gap acidosis seen in methanol poisoning, while lactate, butyrate, and acetate account for the rest of the acidosis. The accumulation of formate in the blood is associated with the onset of clinical symptoms such as anorexia, photophobia, and hyperpnea, and can be correlated with the decrease in carbon dioxide content and the severity of the metabolic acidosis.

Table 96-1. Pharmacokinetic Model to Estimate the Significance of the Ingestion

Example: A 1-year-old boy ingested 5 mL of 100% methanol. The child weighs 10 kg.

Volume of distribution (V_d) = 0.6 L/kg for methanol
Specific gravity of methanol = 0.8 gm/mL
C = dose/V_d
= (5 mL)(0.8 gm/mL)/(0.6 L/kg)(10 kg)
= 0.667 gm/L = 66.7 mg/dL

This calculation can be used for all alcohols with the appropriate specific gravity and V_d

The predilection of methanol for ocular toxicity may be related to higher formate concentrations in the vitreous humor and optic nerve than in the blood. The structural changes in the eye may be caused by the interference of formate with cytochrome oxidase and with Na^+,K^+-ATPase in the optic nerve itself. Optic disk edema can be produced in monkeys by formate infusion, even though a normal systemic pH is maintained with bicarbonate infusion.

Clinical Features

The major toxic signs and symptoms of methanol ingestion are (1) visual symptoms; (2) CNS depression; (3) abdominal pain, nausea, and vomiting; and (4) metabolic acidosis. Methanol itself, like other alcohols, can produce confusion, lethargy, and obtundation. However, methanol is less intoxicating than ethanol so that patients may have toxic methanol levels with little or no evidence of intoxication. The onset of other symptoms varies from 1 to 72 h from the time of ingestion. Nausea, vomiting, and severe abdominal pain are frequently seen, and appear to be due to acute gastritis and pancreatitis. In the study by Bennett et al., 76 percent of patients had evidence of hemorrhagic pancreatitis at postmortem examination. The onset of symptoms correlates with the appearance of metabolic acidosis. Visual complaints such as photophobia, blurred or indistinct vision, or descriptions of looking at a snowstorm occur in almost all symptomatic cases of methanol poisoning. The pupils are frequently dilated and sluggishly reactive or unreactive to light. Hyperemia of the optic disk is evident at the onset of visual disturbances. Papilledema may develop within hours. Microscopic findings include edema of the retinal nerve fiber layer and engorgement of the retinal veins. Optic atrophy and blindness can develop rapidly.

Generalized seizure activity may occur, and mental status may rapidly change from alertness to coma. Although cerebral edema has been described as a classic sign of methanol poisoning, only 10 percent of autopsied patients had evidence of cerebral edema in the series of 323 cases reviewed by Bennett et al. For unclear reasons, the putamen is quite susceptible to hemorrhagic necrosis in methanol intoxication. Residual parkinsonism has been reported in patients recovered from methanol intoxication.

Anion gap acidosis is a hallmark of methanol intoxication and presents when methanol has been metabolized to formate. Methanol poisoning is one of the instances in which a zero plasma bicarbonate can occur and spectacular amounts of bicarbonate may be necessary to prevent severe acidemia. However, normal acid-base status should be expected early in the ingestion of when there is concurrent ethanol consumption. Osmolal gap, the difference between the measured osmolality (mOsm/kg) and the calculated osmolarity (mOsm/L), can be an important early laboratory clue to the diagnosis of toxic alcohol ingestions (see Table 96-2). An elevated osmolal gap suggests the presence in the serum of osmotically active substances (such as methanol, ethylene glycol, isopropanol, ethanol, glycerol, and mannitol) in significant concentration not accounted for by the calculated somolarity. An ethanol level should be obtained simultaneously and can be incorporated into the calculation for serum osmolarity. While an elevated osmolal gap can be helpful in diagnosing the ingestion of methanol and other toxic alcohols, a "normal" osmolal gap does not exclude toxic alcohol ingestion and does not replace direct methanol measurement (see Table 96-3). Methanol levels should be obtained immediately in all potential methanol exposures.

Table 96-2. Calculating Serum Osmolarity

$$\text{Osm cal.} = 2[\text{Na}] + \frac{\text{Glucose(mg/dL)}}{18} + \frac{\text{BUN(mg/dL)}}{2.8}$$

To correct for the presence of ethanol:

$$\text{Add } \frac{\text{ethanol level(mg/dL)}}{4.6}$$

Table 96-3. Pitfalls in a "Normal Osmolal Gap" for Toxic Alcohol Intoxications

Population normals for osmolal gap have not been well standardized and appear to be highly variable (variations reported −7 to 17 mOsm/L)
A change in a gap of 10 mOsm/L can still result from toxic concentrations of methanol and ethylene glycol
Laboratory variations in measurements
Using boiling point elevation osmolality for methanol or other volatile alcohols will negate the results
The osmolal gap declines or disappears as the parent alcohols are metabolized

Treatment

The treatment of methanol poisoning consists of (1) general supportive measures, (2) correction of metabolic acidosis, (3) prevention of conversion of methanol to formate, and (4) elimination of methanol and formate.

Airway, breathing, and circulation must be quickly assessed and supported in all patients. Appropriate substrates such as glucose, thiamine, and naloxone should be administered to obtunded or stuporous patients. Gastric lavage via a nasogastric tube may be indicated if the ingestion was within the last 1 to 2 h. Since methanol has minimal adsorption to charcoal, charcoal has limited utility unless there are coingestants. Cathartics have no role since methanol is quickly absorbed from the gastrointestinal tract.

For metabolic acidosis, administer appropriate bicarbonate to correct the acidemia. Limited data suggest that the correction of acidemia may have some attenuating effects on the ocular toxicity of methanol and may increase formate elimination.

Ethanol therapy is indicated when the clinical diagnosis of methanol intoxication is suspected. Both ethanol and methanol are substrates for alcohol dehydrogenase. But ethanol has 10 times the affinity for alcohol dehydrogenase when compared with methanol. A loading dose and continuous infusion of ethanol (to maintain a serum ethanol concentration at 100 to 150 mg/dL) will prevent the metabolism of methanol (Table 96-4). The formate already generated in the serum will not be affected by ethanol. The rate of metabolism of ethanol is highly variable between individuals and substantially increased in chronic alcoholics, so repeated ethanol assays are necessary to ensure the desired serum concentration. All patients receiving ethanol therapy, but particularly the pediatric patient, should receive glucose supplementation and frequent glucose monitoring because of the potential for hypoglycemia.

Formate metabolism in primates is implemented by a folate-dependent system. According to Noker et al., folinic acid infusion of 2 mg/kg in methanol-poisoned monkeys decreased formate accumulation and reversed the metabolic acidosis. The current recommendation for methanol intoxication is to give folinic acid (1 mg/kg IV), the active coenzyme, as the first dose, and then continue with folate (1 mg/kg) every 4 h for 24 h.

Table 96-4. Ethanol Dosing for Methanol and Ethylene Glycol Intoxications*

Loading Dose	
0.8 gm/kg = 1 mL/kg of 100% ethanol = 10 mL/kg of 10% ethanol†	
Maintenance Dose	
For nontolerant individuals: 130 mg/kg/h to 0.15 mL/kg/h of 100% ethanol (1.5 mL/kg/h of 10% ethanol)	
For tolerant individuals: double the maintenance dose	
If pharmaceutical ethanol is not available, various spirits can be given orally:	
Loading dose	= (200/proof) mL/kg
Maintenance dose‡	= (30/proof)ml/kg/h

* Ethanol concentration for IV use should be ≤ 10%

† Intravenous loading infused over 30–60 min.

‡ Double maintenance dose for tolerant individuals.

Hemodialysis remains the treatment of choice for significant methanol intoxications. Hemodialysis removes methanol, formaldehyde, and formate and corrects the acidosis. During hemodialysis the maintenance ethanol infusion will need to be increased (often doubled) to account for its increased clearance. Appropriate consultation with the nephrologist should be started as soon as possible when the diagnosis of methanol intoxication is entertained. When the diagnosis of methanol intoxication is likely based on the history, symptoms, and supporting laboratory studies, hemodialysis should not be delayed while awaiting the methanol assay. Ethanol infusion should be continued after hemodialysis until the postdialysis methanol level becomes negligible. If the initial methanol concentration is greater than 100 mg/dL, more than one hemodialysis session may be required. Hemodialysis should be instituted (1) if the methanol level is greater than 25 mg/dL, (2) if an acidosis already exists, (3) if there is visual impairment, or (4) if there is renal failure. Peritoneal dialysis is ineffective for the clearance of methanol and its metabolites.

4-Methylpyrazole (4-MP), a potent alcohol dehydrogenase inhibitor, is undergoing clinical evaluation for both methanol and ethylene glycol intoxications. Unlike its parent compound pyrazole, 4-MP has not been demonstrated to cause ocular and hepatotoxic effects in primates and humans. The advantages of 4-MP over ethanol include the lack of sedation, predictable alcohol dehydrogenase inhibition with twice daily oral dosing, and the fact that it is unaffected by hemodialysis. However, 4-MP will not replace hemodialysis in patients with symptoms or acidosis.

ETHYLENE GLYCOL

Ethylene glycol is an aliphatic straight-chain polyalcohol. It is a colorless, odorless, sweet-tasting, nonvolatile liquid that is a component of various commercial products such as detergents, paints, pharmaceuticals, polishes, antifreeze, and coolants. Ethylene glycol has intoxicating effects similar to those of ethanol, and sometimes it is unwisely substituted for ethanol.

Pathophysiology

Ethylene glycol is readily absorbed orally, but not by the lung or skin. The volume of distribution of ethylene glycol is 0.6 to 0.8 L/kg. The lethal dose of ethylene glycol is approximately 1 to 1.5 mL/kg of a 100% solution, although any amount ingested should be regarded as toxic and potentially lethal.

Ethylene glycol is metabolized principally in the liver and excreted by the kidney (Fig. 96-1), and toxicity is due primarily to the accumulation of toxic metabolites: glycoaldehyde, glycolate, glyoxalate, and oxalate. These compounds contain ketoaldehyde groups that inhibit oxidative phosphorylation, protein synthesis, and sulfhydryl-containing enzymes. In addition, calcium oxalate precipitates in the kidneys, brain, liver, blood vessels, and pericardium, causing tissue destruction. A hallmark of ethylene glycol intoxication is severe anion gap metabolic acidosis due to accumulation of glycolate, oxalate, and lactate. Hypocalcemia can result from the precipitation of calcium oxalate crystals.

Ethylene glycol is converted to glycoaldehyde by the action of alcohol dehydrogenase. During this reaction the generation of large amounts of reduced nicotinamide adenine dinucleotide (NADH) can result in lactic acidosis if the NADH/NAD$^+$ ratio is changed. Pyridoxal phosphate and thiamine are cofactors necessary for the conversion of the toxic glyoxalate to the nontoxic metabolites glycine and α-hydroxy-β-ketoadipate, respectively. The plasma half-life of ethylene glycol is about 3 to 6 h. However, metabolites responsible for the toxicity may have half-lives of up to 12 h. Ethanol administration prolongs the half-life of ethylene glycol to approximately 17 h.

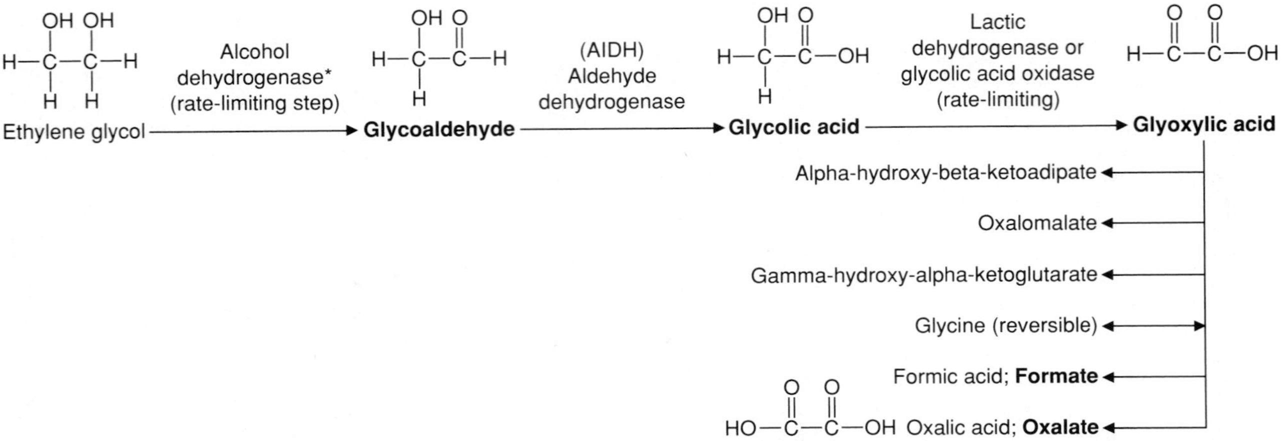

Ethylene glycol → Alcohol dehydrogenase* (rate-limiting step) → **Glycoaldehyde** → (AlDH) Aldehyde dehydrogenase → **Glycolic acid** → Lactic dehydrogenase or glycolic acid oxidase (rate-limiting) → **Glyoxylic acid**

Glyoxylic acid → Alpha-hydroxy-beta-ketoadipate

Glyoxylic acid → Oxalomalate

Glyoxylic acid → Gamma-hydroxy-alpha-ketoglutarate

Glyoxylic acid ↔ Glycine (reversible)

Glyoxylic acid → Formic acid; **Formate**

Glyoxylic acid → Oxalic acid; **Oxalate**

Fig. 96-1. Major pathways of ethylene glycol metabolism. (Toxic metabolites in boldface.) Therapy is aimed at interfering with alcohol dehydrogenase, blocking the conversion of ethylene glycol to glycoaldehyde. (Reproduced with permission from Goldfrank's Toxicologic Emergencies.)

Clinical Features

The major signs and symptoms of ethylene glycol poisoning can be divided into three stages, depending on the amount of ethylene glycol ingested: stage 1, CNS depression; stage 2, cardiopulmonary toxicity; and stage 3, renal toxicity.

Central nervous system symptoms generally appear 1 to 12 h after ingestion, a time that correlates with peak glycoaldehyde production. Ataxia, nystagmus, ophthalmoplegia, papilledema, optic atrophy, myoclonus, focal or generalized convulsions, hallucinations, stupor, and coma may occur. At postmortem, calcium oxalate deposits can be demonstrated in the white matter of the brain, blood vessels, and choroid plexus. There is general edema and widespread petechiae.

A large anion gap metabolic acidosis usually accompanies the development of CNS symptoms. An osmolal gap may be present. However, the osmolal gap may be normal even with significant ethylene glycol poisoning (Table 96-3). Hypocalcemia is sometimes severe enough to induce tetany and QT prolongation on ECG, and may lead to arrhythmias. Myalgia and elevation of creatine phosphokinase levels have also been reported. Nausea, vomiting, and abdominal pain develop in a great number of patients.

Within 12 to 72 h post ingestion, cardiopulmonary symptoms may predominant. Tachycardia, tachypnea, and mild hypertension are frequently reported. In patients with severe toxicity, pneumonia, pulmonary edema, and fulminant cardiac failure occur.

Oligouric renal failure develops within 24 to 72 h if the patient survives the first two stages. Both the aldehyde metabolites of ethylene glycol and oxalic acid have direct renal toxicity. The intratubular deposition of oxalate crystals is widespread (Fig.96-2). Positive birefringent calcium oxalate crystals in the urine are pathognomonic of the diagnosis, although these crystals are frequently absent (especially in the early phase) even in severe poisoning. There are two forms of calcium oxalate crystals. The dihydrate crystals are octahedral or envelope-shaped and can be easily recognized, but they appear only when the urinary calcium oxalate concentration is high. The monohydrate crystals are needle-shaped and are more stable under physiologic conditions. Microscopic hematuria, proteinuria, and renal epithelial cells are also commonly found on urinalysis. Azotemia and anuria follow. The renal failure is frequently reversible with good supportive therapy.

The diagnosis of ethylene glycol intoxication is based on the clinical recognition of symptoms and the identification of a large anion gap metabolic acidosis and osmolal gap. Hypocalcemia and symptoms of hypocalcemia (tetany and QT prolongation), oxalate crystals in the urine, renal dysfunction, and fluorescence of the urine with wood's lamp (fluorescein is present in many antifreezes) are clues that may be helpful to confirm the diagnosis of ethylene glycol poisoning. Serum ethylene glycol measurements are technically more difficult than methanol measurement but should be obtained in all suspected cases. As occurs with methanol, the osmolal gap develops first with normal anion gap. When the parent alcohol molecules are metabolized, the osmolal gap may decrease or disappear while the anion gap increases.

Other laboratory studies that are important for the evaluation of ethylene glycol intoxication include standard electrolytes, glucose, acetone, ethanol, BUN, creatinine, salicylate, osmolality, arterial blood gases, calcium, and magnesium. Methanol overdose as well as alcoholic ketoacidosis should also be considered in the differential diagnosis. Where available, specific toxicology studies, including methanol and ethylene glycol levels, should be obtained.

Treatment

As with methanol, therapy for ethylene glycol intoxication consists of (1) general supportive measures, (2) correction of metabolic acidosis and electrolyte abnormalities, (3) prevention of ethylene glycol metabolism, and (4) removal of ethylene glycol and its metabolites. Treatment must be initiated as soon as the diagnosis is suspected. Any delay in treatment (such as waiting until toxicology results are received) can cause serious or even irreversible complications.

Gastric lavage with a nasogastric tube can be employed if the ingestion has been within the last 1 to 2 h. Activated charcoal should be employed if coingestants are suspected; otherwise ethylene glycol has limited adsorption to charcoal.

The anion gap metabolic acidosis should be corrected by the administration of sodium bicarbonate while monitoring the pH and bicarbonate content. Hypocalcemia can be treated with calcium chloride. Administer thiamine (100 mg) and pyridoxine (1 mg/kg) IV. They are cofactors for the detoxification of ethylene glycol.

Maintain adequate urine output to enhance the renal clearance of ethylene glycol and oxalate. Appropriate fluid therapy should be carried out with close monitoring of renal function and urine output. Loop diuretics may be employed to maintain urine output after appropriate fluid therapy.

Ethanol should be administered to compete for alcohol dehydrogenase, thereby inhibiting the metabolism of ethylene glycol to toxic metabolites. A therapeutic serum ethanol concentration of 100 to 150 mg/dL should be maintained (Table 96-3). As discussed above 4-methylpyrazole has the potential to replace ethanol in the future as a more predictable alcohol dehydrogenase inhibitor for both ethylene glycol and methanol poisonings.

Hemodialysis is indicated if the patient has an acidosis, renal dysfunction, or an ethylene glycol level of 25 mg/dL or greater. Ethanol infusions often need to be doubled during hemodialysis because of

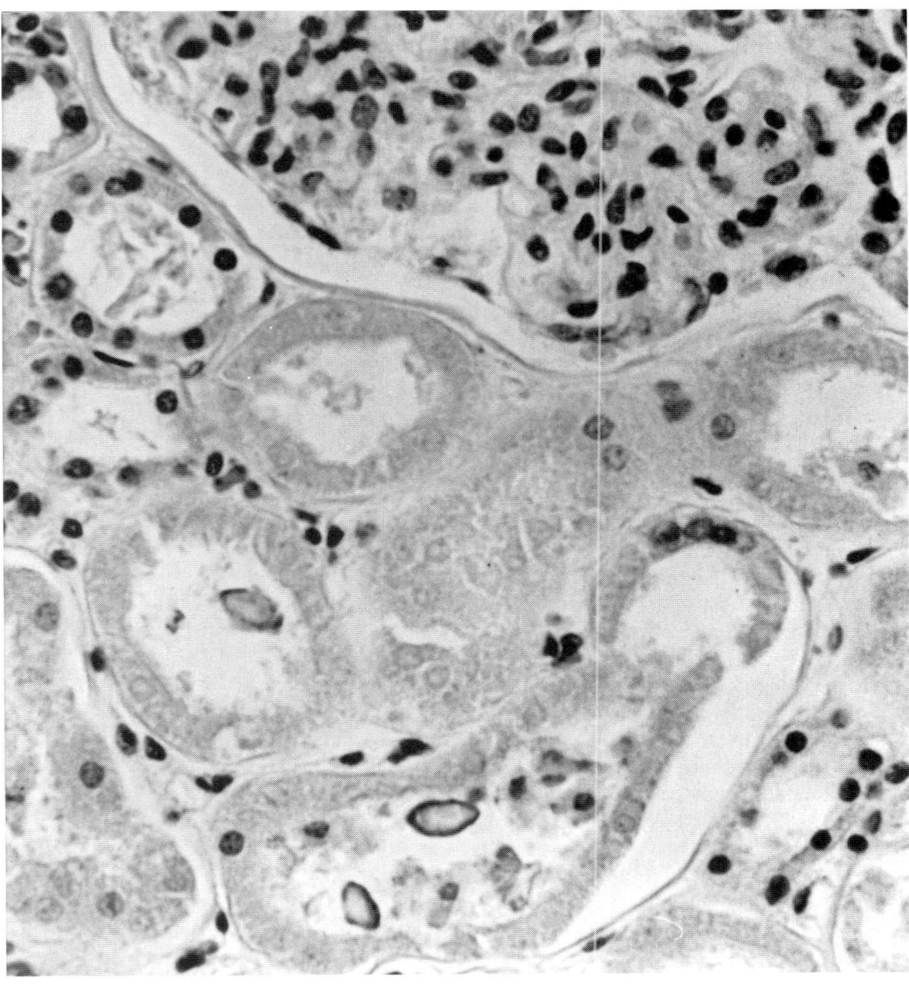

Fig. 96-2. Renal histological findings in a patient with renal failure from ethylene glycol intoxication. Diffuse calcium oxalate crystal disposit in the tubules and tubular necrosis are seen.

increased ethanol clearance. The ethanol infusion should be maintained until the ethylene glycol level approaches zero and there is resolution of the acidosis. Peritoneal dialysis does not play a role in the treatment of ethylene glycol intoxication.

ETHANOL

Ethanol is the most commonly used and abused drug in this country. It is pervasive among all age groups and all races, and represents a tremendous economic and social cost to society. Approximately 42 percent of all traffic fatalities, 69 percent of all drownings, and 23 percent of all suicide deaths are ethanol-related. Total mortalities (medical and nonmedical) attributed to ethanol are estimated to be 100,000 deaths per year.

Pathophysiology

Ethanol is metabolized via three different pathways. The most important pathway is by alcohol dehydrogenase, with NAD^+ as an oxidizing agent converting ethanol to acetaldehyde. Microsomal ethanol-oxidizing systems and catalase account for a small portion of ethanol metabolism. Acetaldehyde is further metabolized by aldehyde dehydrogenase and NAD^+ to acetate. Acetate is finally converted to acetyl-CoA and is metabolized to CO_2 and H_2O in the tricarboxylic acid cycle (TCA cycle).

Ethanol metabolism follows essentially zero-order kinetics. Nontolerant individuals generally metabolize ethanol at 15 to 20 mg/dL per hour, and chronic alcoholics metabolize ethanol at 30 mg/dL per hour.

Ethanol is a direct CNS depressant, probably mediated by altering membrane lipid fluidity or by affecting the benzodiazepine–GABA–chloride complex. The effects of ethanol vary significantly depending on individual tolerance. Although many alcoholics may develop tolerance for some CNS symptoms, respiratory tolerance and the lethal dose are unaltered.

Ethanol is well known to cause metabolic derangements such as hypoglycemia and alcoholic ketoacidosis (AKA); however, the development of these metabolic states is usually multifactorial, and the conditions may be independent for one another. Ethanol oxidation shifts the intracellular redox potential by increasing the $NADH/NAD^+$ ratio, which favors the formation of lactate and β-hydroxybutyrate. A relative state of starvation frequently develops during the drinking binges of alcoholics. Nausea and vomiting from gastritis or pancreatitis further limit food intake and increase dehydration. All of these factors lead to increased fatty acid metabolism for energy, resulting in AKA. Hypoglycemia is related to glycogen depletion from starvation and to the depletion of pyruvate, which is an important intermediate for gluconeogenesis.

Thiamine deficiency is very common in alcoholics. Ethanol intake directly diminishes the absorption of thiamine from the GI tract. The poor nutritional intake of the alcoholic patient further contributes to thiamine deficiency. Thiamine is a cofactor for enzymes in various metabolic pathways: (1) pyruvate dehydrogenase, an enzyme which converts pyruvate into acetyl-CoA, a substrate for the TCA cycle or for fatty acid synthesis; (2) α-ketoglutarate dehydrogenase, an enzyme in the TCA cycle; and (3) transketolase, an enzyme in the pentose phosphate shunt pathway. Thiamine also has an undefined but important role in maintaining neural axonal functions. The result of thiamine deficiency may lead to Wernicke's encephalopathy, peripheral neuropathy, cardiomyopathy (''wet'' beriberi), and metabolic acidosis.

Alcoholics may also have a number of other vitamin and electrolyte deficits because of poor oral intake and GI tract problems. Niacin, folate, magnesium, and potassium may frequently be low and need replenishment. Chronic ethanol usage has direct and indirect deleterious effects on virtually every organ system in the body. However, a review of these effects is beyond the scope of this chapter.

Clinical Features

The clinical features of ethanol intoxication are similar to those induced by sedative-hypnotic agents. The signs of mild intoxication are colored by the individual's basic personality, and can range from euphoria, expansiveness, and loss of self-control to general bad temper. Ataxia, slurred speech, nystagmus, lethargy, and dullness or distortion of sensory perceptions occur next. Tachycardia due to peripheral vasodilation induced by ethanol and dehydration is common. With toxic levels, hypoventilation, hypothermia, and hypotension develop.

Wernicke's encephalopathy should be consider in any alcoholic with an altered mental status. The classic triad consists of ataxia, ophthmaloplegia (nystagmus and sixth nerve palsy), and an altered mental status. These classic findings are, however, neither consistent nor common. Other manifestations of Wernicke's encephalopathy include hypothermia, coma, and hypotension.

Alcohol-drug interactions should be considered when evaluating the intoxicated patient and when prescribing medications. Disulfiram (Antabuse) inhibits aldehyde dehydrogenase, and the inhibition of the enzyme may persist for up to 2 weeks after the last dose of medication. The consumption of ethanol while the patient is on disulfiram results in the accumulation of acetaldehyde. Acetaldehyde is a potent vasodilator resulting in flushing of the skin, nausea and vomiting, and headaches, and in a severe reaction, can lead to hypotension. Reactions similar to disulfiram–ethanol reactions may also result when ethanol is taken with other medications, including metronidazole, chlorpropamide, griseofulvin, and a number of third-generation cephalosporin antibiotics.

Motor vehicle accidents often occur while the driver is under the influence of ethanol. Physical examination of a trauma patient who is intoxicated is often unreliable, as the patient's sensory response to pain is altered. The mechanism of injury may be difficult to reconstruct because the patient's history is unreliable.

The patient who appears to be ethanol-intoxicated must be carefully evaluated for a wide variety of coexisting abnormalities. Head and neck injury, hypoglycemia, electrolyte abnormalities, meningitis, sepsis, myopathy and neuropathy, bone marrow suppression, cardiac myopathy and arrhythmias, GI bleeding, pancreatitis, liver disease, and coingestion of ethylene glycol and methanol are a few of the complications that alcoholics can exhibit. Several mental status and neurologic examinations should demonstrate continued improvement if the patient is only ethanol intoxicated. The alcoholic patient often has more than one disease, and meticulous emergency department evaluation should be the rule.

Treatment

For the patient with uncomplicated intoxication, observation until sober is generally all that is required. Thiamine (100 mg IM or IV) should be administered to all intoxicated patients to prevent thiamine deficiency and Wernicke's encephalopathy. Dextrose 50% should be administered IV since hypoglycemia may mimic ethanol intoxication. There is no evidence that naloxone will reverse the effects of ethanol. The use of fructose does not speed up sobriety and may cause a significant lactate acidosis.

The treatment of Wernicke's encephalopathy is parenteral thiamine. Ophthmaloplegia may reverse quickly with 100 mg thiamine IV. However, other manifestations may last for days, and these patients should be admitted for daily parenteral thiamine therapy (for at least 10 days).

Other supportive measures, such as the replacement of fluid and administration of multivitamins, potassium, and magnesium, should be instituted on a case-by-case basis. Most importantly, patients should be evaluated for concomitant medical problems such as occult trauma and typical and atypical infections. These patients are at risk for a multitude of diseases and disorders, but they are the most difficult patients to evaluate during the period of intoxication.

The physician must recognize the presence of alcohol dependency in any patient who is treated in the emergency department for ethanol intoxication. Intoxicated adolescents should be evaluated for abuse, neglect, and the potential for suicide. Emergency department treatment is not complete until the patient has received counseling in the emergency department and has been referred to an alcohol treatment center upon discharge.

Ethanol Withdrawal

The clinical features now recognized as ethanol withdrawal and delirum tremens (DTs) have been described for hundreds of years.

Pathophysiology

The physiologic basis for ethanol withdrawal is not completely elucidated. Ethanol exerts direct effects on the benzodiazepine–GABA–chloride receptor complex. Ethanol withdrawal may cause substantial decreases in GABA activity. Elevation of norepinephrine plasma concentrations and increase in sympathetic activity account for many of the symptoms of ethanol withdrawal.

Clinical Features

The symptoms and the severity of ethanol withdrawal are highly variable, and depend on the tolerance of the individual and the amount and duration of ethanol usage. Victor and Adams described four independent clinical syndromes associated with ethanol withdrawal: tremors, hallucinations, seizures, and delirium tremens. Because these syndromes can coexist, it is more practical for the clinician to classify ethanol withdrawal symptoms as mild, moderate, or severe.

Table 96-5. Clinical Differentiation of the Toxic Alcohols

Alcohol	Osmolar Gap	Anion Gap	Ketosis	Specific Signs and Symptoms
Methanol	+	+ + +	–	Visual symptoms Papilledema
Ethylene glycol	+	+ + +	–	Renal failure Hypocalcemia Ca oxalate crystals
Isopropanol	+	–	+ + +	Hemorrhagic gastritis and tracheobronchitis

Ethanol withdrawal usually begins within hours after the cessation or diminution of ethanol intake. Mild withdrawal symptoms consist of insomnia, tremors, and irritability. As the symptoms worsen, sympathetic symptoms such as tachycardia, hypertension, and diaphoresis become more prominent. The patient may experience hallucinations, which can be visual, auditory, olfactory, or a combination of several forms. ''Rum fits'' are seizures related to ethanol abstinence. These seizures are almost always grand mal in nature, and 90 percent of patients initiate and terminate such seizures within 7 to 48 h after ethanol abstinence. Status epilepticus is rare and should suggest other etiologies. Patients without an underlying seizure focus will have normal EEGs during periods of intoxication and dependency, but abnormal EEGs during the withdrawal period. In Victor and Brausch's study, approximately a third of the patient with ethanol withdrawal seizures progressed to delerium tremens if untreated.

Delirium tremens is the most severe form of ethanol withdrawal symptomatology, and generally develops about 48 to 100 h after ethanol abstinence. Hyperthermia, tachycardia, hypertension, and significant agitation and altered mental status are prominent. Untreated, delerium tremens can ultimately lead to cardiovascular collapse and death.

Treatment

The goals for the treatment of ethanol withdrawal are (1) to minimize acute morbidity and mortality, (2) to prevent and treat acute withdrawal symptoms, and (3) to facilitate long-term detoxification.

Patients with moderate to severe ethanol withdrawal symptoms should receive treatment and detoxification in an intensive care setting until they are stabilized. Patients with mild ethanol withdrawal symptoms who do not have a previous history of withdrawal seizures, delirium tremens, or other significant withdrawal symptoms, and do not have concomitant medical complications, may be successfully detoxified in a structured outpatient program. Most patients in urban emergency departments will not be candidates for outpatient detoxification because of their frequently associated medical problems, the lack of social support, and the lack of availability of structured detoxification programs in the community.

The most important pharmacologic therapy for these patients is the replacement of ethanol with another cross-tolerant sedative-hypnotic agent. Adequate sedation with prevent or treat sympathetic autonomic responses, agitation, and hyperthermia. Long-acting benzodiazepines such as diazepam are the treatment of choice. Diazepam can be given IV 5 to 10 mg every 10 to 15 min until the patient is sedated. Some patients may require large cumulative doses of benzodiazepines to adequately control their withdrawal symptoms. The IV route of drug administration is preferred in all patients with significant symptoms because of predictable drug delivery and onset of action. Mixing drugs or routes of administration may increase the risk of drug–drug interactions and increased adverse drug effects.

Phenobarbital, a long-acting barbiturate, is an acceptable alternative to benzodiazepines, particularly for patients with ethanol withdrawal and withdrawal seizures. Phenytoin is not effective in preventing withdrawal seizures and its only role remains in the patient with an underlying seizure focus, which may be difficult to define in an emergency setting. Phenothiazines have no cross-tolerance with ethanol and will not treat the withdrawal symptom. Furthermore, they can increase the risk of seizures and hypotension. Ethanol should not be used because of the availability of safer therapeutic agents. β blockers and α agonists have only been studied in patients with mild ethanol withdrawal symptoms. The use of these agents in patients with significant withdrawal symptoms can mask peripheral sympathetic symptoms without preventing central agitation and convulsions.

Concomitant medical and nutritional problems associated with alcoholism should be addressed during treatment. Fluid replacement is essential because of excessive fluid losses from diaphoresis, vomiting, agitation, and hyperthermia. Hypomagnesemia is common and may contribute to the withdrawal symptoms. Magnesium should be replaced in these patients. Thiamine and niacin replacement will prevent and treat Wernicke's encephalopathy and pellagra, respectively. Finally, infections and trauma are common in alcoholics, and a meticulous assessment is required in all patients. With the use of appropriate therapies, the mortality associated with delerium tremens has decreased from 37 percent in 1907 to less than 5 percent in the recent literatures.

ISOPROPANOL

Isopropanol is most commonly found in the home as rubbing alcohol. It is also used as a disinfectant, industrial solvent, cleaning agent, and solvent in cosmetics. Recently, many rubbing alcohol preparations have been changed from isopropanol to ethanol. Isopropanol is less toxic than methanol or ethylene glycol, but more toxic than ethanol.

Pathophysiology

Isopropanol is readily absorbed from the GI tract or by inhalation. Dermal absorption is small except when prolonged and extensive skin contact occurs such as after an isopropanol sponge bath. The volume of distribution is approximately 0.6 to 0.7 L/kg.

The major pathway of metabolism (80 percent) is probably oxidation via alcohol dehydrogenase to acetone. The rest is excreted unchanged via the kidneys. Metabolism follows first-order kinetics, with elimination of about 25 percent per hour. Acetone, a tertiary ketone, is not metabolized by aldehyde dehydrogenase. Acetone is eliminated largely through the kidney, and a smaller amount is exhaled. The elimination of the active metabolite acetone is more prolonged, with a half-life of approximately 29 h. Acetone is responsible for the prolonged symptoms associated with isopropanol intoxication.

Isopropanol is a potent CNS depressant. Animal studies suggest that it is 2 to 3 times as potent as ethanol as a direct CNS depressant. Acetone is also a CNS depressant on the same order of potency as ethanol. Direct GI irritating effects, vasodilatory effects, and myocardial depressant effects from both isopropanol and acetone are responsible for the other manifestations of isopropanol intoxication.

Clinical Features

The major clinical manifestations of isopropanol intoxication are (1) CNS depression, (2) abdominal pain and vomiting, (3) hypotension, and (4) ketosis. In many respects, these manifestations resemble ethanol intoxication, except for the duration of symptoms and significant ketosis.

Central nervous system depression in isopropanol intoxications can persist for 24 h. Gastric irritation occurs early, with nausea, vomiting, and abdominal pain. Severe hemorrhagic gastritis can be a striking feature. Hypotension can result from vasodilation, direct myocardial depression, or hemorrhagic gastritis. Rhabdomyolysis, acute tubular necrosis, and hepatocellular toxicity have also been reported, but probably are accounted for by prolonged hypotension and hypoperfusion of different organs.

The most characteristic and specific laboratory findings are an elevated osmolal gap, acetonemia, acetonuria, and absent acidosis. Acetone is not a ketoacid, and therefore acidosis is not a feature of isopropanol intoxications except when either hypotension or recent starvation is prominent. Significant acidosis should suggest other etiologies such as methanol and ethylene glycol intoxications. Hypoglycemia can result from starvation and an increased NADH/NAD$^+$ ratio. A falsely elevated creatinine is frequently seen because acetone interferes with the colorimetric assay of creatinine.

Treatment

Therapy consists mostly of supportive measures. Lavage can be performed if the ingestion occurred within the last 1 to 2 h. Glucose and thiamine should be given to patients with altered sensorium. Fluid therapy aimed at maintaining adequate circulating volume and urine output is important. These measures will suffice for almost all patients with isopropanol intoxication. Although hemodialysis is effective in removing isopropanol and acetone, it should be considered only if the patient has persistent hypotension and the isopropanol level exceeds 400 mg/dL.

SUMMARY

While the toxic effects of the different alcohols can be distinct, there are also many similarities. Patients that consume one alcohol may have taken another alcohol simultaneously. Accurate evaluation is difficult because of the pattern of initial intoxication is similar for the alcohols. Alcohol-intoxicated patients are also at risk for subtle or occult traumatic injuries and medical disorders. Furthermore, underlying psychological and social issues such as suicidal ideations, negligence, homelessness, and drug dependency must be evaluated to ensure proper disposition.

BIBLIOGRAPHY

Bennett I, Cary F, Mitchell G, et al: Acute methyl alcohol poisoning: A review based on experiences in an outbreak of 323 cases. *Medicine* 32:431, 1953.

Bjorkqvist SE: Clonidine in alcohol withdrawal. *Acta Psychiatr Scand* 52:256, 1975.

Clay KL, Murphy RC, Watkins WD: Experimental methanol toxicity in the primate: Analysis of metabolic acidosis. *Toxicol Appl Pharmacol* 34:49, 1975.

Golber TM, Sanz CJ, Rose HD, et al: Comparative evaluation of treatments of alcohol withdrawal syndromes. *JAMA* 201:113, 1967.

Goldfrank LR, Flomenbaum NE, Lewin NA, et al: Methnaol, ethylene glycol, and isopropanol, in Goldfrank LR, Flomenbaum NE, Lewin NA, et al. (eds.): *Goldfrank's Toxicologic Emergencies*. Norwalk, Connecticut, Appleton and Lange, 1990, pp. 481–496.

Gonda A, Gault H, Churchill D, et al: Hemodialysis for methanol intoxication. *Am J Med* 64:749, 1978.

Horwitz RI, Gottlieb LD, Kraus ML: The efficacy of atenolol in the outpatient management of the alcohol withdrawal syndrome. Result of a randomized clinical trial. *Arch Intern Med* 149:1089, 1989.

Isbell H, Fraser HF: An experimental study of the etiology of "rum fits" and delirium tremens. *Q J Stud Alcohol* 16:1, 1955.

Jacobsen D, Brodesen JE: Studies on ethylene glycol poisoning. *Acta Med Scan* 211:17, 1982.

Jacobsen D, Hewlett TP, Webb R, et al: Ethylene glycol intoxication: Evaluation of kinetics and crystalluria. *Am J Med* 84:145, 1988.

Jacobsen D, McMartin KE: Methanol and ethylene glycol poisonings: Mechanism of toxicity, clinical course, diagnosis and treatment. *Med Toxicol* 1:309, 1986.

Kaim SC, Klett CJ: Treatment of delirium tremens: A comparative evaluation of four drugs. *Q J Stud Alcohol* 33:1065, 1972.

Kayvan-Larijarni H, Tannenberg AM: Methanol intoxication: Comparison of peritoneal dialysis and hemodialysis treatment. *Arch Intern Med* 134:293, 1974.

Keeney A, Mellinkoff SM: Methyl alcohol poisoning. *Ann Intern Med* 34:331, 1951.

Lacourtrue PG, Wason S, Abram A, et al: Acute isopropyl alcohol intoxication: Diagnosis and management. *Am J Med* 75:680, 1983.

Lieber CS: Metabolism and metabolic effects on alcohol. *Med Clin North Am* 68:3, 1984.

Martin-Amat G, McMartin KE, Hayreh SS, et al: Methanol poisoning: Ocular toxicity produced by formate. *Toxicol Appl Pharmacol* 45:201, 1978.

Martinez TT, Jaeger RW, de Castro FJ: A comparison of the absorption and metabolism of isopropyl alchohol by oral, dermal and inhalation routes. *Vet Hum Toxicol* 28:233, 1986.

McMartin KE, Ambre JJ, Tephly TR: Methanol poisoning in human subjects: Role for formic acid accumulation in the metabolic acidosis. *Am J Med* 68:414, 1980.

McMartin KE, Makar AB, Martin G, et al: Methanol poisoning: I. The role of formic acid in the development of metabolic acidosis in the monkey and the reversal by 4-methylpyrazole. *Biochem Med* 13:319, 1975.

Noker PE, Eells JT, Tephly TR: Methanol toxicity: Treatment with folic acid and 5-formyl tetrahydrofolic acid. *Clin Exp Res* 4:378, 1980.

Peterson CD, Collins AJ, Himes JM, et al: Ethylene glycol poisoning. *N Engl J Med* 304:21, 1981.

Reuler JB, Girard DE: Wernicke's encephalopathy. *N Engl J Med* 312:1035, 1985.

Rosenbloom AJ: Optimizing drug treatment of alcohol withdrawal. *Am J Med* 81:901, 1986.

Sampliner R, Iber FL: Diphenylhydantoin control of alcohol withdrawal seizures: Results of a controlled study. *JAMA* 230:1430, 1974.

Swartz RD, Millman RP, Billi JE, et al: Epidemic methanol poisoning: Clinical and biochemical analysis of a recent episode. *Medicine* 60:373, 1981.

Tracy P, Hewlett MS, McMartin KE: Ethylene glycol poisoning: The value of glycolic acid determinations for diagnosis and treatment. *Clin Toxicol* 24:389, 1986.

Underwood F, Bennett WM: Ethylene glycol intoxication: Prevention of renal failure by aggressive management. *JAMA* 226:1453, 1973.

Victor M, Adams RD: The effect of alcohol on the nervous systems. *Res Publ Assoc Res Nerv Ment Dis* 32:526, 1953.

Victor M, Brausch C: The role of abstinence in the genesis of alcoholic epilepsy. *Epilepsia* 8:1, 1967.

Williams HF: Alcoholic hypoglycemia and ketoacidosis. *Med Clin North Am* 68:33, 1984.

Young GP, Rores C, Murphy C, et al: Intravenous phenobarbital for alcohol withdrawal and convulsions. *Ann Emerg Med* 16:847, 1987.

Zilm DH, Sellers EM, Macleod SM, Degani N: Propranolol effect on tremor in alcoholic withdrawal. *Ann Intern Med* 83:234, 1975.

97 COCAINE

Susi Vassallo

Illicit cocaine use is widespread. The Drug Abuse Awareness Network (DAWN) has identified cocaine as the drug of abuse most often involved in emergency department visits. In 1988, it was the second most common cause of drug-related death reported to the AAPCC. Because of the pervasiveness of cocaine use and the increasing numbers of cocaine-related emergencies, the emergency physician must be familiar with the clinical manifestations and management of acute cocaine intoxication, as well as the diverse complications which result from its cardiac, neurologic, and vascular effects.

FORMS OF COCAINE

Cocaine (benzoylmethylecgonine) is a naturally occurring plant alkaloid found in the leaves of the Erythroxylon coca plant. Cocaine sulfate is prepared by crushing the leaves with a hydrocarbon solvent, followed by extraction of the alkaloid with sulfuric acid. This preparation has many plant impurities and undergoes further purification procedures to form the water-soluble cocaine hydrochloride salt, the familiar white powder form in which cocaine was most often sold in the past. Adulterants such as quinine and talc, even strychnine and arsenic, have been used to "cut" the powder, rendering it less potent and more profitable. Cocaine hydrochloride is insufflated or "snorted" intranasally or injected intravenously. This form is not suitable for smoking because it decomposes when burned.

A very different form of cocaine is obtained by dissolving the cocaine hydrochloride in an alkaline solution followed by extraction with ether. Evaporation of the ether yields the pure alkaloidal form of cocaine, called free base. Cocaine free base is also called crack because of the sound made by the crystals when they are heated. Crack, which is almost pure cocaine, is not destroyed by heating and vaporizes at high temperatures, making it suitable for smoking. The crystals of alkaloidal cocaine can be crushed and mixed with tobacco and smoked as a cigarette, or placed in a pipe and "freebased."

PHARMACOLOGY

Cocaine is absorbed from all sites including the mucous membranes, the gastrointestinal tract, and the respiratory tree. The route of administration affects the rapidity of onset of action as well as the duration of effect. Absorption across mucous membranes is relatively slow because cocaine-induced vasoconstriction inhibits its own absorption. The peak effect following intravaginal or intranasal administration occurs within one half hour and may last up to one and one-half hours. Gastrointestinal absorption may peak as late as 90 min and last up to 3 h. Intravenous use and inhalation result in a peak onset of action at 30 s to 2 min and a duration of action of approximately 20 min.

Cocaine has several important pharmacologic effects. Its local anesthetic affects are related to its ability to block sodium ion influx during depolarization of peripheral nerves. This prevents both the initiation and conduction of electrical impulses within nerve cells. In the central nervous system, cocaine blocks the presynaptic reuptake of the neurotransmitters norepinephrine, serotonin, and dopamine, producing an excess of the neurotransmitter at the postsynaptic site. This results in excessive sympathetic stimulation. Tachycardia, hypertension, hyperthermia, agitation, and seizures are a consequence of this adrenergic stimulation. Very high doses of cocaine have depressant effects resulting in hypotension, bradycardia, and coma. Cocaine effects on dopaminergic transmission may be involved in the production of euphoria and the general feeling of well-being which the user seeks. Depletion of dopamine at nerve terminals with long-term use is postulated to cause the dysphoria observed during cessation of cocaine use and the subsequent desire for more drug.

Cocaine is metabolized primarily by plasma pseudocholinesterase to ecgonine methyl ester, an inactive metabolite. Benzoylecgonine is formed by nonenzymatic hydrolysis. Norcocaine is formed by *N*-demethylation. Ecgonine methyl ester and benzoylecgonine are water-soluble metabolites excreted in the urine. Typically, urine toxicology assay for these metabolites will be positive for 24 to 72 h. In chronic cocaine users, urine tests for cocaine metabolites using the highly sensitive techniques of gas chromatography and mass spectrophotometry have been reported to remain positive for up to 2 weeks following discontinuation of the drug. Recently, it has been suggested that individuals with low plasma cholinesterase levels may be at increased risk for toxicity. Lower enzyme activity may result in increased availability of the parent cocaine compound or may increase the percentage of cocaine metabolized by *N*-demethylation to norcocaine, the only known active metabolite.

MEDICAL COMPLICATIONS

Cardiac

Acute myocardial infarction temporarily related to cocaine use is well described in the literature and continues to be of concern to the clinician treating individuals known to use cocaine. Chest pain following the use of cocaine is a frequent emergency department complaint. Despite normal or nondiagnostic ECGs on presentation, 19 percent of patients have been found to have elevated CPK and CPK-MB isoenzyme results. The time from cocaine use to onset of chest pain is reported to vary from immediately to greater than 24 h. A recent study demonstrated episodes of myocardial ischemia during holter monitoring of chronic cocaine users for a period of 2 weeks following withdrawal of the drug. Any person complaining of symptoms which may be consistent with myocardial ischemia must be carefully interviewed in order to assess the possibility of cocaine use. The astute clinician will not be lulled into complacency by a preconceived notion of the kinds of patients at risk for myocardial infarction and/or cocaine use. A history of cocaine use may not be forthcoming without pointed inquiry.

The mechanisms of cocaine-related myocardial injury appear to be multifactorial. Myocardial infarction temporarily related to cocaine use has been reported in individuals with preexisting angina or previous myocardial infarction, as well as patients with no previous history of heart disease and normal coronary arteries demonstrated by selective coronary angiography. Several mechanisms by which cocaine causes myocardial injury have been proposed. First, cocaine directly stimulates the sympathetic nervous system, resulting in an increased blood pressure–heart rate product and increased myocardial contractility. These effects raise myocardial oxygen demand. It is likely that some patients with fixed coronary lesions develop ischemic cardiac injury under circumstances of increased myocardial oxygen demand imposed by cocaine use. Second, cocaine-induced vasospasm may overcome normal myocardial autoregulatory dilatation of vessels and lead to impaired myocardial oxygenation. Third, the angiographic demonstration of coronary artery thrombosis in cocaine-related myocardial infarction has led to speculation that spasm in combination with cocaine-induced intimal injury or effects on platelet aggregation and release of thromboxanes may play a pathogenic role, particularly in patients without underlying coronary artery disease. Nonatherosclerotic intimal proliferation of smooth muscle has been noted in a chronic cocaine user. When acute coronary artery thrombus formation has been demonstrated angiographically, it has responded to intravenous thrombolytic therapy and balloon angioplasty.

Other disorders of the cardiovascular system described in association with cocaine use include atrial and ventricular arrhythmias, myocarditis, aortic rupture, and congestive heart failure. Arrhythmias have been attributed to the increase in circulating catecholamines. In addition, cocaine may also have a quinidinelike effect on myocardial conduction resulting in QT prolongation and QRS widening. Increased shear forces brought on by increased pulse and blood pressure have been implicated in acute aortic rupture. Focal myocardial injury manifest as "contraction band necrosis" has been demonstrated in autopsy studies of chronic cocaine users. This is thought to be related to catecholamine-mediated myocardial injury. An increased risk of endocarditis has been demonstrated in intravenous cocaine users and may be related to endocardial damage caused by cocaine.

Pulmonary

Spontaneous pneumothorax and pneumomediastinum have been reported after inhalation of cocaine vapors. The mechanism for this probably relates to the deep inspiration and breath holding which accompany freebasing. The development of pulmonary infiltrates, fever, and bronchospasm has been called "crack lung" and may be an IgE-mediated entity. Pulmonary infarction has also been reported.

Central Nervous System

Both ischemic and hemorrhagic cerebrovascular accidents have been temporally related to cocaine use. Hemorrhagic strokes may be intraventricular, intraparenchymal, or subarachnoid. Infarcts occur throughout the central nervous system, including the spinal cord and retina. Of 15 cerebral angiograms reported by Levine, 10 (67 percent) were normal. Vasculitis was not suggested by any of the angiographic data. Reported angiographic anomalies include intraluminal clot, stenosis, vasospasm, vasculitis, cerebrovascular malformation, and cerebral aneurysm, occurring in a variety of locations within the cerebral vasculature.

The mechanisms of cocaine-related stroke are undoubtedly similar to those leading to detrimental effects on the heart, including induction of vasospasm and enhanced platelet aggregability. Acute rises in blood pressure predispose to hemorrhagic stroke, especially in patients with cerebral vascular abnormalities. Cardiac arrhythmias or cardiomyopathy may contribute to cerebral embolism.

The clinician should be alert to the possibility of an intracranial event in the cocaine-using patient who presents with headache, seizures, an altered level of consciousness, or persistent agitation. Subtle change in affect, focal neurologic deficits, and many softer signs in the neurologic and mental status examination may suggest intracerebral pathology. Brain abscess and other intracranial infection have resulted from intranasal and intravenous cocaine use.

Obstetrical

The nature of the maternal and fetal risks due to cocaine use during pregnancy have yet to be satisfactorily delineated. Small reported studies suggest a greater incidence of spontaneous abortion, small-for-gestational-age infants, abruptio placenta, and congenital anomalies, as well as abnormal behavior and delayed infant development. Both mother and fetus are at risk for the life-threatening cardiovascular and CNS effects of cocaine. Large animal studies have demonstrated cocaine-induced vascular effects as a cause of maternal hypertension, fetal vasoconstriction, and decreased uteroplacental flow. Hypoxia secondary to decreased uteroplacental blood flow is a significant contributor to fetal distress noted following maternal administration of cocaine.

Renal

Rhabdomyolysis is an expected complication in the cocaine-intoxicated patient, occasionally resulting in acute myoglobinuric renal failure. Muscle breakdown associated with cocaine use may result from motor agitation and hyperthermia. In addition, it is possible that cocaine-induced arterial vasospasm causes muscle ischemia or that cocaine has a direct toxic effect on muscle metabolism. Hypotension, depletion of intravascular volume, and hyperthermia contribute to the development of renal failure. Renal infarction has also been reported with intravenous cocaine use.

Other Cocaine-Related Complications

Ischemic injury and infarction have been reported in almost every organ, including the liver, the bowel, and the skin. Vascular injury resulting in extremity ischemia has resulted from accidental interarterial injection of cocaine. Necrosis of the nasal septum from repeated insufflation of cocaine commonly occurs in chronic users. A multitude of infectious diseases are routinely seen in the cocaine-using population, such as osteomyelitis, hepatitis, thrombophlebitis, abscess formation, sepsis, endocarditis, pneumonia, and acquired immunodeficiency syndrome (AIDS). The incidence of AIDS contracted through intravenous drug use has created a health care crisis of critical proportions. Heightened sexual activity in crack users has also been postulated as a mechanism of sexual transmission of AIDS.

Body Packers and Stuffers

The term "body packer" or "mule" refers to the individual who packages illegal drugs and swallows them as a means of gastrointestinal smuggling. "Body stuffer" refers to the individual who quickly swallows the drug at the moment of arrest in order to conceal possession of the substance. Theoretically, body packers apply more forethought and care to their task and carefully wrap the illicit merchandise in condoms, cellophane, foil, balloons, or the fingers of latex gloves. Rubber bands or ties of some type are used to secure the small packages. Each packet contains a potentially lethal amount of drug. Rupture of a single packet has resulted in rapidly fatal cocaine toxicity. Management of such ingestions is controversial. No controlled clinical studies have been done, and each case presents variations in packaging, contents, time from ingestion, clinical symptoms, and patient cooperation. Various management strategies have been tried including whole bowel irrigation, charcoal, cathartics, ipecac, and endoscopic and surgical removal. In addition to history and physical examination, chest and abdominal x-rays as well as contrast radiography may be helpful.

Topical Cocaine

The application of TAC, the topical anesthetic containing tetracaine 0.5%, adrenaline 0.05%, and cocaine 11.8%, is popular in some emergency departments for the prevention of pain from laceration repair, particularly in children. Cocaine toxicity and fatalities have resulted from systemic absorption, particularly following mucous membrane contact. Cocaine and its metabolites have been demonstrated in the plasma of children receiving TAC for topical anesthesia. Because of the serious complications reported with TAC, great caution must be exercised in its use.

PRESENTATION AND MANAGEMENT

The signs and symptoms of sympathetic overstimulation characterize cocaine intoxication. Hypertension, tachycardia, increased rate of respiration, diaphoresis, hyperthermia, and agitation are classic. Adequate sedation and control of hyperthermia and seizures are the primary initial therapeutic objectives. In addition, adequate fluid support is essential to prevent the renal complications of rhabdomyolysis. Other causes of agitated delirium should be considered while treatment is instituted. Central nervous system infection, intracranial events, sedative-hypnotic withdrawal, hypoglycemic, and other toxic exposures (phencyclidine, amphetamine, anticholinergics, lithium, monoamine oxidase inhibitors, etc.) are part of the differential diagnosis. The literature clearly supports the safety and efficacy of sedation with benzodiazepines. Avoidance of respiratory depression can be achieved by titration with small frequent intravenous boluses of lorazepam or diazepam. Sedation should be achieved concurrent with implementation of cooling measures such as ice water and fans if the temperature is elevated. A soft, flexible rectal temperature probe should be used to monitor temperature and prevent injury to the patient. The use of standard cooling blankets is not adequate in managing temperature elevations in these patients, nor is the use of antipyretics. The use of phenothiazines in this setting may lower the seizure threshold, impair heat loss mechanisms through their anticholinergic effects, and cause hypotension. In the event that the agitated delirium is a result of sedative withdrawal rather than drug toxicity, use of a sedating agent which is not regarded as having significant cross-tolerance with sedative hypnotic agents, such as a phenothiazine or butyrophenone, would leave the condition inadequately treated.

In the great majority of patients sedation with the benzodiazepines will result in control of hypertension and tachycardia as well. Severe hypertension unresponsive to sedation should be treated with nitroprusside or phentolamine. The use of calcium channel blockers may also be beneficial, although definitive study in this setting is yet to be completed. Arguments against the use of β blockers to control hypertension are numerous. Recent work by Lange demonstrated potentiation of cocaine-induced coronary vasoconstriction by β-adrenergic blockade. The vasoconstrictive effects of cocaine in the coronary circulation were reversed by phentolamine. Blockade of peripheral β_2 receptors may result in unopposed α-receptor stimulation, worsening peripheral vasospasm and possibly further increasing blood pressure. Other studies have shown an adverse effect of propanolol on seizures and mortality. Labetolol has been suggested as an alternative to propranolol in treatment of cocaine-induced hypertension. However, when used intravenously labetalol has much greater β-blocking than α-blocking effect, approximately 7 to 1. Its use in the treatment of a pheochromocytoma-mediated hypertensive crisis, a hypercatecholamine condition often compared to the cocaine-induced hypercatecholamine state, resulted in worsened hypertension. Because a significant body of evidence suggests that the use of β blockers may be detrimental in the hypercatecholamine state, the other therapeutic modalities already mentioned (sedation, nitroprusside, phentolamine) are better choices for treatment of most cases of cocaine poisoning. However, β blockers may still be the agents of choice for the treatment of hemodynamically significant tachyarrhythmias in the cocaine-poisoned patient. The use of sodium bicarbonate to treat the quinidinelike effects of cocaine, such as widening of the QRS and prolongation of the QT interval, needs further exploration.

Following control of agitation, myocardial ischemia and infarction should be treated in the standard way with the use of nitrates, β blockers or calcium channel blockers, and thrombolytic agents.

SUMMARY

The treatment of the cocaine-intoxicated patient is an area of continued interest and research. A thoughtful approach to problem-solving based on knowledge of physiology and pharmacology as well as circumspect evaluation of new information will further understanding and provide scientific support of clinical practice. The emergency physician is uniquely placed in the health care system and must respond to the crisis of the moment presented by each patient as well as the greater challenges of these times.

BIBLIOGRAPHY

Brody SL, Wrenn KD, Wilber MM, et al: Predicting the severity of cocaine-associated rhabdomyolysis. *Ann Emerg Med* 19:1137, 1990.

Chasnoff IJ, Burns WJ, Schnoll SH, et al. Cocaine use in pregnancy. *N Engl J Med* 313:666, 1985.

Goldfrank LR, Hoffman RS. The cardiovascular effects of cocaine. *Ann Emerg Med* (in press).

Hoffman R, Smilkstein M, Goldfrank LR. Bowel irrigation and the cocaine body packer: A new approach to a common problem. *Am J Emerg Med* 8:523, 1990.

Hoffman R, Henry GL, Weisman RS, et al. Association between plasma cholinesterase activity and cocaine toxicity. *Ann Emerg Med* 19:467, 1990.

Lange RA, Cigorroa RG, Yancy CW, et al. Cocaine-induced coronary-artery vasoconstriction. *New Engl J Med* 321:1557, 1989.

Levine SR, Brust JCM, Futrell N, et al. Cerebrovascular complications of the use of the "crack" form of alkaloidal cocaine. *N Engl J Med* 323:699, 1990.

Nahas G, Trouve R, Demus JF, et al. A calcium-channel blocker as antidote to the cardiac effects of cocaine intoxication. *N Engl J Med* 313:519, 1985.

Roth D, Alarcon FJ, Fernandez JA, et al. Acute Rhabdomyolysis associated with cocaine intoxication. *N Engl J Med* 319:673, 1988.

Smith HWB, Liberman HA, Brody SL, et al. Acute myocardial infarction temporally related to cocaine use: Clinical, angiographic and pathophysiologic observations. *Ann Intern Med* 107:13, 1987.

Woods JR, Plessinger MA, Clark KE. Effect of cocaine on uterine blood flow and fetal oxygenation. *JAMA* 257:957, 1987.

98
AMPHETAMINES AND AMPHETAMINE-LIKE DRUGS

Donald B. Kunkel

Amphetamine is a generic term used to correctly describe a specific drug (β-phenylisopropylamine) and to loosely refer to a wide variety of chemical entities which may be controlled substances, legal over-the-counter preparations, or illicit street drugs.

Historically, amphetamine itself was first synthesized in 1887, but the first commercially available preparation did not appear until 1932, with the introduction of Benzedrine nasal inhalers. With the observation that amphetamine had powerful central nervous system arousal effects, amphetamine began to be touted for a variety of medical disorders, including availability in tablet form for narcolepsy in 1937. Shortly thereafter, oral amphetamine was placed under FDA control as a prescription drug, but this move failed to curb its growing use during World War II, when military troops and home-front workers were allowed access to almost limitless supplies of the drug. Following a postwar binge of amphetamine use and with the increased use of amphetamines and other drugs during the 1960s, a number of amphetamines were moved to Schedule II classification in 1970. Three factors have tended to thwart this move: (1) continued availability of potent amphetamines via prescription abuse and foreign trafficking, (2) exclusion of certain "amphetamines" (e.g., phenylpropanolamine) from control, and (3) street manufacture of a variety of these drugs.

PHARMACOLOGY

Structurally, the amphetamines are similar to the endogenous catecholamines (epinephrine, norepinephrine) but differ in their usually marked effects on the central nervous system.

Central effects are probably mediated by numerous pathways and receptors, resulting in restlessness, hyperactivity, repetitive or stereotyped behavior, anorexia, and sleep reduction. Advanced stimulation may lead to psychosis and convulsions.

Peripheral effects of amphetamines reflect a largely indirect action via release of endogenous catecholamines. Mixed α and β receptor effects are noted, producing pupillary dilatation, peripheral vasoconstriction, increased metabolism, tachycardia, and bronchodilation, among other effects.

Amphetamines are rapidly absorbed from the gastrointestinal tract and peak plasma levels occur within an hour or two following ingestion. Approximately 30 to 40 percent of amphetamine is metabolized in the liver, and elimination of parent drug and metabolites is renal. Amphetamines may be detected in urine for several days. Because of the high pK_a of amphetamine, an acid urine will hasten the excretion of both parent drug and metabolites. In addition to ingestion of amphetamine, injection, inhalation, and even vaginal routes have been employed.

TOXICITY

Tolerance to amphetamines may dictate to a large degree the severity of reaction to otherwise toxic doses of amphetamine. Blood levels are generally of little value in determining individual prognosis. Following exposure to toxic doses, the following findings may occur:

Neurologic

- Mydriasis, piloerection, and diaphoresis
- Extreme restlessness with repetitive and bizarre behavior
- Choreoathetosis
- Psychosis and delirium
- Coma
- Extrapyramidal syndrome (rare)
- Cerebral vasculitis
- Intracranial hemorrhage

Cardiovascular

- Flushing
- Hypertension
- Tachycardia
- Arrhythmias
- Myocardial infarction
- Circulatory collapse
- Acute and chronic cardiomyopathy
- Polyarteritis nodosa

Gastrointestinal

- Nausea and vomiting
- Diarrhea

Other

- Hyperpyrexia
- Rhabdomyolysis
- Coagulopathies
- Leukocytosis
- Elevated T_4
- Acute pulmonary edema (from smoking methamphetamine)

WITHDRAWAL

In the adult user, abrupt cessation of amphetamine results in abstinence symptoms which are rarely life-threatening, and which peak within 2 to 3 days following discontinuation of drug. Depression and increased appetite are common, along with cramps, nausea, diarrhea, and headache.

Neonatal withdrawal may result in diaphoresis, restlessness, hypoglycemia, and seizures.

MANAGEMENT OF TOXICITY

Following an acute oral exposure, avoid emesis because of the potential for seizures due to the central nervous system effects of amphetamine. Gastric lavage may be indicated, followed by tube instillation of activated charcoal.

Cardiac monitoring may be indicated due to the potential for arrhythmias and myocardial infarction.

Hyperactivity is best managed in a quiet area with decreased sensory input. Diazepam in lesser situations or haloperidol parenterally in cases of extreme hyperactivity or psychosis is currently recommended.

Seizures may be treated with intravenous diazepam. Uncontrollable seizures may require phenytoin, phenobarbital, or even a paralyzing agent (pancuronium).

Aggressive cooling measures may be necessary with hyperthermic states, and paralysis may be appropriate.

Severe hypertension may require the use of a nitroprusside drip. Beta-blocker agents should be used with caution due to the possible precipitation of unopposed alpha effects (hypertension). If used, consideration should be given to concomitant use of a vasodilating agent to control pressor effects.

Theoretically, urinary acidification may hasten excretion of amphetamine, but the clinical effectiveness of this maneuver has not been demonstrated. In addition, urinary acidification is contraindicated in myoglobinuria, where urinary alkalinization is recommended. Urine flow rates should be kept within physiologic parameters, however.

SPECIAL CONSIDERATIONS

Phenylpropanolamine (PPA) is an amphetamine-like substance which was *not* scheduled as a Class II drug by the Controlled Substances Act of 1970. It is commonly available as an over-the-counter agent in many diet and decongestant preparations and is frequently encountered as a component of "look-alike" street drugs in combination with ephedrine, pseudoephedrine, and caffeine. PPA has been known to cause hypertension, seizures, intracerebral hemorrhage, and arrhythmias.

Propylhexedrine was introduced in the Benzedrex inhaler in 1949 as an alternative to the then-abused Benzedrine inhaler containing amphetamine. Propylhexedrine itself became the object of abuse via injection of the contents of the Benzedrex inhaler. A 1979 report listed 12 deaths following intravenous abuse of Benzedrex inhalers in Dallas. Pulmonary edema, foreign body granulomas, fibrosis, and evidence of pulmonary hypertension were frequently noted at autopsy.

"Designer drugs" in the amphetamine group include 3,4-methylenedioxyamphetamine (MDA), 3,4-methylenedioxymethamphetamine (MDMA) ("Adam," "Ecstasy"), 3,4-methylenedioxyethamphetamine (MDEA) ("Eve"), and 4-bromo-2,5-dimethoxyamphetamine (DOB). All these drugs are structurally related to amphetamine and mescaline. Recent deaths attributable to use of MDMA and MDEA have been reported. DOB has been reported to cause diffuse vascular spasm following oral use.

Of growing concern in recent years has been the spectacular rise of methamphetamine as a street drug, with use surpassing that of cocaine in some geographic areas of the United States. Known popularly as "crank" or "ice" (smokable crystalline form), street-origin methamphetamine is commonly manufactured in clandestine laboratories, and the laboratory itself may present explosive and toxic hazards due to the storage and handling of chemicals (see Table 98-1) which are used in the manufacture of methamphetamine. Methamphetamine's effect is almost immediate following intravenous or intranasal use, or when smoked. As compared to cocaine, users report similar effects with methamphetamine when injected or smoked, but the effects of methamphetamine are much longer (4–6 hours) compared to cocaine's duration of action (an hour or less). In addition to the usual amphetamine effects, smoked methamphetamine has been reported to cause acute pulmonary edema, and chronic methamphetamine use seems highly prone to causing psychotic reactions. Lead poisoning has been reported due to abuse of contaminated methamphetamine.

Leaves of the khat shrub are widely used as a stimulant in eastern Africa and the Arabian Peninsula. Cathinone, the active principle in khat leaves, has pharmacologic activity similar to that of amphetamine. Khat may induce a toxic psychosis.

Some common amphetamines are listed in Table 98-2.

Table 98-1. Common Chemicals Used in Illicit MA Manufacture

Reagents
- Aluminum
- Lead Acetate
- Mercuric Chloride
- Potassium Cyanide
- Phosphorous
- Thionyl Chloride
- Hydrochloric Acid
- Hydroiodic Acid
- Sodium Hydroxide

Solvents
- Acetone
- Ethyl Ether
- Ethanol
- Isopropanol
- Methanol
- Pyridine
- Toluene

Precursors
- Benzyl Cyanide
- Benzylchloride
- Dimethylformamide
- Ephedrine
- Formic Acid
- Hydrogen Gas
- Methylamine
- N-methylformamide
- Phenyl-2-Propanone
- Phenylacetic Acid

Table 98-2. Common Amphetamines: Schedule II or III Agents

Generic Name	Common Trade Name(s)
PRESCRIPTION AGENTS	
Amphetamine (racemic)	Benzedrine, Biphetamine
Benzphetamine	Didrex
Dextroamphetamine	Dexampex, Dexedrine, Spancap No. 1
Diethylpropion	Depletite, Tenuate, Tepanil
Fenfluramine	Pondimin
Methamphetamine	Desoxyn, Methampex
Methylphenidate	Ritalin
Phendimetrazine	Bontril, Dyrexan, Melfiat, Prelu-2, SPRX, Statobex, Wehless
Phenmetrazine	Preludin
Phentermine	Fastin, Ionamin, Obephen, Obermine, Phentrol, Unifast
OVER-THE-COUNTER AGENTS (*NOTE: Formulations may vary*)	
Cinnamedrine	Midol (Some formulations)
Desoxyephedrine	Vicks inhaler
Ephedrine	Bronkaid (tablets), Marax, Quibron (elixir), Tedral, Vatronol
Phenylpropanolamine	ARM, Alka-Seltzer Plus, Allerest, Appedrine, Comtrex, Contac, Dexatrim, Dimetapp, Entex, Naldecon, Novahistine (tablets), Extra-Strength Sinutab, Triaminic
Propylhexedrine	Benzedrex inhaler
Pseudoephedrine	Actifed, Ambenyl, Chlortrimeton, Co-Tylenol, Drixoral, Fedahist, Novahistine, Rondec, Sine-Aid, Sudafed, Tussend

Modified from: Linden CH, Kulig KW, Rumack BH: Amphetamines. *Topics Emerg Med* 7:18, 1985. Used by permission.

BIBLIOGRAPHY

Anderson RJ, Garza HR, Garriott JC, et al: Intravenous propylhexedrine (Benzedrex) abuse and sudden death. *Am J Med* 67:15, 1979.

Burton BT: Methamphetamine: drug of the 90's. *Poison Press* 1:1, 1990.

Anderson RJ, Reed WG, Hillis LD, et al: History, epidemiology, and medical complications of nasal inhaler abuse. *J Toxicol Clin Toxicol* 19:95, 1982.

Dowling GP, McDonough ET, Bost RO: "Eve" and "Ecstasy": A report of five deaths associated with the use of MDEA and MDMA. *JAMA* 257:1615, 1987.

Gomolin I: Amphetamines. *Clin Toxicol Rev* 2:1, 1979.

Kulig KW: Amphetamines and related drugs, in Rumack BH (ed): *Poisindex*. Denver, Micromedex, 1987.

Linden CH, Kulig KW, Rumack BH: Amphetamines. *Topics Emerg Med* 7:18, 1985.

Nestor TA, Tamamoto WI, Kam TH, et al: Acute pulmonary edema caused by crystalline methamphetamine. *Lancet* 2:1277, 1989.

Pentel P: Toxicity of over-the-counter stimulants. *JAMA* 252:1898, 1984.

Pentel PR, Asinger RW, Benowitz NL: Propranolol antagonism of phenylpropanolamine-induced hypertension. *Clin Pharmacol Ther* 37:488, 1985.

99
HALLUCINOGENS

Robert S. Hoffman

BACKGROUND AND DEFINITIONS

The group of agents known as hallucinogens comprises a heterogeneous group of synthetic and naturally occurring compounds that share the ability to produce a subjective alteration in reality, such that the individual perceives events that do not truly exist. The term "psychedelic," which is often used interchangeably with hallucinogenic more rigidly refers to those agents that alter perceptual awareness, while allowing the individual to retain the ability to recognize that the experience is not real. Synesthesias, the condition in which a stimulus of one sense is perceived as a sensation of a different sense (such as the ability to hear colors or smell sounds), are common manifestations of the psychedelic experience. These must be distinguished from true hallucinations, where no stimulus is present for the perceived sensation. True drug-induced hallucinations do occur and are usually visual or tactile, which helps to distinguish them from primary psychiatric disorders that are often associated with auditory hallucinations. In this chapter, the term hallucinogen will be used to refer to both those agents capable of producing true hallucinations and the "illusogens" (agents that produce psychedelic phenomena). A discussion of marijuana, which is rarely reported to induce either illusions or true hallucinations, is also included in this chapter.

While the exact frequency of hallucinogen use is unknown, several estimates are available. The 1988 National Institute on Drug Abuse (NIDA) household survey estimates that over 14.5 million Americans have used a hallucinogenic agent at some time in their lives. At present there are almost 800,000 regular hallucinogen users. This should be compared with over 11.5 million regular marijuana users. Among Americans, marijuana is the most commonly used illicit substance.

Although these agents are often employed, acute and severe toxicity requiring evaluation by health care professionals is uncommon, as represented by recent results of the American Association of Poison Control Centers (AAPCC) National Data Collection System. In this data base of over 1.3 million reported human exposures, only 2330 exposures were recorded for marijuana, lysergic acid diethylamide (LSD), phencyclidine (PCP), and mescaline combined, of which over 75 percent were coded as having either none or minor effects. It is almost certain that both the NIDA and AAPCC studies underreport the true incidence of hallucinogen use.

The following sections will discuss the pharmacology, clinical presentation, diagnosis, and management of hallucinogen intoxications. Although this chapter is divided into sections based on individual agents, the emergency physician should concentrate on the similarities among these agents. This will allow for a uniform approach to the management of hallucinogen intoxication.

PCP

PCP is a dissociative anesthetic agent that was evaluated for human use in the 1950s. Originally it was felt to be an ideal agent because it had potent anesthetic and analgesic properties without causing respiratory depression. Unfortunately, it had to be taken off the market because many patients experienced postoperative psychotomimetic effects. Ketamine, a derivative of PCP, is still used in both human and veterinary medicine.

PCP and its chemical congeners (PCE, PCC, PHP, TCP, etc.) are available in powdered form or solution. The individual adds the PCP to tobacco or marijuana cigarettes prior to smoking. Inhalation results in rapid absorption with an onset of symptoms in 2 to 5 min and a peak effect by about 15 min. Although PCP is also absorbed by the gastrointestinal and percutaneous routes, the effects are somewhat delayed. The drug is both highly protein-bound and highly lipid-soluble resulting in a volume of distribution in excess of 6 L/kg. The majority of PCP undergoes liver metabolism to hydroxylated derivatives, leaving about 10 percent of the drug to be excreted in the urine in an unchanged form. Elimination half-lives are variable and have been reported to range from 7 h to 3 days. PCP is a weak base (p*Ka,* 8.5) and can be ion trapped in acid environments.

The clinical spectrum of PCP toxicity is dose-dependent and has been reviewed extensively. At low doses, loss of inhibition, mild agitation, nystagmus, ataxia, emotional lability, and either violent or aggressive behavior are noted. The nystagmus, which is often vertical or rotatory in addition to horizontal, is characteristic of PCP intoxication. Moderate doses of PCP produce muscle rigidity, hypertension, tachycardia, bizarre behavior, and either a regressive or excitatory state. With the most severe intoxications prolonged coma, seizures, and hyperpyrexia may occur. The most reliable findings are nystagmus, hypertension, and tachycardia. PCP is neither a cholinergic nor an anticholinergic agent, thus signs consistent with either syndrome may be present.

Complications often result from both the drug itself, and the behavioral effects that result from intoxication. Consequential trauma has been associated with PCP intoxication, either from the loss of coordination (while driving, for example) or from drug-associated violent behavior. Since the agitation associated with PCP is severe and is seen at low-to-moderate doses, patients who present with stupor or coma should be restrained prophylactically in anticipation of impending agitation. Severe psychomotor agitation results in hyperpyrexia and rhabdomyolysis, which are the two most common complications of PCP intoxication. Rapid control, sedation, and cooling are essential for the prevention of long-term complications (see "General Management"). Although acidification of the urine will increase the elimination of PCP, this increase is minor and insignificant when compared with its risks. As the urine becomes more acidic, myoglobin precipitation increases. Thus, in a severe PCP intoxication (where myoglobinuric renal failure is expected), the attempt to increase drug elimination can increase the complication rate. Since only a minor increase in elimination can be achieved, exposure to the risks of renal failure and systemic acidosis seems unwarranted. Alternatively, since the gastric juices are also acid, some authors have recommended continual nasogastric suction and multiple-dose activated charcoal in severe PCP intoxication. This probably only applies to the comatose patient.

LSD

While searching for a new analeptic agent in the 1930s, a German chemist named Albert Hoffmann noted a similarity between the structures of nikethamide and lysergic acid. The compound LSD-25 (now known as LSD) was synthesized, but its effects were not known until years later when Hoffmann became intoxicated accidentally. The drug culture of the 1960s popularized LSD as the way to achieve an alternative consciousness, or to "turn on and drop out" as it was described.

Although the exact mechanism of action of LSD is unknown, it is generally presumed to achieve some effects through inhibition of serotonergic neurotransmission. This decreases inhibitory tone in higher cortical centers and results in perceptual distortions. In addition, LSD appears to have both agonistic and antagonistic effects on central dopamine receptors, which may be responsible for the sympathomimetic effects seen with intoxication.

Since LSD is a very potent toxin (typical doses range from 25 to 500 μg), it is easily transported and disguised in large quantities. While inhalation, insufflation, and injection are all possible routes of administration of LSD, simple ingestion is the most popular. Solutions of LSD are applied to blotter paper, sugar cubes, or gelatin and consumed in this fashion.

Symptoms begin within 0.5 to 1.5 h and initially consist of a mild sympathomimetic response—mydriasis and minimal elevations of heart rate, blood pressure, respiration, and temperature. Gastrointestinal discomfort, salivation, piloerection, and parasympathomimetic effects also have been described. Neuromuscular weakness may be accompanied by tremor and hyperreflexia. Peak effects occur by 2 h and are associated with synesthesias, illusions, feelings of depersonalization, and possibly true hallucinations. Formal thought content may be disordered, and true paranoia may occur. Symptoms begin to wane by 4 h postingestion and usually resolve by 8 to 12 h postingestion.

Intoxication may be complicated by seizures, central nervous system venoocclusive disease, life-threatening hyperpyrexia, rhabdomyolysis, coagulopathy, and acute psychosis. The latter may persist for days after intoxication and is indistinguishable from other toxic psychoses or schizophrenia, except by association. Several chronic effects of LSD use also have been noted. A "flashback" phenomenon has been described, where the visual effects previously experienced with LSD use return long after drug use has ceased. This effect often is attributed to underlying psychiatric pathology. Also, an increased incidence of chromosomal abnormalities has been reported is association with LSD use. While this increase is real, it does not appear to be more significant than those associated with the use of other hallucinogenic agents. One must conclude that use of all these agents is associated with potential mutagenic effects.

The initial management strategy should concentrate on airway, breathing, and circulation, followed by the life threats—agitation, seizures, and hyperpyrexia. Cooling, sedation, and volume resuscitation usually will suffice. (Details of this approach are given in "General Management.")

MORNING GLORY

The seeds of the morning glory, and other members of the *Convolvulaceae* family, contain mind-altering alkaloids (e.g., D-lysergic acid amide) similar to those found in ergots. While not all morning glory seeds contain these alkaloids, those of *Ipomoea violacea* (also known as *Ipomoea rubrocaerulea*) are perhaps the most well known. *Rivea corymbosa* (known as *Ololiuqui*) is a similar plant that also contains these toxins.

The clinical effects and their management are identical to those seen with LSD. As many as 200 seeds may be required to produce effects similar to 200 μg of LSD. Most symptoms would be expected to resolve within 8 to 10 h.

MESCALINE

Mescaline is obtained from the top ("button") of the peyote cactus (*Lophophora williamsii*). Like many other naturally occurring hallucinogens, mescaline is found in combination with at least 15 other active alkaloids. Although the chemical structure of mescaline is similar to the hallucinogenic amphetamines, it probably acts by altering dopamine and serotonin transmission, similar to psilocybin and the hallucinogenic indoles.

Six to twelve buttons (270 to 540 mg) are required to produce hallucinogenic effects. Nausea, vomiting, blurred vision (from mydriasis), and mild hypertension and tachycardia are present at these doses. Respiratory depression, hypotension, and bradycardia may result from greater ingestions (20 to 60 mg/kg). Symptoms usually progress from nausea and vomiting, which begin within minutes and subside by 2 h postingestion to hallucinations, which peak at 2 h and last for 6 to 12 h. Mescaline has been used as part of religious ceremonies, and it is reported that intoxicated individuals have the ability to transcend space and time. Pronounced tactile, visual, olfactory, auditory, and gustatory hallucinations have all been described.

Similar to intoxications with other hallucinogenic agents, most patients intoxicated with mescaline will not come to medical attention. Many of those that do present to the emergency department will require rest and gentle assurance alone. Gastrointestinal decontamination is of little importance because of the predictable vomiting and rapid absorption. Intravenous hydration and gentle sedation may be indicated when a severe agitated delirium is present (see "General Management"). The sedative of choice is a benzodiazepine—phenothiazines may be associated with an increased risk of flashback phenomenon. Although patients rarely require admission, they may have to remain in the emergency department for several hours until they are stable for discharge.

MUSHROOMS

Hallucinogenic mushrooms fall into one of two categories: those that contain (1) psilocybin or (2) ibotenic acid. Within each category are a variety of genera, many of which commonly grow in the United States. Since mushrooms of different genera often contain the same toxins, while members of the same genus may not, novice mushroom hunters cannot use a characteristic physical attribute (associated with a known hallucinogenic mushroom) to predict reliably the toxicity of a given mushroom. Although excellent references (Linkoff) are available to assist with mushroom identification, the physician should concentrate on clinical scenarios because a sample of the ingested mushrooms rarely is available on presentation.

Psilocybin-containing mushrooms usually belong to the *Psilocybe, Panaeolus,* or *Gymnophilus* genera, which can be found throughout the Pacific Northwest, Texas, Florida and Hawaii. Also known as "magic mushrooms," their use (especially in religious ceremonies) dates back to ancient Aztec times. While many compounds have been isolated from these mushrooms, psilocybin and psilocin are felt to be the active ingredients. These agents are similar in structure to serotonin, and like LSD, they probably produce their effects through modification of serotoninergic transmission.

Psilocybin mushrooms are eaten raw, brewed in a soup or tea, or dried for later use. Intravenous injection of a mushroom extract, although rare, produces more pronounced toxicity. The dose of mushroom required to produce symptoms is quite variable and may depend both on the individual and the potency of the mushrooms. This may also be modified by the presence of food in the gastrointestinal tract. Within 5 to 30 min of ingestion, most patients will note gastrointestinal discomfort. Nausea is common, and vomiting will occur in up to 20 percent of ingestions. While mydriasis is common, other sympathomimetic effects (hypertension and tachycardia) are usually mild if present at all. Hallucinations are indistinguishable in form or content from those induced from mescaline or LSD, and last from 4 to no more than 12 h. Although coma, seizures, and hyperthermia have been reported, they seem to be infrequent findings and seem to be associated with relative dose and body size. Thus, children appear to be more susceptible to these events.

Mushrooms that contain the toxin, ibotenic acid, and its metabolite, muscimol, almost exclusively belong to the genus *Amanita*, examples being the *A. muscaria* and *A. pantherina* species. Ibotenic acid and muscimol are isoxazole compounds that are known to cause distorted visual perception or illusions rather than true formed hallucinations. These toxins appear to act either by modifying γ-aminobutyric acid (GABA), glutamate, or serotonin function. The name "muscimol" has caused some confusion because of its similarity with muscarine. One should note, however, that neither muscarinic nor antimuscarinic (anticholinergic) symptoms are produced characteristically after ingestion of these agents.

The onset of symptoms is quite rapid, with patients describing dizziness, headache, and ataxia within 0.5 to 1.5 h of ingestion. Ingestion of ibotenic-acid-containing mushrooms rarely is associated with gastrointestinal distress, which may help distinguish these from psilocybin ingestions. Symptoms peak by 2 to 4 h, with the addition of visual illusions, muscle twitching, and seizures in the more severe intoxications. The total duration of effect is 6 to 12 h, although rarely, symptoms lasting up to 48 h have been described.

Patients who present to the emergency department have either accidentally ingested these mushrooms or are generally the sicker patients with intentional ingestions. Treatment is largely supportive. Anticonvulsants or sedatives may be required, as dictated by the clinical presentation (see ''General Management'') Both atropine and physostigmine are contraindicated as they may exacerbate toxicity.

NUTMEG

Nutmeg, produced from the evergreen tree *Myristica fragrans,* has a long history of use in foods and herbal remedies. While the spice contains many volatile oils, myristicin is the major component. Pure myristicin cannot produce all the clinical manifestations of nutmeg poisoning. Many of the symptoms can be attributed either to 3, methoxy–4,5–methylenedioxyamphetamine (a myristicin metabolite), or to 3,4,5–trimethoxyamphetamine (a metabolite of *p*-methoxyamphetamine, which is also found in nutmeg). Both of these compounds are hallucinogenic amphetamine derivatives.

About 10 to 50 g of fresh nutmeg (two to nine whole nutmegs) are required to produce symptoms; grinding and drying may reduce toxicity through loss of essential oils.

Within 3 to 6 h after ingestion, patients will notice the onset of nausea, vomiting, and abdominal pain. Cold extremities with weak pulses and shallow respirations may accompany periods of lethargy, delirium, agitation, and hallucinations. Mixed pupillary and skin findings have been described, with neither a true sympathomimetic nor an anticholinergic state predominating. Symptoms usually resolve within 24 h with supportive care alone.

DESIGNER AMPHETAMINES

The term ''designer drug'' refers to a chemical modification of an existing compound that is designed to produce desirable effects while simultaneously circumventing legal restrictions. Until the 1986 Controlled Substances Act was enacted, every new congener of an existing illicit substance had to be ruled on individually. Thus by causing minor chemical alterations, illicit substances temporarily were made legal. While many designer drugs were made in clandestine laboratories, some were the result of legitimate pharmaceutical endeavors. This section only discusses those drugs with amphetamine-like properties, known as designer amphetamines, or more correctly, phenylethylamine derivatives.

The phenylethylamine molecule is the fundamental building block for endogenous and exogenous catecholamines, mescaline, and amphetamine. Modifications of this structure lead to the varying effects on α- and β-adrenergic, dopaminergic, and serotonergic receptors that give individual compounds their specific activities. These compounds either are known by the initials that represent their chemical structures (MDA for methylenedioxyamphetamine) or common names such as ''Adam,'' ''Eve,'' and ''ecstasy.''

Recent attention has been drawn to the compound ecstasy (also called MDMA or 3,4-methylenedioxymethamphetamine) because of its ability to damage serotonergic neurons in experimental animals. Similar effects had been described previously with MDA. The conclusion from both reports appears to indicate that repeated stimulation of serotonergic neurons with chronic drug administration ultimately results in neuron loss and permanent dysfunction.

The clinical effects associated with the use of designer amphetamines are both drug specific and dose dependent. Each agent possesses varying degrees of hallucinogenic and psychomotor effects. Durations of effect range from several hours to 1 to 2 days, depending on the agent and dose ingested. The relative effects of some of these agents have been reviewed extensively by Buchanan and Simpson.

Patients who ingest agents with nonspecific adrenergic and serotonergic effects present with severe psychomotor agitation and generally have other signs of catecholamine excess (sympathomimetic presentations). In contrast, patients who ingest agents with predominantly serotonergic effects present with disorders of thought process and content and usually have limited psychomotor agitation. The complications produced are similar to those associated with amphetamine overdose and include hypertension, hyperpyrexia, seizures, rhabdomyolysis, disseminated intravascular coagulation, adult respiratory distress syndrome, and death. Management is generally supportive, with efforts directed at cooling, sedation, volume resuscitation, and decontamination. (See ''General Management.'')

ANTICHOLINERGICS

Although the blurred vision, dry mouth, and urinary retention associated with anticholinergic intoxications usually are uncomfortable enough to deter their use, a variety of agents have been abused for their potentially hallucinogenic properties. Among these agents jimson weed (*Datura stramonium*) is the most well known. The plant is described as a stout weed found throughout the continental United States, that stands 3 to 4 ft high, and is recognized by its characteristic prickly fruits which contain numerous seeds. While the entire plant contains the toxic alkaloids atropine and scopolamine, the highest concentrations are located in the seeds.

Intoxication is usually achieved by chewing the seeds or leaves or brewing them in a tea. The typical patient is an adolescent or a young adult who presents with hallucinations and a classic anticholinergic syndrome. Severe intoxications may present with significant psychomotor agitation, hyperpyrexia, and seizures requiring pharmacologic therapy. Physostigmine may be useful as an adjunct in these cases. Patients with less significant toxicity may be managed conservatively.

MARIJUANA

Marijuana is the name commonly used to describe the dried flowers and leaves of the plant *Cannabis sativa*. Both marijuana and hashish (the dried resin of the plant) contain the toxin delta,9–tetrahydrocannabinol (THC), whose medicinal qualities were recognized in China more than 4000 years ago. Even today, THC-containing products are available as antiemetics and are being investigated for the treatment of glaucoma and chronic pain syndromes.

The most recent statistics suggest that marijuana is the most commonly used illicit substance, surpassed only by ethanol and tobacco. As such, intoxication is often seen in combination with other agents. For example, marijuana cigarettes routinely are used as vehicles for the delivery of PCP.

While smoking is the preferred route of administration, ingestion and intravenous use also have been described, the latter with catastrophic sequelae. THC levels peak about 7 to 8 min after inhalation and about 45 min after ingestion. Clinical effects, however, lag behind serum levels, with maximal intoxication seen 20 to 30 min after inhalation and as late as 2 to 3 h after ingestion. Intoxication will last 2 to 6 h, depending on dose and route of administration. These and other pharmacokinetic parameters have been reviewed in depth by Seldon.

The exact mechanism of action of THC is unknown. In order to explain marijuana's effects, investigators have postulated the existence of specific THC receptors, nonspecific effects on cell membranes (like the general anesthetics), and interactions with serotonergic, dopaminergic, noradrenergic, and GABA systems. Although the exact mechanism has not been elucidated, the clinical effects are well known. Patients experience a variety of perceptual alterations including mild stimulation, euphoria, and an increased sense of well being, depersonalization, dysphoria, hallucinations, and paranoia. At higher doses, sedation is common. Other effects include conjunctival irritation, dry mouth, hunger (especially for sweets), mild tachycardia, and unsteady gait. The most reliable indicators of acute marijuana intoxication seem to be the unsteady gait and conjunctival injection. Chronic use of marijuana has been reported to have adverse effects on the endocrine, pulmonary, reproductive, and immune systems and is also associated with cognitive dysfunction.

Intoxication with marijuana, as with other hallucinogens, rarely requires acute medical intervention. The patient who presents to the emergency department can be expected to be the uncommon individual with accidental poisoning or one who has suffered from paranoid ideations or associated trauma. Most of these patients can be managed conservatively with hydration and gentle sedation, if indicated. Chronic effects and long-term complications may be addressed through outpatient referral.

DIAGNOSIS

The diagnosis of hallucinogen intoxication may be determined largely from the history and physical examination. Clues to the identification of specific toxins should include: the predominance of sympathomimetic or anticholinergic symptoms, the pupil size and conjunctival appearance, the presence and character of nystagmus, and the association of gastrointestinal symptoms. Although subtle differences may exist in the clinical presentation, the emergency physician should realize that the diagnosis of a specific toxin rarely is required. The exception to this statement should be the identification of a pure anticholinergic poisoning, because of the availability of an antidote (physostigmine). Recognition that mydriasis, dry flushed skin, tachycardia, absent bowel sounds, urinary retention, hyperpyrexia, and central nervous system agitation constitute the anticholinergic toxic syndrome is required.

General toxicologic screening has a limited role in the evaluation of hallucinogen toxicity. While many agents (such as THC and PCP) routinely are screened, others (such as the congeners of PCP and designer amphetamines) can be detected only with sophisticated, expensive techniques. Furthermore, it should be noted that since THC, for example, may be detected in the urine weeks after the last exposure, a positive toxicology screen cannot be used to confirm an acute intoxication with certainty in a habitual user. All that may be concluded from such a result is that the patient was exposed to marijuana within the last several weeks. Routine urine toxicology screening should be discouraged (except for educational or medicolegal reasons) since management rarely is altered by the results, and the tests are expensive and time consuming.

GENERAL MANAGEMENT STRATEGY

The general approach to the patient with suspected hallucinogen intoxication must begin by addressing life-threatening events. After stability of the airway, breathing, and circulation have been assured, the emergency physician should consider the different diagnosis and those manifestations that are most associated with patient morbidity. Meningitis should be suspected in all patients with altered mental status and fever. Prophylactic antibiotics or lumbar puncture is required.

Severe psychomotor agitation is the next most obvious threat. The agitated patient may do physical harm, both to himself and to medical personnel. While physical restraints are indicated, when the patient fights against restraints, the risk for hyperpyrexia and rhabdomyolysis is increased. Thus physical restraints should be used for protection until chemical restraint can be achieved. Intravenous access should be established for hydration and administration of medications, and substrates such as oxygen, glucose, and thiamine should be given.

Controversy exists over the best method of achieving chemical restraint. While the animal literature may assist with theoretically optimal choices for known agents, sound human data are lacking. Patients often abuse substances in combination, and, in any given patient, the choice of agents must be safe and effective not only in treating the suspected toxin, but also in treating the other etiologies included in the differential diagnosis. Popular choices include the use of benzodiazepines (diazepam, lorazepam, or midazolam) and butyrophenones (haloperidol). Benzodiazepines offer several distinct advantages. In most animal models, they are safe and effective. They increase the seizure threshold and are cross-tolerant with sedative hypnotics (that is, they will treat alcohol withdrawal). Butyrophenones may decrease the seizure threshold and can interfere with heat dissipation through their anticholinergic effects. In general, incremental doses of parenteral benzodiazepines should be given with the end point of gentle sedation.

Rapid cooling is indicated when temperatures approach 41°C (105.8°F). Patients should be undressed completely and cooled with a mist of water and a high-velocity fan. Alternatively, ice baths may be used. These techniques may require additional sedation or neuromuscular paralysis as adjunctive therapy. There is no proven role for dantrolene or acetaminophen, and salicylates, phenothiazines, and alcohol baths should be avoided because they may compound the toxicity.

Aggressive gastrointestinal decontamination has a limited role in hallucinogen intoxication but can be used when coingestions are suspected. Orally administered activated charcoal, alone or with a cathartic, usually will suffice. Forced diuresis, acid or alkaline diuresis, hemodialysis, and hemoperfusion have no proven clinical utility with intoxication from any of these agents. Although continual nasogastric suction may be useful in severe PCP intoxication, multiple doses of activated charcoal should achieve similar results without the associated risk of fluid and electrolyte abnormalities. Standard therapy for seizures and rhabdomyolysis should be instituted. When a clear anticholinergic poisoning is present, physostigmine can be administered with great caution.

DISPOSITION

Hospital admission rarely is required for the patient with acute hallucinogen intoxication. The decision to admit should be based largely on clinical grounds. Most patients who present to the hospital will have mild-to-moderate degrees of psychomotor agitation that resolve over brief periods of time or with gentle sedation. As delayed toxicity is not expected in this group of patients, hospitalization is not required. Patients should be admitted, however, if intoxication is accompanied by severe psychomotor agitation, such that either seizures, hyperpyrexia, rhabdomyolysis, or renal dysfunction is present. Other less common manifestations (such as cardiovascular instability) also warrant hospitalization for prolonged observation. A referral for drug-abuse counseling should be available on discharge either from the emergency department or an inpatient service.

BIBLIOGRAPHY

Aaron CK: Lysergic acid diethylamide and other psychedelics, in Goldfrank LR, Flomenbaum NE, Lewin NA, et al (eds): *Goldfrank's Toxicologic Emergencies,* 4th ed. Norwalk, Appleton & Lange, 1990, pp 523–527.

Abraham HD: Visual phenomenology of the LSD flash. *Arch Gen Psychiatry* 40:884, 1983.

Ammirati JF, Traquair JA, Horgan PA: Poisonous Mushrooms of the Northern United States and Canada. Minneapolis, University of Minnesota Press, 1985.

Baldridge EB, Bessen HA: Phencyclidine. *Emerg Med Clin North Am* 8:541, 1990.

Buchanan JF, Brown CR: Designer drugs: A problem in clinical toxicology. *Med Toxicol* 3:1, 1988.

Caldwell J, Sever PS: The biochemical pharmacology of abused drugs: Amphetamines, cocaine and LSD. *Clin Pharmacol Ther* 16:625, 1974.

Curry SC, Rose MC: Intravenous mushroom poisoning. *Ann Emerg Med* 14:900, 1985.

Ellenhorn MJ, Barceloux DG (eds): Phencyclidine, in *Medical Toxicology—Diagnosis and Treatment of Human Poisoning.* New York, Elsevier, 1988, pp. 764–777.

Ellenhorn MJ, Barceloux DG (eds): Plants, mycotoxins, mushrooms, in *Medical Toxicology—Diagnosis and Treatment of Human Poisoning.* New York, Elsevier, 1988, pp. 1209–1352.

Gaddum JH: Antagonism between lysergic acid diethylamide and 5–hydroxytryptamine. *J Physiol* 121:15, 1953.

Glennon RA, Young R: MDA: An agent that produces stimulus effects similar to those of 3,4–DMA, LSD, and cocaine. *Eur J Pharmacol* 99:249, 1984.

Green RC: Nutmeg poisoning. *JAMA* 171:1342, 1959.

Ingram AL: Morning glory seed reaction. *JAMA* 190:107, 1964.

Kapadia GJ, Fayez BNBE: Peyote constituents: Chemistry, biogenesis, and biological effects. *J Pharmacol Sci* 59:1699, 1970.

Klein-Schwartz W, Oderda GM: Jimsonweed intoxication in adolescents and young adults. *Am J Dis Child* 38:737, 1984.

Kuhn DM, White FJ, Appel JB: The discriminative stimulus properties of LSD: Mechanisms of action. *Neuropharmacology* 17:257, 1978.

Lampe KF, McCann MA (eds): *AMA Handbook of Poisonous and Injurious Plants*. Chicago, American Medical Association, 1985, pp. 70–72.

Lincoff GH, Knopf AA: The Audubon Society Field Guide to North American Mushrooms. New York, Chanticleer, 1988.

Litovitz TL, Schmitz BF, Holm KC: 1988 Annual Report of American Association of Poison Control Centers National Data Collection System. *Am J Emerg Med* 7:495, 1989.

Lyles A: LSD: A review. *Pharmacol Alert* 11:1, 1979.

Mace S: LSD. *Clin Toxicol* 15:219, 1979.

McCormick DJ, Avbel AJ, Gibbons RC: Nonlethal mushroom poisoning. *Ann Intern Med* 90:332, 1979.

National Institute on Drug Abuse: National household survey on drug abuse: Population estimates 1988. Washington, DC, US Government Printing Office. DHHS Publication No. (ADM) 89–1636, 1989.

Nutmeg, in *The Lawrence Review of Natural Products*. Levittown, PA, Pharmaceutical Information Associates, September 1987.

O'Grady TC, Brown J, Jacamo J: Outbreak of jimson weed abuse among Marine Corps personnel at Camp Pendleton. *Military Med* 148:732, 1983.

Ohlsson A, Lindgren LE, Wahlen A, et al: Plasma delta–9–tetrahydrocannabinol concentrations and clinical effects after oral and intravenous administration and smoking. *Clin Pharmacol Ther* 28:409, 1980.

Payne RB: Nutmeg intoxication. *N Engl J Med* 269:36, 1973.

Payne RJ, Brand SS: The toxicity of intravenously used marijuana. *JAMA* 223:351, 1975.

Ricaurte G, Bryan G, Straus L, et al: Hallucinogenic amphetamine selectively destroys brain serotonin nerve terminals. *Science* 229:986, 1985.

Ricaurte GA, Forrno LS, Wilson MA, et al: (±) 3,4–Methylenedioxymethamphetamine selectively damages central serotonergic neurons in nonhuman primates. *JAMA* 260:51, 1988.

Saidel DR, Babineau R: Prolonged LSD flashbacks as conversion reactions. *J Nerv Ment Dis* 162:352, 1976.

Selden BS, Clark RF, Curry SC: Marijuana. *Emerg Med Clin North Am* 8:527, 1990.

Simpson DL, Rumack BH: Methylenedioxyamphetamine: Clinical description of overdose, death, and review of pharmacology. *Arch Intern Med* 141:1507, 1981.

Smith JA, Walters G, Johnston D: LSD "flashbacks" as a cause of diagnostic error. *Postgrad Med J* 56:421, 1980.

Spoerke DG, Hall AH: Plants and mushrooms of abuse. *Emerg Med Clin North Am* 8:579, 1990.

100 SALICYLATES

Steven C. Curry

Salicylates are available in both prescription and over-the-counter preparations in many forms, usually as acetylsalicylic acid (aspirin). Oil of wintergreen (methyl salicylate) is an extremely toxic form of salicylate. Sodium salicylate is used as a kerotolytic agent. Many combination analgesics such as Darvon Compound, Percodan, and Fiorinal also contain significant amounts of salicylates.

PATHOPHYSIOLOGY AND CLINICAL FINDINGS

General and Metabolic

Acute ingestions of salicylates are frequently accompanied by gastroenteritis from direct irritation to the gastrointestinal (GI) tract. Rare reports of gastric perforation continue to appear. Upper GI bleeding is frequent, and severe and persistent vomiting can be difficult to control. Renal failure has been rarely reported as a consequence of acute poisoning.

A mixed respiratory alkalosis and metabolic acidosis is usually seen in salicylate poisoning. Salicylate directly stimulates respiratory centers in the brainstem, resulting in respiratory alkalosis. Very high levels of salicylate depress respirations.

Salicylate enhances lipolysis, uncouples oxidative phosphorylation, and inhibits various enzymes involved in energy production and amino acid metabolism. Because oxidative phosphorylation is a major buffer of hydrogen ions, impairment of oxidative phosphorylation by salicylate results in metabolic acidosis. Ketoacids are frequently elevated due to enhanced lypolysis. Elevated circulating lactate concentrations in a minority of patients reflect increased glycolytic activity. The accumulation of other intermediate acids involved in energy metabolism has been suggested to contribute to metabolic acidosis.

Salicylate causes mobilization of glycogen stores, resulting in hyperglycemia. However, salicylate is also a potent inhibitor of gluconeogenesis. Therefore, normoglycemia, hyperglycemia, or hypoglycemia may be noted in salicylate poisoning. Children are more likely than adults to develop hypoglycemia.

Central Nervous System

Confusion, lethargy, convulsions, respiratory arrest, coma, and brain death can all be seen in severe poisoning. Decreased ATP production from uncoupling of oxidative phosphorylation results in acute brain failure and cerebral edema. CSF glucose concentrations can be very low compared with serum glucose levels, and can mimic those of bacterial meningitis. Patients who die from salicylate poisoning in spite of intensive supportive care frequently die a cerebral death. Even patients who die in refractory shock have developed serious neurotoxicity prior to the onset of shock.

Cardiovascular

Cardiac toxicity is due to impaired ATP production, acidosis, electrolyte abnormalities, and, occasionally, significant hyperthermia. Heart failure can occur but is usually not a major problem, except in those near death or in those with preexistent heart disease. Cardiac arrhythmias, including ventricular premature beats, ventricular tachycardia, and ventricular fibrillation, are possible.

Pulmonary

Pulmonary edema can be a major cause of morbidity. Most pulmonary edema is noncardiogenic (adult respiratory distress syndrome), and ARDS complicating acute overdoses is more common in adults than in children. However, overaggressive attempts at a forced diuresis in the treatment of salicylate poisoning can result in hydrostatic pulmonary edema from fluid overload, especially in the elderly with marginal cardiac reserve. Children with inappropriate secretion of antidiuretic hormone are also predisposed to fluid overload and pulmonary edema. In contrast to acute poisoning, in which pulmonary edema is not frequent, chronic salicylate poisoning often results in ARDS.

TOXIC DOSES AND SALICYLATE LEVELS

Some understanding of the absorption, distribution, metabolism, and excretion of salicylate is needed in order to interpret serum salicylate levels appropriately and hence provide optimum care of the patient.

Within a few minutes after absorption, acetylsalicylic acid is converted to salicylate. After ingestion of large amounts of aspirin, peak serum salicylate levels may not be reached for 18 to 24 h, although toxic levels are usually seen within 6 h. A concentration of salicylate that allows continued absorption may form in the stomach. Methyl salicylate, being a liquid, produces peak levels earlier. On the other hand, toxic levels may not be reached for hours after the ingestion of enteric-coated aspirin.

At therapeutic levels, salicylate is mainly cleared by hepatic metabolism. Even at upper therapeutic levels, hepatic enzymes are saturated, leading to zero-order elimination kinetics. In zero-order kinetics, a set amount of the drug is metabolized per unit time, regardless of plasma levels of the drug. This allows accumulation of salicylate and a prolonged elimination of salicylate from the body.

At toxic levels, renal excretion becomes a major route of elimination. Un-ionized salicylate is reabsorbed by the renal tubules, prolonging elimination. Alkaline urine favors the formation of ionized salicylate, which cannot be reabsorbed and is excreted in the urine. Because of zero-order kinetics, dehydration, and acidic urine, days may be required for salicylate levels to decrease by half in untreated patients suffering from salicylate poisoning.

After absorption, salicylate distributes throughout body tissues. At higher salicylate concentrations, a lesser percentage of the drug is protein-bound. As a metabolic acidosis develops, a greater percentage of the free drug is un-ionized and is able to move into tissue. In fact, a drop in pH from 7.4 to 7.2 almost *doubles* the amount of un-ionized drug which is able to diffuse out of the plasma. The decreased protein binding and increased un-ionized fraction of the drug at lower pHs cause a change in the volume of distribution (V_d) of salicylate. Depending on various factors, the V_d can vary over twofold from 0.15 to 0.35 L/kg. Those suffering from chronic salicylate toxicity have large V_d's.

It is this changing V_d that makes it difficult to interpret serum salicylate levels. Because patients can have different V_d's, patients can have tremendous differences in total body burdens (and tissue levels) of salicylate while having the same serum salicylate concentrations. When elevated serum salicylate levels are decreasing in a patient, they can be decreasing not only from metabolism and renal excretion, but also because salicylate is leaving blood, moving into tissues, and causing more toxicity as the V_d increases. It is for these reasons that it is more important to treat the patient than the serum salicylate level. This is especially important in chronic salicylate toxicity, in which severe toxicity may be demonstrated at serum levels that would produce minimal symptoms in acute poisoning.

The acute aspirin ingestion of 150 mg/kg or less is not expected to produce significant toxicity other than, perhaps, vomiting from a gastrointestinal irritation. Acute aspirin ingestions of 150 to 300 mg/kg produce mild to moderate toxicity with hyperpnea, vomiting, diaphoresis, tinnitus, and acid/base disturbances. The ingestion of greater than 300 mg/kg can produce moderate to severe toxicity. If aspirin has been taken within the last 24 h, potential toxicity of an acutely ingested dose is worse.

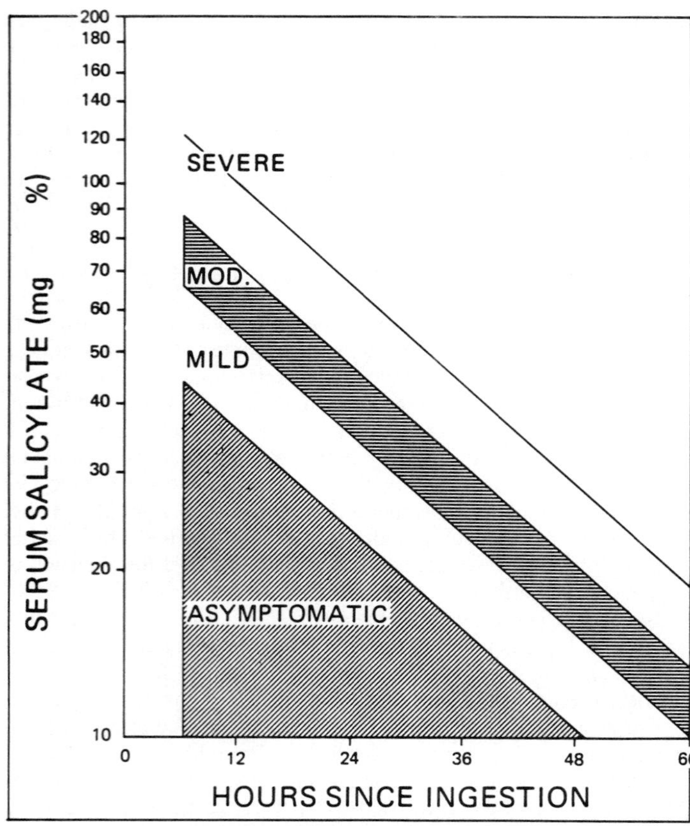

Fig. 100-1. The Done nomogram can be used to assist in determining the likelihood of toxicity. It can only be used after a single, acute ingestion of aspirin in which no salicylate has been taken previously in the last 24 h. Nontoxic levels drawn before 6 h cannot be used to determine degree of toxicity. This nomogram cannot be used in chronic salicylate poisoning or after the ingestion of enteric-coated aspirin. (From Done AK: Salicylate intoxication: Significance of salicylate in blood in cases of acute ingestion. *Pediatrics* 26:800, 1960. Used by permission)

The Done nomogram can be used to *assist* in predicting the degree of toxicity after an *acute, single* ingestion of aspirin in a patient who has not been taking salicylate recently (Fig. 100-1). A serum level should not be plotted on the nomogram unless it was drawn at least 6 h after ingestion. Nontoxic levels drawn before 6 h do not rule out impending toxicity. Symptomatic patients should be treated regardless of where they fall on the Done nomogram. The Done nomogram *cannot* be used in the following instances:

1. In acute ingestions when salicylate has been taken previously within the last 24 h
2. In acute overdoses when salicylate was ingested over several hours
3. In chronic salicylate poisoning
4. After ingestion of enteric-coated aspirin tablets

Chronic salicylate toxicity is the result of excessive therapeutic administration over a period of 12 h or longer. Defining doses that lead to chronic toxicity is difficult. For example, if a patient is dehydrated from an illness, and renal excretion of salicylate has decreased, the drug may accumulate and cause chronic toxicity in doses that otherwise would not cause problems. On the other hand, the chronic ingestion of excessive salicylate doses will cause toxicity in any otherwise healthy person. As discussed below, chronic salicylate poisoning is better described as a syndrome than as a particular dose over a particular period of time.

ACUTE VERSUS CHRONIC POISONING

Acute and chronic salicylate poisoning have several distinct characteristics. The adult patient with acute salicylate toxicity usually presents with vomiting (sometimes hematemesis), abdominal pain, hyperventilation, diaphoresis, dehydration, alkalemia, ketonuria, and a respiratory alkalosis with metabolic acidosis. As the poisoning progresses, acidemia, lethargy, cardiovascular abnormalities, coagulation disorders, hyperthermia, and serious neurotoxicity develop. Pulmonary edema can occur but is not common. As noted earlier, children frequently present with acidemia. In acute poisoning, serum salicylate levels correlate fairly well with the degree of toxicity, which is the basis for the Done nomogram described above.

In contrast to acute poisoning, patients with chronic salicylate toxicity usually do not have significant gastroenteritis, although dehydration can be severe. They are usually brought in by family members because of changes in mentation, including lethargy, disorientation, and hallucinations. Even adults are frequently, but not always, acidemic on presentation. ARDS is common in chronic toxicity. Because patients with chronic toxicity have a large V_d, they present with more serious toxicity at a given serum salicylate concentration compared with an acutely poisoned patient. An elevated prothrombin time is frequently present. Elevated levels of liver enzymes are present in some patients chronically using salicylates, even if chronic toxicity is not present.

Chronic salicylate toxicity must be considered in any patient with unexplained CNS dysfunction, especially in the presence of a mixed acid/base disturbance. Studies have shown that about 50 percent of patients with chronic salicylate toxicity are incorrectly diagnosed at the time of hospital admission. Patients taking carbonic anhydrase inhibitors can develop chronic toxicity while using relatively low doses of salicylates because the carbonic anhydrase inhibitor alkalinizes CSF and acidifies blood, raising the V_d of salicylate and concentrating salicylate in the CNS. The most important point to remember is that, because of a large V_d, *a patient suffering from chronic salicylate toxicity can have a therapeutic serum salicylate concentration.*

The contrast between chronic and acute poisoning is not always clear. The longer one waits after an acute ingestion, the more a patient behaves like a chronically intoxicated one. In a severely, acutely poisoned patient many hours after aspirin ingestion, CNS changes, acidemia, elevated prothrombin time, and significant toxicity in the face of decreasing or normal salicylate levels are signs that are exactly the same as those in a chronically poisoned patient. In these patients it is important to remember to treat the patient and not the serum salicylate level or degree of toxicity as determined by the nomogram.

TREATMENT

GI Decontamination

The administration of activated charcoal alone appears to be superior to induction of vomiting with ipecac. One gram per kilogram of body weight of activated charcoal should be administered to patients who have ingested potentially toxic amounts of salicylate. Cathartics have not been beneficial in animal models of nonenteric-coated salicylate poisoning. There is controversy as to whether repeat doses of activated charcoal enhance salicylate elimination. Persistent and severe vomiting is not unusual in the acutely poisoned patient and frequently limits the use of activated charcoal.

If the serum salicylate level drawn 6 h after ingestion falls in the asymptomatic portion of the Done nomogram, the patient has minimal or no symptoms, and a repeat serum salicylate determination shows that levels are falling, then the patient can be discharged. Patients whose serum salicylate levels are in the mild range can be discharged if they have minimal symptoms, if nausea and vomiting have resolved, and if adequate follow-up can be provided. If nausea and vomiting persist, dehydration may prevent adequate elimination of salicylate and result in worsening toxicity. All other patients should be admitted to the hospital.

The acute ingestion of enteric-coated salicylate deserves special mention. Enteric coating allows a delayed and slower absorption of aspirin. There have been several reports of patients who have ingested toxic amounts of enteric-coated aspirin tablets and have been asymptomatic with nontoxic salicylate levels 6 h after ingestion. These patients then returned hours later with severe toxicity and elevated salicylate levels. Considering the inaccurate histories that frequently accompany overdose victims, anyone who has ingested over 150 mg of enteric-coated aspirin per kilogram should be admitted for observation and serial serum salicylate levels. Adequate follow-up should be ensured for all those who are discharged from the emergency department.

Laboratory Work

In symptomatic patients, blood should immediately be drawn for determination of serum levels of electrolytes, glucose, BUN, creatinine, and salicylate; prothrombin time; and hemoglobin/hematocrit. Arterial blood gases should be measured to determine the type and degree of acid/base imbalance. The differential diagnosis of salicylate poisoning includes theophylline toxicity, caffeine overdose, acute iron poisoning, Reye's syndrome, diabetic ketoacidosis, sepsis, and meningitis. Phenistix, a urine dipstick, used to test for phenylketonuria, detects moderate to large concentrations of salicylate in the urine.

Intravenous Fluids and Urine Alkalinization

Almost all symptomatic patients with salicylate poisoning are dehydrated. Appropriate fluid challenges using saline or colloids should be given rapidly to replenish intravascular volume and produce adequate urine flow. All patients with CNS depression or seizures should be presumed to be hypoglycemic and should receive 50% glucose intravenously if bedside determination of serum glucose is not readily available. After adequate hydration, intravenous fluids should include adequate amounts of sodium and potassium to replenish depleted body stores. Children should never receive plain 5% dextrose in water as an intravenous fluid.

All efforts should be made to keep arterial pH 7.4 or greater. Even the slightest fall in arterial pH results in a greater concentration of unionized salicylate, which can move into tissues to produce worsening of toxicity. The alkalinization of urine is performed to enhance urinary excretion of salicylate.

One excellent study by Prescott et al., has shown that an alkaline urine is more important than a diuresis in enhancing salicylate excretion. However, in the patient who appears to be able to handle a fluid load well, a urine output above normal is desirable. If only maintenance intravenous rates will be used, then 10% glucose should be present in the infusions.

Both bicarbonate *and* potassium are needed to produce an alkaline urine. Even if arterial pH is 7.5, alkaline urine will not be produced if, when reabsorbing sodium, the kidney is preferentially secreting hydrogen ions into the tubular lumen rather than potassium ions. Arterial blood gases, serum electrolytes, and urine pH should be monitored at least every 2 to 4 h in the severely ill patient. This is especially important in preventing hyperkalemia from the administration of large amounts of potassium, and in preventing a fall in arterial pH.

The method I use in producing an alkaline diuresis is to hydrate the patient with normal saline until a good urine output is obtained. Sodium bicarbonate as 1 mEq/kg is given intravenously in boluses until arterial pH is at least 7.5. A continuous intravenous infusion of 1 L 5% dextrose in water to which is added 50 to 100 mmol sodium bicarbonate and 40 mmol potassium chloride is started at three times the maintenance rate. Monitoring of urine pH, serum electrolyte levels, and arterial blood gases at least every 2 to 4 h is performed to fine-tune the infusion, to detect hyperkalemia or hypokalemia, and to detect hyponatremia. Tremendous doses of potassium may be required along with bicarbonate to produce an alkaline urine. If the blood is alkaline, if the serum potassium level is normal, and if the urine is acidic, more potassium is needed. In my experience, it may be necessary to administer as much as 110 mEq of potassium every 4 h to an adult to maintain an alkaline urine. Boluses of sodium bicarbonate are given to keep arterial pH above 7.4. Furosemide can be given if evidence of fluid overload develops, or if urine output does not approach the rate of intravenous infusion in spite of adequate hydration. Serum salicylate levels should be determined every few hours until they are known to be consistently falling.

The use of carbonic anhydrase inhibitors (e.g., acetazolamide) is mentioned only to be condemned. Although acetazolamide alkalinizes urine, it also alkalinizes CSF, trapping salicylate in the CNS. Acetazolamide dramatically increases mortality in animal models of salicylate toxicity.

Dialysis

Hemodialysis greatly enhances the clearance of salicylate from the body. It also has the advantage of correcting fluid and electrolyte abnormalities at the same time. Hemodialysis is indicated in the following cases:

1. In the patient who is deteriorating in spite of supportive care and an alkaline diuresis
2. In the patient who is deteriorating and in whom an alkaline urine cannot be successfully produced (e.g., acidic urine in spite of alkalemic blood and hyperkalemia)
3. In the patient with renal failure
4. In the comatose patient or in one with severe cardiac toxicity
5. In the patient with ARDS in whom the salicylate levels are not rapidly falling

Peritoneal dialysis is not nearly as effective as hemodialysis and should not be used if hemodialysis is available. If peritoneal dialysis is used, the dialysate should contain 5% albumin to enhance salicylate clearance through protein binding.

Neurotoxicity

Except in severe cases, coma usually does not develop after acute ingestions. CNS depression is common in those with chronic toxicity. Seizures should be treated with standard anticonvulsants. Patients receiving intensive support care who go on to die from acute salicylate poisoning frequently die a cerebral death. Shock is usually preceded by serious neurotoxicity. Animal studies indicate that there is a critical CNS salicylate concentration responsible for malignant cerebral edema and mortality. Therefore, *the continued deterioration in level of consciousness in spite of supportive care is an ominous sign and is an indication for immediate dialysis and treatment for cerebral edema.* This is especially true if serum salicylate levels are not rapidly falling. Intravenous mannitol can be effective in controlling severe cerebral edema until salicylate levels have fallen.

General

Parenteral vitamin K_1 can be given for a prolonged prothrombin time. Antacids may be required in the treatment of upper GI bleeding following overdose. Standard antiarrhythmic drugs can be used in treating ventricular arrhythmias. I have seen a case in which ventricular bigeminy was secondary to severe respiratory alkalosis (pH 7.68). Mild sedation and increasing dead space ventilation produced a fall in pH and a resolution of ventricular arrhythmias.

The frequent monitoring of arterial blood gases, serum electrolytes, and urine pH cannot be overemphasized. The acid/base and electrolyte status of the patient suffering from serious salicylate poisoning is constantly changing. Small changes in serum potassium levels or arterial pH can have dramatic effects on the degree of toxicity and on salicylate clearance. With close monitoring of the patient, aggressive support care, and hemodialysis when indicated, death from salicylate poisoning should be a rare occurrence.

BIBLIOGRAPHY

Anderson RJ, Potts DE, Gabow PA, et al: Unrecognized adult salicylate intoxication. *Ann Intern Med* 85:745, 1976.

Curtis RA, Barone J, Giacona N: Efficacy of ipecac and activated charcoal/cathartic: Prevention of salicylate absorption in a simulated overdose. *Arch Intern Med* 144:48, 1984.

Danel V, Henry JA, Glucksman E: Activated charcoal, emesis, and gastric lavage in aspirin overdose. *Br Med J* 296:1507, 1988.

Done AK: Salicylate intoxication: Significance of salicylate in blood in cases of acute ingestion. *Pediatrics* 26:800, 1960.

Gaudreault P, Temple AR, Lovejoy F: The relative severity of acute versus chronic salicylate poisoning in children: A clinical comparison. *Pediatrics* 70:566, 1982.

Gumpel JM: Enteric-coated aspirin overdose and gastric perforation. *Br Med J* 4:287, 1975 (letter).

Heffner JE, Sahn SA: Salicylate-induced pulmonary edema: Clinical features and prognosis. *Ann Intern Med* 95:405, 1981.

Henry AF: Overdoses of Entrophen. *Can Med Assos J* 128:1142, 1983 (letter).

Hill JB: Salicylate intoxication. *N Engl J Med* 288:1110, 1973.

Kwong TC, Laczin J, Baum J: Self-poisoning with enteric-coated aspirin. *Am J Clin Pathol* 80:888, 1983.

Levy G: Clinical pharmacokinetics of aspirin. *Pediatrics* 62:867, 1978.

Prescott LF, Balali-Mood M, Critchley JH, et al: Diuresis or urinary alkalinization for salicylate poisoning? *Br Med J* 285:1383, 1982.

Snodgrass W, Rumack BH, Petereson RG, et al: Salicylate toxicity following therapeutic doses in young children. *Clin Toxicol* 18:247, 1981.

Sweeney KR, Chapron DJ, Brandt JL, et al: Toxic interaction between acetazolamide and salicylate: Case reports and a pharmacokinetic explanation. *Clin Pharmacol Ther* 40:518, 1986.

Temple AR: Pathophysiology of aspirin overdose toxicity, with implications for management. *Pediatrics* 62 (suppl):873, 1978.

Thisted B, Krantz T, Strom J, et al: Acute salicylate self-poisoning in 177 consecutive patients treated in ICU. *Acta Anaesthesiol Scand* 31:312, 1987.

Walters JS, Woodring JH, Stelling CB, et al: Salicylate-induced pulmonary edema. *Radiology* 146:289, 1983.

101
ACETAMINOPHEN POISONING

Christopher H. Linden
Barry H. Rumack

Acetaminophen, also known as paracetamol, is found in hundreds of prescription and nonprescription cough, cold, and pain-relief preparations, either alone or in combination with other drugs such as anticholinergics, antihistamines, barbiturates, caffeine, muscle relaxants, narcotics, phenothiazines, and sympathomimetics. Its widespread availability accounts for the high incidence of both intentional and accidental overdoses. Acetaminophen poisoning may result in potentially fatal hepatic necrosis. The risk of hepatotoxicity can be predicted by a nomogram that relates the plasma acetaminophen concentration to the time of ingestion. Antidotal treatment with *N*-acetylcysteine can prevent or limit hepatic injury in patients with potentially toxic acetaminophen levels if therapy is started within 24 h of an overdose.

Early signs and symptoms of acetaminophen poisoning are nonspecific. They may be subtle and can easily be overlooked or masked by the more dramatic effects of other agents in patients with polydrug poisoning. In addition, biochemical evidence of hepatic injury may not become apparent until 24 to 36 h following overdose. Hence, unless a high index of suspicion is maintained and acetaminophen is routinely included in toxicological screening assays, acetaminophen poisoning may not be discovered until signs of hepatotoxicity develop and it is too late for antidotal therapy to be effective.

PHARMACOLOGY

Acetaminophen (*N*-acetyl-*para*-aminophenol, or APAP) is a nonnarcotic analgesic and antipyretic agent. Its antipyretic activity appears to involve the inhibition of a hypothalamic prostaglandin synthetase and be effected by cutaneous vasodilation. The inhibition of central nervous system and perhaps peripheral prostaglandin synthesis may also be responsible for APAP's analgesic activity.

APAP is available in liquid, tablet, caplet, and suppository formulations. Capsule formulations are no longer marketed. The bioavailability of APAP from suppositories is only 80 percent that from oral formulations. The therapeutic dose is 15 mg/kg every 4 to 6 h in children and 325 to 1000 mg every 4 h in adults. The maximum recommended daily dose is 80 mg/kg in children and 4 g in adults.

Most APAP preparations are rapidly and completely absorbed from the gastrointestinal tract. Peak serum concentrations of 5 to 20 μg/mL occur ½ to 2 h following a therapeutic oral dose. Pharmacological effects are generally observed within 30 min and last about 4 h. The apparent volume of distribution of APAP is 0.9 to 1 L/kg, but tissue concentrations are variable. Rapid uptake by hepatocytes results in relatively high liver concentrations. Since plasma protein binding of APAP, primarily to albumin, is low (5 to 10 percent), APAP does not significantly displace other drugs from such binding sites.

APAP is eliminated primarily by hepatic metabolism. Small amounts are also metabolized by the kidney and during absorption from the gastrointestinal tract. About 90 percent of a therapeutic dose is converted to the inactive glucuronide and sulfate conjugates, which are then excreted (Fig. 101–1). The predominant metabolite in adults is APAP-glucuronide, whereas APAP-sulfate is the major metabolite in neonates. Paralleling maturation of the glucuronidation pathway, there appears to be a gradual transition of APAP metabolism with increasing age. The adult pattern is reached between ages 9 and 12 years. Less than 4 percent of a therapeutic dose is excreted as unchanged APAP, and a similar fraction is conjugated with glutathione by hepatic cytochrome P_{450}-dependent mixed-function oxidases (P_{450}-MFOs) and excreted as mercapturic acid and cysteine conjugates. In adults, the plasma half-life of APAP is approximately 2 h after a therapeutic dose. It is slightly shorter in children and perhaps with repeated administration and is somewhat longer in neonates, the elderly, and those with underlying liver disease.

APAP is a metabolite of two other analgesics, phenacetin and phenazopyridine (Pyridium). Although methemoglobinemia, sulfhemoglobinemia, and hemolytic anemia may occur following the ingestion of these agents, APAP itself does not produce such effects in humans. Other species (e.g., cats and dogs), however, are susceptible to this toxicity, and relatively small doses of APAP may be rapidly fatal if ingested by these common house pets.

MECHANISM OF TOXICITY

The mechanism of APAP-induced hepatotoxicity is unclear. A highly reactive metabolite of APAP (probably *N*-acetyl-*para*-benzoquinonimine) formed during its metabolism by the P_{450}-MFO pathway is thought to cause hepatic necrosis by binding to hepatocyte protein macromolecules (Fig. 101–1). Recent experimental data suggest that free radical formation is not involved in the pathogenesis of hexatoxicity. Although the amount of toxic intermediary formed during the metabolism of therapeutic doses of APAP can be rapidly detoxified by conjugation with hepatic glutathione, the metabolism of toxic doses of APAP eventually depletes glutathione. It also saturates the glucuronide and sulfate conjugation pathways and depletes sulfate stores, effects which may contribute to glutathione depletion by shunting more APAP into the P_{450}-MFO pathway. When glutathione is depleted by more than 70 percent, the capacity of the liver to detoxify the reactive intermediary is exceeded, and hepatic necrosis ensues. Corresponding to the region of greatest P_{450}-MFO activity, a centrilobular distribution pattern of hepatic necrosis is observed on histologic examination.

The minimal dose of APAP capable of causing liver toxicity following acute ingestion is estimated to be 140 mg/kg in children and 7.5 g in adults. However, because of inaccuracies in overdose history, individual differences in hepatic glutathine stores and P_{450}-MFO activity, and the occurrence of spontaneous emesis, only a rough correlation exists between the amount of APAP reportedly ingested and the likelihood of toxicity. In addition, the chronic use of drugs such as antihistamines, phenytoin, barbiturates, and other sedatives that stimulate the P_{450}-MFO system may enhance APAP toxicity. Conversely, the use of drugs such as cimetidine may inhibit this system and protect against APAP toxicity. Children appear to be less susceptible to hepatotoxicity than adults, perhaps because of differences in APAP metabolism.

The effect of ethanol consumption on APAP toxicity is variable. Since ethanol is also metabolized by P_{450}-MFO enzymes (the microsomal ethanol-oxidizing system, or MEOS), it may competitively in-

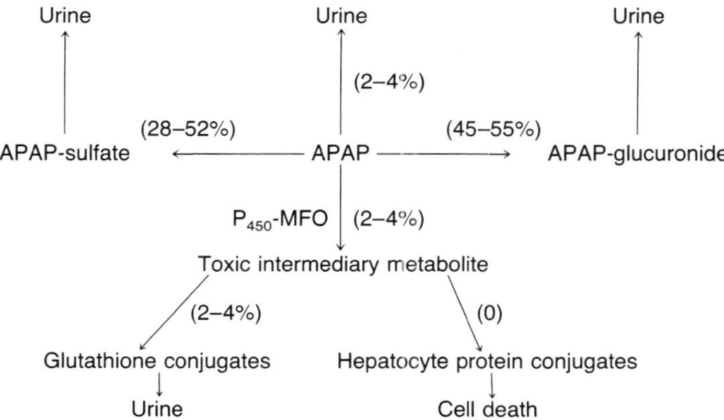

Fig. 101-1. Disposition of acetaminophen and metabolites. Numbers in parentheses refer to disposition following therapeutic doses only.

hibit the metabolism of APAP by this pathway following the acute ingestion of both agents. In this setting, ethanol may lessen the likelihood of APAP-induced hepatotoxicity. Chronic ethanol consumption may induce P_{450}-MFO enzymes yet lead to decreased glutathione stores and P_{450}-MFO activity as a result of coexistent malnutrition. Hence, the effect of chronic ethanol consumption on susceptibility to APAP toxicity is variable.

The central nervous system, cardiac, and renal toxicity that may be observed in APAP poisoning is generally secondary to hepatic failure. There are, however, extremely rare instances where significant renal failure occurs in the presence of only mild hepatotoxicity. Direct nephrotoxicity resulting from the generation of reactive APAP metabolites in the renal medulla is the postulated mechanism.

CLINICAL TOXICITY

The clinical course of patients who became poisoned as a result of a single large overdose can be divided into four stages (Table 101–1). During stage I, nausea and vomiting are frequently present, particularly in children and those with very large overdoses. However, gastrointestinal symptoms may be mild, and some patients are entirely asymptomatic. Since APAP does not cause direct central nervous system (CNS), cardiovascular, or respiratory abnormalities, the ingestion of other drugs should be suspected if such findings are present. An increased anion gap metabolic acidosis associated with high serum lactate levels may be noted in patients with massive overdoses, but this finding is extremely rare.

During stage II, signs, symptoms, and laboratory evidence of hepatic toxicity become apparent. Transient clinical improvement (i.e., resolution of initial gastrointestinal symptoms) may be noted despite the appearance of biochemical abnormalities indicative of hepatitis (i.e., elevated serum transaminase levels). The patient may then develop right upper quadrant abdominal pain with liver enlargement and tenderness. Pancreatitis has also been reported. Oliguria may develop as a result of dehydration or direct APAP-induced renal toxicity (i.e., acute tubular necrosis).

During stage III, the time of peak liver function abnormalities, gastrointestinal symptoms reappear, persist, or worsen. Jaundice may become evident. It is not uncommon for the SGOT (AST) to rise to over 10,000 IU/mL. The SGPT (ALT) may also rise to 100 times the normal level. Lesser elevations in serum alkaline phosphatase and glutathione-*S*-transferase (GST) are often noted. The serum bilirubin level (primarily the indirect fraction) may also increase, and the prothrombin time may become prolonged. Elevation of the serum creatinine and BUN levels along with proteinuria, glycosuria, hematuria, pyuria, and granular casts on urinalysis are seen in patients with renal toxicity. Fetal death and spontaneous abortion have been reported following acute APAP overdose during pregnancy.

Stage IV is characterized by either recovery or progressive deterioration with death from fulminant hepatic failure. In patients who recover, hepatic function returns to normal, and liver biopsies show normal histology (unless underlying liver disease is present). In those who deteriorate, encephalopathy (ranging from confusion to coma), hypoglycemia, elevated serum ammonia levels, renal failure (i.e., hepatorenal syndrome), ECG changes suggestive of myocardial injury, worsening jaundice, and bleeding complications may be noted.

Table 101-1. Stages of Acetaminophen Poisoning

Stage	Time Following Ingestion	Characteristics
I	½–24 h	Anorexia, nausea, vomiting, malaise, pallor, diaphoresis
II	24–48 h	Abdominal pain, liver tenderness, elevated hepatic enzymes, oliguria
III	72–96 h	Peak hepatic enzyme abnormalities, increased bilirubin level and prothrombin time
IV	4 days–2 weeks	Resolution of hepatotoxicity or progressive hepatic failure

A unique syndrome of severe, combined hepatic and renal toxicity has been described in alcoholics following the ingestion of therapeutic or slightly greater doses of APAP. The etiology of this syndrome has been questioned, however, since APAP levels have not been measured to confirm drug exposure. Susceptible patients typically present with jaundice, markedly elevated serum transaminases, coagulopathy, and hypoglycemia. Acute tubular necrosis is also present in up to 50 percent of these patients.

Nonalcoholic patients can also become poisoned following the therapeutic ingestion of multiple excessive doses (small overdoses) of APAP over a short period of time (1 or 2 days). Their clinical course appears to be similar to that of patients who ingest a single large overdose.

PROGNOSTIC FACTORS AND RATIONALE FOR ANTIDOTAL THERAPY

In the setting of APAP poisoning, hepatotoxicity is defined as a serum aminotransferase (AST or ALT) level above 1000 IU/L. Lesser elevations of serum transaminases are not considered clinically significant. The plasma APAP concentration, measured 4 to 24 h after a single large overdose and related to the time of ingestion, is the best predictor of the risk of hepatotoxicity. The Rumack-Matthew nomogram (Fig. 101–2) depicts this relationship. With supportive care alone, patients with APAP levels in the "probable hepatic toxicity" area of the nomogram were reported to have a 14 to 89 percent incidence of hepatotoxicity and a mortality rate of 5 to 24 percent.

At any given time after ingestion, the risk of hepatotoxicity and death increases as the APAP concentration increases. Patients considered to be at high risk are those with APAP levels above a line parallel to that showing the lower limit of probable toxicity and connecting a 4-h APAP level of 300 μg/mL with a 24-h level of 9.4 μg/mL. As originally reported, patients with APAP levels below the lower limit of probable toxicity were not found to be at risk for clinically significant hepatotoxicity. However, because of potential errors in the reported time of ingestion and in the laboratory measurement of plasma APAP concentrations, a safety zone (the area of "possible hepatic toxicity") was created by lowering the probable toxicity line by 25 percent. If a plasma APAP concentration is not readily available, patients should be considered at risk for hepatoxicity if they have ingested more than 7.5 g or 140 mg/kg.

Other predictors of hepatotoxicity include early elevation of ALT, AST, or GST levels (levels greater than twice normal on presentation or within 24 h of overdose); an APAP elimination half-life of more than 4 h; and possibly the presence of severe or persistent phase I gastrointestinal symptoms. In patients who develop hepatotoxicity, a serum bilirubin level greater than 4 mg/dL or a prothrombin time of more than twice normal has been associated with the subsequent occurrence of severe hepatic failure. In contrast, hepatic enzyme concentrations do not appear to correlate with outcome (i.e., higher enzyme levels during phase III are not associated with a poorer prognosis).

The risk of hepatotoxicity in alcoholics who ingest multiple therapeutic or slightly greater doses of APAP is unknown but appears to be low. APAP levels in these patients are not known to correlate with toxicity. Nonalcoholic patients who take multiple small therapeutic overdoses of APAP and have a potentially toxic APAP level on the nomogram (timed with respect to the last dose) are clearly at risk for hepatoxicity. Patients with ingestions of more than 7.5 g or 140 mg/kg over a period of 24 h or less who have elevated but nontoxic APAP levels are probably also at risk, but the degree of risk is unknown.

Following the observation that APAP-induced hepatotoxicity co-

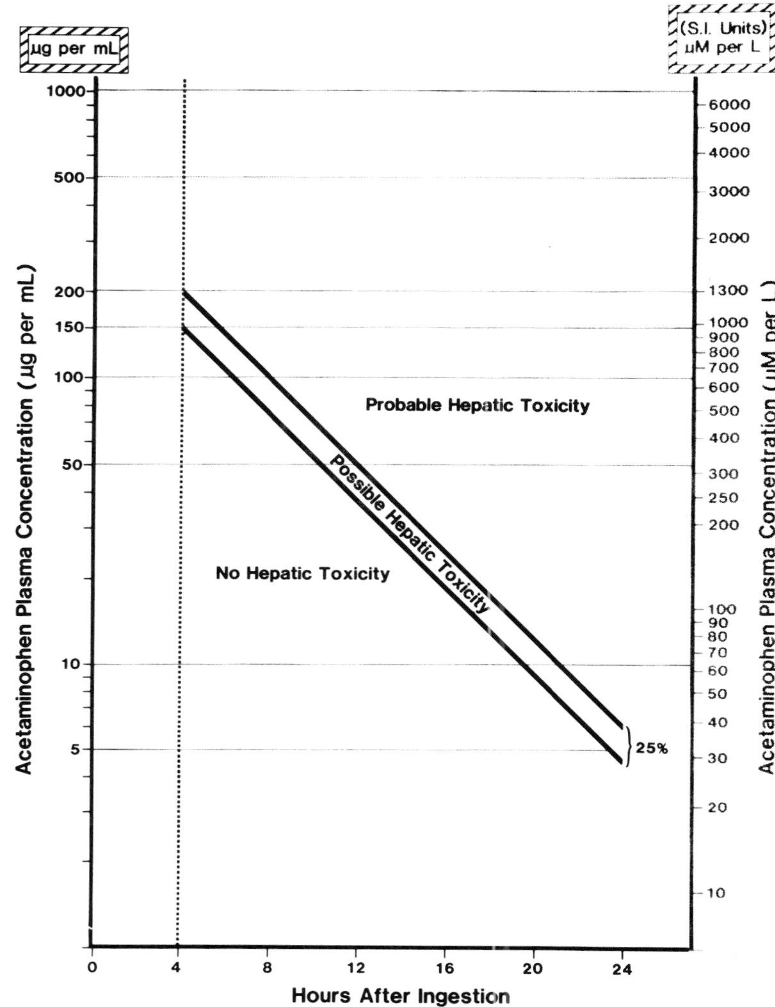

Fig. 101-2. Semilogarithmic plot of plasma acetaminophen levels versus time. (Adapted from Rumack BH, Matthew H: Acetaminophen poisoning and toxicity. *Pediatrics* 55:873, 1975.)

incided with depletion of glutathione, a number of compounds were administered to experimental animals and overdose patients in an attempt to pevent glutathione depletion and the associated liver toxicity. Since glutathione, a three-amino acid protein, does not readily enter cells, a variety of related sulfhydryl-containing compounds were studied. Although cysteamine and methionine were the first compounds to be used with success, *N*-acetylcysteine (NAC) has emerged as the treatment of choice. After entering cells, NAC is metabolized to cysteine, a glutathione precursor. However, the mechanism by which NAC prevents hepatotoxicity is unclear. It may act by increasing the supply of glutathione, combining directly with the toxic intermediary, or by inhibiting the formation of this metabolite. It may also act as a sulfate precursor and prevent saturation of the sulfate conjugation pathway.

The efficacy of NAC in preventing hepatotoxicity and death decreases as the time interval between APAP overdose and the initiation of treatment increases. It also decreases as the risk of toxicity (possible, probable, or high), as identified by plotting the plasma APAP concentration on the Rumack-Matthew nomogram, increases. In patients with APAP levels in the probable risk area of the nomogram, the incidence of hepatotoxicity is 2 to 7 percent if treatment is begun within 8 to 10 h of ingestion, and death is extremely rare. The incidence of hepatotoxicity is 26 to 29 percent if NAC is started 10 to 24 h after ingestion, and the mortality rate is less than 1 percent. In high-risk patients, the incidence of hepatotoxicity is 8 to 10 percent, and the mortality rate is about 1 percent if treatment is begun within 10 h of ingestion. Hepatotoxicity occurs in about 34 percent of high-risk patients initially treated 10 to 16 h after ingestion and in 41 to 82 percent of those in whom treatment is started 16 to 24 h after ingestion. High-risk patients have a mortality of 2 to 3 percent when treatment is initiated more than 10 h after overdosage. In pregnant overdose patients, delayed treatment is associated with an increased incidence of spontaneous abortion and fetal death.

The efficacy of NAC may also be influenced by the dose of NAC. Animal studies have shown that the efficacy of NAC increases as the dose of NAC increases. When NAC is given in doses equal to the amount of APAP administered, it is virtually 100-percent effective in preventing hepatotoxicity as long as treatment is started immediately after the overdose. Such a dose-response effect may explain why oral NAC in a dose of 1330 mg/kg over 72 h and intravenous NAC in a dose of 980 mg/kg over 48 h appear to be more effective than intravenous NAC in a dose of 300 mg/kg over 20 h in late-treated overdose patients. In addition, with shorter treatment, significant amounts of unmetabolized APAP may still be present at the time therapy is terminated. Although differences in efficacy may also be related to the duration of treatment, they are probably not influenced by the route of NAC administration. Intravenous therapy results in higher plasma NAC concentrations than does oral therapy, whereas the oral route would be expected to produce higher hepatic concentrations (since NAC is delivered directly to the liver following absorption into the portal venous circulation). Animal studies indicate comparable potency with the intravenous and oral routes of administration.

GENERAL EVALUATION AND MANAGEMENT

Children accidentally ingesting less than 140 mg/kg of APAP may be managed at home if the history is assuredly accurate. No treatment is necessary if less than 100 mg/kg has been ingested. For those ingesting 100 to 140 mg/kg, ipecac-induced emesis or activated charcoal (AC) is recommended if less than 4 h has passed since the time of ingestion. Intermittent follow-up (i.e., telephone contact) for 12 to 24 h is essential. Persistent gastrointestinal symptoms following induced emesis suggest the possibility of an inaccurate history, and children who develop these findings should be evaluated in person and managed as outlined below.

Children who have accidentally ingested more than 140 mg/kg and all patients who have taken an intentional overdose should be evaluated at a health care facility. Gastric decontamination is recommended for patients presenting within 4 h of overdose. Since food, anticholinergics, and narcotics may decrease gastric motility and delay APAP absorption, decontamination procedures may be useful after a longer interval if these substances have also been ingested.

In contrast to past recommendations, AC is now considered an acceptable method of decontamination. In fact, it may be the treatment of choice for the following reasons. AC effectively adsorbs APAP: 75 to 85 percent is adsorbed at an AC-to-APAP ratio of 4 to 1, and more than 98 percent is adsorbed at a ratio of 8 to 1. AC is more effective than syrup of ipecac in preventing the absorption of therapeutic doses of APAP. With increasing doses of both AC and APAP (at a constant AC-to-APAP ratio), the efficacy of AC in preventing APAP absorption increases, suggesting that AC may be relatively more effective in the overdose setting (provided a high AC-to-APAP ratio can be achieved). Although AC also absorbs NAC and can prevent its absorption, it has a higher affinity for APAP than for NAC, and the concomitant presence of APAP decreases the ability of AC to absorb NAC.

In addition, the simultaneous administration of AC and NAC is rarely necessary. When used to prevent drug absorption, AC is likely to be effective only if given within 4 h of an overdose, at a time when the need for antidotal therapy is not yet known. When AC is given in multiple doses to enhance drug elimination, doses of AC can be alternated with doses of NAC every 2 h. Even if AC and NAC are given together, experimental data suggest a beneficial rather than a detrimental effect. Treatment of animal APAP poisoning with a combination of AC and NAC appears to be just as effective, if not more effective, than treatment with NAC alone. And finally, syrup of ipecac delays the administration of AC, and its emetic effects, when combined with those caused by toxic doses of APAP and therapeutic doses of NAC (see below), may make oral antidotal therapy difficult if not impossible. Hence, syrup of ipecac is best reserved for patients with small overdoses who are unlikely to require antidotal therapy. The combined use of gastric lavage (via a large-bore orogastric tube) and AC may be optimal for the decontamination of comatose patients with mixed ingestions. However, the forcible insertion of a large-bore tube in an awake but uncooperative patient has the potential for serious complications and is not recommended. In such patients, it is easier and safer to insert a small-bore nasogastric tube and give a dose of AC.

The value of cathartics in the treatment of APAP overdose also deserves reconsideration. Although sorbitol is the most effective agent, it has not been shown to prevent drug absorption in simulated APAP overdoses. It is, however, associated with an increased incidence of adverse effects (i.e., nausea, cramping, and diarrhea). Since these effects are similar to those caused by NAC (and may be additive), sorbitol is not recommended. Although adverse gastrointestinal effects are also caused by other cathartics, sulfate salts can be absorbed and can theoretically prevent APAP-induced sulfate depletion. Sodium sulfate is better absorbed than magnesium sulfate, and its absorption is not inhibited by AC. Hence, if a cathartic is used at all, sodium sulfate is suggested as the agent of choice.

The plasma APAP concentration should be measured as soon as possible during the period from 4 to 24 h following an overdose. Since the colorimetric assay may be unreliable, high-pressure liquid chromatography, gas chromatography, or enzymatic immunoassay are the preferred methods of measuring APAP. An APAP level falling above the lower line of the nomogram (i.e., falling in either the possible or probable toxicity areas) indicates the need for NAC therapy. Serial APAP levels are not necessary. Even if a subsequent level is found to be nontoxic by the nomogram, a full course of NAC is indicated.

If an APAP level cannot readily be obtained (i.e., if quantitative analysis is not locally available), antidotal treatment should be initiated on the basis of a history of a potentially toxic ingestion. Treatment can be discontinued if the APAP level, as subsequently reported, is found to be in the nontoxic area of the nomogram. If the time or the amount of a single large ingestion is not known, NAC therapy should be initiated if the APAP level is above 4.4 μg/mL. A second APAP level should be measured 4 h later. Since an APAP half-life of greater than 4 h has been associated with the development of hepatotoxicity, a full course of NAC should be administered if the second APAP level is greater than one-half the initial level.

NAC has not been shown to be effective in altering the course of alcoholics with toxicity resulting from the ingestion of multiple therapeutic or excessive doses. Hence, in these patients APAP levels are useful only to confirm exposure. Patients with ingestions of more than 7.5 g or 140 mg/kg over a period of less than 24 h should receive a full course of NAC if they have a potentially toxic APAP level by the nomogram or an elevated APAP level and an APAP half-life exceeding 4 h.

Patients requiring antidotal therapy should have routine laboratory evaluation, including measurements of amylase, SGOT (AST), SGPT (ALT), bilirubin, prothrombin time, BUN, and creatinine and a urinalysis. These tests should be repeated daily for 3 to 4 days or until values begin to return to normal. Follow-up may be on an outpatient basis once antidotal therapy is complete and the patient is clinically well. Alcoholic patients with hepatotoxicity after therapeutic or excessive doses of APAP require similar laboratory monitoring.

Hepatic or renal failure should be by standard measures. Although hemodialysis and hemoperfusion are capable of removing APAP from the plasma, they have not been shown to prevent poisoning and are not indicated for this purpose. These procedures may, however, be useful for the correction of metabolic abnormalities in patients who develop hepatic or renal dysfunction. Liver transplantation should be considered in those with advanced hepatic failure unresponsive to supportive therapy. It should not be performed prematurely (i.e., within the first week following overdose), since patients often recover despite marked enzymatic abnormalities early in the course of poisoning.

ANTIDOTAL TREATMENT

NAC is given orally in an initial (i.e., loading) dose of 140 mg/kg followed by 17 more (i.e., maintenance) doses of 70 mg/kg every 4 h. This protocol was approved by the U.S. Food and Drug Administration in 1985, and informed consent is no longer necessary. NAC is commercially available in a 20% (20 g/100 mL or 200 mg/mL) or 10% (10 g/100 mL or 100 mg/mL) solution (Mucomyst, Mead Johnson & Company). Since Mucomyst has a foul smell and tastes like rotten eggs, it should be diluted to a 5% solution with one or three parts of a soft drink or fruit juice to increase its palatability. Nausea and vomiting are frequent side effects. Diarrhea may also occur. The dose should be repeated if vomiting occurs within 1 h of administration. Changing the diluent, chilling the solution with ice, further diluting it, administering it slowly or in small aliquots (rather than as a bolus), having the patient sip it through a straw from a covered cup, or giving it by nasogastric or duodenal tube may be tried if repeated vomiting occurs. Metoclopramide (Reglan), 0.1 to 1.0 mg/kg intravenously, or droperidol (Inapsine), 2.5 to 5 mg intravenously or intramuscularly in adults (0.05 to 0.1 mg/kg in children), with further doses as necessary, can also be used to prevent or treat vomiting. NAC should be discontinued if signs of hepatic encephalopathy develop, since the continued administration of this protein could be detrimental. Otherwise, the full 18-dose regimen should be administered. Should delivery occur during the course of treatment of a pregnant patient, a complete course of NAC should be given to the newborn as well as the mother.

Higher than usual doses of NAC may be beneficial in some patients. Since the dose of NAC must be equal to the dose of APAP ingested for optimal efficacy in experimental animals, patients with very large APAP overdoses (e.g., those with acute ingestions of more than 1 g/kg or APAP levels indicating a high risk of hepatotoxicity) might benefit from higher than usual doses of NAC. This can be accomplished by increasing the NAC loading dose or substituting NAC loading doses for the first few maintenance doses. Similarly, since NAC appears to be effective up to 24 h following an overdose, it may have some effect when initiated even later. Hence, patients with APAP levels above 4.4 μg/mL 24 h or more after an overdose may also benefit from antidotal therapy. Since the efficacy of these therapeutic modifications remains to be proven, a poison center or toxicologist should be consulted regarding the treatment of patients with very large ingestions or very late presentations.

Intravenous NAC (300 mg/kg over 20 h) has been used with success in Europe and Canada for a number of years but is not yet approved for general use in the United States. A multicenter clinical study of intravenous NAC (980 mg/kg over 48 h) is currently being conducted in the United States using a dosage schedule identical to the oral protocol but stopping after a total of 12 doses. More information can be obtained by calling the Rocky Mountain Poison and Drug Center at 1-800-525-6115. If it is impossible to administer oral NAC (e.g., if there is active upper gastrointestinal bleeding or concomitant corrosive ingestion) and the patient cannot be transferred to an intravenous NAC study center, Mucomyst can be given intravenously. However, since Mucomyst is not certified as pyrogen-free and is not recommended for intravenous use by the manufacturer, informed consent should be obtained.

BIBLIOGRAPHY

Haber PAL: Acetaminophen, alcohol, and cytochrome P-450. *Ann Intern Med* 104:427, 1986.

Hall AH, Rumak BH: The treatment of acute acetaminophen poisoning. *J Intens Care Med* 1:29, 1986.

Harrison PM, Keays R, Bray GP, et al: Improved outcome of paracetamol-induced fulminant hepatic failure by late administration of acetylcysteine. *Lancet* 335:1572, 1990.

Henretig FM, Selbst SM, Forrest C, et al: Repeated acetaminophen overdosing causing heptotoxicity in children. *Clin Pediatr* 28:525, 1989.

Kaysen GA, Pond SM, Roper MH, et al: Combined hepatic and renal injury in alcoholics during therapeutic use of acetaminophen. *Arch Intern Med* 145:2019, 1985.

Koch-Weser J: Acetaminophen. *N Engl J Med* 295:1297, 1976.

Linden CH, Rumack BH: Acetaminophen overdose. *Emerg Med Clin North Am* 2:103, 1984.

Prescott LF: Paracetamol overdosage: Pharmacological considerations and clinical management. *Drugs* 25:209, 1983.

Renzi FP, Donovan JW, Martin TG, et al: Concomitant use of activated charcoal and *N*-acetylcysteine. *Ann Emerg Med* 14:568, 1985.

Riggs BS, Brunstein AC, Kulig K, et al: Acute acetaminophen overdose during pregnancy. *Obstet Gynecol* 74:247, 1989.

Rumack BH: Acetaminophen overdose in children and adolescents. *Pediatr Clin North Am* 33:691, 1986.

Seeff LB, Cuccherini BA, Zimmerman HJ, et al: Acetaminophen hepatotoxicity in alcoholics: A therapeutic misadventure. *Ann Intern Med* 104:399, 1986.

Smilkstein MJ, Knapp GL, Kulig KW, et al: Efficacy of oral *N*-acetylcysteine in the treatment of acetaminophen overdose: Analysis of the national multicenter study (1976–1985). *N Engl J Med* 319:1557, 1988.

102 IRON

Steven C. Curry

The accidental or intentional ingestion of iron preparations continues to be a common poisoning. Prompt and aggressive management of these patients is needed to prevent mortality and serious morbidity.

PATHOPHYSIOLOGY

About 10 percent of ingested iron, mainly in the ferrous (Fe^{2+}) state, is absorbed each day from the small intestine. Free unbound iron is very toxic to living tissue. Therefore, the body has many mechanisms to keep iron bound to proteins or other macromolecules at all times.

After absorption, iron changes to the ferric (Fe^{3+}) state and is stored in intestinal mucosa complexed to the iron storage protein, ferritin. From the intestinal mucosa, iron is transported to the liver, spleen, and bone marrow for further storage as ferritin, or to the bone marrow and other tissues for incorporation into heme molecules.

Whenever iron is transported in the blood, it is complexed with the protein, transferrin. The total amount of iron with which transferrin can bind is termed the total iron binding capacity (TIBC). Normal serum iron concentrations vary from 50 to 150 μg/dL, while normal TIBCs can range from 300 to 435 μg/dL. Because the TIBC is far in excess of the total serum iron concentration, there normally is no "free" iron circulating in blood.

Excessive iron is directly caustic to the gastrointestinal (GI) tract, resulting in hemorrhagic gastroenteritis with hypovolemia and blood loss. If enough iron is absorbed, systemic and metabolic consequences of iron poisoning develop. Iron mainly accumulates in the liver after overdose, but can have toxic effects in almost any organ, including the kidneys, brain, lungs, and heart. Iron is concentrated in the mitochondria, where it disrupts oxidative phosphorylation and catalyzes the formation of oxygen-free radicals, leading to lipid peroxidation and cell death. Iron, possibly in the form of the ferritin complex, also is able to cause dilation of venules, resulting in venous pooling. Iron increases capillary membrane permeability and causes significant third spacing of fluids. The lactic acidosis seen in iron poisoning is due to various factors, including hypovolemia and tissue hypoperfusion; the hydration of the ferric ion, resulting in the generation of hydrogen ions; and the shift of cells to anaerobic metabolism as oxidative phosphorylation is impaired. An elevated serum iron level is able directly to inhibit serine proteases such as thrombin and cause a coagulopathy, even before the onset of hepatic dysfunction. While isolated hepatic dysfunction can be seen after a significant overdose, multiple organ system failure and death can be seen in severe poisonings.

TOXIC DOSE

When determining the amount of iron ingested, *elemental* iron must be used in calculations. For example, only 20 percent of a 300-mg ferrous sulfate tablet is iron. Ferrous fumarate contains about 33 percent elemental iron, and ferrous gluconate contains about 12 percent elemental iron.

Opinions vary as to what constitutes a toxic dose of iron. Some patients become symptomatic following the ingestion of only 20 mg of elemental iron per kilogram. Serious poisoning can often be seen after the ingestion of greater than 40 mg of iron per kilogram. The unreliability of parents in estimating how many pills their child may have ingested cannot be overemphasized. Obviously, a symptomatic patient requires evaluation and possible treatment regardless of history.

CLINICAL PICTURE

Based on clinical findings, iron poisoning can be divided into various stages. We use four stages for purposes of discussion. *Patients can die in any stage of iron poisoning. They just die for different reasons!*

The first stage of iron poisoning develops within the first few hours after ingestion. It is due to the direct corrosive effects of iron on the GI tract and is characterized by abdominal pain, vomiting, and diarrhea. Hematemesis is not unusual. In this stage, lethargy, shock, and a metabolic acidosis are due to hypovolemia, anemia (GI bleeding), and tissue hypoperfusion.

The second stage, not always seen, may continue for up to 12 h following ingestion. During this stage, toxic amounts of iron are being absorbed into the body. GI symptoms may resolve, and the patient is frequently quiet. The apparent improvement in the patient's condition can be falsely reassuring.

The third stage may appear early in severe poisonings, or may develop hours following the second stage. Toxic amounts of iron have moved from blood into tissues, disrupting cellular metabolism, causing third spacing of fluids, and producing venous pooling of blood. Shock and a metabolic acidosis in this stage of iron poisoning can be due to persistent hypovolemia; anemia; hepatic dysfunction (including hypoglycemia); impaired oxidative phosphorylation; heart failure; and renal failure. Hepatic injury is unusual when serum peak iron levels remain under 500 μg/dL.

The fourth stage develops days to weeks after recovery from iron poisoning. It is characterized by gastric outlet or small bowel obstruction secondary to scarring from the original corrosive injury produced by iron.

TREATMENT

Patients arriving in the emergency department who have remained completely asymptomatic for 6 h after ingestion of iron and who have a completely normal physical examination do not need medical treatment for iron poisoning.

Patients who have a significant ingestion of iron (about 20 mg/kg or greater) should receive gastric lavage. Since ipecac-induced vomiting is confused with signs of serious iron poisoning, it should not be used. There are no data supporting lavage with sodium bicarbonate solutions or supporting administration of phosphates to prevent iron absorption. Cathartics should not be administered to those who already have diarrhea. A plain film of the kidneys, ureters, and bladder (KUB) may reveal iron in the GI tract; however, 50 percent of children who develop serum iron levels in excess of 300 μg/dL have a negative KUB.

Patients who have only minimal symptoms after ingestion do well with supportive care. If the patient remains well after several hours of observation, and a serum iron level drawn 3 to 5 h after ingestion is well below 350 μg/dL, the patient can be discharged. A repeat serum iron determination during observation helps to ensure that iron levels are not rising. A KUB demonstrating iron remaining in the GI tract obviously indicates that serum iron levels may continue to increase. Again, a negative KUB does not preclude a continued rise in serum iron concentration.

Intravenous hydration should be initiated in patients with significant gastroenteritis. A fluid challenge should be given intravenously to those patients with hypotension. Laboratory work should include measurements of serum electrolytes, blood urea nitrogen, serum glucose, coagulation parameters, a complete blood cell count, and serum iron level. Blood gases should be determined in any severely symptomatic patient.

Deferoxamine mesylate is a chelating agent that can remove iron from tissues and can remove free iron from plasma. Deferoxamine combines with iron to form water-soluble ferrioxamine, which is excreted in the urine. The preferred route of administration is as an intravenous infusion at a rate of 15 mg/kg per hour. Higher rates of infusion are recommended in severe cases by some authorities. Hypotension is occasionally seen when deferoxamine is used in acute iron poisoning. Hypotension is thought to be due to vasodilation, possibly from histamine release. This is usually not a problem if infusion rates are kept below 45 mg/kg per hour.

Deferoxamine can be given intramuscularly, but studies in patients with chronic iron overload show that intravenous administration of deferoxamine removes much more iron than intramuscular administration. Furthermore, an intramuscular injection would be expected to produce a higher peak level, making hypotension more likely. Adequate hydration should always be given before deferoxamine is administered intramuscularly. A commonly recommended dose for intramuscular deferoxamine mesylate is 90 mg/kg, up to 1 g, every 8 h.

There are no human data to support a recommendation that the total daily dose of deferoxamine not exceed 6 g in the treatment of acute iron poisoning. In fact, much larger doses have been given without complications. The use of deferoxamine in patients with chronic renal failure and/or chronic iron overload has produced neurotoxicity consisting of hearing loss, decreased visual acuity, and changes in color vision. Such changes have not been reported after the short-term use of deferoxamine in patients suffering from acute iron poisoning. Deferoxamine causes a fall in glomerular filtration rate and renal blood flow in dogs, and case reports suggest the existence of deferoxamine-induced renal failure. A canine study demonstrates the importance of adequate hydration in preventing renal dysfunction from deferoxamine. The use of deferoxamine infusions for several days has been associated with rapidly progressive and fatal pneumonitis/adult respiratory distress syndrome. Again, this has not been reported after short-term use (12 to 24 h) of deferoxamine for the treatment of acute iron poisoning.

Gastric lavage with deferoxamine mesylate is not recommended because tremendous amounts of deferoxamine mesylate would be required to complex with ingested, but yet unabsorbed, iron. Fortunately, most iron is not absorbed following overdose, which is why lesser amounts of deferoxamine can be given parenterally.

To use deferoxamine wisely, one needs to understand the limitations of using serum iron levels as a basis for therapy. Serum iron levels usually peak anywhere from 2 to 6 h after ingestion. Many patients have normal serum iron levels by the time they die from iron poisoning because it is free iron that has moved from blood into *tissues* that causes systemic toxicity. Although deferoxamine can remove free iron from plasma, an important reason for giving deferoxamine is to remove iron from *tissues*.

A serum iron concentration below the TIBC, then, does not mean that deferoxamine would be of no benefit. The determination of a single iron level may not reflect what iron levels have been previously, or what direction iron levels are going. For example, suppose you have just received laboratory results reporting a serum iron concentration of 310 μg/dL and a TIBC of 365 μg/dL. The serum iron concentration may have been above the TIBC earlier, resulting in significant tissue levels of iron. On the other hand, the serum iron concentration may have been rising at the time blood was drawn, and exceeds the TIBC by the time laboratory results return. Furthermore, a recent study demonstrated that commonly used methods to measure TIBC result in a falsely elevated TIBC at toxic iron concentrations. Therefore, elevated serum iron concentrations are accompanied by falsely elevated TIBCs, making interpretation of the relationship between TIBC and serum iron difficult or impossible. Therefore, *one should never wait for results of a serum iron level or TIBC to decide whether to give deferoxamine to a significantly symptomatic patient.* If a patient is severely symptomatic, deferoxamine is probably indicated regardless of the serum iron concentration or TIBC.

Clinical findings can help predict the degree of toxicity. Of all children who vomit, 67 percent have serum iron concentrations greater than 300 μg/dL. Of all children who have a diarrhea stool, 75 percent develop serum iron concentrations greater than 300 μg/dL. Most children with a white blood cell count > 15,000/mm^3, or a serum glucose level > 150 mg/dL, have a serum iron level greater than 300 μg/dL. *Severely poisoned children can still have a normal white blood cell count and a normal serum glucose level.* The appearance of a rosé wine color to the urine after an injection or infusion of deferoxamine is due to ferrioxamine in the urine. The absence of this color is an *unreliable* indicator of lack of significant iron poisoning, and an *unreliable* indicator of lack of need for deferoxamine.

Therefore, the following patients should receive deferoxamine after adequate hydration:

1. Any moderately or severely symptomatic patient (e.g., one with hypotension, severe gastroenteritis, lethargy), even if iron levels are below the TIBC, have not yet returned, or are not available.
2. Any patient whose serum iron level is greater than the TIBC.
3. Any patient with a serum iron level greater than 350 μg/dL.

Our center recommends that deferoxamine be continued until the patient is free of any evidence of systemic iron toxicity *and* serum iron levels are normal or low.

Dialysis and charcoal hemoperfusion can remove some ferrioxamine as well as deferoxamine. It has been recommended that deferoxamine should be continued and dialysis instituted in the face of acute renal failure during acute iron poisoning. However, it appears that increasing urinary elimination of ferrioxamine is not deferoxamine's main mechanism in counteracting iron poisoning. Data suggest that deferoxamine's main protective mechanism is to combine with and inactivate iron by forming ferrioxamine, regardless of how quickly ferrioxamine may be excreted in urine. While it makes sense that deferoxamine should be continued in the face of renal failure, it is not established that dialysis or hemoperfusion should be instituted only to enhance ferrioxamine clearance. When deferoxamine is used in patients with renal failure, the elimination half-life is prolonged markedly (mean value of 25.6 h versus 1 to 4 h in normal patients), and the infusion rate should be decreased appropriately.

PITFALLS IN TREATING IRON POISONING

Several common mistakes are made by those who treat iron poisoning, and these pitfalls are summarized in Table 102-1. Attention has been drawn to several of these in the previous sections, but two others deserve special mention.

Some laboratories use radioimmunoassays to measure serum iron levels. These assays *cannot* measure serum iron concentrations greater than the TIBC. Therefore, if the serum iron level is reported to be close to the TIBC, it is possible that it is really much greater than the TIBC. A colorimetric method is probably the most reliable for measuring serum iron levels after overdose, unless methods using atomic absorption are readily available.

The second important point is that deferoxamine interferes with the determination of serum iron levels, even by colorimetric methods. Once deferoxamine has been given, serum iron level measurements may be falsely depressed by as much as 30 to 50 percent, and possibly more. This is mainly important when the serum iron level exceeds the TIBC, and must be considered when interpreting reports of serum iron

Table 102-1. Pitfalls in Treating Iron Poisoning

- Waiting until results of serum iron levels are returned before administering deferoxamine to moderately or severely symptomatic patients
- Withholding deferoxamine from severely symptomatic patients only because serum iron levels are below the TIBC
- Sending a stage-2 iron poisoning victim home
- Relying only on a negative KUB, a normal WBC, and/or a normal serum glucose level to rule out significant iron ingestion
- Using radioimmunoassays when measuring serum iron
- Not recognizing that deferoxamine causes a falsely low determination of serum iron levels by most laboratory methods

concentrations. At our center we correct for the presence of deferoxamine by adding sodium hydrosulfite. However, this is rarely done at other institutions. This is the main reason why our center recommends that serum iron level measurements be so low before stopping deferoxamine therapy.

BIBLIOGRAPHY

Chang TMS, Barre P: Effect of desferrioxamine on removal of aluminum and iron by coated charcoal haemoperfusion and haemodialysis. *Lancet* 2:1051, 1983.

Dean BS, Krenzelok EP: In vivo effectiveness of oral complexation agents in the management of iron poisoning. *Clin Toxicol* 25:221, 1987.

Evensen SA, Forde R, Opedal I, et al: Acute iron intoxication with abruptly reduced levels of vitamin K-dependent coagulation factors. *Scand J Haematol* 29:25, 1982.

Freedman MH, Grisaru D, Olivieri N, et al: Pulmonary syndrome in patients with thalassemia major receiving intravenous deferoxamine infusions. *Am J Dis Child* 144:565, 1990.

Gevirtz NR, Wasserman LR: The measurement of iron and iron-binding capacity in plasma containing deferoxamine. *J Pediatr* 68:802, 1966.

Jacobs J, Greene H, Gendel BR: Acute iron intoxication. *N Engl J Med* 273:1124, 1965.

Koren G, Bentur Y, Strong D, et al: Acute changes in renal function associated with deferoxamine therapy. *Am J Dis Child* 143:1077, 1989.

Lacouture PG, Wason S, Temple AR, et al: Emergency assessment of severity in iron overdose by clinical and laboratory methods. *J Pediatr* 99:89, 1981.

Leikin S, Vossough P, Mochir-Fatemi F: Chelation therapy in acute iron poisoning. *J Pediatr* 71:425, 1967.

Lovejoy FH: Chelation therapy in iron posioning. *J Toxicol Clin Toxicol* 19:871, 1983.

McEnry JT, Greengard J: Treatment of acute iron ingestion with deferoxamine in 20 children. *J Pediatr* 68:773, 1966.

Peck MG, Rogers JF, Rivenbark JF: Use of high doses of deferoxamine (Desferal) in an adult patient with acute iron overdosage. *J Toxicol Clin Toxicol* 19:875, 1983.

Proudfoot AT, Simpson D, Dyson EH: Management of acute iron poisoning. *Med Toxicol* 1:83, 1986.

Robotham JL, Lietman PS: Acute iron poisoning. *Am J Dis Child* 134:875, 1980.

Stivelman J, Schulman G, Fosburg M, et al: Kinetics and efficacy of deferoxamine in iron-overloaded hemodialysis patients. *Kidney Int* 36:1125, 1989.

Tenenbein M, Kowalskis, Roberts D: Pulmonary toxicity in iron poisoning: Deferoxamine induced? *Vet Hum Toxicol* 32:349, 1990 (abstract).

Tenenbein M, Yatscoff R: Total iron binding capacity (TIBC) in iron poisoning: Who needs it? *Vet Hum Toxicol* 31:343, 1989 (abstract).

Whitten CF, Chen YC, Gibson GW: Studies in acute iron poisoning: II. Further observations on deferoxamine in the treatment of acute iron poisoning. *Pediatrics* 38:102, 1966.

103 HYDROCARBONS

Paul M. Wax

Hydrocarbons are a diverse group of organic compounds consisting primarily of carbon and hydrogen atoms arranged in various aliphatic and aromatic configurations. Products containing hydrocarbons are found in many households and occupational settings. Examples include fuels, lighter fluids, paints, paint removers, glues, cleaning and polishing agents, spot removers, degreasers, lubricants, solvents, and pesticides. Exposure may cause life-threatening toxicity.

CLASSIFICATION

Most hydrocarbons (gasoline, kerosene, etc.) are produced from petroleum distillation which results in predominantly aliphatic (open-chain) mixtures of hydrocarbons of different chain lengths. Chain length determines the phase of the hydrocarbon at room temperature. Short-chain aliphatic compounds, such as methane or butane, are gases; long-chain aliphatic compounds, such as tar, are solids. Intermediate-chain (C5–15) aliphatic compounds are in liquid form and account for most hydrocarbon exposures seen in the emergency department (Table 103-1). Pulmonary toxicity secondary to aspiration is the most common complication from ingesting liquid aliphatic hydrocarbons.

The wood distillates (e.g., turpentine and pine oil) consist mainly of cyclic terpene derivatives and make up another class of hydrocarbons. Gastrointestinal (GI) absorption of wood distillates tends to be greater than that of aliphatic petroleum distillates, increasing the risk for central nervous system (CNS) depression.

Aromatic hydrocarbons (containing a benzene ring, Table 103-2) and halogenated hydrocarbons (aliphatics with a substituted halogen group, Table 103-3) are widely used industrial solvents. Exposure, usually from inhalation, is most often found in substance abusers and in certain occupational settings and may result in significant systemic toxicity. Specific cardiovascular, hepatic, renal, and hematologic effects are attributed to aromatic and halogenated hydrocarbons.

EPIDEMIOLOGY

Hydrocarbon ingestions account for approximately 3 to 10 percent of all accidental childhood poisonings. Ingestions of gasoline, kerosene, lighter fluid, mineral seal oil, and turpentine are most frequent. The 1989 American Association of Poison Control Centers National Data Collection Systems revealed that of the 58,536 hydrocarbon exposures reported to poison control centers, 1602 developed moderate to severe toxicity, and 31 died. These data imply that most hydrocarbon ingestions have a benign clinical course.

DETERMINANTS OF TOXICITY

The toxic potential of hydrocarbons depends on physical characteristics (volatility, viscosity, and surface tension), chemical characteristics (aliphatic, aromatic, or halogenated), presence of toxic additives such as pesticides or heavy metals, route of exposure, concentration, and dose. Viscosity, defined as the resistance to flow, and surface tension, denoting "creeping" ability, both play a major role in determining the aspiration potential. Viscosity is measured in Saybolt Seconds Universal (SSU). Patients ingesting substances with viscosities less than 60 SSU are at greater risk for aspiration than those ingesting substances with viscosities greater than 100 SSU (Table 103-4). Volatility denotes the ability of a substance to vaporize. Inhalation of a highly volatile agent, such as the aromatic hydrocarbons, halogenated hydrocarbons, or gasoline results in systemic absorption and the potential for significant toxicity.

Dermal exposure to hydrocarbons causes local toxicity, and occasionally leads to systemic absorption. Toxicity secondary to intravenous administration of hydrocarbons has been reported. When used intravenously, hydrocarbons may cause pulmonary toxicity by their first-pass exposure to the lungs.

Table 103-1. Common Aliphatic Hydrocarbons

Substance	Commercial Use
Gasoline	Motor fuel
Kerosene	Stove and lamp fuel
Mineral seal oil	Furniture polish
Naphtha	Lighter fluid
Diesel oil	Lubricant
N–Hexane	Plastic cement, rubber cement

PRESENTATION

Toxicity from hydrocarbon exposure can be divided into different clinical syndromes based on the organ system(s) predominately affected. Characteristic presentations usually affect one or more of the following systems: pulmonary, neurologic (central and peripheral), GI, cutaneous, hepatic, cardiac, renal, or hematologic.

Pulmonary

Pulmonary complications, especially aspiration, are the most frequent adverse effects of hydrocarbon exposure. Typically, this involves the accidental childhood ingestion of small amounts of aliphatic hydrocarbon mixtures commonly stored in the household. Aliphatic hydrocarbons have a limited GI absorption, and toxicity results only from aspiration of the low-viscosity hydrocarbons or inadvertent inhalation of the high-volatility hydrocarbons. Although ingestion of aromatic or halogenated hydrocarbons may also result in aspiration, these more typically produce CNS and other systemic toxicity secondary to GI absorption.

Aspiration is not dependent on volume ingested. Experimentally in rats, as little as 0.2 mL instilled intratracheally has caused pneumonitis. In a recent study of childhood ingestions, only 12 percent of 950 patients developed clinical or radiographic evidence of pulmonary toxicity. Pulmonary toxicity does not result from GI absorption but occurs from direct aspiration of the hydrocarbon into the pulmonary tree at the time of ingestion by spreading from the hypopharynx into the airway. There is no evidence that hydrocarbons creep up from the stomach into the airway. Spontaneous vomiting, however, does in-

Table 103-2. Common Aromatic Hydrocarbons

Substance	Commercial Use
Benzene	Chemical intermediate, gasoline (small amount; average, 0.8%)
Toluene	Airplane glue, plastic cement, acrylic paint
Xylene	Solvent, cleaning agent, degreaser

Table 103-3. Common Halogenated Hydrocarbons

Substance	Commercial Use
Carbon tetrachloride	Solvent, refrigerant, aerosol propellant
Chloroform	Solvent, chemical intermediate
Methylene chloride	Paint stripper, varnish remover, aerosol paint, degreaser
Trichloroethylene (TCE)	Spot remover, degreaser, typewriter correction fluid
Trichloroethane (TCA)	Spot remover, degreaser, typewriter correction fluid
Tetrachloroethylene (Perchloroethylene)	Dry cleaning agent, degreaser

Table 103-4. Hydrocarbon Viscosities

Less Than 60 SSU	More Than 100 SSU
Aromatic hydrocarbons	Diesel oil
Gasoline	Grease
Halogenated hydrocarbons	Mineral oil
Kerosene	Paraffin wax
Mineral seal oil	Petroleum jelly
Naphtha	Tar
N–Hexane	
Turpentine	

Source: Ellenhorn MJ, Barceloux DG: *Medical Toxicology*. New York, Elsevier, 1988. Used with permission.

crease the risk of aspiration. Pulmonary toxicity from the inhalation of an aerosolized aliphatic hydrocarbon (kerosene) has also been reported.

Hydrocarbon aspiration causes chemical pneumonitis by direct toxic injury to the pulmonary parenchyma. Destruction of alveolar and capillary membranes results in increased vascular permeability and edema. Altered surfactant function may also contribute. Early distal airway closure and alveolar collapse produces clinical bronchospasm and ventilation–perfusion mismatch. The CNS manifestations seen after ingestion of a poorly GI-absorbed aliphatic hydrocarbon are thought to be from hypoxia secondary to the hydrocarbon-induced pneumonitis and/or direct CNS toxicity following the pulmonary absorption of a volatile hydrocarbon. Studies performed in animals in which hydrocarbons were instilled into the stomach after ligation of the esophagus demonstrate negligible absorption of aliphatic compounds from the GI tract with no evidence of subsequent pneumonitis. Pneumatoceles, pneumothoraces, and/or pneumomediastinum are also associated with hydrocarbon aspiration. Other complications include bacterial superinfection, acute respiratory distress syndrome, and death. Long-term pulmonary dysfunction may occur.

The clinical manifestations of pulmonary aspiration are usually apparent almost immediately upon ingestion. The early effects result from irritation of the oral mucosa and tracheobronchial tree. Symptoms include coughing, choking, gasping, dyspnea, and burning of the mouth. Patients with these symptoms should be assumed to have aspirated until proven otherwise. Physical examination may reveal grunting respirations, retractions, tachypnea, tachycardia, and cyanosis. Fever has been noted on admission in about 30 percent. An odor of the hydrocarbon may be noted on the patient's breath.

Auscultation may be normal, or reveal wheezing, and decreased, or absent breath sounds. Arterial blood-gas analysis may demonstrate a widened alveolar–arterial oxygen gradient or frank hypoxemia. The development of a necrotizing pneumonitis and hemorrhagic pulmonary edema usually occurs within hours in severe aspiration.

Most fatalities from these complications occur within 24 h. With less severe damage, symptoms usually subside within 2 to 5 days except with pneumatoceles and lipoid pneumonias where symptoms may persist for weeks to months.

Although most patients with clinically significant aspiration have abnormal chest x-rays, the time course of radiographic changes varies and correlation with physical examination may be poor. Changes may be seen as early as 30 min after aspiration, but the initial radiograph in the symptomatic patient may be deceptively clear. Radiographic changes usually appear by 4 to 6 h and are almost always present by 18 to 24 h if they are to occur. The infiltrates range in appearance from streaking to flocculent to homogeneous and are usually located in the dependent lobes. Multilobar involvement is more common than single-lobe involvement. Radiographic changes showing only perihilar involvement may also occur. High-viscosity compounds such as lubricants, mineral oil, or tar are not aspirated readily and tend to be nontoxic when ingested. Occasionally, however, aspiration will occur resulting in the development of lipoid pneumonia.

Nervous System

Central

CNS toxicity may result from either a direct toxic response to the systemic absorption of the hydrocarbon, as an indirect result of severe hypoxia secondary to aspiration, or as a result of simple asphyxiation. Systemic absorption usually occurs through the inhalation of highly volatile petroleum distillates which may be absorbed inadvertently, for example as an occupational risk, or deliberately associated with solvent abuse.

Solvent abuse most often occurs in teenagers and younger adults, especially from lower socioeconomic backgrounds and in particular cultures (Native Americans). These patients are described as "huffers" or "baggers" depending on whether they inhale through a rag soaked with the hydrocarbon held to the mouth or rebreathe into a plastic bag containing the hydrocarbon. The act of rebreathing to facilitate inhalation may also contribute to toxicity by producing significant hypercarbia and hypoxia. Commonly abused agents include aromatic hydrocarbons such as toluene (contained in glue and acrylic spray paints), halogenated hydrocarbons such as trichloroethylene (found in typewriter correction fluid), or highly volatile aliphatics such as gasoline.

Many hydrocarbons which affect the CNS are organic solvents and have a natural affinity for the lipid-rich neural tissue. They behave similarly to the inhalational anesthetic agents. Hydrocarbon intoxication may be confused with ethanol inebriation. CNS depression ranges in severity from dizziness, slurred speech, ataxia, and lethargy to obtundation and coma. Depression of the central ventilatory drive may also occur. These effects are usually dose dependent. Although hydrocarbons are CNS depressants, they often have an initial excitatory effect manifested as euphoria, exhilaration, and giddiness, effects sought by those who abuse them. More severe excitatory features include tremor, agitation, and convulsions. Perceptual changes such as confusion, hallucinations, and psychosis may occur.

Chronic CNS sequelae may result from recurrent inhalational exposure to hydrocarbons in the work place or with solvent abuse. These sequelae are seen among house painters and solvent abusers exposed to toluene-containing substances. The syndrome is characterized by recurrent headaches, cerebellar ataxia, and a chronic encephalopathy consisting of tremors, emotional lability, mental status changes, cognitive impairment, and psychomotor impairment. These effects may be transitory or permanent. The development of encephalopathy, ataxia, tremor, chorea, and myoclonus also is associated with the habitual sniffing of leaded gasoline. In this case, symptoms are thought to be secondary to the effects of tetraethyl lead and its toxic metabolites.

Peripheral

Exposure to n–Hexane, methyl n–butyl ketone, and other six-carbon aliphatic hydrocarbons is associated with the development of a characteristic peripheral polyneuropathy caused by demyelinization and retrograde axonal degeneration resembling a dying-back neuropathy. Onset of symptoms may be delayed for months to years after initial exposure. Toxicity is attributed to a metabolite, 2,5–hexanedione produced by the cytochrome P_{450}-mediated biotransformation of the parent compounds. This neurotoxic metabolite is thought to inhibit glutaraldehyde–3–phosphate dehydrogenase which supplies energy for axonal transport. Long, distal nerves seem to be most vulnerable, characteristically producing foot and wrist drop with numbness and paresthesias. The electromyelogram typically shows a decrease in nerve conduction velocity.

GI

Local GI toxicity may occur after hydrocarbon ingestion. Most hydrocarbons act as intestinal irritants, resulting in burning in the mouth and throat, abdominal pain, belching, nausea, vomiting, and diarrhea. Vomiting, which occurs in about one-third of the patients with aliphatic hydrocarbon ingestions, is particularly troublesome because of the increased risk of pulmonary aspiration.

Dermal

Dermal exposure may also result in toxicity. Cutaneous injury is associated most often with the short-chain aliphatic, aromatic, and halogenated hydrocarbons. These agents act as primary irritants and as sensitizers. Clinically, skin findings can range from local erythema, papules, and vesicles to a generalized scarlatiniform eruption and an exfoliative dermatitis. A "huffer's rash" may be noted over the face of patients who chronically abuse the volatile hydrocarbons. Pruritus may also be present. A defatting dermatitis, similar to a chronic eczematoid dermatitis, may occur. Cellulitis and sterile abscesses have been associated with the injection of hydrocarbons. Extensive partial-thickness and full-thickness burns following immersion in hydrocarbons may also occur.

Exposure to heated high-viscosity, long-chain aliphatics, such as tar or asphalt, present a particularly challenging problem because of their association with burns and hyperthermia, and difficulty with decontamination.

Cardiac

Life-threatening arrhythmias, such as ventricular tachycardia and ventricular fibrillation, may be present with systemic absorption of a variety of hydrocarbon compounds. In particular, arrhythmias after exposure to halogenated hydrocarbons and aromatic hydrocarbons are common. The mechanism of toxicity is believed to be secondary to a sensitization of the heart to catecholamines. The term "sudden sniffing death" describes solvent abusers who die suddenly after exertion, panic, or fright. The sudden release of catecholamines in these situations is thought to induce these fatal arrhythmias. Cardiac arrhythmias as a consequence of industrial exposure to volatile hydrocarbons have also been described. Other mechanisms for sudden death include asphyxia, respiratory depression, and vagal inhibition. The use of exogenous catecholamines, such as epinephrine, may precipitate sudden arrhythmias and should be avoided except if required for cardiac resuscitation. There may be a causal relationship between halogenated hydrocarbon exposure and a decrease in myocardial contractility.

Hepatic

Hydrocarbon-induced hepatic damage resulting from halogenated hydrocarbons is well described. Carbon tetrachloride toxicity has been utilized as a model for toxin-induced hepatic dysfunction. As little as 3 mL of carbon tetrachloride has been associated with the development of fatal liver injury. Other halogenated hydrocarbons, such as chloroform, are also associated with liver dysfunction. Free-radical metabolites of these agents that cause lipid peroxidation are apparently responsible for hepatocellular destruction.

Pathologic examination reveals acute fatty degeneration of the liver with areas of centrilobular necrosis. Phenobarbital, ethanol, and other agents which induce cytochrome P_{450} enzymes are contraindicated because of the propensity to increase the production of the toxic metabolites. Liver function tests may be elevated in 24 h after ingestion with the development of liver tenderness and jaundice in 48 to 96 h. Chronic exposure to carbon tetrachloride may be associated with the development of cirrhosis and hepatomas.

Renal and Metabolic

Renal tubular acidosis may occur in patients who abuse toluene-containing substances. Patients present with a nonanion-gap metabolic acidosis, hypokalemia, and hypophosphatemia. The serum potassium may be so low (less than 2 mEq/L) that severe muscle weakness develops, occasionally resulting in quadriparesis. Significant rhabdomyolysis may also result.

Toluene toxicity may also cause a high-anion-gap metabolic acidosis as a result of the accumulation of hippuric acid and benzoic acid metabolites. Proteinuria and renal insufficiency can occur in patients who abuse toluene. Exposure to hepatotoxic halogenated hydrocarbons, such as carbon tetrachloride and trichloroethylene, can cause nephrotoxicity.

Hematologic

Chronic exposure to benzene, the prototypical aromatic hydrocarbon, is associated with an increased incidence of hematologic disorders including aplastic anemia, acute myelogenous leukemia, and multiple myeloma. This association has received much attention because of the extensive use of benzene in the work place. The etiology of these blood dyscrasias is probably not benzene itself but rather a toxic metabolite. While aplastic anemia is associated with glue sniffing, this is most likely due to the benzene fraction of the glue and not the toluene. Reports of hydrocarbon-induced hemolysis and consumptive coagulopathy suggest possible acute effects of hydrocarbons on the hematologic system.

A peculiar complication of methylene chloride exposure is the endogenous production of carbon monoxide (CO) as a byproduct of its metabolism. This is unlike ordinary CO exposure from exogenous sources where maximum carboxyhemoglobin level occurs at the time of exposure. With methylene chloride exposure, carbon monoxide formation may continue after cessation of exposure due to slow release of methylene chloride from the tissues prior to its metabolism to carbon monoxide. When patients exposed to methylene chloride present with CNS and cardiac symptoms, impairment due to significant CO production must be considered.

MANAGEMENT

Not all patients who have ingested hydrocarbons require emergency department evaluation. In Ng's recent retrospective study of 211 patients with hydrocarbon ingestions called to a poison center, less than 1 percent required physician intervention. This suggests that patients who are asymptomatic or quickly become asymptomatic after ingestion can be watched safely at home. This approach of home observation for asymptomatic patients can be supported when the ingestion is accidental, the ingredients are known and do not require GI decontamination, and reliable follow-up can be assured. All symptomatic patients should be referred to the hospital for further evaluation.

GI decontamination is indicated for hydrocarbon ingestions where the hydrocarbon or a toxic additive has good GI absorption and a propensity for significant systemic toxicity. The CHAMP mnemonic (Camphor, Halogenated hydrocarbons, Aromatic hydrocarbons, Metals, Pesticides) is helpful in remembering most situations which require GI decontamination. Ingestion of these substances, whether or not symptomatic, should be referred to the hospital. The use of ipecac in the home is not recommended because of the increased risk of aspiration. An exception to this is the ingestion of benzene where the patient's risk of delayed toxicity following absorption is higher than the risk of aspiration.

For most other hydrocarbon ingestions, ipecac and gastric lavage are of no benefit; supportive care and appropriate treatment of coexisting ingestions are all that is required. The necessity for GI decontamination is dependent on the type of hydrocarbon and route of exposure. The risk of systemic toxicity by intestinal absorption has to be weighed against the risks of aspiration associated with gastric emptying. The majority of hydrocarbon ingestions, consisting of a mixture of aliphatic hydrocarbons (Table 103-1), do not require GI decontamination. These agents have poor GI absorption and their toxicity is limited primarily to pulmonary aspiration. In the typical childhood accidental ingestion, the actual amount ingested is usually about one swallow or about 5 mL. Suicidal ingestions, which involve larger amounts of hydrocarbons, frequently are associated with spontaneous emesis, and further decontamination is usually not required. Some recommend GI decontamination if emesis has not occurred and the dose is > 1 to 2 mL/kg, although this strategy has not been studied.

General principles of poison management apply to the initial approach to patients exposed to hydrocarbons once they reach the hospital. Establishing the airway and maintaining ventilation is the critical first maneuver. The detection of a sweet odor associated with hydrocarbon exposure (especially chloroform and trichloroethylene), may be noted. Glucose, thiamine, and naloxone should be administered in cases of altered mental status. Hypotension should be treated with aggressive fluid resuscitation. Catecholamines, such as dopamine, norephinephrine, or epinephrine, are avoided to prevent precipitating arrhythmias, especially following exposure to halogenated hydrocarbons and aromatic hydrocarbons. Obtaining an electrocardiogram and continued cardiac monitoring is especially important in these situations. The patient needs to be fully undressed to prevent ongoing contamination from hydrocarbon-soaked clothes. Dermal decontamination with soap and water and eye decontamination with saline irrigation should be performed. Protective gloves and aprons should be worn by the staff to prevent possible secondary exposure. Specific antidotal treatment directed at the complications of toxic additives such as organophosphates or heavy metals may also be needed.

Useful diagnostic tests include the chest x-ray and arterial blood gas to detect pulmonary aspiration and hypoxemia. Abdominal x-ray examination may show evidence of chlorinated hydrocarbon ingestions, such as carbon tetrachloride, because of the radiopaque nature of these substances. Tests of liver and renal function should be obtained in all aromatic and halogenated hydrocarbon exposures to check for the development of hepatic and renal injury. A serum lead level may be helpful when evaluating patients with chronic gasoline exposure. A carboxyhemoglobin level is useful to evaluate the extent of endogenous carbon monoxide production following methylene chloride exposure. Routine drug screens are not useful for the detection of hydrocarbons, but as in all intentional ingestions, an acetaminophen level, ethanol level, anion gap, and osmolality may be helpful in assessing for the presence of other coingestants.

The preferred method of gastric emptying for ingestions of CHAMP-type hydrocarbons, significant amounts of wood distillates, or coingestants is controversial. Some recommend ipecac in the alert patient who has an intact gag reflex. Ipecac should never be used in patients with altered mental status or potential for sudden deterioration, such as following a camphor or organophosphate ingestion. Lavage is recommended for significant wood distillate ingestions because of their GI absorption and tendency to cause CNS depression. If the ingestion is limited to liquid preparations only, lavage with a small nasogastric tube should suffice, but if there is a concern about a concomitant solid ingestion, a large-bore orogastric tube is used. In patients with altered mental status, it is preferable to protect the airway with a cuffed endotracheal tube, although in smaller children under 8 years of age, the cuff should be kept inflated only during the period of lavage because of cuff-related injury from prolonged inflation.

Activated charcoal has not been shown to be efficacious in adsorbing hydrocarbon compounds. Charcoal instillation may distend the stomach increasing the risk for vomiting and aspiration. The use of charcoal is not recommended unless a dangerous hydrocarbon (such as benzene or toluene), toxic additive, or coingested absorbable toxin has been ingested.

The use of cathartics to hasten GI transit and facilitate decontamination has no proven efficacy in hydrocarbon ingestions. Many patients will already have diarrhea from the hydrocarbon, and further catharsis is not required. Oil-based cathartics, which had been used in the past to thicken the ingested hydrocarbon in order to increase its viscosity and decrease subsequent risk of aspiration, are contraindicated. They may actually increase GI absorption and are associated with an increased risk of lipoid pneumonia when aspirated.

Nebulized oxygen is helpful in the treatment of pulmonary aspiration. Positive end-expiratory pressure (PEEP) or continuous positive-airway pressure (CPAP) may sometimes be required, but because of the additional barotrauma this creates, one should observe for the development of pneumatoceles or pneumothoraces. Corticosteroids are contraindicated because they impair the cellular immune response and increase the chance of bacterial superinfection. Antibiotics have no proven role in prophylaxis and are usually not required except in cases of continued pulmonary deterioration because of the risk of a superimposed bacterial pneumonitis.

There are few antidotes to counteract the actions of hydrocarbons. *N*-acetyl cysteine and hyperbaric oxygen may have a role in preventing hepatic toxicity after carbon tetrachloride (and possibly chloroform) exposure, but more studies are needed. Hyperbaric oxygen therapy is indicated for patients who develop significant CO toxicity after exposure to methylene chloride. Beta blockers may be useful in the treatment of hydrocarbon-induced malignant arrhythmias. Although extracorporeal removal with hemodialysis, hemoperfusion, or peritoneal dialysis has been attempted for severe intoxications, clinically controlled evidence of efficacy is lacking.

Undoubtedly, the best therapy begins with preventive measures to reduce accessibility of these compounds to young children. Proper labeling of containers which store hydrocarbons, mandatory use of safety closures, and public education on the risks of hydrocarbons also limit the potential for inadvertent hydrocarbon toxicity.

The treatment of tar and asphalt injuries are a particular problem because of the difficulty in removing these substances without causing further tissue injury. De-Solv-It, a surface-active petroleum-based solvent, has proven both nonirritating and effective in removing these agents. Neosporin ointment, although occasionally sensitizing, may also work and is readily available. In some instances, early excision and skin grafting will be required to treat the more significant hot tar burns.

DISPOSITION

Hospitalization is required for patients who have ingested aliphatic hydrocarbons who are symptomatic at the time of evaluation. After a 6-h observation period, asymptomatic patients with a normal chest x-ray may be discharged home. Similar disposition of asymptomatic patients with abnormal chest x-rays has also been suggested if reliable follow-up can be ensured. However some physicians prefer to watch these patients for 24 h in the hospital. Hospitalization is advisable for those who ingest hydrocarbons capable of producing delayed complications (e.g., halogenated hydrocarbons causing hepatic toxicity) and those with toxic additives (organophosphates). All patients taking ingestions with suicidal intent or presenting with complications of solvent abuse should have psychiatric evaluation following medical clearance.

BIBLIOGRAPHY

Abedin Z, Cook RC, Milberg RM: Cardiac toxicity of perchlorethylene (a dry cleaning agent). *South Med J* 73:1081, 1980.

Anas N, Namasonthi V, Ginsburg CM: Criteria for hospitalizing children who have ingested products containing hydrocarbons. *JAMA* 246:840, 1981.

Banner W, Walson PD: Systemic toxicity following gasoline aspiration. *Am J Emerg Med* 3:292, 1983.

Beamon RF, Siegel CF, Landers G, et al: Hydrocarbon ingestion in children: A six-year retrospective study. *JACEP* 5:771, 1976.

Brook MP, McCarron MM, Mueller JA: Pine oil cleaner ingestion. *Ann Emerg Med* 18:391, 1989.

Burk RF, Reiter R, Lane JM: Hyperbaric oxygen protection against carbon tetrachloride hepatotoxicity in the rat. *Gastroenterology* 90:812, 1986.

Demling RH, Buerstatte WR, Perea A: Management of hot tar burns. *J Trauma* 20:242, 1980.

Dice WH, Ward G, Kelly J, et al: Pulmonary toxicity following gastrointestinal ingestion of kerosene. *Ann Emerg Med* 11:138, 1982.

Fortenberry JD: Gasoline sniffing. *Am J Med* 79:740, 1985.

Goldfrank LR, Kulberg AG, Bresnitz EA: Hydrocarbons, in Goldfrank LR, Flomenbaum NE, Lewin NA, et al (eds): *Goldfrank's Toxicologic Emergencies*. Norwalk, Appleton & Lange, 1990, pp 759–768.

Hansbrough JF, Zaputa-Sirvent R, Dominic W, et al: Hydrocarbon contact injuries. *J Trauma* 25:250, 1985.

Hryhorczuk D: 1,1,1-Trichloroethane. *Clin Tox Rev* 10:7, 1988.

Hutchens KS, Kung M: "Experimentation" with chloroform. *Am J Med* 78:715, 1985.

Kirk LM, Anderson RJ, Martin K: Sudden death from toluene abuse. *Ann Emerg Med* 13:68, 1984.

Linden CH: Volatile substances of abuse. *Emerg Med Clin North Am* 8:559, 1990.

Litovitz TL, Schmitz BF, Bailey KM: 1989 Annual Report of the American Association of Poison Control Centers National Data Collection System. *Am J Emerg Med* 8:394, 1990.

Machado B, Cross K, Snodgrass WR: Accidental hydrocarbon ingestion cases telephoned to a regional poison center. *Ann Emerg Med* 17:804, 1988.

Mathieson PW, Williams G, MacSweeney JE: Survival after massive ingestion of carbon tetrachloride treated by intravenous infusion acetylcysteine. *Hum Toxicol* 4:627, 1985.

McGuigan MA: Turpentine. *Clin Tox Review* 8:1, 1985.

Ng RC, Darwish H, Stewart DA: Emergency treatment of petroleum distillate and turpentine ingestion. *Can Med Assoc J* 111:537, 1974.

Perrone H, Passero MA: Hydrocarbon aerosol pneumonitis in an adult. *Arch Intern Med* 143:1607, 1983.

Rioux JP, Myers RAM: Hyperbaric oxygen for methylene chloride poisoning: Report on two cases. *Ann Emerg Med* 18:691, 1989.

Ruprah M, Mant TGK, Flanagan RJ: Acute carbon tetrachloride poisoning in 19 patients: Implications for diagnosis and treatment. *Lancet* 1:1027, 1985.

Shepherd RT: Mechanism of death associated with volatile substance abuse. *Hum Toxicol* 8:289, 1989.

Simpson LA, Cruse CW: Gasoline immersion injury. *Plast Reconstr Surg* 67:54, 1981.

Stratta RJ, Saffle JR, Kravitz M, et al: Management of tar and asphalt injuries. *Am J Surg* 146:766, 1983.

Streicher HZ, Gabow PA, Moss AH, et al: Syndromes of toluene in adults. *Ann Intern Med* 94:758, 1981.

Troutman WG: Additional deaths associated with the intentional inhalation of typewriter correction fluid. *Vet Hum Toxicol* 30:130, 1988.

Wason S, Greiner PT: Intravenous hydrocarbon abuse. *Am J Emerg Med* 4:543, 1986.

Wedlin GP, Jones RR: Parenteral administration of hydrocarbons. *J Toxicol Clin Toxicol* 22:485, 1984.

Wolfsdorf J, Kundig H: Dexamethasone in the management of kerosene pneumonia. *Pediatrics* 53:86, 1974.

Zucker AR, Berger S, Wood LDH: Management of kerosene-induced pulmonary injury. *Crit Care Med* 14:303, 1986.

104
CAUSTIC INGESTIONS

Robert Knopp

Alkalis and acids are the most commonly ingested caustic substances. Devastating injuries to the gastrointestinal tract can result from ingestion of these substances. This discussion will be limited to emergency management.

INCIDENCE

It is estimated that about 5 percent of accidental ingestions involve alkali or acid. Although many substances are involved, sodium hydroxide (lye) is the most frequent cause of severe injuries. The frequency of caustic ingestions is highest in small children; 5000 to 8000 accidental caustic ingestions occur yearly in children under the age of 5 years. Adult ingestion of caustic substances often results in severe injury since the ingestion is usually intentional rather than accidental.

CLASSIFICATION OF CAUSTIC SUBSTANCES

A number of the commonly ingested acid and alkali substances are listed in Tables 104-1 and 104-2. There are two reasons why these substances are the most commonly ingested caustics.

1. Access: Most of these substances are household items located in the kitchen, bathroom, or garage. Easy access is the primary cause of caustic ingestion in small children.
2. Numerous cases exist where caustic substances have been placed in drinking containers (e.g., soda bottles). The patient inadvertently drinks from the container without realizing that the substance is a caustic.

Table 104-1. Common Alkali Substances

Sodium or potassium hydroxide (lye):
Washing powders
Paint removers
Drainpipe and toilet bowl cleaners
Clinitest tablets
Button batteries
Others:
Sodium hypochlorite (Clorox) bleach
Nonphosphate detergents–sodium carbonate
Sodium carbonate (Purex) bleach
Potassium permanganate
Ammonia–metal cleaners or polishes, hair dyes and tints, antirust products, jewelry cleaners
Automatic dishwasher detergents

Table 104-2. Common Acid Substances

Hydrochloric acid:
Metal
Swimming pool cleaners
Toilet bowl cleaners
Sulfuric acid:
Battery acid
Toilet bowl cleaners (sodium bisulfate)
Others [carbolic (phenol), nitric, oxalic, hydrofluoric, aqua regia (mixture of hydrochloric and nitric)]:
Toilet bowl cleaners
Slate cleaners
Bleach disinfectants
Soldering fluxes

PATHOPHYSIOLOGY

Most studies of caustic ingestion have focused on the effects of lye on the gastrointestinal tract. There are very few studies of acid ingestion.

Solid lye ingestion produces deep tissue injury of the esophagus and less frequently the stomach. Ingestion of liquid lye, however, affects the esophagus and stomach with equal frequency. Several mechanisms have been proposed to explain the tissue injury that occurs after lye ingestion. Liquefaction necrosis occurs in tissues after exposure to lye. This is the result of the ability to lye to penetrate deeply into the tissues. The ingestion of liquid lye causes severe tissue injury in seconds, which limits the effectiveness of virtually all nonsurgical treatment. The reaction which occurs when lye comes into contact with the tissues involves the production of heat and resultant tissue injury. Saponification of fat also occurs from lye ingestion but is not a thermal injury.

Ingestion of acids tends to produce a different distribution of gastrointestinal injury. Severe esophageal injury is less frequent; coagulation necrosis occurs which usually is limited to the superficial tissues in the esophagus. The mechanism of injury in acid ingestion is reported to be dehydration and/or excessive heat generation. Injury to the stomach is more frequent and severe. The complications associated with acid ingestion demonstrate a predominance of gastric complications.

Regardless of whether the substance ingested is an alkali or acid, tissue injury is dependent on a number of factors: (1) the nature, volume, and concentration of the substance; (2) contact time with the tissues; (3) presence or absence of stomach contents at the time of ingestion; and (4) tonicity of the pyloric sphincter.

COMPLICATIONS

The major complications from caustic ingestion can be divided into immediate (within 48 to 72 h) and delayed. Immediate complications occur as a result of hyperthermic injury to the tissues. Injury to the larynx, epiglottis, or vocal cords is a potentially catastrophic problem which may cause soft tissue swelling and result in upper airway compromise.

The most frequent serious complication occurring during the first few days after ingestion of lye is perforation of the esophagus or stomach. Morbidity and mortality may occur from hemorrhage or infection.

Delayed complications can occur in both alkali and acid ingestions. Strictures of the gastrointestinal tract represent the most common delayed complication from caustic ingestion. Esophageal strictures occur most commonly after lye ingestion, whereas stricture of the pylorus is most common after acid ingestions.

CLINICAL EVALUATION

Initial assessment of the patient involves the identification and treatment of life-threatening problems (e.g., airway obstruction, hemorrhage). In most instances, however, the patient will present in severe distress from pain, not shock or respiratory distress.

The diagnosis of gastrointestinal injury is usually confirmed by the history of ingestion and a brief examination of the mouth and oropharynx. The absence of oral lesions does not, however, preclude the possibility of esophageal burns. A number of studies have documented cases of alkali ingestion in which esophageal burns are found during endoscopy without any signs or symptoms of oral burns. Thus, endoscopy is warranted in patients who may have ingested caustic materials.

When button battery ingestion is suspected, radiographic examination of the esophagus and stomach is necessary to locate the battery. If it is lodged in the esophagus, prompt removal by endoscopy is indicated. If the battery has reached the stomach, the patient can be followed as an outpatient to assure that the battery will pass within 4 to 7 days. Endoscopic or surgical removal is indicated if the battery will not pass or the patient becomes symptomatic.

The physician should attempt to elicit symptoms associated with ingestion of a caustic substance, such as difficulty in swallowing or pain in the mouth, chest, or abdomen. Physical examination consists of attempting to determine whether signs of overt or impending perforation are present.

MANAGEMENT

Stabilization (See Table 104-3)

Initial management of both acid and alkali ingestions is similar. Respiratory distress may be the primary presenting problem. In one study of 33 consecutive pediatric admissions for caustic ingestions, seven children required immediate or prompt endotracheal intubation for respiratory distress secondary to upper airway injury.

The usual cause of respiratory distress is upper airway obstruction secondary to soft tissue swelling of the larynx, epiglottis, or vocal cords. Unless endotracheal intubation can be accomplished without additional trauma, a cricothyrotomy (or tracheostomy) may be necessary. With soft tissue swelling in the hypopharynx, there is a risk of perforation. Blind nasotracheal intubation in this situation is contraindicated. Although aspiration can occur with caustic ingestions, it has not been documented as a cause of acute respiratory distress.

Arterial blood gases should be obtained and oxygen given if the patient is in shock or respiratory distress. Intravenous access should be established. Central venous cannulation and pressure monitoring are necessary if signs of perforation or shock are present. Blood should be typed and cross matched and baseline hemoglobin determined.

If the patient is complaining of severe pain due to oropharyngeal burns or perforation of the esophagus or stomach, meperidine or morphine may be given intravenously, once the diagnosis has been established. In cases of severe ingestion, after the patient has been stabilized, x-ray films of the chest and abdomen should be obtained for signs of esophageal or gastric perforation.

The patient is given nothing by mouth because of the potential risk of vomiting or aspiration.

Diluents

The use of diluents in the treatment of caustic ingestions has provoked a great deal of controversy. Diluents are used for two reasons: (1) to move any solid alkali material adhering to the oropharynx and esophagus into the stomach where it can be neutralized, and (2) to dilute the caustic material and decrease the degree of tissue injury. Because of the risk of increasing the severity of tissue injury from vomiting, the administration of diluents by prehospital or emergency department personnel should be avoided.

Rumack and Burrington have demonstrated that milk or water is the preferred diluent in solid lye ingestion. They used water, milk, acetic acid, and lemon juice as diluents. Temperatures were recorded before and after each of the diluents was added. Milk was the most effective diluent in reducing the amount of heat generated. Water also appeared preferable to the acidic substances. Because of accessibility, milk and water are probably the best diluents. The current recommendations on product containers also suggest the use of milk or water as diluents. There have, however, been no controlled studies demonstrating their benefit. In summary although diluents are not to be used in the emergency department setting, when ingestions are witnessed, they probably can be used at the time of ingestion.

Table 104-3. General Management: Stabilization

1. ABCs and vital signs
2. O_2 and ABGs if indicated
3. IV
4. CBC and T&C, 4 units
5. Physical examination
6. Analgesia—meperidine or morphine IV
7. X-ray of chest and abdomen
8. NPO

Diluents are of no value in liquid lye ingestion. By the time the patient reaches the emergency department, tissue injury is probably complete. The work of Ritter et al. shows that administering water to patients with gastric burns secondary to liquid lye ingestion may result in vomiting. Reexposure of the esophagus, larynx, and oral cavity to lye could increase tissue injury in these areas.

Alkalis

Recommendations in the older literature and on the labels of a number of alkali products advocate the use of acidic substances as antidotes. Until 1977, some medical literature still supported this idea. Although neutralizing a base with an acid seems logical, such a mixture actually produces an exothermic reaction releasing significant amounts of heat. This heat could produce a thermal injury and increase tissue damage. Therefore, the use of acidic substances such as lemon juice, acetic acid, or vinegar as antidotes is contraindicated.

Acids

Although diluents have been recommended in acid ingestion, no studies have demonstrated their benefit. However, tissue injury may occur rapidly, and by the time the patient reaches the emergency department diluents may have no beneficial effect.

Emesis and Lavage

Gastric lavage or emesis is contraindicated in alkali ingestions. The potential hazards of such treatment are (1) reexposure of the esophagus to the alkali, (2) perforation of injured tissues, and (3) aspiration. Because tissue injury is often present by the time the patient reaches the emergency department, little benefit is gained by attempts to remove any remaining material.

Emesis is contraindicated in acid ingestions. Reexposure of the esophagus to the caustic and possible perforation of the stomach are the primary reasons for not inducing emesis.

Controversy exists regarding the use of gastric aspiration and lavage in acid ingestions; although several authors recommend their use, no studies have been performed which demonstrate the advantages or disadvantages of such treatment. Those who recommend lavage specify that a soft rubber catheter be used and lavage considered only in patients seen soon after ingestion. Others advise against the use of gastric lavage regardless of the circumstances. Until further evidence is available demonstrating the benefit of gastric lavage, it probably should not be used in caustic ingestions.

Cathartics and Charcoal

Cathartics and activated charcoal are recommended in the early management of many overdoses; however, they are contraindicated in ingestions of alkali and acids for the following reasons: (1) alkalis and acids are poorly absorbed by activated charcoal, (2) tissue injury occurs so rapidly that neither cathartics nor charcoal would be of any benefit when the patient reaches the emergency department, and (3) activated charcoal may limit the endoscopist's ability to identify tissue injury.

Steroids

Although opinions vary as to their efficacy, steroids have been used in alkali ingestions to reduce the incidence of esophageal strictures. The use of steroids is based on studies by Spain. He observed that glucocorticoids inhibit fibroplasia and the formation of granulation tissue if given within 48 h of injury. Several studies have demonstrated a decreased incidence of esophageal stricture formation following lye ingestion in animals treated with steroids.

As a result of these studies, glucocorticoids have been given to patients with esophageal injury secondary to alkali ingestion. Unfortunately, no controlled studies exist to demonstrate that steroids decrease the incidence of esophageal stricture formation in humans. Recently, a study by Anderson demonstrated that steroids are not effective in preventing esophageal stricture in children. Clinicians must consider these findings and the complications associated with steroid therapy when deciding whether or not to use steroids. The side effects of long-term steroid administration are well documented, but in treating most caustic ingestions steroids are used only for a period of several weeks. The frequency of steroid-related complications in caustic ingestions has not been adequately studied. Steroids have been reported to cause an increased incidence of suppurative complications in animals as well as an increased risk of esophageal perforation in patients having ingested concentrated solutions of alkali.

Certain contraindications to steroid use must be considered. First, certain medical problems, such as an actively bleeding ulcer, would constitute a contraindication. Second, signs of gastric or esophageal perforation would contraindicate the use of steroids because severe irreversible tissue damage has occurred and steroids may tend to mask signs of perforation. Third, if more than 48 h has elapsed, the ability of steroids to prevent esophageal strictures is markedly reduced.

Prednisone has been recommended for oral treatment in a dose of 1 to 2 mg/kg per day. Most patients, however, will be unable to take oral steroid preparations, and methylprednisolone, 20 mg intravenously every 8 h for patients under the age of 2, and 40 mg every 8 h for patients over the age of 2, has been recommended.

It appears that steroid therapy does not prevent esophageal stricture. Prevention remains the best method for reducing the number of serious complications associated with caustic ingestions.

Antibiotics

Antibiotics have been recommended for alkali ingestions in patients with signs of gastric or esophageal perforation and prophylactically in patients requiring steroid therapy for esophageal burns. There is some evidence that prophylactic antibiotics may be effective in reducing the frequency of suppurative complications associated with steroid therapy. Haller as well as Rosenberg demonstrated that cats and rabbits with esophageal burns from lye ingestion have a higher mortality from infections when treated with steroids alone than with a combination of steroids and antibiotics. Haller reported frequent mortality from aspiration pneumonia in cats treated with steroids alone.

Despite this experimental data, controversy exists over whether prophylactic antibiotics are beneficial, and no clinical studies have been published to resolve this controversy.

TREATMENT IN THE EMERGENCY DEPARTMENT

Treatment decisions regarding adults and older children involve three factors: (1) reliability of the patient, (2) presence or absence of specific symptoms (oropharyngeal, chest or abdominal pain, dysphagia, respiratory distress) or signs (drooling, shock, abdominal tenderness, etc.), and (3) presence or absence of oral burns.

In patients with signs or symptoms of caustic ingestion, endoscopy is required to determine the severity of the burn. Endoscopy is usually performed within 12 to 24 h of the time of injury. Recently, the use of the pediatric endoscope has been advocated as a safer means of evaluating the gastrointestinal tract. In patients with signs of perforation, immediate operative intervention is required and endoscopy deferred.

Institution of steroid therapy is indicated in patients with signs or symptoms of caustic ingestion but no signs of esophageal or gastric perforation. Steroid therapy should be initiated as soon as possible, but withholding steroids until after endoscopy is an acceptable alternative if endoscopy is performed in less than 24 h. Administration of prophylactic antibiotics remains controversial.

A small percentage of patients with no oral burns will have esophageal burns. Therefore, in small children or unreliable adults with no signs or symptoms of caustic ingestion, the decision whether to perform endoscopy and initiate treatment is most difficult. Unless strong evidence exists that the ingestion did not occur or the substance was not caustic, endoscopy should be performed.

BIBLIOGRAPHY

Anderson KD, Rouse TM, Randolph JD: A controlled trial of corticosteroids in children with corrosive injury of the esophagus. *N Engl J Med* 323:637, 1990.

Cello JP, Fogel RP, Boland CR: Liquid caustic ingestion. *Arch Intern Med* 140:501, 1980.

Chodak GW, Passaro E: Acid ingestions. *JAMA* 239:225, 1978.

Friedman EM: Caustic ingestions and foreign bodies in the aerodigestive tract of children. *Pediatr Clin North Am* 36:1403, 1989.

Gandreault P, Parent M, McGuigan MA, et al: Predictability of esophageal injury from signs and symptoms: A study of caustic ingestion in 378 children. *Pediatrics* 71:767, 1983.

Haller JA, Andrews HG, White JJ: Pathophysiology and management of acute corrosive burns of the esophagus: Results and treatment in 285 children. *J Pediatr Surg* 6:578, 1971.

Haller JA, Bachman K: The comparative effect of current therapy on experimental caustic burns of the esophagus. *Pediatrics* 34:236, 1964.

Kirsh MM, Ritter F: Caustic ingestion and subsequent damage to the oropharyngeal and digestive passages. *Ann Thorac Surg* 21:74, 1976.

Moulin D, Bertrand J, Buts J, et al: Upper airway lesions in children after accidental ingestion of caustic substances. *J Pediatr* 106:408, 1985.

Ritter FN, Newman MJ, Newman DE: A clinical and experimental study of corrosive burns of the esophagus. *Ann Otolaryngol* 77:830, 1968.

Rosenberg N, Kunderman PH, Vroman L: Prevention of experimental lye stricture by cortisone: II—control of suppurative complications by penicillin. *Arch Surg* 66:593, 1953.

Rumack BH, Burrington JD: Caustic ingestions: A rational look at diluents. *Clin Toxicol* 11:27, 1977.

Spain DM, Molomut N, Harber A: The effect of cortisone on the formation of granulation tissue in mice. *Am J Pathol* 26:710, 1950.

105
ORGANOPHOSPHATE AND CARBAMATE POISONING

John Tafuri
James Roberts

Currently there exist over 900 chemicals with 25,000 brand names registered in the United States as pesticides and more than 1 billion pounds are produced annually. There are two major classes of insecticides—the organophosphates and the carbamates. The organophosphate compounds are the type of insecticide most commonly associated with serious human toxicity, accounting for over 80 percent of pesticide-related hospitalizations. The more toxic chlorinated hydrocarbon compounds, such as DDT, heptachlor, chlordane, and Kepone, were commonly used in the past but these compounds have been banned from private or commercial use. Organophosphate and carbamate insecticides have become increasingly popular for both agricultural and home use because their unstable chemical structure leads to rapid hydrolysis into harmless compounds with little long-term accumulation in the environment. This widespread use, however, has resulted in increased numbers of human poisonings. The 1989 report of the American Association of Poison Control Centers national data collection system listed 15,424 organophosphate exposures (7 deaths), 5426 carbamate exposures (1 death), and 2958 combined exposures.

Potent organophosphates are the principal toxins found in some nerve gases used in chemical warfare.

PATHOPHYSIOLOGY

Organophosphate insecticides are a class of compounds which avidly and permanently bind to cholinesterase molecules and share a similar chemical structure (Fig. 105-1). Carbamates exhibit similar pathophysiology except that they form a reversible bond with cholinesterase. A list of common commercial organophosphate insecticides is included in Table 105-1, and common carbamate insecticides are given in Table 105-2. Unless otherwise specified, all comments in the following discussion about organophosphates apply to carbamates as well.

The neurotransmitter acetylcholine is present in the terminal endings of all postganglionic parasympathetic nerves, at myoneural junctions, and at both parasympathetic and sympathetic ganglia (Fig. 105-2). Normally, cholinesterases rapidly hydrolyze acetylcholine into inactive fragments of choline and acetic acid after the completion of neurochemical transmission. In humans, the two principal cholinesterases are erythrocyte (RBC) or true cholinesterase (acetylcholinesterase), and serum cholinesterase (pseudocholinesterase). The major toxicity of organophosphate insecticides is related to the covalent binding of phosphate radicals to the active sites of the cholinesterases, transforming the cholinesterases into enzymatically inert proteins. Organophosphates act as irreversible cholinesterase inhibitors. The organophosphate—cholinesterase bond is not spontaneously reversible without pharmacological intervention and after 24 to 48 h of continuous binding, cholinesterase is irreversibly destroyed. The carbamate-cholinesterase bond reverses spontaneously in 4 to 8 h, yielding a normal cholinesterase molecule.

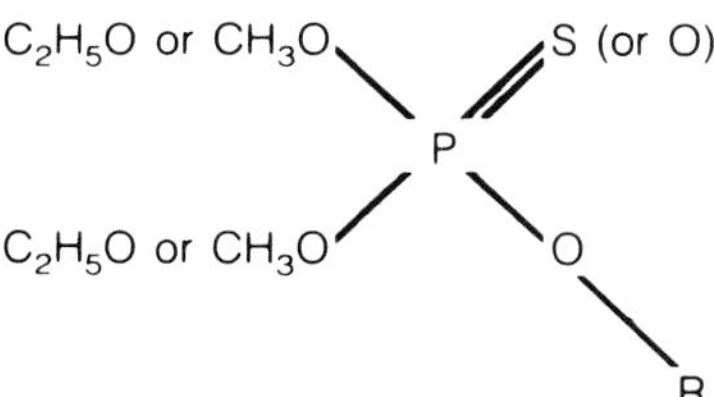

Fig. 105-1. The general chemical structure of organophosphates. (From Tafuri J, Roberts J: Organophosphate poisoning. *Ann Emerg Med* 16:193, 1987. Published with permission.)

Table 105-1. Common Commercial Organophosphate Insecticides*

Highly Toxic	Moderately Toxic
TEPP	Bromophos-ethyl (Nexagan)
Phorate (Thimet)	Leptophos (Phosvel)
Disulfoton (Di-Syston)	Dichlorvos (DDVP, Vapona)
Fensulfothion (Dasanit)	Coumaphos (Co-Ral)
Demeton (Systox)	Ethoprop (Mocap)
Terbufos (Counter)	Quinalphos (Bayrusil)
Mevinphos (Phosdrin)	Triazophos (Hostathion)
Methidathion (Supracide)	Demeton-methyl (Metasystox)
Chlormephos (Dotan)	Propetamphos (Safrotin)
Sulfotepp (Bladafum)	Chlorpyrifos (Lorsban)
Chlorthiophos (Celathion)	
Monocrotophos (Azodrin)	Dioxanthion (Delnav)
Fonofos (Dyfonate)	Isoxathion (Karphos)
Prothoate (Fac)	Phosalone (Zolone)
Fenamiphos (Nemacur)	Thiometon (Ekatin)
Phosfolan (Cyolane)	Heptenophos (Hostaquick)
Methyl parathion (Dalf)	Crotoxyphos (Ciodrin)
Schradan (OMPA)	Cythioate (Proban)
Chlorfenvinphos (Birlane)	Phencapton (G28029)
Ethyl parathion (Parathion)	DEF (De-Green, E-Z-off D)
Azinphos-methyl (Guthion)	Ethion
Phosphamidon (Dimecron)	Dimethoate (Cygon, De-Fend)
Methamidophos (Monitor)	Fenthion (Baytex, Entex)
Dicrotophos (Bidrin)	Dichlorfenthion (Mobilawn)
Isofenphos (Amaze, Oftanol)	EPBP (S-Seven)
Bomyl (Swat)	Diazinon (Spectacide)
Carbophenothion (Trithion)	Phosmet (Imidan, Prolate)
EPN	Formothion (Anthio)
Famphur (Warbex, Bo-Ana)	Profenfos (Curacron)
Fenophosphon (Agritox)	Naled (Dibrom)
Dialifor (Torak)	Phenthoate
Cyanofenphos (Surecide)	Trichlorfon (Dylox, Dipterex)
	Pyrazophos (Afugan, Curamil)
	Fenitrothion (Agrothion)
	Cyanphos (Cyanox)
	Pyridaphenthion (Ofunack)
	Propylthiopyrophosphate (Aspon)
	Acephate (Orthene)
	Merphos (Folex)
	Malathion (Cythion)
	Etrimfox (Ekamet)
	Phoxim (Baythion)
	Pirimiphosmethyl (Actellic)
	Iodofenphos (Nuvanol-N)
	Bromophos (Nexion)
	Tetrachlorvinphos (Gardona, Rabon)
	Temephos (Abate, Abathion)

* Compounds are listed in order of decreasing toxicity. "Highly toxic" compounds have listed LD50 values of less than 50 mg/kg in the rat.

Source: Modified from Morgan DP: *Recognition and management of pesticide poisonings.* U.S. Government Printing Office, Washington, D.C., 1982.

The inhibition of cholinesterase activity leads to the accumulation of acetylcholine at synapses. This causes overstimulation and subsequent disruption of transmission in both the central and peripheral nervous systems, leading to a variety of physiologic and metabolic derangements. Exposure to cholinesterase inhibitors will, therefore, interfere with synaptic transmission in the central nervous system and peripherally at both the muscarinic neuroeffector junctions (postganglionic parasympathetic nerve endings) and nicotinic receptors (autonomic ganglia and skeletal myoneural junctions).

Organophosphates and carbamates produce a similar clinical spectrum of poisoning and have identical pathophysiologic mechanisms.

Table 105-2. Carbamate Insecticides

Aldicarb (Temik)
Aminocarb (Matacil)
Oxamyl (Vydate)
Isolan (Isolan)
Carbofuran (Furadan)
Methomyl (Lannate)
Mexacarbate (Zectran)
Methiocarb (Mesurol)
Dimetilan (Snip, Snipfly)
Propoxur (Baygon)
Carbaryl (Sevin)

However, the carbamates are considered less toxic and have poor CNS penetration. Generally, the carbamates produce a similar but shorter and more benign clinical course.

EXPOSURE

The mode of contact in organophosphate and carbamate poisoning may be quite variable, as these compounds are absorbed efficiently by oral, dermal, conjunctival, gastrointestinal, and respiratory routes. Poisoning commonly occurs as a result of agricultural use, accidental exposure, suicide, and, rarely, homicide. There have been numerous reports of agricultural worker contamination after application on crops, and less frequently among industrial workers who are involved in the manufacture or transport of these chemicals. Nonagricultural workers also have been poisoned after working in areas recently treated for insect control. Low-grade chronic organophosphate poisoning has been reported in pet groomers who are exposed to flea-dip products and in workers who wear clothing contaminated with the insecticide. Children are frequently poisoned while playing in areas recently treated with organophosphates, by playing with instruments used in the chemical's application, or by ingestion. Haddad's experience with organophosphate poisoning within the United States indicates that suicide is the most common mode of contamination, followed by accidental agricultural and industrial contacts and accidental poisoning of children within the home. Mass poisoning secondary to widespread food contamination also has been observed in India, Colombia, Egypt, Singapore, and Mexico. The organophosphates in nerve gases are effectively absorbed through the skin and respiratory tract.

The onset of the signs and symptoms of poisoning may vary with the route and degree of exposure; however, the time interval between exposure and symptoms generally is less than 12 to 24 h. Nerve gases may produce symptoms within seconds of inhalation. It should be noted, however, that certain newer, more lipid-soluble organophosphates, such as dichlorfenthion and fenthion, may not produce cholinergic crisis for up to several days and symptoms may persist for up to several weeks to months with periodic relapses despite adequate therapy, probably because of initial lipid storage and subsequent redistribution.

CLINICAL PRESENTATION

In mild to moderate poisoning with a cholinesterase-inhibiting agent, the patient will typically be alert and oriented, and will complain of a variety of symptoms including headache, dizziness, blurred vision, weakness, incoordination, muscle fasciculation, tremor, diarrhea, abdominal cramping, and occasionally chest tightness, wheezing, and a productive cough (Table 105-3 and 105-5). Any episodes of incontinence, convulsions, or unconsciousness are indicative of severe poisoning. It should be noted that symptoms from a single moderate dose exposure may persist for weeks after initial contact. Chronic intermediate dose exposure may be manifested as nonspecific symptoms including weakness, fatigue, malaise, and anorexia.

Signs and symptoms may be more conveniently understood by differentiating them into the effect of cholinergic excess as it relates to overstimulation of muscarinic, nicotinic, and CNS receptors (Table 105-4). *Muscarinic* overstimulation is manifested as hyperactivity of the parasympathetic system, including miosis; hypersecretion of the salivary, lacrimal, and bronchial glands; bronchoconstriction; nausea; vomiting; diarrhea; urinary and fecal incontinence; and bradycardia. The *nicotinic* effects include muscle fasciculations, cramping, and weakness. In addition, overstimulation of the nicotinic receptors in the sympathetic ganglia may overwhelm parasympathetic stimulation and produce tachycardia, hypertension, and stimulation of the adrenal stimulation, mediated by cholinergic sympathetic ganglia, produces mydriasis, tachycardia, vasoconstriction of blood vessels, slowing of GI motor activity, and bronchodilation. The degree to which either the sympathetic or parasympathetic system will predominate during organophosphate intoxication depends on the type and dose of organophosphate, rate of absorption, and individual physiologic factors.

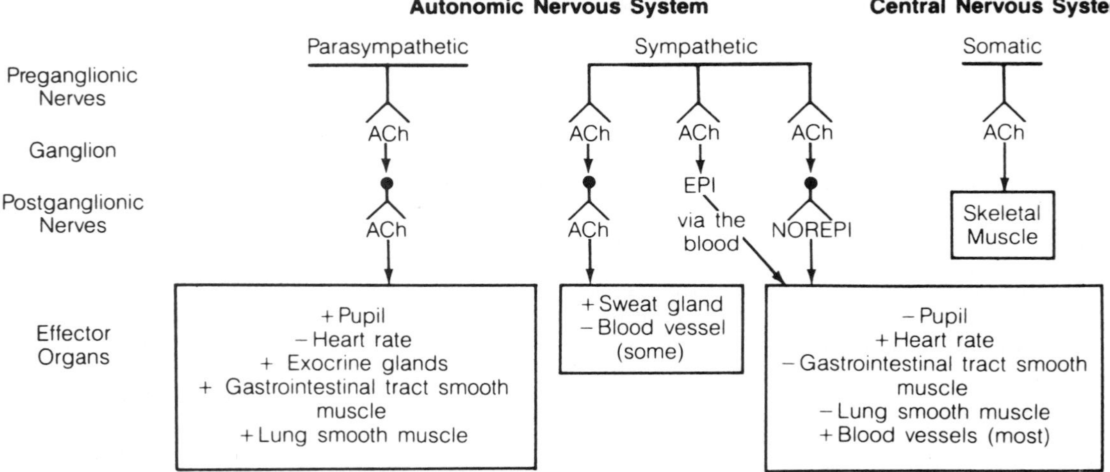

Fig. 105-2. Schematic representation of the human peripheral nervous system. Hyperstimulation of peripheral nerves during organophosphate intoxication will occur at *all* synapses where the neurotransmitter acetylcholine (ACh) is present, including the parasympathetic, and somatic divisions. Parasympathetic stimulation will cause miosis, bradycardia, secretion of the exocrine glands (lacrimal, salivary, bronchial, and pancreatic), hyperactivity of GI smooth muscle, and bronchoconstriction. Sympathetic cholinergic stimulation will cause diaphoresis and perhaps vasodilation within skeletal muscle. Sympathetic adrenergic (EPI = epinephrine, NOREPI = norepinephrine). (From Tafuri J, Roberts J: Organophosphate poisoning. *Ann Emerg Med* 16:193, 1987. Published with permission.)

Table 105-3. Incidence of Clinical and Laboratory Features in Acute Organophosphate Poisoning

Symptom	Whorton (%)	MMWR (%)
Weakness	100	28
Blurred vision	100	48
Nausea	100	38
Headache	79	48
Vomiting	63	—
Abdominal pain	58	—
Dizziness	58	41
Night sweats	37	7
Collapse	11	—
Eye irritation	—	76
Chest pain/SOB	—	21
Skin irritation	—	17
Diarrhea	—	7
Sign		**Hayes (%)**
Constricted pupils		85
Vomiting		59
Salivation excess		58
Respiratory distress		48
Abdominal pain		42
Depressed level of consciousness		42
Muscle fasciculation		40
Diarrhea		37
Diaphoresis		26
Pyrexia		24
Muscle weakness		23
Tachypnea		22
Tachycardia		21
Hypertension		18
Pulmonary edema		16
Smell of poison		11
Bradycardia		10
Restlessness		9
Cyanosis		8
Hypothermia		7
Hypotension		7
Lacrimation		7
Seizures		6
Urinary incontinence		6
Fecal incontinence		5
Conjunctival injection		3
Dilated pupils		2
Laboratory		**Hayes (%)**
Serum cholinesterase (markedly depleted)		97
Neutrophil leukocytosis		46
Proteinuria		19
Glycosuria		14
Hyperglycemia		7
Abnormal ECG (other than bradycardia/tachycardia)		5

Source: From Tafuri J, Robert J: Organophosphate poisoning. *Ann Emerg Med* 16:193, 1987. Published with permission.

medulla. Many authors consider miosis and muscle fasciculations to be the most reliable clinical signs of organophosphate toxicity. Cholinergic excess in the *central nervous system* (CNS) produces varying degrees of delirium, confusion, coma, and seizure activity. The usual cause of death is respiratory failure, which is due to a combination of depression of the CNS respiratory center, weakness of the respiratory muscles, and increased bronchial secretions.

LABORATORY FINDINGS

Routine laboratory studies are nondiagnostic of organophosphate or carbamate poisoning and are typically unremarkable with several occasional exceptions: Nonketotic hyperglycemia, hypokalemia, leukocytosis (both with and without a left shift), elevated serum amylase, glycosuria, and proteinuria are not uncommon findings (Table 105-3). A chest radiograph is usually unremarkable, but may reveal evidence of pulmonary edema in severe cases.

From a pathophysiologic standpoint, one might expect bradycardia to be a universal finding due to vagal (parasympathetic) stimulation by excess acetylcholine. However, since the nicotinic receptors (autonomic ganglia) are also stimulated, there may be a combination of both parasympathetic and sympathetic responses. The ECG may display a variety of abnormalities in acute organophosphate poisoning. Idioventricular rhythms, multiform ventricular extrasystoles, ventricular tachycardia, torsade de pointes, ventricular fibrillation, complete heart block, and asystole have been reported. Classically, cardiac arrhythmias in organophosphate poisoning consist of two phases: first, a transient phase of intense sympathetic tone causing sinus tachycardia, followed by a second phase of extreme parasympathetic tone causing sinus bradycardia, atrioventricular block, and ST- and T-wave abnormalities. Prolongation of the Q-T interval is commonly noted.

Table 105-4. Classification of the Signs and Symptoms of Acute Organophosphate or Carbarmate Poisoning According to Receptor Site and Type

Muscarinic	Nicotinic	Central†
Miosis*	Muscle fasciculations* (striated muscle)	Unconsciousness
Blurred vision	Paralysis	Confusion
Nausea	Muscle weakness	Toxic psychosis
Vomiting	Hypertension	Seizures
Diarrhea	Tachycardia	Fatigue
Salivation	Pallor	Respiratory depression
Lacrimation	Mydriasis (rare)	Dysarthria
Bradycardia		Ataxia
Abdominal pain (cramping)		Anxiety
Diaphoresis		
Wheezing		
Urinary incontinence		
Fecal incontinence		

* Most specific clinical findings.
† Less prominent with carbarmate exposure.
Source: From Tafuri J, Roberts J: Organophosphate poisoning. *Ann Emerg Med* 16:193, 1987. Published with permission.

DIAGNOSIS

The classic clinical presentation of serious organophosphate or carbamate poisoning includes an agitated or comatose patient with diaphoresis, pinpoint pupils, muscle fasciculations, bradycardia, and varying degrees of respiratory distress. There are often increased oral and bronchial secretions with urinary and bowel incontinence. Occasionally the patient will manifest the garliclike odor associated with organophosphates.

The definitive diagnosis of organophosphate insecticide poisoning is established by demonstrating decreased cholinesterase activity in the blood. Carbamate poisoning may be a clinical diagnosis. The two principal human cholinesterases are RBC cholinesterase (true cholinesterase), which is present in nerve tissue and red blood cells, and serum cholinesterase (pseudocholinesterase), which is present in the liver and plasma. Both serum cholinesterase and RBC cholinesterase can and should be measured, although the laboratory results will not be readily available to the emergency physician. RBC cholinesterase is theoretically a more accurate test and is believed to more closely reflect the degree of synaptic cholinesterase activity. The serum (pseudocholinesterase) level is a more sensitive test and is more readily measured by most laboratories, but it may be a less specific indicator of organophosphate poisoning than is the RBC cholinesterase level. Low pseudocholinesterase activity can be seen as a genetic variant and in a number of disease states, such as malnutrition, acute infections, or liver disease. The pseudocholinesterase level will gradually return to normal in days to weeks after exposure without treatment, but regeneration of RBC cholinesterase occurs at a rate of only 1 percent per day or less and can require 3 to 4 months to normalize in severe cases. In mild cases the cholinesterase levels are decreased by 20 to 50 percent of normal, and less than 10 percent cholinesterase activity produces severe clinical manifestations. It should be noted that the quoted normal ranges of cholinesterase levels are quite broad and individuals may manifest some organophosphate toxicity with "normal" (but significantly decreased from baseline) cholinesterase levels. Cholinesterase levels are diagnostic aids only and have no specific value in management of the clinical symptoms. Some laboratories can identify the organophosphates in gastric washings or urine. The laboratory is less useful in the diagnosis of carbamate poisoning, since cholinesterase levels may return to normal in 4 to 8 h after exposure has been terminated.

MANAGEMENT

A history or suspicion of organophosphate or carbamate exposure, coupled with the appropriate findings on physical examination, will direct the specific treatment. Asymptomatic patients require 6 to 8 h observation only. The aim of treatment of seriously poisoned patients consists of vigorous decontamination and respiratory support and the use of specific antidotes. A classification of the degree of poisoning and a guide to treatment are given outlined in Table 105-5.

Establishment of Airway

The initial objective of treatment should be the establishment of an airway and adequate ventilation. The patient with serious organophosphate poisoning commonly presents with respiratory distress secondary to excessive oropharyngeal secretions, bronchospasm, and respiratory muscle paralysis. Acute management in these cases consists of suctioning the copious oropharyngeal secretions and any vomitus. Tracheal intubation and mechanical ventilation are often required in serious poisoning. If the depolarizing neuromuscular blocking agent succinylcholine is used as an aid to intubation, it should be noted that its effect may be quite prolonged due to the inhibition of pseudocholinesterase. It is essential to improve tissue oxygenation as much as possible prior to the administration of atropine in order to minimize the risk of ventricular fibrillation.

Table 105-5. Classification and Treatment of Organophosphate Poisoning

LATENT POISONING

Clinical manifestations: None.
Serum cholinesterase: Greater than 50% of normal value.
Treatment: None. Observation for 6 h to monitor for progression of symptoms.

MILD POISONING

Clinical manifestations: Fatigue, headache, dizziness, numbness of extremities, nausea and vomiting, diaphoresis, excessive salivation, wheezing, abdominal pain, diarrhea. The patient is able to ambulate.
Serum cholinesterase: 20 to 50% of normal value.
Treatment: Atropine 1 mg intravenously and pralidoxime 1 g intravenously.

MODERATE POISONING

Clinical manifestations: Generalized weakness, dysarthria, muscle fasciculations, miosis, and symptoms described in mild poisoning. The patient is unable to ambulate.
Serum cholinesterase: 10 to 20% of normal value.
Treatment: Atropine 1 to 2 mg intravenously every 15 to 30 min until signs of atropinization appear, and pralidoxime 1 g intravenously.

SEVERE POISONING

Clinical manifestations: Marked miosis and loss of pupillary reflex to light, muscle fasciculations, flaccid paralysis, pulmonary rales, respiratory distress, cyanosis. The patient is unconscious.
Serum cholinesterase: Less than 10% of normal value.
Treatment: Atropine 5 mg every 15 to 30 min until signs of atropinization appear. Pralidoxime 1 to 2 g intravenously. If therapy is not followed by improvement, intravenous infusion of pralidoxime at 0.5 g per hour.

Source: Modified from Namba T. Nolte C, Jackrel J, et al: Poisoning due to organophosphate insecticides. *Am J Med* 50:475, 1971.

Atropine

Atropine acts as a physiologic antidote in the state of acetylcholine excess by competitively blocking the action of acetylcholine at muscarinic receptors, thereby ameliorating the excessive parasympathetic stimulation caused by acetylcholinesterase inactivation. Atropine sulfate should be administered intravenously. Repeated doses of atropine should be administered until signs of atropinization (mydriasis, tachycardia, flushing, xerostomia, anhydrosis, etc.) appear. Pupils frequently dilate with atropine therapy but it is difficult to use only pupil size as a clinical guide to adequate atropine therapy. In moderately severe poisoning, adults should receive 2 mg intravenously every 5 to 15 min until adequate atropinization is established. The pediatric dosage is 0.05 mg/kg, repeated every 15 min as necessary.

It is essential to recognize that a severely poisoned individual will exhibit marked atropine refractoriness and may require massive doses, occasionally depleting the hospital's entire supply of the drug. Aggressive therapy is mandatory, as the most common cause of treatment failure is probably *inadequate atropinization.* It should be noted that atropine will have no effect on the nicotinic receptors at skeletal myoneural junctions or within the sympathetic ganglia, although it may be therapeutic for CNS symptoms. Atropine does not hasten the regeneration of the inhibited or destroyed cholinesterases. Glycopyrrolate (Robinul) administered intravenously in doses approximately half those of atropine may be equally effective with fewer CNS side effects.

Decontamination

After initial stabilization, the patient should be decontaminated. This involves the removal of all exposed clothing and vigorous washing of the skin with soap and water. Some suggest a second washing with ethanol and water. It is essential that all personnel who have contact with the patient wear protective clothing and gloves to prevent accidental dermal absorption.

Ipecac, Charcoal, Cathartic

If the patient has ingested a significant amount of organophosphate or carbamate, gastric emptying is indicated. A small taste or sip may not require gastric emptying but oral activated charcoal should be given. Gastric lavage is preferred over ipecac-induced emesis because of the potential for seizures and the delayed onset of ipecac. Ideally, activated charcoal should be added to the lavage fluid and administered again with a cathartic following lavage. The value of multiple doses of oral activated charcoal is unknown, but the regimen is recommended by the authors.

Pralidoxime

After blood samples have been obtained for basic laboratory studies and serum and RBC cholinesterase levels, pralidoxime may be administered. Pralidoxime (Protopam, 2-PAM chloride) is a biochemical antidote for primarily organophosphate intoxication but probably not for pure carbamate poisoning. Pralidoxime reverses the cholinergic nicotinic effects that are unaffected by the use of atropine alone. These nicotinic effects include muscle weakness and fasciculations and stimulation of the sympathetic ganglia. Pralidoxime has also been demonstrated to reactivate the cholinesterase that has been phosphorylated by an organophosphate if it is given with 24 to 36 h of acute exposure. If it is not administered within this period, a change in the organophosphate-enzyme complex may occur, irreversibly destroying the cholinesterase. After this has occurred, restoration of normal function requires the total regeneration of the destroyed cholinesterase molecules, a process which requires weeks.

The beneficial effects of pralidoxime include (1) reactivation of cholinesterase by cleavage of phosphorylated active sites, (2) direct reaction and detoxification of unbounded organophosphate molecules, and (3) an endogenous anticholinergic effect in normal doses. Although pralidoxime is not equally effective against all cholinesterase inhibitors, it has been documented to be efficacious in numerous organophosphate insecticide intoxications. Pralidoxime should be administered, however, regardless of the type of organophosphate involved. Pralidoxime should not be given routinely to asymptomatic patients or in cases of known carbamate exposure with minimal symptoms. There is some concern that pralidoxime may worsen carbamate poisoning or render atropine (the preferred antidote in carbamate poisoning) less effective. In instances of symptomatic mixed carbamate/organophosphate exposure or in cases of unknown exposure with significant symptoms, the use of pralidoxime is warranted.

The initial dose of pralidoxime is 1 g given intravenously over 15 to 30 min. The pediatric dose is 20 to 50 mg/kg given over 15 to 30 min. Subsequent doses may be repeated 1 to 2 h after the initial dose and every 10 to 12 h thereafter as needed. A continuous intravenous infusion of pralidoxime (0.5 g/h in adults and 10 to 20 mg/kg per hour in children) has also been recommended. Reversal of muscle weakness and fasciculations usually begins within 10 to 40 min after administration.

Pralidoxime possesses little inherent toxicity. In normal doses of 1 to 2 g, pralidoxime has been shown to produce no significant side effects in normal subjects when given intravenously, but it has been noted to produce hypertension, headache, electrocardiographic changes, dizziness, and gastrointestinal upset at high doses.

COMPLICATIONS

Acute complications of organophosphate insecticide poisoning which may require urgent treatment include seizure activity and complex ventricular arrhythmias. Seizures may be easily treated with intravenous diazepam or lorazepam until the acute poisoning has resolved. Significant ventricular arrhythmias which are not responsive to lidocaine, bretylium, and/or cardioversion have been shown to be best treated with intravenous isoproterenol and overdrive pacing and continuous cardiac monitoring.

Nonspecific symptoms such as headache, memory impairment, depression, confusion, and peripheral neuropathies may persist for some time following significant exposure but the exact biochemical nature of these impairments is unknown.

BIBLIOGRAPHY

Acute poisoning following exposure to an agricultural insecticide—California. *Morbid Mortal Weekly Rep* 34:464, 1985.

Bardin PG, Van Eeden SF: Organophosphate poisoning: Grading the severity and comparing treatment between atropine and glycopyrrolate *Crit Care Med* 18:956, 1990.

Farrar HC, Wells TG, Kearns G: Use of continuous infusion of pralidoxime for treatment of organophosphate poisoning in children *J. Pediatr* 116:658, 1990.

Haddad L, Winchester J: *Clinical Management of Poisoning and Overdose*, 2d ed. Philadelphia, Saunders, 1983.

Hayes M, Van Der Westhuizen N, Gelfand M: Organophosphate poisoning in Rhodesia. *S Afr Med J* 53:230, 1978.

Kurtz PH: Pralidoxime in the treatment of carbamate intoxication. *Am J Emerg Med* 8:68, 1990.

Morgan D: *Recognition and management of pesticide poisonings*. Washington, D.C., U.S. Government Printing Office, 1982.

Namba T, Nolte C, Jackrel J, et al: Poisoning due to organophosphate insecticides. *Am J Med* 50:475, 1971.

Tafuri J, Roberts J: Organophosphate poisoning. *Ann Emerg Med* 16:193, 1987.

Whorton M, Obrinsky D: Persistence of symptoms after mild to moderate organophosphate poisoning among 19 farm workers. *J Toxicol Environ Health* 11:347, 1983.

106 THEOPHYLLINE

Charles L. Emerman

Theophylline use is complicated by its narrow therapeutic window, with a metabolism that depends on the patient's coincident medical problems and use of other medications. Poisoning was involved in 5,924 exposures, according to the 1988 Annual Report of The American Association of Poison Control Centers while 26 deaths were due to theophylline or methylxanthines. Most consider a theophylline level greater than 20 μg/mL (110 μmol/L) as toxic although side effects may be seen at lower levels. Toxic levels are common in emergency patients with asthma or chronic obstructive pulmonary disease. Fortunately, most have a benign course, requiring little specific therapy. Life-threatening toxicity from theophylline poisoning can result in significant cardiac, neurologic, and metabolic abnormalities. Several modalities are available for treating theophylline toxicity, but indications for use in patients without life-threatening symptoms is controversial.

PHARMACOLOGY

Theophylline and related products (Table 106-1) have a complex mechanism of action that has not been entirely elucidated. Although traditional teaching is that theophylline acts by inhibiting the action of phosphodiesterase, the concentration required for effective in vivo inhibition far exceeds the concentration usually produced by clinical dosages. Others have suggested that theophylline may act by affecting the binding of cyclic AMP, prostaglandin antagonism, modification of intracellular calcium, stimulation of catecholamine release, or adenosine antagonism.

Theophylline is readily absorbed after oral administration, with peak levels occurring 90 to 120 min after ingestion. Oral absorption is enhanced by fasting or ingestion of large volumes of fluid and is decreased following certain foods. Enteric-coated tablets and sustained-released preparations reach peak plasma levels between 6 and 8 h. The newer "once-daily" preparations have an erratic absorption rate, particularly after eating, which may lead to drug "dumping" and elevated theophylline levels. Peak levels are reached within 30 min after intravenous administration of aminophylline. The absorption of intramuscular and rectally administered drug is erratic and unpredictable. Consequently, these routes should not be used.

Theophylline is approximately 60 percent protein bound, with less binding in neonates and patients with cirrhosis. The volume of distribution ranges from 0.3 to 0.7 L/kg with an average of 0.5 L/kg. Theophylline is primary (85 to 90 percent) eliminated by the hepatic P_{450} cytochrome system with the remaining 10 to 15 percent eliminated by urinary excretion. Metabolism generally follows first-order elimination. The half-life is 4 to 8 h in young, healthy, nonsmoking adults; children and smokers have a shorter half-life. A number of factors affect theophylline's half-life, including cigarette use, diet, cardiac or liver disease, and certain medications (Table 106-2).

Table 106-1. Theophylline Content of Related Drugs

Drug	Theophylline Content, %
Aminophylline	80–85
Oxytriphylline	65
Dyphylline	50

Table 106-2. Factors Affecting Theophylline Half-Life

Decreased Half-Life	Increased Half-Life
Carbamazepine	Erythromycin
Phenobarbital	Cimetidine
Phenytoin	Allopurinol
Rifampin	Troleandomycin
	? Oral contraceptives
	Quinolone antibiotics
	Cirrhosis
	Congestive heart failure
	Pulmonary edema
	Pneumonia
	Severe acute obstructive airway disease
	Viral illness in children
Smoking	Obesity
Charcoal broiled foods	Neonates
Children	

TOXIC EFFECTS

Cardiovascular

Even at therapeutic levels (10 to 20 μg/mL), theophylline can cause cardiac side effects. Sinus tachycardia may occur after administration and increased atrial automaticity with premature atrial contractions, atrial tachycardia, multifocal atrial tachycardia, atrial fibrillation, and atrial flutter is seen with increasing frequency with levels above 20 μg/mL. Ventricular arrhythmias with premature ventricular contractions and self-limited runs of ventricular tachycardia may also occur. Sustained ventricular tachycardia may occur in the older patient with chronic overdose with levels of around 40 to 60 μg/mL. Younger patients with acute intentional overdose may tolerate levels above 100 μg/mL without developing life-threatening cardiac effects. Patients with a prior history of arrhythmias may experience a recurrence of arrhythmias with levels < 40 μg/mL. Hypotension has also been associated with acute ingestion, but may also occur, with chronic overmedication.

Neurologic

Even with therapeutic levels, theophylline use can be associated with agitation, headache, irritability, sleeplessness, tremors, and muscular twitching. Seizures, including both generalized tonic-clonic and focal motor, have been reported in patients with therapeutic levels. Patients with a history of epilepsy are particularly susceptible to aminophylline-induced seizures. The incidence of seizures increases with toxic levels. Status epilepticus resistant to treatment can occur as the level rises above 25 μg/mL/. In general, seizures occur at mildly elevated levels only in patients with underlying neurologic deficits. The occurrence of seizures does not appear to correlate with prognosis. Theophylline toxicity has also been associated with hallucinations and psychosis.

Metabolic

Theophylline produces a dose-dependent increase in circulating catecholamines. There is a concomitant increase in glucose, free fatty acids, insulin levels, and white blood cell count. Hypokalemia may occur, with the fall in serum potassium inversely related to the theophylline concentration. Hypokalemia appears to be a particular problem in patients with acute overdose or an acute overdose superimposed on chronic use. B-agonist administration may also be associated with hypokalemia and, with the hypokalemia produced by theophylline overdose, may lead to cardiac arrhythmias. Lactic acidosis and ketosis also occur.

Gastrointestinal

Theophylline has a direct central nervous system effect leading to nausea and vomiting. In addition, theophylline increases gastric acid secretion. Nausea and vomiting can be seen with therapeutic levels, although the incidence of nausea and vomiting increases markedly with levels above 15 μg/mL. Approximately 25% of patients with levels > 20 μg/mL have nausea or vomiting. Gastrointestinal bleeding may also occur, with epigastric pain. Esophageal reflux has also been reported.

TREATMENT

Gastric Elimination

Following acute ingestion of potentially toxic doses of aminophylline or theophylline, gastric emptying should be initiated with gastric lavage. This is probably not indicated for patients whose dose is calculated to raise their levels to less than 30 μg/mL (approximately 15 mg/kg), unless coingestion of other medications is suspected. Administration of ipecac may complicate the use of other therapies for enhancing the elimination of theophylline. In addition, vomiting is usually a prominent symptom in theophylline toxicity. Therefore, the use of ipepac is limited in this syndrome.

Cathartics

Cathartics should be administered to enhance the passage of ingested theophylline through the gastrointestinal tract. Some investigators have found magnesium citrate not to be effective in lowering the theophylline level. Further, there have been reports of magnesium toxicity after magnesium cathartics.

Sorbitol may be a better choice. One hundred milliliters of 70% sorbitol solution can be used either alone or in combination with activated charcoal for patients with potentially toxic ingestions.

Activated Charcoal

Theophylline undergoes hepatobiliary enteric circulation. Administration of repeated doses of activated charcoal at 2 to 4-h intervals significantly decreases theophylline's half-life. Doses of 30 to 60 g should be used in adults. Charcoal may also be administered as a continuous nasogastric infusion at rates of 0.25 to 0.5 g/kg per hour. In patients with markedly elevated theophylline levels, the administration of charcoal is complicated by repeated episodes of emesis. In one study, patients with levels > 50 μg/mL could not tolerate any of their charcoal doses because of repeated episodes of emesis. Patients who cannot tolerate oral administration of activated charcoal should be pretreated with ranitidine.

Ranitidine

Treatment of theophylline toxicity is hindered by the recurrent nausea and vomiting producted by toxic levels. Administration of ranitidine, 50 mg intravenously, is useful when nausea and vomiting are present. This will permit the use of repeated doses of activated charcoal to enhance drug elimination.

Antiepileptics

Diazepam, phenobarbital, and phenytoin have been used in the treatment of theophylline-induced seizures. Unfortunately, status epileticus may be resistant to these modes of therapy. The airway should be protected in patients with theophylline-induced status epileticus, particularly after administration of oral activated charcoal. Patients with status epileticus which is resistant to traditional modes of therapy may require the induction of general anesthesia pending more aggressive measures to lower the serum theophylline level.

Hemoperfusion/Hemodialysis

Although it is less effective than hemoperfusion, hemodialysis may be used for patients with toxicity. The clearance rate induced by hemodialysis is approximately 25 mL/kg per hour. Charcoal hemoperfusion with resin or charcoal filters is more effective than hemodialysis, producing extraction ratios above 0.85 with clearance rates of 120 to 300 mL/kg per hour. The indications for hemoperfusion are controversial (Table 106-3). In the view of some investigators, hemoperfusion is not absolutely indicated at any theophylline level in the absence of life-threatening symptoms such as status epilepticus or resistant ventricular arrhythmias. Others have felt that patients with increased half-lives, advanced age, or theophylline levels above 60 μg/mL may be candidates for hemoperfusion. Young, healthy patients with an acute ingestion may be able to tolerate levels over 100 μg/mL without adverse incident. The decision to use hemoperfusion should be made considering the potential for life-threatening toxicity.

Beta-Blockade

Hypotension or life-threatening cardiac arrhythmias may be an indication for β-blocker therapy when symptoms do not respond to other therapy. The use of β-blockers may be complicated by further cardiac depression or exacerbation of airway obstruction. They should be administered cautiously, in low doses, monitoring for adverse effect. Propanolol may be used, given in 1 mg doses, up to a total of 10 mg. Alternatively, one of the newer, beta-blocker agents such as labetalol or the short-acting esmolol may be used.

Antiarrhythmics

In addition to beta-blockade, cardiac arrhythmias may also be treated with other antiarrhythmics. Verapamil has been effective in animal studies. The use of digoxin, lidocaine, and phenytoin has been reported for treatment of venticular arrhythmias. The contributory effect of hypokalemia should be considered in treating the patient with resistant ventricular arrhythmias and correction of serum electrolyte abnormalities may be effective in terminating recurrent arrhythmias.

INDICATIONS FOR TREATMENT AND ADMISSION

While theophylline toxicity can lead to life-threatening side effects, toxic theophylline levels are common, and most patients tolerate these with only minor toxic manifestations. No good studies have demonstrated that prophylactic use of antiarrhythmics or antiepileptics decreases morbidity or mortality. Similarly, while hemodialysis, hemoperfusion, and oral activated charcoal therapy will enhance theophylline clearance, there is no compelling evidence that their use prevents morbidity or mortality in patients with only mild toxic symptoms or minimally elevated levels.

Table 106-3. Indications for Hemoperfusion

Clinical Conditions	Recommendation
Life-threatening toxicity (i.e., seizures, tachyarrhythmias) not responsible to other therapy	Hemoperfusion clearly indicated
Acute overdose with level > 100 μg/mL	Hemoperfusion possibly indicated
Chronic overdose with level > 60 μg/mL	Hemoperfusion possibly indicated
Elderly patient with prolonged half-life, severe liver or severe cardiac disease, with level between 40 μg/mL and 60 μg/mL	Hemoperfusion controversial
Theophylline level < 30 μg/mL	Hemoperfusion not indicated

On the other hand, ventricular arrhythmias or seizures may occur in patients before the manifestation of other minor toxic effects leading some authors to advocate aggressive therapy. Older patients, with concomitant medical problems are more susceptible to life-threatening theophylline toxicity following chronic over medication than are younger patients with an acute overdose.

As a general guideline, patients with a prior history of seizures or ventricular arrhythmias should be closely monitored until their theophylline level returns to normal. Patients with levels below 25 μg/mL do not require specific therapy other than discontinuation or modification of theophylline administration. Patients with levels above 30 μg/mL should be treated with oral activated charcoal (repeated) and monitored for toxic side effects. Hemoperfusion use is controversial, but may be indicated in older patients with levels above 60 μg/mL or in the younger patient with acute intentional overdose with levels above 100 μg/mL.

PREVENTION

Theophylline toxicity is only rarely a result of intentional overdose. Physician prescribing errors, patient self-overmedication, and variations in plasma clearance due to deteriorating cardiac or hepatic status, smoking cessation, or concomitant administration of drugs that affect theophylline clearance all may lead to elevated levels. Aminophylline infusions should be started using standard guidelines with close monitoring of serum levels. Because the history of outpatient theophylline use has been found to be a poor guide to the serum concentration, loading doses of aminophylline should be calculated using the initial theophylline level. As a rough approximation, each milligram per kilogram of aminophylline will raise the theophylline level by 2 μg/mL. The initial dose of oral theophylline should not exceed 900 mg/day. Patients should be started at a much lower dose (400 mg/day) to avoid the nausea and vomiting frequently accompanying initial theophylline use. Levels should be obtained to monitor therapy. Patients should be cautioned not to alter their medication regimen without physician guidance. Patients being started on erythromycin or cimetidine should have their theophylline dose decreased by approximately 25 percent.

BIBLIOGRAPHY

Baker MD: Theophylline toxicity in children. *J Pediatr* 109:538, 1986.

Bertino JS, Walker JW: Reassessment of theophylline toxicity: Serum concentrations, clinical cords, and treatment. *Arch Intern Med* 147:757, 1987.

Emerman CL, Devlin C, Connors AF: Risk of toxocity in patients with elevated theophylline levels. *Ann Emerg Med* 19:643, 1990.

Goldberg MJ, Park GD, Berlinger WG: Treatment of theophylline intoxication. *J Allergy Clin Immunol* 78:811, 1986.

Greenberg A, Piraino BH, Kroboth PD, et al: Severe theophylline toxicity: Role of conservative measures, anti-arrhythmic agents, and charcoal hemoperfusion. *Am J Med* 76:854, 1984.

Hendeles L, Massanari M, Weinberger M: Update of the pharmacodynamics and pharmacokinetics of theophylline. *Chest* 88:103S, 1985.

Ogilvier I: Clinical pharmacokinetics of theophylline. *Clin Pharmacokinet* 3:267, 1978.

Olson KR, Benowitz NL, Woo OF, et al: Theophylline overdose: Acute single ingestion vs. chronic repeated over-medication. *Ann Emerg Med* 3:386, 1985.

Paloucek FP, Rodvold KA: Evaluation of theophylline overdose and toxicities. *Ann Emerg Med* 17:135, 1988.

Sessler CN: Theophylline toxicity: Clinical features of 116 consecutive cases. *Am J Med* 88:567, 1990.

107
DIGITALIS GLYCOSIDES

Mark A. Kirk

For centuries, digitalis glycosides have been recognized for their medicinal benefits and potential toxicity. Digitalis preparations are used most commonly in the treatment of supraventricular tachyarrhythmias and congestive heart failure. In addition to their availability as pharmaceuticals, cardiac glycosides are also found in plants such as foxglove, oleander, and lily of the valley, as well as the skin of certain toads. It is important that physicians recognize digitalis toxicity because potentially fatal cardiac arrhythmias can develop. Prompt administration of a highly specific antidote, digoxin-specific Fab fragments, can reverse otherwise fatal toxicity.

Digitalis has a narrow margin between therapeutic and toxic effects. Toxicity results from an exaggeration of its therapeutic effects. Digitalis binds to a specific receptor site on the cell membrane, inactivating the sodium–potassium adenosine triphosphate pump (Na^+–K^+-ATPase). This pump concentrates sodium extracellularly and potassium intracellularly to maintain the electrochemical membrane potential so vital to conduction tissues. When Na^+–K^+ ATPase is inhibited, the sodium–calcium exchanger removes accumulated intracellular sodium in exchange for calcium. This exchange increases sarcoplasmic calcium and is the mechanism responsible for the positive inotropic effect of digitalis. Inhibition of the Na^+–K^+-ATPase pump also results in an increase in extracellular potassium. Digitalis increases vagal tone and decreases conduction through the AV node. In toxic doses, these effects result in various bradyarrhythmias. Slowing of the conduction tissue, along with a decreased refractory period of the myocardium, increases automaticity. Intracellular calcium overload creates transient depolarizations, giving rise to triggered arrhythmias.

Digoxin is currently the most widely used digitalis preparation. It is rapidly absorbed from the gastrointestinal tract and is primarily eliminated through renal excretion. It has a volume of distribution of 7 to 10 L/kg. The half-life of a therapeutic dose is 36 to 48 h.

PREDISPOSING FACTORS

Patients may have a variety of predisposing factors that increase their susceptibility to toxicity. End-organ sensitivity is seen with increasing age, ischemic heart disease, electrolyte disturbances (hypokalemia, hypomagnesemia, and hypercalcemia), and hypoxia. Chronic illnesses such as heart disease, renal dysfunction, hepatic dysfunction, hypothyroidism, and chronic obstructive pulmonary disease may increase susceptibility. Drug interactions, most notably quinidine and calcium-channel blockers, potentiate digitalis toxicity.

CLINICAL PRESENTATION AND EVALUATION

Digitalis glycoside toxicity is determined by evaluating the entire clinical picture. The history, physical examination, and laboratory provide important clues, with no single element to exclude or confirm the diagnosis.

When a poisoned patient presents to the emergency department, make every effort to obtain critical information about the patient and the events surrounding the present illness. Determine if toxicity is due to an accidental ingestion, massive intentional ingestion, or chronic toxicity from therapeutic use of digitalis. If the ingestion is intentional, historic information may be inaccurate or incomplete, and coingestants should be suspected. The time of ingestion is extremely helpful in interpreting laboratory information. In addition, current medications and preexisting medical conditions may identify risk factors that potentiate digitalis toxicity. Since various plants contain digitalis glycosides and cause similar toxicity to medicinal forms, attempt to identify any ingested plants accurately.

Carefully evaluate the cardiac, neurologic, and gastrointestinal systems for clues of developing toxicity. Cardiac arrhythmias are nonspecific and may be life-threatening. Suspect digitalis toxicity whenever tachyarrhythmias with AV block or AV block with junctional escape rhythms are identified. The most common arrhythmia is frequent premature ventricular beats, especially in a diseased heart. Bidirectional ventricular tachycardia, a narrow complex tachycardia with right bundle branch morphology, is specific for digitalis toxicity, but is rare.

In addition to cardiac manifestations, gastrointestinal distress, dizziness, headache, weakness, syncope, and seizures may occur. Reported psychiatric symptoms include confusion, disorientation, delirium, and hallucinations. Patients with toxicity have reported seeing yellow–green halos.

Laboratory Evaluation

Serum potassium and serum digoxin levels will assist in providing information necessary to make adequate therapeutic decisions. Acute poisoning of the Na^+–K^+-ATPase pump and a general release of potassium from many tissues results in markedly elevated serum potassium levels. In fact, the serum potassium may be a better indicator of end-organ toxicity and a better prognostic indicator than the serum digoxin level in the acutely poisoned patient. A high incidence of hyperkalemia has been noted in patients with severe acute poisoning. In one case report, a potassium level of 13 mEq/L resulted from acute digitalis toxicity in a previously healthy patient. Hyperkalemia is uncommon in chronically poisoned patients.

Accepted therapeutic serum digoxin levels are 0.5 to 2.0 ng/mL. In most laboratories, the serum digoxin level is not part of the routine toxicologic screen and must be requested specifically.

Serum digoxin levels in both acute and chronic toxicity should be interpreted in the overall clinical context. In acute exposures, digoxin is absorbed into the plasma compartment and then redistributed slowly into the tissue compartment. Hence, severe poisoning may be present *without* high serum digoxin levels. Serum levels are most reliable when obtained after 6 h, when distribution is complete. Patients with clinical evidence of chronic digitalis toxicity show considerable overlap in serum digoxin levels when compared to those without toxicity. A "therapeutic" level does not exclude toxicity, especially when predisposing factors to toxicity are present. Conversely, levels above the upper limits of normal do not always cause toxicity.

A positive serum assay is diagnostic of acute ingestion if the patient has not received digitalis glycosides therapeutically. The rare exception is in the presence of digoxin-like immunoreactive substance that has been detected in neonates and patients with renal insufficiency or hepatic dysfunction. In addition, naturally occurring digitalis glycosides from plants and animals can cross-react with the digoxin assay. The degree of cross-reactivity is unknown, and no correlation has been established between serum levels of these glycosides and toxicity.

Additional laboratory evaluation includes the determination of adequate oxygenation, renal and hepatic function, and electrolyte determinations in addition to potassium. Continuous electrocardiographic monitoring is essential to detect arrhythmias and evidence of hyperkalemia.

Differences in the Presentation of Acute and Chronic Toxicity

A distinct clinical presentation exists for both acute and chronic digitalis glycoside toxicity (Table 107-1). Acute poisoning most often results from accidental or intentional ingestion. There may be an asymptomatic period of several hours prior to development of symptoms. Gastrointestinal symptoms are often the earliest manifestation of toxicity. In

Table 107-1. Clinical Presentation of Digitalis Toxicity

Acute Toxicity
Clinical history: Intentional or accidental ingestion
GI effects: Nausea and vomiting
CNS effects: Headache, dizziness, confusion, coma
Cardiac effects: Predominately supraventricular tachyarrhythmias with AV block bradyarrhythmias
Electrolyte abnormalities: Hyperkalemia
Digoxin level: Marked elevation
Chronic toxicity
Clinical history: Typically an elderly cardiac patient taking diuretics. May have renal insufficiency
GI effects: Nausea, vomiting, diarrhea, abdominal pain
CNS effects: Fatigue, weakness, confusion, delirium, coma
Cardiac effects: Ventricular arrhythmias are common. Almost any ventricular or supraventricular arrhythmia can occur.
Electrolyte abnormalities: Hypokalemia or normal serum K, hypomagnesemia
Digoxin level: Minimally elevated or ''therapeutic'' range

the early period of toxicity, increased vagal tone produces cardiac arrhythmias that are typically bradyarrhythmias, or supraventricular arrhythmias with AV block; however, life-threatening ventricular arrhythmias may develop at any stage in an acute massive ingestion. Acute toxicity most closely correlates with hyperkalemia, and correlates poorly with the serum digoxin level.

Chronic toxicity occurs most typically in the elderly cardiac patient on digoxin and diuretics. Signs and symptoms may mimic more common illnesses such as influenza or gastroenteritis. An altered mental status or psychiatric symptoms may not be recognized as signs of digitalis toxicity. Almost any cardiac arrhythmia may be seen, but ventricular arrhythmias occur more frequently in chronic than in acute poisonings. The serum digoxin level is not an accurate predictor of toxicity and the serum potassium is usually decreased or normal.

MANAGEMENT

The basic emergency department management of any poisoned patient includes general supportive care, treatment of specific complications of toxicity, prevention of further drug absorption, enhanced drug elimination, antidote administration, and safe disposition (Table 107-2). Patients with intentional or accidental ingestions may present with no symptoms. Assume the worst and anticipate life-threatening complications of toxicity. Focus the management of the asymptomatic patient on preventing drug absorption and closely monitoring for development of toxicity. Provide continuous cardiac monitoring, intravenous access, and frequent reevaluations for any patient with a potentially toxic ingestion of digitalis. Toxicity may not develop for several hours after an acute ingestion; therefore, extended observation is required for anyone with a confirmed ingestion. Admission to the intensive care unit (ICU) and frequent reassessment is required for any patient developing signs of toxicity.

Treatment of Life-Threatening Conditions

Approach the symptomatic patient methodically. Ensure a patent airway, adequate ventilation, and effective circulation. Rapidly correct conditions such as hypoxia, hypoglycemia, hypovolemia, and electrolyte abnormalities.

Conventional and antidote therapy are available to treat digitalis-induced arrhythmias. Atropine and cardiac pacing (external and transvenous) have been used successfully in treating bradyarrhythmias. Because of phenytoin's ability to accelerate conduction at the AV node, it has been considered the antiarrhythmic of choice for digitalis-induced ventricular arrhythmias. Both phenytoin and lidocaine depress ventricular automaticity and increase the fibrillation threshold. Bretylium has suppressed arrhythmias effectively in the clinical setting,

Table 107-2. Treatment of Digitalis Glycoside Poisoning

Asymptomatic patients
Obtain accurate history
Continuous cardiac monitoring
Intravenous access
Gastrointestinal decontamination:
Activated charcoal (1 g/kg)
±Gastric lavage
Frequent reevaluation
Fab fragments at bedside (Calculate dose required for emergent use)
Symptomatic patients
ABCs
Intravenous access
Continuous cardiac monitoring
Treat altered mental status
Oxygen
Dextrose (thiamine)
Naloxone
Arrhythmias
Bradyarrhythmias
Atropine (0.5–2.0 mg IV)
Pacemaker (external or transvenous)
Fab fragments (IV infusion)
Ventricular arrhythmias
Fab fragments (IV infusion or bolus)
Phenytoin (15 mg/kg—infuse no faster than 25 mg/min) or lidocaine (1 mg/kg)
Magnesium sulfate (2–4 g IV)
Electrocardioversion (10–25 W-s—use as a last resort)
Cardiac arrest
CPR
ACLS protocols
Fab fragments (IV bolus—give 10 vials if amount ingested is unknown)
Electrolyte abnormalities
Hyperkalemia
Fab fragments (IV infusion or bolus)
Glucose–insulin
Sodium bicarbonate
Potassium resin binder
Hemodialysis
Avoid calcium chloride
Hypomagnesemia
Evaluate renal status prior to replacement
Magnesium sulfate (2–4 g IV)
Gastrointestinal decontamination
Activated charcoal (1 g/kg then 0.5 g/kg every 4–6 h)
±Gastric lavage

although in a digitalis-toxic animal model, it was found to enhance arrhythmias. Class IA antiarrhythmics, such as quinidine and procainamide, are contraindicated because they depress AV nodal conduction, which in turn, may enhance digitalis-induced cardiac toxicity. Intravenous magnesium has been reported to counteract ventricular irritability in digitalis toxicity. Electrocardioversion may induce intractable ventricular fibrillation and should be considered only as a last resort. If necessary, use a low setting (10 to 25 W-s) and prepare to treat resulting ventricular fibrillation. In severe toxicity, conventional treatment may be unsuccessful. When available, Fab is the treatment of choice for those arrhythmias that are life-threatening and do not respond immediately to conventional therapy.

Hyperkalemia may be life-threatening and needs immediate treatment. Treatment includes intravenous administration of dextrose, insulin, sodium bicarbonate, and enteral administration of a potassium-binding resin. Calcium chloride administration in the face of digitalis-induced hyperkalemia may enhance cardiac toxicity and should be avoided. If digitalis-induced hyperkalemia is not rapidly corrected by conventional therapy, then Fab fragments are indicated for reversal.

Gastrointestinal Decontamination and Enhanced Elimination

After initial stabilization, administer activated charcoal to prevent further drug absorption and consider performing gastric lavage. Ipecac has no role in the emergency department management of digitalis glycoside poisoning. Evacuate the stomach with gastric lavage in patients presenting with massive intentional ingestions. When cardiac toxicity is evident, vagal stimulation may worsen bradyarrhythmias or produce asystole, but the presence of cardiac toxicity is not a contraindication to gastric lavage. Activated charcoal effectively adsorbs digitalis glycosides and should be administered to any patient with a potentially toxic ingestion.

Multiple doses of activated charcoal enhance elimination of oral and intravenous digoxin. Although resin binders effectively enhance digitalis elimination, they have no advantage over activated charcoal. Forced diuresis, hemodialysis, or hemoperfusion do not enhance elimination of digitalis.

Antidote Therapy

A unique aspect in the management of digitalis poisoning is the availability of drug-specific antibodies. Digoxin-specific Fab (Digibind) is the IgG fragment of sheep antidigoxin antibodies. Fab fragments distribute widely throughout tissues and remove digitalis from tissue-binding sites. In a series of 150 severely poisoned patients, 90 percent showed reversal or significant improvement in life-threatening arrhythmias and hyperkalemia after Fab-fragment administration. Those patients developing cardiac arrest prior to Fab administration had a 50 percent survival, which is significantly improved from survival by treatment with conventional therapies. Indications for digitalis-specific Fab fragments are (1) ventricular arrhythmias, (2) bradyarrhythmias unresponsive to standard therapy, and (3) hyperkalemia in excess of 5.5 mEq/L.

Fab fragment therapy should be immediately accessible at the bedside to all patients presenting with acute massive ingestions or with risk factors for enhanced toxicity such as old age and preexisting cardiac disease. Serum digoxin levels should not be the sole indication for Fab-fragment administration. Fab fragments have also been reported to be beneficial in treating digitoxin and oleander poisonings.

The Fab fragment dosage is based on an estimation of total body load of digoxin. This can be determined from the serum digoxin level or based on the estimated dose ingested.

$$\text{Total body load} = \frac{\text{serum digoxin level} \times 5.6\ \text{L/kg} \times \text{Patient's wt (kg)}}{1000}$$

$$= \text{milligrams ingested} \times 0.80\ \text{(bioavailability)}$$

It is assumed that an equimolar dose of Fab fragments is required for neutralization. One vial (40 mg) of Fab fragments binds 0.6 mg of digoxin. The number of vials required can be calculated by dividing the total body burden by 0.6. In one series, a mean dose of 480 mg (12 vials) was required to treat 34 seriously digitalis-toxic patients effectively. When the ingested dose is unknown, 10 vials are recommended as initial treatment in life-threatening situations. Fab fragments are administered intravenously through a 0.22-μm filter over 30 min, except in cardiac arrest, where it may be given as a bolus. In many cases, clinical improvement in cardiac rhythm occurs within 1 h of antidote administration. Any patient receiving Fab fragments requires ICU observation for at least 24 h.

Fab fragment administration has resulted in few adverse effects. Cardiogenic shock has been reported in patients dependent upon digoxin for inotropic support. In addition, ventricular response to atrial fibrillation may be increased. Hypokalemia may develop rapidly as digitalis toxicity is reversed. In a series of 150 patients treated with Fab fragments, delayed or acute hypersensitivity reactions were not observed. Since Fab is derived from sheep protein, skin testing should be considered in patients with a strong history of allergies. If cardiac arrest is imminent, Fab fragment infusion should not be delayed for skin testing.

The serum level has no correlation with clinical toxicity following Fab administration because the assay measures bound and unbound digoxin. Minutes after Fab-fragment administration, the free digoxin level falls to zero, but the total serum digoxin level (bound to Fab fragments) increases 10 to 20-fold. The Fab–digoxin complex is eliminated by renal excretion. In the case of renal failure, the complex may persist in the circulation for prolonged periods.

BIBLIOGRAPHY

Antman EM, Wenger TL, Butler VP, et al: Treatment of 150 cases of life-threatening digitalis intoxication with digoxin-specific Fab antibody fragments. *Circulation* 81:1744, 1990.

Bismuth C, Gaultier M, Conso F, et al: Hyperkalemia in acute digitalis poisoning: Prognostic significance and therapeutic implications. *Clin Toxicol* 6:153, 1973.

Rainey PM: Effects of digoxin immune Fab (ovine) on digoxin immunoassays. *Am J Clin Pathol* 92:779, 1989.

Reisdorff EJ, Clark MR, Walters BL: Acute digitalis poisoning: The role of intravenous magnesium sulfate. *J Emerg Med* 4:463, 1986.

Sharff JA, Bayer MJ: Acute and chronic digitalis toxicity: Presentation and treatment. *Ann Emerg Med* 11:327, 1982.

Shumaik GM, Wu AW, Ping AC: Oleander poisoning: Treatment with digoxin-specific Fab antibody fragments. *Ann Emerg Med* 17:732, 1988.

Smith TW, Butler VP, Haber E, et al: Treatment of life-threatening digitalis intoxication with digoxin-specific Fab antibody fragments: Experience in 26 cases. *N Engl J Med* 307:1357, 1982.

Smith TW: Digitalis: Mechanisms of action and clinical use. *N Engl J Med* 318:358, 1988.

Smolarz A, Roesch E, Lenz E, et al: Digoxin specific antibody (Fab) fragments in 34 cases of severe digitalis intoxication. *Clin Toxicol* 23:327, 1985.

Springer M, Olsen KR, Feaster W: Acute massive digoxin overdose: Survival without use of digitalis-specific antibodies. *Am J Emerg Med* 4:364, 1986.

Wenger TL, Butler VP, Haber E, et al: Treatment of 63 severely digitalis-toxic patients with digoxin-specific antibody fragments. *J Am Coll Cardiol* 5:118A, 1985.

Zucker AR, Lacina AJ, DasGupta DS, et al: Fab fragments of digoxin-specific antibodies used to reverse ventricular fibrillation induced by digoxin ingestion in a child. *Pediatrics* 70:468, 1982.

108
BETA BLOCKERS AND CALCIUM CHANNEL BLOCKERS

Peter Viccellio
Mark Henry

CALCIUM CHANNEL BLOCKERS

Pharmacology and Properties of Agents

The selective calcium channel blockers are a pharmacologically and structurally diverse group of drugs. They include the phenyalkylamines (verapamil and gallopamil), the dihydropyridines (nifedipine, nicardipine, and nimodipine), the benzothiazepines (diltiazem), and diphenylpiperazines (cinnarizine and flunarizine). Membrane transport of calcium through "slow channels" during the inward excitation–contraction phase in smooth muscle is blocked by calcium channel blockers. In particular, cardiac muscle and vascular smooth muscle, heavily dependent upon the influx of calcium for contraction, and the cardiac conduction system are affected.

Calcium channel blockers vary in their effect on these cells. Verapamil has its greatest effect on the conduction system, depressing sinus node activity and conduction through the atrioventricular (AV) node, with lesser effects on the myocardium and peripheral vasculature. Nifedipine is virtually a pure peripheral vasodilator at therapeutic doses. Diltiazem is intermediate in its effects between verapamil and nifedipine. Nimodipine is most similar to nifedipine in action but has a special affinity for the cerebral vasculature. These agents have been used as antihypertensive and antianginal agents. Verapamil is also used in the treatment of supraventricular arrhythmias. Nimodipine appears to decrease ischemic neurologic complications associated with subarachnoid hemorrhage Other clinical problems where the use of calcium channel blockers are currently under investigation include irritable bowel syndrome, migraine, arterial peripheral vascular disease, Raynaud's phenomena, and asthma.

Presentation

The predominant symptoms in calcium channel blocker overdose include bradyarrhythmias, myocardial depression, and peripheral vasodilation. Symptoms depend upon the amount and type of calcium channel blocker ingested, its route of ingestion, the patient's disease (particularly cardiovascular), and the presence of other medications or drugs which may modify the presenting symptoms. Patients already receiving, or who concomitantly ingest β blockers, may experience toxicity at lower doses of calcium channel blockers. The clinical presentation can be precipitous, with sudden deterioration of vital signs in an otherwise stable patient. Typically, initial symptoms occur 1 to 5 h postingestion. This may be altered with newer long-acting, slow-absorption preparations. With intravenous administration, symptoms occur within minutes. Patients who respond to initial treatment frequently will experience subsequent deterioration.

Nausea and vomiting are frequent after significant ingestions. Lethargy and coma have been noted. In addition, seizures have been described with overdoses. Whether this is a direct effect of the drug or a consequence of hypoperfusion is unknown. Hyperglycemia can occur and, in some cases, has been a major complication of ingestion. Verapamil, in particular, blocks calcium entry into pancreatic islet beta cells, resulting in impairment of insulin release and hyperglycemia.

In patients treated with intravenous (IV) verapamil to terminate a supraventricular tachyarrhythmia, clinical studies have confirmed that pretreatment with calcium will block the verapamil-induced peripheral vasodilation but will not block the effect at the AV node. Some evidence suggests that binding at the AV node is greater than at other sites. This may explain the difficulty sometimes encountered in treatment of bradyarrhythmias induced by this agent and the frequent need for temporary pacing. In the pregnant woman, verapamil apparently crosses the placenta and may slow the fetal heart rate. The clinical significance of this is unknown. The negative inotropic effect, particularly of verapamil, may precipitate congestive heart failure or pulmonary edema.

Nifedipine is less likely to cause heart block, although this has been reported, and may not be unusual, with serious ingestions. Hypotension is usually primarily due to peripheral vasodilation, and patients typically will develop a tachycardic response to the hypotension. Sublingual nifedipine will cause a drop in the blood pressure within 5 min.

Diagnosis

History and clinical suspicion are generally the only modalities available to the physician confronting this diagnosis. The characteristic presentation of hypotension and sinus bradycardia, sinus arrest, or varying degrees of heart block are characteristic of calcium channel blocker overdoses but are also characteristic of several other drugs, including β-blocker and digoxin overdoses. Care should be exercised in the use of intravenous calcium if digoxin overdose is suspected, given the propensity for calcium to worsen heart block in digoxin toxicity.

Electrocardiographic changes other than varying degrees of block and bradyarrhythmias include prominent U waves, low voltage T waves, and nonspecific ST-TW changes. Block has been reported up to 24 h postpresentation. QT prolongation, although described, is not a usual finding in calcium channel blocker overdoses.

Laboratory Analysis

Routine laboratory analysis should include electrolytes, an arterial blood gas, and an electrocardiogram. Although calcium levels have been recommended, their usefulness is unclear, and levels typically are normal.

The need for routine toxicologic screening should be determined by the treating physician. Because of lack of immediate availability of results, such screens have little use in calcium channel blocker toxicity per se. Routine toxicologic screening often will not test for the presence of calcium blocking agents but may be useful for determining the presence of other agents. Levels of specific agents may be requested should retrospective confirmation be desired by the physician. From cases reported in the literature, serum levels only approximate clinical manifestations.

Management and Treatment

General Management

The treating clinician must keep in mind the potentially abrupt change in clinical status often seen with overdose of calcium channel agents. The patient should be kept in a closely monitored environment, with equipment and drugs available for airway management and treatment of hypotension and bradyarrhythmias.

Evacuation and Elimination

Given the possibility of emetic agents having their peak effect as the patient becomes acutely unstable, the hazards of the use of emetics will outweigh their usefulness and should be avoided unless administered within 30 min of ingestion. In addition, emetics enhance vagal activity and, as such, could worsen bradyarrhythmias.

Gastric lavage may have some use in calcium channel blocker overdose, particularly if performed within the first 30 min. Insertion of the nasogastric tube can cause vagal stimulation, however. Because the clinical picture can change rapidly, meticulous attention to airway protection is mandatory. Lavage should be performed in clinically symptomatic patients after establishment of a secure airway.

Multiple-dose charcoal is recommended increasingly for all suspected overdoses, until clinical symptoms have resolved. There is no clear evidence that multiple-dose charcoal hastens the elimination of calcium channel blockers. Cathartic should be administered with the first dose and subsequently on an as-needed basis. Given the potential for prolonged absorption and delayed clinical symptoms in ingestions of long-acting preparations, some recent articles have promoted whole bowel irrigation for their removal.

Specific/Antidotal

Calcium chloride ($CaCl_2$) 10% 10 to 20 mL (10 to 30 mg/kg in children) is the mainstay of therapy for calcium channel toxicity. Calcium gluconate 10% 0.2 to 0.5 mL/kg per dose (up to 10 mL per dose) also has been used but does not produce as predictable a rise in serum calcium or clinical effect as does calcium chloride. Dosage is based on responses in clinical case reports, and neither the proper dosage, frequency, or maximal safe dose have been established. Calcium should be administered by slow intravenous push over several minutes. Side effects include peripheral vasodilatation with hypotension, particularly with rapid bolus injection; arrhythmia, particularly in those patients taking digoxin; and local tissue necrosis from IV infiltration. Classic symptoms of sustained hypercalcemia have not been described following IV administration in this setting.

The patient may respond dramatically to this agent, although significant overdoses may require treatment with additional agents such as dopamine, epinephrine, norepinephrine, isoproterenol, and pacing. It is possible that a combination of these agents may be synergistic. Subsequent deterioration, if the patient has shown a response, should be treated with repeat doses of $CaCl_2$ or continuous calcium infusion. An infusion of 5 mmol/h has been used with success. Interim measurement of serum calcium has been recommended, but the usefulness and frequency of such monitoring has not been established. Monitoring the QT interval is an inaccurate method for determining calcium serum concentrations.

Hypotension may be reversed by infusion of isotonic fluids, but given the potential for calcium channel blocker induced myocardial depression, fluids should be administered with caution.

Intracellular release of calcium from the sarcoplasmic reticulum in cardiac cells can be triggered by β agonists through mechanisms independent of the transmembrane calcium channels. This pathway is not affected by calcium channel blockade and, to a certain degree, allows an alternative pathway for enhancing contractility in significant overdose. In a similar way, α_1-receptors can stimulate contraction of vascular smooth muscle in calcium channel blockade. Dopamine has been used in patients who have had inadequate or no response to $CaCl_2$ at doses as high as 50 μg/kg per minute. Although dobutamine is an effective inotrope, it lacks a vasopressor effect. Also, epinephrine infusion, norepinephrine, and isoproterenol have been used with some success. Stimulation of peripheral α receptors by α agents may be critical in reversing the calcium channel blocker induced peripheral vasodilation. In addition, recent reports of amrinone suggest that it may have some use.

Care should be exercised in administering isoproterenol to patients with coronary artery disease and in patients with idiopathic hypertrophic subaortic stenosis (IHSS). In patients with known IHSS, α agonists may be useful. The maximal appropriate dose of these agents in significant ingestion has not been established. However, the use of these agents in dosages beyond those normally recommended has been reported commonly in the literature without reports of complication from therapy.

Atropine in doses of 0.5 to 1.0 mg (0.01 mg/kg in the pediatric population) has been used to treat symptomatic bradyarrhythmias. Bradyarrhythmias and heart block in this setting are not predominantly vagally mediated, however, and success has been reported only occasionally with this agent.

Some success has been reported with the use of glucagon for heart block and myocardial depression secondary to calcium channel blockade. The mechanism of action involves pathways independent of calcium channels.

Specific antidotal therapy for calcium channel blockade soon may become available in the United States. The drug 4–aminopyridine directly opposes the effects of verapamil. Animal studies have confirmed an immediate reversal of toxic effects of calcium channel blockade by the infusion of 4–aminopyridine, and reports of dramatic success now exist in the medical literature. It is currently available in the US for investigational purposes only.

Transvenous or external pacing may be necessary in those patients not responding to pharmacologic treatment. Also, for those patients whose hemodynamic status is unstable, monitoring of pulmonary wedge pressures and cardiac output becomes necessary.

Seizures are treated, in standard fashion, with diazepam and phenytoin or phenobarbital, if persistent. Seizures appear to be a consequence of hemodynamic instability, which must be corrected aggressively.

Should a patient with accessory conduction pathways, as with Wolff-Parkinson-White or Lown-Ganong-Levine syndrome, receive therapeutic doses of verapamil for treatment of a supraventricular tachyarrhythmia, the patient may sustain a dangerous acceleration of the rate due to antegrade conduction down the accessory pathway. The treatment of such arrhythmias include cardioversion, procainamide, and possibly lidocaine.

Although reports exist describing the use of dialysis and charcoal hemoperfusion, this is not an established or recommended practice. Theoretically, given the large volume of distribution and significant protein binding of these agents, hemoperfusion would not be expected to play a major role in the treatment of such overdoses.

Range of Toxicity

The minimum range of toxicity has not been clearly established and depends upon the particular drug, coingestions, and the underlying host.

Disposition/Follow-Up

Symptoms of toxicity can recur hours after the patient appears stable. Patients with significant ingestions should be admitted to an intensive care unit and observed until symptoms have resolved completely.

β-BLOCKERS

Pharmacology and Properties of Agents

β-blockers frequently are prescribed for hypertension, ischemic heart disease, cardiac arrhythmias, obstructive heart disease, prevention of migraines, control of glaucoma, and other conditions. Within the adrenergic nervous system, α- and β-receptor sites are activated by catecholamines. Stimulation of β_1-receptors increases the force and rate of myocardial contraction, AV node conduction velocity, and increased renin secretion. Stimulation of β_2-receptors promotes relaxation of smooth muscle in blood vessels, bronchi, and the gastrointestinal and genitourinary tract. In addition, β_2 stimulation promotes glycogenolysis from skeletal muscle and glycogenolysis and gluconeogenesis from liver. The β-blockers act as competitive antagonists to catecholamines at β-receptor sites.

Propranolol was the first β-blocker in widespread use, and much of the clinical and overdose experience was gained from case reports and clinical studies of this drug. Propranolol is a nonselective β-blocker, showing equal affinity for both β_1- and β_2-receptors. Other nonselective β-blockers include nadolol, timolol, and pindolol. Selective β-blockers (β_1-antagonists) show a greater relative affinity for

β_1 over β_2 sites and are less likely to cause bronchospasm or interfere with glucose and glycogen metabolism when administered in low doses. Selective β_1-blockers include metroprolol, atenolol, esmolol, and acebutolol. Labetalol blocks α_1 receptors as well as both β_1 and β_2.

Some β-blockers, such as pindolol and acebutolol, also have β-agonist properties. While their agonist property is weaker than the catecholamines, they are capable of stimulating β-receptors, especially when catecholamine levels are low. These agents are said to have intrinsic sympathomimetic activity.

Other properties of importance in interpreting findings and planning therapy in overdose are membrane stabilizing activity and lipid solubility. Propranolol, labetalol, and pindolol are examples of agents which show membrane stabilizing activity or quinidine-like effects in high doses. Lipid solubility, higher in agents like propranolol and low in agents like atenolol and nadolol, may influence the degree of central nervous system effects and utility of hemodialysis in removing the agent in the overdosed patient.

β-blockers can be administered intravenously, orally, and as ophthalmic preparations. Timolol eye drops have caused systemic toxicity and side effects including respiratory arrest, asthma, congestive heart failure, and depression.

Clinical Presentation

β-blockers are absorbed rapidly from the stomach, and the onset of toxicity after oral overdose can occur from 20 min to 1 to 2 h following ingestion. Long-acting preparations may have delayed manifestations.

A patient presenting with bradycardia, AV block, and hypotension should raise consideration of β-blocker toxicity in the differential diagnosis. Sinus bradycardia, first-degree block, widening of the QRS complex, peaked T waves, and ST changes have been reported. Bradycardia, by itself, is not necessarily helpful as a warning sign since slowing of the heart rate and damping of tachycardia in response to stress is seen with therapeutic levels. Tachycardia, while unusual, has been reported with practolol, pindolol, and sotalol. Cardiac output falls, and hypotension results, from both bradycardia and negative inotropy, which in turn, jeopardizes myocardial perfusion, creating a downward spiral.

Changes in mental status are common, ranging from delirium to coma. Coma occurs often in the setting of cardiovascular collapse. It may be less pronounced in overdoses of drugs with smaller volumes of distribution (atenolol) or cardioselective agents. Grand mal seizures have been commonly reported.

Bronchospasm is not a common manifestation of overdose, although it can occur. Respiratory arrest has been described. Congestive heart failure and pulmonary edema are more apt to occur in the patient with underlying heart disease.

Hypoglycemic reactions in unstable diabetics are problematic. Nonselective β-blockers can impair the recovery from hypoglycemia, and all β-blockers can prevent tachycardia, an important warning sign of hypoglycemia. In overdose, hypoglycemia is reported in children but rare in adults.

Laboratory

An electrocardiogram, cardiac monitoring, blood levels of electrolytes, glucose, and tests for renal and liver function are routine. While it is possible to obtain both qualitative and quantitative levels of β-blocker agents, the turnaround time and the variability of response in individual patients require the clinician to rely on clinical judgment in most cases.

Treatment

General

Following general toxicologic principles and providing supportive care with careful monitoring is the mainstay of treatment. To remove drugs in the stomach, gastric lavage is preferred over emesis because of the rapid absorption and onset of toxicity with these agents. Some recommend that gastric lavage be undertaken with pretreatment with atropine to avoid the potential for increased vagal tone to compound the clinical picture. Charcoal administration is recommended and repeat doses may be of value in management of some agents such as atenolol and nadolol.

Specific/Antidotal

Therapy is directed at countering the effects of β-blockade. Agents used include atropine, catecholamines, and glucagon. Isoproterenol, a pure β-receptor stimulant, may aggravate hypotension by its vasodilatory effects. Agents with β_1-selective properties (dobutamine) or combined α- and β-agonist properties (epinephrine, norepinephrine, and dopamine) may be necessary to maintain blood pressure. The optimal doses of these pressors are unknown, but it may be necessary to exceed usual clinical doses in the treatment of overdoses with these agents.

Intravenous glucagon, which enhances myocardial contractility, heart rate, and AV conduction, may be most useful to counteract the bradycardia, conduction defects, and hypotension. It is considered by many to be the drug of choice in the management of these overdoses. The production of intracellular cyclic AMP is reduced with β-blockade. Glucagon stimulates the production of cyclic AMP through nonadrenergic pathways, which probably explains its efficacy. Success has been noted with a bolus dose of 3 to 10 mg or 50 to 150 μg over 1 min, followed by an infusion of 2 to 5 mg/h.

A pacemaker may be necessary if there is no response to pharmacologic therapy. Fluid replacement to combat hypotension should be administered carefully with arterial pressure and Swan-Ganz monitoring as indicated to help guide therapy. In extremis, prolonged cardiopulmonary resuscitation, balloon pump, and even bypass may be indicated. Resuscitation with discharge from the hospital has followed prolonged efforts at resuscitation.

Seizures can be treated with diazepam and, if necessary, phenytoin and/or phenobarbital. Hypoglycemia should be treated with an infusion of glucose and possibly glucagon. Bronchospasm can be treated with a β_2-agonist and aminophylline.

Charcoal hemoperfusion and dialysis may be indicated for agents with a small volume of distribution, low protein binding, and high level of urinary excretion. Agents such as atenolol, nadolol, and acebutolol are reported to be dialyzable.

Range of Toxicity

As with the calcium channel blockers, the minimum range of toxicity has not been established clearly and depends upon the particular drug, coingestions, and the underlying host.

Disposition/Follow-Up

Patients with significant ingestions should be admitted to an intensive care unit and observed until all symptoms have resolved completely.

BIBLIOGRAPHY

Ellenhorn MJ, Barceloux, DG: *Medical Toxicology: Diagnosis and Treatment of Human Poisoning*. Elsevier, New York, 1988.

Frishman W, Jacob H, Eisenberg E, et al: Clinical pharmacology of the new beta-adrenergic blocking drugs. Part 8. Self-poisoning with beta-adrenoceptor blocking agents: Recognition and management. *Am Heart J* 98:798, 1979.

Goldfrank LR, Flomenbaum NE, Lewin NA, et al: *Goldfrank's Toxicologic Emergencies*, 4th ed. Norwalk, Appleton & Lange, 1990.

Gilman AG, Rall TR, Nies AS, et al: *Goodman and Gilman's The Pharmacological Basis of Therapeutics*, 8th ed. New York, Pergamon, 1990.

Henry M, Kay MM, Viccellio P: Cardiogenic shock associated with calcium-channel and beta blockers: Reversal with intravenous calcium chloride. *Am J Emerg Med* 3:334, 1985.

Horowitz BZ, Rhee KJ: Massive verapamil ingestion: A report of two cases and a review of the literature. *Am J Emerg Med* 7:624, 1989.

Lane AS, Woodwad AC, Goldman MR: Massive propranolol overdose poorly responsive to pharmacologic therapy: Use of the intra-aortic balloon pump. *Ann Emerg Med* 16:103, 1987.

Rumack BH (ed): *POISINDEX Information System*. Denver, Micromedex, 1990.

Weinstein RS: Recognition and management of poisoning with beta-adrenergic blocking agents. *Ann Emerg Med* 13:79, 1984.

Wolff F, Breuker KH, Schlensker KH, et al: Prenatal diagnosis and therapy of fetal heart rate anomalies: With a contribution on the placental transfer of verapamil. *J Perinat Med* 8:203, 1980.

109
BENZODIAZEPINES

George M. Bosse

Benzodiazepines are commonly used pharmacologic agents. Indications for their use include the treatment of anxiety, insomnia, seizures, and alcohol withdrawal. They also are used in conscious sedation as well as general anesthesia. There are 14 different generic benzodiazepines approved for use in the United States today (Table 109-1).

Benzodiazepines are frequent agents of accidental and intentional overdose. The 1988 report by the American Association of Poison Control Centers National Data Collection System indicated that in patients over 17 years of age, benzodiazepines accounted for the highest number of toxic exposures, both as a single agent and in combination with other drugs. While the ingestion of benzodiazepines alone appears to result in relatively few deaths, increased morbidity and mortality does result from mixed overdose. Parenteral administration of benzodiazepines may also result in significant complications, particularly respiratory depression and hypotension.

PHARMACOLOGY

A specific benzodiazepine receptor has been identified in the central nervous system (CNS). Specific peripheral receptor sites also have been identified; however, the predominant clinical effects of benzodiazepines are mediated through the CNS receptors. Although not fully characterized, research supports the concept of a neuronal cell-surface protein complex containing a benzodiazepine receptor, a γ-aminobutyric acid (GABA) receptor, and a chloride channel. GABA is an inhibitory neurotransmitter; effects of stimulation of GABA pathways include sedation, anxiolysis, and striated muscle relaxation. Stimulation of the benzodiazepine receptor appears to increase the sensitivity of the GABA receptor complex to stimulation by GABA. The enhancement of GABA transmission by the administration of benzodiazepines is felt to occur by either increasing the affinity of the GABA receptor for its ligand or improving coupling between the GABA receptor and its associated chloride channel. Increased GABA output leads to inhibitory effects throughout the neuroaxis and the resultant typical clinical effects of benzodiazepines. The presence of an endogenous ligand for the benzodiazepine receptor has been proposed but not conclusively identified.

In general, benzodiazepines are well absorbed from the gastrointestinal tract. The onset of action after oral ingestion is limited more by the rate of absorption from the gastrointestinal tract than by the relatively rapid passage from the blood stream into the brain. With the exception of lorazepam and midazolam, intramuscular injection of benzodiazepines results in unpredictable absorption.

Benzodiazepines are all relatively lipid soluble, with some variation among the different agents. Increased lipid solubility is associated with more rapid diffusion across the blood–brain barrier. After single doses, the more highly lipophilic benzodiazepines have a shorter onset of action but also a shorter duration of activity. This short duration of activity occurs because of rapid egress of drug from the brain and blood stream into inactive tissue storage sites. For this reason, the half-life may not be a good indicator of the duration of action in an acute ingestion. As an example, diazepam is a derivative with a long elimination half-life but relatively short duration of action.

Benzodiazepine derivatives undergo metabolism by hepatic biotransformation through either oxidation or conjugation. Several derivatives are metabolized by both oxidative and conjugative processes. Oxidation often results in active metabolities which prolong the biologic half-life of the parent compounds. Conjugation is a rapid process which results in inactive metabolites. Oxidation is more susceptible to impairment by such factors as disease states (e.g., chronic liver disease), population characteristics (old age), and concurrent treatment with drugs that impair oxidizing capacity (e.g., cimetidine, estrogen, isoniazid, ethanol, and phenytoin). Examples of agents that undergo conjugation primarily include oxazepam, lorazepam, and temazepam. Administration of benzodiazepines that undergo conjugation may be safer in susceptible groups.

Selection of a benzodiazepine for use by a physician depends on the clinical properties of the particular derivative. Although individual drugs are marketed for specific conditions, there is considerable overlap of activity. For this reason, some hospital formulary committees have limited the number of available agents.

Table 109-1. Benzodiazepines Approved for Use in the US

Generic Name	Brand Name	$t\frac{1}{2}$ (h)*	Metabolite Characteristics†
Alprazolam	Xanax	6–26	Inactive
Chloridazepoxide	Librium	5–30	Active
Clonazepam	Klonopin	39	Inactive
Chlorazepate dipotassium	Tranxene	1.1–2.9	Active
Diazepam	Valium	20–70	Active
Flurazepam	Dalmane	2–3	Active
Halazepam	Paxipam	14	Active
Lorazepam	Ativan	9–19	Inactive
Midazolam	Versed	2–5	Inactive
Oxazepam	Serax	5.4–9.8	Inactive
Prazepam	Centrax	0.6–2.0	Active
Quazepam	Doral	25–41	Active
Temazepam	Restoril	10–16	Inactive
Triazolam	Halcion	1.6–5.4	Inactive

* Elimination half-life of parent compound.

† Some of the derivatives listed as having inactive metabolites actually are converted to active compounds. However, rapid metabolism occurs, such that there is no appreciable accumulation of active intermediates.

CLINICAL FEATURES

Pure benzodiazepine overdose is notable for the relative lack of serious morbidity and mortality. Most reported cases of serious toxicity have occurred in the setting of coingestion of other agents or with parenteral administration. However, deaths in isolated overdose have been reported and appear to be more likely with the newer short-acting derivatives such as triazolam, alprazolam and temazepam.

The clinical presentation of benzodiazepine intoxication is nonspecific. Clinical assessment also may be difficult because of the frequent coingestion of other agents. Except for additive effects, drug interactions of benzodiazepines with other sedative hypnotics are unusual.

The nonspecific presentation of benzodiazepine toxicity is similar to other sedative hypnotics. However, other agents can have at least a few distinguishing features. Chloral hydrate is known to precipitate cardiac arrhythmias. Ethchlorvinyl can produce prolonged coma and may be suspected by the presence of a vinyllike odor. Glutethimide may give rise to fluctuating levels of CNS impairment and anticholinergic signs. Barbiturates are more likely than benzodiazepines to produce coma and depressant myocardial effects.

The predominant manifestations of benzodiazepines are neurologic. CNS effects include drowsiness, dizziness, slurred speech, confusion, ataxia, and impairment of intellectual function. Frank coma, particularly if prolonged, is atypical and should prompt suspicion of intoxication with other agents or a nontoxin-related medical condition. The elderly are more prone to manifest the CNS effects of benzodiazepines.

Paradoxic reactions, including excitement, anxiety, aggression, hostile behavior, rage, and delirium, are reported but are uncommon. Although unclear, the etiology of such effects is probably not on an idiosyncratic basis. Benzodiazepines may have a disinhibiting effect, which in the presence of extrinsic factors such as environmental frustration, could lead to such actions as aggressive or hostile behavior. Other effects, which are reported and which have unclear etiologies include headache, nausea, vomiting, chest pain, joint pain, diarrhea, and incontinence.

Uncommonly, respiratory depression and hypotension may occur. This generally occurs with either parenteral administration or in the presence of coingestants. Intravenous administration is more likely to cause serious cardiorespiratory effects with rapid administration of large doses. In addition, the elderly and those with underlying cardiorespiratory disease are more susceptible to adverse effects of IV administration. The use of propylene glycol as a diluent in parenteral preparations of diazepam has also been implicated as a factor in cardiorespiratory arrest.

Extrapyramidal reactions have been associated with the use of benzodiazepines. Various allergic, hepatotoxic, and hematologic reactions also have been reported; however, these are infrequent. In general, benzodiazepines have no long-term organ-system toxicity other than what can be ascribed to indirect effects from CNS or cardiorespiratory depression.

Laboratory data in benzodiazepine ingestion is of limited value. Serum benzodiazepine levels are not indicated routinely as they do not correlate well with the clinical state. Qualitative testing may be helpful, but the laboratory may not test routinely for all available derivatives. Familiarity with laboratory capabilities at the particular institution is essential.

MANAGEMENT

Benzodiazepines often are ingested with other agents, and the history frequently is inaccurate. Therefore, administration of concentrated dextrose, thiamine, and naloxone should be considered in such patients when depressed or altered mental status is present. Induction of emesis should be avoided in benzodiazepine overdose as CNS depression may ensue. Gastric lavage is safer and is recommended if the amount ingested is felt to be large or in coingestions with toxic agents. Activated charcoal binds benzodiazepines effectively and should be administered in most situations. Elimination enhancement by forced diuresis, hemodialysis, or hemoperfusion is not effective, and most patients do not manifest toxicity serious enough to warrant consideration of such measures. The patient should be monitored closely for CNS and respiratory depression. If CNS depression persists or is profound, other agents or conditions must be considered.

To date, the management of benzodiazepine ingestion has been largely supportive in nature. Flumazenil, a unique selective antagonist of the central effects of benzodiazepines, is now in clinical use in several countries outside the United States. Trials investigating the use of flumazenil for reversal of benzodiazepine overdose as well as benzodiazepine-induced conscious sedation and general anesthesia have been conducted in the United States. These results, as well as the non-US experience, have been encouraging. Its use in benzodiazepine toxicity may obviate the need for intubation and respiratory support. Its use as a diagnostic aid in obscure alterations of mental status may reduce the need for expensive and invasive procedures (e.g., computed tomography or lumbar puncture). Potential concerns include the precipitation of withdrawal manifestations in patients receiving chronic benzodiazepine therapy and the possibility of seizures in coingestions of agents that lower the seizure threshold (e.g., tricyclic antidepressants).

BENZODIAZEPINE ABUSE AND DEPENDENCE

Over the last two decades, benzodiazepine abuse and addiction has been a common public concern. Genuine physiologic addiction to benzodiazepines may occur, particularly with prolonged and high doses. However, the abuse potential of benzodiazepines appears to be low in comparison with agents such as cocaine, opiates, and barbiturates. Benzodiazepine abuse usually occurs in individuals with a history of abuse of other psychoactive drugs. Primary drug abuse with benzodiazepines is not common.

Benzodiazepine withdrawal may occur upon abrupt discontinuation and is more likely in patients with prolonged use and high doses. Because of the long biologic half-life of several derivatives, withdrawal manifestations may not occur for several days to over 1 week after the benzodiazepine is discontinued. Unfortunately, it is often difficult to distinguish between withdrawal and underlying symptoms for which the drugs were prescribed initially.

Reported withdrawal manifestations include anxiety, irritability, insomnia, nausea, vomiting, tremor, sweating, and anorexia. Serious manifestations, including confusion, disorientation, psychosis, and seizures, also have been reported. For patients with an acute organic brain syndrome, a history of possible benzodiazepine withdrawal should always be pursued. Withdrawal reactions may be avoided by dose tapering. Treatment of withdrawal reactions may be accomplished by drug substitution or by reintroduction of a benzodiazepine and subsequent tapering.

BIBLIOGRAPHY

Amrein R, Leishman B, Bentzinger C, et al: Flumazenil in benzodiazepine antagonism: Actions and clinical use in intoxications and anaesthesiology. *Med Toxicol* 2:411, 1987.

Greenblatt DJ, Shader RI, Abernathy DR: Current status of benzodiazepines. *N Engl J Med* 309:354, 1983.

Hojer J, Baehrendtz S, Gustafsson L: Benzodiazepine poisoning: Experience of 702 admissions to an intensive care unit during a 14 year period. *J Intern Med* 226:117, 1989.

Litovitz TL, Schmitz BF, Holm KC: 1988 Annual Report of the American Association of Poison Control Centers National Data Collection System. *Am J Emer Med* 7:495, 1989.

Mohler H, Okada T: Benzodiazepine receptor: Demonstration in the central nervous system. *Science* 198:849, 1977.

Noyes R, Garvey MJ, Cook BL, et al: Benzodiazepine withdrawal: A review of the evidence. *J Clin Psychiatry* 49:382, 1988.

Rall TW: Hypnotics and sedatives: Ethanol, in Goodman AG, Rall TW, Nies AS, et al: *Goodman and Gilman's The Pharmacological Basis of Therapeutics,* 8th ed. New York, Pergamon, 1990, pp 345–383.

Roberts JR, Tafuri JA: Benzodiazepines, in Haddad LM, Winchester JF: *Clinical Management of Poisoning and Drug Overdose,* 2d ed. Philadelphia, WB Saunders, 1990, pp 800–820.

Schauben JL: Benzodiazepines. *Top Emerg Med* 7:39, 1985.

Woods JH, Katz JL, Winger G: Use and abuse of benzodiazepines: issues relevant to prescribing. *JAMA* 260:3476, 1988.

110
NONSTEROIDAL ANTIINFLAMMATORY AGENTS

Richard F. Clark

The use of nonsteroidal antiinflammatory agents (NSAIDs) has increased rapidly since their introduction in the 1960s. Today they are prescribed widely for their analgesic, antiinflammatory, and antipyretic properties. Over-the-counter preparations of ibuprofen are now available in the United States, and poisonings involving these medications are becoming more common. In 1988, 29,293 exposures to NSAIDs were reported to the American Association of Poison Control Centers. Of these, only 76 resulted in major outcomes (effects potentially life threatening, lasting longer than 24 h, or resulting in permanent sequelae), and only six (0.02 percent) patients died. Most of these deaths were mixed ingestions. Severe morbidity and mortality associated with ingestions of these products is infrequent.

NSAIDs include both salicylates and nonsalicylates (Table 110-1). This chapter focuses on the nonsalicylate group, of which there are four major classes: acetic acids, fenamic acids, oxicams, and propionic acids. Diflunisal is a difluorophenyl derivative of salicylic acid that produces toxicity in overdose similar to that of members of the nonsalicylate group and will be included in this chapter.

PHARMACOKINETICS

Absorption and Distribution

NSAIDs are rapidly absorbed from the gastrointestinal (GI) tract, with maximum concentrations appearing in the blood within 1 to 2 h. Almost all are greater than 90 percent protein bound and are distributed to about 10 percent of body weight. Only free fractions of NSAIDs (normally less than 1 percent) are available for pharmacologic activity and metabolism. Elderly patients, and those with renal and hepatic disease or congestive heart failure, tend to have less circulating protein to bind free drug. These patients often have elevated levels of free NSAIDs in their circulation and develop adverse reactions at lower doses.

Table 110-1. Trade Names of Common NSAIDs Marketed in the United States

Chemical Class	Compound	Trade Name
Acetic acids		
	Diclofenac	Voltaren
	Indomethacin	Indocin
	Sulindac	Clinoril
	Tolmetin	Tolectin
Propionic acids		
	Fluribuprofen	Ansaid
	Fenoprofen	Nalfon
	Ibuprofen	Motrin, Advil
	Ketoprofen	Orudis
	Naproxen	Naprosyn
	Naproxen sodium	Anaprox
Fenamic acids		
	Mefenamic acid	Ponstel
	Meclofenamate sodium	Meclomen
Oxicams		
	Piroxicam	Feldene
Salicylic acid derivatives		
	Diflunisal	Dolobid

Metabolism and Elimination

NSAIDs can undergo hydroxylation and oxidation but are mostly metabolized through conjugation with glucuronic acid. Renal excretion of unchanged drug is only from 1 to 5 percent. Renal clearance and elimination half-life vary among NSAIDs, producing serum half-lives ranging from 1.5 h for tolmetin to 50 h for piroxicam. The significant difference in half-life is related to clearance rather than volume of distribution. The duration of symptoms after toxic ingestion of NSAIDs such as piroxicam may, therefore, be prolonged.

MECHANISM OF TOXICITY AND CLINICAL PRESENTATION

NSAIDs reversibly block the enzyme cyclooxygenase, interrupting the conversion of arachidonic acid to prostaglandins within cell membranes. Prostaglandins mediate the inflammatory cascade within the body and are responsible for other physiologic actions such as dilating renal blood vessels, inhibiting gastric acid production, stimulating gastric bicarbonate and mucin secretion, and promoting sodium and water excretion. Interference with these physiologic actions leads to the significant adverse drug reaction profile of NSAIDs. All NSAIDs can cause GI intolerance, nephrotoxicity, headache, tinnitus, peripheral edema, and platelet dysfunction in therapeutic doses. Toxic ingestions most often manifest as mild drowsiness and gastrointestinal upset. No toxic syndrome is characteristic of all NSAIDs.

Gastrointestinal

Prostacyclin appears to have cytoprotective effects on gastric mucosa. Inhibition of prostacyclin either chronically or in acute poisonings with NSAIDs may impair this protective mucosal barrier. All available NSAIDs can produce or aggravate peptic ulcer disease and cause nausea, vomiting, and epigastric pain both in therapeutic use and overdose. Elderly patients appear to be more susceptible. The relative risk of GI hemorrhage in patients taking NSAIDs therapeutically may be as much as twice that of the general population.

Indomethacin is suggested to cause GI side effects most frequently among all NSAIDs and has been shown to produce ileal and jejunal ulcers in addition to gastric lesions. The fenamic acids and diclofenac also can induce small bowel erosions, and this may be in part responsible for the high incidence (10 to 25 percent) of diarrhea reported in patients taking these agents.

Acute pancreatitis has been reported in therapeutic use of sulindac. The mechanism of this toxicity is unclear.

Renal

In disease states such as congestive heart failure and cirrhosis, and in volume-contracted patients taking diuretics, renal prostaglandins dilate the renal vasculature to maintain the glomerular filtration rate (GFR). NSAIDs inhibit this compensatory mechanism, resulting in renal vasoconstriction. Although all NSAIDs can produce fluid retention and nephrotoxicity in these patients, indomethacin has been suggested to cause renal insufficiency and hypertension more often at therapeutic doses than other agents.

Renal vasoconstriction may also be responsible for nephrotoxicity following acute NSAID poisonings. Acute renal failure has developed after massive overdoses of fenoprofen and ibuprofen.

A second type of renal toxicity from NSAIDs is the development of hyperkalemia, usually accompanied by a hyperchloremic metabolic acidosis. The etiology is felt to be the inhibition of prostaglandin-dependent secretion of renin and aldosterone, leading to a hyporenin–hypoaldosterone state. These effects may be noted in the absence of alterations in BUN or creatinine. Again, indomethacin is cited most commonly in generating this type of nephrotoxicity.

Finally, a nephrogenic hypersensitivity reaction leading to acute interstitial nephritis has been described with chronic therapeutic doses

Table 110-2. Clinical Findings Reported Following Toxic Ingestions of NSAIDs

Findings	Acetic Acids	Propionic Acids	Fenamic Acids	Oxicams	Diflunisal
Gastrointestinal					
Nausea	‡	‡	†	†	†
Vomiting	‡	‡	†	†	†
Diarrhea	†	*	†		†
Bloody diarrhea			†	†	†
Abdominal pain	‡	‡		*	
Gastritis	*				†
Hematemesis	*	†		*	
Neurologic					
Miosis		†			
Headache	†	†			
Blurred vision		†	*	*	*
Tinnitus	†	†			
Irritability			‡	*	
Drowsiness	‡	‡	†	†	‡
Nystagmus	*	†			
Ataxia		†			
Diplopia	*	†			
Tremor				*	
Agitation	†		‡	*	
Muscle twitching			†	*	
Confusion	†	†		*	
Dizziness	†	†		*	†
Hallucinations			*		
Auditory hallucinations	*				
Respiratory depression	†	†	†		*
Apnea	†	†	†		*
Seizures	†	†	‡	*	
Coma	†	†	†	*	*
Renal					
Hematuria	*	†		*	
Proteinuria	*			*	
Acute renal failure	*	†	*		
Cardiovascular					
Sinus tachycardia	†	†	†	*	†
Bradycardia		*			
Hypotension	*	†	*	*	†
Hematologic					
Abnormal coagulation studies	*	†	*	*	
Leukocytosis	*		*		
Bone marrow aplasia				*	
Laboratory					
Metabolic acidosis	*	‡		*	
Hyperkalemia		*			
Hypokalemia	*	*			
Hypophosphatemia		*			
Hyponatremia				*	
Hypocalcemia				*	
Cross-reacts with salicylate assays					‡
Elevated hepatic enzymes				†	*

* Isolated case report.

† Several case reports.

‡ Frequently reported.

§ *Source:* Adapted from Smolinske SC, Hall AH, Vandenberg SA, et al: Toxic effects of non-steroidal anti-inflammatory drugs in overdose. *Drug Safety* 5:252, 1990.

of some NSAIDs. Most cases have been attributed to the propionic and acetic acids. These patients often present with hematuria and flank pain.

Pulmonary

Aspirin may exacerbate bronchospasm in up to 20 percent of asthmatic patients by inhibiting pulmonary prostaglandins. By the same mechanism, all NSAIDs can cause a spectrum of respiratory toxicity ranging from rhinitis to bronchospasm in susceptible individuals. Aspirin-sensitive asthmatics are prone to bronchospasm when administered NSAIDs. Overdoses of NSAIDs rarely lead to serious pulmonary toxicity. Apnea has been reported in a child after ingesting as few as ten ibuprofen tablets. Noncardiogenic pulmonary edema, a major cause of morbidity in salicylate poisoning, has not been reported after toxic ingestions of NSAIDs.

Hematologic

Aplastic anemia has occurred with the therapeutic use of piroxicam, and hemolytic anemia has been described with long-term use of sulindac and mefenamic acid. The mechanism is unclear. All NSAIDs reversibly inhibit platelet aggregation by altering the balance between thromboxane A_2 and prostacyclin, prolonging the Ivy or template bleeding times.

Hepatic

Many NSAIDs produce a transient rise in liver enzymes through a hypersensitivity response at therapeutic concentrations. The acetic and propionic acids species have demonstrated the highest incidence of hepatotoxicity. Sulindac has been found to cause direct hepatocellular injury and cholestatic jaundice in susceptible individuals. A similar idiosyncratic reaction led to the withdrawal of benoxaprofen from the market.

Dermatologic

Although generalized exanthems and pruritus are the most common cutaneous reactions described by patients receiving NSAIDs, erythema multiforme, Stevens Johnson syndrome (SJS), toxic epidermal necrolysis (TEN), bullous eruptions, photosensitivity, fixed drug eruptions, urticaria, and pustular psoriasis have all been reported. TEN and SJS most frequently are associated with sulindac. Photosensitivity is most common in piroxicam and other NSAIDs with extended half-lives.

Central Nervous System

Headache, drowsiness, tinnitus, and other subtle central nervous system symptoms are noted by patients taking NSAIDs in therapeutic doses. Psychologic effects can be seen with chronic use of most NSAIDs but appear to be described more frequently with indomethacin. Behavioral changes such as depression, confusion, and psychosis have been associated with therapeutic doses of indomethacin. The mechanism of interaction with the central nervous system is unclear, but it has been suggested that prostaglandins may modulate neurotransmitter release in the brain.

Aseptic meningitis has been described with sulindac, ibuprofen, and tolmetin, most often in patients suffering from connective tissue diseases such as systemic lupus erythematosus. Prostaglandin inhibition may not be the etiology of the meningeal leukocytosis since patients have experienced meningitic symptoms related to one NSAID and not others.

Drowsiness, dizziness, and lethargy are common symptoms in acute toxic ingestions of NSAIDs. Although coma and convulsions are rare in most uncomplicated NSAID overdoses, mefenamic acid poisonings are characterized by a relatively high incidence of seizures. Convulsions have occurred following acute mefenamic acid exposures as small as 7.5 g and, in one series, were present in up to 40 percent of acute ingestions where the serum mefenamic acid concentration exceeded the maximum therapeutic concentration. Mefenamic acid-induced seizures are usually self-limited, occur between 2 and 8 h after overdose, and appear unrelated to hypoxia. Propionic and acetic acid derivatives also can produce seizures after massive ingestions.

Adverse Drug Interactions

NSAIDs can alter the effects of other medications by displacing them from protein binding sites. The most serious potential drug interaction involves the concomitant use of oral anticoagulants. Gastritis, peptic ulceration, and inhibition of platelet aggregation caused by NSAIDs increases the risk of GI hemorrhage in these patients.

Most NSAIDs have been found to antagonize the action of antihypertensive agents by promoting sodium and water retention. Ibuprofen and piroxicam are well documented to act in this regard. Indomethacin has been shown to elevate the arterial pressure in hypertensive patients treated with angiotensin-converting enzyme inhibitors, diuretics, and β blockers. Indomethacin, ibuprofen, and piroxicam have also been reported to increase serum lithium concentrations by decreasing tubular lithium secretion.

A summary of the acute toxic effects reported in poisonings with each class of NSAID is presented in Table 110-2.

DIFFERENTIAL DIAGNOSIS

There are few characteristics by which toxic ingestions of NSAIDs can be recognized easily. The nausea, vomiting, and mild CNS depression witnessed most often in NSAID poisonings can be consistent with acute ingestions of many substances. A mild metabolic acidosis can be seen with NSAID toxicity and probably is related to the weak acidity of NSAIDs and their oxidized metabolites. Although dehydration from nausea, vomiting, and diarrhea of any etiology can produce a metabolic acidosis, substances such as methanol, ethylene glycol, aspirin, and iron should be considered in a patient with a metabolic acidosis following an unknown ingestion. A severe metabolic acidosis may also suggest a recent seizure.

Diflunisal can cross-react with the TDx and colorimetric salicylate assays yielding false-positive salicylate levels. GI and central nervous system toxicities associated with diflunisal overdose also can resemble salicylate poisoning. However, classic symptoms of salicylism such as respiratory alkalosis and an elevated-anion-gap metabolic acidosis are not observed in acute toxic ingestions of diflunisal.

TREATMENT

Who to Treat

All patients developing symptoms after an acute ingestion of NSAIDs need evaluation and observation. There are still too few case reports of toxicity from NSAIDs with reliable laboratory data to establish correlation between dose ingested, plasma concentration, and toxic effect. A review of *uncomplicated* ibuprofen ingestions found that no initially asymptomatic patient became symptomatic more than 4 h after ingestion. It therefore seems prudent to observe asymptomatic patients who may have ingested potentially toxic doses of ibuprofen in the emergency department for at least 4 to 6 h. If the patient remains asymptomatic with normal vital signs after this time, they can be medically cleared.

Large reviews also have demonstrated that patients rarely, if ever, develop symptoms with acute *uncomplicated* ibuprofen ingestions of less than 100 mg/kg. Asymptomatic children fitting this description may be observed at home. Mixed ingestions, symptomatic or suicidal patients ingesting any type of NSAID, and those ingesting *potentially* toxic doses of any NSAID or more than 100 mg/kg of ibuprofen should be evaluated medically.

Blood Levels

Assays are available for measuring serum concentrations of NSAIDs. Although a nomogram using serum concentrations has been constructed for acute ibuprofen poisoning, serum concentrations of ibuprofen poorly correlate with the development of toxicity. It is therefore best to treat the patient with respect to clinical presentation alone.

Other laboratory screening may be helpful in symptomatic patients. An arterial blood gas, complete blood count, electrolytes, creatinine, coagulation studies, and hepatic enzymes should be followed. Acetaminophen levels and urine drug screens may be required in patients where mixed ingestions are suspected.

Initial Stabilization

As in any poisoning, initial management of the patient with NSAID toxicity should begin with airway maintenance. Central nervous system depression and apnea may be associated with massive ingestions of NSAIDs, and endotracheal intubation may be necessary.

Vital signs should be monitored closely. Dehydration from vomiting and diarrhea should be treated aggressively. The hypotensive or hypovolemic patient should receive boluses of normal saline solution or Ringer's lactate. In the rare patient with hypotension refractory to intensive fluid resuscitation, a vasopressor such as dopamine or norepinephrine can be added.

All patients with signs of severe toxicity, including hypovolemia or potassium abnormalities, should have continuous cardiac monitoring. Aside from sinus tachycardia, cardiac arrhythmias are not reported routinely following uncomplicated NSAID poisoning but may be observed in association with mixed ingestions, severe electrolyte abnormalities, hypotension, hypoxia, metabolic acidosis, or in patients with preexisting cardiac disease.

Seizures occurring after poisonings with NSAIDs are usually of short duration and self-limited, responding to benzodiazepines and conservative management. Patients with repetitive seizures or status epilepticus can receive phenytoin or phenobarbital in standard doses.

Decontamination

Because NSAIDs are absorbed rapidly, decontamination techniques will likely be of no benefit in patients presenting more than 2 or 3 h after uncomplicated ingestions. In massive poisonings and mixed ingestions, gastric motility can be slowed, prolonging absorption from the GI tract and delaying the onset of symptoms. Late decontamination may benefit these patients.

Syrup of Ipecac

The effects of syrup of ipecac may not only mimic symptoms of NSAID toxicity, but may lead to aspiration if convulsions should occur. Syrup of ipecac is therefore not recommended following NSAID ingestion.

Gastric Lavage

Gastric lavage may be efficacious if performed within the first 1 to 2 h after the ingestion. A large-bore orogastric tube should be utilized when tablets or pills are involved.

Activated Charcoal

Activated charcoal has been shown to bind indomethacin, mefenamic acid, piroxicam, and tolfenamic acid. Charcoal should be administered in doses of 0.5 to 1 g/kg body weight if the patient presents within 4 h of an uncomplicated ingestion. Although the administration of a cathartic with charcoal has been advocated by some authors, this has never been shown to affect the outcome of acute ingestions. Patients often vomit when given sorbitol, and children may become dehydrated from copious diarrhea. It is therefore not recommended to give cathartics with charcoal following NSAID overdose.

Multiple-Dose Activated Charcoal

Enterohepatic recirculation occurs with NSAIDs such as indomethacin, sulindac, and piroxicam. This suggests that multiple doses of activated charcoal may be of benefit in more rapid removal of these drugs. Repeat dosing of charcoal has been found to shorten the elimination half-life of piroxicam from 40 to 20 h in human volunteers. However, the short elimination half-life and mild toxicity following ingestions of most NSAIDs do not indicate a need for repeat doses of charcoal and, again, this therapy has never been shown to affect clinical outcome.

Dialysis, Alkaline Diuresis

Although most NSAIDs have very small volumes of distribution, most are highly protein bound, and procedures for enhancing elimination such as hemodialysis or peritoneal dialysis are unlikely to be of benefit. Urine alkalinization or forced diuresis also is unlikely to affect the clinical outcome in poisonings with these agents since the kidney excretes only a small portion of the absorbed dose unchanged.

Overall Strategy

The key to managing patients poisoned by NSAIDs is supportive care. There are no specific antidotes available to treat NSAID toxicity. Initial stabilization should focus on airway management and volume replacement. Decontamination with gastric lavage and charcoal, or charcoal alone, should be instituted when indicated in patients presenting after acute ingestions of NSAIDs. The lack of dose–response data for toxic ingestions of these medications mandates all asymptomatic patients ingesting potentially toxic doses of NSAIDs be observed in the emergency department for at least 4 to 6 h. Severely ill patients, especially when longer-acting varieties such as piroxicam or sulindac are involved, should be admitted for observation. Renal and hepatic function should be monitored in ingestions of those NSAIDs associated with toxicity to these organs. Oliguric renal failure in the severely poisoned patient may require initial hemodialysis, but recovery of renal function most always occurs over several days. Electrolytes should be monitored with attention to acid–base and potassium abnormalities.

Most severely poisoned patients will have some GI distress. A few may have GI bleeding with hematemesis or guaiac-positive stools. These patients should have liberal volume replacement and endoscopic evaluation as necessary. Antacids or H_2 blockers may be employed for treatment or prophylaxis, but their usefulness in this situation is unproven.

CONCLUSION

Despite the widespread use and over-the-counter availability of NSAIDs, severe toxicity resulting from acute poisonings with these agents is uncommon. Except when massive quantities are ingested, toxicity usually is confined to GI discomfort and mild CNS depression, with rapid resolution in most cases. The mainstay of treatment is supportive care.

BIBLIOGRAPHY

Aaron TH, Murritt ELC: Reactions to acetylsalicylic acid. *Can Med Assoc J* 126:609, 1982.

Abramson SB, Weissmann G: The mechnisms of action of nonsteroidal antiinflammatory drugs. *Arthritis Rheum* 32:1, 1989.

Antal EJ, Wright CE, Brown BL, et al: The influence of hemodialysis on the pharmacokinetics of ibuprofen and its major metabolites. *J Clin Pharmacol* 26:184, 1986.

Balali-Mood M, Critchley JAJH, Proudfoot AT, et al: Mefenamic acid overdose. *Lancet* 1:1354, 1981.

Bigby M, Stern R: Cutaneous reactions to nonsteroidal anti-inflammatory drugs. *J Am Acad Dermatol* 12:866, 1985.

Brater DC: Clinical pharmacology of NSAIDs. *J Clin Pharmacol* 28:518, 1988.

Coles LS, Fries JF, Kraines RG: From experiment to experience: side effects of nonsteroidal anti-inflammatory drugs. *Am J Med* 74:820, 1983.

Court H, Volens GN: Poisoning after overdose with non-steroidal antiinflammatory drugs. *Adverse Drug React Acute Poisoning Rev* 3:1, 1984.

Fox DA, Jick H: Non-steroidal anti-inflammatory drugs and renal disease. *JAMA* 251:1299, 1984.

Fredell EW, Strand LJ: Naproxen overdose. *JAMA* 238:938, 1977.

Hall AH, Smolinske SC, Conrad FL, et al: Ibuprofen overdose: 126 cases. *Ann Emerg Med* 15:1308, 1986.

Harchelroad F, Evans TC, Hobbs E: Ibuprofen blood levels vary. *Ann Emerg Med* 17:186, 1988.

Ivey KJ: Mechanisms of nonsteroidal anti-inflammatory drug-induced gastric damage. *Am J Med* 84(suppl 2A):41, 1988.

Levy RA, Smith DL: Clinical differences among nonsteroidal antiinflammatory drugs: Implications for therapeutic substitution in ambulatory patients. *Drug Intell Clin Pharmacol* 23:76, 1989.

Lewis JH: Hepatic toxicity of non-steroidal anti-inflammatory drugs. *Clin Pharmacol* 3:128, 1984.

Linden CH, Townsend PL: Metabolic acidosis after acute ibuprofen overdosage. *J Pediatrics* 111:922, 1987.

Litovitz TL, Schmitz BF, Holms KC: 1988 Annual Report of the American Association of Poison Control Centers National Data Collection System. *Am J Emerg Med* 6:495, 1989.

McElwee NE, Veltri JC, Bradford DC, et al: A prospective, population-based study of acute ibuprofen overdose: Complications are rare and routine serum levels not warranted. *Ann Emerg Med* 19:657, 1990.

Oates JA, FitzGerald GA, Branch RA, et al: Clinical implications of prostaglandin and thromboxane A2 formation (part 1). *N Engl J Med* 319:689, 1988.

Ragheb M, Ban TA, Buchanan D, et al: Interaction of indomethacin and ibuprofen with lithium in manic patients under a steady state lithium level. *J Clin Psychiatry* 41:397, 1980.

Reeves WB, Foley RJ, Weinman EJ: Renal dysfunction from nonsteroidal anti-inflammatory drugs. *Arch Intern Med* 144:1943, 1984.

Roth SH: Nonsteroidal anti-inflammatory drugs: Gastropathy, deaths, and medical practice. *Ann Intern Med* 109:353, 1988.

Smolinski SC, Hall AH, Vandenberg SA, et al: Toxic effects of nonsteroidal anti-inflammatory drugs in overdose. *Drug Safety* 5:252, 1990.

Somerville K, Faulkner G, Langman M: Non-steroidal anti-inflammatory drugs and bleeding peptic ulcer. *Lancet* 1:462, 1986.

Szczekik A, Gryglewski RJ, Czerniawska-Mysik G: Clinical patterns of hypersensitivity to non-steroidal anti-inflammatory drugs and their pathogenesis. *J Allergy Clin Immunol* 60:276, 1977.

Tan SY, Shapiro R, Franco R, et al: Indomethacin-induced prostaglandin inhibition with hyperkalemia. *Ann Intern Med* 90:783, 1979.

Vale JA, Meredith TJ: Acute poisoning due to non-steroidal antiinflammatory drugs. *Med Toxicol* 1:12, 1986.

Verbeeck RK, Blackburn JL, Loewen GR: Clinical pharmacokinetics of nonsteroidal anti-inflammatory drugs. *Clin Pharmacokinet* 8:302, 1983.

Webster J: Interactions of NSAIDs with diuretics and β-blockers: Mechanisms and clinical implications. *Drugs* 30:32, 1985.

111
CYANIDE

Kathleen Delaney

Cyanide is a potent cellular toxin. As little as 50 mg may cause death in an adult. It has an ancient and infamous history. The ability of extracts of bitter almonds and of cherry laurel leaves to cause fulminant deterioration and death has been known for centuries, although the causative agent was not identified as cyanide until the end of the eighteenth century. State executions by oral administration of extracts of apricot, cherry, or peach pits were an ancient Greek and Roman practice. The first chemist to synthesize hydrogen cyanide gas died dramatically in 1786 when a vial of the gas broke on his laboratory floor. Cyanide has provided a ready means of mass murder and suicide in this century. In 1978 hundreds of people died in Jonestown, British Guyana, following mass cyanide ingestion. Most recently, hydrogen cyanide gas was the reported cause of thousands of civilian deaths in the Iran-Iraq war. Cyanide gas has been used in modern judicial executions in the state of California.

Cyanide is a simple compound of carbon and nitrogen which has many uses in industry and the chemical laboratory. Its wide availability was emphasized by the experience of investigators who found 65 legitimate sources of cyanide in the Chicago area during attempts to trace the source of cyanide used in the infamous Tylenol-substitution poisonings. Cyanide is also found in large amounts in certain nuts, plants, and fruit pits in the form of cyanogenic glycosides. Tobacco smoke has been estimated to contain from 100 to 1600 parts per million (ppm) cyanide, and smokers have been shown to have higher levels of cyanide and thiocyanate, a "detoxified" form of cyanide. Hundreds of fungi and several bacterial species also produce cyanide. Since it is so ubiquitous in nature, animals have evolved biochemical means of detoxifying cyanide. In humans and many other mammals, the enzyme rhodanase detoxifies cyanide by binding it to sulfate to form the less toxic thiocyanate, which is excreted by the kidneys.

SOURCES OF EXPOSURE

Acute cyanide poisoning occurs in a number of settings: (1) accidental occupational poisonings; (2) nonoccupational accidental or suicidal ingestions of cyanide or cyanide-containing products, such as metal polishes or acetonitrile-containing solvents; (3) iatrogenic toxicity due to prolonged exposure to intravenous nitroprusside; and (4) ingestion of plants or foods containing naturally occurring cyanogenic glycosides.

Because of its high reactivity, cyanide is widely used in synthetic laboratory and industrial processes. The most common industrial process used to make cyanide produces hydrogen cyanide gas (HCN) by combining ammonia (NH_3) and methane (CH_4). Commercial quantities of water-soluble salts such as sodium cyanide (NaCN) and potassium cyanide (KCN) are synthesized from hydrogen cyanide gas. Hydrogen cyanide gas is readily liberated when cyanide salts are exposed to acid. Cyanide compounds are both precursors and incidental by-products in the production of plastics, solvents, enamels, high-strength paper, paints, glues, wrinkle-resistant fabrics, herbicides, pesticides, and fertilizers. Hydrogen cyanide gas is produced in large quantities during the manufacture of acrylonitrile, a precursor of many plastic compounds. The affinity of cyanide for metals makes it useful in the extraction of ores, in metal polishing, and in the electroplating industry. It is also used to strip hair from hides in the leather industry. The past widespread use of cyanide as a fumigant resulted in many poisonings. Industrial exposures most commonly occur through inhalation; however, skin exposure to solutions of cyanide salts has also resulted in poisoning. Inadvertent ingestion of cyanide salts while eating in a contaminated work setting has also been proposed as a cause of accidental subacute poisoning in the workplace.

The possibility of cyanide toxicity is frequently overlooked in victims of closed-space fires. Large amounts of hydrogen cyanide may be released when natural and synthetic nitrogen-containing polymers such as wool, silk, polyurethane, or vinyl are burned. Elevated cyanide levels have been reported frequently in victims of smoke inhalation, most often in association with elevated carbon monoxide levels, and have been implicated in fire-related fatalities.

Iatrogenic cyanide poisonings also occur. In the early half of this century, chronic administration of sodium thiocyanate for the treatment of severe hypertension resulted in many cases of poisoning with manifestations similar to cyanide toxicity. Thiocyanate is thought to maintain an equilibrium with free cyanide. As late as 1951, deaths attributed to this therapy were reported. Cyanide toxicity is seen when high levels of sodium thiocyanate accumulate during prolonged administration of nitroprusside.

Adverse physiologic effects due to chronic subacute cyanide exposure have been proposed but are poorly defined. Studies of workers chronically exposed to cyanide have demonstrated a higher incidence of thyroid disease and vitamin B_{12} deficiency. Demyelinating diseases, B_{12} deficiency disorders, and goiter have all been related to the chronic ingestion of linamarin, a cyanogenic glycoside found in the hardy cassava plant. Cassava provides a significant source of carbohydrate to many peoples in the third world. In areas of the world where cassava ingestion is high, goiter and tropical ataxic neuropathy are endemic and plasma and urinary levels of cyanide are elevated.

BIOCHEMICAL TOXICOLOGY

Cyanide binds avidly to many metals. This property, which makes cyanide useful in industry, also accounts for its serious physiologic effects in poisoning. Cyanide disrupts metabolism by binding and inhibiting the function of important metal-containing enzymes, particularly those which contain trivalent ferric (+3) iron. Although cyanide has been shown to inhibit a substantial number of biochemically important enzymes, the most dramatic physiologic effects are produced by its disruption of mitochondrial oxidative phosphorylation through the inhibition of cytochrome A_3, also called cytochrome oxidase. This binding is labile and readily reversible. Cytochrome A_3 catalyzes the final step in electron transport, in which molecular oxygen is reduced to water. Without this enzyme, the body tissues cannot utilize oxygen and only anaerobic metabolism occurs. When poisoning is not rapidly fatal, both hyperglycemia related to disruption of glycogen metabolism and lipid disorders can be demonstrated.

CLINICAL TIME COURSE OF POISONING: ROUTES OF EXPOSURE

The time course and severity of the clinical effects of cyanide are a function of the nature of the cyanide-containing compound, the route of exposure, and the concentration of cyanide to which the patient is exposed. The absorption of cyanide following inhalational exposures to hydrogen cyanide gas is virtually immediate. Symptoms depend on the concentration of inspired gas. Toxicity occurs when the rate of accumulation of cyanide is greater than the rate of detoxification. Several hours of exposure to low concentrations of gas (<50 ppm) cause restlessness, anxiety, palpitations, dyspnea, and headache. Death may occur following prolonged exposure at these levels. Recovery is rapid following removal from exposure. Exposure to 100 ppm may be fatal within 30 min. Serious inhalational exposures lead to severe dyspnea, loss of consciousness, seizures, and cardiac arrhythmias. These may also resolve quickly with supportive care following removal from exposure. Coma and cardiovascular collapse can occur immediately upon exposure to levels of hydrogen cyanide greater than 270 ppm. Survival with aggressive resuscitation has been reported following a 3-min industrial exposure to 500 ppm. Although in most industrial accidents it has been difficult to separate the effects of inhalational absorption from percutaneous absorption, animal studies and studies of human skin have clearly shown that absorption of both cyanide ion (CN^-) and HCN vapor occur through intact skin. In one industrial case reported in the 1950s, a fully protected worker was poisoned when he removed a glove and allowed his hand to contact aqueous HCN.

The onset of symptoms following ingestion of a cyanide salt may occur within minutes, depending on the amount of cyanide ingested and the rate of absorption. Deaths have occurred in adults following the ingestion of as little as 50 mg, and survival has been reported after much larger ingestions with aggressive resuscitation and use of antidotes.

Certain cyanide-containing compounds, such as nitriles or cyanogenic glycosides, require enzymatic breakdown and release of free cyanide before the symptoms of poisoning occur. Acetonitrile is a solvent sold commercially as a nail polish remover. It undergoes hepatic oxidative metabolism which results in the release of hydrogen cyanide. Severe poisoning and death attributed to cyanide poisoning have been reported following latency periods as long as 12 h after ingestion. Amygdalin is a cyanogenic glycoside which is found in particularly high concentrations in apricot pits and bitter almonds. It is the principal constituent of laetrile, a compound popular for nontraditional cancer therapies in the late 1970s. Because the release of cyanide requires hydrolysis of the glycoside by enzymes in the alkaline environment of the small intestine, the progression of symptoms following these ingestions is characteristically slow, with a latency of onset of several hours. Amygdalin does not produce cyanide poisoning when given intravenously.

CLINICAL PRESENTATION OF CYANIDE POISONING

Although isolated individual poisonings with cyanide are relatively rare, it is important that emergency physicians recognize signs of serious poisoning, as specific antidotal treatment is available and effective. The clinical signs and symptoms of cyanide poisoning mimic those of hypoxia, with one exception: patients are not cyanotic. These clinical effects are readily understood based on the effect of cyanide on cytochrome oxidase activity. Blockade of the ability of mitochondria to utilize oxygen produces a state of severe hypoxia despite the presence of oxygen. Anaerobic metabolism is switched on, generating large amounts of lactic acid. Severe, unexplained acidosis is an important clinical clue to the timely diagnosis of cyanide poisoning in case of an "unknown" ingestion. Clinically, the brain is the primary organ affected by cyanide, followed by the heart. After fatal poisoning with cyanide, concentrations are highest in these organs. At the onset of poisoning, there is an inspiratory gasp followed by hyperventilation. Patients complain of breathlessness and anxiety. Symptoms related to anxiety about the exposure may also mimic these initial symptoms of toxicity. During inhalational exposure, these symptoms will resolve following removal from the toxic exposure. Cerebral function is rapidly affected in significant exposures. Loss of consciousness occurs, often associated with seizures. Early cardiac effects include sinus tachycardia, atrial arrythmias, and premature ventricular contractions. Even such severely poisoned patients may recover rapidly and spontaneously when removed from an inhalational exposure. When exposure continues, bradycardia and apnea occur, followed by asystolic arrest. Ventricular tachycardia and fibrillation are uncommon (see Table 111-1). Although small amounts of cyanide bind to the ferrous (+2) form of hemoglobin, there is no significant interference with the ability of hemoglobin to bind oxygen. Therefore, cyanosis does not occur except as a terminal event. The inability to use oxygen leads to decreased oxygen extraction and a concomitant increase in the oxygen content of venous blood. This is manifest as a decrease in the normal arteriolar-venous oxygen [$(A - V)_{O_2}$] difference, a measure of the amount of oxygen extracted by the tissues. This effect may be detected clinically on funduscopic examination as "arteriolized" retinal veins. Accurate determination of the $(A - V)_{O_2}$ gradient requires pulmonary artery sampling and a time-consuming calculation. Although peripheral venous samples do not reflect whole-body oxygen extraction, it is clinically useful to recall that the venous saturation of forearm blood is around 40% in patients breathing room air under normal circumstances. A high forearm venous oxygen saturation would support the diagnosis of cyanide poisoning (see Table 111-2). Cyanide salts are caustic and

Table 111-1. Signs and Symptoms of Acute Cyanide Toxicity

Central nervous system effects
Headache
Drowsiness
Dizziness
Seizures
Coma
Paralysis
Pulmonary effects
Early stage
Dyspnea
Tachypnea
Late stage
Rapid decrease in respiratory rate
Apnea
Pulmonary edema
Cardiovascular effects
Early stage
Hypertension
Tachycardia
Sinus or AV nodal arrhythmias
Late stage
Hypotension
Bradycardia
Asystole
Cardiovascular collapse
Local effects (after oral ingestion)
Burning of the tongue and mucous membranes
Nausea
Gastrointestinal irritation

Source: Adapted with permission from Holland MA, Kozlowski LM.

Table 111-2. Anticipated Laboratory Abnormalities in Cyanide Poisoning

Test	Result	Cause
Serum electrolytes	Elevated anion gap	Lactic acidosis from increased anaerobic metabolism
Arterial blood gas	Metabolic acidosis Normal Po_2	As above
Calculated % O_2 saturation	Normal	
Measured % O_2 saturation	May be decreased*	Small amount of cyanide bound to hemoglobin
Arterial-central venous O_2 difference	Increased (normal is 5 mL O_2/100 mL-blood)	Decreased tissue O_2 utilization
Forearm venous O_2 saturation	Increased (normal is approx. 40%, >90% reported in cyanide cases) ??effect of supplemental oxygen	As above

* A % O_2 saturation gap of 5 points may be significant. Carbon monoxide and hydrogen sulfide also increase the "% O_2 saturation gap."

Source: Adapted with permission from Hall AH, Rumack BH.

may cause oral burns when concentrated solutions or undiluted salts are ingested. A deeply comatose, acidotic patient without evidence of cyanosis or hypoxia on arterial blood gas examination should cause the clinician to think of cyanide. The finding of bright-red retinal vessels, an abnormally elevated venous oxygen saturation, an empty vial of cyanide, oral burns, or the smell of bitter almonds support the diagnosis, although clues of this nature are frequently absent. It is estimated that only 20 to 40 percent of the population can detect the characteristic almond odor of cyanide.

A brief occupational history may provide a clue to the diagnosis of cyanide poisoning in an acutely ill adult. In patients with work-related industrial poisoning, the exposure is usually accidental, and the diagnosis suggested by the patient's job and circumstances. Frequently multiple exposures result from the same incident. Suicidal ingestions of cyanide often occur in patients whose occupations provide access to cyanide salts, such as industrial and research chemists, laboratory technicians, science students, or jewelers. Accidental or suicidal ingestions of cyanide-containing commercial products, such as metal polishes or acetonitrile-containing solvents, have been associated with severe cyanide toxicity. A history of use of herbal or nontraditional cancer therapies would provide a clue to the ingestion of laetrile or other cyanogen-containing preparations. Careful identification of ingestants in asymptomatic patients will prevent the mistaken discharge of a patient who has ingested a compound with delayed toxicity.

DIFFERENTIAL DIAGNOSIS OF CYANIDE POISONING

Cyanide-poisoned patients frequently present to emergency departments without any history of exposure. Cyanide poisoning should always be considered in the comatose, acidotic patient. The differential diagnosis of acidosis in the setting of inhalational exposure includes other cellular toxins such as hydrogen sulfide and carbon monoxide and simple asphyxiants. Hydrogen sulfide is a product of organic decomposition, encountered in septic tanks and sewers, petroleum production, and a number of other occupational settings. The characteristic odor of "rotten eggs" is frequently detectable. The setting of carbon monoxide exposure often suggests that diagnosis, which is readily confirmed by measurement of a carboxyhemoglobin level. The differential diagnosis of acidosis in patients with suspected ingestions includes methanol, ethylene glycol, salicylates, and iron. The slower time course of deterioration and the variable depth of mental status depression frequently help to distinguish the effects of these agents from those of cyanide. Severe isoniazid and cocaine poisoning are also associated with significant acidosis which occurs in the setting of seizures. The initial manifestations of severe intoxication with these agents may be clinically indistinguishable from those of cyanide intoxication.

PHARMACOLOGIC PRINCIPLES OF TREATMENT

Standard therapy for cyanide poisoning in the United States is based on experimental and chemical principles developed by Chen in 1933. Treatment is provided by the Lilly Cyanide Antidote Kit. The kit contains nitrites in two forms, an ampule of amyl nitrite for inhalation, and 10 mL of a 3% solution of sodium nitrite for intravenous infusion. It also contains 50 mL of a 25% solution of sodium thiosulfate. The usual adult dose of sodium nitrite is 300 mg, followed by 12.5 g of sodium thiosulfate. The pediatric dose is 0.33 mL/kg of 10% sodium nitrite and 1.65 mL/kg of 25% sodium thiosulfate. Pediatric dosages of sodium nitrite should be adjusted if anemia is known to be present (see Table 111-3). The amyl nitrite is used to temporize in the prehospital setting or until intravenous access can be obtained and does not need to be administered when sodium nitrite is readily available. Nitrites act quickly and therefore are the first antidote to be used.

The initial rationale for choosing nitrites was based on their capacity to form methemoglobin. Methemoglobin binds avidly to cyanide and prevents its binding to cytochrome oxidase. Although the antidotal efficacy of nitrites is not disputed, their actual mechanism of action has recently been questioned. The formation of methemoglobin is a slow process relative to the rapidity of the therapeutic response to nitrites. In addition, the reversal of cyanide toxicity in animals by nitrites has been demonstrated to occur in the presence of methylene blue, which prevents the formation of methemoglobin. Rapid methemoglobin formers, such as dimethyl-4-aminophenol, which is now used in Germany to treat cyanide poisoning, do not appear to work any faster than sodium nitrite. Many papers imply that a level of methemoglobin of at least 25 percent should be a goal of therapy. This is based on work in dogs, who are much more sensitive to the methemoglobin-forming effects of nitrites than humans. It has been repeatedly demonstrated that the rapid clinical reversal of cyanide toxicity occurs despite the demonstration of only very small amounts of methemoglobin. Since cyanomethemoglobin is not detected by the cooximeter, it is possible that demonstrable methemoglobin levels are low in cyanide poisoning because the methemoglobin is rapidly converted to cyanomethemoglobin or that nitrites are acting through another mechanism. These observations have led to trials of vasodilators in the treatment of cyanide poisoning. Rapid detoxification of cyanide has been reported using solutions of methemoglobin stripped of the red cell walls, so called stroma-free methemoglobin. Nitrites have a potential to cause serious side effects. Their vasodilatory properties can exacerbate hypotension. A single death has been reported secondary to massive methemoglobinemia in an asymptomatic child with an inconsequential cyanide ingestion.

Table 111-3. Treatment of Cyanide Poisoning

Children

1. Amyl nitrite inhaler: crack vial and inhale 30 s/min
2. Administration of IV sodium nitrite and sodium thiosulfate:

Hb, g/100 mL	3% $NaNO_2$ mL/kg	25% $Na_2S_2O_3$, mL/kg
7	0.19	0.95
8	0.22	1.10
9	0.25	1.25
10	0.27	1.35
11	0.30	1.50
12	0.33*	1.65
13	0.36	1.80
14	0.39	1.95

3. May repeat once at one-half dose.
4. Monitor methemoglobin to keep level less than 30%.

Adults

1. Amyl nitrite: crack and inhale 30 s/min.
2. Sodium nitrite: 10 mL IV (10-mL ampule 3% $NaNO_2$ = 300 mg)
3. Sodium thiosulfate: 50 mL IV (50-mL ampule 25% $Na_2S_2O_3$ = 12.5 g)
4. May repeat once at one-half dose.

* Doses in mL/kg of sodium nitrite and sodium thiosulfate for the average child.

Source: Adapted with permission from Hall AH, Rumack BH.

Following the adminstration of sodium nitrite, sodium thiosulfate is given. Studies of the cyanide LD_{50} in animals demonstrate that the therapeutic effect of the combination of sodium nitrite and sodium thiosulfate is greater than the additive effects of both agents alone. Sodium thiosulfate enhances the activity of the body's own detoxification enzyme, rhodanase, by acting as a sulfur donor. Rhodanase removes the cyanide molecule from methemoglobin and transfers it to sulfur, forming thiocyanate which is renally excreted. The rate of this detoxification reaction in humans is limited by the availability of sulfur. (see Fig. 111-1). The speed of the antidotal effect of sodium thiosulfate administration has been noted to be species dependent; very slow in rabbits, intermediate in dogs, and very rapid in sheep. There are limited data on the efficacy of sodium thiosulfate as sole therapy

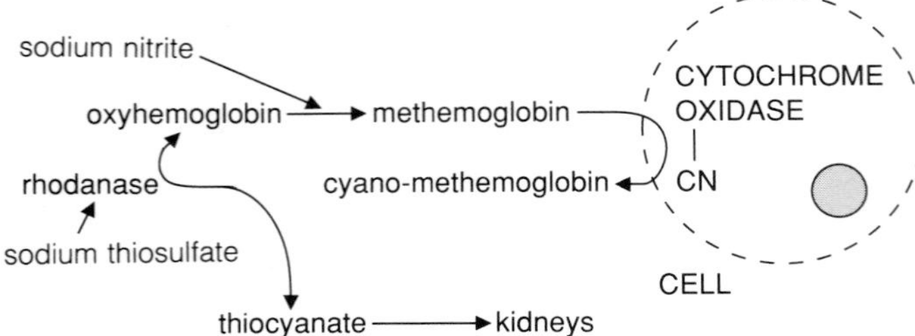

Figure 111-1. Mechanism of action of the nitrite-thiosulfate antidote.

for cyanide poisoning in humans. This is an important question because sodium thiosulfate has very limited toxicity in comparison with the nitrites and may be of value as an empirical therapy in unclear cases.

Administration of 100% oxygen has been clearly shown in animal studies to significantly enhance the therapeutic efficacy of both sodium thiosulfate alone and the nitrite-thiosulfate combination. If the only mechanism of toxicity of cyanide were its binding to cytochrome A_3, then rationally oxygen would not be expected to have any therapeutic effect. Its antidotal action does not appear to be related to any effect on cyanide distribution or the efficacy of rhodanase. It has been proposed that oxygen may affect the binding of cyanide to cytochrome oxidase or the ability to form methemoglobin. Hyperbaric oxygen has not been shown to offer any benefit over 100% oxygen in animal studies. Hyperbaric oxygen has been used, in addition to standard therapies, to treat two severely poisoned cyanide patients. It should not be regarded as a standard of care and should be considered only when standard therapies have failed. The exception to this is the patient with suspected cyanide poisoning who has concomitant carbon monoxide poisoning, discussed below.

Because of the potential side effects of the nitrites, a great deal of effort has been made to develop equally efficacious but less toxic therapies. Many agents bind cyanide and render it nontoxic. Cobalt compounds have a high affinity for cyanide and are less toxic than the cobalt salts, which injure the myocardium. Hydroxocobalamin (vitamin B_{12a}) has been shown to reverse cyanide toxicity in animal models and is used to protect patients on prolonged nitroprusside infusions from cyanide toxicity. Anaphylactoid reactions have been reported with its use. In addition, the huge amounts of the agent needed to neutralize cyanide require large volume infusions in the concentrations currently available. Studies are currently being conducted of a combination of hydroxocobalamin with sodium thiosulfate. This combination has been used successfully in France with minimal side effects. The concurrent use of sodium thiosulfate is thought to "recycle" the hydroxocobalamin binding sites, allowing administration of a smaller dose. Recent studies support this concept. It appears that when only hydroxocobalamin is administered, cyanide is held in the form of cyanocobalamin. When the combination is used, cyanide appears in the form of thiocyanate. This effect has been termed "antidotal synergy."

Dicobalt edetate (Kelocyanor) is the therapeutic agent used as first line treatment of cyanide poisoning in the United Kingdom. It is highly effective as a cyanide antidote but is not devoid of toxicity. Metabolic acidosis and hypotension have occurred in animals, and massive edema and ventricular tachycardia have been attributed to its administration to humans. The toxicity of dicobalt edetate is greater when cyanide is not present, limiting its use as an empirical therapy or in minimally symptomatic patients with cyanide exposure.

4-Dimethylaminophenol (DMAP) is an agent developed in Germany for the treatment of cyanide poisoning. It rapidly produces methemoglobinemia but has not been demonstrated to be more clinically efficacious than sodium nitrite. It does not cause the same degree of hypotension but has been associated with renal failure in experimental animals. Unlike dicobalt edetate, it does not have greater side effects in the absence of cyanide. In practice, most of these agents are used in combination with sodium thiosulfate.

MANAGEMENT DECISIONS: USE OF SPECIFIC ANTIDOTES

Severely poisoned patients have survived with supportive therapy alone, although survival in many cases of massive exposure has undoubtedly been facilitated by specific antidotal therapy. The largest reported ingestion where survival occurred with supportive care alone was 600 mg. Much larger ingestions have resulted in survival when specific antidotes were used. All patients should receive 100% oxygen by mask and be put on a cardiac monitor with an intravenous line in place. Patients with a history of cyanide ingestion should have careful gastric lavage. Ipecac is absolutely contraindicated due to the expected rapid onset of symptoms. Gastric decontamination should never take priority over resuscitation of the symptomatic patient. Superactivated charcoal has been shown to bind small amounts of cyanide and may be useful in decreasing the significance of an ingestion. Patients with inhalational exposures do not require gastric decontamination. Extensive decontamination of the skin should be accomplished in patients with cutaneous exposure, with adequate precautions to protect the staff from skin contamination. Patients with inhalational exposures often evidence recovery following their rescue from the toxic environment. They do not require specific antidotal therapy if significant recovery has occurred prior to reaching medical attention. The decision regarding the administration of the sodium nitrite-thiosulfate antidote is straightforward when faced with a comatose, bradycardic patient with a clear history of cyanide exposure. Hypotension is not a contraindication to sodium nitrite therapy in this setting. At the other end of the spectrum, because of the potential toxicity of the nitrites, it is never appropriate to treat an asymptomatic patient. A patient with mild to moderate symptoms may be closely observed for more serious signs prior to the initiation of treatment. More difficult management decisions arise in (1) patients with smoke inhalation who have, or may have, carbon monoxide exposure as well as suspected cyanide exposure and (2) patients who are comatose and acidotic without any history of cyanide exposure. In these cases, the yet-to-be-developed completely nontoxic antidote would obviously be useful. Empirical administration of nitrites to patients who have, or may have, elevated carboxyhemoglobin levels is contraindicated because of the decreased oxygen carrying capacity caused by simultaneous induction of methemoglobinemia. Since it is not possible to distinguish patients with cyanide poisoning in this setting, the safest and only immediate empirical therapy which is warranted is the administration of 100% oxygen and sodium thiosulfate. If the carboxyhemoglobin level is not elevated and oxygenation is normal in a comatose acidotic victim of smoke inhalation, the sodium nitrite can be given. It can also be given safely in the hyperbaric chamber.

Empirical therapy in the unknown patient with possible toxic ingestion who is comatose and acidotic should include 100% oxygen, 25 mL of 50% dextrose in water, and naloxone, in addition to aggressive supportive care. When cyanide poisoning is considered, empirical administration of sodium thiosulfate is indicated. Consideration should be given to the administration of vitamin B_6 where isoniazid ingestion is a possibility. Following the demonstration of adequate oxygenation and the absence of an elevated carboxyhemoglobin level, sodium nitrite may be administered after the sodium thiosulfate if the diagnosis is strongly entertained. Significant hypotension is a contraindication to empirical administration of sodium nitrite.

LABORATORY EVALUATION

In order to be effective, treatment of cyanide poisoning must be instituted long before confirmatory laboratory studies can be accomplished. Cyanide levels are useful to confirm a clinical diagnosis in retrospect; they cannot be obtained in time to make the diagnosis at the bedside. Because cyanide is sequestered in erythrocytes, whole blood and plasma cyanide levels should be obtained. Cyanide levels do not correlate well with toxicity but will support a diagnosis. Whole-blood levels greater than 2 μg/mL have been associated with fatal poisoning. The arterial blood gas is a rapid and useful test as noted above, as is the determination of oxyhemoglobin and methemoglobin levels on the cooximeter. Some authors have suggested that the demonstration of a gap of 5 percentage points or greater between the calculated and measured oxyhemoglobin levels suggests the presence of an abnormal unmeasured hemoglobin such as cyanhemoglobin. Carbon monoxide, methemoglobin, and hydrogen sulfide will also produce such a gap. Routine electrolytes may reveal elevation of the serum glucose. The absence of an anion gap would exclude the diagnosis of acute cyanide poisoning in a symptomatic patient.

PROGNOSIS

Full recovery is anticipated in many cases of severe poisoning where treatment is initiated rapidly and cardiac arrest has not yet occurred. Recovery despite cardiac arrest has also been reported. Most patients who survive do not suffer neurological injury, although anoxic encephalopathy may ensue.

SUMMARY

Cyanide is a rapidly effective cellular toxin. Central nervous system effects are most pronounced, followed by cardiac effects. Lactic acidosis as a primary manifestation of blocked mitochondrial oxygen utilization is early and pronounced. In critically ill patients, the diagnosis must be considered and treatment initiated solely on the basis of the history and clinical presentation. Treatment in the setting of known or strongly suspected exposure utilizes a combination of oxygen, nitrites, and sodium thiosulfate. Empirical therapy in the United States is limited to administation of oxygen and sodium thiosulfate. Aggressive supportive care is essential in all cases.

BIBLIOGRAPHY

Ballantyne B: Toxicology of cyanides, in Ballantyne B, Marrs TC (eds): *Clinical and Experimental Toxicology of Cyanide*. Bristol, Wright, 1987, pp 40–125.

Barnett HJM, Jackson MV, Spaulding WB: Thiocyanate psychosis. *JAMA* 147:1554, 1951.

Berlin CM: The treatment of cyanide poisoning in children. *Pediatrics* 46:793, 1970.

Caravati EM, Litovitz TL: Pediatric cyanide intoxication and death from an acetonitrile-containing cosmetic. *JAMA* 260:3470, 1988.

Chen KK, Rose CL: Nitrite and thiosulfate therapy in cyanide poisoning. *JAMA* 149:113, 1952.

Cottrell JE, Casthely P, Brodie JD, et al: Prevention of nitroprusside-induced cyanide toxicity with hydroxocobalamin. *N Engl J Med* 15:809, 1978.

Hall AH, Rumack BH: Hydroxycobalamin/sodium thiosulfate as a cyanide antidote. *J Emerg Med* 5:115, 1987.

Hall AH, Rumack BH: Clinical toxicology of cyanide. *Ann Emerg Med* 15:1067, 1986.

Holland MA, Kozlowski LM: Clinical features and management of cyanide poisoning. *Clin Pharmacol* 5:737, 1986.

Homan ERJ: Reactions, processes and materials with potential for cyanide exposure, in Ballantyne B, Marrs TC (eds): *Clinical and Experimental Toxicology of Cyanide*. Bristol, Wright, 1987.

Johnson RP, Mellors JW: Arteriolization of venous blood gases: A clue to the diagnosis of cyanide poisoning. *J Emerg Med* 6:401, 1988.

Johnson WS, Hall AH, Rumack BH: Cyanide poisoning successfully treated without "therapeutic methemoglobin levels." *Am J Emerg Med* 7:437, 1989.

Jones J, McMullen MJ, Dougherty J: Toxic smoke inhalation: Cyanide poisoning in fire victims. *Am J Emerg Med* 5:318, 1987.

Krieg A, Saxena K: Cyanide poisoning from metal cleaning solutions. *Ann Emerg Med* 16:582, 1987.

Lambert RJ, Kindler BL, Schaeffer DJ: The efficacy of superactivated charcoal in treating rats exposed to a lethal oral dose of potassium cyanide. *Ann Emerg Med* 17:595, 1988.

Litovitz T: The use of oxygen in the treatment of acute cyanide poisoning, in Ballantyne B, Marrs TC (eds): *Clinical and Experimental Toxicology of Cyanide*. Bristol, Wright, 1987, pp. 468–472

Marrs TC: The choice of cyanide antidotes, in Ballantyne B, Marrs TC (eds): *Clinical and Experimental Toxicology of Cyanide*. Bristol, Wright, 1987, pp. 382–400.

Nagler J, Provost RA, Parizel G: Hydrogen cyanide poisoning: Treatment with cobalt EDTA. *J Occup Med* 20:414, 1978.

Peden NR, Taha A, McSorley PD, et al: Industrial exposure to hydrogen cyanide: Implications for treatment. *Br Med J* 293:538, 1986.

Symington IS, Anderson RA, Thomson I, et al: Cyanide exposure in fires. *Lancet* July 8, 1978, pp. 91–92.

Ten Eyck RP, Schaerdel AD, Ottinger WE: Stroma-free methemoglobin solution: An effective antidote for acute cyanide poisoning. *Am J Emerg Med* 3:519, 1985.

Way JL: Cyanide intoxication and its mechanism of antagonism. *Ann Rev Tox* 24:451, 1984.

Way JL, Leung P, Cannon E, et al: The mechanisms of cyanide intoxication and its antagonism. *Ciba Foundation Symposium* 140:232, 1988.

112 ANTICHOLINERGIC TOXICITY

Leslie R. Wolf

Because of the frequent use of tricyclic antidepressants, phenothiazines, antihistamines, and antiparkinsonian drugs, anticholinergic toxicity is commonly seen in the emergency department. Many drugs have anticholinergic properties (Table 112-1) that may be mild at therapeutic doses but are life-threatening in overdose. The use and abuse of some plants and mushrooms may also result in anticholinergic toxicity.

PHARMACOLOGIC PROPERTIES

Drug absorption can occur after ingestion, smoking, or ocular use. The rate of absorption varies depending on the drug and the route of exposure. Because cholinergic blockade delays gastric emptying and decreases intestinal motility, absorption and peak clinical effects are often delayed.

The signs and symptoms of anticholinergic toxicity are a result of both central and peripheral cholinergic blockade. Muscarinic acetylcholine receptors predominate in the brain, while nicotinic receptors predominate in the spinal cord. Depending on the drug involved, antagonism of muscarinic, nicotinic, or both receptors may occur. The central effects of cholinergic blockade include agitation, amnesia, anxiety, ataxia, coma, confusion, delirium, disorientation, dysarthria, hallucinations, hyperactivity, lethargy, somnolence, seizures, circulatory collapse, mydriasis, and respiratory failure. The peripheral effects include arrhythmias, tachycardia, decreased bronchial secretions, dysphagia, decreased gastrointestinal motility, hyperthermia, hypo- or hypertension, decreased salivation, decreased sweating, urinary retention, and vasodilation.

CLINICAL PRESENTATION

The classic presentation of patients with anticholinergic toxicity can be remembered as:

Hot as Hades
Blind a a Bat
Dry as a Bone
Red as a Beet
Mad as a Hatter

Clinical characteristics include unreactive mydriasis, hypo- or hypertension, absent bowel sounds, tachycardia, flushed skin, disorientation, urinary retention, hyperthermia, dry skin and mucous membranes, and auditory and visual hallucinations. Patients can also present with seizures or coma. Cardiogenic pulmonary edema may occur secondary to depression of myocardial contraction.

The diagnosis of anticholinergic toxicity must be based on clinical

Table 112-1. Anticholinergic Substances

Antihistamines
- Ethanolamines
  - Dimenhydrinate (Dramamine)
  - Diphenhydramine (Benadryl)
- Ethylenediamines
  - Tripelennamine (Pyribenzamine)
- Alkylamines
  - Chlorpheniramine (Teldrin)
- Piperazines
  - Cyclizine (Marezine)
  - Meclizine (Antivert)
- Phenothiazines
  - Promethazine (Phenergan)

Antiparkinsonian drugs
- Benztropine mesylate (Cogentin)
- Biperiden (Akineton)
- Ethopropazine (Parsidol)
- Trihexyphenidyl (Artane)
- Procyclidine (Kemadrin)

Antipsychotics
- Phenothiazines
  - Chlorpromazine (Thorazine)
  - Thioridazine (Mellaril)
  - Perphenazine (Trilafon)
- Nonphenothiazines
  - Molindone (Moban)
  - Loxapine (Loxitane)

Antispasmodics
- Clidinium bromide (Quarzan, Librax)
- Dicyclomine (Bentyl)
- Methantheline bromide (Banthine)
- Propantheline bromide (Pro-Banthine)
- Tridihexethyl chloride (Pathilon)

Plants
- Deadly nightshade
- Mandrake
- Jimson weed

Belladonna alkaloids, synthetic cogeners
- Atropine (Hyoscyamine)
- Belladonna alkaloid mixtures
- Glycopyrrolate (Robinul)
- Homatropine (Dia-Quel, Malcotran)
- Methscopolamine bromide (Pamine)
- Scopolamine hydrobromide (Hyoscine)

Cyclic antidepressants
- Amitryptiline hydrochloride (Elavil, Amitril, Endep)
- Desipramine hydrochloride (Norpramin, Pertofrane)
- Doxepin hydrochloride (Sinequan, Adapin)
- Imipramine hydrochloride (Tofranil, Pramine)
- Nortriptyline hydrochloride (Aventyl, Pamelor)
- Protriptyline hydrochloride (Vivactil)
- Trimipramine (Surmontil)
- Maprotiline hydrochloride (Ludiomil)
- Zimelidine hydrochloride
- Fluoxetine (Prozac)
- Amoxapine (Asendin)

Ophthalmic products
- Atropine and scopolamine solutions
- Cyclopentolate hydrochloride (Cyclogyl)
- Tropicamide (Mydriacyl)

OTC medications (including antihistamines and belladonna alkaloids)
- Analgesics: Excedrin PM, Percogesic
- Cold remedies: Actifed, Allerest, Coricidin, Dristan, Flavihist, Romex, Sine-Off
- Hypnotics: Compoz, Sleep-Eze, Sominex
- Menstrual products: Pamprin, Premesyn PMS

Skeletal muscle relaxants
- Orphenadrine citrate (Norflex)
- Cyclobenzaprine hydrochloride (Flexeril)

Mushrooms
- *Amanita muscaria*
- *Amanita pantherina*

Source: Adapted from LR Goldfrank.

presentation. The diagnosis may be confused with delirium tremens or an acute psychiatric disorder. Anticholinergic toxicity can be differentiated from delirium tremens and sympathomimetic toxicity by the presence of dry skin and the absence of bowel sounds. Acute psychiatric disorders may have associated tachycardia and tachypnea, but usually the physical exam is normal. Complications from anticholinergic toxicity occur secondary to hyperthermia, arrhythmias, seizures, and circulatory collapse.

Electrocardiographic abnormalities may include QRS prolongation, abnormal conduction, bundle branch block, AV dissociation, and atrial and ventricular tachycardias. Sinus tachycardia is the most common abnormality. Routine laboratory evaluations, including measurement of electrolytes, glucose, and arterial blood gases, should be checked in the presence of abnormal mental status, but should be normal in isolated anticholinergic toxicity. Comprehensive toxicologic screens are of little value in the acute setting, and some anticholinergic agents (e.g., scopolamine) may not be detected. The screen can be used for confirmation, but the diagnosis should be based on clinical findings.

TREATMENT

Conservative, supportive therapy is the mainstay of treatment of anticholinergic toxicity. Evaluation of the airway, breathing, and circulation is a priority. An intravenous line should be established and an ECG monitor placed in any patient with significant symptoms. Because gastrointestinal motility is delayed, gastric emptying may be effective after several hours. Activated charcoal may be useful to decrease drug absorption, particularly with agents that undergo enterohepatic circulation or when the agents ingested are unknown. A cathartic should also be administered.

Hyperthermia should be controlled with conventional therapy. Seizures can be treated with benzodiazepines and barbiturates. Hypertension usually does not require treatment, but conventional therapy should be used if necessary. The treatment of arrhythmias depends on the type and on the causative agent. Standard antiarrythmics are usually effective, but class Ia agents should be avoided due to the quinidine-like effect of many anticholinergic drugs. Agitation can be treated with benzodiazepines. Because of their anticholinergic effects, phenothiazines should be avoided.

The most controversial topic surrounding anticholinergic toxicity is the use of physostigmine. Physostigmine is a tertiary ammonium compound which is a reversible acetylcholinesterase inhibitor that crosses the blood-brain barrier and reverses both central and peripheral anticholinergic effects. Physostigmine may aggravate arrhythmias and seizures and must be used with extreme caution. The indications for its use include the presence of peripheral anticholinergic signs and seizures unresponsive to conventional therapy, uncontrollable agitation, hemodynamically unstable arrhythmias unresponsive to conventional therapy, coma with respiratory depression, malignant hypertension, or refractory hypotension. Physostigmine should only be used in cyclic antidepressant overdose as a last resort, as it may potentiate toxicity and increase mortality. The initial dose of physostigmine is 0.5 to 2.0 mg IV over 5 min. Improvement of central signs usually occurs within 5 to 15 min. The minimal effective dose should be used. Due to rapid elimination, repeat doses may be necessary every 30 to 60 min. Physostigmine use is contraindicated in patients with cardiovascular disease, bronchospasm, intestinal obstruction, heart block, peripheral vascular disease, and bladder obstruction. Patients receiving physostigmine should be on a monitor and observed for cholinergic symptoms (salivation, lacrimation, urination, and defecation).

Patients with mild symptoms of anticholinergic toxicity can be discharged after 6 h of observation, if their symptoms are improving. Patients receiving physostigmine usually require admission for at least 24 h.

JIMSON WEED

Many plants have anticholinergic effects, including deadly nightshade, henbane, mandrake, burdock root, Jimson weed, and others. They are often used for medicinal purposes or brewed in teas. *Datura stramonium,* also known as Jimson weed, is a member of the *Solanaceae* family. It is a common weed that grows to be 3 to 6 ft high and can be found throughout the United States. Its leaves are large, jagged, and have a bitter taste and foul odor. The plant has large white or purple trumpet-shaped flowers that bloom in the late spring and become thorny quadripartite capsules in the fall, filled with black seeds. The entire plant is toxic and contains atropine, hyoscyamine, and scopolamine in various amounts. In the past, Jimson weed was marketed and sold in health food stores in a preparation for the treatment of asthma. Many accidental childhood poisonings from Jimson weed have been reported. Over the past 15 to 20 years, Jimson weed has been involved in inadvertent overdoses in persons experimenting with mind-altering drugs. The plant can be smoked or ingested. Fifty to one hundred seeds contain the equivalent of 3 to 6 mg atropine.

Symptoms of anticholinergic toxicity occur within 2 to 6 h after the ingestion of Jimson weed. As with other agents causing anticholinergic toxicity, patients present with fever, erythema, mydriasis, delirium, hallucinations, tachycardia, and amnesia. The treatment is the same as that described above. Because the seeds may remain in the stomach for prolonged periods, gastric emptying is recommended up to 12 to 24 h after the ingestion of seeds. The most persistent symptom of Jimson weed toxicity is blurred vision, as mydriasis can persist for up to 1 week. Mydriasis can also occur from isolated local contact of Jimson weed with the eye (''cornpicker's pupil'').

BIBLIOGRAPHY

Ellenhorn MJ, Barceloux DG: *Medical Toxicology, Diagnosis and Treatment of Human Poisoning.* New York, Elsevier, 1988.

Goldfrank LR, Flomenbaum NE, Lewin NA, Weisman RS, Howland MA (eds): *Goldfrank's Toxicologic Emergencies,* 4th ed. Norwalk, Appleton & Lange, 1990.

Goldfrank L, Flomenbaum N, Lewin N: Anticholinergic poisoning. *J Toxicol Clin Toxicol* 19(1):17, 1982.

Levy R: Jimson seed poisoning: A new hallucinogen on the horizon. JACEP 6:58, 1977.

Rosen CS, Lechner M: Jimson-weed intoxication. *N Engl J Med* 267:448, 1967.

Savitt DL, Roberts JR, Siegel EG: Anisocoria from Jimsonweed. *JAMA* 255(1):1439, 1986.

Thompson HS: Cornpicker's pupil: Jimsonweed mydriasis. *J Iowa Med Soc* 61:475, 1971.

Vance MA, Ross SM, Millington WR, Blumberg JB: Potentiation of tricyclic antidepressant toxicity by physostigmine in mice. *Clin Toxicol* 11(4):413, 1977.

113
HEAVY METALS

Marsha D. Ford

Acute heavy metal toxicity is a clinical entity that will only occasionally be encountered by the emergency physician yet can be a cause of significant morbidity and mortality if unrecognized and inappropriately treated. Because of their effects on numerous enzymatic systems in the body, the heavy metals often present with protean manifestations primarily affecting four systems: neurologic, gastrointestinal, hematologic and renal. Emergency physicians should be familiar with the common toxic manifestations of the most common metals—lead, arsenic, and mercury—in order to appropriately diagnose poisoned patients and to recognize an initial "index case" in order to prevent others from being poisoned when the metal source is environmental or industrial (see Table 113-1).

LEAD

Lead is the most common cause of chronic heavy metal poisoning and remains a major environmental contaminant. The National Health and Nutrition Examination Survey II, conducted from 1976 to 1980, found that 1.9 percent of persons aged 6 months to 74 years had blood lead levels ≥ 30 μg/dL, with significantly higher levels being found in

Table 113-1. Sources of Heavy Metals

Heavy Metal	Source
Lead	
Inorganic	Soldering; battery burning/reclamation; bronzing; brassmaking; glassmaking; stripping old paint, "deleading" homes; "moonshine" whiskey; liquids in improperly glazed pottery; contaminated herbal medications; indoor shooting ranges; ingestion of paint chips, lead-laden floor dust, lead foreign bodies; lead bullets in abdomen or joint spaces. Workers at risk: jewelers, painters, lead burners and smelters, pipe cutters, pigment makers, printers, welders, pottery makers, radiator repair personnel.
Organic	Leaded gasoline
Arsenic	
Inorganic [arsenite(As^{3+}), arsenate (As^{5+}), elemental]	Insecticides, rodenticides, herbicides; mining smelting/refining; homeopathic medicines; kelp.
Organic	Parasitical medicines (veterinary)
Gas (arsine)	Mining smelting/refining; semiconductor industry; made by mixing acids with arsenic-containing insecticides.
Mercury	
Elemental	Battery and thermometer manufacture; sphygmomanometer repair; dentistry; jewelry and lamp manufacture; photography; mercury mining; manufacture of scientific instruments.
Salts	Taxidermy; fur processing; tannery work; chemical laboratories; manufacture of explosives, fireworks, disinfectants, button batteries, inks, and vinyl chloride.
Organic (methylmercury, ethylmercury, phenylmercury)	Contaminated seafood; embalming; manufacture of drugs, fungicides, bactericides; handling of insecticides; pesticides, coated seeds; manufacture of chloralkali; working with wood perservatives.

blacks and in children from lower socioeconomic groups. Both inorganic and organic forms of lead produce clinical toxicity. Inorganic lead affects the central and peripheral nervous systems, hematopoietic system, kidney, gastrointestinal tract, liver, myocardium, and reproductive capacity. With organic lead intoxication, central nervous system effects predominate.

Inorganic Lead

Pharmacology

Absorption occurs primarily via the respiratory and gastrointestinal tracts, while skin absorption is negligible. In the body, lead distributes into the blood, soft tissues, and bone. Greater than 90 percent of the total body lead is stored in bone, where it easily exchanges with the blood. Excretion of lead occurs slowly; the biologic half-life of lead in bone has been estimated to be 30 years.

Toxicopathology

Like all the heavy metals, lead combines with sulfhydryl groups in proteins, thereby interfering with enzymatic activity. In the hematopoietic system lead interferes with porphyrin metabolism resulting in anemia (see Fig. 113-1). The two enzymes chiefly affected are Δ-aminolevulinic acid dehydratase and ferrochelatase, the latter being the enzyme which catalyzes the transfer of iron from ferritin to protophorphyrin to form hemoglobin. Coexistent iron deficiency may act synergistically with lead toxicity to produce a more profound anemia and, in children, may be more important than lead as the cause of a microcytic anemia. Hemolytic anemia also occurs due to inhibition of red blood cell (RBC) pyrimidine 5′-nucleotidase, an enzyme responsible for clearing cellular RNA degradation products. On a blood peripheral smear, these products produce the RBC basophilic stippling sometimes seen in lead-poisoned patients.

Interference with enzymatic activity in the central nervous system (CNS) produces acute cytotoxicity and cerebral edema. In the peripheral nervous system (PNS), nerves undergo primary segmental demyelination followed by secondary axonal degeneration, primarily of the motor nerves. In the kidney acute lead toxicity affects the proximal tubule, producing a Fanconi-like syndrome with aminoaciduria, glucosuria, phosphaturia, and renal tubular acidosis. Chronic effects include interstitial nephritis and increased uric acid levels due to increased tubular reabsorption of urate. The relationsip between chronic lead toxicity, gout, hypertension, and chronic renal failure remains controversial.

Toxic hepatitis with mildly elevated transaminases, normal bilirubin, and normal alkaline phosphatase can occur. Lead-induced adverse

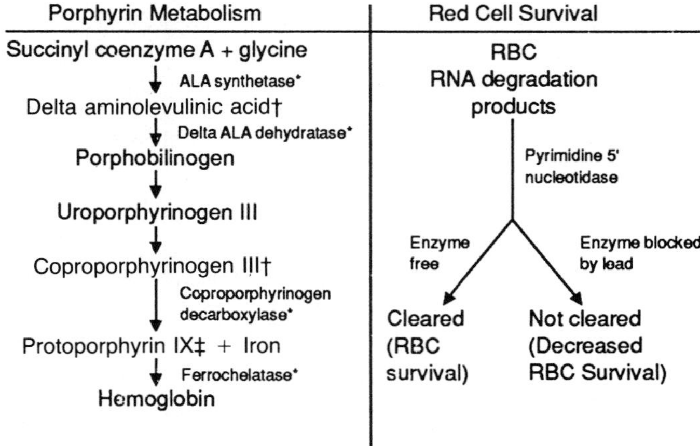

Fig. 113-1. Effects of Lead on the Hematopoietic System. * Enzymes affected by lead; † levels elevated in urine; and ‡ level elevated in RBCs.

effects on the reproductive system include increased fetal wastage, premature membrane rupture, depressed sperm counts, abnormal/nonmotile sperm, and sterility. Chronic lead toxicity can depress free thyroxine levels without producing clinical hypothyroidism.

Clinical Effects

The common signs and symptoms of acute, chronic and delayed toxicity are listed in Table 113-2. A few points bear emphasis. Young children are more susceptible than adults to the effects of lead. Encephalopathy, a major cause of morbidity and mortality, may begin dramatically with seizures and coma or develop indolently over weeks to months with decreased alertness and memory progressing to mania, delirium, and cerebral edema. Gastrointestinal and hematologic manifestations occur more frequently with acute than with chronic poisoning, and the colicky abdominal pains may be associated with concurrent hemolysis. Patients may complain of a metallic taste and have bluish gingival lead lines. Delayed cognitive development can occur in infants and children whose cord and blood lead (PbB) levels are less than the 25 μg/dL level currently accepted as safe by the Centers for Disease Control (CDC). Finally, patients may be asymptomatic in the face of significantly elevated PbB levels.

Diagnosis

History of an exposure—occupational, hobby, environmental, or alcohol-related—is the most important clue to making the diagnosis. The combination of abdominal or neurologic dysfunctions with a hemolytic anemia should raise the suspicion of lead toxicity. Emergency physicians should consider the diagnosis in all children presenting with encephalopathy.

Laboratory studies in the emergency department should focus on evaluation for anemia and examination of bone radiographs in children for "lead bands." The anemia can be normocytic or microcytic, possibly with evidence of hemolysis including an elevated reticulocyte count and increased serum free hemoglobin. The peripheral smear may show basophilic stippling of the RBCs. Both anemia and basophilic stippling occur variably, and their absence does not rule out lead toxicity. Basophilic stippling of RBCs is nonspecific for lead toxicity, as it is also found in arsenic toxicity, sideroblastic anemia, and the thalassemias. In children radiographs of long bones, especially of the knee, may reveal horizontal, metaphyseal "lead bands," which represent failure of bone remodeling rather than deposition of lead.

The definitive diagnosis rests upon finding an elevated PbB level, with or without symptoms, or on a positive chelation provocation test. The PbB level is the best single test for evaluating lead toxicity, but the level may be misleadingly low if the lead exposure was remote. In that case, a calcium disodium versenate ($CaNa_2$-EDTA) provocation test may be necessary to evaluate total-body lead stores. Measuring erythrocyte protoporphyrin (EP) levels may also be useful in screening for chronic, but not acute, toxicity. EP levels rise when the final step in hemoglobin synthesis, which is catalyzed by ferrochelatase, is blocked by lead. The elevated EP levels represent an end-organ effect of lead and have been found to correlate well with PbB levels. Iron deficiency also elevates EP levels and must be ruled out when evaluating an elevated EP level.

Differential Diagnosis

The differential diagnosis of lead toxicity includes causes of encephalopathy such as Wernicke's encephalopathy; withdrawal from ethanol and other sedative-hypnotics drugs; meningitis; encephalitis; human immunodeficiency virus (HIV) infection; intracerebral hemorrhage; hypoglycemia; severe fluid and electrolyte imbalances; hypoxia; arsenic, thallium, and mercury toxicity; and poisoning with cyclic antidepressants, and anticholinergic drugs, ethylene glycol, or carbon monoxide. The abdominal pains can mimic sickle cell crisis or the hepatic porphyrias. Chronic lead toxicity can masquerade as depression, neurosis, hypothyroidism, polyneuritis, gout, iron deficiency anemia, and learning disability.

Management

All patients with appropriate symptoms and an elevated PbB level are classified as lead toxic and should be treated. Fortunately, lead-induced encephalopathy rarely occurs now, but, unfortunately, it remains a major cause of serious morbidity and mortality in lead-toxic patients. Standard life support measures should be instituted and seizures treated with benzodiazepines, phenobarbital, phenytoin, and general anesthesia, if necessary. If abdominal films demonstrate radiopaque flecks consistent with lead, whole-bowel irrigation with a polyethylene glycol electrolyte solution (Colyte, Golytely) should be instituted. The solution should be administered continuously at a rate of 2000 mL/h for adults and 500 mL/h for children until the abdominal radiograph is clear. It will not alter fluid or electrolyte balance in the patient. Fluid administration should be carefully controlled to avoid worsening the cerebral edema. Lumbar puncture may precipitate cerebral herniation

Table 113-2. Clinical Effects of Inorganic Lead Toxicity

System	Acute	Chronic	Late
Central nervous system	Encephalopathy (more common in children); seizures (focal or generalized); confusion, obtundation, coma; papilledema; optic neuritis; vomiting; ataxia. May have complaints listed under Chronic. Normal cerebellar and cranial nerve function.	Headache; irritability; depression, fatigue, behavioral change; memory deficit; apathy; sleep disturbances.	
Peripheral nervous system	Paresthesias. May have some or all findings listed under Chronic.	Motor weakness, including classic wrist drop (peripheral neuropathy rare in children); depressed/absent DTRs; normal sensory function.	
Hematologic	Hypoproliferative and/or hemolytic anemias. Basophilic stippling (uncommon).	Same as in Acute.	
Gastrointestinal	Abdominal pain (colicky).	Abdominal pain (usually not severe, often absent); constipation; diarrhea.	
Renal	Fanconi-like syndrome: aminoaciduria, glucosuria, phosphaturia, renal tubular acidosis.	Interstitial nephritis.	Chronic renal failure; ? hypertension; gout.
Reproductive		Decreased libido; impotence; sterility; abortions; premature births; insufficient and abnormal sperm production.	
Other	Bone pain.	Arthralgias; weakness; weight loss.	

and should be performed carefully, if at all, with the removal of a small amount of cerebrospinal fluid only.

Chelation therapy should be instituted immediately, prior to obtaining laboratory verification of the diagnosis. All chelating agents supply sulfhydryl groups to which the lead attaches. Dimercaprol (British anti-Lewisite, or BAL), 75 mg/m^2, should be administered IM first, followed 4 h later by $CaNa_2$-EDTA, 1500 mg/m^2 per 24 h, in a continuous IV infusion. The BAL administration is continued every 4 h. BAL chelates intracellular as well as extracellular lead and may be administered to patients in renal failure since it is excreted in the bile. It is mixed in peanut oil and must be given IM. $CaNa_2$-EDTA chelates extracellular lead only and may exacerbate lead-induced CNS toxicity in patients with high PbB levels unless preceded by BAL therapy. Continuous IV infusion is the preferred method of delivery. $CaNa_2$-EDTA can cause renal toxicity, and patients should be adequately hydrated to promote diuresis and minimize the risk of this complication. It should not be used in patients with renal failure. Adverse effects of the chelating agents are listed in Table 113-3.

For symptomatic patients without encephalopathy and for asymptomatic patients with elevated PbB levels or provocation tests requiring chelation, the use of BAL and/or $CaNa_2$-EDTA and the dosing schedules are determined by the PbB levels and the presence or absence of symptoms. Children who are symptomatic but not encephalopathic should be treated as above except with doses of BAL, 50 mg/m$_2$, and $CaNa_2$-EDTA, 1000 mg/m^2 per 24 h. Symptomatic, nonencephalopathic adults may be treated with BAL and $CaNa_2$-EDTA or with $CaNa_2$-EDTA alone. In asymptomatic patients, the standards for determining lead toxicity and the necessity for treatment differ for children and adults. The CDC define lead toxicity in children as a PbB level $\geq$ 25 μg/dL in conjunction with an EP level $\geq$ 35 μg/dL. In asymptomatic children, chelation therapy should be performed if the PbB level is $\geq$ 56 μg/dL or if the PbB level is 25 to 55 μg/dL in conjunction with a positive $CaNa_2$-EDTA provocation test. In asymptomatic adults, the guidelines are less rigorous. In workers, a PbB of $<$ 40 μg/dL is accepted as normal, levels of 40 to 50 μg/dL require increased job surveillance, and levels $>$ 50 μg/dL require temporary removal from the job until the PbB drops below 40 μg/dL. Details on therapy for these various groups can be found in standard toxicology references.

Two other chelating agents have been used in lead toxicity. D-Penicillamine is a less effective chelating agent than $CaNa_2$-EDTA but has the advantage of oral administration. It has been used for outpatient therapy in both asymptomatic children and adults with mild PbB elevations. Dimercaptosuccinic acid (DMSA), an experimental analogue of dimercaprol, effectively chelates lead in adults and children. Its advantages include oral administration without increasing lead absorption, no serious adverse effects, and minimal chelation of essential metals. A regional poison control center can assist in patient referral and enrollment in the investigational protocol.

Table 113-3. Adverse Effects of Chelating Agents

Chelating Agent	Adverse Effects
BAL (dimercaprol)	Hypertension Febrile reaction Painful injection Nausea/vomiting, salivation Headache Hemolysis in G6PD-deficient patients BAL-iron complex very toxic
$CaNa_2$-EDTA	Renal toxicity (especially if dehydrated) Can increase CNS levels of lead if given prior to BAL Chelates essential metals (e.g., copper, zinc, iron) Dermatitis Minor: Headache, chills, fever, myalgias, fatigue
D-Penicillamine	Nausea/vomiting Fever Rash Leukopenia, thrombocytopenia Eosinophilia Hemolytic anemia Stevens-Johnson syndrome (Probably safe in penicillin-allergic patients)
DMSA (experimental)	Abdominal gas, pain ? transient elevated AST, alkaline phosphatase

Removal of the source of lead is mandatory for all patients. Patients should not be discharged to their former environments until appropriate deleading and decontamination measures have been accomplished. Family members and coworkers should be evaluated for occult lead toxicity.

A guide for hospitalization would be to hospitalize:

1. All children with symptoms, with a PbB $\geq$ 56 μg/dL or with a positive chelation provocation test.
2. All adults with CNS symptoms.
3. All patients with suspected toxicity when returning to the environment is considered dangerous.

Prognosis

Approximately 85 percent of patients who suffer encephalopathy develop permanent CNS damage including seizures, mental retardation in children, and cognitive deficits in adults. Abdominal colic usually subsides within days after beginning chelation therapy, and other acute manifestations clear within 1 to 16 weeks with therapy. Lead-induced nephropathy may be partially reversible with chelation therapy.

Organic Lead Intoxication

Exposure to tetraethyl lead (TEL), found in leaded gasoline, can occur with gasoline sniffing or in the occupational setting. Tetraethyl lead is metabolized to inorganic lead and triethyl lead. Triethyl lead is the primary toxic product which produces predominantly CNS toxicity. Symptoms range from behavioral changes with irritability, insomnia, restlessness, and nausea/vomiting to tremor, chorea, convulsions, and mania. Muscle, hepatic, and renal damage can occur. Anemia and elevated EP levels are usually not found. PbB levels may be normal or elevated. Therapy consists of removal from the source, symptomatic treatment, and chelation only if the PbB is elevated.

ARSENIC

Arsenic is a nearly tasteless, odorless metal which is the most common cause of acute heavy metal poisoning and the second leading source of chronic heavy metal toxicity. Arsenicals are found in a variety of compounds and industries (see Table 113-1) and continue to be used as tools for homicides and suicides. Inorganic, organic, and gaseous forms exist. Inorganic compounds include arsenite (As^{3+}) arsenate (As^{5+}) and elemental arsenic. Arsine, a gaseous form, has toxicopathologic mechanisms and treatment which differ from those of other arsenical compounds. It will be discussed under a separate heading below.

Pharmacology

Arsenic is well absorbed via the gastrointestinal (GI), dermal, respiratory, and parenteral routes. Due to its water solubility, pentavalent arsenic (arsenate) is more readily absorbed through mucous membranes, for example, the GI tract, than trivalent arsenic (arsenite). Arsenite penetrates the skin more readily due to its increased lipid solubility. After absorption, arsenic localizes in erythrocytes and leukocytes or binds to serum proteins. Within 24 h redistribution into the liver, kidney, spleen, lung, GI tract, muscle, and nervous tissues occurs with subsequent integration into hair, nails, and bone. Excretion is predominantly renal with greater than 50 percent of a dose excreted within 30 h of ingestion. Toxicity of the various forms is partially determined by excretory rates, with the more toxic arsenite being excreted at a slower rate than arsenate or the organic arsenical compounds. Arsenic crosses the placenta and has produced teratogenicity in both animals and humans.

Toxicopathology

Arsenic reversibly binds with sulfhydryl groups found in many tissues and enzyme systems. It blocks oxidative phosphorylation through two distinct mechanisms:

1. Inhibition of the conversions of pyruvate to acetyl coenzyme A (acetyl-CoA) and α-ketoglutarate to succinyl-CoA in the Krebs cycle. Specifically, arsenic blocks the conversion of dihydrolipoate to lipoate, a necessary cofactor in these two conversions. This is the most important toxic mechanism.
2. Substitution of arsenic for phosphate, resulting in the loss of stable phosphoryl compounds with their high-energy phosphate bonds.

Pathologically, acute exposure produces dilation and increased permeability of small blood vessels, resulting in GI mucosal and submucosal inflammation and necrosis, cerebral edema and hemorrhage, myocardial tissue destruction, and fatty degeneration of the liver and kidneys. Subacute or chronic exposure can cause a primary peripheral axonal neuropathy with secondary demyelination.

Clinical Effects

The signs and symptoms of toxicity vary with the form, amount, and concentration ingested and the rates of absorption and excretion of the various arsenical compounds. Arsenite (trivalent) is more toxic than arsenate (pentavalent). Symptoms usually occur within 30 min to several hours of ingestion. Severe gastroenteritis with nausea, vomiting, and cholera-like diarrhea is the hallmark of acute poisoning and may last several days to weeks, frequently necessitating hospitalization. Patients may complain of garlicky breath odor and a metallic taste. Hypotension and tachycardia secondary to volume depletion, capillary leak, and myocardial dysfunction occur in moderate to severe cases. The ECG may demonstrate nonspecific ST- and T-wave changes with a prolonged QTc, although these findings are more common in chronic intoxication. Ventricular tachycardia with a torsade de pointes morphology has been reported. Secondary myocardial ischemia may occur, leading to an erroneous diagnosis of primary myocardial infarction. Acute encephalopathy with delirium, seizures, and coma; pulmonary edema; acute renal failure; rhabdomyolysis; and death may ensue.

Patients with subacute or chronic toxicity typically present with complaints of a peripheral neuropathy, skin rash, or a nonspecific malaise and weakness, often with a history of gastroenteritis occurring 1 to 6 weeks earlier. Survivors of acute poisonings can develop the same problems. The peripheral neuropathy develops in a stocking-glove distribution and is initially sensory, with later motor symptoms. Severe cases can develop an ascending paralysis mimicking Guillain-Barré syndrome. The dermatologic manifestations vary. Hyperpigmentation, hyperkeratosis of the palms and soles, morbilliform rash, and epidermoid cancer have been reported. Mee's lines (1- to 2-mm-wide transverse white lines in the nails) may be seen 4 to 6 weeks after an acute ingestion, while nasal septal perforation has been found in workers exposed occupationally to arsenic. Patients may complain of weakness, muscular aching, abdominal pain, memory loss, personality changes, periorbital and extremity edema, or decreased hearing secondary to sensorineural damage. Chronic encephalopathy with delirium, hallucinations, disorientation, agitation, and confabulation resembling Korsakoff's syndrome has been reported. Chronic exposure to arsenic has been linked with the development of squamous cell and basal skin carcinomas, respiratory tract cancer, hepatic angiosarcoma, and possibly with leukemia.

Diagnosis

Without a history of known exposure to arsenic, the diagnosis must be based on the presenting signs and symptoms and a strong index of clinical suspicion. Physicians rarely encounter arsenic toxicity, and, unfortunately, criminal poisonings often go undetected. The diagnosis of acute arsenic poisoning should be considered in any patient with hypotension of unknown etiology which was preceded by a severe gastroenteritis. The diagnosis of chronic arsenic toxicity should be considered in a patient with a peripheral neuropathy, typical skin manifestations, or recurrent bouts of unexplained gastroenteritis.

An abdominal radiograph may demonstrate intestinal radiopaque metallic flecks in cases of arsenic ingestions. The complete blood count may reveal either a normocytic, normochromic, or megaloblastic anemia and/or a thrombocytopenia. The white blood cell (WBC) count may be elevated in acute toxicity and decreased in chronic cases. A relative eosinophilia, up to 21 percent, and basophilic stippling of the RBCs have been reported. Elevated reticulocyte counts are found in cases with a component of hemolytic anemia. The electrocardiogram often reveals a prolonged QTc interval, especially in cases of chronic poisoning.

Definitive diagnosis depends upon finding elevated arsenic levels in a 24-h urine collection. All urinary measurements of heavy metals should be collected in metal-free containers. Normal urinary arsenic is <0.05 mg/L, and total urinary arsenic excretion in an unexposed patient should not exceed 0.1 mg/24 h. If the baseline urinary level is within normal limits and arsenic intoxication is still suspected, a D-penicillamine mobilization test (25 mg/kg per dose to a maximum 250 mg per dose for four doses) should be performed with concomitant 24-h urine collection for arsenic. Due to the rapid distribution of arsenic in tissues, blood arsenic levels are unreliable.

Different Diagnosis

Arsenic toxicity should be included in the differential diagnosis for septic shock; peripheral neuropathy, including Guillain-Barré syndrome; Addison's disease; patients with the previously mentioned dermatologic manifestations; Korsakoff's syndrome; cholera-like diarrhea; porphyria; other heavy metal, such as thallium, toxicities and unexplained, prolonged malaise and weakness.

Management

Acute arsenical toxicity is a life-threatening illness requiring aggressive management. The first task is to ensure adequate respiratory and circulatory function. Hypotension and arrhythmias are the chief causes of death. Hypotension, usually due to volume depletion, should be managed initially with crystalloid volume replacement. Invasive hemodynamic monitoring followed by further crystalloid and pressor therapy with dopamine or norepinephrine (levarterenol) may be required. Overhydration should be avoided since pulmonary and cerebral edema can occur. Cardiac monitoring should be instituted. Ventricular tachycardia and fibrillation may be treated with lidocaine, bretyllium, and electrical defibrillation as necessary. Isoproterenol, magnesium, and overdrive pacing therapies should be considered for torsade de pointes arrhythmias. Drugs which prolong the QTc, including type IA antiarrhythmics (procainamide, quinidine, disopyramide) should be avoided. Potassium, calcium, and magnesium levels should be monitored and corrected as necessary to prevent further prolongation of the QTc with possible exacerbation of torsade de pointes arrhythmias.

Gastric lavage with a large-bore orogastric tube should be performed in all cases of acute ingestion, and activated charcoal (1 g/kg body weight) and a cathartic should be instilled. Activated charcoal poorly adsorbs arsenic but may be effective if coingestants were taken. Whole-bowel irrigation should be considered if abdominal radiographs reveal intestinal radiopaque materials consistent with arsenic.

Seizures can be treated with benzodiazepines, phenobarbital, phenytoin, and general anesthesia as necessary.

Initial management of chronic toxicity should be directed toward prevention of further arsenic absorption and gastrointestinal decontamination, if appropriate. In cases of suspected homicidal intent, patients should be advised to avoid food and drinks prepared by others, and visitor contact with hospitalized patients should be carefully monitored.

Chelation therapy with BAL should be instituted immediately in all cases of known or suspected acute arsenical poisoning and in proven cases of chronic toxicity. In cases of suspected chronic toxicity with stable symptoms, therapy may be withheld pending diagnosis. BAL doses range 3 to 5 mg/kg IM every 4 h for 2 days followed by 3 to 5 mg/kg every 6 to 12 h. In severe, life-threatening toxicity BAL therapy should be continued until the clinical condition stabilizes and a less toxic oral chelating agent can be substituted. Two chelating agents discussed in the section on lead toxicity, D-penicillamine and the investigational drug DMSA, can also be used to enhance arsenic excretion. D-Penicillamine (100 mg/kg per day with a maximum dose of 2 g for adults and 1 g for children) should be given in four divided doses per day for 5 days. DMSA is given according to an investigational protocol. A regional poison control center can provide information on enrolling a patient in this protocol. During chelation intermittent 24-h urinary arsenic levels should be measured and therapy continued until the urine level falls below 0.05 mg/L per 24 h.

Hemodialysis can remove small amounts of arsenic (2 to 4.5 mg) in patients with acute renal failure but is not indicated otherwise.

Hospitalize:

1. All patients with acute or life-threatening known or suspected arsenic poisoning.
2. All chronically poisoned patients requiring BAL therapy.
3. All patients in whom suicidal or homicidal intent is suspected.

Prognosis and Sequelae

In acute toxicity, prognosis may be influenced favorably by the rapid institution of BAL therapy. Recovery from arsenical neuropathy appears to be related more to initial severity of symptoms than to institution of chelation therapy, although in those patients who do recover, BAL appears to significantly shorten the duration of illness. Often, neurological recovery occurs slowly over months to years. Normalization of hematologic values can occur in the absence of any specific therapy. BAL has a variable effect on the dermatologic manifestations; hyperpigmentation is unresponsive to this therapy.

Arsine

Arsine is a colorless, nonirritating gas encountered in the semiconductor industry, ore smelting, and refining processes and is also produced when arsenic-containing insecticides are mixed with acids. Arsine attaches to sulhydryl groups of hemoglobin, producing an acute hemolytic anemia with resultant jaundice, abdominal pain, and hemoglobinuria-induced acute renal failure. Acute poisonings are managed with blood transfusions, exchange transfusion to remove the nondialyzable arsine, and hemodialysis for the acute renal failure. BAL therapy has no role in the management of arsine toxicity.

MERCURY

Mercury occurs in both inorganic and organic forms. Inorganic compounds are divided further into elemental mercury and mercurous and mercuric salts. Organic mercurials exist as short and long-chained alkyl and aryl compounds. The short-chained alkyls, such as methyl mercury and ethyl mercury, are more toxic to humans. All forms of mercury are toxic but differ in the routes of absorption, constellations of clinical findings, and responses to therapy.

Pharmacology

Elemental mercury is primarily absorbed via inhalation of its vapor but may also be absorbed dermally. Absorption by the gastrointestinal tract is usually negligible. Intramuscular injections of mercury can induce abscess and granuloma formation; delayed systemic toxicity can occur. Intravenous injections have produced mercury pulmonary and systemic emboli. Both mercuric salts and organic mercury are primarily absorbed through the GI tract, with the short-chained alkyl organic compounds being much better absorbed than the aryl organic compounds.

Elemental mercury crosses the blood-brain barrier where it is ionized and trapped in the CNS. Mercuric salts are deposited in the ionized form primarily in the kidney and also in the liver and spleen. The salts do not enter the CNS in consequential amounts. With organic mercury compounds, the highly lipid soluble short-chained alkyls easily cross membranes, accumulating in RBCs, the CNS, liver, kidney, and the fetus. Longer-chained alkyl and the aryl compounds are biotransformed into inorganic mercuric ions in the body. Therefore, toxicity with these compounds more closely resembles inorganic mercury toxicity.

Inorganic and the aryl organic mercurials are eliminated in the urine and feces. The short-chained alkyl compounds are primarily excreted in the bile where they undergo significant enterohepatic circulation.

Toxicopathology

Mercury binds with sulfhydryl groups, affecting a diverse number of enzyme and protein systems. Methylmercury also inhibits choline acetyl transferase, which catalyzes the final step in the production of acetylcholine, and may produce an acetylcholine deficiency.

Clinical Effects

The clinical effects of mercury poisoning depend upon the form and, in some cases, the route of administration. In general, the neurological, gastrointestinal, and renal systems are predominantly affected. The short-chained alkyl compounds, methyl- and ethylmercury, have the most devastating effects on the CNS, followed by elemental mercury, whose primary toxicity is neurological. Both forms of mercury produce erethism, a constellation of neuropsychiatric abnormalities including anxiety, depression, irritability, mania, sleep disturbances, excessive shyness, and memory loss. Tremor, either intention or nonintention, is a common physical finding. The short-chained alkyls produce paresthesias (early sign), ataxia, muscular rigidity or spasticity, and visual and hearing impairment and induce CNS teratogenic effects. Gastrointestinal effects of both elemental and short-chained alkyl compounds are mild. In cases of severe, chronic poisoning with elemental mercury, stomatitis, gingivitis, and excessive salivation are seen. Chronic toxicity of elemental and organic forms may cause renal glomerular and tubular damage.

In contrast, the mercury salts have little to no effect on the CNS but produce a severe corrosive gastroenteritis with abdominal pain which may be followed rapidly by cardiovascular collapse. Renal effects are typical, including acute tubular necrosis within 24 h. Children exposed to all forms of mercury except the short-chained alkyls can develop acrodynia, a condition characterized by a generalized rash, fever, irritability, splenomegaly, and generalized hypotonia with particular weakness of the pelvic and pectoral muscles. Further details of clinical findings are listed in Table 113-4. Swallowing mercury contained in a glass thermometer usually does not produce adverse effects because the mercury is not absorbed from the gastrointestinal tract unless the gastrointestine tract is damaged or contains fistulas.

Diagnosis

A thorough history, including occupational exposures, and typical physical findings, especially tremor or a constellation of signs and symptoms suggesting erethism or acrodynia, may alert the emergency physician to mercury toxicity. Ingestion of mercuric chloride can pro-

Table 113-4. Clinical Effects of Mercury Toxicity

	Inorganic		Organic	
System	**Elemental**	**Salts**	**Short-Chained Alkyls***	**Long-Chained Alkyls, Aryls**
Neurological	Tremor (intention and nonintention), peripheral neuropathy (sensorimotor). Seizures (vapor inhalation).	(−)	Paresthesias (early sign); ataxia; sensory and hearing impairment; constricted visual fields; dysarthria; muscular rigidity or spasticity; seizures (rare); muscle tenderness; and optic atrophy (EM only). MM: Sensorimotor neuropathy.	
Erethism	+	−	+	
GI	Stomatitis, gingivitis, excessive salivation, (severe chronic poisoning). Blue gum line.	Severe gastroenteritis, may be hemorrhagic; abdominal pain, stomatitis, proctitis, colitis.	MM: Rarely symptoms. EM: Nausea/vomiting, abdominal cramps.	Similar to elemental.
Renal	Glomerular and tubular damage (chronic).	Acute tubular necrosis (severe poisoning); proteinuria, hematuria and casts (mild poisoning). Nephrotic syndrome.	MM: − EM: Polyuria, proteinuria.	Similar to elemental.
Pulmonary (inhaled)	Pneumonitis, pulmonary edema, penumothorax, pneumomediastinum.	−	Same as elemental.	Same as elemental.
Skin	Slate-gray pigmentation. Brownish-yellow discoloration of anterior capsule of eye. Allergic dermatitis.	Urticaria, vesication, allergic dermatitis.	Erythroderma, pruritus.	
Teratogenicity	−	−	Cerebral palsy, mental retardation, micrognathia, microcephaly, cleft palate, blindness, chorea, ataxia.	
Acrodynia†	+	+	−	+
Other		Rapid cardiovascular collapse with mercuric chloride.	EM: Severe musculoskeletal pain.	

* MM = methylmercury; EM = ethylmercury.
† Generalized rash with erythema and desquamation of hands, feet and nose; fever, diaphoresis, splenomegaly; hypotonia, irritability, weakness of pelvic/pectoral muscles. Does not occur in newborns or adults.

duce a rapidly fatal course and should be considered in any patient presenting with a corrosive gastroenteritis. Often, however, the diagnosis of mercury toxicity is subtle, arrived at only after many other diagnoses have been investigated.

For all forms of mercury except short-chained alkyls, a 24-h urinary measurement of mercury should be performed. Most unexposed individuals will have levels ≤ 10 to 15 μg/L. A level of > 100 μg/L either before or after therapy indicates meaningful exposure. In cases of chronic toxicity this measurement may be falsely low. Whole-blood mercury levels are less reliable diagnostically. A seafood meal can temporarily elevate the blood level to the toxic range.

Short-chained alkyl mercury compounds are predominantly excreted via the bile, rendering urinary measurements invalid. Laboratory diagnosis rests on finding elevated whole-blood mercury levels, since these compounds concentrate in erythrocytes. Whole-blood mercury levels are normally < 1.5 μg/dL.

Differential Diagnosis

The differential diagnosis of mercury toxicity depends upon the form ingested. Hypothyroidism, apathetic hyperthryroidism, metabolic encephalopathy, senile dementia, adverse effects of therapeutic drugs (such as lithium, theophylline, phenytoin), Parkinson's disease, delayed neuropsychiatric sequelae of carbon monoxide poisoning, lacunar infarction, cerebellar degenerative disease or tumor, and ethanol or sedative-hypnotic drug withdrawal may produce behavioral changes or tremor similar to those caused by elemental mercury. Causes of corrosive gastroenteritis such as iron, arsenic, phosphorus, acids, or alkalis should be considered in the differential diagnosis for mercury salts. Many of the differential diagnoses for elemental mercury also apply to the organic mercury compounds. Cerebral palsy, intrauterine hypoxia, and teratogenic effects of therapeutic and illicit drugs and environmental contaminants should be considered when evaluating an infant thought to be affected in utero by the short-chained alkyl mercury compounds.

Treatment

General therapeutic measures include removal from exposure and supportive therapy. Ingestion of mercury salts should be treated with aggressive gastrointestinal decontamination including instillation of milk or egg whites to bind the mercury, lavage, and activated charcoal. Given the profuse diarrhea which may ensue, a cathartic may not be indicated. A polythiolated resin (commercially unavailable) has been used to bind intestinal methylmercury and interrupt the enterohepatic circulation. Neostigmine may improve motor function in methylmercury-poisoned patients by improving acetylcholine levels.

Both BAL and D-penicillamine may be used for chelation therapy. BAL is the preferred chelator for mercury salts and is administered in a regimen of 3 to 5 mg/kg per dose IM every 4 h for 2 days, then every 6 h for 2 days, followed by every 12 h for 7 days. BAL is contraindicated in methylmercury poisoning due to exacerbation of CNS symptoms. The BAL-mercury complex is dialyzable, and hemodialysis may be helpful in patients receiving BAL who have diminished renal function. D-Penicillamine is used in elemental mercury and less severe cases of mercury salt toxicities. The dose is 100 mg/kg per day, to a maximum of 1 g in four divided doses for 3 to 10 days. D-Penicillamine has been used with variable results in organic mercury poisoning. The experimental chelator DMSA has demonstrated efficacy in binding mercury, including organic forms, and may become the treatment of choice for the short-chained alkyl compounds.

Hospitalize:

1. All patients known or suspected of ingesting mercury salts.
2. All patients known to have or suspected to have inhaled elemental mercury vapor with pulmonary.
3. All patients requiring BAL therapy.

Prognosis and Sequelae

Outcome depends upon the form of mercury and the severity of toxicity. Mild cases of elemental and mercury salt poisoning and very mild cases of organic mercury toxicity may result in complete recovery. Death can occur in severe cases of mercuric chloride poisoning. Most cases of organic mercury poisoning are left with residual neurological deficits.

BIBLIOGRAPHY

General

Goldfrank LR, Flomenbaum NE, Lewin NA, et al (eds): *Goldfrank's Toxicologic Emergencies,* 4th ed. Norwalk, Appleton & Lange, 1990.

Graziano JH: Role of 2,3-dimercaptosuccinic acid in the treatment of heavy metal poisoning. *Med Toxicol* 1:155, 1986.

Halverson, PB, Kozin F, Bernhard GC, et al: Toxicity of penicillamine. *JAMA* 240:1870, 1978.

Lead

Bellinger D, Leviton A, Waternaux C, et al: Longitudinal analysis of prenatal and postnatal lead exposure and early cognitive development. *N Engl J Med* 316:1037, 1987.

Clark M, Royal J, Solar R: Interaction of iron deficiency and lead and the hematologic findings in children with severe lead poisoning. *Pediatrics* 81:247, 1988.

Cory-Slechta D, Weiss B, Cox C: Mobilization and redistribution of lead over the course of calcium disodium ethylenediamine tetraacetate chelation therapy. *J Pharmacol Exp Ther* 243:804, 1987.

Cullen M, Robins J, Eskenazi B: Adult inorganic lead intoxication: Presentation of 31 new cases and a review of recent advances in the literature. *Medicine* 62:221, 1983.

Dillman R, Crumb C, Kidsky M: Lead poisoning from a gunshot wound. *Am J Med* 66:509, 1979.

Graziano JH, Siris ES, Lolacone NJ, et al: 2,3-Dimercaptosuccinic acid as an antidote for lead intoxication. *Clin Pharmacol Ther* 37:431, 1985.

Graziano JH, Lolacono NJ, Meyer P: Dose-response study of oral 2,3-dimercaptosuccinic acid in children with elevated blood lead concentrations. *J Pediatr* 113:751, 1988.

Kapoor SC, Wielopolski L, Graziano JH, et al: Influence of 2,3-dimercaptosuccinic acid on gastrointestinal lead absorption and whole-body lead retention. *Toxicol Appl Pharmacol* 97:525, 1989.

Mahaffey KR, Annest JL, Roberts J, et al: National estimates of blood lead levels: United States, 1976–1980. *N Engl J Med* 307:573, 1982.

McMichael AJ, Baghurst PA, Wigg NR, et al: Port Pirie cohort study: Environmental exposure to lead and children's abilities at the age of four years. *N Engl J Med* 319:468, 1988.

Piomelli S, Rosen JF, Chisolm JJ, et al: Management of childhood lead poisoning. *J Pediatr* 105:523, 1984.

Whitfield CL, Ch'ien LT, Whitehead JD: Lead encephalopathy in adults. *Am J Med* 52:289, 1972.

Arsenic

Eichner E: Erythroid karyorrhexis in the peripheral blood smear in severe arsenic poisoning: A comparison with lead poisoning. *Am J Clin Pathol* 81:533, 1984.

Feldman RG, Niles CA, Kelly-Hayes M, et al: Peripheral neuropathy in arsenic smelter workers. *Neurology* 29:939, 1979.

Fincher RE, Koerker RM: Long-term survival in acute arsenic encephalopathy: Follow-up using newer measures of electrophysiologic parameters. *Am J Med* 82:549, 1987.

Fowler BA, Weissberg JB: Arsine poisoning. *N Engl J Med* 291:1171, 1974.

Gousios AG, Adelson L: Electrocardiographic and radiographic findings in acute arsenic poisoning. *Am J Med* 659, 1959.

Graziano JH, Cuccia D, Friedheim E: The pharmacology of 2,3-dimercaptosuccininc acid and its potential use in arsenic poisoning. *J Pharmacol Exp Ther* 20:1051, 1978.

Greenberg C, Davies S, McGowan T, et al: Acute respiratory failure following severe arsenic poisoning. *Chest* 76:596, 1979.

Kerr HD: Arsenic content of homeopathic medicines. *Clin Toxicol* 24:451, 1986.

Kyle RA, Pease GL: Hematologic aspects of arsenic intoxication. *N Engl J Med* 273:18, 1965.

Petery J, Gross C, Victoria BE, et al: Ventricular fibrillation caused by arsenic poisoning. *Am J Dis Child* 120:367, 1970.

Schoolmeester WL, White DR: Arsenic poisoning. *South Med J* 73:198, 1980.

Mercury

Agocs MM, Etzel RA, Parrish RG, et al: Mercury exposure from interior latex paint. *N Engl J Med* 323:1096, 1990.

Ambre JJ, Welsh MJ, Svare CW, et al: Intravenous elemental mercury injection: Blood levels and excretion of mercury. *Ann Intern Med* 87:451, 1977.

Elhassani SA: The many faces of methylmercury poisoning. *Clin Toxicol* 19:875, 1982–83.

Eyl TB: Organic-mercury food poisoning. *N Engl J Med* 284:706, 1971.

Laundy T, Adam AE, Kershaw JB, et al: Deaths after peritoneal lavage with mercuric chloride solutions: Case report and review of the literature. *B Med J* 289:96, 1984.

Levin SP, Cavender GD, Langoff GD, et al: Elemental mercury exposure: Peripheral neurotoxicity. *Br J Indust Med* 39:136, 1982.

Lilis R, Miller A, Lerman Y: Acute mercury poisoning with severe chronic pulmonary manifestations. *Chest* 88:306, 1985.

McAlpine D, Araki S: Minamata disease: An unusual neurological disorder caused by contaminated fish. *Lancet* 2:629, 1958.

Sketris IS, Gray JD: Mercury poisoning. *Clin Toxicol Consult* 5:10, 1983.

Winek CL, Fochtman FW, Bricker JD, et al: Fatal mercuric chloride ingestion. *Clin Toxicol* 18:261, 1981.

SECTION 11
Environmental Injuries

114
FROSTBITE

Barry Heller

DEFINITIONS AND PATHOGENESIS

Injury due to cold may be generalized, as in hypothermia, or may occur locally, as in frostbite. Local cold injury may occur at temperatures both above and below freezing. Nonfreezing cold injury can be divided into two groups on the basis of exposure to either dry or wet cold.

Trench foot, or immersion foot, occurs with exposure to wet cold for 1 to 2 days, with ambient temperatures above freezing. In this situation, the extremity often develops severe superficial damage resembling partial-thickness burns. Deep tissue destruction in this setting, however, is rare.

Pernio, or chilblain, refers to prolonged exposure of an extremity to dry cold at temperatures above freezing. This is seen most commonly in mountain climbers, and consists of small, superficial, painful ulcerations over chronically exposed areas. These lesions are often associated with hypersensitivity of the surrounding skin, pruritus, and erythema. On occasion, this process may be complicated by extensor tenosynovitis.

Freezing cold injury results in the clinical picture most often referred to as *frostbite.* The pathogenesis of frostbite remains controversial, however, there is evidence for both macrovascular and microvascular processes as well as direct cellular injury. When a body surface comes into contact with cold, there may be superficial tissue freezing to a depth dependent on the intensity and duration of cold exposure. Instantaneous, severe freezing can occur in tissue exposed to volatile hydrocarbons, such as gasoline, at low temperatures. Below this zone of freezing, capillary circulation slows and eventually halts secondary to cold-induced vasospasm and increased viscosity of blood. At this point, certain macrovascular responses have been shown to occur. Initially, the arterioles in the area constrict in an effort to decrease loss of heat at the site of the cold insult. Following this, capillary shunting occurs with arteriole-to-venule flow of blood. This mechanism, known as the "hunting response," is the body's physiologic effort to keep some blood circulating to the cold extremity while minimizing heat loss. However, chilled blood returning from the periphery to the heart may cause a drop in the core temperature as loss of body heat exceeds production capacity. To complicate matters further, the tissues once supplied by the capillaries, which are now being bypassed, remain devoid of oxygen and nutrients. With the inevitable drop in core temperature, shunting stops, allowing the extremity to freeze. This is the ultimate physiologic mechanism of survival; sacrifice of an extremity in order to preserve the core of the organism. It is easy to see how this process can be worsened by shock, panic, and poor physical conditioning.

There is evidence that ice crystals actually form in the extra- and intracellular spaces. The resulting shift of water leads to increased intracellular osmolality, intracellular dehydration, and ultimate denaturation of intracellular proteins. Intracellular ice crystals disrupt cellular architecture and function. Microvascular occlusion also has been shown to occur in the process of local cold injury. Low temperature leads to decreased flow of blood and sludging secondary to increased viscosity. Platelets aggregate, occluding venules, so that within 1 to 2 h capillary and arteriolar vascular beds are damaged. After thawing, protein-rich fluid leaks from the injured vasculature into the interstitial space. This leads to increased tissue pressure, further promoting venous stasis and occlusion, with eventual tissue damage and death.

The areas of the body most likely to suffer local cold injury are those farthest from the body's core, such as earlobes, cheeks, nose, hands, and feet. To prevent local cold injury, the body must be warm enough to supply warm blood to these areas. Adequate clothing and general physical condition of the body as a whole are therefore at least as important as warm covering for the hands and feet. However, local cold injury may occur in the presence or absence of generalized hypothermia.

There are several factors which influence the severity of cold injury. Obviously, the temperature and duration of exposure are of prime importance. Wet cold cools tissue much more quickly than dry cold, and the insulating effect of any piece of clothing is markedly diminished when the clothing is wet. Air movement accelerates heat loss so that the chilling effect of ambient temperature at −7°C (19.4°F) combined with a 72.5-km/h (45-mi/h) wind is identical to that of −40°C (−40°F) temperature on a windless day. Wind speed does not determine final tissue temperature because tissue cannot fall to temperatures below that of the ambient air, but it does greatly promote body and extremity heat loss.

High altitude also has a deleterious effect in terms of temperature regulation. Though blood has not been shown to be more viscous because of high altitude (in spite of increased packed red blood cell volume), water loss from increased respiratory rates can lead to relative dehydration and decreased blood flow. Furthermore, high altitude can lead to hypoxic conditions in the central nervous system, resulting in impaired behavioral responses and mechanisms of adaptation to cold and stress.

CLINICAL FEATURES

The initial clinical response to cold produces reversible skin changes known as "frostnip." The skin becomes blanched and numb, followed by a sudden cessation of cold and discomfort. This sudden loss of cold sensation at the injured location is a fairly reliable sign of incipient frostbite. If heeded instantly, frostnip will not progress to frostbite.

Frostbite has been divided on clinical grounds into as many as four different categories of severity ranging from hyperemia and edema to full-thickness necrosis. However, for purposes of recognition, treatment, and prognosis, two clinical classes of frostbite, *superficial* and *deep,* seem adequate. As frostnip progresses to frostbite, the frozen tissue remains cold to the touch, pale, gray, and bloodless. In superficial frostbite, the skin remains pliable and soft beneath the surface. In deep frostbite, the tissues feel woody and stony. Note, however, that this particular clinical distinction can be made only prior to thawing of the tissues.

In superficial frostbite, large, clear blisters appear in 24 to 48 h. Following this, the skin hardens, blister fluid is resorbed, and the skin blackens into a hard carapace. Within several weeks, a demarcation line occurs between blackened skin and healthy viable tissue. This carapace is in essence a dry gangrene of a very superficial nature (in contrast to that associated with arteriosclerotic-induced gangrene, which may include several tissue layers), peeling off bit by bit over several months and revealing a shiny red skin beneath. This "new" skin will be abnormally tender and hypersensitive to heat and cold. Ultimately it will assume the characteristics of normal skin, but for unknown reasons will remain more susceptible to cold injury and frostbite compared with unaffected skin.

Deep frostbite involves deep structures including, in some cases, muscle, bone, and tendon, because nutritional capillary flow is never returned to these areas. The extremity appears deep purple or red and is cool to the touch. Although sensation and distal function are absent, the patient may be able to move distal parts because proximal muscles and tendons may be functional. In contrast to superficial frostbite, small, dark hemorrhagic blisters appear in 1 to 3 weeks. Edema is slow to form but may persist for months. Eventually, nonviable skin and deep structures demarcate, mummify, and slough.

Prediction of tissue loss may be impossible for several months. However, the appearance of the tissue after initial thawing gives some clues to the severity of tissue damage. In mild or superficial frostbite, after thawing, the skin is sensitive to pinprick, has good color, and is warm to the touch. Furthermore, blisters of clear fluid occur early and extend to the tip of the digits. In deep or severe frostbite, after thawing, the distal portions remain cold and cyanotic. There is late appearance of small, dark vesicles, and failure of vesicles to extend to the volar pads of the distal digits. Once formed, if the blackened carapace corresponds to the original affected part, much tissue loss is unlikely. But if the contour of the pulp of the finger disappears, then the carapace will appear wrinkled, betraying the loss of tissue beneath it.

Laboratory tests are of little value in predicting severity of frostbite. However, recent studies with technetium pertechnetate scanning have shown a good correlation between persistent perfusion defects on scintigraphy and deep tissue damage for which surgical resection is ultimately required. Technetium pyrophosphate scanning can identify nonviable bone with accuracy. A scan at 24 to 48 h after injury, followed by a repeat study at 7 to 10 days, will help to assess the efficacy of initial conservative treatment. If amputation is required, these studies may help to determine the level. Doppler and plethysmographic studies are of some assistance in the differentiation of mild from severe frostbite after thawing. Angiography is best reserved for evaluation of chronic vascular abnormalities associated with freeze-injured tissues.

Early surgical intervention (i.e., amputation) should be delayed until the extent of ultimate tissue loss is clearly demarcated. Even an extremity with deep frostbite may return to near normal, with minimal tissue loss, over a period of several months.

TREATMENT

Frostnip is the only form of frostbite which should be treated at the scene. A site sheltered from the wind is used and the affected part is warmed by hand (without rubbing), by breathing through cupped hands, or by placing frostnipped fingers in the armpit. As the skin rewarms and color returns to normal, the patient will often experience a tingling sensation which heralds return of adequate circulation to the area. The patient may continue working, but all members of the party must watch each other periodically for the signs described above.

Rubbing the affected part with snow or another body part causes skin breakage, increases chances of infection, and, in actuality, does not thaw tissues adequately. Wet or constrictive clothing should be removed. Alcohol is contraindicated until definitive warming can be accomplished and maintained, as alcohol causes increased heat loss on the basis of peripheral vasodilation, while providing a false sense of security.

Rapid rewarming of the frozen part is the single most effective therapeutic measure for preserving viable tissue. This is best accomplished by immersion of the extremity in 42°C circulating water for 20 min or until a distal flush of the extremity is observed. Slow rewarming, in contrast, has been shown to be less effective and to increase tissue damage. Also, dry heat, such as that from a campfire, is very dangerous as a thawing method. Because the frozen part is insensitive, there is a high chance of superficial burning and unnecessary tissue destruction.

Refreezing of thawed tissue drastically increases tissue damage and loss. If a patient develops frostbite on the trail, the extremity should not be thawed until definitive care can be given and maintained so that refreezing does not occur. It is more prudent to walk on a frozen foot to base camp or hospital rather than to thaw the foot first and then begin to hike to safety. Ideally, help should be brought to the victim.

As the definitive thawing is often quite painful, narcotic analgesics should be used liberally and tetanus prophylaxis administered appropriately. If the involved areas are large, intravenous fluid replacement should be considered. Antibiotics should be reserved for situations where infection is present or if there was an open wound on the extremity prior to freezing.

Recently, the breakdown products of arachidonic acid (e.g., thromboxane) have been implicated as mediators of progressive dermal ischemia in cold injury. Research aimed at preventing this breakdown through the use of antiprostaglandin agents, as well as thromboxane inhibitors, has been promising. In some studies, preservation of dermal circulation and increased tissue survival has been demonstrated experimentally and clinically with the use of non-steroidal anti-inflammatory agents (antiprostaglandin) systemically and aloe vera (thromboxane inhibitor) topically.

Local care of the extremity involves several basic principles. White or clear blisters should be debrided, as they contain fluid rich in prostaglandin and thromboxane, both of which are detrimental to damaged underlying tissue. Hemorrhagic blisters, however, reflect structural damage to the subdermal plexus and are left intact to prevent further damage to the vascular supply and to minimize loss of surrounding viable tissue. The injured extremity should be elevated to decrease further edema. With proper cradling of the extremity, it is best to leave it open to air during healing. The digits should be kept apart with soft, dry, absorbent dressings. These same dressings should be used to cover ruptured vesicle sites. Topical antibiotics, such as silver sulfadiazine, may be used, but should not substitute for definitive care of a clinically apparent infection. Weight bearing is proscribed on healing extremities. Whirlpool treatments with warm antibiotic solutions twice daily aid in gentle debridement, reduce the risk of infection, and soften the eschar for physiotherapy (which should include basic active range of motion exercises to prevent stiffness and contractures). Pressure dressings to decrease edema are discouraged as they tend to increase tissue destruction.

Hospitalization should be considered for: (1) those patients with accompanying medical problems such as generalized hypothermia, diabetes, and peripheral vascular disease; (2) frostbite which requires rapid rewarming in the Emergency Department; (3) facial frostbite with significant periorbital swelling; (4) bilateral extremity frostbite, and (5) unilateral extremity frostbite involving more than 65 percent of the glabrous extremity skin.

Again, early surgical intervention is not indicated for three reasons. First, it is impossible to assess the depth of frostbite in early stages. Second, the blackened, mummified carapace is protective to the underlying regenerating tissue. Third, premature surgery has been the most important cause of poor results and unnecessary tissue loss in this disease process. If wet gangrene or infection complicate the process, surgical intervention may be unavoidable.

Escharotomy and fasciotomy have been used in the past. However, since loss of circulation is due to primary vascular damage rather than occluding edema, these procedures are usually not indicated. If the eschar is preventing adequate range of motion, then escharotomy may be helpful.

Sympathectomy to increase blood flow has been advocated by several investigators with varying results. No rigorous study to date has demonstrated increased tissue salvage with this procedure and, thus, it remains controversial. Chemical sympathetic blockade also has been tried but found to be most useful in the chronic vasospastic sequelae of frostbite. Heparin and low-molecular-weight dextran have both been advocated in the treatment of frostbite, but clinical trials have not justified their routine use. Skin grafting procedures may be useful after final tissue loss is evident.

COMPLICATIONS AND SEQUELAE

There are several complications and sequelae of frostbite. Because of tissue and, more specifically, muscle damage, rhabdomyolysis and subsequent renal failure have been reported in several cases of frostbite. These complications should be anticipated and urinalysis and muscle enzyme determinations performed. Subsequent cold injury is more likely in a previously frostbitten extremity. Furthermore, healed frostbitten extremities demonstrate skin that is drier and more easily cracked with subsequent fissuring. This can be treated with moisturizing creams. Permanent depigmentation of the extremity may occur following recovery from frostbite.

Certain radiographic bony changes occur in extremities with a past history of frostbite. Three to six months following frostbite recovery, fine, irregular, punched-out lytic lesions appear at the MCP, MTP, PIP, and DIP joints of the extremities. These may be juxta- or subarticular and may extend into the joint. They are felt to be suggestive of chronic subperiosteal inflammation. Biopsy of the lesions reveals dense fibrous connective tissue. Clinical arthritis with fusiform soft tissue swelling and decreased range of motion may occur in these extremities and may be secondary to the above processes as well as to disuse, direct cold injury to bones and joints, and/or avascular necrosis as a result of thrombosis of digital arteries.

PREVENTION

Obviously, prevention is the best treatment for frostbite. People working or traveling in cold weather or high altitude should be in good general health, assure themselves an adequate diet, dress appropriately, and avoid panic, fatigue, and alcohol consumption. Use of a buddy system to observe for frostnip and treatment is helpful. Frostbite should not be rewarmed on the trail, and frozen feet, once thawed, should not be walked on. Cryotherapy (e.g., ice packs) for various disorders such as sprains or epididymitis, should be used with respect as there have been reports of iatrogenic frostbite to the scrotum, fingers, and toes.

BIBLIOGRAPHY

Bangs C: Hypothermia and frostbite. *Emerg Med Clin North Am* 2:475, 1984.

Bourne M, Piepkorn MW, Clayton F, et al: Analysis of microvascular changes in frostbite injury. *J Surg Res* 40:26, 1986.

Heggers JP, Robson MC, Manavalen K, et al: Experimental and clinical observations on frostbite. *Ann Emerg Med* 16:1056, 1987.

Kyosola K: Clinical experience in the management of cold injuries: A study of 110 cases. *J Trauma* 14:32, 1974.

McCauley RL, Hing DN, Robson MC, et al: A rational approach to frostbite based on the pathophysiology. *J Trauma* 23:143, 1983.

Mills WJ, Jr: Frostbite and hypothermia—current concepts. *Alaska Med* 15:26, 1975.

Vogel JE, Dellon AL: Frostbite injuries of the hand. *Clin Plast Surg* 16:565, 1989.

Ward M: Frostbite. *Br Med J* 1:67, 1974.

Washburn B: Frostbite, what it is—how to prevent it—emergency treatment. *N Engl J Med* 266:974, 1962.

Weatherly-White RCA, Sjostrom B, Paton BR, et al: Pathogenesis of frostbite. *J Surg Res* 4:17, 1964.

115
HYPOTHERMIA

Howard A. Bessen

Hypothermia is defined as a core temperature less than 35°C (95°F). While most commonly seen in cold climates, it may develop without exposure to extreme environmental conditions. Indeed, hypothermia is not uncommon in temperate regions, and may develop indoors during the summer.

PHYSIOLOGY OF TEMPERATURE HOMEOSTASIS

Body temperature may fall as a result of heat loss by conduction, convection, radiation, or evaporation. Conduction is the transfer of heat by direct contact, down a temperature gradient, e.g., from a warm body to the cold environment. Since the thermal conductivity of water is approximately 30 times that of air, the body loses heat rapidly when immersed in water, producing a rapid decline in body temperature.

Convection is the transfer of heat by the actual movement of heated material, for example, wind disrupting the layer of warm air surrounding the body. Convective heat loss increases in windy conditions, a particular hazard for outdoors enthusiasts.

Heat may also be lost by radiation to the environment (primarily from noninsulated body areas) and by evaporation of water. Evaporation of the water contained in exhaled, water-saturated air occurs over a wide range of ambient temperatures, and may be prevented by inhalation of warmed humidified air.

Opposing the loss of body heat are the mechanisms of heat conservation and gain. In general, these are controlled by the hypothalamus; thus, hypothalamic dysfunction may cause an impairment in temperature homeostasis. Heat is conserved by peripheral vasoconstriction and, importantly, by behavioral responses. If behavioral responses such as putting on clothing or coming indoors from a cold environment are impaired for any reason (e.g., drug intoxication or trauma), the risk of hypothermia is increased.

Heat gain is effected by shivering, and by "nonshivering thermogenesis." The nonshivering component of heat production consists of an increase in metabolic rate brought about by increased output from the thyroid and adrenal glands.

HIGH-RISK PATIENTS

Individuals at the extremes of age, and those with an altered sensorium for any reason, are particularly susceptible to developing hypothermia.

The elderly often lose their ability to sense cold; neonates easily become hypothermic because of their large body surface area. Both groups have a limited ability to increase heat production and to conserve body heat. Individuals with an altered sensorium, if unable to carry out the appropriate behavioral responses to cold stress, may develop hypothermia despite otherwise intact thermoregulatory mechanisms.

ETIOLOGY OF HYPOTHERMIA: CLINICAL SETTINGS

Table 115-1 lists the common causes of hypothermia. Nearly all patients will have hypothermia due to one or more of these.

Table 115-1. Causes of Hypothermia: Clinical Settings

"Accidental" (environmental)
Metabolic
Hypothalamic and CNS dysfunction
Drug-induced
Sepsis
Dermal disease
Acute incapacitating illness

"Accidental" hypothermia may be divided into immersion and nonimmersion cold exposure. Exposure to cold environmental conditions may lead to hypothermia even in healthy subjects, especially in wind and rain. Inadequate clothing and physical exhaustion contribute to the loss of body heat. The high thermal conductivity of water leads to the rapid development of immersion hypothermia. Though the rate of heat loss is determined by water temperature, immersion in any water less than 16 to 21°C (60 to 70°F) may lead to hypothermia.

Metabolic causes of hypothermia include various hypoendocrine states (hypothyroidism, hypoadrenalism, hypopituitarism), which lead to a decrease in metabolic rate. Hypoglycemia may also lead to hypothermia; the probable mechanism is hypothalamic dysfunction secondary to glucopenia.

Other causes of hypothalamic and CNS dysfunction (e.g., head trauma, tumor, stroke) may interfere with mechanisms of temperature regulation. Wernicke's disease may involve the hypothalamus; this is a rare but important cause of hypothermia, since it is potentially reversible with parenteral thiamine.

In the United States, the vast majority of hypothermic patients are intoxicated with ethanol or other drugs. Ethanol is a vasodilator, and, because of its anesthetic and CNS-depressant effects, intoxicated subjects neither feel the cold nor respond to it appropriately. Other drugs commonly implicated in the development of hypothermia include barbiturates, phenothiazines, and occasionally insulin.

Sepsis may alter the hypothalamic temperature set point and is a well-known cause of hypothermia. Subnormal body temperature is a poor prognostic factor in patients with bacteremia.

Severe dermal disease may impair the skin's thermoregulatory functions. Significant burns or severe exfoliative dermatitis may prevent cutaneous vasoconstriction and increase transcutaneous water loss, predisposing to the development of hypothermia.

Finally, hypothermia may develop in anyone with an acute incapacitating illness. Thus, patients with severe infections, diabetic ketoacidosis, immobilizing injuries, and various other conditions may have impaired thermoregulatory function, including altered behavioral responses.

PATHOPHYSIOLOGY

In general, body temperatures from 32 to 35°C (90 to 95°F) constitute "mild" hypothermia. In this temperature range, the patient is in an excitation (responsive) stage, in which physiologic adjustments attempt to retain and generate heat.

When temperature drops below 32°C, general excitation gives way to the slowing (adynamic) stage, in which there is a progressive slowdown of bodily functions. Metabolism slows, causing a decrease in both oxygen utilization and CO_2 production. Shivering ceases when body temperature falls below 30 to 32°C (86 to 90°F).

In the initial excitation phase, heart rate, cardiac output, and blood pressure all rise. With decreasing temperature, these all decline. Cardiac output and blood pressure may be markedly depressed by the negative inotropic and chronotropic effects of hypothermia, and further depressed by concomitant hypovolemia.

Hypothermia causes characteristic ECG changes, and may induce life-threatening arrhythmias (Table 115-2). The Osborn (J) wave, a slow, positive deflection at the end of the QRS complex (Fig. 115-1), is characteristic, though not pathognomic, of hypothermia.

Patients are at risk for arrhythmias at body temperatures below 30°C (86°F); the risk increases as body temperature decreases. Although various arrhythmias may occur at any time, the typical sequence is a progression from sinus bradycardia to atrial fibrillation with a slow ventricular response, to ventricular fibrillation, and, ultimately, to asystole. The hypothermic myocardium is extremely irritable, and

Table 115-2. ECG Changes in Hypothermia

T-wave inversions
PR, QRS, QT prolongation
Muscle tremor artifact
Osborn (J) wave
Arrhythmias:
Sinus bradycardia
Atrial fibrillation or flutter
Nodal rhythms
AV block
PVCs
Ventricular fibrillation
Asystole

ventricular fibrillation may be induced by a variety of manipulations and interventions which stimulate the heart, including rough handling of the patient.

Pulmonary effects include initial tachypnea, followed by a progressive decrease in respiratory rate and tidal volume. Cold-induced bronchorrhea, along with a depression of cough and gag reflexes, makes aspiration pneumonia a common complication.

Much attention has been paid to the temperature correction of arterial blood gases in the hypothermic patient, yet the interpretation of blood gases remains a problem. Since the blood gas analyzer warms the blood to 37°C, thus increasing the partial pressure of dissolved gases, the machine will report a higher P_{O_2} and P_{CO_2}, and lower pH, than the actual values at the patient's body temperature. Correction factors and nomograms are available to determine the actual values in the patient's body; however, the optimal or "normal" values in hypothermia are not known. The simplest solution is to use the uncorrected values as if the patient were normothermic; studies suggest that this approach is the most physiologically sound. P_{CO_2} is often quite low secondary to depressed metabolism and decreased CO_2 production, and iatrogenic hyperventilation may lead to marked respiratory alkalosis.

Hypothermia causes a leftward shift of the oxyhemoglobin dissociation curve, potentially impairing oxygen release to tissues. Patients may have minimal oxygen reserves despite diminished oxygen requirements, warranting the administration of supplemental oxygen.

The central nervous system is affected by hypothermia, with a progressive depression of consciousness level with decreasing temperature. Mild incoordination is followed by confusion, lethargy, and coma; pupils may be dilated and unreactive. These changes are associated with a decrease in cerebral blood flow. An even greater decrease in cerebral oxygen requirements may protect the brain against anoxic or ischemic damage.

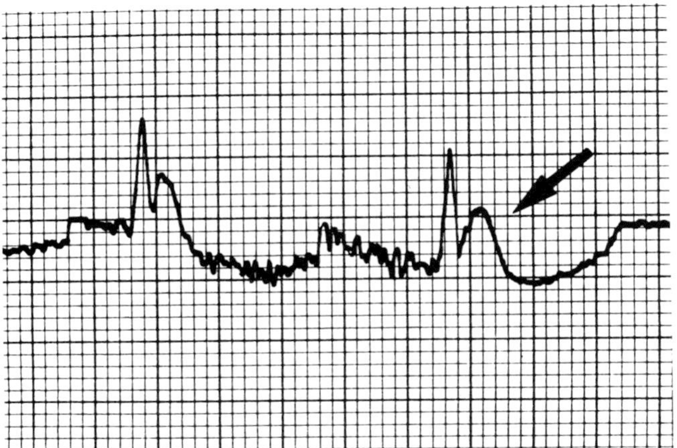

Fig. 115-1. Rhythm strip from patient with temperature of 25°C (77°F), showing atrial fibrillation with a slow ventricular response, muscle tremor artifact, and Osborn (J) wave (arrow).

Hypothermia impairs renal concentrating abilities and induces a "cold diuresis," leading to significant volume losses. Because of this concentrating defect, urine flow and specific gravity are unreliable indicators of intravascular volume and circulatory status. The immobile hypothermic patient is prone to rhabdomyolysis, and acute tubular necrosis may occur because of myoglobinuria and renal hypoperfusion.

Intravascular volume is also lost due to a plasma shift to the extravascular space. The combination of hemoconcentration, cold-induced increase in blood viscosity, and poor circulation may lead to intravascular thrombosis and subsequent embolic complications. Disseminated intravascular coagulation may occur because of release of tissue thromboplastins into the bloodstream, especially when circulation is restored during rewarming.

Endocrine function is fairly well preserved at low body temperatures. Plasma cortisol and thyroid hormone levels are usually normal or elevated unless the patient has a preexisting deficiency. Glucose levels may be normal, low, or elevated. Though hyperglycemia is common due to decreased insulin release as well as decreased glucose utilization, hypoglycemia may occur in up to 40 percent of patients.

Acid-base disturbances are common in hypothermia but follow no uniform pattern. Acidosis may occur due to severe respiratory depression and CO_2 retention and to lactic acid production from shivering and poor tissue perfusion. Alkalosis may result from diminished CO_2 production with low metabolic rates, or from iatrogenic hyperventilation or sodium bicarbonate administration.

Pancreatitis (not only hyperamylasemia but true pancreatic necrosis) may occur in hypothermia. Hepatic function is depressed by cold, so drugs normally metabolized, conjugated, or detoxified by the liver (e.g., lidocaine) may rapidly accumulate to toxic levels.

Finally, local cold injury and frostbite need special attention.

DIAGNOSIS

The diagnosis of hypothermia is often not obvious; exposure to profound cold is *not* necessary to produce hypothermia. Since most standard clinical thermometers record only to 34.4°C (94°F), low-reading glass or electronic thermometers are required to accurately measure the temperature of hypothermic patients. Electronic thermometers with flexible probes can be used to continuously monitor rectal or esophageal temperatures; tympanic thermometers may also be useful.

MANAGEMENT

Treatment includes both general supportive measures and specific rewarming techniques. Therapy begins with careful, gentle handling, since manipulation can precipitate ventricular fibrillation in the irritable hypothermic myocardium.

Controversy has arisen regarding the performance of CPR on an unmonitored patient who appears to be profoundly hypothermic and in cardiopulmonary arrest. Opponents of CPR argue that pulses may be difficult to detect in this setting, and that chest compressions may precipitate lethal arrhythmias. They recommend withholding CPR until the presence of an arrested rhythm (ventricular fibrillation or asystole) is confirmed. Alternatively, withholding CPR in the patient who is truly in cardiac arrest may unnecessarily subject the brain and other organs to prolonged ischemia. This CPR controversy applies only to patients with severe hypothermia, with core temperatures less than 28°C (82°F); practically, it may be difficult to confirm this diagnosis in the field. To avoid inappropriate chest compressions, prehospital care personnel should examine the patient for a full minute before diagnosing pulselessness. If no pulses are detected, most recommend initiating CPR. The optimal rate of chest compressions and ventilations has not been determined.

Oxygen and intravenous fluids should be warmed, and patients should have constant monitoring of their core temperature and cardiac rhythm. If central venous lines are placed, care should be taken to avoid entering and irritating the heart. In general, indications for endotracheal intubation are the same as in the normothermic patient. Concern has been raised regarding induction of arrhythmias during intubation; however, there is a very low complication rate with gentle intubation after oxygenation.

Although arrhythmias in the hypothermic patient may represent an immediate threat to life, most rhythm disturbances (e.g., sinus bradycardia, atrial fibrillation or flutter) require no therapy and revert spontaneously with rewarming. In addition, the activity of antiarrhythmic and cardioactive drugs is unpredictable in hypothermia, and the hypothermic heart is relatively resistant to atropine, pacing, and countershock.

Ventricular fibrillation is often refractory to therapy until the patient is rewarmed. The patient in ventricular fibrillation should receive one or two attempts at electrical defibrillation. If this is unsuccessful, CPR should be instituted and rapid rewarming begun. As the myocardium warms, the rhythm may revert spontaneously or in response to electrical defibrillation.

Drug Therapy

Because a large proportion of hypothermic patients are thiamine-depleted alcoholics (and because Wernicke's disease may cause hypothermia), patients should be given intravenous thiamine. Fifty to 100 mL of 50% dextrose should be administered if a dipstick serum glucose measurement is low or if a rapid test is unavailable.

Administration of antibiotics, steroids, and thyroid hormone must be individualized. Serious, often occult, infections may either precipitate or complicate hypothermia, and a thorough search for infection is indicated. Routine steroid therapy is generally not indicated, but hydrocortisone (100 mg) should be given to the patient with a history of adrenal suppression or insufficiency preceding the hypothermic episode, as well as to the patient with myxedema coma.

Hypothermia and hypothyroidism share many clinical features. While the majority of patients with myxedema coma are hypothermic, only a small minority of hypothermic patients are hypothyroid; thyroid hormone levels are most often normal or elevated. Thyroxine in large doses is necessary for the patient in myxedema coma, but may be harmful to other hypothermic patients. Therefore, thyroid hormone replacement is indicated only in patients with a known history of hypothyroidism, a thyroidectomy scar, or other strong clinical evidence of myxedema coma.

Rewarming Techniques

Modalities available for rewarming are listed in Table 115-3. The choice of method is a matter of controversy. There are no prospective, controlled studies comparing rewarming methods in humans, and each method has its own advantages and disadvantages.

Passive rewarming allows patients to rewarm on their own, using endogenous heat produced by metabolism. Since patients often become hypothermic over a period of hours to days, slow, passive rewarming is physiologically sound, avoiding rapid changes in cardiovascular status and the complications associated with active rewarming methods. However, temperature rises slowly and passive rewarming may be inappropriate for patients with cardiovascular compromise.

Active external rewarming (application of exogenous heat to the body) is often rapidly effective in raising body temperature, and has been used successfully in many patients. However, this method has several potential disadvantages. Application of external heat may cause peripheral vasodilation, returning cold blood to the core. While warming the periphery, this may paradoxically cause central cooling ("core temperature afterdrop"), potentially leading to arrhythmias. Although the mechanism and significance of this afterdrop phenomenon have been questioned, its occurrence with external rewarming has been well documented. The peripheral vasodilation and venous pooling can also lead to relative hypovolemia and hypotension (rewarming shock).

Table 115-3. Rewarming Techniques

Passive rewarming:
Removal from cold environment
Insulation
Active external rewarming:
Warm water immersion
Heating blankets
Heated objects (water bottles, etc.)
Radiant heat
Active core rewarming:
Inhalation rewarming
Heated IV fluids
GI tract lavage
Bladder lavage
Peritoneal lavage
Pleural lavage
Extracorporeal rewarming
Hemodialysis
Cardiopulmonary bypass (partial or complete)
Mediastinal lavage via thoracotomy

Washout of lactic acid from the peripheral tissues may lead to "rewarming acidosis," and an increase in metabolic demands of the periphery before the hypothermic heart can provide adequate tissue perfusion may lead to further tissue hypoxia and acidosis. Finally, resuscitation and monitoring of a patient immersed in warm water are technically difficult.

Active core rewarming has several theoretical advantages. Internal organs including the heart are preferentially rewarmed, decreasing myocardial irritability and returning cardiac function. Peripheral vasodilation is avoided, decreasing the incidence and magnitude of core temperature afterdrop, rewarming shock, and acidosis. However, some internal rewarming techniques are invasive and may be difficult to institute.

Inhalation rewarming—administration of warmed, humidified oxygen through a mask or endotracheal tube—provides a fairly small heat gain, and is not effective for rapid rewarming. This is an important modality, however, as it minimizes heat loss from the lungs, a potential loss of up to 30 percent of the total metabolic heat production. Similarly, IV fluids should be warmed to avoid further cooling by the administration of fluids at room temperature.

GI tract (gastric or colonic) lavage with warmed saline is technically simple, and patients can be lavaged with large volumes of fluid in a short time period. The obtunded hypothermic patient may develop pulmonary aspiration if lavaged with an unprotected airway. In a manner similar to GI tract lavage, the bladder can be lavaged with warm saline solution using a Foley catheter.

Peritoneal lavage affords rapid rewarming. It is widely available, may be instituted rapidly and with little technical difficulty, and has been shown to be effective in both animal studies and human applications. In addition to allowing relatively rapid rewarming, peritoneal dialysis has the potential to remove toxic drugs and correct electrolyte abnormalities. Standard dialysis solution is warmed to 40 to 45°C (104 to 113°F), instilled and then removed; the use of two catheters (one for fluid instillation and one for removal) may increase the rewarming rate.

Pleural lavage using thoracostomy tubes has provided effective rewarming in animal studies and a few human cases. Lavaging the left thoracic cavity delivers heated fluid in close proximity to the heart, potentially allowing rapid cardiac warming. Two thoracostomy tubes (for fluid inflow and outflow) have generally been employed. If this technique is chosen, care must be taken to monitor the net fluid infusion, as increased intrathoracic pressure and tension hydrothorax may complicate the procedure. The risk of precipitating arrhythmias during chest tube insertion is unknown.

Rapid internal rewarming can also be accomplished through an extracorporeal circuit, employing heated hemodialysis or cardiopulmonary bypass. This consists of an arteriovenous shunt with an interposed heat exchanger; most commonly, the femoral vessels are used for vascular access. Full cardiopulmonary bypass using a median sternotomy has also been employed. Profoundly hypothermic patients may be rewarmed in a very short time period with these methods. In addition to allowing rapid rewarming, partial (femoral-femoral) or complete cardiopulmonary bypass provides circulatory support and oxygenation of blood, a great advantage in the management of patients in cardiac arrest or with severe cardiovascular compromise. Specialized equipment and personnel are required, however, and lack of immediate availability often precludes the use of this technique. In addition, the heparinization required for extracorporeal techniques may cause complications in hypothermic trauma patients.

Various diathermy and radiowave techniques, although promising, have had limited use in hypothermic humans.

Finally, mediastinal irrigation using open thoracotomy has been used successfully as a rewarming technique in a few patients. It is possible that these patients could have been resuscitated using less invasive modalities. Thoracotomy has many potential complications, and should only be considered in arrested patients. Even then, indications for this procedure are unclear.

Approach to Rewarming

No prospective controlled studies comparing the various rewarming modalities have been done in humans. Therefore, firm guidelines for therapy cannot be given.

Patients with mild hypothermia, who are still in the "excitation" stage, generally improve spontaneously, as long as endogenous heat production mechanisms are functional. In addition, at temperatures above 30°C (86°F) the incidence of arrhythmias is low, and rapid rewarming is rarely necessary.

By far the most important consideration is the patient's cardiovascular status; a secondary consideration is the presenting temperature. Some feel that patients with a stable cardiac rhythm (including sinus bradycardia and atrial fibrillation) and stable vital signs do not need rapid rewarming, even if the temperature is very low. They recommend passive rewarming and noninvasive internal modalities (e.g., warm moist oxygen and warm IV fluids) in this setting. Others argue that profoundly hypothermic patients, even if currently "stable," are at risk of developing life-threatening arrhythmias. They recommend rapid rewarming until the temperature has reached 30 to 32°C to minimize the time period during which arrhythmias may develop. The relative merits of each approach have not been studied.

Patients with cardiovascular insufficiency or instability, including persistent hypotension and life-threatening arrhythmias, need to be rewarmed rapidly. The best method remains to be definitively determined. Cardiopulmonary bypass offers many advantages but is often unavailable. If extracorporeal rewarming is not available, multiple other rewarming modalities can be used simultaneously.

PROGNOSIS

Many hypothermic patients have severe infections or other life-threatening illnesses. Patients with "uncomplicated" hypothermia (often purely due to cold exposure) have a fairly low mortality rate; patients with significant associated diseases have a much worse prognosis. In terms of ultimate outcome, the underlying disease process is far more important than the initial temperature or the rewarming method chosen. Therefore, evaluation and treatment of these patients must include a search for associated diseases as well as treatment of the hypothermia itself.

The protective effect of hypothermia may have an important influence on prognosis; decreased oxygen requirements can protect the brain and other organs against anoxic and ischemic damage. This means that the usual criteria indicating death or irreversibility of disease are not valid in the hypothermic patient, who may even survive prolonged cardiac arrest without neurologic sequelae.

Hypothermic patients may recover completely after presenting in a rigid, apneic state with fixed and dilated pupils. Recovery has been documented with core temperatures as low as 16°C (61°F), and with cardiac arrest for over 3 h. Death in hypothermia must be defined as a failure to revive with rewarming; resuscitative efforts should be continued until core temperature is at least 30 to 32°C (86 to 90°F).

No one is dead until warm and dead!

BIBLIOGRAPHY

Brunette DD, Sterner S, Robinson EP, et al: Comparison of gastric lavage and thoracic cavity lavage in the treatment of severe hypothermia in dogs. *Ann Emerg Med* 16:1222, 1987.

Clements SD, Hurst JW: Diagnostic value of electrocardiographic abnormalities observed in subjects accidentally exposed to cold. *Am J Cardiol* 29:729, 1972.

Danzl DF, Pozos RS: Multicenter hypothermia survey. *Ann Emerg Med* 16:1042, 1987.

Delaney KA, Howland MA, Vassallo S, et al: Assessment of acid-base disturbances in hypothermia and their physiologic consequences. *Ann Emerg Med* 18:72, 1989.

Gillen JP, Vogel MEX, Holterman RK, et al: Ventricular fibrillation during orotracheal intubation of hypothermic dogs. *Ann Emerg Med* 15:412, 1986.

Lewin S, Brettman LR, Holzman RS: Infections in hypothermic patients. *Arch Intern Med* 141:920, 1981.

Ornato JP: Special resuscitation situations: Near drowning, traumatic injury, electric shock, and hypothermia. *Circulation* 74(suppl 4):23, 1986.

Otto RJ, Metzler MH: Rewarming from experimental hypothermia: Comparison of heated aerosol inhalation, peritoneal lavage, and pleural lavage. *Crit Care Med* 16:869, 875, 1988.

Reuler JB: Hypothermia: Pathophysiology, clinical settings and management. *Ann Intern Med* 89:519, 1978.

Steinman AM: Cardiopulmonary resuscitation and hypothermia. *Circulation* 74(suppl 4):29, 1986.

Zell SC, Kurtz KJ: Severe exposure hypothermia: A resuscitation protocol. *Ann Emerg Med* 14:339, 1985.

116
HEAT EMERGENCIES

Michael V. Vance

It does not take long either to boil an egg or to cook neurones.
(D. Hamilton. *Anesthesia* 31:271, 1976.)

Body temperature is dependent on the balance between heat production and heat loss; it is maintained within narrow limits through a variety of mechanisms. Under normal circumstances, heat production results from exothermic intracellular metabolic processes and absorption of heat from external sources (solar radiation, environmental temperature). Basal metabolic activity normally produces 60 to 70 kcal/h, and solar irradiation under temperate conditions may add 100 to 150 kcal/h. However, strenuous physical exertion may produce up to 900 kcal/h for short periods of time, and severe environmental conditions will contribute to even greater levels of heat gain.

Heat loss is accomplished by radiation, convection, conduction, and evaporation. Responses to core temperature changes are directed by the anterior hypothalamus and are mediated via the endocrine system, the autonomic nervous system, and neuromuscular activity. The primary response to increased core temperature is cutaneous vasodilation, resulting in greater heat transfer from the skin to the atmosphere. However, as ambient temperature approaches body temperature, heat loss becomes increasingly dependent on evaporation of sweat produced by the activity of cholinergic sympathetic nerve fibers. The efficiency of evaporative heat loss is in turn influenced greatly by ambient humidity.

The body's temperature-regulating system generally functions well in the face of diverse metabolic and environmental conditions, and the human system is remarkably capable of adapting to dramatic changes through the process of acclimatization. Acclimatization occurs gradually over a period of days to weeks, and primarily involves alterations of sodium and water balance mediated by aldosterone. When a human being is initially exposed to a hot and humid environment, sodium and water are lost through sweating. In addition, blood is shunted to the skin to aid in heat dissipation. The net result is contraction of the extracellular fluid volume, decreased renal plasma flow, and consequently an increase in aldosterone secretion. The concentration of sodium in urine and sweat then decreases markedly (although potassium losses continue). Sodium retention results in expansion of extracellular fluid volume, and, at some point, acclimatization to the new environment is completed.

Heat cramps, heat exhaustion, and heatstroke develop from the inability to respond adequately to environmental conditions, inadequate correction of fluid and electrolyte deficiencies, and malfunction of the system through exogenous or endogenous causes. While one mechanism may predominate in any particular heat disorder, multiple factors are most commonly responsible.

There is a great deal of overlap and interrelationship among all the heat disorders, and individual patients may present with mixed pictures. A number of predisposing factors are common to all forms of heat-related emergencies (Table 116-1). Obviously, anyone involved in physical exertion in a hot, humid environment, whether indoors or outdoors, is at risk for any of the heat disorders. As ambient temperature or humidity increases, and/or if the level of exercise is increased, the risk of a heat disorder increases proportionately, even among well-acclimatized persons.

Table 116-1. Risk Factors Associated with Heat Emergencies

Age
Infants (greater sweat losses, poorly developed compensatory mechanisms)
Elderly (cardiovascular disease, multiple drug therapies)
Environment
High ambient temperature
High ambient humidity
Occupation
Athletes
Laborers
Military
Pharmacologic factors
Drugs with central effect on hypothalamus:
Phenothiazine model
Drugs with peripheral (anticholinergic) effects on sweat glands
Cyclic antidepressants
Lithium intoxication
Malignant hyperpyrexia following exposure to halothane or succinylcholine; caffeine; severe fluid restriction
Psychological factors
Belief in the invulnerability of the young
Sweat gland abnormalities
Congenital anhidrosis
Cystic fibrosis
Quadriplegia

Certain drugs contribute to the development of heat disorders, particularly those such as the phenothiazines that alter the response of the hypothalamus (most likely through dopaminergic-blocking effects) and those such as the cyclic antidepressants, whose anticholinergic properties may interfere with sweating (Table 116-2).

HEAT CRAMPS

Heat cramps are generally associated with strenuous physical activity. They are characterized by painful spasm of skeletal muscles, including muscles of the extremities and abdomen. The production of large amounts of sweat, which has a high sodium content, coupled with inadequate sodium replacement (typically through drinking tap water or other salt-poor fluid) results in hyponatremia, which probably produces muscle cramps through interference with calcium-dependent muscle relaxation. Another factor which may contribute to the development of heat cramps is hyperventilation, which occurs commonly in association with the heat syndromes. Possibly due to the local accumulation of lactate, hyperventilation produces respiratory alkalosis, and an associated hypokalemia (due to intracellular potassium

Table 116-2. Drugs Associated with Heatstroke

Anticholinergic drugs:	Monoamine oxidase inhibitors:
Atropine	Osocarboxazid (Marplan)
Scopolamine	Nialamide (Niamid)
Benztropine mesylate (Cogentin)	Phenelzine (Nardil)
Phenothiazine derivatives:	Tranylcypromine (Parnate)
Chlorpromazine (Thorazine)	Glutehimide (Doriden)
Mepazine (Pacatal)	Lysergic acid diethylamide (LSD)
Cyclic antidepressants:	Amphetamine
Amitriptyline (Elavil)	Inhalation anesthetic:
Desmethylimipramine (Norpramin)	Ether
Imipramine (Tofranil)	Ethylchloride
Nortriptyline (Aventyl)	Halothane
Protriptyline (Vivactil)	Nitrous oxide
	Suxamethonium chloride (succinylcholine)

Source: Shibolet S, Lancaster MC, Danon Y: Heat stroke: A review. *Aviat Space Environ Med* 47:281, 1976. Used by permission.

shifts) may contribute to the development of muscle cramps, paresthesias, and tetany.

Clinically, body temperature is normal, and there is generally no evidence of dehydration. Laboratory studies may show hyponatremia, hypokalemia, and respiratory alkalosis, as well as hypomagnesemia and hypophosphatemia.

While painful, heat cramps are a benign entity and are effectively treated with rest and oral or intravenous electrolyte replacement. However, episodes of muscular pain due to exertional rhabdomyolysis may be misdiagnosed as heat cramps. Rhabdomyolysis is a potentially serious condition characterized by injury and death of muscle cells, massive elevations of creatine phosphokinase (CPK), myoglobinuria, and possibly renal failure. A potentially lethal complication of exertional rhabdomyolysis is severe hyperkalemia and accompanying dysrhythmias due to the release of potassium from massive muscle cellular disruption.

HEAT EXHAUSTION

Heat exhaustion is characterized by volume depletion. Fluid and electrolyte losses due to sweating coupled with inadequate replacement result in hypovolemia and tissue hypoperfusion.

The signs and symptoms of heat exhaustion are variable. Early complaints of fatigue may progress to light-headedness, nausea and vomiting, severe headache, and, finally, evidence of significant volume depletion with tachycardia, hyperventilation, and hypotension. The body temperature is normal or slightly elevated and there may be profuse sweating.

Laboratory studies will almost universally demonstrate hemoconcentration, although specific electrolyte abnormalities depend on the ratio of fluid and electrolyte losses to intake. Patients who have virtually no fluid intake of any kind will usually have an associated hypernatremia, while those who partially rehydrate with salt-containing fluids may show relatively normal sodium and chloride levels in an isotonic dehydration pattern. Abnormalities in serum potassium and other electrolytes may vary widely, depending on other factors.

The definitive treatment of heat exhaustion is rest coupled with volume replacement. Rapid administration of moderate amounts of intravenous fluids (1 to 2 L of saline solution) may be necessary in occasional patients who demonstrate significant tissue hypoperfusion. The choice of solution is guided by laboratory determinations, but balanced salt solutions may be utilized until specific electrolyte abnormalities are determined to be present.

HEATSTROKE

Heatstroke is defined as the combination of hyperpyrexia [often to 40°C (106°F) or greater] and neurological symptoms. Lack of sweating is not an absolute diagnostic criterion. In contradistinction to heat cramps and heat exhaustion, heatstroke is a true medical emergency which may result in widespread organ system dysfunction and injury, with a potentially high mortality rate.

Risk factors associated with heat emergencies are summarized in Table 116-1. The central nervous system is particularly vulnerable to heatstroke. The clinical onset of heatstroke begins with an alteration of neurological function, frequently manifested by a sudden loss of consciousness with little or no prodrome. Irritability, bizarre behavior, combativeness, hallucinations, or coma may occur. Virtually any neurological abnormality may be present, including plantar responses, pupillary abnormalities, decorticate and decerebrate posturing, hemiplegia, and status epilepticus.

The mixed neurological picture associated with hyperpyrexia may present the emergency physician with a difficult ''chicken-egg'' problem, since cerebrovascular accidents may be accompanied by high fever. However, it cannot be overemphasized that a sudden alteration of consciousness in a setting of heat exposure must suggest the possibility of heatstroke, and prompt measurement of core temperature should follow. There are probably many episodes of early heatstroke that go unrecognized because mental status improves after cessation of exercise and removal of the patient from the hot environment. The patient may never seek medical care, or, if the patient does consult a physician, the core temperature may not be measured or it may have declined by the time of evaluation. In addition, mild cases of heatstroke with cerebral dysfunction may occur at a much lower temperature than expected: in at least one study of volunteers undergoing heat stress, alteration of consciousness was produced when rectal temperature was 39.1°C (102.4°F).

The presence or absence of sweating has classically been one of the important distinctions between true heatstroke and the other heat emergencies. However, while patients with early heatstroke typically demonstrate marked sweating, many patients will at some point lose the ability to sweat and demonstrate the characteristic hot, dry skin. The exact mechanism of the breakdown of the sweating mechanism is unclear, although direct thermal injury to the sweat glands is certainly an important factor. However, whatever the temporal relationship between the onset of clinical heatstroke and the failure of the sweating mechanism, there is no doubt that any abnormality of this organ system is an important contributing factor in the development of heatstroke. While an occasional patient with a rare problem such as congenital absence of sweat glands, cystic fibrosis, or quadriplegia will be encountered, the most common cause of impaired sweating is the administration of medications with anticholinergic properties.

Non-exercise-induced heatstroke may be encountered in the elderly or chronically debilitated patient whose cardiovascular system is unable to meet the metabolic demands of a hot environment. Exercise-induced heatstroke typically occurs in previously healthy persons under a wide variety of circumstances. In a recent year in a large Southwestern city, for example, roofers had the highest incidence of heatstroke but were closely followed by tennis players. Regardless of the environmental setting or the presence or absence of predisposing or contributing factors, elevation of the core body temperature to critical levels results in widespread and disastrous effects on most body tissues. Temperatures in the range of 42°C (107.6°F) and above are associated with a poor prognosis, although clinical signs and symptoms may occur at much lower levels.

The status of the cardiovascular system is an important factor in the development of heatstroke. This is particularly true in the elderly and in other patient populations with preexistent cardiovascular disease. In the patient with a relatively intact cardiovascular response, heat stress will promote heat loss, with an increase in heart rate, cardiac index, and central venous pressure as a response to peripheral vasodilation. However, heart failure, pulmonary edema, and cardiovascular collapse can occur in young, otherwise healthy persons suffering heatstroke. In any age group, the presence of hypotension, decreased cardiac output, and a falling cardiac index indicates a particularly poor prognosis.

Hepatic and renal abnormalities may also be found in patients with heatstroke. Centrilobular necrosis due to direct thermal injury results in abnormal liver function studies, although recovery is to be expected. Jaundice is unusual. Microscopic hematuria, proteinuria, and casts develop rapidly. Severe cases, especially those complicated by hypovolemia and a decreased renal blood flow, may progress to acute tubular necrosis (ATN) and renal failure. Exercise-induced heatstroke is often complicated by rhabdomyolysis, sometimes with massive myoglobinuria and renal failure. This complication may not develop until 2–3 days following the initial injury, and careful monitoring of CPKs and renal function is necessary. Occasionally, a patient may present to the emergency department with the dark urine of myoglobinuria, and historical considerations should include recent heat exposure or heavy exertion.

Widespread hematologic disorders may be apparent both clinically and on laboratory evaluation. Purpura, conjunctival hemorrhages, petechiae, and pulmonary, gastrointestinal, and renal hemorrhages may be present. Coagulation studies may show decreased platelets, hypoprothrombinemia, and hypofibrinogenemia. Thermal injury to the vascular endothelium causes increased platelet aggregation, changes in capillary permeability, thermal deactivation of plasma proteins resulting in a decreased level of clotting factors, and, rarely, disseminated intravascular coagulation or fibrinolysis.

As expected, the fluid and electrolyte abnormalities vary with the onset and duration of the disorder, underlying disease (especially cardiovascular disease), and prior use of medications such as diuretics. The most important consideration with respect to fluid and electrolyte abnormalities in heatstroke is that dehydration and volume depletion may not occur in classic heatstroke, whereas they are common signs of heat exhaustion. Vigorous fluid administration may produce pulmonary edema, especially in the elderly. A myriad of blood gas abnormalities may be encountered, from respiratory alkalosis to severe metabolic acidosis.

Treatment

Once the diagnosis of heatstroke is made or suspected, rapid, aggressive therapy aimed at lowering the body temperature should be initiated immediately by whatever means available, whether in the prehospital or emergency department setting. In the field, remove the patient from external sources of heat; remove clothing; and promote evaporative cooling by applying cool or iced water to the entire skin surface by sponging or splashing, accompanied by fanning either by hand or mechanical means. This should be continued throughout transportation to an emergency receiving facility, and should be continued within the facility as well. There are a number of disadvantages to the use of an iced bath: it is more difficult to handle the patient; peripheral vasoconstriction may decrease heat transfer to the skin surface, although this may be overcome somewhat by vigorous skin massage; and intense shivering may actually increase endogenous heat production.

Intense shivering during any form of cooling therapy may be controlled with diazepam or chlorpromazine. While the latter is known to produce hyperpyrexia itself, this is believed to be due to effects on the hypothalamus and is probably not a significant factor when external, artificial cooling methods are utilized. Hypothermia blankets and ice packs to the groin and axilliae are also useful. Additional methods such as iced water gastric lavage and enemas, iced water peritoneal dialysis, and intratracheal administration of cold helium have also been suggested as methods of promoting heat transfer from the body but are not widely used. Antipyretics such as salicylates have not proved useful in treating heatstroke.

While the rapid reduction of body temperature is the primary goal, additional supportive measures may be established early in the course of treatment, including oxygen therapy in conjunction with endotracheal intubation if necessary. An intravenous line should be established; a central venous pressure line may be preferable, since many patients with true heatstroke do not have large fluid requirements. Early baseline determinations of clotting parameters and electrolyte levels, hepatic and renal studies, and a serum glucose level should be obtained. When blood gases are obtained, inform the laboratory of the patient's body temperature so that the appropriate corrections can be made. Specific complications, such as heart failure, cardiovascular collapse, hepatic or renal failure, and myoglobinemia and myoglobinuria may be treated by standard approaches. Patients with depleted clotting factors must be carefully evaluated. Generally, they can be managed by administering platelets and fresh-frozen plasma.

OTHER CAUSES OF HYPERTHERMIA

In addition to heat syndromes resulting from heat exposure, there are a variety of other causes of hyperthemia. The first indication of many infectious diseases may be a markedly elevated temperature. A patient with severe dehydration may be hyperpyrexic because general hypoperfusion prevents effective dissipation of heat from the skin. Drugs producing an anticholinergic syndrome may cause hyperthermia through a combination of hypothalamic effects and decreased sweating. In fact, these patients, as well as those suffering from cerebrovascular accidents, including stroke and intracerebral or subarachnoid hemorrhage, may exhibit the classic signs of heatstroke: neurological dysfunction, hyperpyrexia, and hot, dry skin. When confronted with such a clinical picture, establishing a definitive diagnosis is difficult. It is most important to begin to aggressively lower the body temperature while awaiting resolution of the diagnostic problem.

Rarely, a person with a combination of underlying muscle disease and exposure to anesthetic agents may develop malignant hyperpyrexia, which is associated with an extremely high mortality. In addition, patients taking neuroleptic agents such as chlorpromazine and haloperidol may develop neuroleptic, malignant syndrome, typically presenting with altered mental status, muscular rigidity, elevated CPK, and hyperthermia. This must be differentiated from the more benign dystonic reactions associated with these drugs and requires admission and frequently prolonged therapy with bromocriptine and/or dantrolene.

BIBLIOGRAPHY

Ellenhorn MJ, Barcelous DG: Medical Toxicology: Diagnosis and Treatment of Human Poisoning. New York: Elsevier Science Publishing Company, 1988.

Goldfrank LR, Flomenbaum NE, Lewin NA, Weisman RS, Howland MA: Goldfrank's Toxicologic Emergencies, 4th ed., East Norwalk, Conn: Appleton & Lange, 1990.

Haddad LM, Winchester JF (Eds.): Clinical Management of Poisoning and Drug Overdose, 2nd ed., Philadelphia: WB Saunders Co., 1990.

General

Costrini A: Emergency treatment of exertional heatstroke and comparison of whole body cooling techniques. Med Sci Sports Exerc 22:15, 1990.

Graham BS, Lichtenstein MJ, Hinson JM, et al: Nonexertional heatstroke. *Arch Intern Med* 146:87, 1986.

Hart GR, Anderson RJ, Crumpler CP, et al: Epidemic classical heat stroke: clinical characteristics and course of 28 patients. *Medicine* 61:189, 1982.

Hubbard RW, Matthew CB, Durkot MJ, et al: Novel approaches to the pathophysiology of heatstroke: the energy depletion model. *Ann Emerg Med* 16:1066, 1987.

Knochel JP: Environmental heat illness. *Arch Intern Med* 133:841, 1974.

Olson KR, Benowitz NL: Environmental and drug-induced hyperthermia. *Emerg Clin North Am* 2:459, 1984.

Tomarken JL, Britt BA: Malignant hyperthermia. *Ann Emerg Med* 16:1253, 1987.

Neuroleptic Malignant Syndrome

Levenson JL: Neuroleptic malignant syndrome. *Am J Psych* 142:1137, 1985.

Rosenberg MR, Green M: Neuroleptic malignant syndrome: review of response to therapy. *Arch Intern Med* 149:1927, 1989.

117
INSECT AND SPIDER BITES

Claude Frazier

IMMEDIATE CONCERNS
• Severe toxic reactions • Anaphylactic shock • Upper airway obstruction

Toxic reactions to multiple stings by members of the order of Hymenoptera and severe systemic reactions to one or two stings or to bites of some other insections such as deerflies, blackflies, horseflies, and kissing bugs can both present an emergency, life-threatening situation. (See Table 117-1 for a listing of harmful anthropods of the United States.) However, fatalities due to biting insects are far rarer than those caused by the venom of Hymenoptera.

Table 117-1. Harmful Arthropods of the United States

Class and Order	Common Name	Bite	Sting
Hexapoda (Insecta)			
Hymenoptera	Bees:		
	Bumblebees		x
	Sweat bees		x
	Honeybees		x
	Wasps:		
	Hornets		x
	Yellow jackets		x
	Ants:		
	Fire ants		x
	Harvester ants		x
Diptera	Mosquitoes	x	
	Deerflies	x	
	Horseflies	x	
	Stable flies	x	
	Blackflies	x	
	Biting midges	x	
Hemiptera	Bedbugs	x	
	Wheel bugs	x	
	Kissing bugs	x	
Coleoptera	Blister beetles		x
Lepidoptera	Puss caterpillars		x
	Browntail caterpillars		x
	Buck mouth caterpillars		x
Siphonaptera	Fleas (human, cat, dog)	x	
Anoplura	Lice, (body, head, pubic)	x	
Arachnida			
Araneida	Black widow spiders	x	
	Brown recluse spiders	x	
Acarina	Mites	x	
	Ticks	x	
Scorpionida	Scorpions		x

Source: Frazier CA: *Insect Allergy*. St. Louis, WH Green, revised edition, 1987, p 421. Used by permission.

HYMENOPTERA STINGS

The normal response to Hymenoptera venom consists of pain, slight erythema, and some edema at the sting site, usually followed by pruritus.

Type of Reaction

Local reaction. A local reaction consists of marked and prolonged edema contiguous with the sting site. Although there are no systemic signs or symptoms, a severe local reaction may involve one or more neighboring joints. The seriousness of a local reaction depends upon the sting location. A local reaction occurring in the mouth or throat can produce airway obstruction. Stings around the eye or on the lid may result in the development of an anterior capsular cataract, atrophy of the iris, lens abscess, perforation of the globe, glaucoma, or refractive changes.

When subsequent local reactions become increasingly severe, the likelihood of future systemic reactions appears to increase and to be great enough, especially if skin tests are positive, to warrant immunotherapy.

Toxic reaction. A toxic reaction should be considered if there is a history of 10 or more stings. While symptoms resemble those of a systemic reaction, there is generally a greater frequency of gatrointestinal disturbance. Vomiting, diarrhea, light-headedness, and syncope are the principal features. There may also be headache, fever, drowsiness, involuntary muscle spasms, edema without urticaria, and occasionally convulsions. Urticaria and bronchospasm are not present. Symptoms usually subside with 48 h. Toxic reactions are believed to be a response to the nonantigenic properties of Hymenoptera venom.

Systemic or anaphylactic reaction. A generalized systemic reaction, whether in response to a single or to multiple stings, may range from the mild to the fatal, and death can occur within minutes. It is believed that the shorter the interval between the sting and the onset of symptoms, the more severe the reaction. Initial symptoms usually consist of itching eyes, facial flushing, generalized urticaria, and dry cough. Symptoms may intensify rapidly with chest or throat constriction, wheezing, dyspnea, cyanosis, abdominal cramps, diarrhea, nausea, vomiting, vertigo, chills and fever, laryngeal stridor, shock, loss of consciousness, involuntary bowel or bladder action, and bloody, frothy sputum. Such a reaction can be fatal within ½ h, sometimes within 10 to 15 min, and, rarely, within 3 to 5 min. Initial mild symptoms can progress swiftly to anaphylactic shock. In addition, severe signs may overrun initial signs so that the physician is faced almost at once with respiratory failure or cardiovascular collapse.

Delayed reaction. A delayed reaction consists of serum-sickness-like symptoms of fever, malaise, headache, urticaria, lymphadenopathy, and polyarthritis that appear 10 to 14 days after a sting. Frequently, the patient has forgotten about the encounter and is puzzled by sudden appearance of symptoms.

Unusual reactions. Infrequently neurological, cardiovascular, and urological symptoms are involved in a reaction to Hymenoptera venom, with signs of encephalopathy, neuritis, vasculitis, and nephrosis. A case of Guillain-Barré syndrome has been reported as a possible consequence of a Hymenoptera sting. Another unusual reaction is intense fear following a sting, with symptoms of faintness, excessive sweating, and an increased heart rate.

Pathophysiology of Systemic Reaction

A generalized systemic reaction to Hymenoptera venom is thought to be IgE-mediated. When an individual predisposed to allergy to bees is stung, there is usually an increase in the production of IgE antibodies, which become attached to the mast cells and basophils. This sensitizes the individual so that a subsequent sting may result in an antigen-antibody interaction that releases pharmacologically active mediators: histamine; the slow reacting substance of anaphylaxis (SRS-A), which is an acidic sulfates ester; and eosinophil chemotactic factors of anaphylaxis (ECF-A). It is these mediators which actually cause tissue damage and systemic symptoms.

The pharmacological effects of histamine are vasodilation, urticaria or angioedema, either an increased or decreased respiratory rate, fall in blood pressure, vomiting, and tenesmus. Histamine is believed responsible for symptoms of bronchoconstriction in a systemic reaction. SRS-A is also believed to be a constrictor of bronchial smooth muscle and may potentiate the effects of histamine. In addition to producing the eosinophil cell increase seen in an allergic reaction, ECF-A may serve to decrease the activity of SRS-A and histamine, and thus be responsible for decreasing the acuteness of the reaction. Platelet-activating factors may contribute to the reaction by platelet aggregation and degranulation.

We do not know the exact role of released bradykinin in the reaction, although we know the response can be contraction of bronchial smooth muscle and increased venular permeability.

Electrophoretic, chromatographic, and fractionating techniques have recently increased our knowledge of the chemical and immunological charactristics of Hymenoptera venoms. These venoms are similar in some substances but differ in others. Honeybee venom contains histmine; wasp venom contains histamine and serotonin; hornet venom contains both histamine and serotonin, as well as acetylcholine. Pharmacologically active amines in the venoms have been identified as histamine, serotonin, acetylcholine, adrenaline, noradrenaline, and dopamine. Melittin and apamin are among the polypeptides, while phospholipase A and hyaluronidase are the major enzymes. The five important allergens in honeybee venom are phospholipase A, hyaluronidase, melittin, acid phosphatase, and diphenylpyraline (Allergen C). There is some controversy as to whether phospholipase A or hyaluronidase is the main allergen.

The venom of other members of Hymenoptera differs from honeybee venom in several respects. Wasp venom contains histamine, 5-hydroxytryptamine, and kinins, while hornet venom contains these fractions plus acetylcholine. As Reisman (1979) points out, this allergenic specificity resides in the fact that bees belong to the super-family Apoidea, while wasps, hornets, and yellow jackets belong to Vespoidea. A common antigen occurs in the body of a wasp and a honeybee, but it is not common to their respective venoms.There is also a common antigen in the body of a bee and a yellow jacket. Cross-reactivity appears to be the greatest between the wasp and yellow jacket, for they share a common body antigen as well as a common antigen in their venom sacs.

The venom of the imported fire ant is distinctive from that of other members of Hymenoptera in that it is mainly alkaloid and is the only venom that demonstrates necrotic activity. The venom is nonproteinaceous and, interestingly, is toxic to other insect species. It also exhibits antibiotic activity, which apparently explains why pustules that form at the sting sites are generally sterile.

Diagnosis

Identification of the offending insect can be difficult, except for the honeybee, which almost invariably leaves its stinger with venom sac attached in the lesion. A careful history is often necessary to distinguish members of Vespoidea from each other, and slides or pictures of the various species can aid the patient in recall. Some questions that can be asked in an effort to identify the offending insect are: Where did the encounter occur? Was a nest noted, and, if so, was it in the ground (yellow jackets), under eaves or windowsills (wasps), in bushes or low-hanging tree limbs (hornets)? Skin tests are not always reliable in identification since most individuals allergic to insects are sensitive to two or three species. This high incidence of cross-reactivity underlines the importance of mixed species extracts in immunotherapy.

If edema persists at the sting site, secondary infection, such as cellulitis, must be considered. Severe local reactions on the foot or ankle can be misdiagnosed as gout if the insect bite is not visible.

Stings by the imported fire ant in the southern region of the United States are distinctive, both because of their groupings of three of four stings in the same general area and because of the typical pustules produced. In any case, few patients forget the painful nature of the event when they blunder into a fire ant mound or accidentally encounter these fierce ants going about their business.

Treatment

If a honeybee's stinger is present in the wound, scrape it out. Never squeeze with fingers or tweezers since this will force more venom from the attached sac into the wound. Remove stingers as quickly as possible in cases of multiple bee stings, for the venom sac of a honeybee continues to pulse even after the bee has torn free, thus pumping more venom into the lesion. Sting sites should be thoroughly washed with soap and water to minimize the possibility of infection. Analgesics may be administered if pain and discomfort are considerable, a likely contingency in the case of multiple stings and toxic reactions.

For local reactions ice packs at the sting site will help delay absorption of the venom and limit edema, while oral antihistamines and analgesics can relieve discomfort. If an extremity is involved and edema is significant, elevation and rest of the affected limb will help limit the reaction's duration, while prednisone 20 to 40 mg orally, daily for several mornings, will reduce swelling. Diphenhydramine hydrochloride, 25 to 50 mg orally, is effective in relieving pruritus. If secondary infection develops, antibiotics will be necessary.

While the initial symptoms of a systemic reaction may be mild, symptoms can intensify rapidly to become life-threatening in a matter of minutes. It is vital to administer epinephrine hydrochloride; 1 : 1000, 0.3 to 0.5 mL for an adult, and 0.01 mL/kg for a child (never more than 0.3 mL). It should be injected subcutaneously and the injection site massaged to hasten absorption of the drug. The patient should then be observed for several hours to ensure that symptoms do not intensify.

More severe symptoms of a systemic reaction, such as chest constriction, nausea, faintness, and pronounced uneasiness, may require a second injection of epinephrine in 10 to 15 min. Antihistamines, such as diphenhydramine, 25 to 50 mg, should be administered intramuscularly.

If bronchospasm develops a secure intravenous line should be established and an infusion of aminophylline administered IV over 20 to 30 min. The adult dose is 500 mg; a child's dose is 5 mg/kg. Blood pressure and heart rate should be monitored closely. Maintain an open airway and administer oxygen as needed. If laryngeal edema is severe and airway obstruction develops, insert an endotracheal tube. Hypotension requires massive crystalloid infusion, and CVP monitoring may be helpful in some cases. Persistent hypotension after massive volume replacement may call for an initial infusion of dopamine, 200 mg in 250 mL of normal saline, at 5 μg/(kg/min), which may be increased gradually to 20 to 50 μg/(kg/min). While steroids are of no help in combating the immediate problem, their administration tends to limit urticaria and edema and may prolong the effects of other measures. Hydrocortisone IV initially, then prednisone, 10 mg daily for 5 to 7 days, may help prevent delayed symptoms of nephrosis or central nervous system damage.

The patient who suffers a severe systemic reaction should be kept under observation for 24 to 48 h and examined for evidence of cardiac problems, bleeding, proteinuria, or neurological complications.

In treating a delayed reaction, it may be necessary to administer prednisone (8 mg for adults, half that dosage for children) at 8 A.M. for 3 days, then discontinue. Oral antihistamines, such as brompheniramine maleate 2 to 4 mg (four times a day for adults and half that for children), may also be of help.

When ant stings or bites result in systemic reactions, especially if the bite is from the fire ant, treatment is the same as for Hymenoptera stings, but since secondary infection is frequent, antibiotics may be necessary even if the reaction is nonallergic. On occasion, scarring is extensive enough to require skin grafts.

Long-Term Management

If skin tests are positive, immunotherapy should be initiated and the patient maintained thereafter on an optimum dose. While the question may become moot if the FDA revokes the license for whole-body extracts in favor of venom extracts, there is still controversy over the relative effectiveness and safety of both methods. Nor has the problem of which patients should undergo immunotherapy been totally resolved. Generally speaking, a rise in IgE levels indicates sensitivity and an increase in IgG levels may indicate protection, but unfortunately this is not always the case. Nor are skin tests and RAST 100 percent reliable in determining the need for patient protection, for patients who present negative results may have been sensitized by the skin tests themselves. Every patient who has had a systemic reaction must be provided with an insect sting kit containing premeasured epinephrine and be carefully instructed in its use.

When immunotherapy with venom extracts is decided upon, the injection schedule may be rapid, with weekly visits until the optimum (for most patients) maintenance dose of 100 μg is reached. A slower schedule may be used, with the advantage of fewer systemic reactions during the process, but the goal should remain 100 μg. It is believed that there are no contraindications to immunotherapy, although pregnancy may require extra caution against the possibility of systemic reactions during treatment.

Since we do not as yet have a foolproof method of determining when a protection level is reached, a patient deemed allergic to Hymenoptera should be kept on maintenance injections indefinitely.

There are several insect sting kits available. Probably the simplest to use is the Ana-Kit, which contains a sterile syringe preloaded with two doses of epinephrine 1:1000, 0.5 mL in each dose with a stop between. The kit also contains a tourniquet, sterile alcohol pads, several antihistamine tablets, and instructions for self-injection. When prescribing this kit, the physician should stress that the patient must not rely on simply taking the antihistamine tablets, since these would not mitigate intensifying symptoms, but should inject the epinephrine subcutaneously at the first sign of a systemic reaction.

A second kit, the Epi-Pen, contains a single self-injecting syringe, spring-loaded, of epinephrine 1:1000. Its advantage is the ease of injection; its disadvantages are that to be on the safe side the patient should carry two kits and there is no way to measure a proper and lesser dosage for children.

Physicians should, as a matter of course, advise their patients who are allergic to insects to wear Medic-alert tags, and they should provide those patients with a list of avoidance measures to prevent being stung (Table 117-1).

Armed with these preventive measures—a medical warning tag and three insect sting kits, one for the home, one for the car, and one to carry in the field—the individual allergic to insects has taken every possible precautionary measure.

MOSQUITO AND FLY BITES

From available evidence, it is apparent that a characteristic sequence of events takes place in all subjects exposed to mosquito bites over a period of time. Human reaction to bites of the mosquito may be classified as follows:

1. Immediate and delayed reactions, both negative
2. Immediate reaction negative; delayed reaction positive
3. Immediate and delayed reactions, both positive
4. Immediate reaction positive and delayed reaction negative

An immediate skin reaction to mosquito bites includes redness, wheal, and itching. A delayed reaction usually consists of edema and a burning pruritus. The immediate reaction tends to be of short duration, whereas a delayed reaction may persist for hours, days, and even weeks.

Hypersensitivity reactions are of three types: tuberculin, urticarial, and eczemoid. Arthus' phenomenon with skin necrosis occurs occasionally. The history of an allergy to mosquito saliva constitutents consists of an increasing reaction to seasonal exposures with more and more pronounced adematous and pruritic lesions, accompanied sometimes by complications such as fever, malaise, generalized edema, severe nausea and vomiting, and necrosis with resulting scarring.

Table 117-2. Prevention of Insect Stings

1. Seek and destroy Hymenoptera nests that may be in the vicinity of the home, outbuildings, and yard. Begin with the advent of warm weather and conduct the searches periodically until the first hard frost. This task, however, should not be undertaken by the insect-allergic individual, but rather by a nonallergic person or by a professional exterminator.
2. Avoid going barefoot or wearing sandals outdoors.
3. When outdoors, wear light colors such as white, tan, khaki, or light green. Do not wear bright colors or flowery prints.
4. Do not use perfumed lotions, aftershaves, or shampoos during the warm months.
5. Cover up with long sleeves and long pants and wear gloves when working outdoors, and refrain from wearing floppy clothing that could entangle an irate stinging insect and from wearing bright jewelry that could attract one. Suede and leather articles may also not only attract but irritate Hymenoptera.
6. Anyone severely allergic to insects should not mow lawns, pick flowers, or clip hedges. Such an individual should be wary when eating outdoors, especially sugary food or drinks, and should avoid areas near garbage cans, littered picnic grounds, or fruit trees where fruit flies rotting on the ground.
7. If confronted by a member or members of hymenoptera, remain calm, never swat or move hastily, but rather retreat as slowly and calmly as possible. If retreat seems impossible, lie on the ground and cover your head with your arms.

Source: Frazier CA: *Insect Allergy*. St. Louis, WH Green, 1969.

Fly Bites

Bloodsucking flies that stab and pierce the skin can cause some degree of pain and, commonly, subsequent pruritus. Several species, such as deerflies, blackflies, horseflies, and sand flies, can produce allergic reactions, although rarely as severe as those produced by Hymenoptera venom. There is also the possibility of myiasis with fly bites, but this, too, is rare in the United States.

The diagnosis of fly bites depends chiefly on the patient's history and a knowledge of the insects that frequent the area of the encounter.

Treatment

Treatment for the more severe normal reactions to insect bites is symptomatic, while treatment of systemic reactions is the same as it is for Hymenoptera venom. Prevention of secondary infection, especially in the case of fly bites, is important, although antibiotics should not be given prophylactically. Oral antihistamines and cyproheptadine or hydroxyzine hyrochloride are helpful in relieving pruritus; trimeprazine tartrate is particularly effective in relieving pruritus of mosquito bites. Use of topical antihistamines runs the risk of contact dermatitis. However, topical steroid ointments are helpful when local reactions are severe or if scarring occurs.

Cold compresses may alleviate localized edema. For severe systemic reactions oral or parenteral steroids may be indicated. While immunotherapy has not proved as successful for mosquito or fly bite allergies as for Hymenoptera allergies, it is well worth the attempt for patients who suffer severe systemic reactions.

FLEA, LICE, AND SCABIES BITES

Flea bites

Bites of fleas, lice, and scabies produce lesions so similar that diagnosis is often difficult. Flea bites are frequently found in zigzag lines, especially on the legs and in the waist area. The lesions have hemorrhagic puncta surrounded by erythematous and urticarial patches. Pruritus is intense, and often, even after the lesions clear, dull red spots persist. Children may develop impetigo as a complication.

The main concern in the treatment of flea bites is the possibility of secondary infection. The lesions should be washed thoroughly with soap and water. For children, keep the fingernails cut short to prevent scratching. To relieve discomfort and itching, starch baths at bedtime (about 1 kg starch to a tubful of water), local application of calamine, cool soaks, and an oral antihistamine such as trimeprazine may be helpful. For severe discomfort, application of a topical steroid cream or spray may be necessary.

If secondary infection develops, a topical antibiotic such as neomycin or polymyxin may be needed.

Lice

Body lice concentrate about the waist, shoulders, axillae, and neck. The lice and their eggs can often be found in the seams of clothing. The lesions begin as small, noninflammatory red spots that quickly become papular wheals. They are so intensely pruritic that their linear scratch marks are diagnostically suggestive of infestation.

The white ova of head lice can be mistaken for dandruff, but unlike dandruff, they cannot be brushed out, for they are glued to the hair itself.

Pubic lice leave bluish spots in the abdomen and thighs, and ova are evident on the shafts of pubic hairs. If sensitization to lice saliva and feces components takes place, delayed reactions may develop. Fever and malaise are possible, and secondary infection may produce enlarged lymph glands. Long periods of infestation may bring a decrease in pruritus and often impart a thick, dry, scaly appearance to the skin. A brownish pigmentation characteristic of vagabond's disease can occur on the neck, shoulders, and back, or can become generalized and include even the mucuous membranes.

Treatment for body lice infestation consists of a thorough application of γ-benzene hexachloride (Kwell) or crotamiton (Eurax), plus sterilization of clothing, bedding, and personal articles. Kwell, however, must be employed with caution for infants and children since it can be absorbed more readily by their skin. It can be toxic to the central nervous system. Eurax should not be employed on raw or weeping areas. Head lice are treated with either of the above medications, daily shampoos, and fine combing the hair. Personal articles should be sterilized.

Scabies

While scabies infestation resemblies that of lice, scabies bites are generally concentrated around the hands and feet, especially in the webs between the fingers and toes. In children, however, the face and scalp may be infested as well. In adults, scabies frequently affects the nipples in females, the penis in males.

The scabies mite, an arachnid like the spider, is a universal pest that appear to follow a 30-year cycle of waxing and waning. During the last several years, there has been an epidemic of scabies infestation in the United States. In general, scabies infestation is more likely to occur by direct contact between the infested individual and the noninfested individual than by indirect contact with clothing and personal articles.

Diagnostically, pruritus is the dominant symptom, although it takes about a month for sensitization to develop and itching to begin. However, a patient who becomes infested, and who is already sensitized, develops inflammation and pruritus within a few hours of contact.

The distinctive feature of scabies infestation is the burrow that the female mite digs into the skin to lay her eggs. Vesicles and papules form at the surface of these zigzag, whitish, threadlike channels that contain small gray spots at the closed ends where the parasite rests. Burrows tend to enlarge and be more visible in children. The burrows can be traced with the hand lens and the female mite scraped out with a needle or razor blade. A thin shaving of skin containing both burrow and mite can be examined under a microscope to establish diagnosis clearly. Unfortunately, the burrows are often disguised by the results of fierce scratching. These distinctive physical findings are then obscured by crusting, eczematization, and secondary infection.

Treatment

Treatment for scabies infestation consists of a thorough application of γ-benzene hexachloride (GBH; Kwell, cream or lotion) from the neck down, following a warm bath with liberal use of soap. The patient should be cautioned to keep the substance from eyes and mucous membranes and to avoid inhaling the vapors. Again, since GBH is toxic, it probably should not be employed for young children or pregnant women. A 5% sulfur ointment can be substituted if necessary, although it is apt to be somewhat odoriferous and messy. It should be applied twice from the neck down, with a 24-h interval between applications, followed each time by a soap and water bath. A third application following the second by 12 h should be effective.

Crotamiton, which is also antipruritic in action, can be applied from the neck down in two applications of 24 h apart and followed 24 to 48 h later by a bath. The safety of its use, too, is somewhat in doubt, and it should be employed with caution.

Even after the scabies mites have been destroyed, lesions and pruritus can persist. No further use of scabicide is needed, but calamine lotion, oral antipruritic agents, and analgesics will help alleviate discomfort. Antiobiotics are only necessary where secondary infection is a problem.

KISSING BUG BITES

Triatoma species, commonly known as conenose or kissing bugs, are found mainly in the southeastern and Pacific coast regions of the United States. They feed on the blood of vertebrate animals, including humans. Their common name derives from their habit of feeding at night on any exposed surface of a sleeping victim, which commonly is the face. Since their bite is relatively painless, the victim is rarely aware of the attack.

Kissing bugs, like bedbugs, live in baseboards, between cracks in walls and floors, and in furniture.

Bites are usually multiple and consist of hemorrhagic papules or bullae if the bites occur on the hands or feet, and large wheals if they are on the trunk.

Diagnostically, kissing bug bites can be differentiated from bedbug bites in that they do not appear to form a linear formation nor do they leave the telltale brown or black patterns of excrement on the bed linen. They can be distinguished from spider bites, since the latter tend to be single lesions, and they usually can be distinguished from erythema multiforme by their unilateral, local distribution.

Treatment

Generally, treatment is symptomatic with cool local applications and mild analgesics to relieve pruritus. Some individuals become highly sensitive to the kissing bug and react with systemic symptoms, which should be treated as previously outlined for Hymenoptera venom. They are enough recorded cases of successful results with immunotherapy for allergy to kissing bugs to make it well worth the attempt for the hypersensitive individual.

CATERPILLAR STINGS

Some caterpillars possess hollow spines among their hairs which contain urticating poison that can cause symptoms ranging from local dermatitis to generalized systemic reactions. The puss caterpillar, larval stage of the flannel moth *Megalopyge opercularis*, is perhaps the most toxic in the United States and is especially hazardous for children who tend to find it intriguing and thus handle it.

Found primarily in the southeastern states and especially in Texas and Florida, the venom of the puss caterpillar has demonstrated hemolytic action in laboratory studies and an ability to increase vascular permeability. It is believed to be proteinaceous in nature.

The dominant feature of the of the puss caterpillar's sting is intense immediate pain, often rhythmic. Local edema and pruritus follow quickly, and a rash of red blotches and ridges develops. The lesions consist of white or red papules and vesicles, and frequently they form a perfect gridlike mark where the caterpillar made contact. The patient may be notably restless and frightened. In addition, generalized symptoms commonly occur with fever and muscle cramps. Shocklike symptoms have also been reported. Within several hours or days, local desquamation may develop. Lymphadenopathy has been described.

Treatment

Treatment should begin with immediate removal of broken-off spines by placing cellophane tape over the sting site. Calcium gluconate, 10 mL of a 10% solution, intravenously, is effective in relieving pain in severe cases, while tripelennamine usually brings relief in milder cases. Generalized symptoms are treated symptomatically.

BLISTER BEETLE STINGS

Blister beetles are found most frequently in the western section of the United States. When disturbed, they exude a vesicating agent, cantharidin, which can penetrate the epidermis to produce irritation and blistering within a few hours of contact. If ingested, cantharidin can produce intense gastrointestinal disturbances with symptoms of nausea, vomitting, diarrhea, and abdominal cramps. Initial contact with the beetle produces a burning, tingling sensation and a mild rash. Within a few hours, flaccid, elongated vesicles and bullae develop.

Treatment

Treatment consists of protecting the bullae from trauma by an occlusive dressing. Large bullae should be drained and an antibiotic ointment applied. If bullae occur on the feet, the patient should be advised to stay off the feet and wet dressings should be applied for 24 to 48 h.

INHALANT ALLERGY TO INSECTS

Allergic respiratory disease can be caused by insect debris in the atmosphere, such as wing scales and chitin.

BIBLIOGRAPHY

Abbudn F: Myiasis in otolaryngology. *Ear, Nose, Throat* 59:32, 1980.

American Academy of Allergy: Monograph on Insect Allergy, 1981.

Baer H, Liu TY, Anderson MC, et al: Protein components of fire ant venom (*Solenopsis invicta*). *Toxixcon* 17:397, 1979.

Feinstein RJ: Ticks. *Dermatologica* 1:13, 1978.

Frazier CA: Biting insect survey: A statistical report. *Ann Allergy* 32:200, 1974.

Frazier CA: Insect stings—a medical emergency. *JAMA* 235:2410, 1976.

Frazier CA: A preventable emergency. *Mil Med* 141:222, 1977.

Geller RG, Yoshida H, Beaven MA, et al: Pharmacologically active substances in venoms of the bald-faced hornet, *Vespula (Dolichovespula) maculata*, and the yellow jacket, *Vespula (Vespula) muculifrons*. *Toxicon* 14:27, 1976.

Hoffman DR: Honeybee venom allergy: Immunological studies of systemic and large local reactions. *Ann Allergy* 41:278, 1978.

Hoffman DR, Shipman WH: Allergens in bee venom. *J Allergy Clin Immunol* 58:551, 1976.

Paull BR, Yungingr JW, Gleich GJ: Melittin: An allergen of honeybee venom. *J Allergy Clin Immunol* 59:334, 1977.

Reisman RE, Arbesman CE, Lazell M: Observations on the aetiology and natural history of stinging insect sensitivity: Application of measurements of venom-specific IgE. *Clin Allergy* 9:303, 1979.

Reisman RE, Lazell M, Doerr J: Insect venom allergy: A prospective cae study showing lack of correlation between immunologic reactivity and clinical sensitivity. *J Allergy Clin Immunol* 68:406, 1981

Systemic reactions to Hymenoptera stings. *Med Lett Drug Ther* 20:54, 1978.

118
REPTILE BITES AND SCORPION STINGS

George Podgorny

SNAKEBITE

Although data concerning the incidence of snakebites in the United States are not available, a reasonable estimate is 8000 bites per year by venomous snakes and twice that number by harmless snakes. North Carolina has the highest incidence of admissions for venomous snakebites in the 48 contiguous states, followed by Arkansas, Texas, Georgia, West Virginia, Mississippi, and Louisiana, all with 10 or more admissions per year per 100,000 population. South Carolina, Oklahoma, New Mexico, and Florida follow.

A bite by a harmless snake is a minor nuisance, but its venomous counterparts can produce serious consequences. Annual mortality from venomous snakebites is about 50.

Most snakebites occur in the sunbelt. Peak months are July and August, followed by June and September, and then May and October. In general, snakes are poikilothermic and hibernate or undergo denning in cool temperatures. Abnormal and unexpected variations in temperature, however, can confuse snakes. Depending on the climate, snakes may be absent for a substantial portion of the year, or be present almost year-round. In areas with four seasons, snakes emerge from hibernation late in spring and reenter in mid-fall. As in all animals, the instinct of fight or flight is present in snakes. Most snakes prefer to retreat rather than fight. Aggressive behavior usually represents an attempt to secure prey or is a defensive maneuver when the snake is unable to retreat. Snakes are more aggressive when emerging from, and immediately preceding, hibernation. Because of relative dehydration and fat loss during hibernation, venomous snakes possess more concentrated and, therefore, more potent venom immediately on emergence from hibernation. The snake's control over its venom-injection apparatus is poorly understood. However, a venomous snake, at the time of biting, may inject varying amounts of venom or none at all.

Although basically nocturnal, snakes more frequently encounter humans between 6 A.M. and 9 P.M. In the outdoor, human exposure occurs during agricultural activity, hiking, hunting, fishing, and professional or amateur study of nature.

Indoor exposure to snakes occurs in zoos and animal research facilities. Bites often occur in the context of amateur snake-keeping and handling activities as the result of carelessness or daring. Certain religious cults and their venomous snake-handling activities provide an additional setting for exposure in some areas of Appalachia.

Handling snakes that appear to be dead may result in a venomous snake bite secondary to postmortem reflex action of the snake's head or even by inadvertently striking fingers against a fang of a preserved snake.

Many venomous snakes, particularly pit vipers, possess long and sharp fangs that can easily penetrate regular clothing. For this reason, humans should protect their extremities when in snake-infested areas.

Identification of Indigenous (Native) Venomous Snakes

Identification of the snake, either dead or alive, is important in order to determine whether it is harmless or venomous (Table 118-1). If the snake is not available, a reliable observer may be able to identify or describe it. If the snake is venomous, it must be determined whether it is a pit viper or coral snake, and, in the case of the former, whether it is a copperhead, cottonmouth, or rattlesnake.

Pit Vipers

Kin to the vipers of the old world, pit vipers are specific to the western hemisphere. The name is derived from the pit, a small indentation halfway between the snake's eye and nostril (Fig. 118-1). This represents a thermoreceptor organ that provides the snake with the ability to locate, track, and approach warm-blooded animals. In addition, all pit vipers possess anteriorly positioned, hollow, retractable fangs on the maxilla (Fig. 118-2). The anlage of the parotid glands produce the venom, and when the glands are squeezed by palatine muscles, the venom flows through ducts into the hollow fangs for injection.

Three additional characteristics of pit vipers aid in distinguishing them. First, they have vertical pupils. Most harmless snakes have round pupils, although some venomous snakes also have round pupils. Second, a pit viper's head is generally triangular in shape or, more precisely, is shaped like an arrowhead. Harmless snakes have oval or egg-shaped heads. Even in the hands of cognoscenti, this can be difficult to discern. A final distinction between pit vipers and harmless snakes lies in the pattern of plates on the snakes' undersides. On a snake's ventral side, somewhat caudad, are whitish, seemingly loose scales called the anal plates. In venomous snakes, scales are arranged in a single row from the anal plate to a point approximately a third of the

Table 118-1. The More Common and Better-Known Indigenous Venomous Snakes of the United States

Family	Genus and Species	Common Name	Geographic Distribution
Crotalidae (pit vipers)	*Crotalus adamanteus* (true rattlesnake)	Eastern diamondback	Eastern seaboard, tidal and adjoining areas from North Carolina to Florida and Gulf coast, Georgia, Alabama, and Mississippi
	C. horridus	Timber	North and northeast except Maine. West of Mississippi into central states and east Texas
	C. viridis	Prairie	Great plains, midwest, and prairie states
	C. atrox	Western diamondback	Texas, Oklahoma, and west into southeastern California
	C. cerastes	Mojave sidewinder	California, Arizona, Utah
	C. scutulatus	Mojave	Southwest Texas to California
	Sistrurus catenatus ("rattlesnake")	Massasauga	Nebraska, Iowa, Colorado, Texas, Arizona
	S. miliarius	Pygmy	North Carolina to Florida, and west to Oklahoma and Texas
	Agkistrodon contortrix	Copperhead	Central Massachusetts to north Florida, west to Illinois and Texas
	A. piscivorus	Cottonmouth (water moccasin)	South Virginia to Florida; west to east Texas, Mississippi valley, Illinois and Indiana
Elapidae (coral snakes)	*Micrurus fulvius*	Eastern	Southeastern North Carolina to tip of florida into Gulf coastal plain, Mississippi valley to central Arkansas, Texas, and adjacent Mexico
	Micruroides euryxanthus	Western (Sonoran) (Arizona)	Southern Arizona, southwest Mexico, and adjacent Mexico

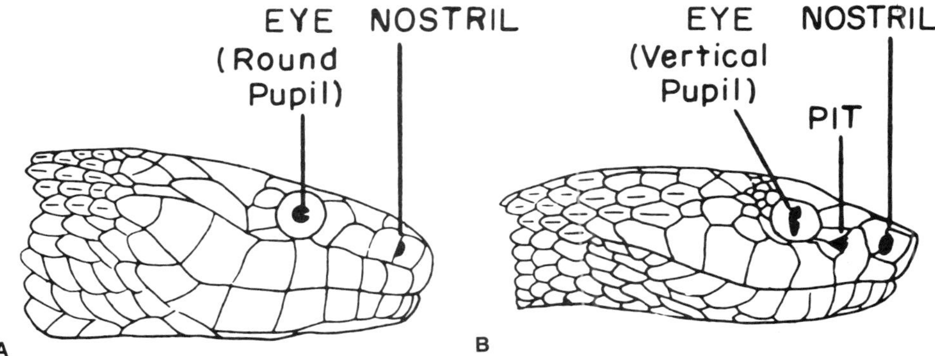

Fig. 118-1. Lateral view of the head of a harmless snake (**A**), and of a pit viper (**B**). (Adapted from Blanchard.)

distance away from the tip of the tail. In most harmless snakes, the scales are arranged in double rows from the anal plate to the tip of the tail.

Three genera of pit vipers are considered. The genus *Crotalus* includes almost all of the true rattlesnakes and is composed of nearly 20 different species and variations. Two "rattlesnakes," the pygmy and the massasauga, belong to the genus *Sistrurus*. All rattlesnakes, when intact and not suffering from congenital malformation, possess characteristic terminal rattles. The number and the size of the rattles do not denote the years of the snake's age; however, they reflect overall longevity. When all the rattles are missing, the tail's end is unexpectedly blunt. Rattlesnakes are present in most of the continental United States (see Table 118-1). Except for the pgymy rattler, rattlesnakes usually grow to a large size, and their bites are potentially fatal.

The third genus of pit vipers, *Agkistrodon,* consists of two species. The water moccasin (*A. piscivorus*), also called cottonmouth because of its white buccal mucosa, is "amphibious." It tends to be smaller than a rattlesnake, but is similar in terms of venom characteristics. The second species, the copperhead (*A. contortrix*), is so called because of the copperlike coloration of the mature adult. It is the most prevalent venomous snake in the United States but fortunately the least venomous of the pit vipers. It is responsible for a substantial number of venomous snakebites, particularly east of the Mississippi.

Coral Snake (Elapidae)

Two species of coral snakes are present in the United States. They are the only representatives of a totally different group of venomous snakes and are kin to cobras and kraits of the old world. The two species closely resemble each other. They are relatively small, shy snakes with a rather distinct pattern of red and black bands that are

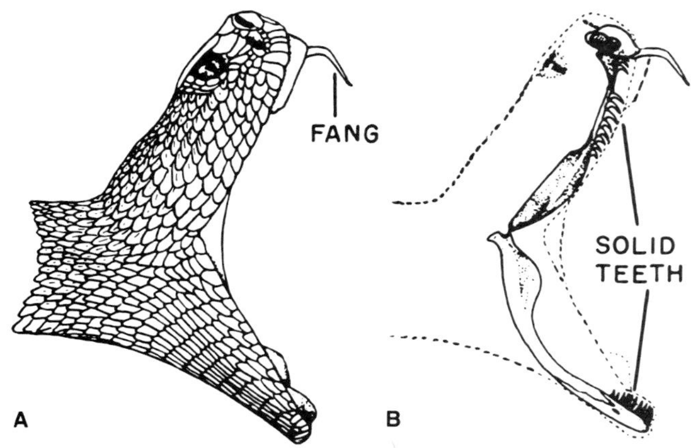

Fig. 118-2. Lateral view of a head of a snake (rattlesnake) showing exposed fangs approximately in striking position. **A.** Tissues intact as in a live snake. **B.** Position of the tooth-bearing bones. (Adapted from Pope.)

wider than the interspaced yellow rings. This has given rise to the following mnemonic rhyme: "Red on yellow, kill a fellow—coral snake. Red on black, venom lack—harmless snake." The more plentiful of the species, the eastern coral snake (*Micrurus fulvius*), has a black snout with the previously described coloration of the body.

Most of the head is black in the Arizona or Sonora coral snake (*Micruroides euryxanthus*), but the rest of its coloration is similar to the eastern coral snake (yellow rings may be narrower or paler).

Variables Influencing Severity of Venomous Snakebite

Snake Variables

The size and vitiation of the snake govern the type, quantity, and quality of venom available. The larger the snake (of the same species), the more venom it possesses and has available for injection. A hungry, disturbed, and alert snake is deadlier. The angle of bite is significant, and so is its depth and the duration of the time of penetration of one or both fangs.

Snake venoms are highly complex biochemical compounds. The following components have been identified:

1. Blood coagulants, such as thrombin or prothrombin-like substances, anticoagulants, and agglutinins, which affect coagulation and red blood cells.
2. Cytolysins, proteolysins, and antibactericidin, which affect cellular blood components as well as the endothelium of the vessels. Antibactericidin contributes to suppuration, paralyzing the phagocytic activity of the white blood cells.
3. Neurotoxins A and B, which affect the nervous system, particularly the cardiorespiratory centers and higher central nervous system; neurotoxin B also affects the myoneural junction.
4. Cholinesterase and anticholinesterase, which affect the myoneural junction.
5. Cardiotoxin, which stimulates the heart.
6. Hyaluronidase, which facilitates the tissue spread of the venom.
7. Proteolytic enzymes.
8. Phospholipases.

The presence and mix vary depending on the type of snake. For instance, the venom of pit vipers is high in the hemopathic components, while venom from the coral snake is rich in neurotoxins.

Victim Variables

The size of the victim is important; children and infants are more vulnerable. The condition of the victim will seriously affect the outcome. Hypertension, diabetes, advanced age, debility, or coagulation disorders are aggravated by a venomous snakebite. Individuals with bleeding tendencies, such as hemophilia, or those on anticoagulant therapy, with active peptic ulcers, or with open wounds are susceptible to bleeding secondary to envenomation. Women who are menstruating may bleed excessively after a pit viper bite. Those who have endometriosis may bleed excessively and develop severe pain. Abortions in pregnant women who have been bitten by pit vipers have been reported.

The location of the bite is of great importance. Snakebites on the head and trunk are from two to three times more dangerous than those on the extremities. Venomous bites on the upper extremities are more serious than those on the lower extremities. Incidental penetrations of fangs and injection of venom into a blood vessel are usually catastrophic.

Clinical Features

It is safe to assume that the bite is venomous if one or two fang marks are present. Rarely three or four marks may be present. Absence of fang marks is presumptive evidence of a harmless snakebite or an unsuccessful attempt by the pit viper without penetration. Fang marks separated by 15 mm or more indicate a bite by a very large snake, while those separated by less than 8 mm point to a smaller snake. A coral snake bite may present an atypical pattern.

Signs and Symptoms

If the offending snake cannot be identified, the symptoms and signs are the only remaining criteria of severity. They are divided into hemopathic, neurotoxic, and systemic manifestations.

Hemopathic Manifestations

Swelling, edema, ecchymoses, extravasation of blood, and bleeding from kidneys, lungs, peritoneum, rectum, and vagina may occur owing to endothelial damage of small vessels and lymphatic channels.

Changes in red blood cells and their ability to transport oxygen may result in bleeding, drop in hemoglobin, and tissue anoxia leading to necrosis. There may be local bleeding from areas such as the endometrium or urinary tract or bleeding from pathological foci, such as peptic ulcers, because of impaired coagulation mechanisms. Hypofibrinogenemia, with or without thrombocytopenia, disseminated intravascular coagulation, or fibrinolysis can occur.

While hemopathic and systemic signs, including swelling, edema, and pain predominate with pit viper bites, neurologic signs may also occur.

Neurotoxic Manifestations

The effects of neurotoxins A and B on the central nervous system are manifested by dysphagia, convulsions, and psychotic behavior. The myoneural junction is also affected by neurotoxin B, which results in locomotor disturbances, manifested by weakness of the muscles, fasciculation, paresthesia, and, in very extreme cases, paralysis. Neurologic signs predominate with coral snake and cobra bites.

Systemic Effects

General systemic signs and symptoms of venomous snakebite include elevation or depression of the temperature, nausea, vomiting, diarrhea, pain, and restlessness. Although tachycardia is common, severe bradycardia may develop. The pathogenesis of the bradycardia is obscure. Renal failure from acute tubular necrosis or bilateral cortical necrosis has been reported.

Unless obvious signs and symptoms of venomous snakebite are present, the differential diagnosis may be difficult. Consideration should be given to bites of chiggers, occasionally of tarantulas, and some insects. Frequently, individuals with two chigger bites which are about 1 cm apart seek medical treatment claiming that they have sustained a snakebite. Only in that context is the differential diagnosis necessary; certainly, the symptomatology is not related. Factitious "fang marks" are seen occasionally in supervised group environments such as summer camps, military installations, and correctional institutions.

Treatment

First Aid

Victim should be placed supine to rest, as rest decreases metabolism, spread, and absorption of venom. When practical, the bitten part should be immobilized in a dependent position. The victim should be reassured and supported. Prehospital measures should include infusion of isotonic intravenous fluids and the patient should be transported to a medical facility that has the appropriate antivenin available.

Guidelines for the treatment of pit viper bites, including surgical, medical, and anticipatory measures, are listed in Table 118-2.

Antivenin is available by prescription only and its use and storage by laypersons remain controversial. Therefore, the decision to issue antivenin to a nonphysician should be made on the basis of the circumstances of the environment, the logistics of communication with and transportation to a medical facility and personnel, and the ability of the individual to properly use and administer the antivenin. Proper information, training, and standing orders ought to be available to the EMS personnel. Physician supervision should be readily available, particularly in situations where life or limb are endangered. Prior knowledge of the location of facilities that store type-specific antivenin should be publicized to EMS and law enforcement personnel. In cases of severe envenomation, speedy transport and resuscitative measures in transit should be implemented.

Table 118-2. Guidelines for Treatment of Pit Viper Bite

Grade of Envenomation	Symptoms and Signs within 2 to 5 h	Surgical Measures	Medical Measures	Anticipatory Measures
I Minimal	Moderate pain, edema 2.5–15 cm, erythema, no systemic symptoms	Cleansing and debridement	Antibiotic, tetanus prophylaxis, antihistamine	Type and cross-match blood, CBC, urinalysis, clotting time
II Moderate	Severe pain, tenderness, edema 25–40 cm, erythema, petechiae, vomiting, fever, weakness	Cleansing and debridement	As above, plus IV antivenin infusion in selected cases of bites of rattler and cottonmouth	As above; also be ready to treat hemorrhage, test for horse serum sensitivity
III Severe	Widespread pain, tenderness, edema 40–50 cm, ecchymosis, systemic signs, vertigo	Cleansing and debridement	As above; also IV antivenin, follow coagulation parameters, and give calcium gluconate if indicated for seizures	As above; also be ready to intubate and support respiration if needed
IV Very severe	Rapid swelling, ecchymosis, CNS symptoms, visual disturbance, shock, convulsions	Cleansing and debridement	IV antivenin in massive doses, blood transfusions	As above; also watch for cardiac arrest, renal failure, compartment syndrome in extremities

Medical Measures

Treatment should be directed toward general life support. Intravenous isotonic fluids should be administered. Blood samples should be sent immediately for typing and cross-matching, which may become difficult as envenomation progresses. In severe cases, intubation and ventilatory support are necessary.

Blood transfusions may be necessary if bleeding is severe. Intravenous calcium gluconate, 10 mL of a 10% solution, has been recommended for the treatment of seizures, although the mode of action is obscure, and controlled studies of its effectiveness are not available. Cardiac arrhythmias are treated in the usual manner. Antihistamines are helpful for itching and urticaria.

Close evaluation of the symptoms, signs, and condition of the victim is necessary. The presence and extent of ecchymoses, discoloration, vesicle formation, and edema should be recorded. Marking progression of edema on the limbs is useful and can be done along with periodic measurement of the circumference of both limbs at predetermined points.

Clinical laboratory determinations including CBC; platelet count; BUN, creatinine, and electrolyte levels; coagulation profile; blood type and cross-match; and urinalysis should be obtained.

Appropriate tetanus prophylaxis should be administered.

Snakebites are notorious for becoming infected. The microorganisms represent a mixed flora both gram-positive and gram-negative. Broad-spectrum antibiotics (cephalosporins or tetracyclines) are indicated pending culture and sensitivity determination.

Antivenin

Antivenin neutralizes the snake venom. There are two types produced in the United States and approved by the FDA. Antivenin (Crotalidae) made by Wyeth Laboratories is polyvalent against the pit viper venoms of North and South America. It is supplied as a powder to be mixed with sterile water and comes in a self-contained kit with instructions. Crotalidae antivenin is prepared from hyperimmune equine serum of horses exposed to venoms of the eastern diamondback rattlesnake, western diamondback rattlesnake, tropical rattlesnake, and fer-de-lance. These venoms contain basic antigens common to most of the pit vipers of the Americas, including rattlesnakes and moccasins of the United States, Japan, and Korea, and of the fer-de-lance and bushmaster.

A second type made by Wyeth Laboratories is specific against the eastern coral snake bite. There is no evidence that this antivenin is of any value in the treatment of Arizona coral snake bites, which are extremely rare.

All antivenins are made from horse serum. The patient should not be skin tested until a decision to administer antivenin has been made, because theoretically protein sensitivity could be induced by the skin test. Testing can be accomplished by the intradermal injection of 0.2 mL of horse serum diluted 1 : 10 or 1 : 100 depending on whether the patient has a possible history of sensitivity to equine serum. Appearance of a wheal with or without pseudopods, erythema, and severe itching within 15 to 30 min suggests a positive reaction. Epinephrine for subcutaneous injection should be immediately available to counteract any untoward event.

Horse Serum Sensitivity

The question of whether to give horse serum-based antivenin to those who show evidence, or have a history, of allergy to horse serum remains a problem. Clinical judgment should be used to weigh the advantages and disadvantages of administering antivenin in light of the severity of the venomous snake bite. Not only potential mortality, but morbidity and later complications should enter into clinical consideration. Guidelines for antivenin administration are listed in Table 118-3. Wingert and Wainschel have described a method for intravenous infusion in severely envenomated patients with sensitivity to horse serum, consisting of 50 mg of diphenhydramine IV, followed by slow IV infusion of antivenin.

Table 118-3. Guidelines for Antivenin Administration

Grade of Envenomation		Dose
I	Minimal	None
II	Moderate	20–mL (2–4 vials)*
III	Severe	50–90 mL (5–9 vials)
IV	Very severe	100–150 mL or more (10–15 or more vials)

* Use of antivenin here is controversial—use clinical judgment.

Source: Data from Antivenin (Crotalidae) Polyvalent package insert. Wyeth Laboratories, Philadelphia, PA.

Antivenin is necessary for severe envenomation, but for minimal envenomation, the risks of administration may outweigh the benefits. Complications of antivenin administration are serum sickness, which develops nearly universally in those receiving seven ampoules or more of antivenin; radiculitis or other neuropathies; and, of course, anaphylaxis. Do not give antivenin if a patient is definitely sensitive to horse serum and the pit viper bite is within grades I or II. However, in grades III or IV, particularly in a child or infant, lack of antivenin therapy could be fatal.

Administration and Dose

Antivenin is packaged in vials of 10 mL each. Anywhere from 5 to 15 or more vials may be used depending on the severity of the bite and the type for snake involved. Compared with adults, in similar circumstances, children should be given proportionately more since the aim is to neutralize the venom, and they have received a greater amount of venom per kilogram of body weight. Antivenin should be given within 4 h of the bite; 12 h after the bite the use of antivenin is of uncertain value.

Antivenin should be administered as an isotonic intravenous infusion and regulated according to the advance or recess of the swelling and other symptoms. It should never be injected into the area of the bite.

In most instances, bites of rattlesnakes and water moccasins should be treated with antivenin unless there is a contraindication or the bite is not considered to be severe enough to warrant antivenin administration. As a rule, the bite of the copperhead is self-limiting and will not require antivenin or treatment. Exceptions would be cases involving an unusually large snake, multiple bites, or a small or debilitated victim.

Helpful Hints

1. Absence of fang marks precludes envenomation.
2. In presence of venom injection, the fang marks continue oozing nonclotting blood.
3. Marks without bleeding or with clotted blood probably represent a lack of envenomation or an insect bite or are factitious.
4. Very soon after a pit viper bite, mild ecchymoses appear around the fang marks.
5. Immediate severe burning pain is characteristic of pit viper bite.
6. Absence of microhematuria after a pit viper bite is a good prognostic sign indicating lack of severe envenomation.

Surgical Measures

Infrequently, compartment syndrome may follow venomous snakebites. The volar compartment of the forearm and the thenar compartment of the hand are frequently involved in the upper extremity. Compartments of the leg can also be involved. Compartment syndromes more often than not occur in children and adults of small size. If increased, compartment pressure jeopardizes the blood supply of the distal portion of the limb or digit.

Compartment pressures should be measured, and when 30 mmHg or higher fasciotomy should be performed. The appearance of the muscle beneath the fasciotomy incision may be misleading, and any debridement should be carried out in a very conservative fashion. In several days the fasciotomy should be closed, preferably by primary repair.

Fasciotomy per se will have no specific affect on the outcome of the snakebite as a systemic problem. Antivenin will have to be used if indicated. Reports of definitive treatment of pit viper bites by fasciotomy with and without steroids have not gained acceptance.

Incision of the skin of the lateral and medial aspects of a bitten finger may relieve swelling and pain in the finger.

In this author's opinion, excision of the local soft tissues should be undertaken only if envenomation is severe; if the bite is on the trunk; if no antivenin is available; if no more than 1 h has elapsed from the time of the bite; and if no anatomical contraindications exist. It should be carried out by, or in consultation with, a surgeon. The skin and subcutaneous tissue should be excised in a radius of 3 to 4 cm from the fang marks and deep to the fascia. In 72 h, apply a split-thickness skin graft unless the recipient site is infected. The skin of the excised specimen, if intact, can be removed and preserved as full- or split-thickness graft for later use. Huang et al. have reported good success with early excision, under 2 h, even with involvement of upper or lower extremities or digits.

Consultation Service

A national index is maintained by the Arizona Poison Control Center (1-800-362-0101) for locating type-specific antivenins to use in exotic venomous snakebites. The international Antivenin Index lists medical consultants and internationally available antivenins and the species against which they are effective.

Other Modalities

Proper application of tourniquets for snakebite is difficult and probably ineffective. An arterial tourniquet will cause distal ischemia. A venous tourniquet causes venous stasis unless released every 10 min. Most venom absorption is through lymphatic channels. In order to be effective, a lymphatic tourniquet is also an arterial tourniquet. There are no data that support the effectiveness of tourniquets. Insignificant envenomations do well regardless of treatment, and serious snakebites will not be helped by a tourniquet and require antivenin.

Incision and suction became popular because it was believed that there is a venom "pool" underneath the fang mark. However, pit viper fangs are long and curved. The venom is not deposited beneath the fang mark, but rather along a circle where the radius equals the length of the arc of the fang. In order to reach such a venom "pool," it is necessary to incise the arc, not necessarily through the fank marks. Cruciate incisions through the fang marks heal poorly, leaving unsightly retracted central scars. Furthermore, in significant snakebites, penetration of the fangs is deep, and the venom is deposited, not subcutaneously, but in the deeper tissues and often in the muscles. In the fingers, hand, and wrist as well as in the toes, foot, and ankle, where most venomous snakebites occur, venom is deposited deep into the skin and subcutaneous tissues. To incise deeply causes additional complications. If incision is done at all, must be done by an individual fully aware of anatomy and proper technique. Incisions should be linear and along the long axis of the limb and should not cross blood vessels, nerves, or tendons. Incisions must be deep enough to reach the "venom pool."

Suction can be done by the patient or rescuer provided there are no fresh defects in the oral mucosa or tongue. Some local anesthesia will result from contact with the venom. There are various suction devices available, which in the experience of this author have not been very useful.

If incision and suction are to be of any value, they must be done within 15 min of the bite, adequately performed, and later cleansed and debrided. For mild snakebite, incision and suction are unnecessary. For potentially fatal snakebite, antivenin is necessary, and incision and suction are of little, if any, value.

Cryotherapy or immersion of the limb in ice water (not saline) may jeopardize the injured limb because of cold-mediated vasocontriction, or frostbite, and has not been demonstrated to inhibit the destructive effects of venom. It is contraindicated in the management of snakebite.

Sullivan and Russell at the University of Arizona have been able to demonstrate both in vivo and in vitro the efficacy of immunopurified polyvalent IgG (T) antibodies. This product may be more efficacious than the currently available antivenin and particularly less likely to produce anaphylaxis and serum sickness.

Local injection of lidocaine or procaine may help relieve pain, but the local injection of epinephrine is contraindicated because it further potentiates tissue ischemia. Steroids are indicated later for the management of serum sickness, but have no role in the management of acute envenomation.

Complications

One major mistake made in treating snake bite is not giving enough antivenin. Tissue necrosis and slough are frequently results of inadequate treatment of the pit viper bite. In the absence or delay of administration of specific antivenin, extensive vasculitis, necrosis, and sloughing of the skin and subcutaneous tissues may occur.

Fibrosis can result secondary to the bites of rattlesnakes and water moccasins. Bites of the hand, both on the dorsum and on the palm, are particularly susceptible to later fibrosis and contractures. Limitations of motion, both in flexion and extension, are frequently seen. Fibrosis is a component of healing and scarring. Snakebite victims taking β-blockers are more susceptible to anaphylaxis secondary to antivenin.

The second major mistake is giving antivenin unncessarily.

In rare cases of disseminated intravascular clotting that may be a complication of venomous snakebites, heparin should be utilized.

Immunization

Periodic reports in quasiscientific and lay literature indicate that certain individuals who have been bitten frequently by venomous snakes develop active immunity and, in addition, their serum confirms passive immunity. Such reports are at best anecdotal and frequently charged with emotion. Several controlled attempts to produce immunity in humans have failed. At least two individuals known to the author who have sustained many venomous snakebites became just as ill or worse with subsequent bites as they did with earlier ones.

Reports of application of pressure devices, as well as of electric shock immediately to the bite site or the extremity are yet to be scientifically validated.

Coral Snakes

Coral snakes have short, fixed anterior fangs. Therefore, they need greater leverage to puncture the skin and a longer period to inject their venom. Coral snake venom has a blocking action on acetylcholine receptor sites and may be responsive to treatment with neostigmine. The early signs of coral snake bite are slurred speech, ptosis, dilated pupils, dysphagia, and myalgia. Frequently symptoms are not evident until a few hours after the bite.

Delayed symptoms of coral snake bite include euphoria, drowsiness, strabismus, excessive salivation, confusion, and vomiting. When not treated, death results within 8 to 24 h, due to progressive paralysis, and respiratory arrest secondary to central nervous system inhibition, ending in cardiorespiratory arrest.

Absorption of coral snake venom is rapid, and fixation is at the myoneural junction. Mechanical measures of tourniquet, incision, and suction are not of value in retarding absorption.

A specific antivenin prepared in horse serum is available against the eastern coral snake. It is of no value against the venom of the Sonoran coral snake. Testing for sensitivity to horse serum is mandatory and should the snake bite be potentially fatal, only the use of antivenin will be lifesaving. Recent experience using edrophonium (Tensilon) test to counteract neurotoxic envenomation by the Philippine cobra (*Naja naja*) indicates that anticholinesterases may be of benefit in management of neurotoxic snake envenomation, such as neostigmine 2.5 mg every 30 to 60 min.

Harmless Snakes

Bites of harmless snakes are significant only as contaminated puncture wounds. Harmless snakes have several rows of teeth, and frequently the imprints of the teeth are seen on the skin of the victim. Cleansing, debridement, and administration of tetanus prophylaxis, as indicated, usually suffice. The use of broad-spectrum antibiotics may be indicated because the mouth of the snake harbors many organisms. Infrequently, the bite of a harmless snake will produce swelling, itching, and erythema. This is an allergic reaction to the snake's saliva, and an antihistamine will quickly relieve the symptoms.

Recent reports indicate that a few types of snakes, so far considered harmless, produce small amounts of low-toxicity venom and cause a mildly symptomatic bite. The following snakes have been implicated: lyre (*Trimorphodon*), vine (*Oxybelis*), and garter (*Thamnophis*). Treatment of the local symptoms is sufficient.

GILA MONSTER BITE

The Gila monster (*Heloderma suspectum*) is a sluggish, shy lizard that lives in the southwest and, in undergoing evolutionary changes, has developed eight venomous glands in the floor of its mouth. The venom is secreted into the oral cavity and then flows along the teeth, which are grooved posteriorly. Because of this rather primitive and ineffective injection apparatus, these lizards have to hang on tenaciously and chew on the soft tissues to introduce a sufficient amount of venom to immobilize the prey. To detach the monster from the victim, introduce a hemostat, stick, or spoon between the jaws posteriorly and pry them apart.

The venom primarily contains neurotoxins, and produces pain, edema, and a mostly local reaction. Reports of death secondary to the bite are not substantiated. There is no antivenin available for a Gila monster bite. Use of a venous tourniquet soon after the bite, local measures, and tetanus protection are indicated treatments. There is some evidence that meperidine may be synergistic with the venom; thus it is contraindicated for pain. Anaphylaxis has been reported. Broad-spectrum antibiotics such as cephalosporins are indicated.

SCORPION STINGS

The only significant group of Arizona scorpions are those belonging to the *Centruroides*. The primary offending species are *C. sculpturatus*, now renamed *C. exilicauda*. This scorpion often has different common names such as the bark scorpion, yellow scorpion, or whip scorpion. It is a relatively slender scorpion with a slim tail. Its telson has a significant protuberance at the base. Adults may be from light yellow to straw color sometimes with darker stripes along the back of the trunk and may reach a size of 52 to 60 mm.

Scorpions prefer moisture and coolness and are frequently found in the bark of fallen trees, under moist ground cover, or in tents or camping equipment.

Most scorpion stings are allergenic rather than venomous. The sting causes a sharp, burning sensation lasting for a few minutes. Some species produce marked local edema that resolves over a day or two. However, the sting of *C. exilicauda* causes primarily systemic rather than local effects, and three to four deaths occur annually in the United States. The symptoms include restlessness, hyperactivity, fasciculation, and excessive salivation and lacrimation.

Treatment

In the absence of a systemic reaction, no danger exists from scorpion stings. Cleansing, tetanus prophylaxis, and antihistamines are adequate treatments. For bites with systemic reactions, general life support measures, antihistamines, and atropine to counteract the parasympathomimetic effects are indicated. Specific antivenin for *C. exilicauda* is available in scropion-infested areas of the southwest, but as of this writing, it has not yet been approved by the Federal Drug Administration.

BIBLIOGRAPHY

Kunkel DB: Bites of venomous reptiles. *Emerg Med Clin North Am* 2:563, 1984.

Nelson BK: Snake venomation, incidence, clinical presentation and management. *Med Toxicol* 4:17, 1989.

Podgorny G: Treatment of snake bite, in Haddad LM, Winchester JF (eds): *Clinical Management of Poisoning and Drug Overdose*. Philadelphia, Saunders, 1983.

Russell F, Minoo B Madon: Introduction of the scorpion *Centruroides exilicauda* into California and its public health significance. *Toxicon* 22:658, 1984.

Streiffer RH: Bite of the venomous lizard, the Gila monster. *Postgrad Med* 79:279, 1986.

Sullivan JB: Immunotherapy in the poisoned patient: overview of present applications and future trends. *Med Toxicol* 1:47, 1987.

Watt G, Theakston R, Hayes C, et al: Positive response to edrophonium in patients with neurotoxic envenomation by cobras. *N Engl J Med* 315:1444, 1986.

119 TRAUMA AND ENVENOMATIONS FROM MARINE FAUNA

Paul S. Auerbach

Although noxious marine organisms are concentrated predominantly in warm temperate and tropical seas, particularly in the Indo-Pacific region, hazardous animals may be found as far north as latitude 50°. Dangerous marine animals can be divided into four groups: (1) traumatogenic; (2) stinging; (3) poisonous on ingestion; and (4) shocking. *Oral toxins* are poisonous to eat and include bacterial poisons and products of decomposition. *Parenteral toxins* are venoms produced in specialized glands and injected mechanically with traumatogenic devices, such as spines or teeth. *Crinotoxins* are venoms produced in specialized glands, typically as slimes or gastric secretions, and administered without the aid of traumatogenic devices. Thus, the emergency physician may encounter subsets of trauma (hemorrhage, lacerations, foreign bodies), infections, envenomations, and obscure poisonings.

BACTERIOLOGY OF THE MARINE ENVIRONMENT

Ocean water provides a saline milieu for microbes. Although the greatest number and diversity of bacteria are found near the ocean surface, diverse bacteria and fungi are found in marine silts, sediments, and sand. Microbes are most abundant in areas that have the greatest numbers of higher life forms. Marine bacteria are generally halophilic, heterotrophic, motile, and gram-negative rod forms. In addition, microalgae, protozoa, yeasts, and viruses have been identified in, or cultured from, seawater, marine sediments, marine life, and from marine-acquired or marine-contaminated infected wounds or body fluids of septic victims. Because special media may be necessary for culture and sensitivity testing, in the setting of wound infection or sepsis, the clinician should alert the laboratory that a marine-acquired organism may be present. Unusual pathogens include *Acinetobacter lwoffi, Alteromonas haloplanktis, Bacillus subtilis, Bacteroides fragilis, Clostridium perfringens, Edwardsiella tarda, Erysipelothrix rhusiopathiae, Micrococcus sedentarius, Mycobacterium marinum, Providencia stuartii, Pseudomonas* species, and diverse *Vibrio* species, including *V. alginolyticus, V. cholerae, V. damsela, V. fluvialis, V. furnissii, V. harveyi, V. hollissae, V. parahaemolyticus, V. pelagius II, V. mimicus, V. splendidus I,* and *V. vulnificus.*

TREATMENT OF INFECTIONS

The objectives for the management of infections from marine microorganisms are to recognize the clinical condition, culture the organism, and provide antimicrobial therapy. There is no advantage to quantitative wound culture prior to the appearance of a wound infection. Minor abrasions or lacerations (e.g., coral cuts or superficial sea urchin puncture wounds) do not require the administration of prophylactic antibiotics in the normal host. Persons who are chronically ill (e.g., with diabetes, hemophilia, or thalassemia) or immunologically impaired (e.g., who have leukemia or AIDS or who are undergoing chemotherapy or prolonged corticosteroid therapy), or who suffer from serious liver disease (e.g., who have hepatitis, cirrhosis, or hemochromatosis, particularly those with elevated serum iron levels) should be placed immediately after injury on oral trimethoprim-sulfamethoxazole or ciprofloxacin. These persons appear to have an increased risk for serious wound infection and bacteremia. The appearance of an infection indicates the need for prompt debridement, foreign body removal and antibiotic therapy.

Wounds at especial risk for infection include large lacerations, serious burns, major envenomations, deep puncture wounds, or a retained foreign body. Infected wounds should be cultured for aerobes and anaerobes. If rapidly progessive cellulitis or myositis develops, infection from *Vibrio parahaemolyticus* or *V. vulnificus* should be considered, particularly in the presence of chronic liver disease. If a wound infection is minor and has the appearance of a classic erysipeloid reaction (*Erysipelothrix rhusiopathiae*), penicillin, cephalexin, or erythromycin should be administered.

Management of marine-acquired infections should include therapy directed against *Vibrio* species. Third-generation cephalosporins (e.g., cefoperazone) provide excellent coverage; first- and second-generation cephalosporins appear to be less effective in vitro. Other antimicrobials that are efficacious in vitro against gram-negative marine bacteria include imipenem-cilastatin, trimethoprim-sulfamethoxazole, tetracycline, azlocillin, mezlocillin, gentamicin, tobramycin, chloramphenicol, piperacillin, and, in clinical observation, ciprofloxacin.

BITES, LACERATIONS, AND PUNCTURES

Approximately 32 of the at least 350 species of sharks have been implicated in the 50 to 100 shark attacks (with six to ten deaths) reported annually worldwide. Another 35 to 40 species are considered potentially dangerous. The danger to humans is a combination of size, aggression, and dentition. The first contact with a shark may be a "bumping," which is an attempt by the shark to wound the victim prior to the definitive strike. Severe skin abrasions from the shark skin denticles can occur in this manner. The jaws of the shark are crescent-shaped and contain rows or series of razor-sharp ripsaw teeth. Incredibly, the biting force of some sharks is estimated at 18 tons per square inch. Severe shark bites result in massive tissue loss, hemorrhage, severe fractures, shock, and death. Broken ribs are often accompanied by intrathoracic, intraperitoneal, and retroperitoneal injuries. Wounds are fatal in 15 to 25 percent of attacks. The major causes of death are due to hemorrhage and drowning.

Other marine animals that bite or puncture without envenomation include the barracuda, moray eel, sea lion, polar bear, needlefish, giant grouper, and crocodile. The injuries are a combination of crush, puncture, and laceration. Because *Clostridia* species can be cultured from ocean water, tetanus toxoid, 0.5 mL IM, and tetanus immune globulin, 250 to 500 units IM, must be given. Extensive and complicated wounds are often best managed by operative debridement. If treated in the emergency department, vigorous irrigation, removal of foreign bodies, and loose closure, possibly with drain placement, are necessary.

Multiple small puncture wounds are common following moray eel bites; the hand is most commonly involved. If the eel remains attached to the victim, the jaws may need to be broken or the animal decapitated for release. Wounds should be explored to located retained teeth. The risk for infection is high, so puncture wounds should be left unsutured and prophylactic antibiotics given.

Coral cuts are probably the most common injuries sustained underwater. The initial reaction to a coral cut is stinging pain, erythema, and pruritus, most commonly on the hands, forearms, elbows, and knees. A break in the skin may be surrounded by an erythematous wheal within minutes, which fades over 1 to 2 h. The local reaction of red, raised welts and local pruritus is called "coral poisoning." With or without prompt treatment, this may progress to cellulitis with ulceration and tissue sloughing. The wounds heal slowly (3 to 6 weeks) and result in prolonged morbidity. In an extreme case, the victim develops cellulitis with lymphangitis, reactive bursitis, local ulceration, and wound necrosis. Coral cuts should be promptly and vigorously irrigated to remove all foreign matter. Any fragments that remain can become embedded and increase the risk for infection or foreign body granuloma. If stinging is a major symptom, there may be an element of envenomation by nematocysts. A brief rinse with diluted acetic acid (vinegar) or isopropyl alcohol 20% may diminish the discomfort (after the initial pain from contact with the open wound). If a coral-induced laceration is severe, it should be closed with adhesive strips rather than sutures if possible; preferably, it should be debrided sharply each day for 3 to 4 days. The preferred approach to wound care is to apply twice-daily sterile wet-to-dry dessings, utilizing saline or dilute antiseptics (povidone-iodine solution, 1 to 5%). Alternatively, a nontoxic topical antibiotic ointment (bacitracin or polymyxin B–bacitracin–neomycin) may be used sparingly, covered with a nonadherent dressing. A final approach is to apply full-strength antiseptic solutions, followed by powdered topical antibiotics, such as tetracycline. No method has been supported by a prospective trial.

ENVENOMATIONS

Sponges

There are approximately 4000 species of sponges, which are composed of horny but elastic skeletons. Embedded in the connective tissue matrices are spicules of silicon dioxide or calcium carbonate. Secondary coelenterate inhabitants are responsible for the dermatitis and local necrotic skin reaction termed *sponge diver's disease*. A number of sponges produce crinotoxins that may be direct dermal irritants, such as subcritine, halitoxin, and okadaic acid.

Two general syndromes, with minor variations, are induced by contact with sponges. The first is a pruritic dermatitis similar to plant-induced allergic dermatitis. Within a few hours after skin contact, the reactions are characterized by itching and burning, which may progress to local joint swelling, soft tissue edema, vesiculation, and stiffness, particularly if small pieces of broken sponge are retained in the skin near the interphalangeal or metacarpophalangeal joints. The skin may become mottled or purpuric. Untreated and mild reactions will subside within 3 to 7 days. With large skin surface area involvement, the victim may complain of fever, chills, malaise, dizziness, nausea, and muscle cramps. Bullae may become purulent. Systemic erythema multiforme or an anaphylactoid reaction may develop a week to 14 days after a severe exposure.

The second syndrome is an irritant dermatitis and follows the penetration of small spicules of silica or calcium carbonate into the skin. Crinotoxins enter microtraumatic lesions caused by the spicules. In severe cases, surface desquamation of the skin may follow in 10 days to 2 months. There is no medical intervention that can retard this process. Recurrent eczema and persistent arthralgias are rare complications.

Because it is usually impossible to distinguish clinically between the allergic and spicule-induced reactions, it is safest to treat for both. The skin should be gently dried. Spicules should be removed, if possible, using adhesive tape or a facial peel. Beginning as soon as possible, apply dilute (5%) acetic acid (vinegar) soaks for 10 to 30 min three to four times daily to affected areas. Isopropyl alcohol 40 to 70% is a reasonable second choice. Although topical steroids may help to relieve the secondary inflammation, they are of no initial value. If steroids are applied before the vinegar soak, they appear to worsen the primary reaction. Delayed primary therapy or inadequate decontamination may result in the persistence of bullae. Erythema multiforme may require the administration of systemic corticosteroids, beginning with a moderately high dose (prednisone, 60 to 100 mg) tapered over 2 to 3 weeks. Following initial decontamination, a mild emollient cream or steroid preparation may be applied to the skin. If the allergic component is severe, systemic corticosteroids (prednisone, 40 to 80 mg, tapered over 2 weeks) may be beneficial. Severe itching may be controlled with an antihistamine.

Coelenterates

Coelenterates are an enormous group, comprising approximately 9000 species, at least 100 of which are dangerous to humans. Coelenterates, which possess the venom-charged stinging cells called nematocysts, are *cnidaria*. Cnidaria can be divided into three main groups: (1) hydrozoans, e.g., Portuguese man-of-war; (2) scyphozoans, e.g., true jellyfish; and (3) anthozoans, e.g., anemones. The stinging organelles are located on the outer surfaces of the tentacles or near the mouth and are triggered by contact with the victim's body surface. The sharp tip of the thread tube enters the victim's skin and envenomation occurs. The thread penetrates the upper dermis, where the viscous venom diffuses into the general circulation.

Contact with the nematocysts of a feather hydroid induces a mild reaction, which consists of instantaneous burning, itching, and urticaria. If the exposure is brief, the skin rash may not be noticeable or may consist of a faint erythematous miliary irritation. A second variety of envenomation consists of a delayed papular, hemorrhagic, or zosteriform reaction with onset 4 to 12 h after contact. Rarely, erythema multiforme or a desquamative eruption may develop. Systemic manifestations are rarely reported and are associated with large areas of surface involvement.

The stony, hydroid, and corallike *Millepora* species (*M. alcicornis*), or fire corals, are widely distributed in shallow tropical waters. From numerous minute surface gastropores protrude tiny nematocyst-bearing tentacles. Immediately following contact with fire coral, the victim suffers burning or stinging pain, with rare central radiation. Intense and painful pruritus follows within seconds. Over the course of 5 to 30 min, urticarial wheals develop, marked by redness, warmth, and pruritus. The wheals become moderately edematous and reach a maximum size in 30 to 60 min. The lesions resolve over 3 to 7 days, occasionally leaving an area of hyperpigmentation that may require 4 to 8 weeks to disappear. The pain generally resolves without treatment in 30 to 90 min. In the case of multiple stings, regional lymph nodes may become inflamed and painful.

The Atlantic Portuguese man-of-war (*Physalia physalis*) inhabits the surface of the ocean. It is constructed of a floating sail (pneumatophore) from which are suspended multiple nematocyst-bearing tentacles, which may measure up to 30 m in length. The smaller Pacific bluebottle (*Physalia utriculus*) usually has a single fishing tentacle which attains lengths of up to 15 m. Detached moistened tentacles, often found by the thousands fragmented on the beach, carry live nematocysts capable of discharging for months. Air-dried nematocysts may retain considerable potency, even after weeks.

The scyphozoan group of animals comprises the larger medusae or jellyfish. These creatures are armed with some of the most potent venoms in existence. The extreme example of envenomation occurs with the Indo-Pacific box jellyfish (*Chironex fleckeri*). Death is attributed to hypotension, profound muscle spasm, muscular and respiratory paralysis, and subsequent cardiac arrest. The overall mortality following box jellyfish stings approaches 15 to 20 percent. Most stings are minor; severe reactions or death follow skin contact with tentacles in excess of 6 to 7 m. The sting is immediately intensely painful, and the victim usually struggles purposefully for only a minute or two prior to collapse. The toxic skin reaction may be quite intense, with rapid formation of wheals, vesicles, and a darkened reddish-brown or purple whiplike flare pattern with stripes of 8 to 10 mm in width. With major stings, skin blistering occurs within 6 h, with superficial necrosis in 12 to 18 h. On occasion, a pathognomonic "frosted" appearance with transverse cross-hatched pattern may be present.

There is a considerable phylogenetic relationship between all stinging species. Any victim in distress pulled from marine waters should be carefully examined for a cutaneous lesion(s) that may provide the clue to a coelenterate envenomation. Untreated, minor-to-moderate skin lesions resolve over 1 to 2 weeks, with occasional residual hyperpigmentation for 1 to 2 months. Moderate and severe envenomations are compounded by systemic symptoms, which may appear immediately or be delayed by several hours (Table 119-1).

Anemones are attractive creatures often found in tidal pools, where the unwary will brush up against them or inquisitively touch them. Like other coelenterates, they possess tentacles loaded with one of

Table 119-1. Signs and Symptoms of Coelenterate Envenomation

Nervous System	*Musculoskeletal*
Headache	Arthralgias
Nightmares	Myalgias
Diminished touch and temperature sensation	Muscle cramps and spasms
Vertigo	Paralysis
Ataxia	Aphonia
Mononeuritis multiplex	*Allergic*
Parasympathetic dysautonomia	Anaphylaxis
Delirium	Laryngeal edema
Seizures	Bronchospasm
Coma	*Miscellaneous*
Cardiovascular	Chills
Hypotension	Fever
Brady- and tachyarrhythmias	Malaise
Pulmonary edema	Hemolysis
Ventricular fibrillation	Acute renal failure
Cyanosis	Nausea, vomiting, diarrhea
Eye-Ear-Nose-Throat	*Dermatologic*
Rhinitis	Urticaria
Dysphagia	Erythema
Hypersalivation	Bullae and vesicles
Thirst	
Conjunctivitis	
Chemosis	
Corneal ulcers	
Lacrimation	

two variations of the nematocyst. The dermatitis caused by contact is similar in all regards to that from fire coral or a small man-of-war. If the envenomation is severe, intense local hemorrhage, vesiculation, necrosis, skin ulceration, and secondary infection may occur.

Therapy for coelenterate envenomation is directed at stabilizing the airway, ventilation, and hemodynamics; detoxifying the venom; and providing symptomatic treatment, including alleviating pain. Nematocysts still attached to the victim must be detoxified to prevent continued envenomation. All victims with systemic signs or symptoms should be observed for at least 8 h, as rebound of symptoms can occur. *Chironex fleckeri* produces the only coelenterate venom for which there is a specific antidote.

The following steps are necessary for detoxification:

1. Immediately rinse the wound with sea water, *not with fresh water*. Do not rub the wound with a towel or clothing. Remove the gross tentacles with forceps or a well-gloved hand. The keratinized palm of the hand is relatively protected. A cold pack may be applied if its external surface is dry.
2. *Acetic acid (vinegar)* 5% is the treatment of choice to inactivate the toxin. An alternative is isopropyl alcohol (40 to 70%). Perfume, aftershave lotion, or high-proof liquor are less efficacious and may be detrimental. The detoxicant should be applied continuously for at least 30 min or until there is no further pain. Vinegar will not alleviate the pain from a *Chironex* sting, but interrupts the envenomation. There is some evidence that alcohol may stimulate the discharge of nematocysts in vitro; the clinical significance is as yet undetermined.
3. Once the wound has been soaked with vinegar or alcohol, the easiest way to remove the remaining nematocysts is to apply shaving cream or a paste of baking soda, flour, or talc and to shave the area with a razor.

After detoxification, local anesthetic ointments or mild steroid lotions may be soothing. Patients should receive standard tetanus prophylaxis. Wounds should be checked at about 3 and 7 days after injury for infection. Ulcerating lesions should be cleaned three times a day and covered with a thin layer of nonsensitizing antiseptic ointment.

Stingrays, Scorpionfish, Sea Urchins, and Starfish

Puncture wounds created by venomous spines create injuries which vary according to the potency of the venom and number of punctures.

The stingrays are the most commonly incriminated group of fishes involved in human envenomations. The venom organ of stingrays consists of one to four venomous stings on the dorsum of an elongate, whiplike caudal appendage. When an unwary human handles, corners, or steps on a ray, the tail reflexly whips upward and accurately thrusts the caudal spines into the victim, producing a puncture wound or jagged laceration, which is also an envenomation. On occasion, the entire spine tip is broken off and remains in the wound. Envenomation causes immediate local intense pain, edema, and variable bleeding. The pain may radiate centrally, peaks at 30 to 60 min and may last for up to 48 h. The wound is initially dusky or cyanotic and rapidly progresses to become erythematous and hemorrhagic, with rapid fat and muscle hemorrhage and necrosis. Systemic manifestations include weakness, nausea, vomiting, diarrhea, diaphoresis, vertigo, tachycardia, headache, syncope, seizures, inguinal or axillary pain, muscle cramps, fasciculations, generalized edema (with truncal wounds), paralysis, hypotension, arrhythmias, and death.

Scorpionfish follow stingrays as perpetrators of piscine stings. Distributed in tropical and, less commonly, in temperature oceans, several hundred species are divided into three groups typified by different genera on the basis of venom organ structure: (1) *Pterois* (zebrafish, lionfish, and butterfly cod), (2) *Scorpaena* (scorpionfish, bullrout, and sculpin), and (3) *Synanceja* (stonefish). Other venomous fish that sting in a manner similar to scorpionfish include catfish, surgeonfish, weeverfish, horned sharks, toadfish, ratfish, rabbitfish, stargazers, and leatherbacks. With regard to scorpionfish, the venom organs consist of 12 to 13 dorsal, two pelvic, and three anal spines, with associated venom glands. Although they are frequently large, plumelike, and ornate, the pectoral spines are not associated with venom glands.

Scorpionfish venom has been likened in potency to cobra venom. Its principal action appears to be direct muscle toxicity, resulting in paralysis of cardiac, involuntary, and skeletal muscles. The presentation of injury is similar to the stingray envenomation. Scorpionfish stings vary according to the species, with a progression in severity from the lionfish (mild) through the scorpionfish (moderate-severe) to the stonefish (severe–life threatening). Pain is immediate and intense, with radiation centrally. Untreated, the pain peaks at 60 to 90 min and persists for 6 to 12 h. In the case of the stonefish, the pain may be severe enough to cause delirium and may persist at high levels for days. The wound and surrounding area are initially ischemic and then cyanotic, with more broadly surrounding areas of erythema, edema, and warmth. Vesicles may form. Rapid tissue sloughing and close surrounding areas of cellulitis may develop within 48 h. Systemic effects are similar to those of coelenterate envenomation.

The venom apparatuses of sea urchins consist of the sharp, brittle, and venom-filled spines or the triple-jawed globiferous pedicellariae. Venomous spines inflict immediate and intensely painful stings. Burning pain rapidly evolves into severe local muscle aching with erythema and swelling of the skin surrounding the puncture sites. Frequently, spines break off and lodge in the victim. If a spine enters a joint, it may rapidly induce severe synovitis. If multiple spines have penetrated the skin, particularly if they are deeply embedded, the victim may rapidly develop systemic symptoms which include nausea, vomiting, paresthesias, numbness and muscular paralysis, abdominal pain, syncope, hypotension, and respiratory distress. Pedicellariae can cause more severe symptoms, creating immediate intense and radiating pain, local edema and hemorrhage, malaise, weakness, paresthesias, hypesthesia, arthralgias, aphonia, dizziness, syncope, generalized muscular paralysis, respiratory distress, hypotension, and, rarely, death.

The carnivorous starfish *Acanthaster planci* is a particularly venomous species. The sharp, rigid, and venomous aboral spines of this animal may grow to 4 to 6 cm. As the spines enter the skin, they carry venom into the wound, with immediate pain, copious bleeding, and mild edema. The wound may become dusky or discolored. Multiple puncture wounds may result in acute systemic reactions, which include paresthesias, nausea, vomiting, lymphadenopathy, and muscular paralysis.

For stings from marine animal spines, the success of therapy is related to the rapidity with which it is undertaken. The wound should be irrigated *immediately* with whatever cold diluent is at hand. If sterile saline or water is not available, tap or ocean water may be used. In a rapid primary exploration of the wound, any visible pieces of the spine or integumentary sheath should be removed. As soon as possible, the wound should be soaked in nonscalding hot water to tolerance (113°F or 45°C) for 30 to 90 min. During the hot water soak, the wounds should be explored and foreign material removed. Cryotherapy can be disastrous.

Pain control should be initiated during the first debridement or soaking period. Narcotics may be necessary. Local infiltration of the wound with lidocaine without epinephrine or a regional nerve block may be very useful.

After the soaking procedure, the wound should be prepared in a sterile fashion, reexplored, and thoroughly debrided. Soft tissue radiography should be employed to visualize calcified matter. Wounds should remain open for delayed primary closure or sutured loosely around adequate drainage. Prophylactic antibiotics are recommended because of the high incidence of ulceration, necrosis, and secondary infection. If a victim is to be treated and released, he or she should be observed for at least 4 h for systemic side effects.

A stonefish antivenin is manufactured by the Commonwealth Serum Laboratories, Melbourne, Australia. In cases of severe systemic reactions from stings of *Synanceja* species, and rarely from other scorpionfish, it is administered intravenously.

With regard to sea urchins, any pedicellariae that are still attached to the skin must be removed. This may be accomplished by the application of shaving foam and gently scraping with a razor. Embedded spines should be removed with care, as they are easily fractured. All thick spines should be removed due to the risk of infection, foreign body encaseation granuloma, or dermoid inclusion cyst. External percussion to achieve fragmentation is not advised. If the spines have acutely entered into joints or are closely aligned to neurovascular structures, they should be removed as soon as possible after the injury. If the spine has entered into an interphalangeal joint, the finger should be splinted until the spine is removed to limit fragmentation and further penetration. The granulomas caused by retained sea urchin spine fragments generally appear 2 to 12 months after the initial injury. The lesion may be removed surgically. Intralesional injection with triamcinolone hexacetonide is less efficacious.

BIBLIOGRAPHY

Auerbach PS, Yajko DM, Nassos PS, Kizer KW, McCosker JE, Geehr EC, Hadley WK: Bacteriology of the marine environment: Implications for clinical therapy. *Ann Emerg Med* 16:643, 1987.

Auerbach PS, McKinney HE, Rees R, Heggers J: Analysis of vesicle fluid following the sting of the lionfish *Pterois volitans*. *Toxicon* 12:1350, 1987.

Auerbach PS: Clinical therapy of marine envenomation and poisoning, in Tu AT, (ed): *Handbook of Natural Toxins*, (vol. 3), *Marine Toxins and Venoms*, New York, Dekker, 1988, pp 493–565.

Auerbach PS, Halstead BW: Hazardous aquatic life, in Auerbach PS, Geehr EC (eds): *Management of Wilderness and Environmental Emergencies*, 2d ed, St. Louis, Mosby, 1989, pp 933–1028.

Burnett JW, Calton GJ: Jellyfish envenomation syndromes updated. *Ann Emerg Med* 16:1000, 1987.

Fenner PJ, Williamson JA, Blenkin JA: Successful use of *Chironex* antivenom by members of the Queensland Ambulance Transport Brigade. *Med J Aust* 151:708, 1989.

Fenner PJ, Williamson JA, Skinner RA: Fatal and non-fatal stingray envenomation. *Med J Aust* 151:621, 1989.

Kizer KW, McKinney HE, Auerbach PS: Scorpaenidae envenomation: a five-year poison center experience. *JAMA* 253:807, 1985.

Shiomi K, Yamamoto S, Yamanaka H, Kikuchi T: Purification and characterization of a lethal factor in venom from the crown-of-thorns starfish (*Acanthaster planci*). *Toxicon* 26:1077, 1988.

120 HIGH ALTITUDE MEDICAL PROBLEMS

Peter H. Hackett

Over 40 million visitors to the western United States went to altitudes over 2400 m (8000 ft) in 1989, and tens of thousands traveled to other high altitude locations in Alaska, Europe, Asia, South America, and Africa. Physicians working or traveling in or near these locations therefore are increasingly likely to encounter persons ill with a high altitude illness or suffering an untoward effect of altitude on a preexisting condition. Although the focus of this chapter is hypoxia-related problems, patients in the mountain environment also may require care for associated illnesses such as hypothermia, frostbite, trauma, ultraviolet keratitis, dehydration, and lightning injury, which are covered elsewhere in this text.

High altitude is a hypoxic environment. Since the concentration of oxygen in the troposphere remains constant at 21 percent, the partial pressure of oxygen decreases as a function of the barometric pressure (Fig. 120-1). In Denver (1610 m), air pressure is 17 percent less than at sea level and therefore contains 17 percent less oxygen. The air of Aspen, Colorado (2438 m) has 26 percent less oxygen, and the barometric pressure on top of Mt. Everest is merely one-third that of sea level. Paul Bert, in his classic experiments of the late 19th century, showed that supplemental oxygen prevented symptoms of altitude illness during hypobaric exposure and concluded that hypoxia, not hypobaria, was responsible for illness.

For purposes of discussion, the range of high altitude may be divided based on physiological effects. From 1500 to 3500 m above sea level (4900 ft to 11,500 ft) is considered *high altitude;* decreased exercise performance and increased ventilation (lower arterial P_{CO_2}) occur, without a major impairment in arterial oxygen transport, even though altitude illness is common with abrupt ascent to over 2500 m (8200 ft). *Very high altitude* encompasses the range of 3500 to 5500 m (18,000 ft), where maximum arterial oxygen saturation falls to less than 90 percent ($Pa_{O_2} < 60$ mmHg), and extreme hypoxemia may occur during exercise, sleep, and altitude illness. Abrupt ascent to these altitudes may be dangerous; a period of acclimatization is required. *Extreme altitude,* over 5500 m, is accompanied by severe hypoxemia and hypocapnia, and abrupt ascent precipitates illness in nearly all individuals. At this altitude, progressive physiologic deterioration eventually outstrips acclimatization; no human habitations are higher.

ACCLIMATIZATION TO HIGH ALTITUDE

Persons rendered acutely hypoxic become dizzy, faint, and rapidly unconscious if hypoxic stress is sufficient. These same individuals, given days to weeks to develop the exact same degree of hypoxia, are able to function quite well. While the fundamental process of this acclimatization takes place in the metabolic machinery of cells and mitochondria, acute "struggle" responses are critical while allowing the cells time to adjust.

Ventilation

Defense of alveolar P_{O_2} through increased ventilation is the primary initial adaptation. The hypoxic ventilatory response (HVR) is effected by the carotid body, which senses a decrease in arterial oxygenation and inputs to the central respiratory center in the medulla to increase ventilation. The vigor of this inborn response is related to successful acclimatization. Respiratory depressants or stimulants may affect HVR, as does chronic hypoxia, which eventually blunts the response. A low hypoxic drive may allow extreme hypoxemia to develop during sleep. The initial hyperventilation is quickly attenuated by respiratory alkalosis, which acts as a brake on the respiratory center. As renal excretion of bicarbonate compensates for the respiratory alkalosis, pH returns toward normal, and ventilation continues to increase. This process of maximizing ventilation, termed ventilatory acclimatization, culminates after 4 to 7 days at a given altitude. With continuing ascent to higher altitudes, the central chemoreceptors reset to progressively lower P_{CO_2} values, and the completeness of acclimatization can be gauged by the arterial P_{CO_2}. Acetazolamide, which forces a bicarbonate diuresis, greatly facilitates this process. An appreciation of the normal values for blood gases and acid-base status with acclimatization at various altitudes is necessary in order to distinguish abnormalities (Table 120-1).

Blood

The hematopoietic response to altitude was first observed in 1890 by Viault. We now know that within 2 h of ascent to altitude, erythropoietin is increased in plasma and, over days to weeks, results in increased red cell mass. This adaptation has no importance during initial acclimatization when altitude illness develops and, when excessive, results in chronic mountain polycythemia. Shifts in the oxyhemoglobin dissociation curve are thought to be minimal *in vivo* at altitude, since the increase in 2,3-diphosphoglyceric acid, which is proportional to the severity of hypoxia and shifts the curve to the right, is offset by the alkalosis, which shifts the curve to the left. Naturally occurring left-shifted hemoglobin is an advantage at high altitude.

Fluid Balance

Peripheral venous constriction on ascent to altitude causes an increase in central blood volume, which triggers baroreceptors to suppress antidiuretic hormone (ADH) and aldosterone and induce a diuresis. Combined with the bicarbonate diuresis from the respiratory alkalosis, this can result in decreased plasma volume and hyperosmolality (serum osmolality of 290 to 300, which the body appears to permit by a reset

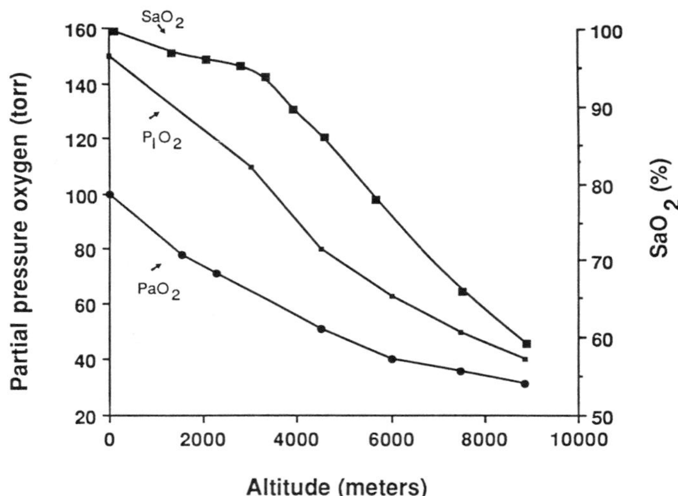

Fig. 120-1. Increasing altitude results in a fall of inspired P_{O_2} (PI_{O_2}), arterial P_{O_2}(Pa_{O_2}), and arterial oxygen saturation (Sa_{O_2}). *Note:* (1) the difference between inspired and arterial P_{O_2} narrows at high altitude and (2) Sa_{O_2}% is well maintained while awake until nearly 4000 m. (From Hackett, Roach, and Sutton, *Management of Wilderness and Environmental Emergencies*. St. Louis, Mosby, 1988. Used by permission.)

Table 120-1. Blood Gases and Altitude

Altitude (meters)	Pa_{O_2} (mmHg)	Sa_{O_2}%	Pa_{CO_2} (mmHg)
Sea level	90–95	96	40
1524 (5000 ft)	75–81	95	32–33
2286 (7500 ft)	69–74	92–93	31–33
4572 (15,000 ft)	48–53	86	25
6096 (20,000 ft)	37–45	76	20
7620 (25,000 ft)	32–39	68	13
8848 (29,029 ft)	26–33	58	9.5–13.8

Source: Hackett, Roach, and Sutton. *Management of Wilderness and Environmental Emergencies.* St. Louis, Mosby, 1988. Used by permission.

of the osmol center of the brain. Clinically, diuresis and hemoconcentration is considered a healthy response.

Cardiovascular

Stroke volume is decreased initially, and an increased heart rate maintains cardiac output. Maximum exercising heart rate declines at altitude proportional to the decrease in V_{O_2} max. Cardiac muscle in healthy persons is able to withstand extreme levels of hypoxemia ($Pa_{O_2} < 30$ mmHg) without evidence of ST segment changes or ischemic events. Blood pressure is mildly elevated on ascent secondary to increased sympathetic tone.

The pulmonary circulation constricts with exposure to hypoxia. This is an advantage during regional alveolar hypoxia, such as pneumonia, but is a disadvantage during the global hypoxia of altitude exposure. As a result, pulmonary pressure increases. This degree of hypertension is quite variable, with those having a hyperreactive response much more susceptible to high altitude pulmonary edema.

Cerebral blood flow transiently increases on ascent to altitude (despite the hypocapnic alkalosis), which increases oxygen delivery to the brain. This response, however, is limited by the increase in cerebral blood volume, which may increase intracranial pressure and produce and/or aggravate symptoms of altitude illness.

Effects on Exercise

Exercise capacity, as measured by maximum oxygen consumption, drops dramatically on ascent to altitude, approximately 10 percent for each 1000-m altitude gain above 1500 m. During acclimatization, submaximal endurance increases appreciably after 10 days, but V_{O_2} max does not. The mechanism of the decrement is probably lack of adequate oxygen supply to the muscle cells due to the low driving pressure for diffusion of oxygen from the capillary.

Limitations

There are limits to acclimatization. Even those who are by nature good acclimatizers cannot tolerate the hypoxia of extreme altitude for long. Miners from South America report that they cannot live at altitudes above 5800 m because of weight loss, increasing lethargy, poor quality sleep, weakness, and headache. High altitude mountaineers cannot survive for more than a few days above 8000 m without supplemental oxygen because of more acute deterioration in physiologic functioning. Considerable weight loss, both of fat and lean body mass, are unavoidable at extreme altitude, and help contribute to demise. Other factors limiting ability to acclimatize to extreme altitude include right ventricular strain from excessive pulmonary hypertension, intestinal malabsorption, impaired renal function, polycythemia and microcirculatory sludging, and prolonged cerebral hypoxia. Even at more modest altitudes, some individuals are very slow or poor acclimatizers for reasons not entirely known but, at least in part, due to poor carotid body function and inadequate ventilation.

Sleep at High Altitude

Sleep stages III and IV are reduced at altitude while sleep stage I is increased. More time is spent awake, with a significant increase in arousals, but only slightly less rapid eye movement (REM) time. The frequent arousals are a common source of bitter complaints from skiers and others, but they are innocuous and improve with time at altitude. The typical periodic breathing (Cheyne-Stokes) in those sleeping above 2700 m (9000 ft) consists of 6- to 12-s apneic pauses interspersed with cycles of vigorous ventilation. Interestingly, the frequent awakenings are not necessarily related to the sleep periodic breathing, and neither are they related to acute mountain sickness. Presumably, the mechanism of the lighter sleep is related to cerebral hypoxia. Quality of sleep and also arterial oxygenation during sleep improves with acclimatization and with acetazolamide.

HIGH ALTITUDE SYNDROMES

High altitude syndromes of primary concern are those problems attributed directly to the hypoxia: acute hypoxia, acute mountain sickness, pulmonary edema, cerebral edema, retinopathy, peripheral edema, sleeping problems, and a group of neurologic syndromes. The other syndromes, not necessarily related to hypoxia, include thromboembolic events (which may be attributable to dehydration, prolonged incapacitation, polycythemia, and cold), high altitude pharyngitis and bronchitis, and ultraviolet keratitis. Although the different hypoxic clinical syndromes overlap, all share a fundamental mechanism, all are seen in the same setting of rapid ascent in unacclimatized persons, and all respond to the same essential therapy: descent and oxygen.

Acute Hypoxia

The syndrome of acute hypoxia occurs in the setting of sudden and severe hypoxic insult, such as accidental decompression of a pressurized aircraft cabin or a failed oxygen system in a pilot or high altitude mountaineer. Sudden overexertion precipitating arterial desaturation, acute onset of pulmonary edema, carbon monoxide poisoning, and sleep apnea may result in relatively acute hypoxia as well. Unacclimatized persons become unconscious at an arterial oxygen saturation of 50 to 60 percent, an arterial P_{O_2} of less than about 30 mmHg, or a jugular venous P_{O_2} less than 15 mmHg. Acute hypoxia is reversed by immediate administration of oxygen, rapid descent, and correction of the underlying cause such as removal of the carbon monoxide source or repair of the oxygen delivery system. Symptoms of acute hypoxia reflect the sensitivity of the central nervous system (CNS) to this insult: dizziness, light-headedness, and dimmed vision progressing to loss of consciousness. Hyperventilation has been shown to increase the time of useful consciousness during acute alveolar hypoxia.

Acute Mountain Sickness (AMS)

Incidence

AMS occurs in the setting of more gradual and less severe hypoxic insult than with acute hypoxic syndrome. Its incidence varies by location, depending on ease of access, rate of ascent, and sleeping altitude reached. A recent study at 2100 m (6900 ft) found a 25 percent incidence of AMS in physicians attending a continuing-education meeting in Colorado. Other studies at resorts between 2220 and 2700 m (7200 and 9000 ft, respectively) claimed an incidence between 17 and 40 percent, and a sleeping altitude of 2750 m (9000 ft) seemed to be a threshold for increased attack rate. Approximately 40 percent of trekkers in Nepal on the path to Mt. Everest suffer AMS, while climbers on Mt. Rainier have the very high incidence of 70 percent because of the rapidity of ascent.

Susceptibility

In addition to rate of ascent and sleeping altitude, inherent factors determine individual susceptibility to acute mountain sickness. Factors identified so far are low hypoxic ventilatory response and low vital capacity. Age has a small influence on incidence, with children being somewhat more susceptible. Women are just as likely, if not more so, to develop mountain sickness but appear to have less pulmonary edema. Susceptibility to AMS is generally reproducible in an individual or repeated exposures. Persons living at intermediate altitudes of 1000 to 2000 m already are acclimatized partially and do much better than lowlanders upon ascent to higher altitudes. There is no relationship of susceptibility to AMS and physical fitness.

Clinical Presentation

The diagnosis of AMS is based on the setting, symptoms, and physical findings. The setting is rapid ascent of an unacclimatized person to 2000 m (6600 ft) or higher. Typically, the person on arrival feels lightheaded and slightly breathless, especially with exercise. One to six h later, but sometimes delayed for 1 day or more (and especially after a night's sleep), the typical symptoms of mild AMS develop; they are similar to an alcohol hangover. The headache usually is described as bifrontal and worsened with bending over and the valsalva maneuver. Gastrointestinal symptoms include anorexia, nausea, and sometimes vomiting, and the chief constitutional symptoms are lassitude and weakness. The person with AMS is often irritable and wants to be left alone. Sleepiness and a deep inner chill, especially in a cold environment, also are common. If the illness progresses, the headache becomes more severe, and vomiting, oliguria, and increased dyspnea develop. Lassitude may progress to the victim requiring assistance for eating and dressing. The most severe form of AMS, high altitude cerebral edema (HACE), is heralded by onset of ataxia and altered level of consciousness; coma may ensue within 12 h if treatment is delayed.

Physical findings in mild AMS are nonspecific. Heart rate and blood pressure are variable, and usually in the normal range, although postural hypotension may be present. Localized rales are detectable in up to 20 percent of persons with AMS. Fever is unusual except in the presence of pulmonary edema. Funduscopy reveals venous tortuosity and dilatation, and retinal hemorrhages are common over 5000 m or in those with pulmonary and cerebral edema. Fluid retention is a hallmark of AMS, in contrast to the usual diuresis of acclimatization, and may result in peripheral edema, especially of the face. Differential diagnosis in this setting includes hypothermia, carbon monoxide poisoning, pulmonary or CNS infection, dehydration, and exhaustion.

The natural history of AMS at a Colorado resort (3000 m or 10,000 ft) recently was documented. Mean duration of symptoms was 15 h, with a range to 94 h, despite the fact that one-half of those with symptoms self-medicated. At higher sleeping altitudes, the illness may last much longer, even weeks if untreated, and is more likely to progress to pulmonary or cerebral edema. Eight percent of those with AMS at 4243 m (14,000 ft) in Nepal developed cerebral or pulmonary edema, or both.

Pathophysiology

AMS is due to hypobaric hypoxia, but the exact sequence of events leading to illness is unclear. Figure 120-2 offers a schema for the pathophysiology. The symptoms indicate a neurologic etiology and elevated cerebrospinal fluid pressure; scans confirming cerebral edema have been obtained in persons severely ill. Whether the more common mild illness of headache, anorexia, and malaise is due to mild cerebral edema has yet to be confirmed, but seems likely. Two types of cerebral edema have been proposed. One is cytotoxic edema, due to failure of the sodium-potassium pump with subsequent intracellular accumulation of sodium and water. The other is a vasogenic edema, due to a leaky blood-brain barrier.

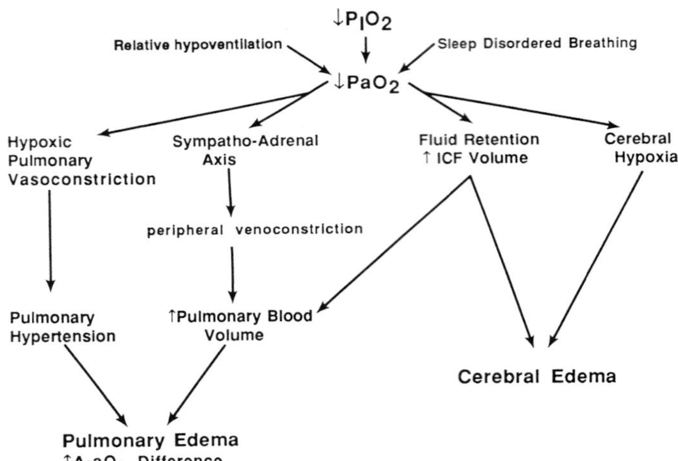

Fig. 120-2. A schema of pathophysiology for high altitude illness. (From Hackett and Roach, *Ann Emerg Med* 16:980, 1987. Used by permission.)

No direct evidence for cytotoxic edema in humans at altitude has been reported, but a large shift of fluid into the total intracellular space, presumably including the brain, was demonstrated to take place over the first 3 days at altitude, when AMS occurs. The time required for fluid shift and overhydration of the brain may explain the time lag in onset of symptoms, which distinguishes AMS from acute hypoxia. In support of the vasogenic theory, white-matter brain edema on magnetic resonance imaging (MRI) recently was demonstrated in persons with high altitude cerebral edema, and it may also occur in AMS. The leaky blood-brain barrier is due either to loss of autoregulation and overperfusion or to hypoxia-induced increased permeability. The fact that corticosteroids so effectively treat AMS also supports the notion of vasogenic edema, since this is the only type of cerebral edema responsive to steroids. Further research is likely to reveal that brain swelling is due to both cytotoxic and vasogenic mechanisms.

The cerebral edema, interstitial pulmonary edema, peripheral edema, and the antidiuresis observed in AMS all point to an abnormality of water handling by the body. The mechanism is thought to be increased renin-angiotensin, aldosterone, and ADH in contrast to the normal ADH and aldosterone suppression at high altitude and usual diuresis. A decrease in glomerular filtration also has been observed. The effectiveness of diuretics in prevention and treatment of AMS reinforces the importance of fluid retention in the pathophysiology.

Relative hypoventilation due to a sluggish hypoxic ventilatory response is a characteristic of AMS-susceptible individuals and has been linked to fluid retention. Hypoventilation, of course, results in greater hypoxic stress and is equivalent to being at a higher altitude. Higher P_{CO_2} and lower P_{O_2} also increase cerebral blood flow and aggravate brain swelling. Less hypocapnia also may reduce the stimulus for bicarbonate diuresis and aggravate fluid retention.

Treatment (Table 120-2)

Descent and Oxygen

The goals of treatment are to prevent progression, abort the illness, and improve acclimatization; early diagnosis is essential. Initial clinical presentation does not predict eventual severity, and all persons with AMS must be observed carefully for progression. The three principles of treatment are (1) to not proceed to a higher sleeping altitude in the presence of symptoms, (2) to descend if symptoms do not abate or become worse despite treatment, and (3) to descend and treat immediately in the presence of a change in consciousness, ataxia, or pulmonary edema. Mild AMS is self-limited and generally improves with an extra 12 to 36 h of acclimatization if ascent is halted. Descent is the definitive treatment for all forms of altitude illness, although it is not always an option, nor always necessary. Remarkably, a drop in altitude of only 500 to 1000 m usually is effective promptly. Evacuation to a hospital or to sea level is unnecessary except in the most severe cases. To simulate descent, portable hyperbaric bags are being used in various locations to treat AMS. The patient is inserted into the fabric chamber, and a pressure of 2 psi is achieved by means of a manual or automated pump; the pressure is equivalent to a drop in altitude of 1500 m (5000 ft). A valve system creates sufficient ventilation to avoid CO_2 accumulation or O_2 depletion.

Oxygen effectively relieves symptoms, but it often is unavailable in the field and generally reserved for moderate to severe AMS in order to conserve supplies. Oxygen promptly relieves headache, dizziness, and most other symptoms, although ataxia may resolve more slowly. Nocturnal low flow oxygen (0.5 to 1 L/min) is particularly helpful and efficient. The combination of oxygen and descent provides optimal therapy, especially in more severe cases.

Medical Therapy

Pharmacologic treatment offers an alternative to descent or oxygen in mild to moderately severe AMS. Acetazolamide is very helpful in speeding acclimatization and aborting illness, especially when used early. The drug acts by inhibiting the enzyme carbonic anhydrase, slowing the hydration of carbon dioxide to hydrogen and bicarbonate ions. In the kidney, acetazolamide reduces reabsorption of bicarbonate, causing a bicarbonate diuresis and metabolic acidosis, which stimulates ventilation. The drug essentially mimics the process of ventilatory acclimatization. As a result, arterial P_{O_2} is higher, and sleep oxygenation remains high and stable, without periods of apnea (Fig. 120-3). The drug also maintains cerebral blood flow despite greater hypocapnia, and because of its diuretic action, it counteracts the fluid retention of AMS. Many trials have shown its value for prevention; although widely used empirically for treatment, controlled studies have been hindered by the reluctance of ill persons to enroll in placebo trials. Current indications for acetazolamide are (1) a history of altitude illness, (2) abrupt ascent to over 3000 m (10,000 ft), (3) for treatment of AMS, and (4) bothersome sleep periodic breathing. The dosage regimen varies; 5 mg/kg per day in two or three divided doses is sufficient, whether for prevention or treatment. An extended-release formulation of acetazolamide, 500 mg 24 h, is a convenient regimen. Treatment should be continued until symptoms of AMS resolve, and then the drug should be restarted if symptoms return. Since the drug acts by improving acclimatization, fear of masking serious illness is unwarranted. Common side effects of acetazolamide include peripheral paresthesias and sometimes nausea or drowsiness, and the usual precautions of sulfa drugs apply to acetazolamide because of the sulfhydryl moiety. Since the drug inhibits the instant hydration of CO_2 on the tongue, the carbon dioxide in carbonated beverages can be tasted, ruining the flavor of beer and other drinks.

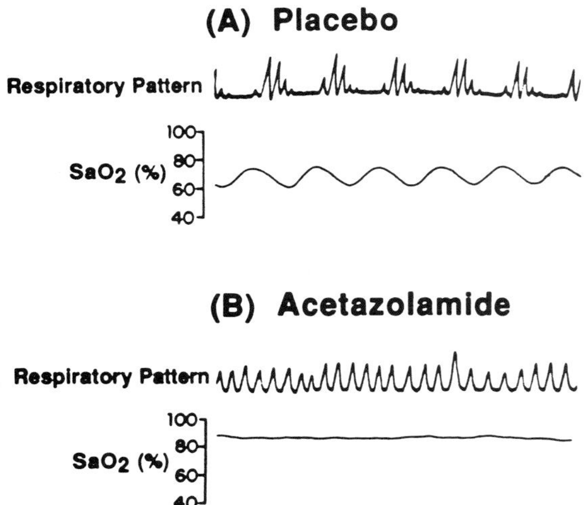

Fig. 120-3. Respiratory patterns and arterial oxygen saturation (Sa_{O_2}%) with placebo and acetazolamide in two sleep studies of a subject at 4400 m. (From Hackett and Roach, *Ann Emerg Med* 16:980, 1987. Used by permission.)

Symptomatic treatment of AMS is sometimes sufficient. Aspirin 650 mg or acetaminophen 650 to 1000 mg (with or without codeine) can be given for headache. Prochlorperazine 5 to 10 mg intramuscularly is useful for nausea and vomiting and has the advantage of augmenting the hypoxic ventilatory response. The short-acting benzodiazepines such as triazolam 0.25 mg and temazepam 15 mg also can be used to treat the complaint of frequent wakening, but they are potentially dangerous in ill persons because of respiratory depression and may decrease oxygenation even in persons acclimatizing well. A combination of acetazolamide and benzodiazepine may work very well.

Dexamethasone 4 mg PO, IM, or IV every six h is quite effective therapy for mountain sickness, but it is best reserved for moderate to severe AMS, since it may be associated with significant side effects and does not aid acclimatization, sometimes resulting in rebound symptoms when discontinued. The mechanism of action of dexamethasone may be to reduce vasogenic edema, to lower intracranial pressure, or to act as an antiemetic and mood elevator. The use of acetazolamide to speed acclimatization and a brief course of dexamethasone to treat illness can be a useful combination. The use of diuretics is reasonable because of the fluid retention associated with mountain sickness. Furosemide 20 to 40 mg every 12 h until improved was reported effective by the Indian army, although other investigators have not been enthusiastic about its use because of concerns for avoiding hypovolemia, hypotension, and incapacitation.

Prevention

Graded ascent with adequate time for acclimatization is the best prevention. A recommendation for those visiting medium altitude resorts in the western United States is to spend a night at an intermediate altitude of 1500 to 2000 m (Denver or Salt Lake City) before sleeping at altitudes above 2500 m (8200 ft). Mountaineers and trekkers should avoid abrupt ascent to sleeping altitudes over 3000 m and then allow two nights for each 1000-m altitude gain in camp altitude, starting at 3000 m. Other preventative measures include avoiding overexertion, alcohol, and respiratory depressants, and eating a high carbohydrate diet. Acetazolamide is a useful prophylactic agent for those with a history of AMS or for forced abrupt ascent without acclimatization stages. The drug should be started 24 h before the ascent and continued for the first 2 days at altitude. The medication then can be discontinued and started again if illness develops. Acetazolamide can be expected to reduce the symptoms of AMS by approximately 75 percent in persons ascending rapidly to sleeping altitudes of over 2500 m. An alternative for those allergic to sulfa is dexamethasone 4 mg every 12 h starting the day of ascent and continuing for the first 2 days at altitude.

Neurologic Syndromes of High Altitude

Until recently, most neurologic events at high altitude were attributed to HACE or AMS. Clearly, this has been a diagnostic oversimplification. Other syndromes now recognized as related to high altitude include altitude syncope, cerebrovascular spasm (migraine equivalent), cerebral arterial or venous thrombosis (infarct), transient ischemic attack, and cerebral hemorrhage. These syndromes are characterized by more focal neurologic findings than in cerebral edema, though differentiation in the field may be impossible.

Other problems may be due to exacerbation or unmasking of underlying disease, such as previously asymptomatic brain tumors and epilepsy. Presumably, space-occupying lesions become symptomatic because of increased brain volume at altitude. Hyperventilation (hypocapnic alkalosis), which is commonly used to induce seizure activity on electroencephalography, may explain unmasking of a seizure disorder at altitude, while changes in cerebral blood flow may exacerbate vascular lesions. Even generalized encephalopathy or coma, considered the hallmark of HACE, may be due to factors other than edema. Indeed, unconsciousness from acute hypoxia at sea level clearly is not due to edema, but rather to neurotransmitter failure, similar to the neuroglycopenia of insulin reactions.

High Altitude Cerebral Edema (HACE)

HACE is defined clinically as the presence of progressive neurologic deterioration in someone with AMS or high altitude pulmonary edema (HAPE). It is characterized by altered mental status, ataxia, stupor, and progression to coma if untreated. Headache, nausea, and vomiting are not always present. Because of raised intracranial pressure, focal neurologic signs such as third and sixth cranial nerve palsies may result from distortion of brain structures or by extraxial compression.

HACE is usually associated with pulmonary edema. Pathologically, necropsies have described severe, diffuse cerebral edema with multiple small hemorrhages and sometimes thrombosis.

The treatment of HACE is the same as for severe AMS: oxygen, descent, and steroids (Table 120-2). Descent is the highest priority. Acetazolamide may be an adjunct, but immediate reversal of the illness is the goal; improving acclimatization comes later. In acutely ill patients who cannot descend, the combination of steroids, supplemental oxygen, and a hyperbaric bag is optimal therapy, but rarely available. Comatose patients require additional airway management, bladder drainage, and other coma care. For coma, the use of hyperventilation to decrease intracranial pressure is a reasonable approach, keeping in mind that the P_{CO_2} is already low and pH high in these individuals. Additional acute hyperventilation could produce cerebral ischemia; monitoring of arterial blood gases and, if available, cerebral blood velocities by transcranial Doppler ultrasonography may be advisable. Loop diuretics such as furosemide 40 to 80 mg or bumetanide 1 to 2 mg may help reduce brain overhydration, but hypoperfusion must be avoided. Hypertonic solutions of saline, mannitol, or urea have been used too infrequently to establish clinical guidelines. In the hospital setting, mannitol in a patient who does not respond immediately is worth considering. Coma may persist for days, even for weeks after evacuation to lower altitude, and the patient may still recover, sometimes with permanent sequelae. Persistent coma is unusual, however, and mandates exclusion of other possible etiologies.

Table 120-2. Suggested Treatment of High Altitude Illness

Mild AMS	Stop ascent Descend to lower altitude or acclimatize at same altitude Acetazolamide 125–250 mg b.i.d. to speed acclimatization Symptomatic treatment as necessary with analgesics and antiemetics
Moderate AMS	Immediate descent for worsening symptoms Low flow oxygen if available Acetazolamide 250 mg b.i.d. and/or dexamethasone 4 mg q 6 h Hyperbaric therapy
HACE	Immediate descent or evacuation Oxygen 2–4 L/min Dexamethasone 8 mg PO, IM, or IV, then 4 mg q 6 h Hyperbaric therapy if cannot descend
HAPE	Immediate descent or evacuation Oxygen 4 L/min Nifedipine 10 mg PO or 30 mg q 4–6 h extended-release q 6 h if no oxygen or descent Hyperbaric therapy if cannot descend Continuous positive airway pressure Minimize exertion and keep warm
Periodic Breathing	Acetazolamide 125 mg at bedtime as needed

Cerebrovascular Syndromes of Altitude

Strokes, due both to infarct and hemorrhage in the arterial circulation, as well as venous thrombosis have been reported in young healthy persons at altitude who otherwise would not be considered at risk for such conditions. Transient ischemic attack, cortical blindness, and various focal neurologic signs such as hemiparesis or hemiplegia of a transient nature also occur. Since these latter events are reversible, they suggest etiologies such as vasospasm, watershed hypoxia between arterial zones, or transient ischemia attack.

Differentiation of the various neurologic syndromes may be impossible in the field, and treating as if cerebral edema were present may be reasonable, with a rapid descent to lower altitude, oxygen, and steroids, and evacuation to a hospital if symptoms persist despite treatment. Fortunately, focal neurologic signs usually resolve spontaneously and do not recur upon reascent. However, a thorough cerebrovascular evaluation before advising reascent may be prudent.

High Altitude Pulmonary Edema (HAPE)

HAPE is the most lethal of the altitude illnesses. Since the condition is easily reversible with descent and oxygen, the cause of death is usually lack of early recognition, misdiagnosis, or inability to descend to a lower altitude.

Epidemiology

The incidence of HAPE varies from less than one in 10,000 skiers in Colorado to 2 to 3 percent of climbers on Mt. McKinley and was reported as high as 15 percent in some regiments in the Indian army who were airlifted to high altitude during the Indian/Chinese war. Children appear more susceptible; women appear less susceptible than men. Risk factors include heavy exertion, rapid ascent, cold, excessive salt ingestion, use of sleeping medication, and a previous history indicating inherent individual susceptibility.

Clinical Presentation (Table 120-3)

Early in the course of illness, when the edema is still interstitial or localized, the victim develops a dry cough, decreased exercise performance, dyspnea on exertion, increased recovery time from exercise, and localized rales, usually in the right midlung field. Late in the course of the illness, there develops tachycardia, tachypnea, and dyspnea at rest, marked weakness, productive cough, cyanosis, and more generalized rales. As hypoxemia worsens, consciousness becomes impaired. Victims usually become comatose and then die. Early diagnosis is critical, and decreased exercise performance and dry cough is enough to raise the suspicion of early HAPE. The typical victim is strong and fit and may or may not have symptoms of AMS before onset of HAPE. The condition typically worsens at night and is noticed most commonly on the second night at a new altitude. Unfortunately, rales may not be audible in 30 percent of persons with HAPE at rest but can be elicited immediately after a short bout of exercise. Fever up to 38.5°C is common, and tachycardia and tachypnea generally correlate with the severity of illness. On cardiac auscultation, a prominent P2 and right ventricular heave may be appreciated. ECG generally reveals right axis deviation and a right ventricular strain pattern consistent with acute pulmonary hypertension. Chest x-ray findings progress from interstitial to localized alveolar to generalized alveolar infiltrates as the illness progresses from mild to severe.

Pathophysiology

The pioneering work of Hultgren established HAPE as a noncardiogenic edema. Left ventricular function is normal. Left ventricular

Table 120-3. Severity Classification of HAPE

Grade	Symptoms	Signs	Chest Film
1 Mild	Dyspnea on exertion, dry cough fatigue while moving uphill	Heart rate (HR) (rest) < 90–100, respiratory rate (RR) (rest) < 20, Dusky nailbeds, Localized rales, if any	Minor exudate involving less than one-fourth of one lung field
2 Moderate	Dyspnea, weakness, fatigue on level walking, raspy cough, headache, anorexia	HR 90–100, RR 16–30, cyanotic nailbeds, rales present, ataxia may be present	Some infiltrate involving 50% of one lung or smaller area of both lungs
3 Severe	Dyspnea at rest, productive cough, orthopnea, extreme weakness	Bilateral rales, HR > 110, RR > 30, Facial and nailbed cyanosis, ataxia, stupor, coma, blood-tinged sputum	Bilateral infiltrates > 50% each lung

Source: Hultgren HN: High altitude pulmonary edema, in Staub NC (ed): *Lung Water and Solute Exchange.* New York, Marcel Dekker, 1978, pp 437–469.

end diastolic pressure, wedge pressures, and left atrial pressures are low to normal, cardiac output is low, and pulmonary vascular resistance and pulmonary artery pressure are markedly elevated. The exact cause of the edema is still unclear. Pulmonary hypertension is an essential component, and persons with a history of HAPE have been shown to have exaggerated pulmonary pressor responses to hypoxia. Whether this represents one end of a normal distribution or a pathologic subpopulation is unknown. However, not all persons with pulmonary hypertension develop HAPE; another factor must also be present, which induces a change in capillary membrane permeability. Pulmonary venous constriction, fibrin and platelet thrombi, and uneven arterial vasoconstriction leading to overperfusion of some areas of the vasculature have all been proposed. Predisposed individuals have a low hypoxic ventilatory response, an abnormal pulmonary circulation, and tend to suffer HAPE on repeated exposures.

Treatment

The key to successful treatment of HAPE (Table 120-2) is early recognition, since the condition in its early stage is easily reversible. The optimal therapy depends upon the environmental setting, evacuation options, availability of oxygen or hyperbaric units, and ease of descent. Immediate descent is the treatment of choice, but this is not always possible. During descent, exertion by the victim must be minimized. Reports of victims dying during descent probably are related to overexertion offsetting the benefit of lower altitude. With descent, oxygen is unnecessary except in severe cases. Oxygen provides excellent results and can completely resolve pulmonary edema without descent to a lower altitude, but may require 36 to 72 h to do so. Such quantities of oxygen rarely are available to trekking, mountaineering, and skiing groups, but they may be available at ski resorts or medical facilities. Oxygen immediately lowers pulmonary artery pressure and improves arterial oxygenation. Its use is life saving when descent is not an option; in such cases, rescue groups should make delivery of oxygen to the victim the highest priority.

Bed rest may be adequate for very mild cases, and bed rest with supplemental oxygen may suffice for moderate illness, as long as the safety of the patient can be assured by the presence of a medical facility, adequate oxygen, or immediate descent capability should the patient's condition deteriorate. Since cold stress elevates pulmonary artery pressure, the patient should be kept warm. The use of an end expiratory pressure mask has been shown to improve gas exchange in persons with HAPE and may be a useful adjunct.

Since oxygen and descent are so effective, experience with drugs has been limited. Morphine and furosemide were used with good results by the Indian army, and both seem physiologically reasonable since they augment venous pooling, reduce pulmonary blood flow, and therefore reduce hydrostatic force for fluid extravasation in the lung. However, patients with HAPE often are dehydrated intravascularly, and caution must be exercised to avoid hypotension. Recently, nifedipine, either 10 mg capsule or 30 mg extended-release formulation orally was reported to be of clinical benefit, to reduce pulmonary artery pressure by 30 to 50 percent, and to increase arterial oxygen saturation. The mechanism presumably is by lowering pulmonary pressure and, therefore, the pressure gradient for flux of fluid across the membrane. Hypotension is a potential problem with nifedipine, and the results are not nearly as dramatic as with oxygen or descent, which still remain the treatments of choice.

Hospitalization may be warranted for severe cases that do not respond immediately to descent, especially if cerebral edema is present. Intubation, high FI_{O_2}, and positive end-expiratory pressure ventilation are rarely required. Antibiotics are indicated for coexisting infection when present. Occasionally pulmonary artery catheterization is useful to exclude a cardiac component to the edema in persons with heart disease. The patient with HAPE who does not make the usual rapid improvement should be evaluated for pulmonary emboli, mediastinal pulmonary artery obstruction, or other pulmonary circulatory abnormalities, such as congenital absence of a pulmonary artery. Adequate discharge criteria are progressive clinical and radiographic improvement, and an arterial P_{O_2} of 60 mmHg or arterial oxygen saturation greater than 90 percent. Residua such as fibrosis and impaired pulmonary function tests have not been reported. Patients are advised to resume activities gradually and are warned that they may feel weak for 1 to 2 weeks. An episode of HAPE is not a contraindication to subsequent ascent, but patients should be advised on staged ascent, acetazolamide prophylaxis, and recognition of early signs and symptoms.

Reentry Pulmonary Edema

A rather high incidence of HAPE, especially in children, has been reported in residents of high altitude who sojourn to a lower altitude and then suffer HAPE when returning home. In Peru, Hultgren found a prevalence of 6.4 per 100 exposures in the 1 to 20-year-old age group, and 0.4 per 100 exposures in persons over 21. Reports have also been published from Leadville, Colorado. The mechanism is thought to be more vigorous pulmonary vasoconstriction and pulmonary hypertension upon reexposure to hypoxia because of increased muscularization of pulmonary arterioles.

Peripheral Edema

Swelling of the face and distal extremities is common at high altitude. Peripheral edema was reported in 18 percent of trekkers at 4200 m in Nepal and was twice as likely in women. It was often associated with AMS, but not necessarily. The presence of peripheral edema should raise suspicion of altitude illness and prompt a thorough examination for pulmonary and cerebral edema. The problem can be treated with diuretics, but if left untreated, it will resolve spontaneously with descent. The mechanism is presumably similar to that of the fluid retention of AMS but with edema formation peripherally rather than in the brain and lung.

High Altitude Retinopathy

Retinal abnormalities described at high altitude include retinal edema, tortuosity and dilatation of retinal veins, disc hyperemia, retinal hemorrhages, and, rarely, cotton-wool exudates. Retinal hemorrhages are asymptomatic, except for rarely occurring macular hemorrhages, and are not considered an indication for descent unless visual changes are present. They resolve spontaneously in 10 to 14 days. Hemorrhages are common above a sleeping altitude of 5000 m and occur at lower altitudes in persons with altitude illness.

High Altitude Pharyngitis and Bronchitis

Most unacclimatized persons exercising at altitudes over 2500 m develop a dry, hacking cough. With exposure to extreme altitudes for prolonged periods of time, a purulent bronchitis and a painful pharyngitis become nearly universal. These problems may not be of an infectious nature; high volumes of dry, cold air through the lungs may induce respiratory heat loss and cause purulent secretions on that basis alone. Bronchospasm may also be triggered by respiratory heat loss. Severe coughing spasms can result in cough fracture of the ribs.

Pharyngeal membranes become dry, painful, and cracked because of the dehydration and high ventilation. Mucosal cracks may be an entry for pathogens, or the erythema and dryness may cause discomfort strictly on a mechanical basis. Antibiotics generally are not helpful, supporting the concept of a noninfectious etiology. Breathing of steam, ingesting hard candies or lozenges to increase salivation, and forcing hydration may provide some benefit with systemic analgesics as necessary. A silk Balaclava or similar material across the nose and mouth that is sufficiently porous to allow large volume ventilation but trap some moisture and heat helps ameliorate these bothersome high altitude conditions.

Chronic Mountain Polycythemia (CMP)

Monge's disease, also called chronic mountain sickness or CMP, has now been recognized in all high altitude locations of the world. Both long-term high altitude residents and lowlanders who relocate to high altitude may develop this condition after variable length of residence. The incidence is much higher in males and increases with age. The disease is characterized by excessive polycythemia for a given altitude, which causes symptoms such as headache, muddled thinking, difficulty sleeping, impaired peripheral circulation, drowsiness, and chest congestion. The diagnosis is made by the characteristic symptoms and a hemoglobin value greater than expected for the altitude, generally over 20 to 22 g/dL. Any problem causing hypoxemia at sea level causes greater hypoxemia at altitude, and the etiology of CMP can be traced to problems such as chronic obstructive pulmonary disease (COPD) and sleep apnea in 50 percent of patients. The etiology of pure CMP is attributed to idiopathic hypoventilation on the basis of diminished respiratory drive.

Therapy includes phlebotomy, relocation to lower altitude, or home oxygen use. Respiratory stimulants such as acetazolamide (250 mg twice a day) and medroxyprogesterone acetate (20 to 60 mg/day) have also been employed successfully. The response to respiratory stimulants supports the role of hypoventilation in this disorder.

Ultraviolet Keratitis (Snow Blindness)

Ultraviolet light (UVA and UVB) penetrates the atmosphere to a greater degree at high altitude because of less cloud cover, less water vapor, and less particulate matter in the air. Radiation increases roughly 5 percent for every 300 m (1000 ft) gained, and it is exacerbated by reflection back from snow. UV radiation below 300 nm (UVB) is absorbed by the cornea, and high exposure levels can cause corneal burns in 1 h, although symptoms do not become apparent for 6 to 12 h. The typical symptoms of photokeratitis are severe pain, a foreign body or gritty sensation, photophobia, tearing, marked conjunctival erythema, chemosis, and eyelid swelling. UV keratitis generally is self-limited and heals within 24 h, but the condition is sufficiently painful to warrant systemic analgesics. Cold compresses may also provide some relief, and eye patches may be necessary for comfort. Prevention is obviously of great importance, since this condition can be disabling, especially in hazardous terrain. Adequate sunglasses should transmit less than 10 percent of UVB light. Side shields are necessary if traveling on snow, and polarizing lenses help by absorbing glare. Makeshift protection can be fashioned by cutting narrow horizontal slits in cardboard, foam, or any available material (Eskimo sunglasses).

ILLNESSES AGGRAVATED BY HIGH ALTITUDE

Chronic Lung Disease

COPD patients ascending to altitude often report increased dyspnea and reduced exercise ability. Obviously, those with hypoxemia, pulmonary hypertension, disordered control of ventilation, and sleep disordered breathing at sea level will have greater problems at altitude because of the greater alveolar hypoxia. Such patients may require supplemental oxygen at altitude when they do not at sea level (and avoid having to descend), and oxygen-dependent patients at sea level may need to increase the FI_{O_2}. The required FI_{O_2} can be calculated by multiplying low-altitude FI_{O_2} by the ratio of low altitude barometric pressure divided by high altitude barometric pressure. This will ensure the delivery of the same partial pressure of oxygen as at low altitude. There are no data to suggest that persons with COPD are more likely to develop AMS or HAPE, although such persons may be self-selected to avoid travel to high altitude locations. In fact, persons with mild to moderate COPD already are partially acclimatized and may do well at modest altitude, as suggested by Graham and Houston. High altitude per se does not exacerbate asthma, and persons with chronic bronchospasm often report easier breathing at high altitude, due to lower air density and/or cleaner air.

Arteriosclerotic Heart Disease (ASHD)

The healthy heart and cardiovascular system tolerates even extreme hypoxia very well. Numerous ECG studies, echocardiograms, heart catheterizations and exercise tests do not demonstrate cardiac ischemia or cardiac dysfunction in healthy persons at high altitude, even when arterial P_{O_2} was less than 30 mmHg. Those with arteriosclerotic disease may not have the same adaptive capabilities and intuitively seem more likely to suffer from acute cardiac events. Epidemiologic data, however, do not support this supposition. Morbidity and mortality from arteriosclerotic heart disease is reduced in persons with long-term residence at high altitude, and visitors apparently do not have increased risk of acute myocardial infarction. Recent work, however, suggested earlier onset of angina at high altitude compared with sea level. Congestive heart failure (CHF) may worsen in tourists arriving at the medium altitude of ski resorts, and it is related apparently to fluid retention rather than depressed ventricular function from hypoxia. Patients with CHF should therefore maintain or increase their diuretic regimen during travel to high altitude, and clinicians may want to consider low flow oxygen during sleep for CHF patients, at least for the first few nights. Patients' status postcoronary artery bypass grafting have trekked to altitudes over 5000 m without problems, the issue of safety having generated much debate. Overall, high altitude does not impose as much stress on the heart as would seem intuitively obvious. Further study will more clearly define subcategories of cardiac patients at risk.

Ascent to altitude produces a mild increase in blood pressure in normotensive persons, secondary to increased sympathetic tone; the matter has not been studied in hypertensives. Patients should continue hypertensive medications at altitude. No data suggest that hypertensives are more likely to succumb to any of the altitude illnesses, and in general, hypertension would not seem to be a contraindication to altitude exposure.

Sickle Cell Disease

Even the modest simulated altitude of a pressurized aircraft (1500 to 2000 m) may cause persons with hemoglobin SC and sickle-thalassemia to have a vasoocclusive crisis. High altitude exposure without supplemental oxygen is considered a contraindication in these persons. Sickle cell trait is not considered an increased risk, although splenic infarction syndrome during heavy exercise at altitude has been reported in those with trait.

Pregnancy

Pregnant residents of high altitude have an increased prevalence of hypertension, low-birth-weight infants, and neonatal hyperbilirubinemia. However, an increased incidence of pregnancy complications in lowlanders who visit high altitude has not been reported. The normal P_{O_2} of the fetus is 29 to 33 mmHg, and the mild maternal hypoxia induced by traveling to resort-type altitudes does not generate significantly more hypoxic stress. Until more data become available, pregnant patients should not be advised to curtail reasonable activities they wish to undertake. Perhaps of more concern than mild hypoxia is the fact that high altitude locations are often remote from medical facilities, and patients need to be aware that without access to sophisticated medical care, complications could have more serious consequences than at home.

BIBLIOGRAPHY

Bert P: *Barometric Pressure*. Bethesda, MD, Undersea Medical Society, 1978.

Blume FD, Boyer SJ, Braverman LE, et al: Impaired osmoregulation at high altitude. *JAMA* 252:524, 1984.

Dean AG, Yip R, Hoffmann RE: High incidence of mild acute mountain sickness in conference attendees at 10000 foot altitude. *J Wilderness Med* 1:86, 1990.

Fasules JW, Wiggins JW, Wolfe RR: Increased lung vasoreactivity in children from Leadville, Colorado after recovery from high altitude pulmonary edema. *Circulation* 72:957, 1985.

Hackett PH, Rennie ID: Rales, peripheral edema, retinal hemorrhage and acute mountain sickness. *Am J Med* 67:214, 1979.

Hackett PH, Rennie ID, Hofmeister SE, et al: Fluid retention and relative hypoventilation in acute mountain sickness. *Respiration* 43:321, 1982.

Hackett PH, Rennie ID, Levine HD: The incidence, importance, and prophylaxis of acute mountain sickness. *Lancet* 2:1149, 1976.

Hackett PH, Roach RC: Medical therapy of altitude illness. *Ann Emerg Med* 16:980, 1987.

Hackett PH, Roach RC: High altitude pulmonary edema. *J Wilderness Med* 1:3, 1990.

Hultgren HN, Lopez CE, Lundberg E, et al: Physiologic studies of pulmonary edema at high altitude. *Circulation* 29:393, 1964.

Hultgren HN, Marticorena E: High altitude pulmonary edema: Epidemiologic observations in Peru. *Chest* 74:372, 1978.

Hultgren HN, Spickard WB, Hellriegel K, et al: High altitude pulmonary edema. *Medicine* 40:289, 1961.

Johnson TS, Rock PB: Acute mountain sickness. *N Engl J Med* 319:841, 1988.

Karliner JS, Sarnquist FH, Graber DJ, et al: The electrocardiogram at extreme altitude: Experience on Mt. Everest. *Am Heart J* 109:505, 1985.

King SJ, Greenlee R, Goldings HJ: Acute mountain sickness (Letter). *N Engl J Med* 320:1492, 1989.

Levine BD, Yoshimura K, Kobayashi T, et al: Dexamethasone in the treatment of acute mountain sickness. *N Engl J Med* 321:1707, 1989.

Mahoney BS, Githens JH: Sickling crisis and altitude: Occurrence in the Colorado patient population. *Clin Pediatr* 18:431, 1979.

Mairbaurl H, Schobersberger W, Oelz O, et al: Unchanged in vivo P50 at high altitude despite decreased erythrocyte age and elevated 2, 3 diphosphoglycerate. *J Appl Physiol* 68:1186, 1990.

Montgomery AB, Mills J, Luce JM: Incidence of acute mountain sickness at intermediate altitude. *JAMA* 261:732, 1989.

Moore LG: Altitude aggravated illness: Examples from pregnancy and prenatal life. *Ann Emerg Med* 16:965, 1976.

Mortimer EA, Monson RR, MacMahon B: Reduction in mortality from coronary heart disease in men residing at high altitude. *N Engl J Med* 296:581, 1977.

Oelz O, Maggiorini M, Ritter M, et al: Nifedipine for high altitude pulmonary edema. *Lancet* 2:1241, 1989.

Reite M, Jackson D, Cahoon RL, et al: Sleep physiology at high altitude. *Electroencephalogr Clin Neurophysiol* 38:463, 1975.

Schoene RB, Roach RC, Hackett PH, et al: High altitude pulmonary edema and exercise at 4400 meters on Mt McKinley: Effect of expiratory positive airway pressure. *Chest* 87:330, 1985.

Sophocles AM: High-altitude pulmonary edema in Vail, Colorado, 1975–1982. *West J Med* 144:569, 1986.

Sutton JR, Houston CS, Marsell AL, et al: Effect of acetazolamide on hypoxemia during sleep at high altitude. *N Engl J Med* 301:1329, 1979.

Viault F: On the large increase in the number of red cells in the blood of the inhabitants of the high plateaus of South America, in West JB (ed): *High Altitude Physiology*. Stroudsberg, PA, Hutchinson Ross, 1981, pp 333–334.

Vock P, Fretz C, Franciolli M, et al: High-altitude pulmonary edema: Findings at high-altitude chest radiography and physical examination. *Radiology* 170:661, 1989.

Wohns RN: High altitude cerebral edema: A pathophysiological review. *Crit Care Med* 9:880, 1981.

121
DYSBARISM

Kenneth W. Kizer

DYSBARIC DIVING CASUALTIES

There are now over 3 million recreational scuba[1] divers in the United States, and over 300,000 new sport divers are certified each year. In addition, diving has become an integral part of many commercial, scientific, and military professions (Table 121-1).

The health problems associated with diving are due to the hazards of the aquatic environment and the breathing of compressed gases at higher than normal atmospheric pressure. Table 121-2 categorizes a number of diving-related medical problems.

Physical Principles

Pressure

Many adverse physical conditions are encountered in the underwater environment. These include cold, wetness, changes in light and sound conduction, increased density of the surrounding environment, and increased atmospheric pressure. Of these, the indirect or direct effects of pressure account for the majority of serious diving medical problems.

Pressure is force per unit area and is measured in a number of different units (Table 121-3). The weight of air at sea level is equal to 14.7 lb/in^2 (psi) or 1 atm absolute (ATA). Under water, pressure increases because of the weight of the water. Since water is much denser than air, large changes in pressure will accompany small fluctuations in depth. Thus (Table 121-4), at a depth of 33 ft of seawater (fsw) the pressure is 2 ATA, and at 165 fsw it is 6 ATA.[2] The proportionate change in pressure per unit depth is greatest near the surface and progressively diminishes with increasing depth. Since fresh water is less dense than saltwater, it takes a depth change of 34 ft of fresh water (ffw) to change the pressure 1 ATA. Scuba diving is generally done at pressure of less than 6 ATA, with the overwhelming majority in the 2- to 4-ATA range.

Since body tissues are composed mostly of water, which is not compressible, they are not directly affected by pressure changes. However, gases are compressible, and, consequently, gas-filled organs of the body are directly affected by pressure changes.

Table 121-1. Types of Commercial Diving

Recovery of natural resources:	Construction:
Oil and natural gas	Piers and harbors
Minerals	Bridges and tunnels
Fish and shellfish	Dams
Pearls, corals, and shells	Underwater photography and motion picture production
Algae (e.g., kelp or limu)	
Wood (logging)	Marine studies:
Aquaculture	Biology
Salvage operations	Geology
Maintenance and repair work:	Archeology
Ship hulls	Other sciences
Nuclear power plants	Rescue and recovery operations
Bridges and tunnels	Sport diving instructors and tour guides
Piers and harbors	
Aquariums	

[1] *Scuba* is an acronym for *s*elf-*c*ontained *u*nderwater *b*reathing *a*pparatus.

[2] In diving and hyperbaric medicine the most commonly used units of pressure and depth are ATA and fsw.

Table 121-2. Primary Problems in Diving Medicine

1. Environmental exposure problems:
   a. Motion sickness
   b. Near drowning and other immersion syndromes
   c. Hypothermia and heat illness
   d. Sunburn and other actinic radiation syndromes
   e. Irritant dermatitides
   f. Infectious diseases
   g. Mechanical trauma
2. Dysbarism:
   a. Barotrauma
   b. Dysbaric air embolism
   c. Decompression sickness
   d. Dysbaric osteonecrosis
   e. Hyperbaric cephalgia
3. Breathing gas-related problems:
   a. Nitrogen or other inert gas narcosis
   b. Hypoxia
   c. Oxygen toxicity
   d. Hypo- or hypercarbia
   e. Carbon monoxide poisoning
   f. Nitrogen oxide toxicity
   g. Lipoid pneumonitis
   h. High-pressure nervous syndrome
   i. Cutaneous isobaric counterdiffusion
4. Hazardous marine life
   a. Envenomations
   b. Animals that inflict trauma
   c. Toxic ingestions
5. Miscellaneous:
   a. Hearing loss
   b. Carotogenic blackout
   c. Panic and other psychological problems

Source: Adapted from Kizer KW: Management of dysbaric diving casualties. *Emerg Med Clin North Am* 1:659, 1983. Used by permission.

Gas Laws

Diving physiology is largely explained by three gas laws.

The first is Boyle's law, which states that the volume of a gas is inversely proportional to its pressure at a constant temperature. This is expressed by the equation.

$$PV = K$$

where P is pressure, V is volume, and K is a constant. Thus, as shown (Table 121-4), when the pressure is doubled the volume of a unit of gas is halved, and conversely. Boyle's law explains the basic mechanism of all types of barotrauma.

The second is Dalton's law, which states that the pressure exerted by each gas in a mixture of gases is the same as it would exert if it alone occupied the same volume, or, alternatively, the total pressure of mixture of gases is equal to the sum of the partial pressures of the

Table 121-3. Pressure Equivalents

1 atmosphere absolute (ATA)	= 33 ft seawater (fsw)*
	= 5.5 fathoms seawater
	= 34 ft freshwater (ffw)
	= 14.7 psi
	= 760 mmHg
	= 29.9 inHg
	= 1.033 kg/cm^2
	= 1.013 bar
	= 10.06 m
	= 0 atm gauge

* 1 fsw = 0.445 psi = 0.0303 atm.

Source: From Kizer KW: Management of dysbaric diving casualties. *Emerg Med Clin North Am* 1:659, 1983. Used by permission.

Table 121-4. Pressure-Volume Relationships According to Boyle's Law

	Depth, fsw	Gauge Pressure, atm*	Absolute Pressure, atm	Gas Volume, %	Bubble Diameter,† %
Air	0	0	1	100	100
Seawater	33	1	2	50	79
	66	2	3	33	69
	99	3	4	25	63
	.	.	.	.	.
	.	.	.	.	.
	.	.	.	.	.
	165	5	6	17	54

* Gauge pressure is always 1 atm less than absolute pressure.

† Bubble diameter is probably more important than volume in consideration of the ability of recompression to restore circulation to a gas-embolized blood vessel.

Source: Adapted from Kizer KW: Management of dysbaric diving casualties. *Emerg Med Clin North Am* 1:659, 1983. Used by permission.

component gases. This is mathematically stated as

$$P_t = P_{O_2} + P_{N_2} + P_x$$

where P_t is the total pressure, P_{O_2} is the partial pressure of oxygen, P_{N_2} is the partial pressure of nitrogen, and P_x is the partial pressure of the remaining gases in the mixture. This law explains why the partial pressures of component gases in a mixture change proportionately to changes in ambient pressure even though their absolute concentrations remain constant. This law is fundamental to the understanding of decompression sickness and other breathing gas-related problems.

Henry's law states that the amount of gas dissolved in a given volume of fluid is proportional to the pressure of the gas with which it is in equilibrium. The formula is

$$\%X = \frac{P_X}{P_t} \times 100$$

where $\%X$ is the amount of gas dissolved in a liquid, P_X is the partial pressure of gas X and P_t is the total atmospheric pressure. This law explains why more inert gas, e.g., nitrogen, dissolves in the diver's body as ambient pressure is increased with descent and, conversely, is released from tissue with ascent.

Direct Effects of Pressure—Barotrauma

The pressure-related diving syndromes can be divided into problems caused by the mechanical effects of pressure, i.e., barotrauma, and problems caused by breathing gases at elevated partial pressures, i.e., gas toxicities and decompression sickness.

Barotrauma is the most common affliction of divers. It is defined as tissue damage resulting from contraction or expansion of gas spaces which occurs when the gas pressure in the body, or its compartments, is not equal to ambient pressure. For purposes of discussion, barotrauma can be viewed according to whether it occurs during descent or ascent.

Barotrauma of Descent

Barotrauma of descent, or "squeeze," as it is known in common diving parlance, results from the compression of gas in enclosed spaces as ambient pressure increases with underwater descent. Gas pressure in the various air-filled spaces of the body is normally in equilibrium with the environment; however, if something obstructs the portals of gas exchange, pressure equalization is precluded. If the air-filled space is not collapsible, the resulting pressure imbalance will cause tissue distortion, vascular engorgement and muscosal edema, hemorrhage, and other tissue damage. The ears and paranasal sinuses are most likely to be affected by such a process.

Aural barotrauma is the most common type of barotrauma and is a major cause of morbidity among divers, experienced by essentially all divers at one time or another. There are three main types of aural barotrauma, depending on which part of the ear is affected, and they may occur singly or in combination.

The first type involves the external auditory canal and is generally referred to as *external ear squeeze,* or *barotitis externa.* The external ear canal normally communicates with the environment and, consequently, the air in the canal is replaced by water when a diver is submerged. However, if the external ear canal is occluded (e.g., by cerumen, foreign bodies, exostoses, or earplugs), water entry is prevented, and compression of the enclosed air with descent will have to be compensated for by tissue collapse, outward bulging of the tympanic membrane, or hemorrhage. This is typically manifested by pain and/or bloody otorrhea. Physical examination may reveal petechiae or blood-filled cutaneous blebs along the canal, along with erythema or rupture of the tympanic membrane. Treatment involves keeping the canal dry, prohibition of swimming or diving until healed, and, in special cases, antibiotics and analgesics.

The next and by far the most common type of aural barotrauma is *middle ear squeeze,* or *barotitis media.* This results from a failure to equalize the middle ear and environmental pressures because of occlusion or dysfunction of the eustachian tube.

The eustachian tubes normally open and allow equalization of middle ear pressure when the pressure difference between the middle ear and pharynx reaches about 20 mmHg. This can be facilitated by yawning, swallowing, or utilizing various autoinflation techniques (e.g., the Valsalva or Frenzel maneuvers). If middle ear pressure equalization is not achieved, the diver will notice discomfort or pain when the pressure differential reaches 100 to 150 mmHg or, roughly, when there has been a 20 percent reduction in middle ear gas volume. As the pressure differential is increased, mucosal engorgement and edema, hemorrhage, and inward bulging of the tympanic membrane develop. Eventually, these will be inadequate to compensate for the gas volume contraction, and the tympanic membrane ruptures. Fortunately, this is uncommon.

A number of factors may cause eustachian tube blockage or dysfunction, e.g., mucosal congestion secondary to upper respiratory infection, allergies, or smoking; mucosal polyps; excessively vigorous autoinflation maneuvers; and previous maxillofacial trauma. Persons with such conditions are at increased risk of middle ear barotrauma.

Divers having a middle ear squeeze usually complain of ear fullness or pain. As would be expected from the way that pressure changes with depth (Table 121-4), most problems occur near the surface. The pain is substantial and usually causes the diver to abort the dive. If not, it will continue to worsen until the eardrum ruptures, at which time the diver may feel air bubbles escaping from the ear and experience disorientation, nausea, and vertigo secondary to the caloric stimulation of cold water entering the middle ear. This sequence has been responsible for cases of panic and near drowning.

The otoscopic appearance of the tympanic membrane in cases of middle ear squeeze varies according to the severity of the injury and can be graded according to the amount of hemorrhage in the eardrum, with grades running from 0 (symptoms only) to 5 (gross hemorrhage and rupture). Physical examination may also disclose blood around the nose or mouth and a mild conductive hearing loss, which is usually only temporary.

Treatment of middle ear squeeze involves abstinence from diving until the condition has resolved and use of decongestants, which may be combined with antihistamines if there is an allergic component to the eustachian tube dysfunction. A combination of oral and long-acting spray decongestants is usually most efficacious. Antibiotics should be used when there is a tympanic membrane rupture or a preexisting infection, or after diving in polluted waters. No diving should be done until a perforated eardrum has healed. Oral analgesics or topical aural anesthetics may be needed for a couple of days. In general, eardrops should not be used when there is a tympanic membrane perforation. Ideally, an audiogram should be obtained in anyone having more than a trivial squeeze, and serial audiograms should be obtained in patients having hearing loss. Most middle ear squeezes will resolve without complication in 3 to 7 days. Prevention is preferable; a diver should refrain from diving when unable to easily equalize pressure in the ears and should heed warning signs of ear pain.

Although less common, the third type of aural barotrauma, *inner ear barotrauma,* is much more serious than middle ear barotrauma because of possible permanently disabling injury to the cochleovestibular system. Inner ear barotrauma typically results from the sudden or rapid development of markedly different pressures between the middle and inner ear, such as may occur as a result of an overly forceful Valsalva maneuver intended to equalize the pressure in the middle ear or an exceptionally rapid descent during which the middle ear pressure is not equalized.

Patients with inner ear barotrauma typically are quite symptomatic, having a feeling of fullness or "blockage" of the affected ear, nausea, vomiting, nystagmus, diaphoresis, disorientation, or ataxia. The classic triad of symptoms indicating inner ear barotrauma is roaring tinnitus, vertigo, and deafness. The onset of these symptoms may occur soon after the injury or may be delayed many hours, depending on the specific type of inner ear injury and the diver's activities during and after the dive. Findings on physical examination may be normal or may reveal signs of middle ear barotrauma or vestibular dysfunction, and audimetry may demonstrate a mild to severe sensorineural hearing loss. Any scuba diver with a hearing loss or vestibular symptoms following a nondecompression dive should be considered to have inner ear barotrauma until shown otherwise.

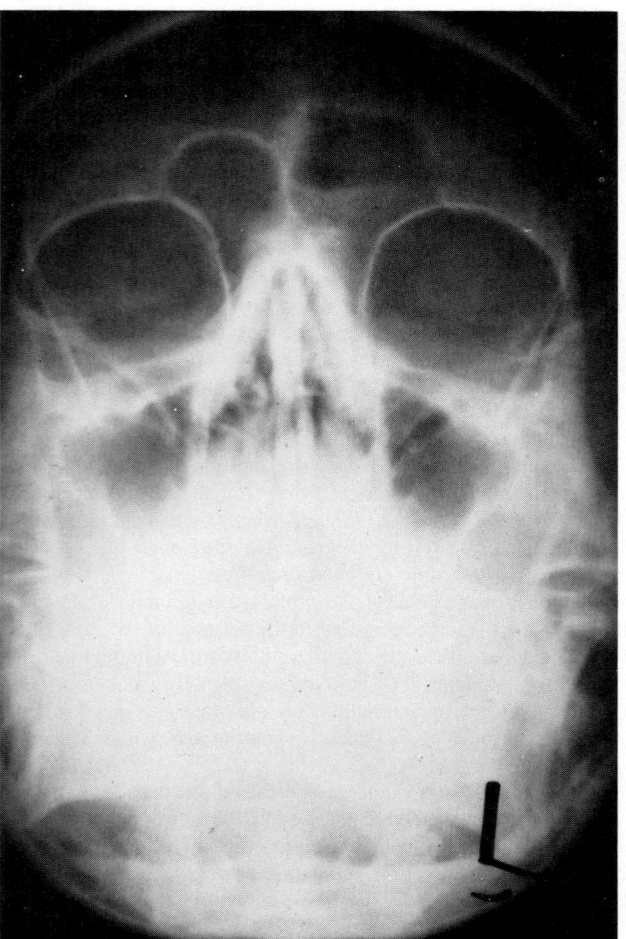

Fig. 121-1. Radiograph showing an air-fluid level in the left frontal sinus from a sinus squeeze. (Photograph by KW Kizer.)

Clinically, there appear to be four categories of or mechanisms for these injuries: (1) hemorrhage within the inner ear (especially in the basal turn of the cochlea); (2) rupture of the Reissner's membrane, resulting in mixing of endolymph and perilymph; (3) fistulation of the round or oval window; and (4) a mixed injury involving a combination of any or all of the other three. Injury to the membranous labyrinth may be either implosive or explosive.

Hemorrhage within the inner ear usually is associated with findings of middle ear barotrauma, no or transient vestibular symptoms, and a diffuse mild to severe sensorineural hearing loss (SNHL). Treatment of these patients should consist of bedrest with head elevated, avoidance of strain or strenuous activities, and symptomatic measures, as needed. The potential for full recovery is excellent, with the hearing loss usually completely resolved in 3 weeks to 3 months.

Manifestations of a tear in Reissner's membrane are similar to those of inner ear hemorrhage, although a persistent localized SNHL remains commensurate with the area of membrane tear. Treatment is similar to that of inner ear hemorrhage.

Inner ear fistulas typically present with a mild high-frequency SNHL or a marked cochleovestibular deficit and no or little evidence of middle ear barotrauma. Initially, these should be treated with bed rest, avoidance of strain, and other symptomatic measures, as needed. Deterioration of hearing or vestibular symptoms or persistence of significant vestibular symptoms after a few days indicates the need for surgical exploration and repair. Some authorities, however, recommend immediate tympanotomy if severe symptoms are present initially. Importantly, recompression is contraindicated unless decompression sickness or air embolism is also suspected to be present.

Any of the paranasal sinuses may fail to equalize pressure during descent. Manifestations of sinus squeeze include a sensation of fullness or pressure in the affected sinus, pain, or hemorrhage. Predisposing conditions for barosinusitis include upper respiratory infections, sinusitis, nasal polyps, or anything else that impairs the free flow of air from sinus cavity to nose. The maxillary and frontal sinuses are most often affected (Fig. 121-1). Treatment for sinus squeeze is much the same as for middle ear squeeze, although antibiotics are usually indicated in cases involving the frontal sinuses.

Squeeze can also affect any other gas space that does not equilibrate with ambient pressure. For example, conjunctival and scleral hemorrhage may result if the diver fails to exhale into the mask during descent, resulting in telltale erythema, ecchymosis, and petechiae of the part of the face enclosed by the face mask—i.e., "face mask squeeze." If an area of skin is tightly enclosed by a dry diving suit a "suit squeeze" may occur. Although the appearance of these injuries may be spectacular, no special treatment is required, and they usually resolve in a few days.

Another special kind of squeeze may occur in divers who, while holding their breath, descend below the depth at which their total lung volume is reduced to less than residual volume. As occurs in other types of barotrauma of descent, the underventilated lung air spaces fill with tissue fluids and blood in an attempt to relieve the negative pressure. Clinical manifestations include chest pain, cough, hemoptysis, dyspnea, and pulmonary edema. Treatment includes administration of 100% oxygen, fluid replacement, and other supportive measures as clinically indicated. Because of the intrinsic lung injury and consequent potential for gas embolism, positive-pressure breathing (e.g., PEEP or CPAP) should be avoided if possible. Very few divers attempt to free-dive to depths likely to cause lung squeeze, and it is rarely seen.

Barotrauma of Ascent

If there has been adequate equilibration of the pressure in the body's air-filled spaces during descent, the gas in those spaces will expand according to Boyle's law as ambient pressure decreases with ascent. The resulting excess gas is normally vented to the atmosphere. However, if this is prevented by obstruction of the air passages, the expanding gases will distend the tissues surrounding them; the resulting damage is known as *barotrauma of ascent* and is the reverse process of squeeze.

Although the ears and sinuses may be affected by barotrauma of ascent, this is unusual, since impediment of air egress is unlikely if pressure equalization is achieved with descent. However, middle ear barotrauma of ascent, or *reverse squeeze,* can occur, especially in divers having upper respiratory congestion treated with a short-acting nasal spray whose vasoconstrictive effect wears off while the diver is submerged. Similarly, *alternobaric vertigo* (ABV) resulting from unequal vestibular stimulation due to asymmetric middle ear pressure may occur during ascent. Although usually only transient, ABV may be severe enough to cause panic. Rarely, it may last for several hours after a dive.

Three other types of barotrauma of ascent should be discussed. The first of these may occur with either ascent or descent, although more commonly with ascent, and is known as *barodontalgia,* or, less accurately, "tooth squeeze." Several specific conditions are associated with this problem (e.g., pulp decay, peridontal infections, or recent extraction sockets or fillings), but it may be due to anything that causes a pressure disequilibrium in an air-filled space in or about a tooth. Although rare and usually self-limited, anyone presenting with a toothache after diving should be referred for dental evaluation after maxillary sinus squeeze has been excluded.

Another unusual type of barotrauma of ascent is gastrointestinal barotrauma, which is also known as *aerogastralgia,* or "gas in the gut." This occurs most commonly in novice scuba divers, who are more prone to aerophagia, and is caused by expansion of intraluminal bowel gas as ambient pressure is decreased during ascent. Other predisposing conditions include repeated performance of the Valsalva maneuver in the head-down position (which forces air into the stomach), drinking carbonated beverages or eating a heavy meal before diving (especially one containing legumes or other flatogenic substances), or chewing gum while diving. Symptoms of gastrointestinal barotrauma include abdominal fullness, colicky abdominal pain, belching, and flatulence. It is rarely severe because most divers will readily vent any excess bowel gas during ascent; however, it has been know to cause syncope and shocklike states. Actual gastric rupture from GI barotrauma has occurred, but this is exceedingly rare.

The last and most serious type of barotrauma of ascent is pulmonary barotrauma (PBT). Several different injuries can result from PBT of ascent, and these are collectively referred to as the pulmonary overpressurization syndrome (POPS), or "burst lung" (Table 121-5).

Diving equipment is designed to deliver compressed gas to the diver at the same pressure as the surrounding environment, e.g., at 33 fsw the diver breathes gas at 2 ATA. Consequently, the compressed gas will expand during ascent according to Boyle's law, and the diver must allow the expanding gas to escape from the lungs, or it will rupture and dissect into the surrounding tissue. The resultant injury will depend on the location and amount of escaped gas. Overt symptoms may appear immediately upon surfacing or may be delayed for several hours. Mediastinal or subcutaneous emphysema are the most common forms of the POPS. The patient usually presents with gradually increasing hoarseness, neck fullness, and substernal chest pain several hours after diving. Dyspnea, dysphagia, syncope, and other symptoms may be present as well. The history is usually diagnostic, although radiographs are indicated to verify the location of gas and exclude the presence of a pneumothorax (Fig. 121-2).

Table 121-5. Manifestations of Pulmonary Barotrauma

1. Pneumomediastinum
2. Subcutaneous emphysema
3. Pneumopericardium
4. Pneumothorax
5. Pulmonary interstitial emphysema
6. Pneumoperitoneum
7. Diffuse alveolar hemorrhage
8. Gas embolism
   a. Brain
   b. Heart
   c. Visceral

The development of a pneumothorax while diving is serious, for intrapleural gas cannot be released to the environment and is likely to progress to tension pneumothorax during ascent, leading to syncope, shock, or unconsciousness upon surfacing.

Except for pneumothorax, which may require needle aspiration or tube thoracostomy, treatment of uncomplicated pulmonary overpressurization typically requires only observation, rest, and, sometimes, supplemental oxygen. Recompression is necessary only in extremely severe cases.

Air Embolism

The most feared complication of PBT is air embolism. Indeed, dysbaric air embolism (DAE) is one of the most dramatic and serious injuries associated with diving and is a major cause of death and disability among sport divers.

DAE results from the entry of gas bubbles into the systemic circulation through ruptured pulmonary veins. After passing through the heart, bubbles lodge in small arteries, occluding the more distal circulation. The resulting manifestations will depend on the location of the occlusion, and, depending on the site, even minute quantities of gas can have disastrous consequences.

DAE usually presents immediately after a diver surfaces, at which time the high intrapulmonic pressure resulting from lung overexpansion is relieved, which allows bubble-laden blood to return to the heart. Although the classic history is that the diver ascends rapidly because of running out of air, panic, or some similar circumstance, this is not always the case, and localized overinflation may also result from focally increased elastic recoil of the lungs in some divers.

The presenting manifestations of DAE are usually dramatic. Coronary occlusion and cardiac arrest may occur, although the brain is by far the most often affected organ. The neurological manifestations are typical of an acute stroke, such as meno- or multiplegia, focal paralysis, sensory disturbance, blindness, deafness, vertigo, dizziness, confusion, convulsions, or aphasia. Asymmetric multiplegias are the most common presentation, and the differentiation of DAE from severe neurologic decompression sickness is often impossible. Sudden loss of consciousness upon surfacing should always be assumed to be due to gas embolism until proved otherwise. Other reported clinical findings such as visualization of bubbles in the retinal arteries or Libermeister's sign (a sharply circumscribed area of glossal pallor) are exceedingly rare.

Some patients with very severe initial neurological symptoms may improve spontaneously. The mechanism of spontaneous recovery is not clear. Nonetheless, such patients should still be referred for recompression since even subtle dysbaric injuries may become irreversible without definitive care. Before recompression, pneumothorax should be ruled out.

Indirect Effects of Pressure

Nitrogen narcosis and decompression sickness may develop as a result of breathing gases at higher-than-normal atmospheric pressure.

Nitrogen Narcosis

Nitrogen and other lipid-soluble inert gases have an anesthetic effect at elevated partial pressures. The narcotic effects are similar to those of alcohol and become evident in most divers between 70 and 100 fsw. Many divers are so markedly impaired at 200 fsw that they can

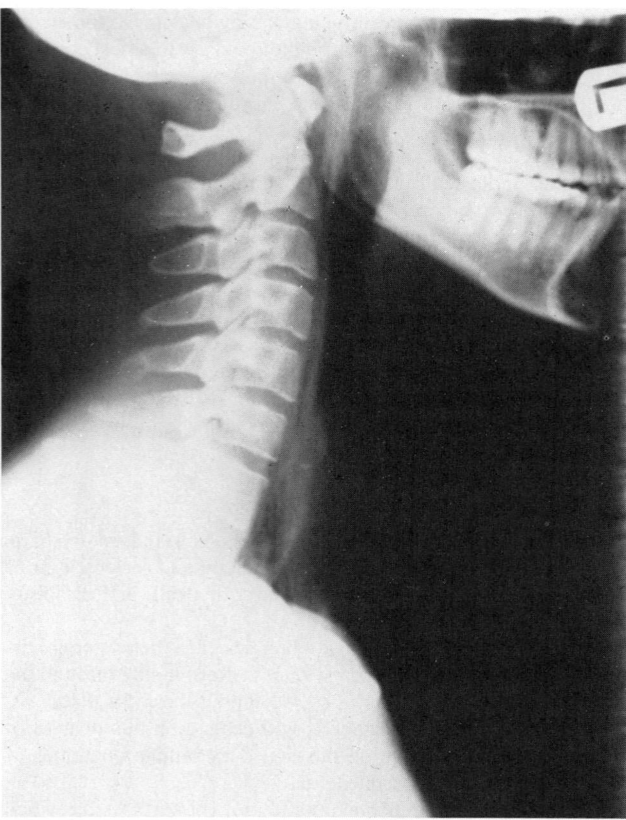

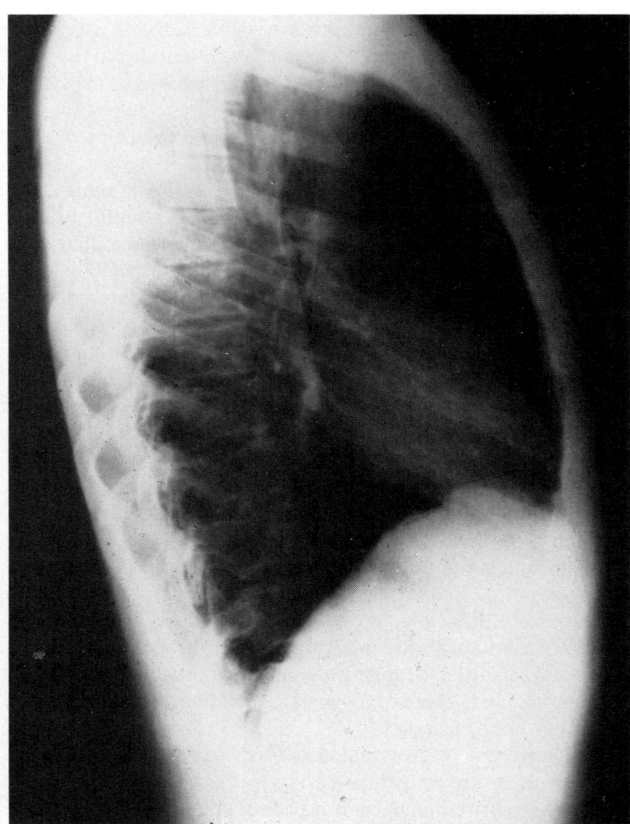

Fig. 121-2. Radiographs showing air dissecting through the mediastinum and into the neck from pulmonary barotrauma. (Photograph by KW Kizer.)

do no useful work, and at depths over 300 fsw unconsciousness ensues. Although narcotic effects are reversed as the P_{N_2} decreases with ascent, nitrogen narcosis is not an uncommon precipitating factor in diving accidents and may impair a diver's memory of the circumstances leading up to the accident.

Decompression Sickness

Decompression sickness is a multisystem disorder resulting from the liberation in inert gas from solution with the formation of gas bubbles in blood and body tissues when ambient pressure is decreased. The critical factor in its pathogenesis is increased tissue absorption of inert gas, which in most diving situations is nitrogen.

As an air-breathing diver descends, ambient pressure increases, and a positive gradient of nitrogen from alveoli to blood to tissue develops. After a time at depth this gradient will diminish, eventually becoming zero as a new equilibrium is reached. The time that it takes for the new equilibrium to be achieved will depend on the alveolar-to-tissue inert gas gradient, the tissue blood flow, and the ratio of blood-to-tissue inert gas solubility. Consequently, the rate at which a diver reaches a new inert gas equilibrium will be an exponential function of the diffusion and perfusion characteristics of the different tissues.

The tissue absorption of increased gas is the first step to decompression sickness (DCS), but it is only when ambient pressure is decreased too rapidly to allow the diffusion of inert gas from tissues that DCS occurs.

The pathophysiology of decompression sickness consists of both mechanical and biophysical effects of bubbles (Fig. 121-3). The major mechanical effect of bubbles in DCS is vascular occlusion; however, the bubbles in DCS form primarily in the venous circulation and thus impair venous return. However, the bubbles in DCS can form any-

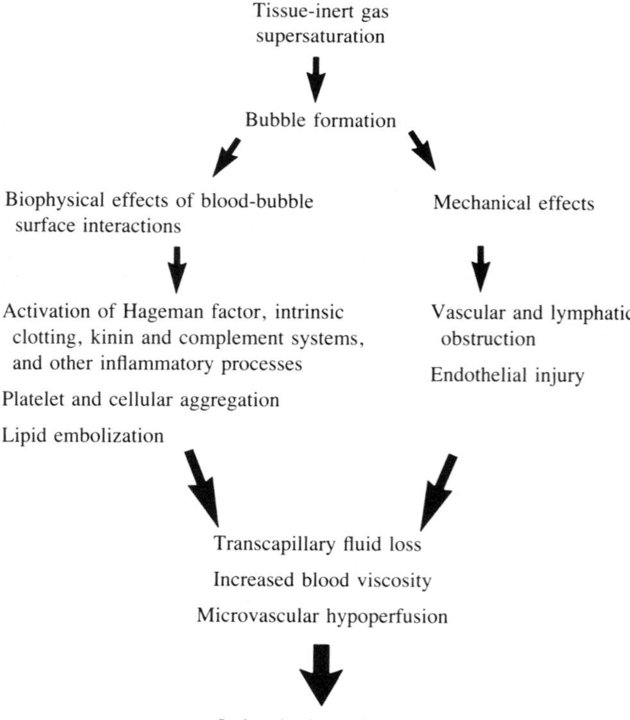

Fig. 121-3. Schematic representation of the pathogenesis of decompression sickness. (Adapted from Kizer KW: Management of dysbaric diving casualties. *Emerg Med Clin North Am* 1:659, 1983. Used by permission.)

where, such as in lymphatics, or intracellularly or extravascularly. Lymphedema, cellular distension and rupture, and intercellular dislocation can all compound the effects of vascular occlusion. Also, venous gas emboli may cause paradoxical arterial embolization via intrapulmonic and intracardiac shunts. Indeed, it is now clear that some dysbaric cerebral injuries are due to paradoxical embolization through previously unrecognized right-to-left intracardiac shunts that may only be open during abnormal pressure conditions found during diving. In two recently reported series, 60 to 80 percent of serious neurologic decompression sickness patients had paradoxical shunting. Such paradoxical embolization may explain the high frequency of apparent combined decompression sickness/air embolism noted in some series.

Bubbles also exert a variety of biophysical effects due to blood-bubble surface interaction. In essence, bubbles are viewed by the immune system as foreign matter and incite an inflammatory reaction. The key step in the process is activation of the Hageman factor, which, in turn, activates the intrinsic clotting mechanisms and kinin and complement systems, which results in platelet activation, cellular clumping, lipid embolization, increased vascular permeability, interstitial edema, and microvascular sludging. The net effect of all these processes is decreased tissue perfusion and ischemic injury.

The clinical manifestations of decompression sickness are protean (Table 121-6), but the joints and spinal cord are most often affected. Technically, the term *bends* refers only to the musculoskeletal form of DCS, but it is commonly used to mean any type of DCS. The various forms of DCS have also been arbitrarily categorized as either types I or II, with type I referring to the mild forms of DCS (skin, lymphatic, and musculoskeletal systems) and type II including the neurological and other serious types. Although this latter categorization is firmly entrenched in the literature, it is clinically more meaningful to refer to the systems affected when discussing patients with DCS.

Cutaneous manifestations include pruritus, subcutaneous emphysema, and scarlatiniform, erysipeloid, or mottled rashes. Localized swelling or peau d'orange may result from lymphatic obstruction.

Periarticular joint pain is typically described as a deep, dull ache, although it may be throbbing or sharp. There may be a vague area of numbness or dysesthesia around the affected joint. Movement of the affected extremity usually aggravates the pain, but inflation of a blood pressure cuff around the involved joint may relieve the pain for as long as the cuff is inflated. The shoulders and elbows are most often affected in scuba divers, although essentially any joint may be involved.

Neurologic DCS may be manifest by a vast array of symptoms and signs, and essentially any symptom is compatible with neurologic DCS. Classically, however, neurological DCS involves the lower thoracic, lumbar, and sacral portions of the spinal cord and produces paraplegia or paraparesis, lower-extremity paresthesias, and bladder dysfunction. Historically, urinary retention was such a frequent manifestation of spinal cord DCS that a urethral catheter used to be part of the diver's standard equipment. Recently, Hallenbeck et al. have convincingly demonstrated that at least some cases of spinal cord DCS result from venous infarction of the cord due to obstruction of venous drainage in the epidural vertebral venous plexus.

Table 121-6. Forms of Decompression Sickness

1. Cutaneous ("skin bends")
2. Lymphatic
3. Musculoskeletal (the "bends" or pain-only bends)
4. Neurologic
    a. Spinal cord
    b. Cerebral
    c. Cerebellar (the "staggers")
    d. Inner ear
    e. Peripheral nerves
5. Pulmonary (the "chokes")
6. Cardiovascular (decompression shock)
7. Visceral

Pulmonary DCS results from massive venous air embolization and usually does not become symptomatic until at least 10 percent of the pulmonary vascular bed is obstructed. Signs and symptoms include chest pain, cough, dyspnea, shock, and pulmonary edema. The clinical course is often fulminant and downhill.

Many divers develop intravascular bubbles but no apparent illness; these have been called "silent bubbles" and their clinical significance is unclear.

A variety of laboratory abnormalities may be demonstrated in DCS, but most of them have little clinical relevance to acute care.

Dysbaric casualties should be rapidly referred for hyperbaric treatment. However, the patient should also be evaluated for lifethreatening nondysbaric injuries and, if present, resuscitation commenced.

Since intravascular volume depletion and hemoconcentration are common in serious DCS, fluid replacement should be an integral part of therapy.

Treatment of Diving Casualties

The Diving Accident History

Most diving problems can be properly diagnosed by history and physical examination alone. The specific diving accident history should encompass the following basic points.

1. The type of diving engaged in and the equipment used. Some kinds of diving or certain types of equipment are associated with specific problems, e.g., hypercarbia or oxygen toxicity with rebreathing apparatus. Always make sure that the patient was actually breathing compressed air before sending for recompression treatment.
2. The number, depth, bottom time, and surface interval between repetitive dives for all dives in the 48 to 72 h preceding symptom onset. Even though this information may not be especially meaningful to you, having it available will facilitate communication with the diving medicine consultant, who will want to ascertain whether required decompression steps were omitted.
3. In-water decompression. Again, this is relevant to the determination of the likelihood of the diver having DCS.
4. In-water recompression. Except in very unusual situations using 100% oxygen, full face mask, and other specialized support, in-water recompression should not be attempted. Recompression with compressed air should never be done, for it almost always leaves the diver in a worse condition than originally and is fraught with other hazards.
5. Site of diving (e.g., ocean, lake, or quarry) and environmental conditions (e.g., water temperature, amount of current) associated with the dive. Other things being equal, DCS is more likely to occur after diving in cold water, but nondysbaric problems related to the environment (e.g., motion sickness) must be excluded.
6. Primary diving activity (e.g., spearfishing, photography). DCS is more likely after an arduous dive.
7. Presence of predisposing factors. A number of factors have been anecdotally related to the development of DCS. These include advanced age (decreased tissue perfusion), obesity (increased absorption of inert gas), dehydration, recent alcohol intoxication, cold water (decreased peripheral perfusion), vigorous underwater exercise (increased gas uptake), local physical injury (decreased local perfusion), and multiple repetitive dives in unacclimatized individuals (gradual buildup of inert gas).
8. Dive complications. These include running out of air, marine animal envenomation, mechanical trauma, or some other unexpected event. Musculoskeletal pain may be due to overexertion or muscle strain, and numbness in an extremity may be from a jellyfish sting rather than DCS.
9. Predive and postdive activities. Activities such as jogging and unpressurized airplane travel after diving may precipitate DCS.

Likewise, trivial dysbaric symptoms may become severe after similar activities.

10. Onset of symptoms. Certain conditions are more likely to occur at given times in the dive profile, and a differential scheme can be derived on the basis of time of symptom onset.

Differential Diagnosis of Diving Accidents

In general, a scuba dive can be divided into five stages, each of which is associated with characteristic problems.

The Predive Surface Phase

The predive surface phase includes all activities prior to going underwater and beginning to breathe compressed air. This often involves considerable surface swimming to the dive site. The most often encountered problems during this phase of the dive are motion sickness, hyperventilation, mechanical trauma, near drowning, and untoward marine animal encounters.

Descent Phase

The primary problems associated with descent are the squeeze syndromes, especially aural barotrauma, although inner ear barotrauma and ABV may also occur. Similarly, carbon monoxide poisoning, hypoxia, or other breathing gas problems may develop early in the dive.

At-Depth or Bottom Phase

Overall, few problems occur ''on the bottom,'' and the most likely ones are mechanical trauma or encounters with dangerous marine life. Nitrogen narcosis may contribute to an underwater accident. Inner ear barotrauma or gas mixture problems may first become symptomatic at this time.

Ascent Phase

Again, barotrauma is the problem most often encountered with ascent, although much less frequently than during descent. The relationship of POPS, ABV, and inner ear barotrauma with ascent have already been discussed. Gas mixture problems may become manifest at this time, and hypercarbia can be experienced toward the end of a dive. Decompression sickness may occasionally occur while a diver is still submerged; if this happens it usually implies a very serious problem.

Postdive Surface Phase

The postdive surface phase is divided into immediate (within 10 min of surfacing) and delayed (after 10 min). Any symptom occurring in the immediate postdive phase should be considered an air embolism until shown otherwise. Any symptom which begins more than 10 min after the dive should be viewed as decompression sickness until otherwise explained. More than half of all DCS patients will become symptomatic in the first hour after surfacing, with most of the rest experiencing symptoms within 6 h. A very few patients (1 to 2 percent) may first note their symptoms 24 to 48 h after diving. Other problems that may be first noted in the delayed postdive phase include mild forms of the POPS, sequelae of barotrauma, inner ear barotrauma, motion sickness, exhaustion, irritant or venomous dermatoses, and nondysbaric conditions related to physical activity.

Immediate Management

The victim should be rescued from the water and life-support measures begun as needed. Hypothermia should be considered an aggravating factor in every aquatic accident victim.

If DAE is suspected, it is recommended that the patient be maintained supine in the field and during transport. Placement in the Trendelenburg or Durant positions is no longer recommended because of the uncertain benefit of such maneuvers, and concerns about causing or aggravating cerebral edema (especially if left in the head-down position for longer than 30 to 60 min) and the increased respiratory difficulty attendant to being in such positions.

Supplemental 100% oxygen should always be given as soon as possible, being best administered by mask at 6 to 8 L/min. This facilitates offgassing of the nitrogen bubbles and improves oxygenation of damaged tissues.

Depending on local circumstances, patients with suspected DAE or DCS may be taken directly to the recompression chamber (Fig. 121-4) or may need emergency department intervention. Whichever the case, transportation should be an expeditious as possible. If air transportation is used, the patient should be subjected to the least possible pressure reduction so as not to cause any further gas expansion. Either a low-flying helicopter or light airplane, capable of flight at 1000 ft or less, should be used. Alternatively, aircraft that can be pressurized to 1 ATA (e.g., Lear jet, Cessna Citation, or C-130 Hercules) can be used.

Advanced life support drugs should be administered according to the victim's condition and standard protocols. In general, most DCS victims will be at least mildly volume depleted, so parenteral and oral (if the patient is alert) fluids should be given at a brisk rate unless they are contraindicated for other reasons.

Although high-dose parenteral corticosteroids have been widely recommended, and, typically, used, in the past two decades as an adjunct to recompression treatment of both neurologic decompression sickness and dysbaric air embolism, there is little evidence to support their use. The use of glucocorticoids became prevalent based on the belief that they were beneficial in the treatment of cerebral edema, shock, and other conditions pertinent to decompression sickness, but their benefit in many of these other conditions is now questioned. A few anecdotal cases suggesting that steroids are beneficial, either alone or with other pharmacologic interventions combined with standard recompression therapy, have been reported, but there have been no published clinical series or controlled trials demonstrating their efficacy. In contrast, recent controlled studies of high-dose parenteral dexamethasone or methyl prednisolone in decompression sickness–affected dogs showed that the use of glucocorticoids as an adjunct to conventional hyperbaric oxygen treatment produced no benefit and even suggested that the steroid-treated animals did less well.

If the need for recompression or the location of the nearest hyperbaric treatment facility is uncertain, assistance is available 24 h/day through the National Diving Alert Network at Duke University (919-684-8111).

Hyperbaric Treatment

Pressure and oxygen are the keystones of treatment for DCS and DAE and should be administered according to well-established protocols.

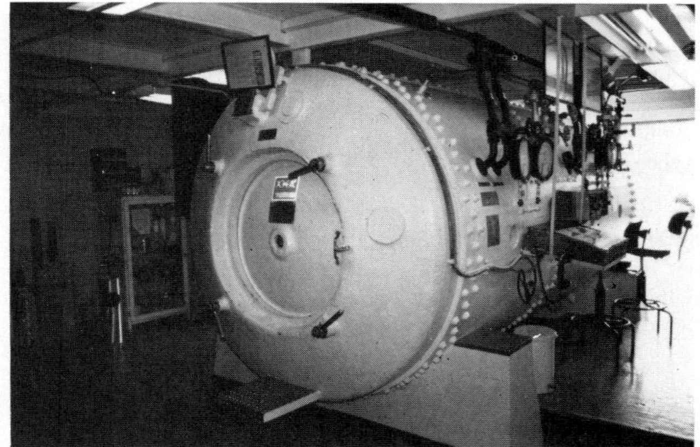

Fig. 121-4. Typical multiplace recompression chamber. The two compartments can be pressurized independently of each other up to at least 6 ATA, and as many as 12 persons can be seated in the chamber. (Photograph by KW Kizer.)

Various types of hyperbaric chambers may be utilized for treatment, and the relative merits of one type or another need not be recounted here.

The outcome of recompression treatment will, of course, depend on the severity of the disease, the delay in commencing hyperbaric treatment, and the victim's health prior to the accident. Overall, 80 to 90 percent success rates have been reported from a variety of sources, and even though recompression is generally believed to be more likely to be beneficial the sooner that it is commenced after the onset of symptoms, it should not be refused to someone who presents 2, 3, or more days after an accident, for dramatic recoveries have been reported after treatment delays of 10 days or longer. It is not possible to determine in advance what the effect of a delay in recompression will be for any individual patient.

Postrecompression Evaluation

Since recompression treatment does not always result in complete resolution of dysbaric neurologic injury and since occasional situations arise when the differential diagnosis of acute diving-related neurologic dysfunction includes intracranial hemorrhage, trauma, or other non-dysbaric injury, it is sometimes important to be able to characterize the site, extent, and origin of central nervous system lesions beyond what can be achieved by the traditional means of history and physical examination.

Both computerized tomography (CT) and magnetic resonance (MR) imaging have been used in this regard. Regrettably, conventional CT has not been found to be an efficient investigative tool for the post-treatment evaluation of decompression sickness, and CT imaging of spinal cord lesions (which constitute the majority of neurologic decompression sickness) is not feasible. In contrast, limited clinical data support the feasibility and efficacy of MR imaging of these conditions, especially when intracranial injury is present.

BLAST INJURY

The phenomenon of blast injury has been recognized for as long as humans have used explosives, although it has been mainly a wartime concern. However, in the past few decades there has been a dramatic increase in the incidence of peacetime civilian explosive blast injuries because of the popularity of the homemade bomb as a vehicle of social protest and the continued hazard of explosions in mining, grain storage, and other industries. In addition, blast injuries remain a prominent cause of fire-related morbidity.

Blast Physics and Terminology

Explosives are materials which are rapidly converted into gases when detonated. *Blast* and *blast injury* are, respectively, general terms used to describe this gaseous decomposition and the damage occurring in an organism subjected to the pressure field produced by an explosion.

Blasts are characterized by the release of large quantities of energy in the form of pressure and heat, with the exact amount depending on the type and amount of explosive. If the explosion in confined within some sort of casing, e.g., a bomb, the pressure will rupture the housing and eject the resulting fragments at high velocity. The remaining energy is transmitted to the surrounding environment in the form of a blast wave, blast winds, ground shock, and fire.

The *blast wave* begins as a single pulse of increased pressure that rises to peak levels within a few milliseconds and then rapidly falls to a minimum pressure that is lower than the original atmospheric pressure (Fig. 121-5). It is propagated outward radially from the explosion, with the sharply marginated periphery of the sphere becoming the blast, overpressure, or shock wave, as it has been variously called. The duration and level of the high pressure peak depends on the nature of the explosive, the conducting medium, and the distance from the detonation point. This blast wave pressure peak determines the *overpressure* that an object in its path is subjected to and is the main

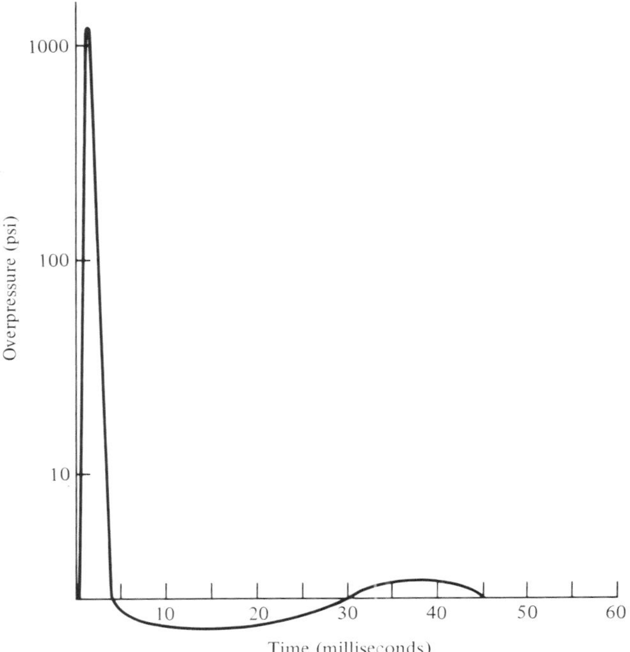

Fig. 121-5. The general form of a blast wave − 700 mmHg (−14.7 psi).

determinant of primary blast injury. Conversely, the negative pressure wave, or suction of the blast wave, lasts several times longer than the high-pressure wave but can never be greater than −700 mmHg (−14.7 psi). Representative pressure effects are listed in Table 121-7.

The rapidly expanding gases from an explosion also displace air, causing it to move away at very high velocity and produce transient *blast winds* that travel immediately behind the shock front of the blast wave. The blast wave may also accelerate loose objects (e.g., people) through the air, causing acceleration-decleration injuries. In the immediate vicinity of an explosion this *windage* can cause atomization, or total disintegration, of a body, evisceration, or traumatic amputations, depending on the force of the explosion. Illustrative of the force of such winds, an overpressure of about 5200 mmHg (100 psi) produces a blast wind having a velocity of about 2400 km/h (1500 mi/h).

In addition to the amount and duration of overpressure caused by an explosion, the overall effect of the blast wave will also depend on the exact waveform of the overpressure (i.e., its rise time), the victim's body mass and orientation to the explosion, the presence of deflecting and reflecting surfaces in the environment, and the medium through which the shock wave is conducted. For example, because of the greater density of water and its relative incompressibility, blast waves produced by underwater explosions travel much faster and farther than those produced by above-ground explosions. Consequently, blast injuries in water occur at greater distances from the detonation point and tend to be more severe. Underwater blast injury has other peculiarities, too, but these are beyond the scope of this discussion.

Table 121-7. Selected Pressure Effects

Pressure, psi*	Effect
5	Possible tympanic membrane rupture
15	50% incidence of tympanic membrane rupture
30	Possible lung injury
75	50% incidence of lung injury
100	Possible fatal injuries
200	Death more likely than not

* 1 psi = 51.7 mmHg.

Categories and Manifestations of Blast Injury

Explosive blast injuries can be divided into four categories (Table 121-8).

Primary Blast Injury

Type I, or *primary, blast injury* results directly from the sudden changes in environmental pressure caused by the blast wave. Tissues vary in their susceptibility to primary blast injury, with homogeneous or solid tissues being at least risk because they are essentially noncompressible and merely vibrate as a whole when subjected to a blast wave. Conversely, gas-filled organs are compressible and have tissue-gas interfaces, which means that displacement occurs wherever tissues of different densities interface, resulting in tissue distortion and tearing. Thus, primary blast injury mainly affects organs containing air and causes the most severe damage at the junctions between tissues, where loose, poorly supported tissue is displaced beyond its elastic limit.

There are three general mechanisms where a blast shock wave can damage living tissue. The first of these is known as *spalling* and occurs when a shock wave traveling through a medium of higher density (e.g., liquid) passes into a medium of lower density (e.g., gas), creating a negative reflection at the interface and, thus, fragmenting the surface of the heavier medium. This is analogous to hitting the outside of a rusty bucket with a hammer, which causes flakes to come off inside the bucket.

The second mechanism is implosion of gas-filled spaces as the high pressure in the surrounding fluid or solid compresses these spaces. Similarly, because there is a pressure differential between the air-filled and vascular spaces, blood and fluid are forced into the air-filled spaces. This mechanism is of particular importance in the lungs, where it contributes to pulmonary hemorrhage. In addition, as the negative pressure wave follows the initial positive pressure, smaller internal secondary explosions occur as the compressed gas reexpands.

Third, tissues of different densities will be accelerated and decelerated at different rates relative to each other, producing shearing forces that can tear or otherwise damage the tissue.

The organs most vulnerable to primary blast injuries are the ears, lungs, central nervous system, and gastrointestinal tract. Abdominal visceral injury is relatively rare in air blast casualties but is of considerable concern in persons exposed to underwater blasts.

Otolaryngologic Manifestations

The ears are most often affected by explosive blasts, with hearing loss being the primary manifestation. Hearing can be damaged by one of three ways. First, the tympanic membranes may rupture. This usually occurs in adults at a pressure differential between the middle and external ears of around 360 mmHg (7 psi), and most often presents as a linear perforation of the pars tensa. The second way is dislocation of the ossicles, which may accompany tympanic membrane rupture or occur as the sole injury. Finally, deafness may result from blast effects on the inner ear, causing perilymph fistula and other damage. In addition to hearing loss, primary symptoms of inner ear damage include vertigo and tinnitus.

The paranasal sinuses are also susceptible to blast injury, usually manifesting barotraumatic damage similar to the squeeze syndromes that occur with compressed air diving.

Table 121-8. Categories of Blast Injury

Category	Injury Caused by	Primary Target Organs
I. Primary blast injury	Blast wave	Ears, lungs, GI tract, CNS
II. Secondary blast injury	Victim struck by flying debris	Integument, CNS, eyes, musculoskeletal system
III. Tertiary blast injury	Bodily displacement, i.e., victim impact with stationary objects	Abdominal viscera, CNS, lungs, integument, musculoskeletal system
IV. Miscellaneous	Inhalation of dust or toxic gases, thermal burns, radiation, other	Lungs, integument, eyes

Pulmonary Manifestations

The lungs are generally the organs most severely affected by blast injury, and these injuries are likely to present a threat to life. (Of course, the severe injuries resulting from windage in the immediate vicinity of the explosion are also life-threatening.) The blast wave causes widespread alveolar damage because of its effects on tissue-gas interfaces, producing interstitial and intraalveolar hemorrhage and edema, parenchymal and pleural lacerations, and alveolar-venous fistulas. Because of the widespread nature of this damage a variety of specific injuries may be found, including pulmonary edema, pneumothorax and other extraalveolar air syndromes, and air embolism. Similarly, pulmonary contusions result from compression of the lung between the spine, thoracic wall, and rising diaphragm, as well as from being thrown against solid objects in the environment.

The actual symptoms experienced by victims of blast lung injury will vary with the severity and nature of their specific injuries, but, in general, they will present with dyspnea and other signs of pulmonary insufficiency, chest pain, hemoptysis, rales, rhonchi and other signs of pulmonary edema or hemorrhage, as well as symptoms of the pulmonary overpressurization syndrome.

Gastrointestinal Manifestations

Blast injuries to the stomach and bowels are due to damage at tissue-gas interfaces, producing hemorrhage into the wall and lumen along with perforations, which tend to be multifocal. Since the large bowel usually contains more gas than the small bowel, it tends to be more severely affected. Common clinical manifestations include abdominal pain, melena, signs of peritonitis, and free air in the abdomen. Evisceration and other gross damage may be found in victims who were very close to the detonation site, but these types of injury are nearly always fatal.

Neurological Manifestations

Blast injuries of the central nervous system are of two main types. First are the direct shock wave effects, which produce a concussion syndrome and various types of intra- and extraaxial hemorrhage, and second are the effects of cerebral air embolism. As with dysbaric diving casualties, the actual neurological manifestations of air embolism vary.

Other Categories of Blast Injury

Type II, or *secondary, blast injuries* are due largely to the blast wind and result from the victim being struck by flying debris. Conversely, *type III,* or *tertiary, blast injuries* are those that result from the victim being displaced through space by the blast wind and impacting a stationary object; this sudden deceleration usually causes more harm than the acceleration through space. *Type IV blast injuries* include a wide variety of injuries resulting from inhalation of dust and toxic gases, exposure to radiation, thermal burns, and so on.

The myriad number of bodily insults that can result from these latter types of blast injury are far too numerous to list here. Of particular concern, though, are the traumatic amputations, occurring in about 25 percent of severely wounded victims, and liver, spleen, or other visceral injury produced from the acceleration-deceleration forces of the blast wind. Likewise, bomb casing fragments or missiles such as nails, nuts and bolts, screws, ball bearings, etc., can cause high-velocity missile injuries.

Management of Blast Casualties

Blast injury victims should be managed in the same manner as any multiple trauma victim, except that particular attention should be directed to the respiratory system. This includes giving special attention to maintenance of a patent airway (especially when maxillofacial, cervical spine, or other head and neck injuries are present), administering supplemental oxygen, judiciously using intravenous fluids and analgesics, evacuating pneumo- and hemothoraxes, and promptly implementing mechanical ventilation if signs of respiratory failure or inadequate oxygenation are present. Although positive pressure ventilation may be necessary to maintain adequate oxygenation, its use is fraught with hazard, since the diffuse alveolar-capillary damage present in blast lung greatly increases the risk of causing extraalveolar extravasation of air, including air embolism.

Systemic air embolization presents particular problems in the management of blast casualties, since the effects on the brain, heart, and viscera caused by air emboli may be indistinguishable from other types of injury. Yet, the preferred therapy for air embolism is hyperbaric oxygen treatment (HBOT), which may not be readily available or may be impractical because of coexistent injuries or other logistical problems. Whenever possible, though, HBOT should be implemented as expeditiously as possible, being given in a manner similar to the treatment of dysbaric diving casualties, since it is usually very effective in reversing cerebral or coronary injuries.

Tympanic membrane rupture and other otolaryngologic trauma, as well as most other types of blast injury, should be treated essentially the same as they are treated when due to other causes. Closed abdominal injuries are always of particular concern and should be treated according to the patient's signs and symptoms, with prompt surgical exploration being undertaken whenever there are signs of peritonitis or peritoneal free air. Abdominal visceral injuries should be especially looked for in victims of underwater explosion. Lacerations, fractures, amputations, and missile wounds should be treated in the usual manner, except for delayed primary closure being the generally preferred method of wound management.

Explosions in confined spaces typically produce worse injuries than those occurring in the open because of the greater likelihood of inhalation injury from dust, smoke, and toxic gases. Again, though, the inhalation injury is treated essentially the same as that resulting from other circumstances.

Since primary blast injuries may not always be present when the victim is first evaluated, all blast-injured patients should be closely observed for at least 6 to 12 h after the accident. This is particularly true if there is perforation of the eardrums, which is generally an indication of significant exposure to high pressure.

BIBLIOGRAPHY

Dysbaric Diving Casualties

Bove AA: The basis for drug therapy in decompression sickness. *Undersea Biomed Res* 9:91, 1982.

Colebatch HJM, Smith MM, Ng CKY: Increased elastic recoil as a determinant of pulmonary barotrauma in divers. *Respir Physiol* 26:55, 1976.

Cramer FS, Heimbach RD: Stomach rupture as as result of gastrointestinal barotrauma in a scuba diver. *J Trauma* 22:238, 1982.

Gillen HW: Symptomatology of cerebral gas embolism. *Neurology* 18:507, 1968.

Hallenbeck JM, Bove AA, Elliott DH: Mechanisms underlying spinal cord damage in decompression sickness. *Neurology* 25:308, 1975.

Kizer KW: Delayed treatment of dysbarism; a retrospective review of 50 cases. *JAMA* 247:2555, 1982.

Kizer KW: Dysbaric cerebral air embolism in Hawaii. *Ann Emerg Med* 16:535, 1987.

Kizer KW, Goodman PG: Radiographic manifestations of venous air embolism. *Radiology* 144:35, 1982.

Lundgren CEG, Tjernstrom O, Ornhagen H: Alternobaric vertigo and hearing disturbances in connection with diving: An epidemiologic study. *Undersea Biomed Res* 1:251, 1974.

Parell GJ, Becker GD: Conservative management of inner ear barotrauma resulting from scuba diving. *Otolaryngol Head Neck Surg* 93:393, 1985.

Blast Injury

Benzinger T: Physiological effects of blast in air and water, in *German Aviation Medicine, World War II*, vol II. Washington, DC, U.S. Government Printing Office, 1950, pp. 1225–1259.

Caseby NG, Porter MF: Blast injuries to the lungs: Clinical presentation, management and course. *Injury* 8:1, 1976.

Clemedson CJ: Blast injury. *Physiol Rev* 36:336, 1956.

Hadden WA, Rutherford WH, Merrett JD: The injuries of terrorist bombing: A study of 1532 consecutive patients. *Br J Surg* 65:525, 1978.

Huller T, Bazini Y: Blast injuries of the chest and abdomen. *Arch Surg* 100:24, 1970.

Kerr AG: Trauma and the temporal bone—the effects of blast on the ear. *J Laryngol Otol* 94:107, 1980.

Pahor AL: Blast injuries to the ear: An historical and literary review. *J Laryngol Otol* 93:225, 1979.

Pahor AL: The ENT problems following the Birmingham bombings. *J Laryngol Otol* 95:399, 1981.

Rawlings JSP: Physical and pathophysiological effects of blast. *Injury* 9:313, 1977.

Roy D: Gunshot and bomb blast injuries: A review of experience in Belfast. *J Roy Soc Med* 75:542, 1982.

122 NEAR DROWNING

Bruce E. Haynes

Drowning, like other causes of accidental death, often strikes young, otherwise healthy individuals, and prevention is the most important way to reduce these unnecessary deaths. The patient's prognosis after near drowning depends on the speed of rescue and resuscitation, emphasizing the role of emergency medical care.

DEFINITIONS

Almost as many definitions of drowning exist as authors in the field. One approach is to define drowning as death from suffocation after submersion, while those who suffer near drowning survive, at least temporarily, after suffocation by submersion. A few use the more generic term *immersion syndrome* to highlight the blurred margins between the two entities, although this term has also been used to refer to sudden death after immersion in cold water. Postimmersion syndrome, or secondary drowning, refers to the deterioration of a seemingly well patient after immersion.

EPIDEMIOLOGY

About 4500 people die of submersion in the United States each year, making drowning the third leading cause of accidental death. Many more—the exact number is uncertain—experience serious submersion episodes; it has been estimated 10 percent of young boys survive these incidents.

Freshwater drowning, especially in pools, is more common than saltwater drowning, even in coastal areas. There is a bimodal age distribution, with large numbers of deaths among children under age 4 and then later among teenagers, although risk climbs again in the elderly from bathtub drowning.

Alcohol or drug use by victims or by supervising adults often plays a role in drowning and boating accidents; trauma, especially to the lower cervical spine, results in some cases. Poor swimming skills, combined with children oblivious to dangerous situations, causes numerous drownings, and swimming lessons can be targeted at ethnic groups who need them. Hypothermia, hyperventilation before underwater swimming, or seizure disorders are also factors. Patients with seizure disorders must receive careful supervision if swimming and should, depending on seizure control, probably bathe in showers or tubs with open drains and plastic stalls. This patient education is important when first-time seizure patients are discharged from emergency departments.

Drowning deaths should be prevented by adequate, well-maintained fencing with self-locking gates that surrounds pools themselves, rather than simply isolating the backyard, leaving access to the pool from the house and yard. Drowning occurs extraordinarily rapidly, and caretakers must be taught that attention to children must not be diverted by chores, socializing, telephone calls, or other seemingly momentary distractions. Cardiopulmonary resuscitation (CPR) is frequently not started by rescuers, and pool owners should be encouraged to learn CPR and have telephones in the pool area.

CLINICAL COURSE

Respiratory failure and ischemic neurologic injury are the threats to life after submersion, although associated injuries are occasionally severe. After the initiating event, panic frequently supervenes, followed by struggling in the water and desperate breath holding or hyperventilation. These soon lead to vomiting and aspiration of water and emesis. "Dry drowning" without aspiration results from laryngospasm and glottal closure and is thought to be responsible for 10 to 15 percent of deaths. Whatever the mechanism, the final common pathway is profound hypoxemia.

While both seawater and fresh water wash surfactant out of alveoli, fresh water also changes the surface tension properties of surfactant. Surfactant loss leads to atelectasis, ventilation-perfusion mismatch, and breakdown of the alveolar capillary membrane. Hypoxemia follows aspiration of small amounts of water and is seen experimentally with aspiration of 2.2 mL/kg of either fresh water or salt water. Contributing to hypoxemia may be aspiration of bacteria, algae, sand, particulate matter, emesis, and chemical irritants. Noncardiogenic pulmonary edema results from direct pulmonary injury, surfactant loss, inflammatory contaminants, and cerebral hypoxia.

Poor perfusion and hypoxemia lead to metabolic acidosis in a majority of patients; yet perhaps as a result of the young age of most victims, the cardiovascular status is remarkably stable. Blood volume shifts depend on the nature and quantity of the fluid aspirated, although life-threatening changes are unusual, since most human drowning victims aspirate quantities of water far below those which produce significant disturbances. Electrolyte abnormalities in near-drowning patients are seldom significant, and hematologic values are usually normal, although the clinician will occasionally see hemolysis resulting in anemia. Rarely, disseminated intravascular coagulation will occur.

Renal function is usually adequate, although proteinuria may occur and hemoglobinuria can follow hemolysis. Acute tubular necrosis can result from hypoxia or myoglobinuria.

THERAPY

Prehospital Care

Treatment of near drowning begins at the scene with rapid, cautious removal of the victim from the water (Table 122-1). Spinal precautions should be observed if the mechanism of injury, such as diving or surfing, raises suspicion of such injury. The vast majority of spinal injuries are to the lower cervical spine after diving, and burst fractures predominate. Clues to spinal injury may be paradoxical respiration, flaccidity, priapism, unexplained hypotension or bradycardia. Lifeguards and emergency medical technicians should maintain spinal precautions during rescue if possible. Initial history may be unreliable, and the physician should have a low threshold for obtaining cervical spine x-rays.

A patent airway must be maintained and ventilation assisted as needed; all patients should receive supplemental oxygen. Cardiopulmonary resuscitation should be started on any arrested patient with even a remote possibility of success. Sodium bicarbonate should be considered in unstable patients, and any patient with a significant episode, including those asymptomatic at the scene, should be transported to the hospital for evaluation.

In-water CPR is generally ineffective and dangerous for the rescuer, and should not be attempted unless a firm, stable surface is available. Postural drainage or the abdominal thrust (Heimlich maneuver) is of unproven efficacy in removing water from the lungs or improving oxygenation. No drainage procedure appears to significantly affect oxygenation in experimental preparations; human near-drowning victims aspirate small quantities of water, and there is little evidence that aspirated water interferes with ventilation. Field limitations to postural drainage include the danger of aspiration from an uncontrolled airway,

Table 122-1. Prehospital Care of Near-Drowning Victims

Rapid, cautious rescue
Spinal precautions
Cardiopulmonary resuscitation, with administration of dextrose and naloxone (if indicated)
Supplemental oxygen on all patients
Transport all patients

interruption of ventilation or CPR, the danger of spinal injury, and the possibility of aggravating other undiagnosed injuries. An appropriate maneuver for airway obstruction should be employed only if ventilation is obstructed.

Hospital Care

Hospital evaluation and care of drowning victims emphasizes initial resuscitation, evaluation of associated injuries, treatment of respiratory failure, and measures to protect the brain from hypoxic insult (Table 122-2).

While patient survival in a persistent vegetative state is a concern, substantial numbers of patients, predominantly children, requiring CPR on emergency department arrival have survived with good outcomes, and physicians should err on the side of providing resuscitation. Life support can always be withdrawn in the intensive care unit once the medical and social picture is clearer.

On the victim's arrival in the emergency department adequate oxygenation should be assured, the integrity of the patient's cervical spine should be confirmed if necessary, and associated injuries should be sought. Pulmonary insufficiency may be indicated by dyspnea, tachypnea, or use of accessory muscles of respiration. Physical examination may reveal wheezing, rales, or rhonchi, although the chest may be completely normal to auscultation after aspiration.

All patients should receive supplemental oxygen during evaluation, and those with more than mild symptoms should be on 100% O_2 until adequate oxygenation is documented. If high-flow oxygen (40 to 50%) cannot maintain the arterial P_{O_2} greater than 60 mmHg in adults or 80 mmHg in children, the patient should be intubated and mechanical ventilation employed.

Intubated patients generally require positive end-expiratory pressure (PEEP) or continuous positive airway pressure (CPAP). Muscular paralysis will be needed in some patients, and hyperventilation to a P_{CO_2} of 30 may help control cerebral edema.

Occasionally, a patient may require only increased oxygenation and CPAP without mechanical ventilation. Only patients who are alert and unlikely to vomit are candidates for mask CPAP ventilation.

Those patients whose temperatures register at the low end of standard thermometers need further investigation. A hypothermia thermometer is best, but emergency departments can usually obtain low-reading thermometers from their clinical laboratory or operating room. Hypothermia can immobilize a swimmer, resulting in drowning, may cause primary ventricular fibrillation, or may be responsible for a variety of adverse metabolic effects. Severe hypothermia often indicates prolonged submersion and is a bad prognostic sign. Despite this, individuals have survived after prolonged submersion (up to 40 min) in cold water. These patients have body temperatures less than 30°C (86°F) after submersion in water less than 20°C (68°F). The nature of the protective effect of hypothermia is unclear, it may be general slowing of metabolism or preferential shunting of blood to the brain, heart, and lungs (diving reflex). The similarity between severe hypothermia and death has led to the aphorism that no one is dead until warm and dead. Near-drowning victims who are hypothermic should be warmed to at least 30 to 32.5°C (86 to 90°F) before resuscitation efforts are abandoned.

Table 122-2. Hospital Care of Near-Drowning Victims

Clear cervical spine
Laboratory studies:
- CBC, electrolytes, glucose, clotting studies, urinalysis
- Arterial blood gases, pulse oximetry
- Chest x-ray
- Electrocardiogram

Pulmonary support:
- Supplemental oxygen on all patients
- High-flow O_2 as needed
- Intubation and positive pressure (PEEP, CPAP)

Nasogastric tube
Foley catheter
Monitor:
- Oxygenation
- Acid-base balance
- Temperature
- Volume status

Evaluate and treat:
- Associated injuries
- Specific conditions: hypoglycemia, hypothermia, etc.

Appropriate laboratory data should be obtained (Table 122-2). A baseline Gram's stain and culture of the trachea will be useful in intubated patients. Direct measurement of oxygenation and acid-base status by arterial blood-gas analysis and on-line pulse oximetry guide pulmonary therapy and the need for sodium bicarbonate.

Roentgenograms of the chest may be normal after a significant near-drowning incident or may show generalized pulmonary edema (Fig. 122-1), perihilar infiltrates, or other patterns. Chest films do not necessarily correlate with arterial P_{O_2}, making direct measurement of arterial blood gases important, although many patients with significantly abnormal films will require intubation.

If not given in the field, an initial dose of 1 mEq/kg of $NaHCO_3$ may be administered while awaiting blood-gas analysis if the patient is unstable. Standard treatment of bronchospasm, electrolyte imbalance (especially hypoglycemia), seizures, hypothermia, arrhythmias, and hypotension should be undertaken as needed. Some patients may need fluid resuscitation in the face of noncardiogenic pulmonary edema. To avoid inducing arrhythmias, central venous catheters, if used, should not enter the heart in hypothermic patients. A nasogastric tube will empty the stomach and help prevent vomiting, and a Foley catheter will help to monitor urine output.

Neither antibiotics nor steroids alter the course of aspiration pneumonia or pulmonary edema in drowning, and they should not be given prophylactically.

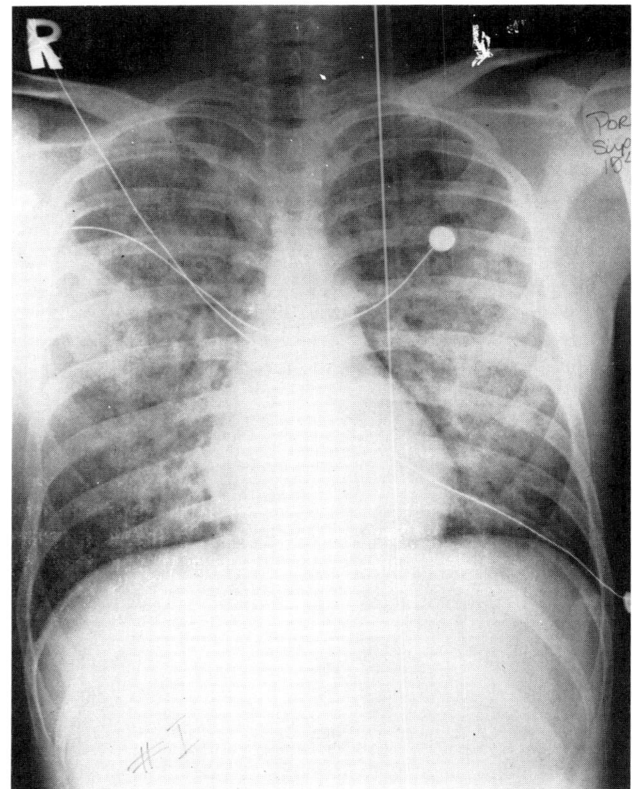

Fig. 122-1. Chest roentgenogram of near-drowning patient demonstrating diffuse noncardiogenic pulmonary edema.

PROGNOSIS AND CEREBRAL RESUSCITATION

Statistics on survival and the incidence of severe neurologic deficits after near drowning are difficult to interpret. They vary with regard to definitions, patient age, water temperature, treatment regimens, and many other variables. Almost all patients who are alert and fully conscious will survive without sequelae, as will the vast majority of victims who are obtunded but have a purposeful response to pain. Allman et al. reported that 24 percent of their intensive care unit (ICU) patients who required full CPR and had an initial Glasgow Coma Scale (GCS) of 3 in the referring emergency department survived with intact neurologic function. Patients whose GCS remained 3 in the intensive care unit either died or survived in a vegetative state, while those with a GCS in the ICU of 4 to 5 were divided between intact survivors and those who died or survived in a vegetative state. Patients with a GCS over 5 in the ICU were unlikely to die of neurologic complications.

Regimens based on the principles of cerebral resuscitation have been used in seriously ill patients, including moderate dehydration by fluid restriction and diuretics, mechanical ventilation with mild hypocapnia ($P_{CO_2} = 30$), hypothermia to 30°C (86°F), muscular paralysis, use of corticosteroids, and barbiturate coma. There is little evidence that the regimen improves outcome, and barbiturate coma has been shown to be ineffective in independently improving outcome.

Intracranial pressure (ICP) monitoring is employed frequently in pediatric near-drowning victims. Patients who develop intracranial hypertension (ICP $>$ 20 mmHg) almost always die or are left in a persistent vegetative state; unfortunately, ICP monitoring cannot distinguish between those with normal ICP who will survive intact and those who will survive in a vegetative state. Not all flaccid patients with fixed, dilated pupils have elevated intracranial pressure.

Routine measures such as muscular paralysis and hyperventilation are easily, and for the most part safely, accomplished in the emergency department, while techniques requiring close monitoring should be reserved for the ICU.

DISPOSITION

Most older reports on drowning recommend admission and monitoring of all near-drowning victims. This recommendation arose from descriptions of "secondary drowning" in which 2 to 25 percent of near-drowning patients deteriorated significantly or died after a seemingly successful rescue and/or resuscitation. Most of the patients in these reports, however, simply had pulmonary insufficiency that progressed and symptoms or signs that today would be discovered easily by an adequate evaluation. The decision of whom to admit must focus on those at risk for pulmonary insufficiency or other complications.

Patients at risk have undergone a "significant" episode and display symptoms such as coughing, dyspnea, or tachypnea, or have historical factors such as unconsciousness in the water. Occasionally, patients who suffered transient severe hypoxia or who have underlying cardiovascular disease will fall into the same group.

The physician's approach should depend on the patient's symptoms and the results of screening examinations. For convenience, patients may be separated into four groups, although one should take particular care in evaluating young children. One group will have no evidence of significant submersion and may be discharged quickly. Chest roentgenograms and arterial blood gas determinations are unnecessary in the face of a benign history, but the studies or pulse oximetry may lend weight to the decision to discharge.

A second group will be asymptomatic or have mild symptoms after a significant episode. They can frequently be observed in the emergency department for several hours and then discharged if their social situation allows adequate follow-up. The third group will have mild to moderate hypoxemia corrected by oxygen therapy. These patients are admitted and then discharged when the hypoxemia resolves if no complications ensue.

The final group is composed of patients who require intubation and mechanical ventilation whose prognosis usually depends more on their neurologic status than on their pulmonary injury, unless they develop serious aspiration pneumonia or progressive, irreversible lung injury.

SUMMARY

Near drowning is a common cause of accidental death, particularly in younger people. Prevention is the key, although emergency medical care is crucial for rapid, safe rescue and resuscitation. Emergency department care focuses on identifying and treating aspiration and resulting respiratory failure. Concurrent problems such as hypotension and hypothermia must be treated.

BIBLIOGRAPHY

Allman FD, Nelson WB, Pacentine GA, et al: Outcome following cardiopulmonary resuscitation in severe pediatric near-drowning. *Am J Dis Child* 140:571, 1986.

Modell JH, Calderwood HW, Ruiz BC, et al: Effects of ventilatory patterns on arterial oxygenation after near-drowning in sea water. *Anesthesiology* 40:376, 1974.

Modell JH, Graves SA, Ketover A: Clinical course of 91 consecutive near-drowning victims. *Chest* 70:231, 1976.

Nussbaum E, Maggi JC: Pentobarbital therapy does not improve neurologic outcome in nearly drowned, flaccid-comatose children. *Pediatrics* 81:630, 1988.

Pearn JH, Bart RD, Yamaoka R: Neurologic sequelae after childhood near-drowning: A total population study from Hawaii. *Pediatrics* 64:187, 1979.

Pratt FD, Haynes BE: Incidence of "secondary drowning" after salt water submersion. *Ann Emerg Med* 15:1084, 1986.

Ruiz BC, Calderwood HW, Modell JH, et al: Effect of ventilatory patterns on arterial oxygenation after near-drowning with fresh water. A comparative study in dogs. *Anesth Analg* 52:570, 1973.

123
BURNS AND ELECTRICAL INJURIES

Alan R. Dimick

BURNS

Approximately 2 million persons per year will seek medical treatment for a burn injury in the United States. Of these, 100,000 will sustain a life-threatening injury requiring hospitalization, and 20,000 will die either directly as a result of the burn or of complications. Deaths due to inhalation injuries resulting from the 750,000 annual residential fires, which result in 57 percent of the deaths from fire, could be decreased by the installation of smoke detectors. Burns due to heat or flame are frequently associated with concomitant clothing fire. The use of wood-burning fireplaces or stoves and the use of kerosene heaters to warm homes contribute to the increased incidence of residential fires and concomitant burn injury.

Pathophysiology

A burn is the result of the impact of heat on the skin and underlying tissues. Burns are classified in terms of depth as first-degree, second-degree, and third-degree. Third-degree burns are full-thickness burns, which usually require skin graft. First- and second-degree burns are partial-thickness burns, which usually heal without surgery. However, if second-degree burns become infected, they convert to third-degree burns. Burns are also classified by cause, size, extent of body surface area damaged, age of patient, and other complicating trauma or chronic illness. Of all these factors, the most important contributors to morbidity and mortality are patient age and extent of injury, particularly the extent of third-degree burn. In 1990 the American Burn Association (ABA) devised criteria for the referral of patients with burn injuries to burn centers. The ABA recommends that questions concerning specific patients be resolved by consultation between the referring physician and the burn center physician. The ABA criteria for burn center referral include the following:

1. Second- and third-degree burns of greater than 10 percent of the total body surface area (TBSA) in patients under 10 or over 50 years of age
2. Second- and third-degree burns of greater than 20 percent of the TBSA in other age groups
3. Second- and third-degree burns that involve the face, hands, feet, genitalia, perineum, and major joints
4. Third-degree burns of greater than 5 percent of the TBSA in any age group
5. Electrical burns, including lightning injury
6. Chemical burns
7. Burn injury with inhalation injury
8. Burn injury in patients with preexisting medical disorders that could complicate management, prolong recovery, or affect mortality
9. Any patients with burns and concomitant trauma (e.g., fractures) in which the burn injury poses the greatest risk of morbidity or mortality (If the trauma poses the greater immediate risk, the patient may be treated initially in a trauma center until stable before being transferred to a burn center; physician judgment is necessary in such situations and should be in concert with the regional medical control plan and triage protocols.)
10. Hospitals without qualified personnel or equipment for the care of children should transfer children with burns to a burn center with these capabilities
11. Burn injury in patients who will require special social or emotional and/or long-term rehabilitative support, including cases involving suspected child abuse, substance abuse, and so on

The extent of injury to an adult is estimated using the rule of nines (Fig. 123-1). On figures representing the anterior and posterior outlines of the body, the patient's burned areas are diagramed, with partial- and full-thickness areas marked differently. The head and neck are 9 percent of the TBSA, the arms and hands are 9 percent, and the thighs and legs are 18 percent. The anterior trunk from the clavicles to the pubis and the posterior trunk from the root of the neck to and including the buttocks are each 18 percent. The perineum constitutes 1 percent of the TBSA. Thus, a patient with the anterior trunk (18 percent TBSA), perineum (1 percent BSA), and left thigh circumferentially burned (9 percent TBSA) would have a total injury of 28 percent TBSA.

The Lund and Browder chart (Fig. 123-2) is used in infants and young children because it corrects for changes due to growth. For example, in the adult the head is 9 percent of the TBSA, but the head of the newborn is 18 percent of the TBSA.

On the same diagram, it is also possible to note other injuries, such as fractures, abrasions, lacerations, and so forth, that have occurred. These charts are a part of the patient's medical record.

The depth of a burn is dependent upon the extent of tissue destroyed. First-degree burns involve minimal tissue destruction of the outer layers of the epidermis, are red and painful, and are slightly edematous. They usually heal within 7 days with the characteristic peeling of dead skin.

Second-degree burns occur when the tissue damage extends into the dermis but hair follicles, sweat glands, and other adnexal structures are left. These structures are lined with epithelium, and it is from them that the epithelium proliferates to cover the area of skin loss. Epithelial coverage usually takes 14 to 21 days. Second-degree burns are characterized by blisters and have red or whitish areas extremely painful to touch. When the blisters are removed, they leave a bright-red moist surface.

Third-degree burns present either a charred or a pearly white surface. Due to the destruction of all layers of the skin including the nerve endings, the area is insensitive to pain or touch. The only definitive sign of a third-degree burn is a translucent surface in the depths of which thrombosed veins are visible. Since complete destruction of all skin layers has occurred, full-thickness burns heal only with skin grafting or scarring.

Burns resulting from fires in an enclosed space, or where toxic

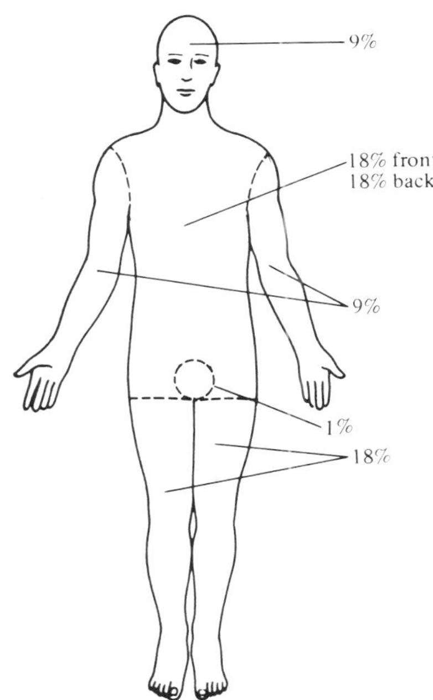

Fig. 123-1. Rule of nines.

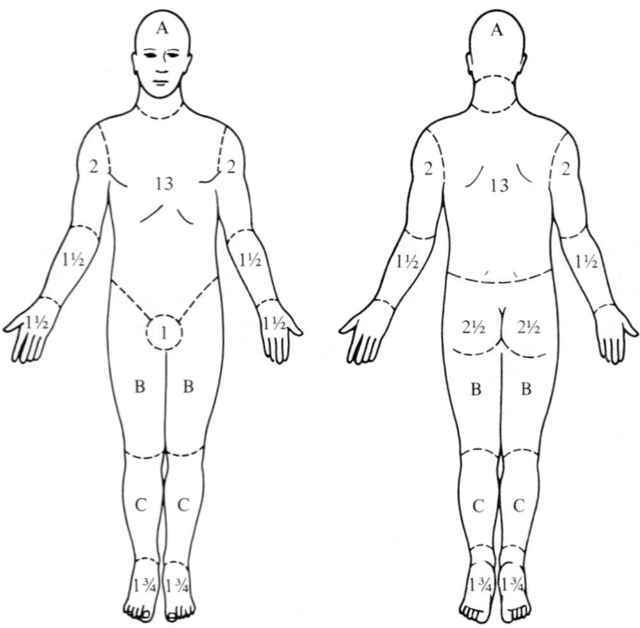

Relative Percentages of Areas Affected by Growth (Age in Years)

	0	1	5	10	15	Adult
A: half of head	$9\frac{1}{2}$	$8\frac{1}{2}$	$6\frac{1}{2}$	$5\frac{1}{2}$	$4\frac{1}{2}$	$3\frac{1}{2}$
B: half of thigh	$2\frac{3}{4}$	$3\frac{1}{4}$	4	$4\frac{1}{4}$	$4\frac{1}{2}$	$4\frac{3}{4}$
C: half of leg	$2\frac{1}{2}$	$2\frac{1}{2}$	$2\frac{3}{4}$	3	$3\frac{1}{4}$	$3\frac{1}{2}$

Second degree ____________ and

Third degree ____________ =

Total percent burned ___

Fig. 123-2. Classic Lund and Browder chart.

chemicals or plastics are involved, can be associated with upper and lower respiratory tract injury. Facial burns, singed facial or nasal hairs, sooty sputum, and respiratory distress or wheezing are clinical signs of such injury. Tracheobronchial edema, ulceration, or bronchospasm can result from steam or chemical inhalation. Alveolar damage is usually due to chemicals in the inhaled smoke and fumes. Edema and loss of integrity of the alveolocapillary membrane result in hypoxia or pulmonary edema.

Prehospital Care

The emergency medical system should have a triage burn protocol based on the severity and complexity of the burn. In general, referral patients with burn injuries should follow the recommendations of the ABA, as mentioned earlier. Minor burns may be treated in an emergency department, clinic, or physician's office.

The patient should be evaluated with regard to airway, breathing, and circulation, followed by a survey for hidden trauma. After this, the patient should be wrapped in a clean dry sheet. Ointment or cream should not be applied, and wound contamination must be minimized.

Ice should never be placed directly on the burn wound because cold injury can increase the depth of the wound. Small burns can be covered with (iced) water or saline, but ice should not come in contact with the wound. For larger burns, the use of iced saline can result in hypothermia and should be avoided. Intravenous fluids and pain medication should be determined by emergency medical service personnel in consultation with the medical control physician; such decisions are influenced by transport time.

All patients should receive oxygen during transport. The patient should be kept warm, with airway, vital signs, and level of consciousness monitored during transport. In urban areas the patient may be transported directly to the designated burn center if the magnitude of burn indicates the need for specialized care. In suburban and rural areas transport should be initially to the nearest emergency facility capable of stabilizing the burn patient. Referral to a regional burn center may subsequently be necessary.

EMERGENCY DEPARTMENT CARE

Airway, breathing, and circulation should be assessed. Examination for hidden trauma is important. If pulmonary injury due to smoke inhalation is suspected, or if there are severe burns to the face which may result in edema and upper airway obstruction, tracheal intubation is necessary. Facial swelling and upper airway obstruction should be anticipated. Early intubation is essential before swelling obliterates the landmarks and makes it impossible. The mortality of patients undergoing emergency tracheostomy greatly exceeds the complications from tracheal intubation.

Chest x-ray films and arterial blood gas levels must be obtained to evaluate alveolar function. Fiberoptic bronchoscopy should be done to evaluate the trachea and bronchi. Hypoxia is treated by intubation, delivery of high concentrations of oxygen, and positive-pressure ventilation with frequent monitoring of arterial blood gas levels. Carboxyhemoglobin levels should also be determined. The intravenous line should be established above the waist even if it is necessary to go through the wound itself. A central venous line is not usually necessary during the initial phases of resuscitation, but a large-bore line (18 gauge or better) is essential, since flow is dependent on the diameter of the catheter.

As a result of the burn injury, there is vasodilatation and leakage of plasma through all capillaries in burned tissues. The bigger the area burned, the more extensive the loss of vascular volume. Thus, early management includes the administration of adequate amounts of lactated Ringer's solution to expand the vascular volume. Several formulas are recommended for treating burn shock (Table 123-1).

The National Institutes of Health burn care consensus conference was held in 1978, and its proceedings were published in the November 1979 issue of the *Journal of Trauma.* This conference recommended the consensus fluid formula given in Table 123-1. The initial use of Ringer's lactate for the resuscitation of all burn patients was recommended.

In patients requiring hospital admission, a urinary catheter should be inserted and the hourly urine volume monitored. Intravenous fluids should be regulated to maintain a urine output of 30 to 50 mL/h in adults and 1 mL/kg per hour in children weighing less than 30 kg.

Keeping the patient warm while evaluating the extent of the injury is of great importance in the major burn patient, as hypothermia rapidly

Table 123-1. Current Formulas Recommended for Treating Burn Shock in First 24 h

Parkland formula:

Give 4 mL of lactated Ringer's solution per kilogram body weight per percentage of BSA burned.

Give one-half this amount in first 8 h, and one-half in next 16 h post burn.

Brooke formula:

Give 3 mL of lactated Ringer's solution per kilogram body weight per percentage of BSA burned.

Give one-half this amount in first 8 h, and one-half in next 16 h post burn.

Consensus fluid formula:

Give 2–4 mL of lactated Ringer's solution per kilogram body weight per percentage of BSA burned.

Give one-half this amount in first 8 h, and one-half in next 16 h post burn.

develops. In major and moderate burns neither cool water nor ice should be applied to the burns.

Small doses of morphine (2 to 4 mg) should be given intravenously to alleviate pain and anxiety unless contraindicated by other injuries. Intramuscular injections other than tetanus prophylaxis should be avoided because of poor and irregular absorption from the muscle in shock states.

Tetanus toxoid, 0.5 mL booster, should be given intramuscularly in all burn patients. Where any doubt of previous immunization exists, 250 units of human hyperimmune tetanus globulin should be given intramuscularly in the opposite extremity. In the patient with small burns where compliance does not appear to be a problem, 0.5 mL of tetanus toxoid may be given with a repeat dose 2 weeks later.

Since shock produces gastric distension with accompanying ileus, a nasogastric tube should be inserted in patients with moderate and major burn injury. Air swallowing due to apprehension and fear can also result in severe gastric distension. For aeromedical transfer, the stomach must be decompressed to avoid rupture during transfer.

Prophylactic antibiotics are not recommended by most burn centers because of the development of resistant bacteria.

Laboratory data including a complete blood cell count; urinalysis; and measurement of levels of serum electrolytes, glucose, blood urea nitrogen, creatinine, arterial blood gases, and carboxyhemoglobin should be obtained.

Debridement of the burn wound should be accomplished by gentle washing of the surface with a mild soap or detergent. Sharp debridement of loose tissue and all blisters should be done. Blister fluid recently has been shown to contain vasospastic agents which potentiate tissue ischemia. Therefore, blister fluid should be removed as soon as possible.

Following wound cleansing, a topical antibacterial agent such as silver sulfadiazine should be used. The agent should be applied over the affected area in a 1/16-in.-deep layer. Occlusive cotton gauze dressing should be applied to cover the wound.

A circumferential burn of the arms or legs may compromise the vascular supply to the hands or feet due to edema under the burn eschar, which is tough and unyielding. The Doppler flow probe is extremely useful in determining the presence of pulses in the extremities. An escharotomy may be necessary if distal pulses are diminished or absent. The incision should be made through the eschar so that fat bulges through the wound. Escharotomies may be performed on the lateral or medial surfaces of the legs and arms and if necessary continued onto the dorsum of the hand or foot in a Y-shaped fashion. One limb of the Y goes to the web space between the first and second digits, and the other limb to the web space between the fourth and fifth digits. The fingers should not have escharotomies even if they are severely burned.

If the chest is burned circumferentially, mechanical restriction to respiration may occur because of collection of edema fluid under the tough eschar. This requires relief by escharotomy of the chest wall with an incision in the anterior axillary line commencing at the second rib and ending at the top of the twelfth rib (Fig. 123-3). The superior and inferior angles of these incisions should be joined by an incision perpendicular to the long axis of the body. Thus, a floating square of tissue is defined that moves with respiration and alleviates restriction to ventilation.

Outpatient Management

Minor burns (10 percent of the body surface or less) are not at a significant risk of infection, and topical antimicrobial agents may or may not be used. Blisters should be removed and debrided, or at least the fluid evacuated. Such small burns can be dressed with fine mesh gauze, with or without medication, and covered with a dry dressing held in place with an elastic gauze dressing. The dressing should be inspected at least every 3 to 5 days. If the outer dressing is soaked, it should be removed. If the inner dressing is intact with no evidence of suppuration, a new outer dressing is then applied.

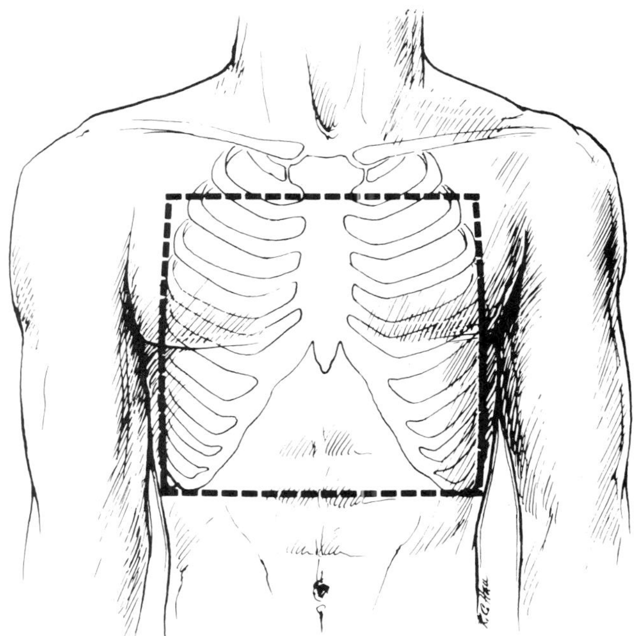

Fig. 123-3. In escharotomy of the chest wall, the constricting eschar that may impair ventilation is cut and a floating square of tissue is defined.

ELECTRICAL INJURIES

High-voltage electrical injuries are uncommon, affecting primarily skilled industrial workers or the curious infant who plays with an electric outlet or bites an electric cord.

In the curious infant or child and in patients injured in using electric appliances in the bathroom, alternating current in which the flow of electrons switches from positive to negative at 60 Hz is the cause of the injury. Alternating current produces entrance and exit wounds of approximately the same size. Children with burns of the lips should be observed carefully for subsequent rupture of the labial artery 3 to 5 days post injury.

In the industrial environment, direct current, in which the electrons flow in one direction with one positive lead and one negative lead, is the most common cause of injuries. Direct current produces a small entrance wound and a much larger exit wound.

These exit and entrance wounds are local lesions with a central area appearing charred, a middle zone of whitish to gray coagulation necrosis, and an outer area of brighter-red, edematous damaged tissue.

Electricity flows from the point of contact to the ground, producing heat directly proportional to the distance between these two points and the resistance of the tissues in between. The effects of electric passage are generally worse with alternating current than with direct current. The current follows the lines of least resistance in the body. Skin has a high resistance in the dry state. Nerve, blood vessel, muscle, and bone exhibit greater resistance and, therefore, incur greater damage in the reverse order of the listing.

Electrical injury has been likened to crush injury because the systemic effects are often similar. If muscle is injured, myoglobin is released systemically. The greatest threats to life are cardiac arrhythmias, renal failure secondary to the precipitation of myoglobin and hemoglobin in the kidneys, and electrolyte abnormalities such as hyperkalemia and hypocalcemia due to massive muscle breakdown.

Any or all of the major organs may be damaged. After first ensuring that the patient has adequate airway, breathing, and circulation, a baseline 12-lead ECG is indicated in all electrical injuries, with subsequent cardiac monitoring for at least 24 h. The electricity may cause thrombosis of any blood vessel in the body. Therefore, a thorough review of all body systems is indicated, since initially it is not possible to assess the full extent of tissue injury caused by the electricity. Electrical injury may cause progressive intravascular thrombosis, which may occur over a period of several days, causing progression of tissue destruction.

After the safe extrication of the patient at the scene of injury, an immediate evaluation of airway, breathing, and circulation should be done. Cardiac monitoring is essential. If the patient is stable, a survey for other injuries should be made, since fractures and dislocations, especially of vertebrae and long bones, often accompany electrical injury. A cervical collar should be applied and the patient placed on a backboard until spinal injury has been excluded. The establishment of a large-bore intravenous line with Ringer's lactate is necessary. Fluid replacement must be vigorous, utilizing central venous pressure and urine output monitoring. An osmotic diuretic such as mannitol should not be used to treat myoglobinuria until it is certain that intravascular volume has been adequately replaced. One ampule of mannitol (12.5 g) is given as a bolus intravenously, and then one ampule is placed in each subsequent bottle of intravenous fluids until the pigment clears from the urine. Blood studies should include a complete blood cell count, and measurement of levels of plasma and urine myoglobin, serum electrolytes, cardiac enzymes, and arterial blood gases. Cardiac monitoring is employed for the first 24 h. X-ray films of injured areas to rule out fracture should be obtained. Tetanus prophylaxis is necessary. Debridement of dead tissue should be extremely conservative, as the true extent of the injury is unknown at initial evaluation. In particular, debridement of lesions of the hands, fingers, and face should never be attempted in the emergency department.

Burn center referral is often necessary for electrical burns, as considerable injury to deeper neurovascular and musculoskeletal structures may not be obvious until several days post injury.

BIBLIOGRAPHY

American Burn Association: Hospital and prehospital resources for optimal care of patients with burn injury: Guidelines for development and operation of burn centers. *J Burn Care Rehab* 11:98, 1990.

Arturson MG: The pathophysiology of severe thermal injury. *J Burn Care Rehab* 6:129, 1985.

Davies JWL: Toxic chemicals versus lung tissue. *J Burn Care Rehab* 7:213, 1986.

Demling RH: Burns. *N Engl J Med* 313:1389, 1985.

Dimick AR, Potts LH, Shaw SE, et al: Ten year profile of 1,271 burn patients. *J Burn Care Rehab* 6:431, 1985.

Frank HA, Wachtel TL (eds): Thermal injuries. *Top Emerg Med* 3:3, 1981.

Haponik EF, Munster AM (eds): *Respiratory Injury: Smoke Inhalation and Burns*. New York, McGraw-Hill, 1990.

Haynes BW: Emergency department management of minor burns. *Top Emerg Med* 3:3, 1981.

Matthews JB, Jelenko C III: Psychosocial support of the burn patient, his family, and the burn team. *Life Sup Nurs* 2:13, 1979.

Rouse RF, Dimick AR: The treatment of electrical injury compared to burn injury: A review of pathophysiology and comparison of patient management protocols. *J Trauma* 18:43, 1978.

Shires GT, Black EA (eds): Proceedings of the NIH Consensus Development Conference in supportive therapy in burn care. *J Trauma* 19:855, 1979.

Shires GT, Black EA (eds): Second conference on supportive therapy in burn care. *J Trauma* 21:665, 1981.

124
CHEMICAL BURNS

Marcus L. Martin
Fred P. Harchelroad, Jr.

Chemical burns occur in the home, industry, agriculture, school and research laboratories, and military settings and as a result of civilian assaults, hobby accidents, and other accidents. Chemical burns also occur as a result of innocent application of products for medical purposes and for hair and skin care.

More than 25,000 products are capable of producing chemical burns. Both occupational exposure and our contact with numerous chemicals during daily life contribute to the large number of chemical injuries to the skin. There are no good epidemiologic data on the incidence of toxic cutaneous exposure in the nonoccupational setting. However, about 40 percent of all occupationally related diseases reported concern the skin, and about 25 percent of these are due to chemical burns.

Common household chemical burns are caused by lye (drain cleaners, paint removers, urine sugar reagent test tablets), phenols (deodorizers, sanitizers, disinfectants), sodium hypochlorite (disinfectants, bleaches), and sulfuric acid (toilet bowl cleaners). In industries, chemicals are used for cleaning, tanning, curing, extracting, preserving, soldering, and other functions. The most commonly used industrial acids are tungstic, picric, sulfosalicylic, tannic, formic, sulfuric, acetic, cresylic, trichloroacetic, chromic, hydrochloric, and hydrofluoric acids. Widely used alkalis are the hydroxide salts of sodium, potassium, ammonium, lithium, barium, and calcium. White phosphorus used in munitions was the most common cause for chemical burns to military personnel during armed conflict times in the 1960s. White phosphorus is also found in rodenticides and pesticides.

The body sites most often burned by chemicals are the face, eyes, and extremities. Less than 5 percent of patients admitted to major burn centers suffer from chemical burns. In general, chemical burn average sizes are small, and mortality rate is lower than for thermal burns, but wound healing and hospital stay times are higher.

PATHOPHYSIOLOGY

The skin interfaces with the external environment and constitutes a barrier and a transition zone between the internal and external milieus. The outer stratum corneum layer of the skin functions as an excellent barrier against certain chemical agents, whereas others may penetrate readily. The skin contains three main layers: an outer layer of epithelial tissue (epidermis), a loose connective tissue layer (dermis), and a variable-thickness inner layer containing adipose and connective tissue (hypodermis or panniculus adiposus).

Chemicals can produce burns, dermatitis, allergic reaction, thermal injury, or systemic toxicity. Pathophysiologically, burns produced by all chemicals are similar. The skin has a limited variety of toxic responses, corresponding to the major patterns of possible structural or functional changes. Toxic reactions are described mainly on the basis of morphologic rather than functional responses. There are morphologic, physiologic, and biochemical protective mechanisms and elements in the skin which include the epidermal barrier, eccrine sweating, phagocytic cells, metabolic detoxification, immunologic processes, and melanin pigmentation. However, these vary on a phenotypic basis and may be affected by systemic or local disease.

Skin damage by chemicals may demonstrate the classic manifestations of thermal injury (erythema, blistering, or full-thickness loss); however, the acute injury may be deceptively mild, only to be followed by extensive skin damage and systemic toxicity. A superficial (first-degree) burn causes capillary and arterial dilatation. Initially, this involves only the superficial vessels, but then extends to the deeper subcutaneous vessels by both direct and reflex action. This tissue hyperemia and congestion results in symptoms of itching, burning, or pain. More extensive inflammatory reactions result in an outpouring of fluid into the extracellular space causing edema and vesicle or bulla formation characteristic of partial-thickness (second-degree) burns. Continued chemical damage through the dermis or into the hypodermis results in a full-thickness (third-degree) burn.

Tissue damage is determined by:

- Strength/concentration of the agent
- Manner of contact
- Quantity of agent
- Duration of contact
- Mechanism of action
- Extent of penetration

Factors enhancing percutaneous absorption of chemical are: body site (areas of thin skin, i.e., genitalia, face; chemical contact between skin folds; amount of surface area exposed); integrity of skin (traumatized skin; elderly skin; decreased lipid; dehydration; inflammation); nature of the chemical (lipid solubility; pH; concentration) and occlusion (garments; occlusive dressings).

The majority of chemical burns are caused by acids or alkalis. At similar volumes and manner of contact, alkalis usually produce far more tissue damage than acids. Acids in general cause coagulation necrosis with protein precipitation. Tough leathery eschar may form with development of underlying ulcers. The eschar limits spread of the agent. Heat may be released during reaction of acid with skin. Alkalis produce liquefaction necrosis with loosening of material which allows deeper penetration of the unattached chemical into tissue. Since not all chemicals causing burns can be considered as acid or alkali, a useful classification by C. Jelenko groups chemicals by the manner in which they damage protein:

1. Oxidizing agents: Damage is produced when a chemical becomes oxidized in contact with tissue. Often a toxic moiety is released during this reaction.
2. Corrosives: Extensive protein denaturation is produced, resulting in soft eschar and shallow, indolent ulcers.
3. Reducing agents: Protein denaturation is produced by binding of free electrons in tissue protein.
4. Desiccants: Severe cellular dehydration is produced, and thermal injury occurs due to exothermic reaction.
5. Vesicant: Blisters are produced, tissue amines are liberated, local ischemia and anoxic tissue damage and pandermic inflammation occurs.
6. Protoplasmic poisons: Protein is denatured by salt formation or by metabolic competition/inhibition (i.e., binding calcium or other inorganic ions necessary for tissue viability and function).

GENERAL APPROACH

The goal of treatment is to minimize any area of irreversible injury and maximize salvage of the zone of reversible damage. Hydrotherapy is the cornerstone of initial treatment for chemical burns with few exceptions. Chemical agents may continue to damage tissue until they are removed or inactivated. The first priority is to stop the burning process. Immediate removal from the offending chemical, removal of garments, and counteraction of the chemical remaining on the body by dilution, debridement, or neutralization are important measures. Dry chemical particles such as lime should be brushed away before irrigation. Initially sodium metal and related compounds should be covered with mineral oil or excised, since water can cause a severe exothermic reaction. Dilution of phenol (carbolic acid) with water may enhance penetration. For the most part, however, use of water or saline to irrigate a chemical burn should not be delayed while searching for a neutralizing agent and should begin at the scene of the accident. In general, the earlier the irrigation, the better the prognosis.

The amount of elapsed time to initiate dilution or removal of chemical agents relates to the depth and degree of injury. Wounds irrigated 3 min after contact with some chemicals have a twofold greater chance of becoming full-thickness burns than wounds irrigated within 1 min of chemical contact. When using agents to neutralize a chemical burn, additional tissue injury may occur through heat production. In some cases, heat of dilution may be produced using water irrigation, but copious amounts will decrease the rate and amount of chemical reaction and dissipate the heat. Irrigation should be maintained at a gentle flow to avoid driving the chemical deeper into tissue or splashing chemical into the victim's or rescuer's eyes. The time required for irrigation varies; irrigation may need to be continued for hours in the case of alkali burns. Use of pH litmus paper may help determine continued presence of alkali or acid in burn wounds.

After irrigation and debridement of remaining particles and devitalized tissue, antimicrobial agents should be used and tetanus immunization should be updated as needed. Other than measures specific for a particular chemical burn, treatment following initial therapy is basically the same as for thermal burns. Patients sustaining chemical burns require the same aggressive fluid replacement as those with thermal burns. Analgesics may be needed, and, in the case of allergic responses to chemicals, antihistamines, steroids, and epinephrine may be required. Hemodialysis may be required in cases of severe systemic toxicity and renal failure. Autografts, heterografts, homografts, or synthetic material may be necessary for full-thickness burns. Hyperbaric oxygen may be utilized to assist healing of resistant burn wounds.

SPECIFIC CHEMICALS

Acids

With the exception of hydrofluoric acid, strong acids produce coagulation necrosis as a result of the desiccating action of the acid on proteins in the superficial tissue. Injury severity is related to certain physical characteristics of the acid. Most substances with a pH less than 2 are strong corrosives. Other important factors increasing the tissue-damaging properties of acids include concentration, molarity, and complexing affinity for hydroxy ions. The higher each of these factors is, the greater the tissue damage. Contact time with the skin is the most important feature of chemical burns which health care professionals may alter. Instantaneous skin decontamination of 18 *M* sulfuric acid will cause no burn; however, a 1-min exposure can cause full-thickness skin damage. Examination of the patient with a significant chemical burn from these acids should not be limited to observation of the skin because several of these acids are respiratory and mucous membrane irritants as well. Furthermore, skin absorption of some compounds may occur and result in systemic signs and symptoms. The most commonly used acids are listed in Table 124-1.

Table 124-1. Chemicals That Cause Burns

Agent	Use	Initial Treatment
Acetic acid	Permanent wave neutralizers, printing, dyeing, hat making	Water irrigation
Alkyl mercury compounds	Disinfectants, fungicides, wood preservatives	Water irrigation & prompt removal of blister fluid and overlying skin to prevent intoxication
Cantharides ("Spanish fly")	Veterinary aphrodisiac	Water irrigation
Chromic acid	Microelectronics/microinstruments, photography, metal cleaning and plating, leather tanning, cement manufacture	Water irrigation
Cresol (Lysol)	Disinfectant	Water irrigation
Creosote	Fungicides, wood preservative	Water irrigation
Cresylic acid	Industry	Water irrigation
Dimethyl sulfoxide (DMSO)	Topical treatment for sprains, arthritis	Water irrigation
Diquat dibromide	Herbicides	Water irrigation
Formic acid	Airplane-glue making	Water irrigation
Hydrocarbons	Industry, commerce	Water irrigation
Hydrochloric acid (muriatic acid)	Bleaching agents, metal cleaning, chemistry laboratories, fire proofing material, semiconductor industry	Water irrigation
Hydrofluoric acid	Microelectronics/microinstruments, petroleum refining, glass etching/frosting, metal etching, rust removal, dyes, plastics, germicides, leather tanning	Water irrigation Calcium gluconate
Lime	Agriculture Cement	Brush off, water irrigation
Lyes (alkalis) KOH, NaOH, NH_4OH, LiOH, $Ba_2(OH)_3$, $Ca(OH)_3$	Industrial cleansers, washing powders, drain cleaners, paint removers, urine sugar reagent tablets, portland cement	Water irrigation
Metals	Industry	Cover with mineral oil, excision
Mustard gas	Chemical warfare	Water irrigation/mineral oil
Nitric acid	Electroplating, engraving, fertilizer manufacturing, casting iron/steel	Water irrigation
Oxalic acid	Leather tanning, blueprint paper	Water irrigation, IV calcium gluconate
Phenols (carbolic acid)	Dyes, deodorizers, sanitizers, disinfectants, cosmetics, plastics manufacture, agriculture	Water irrigation, PEG/IMS or glycerol, or isopropyl alcohol
Phosphoric acid	Metal cleaning, disinfectants, rust proofing	Water irrigation
Picric acid	Industry	Water irrigation
Potassium permanganate	Disinfectants, bleach, deodorizers, medical	Water irrigation
Sodium hypochlorite (Clorox)	Cleanser	Water irrigation
Sulfosalicylic acid	Industry	Water irrigation
Sulfuric acid	Casting iron/steel, chemistry laboratories	Water irrigation
Tannic acid	Industry	Water irrigation
Trichloracetic acid	Industry	Water irrigation
Tungstic acid	Industry	Water irrigation
White phosphorus	Warfare incendiary, insecticides, rodent poison, fertilizers	Water irrigation, 1% copper sulfate irrigation

Acetic Acid

The dilute (< 40%) acetic acid solution found in hair wave neutralizer solutions is perhaps the most common cause of chemical burns to the scalp in women. Prolonged contact, especially with an already damaged scalp, may cause a partial thickness burn which heals slowly because of the constant bacterial flora on the hair. Initial treatment is copious water irrigation. As trimming the hair is not a viable option in these patients, oral antibiotics are often given if the entire scalp is involved.

Phenol

Phenol (carbolic acid), a corrosive organic acid used widely in industry and medicine, denatures proteins and causes chemical burns characterized by a white- or brown-colored coagulum that is relatively painless. Its unpleasant, acrid odor, detectable in air at 0.047 parts per million, and its low volatility help prevent airborne exposure. Though commercially available in concentrations of 1 to 90%, even dilute solutions of 1 to 2% phenol may cause a burn if contact is prolonged. Hexylresorcinol is a bactericidal phenol derivative. Chemically related phenolic compounds that induce skin damage include cresol, creosote, and cresylic acid.

Coagulation necrosis of the involved area is common. Necrotic tissue may delay absorption temporarily, but phenol may become entrapped under the eschar. Contaminated clothing should be removed and water lavage begun immediately. Water lavage alone may be ineffective, presumably because the necrotic coagulum inhibits water penetration to the deeper layers. Paradoxically, dilute phenol penetrates tissue more readily than when concentrated.

More effective decontamination has been demonstrated with a 5- to 10-min swab with a combination of polyethylene glycol 300 (PEG 300) and industrial methylated spirits (IMS) in a 2:1 mixture. This should not only reduce the extent of cutaneous corrosion but also decrease systemic toxicity. The PEG 300 is mixed with the IMS to form a more liquid (and therefore easier to use) formulation. However, the viscous PEG 300 or PEG 400 may be used alone, and, indeed, glycerol is an acceptable substitute if the PEG 300/IMS mixture is not available. The use of an isopropyl alcohol rinse may be superior to PEG/IMS or water alone in removing phenol. The advantage of isopropyl alcohol is its easy availability.

Chromic Acid

The toxicity of chromium compounds is related to the powerful oxidizing action of the hexavalent compounds (Cr^{6+}). The chromate ion in chromic acid will produce a chronic penetrating ulcerating lesion of the skin. Associated signs and symptoms are conjunctivitis, lacrimation, ulceration of the nasal septum, and systemic chromium toxicity. A 10 percent total body surface area cutaneous burn caused by chromic acid was fatal due to systemic toxicity. Any acute skin exposure to chromic acid should be treated with copious water irrigation and observation for systemic effects.

Formic Acid

Formic acid in 60% solution is used by airplane-glue makers, cellulose formate workers, and tanning workers. Formic acid produces coagulation necrosis of the skin. Treatment includes immediate decontamination and irrigation with water. Open lesions should be treated like any damaged skin: with debridement of devitalized tissue, prevention of further damage and infection, and skin grafting if the defect is full thickness and of a size requiring closure.

Hydrochloric and Sulfuric Acids

The dermal toxicity of hydrochloric and sulfuric acid is so well recognized that early decontamination and water irrigation usually prevent severe burns to the skin. These acids can turn the skin dark-brown or black when burned. Toilet bowl cleaners may contain 80% solutions of sulfuric acid. Some drain cleaners may be 95 to 99% sulfuric acid solutions. Munitions, chemical, and fertilizer manufacturers commonly use 95 to 98% sulfuric acid solutions in their industrial processes. Automobile battery fluid is 25% sulfuric acid. Most household bleaches are only 3 to 6% hypochlorite solutions, which though acidic, cause little damage unless they are in contact with skin for a prolonged time. Treatment is the same as for formic acid burns.

Nitric Acid

Nitric acid is used in industry for casting iron and steel, electroplating, engraving, and fertilizer manufacturing. Upon contact with skin, nitric acid can produce tissue damage by oxidation and may turn the skin a yellowish color as it is burned.

Hydrofluoric Acid

Hydrofluoric acid (HF) is unique among the corrosives in its mechanism of action and degree of toxicity. HF acts like alkalis and will cause progressive tissue loss, including bony destruction. Hydrofluoric acid, considered a protoplasmic poison, penetrates the skin, dissociates, and releases fluoride ions. Fluoride ions immobilize intracellular calcium and magnesium and poison cellular enzymatic reactions. Potassium permeability is increased and results in spontaneous depolarization of nerve tissue and pain.

Industrial applications include use in production of high-octane fuel; etching and frosting glass; semiconductors; microelectronics/microinstruments; germicides; dyes; plastics; tanning; and fireproofing material and use in cleaning stone and brick buildings. It is also a very effective rust remover.

HF rapidly penetrates the skin and causes both local and systemic toxicity. Its systemic effects include hypocalcemia, hypomagnesemia, and hyperkalemia. The dermal effects may not be immediately noted and appear to be more related to the concentration of HF than to the duration of exposure. Solutions greater than 50% produce immediate pain and tissue destruction; solutions less than 20% may not produce signs and symptoms until 12 to 24 h after exposure. The skin may develop a blue-gray appearance with a surrounding region of erythema.

Unlike the treatment of dermal injury caused by other acids, the treatment of HF burns consists of two phases. The first is immediate and copious water irrigation of the affected skin for 15 to 30 min. This may be the only treatment that is needed if the HF solution is less than 20% concentrated, the duration of exposure was very brief, and decontamination is begun immediately. Unfortunately, this is rarely the case. Severe, persistent pain denotes a more serious injury requiring the second phase of treatment.

The second phase of treatment is aimed at detoxifying the enzyme-poisoning fluoride ion. Two ions, calcium (Ca^{2+}) and magnesium (Mg^{2+}) have been shown to be beneficial in binding the fluoride and curtailing its toxic effects. However, the overwhelming clinical experience to date has been with the use of calcium gluconate, and it should be considered the agent of choice at present. Three therapeutic modalities are available for using calcium gluconate: topical, subcutaneous/intradermal injection, or intraarterial infusion.

A calcium gluconate gel made of either Surgilube or dimethylsulfoxide (DMSO) in a 2.5 to 10% concentration may be applied directly to the affected area. The main limitation of topical therapy is the impermeability of the skin to calcium. Penetration into the dermis and subcutaneous tissues may be enhanced if the formulation with DMSO is used. The topical therapy can be utilized in the outpatient setting, and industries utilizing HF should keep this topical formulation on hand for emergency use.

Subcutaneous and intradermal injection of a 10% calcium gluconate solution through a 30-gauge needle into the HF-burned skin is the most widely used treatment. A maximum dose of 0.5 mL of 10% calcium gluconate per square centimeter of burned skin is recommended. Pain relief is near immediate, and indeed, the elimination of pain may be used as a guide for further therapy. Recurrence of pain indicates the need for further therapy. Unfortunately, injection therapy has several disadvantages: (1) only limited amounts of calcium are delivered to the tissue, (2) hyperosmolarity and inherent toxicity of free calcium ions cause more pain initially, and more tissue damage is possible if calcium is not bound to fluoride; (3) vascular compromise can result if too much fluid is injected, especially into digits; and (4) rapid penetration of HF beneath the nail requires nail removal to administer the calcium gluconate into the nail bed adequately.

Intraarterial infusion of calcium gluconate may be used to prevent tissue necrosis and stop the pain associated with HF burns. This should be performed as soon as possible after the initial burn, preferably within 6 h of insult. An intraarterial catheter should be placed in the appropriate vascular supply (the brachial artery if the entire hand is affected) and connected to a three-way stopcock to which is attached an arterial pressure monitoring device and the infusion syringe of calcium gluconate. A 50-mL syringe may be filled with 10 mL of a 10% calcium gluconate solution and 40 mL of 5% dextrose. This should be infused over 2 to 4 h. The arterial pressure monitoring device ensures that the catheter has not dislodged from the lumen of the cannulated artery. Infusion of the calcium solution into the deep tissues may cause further tissue damage. Repeat infusion may be needed if pain recurs within 4 h. This intraarterial infusion avoids the disadvantages of local infiltration therapy; however, it has its own disadvantages: an invasive vascular procedure (1) may result in arterial spasm or thrombosis and (2) requires more time and resources, including hospital admission.

Ocular exposure to HF requires water irrigation for at least 30 min. Treatment with calcium chloride or magnesium chloride by subconjunctival injection or irrigation may increase corneal damage.

Systemic toxicity related to dermal HF exposure has resulted in death. This appears to be related to myocardial irritability and subsequent ventricular fibrillation as a result of systemic acidosis, hyperkalemia, hypomagnesemia, and hypocalcemia. Cardiac monitoring, intravenous access, and electrolyte monitoring should be performed in all significant HF dermal burns.

Oxalic Acid

Oxalic acid is used for leather tanning and blueprint paper. Like hydrofluoric acid, it poisons enzymatic processes. Oxalic acid binds calcium and prevents muscle contraction. The burn wounds should be irrigated with water, intravenous calcium may be required. Serum electrolytes and renal function should be checked, and cardiac monitoring should be performed after serious dermal exposure.

ALKALIS

Alkalis penetrate the skin much more deeply and longer than acids, causing liquefaction necrosis of the tissue with danger of further toxicity from systemic absorption. Wounds may look superficial initially and in 2 to 3 days become full-thickness burns. Alkalis combine with protein and lipids in tissue to form soluble protein complexes and soaps which permit further passage of hydroxyl ions deep into tissue. Soft, gelatinous, friable, brownish eschars are often produced. Strong alkalis have a pH $\geq$ 12.

Lyes

Strong, corrosive alkalis termed "lyes" include ammonium, barium, calcium, lithium, potassium (caustic potash), and sodium (caustic soda) hydroxides. Lyes are widely used in industry and also found in home products such as drain and toilet cleaners, washing powders, and paint removers. The urine sugar reagent tablet Clinitest contains anhydrous sodium hydroxide. As a mode of assault, lyes cause lower mortality than gunshot wounds or stabbings, but victims often suffer long-term pain and cosmetic scarring and blindness. Lyes are extremely corrosive and penetrating, and burns require copious irrigation for long periods.

Lime

Lime (calcium oxide) is found in agriculture products and cements. It is converted by water to the alkali calcium hydroxide. Contact with lime draws water out of the skin. All dry particles should be brushed away prior to irrigation. Paradoxically, a small amount of water may generate an exothermic reaction with tissue injury secondary to calcium hyroxide formation. A large amount and strong stream of water taking care to avoid splashing in eyes should be used and will permit dissipation of heat. There is considerable variability of lime content in different grades of cement, with fine to textured masonry cement having more than concrete.

Portland Cement

Portland cement, which accounts for a major proportion of the cement used in the United States, is a mixture of sand, lime, and other metal oxides. In the presence of water, calcium hydroxide, sodium hyroxide, and potassium hydroxide may all be formed. Workers who kneel in wet cement or get cement in their boots may discover burns hours after initial contact. In addition, skin may become irritated from gritty material, and a contact dermatitis may develop in individuals sensitive to the chromate contained in the material.

Metals

Burns due to molten metal occur in foundry workers. Molten metal may spill or splash on body parts and may run down into the boots of workers. Elemental metals, sodium, lithium, potassium, magnesium, aluminum, and calcium may all cause burns. When exposed to air, some elemental metals spontaneously ignite. Water is generally contraindicated in extinguishing burning metal fragments embedded in the skin because the explosive exothermic reaction that may result can lead to significant tissue injury. Burning metal may be extinguished with a class D fire extinguisher or smothered with sand. Covering metal fragments with mineral oil, however, appears to be the favored treatment method. Wound debridement should include excision of metal fragments which cannot be wiped away. Metal fragments should be placed in mineral oil to prevent further accidents.

OTHERS

Hydrocarbons

Hydrocarbons will cause a fat-dissolving corrosive injury to the skin. In our present petroleum-dependent society, gasoline is a common agent of burns. Patients sustaining gasoline immersion burns usually have undergone some other traumatic insult (i.e., a motor vehicle accident). Gasoline is a complex mixture of alkanes, cycloalkanes, and aromatic hydrocarbons. The hydrocarbon chemical burn resembles either a thermal scald or a partial-thickness burn. Full-thickness burns secondary to prolonged contact with gasoline have been reported. Topical gasoline exposure in cold weather can result in frostbite of the digits due to rapid evaporation of gasoline resulting in heat loss from the skin. Any potential for systemic effects of the involved hydrocarbon (or what it was a solvent for) must be recognized, as this may expose the patient to greater morbidity than the skin damage. Dehydration of the skin associated with solvent contact contributes to injury. Treatment involves decontamination and otherwise management is as for a thermal burn.

Hot tar is derived from long-chain petroleum and coal hydrocarbons. Roofing tars and asphalt are heated to temperatures in excess of 500°F and the burns sustained are usually thought of more as thermal than chemical. Liquefaction injury to tissue can occur. Though the surface area size of the burn is usually small, solidified material, stuck to skin and hair is hard to remove. The tar should be cooled to prevent continued thermal injury. Manual mechanical debridement can be painful and destructive to skin structures. Polyoxylene sorbitan (polysorbate) contained in neosporin is an emulsifying agent that can be used to remove tar. De-solv-it, a citrus and petroleum distillate, is also reported effective in tar removal. The use of mayonnaise topically has been reported as a home remedy utilized in a similar fashion.

DMSO, Cantharides, and Mustard Gas

DMSO, cantharides, and mustard gas are considered to be vesicant agents. Skin burns with edema and blister formation can occur due to production of ischemia and anoxic necrosis at the site of contact. DMSO is a water-soluble organic solvent that has been used industrially since the 1940s. General therapeutic interest in DMSO began in the 1960s, when it was used by thousands of patents topically for sprains, bruises, minor burns, and arthritis. Its use has declined substantially because of eye toxicity, although it is still used for research and some clinical problems. Cantharides, "Spanish fly," is used as a veterinary aphrodisiac and occasionally by human beings as well for its supposed aphrodisiac effects. Mustard gas is a war gas that is unlikely to be seen in civilian practice. Burns resulting from vesicants should be irrigated copiously with water or saline. Mineral oil is also recommended for mustard gas burns.

Potassium Permanganate

Potassium permanganate is an oxidizing agent which is mildly irritating in dilute solution but in concentrated solution can produce dermal burns with a thick, brownish-purple eschar of coagulated protein. Burns should be copiously irrigated.

Alkyl Mercury Compounds

Alkyl mercury compounds are reducing agents used in disinfectants, fungicides, and wood preservatives. Alkyl mercury can produce dermatitis or burn lesions. Lesions typically are erythematous with blister formation. The blister fluid is high in metallic mercury content. The burning process continues as long as the agent remains in contact with skin. Partial-thickness burns deepen if the blister fluid is allowed to remain. The treatment is to debride, and remove blister fluid, and irrigate copiously.

Diquat Dibromide

Full-thickness skin burns have been reported to occur after prolonged exposure to the herbicide diquat dibromide. These burns were treated with skin grafting. It is unknown if earlier therapy would have prevented the chain of events.

Lacrimators (Chloroacetophenone and Chlorobenzylidenemalonitrile)

Lacrimators (tear gas) such as chloroacetophenone and chlorobenzylidenemalonitrile will cause skin and mucosal irritation and contact dermatitis. The epidermal injury is limited, in contrast to the possible pulmonary parenchymal damage. Burns to the skin are treated with standard water irrigation. Ocular irritation likewise is treated with copious water irrigation, followed by slit-lamp examination for evidence of corneal damage. Structural damage to the cornea occurs only at high concentrations of these lacrimators.

White Phosphorus

White phosphorus is a chemical used as an incendiary and in insecticides, rodenticides, and fertilizers. It can ignite spontaneously when exposed to air and is rapidly oxidized to phosphorus pentoxide. White phosphorus is commonly found in hand grenades and other warfare munitions and thus is implicated in wartime and accidental burns to military personnel. In munitions, white phosphorus is solid in form, but some of it may liquefy with detonation. Burns may be caused by liquid or solid forms. White phosphorus burns may be complicated by multiple traumatic injuries as a result of shell fragments and the force of weapon explosions. Because of its many uses, white phosphorus burns also occur in civilians.

Flaming droplets of inorganic phosphorus may embed beneath the skin. The heat of reaction can be directly destructive to tissue. Particles continue to oxidize slowly until either debrided, neutralized, or completely oxidized. Contaminated clothing should be removed. Debride visible particles and irrigate the burns copiously with normal saline or water. A brief rinse with 1% copper sulfate solution may be helpful. Copper sulfate combines with phosphorus to form a dark-copper phosphide coating on the particles which make them easier to see and debride and also impedes further oxidation. After copper sulfate use, the burn should be irrigated again to remove copper and prevent systemic copper toxicity.

OCULAR BURNS

Chemical burns to the eyes are common and considered true ocular emergencies requiring immediate treatment. Typically, chemical burns to the eye occur in the industrial setting, in laboratories, or as a result of accidents such as battery explosion and intentional assaults. Early signs and symptoms of eye burns include tearing, rubbing, redness, pain, and blepharospasm. Conjunctivas, if severely injured, may appear pale due to ischemia. Swelling of the corneal epithelium, clouding of the anterior chamber, pupillary dilatation, and corneal ulceration may all occur.

If the nature of the chemical is not known, pH paper should be used to determine the presence of acid or alkali. Acid quickly precipitates the superficial tissue proteins of the eye, but penetration is generally limited by local buffering and barrier effects. The damage sustained secondary to acid burns in most cases is immediate and limited to the area of contact. The posterior segment of the eye rarely suffers injury, and there are usually no late effects such as cell disruption or tissue softening.

Alkali burns are much more serious, and results are frequently unsightly and disastrous. In general, the higher the pH of the alkali, the more damage occurs. In a short period of time, strong alkali can penetrate the cornea, anterior chamber, and the retina with destruction of all sensory elements, thus causing complete blindness. Alkali combines with cellular membrane lipids, resulting in cell disruption and tissue softening. Severe disruption of stromal mucopolysaccharides of the cornea occurs. The penetration of alkali can continue for hours to days. An opaque, marbled appearance of the cornea and even perforation may occur with deep injury. Conjunctival and scleral blood vessels and collecting veins of the anterior chamber may be destroyed, leading to secondary glaucoma.

Chronic inflammation of the iris and ciliary body (iridocyclitis) and adhesions between lens and iris (posterior synechiae) are complications. Other complications of eye burns include ectropion (lid deformity), cataract formation, scarring and marked revascularization of the cornea, and scarring of both palpebral and bulbar conjunctiva with resulting adhesions between the lids and globe (symblepharon).

Treatment of eye burns should begin immediately with the rare exception of burns from chemicals that react violently with water. Immediate treatment is copious and continuous irrigation at the scene, in transport, and at the hospital. Time should not be wasted in search for a neutralizing substance. Special eye-irrigating kits may be used, but in general IV tubing set up using 1 to 2 L of normal saline for 1-h continuous irrigation is the minimum treatment, particularly for alkali burns.

Acid burns may not require as much volume or treatment time. Twenty-four hours or more of continuous irrigation for alkali burns has been recommended by some. Checking the pH in the conjunctival sac to see if it has returned to normal may be helpful in determining need for further irrigation (tears have a pH between 7.3 to 7.7). The eyelid may have to be held open manually or with retractors due to severe orbicularis spasm. The eyelids should be everted if they are not too edematous. All particulate matter should be removed using a moistened cotton applicator or forceps.

Pain control with topical anesthetics initially and subsequent systemic analgesics may be necessary. Cycloplegics, mydriatics, and antibiotics should be used and the use of an eye patch may encourage corneal reepithelialization. The patient should be hospitalized and ophthalmology consultation obtained for severe burns.

Another treatment modality is the use of collagenase inhibitors such as cysteine and acetylcysteine (Mucomyst) to prevent loss of corneal stroma which occurs with liberation of collagenase from injured corneal and conjunctival epithelium. Topical steroids may reduce iridocyclitis but may also exacerbate collagenase-induced corneal ulceration. Use of scleral contact lens may reduce adhesions and scarring. Agents to reduce intraocular pressure should be used if glaucoma develops. Paracentesis may be required in severe alkali burns to introduce sterile phosphate buffer solution into the anterior chamber in attempt to reduce the pH of the inner eye. Surgery to the eye is usually not indicated during the early phase of burn management unless for corneal grafting following corneal perforation. Blepharoplasty, keratoplasty, or keratoprosthesis may be eventually required.

IATROGENIC CHEMICAL BURNS

Iatrogenic chemical burns have been caused by the use of potassium permanganate for dermatologic problems at an inappropriately high concentration. DMSO used as a transcutaneous vehicle for minor sprains has caused burns. Patients in the operating room may develop burns from skin prep solutions. Thimerosal, which has a high mercury content, is the most common agent implicated. Mechanical abrasion of the skin from scrubbing and from pooling of the skin prep agent under the torso or tourniquet predisposes to burns. Blister formation, skin sloughing, and eschar development has been reported in neonates when isopropyl alcohol pledgets were substituted for conducting paste beneath limb ECG electrodes.

SYSTEMIC TOXICITY

Death early after severe chemical burns is usually related to hypotension, acute tubular necrosis, and shock as a result of fluid loss. However, systemic toxicity and subsequent morbidity and mortality may also occur with some chemicals which are absorbed through denuded dermis. Acidosis, hypotension, and shock can occur with significant absorption of acids. Hypocalcemia has been reported with both oxalic acid and hydrofluoric acid burns. Profound hypocalcemia and hypomagnesemia may be accompanied by hyperkalemia, cardiac arrhythmias, and sudden death. Tannic acid, chromic acid, formic acid, picric acid, and phosphorus may cause hepatic necrosis and nephrotoxicity. Cresol can cause methemoglobinemia and massive hemolysis. Gasoline immersion with large surface area exposure and absorption of hydrocarbon aromatic components may result in severe pulmonary, cardiovascular, neurologic, renal, and hepatic complications. The gasoline lead additives such as tetraethyl and tetramethyl can cause lead encephalopathy. Carburetor cleaning solvent containing phenol and methylene chloride may cause renal and hepatic failure. Phenol (carbolic acid) when absorbed can lead to intravascular hemolysis, cardiovascular, pulmonary, and central nervous system toxicity. The use of phenol as a skin disinfectant by medical personnel in the 1800s caused chronic toxicity (carbolic marasmus) characterized by weight loss, vertigo, salivation, and increased skin and scleral pigmentation.

Sodium nitrate and potassium nitrate can cause a severe toxic methemoglobinemia from absorption with refractory cyanosis. Significant absorption of dichromate solution can result in liver failure and acute tubular necrosis and death despite hemodialysis.

Just as with thermal burns, overwhelming sepsis can be a systemic complication with chemical burns.

CONCLUSION

Although chemical burns are not a frequent problem in many emergency departments, certain unique characteristics, particularly in the initial stages of treatment, justify considering them separately from the other types of burns.

The diversity of chemical agents and the increasing number of new products present a challenge for emergency treatment of chemical burns. Use of protective garb by individuals handling chemicals and cautionary labeling of hazardous chemicals and awareness of first-aid measures are essential. Maintenance of information and treatment protocols by regional poison centers and emergency departments is also of utmost importance. The mainstay of treatment for most, but not all, agents will continue to be early irrigation with copious water. Proper management for some specific chemicals requires identification and knowledge of their toxic actions. After initial treatment measures, basic burn care principles should be followed and appropriate consultation should be obtained as needed.

BIBLIOGRAPHY

Caravati EM: Acute hydrofluoric acid exposure. *Am J Emerg Med* 6:143, 1988.

Carney SA, Hall M, Lawrence JC, et al: Rationale of the treatment of hydrofluoric acid burns. Br J Ind Med 31:317, 1974.

Curreri PW, Asch MJ, Pruitt BA: The treatment of chemical burns: Specialized diagnostic therapeutic, and prognostic considerations. J Trauma 10:634, 1970.

Emmett EA: Toxic responses of the skin, in Klaassen CD, Amdur MO, Doull J (eds): *Cassaret and Doull's Toxicology: The Basic Science of Poisons.* New York, Macmillan, 1986, pp 412–423.

Goldberg MF, Paton D: Ocular emergencies, In Peyman GA, Sanders DR, Goldberg MF (eds): *Principles and Practice of Ophthalmology.* Philadelphia, Saunders, 1980, pp. 2425–2512.

Guzzardi LJ: Chemical injuries to skin, in Rosen P, Baker FJ, Barkin RM, et al: *Emergency Medicine: Concepts and Clinical Practice.* St. Louis, Mosby, 1988, pp 617–620.

Hansbrough JF, Zapata-Sirvent R, Dominic W, et al: Hydrocarbons contact injuries. *J Trauma* 25:250, 1985.

Jelenko C: Chemicals that "burn." *J Trauma* 14:65, 1974.

Konjoyan TR: White phosphorus burns: Case report and literature review. *Military Med* 148:881, 1983.

Leonard LG, Scheulen JJ, Munster AM: Chemical burns: Effect of prompt first aid. *J Trauma* 22:420, 1982.

Luterman A, Curreri PW: Chemical burn injury in Boswick JA (ed): *The Art and Science of Burn Care.* Rockville, MD, Aspen, 1987, pp 233–239.

Stewart CE: Chemical skin burns. *AFP* 31:149, 1985.

Vance MV, Curry SC, Kunkel DB, et al: Digital hydrofluoric acid burns: Treatment with intraarterial calcium infusion. *Ann Emerg Med* 15:890, 1986.

125 LIGHTNING INJURIES

Mary Ann Cooper

Lightning injuries have little relation to injuries from high-voltage electricity or other burn mechanisms. While lightning is an electrical phenomenon and follows the same laws of physics governing electricity, the substantial differences in the properties of a lightning strike account for the differences in the types and severity of injuries seen. Treating victims of natural electricity as though they were victims of human-generated electricity may cause significant morbidity and mortality. Lightning kills approximately 100 to 200 persons annually in the United States, more than most other natural disasters combined.

PATHOPHYSIOLOGY OF LIGHTNING INJURY

The voltage of lightning may vary from a few million to 2 billion V, usually averaging about 10 to 30 million V for most strikes. The current may reach from 2000 to 300,000 A. Normal human-produced-electricity exposures are much lower, seldom exceeding 70,000 V in the most devastating cases. Lightning, being more like a direct current, acts as a massive cosmic countershock, causing asystole and respiratory arrest, unlike the more common alternating current of human-produced electricity, which tends to cause venticular fibrillation.

The factor that seems to make the greatest difference in the injury complex is the duration of the electrical exposure. With generated electricity, the contact tends to be prolonged, with resulting skin breakdown and sustained flow of electric current internally, causing extensive, deep internal damage to muscles, blood vessels, nerves, and other structures.

Lightning, on the other hand, normally has a duration of from 0.1 to 10 ms. The exposure is rarely long enough to cause breakdown of the skin, the primary insulator of the body to current flow. The current instead passes over the outside of the body, the so-called flashover phenomenon, similar to the current flow along the outside of a metal conductor. The majority of the current thus passes outside the body. If the victim is wet from sweat or rainwater, the flow of current may cause secondary first- and second-degree burns as the fluid in the sweat lines is turned into steam. In addition, the clothes may be exploded off by the sudden expansion of the water turning into steam under them. Because of the flashover phenomenon, true entry and exit burns are rare and internal injuries normally encountered with high-voltage electrical burns occur in less than 10 percent of cases.

MECHANISMS OF INJURY

There are six main mechanisms of injury with lightning injury:

1. Direct strike
2. Contact voltage
3. Side flash or splash
4. Ground or stride voltage
5. Thermal burning
6. Blunt injury

Direct strike is self-evident. Contact voltage occurs when the victim is touching an object, such as a tent pole or a tree, that is struck by lightning. Side flash or splash occurs when lightning hits a tree, building, or other relatively high resistance object and splashes off to a victim that may offer less resistance to the current flow. Side flashes may also occur from other people, which is why persons should not stand close together or under trees in thunderstorms. Ground current, step voltage, or stride voltage injury occurs when the victim has one leg or some other portion of the body touching the ground closer to the strike point than another part of the body. This produces a potential difference between the parts and may cause a current to flow between them or around them. Thermal burning may occur when metal objects worn by the victim become super-heated or when lightning ignites the clothing.

Blunt injuries may occur from a number of mechanisms. The victim may be thrown a distance by the strike and suffer blunt injuries. In addition, lightning has an explosive effect in that as it passes through the atmosphere it heats the air channel through which it passes to 8000°C. This causes rapid expansion, a shock wave later heard by bystanders as thunder, and then an almost equally rapid implosion of air as the channel quickly cools to 1500 to 2000°C. Several cases of contusion, blunt injury, fractures, and dislocations have been reported.

It is not unusual for multiple victims to be injured by a single strike. They may show many different levels and mechanisms of injury. In addition, since lightning can strike twice in the same place, rescuers should be aware of continuing danger if rescue takes place in the middle of the thunderstorm.

DIFFERENTIAL DIAGNOSIS

In the past, lightning injuries have been confused with seizures, subarachnoid hemorrhages and other cerebral vascular catastrophies, cardiac arrhythmias and myocardial infarction, assaults, spinal cord and head injuries, and heavy metal poisoning. Points that may be helpful in distinguishing the diagnoses are

1. History of a recent thunderstorm
2. Outdoor occurrence of the accident
3. Tympanic membrane injury
4. Younger age of the victims
5. Multiple victims
6. Superficial linear or punctate burns or pathognomonic arborescent patterns
7. Partial or complete clothing disintegration

INJURIES AND THEIR TREATMENT

Injuries vary with the part of the body or body system involved with the lightning strike. Despite the flashover phenomenon, a small amount of current may still leak through the body, or perhaps be induced in the body. While studies have shown that lightning injuries usually have only a 20 to 30 percent mortality, morbidity and permanent sequelae are common in up to two-thirds of the survivors.

Cardiorespiratory System Injuries

The almost universal cause of death is cardiac arrest. Lightning acts as a massive countershock, sending the heart into asystole that is usually temporary in the otherwise healthy young adults that are most often its victims. Unfortunately, the respiratory arrest that often accompanies the cardiac arrest may last significantly longer than the cardiac event, often causing enough hypoxia that the heart goes into a secondary arrest from arrhythmias and eventually into ventricular fibrillation. Triage of multiple victims should take this phenomenon into account. If the victim is moaning and groaning and showing some signs of life, then at least a degree of stability of the vital signs can be presumed, and recovery, even with sequelae, is the rule. Those without signs of life, on the other hand, may still potentially be resuscitated with appropriate intervention, including cardiopulmonary resuscitation.

Elevation of the creatine phosphokinase cardiac (MB) fraction, electrocardiographic evidence of ischemia and injury, arrhythmias, myocardial necrosis on necropsy, and both immediate and delayed pulmonary edema have been reported. Cardiac damage may be from a number of mechanisms including arterial spasm, direct myocardial damage, and blunt injury. Pulmonary contusion, rib fractures, and other evidence of blunt injury have also been reported.

Advanced cardiac life support protocols do not need to be modified for victims of lightning injury. Treatment of arrhythmias is standard. All victims should have an electrocardiogram and, because of the reports of delayed congestive heart failure, should probably be monitored for several hours. Asymptomatic patients may still go on to have serious cardiac dysfunction. Victims should also have serial cardiac enzymes if there is evidence of damage or if there is chest pain. The use of prophylactic lidocaine and other antiarrhythmic agents may be efficacious but has not been tested. Other critical care and supportive therapy, as indicated by the patient's status, should be given.

Of patients who present to the emergency department with vital signs, a few may exhibit transient hypertension which need not be treated.

Burns

Burns from lightning are usually superficial and minor unless the patients have suffered significant thermal burns from the ignition of their clothing. Burns which do occur may be treated in the standard fashion. Because the burns usually are so superficial, deep muscle damage and the resulting myoglobinuria is rare but should be tested for. Fluid loading, the use of mannitol and other diuretics to take care of myoglobinuria, and fasciotomies and escharotomies are rarely required. In fact, fluid loading may further complicate a patient with cerebral edema and should be done cautiously, if at all, unless the patient is in shock for other reasons. Tetanus prophylaxis should be instituted according to the patient's immunization status.

Neurologic Injuries

In addition to cardiac complications, neurologic signs and symptoms are usually the most worrisome. Almost two-thirds of severely injured patients present with lower extremity paralysis, and one-third with upper extremity paralysis. The extremities appear cold, lifeless, mottled, insensitive, and pulseless. While this is usually due to vascular spasm and sympathetic instability and resolves in a few hours, some patients will have permanent paresis and paresthesia. A complete neurologic exam with serial updates is mandatory. Direct or blunt injury to the spinal cord should be ruled out if the symptoms do not resolve.

Seizures may occur as a presenting or complicating event. Any hypoxia should be corrected and seizures treated in the standard fashion, including ruling out intracranial lesions such as subdural and epidural hematomas. A patient with a decreasing level of consciousness should have immediate computed tomography.

A patient who presents unconscious and unresponsive has a grave prognosis. Coma may be a result of prolonged hypoxia prior to resuscitation but may also be a result of closed head injury. Fluid restriction should be the rule, and computed tomography is indicated to rule out a surgically correctable lesion. Hypothermia should also be considered as a cause of coma since many of these patients are wet and have a significant potential for hypothermia.

It is not uncommon for the alert victim to be somewhat confused for a few days or have permanent amnesia for the events of the first few days after the shock, similar to a patient who has had electroconvulsive shock therapy. A few have even reported permanent personality changes and psychiatric illness after the strike.

A victim may also have permanent neurologic sequelae of paraplegia, hemiplegia, paresis, neuritis and neuralgia, trouble with fine calculations or other mental functions, difficulty with balance, insomnia, panic attacks, intermittent sympathetic activity, chronic subdural hematoma, aphasia, and symptoms of post-traumatic stress disorder.

Table 125-1. Minimum Laboratory Examinations for Lightning Victims

CBC
UA for myoglobin, if present; BUN, creatinine
Cardiac isoenzymes
ECG, monitor
Appropriate x-rays, including CT scan if decreasing LOC

Eyes

Cataracts are common and may occur either at the time of the injury or up to 2 years after the incident. Optic nerve damage, retinal separation and perforation, uveitis, and iritis have all been reported. As a result of some of these, dilated unresponsive pupils cannot be taken as a sign of brain death in lightning victims.

Ears

Over 50 percent of lightning victims have tympanic membrane rupture, either unilateral or bilateral, which may be from the concussive force, from basilar skull fracture, or a direct burn. It is often missed because the physician forgets to look for it and does not expect it. Treatment consists of removal of blood and debris. Surgical repair of any defects is usually done at a later date after ossicular necrosis, disruption, and other injuries have had a chance to mature to the point of proper evaluation and intervention. The physician should also be alert to the possibility of a cerebrospinal fluid leak.

Musculoskeletal System

Fractures of the scapulae, clavicles, skull, and long bones have been reported but seem to be less common with lightning injuries than with high-voltage electrical injuries. Dislocations may also occur. Blunt injuries should always be sought because of the mechanisms of injury already mentioned.

Fetal Survival

Roughly half of the lightning strikes in pregnancy result in fetal wastage, one-fourth in neonatal death, and one-fourth in healthy living children with no signs of any injury. Outcome predictions based on the trimester in which the strike occurred or other factors cannot be made because of the extremely low number of cases reported.

Laboratory Examinations

Minimum laboratory examinations are listed in Table 125-1. More extensive laboratory analysis, x-rays, and monitoring may be indicated depending on the severity of the injury and presenting symptoms and signs of the patient.

BIBLIOGRAPHY

Andrews CJ, Darveniza M: Telephone-mediated lightning injury. An Australian survey. *J Trauma* 29:665, 1989.

Bellucci RJ: Traumatic injuries of the middle ear. *Otolaryngol Clin North Am* 16:633, 1983.

Chia BL: Electrocardiographic abnormalities and congestive cardiac failure due to lightning stroke. *Cardiology* 68:49, 1981.

Cooper MA: Prognosis signs for death in patients seriously injured by lightning. *Ann Emerg Med* 9:134, 1980.

Cwinn AA, Cantrill SV: Lightning injuries. *J Emerg Med* 2:379, 1985.

Jackson SHD, Parry DJ: Lightning and the heart. *Br Heart J* 43:454, 1980.

McCrady-Kahn VL, Kahn AM: Lightning burns. *West J Med* 134:215, 1981.

Peters WJ: Lightning injury. *Can Med Assoc J* 128:148, 1983.

126
CARBON MONOXIDE POISONING

Earl J. Reisdorff
John G. Wiegenstein

Carbon monoxide (CO) is the single leading cause of toxin-related death in the United States. It causes 3800 accidental and suicidal deaths annually. The incidence of nonlethal CO poisoning is not established. CO is a colorless, odorless, nonirritating gas. Its specific gravity is 0.97 relative to air, so it does not stratify. CO has a high affinity for hemoglobin. It reversibly displaces oxygen from hemoglobin to produce carboxyhemoglobin (COHb), resulting in tissue hypoxia.

The symptoms of CO poisoning are protean and vague, resulting in a high rate of misdiagnosis. Correct treatment requires aggressive oxygen therapy and using hyperbaric oxygen (HBO) when necessary.

SOURCES

Carbon monoxide is endogenously produced during the metabolism of heme pigments. When protoporphyrin is converted into bilirubin, CO is released. This generates 75 percent of the endogenous production of CO, producing a serum COHb level of less than 1.0. This level varies during the menstrual cycle and pregnancy. Higher levels (4 to 6 percent) are seen with acute hemolytic anemia due to the accelerated metabolism of hemoglobin. CO is eliminated primarily unchanged during pulmonary respiration, though a small amount is metabolized to CO_2.

Exogenous CO is produced by the incomplete combustion of organic fuels. Gas-powered engines produce significant amounts of CO. Other sources include furnaces, home water heaters, gas heaters, pool heaters, wood stoves, kerosene heaters, indoor charcoal fires, and Sterno fuel. Industrial sources include steel foundries, pulp paper mills, and plants producing formaldehyde and coke. Fire fighters are at high risk, and most immediate deaths from building fires are due to CO poisoning. All patients from a fire scene must, therefore, be evaluated for CO toxicity.

Tobacco smoke is a significant source of CO. Serum COHb levels in smokers are usually between 5 and 15 percent, but may reach 20 percent. These levels can compromise patients with preexisting cardiopulmonary disease. Furthermore, CO toxicity from cigarette smoking has been implicated as a major factor in atherogenesis. It is also known to be a precipitating factor in angina, myocardial infarction, and cardiac arrhythmias. Smoke released from the tip of the cigarette contains 2.5 times more CO than the inhaled smoke. Cigarette smoking in poorly ventilated rooms can cause CO toxicity in the exposed nonsmoker.

Methylene chloride is found in many paint removers and its vapors are readily absorbed through the lungs. In the liver it is converted into CO. Since methylene chloride is stored in tissues and gradually released, the CO elimination half-life in patients exposed to this substance is twice that of inhaled CO.

PATHOPHYSIOLOGY

The pathophysiology of CO poisoning is not completely understood. Laboratory studies have yielded conflicting results. Nevertheless, four mechanisms explaining the toxic effects of CO have been proposed: (1) tissue hypoxia, (2) shift in the oxygen-hemoglobin dissociation curve, (3) direct cardiovascular depression, and (4) inhibition of cytochrome A_3.

Tissue Hypoxia

Carbon monoxide readily crosses the pulmonary alveolar membrane. It acts as a competitive inhibitor of oxygen binding by reversibly coupling with hemoglobin. The affinity of CO for hemoglobin is 240 times greater than the affinity of oxygen for hemoglobin. This results in high serum COHb levels from exposures to environments with relatively low partial pressures of CO. When inhaled air contains 0.01% CO, the resulting serum COHb level is 10 percent. The net effect of COHb production is a reduction of the oxygen-carrying capacity in the blood. This produces tissue hypoxia, the predominant toxicologic property of CO.

Shifting the Oxygen-Hemoglobin Curve

The tissue hypoxia caused by the formation of COHb does not adequately explain the toxic effects of CO. Hemoglobin has four binding sites for oxygen. When CO binds to one of these sites, the remaining three oxygen molecules are held more tightly by the hemoglobin molecule. This shifts the oxygen-hemoglobin curve to the left, further reducing the amount of oxygen available at the cellular level.

Cardiovascular Depression

The extravascular compartment stores 10 to 15 percent of the total body CO. This portion is bound to hemeproteins including cytochrome P_{450}, cytochrome A_3, and myoglobin. Most of the extravascular CO is bound to myoglobin. Carboxymyoglobin levels are markedly increased in the presence of hypoxia and high serum COHb concentrations. Since carboxymyoglobin dissociates slower than COHb, a rebound increase of the serum COHb level may occur after treatment. After the serum COHb decreases, the myoglobin releases the bound CO, causing an increase in the serum COHb concentration.

Carbon monoxide preferentially binds to cardiac myoglobin at a 3:1 ratio compared to skeletal myoglobin. Carboxymyoglobin reduces the amount of oxygen available to the myocardium and may result in myocardial depression. A decrease in myocardial performance may result in hypotension and cerebral ischemia.

Inhibition of Cytochrome A_3

Carbon monoxide may also bind to cytochrome P_{450} and cytochrome A_3. The significance of cytochrome P_{450} binding is not known. CO inhibits the cytochrome oxidase system in vitro, leading to a depression of mitochondrial respiration. This inhibition of the cytochrome system may explain the profound neurologic depression which may persist long after COHb levels have been lowered to "nontoxic" levels.

Oxygen has a nine times higher affinity for cytochrome A_3 than has CO. Opponents to the cytochrome-inhibition theory contend that the low affinity of CO for cytochrome A_3 prohibits sufficient binding of CO to cytochrome to cause inhibition of cellular respiration. Prolonged exposure to CO in a hypoxic environment, however, can lead to moderate CO-cytochrome binding, suppressing mitochondrial respiration. A recent study shows that small amounts of dissolved CO can inhibit cellular respiration in a nonhypoxic system.

CLINICAL PRESENTATION

The manifestations of CO poisoning are often vague, leading to frequent misdiagnoses with subsequent delays in therapy. Initial symptoms commonly include headache, dizziness, weakness, and nausea. CO poisoning is often misdiagnosed as "flu," gastroenteritis, and psychiatric disorders. It is confused less frequently with stroke, migraine, delirium tremens, myocardial ischemia, cerebral tumor, atypical pneumonia, epilepsy, and cholecystitis.

Routine CO screening of emergency patients during the winter months revealed a 2.8 percent incidence of elevated CO levels. With patients complaining of headache during colder months, a similar incidence was found.

In addition, physicians were unable to predict elevated COHb levels in patients. At the scene of the exposure, COHb levels correlate fairly well to symptoms (see Table 126-1). When patients are removed from

Table 126-1. Signs and Symptoms at Various Carboxyhemoglobin Concentrations

COHb Level, %	Signs and Symptoms
0	Usually none
10	Frontal headache
20	Throbbing headache, dyspnea with exertion
30	Impaired judgment, nausea, dizziness, visual disturbance, fatigue
40	Confusion, syncope
50	Coma, seizures
60	Hypotension, respiratory failure
70	Death

CO or have been breathing 100% oxygen, there is a poor correlation between COHb levels and the clinical manifestations. Despite "non-toxic" COHb levels after treatment, patients may still demonstrate signs of severe poisoning. Patients may lapse into coma and die without intermediary symptoms when exposed to high levels of CO. Low-level exposures over a long period of time may be more harmful than high-level exposures over a brief time, though COHb levels may be similar. It is therefore important that a serum sample be drawn by emergency medical personnel at the scene. The field specimen COHb level will correlate best with the clinical presentation.

SYSTEMIC MANIFESTATIONS

Cardiac

Although CO poisoning affects every organ system (see Table 126-2), the brain and heart, having the highest metabolic requirements, are most susceptible to CO toxicity. Most deaths from CO exposure result from cardiac arrhythmias. When coronary artery disease is present, a low serum COHb level can produce myocardial ischemia and infarction. Myocardial ischemia is most prominent in the subendocardial and subepicardial regions of the ventricles. This may produce papillary muscle dysfunction, abnormal ventricular wall motion, and mitral valve prolapse. The electrocardiogram often reflects ischemia, showing ST-segment and T-wave abnormalities. Atrial flutter, atrial fibrillation, premature ventricular tachycardia, and conduction system disturbances are also seen. The ventricular fibrillation threshold is lowered by CO. Pathologic changes associated with CO toxicity include focal leukocyte infiltration, punctate hemorrhage, myocardial necrosis, and mural thrombi with coronary artery embolization. These often resolve completely in 1 to 2 weeks. More severe lesions are seen with preexisting coronary artery disease.

Ophthalmologic

Visual disturbances are frequent and correlate well with the duration of exposure. Funduscopic examination may reveal flame-shaped retinal hemorrhages. They are caused by hypoxia and may be unilateral. The hemorrhages often resolve without visual deficit. A more sensitive indicator of CO toxicity is the presence of red retinal veins. These may be seen before the mucous membranes become erythematous and appear at lower COHb levels. Blindness is infrequent and is usually temporary.

Dermatologic

The classic "cherry-red" skin of CO poisoning is rarely seen; more often, victims are pale or cyanotic. Dermal necrosis with bullae formation may occur anywhere, but especially at pressure point areas in the comatose patient and over areas of myonecrosis. Myonecrosis from pressure or prolonged tissue hypoxia may cause rhabdomyolysis, a potential cause of renal failure. Other dermal changes include sweat gland necrosis, alopecia, edema, and erythematous patches.

Table 126-2. Reported Complications of Carbon Monoxide Poisoning

System Involved	Complication
Neuropsychiatric	Coma, seizures, agitation, leukoencephalopathy, cerebral edema, behavioral disorders, decreased cognitive ability, Tourette-like syndrome, mutism, fecal and urinary incontinence, parietal lobe dysfunction, ataxia, muscular rigidity, parkinsonism, peripheral neuropathy, psychosis, memory impairment, gait disturbance, abnormal EEG, personality changes
Cardiovascular	Angina, tachycardia, ST-segment changes, hypotension, arrhythmias, myocardial infarction, heart block
Pulmonary	Pulmonary edema and hemorrhage, unilateral diaphragmatic paralysis
Ophthalmologic	Flame-shaped retinal hemorrhages, decreased light sensitivity, decreased visual acuity, cortical blindness, retrobulbar neuritis, papilledema, paracentral scotomas
Vestibular and auditory	Central hearing loss, tinnitus, vertigo, nystagmus
Gastrointestinal	Vomiting, diarrhea, hepatic necrosis, hematochezia, melena
Dermatologic	Bullae, alopecia, sweat gland necrosis, "cherry-red" skin color (rare), edema, cyanosis, pallor, erythematous patches
Hematologic	Disseminated intravascular coagulation, thrombotic thrombocytopenic purpura, leukocytosis
Musculoskeletal	Rhabdomyolysis, myonecrosis, compartment syndrome
Renal	Acute renal failure secondary to myoglobinuria, proteinuria
Metabolic	Lactic acidosis, nonpancreatic hyperamylasemia, diabetes insipidus, hyperglycemia, hypocalcemia
Fetal	Death, cerebral atrophy, microcephalus, low birth weight, psychomotor retardation, seizures, spasticity

Other

Other physiologic effects of CO poisoning include noncardiogenic pulmonary edema, bowel ischemia, hepatic failure, vestibular dysfunction, hearing loss, disseminated intravascular coagulation, and thrombotic thrombocytopenic purpura.

Fetal

Of all patients receiving HBO in New York City, 10 percent are pregnant. In pregnancy, the fetus is particularly susceptible, as CO readily crosses the placenta. During exposure, fetal COHb levels lag behind the maternal level, achieving equilibration after 14 to 24 h. After equilibration with maternal blood, fetal COHb levels are 10 to 15 percent higher than maternal levels. In addition, because of the fetal oxygen-hemoglobin dissociation curve, small amounts of COHb can markedly decrease the fetal oxygen tension and content. The normal fetal Pa_{O_2} is about 20 mmHg, with an oxygen content of 12 mL/dL. Fetal elimination of CO is prolonged, resulting in a fetal CO elimination half-life that is three and a half times longer than that of the mother. Pregnant women should receive more aggressive and prolonged oxygen therapy. Longo suggests that the mother should receive oxygen for a period five times longer than the time period needed to complete just the maternal course of therapy. For example, if 4 h is required to completely treat the mother, an additional 20 h of oxygen treatment is required. Fetal heart tones should be obtained and cardiotachodynomanometry instituted at 20 weeks' gestation or greater. Up to 80 percent of children born to women surviving CO poisoning have neurologic sequelae. In addition, CO is teratogenic and causes lower-birth-weight infants. Fetal death has occurred in as many as 50 percent of cases of nonlethal maternal poisoning. Fetal demise may be seen immediately, or be delayed. Fetal outcome roughly correlates to maternal symptoms at the time of CO exposure; there is no relationship between fetal death and maternal HbCO concentrations.

Pediatric

Children make up 37 percent of patients receiving HBO therapy; children less than 5 years old account for 25 percent of victims receiving HbCO. Among acutely exposed children, as many as 17 percent die and 48 percent require cardiopulmonary resuscitation (CPR). Most childhood deaths from CO poisoning are fire-related. Newborns are more susceptible to the effects of CO poisoning due to a higher fetal hemoglobin concentration which shifts the oxygen-hemoglobin curve to the left.

In children, in whom nausea is a common complaint, CO toxicity is frequently misdiagnosed as acute gastroenteritis; in young infants it can be confused with colic. Children are frequently affected by riding in the back seats of cars with faulty exhaust systems. In fact, children riding in the same vehicle can have different symptoms with the same HbCO levels, or have markedly different HbCO levels from the same exposure. CO toxicity has been implicated as the cause for some cases of sudden infant death.

The treatment of CO toxicity for children is similar to that for adults; however, myringotomy is more commonly performed in children undergoing HBO therapy.

Neurologic

Since the brain has high oxygen requirement, most acute symptoms are related to the central nervous system (CNS). In a mass exposure of 184 victims, the most common complaints were headache (90 percent), dizziness (82 percent), and weakness (53 percent). The most significant pathologic changes of the brain seen with CO poisoning are white matter lesions. These include white matter demyelination, edema, focal and laminar necrosis, and petechiae. Lesions of the hippocampus are reported in half of the cases. Gray matter lesions also occur in the watershed area between the anterior and middle cerebral arteries. The characteristic pathologic injury of CO poisoning is bilateral lesions of the globus pallidus. These lesions are seen with other hypoxic-ischemic insults and may be unilateral or asymmetric. The globus pallidus lesions cannot be entirely explained by the hypoxic effect of CO. The lesions are most likely the result of hypoxia with concomitant ischemia. This area has relatively low oxygen requirements, protecting it from pure hypoxia, but it has a poor blood supply, making it vulnerable to hypoperfusion. Low-density lesions of the globus pallidus demonstrated on CT scan are associated with a high incidence of neurologic sequelae.

Neurologic abnormalities are frequent in acute poisoning (Table 126-2). The most common neurologic complaints are headache, dizziness, agitation, stupor, seizures, and coma. Other aberrations include behavioral disorders, decreased cognitive ability, gait disturbance, parkinsonism, mutism, tic disorders, and impairment of parietal lobe functions. Long-term psychiatric and neurologic sequelae are grossly apparent in 11 percent of survivors. Memory impairment occurs in up to 43 percent. The most common personality change, "affective incontinence," is characterized by emotional lability and may be a consequence of damage to the hippocampus. Resolution of the neurologic sequelae, when it occurs, may take 2 years. These deficits may be permanent.

A syndrome of delayed neurologic sequelae has been described. Delayed sequelae usually occur after coma from a prolonged exposure. The patient recovers, has a symptom-free interval, then undergoes rapid neurologic deterioration. In 10 to 30 percent of poisonings, neuropsychiatric symptoms will appear within 2 to 3 weeks after exposure. The common symptoms are mental deterioration, urinary and fecal incontinence, and gait disturbance. Complete recovery occurs in two-thirds. Older patients are at greater risk for developing delayed sequelae. Diffuse demyelinization of white matter is associated with delayed deterioration. More aggressive oxygen therapy may reduce the incidence of sequelae.

EVALUATION AND LABORATORY STUDIES

The diagnosis of CO poisoning is based primarily on the history. If patients have been removed from the CO-containing environment and given 100% oxygen, COHb levels may be deceptively normal. A high index of suspicion for CO poisoning is required, particularly in patients with nonspecific complaints during the winter months.

The evaluation of the CO poisoning victim must be guided by the situation. For example, the fire victim must be inspected for thermal airway injury, cyanide toxicity, or other toxic gas inhalation. When evaluating those attempting suicide, a routine drug screen and measurement of ethanol, phenobarbital, salicylate, and acetaminophen levels may be required. Asymptomatic individuals with minor exposure do not require as extensive evaluations.

A carboxyhemoglobin level should be obtained in all cases. This should not delay the administration of 100% oxygen. Levels should be obtained by a modified spectrophotometric blood gas analyzer or, less accurately, by measuring expired CO concentration with a handheld breath analyzer. A high expired CO concentration or serum COHb level confirms CO poisoning, but a low level does not exclude the diagnosis.

An arterial blood gas measurement will typically reveal a normal Pa_{O_2}. The Pa_{O_2} is a measurement of the dissolved oxygen in arterial blood, not the amount of oxygen bound to hemoglobin. Many blood gas analyzers calculate the percentage of oxygen saturation based on the Pa_{O_2}. Since the amount of oxygen dissolved in the blood is not affected by CO, the calculated oxygen saturations are falsely high when compared to those directly measured by oximetry. This "saturation gap" is characteristic of CO poisoning.

An ECG should be performed on patients with cardiac symptoms, coronary artery disease, altered mental status, or a COHb level greater than 10 percent. The ECG is often abnormal. Sinus tachycardia and ST-segment changes are the most frequently seen aberrations, although almost any abnormality may be present.

Serial creatine phosphokinase (CPK) and lactic dehydrogenase (LDH) levels assist in determining myocardial damage. The CPK is frequently elevated. Isoenzymes, especially of the CPK, differentiate rhabdomyolysis from cardiac necrosis or infarction. In addition, a urinalysis may reveal myoglobinuria.

Fire victims must have a chest radiograph taken. Though frequently normal acutely, it serves as a valuable baseline study. Cyanide levels can be obtained but are of limited value. Assays for other toxic inhalants, such as acrolein, phosgene, or gaseous hydrogen chloride, are unavailable. Spirometry and fiberoptic bronchoscopy may be required.

Alcohol is frequently consumed with both suicidal and accidental CO poisoning, sometimes making a rapid diagnosis difficult. Therefore, a blood alcohol level should be measured. If a suicide attempt is suspected, a drug screen may be sent for analysis. In addition, quantitative aspirin, phenobarbital, and acetaminophen levels should be obtained.

Other laboratory tests assist in confirming CO poisoning. A routine complete blood count (CBC) may show a leukocytosis. Determination of arterial blood gas and electrolyte levels may demonstrate an anion gap acidosis. The acidosis results from lactic acid production. Abnormalities are commonly seen with measurements of the blood glucose, amylase, and transaminases. These findings, however, are of limited clinical significance.

The neurologic evaluation should include psychometric testing in all CO-poisoned patients. CT scan abnormalities suggest a poor neurologic outcome. The CT scan may reveal the characteristic hypodense lesions of the globus pallidus. It may also demonstrate cerebral edema, necrosis, and white matter defects. Magnetic resonance imaging is more sensitive, demonstrating lesions not seen on CT scan. Electroencephalographic studies typically show generalized slow wave activity and, rarely, focal epileptiform activity.

TREATMENT

In treating CO-poisoned patients one should remove the victims from the CO-containing atmosphere, keep them at rest to minimize oxygen requirements, and immediately administer 100% oxygen. A simple mask which allows for mixture with room air is not adequate. A mask with a bag reservoir is required to deliver a high FI_{O_2}. The mask should fit tightly. The serum elimination half-life of COHb when breathing room air is 520 min, compared to 80 min when breathing 100% oxygen. Oxygen therapy should not be discontinued until the patient is asymptomatic and the COHb level is less than 10 percent.

HBO therapy is recommended for very severe cases. HBO is delivered in monoplace or multiplace chambers. The multiplace chamber permits treatment of multiple patients simultaneously and provides room for staff and accessory equipment, e.g., ventilators. A typical treatment consists of 100% oxygen at 2.8 atm pressure for 46 min. A second treatment is given in 6 to 8 h if symptoms persist. With HBO therapy, the elimination half-life of CO is reduced to 23 min. When HBO is used to treat methylene chloride–induced CO toxicity, the CO half-life changes from 13.0 h at room air to 5.8 h.

With HBO therapy at 3 atm pressure, the amount of oxygen dissolved in the blood is increased to 6.9 vol percent. This amount is sufficient to meet the demands of cerebral metabolism independent of the COHb concentration. HBO therapy also reduces the amount of cerebral edema. Proponents of HBO contend that this decreases the incidence of delayed neurologic sequelae. There are no adequate studies comparing 100% oxygen delivered by mask to HBO therapy.

As many as 10 percent of patients requiring HBO therapy are pregnant. Animal studies have raised concerns regarding the potential adverse effects of high partial pressures of oxygen on the fetus, but the pressures and durations used were greater than those used in humans. The Soviets have the largest experience with HBO in pregnancy. They found a decrease in perinatal complications and mortality. The greatest advantage of HBO over 100% normobaric oxygen is that it reduces the time required to decrease fetal HbCO. Given the safety of HBO and the danger of CO toxicity to the fetus, many recommend liberal use of HBO in pregnant women.

Since transferring a patient to a hyperbaric facility can be difficult, telephone consultation with the nearest hyperbaric chamber facility is helpful. The nearest hyperbaric chamber can be located by calling Divers Alert Network at Duke University (1-919-684-8111).

During HBO therapy patients often experience otalgia and sinus discomfort; however, tympanic membrane rupture and epistaxis are rare. A significant number of patients will also experience seizures (6 percent) and vomiting (6 percent).

The following are possible considerations for HBO use:

1. History or presence of coma
2. COHb level greater than 25 percent at any time (maternal COHb greater than 20 percent) and vomiting (6 percent)
3. Symptoms persisting after 4 h of 100% oxygen therapy (including abnormal psychometric testing and tachycardia)
4. Delayed neurologic sequelae
5. pH < 7.20
6. Neonates
7. Pregnancy

The role of nitrites with mixed cyanide and CO exposures is not clearly defined and is theoretically harmful. The nitrites given to treat cyanide toxicity cause methemoglobinemia. This shifts the oxygen-hemoglobin dissociation curve further to the left, exacerbating tissue hypoxia. If the patient has been removed from the source and presents to the emergency department alive, sodium thiosulfate, 12.5 g intravenously, will detoxify the cyanide.

Cerebral edema should be treated with mannitol and by elevation of the head of the bed. Hyperventilation should be used in severe cases. The efficacy of steroids is debated.

Correcting the metabolic acidosis may be harmful; a mild acidosis is often a normal compensatory response. A low pH shifts the oxygen-hemoglobin dissociation curve to the right, increasing oxygen unloading to the tissue. Alkalinization will shift the oxygen-hemoglobin curve to the left, further reducing tissue availability of oxygen and exacerbating the toxic effect of CO. Nevertheless, if the pH is less than 7.20, cardiovascular performance is compromised, and judicious alkalinization is required.

Many authors empirically recommend rest for 3 to 6 weeks after severe exposure. Being at rest reduces oxygen requirements, minimizing the risk of delayed neurologic sequelae.

Other reported therapies include hypothermia and carboxygen. Carboxygen is a 5% carbon dioxide and 95% oxygen mixture and offers no therapeutic advantage over 100% oxygen. Hypothermia is harmful, because it reduces tissue uptake of oxygen and increases CO affinity for hemoglobin. The oxygen-carrying blood substitute Fluosol-DA may have a role in treatment. All patients should be followed for neuropsychiatric sequelae.

PROGNOSIS

Many variables, such as age, smoking habit, existing cardiopulmonary disease, severity of exposure, prior state of health, and form of therapy, influence outcome. Coma, cardiac arrest, metabolic acidosis, and high COHb levels have been associated with poor neurologic outcome. These factors, however, are inconsistent predictors of outcome and therefore are of limited value. Abnormal CT findings are associated with neurologic sequelae. Almost all patients with abnormal CT scans will have persistent neurologic deficits.

BIBLIOGRAPHY

Binder JW, Roberts RJ: Carbon monoxide intoxication in children. *Clin Toxicol* 16:287, 1980.

Burney RE, Wu SC, Nemiroff MJ: Mass carbon monoxide poisoning: Clinical effects and results of treatment in 184 victims. *Ann Emerg Med* 11:394, 1982.

Cramer CR: Fetal death due to accidental maternal carbon monoxide poisoning. *J Toxicol Clin Toxicol* 19:297, 1982.

Longo LD: The biological effects of carbon monoxide on the pregnant woman, fetus, and newborn infant. *Am J Obstet Gynecol* 129:69, 1977.

Margulies JL: Acute carbon monoxide poisoning during pregnancy. *Am J Emerg Med* 4:516, 1986.

Myers RAM: Carbon monoxide poisoning. *J Emerg Med* 1:245, 1984.

Myers RAM, Snyder SK, Emhoff TA: Subacute sequelae of carbon monoxide poisoning. *Ann Emerg Med* 14:1163, 1985.

Peirce EC, Kaufmann H, Bensky WH, et al: A registry for carbon monoxide poisoning in New York City. *Clin Toxicol* 26:419, 1988.

Piatt JP, Kaplan AM, Bond GR, et al: Occult carbon monoxide poisoning in an infant. *Ped Emerg Care* 6:21, 1990.

Van Hoesen KB, Camporesi EM, Moon RE, et al: Should hyperbaric oxygen be used to treat the pregnant patient for acute carbon monoxide poisoning? *JAMA* 261:1039, 1989.

127 ACUTE EXPOSURE TO TOXIC AGENTS

Constance J. Doyle

Acute exposure to hazardous materials is a very probable event in today's society. Workplace accidents can result in acute exposure to hazardous materials. Health morbidity can occur from both acute accidental and chronic, long-term exposure.

The U.S. Department of Transportation lists seven major classes of hazardous materials, with 2750 subcategories. The Association of American Railroads lists eight classes of hazardous materials, including explosives, gases, flammable and combustible liquids, flammable solids, oxidizers and organic peroxides, poisons, radioactive materials, and corrosives.

Transportation accidents result in non-work- or work-related exposures. In addition, all emergency personnel may be at risk of exposure. The emergency physician and poison control centers may be called upon to access data to help emergency personnel care for patients and to aid in evacuation decisions. Problems resulting from trauma from the initial incident or the subsequent fire, smoke, or explosion may pose additional hazards. Tens of thousands of chemical substances are produced, transported, and stored throughout the United States. CHEMTREC has logged over 55,000 calls for hazardous materials emergency assistance in the past year.[1]

PLANNING

Every emergency department should have a hazardous materials plan to include on-site prehospital decontamination, decontamination at the hospital, types of protective equipment available, decontamination equipment, decontamination location, and personnel responsible for the decontamination and treatment process. Responsibilities for decontamination, triage, and treatment should be written into the plan.

Medical control should be involved early to access toxicity data and to ensure that proper safety equipment is used and that decontamination begins on site if necessary. Hazardous materials patient-care protocols should be clearly outlined. Guidebooks and resource lists of telephone numbers for information and equipment should be available to medical control and rescue personnel at the scene of a hazardous materials emergency.

DECONTAMINATION

If possible decontamination should occur at the site of the chemical incident and the contaminated material should not leave the site until environmental cleanup personnel arrive. With injuries necessitating medical treatment, one must simultaneously treat the injury, effect rapid decontamination, and avoid exposing others to the contaminated material. Rescue personnel should wear protective clothing and/or respiratory protection as dictated by the toxicity of the chemical involved. If such protection is unavailable, firefighters in "full turnout gear" may be used.

With attention to airway and cervical spine precautions if indicated, the patient should be washed rapidly with water from a nearby hose, or *clean* orchard sprayer, or buckets of water. Only lifesaving treatment should be carried out in the immediate "hot" area of the spill. After the patient is washed and wrapped in clean blankets, advanced life support (ALS) measures should be instituted. Transportation in a non-ALS vehicle saves ALS vehicles from being out of service for decontamination.

The ideal decontamination facility has a separate entrance from the outside and contains a shower, separate wastewater collection, and separate air venting. If a contaminated patient uses the decontamination room, staff need protective clothing and/or self-contained breathing apparatus. If this is not available, firefighters in full turnout gear working in self-contained breathing apparatus can assist.

PATTERNS OF INJURY

Most industrial and transportation exposures are either by inhalation or dermal exposure with or without systemic toxicity. Some chemicals on the skin can vaporize and result in a simultaneous inhalation injury.

Cutaneous injury results from materials contacting the skin. A contact dermatitis, a chemical burn, or allergic reaction may result. Some chemicals penetrate the superficial skin layers, such as the deep burns that result from hydrofluoric acid. Others may be absorbed systemically, or volatilize and be inhaled, causing systemic symptoms. Decontamination of the skin and/or eye with copious amounts of water prevents further exposure. There are rare agents that react violently with water, such as chlorosulfonic acid, titanium tetrachloride, and calcium oxide, or that are insoluble in water, such as phosphorus. These should be wiped off with a dry cloth, and all clothing removed. References should be consulted for specific decontamination procedures for these agents.

Inhalation of volatile chemicals or their products of combustion can result in asphyxiation, irritation, systemic absorption, or a combination of these (see Table 127-1). Asphyxiants cause toxicity by replacing oxygen in the lungs. Biologically inert substances such as nitrogen, methane, and carbon dioxide are examples. Chemical asphyxiants interfere with tissue oxygenation by preventing the delivery of oxygen to the cell or by inhibiting the use of oxygen at the cellular level. Examples include carbon monoxide and cyanide. Both types of asphyxiant gases cause little direct lung damage but can have a profound effect on the neurologic, metabolic, and cardiovascular systems secondary to the hypoxia they cause.

Irritant gases act directly on the mucosa of the respiratory tree. The location of the pulmonary damage depends on their water solubility. Ammonia, very water soluble, is absorbed in the upper airway and produces such signs of upper airway irritation as cough, laryngeal edema, and pharyngitis. Phosgene, which has little water solubility, reaches the lower airways and causes pneumonitis and pulmonary edema. Gases with intermediate solubility cause upper airway symptoms if exposure is brief. If exposure is prolonged, lower respiratory symptoms predominate.

A fourth class of gases, such as hydrogen sulfide, methylated halogens, and metal fumes, act both as irritants and asphyxiants. Smoke includes multiple products of combustion, including carbon monoxide. Toluene diisocyanate, hydrocyanic acid, acrolein, ammonia, acetic acid, and formic acid are common products produced by burning nylon and plastics. Thermal injury from heat and irritation from inhaled soot add to injury. Immediate application of 100% oxygen must be done

Table 127-1. Classification of Noxious Gases

Asphyxiants, simple:
Carbon dioxide, nitrogen, hydrocarbons, helium, argon, neon, hydrogen, ethane, acetylene
Asphyxiants, chemical:
Carbon monoxide, cyanide, hydrogen cyanide, acetonitrile, acrylonitrile
Irritants:
Ammonia, phosgene, nitrogen dioxide, hydrogen halides, acrolein, methyl bromide, ethylene oxide, fluorine, nitric acid, sulfur dioxide
Combined asphyxiants and irritants:
Hydrogen sulfides, metal fumes, metallic oxides, aromatic hydrocarbons, ozone, paraquat, methylated halogens

[1] Computer modem access numbers for chemical information data banks should also be available.

until carbon monoxide inhalation is ruled out and complete respiratory evaluation has been done.

Hemoglobinopathies, such as carboxyhemoglobinemia, sulfhemoglobinemia, and methemoglobinemia, result from exposures to chemicals that impair oxygen transport by hemoglobin. Symptoms include dizziness, headache, nausea and vomiting, disorientation, seizures, and coma. Cardiac toxicity including tachycardia, arrhythmias, myocardial infarction, and cardiovascular collapse is present in carbon monoxide poisoning. Methemoglobinemia, sulfhemoglobinemia, and cyanide poisoning present with cyanosis unresponsive to oxygen therapy. Organophosphate poisoning presents with a syndrome of salivation, lacrimation, urination, and defecation (SLUD) as well as sweating, bronchospasm and pulmonary edema, and CNS symptoms such as restlessness, ataxia, convulsions, and respiratory and circulatory depression. Metal fume fever occurs when volatilized metals are inhaled and produces chills, fever, muscle ache, headache, fatigue, and dry throat. It is found in metal workers, welders, foundry workers, and shipyard workers.

INITIAL STABILIZATION

Treatment of chemical injuries includes initial hazard assessment, and protection of rescuers with proper clothing and respiratory protection. Early decontamination not only mitigates some effects of some toxic substances, but also contains environmental hazards to prevent further spread.

Immediate attention to airway is paramount, along with stabilization of the cervical spine if there is concern about trauma. If there are highly toxic fumes, an open bag-valve-mask respirator should not be used. A demand valve or a closed system with 100% oxygen ensures that no additional fumes are ventilated into the patient's airway. After the airway and breathing are established, exsanguinating hemorrhage is controlled, any sucking chest injury is sealed, and tension pneumothorax is relieved. When the patient has been exposed to fumes, and/or has CNS alteration, 100% oxygen should be administered pending full respiratory investigation.

In the absence of a specific antidote, all medical care is supportive. This includes a meticulous history of the exposure, including agent, length of exposure, route, interval since the exposure, and associated trauma including that from fire and explosion. Was the exposure in an enclosed space? Were any unusual odors noted? Long-term and delayed effects of an exposure should be checked in available references to counsel the patient and to anticipate delayed medical consequences that may mean that the patient needs close medical supervision. The patient's prior health status and any previous similar injuries or episodes must be documented since some cases may involve compensation claims.

A physical examination with careful attention to signs of covert trauma must be done. Intravenous lines with crystalloid are started, and blood should be drawn for definitive testing. Pulse oximetry can give an immediate estimate of oxygen saturation while other tests are completed. Arterial blood gas and carboxyhemoglobin measurements must be done for anyone with an inhalation injury due to fire, smoke, and/or explosion and any unknown inhalation. Blood and/or urine for specific toxicologic screens should be sent. Supportive treatment should proceed without waiting for definitive laboratory test results to return.

Cutaneous injury is treated with copious washing and treatment of the specific injury present. Burns are treated by stopping the burning process with removal of the agent and any burning clothing and debris. Strong alkali burns are irrigated under running water for prolonged periods. Burns are then cleaned, debrided, and dressed. Consultation with a burn surgeon should be considered in all but the most minor chemical burns. Contact dermatitis and local allergic reactions should be treated with standard agents to reduce swelling, itching, and irritation. Systemic toxicity from injury to the skin is related to the lipid solubility of the material and to inhalation of vapors from volatilized substances.

Strong alkali burns of the eye require immediate, on-site irrigation with normal saline solution of running water, and irrigation must continue en route and in the emergency department. Other eye exposures should be irrigated copiously with the goal of bringing the pH of the lacrimal fluid to 7.0. Topical anesthetic may be used but should not delay copious irrigation. Surface pH testing in alkali exposure is inadequate since residual alkali may persist in the tissues and act as a reservoir. A thorough eye examination should follow to check for abrasions, imbedded foreign bodies, visual acuity, and fundal integrity. Consultation with an ophthalmologist ensures that complications and problems are addressed.

Examination of the patient with inhalation injury should include examination of the entire respiratory tree. Singed nasal vibrissae and soot in the posterior pharynx indicate inhaled smoke and hot gases. Cough and change in voice may indicate upper airway irritation. The presence of stridor and the use of accessory muscles should be noted. Tachypnea, respiratory rate, and dyspnea as well as wheezing, rales, and rhonchi should be noted. Patients with inhalation injuries receive supportive treatment dependent on signs and symptoms uncovered during the physical and laboratory examinations. Unless symptoms are very mild and only involve the nose and pharynx, oxygen should be started while a history and physical examination are completed.

If CNS signs or respiratory distress are present, 100% oxygen is started until carbon monoxide inhalation can be ruled out, since oxygen is the specific antidote. Humidification aids in tracheobronchitis, and bronchospasm is treated with nebulized β agonists and subcutaneous terbutaline or epinephrine. Aminophylline can be added, if needed.

If pulmonary edema develops, aggressive use of diuretics and vasodilators is indicated. Respiratory failure may require ventilatory support including mechanical ventilation and positive end-expiratory pressure.

Baseline ECG, chest x-ray, and arterial blood gas and carboxyhemoglobin levels are minimum studies. Other studies depend on the patient's signs, symptoms, and previous medical history. Patients with thermal injury to the airway may need laryngoscopy, bronchoscopy, or intubation if severe laryngeal or tracheal injury is present. Pulmonary function tests may add additional information about parenchymal involvement and will provide important baseline values if long-term follow-up is necessary. The use of prophylactic antibiotics in the absence of pneumonia and the use of steroids are controversial.

Criteria for admission to the hospital include anticipated delayed effects from a particular chemical; hypoxia; a carboxyhemoglobin level above 15 to 20 percent, or lower with systemic symptoms; dyspnea in room air; thermal injury; evidence of lower airway injury; tracheobronchitis; pulmonary edema; pneumonia; and severe upper airway irritation which may progress to obstruction. Systemic signs may be due to hypoxia or systemic toxicity and should be treated supportively.

ENTITIES WITH SPECIFIC ANTIDOTES

Carbon Monoxide (See Chap. 126)

Cyanide

Cyanide is used in industry in electroplating, silver recovery from x-ray film, ore extraction, in fumigation, and as a fertilizer. It is one of the products of combustion from burning nylon and polyurethane.

Cyanide is absorbed through the lung and interferes with the cytochrome oxidase system. It is a rapidly acting poison, and a strong index of suspicion must be maintained. The antidote should be administered promptly when the diagnosis is suspected. Symptoms include weakness, dizziness, and headache, rapidly progressing to dyspnea and unconsciousness. There may be an odor of bitter almonds on the breath or on the body, but 20 to 40 percent of the population is unable to detect this odor. Bright-red venous blood may be present in early stages and may not be present in later stages. Blood should be drawn for arterial blood gases and measurement of electrolytes, lactate, pyruvate, and carbon monoxide. Cyanide levels from blood and lavage fluid in ingestions should be tested for, but treatment should not be held pending results.

Treatment of symptomatic patients uses the specific antidotes contained in the Lilly Cyanide Poison Kit (amyl nitrite, sodium nitrite, and sodium thiosulfate). The object of treatment is to induce methemoglobinemia. Methemoglobin combines with cyanide to become cyanmethemoglobin, thus unbinding the cytochrome oxidase system. Methemoglobin levels can be helpful if more than one dose of sodium nitrate is needed. One should not wait for cyanide levels to begin treatment. Lactic acidosis with a high ion gap may suggest that cyanide poisoning has occurred. Initially, 100% oxygen is started to support respiration. Intubation may be necessary. Rapid decontamination and removal of any contaminated clothing is essential. If there has been ingestion, rapid lavage followed by charcoal and cathartic is instituted but *should not delay* antidote administration. A pearl of amyl nitrite is crushed and held under the patient's nose or intake valve of an Ambu bag for about 15 to 30 s out of each minute, and 10 mL of a 3% solution of sodium nitrite is injected over a 3- to 5-min period. The dosage for children is approximately 0.33 mL/kg and varies with hemoglobin level. Blood pressure is carefully monitored, and the patient is treated with vasopressors if necessary.

Sodium thiosulfate is given to form thiocyanate, which can be excreted by the kidneys. The initial dose of a 25% solution is 50 mL intravenously. The dose for children is 1.6 mL/kg. If signs of poisoning recur or recovery is not evident, repeat injections of sodium nitrite and sodium thiosulfate are needed in 1 h.

Hydrogen Sulfide

Hydrogen sulfide poisoning is similar to cyanide poisoning, and hydrogen sulfide binding of the cytochrome oxidase system can be displaced by sodium nitrite induction of methemoglobin. Amyl nitrite and sodium nitrite are used, but sodium thiosulfate is not. Hydrogen sulfide is found in natural gases, sulfur springs, and decaying materials. There are multiple descriptions of rescuer morbidity and mortality with this material. H_2S has a rotten egg odor, but one quickly gets olfactory fatigue and may not be aware of continued exposure.

Organophosphate Insecticides and Carbamate Insecticides

Organophosphate insecticides are prevalent in farming and in weaker household insecticide preparations. These compounds inhibit acetylcholinesterase in the nervous system, and acetylcholine accumulates at the myoneural junction and synapses.

These agents produce excessive salivation, lacrimation, urination, and defecation (SLUD), and bronchorrhea, sweating, wheezing, bradycardia, muscular weakness, cramping, and respiratory and circulatory collapse.

Treatment is begun with respiratory support, decontamination of the patient, and removal of all the patient's clothing. Clothing should be isolated and discarded. Fumes from clothing are a hazard to emergency personnel. The patient should be washed at least three times with soap and water. Respiratory status should be monitored and adequate oxygenation ensured. Atropine in large doses of 2 to 5 mg is given intravenously every 15 to 30 min until there are signs of dry mouth, flushing, tachycardia, and dilated pupils. A test dose of 1 to 2 mg (0.01 mg/kg for children) may be given. If this dose produces atropinization, organophosphate poisoning is unlikely.

Atropine needs to be continued at least 12 to 24 h and may be needed for several days. Adrenergic amines, aminophylline, physostigmine, phenothiazines, morphine, succinylcholine, or reserpine should not be used. Treatment of carbamate insecticide poisoning is with atropine alone.

Because muscular weakness and fasciculation are not reversed with atropine, another specific antidote must be used if symptoms are present. Pralidoxime, or 2-PAM (Protopam), is given in doses of 1 g diluted in dextrose and water and infused over 15 to 30 min except when carbamate insecticides are the offending agents. If severe symptoms persist, the dosage may be repeated in 1 to 2 h and again in 6 to 8 h if symptoms persist.

Methemoglobinemia

Methemoglobinemia is caused by abnormal hemoglobin or exposure to various nitrates, including nitroglycerin, explosives, aniline dye derivatives, and some sulfonamides. Brown color of arterial blood, and cyanosis that does not clear with oxygenation, are clues to the diagnosis. There may be marked cyanosis with little respiratory distress.

Treatment is supportive with oxygen administration, and decontamination with soap and water if exposure was dermal. A 1% solution of methylene blue in doses of 0.1 to 0.2 mL/kg or 1 to 2 mg/kg is given intravenously over 5 min in patients with methemoglobin levels over 30% or with symptomatic angina, arrhythmias, hypotension, seizures, or coma. The dose may be repeated in 1 h if necessary if severe cyanosis persists. Exchange transfusions and hyperbaric oxygenation have been used in very severe cases.

Hydrofluoric Acid

Hydrofluoric acid is a strong inorganic acid which can penetrate intact skin and cause coagulation necrosis of subcutaneous fat. It causes severe pain which may be out of proportion to the visible injury. The onset of pain is often delayed, and the patient may present with severe burning hours after the exposure. Severe damage can occur to subcutaneous structures including muscle and bone.

Calcium will precipitate the fluoride ion (Table 127-2). A 2.5% calcium gluconate gel should then be applied and massaged into the skin using pain relief as an end point. Subcutaneous injection of 10% calcium gluconate may be used with a maximum of 0.5 mL per digit. Nails may need to be removed or alternative treatment of interarterial calcium gluconate considered. If regional anesthesia is used, the end point of pain relief is obscured. Narcotic analgesia may be necessary. Systemic calcium replacement may also be necessary in severe cases. Consultation with a burn surgeon is necessary for severe burns, circumferential burns, burns of nail plates, and burns which do not respond to simple treatment.

Phenol

Phenol, or carbolic acid, and its derivatives are used as deodorizers, disinfectants, and sanitizers. It is absorbed through the skin and causes liver and kidney damage, as well as CNS depression. On contact it denatures protein and causes intense pain and burning and may form an eschar which traps the phenol in the subcutaneous tissues. Gangrene may develop. Dinitrophenol and hydroquinone can cause methemoglobinemia.

Management includes immediate washing with water and olive oil. If an eschar was formed, washing with glycerol may be indicated.

Table 127-2. Topical Therapy for Hydrofluoric Acid Burns

Calcium gluconate gel
Surgical lubricant 4.25 oz (120 g) and 30 mL of 10% calcium gluconate (3 g)
Surgical lubricant, 5-oz tube, 3.5 g calcium gluconate
H-F antidote gel, Pharmascience, Inc., Quebec, Canada
Zephiran solution

BIBLIOGRAPHY

Burgess WA: *Recognition of Health Hazards in Industry: A Review of Materials and Processes*. New York, Wiley, 1981.

Doyle CJ: Hazardous chemicals, *Emerg Med Clin North Am* 1:653, 1983.

Goldberg MJ, Spector R, Park GD, et al: An approach to the management of the poisoned patient. *Arch Intern Med* July 1986, p 1381.

Goldfrank LR, Flomenbaum NE, et al: *Toxicologic Emergencies,* 4th ed. Norwalk, Conn, Appleton and Lange, 1990.

Guzzardi L: Toxic products of combustion. *Top Emerg Med* 7:45, 1985.

Haddad LM: The organophosphate insecticides, in Haddad LM, Winchester JF (eds): *Clinical Management of Poisoning and Drug Overdose,* Philadelphia, Saunders, 1990, pp 1076–1087.

Hall AH, Rumack BH: Cyanide, in Haddad LM, Winchester JF (eds): *Clinical Management of Poisoning and Overdose,* Philadelphia, Saunders, 1990, 1103–1111.

Hedges JR: Acute noxious gas exposure. *Curr Top Emerg Med* 2:59, 1978.

Johnson WS: Cyanide poisoning successfully treated without therapeutic methemoglobin levels. *Am J Emerg Med* 7(4):437, 1989.

Johnston BD: Inhalation injuries, in *Management of Wilderness and Environmental Emergencies*. New York, Macmillan, 1983, pp. 585–605.

Kizer KW: Toxic inhalations. *Emerg Med Clin North Am* 2:649, 1984.

Maibach HI: *Occupational and Industrial Dermatology* 2d ed, Chicago, Year Book, 1987.

Noji EK, Kelen GD: *Manual of Toxicologic Emergencies,* Chicago, Year Book, 1989.

Proctor NH, Hughes JP: *Chemical Hazards of the Workplace,* 2d ed. Philadelphia, Lippincott, 1988.

Rumack B et al: Poison index, Micromedex Denver Colorado exp 11/90.

Student PJ, *Emergency Handling of Hazardous Materials in Surface Transportation*. Washington, DC, Bureau of Explosives, 1981.

Stutz DR, Ricks RC, Olsen MF: *Hazardous Materials Injuries: A Handbook for Pre-Hospital Care*. Greenbelt, Maryland, Bradford Communications, 1982.

Stair T: Carbon monoxide, in Haddad LM, Winchester JF (eds): *Clinical Management of Poisoning and Drug Overdose*. Philadelphia, Saunders, 1990, pp 1233–1234.

Upfal M, Doyle CJ: Medical management of hydrofluoric acid exposure. *J Occup Med* 32(8):726, 1990.

US Department of Transportation: *Hazardous Material—Emergency Response Guidebook*. Washington, DC, DOT-P 5800.3, 1991.

Vicas IM, Whitcraft DD: Hydrogen sulfide and carbon disulfide, in Haddad LM, Winchester JF (eds): *Clinical Management of Poisoning and Drug Overdose*. Philadelphia, Saunders, 1990, pp 1244–1252.

128
RADIATION INJURIES

H. Arnold Muller

We cannot see, smell, feel, or hear radiation, yet it captured our attention during the 1979 Three Mile Island accident. And on April 26, 1986, the worst commercial nuclear power plant disaster in history occurred with the explosion and fire at the Chernobyl No. 4 nuclear power plant in the Soviet Union. In terms of the amount of radioactivity released into the environment, the size of the affected area, long-term consequences, the numerous acute injuries, and 29 known deaths, the Chernobyl accident was the most significant nuclear event since the bombing of Hiroshima and Nagasaki.

Some elements of radiation physics, common sources of radiation (Table 128-1), the tissue effects of radiation, the signs and symptoms of radiation injury, and the evaluation and therapy of radiation injuries and exposure will be briefly covered in this chapter.

Table 128-1. Common Sources of Radiation

Source	Whole Body, mrem/yr	Dose Rate
Natural Sources:		
Radon	200	
Natural background radiation	35	
Air	5	
Building materials	34	
Food	25	
Ground	11	
Medical	50	
Total	360	
Technological Sources:		
Coast-to-coast jet flight		5 mrem/round trip
Color television		1 mrem/yr
AP chest film		10 mrem/film

Source: Linnemann RE: *Background Information on Radiation.* April 4, 1979. San Jose, California, General Electric Nuclear Energy Group. Used by permission. Above table has been altered with permission of Dr. Linnemann to reflect more recent information regarding common sources of radiation.

PATHOPHYSIOLOGY

Radiation may be classified as *ionizing* or *nonionizing*. Ionizing radiation is produced by nuclear weapons and reactors, radioactive material, and x-ray machines. The term *ionizing* is derived from the effect that such radiation produces when it interacts with matter, that is, it causes atoms to convert to ions as a result of the atoms' loss or gain of electrons. Biological function may be affected if such ionized atoms are in the human body. On the other hand, light, radio waves, and microwaves are examples of *nonionizing radiation*.

Radiation is either *particulate* or *electromagnetic*. Electromagnetic radiation occurs in waveform and has no mass or charge. It belongs to a family of radiant energies that is described by wavelengths. Electromagnetic radiations, in order of decreasing energy content are γ rays, x-rays, ultraviolet rays, visible rays, infrared rays, microwaves, and radio waves. Both γ waves and x-rays are electromagnetic radiations that can cause ionization. The electrons lost from atoms act as secondary particles and produce additional ionizations. X-rays differ from γ rays only in that x-rays are produced outside the nucleus of an atom; γ rays are emitted from the nucleus. Both travel great distances and readily penetrate body cells. X-rays and γ rays can easily be detected by Geiger-Müller (GM) counters.

Although α and β particles are not electromagnetic, they do cause ionization. The α particle consists of two protons and two neutrons (identical to a helium atom without electrons) that are emitted from the nucleus of a radioactive atom. The α particles travel only a few centimeters and are completely stopped by paper or the keratin layer of the skin. The β particle is an electron emitted from the nucleus of a radioactive atom. They travel up to a few meters in air but barely penetrate the skin. Both α and β particles are harmful, however, if they contaminate wounds or are ingested or inhaled. Contamination of the body surfaces by α and β particles can be detected by counters.

Energy deposited by radiation per unit of mass is referred to as the *dose*. A *rad* (*r*adiation *a*bsorbed *d*ose) is 100 ergs of energy deposited in 1 g of material. The Standard International Unit (SI) for dose is the Gray (Gy): 1 Gy = 100 rad; 1 cGy = 1 rad. The rem (*r*oentgen *e*quivalent *m*an) is a calculated radiation unit of dose equivalent in which the absorbed dose in rad (or Gy) is multiplied by a quality factor to account for the biological effectiveness of different types of radiation. The SI unit for dose equivalent is the Sievert (Sv). 1 Sv = 100 rem; 1 cSv = 1 rem. We generally use the term *rem* or *millirem* (mrem) when referring to the exposure of biological systems. For x-rays, γ rays, and β particles, the rad and the rem and the Gray and the Sievert are equivalent. A given rad dose from neutrons of α particles produces up to 20 times as much biological damage as the same dose in rad from x-rays or γ rays. The whole body dose of ionizing radiation that will kill half of those who are exposed is approximately 400 rem (4 Sv). At about 600 rem (6 Sv) the mortality has been nearly 100 percent. Mental retardation has been associated with radiation doses as low as 5 rem to the fetus during the eighth to fifteenth week of gestation. The human average annual "normal" exposure to radiation in the United States from all sources, including radon, is approximately 360 mrem. A person or object exposed to radiation, other than high-dose neutron radiation, does not become radioactive. It is only the presence of contamination, or radioactive dirt, that poses risk to personnel rendering treatment.

Equivalent doses received over a long time are less harmful than those received over a short period of time. For example, 100 rem delivered over 1 year is much less harmful than 100 rem delivered in 1 s. The radiation dose from a point source of radiation decreases inversely as the square of the distance from the source.

The biological effects of radiation are a consequence of ionization. Free radicals are formed from water and can cause DNA and RNA strands to be broken. Cell and chromosomal changes may be minor and not pose a hazard to the organism. They may result in aberrations that are passed on to subsequent generations, or they may result in cell death, or the inability to replicate.

CLINICAL FEATURES

The most prominent systemic signs and symptoms of high [$>$ 100 rem (1 Sv)] whole body radiation exposure are malaise, nausea, vomiting, and diarrhea; seizures; erythema of the skin; and later, bleeding, anemia, and infection. Nausea and vomiting occasionally occur at about 100-rem exposure (Table 128-2). If they develop within 2 h of exposure, it suggests a dose of more than 400 rem; after 2 h exposure, less than 200 rem; if none after 6 h exposure, less than 50 rem. Erythema, local or generalized, indicates skin exposure greater than 300 rem; diarrhea indicates exposure of the gastrointestinal tract to greater than 400 rem; and seizures indicate central nervous system exposure greater than 2000 rem. Lymphocyte counts are useful prognostically. If after 48 h the lymphocyte count is $>1200/mm^3$, the prognosis is good; 300 to 1200, fair; less than $300/mm^3$, poor. Bleeding, anemia, and infection may occur after a latent period of 20 to 30 days.

Erythema and brawniness of the skin develop in a few hours and progress over days, just as with a thermal burn. Radiation burns are initially less painful than thermal burns. Loss of hair, vesiculation, and ulceration may eventually develop if the dose is high enough.

Table 128-2. Dose-Effect Relations Following Acute Whole Body Irradiation (X- or γ-Ray)

Whole Body Dose, rad	Clinical and Laboratory Findings
5–25	Asymptomatic. Conventional blood studies are normal. Chromosome aberrations detectable.
50–75	Asymptomatic. Minor depressions of white cells and platelets detectable in a few persons, especially if baseline values established.
75–125	Minimal acute doses that produce prodromal symptoms (anorexia, nausea, vomiting, fatigue) in about 10–20% of persons within 2 days. Mild depressions of white cells and platelets in some persons.
125–200	Symptomatic course with transient disability and clear hematologic changes in a majority of exposed persons. Lymphocyte depression of about 50% within 48 h.
240–340	Serious, disabling illness in most persons with about 50% mortality if untreated. Lymphocyte depression of about $\geq$ 75% within 48 h.
500+	Accelerated version of acute radiation syndrome with GI complications within 2 weeks, bleeding, and death in most exposed persons.
5000+	Fulminating course with cardiovascular, GI, and CNS complications resulting in death within 24–72 h.

Source: Mettler FD: Emergency management of radiation accidents. *JACEP* 7:302, 1978. Used by permission.

Following radiation exposure the likelihood of significant systemic effects can be estimated based on time of onset of nausea, vomiting, and diarrhea; changes in lymphocyte count; and knowledge of the accident, the radiation source, the dose readings at the site of the accident, and the duration of exposure.

Often a health physicist at the scene of an industrial accident is able to provide some indication of dose. Severity of symptoms varies and does not correlate with dose, but onset following exposure does. The earlier signs and symptoms develop, the higher the dose and the worse the prognosis. Initial symptoms (nausea, vomiting, and general malaise) generally subside within a few hours to several days and are followed by a latent period of 1 or more weeks. In general, if exposure is less than 125 rem, prognosis is good. For patients with doses less than 200 rem, probably nothing more than symptomatic treatment is needed, and recovery should occur. Those with exposure of 200 to 1000 rem should be promptly placed into a reverse isolation atmosphere. Further treatment need is probable to certain, and aggressive treatment can make a great difference in patient survival. Other than prompt external and internal body decontamination of radioactive material, and fluid replacement, when indicated, there is no *emergency* treatment specific to radiation exposure that will make any difference in long-term survival. Whatever symptoms occur should be treated symptomatically.

Following exposure to radiation, the exposed population is at risk for delayed complications such as leukemia and thyroid carcinoma. Contraception should be practiced for several months to avoid congenital defects in offspring.

TREATMENT

Initial treatment of radiation-exposed patients must first involve management of life-threatening injuries: airway impairment, bleeding, and circulation impairment. Patients who have been irradiated, that is, subjected to a high flux of γ rays or x-rays, are not radioactive. As such, no radiation is detected on the patient's body or clothes. Any tissue damage occurs instantaneously and will manifest itself in time. An irradiated person may sustain local or total body exposure. Following immediate management of life-threatening injuries, the patient should be checked with a GM counter for surface contamination, and it should be determined whether radioactive material has been ingested or inhaled. The GM counter is very useful for detecting β and γ radiation. If used to detect α radiation, it must contain a special window because of the low penetrating power of α particles. The health physicist at the site should be contacted so that data regarding dose, nature of exposure, type of radiation, and duration of exposure can be obtained. A hotline to the regional decontamination area is most helpful for these and similar calls.

Treatment protocol is as follows. Cover open wounds, remove the patient's clothing, and deposit contaminated material in closed receptacles. Protect open wounds to avoid contamination while washing or disrobing the patient. Next, wash the patient with soap and water. If the patient is on a drainage table, contaminated water can be collected in containers. If radioactive material in the form of solid particles, liquid, or dust is inhaled or ingested or contaminates an open wound, then incorporation has occurred. Since such material will irradiate internal tissues and may well cause extensive cellular damage, and since some radioactive elements may become permanently incorporated in the body's molecules, immediate treatment (decorporation) is indicated. Chelating agents provide an ion-exchange matrix that results in formation of an excretable stable complex containing the radioactivity. Radioactive actinide isotopes can be chelated effectively and subsequently excreted when diethylenetriaminepentaacetic acid (DTPA) is administered. Such action should be taken within 1 h of internal contamination. Chelating agents are useful only for transuranics and certain heavy metals. They would probably only be needed for accidents near a fuel-processing or military weapons facility. Although nuclear medicine departments may have stock DTPA solutions, they are too dilute to be useful as chelating agents for the removal of internal radioactive contamination. DTPA may be ordered from the Radiation Emergency Assistance Center/Training Site (REAC/TS) at Oak Ridge, Tennessee. If one anticipates the possible future need for DTPA, a request for current acquisition of it should be made to REAC/TS. DTPA is itself dangerous to use.

Primary wound closure is acceptable if successful decontamination is possible; however, if, in spite of irrigation and cleansing, a significant amount of contamination is retained in a wound, the wound should be left open for 24 h. Much of the remaining contamination will be freed up by bleeding and exudate and can then be removed by debridement. If an extremity is severely contaminated and adequate decontamination is not possible, the question of amputation may be raised. In general, unless the extremity is so severely traumatized that functional recovery is unlikely or unless contamination by radionuclides is so severe that extensive and severe radiation-induced necrosis can be expected, amputation is rarely indicated. The dictum is, decontaminate, but do not mutilate.

Though amputation is rarely required, one should aggressively debride and surgically decontaminate. Such procedures can usually be done without endangering a functional recovery. As surgical instruments become contaminated, they should be removed from the surgical field in order to prevent extension of contamination.

For contamination by plutonium or another long-lived α emitter for which DTPA is an effective chelating agent, treatment locally and intravenously is indicated promptly, preferably prior to surgical decontamination.

Potassium iodide effectively blocks the uptake of radioactive iodine by the thyroid if it is given within a few hours of exposure. The National Council on Radiation Protection and Measurements recommends treatment to protect the thyroid when the dose is, or is expected to be, 10 to 30 rem. Persons 1 year of age or older should receive 130 mg of potassium iodide by mouth daily for 14 days. The dose for children less than 1 year of age is 65 mg. Antacids in the stomach precipitate many metals in the form of insoluble hydroxides, and cathartics can shorten the internal transit time of such material. Aluminum phosphate gel (100 mL) reduces the intestinal absorption of radioactive strontium by 85 percent, and barium sulfate precipitates radium.

A baseline complete blood cell count, differential blood cell count, and platelet count should be done during this initial treatment phase. For patients who have received >200 rem, protective isolation is indicated, and blood transfusions may be necessary later. Bone marrow depression is usually evident 20 to 30 days after exposure. Appropriate cultures, antibiotic therapy as soon as there is evidence of infection, prophylaxis against fungal infections, and HLA typing of the patient and family members are all indicated in serious cases.

Radiation burns are like electrical burns in that physical findings may be minimal initially. For β-particle burns, excision followed by full-thickness grafting may be necessary.

Patients from a radiation accident scene may also have been exposed to chemical hazards. Thus, beryllium, which is present in many nuclear weapons, may be released as fumes and smoke, which in turn may cause respiratory distress, nervousness, and fever. Contamination of open wounds with beryllium results in greatly delayed wound healing. Treatment of the pulmonary problem includes, in addition to oxygen, ethylenediaminetetraacetic acid (EDTA), or another effective chelating agent.

Lead, used in nuclear weapon devices for shielding, on burning releases toxic fumes which can cause pneumonitis and dermatitis. Dermatitis and delayed-onset pneumonitis may also occur as a result of the inhalation of fumes from the combustion of plastics, which are used in most nuclear devices.

Finally, if a U.S. nuclear weapon were to accidentally detonate, such detonation would in all probability be incomplete. It would, however, be associated with blast effects, fires, and the spread of radioactive material. Unexploded pieces of the explosive might be scattered around an accident site. Such pieces frequently look like natural rock and should not be touched or moved unless absolutely necessary for evacuation of casualties.

DECONTAMINATION IN THE EMERGENCY DEPARTMENT

Advance notice of the arrival of a radiation-injured patient is important so that the emergency department can be prepared. Given such notice, emergency personnel can also advise on prior decontamination in the field.

Every nuclear facility must have identified primary and tertiary referral facilities. It is necessary to develop and maintain open channels of communication between the nuclear facility and the emergency department so that each will be prepared in times of individual injury or major accident. One should not rely on telephone communication being available within the hospital or between the hospital and other facilities in the event of a major nuclear accident or disaster. A predetermined plan involving backup radio communication is advised. Periodic exercises in which the facility is suddenly faced with the hypothetical need to treat a few or hundreds of irradiated and/or radioactive-contaminated patients is the best means to ensure the capability of dealing with such problems.

In the emergency department, a designated area, the radiation emergency area, preferably with a separate entryway, should be available for the management of patients with radiation exposure. Contamination should be prevented by covering the floor with plastic or paper sheets and providing an isolated radiation emergency area. Patients and personnel should be monitored for evidence of contamination. Personnel treating or attending the patient must be gowned and wear caps, masks, foot covers, double gloves, and personnel monitoring devices (i.e., film badge, thermoluminescent dosimeter badge, and/or pocket dosimeters).

In rare cases it may also be necessary to provide a lead shield to protect personnel, especially in cases in which there are highly contaminated foreign bodies. Exposure can also be minimized by decreasing exposure time (several people would share care of a patient) and maintaining a distance from the patient whenever possible. Those providing care should not be exposed to more than 5000 mrem except to save a life. The National Council on Radiation Protection has established that a once-in-a-lifetime exposure to 100,000 mrem for purposes of saving a life is acceptable and will result in no undue morbidity. Individuals not involved in the treatment should be kept away from the roped-off area. All attendant personnel should be monitored and decontaminated and their garments appropriately disposed of following completion of their involvement in the treatment process. Everyone working in the radiation emergency area must remain there, and traffic should never move in the reverse direction without first being appropriately monitored. Ambulance personnel and their vehicle(s) should also be checked for the presence of contamination before leaving the facility.

PREHOSPITAL DECONTAMINATION

R. E. Linnemann suggests an order of priority for treating a number of individuals involved in radiation accidents:

1. Injured and contaminated patients
2. Patients with certain types of internal contamination
3. Patients exposed only to external total body radiation
4. Patients exposed only to external local body radiation

If treatment of great numbers of radiation-exposed and contaminated patients is necessary, different modes of treatment may be indicated. Home treatment with showers or garden hoses should be considered, as should treatment at nearby facilities such as schools. An alternative decontamination facility within the hospital should be such that ready access and shelter available from fallout may be provided for a large number of contaminated patients. Triage should be performed to identify those who may require decontamination. Those found to be contaminated should pass through a disrobing area and a shower, and ultimately be garbed with hospital gowns and reassessed for residual contamination. Again, resuscitation and stabilization always take precedence over decontamination.

Under these circumstances all available GM counters and dosimeters would be commandeered. Provision should be made for initial and follow-up treatment of any injuries. One should also consider establishing a large holding area, with subsequent transfer, if necessary, to other institutions where there is no area-wide radiation risk.

THE EVACUATION DILEMMA

Emergency physicians should be aware of the burden carried by local and state government officials who must make evacuation decisions. A population should be evacuated if the estimated per capita whole body radiation dose will be 5000 mrem or more. However, the present methods of dose assessment have a great range of uncertainty. The timing of a decision to evacuate may be crucial. Thus, officials fail if they wait too long, that is, until dangerous levels of radiation are present in populated areas, and they fail, too, if an unnecessary evacuation is ordered, for there are many risks inherent in an evacuation including adverse effects on moving hospitalized patients, panic reactions, and injuries and death from automobile crashes.

HOSPITAL EVACUATION

It is conceivable that internal hospital evacuation may be necessary in the event of radiation threat. Emergency radiation disaster plans should include designation of preselected sites within the hospital which afford the most protection for patients and health care personnel. Such sites are usually at ground level or below. As much "concrete" as possible should be placed between personnel and the environment. Provision should be made for ensuring appropriate medical equipment, food, medications, and electric power and heat at the new care site (Table 128-3). Consideration should be given to shutting off fans and air conditioning during the critical exposure period (plume phase).

Table 128-3. Emergency Supplies for Use in Radiation Emergencies

1. Radiation detection instruments including Geiger-Müller counters, spare batteries, film badges, ring badges, self-reading dosimeters
2. Surgical scrub suits
3. Surgical gowns
4. Surgical caps
5. Surgical masks
6. Surgical gloves
7. Plastic shoe covers
8. Adhesive tape
9. Plastic sheets and bags
10. Step-off pads
11. Plastic containers for collection of decontamination fluids
12. Decontamination stretcher
13. Roll of plastic floor covering for use in the hallway
14. Radiation "mark off" rope
15. Radioactive signs and labels
16. Filter paper for smears
17. Clipboard, paper, and pens
18. Assorted containers for sample collection

The duration of such an evacuation would be related to the type of radiation and its half-life, atmospheric conditions, availability of supplies, and the condition of the patients.

External evacuation in the event of a radiation threat can be even more chaotic if not properly planned. One central source must provide for the evacuation needs of the hospitals in the area and determine the availability of off-site hospitals. Such an external evacuation would entail the need to categorize patients, effect discharge of ambulatory patients if possible, and provide clinical summaries plus radiographs and reports, a listing of medications and treatments needed, and a 24-h supply of food, water, and medications. Categorized patients would be taken to different and appropriate facility staging areas within the facility to await their external evacuation.

LESSONS LEARNED FROM CHERNOBYL

In the Three Mile Island incident, two workers received 3 to 4 rem total body dose and several received β radiation skin exposure of about 300 rem. No acute injury resulted in any of these cases. By contrast, 203 people were hospitalized and 29 died of radiation exposure as a result of the Chernobyl accident.

The lesson: build safe nuclear power plants. The Chernobyl #4 reactor, unlike U.S. nuclear power plants, contained a large mass of combustible material (2700 tons of graphite) and had much less contamination protection than do U.S. reactors.

A radiation disaster plan should include provision for (1) on-site triage, (2) a nearby hospital prepared for secondary triage, further decontamination, and treatment of life-threatening injuries, and (3) identified tertiary care radiation injury treatment centers to deal with contaminated injuries, including those of burn patients and patients in the advanced hematologic and immune system–suppressed states.

Based on the Chernobyl experience most patients receiving less than 400 rem whole body radiation can be expected to recover, if provided with optimal supportive care. Indeed, survival following a dose of 600 rem now appears possible.

The human immune system is vulnerable between 150 and 200 rem. At total body radiation exposures between 200 and 1500 rem, marrow damage is a major cause of death. And at higher doses, survival is limited by damage to skin, liver, lung, and gastrointestinal tract. At 5000 rem (50 Gy), death occurs in less than 2 days from central nervous system vasculitis.

Inhalation of particulate radioactivity can be significantly reduced (a factor of 3 to 5) by breathing through several layers of moistened handkerchiefs, although the method is almost ineffective against gaseous radioiodines.

Emergency physicians might be faced with evaluating patients at times other than after acute exposure. In that context, the following points are important: granulocytopenic patients who develop fever require treatment with antibiotics, generally with those that cover enteric bacteria. Acyclovir is helpful in treating oral herpes simplex infection, which is apt to recrudesce following radiation exposure. If fever persists in a patient being treated with antibiotics, one should think of the possibility of systemic fungal infections and consider treating with amphotericin B.

Thermal burns and significant musculoskeletal and visceral injuries, if present, contribute significantly to radiation-related deaths. Physical radiation monitoring devices may prove inadequate, as they did at Chernobyl, in a nuclear accident. The devices may be destroyed, or they may not have been designed for the high levels of radiation encountered.

At Chernobyl biological dosimetry was used for dose assessment. Thus, serial measurements of granulocyte and lymphocyte levels as well as analyses of blood and bone marrow cell chromosomes for dicentrics, tricentrics, and rings were performed. In the case of cell chromosome analyses, the number of changes per cell is linearly related to exposures between 15 and 600 rem. The time elapsed between exposure and the onset of nausea and/or vomiting was also used for dose assessment purposes.

The world's ongoing need for nonfossil energy sources is borne out by the choices of other nations. The Japanese are building 100 more nuclear reactors, the Soviets have doubled their commitment, and 74 percent of France's power generation is from nuclear plants.

SPECIAL ASPECTS OF RADIATION ACCIDENTS AND DISASTERS

In the absence of nuclear war or nuclear power plant disaster, such as occurred at Chernobyl, it is unlikely that most hospitals will receive any patients who have been involved in life-threatening radiation accidents. It is more likely that a given hospital's emergency department personnel will be called upon to handle a patient with routine injuries complicated by inadvertent radiation exposure or the presence of low-level radioactive contamination. Such a circumstance might result from an accident involving transportation of radioactive materials.

Linnemann reported in 1983 that radiation injuries are an infrequent medical event. And despite the Chernobyl accident, that remains true, even though there are ever-increasing production and use of radiation-producing machines, radioactive products, nuclear plants, and nuclear weapons. Thus, as of 1988, worldwide there had been 69 peacetime deaths secondary to radiation exposure. And of these 69, 9 were in the United States. No significant injuries or deaths due to radiation overexposure have occurred in the U.S. commercial nuclear power industry since its inception in 1957. L. L. Richter and coworkers report that the majority of industrial radiation accidents involve personnel radiated from high-activity sealed sources used in radiography. Nevertheless, as we plan for the more likely minor radiation accident, we must recognize that it is possible that the United States might sustain a terrorist attack with a nuclear weapon or suffer the accidental discharge and detonation of a nuclear weapon by another nation. An all-out exchange of thermonuclear weapons would not likely leave enough medical facilities and staff to provide an effective response, nor would any medical response under such conditions be apt to be sustainable.

Whatever the basis for a radiation accident or disaster, prior communication, instruction, and staff exercises are the best preparation for any eventuality. As a corollary, ongoing communication with staff during an exercise or "real life" accident or disaster is a must. The role of the public relations department is very important, for it is such personnel who, under such circumstances, deal with the media and the public.

In addition to your own staff and others who are experienced and knowledgeable about radiation, there are other individuals and organizations, private, state, and federal, willing and able to promptly respond to your call for aid. REAC/TS can be contacted 24 hours a day for radiation accident assistance at (615) 576-1004 and Radiation Management Consultants (RMC) may be contacted at (215) 537-0672.

Nuclear facilities do not "blow up" like nuclear bombs. It is physically impossible. Rather, a nuclear plant accident is more apt to be associated with a potentially large number of people being slightly exposed, slightly contaminated, and very anxious.

Finally it should be realized that rarely do radiation accident victims just walk in off the street. The use of hazardous quantities of radioactive materials or radiation producing machines require licensure or registration and individuals knowledgeable in radiation safety. Such individuals should be available to advise physicians, at least initially.

BIBLIOGRAPHY

Becker DV: Reactor accidents. *JAMA* 258:649, 1987.

Benson JM: Radiation safety. *J Fam Practice* 15:435, 1982.

Bores RJ: The scope of Nuclear Regulatory Commission requirements for arrangements for contaminated injured individuals. *Bull NY Acad Med* 59:956, 1983.

Champlin RE: Radiation accidents and nuclear energy: Medical consequences and therapy. *Ann Intern Med* 109:730, 1988.

DeMuth WE, Miller KL: A perspective on Three Mile Island. *Contin Educat Fam Physician* 17:18, 1982.

Geiger HJ: The accident at Chernobyl and the medical response. *JAMA* 256:609, 1986.

Hendee WR: Management of individuals accidently exposed to radiation or radioactive materials. *Semin Nucl Med* 16:203, 1986.

Leonard RB, Rucks RC: Emergency department radiation accident protocol. *Ann Emerg Med* 9:462, 1980.

Linnemann RE: Initial management of radiation injuries. *J Radiat Protect* 5:1, 1980.

Linnemann RE: Medical and public health consequences of the off-site release of radiation. Presented at the Medical Planning and Protocols for Nuclear Accidents Seminar at Lincolnshire, Illinois, September 1983.

Linnemann RE: Radiation injuries. Presented at the Medical Planning and Protocols for Nuclear Accidents Seminar, Lincolnshire, Illinois, September 1983.

Linnemann RE: Medical experience and preparedness for handling radiation injuries. *J Med Assoc Georgia* 78:95, 1989.

Management of Persons Accidently Contaminated with Radionuclide, report 65. National Council on Radiation Protection and Measurements. April 1980.

Milroy WC: Management of irradiated and contaminated casualty victims. *Emerg Med Clin North Am* 2:667, 1984.

National Council on Radiation Protection and Measurements, Ionizing Radiation Exposure of the Population of the United States, NCRP Report of 93. National Council on Radiation Protection and Measurements, Bethesda, MD, 1987.

Otake H, Schull WJ: In utero exposure to a bomb radiation and mental retardation: A reassessment. *Br J Radiol* 57:409, 1984.

Perry AR, Iglar AF: The accident at Chernobyl: Radiation doses and effects. *Radiol Technol* 61:290, 1990.

Richter LL, Berk LW, Teates CD, et al: A systems approach to the management of radiation accidents. *Ann Emerg Med* 9:303, 1980.

Saenger EL: Radiation accidents. *Ann Emerg Med* 15:1061, 1986.

VanRensburg LCJ, et al: Possible radiation injury at Koeburg Nuclear Power Station. *SAMT* 70:487, 1986.

Young RW: Chernobyl in retrospect. *Pharmacol Therapy* 39:27, 1988.

129 MUSHROOM POISONING

Christopher H. Linden
Barry H. Rumack

Mushrooms, also known as toadstools, are the visible fruit of certain fungi. Of the thousands of species known to exist, only about 100 can cause serious illness, and only about 10 are responsible for fatal poisoning. Parallel with the increased popularity of foraging for edible wild mushrooms, the incidence of mushroom poisoning has risen in recent years. Of the thousands of ingestions of potentially toxic mushrooms reported annually in the United States, however, only a few hundred result in significant morbidity or death.

Poisoning is most common during the late summer and early fall, since wild mushrooms are most abundant during these seasons. It most often occurs when amateur foragers (and their friends and relatives) mistake poisonous species for edible ones. *Amanita phalloides* (the "death cap") and *A. virosa* (the "destroying angel") are the species responsible for most fatalities. Young children who accidentally ingest a wild mushroom rarely become seriously ill (unless they partake of a mushroom meal served to them by adults), probably because uncooked wild mushrooms are generally not very palatable. Recreational drug users may experience untoward effects after intentionally ingesting hallucinogenic mushrooms. They may also become poisoned by phencyclidine (PCP) or lysergic acid diethylamide (LSD), since edible mushrooms laced with these chemicals are frequently sold on the street as psychoactive species. Although hallucinogenic mushrooms are most commonly ingested (usually as dried or fresh mushroom pieces but occasionally after brewing as a tea), they are sometimes snorted, smoked, or injected intravenously. The inhalation of vapors evolved during the boiling (i.e., attempted detoxification) of some species of wild mushrooms can also cause poisoning.

Under certain circumstances, or in susceptible persons, poisoning can occur after the ingestion of normally edible mushrooms. Some species of edible mushrooms cause an adverse reaction if ingested with ethanol. Mushrooms can become contaminated with bacteria or chemicals (e.g., insecticides). The common grocery store mushroom, *Agaricus bisporus,* can cause unpleasant gastrointestinal effects in individuals who are inherently intolerant to this species.

There are no easy rules for differentiating poisonous from edible species. That boiling, drying, or salting a poisonous mushroom will detoxify it are common misconceptions. Correctly identifying a mushroom as edible or poisonous requires careful analysis of its morphologic features by an experienced mycologist.

Toxic and nontoxic species may be found growing side by side, they may be gathered and eaten together, and the mushroom available for identification may not be the one (or the only one) ingested. The appearance and toxicity of a given species of mushroom may vary depending on such factors as mushroom maturity, geographic location, and growing conditions. Poisonous strains of reportedly edible mushrooms may exist. The treatment of poisoning by one species of mushroom may be harmful if another species or condition is the true source. For these reasons, it is the clinical presentation that ultimately determines the diagnosis and the appropriate treatment.

PHARMACOLOGY

Poisonous mushrooms can be divided into eight different groups based on their principal toxins and the nature and time of onset of clinical toxicity (Table 129-1). *Amatoxins* are bicyclic octapeptides which act by inhibiting RNA polymerase II and thus interfere with DNA and RNA transcription. The resultant disintegration of nucleoli and disruption of protein synthesis ultimately causes potentially fatal intestinal, hepatic, and renal tubular necrosis. Intestinal effects may be mediated or enhanced by cyclic heptapeptides (phallotoxins) also present in species containing amatoxins. Amatoxins are rapidly absorbed, metabolized, and excreted in bile and urine. They are not significantly bound to plasma proteins and do not cross the placental barrier. Metabolic activation of amatoxins by hepatic cytochrome P_{450} microsomal enzymes may be involved in the pathogenesis of poisoning. Amatoxins are heat stable and nonvolatile; boiling, cooking, or drying mushrooms containing these toxins does not affect their potency.

Gyromitrins are hydrazones whose hydrazine metabolites (e.g., *N*-methyl-*N*-formylhydrazine and *N*-monomethyl-hydrazine, MFH and MMH) can oxidize hemoglobin, inhibit glutamic acid decarboxylase, and cause fatal hepatitis and, possibly, interstitial nephritis. The oxidization of hemoglobin could potentially cause methemoglobinemia and Heinz body hemolytic anemia. Inhibition of glutamic acid decarboxylase results in decreased γ-aminobutyric acid (GABA) synthesis. Low central nervous system (CNS) levels of this inhibitory neurotransmitter may be responsible for the neurologic toxicity of gyromitrins. Hepatic damage may result from a direct interaction between gyromitrins and mixed function oxidase enzymes.

These toxins are eliminated primarily by hepatic metabolism, with lesser amounts excreted unchanged in the urine. Small amounts also undergo pulmonary excretion. Since gyromitrins are volatile, boiling or drying reduces the toxicity of gyromitrin-containing mushrooms. Such processing does not, however, necessarily render them harmless.

Orellanine and orelline are bipyridine cyclopeptides which can inhibit renal alkaline phosphatase, decrease adenosine triphosphate production, and cause a tubulointerstitial nephritis. Their biological disposition is unclear. Heating or drying mushrooms containing these toxins does not reduce their toxicity.

Coprine is a glutamine derivative whose metabolite(s) appear to act by inhibiting alcohol dehydrogenase or dopamine decarboxylase. If ingested with ethanol, mushrooms containing coprine can cause β-adrenergic stimulation similar to that which results from disulfiram-ethanol reactions. Coprine and its metabolites are metabolized by the liver and excreted in urine. These toxins are not destroyed by heat.

Ibotenic acid and muscimol are isoxazole derivatives which are similar to GABA in structure. They interact with multiple central and peripheral neurotransmitters and neuroreceptors causing hallucinations and manifestations of inhibited cholinergic activity. Mushrooms containing ibotenic acid and muscimol may also contain pharmacologically insignificant amounts of muscarine. Ibotenic acid and its metabolite, muscimol, are eliminated primarily by hepatic metabolism. These toxins and their inactive metabolites are excreted in the urine. Boiling or cooking does not affect the toxicity of mushrooms containing these chemicals, but drying may reduce their potency.

Muscarine, an aminofuran alkaloid, acts by stimulating peripheral parasympathetic (cholinergic) neurons. It also may have histamine-releasing or receptor-stimulating activity. Muscarine is eliminated primarily by hepatic metabolism. The parent chemical and its metabolites are excreted in the urine. Muscarine is heat stable and nonvolatile.

Psilocybin and psilocin are dimethyltryptamines, similar in structure to serotonin. Interactions with CNS neuroreceptors appear to be responsible for their hallucinogenic and sympathomimetic activity. Psilocybin undergoes hepatic metabolism to the more active psilocin. Psilocin is eliminated primarily by metabolism, with small amounts excreted unchanged in the urine. Cooking or drying mushrooms containing these chemicals does not detoxify them.

Miscellaneous/unidentified toxins probably act locally on the gastrointestinal tract as mucosal irritants or motility stimulants.

For most toxins and mushrooms, the minimal dose that will result in human poisoning is unknown. Hence, it is prudent to assume that all intentional ingestions (i.e., mushroom consumption for food or hallucinogenic effects) and all accidental ingestions of more than one mushroom are capable of causing poisoning.

Table 129-1. Classification of Poisonous Mushrooms

Principal Toxin	Genus (Species)*	Clinical Toxicity†	Onset‡
Amatoxins	*Amanita* (*bisporigia, ocreata, phalloides, suballiacae, tennifolia, verna, virosa*); *Conocybe* (*filaris*); *Galerina* (*autumnalis, marginata, vererata*); *Lepiota* (*helveola*)	Hepatitis Renal tubular necrosis	Late
Gyromitrins	*Gyromitra* (*brunnea, caroliniana, fastigiate, infula, umbigna*); *Paxina* (*involutus*); *Sarcosphaera* (*coronaria*)	Hepatitis CNS depression/stimulation Hemolysis ?Methemoglobinemia	Late
Orellanine/orelline	*Cortinarius* (*calisteus, cinnamomeus, gentilis, orellanus, rainierensis, semisanguineus, speciosissimus*)	Tubulointerstitial nephritis	Late
Coprine	*Clitocybe* (*calvipes*); *Coprinus* (*atramentarius*)	Disulfiram-ethanol-like reaction	Early
Ibotenic acid/ muscimol	*Amanita* (*cokeri, cothurna, gemmata, musaria, pantherina*)	Hallucinations Anticholinergic effects	Early
Muscarine	*Boletus* (*calopus, luridus, pulcherrimus, satanas*); *Clitocybe* (*cerbissata, dealbata, illudens, and rivulosa*); *Inocybe* (*fatigata, geophylla, lilacina, patuoillardi, purica, rimosus*); *Omphalotus* (olearius)	Cholinergic effects	Early
Psilocybin/psilocin	*Conocybe* (*cyanopus*); *Gymmopilus* (*auruginosa, spetabilis, validipes*); *Psilocybe* (*balocystis, caerulescens, cubensis, cyanescens, fimentaria, mexicana, semilanceata, silvatica*); *Strophans* (*coronilla*)	Hallucinations Sympathomimetic effects	Early
Miscellaneous/ unidentified	*Boletus, Chorophyllum, Entoloma, Gomphius, Hebeloma, Lacterius, Omphalotus, Paxillus, Pholiota, Ramaria, Russula, Tricholoma,* and *Verpa* species	Gastroenteritis	Early

* Partial listing (other toxic species may exist).

† Includes gastroenteritis in virtually all cases of mushroom poisoning.

‡ Late indicates effects begin more than 6 h after ingestion, whereas early indicates onset within 3 h of ingestion.

CLINICAL TOXICITY

Regardless of group, initial symptoms of mushroom poisoning consist of nausea, vomiting, diarrhea, and abdominal cramps. The time of onset and severity of these symptoms and the nature and severity of subsequent toxicity differ from group to group. The severity of poisoning may also reflect differences in the amount of toxin ingested or absorbed, in individual susceptibility, or in toxin metabolism.

Amatoxin poisoning has a delayed onset. Nausea, vomiting, thirst, colicky abdominal pain, and profuse diarrhea typically begin abruptly 6 to 24 h (up to 48 h) after the ingestion of mushrooms containing these toxins (Table 129-1). The emesis and diarrhea may be bloody. Gastrointestinal effects tend to be more severe and prolonged than those caused by other groups. Severe dehydration with hypotension, tachycardia, and oliguria can occur. Laboratory findings may include acidosis, hyperamylasemia, hypoglycemia, leukocytosis, increased BUN and creatinine, and abnormalities of serum sodium and potassium due to fluid and electrolyte losses. The hematocrit may decrease as a result of blood loss or increase as a result of hemoconcentration.

Gastrointestinal symptoms may last 12 to 24 h and be terminated by a period of apparent improvement, or they may continue unabated. Adynamic ileus can occur. One to three days following ingestion, liver enzymes, bilirubin, and the PT and PTT may begin to rise. Right upper quadrant pain, liver enlargement and tenderness, jaundice, hypoglycemia, coagulopathy, cardiomyopathy, asterixis, encephalopathy, seizures, coma, and other features of hepatic failure may ensue. Concomitant renal failure with increasing levels of BUN and creatinine, oliguria, hematuria, and proteinuria may be noted. Kidney dysfunction can occasionally occur without significant hepatotoxicity.

Most patients with amatoxin poisoning recover slowly over a period of 1 or more weeks. In severe cases, progressive hepatic failure may end in death (most commonly about 7 days after mushroom ingestion).

Gyromitrin poisoning also has a delayed onset. Gastrointestinal symptoms typically begin 6 to 8 h (sometimes as long as 24 h) after the ingestion of certain species (Table 129-1). They tend to be mild to moderate in severity and duration and are often accompanied by agitation, ataxia, hyperreflexia, muscle cramps, vertigo, and weakness. A severe headache is typically present. Gyromitrin poisoning can also occur following the inhalation of vapors during the cooking of mushrooms containing these toxins.

In severe cases, dehydration and biochemical evidence of hepatitis, sometimes progressing to hepatic failure, may ensue. Laboratory findings are similar to those seen in amatoxin poisoning but are usually less pronounced. Additional complications may include hemolysis with anemia and hemoglobinuria, and renal failure. Hypoglycemia and methemoglobinemia have been observed in experimental animal poisoning. In severe cases, recovery often takes several weeks. Fatalities are rare.

Orellanine and orelline poisoning is even more slow and insidious in onset. Gastrointestinal symptoms are typically mild, transient, and do not occur until 1 to 3 days after the ingestion of mushrooms containing these toxins (Table 129-1). Constipation, rather than diarrhea, is often present. Patients frequently do not seek medical attention until 3 days to 3 weeks after ingestion, when they develop renal toxicity. Anorexia, chills, headache, malaise, night sweats, back pain, polyuria or oliguria, and thirst (often intense and burning) are the usual presenting complaints. Examination may reveal flank tenderness. Typical laboratory findings include increased BUN and creatinine, albuminuria (sometimes massive), hematuria, and red cell casts in the urine. Renal failure may be permanent and is potentially fatal. In most cases, renal function returns to normal, or near normal, over a period of several weeks to several months.

Coprine poisoning occurs only if ethanol is consumed within several hours to several days of the ingestion of certain normally edible mushroom species (Table 129-1). If the interval between mushroom and ethanol ingestion is longer than 24 h, patients may not relate the two events and the cause of symptoms may not be appreciated. Symptoms typically begin within a half hour of ethanol ingestion and last 3 to 6 h. The severity of poisoning appears to correlate directly with the quantity of mushrooms ingested and inversely with the time interval between mushroom and ethanol ingestion.

Gastrointestinal symptoms can occur abruptly and be severe. Other manifestations of the coprine-ethanol reaction include agitation, confusion, diaphoresis, dyspnea, flushed skin, headache, hypotension (supine or orthostatic), chest tightness, palpitations, tachycardia, paresthesias, vertigo, and weakness. Arrhythmias (atrial fibrillation and premature atrial and ventricular beats) have been reported.

Ibotenic acid and muscimol poisoning is typically associated with the recreational use of certain species of mushrooms (Table 129-1) for their mind-altering effects. Symptoms usually begin 20 min to 2 h following mushroom ingestion. Although vomiting can occur, gastrointestinal effects are often absent. Drowsiness, dizziness, and lethargy may be followed by agitation, ataxia, confusion, delirium, euphoria, hallucinations, and psychosis. The level of consciousness may fluctuate. Coma and seizures can occur in severe cases. Hallucinations are characteristically visual (e.g., misperceptions of color and shape) and tend to be illusionary. Anticholinergic effects such as dry skin, fever, mydriasis, myoclonus, hypertension, and tachycardia may also present. Except for a headache, which may last several days following acute intoxication, symptoms rarely last more than 8 h.

Muscarine poisoning typically begins 15 min to 2 h after the ingestion of mushrooms containing this toxin (Table 129-1). Gastrointestinal symptoms are usually mild to moderate in severity. They are often associated with manifestations of cholinergic hyperactivity such as blurred vision, diaphoresis, headache, lacrimation, miosis, salivation, and urinary frequency. Skin flushing may sometimes be noted. Bradycardia, hypotension, seizures, and wheezing can occur in severe cases. Transient increases in hepatic enzymes have also been reported. Symptoms usually last from 2 to 10 h.

Psilocin and psilocybin poisoning occur primarily in the setting of the recreational use of certain psychoactive mushroom species (Table 129-1). Symptoms begin 30 to 60 min after ingestion and include ataxia, blurred vision, confusion, dysphoria, hallucinations, incoordination, paresthesias, and weakness. If present, nausea and vomiting are usually mild and transient. Hallucinations are most often visual, but they can also be auditory or tactile. Although psychic effects are usually perceived as pleasant, ''bad trips'' with aggressive, irrational, and suicidal behavior can occur. Physical manifestations, usually mild, may include hyperreflexia, hypertension, mydriasis, and trachycardia. Symptoms rarely last longer than 4 to 6 h following ingestion, but ''flashbacks'' may occur for months following acute intoxication.

Severe poisoning can result in coma, hyperthermia, seizures, and death. It occurs primarily in children and follows ingestion. Severe poisoning may also occur in adults following the intravenous injection of mushroom extracts. Manifestations of poisoning by this route may include arthralgias, cyanosis, chills, fever, and myalgias. Laboratory findings may include hypoxia, mild methemoglobinemia, and biochemical evidence of hepatorenal dysfunction.

Miscellaneous/unidentified toxins are present in a variety of mushrooms (Table 129-1). They cause poisoning of variable duration and severity. Gastrointestinal symptoms may begin 30 min to 6 h after mushroom ingestion and last 4 to 48 h. They are usually mild, but gastrointestinal fluid losses can sometimes lead to dehydration. Bloody diarrhea may occasionally be present. Infrequent complaints include chills, diaphoresis, dyspnea, headache, myalgias, light-headedness, carpopedal spasm, paresthesias, and weakness.

DIAGNOSTIC EVALUATION

A high index of suspicion is necessary in order to avoid missing the diagnosis of mushroom poisoning. There may be nothing to suggest that what first appears to be a self-limited gastrointestinal process such as viral gastroenteritis or food poisoning may progress to a more serious or even fatal illness unless a history of mushroom ingestion is elicited. By routinely including mushroom poisoning in the differential diagnosis of ''gastroenteritis,'' subsequent morbidity and mortality may be averted.

When a history of mushroom ingestion is available, the time of ingestion, the number of mushrooms and mushroom species that were consumed, who else ate them, and the nature, severity, and time of onset of symptoms should be determined. The clinical course and manifestations of poisoning can be used to presumptively identify the offending toxin. Although gastrointestinal symptoms are nonspecific, the time between mushroom ingestion and their onset depends on the toxin involved and is a useful parameter.

An interval of more than 6 h between mushroom ingestion and the onset of symptoms suggests amatoxin, gyromitrin, or orellanine/orelline poisoning; an interval of less than 6 h suggests coprine, ibotenic acid/muscimol, muscarine, psilocin/psilocybin, or miscellaneous/unidentified toxin poisoning. This distinction is important because it differentiates mushrooms which are cytotoxic and can cause permanent organ damage with serious or fatal consequences from those which are physiotoxic and cause only transient autonomic and central nervous system dysfunction.

Both the very young and the elderly appear to be more susceptible to fluid and electrolyte disturbances secondary to vomiting and diarrhea than those of intermediate age. Small children also appear to be more sensitive to other effects of ingested toxins, and the elderly are more likely to have underlying health problems which could adversely effect the outcome of poisoning. The method of mushroom preparation sometimes influences the severity of poisoning. Cooking can decrease the toxicity of mushrooms containing gyromitrins, but it can also generate toxic vapors.

The physical exam should initially be directed toward assessing the patient for potential dehydration. Orthostatic vital signs should be routinely measured. The pulse, blood pressure, temperature, pupil size, neuromuscular function, and skin characteristics should also be evaluated for signs of cholinergic, anticholinergic, or sympathetic stimulation. The level of consciousness and mental status should be documented with particular attention to the presence or absence of hallucinations. A general cardiopulmonary exam should be performed. The abdomen should be examined for tenderness and bowel sounds. The presence or absence of jaundice and flank pain should be noted. If signs of peritoneal irritation are present, a diagnosis other than mushroom poisoning should be considered. Any available stool or vomitus should be tested for the presence of occult blood.

In patients with moderate or severe gastrointestinal symptoms or signs of dehydration, routine laboratory tests should include a complete blood count, electrolytes, BUN, creatinine, glucose, and urinalysis. If symptoms began more than 6 h after mushroom ingestion or if ingestion of a cytotoxic species is suspected or confirmed by mushroom identification, a serum amylase level and liver function tests (i.e., SGOT/AST, SGPT/ALT, bilirubin, PT/PTT) should also be obtained. Toxicology screening may be useful to rule out other etiologies of poisoning. Except for psilocin, however, mushroom toxins cannot be identified by routine urine testing. Specific assays can detect other toxins but they are not routinely available. Abdominal x-rays can confirm the diagnosis of an ileus but are not otherwise helpful. Cardiac rhythm analysis by monitor or EKG should be performed in patients with chest pain, hypotension, palpitations, respiratory symptoms, or an abnormal cardiopulmonary finding.

If a sample of the ingested mushroom can be obtained, analysis of the shape, texture, and color of the pileus (cap), gills, stipe (stem), base, and spores can be used to identify its genus and species and hence the offending toxin. The odor, food substrate (e.g., soil, wood, dung, or another mushroom), habitat, geographic location, and the season of harvest are also helpful. It is best to have the mushroom examined by a competent mycologist. Prior arrangements will prevent confusion and costly or even fatal delays when an emergency arises. Mycologists may be located through university botany departments, botanical gardens, mycological societies and clubs, and poison centers. A listing of state mycological societies and color photographs of common poisonous mushrooms (and their spores) may be found in *Poisindex*.

If a mycologist is not physically available to examine the mushroom, the mushroom can be sent to one. When shipping a mushroom, it should first be dried in air, by hot light, hairdryer, or in an oven (microwaves excluded) at 95°C (200°F). It should be shipped in a paper container rather than a plastic one to avoid decomposition. Alternatively, the physician may describe the mushroom to the mycologist or attempt to identify the mushroom utilizing one of the many available field guides.

When a sample of the mushroom is not available, identification may still be possible by microscopic examination of spores recovered from the patient's vomitus, gastric aspirate, or stool. Spores may also be found on the gills of a partially eaten mushroom or on the dish from which the mushroom was served. The specimen should be suspended in a drop of water, placed on a slide with a coverslip, and examined using an oil immersion lens. Spores are oval or popcorn-kernel-shaped and are similar in size to red blood cells (8 to 20 μm). The parent mushroom may be identified by comparing observed spore features (e.g., color, size, shape, surface texture, wall thickness, presence or absence of an apical pore) with those found in photographs and descriptions in reference texts.

If no spores are seen on direct smear, the sample can be filtered through cheesecloth, using water as an emulsifier, certrifuged for 10 min, and reexamined. If spores are still not seen, the sediment can be heat-fixed to the slide and stained with 1% acid fuchsin. This gives spores a vivid-red appearance. Spores may also be stained with Meltzer's solution, which can be made by dissolving 1.5 g of potassium iodide, 0.5 g of iodine, and 20 g of chloral hydrate in 20 mL of water. The resulting spore wall color is characteristic of a given species of mushroom and may be helpful if the spore cannot be positively identified by its other characteristics.

GENERAL MANAGEMENT

Treatment begins with supportive care. Airway management, ventilatory support, oxygenation, and correction of hemodynamic instability are the highest priorities. Attention should then be focused on gastrointestinal decontamination.

A bolus of glucose should be given to patients with altered mental status, and acid-base and electrolyte abnormalities should be corrected. Except when using atropine for cholinergic poisoning, antiemetics and antispasmodics should be avoided, since such therapy may delay spontaneous evacuation of stool or vomitus and lead to increased toxin absorption.

Activated charcoal (0.5 to 1 g/kg orally or by nasogastric tube) is recommended for gastrointestinal decontamination in all patients. In the absence of spontaneous diarrhea, a cathartic such as sorbitol should be administered along with activated charcoal. Syrup of ipecac can be used for the home treatment of children with accidental ingestions. In addition to a dose of charcoal, whole bowel irrigation (e.g., 0.5 to 2 L/h of a Colyte or Golightly bowel prep solution orally or by nasogastric tube) should also be considered if the ingestion of a cytotoxic species is suspected and treatment can be accomplished within 24 h of ingestion. Multiple-dose activated charcoal therapy (i.e., repeated dosing every 2 to 4 h during the first 48 h after ingestion) may enhance the elimination of previously absorbed toxins and is also recommended.

Patients with potential amatoxin, gyromitrin, or orellanine/orelline poisoning and those with moderate to severe poisoning caused by other mushroom toxins should be admitted for observation and/or treatment. Other patients can be discharged from the emergency department if they remain or become asymptomatic after a 4- to 6-h period of observation and treatment. Those who are discharged should be instructed to return promptly if symptoms reoccur. Patients who intentionally ingest hallucinogenic mushrooms should be referred for drug abuse counseling.

TOXIN-SPECIFIC TREATMENT

A number of toxin elimination measures, metabolic antidotes, and physiologic antagonists have been used in the treatment of specific types of mushroom poisoning. Unfortunately, there are few if any controlled trials documenting the efficacy of these measures.

Specific interventions that may be helpful in the treatment of *amatoxin* poisoning include forced diuresis, charcoal hemoperfusion, high-dose penicillin, high-dose cimetidine, liver transplantation, and possibly hyperbaric oxygen therapy, high-dose ascorbic acid, and *N*-acetylcysteine. Silibinin and aucubin may also be effective, but they are not yet available for human use in the United States. Corticosteroids and thioctic acid are of no benefit and are no longer recommended.

Forced diuresis and charcoal hemoperfusion may enhance amatoxin elimination. Diuresis (i.e., maintaining a urine output of 2 to 4 mL/kg per hour) using normal saline is likely to be effective only if employed during the first 10 h following ingestion. Hemoperfusion is likely to be effective only if undertaken within 24 h (or possibly 48 h) of ingestion. Whether it offers any advantage over multiple doses of oral charcoal is unknown. Hemoperfusion may also be used supportively (i.e., for the correction of metabolic and neurologic abnormalities associated with severe liver failure). Hemodialysis does not enhance amatoxin elimination, but it can be used as a supportive procedure in patients with renal failure.

Penicillin is thought to act by inhibiting the uptake of amatoxin by hepatocytes. It may also act by sterilizing the gut and inhibiting the bacterial production of GABA, a neurotransmitter thought to be involved in the pathogenesis of hepatic encephalopathy. Recommended doses of penicillin G (benzyl penicillin) range from 0.2 to 0.6 mg/kg per day (in divided doses) for 2 to 3 days following mushroom ingestion. Hyperbaric oxygen therapy may enhance the efficacy of penicillin and is reasonable to employ as an adjunctive measure if it is easily and readily available.

Large doses of cimetidine prevent amatoxin-induced hepatic damage in experimental animals. Cimetidine appears to act by inhibiting hepatic cytochrome P_{450} enzymes, since other H_2 blockers are not as effective. Since therapeutic doses of this drug are known to inhibit cytochrome P_{450} enzymes in humans, maximal recommended adult doses (600 mg intravenously every 6 h) might be beneficial if given during the first 2 to 3 days after mushroom ingestion. High-dose ascorbic acid enhances the efficacy of cimetidine in experimental amatoxin poisoning. Hence, adjunctive therapy with maximal human doses of this vitamin (i.e., 10 to 40 mg/kg per day orally or intravenously in divided doses) might also be helpful.

N-Acetylcysteine (Mucomyst) might also be effective in amatoxin poisoning since amatoxin metabolites generated by cytochrome P_{450} enzymes appear to be involved in the pathogenesis of hepatoxicity. Although it is not effective in experimental animals when given in a single dose, a regimen similar to that used in the treatment of human acetaminophen poisoning might be beneficial.

Silibinin, a milk thistle extract, appears to be effective in preventing hepatotoxicity when given intravenously in doses of 20 to 50 mg/kg per day for 2 to 4 days. Its active component, silymarin, may inhibit the uptake of amatoxins by hepatocytes. Silibinin is currently being studied in clinical trials in Europe. Dietary preparations of silibinin (sold in health food stores in the United States) may also be effective, but the therapeutic oral dose is unknown. Aucubin, an iridoid glycoside obtained from the plants aucuba japonica and picrorhiza kurroa, may also be an effective antidote, but it has only been studied in animals.

In addition to standard treatments of hepatic failure, liver transplantation has been used with success in patients with severe amatoxin poisoning. It should not be performed prematurely, however, as some patients spontaneously recover despite having marked hepatic dysfunction during the first week after mushroom ingestion.

Specific treatments that may be helpful in patients with *gyromitrin* poisoning include pyridoxine, benzodiazepines, diuresis, blood transfusions, and possibly methylene blue. As in isoniazid poisoning, pyridoxine may reverse the inhibition of glutamic acid decarboxylase by substituting for pyridoxal phosphate, the enzyme's cofactor. It may be effective in reversing neurologic toxicity. The recommended dose is 25 mg/kg, given intravenously over 15 to 30 min. The dose can be repeated up to four times in 24 h if symptoms persist or recur. Higher doses are unlikely to be of additional benefit and may result in pyridoxine toxicity. Benzodiazepines may also be used to control agitation and neuromuscular hyperactivity.

Maintenance of a normal or brisk urine output may enhance hemoglobin excretion and prevent associated renal dysfunction in patients with hemolysis. Red blood cell transfusions might also be necessary. Although probably only a theoretical concern, significant methemoglobinemia (i.e., levels above 30 percent or lower levels associated with hypoxic or ischemic manifestations) could require treatment with intravenous methylene blue (0.1 to 0.2 mL/kg of a 1% solution).

The treatment of *orellanine/orelline* poisoning consists primarily of maintaining fluid and electrolyte homeostasis and temporary or chronic support of renal function using dialysis. Charcoal hemoperfusion may enhance toxin elimination. It is probably most effective if started within 2 days of mushroom ingestion but may be of some benefit up to 1 week after ingestion. Whether hemoperfusion is superior to repeated oral doses of charcoal is unknown.

In patients with *coprine-ethanol reactions,* dopamine or norepinephrine may be required for the treatment of hypotension unresponsive to fluid administration. Pharmacologic therapy may also be required for tachyarrhythmias. β Blockers are the most theoretically attractive choice, but any antiarrhythmic drug may be used. Myocardial ischemia and infarction should be treated with standard measures.

Patients with *ibotenic acid/muscimol* poisoning may require control of neuromuscular hyperactivity. Reassurance and a quiet atmosphere may be effective in calming agitated patients. If necessary, restraint should be accomplished by pharmacologic rather than physical measures. Benzodiazepines are preferable to neuroleptic agents since the latter may lower the seizure threshold. Physostigmine may also be tried, but only if EKG analysis reveals sinus tachycardia with normal PR, QRS, and QT intervals and peripheral anticholinergic findings are also present. It is given as a slow intravenous bolus over several minutes in an initial dose of 1 to 2 mg in adults and 0.5 mg in children. The dose may be repeated if the response is incomplete or transient. Seizures should be treated with standard anticonvulsants.

Specific treatments that may be helpful in patients with *muscarine* poisoning include atropine, inhaled bronchodilators (i.e., β_2 agonists), and possibly antihistamines. Atropine is effective in decreasing excessive pharyngeal or pulmonary secretions. It may also be used to treat hypotension unresponsive to fluid administration when it is accompanied by bradycardia. Atropine is also effective in treating gastrointestinal cramps, vomiting, diarrhea, and diaphoresis. However, it should not be used solely for this purpose unless there is a clear history of ingestion of mushrooms containing muscarine, since ibotenic acid/muscimol poisoning may be exacerbated by atropine. The usual dose of atropine is 0.5 to 1.0 mg in adults and 0.01 mg/kg in children, given intravenously. Similar or smaller doses may be repeated as necessary until secretions are controlled or tachycardia develops.

Inhaled bronchodilators (e.g., albuterol, isoetharine, or metaproterenol) may be useful as an adjunctive therapy in patients with wheezing. Antihistamines (both H_1 and H_2 receptor antagonists) are also of theoretical value in the treatment of effects possibly mediated by histamine (e.g., wheezing, hypotension, and flushing).

The treatment of *psilocin/psilocybin* poisoning includes reassurance, avoidance of unnecessary stimulation, and pharmacologic control of behavioral, physiological, and CNS hyperactivity as described for ibotenic acid/muscimol poisoning. Sedative and therapeutic paralysis as well as physical cooling measures may be necessary for the treatment of hyperthermia.

Supportive therapy is all that is necessary for the treatment of patients poisoned by *miscellaneous/unidentified* mushroom toxins.

BIBLIOGRAPHY

Caley MJ, Clark RA: Cardiac arrhythmia after mushroom ingestion. *Br Med J* 2:1633, 1977.

Curry SC, Rose MC: Intravenous mushroom poisoning. *Ann Emerg Med* 14:900, 1985.

Floersheim GL: Treatment of human amatoxin mushroom poisoning: Myths and advances in therapy. *Med Toxicol* 2:1, 1987.

Klein AS, Hart J, Brems JJ, et al: *Amanita* poisoning: Treatment and the role of liver transplantation. *Am J Med* 86:187, 1989.

Lampe KF: Differential diagnosis of poisoning by North American mushrooms, with emphasis on *Amanita phalloides*-like intoxication. *Ann Emerg Med* 16:956, 1987.

Lincoff G, Mitchell DH: *Toxic and Hallucinogenic Mushroom Poisoning: A Handbook for Physicians and Mushroom Hunters.* New York, Van Nostrand Reinhold, 1977.

McCormick DJ, Aubel JJ, Gibbons MC: Nonlethal mushroom poisoning. *Ann Intern Med* 90:332, 1979.

McDonald A: Mushrooms and madness: Hallucinogenic mushrooms and some psychopharmacological implications. *Can J Psychiatr* 25:586, 1980.

Miller OK: *Mushrooms of North America.* New York, Dutton, 1980.

Mitchell DH: *Amanita* mushroom poisoning. *Ann Rev Med* 31:51, 1980.

Schneider SM, Borochovitz D, Krenzelok EP: Cimetidine protection against alpha-amanitin hepatoxicity in mice: A potential model for the treatment of *Amanita phalloides* poisoning. *Ann Emerg Med* 16:1136, 1987.

Short AIK, Watling R, MacDonald WK: Poisoning by *Cortinarius speciosissimus. Lancet* 2:942, 1980.

Vesconi S, Langer M, Iapichino G, et al: Therapy of cytotoxic mushroom intoxication. *Crit Care Med* 13:402, 1985.

130
POISONOUS PLANTS

David C. Michener
Rodger Keller
Robert F. Kowalski

Plants have evolved an extraordinarily complex and diverse array of secondary metabolites that are toxic to the animals (especially insects) that feed on them. That some of these compounds are toxic to humans is inconsequential from an evolutionary perspective. The presence and distribution of pyrrolizidine alkaloids, nonprotein amino acids, cyanogenic and cardiac glycosides, glucosinolates, iridoids, sesquiterpene lactones, saponins, sterols (including estrogens and other vertebrate sex hormones; insect moulting hormones), and tannins vary by plant division (phylum), family, genus, and even within an individual plant both by season and by tissue. As a result, reports from the chemical and ecological literature on the presence or distribution of such compounds in roots, foliage, or fruits may be difficult to place in a clinical context. Since toxic compounds are ubiquitous in noncrop plants (an aspect of domestication is selection for palatability), we focus only on those plants that are reported ingestions with emphasis on the subset that are generally considered to be dangerous to humans.

The tables (Tables 130-1 and 130-2) and descriptions are intended only to allow an initial decision whether the plant involved (determined either by samples or from rough narratives) is the plant featured and whether the toxic parts have been encountered. Good color photographs, although no substitute for a knowledgeable consultant, can be found in the books by Graf, Lampe and McCann, and Westbrooks and Preacher cited in the bibliography of this chapter and may help nonbotanists eliminate candidate plants. Scientific names, family names, and toxins are listed to facilitate cross referencing.

A complex array of herbicides, insecticides, fertilizers, fungicides, and phytohormones are often applied to cultivated plants, especially to their leaves. These organics and/or their "inert" carriers may be the cause of or may confound symptoms.

Table 130-1 lists the "little red berries" most likely to be ingested by children or, from our experience, to be encountered in North America. The most toxic plants are marked(!). Since brightly colored fruits have coevolved with their seed dispersers (primarily birds, occasionally other vertebrates such as turtles), it is noteworthy how few are truly dangerous rather than just unpleasant to humans. *Note that fleshy pulp may be essentially harmless while the seeds, if chewed, may be severely toxic.* This is especially true in *Taxus* and to a lesser extent for many cultivated members of the Rosaceae including apples, apricots, cherries, and pears.

Specific Toxic Plants & Management

Approximately 10 percent of calls to poison control centers concern plants. Fortunately, in most cases, patients are asymptomatic or have a mild gastrointestinal irritation. However, in some cases, plants and plant products can be extremely toxic. When treating patients with plant ingestions, one must remember to treat the patient and not the plant.

The effects seen may be those of pesticides, fertilizers, or adjacent plants, as stated above. The following recommendations for general management of plant ingestions do not include mushroom ingestion or contact dermatitis, which are covered elsewhere in this study guide.

Initial Management

Initial management of plant ingestions is similar to that of other poisonings. However, emergency physicians should be aware that there are a few specific plant ingestions in which standard detoxification procedures are not indicated.

Ipecac, in standard doses, may be used to induce emesis. However,

Table 130-1. "Little Red Berries" of North America Likely to Be Ingested by Children

Scientific Name	Common Names	Family	Key*
!*Abrus precatorius*	Rosary pea	Fabaceae	v
!*Actaea rubra*	Red baneberry	Ranunculaceae	h
Amelanchier spp.	Shad. rowan	Rosaceae	s/t
Arisaema triphyllum	Jack-in-the-pulpit	Araceae	h
Berberis spp.	Barberries	Berberidaceae	s
Capsicum spp.	Ornamental peppers	Solanaceae	h
Celastrus scandens	Bittersweet	Celastraceae	v
!*Convallaria majalis*	Lily-of-the-valley	Liliaceae	h
Cornus spp.†	Dogwoods	Cornaceae	s/t
Cotoneaster spp.†	Cotoneasters	Rosaceae	s
Crataegus spp.	Hawthorns	Rosaceae	t
!*Daphne mezereum*	Daphne	Thymeliaceae	s
Elaeagnus spp.	Autumn and Russian olives	Elaeagnaceae	s
!*Ilex* spp.†	Hollies	Aquifoliaceae	s/t
Lonicera spp.†	Honeysuckles	Caprifoliaceae	s/v
Magnolia spp.	Magnolias	Magnoliaceae	s/t
Malus spp.	Apples and crabapples	Rosaceae	t
Prunus spp.†	Bird and wild cherries	Rosaceae	s/t
Pyracantha	Firethorns	Rosaceae	s
Rhamnus spp.†	Buckthorns	Rhamnaceae	s/t
Schinus spp.†	Pepper trees	Anacardiaceae	s/t
Smilacina racemosa	False Solomon's seal	Liliaceae	h
!*Solanum* spp.†	Nightshades	Solanaceae	h/v
Sorbus spp.	Mountain ashes	Rosaceae	s/t
!*Taxus* spp.	Yews	Taxaceae	s/t
Viburnum spp.†	Viburnums	Caprifoliaceae	s/t

* h = herb, s = shrub, t = tree, v = vine; combinations allowed.

† Fruits may also be black, blue, or purple, especially with age.

! Generally considered to be dangerous; see text.

Table 130-2. Seasonally Common Houseplants and Decorative Materials

Scientific Name	Common Names	Family
THANKSGIVING–NEW YEARS		
Capsicum annuum	Ornamental pepper	Solanaceae
Celastrus scandens	Bittersweet	Celastraceae
Chrysanthemum spp.	Chrysanthemums	Asteraceae
Euphorbia pulcherrima	Poinsettia	Euphorbiaceae
!*Ilex* spp.	Hollies	Aquifoliaceae
Phoradendron	Mistletoes	Loranthaceae
Solanum pseudocapsicum	Jerusalem cherry	Solanaceae
EASTER–PASSOVER		
Crocus spp.	Crocus	Iridaceae
!*Convallaria* spp.	Lily-of-the-valley	Liliaceae
Cyclamen spp.	Florists' cyclamen	Primulaceae
Hyacinthus spp.	Hyacinths	Liliaceae
Lilium spp.	Lilies	Liliaceae
Narcissus spp.	Daffodils	Liliaceae
Tulipa spp.	Tulips	Liliaceae

! Generally considered to be dangerous; see text.

if vomiting and diarrhea have already ensued, its use is not necessary. In two specific plant ingestions, use of ipecac is contraindicated:

1. The jequirity bean (*Abrus precatorius*), which is strongly alkaline and may cause esophageal and pharyngeal burns similar to caustics.
2. The poison hemlocks (*Conium* or *Circuta* species), which may cause seizures.

If the emesis is not successful, the use of lavage may be helpful for large ingestions. However, most plant ingestions are of small quantities, and lavage may not be of benefit. The use of lavage depends on clinical judgment. Activated charcoal with a cathartic in standard doses may be the safest detoxificant, especially if the plant cannot be identified.

Hypotension should be treated with intravenous fluids and the patient placed in the Trendelenburg position. In severe cases, vasopressors may be needed.

If seizures ensue, standard management with diazepam is indicated. If seizures are not controlled, phenytoin or phenobarbital may be used.

Hallucinations may be caused by ingestion of certain plant parts (i.e., morning glory seeds, Convolvulus, and Ipomea). Patients may also exhibit nicotinic, cholinergic, or anticholinergic symptoms for which treatment is specific. In most cases, a calm, quiet environment with friends or family is helpful.

If the patient is uncontrollable and dangerous to himself or herself or others, the use of diazepam for sedation is indicated.

Prolonged vomiting and diarrhea secondary to plant ingestions may require intravenous (IV) fluids and monitoring of electrolytes.

Based on the patient's symptoms in most cases, a period of observation in the emergency department is the best diagnostic procedure. The use of the laboratory for identification in plant ingestions is usually not helpful. However, if an emergency department has access to consultation with botanical experts, macro- and microscopic examination of plant products from gastric contents may be helpful in identification. Specific management for every plant ingestion is beyond the scope of this chapter. There are several references available that every emergency department should have access to.

COMMONLY INGESTED PLANTS, EFFECTS, AND MANAGEMENT

Abrus precatorius

There is usually a delay in symptoms from hours to a few days, depending on the amount ingested or chewed. There may be nausea, vomiting, diarrhea, and occasionally ulcerations in the pharynx, esophagus, stomach, and ileum. An ileus may develop. There also may be massive fluid with electrolyte loss.

Management

Treatment is mainly supportive with fluid and electrolyte replacement. However, ingestion of one chewed seed may be fatal even with intensive care.

Actaea

There is hypersalivation with blisters and ulcers to the oropharynx. Bloody vomiting and diarrhea occur with abdominal pain secondary to cramping. Renal injury occurs, starting with polyuria, dysuria, and hematuria, and followed by oliguria. Central nervous system symptoms such as dizziness, confusion, and syncope with seizures may occur 30 min after ingestion. Hallucinations were reported in one case.

Management

Lavage should be instituted if a large amount has been ingested, followed by the use of a demulcent (egg white in milk), and monitoring of fluids, electrolytes, and renal function with appropriate replacement.

Aloe

A marked catharsis occurs 6 to 12 h after ingestion. Alkaline urine may turn red. Large doses may cause nephritis.

Management

Fluids may be necessary. Otherwise, no therapy is usually required. Symptomatic treatment of pain may be instituted.

Capsicum

Children may experience painful, but harmless, irritation to the oropharynx. Exposure to skin may cause erythema, but not blistering.

Management

No therapy is usually required. Symptomatic treatment of pain may be instituted.

Conium

This is similar to nicotine poisoning. There is an onset of irritation to the oropharynx with nausea, salivation, and vomiting. Headache, thirst, diaphoresis, mydriasis and light-headedness may occur. Severe cases may have seizures, coma, and death, secondary to pulmonary failure.

Management

Treatment is symptomatic with administration of activated charcoal slurry after vomiting ceases.

Lily of the Valley (*Convallaria*)

Oropharyngeal pain, nausea, vomiting, diarrhea, abdominal pain, and cramping may develop. Digitalis-type toxicity depends upon the amount ingested and may take hours to express itself. Toxic effects are usually conduction defects, sinus bradycardia, and hyperkalemia. Arrythmias are uncommon, except for escape beats.

Management

Standard detoxification procedures may be performed. One should monitor electrocardiogram and serum potassium. Atropine or cardiac pacing may be required for conduction defects. If rhythm disturbances ensue, phenytoin is the drug of choice. Hemodialysis and forced diuresis are not helpful.

Daphne

Ingestion produces blistering and swelling of the entire oropharynx with salivation and dysphagia. Other later symptoms include thirst, vomiting, bloody diarrhea, and abdominal pain. Renal damage, hypovolemia, and electrolyte imbalance may occur.

Management

This ingestion is potentially lethal. Airway must be maintained along with monitoring fluid and electrolytes. Symptoms may last for days.

Datura

Ingestion may cause anticholinergic symptoms, including dry mouth, mydriasis, erythema, tachycardia, delirium, hallucinations, fever, hypertension, decrease in peristalsis, and urinary retention.

Management

As for anticholinergic poisoning.

Dieffenbachia

Mastication causes sudden, severe pain. It is occasionally followed by swelling of the oropharynx and bullae formation. The name "dumbcane" came about because in severe cases, speech is affected. Swallowing of the plant causes laryngeal edema, but this is not common because severe pain usually prevents swallowing. The swelling and pain may last for days and cause necrosis of the oral mucosa.

Management

The swelling and pain in the oropharynx resolve over time without intervention. Cool oral fluids may give some symptomatic relief. Judicious use of analgesics may be indicated. Systemic poisoning is not produced by the insoluble oxalates in these plants.

Euphorbia

Contact dermatitis may occur and may be corrosive. Conjunctivitis may occur with contamination to the eyes. Vomiting may follow after ingestion.

Management

If vomiting is present, patients should have electrolytes monitored and appropriate intravenous fluids given.

Ilex

Nausea, protracted vomiting and occasional diarrhea occurs after ingestion of berries.

Management

This includes monitoring of electrolytes and use of intravenous fluids to prevent dehydration. This is especially important in children.

Laportea and Urtica

These nettles rapidly cause an intensive burning sensation when contacted; they are unlikely to be held long enough to be eaten.

Management

Standard treatment with antihistamines is usually helpful.

Lonicera

The old European literature reports of deaths and toxicity due to *Lonicera* may be in error; the fruits are generally considered innocuous in the United States.

Nerium oleander

See "*Convallaria.*"

Philodendron

See "Dieffenbachia."

Phytolacca

Two to three h after ingestion, nausea, abdominal cramping, vomiting, diaphoresis, and diarrhea develop. These symptoms may last for 48 h.

Management

This includes monitoring of electrolytes with appropriate replacement. Pain may also be treated.

Rhododendron

Severe intoxications have occurred from chewing leaves and from eating honey made from rhododendron nectar. Upon ingestion, there is an initial burning sensation in the oropharynx. This is followed hours later by salivation, vomiting, diarrhea, and paresthesias. Other complaints include cephalgia, weakness, and decreased vision. In severe cases, bradycardia may develop followed by hypotension, coma, and seizures, leading to an increase in morbidity and mortality.

Management

Respiratory and fluid therapy are essential. If bradycardia ensues, atropine may be indicated. Hypotension is treated by intravenous fluids, Trendelenburg positioning, and ephedrine, if necessary. Cardiac telemetry is required. Complete recovery can be expected in 24 h.

Ricinus

Nausea, vomiting, and diarrhea ensue several hours after ingestion. Other symptoms are the result of fluid and electrolyte loss and bowel dysfunction.

Management

Fluid and electrolyte replacement are indicated. Parenteral alimentation may be necessary in severe cases. Fatalities have been recorded with the ingestion of two to six seeds.

Solanum

This is rarely toxic in adults. However, fatal ingestions have taken place in children. Gastrointestinal upset, oropharyngeal irritation, fever, and diarrhea occur after ingestion. The clinical picture is similar to bacterial gastroenteritis. There is a latent period after ingestion of several hours, and the symptoms may last for days.

Management

Supportive care with monitoring of fluids and electrolytes is indicated.

Taxus

Within 1 h after ingestion, light-headedness, dry oropharynx, mydriasis, abdominal cramping, salivation, and vomiting may occur. Facial pallor, circumoral cyanosis, and a rash may appear. Generalized weakness followed by coma is seen in severe intoxications. Cardiopulmonary symptoms include bradycardia, hypotension, dysrhythmias, and dyspnea. Death is secondary to cardiac or respiratory failure. Anaphylaxis may occur from chewing the needles.

Management

Routine decontamination with lavage followed by oral administration of activated charcoal is indicated. Cardiac monitoring is necessary. A cardiac pacemaker and appropriate respiratory therapy may be indicated. Standard treatment for anaphylaxis, if present, with epinephrine fluids and respiratory support is indicated.

Descriptions of Commonly Ingested Plants

***Abrus precatorius* L.** Common names: Coral-bead, crabs'-eye, jequerity, licorice vine, love bean, prayer bean, precatory bean, rosary pea, weather vine. Family: Leguminosae (Fabaceae). Note: Dangerous with known fatalities; ingestion and chewing of one of these brightly colored beans exceeds lethal dose for adults; toxin soluble in saliva has killed children. Seeds resemble small sugar candies and are used in native American necklaces and rosaries purchased by unsuspecting tourists. Toxins: Abrin, one of the most lethal toxins known. Presence: Seeds; fatality in children known from chewing seeds without swallowing seeds. Grows: Outdoors in tropical United States (including Hawaii). Description: Vine to 6 m spread, leaves small, alternate, pinnate; flowers pealike, rose, purple, or white; seeds rather uniform in size, about 7 mm (5 to 10 mm) long, shiny, two-thirds orange-red and one-third black, seed attachment scar in the black zone (colors fade with age); seeds produced in papery, hairy pods.

***Actaea rubra* (Ait.) Willd., *Actaea pachypoda* Ell.** Common names: baneberry, doll's eyes, necklaceweed, red baneberry. Family: Ranunculaceae. Note: Generally considered dangerous. Toxins: Protoanemonin; destroyed by drying or cooking. Presence: In berries and roots; berries only likely to be ingested by children. Grows: Forested, temperate North America, unusual but present in wildflower gardens, otherwise rarely grown. Description: Perennial from stout root; leaves compound through multiple divisions; leaflets cleft and toothed; fruits berry-like, red (white with black spot in *Actaea pachypoda*) usually with 5 to 15 seeds.

***Aloe barbadensis* Mill.** Common names: aloe vera, Barbados aloe, burn plant, curacoe, medicinal aloe. Family: Liliaceae. Toxins: Some of the more than 200 species of *Aloe* contain unspecified cathartic and irritating compounds. Presence: leaves. Grows: Common houseplant in northern regions, grown outdoors in subtropical and desert regions. Description: Clump-forming succulent; leaves yellow-green, may be speckled when young, to 30 to 50 cm long at maturity; flowers yellowish on stalks to 1 m long.

***Capsicum annuum* L.** Common names: pepper (banana, bell, green, hot, ornamental, red, sweet, etc.). Family: Solanaceae. Note: Generally considered nontoxic (common green peppers of grocery stores), but some ornamental and "hot" cultivars may cause severe irritation if ingested or contacted. Toxins: Capsicine. Presence: fruits and seeds. Grows: Common vegetable and house plants cultivated for both edible and ornamental fruits. Description: perennial herb (treated as an annual in cold climates) with alternate, simple leaves; fruits inflated, green, red, yellow, purple, or white.

***Chlorophytum comosum* (Thunb.) Jacques.** Common names: Ribbon plant, spider plant, walking plant. Family: Liliaceae. Note: Generally considered nontoxic but is among the 25 most frequently ingested houseplants. Grows: Common houseplant in north, used as a ground cover in shade in tropics. Description: Clump-forming perennial with broad grassy leaves (these often variegated with a white to yellow-green stripe); in pot culture often with pendant young plants on the ends of flexible stems; flowers small, white to yellow on long scapes.

***Conium maculatum* L.** Common names: fool's parsley, poison hemlock, poison parsley, spotted hemlock, spotted parsley, winter fern. Family: Apiaceae (Umbelliferae). Note: Dangerous with known fatalities. Toxins: Alkaloids, especially coniine and derivatives. Presence: Whole plant; roots and seeds most likely ingested by adults mistaking it for edible wild carrots or anise seed. Grows: An escaped weed of waste and moist places throughout temperate North America. Description: Large, branching biennial herb to more than 2 m tall from solid taproot; stems hollow; leaves pinnately and repeatedly compound; flowers small, white, in clusters.

***Convallaria majalis* L.** Common names: Lily-of-the-valley. Family: Liliaceae. Note: Generally considered dangerous. Toxins: Cardiac glycosides. Presence: Throughout plant; also water in vases when these are used as cut flowers. Outdoors the berries and indoors the vase water have been ingested by children. Grows: Cultivated garden perennial throughout temperate North America; often forced in pots indoors for flowers. Description: Low perennial herb from creeping underground rootstock, leaves usually two or three, oblong, entire; flowers white, bell-like, fragrant, pendant from scape; fruits orange to red pulpy berries with few seeds.

***Crassula argentea* (Thunb.).** Common names: Chinese rubber plant, dollar plant, jade plant, jade tree. Family: Crassulaceae. Note: Generally considered nontoxic; leaves commonly ingested by children. Grows: Common houseplant, used outdoors in subtropics. Description: Sturdy succulent-stemmed perennial, ultimately a shrub, with thick, oval, succulent leaves that may be striped with red or white; flowers small, white, star-shaped, in many-flowered clusters.

***Daphne mezerium* L.** Common names: Daphne. Family: Thymeliaceae. Note: Dangerous; 10 to 12 fruits can be lethal for children; 30 percent mortality reported for ingestions. Toxins: Daphnetoxin and mezerein. Presence: All parts; ingestion of fruits is the rare but expected exposure. Grows: Uncommon ornamental shrub of temperate North America; grown for its intensely fragrant flowers. Description: Small shrubs often less than 1 m tall with relatively thick stems; leaves alternate and simple, elliptical; flowers white to purple, flowering before leaves are present; fruits bright red to yellow.

***Datura* species (including *Brugmansia* sp.).** Common names: angel's trumpet, horn-of-plenty, indian apple, Jimson weed, thorn apple. Family: Solanaceae. Note: Dangerous, potentially lethal; cultivated for millenia for ornament and hallucinogens. Toxins: Alkaloids; atropine, hyoscyamine. Presence: All parts including nectar; leaves smoked or seeds eaten by adults seeking a "high." Grows: These are occasionally garden plants of temperate zone, also as escaped weeds of subtropical and tropical states. Description: Rank, short-lived perennials and annuals with coarse, soft, alternate leaves foul-smelling when crushed; flowers medium to large funnels, white to yellow usually extremely fragrant lasting one to a few days; fruits a spiny (sometimes smooth) pepper-like pod.

***Dieffenbachia* species (over 30).** Common names: dumbcane, dumb plant, mother-in-law's tongue. Family: Araceae. Note: Members of the Araceae possess raphides: numerous needle-shaped crystals of calcium oxalate that are physically ejected by turgor pressure when the cell containing them is disturbed. The immediate and intense reaction is due to this physical assault. If leaves are chewed, the swelling may become so intense the individual cannot speak and is rendered "dumb." Toxins: Calcium oxalate crystals; proteolytic enzymes also reported to be present. Presence: Primarily leaves, ingested by both children and adults; stems equally noxious if chewed. Grows: One of the most common house and office plants; common outdoors in tropical climates. Description: Long-lived erect perennial herbs to shrubs over 1 m tall with large entire leaves; numerous cultivars with variegated leaves; flowers and fruits uncommon in indoor culture.

***Euphorbia pulcherrima* Willd.** Common names: Christmas flower, poinsettia. Family: Euphorbiaceae. Notes: Foliage and latex of this species evidently harmless but cause for numerous inquiries; other species (2000 are known) can cause dermatitis. Grows: Common houseplant forced for Christmas displays; used outdoors in tropical states. Description: Shrub to 3 m tall with alternate, toothed leaves; floral bracts red, pink, orange, or white (commonly mistaken for petals); flowers insignificant, in a complex structure.

***Ficus* species (over 800 species).** Common names: banyan, botree, climbing figs, figs, rubber tree, weeping fig. Family: Moraceae. Notes: One of the top 25 causes of ingestion inquiries; most generally considered to be nontoxic. Grows: Common house and office shrubs and trees; very common outdoors in tropical regions. Description: Trees and shrubs with often thick, evergreen leaves; leaf size and lobing quite variable between species.

***Ilex* species (400 species).** Common names: American holly, cassena, dahoon, English holly, holly, inkberry, possum haw, winterberry, yaupon. Family: Aquifoliaceae. Note: Dangerous: 20 to 30 berries can be fatal to children; native American Indians used infusions of *Ilex vomitoria* berries to promote vomiting. Toxins: Uncertain; saponins in some cases. Presence: Berries only; leaves are used as a tea substitute. Grows: Native or cultivated plants throughout North America except in very arid or northern climates. Description: Trees and shrubs with often prickly evergreen leaves (some species with simple deciduous or evergreen leaves); fruits bright red, yellow, or black. Common Christmas decoration.

***Laportea* and *Urtica* species.** Common names: bull nettle, stinging nettle, wood nettle. Family: Urticaceae. Toxins: histamines(?). Presence: Leaves and stems. Grows: Moist woods and fields in temperate North America. Description: Short to tall perennial herbs; leaves alternate, somewhat heart-shaped (*Laportea*) or elongate (*Urtica*), covered with short, stiff, stinging glandular hairs; flowers minute, clustered near leaf bases.

***Lonicera* species (200 species).** Common names: honeysuckle, woodbine. Family: Caprifoliaceae. Generally considered nontoxic. Grows: Common ornamental and native shrubs and vines found throughout temperate North America; shrubs especially common in colder regions. Description: Shrubs and vines with opposite and usually entire leaves; flowers white, cream, yellow, or red; fruits paired, red (rarely yellow or blue), often translucent.

***Nerium oleander* L.** Common names: oleander, rose bay. Family: Apocynaceae. Note: Dangerous with known fatalities; all plant parts, smoke from plants, vase water from cut flowers. Notorious for poisoning food if stems used to roast hot dogs, marshmallows, etc. Toxins: Cardioactive glycosides. Presence: Entire plant. Grows: Subtropical to tropical states; grown as a tub or garden room plant in colder climates. Very common highway planting in central and southern California. Description: Large shrub to over 5 m; leaves narrow, opposite (or often in threes), evergreen; flowers in terminal clusters, white, yellow, red, or purple.

***Philodendron* species (275 species).** Common names: Philodendron. Family: Araceae. Note: The most common houseplant and leading cause of infant exposures due to leaf ingestion; see *Dieffenbachia*. Description: Perennial tropical vines tolerant of low light levels (as homes and offices); leaves heart-shaped to oval, thick, evergreen; flowers and fruits uncommon in cultivation.

***Phytolacca americana* L.** Common names: inkberry, phytolacca, pigeonberry, poke, pokeweed, salat. Family: Phytolaccaceae. Toxins: Triterpenes. Presence: Roots, leaves, and berries; however, cooked roots, greens, and berries (for pies) are featured in some Appalachian and Southern recipes; commercially canned greens are marketed as ''salat''; adult poisonings result from improper cooking of fresh roots or use of raw greens. Grows: Common weed of disturbed places and fencerows in eastern North America. Description: Rank perennial from fleshy rootstock growing to over 3 m tall (often mistaken for a shrub); leaves alternate, elliptical, often with purplish tinge; berries succulent, bright purplish-black with intense purplish-red stain.

***Pyracantha* species (10 species).** Common names: firethorn, pyracantha. Family: Rosaceae. Note: Generally considered nontoxic but one of 25 most commonly ingested berries. Grows: Ornamental shrub throughout temperate North America. Description: Multiple trunked thorny shrub to over 3 m tall, leaves alternate, linear to elliptical, deciduous to semievergreen (depending on climate); fruits orange to red, shaped like miniature apples.

***Rhododendron* species (over 500 species).** Common names: azalea, rhododendron. Family: Ericaceae. Toxins: Andromedotoxins. Presence: Leaves, flowers, and their honey; children known to chew leaves; adults may experiment with flowers in foods. Grows: Common ornamental and native shrubs in temperate North America except for the Great Plains and arid Southwest. Common houseplants. Description: Evergreen to deciduous shrubs with simple, alternate and often glossy leaves; flowers bellshaped to flaring, in most colors but blue.

***Rhus*.** See *Toxicodendron*.

***Ricinus communis* L.** Common names: castor bean, castor-oil plant. Family: Euphorbiaceae. Note: Dangerous with known fatalities. Toxins: Ricin, one of the most toxic compounds known. Seeds used in necklaces in tropical America and purchased by unsuspecting tourists. Presence: Concentrated in seeds but present in most of plant. Grows: Cultivated throughout North America. Description: Rank annual to 4 m, widely grown both as an ornamental and for the oil extracted from the seeds; variable in size and coloration (dull green to bronze/red), colors brightest in new growth; leaves large, star-shaped; flowers in upper leaf axils, small; seed pods usually brightly colored, densely hairy to prickly, borne in tight clusters; seeds quite variable, oval, with a white to gray nodule at the smaller end; seed coloration intricately marbled or striped, silver, gold, brown, and black.

***Schefflera* species (including *Brassaia*).** Common names: Australian umbrella tree, dwarf schefflera, umbrella tree. Family: Araliaceae. Notes: Generally considered nontoxic but a leading cause of ingestion inquiries. Grows: Common house and office plant; used outdoors in subtropics. Description: Shrubs to trees with shiny, dull to dark green, alternate, palmately compound leaves (leaflets arranged in a circle on a common leaf stalk).

***Solanum* species.** Common names: deadly nightshade, eggplant, Jerusalem cherry, nightshade, potato, woody nightshade. Family: Solanaceae. Note: Some species dangerous and potentially lethal; over 2000 species of mostly tropical herbs, shrubs, small trees, and vines and thus extremely variable. Includes the potato and eggplant as well as attractive houseplants and toxic weeds; the foliage is often malodorous when crushed; the fruits of some species are frequently ingested by children. Toxins: Solanine, glycoalkaloids. Presence: Foliage, fruits (especially immature), green skins of potatoes. Grows: Common in gardens and as weeds. Descriptions: (1) *S. dulcamara* L., deadly nightshade. Perennial weedy vine to 5 m; leaves alternate, lobed or divided, hairy; flowers star-shaped, purple; fruits red, produced in clusters, egg-shaped, about 1 cm long. (2) *S. nigrum* L., black nightshade. Low spreading annual; leaves glossy, shallowly lobed to entire; flowers white, star-shaped arising from leaf axils; fruits green becoming black. Cultivated forms as ''garden huckleberry'' leaves are edible when cooked and fruits when ripe; wild types reportedly toxic. (3) *S. pseudocapsicum* L., Jerusalem cherry. Unlike the previous two species, this is most commonly encountered as a winter houseplant and grown outdoors in subtropics. Shrub to 1.5 m, pot plant often less than 50 cm; leaves small, oblong, dull green; flowers small, star-shaped, white; fruits orange-red about 1.5 cm long, spherical.

***Taxus* species (10 species).** Common names: Yew. Family: Taxaceae. Note: Dangerous with known fatalities especially if ingestion of ''berries'' (actually a modified cone structure) is accompanied by chewing of seeds. Toxins: Taxine alkaloids. Presence: Foliage and seeds (but not the fleshy red aril = ''berry'' pulp). Grows: Common ornamentals and one uncommon native in temperate North America often clipped for hedges, foundation plantings, etc. Description: Shrubs to small trees with flat dark-green evergreen needles; cones highly modified and commonly called ''berries'' but technically a fleshy red aril surrounding the naked seed.

BIBLIOGRAPHY

Andrews J: *Peppers. The Domesticated Capsicums*. Austin, University of Texas Press, 1984.

Bailey Hortorium staff: *Hortus Third*. New York, Macmillan, 1976.

Graf AB: *Exotica*, series 4 (2 vols). East Rutherford, Roehrs, 1982.

Harborne JB: *Introduction to Ecological Biochemistry,* 2d ed. London, Academic, 1982.

Keeler RF, Tu AT (eds): *Handbook of Natural Toxins,* vol 1, *Plant and Fungal Toxins.* New York, Dekker, 1983.

Kingsbury JM: The evolutionary and ecological significance of plant toxins, in Keeler RF, Tu AT: *Handbook of Natural Toxins,* vol 1, *Plant and Fungal Toxins.* New York, Dekker, 1983, pp 675–706.

Lampe KF, Fagerstrom R: *Plant Toxicity and Dermatitis. A Manual for Physicians.* Baltimore, Williams & Wilkins, 1968.

Lampe KF, McCann MA: *AMA Handbook of Poisonous and Injurious Plants.* Chicago, American Medical Association, 1985.

Levey CK, Primack PB: *A Field Guide to Poisonous Plants and Mushrooms of North America.* Brattleboro, Stephen Green, 1984.

Litovitz TL, Schmitz BF, Holm KC: 1988 Annual Report of the American Association of Poison Control Centers National Data Collections System. *Am J Emerg Med* 7(5):495, 1988.

Rumack BH (ed): *Poisonindex,* vol 67. Micromedex, Inc., 1991.

Smith PM: *The Chemotaxonomy of Plants.* New York, Elsevier, 1976.

Westbrooks RG, Preacher JW: *Poisonous Plants of Eastern North America.* Columbia, University of South Carolina Press, 1986.

Willis JC, Shaw HKA: *A Dictionary of the Flowering Plants and Ferns,* 8th ed. Cambridge, Cambridge University Press, 1973.

SECTION 12
Endocrine Emergencies

131
HYPOGLYCEMIA

Gene Ragland

Glucose is the main energy source of the brain, and prolonged, severe hypoglycemia has been reported to cause brain damage and death. The blood glucose level at which hypoglycemia occurs is variable but has been generally accepted as <50 mg/dL. Hypoglycemia occurs most often in insulin-dependent diabetics as a complication of insulin therapy and accounts for 3 to 7 percent of deaths in patients with insulin-dependent diabetes mellitus. Treatment includes the administration of glucose, in most instances, and the outcome is usually favorable.

CNS GLUCOSE DEPRIVATION

The central nervous system (CNS) depends upon glucose as its sole source of energy, except under conditions of prolonged starvation, when it can utilize ketones to meet energy needs. Hypoglycemia can be defined as a fall in blood glucose concentration to a level that elicits symptoms due to glucose deprivation in the CNS. The symptoms of hypoglycemia are therefore due to CNS dysfunction. When hypoglycemia occurs suddenly, the symptoms are classified as adrenergic or sympathomimetic and include diaphoresis, pallor, tremulousness, tachycardia, palpitations, visual disturbances, mental confusion, weakness, and light-headedness. Hypoglycemia may also develop slowly so that the signs of acute hyperepinephrinemia are not seen. The usual clinical picture is that of more-prolonged CNS glucose deprivation. These symptoms are classified as neuroglycopenic and include fatigue, confusion, headache, memory loss, seizures, and coma.

The actual level of blood glucose that causes CNS deprivation and produces symptoms is highly individual. The glucose level may be influenced by factors such as age, sex, weight, dietary history, physical activity, emotion, and coexisting disease. Many reports exist of asymptomatic individuals with plasma glucose levels of 35 mg/dL or lower and of individuals who are symptomatic with glucose levels in the "normal" range. The actual value of plasma glucose that defines hypoglycemia is somewhat arbitrary. The clinical state of the patient must be correlated with the glucose determination.

GLUCOSE HOMEOSTASIS

Glucose homeostasis in humans involves a complex, dynamic synchronized interaction of neural and hormonal factors. The primary glucoregulatory organs are the liver, the pancreas, the adrenal glands, and the pituitary gland, and glucose homeostasis is maintained by the interaction of insulin, glucagon, catecholamines, glucocorticoids, and growth hormone from these organs. This interaction is largely determined by glucose intake and varies in the fed and the fasting state. During the fed state, glucose intake stimulates the release of insulin, which initiates tissue uptake and storage of fuels. During fasting, low insulin levels initiate the mobilization of stored fuels from tissue sources.

The fed state begins with the ingestion of food and extends for 2 to 3 h. The fasting state begins 3 to 4 h after eating. Because of the human's continuous energy needs but intermittent food intake, fuel for use between feedings and during fasting must be stored. The major forms of stored fuel are glycogen in the liver, triglycerides in adipose tissue, and protein in muscle.

Following food intake and absorption from the gut, glucose stimulates the release of insulin from pancreatic β cells. Insulin promotes the uptake of glucose by the liver; the glucose is converted to glycogen and stored in that form. Insulin also acts on the liver to decrease glucose output by inhibiting glycogenolysis (breakdown of glycogen to glucose) and gluconeogenesis (formation of glucose from precursors). Insulin promotes the storage of other energy sources by restraining lipolysis and enhancing lipogenesis in adipose cells and by promoting the uptake of amino acids into muscle protein and inhibiting proteolysis.

In the fasting state, the most readily available source of glucose is hepatic glycogen, which is utilized first. Hepatic glycogenolysis is enzyme-mediated and is stimulated by glucagon and catecholamines. This glycogen reserve is depleted in 24 to 48 h, and other fuel stores must be mobilized if fasting is prolonged. As hepatic glycogen stores are exhausted, blood glucose and plasma insulin levels decrease. The inhibitory action of insulin on lipolysis and proteolysis is removed, and alternative fuel stores can be mobilized and utilized.

During fasting, after several hours' worth of liver glycogen has been utilized, gluconeogenesis becomes the primary source of blood glucose needed for brain metabolism. Gluconeogenesis occurs primarily in the liver. Amino acids, principally alanine, are mobilized from the muscles via proteolysis. This process is facilitated by low insulin levels and mediated by glucocorticoids from the adrenal glands. Glucagon aids the conversion of amino acids to glucose in the liver. Lactate, from recycled glucose, and glycerol, from fat breakdown, can also be transformed to glucose but are minor sources of energy. During nonprolonged overnight fasting, 90 percent of gluconeogenesis occurs via proteolysis and conversion of amino acids to glucose. In starvation states, the kidneys play an important role in gluconeogenesis.

Fat stores are a major source of energy. Fat is stored as triglycerides (free fatty acids plus glycerol), and this process is promoted by insulin. Lipolysis can occur with low insulin levels and is enhanced by epinephrine and growth hormone. When triglycerides are broken down, free fatty acids (FFA) and glycerol are released. Most tissues, except brain and formed blood elements, can utilize FFA as a source of energy. This mechanism allows the body to conserve glucose for use in the CNS and to spare protein from breakdown for conversion to glucose. Additionally, the released glycerol can be converted to glucose in the liver. Growth hormone stimulates the preferential use of fat over glucose.

In brief summary, glucose homeostasis involves a complex interaction between insulin and the counterregulatory hormones glucagon, catecholamines, glucocorticoids, and growth hormone. The action of insulin depends upon its concentration, which is determined by the level of blood glucose through a sensitive feedback loop. In the fed state, insulin acts to convert glucose to stored energy and inhibits the release of other fuel stores. The glucose concentration during the transition from a fed to a fasting state depends upon the relative balance between glucose use and glucose production. The CNS is the primary consumer of glucose. The production of glucose during a brief fast occurs through glycogenolysis. When the fast is more than a few hours, such as overnight, gluconeogenesis is the primary mechanism responsible for glucose production. Hypoglycemia may result from disease of any of the glucoregulatory organs or as a breakdown of normal glucose homeostasis.

PATHOGENESIS

Hypoglycemia has been classified in a variety of ways. Table 131-1 lists the common causes of hypoglycemia seen in the emergency department and divides these into spontaneous and induced causes. This classification is arbitrary, and overlap occurs.

Spontaneous Hypoglycemia

Fed Hypoglycemia

Hypoglycemia occurring during the fed state has also been termed *reactive* and *postprandial hypoglycemia*. Fed hypoglycemias are characterized by normal fasting serum glucose levels with a decline to hypoglycemic levels within 6 h of a glucose load. Most commonly fed hypoglycemia occurs several hours after eating, usually in the late morning or the late afternoon. The critical period in which hypoglycemia may develop is during the transition from the fed to the fasting state, between 2 and 4 h after the ingestion of glucose. Diagnosis is supported by an abnormal 6-h glucose tolerance test (GTT) when the nadir of the plasma glucose level occurs with symptoms.

Alimentary

The major causes of fed hypoglycemia are alimentary causes, early diabetes mellitus, and idiopathic. Following partial or total gastrectomy, gastrojejunostomy, or pyloroplasty, 5 to 10 percent of the patients may develop symptomatic hypoglycemia $1\frac{1}{2}$ to 3 h after a meal. The cause appears to be rapid gastric emptying and an exaggerated insulin response. A correlation of hypoglycemia with peak insulin levels has been shown.

Postgastrectomy hypoglycemia is not the same as dumping syndrome, which is due to rapid dilution of a hyperosmolar load in the jejunum and produces symptoms of weakness, pallor, nausea, epigastric discomfort, palpitations, dizziness, and diarrhea. These symptoms occur within 10 min after a meal, subside within 1 h, and are not due to hypoglycemia. Alimentary hypoglycemia in the absence of gastrointestinal (GI) surgery has been described. Patients with this entity may have a gut defect with rapid glucose absorption, or release of gut factors that stimulate insulin secretion. Treatment of alimentary hypoglycemia is aimed at minimizing insulin release by decreasing the amount of ingested carbohydrate.

Table 131-1. Causes of Hypoglycemia

Spontaneous	Induced
Fed—reactive—postprandial	Insulin
Alimentary	Factitious
Early diabetes mellitus	Sulfonylureas
Idiopathic	Alcohol
Fasting	Miscellaneous drugs
Islet-cell tumor of pancreas (insulinoma)	Posthyperalimentation or -hemodialysis
Extrapancreatic neoplasms	
Endocrine-related	
Pituitary insufficiency	
Adrenal insufficiency	
Glucagon deficiency	
Thyroid insufficiency	
Hepatic disease	
Miscellaneous	
Sepsis	
Chronic renal failure	
Starvation	
Autoimmune	
Exercise	
Artifactual	

Early Diabetes

Spontaneous hypoglycemia occurring 3 to 5 h after a meal may be seen as an early manifestation of maturity-onset (type II) diabetes. It is postulated that there is a delay in the early release of insulin with subsequent excessive insulin secretion in response to the initial hyperglycemia. The symptoms are usually brief and mild, lasting 15 to 20 min. A family history of diabetes is usual.

Idiopathic

Idiopathic hypoglycemia is probably rare and may simply reflect the transition in intermediary metabolism between the fed and fasting state. It is diagnosed far more often than justified. It is usually described as occurring 2 to 4 h after meals or with minor deprivation of food such as a missed meal. The patient is often a healthy young adult with no known underlying cause of hypoglycemia. Symptoms of sweating, shakiness, weakness, light-headedness, numbness, confusion, and anxiety are commonly reported and may lead the physician to obtain a 6-h GTT. If the blood glucose level goes below 50 mg/dL, the patient is diagnosed as having hypoglycemia and placed on a high-protein, low-carbohydrate diet.

Many question the diagnosis. A blood glucose level below 50 mg/dL during a 6-h GTT is not uncommon in normal individuals. Several investigations of patients with idiopathic hypoglycemia have shown a poor correlation between symptoms and the blood glucose levels. If the serum glucose level is less than 50 mg/dL and is associated with spontaneous symptoms, the diagnosis should be considered and the patient referred for further evaluation.

According to the American Diabetes Association, the following are criteria for the diagnosis of idiopathic hypoglycemia: the occurrence of documented low blood sugar; the particular symptoms of which the patient complains must be shown to be due to low blood sugar; the symptoms must be relieved by the ingestion of food or sugar; and the particular kind of hypoglycemia causing symptoms must be established.

Fasting Hypoglycemia

Fasting hypoglycemia is by far the most important hypoglycemic state for the emergency physician to recognize. Fasting hypoglycemia often reflects serious underlying organic disease. Hypoglycemia may develop slowly so that the signs of hyperepinephrinemia may not be seen, and the patient may simply lapse into coma.

By definition, fasting hypoglycemia begins 5 to 6 h after a meal. Most patients with a disorder that causes fasting hypoglycemia develop low glucose levels during a 24-h fast. Occasionally a 72-h fast is required to establish or rule out this diagnosis. Not uncommonly, the patient is difficult to arouse in the morning following an overnight fast. Evaluation of the cause of this type of hypoglycemia requires hospitalization.

Islet-cell Tumor of the Pancreas

Hypoglycemia due to insulinoma may occur in the fasting or the fed state. In 80 percent of the cases, the tumor is small, single, and nonmalignant and is located anywhere within the pancreas. About 10 percent of the patients have multiple tumors and also a high association with multiple endocrine neoplasia (MEN), type I. The remaining 10 percent have metastatic malignant insulinoma.

Insulinoma occurs somewhat more often in women in the later decades of life (40 to 70 years). Most of the patients have symptoms consisting of various combinations of sweating, palpitations, weakness, diplopia, and blurred vision. Confusion or abnormal behavior is seen in 80 percent of the cases. Coma or amnesia for the hypoglycemic episode occurs in about half the patients and seizures in 12 percent. Symptoms occur at irregular intervals, more often in the late afternoon or early morning before breakfast and may be induced by exercise. The symptoms are of varying duration and are alleviated by food in the majority of instances. The interval between the appearance of the first hypoglycemic symptoms and the diagnosis of insulinoma is usually months (19 months) and may be years. Many of these patients are diagnosed to have a neurologic abnormality such as a convulsive disorder, a cerebrovascular accident, a brain tumor, or narcolepsy, or they may be thought to have a psychiatric problem such as psychosis or hysteria. Some patients have been diagnosed to have Adams-Stokes attacks.

In one series of 78 patients with insulinoma, 38 (49 percent) were evaluated in an emergency department because of CNS symptoms. Twenty patients were identified as hypoglycemic, and eight of those were immediately admitted to rule out hyperinsulinism. Eight patients did not have a blood glucose determination, and the remaining ten patients had various neurologic or psychiatric diagnoses. For 15 of these patients (39 percent) their presentation to the emergency department was for their first symptomatic episode.

The hypoglycemia of insulinoma is thought to be due to excess insulin secreted by the tumor. The diagnosis is made by the demonstration of hypoglycemia and hyperinsulinemia at the time of spontaneous symptoms. A prolonged fast (72 h) may be required to provoke hypoglycemia, but most patients (75 to 90 percent) develop it before 24 h of fasting. A variety of provocative tests based upon the administration of insulin secretagogues, and several suppression tests utilizing insulin inhibitors, can be used as diagnostic aids. The ratio of immunoreactive insulin to glucose (IRI/G) can be determined to see if the insulin level is inappropriate to the concomitant level of blood glucose.

The differential diagnosis of insulinoma includes surreptitious self-administration of insulin. In an insulin-dependent diabetic, factitious hypoglycemia from excess insulin administration can be diagnosed by the determination of C-peptide levels. Proinsulin is converted to insulin and C peptide in the pancreatic β cells, and these two peptides are secreted in equimolar concentrations. If insulin is endogenously produced, the insulin and the C-peptide levels correspond. If insulin is exogenously administered, the insulin level is elevated but the C-peptide level is low. In patients who are not insulin-dependent diabetics, the presence of insulin antibodies in the serum points to the self-administration of insulin. These antibodies may not be detectable before 6 weeks to 2 months of exogenous insulin administration.

The treatment of insulinoma is surgical excision of the tumor, and this is curative in most cases. In those patients in whom surgical therapy is not feasible or curative or in whom surgery must be delayed, drug treatment and diet can be used. More frequent feedings using slowly absorbable forms of carbohydrate are indicated. Benign tumors can be treated with diazoxide and a natriuretic diuretic. Diazoxide acts to directly inhibit the release of insulin by the β cells and has an extrapancreatic hyperglycemic effect. The diuretic prevents edema caused by diazoxide-induced sodium retention. With malignant insulinoma, streptozotocin is the most effective antitumor agent to date.

Extrapancreatic Neoplasms

Hypoglycemia may be associated with, and caused by, neoplasms of virtually every histopathologic type. Hypoglycemia-causing tumors may be unsuspected and discovered during systemic evaluation of a patient with fasting hypoglycemia; or hypoglycemia may occur as a late or preterminal event in a patient with known neoplasia.

Mesenchymal tumors are the most common tumors of nonpancreatic origin associated with tumor hypoglycemia. Thoracic and retroperitoneal tumors, especially fibrosarcomas and mesotheliomas, are most common. Mesenchymal tumors are slow-growing and large and may be massive (20 kg or more). Other endocrinopathies may be present because of the ectopic production of a variety of hormones by these tumors. The presenting signs and symptoms may include profound hypoglycemia, depressed cerebral function, weight loss, and a large intrathoracic or intraabdominal mass.

Epithelial and endothelial tumors involving the lung, breast, kidney, ovary, and GI tract can cause hypoglycemia. The epithelial tumors most often associated with hypoglycemia are hepatic carcinomas, adrenocortical neoplasms, and carcinoid tumors. Hepatic carcinomas are invariably large, occur more commonly in men than women (4 to 1), and usually have a rapid clinical course with a fatal outcome in 1 to 6 months. Hypoglycemia occurs as a terminal or a preterminal event. Adrenocortical neoplasms are usually malignant and large. Carcinoid tumors develop from cells of the amine precursor uptake and decarboxylation (APUD) series and may occur in a variety of locations. These tumors are slow-growing and elaborate a variety of biologically active substances. They are capable of producing hypoglycemia as well as the carcinoid syndrome. Diagnosis is made by the demonstration of increased 5-hydroxyindoleacetic acids (5-HIAA) in a 24-h urine collection.

Tumor hypoglycemia is a heterogeneous disorder that no single mechanism can satisfactorily explain. Some tumors secrete substances with insulinlike biological activity. Other causes of tumor hypoglycemia include increased utilization of glucose by the tumor, decreased gluconeogenesis from cachexia and depletion of substrates, liver impairment due to metastasis or tumor products, or depression of glucagon secretion and activity. Regardless of the mechanism, the treatment is intravenous or oral glucose replacement.

Endocrine-Related

The crucial role of the counterregulatory hormones in the maintenance of glucose homeostasis has been reviewed. Deficiency of any of these hormones could result in hypoglycemia. Catecholamine deficiency has not been documented to cause hypoglycemia, but deficiency of glucagon, glucocorticoids, and growth hormone has. Glucagon or pancreatic α-cell deficiency is a rare cause of hypoglycemia. Glucocorticoid deficiency as a cause of fasting hypoglycemia is seen with primary or secondary adrenal insufficiency. Hypoglycemia is more pronounced with secondary adrenal insufficiency (hypopituitarism) because of concomitant growth hormone and glucocorticoid deficiencies. Patients with growth hormone deficiency may have fasting or fed hypoglycemia even when growth hormone deficiency is not accompanied by deficits in other pituitary hormones. Another endocrine-related cause of hypoglycemia is thyroid hormone deficiency, especially when severe enough to cause myxedema coma.

Hepatic Disease

Diffuse, severe liver disease, in which 80 to 85 percent of the liver is functionally impaired or destroyed, may result in hypoglycemia due to impaired glycogenolysis and gluconeogenesis. Diseases such as acute hepatic necrosis, acute viral hepatitis, Reye syndrome, and severe passive congestion have been implicated. Metastatic or primary liver neoplasia may cause hypoglycemia if a large portion of the liver is involved, but liver metastases usually do not produce hypoglycemia. Hypoglycemia has been described as part of the syndrome of fatty liver of pregnancy. An association between hypoglycemia and the HELLP syndrome (hemolysis, elevated liver enzyme levels, and low platelet count) has also been reported. A spectrum of hepatic damage ranging from preeclampsia to HELLP syndrome to acute fatty liver may occur in pregnancy. All ill women in the third trimester should have glucose level determinations. Chronic liver disease only rarely is a cause of hypoglycemia. Patients with hepatic failure severe enough to cause hypoglycemia are often in a coma. Hypoglycemia as a cause of coma may be missed if it is assumed that coma is due to hepatic encephalopathy.

Miscellaneous

Hypoglycemia has been described in a wide variety of other clinical situations. Sepsis can cause hypoglycemia, more often in elderly patients with underlying liver and renal disease. It has also been described in a 6-month-old patient with *Neisseria* meningitis and in other patients in whom no cause for hypoglycemia other than sepsis was present. Spontaneous, fasting hypoglycemia with chronic renal failure in diabetic and non-diabetic patients is well-documented. The pathogenesis is poorly understood, but is often accompanied by severe lactic acidosis.

Starvation-related hypoglycemia is occasionally seen. The majority of the case reports on starvation hypoglycemia involve children with kwashiorkor, but adult cases, especially associated with anorexia nervosa, have been described. Hypoglycemia can be severe and refractory to therapy. The mechanisms are obscure, but include the failure of gluconeogenesis due to the depletion of fat and protein stores, or abnormally increased cellular glucose consumption. An infusion of 20% dextrose and lactated Ringer's solution containing hydrocortisone is used to treat this condition.

Fasting and fed autoimmune hypoglycemia has been described. The presence of anti-insulin antibodies in patients not known to have received insulin injections has been confirmed in several reports. The mechanism is thought to be dissociation of insulin-antibody complexes with the release of sufficient amounts of free insulin to cause hypoglycemia. Saturation of the insulin-binding capacity with the continued release of insulin from the pancreas has also been suggested. Additionally, hypoglycemia associated with antibodies to the insulin receptor has been identified. These autoantibodies may mimic the bioactivity of insulin on target tissues, causing hypoglycemia.

Prolonged exercise may result in hypoglycemia. With intense, continued exercise (longer than 90 min), liver glycogen stores are depleted, and the rate of glucose production may fail to keep pace with the rate of glucose use, resulting in a fall in the blood glucose concentration. With the current popularity of endurance training, a patient with exercise-induced hypoglycemia could present to the emergency department.

Artifactual hypoglycemia may occur in conditions in which either the leukocyte or lymphocyte count is markedly increased (>60,000 mm^3, regardless of the underlying disease). This is thought to be due to continued glycolysis by the large number of leukocytes or lymphocytes between the time the blood is drawn and the time the glucose determination is made. Artifactual hypoglycemia has been reported in various leukemias, with nucleated red blood cells during a hemolytic crisis, and in polycythemia rubra vera. True hypoglycemia has been reported in terminal leukemia and must be distinguished from artifactual hypoglycemia, which is asymptomatic. The refrigeration of blood samples and the addition of an antiglycolytic agent, such as sodium fluoride, decreases glucose consumption by the white blood cells.

Induced Hypoglycemia

Induced hypoglycemia is almost always due to drugs, commonly insulin, sulfonylureas, alcohol, and salicylates. During the first 2 years of life, salicylates account for most cases of drug-induced hypoglycemia. During the next 8 years, alcohol is the most likely cause. In patients 11 to 30 years of age, two-thirds of all comas have been caused by sulfonylureas or insulin, with half of these occurring in nondiabetic young women attempting suicide. Alcohol alone or in combination with insulin is a common cause of hypoglycemic coma in patients between 30 and 50 years of age who have drug-related hypoglycemia. Hypoglycemia caused by sulfonylurea agents is more likely after 60 years of age.

Factors predisposing to drug-induced hypoglycemia include restricted carbohydrate intake and renal or hepatic disease.

Insulin-Induced

Insulin reaction in the diabetic patient is by far the most common cause of hypoglycemia seen in the emergency department.

Multiple factors affect the severity and the frequency of insulin reactions. The severity of the diabetes is directly related to the incidence of insulin reactions. Those with the least endogenous insulin have the widest variation in blood glucose levels. It is well-documented that the counterregulatory hormones increase in response to insulin-induced hypoglycemia.

Recent investigations concerning the role of the counterregulatory hormones in the prevention or correction of hypoglycemic reactions in insulin-dependent diabetic patients have shown that glucagon is the primary hormone protecting against hypoglycemia. Epinephrine is not normally critical but becomes so when glucagon is deficient. The effects of cortisol and growth hormone require several hours to occur, and thus they are not factors in rapid counterregulation of hypoglycemia but are more important in recovery from prolonged hypoglycemia.

Patients who have been diabetic for less than 2 years generally have an intact defense against hypoglycemia with a normal glucagon and epinephrine response. Most patients with insulin-dependent diabetes acquire a deficiency in glucagon secretory response during hypoglycemia. This defect is almost universally present after 5 years of diabetes. These patients are dependent upon epinephrine to promote recovery from hypoglycemia. Deficient epinephrine secretion as a result of adrenergic neuropathy or blockade with the use of a nonselective β-adrenergic antagonist places these patients at increased risk of prolonged, severe hypoglycemic reactions.

Some other factors that may precipitate hypoglycemia in an insulin-dependent diabetic patient include exercise, emotions, late meals, undereating of carbohydrates, alcohol ingestion, errors of insulin dosage, erratic absorption of insulin from subcutaneous sites, and overtreatment with insulin. Of these factors, overtreatment with insulin deserves further discussion. Excess insulin dosage may occur because of a physician error or when a patient attempts too-rigid control, especially when glucosuria is used as the principal indicator for the insulin dose. Following the classic report by Somogyi, excess insulin as a cause of hypoglycemia, nocturnal hypoglycemia, and rebound hyperglycemia has been well-documented and is fairly common in adults and children.

Nocturnal hypoglycemia is often difficult to recognize clinically. It is most likely to be associated with the use of long-acting insulin preparations taken once daily. Suggestive features include lethargy, depression, night sweats, nightmares, morning headaches, seizures, hepatomegaly due to glycogen accumulation, and acquired tolerance to high doses of insulin. Polyuria, nocturia, or enuresis despite increasing insulin dosage, excessive appetite, weight gain, mood swings, and frequent bouts of rapidly developing ketoacidosis are additional clues to the recognition of insulin overdosage (see Table 131-2). Fasting early-morning blood glucose levels may be normal in spite of nocturnal hypoglycemia. They may also be elevated and lead to an increase in the insulin dose and a worsening of the symptoms. Recent clinical studies have challenged the hypothesis that nocturnal hypoglycemia causes clinically important fasting hyperglycemia in patients with in-

Table 131-2. Clinical Clues of Nocturnal Hypoglycemia

1. Lassitude, depression, difficulty with waking in morning
2. Early morning headaches or irritability
3. Night sweats, nightmares
4. Polyuria, nocturia, enuresis in children
5. Convulsions
6. Increased appetite and weight gain
7. Hepatomegaly
8. Morning ketonuria without glucosuria or disproportionate to glucosuria
9. Worsening of symptoms with increased insulin dose
10. Insulin dose greater than 1.0 unit/kg of body weight per day

sulin-dependent diabetes mellitus. When insulin-dependent diabetic patients are brought to the emergency department with early morning hyperglycemia or with symptoms of undetermined cause, follow-up arrangements should be made with their physicians through personal communication.

Another cause of early morning hyperglycemia is the dawn phenomenon. This condition has been described in insulin-dependent and non-insulin-dependent diabetic patients and in nondiabetics. It is characterized by an abrupt increase in fasting levels of plasma glucose between 5 and 9 A.M. in the absence of antecedent hypoglycemia. This phenomenon is extremely common, occurring in the vast majority of those patients who have been studied. The mechanism is unknown. Elevated glucose levels occur irrespective of insulin levels and may reflect a circadian variation in glucose tolerance.

Clinically, it is important to distinguish among the Somogyi phenomenon, the dawn phenomenon, and simple waning of previously injected insulin as a cause of early morning hyperglycemia, as treatments differ. Management of the Somogyi phenomenon consists of reducing insulin doses and providing late-evening carbohydrate to avoid hypoglycemia. Treatment of the dawn phenomenon and insulin waning generally consists of adjusting the evening dose of intermediate- or long-acting insulin to provide additional coverage in the early morning hours. Attribution of early-morning hyperglycemia to an incorrect cause could result in inappropriate treatment. A coordinated management effort between the emergency physician and the patient's personal physician is important in such cases.

The question of rigid or tight control of diabetes is even more vital following a policy statement from the American Diabetes Association in 1976 calling for "a serious effort to achieve levels of blood glucose as close to those in the nondiabetic state as feasible." This therapeutic goal is based upon the belief that the long-term vascular complications of diabetes, particularly retinopathy and nephropathy, are decreased by reduction of the blood glucose concentration. To this end, newer methods for tight diabetic control have been introduced. These include home blood glucose monitoring with multiple insulin injections (two or three times a day) based upon glucose levels, continuous subcutaneous insulin infusion using a portable pump, and the development of an artificial pancreas.

Several authors have cautioned against too-rigid control. In spite of the efficacy of home blood glucose monitoring and the apparent effectiveness of the infusion pump, complications have been reported. Results from the Diabetes Control and Complications Trial, a large, multicenter study comparing intensive insulin therapy with standard treatment regimens for insulin-dependent patients, indicate that the incidence of severe hypoglycemia or coma is approximately three times higher in patients receiving intensive therapy.

Several authors have recently stressed that the glycemic goals for insulin-dependent diabetic patients must be individualized. Intensive insulin therapy should be utilized only in those patients who are apt to benefit from such regimens and who are at relatively low risk of sustained hypoglycemia. Individuals whose life expectancy is reduced by advanced age, life-shortening disorders, and end-stage diabetic complications are unlikely to obtain long-term benefits from rigorous glucose control. Additionally, those patients with defective glucose counterregulation from deficient glucagon and epinephrine responses are not candidates for meticulous control.

It is important to prevent hypoglycemic reactions in the insulin-dependent diabetic patient. Studies with continuous blood glucose sampling in type I diabetics have suggested that less than a third of all hypoglycemic episodes are symptomatic.

The emergency physician must be prepared to identify and advise the diabetic patient who drives a motor vehicle and is prone to hypoglycemic reactions, especially neuroglycopenic ones. One survey of 250 insulin-dependent diabetic patient drivers identified 34 percent with severe or frequent hypoglycemia in the preceding 6 months, during which they had been driving regularly. Thirty-four patients (13.6 percent) had been involved in a driving accident since commencing treatment with insulin, and 13 of those patients were aware that hypoglycemia had been an important causal factor. Another survey of 85 young diabetic patients identified 5 percent who experienced unexpected hypoglycemic reactions while driving or operating machinery.

The emergency physicians must directly question the insulin-dependent diabetic driver about unexpected hypoglycemic reactions. If any have occurred, the patient should be instructed to self-monitor the blood glucose level just before driving and at 1- to 2-h intervals on long trips. The blood glucose level should be maintained at about 200 mg/dL, and the patient should take supplemental feedings whenever the glucose falls below that level. Patients subject to unexpected hypoglycemia should have sugar and glucagon available in the vehicle and should drive accompanied by an informed person who can administer them. Finally, the hypoglycemia-prone patient must avoid alcohol and all medications that may cause or potentiate hypoglycemic reactions.

A cooperative effort between the patient, the patient's primary physician, and the emergency physician is essential for the appropriate follow-up of a diabetic patient presenting to the emergency department.

When a diabetic patient is brought to the emergency department with depressed cerebral function or in coma, rapid differentiation between hypoglycemia and ketoacidosis must be made (see Table 131-3). Testing a drop of blood with a glucose reagent strip reliably allows differentiation between high and low blood glucose levels within minutes. If there is still uncertainty about the cause, 50 mL of a 50%

Table 131-3. Differential Diagnosis of Coma in a Known Diabetic Patient

	Hypoglycemia	**Ketoacidosis**
History	Insufficient food, excess insulin, excess exercise	Insufficient insulin, infection, gastrointestinal upset
Onset	Following *short-acting insulin:* Sudden, a few hours after injection Following *long-acting insulin:* Relatively slower, many hours after injection	Gradual over many hours
Course	Anxiety, sweating, hunger, headache, diplopia, incoordination, twitching, convulsions, coma (headache, nausea, and haziness especially following long-acting insulin)	Polyuria, polydipsia, anorexia, nausea, vomiting, labored deep breathing, weakness, drowsiness, possible fever and abdominal pain, coma
Physical findings	Pale moist skin, full rapid pulse, dilated pupils, normal breathing, blood pressure normal or elevated, overactive reflexes, positive Babinski sign	Florid, dry skin. Kussmaul breathing with acetone odor, decreased blood pressure, weak rapid pulse, soft eyeballs
Laboratory findings	Second urine specimen sugar- and ketone-free, low blood sugar, normal serum CO_2	Urine contains sugar and ketone bodies; high blood sugar, low serum CO_2

Source: Ensinck JW, Williams RH: Disorders causing hypoglycemia, in Williams RH (ed): *Textbook of Endocrinology*, 6th ed, Philadelphia, Saunders, 1981, p 873.

glucose solution should be given intravenously after blood has been obtained for appropriate studies. The hypoglycemic patient benefits, and the patient in ketoacidosis is not unduly harmed.

Factitious Hypoglycemia

An occasional emotionally unstable patient surreptitiously administers insulin or an oral hypoglycemic drug to induce hypoglycemia and simulate organic disease. These patients may be medical personnel or diabetic, or they may be related to someone who is diabetic or in the medical profession. These patients often exhibit erratic patterns of hypoglycemia and usually deny drug misuse even when confronted directly. The use of insulin or oral hypoglycemic agents causes hyperinsulinemia, which may be mistaken for an insulinoma. Factitious hypoglycemia resulting from oral hypoglycemics can be diagnosed by detecting sulfonylurea agents in the blood. Proinsulin and C-peptide determinations are not useful for ruling out factitious hypoglycemia due to ingestion of sulfonylurea agents. Those drugs stimulate the pancreas to secrete insulin, and equivalent amounts of C-peptide and insulin are present. Additionally, no insulin antibodies are present. Because the second-generation sulfonylurea agents are more potent, smaller doses are used and the plasma levels are not very high. Differentiating between surreptitious ingestion of these agents and insulinoma may be difficult.

Insulin antibodies may be detected in the serum of patients who claim to have never used insulin if the insulin has been administered for 6 to 8 weeks. The measurement of C-peptide levels is indicated if insulin antibodies are not detected or if a diabetic patient is suspected of factitious hypoglycemia. The C-peptide levels are low if the source of the insulin is exogenous and high in cases of endogenous hyperinsulinemia.

Sulfonylureas

The sulfonylureas are commonly used as oral hypoglycemic agents and include the first-generation agents chlorpropamide, tolbutamide, acetohexamide, and tolazamide. Second-generation sulfonylurea drugs are glyburide and glipizide. These newer drugs have a greater hypoglycemic effect per milligram than older agents. All sulfonylurea drugs stimulate the release of insulin from the pancreas with a subsequent decrease in hepatic glucose output. These agents are commonly used to treat mild, type II diabetes. Hypoglycemic reactions may be profound, prolonged, and life-threatening. Sulfonylurea overdose and surreptitious self-administration may also produce hypoglycemia. Encephalopathy from recurrent hypoglycemic reactions induced by oral hypoglycemic drugs has been reported.

Other drugs may potentiate the hypoglycemic effect of sulfonylurea agents. Alcohol, salicylates, sulfonamides, bis-hydroxycoumarin, and phenylbutazone should be avoided in patients on sulfonylureas. All the sulfonylurea compounds have caused hypoglycemia, but chlorpropamide is responsible for most cases. Hypoglycemia due to chlorpropamide has occurred during normal food intake, with intact renal function, and at ordinary dosages. Chlorpropamide causes the most prolonged hypoglycemia of all sulfonylurea drugs. Its half-life in the serum is 36 h, and 3 to 5 days are required for complete elimination from the body. Severe and prolonged hypoglycemia due to glyburide has also been described.

Sulfonylurea-induced hypoglycemia may be refractory to treatment by intravenous glucose alone. This is particularly true in nondiabetic patients in whom insulin-release mechanisms are intact. Infused glucose stimulates insulin release, which may further lower the blood glucose level. Diazoxide, 300 mg by slow intravenous infusion over a 30-min period, repeated every 4 h, has been successful in raising the blood glucose to supranormal levels without causing hypotension. All patients with sulfonylurea-induced hypoglycemia require hospitalization and prolonged treatment.

Alcohol

Alcohol-induced hypoglycemia is usually seen in malnourished chronic alcoholics. It may also occur in spree drinkers, in occasional drinkers who have missed a meal or two, and in children and adolescents. Severe alcoholic intoxication and hypoglycemic coma has also been reported from continuous sponging of a febrile child with rubbing alcohol.

Patients with alcohol-induced hypoglycemia usually present in coma or semicoma 2 to 10 h after alcohol ingestion. The presenting physical findings may include hypothermia, tachypnea, and the smell of alcohol on the breath. The absence of alcohol fetor does not rule out alcohol as a cause of hypoglycemia or coma. Most patients are unresponsive except to deep pain stimulation. Convulsions are a particularly frequent occurrence in children with alcoholic hypoglycemia. Laboratory findings, in addition to hypoglycemia, usually include an elevated blood alcohol level, ketonuria without glucosuria, and mild acidosis.

Alcohol-induced hypoglycemia is attributed primarily to the inhibition of gluconeogenesis during alcohol metabolism. Ethyl alcohol is metabolized primarily in the cytoplasm of the liver cells, utilizing nicotinamide adenine dinucleotide (NAD) as the hydrogen acceptor. During this process the rate of NAD reduction exceeds the rate of NADH oxidation, and the NADH/NAD ratio increases severalfold. The NAD available for those oxidation-reduction reactions necessary to sustain gluconeogenesis is thus decreased, and the level of plasma glucose subsequently falls. The chronic alcoholic with reduced caloric intake and depleted liver glycogen stores has no glucogenic reserve, and hypoglycemic coma results. The mechanism by which alcohol induces hypoglycemia in the well-fed person is less well defined.

Treatment with intravenous glucose is usually sufficient to correct alcohol-induced hypoglycemia. Thiamine should be given before glucose in chronic or suspected alcoholics. Glucagon is not recommended in the chronic alcoholic, as liver glycogen stores are usually exhausted.

Miscellaneous Drugs

Several other drugs should be mentioned in relation to drug-induced hypoglycemia. Salicylate-induced hypoglycemic coma in children can occur with overtreatment of febrile illnesses with aspirin, and from accidental overdose. Salicylate toxicity and hypoglycemia should be considered in any child with coma, convulsions, or cardiovascular collapse. Salicylate-related hypoglycemia in adults most often occurs when aspirin is used in conjunction with other compounds that lower the levels of glucose. Propranolol has been reported to precipitate hypoglycemia, and several authors have expressed concern over the use of β-adrenergic blockers in diabetic patients. They believe that β blockers may mask the adrenergic symptoms of hypoglycemia and increase the risk and the severity of hypoglycemic reactions. Experimental and clinical evidence is contradictory. Some researchers find that β blockers potentiate insulin-induced hypoglycemia and delay the blood glucose recovery after hypoglycemic reactions, while others have disputed these findings. The β blockers are widely used among diabetic patients for the treatment of angina and hypertension. Cardioselective β blockers have been recommended when diabetic patients require β-blocking drugs. The possible induction, potentiation, or masking of hypoglycemia by β-blocking drugs in diabetics should be considered.

A wide variety of drugs have been found to cause hypoglycemia in isolated instances (Table 131-4). Disopyramide-induced hypoglycemia has been reported increasingly since 1978 and usually occurs in elderly patients who are poorly nourished and have mild abnormalities in glucose homeostasis.

A final cause of induced hypoglycemia is the sudden cessation of a high-concentration glucose infusion. Hypoglycemia from this cause may occur in patients receiving hyperalimentation or hemodialysis. An occasional patient undergoing outpatient hemodialysis may be

Table 131-4. Potentially Hypoglycemic Agents

Acetaminophen	Lithium
Amphetamine	Manganese
Aspirin	Monoamine oxidase inhibitors
Chloramphenicol	Onion extract
Dextropropoxyphene	Orphenadrine
Dicumarol	Oxytetracycline
Disopryamide	Pentamidine
Ethylenediaminetetraacetate	Phenothiazines
Halofenate	Phenylbutazone
Haloperidol	Propranolol
Hypoglycin (akee nut)	Quinine
Kerola (herb)	Sulfa drugs

Source: Malouf R, Brust JCM: Hypoglycemia: Causes, neurological manifestations, and outcome. *Ann Neurol* 17:421, 1985.

brought to the emergency department with hypoglycemia due to this reason.

Hypoglycemia of Infancy and Childhood

Hypoglycemia is relatively common in the pediatric age group. Many of the disorders already discussed cause hypoglycemia in neonates and children, but several metabolic and/or inherited abnormalities which can result in hypoglycemia occur exclusively in this age group. Only selected aspects of pediatric hypoglycemia will be mentioned.

Neonatal hypoglycemia occurs in approximately 4 infants per 1000 live births. The infant may be asymptomatic or have various symptoms consisting of limpness, tremors, irritability, convulsions, apnea, cyanosis, abnormal cry, and bradycardia. In the emergency setting, the infants at greatest risk of hypoglycemia are those born to diabetic mothers, especially if the mothers are on insulin or oral hypoglycemics, and infants born to mothers taking narcotics. Hypoglycemia also occurs in neonates in association with erythroblastosis fetalis, prematurity or postmaturity, hypoxia during delivery, and small size in relation to the gestational age. All neonates with plasma glucose levels less than 40 mg/dL, or infants suspected of hypoglycemia, should be treated with intravenous glucose infusion and referred to their pediatrician for hospitalization and evaluation.

The most common hypoglycemia in childhood is ketotic hypoglycemia, which accounts for more than half of all the cases. The precise mechanism of the hypoglycemia is unknown, but the underlying defect is probably present at birth. Manifestations of ketotic hypoglycemia do not occur until the child is stressed with caloric deprivation. Boys are affected twice as often as girls, and the onset is usually between 18 months and 5 years of age. The attacks are episodic, occurring in the morning or during periods of illness, vomiting, or deprivation of food. Ketonuria is frequently associated with the hypoglycemia. The hypoglycemic episodes respond promptly to the administration of glucose, and spontaneous remission of this disorder occurs by 8 to 10 years of age.

CLINICAL PRESENTATION

The clinical manifestations of hypoglycemia vary widely. Some patients are asymptomatic even though the hypoglycemia is significant. As glucose is the main source of energy for the brain, it is not surprising that most symptomatic hypoglycemia produces neurologic and mental dysfunction. The sympathomimetic symptoms of sudden hypoglycemia, and the neuroglycopenic symptoms, reflective of a gradual lowering of the blood glucose level, were described earlier.

Hypoglycemia can cause other neurologic manifestations such as cranial nerve palsies, paresthesias, and transient hemiplegia. Hemiplegia may be due to spontaneous or induced hypoglycemia. The paralysis is usually abrupt in onset, is associated with extensor plantar responses, and may last a few hours to a few days. This phenomenon is thought to be due to decreased glucose perfusion of a selected area of the brain because of arteriosclerotic narrowing of a blood vessel. Hypoglycemic hemiplegia has also been described in children and adolescents, however. Additional neurologic abnormalities due to hypoglycemia include diplopia, clonus, and decerebrate posturing. In the absence of neuronal damage, these neurologic deficits should reverse with the administration of glucose.

Moderate hypothermia may occur with hypoglycemia and can be a useful clue in cases of unsuspected hypoglycemia. Sweating, peripheral vasodilatation, hyperventilation, and reduced heat production contribute to hypoglycemic-induced hypothermia. When hypoglycemia is accompanied by elevated temperature, infection, dehydration, or cerebral edema may be the cause.

Unsuspected hypoglycemia may masquerade as neurologic, psychiatric, or cardiovascular disorders. Hypoglycemia has been misdiagnosed as a cerebrovascular accident, a transient ischemic attack, a seizure disorder, a brain tumor, narcolepsy, multiple sclerosis, psychosis, hysteria, depression, and Adams-Stokes attacks. Particular care should be exercised when dealing with these entities so that hypoglycemia is not missed.

Evaluation of Hypoglycemia

The ability to detect and evaluate hypoglycemia in the emergency department is limited. A history, a physical examination, selected x-ray studies, and laboratory studies, such as random glucose and urine chemistries, are the main investigative tools available to the emergency physician. One test that could assist in the diagnosis of suspected transient hypoglycemia is the cerebrospinal fluid glucose analysis. Gruber has reported that the CSF glucose level lags behind the blood glucose level during the return to the normal range. The delay in the return to a baseline level may be as much as 4 to 6 h. Transient hypoglycemia could be reflected in a low CSF glucose level at a time when the blood glucose concentration is normal. Other laboratory studies, such as a 6-h GTT, and measurement of the levels of insulin, insulin antibodies, and C peptides, should be obtained in conjunction with the patient's primary physician.

Fed hypoglycemic reactions are suspected based upon the proximity of the symptoms to eating, especially when a repetitive pattern is evident. A history of gastric surgery or relatives with diabetes may be obtained. A 6-h GTT may confirm this diagnosis. If idiopathic hypoglycemia is suspected, home blood glucose monitoring or random blood glucose levels obtained at the time of the symptoms are indicated. Fasting hypoglycemia may occasionally be detected in the emergency department if the patient presents in a fasting state or if a random blood glucose level is low. Patients suspected of having fasting hypoglycemia should be admitted to the hospital for evaluation.

The plasma glucose levels should be determined in all patients who are comatose, have a seizure, have a disturbance of sensorium, have taken a drug overdose, smell of alcohol, or have "funny spells" that are undefined. Random glucose levels should be determined in all diabetic patients with clinically significant complaints.

TREATMENT

Many aspects of treating hypoglycemia have been discussed in conjunction with specific disorders. The armamentarium of the emergency physician in combating hypoglycemia consists of intravenous or oral glucose solutions, glucagon, and hydrocortisone.

Outpatient treatment of insulin reactions can often be self-administered by the ingestion of glucose. One study recommends 20 g of D-glucose as most efficacious, correcting moderate to severe hypoglycemia in 20 min without causing prolonged hypoglycemia. See Table 131-5 for a list of common sources of D-glucose.

Diabetic adults in coma, or other patients who have coma of uncertain cause, should be given 50 mL of a 50% glucose solution by intravenous

Table 131-5. Common Sources of 20 g of D-Glucose

Food	Amount
Kool-Aid with sugar	13.4 fl oz*
Coke	13.3 fl oz†
Orange soda (Fanta)	10.0 fl oz†
Ginger ale (Fanta)	15.5 fl oz†
Tang (orange with sugar)	12.0 fl oz*
Hershey milk chocolate bar	2.5 fl oz‡
Gelatin sweetened with sugar	6.4 oz
Orange juice	12.0 fl oz*
Apple juice	12.0 fl oz*
Banana (flecked)	6.4 oz§

* One cup equals 8 oz.
† One can equals 12 oz.
‡ One bar equals 1.45 oz.
§ One large or two small bananas equal 7 oz.
Source: Brodows RG, Williams C, Amatruda JM: Treatment of insulin reactions in diabetics. *JAMA* 252:3378, 1984.

bolus, after blood has been obtained for appropriate studies. In confirmed hypoglycemia, a follow-up infusion of a 5, 10, or 20% glucose solution should be started. Continuous intravenous glucose for 4 to 6 h is needed for most hypoglycemic reactions. Prolonged therapy may be indicated in some cases, and knowledge of the cause of the hypoglycemia should guide the duration of treatment. Care must be taken not to discontinue the glucose infusion too soon, as the hypoglycemia may recur.

The glucose level with the infusion running should be 100 mg/dL or greater. The blood glucose level should be monitored every 2 to 3 h. If the first liter of glucose solution fails to establish and maintain elevated glucose levels, 100 mg of hydrocortisone and 1 mg of glucagon should be added to each liter of infusate for as long as necessary. Persistent hyperglycemia, maintained by slow administration of 5% glucose, is a sign that the glucose infusion may be withdrawn. After intravenous therapy has been discontinued, the blood glucose level should be determined in every patient discharged from the emergency department. Patients should be instructed to continue oral carbohydrate intake and to return if any symptoms of hypoglycemia recur.

The required duration of continuous glucose infusion is unpredictable. Most diabetic patients with insulin reactions respond fairly rapidly to intravenous glucose. Similarly, alcohol-induced hypoglycemia usually responds quickly to glucose administration. Sulfonylurea-induced hypoglycemia can be prolonged and may not respond to intravenous glucose alone. Diazoxide as adjunctive therapy may be required. All patients with sulfonylurea hypoglycemia should be admitted to the hospital.

Glucagon is effective adjunctive therapy in selected cases. Glucagon increases glucose production by the liver providing that glycogen stores are adequate. Glucagon can be administered intramuscularly, subcutaneously, or intravenously in 0.5- to 2.0-mg doses. It is effective in 10 to 20 min and may be repeated twice. If glucagon is given intravenously, continuous infusion should be used because of glucagon's short half-life in the circulation. Glucagon is not effective in the treatment of alcohol-induced hypoglycemia in chronic alcoholics because of the depletion of liver glycogen stores.

If a patient does not respond clinically to intravenous glucose, glucagon or hydrocortisone should be considered and other causes of coma should be investigated.

BIBLIOGRAPHY

Arky R: Pathophysiology and therapy of the fasting hypoglycemias. *DM* February 1968, p 3.

Aynsley-Green A: Hypoglycemia in infants and children. *Clin Endocrinol Metab* 11:159, 1982.

Campbell PJ, Gerich JE: Mechanisms for prevention, development, and reversal of hypoglycemia. *Adv Intern Med* 33:205, 1988.

Deckert T, Poulsen JE, Larsen M: Prognosis of diabetics with diabetes onset before the age of thirty one. I. Survival, causes of death, and complications. *Diabetologia* 14:363, 1978.

Exton JH: Gluconeogenesis. *Metabolism* 21:945, 1972.

Field JB: Hypoglycemia. *Endocrinol Metab Clin North Am* 18:March 1989.

Gerich JE: Oral hypoglycemic agents. *N Engl J Med* 321:1231, 1989.

Malouf R, Brust JCM: Hypoglycemia: Causes, neurological manifestations, and outcome. *Ann Neurol* 17:421, 1985.

Service FJ, Dale AJD, Elveback LR, et al: Insulinoma: Clinical and diagnostic features of 60 consecutive cases. *Mayo Clin Proc* 51:417, 1976.

Yager J, Young RT: Non-hypoglycemia is an epidemic condition. *N Engl J Med* 291:907, 1974.

132 DIABETIC KETOACIDOSIS

Gene Ragland

Diabetic ketoacidosis occurs exclusively in the diabetic population. It is characterized by hyperglycemia and ketonemia. A relative deficiency of insulin and a concurrent excess of stress hormones are responsible for the metabolic derangement. Therapy includes the replacement of insulin using low doses administered with various techniques.

PATHOGENESIS

The major metabolic abnormalities that occur during diabetic ketoacidosis are hyperglycemia and ketonemia. The metabolic derangements can be explained by relative insulin insufficiency and stress hormone excess. Insulin is the prime anabolic hormone and is responsible for the metabolism and storage of carbohydrates, fats, and proteins. The stress hormones, or counterregulatory hormones, are glucagon, catecholamines, cortisol, and growth hormone.

Insulin

Ingested glucose is the primary stimulant of insulin release from the β cells of the pancreas. Insulin acts on the liver to facilitate the uptake of glucose and its conversion to glycogen. Insulin inhibits glycogen breakdown (glycogenolysis) and suppresses gluconeogenesis. The net effect of these actions is to promote the storage of glucose in the form of glycogen.

Insulin's effect on lipid metabolism is to increase lipogenesis in the liver and adipose cells and simultaneously to prevent lipolysis. Insulin promotes the production of triglycerides from free fatty acids and facilitates the storage of fat. The breakdown of triglycerides to free fatty acids and glycerol is inhibited by insulin. The overall result is the conversion of glucose to stored energy as triglycerides.

Insulin's action in protein metabolism is to stimulate the uptake of amino acids into muscle cells and to mediate the incorporation of amino acids into muscle protein. It prevents the release of amino acids from muscle protein and from hepatic protein sources.

Deficiency in the insulin-secretory mechanism of the β cells of the pancreas is the predominant lesion in diabetes mellitus. This defect results in insulin lack that may be partial or total.

Absolute insulin lack is rare but may be found in juvenile diabetic patients. In the typical maturity-onset diabetic patient, secretory failure involves primarily the initial rapid-release phase of insulin secretion. Minimal insulin inadequacy causes a decrease in the storage of body fuels, and β-cell failure is evident only by the abnormal response to a glucose load—abnormal glucose tolerance test. With more severe failure of insulin secretion, not only is fuel storage impaired, but fuel stores are mobilized during fasting, resulting in hyperglycemia. The increase in the blood glucose level is due to increased glycogenolysis and may elicit an increase in insulin secretion if β-cell reserve is present. The glucose metabolism and concentration may then return to normal.

When there is an absolute or relative failure in insulin secretion, hyperglycemia does not produce increased insulin activity. Loss of the normal physiologic effects of insulin results in catabolism, and hyperglycemia and ketonemia occur.

Stress Hormones

During insulin insufficiency, glucose transport into the cells is inhibited. The physiologic response to cellular starvation and other stresses is to increase the hormones glucagon, catecholamines, cortisol, and growth hormone. These hormones are grouped as counterregulatory hormones because of their anti-insulin effects. The relative roles of each and their mechanisms of action in diabetic ketoacidosis have not been completely elucidated. However, glucagon in excess has been implicated as the main hormone contributing to hyperglycemia and ketonemia. Excess counterregulatory hormone secretion, in conjunction with relative insulin deficiency, is essential to the development of diabetic ketoacidosis. This is shown by the failure of diabetic animals to develop ketoacidosis in the absence of counterregulatory hormones, the elevation of at least one hormone in every case of diabetic ketoacidosis, a delay or reduction of ketoacidosis with pharmacologic blockade of individual stress hormones, and an increase in ketogenic activity when each of the counterregulatory hormones is infused in high physiologic concentrations. No correlation has been reported between the plasma level of insulin during diabetic ketoacidosis and the severity of the ketoacidosis. Finally, the association between antecedent stress and diabetic ketoacidosis has long been recognized. Secretion of the counterregulatory hormones characterizes all major forms of stress.

The counterregulatory hormones are catabolic and, in general, reverse the physiologic processes promoted by insulin. They affect carbohydrate metabolism by increasing glycogenolysis and gluconeogenesis, thereby raising the blood glucose level. Lipolysis is stimulated by glucagon and catecholamines, and this results in increased free fatty acids for conversion to ketones. Protein breakdown is accelerated and provides amino acids for gluconeogenesis. The net effect of relative insulin insufficiency and excess counterregulatory hormones is hyperglycemia and ketonemia (Figure 132-1).

Hyperglycemia occurs earlier than ketonemia during diabetic ketoacidosis. Glucose is underutilized because of insulin lack and overproduced because of enhanced glycogenolysis and gluconeogenesis. Gluconeogenesis is faciliated by increased levels of glucogenic precursors such as glycerol and amino acids resulting from unopposed lipolysis and proteolysis.

Ketonemia occurs because of increased lipolysis and ketogenesis. Insulin deficiency and excess stress hormones lead to the breakdown of triglycerides and the release of large amounts of fatty acids into the circulation. These fatty acids are assimilated in the liver, where they are converted to ketone bodies. The peripheral utilization of ketones is decreased during insulin insufficiency, and they accumulate in the usual 3:1 ratio (β-hydroxybutyrate to acetoacetate).

PRECIPITATING FACTORS

Factors known to precipitate diabetic ketoacidosis include omission of daily insulin injections and a variety of stressful events, such as infections, stroke, myocardial infarction, trauma, pregnancy, hyperthyroidism, and pancreatitis. However, in many patients, there is no clear precipitating cause.

CLINICAL PRESENTATION

Most of the clinical manifestations of diabetic ketoacidosis are related to the biochemical derangements. Hyperglycemia causes an increased osmotic load, and intracellular water is lost because cellular membranes are not freely permeable to glucose. Osmotic diuresis produces total body fluid depletion. Dehydration, hypotension, and reflex tachycardia are consequences. Osmotic diuresis also causes loss of sodium, chloride, potassium, phosphorus, calcium, and magnesium. The serum sodium level may be further decreased by a dilution effect of hyperglycemia. The dilutional effect is a serum sodium decrease of about 5 mEq/L for every 180 mg/dL increase of blood glucose. Electrolyte loss may be worsened by repeated bouts of vomiting.

Dissociation of hydrogen ions from circulating ketone bodies is responsible for the development of acidosis and the fall in the serum bicarbonate level. Some of the ketone bodies are oxidized to acetone, a neutral, soluble, volatile substance that causes the characteristic fruity odor on the breath of a patient with ketoacidosis. Hepatomegaly due

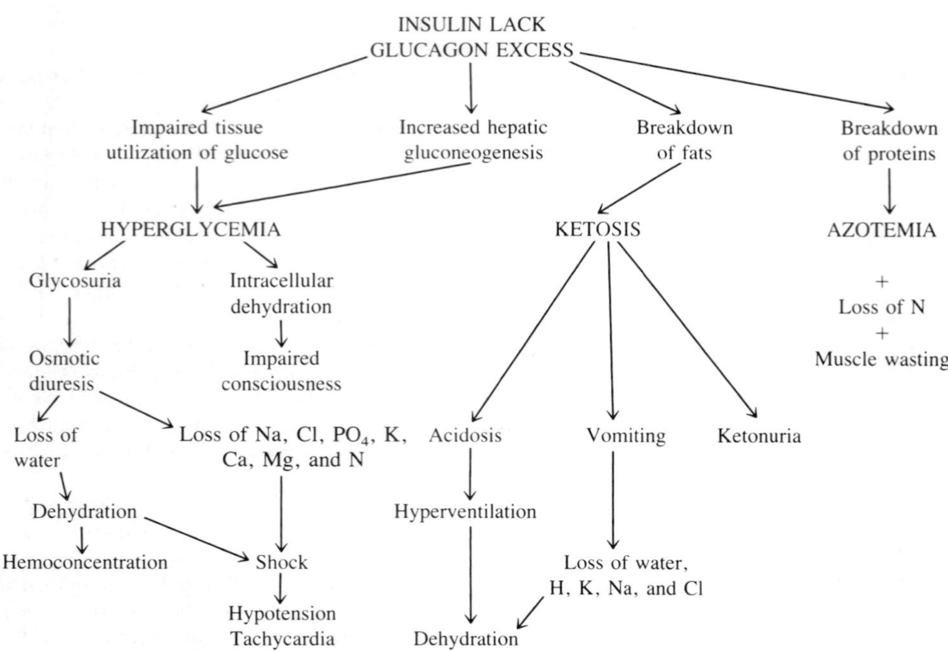

Fig. 132-1. Metabolic consequences of insulin lack, accelerated by glucagon excess. (From Baruh S, Sherman L, Markowitz S: Diabetic ketoacidosis and coma. *Med Clin North Am* 65:117, 1981. Used by permission.)

to accumulation of fat within the liver may occur and should resolve with reversal of ketogenesis.

Acidosis produces other clinical consequences. Compensatory hyperventilation is commonly seen. Exchange of H^+ ions for K^+ across the intracellular membrane is partially responsible for the elevated serum potassium level seen in patients in diabetic ketoacidosis. Peripheral vasodilatation and vascular collapse can result from acidosis.

There is no apparent correlation between the state of consciousness of the patient and the degree of ketonemia, hyperglycemia, electrolyte imbalance, or acidosis. The most direct correlation is with serum osmolality. Some degree of mental confusion or coma is more likely with serum osmolality levels above 340 mOsm/kg.

Nausea, vomiting, and abdominal pain are common presenting complaints. The cause of these disturbances is not clear. Gastric dilatation, paralytic ileus, and abdominal tenderness may be present. Although pancreatitis may develop as a result of ketoacidosis, the diagnosis is difficult since the serum amylase level and the amylase clearance can be elevated in both conditions. Of course, the reverse can occur, so that acute inflammatory or hemorrhagic pancreatitis can result in ketoacidosis. In general, abdominal signs and symptoms should disappear with the resolution of ketoacidosis, and carefully repeated evaluation is necessary to rule out a serious intraabdominal disorder.

Inappropriate normothermia can occur, so that infection must be presumed even in the absence of fever.

Diabetic ketoacidosis may develop rapidly or over a few days. If the patient is able to maintain an adequate fluid and salt intake, a state of compensated ketosis may develop. During the early stages of ketoacidosis or when nausea and vomiting occur, the patient may decrease or omit insulin, thus hastening full-blown diabetic ketoacidosis. The typical patient has nausea, vomiting, abdominal pain, weight loss, dehydration, hypotension, tachycardia, hyperventilation or Kussmaul's respirations, and the odor of acetone on the breath.

LABORATORY

Laboratory abnormalities that are always present during diabetic ketoacidosis include elevated levels of blood glucose, β-hydroxybutyrate, and acetoacetate. Similarly, glucosuria and ketonuria are consistent findings. A decreased pH, low serum bicarbonate level, and decreased P_{CO_2} are present because of metabolic acidosis with respiratory compensation.

The serum sodium level is variable. More water is lost than solutes, and even if the serum sodium level is low, the patient is hypertonic. Initially, the serum potassium level is usually elevated or normal, but it falls as the acidosis is corrected and potassium shifts intracellularly. The serum chloride level may be low if excessive vomiting has occurred. An increased anion-gap acidosis is present because of ketonemia.

The diagnosis of diabetic ketoacidosis should be suspected based upon the clinical presentation previously described. Confirmatory laboratory findings include a blood glucose level greater than 300 mg/dL, a bicarbonate level less than 15 mEq/L, a serum acetone level greater than 2:1 dilution, and a pH less than 7.3. Venous blood should be drawn for a complete blood cell count and determinations of serum glucose, electrolytes, blood urea nitrogen (BUN), creatinine, phosphorus, calcium, magnesium, and acetone. Arterial blood gases are essential. Urinalysis and a chest roentgenogram to search for infection, and an ECG to identify acute myocardial infarction and hyperkalemia, are necessary.

Differential Diagnosis

The differential diagnosis of metabolic coma in a diabetic patient includes hypoglycemia, nonketotic hyperosmolar coma, alcoholic ketoacidosis, and lactic acidosis. A rapid differentiation can be made in the emergency department (Figure 132-2). The result of the analysis of blood gases should be available in a few minutes, and acidosis, if present, will be confirmed. While the physician is awaiting other

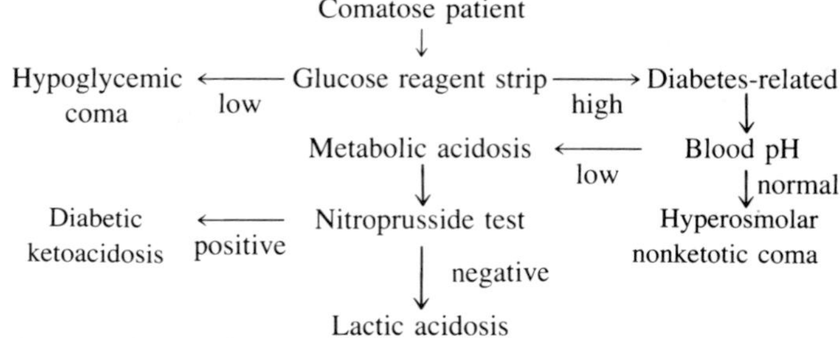

Fig. 132-2. Differential diagnosis of metabolic causes of coma in a diabetic patient. (Adapted from Skillman TG: Diabetic ketoacidosis. *Heart Lung* 7:598, 1978. Used by permission.)

laboratory results, a drop of blood can be tested for blood glucose and serum ketones.

Reagent strips that measure blood glucose levels can be interpreted visually, or can be read in a reflectance meter. Visual interpretation identifies a range but not a precise number, and this method reliably distinguishes between hyperglycemic and hypoglycemic levels. Semiquantitative estimation of serum ketones can be made by testing a drop of blood with a nitroprusside-impregnated tablet. The nitroprusside reaction measures acetoacetate but not β-hydroxybutyrate. This test can be misleading if most of the serum ketones are in the form of β-hydroxybutyrate. Additionally, lactic acidosis may occur simultaneously with diabetic ketoacidosis. Measurement of serum lactate levels may be indicated to determine the contribution of lactic acid to the metabolic acidosis. Finally, in mixed acid-base disturbance, the pH may not accurately reflect the degree of acidosis. The anion gap can assist in identifying unmeasured acids.

TREATMENT

Once the diagnosis of diabetic ketoacidosis has been established, therapy must be started immediately. Specific therapeutic goals include rehydration, correction of electrolyte and acid-base imbalance, reversal of the metabolic consequences of insulin insufficiency, treatment of precipitating causes, and avoidance of complications.

A variety of therapeutic approaches are advocated. Regardless of the approach used, frequent monitoring of the effects is essential. The levels of blood glucose, ketone bodies, potassium, and carbon dioxide should be determined every 1 to 2 h until recovery is well-established. A flow sheet to record vital signs, level of consciousness, intake and output, therapeutic measures, and blood chemistry determinations is recommended. Complete clearing of hyperglycemia and ketonemia usually requires 8 to 16 h.

Fluid Administration

Rapid fluid administration is the most important initial step in the treatment of diabetic ketoacidosis. The average patient in diabetic ketoacidosis has a water deficit of 5 to 10 L and a sodium deficit of 450 to 500 mEq. Normal saline is the most frequently recommended fluid for initial rehydration even though the extracellular fluid of the patient is hypertonic. The normal saline does not provide "free water" to correct intracellular dehydration, but it does prevent a too-rapid fall in extracellular osmolality and excessive transfer of water into the central nervous system (CNS). Most authors favor alternating the administration of normal saline with the administration of half-normal saline.

The first liter of fluid should be administered rapidly, usually over ½ to 1 h. During the first 3 to 4 h, 3 to 5 L of fluid may be required. The blood glucose level and ketone body concentration fall after fluid administration and before implementation of any other therapeutic modality. With rehydration, tissue perfusion is restored, improving the effectiveness of insulin, and renal blood flow increases, allowing the excretion of ketone bodies.

The fluid should be changed to a hypotonic solution after the initial replacement of intravascular volume or if the serum sodium level is 155 mEq/L. Central venous pressure or pulmonary artery wedge pressure should be monitored during fluid replacement in the elderly patients or those with heart disease.

Bicarbonate

Sodium bicarbonate is given to correct the negative effects of acidosis. At a pH of 7, peripheral vasodilatation, decreased cardiac output, and hypotension can occur. Respiratory and CNS depression can occur with severe acidosis (pH less than 6.8).

The hazards of excessive alkali replacement can outweigh the potential benefits. These include paradoxical spinal fluid acidosis, hypokalemia, impaired oxyhemoglobin dissociation, rebound alkalosis, and sodium overload.

It has been established that cerebrospinal fluid (CSF) acidosis is deleterious to brain function. Systemic acidosis per se does not cause mental aberration as long as the CSF is protected against large pH changes. When sodium bicarbonate is administered in large doses, the carbon dioxide loss is diminished, and extracellular fluid and levels of carbon dioxide and bicarbonate increase. Carbon dioxide diffuses freely across the blood-brain barrier, but bicarbonate diffuses into the CSF much more slowly. The difference in the rates of movement into the spinal fluid results in an increase in CSF carbonic acid, a fall in CSF pH, and paradoxical spinal fluid acidosis.

Alkali administration causes a shift of potassium intracellularly. In a patient who already has total body potassium depletion, severe hypokalemia could result. During acidosis, the oxyhemoglobin dissociation curve shifts to the right, facilitating the off-loading of oxygen at the tissue level. This beneficial effect of acidosis could be lost with sudden restoration of the pH toward normal. Final complications of excessive sodium bicarbonate administration include overcompensated rebound alkalosis and sodium overload.

Current recommendations are to administer sodium bicarbonate in modest amounts, i.e., 44 to 100 mEq, when the pH is less than 6.9 for adults. Some studies have shown that use of bicarbonate therapy in patients with diabetic ketoacidosis has provided no beneficial effects in terms of clinical recovery or biochemical variables, even with a pH as low as 6.9. Hydrogen ion production ceases when ketogenesis stops; excessive hydrogen ions are eliminated through the urine and through the respiratory tract, and ketone body metabolism results in the endogenous production of alkali.

Potassium

The deficiency of total body potassium is created by insulin deficit, acidosis, diuresis, and frequent vomiting. The potassium deficit is about 5 to 10 mEq/kg. The initial serum potassium level is usually normal or high because of a deficit of body fluid, diminished renal function, and intracellular exchange of potassium for hydrogen ions during acidosis. Initial hypokalemia indicates severe total body potassium depletion, and massive amounts of potassium for replacement are required during the next 24 h.

The goals of potassium replacement are to maintain a normal extracellular potassium concentration during the acute phases of therapy and to replace the intracellular deficit over a period of days or weeks. With initiation of therapy for diabetic ketoacidosis, the serum potassium concentration falls. This is due to dilution of extracellular fluid, correction of acidosis, increased urinary loss of potassium, and the action of insulin in promoting reentry of potassium into the cells. If these changes occur too rapidly, precipitous hypokalemia may result in fatal cardiac arrhythmias, respiratory paralysis, and paralytic ileus. These complications are avoidable if the pathophysiology is understood and the effects of therapy are frequently monitored.

The ability of insulin to drive potassium into the cells is directly proportional to the insulin concentration. Low-dose insulin therapy provides greater stabilization of the extracellular potassium concentration during the early stages of therapy.

Early potassium replacement is now a standard modality of care. Some authors recommend that small doses of potassium (20 mEq) be added to the intravenous fluid given initially. Others favor administering potassium within the first 2 to 3 h, when insulin therapy is initiated, or after volume expansion has been accomplished. If oliguria is present, renal function must be evaluated and potassium replacement must be decreased. Potassium determinations every 1 to 2 h and continuous ECG monitoring for changes reflecting the potassium concentration should be employed. From 100 to 200 mEq of potassium during the first 12 to 24 h is usually required. Occasionally, as much as 500 mEq of potassium may be necessary.

Insulin

Familiarity with a particular insulin replacement regimen, continuous monitoring, and attention to detail are the most important factors in successfully treating a patient in diabetic ketoacidosis. The amount and route of insulin administration are of secondary importance.

Large doses of insulin are not required to reverse the metabolic derangements of diabetic ketoacidosis and hypoglycemia, osmotic disequilibrium, and hypokalemia are more frequent with large-dose insulin therapy.

Low-dose insulin techniques for treatment of diabetic ketoacidosis are simple, safe, and effective. Techniques for continuous intravenous infusion and intramuscular, subcutaneous, and intravenous bolus therapy have been developed. Blood insulin concentrations of 20 to 200 μU/mL inhibit gluconeogenesis and lipogenesis, stimulate the uptake of potassium by peripheral tissues, and achieve maximum rates of fall of blood glucose concentrations. A continuous insulin infusion of 1 U/h raises the plasma insulin concentration by 20 μU/mL. Similarly, 5 U/h produces a therapeutic level of 100 μU/mL. This level is generally sufficient to achieve normal metabolic homeostasis. The half-life of insulin given intravenously is 4 to 5 min, with an effective biological half-life at the tissue level of approximately 20 to 30 min.

Hypoglycemia using low-dose insulin techniques is almost nonexistent as long as monitoring is done carefully. With low-dose insulin therapies and proper potassium replacement, the occurrence of hypokalemia is less than 5 percent. The more gradual, even insulin effect achieved by low-dose therapy avoids rapid osmotic fluid shifts and the development of cerebral edema.

All low-dose insulin techniques are effective in reversing the metabolic consequences of insulin insufficiency (Figure 132-3). In continuous intravenous infusion of low doses of insulin, 5 to 10 units of regular insulin are administered per hour. The effect of insulin begins almost immediately after the initiation of the infusion, and a "priming" intravenous bolus is not required. Continuous insulin administration ensures that a steady blood concentration is maintained in an effective range, and this technique allows flexibility in adjusting the insulin dose. When the infusion is stopped, the insulin already in the blood is quickly degraded, providing greater control of the amount of insulin given in comparison with the intramuscular or subcutaneous routes.

Serious complications with continuous intravenous low-dose insulin infusion are minimal. The main disadvantage is that it requires an infusion pump and frequent monitoring to ensure that insulin is being administered in the desired amount. A separate intravenous site for the insulin infusion is desirable but not required.

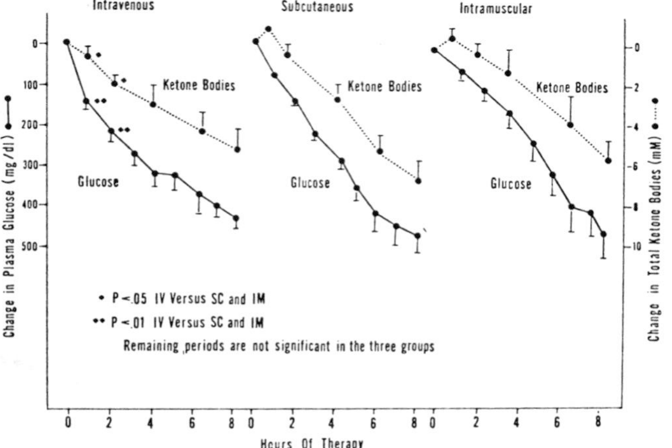

Fig. 132-3. Change in levels of plasma glucose and total ketone bodies (β-hydroxybutyrate plus acetoacetate) after intravenous, subcutaneous, or intramuscular low-dose insulin therapy (15 patients in each group). (From Fisher JN, Shahshahani MN, Kitabchi AE: Diabetic ketoacidosis: Low-dose insulin therapy by various routes. *N Engl J Med* 297:238, 1977. Used by permission.)

The technique of low-dose intramuscular or subcutaneous insulin therapy is better suited to a hospital environment in which constant nursing supervision is not always possible. The main disadvantage to this approach, more marked with the subcutaneous route, is that insulin absorption may be erratic in a hypotensive, peripherally vasoconstricted patient. Erratic absorption may result in a delay in achieving adequate insulin levels. Further, delayed absorption can produce deposits of insulin that may later be absorbed, causing hypoglycemia. These problems can largely be eliminated by ensuring adequate hydration of the patient and by using small enough doses of insulin to preclude accumulation of large insulin deposits.

The onset of action of insulin given intramuscularly is delayed in comparison with that of insulin given intravenously. The most current protocols recommend an initial dose of 20 units of insulin intramuscularly, intravenously, or divided between these routes, followed by 5 to 10 U/h intramuscularly. The half-life of insulin given intramuscularly is 2 h. Hourly injections produce a continuous, effective blood concentration of insulin.

There are common problems with insulin therapy regardless of the technique used. The incidence of nonresponders to low-dose therapies is 1 to 2 percent. Infection is the main reason for failure to respond to low-dose insulin therapy. If the patient fails to respond to low-dose insulin therapy in the first hour, most protocols recommend doubling the infusion rate or administering an intravenous bolus of insulin. The insulin dose is increased in a similar fashion each hour until a satisfactory response is achieved.

Glucose should be added to the intravenous fluid when the blood glucose concentration falls to 250 mg/dL. Insulin therapy should not be stopped just because the blood glucose level declines but should be continued until the ketonemia and acidosis have cleared. Intravenous insulin should not be abruptly discontinued. An overlap period in which subcutaneous insulin is given should precede discontinuation of the insulin infusion.

Phosphate Replacement

The role of phosphate replacement during the treatment of diabetic ketoacidosis remains controversial. Hyperphosphatemia is the initial finding in most cases of diabetic ketoacidosis. However, one author estimates that up to 90 percent of patients have acute hypophosphatemia within 6 to 12 h after initiation of therapy for diabetic ketoacidosis. The decrease is primarily due to a sudden shift of phosphate from the extracellular to the intracellular compartment following insulin administration and accelerated glucose storage. Phosphate is found in all body tissues, and this sudden shift deprives them of this essential constituent. Hypophosphatemia is usually most severe 24 to 48 h after the start of insulin therapy.

Phosphate plays an integral part in the conversion of energy from adenosine triphosphate (ATP) and in the delivery of oxygen at the tissue level through 2,3-diphosphoglyceric acid (2,3-DPG). In addition, many important enzymes, cofactors, and biochemical intermediates depend upon phosphate. Acute phosphate deficiency has been associated with a variety of clinical disorders including neuromuscular paralysis leading to respiratory failure and possibly myocardial dysfunction.

Acute hypophosphatemia can be corrected by intravenous or oral administration of phosphorus. Several oral forms are available but may cause diarrhea and be erratically absorbed. A commercial intravenous preparation (KH_2PO_4 plus K_2HPO_4) containing K^+ at a concentration of 4 mEq/mL and phosphorus at a concentration of 96 mg/mL can be used. Five milliliters of this commercial potassium phosphate preparation added to 1 L of intravenous fluid provides approximately 20 mEq of K^+ and 480 mg of PO_4^{2+}.

Hypophosphatemia is not associated with untoward consequences until a serum concentration of less than 1.0 mg/dL is reached. Phosphorus supplementation is not indicated and should not be given as long as the level remains above this concentration. Some authors have recommended the use of potassium phosphate salts instead of potassium chloride as a means of potassium replacement during therapy for diabetic ketoacidosis. Early routine use of potassium phosphate solutions to replace potassium should be discouraged. The need for phosphorus replacement, if at all, occurs several hours after therapy for diabetic ketoacidosis has begun, and potassium is usually required much sooner.

Several undesirable side effects from phosphate administration have been reported. These include hyperphosphatemia, hypocalcemia, hypomagnesemia, metastatic soft tissue calcifications, and hypernatremia and dehydration from osmotic diuresis. The serum phosphate level should be monitored during treatment of diabetic ketoacidosis, but the case for routine phosphate replacement has not been made.

COMPLICATIONS AND MORTALITY

Complications related to the disease state include aspiration of gastric contents by an unconscious patient, vascular stasis and deep vein thrombosis, and disseminated intravascular coagulation (DIC). Rhabdomyolysis during diabetic ketoacidosis has also been recently reported. Protection of the airway and evacuation of gastric contents are indicated in an unconscious patient. Prophylactic heparin therapy may help to prevent thrombotic complications.

Major complications related to the therapy of diabetic ketoacidosis include hypokalemia, paradoxical spinal fluid acidosis, and cerebral edema. These complications are largely preventable. The goal of therapy of diabetic ketoacidosis is to produce a gradual, even return to normal metabolic balance. Rapids shifts of the levels of water, electrolytes, and other solutes can be avoided by using isotonic saline as the initial intravenous fluid, refraining from excessive bicarbonate administration, replacing potassium early in the course of treatment, and using low-dose insulin techniques. Above all, a basic understanding of the pathophysiology of diabetic ketoacidosis, constant monitoring of the patient, and attention to detail are essential to prevent complications of treatment.

In general, the greater the presenting serum osmolality, blood urea nitrogen (BUN), and blood glucose concentration, the greater the mortality. There is also increased mortality for patients presenting with a serum bicarbonate level of less than 10 mEq/L.

Of the factors responsibile for precipitating diabetic ketoacidosis, infection and myocardial infarction are the main contributors to high mortality. Half the patients in diabetic ketoacidosis die when myocardial infarction is the precipitating event. Additional factors that reduce the chances of survival include old age, severe hypotension, prolonged and severe coma, and underlying renal and cardiovascular disease.

BIBLIOGRAPHY

Alberti KGMM, Christensen NJ, Iversen J, et al: Role of glucagon and other hormones in development of diabetic ketoacidosis. *Lancet* 1:1307, 1975.

Albert KGMM, Hockaday TDR: Diabetic coma: A reappraisal after five years. *Clin Endocrinol Metab* 6:421, 1977.

Becker DJ, Brown DR, Steranka BH, et al: Phosphate replacement during treatment of diabetic ketosis: Effects on calcium and phosphorus homeostasis. *Am J Dis Child* 137:241, 1983.

Fisher JN, Kitabchi AE: A randomized study of phosphate therapy in the treatment of diabetic ketoacidosis. *J Clin Endocrinol Metab* 57:177, 1983.

Fisher JN, Shahshahani MN, Kitabchi AE: Diabetic ketoacidosis: Low-dose insulin therapy by various routes. *N Engl J Med* 297:238, 1977.

Foster DW, McGarry JD: The metabolic derangements and treatment of diabetic ketoacidosis. *N Engl J Med* 309:159, 1983.

Kitabchi AE: Low-dose insulin therapy in diabetic ketoacidosis: Fact or fiction? *Diabetes Metab Rev* 5:337, 1989.

Krane EJ: Diabetic ketoacidosis: Biochemistry, physiology, treatment, and prevention. *Pediatr Clin North Am* 34:935, 1987.

Kreisberg RA: Diabetic ketoacidosis: An update. *Crit Care Clin* 5:817, 1987.

Page MM, Alberti KGMM, Greenwood R, et al: Treatment of diabetic coma with continuous low-dose infusion of insulin. *Br Med J* 2:687, 1974.

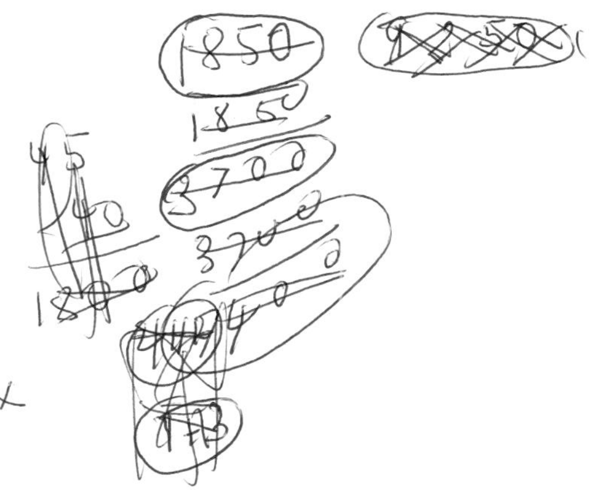

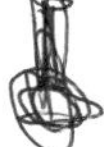

133
ALCOHOLIC KETOACIDOSIS

Gene Ragland

Alcoholic ketoacidosis is characterized by an anion gap acidosis due to high levels of ketoacids. It occurs exclusively in relation to alcohol abuse but not just in chronic alcoholics. It has been reported in first-time drinkers whose food intake is minimal.

The true incidence is unknown, and the frequency is probably directly related to the incidence of alcoholism in a population.

PATHOGENESIS

Several mechanisms have been postulated. In one explanation, ketosis results from increased mobilization of free fatty acids from adipose tissue coupled with simultaneous enhancement of the liver's capacity to convert these substrates into acetoacetate and β-hydroxybutyrate.

During the metabolism of alcohol in the liver the rate of nicotinamide adenine dinucleotide (NAD) reduction exceeds the rate of mitochondrial NADH oxidation, causing a decrease in available NAD. This state persists for a few days in spite of no further alcohol consumption. An NAD-dependent step in the oxidation of fatty acids in the mitochondria of the hepatocyte is displaced in favor of ketone body formation.

During alcoholic ketoacidosis insulin levels are low, whereas levels of cortisol, growth hormone, glucagon, and epinephrine are increased, possibly as a result of alcohol-induced hypoglycemia. This hormonal milieu promotes lipolysis, which increases the levels of free fatty acids available for conversion to ketones.

Additional mechanisms that may contribute to ketosis include the conversion of acetate, an alcohol breakdown product, to ketones; alcohol-induced mitochondrial structural changes which enhance the rate of ketosis; and mitochondrial phosphorus depletion, which inhibits the utilization for NADH and increases ketone body formation. Finally, vomiting and starvation superimposed on chronic malnutrition also contribute to ketoacidosis.

CLINICAL PRESENTATION

The usual history is one of heavy alcohol consumption or binge drinking with decreased or absent food intake for several days. Food and alcohol intake are usually terminated by nausea, protracted vomiting, and abdominal pain occurring 24 to 72 h before presentation. It is during this period that ketoacidosis develops.

Clinically the patient appears acutely ill with dehydration, tachypnea, tachycardia, and diffuse abdominal pain. Most patients are alert, but they may be mildly disoriented or occasionally comatose.

There are no specific physical findings. Evidence of dehydration such as hypotension, orthostatic changes in blood pressure, tachycardia, and decreased urine output may be present. The temperature varies from hypothermia to mildly elevated. Abdominal pain due to non-specific causes or due to gastritis, pancreatitis, or hepatitis is common. Sepsis, meningitis, pyelonephritis, or pneumonia may be present, and delirium tremens may develop.

LABORATORY

Alcohol levels are usually low or undetectable, as the alcohol intake is decreased or discontinued during the period of anorexia and vomiting. Essential to the diagnosis of alcoholic ketoacidosis is a large anion gap due to high levels of serum ketones. Most patients have a blood pH reflective of the underlying metabolic acidosis, but many may present with normal or alkalemic pH values.

Acid-Base Balance

Fulop and Hoberman compared typical laboratory data from patients with diabetic ketoacidosis with data from patients with alcoholic ketoacidosis (Table 133-1). The alcoholic patients tended to have a higher blood pH, lower levels of serum K^+ and Cl^-, and a higher level of plasma HCO_3^- than the diabetic patients. This difference is attributed to the severe recurrent vomiting experienced by the alcoholic patients. Vomiting causes chloride depletion and metabolic alkalosis. In addition, respiratory alkalosis may occur secondary to fever, sepsis, or alcohol withdrawal and further increases the blood pH.

Ketones

The anion gap $[Na^+ - (Cl^- + HCO_3^-) = 12 \pm 4$ mEq/L] in the patient groups is very similar and is due primarily to high levels of β-hydroxybutyrate and to a lesser extent to lactic acid accumulation. The principal ketones are acetoacetate and β-hydroxybutyrate. These ketones are intermediates in the oxidation of fatty acids; they are normally produced in equal amounts and are not normally detectable in the serum. Acetoacetate and β-hydroxybutyrate are a redox pair and are interconverted by an oxidation-reduction reaction with NAD and NADH as cofactors. In alcoholic ketoacidosis, perhaps because of lack of NAD, β-hydroxybutyrate accumulates to levels several times higher than the levels of acetoacetate. Acetone is a volatile, neutral ketone that is formed from acetoacetate by irreversible spontaneous decarboxylation. Its presence reflects the level and duration of acetoacetate elevation and is indicative of a sustained, severe acidosis.

Nitroprusside Test

The nitroprusside test is used to detect the presence of ketones in serum and urine. This is a semiquantitative test that gives a reaction with acetoacetate, is less sensitive to acetone, and does not detect β-hydroxybutyrate at all. There is no practical test that measures β-hydroxybutyrate levels. In most series on alcoholic ketoacidosis, the nitroprusside test has shown moderate or large ketonemia or ketonuria. But in a significant minority of patients, the reaction may be weakly positive or negative even though ketoacidosis, because of high levels of β-hydroxybutyrate, is pronounced. Reliance on this test alone as a measure of ketoacidosis may lead to failure to recognize the presence of ketoacidosis or to an underestimation of the severity of the ketoacidosis.

Glucose

The blood glucose level in alcoholic ketoacidosis varies from hypoglycemia to mild elevation. In most series it is normal or slightly increased. Glucosuria is usually mild or absent. A subset of alcoholic patients in whom hypoglycemia and ketoacidosis are coexistent has been described.

The pathogenesis of alcohol-induced hypoglycemia includes acute starvation, depletion of liver glycogen stores because of chronic malnutrition, and inhibition of gluconeogenesis because of alcohol-induced alteration of the NAD/NADH ratio. Alcohol also causes decreased peripheral utilization of glucose, and this acts to balance the glucose-depleting processes. Devenyi asks if alcoholic hypoglycemia and alcoholic ketoacidosis are sequential events of the same process. He theorizes that alcohol-induced hypoglycemia occurs first, causing increased levels of cortisol, growth hormone, glucagon, and epinephrine; this may correct the hypoglycemia and mobilize free fatty acids, which are converted to ketones. If this theory is correct, the diagnosis of alcoholic hypoglycemia or alcoholic ketoacidosis may depend upon the point in this process at which the disorder is detected.

DIAGNOSIS

The diagnosis of alcoholic ketoacidosis is easily established in those patients with an antecedent history of alcohol intake, decreased food

Table 133-1. Comparison of Admission Laboratory Data in Patients with Diabetic Ketoacidosis and Alcoholic Ketosis*

	Diabetic Ketoacidosis		
Variable†	**Oh and Co-workers (N = 35)**	**Our Series (N = 27)**	**Alcoholic Ketoacidosis (N = 18)**
Blood pH	7.07 ± 0	7.17 ± 0.02	7.35 ± 0.05
Serum Na^+	135.5 ± 1.6	133.0 ± 1.2	135.2 ± 1.6
Serum K^+		4.9 ± 0.2	4.1 ± 0.3
Serum Cl^-	101.0 ± 1.4	97.3 ± 1.1	90.9 ± 3.9
Plasma HCO_3^-	9.4‡	6.7 ± 0.6	16.5 ± 2.4
Δ HCO_3^-	14.6	17.3 ± 0.6	7.5 ± 2.4
Anion gap§	26.1	28.9 ± 1.1	27.8 ± 2.5
Plasma lactate	2.7 ± 0.3	2.1 ± 0.1	3.9 ± 1.2
Plasma β-hydroxybutyrate	10.3 ± 0.3	10.8 ± 0.6	9.3 ± 1.1
Plasma lactate + β-hydroxybutyrate	13.0	12.9 ± 0.6	13.2 ± 1.6
Excess anion gap¶	14.1	17.0 ± 1.1	15.8 ± 2.5

* Data given as mean ± SEM.

† All units except blood pH are in mEq/L.

‡ This and all succeeding values in this column refer to 15 patients.

§ Calculated as serum $Na^+ - (Cl^- + HCO_3^-)$.

¶ Calculated as anion gap − 12 mEq/L.

Source: Fulop M, Hoberman HD: Diabetic ketoacidosis and alcoholic ketoacidosis. *Ann Intern Med* 91:796, 1979.

intake, vomiting, and abdominal pain, and laboratory findings of metabolic acidosis, a positive nitroprusside test, and a low or mildly elevated glucose level.

Several factors may contribute to the failure to recognize this metabolic disorder. The blood alcohol level may be zero, and, in the absence of a history of alcohol intake, this diagnosis may not be considered. The nitroprusside test may be weakly positive or negative in spite of significant ketoacidosis. The pH may be mildly acidotic, normal, or even alkalemic in the face of pronounced metabolic acidosis. There are no specific physical findings which suggest the diagnosis of alcoholic ketoacidosis. Alcoholic patients may have a variety of alcohol-induced associated illnesses which may obscure or distract from this diagnosis. Mental confusion or coma may be incorrectly attributed to alcoholic intoxication or other causes if the appropriate laboratory studies are not performed or if they are incorrectly interpreted.

Diagnostic Criteria

Soffer and Hamburger's criteria to define alcoholic ketoacidosis are a serum glucose level less than 300 mg/dL, a recent history of alcohol intake with a relative or absolute decline in ethanol consumption 24 to 72 h before hospitalization, a history of vomiting, and a metabolic acidosis for which other causes, such as diabetic ketoacidosis, lactic acidosis, renal failure, or drug ingestion, are excluded by clinical observations or laboratory studies. A positive serum nitroprusside test, because of its limitations, is not a criterion for diagnosis.

Differential Diagnosis

A positive nitroprusside test and a very low plasma bicarbonate concentration suggest ketosis with a high level of β-hydroxybutyrate. The combination of a barely positive nitroprusside test and a low plasma bicarbonate concentration signifies either a very reduced state with high concentrations of β-hydroxybutyrate or else a coincidental lactic acidosis. The measurement of serum lactate levels aids in this differential diagnosis.

The entity with which alcoholic ketoacidosis is most often confused is diabetic ketoacidosis. The magnitude of ketoacidosis is equal in these two disorders. It is important to make the proper distinction, as the treatment of each entity is different. In diabetic ketoacidosis, hyperglycemia and glycosuria are present. The serum glucose level in alcoholic ketoacidosis varies from hypoglycemia to mild elevation, and glucosuria is usually mild or absent. This differential diagnosis can be made in the emergency department.

TREATMENT

Therapy of alcoholic ketoacidosis is simple and effective and consists of the intravenous administration of a glucose and saline solution. Patients given only saline improve, but not as rapidly as those who are also given glucose. Thiamine, 50 to 100 mg intravenously, should be given before the glucose to prevent precipitation of Wernicke's disease. Reversal of ketoacidosis usually occurs in 12 to 18 h.

Restoration of intravascular volume is best accomplished by alternating infusions of glucose-containing normal and half-normal saline. Volume repletion is necessary to correct insulin-release inhibition by adrenergic nerve endings in the islets of Langerhans as well as by circulating catecholamines. Glucose infusion stimulates insulin release, and insulin inhibits lipolysis and terminates ketoacid production. Glucose may inhibit further ketoacid production by increasing oxidation of accumulated NADH via glucose-induced uptake of phosphorus by the hepatic mitochondria.

Exogenous administration of insulin is not indicated in treatment of alcoholic ketoacidosis; this aspect of therapy differs from therapy of diabetic ketoacidosis. Inappropriate administration of insulin to a patient with a normal or low glucose level could be dangerous.

Administration of sodium bicarbonate is usually not required. As ketoacid levels fall, plasma bicarbonate levels increase, and the pH returns to normal. A small amount of bicarbonate may be indicated if the pH is less than 7.1 or if the patient is clinically deteriorating as evidenced by a weak, rapid pulse, hypotension, or inability to compensate by hyperventilation because of weakness. The role of phosphorus replenishment in therapy of alcoholic ketoacidosis is not clear.

With recovery and reversal of the acidosis, β-hydroxybutyrate is converted to acetoacetate. As this process occurs, the nitroprusside test becomes more positive because of higher levels of acetoacetate. This factitious hyperketonemia may cause the uninformed clinician unnecessary concern, as it appears that the ketoacidosis is worsening. Clinical improvement of the patient and increasing blood pH values are more reliable parameters of recovery than the nitroprusside test.

The survival rates of patients with alcoholic ketoacidosis are good. Those patients that die usually do so because of other complications of chronic alcoholism. A thorough search for and treatment of associated alcoholic disorders is essential. Recurrent episodes of alcoholic ketoacidosis after subsequent alcoholic debauch are not uncommon.

BIBLIOGRAPHY

Cooperman MT, Davidoff F, Spark R, et al: Clinical studies of alcoholic ketoacidosis. *Diabetes* 23:433, 1974.

Devenyi P: Alcoholic hypoglycemia and alcoholic ketoacidosis: Sequential events of the same process? *Can Med Assoc J* 127:513, 1982.

Dillon ES, Dyer WW, Smelo LS: Ketone acidosis in nondiabetic adults. *Med Clin North Am* 24:1813, 1940.

Fulop M, Ben-Ezra J, Bock J: Alcoholic ketosis. *Alcoholism: Clin Exp Res* 10:610, 1986.

Fulop M, Hoberman HD: Alcoholic ketosis. *Diabetes* 24:785, 1975.

Jenkins DW, Eckel RE, Craig JW: Alcoholic ketoacidosis. *JAMA* 217:177, 1971.

Levy LJ, Duga J, Girgis M, et al: Ketoacidosis associated with alcoholism in nondiabetic subjects. *Ann Intern Med* 78:213, 1973.

Miller PD, Heinig RE, Waterhouse C: Treatment of alcoholic acidosis—The role of dextrose and phosphorus. *Arch Intern Med* 138:67, 1978.

Platia EV, Hsu TH: Hypoglycemic coma with ketoacidosis in nondiabetic alcoholics. *West J Med* 131:270, 1979.

Soffer A, Hamburger S: Alcoholic ketoacidosis: A review of 30 cases. *J Am Med Wom Assoc* 37:106, 1982.

134 NONKETOTIC HYPEROSMOLAR COMA

Gene Ragland

Nonketotic hyperosmolar coma is characterized by severe hyperglycemia, hyperosmolality, and dehydration, but no ketoacidosis. This metabolic derangement occurs primarily in diabetics but may occur in nondiabetics under certain circumstances. Many names have been used to identify this entity, but the term *nonketotic hyperosmolar coma* is used in this chapter.

This syndrome shares many features with diabetic ketoacidosis, including hyperglycemia and hyperosmolality, but the lack of ketoacidosis is its main distinguishing feature. Nonketotic hyperosmolar coma is much less common than diabetic ketoacidosis. Nonketotic hyperosmolar coma and diabetic ketoacidosis are part of a continuum, and when present in pure form, they represent the opposite ends of a spectrum with regard to lipid mobilization. In general, a patient with nonketotic hyperosmolar coma has a blood glucose concentration greater than 800 mg/dL, usually 1000 mg/dL or more, a serum osmolality greater than 350 mOsm/kg, and a negative test for serum ketones. By comparison, the average blood glucose level of a patient in diabetic ketoacidosis is usually less than 600 mg/dL, the serum osmolality is rarely above 350 mOsm/kg, and the test for serum ketones is strongly positive.

Nonketotic hyperosmolar coma occurs most commonly as the initial manifestation of adult-onset diabetes. Most known diabetics who develop this syndrome have mild, maturity-onset diabetes controlled by diet or oral hypoglycemic agents. A small minority of insulin-dependent patients on parenteral therapy develop nonketotic hyperosmolar coma. Both extremes—nonketotic hyperosmolar coma and diabetic ketoacidosis—have been reported to occur in the same patient.

PATHOGENESIS

Any explanation of the pathogenesis of nonketotic hyperosmolar coma must explain why extreme hyperglycemia develops and why ketoacidosis does not. Neither of these questions has been answered with certainty. Simply put, extreme hyperglycemia develops because ketoacidosis does not. The failure of ketoacidosis to occur allows the underlying process to continue unrecognized and much higher levels of glucose to result.

When a patient with mild, maturity-onset diabetes is subjected to stress, the β cells of the pancreas respond to the increased glucose concentration by increasing the secretion of insulin. Continued diabetogenic stress eventually exhausts the insulinogenic reserve of the β cells, and plasma insulin levels fall. Because of the increased insulinogenic capacity of the patient with mild diabetes, higher levels of blood glucose occur before this reserve is depleted. If the patient is receiving insulin therapy, supplemental insulin allows additional time for β-cell recovery and further prolongs the time required for exhaustion of the insulin reserve. In addition, elevated levels of glucagon may promote gluconeogenesis in the liver, resulting in massive hyperglycemia.

The reason ketoacidosis does not occur is not well understood, and explanations conflict. Some have found low levels of free fatty acids (FFAs), with normal insulin, glucocorticoid, and growth hormone levels. They believe that inhibition of lipolysis occurs because of relatively higher circulating insulin levels or lower lipolytic hormone levels than are present with diabetic ketoacidosis. When lipolysis is inhibited, the precursors required for ketone body formation are not released and ketoacidosis does not develop. It is known that the quantity of insulin required to inhibit lipolysis in adipose tissue is less than the quantity required to promote the utilization of glucose by peripheral tissues. Ketoacidosis may not develop because there is enough circulating insulin to inhibit lipolysis but an insufficient amount to protect against the development of hyperglycemia.

Others have reported similar high FFA levels and low circulating insulin levels in both nonketotic hyperosmolar coma and diabetic ketoacidosis. Additionally, glucagon and glucocorticoids (cortisol) have been found to be increased to the same extent in both conditions. These authors conclude that in nonketotic hyperosmolar coma the FFAs are mobilized to the same extent as in diabetic ketoacidosis, but that the intrahepatic oxidation of the incoming FFAs is directed along nonketogenic metabolic pathways, such as triglyceride synthesis, because of an insulinated liver. Prehepatic and posthepatic insulin levels have been measured. In diabetic ketoacidosis, both pre- and posthepatic insulin levels are low, but in nonketotic hyperosmolar coma, prehepatic insulin levels twice the posthepatic ones have been found. Subscribers to this theory conclude that the liver is selectively bathed in insulin while the periphery is in a "diabetic" state. They conclude that the available insulin exerts its antiketogenic effect at the hepatic and not the adipocyte level.

Regardless of the pathogenesis of nonketotic hyperosmolar coma, the effect of hyperglycemia in producing osmotic diuresis and fluid and electrolyte imbalance is understood. When relative insulin insufficiency develops in the diabetic patient, osmotically active glucose is located in the extracellular fluid compartment. During insulin insufficiency the cell membrane is not freely permeable to glucose, and water is drawn from the intracellular compartment into the extracellular compartment in an attempt to achieve equal osmolality. The presence of large amounts of glucose in the extracellular compartment tends to preserve that compartment at the expense of cellular volume. Relative expansion of the extracellular fluid volume may protect against hypotension until late in the course of nonketotic hyperosmolar coma.

In addition to the internal shifts in body fluids, an osmotic diuresis also occurs. Normally, antidiuretic hormone (ADH) from the posterior pituitary gland acts to maintain water balance. With severe hyperglycemia, glycosuria produces an increased volume and rate of urine flow through the kidneys. Despite maximum levels of ADH, water can no longer be maximally reabsorbed, and an increased volume of urine results. Total body water is decreased and serum osmolality is increased. Fluid losses during nonketotic hyperosmolar coma range from 8 to 12 L.

Sodium balance is also upset by osmotic diuresis. Sodium reabsorption normally occurs in the distal tubules, mediated by the renin-angiotensin system. The concentration gradient against which sodium must be actively transported into the distal tubules is increased as water reabsorption diminishes. Thus a large proportion of the filtered sodium remains unabsorbed and passes into the urine. Nevertheless, the water loss during osmotic diuresis is greater than the sodium loss, and the patient becomes hypertonic relative to sodium. Prolonged diuresis results in hypovolemia and hypertonic dehydration.

Total body potassium depletion is also a consequence of osmotic diuresis. The distal tubules are under maximal stimulation by aldosterone, and some sodium is reabsorbed in exchange for potassium. Because of the longer duration of osmotic diuresis with nonketotic hyperosmolar coma, potassium depletion is greater than that which occurs with diabetic ketoacidosis and may reach 400 to 1000 mEq. Potassium depletion may not become evident until the patient is rehydrated. Other solutes such as magnesium and phosphate are also lost during osmotic diuresis (see Fig. 134-1).

CLINICAL PRESENTATION

Nonketotic hyperosmolar coma is most common in the middle-aged or elderly and occurs most commonly in diabetics, although the ma-

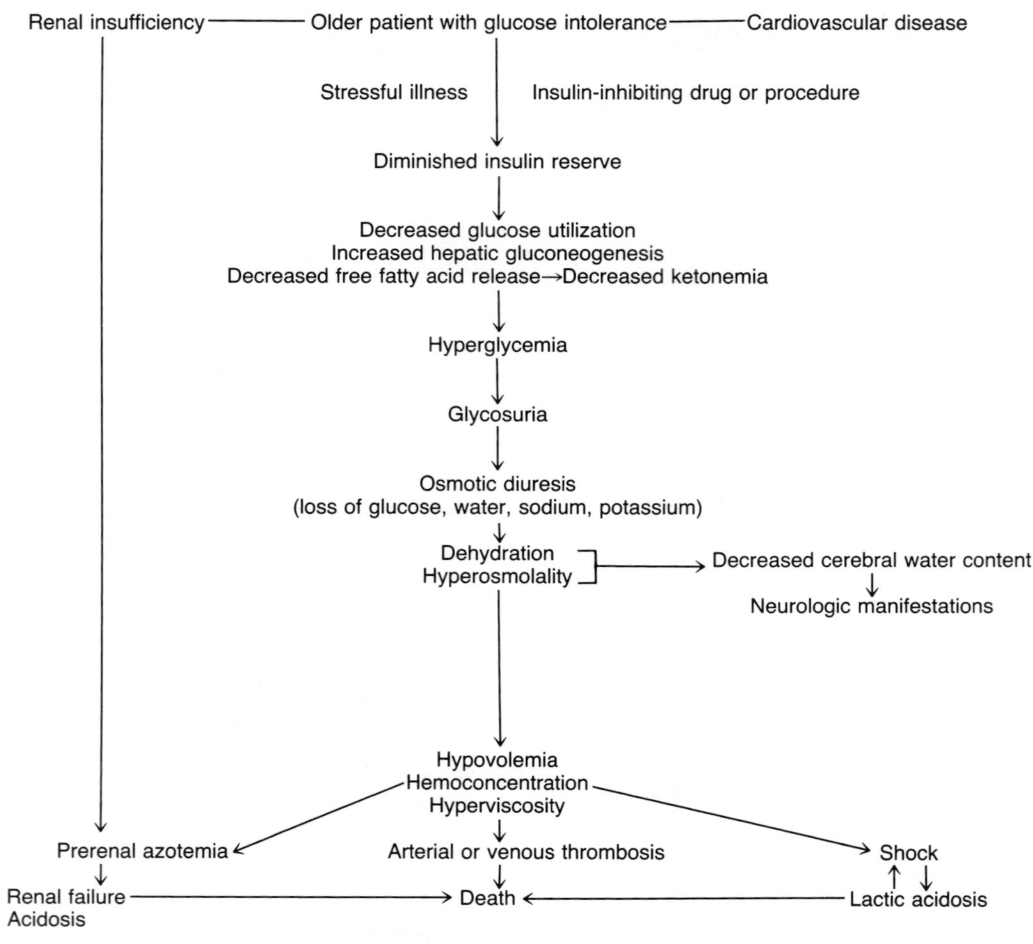

Fig. 134-1. Pathophysiology of nonketotic hyperosmolar coma. (From Grace TW: Hyperosmolar non-ketotic diabetic coma. *Am Fam Physician* 32:119, 1985. Used by permission.)

jority are undiagnosed at the time of presentation. Patients who depend upon others to meet their needs, such as infants, nursing home patients, and the mentally retarded, are particularly vulnerable to its insidious onset. Inaccessibility to water coupled with an inability to communicate masks the early signs and symptoms.

Precipitating Factors

Minor upper respiratory infection or gastroenteritis is capable of precipitating diabetic ketoacidosis, but an illness of greater magnitude is usually required before nonketotic hyperosmolar coma results. Infection is a common precipitating cause, especially gram-negative pneumonias. Other precipitating illnesses include myocardial infarction, cerebrovascular accidents, gastrointestinal (GI) hemorrhage, acute pyelonephritis, acute pancreatitis, uremia, subdural hematomas, and peripheral vascular occlusion. Chronic renal and cardiovascular disease is common.

Various drugs have been linked to the onset of nonketotic hyperosmolar coma (Table 134-1). Most are dehydrating agents or have side effects of impairing insulin release from the pancreas or of interfering with the peripheral action of insulin. Thiazide diuretics and diazoxide possess both characteristics and are well-recognized causes of nonketotic hyperosmolar coma. Other drugs causally related to this syndrome include corticosteroids, phenytoin, mannitol, cimetidine, propranolol, calcium channel blockers, and immunosuppressive agents.

Clinical situations that can result in severe dehydration or an excessive glucose load or both may produce this syndrome in nondiabetic patients. These include extensive burns, heatstroke, hypothermia, peritoneal or hemodialysis with a hypertonic glucose solution, and hyperalimentation; these causes are most commonly seen in hospitalized patients.

An occasional patient may have a history of ingesting enormous quantities of sugar-containing fluids. This patient is usually alert and has a lesser degree of dehydration than the usual patient with nonketotic hyperosmolar coma.

Table 134-1. Drugs and Procedures that May Cause Hyperosmolar Coma

Hydrochlorothiazide and other thiazide diuretics	Cimetidine (Tagamet)
Chlorthalidone (Hygroton, Thalitone)	Propranolol (Inderal)
Furosemide (Lasix)	Asparaginase (Elspar)
Ethacrynic acid (Edecrin)	Immunosuppressive agents
Diazoxide (Hyperstat, Proglycem)	Mannitol
Calcium channel blockers	Peritoneal dialysis
Glucocorticoids	Hemodialysis
Phenytoin (Dilantin)	Intravenous hyperosmolar alimentation
Chloropromazine (Thorazine)	

Source: Grace TW: Hyperosmolar non-ketotic diabetic coma. *Am Fam Physician* 32:119, 1985.

The prodromal period during the development of nonketotic hyperosmolar coma is longer than that for diabetic ketoacidosis. Metabolic changes occur over many days to several weeks. Symptoms of polyuria, polydipsia, and increasing lethargy are almost always present but may not be appreciated. Failure to develop ketoacidosis and its clinical manifestations may allow the underlying process to go unrecognized until stupor or coma develops. Decreased responsiveness is the main reason patients receive medical attention.

Physical Findings

There are no specific physical findings. Virtually all are significantly dehydrated. Fever, hypotension, and tachycardia may be present. Shock is especially common if gram-negative pneumonia is present. Respirations are variable. Kussmaul's breathing is not a feature of uncomplicated nonketotic hyperosmolar coma, but hyperventilation may be present if the patient is acidotic for other reasons. Shallow respirations with hyperpnea and tachypnea are usual. The smell of acetone on the breath is absent.

The most prominent physical findings are neurologic (Table 134-2). Almost all patients exhibit some disturbance in mentation, ranging from inappropriate response to confusion, drowsiness, stupor, or coma. The higher the osmolality, the greater the obtundation. The average osmolality for a comatose patient with nonketotic hyperosmolar coma is 380 mOsm/kg. Depression of the sensorium does not correlate with the glucose concentration or with the pH of the plasma or cerebrospinal fluid.

The most common focal signs are hemisensory deficits or hemiparesis or both. Approximately 15 percent of the patients exhibit seizure activity, usually of the focal motor type (85 percent). Grand mal seizures can occur. Tremors, fasciculations, and a variety of other neurologic abnormalities including aphasia, hyperreflexia, flaccidity, depressed deep tendon reflexes, positive plantar response, and nuchal rigidity may be seen. In one series by Arieff and Carroll, 12 of 33 patients with nonketotic hyperosmolar coma were initially diagnosed as "probably acute stroke." This diagnosis was not confirmed in any of the patients.

Considering the age of the patient population and the frequency of neurologic findings, it is not surprising that the misdiagnosis of stroke or organic brain syndrome is common. Nonketotic hyperosmolar coma must be suspected in every elderly, dehydrated patient wih glucosuria or hyperglycemia, especially if they are mild diabetics and receiving diuretic drugs or glucocorticoids.

Laboratory

Confirmation of the diagnosis is with laboratory findings. The essential tests are blood glucose levels, calculated and measured serum osmolality, and serum ketone levels. A reasonable approximation of the blood glucose and serum ketone levels can be made promptly at the bedside by use of the nitroprusside test and glucose reagent strips. Additional tests should include a complete blood cell count and levels of electrolytes, blood urea nitrogen (BUN), creatinine, and arterial blood gases.

Serum electrolytes display a variable pattern. Serum sodium values usually range from 120 to 160 mEq/L, but because water is lost in excess of sodium through osmotic diuresis, the patient is almost always hypertonic. There is a sodium decrement of 1.6 mEq/L for every 100 mg/dL increase in blood glucose. Total body potassium depletion is usually severe. Potassium loss in nonketotic hyperosmolar coma is greater than that with diabetic ketoacidosis because of the longer duration of osmotic diuresis, GI loss, and prior diuretic use.

The BUN level is almost always elevated because of extracellular volume depletion and underlying renal disease. The initial BUN level is elevated out of proportion to the creatinine level. Ratios of BUN to creatinine may be 30:1. Prerenal azotemia resolves with volume replacement, but most patients have underlying chronic renal impairment.

Metabolic acidosis due to the accumulation of ketone bodies is not a feature of nonketotic hyperosmolar coma, but metabolic acidosis due to other causes can occur. In most series, 30 to 40 percent of the patients have a mild metabolic acidosis attributed to accumulation of lactic acid or due to uremia. However, in a significant number of these cases, no cause of the acidosis can be identified. Striking elevations of creatine phosphokinase (CPK) in patients with nonketotic hyperosmolar coma have been reported and are attributed to the complication of rhabdomyolysis. This condition as a complication of severe hyperosmolality has been reported.

Because of the frequency of underlying chronic disease and precipitating illnesses, a search for a precipitating cause must be made. Urinalysis, chest roentgenogram, ECG, and cultures of the blood, urine, and sputum should be performed. Because of the frequency of fever and neurologic signs, including nuchal rigidity, a CT scan and lumbar puncture may be necessary. Typical findings in the spinal fluid include a normal opening pressure, a markedly elevated glucose level (usually 50 percent of the serum value), a normal or slightly elevated protein level, and an osmolality identical to that of the serum.

Table 134-2. Neurologic Manifestations of Nonketotic Hyperosmolar Coma

Diffuse	*Focal*
Seizures	Focal seizures
Lethargy	Todd's paralysis
Confusion	Hemisensory loss
Delirium and hallucinations	Hemiparesis
Stupor	Babinski's reflex
Coma	Aphasia
	Hemianopsia
	Tonic eye deviation
	Nystagmus
	Hyperreflexia
	Choreoathetosis or ballism

Source: Grace TW: Hyperosmolar non-ketotic diabetic coma. *Am Fam Physician* 32:119, 1985.

TREATMENT

Attention to detail and constant monitoring are necessary. Serial measurements of glucose, electrolyte, and serum osmolality levels are essential. A flow sheet to record therapeutic measures and patient response is recommended. The specific goals of therapy of nonketotic hyperosmolar coma include correction of hypovolemia and dehydration, restoration of electrolyte balance, and reduction of serum glucose and hyperosmolality levels. Reasonable end points that can usually be achieved within 36 h are a blood glucose level of 250 mg/dL, a serum osmolality of 320 mOsm/kg, and a urine output of at least 50 mL/h.

Fluids

No agreement exists on the composition of the initial replacement fluid. Some authors advocate the use of isotonic saline (0.9% NaCl), and others recommend the use of half-normal saline (0.45% NaCl). Those who advocate isotonic saline believe that the most immediate threat to life is hypovolemic shock. Even though the patient has lost water in excess of solute and is hypertonic, normal saline is still hypotonic to the patient with nonketotic hyperosmolar coma. Normal saline corrects the extracellular volume deficit, stabilizes the blood pressure, and maintains adequate urinary flow. Once this has been achieved, hypotonic saline can be administered to provide free water for correction of intracellular volume deficits.

Those who recommend half-normal or hypotonic saline as initial fluid therapy argue that any osmotically active solute in the replacement fluid prolongs and enhances the hyperosmotic state. Further, since the patient has lost water in excess of solute, a hypotonic solution is the logical replacement.

All authors agree that if the patient is in hypovolemic shock, isotonic saline should be given until volume has been restored. Most agree that if the patient has significant hypernatremia (155 mEq/L) or hypertension, hypotonic saline should be the initial fluid of choice.

Rarely a patient has hyperglycemia, hyponatremia, and a low or normal osmolality. This indicates a significant excess of water, probably due to the ingestion of enormous quantities. The use of hypotonic saline in this setting can precipitate water intoxication.

There are no controlled studies that compare the advantages of isotonic solutions with those of hypotonic solutions in the initial management of nonketotic hyperosmolar coma. Regardless of the fluid used, there are guidelines to determine the rate and amount of fluid administration.

The average fluid deficit in nonketotic hyperosmolar coma is usually between 20 and 25 percent of total body water (TBW), or 8 to 12 L. In elderly subjects, it is assumed that 50 percent of the body weight is due to TBW. By using the patient's usual weight in kilograms, normal TBW and water deficit (20 to 25 percent of TBW) can be calculated. One-half of the estimated water deficit should be replaced during the first 12 h and the balance during the next 24 h. Ongoing insensible and urinary losses should also be replaced.

The fluid should be infused at a rate determined by the individual needs of the patient, but in general it should be given rapidly until the blood pressure is stable and the urine output is adequate. Fluid administration is subject to the usual considerations of renal and cardiovascular status.

Electrolytes

Electrolyte replacement is an essential part of therapy for nonketotic hyperosmolar coma. In the average patient, for every liter of body water lost, 70 mEq of monovalent ions is concomitantly lost. That translates into 300 to 800 mEq of sodium and potassium that usually needs to be replaced.

The sodium deficit is replenished by the administration of normal saline (154 mEq of sodium per liter) or half-normal saline (77 mEq of sodium per liter). Potassium replacement, as with diabetic ketoacidosis, should be started early in the course of treatment. Potassium supplement should be started within 2 h of the institution of fluid and insulin therapy or as soon as adequate renal function has been confirmed. Most authors recommend the infusion of KCl at a rate of 10 to 20 mEq/h during the acute phase of therapy (24 to 36 h). Potassium should be added to the initial intravenous fluid if the patient presents with hypokalemia. Magnesium levels should be obtained and replacement given if the level is low. Caution is necessary in the presence of renal dysfunction.

Insulin

Traditionally it has been taught that the insulin requirement of a patient with nonketotic hyperosmolar coma is less than that of a patient with diabetic ketoacidosis. The difference in insulin requirement was attributed to decreased insulin resistance in the patient with nonketotic hyperosmolar coma because of the absence of acidosis.

Changing concepts have led to a reappraisal of insulin therapy, and continuous intravenous infusion of low doses of insulin and intermittent intramuscular injections of low doses of insulin are effective therapy.

Five to ten units of regular insulin per hour should be given by continuous intravenous infusion or by intramuscular injection. If the intramuscular route is chosen, 20 units of regular insulin can initially be administered intramuscularly or by intravenous bolus. Often no additional insulin is required after the initial dose. No insulin should be given after the blood glucose level reaches approximately 300 mg/dL.

The reasons for not using large doses of insulin when treating nonketotic hyperosmolar coma are even more compelling than those stated for diabetic ketoacidosis. In addition to producing a more gradual reduction of the glucose concentration, thus avoiding hypoglycemia, hypokalemia, and cerebral edema, low-dose insulin techniques may help to avoid vascular collapse and renal shutdown in the patient with nonketotic hyperosmolar coma.

A high glucose concentration in the extracellular fluid compartment protects that compartment against hypovolemia at the expense of intracellular water. If the concentration of glucose is rapidly lowered by the administration of large doses of insulin, insufficient extracellular osmotic solute may result in a net intracellular shift of large volumes of water, producing hypovolemia and vascular collapse. Similarly, osmotic diuresis induced by hyperglycemia acts to protect the kidney against acute tubular necrosis (ATN) in the presence of reduced renal perfusion. If the blood glucose concentration is rapidly reduced, the osmotic diuresis decreases, and ATN may result. Acute tubular necrosis after institution of large-dose insulin therapy was reported in 5 of 30 patients in the series studied by Arieff and Carroll.

Glucose

Glucose should be added to the intravenous solution when the blood glucose level declines to 250 mg/dL. It is at this level that further rapid lowering of the blood glucose concentration may result in cerebral edema. Cerebral edema can be recognized clinically by the sudden onset of hyperpyrexia, hypotension, and deepening of coma in spite of biochemical improvement. Though cerebral edema during treatment of nonketotic hyperosmolar coma is rare, it is invariably fatal and can be prevented.

Additional Treatment

The role of phosphate replacement during treatment of nonketotic hyperosmolar coma is controversial. The plasma phosphorus level should be monitored during therapy, but a case for routine phosphate infusion has not been made convincingly.

Patients with nonketotic hyperosmolar coma are at risk for the development of arterial and venous thrombosis. Low-dose prophylactic heparin therapy should be considered.

Seizures are usually due to hyperosmolality and electrolyte abnormalities, but CNS mass lesions and meningitis or encephalitis should be considered. Unless the patient has an underlying seizure disorder or has status epilepticus, specific treatment for single seizures is not necessary. Phenytoin may precipitate nonketotic hyperosmolar coma and should be given with caution.

BIBLIOGRAPHY

Arieff AI, Carroll HJ: Cerebral edema and depression of sensorium in nonketotic hyperosmolar coma. *Diabetes* 23:525, 1974.

Arieff AI, Carroll HJ: Nonketotic hyperosmolar coma with hyperglycemia: Clinical features, pathophysiology, renal function, acid-base balance, plasma-cerebrospinal fluid equilibria and the effects of therapy in 37 cases. *Medicine* 51:73, 1972.

Beigelman PM: Severe diabetic ketoacidosis (diabetic "coma"): 482 episodes in 257 patients; Experience of three years. *Diabetes* 20:490, 1971.

Bendezu R, Wieland RH, Furst BH, et al: Experience with low-dose insulin infusion in diabetic ketoacidosis and diabetic hyperosmolarity. *Arch Intern Med* 138:60, 1978.

Feig Pu, McCurdy DK: The hypertonic state. *N Engl J Med* 297:1444, 1977.

Gerich JE, Martin MM, Recant L: Clinical and metabolic characteristics of hyperosmolar nonketotic coma. *Diabetes* 20:228, 1971.

Gordon EE, Kabadi UM: The hyperglycemic hyperosmolar syndrome. *Am J Med Sci* 271: 252, 1976.

Keller U, Berger W, Ritz R, et al: Course and prognosis of 86 episodes of diabetic coma: A five year experience with a uniform schedule of treatment. *Diabetologia* 11:93, 1975.

Podolsky S: Hyperosmolar nonketotic coma in the elderly diabetic. *Med Clin North Am* 62:815, 1978.

Sament S, Schwartz MB: Severe diabetic stupor without ketosis. *S Afr Med J* 31:893, 1957.

135
LACTIC ACIDOSIS

Gene Ragland

Lactic acidosis is the most common metabolic acidosis. It occurs in association with a wide variety of underlying processes and may represent a well-tolerated, physiologic event or a life-threatening, pathologic condition. Lactic acidosis is classified based upon oxygen supply to the tissues. Type A is that clearly associated with clinically evident hypoperfusion or hypoxia, and type B includes all other forms, those in which there is no evidence of tissue anoxia. Lactic acidosis is often diagnosed during the evaluation of an anion gap acidosis. Treatment is directed toward identification and correction of the underlying disorder and restitution of normal acid-base equilibrium.

PHYSIOLOGY

Lactate Homeostasis

Lactate is a metabolic product of anaerobic glycolysis and under normal conditions is in equilibrium with its immediate precursor, pyruvate. The basal production of lactate in a 70-kg person is approximately 1300 mEq/day, and the normal lactate concentration in extracellular fluid is about 1 mEq/L. The maintenance of lactate homeostasis is a complex, dynamic process involving interorgan balance between lactate production and utilization. Virtually all body tissues are capable of producing lactate, but skeletal muscle, erythrocytes, brain, skin, and intestinal mucosa are the most active. The utilization of lactate takes place in the liver and kidneys and to a lesser extent in the heart and skeletal muscle. Lactate is primarily disposed of in the liver and kidneys via gluconeogenesis, a process that requires the conversion of lactate back to pyruvate.

Lactate Production

Lactate is formed from pyruvate as an end product of anaerobic glycolysis. This oxidation-reduction reaction requires reduced nicotinamide adenine dinucleotide (NADH) and hydrogen ion (H^+) and is catalyzed by lactate dehydrogenase (LDH). This reaction is expressed by the equation

$$\text{Pyruvate} + \text{NADH} + \text{H}^+ \overset{\text{LDH}}{\rightleftharpoons} \text{Lactate} + \text{NAD}$$

The equilibrium of this reaction strongly favors the formation of lactate. The normal ratio of lactate to pyruvate is 10:1. Lactate is a metabolic blind end; it cannot be utilized in any other intracellular reactions and must be converted back to pyruvate for gluconeogenesis or oxidation to CO_2 and H_2O via the Krebs cycle. The result of this biochemical reaction is to produce energy in the form of adenosine triphosphate (ATP) and to oxidize NADH to NAD. A small amount of lactic acid is produced even at rest and under aerobic conditions. In the presence of oxygen and essential cofactors, lactate is converted back to pyruvate; it does not accumulate and maintains equilibrium with pyruvate.

A variety of factors may alter this normal process. The concentration of lactate in the cytosol depends primarily upon the concentration of pyruvate, the intracellular redox state (NADH/NAD), and the intracellular pH. The net effect of these multiple factors determines the intracellular concentration of lactate.

Pyruvate

Since lactate can be eliminated only by conversion back to pyruvate, lactate concentration is intimately interrelated to the fate of pyruvate. Pyruvate is a key intermediary at the junction of several important pathways. The major sources of pyruvate are glycolysis, in which pyruvate is formed from the oxidation of glucose, and transamination, a process by which pyruvate can be derived from amino acids, especially alanine. Pyruvate may be utilized via gluconeogenesis in which pyruvate is a substrate in the formation of glucose, and mitochondrial oxidation, in which pyruvate enters the mitochondria for oxidation to CO_2 and H_2O. A variety of factors may alter these normal pathways. For example, rapid glycolysis can be induced by alkalosis, protein catabolic states may increase transamination, metabolic poisons may impair mitochondrial function, or key enzymes and cofactors may be inactivated or unavailable. The concentration of pyruvate, and thus the concentration of lactate, depends upon the net production and consumption of pyruvate by these various routes.

Redox State

The intracellular redox state is a critical factor in determining the concentration of lactate. The availability of oxygen at the tissue level is an important determinant of the cellular redox. During prolonged anaerobic conditions, lactate cannot be reoxidized back to pyruvate because of a lack of NAD. Normally, NADH can be reoxidized to NAD within the mitochondria via the electron transport chain coupled with oxidative phosphorylation. Electron transport abruptly ceases during anoxia. NAD is not available for lactate conversion, and lactate accumulates. This mechanism is thought to be operative during type A lactic acidosis. Other factors may alter the cellular redox, and consequently, alterations in the NADH/NAD ratio do not solely reflect tissue oxygenation.

Intracellular pH

A third major determinant of lactate concentration within the cytosol is the intracellular hydrogen ion concentration. Changes in the intracellular pH affect enzymatic reactions, lactate transport, and the lactate/pyruvate ratio. Some of these effects may counterbalance each other. In general, a fall in pH causes decreased lactate production, whereas an increase in pH causes increased lactate concentration. One important aspect of a change in intracellular pH is its effect on the liver. As the pH declines, lactate uptake by the liver decreases. Additionally, when the pH is 7.0 or less, the liver becomes an organ of lactate production instead of lactate clearance.

Lactate Utilization

The liver and kidneys are the major organs that consume lactate. Gluconeogenesis is the main pathway utilized by these organs in lactate removal. This process utilizes the hydrogen ions produced during the formation of lactic acid and this acts to maintain acid-base balance. The liver normally clears more than half the total daily lactate load, and the kidneys remove approximately 30 percent. Some researchers believe that the kidneys have a negligible role in lactate clearance and that other extrahepatic sites are more important. Of the approximately 1300 mEq of lactate produced each day, 60 to 70 mEq of lactate is extracted by the liver every 2 h. The hydrogen ion that is consumed by the liver during this period is roughly equivalent to the total amount of hydrogen ion excreted daily by the kidneys. By virtue of the liver's ability to clear lactate, the role of the liver in the maintenance of the overall acid-base balance is very important. In addition, the liver has a large reserve capacity to extract lactate; this has been estimated to be as high as 3400 to 4000 mEq/day. Obviously, any situation which converts the liver from a lactate-consuming to a lactate-producing organ results in serious acid-base disturbance. Lactic acid clearance by the liver may be reduced with decreased hepatic blood flow or parenchymal hypoxia.

The kidneys carry out their role in lactate clearance primarily through gluconeogenesis, not excretion. The renal threshold for lactate is about

7 to 10 mEq/L, so the amount of lactate excreted by the kidneys at normal plasma levels is negligible. The kidneys may also dispose of lactate through oxidation, but this is not the preferred pathway. At a pH of less than 7.1, lactate uptake by the kidneys may be decreased, and at a pH of 7.0 or below, the kidneys—like the liver—may produce lactic acid.

Skeletal and cardiac muscle is capable of extracting some lactate from the circulation. The relative role of these sites of lactate clearance is not clear. Lactate utilization by skeletal muscle may depend on the concentration of lactate and whether the muscle is active or at rest.

Lactic Acidosis

Lactic acidosis can be thought of as an imbalance between the rate of production of lactate by tissues active in glycolysis and the rate of utilization by tissues active in gluconeogenesis. Disagreement exists over whether the primary mechanism responsible for lactic acidosis is overproduction or underutilization.

Lactic acid is a strong organic acid that is almost completely dissociated at physiologic pH. The ratio of lactate ion to undissociated lactic acid at a pH of 7.4 is more than 3000 : 1. For each milliequivalent of lactic acid produced, equal amounts of hydrogen ion and lactate are liberated. Hydrogen ions are initially buffered by bicarbonate and other buffers and then consumed during the utilization of lactate via gluconeogenesis or oxidation. Acid-base balance is therefore maintained. Under circumstances of increased lactic acid production and/or decreased lactic acid utilization, body buffers are saturated by the excess hydrogen ions. When this is of sufficient magnitude, acidosis results. Whether the resultant lactic acidosis is clinically significant depends upon the underlying process responsible for the lactic acid accumulation and the preexistent acid-base status.

Diagnosis

Lactic acidosis is a metabolic acidosis caused by the accumulation of lactate and hydrogen ion. It is accompanied by an elevated blood lactate concentration, but there is no consensus on what level of lactate defines lactic acidosis. The normal plasma lactate level is 0.5 to 1.5 mEq/L. In general, a lactate concentration of 5 to 6 mEq/L is considered indicative of significant acid-base disturbance. Some authors have included demonstration of a reduced arterial pH, ≤ 7.35, as a criterion for diagnosis. However, if there is a coexistent alkalosis, the pH could be normal or even alkalemic in the face of significant lactic acidosis.

The presence of hyperlactemia per se does not mean that the patient has clinically significant lactic acidosis. Many situations encountered clinically may result in elevation of blood lactate levels but not produce significant clinical consequences. Exercise; hyperventilation; infusions of glucose, saline, or bicarbonate; and injections of insulin or epinephrine may all cause elevation of lactate levels without clinical manifestations. Plasma lactate concentrations after vigorous exercise or maximum work have been reported to reach 14 to 30 mEq/L. In patients with grand mal seizures, levels of 12.7 mEq/L have been recorded. In spite of these high levels, the lactate production is self-limited, and the lactate is rapidly cleared from the circulation without untoward consequences. Persistent elevation of lactate levels may occur with chronic disorders such as severe congestive heart failure, pulmonary disease, liver disease, and diabetes mellitus. These levels are generally well-tolerated. To identify the patient in whom an increased lactate level is significant, the physician must assess the clinical state and correlate it with the extent to which increased lactate and hydrogen ion levels contribute to clinical abnormalities.

A presumptive diagnosis of lactic acidosis can be made in many instances. This diagnosis is based upon the recognition of an anion gap acidosis in a patient with a clinical disorder in which lactic acidosis is known to occur. For this impression to be confirmed, other causes of an increased anion gap metabolic acidosis must be excluded, and the plasma lactate concentration must be shown to be elevated.

Anion Gap Acidosis

The anion gap is generally determined by subtracting the concentration of chloride plus bicarbonate ions from the concentration of sodium ion: $Na^+ - (Cl^- + HCO_3^-)$. The normal value is 12 mEq/L ± 4. Any value greater than 16 mEq/L suggests the presence of an "unmeasured ion," usually an accumulation of organic anions. Most patients with lactic acidosis have an anion gap that averages 25 to 30 mEq/L. The major causes of anion gap acidosis in addition to lactic acidosis include diabetic ketoacidosis, uremic acidosis, alcoholic ketoacidosis, and ingestion of the toxins salicylate, methanol, ethylene glycol, paraldehyde, or cyanide (Table 135-1). Laboratory determinations of the levels of arterial blood gases, electrolytes, glucose, blood urea nitrogen, creatinine, and lactate, and liver function studies and appropriate drug screens, should help establish the correct cause of acidosis.

Particular caution should be used with diabetic and alcoholic patients to ensure that the unmeasured anion is correctly identified. The major organic anion in diabetic and alcoholic ketoacidosis is β-hydroxybutyrate, which is not measured by the serum nitroprusside test. Lactic acidosis and ketoacidosis may occur simultaneously. If lactate levels do not account for the entire increase in the anion gap, ketoacidosis should be suspected, even with a negative acetone test. The bicarbonate level may provide additional help with this differential point. In uncomplicated diabetic ketoacidosis, the increase in the anion gap is identical to the decrease in the bicarbonate concentration, whereas in lactic acidosis, the increase in the anion gap is usually greater than the decrease in the bicarbonate concentration.

Clinical Presentation

The clinical findings in lactic acidosis are nonspecific. The onset may be abrupt, often occurring over several hours. Generally the patient appears ill. Hyperventilation or Kussmaul's respiration is the most constant feature. The level of consciousness may vary from lethargy to coma. Vomiting and abdominal pain sometimes occur. Hypotension and evidence of hypoxia occur with type A lactic acidosis but not with type B.

Laboratory abnormalities that occur during lactic acidosis include elevated lactate levels, increased anion gap, hyperkalemia, decreased biocarbonate levels, and decreased pH unless altered by compensatory alkalosis. Serum potassium concentrations are most likely to be elevated in those patients with underlying renal insufficiency or tissue destruction. Marked hyperphosphatemia and hyperuricemia may be seen. The white blood cell count is usually elevated and may reach leukemoid proportions. Hypoglycemia has also been reported, especially in conjunction with liver disease.

Classification of Lactic Acidosis

Lactic acidosis is classified on clinical grounds and occurs in two principal clinical settings. According to Cohen and Woods' classification, type A lactic acidosis occurs with clinically evident tissue anoxia, such as during shock or severe hypoxia. Type B lactic acidosis includes all other forms, those in which there is no evidence of tissue anoxia (Table 135-2). Spontaneous or idiopathic lactic acidosis has been described but is now felt to be nonexistent. Recognition of an increasing array of disorders in which lactic acidosis can occur without evident tissue anoxia has virtually eliminated this category. A new

Table 135-1. Causes of Increased Anion Gap Metabolic Acidosis

Increased endogenous organic acids:	Ingestion of toxins:
Diabetic ketoacidosis	Salicylates
Alcoholic ketoacidosis	Methanol
Lactic acidosis	Ethylene glycol
Decreased excretion of organic and inorganic acids:	Paraldehyde
Renal failure (uremia)	Cyanide

Table 135-2. Classification of Lactic Acidosis

Type A:
- Clinically evident tissue anoxia (e.g., shock, hypoxia)

Type B:
1. Various common disorders:
   - Diabetes mellitus
   - Renal failure
   - Liver disease
   - Infection
   - Leukemia and certain other malignant conditions
   - Convulsions
2. Drugs, toxins:
   - Biguanides (phenformin)
   - Ethanol
   - Fructose and other saccharides
   - Methanol
   - Various other drugs
3. Hereditary forms:
   - Type I glycogen storage disease
   - Fructose-biphosphatase deficiency
   - Subacute necrotizing encephalomyelopathy (Leigh's syndrome)
   - Methylmalonic aciduria
   - Others

Source: Adapted from Cohen RD, Woods HF: *Clinical and Biochemical Aspects of Lactic Acidosis*. Oxford, Blackwell, 1976.

metabolic disorder, D-lactic acidosis, has been described. It occurs in patients with anatomically or functionally shortened small bowel. Bacterial fermentation produces D-lactic acid, which can be absorbed and cause an increased anion gap acidosis and stupor or coma. The plasma levels of L-lactate are normal. Treatment with neomycin or vancomycin results in correction of the metabolic abnormalities.

Type A Lactic Acidosis

This is the most common form of lactic acidosis seen in the emergency department and is most often due to shock. Hemorrhagic, hypovolemic, cardiogenic, or septic shock have been shown to cause lactic acidosis. The pathogenesis of lactic acidosis during shock is inadequate tissue perfusion with subsequent anoxia and lactate and hydrogen ion accumulation. Clearance of lactate by the liver is reduced because of decreased splanchnic and hepatic artery perfusion, and hepatocellular ischemia. At a pH of around 7.0 or less, the liver and kidneys may become organs of lactate production.

The association between shock and lactic acidosis is so common that a presumptive diagnosis can be made in a critically ill patient in shock who suddenly develops severe hyperventilation and an increased anion gap acidosis. Treatment should be directed toward correction of the cause of shock. In general, the higher the lactate level, the higher the mortality.

Hypoxia may also cause type A lactic acidosis. The hypoxia must be acute and severe. Adaptations such as polycythemia, diminished hemoglobin affinity for oxygen, and increased tissue extraction of oxygen protect patients with chronic, stable lung disease from developing lactic acidosis.

These patients may not develop significant lactic acidosis until an arterial P_{O_2} of 30 to 35 mmHg is reached. In patients with a diminished ability to compensate for a respiratory insult, lactic acidosis may arise at considerably higher arterial oxygen tensions. Acute asphyxiation, pulmonary edema, status asthmaticus, acute exacerbation of chronic obstructive pulmonary disease, and displacement of oxygen by carboxyhemoglobin, sulfhemoglobin, or methemoglobin have been associated with lactic acidosis.

Type B Lactic Acidosis

Type B lactic acidosis includes all forms in which there is no clinical evidence of tissue anoxia. This form may occur abruptly, over a few hours. The diagnosis may be missed or delayed because of no clear antecedent event, or because of lack of familiarity with the disorders associated with type B lactic acidosis. The mechanisms by which these disorders predispose to lactic acidosis are not well understood. By definition, the cardiovascular function is not impaired and the blood pressure is not decreased. Subclinical, regional underperfusion of tissue has been suggested as a possible cause. In many cases of severe type B lactic acidosis, circulatory insufficiency may occur after a few hours, making this condition clinically indistinguishable from type A lactic acidosis. Type B lactic acidosis is divided into three subgroups.

Type B_1

Type B_1 lactic acidosis comprises those cases that occur in association with other medical disorders such as diabetes, renal and hepatic disease, infection, neoplasia, and convulsions. There is no clear causal relation between diabetes and lactic acidosis, but the association between them has been noted by many authors. Massive hepatic necrosis and cirrhosis are associated with lactic acidosis. Decreased lactate clearance by the liver because of insufficient liver tissue for gluconeogenesis may be the cause. Acute and chronic renal insufficiency is commonly associated with lactic acidosis but is probably not a cause in its own right. Some patients with severe infections, especially bacteremia, develop lactic acidosis for unknown reasons. Myeloproliferative disorders such as leukemia, multiple myeloma, generalized lymphoma, and Hodgkin's disease are associated with lactic acidosis. Grand mal seizures may result in lactic acidosis because of muscular hyperactivity and probably hypoxia. Lactic acidosis in Reye's syndrome has been reported. A close correspondence between the stage of coma and lactate levels has been noted.

Type B_2

This subgroup includes cases of lactic acidosis due to drugs, chemicals, and toxins. This category was formerly dominated by the oral hypoglycemic agent phenformin, which has been withdrawn from U.S. markets. Ethanol is currently the most common drug associated with lactic acidosis. During the oxidation of alcohol, NADH levels increase, causing utilization of the pyruvate-lactate pathway for the reoxidation of NADH. This reaction produces a moderate increase in the lactate level. In the presence of other causes of lactic acidosis, ethanol ingestion may cause increased acidosis. Other drugs associated with lactic acidosis include fructose; sorbitol; excess amounts of epinephrine and other catecholamines; methanol; and possibly salicylates. Many other drugs have also been implicated as causally related to lactic acidosis.

Type B_3

This form of lactic acidosis is rare and is due to inborn errors of metabolism such as type I glycogen storage disease (glucose-6 phosphatase deficiency) and hepatic fructose-biphosphatase deficiency. These congential lactic acidoses include defects in gluconeogenesis, the pyruvate dehydrogenase complex, the krebs cycle, and cellular respiratory mechanisms.

Treatment

The basic therapeutic goals in treatment of lactic acidosis are to identify and correct the underlying cause of the lactic acid accumulation and to counteract the deleterious effects of the acidosis.

The specifics of therapy depend upon the cause. Shock and hypoxia must be corrected as soon as possible. Adequate ventilation is imperative. Restoration of blood pressure, cardiac output, and tissue perfusion with well-oxygenated blood is essential. Volume replacement with fluids, plasma expanders, or blood, as indicated, should be instituted. Vasopressors should probably be avoided as they may decrease tissue perfusion and worsen the acidosis. Low cardiac output states should be treated with inotropic compounds along with afterload-reducing agents. Catecholamines are glycogenolytic and may enhance lactic acid production. In type B lactic acidosis, the underlying disorder may not be readily identifiable or amenable to therapy. Drugs known to be associated with lactic acidosis should be discontinued, and infection must be aggressively treated.

Sodium bicarbonate

Treatment of acidosis with intravenous sodium bicarbonate ($NaHCO_3$) has been a mainstay of therapy for lactic acidosis. The purpose of this therapy is to reverse the untoward effects of acidosis and allow time for other therapeutic modalities to correct the cause of the acidosis. If the cause of lactic acidosis can be quickly corrected, such as with respiratory failure or pulmonary edema, alkali therapy may not be needed. The undesirable effects of acidosis include depression of myocardal contractility and decreased cardiac output at a pH below 7.1. Arteriolar dilatation and hypotension may occur when the blood pH falls below 7.0. Additionally, a pH below 7.0 impairs hepatic utilization of lactate and may induce production of lactate by the liver and kidneys. These effects may be the cause of the cardiovascular collapse that occurs during the course of type B lactic acidosis.

Several authors have suggested that alkali administration may not only lack benefit but actually be deleterious in the treatment of lactic acidosis. This position is based upon experimental animal studies and the reevaluation of the use of sodium bicarbonate in the treatment of such conditions as diabetic ketoacidosis and cardiopulmonary arrest. This question will most likely remain unresolved for some time. Until an efficacious alternative is identified, sodium bicarbonate will continue to be used in conjunction with cause-specific measures.

In general, sodium bicarbonate should be given when the pH is 7.1 or less. The smallest possible amount of bicarbonate that will return the systemic pH to hemodynamically safe levels (e.g., pH of 7.2) should be used. Frequent monitoring of the acid-base status during bicarbonate therapy is essential for appraisal of additional bicarbonate requirements. Some undesirable effects of sodium biacarbonate include fluid and sodium overload, hyperosmolarity, alkaline overshoot which could increase lactate production, displacement of the oxyhemoglobin dissociation curve to the left, and paradoxical cerebrospinal fluid acidosis.

The approximate dose of bicarbonate required to correct the acidosis can be calculated from the following formula:

$$HCO_3 \text{ deficit} = (25 \text{ mEq/L } HCO_3 - \text{measured } HCO_3) \times 0.5(\text{body weight in kg})$$

This equation is based upon the assumption that bicarbonate distributes in a space equal to 50 percent of the body weight in kilograms. The apparent space of distribution for bicarbonate is enlarged in hypobicarbonatemic states; thus, using 50 percent body weight to calculate the space for distribution of bicarbonate may underestimate the bicarbonate requirements.

Some patients may require massive amounts of sodium bicarbonate to correct acidemia. Those unable to tolerate fluid and sodium overload can be treated with a bicarbonate infusion, potent loop diuretic, or tris(hydroxymethyl)aminomethane (THAM). Hyperosmolarity can be reduced by adding 3 to 4 ampoules of $NaHCO_3$ (44 mEq/L) to 1 L of 5% dextrose and water. This solution provides 132 to 176 mEq/L, respectively. Use of a potent loop diuretic creates intravascular space for fluid and sodium. A diuretic should be given in whatever dose is required to maintain a brisk diuresis (300 to 500 mL/h). Urinary sodium and potassium losses can be measured and replaced along with the urinary volume loss on an equal basis.

Oliguric patients require hemodialysis to permit administration of large amounts of sodium bicarbonate. Standard dialysis baths can be replaced by a bicarbonate bath so that the fluid and sodium chloride removed by the hypertonic solution can be replaced as the bicarbonate salt. Hemodialysis and peritoneal dialysis remove lactate. As there is no evidence that lactate ion per se is harmful, this approach is unnecessary. Removal of lactate, however, can minimize the rebound alkalosis that often occurs after correction of the acidosis.

There is often a delay of many hours between the return of the pH to the normal range and a fall in the blood lactate level. The bicarbonate infusion can be decreased after several hours of a normal pH. If the pH begins to drop, the bicarbonate infusion can be increased. When the pH stabilizes in an acceptable range, the infusion can be discontinued. As always, the clinical status of the patient is the best parameter to follow during recovery.

Additional Treatment

A variety of other therapies have been advocated in treatment of lactic acidosis. These include insulin, glucose, thiamine, methylene blue, vasodilator drugs such as sodium nitroprusside, carbicarb, and the experimental drug dichloroacetate. Most authors do not favor the use of insulin, or insulin in conjunction with glucose, in treatment of lactic acidosis. Insulin may be indicated in a diabetic patient with concomitant lactic acidosis or in a diabetic with an unexplained increased anion gap acidosis. Insulin therapy in these instances should be based upon individual need. Glucose infusion in the setting of hypoglycemia and lactic acidosis has been reported to correct the lactic acidosis.

Thiamine is a necessary cofactor for the enzyme that catalyzes the first step in the oxidation of pyruvate. This vitamin should be given to alcoholic patients with lactic acidosis, but a role for thiamine therapy in other patients has not been established. Methylene blue is a redox dye that is capable of accepting H^+ and thereby oxidizing $NADH_2$ to NAD^+ and theoretically limiting the conversion of pyruvate to lactate. Clinical trials have not supported the benefit of this drug. Vasodilator therapy is based upon the premise that tissue perfusion improves with reduced peripheral vascular resistance and increased cardiac output. The value of vasodilator agents in treatment of lactic acidosis remains to be proved.

Carbicarb is an equimolar solution of sodium bicarbonate and sodium carbonate. This mixture buffers hydrogen ion without the net generation of CO_2. Carbicarb also consumes excess CO_2 to yield more bicarbonate buffer. The deleterious effect of an increase in tissue P_{CO_2} is avoided. Experimentation with carbicarb is ongoing and no clear clinical benefit has been demonstrated.

Dichloroacetate (DCA) is an experimental drug that increases the activity of pyruvate dehydrogenase, and this promotes the oxidation of glucose, pyruvate, and lactate and thus reduces blood lactate levels. Since oxygen is required for this metabolic process, DCA has no role in treatment of type A lactic acidosis. Its role in therapy for type B lactic acidosis may be limited by the increased ketosis and neurologic complications that occur with its use.

The fact that so many experimental therapies have been tried in lactic acidosis reflects the poor outcome of this disorder with the use of current treatment. The mortality of patients with type A lactic acidosis is approximately 80 percent; with type B it is 50 to 80 percent. Earlier recognition and correction of the underlying disorder responsible for the lactic acidosis is the best hope for reduction of this high mortality.

BIBLIOGRAPHY

Cohen RD, Woods, HF: *Clinical and Biochemical Aspects of Lactic Acidosis*, Boston, Blackwell Scientific Publications, Inc, 1976.

Harken AH: Lactic acidosis. *Surg Gynecol Obstet* 142:593, 1976.

Huckabee WE: Abnormal resting blood lactate. II. Lactic acidosis. *Am J Med* 30:840, 1961.

Kreisberg RA: Pathogenesis and management of lactic acidosis. *Annu Rev Med* 35:181, 1984.

Mizock BA: Lactic acidosis. *Dis Mon* 35:233, 1989.

Narins RG, Cohen JJ: Bicarbonate therapy for organic acidosis: The case for its continued use. *Ann Intern Med* 106:615, 1987.

Oh MS, Phelps KR, Traube M, et al: D-lactic acidosis in a man with the short-bowel syndrome. *N Engl J Med* 301:249, 1979.

Oliva PB: Lactic acidosis. *Am J Med* 48:209, 1970.

Park R, Arieff AI: Lactic acidosis: Current concepts. *Clin Endocrinol Metab* 12:339, 1983.

Stacpoole PW, Lorenz AC, Thomas RG: Dichloroacetate in the treatment of lactic acidosis. *Ann Intern Med* 108:58, 1988.

136
THYROID STORM
Gene Ragland

Thyroid storm is a rare complication of hyperthyroidism in which the manifestations of thyrotoxicosis are exaggerated to life-threatening proportions. Thyroid storm is most often seen in a patient with moderate to severe antecedent Graves' disease and is usually precipitated by a stressful event. It must be suspected and treated based upon a clinical impression, as there are no pathognomonic findings or confirmatory tests.

Hyperthyroid patients who are undiagnosed or undertreated are at risk for this complication. The duration of uncomplicated thyrotoxicosis preceding the onset of storm varies from months to years. A majority of the patients have had symptoms of hyperthyroidism for fewer than 24 months. It is not possible to predict accurately which thyrotoxic patient will develop storm as there is no predisposition by age, sex, or race.

PRECIPITATING FACTORS

A wide variety of factors have been reported as precipitating events. Thyroid surgery for treatment of hyperthyroidism used to be the most common cause of storm. Medically identified causes of thyroid storm are numerous and now predominate over surgical ones. Infection, especially pulmonary infection, is the most common precipitating event. In diabetic patients, ketoacidosis, hyperosmolar coma, and insulin-induced hypoglycemia have provoked storm. Events known to increase the levels of circulating thyroid hormones and initiate storm in susceptible persons, include premature withdrawal of antithyroid drugs, administration of radioactive iodide, use of an iodinated contrast medium during x-ray study, thyroid hormone overdose, administration of a saturated solution of potassium iodide to patients with nontoxic goiters, and vigorous palpation of the thyroid gland in thyrotoxic patients. Additional events implicated as causes of storm include vascular accidents, pulmonary emboli, toxemia of pregnancy, and emotional stress. Finally, hospitalization may lead to storm because of the rigors of diagnostic procedures.

PATHOGENESIS

The exact pathogenesis of thyroid storm has not been defined. It is attractive to attribute storm to excess thyroid hormone production or secretion. The results of thyroid function studies are elevated in the vast majority of patients during storm, but the values are not significantly different from those found in uncomplicated thyrotoxicosis. An increase in free triiodothyronine (T_3) or free thyroxine (T_4) levels has been suggested as causative of storm. But storm has occurred in the absence of elevated free T_3 or T_4 levels. Something in addition to excess amounts or forms of thyroid hormones must occur during storm.

Adrenergic hyperreactivity due to either patient sensitization by thyroid hormones or altered interaction between thyroid hormones and catecholamines has been suggested. Plasma levels of epinephrine and norepinephrine are not increased during thyroid storm. The exact role of catecholamines in storm awaits further study.

Altered peripheral response to thyroid hormone, causing increased lipolysis and overproduction of heat, is another theory. This theory maintains that excessive lipolysis due to catecholamine-thyroid hormone interaction results in excessive thermal energy and fever. Finally, exhaustion of the body's tolerance to the action of thyroid hormones, leading to "decompensated thyrotoxicosis," is a long-standing viewpoint. This implies an altered response to thyroid hormones rather than a sudden increase in their concentration.

CLINICAL PRESENTATION

Thyroid storm is a clinical diagnosis as there are no laboratory studies that distinguish it from thyrotoxicosis. Although the clinical presentation is extremely variable, there are clues to diagnosis. A history of hyperthyroidism, eye signs of Graves' disease, widened pulse pressure, and a palpable goiter are present in most patients who develop thyroid storm. However, the history may be unobtainable and the usual features of Graves' disease absent, including no obvious goiter in up to 9 percent of patients with Graves' disease.

Diagnostic Criteria

The generally accepted diagnostic criteria for thyroid storm are a temperature higher than 37.8°C (100°F); marked tachycardia out of proportion to the fever; dysfunction of the CNS, cardiovascular system or gastrointestinal (GI) system; and exaggerated peripheral manifestations of thyrotoxicosis.

The signs and symptoms of storm usually occur suddenly, but there may be a prodromal period with subtle increases in the manifestations of thyrotoxicosis.

Signs and Symptoms

The earliest signs are fever, tachycardia, diaphoresis, increased CNS activity, and emotional lability. If the condition is untreated, a hyperkinetic toxic state ensues in which the symptoms are intensified. Progression to congestive heart failure, refractory pulmonary edema, circulatory collapse, coma, and death may occur within 72 h.

Fever ranges from 38°C (100.4°F) to 41°C (105.8°F). The pulse rate may range between 120 and 200 beats per minute but has been reported as high as 300 beats per minute. Sweating may be profuse, leading to dehydration from insensible fluid loss.

Central nervous system disturbance occurs in 90 percent of patients with thyroid storm. Symptoms vary from restlessness, anxiety, and emotional lability, manic behavior, agitation, and psychosis, to mental confusion, obtundation, and coma. Extreme muscle weakness can occur. Thyrotoxic myopathy can occur and usually involves the proximal muscles. In severe forms, muscles of the more distal extremities and muscles of the trunk and face may be involved. About 1 percent of patients with Graves' disease develop myasthenia gravis, producing an occasional confusing clinical situation. The response of thyrotoxic myopathy to edrophonium (Tensilon test) is incomplete, unlike the complete response that occurs with myasthenia gravis. Hypokalemic periodic paralysis may also occur in patients with thyrotoxicosis.

Cardiovascular abnormalities are present in 50 percent of the patients regardless of underlying heart disease. Sinus tachycardia is usual. Arrhythmias, especially atrial fibrillation, but also including premature ventricular contractions and, rarely, complete heart block, may be present. In addition to increased heart rate, there is increased stroke volume, cardiac output, and myocardial oxygen consumption. Pulse pressure is characteristically widened. Congestive heart failure, pulmonary edema, and circulatory collapse may be terminal events.

Gastrointestinal symptoms develop in most patients in storm. Before the onset of storm, a history of severe weight loss is usual. Diarrhea and hyperdefecation seem to herald impending storm and can be severe, contributing to dehydration. During storm, anorexia, nausea, vomiting, and crampy abdominal pain may occur. Jaundice and tender hepatomegaly due to passive congestion of the liver, or even hepatic necrosis, have been reported. Jaundice is a poor prognostic sign.

LABORATORY

There are no laboratory tests that confirm thyroid storm. Serum levels of T_3 and T_4 are usually elevated but do not distinguish uncomplicated hyperthyroidism from thyroid storm. Radioactive iodine (RAI) uptake during storm is frequently quite high but on occasion can be below the mean range found in patients with uncomplicated thyrotoxicosis.

A rapid 1- to 2-h RAI uptake study, after β-blocking agents have been started but before treatment with antithyroid drugs and iodides, has been recommended. This test should not be performed in an acutely ill patient as it delays therapy. Others have recommended a 15-min dynamic flow study of the thyroid using ^{99m}Tc-pertechnetate. Although this test may demonstrate a hyperactive thyroid gland, it cannot resolve whether storm is present or not.

Routine laboratory data during thyroid storm show wide variation. Nonspecific abnormalities in the complete blood cell count, electrolyte levels, and liver function studies may be found. Bacterial infection may be reflected only by a leftward shift in the differential white count without elevation in the total white cell count. Hyperglycemia (>120 mg/dL) is common, and hypercalcemia is occasionally present. One series reported all patients to have low cholesterol levels with a mean value of 117 mg/dL. Plasma cortisol levels have been observed to be inappropriately low for the degree of stress, suggesting a lack of adrenal reserve.

APATHETIC THYROTOXICOSIS

Apathetic thyrotoxicosis is a rare, distinct form that usually occurs in the elderly and is frequently misdiagnosed. These patients may develop thyroid storm without the usual hyperkinetic manifestations and may quietly lapse into coma and die. There are some salient clinical characteristics which are helpful in establishing this diagnosis. The patient is generally in the seventh decade or older, with lethargy, slowed mentation, and placid apathetic facies. Goiter is usually present but may be small and multinodular. The usual eye signs of exophthalmos, stare, and lid lag are absent, but blepharoptosis (drooping upper eye lid) is common. Excessive weight loss and proximal muscle weakness are usual. These patients generally have had symptoms longer than nonapathetic thyrotoxic patients.

"Masked" thyrotoxicosis occurs when signs and symptoms referable to dysfunction of one organ system dominate and obscure the underlying thyrotoxicosis. Signs and symptoms referable to the cardiovascular system tend to mask thyrotoxicosis in apathetic patients. These patients frequently present with atrial fibrillation and congestive heart failure. In one series of nine patients, the diagnosis of hyperthyroidism was unsuspected in each case because of the predominance of cardiovascular symptoms. Congestive heart failure in this setting may be refractory to the usual therapy unless the underlying hyperthyroidism is diagnosed and treated.

The pathogenesis of an apathetic response to thyrotoxicosis is not understood. Age alone is not the determining factor, as apathetic thyrotoxicosis has been described in the pediatric age group. A high index of suspicion must be maintained for this diagnosis.

TREATMENT

The importance of early treatment of thyroid storm based upon the clinical impression cannot be overemphasized. Before the therapy is begun, blood should be drawn for free T_4 index or free T_4 assay and free T_3 and cortisol levels, a complete blood cell count, and routine chemistries. Appropriate cultures in search of infection are indicated.

Specific therapeutic goals can be divided into five areas; general supportive care, inhibition of thyroid hormone synthesis, retardation of thyroid hormone release, blockade of peripheral thyroid hormone effects, and identification and treatment of precipitating events. Each of these goals must be pursued concurrently.

General Supportive Care

Adequate hydration with intravenous fluids and electrolytes to replace insensible and GI losses is indicated. Supplemental oxygen is needed because of increased oxygen consumption. Hyperglycemia and hypercalcemia usually improve with fluid administration but occasionally require specific therapy. Fever should be controlled through the use of antipyretics and a cooling blanket. Aspirin should be used with caution or not at all during storm because salicylates increase free T_3 and T_4 levels because of decreased protein binding. This objection to the use of aspirin is theoretical, as no untoward clinical effect from aspirin use has been demonstrated. Caution should also be exercised in the use of sedatives during thyroid storm. Sedation depresses the level of consciousness and reduces the value of this parameter as an indicator of clinical improvement. Sedation may also cause hypoventilation.

Congestive heart failure should be treated with digitalis and diuretics even though congestive failure due to hyperthyroidism may be refractory to digitalis. Cardiac arrthythmias are treated with the usual antiarrhythmic agents. Atropine should be avoided, as its parasympatholytic effect may accelerate the heart rate. Atropine also may counteract the effect of propranolol.

Intravenous glucocorticoids equivalent to 300 mg of hydrocortisone per day should be given. The role of the adrenal glands in the pathogenesis of thyroid storm is uncertain, but the use of hydrocortisone has been reported to increase the rate of survival. Dexamethasone offers an advantage over other glucocorticoids as it decreases the peripheral conversion of T_4 to T_3.

Inhibition of Thyroid Hormone Synthesis

The antithyroid drugs propylthiouracil (PTU) and methimazole act to block the synthesis of thyroid hormone by inhibiting the organification of tyrosine residues. This action begins within 1 h after administration, but a full therapeutic effect is not achieved for weeks. An initial loading dose of PTU, 900 to 1200 mg, should be given, followed by 300 to 600 mg daily for 3 to 6 weeks or until the thyrotoxicosis comes under control. Methimazole, 90 to 120 mg initially followed by 30 to 60 mg daily, is an acceptable alternative. Both preparations must be given orally or via a nasogastric tube, as no parenteral form is available. The PTU has an advantage over methimazole because it inhibits the peripheral conversion of T_4 to T_3 and produces a more rapid clinical response. Although these drugs inhibit the synthesis of new thyroid hormone, they do not affect the release of stored hormone.

Retardation of Thyroid Hormone Release

Iodide administration promptly retards thyroidal release of stored hormones. Iodide can be given as strong iodine solution, 30 drops orally each day, or as sodium iodide, 1 g every 8 to 12 h by slow intravenous infusion. Iodide should be administered 1 h after the loading dose of antithyroid medication to prevent utilization of the iodide by the thyroid in the synthesis of new hormone.

Blockade of Peripheral Thyroid Hormone Effects

Adrenergic blockade is a maintstay of therapy for thyroid storm. Currently, the β-adrenergic blocking agent propranolol is the drug of choice. In addition to reducing sympathetic hyperactivity, propranolol also partially blocks the peripheral conversion of T_4 to T_3.

Propranolol can be given intravenously at a rate of 1 mg/min with cautious incremental increases of 1 mg every 10 to 15 min to a total dose of 10 mg. The effects of the drug in controlling cardiac and psychomotor manifestations of storm should be seen in 10 min. The lowest possible dose required to control thyrotoxic symptoms should be used, and this dose can be repeated every 3 to 4 h as needed. The oral dose of propranolol is 20 to 120 mg every 4 to 6 h. When given by mouth, propranolol is effective in about 1 h. Propranolol has been used successfully in treatment of thyroid storm in childhood. Younger patients may require a dosage as high as 240 to 320 mg/day orally.

The usual precaution of avoiding propranolol in patients with bronchospastic disease and heart block should be observed. Electrocardiographic evaluation for conduction disturbance should occur before the administration of propranolol. In patients with congestive heart failure, the benefit of slowing the heart rate and controlling certain arrhythmias must be weighed against the risk of depressing myocardial contractility with β-adrenergic blockade. Urbanic believes the benefit outweighs the risk in this situation but recommends administration of digitalis before propranolol.

Guanethidine and reserpine also provide effective autonomic blockade and are alternatives to propranolol. Guanethidine depletes catecholamine stores and blocks their release. When given 1 to 2 mg/kg per day orally (50 to 150 mg), it is effective in 24 h, but it may not have its maximum effect for several days. Toxic reactions are cumulative and include postural hypotension, myocardial decompensation, and diarrhea. It has an advantage over reserpine because it does not cause the pronounced sedation observed with that drug.

Reserpine acts to deplete catecholamine stores. As the initial dose, 1 to 5 mg is given intramuscularly, followed by 1 to 2.5 mg every 4 to 6 h. Improvement may be seen within 4 to 8 h. Side effects include sedation; psychic depression, which can be severe; abdominal cramping; and diarrhea.

Finally, a thorough evaluation for a precipitating cause of thyroid storm should be made. The treatment of thyroid storm should not be delayed by this evaluation, which may have to wait until the patient is at least partially stabilized.

Following the initiation of therapy, symptomatic improvement should occur within a few hours, primarily due to adrenergic blockade. Resolution of thyroid storm requires degradation of the already-circulating thyroid hormones, whose biological half-life is 6 days for T_4 and 22 h for T_3. Storm may last from 1 to 8 days, with an average duration of 3 days. If conventional therapy is not successful in controlling storm, alternative therapeutic modalities include peritoneal dialysis, plasmapheresis, and charcoal hemoperfusion to remove circulating thyroid hormone. Following recovery from thyroid storm, radioactive iodine therapy is the treatment of choice for hyperthyroidism. The mortality in untreated thyroid storm approaches 100 percent. Decreased mortality has occurred with the use of antithyroid drugs. Underlying illness is the cause of death in many cases. Prevention of thyroid storm is the ultimate solution to reduce mortality.

BIBLIOGRAPHY

Cooper DS: Antithyroid drugs. *N Engl J Med* 311:1353, 1984.

Davis PJ, Davis FB: Hyperthyroidism in patients over the age of 60 years: Clinical features in 85 patients. *Medicine* 53:161, 1974.

Dillon PT, Babe J, Meloni CR, et al: Reserpine in thyrotoxic crisis. *N Engl J Med* 283: 1020, 1970.

Levey GS: Catecholamine sensitivity, thyroid hormone and the heart. *Am J Med* 50:413, 1971.

Mazzaferri EL, Reynolds JC, Young RL, et al: Propranolol as primary therapy for thyrotoxicosis: Results of a long-term prospective study. *Arch Intern Med* 136:50, 1976.

Mazzaferri EL, Skillman TG: Thyroid storm: A review of 22 episodes with special emphasis on the use of guanethidine. *Arch Intern Med* 124:684, 1969.

Thomas FB, Mazzaferri EL, Skillman TG: Apathetic throtoxicosis: A distinctive clinical and laboratory entity. *Ann Intern Med* 72:679, 1970.

Urbanic RC, Mazzaferri EL: Thyrotoxic crisis and myxedema coma. *Heart Lung* 7:435, 1978.

Waldstein SS, Slodki SJ, Kaganiec GI, et al: A clinical study of thyroid storm. *Ann Intern Med* 52:626, 1960.

White GH: Recent advances in routine thyroid function testing. *CRC Crit Rev Clin Lab Sci* 24:315, 1987.

137
HYPOTHYROIDISM AND MYXEDEMA COMA

Gene Ragland

Myxedema coma is a life-threatening expression of hypothyroidism in its most severe form. It occurs most often during the winter months in elderly women with long-standing, undiagnosed, or undertreated hypothyroidism. It may be precipitated by infection or other stresses, and the diagnosis must be suspected based upon the clinical presentation. Treatment should be prompt and requires the administration of thyroid hormone in large doses. The mortality is greater than 50 percent in spite of optimum therapy.

CAUSES OF HYPOTHYROIDISM

Hypothyroidism is a chronic systemic disorder characterized by progressive slowing of all bodily functions because of thyroid hormone deficiency. The prevalence of hypothyroidism is about 1 percent in women and 0.1 percent in men. After age 60, the prevalence may be as high as 6 to 7 percent in women. Thyroid hormone is secreted in response to stimulation of the thyroid gland by thyroid-stimulating hormone (TSH) from the anterior pituitary gland. The TSH release is promoted by thyrotropin releasing hormone (TRH) from the hypothalamus. Therefore, thyroid failure may be primary, due to intrinsic failure of the thyroid gland, or secondary, due to disease or destruction of the hypothalamus or pituitary gland (Table 137-1).

Primary Hypothyroidism

Primary thyroid failure is by far the most common cause, accounting for 95 percent of the cases of hypothyroidism. The most common cause of hypothyroidism in the adult is treatment of Graves' disease by radioactive iodine or subtotal thyroidectomy. Postoperative hypothyroidism is usually evident within 12 to 15 months after surgery. The incidence of hypothyroidism following destruction of thyroid tissue with radioiodine increases progressively with time. The development of hypothyroidism as a consequence of surgical or radioiodine therapy may take years or decades. If hypothyroidism develops, these patients are committed to replacement thyroid hormone therapy for life.

Autoimmune thyroid disorders are the next most common cause of hypothyroidism. These include primary hypothyroidism and Hashimoto's thyroiditis. Primary hypothyroidism is thought to be the end result of an autoimmune destruction of the thyroid gland and produces thyroid failure because of glandular atrophy. Hashimoto's thyroiditis is the most common cause of goitrous hypothyroidism in areas with adequate iodine and may cause hypothyroidism because of defective hormone synthesis. There is clinical and immunologic overlap of these entities. Other causes of primary thyroid failure are rare and include iodine deficiency, antithyroid drugs such as lithium and phenylbutazone, spontaneous hypothyroidism from Graves' disease, and congenital causes.

Table 137-1. Differentiation of Primary and Secondary Myxedema*

Primary (Thyroid)	Secondary (Pituitary)
Previous thyroid operation	No previous thyroid operation
Obese	Less obese
Goiter present	No goiter present
Hypothermia more common	Hypothermia less common
Increased serum cholesterol	Normal serum cholesterol
Voice coarse	Voice less coarse
Pubic hair present	Pubic hair absent
Sella turcica normal	Sella turcica may be increased in size
Plasma cortisol level normal	Plasma cortisol level decreased
Skin dry and coarse	Skin fine and soft
Heart increased in size	Heart usually small
Normal menses and lactation	Traumatic delivery, no lactation; amenorrhea
No response to TSH	Good response to TSH
Good response to levothyroxine without steroids	Poor response to levothyroxine without steroids
PBI $< 2\mu g/dL$	PBI $> 2\mu g/dL$
Serum TSH increased	Serum TSH decreased

* TSH signifies thyroid-stimulating hormone; PBI, protein-bound iodine.

Source: Senior RM, Birge SJ: The recognition and management of myxedema coma. *JAMA* 217:61, 1971.

Secondary Hypothyroidism

Secondary thyroid failure accounts for 5 percent of the cases of hypothyroidism. Pituitary tumors, postpartum hemorrhage, or infiltrative disorders, such as sarcoidosis, may result in secondary thyroid failure. There are clinical and historical differences that distinguish primary thyroid insufficiency from pituitary failure (see Table 137-1.) This differential diagnosis is difficult on clinical grounds and requires laboratory evaluation. In general, the TSH level is high in primary hypothyroidism and low or normal in secondary hypothyroidism. Disease of the hypothalamus may cause failure to secrete TRH and may result in thyroid failure. This condition has been termed *tertiary hypothyroidism*. A few hypothyroid patients have been identified who have presumed hypothalamic disease and respond to TRH administration by increasing TSH above baseline levels.

Clinical Presentation

All patients who develop myxedema are hypothyroid, but not all hypothyroid patients have myxedema. Hypothyroidism is a graded phenomenon with various signs and symptoms along the clinical spectrum. With moderate to severe hypothyroidism, a nonpitting, dry, waxy swelling of the skin and subcutaneous tissue may occur, resulting in a puffy face and extremities. The term *myxedema* refers to this particular presentation of hypothyroidism.

The signs and symptoms of mild hypothyroidism may be subtle and the diagnosis difficult. With advanced hypothyroidism, the patients present with characteristic features. Typically, they complain of fatigue, weakness, cold intolerance, constipation, and weight gain without an increase in appetite. Muscle cramps, decreased hearing, mental disturbances, and menstrual irregularities are additional symptoms. Cutaneous features noted on physical examination include dry, scaly, yellow skin, puffy eyes, thinning of the eyebrows, and scant body hair. The voice may be deep and coarse and the tongue thickened. Paresthesia, ataxia, and prolongation of the deep tendon reflexes are characteristic neurologic manifestations. Bell's palsy due to hypothyroidism has been reported. In advanced cases, delusions, hallucinations, and psychosis (myxedema madness) may occur. Abdominal distension and fecal impaction may be present. Cardiac findings include bradycardia, enlarged heart, and low voltage on ECG. Mild hypertension rather than hypotension is the rule. Hypertension in conjunction with hypercholesterolemia may contribute to coronary artery disease and angina pectoris. A surgical scar on the neck may be present, but a palpable goiter is uncommon.

Diagnosis of hypothyroidism in a patient with these signs and symptoms can be made essentially on clinical grounds. Abnormally low levels of thyroid hormones confirm the diagnosis. Serum TSH levels should also be measured, and elevated levels are virtually diagnostic of primary hypothyroidism. If the disease is not treated, death follows a progressive intensification of these signs and symptoms. The time from onset to death varies between 10 and 15 years. Appropriate therapy is L-thyroxine in an average maintenance dosage of 0.1 to 0.3 mg once daily. The dosage must be individualized and may be higher or lower. Other thyroid preparations are available and acceptable as replacement thyroid hormone therapy.

MYXEDEMA COMA

Myxedema coma is a rare complication of hypothyroidism. The incidence is greater in women than men, and approximately half the patients are between 60 and 70 years old. A patient with undiagnosed hypothyroidism may develop coma as the initial manifestation. More commonly, the disease progresses insidiously, and coma develops when the patient is subjected to stress.

Precipitating Factors

A precipitating factor can be found in most cases of myxedema coma. Exposure to a cold environment is a significant antecedent occurrence with pulmonary infection and heart failure the most frequent precipitating events. Other stresses reported to initiate coma include hemorrhage, cerebrovascular accident, hypoxia, hypercapnia, hyponatremia, hypoglycemia, and trauma.

Significantly, it has been observed that more than 50 percent of the patients whose cases were reported in the literature lapsed into coma after admission to the hospital. In this setting, the stress of diagnostic and therapeutic procedures, acquisition of nosocomial infections, and the administration of certain drugs have been implicated as causative factors. Hypothyroid patients metabolize drugs more slowly than normal persons, and narcotics, anesthetics, phenothiazines, and other tranquilizers or sedatives have been reported to induce coma. Disastrous results may occur in a patient with advanced hypothyroidism and myxedema madness whose psychosis is treated with phenothiazines. The β-blocking drugs may cause myxedema coma by reducing thyroid hormone levels through peripheral conversion of thyroxine to triiodothyronine. Amiodarone-induced hypothyroidism leading to myxedema coma has been reported. Caution must be used when administering drugs, even in normal amounts, to hypothyroid patients. A final drug-related cause of myxedema coma is the failure to take necessary replacement thyroid hormone medication.

Clinical Presentation

The diagnosis of myxedema coma may easily be made in a patient who presents with the previously described general appearance and physical findings and with a history of previous thyroid hormone medication, radioactive iodine therapy, or subtotal thyroidectomy. Unfortunately, the diagnosis is not always that easy. A wide variety of clinical and laboratory abnormalities occur and may tend to occupy the physician's attention. Coma may be attributed to hypothermia, respiratory failure, and CO_2 narcosis; electrolye imbalance and hyponatremia; hypoglycemia; congestive heart failure; stroke; drug overdose; and other causes. Indeed, any of these disorders may lead to or worsen coma in the hypothyroid patient, but unless the underlying thyroid failure is diagnosed and treated, therapeutic efforts are unsuccessful. The overall clinical picture must be correlated and the diagnosis of myxedema coma considered.

Hypothermia

Hypothermia, unaccompanied by sweating or shivering, is typical of patients in myxedema coma and occurs in 80 percent of the cases. Approximately 15 percent have a temperature of 29.5°C (85°F) or less. A normal or elevated temperature suggests underlying infection. It is not coincidental that most patients develop myxedema coma during the winter, as normal thermogenesis is impaired in hypothyroidism.

This important diagnostic sign may be missed if a low-reading thermometer is not used or if the mercury in the thermometer is not shaken down. Hypothermia should be treated by gradual rewarming at room temperature. Too-rapid rewarming may cause peripheral vasodilation and circulatory collapse.

Respiratory Failure

Hypoventilation, hypercapnia, and hypoxia are common in patients with myxedema coma and may be the cause of death in many instances. Multiple factors have been implicated as causes of respiratory failure. Impaired respiratory mechanics due to dysfunction of the muscles of the respiratory system may lead to alveolar hypoventilation, hypercapnia, and hypoxia, and loss of responsiveness of the respiratory center to these stimuli. With thyroid hormone replacement hypoxic ventilatory drive is increased but hypercapnic ventilatory drive is not.

Additional factors that may further impair pulmonary function include obesity, congestive heart failure, pleural effusions, ascites, parenchymal lung involvement by myxedematous infiltrate, enlarged tongue, and changes in the airway, which may occur over its entire length. Airway obstruction due to myxedematous infiltration of the laryngeal mucosa has been reported. Patients should be evaluated by chest roentgenography and arterial blood gas levels, and require close monitoring. Drugs that may further depress respirations should be avoided. Mechanical ventilation may be required, and initial tracheostomy has been recommended because of the long recovery time for normal ventilatory function.

Hyponatremia

Water retention with hyponatremia and hypochloremia is another common finding in myxedema coma. Hyponatremia is dilutional, due to extracellular volume expansion and impaired ability to excrete a water load. Several mechanisms to account for the hyponatremia have been proposed. These range from deficiency of adrenal cortical hormones to decreased water delivery to the distal nephron to inappropriate secretion of antidiuretic hormone. Regardless of the etiology, hyponatremia is a potentially grave complication that can lead to water intoxication, brain edema, and death.

Conventional therapy is fluid restriction, but hypertonic saline is recommended if the serum sodium level is less than 115 mEq/L. A convincing case for a different therapeutic approach utilizing hypertonic saline, furosemide, and thyroid hormone has been presented. A review of the 24 hyponatremic-hypothyroid patients described in the literature since 1953 showed the serum sodium levels to range from 120 to 129 mEq/L in 8 patients and from 110 to 119 mEq/L in 10 patients, and to be less than 110 mEq/L in 6 others. All 6 patients treated with hypertonic saline survived, while 13 out of 18 who did not receive this treatment died. Intravenous furosemide induces negative water balance, while hypertonic saline replaces urinary sodium losses. Extreme caution must be used to avoid heart failure during the administration of hypertonic saline.

Cardiovascular System

The cardiovascular system is altered in structure and function with advanced hypothyroidism. Hypotension, cardiac enlargement detectable on x-ray films, and bradycardia are the most significant abnormalities to occur during myxedema coma. Thyroid hormones and sympathomimetic amines act synergistically to maintain left ventricular performance and vascular tone. Hypotension may result from a decreased synergistic effect due to thyroid hormone deficiency. Left ventricular dysfunction and hypotension are usually corrected by thyroid hormone replacement. Vasopressors do not work well in the absence of thyroid hormone and should be used, with caution, only in cases of severe hypotension unresponsive to other therapy. Ventricular arrhythmias may occur because of the synergistic actions of simultaneously administered thyroid hormone and vasopressors on a myxedematous myocardium.

Cardiomegaly is common, and is thought to be due to either pericardial effusion or underlying heart disease and not to ventricular dilation induced by hypothyroidism. The presence or absence of cardiomegaly on x-ray film is not a reliable indicator of a pericardial effusion, and echocardiography is the best way to identify a pericardial effusion. In spite of the frequency of pericardial effusions, cardiac tamponade in myxedema coma is rare because of the slow formation of the effusion and the ability of the pericardium to distend. Most pericardial effusions resolve with thyroid hormone replacement, but some may require pericardiocentesis or pericardial fenestration.

Sinus bradycardia is the most common electrocardiographic abnormality during myxedema coma. Other findings include low voltage, flattening or inversion of the T waves, and prolongation of the PR interval. In spite of impaired cardiac contractility, pericardial effusions, and conduction disturbances, congestive heart failure is unusual in myxedema coma and probably reflects underlying heart disease.

Nervous System

Coma is the terminal expression of neurologic dysfunction in myxedema and may be directly due to a lack of thyroid hormone in the brain. A variety of neurologic symptoms premonitory of myxedema coma do occur. Psychiatric disorders include slowed mentation, memory loss, personality changes, hallucinations, delusions, and psychosis. Cerebellar ataxia, intention tremor, nystagmus, and difficulty with coordinated movements may occur. Twenty-five percent of those who develop myxedema coma initially present with grand mal seizure. Many of the neuropsychiatric abnormalities improve with thyroid hormone replacement, but permanent dementia may remain after treatment. The role of hypothermia, CO_2 narcosis, cerebral edema, and other metabolic disturbances in the genesis of coma must not be overlooked.

Gastrointestinal System

Patients with myxedema may have abdominal distension due to ascites, paralytic ileus, or fecal impaction. Acquired megacolon is almost uniformly observed and has been the cause of unnecessary abdominal surgery. Urinary retention may occur, causing lower abdominal discomfort from a distended bladder. The weight gain that occurs with hypothyroidism is due to accumulation of some adipose tissue and retention of fluid. Patients with myxedema coma may be emaciated because of long-standing illness and decreased food intake. The treatment of abdominal complications consists of thyroid replacement and conservative measures such as nasogastric aspiration and enemas.

Laboratory

Although some laboratory findings are characteristic of myxedema coma, only thyroid function tests can confirm hypothyroidism. Serum thyroxine level (free T_4 index or free T_4 assay), triiodothyronine resin uptake (T_3 RU), and TSH levels should be measured. The results of these tests will not be available for use in the emergent situation but can later be used to support the clinical impression.

Characteristic laboratory abnormalities of myxedema coma already mentioned include hypoxemia, hypercapnia, hyponatremia, and hypochloremia. Serum potassium levels are extremely variable. Blood glucose levels are generally in the normal range, but severe hypoglycemia can occur. Hypercalcemia is rare, but hypocalcemia can occur in thyroidectomized patients in whom the parathyroids have been removed.

Bacterial infection may be reflected only by a leftward shift in the differential white blood cell count without appreciable elevation of the total white cell count.

Elevated serum cholesterol levels occur in approximately two-thirds of myxedematous patients. Malnutrition may lower the serum cholesterol level in some cases. Carotenemia has also been reported and may be the cause of the yellowish skin discoloration. Occasionally, striking elevations of the levels of muscle enzymes such as creatine kinase (CPK), serum glutamic-oxaloacetic transaminase (SGOT), lactate dehydrogenase (LDH), and fructose-biphosphate aldolase may be present. The elevations are thought to be due to changes in membrane permeability in skeletal muscle rather than to muscle destruction. The concentrations of these enzymes fall quickly when thyroid hormone is replaced. Finally, in most hypothyroid patients the CSF protein level is elevated to 100 mg/dL or more. The CSF pressure may occasionally be increased to over 400 mmH_2O. The significance of these CSF abnormalities remains obscure.

TREATMENT

Patients with myxedema coma are critically ill with a multiplicity of precarious and complex management problems. Specific therapy requires the administration of large doses of thyroid hormone. This decision must be based upon clinical judgment and made with extreme caution. The recommended dose of thyroid hormone could be fatal to the euthyroid comatose patient and harmful to the patient with ordinary myxedema. Every attempt to rule out causes of coma unrelated to hypothyroidism must be made first.

Supportive Therapy

Coma in myxedema may be primary, from a cerebral lack of thyroid hormone, or secondary, due to complications or precipitating causes. Treatment of the secondary causes of coma already mentioned includes oxygen administration and ventilatory support for respiratory failure, avoidance of drugs that may further depress respiratory or metabolic function, gradual rewarming of hypothermic patients, correction of hyponatremia by fluid restriction or hypertonic saline and furosemide, correction of hypoglycemia by glucose infusion, and treatment of hypotension with thyroid hormone and vasopressors, as needed. A thorough search for precipitating causes of coma should be made. Antibiotics are indicated for underlying infection. Additional adjunctive therapy is hydrocortisone, 300 mg/day, to protect against adrenal insufficiency.

Thyroid Hormome

Thyroid hormone replacement is the most critical and specific aspect of therapy for myxedema coma. The treatment already mentioned is largely supportive and is not fully effective until adequate thyroid hormone is given. Disagreement exists over the type, doses, and route of thyroid hormone administration.

Intravenous thyroxine is the drug of choice of most authors. It has been shown to be fully effective within 24 h with an onset of action in 6 h. The initial intravenous dose is 400 to 500 μg infused slowly; this is followed by 50 to 100 μg IV daily. Following the initial dose, some authors recommend no further thyroxine therapy until 3 to 7 days later. Once-daily therapy allows a smooth rise in hormone levels, as the turnover rate for L-thyroxine is about 10 percent per day. An oral dosage of thyroxine, 100 to 200 μg/day, can be started when possible. Cardiac arrest following the intravenous administration of L-thyroxine has been reported. The dose of thyroxine should be reduced in the face of cardiac ischemia or arrhythmias.

Triiodothyronine is an effective drug for treatment of myxedema coma. It has a more rapid onset of action than thyroxine but a shorter half-life. Repeated doses are required, which may cause abrupt cyclic changes in metabolic status. In addition, triiodothyronine must be administered orally or via nasogastric tube and has less predictable absorption by this route. In spite of these drawbacks, triiodothyronine, 12.5 to 25 μg every 6 to 8 h, can be used. Doses as low as 2.5 μg have been shown to be effective in treatment of myxedema coma. Overall clinical improvement should be seen in 24 to 36 h.

BIBLIOGRAPHY

Catz B, Russell S: Myxedema, shock and coma: Seven survival cases. *Arch Intern Med* 108:407, 1961.

Forester CF: Coma in myxedema. *Arch Intern Med* 111:734, 1963.

Holvey, DN, Goodner CJ, Nicoloff JT, et al: Treatment of myxedema coma with intravenous thyroxine. *Arch Intern Med* 113:89, 1964.

Maclean D, Giffiths PD, Browning MCK, et al: Metabolic aspects of spontaneous rewarming in accidental hypothermia and hypothermic myxedema. *QJ Med* 63:371, 1974.

Mitchell JM: Thyroid disease in the emergency department: Thyroid function tests and hypothyroidism and myxedema coma. *Emerg Med Clin North Am* 7:885, 1989.

Ridgway EC, McCammon JA, Benotti J, et al: Acute metabolic responses in myxedema to large doses of intravenous L-thyroxine. *Ann Intern Med* 77:549, 1972.

Sanders V: Neurologic manifestations of myxedema. *N Engl J Med* 266:547 and 599, 1962.

Shalev O, Naparstek Y, Brezis M, et al: Hyponatremia in myxedema: A suggested therapeutic approach. *Isr J Med Sci* 15:913, 1979.

Urbanic RC, Mazzaferri EL: Thyrotoxic crisis and myxedema coma. *Heart Lung* 7:435 1978.

Zwillich CW, Pierson DJ, Hofeldt FD, et al: Ventilatory control in myxedema and hypothyroidism. *N Engl J Med* 292:662, 1975.

138
ADRENAL INSUFFICIENCY AND ADRENAL CRISIS

Gene Ragland

Adrenal insufficiency consists of decreased levels of or absent hormones produced by the adrenal glands and results from structural or functional lesions of the adrenal cortex or the anterior pituitary gland. Deficit of adrenal hormones may manifest clinically as a chronic, insidious disorder, or as an acute, life-threatening emergency. Therapy of adrenal insufficiency is specific and includes replacement of the deficient hormones.

Chronic adrenal insufficiency is due to a variety of causes. It may be primary (Addison's disease), due to failure of the adrenal glands. It may also occur secondarily because of failure of the hypothalamus or pituitary gland (hypopituitarism) or because of iatrogenic adrenal suppression from prolonged steroid use. Acute adrenal insufficiency (adrenal crisis) may result from certain acute events, or when a person with chronic adrenal insufficiency is subjected to stress and exhausts reserve adrenal hormones, or when replacement hormone medication is discontinued.

PATHOPHYSIOLOGY OF THE ADRENAL GLANDS

The adrenal glands are divisble into the cortex and medulla. The adrenal cortex is essential for life and produces glucocorticoid, mineralocorticoid, and androgenic steroid hormones. The medulla secretes the catecholamines epinephrine and norepinephrine, largely under neural control. No definite clinical condition has been ascribed to hypofunction of the adrenal medulla. Most of the manifestations of adrenal insufficiency occur when the physiologic requirement for glucocorticoid and mineralocorticoid hormones exceeds the capacity of the adrenal glands to produce them.

Cortisol

The major glucocorticoid is cortisol, which is secreted in response to direct stimulation by adrenocorticotropic hormone (ACTH) from the anterior pituitary gland. Secretion of ACTH is governed by the hormone corticotropin-releasing factor (CRF) from the hypothalamus. This normally occurs with a diurnal rhythm, with the highest levels in the morning and the lowest levels in the late evening. Upon stimulation by ACTH, the adrenal glands respond in minutes to secrete cortisol in direct proportion to the ACTH concentration. Cortisol is normally secreted at the rate of 20 to 25 mg/day. Through negative feedback inhibition, the plasma cortisol level acts to suppress ACTH release.

By an undefined mechanism, stress factors such as anoxia, trauma, infections, and hypoglycemia can also trigger CRF and ACTH release and produce cortisol levels several times normal. The release of CRF in response to stress is resistant to suppression through negative feedback inhibition.

Cortisol is a potent hormone and affects the metabolism of most body tissues. In general, cortisol acts to maintain blood glucose levels by decreasing glucose uptake at extrahepatic sites and by providing precursors for gluconeogenesis via protein and fat breakdown. Cortisol governs the distribution of water between extracellular and intracellular compartments and possesses a minor sodium-retaining effect. It also acts to enhance the pressor effects of catecholamines on heart muscle and arterioles. In supraphysiologic amounts, cortisol inhibits inflammatory and allergic reactions. Finally, through negative feedback inhibition, cortisol suppresses the secretion of ACTH and melanocyte-stimulating hormone (MSH) from the anterior pituitary gland.

Aldosterone

The major mineralocorticoid is aldosterone. The renin-angiotensin system and plasma potassium concentration regulate aldosterone through negative feedback loops. These mechanisms are probably of equal importance and far more important than the minor aldosterone-stimulating effect of ACTH.

Aldosterone acts to increase sodium reabsorption and potassium excretion, primarily in the distal tubules of the kidneys. Other tissue effects of aldosterone are minor in comparison with its regulation of sodium and potassium levels.

Androgens

Androgenic hormone production by the adrenal glands is regulated by ACTH and is trivial in comparison with the production of these hormones by the gonads.

PRIMARY ADRENAL INSUFFICIENCY

Idiopathic

Primary adrenal insufficiency, or Addison's disease, is due to disease or destruction of the adrenal cortex and has a wide variety of causes (see Table 138-1). Approximately 90 percent of the adrenal cortex must be involved before clinical manifestations of adrenal failure result. Idiopathic atrophy of the adrenal glands is the leading cause of chronic adrenal insufficiency. Idiopathic adrenal insufficiency has been further divided into autoimmune (70 to 75 percent) and truly idiopathic (25 to 30 percent).

There is an overwhelming association between idiopathic adrenal insufficiency and other autoimmune diseases. Associated diseases include diabetes mellitus, Hashimoto's thyroiditis, pernicious anemia, and primary ovarian failure. Other investigators have reported frequent association with hypoparathyroidism, chronic active hepatitis, malabsorption, chronic mucocutaneous candidiasis, alopecia, and vitiligo.

Infiltrative or Infectious

Adrenal tuberculosis has declined in frequency as a cause of Addison's disease but is still reported to be a cause in 17 to 21 percent of the cases. Fungal infections and other infiltrative processes are infrequent causes of adrenal insufficiency during active, disseminated disease. Adrenal insufficiency as a complication of the acquired immunodeficiency syndrome (AIDS) has been reported. Infectious infiltration of

Table 138-1. Pathogenesis of Primary Adrenal Insufficiency

1 Primary, chronic
- *a* Idiopathic (autoimmune)
- *b* Infiltrative or infectious
  - (1) Tuberculosis
  - (2) Fungal infections
  - (3) Sarcoidosis
  - (4) Amyloidosis
  - (5) Hemochromatosis
  - (6) Acquired immunodeficiency syndrome (AIDS)
  - (7) Neoplastic (metastatic) disease
  - (8) Adrenoleukodystrophy
- *c* Hemorrhage or infarction
- *d* Bilateral adrenalectomy
- *e* Drugs
- *f* Congenital adrenal hyperplasia
- *g* Congenital unresponsiveness to ACTH

2 Primary, acute
- *a* Hemorrhage (adrenal apoplexy)
  - (1) Fulminant septicemia
  - (2) Newborn
  - (3) Anticoagulants
- *b* Discontinuation of replacement steroids

the adrenal glands with *Mycobacterium avium* or *M. intracellulare* or with cytomegalovirus may have caused the adrenal failure. Metastatic carcinoma in the adrenal glands is a relatively frequent finding at autopsy in patients with certain carcinomas, but it only rarely causes adrenal insufficiency.

Bilateral Adrenal Hemorrhage

Bilateral adrenal gland hemorrhage (adrenal apoplexy) is rare. In general, patients with a serious underlying condition whose adrenal glands are stressed are at risk for this complication. Stress-stimulated adrenal glands are hemorrhage prone. The association between adrenal hemorrhage and anticoagulant therapy with heparin and dicumarol is well established. Adrenal hemorrhage in this setting is most likely to occur between the third and eighteenth day of anticoagulation. Sudden deterioration with hypotension and pain in the flank, costovertebral angle, or epigastrium should suggest this disastrous event. Associated findings may include fever, nausea, vomiting, and disturbed sensorium. Computed tomography and ultrasound can assist in establishing this diagnosis. Other stressful events that have been associated with adrenal hemorrhage include surgery, trauma, burns, convulsions, pregnancy, and adrenal vein thrombosis.

Adrenal crisis as a consequence of adrenal hemorrhage also occurs with overwhelming septicemia and in the newborn. Fulminant septicemia with meningococcus, pneumococcus, staphylococcus, streptococcus, *Haemophilus influenzae,* and gram-negative organisms has been reported to cause adrenal hemorrhage. The Waterhouse-Friderichsen syndrome is a life-threatening disorder resulting from overwhelming septicemia due to meningococcemia. The patient is acutely ill and has shaking chills, severe headache, and a petechial rash that may progress to extensive purpura. Bilateral adrenal gland hemorrhage frequently occurs with this disorder. Vascular collapse and death may result unless the patient is promptly treated.

Miscellaneous

Another cause of primary adrenal failure is bilateral adrenalectomy for metastatic breast or prostate cancer or for Cushing's syndrome. Following such a procedure the patient is totally dependent upon replacement corticosteroids for life. Chemotherapeutic agents such as mitotane (*o,p'*-DDD) used in treatment of Cushing's disease can produce adrenal failure. Other drugs such as methadone, rifampin, and ketoconazole have been reported to cause adrenal insufficiency. Finally, rare congenital and inherited disorders can cause adrenal insufficiency.

Clinical Presentation

The clinical manifestations of chronic adrenal insufficiency develop gradually with subtle signs and symptoms that provide a diagnostic challenge. The clinical presentation of Addison's disease can be explained on the basis of a deficiency of cortisol and aldosterone and a lack of feedback suppression of ACTH and MSH.

Cortisol deficiency manifests clinically with anorexia, nausea, vomiting, lethargy, hypoglycemia with fasting, and inability to withstand even minor stresses without shock. The ability to excrete a free water load is also impaired and can lead to water intoxication. Lack of aldosterone results in impaired ability to conserve sodium and excrete potassium. The patient with aldosterone deficiency presents with sodium depletion, dehydration, hypotension, postural syncope, and decreased cardiac size and output. Renal blood flow is decreased, and azotemia may develop. Hyperkalemia is commonly seen but rarely is severe. Lack of suppression of ACTH and MSH secretion occurs because of deficient cortisol levels and results in increased pigmentation.

The overall clinical picture of a patient with Addison's disease is that of one who is weak and lethargic, with loss of vigor, and fatigue on exertion. The patient may have a feeble tachycardic pulse. Postural hypotension and syncope are common. In spite of hypotension, the extremities usually remain warm. Heart sounds may be soft or almost inaudible on auscultation.

Gastrointestinal (GI) symptoms are a prominent feature of chronic adrenal insufficiency and include anorexia, nausea, vomiting, weight loss, abdominal pain, and sometimes diarrhea.

Cutaneous manifestations of Addison's disease include increased brownish pigmentation over exposed body areas such as the face, neck, arms, and dorsum of the hands, and over friction or pressure points such as the elbows, knees, fingers, toes, and nipples. Pigmentation of mucous membranes, darkening of nevi and hair, and longitudinal pigmented bands in the nails may be seen. Vitiligo, mucocutaneous candidiasis, and alopecia may occur with Addison's disease that has an autoimmune cause. Women with Addison's disease may exhibit decreased growth of axillary and pubic hair because of adrenal androgen deficiency. This is not seen in men because of adequate testicular androgen.

Mentally these patients vary from alert to confused. Unconsciousness is rare unless the condition is preterminal. The sensory modalities of taste, olfaction, and hearing may be increased. Hyperkalemic paralysis is a rare, emergent complication of adrenal insufficiency; the patient presents with a rapidly ascending muscular weakness which leads to flaccid quadriplegia. Treatment of this complication consists of the intravenous administration of glucose and insulin or bicarbonate.

Laboratory

The usual laboratory findings in patients with primary adrenal insufficiency include hyponatremia, hyperkalemia, hypoglycemia, and azotemia. Hyponatremia is usually mild to moderate, and severe hyponatremia (<120 mEq/L) is rare. Hyperkalemia is usually mild, and the potassium level rarely exceeds 7 mEq/L. Initial potassium levels may be normal or low if protracted vomiting has occurred. Rarely, hyperkalemia may be severe and cause cardiac arrhythmia or paralysis.

Hypoglycemia, especially with fasting, is a characteristic finding. Moderate elevation of the blood urea nitrogen (BUN) level may occur because of dehydration secondary to aldosterone deficiency. Azotemia is usually reversible with rehydration.

Electrocardiographic changes include flat or inverted T waves, a prolonged QT interval, low voltage, a prolonged PR or QRS interval, and a depressed ST segment. The ECG changes reflective of hyperkalemia may also be present. The chest x-ray film may show a small, narrow cardiac silhouette due to decreased intravascular volume. A flat plate film of the abdomen may show adrenal calcification, which is most commonly due to tuberculosis but may occur with infection or hemorrhage.

SECONDARY ADRENAL INSUFFICIENCY

Secondary adrenal insufficiency may be due to disease or destruction of the hypothalamus or pituitary gland, resulting in impaired capacity of the pituitary to secrete ACTH. Those disorders responsible for secondary adrenal failure are listed in Table 138-2.

The most common cause of secondary adrenal insufficiency and adrenal crisis is iatrogenic adrenal suppression from prolonged steroid use. Rapid withdrawal of steroids from patients with adrenal atrophy secondary to chronic steroid use may result in collapse and death, especially under circumstances of increased stress. Exogenous administration of glucocorticoids may cause hypothalamic-pituitary-adrenal (HPA) suppression and subsequent adrenal atrophy. This complication has been reported to occur not only with oral steroids but also with those given by the intrathecal, topical, and inhalant routes.

The mechanism of continued adrenal atrophy following discontinuation of exogenous steroids may be a failure of normal diurnal release of CRF. Stress-induced release of ACTH may remain intact, but the

Table 138-2. Pathogenesis of Secondary Adrenal Insufficiency

1 Secondary, chronic
  a Pituitary tumor (chromophobe adenoma, craniopharyngioma, hamartoma, meningioma, glioma)
  b Pituitary hemorrhage or vascular accident
  c Postpartum pituitary infarction (Sheehan's syndrome)
  d Infiltrative and granulomatous disease
    (1) Sarcoidosis
    (2) Hemochromatosis
    (3) Histiocytosis X
  e Internal carotid artery aneurysm
  f Head trauma (basilar skull fracture)
  g Infection (meningitis, cavernous sinus thrombosis)
  h Hypophysectomy
  i Pituitary gland irradiation
  j Isolated ACTH deficiency
2 Secondary, acute
  a Iatrogenic HPA suppression due to steroid therapy
  b Discontinuation of replacement steroids.

atrophic adrenal glands are unable to secrete sufficient cortisol to meet the physiologic requirements in response to stress. The shortest time interval or the smallest dose at which HPA suppression occurs is unknown. Any patient who has been on dosages of glucocorticoids equivalent to 20 to 30 mg of prednisone per day for a week or more should be suspected of having HPA suppression.

Following prolonged supraphysiologic dosages of steroids, it may take up to 6 to 12 months for recovery of HPA function when steroids are withdrawn completely. Until complete recovery has occurred, it is wise to assume the patient will need basal steroid therapy and supplementary therapy during intercurrent illness or stress. Adrenal suppression must be suspected based upon the history of prior steroid use. When in doubt about the HPA status of a seriously ill or deteriorating patient, steroids should be given.

Clinical Presentation

Significant clinical and laboratory differences exist between patients with primary and those with secondary adrenal insufficiency. With secondary adrenal failure, the capacity of the pituitary to secrete ACTH is impaired. The level of aldosterone is largely unaffected because of its regulation by the renin-angiotensin system and the plasma potassium concentration. The clinical manifestations of secondary adrenal failure are due to insufficiency of cortisol and adrenal androgens. In addition, insufficiency of other anterior pituitary hormones such as growth hormone, thyroid hormone, and gonadotropic hormone may cause clinical abnormalities.

Patients with secondary adrenal insufficiency are better able to tolerate sodium deprivation without developing shock. This is true because of intact aldosterone secretion. Hyponatremia, hyperkalemia, and azotemia are not prominent features of secondary failure. Hypoglycemia, however, may be more common in patients with hypopituitarism because of concomitant growth hormone deficiency. Hyperpigmentation does not occur with secondary failure because ACTH and MSH are eliminated at their source, the pituitary gland. Finally, with secondary failure, men as well as women may exhibit signs of androgen deficiency because of insufficient gonadotopic hormone from the pituitary.

DIAGNOSIS

Differentiation of primary from secondary adrenal failure on other than clinical grounds requires in-hospital evaluation. Primary adrenal insufficiency is diagnosed by demonstrating a low baseline plasma cortisol level and failure to increase this level in response to exogenous administration of ACTH. Failure to respond to ACTH stimulation occurs because the adrenal cortex is damaged or destroyed and has no functional capacity to respond. Secondary adrenal insufficiency is diagnosed by demonstrating low plasma cortisol and urinary metabolite levels that increase in a stepwise fashion with repetitive ACTH stimulation over a period of days. A variety of tests to assess the integrity of the HPA axis are available.

A rapid screening test can reliably distinguish patients with normal adrenal function from those with adrenal insufficiency. This test is based on the fact that adrenal response to a single injection of ACTH is maximal within 1 h. Plasma for measurement of baseline cortisol level is drawn, and then 25 units of corticotropin (synthetic ACTH) is administered subcutaneously, intramuscularly, or intravenously. Another plasma cortisol level is obtained 30 to 60 min later. Normal persons should respond with a doubling of the baseline cortisol level. Patients with primary adrenal insufficiency show no increase in plasma cortisol levels, whereas those with secondary adrenal failure may show no, or a slight, response to corticotropin. A normal response is defined by a peak cortisol value of greater than or equal to 20 μg/dL. However, both falsely normal and abnormal rapid ACTH test results have been reported. This test should be used as a screening test, or to assess adrenal reserve in patients previously receiving steriods, but not as a diagnostic test for adrenocortical failure. A more prolonged period of ACTH stimulation is necessary to confirm adrenal failure and to reliably distinguish primary from secondary adrenal insufficiency.

TREATMENT

Glucocorticoid

Therapy of primary adrenal insufficiency consists of replacement of cortisol and aldosterone, and, on occasion, supplemental androgen therapy in the female patient. The usual maintenance dosage for glucocorticoid replacement varies from 20 to 37.5 mg of cortisol per day. Various preparations may be used (see Table 138-3 for steroid equivalents). A generally accepted dosage schedule is 25 mg of cortisone acetate or 5 mg of prednisone in the morning, followed by 12.5 mg of cortisone or 2.5 mg of prednisone in the afternoon. This simulates the normal diurnal variation of cortisol secretion. A few patients, especially large active men, may require a total daily dose of 50 mg of cortisone or 10 mg of prednisone for optimum response.

Mineralocorticoid

Mineralocorticoid replacement in patients with primary adrenal insufficiency can be achieved by administration of the synthetic mineralocorticoid fludrocortisone acetate (Florinef), 0.05 to 0.2 mg/day orally. This dosage should be appropriately reduced in patients in whom hypertension develops. It is also important for the patient with Addison's disease to maintain an adequate dietary salt intake.

Androgen

The woman with primary adrenal insufficiency may show signs of androgen deficiency such as decreased growth of axillary and pubic

Table 138-3. Steroid Equivalents

Drug	Equivalent Dose, mg	Na^+ Retention
Short-acting		
Cortisone	25	2+
Hydrocortisone (cortisol)	20	2+
Prednisone	5	1+
Prednisolone	5	1+
Methylprednisolone	4	0
Intermediate-acting		
Triamcinolone	4	0
Long-acting		
Dexamethasone	0.75	0
Betamethasone	0.6	0

hair. Supplemental androgen therapy can be achieved with 2 to 5 mg of fluoxymesterone (Halotestin) orally per day.

Secondary Insufficiency

Treatment of secondary adrenal insufficiency differs from that of primary adrenal insufficiency with regard to mineralocorticoid and androgen replacement. Patients with secondary adrenal failure usually do not require mineralocorticoid therapy and can maintain salt and fluid balance with a diet generous in sodium chloride. In the presence of hypotension, however, supplementary fludrocortisone acetate, 0.05 to 0.1 mg/day, is indicated. Evidence of androgen insufficiency may occur with male and female patients with hypopituitarism. Sufficient androgen in the female patient can be achieved with 2 to 5 mg of fluoxymesterone orally per day. Larger dosages of this preparation or long-acting testosterone (Depo-Testosterone) can be used in the male patient.

ADRENAL CRISIS

Adrenal crisis is an acute, life-threatening emergency that must be suspected and treated based upon clinical impression. It is due primarily to cortisol insufficiency and to a lesser extent, aldosterone insufficiency, and occurs when the physiologic demand for these hormones exceeds the capacity of the adrenal glands to produce them.

Adrenal reserve may be exhausted in patients with chronic adrenal insufficiency when they are subjected to intercurrent illness or stress. A variety of conditions may precipitate crisis in this setting; these include major or minor infections, trauma, surgery, burns, pregnancy, hypermetabolic states such as hyperthyroidism, and drugs, especially hypnotics or general anesthetics. Adrenal crisis may also occur in patients with chronic adrenal failure if the patient fails to or is unable to take replacement steroid medication. The most common cause of adrenal crisis is abrupt withdrawal of steroids from a patient with iatrogenic adrenal suppression due to prolonged steroid use. Finally, bilateral adrenal gland hemorrhage from fulminant septicemia or other causes can produce adrenal crisis.

Clinical Presentation

The clinical manifestations of adrenal crisis are due primarily to insufficiency of cortisol and to a lesser extent, insufficiency of aldosterone. Patients appear acutely ill. They are profoundly weak and may be confused. Hypotension, especially postural hypotension, is usual. Circulatory collapse may be profound. The pulse is feeble and rapid, and heart sounds may be soft. Temperature elevation is common but may be due to underlying infection. Anorexia, nausea, vomiting, and abdominal pain are almost universal. The abdominal pain may be severe, simulating an acute abdomen. Patients in crisis may exhibit increased motor activity which can progress to delirium or seizures.

Laboratory findings vary. The serum sodium level is usually moderately decreased but may be normal. Potassium levels may be normal or slightly increased. Rarely the potassium concentration may be markedly increased, and this can cause cardiac arrhythmias or hyperkalemic paralysis. Hypoglycemia is characteristic and can be severe.

Treatment

Treatment must be instituted promptly based upon clinical impression and should not be delayed for confirmatory testing of adrenal function. Therapeutic measures in treatment of adrenal crisis include replacement of fluids and sodium, administration of glucocorticoid, correction of hypotension and hypoglycemia, reduction of hyperkalemia, and identification and treatment of a precipitating cause of the crisis.

Fluids

A rapid infusion of 5% dextrose and isotonic saline should be started immediately. This acts to correct dehydration, hypotension, hyponatremia, and hypoglycemia. The extracellular volume deficit in the average adult in adrenal crisis is approximately 20 percent, or 3 L. The first liter should be given over 1 h, and 2 or 3 L may be required during the first 8 h of therapy. The functional capacity of the cardiovascular system is reduced with adrenal insufficiency, and the usual precautions with the rapid administration of saline should be observed.

Steroids

A water-soluable glucocorticoid should be administered promptly. As soon as the diagnosis of adrenal crisis is entertained, 100 mg of hydrocortisone sodium succinate (Solu-Cortef) or phosphate should be given in an intravenous bolus. In addition, 100 mg of hydrocortisone should be added to the intravenous solution. Usually, 200 mg of hydrocortisone is given every 6 h during the first 24 h of therapy. Glucocorticoid therapy acts to correct hypotension, hyponatremia, hyperkalemia, and hypoglycemia.

Mineralcorticoid therapy is not required during initial treatment of adrenal crisis. High dosages of hydrocortisone provide sufficient mineralocorticoid effect. As the total dosage of glucocorticoid is reduced below 100 mg/24 h, many patients need supplementary mineralocorticoid, which can be provided as desoxycorticosterone acetate (Percorten), 2.5 to 5.0 mg intramuscularly one or twice daily. If hypotension persists despite adequate volume and corticosteroid replacement, additional corticosteroid can be given and other causes of hypotension should be investigated. Vasopressors may be needed to correct hypotension. Adrenal hemorrhage should be considered, especially if the patient is receiving anticoagulants.

Simultaneous Treatment and Testing

It is possible to treat adrenal crisis and to perform simultaneous, confirmatory diagnostic testing for adrenal insufficiency. Physiologic saline is administered, but instead of hydrocortisone, 4 mg of dexamethasone is added to the infusion. Additionally, 25 units of corticotropin is added to the solution and this liter is infused in the first hour. Blood for plasma cortisol assay is obtained before and at the completion of the infusion. A 24-h urine collection for measurement of 17-hydroxycorticosteroid (17-OHCS) is collected. Additional corticotropin is added to subsequent intravenous solutions so that at least 3 units is infused each hour for 8 h. A third blood specimen for cortisol assay is obtained between the sixth and eighth hours of intravenous therapy.

If the patient has primary adrenal insufficiency, all plasma cortisol levels are low (<15 μg/dL), and the urinary 17-OHCS is also low, confirming the inability of the adrenals to respond to ACTH stimulation. An adequate rise in the plasma cortisol level excludes the diagnosis of adrenal insufficiency. A response indicative of partially intact adrenocortical reserve excludes the diagnosis of primary adrenal failure in favor of secondary adrenal insufficiency, but further testing is required to confirm this diagnosis. Other methods for simultaneous diagnosis and treatment have been described.

The adrenal crisis should begin to resolve favorably within a few hours after initiation of appropriate therapy. Intensive treatment and monitoring should continue for 24 to 48 h. Once the patient's condition has stabilized, the transition to an oral maintenance program can begin. Usually, 7 to 10 days are required for this transition.

The main causes of death during adrenal crisis are circulatory collapse and hyperkalemia-induced arrhythmias. Hypoglycemia may contribute to demise in some cases. With prompt recognition and appropriate treatment, most patients in adrenal crisis should do well.

BIBLIOGRAPHY

Addison T: On the constitutional and local effects of disease of the supra-renal capsules. *Med Classics* 2:244, 1937.

Axelrod L: Glucocorticoid therapy. *Medicine* 55:39, 1976.

Irvine WJ, Barnes EW: Adrenocortical insufficiency. *Clin Endocrinol Metab* 1:549, 1972.

Kozak GP: Primary adrenocortical insufficiency (Addison's disease). *Am Fam Physician* 15(5):124, 1977.

Nerup J: Addison's disease—clinical studies. A report of 108 cases. *Acta Endocrinol* 76:127, 1974.

Sampson PA, Brooke BN, Winstone NE: Biochemical confirmation of collapse due to adrenal failure. *Lancet* 1:1377, 1961.

Tapper ML, Rotterdam HZ, Lerner CW, et al: Adrenal necrosis in the acquired immunodeficiency syndrome. *Ann Intern Med* 100:239, 1984.

Thorn GW, Lauler DP: Clinical therapeutics of adrenal disorders. *Am J Med* 53:673, 1972.

Tyler FH, West CD: Laboratory evaluation of disorders of the adrenal cortex. *Am J Med* 53:664, 1972.

Xarli VP, Steele AA, David PJ, et al: Adrenal hemorrhage in the adult. *Medicine* 57:211, 1978.

SECTION 13
Hematologic and Oncologic Emergencies

139
APPROACH TO THE BLEEDING PATIENT

Daniel Esposito

SIGNS OF BLEEDING DIATHESIS

Trauma and tissue injury remain the most common causes of local bleeding. The following clinical findings should alert the physician to consider and evaluate the possibility of an underlying bleeding disorder:

- Inordinately profuse or prolonged bleeding after minor injury
- Spontaneous bleeding into joints (hemarthrosis) and deep subcutaneous tissues (hematomas)
- Concurrent multisystem or multisite bleeding
- Delayed bleeding several hours after trauma or surgery
- Diffuse petechiae, ecchymoses, or both
- Spontaneous bleeding from mucous membranes, such as the conjunctivae, or oral, rectal, and vaginal mucosa, may indicate a severe bleeding diathesis that may ultimately be complicated by CNS hemorrhage

GENERAL CONSIDERATIONS OF HEMOSTASIS

Hemostasis involves the synergistic interaction of four essential systems: vascular integrity, platelets, coagulation factors, and fibrinolysis. The complexity of the clotting mechanism is often overexaggerated. Table 139-1 outlines this concept and reviews clinical and laboratory features. The hybrid disorders—von Willebrand's disease and disseminated intravascular coagulation (DIC)—involve abnormalities in both platelets and clotting factors.

Vascular Bleeding

The primary defect is in either the blood vessel wall (inflammation) or the supportive connective tissue. Bleeding tends to be from smaller blood vessels. Increased vascular friability related to age (senile purpura) or steroid therapy has its genesis in diminished connective tissue support.

Platelets

Platelets participate at several levels of hemostasis by organizing at the site of vascular injury, by releasing adenosine 5′-diphosphate

Table 139-1. Clinical and Laboratory Signs of Bleeding Disorders

Disorder	Clinical Stigmata	LABORATORY STUDIES Abnormal	LABORATORY STUDIES Normal	Miscellaneous Condition
Vascular bleeding	Purpura (petechiae) Telangiectasia of skin and mucous membranes (Osler-Weber-Rendu disease) Perifollicular bleeding in scurvy Prolonged traumatic bleeding	Prolonged bleeding time Positive tourniquet test may be present in vasculitis	Normal platelet count Normal PT Normal PTT	Vasculitis Allergy to drugs, chemicals Infections Immune diseases Hereditary telangiectasis Scurvy Abnormal connective tissue
Platelet disorders	Purpura GI bleeding GU bleeding Epistaxis	Prolonged bleeding time Low platelet count in thrombocytopenia Normal platelet count in thrombopathy von Willebrand's disease	Normal PT Normal PTT	Thrombocytopenia Primary hemorrhage Thrombocythemia von Willebrand's disease Abnormal platelet function Thrombocytopathy Bernard-Soulier Glanzmann's
Coagulation factor disorders	Hemarthrosis Delayed bleeding Prolonged traumatic bleeding Deep intramuscular bleeding Male predominance	PT PTT Specific factor assay	Normal platelet count Normal bleeding time Normal thrombin time except with heparin and fibrinogen disorders	Hemophilia Sodium warfarin therapy Heparin therapy Vitamin K deficiency Congenital hypo- + dysfibrinogenemia von Willebrand's disease (VIII)
DIC and fibrinolysis	Delayed bleeding in fibrinolysis Diffused skin and mucous membrane bleeding Stigmata of chronic liver disease may be present	Variable prolongation in PT and PTT Low platelet count Low fibrinogen level Elevated fibrin degradation products		DIC—see Chapter 140 Primary fibrinolysis Liver disease Streptokinase and urokinase therapy Tissue plasminogen activator (TPA)

(ADP) that induces further aggregation; and by releasing platelet factor II and phospholipid which catalyze clotting. As in vascular bleeding, abnormal platelet number or function tends to cause small vessel bleeding (purpura).

Coagulation Factors and Clotting

Figure 139-1 outlines the intrinsic and extrinsic clotting cascades and schematizes the coagulation factors involved with the common coagulation screening tests. Tissue injury activates both pathways concurrently and both systems may participate in producing an insoluble fibrin clot. With isolated (e.g., hemophilia) or combined (e.g., sodium warfarin-therapy) with decreased factor (II, VII, IX, X) deficiencies, bleeding tends to be from larger blood vessels.

Fibrinolysis

The clotting process converts plasminogen to plasmin, a proteolytic enzyme that cleaves fibrin polymers into fibrin degradation (split) products and acts to lyse thrombi. Excessive fibrinolysis is the exaggeration of this homeostatic, thrombolytic mechanism and can produce bleeding by functionally altering other coagulation factors or by inducing excessive consumption of clotting factors as in DIC. The current use of streptokinase and urokinase (plasminogen activators) as thrombolytic agents in acute pulmonary embolism and myocardial infarction can be complicated by generalized bleeding from hyperfibrinolysis and hypofibrinogenemia.

LABORATORY INTERPRETATION

The screening battery is outlined in Table 139-2. Interpretations of the platelet count, prothrombin time (PT), and partial thromboplastin time (PTT) are discussed below.

Table 139-2. Bleeding Screening Tests

Type of Bleeding	Screening Test	Adjunctive
Vascular	Platelet count	Tourniquet test
Platelet	Platelet count	Bleeding time
Clotting	Prothrombin time (PT)	Fibrinogen level
Fibrinolysis	Partial thromboplastin time (PTT)	Factor assays

Platelet Count

Spontaneous bleeding generally does not occur if the platelet count exceeds 50,000 per cubic millimeter. Life-threatening CNS hemorrhage may occur spontaneously with platelet counts below 10,000 per cubic millimeter. If a platelet count is not available, an estimate of the number can be made by scanning the peripheral blood smear. In general, each platelet per oil immersion field represents 10,000 to 15,000 platelets per cubic millimeter. Platelet clumping on the smear may yield a factitiously low estimate.

Prothrombin Time Prolongation

The prothrombin time is the time required to induce clot formation in citrated plasma after the addition of tissue thromboplastin and calcium. Control values are in the 10- to 12-s range and are considered significantly prolonged when the patient's value is greater then 3 to 4 s above control. As illustrated in Fig. 139-1 the PT can be affected by abnormalities in factors I, II, V, VII, or X and is normal in hemophilia. The PT is a valuable, reproducible study and an isolated prolongation (with a normal PTT) suggests sodium warfarin therapy, vitamin K deficiency, or liver disease.

Partial Thromboplastin Time Prolongation

The PTT measures the intrinsic pathway of coagulation. It is the time necessary to induce clot formation in citrated plasma after the addition of calcium and contact with a surface (with kaolin activation it is called "activated" PTT). The control range is 25 to 35 s and varies widely depending on laboratory methodology. Significance is attributed to prolongations of 8 to 10 s above control. Isolated prolongation of the PTT suggests deficiency of factors VIII, IX, or XI or heparin effect.

Prolongation of PT and PTT

Significant abnormalities in the common pathway (Fig. 139-1) may prolong both the PT and PTT. Since heparin acts primarily by inhibiting thrombin and factor X, heparin overdose can affect both studies. Similarly, sodium warfarin overdose may depress factors II, VII, IX, and X, affecting both pathways. In DIC, the rate of clotting factor consumption exceeds that of production (particularly fibrinogen, factor V, and factor VIII), and the additive antithrombin effect of fibrin-split products may prolong the PT and PTT.

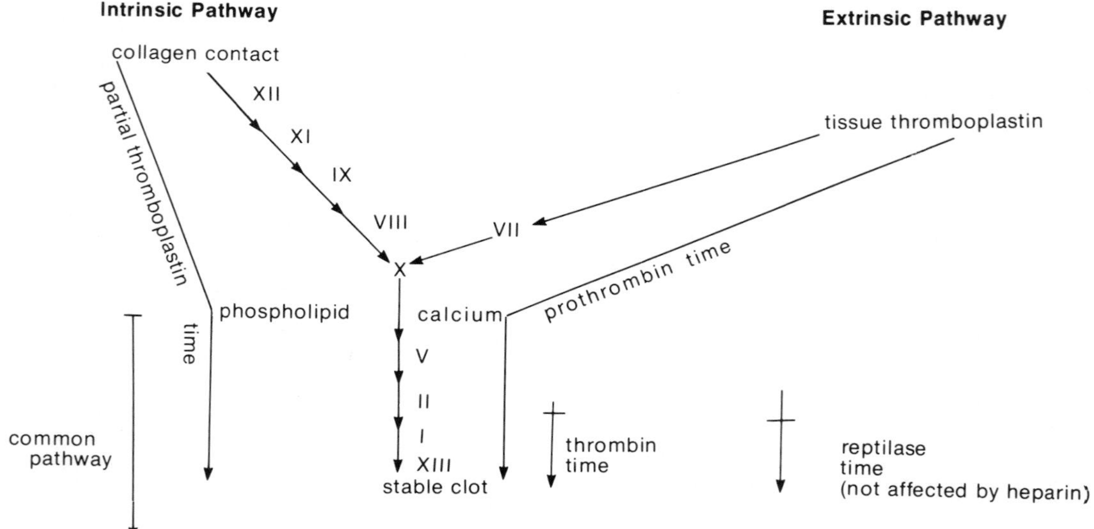

Fig. 139-1. Schema of intrinsic and extrinsic mechanisms of blood coagulation.

Thrombolytic therapy prolongs the partial thromboplastin time and the thrombin time, but both tests are also prolonged by heparin. However, the laboratory lytic state correlates poorly with clinical bleeding. With continued bleeding, assays for fibrinogen, fibrin degradation products, and factors V and VIII can aid in replacement therapy.

DIC Screen (See Chapter 140, "Acquired Bleeding Disorders.")

Because of the clinical importance of DIC, many laboratories are now establishing composite tests for defining the presence of intravascular coagulation:

Prolonged PT
Decreased fibrinogen level
Decreased platelet count
Increased fibrin degradation products

BIBLIOGRAPHY

Bennett JS: Blood coagulation and coagulation tests. *Med Clin North Am* 68:557–576, 1984.

Gregory SA, McKenna R, Sassetti RJ et al: Hematologic emergencies. *Med Clin North Am* 70:1129–1149, 1986.

140
ACQUIRED BLEEDING DISORDERS

Daniel Esposito

THROMBOCYTOPENIA

Acquired disorders that may underlie an abnormally low platelet count fall into two general categories: decreased platelet production and increased destruction. The list of etiologic agents is long and should be reviewed in a reference text. The more commonly encountered conditions include:

Decreased bone marrow production
- Aplastic anemia
- Malignant replacement of the bone marrow (leukemia, carcinoma, etc.)
- Drug suppression of the bone marrow (chemotherapy, radiation, alcohol, etc.)
- Infectious suppression (measles, tuberculosis)
- B_{12} and folic acid deficiency

Increased peripheral destruction
- Immune [idiopathic thrombocytopenic purpura (ITP), systemic lupus erythematosus, drug-induced, infectious mononucleosis, HIV-induced, etc.]
- Disseminated intravascular coagulation (DIC)
- Hypersplenism
- Thrombotic thrombocytopenic purpura

The bleeding tendency is greatest when the platelet count is below 50,000 per cubic millimeter. Fatal, spontaneous bleeding may occur when the platelet count is below 10,000 to 20,000 per cubic millimeter. Large platelets (megathrombocytes) on the peripheral blood smear may reflect increased bone marrow production and imply a peripheral destructive process. Young, large platelets appear to be functionally hyperactive and may explain why patients with immune destruction tend to tolerate lower platelet counts than those with marrow failure. The demonstration of megakaryocytes and increased platelet destruction on bone marrow examination is important in excluding bone marrow failure as a cause of severe thrombocytopenia.

Management

Stabilization of intravascular volume and maintenance of circulating hemoglobin should receive priority in any bleeding patient. Platelet transfusion is most effective when decreased platelet production is the underlying cause (i.e., normal peripheral survival). In general, one can assume an increment in the platelet count of 10,000 per cubic millimeter per unit of transfused platelets. Although platelet survival may be markedly shortened in peripheral destructive processes (particularly immune thrombocytopenia), and platelet transfusion as maintenance therapy is only slightly indicated, the patient with life-threatening bleeding should receive exogenous platelets as emergency therapy. Antibody suppressive therapy with corticosteroids and other immunosuppressive agents requires several days to improve platelet counts in the immune thrombocytopenias and is not commonly utilized in the emergency department.

The intravenous administration of purified human immunoglobulin (IV Ig) is a new approach designed to competitively inhibit the thrombocytopenic effect of antiplatelet antibody in ITP. It has been used successfully in acute childhood, adult, and pregnancy-related ITP and is generally reserved for children with active bleeding or adults with ITP refractory to steroids.

HYPOPROTHROMBINEMIA

Sodium Warfarin Therapy and Vitamin K Deficiency

Prothrombin is a glycoprotein produced by the liver under the influence of vitamin K and is converted to thrombin in the common pathway of the coagulation sequence. Congenital prothrombin deficiency is exceedingly rare and bleeding due to abnormalities of prothrombin production is generally related to vitamin K deficiency, sodium warfarin therapy, or hepatic insufficiency. The multifactorial pathogenesis of bleeding in liver disease will be treated as a separate subject.

Fat-soluble vitamin K is necessary for the hepatic production of factors II, VII, IX, and X. Dietary and biliary insufficiency, as well as intestinal fat malabsorption, may lead to a bleeding diathesis characterized by a prolonged prothrombin time (PT) [variable prolongation of the partial thromboplastin time (PTT)] that reverses with parenteral vitamin K therapy.

Coumarin derivatives (warfarin or Coumadin, and dicumarol) are competitive inhibitors of vitamin K. Their anticoagulant properties may be enhanced by a variety of drugs through protein displacement (phenylbutazone, clofibrate, indomethacin, etc.) or by metabolic inhibition (allopurinol, chloramphenicol, nortriptyline). With therapeutic doses, the PT is 2 to 2½ times the control value and the PTT is generally normal. Otherwise, minor trauma may induce bleeding which, if uncontrollable by local compression, may require discontinuing the medication and reversal with vitamin K (oral or parenteral). The dose of vitamin K is 5 to 25 mg parenterally. The most common dose given is 10 mg either IM or IV. If given IV, it must be administered slowly at the rate of 1 mg/min. Sodium warfarin overdose may produce fatal, spontaneous bleeding with prolongation of both the PT and PTT. Clinical judgment should dictate the need for volume-red cell replacement and emergency fresh-frozen plasma infusion (see Chapter 143, "Blood Transfusion—Components and Practices").

LIVER DISEASE

Many factors may be responsible for abnormal (atraumatic) bleeding in acute and chronic liver disease. All four general categories of hemostasis may be individually or simultaneously affected as shown in the following outline:

Vascular
- Trauma
- Peptic ulcer disease and alcoholic gastritis
- Variceal bleeding in portal hypertension
- Hemorrhoids

Platelets (thrombopenia)
- Alcoholic bone marrow suppression
- Hypersplenism
- Folic acid deficiency
- DIC

Clotting factors
- Vitamin K deficiency and malabsorption
- Insufficient production of factors I, II, V, VII, IX, X
- Chronic consumption coagulopathy (DIC)

Hyperfibrinolysis
- Hepatic inability to deactivate plasmin
- Inhibition of coagulation by circulating fibrin-split products
- Hypofibrinogenia

Bleeding in the presence of liver disease is, therefore, complex and requires diligent laboratory and clinical efforts to determine the nature and site of bleeding, degree of volume loss, and relative contribution of platelet and clotting factor abnormalities. The battery of laboratory studies should include: platelet count, PT, PTT, and fibrinogen level. Fibrin-split products may be obtained as a supportive test.

HYPOFIBRINOGENEMIA

Congenital hypofibrinogenemia and dysfibrinogenemia are rare, and clinical manifestations are variable (thrombosis, bleeding, wound dehiscence, or asymptomatic). Acquired hypofibrinogenemia is rarely an isolated phenomenon and is generally a composite feature of advanced liver disease, DIC, primary fibrinolysis, or increased fibrinolysis due to streptokinase/urokinase therapy. Prolongation of the PT, PTT, thrombin, and reptilase times may vary relative to the degree of fibrinogen level depression. Therapy is directed at the underlying etiology and replacement therapy with cryoprecipitate is utilized in the seriously bleeding patient. Pooled, fibrinogen concentrates have a high incidence of hepatitis transmission.

DISSEMINATED INTRAVASCULAR COAGULATION (DIC)

DIC is a clinical syndrome characterized by diffuse bleeding from the skin, mucous membranes, and viscera. Widespread activation of the clotting mechanism results in consumption of the circulating clotting factors and platelets available for hemostatic homeostasis. When the rate of utilization exceeds production, diffuse bleeding ensues.

Any condition accompanied by significant tissue destruction can trigger and sustain unbridled intravascular clotting (e.g., burns, trauma, crush injury, malignant, fetal death in utero, gangrene). In addition to tissue necrosis, DIC can be a sequela of drug reactions, amniotic fluid emboli, transfusion reactions, liver disease, and a host of infectious diseases.

The diagnosis of DIC may not always be achieved with absolute certainty (particularly in liver disease, TTP, etc.), however, the laboratory triad of prolonged prothrombin time, thrombocytopenia, and hypofibrinogenemia should signal its possible presence in the patient with multisite bleeding. Supportive laboratory evidence of DIC includes demonstration of elevated fibrin-split products and microangiopathic hemolytic anemia with fragmented red blood cells on peripheral blood smear.

Primary therapy should be directed at the underlying cause when readily identifiable (sepsis, pregnancy, drug, or transfusion therapy), and early recognition and correction of hemodynamic instability through volume and red cell replacement are essential. Current consensus favors clotting factor (fresh frozen plasma), fibrinogen (cryoprecipitate or fresh frozen plasma), and platelet replacement in the uncontrollably bleeding patient, rarely in association with intravenous heparin therapy.

The continuous use of heparin to interrupt inappropriate coagulation activity may be effective prophylaxis in certain chronic DIC states such as carcinoma and acute progranulocytic leukemia.

THROMBOLYTIC AGENTS

The ultimate effect of thrombolytic agents is the conversion of plasminogen to plasmin. Tissue-type plasminogen activator and single-chain urokinase generate plasmin primarily on fibrin surfaces. Streptokinase combines with plasminogen both in the circulation and on fibrin surfaces. Although acylated plasminogen-streptokinase activator complex is somewhat fibrin-specific, its systemic action is similar to that of streptokinase.

Bleeding is the commonest complication of thrombolytic therapy and is most often associated with invasive procedures, although spontaneous GI and CNS bleeding can occur. Bleeding is multifactorial, due to vascular injury, hypofibrinogenemia, fibrin degradation products, platelet dysfunction, and depletion of other coagulation factors, notably Factors V and VIII.

Bleeding can begin from 30 minutes to several hours after the initiation of thrombolytic therapy. The thrombin time, partial thromboplastin time, and fibrinogen level can be used to monitor the lytic state.

Initial treatment of bleeding consists of manual pressure to venipuncture sites, volume expansion, and discontinuation or reversal of heparin. Continued and severe bleeding can be managed by infusion of packed red blood cells, cryoprecipitate, and platelet and fresh frozen plasma infusion.

BIBLIOGRAPHY

Bussel JM, Hilgartner MW: The use and mechanism of action of intravenous immunoglobulin in the treatment of immune haematologic disease. *Br J Haematol* 56:1, 1984.

Eisenstaedt R: "Blood Component Therapy in the Treatment of Platelet Disorders." Seminars in Hematology. Jan. 1986, 23:1–7.

George JN, Shattil SJ: "The Clinical Importance of Acquired Abnormalities of Platelet Function." NEJM Jan 3, 1991, 324:27–38.

Hirsch J: Heparin. *N Engl J Med* 324:1565, 1991.

Kwaan HC. "Clinicopathologic Features of Thrombotic Thrombocytopenic Purpura." Seminars in Hematology, April 1987, 24:71–81.

Linnik W, Tintinalli J, and Ramos R: "Associated Reactions during and Immediately after RTPA Infusion." Ann Emerg Med, Mar 1989, 18:234–239.

Sone DC, Califf RM, Topol EJ, et al: "Bleeding during Thrombolytic Therapy for Acute Myocardial Infarction: Mechanisms and Management." Ann Int Med Dec 1989, 15:1010–1022.

Zon LI, Groopman JE: "Hematologic Manifestations of the Human Immune Deficiency Virus (HIV)." Seminars in Hematology, July, 1988, 25:208–218.

141 HEMOPHILIA

Ronald Sacher

The hemophilias comprise a group of hereditary bleeding disorders that have in common a disturbance in intrinsic coagulation. These may be further subdivided into hemophilia A (classic hemophilia), hemophilia B (Christmas disease), and von Willebrand's disease.

GENERAL CONSIDERATIONS AND CLINICAL SYNDROMES

Classic hemophilia is a deficiency of normal functional factor VIII, Christmas disease is a deficiency of normal functional factor IX, and von Willebrand's disease is a deficiency of both antigenic and functional factor VIII and von Willebrand cofactor. The factors of the intrinsic coagulation pathway are measured by the partial thromboplastin time (PTT). Factors VIII and IX are unique and important components of the intrinsic pathway, and their deficiency is associated with prolongation of the PTT. The other factors unique to the intrinsic pathway, namely, factors XII and XI, may also be genetically absent, but these deficiencies constitute much less frequent and less severe clinical entities.

The prothrombin time (PT) measures the extrinsic coagulation pathway, and factor VII is unique to this system. It is obvious that certain factors, such as X, V, II, and I, are common to both pathways. Thus a deficiency of factor VIII or IX would produce a prolonged PTT and a normal PT. This is a hallmark of the hemophilias. Obviously, identification of the deficient factor is essential to specifically define the type of hemophilia that is present. Identification also affects specific treatment. The thrombin time (TT) measures thrombin-fibrinogen interaction. This test is always prolonged with heparin therapy or in cases of disseminated intravascular coagulation (DIC). It is, however, normal in hemophilia.

Genetic Types

Classic Hemophilia (Hemophilia A)

Hemophilia A is a sex-linked genetic disorder resulting in deficiency of factor VIII coagulant activity. The deficiency is often defined as severe (less than 2 percent activity), moderate (2 to 5 percent activity), and mild (5 to 30 percent activity), depending on the level of factor VIII present. Only about 50 percent of severe hemophilia patients have a positive family history.

Christmas Disease (Hemophilia B)

Hemophilia B is a sex-linked genetic disorder resulting in a deficiency of factor IX coagulant activity. Severe, moderate, and mild forms also exist. More than 75 percent of patients give a family history of hemophilia. It is clinically indistinguishable from hemophilia A.

von Willebrand's Disease

This disorder is an autosomal genetic disease resulting in a deficiency in factor VIII coagulation activity (VIII-C), immunologic activity vWF-antigen (vWF:Ag), and the von Willebrand factor activity (vWF:activity). The latter is the factor that corrects the platelet dysfunction found in von Willebrand's disease (see Table 141–1 for laboratory diagnosis of hemophilia).

This disorder is usually transmitted as an autosomal dominant with variation in expression of the disorder.

Clinical Syndromes of Hemophilia

Mild Disease

Mild disease may not be diagnosed until adult life, although very often the patients give a history of minor, but recurrent, bleeding episodes in early life. Serious bleeding, however, rarely follows mild trauma but occurs following dental extractions, tonsillectomy, and other surgical challenges or severe trauma. Female carriers may easily bruise, producing cosmetically disturbing ecchymoses, and have excessive menstrual flow. Patients with mild factor VIII or IX deficiency may occasionally have a normal PTT.

Moderate and Severe Disease

Moderate and severe disease usually presents in infancy or early childhood. The disease may become apparent following circumcision. In infants learning to walk, falling may produce recurrent and severe muscle hematomas, lip lacerations, or tongue biting, leading to severe bleeding episodes. Dental procedures may provoke severe bleeding. Hematuria may occur in adolescence and adulthood and may be spontaneous or associated with physical activity. The characteristic hemarthroses and muscle hematomas occur when the child is walking well, and the peak incidence is in schoolboys and adolescents.

Muscle hemorrhages are associated with stiffness and pain before the cardinal signs of swelling and warmth become apparent, Retroperitoneal hematomas may be difficult to diagnose, and the patient may have groin pain at the insertion of the psoas muscle due to hemorrhage down the fascial planes.

Joint hemorrhages are usually recognized by a sensation of joint fullness and limitation of range of movement. Pain and swelling become apparent. Knees, elbows, ankles, hips, and shoulders are affected in decreasing order of frequency. Chronic arthropathy may occur if treatment and consequently resolution of hemorrhage is delayed. Recurrent hemorrhages lead to synovial hypertrophy, chronic inflammation with fibrous adhesions, and joint ankylosis. Severe deformities can occur.

MANAGEMENT

Acute Medical Management

Replacement Therapy

Specific identification of the deficient factor is essential to proper management. All coagulation factors are present in fresh-frozen

Table 141–1. Laboratory Diagnosis of Hemophilia

	PT*	PTT*	Factor* VIII-C	von Willebrand Factor Antigen (vWF:Ag)	Ristocetin Platelet Aggregation (vWF activity)	Bleeding Time	Factor IX
Hemophilia A	N	↑	↓	N	N	N	N
Hemophilia B	N	↑	N	N	N	N	↓
von Willebrand's (C)	N	↑	↓	↓	↓	↑	N

* See text for explanation of abbreviations.

Note: N = Normal; ↑ = prolonged ↓ = decreased.

plasma, which can be given in a situation where the specific abnormality is unknown. However, the deficient individual usually requires a substantial amount of replacement therapy to achieve hemostasis, and volume overload may be a problem. The average patient has approximately 40 mL of plasma per kilogram of body weight. Each 1 mL of normal plasma has 1 unit of factor activity. Therefore, 40 units per kg factor VIII will raise the factor VIII level to 100 percent. The emergency physician should be able to calculate the amount of a given factor necessary to raise the patient's factor activity to the desired percentage of normal. Depending on whether bleeding is mild to severe, one may wish to raise the plasma level to 50 to 100 percent of predicted normal (see Table 141–2). Since the half-life of the antihemophilic factors is only 12 h, the patient may need to be treated repeatedly, depending on the site, severity, and persistence of bleeding.

Desmopressin acetate is an antidiuretic hormone affecting renal water conservation and is a synthetic analogue of the natural hormone argenine vasopressin. D-Amino-8, D-anginine vasopressin (DDAVP) is more potent at raising plasma levels of factor VIII activity in patients with hemophilia A and von Willebrand's disease type 1. The usual dose is 0.4 μg/kg, which induces a rapid elevation in factor VIII levels in these patients. The effect is evident within 30 min, reaching a maximum at 90 min to 2 h. Factor VIII coagulant activity responds to a greater degree than vWF:Ag and vWF activity. The compound is infused over a 10- to 15-min period in saline, while blood pressure is monitored closely. Most patients experience facial flushing, and some may experience blood pressure elevation. Increase in factor VIII plasma levels of 300 to 400 percent of the initial concentration can be seen after infusion.

Cryoprecipitate was, until recently, the therapeutic product of choice for most patients with mild classic hemophilia (5 to 30 percent factor VIII activity) and for patients with von Willebrand's disease. In view of the potential for transfusion-transmitted viral diseases when blood products are used, alternative strategies have been developed. The use of DDAVP, 0.4 μg/kg, almost always achieves factor VIII levels adequate for hemostatis in these patients. This agent is a vasopressin analogue and therefore is not associated with infectious disease transmission. Unfortunately, DDAVP is not effective in severe, or in most cases of moderate, hemophilia, or in severe and type IIB von Willebrand's disease. The latter is an unusual form of von Willebrand's disease and diagnosis requires an extensive evaluation by a hematologist.

Fresh-frozen plasma or cryoprecipitate may also be used in the treatment of von Willebrand's disease. Plasma may also be used to treat mild factor VIII or IX deficiency. Its use is limited by the volume needed since only 10 to 15 mL/kg is safely given in one dose with an expected rise of 20 to 30 percent in clotting factor activity.

The use of concentrates has made management of moderate or severe disease more practical. The dose of concentrate must be adjusted to the severity of the hemorrhage. Minor bleeding can be managed by a single infusion of several bags of cryoprecipitate in the emergency department. The patient is instructed to return if bleeding recurs. Cryoprecipitate is rich in factor VIII and contains approximately 5 to 10 units of factor VIII activity per milliliter. Single cryobags derived from a single donor contain about 10 mL total volume, i.e., 50 to 100 units of factor VIII activity per bag of cryoprecipitate.

Heat- or detergent-treated factor VIII concentrates are available in different total strengths. These concentrates are derived from pooled plasma, lyophilized, and then reconstituted with sterile water. The total activity is indicated on the container. The major advantage is that less volume is needed; however, since this product is derived from pooled plasma, it carries a greater risk of hepatitis and formerly, AIDS. Heat and detergent treatment inactivates human immune deficiency virus (HIV), the causative agent of AIDS. Nevertheless, all the donors are tested and are negative for antibodies to HIV. Concentrates are more expensive. The approximate number of units per milliliter can vary considerably from preparation to preparation.

Lyophilized concentrates of factors II, VII, IX, and X (prothrombin complex) are used primarily for the treatment of factor IX deficiency. The complex is not separated for technical reasons and carries a higher risk of infectious disease transmission as well as thrombotic activity. Average factor IX activity is 20 units/mL concentrate.

The recently introduced monoclonal antibody purified factor VIII

Table 141–2. Treatment Schedule for *Severe* Hemophilia (< 1% of Factor Present) without an Inhibitor*

Disorder	Degree of Hemorrhage	Initial Dose of Concentrate, Units of Factor Activity per kg	Subsequent Doses	
Hemophilia A, classic hemophilia (factor VIII deficiency)	Minor Hemarthrosis Muscle hematoma Mild hematuria	18	10 units/kg q 8–12 h	Until objective bleeding and pain revolves; single doses may be sufficient.
	Moderate	26	14 units/kg q 8–12 h	7–10 days to permit adequate healing
	Severe Life-threatening surgical procedure Major trauma Head injury	35	18 units/kg q 8–12 h	7–10 days to permit adequate healing
Hemophilia B, Christmas disease (factor IX deficiency)	Minor Hemarthrosis Muscle hematoma Mild hematuria	25	5 units/kg q 12–24 h	Until objective bleeding and pain resolve; single dose may be sufficient.
	Moderate	35	8 units/kg q 12–24 h	7–10 days to permit adequate healing
	Severe	45	10 units/kg q 12–24 h	7–10 days to permit adequate healing
	Life-threatening surgical procedure Major trauma Head injury			

* Cryoprecipitate contains about 80 units of factor VIII activity per bag.
Factor VIII and factor IX heat-treated concentrates contain a value printed on the label.
Fresh-frozen plasma contains 1 unit of factor IX or factor VIII per mL.

concentrates appear to be the purest and safest form of factor VIII preparation available. These ultrapure and presumably safer products are becoming the standard of treatment in newly diagnosed hemophiliacs despite their substantially greater cost. Although it may seem that these factor VIII products could be reserved for new cases of hemophilia or patients with low levels of viral exposure, they are now being used very generally. Clinical trials are currently underway to assess the effectiveness of recombinant factor VIII which may prove useful in the future. They are, however, currently unavailable for general use.

Dosages and treatment schedules are outlined in Table 141–2.

Additional Features in Management

Local care, using ice packs and immobilization with an elastic bandage, can limit muscle hematomas and hemorrhage under the skin. Hemarthroses generally only occur in severe hemophilias and almost never in von Willebrand's disease. Temporary splinting is necessary to avoid further trauma, limit swelling, and help relieve pain.

Appropriate analgesia is important in the hemophilias. An increasing list of analgesics contain aspirin and should be avoided since they inhibit platelet aggregation and compound the hemostatic problem. Propoxyphene, acetaminophen, and codeine may be used as alternatives. Intramuscular injections must be avoided.

Anti-inflammatory agents, most specifically steroids, are used in hematuria, acute hemarthrosis, and chronic synovitis. The dosage is usually 1 mg/kg per day.

Special Considerations

Occasionally patients with severe hemophilia fail to respond to appropriate replacement therapy. These patients may constitute the small, but therapeutically complicated, group of patients with circulating anticoagulants (inhibitors). Hematologic consultation is advised for the management of this serious problem.

Current estimates are that about 90 percent of severely affected classic hemophilic patients have antibodies to HIV. Most of these patients, however, do not have clinical AIDS. The major cause of death in hemophilic patients is no longer hemorrhage and continues to be the complications of blood component–derived infections.

BIBLIOGRAPHY

Brettler DB, Levine PH: Factor concentrates for the treatment of hemophilia: Which one to choose? Blood 73:2067, 1989.

Hougie C: Disorders of hemostasis, in Williams WJ, Beutler E, Erslev AJ, Lichtman MA (eds): *Hematology,* 3d ed. New York, McGraw-Hill, 1983, pp 1381–1397.

Kasper CK: Hematologic treatment of hemophilia dn von Willebrand's disease, in Luban NLC and Kolins J (eds): *Hemotherapy in Childhood and Adolescence.* Arlington, Va, American Association of Blood Banks, 1985, pp 53–68.

Lusher JM: Desmopressin acetate (DDAVP); Its use in disorders of hemostasis. *Thromb Haemost* 6:385, 1984.

McDougall JS, Martin LS, Cort SP, et al: Thermal inactivation of AIDS virus, HTLV-III-LAV, with special reference to anti-hemophilic factor. *J Clin Invest* 76:875, 1985.

Roberts HR, Jones MR: Hemophilia and related conditions—Congenital deficiencies of prothrombin (factor II), factor V, and factors VII to XII, in Williams WJ, Bentler E, Erslev AJ, Lichtman MA (eds): *Hematology,* 4th ed. New York, McGraw-Hill, 1990, pp 1453-1473.

Ruggeri ZM, Zimmerman TS: von Willebrand factor and von Willebrand's disease. *Blood* 70:895, 1987.

White GC, McMillan CW, Kingdon HS, et al: Use of recombinant antihemophilic factor in the treatment of two patients with classic hemophilia. *N Engl J Med* 320:166, 1989.

142 SICKLE CELL ANEMIA

Daniel Esposito

Sickle cell anemia is a qualitative hemoglobinopathy inherited as an autosomal dominant trait with an approximate gene frequency in black Americans of 8 percent.

GENERAL

Pathogenesis

The biochemical abnormality of sickle hemoglobin is due to the substitution of B_6 valine for glutamic acid in the hemoglobin chain. This single substitution is responsible for the susceptibility of deoxygenated sickle hemoglobin to polymerize and aggregate, which, in turn, induces red cell deformation.

By virtue of their shape change, sickled erythrocytes are unable to freely pass through the microvasculature and this ongoing process of thrombosis and hemolysis is largely responsible for the clinical expressions of ischemia, infarction, chronic hemolytic anemia, and multisystem compromise.

Patients with sickle cell disease (homozygous-SS) have a clearly defined increased susceptibility to infection. Functional hyposplenism and autosplenectomy result from repeated erythrocyte stasis, thrombosis, and splenic infarction during childhood as a direct extension of the sickling process. Apart from diminished splenic and reticuloendothelial phagocytic function, deficient oposonin activity against pneumococci and *Salmonella,* as well as defective granulation and polymorphonuclear mobility, appear additive in predisposing to infectious complications.

Sickle Disease Variants

In populous urban settings the diagnosis of sickle cell anemia and related hemoglobinopathies is often first considered and evaluated in the emergency department.

Sickle Cell Anemia (Homozygosity) Hb SS

The most severe form of sickle syndromes occurs in the homozygous state, when 75 to 95 percent of circulating hemoglobin is of the sickle variety. Because of the likelihood of focal or disseminated microcirculatory thrombosis (crisis) with high sickle hemoglobin concentrations, the homozygous state should be considered in children who have unexplained bone pain, severe hemoloytic anemia, jaundice, or recurrent left upper quandrant pain associated with splenic infarctions. The degree of severity varies and the age at onset of symptoms may range from 6 months to 15 years.

Sickle Cell Trait (Heterozygosity) Hb AS

When the sickle gene is inherited from one parent and normal hemoglobin A from the other, one expects only partial expression of the abnormal gene. Erythrocytes will then contain both hemoglobin A and S in variable proportions depending on their synthetic rates. Since less than 50 percent of circulating hemoglobin is subject to sickling, the severe vasoocclusive and hemolytic manifestations do not occur.

Doubly Heterozygous (Heterozygous for S, Heterozygous for Another Abnormal Hemoglobin)

The most commonly encountered doubly heterozygous conditions are Hb SC, Hb SB thalassemia, Hb SD, and Hb S-fetal persistence. Patients may have severe systemic complications of sickle cell disease or may lead relatively asymptomatic lives. Distinction from sickle cell disease can only be accomplished with hemoglobin electrophoresis. Initial symptoms may manifest relatively late in life and the diagnosis often overlooked until the second to third decade. Recent attention to Hb SC disease and pregnancy complicated by bone marrow infarction and fat emboli further underscores the need to maintain awareness of sickle disease variants.

DIAGNOSIS AND TREATMENT

Laboratory Diagnosis

Depression of the hematocrit and hemoglobin level due to sickle cell trait is uncommon; however, significant anemia, usually with a chronically elevated reticulocyte count, is invariably present in homozygous sickle cell disease. The hemolytic anemia serves as a constant bone marrow stimulus, and as a result elevated leukocyte and platelet counts are present in the "steady state" and serve little value in assessing the presence of infection. The diagnosis of sickle cell anemia is confirmed by the demonstration of sickle hemoglobin by electrophoretic separation.

The emergency physician can be relatively sure of the diagnosis if irreversibly sickled red cells are present on the peripheral blood smear. Since erythrocytes are exposed to oxygen during blood smear preparation, sickled red cells may revert to their normal shape. Irreversibly sickled cells on peripheral smear generally indicate homozygous disease or doubly heterozygous variants and are not seen in Hb AS patients. Most of the currently available screening tests for sickle hemoglobin (Sickledex, SickleScrene, Sik-L-Stat, SCAT) rely on the insolubility of sickle hemoglobin in a reduced environment. The turbidity thus produced constitutes a positive test, but does not distinguish between sickle trait or disease.

Clinical Manifestations and Management

Having considered the pathogenetic mechanisms of microcirculatory thrombosis, ischemia, and infarction, one can readily appreciate the panorama of systemic illness and organ dysfunction that befalls the homozygous sickler. The long-term deleterious effects of anemia and ischemia can produce a spectrum of chronic disorders, including progressive optic atrophy and blindness due to repeated vasoocclusion, hemorrhage, and neovascularization; chronic organic brain syndrome with epileptic foci; respiratory insufficiency with cor pulmonale; chronic congestive heart failure; progressive renal insufficiency and the nephrotic syndrome; and chronic, recurrent, ischemic leg ulceration.

Sickle cell crisis, acute respiratory insufficiency, arthropathy, and priapism are acute problems that are often encountered in the emergency department.

Sickle Cell Crises

Sickle cell crises include thrombotic crisis (vasoocclusive-infarctive); hemolytic crisis, exaggeration of the steady-state hemolytic process manifested as a dramatic fall in the hematocrit with concomitant jaundice; aplastic crisis, which is often induced by concurrent infectious suppression of the bone marrow or folic acid deficiency with life-threatening depression of the hematocrit and reticulocyte count; and sequestration crisis, an uncommon feature of childhood sickle cell disease, clinically manifested as sudden painful enlargement of the liver and spleen with associated pancytopenia.

Thrombotic sickle crisis, which is universally more common than hemolytic or aplastic crisis, implies a sequential progression of pathological, symptomatic events that culminate in a clinical state of unremitting pain, prostration, and anxiety. Initially, gnawing pain may develop locally in the tibia, periarticular areas, back, abdomen, or chest. Paroxysmal pain may last only a few hours and subsequently recur with greater intensity and duration. "Impending" crisis seemingly refers to the sickle patient who has vague discomfort, a paucity of physical findings, and symptoms that initially appear easily manageable with fluid therapy and analgesics. The experienced emergency physician has no doubt seen this patient return several times in a 48- to 72-h period prior to the ultimate development of crescendo pain necessitating hospitalization. Thrombotic crisis is a clinical diagnosis before it is a laboratory one and recent reports of elevated α-hydroxybutyrate dehydrogenase as a laboratory earmark of crisis have not, as yet, been substantiated. An element of increased hemolytic activity is commonly present and when baseline data are available, there may be an elevated reticulocyte count and a hematocrit below that of the patient's steady state. Laboratory studies should be further directed at identifying possible precipitating factors, including pneumonia, urinary tract infection, pharyngitis, acidosis, and dehydration.

Analgesics, rehydration, correction of acidosis, and treatment of infection remain as mainstay therapy for vasoocclusive crisis. Supplemental oxygen is advised but does little to improve oxygen tension in the stagnating microenvironment. Red cell transfusion should be reserved for significantly anemic patients (hematocrit less than 17 to 18 percent) as liberal transfusion to a hematocrit greater than 30 percent may increase whole blood viscosity and promote further sludging and vasocclusion. Continued supplemental folic acid is indicated to meet the exaggerated red cell turnover rate. Antisickling agents (urea, sodium cyanate) have not proven clinically useful.

Acute Respiratory Insufficiency

Acute pulmonary manifestations include bacterial and *Mycoplasma* pneumonias, thromboembolism, in situ pulmonary thrombosis, and acute pulmonary hypertension. Bone marrow infarction and pulmonic fat emboli have been described in Hb SS and Hb SC disease.

Central Nervous System

Acute neurological manifestations of sickle cell disease are primarily related to vascular occlusion, although narcotic overdose and withdrawal syndromes should also be considered in the individual with an altered sensorium. Subarachnoid hemorrhage, hemiplegia, and convulsions are the most common manifestations. Current therapeutic trends favor long-term transfusion programs in an effort to prevent irreversible cerebral damage. If stupor and coma are present, suspect severe anemia and aplastic crisis.

Arthropathy

It is convenient to consider an acutely tender and inflamed joint as another manifestation of thrombosis (synovial or periarticular); however, aseptic necrosis, septic arthritis, osteomyelitis, hemarthrosis, and gout are frequently responsible. When fever and monoarticular involvement coexist, diagnostic arthrocentesis may be necessary.

Priapism

Penile engorgement prolonged beyond several hours is uncommon but may occasionally occur in both sickle cell disease and sickle trait. Analgesia and ice compresses aid in relieving corpus cavernosal engorgement and urological consultation should be requested immediately.

Hematuria

Painless, gross hematuria is a common clinical feature of sickle cell trait and sickle disease. Relative hyperosmolarity of the renal medulla favors in situ sickling and subsequent papillary necrosis. Severe necrosis and substantial tissue sloughing may rarely obstruct the ureteropelvic junction, producing acute flank pain with hematuria.

Narcotic Drug Addiction

Chronic pain associated with chronic disease states is associated with narcotic use and abuse. It is not surprising that many adult sickle cell patients are addicted to oral and occasionally intravenous narcotic analgesics. The emergency physician should be alerted to the possibility of narcotic withdrawal syndromes. These include nonspecific abdominal pain, emotional lability attended by either hyperactivity or lethargy, malingering, or delirium. Narcotic overdose can be generally recognized by the clinical triad of pinpoint pupils, stupor, and a favorable response to intravenous naloxone.

GLUCOSE-6-PHOSPHATE DEHYDROGENASE (G-6-P-D) DEFICIENCY

Hereditary G-6-P-D deficient hemolytic anemias can occur in two variants: Black (X-linked) and non-Black (favism, as seen in India, Asia, and the Mediterranean countries—an Autosomal recessive disease). Eleven percent of black males may be homozygous and up to twenty-two percent of black females heterozygous. Hemolytic episodes may be severe in oxidative stresses such as acute viral infections, quinine-naphthalene medication exposures, etc. The clinical features of acute severe hemolysis include severe asthenia and dyspnea from acute anemia, jaundice, and marked pallor.

Non-black variants (favism) tend to be more severe. Screening tests for G-6-P-D deficiency are qualitative in nature and essentially screen for the presence of Heinz bodies. Quantitative G-6-P-D tests are more accurate. However, shortly after acute hemolysis, G-6-P-D screens may be spuriously negative since young RBCs (reticulocytes) contain more G-6-P-D. The older, G-6-P-D deficient RBCs are already cleared from the circulation by hemolysis.

Acute hemolytic episodes are treated with red cell transfusion as indicated clinically. Avoidance of oxidative medications such as chloroquin, quinines, sulfonamides, etc. is particularly important in suspected black males.

BIBLIOGRAPHY

Sickle Cell Anemia

Alavi JB: Sickle cell anemia: pathophysiology and treatment. *Med Clin North Am* 68:545, 1984.

Hillner BE, Smith TJ: Glucose-6-phosphate dehydrogenase deficiency. *N Engl J Med* 324:169, 1991.

Horberg A, Ernst J, Uddin DE: Sickle cell trait and glucose-6-phosphate dehydrogenase deficiency: Effects on health and military performance in black navy enlistees. *Arch Intern Med* 141:1485, 1981.

Kork JA, Posey DM, Schumacher HR, et al: Sickle-cell trait as a risk factor for sudden death in physical training. *N Engl J Med* 317:781, 1987.

Leikin SL, Gallagher D, Kinney TR, et al: Mortality in Children and Adolescents with Sickle Cell Disease. *Pediatrics* 84:500, 1989.

G-6-P-D Deficiency

Beutler E, Blume KG, Lohr GW, et al: (1979) International committee for standardization in Haematology. Recommended screening test for glucose-6-phosphate deficiency. *Br J Hematol* 43:465, 1979.

Shannon K, Buchanan GR: Severe hemolytic anemia in black children with glucose-6-phosphate dehydrogenase deficiency. *Pediatrics* 70:364, 1982.

Cowan MJ, Amman AJ: *Clinics in Hematology–Enzymopathies.* 10:152, 1981.

143
BLOOD TRANSFUSION—COMPONENTS AND PRACTICES

Steven J. Davidson

BLOOD COMPONENTS—DESCRIPTIONS AND INDICATIONS

Whole blood consists of cellular and noncellular components. Cellular components include red cells, platelets, and granulocytes. Noncellular components include albumin, plasma protein fraction (PPF), fresh-frozen plasma (FFP), cryoprecipitate, and other soluble coagulation factors. Component transfusion, rather than whole blood transfusion, is preferred to correct a specific physiologic deficiency and to make the most efficient use of a limited resource.

The emergency physician will most frequently use red blood cell (RBC) concentrates and will have secondary needs for FFP coagulation factor concentrates, platelets, albumin, and PPF. Whole blood transfusions are currently rarely used, generally only for infant transfusion.

Transfusion of all but the chemically and heat-treated components (albumin, PPF) carries with it the risk of hepatitis. Other infectious illness, including acquired immunodeficiency syndrome (AIDS), can also be transmitted by blood transfusion. Incompatibility, isoimmunization, and allergic and toxic reactions are all potential complications.

Whole Blood

Even whole blood is no longer "whole" at the time of administration. Within 24 h of initiating storage in citrate-phosphate-dextrose (CPD) or citrate-phosphate-dextrose-adenine (CDPA-1) solutions, blood stored at 4°C (39.2°F) has no functioning granulocytes, and only 50 percent of the functional activity of platelets and coagulation factor VIII remains. Both platelet function and factor VIII activity are negligible by 72 h.

Continued refrigerated storage of whole blood causes a 50 percent reduction in factor V at 3 to 5 days and increased affinity of hemoglobin for oxygen at 4 to 6 days with decreasing RBC viability and deformability beginning at about the same time. About the fifth day, hydrogen ion, ammonia, and potassium concentrations begin to rise and microaggregates of platelets, fibrin, and leukocytes collect rapidly. Viability of at least 70 percent of the administered RBCs at 24 h is the standard by which all storage of blood products is judged. CPD permits 21-day storage, and CPDA-1 permits 35-day storage to meet this standard. Decreased RBC deformability limits the ability of RBCs to travel through capillaries in tissues, and increased RBC oxygen affinity reduces tissue oxygenation. These latter effects are reversed 24 to 48 h after the RBCs are returned to the more "natural" environment of the vascular tree. Detriments to the use of whole blood include limited concentrations of labile clotting factors; excessive accumulations of metabolic by-products; volume overload; contamination with viruses or bacteria; and exposure to antigens. Usually, RBC concentrates and crystalloid infusions suffice when volume and RBC mass repletion are necessary. In massive transfusion, however, fresh whole blood, when available, is appropriate, and autotransfusion may also be a helpful adjunct in these circumstances.

Cellular Concentrates

Packed Red Blood Cells

Packed red blood cells (PRBCs) are transfused when RBC mass repletion is the primary aim. They are prepared in closed systems to a hematocrit no greater than 80 and have a 21- to 35-day refrigerated shelf life depending on the storage medium. PRBCs and crystalloid solutions are ideal volume and RBC repletion fluids in the overwhelming majority of emergency transfusions. The infusion rate is maximized by using wide tubing and a large-bore infusion catheter, and by diluting the blood with warmed normal saline solution. Infusing warm, rather than cold, blood also reduces the patient's metabolic workload and the risk of hypothermia.

PRBCs do not provide volume repletion or noncellular coagulation factors, and crystalloid infusions are necessary to replace lost circulating volume. Approximately 10 percent of the original donor plasma remains in each unit of PRBCs; but except in exchange or massive transfusions, hepatic synthesis of coagulation proteins rapidly replenishes intravascular stores.

The advantages to the use of PRBCs include (1) decreased burden of citrate, ammonia, and organic acids, (2) reduced risk of alloimmunization, since fewer antigens are infused, and (3) reduced risk of volume overload when multiple units are infused.

Washed Red Blood Cells

Washed RBCs provide a pure PRBC unit with a 24-h shelf life. They are most often utilized for patients with known allergic reactions to platelet, granulocyte, or plasma antigens and are rarely used in the emergency service.

Platelets

Platelets are administered for bleeding resulting from thrombocytopenia or inadequate platelet function. A platelet pack increases the platelet count by 4000 to 8000 in a 70-kg patient, and 10 packs are generally given at a time. ABO matching is not necessary, although HLA matching may be performed in special circumstances. In surgical or trauma patients with normal platelet function, platelet counts of 40,000 to 100,000/mm^3 may result in bleeding correctable by platelet administration. Spontaneous bleeding is uncommon with platelet counts above 20,000/mm^3 but is frequent and severe at platelet counts below 10,000/mm^3.

Noncelluar Components

Fresh Frozen Plasma (FFP)

Fresh frozen plasma contains all noncellular coagulation factors in near-normal levels. Units come from a single donor, are approximately 250 mL in volume, are thawed to order, and are ABO-matched prior to transfusion. Since hepatitis and other disease transmission risks are identical to those of whole blood and PRBCs, FFP should not be used for simple colloid volume replacement or expansion.

A recent National Institutes of Health consensus conference concluded that FFP is the most overutilized blood product. The only unequivocal indication for FFP is the correction of clinically significant deficiencies of clotting factors. For example, FFP might be transfused to a patient who is taking warfarin and who has significant bleeding or needs immediate surgery. Even in this case, however, it is inefficient since coagulation factors are not concentrated in FFP. Cryoprecipitate (see below) is a more rational choice to correct a deficiency in the factors it contains. For the patient with an acute, undiagnosed bleeding disorder, FFP is the only source of all noncellular coagulation factors. At the risk of volume overload, FFP given in adequate volume will correct any deficiency. However, once a diagnosis is made, the specific factor that is deficient should be given.

Prophylactic administration of FFP should be discouraged. Historically, many practitioners administered 1 unit of FFP for every 5 to 6 units of PRBCs. Apparently, a concern regarding "dilutional coagulopathy" drove this practice. However, the mathematics of exchange transfusion demonstrate the irrationality of this practice. Furthermore, evaluation in individual patients seldom demonstrates consistent findings—a situation typical of the clinical environment. Some patients bleed abnormally, while others do not. The coagulation abnormalities of those who do bleed abnormally cannot be explained by dilution alone. Fibrin-split products found in the blood of these patients, and limited transient response to coagulation factor repletion, suggests consumption of clotting factors as found in disseminated intravascular coagulopathy.

Specific Factor Therapy

Classic hemophilia (a factor VIII deficiency, also known as hemophilia A) accounts for approximately 85 percent of patients with congenital coagulation factor abnormalities. Most patients are aware of the diagnosis and their usual therapeutic requirements. Treatment of this disorder is replacement of the specific factor deficiency through the use of cryoprecipitate, usually obtained through standard blood bank resources. Recently, a commercially available factor VIII product produced through the use of recombinant DNA technology has become available. As it is highly standardized in factor VIII content, there is an apparent advantage to its use, especially since there is no risk of transmission of hepatitis or HIV. However, its cost is substantially greater than cryoprecipitate and this marketplace concern currently limits its use. At the time of this writing, a bill has been introduced in Congress to fund the use of this product for hemophiliacs in the future.

Cryoprecipitate is prepared by first freezing individual units of plasma and then thawing at 4°C (39.2°F). The small amount of protein precipitated in the process is rich in factor VIII and fibrinogen. When packaged separately and provided as individual units, it is commonly known as cryoprecipitate. Cryoprecipitate does not require crossmatching prior to administration. Factor VIII potency may vary significantly between units of cryoprecipitate. Thus, cryoprecipitate is commonly administered in multiple packs based on the usual requirements for the extent of the injury being treated. The most common error made by the treating physician is not wrongly estimating the total dose but rather failing to initiate treatment early enough and to continue adequate treatment through the course. The goal is to raise factor VIII levels sufficiently to assume adequate function according to the specific clinical situation. For example, early superficial hematomas may be treated by raising factor VIII levels to 25 percent, while deep muscle hematomas or dental bleeding may require levels of 50 percent. Treatment of a hemophiliac patient with intracranial bleeding or serious trauma requires levels of up to 80 percent. Fibrinogen is also present in large quantities in cryoprecipitate. The rare individual with congenital hypofibrinogenemia may be treated with cryoprecipitate.

Factor IX deficiency (Christmas disease, hemophilia B) is a far less common congenital coagulopathy. Formerly available commercial products to treat episodes contained all the Vitamin K–dependent coagulation factors, including factors II, VII, IX, and X. These products, prepared from pooled plasma collected from paid donors, carried the risk of disease transmission, and so are no longer available. FFP is generally substituted. A recombinant DNA product may become available in the future.

Albumin and Plasma Protein Fraction

Colloid administration for maintenance or restoration of oncotic pressure remains controversial. Both albumin and PPF are chemically and heat-treated to eliminate the risk of hepatitis transmission. Albumin is available as a 25% "salt-poor" preparation (which in reality contains 160 mEq of sodium per liter) hyperoncotic to plasma, and a 5% buffered solution isooncotic to plasma. The typical 25-mL ampule (12.5 g) has an oncotic effect approximately equal to 1 unit of FFP. Plasma protein fraction contains 88 percent albumin and 12 percent globulins. It is isoosmotic with plasma, containing 130 to 160 mEq of sodium per liter. Current methods of preparation have eliminated the risk of hypotension due to the presence of prekallikrein activator.

Immune Globulins

Immune globulins such as tetanus (Hypertet), hepatitis B (H-BIG), and rabies (Hyperab) are prepared by hyperimmunizing donors who undergo plasmapheresis. Immune serum globulin is prepared by routine fractionating of plasma separated from whole blood. Hyperimmunized donors are not used. It is often used in an attempt to modify or prevent viral illnesses such as rubella, poliomyelitis, or rubeola, and to treat acquired or congenital hypo- or agammaglobulinemias. It is sometimes suggested for prophylaxis following inadvertent needle-stick exposure. The nature of the separation and processing of immune serum globulin precludes any risk of hepatitis or AIDS transmission.

BLOOD TRANSFUSION PRACTICES

Absolute identification and documentation of blood specimen, patient, and donor unit are essential. The following criteria are useful for identifying patients who require typing and crossmatching for donor units:

1. Shock
2. Observed 100-mL or greater blood loss
3. Gross gastrointestinal bleeding
4. Hemoglobin level less than 10 mg/dL, or hematocrit less than 30
5. Probability of a blood-losing operation (e.g., laparotoy for trauma, ectopic pregnancy, etc.)

There are no guidelines for determining the appropriate number of units to prepare for any given patient. The number of units requested is a clinical judgment, based upon an estimate of ongoing and future losses. For patients who do not fulfill any of the above criteria, blood typing and a screen for atypical antibodies suffice as long as the antibody screen is negative. In the event that it is not, the clinician should be notified by the blood bank so that the ordering of blood for crossmatching may be considered.

Blood Administration Devices

Patients who receive blood in the emergency service are likely to have multiple units transfused. The use of micropore filters, bloodwarming systems, pressure infusion pumps, and special tubing can contribute positively to the outcome.

Blood can be administered with large-bore intravenous extension tubing, or with Y-type administration sets that have one inlet for the blood and another for the intravenous solution. Warmed saline solution can be run through one arm of the Y, and when blood is infused, it is warmed and diluted by the saline so as to flow faster. Calcium- or glucose-containing solutions should not be used. Normal saline rather than hypotonic saline solutions should be used to prevent RBC lysis.

Micropore filters, available in 20- to 40-μm pore sizes, should be used to filter microaggregates of platelets, fibrin, and leukocyte fragments. They slow the rate of transfusion, but earlier concern about precipitating thrombocytopenia is unwarranted since packed RBCs contain no platelets in any case.

The energy and oxygen demand placed on a patient to warm a blood volume from 4 to 37°C (39.2 to 98.6°F) is significant, and potentially life-threatening hypothermia can occur with massive transfusion. All too often, the patient is unclothed during resuscitation, massively transfused, and subsequently subjected to a surgical procedure in an air-conditioned operating room. Warming of the blood and other fluids tends to be overlooked.

Current warming systems operate by maintaining a thermostatically controlled water bath or heating plate through which blood in a closed tubing system, designed to expose a maximum surface area, is circulated. The major deficiency with these systems is the reduction in rate of flow through the system and thus reduced rate of infusion. Pressurized infusion systems may assist with the maintenance of adequate flow and to some extent offset this liability of warming systems.

Pressure infusion devices operate by applying pneumatic pressure of no more than 300 torr (mmHg) to the blood bag. Systems should be closed to utilize such pressure infusion devices, and any puncture of a port in the system will likely result in leakage upon pressurization.

Recently, warming devices with high-flow, large-bore manifolds and heat exchangers, utilizing high-volume counter-current flow of thermostatically regulated warmed water, have become available. These systems are expensive, but quite effective at warming large quantities of blood while maintaining high rates of flow. The most widely available of these, the Fluid Warmer, is made by Level-1 Technologies.

An alternative, readily available approach in most emergency departments, however, is to warm the sterile normal saline solution to approximately 43.3°C (110°F) in a thermostatically controlled oven or standard microwave oven. The warmed saline solution may then be used to dilute cold-packed RBCs, warming the entire infusion toward a more physiologic temperature.

Emergency Release of Blood

The administration of type-specific but incompletely crossmatched blood or type O blood carries a risk of transfusion reaction, yet may be lifesaving.

When possible, the additional 5 min necessary to secure type-specific, rather than universal, donor blood for emergency transfusion is preferred. However, the clinical decision to use incompletely crossmatched or universal donor blood is justifiable in the following circumstances:

1. Exsanguinating hemorrhage with no or insufficient initial response to the rapid infusion of crystalloid volume expanders
2. Profound shock resulting from exsanguination in patients with cardiopulmonary, cerebral, or vascular disease
3. Profound shock from blood loss in infants and small children, due to their smaller blood volume
4. Any situation in which the typical additional delay of 20 to 30 min for crossmatched blood would further endanger the patient

The civilian use of type O universal donor blood is less widely practiced. Military experience in the use of group O PRBCs documents the safety of its use in a young male population. Nearly 0.25 million units were transfused in a 20-month period during the Vietnam conflict. Only 1 of the 24 hemolytic transfusion reactions resulting was due to something other than misidentification of donor blood. Smaller-scale civilian population studies have shown a small risk of transfusion reactions in previously transfused individuals and in parous women.

All the military studies utilized Rh-positive blood, since only men were transfused and large quantities of Rh-negative blood are unavailable. The civilian studies and most civilian practice call for the use of Rh-negative blood, since demand is far more episodic and local stores can more easily be replenished. In any case, whether one uses Rh-positive type O in men, Rh-negative in women, or Rh-negative in all patients requiring critically urgent transfusions, only PRBCs should be transfused so as to limit the volume of antibody-containing plasma transfused. Type-specific crossmatched PRBCs should be given as soon as available unless more than 4 units of universal donor blood has already been transfused.

Neither fluorocarbons nor pyridoxilated hemoglobin polymer have yet been shown to be effective substitutes for RBCs.

Autotransfusion

As practiced in the emergency unit, autotransfusion is the collection of shed blood from the thorax or peritoneal cavity and reinfusion into the same patient. Reinfusion of blood shed intraperitoneally is usually done with cell washing and antibiotic administration.

Hemothorax blood is drained through a chest tube, and then screen-filtered to remove gross clot and debris. CPD solution may be added, either by premeasurement or simultaneously with the collection of blood, to inhibit coagulation in the system. The blood may be reinfused through a micropore filter.

Autotransfusion provides a rapidly available, warm, type-specific source of blood for the patient in urgent need. Blood collected from the chest has functioning white cells and near-normal levels of all noncellular coagulation factors except fibrinogen. Platelets are apparently altered in the collection process, and those few which pass through the micropore filter do not function normally.

Complications of autotransfusion are rare and mostly dose-related. Reinfusion of less than 4000 mL of autotransfused blood is rarely associated with clinical complications. Hemoglobinemia and hemoglobinuria occur in various degrees after autotransfusions. In most reported series, they have not been associated with renal failure. Disseminated intravascular coagulation (DIC) has been a reported complication, and dilutional coagulopathy can result after autotransfusion of larger amounts.

Massive Transfusion

Massive transfusion is transfusion of one-half of the patient's blood volume at one time or transfusion of total blood volume in a 24-h period. Complications of massive transfusion are coagulopathies, hypothermia, adult respiratory distress syndrome (ARDS), hypocalcemia, and citrate toxicity. Coagulopathies can result from dilution of labile clotting factors and platelet destruction, and from DIC. However, the mathematics of exchange transfusion demonstrate that 37 percent of the circulating volume originally present is still present after a 10-unit transfusion of PRBCs and supplemental crystalloid.

The deficiencies of factors VIII and V present in all refrigerated blood are rapidly made up by liver-maintained stores. Even when huge quantities of blood are transfused, the liver will rapidly correct for dilution by rapid synthesis. Indeed, factors V and VIII are particularly well maintained, regardless of their depletion in refrigerated blood. Massively transfused patients with clinically significant bleeding and impaired hemostasis invariably have deficits much greater than can be explained by the dilution, and thus routine, "prophylactic" administration of FFP is unwarranted. However, a massively transfused and bleeding patient may well require supplementation with FFP.

Dilutional thrombocytopenia should be anticipated after transfusion of more than one blood volume in less than 6 h. Ten platelet packs should be given if continued transfusion is anticipated.

Cold blood can cause hypothermia, which increases the metabolic workload and depresses cardiac function. In massive transfusion, blood must be warmed as it is infused.

Microaggregates contained in refrigerated blood have been implicated in posttraumatic and posttransfusion adult respiratory distress syndrome. A dose-related effect has been postulated. Micropore filtration relieves the lung of the burden of removing microaggregates from the circulation.

Citrated blood infusion at rates greater than 1 mL/kg per minute is rarely associated with perioral tingling and carpopedal spasm. At greatest potential risk are infants and those with hepatic dysfunction.

Citrate chelates ionized calcium, and this effect continues until the citrate is metabolized. Myocardial depression has been demonstrated at ionized calcium levels one-third of normal. Total calcium levels are variable and in hemorrhagic shock are unreliable predictors of the need for calcium supplementation.

Calcium supplementation is not routinely necessary for massively transfused patients but could be considered for the patient who is not responding to adequate volume replacement or who has acute heart failure. Electrocardiographic monitoring of the QT interval is not useful in determining the need for calcium. When used, 5 to 10 mL of calcium gluconate should be given slowly intravenously at a site distant from the blood transfusion.

Immediate Transfusion Reactions

Immediate transfusion reactions are classified as febrile, allergic, and hemolytic.

Febrile Reactions

Febrile reactions, the most common reactions, are characterized by the development of fever, chills, and malaise. They rarely progress to hypotension or respiratory distress. Febrile reactions are thought to be the result of the infusion of platelets and leukocytes to which the recipient has antibodies. The use of leukocyte-poor blood or washed PRBCs for this type of reaction prevents its occurrence.

Once a febrile reaction is recognized, the transfusion should be terminated, since it is impossible to differentiate on clinical grounds between a simple febrile reaction and the more serious immediate intravascular hemolytic transfusion reaction. Anesthetized patients, infants incapable of shivering, and unconscious patients do not demonstrate, and obviously do not report, the symptoms of a febrile reaction. A search for RBC destruction (described below) should immediately ensue.

Allergic Reactions

True anaphylactic reactions to blood transfusion are rare, occurring approximately once in 20,000 transfusions. The genetically IgA-deficient recipient is most at risk. Patients with a history of multiple allergies should be carefully observed during transfusion. Patients with a history of previous allergic reaction to transfusion should be premedicated with antihistamines. Ideally, these patients should be given washed PRBCs or blood from IgA-deficient donors.

The treatment of immediate hypersensitivity reaction to blood is the same as the treatment of any anaphylactic reaction: epinephrine, fluids, and antihistamines. The transfusion should be stopped immediately.

Hemolytic Reactions

Intravascular hemolysis, the most serious immediate reaction, is most often the result of misidentification of patient, specimen, or blood unit. This antibody-mediated reaction results in the rapid destruction of transfused RBCs within minutes of administration. The resulting release of free hemoglobin produces hemoglobinemia, hemoglobinuria, depletion of haptoglobin, and subsequent elevation of the bilirubin level. Clinical manifestations include fever, chills, low back pain and other myalgias, and a burning sensation at the site of infusion and along the vein centrally. Later manifestations include a feeling of breathlessness or chest tightness, hypotension, and bleeding. Anesthetized and unconscious patients may manifest only hypotension, bleeding, and hemoglobinuria. The damaged RBCs activate complement, leading to DIC, renal failure, or respiratory failure.

Laboratory evaluation includes determination of haptoglobin and free hemoglobin in blood serum, hemoglobin in urine, direct and indirect Coombs' test, and coagulation and renal-function profiles. A quick, simple screen can be performed by saving a complete blood count tube and centrifuging it. A pale pink color suggests a free hemoglobin level of 50 to 100 mg/dL. A pale brown color may be evident at levels as low as 20 mg/dL. This "naked eye" screen does not supplant the need for full laboratory evaluation.

Treatment begins with discontinuing the current transfusion and instituting crystalloid infusion. Furosemide in 80- to 100-mg doses intravenously increases renal cortical blood flow and helps protect renal function. Mannitol, which increases urine flow by decreasing tubular absorption, does not improve renal blood flow and therefore should not be used. Large amounts of fluids must be administered to maintain intravascular volume. Urinary output should be maintained at 0.5 to 1.0 mL/kg per hour. Following central venous pressures or pulmonary capillary wedge pressures ensures that volume depletion is not mistaken for renal failure subsequent to the hemolytic transfusion reaction.

Delayed Reactions

Extravascular hemolysis is the commonest type of delayed transfusion reaction. An unexplained decrease in hemoglobin days after transfusion is the most common clinical manifestation of delayed extravascular hemolytic transfusion reactions. Transfused RBCs become coated by nonagglutinating antibodies and are removed by tissue-bound macrophages, primarily in the spleen.

Treatment includes fluid administration and redetermination of the transfusion compatibility of all blood units destined for transfusion to the patient. Blood specimens for the determination of hemoglobin, bilirubin, and haptoglobin levels help to differentiate between extravascular and intravascular hemolysis. Repeat searches for atypical antibodies may now reveal the presence of a previously undetected antibody as a result of the anamnestic immunologic response.

Infections

Infections resulting from blood transfusion include hepatitis, human immunodeficiency virus (HIV), HIV-2, HTLV-I, HTLV-II, cytomegalovirus (CMV), Epstein-Barr virus, syphilis, and malaria. Viral hepatitis is the most common and most severe infectious complication, occurring at a rate of 30,000 cases per year and resulting in perhaps 1500 to 3000 deaths annually.

Antibody to the hepatitis B virus can be tested for directly; however, the non-A, non-B hepatitis virus is not directly detectable by current screening methods. The use of indirect screening tests for blood units to determine the presence of chronically elevated liver enzymes, in particular alanine amino transferase (ALT), once widely debated, has been implemented because of the growing concern about the safety of the blood supply. The loss of 6 percent of the currently available units for transfusion has still further strained the already stressed blood supply system.

No therapeutic or prophylactic modality has been shown effective in avoiding posttransfusion hepatitis. Prophylactic administration of immune serum globulin may reduce the risk in patients receiving multiple transfusions, but extensive washing of red blood cells has not been useful.

Human immunodeficiency virus, the causative agent in acquired immunodeficiency syndrome (AIDS), and related retroviruses (HIV-2, HTLV-I, HTLV-II) have become a concern only in the last decade. The rapid development and implementation of serologic testing for HIV has been a major stride in control of disease transmission. All single-donor blood products transfused since 1985 have been screened by such tests. Since viremia is present prior to the development of antibody, not all infected units are excluded by testing. The continuing use of guidelines excluding donors at high risk, in conjunction with serologic testing, has reduced the risk of transmission of HIV to between 1 in 100,000 and 1 in 1,000,000. The next generation of assays, which will identify specific viral antigens of HIV in blood, will reduce the risk even further. Testing for antibody to HTLV-I, a leukemia virus, has recently been implemented and concern about transmission of a second AIDS virus (HIV-2) may lead to testing for its antibodies.

Cytomegalovirus and the Epstein-Barr virus can also be transmitted by transfusion. A serologic test for antibody to cytomegalovirus has been approved and is being implemented for screening. However, since most normal adults have antibody to CMV, units are not automatically screened and excluded from the blood supply. Rather, CMV seronegative units are sought and reserved for immunocompromised patients such as seronegative organ-transplant recipients, premature neonates, and seronegative pregnant women.

Syphilis may be transmitted by fresh, untested blood units, but this is rare since all banked blood is tested for its presence and *Treponema pallidum* will not survive in citrated blood for more than 2 or 3 days. Malaria is rarely transmitted since blood is not accepted from donors who have traveled in endemic areas 6 months prior to the donation or who have ever contracted the disease.

BIBLIOGRAPHY

Alter HJ, Purcell RH, Shih JW, et al: Detection of antibody to hepatitis C virus in prospectively followed transfusion recipients with acute and chronic non-A, non-B hepatitis. *N Engl J Med* 321:1494, 1989.

Barnes A: Transfusion of universal donor and uncrossmatched blood: Surgical hemotherapy. *Bibl Haematologica* 46:132, 1980.

Bove Jr: Transfusion-transmitted diseases: Current problems and challenges, in *Progress in Hematology*, vol XIV. New York, Grune and Stratton, 1986, pp 123–147.

Charache S: Problems in transfusion therapy. *N Engl J Med* 322:1666, 1990.

Clarke JR, Davidson SJ, Bergman GE, et al: Blood ordering for emergency department patients. *Ann Emerg Med* 9:2, 1980.

Collins JA: Current status of blood therapy in surgery. *Adv Surg* 22:75, 1989.

Jurkovich GJ, Moore EE, Medina G: Autotransfusion in trauma: A pragmatic analysis. *Am J Surg* 148:782, 1984.

Marsaglia G, Thomas ED: Mathematical consideration of cross circulation and exchange transfusion. *Transfusion* 11:216, 1971.

Mollison PL, Engelfriet CP, Contreras M: *Blood Transfusion in Clinical Medicine,* 8th ed. St. Louis, Blackwell, 1987.

Oberman H, Chaplin H, Polesky HF, et al (eds): *General Principles of Blood Transfusion*. Chicago, American Medical Association, 1985.

Shulman IA: Adverse reactions to blood transfusion. *Tex Med* 85:35, 1989.

144
EMERGENCY COMPLICATIONS OF MALIGNANCY

Daniel Esposito

The increasing prevalence of malignant disease and the escalating frequency of complications resulting from local tumor effects, as well as from the adverse effects of medical treatments, demand that the emergency physician be able to recognize potential life-threatening situations and initiate appropriate therapy. Most of the clinical problems are in themselves sufficient grounds for immediate hospitalization.

The widespread use of combination chemotherapy and radiotherapy in both inpatient and outpatient arenas underlies the likelihood of emergency department exposure to the hemorrhagic and infectious complications of myelosuppression. Many tumors produce similar syndromes by virtue of local compressive effects (spinal cord compression, upper airway obstruction, etc.). Other situations will be unique to certain tumors (e.g., the hyperviscosity syndrome of multiple myeloma-macroglobulinemia). The situations considered imminently life-threatening are outlined in Table 144-1 with the intention of correlating pathogenic mechanisms with acute local or systemic compromise. A listing of the more frequent associated malignancies will be presented with each subtopic.

ACUTE SPINAL CORD COMPRESSION

Multiple myeloma
Non-Hodgkin's and Hodgkin's lymphomas
Carcinoma of lung
Carcinoma of prostate
Carcinoma of breast

Spinal cord compression can result from bleeding, infection, or fracture. It may be the first sign of a neoplasm, or can complicate preexisting metastatic disease. The incidence is estimated at > 5 percent, and repeated occurrences in the same patient have been reported. Ischemic dysfunction of the spinal cord due to extrinsic compression occurs most commonly with multiple myeloma and lymphoma. It is uncommon and is generally suspected in individuals with previously documented malignancy who develop paraparesis, paraplegia, sensory deficits, or urinary incontinence. Spinal cord compression may also present as acute urinary retention. All patients with acute urinary retention should have a careful neurological examination, including assessment of reflexes, motor and sensory function, rectal sphincter tone, and gait, to rule out spinal cord compression. Pain localized to involved vertebrae may be present and intensified by local percussion during the physical examination. However, as is often the case in lymphomas, if lytic bony lesions are not present, local pain is absent and the patient may have only a sensory-level or distal flaccid paralysis. Hypoesthesia, lower extremity weakness, or gait disturbance are early symptoms and should alert the emergency physician. Early treatment may avert progression to paraplegia and prevent sphincter loss.

Table 144-1. Emergency Complications of Malignancy

RELATED TO LOCAL TUMOR COMPRESSION
1. Acute spinal cord compression
2. Upper airway obstruction
3. Malignant pericardial effusion with tamponade
4. Superior vena cava syndrome
RELATED TO BIOCHEMICAL DERANGEMENT AND SYSTEMIC COLLAPSE
1. Hypercalcemia of malignancy
2. Syndrome of inappropriate ADH (SIADH)
3. Hyperviscosity syndrome
4. Adrenocortical insufficiency with shock
RELATED TO MYELOSUPPRESSION AND INFECTION
1. Granulocytopenia and sepsis
2. Immunosuppression and opportunistic infections
3. Thrombocytopenia and hemorrhage
4. Anaphylaxis and transfusion reactions

The emergency physician's role includes not only suspicion and recognition of cord compression but also institution of measures to prepare the patient for potential emergency surgery. This would include assessment of fluid status, clotting parameters, anemia, and cardiorespiratory systems. CT scanning of the thoracolumbar spine may demonstrate the level of compression. Myelography is definitive. Decadron, 10 mg IV, or Solumedrol, 30 mg/kg IV, as recommended for acute traumatic spinal cord injury, should be given. Emergency surgical decompression or emergency radiotherapy is necessary to prevent irreversible neural damage.

UPPER AIRWAY OBSTRUCTION

Carcinoma of larynx
Thyroid carcinoma
Lymphoma
Metastatic lung carcinoma

Acute upper airway obstruction is generally associated with aspiration of foreign bodies or food elements, with epiglottis, or with other oropharyngeal infections. Malignancy-related obstruction to airflow is more insidious and often attended by voice change. This is generally a late manifestation of tumors arising in the oropharynx, neck, and superior mediastinum. Acute compromise is uncommon unless infection, hemorrhage, or inspissated secretions supervene. Rapidly growing tumors such as Burkitt's lymphoma and anaplastic carcinoma of the thyroid are capable of compromising airflow within weeks and should be suspected in afebrile individuals with laryngeal stridor and palpable anterior neck masses.

Fiberoptic or direct laryngoscopy is usually necessary to evaluate lumen size, as local anatomy is generally greatly distorted. Lateral soft-tissue x-rays are of value in assessing laryngotracheal patency. Establishment of an effective airway is primary and surgical tracheostomy may be required prior to the intitiation of radiotherapy.

MALIGNANT PERICARDIAL EFFUSION WITH TAMPONADE

Malignant melanoma
Hodgkin's lymphoma
Acute leukemia
Carcinoma of lung
Carcinoma of breast
Carcinoma of ovary
Radiation pericarditis

Malignant involvement of the pericardium may give rise to chronic cardiac tamponade by inducing the formation of hemorrhagic malignant effusions. The hemodynamic consequences of such effusions are a function of the volume as well as the rapidity of accumulation. Large collections (greater than 500 mL) may be well tolerated if development is slow. If sudden intrapericardial bleeding occurs, the emergency physician may be confronted with acutely ill individuals with hypotension and dyspnea. Malignant involvement of the myocardium may also be present and contribute to reduced cardiac output. Significant fluid accumulations can occur from radiotherapy-induced pleuropericarditis, most commonly in patients treated with mediastinal irradiation for Hodgkin's lymphoma.

The classical clinical features of cardiac tamponade include: (1) hypotension with narrow pulse pressure; (2) jugular venous distension; (3) diminished amplitude of heart sounds (quiet heart); (4) pulsus paradoxus of greater than 10 mmHg; (5) low QRS voltage on EEG; and (6) cardiomegaly on chest radiograph with obscuration of the cardiophrenic angles. Neck vein distension and hypotension in acutely ill patients can also occur with massive pulmonary embolism or acute superior vena caval obstruction and should be considered in the differential diagnosis.

Confirmation of the diagnosis is most readily obtained by echocardiography. Emergency percutaneous pericardiocentesis may be necessary and life-saving if profound vascular collapse is present. This may provide time for more definite treatment, such as pericardectomy, pericardial window surgery, radiotherapy, or intrapericardial chemotherapy. The risks of aggressive management must be weighed against the benefits of such treatment modalities in patients otherwise terminally ill from widespread metastases.

SUPERIOR VENA CAVA SYNDROME

Small-cell (oat-cell) carcinoma of lung
Squamous cell carcinoma of lung
Lymphoma

The superior vena cava syndrome is frequently a de novo diagnosis first established in the emergency department. A history of previously documented malignancy is often lacking and patients may seek medical attention because of the insidious and progressive nature of their symptoms. Obstruction to blood flow in the superior vena cava elevates venous pressure in the arms, neck, face, and cerebrum. Patients with moderate obstruction complain of headache, edema of the face and arms, or a nondescript feeling of head congestion and fullness in the neck and face. As venous pressure rises, intracranial pressure also rises and syncope may ensue. Critical intracranial pressure elevations are a true medical emergency and are usually associated with bilateral papilledema.

On physical examination, neck vein and upper chest vein distension may be apparent. Facial plethora and telangiectasia often are promient, but edema of the face and arms is generally subtle. Papilledema on fundoscopic examination indicates critical intracranial pressure and justifies early diuretic therapy. When tumefaction is located in the superior mediastinum, a palpable mass due to direct tumor extension can occasionally be appreciated in the supraclavicular space. Chest x-ray will demonstrate an enlarged mediastinum and possibly an isolated primary lesion in the lung parenchyma.

Prompt administration of diuretics and corticosteroids may help reduce venous pressure prior to initiation of mediastinal irradiation. Furosemide (Lasix), 40 mg intravenously, and methylprednisolone (Solumedrol), 80 to 120 mg intravenously, are frequently used to reduce intracerebral edema. In advanced disease radiotherapy to improve cardiodynamics is frequently necessary before tissue diagnosis can be obtained.

HYPERCALCEMIA OF MALIGNANCY

Multiple myeloma
Bony metastases from carcinoma of breast, prostate, or lung
Humoral-induced non-Hodgkin's lymphoma and adult T-cell lymphoma-leukemia

Mild elevations of serum calcium are well tolerated and produce little in the way of symptoms. However, when serum calcium levels rise rapidly or exceed ionic thresholds, cardiac, neural, and muscular electrophysiology may be greatly altered and sudden death can occur. A number of mechanisms have been identified that promote release of bony calcium into the circulation. Bony involvement with myeloma or carcinoma of the breast, prostate, or lung will release calcium by local matrix destruction. Squamous cell carcinoma of the lung may produce a parathormone-like substance, and an osteoclast activating factor has been associated with non-Hodgkin's lymphoma (diffuse histiocytic) and retrovirus adult T-cell lymphoma-leukemia.

Approximately 40 percent of patients with multiple myeloma will have hypercalcemia. An often encountered clinical triad includes back pain, constipation, and an insidious depression in the level of consciousness. Hypercalcemia from any cause may induce hypertension, constipation, and an altered sensorium. Elevated ionic (nonbound) calcium is responsible for neuromuscular dysfunction and therefore, serum calcium levels should be interpreted in concert with phosphorus, serum albumin, and blood pH determinations. The Q-T interval of the electrocardiogram may shorten as the serum calcium rises.

The majority of patients with malignancy-induced hypercalcemia will improve with saline infusion and intravenous furosemide (1 to 2 L saline load and 80 mg of IV furosemide). This will promote renal calcium excretion but depends upon adequate renal function and glomerular filtration. Because renal insufficiency is a common accompaniment in myeloma, assessment of blood urea nitrogen and creatinine levels is important to ensure both adequacy of response and avoidance of iatrogenic fluid overload. Hemoconcentration and dehydration may additionally aggravate elevating calcium. Short-term use of glucocorticoids may be life-saving in neoplastic hypercalcemia and should be used empirically in comatose or obtunded patients with serum calcium levels greater than 13. Mithramycin has been extremely effective in lowering serum calcium by reducing bone resorption. Doses of 15 to 25 μg/kg intravenously may rapidly reduce critical hypercalcemia.

SYNDROME OF INAPPROPRIATE ADH

Malignancy of the brain, lung, pancreas, duodenum, thymus, prostate
Lymphosarcoma

Ectopic secretion of antidiuretic hormone (ADH) may come from a variety of maligancies, but in any case the end result is the syndrome of inappropriate ADH (SIADH), which consists of serum hyponatremia, less than maximally dilute urine, excessive urine Na excretion (>30 mEq/L), and normal renal, adrenal, and thyroid functions. Treatment is aimed at removing the source of ADH secretion. Water restriction usually raises the serum sodium over a period of several days. The intravenous infusion of 100 to 250 mL of hypertonic saline solution (3 percent) may be necessary in the face of hyponatremic-induced seizures or cardiac arrhythmias.

HYPERVISCOSITY SYNDROME

Multiple myeloma
Waldenström's macroglobulinemia
Chronic myelocytic leukemia

Viscosity is the flow-resisting characteristic of fluids. Marked elevations in certain serum proteins will produce sludging and a reduction in microcirculatory perfusion. IgA myeloma components and IgG subtype 3 proteins have a tendency to polymerize, leading to symptomatic hyperviscosity. Macroglobulinemia is the most common cause for hyperviscosity by virtue of the high molecular weight and high intrinsic viscosity of IgM proteins. Serum viscosity relative to water is normally

1.4 to 1.8 and symptoms develop at viscosities greater than 5 times that of water.

Fatigue, headache, anorexia, and somnolence are early nonspecific symptoms. As blood flow slows, microthromboses may occur, with the advent of local symptoms such as deafness, visual disturbances, and jacksonian or generalized seizures. The diagnosis of hyperviscosity must be considered in the emergency department when patients with unexplained stupor or coma are found to have anemia, with rouleau formation on the peripheral blood smear. The most readily appreciated physical findings are in the ocular fundi and include "sausage-linked" retinal vessels, hemorrhages, and exudates. Laboratory evaluation should include coagulation, renal, and electrolyte profiles. Hypercalcemia can coincide, and when M-component protein concentrations are high, "factitious" hyponatremia due to the displacement phenomenon may also be present. A clue to the presence of hyperviscosity may be the laboratory's inability to perform chemical tests because of serum stasis in the analyzers, undoubtedly due to "too thick" blood. Serum viscosity and protein electrophoresis determinations are diagnostic.

The emergency physician's role is predominantly suspicion and recognition of the syndrome in patients with unexplained stupor and coma. Hyperviscosity is generally a presenting manifestation of certain plasma cell dyscrasias and a history of previously documented disease is often lacking. Initial therapy is rehydration followed by emergency plasmapheresis. When coma is present and the diagnosis rapidly established, a temporizing measure may be a two-unit phlebotomy with saline infusion and replacement of the patient's red cells.

The hyperviscosity syndrome associated with massive leukocytosis of chronic myelogenous leukemia is rheologically similar to the hyperviscosity syndrome of dysproteinemias. Altered mental status and vascular stasis occur because of white cell aggregation in the microcirculation. This is readily diagnosed from the complete blood count and white counts may be greater than several hundred thousand. The treatment consists of urgent leukapheresis and alkylating-agent chemotherapy.

ADRENAL INSUFFICIENCY AND SHOCK

Carcinoma of the lung
Carcinoma of the breast
Malignant melanoma
Retroperitoneal malignancies
Withdrawal of chronic steroid therapy

Adrenal insufficiency may be related to adrenal gland replacement by metastic tumors or to adrenocortical suppression by chronic therapeutic corticosteroid administration and its abrupt cessation. In either case, maximal adrenal function may be inadequate to support the individual when stressed by infection, dehydration, surgery, or trauma. Adrenal crisis and shock with vasomotor collapse may be sudden and fatal. The differential diagnosis of cancer patients with fever, dehydration, hypotension, and shock would more frequently include sepsis and hemorrhagic shock. Adrenal crisis is less common than bleeding and sepsis but empirically covered with intravenous corticosteroids.

Laboratory clues to the possible concomitant presence of adrenal insufficiency may be mild hypoglycemia, hyponatremia, hyperkalemia, and eosinophilia. Azotemia is, however, nonspecific and is often present in dehydration from any cause. In suspected cases, a serum cortisol should be drawn prior to steroid treatment.

Normal adrenal glands maximally produce approximately 300 mg per day of hydrocortisone when stressed. This has served as a guideline for replacement therapy. Adrenalectomized individuals are maintained on average doses of 35 to 40 mg of hydrocortisone per day and this is increased during potential stress. Appropriate emergency doses of hydrocortisone (Solucortef) would be 250 to 500 mg intravenously. Somewhat larger doses have been employed in septic shock.

GRANULOCYTOPENIA, IMMUNOSUPPRESSION, AND INFECTION

Overwhelming infection is a common cause of death in the immunocompromised host. A variety of factors may contribute to increased susceptibility to infection in cancer patients. Important factors include:

1. Malnutrition and cachexia
2. Granulocytopenia
3. Impaired humoral immunity and antibody production, as in chronic lymphocytic leukemia or multiple myeloma
4. Altered cellular immunity, as in Hodgkin's and other lymphomas
5. Postsplenectomy susceptibility to serious pneumococcal infections
6. Reactivation tuberculosis with concurrent corticosteroid therapy
7. Polymicrobial enteric sepsis from bowel organism entry; carcinoma of colon or mucosal damage from chemotherapy
8. Nosocomial infections transmitted through blood transfusion and blood products
9. Immunosuppression and myelosuppression of chemotherapy

Both the frequency of infection and the mortality rate increase significantly when the circulating granulocyte pool is below 1000 to 1500 per cubic millimeter. Cancer patients are at risk for a variety of bacterial, viral, and fungal infections. Frequently encountered infections include pneumococcal sepsis and pneumonia; *Staphylococcus aureus* infection; enteric gram-negative pneumonia or sepsis, including *Pseudomonas* infections; and localized or disseminated varicella zoster viral and cytomegaloviral infections. Immunosuppression predisposes to invasion by organisms that are normally held at bay by host defenses and biocompetition from normal body flora. Such opportunistic infections include *Pneumocystis carinii* pneumonia (protozoal), disseminated candidiasis, aspergillosis, cryptococcal meningitis, pulmonary nocardiosis, and histoplasmosis.

Fever in the presence of malignancy is often difficult to define on clinical grounds alone. The emergency physician should assume an infectious etiology and initiate appropriate laboratory studies and cultures. Life-treatening gram-negative sepsis with hypotension should be aggressively treated after appropriate cultures. Fluids, antibiotics, and intravenous corticosteroids are advised. The choice of antibiotics has been a subject of debate and is indeed becoming a medical subspecialty in itself. However, few bacterial organisms would be missed with regimens containing a second- or third-generation cephalosporin (cefazolin, cefoxitin, cefoperazone, cefotaxime) and an aminoglycoside (gentamicin, tobramycin, amikacin). Anaerobic coverage may be added (clindamycin) if peritonitis or abdominal symptomatology exists.

THROMBOCYTOPENIA AND HEMORRHAGE

Thrombocytopenia results from decreased bone marrow platelet production or increased peripheral destruction. Malignancy-associated thrombocytopenia is more commonly related to decreased production because of radiochemotherapeutic suppression (toxic myelophthisis), marrow replacement with tumor cells (malignant myelophthisis), or infectious suppression. Platelets may be rapidly destroyed in the peripheral blood when disseminated intravascular coagulation complicates malignancy. Autoimmune peripheral platelet destruction has commonly accompanied chronic lymphocytic leukemia and the lymphomas. Hypersplenism may also contribute to decreased platelet survival.

Spontaneous bleeding can occur when the platelet count is below 10,000 per cubic millimeter. The most frequent sites of hemorrhage are the gastrointestinal and genitourinary tracts; however, epistaxis may be a severe and significant management problem in the emergency department. Central nervous system hemorrhage may produce focal neural deficits or catastrophic decerebration. (See Chapters 140–142 on bleeding disorders.)

BIBLIOGRAPHY

Balducci L, Parker M, Sexton W, et al: Pharmacology of antineoplastic agents in the elderly patient. *Seminars in Oncology* 16:76, 1989.

Ebie N, Ryan W, Harris J: Metabolic emergencies in cancer medicine. *Med Clin North Am* 70:1151, 1986.

Ehrke MJ, Mihich E, Berd D, et al: Effects of anticancer drugs on the immune system in humans. *Seminars in Oncology* 16:230, 1989.

Oncologic emergencies. *Seminars in Oncology*. 16:461, 1989. (Entire issue is devoted to oncologic emergencies).

Tintinalli JE: Acute urinary retention as a presenting sign of spinal cord compression. *Ann Emerg Med* 16:1235, 1986.

SECTION 14
Neurology

145
THE NEUROLOGICAL EXAMINATION

Gregory L. Henry

The individual components of the nervous system can be easily tested and analyzed in a simple but structured fashion. It is common for the less organized examiner to spend a vast amount of time and yet obtain little information. The object of this discussion is to lay the groundwork for the diagnosis and treatment of neurological problems in the emergency department.

A systematic approach for performing the neurological examination must be accompanied by an equally thorough method for recording the examination findings. It is not adequate to write, "Neuro within normal limits." The pertinent positive and negative findings should be recorded on the chart, with degree of elaboration depending on the patient's chief complaint.

The press of patient care duties in the emergency department mandates that the basic areas of examination be approached quickly and directly. Further tests in any specific area should be prompted by positive findings.

The object of the neurological examination is to answer two questions: "Where is it?" and "What is it?" The first question usually refers to the level of the nervous system involvement: peripheral nerve, spinal cord, cerebellum, brainstem, or cerebral hemisphere. A disease can involve a number of these areas, and a patient can have more than one disease, so that all data must be synthesized before any conclusions are reached. For example, the chronically demented patient is the one most likely to fall and develop an acute subdural hematoma. The answer to the question "Where is it?" is obtained chiefly by objective data from the neurological examination.

The question "What is it?" is asked to determine the mechanism by which the nervous system is being compromised. As a general rule, this question is best answered by history.

HISTORY

Entities with rapid onset in seconds to minutes and with distinct neurological signs and symptoms are almost invariably vascular in nature. Such vascular events may be large, with huge deficits at the onset, or may represent multiple small infarcts with accumulation of deficits which lead to more and more progressive neurological decline.

The nervous system, however, frequently has warning that a vascular catastrophe is imminent. The transient ischemic attack is such a warning signal. Transient ischemic attacks should be viewed as prestroke lesions and treated aggressively as an emergency medical problem.

A history obtained from family and friends is essential to determine the patient's premorbid level of function. It is not adequate to ask the family if the patient was "all right" prior to presentation to the emergency department. Many families have an unusual perception of what normal mental status and function is, and these perceptions must be carefully determined. It is helpful to have a family member in the room with the patient to assist in monitoring the veracity of the patient's statements. Most patients with a history of progressive downhill function over weeks to years are affected with degenerative disease or some chronic dementing process. If the patient has had a slow downhill course with little change in mental status, it is unlikely that a definitive diagnosis will be made in the emergency department. The emergency physician should always beware of the patient with mild to moderate CNS impairment who presents with sudden deterioration over 2 or 3 days. Such a patient is a prime candidate for a subdural hematoma, CNS infection, dehydration, or some other toxic metabolic condition, including overmedication. Patients with rapidly fluctuating, nonfocal neurological signs should be considered to have a primarily metabolic insult until proved otherwise.

Multiple sclerosis is, as always, nebulous and difficult to diagnose. There is no definitive test for this disease, but it may be suspected in patients who have rapidly changing multiple focal neurological findings which are unrelated to a specific anatomic site.

SCREENING EXAMINATION

A basic neurological screening examination should be employed for all patients with general neurological complaints. It consists of evaluating six areas: (1) mental status, (2) cranial nerves, (3) motor response, (4) sensory response, (5) coordination (cerebellar function and gait), and (6) reflexes. Each area is described below, and the areas evaluated and tests employed are summarized in Table 145-1.

Mental Status

Examination of mental status is performed simply by speaking with the patient. In the emergency department detailed tests for hemispheric function are not necessary in a patient who is conversing normally, is making reasonable responses to questions, and is well oriented. Anything more than observation of simple speech, reasoning power, and normal communications skills is out of the realm of a screening examination. If subtle mental status changes are suspected, more involved testing is required. The brain is divided into a right and left half. In the vast majority of human beings, the left-sided brain is dominant. Dominant functions include speech, mathematical ability, and certain other communications skills. It is more difficult to test nondominant hemisphere functions. The nondominant hemisphere is involved with spatial orientation, sound localization, and body self-image. Specific tests for these areas need be performed only if initial screening evaluation reveals difficulties.

Table 145-1. Neurological Screening Examination

Area	Test
Mental status	Normal orientation, speech
Cranial nerves	Funduscopic, extraocular movements and pupillary response, visual fields, corneal reflexes, and facial muscular strength
Motor	Four basic muscle groups, tone, drift, heel-and-toe walking
Sensory	Cold and vibration on areas indicated by patient or on distal extremities
Coordination (gait)	Observation of gait, and finger-to-nose testing
Reflexes	Deep tendons—knees, ankles, elbows, and wrists; degenerative reflexes—Babinski's signs, snout, grasp, and root

Cranial Nerves

Tests for intact brainstem function are concerned chiefly with the second through seventh cranial nerves.

Mass lesions that are causing pressure either directly or indirectly on the diencephalon can alter the visual fields and pupillary response to light. Insidious tumors of the cerebral hemispheres which may have very few gross neurological findings, can cause early changes in the visual fields. An intact pupillary response to light requires both reception by the second cranial nerve and motor outflow from the third cranial nerve. Visual fields can be tested simply by having the patient look at the examiner's nose from an arm's length distance. With both arms extended and the elbows at right angles, the examiner quickly flicks both index fingers at the same time. The patient is then asked which finger moved. If the patient responds that both fingers moved, gross bitemporal lesions can be eliminated. This test should be performed to evaluate all four quadrants of vision.

Midbrain and pontine dysfunction can be detected by following extraocular movements. The extraocular muscles are innervated by the third, fourth, and sixth cranial nerves. The nuclei for these nerves cover a large area in the pons and midbrain, making them good indications of brainstem function. The patient is asked to follow the examiner's light into the six cardinal positions of gaze, making sure that the eyes are put through the full range of motion. The patient can also be observed simultaneously for nystagmus. Any abnormal findings should prompt a more detailed examination.

The fifth cranial nerve has extensive motor and sensory functions. The corneal reflex is often affected in hemispheric disease long before general facial sensation or the muscles of mastication are involved. Corneal sensation is tested by lightly touching the cornea with a small wisp of cotton. To do this, the patient must look opposite to the direction from which the examiner approaches. Scleral or lid response does not count, and only by touching the cornea can this sensation be tested. Unilateral depression of the corneal reflex is objective evidence of intracranial disease.

Seventh nerve function is commonly tested by having a patient smile or show the teeth. While considerable emphasis has been placed on the significance of asymmetry of the nasolabial folds, many people have slight asymmetry. A better test for facial strength is to ask the patient to squeeze the eyes tightly, and observe the degree to which the eyelashes are buried. Then, try to open the patient's eyes against such resistance. Another test is to have the patient purse the lips as in a whistle. Upper motor neuron lesions are characterized by unilateral weakness of the lower half of the face, while peripheral lesions involve the entire half of the face.

The eighth cranial nerve rarely requires testing in the emergency department unless there are specific complaints related to vertigo or hearing difficulties. Whenever questions with regard to the eighth cranial nerve function are raised, tests of both the vestibular and cochlear portions of the nerve are necessary. Speech reception testing by whispering numbers and words, as well as tuning fork evaluation for both the standard Weber and Rinne responses, is usually sufficient to separate out gross hearing abnormalities.

Tests for the ninth, tenth, eleventh, and twelfth cranial nerves are not important in the emergency department. There are no acute diseases which will manifest themselves with findings only in these areas, and in a rapid neurological screening examination they are of little value. Lower cranial nerve testing is important, however, if screening examination findings are referable to other cranial nerves.

Motor Response

Evaluation of general muscle strength, tone, and symmetry is the objective of the screening examination. Have the patient lie on the back so that the legs and arms can be observed. To check tone, quickly lift the knee off the cot and observe the actions of the foot. The normal response is to drag the heel along the bed as the knee is quickly jerked upward. If the leg comes up as a single unit, tone is probably increased. Gross bulk is estimated by observing the muscles of the calf and upper arm for mass, asymmetry, or fasciculations.

As a general rule, muscles essential in maintaining the body's normal posture have bilateral innervation and are less useful for determining lateralized weakness. In the upper extremities, the dorsiflexors of the wrist and the extensors of the forearm at the elbow have sufficiently uncrossed fibers to be useful in examination. In the lower extremities, evaluation of the dorsiflexors of the great toe and the flexors of the lower leg at the knee is all that is required to get a general idea of focal weakness.

An extremely sensitive indicator of focal weakness is testing for drift. In this examination, the patient is asked to extend both arms in front of the body, with the palms up and eyes closed. The patient is then carefully observed to see if there is any movement of one arm downward while the eyes remain closed. This test can be especially helpful in the minimally cooperative patient who is exhibiting give-way weakness on specific muscle testing. Another exceptionally good test for gross strength is to have the patient walk on the heels and then on the toes. This requires intact muscular strength.

Sensory Response

Testing sensation is the least exacting and least informative part of the neurological screening examination. If the patient has an area of decreased sensation, it is probably best to have the patient outline that area before attempting to isolate the lesion. If a definitive nerve root or peripheral nerve is outlined, direct testing for sensation should confirm the diagnosis.

A much more useful system in the emergency department is to think of sensory and motor loss in terms of patterns. Whenever sensation is found to be lacking in the "stocking/glove" distribution, peripheral nerve lesions should be considered. Loss of either motor or sensory response in the upper extremities and across the chest in a cloak or capelike distribution is often associated with lesions in the spinal column. Syringomyelia, a degenerative disease process, may present in such a fashion. More important to the emergency physician is that traumatic central cord syndrome of the cervical cord may likewise present with a capelike distribution. Loss of all sensation below a specific vertebral level defines a spinal cord injury. A mixed picture may be seen with only partial cord involvement, as in the Brown-Séquard syndrome. Loss of sensation on one side of the body or the other denotes a lesion high in the central nervous system before entering into brainstem structures. Areas of alternating hemianesthesia or hemiplegia, that is, facial findings on one side and lower body findings on the opposite side, always indicate a lesion in the brainstem itself.

In the patient who does not have a specific sensory complaint, testing with a cold stethoscope, reflex hammer, or tuning fork is probably as accurate as any other method. Remember that sensory loss confined to one-half of the body usually involves a CNS lesion and most often is a hemispheric problem. If there is some decrease in response to vibratory sensation or hot and cold in either the hands or the feet, compare the lower extremities with each other, and against the upper extremities. Peripheral neuropathies tend to be symmetrical and show increasing sensation as one moves proximally along the limb. In symmetrical metabolic peripheral neuropathies there should be approximately the same level of nerve loss in both lower and upper extremities, and the legs tend to be involved earlier than the hands and arms.

The Romberg test requires explanation. A properly performed Romberg examination should be done with the patient standing and unsupported by any aids. With the feet together and arms at the side, the patient is asked to stand with the eyes open. If a patient cannot stand with the eyes open, the problem is usually related to one of cerebellar coordination. If the patient is able to stand with the eyes open but has difficulty in holding this position with the eyes closed, the problem is not one of coordination but one of sensation, with abnormality in position sense. This usually indicates involvement of posterior column function or may be seen as an isolated finding or as part of a general peripheral neuropathy.

Coordination (Gait)

This part of the neurological examination is frequently referred to as *cerebellar testing*. In truth, it is difficult to isolate the cerebellum because many areas are responsible for coordinating motor activity. Observing the patient's stance and gait is useful for testing both motor function and coordination. A broad-based, unsteady gait suggests cerebellar dysfunction. Patients with midline cerebellar lesions may have difficulty sitting up in bed without help. One good test for peripheral cerebellar lesions is finger-to-nose testing. Ask the patient to be precise, and to touch the tip of your finger to the tip of his or her nose in rapid sequence. Development of oscillation the last few inches before touching the target is abnormal. Hysterical patients commonly produce wide oscillations from the moment they begin the motor task, or always touch precisely off the target.

Reflexes

Both deep tendon and regressive reflexes can be rapidly tested. Asymmetry of response is the significant finding. The patient with brisk reflexes in all extremities, and no other signs of neurological disease, probably has a normal variant. Likewise, the patient who essentially has no deep tendon reflexes without other neurological findings is probably exhibiting a baseline state. A change, however, in the threshold required to elicit a reflex or clonus on one side of the body suggests a lateralizing lesion high in the CNS. A difference in reflexes between the arms and the legs suggests a lesion involving the spinal cord. Depression of reflexes in only one limb, while the other is symmetrical, is consistent with a root or peripheral nerve lesion. The various reflexes and their nerve roots of innervation are listed in Fig. 145-1.

Pathological reflexes, such as Babinski's reflex and snout, root, and grasp reflexes, indicate a lack of inhibition from higher cortical centers to primitive stereotype responses. Babinski's reflex, which is elicited by stroking the lateral aspect of the foot, is the most commonly used,

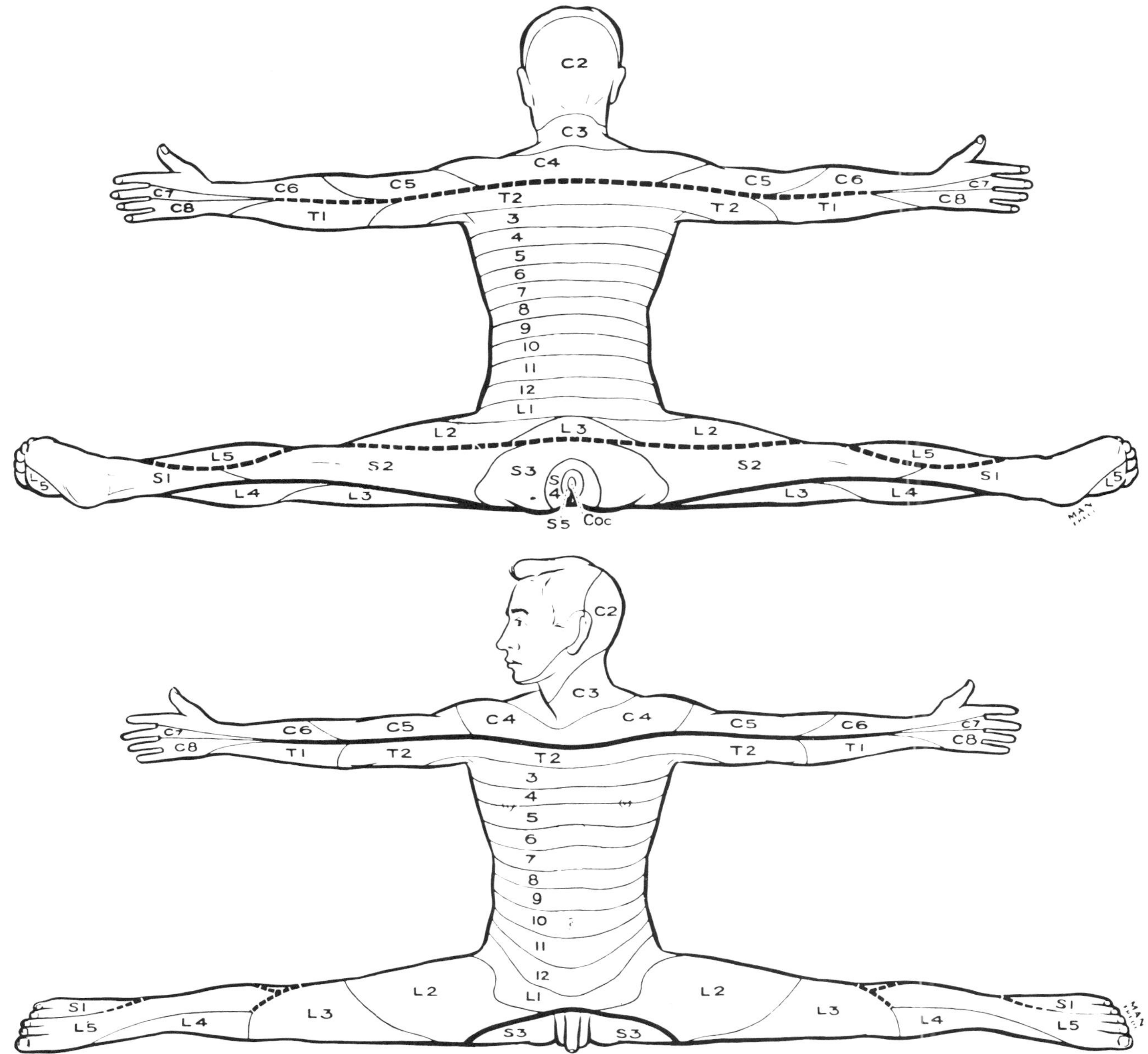

Fig. 145-1. Nerve root origin of various reflexes. (From Haymaker W, Woodhall B: *Peripheral Nerve Injuries: Principles of Diagnosis*, 1st ed. Philadelphia, Saunders, 1945, p. 16. Used by permission.)

Table 145-2. Diagnostic Neurological Tests Correlated with Specific Abnormal Neurological Complaints

Presenting Signs, Symptoms	Accessory Tests	Presenting Signs, Symptoms	Accessory Tests
Confusion, delirium, paucity of affect	Basic neurological examination plus: Formal mental status testing Aphasia testing Psychological testing Thought process and content evaluation (remember that the patient with decreased affect may be psychologically depressed, so try to obtain a measure of thought content) Snout, grasp, root, Babinski's reflexes Physical examination of head, supple neck	Dizziness	Basic neurological examination plus: Orthostatic vital signs taken on both arms Enough history should be taken to divide the patient into those with: Vertigo—positional and cold water caloric testing Syncope—cardiac examination, ECG, perhaps in-house monitoring
Blurred, dim, absent, or double vision	Basic neurological examination plus: Visual acuity and light perception Optokinetic nystagmus—in blindness Red glass testing—diplopia Careful fundoscopic examination Careful auscultation of head and eyes	Coma	Completely separate examination: Level of consciousness Respirations Doll's eye movements or caloric testing Pupillary responses Motor responses and general physical examination
Headache	Basic neurological examination plus: Auscultation of head and neck Careful palpation of the head and neck, particularly the temporal arteries; hypertension	Trauma	Coma: go directly to coma protocol Awake: do limited examination Fine-motor movements Drift Do not put patients through major testing until cervical spine x-ray films are reviewed; the ABCs (airway, breathing, and circulation) precede all else in traumatized patients
Focal weakness	Basic neurological examination plus: Systematic testing of each nerve root or peripheral nerve involved in both motor and sensory function Hemispheric testing	Back pain without history of direct trauma	Basic neurological examination, plus: Straight-leg raising Anal wink Expanded motor, sensory, reflex examinations Gait
Nonfocal weakness	Basic neurological examination plus: Test for muscle fatigue, including lid lag and drift (suspect myasthenia gravis, Lambert-Eaton syndrome, alcoholic myopathy)		

and is a good lateralizing sign. The presence of snout, root, and grasp reflexes indicates diffuse, bilateral hemispheric disease.

Depending on the chief complaint of the patient and positive findings in the neurological examination, a more thorough examination may be necessary. Some aspects of such an examination require special training, but frequently you can further delineate the patient's problems by just a few simple testing procedures. Listed in Table 145-2 are various presenting complaints and the accessory tests that can aid the emergency physician in making a diagnosis.

BIBLIOGRAPHY

DeJong RN: Case taking and the neurological examination, in Baker AB, Baker LH: *Clinical Neurology*. Hagerstown, Harper & Row, 1977, vol 1, chap 1, pp 1–83.

Henry G, Little N: *Acute Neurologic Emergencies: A Symptom Oriented Approach*. New York, McGraw-Hill, 1985.

Plum F, Possner JB: *The Diagnosis of Stupor and Coma*, 3rd ed. Philadelphia, Davis, 1980.

Schaffner MH, Jelenko C III: Rapid orthopedic and neurologic evaluation. *Ann Emerg Med* 9:103, 1980.

Weiner HL, Levitt LD: *Neurology for the House Officer*, 2nd ed. Baltimore, Williams & Wilkins, 1978.

146 HEADACHE

Gwendolyn L. Hoffman

Headache is a common presenting complaint to the emergency department. Approximately 40 percent of all Americans have a significant headache at some time, with 10 percent of the population seeing a physician episodically for headaches. The pain can originate extracranially from the skin, fat, muscle, blood vessels, periosteum, and fascial planes of the neck. It can also originate intracranially, from the great venous sinuses, their tributaries, the dura at the base of the skull, the dural arteries, the falx cerebri, and the large arteries at the base of the brain, all of which have pain fibers. Actual brain parenchyma, most of the dura, the arachnoid, and the pia mater are incapable of producing painful stimuli. The fifth cranial nerve is responsible for pain arising from above the tentorium and serves most of the facial areas. The ninth, tenth, and eleventh cranial nerves and upper cervical spinal nerves serve the region below the tentorium; pain is often referred to the neck and back of the head.

The pain-sensitive structures of the head and neck are affected by the following pain-producing mechanisms: distension, dilation, inflammation, tension, and traction. The emergency physician must distinguish serious and life-threatening presentations from those that are less serious. This is best accomplished by a directed history and physical examination supported by ancillary testing.

CLINICAL EVALUATION

History

Basically three categories of headache patients will present to the emergency department.

1. The chronic headache patient who has been thoroughly evaluated and presents for pain control with no change in the headache pattern.
2. The person who has never been evaluated and presents with a first severe headache.
3. The patient with prior history of evaluated headaches who now presents with a change in the quality and intensity or character of the headache.

No matter what category the patient is in, a determination of the time, location, and quality of the pain must be made.

Time. One of the most important things to determine is the speed of onset. A sudden onset of severe headache, especially associated with other symptoms, is suggestive of a serious illness such as subarachnoid hemorrhage. Any preceding event such as strenuous exercise or sexual intercourse should be noted. The regularity and length of the headaches, associated with any prodromal symptoms, and correlation with food, drugs, and menstrual cycle should be noted.

Location. The site of the headache may also be helpful in diagnosis. Approximately two-thirds of migraine headaches are unilateral. Tension headaches may be bilateral or circumferential. A headache always in the same location may be suggestive of a mass lesion.

Quality. A throbbing, pulsatile headache tends to be of vascular origin with dilation of extracranial arteries. The blood running through the arteries causes them to distend, exacerbating the pain. A deep, piercing, intense unilateral pain is often seen with cluster headaches. A transient shocklike pain in the distribution of the fifth cranial nerve is seen with trigeminal neuralgia.

Physical Examination

Hypertension is usually seen with subarachnoid hemorrhage. Tachycardia may be seen with severe pain. Tachypnea is possible with headaches associated with anoxia, such as carbon monoxide poisoning. Fever may indicate meningitis, brain abscess, or encephalitis.

In funduscopic examination, spontaneous venous pulsations as viewed in the upright patient indicate normal intracranial pressure. This is an important finding especially if later lost. Papilledema indicates increased intracranial pressure. Subhyaloid or preretinal hemorrhages are diagnostic of subarachnoid hemorrhage. Acute hemorrhages and exudates may be seen with hypertensive encephalopathy.

Palpation of the head conveys a sense of thoroughness to the patient. In addition the finding of tenderness may be related to trauma or muscle spasm. Tenderness in the temporal arteries is important in the elderly since it may indicate temporal arteritis. Tenderness in the areas of the sinuses, teeth, and fifth cranial nerve may also be helpful in making a diagnosis.

Stiffness indicates irritation of the meninges. To check for it the patient should be relaxed and in the supine position. With the patient relaxed, the examiner flexes the neck to determine whether there is involuntary resistance.

A sensitive sign of unilateral weakness is ''drift'' in one of the outstretched, palm-up arms of the patient. Abnormal gait, inability to touch finger to nose, and tandem walk may be the only clues to a posterior fossa mass.

Ancillary Tests

CT scanning has replaced the skull x-ray for diagnostic evaluation. It can discover, define, and locate any causative lesion, and is approximately 90 percent accurate in locating subarachnoid blood.

Lumbar puncture is necessary to identify intracranial infection, or to detect subarachnoid blood not evident on CT scanning. Magnetic resonance imaging (MRI), visual evoked potential, and noninvasive transcranial Doppler ultrasound are not emergency department tests, but may be required for elective evaluation.

The laboratory studies ordered will depend on the clinical differential diagnosis. For example, a CBC may be ordered if meningitis is suspected, or an ESR if temporal artery dysfunction is suspected.

PATHOPHYSIOLOGY

Based on the mechanism by which pain is produced, headache may be classified into four categories: (1) vascular, (2) muscular contraction and traction, (3) inflammatory, and (4) those due to idiopathic cranial neuralgias. Those due to idiopathic cranial neuralgias are not associated with pathologic changes.

Vascular Headaches

Migraine Headaches

Migraine syndromes are characterized by recurrent attacks of headache that vary widely in intensity, frequency, and duration. Attacks tend to be unilateral. They may be associated with anorexia, nausea, and vomiting, and are often familial. Chocolate, nuts, cheese, alcohol, or monosodium glutamate may precipitate them as well as air pollution, perfumes, fatigue, stress, oversleeping, and use of vasodilators. They may be preceded by or associated with neurologic and mood disturbances. Women are affected slightly more than men with a definite relationship to the menstrual period. The attacks often begin in childhood but may not start until after puberty.

The underlying etiology of all migrainous attacks is the same. First, there is vasoconstriction of the intracranial arteries resulting in reduced cerebral blood flow. This can be caused by neurogenic factors such as stress, causing spasm of the cerebral arteries, or systemically by serotonin, causing vasoconstriction of the innervated vascular system. This results in an aura, the type of which is dependent on the area of ischemia. Serotonin absorbed by blood vessels and tissues interacts with other vasoactive substances such as histamine, tyramine, bradykinins, free fatty acids, and prostaglandins to produce sterile perivascular inflammation. Metabolism of the serotonin causes a rapid drop in blood serotonin with a rebound effect of vasodilation of the arteries and constriction of the capillary vessels. The combination of the arterial distension and inflammation gives rise to the pain.

Types of Migraine

Classic Migraine

This pattern occurs in approximately 15 percent of patients with migraine and is characterized by a sharply defined prodrome lasting up to 60 min. The symptoms are usually constant in a given patient but vary among patients. The most common symptoms are visual, including scintillating scotoma and homonymous hemianopsia and photophobia. Tingling of the lips, face, or hands, extremity weakness; or mild aphasia may occur. Nausea and vomiting occur at the peak of the throbbing headache, which usually lasts 6 to 12 h.

Common Migraine

This is the most frequent migraine syndrome and accounts for 80 percent of vascular headaches. In contrast to classic migraine there are no sharply defined neurologic symptoms. Vague prodromes such as irritability may precede the slowly evolving headache by hours or days. In addition to a positive family history, two of the following should be present: nausea with or without vomiting, unilateral pain, throbbing quality, photophobia, and increase with menses.

Ophthalmoplegic Migraine

Ophthalmoplegic migraine, which is usually seen in young adults, is relatively rare. The third cranial nerve, followed by the sixth and fourth is usually involved. The patient presents with a dilated outwardly deviated eye with ptosis. The pain is moderate in intensity and ipsilateral with the ophthalmoplegia.

Hemiplegic Migraine

Hemiplegic migraine is uncommon. It is characterized by unilateral motor and sensory symptoms ranging from mild hemiparesis to full hemiplegia. The symptoms may persist longer than the headache and should be a diagnosis of exclusion.

Cluster Headache

This type of headache is seen in males, predominantly in middle adulthood. It consists of unilateral intense ocular or retroocular pain lasting less than 2 h but occurring several times a day for periods of weeks to months. There is facial flushing, forehead sweating, lacrimation, rhinorrhea, and conjunctival injection on the side of the pain. An associated ipsilateral Horner's syndrome can also be seen. The pain is incapacitating, with the patient pacing, rocking, and holding his head. The headache may follow the ingestion of alcohol or the use of histamine-containing compounds. The pathogenesis of the pain is not clearly understood but may be the result of vasoactive substances released from mast cells.

Treatment

For the treatment of migraine one must consider general, abortive, acute, and preventive measures.

General treatment consists of avoiding identifiable triggering factors such as chocolate and alcohol.

Abortive treatment is accomplished by giving ergotamines. The best absorbed route of administration is by inhalation or rectally. Ergotamines are contraindicated in patients with peripheral vascular disease, hypertension, coronary artery disease, and pregnancy. Dihydroergotamine, 1 mg given parenterally, is as effective as ergotamine and does not cause peripheral arterial constriction. Two other agents, propranolol (40 to 120 mg over 24 h) and the nonsteroidal antiinflammatory agent (NSAIA) naproxen (750 to 1250 mg over 24 h), have been effective for abortive treatment.

For acute treatment of nausea, vomiting, and dehydration, sedatives, antiemetics, and rehydration are indicated. Prochlorperazine, 5 mg, followed by dihydroergotamine, 0.75 mg IV, can be given over a period of 2 to 3 min. Dihydroergotamine, 0.5 mg, can be repeated in 30 min if needed. However, ergotamines should not be given if there are neurologic defects such as scotomata hemiplegia, aphasia, etc. Prochlorperazine edesylate, 10 mg IV, has been found to relieve pain as well as nausea and vomiting. If the attack is prolonged (status migrainosus), dexamethasone, 8 to 10 mg IV, is helpful and lessens the need for narcotics. Finally, a narcotic such as meperidine, combined with an antiemetic, may be necessary. Ketorolac, a new parenteral NSAIA, may be tried, although its effectiveness has not been established.

Preventive treatment is indicated for those with debilitating headaches who do not respond to abortive therapy. β Blockers, in particular propranolol, atenolol, timolol, metaprolol, and nadolol, are useful. Calcium channel blockers are effective and also relieve the prodromal symptoms. Nimodipine, verapamil, and nifedepine have the most success. Serotonin antagonists such as cyproheptadine and methysergide are effective. However, methysergide is not a drug of choice due to its potential serious side effects. Tricyclics, especially amitriptyline, nortriptyline, and doxypen, reduce the frequency and duration of headaches. Nonpharmacologic therapies such as biofeedback, behavioral counseling, and transcutaneous electrical nerve stimulation alone or with drugs have had varied success. Also, MOA-inhibiting antidepressants, particularly phenelzine, can be effective. Nonsteroidal antiinflammatory agents, especially naproxen, are also effective in prevention.

The treatment for cluster headaches is similar to that for other migraines, although β blockers are not used. Additionally, lithium carbonate and prednisone are helpful preventive measures. Inhalation of 100% oxygen has been helpful during an acute attack. Instillation of 5 to 10% cocaine solution or 4% lidocaine solution into the ipsilateral nostril is also effective.

Nonmigrainous Vascular Headaches

These nonrecurrent, throbbing headaches are not associated with specific functional losses. Presenting symptoms may be similar to those in a migrainous attack, but the pain is bicranial rather than unicranial.

Toxic Metabolic Headaches

Toxic metabolic headaches are caused by vasodilatation of the pain-sensitive arteries often combined with a lowering of the pain threshold by the toxic metabolic substance itself.

Fever greater than 102°F (38.8°C) is the most common cause. Tyramine-containing foods such as ripe cheeses, as well as foods containing monosodium glutamate and sodium nitrate, may precipitate toxic metabolic headaches. Toxic metabolic headaches can also occur with withdrawal from vasoconstricting beverages such as coffee, tea, and cola. The classic alcohol-related hangover headache results from the breakdown of ethanol to acetaldehyde, a potent vasodilator.

Common medications such as oral contraceptives, indomethacin, and nitroglycerin can result in headache. Insulin-dependent diabetics may experience a throbbing headache as an early symptom of hypoglycemia.

Hypoxia and hypercapnia are both potent cerebral vasodilators. Carbon monoxide produces cellular hypoxia with headache presenting when carboxyhemoglobin levels are greater than 20 percent. High-altitude headaches may occur in nonacclimated mountain climbers at 10,000 to 12,000 feet above sea level.

After a generalized seizure, postictal distension of the vasculature with resultant headache may occur. The patient may identify this as a part of the usual postictal state, but if the pain is described as being different from what is usually experienced, further investigation is needed.

Acute anemia secondary to blood loss can result in headache due to vasodilation and a relative oxygen deficiency.

Definitive treatment of most toxic metabolic headaches is removal of the cause with analgesic supplementation as needed.

Hypertensive Headaches

These throbbing occipital headaches do not generally occur until the diastolic pressure exceeds 130 mmHg. Hypertension is an overdiagnosed cause of headaches, but if the headache is due to hypertension, control of the blood pressure with appropriate antihypertensive agents will alleviate the headache.

Muscular Contraction and Traction Headaches

Tension Headaches

Muscular contraction headaches are characterized by sustained contraction of the deep neck muscles and muscles of mastication. They are associated with constant, nonthrobbing, viselike bilateral pain with focal areas of pain in the bioccipital regions, the bitemporal region, and the vertex of the head. On examination there will be scalp tenderness as well as muscle spasms of involved muscles. Treatment consists of mild analgesics such as acetaminophen and aspirin. Relaxation techniques and biofeedback are also helpful. If the headache becomes chronic in nature, amitriptyline is helpful.

Traction Headaches

Traction headaches are secondary to direct pressure, traction, or displacement of pain-sensitive structures, especially blood vessels.

Mass Lesions

Mass lesions can be in the subdural and epidural spaces or in the brain parenchyma itself.

Subdural hematoma is characterized by depression of mental status out of proportion to focal findings with a headache of variable quality. A chronic subdural hematoma is often seen in the elderly after previous forgotten minor injury; it may also be atraumatic. Patients with an acute subdural hematoma are often too obtunded to complain of headache. Diagnosis is by CT scanning followed by neurosurgical consultation.

Epidural hematoma may progress to uncal herniation. There is usually a history of trauma and a brief episode of unconsciousness, followed by consciousness with headache. There is usually a fracture line through the middle meningeal groove. Diagnosis is by CT scan with an urgent neurosurgical consultation.

Brain tumors above the tentorium produce pain referred to the frontal region or vertex. Subtentorial lesions cause pain in the occipital region. An index of suspicion is raised if there is pain upon awakening, if the pain is worse with the Valsalva maneuver, and if there is a new or unfamiliar headache associated with nausea and vomiting. The initial examination may be without focal findings. Follow-up must be arranged and diagnosis can be made by CT scan with contrast.

Postconcussive Headaches

Postconcussive headaches may follow trauma within hours to days. There can be associated vertigo, nausea and vomiting, difficulty with concentration, and mood alterations. The physical examination and CT scan are normal. These headaches are usually self-limiting, but NSAIAs may be beneficial. The prognosis is excellent.

Subarachnoid Hemorrhage

The most common etiology of headache due to subarachnoid hemorrhage is bleeding from an intracranial aneurysm. In a younger person, bleeding is more likely to be from an arteriovenosus malformation. The onset is sudden and the pain is intense. It is often described as "the worst headache" of the patient's life. Loss of consciousness may occur. Meningismus develops as well as signs of increasing intracranial pressure such as vomiting. If CT scanning does not locate the source of bleeding, a lumbar puncture must be performed. Cerebral edema can be controlled by the usual measures of hyperventilation and hypocapnia. Nimodipine can be used to reduce spasm. Urgent neurosurgical consultation is required.

Postlumbar Puncture

The size of the needle used, the amount of fluid withdrawn, and the number of punctures done are causative factors in this bicranial, pulsatile, frontal headache, which is exacerbated by the upright position. Rest, analgesics, avoidance of lifting, and adequate hydration are both prophylactic and treatment modalities. A steroid burst may be beneficial in severe cases.

Pseudotumor Cerebri (Benign Intracranial Hypertension)

The usual patient with benign intracranial hypertension is a young, obese female with irregular menstrual cycles or amenorrhea. She presents with visual complaints and a nonspecific, often severe, headache. On physical examination, papilledema is found. CT scanning reveals slitlike ventricles and no mass effect. Treatment consists of repeated lumbar puncture to relieve the pressure, which can be above 500 mm H_2O, and steroids.

Brain Abscess

The findings in cases of headache due to brain abscess will be similar to those for other space-occupying lesions, but the patient will also have a history of fever and possibly sinusitis. Diagnosis is made by CT scanning.

Inflammatory Headaches

Temporal Arteritis (Giant Cell Arteritis)

Temporal arteritis is a disease in which the branch of the external carotid artery, most frequently the temporal arteries, become infiltrated with lymphocytes, plasma cells, and multinucleate giant cells. It is a disease of people over 50 years of age, and women are affected four times more frequently than men. Frequently it is associated with polymyalgia rheumatica. The headache is unilateral or bilateral, with a piercing or burning quality. Frequent jabs, often excruciating, are experienced at night. The inflamed artery is tender and pulseless, and can sometimes be rolled between the fingers and the skull. An ESR of over 50 mm/h (by the Westergren method) with the above findings is essentially pathognomonic. Biopsy of the involved artery will yield a definitive diagnosis. Treatment should not be withheld while awaiting diagnosis, because blindness is the most common sequela and can develop rapidly secondary to ischemic pathologic papillitis. Treatment is with long-term steroids, but NSAIAs may be beneficial for management of the initial pain.

Meningitis

Headache due to meningitis usually involves the entire head with associated fever and evidence of meningismus.

Sinusitis

Acute infections of the nasal, perinasal, and mastoid sinuses may be associated with severe headaches, along with other symptoms. The pain is either stabbing or aching. It is made worse by bending or coughing, and lessens when the patient is supine.

Headaches Due to Idiopathic Cranial Neuralgias

Trigeminal neuralgia is the most common type of idiopathic cranial neuralgia. It usually occurs in people over 50 years old, and females are twice as likely to be affected as males. The pain is invariably unilateral, on the right side of the face, usually within the second and third branches of the fifth cranial nerve. It is sudden-onset, brief, severe, and lancinating. It may occur in intervals lasting from seconds to a few minutes and characteristically is worse on some occasions than on others.

Trigger points for the pain are usually around the lips, ala nasae, nasal labial fold, or upper eyelid, and an attack is precipitated when these points are stimulated by pressure, facial movements, or even emotional excitement. The simple acts of shaving, teeth brushing, face washing, eating, or drinking can cause an attack.

In the emergency department a parenteral analgesic may be necessary. Medical treatment on an outpatient basis consists of carbamazepine in dosages of 100 mg twice a day to 200 mg three times a day. If medical treatment fails, progressive sectioning of the sensory roots can be accomplished by a neurosurgeon.

Miscellaneous Causes of Headaches

Temporomandibular joint syndrome (Kostin's syndrome) is usually secondary to periarticular spasm of muscles used in mastication. It may be secondary to an overbite, recent dental work, dentures, nocturnal grinding of teeth, or chewing. Besides a headache there may be pain in the ipsilateral ear. Antiinflammatory medication will help the headache, but definitive therapy must be prescribed by a dentist or oral surgeon.

Acute narrow-angle glaucoma may cause a piercing pain in and around the orbit often accompanied by nausea and vomiting. The eye will be injected with decreased visual acuity. The cornea may be edematous and the pupil mid-position. Schiotz tonometry will reveal an elevated pressure.

Iritis presents with photophobia, ocular pain, poorly reactive pupil, decreased visual acuity, and perilimbal injection. Slit lamp examination will show cells and flare of the anterior chamber.

Patients with optic neuritis present with decreased visual acuity, pain on motion of the eye, a tender globe, and a Marcus Gunn pupil. Ophthalmologic consultation is necessary.

Eye strain as a cause of headache is overdiagnosed but can be the etiology when the refractive error is hyperopia in which the cellular body is in a continuous state of accommodation and muscle spasm. Mydriatics will help relieve the pain.

BIBLIOGRAPHY

Diamond S, Medena J: Review article: Current thoughts on migraines. *Headache* 20:208, 1980.

Edmeads J: Emergency management of headache. *Headache* 28:677, 1988.

Gallagher RM: Emergency treatment of intractable migraine. *Headache* 26:74, 1986.

Jones J, Sklar D, Dougherty J, et al: Randomized double-blind trial of intravenous prochlorperazine for the treatment of acute headache. *JAMA* 261:1174, 1989.

Kuhn MJ, Shekar PC: A comparative study of magnetic resonance imaging and computed tomography in the evaluation of migraine. *Comput Med Imaging Graphics* 14:149, 1990.

Kumar K, Cooney T: Vascular headache. *J Gen Int Med* 3:385, 1988.

Little N: Acute head pain, in Henry G (ed): *Neurologic Emergencies.* Philadelphia, Saunders, 1987, pp 687–698.

Marsters JB, Good PA, Mortimer MJ: A diagnostic test for migraine using the visual evoked potential. *Headache* 28:526, 1988.

Ramadan NM, Halvorson HH, VandeLinde A, et al: Low brain magnesium in migraine. *Headache* 29:592, 1989.

Sjaastad O: Cluster headache and its variants. *Headache* 28:667, 1988.

Solomon S, Guglielmo CK, Smith CR: Common migraine: Criteria for diagnosis. *Headache* 28:126, 1988.

Thie A, Spitzer K, Lachenmayer L, et al: Prolonged vasospasm in migraine detected by noninvasive transcranial doppler ultrasound. *Headache* 28:183, 1988.

147
STROKE SYNDROMES AND LATERALIZED DEFICITS

Gregory L. Henry

Patients frequently present to the emergency department with an acute specific loss of neurological function. When such lesions are specific to a region or side of the body, the patient is considered to have a lateralized neurological deficit. Lateralized deficits of the central nervous system may be caused by multiple diseases but are usually mediated through compromise of vascular supply or acute bleeding. The systematic approach to these patients quickly rules out peripheral nerve involvement or spinal cord disease. Since compromise of vascular supply and neurovascular accidents compose the majority of the lateralized deficits, the stroke syndromes will be used as the prototype for the discussion. Later in the chapter differential diagnosis of lateralizing lesions will be discussed.

STROKE

Stroke is one of the most common neurological problems seen in an emergency department. The full-blown anterior circulation stroke syndromes are usually recognized without difficulty, but the more subtle forms of stroke, often characterized by a confusing and unpredictable picture, may baffle even the most experienced examiner. A careful delineation of the underlying mechanism involved and the regions of the brain affected are of absolute necessity for both initiating treatment and making reasonable judgments with regard to prognosis.

In truth, cerebrovascular disease of any type is not a neurological disease, in the strictest sense of the term. Stroke syndromes include not only infarcts and hemorrhages, but also the entire gamut of local or systemic vascular and perivascular disease. Any disease process that impedes regional cerebral blood flow may present as a typical stroke. Examples of diverse entities resulting in stroke are malaria, trichinosis, intracerebral hematoma, and neoplasms.

As with most neurological problems, with stroke a thorough history is important to define the etiology, and the physical examination will be the best guide to the anatomic location. Because of the waxing and waning character of cerebrovascular disease, it is essential to question both the patient and the patient's family members for an accurate description of the signs and symptoms. Frequently, signs and symptoms will change or disappear by the time the patient is seen in an emergency department, and many decisions will have to be made on the basis of history alone. A good example is the patient with a transient ischemic attack (TIA). This disorder is characterized by the absence of permanent neurological deficits, but can be amenable to a number of modes of therapy. Failure to make the diagnosis because of a lack of hard physical findings may result in a return visit because of a completed stroke. The diagnosis of a TIA must frequently be made by history alone. The patient who relates the story of a transient neurological deficit which corresponds to a common vascular distribution should be highly suspect. Posterior circulation (brainstem) TIAs are frequently anticoagulated with aspirin and investigated on a routine basis. Anterior circulation (cortical) TIAs require aggressive investigation with computed tomographic (CT) scanning to rule out mass lesions and then with either Doppler ultrasound or various angiographic techniques to evaluate vascular status.

The first part of this discussion will relate the various disease entities that affect the vasculature of the brain. The second part will describe the most common presenting complaints and specific syndromes with which the emergency physician is most often confronted. It will also include a differential diagnosis and historical and physical examination tips that may lead to the correct diagnosis for each presenting complaint.

CEREBROVASCULAR LESIONS

Pathophysiology

The neurons of the brain require an uninterrupted supply of glucose and oxygen for metabolism because the brain cannot store these substances to any great degree. A decrease in the cerebral circulation will cause neuron dysfunction due to a decrease in supply of these two basic nutrients.

Blood reaches the brain through the four major vessels in the neck: two carotid and two vertebral arteries. Approximately 80 percent of the cerebral blood volume, referred to as the *anterior supply,* is handled by the carotid arteries. The remaining 20 percent, referred to as the *posterior circulation,* comes through the vertebrobasilar system. The anterior circulation is generally considered to supply most cortical and deep gray matter structures, as well as the optic nerves and retinas. The vertebral arteries, which are branches off the subclavian arteries, enter the skull through the foramen magnum and then combine near the pontomedullary junction to form the basilar artery, which has multiple fine branches. The vertebrobasilar system supplies nourishment to the upper spinal cord, brain stem, cerebellum, and certain deep gray matter structures. These two systems are interconnected at various levels, the principal one being the arterial circle of Willis. There is considerable individual variation in collateral blood supply, a fact that accounts for individual variation in symptoms with similar anatomic lesions.

Ischemia and Infarct

In the emergency department, the physician is usually confronted with two types of ischemic problems: thrombotic occlusion of a vessel as a primary process and occlusion of a vessel due to an embolus from a distant source. A third mechanism is external compression of a vessel due to hemorrhage or due to the progressive enlargement of a mass lesion. Compressive occlusion, however, usually is associated with a long history and does not result in sudden onset of symptoms.

Thrombotic Ischemia

Primary thrombotic ischemia may be due to atherosclerosis or vasculitis, such as giant cell arteritis or systemic lupus erythematosus. Thrombosis may also develop when constituents of blood are too viscous to traverse the arteriolar and capillary systems. Acute infectious process characterized by arteritis, such as syphilis or trichinosis, may mimic the atherosclerotic-type ischemic syndrome. Arterial occlusive disease outside the central nervous system or low-cardiac-output states may cause decreased cerebral blood flow. Disease of the aorta or cranial arteries, such as Takayasu's aortitis and aortic arch aneurysms, as well as mechnical problems, such as arthritis of the cervical spine, may contribute to cerebral ischemia.

On a statistical basis, however, the most common causes of infarction are atherosclerosis and embolism. There is still considerable debate over what the most common source of cerebral ischemic lesions is, but the emboli from atherosclerotic plaques in the internal carotid arteries may be the most common source of vascular occlusive disease. It is clear from autopsy studies that small cystic or lacunar infarcts are the most common form of cerebral infarction. The brain receives approximately 20 percent of the entire cardiac output and therefore is continually showered with any and all foreign material that may be present in the bloodstream. Many of these very minute infarcts are in relatively silent areas of brain function and may therefore go unnoticed.

Cerebral Embolism

Cerebral embolism is the term used to describe the occlusion of any intracranial vessel by a fragment of foreign substance arising outside of the CNS. The reason for occlusion may vary tremendously, but once it has taken place, the pathological process is the same. Vascular stasis is followed by edema, which, in a short time, leads to cell death and necrosis. The majority of emboli that reach the brain are sterile and are believed to arise from the large vessels of the neck and the heart. Air embolism following thoracic injury, and fat embolism following long bone injuries, are well documented. Bacterial and fungal emboli may result from endocarditis, sepsis, or from a focus of infection anywhere in the body. In adults, a mural thrombus from atrial fibrillation or myocardial infarction can result in an embolus. Transient ischemic attacks are most likely due to showers of microemboli from plaques in the great vessels of the neck.

The origin of an embolus is of more than academic interest. Treatment of emboli of cardiac origin is accomplished with heparin and warfarin. There is no evidence to suggest that emboli of noncardiac origin are improved by any drugs other than aspirin.

Intracranial Hemorrhage

Intracranial hemorrhage may be the result of bleeding in multiple locations anywhere in the cranial vault. Bleeding can develop in the epidural, subdural, subarachnoid, intraparenchymal, and intraventricular spaces. Traumatic lesions of the middle meningeal artery are the usual source of epidural or extradural hematomas. Subdural hematomas may be the result of either traumatic or spontaneous bleeding from the veins that lie in the subdural space. Subarachnoid bleeding is usually due to rupture of a saccular aneurysm in the cerebral network, or less often, an arteriovenous (AV) malformation.

The majority of hemorrhages into the brain substance are produced by rupture of the arteriolar aneurysms that may be the result of hypertension or congenital malformations. Cerebral hemorrhages have been, to a much lesser extent, associated with certain blood dyscrasias, neoplasms, infections, and anticoagulants. Unlike embolic or thrombotic strokes, intracerebral hemorrhages, particularly the hypertensive variety, may be fatal in up to 80 percent of cases.

Incidence of Cerebrovascular Accidents

Cerebrovascular accidents (*CVA*s) of all types occur in definable patient populations. The term is general, and refers to a variety of cerebral vascular problems. Pale infarcts, embolic lesions, and hemorrhages into the parenchyma of the brain, as well as hemorrhages into the subarachnoid and dural spaces, are all CVAs. Embolic and thrombotic lesions are more likely to occur in patients with the following problems:

- TIAs
- Hypertension
- Clinical evidence of atherosclerosis
- Cardiac abnormalities
- Diabetes mellitus
- Elevated blood lipids, cigarette smoking, erythrocytosis, and gout

There is good evidence that up to 70 percent of patients who have anterior circulation TIAs will develop cerebral infarction or recurrent TIAs within 2 years. The TIA should be considered presumptive evidence of an impending cerebrovascular accident and should be treated aggressively. Hemorrhagic lesions such as aneurysmal bleeding and spontaneous interparenchymal rupture have a strong correlation with hypertension. Since atherosclerosis is a systemic illness, it can be assumed that the process is occurring in cerebral vessels as well.

Those patients with angina pectoris and intermittent claudication of the legs are at increased risk for stroke. Arterial bruits over the carotid arteries can be associated with hemodynamically significant stenosis (i.e., greater than 70 percent) in 90 percent of cases, making this a significant finding. Patients with congenital heart disease, such as septal defects and valvular disease, and those with atrial fibrillation, particularly in conjunction with thyroid disease, have a higher incidence of embolic stroke. Diabetics are prone to stroke because of accelerated atherosclerosis, hypertension, and peripheral vascular disease. Patients with elevated lipid levels, a history of cigarette smoking, erythrocytosis, and gout are also predisposed to stroke.

Clinical Features

When evaluating a patient with an acute lateralizing lesion, the emergency physician should be able to define the time course of the illness and current status of the disease and be able to establish a time frame under which the rest of the workup should be accomplished.

Emergency department evaluation of the potential stroke victim should include a general physical examination, with particular attention to the patient's neurological status. A patient's vital signs are paramount and may suggest that a hypertensive hemorrhage has occurred. A thorough examination of the patient's head and neck with proper movement precautions is important to rule out trauma. By careful auscultation of the head, eyes, and carotid arteries, bruits suggestive of AV malformations or vascular stenosis may be detected. A good cardiac examination and ECG are necessary to evaluate valvular disease and rhythm abnormalities.

The neurological examination should be directed toward determination of the anatomic regions involved. Even in the comatose patient, signs of lateralization should be sought by checking the patient's withdrawal response to noxious stimuli. Hemiparesis, paraparesis, or even quadriparesis can be detected by noting whether the motor response is unilateral, whether the upper extremity responses are greater than those of the lower extremities, or whether facial grimacing and head and neck movement are present but movement of the extremities is absent. Conjugate deviation of the eyes and pupillary changes will help to determine if lateralization is present. Conjugate deviation of the eyes is often present in patients with large cerebral lesions. Remember that the eyes look toward the lesion in major hemispheric abnormalities, and away from the lesion in brainstem abnormalities. Check for nuchal rigidity and abnormal plantar responses.

A reasonable clinical impression can usually be formulated after initial history taking and physical examination. It is of utmost importance to try to distinguish hemorrhage from infarct, as the therapy for these two lesions is markedly different.

Obtain baseline laboratory studies, including ECG, CBC, PT, and PTT. Skull roentgenograms are no longer routinely obtained, and are generally of little value in diagnosis of the lesion.

CT scanning has become the procedure of choice in differentiating the acute bleed from the cerebral infarct. It demonstrates virtually all instances of supratentorial hemorrhage and most cerebellar hemorrhage as well. The CT scan is not without error in detecting smaller hemorrhages, but in those circumstances where spinal tap may be hazardous, such as in the patient with a large supratentorial mass lesion, it may be of great value to the patient. Arteriovenous malformations and aneurysms may be completely missed by CT scanning.

Angiography is an alternative for those patients in whom there is a question about the etiology of the lesion. If hemorrhage is not suspected, and if no specific therapy such as anticoagulation or surgery is anticipated, emergent angiography is probably not indicated.

Traditionally, the examination of CSF obtained by lumbar puncture has been carried out early in suspected cases of intracerebral and subarachnoid hemorrhage due to the high incidence of blood in the CSF. A negative finding was thought to reassure the treating physician about to begin anticoagulant therapy on a stroke in progress. This is not necessarily true, as some intracerebral bleeding does not communicate with the subarachnoid space. If a CT scan is positive for bleeding, there is no need for lumbar puncture. In the face of a normal CT scan and a strong suspicion of bleeding the lumbar puncture becomes important. When looking for blood in CSF it is best to check cell counts in the first and last tubes. Minimal RBCs seen in the first tube and clearing by the last tube can be regarded as traumatic. RBCs which remain stable or increase are indicative of bleeding in the CSF.

In patients who have had symptoms for more than 6 h, the CSF should be checked for xanthochromia.

A suspected acute vascular event requires an acute vascular diagnosis either by CT scan or angiography. One CT scan may not be enough. Pale infarcts can convert to hemorrhagic ones when necrosis occurs. It is suggested that a repeat CT scan be done within 2 to 4 days and before starting patients on anticoagulant or antiplatelet therapy. Even in the case of the patient with rapid onset of headache, nuchal rigidity, and obtundation, and with no lateralizing findings and no history of trauma, a lumbar puncture is probably not needed to confirm the diagnosis of subarachnoid hemorrhage. If a patient has focal findings that strongly suggest a mass CNS lesion, such as subdural hematoma or brain abscess, the lumbar puncture should be deferred if other studies are available. A lumbar puncture is also contraindicated if cerebellar hemorrhage is suspected. In that case, a CT scan or angiogram should be obtained. MRI scans are becoming more readily available. They are often more sensitive to small pale infarcts than CT scans. However, they will frequently miss early bleeding, and therefore CT scanning should still be considered the early diagnostic modality of choice.

Treatment

Thrombotic and Embolic Stroke

Definitive diagnosis and therapy of thrombotic and embolic vascular problems are usually not initiated in the emergency department. There are some general measures, however, that all emergency physicians can take to expedite patient recovery.

Avoid rapid lowering of the blood pressure in the first 10 days, unless the pressure is in a critically high range, usually a diastolic pressure above 130 mmHg. Many authors now suggest that diastolic pressures even in the 120 mmHg range should be watched for several days before starting the patient on antihypertensives. Then it is advisable to lower the patient's diastolic pressure to only the 100-mgHg range. If hypotension is present on initial examination, it should be corrected by the appropriate means.

Carefully monitor the routine use of intravenous fluids in stroke patients. Assuming that the patient presents in a normal state of hydration, only maintenance fluids are required. Excessive amounts of free water may increase cerebral edema and actually add to the area of infarction. Standard nursing care, such as protecting the patients from aspiration and frequent turning to prevent decubiti, is as important in the emergency department as in nursing units.

For most patients with TIAs or small CVAs, aspirin should be considered the cornerstone of therapy at this time. Aspirin has clearly been shown to reduce both anterior circulation TIAs and CVAs. Aspirin can reduce the total number of posterior circulation TIAs, but there is no evidence that aspirin or any other drug has any effect on the incidence of posterior circulation CVAs.

The specific therapy for thrombotic and embolic stroke includes antiplatelets and various surgical procedures. There is much controversy about the role of anticoagulant therapy in stroke patients, but the following guidelines may be helpful:

1. Patients experiencing TIAs, particularly crescendo TIAs, are highly prone to developing completed strokes. This group of patients should be aggressively investigated, and if no surgically correctible lesions are found, a course of oral antiplatelets should be considered.
2. For the stroke in evolution, defined as documented progressive neurological involvement, most authorities still advocate the immediate institution of intravenous heparin therapy to prevent further damage. However, it should be noted that there is little evidence of truly improved outcomes over aspirin. Of course, it must be certain that a mass intracerebral lesion or hemorrhage is not present. CT scanning or angiography may be done, and if no surgically correctible lesions are found, the patient may be switched to oral medications. Current studies using steptokinase, tissue plasminogen activators, and APSAC, are continuing but as yet are not beyond the investigational stage. Until studies become available documenting positive results, thrombolytic therapy should be considered investigational only.

Vasodilators have long been used in the treatment of cerebrovascular disease without convincing evidence of their benefit. Amyl nitrate, papaverine hydrochloride, isoxsuprine hydrochloride, acetazolamide, carbon monoxide, and several other agents increase cerebral blood flow in normal tissue, but there is no evidence that these agents alter the course of ischemic strokes or prevent TIAs. Many investigators believe that the dilation of blood vessels in the remaining normal tissue may actually cause an intracerebral "steal" syndrome, thus reducing the perfusion pressure to already ischemic areas. Biorheological therapy by reducing blood viscosity is still investigational. Medications such as pentoxifylline (Trental) and ancrod have been tried with limited success.

A certain percentage of patients with cerebral infarction will develop seizures, but there is no reason to give prophylactic anticonvulsants to these patients in the emergency department.

Corticosteroids have been found to be of little benefit in cerebral infarction states. It is usually wise to withhold corticosteroids unless the patient has definite signs of increased intracranial pressure or evidence of uncal herniation. Although there was initial hope for prostaglandin-based drugs such as prostayclin, clinical tests have not found them to be of any benefit.

Surgery for embolic and thrombotic lesions is certainly not the province of the emergency physician, but remember that carotid endarterectomy is still the most commonly performed surgical procedure for ischemic cerebrovascular disease. In many series, if surgically approachable lesions of the carotid arteries were corrected, the incidence of completed stroke was reduced. Newer procedures for cerebral artery revascularization, such as anastomosis of the temporal artery to the middle cerebral artery, or saphenous vein bypass of various cerebral arteries, have not yet been shown to be effective.

There is little to offer the completed cerebral stroke patient. Aspirin, however, may reduce the incidence of further strokes.

Hemorrhagic Stroke

Emergency treatment of hemorrhagic strokes follows the same basic rules for therapy of thrombotic and embolic lesions. It is perhaps of even greater importance in hemorrhagic stroke, however, to ensure that the blood pressure is lowered to 100 to 110 mmHg diastolic within a reasonable period of time, without subjecting the patient to hypotension. Unlike thrombotic strokes, where blood pressures above the normal range can be allowed to persist, it is generally considered that blood pressure in hemorrhagic stroke should be brought within acceptable levels according to the patient's age.

Generally there is considerable cerebral edema with hemorrhagic lesions, and mannitol or urea should not be withheld if there is evidence of herniation or progressive obtundation. Because of their transient effects, mannitol and urea are not useful in the long-term management of cerebral edema secondary to intracerebral hemorrhage. These agents are beneficial when given just before neurosurgery in an effort to reverse herniation.

Clotting abnormalities, either intrinsic or secondary to anticoagulant therapy, should be vigorously sought and corrected by administering the appropriate clotting factors or by reversing the chemical anticoagulants present.

Surgical therapy for intracerebral hematomas is highly case-dependent at this point. There is clear evidence, however, that evacuation of a hematoma in the cerebellum can be lifesaving to the patient. If an intracerebellar hematoma is suspected, a CT scan should be obtained immediately and a neurosurgeon consulted. Under no circumstances should a lumbar puncture be performed on a suspected cerebellar hematoma.

In many centers it was once standard therapy to administer antifibrinolytic agents to patients with subarachnoid hemorrhage. ϵ-Aminocaproic acid (Amicar) was the agent most commonly used. There is no statistical evidence that antifibrinolytic agents help, and such medications have now lost popularity. Nimodipine, a calcium channel blocker, has proven effective in reducing vasospasm of the cerebral vessels if started within the first 72 h after the hemorrhage occurs. There is no indication for its use in nonhemorrhagic CVAs.

SPECIFIC CEREBROVASCULAR SYNDROMES

Now that we have considered the pathophysiology of the various types of lesions that can compromise the cerebrocirculation and have described a general approach to assessment and management of these problems, we will review the most common presenting syndromes with which the emergency physician will be confronted. The vascular anatomy of the brain varies minimally from patient to patient, but the collateral circulation is variable. Therefore, a specific patient may have only a portion of the syndromes herein discussed.

Ischemic Stroke Syndromes

Middle Cerebral Artery Syndromes

Occlusion of the middle cerebral artery is usually by embolic phenomena. The clinical picture includes contralateral hemiplegia and hemianesthesia, contralateral homonymous hemianopsia with impairment of conjugate gaze in the direction opposite the lesion, aphasia with dominant involvement, and constructional apraxia and anosognosia with nondominant hemisphere involvement. The usual occlusion, however, involves only the branches of the middle cerebral artery, resulting in incomplete syndromes. Arm involvement is usually greater than leg involvement, and varying forms of aphasia occur with the involvement of the dominant hemisphere.

Anterior Cerebral Artery Syndromes

With the involvement of the anterior cerebral artery, there is frequently paralysis of the contralateral foot and leg and contralateral center loss, with contralateral gegenhalten, abulia, gait apraxia, and urinary incontinence.

Posterior Cerebral Artery Syndromes

The posterior cerebral artery supplies blood to the occipital cortex and branches that supply upper midbrain structures. These patients may have contralateral homonymous hemianopsia or quadrantanopsia, memory loss, dyslexia without agraphia, contralateral hemiparesis, contralateral hemisensory loss, and ipsilateral third-nerve palsy with contralateral hemiplegia.

Vertebrobasilar Syndromes

Vertebrobasilar Lesions

The vertebrobasilar arteries are subject to both atherosclerotic narrowing and embolic phenomena. Since the vertebral system supplies the posterior portions of the brain, including the cerebellum and brain stem, deficits resulting from occlusion of these arteries are predictable. These include ipsilateral ataxia, contralateral hemiplegia with sensory loss, ipsilateral horizontal gaze palsy with contralateral hemiplegia, ipsilateral peripheral seventh-nerve lesions, internuclear ophthalmoplegia, nystagmus, vertigo, nausea and vomiting, and deafness and tinnitus. Simple labrynthitis may be manifest by nystagmus, nausea, and vomiting but should not present any other brainstem or cerebellar signs or symptoms.

Basilar Artery Occlusion

Occlusion of the basilar artery in itself usually gives rise to such severe bilateral signs as quadriplegia, coma, and the locked-in syndrome. In the locked-in syndrome, the patient has a lesion of the tectual pons that knocks out all motor function except upward gaze.

Cerebellar Infarcts

Cerebral infarcts usually produce dizziness, nausea, vomiting, nystagmus, and the inability to stand or walk if midline cerebellar functions are involved. The patient should be observed carefully, and if cerebellar swelling is causing a rapid downhill course, the patient should undergo emergency decompression of the posterior fossa.

Lacunar Infarction

In 1967, Fisher outlined a series of specific brain stem infarctions that were due to small microinfarcts referred to as *lacunar infarctions*. These small cystic infarcts occur principally in the deep gray matter and brain stem and result in some discernible patterns. There are four specific lacunar infarct states that have been delineated. They are

1. The clumsy hand dysarthria syndrome due to a small lesion in the midpons.
2. Leg paresis and ataxia due to a lesion in the pons or internal capsule resulting in ataxia and weakness in one leg.
3. A pure sensory stroke, resulting from a lesion in the thalamus. This usually results in a sensory loss in the face, arm, or leg with no hemiplegia or other signs.
4. Pure motor hemiplegia due to a lesion in the pons or internal capsule with paralysis of the arm, face, and leg without sensory loss. In a right hemiplegia, no aphasia is found. In a left hemiplegia, no parietal lobe findings are evident.

Lacunar infarct states are found in hypertensive patients, and control of hypertension is the principal mode of therapy. Aspirin, although frequently given, may be of minimal benefit. Many patients have relatively transient deficits, and with proper care return to good function.

The scope of this text does not permit a thorough review of all the various brain stem stroke syndromes. Suffice it to say, the majority of brain stem stroke lesions are due to lesions in the vertebrobasilar system, and accurate anatomic localization is possible because of the relatively precise and localized neuroanatomy of the region. There are multiple eponymic syndromes, such as Wallenberg's, Weber's, and Parinaud's syndromes, that are associated with the brain stem, but the important feature to remember is that for alternating symptoms, i.e., lesions on one side involving the cranial nerves on one side of the brain stem, and sensory or motor problems on the opposite side of the body, the lesion must involve the descending tracts after they have left the cortex and internal capsule and before they have decussated in the lower medulla. In this way, a patient may exhibit findings of the cranial nerves on one side of the body and motor and sensory findings below the level of the foramen magnum on the opposite side of the body. Finer articulations are amply discussed in currently available texts.

Transient Global Amnesia

Ischemia to hippocampal and amygdaloid structures may result in a much underdiagnosed syndrome known as *transient global amnesia*. This syndrome usually occurs in patients who are over 60 and is characterized by an abrupt loss of the ability to recall recent events or record new memories; however, there is usually very good memory of past events. During the episode, the patient is usually able to perform highly complex tasks, even arithmetic, and speech is usually unimpaired. Most patients recover completely, and it is questionable whether their symptoms represent the same prognostic values as do other TIAs.

Hemorrhagic Syndromes

Subarachnoid Hemorrhage

Subarachnoid hemorrhage usually results from rupture of a saccular aneurysm. It occurs at sites of arteriolar bifurcation or branching. The majority of patients who experience ruptured aneurysms are between the ages of 36 and 65 years of age. Patients with polycystic kidneys and coarctation of the aorta are known to have a higher incidence of subarachnoid aneurysmal hemorrhage. Unlike thrombotic and embolic lesions that frequently present with TIAs, aneurysms are usually asymptomatic until they rupture.

Typically, the onset is marked by an extremely severe headache that the patient describes as the worst headache ever experienced. The patient usually does not lose consciousness at this point, but may have a rapid onset of stupor progressing to coma, without focal lateralizing signs. The patient's general physical examination and neurological examination may be normal, except for signs of increased meningeal irritation.

Hypertensive Intracerebral Hemorrhage

The hypertensive intracerebral hemorrhage syndromes likewise have a fairly characteristic presentation. Hypertensive hemorrhage almost always proceeds from the small penetrating vessels of the brain that have been damaged by hypertension and usually arises in the following locations, in decreasing order of frequency: putamen, thalamus, pons, and cerebellum. Hemorrhages that are due to anticoagulants or a bleeding diathesis usually involve areas such as the frontal, temporal, parietal, or occipital lobes, which are sites rarely involved with hypertensive hemorrhage.

Hemorrhage of the putamen often presents a picture indistinguishable from middle cerebral artery occlusion, with contralateral hemiplegia, hemianesthesia, homonymous hemianopsia, aphasia, or hemineglect, depending upon the hemisphere involved. There is usually greater depression of consciousness in the patient with putamenal hemorrhage than in the patient with standard middle cerebral artery occlusions.

Thalamic hemorrhage produces contralateral hemiparesis with contralateral hemianesthesia. The sensory loss is usually considerably greater than the motor deficit. Occasionally there is restriction of the upward gaze or skewed deviation of the eyes without visual field defect.

Pontine hemorrhage usually results in pinpoint pupils that are minimally reactive to light, and decerebrate posturing. Patients rapidly progress to coma and lack normal oculovestibular reflexes when caloric testing is performed.

Of all the hemorrhagic or occlusive diagnoses, cerebellar hemorrhage is the most important to make. The patient typically develops sudden dizziness and vomiting, with marked truncal ataxia. The patient is unable to stand and walk but is otherwise alert and oriented. No hemispheric abnormalities are noted. There may be findings associated with compression of the ipsilateral pons, such as ipsilateral sixth-nerve palsy and parapontine gaze center abnormalities, and facial weakness. The patient rapidly progresses to coma, and frequently death results from brain stem compression. This is a treatable form of hemorrhage, and if diagnosed early, it may be relieved by surgical decompression and evacuation of the hematoma, which may restore the patient to near normal function.

DIFFERENTIAL DIAGNOSIS OF PRESENTING COMPLAINTS

Few patients present to an emergency department complaining of a specific disease. Therefore, a standard system of evaluation is necessary to take a general symptom complaint unrelated to a specific etiology. This section will be presented in a schematic form to make it more useful in the emergency department.

Right-Sided Weakness

Cortical Localization

If aphasia is present, the lesion must have a cortical component. Check the patient's ability to name objects, repeat sentences, read, comprehend, and carry out commands. Remember that all right-handed patients, and perhaps 70 to 80 percent of all left-handed patients, are left-hemisphere-dominant.

Cortical Sensory Loss

Cortical sensory loss manifests as loss of two-point discrimination, graphesthesia, and/or stereognosis.

Loss of sensation in the face and arm more than in the leg strongly suggest middle cerebral artery distribution in the cortex.

Eye Deviation

The eyes deviate toward the hemisphere involved and away from the hemiparesis. Field defect is usually present.

Subcortical Localization

Examples of subcortical lesions include lesions of the internal capsule, basal ganglion, or thalamus. The face, arm, and leg are equally involved.

Signs of subcortical localization include the following: no aphasias, abnormal posturing, extremely dense sensory loss, and eye deviation may be the same as in cortical lesions.

Left Brain Stem

Symptoms associated with left-sided brain stem lesions are as follows:

Right hemiplegia with left-sided brain stem signs, such as cranial nerve palsies on the left side of the face.
Cerebellar signs, with abnormal finger-to-nose, rapid alternating movement on the left, and weakness on the right Nystagmus that is most marked when the patient looks toward the side of the lesion
Possible hearing loss
Alternating sensory findings, with sensory loss and weakness on the right side of the body, and sensory loss on the left side of the face, due to involvement of the different tracts for each area
Dysarthria
Tongue deviation
Abnormal gaze palsies resulting in difficulty looking to the left

Spinal Cord Lesions

With spinal cord lesions, there is no involvement of the face, and no aphasias, dysphasias, or dysarthrias. Paralysis is on the same side as the lesion, but pain and temperature sensation may be on the opposite side of the weakness, i.e., Brown-Séquard syndrome.

A sensory level to pinprick is evident. Bladder and bowel disturbances may be noted.

Differential Right-Sided Weakness—Numbness

1. Vascular—thrombotic, hemorrhagic, AVM, subarchnoid hemorrhage, TIA, venous infarct, carotid or intracerebral lesion
2. Subdural hematoma, epidural hematoma
3. Tumor, primary or metastatic
4. Brain abscess
5. Cardiac disease—low flow states and arrhythmias
6. Seizure disorder—postictal paralysis (Todd's paralysis)
7. Bell's palsy—peripheral seventh nerve, face
8. Vascular migraine headache
9. Metabolic—rare cause of focal findings
10. Functional—psychiatric

Left Hemiplegia

In the majority of patients, the nondominant hemisphere is the right hemisphere, which controls the left half of the body. Therefore, assessment of the left hemiplegia basically involves testing of nondominant, or right hemispheric, function. If the lesion is cortical, check for denial of the lesion by answering the following questions:

Does the patient ignore the left side? Or do such patients fail to recognize body parts as being their own?
Does the patient extinguish double simultaneous stimulation by suppressing one part of the body?

Additional questions that are helpful in evaluating nondominant hemisphere function are as follows:

Does the patient exhibit constructional apraxia? Can the patient draw a simple map and name and locate areas on it? Can the patient also draw a clock and fill in the numbers?
Does the patient have spatial disorganization with respect to the room?
Is there a decrease in persistence in completing tasks that are assigned?

All of the above indicate involvement of the nondominant hemisphere. In addition, note findings that are common to both hemispheres, such as quadrantanopsias and weakness in the arm greater than the leg. Subcortical, brain stem, and spinal cord findings are the same as noted in the section on right-sided weakness, except they would be on the left side.

Left-Sided Weakness and Numbness

The entire list of differential diagnoses listed under right-sided weakness are applicable to left-sided weakness.

BIBLIOGRAPHY

Biller J, Bruno A, Adams HP, et al: A randomized trial of aspirin or heparin in hospitalized patients with recent transient ischemic attacks: A pilot study. *Stroke* 20:441, 1989.
Cerebral Embolism Study Group: Immediate anticoagulation of embolic stroke: Brain hemorrhage and management options. *Stroke* 15:799, 1984.
Pellegrino TR: Vascular syndromes. *Emerg Med Clin North Am* 5:751, 1987.
Toronto Cerebral Vascular Study Group: Risk of carotid enarterectomy. *Stroke* 17:848, 1986.
United Kingdom Transient Ischemic Attacks (UK-TIA): Aspirin trial. Interim results. *Br Med J* 296:316, 1988.
Whisnant JP, Matsumoto N, Elvevack LR: The effect of anticoagulant therapy on the prognosis of patients with transient cerebral ischemic attacks in a community—Rochester, Minnesota, 1955–1969. *Mayo Clin Proc* 48:844, 1973.

148
VERTIGO AND DIZZINESS

Neal Little

Complaints of dizziness and light-headedness are among the most common in emergency medicine, and their evaluation can test the problem-solving ability of the physician. Dizziness itself may not be life-threatening, but it is usually bothersome and potentially disabling. The primary challenge to the emergency physician is establishing what a given patient means by "dizziness," which is an ambiguous, nonmedical, subjective term. It may be used to articulate a sensation of weakness, unsteadiness, giddiness, malaise, instability, swimming in the head, faintness or near faintness, or a disturbance of mentation. A variety of disorders affecting the central nervous system, ears, cardiovascular system, eyes, and psyche may all produce dizziness, and thus a systematic approach is imperative.

Vertigo is used to refer to an illusion of motion where no motion exists. Either the patient or the environment seems to be moving. Movement is classically described as spinning or whirling, but may also be described as rocking, staggering, or swaying, or as a sensation of "impulsion," where the person feels as though he or she is being pulled to one side or to the ground as if by a magnet. The distinction between a feeling that the patient is moving versus a feeling that the environment is moving (subjective versus objective vertigo) is rarely useful. Oscillopsia, a visual illusion that objects in the environment are moving, may occur.

Syncope means a transient loss of consciousness, with rapid return to normal, on the basis of diminished cerebral blood flow, oxygen, or glucose. *Near syncope* is an impending loss of consciousness, or a "gray-out" feeling.

When the subjective complaint of dizziness is not well defined and cannot be classified as vertigo or near syncope, the term ill-defined dizziness is often used.

PATHOPHYSIOLOGY

Spatial orientation is determined by the interaction between the visual, labyrinthine, and proprioceptive systems and the integration of impulses by the central nervous system. Dysfunction in either the pathways that integrate those systems or the sensors themselves may be the cause of disordered sensations of spatial orientation, position, and motion.

The visual system, consisting of the eyes, the optic pathways, and the visual cortex create for the person a visual-spatial orientation. The labyrinthine system consists of the otoliths, which primarily produce an orientation to gravity, and the semicircular canals, which produce an orientation to movement or the tilt of the head. The semicircular canals are filled with fluid and lined by hair cells. Movement of the fluid causes movement of the hair cells, which results in a change in afferent vestibular nerve impulses. There is a balanced vestibular neuronal input to the brain stem from both vestibular nerves. Alteration of input from one is perceived as motion. The proprioceptors in the joints and muscles of limbs and neck relate movement and the tilt of the head to that of the body and also sense body position when lying, walking, or sitting.

The integrative structures involved in mediating the sensory input from the receptor systems are the cerebellum, the brain stem (primarily the vestibular nuclei and the medial longitudinal fasciculus), the basal ganglia (red nuclei), and the cerebral cortex (temporal and parietal lobes). Dizziness can occur as a result of dysfunction in one or all of the receptor systems or the mediating structures.

The pathophysiologic mechanisms that can affect these structures include all of the processes which affect the nervous system in general, including vascular, metabolic-nutritional, toxic, neuronal, and psychogenic.

Age-related changes that can contribute to dizziness or vertigo include diminished labyrinthine hair cells, diminished labyrinthine nerve fibers, diminished visual, auditory, and proprioceptive sensations, and diminished integrative abilities.

Nystagmus due to injury to the vestibular system is a to-and-fro movement of the eyes that has a slow component (due to vestibular-ocular reflex) and a fast component. It is named for the fast component. Excitation of one semicircular canal produces eye movement away from that canal (vestibular-ocular reflex). The cortex exerts a quick corrective movement in the opposite direction, resulting in nystagmus. Ocular fixation tends to suppress nystagmus of peripheral vestibular origin. The normally balanced input from the semicircular canals of both ears results in no net eye movement. Most peripheral (vestibular) disorders result in inhibition of one more semicircular canals, and thus nystagmus beating with the quick phase away from the affected ear. Patients with peripheral vertigo feel that the environment is spinning in the direction of the fast component, or that their bodies are spinning in the direction of the slow component. Vestibular nystagmus occurs in the plane of the affected semicircular canal and may be either horizontal or torsional-vertical. Strictly vertical nystagmus is rarely the result of vestibular involvement and usually points to a brain stem origin.

ETIOLOGY AND CLINICAL MANIFESTATIONS

The major characteristics of central and peripheral vertigo are given in Table 148-1. The etiologies of vertigo are classically separated into *peripheral vertigo,* which is caused by disease processes affecting structures peripheral to the brain stem (eighth nerve, vestibular apparatus), and *central vertigo,* which is caused by processes affecting structures central to the brain stem (cerebellum).

Peripheral Vertigo

The vast majority of patients with vertigo seen in emergency practice have peripheral vertigo. Peripheral vertigo is characterized by an intense vertiginous or whirling feeling, often accompanied by profound associated symptoms such as nausea, vomiting, sweating, pallor, diarrhea, and alteration of blood pressure and pulse. Impulsion is very strongly suggestive of peripheral vertigo. These symptoms may be of abrupt onset. Peripheral vertigo may be dramatically influenced by position change, greatly worsened by movement or by the assumption of certain positions of the head, and is extremely distressing to the patient. The symptoms of patients with peripheral vertigo resemble those of classic motion sickness.

Table 148-1. Characteristics of Vertigo

Peripheral origin
Intense spinning, swaying or impulsion
Nausea, vomiting, possibly diarrhea
Diaphoresis
Aggravated by change of position, movement
Possible tinnitus, hearing loss
Acute onset
Fatiguable, unidirectional nystagmus
Nystagmus inhibited by ocular fixation
Central origin
Ill-defined, less intense vertigo
Not positionally related, concomitant brain stem or cerebellar signs and symptoms (diplopia, dysphagia, facial numbness or weakness, ataxia, hemiparesis)
Nystagmus not inhibited by ocular fixation
Nonfatiguable, multidirectional nystagmus

Disorders Causing Peripheral Vertigo

Vestibular Neuronitis

Vestibular neuronitis is characterized by peripheral vertigo without hearing loss. If tests of cochlear function are done, they show no abnormality. Patients may complain of fullness in the ear or tinnitus. Positional nystagmus occurs in one-third of cases. Caloric vestibular testing is usually abnormal on one side. This illness is of suspected viral origin and may occur in epidemics. It may be a mild viral encephalitis affecting the brain stem or a neuronitis affecting the vestibular nerve. The exact site of the lesion is not known. Patients typically complain of acute onset and severe symptoms. The vertigo is worsened by any movement of the head. It may last for days, and residual symptoms may persist for weeks. Most cases of casually diagnosed labyrinthitis probably fall into this category.

Labyrinthitis

Labyrinthitis is characterized by peripheral vertigo associated with hearing loss. While the etiology of many cases of labyrinthitis is a presumed viral infection, there is no proof of this. Occasional cases occur in association with mumps and measles. Bacterial labyrinthitis is an extremely rare condition usually associated with long-standing otitis media with fistula, meningitis, mastoid disease, dermoid tumor, or postsurgical infection. Bacterial labyrinthitis is potentially devastating and requires appropriate antibiotic therapy.

If there is a perilympathic leak from a fistula at the round or oval window, pneumatic changes in the middle ear may be transmitted to the labyrinthine apparatus and cause subjective vertigo. This may occur as a result of trauma. Patients with perilymphatic fistula complain of intermittent or positional vertigo exacerbated by straining, sneezing, and coughing, which may also cause such a fistula. Fluctuating hearing loss occurs. Hennebert's sign, which is subjective vertigo and nystagmus induced by pneumatic otoscopy, is diagnostic.

Menière's disease is a condition characterized by recurrent attacks of severe vertigo, vomiting, and prostration, and usually associated with progressive deafness and tinnitus. It tends to run a recurrent and protracted course over time associated with less severe attacks of vertigo and progressively more severe deafness. It occurs in middle age, and in men and women equally. While little is known about the underlying etiology, there is a gross dilatation of the endolymphatic system of the internal ear.

The typical history in Menière's disease is that of a patient over the age of 50 with slowly progressive tinnitus and deafness in one or rarely both ears over months to years who suddenly develops severe vertigo. It may occur so suddenly that the patient falls. More commonly, it worsens over several minutes. There is an intense sensation of rotation, more commonly of the surroundings than of the patient. nausea and vomiting are common and may be severe. The pulse may be rapid or slow, and the blood pressure raised or lowered. Occasionally patients may develop diarrhea. There may be profound diaphoresis. Preexisting deafness and tinnitus, usually unilateral, may become intensified. The attack may last from half an hour to many hours with gradual offset. The patient is frequently unable to stand or walk and may be unsteady and staggering on attempted ambulation. Between attacks, deafness, usually unilateral, is found. The attacks often occur at regular intervals separated by weeks to years. The severity of the attacks tends to diminish and finally cease as deafness increases. A similar picture may be produced by tertiary syphilis. Tumors at the cerebellopontine angle, such as acoustic schwannoma, may produce progressive unilateral hearing loss and vertigo and simulate Menière's disease.

Drug Effects

A variety of drugs affect the inner ear. Most affect both vestibular and cochlear mechanisms, but the degree to which they affect them is variable. Aspirin in toxic doses affects predominantly cochlear function and produces tinnitus and hearing loss, but little vertigo. Aminoglycosides may produce vestibular neuroepithelial damage before any cochlear damage is evident. Anticonvulsants such as phenytoin may produce exclusively vestibular symptoms. Drugs which affect the inner ear are listed in Table 148-2.

Table 148-2. Drugs and Chemicals Affecting the Inner Ear

Antibiotics	Cytotoxic agents
Aminoglycosides	Vinblastine
Erythromycin	Cisplatin
Minocycline	Nitrogen mustard
Diuretics	Anticonvulsants
Ethacrinic acid	Phenytoin
Furosemide	Barbiturates
Bumetanide	Carbamazepine
Nonsteroidal anti-inflammatory agents	Ethosuccimide
Salicylates	Others
Ibuprofen	Quinine
Naproxen	Chloroquine
Indomethacin	Propylene glycol
	Ethanol
	Methanol
	Mercury

Benign Positional Vertigo

Benign positional vertigo is a syndrome in which patients have repeated attacks of vertigo precipitated by changes in posture, typically a sudden turning of the head as in rolling over in bed. There is no acute hearing loss or tinnitus. It is a very common cause of vertigo, and the most common cause in the elderly. The attacks usually last a few seconds to minutes, and usually subside within a few weeks. Nylen-Barany (Hallpike) testing is diagnostic, and distinguishes between peripheral and central vertigo (Table 148-3). Benign positional vertigo is also known as Barany's vertigo, and is thought to result from calcium carbonate crystals which have detached from the otoconia of the utricle and fallen against the cupula of the posterior semicircular canal.

Eighth-Nerve Lesions

Eighth-nerve lesions, such as acoustic schwannomas or meningiomas, may affect the eighth nerve and produce vertigo. Typically, this gradual-onset vertigo is preceded by hearing loss, and there may be other symptoms to suggest involvement of the cerebellopontine (CP) angle, such as a constant unsteadiness or ataxia and a chronically progressive course. Patients with unilateral sensorineural hearing loss, including those who seem to have Menière's disease, should be evaluated for cerebellopontine angle tumor.

Cerebellopontine Angle Tumor

Many patients with tumors at the CP angle, such as meningiomas and dermoids, exhibit chronic deafness and disequilibrium, and occasion-

Table 148-3. Nylen-Barany (Hallpike) Maneuver

Test: Patient is in sitting position on stretcher. Clinician supports head and has patient rapidly assume supine position, first with head straight, then with head turned 45 degrees left, then 45 degrees right.

Findings with peripheral vertigo:
- Vertigo and nystagmus produced, latency 2–20 s
- Duration less than 1 min
- Unidirectional nystagmus
- Nystagmus and vertigo fatigue with repeated testing
- Even straight head position may elicit vertigo (Barany's)

Findings with central vertigo
- Latency of nystagmus, none
- Nystagmus nonfatiguing, multidirectional
- Duration greater than 1 min

ally vertigo. They may demonstrate ipsilateral impairment of the corneal reflex, facial weakness, and cerebellar signs on the involved side.

Posttraumatic Vertigo

The delicate labyrinthine membranes are susceptible to accelerational forces, and head trauma may result in unilateral contusion or concussion to the labyrinth. After cerebral concussion, up to 20 percent of people develop vertigo. *Acute posttraumatic vertigo* caused by labyrinthine concussion begins immediately after head injury and results in continuous vertigo, nausea, and vomiting. Symptoms usually improve over the first few days, with gradual resolution over a few weeks. *Posttraumatic positional vertigo* may develop days to weeks after injury, and may replace the constant vertigo of acute posttraumatic vertigo. Symptoms are precipitated by changes in head position, as with benign positional vertigo. Symptoms tend to resolve over months, and most are gone by 2 years post injury.

Benign Paroxysmal Vertigo of Childhood

A condition of severe brief attacks of vertigo in children, usually under the age of 3 years, benign paroxysmal vertigo of childhood, is generally self-limited, resolving spontaneously within months to a few years. It is felt to be labyrinthine in origin and of unknown etiology. Because vertigo may represent the aura of a seizure, EEG might be considered in very selected cases of childhood vertigo.

Disorders Causing Central Vertigo

Central vertigo is characterized symptomatically by a much less dramatic vertiginous feeling than peripheral vertigo and is not exacerbated by motion or by assuming specific positions. Typically, central vertigo is not an intense feeling, and has little or no associated nausea, vomiting, pallor, or diaphoresis. The onset is gradual. The nystagmus characteristic of central vertigo may be present in the absence of the subjective sensation of vertigo. Central vertigo is produced by conditions that affect the cerebellum and brain stem. All conditions that affect the brain stem and cause vertigo typically have other brain stem signs associated with them, such as dysphagia, dysarthria, ataxia, diplopia, facial numbness, bilateral limb weakness, or bilateral visual blurring. Oscillopsia may occur.

Conditions producing central vertigo affect the brain stem and cerebellum. Hearing is characteristically unimpaired, and tinnitus is rare. Cerebellar infarction and hemorrhage may result in central vertigo. The typical history of cerebellar hemorrhage is acute vertigo and ataxia, with or without nausea and vomiting, and with or without acute headache. Less typically there may be conjugate eye deviation to the side opposite the hemorrhage, or a sixth-nerve palsy. The patient with cerebellar hemorrhage may not be able to sit without support, although casual neurologic testing done only in the supine position or a supported position may not be abnormal. Cerebellar infarction may present in a similar fashion. Vertigo from cerebellar disease may be described as recurrent front-to-back or side-to-side movement, which may be evoked by position change.

Conditions affecting the brain stem can produce vertigo as part of their clinical symptomatology, particularly lateral medullary infarction (Wallenberg's syndrome), which consists of vertigo; ipsilateral paralysis of the soft palate, pharynx, and larynx with dysphagia and dysphonia; ipsilateral facial numbness with loss of corneal reflex; ipsilateral Horner's syndrome; and ipsilateral cerebellar asynergia and hypotonia. Sixth-, seventh-, and eighth-nerve lesions have been reported with vertigo, nausea and vomiting, nystagmus, and hiccups. There is contralateral loss of pain and temperature on the limbs and trunk.

Transient ischemic attacks affecting the brain stem may produce similar short-lasting symptoms and positional nystagmus, but by definition must include more than simply vertigo. Other structures in the brain stem must be affected in order to render the diagnosis.

Neoplasms of the fourth ventricle, typically ependymomas in young patients and metastases in elderly patients, can likewise affect the brain stem.

Multiple sclerosis, with its myriad manifestations, may produce isolated lesions in the brain stem, producing vertigo and other brain stem findings. Marked nystagmus with little no vertigo should suggest a brain stem origin.

Miscellaneous Causes of Vertigo

Physiologic vertigo, as in motion sickness, results from mismatched vestibular, visual, and somatosensory input. Similar mismatch may occur when the visual sensation of motion, as in watching a movie of an automobile chase, is not accompanied by matching vestibular input.

Vertigo may occur on a psychogenic basis, typically as a long-standing vertiginous feeling unaffected by motion and position and without associated nausea or vomiting. As a prodrome to seizure, a cortical focus may produce transient vertigo prior to the seizure. This is very rare. Rare ocular causes of vertigo include watching a rapidly moving series of objects, such as the car or train from a stationary position or telephone poles from a moving car, inducing a sensation of vertigo and motion sickness. Recent ophthalmoplegia may cause brief vertigo. Serous labyrinthitis due to otitis media may produce vertigo.

The blood supply to the inner ear is not supported by a collateral circulation, and is tenuous. However, direct evidence for reduced blood flow to the inner ear as a cause of vertigo is lacking. While it is postulated that vertigo may occur as a result of imbalanced proprioceptive input due to cervical muscle lesions, its clinical occurrence is doubtful. Basilar migraine may cause throbbing occipital headache, visual hallucinations, vertigo, tinnitus, dysarthria, and drop attacks.

Disequilibrium Syndrome

Disequilibrium syndrome consists of an ill-defined dizziness as a result of multiple sensory abnormalities. There is a chronic mismatch of input from the body systems providing spatial orientation. The patient, typically elderly, may have diminished vision, diminished hearing, and diminished proprioceptive, cerebellar, or peripheral neurologic function. The disequilibrium may be exaggerated or precipitated by sudden worsening in one or more of these sensory modalities, and typically worsens at night when diminished ambient lighting reduces visual input. Unfamiliar situations and surroundings may exacerbate the symptoms. Sedative medications can exaggerate or precipitate the problem. Typically these patients have multiple etiologies for near syncope as well; at times it is difficult to establish a precise diagnosis.

Ill-Defined Light-Headedness

Patients with ill-defined light-headedness frequently cannot characterize their symptomatology in any way that is useful for the physician. They may have concomitant complaints of generalized fatigue or aching and nonfocal weakness. It is very difficult to ascribe a specific etiology to these subjective complaints.

Hyperventilation Syndrome

Some patients with dizziness or light-headedness may suffer from a primary hyperventilation syndrome. Reproduction of their symptoms with directed hyperventilation aids in the diagnosis. Primary hyperventilation must be distinguished from hyperventilation secondary to a variety of medical disorders or insufficient oxygenation.

Anxiety

Anxiety itself may produce dizziness characterized by disequilibrium. Many times the dizziness has been present for very long periods of time, there is no clear relationship to any exacerbating or precipitating factors, and the history and physical and neurologic examinations do not reveal any recognizable pattern. It is sometimes difficult to isolate other possible causes of dizziness when the patient presents with a host of symptoms seemingly precipitated by anxiety.

Near Syncope

Patients with near syncope may complain of dizziness. On detailed questioning, it can usually be elicited that patients have a feeling that they would pass out if the symptomatology became worse. The causes of syncope and near syncope are essentially identical and only differ in magnitude. Near syncope may be produced by orthostatic, autonomic, reflex, and cardiac mechanisms, or by hypoglycemia. Possible orthostatic causes include volume depletion, poor conditioning, venous insufficiency, peripheral neuropathy including that produced by diabetes mellitus, and the effects of antihypertensive, vasodilating, and anti-Parkinson drugs. Preganglionic autonomic dysfunction, such as that presenting with Shy-Drager syndrome, may produce a near syncopal feeling. Reflex causes include a hyperactive carotid sinus, micturition, cough, and swallow syncope. Vasovagal syncope is actually less common in elderly patients and may be associated with multiple causes for stress or prolonged bed rest. Cardiac mechanisms for syncope include mechanical causes, such as valvular disease or subaortic stenosis, and arrhythmias.

DIAGNOSIS

History

Most causes of vertigo are benign, but potentially disabling. Some forms of dizziness may represent life-threatening emergencies, e.g., arrhythmia. Since the primary problem in the diagnosis of a patient with dizziness is establishing a precise definition of the patient's symptomatology, the history is of paramount importance. There is nowhere that the classic neurologic approach to the patient (defining the nature of the disturbance first and its localization second) is more important.

Even though the symptoms may be very difficult for the patient to describe, it is important not to ask leading questions or to suggest to the patient what the symptoms might mean because patients may incorporate the words used by the examiner into the description of their symptoms, whether they fit or not. In general, patients must be given time to elaborate exactly what the subjective feeling of dizziness means to them. At some point it must be established whether or not they have a vertiginous feeling. Whether the feeling is that of syncope should be determined, as well as the relationship to movement, head position, and particular postures.

The temporal profile at onset, such as the rate of development of symptoms and the duration of symptoms, should be elicited. The time of day of any worsening of symptoms should be elicited. All associated symptoms, such as nausea, vomiting, blurriness or double vision, tinnitus, focal or generalized weakness, numbness, visual loss, palpitations, and loss of consciousness should be noted. Past medical facts of most importance are the use of medications, both prescribed and over the counter, any history of trauma, and a history of similar episodes.

Physical Examination

The physical examination should focus on several areas. Bedside tests of hearing and physical examination of the ears should be done. Eye movements, with particular emphasis on nystagmus, both direction and fatigue, should be evaluated. The details of cranial nerve testing are important, particularly eighth-nerve function; the cranial nerves most closely associated with the eighth nerve, specifically fifth-nerve function, including corneal reflex; seventh-nerve function; and ninth- and tenth-nerve function (gag reflex, swallowing). Of particular importance on the motor examination is testing of coordination, such as finger-to-nose testing or rapid alternating movements. Gait testing and an evaluation of the patient's ability to sit without support, as a test for truncal ataxia, may be necessary. Orthostatic vital signs should be checked.

Perhaps the best bedside test of hearing is that of the soft whispered voice. One masks the ear not being tested with light pressure on the external canal or by rubbing the fingers in front of it and whispers names or letters in the unmasked ear that the patient must repeat. If there is a decrease in hearing, then Webber's and Rinne's test may be done to help distinguish between conductive and neurosensory loss.

Of particular importance in the evaluation of the potentially vertiginous patient is the Nylen-Barany maneuver outlined in Table 148-3. The type and duration of nystagmus are noted. In addition to the findings noted in the table, peripheral vertigo is more likely than central vertigo to be associated with nausea and vomiting and relatively severe symptoms (Table 148-1).

Other tests can be done as indicated by the initial history and physical examination. Drachman's dizziness stimulation battery is given in Table 148-4.

Of particular importance on the cardiac exam is to note the rate and rhythm of the heart and to evaluate for evidence of valvular heart disease.

Laboratory Evaluation

Laboratory testing is selected based on the history and physical examination. Glucose testing in particular may be a productive test in patients with disequilibrium syndrome. Diabetes is one major cause of diminished peripheral neurologic function. In patients with typical peripheral vertigo and little else to suggest other medical problems, laboratory testing is not needed. In patients with presyncopal feeling, cardiac rhythm monitoring may be in order. Depending upon the physical examination, other testing to detect cardiac etiology may be indicated, such as echocardiography, ambulatory cardiac rhythm monitoring, etc. In the evaluation of long-term hearing loss with vestibular dysfunction, serologic testing for syphilis is commonly done.

When cerebellar hemorrhage or infarction is suspected, CT scanning should be considered. If tumor at the CP angle is a possibility, CT scanning may be done, although MRI is more sensitive. Patients with suspected central vertigo will require an imaging study and neurologic consultation. Most patients with peripheral vertigo and no suspicion of eighth-nerve lesion or CP angle tumor do not require an urgent imaging study.

TREATMENT

The principle of most importance in emergency department management is to firmly establish the nature of the patient's dizziness. Virtually all of the medications that are useful for peripheral vertigo will result in worsening symptoms of patients with disequilibrium syndromes or ill-defined light-headedness.

There are multiple medications used in the emergency department and outpatient management of peripheral vertigo. Antihistamines have been known to be effective for the treatment of peripheral vertigo for 40 years. Not all antihistamines are useful, and their peripheral potency as antihistamines does not correlate with suppression of vertigo. The most useful ones have anticholinergic properties. Antihistamines may act both centrally, at the brain stem level, and peripherally, within the labyrinthine apparatus. Anticholinergics such as atropine and scopolamine are also quite effective. The efferent nerves of the vestibular sensory cells are cholinergic, and thus affected by anticholinergics.

Table 148-4. Drachman's Dizziness Battery

Blood pressure lying and standing
Valsalva maneuver
Head turn—standing with eyes open
Sudden turn when walking
3 min hyperventilation
Nylen-Barany testing

Table 148-5. Drugs used for Vertigo of Peripheral Origin

Antihistamines
Diphenhydramine
Dimenhydrinate
Cyclizine
Meclizine
Promethazine
Anticholinergics
Atropine
Scopolamine
Antiemetics
Hydroxyzine
Promethazine
Sedatives
Diazepam
Chlordiazepoxide
Calcium channel blockers
Flunarizine

The central effects of anticholinergics may also mediate their action. Diazepam acts centrally on the lateral vestibular nucleus and is useful in acute peripheral vertigo. More recently the calcium channel blocker flunarizine has been found useful in the management of vertigo. Other commonly used antiemetics, such as chlorperazine and chlorpromazine, are of little use in relieving patients with vertigo. Hydroxyzine and promethazine, however, with their antihistaminic activity, are. Effective agents for the management of peripheral vertigo are listed in Table 148-5.

Most patients need reassurance that the symptoms, while overpowering, are self-limiting, are not a reflection of serious pathology, and are not a serious threat to their health. An explanation that symptoms are caused by an imbalanced input from the two ears, and that the nervous system will accommodate to it, is helpful. The component of management that usually requires little explanation for the vertiginous patient is that of either bed rest or resting in a position of comfort and a slowing of all movements so as to not precipitate the vertiginous feeling. Visual fixation on a nearby object may inhibit vertigo of peripheral origin and is preferable to lying with closed eyes.

The efficacy of the many regimens used in the chronic treatment of Menière's disease (low salt diet, ammonium chloride, diuretics, glycerol) has not been proved. Acute management is the same as for other forms of peripheral vertigo. Surgical destruction of the labyrinth or endolymphatic shunt can be done in the long-term management of Menière's disease.

Benign positional vertigo (Barany's) is treated with the same medications as other peripheral disorders, but is seldom very responsive. Some advocate repeated head movement to provoke attacks, fatiguing the response and or dispersion of the otolithic fragments.

In cases of disequilibrium syndrome, if no specific causes are found, one might consider withdrawal of any sedative or hypnotic medications. If the problem appears to be one of multiple sensory deficit syndrome, consideration of changes in ambient light, especially later in the day, and changing some factors in the surroundings may be indicated.

Emergency department management of patients with near syncope is similar to that for those with syncope (see Chap. 13).

For ill-defined light-headedness, when it is impossible to place the patient in a better-defined category of dizziness and when preliminary emergency department testing does not indicate any specific pathology, it is best to avoid medications used for vertigo.

SUMMARY

The evaluation of the dizzy patient is a challenge to the skills of the physician. An initial open-ended history is important to define the clinical symptomatology precisely, without suggesting a particular entity. Precision in history taking will be rewarded by narrowing the field of potential insults causing symptoms. A thorough neurologic examination, with particular emphasis upon nystagmus, must be done. If vertigo is indeed the problem, one must separate peripheral (benign) causes from more ominous central causes. Recognition that symptoms may be quite disabling yet reflect benign processes may be reassuring to the patient. Careful selection of medications for vertigo can only be done when the syndrome is precisely defined and should be avoided unless the diagnosis of peripheral vertigo is established.

BIBLIOGRAPHY

Adams, RD: *Principles of Neurology*, 4th ed. New York, McGraw Hill, 1989, p 238.

Bannister, R: *Brain's Clinical Neurology*, 6th ed. New York, Oxford, 1985, p 75.

Brandt T, Daroff RB: The multisensory physiological and pathological vertigo syndromes. *Ann Neurol* 7:195, 1980.

Drachman DA, Apfelbaum RI, Posner JB: Dizziness and disorders of equilibrium, panel 8. *Arch Neurol* 36:806, 1979.

Drachman DA, Hart CW: An approach to the dizzy patient. *Neurology* 22:323, 1972.

Herr RD, Zun L, Mathews JJ: A directed approach to the dizzy patient. *Ann Emerg Med* 18:664, 1989.

Mohr DN. The syndrome of paroxysmal positional vertigo, a review. *West J Med* 145:645, 1986.

Norris CH: Drugs affecting the inner ear: A review of their clinical efficacy, mechanisms of action, toxicity, and place in therapy. *Drugs* 36:754, 1988.

Olsky M, Murray J: Dizziness and fainting in the elderly. *Emerg Med Clin North Am* 8:295, 1990.

Olsson JE, Atkins JS: Vestibular disorders, *Otolaryngol Clin North Am* 20:83, 1987.

Scheinberg, P: *An Introduction to Diagnosis and Management of Common Neurologic Disorders*, 3d ed. New York, Raven, p 99.

Slater R: Vertigo: How serious are recurrent and single attacks? *Postgrad Med*. 84:58, 1988.

Swanson, PD: *Signs and Symptoms in Neurology*. Philadelphia, Lippincott, 1984, p 123.

Todd PA, Benfield P: Flunarizine: A reappraisal of its pharmacological properties and therapeutic use in neurological disorders. *Drugs* 38:481, 1989.

Weiss HD: Dizziness, in Samuels M (ed): *Manual of Neurologic Therapeutics*, 2d ed. Boston, Little, Brown, 1982, chap 4.

149 SEIZURES AND STATUS EPILEPTICUS IN ADULTS

Thomas R. Pellegrino

A seizure may be defined as an episode of abnormal neurologic function caused by an abnormal electrical discharge of brain neurons. Note that the seizure is the clinical attack experienced by the patient; some patients with "epileptic" electroencephalographic (EEG) discharges may not experience any clinical symptoms. Conversely, some seizure-like clinical episodes may be due to causes other than abnormal brain electrical activity; such attacks, however impressive, are not true seizures.

The term epilepsy denotes a clinical condition in which an individual is subject to recurrent seizures; it implies a more or less fixed condition of the brain responsible for the seizures. Ordinarily, the term epileptic is not used to refer to an individual with recurrent seizures caused by reversible conditions such as alcohol withdrawal, hypoglycemia, or other metabolic derangements.

The occurrence of one or more seizures indicates abnormal function of cerebral neurons. When this occurs in patients who are otherwise normal and in whom no evident cause for the attacks can be discerned, the seizures are referred to as primary or idiopathic. Seizures which occur as a consequence of some other identifiable neurologic condition are referred to as secondary or symptomatic.

Seizures are very common; approximately 1 to 2 percent of persons are subject to recurrent seizures. About 10 percent of individuals will experience at least one seizure during their lives. It is important to note that any individual can be caused to have a seizure under appropriate conditions. Electrical stimulation of the brain, convulsant drugs, profound metabolic disturbances, or a sharp blow to the head may induce seizures in otherwise normal individuals. Such attacks are generally self-limited, and such persons are not considered to have a seizure disorder or epilepsy. From such otherwise normal persons, there extends a continuum which includes, at its other extreme, persons who have frequent recurrent seizures without discernible cause.

The precise mechanisms involved in generating clinical seizures remain unknown, despite intense investigation. The process appears to require both intense and prolonged neuronal electrical discharges and failure or inhibition of normal protective mechanisms, but the molecular mechanisms underlying the events remain unclear. Once the seizure discharge begins, it may remain localized, it may spread to involve nearby populations of neurons, or it may spread rapidly to involve the entire cerebral cortex. The mechanisms by which these electrical discharges cause clinical seizures remain unknown. As mentioned earlier, EEG tracings frequently demonstrate electrical seizure discharges without any associated clinical signs.

SEIZURE CLASSIFICATION

Over the years, many attempts have been made to provide a clinically useful classification of seizure types, both to facilitate communication among physicians and provide a basis for treatment decisions. Seizures may be classified based on the observed clinical features of the attacks, on their presumed etiologies, on EEG findings, on their clinical context, or on some combination of these.

The simplest scheme is to identify seizures as "big ones, little ones, and funny ones," a tradition maintained in the terms "grand mal, petit mal, and psychomotor." Unfortunately, these common terms are neither precise nor very informative. While commonly used informally, they have been largely replaced for most purposes by more formal terminology proposed by the International League Against Epilepsy. In this scheme, seizures are divided into two major groups; generalized seizures and focal seizures. (Table 149-1).

Generalized seizures are thought to be caused by nearly simultaneous activation of the entire cerebral cortex, perhaps caused by an electrical discharge originating deep in the brain and spreading outward. The attacks begin with abrupt loss of consciousness. This may be the only clinical manifestation of the seizures (as in absence attacks), or there may be a variety of motor manifestations (myoclonic jerks, drop attacks, tonic posturing, clonic jerking of the body and extremities, etc.) Motor activity, when present, typically involves all four extremities and is symmetrical (from side to side). Although generalized seizures may be preceded by several hours or days or prodromal symptoms (irritability, tension, isolated myoclonic jerks, etc.), true sensory auras do not occur in generalized seizures. The most familiar varieties of generalized seizures are absence (petit mal) and tonic-clonic (grand mal) attacks.

Petit mal attacks are very brief, generally lasting only a few seconds. The patients abruptly lose consciousness and seem "out of contact." Current activity ceases. They may stare and may have twitching of their eyelids; they do not respond to voice or to other stimulation. They do not fall or exhibit involuntary movements, and they do not lose continence. The attacks cease abruptly, and the patients are able to resume their previous activity with no postictal symptoms. Both patients and witnesses may be unaware that anything has happened. Classic petit mal attacks are virtually limited to school-age children and are often attributed by parents and teachers to daydreaming or not paying attention. The attacks may be very frequent, sometimes occurring 100 or more times daily, and may result in poor school performance. Petit mal attacks may occur alone or be associated with other kinds of seizures, especially as the child enters their adolescent or teenage years. Petit mal attacks usually resolve as the child matures, and true absence attacks are unusual in adults. It is usually incorrect to refer to minor seizures in adults as petit mal. Similar attacks in adults are more likely to be minor complex partial seizures. The distinction is important, since the causes and treatment of the two types of seizures are quite different.

Grand mal attacks are among the most dramatic of medical events. The true generalized grand mal attack begins with an abrupt loss of consciousness; there is usually no warning, and true auras do not occur. The patient suddenly becomes rigid, with trunk and extremities extruded and falls to the ground. Patients are apneic during this period and may be deeply cyanotic; they often urinate or defecate and may vomit. As the rigid (tonic) phase of the attack subsides, there is increasing coarse trembling which evolves into rhythmic (clonic) jerking

Table 149-1. Classification of Seizures

Generalized seizures (consciousness always lost)
Absence seizures (petit mal)
Myoclonic seizures
Tonic seizures
Clonic seizures
Tonic-clonic seizures
Atonic seizures
Partial (focal) seizures
Simple (elementary), no alteration of consciousness
Motor seizures
Sensory seizures
Autonomic seizures
Complex (psychomotor or temporal lobe seizures) consciousness impaired
With psychic, cognitive, or affective symptoms
With automatisms
Partial seizures (elementary or complex) with secondary generalization
Unclassified (due to inadequate information)

of the trunk and extremities. As the attack ends, the patient is left flaccid and unconscious, often with deep rapid breathing. Typical attacks last from 60 to 90 s (occasionally longer). Bystanders generally grossly overestimate the duration of the attack. Consciousness returns gradually, and postictal confusion and fatigue may last several hours or longer.

Partial (focal) seizures are due to electrical discharges which begin in a localized region of the cerebral cortex; the discharge may remain localized or may spread to involve nearby cortical regions or to the entire cortex. Focal seizures are generally thought to be secondary or symptomatic seizures; their occurrence often implies a focal structural lesion of the brain. It is often possible to deduce the likely location of the initial cortical discharge from the clinical features at the onset of the attack. Unilateral tonic or clonic movements (often limited to one extremity) suggest a focus in the motor cortex. Tonic deviation of the head and eyes (usually to the side *away* from the discharge) suggests a frontal lobe focus. Sensory hallucinations (e.g., paresthesias or numbness) suggest a discharge in the sensory cortex. Visual symptoms, especially flashing lights or distortions of vision, suggest an occipital focus. Bizarre olfactory or gustatory hallucinations suggest a focus in the medial temporal lobe. Such sensory phenomena are often the initial symptoms of attacks which then become more widespread. The auras which may precede other kinds of seizures are examples of such focal sensory seizures; the presence of an aura implies that the attack is a focal seizure. In simple or elementary focal seizures, the seizure remains localized, and consciousness and mentation are not affected.

Complex partial seizures are focal seizures in which consciousness and mentation are affected. They are caused most often by a focal discharge originating in the temporal lobe and are sometimes referred to as temporal lobe seizures. Because of their psychic content and automatisms, they are sometimes referred to as psychomotor seizures. Often thought to be rare, they are in fact quite common.

Because of their frequently bizarre symptoms and psychic features, complex partial seizures are commonly misdiagnosed as psychiatric problems. Their symptoms may include visceral symptoms, hallucinations, memory disturbances, dream-like states, automatisms, and affective disorders. Visceral symptoms often consist of a sensation of "butterflies" beginning in the stomach or epigastrium, rising up through the chest to the face. Other visceral auras include nausea or abdominal pains. Hallucinations may involve any sensory modality including smell, taste, hearing, or vision. There may be complex distortions of perception such that objects may appear to change color, shapes may be distorted, or objects may appear larger, smaller, closer, or more distant than they really are. The perception of time is commonly distorted; patients cannot usually estimate the length of the attack and may describe time as passing very slowly or standing still. Rarely, the passage of time seems accelerated. Memory disturbances may include déjà vu, a sense of familiarity in an unfamiliar environment, or jamais vu, a sense of unfamiliarity or strangeness in familiar surroundings. Patients may experience brief "reruns" of past experiences. Automatisms are typically simple, repetitive, purposeless movements such as lip smacking, fiddling with clothing or buttons, or repeating short phrases. More complex behaviors may occur, but well organized, purposeful activity is very rare. Affective disorders may include intense sensations of fear, paranoia, depression, or rarely, elation or ecstasy.

A focal seizure discharge may spread to involve both hemispheres, mimicking a typical generalized seizure. For purposes of classification, diagnosis, and treatment, such attacks are regarded as focal seizures. In some patients, the discharge may spread so rapidly that no focal symptoms are evident, and the correct diagnosis may depend on demonstration of the focal discharge on an EEG recording. In many cases, however, a very careful history will reveal focal symptoms at the onset of the attack and allow a correct diagnosis. The distinction is very important since, as noted previously, the diagnosis of the focal seizure disorder should prompt a search for an underlying structural lesion.

CLINICAL EVALUATION OF SEIZURE PATIENTS

History

The first and most important step in evaluating a seizure patient is to determine if the attack was truly a seizure. Unfortunately, it is common practice to use a diagnosis of "rule out seizure" in patients who have had any transient spells for which no more specific diagnosis is available. This practice is to be condemned, not only for being intellectually and diagnostically sloppy, but also because of the consequences to the individual of being erroneously labeled a seizure patient. There may be serious adverse effects on employability, driving privileges, insurability, etc. Also, it should be remembered that all anticonvulsant drugs are more or less toxic. An erroneous or hasty diagnosis of epilepsy may expose the patient to substantial harm with no prospect of benefit, not to mention delaying appropriate treatment for the correct diagnosis. A basic rule is that "everything which falls down and shakes is not a seizure." There are many episodic disturbances of neurologic function which may be mistaken for seizures by the unwary physician (Table 149-2). A complete review of these conditions would too lengthy for inclusion here but several of the more important possibilities should be mentioned.

Syncope usually is attended by premonitory symptoms such as pallor, diaphoresis, and a "graying out" of vision. Patients often are aware that they are going to pass out and can clearly describe the onset of the attacks. Syncope may be attended by injury or incontinence; in addition, some patients may experience some myoclonic jerks, especially if they are prevented from falling.

Narcolepsy is characterized by brief attacks of uncontrollable daytime sleepiness. Patients are able to feel their attacks coming on and can sometimes control them with judiciously timed naps. An associated symptom is cataplexy, characterized by a sudden brief loss of postural muscle tone. The patient collapses but remains fully conscious; there are no involuntary movements. The attacks are often triggered by emotional upset, laughter, crying, etc.

Movement disorders such as myoclonic jerks, tremors, or tics may occur in a variety of neurologic disorders. Consciousness is always preserved during these movements; the movements, though involuntary, often can be suppressed temporarily by the patient.

Hyperventilation syndrome is very common and is often misdiagnosed as a seizure disorder. A careful history normally will reveal the gradual onset of the attacks with shortness of breath, anxiety, and perioral numbness. Such attacks may progress to involuntary spasm of the extremities and even loss of consciousness. The attacks often are reproduced easily in the emergency room or office by asking the patient to overbreathe.

Psychogenic seizures are very common and may be extremely difficult to distinguish from true seizures. This diagnosis should be suspected when seizures occur regularly in response to emotional upset or when seizures only occur with witnesses present. The attacks are often very bizarre and highly variable. Patients often are able to protect themselves from noxious stimuli during the attack. Incontinence and injury are very rare, and there is often no postictal confusion. In some

Table 149-2. Paroxysmal Disorders: Differential Diagnosis

Seizures
Syncope
Narcolepsy/cataplexy
Movement disorders
Hyperventilation syndrome
Psychogenic seizures
Paroxysmal vertigo
Rage attacks, fugue states
Transient ischemic attacks
Migraine

cases, accurate diagnosis may require prolonged EEG monitoring to demonstrate the presence of normal EEG activity during an attack.

A careful history of the details of the attack usually will allow a diagnosis to be made with a high degree of certainty. The history should be obtained from the patient, if possible, and from any bystanders who actually witnessed the attack. Be very wary of accepting a diagnosis of seizure from witnesses, including other physicians. Also, do not assume that a given episode was a seizure, even if the patient has a history of seizures. The original diagnosis may be incorrect, or the patient may have experienced another kind of attack. In each case, try to get a detailed description of the attack, and draw your own conclusions.

Try to determine how the attack began. Was there any aura? Did the attack begin abruptly or gradually? Ask about staring, lip smacking, blinking, breath holding, etc. Ask about motor activity as the attack progressed. Determine if motor activity was local or generalized, symmetrical or not. Did the motor activity begin in one part of the body and then spread? Finally, ask about the duration of the attack and about any postictal confusion or lethargy. Ask the patient if they have any recollection of the attack. Clinical features which help to distinguish seizures from other kinds of attacks include:

1. Abrupt onset and termination. Although some focal seizures are preceded by auras which last 20 to 30 s (or more), most attacks begin abruptly. Attacks which develop over several minutes, or longer, should be regarded with suspicion. Most seizures last only 1 or 2 min, occasionally more. Be wary of an attack which lasts 30 min or several hours or longer.
2. A true sensory or other aura, if present, is helpful in recognizing focal (especially complex partial) seizures. Absence of an aura is not helpful.
3. True seizures are generally stereotyped. Attacks may vary in intensity or duration, of course, but the basic features will be consistent. There are patients who have more than one type of seizure, but each type will maintain its own pattern. Be very wary if the attacks are highly variable and inconsistent.
4. Lack of recall. Except for simple partial seizures, patients usually cannot recall the details of an attack, the responses and acts of bystanders, etc. Be wary of attacks in which the patient "could hear everyone talking but could not respond."
5. True seizures are not generally provoked by environmental cues or stimuli. There are rare cases of true reflex epilepsy, and seizures may be provoked by sleep deprivation, drugs, or alcohol withdrawal. True seizures, however, are not provoked by emotional distress, being yelled at by parents, etc.
6. Movements or behavior during the attack generally is purposeless or inappropriate. Occasional rare exceptions have been described, but popular literature to the contrary, persons do not rob banks, engage in direct violence, or carry out other coherent, purposeful activity during seizures.
7. Most seizures, except for simple absence attacks (petit mal) or simple partial seizures, will be followed by a period of postictal confusion and lethargy. Be very wary of a dramatic convulsion followed immediately by normal mental function.

Although a clinical diagnosis of seizures often can be made with a high degree of certainty, there are some occasions when the diagnosis is not convincing. In such cases, it is better to admit uncertainty and not use the label seizure or begin inappropriate and potentially hazardous treatment. In such cases, multiple EEG recordings, prolonged EEG monitoring, and evaluation by a neurologist all may be necessary to establish a diagnosis.

Once it is decided that the patient actually has had a seizure, the next step is to determine the clinical context in which the attack occurred. In the case of a patient with a previously documented and evaluated seizure disorder who has had a typical attack, little further evaluation is required. If the patient is receiving anticonvulsant medication, ask about any recent changes in medication, missed doses, etc. Even a single missed dose may result in a marked drop in blood levels of medication and result in a seizure. Ask about a recent change from brand-name to generic medication or from one generic formulation to another. Other possible factors which might provoke a seizure include sleep deprivation, alcohol withdrawal, and use of other drugs.

If there is no previous history of seizures, a much more detailed history is needed. Ask about any symptoms that might suggest previous unwitnessed or unrecognized seizures: blank spells or staring spells in school, involuntary movement, unexplained injuries, nocturnal tongue biting, and enuresis. Ask about any other neurologic symptoms, such as mental retardation, delayed development, progressive headache, head trauma, and focal symptoms. Inquire into any systemic illness: cancer, hypo- or hyperglycemia, electrolyte abnormalities, drug ingestion (licit and illicit), and alcohol use. Finally, ask about any family history of seizures or other neurologic illness (Table 149-3).

Physical Examination

The general physical examination should be directed toward discovering any injuries that might have resulted from the seizure and any systemic illness which might have caused the attack. Seizures may cause injuries such as fractures, sprains, and bruises; posterior dislocations of the shoulder are common and often overlooked. Look for tongue lacerations and broken teeth or any suggestion of aspiration. Look also for any dysmorphic features or birthmarks.

The neurologic examination should evaluate the patient's level of consciousness and mentation. Mental status should be followed closely with serial examinations. Profound obtundation which improves steadily is probably benign, while progressive deterioration should cause great concern. Search for any signs of increased intracranial pressure and any signs of focal weakness or reflex changes. Focal signs following a seizure, even if transient, strongly suggest a focal seizure.

Laboratory Examination

Blood Chemistry

There are no standard or routine laboratory studies to be obtained in seizure patients; the need for such studies must be assessed on an

Table 149-3. Some Causes of Secondary Seizures

Intracranial etiologies
Trauma (recent or remote)
Infection (meningitis, encephalitis, abscess)
Vascular lesion (stroke, arteriovenous malformation, vasculitis)
Mass lesions (neoplasma, subdural hematoma)
Degenerative disease
Extracranial etiologies
Anoxic-ischemic injury (e.g., cardiac arrest, severe hypoxemia)
Endocrine/electolyte disorders
Hypoglycemia
Hyperosmolar states
Hyponatremia
Hypocalcemia, hypomagnesemia (rare)
Toxins and drugs
Cocaine, lidocaine
Antidepressants
Theophylline
Alcohol withdrawal
Barbiturate withdrawal
Benzodiazepine withdrawal
Anticonvulsant withdrawal
and *many* others
Eclampsia of pregnancy (may occur postpartum)
Hypertensive encephalopathy

individual basis. In a patient with a well-documented seizure disorder who has had a single unprovoked seizure, no laboratory studies may be needed. Anticonvulsant drug levels may be helpful but should be interpreted with caution.

In the case of a patient with a first seizure or when the history is unclear, more extensive studies may be helpful. Arterial blood gas studies may demonstrate a metabolic acidemia following a major convulsion; similarly, muscle enzyme levels (e.g., creatine kinase) may be elevated. Serum electrolytes, glucose, blood urea nitrogen (BUN) and creatinine, calcium and magnesium, and a toxicology screen may be indicated depending on the clinical context. Blood prolactin levels may be evaluated for a brief period (30 to 60 min) immediately after a true seizure (but not after pseudoseizures) and are sometimes helpful in confirming that an attack was a true seizure. A normal prolactin level is not helpful. The presence of anticonvulsant drugs in the blood of a patient from whom no history is available suggests (but does not prove) the presence of a seizure disorder.

Anticonvulsant drug levels must be interpreted with caution. The usual therapeutic and toxic levels indicated in laboratory reports are helpful only as very rough guides. The therapeutic level of a drug is that level which provides adequate seizure control without unacceptable side effects; a phenytoin level of only 8 μg/mL may be therapeutic if a patient is having only occasional seizures and if higher levels cause symptoms of toxicity. Similarly a toxic level is one which causes symptoms of intoxication. A phenytoin level of 15 μg/mL (or less) may be toxic in a given patient. Conversely, a phenytoin level of 24 μg/mL may result in excellent seizure control and be well tolerated. A marked change in previously stable drug levels may indicate noncompliance, a change in medication (e.g., from one brand to another), malabsorption of a drug (as in severe diarrhea or vomiting), or ingestion of a competing drug.

Radiographic Studies

In the case of a patient with a known seizure disorder, radiographic studies usually are not needed. There is no rational basis for the common practice of obtaining routine CT scans on each patient who presents to the emergency department after a seizure.

In the case of a patient with a first seizure, CT scanning may be appropriate to look for evidence of a structural lesion responsible for the attack. Whenever possible, such scans should be done both without and with contrast enhancement, since many important processes, such as metastatic or primary tumors or vascular anomalies, may be missed on noncontrast studies. In most cases, the scan may be delayed until the patient has recovered and the results of BUN and creatinine levels are available, and the patient has been asked about any relevant allergies. Emergency scanning is only necessary in a patient whose condition is deteriorating.

Magnetic resonance (MR) scanning is substantially more sensitive than CT in detecting subtle alterations of brain structure, and it is often the study of choice in the evaluation of patients with seizures. Especially in patients with uncomplicated first seizures, it is reasonable to omit the CT scan and obtain an MR scan instead. Consultation with a radiologist may be helpful in choosing the best approach and avoiding unnecessary examinations.

Other radiographic studies may be indicated in some cases. Chest x-rays may reveal primary or metastatic tumors or evidence of aspiration. Skull x-rays may reveal fractures or other bony lesions (though CT scanning is often superior). Special examinations such as angiography may be helpful in some cases but are rarely included in an emergency department evaluation.

EEG

The EEG may be very helpful in the evaluation of patients with seizures. It is sometimes said that the only way to be certain of the diagnosis of epilepsy is to record an attack and demonstrate the characteristic electrical discharge. More commonly, the EEG provides support for the diagnosis of seizures by recording interictal EEG discharges without clinical accompaniment; the EEG can help distinguish focal from generalized seizures and may indicate an underlying disturbance of cerebral function. However, a normal interictal EEG does not exclude the diagnosis of epilepsy. An EEG obtained shortly (within hours) after a clinical attack may demonstrate postictal slowing of EEG rhythms and support the clinical impression that the attack was a true seizure. Finally, the EEG findings may be very helpful in identifying specific epileptic syndromes.

The diagnostic yield of EEG recordings can be increased by appropriate patient preparation (especially sleep deprivation) or by activation techniques such as hyperventilation, photic stimulation, and sleep recordings. More elaborate examinations such as 24-h recordings or video-EEG recordings, also may be used. Consultation with a neurologist can help ensure that the appropriate studies are chosen and inappropriate and unnecessary studies avoided.

TREATMENT

Appropriate emergency treatment of a patient with seizures will vary depending on the specific clinical situation. It should be stressed that the first step in providing appropriate treatment is to make an accurate diagnosis; only in patients with status epilepticus is it sometimes necessary to initiate treatment before diagnostic evaluation has been completed. Certain general measures should be taken for any seizure patient. Vital functions should stabilized; in unconscious patients, it may be necessary to secure the airway. Emptying the stomach will reduce the risk of aspiration and remove any unabsorbed drugs or toxins in the case of ingestion. Standard measures for management of any unconscious patient should be employed.

Definitive management of the patient with seizures should begin, if possible, with treatment of any underlying condition causing the attacks. Seizures caused by hypoglycemia, hyperosmolar states, or hyponatremia, for example, should be treated by managing the metabolic derangement. Anticonvulsant drugs are not indicated and usually are ineffective. In most patients, of course, no such specific cause is present, or if present, may not be amenable to immediate direct treatment. In these patients, anticonvulsant drug therapy is appropriate.

With regard to the specific management of seizures, four clinical scenarios will be reviewed: the patient who is actually having a seizure, the patient with previous epilepsy who has had a recent seizure, the patient with a first seizure, and the patient in status epilepticus.

The Acute Seizure

There is little to be done during the course of an actual seizure other than to protect the patient from injury. Gentle but firm restraint should be used to prevent falls. If possible the patient should be turned to one side to reduce the risk of aspiration should vomiting occur. It is usually not possible to get a bite block between the teeth without using considerable force; there is little point in risking damage to teeth in order to prevent tongue biting. If a bite block is used, be certain that it cannot be aspirated or swallowed. It is usually not necessary or even possible to ventilate a patient during a seizure effectively, but once the attack subsides, it is appropriate to make sure the airway is clear. There is no indication for intravenous anticonvulsant medications during the course of an uncomplicated seizure.

Patients with Previous Seizures

Proper management of a patient with a well-documented seizure disorder who presents after one or more seizures depends on the particular circumstance of the case. Ask about any changes in routine or regimen which might have caused the seizure, such as sleep deprivation, excessive alcohol intake (or alcohol withdrawal), or medication changes. Many such seizures occur because of failure to take anticonvulsant medication as prescribed. Review of the pharmacologic properties of

Table 149-4. Properties of Commonly Used Anticonvulsant Drugs

Drug	Oral Dose (mg/day)*	Therapeutic Level (μg/mL)†	Days to Reach Steady State‡	Serum Half-life (h)	Average Monthly Cost§
Phenytoin	300–400	10–20	5–10	24 ± 12	$ 14.00
Carbamazepine	800–1200	8–12	2–4	12 ± 3	$ 50.00
Phenobarbital	90–120	15–40	15–20	96 ± 12	$ 4.00
Primidone	150–1000	8–12	2–4	12 ± 3	$ 15.00
Valproic acid	1500–3000	50–150	2–4	12–18	$112.00
Ethosuximide	750–1000	40–100	5–7	24–36	$ 54.00

* Daily dose must be individualized for each patient. Drug-drug interactions may dramatically change daily doses in patients receiving multiple drugs.

† See text for definition of therapeutic and toxic levels. Serum levels are for rough guidance *only*.

‡ Indicates times required to establish stable serum level after any change in dose.

§ Average retail cost for brand-name (nongeneric) preparations.

commonly used anticonvulsant drugs (Table 149-4) shows that several of them have very short serum half-lives. This means that missing even a single dose may result in a sharp drop in serum levels and recurrence of seizures. If anticonvulsant levels are very low, supplemental doses may be given and the patient restarted on their regular regimen. If no supplemental medication is given, several days may be required for steady-state blood levels to be reestablished. During that time the patient will be at increased risk for further seizures.

If anticonvulsant levels are adequate and the patient has had a single attack, treatment usually is not needed since even well-controlled patients may have occasional breakthrough seizures. If there has been a recent increase in the frequency of breakthrough seizures, a change in medication may be needed. This decision usually does not need to be made in the emergency department, and the patient can be referred to their regular physician for definitive management. If it is decided to increase the patient's maintenance dose of medication, only very small increments should be made, and close follow-up should be provided since even small dose changes may result in dramatic increases in serum levels of drugs.

The Patient with a First Seizure

There is considerable controversy regarding the management of a patient who has had a first seizure. The goal of anticonvulsant treatment is to prevent recurrent seizures; the need for treatment therefore is determined by the probability that the patient will have further seizures. Published studies suggest the risk of recurrence is between 30 and 70 percent in unselected patients. Most recurrent attacks will occur within 1 year after the first seizure. The effectiveness of anticonvulsant drugs in reducing the risk is a matter of considerable debate.

Many authorities recommend withholding treatment after a single uncomplicated generalized seizure if clinical evaluation does not suggest any treatable cause for the seizures and the neurologic examination is normal. In such patients, the risk of recurrence is low, and the costs and risks of anticonvulsant treatment often can be avoided. Recurrent seizures, if they occur, are likely to pose little direct risk to the patient. The patient should be advised of the usual precautions to reduce the risk from subsequent seizures if they do occur.

The risk of recurrence is much greater in patients who have had a previous seizure, in those whose seizures have a focal onset, in patients with an abnormal neurologic examination, or patients with other evidence of underlying central nervous system (CNS) disease (structural lesions, congenital lesions, or infections). In these individuals, anticonvulsant therapy is appropriate. Either phenytoin or carbamazepine are appropriate; both are about equally effective, and the choice can be based on cost, convenience, side effects, and physician preference (Table 149-5).

It is rarely necessary to make an immediate decision on the need for anticonvulsant treatment. Most such patients can be referred safely to a neurologist or other specialist for definitive evaluation.

A patient who has had a first seizure or an epileptic with breakthrough seizures should take precautions to minimize the risks from further seizures. Such individuals should avoid swimming unless a competent lifeguard is present. They should be very cautious about working with hazardous tools or machinery or on unprotected heights and scaffolding. Driving an automobile raises several special problems; laws vary from state to state, so that the emergency room physician must know the local regulations, including any requirements that the physician notify authorities about patients with seizures.

Alcohol Withdrawal Seizures

The management of seizures in alcoholic patients remains controversial. It is important to distinguish among patients who experience seizures only in the setting of alcohol withdrawal and patients with epilepsy whose seizures are exacerbated by alcohol withdrawal. Most authorities agree that patients whose seizures occur only in the setting of alcohol withdrawal usually do not require specific anticonvulsant therapy. Use of benzodiazepines in doses adequate to manage withdrawal will usually afford adequate protection. Exceptions would be patients with a history of severe or prolonged alcohol withdrawal seizures or patients with very frequent or persistent seizures (status epilepticus). Patients with epilepsy exacerbated by alcohol withdrawal should be managed as any other seizure patient with recurrent seizures.

STATUS EPILEPTICUS

Status epilepticus is characterized by seizures which occur so frequently that each attack begins before the patient has recovered from the previous attack. Attacks may occur every 20 to 30 min or more with the patient remaining postictal between attacks, or they may be very frequent or virtually continuous. Status epilepticus may be lethal with mortality as high as 20 percent. Its prognosis depends on the underlying cause of the seizures, their frequency and severity, and any secondary injury. Death may result from anoxia, cardiovascular collapse, trauma, or renal failure. In addition, uncontrolled seizures per se may result in permanent neuronal injury if not controlled within 1 h.

Table 149-5. Anticonvulsant Drugs: Indications

Generalized seizures	
Absence seizures:	Ethosuximide (1st) Valproic acid (2nd)
Myoclonic seizures:	Valproic acid
Tonic-clonic seizures:	Carbamazepine or phenytoin (1st) Phenobarbital or primidone (2nd) Valproic acid (3rd)
Partial seizures: (simple or complex, with or without generalization)	
	Carbamazepine or phenytoin (1st) Phenobarbital or primidone (2nd) Valproic acid (3rd)

Appropriate management of the patient with status epilepticus requires attention to several general measures and specific anticonvulsant therapy.

General Measures

Evaluation and initial management should be done simultaneously. The history and physical examination should pay special attention to any evidence for head trauma, CNS infection, drug or alcohol use, systemic illness, and previous seizure activity. The patient should be protected against injury; restraints, if necessary, should be used with great caution to avoid causing injury. A large-bore intravenous (IV) line should be established. If there is any concern about adequacy of ventilation or status of the airway, early endotracheal intubation should be done. A nasogastric tube may be used to empty the stomach. Initial blood work should include blood glucose and electrolytes, and where indicated, toxicology screens, blood-gas studies, and anticonvulsant drug levels. Emergency lumbar puncture is rarely indicated (and is likely to be difficult to do until the seizures are controlled). If bacterial meningitis is a serious concern, empiric antibiotic therapy should be started until the lumbar puncture can be done safely. Radiographic studies (such as a CT scan) generally will have to be delayed until the seizures are controlled. Thiamine (100 mg IV) and dextrose (25 to 50 g IV) should be given as soon as the IV line is established.

Anticonvulsant Drugs

The choice of an appropriate drug regimen depends on the frequency and intensity of the seizures. The drugs most commonly used in the initial therapy of status epilepticus are the benzodiazepines (diazepam or lorazepam), phenytoin, and phenobarbital (Table 149-6).

Benzodiazepines are used only when immediate control of the seizure is required. The usual drug of choice is diazepam, 5 to 20 mg, given by slow (5 mg/min) IV infusion. Both respiratory depression and hypotension may occur; both are especially likely in a patient who has taken barbiturates or other sedatives (such as alcohol). The anticonvulsant action of diazepam is very brief (often only 15 or 30 min). If used, it must be followed immediately by a major anticonvulsant (usually phenytoin). Do not wait for seizures to recur. An alternative benzodiazepine is lorazepam. A dose of up to 0.1 mg/kg may be given by slow IV infusion (not greater than 2 mg/min). (Lorazepam has not been approved by the Food and Drug Administration for this indication.) Lorazepam is said to cause less respiratory depression and to have a longer duration of action and is considered the drug of choice by some authorities. There is no reason to use both diazepam and lorazepam in the same patient.

Table 149-6. Management of Status Epilepticus

General measures
- Establish/maintain airway
- Thiamine 100 mg IV
- Dextrose 25–50 g IV

Standard regimen
- Diazepam 5 mg IV (repeat is necessary q 5 min to total of 20 mg) or lorazepam (up to 0.1 mg/kg) and
- Phenytoin 18 mg/kg IV at 25 mg/min
- *If not effective, then:*
- Phenobarbital IV 100 mg/min to total of 10 mg/kg or seizures are controlled.
- *If not effective, then:*
- Phenobarbital 50 mg/min to total (including previous doses) of 20 mg/kg or seizures are controlled.
- *If not effective, then:*
- Phenobarbital 50 mg/min to total (including previous doses) of 30 mg/kg or seizures are controlled.
- *If not effective, then:*
- Consider barbiturate coma, general anesthesia, or diazepam drip

Alternative regimen
- Phenobarbital 100 mg/min IV to total of 10 mg/kg or seizures are controlled.
- *If not effective, then:*
- Phenytoin 18 mg/kg IV (at dose of 25–50 mg/min) and phenobarbital 50 mg/min to total dose of 20 mg/kg or seizures are controlled.
- *If not effective, then:*
- Phenobarbital 50 mg/kg to total dose (including previous doses) of 30 mg/kg or seizures are controlled.
- *If not effective, then:*
- Consider barbiturate coma or general anesthesia

Phenytoin is the most important drug in the management of status epilepticus. It can be used as primary therapy in all patients except those in whom benzodiazepines must be used or in whom it is contraindicated. The loading dose is 18 mg/kg given IV at a rate not to exceed 50 mg/min, although much slower rates may be needed in elderly patients. Note that doses in excess of the traditional 1 g may be needed in some patients. Phenytoin must not be mixed with any glucose-containing IV fluid and should never be given intramuscularly. Adverse effects of phenytoin include hypotension and decreased myocardial contractility; the drug may cause atrioventricular (AV) block or aggravate preexisting AV block (by increasing the refractory period of the AV node and slowing conduction). The patient should be monitored carefully during and shortly after the infusion. If necessary, the infusion may be slowed or, rarely, even discontinued. Phenytoin is contraindicated in the presence of second- or third-degree heart block.

Phenobarbital usually is used as a second-line drug in patients in whom full loading doses of phenytoin have failed to control seizures. An effective regimen is to give a loading dose of 10 mg/kg at a rate of 100 mg/min. If this is ineffective, an additional 10 mg/kg is given at the rate of 50 mg/min. Occasionally, even larger total doses phenobarbital (up to 30 mg/kg) may be needed. Respiratory depression is common, particularly at higher doses or when benzodiazepines have been used. Endotracheal intubation and ventilator support usually are needed.

Phenobarbital may be used as initial therapy in patients with status epilepticus. In a recent prospective study, initial treatment with phenobarbital was found to be more effective and easier to use than regimens using diazepam and phenytoin. Shaner et al. suggest beginning treatment with phenobarbital 100 mg/min IV to a total dose of 10 mg/kg. If not effective, loading with phenytoin (18 mg/kg) is begun at 40 mg/min, and phenobarbital is continued at 50 mg/min to a total dose of 20 mg/kg or until seizures are controlled. If necessary, phenobarbital 50 mg/min is continued to a total dose of 30 mg/kg. If seizure control is not obtained, general anesthesia should be considered.

Refractory Status Epilepticus

The standard regimens of benzodiazepines, phenytoin, and phenobarbital will suffice to control status epilepticus in most patients. In a few cases (generally patients with structural lesions or CNS infections), seizures will continue even after such treatment. Various approaches have been advocated, including IV infusions of lidocaine (2 to 4 mg/min) or diazepam (up to 8 to 10 mg/h). Intravenous infusions of paraldehyde have also been used. The easiest and most direct approach is to obtain general anesthesia with IV barbiturates. Pentobarbital 5 to 15 mg/kg is given initially, followed by a constant infusion of 1 to 3 mg/h. When used in the intensive care unit, continuous EEG monitoring is needed to assess response and guide dosage, and consultation from an anesthesiologist and neurologist should be obtained.

Neuromuscular blocking agents (usually pancuronium or vecuronium) are sometimes helpful. These drugs will abolish tonic-clonic movements and may facilitate ventilation and other measures; they have no effect on abnormal neuronal activity. EEG monitoring is necessary to assess the effectiveness of anticonvulsant therapy when neuromuscular blockers are utilized.

BIBLIOGRAPHY

Adams RD, Victor M: *Principles of Neurology*, ed 4. New York, McGraw-Hill, 1989, pp 249–272.

Commission on Classification and Terminology of the International League Against Epilepsy: Proposal for revised clinical and electroencephographic classification of epileptic seizures. *Epilepsia* 22:489, 1981.

DeLorenzo RJ: The Epilepsies, in Bradley WG, Daroff RB, Fenichel GM, et al (eds): *Neurology in Clinical Practice: Principles of Diagnosis and Management.* Boston, Butterworth-Heinemann, 1991, pp 1443–1477.

Fernandez R, Samuels MA: Epilepsy, in Samuels MA (ed): *Manual of Neurology: Diagnosis and Treatment,* ed 4. Boston, Little, Brown, 1991.

Levy RH, Dreifus FE, Mahson RH, et al (eds): *Antiepileptic Drugs,* ed 3. New York, Raven, 1989.

Lowenstein DH, Aminoff MJ, Simon RP: Barbiturate anesthesia in the treatment of status epilepticus: Clinical experience with 14 patients. *Neurology* 38:395, 1988.

McMicken DB: Evaluation and treatment of seizures in the alcohol-dependent patient. *Critical Decisions in Emergency Medicine* 3:8, 1988.

Porter RJ, Mattson RH, Cramer JA, et al (eds): *Alcohol and Seizures: Basic Mechanisms and Clinical Concepts.* Philadelphia, Davis, 1990.

Shaner DM, McCurdy SA, Herring MO, et al: Treatment of status epilepticus: A prospective comparison of diazepam and phenytoin versus phenobarbital and optional phenytoin. *Neurology* 38:202, 1988.

Treiman DB: Status epilepticus, in Johnson RT (ed): *Current Therapy in Neurologic Disease,* ed 2. Toronto, Decker, 1987, pp 38–42.

Yerby MS, Van Belle G, Friel PN, et al: Serum prolactins in the diagnosis of epilepsy: Sensitivity specificity and predictive value. *Neurology* 37:1224, 1987.

150 ACUTE PERIPHERAL NEUROLOGICAL LESIONS

Gregory L. Henry

There is no problem more frustrating or confusing for the busy emergency physician than a patient who is complaining of generalized weakness or nonspecific ailments in an extremity. These types of problems can be extremely time-consuming and produce very few results unless the physician has a logical and systematic approach to examination and treatment. Four basic guidelines for evaluation are given below.

First, most peripheral neuropathies and myopathies are slowly developing processes with a good history of downhill progression. Family members and the patient should be consulted to determine if the process is acute or chronic. Diffuse, bilateral nerve-muscle lesions are those that evolve over a few hours to days (or at least worsen acutely) and that do not involve severe changes in mental status, at least as their predominant symptomatology.

Second, peripheral nerve lesions must be separated from central nervous system disease. For example, patients with numbness and aching in the right hand may be so occupied with this symptom that they fail to realize they are also having trouble with word finding and facial numbness. If it absolutely essential that by history and physical examination a search is made which will exclude lesions of the central nervous system (see Table 150-1).

Third, of all examinations done in medicine, motor and sensory examinations are often the most imprecise. When unsure as to the cause of specific symptom, it is prudent to advise the patient to return should the symptoms worsen. A brief emergency department evaluation is not the basis for diagnosis of hysteria or functional disorder.

Fourth, reflexes are notoriously difficult to evaluate in the amount of time generally available in the emergency department. A few general statements, however, can be made.

Hyperreflexia in the face of down-going toes and no other pathological reflexes is probably a normal variant. Lesions such as previous stroke, multiple sclerosis, cerebral palsy, and amyotrophic lateral sclerosis may all give hyperreflexia, but these lesions are usually quickly separated out by history and physical examination.

Table 150-1. Focal Weakness

Area of Weakness	Location
Contralateral face, arm, leg (hemiplegia)	Cortex, internal capsule, rarely brainstem
Ipsilateral face, contralateral arm and leg	Brainstem
Bilateral arm and leg without neck and head (quadriplegia)	Cervical spinal cord, rarely medulla or pons
Arms bilaterally without involvement of the head, neck, or legs (diplegia)	Central cord syndrome or syringomyelia of the cervical spinal cord
Legs bilaterally without involvement of upper body or head (paraplegia)	Thoracic or lumbar spinal cord
Ipsilateral weakness one leg, with contralateral leg decreased pin and temperature sensation	Hemisection spinal cord (Brown-Séquard syndrome)
Unilateral or bilateral single dermatome weakness with associated sensory changes	Spinal-nerve-root lesion
Specific peripheral nerve, with associated sensory findings	Isolated peripheral nerve
Isolated arm or leg (monoplegia)	Pons, occasionally central cortex, spinal cord; small lesion, extremely rare

Source: Henry G, Little N: *Neurologic Emergencies: A Symptom Oriented Approach.* New York, McGraw-Hill, 1985. Used by permission.

In the hyporeflexic patient the situation is more difficult. *The patient who is truly areflexic—that is, no reflexes—usually has a neuropathic as opposed to a myopathic disorder.* However, hyporeflexia may be a normal variant, a sign of spinal shock, a sign of acute cerebral vascular accident, or may accompany a variety of myopathies and neuropathies, and is therefore a nonspecific finding.

Keeping in mind the order and extent of the physical examination described in Chapter 145, "The Neurological Examination," and with the above basic guidelines, we are ready to construct the differential diagnosis of acute peripheral problems.

It is beyond the scope of this chapter to discuss the myriad diseases that produce myopathies and neuropathies. We will concentrate on those entities that are both common and acute. No attempt will be made to describe the chronic disease processes that can usually be segregated out by history.

ACUTE TOXIC NEUROPATHIES

Bacterial Illnesses

Overwhelming bacterial sepsis may cause generalized weakness and lack of motor coordination, but only a limited number of bacterial illnesses will present early with severe peripheral neurological findings. These are diphtheria, botulism, and tetanus.

Diphtheria

Infections with *Corynebacterium diphtheriae* are usually characterized by an acute onset, exudative pharyngitis, high fever, and malaise. The organism gives off a powerful exotoxin that acts directly on the heart, kidneys, and the nervous system. The most common presenting neurological problem with diphtheria is mononeuritis or a mononeuritis multiplex. For example, neurological involvement of the palate with difficulty in speaking and changing quality of voice can occur. The most commonly observed paralyses, however, involve the intrinsic and extrinsic muscles of the eye, producing ptosis, strabismus, and problems in accommodation. When the limbs are involved, the patient is critically ill and has bilateral flaccid weakness or paralysis accompanied by absent deep tendon reflexes and, in longstanding cases, atrophy. Sensory involvement is rare. However, bladder and rectal sphincter muscles may be involved, producing urinary retention, overflowing incontinence, and incompetent anal sphincter tone. The ascending transverse myelitis of the Guillain-Barré type has been recorded with cases of diphtheria. Although diphtheria has been considered a rare disease in North America over the past 40 years, pockets of nonimmunized and poorly immunized patients do exist. Recent immigrants, the poor, and religious sects that do not have children immunized should all be considered at risk.

Botulism

Botulism toxin is a preformed toxin, elaborated by *Clostridium botulinum,* an anaerobic gram-positive bacillus that affects both striated and smooth muscle. The toxin exerts its effect principally at the myoneural junction, without direct toxicity to the muscle fibers or the peripheral nerve itself. The principal mode of action is in prevention of the release of acetylcholine. There are at least seven major toxins, but toxins A, B, and E are the ones primarily causing disease in humans.

The principal source of botulism in the United States is food which has been inadequately prepared. There are no definitive telltale signs or smells of the organism so that it may exist in food which are normal on inspection. The neurological symptoms usually appear in 24 to 48 h after ingestion of contaminated foods and may or may not be preceded by nausea, vomiting, and diarrhea. The most common early presenting neurological complaints are related to eye and bulbar musculature.

Symptoms spread very rapidly, however, to involve all the muscles of the trunk and extremities. The smooth muscle of the intestine and the bladder may occasionally be involved, resulting in ileus and acute urinary retention. Good mental status is maintained until the patient is terminal.

It is important to differentiate botulism from diphtheria or Guillain-Barré syndrome. Gullain-Barré syndrome is an ascending transverse myelitis and does not usually begin with involvement of bulbar musculature. Diphtheria is an acute febrile illness, with psuedomembranous oropharyngitis and cardiac involvement. With rapid deterioration, botulism may occasionally be confused with undiagnosed myasthenia gravis. The two are easily differentiated with the edrophonium chloride (Tensilon) test. Botulism should not improve with the administration of cholinesterase inhibitors.

A variant form of botulism, infant botulism, has recently had a resurgence. In almost 40 percent of affected infants, the source of the botulism can be traced to raw honey containing botulinum spores. Children affected with this disease may exhibit lethargy and failure to thrive, eventually leading to paralysis and death. It is almost always insidious in infants because of the extremely small amounts of botulinum toxin ingested along with the honey.

After diagnosis and respiratory support, further treatment of botulism patients is usually carried out in the intensive care unit. As with all ingested toxins, removal of the remaining offending agent by gastric lavage, activated charcoal, and instillation of cathartics is advised. The decision to use botulinum antitoxin is usually made following consultation with infectious disease specialists.

Tetanus

Tetanus is described more fully in Chapter 83. The symptoms of tetanus are due to the toxin elaborated by *Clostridium tetani*. Tetanus may cause local tetany where it diffuses through the perineural tissues at the site of innoculation. More commonly, however, the patient will have generalized tetanus 5 to 10 days after inoculation. The most common presenting symptom is trismus, but it is usually rapidly followed by neck stiffness, rigidity of the back muscles to the point of opisthotonos, and a characteristic tight rigid facial expression that is referred to as *risus sardonicus*.

There are no specific blood, urine, or cerebral fluid abnormalities that will confirm the diagnosis. The combination of rapidly progressive trismus, persistent truncal and extremity tetany, risus sardonicus, and intermittent convulsions give little problem in formulating a differential diagnosis. Strychnine can produce tetany and convulsions, but pronounced muscle relaxation between convulsions is characteristic of strychnine poisoning.

METALLIC POISONS

Poisoning by metallic compounds usually results in prominent central nervous system as well as peripheral nervous system findings. It is impossible to mention all the various types of metallic poisoning syndromes, but arsenic and lead poisoning are worth reviewing. Arsenic is still found in insecticides, rat poisons, and herbicides, and in certain medicinal compounds. Acute gastrointestinal irritation with vomiting and diarrhea are usually presenting signs following ingestions of large amounts of arsenic. In patients receiving lower doses, however, polyneuritis may be one of the presenting complaints. In such cases, a history of occupational exposure is absolutely necessary.

Lead poisoning usually results from accidental and industrial, toxic exposure. Lead may be absorbed through the skin or the lungs, or ingested through the gastrointestinal tract. In severe acute lead poisoning the principal symptoms are acute weakness, prostration, and abdominal pain. In those patients who have received chronic smaller doses of lead, a peripheral motor neuropathy is common. These patients will have sensory findings but may have pronounced distal weakness.

Organic Compounds

Neuromuscular toxic effects can result from a wide variety of organic compounds. The alcohols, phenothiazines, and aminoglycoside antibiotics are discussed here.

Ethanol, methanol, and other alcohols may produce long-standing, slowly progressive peripheral neuropathies, predominantly sensory. Myopathies can be present as well. Acute intoxication with these agents usually causes pronounced central nervous system effects.

The phenothiazines may produce local dystonias even though the mechanism is central. Buccolingual dyskinesias caused by phenothiazine derivatives should be well known to emergency physicians. Often these are not seen in persons taking chronic psychiatric medication, but in those receiving small amounts of phenothiazines for symptoms such as nausea and vomiting, or in those who abuse street drugs.

Neuromuscular blockade can be enhanced by aminoglycoside antibiotics. This is usually encountered in hospitalized patients, especially postoperatively.

Tick Paralysis

Tick paralysis is also discussed in Chapter 87. Tick paralysis is a reversible, rapidly progressive ascending paralysis in which neuromuscular end-plate conduction is affected without morphologic changes. The symptoms of tick paralysis are almost identical to those of Guillaine-Barré syndrome. Flaccid paralysis begins at the extremities and trunk and moves up to involve the bulbar musculature. There are no specific blood, urine, or cerebrospinal fluid changes to aid in the diagnosis. The diagnosis of tick paralysis is made by finding the tick after a thorough examination of the body, including the hairy areas. Formerly, acute poliomyelitis would also be considered in the differential diagnosis of tick paralysis and Guillain-Barré syndrome. However, polio can usually be differentiated from the other two types of paralysis by their lack of fever or neck stiffness, or of cellular and protein changes in the cerebrospinal fluid.

Metabolic Neuropathy

The majority of nutritional and metabolic neuropathies have a slow onset, are progressive, and are clearly beyond the scope of the emergency physician. There are, however, several variants that may occur in a rapid fashion and are thus worth considering in a differential diagnosis: hyperinsulinism, gout, and acute intermittent porphyria. In contrast to diabetic neuropathy, which is symmetric and slow in onset, hyperinsulinism associated with pancreatic tumors may produce acute paresthesia, impaired sensation, muscle weakness, and hyporeflexia. It is usually seen in conjunction with symptomatic hypoglycemia.

During gouty attacks there may be a sudden onset of generalized extremity neuropathy or neuropathies, particularly of the lumbar plexus. The neuropathies seem to disappear when symptoms of gout are controlled.

Acute intermittent porphyria is characterized by psychosis, abdominal pains, and polyneuropathy of the Gullain-Barré type.

Neuropathy of Guillain-Barré

Today, the neuropathy of the Landry-Guillain-Barré disease is thought to be not a disease but a symptom complex that may follow many infectious diseases, exposure to toxins, and collagen vascular diseases. This syndrome usually follows an acute febrile episode or an acute metabolic problem by days or weeks and may be rapidly progressive. Persons in the third to fourth decades are most frequently affected, but it may occur in young children and in older adults.

The usual pattern of presentation is that of an ascending transverse myelitis. The lower extremities are usually involved first and are more severely affected than the upper extremities. The bulbar musculature, however, may be involved partially or totally. Although paralysis usually reaches the maximum within a week, in some patients maximum paralysis is reached within hours. This is considered to be a motor neuron disease, but sensory symptoms are not uncommon and radicular pain is often noted. Although paralysis is rapid in onset, recovery may take a month to years, but it is usually complete.

In the emergency department differential diagnosis is difficult. Frequently the patient gives a vague history of weakness in the lower extremities without any other antecedent history. Since this is a motor neuron disease, reflex arcs are often affected early. A patient who has weakness and loss of lower extremity reflexes should be considered to have Guillain-Barré disease until proved otherwise. Acute exacerbations of lead poisoning, porphyria, botulism, and diphtheria may all enter into the differential diagnosis and must be separated out by history and other pertinent clinical findings.

ACUTE MYOPATHIES

Like neuropathies, most myopathies, particularly in young people, progress slowly. The rapidly progressive acquired myopathies are relatively few in number, and a reasonable differential diagnosis can be made in the emergency department.

The first task is to differentiate neuropathies from myopathies. Neuropathies tend to give distal symptoms, first with pronounced distal weakness progressing proximally. With myopathies, large muscle and central muscle groups are frequently affected at the same time as distal muscle groups, so diffuse or predominantly proximal weakness is a striking finding. A second important clue in differentiating neuropathies and myopathies is that myopathies rarely include sensory symptoms. There may be aching in the involved musculature, but the paresthesias and decreased sensation are not noted. A third differentiating feature is the fact that in myopathies, despite rather pronounced weakness, the patient will maintain deep-tendon reflexes until the disease process is extremely advanced.

Laboratory testing is usually more fruitful for the emergency physician in myopathies as opposed to neuropathies. Elevated leukocyte count, sedimentation rate, and elevated muscle enzymes along with normal spinal fluid parameters characterize myopathies.

Polymyositis Syndrome

It is of little value for the emergency physician to subclassify acute polymyositis into its multiple causes. Polymyositis is more a syndrome than a specific disease. This form of myopathy, however, usually evolves rapidly, and, within weeks of onset, the patient has pronounced symptoms. In severe cases, however, severe weakness may develop over several days. Most patients have muscular pain and tenderness. A significant number also have dysphasia. Accompanying signs and symptoms, such as arthralgia, fever, and Raynaud's phenomenon, all lend credence to the diagnosis of polymyositis. After the polymyositis syndrome is suspected, investigation is necessary to isolate the various treatable causes. Such a complex workup is beyond the scope of emergency diagnosis.

Many infections, including trichinosis and toxoplasmosis, and many viral entities have been associated with polymyositis. All the collagen vascular diseases except periarteritis nodosa have also been implicated. Endocrinopathies, including both hyperthyroidism and hypothyroidism as well as adrenal cortical and parathyroid lesions, are part of the differential diagnosis. Steroids, which are used in treating many forms of polymyositis, can actually exacerbate the problem. Several of the drugs used to treat malaria and other protozoan infection have been associated with polymyositis. This can be confusing, as malaria itself can cause polymyositis. In approximately 10 percent of adults, polymyositis is a remote manifestation of carcinoma. There is no specific emergency department therapy for polymyositis, and use of steroids should await correct diagnosis.

Alcoholic Myopathy

Along with the well-known alcoholic peripheral neuropathy and the propensity to develop other skeletal disorders, alcoholics are prone to at least one type of unique myopathic syndrome. During prolonged periods of heavy alcohol intake, an alcoholic may have severe muscle tenderness and swelling, muscle cramps, and severe weakness. Signs and symptoms may be generalized or focal. This syndrome represents the acute diffuse necrosis of skeletal muscle fibers all in one stage of degeneration, or acute rhabdomyolysis. Muscle degeneration can lead to life-threatening hyperkalemia or hypocalcemia and secondary binding without released intracellular PO_4, and myoglobinuria can cause renal failure. In the alcoholic with acute muscle pain and weakness, serum electrolyte levels, muscle enzymes, and urinalysis for myoglobin are necessary. Although most patients recover within several weeks, return to normal motor functions may take many months.

Myasthenia Gravis

Myasthenia gravis is not a true myopathy, but the presenting symptoms and examination features closely resemble those of the other myopathic diseases. It is discussed in detail in Chapter 152.

Acute Periodic Paralysis

The most bizarre of the acute weakness syndromes is the acute periodic paralysis. There are three basic types or primary forms: hyperkalemic, and normokalemic. The exact mechanisms of these types have not been fully delineated, but an abnormal number of mitochondria and abnormalities in the sarcoplasmic reticulum have been noted by electron microscopy.

This disease is rarely suspected before the ninth or tenth attack. Periodic paralysis occurs predominantly in males (by 4 : 1 or 5 : 1 ratio), and generally the onset is between the seventh and twenty-first years of life.

Interestingly, the patient may often be awakened from sleep by the weakness. A history of extreme physical exertion on that day is important in establishing the diagnosis. Cold weather, large meals, trauma, and surgery may provoke an attack. Some patients will have the attacks on a regular basis, almost daily; others will have only a limited number throughout their lifetime. But the usual story is one of sudden extreme weakness without associated pain. Patients will give a history of being normal before and after the episodes, which usually last 1 or 2 h. Episodes may be so severe that patients will fall while walking or gag while eating.

An in-depth discussion of the various forms of periodic paralysis and paramyotonia congenita is beyond the scope of this basic review, but an understanding of these attacks should alert the emergency physician to consider the diagnosis, obtain a serum potassium level, and provide referral to a neurologist.

NONMYASTHENIC SYNDROMES OF MALIGNANCY

As the average age of the population increases, there will by sheer weight of numbers be more interaction between emergency physicians and patients suffering from or being treated for various forms of cancer. Many acute side effects of cancer or its treatment are due to local disease extension or metastasis. The following entities, however, are unrelated to the tumor mass itself but represent the remote effects of the tumor or its treatment: Eaton-Lambert syndrome, effects of drugs and radiation, cerebellar degeneration, polymyositis, and acute dementia.

Lambert-Eaton Syndrome

For a number of years it has been recognized that there is abnormal neuromuscular transmission associated with certain malignancies, particularly oat-cell carcinoma of the lung. This syndrome, when first described by Eaton and Lambert, was thought to be a mild variant form of myasthenia gravis. However, as the syndrome became more fully delineated, it was clear that the differences between the two were multiple. In the Eaton-Lambert syndrome the patient will occasionally have aching muscle pain and will rarely be as weak as the patient with myasthenia gravis. There is less fluctuation of weakness and strength than found in myasthenia gravis. The cranial nerves are almost always spared in the Lambert-Eaton syndrome.

A rather remarkable finding is the fact that unlike myasthenia gravis, which gets worse with repeated activity, with the Lambert-Eaton syndrome grip strength actually improves with repeated activity. There is no response to edrophonium.

Drugs and Radiation Therapy

For cancer patients currently under treatment, medications and dosage schedules must be carefully reviewed to determine the cause of weakness. Many chemotherapeutic agents are metabolic poisons and this may be the reason for the patient's weakness. *Steroids may produce a polymyositis syndrome.* Many tumors are treated with radiation. If the spinal column is involved, transverse myelitis may develop very suddenly from months to even years later. This is a true medical emergency. The differential diagnosis is radiation myelitis, or a compressive lesion due to metastasis. Emergency neurosurgical consultation and myelography are often necessary.

Another and yet unexplained remote effect of cancer is acute weakness and cerebral degeneration. Patients have a rapid history of deterioration with inability to walk and control the upper extremities, and there is evidence of pancerebellar involvement.

Polymyositis

Polymyositis may be a remote effect of carcinoma. Occult malignancy will be discovered in about 10 percent of adults with polymyositis.

MONONEURITIS MULTIPLEX

Acute temporal arteritis is probably the prototype for this disorder. The principle lesion is infarction of peripheral nerves due to arteritis in the vasa vasorum of the peripheral nerves. It occurs in diabetic patients and those with collagen vascular disease. The patient may complain of a specific peripheral nerve lesion in the right arm, another one in the left leg, and still another in the region of the cervical plexus. On specific testing, perfectly anatomic localizations can be delineated and usually the underlying disease has already been diagnosed. Treatment with steroids may be indicated.

SPECIFIC ISOLATED PERIPHERAL NERVE LESIONS

Herpes Zoster

Herpes zoster represents the most important infection that clinically presents as an isolated peripheral nerve lesion. Herpes as a whole tends to present as an independent condition, but it may be associated with surgical procedures, diabetes, and occasionally trauma. Elderly and immunocompromised patients are at the greatest risk of developing herpes zoster. Younger adults who develop the disease should be considered at high risk for having an underlying illness. Extreme pain, which is generally in a dermatomal distribution, usually precedes the skin lesions by several days. The dermatomes most often affected are the thoracic, followed by the trigeminal nerve, lumbar plexus, and finally the cervical plexus. Although herpes produces principally sensory involvement, motor dysfunction may be seen in up to 25 percent of patients. Although the sensory disturbances and skin lesions usually abate with time, the motor disturbances seen with herpes do not usually completely resolve. Herpes zoster may involve the cranial nerves. Skin lesions in the various divisions of the seventh cranial nerve are frequently seen. Tympanic membrane and corneal involvement may be seen as part of the Ramsay Hunt syndrome. Whenever corneal lesions are suspected, ophthalmologic consultation for consideration of antiviral medications is appropriate. The role of steroids following the initial phase of the lesions is controversial. Current treatment consists of oral acyclovir, 200 mg 5 times a day, for 10 days. Patients do not require admission unless the disease is disseminated, or unless patients are immunocompromised or receiving steroids or chemotherapy. As acyclovir can cause interstitial nephritis, creatinine and BUN should be obtained before beginning acyclovir.

Allergic Neuropathy

An unusual phenomenon that is seen approximately nine times more in males than in females is an allergic neuropathy following the injection of immunologic materials, usually tetanus toxoid. The neurological complications usually develop about 2 days after signs of generalized serum sickness. Although central nervous system signs are reported, the most common neurological complication is a motor peripheral neuropathy involving the branchial plexus. It may or may not be bilateral. A single nerve such as the radial or optic nerve may be involved.

Vascular Peripheral Nerve Lesions

Volkmann's Paralysis

Volkmann's ischemic paralysis is the prototype for vascular peripheral nerve lesions. The paralysis is due primarily to injury to the nutrient vessels of a peripheral nerve, but it can be iatrogenically induced by a tight-fitting cast. During the first few hours, severe pain is the principal symptom. As the disease process progresses, nerves and muscles undergo extensive fibrosis with resultant contractures and impairment of both motor and sensory functions.

Tic Douloureux

Tic douloureux, or trigeminal neuralgia, should be mentioned here. There is probably no one explanation for the source of pain in trigeminal neuralgia. It is believed by many that pulsations from a branch of the basilar artery serve as irritants and decrease the trigeminal nerve's threshold for pain. The symptom is severe lancinating pain usually confined to the area of distribution of the third portion of the trigeminal nerve. Often multiple portions of the trigeminal nerve will be involved, but bilaterality is unusual. Such pain usually presents little problem in differential diagnosis, but treatment may be difficult. During acute attacks opiates are helpful. It is inappropriate for the emergency physician to initiate chronic therapy without consulting the physician who will follow the patient.

Ninth-nerve neuralgia, or glossopharyngeal tic, is less common. Although rare, this disorder is characterized by intense pain localized to the area of the ear and throat on the affected side. Pain may radiate to the posterior third of the tongue, tonsillar pillars, and the oropharynx and larynx. The most common irritants that initiate this unusual pain are swallowing, talking, or chewing. Unlike tic douloureux, the pain of glossopharyngeal neuralgia may last for longer periods of time and usually tends to come in waves or clusters at a particular time of the year. There is no single theory as to the cause of glossopharyngeal neuralgia, but a vascular etiology is hypothesized.

Cranial Nerve Neuropathy

The cranial nerve neuropathies represent a separate subcategory of specific isolated nerve lesions. The general maxim from neurology and ear, nose, and throat surgery is that any cranial nerve neuropathy may represent a tumor until proved otherwise. In all practicality, however, most cranial nerve neuropathies seen by the emergency physician are more likely to be vascular or idiopathic lesions of sudden onset. It is beyond the scope of this discussion to detail each cranial neuropathy, but because the seventh nerve is frequently involved in both traumatic and infectious conditions and is the most commonly involved with idiopathic dysfunction, it will be discussed here.

The seventh cranial nerve, or facial nerve, has two principal divisions as it leaves the brainstem. These are a motor root and the nervus intermedius, which functions to supply taste to the anterior two thirds of the tongue and automatic fibers to the salivary and lacrimal glands. Above the brainstem, the seventh nerve has both crossed and uncrossed fibers, while below the seventh nerve nucleus fibers are uncrossed. If a patient retains muscular strength in the forehead and upper face but not the lower face, the lesion is probably central, i.e., in the brainstem or above. If the patient has weakness of the forehead, around the eyes, and lower face, this probably represents a lower neuron involvement of type usually seen with Bell's palsy. Taste may be affected by involvement of the chorda tympani nerve but is of little clinical value since taste is very difficult to test in the outpatient setting.

Bell's Palsy

Bell's palsy is not a specific disease but represents a constellation of symptoms of multiple etiologies. The exact location of the disorder along the seventh nerve or in the brainstem can often be ascertained by careful physical examination. It is important to localize the level of involvement to determine if a structural lesion or idiopathic Bell's palsy is present. Lesions in the tegmentum of the brainstem involve the nucleus of the seventh nerve and almost invariably have an accompanying sixth-nerve palsy. Lesions of the seventh nerve at the point of emergence from the brainstem frequently have associated auditory components due to involvement of the eighth nerve as well. If the lesion is peripheral to the lateral geniculate ganglion, lacrimal fibers are spared and there is usually an excess collection of tears in the conjunctival sac on that side. Beyond the point where the chorda tympani nerve arises, autonomic functions are no longer involved, and a lesion beyond the stylomastoid foramen results in motor weakness and is characteristic of Bell's palsy. Jaw pain or external ear pain is also a common complaint.

Once the diagnosis of idiopathic Bell's palsy has been established, the next problem is treatment. There is a considerable growing body of evidence that high-dose steroid therapy in short bursts may be of benefit in treatment of Bell's palsy. If steroids are given, they should be prescribed in consultation with an otolaryngologist or neurologist who can also initiate electrostimulatory therapy for the patient's muscles while waiting for recovery of the seventh nerve. There is a small but firm group who advocate unroofing the cranal of the seventh nerve if recovery has not occurred after approximately 6 weeks. However, 98 percent of patients with Bell's palsy recover at least partial function, and operative intervention should be reserved for those patients with prolonged or severe difficulty. It should be remembered that Bell's palsy is a diagnosis of exclusion. Other disease processes such as parotid tumors, lesions of the middle ear, cerebellopontine angle tumors, eighth-nerve lesions, and vascular disease can all begin as isolated lesions of the peripheral seventh nerve.

TRAUMA AND NERVE COMPRESSION SYNDROMES

Spinal Cord Compression

Lesions along the cord may produce distinct isolated neurological syndromes. One of the emergency problems is compression of the spinal cord. This may occur as a result of trauma, herniation of intervertebral disks, primary or metastatic tumors, AV malformations, radiation myelitis, or cysts. It is important to remember that acute spinal cord compression is often associated with areflexia. Cremasteric reflexes, anal sphincter tone, and motor activity in the extremities all help to localize the lesion. Emergency neurosurgical consultation and myelography are indicated.

Root and Trunk Syndromes

The peripheral nerve is the endpoint in a long process of combinations and divisions of nervous tissues. After exiting the cord in the cervical upper thoracic and lumbar regions, nerve roots at each particular level combine with other nerves to form plexuses. Plexuses then form major and minor trunks which divide to form specific peripheral nerves. Therefore, depending on the lesion along the nerve, different symptoms can result. The patient with a C6 root lesion will have a different distribution in the hand than a patient with a medial nerve injury. When evaluating isolated complaints, do not overlook the possible multiple levels at which a nerve might be involved.

Specific Peripheral Nerve Neuropathies

These is not adequate room to list all the various nerve root compression syndromes that the emergency physician might encounter. Two texts are absolutely essential: *Aids to the Investigation of Peripheral Nerve Injuries,* which was first published in 1942 as an aid to British trauma surgeons and has stood the test to time as an excellent reference for acute neuromuscular problems, and *Peripheral Entrapment Neuropathies,* by H. P. Kopel and W. A. Thompson, which carefully reviews the physical findings in entrapment disorders and lists possible locations on the nerve where they are involved. Table 150-2 gives a brief overview to the common nerve entrapments and their symptomatology.

Common Nerve Entrapments

The most common causes of acute mononeuropathies are usually traumatic, following fractures, dislocations, or acute soft tissue swelling. A mononeuropathy can be a result of repetitive motor activity that causes increased connective tissue in small spaces. It should be remembered that with high-velocity missile injuries, direct contact with a nerve is not necessary to produce palsy. Besides trauma, causes of entrapment neuropathies include any inflammation or degeneration in

Table 150-2. Nerve Entrapment Syndromes

Nerve Entrapment Syndromes	Signs and Symptoms
Carpal tunnel syndrome (median nerve)	Tingling in the hand—first, second, third, and one-half of fourth digit; late muscular wasting, thenar area
Pronator syndrome (median nerve at the muscle)	Pain from the elbow to the wrist; weakness of the thenar muscles
Ulnar nerve-wrist	Paresthesia, fourth and fifth fingers; atrophy, intrinsic muscles of the hand
Ulnar nerve-elbow	Same as ulnar nerve–wrist, plus decreased strength in ulnar deviation of the hand at the wrist
Radial nerve	Weakness of the finger extension and wrist extension
Lateral cutaneous of the thigh	Numbness in the lateral part of the thigh
Posterior tibial (tarsal tunnel)	Numbness of the sole of the foot; decreased sensation
Bell's facial-nerve palsy	Weakness of facial musculature all divisions of the seventh cranial nerve ipsilateral to the lesion

Source: Henry G, Little N: *Neurologic Emergencies: A Symptom Oriented Approach.* New York, McGraw-Hill, 1985. Used by permission.

and around tight canals where nerves must pass. This is frequently seen in patients with rheumatoid arthritis, myxedema, thyroid disease, amyloidosis, and pregnancy.

BIBLIOGRAPHY

Aids to the Investigation of Peripheral Nerve Injuries. London, H. M. Stationery Office, 1942.

Henry G, Little N: *Neurologic Emergencies: A Symptom Oriented Approach* New York, McGraw-Hill, 1985.

Kopel HP, Thompson WA: *Peripheral Entrapment Neuropathies*. Baltimore, William & Wilkins, 1963.

Soffer D, Feldman S. Alter M: Epidemiology of Guillain-Barré syndrome. *Neurology* 28: 686, 1978.

151 DEMYELINATING DISEASES

Richard F. Edlich

The demyelinating diseases comprise a group of diseases that share the common pathological feature of central nervous system dysfunction caused by damage to the myelin sheaths covering axons. They can be classified into two basic types. In the first group, myelin loss occurs in the absence of an inflammatory reaction and includes genetic defects in myelin metabolism, toxin-induced injury (e.g., carbon monoxide), and opportunistic viral infection of oligodendrocytes (e.g., progressive multifocal leukoencephalopathy). In the other group, the demyelinating diseases exhibit focal or patchy destruction of the myelin sheaths in the central nervous system in the presence of an inflammatory process. In this latter group, three demyelinating diseases can be distinguished by the clinical history, physical findings, and pathologic examination. These are multiple sclerosis (MS), acute disseminated encephalomyelitis (ADE), and acute necrotizing hemorrhagic encephalomyelitis (ANHE).

MS

MS is an inflammatory disease of the central nervous system that has its primary effect in the oligodendroglial cells, which are responsible for the production and maintenance of the myelin sheaths covering the axons. The key pathologic lesion in MS is the plaque, which is a more or less circumscribed lesion, varying in size from a few to many cubic centimeters, oriented around venules. The characteristic findings in the plaque are primary destruction of myelin with relative preservation of axons and gliosis. Conduction of nerve impulses along axons without myelin is slowed; this defect in nerve conduction is enhanced by hyperthermia. The plaques are present in scattered areas of the white matter of the central nervous system, with a predilection for the periventricular areas of the cerebrum and subpially, and within the brain stem, spinal cord, and optic nerves. The acute lesions usually contain inflammatory infiltrates with lymphocytes at the site of subsequent demyelination.

This disease presents as recurrent attacks of a focal neurologic disease. The presence of clinical remissions remains the clinical rule. Only 30 percent of MS patients experience a progressive course, which is more common in older patients with disease predominantly in the spinal cord. A progressive course from disease onset in the younger patient should make one doubt the diagnosis of MS, suggesting the presence of a degenerative disease or tumor. In addition, the disease should be disseminated over time and location within the nervous system.

MS is the leading cause of neurologic morbidity and mortality among young adults. An estimated 123,000 people in the continental United States have MS. The average age of onset of MS is in the third and fourth decades. Women are affected by MS more commonly than are men. The female-to-male incidence ratio may be as high as 2.5:1. The prevalence rate in the white population is 62 per 100,000 people, compared with 31 per 100,000 people in the nonwhite population. This disease is uncommon in Orientals. Generally, MS is more common in people who live in the northern and southern temperate latitudes than in the more equatorial regions. It has long been recognized that there is a familial incidence of MS; approximately 10 percent of MS patients have an affected relative. Anecdotal evidence and small case series have suggested an association of MS with myasthenia gravis, systemic lupus erythematosus (SLE), ankylosing spondylitis, ulcerative colitis, brain tumor, thyroid disease, scleroderma, diabetes mellitus, and cancer. Interpretation of these reports is difficult given the nature of these studies, especially in the nonpopulation selection of cases.

Clinical diagnostic criteria remain the standard method of diagnosis of MS, and require, in essence, the demonstration that a patient of an appropriate age has had at least two episodes of neurological disturbances implicating necessarily two distinct sites in the white matter. In the latter circumstance, the diagnosis can be made with greater than 95 percent certainty. In recent years, clinical assessment has been supplemented by a number of tests (imaging and evoked potentials), which facilitate the identification of multiple sites of damage in the central nervous system or demonstrate the existence of characteristic immunological abnormalities (cerebrospinal fluid [CSF] electrophoresis). However, none of these tests are specific for MS, and the data they provide must be interpreted in light of the clinical picture.

Clinical Manifestations

The spectrum of clinical symptoms and signs caused by MS is very wide. MS can be viewed as the ''great imitator'' in neurologic disease. The first episode of MS presents as more than one symptom or sign in the majority (55 percent) of cases; the remaining cases become evident as a single sign or symptom. The first symptom of MS in 10 to 30 percent of the cases is optic neuritis. Patients with optic neuritis present with a history of loss of central vision with pain on movement of the globe of one eye. If the demyelinating lesion is located anteriorly in the nerve, there is swelling of the optic disk (papillitis) that may be ophthalmoscopically indistinguishable from papilledema. When the demyelination is located posteriorly (retrobulbar optic neuritis), the disk appears normal, but the patient has visual symptoms and signs. Both types of optic neuritis are followed by optic nerve atrophy detected as abnormal pallor of the optic disk. Follow-up of patients with isolated optic neuritis demonstrates that approximately 50 percent develop clinical MS. The interval between onset of optic neuritis and the development of MS is usually within 10 years, although it can be as long as 35 years.

Symptoms and signs of neurologic dysfunction, arising from the brainstem, cerebellar, and spinal cord lesions, are common in MS. Diplopia may occur either due to internuclear ophthalmoplegia or lesions of either the third, fourth, or sixth cranial nerves. An acute bilateral internuclear ophthalmoplegia in a young adult due to lesions in the medial longitudinal fasciculus bilaterally is almost diagnostic of MS. With attempted gaze to one side, the adducting eye is unable to move beyond the midline, and coarse nystagmus occurs in the abducting eye. Gaze to the opposite side causes similar clinical signs. Despite loss of adduction on lateral gaze, convergence frequently is preserved. Consequently, patients with an acute bilateral internuclear ophthalmoplegia have horizontal double vision on lateral gaze in either direction with minimal or no diplopia on primary gaze. Other possible causes of bilateral internuclear ophthalmoplegia are systemic lupus erythematosus, metastatic cancer, and arteriovenous malformation. Unilateral internuclear ophthalmoplegia also may be due to MS, a vascular disease, or a tumor. A lesion in the medial longitudinal fasciculus unilaterally causes loss of adduction of the eye on the side of the lesion in conjunction with nystagmus of the abducting eye. The eye that is unable to adduct with gaze to one side can adduct with convergence.

Lesions in the brain stem, affecting the third, fifth, seventh, and eighth cranial nerves, can occur in MS. When the seventh nerve is involved, there may be a unilateral peripheral facial nerve palsy that almost never causes changes in taste. The descending root of the fifth cranial nerve may be involved producing unilateral facial numbness, paresthesia, or pain. Paroxysmal unilateral facial pain indistinguishable from trigeminal neuralgia (tic douloureux) without concomitant sensory loss occurs in approximately 2 percent of MS cases. Vertigo, vomiting, and nystagmus due to lesions near the vestibular complex are noted in nearly 30 percent of the MS patients sometime during their illness. Clinical experience suggests that deafness is rare. Lesions in the cerebellum result in ataxia, scanning monotonous speech, and intention tremor.

Spinal cord lesions in MS may involve the lateral corticospinal tracts, lateral spinothalamic tracts, and dorsal columns. Most MS patients will have abnormalities in the motor systems, largely in the corticospinal tracts, which result in features of upper motoneuron dysfunction characterized by paresis, spasticity, hyperreflexia, clonus, Babinski response, and loss of abdominal reflexes. Posterior column lesions produce a decrease in joint-position and vibration sense. The sensory useless hand is an uncommon, but characteristic symptom of MS due to a lesion in the lateral portion of the posterior columns of the cord. The patient will have reduced or absent vibratory sense, two-point discrimination, and joint-position sense in a single upper extremity. Spinothalamic tract involvement, as evidenced by diminution of pain and temperature sensation, occasionally is encountered in MS patients. A small proportion of MS patients develop painful tonic spasms in all muscles of the limb due to spinal cord lesions. Patients with MS frequently complain of a symptom of tingling down the back and into the leg that has an electric shock-like quality produced by flexion of the neck (Lhermitte's sign).

Beyond the well-recognized abnormalities of the somatic neural component of the spinal cord in MS, the spinal cord involvement in MS can produce dysautonomias that can be as devastating as their somatic counterparts. These dysautonomias involve primarily the vesiculourethra, gastrointestinal tract, and sexual function. The severity of dysautonomias in MS is related to the severity of disease, and this is particularly evident in relation to spastic weakness due to damage to the corticospinal tracts. From a practical point of view, vesicourethral dysfunction in MS can be categorized as failure to store urine, failure to empty urine, or a combination of these with detrusor-external sphincter dyssynergia (DESD). Three major risk factors that predispose patients with MS to grave urologic complications are the presence of an indwelling catheter, the presence of DESD in men, and the presence of poor bladder compliance with associated high detrusor pressures (greater than 40 cmH_2O). These urologic abnormalities have been associated with considerable morbidity and mortality. Death in 55 percent of MS patients who have undergone autopsy could be directly attributable to hydronephrosis, pyelonephritis, or septicemia arising from the upper urinary tract. Severe constipation and sexual dysfunction frequently accompany urinary bladder dysfunction in patients with advanced MS. Dysautonomias involving the cardiorespiratory systems rarely are encountered in MS patients with severe neurologic dysfunction.

On rare occasions, severe spinal cord lesions herald the advent of MS. They can result in either complete or incomplete loss of function and are called transverse myelitis. Much more frequent causes of acute transverse myelitis are postinfectious vasculomyelopathy and complications from various vaccinations. When there is evidence of a fairly circumscribed level of neurologic deficit, mechanical compression of the spinal cord must always be considered. The association of acute transverse myelitis with concomitant acute bilateral optic neuritis is sometimes referred to as Devic's syndrome. This latter ill-defined symptom complex is considered by some to be an entity distinct from that of MS.

Even though cerebral MS is seen in fewer than 5 percent of the patients, it is the most disabling and tragic form of MS with serious deterioration of intellect. The most frequent subtle cerebral symptom is depression. Euphoria is associated with widespread cerebral disease, dementia, and pseudobulbar palsy. Up to 5 percent of patients with MS have seizures. Some of these seizures are focal and caused by subcortical lesions.

The adverse effects of elevated core temperature on the neurologic signs and symptoms of MS have been well known for more than 50 years. Many patients with MS experience worsening of their neurologic deficits with exercise and other states of induced hyperthermia. The physiological basis for the adverse effects of increased core temperature on the neurologic symptoms in MS involves a blocking of impulse conduction in a demyelinated nerve. There is growing evidence that significant elevation in core body temperature is not without risk in MS patients, either precipitating permanent neurologic deficits or exposing the patients to circumstances that predispose to serious injury.

Clinical Course

Most young patients (more than 40 percent) have a relapsing and remitting course in which recovery after each episode is complete. The frequency of relapses is unpredictable. Thirty percent of the MS patients have a chronic, progressive course from the onset, which is encountered frequently in older men. At least 20 percent of MS patients have a benign course and have a normal life span of relatively unencumbered physical activities. Fewer than 5 to 10 percent of the patients have a very malignant clinical course that is fulminant and fatal within weeks to months. In general, symptoms that appear acutely and those involving the sensory pathways and/or cranial nerves have a more favorable prognosis than those developing insidiously with either motor deficits or cerebellar dysfunction.

Pregnancy, immunization, overexertion, stress, and infection have been implicated as factors that influence the course of the disease. The MS relapse rate during pregnancy was one-half that expected. This protective effect of pregnancy must be weighed against an increased relapse rate (two to six times) after delivery. Upper viral respiratory tract infections appeared to act as trigger in producing MS exacerbation. Prospective studies have shown that immunization (e.g., influenza, measles, or poliomyelitis vaccines) did not significantly alter the MS relapse rate. Similarly, overexertion and stress did not enhance the relapse rate.

Diagnostic Tests

Paraclinical evidence of multiple sites of involvement is produced by special procedures. The lesion detected may or may not have produced symptoms or signs in the past; in the latter case, the lesion is considered subclinical. Magnetic resonance imaging (MRI) is the recommended imaging technique for obtaining evidence to support the diagnosis of MS (Fig. 151-1). The typical MRI abnormalities of MS are multiple discrete lesions located in the supratentorial white matter, especially in the periventricular area. Lesions are detected less commonly in the cerebellum and brain stem. With further technologic advancements, the imaging of spinal cord and optic nerves should become more reliable. The MRI detects abnormalities consistent with MS in 70 to 95 percent of MS patients. Enhancements of the lesions may be detected by the contrast agent gadolinium, indicating the presence of acute lesions with breakdown of the blood-brain barrier. While computed tomography (CT) is not as sensitive as MRI in the detection of MS lesions, it does reveal a wide variety of findings. It provides a reliable assessment of cerebral atrophy and ventricular enlargement and detects low-density focal lesions in the cerebrum, brain stem, or optic nerves.

Evoked-response testing measures the electric response to stimulation of a sensory pathway, recorded through surface electrodes, then amplified and subjected to signal averaging. It is a sensitive method to detect slowed conduction of visual, auditory, or somatosensory impulses. One or more evoked response tests will reveal a slowing of conduction in approximately 80 percent of the MS patients.

In addition, CSF examination in MS patients is used to support the diagnosis. The CSF has a normal cell number in most patients. While slight increases in cell counts have been reported, cell counts greater than 50 cells/mm^3 are rare. The cells in the CSF are usually T lymphocytes. Immunocytochemical analysis of the CSF can differentiate benign from malignant lymphoproliferation. The protein concentration is increased in approximately 25 percent of the MS patients. The most characteristic CSF finding in MS is an increase in immunoglobulin (IgG) caused by synthesis of IgG in the central nervous system. The

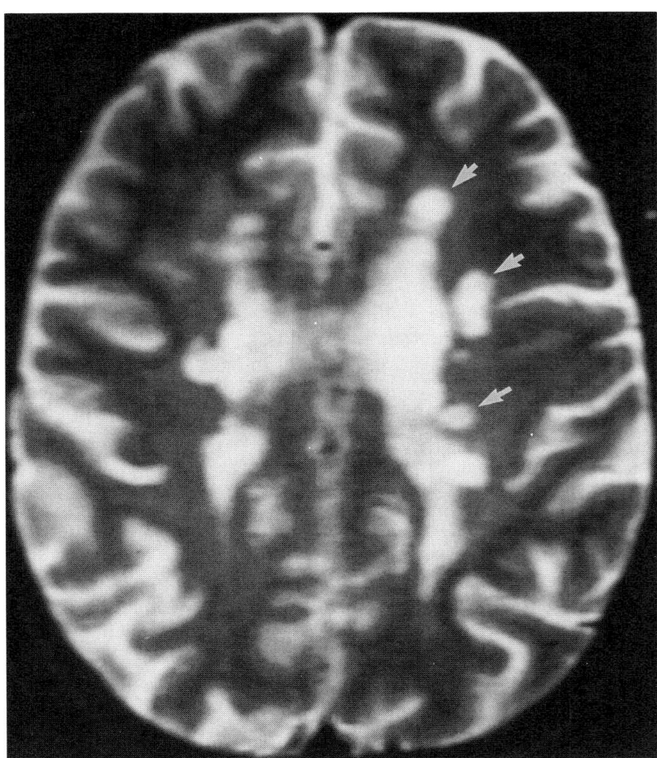

Fig. 151-1. A magnetic resonance image from a patient with MS. Multiple lesions of the white matter (arrows) in the periventricular areas support the diagnosis of MS in a patient with an appropriate history and physical findings.

sensitivity of this measurement can be enhanced by measuring IgG and albumin in the CSF and serum to allow calculation of a CSF IgG index:

$$\text{CSF IgG index} = \frac{(\text{CSF IgG/CSF albumin})}{(\text{serum IgG/CSF serum albumin})}$$

An index greater than 0.77 is considered abnormal and is encountered in 80 to 90 percent of the patients with MS. When CSF IgG is subjected to isoelectric focusing or electrophoresis, it fractionates into oligoclonal bands. Within the CSF, myelin basic protein or its fragments are also detected in the CSF of MS patients.

Before lumbar puncture, clinical assessment for the presence of raised intracranial pressure, encountered in other diseases whose signs and symptoms may mimic those of MS (e.g., cerebral abscess or brain) is mandatory. A history of progressive headache associated with mental changes and the development of localizing neurologic signs and papilledema are reliable manifestations of increased intracranial pressure. Plain skull x-rays should be obtained before lumbar puncture to search for displacement of a calcified pineal gland.

Differential Diagnosis

Patients with other neurologic diseases may at times resemble patients with MS to the extent that they satisfy many of the clinical criteria for MS. A list of the clinical features that cast doubt on the diagnosis of MS include the following: (1) absence of eye findings (optic nerve involvement or extraocular movement abnormalities), (2) absence of clinical remissions, especially in young patients, (3) localized disease (posterior fossa, craniocervical junction, or spinal cord), (4) absence of CSF abnormalities, and (5) atypical clinical features (absence of sensory findings and bladder involvement). The frequency of misdiagnosis even in MS specialty clinics has been estimated to be at least 10 percent. In the past, this error rate may not have had the serious consequences that it may have today, because such a patient may now be treated inappropriately with a variety of therapeutic agents or may be entered into therapeutic trials of new agents. Consequently, it is inappropriate to make the diagnosis based upon emergency department evaluation.

Clinical features common in MS patients may be seen in patients with SLE. Clinically, SLE and MS have several features characteristic of diseases with histocompatibility antigen (HLA) gene products including a chronic and/or relapsing course, an inflammatory component, and a weak familial propensity. Although there are no figures reported for the percentage of patients with SLE who have central nervous system involvement as the sole manifestation of their disease, there are reports of patients with neurologic symptoms resembling MS who later developed SLE. Similarly, there are patients who present with symptoms suggesting SLE who develop MS. In some of these patients, the diagnosis remains obscure for a long time, and the term lupoid sclerosis has been applied. Based on the American Rheumatism Association's criteria, a diagnosis of SLE rests on serologic findings (elevated antinuclear antibody and positive anti-DNA antibodies) and a specific pattern of organ involvement.

Spirochetal organisms also may cause a disease whose neurologic manifestations may mimic some aspects of MS. The best clinical marker of acute Lyme disease is a characteristic skin lesion, erythema chronicum migrans. In many patients, infection progresses to chronic Lyme disease, a spectrum of clinical signs and symptoms characterized by neurologic dysfunction and persistent musculoskeletal and cardiac disease. The diagnosis of acute Lyme disease usually depends on the measurement of serum antibodies to *Borrelia burgdorferi*. However, the presence of the chronic form of the disease cannot be excluded by the absence of antibodies. A T-cell blastogenic response to *B. burgdorferi* is evidence of infection in seronegative patients with clinical signs of Lyme disease.

In Lyme disease, the central nervous system acts as an immunologically distinct compartment in which specific antibody synthesis occurs independent of its production in the remainder of the body. For this reason, just as in other infections, demonstration of intrathecal production of specific antibodies provides a reliable indicator of *B. burgdorferi* infection in the central nervous system.

The differential diagnosis of neurosyphilis is extensive. With the many efforts to develop more sensitive and specific tests for syphilis, it seems ironic that the current screening tests for this disease are the nonspecific nontreponemal tests. Antigens for these tests, traditionally termed cardiolipin or reagin, contain cardiolipin, cholesterol, and lecithin. Of the nontreponemal tests, the Venereal Disease Research lab (VDRL) is the only test recommended for use with CSF. As the length of the latent stage of syphilis increases, the serum titer for the nontreponemal tests decreases. Approximately 30 percent of individuals with latent syphilis will have nonreactive nontreponemal test results. Asymptomatic neurosyphilis should not be diagnosed by a reactive CSF VDRL alone. Other diagnostic criteria for neurosyphilis include reactive serum nontreponemal or treponemal test results, or both, five or more lymphocytes per cubic millimeter of CSF, and CSF total protein of greater than or equal to 45 mg/dL.

Human immunodeficiency virus (HIV) infections also can present with relapsing and remitting symptoms that mimic MS. The close temporal association between the onset of the neurological disease and the demonstration of HIV-1 seropositivity in these patients suggests a causal relationship. Several recent studies have indicated that in addition to its ability to induce leukemia, human T-lymphotrophic virus type I (HTLV-I) also may play an important role in certain disorders of the central nervous system whose clinical manifestations may mimic MS. The progressive spastic paraparetic form of MS seen in white men is virtually identical to tropical spastic paraparesis of HTLV-I associated myelopathy, which is widely distributed in Africa, the Caribbean, and southern Japan. This disease clearly is associated with and probably caused by HTLV-I, and a clear-cut viral isolation has now been reported by several groups. Ninety-five percent of specimens from patients with tropical spastic paraparesis were repeatedly reactive for antibodies to HTLV-I by enzyme immunoassay.

It is well recognized that cobalamin deficiency may present as a neurologic disorder in the absence of anemia or elevated erythrocyte mean corpuscular volume. Even a high serum cobalamin level or a normal result on the Schilling test occasionally may be associated with a neuropsychiatric disorder caused by cobalamin deficiency. In patients with equivocal findings, high serum levels of methylmalonic acid and total homocysteine that return to normal after therapy provide useful confirmatory evidence of a deficiency of cobalamin. The availability of these tests should make it possible to screen individuals with unexplained neuropsychiatric disorders for cobalamin deficiency. If such tests are unavailable, a course of intramuscular cobalamin therapy is recommended, even in doubtful cases.

Treatment

Treatment of MS has focused on three aspects of management: amelioration of an acute exacerbation, slowing the progression of the disease, and relief of symptoms. Adrenocorticoids (initially as corticotropin [ACTH] and subsequently as synthetic steroids) were the first antiinflammatory or immunosuppressive drug used to treat exacerbations. A double-blinded placebo controlled trial of ACTH showed a slightly more rapid improvement in the month following institution of therapy. A short-term (5 days) high-dose (500 mg) course of pulsed intravenous methylprednisone, followed by an oral tapering course of prednisone for 3 weeks, recently has been reported to be beneficial in acute exacerbations of MS. However, it is not known if the long-term recovery of function is any different whether steroids are given or not. Long-term daily or alternate-day steroids are not recommended.

Immunosuppressive therapy with several drugs (azathioprine or cyclophosphamide) is encouraging in that statistically significant results have been obtained, but disappointing by immediate or late adverse effects. When indicated, the MS patient should be treated in a medical center that is experienced in the use of immunosuppressive agents and involved in well-designed clinical trials with these agents.

While the physician cannot cure or reliably alter the long-term course of the disease, advances in the understanding of the pathophysiology of central nervous system dysfunction has enabled physicians to improve dramatically the symptomatic management of MS. Of primary importance in the management of MS urinary dysfunction is to preserve the integrity of the upper urinary tract. Consequently, the initial steps in the detection of urologic dysfunction in MS patients is a careful history and physical examination, followed by a microscopic analysis of the Gram's stain of unspun urine. When bacteria are detected, cultures of the urine are indicated. Symptomatic patients usually complain of either irritative bladder symptoms with urgency, frequency, and incontinence or obstructive bladder symptoms with hesitancy, flow decrease, and retention or as a combination of both. Because the likelihood of infection is associated with excessive postvoiding residual (PVR) urine, all MS patients should have serial PVR urine determinations during the course of their disease. History alone is inadequate in identifying those MS patients who are emptying their bladder incompletely. The PVR urine can be determined accurately either by catheterization using aseptic technique or by ultrasonography after the patient has voided.

The treatment of the urologic dysfunction will depend on the magnitude of PVR urine and the patient's symptomatology. If the MS patient presenting to emergency department has symptomatic voiding or evidence of bacteriuria, a PVR urine determination is indicated. When the residual urines are either greater than 100 mL or more than 20 percent of the voided volume, the treatment of choice is intermittent catheterization by the clean technique. When the bladder does not empty completely with a PVR urine volume of less than 100 mL, the treatment will depend on the patient's symptomatology. In the symptomatic patient, appropriate and effective pharmacologic therapy can be instituted based on specific findings from the urodynamic evaluation by the urologist.

Acute urinary tract infections may be asymptomatic, may produce nonspecific symptoms, or may produce specific symptoms. Patients with dysuria, frequency, urgency, and suprapubic pain usually have cystitis without systemic manifestations. Prominent systemic signs and symptoms, like fever over 39.2°C (103°F), nausea, vomiting, and costovertebral angle tenderness usually indicate renal infection. However, some patients with significant bacteriuria from either cystitis or renal infection are asymptomatic. In addition, urinary tract infections may aggravate seemingly unrelated neurologic symptoms, such as lower extremity weakness or spasticity in MS patients. Consequently, any change in neurologic symptoms in an MS patient should lead to the consideration of urinary tract infection. For this reason, frequent surveillance cultures are helpful in monitoring the patient. When infection occurs, antibiotic treatment is indicated, and treatment should be individualized to the organism and its sensitivity. The recommended duration of treatment is debated. There is growing evidence that short periods of therapy (single-dose therapy) are effective in uncomplicated cystitis. However, the MS patient may respond more favorably to the more conventional 10-day course of therapy in the presence of the concomitant urodynamic abnormalities. Although recurrent urinary tract infection may reflect an inadequately treated infection, chronic infection may indicate significant structural pathology (e.g., calculi or abscess) that warrant further diagnostic study.

In many infections, fever is a prominent, and often the only, manifestation of disease. Because fever ordinarily does little harm and imposes no great discomfort to most patients, antipyretic drugs are rarely necessary and may mask the effect of a specific therapeutic agent on the natural course of the disease. However, lowering the body temperature is of vital importance in the febrile MS patient. Small increases in the body temperature of MS patients can worsen existing signs and symptoms as well as produce additional neurologic manifestations. Because the endogenous hyperthermia of clinical infections worsens the neurologic deficits in patients with MS, lowering the elevated body temperature with antipyretics is prudent. Many other symptoms of MS, which can be ameliorated by appropriate therapy, include gait dysfunction, fatigue, tremors, constipation, seizures, and bowel symptoms. Management of these symptoms is optimal in an MS comprehensive care center with its multidisciplinary staff, rather than the emergency department. An MS comprehensive care center will be able to coordinate effectively the delivery of a uniform standard of care in keeping with modern management guidelines.

When MS patients are subjected to diseases or injuries that warrant surgical intervention, special considerations in the management of these patients are warranted. Anesthesia and surgery may have an adverse effect on patients with MS, but the unpredictable course of the disease and the capriciousness of the signs make confirmation of a definite causal relationship difficult. Before surgery, the patient's respiratory function must be assessed. Failure of spontaneous ventilation may occur in MS patients. Some MS patients have a labile autonomic nervous system that may precipitate hypotension during anesthesia and surgery. Because the autonomic nervous system of the gastrointestinal tract may be affected, MS patients may have gastric and intestinal atony with constipation, bloating, and fecal incontinence. This delayed emptying of the stomach is an invitation to aspiration and subsequent pneumonia during intubation. The use of preoperative medications to enhance gastric motility, followed by rapid-sequence intubation minimizes the chance for aspiration pneumonia. The patient must be searched for infective foci that may predispose to wound infection and pyrexia. Because pyrexia may precipitate an exacerbation, surgery should be postponed, when feasible, until the patient is free from infection.

There is no direct evidence that any of the currently used volatile anesthetic agents have a deleterious effect on the course of this disease. There are also no reports of abnormal responses to nondepolarizing muscle relaxants in MS. Usual doses of alcuronium, D-tubocurarine, and gallamine were tolerated well. Although there is one report of hyperkalemia following succinylcholine, the absence of others suggests low vulnerability and incidence of succinylcholine-induced hyperkalemia in MS patients. The increased incidence of epilepsy in MS patients argues against the use of anesthetic agents that may precipitate seizures. For instance, due to the association of convulsive electroencephalographic activity with enflurane anesthesia, this anesthetic agent should be avoided in MS patients. Because an elevation in body temperature appears to be the normal response to all but the least traumatic procedures, the prophylactic use of antipyretics may be of value.

For 40 years, it has been advocated that spinal anesthesia should be avoided in patients with MS. However, it is fair to state that there is a difference of opinion about the use of regional anesthesia in MS patients, and epidural anesthesia has been successfully used in obstetrical patients with MS.

ADE

ADE or postinfectious encephalomyelitis is an inflammatory and demyelinating disorder that may follow a viral illness, particularly the common childhood exanthems, vaccination, or occur without a recognized antecedent. This disease has been described after rabies vaccination with a vaccine containing brain tissue and and after vaccination against small pox; it begins approximately 10 days to 3 weeks after the vaccination. When the disorder is related to an antecedent viral infection, it usually occurs 6 to 10 days after the origin of the other systemic symptoms. The disease is believed to be immunologically mediated and resembles clinically the experimental disease allergic encephalomyelitis.

Clinically, the disorder is characterized by an acute or subacute illness with fever, headache, and delirium that progresses to seizures and coma. Typically, clinical features are multifocal neurologic signs that include optic neuritis, myelitis, ataxia, hemiparesis, and cranial nerve palsies. There is often a diffuse encephalopathic disturbance with bilateral simultaneous optic neuritis or a severe transverse myelitis. The CSF demonstrates a marked increase in lymphocytes (10 to 100 cells/mm^3), protein (50 to 100 mg/dL), and usually IgG. Oligoclonal bands are present in ADE but disappear after the patient recovers. The MRI reveals multifocal asymmetric white-matter lesions, indistinguishable from those seen in MS. Serial MRIs are helpful in distinguishing monophasic ADE from polyphasic MS. New lesions should not be expected in ADE, providing there is a sufficiently long period of follow-up. The mortality is 20 percent, and many of the survivors have neurologic deficits. High-dose glucocorticoid therapy is the treatment of choice.

ANHE

ANHE is a rare disease that affects young adults and follows an upper respiratory tract infection. The clinical course is characterized by three phases. The first phase is the prodromal period, which averages 5 days and may simulate an upper respiratory infection with mild coryza, sore throat, hoarseness, and a cough. Bronchopneumonia occasionally may follow. The second phase, lasting 1 to 7 days, represents the recovery from the prodromal phase, with the patient returning to normal activities. The third phase is heralded by the acute onset of variable neurologic signs and symptoms such as headache, nausea, vomiting, fever, stiff neck, malaise, confusion, hemiparesis, hemiplegia, and even quadriplegia. Cranial nerve palsies, variable sensory abnormalities, convulsions, and urinary incontinence have been reported. The condition deteriorates in most patients to coma and finally death. The pathologic findings include destruction of one or both hemispheres. The histologic examination resembles ADE with perivenular foci of demyelination of comparable age with intense polymorphonuclear infiltration. The vessels are partially necrotic with hemorrhagic extravasation. The CSF examination discloses polymorphonuclear pleocytosis of up to 2000 cells/mm^3 and marked increase in protein.

The outcome usually is fatal within 10 days to 2 weeks. However, a few survivors have been reported in recent years. The gravity of the clinical course is related to evidence of increased intracranial pressure that must be reduced promptly. The initial use of steroids and dehydrating agents (osmotic diuretics) in sufficient dosages and for an adequate period followed, if necessary, by a large surgical decompression seems to be the appropriate therapeutic regimen for ANHE. Surgical decompression is recommended because it not only relieves intracranial pressure and prevents transtentorial herniation, but also it establishes a diagnosis by obtaining a specimen for histologic examination.

This clinical pathologic entity bears a resemblance to a hyperacute form of experimental allergic encephalomyelitis that can be induced in animals by administration of endotoxin, pertussis vaccine, or its histamine-sensitizing factor coincident with or shortly after the injection of myelin as the adjuvant.

This research was supported by a generous gift from Charles H. Ross, Jr., Rumson, New Jersey.

BIBLIOGRAPHY

Multiple Sclerosis

Bellian KT, Devlin PM, Zimmer CA, et al: Concurrence of multiple sclerosis and Hodgkin's disease. *J Emerg Med* (In press).

Edlich RF, Muir A, Persing JA, et al: Special considerations in the management of a patient with multiple sclerosis and a burn injury. *J Burn Care Rehab* 12:102, 1991.

Edlich RF, Westwater JJ, Lombardi SA, et al: Multiple sclerosis and asymptomatic urinary tract infection. *J Emerg Med* 8:25, 1990.

Ransohoff RM: Multiple sclerosis: New concepts of pathogenesis, diagnosis, and treatment. *Compr Ther* 15(3):39, 1989.

Rodriguez M: Multiple sclerosis: Basic concepts and hypothesis. *Mayo Clin Proc.* 64:570, 1989.

Rudick RA, Schiffer RB, Schwetz KM, et al: Multiple sclerosis: The problem of incorrect diagnosis. *Arch Neurol* 43:578, 1986.

Acute Disseminated Encephalomyelitis

Kesslring J, Miller DH, Robb SA, et al: Acute disseminated encephalomyelitis. *Brain* 113:291, 1990.

McHugh K, McMenamin JB: Acute disseminated encephalomyelitis in childhood. *Irish Med J* 80:412, 1987.

Acute Necrotizing Hemorrhagic Encephalomyelitis

Hwang C-C, Chu N-S, Chen T-J, et al: A hemorrhagic leucoencephalitis with a prolonged clinical course. *J Neurol Neurosurg Psychiatry* 51:870, 1988.

Litel G, Ehni G: Acute hemorrhagic leukoencephalitis: Treatment with corticosteroids and dehydrating agents. *J Neurosurg* 33:445, 1970.

152
DISORDERS OF NEUROMUSCULAR TRANSMISSION

Lawrence H. Phillips II
Richard F. Edlich

INTRODUCTION

Disorders of neuromuscular transmission are characterized by fatigable weakness in a child or adult. The pathophysiology of these disorders relates to a disturbance of neuromuscular transmission at the myoneural junction (motor end plate) of skeletal muscle. A classification of these disorders divides them into autoimmune [myasthenia gravis (MG) and Eaton-Lambert-myasthenic syndrome], genetic, toxic (botulism), and drug-induced forms. The onset of symptoms of the genetic form occurs in the newborn period or infancy, and the symptoms are caused by either presynaptic defects [abnormal acetylcholine (Ach) resynthesis or mobilization, abnormal Ach release], or postsynaptic defects [end-plate acetylcholinesterase (AChE) deficiency, reduced number of acetylcholine receptors (AchR), impaired function of AchR, and slow channel syndrome]. These genetic forms are not caused by antibodies to AchR.

MYASTHENIA GRAVIS

Myasthenia gravis is an uncommon disease which produces varying degrees of muscle weakness. It is an autoimmune disease classified as a disorder of neuromuscular transmission because the cause for weakness is an antibody-mediated depletion of AchR at the muscle end plate. Patients with this disorder may develop acute changes in their condition which can be life-threatening if they are not recognized and treated.

The average annual incidence of MG is approximately 2 to 5 cases per million population. The estimated point prevalence is 5 to 10 cases per 100,000 population. The disease occurs in all ages, with a 2 to 1 female to male ratio. The peak prevalence is in the third decade of life for females and in the fifth or sixth decade for males, thus producing a bimodal distribution.

Pathophysiology

Myasthenia gravis is the prototypical autoimmune disease, and probably more is understood about its pathogenesis than any other autoimmune disorder. Investigations have shown that there is a circulating antibody against the AchR in the sera of myasthenics. This antibody has been demonstrated to bind with the AchR at the motor end plate. The bound antibody mobilizes complement and produces a cascade of destructive events which end in a marked reduction in the number of AchRs.

In the normal motor end plate, there is a large redundancy of AchR. This produces a safety margin for neuromuscular transmission, which can only be exceeded under extraordinary conditions, such as repetitive activation of the motor nerve terminal at sustained high rates. In the case of myasthenic end plate, the safety margin is markedly reduced. The result is that repeated activation of an affected muscle fiber at even low rates will exceed the safety margin and the fiber will become refractory to additional nerve impulses. This phenomenon is the basis for the clinical hallmark of MG, fatigable weakness. In muscles that are affected, the reduced safety margin will result in a certain number of muscle fibers being refractory to nerve impulses after an initial period of activation. Thus an initially strong muscle contraction will rapidly become weaker with repeated contractions.

Myasthenia gravis is frequently only one of several autoimmune diseases which may coexist in a patient. The association of MG with other recognized autoimmune diseases such as rheumatoid arthritis, pernicious anemia, systemic lupus erythematosus, sarcoidosis, and thyroiditis provides further support for the belief of its autoimmune etiology. The interaction of MG with some of the other autoimmune disorders can become clinically important. For example, the hyperthyroid phase of autoimmune thyroiditis can be associated with an increase of muscle weakness due to MG.

Approximately 10 to 25 percent of patients with MG have an associated thymoma, and 30 to 59 percent of patients with thymoma will develop clinical MG. Although thymomas are most commonly benign tumors, they are associated with a more severe form of MG. Frequently, control of the disease can only be attained after removal of the thymic tumor.

Clinical Manifestations

The clinical hallmark of MG is muscle weakness, usually with some component of fatigability. Most patients will have demonstrable weakness present throughout the day. They typically observe that their strength improves after a period of resting, and weakness of a particular muscle group will increase after sustained or repetitive use.

A typical pattern of evolution of muscle weakness affects the majority of patients. Most frequently the first muscles to become weak are the extraocular muscles, although weakness in other muscle groups, such as the bulbar muscles, may be the presenting symptom. The initial symptoms of the disease are usually either diplopia or eyelid ptosis, frequently fluctuating from side to side over the course of the day or from day to day. In approximately 20 percent of patients, the disease remains confined to the extraocular muscles throughout its course. The typical course is for weakness of other muscle groups to develop within months of the ocular symptoms.

Symptoms of the disease are frequently influenced by environmental, emotional, and physical factors. Bright light will often exacerbate ptosis and diplopia, and heat may increase muscle weakness. Emotional stress can increase or decrease the severity of the disease. Viral illness, surgery, menses, pregnancy, immunization and other physical factors all may precipitate a change in the expression of MG, although not in a predictable direction. Changes in strength associated with these factors are usually transient, lasting only as long as the precipitating cause.

When limb muscles become symptomatic, proximal muscles are typically weakest. The most severe manifestation of the disease produces weakness of respiratory muscles, precipitating a life-threatening situation, the *myasthenic crisis*. Myasthenic crisis occurs in a severe MG patient who is either not being treated or is being undertreated because of insufficient medication or drug resistance. Improved treatment of myasthenic crisis has resulted in a dramatic decrease in the mortality of MG, but this remains the most likely cause of death from the disease. Disease progression is most rapid within the first 3 years, and more than one half of the deaths occur within this period. Spontaneous remissions lasting from weeks to years have been noted.

Diagnostic Tests

In the generalized form of MG, the diagnosis is generally not difficult. The combination of ocular, bulbar, and limb weakness which fluctuates during the day and decreases with resting is so typical of the disease that few other disorders need to be considered in the differential diagnosis. The patients who present with disease limited to ocular muscles, particularly when it is mild, sometimes present a diagnostic challenge. Patients who have minimal ocular signs and symptoms and more severe weakness in other muscle groups are particularly difficult to diagnose with certainty. A variety of laboratory and bedside tests have been devised to supplement the clinical examination and provide more certainty about the diagnosis.

Anticholinesterase Tests

The diagnosis of MG can be confirmed at the bedside, often very dramatically, through the use of the edrophonium test. Edrophonium chloride is administered as an intravenous bolus while the patient's muscle strength is tested. Edrophonium chloride is an AchE inhibitor, which prevents rapid breakdown of Ach at the myoneural junction. It acts within a few seconds, and its pharmacologic effect of improving muscle strength is dramatic but transient, lasting 5 to 10 min. A positive result is a definite increase in strength of a previously weak muscle which lasts for several minutes. Muscle weakness then slowly returns. In adults, 1 to 2 mg of the drug is injected intravenously to identify the occasional patient who is hypersensitive to the drug, with the occasional appearance of muscular fasiculations and respiratory depression. This drug must be given cautiously to patients with cardiac disease because it may cause sinus bradycardia, AV block, and rarely cardiac arrest. Atropine is an effective antidote for the muscarinic effects of edrophonium chloride, but is of no value in counteracting the nicotinic effects on the motor end plate that might result in secondary partial paralysis of skeletal muscles. If there are no untoward cholinergic effects in 30 s, a larger dose of 5 to 8 mg is administered. The usual intravenous dose in children is 0.15 mg/kg of body weight, not to exceed 10 mg per dose; a test dose of one-tenth of the total dose is administered first to test for hypersensitivity. Intramuscular neostigmine in adults, 0.5 to 1.0 mg, acts maximally in about 30 min, allowing a more prolonged evaluation of changes in the clinical status.

Special considerations are in order for the use of edrophonium chloride in the emergency department. Only ocular myasthenics or those with mild generalized disease should be tested in the emergency department. Patients with bronchial asthma or cardiac arrhythmia should not be evaluated in the emergency department, but rather in a hospital setting that can appropriately treat increased tracheobronchial secretions and cardiac arrhythmia.

The value of edrophonium chloride testing may be negated if the test is not performed carefully. Particular care must be taken to select weak muscles for evaluation prior to administration of the drug. While some suggest that reversal of eyelid ptosis is the only reliable indicator of a positive test, other muscles can be monitored. The performance of the test in a double-blind fashion is the most reliable strategy to follow. The examiner must have an assistant draw up the edrophonium chloride and an inactive solution, such as normal saline, in identical, coded syringes. The contents of the two syringes are administered sequentially, and the examiner and the patient independently rate the effect of the two agents, prior to breaking the code. Caution must be used in interpreting the results of even a clearly positive test, because other diseases (e.g., amyotrophic lateral sclerosis, Guillain-Barré syndrome, lesions in the cavernous sinus, and Eaton-Lambert-myasthenic syndrome) may, at times, produce a response to edrophonium chloride. Additionally, patients with neurasthenia may have a temporary improvement in strength.

Electromyography

Electromyographic testing has two roles in the diagnosis of MG. The first is to confirm the diagnosis through demonstration of the typical findings of abnormal neuromuscular transmission. The second is to exclude the presence of other diseases, which may form part of the differential diagnosis. The typical electrophysiologic hallmark of a defect of neuromuscular transmission is a decrement in the amplitude of the compound muscle action potential in response to repetitive nerve stimulation.

Serologic Tests

The most specific test for MG is the demonstration of AchR antibodies in the serum. Although there are cases of other disorders associated with the presence of circulating AchR antibodies, a positive antibody test in a patient with clinically suspected MG is diagnostic of the disease. Unfortunately, the assay is relatively insensitive in milder forms of the disease. In ocular MG, fully one-third of patients will not have demonstrable AchR antibodies. Striated muscle antibodies also occur in MG patients, but their role is not known.

Because there is no single test that is absolutely reliable in the diagnosis of the disease, a battery of tests is usually used. As in most other diseases, one should be prepared to use the information obtained from a diagnostic test to guide further management. Fortunately, when MG is the most severe and requires therapeutic intervention, diagnostic testing usually provides unequivocal evidence for the presence of the disease. In other words, if diagnostic tests, particularly electromyography and AchR antibody tests, do not support the diagnosis in a patient with severe weakness, some other disease is most likely present.

A relatively small number of diseases can present signs and symptoms that mimic MG; they include mitochondrial myopathy, oculopharyngeal muscular dystophy, inflammatory myopathies, amyotrophic lateral sclerosis, periodic paralysis syndromes, and neurasthenia. In general, these diseases are rarer than MG.

Treatment

The treatment of MG must be tailored to the needs of the patient. Because the spectrum of the disease can vary from mild ocular weakness to severe, life-threatening generalized weakness, a variety of treatment strategies are used.

Acetylcholinesterase Inhibitors and Myasthenic Crisis

This class of drugs has been the mainstay of symptomatic therapy of MG since the discovery of their effectiveness in the 1930s. They are generally the least dangerous and easiest to regulate of the therapies available. The most commonly used preparation is pyridostigmine bromide. A standard 60-mg dose typically has onset of effect within 30 min to 1 h of administration. The peak drug effect is at 1½ to 2 h, and the effect of the dose disappears within 4 h. Various dosage strategies are used, but the typical patient will take 60 mg three to four times per day, often taking each dose prior to a meal. Other preparations have shorter (neostigmine bromide) or longer (ambenonium chloride) durations of therapeutic effect.

The side effects of anticholinesterase therapy are generally related to peripheral cholinergic excess because the drugs do not penetrate the blood-brain barrier well. The drugs work at muscarinic as well as nicotinic synapses, producing symptoms of abdominal cramping, excessive sweating, lacrimation, and, infrequently, cardiac arrhythmia. Most patients tolerate or adapt to the muscarinic side effects after a period of adjustment. When side effects are intolerable, supplemental doses of anticholinergic drugs, such as atropine sulfate, can be given concurrently with each dose of cholinesterase inhibitor.

The major complication of the use of cholinesterase inhibitors is the development of muscle weakness as a consequence of depolarization block of neuromuscular transmission. This typically occurs in the setting of overdosage of the drug, and is particularly likely to occur in patients with more severe degrees of weakness and larger dosage requirements. Distinction of "cholinergic crisis" from "myasthenic crisis" is sometimes difficult. An edrophonium test performed at the time of expected peak effect of a dose of pyridostigmine may help to distinguish between the two. If the patient becomes stronger after intravenous edrophonium, the patient is undermedicated. If, on the other hand, the patient becomes weaker, a condition of cholinergic blockade of neuromuscular transmission can be inferred. In the latter case, treatment consists of withdrawal of drug until a clear response to edrophonium returns. A return of response may not occur for several days, and many patients require in-hospital monitoring during this time. Patients who have increasing difficulty in breathing, feeding, and handling tracheobronchial secretions and are refractory to relatively high doses of AChE are best treated by drug withdrawal, respiratory support, and intravenous fluids in an intensive care setting.

Thymectomy

The thymus is normal or involuted in 20 percent of patients with MG; the remaining 80 percent have either hyperplasia (65 percent) or thymoma (15 percent). Thymomas tend to occur from the fourth decade onward. Approximately 60 percent are well encapsulated and benign; the other 40 percent are locally invasive and typically spread in a subpleural distribution. Distant metastases are rare. Plain radiography is the simplest technique for identifying thymoma. Computed tomography (CT) and magnetic resonance imaging (MRI) may diagnose small tumors in a few additional patients and successfully negate the possibility in others. Additionally, CT or MRI can identify discontinuous or aberrant thymic tissue and help guide surgical resection in patients undergoing thymectomy. The practice in most centers today is to advocate thymectomy for all MG patients as early in the course of the disease as possible. Exceptions would be patients with mild disease whose symptoms are controlled adequately with anticholinesterase medication, patients with a contraindication to surgery, and elderly patients.

Immunosuppressive Drug Therapy

Patients with the more severe manifestations of the disease generally require some form of immunosuppression. The drug which has been used most frequently in the United States for initial immunosuppression is prednisone. Various dosing strategies are used, but most call for high doses tapered slowly over periods of 2 or more years. Initiation of steroid therapy should be done cautiously, because approximately 10 percent of patients will experience a pronounced increase of weakness within the first 21 days after first exposure to high doses of the drug. The usual response to prednisone is, however, rapid and sustained improvement in strength shortly after beginning the drug. The morbidity of steroid-associated side effects is substantial, and a risk-benefit analysis for steroid therapy should be done for each patient prior to beginning therapy.

In the United States other immunosuppressive drugs, mainly azathioprine, have been used to supplement the therapeutic effect of prednisone and to allow lowering its dose. In some American centers and in Europe, however, azathioprine has been used as the primary modality of therapy. The usual effective dose is in the range of 2 to 3.5 mg/kg of body weight. The onset of therapeutic effect of the drug is often several months, and supplementary therapy, such as plasma exchange, is therefore often necessary. Drug toxicity is primarily on the bone marrow and liver. Initial treatment requires frequent monitoring of blood counts and liver function because some patients may have idiosyncratic reactions at even very low dosage levels. An additional drug undergoing testing in the United States is cyclosporine. Its primary use appears likely to be for supplementation of prednisone therapy.

Plasmapheresis

Plasma exchange involves the removal of the antibody-rich plasma from the blood and replacing it with an inactive protein substitute. In MG, a course of plasma exchange, usually 4 to 6 sessions, is marked by dramatic, rapid improvement in strength. Unfortunately, if therapy is not supplemented by immunosuppressive drugs, weakness returns within days to several weeks after the plasma exchange is ended. In some centers, particularly difficult to control cases are sometimes treated with a regimen of a weekly session of plasma exchange in addition to immunosuppressive drug therapy. In most centers, however, the use of plasma exchange is reserved for treatment of acute myasthenic crisis. A secondary indication is to use plasma exchange to improve strength rapidly in preparation for thymectomy.

Drug Interactions

A number of medications have the potential to increase weakness in patients with MG. Although no drug is absolutely contraindicated, several are known to be particularly hazardous and should be used with proper precautions. A partial listing of drugs which are known to produce increased weakness or to have an exaggerated effect are listed in Table 152-1. When it is necessary to use any of the drugs listed in Table 152-1 for a patient with MG, one should be prepared to deal with increased muscle weakness that may result.

Various antibiotics are known to produce neuromuscular blockade. The aminoglycosides are particularly likely to produce increased weakness in MG. The clinical situation will arise, nevertheless, where the choice of antibiotic to use takes precedence over concern about neuromuscular blockade. In this situation, special care should be taken to monitor the strength of the patient with MG. The increased weakness produced by systemically administered antibiotics is usually not marked, and strength reverts to baseline after discontinuation of the drug.

The neuromuscular blocking agents must be used with great caution. Patients with MG are already suffering from partial neuromuscular blockade, and they may not need any neuromuscular blockers to achieve adequate levels of surgical muscle relaxation. If a patient does not achieve adequate relaxation with general anesthesia alone, very small doses of neuromuscular blockers should be given. If normal doses are used, the effect is usually markedly prolonged, and the patient will likely require prolonged intubation postoperatively.

TRANSITORY MYASTHENIA GRAVIS (TMG)

Transitory myasthenia gravis is noted in 10 to 15 percent of the offspring of MG mothers. It is of interest that the affected and unaffected infants exhibit the same high titer of AchR antibodies as their mothers. However, infants are affected only when they produce antibodies independently, either because of adoptive transfers of immunocytes from the mother or perhaps because fetal AchR damaged by maternal antibodies triggers a transient immune response in infants. Difficulty feeding and generalized hypotonia are the major clinical features of TMG. Symptoms frequently begin within hours after birth, but can be delayed until the third postnatal day. Respiratory insufficiency is uncommon. Recovery is complete, and infants with TMG do not develop MG later in life. The diagnosis of TMG is made by demonstrating high serum concentrations of AchR antibodies in the newborn and temporary reversal of weakness after a subcutaneous injection of edrophonium chloride.

Newborns with severe generalized weakness and respiratory distress may require exchange transfusions. For those who are less impaired, intermittent intramuscular injections of anticholinesterase prior to feeding may provide sufficient improvement.

LAMBERT-EATON MYASTHENIC SYNDROME

Lambert-Eaton myasthenic syndrome is an antibody-mediated decrease in the number of Ach release sites on motor nerve terminals. The clinical hallmark is proximal muscle weakness, particularly of the lower extremities, which may decrease with repetitive activation of the muscle. Patients rarely have weakness of extraocular or respiratory muscles. In addition to the pattern of weakness, which differs from MG, tendon stretch reflexes are markedly diminished or absent. Patients also have autonomic symptoms, principally dry mouth, as a consequence of decreased cholinergic transmission at peripheral autonomic synapses.

Table 152-1. Drugs That Should Be Used with Caution in Myasthenia Gravis

Steroids	Antibiotics (*cont.*)	Cardiovascular (*cont.*)
ACTH*	Colistin	Pindolol
Methylprednisolone*	Lincomycin	Lidocaine
Prednisone*	Clindamycin	Dilantin
Anticonvulsants	Tetracycline	Trimethaphan
Dilantin	Oxytetracycline	Local anesthetic
Ethosuximide	Psychotropics	Lidocaine*
Trimethadione	Chlorpromazine*	Procaine*
Paraldehyde	Lithium carbonate*	Narcotics
Magnesium sulfate	Amitriptyline	Morphine
Barbiturates	Droperidol	Dilaudid
Antimalarials	Haloperidol	Codeine
Chloroquine*	Imipramine	Pantopon
Quinine*	Paraldehyde	Meperidine
IV fluids	Trichlorethanol	Endocrine
Na lactate solution	Antirheumatics	Thyroid
Antibiotics	D-Penicillamine	replacement*
Aminoglycosides	Colchicine	Eyedrops
Neomycin*	Chloroquine	Timolol*
Streptomycin*	Neuromuscular blocking	Ecothiopate
Kanamycin*	agents	Others
Gentamicin	Tubocurarine	Amantadine
Tobramycin	Pancuronium	Diphenhydramine
Dihydrostreptomycin*	Gallamine	Emetine
Amikacin	Dimethyltubocurarine	Diuretics
Polymyxin A	Succinylcholine	Muscle relaxants
Polymyxin B	Cardiovascular	CNS depressants
Bacitracin	Quinidine*	Respiratory depressants
Sulfonamides	Procainamide*	Sedatives
Viomycin	β-blockers	Procaine*
	Propranolol	Tranquilizers

* Case reports exist implicating this drug in severe exacerbations of MG.
Source: Adapted from Adams SL, Mathews J, Grammer LC: Drugs that may exacerbate myasthenia gravis. *Ann Emerg Med* 13:532, 1984.

The syndrome is slightly more common in men than women. Approximately 30 to 50 percent of the patients have a malignant neoplasm, more commonly oat-cell carcinoma of the lung. The disease may precede or follow the discovery of the tumor.

On electromyography, the compound muscle action potential evoked by a single nerve stimulus in a resting muscle is abnormally small. Repetitive stimulation at 2 Hz results in a further fall in the amplitude of successive motor responses. Brief exercise of the muscles or stimulation at frequencies higher than 10 Hz for a brief period markedly facilitates the amplitude of the response to normal levels.

There is ample evidence that Lambert-Eaton myasthenic syndrome is an autoimmune disease. This evidence is based, in part, on its responsiveness to corticosteroids, as well as other immunosuppressants and plasmapheresis. Furthermore, nonneoplastic Lambert-Eaton myasthenic syndrome is associated with autoimmune diseases and organ-specific antibodies. The most compelling evidence for an autoimmune cause of both neoplastic and nonneoplastic Lambert-Eaton myasthenic syndrome is the passive transfer of the main electrophysiologic features of the disease from humans to mice.

The most effective treatment of nonneoplastic cases of Lambert-Eaton myasthenic syndrome is combined therapy with prednisone and azathioprine. Acetylcholinesterases have limited effectiveness.

BOTULISM

Botulism is a rare neuroparalytic disease caused by a potent polypeptide toxin elaborated by *Clostridium botulinum*. The disease occurs in three forms: food-borne, wound, and infantile. The food-borne disease is caused by ingesting food containing the toxin that has not been cooked at a high enough heat for long enough to denature the toxin. It is most commonly produced by consumption of improperly canned food. Typically, more than one case of the disease occurs because the contaminated food is usually consumed as part of a common meal shared by several individuals. In infantile botulism, organisms in the gut produce toxin which is systemically absorbed. Wound botulism should be considered in any patient with a wound and/or a chronic history of drug abuse associated with a progressive descending symmetric paralysis. The organisms contaminating the wound produce a toxin that is systemically absorbed.

The clinical manifestations of botulism resemble Lambert-Eaton myasthenic syndrome more than MG because the toxin impairs release of Ach from motor terminals. Symptoms of infantile botulism are poor suck, constipation, listlessness, regurgitation, and generalized weakness. Cranial nerve deficits appear, manifested by a flaccid facial expression, ptosis, and ophthalmoplegia. Adults present with complaints of nausea, vomiting, blurred vision, and dysphagia, which are followed by a descending symmetric muscle weakness and respiratory insufficiency. Impairment of cholinergic function is encountered and may result in constipation, urinary retention, and reduced salivation and lacrimation.

Diagnosis depends on epidemiologic, clinical, and electrophysiologic findings, and may be confirmed by the finding of the toxin and/or organism in the food, stool, or wound. Diminished amplitude of the evoked muscle action potential with facilitation reaching normal amplitude after exercise or repetitive stimuli is a classic electromyographic finding in botulism.

Precipitous respiratory failure is the most serious threat to the patient. Early elective intubation and the use of ventilatory assistance can be lifesaving. Although the effectiveness of antitoxin therapy remains uncertain, its use is recommended. Because most infants are no longer acutely ill when the diagnosis is established, antitoxin is rarely administered. If ileus is profound, nasogastric suction and parenteral nutrition may be necessary. The use of antitoxin, respiratory support, and parenteral nutrition has reduced fatality rates from 60 to 25 percent over the last 30 years. In addition to the above therapies, wound excision is mandatory for wound botulism.

DRUG-INDUCED DISTURBANCES IN NEUROMUSCULAR TRANSMISSION

Drugs resulting in neuromuscular transmission disturbances affect either pre- or postsynaptic mechanisms or both. These drugs, given parenterally or in cathartics, limit the safety margin of neuromuscular transmission (Table 152-1). Such drug-induced disturbances in neuromuscular transmission cause symptoms that resemble those of MG: prominent extraocular muscle weakness and ptosis and variable degrees of facial, bulbar, and generalized muscular weakness. Respiratory paralysis may occur early and be severe. However, overt MG symptoms do not appear unless an overdose of the drug has been administered or hepatic or renal elimination of the drug is impaired. These same drugs may also enhance the activity of neuromuscular blocking agents used during surgical procedures and thereby delay recovery of strength.

Our research has been supported in the past by a generous gift from the Charles Edison Fund, East Orange, New Jersey.

BIBLIOGRAPHY

Adams SL, Matthews J, Grammer LC: Drugs that may exacerbate myasthenia gravis. *Ann Emerg Med* 13:532, 1984.

Arnon SS: Infant botulism. *Annu Review Med* 31:541, 1980.

Dowell VR Jr: Botulism and tetanus. Selected epidemiologic and microbiologic aspects. *Rev Infect Dis* 6(suppl 1):S202, 1984.

Engel AG: Myasthenia gravis and myasthenic syndromes. *Ann Neurol* 16:519, 1984.

Howard JF Jr: Adverse drug effects on neuromuscular transmission. *Semin Neurol* 10:89, 1990.

Keesey JC: Electrodiagnostic approaches to defects of neuromuscular transmission. *Muscle Nerve* 12:613, 1989.

Misulis KE, Feichel GM: Genetic forms of myasthenia gravis. *Pediatr Neurol* 5:205, 1989

Moore DR: Imaging in myasthenia gravis. *Clin Radiol* 40:115, 1989.

Newsome-Davis J, Murray NMF: Plasma exchange and immunosuppressive drug treatment in Lambert-Eaton myasthenia gravis. *Neurology* 34:480, 1984.

Phillips LH II, Melnick PA: Diagnosis of myasthenia gravis in the 1990's. *Semin Neurol* 10:62, 1990.

Seybold ME: The office Tensilon test for ocular myasthenia gravis. *Arch Neurol* 43:842, 1986.

Swift TR: Disorders of neuromuscular transmission other than myasthenia gravis. *Muscle Nerve* 4:334, 1981.

153
MENINGITIS, ENCEPHALITIS, AND BRAIN ABSCESS

Charles Rennie III

MENINGITIS

The symptom complex of meningitis spans a wide spectrum, which ranges from the mild manifestations of some of the viral meningitides to the fulminant course of some of the bacterial variants. Astute recognition of symptoms and aggressive management are keys to limiting morbidity and mortality. The mortality of untreated bacterial meningitis exceeds 90 percent; with early appropriate therapy it can be brought down to 10 to 20 percent. Sequelae, too, are significant (up to 70 percent in patients with bacterial meningitis) but also can be decreased with prompt therapy.

The primary etiologies of meningitis in the United States are bacterial and viral (with approximately 5000 cases per year being reported to the Centers for Disease Control but the actual number being substantially higher). Less common etiologies include fungal, chemical, and neoplastic mechanisms. As a result of increasing numbers of patients with acquired immunodeficiency syndrome, however, fungal etiologies are becoming more common and once-rare forms of bacterial and viral meningitis are also increasing dramatically in frequency.

Clinical Presentation

Both viral and bacterial meningitis may present either acutely (symptoms for less than 24 h) or subacutely (symptoms for 1 to 7 days). While bacterial meningitis more often presents acutely (25 percent versus 5 percent for viral), this cannot be used to distinguish the two etiologies. One should suspect meningitis in any patient with an altered level of consciousness, unexplained personality changes, unexplained seizures, severe unexplained headache, neck stiffness, unexplained fever, or new-onset focal neurological deficits. These symptoms tend to occur more commonly with bacterial meningitis (see Table 153-1). Approximately 80 to 90 percent of patients with bacterial meningitis will have some alteration in level of consciousness, as opposed to only 25 to 50 percent of patients with viral meningitis. Seizures occur in approximately 30 percent of patients with bacterial and approximately 5 percent of patients with viral meningitis. Focal neurological deficits occur in up to 50 percent of patients with bacterial (30 percent cranial, 20 percent peripheral) but in less than 10 percent with viral meningitis. Headache, meningeal irritation, and fever are the most frequent concomitants. Headache is usually a prominent symptom in both forms, although its absence does not exclude the diagnosis. Meningeal irritation is slightly more common in bacterial than in viral meningitis (80 percent versus 60 to 70 percent) but again is common in both. Both forms usually present with fever, but that of the bacterial infection tends to be higher [approximately 80 percent over 38.9°C (102°F) versus 30 to 40 percent for the viral infection].

No group of symptoms is classic; many variations can occur. As with many other diseases, the very young and the elderly may present atypically and with considerably fewer symptoms. The very young patient may present with symptoms as ill-defined as irritability and poor feeding, with or without projectile vomiting. The elderly patient may present with nothing more than lethargy.

If the presentation is acute, the initial physical examination should be rapid, include a neurological evaluation and identification of drug allergies, and be directed toward initiating therapy within the first 30 min. Here, the focus is toward determining the presence of papilledema and/or a focal neurological deficit, either of which would be an indication for an emergency computed tomographic (CT) scan prior to a lumbar puncture (LP). If neither of the above contraindications is present, an LP should be performed and antibiotics initiated empirically based upon age and host factors. If meningitis is clinically suspected, and a CT scan is required prior to lumbar puncture, antibiotics should be administered before the CT scan. Treatment should not be withheld during diagnostic procedures.

The complete physical examination, even though interrupted to begin therapy, should be thorough. Key aspects include not only those mentioned above but evidence of nuchal rigidity, Brudzinski's sign (flexion of hips and knees produced by passive neck flexion), and Kernig's sign (pain on passive extension of the knee past 120° with the hips flexed). A thorough neurological examination, including mental status, cranial nerve, and peripheral sensory and motor examinations, must be performed. In infants the fontanelles must be palpated. A search for possible sources of infection, including skin, ears, sinuses, posterior oropharynx, genitourinary tract, and chest is likewise important, since it may influence the choice of antibiotics. The presence of a rash also should be noted.

It is not uncommon for patients with viral meningitis (especially that due to the enteroviruses) to have a concomitant maculopapular eruption. A petechial, purpuric, or ecchymotic rash suggests meningococcemia, although petechial reactions may also be produced by *Streptococcus pneumoniae, Haemophilus influenzae,* or *Staphylococcus aureus.*

Diagnosis

Lumbar Puncture

Although laboratory studies are useful, the most critical test is a detailed examination of the cerebrospinal fluid (CSF) obtained from a lumbar puncture. In adults, four tubes totaling 12 to 15 mL are usually withdrawn. A number of important considerations are involved in the LP and the examination of the CSF. These are detailed below and in Table 153-2.

Opening Pressure

The normal opening pressure (OP) is 150 ± 33 mmH_2O, with 95 percent between 94 and 216. It tends to be higher in patients with

Table 153-1. Clinical Findings in Meningitis

	Bacterial	Viral
Acute presentation (symptoms <24 h)	25%	5%
Headache	Prominent	Prominent
Meningeal signs	80%	60–70%
Fever	Common: 80% >38.9°C (102°F)	Common: 30–40% >38.9°C (102°F)
Alteration in mental status	80–90%	25–50%
Seizures	30%	5%
Focal neurological deficits	50%	<10%

Table 153-2. CSF Findings in Bacterial and Nonbacterial Meningitis

Parameter	Normal	Bacterial	Viral
Opening pressure (mmH_2O)	150 ± 33	Mean 307	Normal to sl ↑
Protein (mg/dL)	39 ± 10	>150	<100
CSF/serum glucose ratio	0.6 (infants 0.81)	<0.4	0.6
Cell count (cells/mm^3)	<3 (mononuclear)	>500 (PMNs predominate)	<100 (mononuclear leukocytes predominate)
Gram stain	No organisms	Positive 70–90%	No organisms

bacterial meningitis (the mean was 307 mmH_2O and the range 50 to 600 mmH_2O in one series of 106 patients), although papilledema is rare. Of patients with elevated pressures, one-third return to normal within 48 h and another third within 6 days. If papilledema or focal neurological deficits are present, antibiotics should be given empirically, and an emergency head CT scan should be done before lumbar puncture. If papilledema is absent but the OP is markedly elevated, the examiner can take a small amount of fluid, withdraw the needle (the damage has probably already been done), and initiate measures to decrease intracranial pressure (intubation, hyperventilation, mannitol).

Tentorial herniation may be manifested by fixed, dilated pupils, decerebrate or decorticate posturing, Cheyne-Stokes respirations, or cranial nerve deficits. Should this occur at any point during the LP, immediate measures must be taken to lower intracranial pressure.

Protein

Normal CSF protein is 38 ± 10 mg/dL (95 percent between 18 and 58). In viral meningitis protein is usually less than 100; in bacterial meningitis it is usually greater than 150, although there is considerable overlap. Protein also may be elevated in acute chemical meningitis. Normal values are somewhat higher (mean 90 mg/dL) in infants less than 6 months old owing to the immaturity of the bloodbrain barrier. If blood is present in the CSF (traumatic LP or subarachnoid hemorrhage), the protein level may be elevated by 1 mg/dL for each 1000 red blood cells (RBCs). Several medications, including ethanol and phenytoin, may increase CSF protein. Protein and glucose determinations are generally made on the second tube of CSF.

Glucose

The normal steady-state CSF/serum glucose ratio is approximately 0.6. Both the entry and exit of glucose into and out of the CSF is determined by carrier-mediated diffusion. Infants less than 6 months of age have a mean ratio of 0.81, which is due to immaturity of this carrier system. If the serum glucose level changes abruptly, approximately 2 to 4 h is required for the CSF glucose level to equilibrate. Because of the saturation kinetics of the carrier exchange, the ratio decreases at higher serum glucose levels; at a serum glucose level of 700 mg/dL the ratio is about 0.4. Glucose levels are generally normal in aseptic meningitis, viral encephalitis, brain abscesses, and subdural empyemas. They are often less than 40 in bacterial, fungal, and tubercular meningitis. Late in these entities, the glucose level may be profoundly depressed (less than 20). Hypoglycorrhachia is also seen in 15 to 20 percent of patients with subarachnoid hemorrhages, a low being reached 1 to 8 days posthemorrhage. The mechanism for this is unclear.

Cell Count

The normal cell count in the adult CSF is 0 to 5 mononucleated cells per cubic millimeter. In neonates it ranges up to 30 cells per cubic millimeter [60 percent polymorphonuclear leukocytes (PMNs) and 40 percent mononuclear cells]. In a traumatic tap or after a subarachnoid hemorrhage, one white blood cell (WBC) may be subtracted from the total WBC count in the CSF for each 1000 RBCs present. Classically, bacterial meningitis patients have more than 500 WBCs per cubic millimeter, with a preponderance of PMNs, while patients with viral meningitis have fewer than 100 WBCs per cubic millimeter, with mononuclear leukocytes predominant; unfortunately, presentations often do not fit this picture. About 10 percent of patients with bacterial meningitis will have less than 50 percent PMNs, while 10 percent of patients with viral meningitis will have more than 90 percent PMNs and 30 to 40 percent will have more than 50 percent PMNs. The initial LP examination in patients with viral meningitis may show a majority of PMNs, but within 12 h approximately 90 percent of these patients will show a mononuclear leukocyte-predominant pleocytosis. One may see very low cell counts early in the course of meningitis, particularly with that caused by *Neisseria* or *H. influenzae* but also with overwhelming pneumococcal meningitis. In general, PMNs predominate not only in bacterial meningitis but also in subdural empyemas, ruptured brain abscesses, and chemical meningitis. Viral meningitis, tubercular meningitis, parameningeal osteomyelitis, collagen-vascular disease with CNS manifestations, syphilitic menigitis, viral encephalitis, meningeal neoplasms (and carcinomatosis), and cryptococcal and other fungal meningitides generally show a predominance of mononuclear leukocytes.

If RBCs are seen in the CSF, the most likely cause is either a traumatic LP or a subarachnoid hemorrhage. Cell counts should be done on the first and fourth tubes; approximately equal counts are strongly suggestive of hemorrhage.

On occasion the supernatant liquid of centrifuged CSF may be xanthochromic (a characteristic pink or yellow color). This is due to one of three pigments—oxyhemoglobin, bilirubin, or methemoglobin—which result from the breakdown of RBCs. Therefore, fresh CSF from a traumatic tap should not be xanthochromic. Oxyhemoglobin, which is pink and results from RBC lysis, appears within 4 h of hemorrhage and resolves after 8 to 10 days. Methemoglobin is brownish yellow and results from blood encapsulated in a subdural or intracerebral hematoma. Bilirubin is derived from both RBC lysis and hyperbilirubinemia. In the former it appears at about 10 h and resolves after 2 to 4 weeks. In premature infants xanthochromia due to bilirubin is normal and represents only immaturity of the blood-brain barrier. Xanthochromia may also be caused by hypercarotenemia or markedly elevated CSF protein (>150 mg/dL).

Search for Organisms

The first test to be performed in a search for organisms is the Gram stain of the centrifuged specimen (generally from the third tube of CSF taken). This should generally yield organisms in 70 to 90 percent of cases (87 percent as shown in one large series of meningitides caused by common bacterial pathogens—*H. influenzae,* meningococci, and pneumococci). The yield is somewhat lower (50 percent) for gram-negative enteric pathogens and lower still (30 percent) for *Listeria.* False-negative results may also occur when the bacterial count in the CSF is less than 1000 per cubic millimeter. With select bacteria such as *H. influenzae* and *S. pneumoniae,* organisms can be identified via a Neufeld's reaction test with specific antisera that yield capsular swelling reactions.

If appropriate, an acid-fast stain also should be performed to search for mycobacteria. Specimens to be examined for the possible presence of fungi should be centrifuged and the sediment examined in India ink and/or 10 percent potassium hydroxide. However, several recent papers, most notably that of McGinnis, detail the low yield of this procedure; *Cryptococcus neoformans,* the most common of the fungal isolates, was detected on the first LP in only 26.3 percent of 19 patients ultimately demonstrated to have cryptococcal meningitis. Repeat LPs raised this figure to only about 50 percent. Some recent papers emphasize the need for culturing large volumes of CSF (at least 5 mL), and there are numerous case reports of fungi being recovered only after 15- to 30-mL samples were cultured. These papers downplay the importance of "wasting" CSF on centrifugation and India ink stain.

Aerobic cultures should be sent routinely to the laboratory. Martin recommends using two blood agar plates, a chocolate agar plate, and a tube of tryptic soy broth. Anaerobic cultures need not be sent routinely (anaerobic isolates from positive CSF cultures run less than 10 percent) but should be sent in cases of antecedent trauma; previous CNS surgeries such as shunts, craniotomies, and laminectomies; head and/or neck infection or neoplasm; or concomitant or antecedent anaerobic infections or sepsis elsewhere in the body. Aerobic cultures should be held for 4 days before being discarded as negative; if the patient was on antibiotics before the cultures were made, they should be held for 1 week. If any suspicion of bacterial meningitis exists, multiple blood cultures and cultures of any underlying foci of infection should be obtained.

Over the past decade a number of additional diagnostic modalities have been proposed and utilized with varying success. CSF lactate levels have been utilized as a diagnostic adjunct but pose two problems. First, although CSF lactate is elevated to ≥35 mg/dL in 90 to 95 percent of cases of confirmed bacterial meningitis, it is also elevated in 20 to 30 percent of patients with presumed viral meningitis. Second, there is a high rate of false positives: craniotomies, CNS ischemia and/or anoxia, subarachnoid hemorrhages, intracranial neoplasms, and even closed-head injury can all elevate CSF lactates.

Countercurrent immunoelectrophoresis (CIE), formerly the most widely used of the newer diagnostic modalities, has been superseded in popularity by the more rapidly performed and more sensitive latex agglutination. Both cover the same bacteria (*H. influenzae* group B, *S. pneumoniae,* and *N. meningitidis* groups A and C). Although false positives are rare with CIE, false negatives are generally more frequent than with latex agglutination.

Latex agglutination has approximately 90 percent sensitivity in detecting *H. influenzae* group B and 60 to 80 percent sensitivity in detecting *S. pneumoniae and N. meningitidis* groups A and C. No tests exist for *N. meningitidis* group B. In general, this technique is more rapid and more sensitive than CIE. It is useful in early or partially treated meningitis, where a Gram stain may be negative, and in confirming the results of a Gram stain in select bacterial meningitides.

Enzyme immunoassays also have been attempted with several bacteria. Although highly sensitive and requiring only dilute antisera, they are somewhat cumbersome and require 3 to 6 h to complete.

C-reactive protein (CRP) determinations, recently introduced, also show a fairly high accuracy in differentiating bacterial from viral meningitis.

Treatment

Acute bacterial meningitis is a severe disease with a fulminant course and a significant mortality. For patients with acute presentations antibiotics should be instituted within 30 min. If the patient exhibits focal neurological deficits or papilledema, antibiotics should be initiated immediately according to age and host defense status (see below) and the patient should receive an emergency CT scan prior to LP. If the patient shows neither focal deficits nor papilledema, an LP should be performed and the patient started immediately on antibiotics appropriate for age and host defense status *without waiting for the Gram stain.* Antibiotics can be changed later according to the results of the Gram stain and culture.

Subacute presentations allow for a slightly greater workup before initiating therapy. Here, therapy should be instituted within 2 h of presentation, which allows time to evaluate the Gram stain.

In initiating empirical therapy in patients with suspected bacterial meningitis, it is important to know which organisms predominate in which types of patient (Table 153-3).

Of those adults who are eventually diagnosed as having *S. pneumoniae* meningitis, 30 percent give a history of otitis or mastoiditis and 25 percent give a history of antecedent pneumonia. Other host factors are likewise (but by no means in all circumstances) linked with certain organisms. Alcoholics are prone to *S. pneumoniae* and *Listeria monocytogenes.* Patients with CNS shunts tend to develop staphylococcal infections. Patients with splenic dysfunction are prone to *S. pneumoniae* and *H. influenzae* infections. Staphylococci, *S. pneumoniae,* and gram-negative rods predominate in patients with recent craniotomies. Hospital-acquired meningitis is often secondary to infection with gram-negative rods. Elderly patients have an increased incidence of gram-negative meningitis.

In the emergency department, initial antibiotic treatment for meningitis must be selected without knowledge of the causative organism. The Gram stain (if available when treatment is initiated) may be used to help direct therapy but should not be relied upon exclusively. Patient age, host factors, and immune status should also be considered in selecting appropriate initial therapy.

Table 153-3. Common Etiologies of Bacterial Meningitis in Adults

Host Factors	Organism
Adult	*N. meningitidis*
	S. pneumoniae
	Group A streptococci
Alcoholics	*S. pneumoniae*
	L. monocytogenes
	H. influenzae
	Gram-negative rods
CNS shunt	*S. aureus*
Splenic dysfunction	*S. pneumoniae*
	H. influenzae
Recent craniotomy	Staphylococci
	S. pneumoniae
	Gram-negative rods

Recommended antibiotic regimens for suspected bacterial meningitis vary among authors, but in general there is broad agreement. In infants under 2 months of age (group B streptococci, gram-negative rods), either ampicillin and gentamicin or ampicillin and a third-generation cephalosporin are the drugs of choice. From age 2 months until approximately 15 years (*H. influenzae, S. pneumoniae, N. meningitidis*), either ampicillin and chloramphenicol or a third-generation cephalosporin is appropriate. For patients between 15 and 60 years of age with no special host factors, penicillin G remains the agent of choice. In patients over 60 years of age, gram-negative organisms again become a consideration, and appropriate therapy is either ampicillin and gentamicin or ampicillin and a third-generation cephalosporin. Both immunocompromised patients and patients at particular risk for staphylococcal infections should be covered with a penicillinase-resistant penicillin. Antibiotics should subsequently be titrated to culture results.

For the patient with a history of an anaphylactic reaction to penicillin, alternatives are vancomycin, for suspected gram-positive organisms, and chloroamphenicol, for broader gram-positive and gram-negative coverage.

Of the antibiotics above, only third-generation cephalosporins penetrate the blood-brain barrier well. Penicillins penetrate the normal blood-brain barrier poorly, but their penetration is increased under conditions of inflammation. Aminoglycosides penetrate poorly under any condition, but they are in part redeemed by their small mean inhibitory concentrations. Although third-generation cephalosporins penetrate well, first- and second-generation cephalosporins penetrate poorly.

Initial enthusiasm over the use of third-generation cephalosporins was based on limited data. Increased experience has borne out this enthusiasm. Cefotaxime has demonstrated effectiveness against pneumococci, meningococci, *H. influenzae,* group B streptocci, *E. coli,* and *Klebsiella;* it is not, however effective against *Pseudomonas aeruginosa,* enterococci, or *Listeria.* None of the third-generation cephalosporins are effective against enterococci or *Listeria.* Only ceftazidime appears to be effective against *Pseudomonas aeruginosa,* but its record against pneumococci is spotty.

Other Considerations

A number of difficult questions face the emergency physician in treating the meningitis patient. What if the LP is normal? Could the patient still have meningitis? The answer is yes, although such cases are rare. All such patients have shown clinical signs strongly suggestive of meningitis. A repeat LP in 8 to 36 h will generally show infection. Patients in whom the diagnosis is suspected should be admitted and observed and/or treated. A repeat LP should be performed in 8 to 12 h. If suspicion is high, antibiotic therapy should be initiated empirically prior to the second LP.

When is a repeat LP indicated? Several circumstances (other than that cited above) dictate a repeat LP: (1) a lapse of 24 to 48 h after initiating antibiotic therapy, at which time the culture and Gram stain should be negative, (2) an initial LP in suspected viral meningitis (untreated) that shows a predominance of PMN leukocytes (90 percent will show lymphocyte predominance within 12 h), and (3) failure of any meningitis patient to improve or doubtfulness of the diagnosis.

What about patients who have received prior antibiotics (up to 50 percent in some series)? This has little effect on the overall WBC count but may decrease the number of PMNs to the "aseptic" meningitis range. The yield for the Gram stain and culture will decrease by 10 to 20 percent and that for blood cultures will decrease by 50 percent.

Under what circumstances can patients with presumed viral meningitis be sent home from the emergency department? The diagnosis of viral meningitis is usually made from both the LP and the clinical setting; generally the LP is typical and the patients are often young, present particularly in the early fall, and may have associated viral symptoms. Unfortunately, the symptoms overlap the clinical picture of bacterial meningitis, and 10 percent of patients with viral meningitis progress to severe symptoms. Only the most reliable of patients with clear-cut symptomatology should be managed as outpatients, and even these should be followed closely. If even slight doubt exists as to the diagnosis, the patient should be admitted and observed.

Finally, what should be done for those patients when it is necessary to transfer them to another facility? Any patients who show evidence of increased intracranial pressure or focal neurological deficits should not be transferred. Those who are transferred should have an LP performed and CSF and other appropriate cultures taken and should be started on antibiotics. Cultures should either be sent with the patient (if practical) or incubated at the transferring institution. At least one spare tube of CSF should be sent with the patient.

Summary

Meningitis represents a potentially high-morbidity, high-mortality group of diseases which challenges the emergency physician to provide rapid diagnosis and effective therapy. Patients who present with acute, fulminant symptoms should have antibiotics initiated within 30 min and prior to the LP; the choice and dosage of antibiotics should be determined by age and host factors and will require later adjustment based on CSF findings. Patients with more indolent symptoms should have antibiotics initiated within 2 h, which allows time for CSF examination prior to initiating therapy. Patients with neurological deficits or elevated intracranial pressure should receive an immediate CT scan after antibiotics are initiated empirically and before LP. No constellation of signs or symptoms is pathognomonic of either bacterial or viral meningitis; indeed, the symptoms overlap enormously. Perhaps the greatest aid in differentiating the forms of meningitis lies in thorough examination of the CSF. Newer laboratory methods hold promise for improving identification of specific bacterial agents.

ENCEPHALITIS

Like meningitis, encephalitis encompasses a wide spectrum of symptoms. Common to all, however, is some involvement of the cerebrum, cerebellum, or brain stem in the infectious process. Significant overlap exists with the symptoms of bacterial meningitis.

Encephalitis may be caused by a number of organisms, including viruses such as herpes simplex (HSV), arboviruses such as eastern equine encephalitis virus (EEE), Western equine encephalitis virus (WEG), St. Louis encephalitis virus and California encephalitis virus, *Mycolasma, Toxoplasma, Coccidioides, Cryptococcus, Treponema pallidum, Borrelia burgdorferi, Naegleria,* and *Mycobacterium.* The site of effect may vary widely; for instance, rickettsiae show a predilection for vascular endothelium (with ensuing vasculitis), while HSV tends to affect the medial tempoıal and orbital frontal lobes. Approximately 2000 cases of encephalitis are reported in the United States annually.

Clinical Presentation

The clinical presentation of encephalitis overlaps that of meningitis. An alteration in level of consciousness is invariably present, and may range from mild lethargy to stupor and focal neurological signs. Seizures are common, and ataxic gait disturbances may be seen. A large percentage of patients with bacterial meningitis will also have some alteration in level of consciousness, with a 30 percent incidence of seizures and a 30 percent incidence of focal neurological deficits. Encephalitis can rarely present with gross derangement of the hypothalamopituitary axis and symptoms such as hypothermia or inappropriate antidiuretic hormone secretion. Time course of symptoms is of little use in differentiating the two entities. Systemic exanthems (such as viral exanthems or those of Lyme disease) may be helpful but are rarely definitive. Because differentiation from acute bacterial meningitis is extremely difficult, presumptive therapy should be initiated as for bacterial meningitis prior to completion of workup.

Laboratory Studies

Laboratory studies are directed to identify metabolic or toxic encephalopathies. A CT scan is imperative but should not delay treatment. As with meningitis, CSF examination is also critical, where no contraindication to lumbar puncture exists. CSF protein is usually elevated, although glucose is normal. Depressed glucose levels should raise the index of suspicion for tubercular or other bacterial infections. A CSF pleocytosis is generally present, with mononucleated cells predominating. Approximately 90 percent will show cell counts of $<500/mm^3$. Significant red blood cell counts are found with HSV and *Naegleria.* Gram stain and culture should be done and acid-fast bacillus stain and India ink preparations should be performed where indicated. Blood should be drawn acutely for antibody levels if definitive diagnosis is to be pursued, as well as at intervals throughout the course of the disease. Brain biopsy was formerly recommended to exclude HSV (the only treatable viral pathogen) but has fallen into disfavor due to the morbidity of the procedure and the relatively low toxicity of acyclovir.

Treatment

If bacterial meningitis is in the initial differential diagnosis, immediate treatment should be initiated as outlined in the discussion of meningitis. Treatment for other causes of encephalitis is dictated by the etiology: bacterial, fungal, protozoal, toxic, and endocrine-metabolic. Of these only the toxic and endocrine-metabolic types are readily amenable to diagnosis and initiation of therapy in the emergency department. Treatment of viral encephalitis is supportive with the exception of HSV, which is treated with acyclovir.

BRAIN ABSCESS

Brain abscess represents another entity whose clinical presentation significantly overlaps that of meningitis. Etiologies include (1) direct extension of contiguous infection, (2) open CNS trauma, (3) hematogenous spread, and (4) idiopathic. The first etiology is the most common, with otic, nasal, and paranasal sources predominating. Otic etiologies have dropped significantly in developed countries over the past 20 years.

In the past, staphylococci and streptococci were believed to be the most common etiologic agents. Recent attention to proper anaerobic culture technique, however, has demonstrated that anaerobes, particularly anaerobic streptococci, *Bacteroides,* and *Fusobacterium,* play a major role.

Symptoms of brain abscess reflect more the space-occupying nature of the disease than the infectious aspect. Headache (75 percent) predominates, with over 50 percent of patients showing focal neurologic deficits and 30 percent presenting with seizures. Fever (50 percent) is less common than in meningitis. Duration of symptoms varies widely, but tends to be somewhat longer than in meningitis.

The study of choice is CT scan if brain abscess is suspected. Lumbar puncture is contraindicated, and has been associated with a deleterious outcome in multiple series. Few studies examine penetration of antibiotics into or efficacy of antibiotics in brain abscesses. Penicillin remains the standard of treatment, in combination with either chloramphenicol or metronidazole. The drawbacks of chloramphenicol include bacteriostatic action and evidence for degradation in other types of abscesses. Metronidazole has high abscess concentration and there is some evidence for decreased mortality with its use, but it may have CNS side effects. Prompt neurosurgical consultation is imperative.

BIBLIOGRAPHY

Bolan G, Barza M: Acute bacterial meningitis in children and adults. *Med Clin North Am* 69:231, 1988.

Chun CH, Johnson JD, Hafstetter M, et al: Brain abscesses: A study of 45 consecutive cases. *Medicine* 65:415, 1986.

Cherubin C, Eng R: Experience with the use of cefotaxime in the treatment of bacterial meningitis. *Am J Med* 80:398, 1986.

Feigin RD, Shakelford PG: Value of repeat lumbar puncture in the differential diagnosis of meningitis. *N Engl J Med* 289:571, 1973

Gorse GJ, Thrupp LD, Nudleman KL, et al: Bacterial meningitis in the elderly. *Arch Intern Med* 144:1603, 1984.

Martin WJ: Rapid and reliable techniques for the laboratory detection of bacterial meningitis. *Am J Med Infect Dis Symp* 76:119, 1983.

Marton KI, Gean AD: The spinal tap: A new look at an old test. *Ann Intern Med* 104:840, 1986.

McGinnis MP: Detection of fungi in cerebrospinal fluid. *Am J Med Infect Dis Symp* 76:129, 1983.

Rubin RH, Hooper DC: Central nervous system infection in the compromised host. *Med Clin North Am* 69:281, 1985.

Sippel JG, Hider PA, Controni G, et al: Use of the Directigen latex agglutination test for detection of *Haemophilus influenzae, Streptococcus pneumoniae, and Neisseria meningitidis* antigens in cerebrospinal fluid from meningitis patients. *J Clin Microbiol* 20:884, 1984.

SECTION 15
Eye, Ear, Nose, Throat, and Oral Surgery

154
OCULAR EMERGENCIES

Roland Clark

Prompt recognition and management of ocular emergencies is mandatory for the preservation of visual function. Nonmedical staff should be trained to bring the following actual and potential ocular emergencies to the immediate attention of the clinical staff:

1. Sudden visual loss
2. Severe eye pain
3. Chemical eye injury
4. Any severe blunt or penetrating eye injury

Emergency physicians should be prepared to initiate early management. Many cases may be managed definitively in the emergency department. Firm referral patterns with the ophthalmology staff should be established so that emergency consultation will be available rapidly when necessary.

EYE EXAMINATION

History

In the acute situation, history taking is simultaneous with treatment. In any event, a history relative to the presenting complaint should be recorded. A past history of ocular problems and congenital ocular defects should be identified. In cases in which an intraocular foreign body may be present, a close inquiry should be made into the history of activities involving striking metal on metal.

Physical Examination

A determination of the best corrected visual acuity is the first step in any eye examination. If eyeglasses are normally worn, then the test should be conducted with eyeglasses in place. This examination should be performed prior to any other procedures. If the eyeglasses are not available, a pinhole occluder may be used to approximate the lens correction. While a Snellen eye chart is preferable, any printed material will do for testing as long as the examiner notes the testing material (i.e., newsprint, headlines, etc.).

Occasionally a patient with severe visual deficit may be unable to read any printed material. In this case, the patient may be able to count fingers or perceive hand motion, or may only be able to perceive light. This should be recorded.

Examination of the cornea should be done with magnification, and the slit lamp is the preferred examining instrument. Following initial examination of the eye, a small quantity of fluorescein may be instilled into the eye and the area then examined with cobalt blue filtered light. Areas of damaged epithelium will stain a brilliant yellow-green, whereas fluorescein is ordinarily orange. Fluorescein-coated strips of paper should be used rather than fluorescein solution, since the solution is an excellent culture medium for *Pseudomonas aeruginosa*.

The lids, cornea, anterior chamber, iris, and lens should be examined with the penlight. At the same time the direct and consensual pupillary response to light should be tested. The extraocular movements should be tested in the six cardinal positions of gaze, and any nystagmus noted. Next, the disk, vessels, peripheral retina, and vitreous should be examined with a direct ophthalmoscope. The vitreous is evaluated by setting the ophthalmoscope lens wheel at approximately + 10. This brings the point of focus forward from the retina toward the lens and thus brings objects in the vitreous body into focus.

The optic disk should be examined to see that the outline is crisp and clear. The central optic cup normally accounts for less than one-third of the total diameter of the disk. To obtain a good view of the peripheral retina, it is necessary to dilate the pupil. Paradrine or 2.5% phenylephrine (Neo-Synephrine) are best for this in the emergency setting. Prior to instilling a mydriatic, the examiner should be certain that serial evaluation of pupillary function is not necessary for following a brain-injured patient.

The retinal venules are somewhat larger than the arterioles, the normal ratio being about 3:2. The examiner should be alert for either marked dilation of the veins or narrowing of the arterioles.

Visual fields should be evaluated when there is suspicion that a field defect may be present. Optic neuritis, branch retinal arterial occlusion, retinal detachment, and open-angle glaucoma all have associated visual field defects. Confrontation examination offers a simple screening test which will give an estimate of the visual fields and detect larger field defects. Patient and examiner are seated opposite one another approximately 1 m apart. To test the right eye, the patient's left eye and examiner's right eye are occluded. The patient is instructed to look directly at the examiner's pupil. The examiner extends one or two fingers in each visual field, the patient is instructed to indicate when the correct number of fingers can be identified, as field defects are noted.

Intraocular pressure should be measured if glaucoma is suspected. The technique for using the Shiötz tonometer, which is inexpensive and readily available, is easily learned. The instructions enclosed with the tonometer should be followed carefully. The conversion table is used to translate the scale readings on the tonometer to millimeters of mercury. With the 5.5-g weight in place, a scale reading of 4 or more is equal to about 20 mmHg or less (i.e., normal). The scale readings are inversely related to the pressure; i.e., low scale readings indicate high pressure and high scale readings indicate low pressure.

Three other devices are commonly used to measure intraocular pressure: the Goldman applanation tonometer; the air-puff tonometer; and the Tono-Pen, a small hand-held device.

The Goldman applanation tonometer is extremely accurate and is the standard by which other tonometers are measured. It is mounted on the slit lamp and intraocular pressures read directly from the device. However, the applanation tonometer is quite expensive, and accurate use requires considerable skill and practice.

Like the applanation tonometer, the Tono-Pen requires actual contact with the eye. It is light in weight, easily mastered, and provides a direct digital reading of intraocular pressure.

The air-puff tonometer is also easily mastered and enjoys the advantage of requiring no direct contact with the eye.

COMMON PRESENTING SYMPTOMS

Redness

Conjunctivitis

Bacterial Conjunctivitis

The most common presenting symptoms of bacterial conjunctivitis are redness and subjective sensation of multiple fine granular foreign bodies (''grittiness''). Bacterial conjunctivitis is rarely painful. It is characterized by a mucopurulent discharge of the lids and lashes which may be profuse enough to mat the lids together. Visual acuity is rarely affected. Pupillary reaction and funduscopic examination are unremarkable. Determination of the intraocular pressure should be deferred until the infection has been cleared.

Staphylococcal Allergic Conjunctivitis

This is a special case of bacterial conjunctivitis. It is characterized by small white ulcers at the limbus (staphylococcal marginal ulcers). It is postulated that the disorder is due to an allergy to the staphylococcal toxin.

Treatment with topical 10% sulfacetamide drops or ointment is ordinarily effective for most cases of bacterial conjunctivitis. Ointment should not be prescribed for adults because it blurs vision. Drops should be instilled every 2 h while the patient is awake. Clearing can be expected in 3 to 5 days. For more serious infections, tobramycin (Tobrex) is indicated. For serious infections which require a broad spectrum of coverage, erythromycin tid and tobramycin every 2 h is very effective. In the case of staphylococcal allergic conjunctivitis, a dilute corticosteroid is often added to abbreviate the treatment program. In any event, 3 to 5 days of treatment are usually sufficient. Patching should be avoided.

Viral Conjunctivitis

Redness and subjective symptoms of itching and irritation usually fail to distinguish bacterial from viral conjunctivitis. Viral conjunctivitis is most frequently bilateral, while bacterial conjunctivitis may be unilateral. Moreover, the discharge of viral conjunctivitis is often watery, while that of bacterial conjunctivitis is purulent. However, it is often difficult, if not impossible, to distinguish between the two on the basis of symptoms or clinical appearance alone. As a practical matter then, most conjunctivitis is treated with a topical antibiotic. The risks are few and the rewards may be great. Combination antibiotics are frequently used. One common formulation combines neomycin, polymyxin, and bacitracin. While the use of this combination is not contraindicated, the physician should recognize that neomycin may produce a hypersensitivity dermatitis in as many as 15 percent of patients.

Ordinarily the nonophthalmologist need not make a great effort to distinguish between the various kinds of viral conjunctivitis, although one should recognize that the adenoviruses are common offenders. However, there are certain viral entities that should be recognized clinically. They include the following.

Herpes Zoster Conjunctivitis

This conjunctivitis frequently has its onset as a typical viral conjunctivitis. Since this organism is the same one that causes common shingles, the condition is presumed to be an infection of the nerve root. Consequently, it is almost always uniocular. This infection usually originates from a dermatitis in the distribution of the fifth cranial nerve, which leads to an extensive dermatitis very similar to shingles. Occasionally the cornea alone is involved. The nasociliary nerve supplies both the tip of the nose and the cornea. Thus, if the tip of the nose is involved the cornea will probably also be involved. With ocular involvement there is often a keratitis (inflammation and disruption of the cornea) and anterior uveitis (inflammation of the anterior segment of the eye). The keratitis can lead to catastrophic loss of vision. No specific therapy is truly effective, but large doses of topical and systemic steroids may be helpful for eye involvement. Therapy with some of the newer antiviral agents has shown promising results.

Epidemic Keratoconjunctivitis

Epidemic keratoconjunctivitis is a highly contagious eye infection caused by an adenovirus (type 8). It is characterized by a diffuse conjunctivitis which produces marked discomfort. Tender ipsilateral preauricular lymph nodes appear a few days after the onset of symptoms. Approximately 1 week after the onset of symptoms a keratitis appears which is characterized by widely scattered subepithelial infiltrates. Epidemics are frequently traced to contaminated medical instruments. No specific therapy is indicated, but topical antibiotics may prevent secondary infection.

Allergic Conjunctivitis

Pollens, high smog levels, and other environmental hazards frequently cause or aggravate allergic conjunctivitis. Vernal conjunctivitis, which usually occurs in the spring or fall, is a typical form of this problem. It is characterized by huge cobblestone papillae under the upper lid, itching, and tearing. A contact (allergic) conjunctivitis frequently occurs in postoperative cataract patients and other patients using eye drops. Common offenders are neomycin and atropine.

One particular subset of allergic conjunctivitis is due to reaction to insect protein. In the summer months it is common for small gnats and other flying insects to lodge as conjunctival foreign bodies. The reaction to them is frequently dramatic. Chemosis (swelling of the bulbar conjunctiva) may assume alarming proportions. The upper and lower lids may also swell dramatically. The conjunctiva is usually pale rather than red, and the eye may be very pruritic. The presentation is usually uniocular.

Treatment of allergic conjunctivitis consists of topical antihistamines, vasoconstrictors, and dilute corticosteroids when indicated. Combinations of antihistamines and decongestants are particularly helpful. If no treatment is administered, the problem will usually resolve spontaneously in 24 to 48 h. Removal of the allergen, as in the case of an insect foreign body, is essential.

Chemical Conjunctivitis

Alkali Burns

A burn produced by sodium hydroxide (lye) or other alkali is one of the few absolute ocular emergencies. The eye should be irrigated immediately at the scene with tap water for 15 to 20 min. Telephone questions to the emergency department regarding chemical burns of the eye should be relayed to the nursing staff on an emergency basis. The universal advice should be prompt and copious irrigation with water prior to beginning transport to the hospital. Irrigation should continue in the emergency department with water or saline. Alkalis produce a liquefaction necrosis of the conjunctiva and cornea. Consequently, their corrosive action is unobstructed and they continue to dissolve soft tissue until removed. Hospital treatment may consist of irrigation for hours or days depending on the extent of the burn. Alkali burns of the eye should be seen immediately by an ophthalmologist.

Acid Burns

Acid burns are extremely irritating and can be very serious. However, acids generally produce a coagulation necrosis of the cornea, and their invasion is limited by the coagulum formed in the process. Immediate copious irrigation is still indicated, as is ophthalmologic consultation.

Foreign Bodies

Conjunctival Foreign Bodies

Foreign bodies that adhere to the conjunctiva should always be suspected as a cause of redness, pain, or tearing of the eye. An examination under magnification is indicated, and slit-lamp examination is preferred. Foreign bodies in the inferior cul-de-sac are usually quite apparent. Examination of the everted upper lid will reveal foreign bodies adherent to the conjunctival surface of the tarsal plate. After the foreign body has been identified, a drop of proparacaine hydrochloride should be instilled and the object removed with a cotton-tipped applicator.

Occasionally double eversion is indicated. To accomplish this, the lid is first singly everted. Using a lid elevator, the lid is everted once more to view the superior cul-de-sac. Alternatively, the conjunctiva of the superior cul-de-sac may be prolapsed into view by exerting firm pressure with cotton-tipped applicator after the upper lid has been singly everted.

Small abrasions require no further treatment other than reassurance. Double patching of larger abrasions will usually relieve a great deal of pain, but oral pain medication may be necessary.

Corneal Foreign Bodies

Corneal foreign bodies are a common problem and often cause a great deal of pain and redness. After the examination is completed, a drop of proparacaine hydrochloride should be instilled and the object removed with a corneal spud, burr, or sterile hypodermic needle. This is best accomplished under slit-lamp magnification. After the foreign body is removed, antibiotics should be instilled and the eye doubly patched. Oral pain medication may be necessary, and the patient should be rechecked in 24 to 36 h.

Rust rings are usually present if a ferrous foreign body has been embedded for more than a few hours. The rust ring should be removed with the aid of the slit lamp. A battery-powered rust ring remover greatly facilitates this task. The rust ring should be removed completely, as persistence of the particles may cause recurrent ocular symptoms.

Occasionally the emergency physician may find it impossible to remove all of the rust particles or the rust ring. In this case it is acceptable practice to instill a drop of antibiotic and snugly double-patch the eye. Over time, softening of the corneal epithelium will occur, and the following day the remaining foreign material can be removed more easily.

Corneal foreign bodies which have been present for more than an hour or so will frequently provoke a mild iritis characterized by photophobia and dull ocular pain. A drop of a short-acting cycloplegic such as cyclopentolate 1% will do much to relieve ciliary spasm and pain.

Because of the rich vascular and nerve supply at the limbus (corneal-scleral junction), simple drop anesthesia may not be sufficient for foreign-body removal. A cotton-tipped applicator may be saturated with the anesthetic solution, then gently held against the area to be anesthetized for about 10 s. This will produce a profound anesthesia which is more than adequate for minor operative procedures.

Eyelashes

Eyelashes are common ocular foreign bodies that usually settle in the inferior cul-de-sac. Occasionally the lash may lodge in the inferior punctum. In this case the patient usually has a medial conjunctivitis, with the temporal side clear. To avoid missing this common diagnosis, always check the puncta of the reddened eye.

Blepharitis

Blepharitis is a common condition characterized by chronic inflammation of the lid margins and occasionally the conjunctiva. Slit-lamp examination reveals scaling and a "greasy" appearance to the lid margins which are particularly prominent around the base of the lashes.

The condition is usually attributed to a staphylococcal infection of the skin and oil glands immediately adjacent to the lash follicles. Treatment consists of topical instillation of sulfacetamide drops in combination with a steroid, and application of antibiotic ointment to the lid margins on retiring. This often can be facilitated by carefully scrubbing the lash margins with baby shampoo (nonirritating) to remove oil and scales.

Corneal Ulcer

With a corneal ulcer the eye is usually reddened and extremely painful. Slit-lamp examination will reveal a localized white flocculent infiltrate of the cornea. A hypopyon is a frequently associated finding which is characterized by the accumulation of a white inflammatory exudate in the anterior chamber. Corneal destruction and perforation are the major hazards. No topical medications of any kind should be administered until cultures have been obtained. Immediate ophthalmologic consultation and admission to the hospital are mandatory.

Subconjunctival Hemorrhage

Subconjunctival hemorrhage is an extremely common condition characterized by objective findings of a very reddened eye with virtually no subjective complaints. The cause is the rupture of a small vessel beneath the bulbar conjunctiva. The objective appearance is characteristic. The bulbar conjunctiva is blood red and has a striking appearance. The condition is usually called to the attention of the patient by a concerned observer.

Rupture of these blood vessels is usually benign. Common causes include trivial trauma, foreign bodies, or violent Valsalva maneuvers such as coughing or straining. Important differential considerations include hypertension and blood dyscrasias.

A patient who has not experienced this condition before is often terrified about impending blindness. After the other causes of subconjunctival hemorrhage have been eliminated, the patient may be reassured that the hemorrhage will resolve spontaneously in 10 to 14 days.

Ultraviolet Keratitis—Corneal Flash Burn

Virtually all ultraviolet radiation is absorbed by the cornea, and the majority is absorbed by the corneal epithelium. Especially intense sources of ultraviolet radiation include arc welding and reflected sunlight. "Welders' blindness" and "snow blindness" are both manifestations of excessive ultraviolet radiation to the corneal epithelium. Symptoms include intense pain, burning, blurred vision, and epiphora.

Slit-lamp examination reveals a diffuse punctate keratopathy, which is best seen by fluorescein staining and cobalt blue illumination under slit-lamp magnification. The examiner will note multiple pinpoint-sized areas of staining. These represent swollen and ruptured corneal epithelial cells. The experienced examiner will note diffuse corneal haziness under slit lamp, even without the use of fluorescein.

Management consists of topical anesthesia to facilitate examination, followed by snug double patching and systemic analgesia. The rapid healing properties of the cornea result in only slight irritation after 24 to 36 h of patching.

Indiscriminate use of topical anesthetics has led to grave consequences. Most of the topical anesthetics are cellular toxins in higher doses, and repeated administration will retard healing of the corneal epithelium. Furthermore, because anesthesia deprives the cornea of its normal protective reflexes, additional damage will almost surely follow. Permanent damage to the corneal stoma may then result from the increasingly frequent instillations of topical anesthetics that subsequently become necessary. Visual disability may ensue. Thus prescribing or dispensing topical anesthetics under those circumstances is absolutely contraindicated; firm double patching and adequate levels of systemic analgesia are the only rational modes of treatment.

Miscellaneous

Hordeolum (Stye)

A hordeolum is an acute inflammation of the meibomian glands, usually of the upper lid. Hordeola usually present as pustular vesicles at the lid margin.

Initial treatment consists of warm compresses and topical antibiotics. Surgical intervention is occasionally necessary and consists either of drainage of the gland at the lid margin or eversion and incision with drainage of the gland from the posterior surface of the lid.

Chalazion

A chalazion is a chronic granulomatous inflammation of a meibomian gland, also most commonly of the upper lid. This condition usually presents as an uninflamed and nontender nodule of the lid several millimeters from the lid margin. The treatment for this is surgical and consists of curettage of the substance of the gland.

Acute Eye Pain

Acute Iritis

Acute inflammation of the anterior segment of the eye may be divided into two broad categories, traumatic and nontraumatic. Traumatic iritis will be discussed in a subsequent section. Nontraumatic iritis has a number of causes, and a complete discussion of the differential diagnosis is beyond the scope of this text. However, the emergency physician should be able to recognize the basic symptom complex and initiate management.

The onset of symptoms usually occurs over a period of hours. Symptoms include blurred vision, photophobia, and dull ocular pain, which is usually referred to the brow or temporal area.

Physical examination reveals a reddened and painful eye. The pupil is often constricted, and direct and consensual photophobia is apparent on penlight examination. Close examination may reveal ciliary flush, a diffuse reddening of the sclera at the limbus. Visual acuity is usually decreased, and intraocular pressure is decreased in the affected eye. Slit-lamp examination will reveal flare and cells in the anterior chamber. This is best seen with reduced room illumination and high magnification.

Management consists of cycloplegics and topical steroids. Cycloplegia with cyclopentolate or homatropine markedly reduces ciliary spasm and pain, and steroids tend to reduce the inflammatory response of the anterior segment. Untreated inflammation of the anterior segment can lead to posterior synechiae (adhesions of the posterior leaf of the iris to the anterior lens capsule) or anterior synechiae (inflammatory attachment of the anterior iris leaf to the posterior corneal surface). These conditions produce a visual and cosmetic defect and can lead to secondary glaucoma. Patients with iritis should be referred to an ophthalmologist for a detailed evaluation.

Acute Angle Closure Glaucoma

Congenital narrowing of the anterior chamber angle is the underlying cause of acute angle closure glaucoma. Under a variety of circumstances the angle between the anterior iris leaf and posterior surface of the cornea may close completely, thus preventing the exit of the aqueous humor. Despite the elevated intraocular pressure, the ciliary body continues to produce aqueous humor and the intraocular pressure rises precipitously.

An acute angle closure may be precipitated in susceptible individuals by moving from daylight to a darkened environment, e.g., a movie theater, or iatrogenically by the administration of mydriatics. The latter situation may be a beneficial diagnostic maneuver. The characteristic symptom is a unilateral dull, aching ocular pain, which is frequently accompanied by nausea and vomiting. Vision is blurred, with halos seen around lights. Physical examination will demonstrate a diffusely reddened and congested eye with reduced visual acuity. The cornea is often hazy, and the pupil is mid-dilated and fixed to light. Intraocular pressures are extremely high, frequently 50 mmHg or greater.

Emergency management is directed at reducing the intraocular pressure by two routes: decreasing production of aqueous and facilitating aqueous outflow. Two drugs, parenterally administered acetazolamide (Diamox) and topical timilol 0.5% (Timoptic), decrease intraocular pressure by decreasing the formation of aqueous. Acetazolamide, 500 mg, is administered parenterally and timilol is given as one drop initially followed by a second drop in about 10 min.

Timilol is a nonselective β-adrenergic receptor blocking agent. Consequently, it should be used with great caution in patients with chronic obstructive pulmonary disease or heart disease. Newer cardioselective drugs such as betaxolol (Betoptic) may offer a greater margin of safety for pulmonary patients.

Administration of hyperosmotic agents decreases the intraocular volume, deepens the anterior chamber angle, and facilitates aqueous outflow, often dramatically reducing intraocular pressure. Oral administration of glycerol as a 50% solution given at a dosage of 1 mL/kg will provide an adequate osmotic load. Because glycerol is extremely sweet, it is usually given over ice with a tart lemon flavoring.

If nausea and vomiting prevent oral administration, intravenous mannitol, 1.0 to 2.0 g/kg, may be given. Both agents are osmotic diuretics. Both expand the intravascular volume and may precipitate congestive heart failure in susceptible patients.

Aqueous outflow may also be facilitated by administration of a miotic such as pilocarpine. A drop of 1 or 2% pilocarpine may be given every 15 min for the first hour followed by a drop every 30 to 60 min thereafter. The mid-dilated pupil places the posterior surface of the iris border in close contact with the anterior lens capsule. Aqueous in the posterior chamber may be unable to pass through the pupil to enter the anterior chamber (pupillary block). As a result, the iris bulges forward (iris bombé), further closing the anterior chamber angle.

When miosis is achieved, the pupillary block is relieved and aqueous flows forward into the anterior chamber and out through the trabecular meshwork. However, at elevated intraocular pressures the iris is rendered relatively ischemic and nonresponsive to miotics. Only when the intraocular pressure falls does miosis occur.

Definitive treatment consists of either peripheral laser iridotomy or surgical peripheral iridectomy once the attack has been stemmed.

Open Angle Glaucoma

Open angle glaucoma is a chronic condition of elevated intraocular pressure. Constant elevation of intraocular pressure damages the optic nerve. Physical findings include elevation of the intraocular pressure, an increase in the optic cup/disk ratio, and arcuate scotomas emerging from the physiologic blind spot. Marked constriction of the peripheral visual fields with sparing of central vision is characteristic of late-stage chronic open angle glaucoma. Chronic glaucoma is not an ocular emergency; it is mentioned here to distinguish it from acute angle closure glaucoma.

Herpes Simplex Keratitis

The viral agent responsible for herpes simplex keratitis is herpes simplex virus. It produces an acute infection of the corneal epithelium, which is characterized by localized ocular pain frequently described as a foreign body sensation. Visual acuity is reduced if the lesion happens to fall on the visual axis. The eye is diffusely reddened, and slit-lamp examination of the unstained cornea may reveal a localized area of haziness. Fluorescein staining will often demonstrate a dendrite figure, a branching pattern that resembles the outline of a forked lightning bolt.

Treatment consists of topical administration of antiviral agents and cycloplegics to reduce anterior chamber reaction. Steroids prescribed to quiet a ''simple conjunctivitis'' can lead to a rapid progression of herpes simplex keratitis and should never be prescribed in the emergency department. Ophthalmologic consultation is mandatory since progressive herpes simplex keratitis can lead to destruction of the cornea and grave visual disability.

Acute Visual Loss

Central Retinal Artery Occlusion

Acute occlusion of the central retinal artery is most commonly the result of atherosclerosis and its various manifestations: thrombosis, thromboemboli, and vasospasm. The patient experiences sudden monocular, painless loss of vision. Branch arterioles may be similarly affected, leading to sudden reduced vision and segmental visual field defects. Gross physical findings consist principally of a normal-appearing but sightless eye. Examination of the fundus reveals a very pale retina with a small pink dot in the vicinity of the fovea. Often no retinal arteries are visible.

Central retinal artery occlusion is an absolute ophthalmic emergency, and the prognosis is extremely grave. Vigorous digital massage of the globe and/or anterior chamber paracentesis may reduce the intraocular pressure enough to allow atheromas to move peripherally. Paracentesis should only be performed by an ophthalmologist. Immediate emergency ophthalmologic consultation is mandatory.

Central Retinal Vein Occlusion

A rigid atheromatous artery immediately adjacent to the central retinal vein may ultimately exert sufficient pressure to collapse the vein wall. This gradual process leads to occlusion of the vein. Symptoms are usually confined to uniocular painless decrease of vision, though some visual function may persist. Fundus examination will reveal a chaotically blood-streaked retina with prominent dilated and congested veins. Management is beyond the scope of the nonophthalmologist, and consultation is mandatory.

Retrobulbar Neuritis

The usual presenting complaint in retrobulbar neuritis is loss of central vision in the affected eye. Peripheral vision is usually preserved, and visual field examination will define the degree of involvement. Other than loss of central vision, the physical examination findings are usually totally unremarkable. The diagnosis of multiple sclerosis is associated with retrobulbar neuritis in approximately 25 percent of cases.

Eclipse Burn (Sun Gazer's Retinopathy)

Accidental or prolonged (unprotected) viewing of the sun causes sun gazer's retinopathy. Certain abnormal psychiatric states, or abuse of hallucinogenic or other mind-altering drugs, such as PCP (phencyclidine), predispose to so-called sun gazing. For uncertain reasons such persons may gaze directly at the sun with the unprotected eye for a prolonged period. Most ultraviolet light is absorbed by the ocular media. Lower-frequency radiation is transmitted to the retina, and direct viewing of luminous objects can produce photocoagulation of the macula. The result is reduction of central retinal (macular) vision. Visual acuity under these circumstances is reduced. Confrontation visual field examinations may not reveal this small defect. Funduscopic examination will demonstrate discrete disruption of the retina in the area of the macula.

Amaurosis Fugax

Sudden temporary interruption of the blood supply to the retina will produce the fleeting uniocular visual loss termed *amaurosis fugax*. The duration of visual loss may vary from only a few seconds to several minutes. By definition, complete visual function returns to the affected eye.

This phenomenon is caused by minute emboli of the central retinal artery, usually secondary to extracranial atherosclerosis. This alarming symptom should alert the physician and patient to the need for a diligent search for the treatable atherosclerotic disease.

Retinal Detachment

Spontaneous retinal detachment is painless. The patient experiences the gradual lowering or raising of a curtain over the visual field of the affected eye. A careful history will often reveal prodromal symptoms such as the perception of flashing lights in the peripheral visual field at night or the drifting of "spider webs" or "coal dust" across the visual field. The former symptom is due to mechanical trauma of the retina, while the latter two are a result of small vitreous hemorrhages drifting across the visual axis.

The retina detaches as the result of the seepage of the fluid portion of the posterior vitreous body through the retinal tear, causing separation of the loosely applied retina, much as water seeps behind wallpaper and strips it away from the wall.

Examination with a direct ophthalmoscope may reveal the undulating gray detached retina. Occasionally, vitreous hemorrhages resulting from rupture of retinal vessels bridging the tear will be noted as well. A diligent search with the indirect ophthalmoscope will usually demonstrate the retinal tear that is responsible for the detachment.

Initial management consists of preventing further retinal detachment when possible. As long as the macula remains attached, there is an excellent chance of preserving central retinal vision. If the detachment is inferior, the patient should rest in bed with the head elevated; if the detachment is superior, the patient should lie flat in bed. Prompt ophthalmologic consultation is indicated.

Hysterical Blindness

A variety of psychological factors may precipitate subjective complete loss of vision. The patient may be remarkably calm despite the gravity of this complaint, and the physician may note a variety of other clues that would suggest nonorganic visual loss. With the exception of the loss of subjective vision, the physical examination is unremarkable. Direct and consensual pupillary examination is normal, and the fundus has a normal appearance. Use of an optokinetic drum or strip will usually elicit optokinetic nystagmus, confirming an intact visual pathway. Management is by supportive referral for psychiatric evaluation.

TRAUMA

Lid Lacerations

Wounds that involve only the skin of the lid have an excellent prognosis. Closure may be accomplished with very fine (6-0 or 7-0) suture material. Ordinarily, nonabsorbable material such as nylon should be used. However, suture removal may be very difficult with small children. Absorbable sutures may be used in these cases, although some skin reaction may occur. In 7 to 10 days any remaining sutures may be brushed away. Healing occurs rapidly due to the rich blood supply, and nonabsorbable sutures may be removed within 3 days.

There are at least five anatomic areas where more than the usual level of anatomic knowledge and suturing skill are necessary. These are discussed below.

Lacrimal canaliculi. The horizontal limbs of the lacrimal canaliculi traverse the lid from the lacrimal puncta to the common canaliculi. The canaliculi lie about 1 mm beneath the lid margin. Any wound that affects the lid margin between the punctum and medial canthus has a high probability of damaging the canalicular apparatus.

Levator. Deep transverse lacerations of the upper lid threaten the levator mechanism. The presence of ptosis suggests involvement of the levator palpebrae tendon, and prompt ophthalmologic consultation is indicated. A careful search for any signs of ptosis must be made when the anatomy of the wound suggests this possibility.

Orbital septum. Deep wounds of the upper lid may violate the orbital septum, which runs between the tarsus and the superior orbital rim. When this occurs, there is a high potential for: (1) prolapse of orbital fat, leading to a cosmetically unacceptable outcome; and (2) orbital cellulitis. The septum must be surgically closed, and prophylactic systemic antibiotics are indicated.

Canthal tendons. Penetrating wounds of the medial and lateral canthi may interrupt the canthal tendons. This will lead to a cosmetically unacceptable shortening of the palpebral fissure. Repair is technically difficult and should be performed by an ophthalmic surgeon.

Lid margins. Through-and-through wounds of the lid margin and tarsal plate require meticulous realignment of the structures for a cosmetically acceptable result. If more than about 1 mm of the tarsal plate is lacerated, a complex three-layer closure is required.

Corneal Abrasions

Corneal abrasions are extremely common, and the history will usually define the problem. The affected eye is painful, and epiphora is common. Slit-lamp examination with fluorescein staining will reveal the abraded areas. Myriad extremely fine linear abrasions of the superior third of the cornea (the "ice rink sign") suggest the presence of a foreign body under the upper lid.

Removal of all foreign material, instillation of a topical antibiotic, and firm double patching are indicated for larger abrasions. However, corneal abrasions from contact lenses are usually not patched because patching may predispose to infection. If photophobia and signs of iritis are present, a short-acting mydriatic is indicated. Mydriasis and double patching usually control pain, although systemic analgesics are occasionally required.

Corneal Lacerations

Recognition of small corneal lacerations may be difficult at times. Often slit-lamp examination may be required to identify even a full-thickness laceration. Clues include a "teardrop"-shaped pupil due to prolapse of the iris, and flattening of the anterior chamber resulting from loss of aqueous. Occasionally small fragments of black iris pigment may be present at the lips of the wound. They may be mistaken for foreign bodies. The eye should be protected with a rigid metal eye shield. Repair should occur in the operating room under microscopic control.

Perforation of Globe

Penetrating wounds of lids should raise a suspicion of an occult perforation of the globe. The sclera is particularly thin under the rectus muscles, and this is the area of highest risk.

Even though the perforation may not be visible, visual acuity is usually reduced, the globe is soft, and there may be vitreous hemorrhage visible on ophthalmoscopic examination. A rigid metal eye shield will protect the globe from inadvertent pressure with resulting extrusion of the contents of the globe. Immediate ophthalmologic consultation is indicated.

Hyphema

Small hyphemas (hemorrhages in the anterior chamber) may go unnoticed without slit-lamp examination. Larger hyphemas which do not resolve may lead to secondary glaucoma and blood staining of the corneal endothelium. Although initial hyphemas may be insignificant, recurrences are often more severe, and the complication rate increases dramatically. Even if the initial eye examination is normal, individuals with severe blunt ocular injury, such as an injury caused by a racquetball or tennis ball, should be advised to return to the emergency department for symptoms such as blurred vision or ocular pain. Follow-up examination is advised in 24 h.

Management is directed toward enhancing absorption of blood and prevention of recurrence. Bed rest is necessary, while the use of patches, midriatics, and topical steroids will vary with the preference of the individual ophthalmologist.

Traumatic Dislocated Lens

Blunt trauma to the globe may disrupt the zonules and result in dislocation of the lens. The lens usually falls backward into the vitreous cavity, although it may prolapse into the anterior chamber. In either case visual acuity is markedly reduced. Certain collagen disorders, such as Marfan's syndrome, predispose to spontaneous dislocation of the lens. With a high degree of suspicion on the part of the examiner, adequate slit-lamp and funduscopic examination will confirm the diagnosis.

Blowout Fracture of the Orbit

Blunt trauma to the globe transmits hydraulic forces throughout the entire orbital cavity. The floor and medial wall of the orbit are particularly fragile and subject to fracture. When the floor of the orbit is fractured under these circumstances, orbital contents such as the inferior rectus muscle and orbital fat may prolapse through the fracture and become trapped. The infraorbital nerve traverses the floor of the orbit and is also frequently involved. Symptoms include pain and diplopia on upward gaze. Physical examination may reveal enophthalmos and hypesthesia in the distribution of the infraorbital nerve. Paralysis of upward gaze will produce marked diplopia in the upper visual fields. Virtually every "black eye" should have orbital x-rays, and the preferred view is a modified stereo Waters' view. Initial management is conservative, and ophthalmologic referral is necessary.

Traumatic Retinal Detachment

A history of significant blunt ocular trauma should lead to a diligent examination of the entire retina for signs of retinal tears. Early recognition and therapy of the torn retina will prevent retinal detachment. Examination of the peripheral retina requires more skill in the use of the indirect ophthalmoscope and/or the Goldman contact lens. Findings of even a small amount of vitreous hemorrhage should raise suspicions of a traumatic retinal tear and lead to prompt ophthalmologic referral.

Intraocular Foreign Body

A history of work that involves pounding metal on metal should immediately raise the suspicion of an intraocular foreign body. The initial injury may be painless, and symptoms may not present for a day or more after the initial incident. Decreased visual acuity and dull, nonlocalizing ocular pain are usually the first complaints.

Small intraocular foreign bodies may leave only a minute wound on the lid or globe. The examiner should also search carefully for minute perforations of the iris leaf or early cataract formation resulting from violation of the lens capsule. A careful funduscopic examination after dilation of the pupil may reveal the foreign body.

Metallic foreign bodies may be visible on plain x-ray films of the orbit, although specific localizing views may be necessary. Ultrasonic or computed tomographic (CT) scanning of the globe and orbit are very helpful in the precise localization of foreign bodies.

Virtually all intraocular foreign bodies must be removed. Innovations in the surgical approach to the vitreous body have greatly improved the prognosis for this injury.

Traumatic Iritis

Blunt ocular trauma followed by poorly localized, aching ocular pain, photophobia, and decreased visual acuity suggests a diagnosis of traumatic iritis. The pupil is constricted and a deep ciliary flush is usually present. Slit-lamp examination reveals cells and flare in the anterior chamber. Direct and consensual photophobia are due to iris and ciliary body irritability. Intraocular pressure is frequently lower than in the uninjured eye.

Initial treatment consists of topical short-acting cycloplegics and dilute steroid drops. Cycloplegia is a useful diagnostic tool as it will dramatically decrease ocular pain and photophobia secondary to iritis.

Traumatic Mydriasis

Blunt ocular trauma may selectively impair the function of parasympathetic innervation to the iris leaf and thereby result in mydriasis. This may be a local effect on the globe or may represent trauma to the ciliary ganglion located deep in the orbit. In either case the condition is usually temporary and management consists of recognition and appropriate ophthalmologic referral.

DIAGNOSTIC DILEMMAS

Ophthalmic Migraine Manifestations

Migraine headache may present with ophthalmic symptoms manifested by visual phenomena. The patient may complain of objects taking on a ''silvery''; or ''shimmering'' appearance. This is frequently followed by the development of a scotoma, often described as a ''fortification scotoma,'' in which the margin of the visual field defect is jagged or serrated in appearance. The scotoma may persist for several hours or even for a day or more. The usual course leads to complete resolution. Rarely, there may be a persistent peripheral scotoma after resolution of the migraine event.

Unilateral Dilated Fixed Pupil

The differential diagnosis of unilateral dilated fixed pupil is based on either a significant neurologic event or the accidental (or intentional) instillation of a cycloplegic. To resolve this question, one drop of 2% pilocarpine is placed in the dilated eye and the instillation is repeated in 5 min. If at the end of 20 min the pupil is still fixed and dilated, the patient has instilled a cycloplegic.

Spasm of Accommodation

The hysterical or extremely anxious patient may occasionally present with what amounts to a full-blown manifestation of the near reflex. That is, the pupils are constricted, the eyes are convergent, and accommodation is at a maximum. The patient complains of blurred vision, particularly at a distance. Treatment should be directed at the underlying anxiety, although a drop of a short-acting cycloplegic in each eye may break the cycle.

Tunnel Vision

''Gun barrel,'' or tunnel, vision is another manifestation of hysteria or anxiety. The patient complains of loss of all the visual field with the exception of the central area. A tangent-screen visual field examination will reveal a dense scotoma of all but the central visual field. If the scotoma is truly physiologic and not hysterical in origin, then doubling the distance between the examinee and the tangent screen will double the size of the central visual field. With hysterical tunnel vision the visual field size will remain unchanged.

OPHTHALMIC MEDICATIONS

Anesthetics

Proparacaine. Proparacaine has a rapid onset of action. Its duration of action is approximately 20 min, and the depth of anesthesia produced is adequate for most minor ocular procedures.

Tetracaine. This drug is somewhat more irritating than proparacaine and is less commonly used for ordinary office procedures. The onset of action is more delayed, the depth of anesthesia is greater, and the duration maybe 1 h or more.

Cocaine. Topical cocaine is an excellent anesthetic and profound vasoconstrictor. Hence it is quite useful for minor surgical procedures. However, cocaine softens the corneal epithelium to the point where even minor corneal trauma may desquamate the entire surface.

Mydriatics and Cycloplegics

Tropicamide. Tropicamide is a mydriatic-cycloplegic with onset in 15 to 20 min. Its duration of action is fairly brief, and accommodation and pupillary reaction usually return within 1 to 2 h.

Cyclopentolate. Cyclopentolate is a somewhat more potent cycloplegic than tropicamide, with a longer duration of action.

Homatropine. Homatropine is a mydriatic-cycloplegic with a duration of action of 2 or 3 days.

Atropine. Atropine is a very long lasting mydriatic-cycloplegic with a duration of up to 2 weeks.

Phenylephrine. Phenylephrine (Neo-Synephrine) solution is supplied in strengths of 2.5 and 10%, although the 2.5% solution is adequate for most purposes. Phenylephrine is essentially a pure mydriatic with a rapid onset and a duration of action of 2 or 3 h.

Miotics

Miotics are used almost exclusively for the treatment of glaucoma. Pilocarpine is one of the most commonly used and is usually instilled four times a day in strengths varying from $\frac{1}{8}$ to 4%.

Antibiotics

Sulfacetamide. As the 10% solution or ointment, sulfacetamide is a relatively nonirritating and effective broad-spectrum antibiotic for the management of most external ocular infections.

Chloramphenicol. Chloramphenicol remains one of the most effective broad-spectrum antibiotics available for topical use. Most common gram-positive and gram-negative ocular pathogens are sensitive to chloramphenicol. Unfortunately, bone marrow depression and aplastic anemia have been reported with its ocular use.

Gentamicin. This drug is particularly useful in the management of infections due to penicillin-resistant staphylococci and many of the gram-negative organisms.

Neomycin. While neomycin is effective against many gram-negative organisms, skin sensitivity, manifested by an erythematous, pruritic scaling dermatitis, may appear in as many as 10 to 15 percent of patients.

Tobramycin. Supplied as the 0.3% solution or ointment, tobramycin is effective against a broad range of staphylococci, streptococci, and numerous gram-negative organisms.

Erythromycin ointment. This excellent broad-spectrum antibiotic is well-tolerated and widely used.

Steroids

Although reduction of the inflammatory response may be of great value from the standpoint both of comfort and of altering the pathophysiology of a disease process, steroid use should be limited to those cases which are seen in consultation with an ophthalmologist. A principal risk of topical steroid administration is acute exacerbation of ocular infections. In the case of herpes simplex keratitis, deep stromal scarring or corneal perforation may result from steroid use. Long-term administration for any reason may lead to glaucoma.

Miscellaneous

Acetazolamide. Acetazolamide, a carbonic anhydrase inhibitor, markedly reduces the output of aqueous by the ciliary body. Its principal use is in the management of acute angle closure glaucoma.

Glycerol. Orally administered glycerol acts as a hyperosmotic agent. Shortly after administration there is a notable reduction in intraocular pressure. Its ophthalmic use is ordinarily limited to the management of acute angle closure glaucoma.

TREATMENT TECHNIQUES

Eye Patch

A snugly fitting eye patch is appropriate treatment for larger abrasions of the cornea. The pressure of the patch reduces pain, and, because the lid margin is immobilized, recurrent irritation of the damaged cornea by the lid margin is eliminated.

Double patching is the most common technique. The first patch is folded and applied against the closed eyelid. The second patch is then placed over the first. The bulk of this dressing fills the orbital recess so that when it is correctly taped in place moderate pressure is applied directly to the eye. The patch is commonly taped in place with three parallel strips of 1-in tape extending diagonally from the central forehead to the lateral cheek.

Eye Shield

Use of an eye shield is dictated by the fact that any pressure or contact with the globe must be avoided in cases where there is some question of interruption of the globe's integrity. If the globe is unprotected, accidental pressure may cause its contents to extrude through the wound. The eye shield provides this mechanical barrier of protection.

Foreign Body Removal

Conjunctival Foreign Bodies

Under ordinary circumstances conjunctival foreign bodies are easily removed with a cotton-tipped applicator after topical anesthesia. The examiner should search diligently for any remaining material after the first foreign body has been removed. The upper lid should be everted and the tarsal plate examined closely in every case.

Corneal Foreign Bodies

The slit lamp should be used when removing foreign bodies from the cornea whenever possible. After adequate topical anesthesia, an attempt should be made to sweep away the foreign body with a cotton-tipped applicator.

If the cotton-tipped applicator fails, the foreign body must be removed by a sharp instrument. The most useful instrument is a sterile hypodermic needle used *bevel down* to prevent the tip from burying itself deeply in the corneal stroma. With magnification the foreign body can be meticulously dissected from the corneal surface.

Ferrous foreign bodies present a special problem. After the iron-containing particle has been present in the cornea for a few hours, a rust ring will develop. This should be removed along with the foreign body as it can produce recurrent irritation and permanent corneal staining. The rust ring can be removed with a sterile hypodermic needle. However, a small, electrically driven spherical corneal burr is particularly useful for quick and neat removal.

MISCELLANEOUS OPHTHALMIC PROBLEMS

Contact Lenses

Hard Corneal Contact Lenses

Occasionally, hard contact lenses will become "lost" somewhere in the conjunctival cul-de-sac. If the lens is not tinted, magnification and topical anesthesia may be necessary to find and retrieve it. Once visualized, the lens can easily be removed with a small rubber suction device designed for that purpose. All comatose patients should be examined for the presence of contact lenses, and they should be removed if present.

Soft Contact Lenses

These lenses may contain 60 percent or more water. If they become desiccated, they become brittle and are virtually impossible to remove intact. Repeated instillations of normal saline solution (without additives) will usually hydrate the lens sufficiently so that it can be removed. The removal technique consists of "pinching" the lens off the surface of the eye. Fluorescein stain should be avoided as these lenses readily and permanently absorb this stain. If eye pain or redness is present, both hard and soft corneal contact lenses should be removed and should not be reinserted until the eyes have been evaluated.

Intraocular Lens Implants

An increasing number of cataract patients have undergone lens implantation following cataract removal. These lenses have dramatically reduced the visual distortion previously associated with the use of heavy spectacle lenses for correction. The implanted lenses are held in place by a variety of methods, including loops, clips, sutures, and pins.

The most common complication seen in the emergency department is dislocation of the lens. This may result from pupillary dilation in a darkened environment or from minor direct trauma to the eye. Management consists of prescribing bed rest for the patients and contacting the ophthalmic surgeon. The surgeon will probably dilate the pupil, gingerly tap the front of the eye to pop the loop back under the iris, and then constrict the pupil with pilocarpine. Occasionally reoperation is necessary.

BIBLIOGRAPHY

Armstrong TA: Evaluation of the Tono-Pen and the Pulsair tonometers, *Am J Ophthalmol* 109:716, 1990.

Cinotti AA: *Handbook of Ophthalmologic Emergencies,* ed 3. New York, Elsevier, 1985.

Epstein DL, Pavan D: Glaucoma, in Pavan D (ed): *Manual of Ocular Diagnosis and Therapy,* ed 2. Boston, Little, Brown, 1985.

Havener WH: *Synopsis of Ophthalmology: The Ophthalmology Book,* ed 6. St. Louis, Mosby, 1984.

Johnson DH, et al.: Glaucoma: An overview. *Mayo Clin Proc* 61:59, 1986.

Kooner KS: Management of acute elevated intraocular pressure: II. Treatment. *Ann Ophthalmol* 20:87, 1989.

Rich R, Lowe RF, Reyes A: Therapeutic overview of angle-closure glaucoma, in Rich R, Shields MB, Krupin T (eds): *The Glaucomas,* St. Louis, Mosby, 1989.

155
OTOLARYNGOLOGIC EMERGENCIES

Frank I. Marlowe

OTOLOGIC EMERGENCIES

Otalgia

Ear pain can usually be explained on the basis of the ear examination if there is evidence of otitis externa or media. When it cannot, sources of referred pain must be considered and sought to explain the pain. Cranial nerves V, VII, IX, and X and cervical nerves II and III supply sensation to the ear. The cervical nerve supply may be the source of referred pain in cervical arthritis and occipital neuralgia, but the cranial nerves are most likely to be associated with referred pain. Pain from the temporomandibular joint, mandibular teeth, or tongue may be referred to the ear by the trigeminal nerve. Herpes zoster oticus and Bell's palsy may cause otalgia by the facial nerve. The glossopharyngeal or vagus nerves may be the source of otalgia from tonsillitis, cancer of the tonsil, or foreign bodies of the hypopharynx, larynx, or cervical esophagus.

The management of otalgia is treatment of the underlying conditions, plus analgesics. If no cause for ear pain is found, treatment with analgesics and local heat is prescribed. Ear-nose-throat (ENT) consultation is necessary if pain persists.

Infections

Otitis Externa

The signs and symptoms of otitis externa are itching, pain, and discharge from the ear, with an intact drum. If the swelling is severe, hearing loss may be included. Pain may be severe and made worse by pressing on the tragus or by moving the auricle. Occasionally the entire auricle may be swollen and red, and tender enlarged lymph nodes can be palpated over the mastoid process, parotid area, and upper neck.

Treatment consists of cleaning the external ear canal by suctioning, or with a cotton-tipped applicator, and applying an antibiotic-steroid otic solution for 1 week; if desired, a $\frac{1}{4}$-in wide ribbon gauze moistened with an antibiotic solution can be inserted into the ear canal. Any one of the newer generation cephalosporins should be given if the auricle is enlarged and red or if there is lymphadenopathy. Drainage from the ear canal should always be cultured before initiating antibiotics. The patient should be told that symptoms will continue for 24 to 48 h before they improve, even though the treatment has been started. Malignant external otitis should be suspected in the diabetic patient with external otitis that does not clear rapidly by routine measures. These severe forms of otitis externa may lead to cartilage and bone destruction, and otologic consultation and hospitalization are necessary.

Furuncle

Furuncles of the ear canal cause pain until they spontaneously rupture and drain. Examination reveals a localized area of redness and tenderness at the external meatus.

The treatment is as for external otitis, along with incision and drainage.

The presenting sign of a preauricular sinus is usually a dimple in the preauricular area. Infection or abscess formation may occur if a cyst develops. Treatment is local heat application and 400,000 units of penicillin intramuscularly qid, or 250 mg of penicillin VK four times a day orally if outpatient treatment is indicated. Incision and drainage are necessary if the cyst is fluctuant, with delayed surgical removal of the cyst or sinus when the infection has resolved.

Bullous Myringitis

Bullous myringitis may be of viral or mycoplasmal origin and causes persistent pain and, possibly, mild hearing loss. The tympanic membrane has blisters that may contain clear or hemorrhagic fluid. Bullous myringitis is treated by analgesics, application of local heat and possibly with erythromycin or tetracycline antibiotics. If the pain is severe, the bullae may be ruptured by an otologist. If underlying otitis media is present, it should be treated.

Otitis Media

The symptoms of acute suppurative otitis media are fever, pain, and hearing loss. There will be a discharge if the tympanic membrane has ruptured. The tympanic membrane appears red with engorgement of the vessels, bulging, and thickening.

The treatment is ampicillin or amoxicillin for children up to adolescence and penicillin for older teens and adults, for 10 days. Cephalosporin antibiotics may be used if response to the penicillins is not prompt. Antibiotic-containing eardrops are indicated only when the tympanic membane is ruptured and drainage is present in the ear canal. Topical heat and systemic analgesics are preferred to analgesic eardrops for the control of pain. Acute otitis media is discussed further in Chapter 14f, "Upper Respiratory Emergencies."

Myringotomy is indicated for severe pain, marked toxicity, and high fever, and complications such as facial nerve paralysis, meningitis, or brain abscess.

Chronic otitis media is treated by cleaning and suctioning of the ear, systemic antibiotics, and antibiotic-steroid eardrops. The patient should be referred to an otologist for further evaluation and treatment. A patient with chronic otitis and a cholesteatoma who has facial nerve paralysis, vertigo, or possible intracranial complications should have emergency referral to an otologist.

Sudden Hearing Loss

Sudden hearing loss may occur as a result of lesions of the external ear (impacted cerumen), middle ear (fluid, blood, or pus in the middle ear), or inner ear (Ménière's disease, labyrinthitis, and syphilis). It can result from lesions of the internal auditory meatus or cerebellopontine angle, or from vascular spasm or occlusion. Most often, sudden deafness is idiopathic and is presumed to be of viral or vascular origin.

Vascular causes of sudden hearing loss are presumed to involve vasospasm or hypercoagulation states. The hearing loss may be mild or moderate, but more frequently it is severe or total. The mechanism of sudden hearing loss with a viral cause is unknown.

No specific therapy of proven value is available, but a patient with sudden deafness should be evaluated on an emergency basis by an otologist.

Trauma

Hematoma

Hematomas of the ear usually occur as a result of blunt trauma and are particularly common in wrestlers and boxers. Bleeding occurs between the cartilage and its covering perichondrium. Treatment of a hematoma is aseptic drainage by aspiration or incision. A mastoid-conforming dressing should be applied after drainage. Complications include reaccumulation of the hematoma, deformity, and infection. Reaccumulation requires repeated aspiration or drainage. The cauliflower deformity results from the gradual replacement of the untreated hematoma by fibrous tissue, new cartilage formation, and calcification.

Perichondritis is characterized by a swollen, red, and tender auricle. The causative organism is frequently *Pseudomonas,* and the condition is best treated urgently by an otologist.

Foreign Body of the Ear

Children are particularly prone to acquire foreign bodies of the ear. Animate objects must be stupefied or killed before removal. Place a cotton tampon, well moistened with ether, at the external auditory meatus. After 5 min any insect will be stupefied. Then irrigate to flush the insect out.

Occasionally attempts to remove the object result in pushing it beyond the isthmus, the junction of the cartilaginous and bony portions of the canal. In patients in whom the object is lodged beyond the isthmus, removal may require general anesthesia. If the foreign body is distal to the isthmus, it may be grasped with a microforceps and removed. A larger object is removed by placing a hook or loop behind it and pulling it out. In some instances a stream of water may be directed superiorly to push the object out. However, vegetable foreign bodies should not be irrigated, as they will swell. Unless the child is calm during foreign body removal, it is best to use general anesthesia. Many instances of traumatic injury to the tympanic membrane or the ossicles have been recorded because a child jumped during an attempt to remove a foreign body.

Thermal Injuries

With prolonged exposure to extreme cold, the upper and outer edge of the auricle becomes waxy and white and may feel hard and cold. These signs, associated with loss of sensation, are diagnostic of frostbite. Frostbite is treated by rapid rewarming, with warm irrigations or application of warm compresses, at a temperature between 42 and 44°C (107.6 and 111.2°F), for not more than 20 min. Analgesics are necessary since the thawing process is usually painful. Avoid reexposure.

Contact with hot water bottles, hot liquids, or electric currents may result in burns of various degrees. Severe burns require cleansing of the wound by strict aseptic technique, using detergent skin cleanser and saline solution. After thorough cleansing, excise all devitalized tissue and blisters. Apply silver sulfadiazine cream and a thick mastoid dressing. Tetanus toxoid, antibiotics, and analgesics are indicated.

Chemical Injuries

Strong acids or alkalis produce a burn on immediate contact. Treatment consists of copious irrigation. Bathe the ear and the ear canal with saline or sterile water. Let the liquid remain for 2 or 3 min then aspirate and dry the auricle. Repeat this procedure three or four times, and thoroughly dry the ear and canal.

Traumatic Perforations

Perforations of the tympanic membrane may occur from a penetrating object such as a pencil or cotton-tipped applicator or after blunt trauma from an explosion.

In general, perforations heal spontaneously without specific treatment other than avoiding water in the ear. Careful follow-up is necessary. If the ear is contaminated, either from swimming pool water or by a penetrating object, administer a systemic antibiotic such as penicillin. Facial nerve palsy, hearing loss, or vertigo necessitate immediate ENT consultation. Otherwise, follow-up in a few days is sufficient.

Barotitis

Barotitis may occur following barometric pressure changes such as those associated with flying or scuba diving. The sensation of a blocked ear and pain are the common complaints. Examination usually reveals a hemorrhagic or hyperemic tympanic membrane and fluid in the middle ear.

Barotitis is treated by analgesics, oral decongestants, topical nasal sprays, and middle ear inflation. Antibiotics should be given if secondary infection develops. Myringotomy is indicated if the pain is extremely severe and unrelenting, or if the fluid fails to resolve on medical therapy.

SALIVARY GLAND PROBLEMS

Acute inflammation of the salivary glands presents as painful swelling in the parotid or submandibular areas, often occurring at meal time. It is most often encountered in an acute suppurative form in elderly, dehydrated, or diabetic patients, and the diagnosis is most often made by examination of the oral cavity that shows purulent drainage from the parotid (Stensen's) duct or the submandibular (Wharton's) duct. Treatment consists of hydration, appropriate antibiotic treatment, guided by culture and sensitivity studies, and rarely incision and drainage.

It is not uncommon for lesser degrees of swelling, pain, and tenderness to occur secondary to a stone in the duct (sialolithiasis). The symptoms are usually intermittent, recurrent, and may be associated with a palpable thickening along the course of the duct. Often the stone is radiolucent and does not visualize on plain radiographs. Uncomplicated sialolithiasis is treated symptomatically and with tart lozenges to encourage salivation. Antibiotics are not necessary. Most stones eventually pass spontaneously, but referral to an otolaryngologist should always be given. Persistent obstruction may require probing and dilation of the ducts, contrast radiographic studies (sialograms) and excision of the stone and/or the gland.

In rare instances, inflammation of the submandibular glands may involve the sublingual space with a severe cellulitis (Ludwig's angina) and may threaten airway obstruction. This is an emergency that may require immediate airway control and drainage by incision.

POSTADENOTONSILLECTOMY BLEEDING

Bleeding following tonsillectomy and/or adenoidectomy may be classified as immediate (first 24 hours) or delayed (usually at 5–7 days). It is more common following tonsillectomy than adenoidectomy alone and its occurrence has steadily declined in recent times, probably due to restrictions on the use of salicylate analgesics and to better operative techniques. There is early evidence that tonsillectomy by electrocautery or "hot" technique carries with it a reduced incidence of postoperative bleeding. The emergency management of this type of oral or nasal bleeding is largely supportive and consists of efforts to control bleeding with pressure if possible, avoid airway obstruction by blood clots, and maintain blood pressure with parenteral fluids or blood as necessary. Definitive care of this problem is best left to the otolaryngologic surgeon and may require packing, surgical control by coagulation or suture ligature, or specific vessel ligation, usually under general anesthesia.

ACUTE UPPER AIRWAY OBSTRUCTION

Obstruction of the airway is one of the most demanding emergency problems the physician may encounter. Orderly and prompt evaluation followed by appropriate treatment can be lifesaving.

Signs and Symptoms

The most important signs and symptoms of upper respiratory obstruction are shortness of breath and stridor. Stridor may be either expiratory or inspiratory and tends to be more marked in laryngeal disorders. In general, inspiratory stridor is associated with obstruction of the supraglottic or glottic larynx, while expiratory stridor is associated with subglottic obstruction. Other signs and symptoms that may be present are hoarseness or change in voice, difficulty in speaking, difficulty in swallowing either food or oral secretions, or loud wheezing.

History

A brief, but carefully obtained, history is probably the most important single contribution toward an etiologic diagnosis of upper airway obstruction. It is of prime importance to establish the time of onset; the activities surrounding the onset, such as eating or holding something in the mouth; and whether the obstruction is associated with systemic symptoms such as fever, cough, swollen glands in the neck, weakness, nausea, or vomiting.

Examination

Examination of the patient with acute upper airway obstruction may, of necessity, be brief, but this does not preclude its being thorough. The oral cavity must be examined with particular attention to the tongue, looking for inflammation or swelling. Similar examination of the area of the tonsils, the uvula, and the hypopharynx must be employed.

The neck must be examined for evidence of trauma such as abrasion, hematoma, ecchymosis, or crepitus, or for evidence of inflammation such as tenderness and lymphadenopathy. Auscultate the chest and neck to localize the source of stridor or wheezing and to identify pulmonary disorders such as asthma or pneumothorax.

Differential Diagnosis

The causes of acute upper airway obstruction may be grouped into several categories: foreign bodies, trauma, irritants and corrosives, and inflammatory conditions including infections.

Foreign Bodies

Respiratory obstruction from a foreign body most often occurs in children, who are particularly prone to aspirating objects such as beans, buttons, beads, or parts from small toys that become lodged in the larynx, but does also occur in adults.

If the foreign body lodges in the upper airway at the larynx or above, the presenting symptoms are usually marked stridor and respiratory distress. Indeed, total airway obstruction may occur, and profound asphyxia may be present. Wheezing is present if the aspirated foreign body passes the epiglottis and lodges in one of the main bronchi. Wheezing may be unilateral, but may be heard in both lung fields. Aspiration of a foreign body should be considered in any patient who has a rapid, sudden onset of wheezing or inspiratory stridor without prior upper respiratory tract infection and with no past history of wheezing events.

The diagnosis is made largely on the characteristic history of sudden onset of obstructive symptoms, associated with coughing or choking spells.

If the foreign body is suspected to be in the lower airway and the respiratory status is stable, both inspiratory and expiratory roentgenograms of the chest should be obtained. A plain film may demonstrate air trapping on the affected side. Inspiration and expiration views may demonstrate shift of the mediastinum away from the affected side. A better evaluation of the chest can be made under the fluoroscope if an esophageal foreign body is suspected. Both anteroposterior and lateral views of the chest should be obtained. The aspirated object may be of sufficient radiodensity to be visualized. Even if the object is not radiopaque, air in the stomach may be regurgitated up the esophagus and thus outline the foreign object.

If the obstruction is of mild degree, it is important to refrain from doing anything that might convert a mild or partial obstruction to a total one. If the foreign body is visible in the pharynx, it can be removed. Removal under direct visualization with a laryngoscope or bronchoscope may be necessary.

Recurrent or persistent pneumonia may develop distal to a foreign body obstruction in the lower airways.

Epiglottitis

Acute epiglottitis is characterized by the abrupt onset of rapidly progressive respiratory obstruction, usually in a child aged 2 to 8 years, most commonly caused by *Haemophilus influenzae*, type B, but it is being reported with increasing frequency in adults also.

The clinical course is often characterized by the abrupt onset of severe sore throat, followed by pooling of pharyngeal secretions; drooling and dysphagia; fever that may reach 40.5°C (105°F); and rapid development of dyspnea and stridor. In most cases there is an upper respiratory tract infection prodrome. In over 50 percent of the cases, this may be present for as long as 12 to 24 h preceding the onset of recognizable symptoms. Restlessness, cyanosis, and exhaustion can rapidly develop. The patients entire effort is directed toward obtaining enough air, and quiet breathing provides more air than struggling. The chin is frequently thrust forward, and the patient resists all efforts to be placed on his or her back. Air hunger may be marked, and suprasternal and infrasternal retractions are commonly present. The voice may be muffled or hoarse, but there is a striking absence of expiratory wheezing or the barking cough of croup.

Examination, which is best carried out with the patient in the sitting position, reveals a cherry-red, markedly swollen epiglottis. Complete respiratory arrest has been noted to occur suddenly, provoked by such seemingly innocuous events as attempting to visualize the laryngopharynx or drawing a blood sample. There is some evidence that inspection of the oral cavity is safe in the well-oxygenated patient, and a short period of high-flow oxygenation by face mask seems to be a worthwhile precautionary measure. The diagnosis can often be made on the basis of a soft tissue lateral roentgenogram of the neck. The epiglottis will appear as a thumb-shaped object on the lateral neck film (Fig. 155-1). A normal epiglottis will appear slim, like the distal phalanx of the little finger. However, the best method for rapid diagnosis is direct visualization.

Instruments for immediate intubation, such as a laryngoscope and endotracheal tubes of the appropriate size, and/or a rigid bronchoscope, should be readily available. With this preparation, a gentle attempt is made to visualize the epiglottis with a tongue blade that is directed

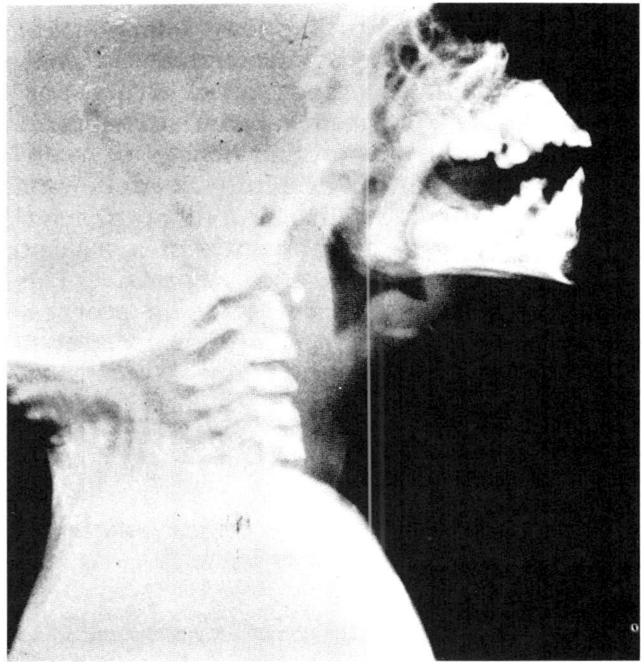

Fig. 155-1. The diagnosis of epiglottitis is confirmed by lateral neck film that shows an enlarged epiglottis obstructing the airway. (*Courtesy of The Children's Hospital Center of Akron, Ohio.*)

inferiorly and not placed near the base of the tongue or pushed posteriorly.

Some authors have suggested that once the presumptive diagnosis of acute epiglottitis is made, all examinations should be carried out in the operating room. The exact cause of respiratory arrest, which can occur with dramatic suddenness, is uncertain, but some authors have suggested that the swollen epiglottis is drawn like a plug into the glottis, and the increased respiratory efforts serve only to impact the structure further. Other authors believe that the inflamed larynx is more prone to laryngospasm or that respiratory arrest results merely from rapidly progressing fatigue. Regardless of the exact mechanism, sudden arrest can and does occur, and if no artificial airway has been established, the patient dies.

Establishment and maintenance of an artificial airway is the primary and crucial part of the management of acute epiglottitis. With an experienced anesthesiologist available, immediate oral or nasal endotracheal intubation is carried out. An alternative, which is much less desirable, is positive-pressure oxygenation by mask as a temporizing measure. If the supraglottic structures are so swollen as to prevent passage of an endotracheal tube, a bronchoscope is introduced to secure an airway. A tracheostomy may then be performed in an orderly fashion over the bronchoscope. In the final analysis, the method of treatment is largely determined by the facilities and the personnel available at the treatment center, and both intubation and tracheostomy are employed under appropriate circumstances with excellent results.

The medical treatment of acute epiglottitis includes broad-spectrum antibiotics, most commonly ampicillin (100 to 200 mg/kg) in divided doses, fluids, humidification and oxygenation, and possibly the use of steroids for their anti-inflammatory effect in reducing laryngeal edema.

Trauma

Obstruction secondary to trauma may be due to direct trauma to the larynx or neck. Indirectly, obstruction may occur from bleeding in the pharynx or from a hematoma in the parapharyngeal structures, or from occlusion by the tongue. Relief of the obstruction may involve a measure as simple as suctioning out the upper airway or altering the position of the patient's head so that obstructing tissues resume a more normal position. Grasping and fixation of obstructing tissues is frequently an excellent means of counteracting the obstructive effect of injured tissues.

The possibility of an injury to the cervical spine should be considered at all times, since extension of the neck in an attempt to place an airway or perform endotracheal intubation can lead to paralysis.

In some forms of direct trauma to the larynx, such as may occur in high-speed vehicular accidents in which the neck strikes the dashboard, marked respiratory distress may occur with little evidence of laryngeal injury. This most often is a result of bilateral vocal cord paralysis from a shearing injury to the recurrent laryngeal nerves in their position posterior to the cricothyroid joint articulation. There seems to be some misconception regarding unusual difficulty in intubating patients with vocal cord paralysis, but this is easily accomplished and is the initial treatment of choice. In some types of direct laryngotracheal injury, the extent of trauma may make nasal or endotracheal intubation impossible, and cricothyrotomy or tracheostomy may be necessary.

Irritants and Corrosives

Damage to the pharyngeal, laryngeal, and cervical tracheal mucous membranes can occur from steam, irritant gases (such as chlorine), corrosive liquids, burning gases, or hot air from a fire.

Examination may reveal burns of the oral mucous membranes, as seen in children with lye ingestions, and the assumption must be made that burns have occurred further down in the aerodigestive tract until proven otherwise. Nasotracheal intubation is often done early, before the development of severe airway edema that can make intubation difficult or impossible. Otherwise, oxygenation and the use of steroids and antibiotics may be sufficient.

Angioneurotic Edema

The rapid and sudden onset of respiratory obstruction secondary to angioneurotic or allergic inflammatory edema may be quite striking and frightening for both the patient and physician. It is most likely to occur in an individual with a history of allergies and may follow the ingestion of foods such as shellfish, chocolate, peanuts, or strawberries, or it may be idiopathic. Examination may reveal massive edema of the tongue, or edema of the palate and uvula to such a degree that the uvula may resemble a large white grape (uvular hydrops). Edema may also involve the epiglottis or larynx.

Treatment is administration of oxygen, epinephrine, and corticosteroids, and the response is usually rapid and dramatic. For uvular edema, topical epinephrine may be helpful; also, multiple scratches with a needle or knife blade on the uvula are almost always effective. In extreme or repetitive cases the tip of the uvula may be amputated by an otolaryngologist.

Peritonsillar, Retropharyngeal, and Parapharyngeal Abscess

These complications of pharyngitis, tonsillitis, or adenoiditis can cause airway obstruction. They are characterized by throat pain and swelling, fever and toxicity, and prior upper respiratory infection. Emergency otolaryngologic consultation is required. Treatment consists of antibiotics and incision and drainage of the abscess.

Peritonsillar Abscess

Peritonsillar abscesses are rare in young children and most common in adolescents and young adults. The patient has a history of tonsillitis that was untreated or treated by a single injection of penicillin. The pain then localizes to one side, and the patient begins to have drooling, alteration of voice, referred ear pain, and trismus. Fever and leukocytosis are present. On examination the tonsil is found to be pushed down medially toward the midline or beyond, displacing the uvula.

Treatment consists of incision and drainage, which in mild cases may consist of aspiration with a large-bore needle and syringe (18 gauge), or in more severe cases may require the use of a sharp blade and the insertion of a long-handled forceps, with spreading to allow adequate drainage. If significant improvement is obtained, there is no embarrassment of the airway, and the patient is able to swallow, treatment as an outpatient may be carried out with oral administration of penicillin. However, hospitalization is frequently required for the administration of parenteral fluids and antibiotics, as the patient is usually unable to swallow. A recent trend has developed toward tonsillectomy within the first 24 h after antibiotic coverage has been established, as a means of the most definitive drainage of any abscess (so-called abscess tonsillectomy).

Retropharyngeal Abscess

A retropharyngeal abscess usually occurs in a child less than 4 years of age. There is usually a history of upper respiratory tract infection. The signs and symptoms include fever, difficulty in breathing and swallowing, enlarged cervical nodes, and a stiff neck. Intraoral examination will show fullness or a mass in the posterior pharyngeal area. Palpation must be carefully done to avoid rupturing the abscess. A lateral soft tissue roentgenogram will help to confirm the diagnosis.

The treatment of retropharyngeal abscess consists of incision and drainage, which are most often done transorally under satisfactory general anesthesia and intubation. This is followed with antibiotic therapy and invariably requires hospitalization.

Parapharyngeal Abscess

The infection localizes in a space bounded by the pterygomandibular raphe, prevertebral fascia, hyoid bone, and base of the skull. The symptoms include marked trismus, fever, painful swallowing, altered voice, and stiff neck. On examination there will be pharyngeal swelling and displacement of the tonsil (but usually with little redness or other signs of tonsillar infection), and external swelling in the parotid regions. Trismus with an internal and external bulge should suggest this diagnosis.

Treatment of parapharyngeal abscess is similar to that for retropharyngeal abscess. However, the incision and drainage are more often done by a lateral approach through the neck.

Miscellaneous Cases

Acute upper airway obstruction may also be noted secondary to congenital anomalies. These may occur above the larynx, such as in choanal atresia (the newborn is usually an obligate nasal breather), or with malformations of the tongue. At the level of the larynx there may be webs, cysts, or atresia of the various cartilages. Below the level of the larynx there may be a tracheoesophageal fistula, vascular rings, or abnormalities of the greater vessels.

Bilateral vocal cord paralysis secondary to dysfunction of the recurrent laryngeal nerves may acutely impair the upper airway. This is most common following thyroid surgery, but it can occur following general anesthesia for any operative procedure, or it may be idiopathic. Inability to abduct the vocal cords may also occur in cricoarytenoid arthritis, or in conditions producing laryngeal tetany or spasm. The onset of the obstruction may be acute, or slow and insidious.

Cysts and neoplasms of the upper respiratory system can produce airway obstruction, and though usually slow-growing, the obstruction may appear acute at the time of presentation. Included in this group are benign neoplasms, such as subglottic hemangioma, and the more common malignant lesions of the larynx, as well as benign cysts such as dermoids and laryngoceles.

Management of Airway Obstruction

Endotracheal Intubation

The most rapid method for establishing an airway is endotracheal intubation. Properly executed, it is done without anesthesia and often averts the necessity for a tracheostomy. Following intubation, anesthesia may be administered while an orderly tracheostomy is performed. There are only rare instances, such as massive facial trauma or direct trauma to the larynx, in which intubation is not possible. This situation might also prevail in the case of impacted foreign body.

Cricothyrotomy (Laryngotomy)

Where endotracheal intubation is not possible, an obstructed airway is best relieved by making an opening through the cricothyroid membrane. This may be done with a large-bore needle, or with a host of other devices designed for this purpose.

In the absence of these special devices, an incision is made into the cricothyroid membrane with a small surgical blade, and the opening maintained with any device at hand.

Emergency Tracheostomy

This procedure is carried out only when the obstruction is too severe to allow time for an orderly tracheostomy, when facilities are unavailable for insertion of a bronchoscope or endotracheal tube, and when the patient cannot survive more than a few minutes without brain damage. The operation is fraught with difficulty, associated with high risk of complications, and to be avoided at all costs by appropriate preplanning.

BIBLIOGRAPHY

Otologic Emergencies

Ballenger JJ: *Diseases of the Nose, Throat and Ear,* ed 12. Philadelphia, Lea & Febiger, 1977.

DeWeese DD, Saunders WH: *Textbook of Otolaryngology,* ed 5. St. Louis, Mosby, 1977.

Newman MH, Olson NR, Singleton EF: *Handbook of Ear, Nose and Throat Emergencies.* Flushing, Medical Examination Publishing, 1973.

Snow JB Jr: *Introduction to Otorhinolaryngology.* Chicago, Year Book, 1979.

Acute Upper Airway Obstruction

Allen T: Suspected esophageal foreign body: Choosing appropriate management. *J Am Coll Emerg Physicians* 8:101, 1979.

Cantrell RW, Bell RA, Morioka WT: Acute epiglottitis: Intubation versus tracheostomy. *Laryngoscope* 88:994, 1978.

Daniidis J, Symeonidis B, Triaridis K, et al: Foreign body in the airways: A review of 90 cases. *Arch Otolaryngol* 103:570, 1977.

Hunsicker RC, Gartner WS: Fogarty catheter technique for removal of endobronchial foreign body. *Arch Otolaryngol* 103:103, 1977.

Liscott MS, Horton WC: Management of upper airway obstruction. *Otolaryngol Clin North Am* 12:351, 1979.

Strome M: Tracheobronchial foreign bodies: An updated approach. *Ann Otol Rhinol Laryngol* 86:649, 1977.

156
NASAL EMERGENCIES AND SINUSITIS

Frank I. Marlowe

EPISTAXIS

The most frequent cause of epistaxis is spontaneous erosion of the superficial mucosal blood vessels situated near the anterior end of the nasal septum. Less commonly, bleeding originates from the branches of the ethmoidal arteries (resulting in bleeding from the roof of the nasal chamber or posterior septum), or sphenopalatine arteries (manifested by postnasal or lateral nasal wall bleeding). Local factors associated with nasal hemorrhage include ulcerations that result from excessive nasal dryness (nose picker's ulcer), nasal septal perforations, nasal trauma, nasal tumors, and hereditary hemorrhagic telangiectasia (Osler-Weber-Rendu disease).

Systemic diseases associated with epistaxis include hypertension, arteriosclerosis, blood dyscrasias, and coagulation disorders. Recognition and control of such associated conditions are important in successful management of the nosebleed.

General management of the severe nosebleed consists of maintaining the vital signs; obtaining a complete blood cell count, platelet count, prothrombin time, and partial thromboplastin time; and stopping the bleeding. The patient should be in the sitting position when examined to prevent swallowing and aspiration of blood. Instruct the patient to blow his or her nose of remaining blood. Using a headlight and nasal speculum, inspect the septum, floor, and lateral wall of both sides of the nose to determine the site of bleeding. Topical vasoconstrictors can be applied in an effort to locate the bleeding point.

Anterior Epistaxis

Usually bleeding is from Kiesselbach's plexus (anterior inferior part of the nasal septum). Active bleeding can be controlled temporarily by pinching the nose for 4 to 5 min. After the active bleeding is controlled, the point may be cauterized with a silver nitrate bead or by electrocautery.

If bleeding cannot be controlled or if the source of bleeding is not accessible to cauterization, anesthetize the nasal chamber with a topical anesthetic such as 4% lidocaine or 2% cocaine and insert nasal packing. When packing is necessary, a properly sized Nasostat hemostatic nasal balloon or continuous strips of ½-in petrolatum gauze inserted under direct vision can be used to stop the bleeding.

The Nasostat hemostatic nasal balloon is a disposable cuffed tube. First the cuff is inflated with 15 to 20 mL of air to make sure the bleeding stops. Then the air is removed and sterile saline is instilled. The Nasostat controls hemorrhage by exerting mechanical pressure on the site of the bleeding that may be in the anterior, middle, or posterior part of the nasal chamber.

The conventional nasal pack consists of petrolatum gauze strips that are placed in layers, starting either in the floor or roof of the nasal chamber, until the nasal chamber is tightly filled. To avoid displacement of the nasal septum to the opposite side, resulting in loosening of the pack, the other nostril may also be packed.

Whenever a nasal packing of any sorts is used, the patient can be placed on a broad-spectrum antibiotic such as ampicillin until the packs are removed. Sinusitis and, rarely, toxic shock syndrome can be complications. A patient with anterior packing can be treated as an outpatient if the medical condition permits, and should be seen again in 24 h.

Posterior Epistaxis

If the bleeding site is in the nasopharynx or posterior end of the nasal chamber, it may be necessary to insert a posterior nasal pack. Posterior packs can be applied by using a gauze pack, Foley catheter, or Nasostat.

The patient with a posterior bleed should be admitted to the hospital for further care and evaluation. Humidified air, antibiotics, and analgesics are generally necessary.

Posterior Gauze Pack

A satisfactory gauze pack can be fashioned by securing three strings of heavy suture material to a rolled 4 in × 4 in gauze sponge. The pack is inserted as follows (Fig. 156-1).

- Anesthetize the nasal chambers.
- Spray the oropharynx with 4% lidocaine or 5% cocaine.
- Insert the tips of two red rubber catheters, size Fr 8 or Fr 10, through the nostrils into the oropharynx.
- Grasp the tips of the catheters with a straight hemostat and pull them out of the mouth. (Now the tips of the catheters are out of the mouth and the ends are in the nostrils.)
- Fasten the ends of two of the strings to the tips of the catheters.
- Pull the ends of the catheters, which are in the nostrils, and make sure that you have fastened the strings to the proper tip on each side. By pulling of the catheters simultaneously the posterior pack is directed into the mouth and then into the oropharynx. The packing is placed in the nasopharynx by pushing with the second and third fingers of the right hand, directing the packing behind the palate, while simultaneously pulling on the string from the bleeding nostril with the left hand.
- Strings from the right and left nostrils are tied on a gauze roll that is placed over the nasal columella. The third string of the posterior pack, which is in the mouth, is taped to the cheek. This string is to facilitate later removal of the packing from the nasopharynx and mouth.
- Anterior nasal packing should then be performed unilaterally or bilaterally.

Foley Catheter Balloon Tamponade

The insertion of a Foley catheter into the nasopharynx is as follows:

- Anesthetize the anterior nasal chambers as before.
- Insert a Foley catheter, Fr 10 to Fr 14 with a 20- to 30-mL bag, into the side that bleeds, advancing it along the floor of the nose until you see the catheter tip in the pharynx.
- Inflate the balloon with air or saline up to 20 mL, and then pull to lodge it in the nasopharynx.
- Ask the patient or the nurse to pull moderately on the catheter while you pack strips of petrolatum gauze in both nostrils.
- Wrap one or two 4 in × 4 in gauze sponges around the stem of the catheter to close the anterior nasal opening. Pull moderately to make sure the bag has not slipped into the oropharynx.
- Keep the Foley catheter in place by putting a Montgomery or Hoffman clamp around the stem of the catheter and on the 4 in × 4 in gauze sponges. Avoid excessive pull on the catheter and avoid pressure on the nasal skin.

NASAL TRAUMA

Fracture

The nasal bones make up the upper one-third of the nasal pyramid, and the lower two-thirds is made of cartilage. The midline dorsal support is provided by the cartilaginous septum, and the lateral nasal vault is supported by paired upper and lower lateral cartilages. In severe trauma the septum may be fractured or displaced from its attachment to the nasal floor.

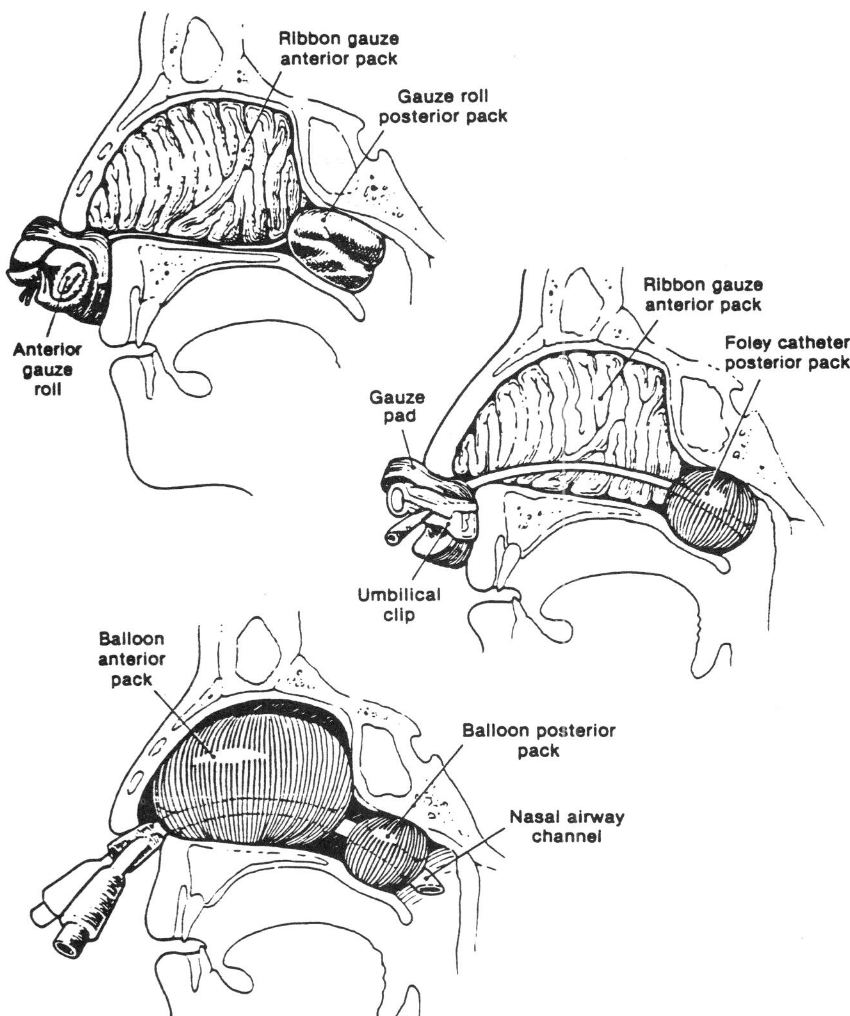

Fig. 156-1. Packing for posterior epistaxis; three materials. [From Silfen EZ, Merida MA, Stair TO (ed): *Eye, Ear, Nose, Mouth, and Throat Emergencies.* Rockville, MD, Aspen Systems Corp., 1986, p 92. Used by permission.]

In evaluating nasal trauma, note any history of preexisting nasal deformity or surgery.

Frontal Nasal Trauma

Frontal nasal trauma displaces the nasal bones inward and downward, resulting in flattening and widening of the osseous dorsum. If the displacement is severe, the medial palpebral ligament may be displaced, leading to an increase in the intercanthal distance. Frontonasal fractures may also be associated with damage to the lacrimal duct, the ethmoid and frontal sinuses, the orbital margins, and the cribriform plate.

Lateral Nasal Trauma

Lateral nasal trauma displaces the nasal bones inwardly on the side of the applied force with outward displacement of the opposite nasal bone, resulting in step deformities between the nasal bone fragments or the nasal bone and the maxilla.

Unrecognized or untreated nasal fractures in children may lead to serious disturbances in nasal growth and contour and are often overlooked. In small children, the external nasal structures are elastic and more resistant to fracture, but septal dislocation is common. If nasal fracture or dislocation is suspected, early treatment is necessary.

Edema, hemorrhage, and discoloration of tissues make it difficult to detect fractures and lacerations of the intranasal structures. To properly evaluate such injuries, carefully remove clots and debris and use a vasoconstrictor to shrink the mucous membrane. Mucosal lacerations commonly occur at the junctions of the cartilaginous and bony pyramid. Because of edema, accurate assessment of hematomas and lacerations may be especially difficult if the patient is seen hours after the injury. Edema of the lips, periorbital ecchymosis, and subconjunctival hemorrhage commonly accompany a nasal fracture. Subcutaneous emphysema is not uncommon. Movement of fragments with crepitation or pain may be prominent features, but it may be difficult to elicit fracture movement if the fragments are impacted. The most reliable guide in assessing nasal deformity is palpation of the nasal contour. Roentgenograms are obtained to confirm the diagnosis.

Early reduction of nasal fractures may be possible if swelling does not preclude an accurate assessment of nasal contour. Reduction of simple fractures should be done when the swelling subsides. Treatment of complex fractures, fractures associated with fractures of other facial bones, can be done in 7 to 10 days whenever the condition of the patient permits.

Complications are the development of a septal hematoma, CSF rhinorrhea, and hemorrhage. Bleeding may occur into the space between the septal cartilage and perichondrium. Such subperichondrial hematomas appear as a soft unilateral or bilateral swelling of the nasal septum. Unless drained, the hematoma may result in aseptic necrosis of the septal cartilage or predispose to formation of a septal abscess. Drainage of nasal septal hematomas should be performed on an emergency basis by an otolaryngologist.

Cerebrospinal fluid rhinorrhea is characterized by clear nasal discharge. The rhinorrhea is usually unilateral and is increased by having the patient lean forward or by compression of the jugular vein. Neurosurgical consultation is required if CSF rhinorrhea is suspected, and nasal packing should be avoided if at all possible.

Nasal bleeding following trauma may be profuse, but it is generally of short duration. Hemorrhage that fails to cease spontaneously is best controlled by nasal packing.

Foreign Bodies

Nasal foreign bodies are the most common cause of unilateral nasal obstruction and rhinorrhea in children. The discharge is characteristically foul and may be temporarily controlled with antibiotics. There is always danger of aspiration of the foreign body into the lower respiratory tract.

Proper illumination and proper instruments are essential for safe removal. Suction secretions from the nostril, spray the nose with 1% phenylephrine, and visualize the object. Irregularly shaped foreign bodies may be gripped with a small alligator forceps, but round or smooth foreign bodies are best removed by a small hooked instrument that is used to engage the posterior end of the foreign body. Do not push the foreign body back into the nasopharynx because of the danger of aspiration. If the patient is uncooperative and cannot be restrained, general anesthesia may be required.

SINUSITIS

Acute paranasal sinusitis usually is precipitated by an acute viral respiratory tract infection. Swelling of the nasal mucous membrane produces obstruction of the ostium of the paranasal sinus; the oxygen in the sinus is resorbed, and relative negative pressure in the sinus develops and causes pain. This condition is spoken of as vacuum sinusitis. If the vacuum is maintained, a transudate of serum from the vessels of the mucous membrane occurs and fills the sinus. Bacteria may enter the sinus and cause a suppurative sinusitis. The causative organisms in acute sinusitis are generally gram-positive cocci, while in an acute exacerbation of chronic sinusitis, they are generally anaerobic or gram-negative organisms.

Acute maxillary sinusitis causes pain in the maxillary area, and toothache; frontal sinusitis produces frontal headache; ethmoid sinusitis causes pain in the retroorbital area and between the eyes, and frontal headache; and pain from sphenoid sinusitis is less well localized and may be referred to the frontal or occipital area. Fever and chills suggest extension of the infection beyond the sinus. Physical examination shows yellow or green purulent rhinorrhea, the mucous membrane of the nose is red and swollen, and there may be tenderness and swelling over the involved sinus.

Radiopacity of the paranasal sinuses due to a swollen mucous membrane or retained pus in the sinus usually is evident, although sinus films may on occasion be normal (Figs. 156-2, 156-3).

Treatment includes antibiotics, drainage, and analgesics. The antibiotic of choice in acute sinusitis is penicillin, with erythromycin a second choice. In chronic sinusitis a broad-spectrum antibiotic such as ampicillin or a cephalosporin may be more effective.

Drainage can be improved by a topical vasoconstrictor such as ¼% phenylephrine. Systemic vasoconstrictors, e.g., ephedrine hydrochloride, pseudoephedrine, or phenylpropanolamine may be prescribed in conjunction with topical ones.

Complications of maxillary sinusitis are caused by uncontrolled spread of infection. Ethmoid sinusitis frequently is complicated by orbital cellulitis and abscess, especially in children. Redness and swelling of the eyelid, proptosis, and displacement of the globe laterally and inferiorly are signs of abscess formation. Orbital abscess and cellulitis are true emergencies and require inpatient treatment, systemic antibiotics, and drainage where indicated.

Frontal sinusitis may cause osteomyelitis of the posterior table of the frontal bone leading to meningitis, epidural abscess, subdural empyema, and brain abscess, or may destroy the anterior table and produce a large forehead abscess (Pott's puffy tumor). If frontal sinusitis fails to respond promptly to systemic antibiotics, the patient should be admitted to the hospital.

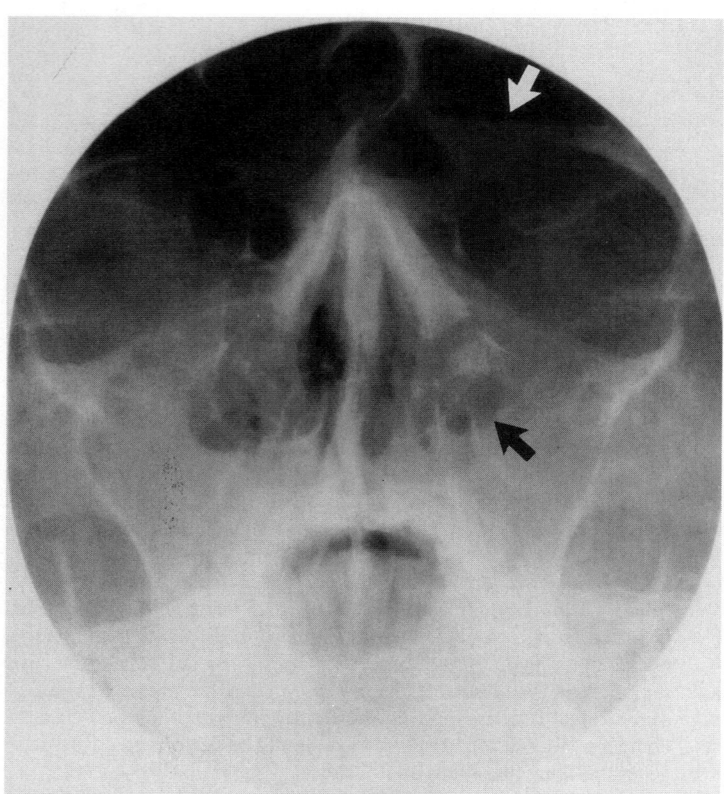

156-2. Upright Water's view showing acute frontal sinusitis with air fluid levels (white arrow) and chronic bilateral maxillary sinusitis with cloudiness of both antra due to marked mucosal thickening (black arrow).

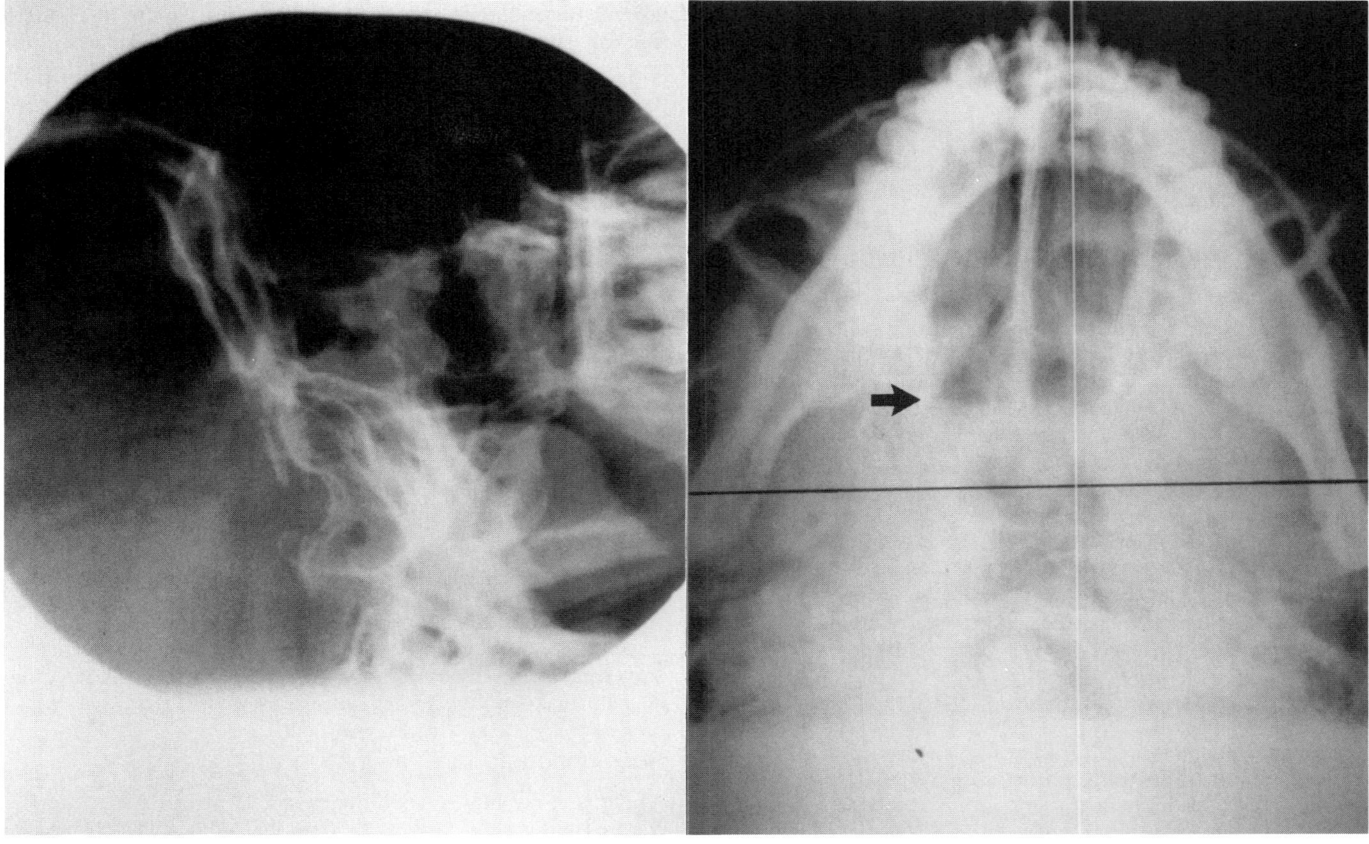

A B

Fig. 156-3. Lateral (**A**) and submental vertex (**B**) views showing an air fluid level (arrow) in the sphenoid sinus in acute sphenoid sinusitis.

Barosinusitis

Barosinusitis results when a significant pressure differential develops between the atmosphere and the paranasal sinus cavity. Rapid descent in an aircraft and rapid ascent from underwater depths are common factors. Inflammatory, allergic, or neoplastic processes may obstruct air flow in and out of the sinus, and gases within the sinus are slowly absorbed. Intense pressure differentials result in mucosal edema, intrasinus hemorrhage, or transudation, which are apparent on sinus roentgenograms. Relief of the pain may be dramatic as the sinus ostium opens. If spontaneous drainage does not occur, topical nasal vasoconstrictors are indicated.

BIBLIOGRAPHY

Goldstein E, Gottlieb MA: Roentgeno-oddities. *Oral Surg* 12:129, 1954.

Hunter KM: Foreign body in the nasal fossa. *Oral Surg* 41:805, 1976.

Katz HP, Katz JR, Bernstein M, et al: Unusual presentation of nasal foreign bodies in children. *JAMA* 241:1496, 1979.

Proctor DF, Anderson IB, Lundqvist G: Clearance of inhaled particles from the human nose. *Arch Intern Med* 131:132, 1973

Walike JW, Chinn J: Evaluation and treatment of acute bleeding from the head and neck. *Otolaryngol Clin North Am* 12:455, 1979.

Yarington CT: Sinusitis as an emergency. *Otolaryngol Clin North Am* 12:447, 1979.

157
MAXILLOFACIAL FRACTURES

Barry H. Hendler

GENERAL PRINCIPLES OF FRACTURE MANAGEMENT

The patient's general medical condition must always be the primary concern in the immediate posttraumatic phase of facial injury. It is rare for a patient to die as a direct result of maxillofacial injuries, yet because of the alarming nature, grotesqueness, and apparent severity of facial injuries, personnel may give these injuries priority over more critical problems.

In the absence of gross soft tissue injury, facial fractures are most often treated several days after initial assessment when an accurate plan for reduction can be developed through definitive radiological evaluation and patient assessment and the soft tissue swelling resolves. Three basic principles of treatment are (1) preservation of life; (2) maintenance of function, specifically the masticatory apparatus; and (3) restoration of appearance.

Maxillofacial Fractures

An arbitrary dividing line in fractures of the jaws is at the level of occlusal contact of the teeth. Fractures above this level involve the multiple bones making up the framework of the middle third of the face, specifically the zygoma, zygomatic arch, maxilla, and nasal and orbital bones. Fractures below this level involve the mandible and its articulations, the bilateral temporomandibular joints (TMJ). In the middle third of the face, displacement is produced primarily by trauma itself, while in the mandible the pull of the attached muscles is a major cause of distraction of the fractured segment.

MANDIBULAR FRACTURES

The classic signs and symptoms of fracture of the mandible are (1) history of trauma; (2) malocclusion; (3) pain; (4) abnormal mobility or crepitus of the fracture segments; (5) interference with function and decreased range of motion; (6) deformity, either facial deformity or deformity of the dental arches; (7) deviation on opening; (8) swelling and ecchymosis; (9) mental nerve anesthesia; and (10) radiological confirmation.

As with any facial fracture, the primary consideration in the treatment of fractures of the mandible is the assessment and treatment of the general condition of the patient. Mandibular fractures are rarely treated at the time of injury in the absence of gross soft tissue wounds.

There are several approaches to the examination of a patient to make the diagnosis of mandibular fracture. Extra- and intraoral examinations, as well as a radiological survey, are required to complete the assessment of mandibular trauma.

Examination and Diagnosis

Extraoral Examination

This will usually reveal unilateral or bilateral swelling, deformity, and ecchymosis associated with the ascending ramus or body of the mandible or both. The mandible should be palpated beginning at the mandibular condyle and proceeding along the entire length of the mandibular border, and any tenderness or break in contour of the posterior or inferior border should be noted. Point tenderness is pathognomonic of fracture and frequently a step deformity may be noted at the inferior border. Bilateral inferior alveolar nerves run through the inferior alveolar canal of the mandible and terminate as the mental nerves that supply sensation to the lower lip. Numbness of the lower lip on one or both sides is a strong indication of mandibular fracture.

Intraoral Examination

Bloodstained saliva will be evident in the mouth shortly after injury and if sufficient time has elapsed prior to examination, a marked fetor oris may be noted. The lower dental arch should be examined for disruption of arch continuity, gross malalignment of the teeth should be noted, and the teeth inspected for looseness. Malocclusion may indicate mandibular fracture. In cases where abnormal occlusion is suspected to have existed prior to the fracture, careful inspection of the wear facets on the teeth should be made. More simply, the patient should be asked to bite on the back teeth as if chewing, and tell the examiner if the bite has changed.

Movement of the mandible is also important. The patient should place the mouth through a full range of motion, with protrusion, lateral excursion, opening and closing, and any limitation of motion or associated pain should be noted. Unilateral subcondylar fractures will cause the mouth to deviate toward the side of fracture on maximum opening. The buccolingual sulcus of the mandible and the mucobuccal and labial gutters should be palpated and these areas examined for tenderness or alteration in contour, break in continuity of the mucosa, or existence of ecchymoses or a sublingual hematoma. A large sublingual hematoma can compromise the airway.

Roentgenographic Examination

A routine x-ray film series of the mandible involves three views: a posteroanterior (PA) view of the face and skull, and right and left lateral oblique views. The whole outline of the mandible is visible in the PA view, but owing to the superimposition of the zygomatic bone and the mastoid process, it may be impossible to accurately interpret the region of the condylar head. In the lateral oblique views, the outline of the mandible may be visualized from the first premolar to the condyle. In all cases, films of both sides of the mandible should be obtained to rule out bilateral or multiple fractures.

Perhaps the best roentgenogram for suspected fracture of the mandible is the panoramic view of the maxilla and mandible. This view is essentially a clear curved surface tomogram at the level of the facial bones taken by an x-ray beam moving around the head. The problem areas that frequently occur in interpretation with the PA and lateral oblique views are virtually eliminated.

Classification of Mandibular Fractures by Region

By site, the most common area of fracture is the angle of the mandible, followed closely by the condyle, molar, and mental regions. The symphysis is least frequently fractured due to the thickness of this area.

Alveolar Fractures

The most common type of mandibular fracture is a fracture of the alveolus, or tooth-bearing segment of the mandible. Alveolar fractures are most frequently observed in the anterior or incisor region, since this area is more directly exposed to trauma. Viable teeth should be preserved even if they have been avulsed, and no segments of alveolus should be removed if they are firmly attached to mucoperiosteum (Fig. 157-1). Injudicious debridement of the oral cavity will leave the patient with large defects in the alveolus that cannot be corrected prosthetically. Direct pressure should be applied with gauze sponges to the attached dental segments and they should then be covered with a saline-soaked sponge. Most alveolar fractures can then be stabilized with wires or arch bar fixation.

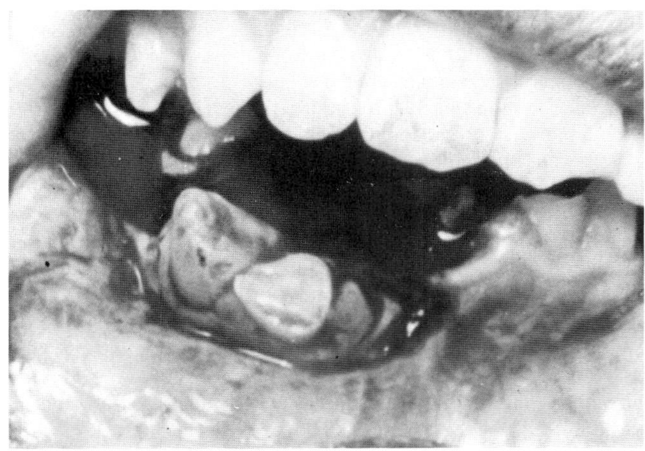

Fig. 157-1. Alveolar fracture with avulsed teeth. Preservation of supporting bone and viable teeth is an important early consideration.

Condyle Fractures

Unilateral fractures of the condyle will cause the jaw to deviate toward the side of fracture on maximum opening. In a bilateral subcondylar fracture the patient usually has an anterior bite, occlusion on the posterior molars, and no contact of the incisor teeth.

Symphysis Fractures

Fractures of the mandibular symphysis are easily noted by observation of displacement of the lower incisor teeth, disruption of arch continuity, and the ease with which segments can be moved on bimanual palpation. Bilateral fracture in the mental region can result in loss of anterior tongue support with possible acute airway obstruction (Fig. 157-2).

Angle and Body Fractures

Unfavorable angle fractures are usually acted upon by muscle pull of the pterygomasseteric sling causing the proximal fragment to ride superiorly. This is best found by roentgenographic examination.

Edentulous Fractures

Since many teeth may be missing in one or more of the fragments and the occlusion may be difficult to evaluate, the only way to accurately diagnose edentulous or partially edentulous mandibular fractures is by roentgenography. Always salvage dentures from the edentulous who has sustained facial fractures. The dentures can not only be used to splint bony fragments, but they may also help maintain occlusal vertical dimension.

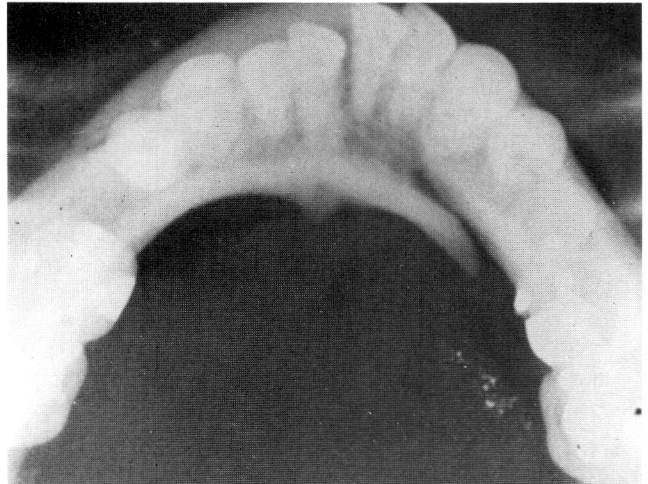

Fig. 157-2. Occlusal view of the mandible showing symphysis fracture with telescoping fragments.

Treatment

Most mandibular fractures can be reduced and fixed in position by wiring upper and lower teeth in occlusion. Nonviable, loose teeth in the fracture site should be removed unless essential for splinting and alignment of the fractures. When many teeth are missing in any or all of the fragments, the problem is more complex but still lends itself to surgical management.

All dental appliances (bridges, etc.) may be utilized in intraoral fixation of fractures and should be preserved for the oral surgeon.

When there are teeth on either side of the fracture site that can be brought into satisfactory occlusion with opposing maxillary teeth, a closed reduction is indicated. When the fracture line is unfavorable and posterior to the last tooth in the dental arch, or in a large edentulous segment, open reduction is most often required.

The use of rigid internal fixation for mandibular fixation has become increasingly useful with the development of mini-plates that are both safe and effective, as well as cosmetically acceptable. The goal of rigid internal fixation is the early pain-free mobilization of the fractured mandible without jeopardizing healing. Rigid fixation affords absolute stabilization through absence of motion between the fractured ends or between the plate and bone enabling the patient to eat with intermaxillary fixation almost immediately after surgery.

Tetanus prophylaxis must be instituted in any case of mandibular fracture where soft tissue injuries exist and there is a risk of contamination. Since most mandibular fractures are compounded intraorally, the risk of infection is always present. Antibiotic therapy is indicated with penicillin or a cephalosporin, the current drugs of choice. However, decision on antibiotic maintenance therapy should be made in consultation with the patient's surgeon.

MIDFACIAL FRACTURES

Since fractures of the midface can be divided into several categories by anatomic region, each type of fracture will be discussed individually. Obviously these fractures can occur in any and all combinations depending on the multiplicity and direction of force. Once the patient is stabilized, immediate treatment of midfacial and mandibular fractures is mainly supportive. Avulsed or partially avulsed teeth should be preserved and reimplanted as soon as possible, preferably within an hour if completely avulsed. In the balance of gross overlying soft tissue injuries, most fractures can be reduced in several days when swelling resolves and facial incisions can be placed more aesthetically.

Zygomatic Arch

Isolated fractures of the zygomatic arch are uncommon, because the force must be directly over the midlateral position of the arch to break it.

Clinical Features

A facial dimpling or depression over the affected region of the zygomatic arch may be evident. This depression may be palpated to elicit point tenderness. In addition, owing to mechanical impingement of the coronoid process of the mandible by the inwardly fractured arch, the patient may not be able to open the mouth or, rarely, may have a partially open mouth and be unable to close it or move it in lateral excursion.

Radiological Examination

The zygomatic arches are best visualized by a modified basal view of the skull. Other names for the survey include submentaloccipital, submental-vertical, or jug-handle view of the skull (Fig. 157-3).

Treatment

Treatment of zygomatic arch fractures is usually delayed. Criteria for surgical intervention are residual cosmetic deformity or restriction of mandibular motion. Frequently several days elapse for resolution of facial swelling before surgery is contemplated.

Zygoma or Zygomatic-Maxillary Complex

The zygoma has major articulations with the frontal bone, maxilla, zygomatic process of the temporal bone, and lateral wall of the sinus, and it is usually subjected to multiple fractures at or near these articulations. A blow to the zygomatic prominence is unlikely to shatter the bone, but probably will result in a line of fracture at the frontal zygomatic suture line; the zygomaticomaxillary suture line or infraorbital rim; the lateral wall of the maxillary sinus at the buttress of the zygoma; or at the zygomatic arch slightly behind the suture, between the short temporal process of the zygomatic bone and the longer zygomatic process of the temporal bone.

Frequently the central portion of the orbital floor will also fracture as part of the zygomaticomaxillary complex. A comminuted depressed fracture may lead to serious complications with entrapment of extraocular muscles. This type of orbital floor fracture should not be confused with the blowout type of orbital fracture.

A pure blowout is caused by direct intraocular trauma, forcing the eye posteriorly, at which time a plunger effect takes place upon the surrounding structures, particularly the relatively incompressible periorbital fat. The dense, strong, laterally angled outer wall of the orbit resists this force that is reflected downward on the thin bone of the floor of the orbit. The bone is forced into the underlying cavity of the maxillary antrum, thus the term *orbital blowout*. Extraocular muscle entrapment may occur with this type of fracture.

Clinical Features

The major clinical signs of a fracture of the zygomatic bone or zygomaticomaxillary complex are (1) edema of the cheek and periorbita; (2) facial flattening shortly after injury or after initial edema subsides; (3) circumorbital or subconjunctival ecchymosis; (4) unilateral epistaxis; (5) anesthesia of the cheek, upper lip, teeth, and gum; (6) step deformity and tenderness over the inferior orbital margin, the frontal zygomatic suture line area, the zygomatic arch, and the lateral wall of the maxillary sinus (intraorally in the region of the zygomatic buttress); (7) diplopia with possible asymmetry of the ocular levels; (8) limitation of mandibular movement; and (9) emphysema of the overlying tissues.

Within 2 or 3 h of injury, the underlying skeletal deformity will be masked by edema. Therefore a great number of these injuries remain undiagnosed until swelling subsides so that resultant disfigurement can be evaluated.

A characteristic flattening of the upper part of the cheek can be seen, either immediately following injury or after the acute phase of edema has subsided, usually in 3 to 5 days (Fig. 157-4).

Palpation, beginning at the medial aspect of the superior orbital margin, will often elicit step deformities at the infraorbital rim and at the frontal zygomatic suture area. The tip of the index finger should be carefully passed around the entire orbital rim. Owing to the thinness of the overlying tissue, step defects are usually easily palpated. Then palpation should proceed along the prominence of the zygoma and along the zygomatic arch. Point tenderness at the fracture sites is usually elicited.

Circumorbital ecchymosis and severe lateral subconjunctival hemorrhage are often present. Carefully examine the pupillary level on both sides to detect unilateral depression of the ocular level. Visual acuity and the range of ocular movement should be tested. Complaints of diplopia or blurring of vision should be noted.

Limitation of mandibular movement may be a result of mechanical obstruction by the depressed zygomatic bone or arch. Intraorally, ecchymosis of the upper buccal sulcus is often evident. Anesthesia of the teeth, gum, cheek, upper lip, and lateral ala nasi on the affected side is caused by injury to the infraorbital nerve at the zygomatico-

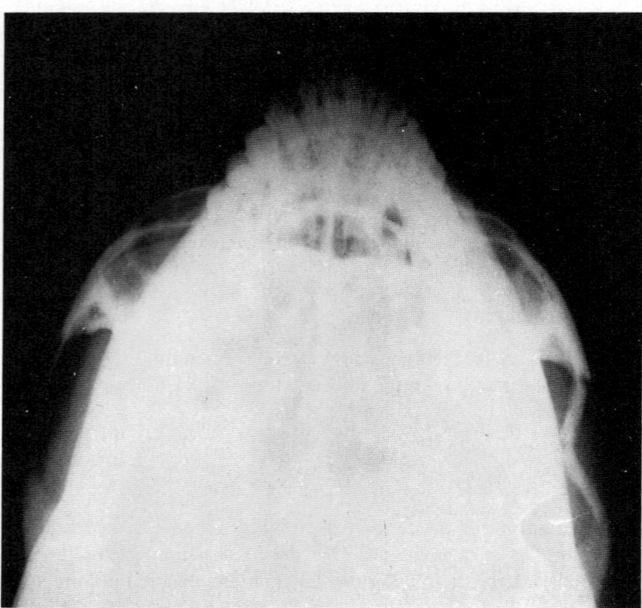

Fig. 157-3. Basal view of skull demonstrating unilateral fracture of the zygomatic arch.

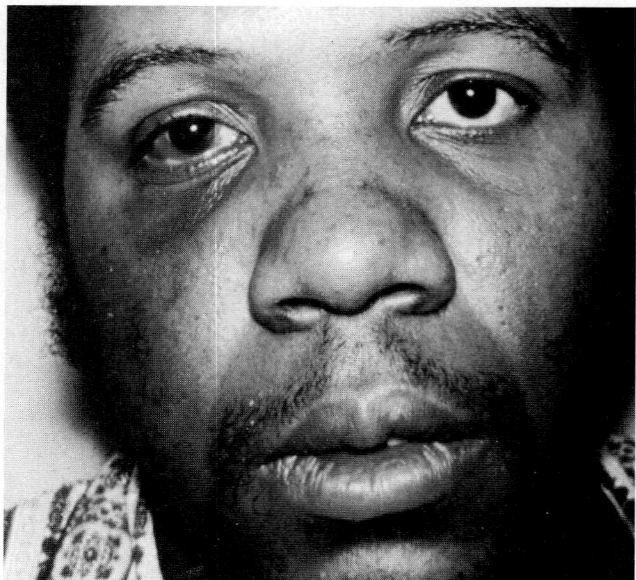

Fig. 157-4. Clinical presentation of fractured zygoma. Note facial flattening and lateral subconjunctival hemorrhage.

maxillary fracture site. Subcutaneous emphysema may be caused by fracture of the lateral antral wall at the zygomatic buttress. Unilateral epistaxis may occur, but this usually ceases spontaneously.

Radiological Examination

The Waters' projection and a basal view of the skull are most important in the initial evaluation of fractures of the zygomatic bone. The Waters' or occipitomental projection, commonly used to visualize the maxillary sinus, offers complete visualization of three of the four areas that commonly fracture and displace in zygomaticomaxillary complex injuries: the frontozygomatic suture area; the zygomaticomaxillary or infraorbital area; and the lateral wall of the maxillary sinus. The presence of opacity or an air-fluid level in the sinus may signify antral hemorrhage secondary to trauma.

A basal view of the skull demonstrates the fourth point of fracture at the zygomatic arch. This view can also demonstrate inward displacement of the prominence of the zygoma and confirm intrusion or rotation of that bone in relation to the undisplaced zygoma on the opposite side. Further evaluation can be obtained through orbital tomograms that confirm fractures at the aforementioned articulations, as well as suspected fractures of the floor of the orbit. Frequently, herniation of orbital contents through the roof of the maxillary antrum can be seen on tomography (see section on CT in maxillofacial trauma).

Treatment

The treatment is surgical through a number of approaches, the most common of which is open reduction and wire fixation or antral packing.

Again, rigid fixation can be used, especially when the surgeon's goals are to promote stabilization after anatomic reduction or to avoid intermaxillary fixation. Absolute stabilization is helpful after reduction of midface fracture in that it permits undisturbed healing. Rigid internal fixation applies forces that will exceed the functioning forces at all times with direct bone contact.

Orbital Floor Fractures

Fracture of the orbital floor may occur as a component of a massive zygomaticomaxillary complex fracture, which usually causes comminution of the thin orbital floor, or as an isolated fracture—the less common orbital blowout fracture—caused by a very rapid increase in intraorbital pressure. The force producing a blowout fracture is usually delivered by a blunt object directed at the globe and lids (e.g., a fist or ball) that is slightly larger than the orbital inlet and penetrates the orbital space for only a short distance. The sudden increase in pressure fractures the bony orbit at areas of weakness, usually at the orbital floor or the medial wall.

Direct entrapment of extraocular muscles is rare. In some instances a large volume of orbital soft tissue may protrude into the maxillary sinus, lowering the globe level, and if the soft tissue is not retrieved and the orbital floor reconstructed, orbital mobility will be impaired.

Clinical Features

The two most common presenting ocular problems from orbital floor injury are diplopia and lowering of the globe. Diplopia occurs particularly in zygomaticomaxillary fractures when the thin orbital floor is fractured and comminuted as the stronger zygomatic complex is depressed downward and medially.

Evaluation of the orbit and contents is best performed before periorbital swelling has occurred, if possible. Corneal abrasions or scleral tears must be sought and foreign bodies on the ocular surface carefully removed. Having determined that there is no penetrating injury to the globe, evert the upper lid and check the conjunctival cul-de-sac for foreign material. Retinal function should be assessed by visual acuity testing, reactivity to light and accommodation, and ophthalmoscopy. Also evaluate extraocular muscle function. Diplopia may follow soft

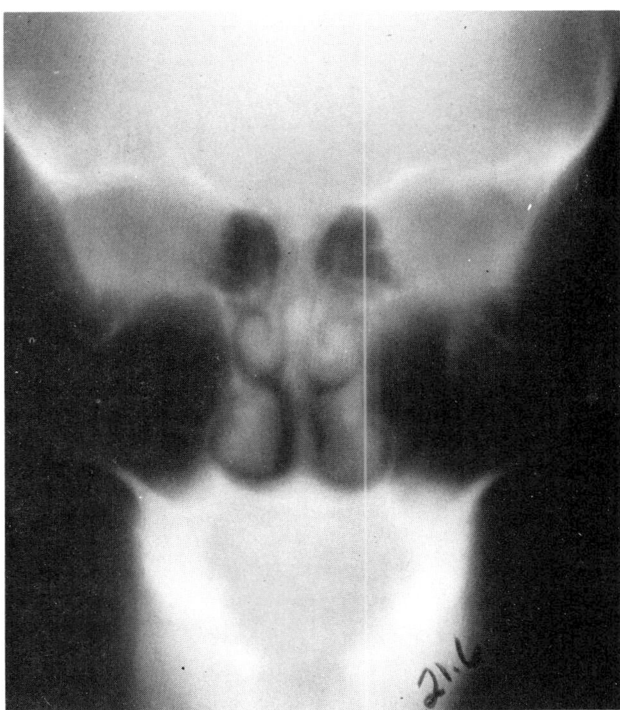

Fig. 157-5. Orbital tomogram showing classical "teardrop" herniation of orbital tissue into the maxillary sinus.

tissue entrapment of the inferior rectus or oblique muscles, disruption of muscular attachments, interruption of muscle innervation, orbital hemorrhage, or edema. Carefully inspect the anterior chamber of the eye for presence of a hyphema. Such hemorrhage, secondary to torn blood vessels in the peripheral iris, can cause blindness if not treated.

X-Ray Findings

Diagnostic studies should include Waters' view x-rays and tomograms. On x-ray, the orbital floor may appear fragmented and displaced bony fragments may be seen in the maxillary sinus. In orbital floor fractures, orbital soft tissue may be seen protruding into the upper portion of the maxillary sinus (Fig. 157-5). In either fracture there may be emphysema of the soft tissues of the orbit. The soft tissue shadow on the x-ray usually appears as a semilunar mass protruding into the upper half of the maxillary sinus.

Treatment

The goal of treatment of orbital floor fractures is to relieve restricted extraocular muscle function and elevate the lowered globe. This can be accomplished through an infraorbital approach, which permits direct inspection of the floor, removal of the small pieces of comminuted bone, and reconstruction of the orbital floor with an implant of alloplastic material or autogenous bone or cartilage.

MAXILLARY FRACTURES

Fractures of the alveolar process alone are the most common form of maxillary fracture and have been previously discussed.

Le Fort Fractures

The characteristic of most maxillary fractures is a separation of attachments to the bony framework of the face or the skull. Studies by the French scientist, René Le Fort, at the turn of the century, produced the Le Fort classification of midfacial maxillary fractures (Fig. 157-6).

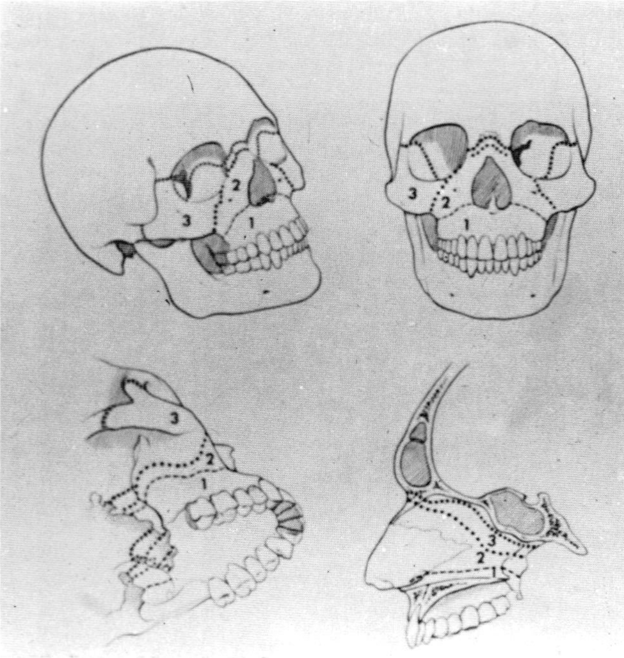

Fig. 157-6. Schematic of midfacial fracture lines: Le Fort I, II, and III. (From Dingman RO, Natvig P: *Surgery of Facial Fractures*. Philadelphia, Saunders, 1964, p. 248. Used by permission.)

Le Fort I or Horizontal Maxillary Fracture

As in all the Le Fort-type fractures, a free-floating jaw is encountered. The horizontal fracture is one in which the body of the maxilla is separated from the base of the skull above the level of the palate, and below the attachment of the zygomatic process. The fracture line runs from the lateral nasal apertures, along the lateral wall of the maxillary sinuses bilaterally, and across the pterygomaxillary tissue to the lateral pterygoid plates.

Diagnosis of Le Fort I Fractures

Many horizontal maxillary fractures are not significantly displaced and their diagnosis may be missed. Displacement is dependent upon the force of the blow and the muscular pull. Diagnosis is most easily made by grasping the alveolar process and anterior teeth between the thumb and forefinger and causing a forward-backward motion. The visualization of movement of the entire upper dental arch means that the patient has, at the very least, a Le Fort I fracture. Roentgenographic survey often does not establish the diagnosis.

Le Fort II or Pyramidal Fracture

The pyramidal fracture consists of vertical fractures through the facial aspects of the maxilla extending upwards to the nasal and ethmoid bones. The fractures extend through the maxillary sinuses and the infraorbital rims bilaterally across the bridge of the nose.

Clinical Features

The entire midface, nose, lips, and eyes are swollen. Bilateral subconjunctival hemorrhage is present and there is often blood in the nares. If clear fluid is seen in the nose, cerebrospinal rhinorrhea must be differentiated from mucus extravasation. A Dextrostix reagent strip can be applied to the fluid as a test for glucose, or a sample of fluid can be taken for glucose analysis. An empirical test consists of collecting some of the fluid on a cloth and if it stiffens on drying, it is mucus. Any patient with suspected cerebrospinal rhinorrhea should be evaluated by the neurosurgical service prior to obtaining a consultation with the oral and maxillofacial surgery service. Cerebrospinal rhinorrhea is a result of fracture of the cribriform plate of the ethmoid bone. It is for this reason that a clinical examination for suspected Le Fort II fracture must be done gently with as little movement as possible. However, the diagnosis of Le Fort II fracture can usually be confirmed by grasping the premaxilla, as with the Le Fort I fracture, in conjunction with palpation of the base of the nose (Fig. 157-7).

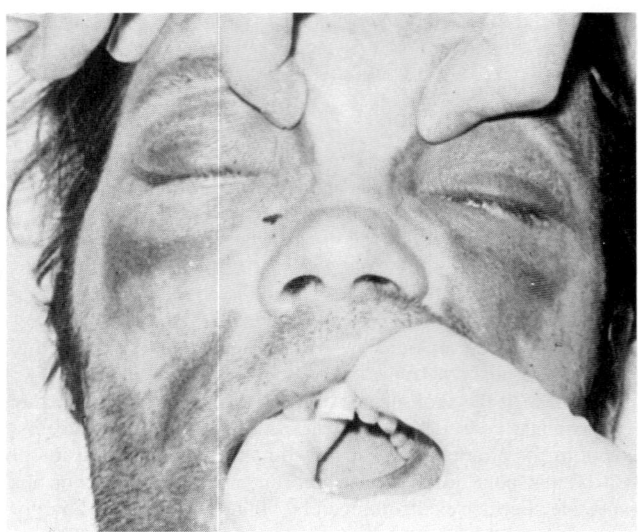

Fig. 157-7. Method of examination for Le Fort II fractures of maxilla.

Radiological Examination

The diagnosis of Le Fort II fracture is usually confirmed by a Waters' view roentgenogram for evaluation of the infraorbital rims bilaterally, together with bilateral orbital tomograms. Films of the nasal bones should also be ordered.

Le Fort III Fracture or Craniofacial Dysjunction

The Le Fort III fracture extends through the frontozygomatic suture lines bilaterally, across the orbits, and through the base of the nose and the ethmoid region (Fig. 157-8). The lateral rim of the orbit is separated and the infraorbital rim may be fractured, along with associated fractures of the zygoma. A pyramidal or horizontal fracture may also be present.

Clinical Features

A characteristic "dishface" may be evident because of retroposition of the entire midface at a 45° angle, along the base of the skull. On profile, the face appears spooned-out in the nasal area and the patient often has an anterior open bite. As the face is repositioned by the force of impact, the teeth in contact on occlusion are the posterior molars while there is no contact of the anterior or incisor teeth. Cerebrospinal rhinorrhea is more common than with the Le Fort II fracture. Palpation should be done gently (Fig. 157-9). If movement of the midface and zygoma occur concurrently, LeFort III fracture is confirmed.

Radiological Examination

A Waters' view roentgenogram and bilateral orbital tomograms confirm the diagnosis.

Treatment

The usual treatment of midfacial fractures is to support the sagging face and restore normal occlusion. The bones of the face must be mobilized and displacements of the zygoma, lacrimal, and other facial bones corrected. Fractures of the nasal bones are usually treated by

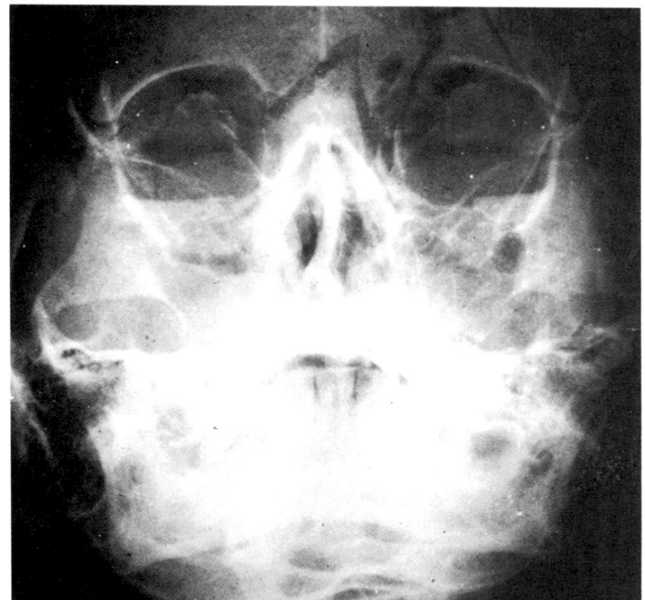

Fig. 157-8. Waters' view roentgenogram of Le Fort III fracture. Note bilateral fracture at the frontozygomatic area and the craniofacial dysjunction.

closed reduction with intranasal reduction and manual molding. Tetanus toxoid and antibiotic prophylaxis should be administered.

NASO-ORBITAL INJURIES

Occasionally, a nasal fracture may traumatize a small vessel (e.g., the anterior ethmoid artery), which may bleed and obscure the nasal airway. An anterior nasal pack inserted for 10 to 15 min can often control anterior bleeding. For posterior nasal bleeding, a Foley catheter with a 30-mL balloon can be inserted through the nose into the nasopharynx, inflated with 10 to 20 mL of saline, and then pulled forward. If this fails to control the bleeding, a posterior nasal pack may be placed, supplemented by an anterior pack.

Nasal fractures should be reduced as soon as possible, unless the patient has more urgent injuries. The key to good reduction is adequate local anesthesia. Once the fracture is reduced, stabilize the nose using a splint. Every attempt should be made to return a displaced cartilaginous septum onto the vomerine groove. A nonreduced septum can distort the shape of the nose at a later date despite adequate nasal bone reduction.

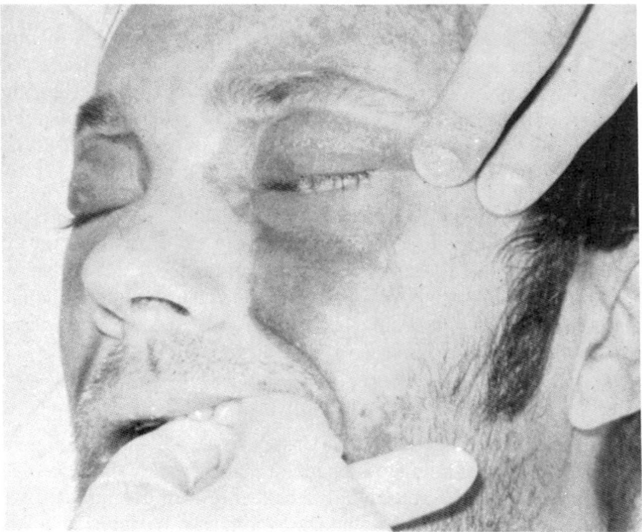

Fig. 157-9. Movement of zygomas on examination indicates probable Le Fort III fracture.

Close all lacerations of the nasal mucosa to prevent nasal webbing. This holds true especially for lacerations near the internal valve, that is, between the upper lateral cartilage and the nasal septum. Even a small change in the diameter of this internal nasal opening causes a great change in airflow through the nose.

Blunt trauma to the naso-orbital area may cause disruption of the interorbital area and detachment of the medial canthal ligaments. Because of the resilience of the lateral canthal ligament, increased intercanthal distance, or telecanthus, will result. It is not uncommon to see an intercanthal distance of 40 or 45 mm in naso-orbital injuries in the white adult, as opposed to the usual intercanthal distance of approximately 35 mm. The medial canthal ligament is normally attached to the anterior and posterior lacrimal crests of the lacrimal bone; the majority of the attachments are to the anterior lacrimal crest. Between these two leaves of the medial canthal ligament the nasolacrimal duct passes through in the nasolacrimal fossa. In naso-orbital injury the medial portion of the palpebral fissure assumes an almond configuration, in contrast to its normal elliptical shape.

Clinical Signs

The triad of a widened bridge of the nose, telecanthus, and an almond-shaped palpebral fissure following trauma to the midface area should lead the clinician to suspect a nasal skeleton fracture along with disruption of the medial canthal ligaments.

X-Ray Studies

Radiographic examination should include Waters' projection, x-ray of the paranasal sinuses, and tomograms when indicated.

COMPUTED TOMOGRAPHY IN MAXILLOFACIAL TRAUMA

The use of computed tomography (CT) in the evaluation of maxillofacial injuries has been extremely helpful in assessing orbital fractures, midfacial trauma, and potential airway obstruction. This technique not only can be used when conventional techniques fail but actually offers some distinct advantages as a primary assessment tool.

The advantages are

1. Soft tissues are clearly displayed and related to the bony framework so that exact margins of lesions can be defined.
2. Both axial and coronal views are available as well as sagittal reconstruction.
3. Blurring does not occur as with conventional tomograms.
4. There is approximately 40 percent less radiation exposure than with the latter.
5. Density determination and identification (e.g., blood, pus, muscle) of tissues are possible by measuring their absorption values.
6. It is the diagnostic modality of choice in the assessment of intracranial lesions.

Orbital and Midfacial Fractures

Fractures of this region are often complicated by edema, making initial clinical assessment of bony injury difficult. Since the bones are thin and lie in various planes, superimposition often occurs and may be further obscured by the dense cranial base.

Fractures of the cribriform plate of the ethmoid can be identified, which is especially important in the diagnosis of cerebrospinal fluid leakage. In addition, persistent leaks can be evaluated by the intrathecal placement of metrizamide (Fig. 157-10).

CT is the only technique that clearly shows the complete skeletal

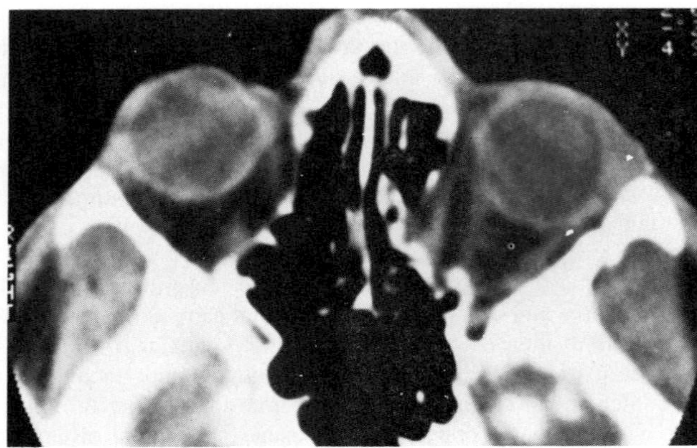

Fig. 157-10. Orbital CT scan showing enophthalmos and fracture of the medial wall of the orbit. Note that the extraocular muscles can also be visualized.

distortion often occurring in middle third fractures. The amount of comminution and degree of displacement, especially at the posterior aspects of the maxilla, are often unobtainable by a routine radiographic study.

DISTURBANCES OF THE TEMPOROMANDIBULAR JOINT

Dislocation of the Mandible

Acute dislocation causes considerable pain, discomfort, and swelling. The anatomic structure of the TMJ fossa and anterior articular eminence of that fossa may predispose to dislocation. The weakness of the connective tissue capsule forming the temporomandibular ligaments also may be a predisposing factor. The capsule may have loose attachments, may be excessively stretched, and more rarely, may be torn. Dislocation is generally caused by trauma to the chin while the mouth is in the open position, but it may occur while yawning, laughing excessively, or opening the mouth widely to chew food. Dislocation can also occur by overstretching the mouth while the patient is under general anesthesia. In addition, hysterical dislocations have been recorded.

Clinical Features

In an acute dislocation, the condyle becomes locked anterior to the articular eminence and is prevented from sliding back by muscular trismus. The external pterygoid, masseter, and internal pterygoid muscles then go into spasm. Characteristically the patient has the mouth open, and is unable to close the anterior teeth. Bilateral dislocation will thus present with an anterior open bite, but if the dislocation is unilateral, the jaw is displaced toward the unaffected side. The head of the condyle may produce swelling in front of the ear below the zygomatic arch. Since the jaw is locked in an open position, talking and swallowing are difficult. Examination of the TMJs will demonstrate the condyle in front of the anterior articular eminence of the joint fossa.

Radiological Examination

The roentgenogram may be an important aid in differentiating dislocation from fracture of the condyle, since these conditions may produce similar occlusal disturbances. It should be obtained prior to reduction to assure that no fracture is present.

Treatment

Temporomandibular joint dislocation can usually be successfully treated by manual manipulation. Occasionally, owing to the intensity of the muscle spasms, the muscles of mastication may have to be injected with a local anesthetic solution to enable them to relax. More frequently, 10 mg of diazepam is injected slowly to aid in muscle relaxation and to allay some of the anxiety of the patient during the relocation procedure.

The manipulation consists of grasping the mandible with both hands, one on each side, with the physician facing the patient, thus reversing the process of dislocation. The patient should be in a sitting position with the physician straddling the patient's knees. The thumbs are then wrapped in gauze and placed on the occlusal surfaces of the posterior teeth with the fingertips placed around the inferior border of the mandible in the region of the mandibular angles. Downward pressure is then exerted while the jaw is opened wide to free the condyle from the stuck position anterior to the eminence. The chin is then pressed back after it has been forced down so that the mouth is closed while the condyle returns to the fossa. Since the jaw may snap back quickly, the gauze protects the physician's thumbs from injury.

After reduction of an acute dislocation, the patient is cautioned against further wide excursions of the mandible, and placed on a soft diet for 1 week. Analgesics and muscle relaxants help override the acute phase of trauma.

In chronic dislocations, or in acute recurrences, a Barton bandage is applied for 1 week to prevent the patient from opening the jaw widely. In severe cases, intermaxillary wiring and fixation may be applied to restrict and control jaw motion during healing. Chronic dislocation may occasionally require surgical intervention, with most procedures aimed at recontour of the articular eminence to prevent dislocation or eliminate locking.

Temporomandibular Joint Dysfunction

The TMJ dysfunction syndrome, usually referred to as myofascial pain dysfunction, is a form of fibrositis that accounts for the majority of patients who seek treatment for TMJ pain. The diagnosis is suspected when an adult patient, usually female, presents with pain in the region of the jaw, earache, "popping" or crepitus, and difficulty with chewing or opening the mouth. Other symptoms include burning sensation in the tongue or roof of the mouth, bruxism, tinnitus, and vertigo. Clinical evidence suggests that pain in the neck, shoulders, arms, and fingers may be related to disorders in the cervical spine that may be associated with temporomandibular disorders. Muscle pain often affects the temporalis, the masseter, and muscles of the occipital areas and the neck.

Physical examination of the TMJ may elicit tenderness on palpation of the joint capsule and of the muscles of mastication. Patients with TMJ disorders fall into three diagnostic categories:

1. Those with joint abnormalities resulting from trauma or from conditions such as ankylosis, synovitis, arthritis, and neoplasm;
2. Those with structural defects of the articular disc (meniscus), ligaments of the disc, condyles, glenoid fossae, or articular tubercles;
3. Those who present with pain or restricted jaw motion but do not have evidence of organic disease or structural defects.

No clear etiology has been established. It is believed that the disease is a neuromuscular disturbance and that occlusal factors are contributory in nature. In addition to irregularities of the teeth and occlusion, factors such as trauma, psychic tension, and neuromuscular habits, such as bruxism and clenching of teeth, are all considered to play a major role in the development of this syndrome.

Clinical Features

Typically, the patient with the TMJ syndrome will have unilateral facial pain, mainly around the immediate region of the joint. The pain is of a dull, aching character that intensifies toward evening because of the use of the jaw during the day. Pain may be referred to the temporal, supraorbital, occipital, and cervical regions.

Commonly, the patient will have acute otalgia mimicking external otitis or otitis media, yet the otologic examination is negative. Inability to open the mouth widely is another complaint. The mouth may deviate on opening toward the side of the mandibular dysfunction or facial pain. Stiffness of the jaw generally worsens with use. Myofascial spasm or trismus may also be associated with clicking of the affected joint.

Clinical examination will usually reveal acute tenderness over the lateral capsular ligament of the TMJ, anterior to the external auditory canal. Placing the fingers on the joint and having the patient open and close the mouth will elicit this tenderness. The masseter and the internal pterygoid muscles may also be tender.

Radiological Examination

Radiological diagnosis is usually unrewarding. TMJ films are taken in the open and closed position. It is uncommon to find irregularities of the joint unless the patient has temporomandibular degenerative joint disease. In that case, osteophyte proliferation and flattening out or erosions of the head of the condyle are characteristic changes.

Treatment

The TMJ syndrome is treated by physiotherapy, dietary restrictions, analgesics, muscle relaxants, and occlusive therapy. Warm, moist compresses should be applied to the affected side of the face for 15 min four times a day for 7 to 10 days. A pureed diet should be followed for 1 to 2 weeks. Analgesics and muscle relaxants help disrupt the pain-muscle spasm-pain cycle.

It is surprising how often relief can be obtained by placing the upper and lower jaws in their proper occlusal relationship and maintaining the joint in its maximum rest position. When the acute phase has subsided, or as an adjunct to the treatment of the acute phase, the patient should be referred for a dental consultation for equilibration of occlusion, and for possible construction of bite splints to disarticulate the posterior teeth and help relieve muscle spasm.

Direct intraarticular injection of steroids is beneficial in many patients who do not respond to conservative therapy, if they show signs of synovitis.

Internal Derangements of the TMJ

In internal derangements and dislocation of the TMJ the menisci become displaced because of tears, perforation, or stretching of the posterior attachments. The term *internal derangements of the TMJ* refers to any disturbance between the articular components in the joint proper. It implies a localized structural derangement that interferes with the smooth function of the joint. It has been adopted in the last few years mainly for changes in the disc-condyle relationship. The disc is most commonly displaced in an anteromedial direction. It often produces pain and/or functional disturbances in the masticatory system. It is most common in young adults, particularly women. The patient often hears a click in the ear with each mouth opening. The joint may lock in the closed position, severe pain inhibiting opening of the mouth. Range of motion of the jaw is limited and with opening of the mouth there may be deviation to the affected side.

Determine whether the click is accompanied by pain. Patients with internal derangements frequently experience an increase in pain before the click followed by a decrease in pain afterward. It is important to notice whether the noise changes, whether it occurs more or less frequently or later during opening, or whether it gets louder or changes otherwise. Changing joint noise may indicate the presence of an active etiologic factor and progression of the disorder. Crepitus is generally considered to represent advanced disease and occurs as a result of movement across irregular surfaces. Internal-derangement patients typically report having previously had a clicking TMJ followed by a period of no joint noise (associated with locking) and then a grating or grinding noise. Frequently crepitus indicates a perforation of the disc or its attachments. This is especially true when degenerative changes are observed in the radiographs. Limited range of movement presents in three forms that usually occur together: opening, protrusive, and lateral movements. Normal opening is 35–50 mm when measured from the tip of the upper to lower incisors. When the disc is anteriorly displaced and does not reduce to a normal position during opening, the patient has limited opening (closed lock). The closed lock condition may be either intermittent or persistent. With intermittent closed lock, the patient usually reports that their jaw suddenly catches or gets stuck. If pain is present, it generally is reported to be worse during the closed lock condition. Disc position is most easily determined with an MRI. Treatment may be surgical via arthroscopy or open arthroplasty.

Osteoarthritis (OA or DJD)

Middle-aged to elderly patients with TMJ osteoarthritis complain of pain and crepitus in the jaw. The latter is evident on movement of the jaw and is worse at the end of the day. Tenderness and spurs may be noted. Conventional roentgenographs show thinning and loss of cortical bone, flattening of the joint contour and spurs in established disease. The roentgenograph is usually sufficient for diagnosis, but a CT scan may be required.

Rheumatoid Arthritis (RA)

Rheumatoid arthritis of the TMJ is almost always part of a generalized arthritic process but it may be the chief complaint, overshadowing other joints. The joint is limited in motion, tender and perhaps swollen. Roentgenographs show erosion of the head and neck of the condyle, flattening of the joint surface, and joint space narrowing. CT scans are particularly useful in the evaluation of RA.

SPREAD OF ODONTOGENIC INFECTION—FASCIAL PLANES OF HEAD AND NECK

Periapical, Periodontal Infections

Acute infections of the oral cavity and jaws run the gamut from minor to life-threatening. The most common infection is the periapical abscess or the acute alveolar abscess that usually begins in the periapical region as a result of nonvitality or degeneration of the pulp of a tooth. These infections are usually easily treated with endodontics or extraction. Periodontal abscesses adjacent to the crowns of teeth can cause acute suppuration and swelling of the marginal gingiva.

Treatment

Superficial drainage of these abscesses, as well as ongoing periodontal therapy, is usually sufficient treatment.

Pericoronal Infection

Impacted third molar teeth commonly present with pericoronal infection, which can occur at any time throughout life. The most usual periods of pericoronal infection occur in early adulthood when food debris or microorganisms are trapped between the gingival or gum tissue and the crown of an impacted or partially erupted tooth, causing acute swelling of the adjacent tissues.

Treatment

Pericoronal infection is generally best treated by irrigation with sterile saline solution, warm salt rinses for 24 to 48 h, and antibiotics.

As in all minor dental-associated infections, oral phenoxymethyl penicillin in dosages of 250 to 500 mg four times a day is the drug of choice and erythromycin in the same dosages if the patient is allergic to penicillin. In many instances, however, the progression of oral infection may cause acute facial cellulitis.

Facial Cellulitis

The severity of cellulitis depends upon the virulence of the organism, the resistance of the host, and the location and spread of infection through the fascial compartments.

The fascial spaces are formed by a deep cervical fascia that consists of the superficial and investing layer, the pretracheal layer, the prevertebral layer, and the carotid sheath. The superficial and investing layer surrounds the neck. Inferiorly, the fascia is attached from the clavicle, sternum, and the spine of the scapula, to the inferior border of the mandible, zygomatic arch, mastoid process, and superior nuchal line of the occipital bone. Anteriorly, it blends to be attached to the symphysis menti and the hyoid bone. Posteriorly, it is attached to the ligamentum nuchi and the spine of the seventh cervical vertebra. The fascia splits as it attaches to the inferior border of the mandible. It thus encloses the parotid gland and masseter and internal pterygoid muscles in the region of the ascending ramus. This split forms the masticator space.

Masticator Space Infection

Spread of infection, particularly in lower molar teeth, commonly invades the area between the internal pterygoid and masseter muscles. This space communicates superiorly above the level of the zygomatic arch into the superficial and deep temporal pouches. Since the mandibular periosteum is firmly attached inferiorly, infection tends to spread into the masticator space, and its extension inferiorly into the neck is prevented by the fascial reinforcement.

Clinical Features

Clinically, masticator space infection is dominated by trismus, pain, and swelling, usually within a few hours of acute onset (Fig. 157-11). The clinical signs increase rapidly to reach a peak in 3 to 5 days. Trismus is intense owing to severe irritation of both the masseter and internal pterygoid. As a result, visualization of the oral pharynx is often impossible, making intraoral evaluation of the source of infection extremely difficult. Patients with this infection require immediate hospital admission.

Treatment

High-dose intravenous antibiotic therapy, generally 15 to 20 million units of penicillin daily, or 600 to 900 mg of clindamycin q 8 h if anaerobes are suspected, is the treatment of choice. Cephalosporins such as cephazolin sodium 1 to 2 g IV q 8 h may also be used.

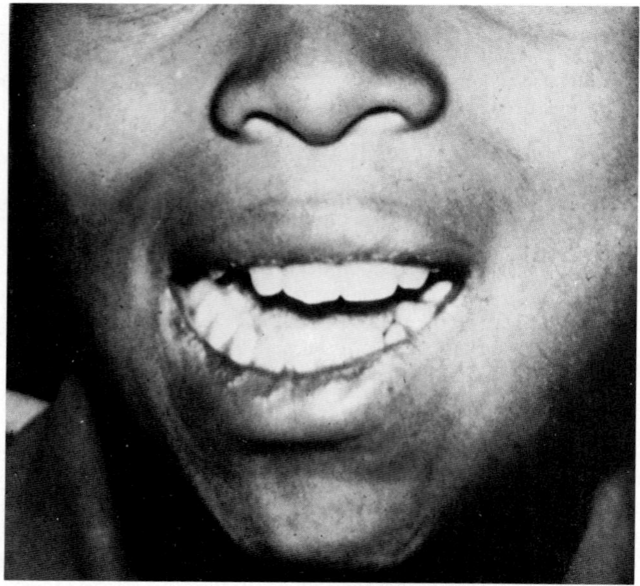

Fig. 157-11. Masticator space infection with trismus.

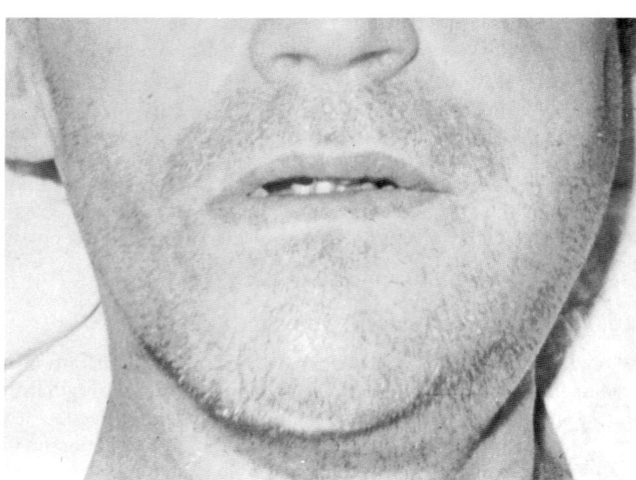

Fig. 157-12. Combined fascial space infection involving the masticator, parapharyngeal, and temporal spaces.

Parapharyngeal Space Infection

The lateral pharyngeal space or parapharyngeal space is deeply situated fascial space lying lateral to the pharynx and medial to the masticator space. It extends from the base of the skull to the level of the hyoid bone and is bound medially by the superior constrictor of the pharynx, laterally by the mandible and the internal pterygoid muscle, superiorly by the petrous portion of the temporal bone, and inferiorly by the submandibular gland and the posterior belly of the digastric muscle.

Infections of the parapharyngeal space are extremely serious (Fig. 157-12). This space is often involved by infections from the palatine tonsils, mastoid air cells, parotid gland, deep cervical lymph nodes, and teeth. Spread of dental infection directly from the masticator space is a common presentation.

Clinical Features

The clinical picture is marked by rapid onset, high fever, and marked swelling, usually obliterating the inferior border of the mandible and the lateral neck. There is severe pain due to the accumulation of pus and tissue fluid between the internal pterygoid and superior constrictor of the pharynx. The patient has marked trismus, difficulty swallowing, and there may be respiratory distress. Visualization of the posterior pharyngeal wall and soft palate is difficult or impossible. A further complication is mediastinal extension, so that hospital admission with a stat CT scan is mandatory to assess this potential.

Treatment

Treatment of this condition is vigorous antibiotic therapy [see section on masticator space infection (above) for drugs and dosages], careful observation of the airway, and incision and drainage. External incision is usually preferred because of the easy access to the submandibular, masticator, and parapharyngeal spaces through one incision. Tracheostomy may be necessary.

Ludwig's Angina

Ludwig's angina is a bilateral boardlike swelling involving the submandibular, submental, and sublingual spaces with elevation of the tongue. It is most often secondary to infection of the lower second

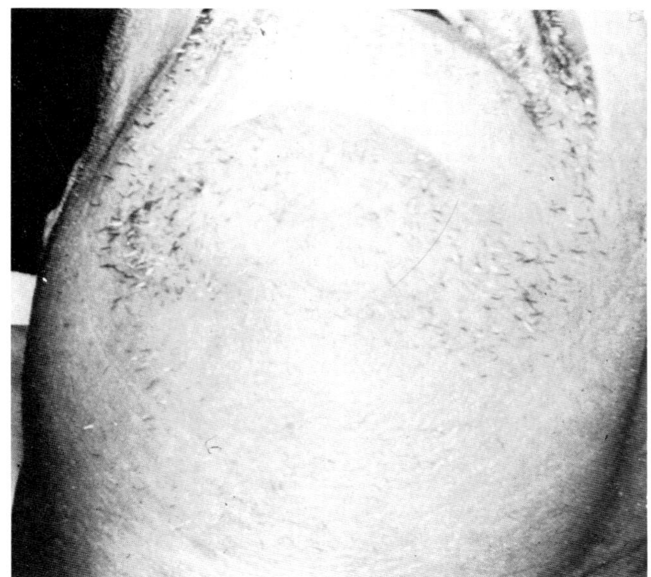

Fig. 157-13. Ludwig's angina.

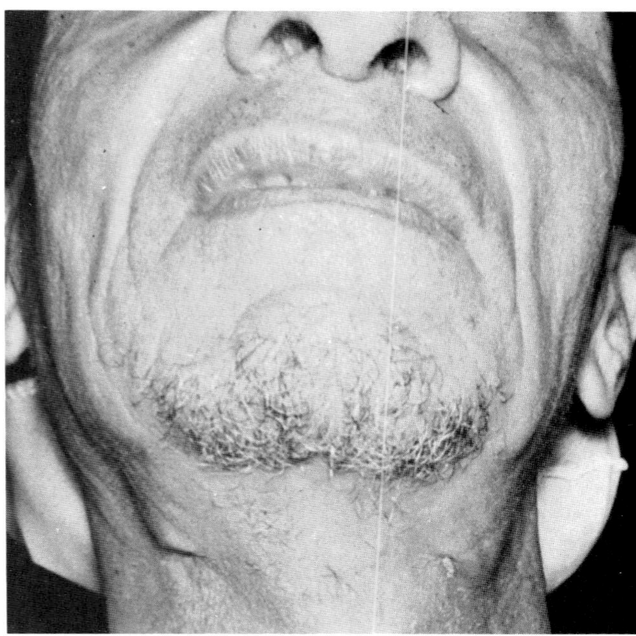

Fig. 157-14. Postoperative view of Ludwig's angina in Fig. 157-13.

and third molars. Brawny induration is characteristic and there is no fluctuance present.

Predominant organisms are hemolytic streptococci, *Staphylococcus*, or mixed aerobes and anaerobes. The presence of anaerobes accounts for gas in the tissues.

Clinical Features

Chills, fever, difficulty in swallowing, stiffness of tongue movements, and trismus are common presenting signs (Figs. 157-13 and 157-14). Respiration becomes increasingly difficult as the tongue is elevated and the oral pharynx becomes occluded; the larynx may become edematous.

Treatment

Treatment consists of high-dose intravenous antibiotic therapy [see section on masticator space infection (above) for drugs and dosages], and tracheostomy may be necessary. Incision and drainage superficial and deep to the mylohyoid muscle and medial to the mandible may be required if antibiotic therapy is not successful. As in parapharyngeal space infection, mediastinal extension can occur.

BIBLIOGRAPHY

Helms CA, Katzberg RW, Morrish R, et al: Computed tomography of the temporomandibular joint meniscus. *J Oral Maxillofacial Surg* 41:512, 1983.

Hendler BH: Maxillofacial trauma in the emergency unit. *Current Topics Emerg Med* 2:00, 1985.

Hendler BH, Quinn PD: Fatal mediastinitis secondary to odontogenic infection. *J Oral Surg* 36:308, 1978.

Hendler BH, Wagner D: Problem—blow to the jaw, trauma rounds. *Emerg Med* 5:60, 1973.

Hendler BH, Wagner D: Injury to the lip and oral mucosa, trauma rounds. *Emerg Med* 6:278, 1974.

Le Fort R: Étude experimentale sur les fractures de la machoire supérieure. *Rev Chir* (Paris) 23:360, 479, 1901.

Rowe NL, Williams JL: *Maxillofacial Injuries,* 2d ed. New York, Churchill Livingstone, 1985, vols I, II.

158 GENERAL DENTAL EMERGENCIES

James T. Amsterdam

There are four categories of general dental emergencies of importance to the emergency physician: (1) oral-facial pain, primarily of odontogenic origin; (2) dentoalveolar trauma; (3) hemorrhage; and (4) oral medicine emergencies including oral manifestations of systemic disease. An understanding of the anatomy of the tooth and attachment apparatus is essential for the recognition and management of these emergencies.

ANATOMY OF THE TEETH

A tooth is a homogeneous body of dentin, a microporous structure which surrounds a central pulp—the neurovascular supply—from which it is nourished and was initially derived. The pulp continuously lays down additional dentin throughout life. The coronal portion of the tooth is that part which is normally seen in the mouth and is covered by enamel; the root portion serves to anchor the tooth and is covered with cementum, a substance which is much softer than enamel.

Thirty-two teeth are generally found in the permanent dentition, consisting of four types of teeth—incisors, canines, premolars, and molars. Beginning from the midline and counting backward, the normal dental anatomy will consist of one central incisor, one lateral incisor, one canine, two premolars, and three permanent molars. The third molar is commonly referred to as the *wisdom tooth*. *Agenesis* or absence of any of these teeth or additional (*supernumerary*) teeth can occur. It is best for the emergency physician simply to describe the type of tooth and location involved in a particular emergency, e.g., an upper right second premolar or a lower left canine. Useful dental nomenclature consists of the following:

Facial: Referring to that part of a tooth that faces the oral vestibule
Incisors to canines: Labial
Premolars to molars: Buccal
Oral: Referring to that part of a tooth that faces the tongue (lingual) or palate (palatal)
Approximal: Referring to the contacting areas of adjacent teeth; those closest to the midline are mesial, those toward the posterior aspect of the mouth are distal
Occlusal: Referring to the biting surfaces of the premolars and molars
Incisal: Referring to the biting surface of the incisors and canines
Apical: Referring to the tip of the root
Coronal: Toward the biting surface of the tooth

THE NORMAL PERIODONTIUM

The normal periodontium is divided into two major components, the gingival unit and the attachment apparatus.

The *gingival unit* is composed of the soft tissues investing the teeth and the alveolar bone. The *gingiva* is covered by a stratified squamous keratinized epithelium. It extends from the free gingival margin to the mucogingival junction. Apical to the mucogingival junction is the *alveolar mucosa,* which is covered by nonkeratinized, stratified squamous epithelium and is continuous with the mucosa of the lip and cheek.

In healthy individuals, the gingiva is attached tightly to the tooth, except for a 2- to 3-mm cuff of tissue surrounding the neck of the tooth (*gingival sulcus*), bounded on one side by enamel and on the other by a continuation of the gingival epithelium. The *attachment apparatus* or anchoring mechanism consists of the cementum covering the root, the alveolar bone surrounding the root, and the periodontal ligament. The periodontal ligament is composed of collagen fibers that insert on one end in the alveolar bone and on the other end in the cementum forming a fibrous attachment, not a calcific union. The anatomy of the dental unit (crown and root) and the periodontium are illustrated in cross section in Fig. 158-1.

ORAL AND FACIAL PAIN

If pain is of odontogenic (tooth) origin, patients usually will be able to localize the pain. The emergency physician should also recognize nonodontogenic causes for facial and oral pain (e.g., temporomandibular joint disturbances, Bell's palsy) and consider ischemic heart disease in the adult presenting with mandibular pain of unclear etiology.

Odontogenic Pain

Tooth Eruption

The earliest pain of odontogenic origin is associated with eruption of the primary teeth in the infant. Although there is some controversy over whether diarrhea and low-grade fever are associated with tooth eruption, an infant with dental pain may refuse to eat or drink and become dehydrated. Management is directed toward (1) pain control, (2) control of diarrhea if present, and (3) adequate hydration. Topical application every 15 to 30 min of a swab dampened with paregoric or any other oral topical anesthetic (benzocaine) agent may be a useful method of analgesia. Adult patients may suffer from pain associated with erupting teeth, most commonly third molars. The gingiva surrounding crowded, malerupted or impacted third molar teeth has a tendency for food impaction and subsequent inflammation, termed *pericoronitis*. Local therapy consists of saline irrigation and mouth rinses; if fluctuance and pus are present, incision and drainage may be useful. If local infection, fever, or malaise are evident, phenoxymethyl penicillin or erythromycin, 250 to 500 mg qid, are prescribed. Once local inflammation has resolved, definitive treatment involves the surgical removal of these teeth. Therefore, referral to an oral and maxillofacial surgeon in 24 to 48 h is important.

Dental Caries

The most common odontogenic pain, *odontalgia* or *toothache,* is associated with a carious tooth. A history of sudden or gradual onset of sharp to dull throbbing pain localized to a specific area of the mouth, aggravated by changes in temperature or possibly relieved by cool temperature, is consistent with caries. Such a history is consistent with pulp involvement and may indicate that the tooth is abscessed (periapical abscess). The pain may be generalized or referred to other areas such as the ear, temple, eye, neck, or even opposite jaw. Physical examination frequently will reveal a grossly decayed tooth (or teeth), or there may be no apparent pathology. Localization is most easily accomplished by percussing individual teeth with a tongue blade; if abscessed, sharp pain is elicited when the tooth is tapped. Treatment is with analgesics such as codeine, acetaminophen-codeine combinations, or even, on occasion, parenteral narcotic analgesics. Patients who have undergone endodontic treatment may experience exquisite pain secondary to instrumentation during therapy and/or the build-up of gas in the tooth after it has been sealed (pericementitis) which may be unrelieved by any analgesic; a general dentist or endodontist should be notified so that the tooth can be reopened.

Any associated oral or facial swelling secondary to abscessed teeth may produce pain. Swelling may range from a parulis (a small swelling in the gingiva opposite an abscessed tooth) to subperiosteal extension or a facial cellulitis. Fluctuant swellings require incision and drainage, antibiotics, and warm saline rinses every 2 h until seen the following day for definitive treatment.

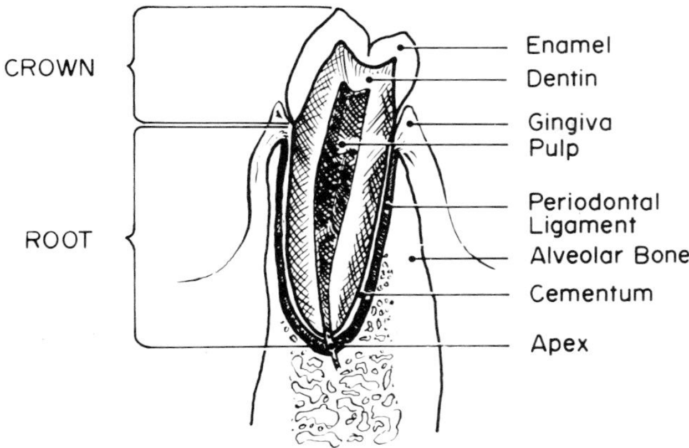

Fig. 158-1. The dental anatomic unit and attachment apparatus.

Postextraction Pain

Pain experienced within 24 h of an extraction, termed *periosteitis,* responds well to analgesics. Severe pain associated with a foul odor and taste in the mouth 2 to 3 days after an extraction is termed *alveolar osteitis* ("dry socket"). This pain is often excruciating and not relieved by oral analgesics. The pathophysiology is due to a combination of loss of the healing blood clot and a localized infection (localized osteomyelitis). Treatment consists of irrigation of the socket and the application of a medicated dental packing, or simply 1 in. of iodoform gauze slightly dampened with eugenol or Campho-Phenique which may be performed by the emergency physician. The patient should be seen by a dentist in 12 to 24 h.

Periodontal Emergencies

Periodontal Abscess

A swelling of the gingiva secondary to entrapment of plaque and debris in a so-called *pocket* (space between the tooth and the gingiva) is termed a *periodontal abscess* and may result in severe pain. Abscesses of this nature usually respond to local therapy consisting of warm saline irrigation and antibiotics (phenoxymethyl penicillin, 250 mg po qid; if allergic to penicillin and not pregnant, tetracycline 250 mg po qid). Larger abscesses may require incision and drainage.

Acute Necrotizing Ulcerative Gingivitis

Acute necrotizing ulcerative gingivitis (ANUG) is an acute destructive disease of the periodontium found most often in adolescents and young adults. ANUG is the only periodontal lesion in which bacteria (*Fusobacteria,* spirochetes) actually invade nonnecrotic tissue. Patients complain of generalized gingival pain associated with a foul taste and odor. Signs that may be present are fever, malaise, and regional lymphadenopathy. On physical examination the gingiva appears edematous and fiery red; the interdental papillae (tissue between the teeth) are edematous, ulcerated, and covered with a grayish pseudomembrane.

ANUG is initially managed with antibiotics (tetracycline 250 mg po qid, preferred; or phenoxymethyl penicillin, 250 mg po qid), warm saline rinses, as well as the application of topical local anesthetic agents such as viscous lidocaine or 10% carbamide peroxide in a specially prepared anhydrous glycerol. Symptomatic improvement is impressive; however, the potential complication of destruction of underlying alveolar bone requires dental follow-up.

Oral Medicine Emergencies

Although it is beyond the scope of this chapter to discuss the myriad of oral medicine emergencies which may result in pain, there are several important classes that represent common problems.

Oral Lesions

Patients frequently present because of pain from oral lesions. It is often difficult to distinguish a primary herpetic gingivostomatitis from recurrent infection, herpangina, or herpes zoster. Such ulcerations when recognized are often best treated palliatively in the emergency department with topical anesthetic agents, e.g., viscous xylocaine and the application of warm saline rinses. Some are now advocating the use of oral acyclovir for primary herpetic infections in the adult. Its use should certainly be considered in the immune-compromised patient. These lesions are usually secondarily infected and since much of the pain is due to the secondary infection itself, the prescription of antibiotics (erythromycin 250 mg qid or phenoxymethyl penicillin 250 mg qid) is often appropriate. In most circumstances, the prescription of topical or systemic corticosteroid preparations should be avoided. Although steroids have been useful in treatment of erythema multiforme, their use with viral oral infection is not indicated. Owing to the complexity of the differential diagnosis of oral vesicular lesions, definitive treatment is best managed by a dentist or oral and maxillofacial surgeon.

Paroxysmal Pain of Neuropathic Origin

Tic douloureux, or trigeminal neuralgia, is the most common cause for paroxysmal pain of neuropathic origin involving the trigeminal (fifth) cranial nerve. The diagnosis is made primarily on history. Patients report a paroxysmal pain, i.e., an episode of sudden pain separated by pain-free periods, which is recurrent, excruciating, normally of short duration, and resembling the pain due to a severe electric shock. The key to the diagnosis is the fact that the pain follows the anatomical distribution of the cranial nerve involved. Often, a similar pain can be initiated by minor sensory stimuli to areas called *trigger zones* that consistently reproduce the pain. Tic douloureux may respond well to the administration of carbamazepine (100 mg bid initially and gradually increased if needed to a maximum dose of 1200 mg daily). The pain of tic douloureux may not necessarily be idiopathic, as it may be the result of a tumor, such as a cerebellopontine angle tumor (e.g., acoustic neuroma); a nasopharyngeal carcinoma; or a manifestation of multiple sclerosis. Any patient in whom the diagnosis of tic douloureux is made requires a careful neurologic examination, a referral to a dentist to rule out oral pathology, and a referral to a neurologist to rule out intracranial pathology.

Nonparoxysmal pain of neuropathic origin may develop (1) in patients who have suffered for a long time from tic douloureux; (2) secondary to surgical trauma along the distribution of the fifth cranial nerve, most frequently the mandibular branch; or (3) in association with viral infections, drugs, or heavy metal intoxication. Other neuropathies, such as alcoholic and diabetic sensory neuropathies, may affect the oral cavity as well.

Other

The differential diagnosis of oral facial pain includes cluster headache, temporal arteritis, and polymyalgia rheumatica. Referred pain from an ischemic myocardium must be considered in the differential diagnosis of jaw pain.

Oral Manifestations of Systemic Disease

Several systemic diseases are associated with important oral manifestations, often as the first manifestation.

Diabetes Mellitus

Acute gingival abscesses and sessile or pedunculated gingival proliferations (granulation tissue that protrudes from under the gingiva, producing a red-gingival hypertrophy) occur frequently in diabetics. Dry burning mouth, gingival tenderness, lip dryness, spontaneous gingival bleeding, and tooth mobility may be seen. Chronic oral disease, particularly periodontal disease, may contribute to out-of-control diabetes.

Collagen Vascular Disease

Systemic lupus erythematosus (SLE) may be associated with large intraoral necrotic ulcerations which may become secondarily infected.

Scleroderma may present with a characteristic facies or thickening of the periodontal ligament on x-ray. Midline lethal granuloma or Wegener's granulomatosis may present with large palatal ulcerations. All ulcerations of the oral cavity which do not respond to palliative treatment warrant biopsy within 7 to 10 days.

Granulomatous Disease

Rarely, tuberculosis may manifest itself orally as granulomatous ulcerations. Other infections such as actinomycosis must be ruled out. These lesions may frequently be confused with syphilitic ulcerations in the oral cavity, with the tongue and tonsil areas being common locations.

A more benign and common entity is a pedunculated or sessile mass, termed *pyogenic granuloma*. This is a proliferation of highly vascularized connective tissue in response to nonspecific infection seen on the gingiva. A specific pyogenic granuloma, occurring primarily during pregnancy, is referred to as a *pregnancy tumor* (Fig. 158-2). The tumor is benign and frequently recurs if removed during pregnancy. If the tumor does not regress 2 to 3 months postpartum, definitive removal is indicated.

Blood Dyscrasias

Acute leukemia, particularly the acute granulocytic form, causes massive infiltration of leukemic cells into the gingival tissues, resulting in a hyperplastic gingivitis so marked as to almost cover the teeth; it is edematous and bluish in color. Chronic leukemia rarely causes oral disorders.

Oral complications that occur during the disease include gingival hemorrhage, local infection, marked discomfort, and loss of appetite. During the acute phase of the disease, only those procedures necessary to alleviate the discomfort and hemorrhaging should be performed (Fig. 158-3).

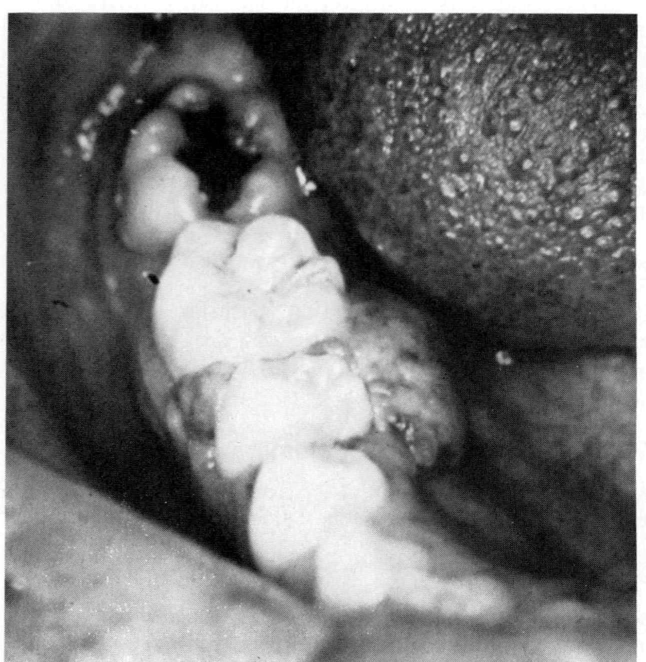

Fig. 158-2. Pyogenic granuloma.

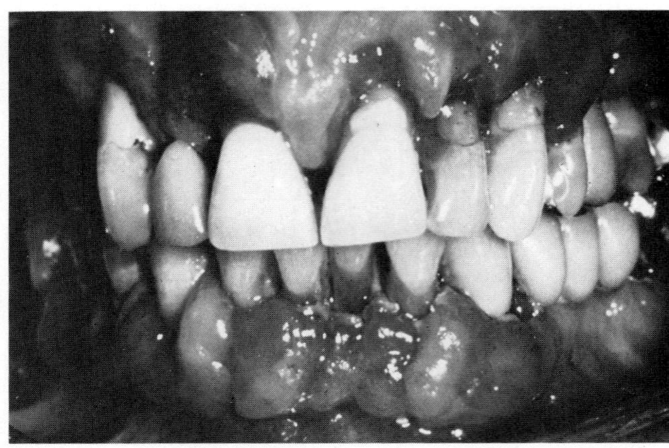

Fig. 158-3. Oral manifestations of leukemia.

Intraoral signs and symptoms of thrombocytopenic purpura consist of gingival bleeding, intramucosal hemorrhages, and prolonged bleeding from trauma. In addition, gingival hypertrophy has been reported.

Phenytoin Hyperplasia

Phenytoin hyperplasia of the gingiva occurs in approximately 40 percent of patients and is more prevalent in younger patients. Its severity may be unrelated to either dosage or blood levels. The initial appearance of hyperplasia is an enlargement of the interdental papillae, which encroaches on the crowns of the teeth with the marginal gingival tissue lobulated, firm, and pale pink in color. Inflammation secondary to local irritants alters the appearance of the hyperplastic gingiva and responds to improved oral hygiene. Surgical removal of tissue is effective, but hyperplasia recurs if the drug is continued. A similar reaction can be associated with nifedipine.

Acquired Immunodeficiency Syndrome

There are numerous intraoral manifestations of acquired immunodeficiency syndrome (AIDS). Many of these are exaggerated responses to the viral conditions described above. Viral conditions that are potentially life-threatening may respond to intravenous acyclovir. Oropharyngeal thrush is perhaps one of the most common and perhaps earliest manifestations of AIDS, and this diagnosis should be suspected in any adult patient who presents with this condition. Periodontal conditions that are seen in the AIDS patient include a variety of advanced periodontitis very similar to the clinical picture of the patient with leukemia in Fig. 158-3 as well as isolated areas of gingival recession (a relatively nonspecific finding) or unusual gingival pigmentation.

DENTOALVEOLAR TRAUMA

The simplest type of dental trauma involves the fracture of anterior teeth. The management of dental fractures is based on (1) the extent of the fracture in relation to the pulp of the tooth, and (2) the age of the patient. A classification, the Ellis system, has been developed to describe the fracture anatomy of teeth. However, the emergency physician may also use a descriptive classification of traumatic injuries to teeth and supporting structures as advocated by Johnson (Fig. 158-4).

Fractures

The Ellis class I fracture involves only the enamel portion of the tooth. This is generally a minor problem and requires immediate intervention

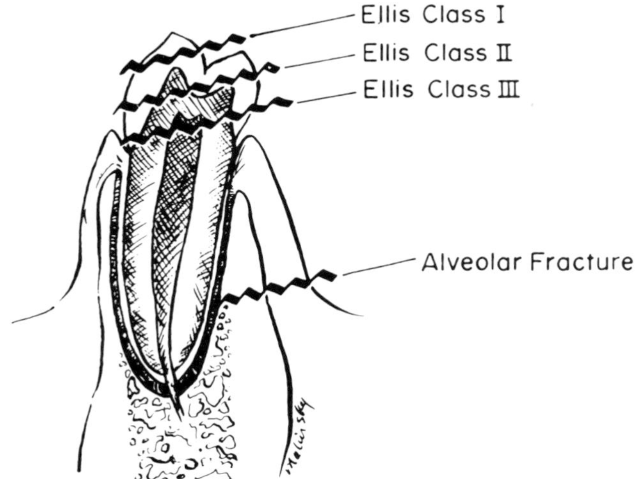

Fig. 158-4. Ellis classification for fractures of anterior teeth.

only if a sharp piece of tooth is causing trauma to soft tissues. In such situations, the rough edge may be smoothed with something as simple as an emery board and/or referred to a general dentist for cosmetic restoration.

The Ellis class II fracture is a more complicated fracture involving not only the enamel but also exposure of dentin. The patient may complain of sensitivity to heat, cold, or even air. Immediate treatment of the Ellis class II fracture is dictated by the age of the patient, since less dentin is present in younger patients (under 12 years). Passage of microorganisms through the microtubules of exposed dentin can contaminate the pulp.

The management of Ellis class II fractures in younger patients requires the immediate placement of a calcium hydroxide dressing on the exposed dentin which is then covered with dry gauze or tinfoil. The patient requires dental referral within 24 h. Older patients (12 to 14 years) who have a greater dentin to pulp ratio may be advised to avoid extremes in temperature and to seek dental care the following day. Patients with severe Ellis class II fractures (which may be recognized by a pinkish tinge to the dentin) should be treated as younger patients. Analgesics may also be required. The correct management of Ellis class II fractures may obviate the need for root canal therapy. The emergency physician should warn any patient who has sustained trauma to the anterior teeth, no matter how minor, that disruption of the tooth's neurovascular supply may have occurred; long-term complications may be pulpal necrosis or resorption (dissolving) of the tooth.

Ellis class III fractures of the teeth involve, in addition to fracture of enamel and the exposure of dentin, the actual exposure of the pulp. These fractures may be differentiated from Ellis class II fractures by gently wiping a tooth clean with a piece of gauze to eliminate the possibility of blood from soft tissue trauma. The tooth is then examined for any red blush of dentin or frank drop of blood. A patient may complain of exquisite pain or no pain if the neurovascular supply is disrupted. Ellis class III fractures are true dental emergencies and require immediate attention from a general dentist or endodontist since delay in treatment may result in significant pain and probably abscess formation. If a dentist is not immediately available, the tooth may be temporarily covered with tinfoil so as to minimize pulpal irritation and pain. Analgesics should be prescribed and the patient should see a dentist as soon as possible. The emergency physician would be ill-advised to introduce any instrument into the tooth for the removal of pulpal tissue since instrument breakage or tooth fracture may result, making endodontic treatment difficult or impossible. Over-the-counter topical dental analgesic preparations should neither be prescribed nor applied in the adult. Although these agents may give the patient temporary relief from pulpal pain, they often cause severe soft tissue irritation and sterile abscesses. In all cases of tooth fracture, soft tissue should be palpated for tooth fragments and radiographed if swelling limits the examination.

Subluxated and Avulsed Teeth

The same force which may have resulted in the fracture of anterior teeth may also result in actual loosening of the tooth, termed subluxation. A traumatized tooth should always be examined for subluxation with use of finger pressure or the application of gentle rocking pressure with two tongue blades on each side of the tooth. A more subtle indication that teeth have been traumatized is the appearance of blood in the gingival crevice of the tooth. Minimally mobile teeth heal well with a soft diet for 1 to 2 weeks. Grossly mobile teeth require prompt stabilization. As a temporizing procedure for teeth which are very loose, it is often useful to have the patient bite gently on a piece of gauze to keep the tooth in place pending examination by a dentist or oral-maxillofacial surgeon.

A tooth that has been completely avulsed from the socket is a true dental emergency. If the patient is unaware of the location of the missing tooth, x-rays should be taken to determine if the missing tooth has been forced beneath the gingiva. Intruded primary ("baby") teeth are allowed to erupt for 6 weeks. Permanent teeth are surgically repositioned with a forceps and stabilized. Failure to diagnose intruded teeth may result in cosmetic deformity or infection. The management of an avulsed tooth depends upon the age of the patient and the length of time that the tooth has been absent from the oral cavity. Avulsed primary anterior teeth in the pediatric patient (ages 6 months to 5 years) are not replaced into their sockets. Replanted primary teeth have a high tendency to ankylose or fuse to the bone itself, resulting in facial deformity.

A permanent tooth should be replaced in its socket as soon as possible if avulsion is less than 2 to 3 h. A percentage point for successful replantation is lost each minute that the tooth is absent from the oral cavity. When a call is received about an avulsed tooth, determine the age of the patient. If it appears that the tooth is permanent, the parent or patient should be instructed to quickly rinse the tooth under running tap water, holding it by the crown portion *only*, and to replant it immediately back in its socket. If actual replantation is not possible, the patient should be advised to bring the tooth to the emergency department as quickly as possible in moist gauze or, preferably, a glass of milk. Ideally, the patient may also be allowed to place the tooth in his or her own mouth to bathe in saliva, with care taken not to swallow the tooth.

New advances have been made in the development of a more ideal storage and transport media for avulsed teeth. When a tooth is avulsed from its socket, periodontal ligament fibers remain attached to both the tooth and the socket. Key to successful replantation is the survival of the remaining periodontal ligament fibers on the root. Milk is an acceptable storage medium due to its osmolarity and essential ion concentration of Ca^{2+} and Mg^{2+}. However, it is now known that the best storage and transport medium is Hank's solution, which is a pH-balanced cell culture medium. This solution is commercially available in the Tooth Preserving System (TPS, Biological Rescue Products, Inc.). It has also been found that Hank's solution can maintain the viability of the periodontal ligament cells for 4 to 6 h or longer. Finally, if the tooth has been avulsed for longer than 30 min, placement of the tooth in the Hank's solution for 20 to 30 min helps restore cell viability. The use of the TPS system is illustrated in Fig. 158-5. The tooth is dropped in a basket and immersed in the Hank's solution; at the time of removal, the basket is lifted out of the solution and tipped over on the padded lid for retrieval.

If the tooth has not been replanted by the time the patient reaches the emergency department, it should be held by the crown at all times,

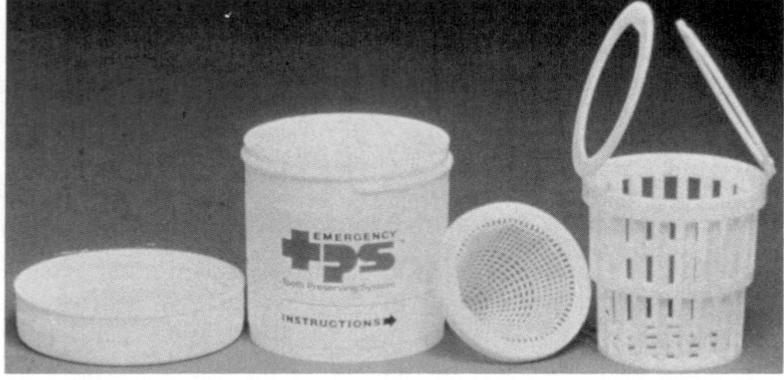

A

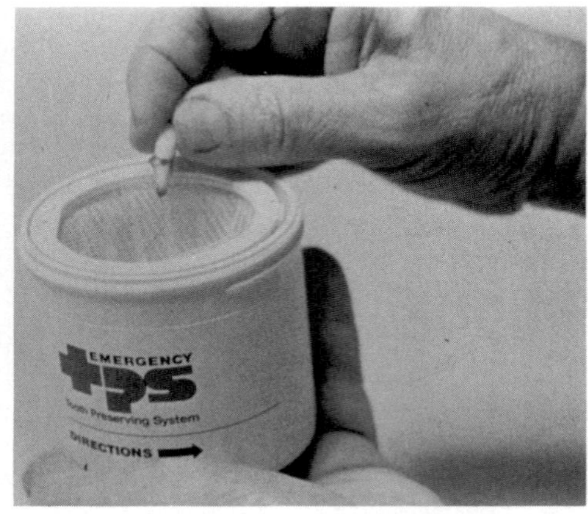

B

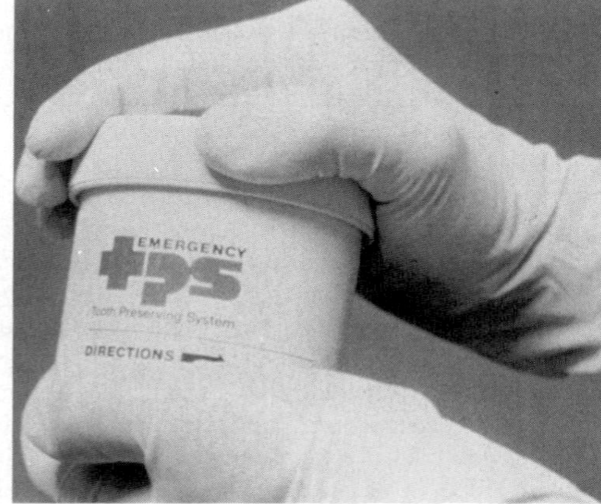

C

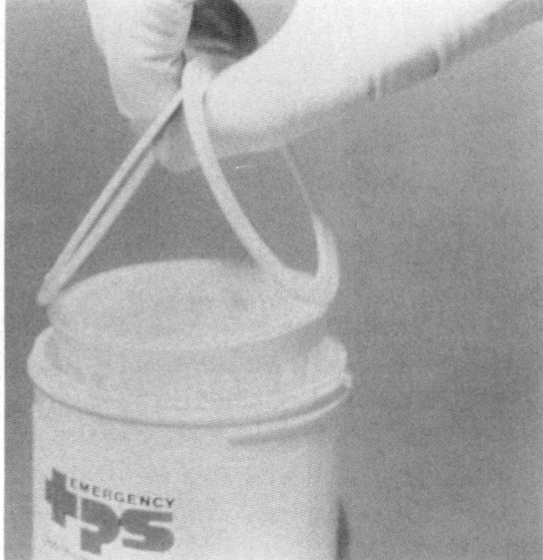

D

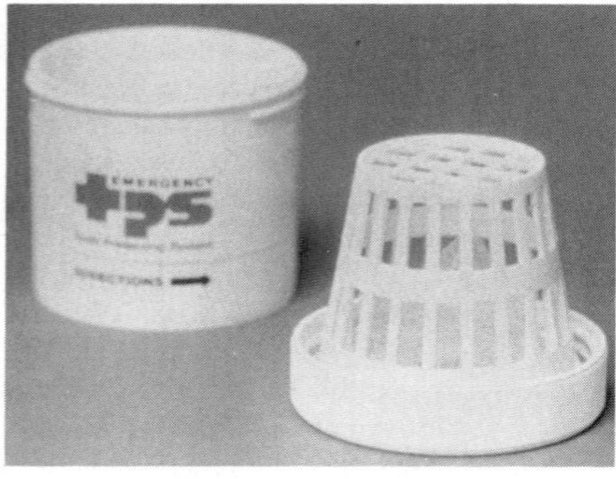

E

Fig. 158-5. A. The Tooth Preserving System (TPS).**B.** Each avulsed tooth is dropped into a separate TPS container of Hank's solution. **C.** The lid is tightly secured. The container can be gently swirled to clean the tooth. **D.** The tooth is removed from the container by lifting up the basket. **E.** The tooth is retrieved by turning the basket over onto the cushioned interior lining of the lid. (Courtesy of Paul Krasner, D.D.S., Biological Rescue Products, Inc., 566 High Street, Pottstown, PA., 19464.)

rinsed under saline or running water, or rinsed in the TPS system but *not* scrubbed (so as to conserve as many of the remaining periodontal ligament fibers as possible for reattachment) and replanted into the socket. If absent longer than 30 min, placement in the TPS system should be considered prior to replantation. If a blood clot prevents replantation, or in the case of long time intervals since avulsion, the clot should be quickly suctioned or debrided under local anesthesia and then the tooth should be replanted.

Avulsed teeth require immediate stabilization or they will exfoliate; biting on gauze is a temporizing measure. Though stabilization is normally performed by the general dentist or oral-maxillofacial surgeon, there are situations where stabilization may be performed by the emergency physician. Indications would be a single avulsed tooth which has been placed back into the socket with satisfactory alignment, e.g., no prematurity of occlusion on jaw closure. Any tooth stablized by the emergency physician should be evaluated by the general dentist or oral-maxillofacial surgeon within 24 h.

Several techniques are at the disposal of the emergency physician for stabilization of subluxated or avulsed teeth. A simple method described by Medford involves the application of a periodontal dressing (''Coe-Pak'') which consists of zinc oxide and a catalyst that set when mixed to a semihard consistency. When molded over the reimplanted tooth and adjacent teeth, 24 h of stabilization can be achieved.

Alveolar Fractures

Avulsed teeth are stabilized for approximately 10 days to 2 weeks and then placed back into function to avoid ankylosis. When there are concomitant alveolar fractures, the stabilization of avulsed or subluxated teeth serves to stabilize the alveolar bone; stabilization is then left for a minimum of 6 weeks. Indiscriminate loss of alveolar bone will lead to more difficult prosthetic restoration of this area than the removal of any ankylosed tooth. Generally, prophylactic antibiotics, e.g., phenoxymethyl penicillin, 250 to 500 mg qid, are used when avulsed teeth are reimplanted in the oral cavity and appropriate tetanus prophylaxis should also be instituted.

Soft Tissue Injury

Closure of associated laceration of the gingiva, mucosa, lips, and other facial soft tissues is performed after the teeth have been stabilized in the oral cavity. Stabilization of these teeth involves various methods of wiring or application of plastic materials or both, all of which require stretching of soft tissues, especially the lips and oral mucosa. Thus, carefully placed sutures will simply be torn and increase the soft tissue injury. The emergency physician should await final stabilization of the dentoalveolar component before instituting soft tissue closure and plastic repair.

Oral Lacerations

Oral lacerations can involve either the lips, mucosa, gingiva, hard palate, tongue, or combinations of each. If lip lacerations are associated with intraoral injuries, the intraoral injuries should be managed first and a new sterile instrument tray used for the skin closure.

Gaping intraoral mucosal lacerations (greater than 1.5 cm) tend to become ulcerated, secondarily infected, and heal in a fibrotic manner resulting in a lump of tissue that is subject to repeated trauma unless sutured. Mucosal lacerations should be inspected carefully for debris, crushed and nonviable tissue should be removed, the wound copiously irrigated, and closed with 4–0 chromic suture material. Black silk suture (4–0) is an acceptable alternative and easier to use but will require removal in 7 to 10 days. Good tissue approximation is preferred to a watertight seal so that drainage can occur should the wound become infected. Extensive mucosal lacerations or those involving large amounts of crushed tissue are best covered with antibiotics (phenoxymethyl penicillin or erythromycin 250 mg po qid) based on clinical experience although there are not much data to support the practice.

Tongue Lacerations

Tongue lacerations greater than 1 cm should be closed with either 4–0 black silk suture or 4–0 chromic. If one finds a laceration of the dorsum of the tongue, the ventral surface should be carefully inspected for additional lacerations from the teeth. Careful attention must be paid to detail in approximating the edges of the wound in a laceration of the dorsum of the tongue. Reepithelialization across the wound margin is desired; if the wound edges are not well approximated, the epithelium will marginate downward to the base of the wound on each side and result in a "bifid" tongue appearance. A bifid tongue results in cosmetic as well as functional deformity and will require revision. Even in the best of hands, this is a potential complication of a tongue laceration, and the patient should be so advised. Extensive lacerations of the mucosal surface of the tongue warrant antibiotic treatment similar to other intraoral mucosal lacerations.

Palate Lacerations

Palatal lacerations may involve either the hard or the soft palate. Soft palate injuries occur commonly in children who fall with a pointed object in their mouth. These lacerations should be treated as puncture wounds. Gaping skin edges can be loosely approximated with 5–0 chromic, but for the most part the wound should be allowed to drain. Injury to the retropharynx should be considered. Prophylactic antibiotic coverage is recommended with the same rationale as that for other intraoral mucosal injuries.

Good patient control is necessary for management of these wounds. An intraoral bite block is a very useful adjunct and makes the procedure more comfortable for the patient. Very young and uncooperative patients who require closure of the wound need sedation and may even require repair in the operating room. Lacerations of the hard palate are difficult to close since this tissue is not very mobile. Closure can be performed with a 4–0 or 5–0 silk or chromic suture using a fine needle. Abrasions of the palate can heal by granulation; a dental emollient paste such as Orabase can be prescribed for comfort. Palatal lacerations tend not be become infected.

Lip Lacerations

Lacerations of the lip require meticulous closure, especially if the vermilion border is involved. As with any facial skin closure, suture removal should occur within 4 to 5 days to avoid suture marks. However, due to the musculature of the lips, premature wound separation can occur with deep lacerations. Therefore, when lip lacerations involve deep subcutaneous tissue and muscle, these structures should be approximated with a resorbable material (5–0 polyvicryl). The skin is then closed with a 6–0 nylon monofilament material. If the vermilion border of the lip is involved, the first step is to approximate the border as precisely as possible. The remainder of the closure is then accomplished. If possible, the suture through the vermilion border itself should be removed (making sure that the wound remains approximated) so that no suture mark will appear on the vermilion border itself. The patient should keep the wound clean with hydrogen peroxide wipes and maintain a layer of triple antibiotic ointment on the wound. Caution should be exercised not to distend the lips with such activity as laughing, yawning, or trying to examine the injury at home.

Controversy surrounds the management of the through-and-through laceration involving communication between the skin and the oral cavity. Some advocate not closing the intraoral component. It is this author's recommendation that if the mucosal laceration meets the criteria specified above, then it should be approximated. Through-and-through wounds should be irrigated well. The patient should be instructed in the use of saline rinses at home. Some well-controlled studies support the practice of prescribing antibiotics (phenoxymethyl penicillin or erythromycin 250 mg qid) as a prophylactic measure. These patients should have the wound checked in 48 to 72 h for infection. Care must be taken not to misinterpret normal mucosal edema associated with initial wound healing for infection. The need for tetanus prophylaxis should be considered with all oral and intraoral lacerations.

HEMORRHAGE

Spontaneous Hemorrhage

Oral hemorrhage may be spontaneous from gingiva. The history should include inquiry as to recent dental scaling or prophylaxis. If this history exists, bleeding usually responds to peroxide mouth rinse and local pressure with gauze compresses. Spontaneous gingival hemorrhage may also be the initial presentaton of a systemic process, such as leukemia or coagulopathy. Extent of the hemorrhage, age of the patient, and results of general examination determine the need for laboratory testing.

Hemorrhage Secondary to Extraction

Bleeding secondary to dental extraction is usually controlled by having the patient apply sustained pressure by biting gauze. Spitting, smoking cigarettes, and the use of straws create a negative pressure intraorally that exudes blood clots from sockets and aggravates postextraction bleeding.

If the bleeding fails to respond to gauze pressure and there are large clots present, the clots should be wiped from the oral cavity, the socket suctioned, and gauze pressure attempted once again. If this is unsuccessful, local anesthesia consisting of 2% lidocaine with 1:100,000 or 1:50,000 epinephrine may be infiltrated in the area of the socket and gingiva, and gauze pressure reapplied for 20 min. If oozing persists, a small piece of absorbable gelatin sponge can be placed in the socket and secured with one or two 3–0 black silk sutures.

If there is sustained, vigorous oozing after all of the above procedures, a screening coagulation profile consisting of a CBC, platelet count, PT, and PTT should be drawn, since postextraction hemorrhage is often the initial manifestation of a coagulopathy. In some instances, postextraction bleeding is due to improper surgical technique or flap design, and lack of a sufficient number of sutures for hemostasis. Flaps may be sutured together and gauze pressure applied.

Postoperative Hemorrhage

In case of bleeding after periodontal surgery, the emergency physician should contact the periodontist, for periodontal packs placed during surgery are extremely important to wound healing and incorrect placement can result in treatment failure.

BIBLIOGRAPHY

Amsterdam J: Dental emergencies, in Rosen P, Baker F, Braen G, et al (eds): *Emergency Medicine: Concepts and Clinical Practice,* 2d ed. St. Louis, Mosby, 1987, pp 1051–1067.

Amsterdam J, Hendler B, Rose L: Dental emergencies, in Roberts J, Hedges J (eds): *Clinical Procedures in Emergency Medicine*. Philadelphia, Saunders, 1986, pp 946–977.

Amsterdam J, Hendler B, Rose L: Dental emergencies, in Schwartz G, Safer P, Stone J, et al (eds): *Principles and Practice of Emergency Medicine,* 2d ed. Philadelphia, Saunders, 1986, pp 1557–1585.

Blomlof L: Milk and saliva as possible storage media for traumatically exarticulated teeth prior to replantation, *Swed Dent J* 8 (suppl):1, 1981.

Johnson R: Descriptive classification of trauma: The injuries to the teeth and supporting structures. *J Am Dent Assoc* 102:195, 1981.

Kristerson L, Soder PO, and Otteskog P: Transport and storage of human teeth in vitro for autotransplantation and replantation, *J Oral Surg* 34:13, 1976.

Kruger GO: *Textbook of Oral and Maxillofacial Surgery,* 6th ed. St. Louis, Mosby, 1984.

Lindskog S, Blomlof L: Influence of osmolality and composition of some storage media on human periodontal ligament cells, *Acta Odontol Scand* 40:435, 1982.

Lynch M (ed): *Burket's Oral Medicine,* 8th ed. Philadelphia, Lippincott, 1984.

Medford HM: Temporary stabilization of avulsed teeth. *Ann Emergy Med* 11:490, 1982.

SECTION 16
Skin and Soft Tissue Emergencies

159
TOXICODENDRON DERMATITIS

Thomas A. Chapel

Kligman states that the *Toxicodendron* species—poison ivy, poison oak, and poison sumac—are responsible for more cases of allergic contact dermatitis in the United States than all other allergens combined. Fisher estimates that at least 70 percent of the population of the United States if casually exposed to the plants would develop allergic contact sensitivity to the *Toxicodendron* species, and the percentage would be even greater if contact were more prolonged. Dark-skinned individuals seem less susceptible than others to *Toxicodendron* dermatitis, and elderly persons are not as susceptible to poison ivy as younger people are.

CHARACTERISTICS OF *Toxicodendron* spp.

Poison ivy and poison oak are the principal causes of plant dermatitis in North America. Poison ivy occurs throughout the United States, while poison oak is more common on the west coast. In the United States there are two species of poison oak, *Toxicodendron diversilobum* (western poison oak) and *T. toxicarium* (eastern poison oak). There also are two species of poison ivy, *T. rydbergii,* a nonclimbing subshrub, and *T. radicans,* which may be either a shrub or a climbing vine. One species of poison sumac, *T. vernix,* occurs in the United States. It grows as a coarse, woody shrub or as a tree and is found in wooded, swampy areas.

All species of poison oak and poison ivy have leaves with three leaflets, and poison sumac has 7 to 13 leaflets per leaf. The *Toxicodendron* species can also be recognized by their U- or V-shaped leaf scars, typical lenticels, and flowers and fruit that arise in the angle between the leaf and the branch. Off-white mature fruit is borne on a doubly branched structure called a *panicle*.

The leaves, stems, seeds, flowers, berries, and roots of the *Toxicodendron* species contain a milky sap which darkens to the appearance of black lacquer on exposure to the air. The black deposit is present where plants have been injured, and its presence proves that a suspicious plant is a toxicodendron. This characteristic can be used by novices or persons working with unfamiliar vegetation to identify these plants. Guin suggests that several leaves from the plant in question be crushed on a sheet of white paper. The sap stain from poison ivy, poison oak, and poison sumac darkens markedly within a few minutes. This black spot test is used only to augment classic methods of plant identification, and care must be taken to avoid contamination of fingers and clothing with sap.

THE DERMATITIS-PRODUCING FACTORS OF THE *Toxicodendron* SPECIES

The antigenic oleoresin of *Toxicodendron* species is easily extracted from plant sap with alcohol and other solvents. The residue left after evaporation of the solvent is called *urushiol,* and its dermatitis-producing principle is pentadecylacatechol. The *Toxicodendron* species share similar antigens, and therefore cross-sensitivity exists between poison ivy, poison oak, and poison sumac.

Urushiol oxidizes and with complete oxidation is rendered nonallergenic. The speed of the breakdown is promoted by moisture and heat. The antigenic film on clothing or other objects may become inactive within 1 week in a hot, humid environment, while the substance remains allergenic for much longer periods in a dry atmosphere. Washing with soap and water rapidly destroys the antigen. The allergenicity of the oleoresin is maximal in fresh plants and diminishes as the plant ages. However, sensitive individuals must avoid handling plants of any age, for even withered leaves produce contact dermatitis.

The persistence of the allergen permits its spread by contaminated fingers, clothing, tools, animals, and sports equipment. Smoke carrying particles of the plant can, and often does, disseminate the disease. However, complete incineration of the plant destroys the allergen.

Toxicodendron antigen may remain under a person's fingernails for several days unless deliberately removed by thorough cleansing. Scratching with antigen-contaminated fingers disseminates the dermatitis to the face, genitals, and covered areas. The dermatitigenic effect of minute amounts of allergen in highly sensitized individuals is astonishing. Kligman contaminated the thumb of a nonsensitized subject with the juice from crushed leaves. The thumb was then pressed onto the back of a nonsensitized subject 99 times, then once onto the back of a highly sensitive individual. This sequence was repeated four more times. The fifth contact on the highly sensitive individual caused a slight dermatitis, even after 500 impressions.

PRESENTATION AND DIAGNOSIS

Clinical Features

Toxicodendron antigen enters the skin rapidly, and in order to prevent a reaction the sap must be totally removed within 30 min after exposure. Under ordinary circumstances such prophylaxis is impossible. Contact dermatitis in susceptible people generally develops within 2 days following exposure. However, Fisher reports that in a few cases the eruption appears 8 h after exposure, and, rarely, the interval may exceed 10 days.

The temporal difference in onset of the eruption and variations in the clinical expression of toxicodendron dermatitis depend upon the patient's degree of sensitivity, the amount of contact with the allergen, and the regional variations in cutaneous reactivity. Mildly sensitive persons can probably withstand casual exposure to the plant without difficulty. Some individuals develop simple erythema, others erythema and papules, and yet others erythema, papules, vesicles, and bullae. The dermatitis usually begins with pruritus and redness. Streaks of erythema or papulovesicles in linear arrangement soon appear (Figs. 159-1 and 159-2). The linear configuration of some lesions is highly suggestive of toxicodendron dermatitis; it is produced by portions of the plant rubbing across the skin or by dissemination of the allergen by scratching with contaminated fingernails. A common myth is that the disorder is spread by rupturing vesicles. However, blister fluid contains no antigen, and therefore it cannot transmit the dermatitis.

The eruption usually disappears without a trace, but leukodermia or hyperpigmentation are occasional sequelae. Urticaria and erythema multiforme infrequently occur as a result of systemic absorption of toxicodendron antigen.

Laboratory findings in patients with poison ivy dermatitis are minimal. Leukocytosis and eosinophils of 5 to 10 percent occur in a small percentage of patients with severe dermatitis.

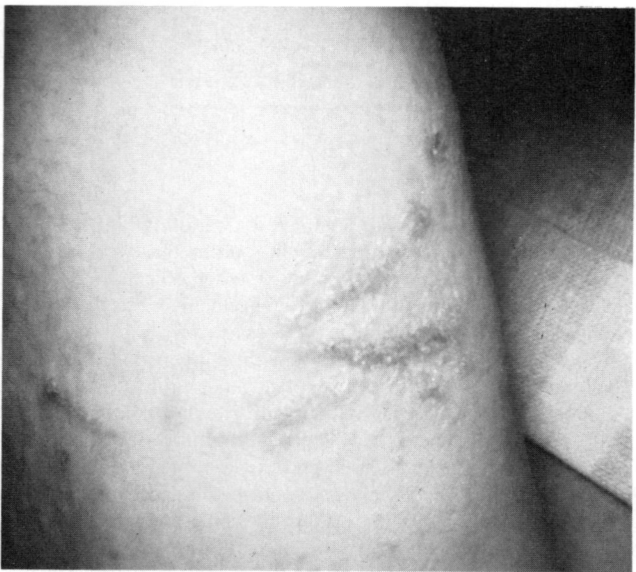

Fig. 159-1. Erythematous, edematous papules and vesicles of the poison ivy in typical linear arrangement.

Differential Diagnosis

Toxicodendron dermatitis is quite distinctive, but occasionally it may be confused with contact dermatitis of other origin. A mimic is phytophotodermatitis caused by lime, parsley, celery, figs, and buttercups. Juices from these plants contain psoralens, which are activated by long-wave ultraviolet light and produce a phototoxic eruption. The eruption consists of striate lesions and irregularly liner bullae in sun-exposed areas. The blisters usually heal with pigmentation that lasts for months. Poison ivy dermatitis is not photoactivated, and it can be distinguished from phytophotodermatitis by lesions that occur on both covered and uncovered areas of the body.

TREATMENT

Treatment of toxicodendron dermatitis is determined by the severity of the eruption. Mild dermatitis consisting of erythema, edema, and papules limited to a few anatomic regions can be managed with shake lotions such as calamine or steroid sprays, creams, or lotions. Compresses or soaks with cold or moderately hot water bring temporary relief from pruritis, and antihistaminics by mouth effectively control persistent itch.

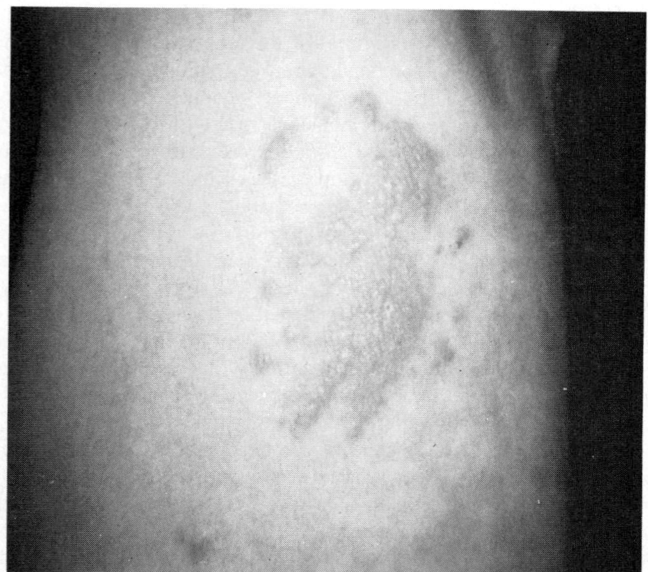

Fig. 159-2. Plaque of poison ivy dermatitis with streaks of erythema and papulovesicles.

More aggressive treatment is required for moderate and severe dermatitis with vesicles and bullae distributed over large areas of the body's surface. Compresses with cool aluminum sulfate diluted 1:10 (Domeboro) help dry lesions and minimize itch. Compresses are applied for 30 to 60 min two to three times each day until blisters dry. Large bullae can be aseptically aspirated with roofs left intact. Potassium permanganate baths aid in drying ruptured blisters. The patient dissolves one-half tablespoon of potassium permanganate crystals in a tub of lukewarm water and soaks for 15 to 20 min each day. Baths with colloidal oatmeal (Aveeno), mixed 1 cupful per tub of water, are also soothing. The pruritus accompanying severe dermatitis should be treated with antihistaminics in full therapeutic doses.

Systemic corticosteroids are effective in bringing relief and are often used if there are no contraindications. If corticosteroids are used, they should be initiated at a level equivalent to 40 to 60 mg of prednisone daily, gradually tapered over a 2- to 3-week period, and then discontinued. Shorter courses of corticosteroids should be avoided as they are frequently associated with a rebound exacerbation of the dermatitis.

The speed with which the eruption heals depends upon the severity and the extent of the cutaneous injury. Mild dermatitis often disappears within 7 to 10 days, while severe eruptions often require 3 or more weeks for normalization.

PROPHYLAXIS

The salient points of toxicodendron dermatitis must be explained carefully to patients, and common myths should be dispelled. The best prophylaxis against recurrent dermatitis is avoidance of the *Toxicodendron* species. This requires that patients recognize poison ivy and related species. Display posters and illustrated pamphlets are helpful teaching aids in educating patients. Persons allergic to the *Toxicodendron* species may have cross reactions to Japanese lacquer and cashew nut trees, the mango, and the marking nut tree of India. Contact with these items also should be avoided.

Individuals exposed to toxicodendrons should wash the entire body with soap and water and carefully clean their fingernails. Clean clothing should be worn, and contaminated clothing laundered. Poison ivy, poison oak, and poison sumac growing in areas of unavoidable contact should be destroyed with herbicides or removed physically to prevent future reexposure.

Epstein and associates advise highly sensitive individuals at increased risk of reexposure because of work or hobbies to try hyposensitization. Hyposensitization requires oral administration of very large doses of urushiol over a 4- to 8-month interval. Unfortunately, hyposensitization lasts no more then several months after the last dose of oil.

BIBLIOGRAPHY

Epstein WL: The poison ivy picker of pennypack park: the continuing saga of poison ivy. *J Invest Dermatol* 88:7, 1987.

Epstein WL: Rhus dermatitis. *Pediatr Clin North Am* 6:843, 1959.

Epstein WL: Topical prevention of poison ivy/oak dermatitis. *Arch Dermatol* 125:499, 1989.

Epstein WL, Byers VS, Baer H: Induction of persistent tolerance to urushiol in humans. *J Allergy Clin Immunol* 68:20, 1981.

Fisher AA: The poison "rhus" plants. *Cutis* 1:230, 1965.

Kligman AM: Poison ivy (Rhus) dermatitis. An experimental study. *Arch Dermatol* 77:149, 1958.

Guin JD: The black spot test for recognizing poison ivy and related species. *J Am Acad Dermatol* 2:332, 1980.

Guin JD, Gillis WT, Beaman JH: Recognizing the *Toxicodendron* (poison ivy, poison oak, poison sumac). *J Am Acad Dermatol* 4:99, 1981.

Maibach HI, Epstein WL: Plant dermatitis: Fact and fancy. *Postgrad Med* 35:571, 1964.

Resnick SD: Poison-ivy and poison-oak dermatitis. *Clin Dermatol* 4:208, 1986.

160
EXFOLIATIVE DERMATITIS

Thomas A. Chapel

Exfoliative dermatitis refers to a condition in which most or all of the skin surface is involved with a scaly erythematous dermatitis. Males are afflicted with the condition twice as often as females, and at least 75 percent of the patients are over the age of 40. The widespread inflammatory exfoliation often is accompanied by immediate or delayed effects in other organ systems.

ETIOLOGY AND PATHOGENESIS

Exfoliative dermatitis is a cutaneous reaction produced in response to a drug or chemical agent or to an underlying cutaneous or systemic disease. The etiologic classification and relative incidence of the more common underlying conditions are listed in Table 160-1. Aside from acute exacerbation of a preexisting dermatosis or generalized exposure to a contact allergen, the mechanisms responsible for exfoliative dermatitis are not known. However, it has been postulated that drug-induced exfoliative dermatitis may be mediated by an excessive number of drug-sensitized suppressor-cytotoxic T lymphocytes and may represent a disorder of immunoregulatory T cells.

Exfoliative dermatitis can have an abrupt onset when related to a drug or contact allergen or to malignancy. Outbreaks arising from an underlying cutaneous disorder usually evolve more slowly, and the identifiable features of the underlying disease may be lost. However, careful observation and a thorough physical examination can sometimes uncover changes characteristic of the primary disease.

In a study of 101 cases, Abrahams et al. found that exfoliative dermatitis tends to be a chronic condition, with a mean duration of 5 years and a median duration of 10 months. A shorter course often follows suppression of the underlying dermatosis, discontinuation of inciting drugs, or avoidance of the inciting allergen. Exfoliative dermatitis with no associated discernible cause can continue for 20 or more years. Death may occur and in general is attributable to hepatocellular damage from severe drug reactions or to underlying malignancies.

There is generalized erythema and warmth of the skin, accompanied by scaling or flaking of the epidermis. The patient usually has a low-grade fever and often complains of pruritus, a chilly sensation, and tightness of the skin. Chronic inflammatory exfoliation produces many changes, such as dystrophic nails, thinning of scalp and body hair, and patchy or diffuse postinflammatory hyperpigmentation or, less commonly, hypopigmentation. Gynecomastia and generalized lymphadenopathy are common in longstanding cases.

Active erythroderma is complicated by excessive heat loss, impairment of temperature regulation, and sometimes hypothermia. The widespread cutaneous vasodilation can cause increased cardiac output. In marginally compensated patients the hemodynamic changes may produce a high-output cardiac failure with dyspnea and dependent edema. Splenomegaly occurred in 3 to 14 percent of the 236 cases reported by Abrahams et al. and Nicolis and Helwig. When associated with exfoliative dermatitis, splenomegaly suggests an underlying leukemia or lymphoma.

The disruption of the epidermis results in increased transepidermal water loss, and continued exfoliation can result in significant protein loss and negative nitrogen balance. Steatorrhea sometimes results from the widespread inflammatory exfoliation, but the enteropathy resolves with improvement of the exfoliative dermatitis. The serum albumin level is lowered because of steatorrhea, cutaneous scaling, and plasma dilution arising from cardiovascular alterations.

Table 160-1. Causes of Dermatitis

Disease	Range of Reported Incidence, %
Generalized flares of preexisting cutaneous disease:	25–40
Psoriasis	
Atopic dermatitis	
Seborrheic dermatitis	
Lichen planus	
Pemphigus foliaceus	
Pityriasis rubra pilaris	
Contact dermatitus	
Drugs	3–10
Lymphoma, leukemia, solid tumors	10–40
Idiopathic	15–45

DIAGNOSIS AND TREATMENT

Differential Diagnosis

The various ichthyoses may mimic exfoliative dermatitis; however, the presence of ichthyosis in other family members, the lifelong presence of disease, and the morphologic detail in scale and anatomic distribution make differentiation easy.

Clinical Evaluation and Treatment

A patient with a newly diagnosed case of exfoliative dermatitis or one who is experiencing an acute exacerbation should be hospitalized for dermatologic nursing care, supportive treatment, and investigative studies. Considerable effort must be made to determine the underlying etiology by a careful history of previous cutaneous disease and of recent drug use, and laboratory tests to establish whether there is possible association with leukemia, lymphoma, or solid tumor. A cutaneous biopsy is indicated, and if there is significant lymphadenopathy, lymph nodes should likewise be biopsied. The patient should also be evaluated for cardiac failure and intestinal dysfunction.

Some patients respond to topical application of corticosteroid cream or ointment and oral antihistamines to control pruritis. However, many require systemic corticosteroids beginning with 40 to 60 mg of prednisone each day. If no response is observed, the dose may be increased by 20 mg. With a favorable response the dose is gradually tapered over weeks or months and eventually discontinued. When systemic steroids are used, the patient can apply bland lotions or creams rather than topical corticosteroid preparations. Tepid colloidal baths, such as cornstarch or oatmeal powder suspension, are of some benefit.

SUMMARY

Exfoliative dermatitis is a cutaneous reaction produced in response to a drug or chemical agent or to an underlying cutaneous or systemic disease. It can be abrupt or insidious in onset. Clinically, it is characterized by generalized erythroderma and flaking or scaling of the epidermis.

Treatment includes control of the underlying cutaneous disorder, avoidance of the inciting drugs or allergen, or treatment of the underlying malignancy. Topical steroids and antipruritic agents may provide relief in many cases, but for more serious disorders systemic corticosteroids may be necessary.

BIBLIOGRAPHY

Abrahams I, McCarthy J, Sanders S: 101 Cases of exfoliative dermatitis. *Arch Dermatol* 87:96, 1963.

Hasan T, Jansen CT: Erythroderma: A follow-up of 50 cases. *J Am Acad Dermatol* 8:836, 1983.

Nicolis GD, Helwig EB: Exfoliative dermatitis: A clinicopathologic study of 135 cases. *Arch Dermatol* 108:788, 1973.

Wong KS, Wong SM, Tham SM, et al: Generalized exfoliative dermatitis—a clinical study of 108 patients. *Ann Acad Med* 17:520, 1988.

161
ERYTHEMA MULTIFORME

Thomas A. Chapel

PATHOLOGY AND CLINICAL CHARACTERISTICS

Erythema multiforme represents a spectrum of disease that ranges from trivial cutaneous lesions to severe, sometimes fatal, multisystem illness. Tissue reaction is of variable expression, yet the histologic features are sufficiently characteristic to differentiate this disorder from other erythematous and vesiculobullous eruptions. The histopathologic spectrum of erythema multiforme has been described by Bedi and Pinkus. Bullae are subepidermal, and epidermal cell necrosis is often noted. The dermis is usually edematous, and a lymphocytic infiltrate is often present about the capillaries and venules of the upper dermis. The disorder is a hypersensitivity reaction precipitated by many agents and conditions (Table 161-1).

Recent data suggest an important role for circulating immune complexes. Direct immunofluorescence studies of erythema multiforme skin lesions have shown deposits of complement components and immunoglobulin in the superficial dermal blood vessels or at the dermal-epidermal junction, and immune complexes have been detected in serum samples of patients with erythema multiforme.

Infections are generally more important as the cause in children, while drugs (Fig. 161-1) and malignancies (Fig. 161-2) are more often implicated in adult cases. About half the cases lack an identifiable cause. Many cases of erythema multiforme occur during epidemics of atypical pneumonia, adenovirus infection, and histoplasmosis.

The disorder occurs at any age, affects males twice as often as females, and is most common in the spring and the fall. The morphology of the cutaneous lesions is variable; they can be macular, urticarial, or vesiculobullous. The skin lesions typically begin as erythematous macules or urticarial-like plaques, and they often contain scattered petechiae. Unlike true hives, the urticarial lesions of erythema multiforme are not usually pruritic. Vesiculobullous lesions develop centrally within preexisting macules, papules, or wheals (Figs. 161-3 and 161-4). Blistering of the mucous membranes occurs in about a quarter of cases, and at times it represents the sole expression of the disease.

Table 161-1. Common Causes of Erythema Multiforme

Associated infectious diseases
Herpes simplex infection, types I and II
Mycoplasma pneumonia
Influenza
Mumps
Psittacosis
Cat-scratch disease
Typhoid fever
Diphtheria
Lymphogranuloma venereum
Histoplasmosis
Cholera
Drugs commonly implicated
Sulfonamides
Oral hypoglycemic agent: chlorpropamide
Pyrazolone derivatives: phenylbutazone, oxyphenbutazone, phenazone
Phenytoin and related anticonvulsants
Barbiturates
Penicillins
Carbamazepine
Malignancy with or without radiation therapy
Carcinoma
Lymphoma

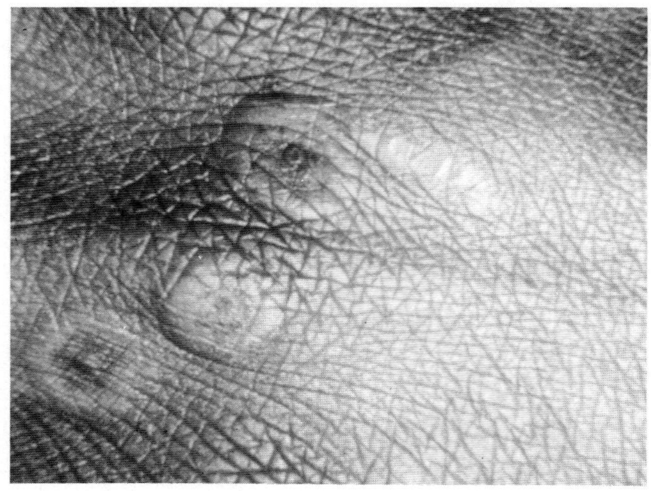

Fig. 161-1. Erythema multiforme secondary to heroin snuff.

The characteristic iris lesions of erythema multiforme are erythematous plaques with dusky centers and bright red borders, resembling the bull's-eye of a target (Fig. 161-5).

The eruption has a predilection for dorsum of the hands, palms, soles, and extensor surfaces of the extremities. Lesions tend to appear in crops over a period of 2 to 4 weeks, and, rarely, over many months. The individual lesions heal in 7 to 10 days without scarring unless the site is secondarily infected. However, in dark-skinned patients post-inflammatory hyperpigmentation or hypopigmentation is common. When associated with herpes simplex virus, erythema multiforme can recur 5 to 7 days after each viral relapse and with drug incitant can recur upon repeat exposure.

The Stevens-Johnson eponym is reserved for the most severe bullous form of erythema multiforme. It is frequently preceded by a prodrome of variable symptoms, such as fever, malaise, myalgias, and arthralgias, which probably stem from an underlying infectious disease. The mucocutaneous lesions have abrupt onset and are associated with marked constitutional symptoms and multisystem pathology. The mucosal surfaces of the lips, cheeks, palate, eyes, urethra, vagina, nose, and anus are involved (Fig. 161-6). In severe cases the linings of the

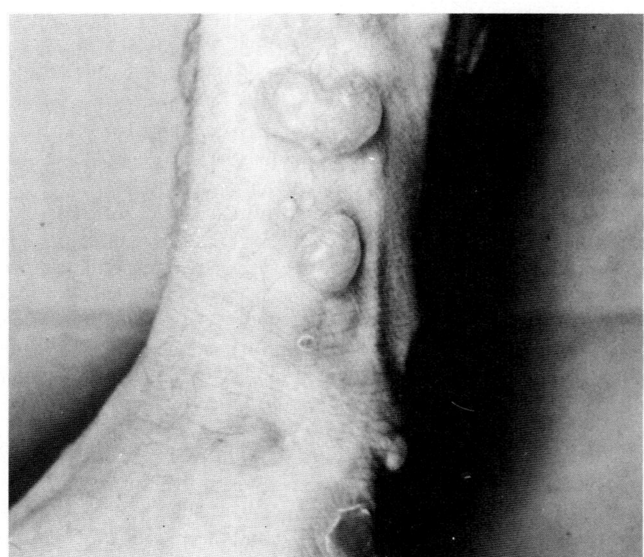

Fig. 161-2. Erythema multiforme bullosum secondary to cancer of the stomach.

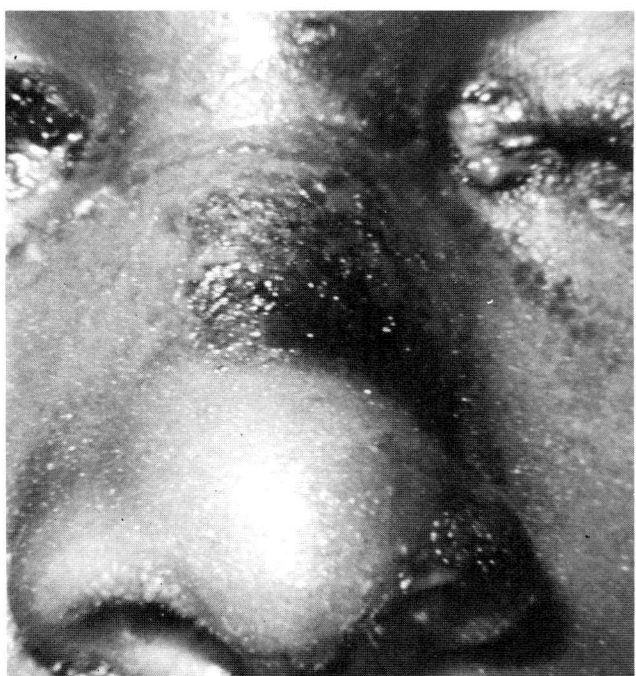

Fig. 161-3. Bullous erythema multiforme of the face.

pharynx, tracheobronchial tree, and esophagus are also affected. The lesions begin as blisters, which rupture to leave shreds of necrotic grayish-white epithelium and blood-crusted denuded bases. Patients are often unable to eat because of the painful stomatitis. The eyes have a catarrhal or purulent conjunctivitis, and vesicles are sometimes observed on the conjunctivae.

The Stevens-Johnson syndrome has substantial morbidity and a mortality of 5 to 10 percent. Denuded surfaces are susceptible to secondary

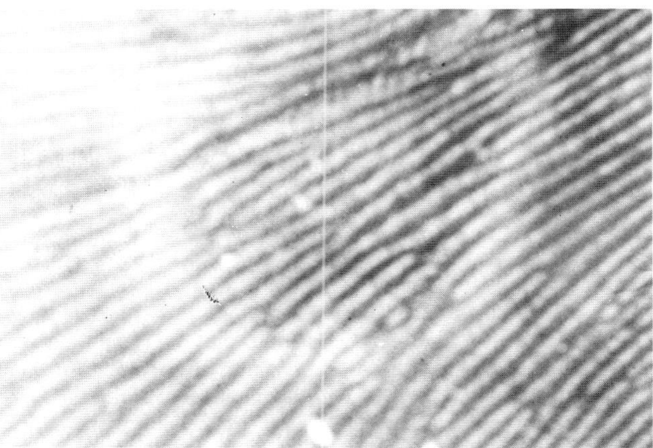

Fig. 161-5. Erythema multiforme lesions tend to appear in crops over a period of 2 to 4 weeks.

bacterial infection, and, when untreated, these can lead to scar formation. Nails may occasionally be shed, balanitis can lead to scarred attachment of the foreskin to the glans, and vulvovaginitis can lead to stenosis of the vagina. Hematuria, renal tubular necrosis, and progressive renal failure can occur but are rare. More common are significant ocular sequelae, including corneal ulceration, anterior uveitis, panophthalmitis, corneal opacities, and blindness.

Differential Diagnosis

Conditions to be differentiated include the migratory annular erythemas such as erythema annulare centrifugum; toxic erythemas of infectious or drug origin; blistering disorders such as bullous pemphigoid, pemphigus vulgaris, herpes gestationis; and the cutaneous and systemic vasculitides. Erythema multiforme has also been seen in association with erythema nodosum and toxic epidermal necrolysis.

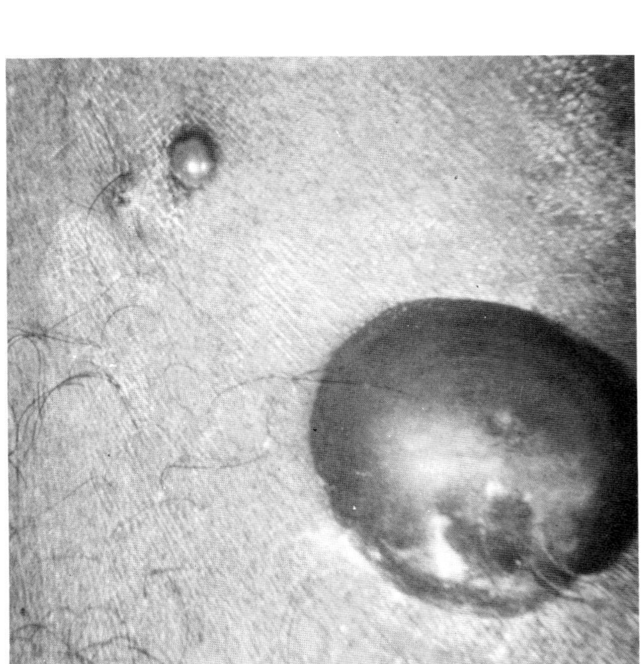

Fig. 161-4. Erythema multiforme bullosum lesions are usually annular and sharply demarcated from normal skin.

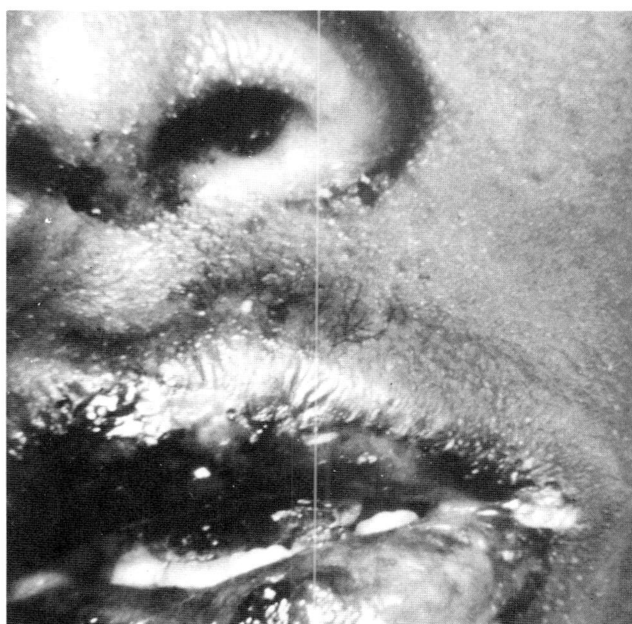

Fig. 161-6. Bullous erythema multiforme of the mouth, a commonly involved orifice.

DIAGNOSIS AND TREATMENT

The clinical features are usually distinctive enough to permit a diagnosis, but a skin biopsy should be obtained in equivocal cases. Because erythema multiforme is a pattern reaction, appropriate investigative studies should be undertaken to determine the underlying cause, and all drugs of potential etiologic significance must be stopped. Respiratory failure can develop secondary to mucosal sloughing. While renal complications are uncommon, kidney function should be monitored.

Patients with limited disease can be treated on an outpatient basis with topical corticosteroids. However, those with severe mucous membrane involvement require hospitalization, preferably in a burn unit, where fluids and electrolytes can be managed and frequent secondary bacterial infections controlled. Ophthalmologic consultation is necessary if there is eye involvement. Relief from painful stomatitis can sometimes be achieved with diphenhydramine hydrochloride elixir or viscous lidocaine held in the mouth for 3 to 5 min before expectorating. Systemic corticosteroids give symptomatic relief but are of unproven value in influencing the duration and outcome of the disease. Indeed, many authorities believe that systemic corticosteroid therapy is contraindicated in the treatment of Stevens-Johnson syndrome.

BIBLIOGRAPHY

Bedi TR, Pinkus H: Histopathological spectrum of erythema multiforme. *Br J Dermatol* 95:243, 1976.

Bianchine JR, Macaraeg P, Lasagna L, et al: Drugs as etiologic factors in the Stevens-Johnson syndrome. *Am J Med* 44:390, 1968.

Bluefarb SM, Szanto P: Erythema multiforme associated with acute renal tubular necrosis. *Arch Dermatol* 92:367, 1965.

Comaish JS, Kerr DNS: Erythema multiforme and nephritis. *Br Med J* 2:84, 1961.

Ginsburg C: Stevens-Johnson syndrome in children. *Pediatr Infect Dis* 1:155, 1982.

Imamura S, Yanese K, Teniguchi S, et al: Erythema multiforme: Demonstration of immune complexes in the sera and skin lesions. *Br J Dermatol* 102:161, 1980.

Kazmirowski JA, Peizner DS, Wuepper MD: Herpes simplex antigen in immune complexes of patients with erythema multiforme. *JAMA* 247:2547, 1982.

Marvin JA, Heimbach DM, Engrav LH, et al: Improved treatment of the Stevens-Johnson syndrome. *Arch Surg* 119:601, 1984.

Prendiville JS, Hebert AA, Greenwald MJ, et al: Management of Stevens-Johnson syndrome and toxic epidermal necrolysis in children. *J Pediatr* 115:881, 1989.

Shelly WB: Herpes simplex virus as a cause of erythema multiforme. *JAMA* 201:153, 1967.

162
TOXIC EPIDERMAL NECROLYSIS
Thomas A. Chapel

Toxic epidermal necrolysis, also called the *scalded skin syndrome,* is composed of two distinct clinicopathologic entities: one associated with staphylococcal infection and the other due to a drug or chemical agent. Both forms are characterized by the sudden appearance of patches of intense, tender erythema that is followed by widespread loosening of skin and denudation to a glistening base.

The first form is called the *staphylococcal scalded skin syndrome* and usually afflicts children under the age of 5 years (Fig. 162-1). The disorder is associated with an underlying staphylococcal infection and is due to the production of a toxin that cleaves the epidermis beneath the stratum granulosum. The exact mode of action of the toxin is unknown, although studies suggest an intercellular target or a specific receptor-toxin interaction. Because the cleavage plane is intraepidermal, fluid loss may not be extreme, and despite widespread exfoliation the mortality is less than 5 percent.

CLINICAL FEATURES

Staphylococcal scalded skin syndrome comprises a spectrum of skin lesions ranging from localized bullous impetigo to generalized exfoliation. The disease begins as tender, erythematous patches of scarletiniform lesions that often follow an upper respiratory tract infection or purulent conjunctivitis. The initial lesions are characteristically distributed on the periorificial areas of the face, the neck, the axillae, and the groin. At this stage lateral pressure on the skin causes separation of the epidermis from the dermis (positive Nikolsky's sign). Large flaccid bullae sometimes develop, and within 24 to 48 h the epidermis spontaneously separates in rumpled sheets revealing a moist, erythematous base. Despite widespread exfoliation of the skin, the mucous membranes are not involved. The denuded bases dry rapidly leading to a postinflammatory desquamation that resolves in 5 to 7 days.

The form caused by a drug or chemical agent occurs chiefly in adults and is characterized by separation of the skin at the dermoepidermal junction (Fig. 162-2). The involved epidermis is necrotic, but little infiltrate is seen in the dermis. The lesions of the scalded skin syndrome are widespread, and the mucous membranes are commonly involved (Figs. 162-3 and 162-4). At times, the skin lesions may resemble those of erythema multiforme. The complete loss of the epidermis is associated with slow healing, and reepithelialization takes 1 to 3 weeks. Drug-related toxic epidermal necrolysis carries a 5 to 50 percent mortality due to fluid loss and secondary infection (Table 162-1)

Differential Diagnosis

Clinically, toxic epidermal necrolysis may be confused with pemphigus vulgaris, thermal or chemical burns, and severe erythema multiforme. Patients with a graft-versus-host reaction may have a reaction like the drug-induced form of toxic epidermal necrolysis.

DIAGNOSIS

The morphology of toxic epidermal necrolysis is sufficiently distinct to permit clinical diagnosis. However, the age of the patient is not an absolute indicator of the underlying cause. A history of drug usage or chemical exposure and the results of bacterial culture and skin biopsy allow differentiation of the two forms. Amon and Dimond have suggested methods for more rapid differentiation. The level of separation in the cutaneum can be determined by examining the cells from denuded areas or by examining frozen sections of bullae roofs.

The first technique involves scraping the denuded bases with a no. 15 sterile surgical blade. The material collected is smeared on a clean glass slide and examined. In the staphylococcal scalded skin syndrome, a few acantholytic keratinocytes will be evident, while in the nonstaphylococcal type, inflammatory cells, cellular debris, and basal cell keratinocytes will be present.

The second technique involves histologic examination of a frozen section of skin peeled from a fresh lesion of toxic epidermal necrolysis. In the drug-induced form of the disorder, the split is at the dermal-epidermal junction and a full thickness of epidermis is present, while in the staphylococcal scalded skin syndrome only stratum corneum and a few granular cells are seen.

The growth of *Staphylococcus aureus* on cultures obtained from the conjuctiva, nose, throat, perineum, and skin strongly suggests an infectious cause. Definitive diagnosis is made by excisional or punch biopsy specimen of involved skin.

TREATMENT

A patient with toxic epidermal necrolysis has temporarily lost his or her skin barrier against percutaneous water loss. Adults with toxic necrolysis lose an average of 2 to 4 L/day by evaporation for the first 9 days. In general, greater losses of plasma occur within the first few days, whereas water loss predominates later in the course. At any rate, volume and electrolyte replacement should be done in the emergency department if there are signs of hypovolemia. The possibility of septic shock should also be considered in the different diagnosis of hypotension.

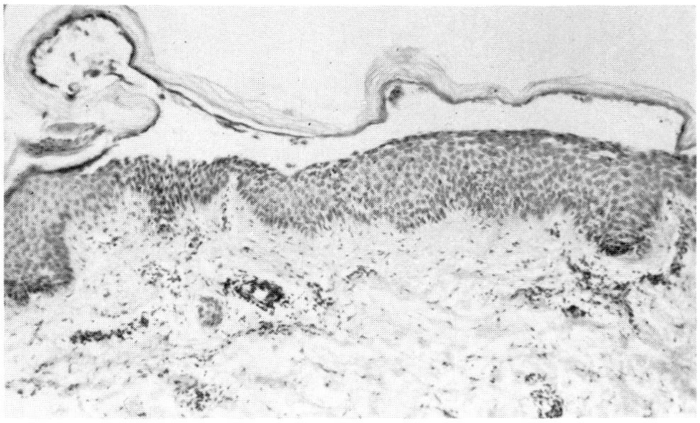

Fig. 162-1. Staphylococcal scalded skin syndrome.

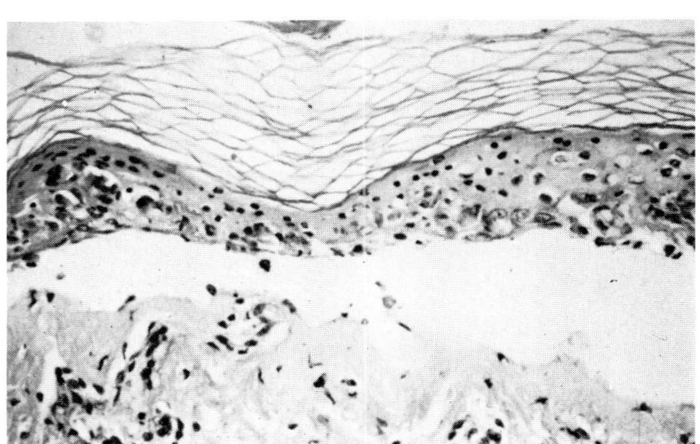

Fig. 162-2. Drug-induced toxic epidermal necrolysis.

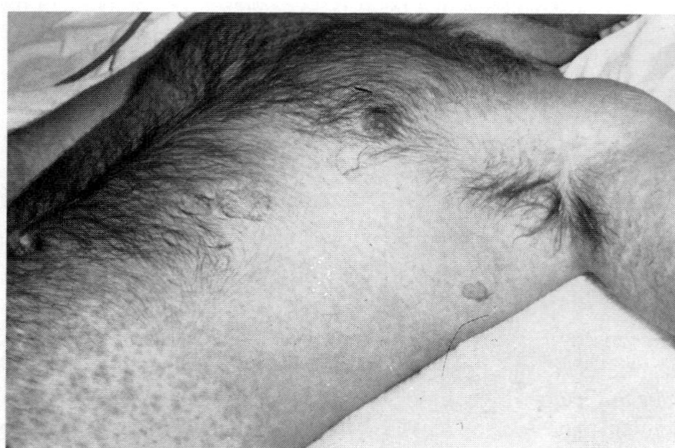

Fig. 162-3. Toxic epidermal necrolysis secondary to a sulfone.

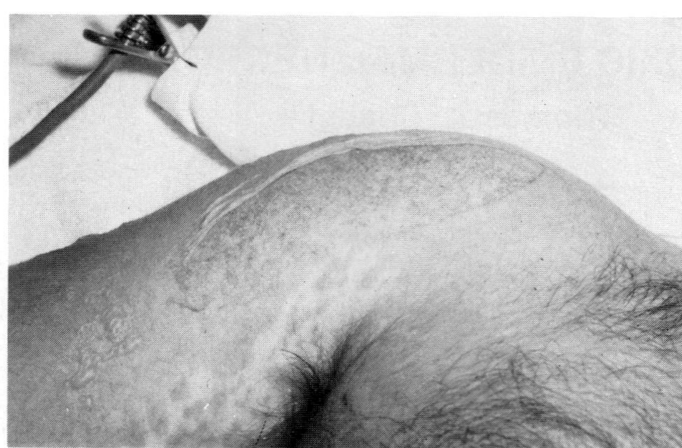

Fig. 162-4. Closeup view of toxic epidermal necrolysis secondary to a sulfone.

Staphylococcal scalded skin syndrome should be treated with an oral or intravenous penicillinase-resistant penicillin, even though antibiotic therapy does not seem to alter the course of the cutaneous disease. Corticosteroids are contraindicated in staphylococcal scalded skin syndrome. Their value has not been proved in drug-related toxic epidermal necrolysis.

Until barrier function is restored, the lesions of toxic epidermal necrolysis are treated as second-degree burns. Patients with less than 10 percent loss of skin usually can be treated successfully with tub baths of potassium permanganate or dressings soaked in 0.5 percent silver nitrate. Silver sulfadiazine and mafenide acetate creams should be avoided because sulfonamide drugs are often the cause of toxic epidermal necrolysis and becuase these drugs delay epithelialization. Antibiotics in drug-induced toxic necrolysis are reserved for treating disease caused by identified pathogens. If the eyes are involved, an ophthalmologist should be consulted.

Patients with more than ten percent loss of skin should be admitted to the burn unit. Intensive supportive care available in burn units coupled with newer grafting techniques using cadaver allografts, porcine xenografts and hydrocolloid dressings have reduced morbidity and mortality.

SUMMARY

There are two forms of toxic epidermal necroylsis, or scalded skin syndrome. The staphylococcal scalded skin syndrome generally occurs in children and, if appropriately treated, carries a favorable prognosis. The adult form is caused by a drug or chemical agent and carries a 5 to 50 percent mortality due to fluid loss and secondary infection.

The age of the patient is not an absolute indicator of the cause. The two types are differentiated by a history of drug usage or chemical exposure and by the results of bacterial culture and skin biopsy.

The lesions are treated as second-degree burns. The form associated with staphylococcal injection is treated with antibiotics, and steroids are contraindicated. Patients with the drug-related form are most appropriately cared for in the burn unit.

BIBLIOGRAPHY

Amon RB, Dimond RL: Toxic epidermal necrolysis: Rapid differentiation between staphylococcal-induced disease and drug-induced disease. *Arch Dermatol* 111:1433, 1975.

Birke G. Liljedahl S, Rajka G: Lyell's syndrome: Metabolic and clinical results of a new form of treatment. *Acta Derm Venereol (Stockh)* 51:199, 1971.

Elias PM, Fritsch P, Dahl MV, et al: Staphylococcal toxic epidermal necrolysis: Pathogenesis and studies on the subcellular site of action of exfoliation. *J Invest Dermatol* 65:501, 1975.

Elias PM, Fritsch P, Epstein EH Jr: Staphylococcal scalded skin syndrome: Clinical features, pathogenesis, and recent microbiological and biochemical developments. *Arch Dermatol* 113:207, 1977.

Lillibridge CB, Melish ME, Glasgow LA: Site of action of exfoliative toxin in the staphylococcal scalded skin syndrome. *Pediatrics* 50:728, 1972.

Lyell A: Toxic epidermal necrolysis: The scalded skin syndrome. *J Contin Ed Dermatol* 16:15, 1978.

Rudolph RI, Schwartz W, Leyden JJ: Treatment of staphylococcal toxic epidermal necrolysis. *Arch Dermatol* 110:559, 1974.

163 CUTANEOUS ABSCESSES

Harvey W. Meislin

Soft tissue infections and cutaneous abscesses are common emergency department problems, accounting for up to 5 percent of all visits. The time-honored treatment has been surgical incision and drainage.

BACTERIOLOGY

The bacteria in cutaneous abscesses, in general, reflect the skin flora of the anatomic area of the body that is involved. Thus, abscesses originating from mucous membranes (e.g., oral cavity, vagina, and rectum) reflect the anaerobic and aerobic flora of the mucosa; abscesses on the other areas of the body reflect skin flora. Anaerobic bacteria are part of the normal flora of the skin and all mucous membranes, including the mouth, vagina, urethra, and colon. In the oral cavity, anaerobes outnumber aerobes 10:1. In the distal colon, this ratio is increased to greater than 1000:1; and 20 to 30 percent of the wet weight of stool is a solid mass of living bacteria, nearly all of which are anaerobic. Anaerobes are commonly seen in abscesses, usually in mixed cultures, and primarily in the perineal areas. Their importance in infection of the central nervous system (CNS) the intraabdominal cavity, and the respiratory system is well documented.

Bacteroides fragilis (Table 163-1) is in general the only anaerobe resistant to penicillin and the most common gram-negative anaerobe in human feces. It is most common in abscesses involving the perineal region. Anaerobic abscesses are usually mixed. *Escherichia coli* and *Neisseria gonorrheae* are not commonly seen in cutaneous abscesses in any location.

Staphylococcus aureus is the most prevalent aerobe in cutaneous abscesses. In several recent studies, *S. aureus* was found in about one-fourth of all abscesses and was almost always isolated in pure culture. It was, however, isolated much less frequently than clinically expected (less than 50 percent of the time; Table 163-2). Two-thirds of all *S. aureus* infections were seen in abscesses from the upper torso (the head, neck, axilla, and trunk area). This organism has a well-recognized propensity for abscess formation, and its potential for abscess formation is not as dependent on synergistic bacterial mixtures as is that of anaerobes. Outpatient infections with *S. aureus* showed a 97-percent resistance to penicillin G.

Proteus mirabilis, a normal inhabitant of feces, is the most common gram-negative aerobe found. It is seen mainly in cutaneous abscesses of the upper torso (Table 163-3). The reason for this in not clear, since *P. mirabilis* is not a normal inhabitant of the skin of the upper torso.

Escherichia coli, the most common aerobe seen in stool and intraabdominal abscesses, is cultured rarely from any cutaneous abscess, occasionally from perineal abscesses. It is a common misconception that foul-smelling pus is due to *E. coli* or other enteric aerobes; in fact, the pus of an *E. coli* abscess is odorless. The foul odor of abscesses in the perirectal area is due to the presence of anaerobic bacteria.

Drug abuse-related abscesses may have more cellulitis, induration, and regional node involvement. Moreover, their course is often more rapid from the onset. This clinical picture is most likely due to the injection of chemical irritants, not only from the drug itself but from other adulterants, occasionally resulting in sterile abscesses.

GRAM STAINS

The Gram-stained smear is a reliable, quick, and readily available method of identifying offending pathogens from soft tissue infections. With this method of presumptive identification, a rational choice of an appropriate antibiotic may be made before culture results are known. Unfortunately, the Gram-stained smear of an abscess does not differentiate aerobes from anaerobes. However, three specific patterns of Gram-stain morphology are consistently helpful:

1. If a Gram-stained smear of pus (carefully aspirated from an abscess cavity) shows only large gram-positive cocci in grapelike clusters, the abscess is almost certainly infected with *S. aureus,* which has been shown to exist most often in pure culture.
2. Gram-stained smears that show no bacteria at all are most likely from a sterile abscess.
3. A mixed Gram-stained pattern, with combinations of gram-positive and gram-negative cocci and rods, is indicative of a mixed aerobic and anaerobic infection.

CLINICAL PRESENTATION

The etiology of an abscess should be sought. Extremity abscesses are usually associated with interruptions of the integrity of the normally protective epithelium. Ultrasound is a useful technique for localizing subcutaneous and intramuscular abscesses as well as foreign bodies. Perirectal abscesses commonly arise from anal crypts; pilonidal abscesses result from infection secondary to an ingrown hair or plugging of small tears in the skin, and vulvovaginal abscesses result from obstructed Bartholin's glands. In general, men present with head and neck, perirectal, and extremity abscesses; women with axillary, vulvovaginal, and perirectal abscesses.

Patients most frequently complain of localized pain and swelling around the abscess. Most date the onset of symptoms within the preceding week. Patients frequently attempt self-treatment by repeatedly squeezing or pinching the abscess soon after its presence is noted and may come to the physician with a traumatized, inadequately drained lesion.

Table 163-1. Frequency of Isolation of *Bacteroides fragilis*

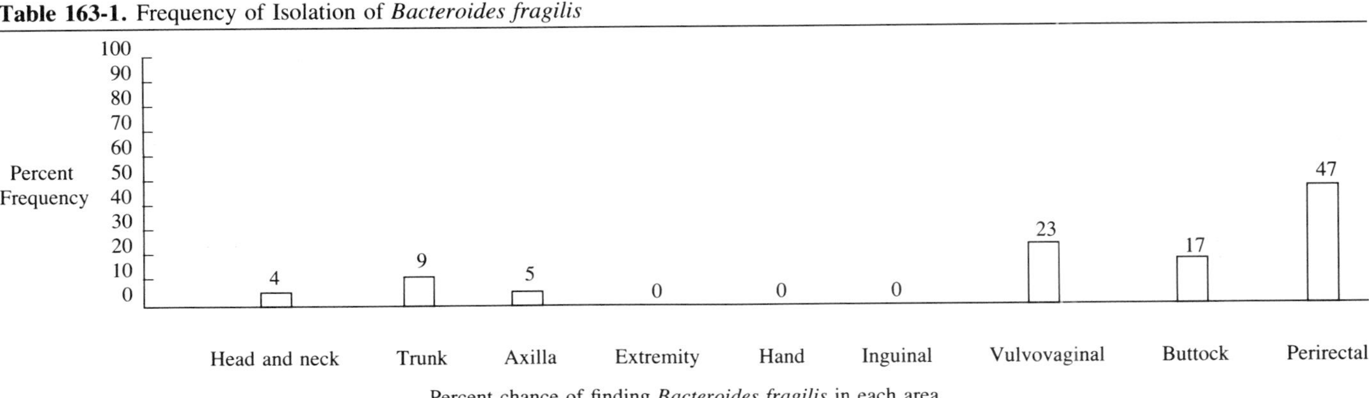

Table 163-2. Frequency of Isolation of *Staphylococcus aureus*

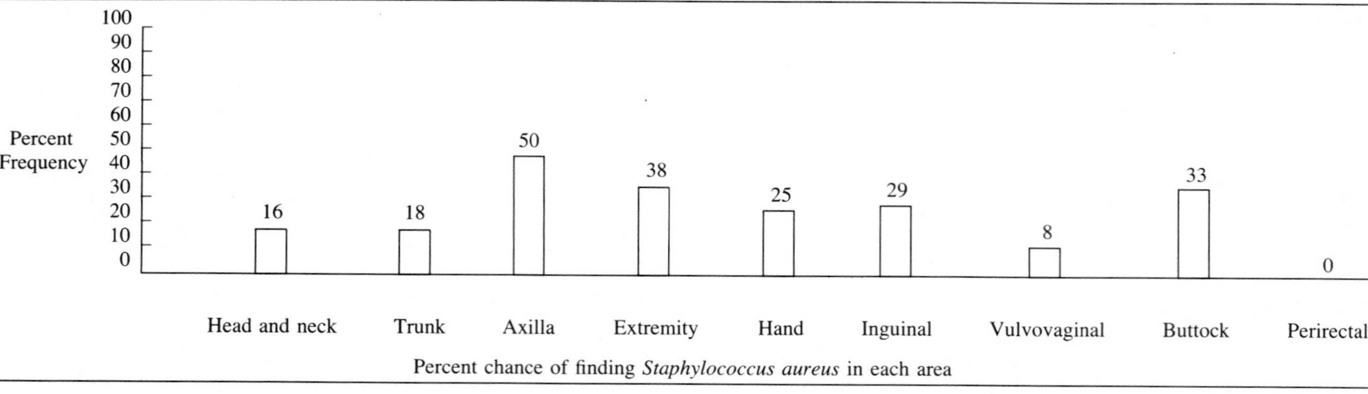

Table 163-3. Frequency of Isolation of *Proteus mirabilis*

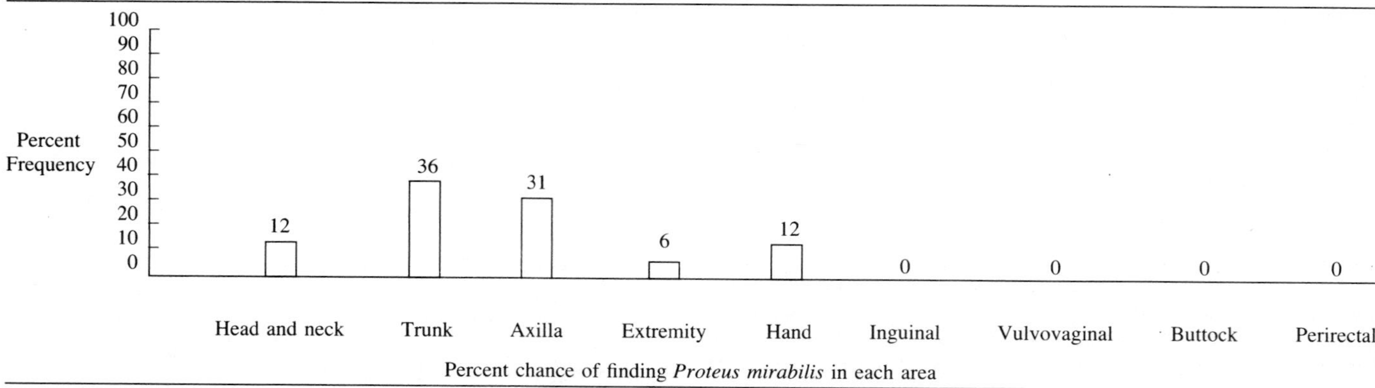

Most normal patients who have cutaneous abscesses have little evidence of systemic toxicity. Although a slight tachycardia is common, it may be due to pain or anxiety as well as to the direct toxic effects of the infection. Induration, cellulitis, lymphedema, lymphangitis, and regional lymphadenopathy may be present. Fever is rare. In fact, fever in a patient with a cutaneous abscess may indicate an infection that is not localized. Similarly, fever may be evidence of compromise in the natural host defenses, which could predispose the patient to systemic infection. The physician should look for evidence of trauma, thermal injury, neoplasms (especially leukemia), diabetes mellitus, vascular insufficiency, collagen vascular disease, corticosteroid therapy, and chemotherapy, all of which lower the body's ability to combat infection.

Some patients, despite adequate treatment, may return with nonhealing or frequently recurring abscesses. Lower abdominal abscesses or abscesses in the perineal area may suggest the presence of an undiagnosed inflammatory bowel disease; 10 percent of patients with Crohn's disease have complications of perirectal abscesses and fistulas. Frequently recurring abscesses in the axillary and inguinal areas may be a sign of hidradenitis suppurativa. Likewise, nonhealing or recurring abscesses may be caused by any of the factors listed above that diminish natural host defenses. Abscesses given special significance are

Furuncle: a deep-inflammatory nodule evolving from a superficial folliculitis. The abscess is thin walled, purulence is usually present, and skin flora predominates.

Carbuncle: an extensive process of deep abscesses that interconnect and extend into the subcutaneous tissue. Predisposing factors include folliculitis; diabetes; steroid usage; heavy perspiration; obesity; and areas of friction, especially the back of the neck.

Hidradenitis suppurativa: chronic suppurative abscesses in the apocrine sweat glands of the axilla and/or groin. Females predominate, and there is an association with obesity, excessive perspiration, shaving, and poor hygiene. The disease is chronic, producing a malodorous discharge, and often heals with scarring. Skin flora predominate, but overgrowth with *Proteus mirabilis* and other mixed aerobes and anaerobes is common. Incision and drainage is the usual treatment for acute disease; chronic processes often need extensive surgical debridement of the apocrine gland areas.

Bartholin's cyst: an abscess occurring secondary to an obstructed Bartholin's duct. The microflora of the purulence usually is typical of vaginal flora. Incision and drainage should take place on the mucosal side of the cyst; marsupialization of the cyst will prevent recurrence.

Pilonidal abscesses: occur in the gluteal fold area and result from disruption of the epithelial surface, with plugging of the resultant cavity with hair or keratin. These are cutaneously borne abscesses and do not originate from the rectal crypts. Thus, the bacteriology of these abscesses is typical of cutaneous surfaces. The patient presents with a painful mass in the gluteal fold. Superficial abscesses should receive incision and drainage typical of cutaneous abscesses. Chronic and deep abscesses are often treated with deep surgical debridement and excision of cysts, sinuses, and granulation tissue.

Perirectal abscess: abscesses originating in the anal crypts and burrowing through the ischiorectal space. The abscesses are named according to where purulence accumulates, for example, perianal, perirectal, ischiorectal, and supralevator (pelvirectal). Fecal flora predominates, and fistula formation is common. Many of these abscesses can be drained in the outpatient setting; however, if the process is extensive or difficult to drain because of pain or location, drainage in the operating suite under appropriate anesthesia is indicated.

TREATMENT

The primary treatment for the localized cutaneous abscess in an otherwise healthy, nontoxic patient is incusion and drainage alone. Most

Table 163-4. Treatment of the Cutaneous Abscess

Normal host defenses:
Incision and drainage
No culture or Gram-stained smear
No antibiotics
High-risk patient (septic, immunosuppressed, diabetic, special locations):
Incision and drainage
Culture and Gram-stained smear
Antibiotics

patients, if treated properly, do not require antibiotics (Table 163-4). Taking cultures or preparing Gram-stained smears of the abscess, while providing definitive information about the infection's cause, is not necessary for a successful outcome in these patients.

Incision and Drainage

It is common to underestimate the extent of the abscess and the amount of pus that needs to be evacuated, especially in perineal and extremity abscesses, where tense induration alone, without fluctuance, may be the only clue to the presence of underlying pus. A physician who is uncertain about whether a subcutaneous infection is a simple cellulitis or an abscess should attempt needle aspiration of the area. Any amount of aspirated pus is significant, since it indicates the presence of an abscess that usually demands surgical drainage. If no pus is aspirated, the infection is probably a cellulitis that has not yet loculated. These infections may be treated with frequent warm soaks and an antibiotic whose spectrum covers the common skin flora of the area involved. The efficacy of antibiotics in the treatment of cellulitis has not been documented. However, if antibiotics are used, a specimen for culture and a Gram-stained smear may be obtained by injecting 1 mL of sterile oxygen-free saline solution (nonbacteriostatic) into the cellulitis area; the saline solution is then reaspirated for examination. Patients must be followed until the process is resolved, since some infections proceed to abscess formation despite the use of antibiotics.

Incision and drainage are unavoidably painful. Local anesthesia, properly used, anesthetizes only the dermal roof of the abscess. Large volumes of anesthetic infiltrated around the abscess only increase the swelling, ultimately causing more pain and further compromise to the blood supply. Regional blocks may provide anesthesia for the drainage of extremity abscesses. It is often comforting to the patient, as well as facilitating for the physician, to premedicate the patient with intramuscular opiates 30 to 40 min prior to the procedure. For a 70-kg patient, a dose of 50 to 150 mg of meperidine hydrochloride or 5 to 10 mg of morphine sulfate with 25 to 50 mg of narcotic potentiator such as promethazine hydochloride or hydroxyzine should be adequate. Intravenous diazepam can also be used, and a 50 percent nitrous oxide/50 percent oxygen mixture can provide analgesia in selected patients.

The decision to drain an abscess in the emergency department as opposed to the operating suite depends upon the ability to achieve adequate anesthesia, the depth of the abscess, and the ability of the patient to recover on an outpatient basis. Most localized cutaneous abscesses can be incised and drained in the emergency department. Deep abscesses that extend below the subcutaneous fascia, those located near neurovascular bundles, those requiring extensive debridement, and those in which analgesia is not satisfactory should be drained in the operating suite. Likewise, perianal abscesses that extend to the supralevator muscle or into the ischiorectal space or rectum must be drained in the operating suite.

The patient should be positioned to allow complete visualization of the abscess site. For vulvovaginal abscesses, the patient should be placed in the lithotomy position. Perirectal and pilonidal abscesses are best treated with the patient in a knee-chest, Sims's, or prone position. Wide adhesive tape extending from the buttock fold to the table edge may be used to retract the buttock to ensure adequate exposure. The involved site is widely scrubbed with povidone-iodine and surgically draped. If no regional block is used, the skin though which the incision will be made should be anesthetized with 1 percent lidocaine or ethyl chloride spray over the extent of the fluctuance or, if no fluctuance is evident, over the central area of induration. If anaerobic cultures are needed, pus should be aspirated either percutaneously or immediately after the incision is made to prevent prolonged exposure to air.

An incision with a No. 11 scalpel blade is made through the skin and into the abscess cavity, extending along the full length of the fluctuance in the plane of the natural skin fold. Elliptical excision of the roof of the abscess cavity will prevent premature closure of the skin surface. Bartholin's abscesses should be incised through the mucosal rather than the cutaneous surface. Pus should flow freely, providing adequate material for culture and a gram-stained smear. An abscess is not a simple sphere but includes fingerlike networks of loculated granulation tissue and pus, extending outward along planes of least resistance. Hence, the cavity should be probed radially to break up loculated pockets of pus and thoroughly irrigated with saline solution until all pus and necrotic debris have been removed. Extreme caution should be used in areas such as the groin and neck, where large and important neurovascular structures are in close proximity. The abscess may then be loosely packed from the skin to its depth with a plain gauze wick. Tight packing of an abscess does not allow drainage and may impede the healing process. It is not necessary to use iodoform gauze. Finally, a dry, absorbent dressing is applied. The perineal area is an especially difficult region in which to maintain an adequate dressing. A sanitary napkin seems to work well with both anterior and posterior abscesses in this area. If the gauze packing inadvertently becomes dislodged, the patient should be instructed not to replace it but rather to begin warm sitz baths for 20 to 30 min four times daily.

The abscess is rechecked in 48 h, except for facial abscesses, which are rechecked in 24 h, when the packing is removed. Patients who show minimal drainage, resolution of the surrounding cellulitis, and formation of healing granulation tissue should be instructed to begin warm soaks. Those patients who show continued drainage should have their abscesses repacked and then rechecked in 24 to 48 h. At the time that the infection shows clear signs of healing, no further follow-up is indicated.

The use of antibiotics (Table 163-4) prior to and following incision and drainage has been considered in patients (1) with toxicity and a significant fever; (2) with an abscess in the mastoid area or the central triangle of the face, that is drained by the cavernous sinus; (3) with systemic disease or vascular compromise; or (4) taking immunosuppressive drugs or chemotherapy.

For such patients, a tentative identification of the invading bacteria may be made by (1) correlating the abscess site with the known bacteriologic data for similar sites to indicate the expected microflora of the abscess (in general, the microbial flora of a cutaneous abscess reflects the microflora of the skin and mucous membrances of that area); (2) finding foul-smelling pus, which often indicates the presence of anaerobes; and (3) preparing a Gram-stained smear of pus, which may identify sterile abscesses, mixed aerobic and anerobic abscesses, and abscesses infected with *S. aureus*.

Once tentative bacteriologic identification has been made, the most appropriate antibiotic can be chosen (Table 163-5). If antibiotics are used for abscesses in the axilla, head, neck, and extremities, an oral antistaphylococcal drug, such as dicloxacillin, erythromycin, cefoxitin, or clindamycin, is required.

Cephalosporins also are effective against *P. mirabilis*. Patients with suspected bacteremia should have blood cultures obtained and should be hospitalized. Drug abuse-related abscesses often contain penicillin-sensitive anaerobes, and *S. aureus* is seen less than one-fourth of the time.

In patients treated with antibiotics, aerobic and anaerobic cultures may be obtained to identify the specific bacteriologic spectrum of the abscess so that the antibiotic choice can be modified if indicated.

Table 163-5. Oral Therapy of Superficial Soft Tissue Infections

Streptococcus, group A:	
Penicillin V (phenoxymethyl penicillin)	250–500 mg q.i.d.
Erythromycin	500 mg–1 g q 6 h
Staphlococcus aureus:	
Cloxacillin	250–500 mg q 8 h
Dicloxacillin	125–500 mg q 6 h
Erythromycin	500 mg–1 g q 6 h
Clindamycin	150–450 mg q 6 h
Cephradine	250–500 mg q 6 h
Cephalexin	250–500 mg q 6 h
Amoxicillin/clavulanate	250–500 mg q 8 h
Haemophilus influenzae:	
Cefaclor	250–500 mg q 8 h
Cephradine	250–500 mg q 6 h
Cephalexin	250–500 mg q 6 h
Amoxicillin/clavulanate	250–500 mg q 8 h
Trimethoprim/sulfamethoxazole	160 mg TMP/800 mg SMX b.i.d.

Tetracycline is a poor first choice, since many anaerobes are resistant to it. Antibiotics for abscesses of the perineal region include gram-negative (aminoglycoside) and anaerobic coverage (clindamycin). Newer-generation cephalosporins may provide such coverage in a single drug.

BIBLIOGRAPHY

Anderson DK, Perry AW: Axillary hidradenitis. *Arch Surg* 110:69, 1975.

Brook I, Finegold SM: Aerobic and anaerobic bacteriology of cutaneous abscesses in children. *Pediatrics* 67:891, 1981.

Eisenhammer S: The anorectal fistulous abscess and fistula. *Dis Colon Rectum* 9:91, 1966.

Finegold SM, Bartless JG, Chow AW, et al: Management of anaerobic infections. *Ann Intern Med* 83:375, 1975.

Ghoneim ATM, McGoldrick J, Blick PWH, et al: Aerobic and anaerobic bacteriology of subcutaneous abscesses. *Br J Surg* 68:498, 1981.

Ginsberg MJ, Ellis GL, et al: Detection of soft tissue foreign bodies by plain radiography, xerography, computed tomography, and ultrasonography. *Ann Emerg Med* 19:701, 1990.

Gorbach SL, Bartlett JG: Anaerobic infections. *N Engl J Med* 290:1177, 1974.

Llera JL, Levy RC, Staneck JL: Cutaneous abscesses: Natural history and management in an outpatient facility. *J Emerg Med* 1:489, 1984.

Meislin HW, Lerner SA, Graves MH, et al: Cutaneous abscesses: Anaerobic and aerobic bacteriology and outpatient management. *Ann Intern Med* 87:145, 1977.

Meislin HW, McGehee MD, Rosen P: Management and microbiology of cutaneous abscesses. *J Am Coll Emerg Phsycians* 75:5, 1978.

Powers RD: Diagnosis and management of skin and soft tissue infections. *Emerg Med Rep* 11:229, 1990.

Simms MH, Curran F, Johnson RA, et al: Treatment of acute abscesses in casualty department. *Br Med J* 284:1827, 1982.

Vincent LM: Ultrasound of soft tissue abnormalities of the extremities. *Radiol Clin North Am,* 26:131, 1988.

164
SOFT TISSUE INFECTIONS

J. Stephan Stapczynski

TETANUS

Tetanus is a potentially lethal neuroparalytic disease caused by tetanospasmin, an exotoxin elaborated by *Clostridium tetani*. Tetanus is a rare disease in the United States—only 58 cases were reported during 1990—but in developing countries, tetanus remains a major health problem. Tetanus has a reported mortality of 21 percent in the United States, but mortality can be over 40 percent in developing countries. *Clostridium tetani* is a gram-positive anaerobic rod, ubiquitous in nature, found primarily in the soil and feces of many animals, including humans. The organism cannot invade healthy tissue; it requires the proper anaerobic conditions for the spores to convert into toxin-producing vegetative forms.

Tetanospasmim is a protoplasmic protein, with a molecular weight of approximately 67,000, released when vegetative forms of *C. tetani* autolyze. The toxin enters peripheral nerve endings and ascends the axons to reach the spinal cord and brain, where it irreversibly binds to and affects four areas of the nervous system. The major effect is at the level of the anterior horn cells of the spinal cord, where it impairs transmission of the inhibitary interneurons, releasing the normal supression of muscular antagonists and leading to marked neuromuscular irritability and generalized spasms. The toxin stimulates the sympathetic nervous system, producing sweating, labile blood pressure, peripheral vasoconstriction, and tachycardia. Tetanospasmin inhibits release of acetylcholine at the myoneural junction. Toxin also binds to cerebral gangliosides, which is probably the cause of the true seizures seen in some cases. There is no direct effect on the sensorium or sensory function.

Adults at highest risk for tetanus are the elderly, intravenous drug abusers, and those with decubiti or diabetic ulcers. Neonates and intravenous drug abusers have a higher case mortality than other patients.

Clinical Features

In tetanus, trismus is the presenting symptom in over 50 percent of cases. The severity of tetanus varies inversely with the incubation period. In mild cases the incubation period is longer than 10 days, stiffness is mild and may stay confined to an isolated muscle group (localized tetanus), true dysphagia or spasms never occur, and the case mortality is low. Patients with moderate cases experience a shorter incubation period, true dysphagia, and paroxysmal spasms but do not develop respiratory difficulty during attacks. Severe cases involve pronounced spasms with respiratory difficulty: glottal spasm may develop during these attacks, causing respiratory arrest.

Differential Diagnosis

The diagnosis of tetanus is based on the clinical picture—no specific ancillary test exists to make the diagnosis. Strychnine poisoning may mimic tetanus, with opisthotonus and seizures, but the signs of strychnine poisoning resolve quickly with supportive care, and the poison is detectable in the urine. Other diseases may mimic parts of the clinical picture of tetanus: acute dystonic reaction to phenothiazines, hypocalcemic tetany, meningitis and encephalitis, early rabies, epileptic seizures, narcotic withdrawal, or localized head and neck infections.

Treatment

Emergency management should include the following:

1. Asphyxia is the most preventable cause of death. Maintaining the airway with endotracheal intubation and mechanical ventilation is necessary in severe cases.
2. Muscular spasms should be controlled with diazepam IV, titrated as needed. Very large doses may be required.
3. Neuromuscular blockade may be necessary to produce the full clinical benefit of mechanical ventilation. Nondepolarizing agents, such as vecuronium or pancuronium, are recommended.
4. Marked variations in blood pressure and heartache due to autonomic nervous system dysfunction may require pharmacologic treatment. Various agents used for this purpose include phenothiazines, general anesthetics, β- and α-adrenergic antagonists, magnesium sulfate, intrathecal baclofen, and morphine. No single agent is consistently effective, and treatment must be adjusted according to the patient's course.
5. Further toxin production should be diminished, and early, aggressive surgical debridement of the causative wound makes theoretical sense, although there is no clear evidence about the effect of the timing and extent of debridement.
6. Any remaining unbound toxin should be neutralized with 3000 to 10,000 units of human tetanus immune globulin [TIG (h), (Hyper-tet)] IM. There is no advantage to infiltrating the wound site with TIG. Studies in other countries suggest that intrathecal administration of TIG, particularly in neonatal tetanus, is associated with a lower case mortality than intramuscular administration.
7. High doses of antibiotics directed against the causative organism are often recommended, although there is no clear evidence of their value. Penicillin G, 4 to 6 million units per day IV, is usually recommended, with metronidazole a good alternative.
8. Patients should be in as quiet a room as possible; any stimulation, including noise, may precipitate generalized spasms and cardiovascular instability.
9. Clinical tetanus does not produce immunity; the first dose of tetanus toxoid should be given in the emergency department.
10. If an acute dystonic reaction is a diagnostic possibility, a test dose of diphenhydramine (50 mg) or benztropine mesylate (2 mg IV) can be given to exclude this diagnosis.

Wound Management

Proper wound care includes cleaning, irrigation, debridement, and removal of foreign bodies from all wounds, even ocular wounds and minor puncture wounds, abrasions, and burns. Since tetanus occasionally occurs after trivial wounds or even without any detectable skin break, the concept of a clean wound without risk of tetanus is debatable. Current recommendations of the Public Health Service Advisory Committee on Immunization Practices for Tetanus prophylaxis in wound management are given in Table 164-1. For children less than 7 years old, diphtheria-tetanus-pertussis vaccine (DTP)—DT if pertussis vaccine is contraindicated—is preferred to tetanus toxoid alone. For those over 7 years old, tetanus-diphtheria toxoid (Td) is preferred to tetanus toxoid alone.

The major hazard of too-frequent (e.g., annual) tetanus toxoid administration is the development of an Arthus-type hypersensitivity reaction, generally beginning 2 to 8 h after injection. Systemic reactions such as uticaria or angioneurotic edema have been rarely reported. The only contraindication to the use of tetanus toxoid is a history of neurologic or severe hypersensitivity reactions; local adverse effects alone do not preclude use. For unimmunized patients older than 7 years complete protection is afforded by three doses of Td. The second dose is given at 4 to 8 weeks and the third dose at 6 to 12 months.

Table 164-1. Summary Guide to Tetanus Prophylaxis in Routine Wound Management, 1985

	Clean, Minor Wounds		All Other Wounds	
	Td	**TIG**	**Td**	**TIG**
Uncertain or <3 doses	Yes	No	Yes	Yes
3 or more doses and <5 years since last dose	No	No	No	No
3 or more doses and 5–10 years since last dose	No	No	Yes	No
3 or more doses and >10 years since last dose	Yes	No	Yes	No

Source: ACIP: Diphtheria, tetanus, pertussis: Guidelines for Vaccine prophylaxis and other preventive measures. *MMWR* 34:405, 419, 1985.

GAS GANGRENE

Clostridial myonecrosis, or *gas gangrene,* is a rapidly progressive soft tissue infection with muscle necrosis, gas production, and systemic toxicity. It is caused by one of seven species of histotoxic *Clostridia,* with *C. perfringens* being the most common isolate. In the most common presentation of this disease, clostridial spores contaminate wounds when trauma produces an anaerobic environment appropriate for the development and growth of the toxin-producing vegetative forms. A less common presentation is spontaneous clostridial myonecrosis; this presumably results from bacteremic spread of the organism from the bowel to skeletal muscle. In the United States, it has been estimated that there are over 1000 civilian cases of clostridial myonecrosis each year, with an overall case mortality of around 30 percent. However, mortalities are significantly higher for patients with either truncal involvement or a spontaneous presentation.

Clinical Presentation

The incubation period is typically short, usually less than 3 days. The onset is acute, the first symptom being a sense of heaviness or weight in the muscle, followed rapidly by severe pain. Systemic toxicity is present, manifested by tachycardia, poor skin perfusion, and alterations in sensorium but usually only a slight elevation in temperature. At this early stage the primary wound is usually not pyogenic and crepitance is minimal. Within hours, a thin, brownish exudate develops and the skin becomes discolored. The discharge contains red cells and clostridia but very few white cells. Gas begins to develop within the muscle and is detected by palpable crepitance or by air visible on x-ray films. Large cutaneous bullae filled with purple fluid may eventually appear. Bacteremia occurs in only 15 percent or less.

Differential Diagnosis

Other rapidly spreading gas-forming soft tissue infections may be confused with gas gangrene: crepitant cellulitis, synergistic necrotizing cellulitis, necrotizing fasciitis, acute streptococcal hemolytic gangrene, and streptococcal myositis. While these syndromes may have a distinctive picture in their pure state, in practice it is often difficult to make a firm clinical diagnosis. Surgical exploration of the involved fascia and muscle is mandatory for correct diagnosis. In the early stage of gas gangrene the muscles are edematous and pale and still bleed when cut. Later, contractility is lost and dissection reveals beefy red, nonbleeding muscle tissue with gas bubbles between the fibers. Gram stain of the exudate or muscle tissue shows the gram-positive rods and very few leukocytes.

Treatment

Emergency management should include the following:

1. Immediate resuscitation requires volume expansion and blood to counteract shock and replenish red cells lost to hemolysis.
2. Antibiotics are recommended to suppress the spread of infection and treat bacteremia; they are also clearly beneficial in animal models of gas gangrene. Penicillin G, 10 to 30 million units per day IV, is the drug of choice, with chloramphenicol, 4 g/day, the alternative in penicillin-allergic patients. Some histotoxic clostridia are resistant to tetracycline. Prior to surgery other gas-forming soft tissue infections may be a diagnostic possibility. Antibiotics to treat possible infection with anaerobes (clindamycin or chloramphenicol), gram-negative rods (aminoglycosides), or staphylococci (semisynthetic penicillinase-resistant penicillin or vancomycin) should be given prior to surgery. The combination of cefoxitin, 80 to 160 mg/kg per day, and gentamicin, 2 to 4 mg/kg per day, IV in divided doses, provides adequate coverage in this situation.
3. Surgical debridement is the second therapeutic modality in animal models and clearly beneficial in humans. However, the timing of surgery is less clear. Obviously it makes sense to remove infected tissue as soon as possible, but some recommend waiting until after the first hyperbaric oxygen (HBO) treatment. There is no conclusive evidence about which should be done first. It seems reasonable that if HBO therapy can be started within 1 h, it should be done and surgery should follow. When there is significant soft tissue swelling that creates a compartment syndrome, decompressive fasciotomy should be done as soon as possible, before HBO therapy.
4. Hyperbaric oxygen therapy is the third therapeutic modality proven useful in animal models. Elevated partial pressures of oxygen can stop toxin production and can even be bacteriocidal to in vitro cultures of *C. perfringens;* the effect is believed to hold also in tissues. Centers which use HBO treatment believe that such therapy limits tissue necrosis, allows better demarcation between viable and nonviable tissue at surgery, and reduces mortality from systemic toxicity. Treatments are usually given with 100% oxygen at 3 atm for 90 min, with two or three treatments planned during the first 24 h.
5. Tetanus prophylaxis should always be given.
6. Prevention of gas gangrene is best accomplished by care of the primary wound. There is evidence that prophylactic penicillin at the time of initial injury might reduce the incidence of clostridial infection, but protection is not absolute.
7. The responsibility of the emergency physician is to recognize this very serious infection, initiate the resuscitation, and deliver the patient to wherever definitive care can be rendered.

CELLULITIS

Cellulitis is an inflammatory infection of the subcutaneous tissues, usually due to staphylococci and/or streptococci or, in young children, *Haemophilus.* In the preantibiotic era, simple cellulitis had up to a 25 percent mortality.

Clinical Features

Simple cellulitis usually presents with local erythema and tenderness. Occasionally, spreading lymphangitis and regional lymphadenopathy are seen. If cellulitis is not treated at this stage, induration and suppuration may develop. Fever, leukocytosis, or bacteremia is unusual in previously healthy individuals with simple cellulitis. The microbial evaluation of patients with cellulitis can be done using (1) cultures taken from obvious ports of entry or discharge, (2) cultures obtained from aspiration of involved subcutaneous tissue, (3) blood cultures, and (4) immunologic evidence of bacterial involvement. The frequency of pathogen isolation when these techniques are used depends on the clinical presentation (Table 164-2). In most patients with simple cellulitis, cultures are of little value because the disease is readily treatable with antibiotics.

Table 164-2. Approximate Incidence of Pathogen Isolation in Previously Healthy Patients with Cellulitis

	Cultures	
	Aspiration, %	**Blood, %**
Extremity or truncal cellulitis with intact skin	10–40	<5
Extremity or truncal cellulitis with broken skin or purulence	80–90	<5
Facial cellulitis in children	40	40–80

Treatment

1. Adults with cellulitis of the head or neck should probably be admitted to the hospital for intravenous antibiotic therapy. A penicillinase-resistant penicillin, cephalosporin, vancomycin, ampicillin-sulbactam, or ticarcillin-clavulanate should be used.
2. Adults with cellulitis of either the trunk or an extremity can usually be treated as outpatients with either an oral penicillinase-resistant penicillin, cephalosporin, erythromycin, trimethoprim-sulfmethoxazole, or amoxicillin-clavulanate.
3. Patients with high fever, systemic toxicity, poor host resistance (e.g., that due to diabetes, alcoholism, or immunosuppression), or underlying skin disease should be treated in the hospital with intravenous antibiotics.

ERYSIPELAS

Erysipelas is a distinctive variety of cellulitis caused by group A streptococci. This has become a rare disease in temperate climates, where it is usually found on the face or scalp of infants, the elderly, and patients with predisposing skin ulcers. In tropical zones, it appears to occur more on the legs, perhaps due to walking barefooted.

Clinical Features

Erysipelas starts with the appearance of a small, raised, red, and painful plaque. The lesion expands slowly over several days to reach a maximal size around 10 to 15 cm. A sharp and distinct advancing edge is characteristic. With facial involvement, severe systemic toxicity, high fever, leukocytosis, and bacteremia are common. With lower extremity involvement, fever occurs just as commonly, but systemic toxicity and bacteremia occur much less frequently. During convalescence, the rash desquamates. Untreated cases have a mortality reported as high as 40 percent.

Treatment

1. Generally, patients with erysipelas should be admitted to the hospital, especially if the face is involved. The affected part should be elevated, if possible, to reduce soft tissue swelling.
2. Penicillin G, 4 to 6 million units per day, should be given intravenously. Erythromycin or cephalosporins can be used in penicillin-allergic patients. Clinical improvements is usually seen within 24 h.

BIBLIOGRAPHY

Tetanus

ACIP: Diphtheria, tetanus, pertussis: Guidelines for vaccine prophylaxis and other preventive measures. *MMWR* 34:405, 419, 1985.

Centers for Disease Control: Tetanus—United States, 1987 and 1988. *JAMA* 263:1192, 1990.

Jagoda A, Riggio S, Burguieres T: Cephalic tetanus: A case report and review of the literature. *Am J Emerg Med* 6:128, 1988.

Percy AS, Kukora JS: The continuing problem of tetanus. *Surg Gynecol Ob* 160:307, 1985.

Powles AB, Ganta R: Use of vecuronium in the management of tetanus. *Anaesthesia* 40:879, 1985.

Wright DK, Lalloo UG, Nayiager S, et al: Autonomic nervous system dysfunction in severe tetanus. Current perspectives. *Crit Care Med* 17:371, 1989.

Gas Gangrene

Cline KA, Turnball TL: Clostridial myonecrosis. *Ann Emerg Med* 14:459, 1985.

Hart GB, Lamb RC, Strauss MB: Gas gangrene. *J Trauma* 23:991, 1983.

Cellulitis and Erysipelas

Carter S, Feldman WE: Etiology and treatment of facial cellulitis in pediatric patients. *Pediatr Infect Dis* 2:222, 1983.

Lutomski DM, Trott AT, Runyon JM, et al: Microbiology of adult cellulitis. *J Fam Pract* 26:45, 1988.

Shimoni Z, Flatau E, Turgeman Y, et al: Changing pattern of erysipelas. *Isr J Med Sci* 20:242, 1984.

SECTION 17
Rheumatology and Allergy

165
MUSCULOSKELETAL DISORDERS IN ADULTS AND CHILDREN

Mary Chester Morgan
Carol Godoshian Ragsdale

Life-threatening complications are rare in rheumatology. Nevertheless, certain manifestations can result in serious morbidity and, if not recognized and managed promptly, mortality. Rheumatologic emergencies may resemble benign complaints in general medicine, but require special diagnostic consideration.

Nonemergency musculoskeletal complaints are abundant in the walk-in clinic or emergency department. The proper management of musculoskeletal disorders may require knowledge of joint and bursa anatomy as well as proficiency in aspiration and synovial fluid analysis.

This chapter provides an overview of emergencies in rheumatology and a guide to management of common musculoskeletal problems.

RHEUMATIC EMERGENCIES ASSOCIATED WITH RISK OF MORTALITY

The Respiratory System

Life-threatening respiratory compromise occurs via two major mechanisms in rheumatic diseases: difficulty ventilating due to airway obstruction and impaired ventilation due to weakness. Patients with airway involvement from relapsing polychondritis occasionally present to the emergency department with trouble breathing. This inflammatory disease affecting cartilage usually begins with abrupt-onset pain, redness, and swelling of the ears or nose. The airway is affected in roughly 50 percent of patients, causing inflammation, destruction, and ultimate collapse of the tracheobronchial cartilage. Patients report throat tenderness over cartilagenous structures and hoarseness. Less commonly they experience shortness of breath, cough, or stridor. Repeated episodes may ultimately cause asphyxiation. Pulmonary function studies are more reliable than bronchoscopy in detecting airway obstruction. Emergency tracheostomy may be helpful, depending upon the level and extent of airway compromise. Hospitalization for careful observation and administration of high-dose steroids is appropriate during acute inflammatory episodes.

Rheumatoid arthritis (RA) is a more common cause of dysfunction of the paired cricoaretynoid joints than are trauma or infection. Although most cases involving RA are asymptomatic, patients may complain of pain with speaking or swallowing, hoarseness, or stridor. If the joints become fixed in a closed position, airway compromise mandates emergency tracheostomy. Presentation with the signs above is an urgent indication for direct laryngoscopy.

This chapter is dedicated to Thomas M. Harrington, M.D., an outstanding teacher and clinician whose contagious curiosity and enthusiasm for rheumatic diseases has enticed many a resident to pursue the field of rheumatology. On behalf of all of us converts, thank you!

The respiratory muscles may be impaired by inflammatory muscle disease. In dermatomyositis and polymyositis respiratory insufficiency is uncommon at presentation, but the muscle impairment may tend to respiratory insufficiency in poorly controlled or chronic disease. Patients should be observed for nasal flaring, for they may be too weak to generate intercostal retractions. Children may present with agitation; they prefer a 45° upright position and may become anxious when flat. Chest x-rays are normal or show ''high-riding'' diaphragms unless pulmonary involvement or an aspiration pneumonitis coexists. Admission for disease control and stabilization is indicated in any patient with inflammatory muscle disease and respiratory impairment. The clinical course can be followed at bedside with measurement of peak inspiratory and expiratory forces. As small children may not cooperate for pulmonary function tests, frequent blood gas evaluation may be necessary.

Pleurisy is common in RA and systemic lupus erythematosus (SLE). It may be asymptomatic in RA, but roughly half of lupus patients have signs and symptoms of pleurisy during the course of their disease. All effusions in rheumatic disease patients should be tapped to exlude other etiologies. Rheumatoid pulmonary effusions characteristically have very low glucose levels, but so do effusions associated with indolent infections such as tuberculosis. Rheumatic, infectious, and malignant effusions are often exudative, and either polymorphonuclear or mononuclear cells may predominate. Nonsteroidal anti-inflammatory agents (NSAIAs—e.g., indomethacin, 25 to 50 mg tid) and antimalarials [hydroxychloroquin, 200 mg bid (6 mg/kg)] usually suffice. Prednisone in low doses is reserved for patients who do not respond to this regimen.

Pulmonary hemorrhage can complicate Goodpasture's disease, SLE, hypersensitivity vasculitis, and Wegener's granulomatosis due to vasculopathic or vasculitic lung involvement. Ankylosing spondylitis (upper lobes), scleroderma, and (rarely) RA and other rheumatic diseases can lead to pulmonary fibrosis. Patients may present with abrupt decompensation with a history of a well-tolerated slow decline. Table 165-1 summarizes respiratory manifestations in rheumatic diseases.

The Heart

The heart is affected in many rheumatic diseases, with potential involvement extending from the pericardium to the endocardium. Of the rheumatic diseases, RA and juvenile rheumatoid arthritis (JRA) are the ones most often associated with pericarditis. Pericarditis is usually asymptomatic, but occasional patients with chest pain attributed to costochondritis may have symptomatic pericarditis. Their chest pain is characteristically positional, and a pericardial rub is usually heard. Systemic lupus erythematosus often causes symptomatic pericarditis, particularly in the elderly. Patients also report symptoms typical of a flare, such as rash, oral ulcers, or joint pain. Symptoms tend to be consistent from one flare to the next, and therefore a thorough review of systems is key. When symptomatic pericarditis is diagnosed, malignancy and infection must be considered and excluded if clinically indicated. Treatment is similar to that for pleurisy above. Indomethacin should not be given to patients under the age of 14. Most children and some adults with pericarditis require prednisone. Pericardial tamponade and constrictive pericarditis from either RA or SLE are uncommon.

While therapy has greatly improved long-term survival in lupus,

Table 165-1. Respiratory Manifestations of Rheumatic Disease

Disease	Common	Infrequent	Rare
SLE	Serositis, effusion	Infiltrate	Hemorrhage, "shrinking lungs," fibrosis
RA and JRA	Nodules, effusion	Pulmonary fibrosis	Cricoarytenoid obstruction
Spondyloarthropathies		Pulmonary fibrosis	
Relapsing polychondritis	Airway obstruction	Tracheobronchial collapse	
Polymyositis and dermatomyositis		Hypoventilation with hypoxemia, respiratory failure	
Scleroderma	Pulmonary fibrosis	Pulmonary hypertension	
Vasculitide's Wegener's granulomatosis	Sinusitis, nasal ulcers, pulmonary nodules, infiltrate		
	Bronchospasm, hemoptysis	Hemorrhage	

Table 165-2. Causes of Precordial Chest Pain in Rheumatic Diseases

Pericarditis, pancarditis
Angina, myocardial infarction
Costochondritis
Vertebral compression (thoracic radiculopathy)
Dermatomal herpes zoster

late mortality from premature atherosclerotic disease is being recognized. Precordial chest pain in lupus is not always due to serositis, particularly with long-standing disease, and angina should be considered. Other causes of precordial pain are listed in Table 165–2.

Myocardial infarction in rheumatic diseases is not usually related to underlying disease. The noteworthy exceptions are Kawasaki disease and polyarteritis nodosa. Some patients with scleroderma have cold-induced vasospastic angina. Kawasaki disease mostly affects children younger than 5 years. They present with fever, oropharyngeal erythema, conjunctival injection, cervical adenopathy, and edema and erythema of the palms and soles. Rashes can be scarlatinaform, morbilliform, multiform, or purpuric. Ten to fourteen days after onset the fingers and toes desquamate. Without proper therapy, 20 percent of patients develop coronary artery aneurysms and 2 to 3 percent die from myocardial infarction during the resolution of the acute disease. With IV gamma globulin and aspirin therapy, aneurysm and myocardial infarction are much less likely to occur. Recommendations for treatment and observation vary, but we recommend hospitalization and observation as IV gamma globulin is administered, with discharge following resolution of fever. A pediatric rheumatologist or cardiologist should be consulted for management and discharge planning. Some children with a history of Kawasaki disease have symptomatic coronary insufficiency years after resolution of the acute disease, with angina, exercise intolerance, or myocardial infarction. Table 165-3 lists the diagnostic criteria for Kawasaki disease. Fever and four of the remaining five manifestations listed in the table must be present for a diagnosis.

Polyarteritis nodosa is an arteritis affecting the skin (nodular, urticarial, or multiform rashes), gut (abdominal angina), and kidneys (hypertension, hematuria). The coronary arteries are commonly involved. Coronary artery involvement is usually clinically silent, but myocardial infarction can occur no matter what the patient's age.

Acute rheumatic fever remains an important cause of pancarditis. Acute rheumatic fever follows streptococcal pharyngitis within a few weeks. It is heralded by rapid development of fever and acute polyarthritis (in adults) or migratory arthritis (in children). A few patients have a more insidious onset. Supportive clinical clues are the presence of subcutaneous nodules, chorea, or erythema marginatum, but only a third of patients will have one of these major manifestations.

Diagnosis is based on documenting the clinical involvement and antecedent streptococcal infection. The throat should be cultured and antistreptolysin O (ASO) or streptozyme titers determined at intervals to document a changing titer. Other baseline tests include serial chest x-rays, echocardiograms and ECGs to monitor the carditis, and acute phase reactants (erythrocyte sedimentation rate, C-reactive protein). The fever and arthritis respond rapidly and completely to salicylate therapy, but salicylates should be withheld until the diagnosis is clear. Patients should be placed at bed rest until clinical and laboratory parameters begin to return to normal.

Rheumatic fever is only one of the diseases associated with migratory arthritis. Bacterial endocarditis or septicemia due to common bacterial pathogens and the prodromal phase of pulmonary mycoplasma or fungal infections must be considered. Children with Schöenlein-Henoch purpura and cefaclor (Ceclor) serum sickness often have migratory articular and periarticular involvement. Stage II Lyme disease can be manifested by migratory articular involvement, with individual joints resolving over hours to days. Often young adults with polyarthritis are empirically treated with intravenous penicillin for disseminated

Table 165-3. Diagnosis of Kawasaki Disease

Fever persisting 5 days or more
Conjunctival injection (not exudative)
Cervical adenopathy (one node or group of nodes >1.5 cm)
Rash (polymorphous, not vesicular or pustular)
Oropharyngeal involvement
Dry, red, cracked lips
Strawberry tongue
Diffuse pharyngeal erythema
Hand and foot involvement
Erythema of palms and soles
Edema of hands and feet
Desquamation of fingers and toes

Source: Sekiguchi M, et al: In Yu PN, Goodwin JF (eds): Progress in Cardiology, ed. 13. Philadelphia, Lea & Febiger, 1985, p.97.

Table 165-4. Conditions Associated with Migratory Arthritis

Rheumatic fever
Subacute bacterial endocarditis
Schöenlein-Henoch purpura
Cefaclor hypersensitivity (children)
Septicemia
Staphylococcal
Streptococcal
Meningococcal
Gonococcal
Pulmonary infection
Mycoplasmosis
Histoplasmosis
Coccidioidomycosis
Lyme disease

Table 165-5. Cardiac Manifestations of Rheumatic Diseases

Disease	Common	Infrequent	Rare
SLE, RA, JRA	Pericarditis	Angina, myocarditis	Tamponade, constrictive pericarditis
Ankylosing spondylitis		Aortic stenosis, aortic insufficiency, aortic dissection	Drop attacks
Relapsing polychondritis		Aortic insufficiency, aortic dissection	
Polymyositis and dermatomyositis		Arrhythmias, myocarditis	
Scleroderma		Angina	Cor pulmonale
Vasculitis		Angina, MI	

gonococcus (GC) until a streptococcal infection is confirmed. The arthritis of acute rheumatic fever does not respond to antibiotic therapy; therefore prompt improvement suggests the diagnosis of GC. Table 165-4 summarizes the diagnostic possibilities in patients with migratory arthritis.

Valvular heart disease is a recognized extraarticular manifestation of the seronegative spondyloarthropathies, particularly ankylosing spondylitis. Fibrotic changes of the aortic valve are usually asymptomatic, with dysfunction occurring more often in patients with longstanding, severe disease. Scar tissue also may impair cardiac conduction, leading to drop attacks. Relapsing polychondritis can affect the valves, causing aortic insufficiency and aneurysm. This may develop early after diagnosis and has a grave prognosis. Table 165-5 summarizes cardiac involvement in rheumatic diseases.

Adrenal Insufficiency in Corticosteroid-Treated Patients with Rheumatic Diseases

Rheumatic disease patients on corticosteroids are usually instructed to seek urgent medical care if an illness like gastroenteritis prevents taking or absorption of prednisone. In general, administration of stress corticosteroids once a day during an acute illness does not worsen the course of any rheumatic disease, even if the dose is much larger than the usual daily dose. A large dose of corticosteroid may be problematic for diabetic patients, but no more so than the condition that has caused vomiting. Other medications used to treat rheumatic diseases are safely stopped for a brief bout of stomach flu. These include NSAIAs, cyclophosphamide or chlorambucil, methotrexate, hydroxychloroquin (Placquenil), and calcium channel blockers if they are only used to treat Raynaud's phenomenon.

Rarely, patients treated with steroids in the recent past (18 months) have developed adrenal insufficiency. They may have early symptoms of weakness, depression, fatigue, and postural dizziness, or late life-threatening vomiting. The serum chemistries will not reveal hyponatremia or hyperkalemia in patients with adrenal insufficiency after prednisone withdrawal because that steroid has no mineralocorticoid activity. If adrenal insufficiency is a remote possibility, stress steroids should be administered. Dexamethasone is preferable, since that steroid does not interfere with assays of other adrenal steroids during subsequent diagnostic testing. Prior to the administration of stress steroids, a cortisol level should be drawn in the emergency room. Under stress, normally functioning adrenal glands generate a cortisol level in excess of 20 μg/dL (see Ch. 138).

RHEUMATIC PRESENTATIONS WITH HIGH RISK OF MORBIDITY

Hypertension

Hypertension can complicate polyarteritis or SLE with renal involvement or RA with drug-induced renal toxicity (fluid retention, nephritis, or renal papillary necrosis), but malignant hypertension is a complication of systemic sclerosis (scleroderma). Hypertensive renal crisis was the leading cause of death in scleroderma until the advent of angiotensin-converting enzyme inhibitors. The most susceptible patients have rapidly progressive skin changes, and present within the first few years of diagnosis with complaints related to hypertension. Laboratory studies reveal rapidly progressive renal insufficiency and a microangiopathic hemolytic anemia. The hypertension results from sclerosis and impaired renal glomerular perfusion causing hyperreninemia. Dehydration from gastroenteritis or diuretics may precipitate the crisis. These patients should be hospitalized and promptly treated with captopril. Any intervention such as diuretics that might exacerbate volume contraction and the underlying pathophysiology should be avoided.

The Cervical Spine and Spinal Cord

Cervical spine disease and its neurologic risk is well recognized in RA and ankylosing spondylitis. Pannus formation and destruction of ligamentous supporting structures may lead to atlantoaxial subluxation; an atlantodental distance in excess of the normal 3.5 mm seen in a lateral flexion view suggests instability (in children under 12, 4 mm of widening is normal). Cord compression may occur acutely following a trivial injury or be more insidious. Subtle clues include a change in bowel or bladder function, new weakness, numbness, or paresthesias. Instability may lead to cranial migration of the odontoid. Complaints relating to vertebral insufficiency (e.g., vertigo) may be reported. Lhermitte's sign, an electric shock sensation radiating down the back on neck flexion, is a classic indication of cervical spine instability. Strength may be difficult to assess in arthritis, so subtle differences in reflexes are particularly informative. Lateral cervical spine films in flexion are essential in evaluating these patients. Neck flexion should not be forced, but rather studied at a degree considered comfortable by the patient.

The ankylosed, inflexible cervical spine in a patient with a seronegative spondyloarthropathy (e.g., ankylosing spondylitis) is susceptible to fracture with minor trauma. A whiplash-type injury or a blow from behind may result in new neck pain in an ankylosed area. The complaint of new neck pain requires a careful history and examination, with attention to possible trauma to the neck and evidence of peripheral nerve damage. Fractures are most commonly transverse through a disk space, leading to high risk of dislocation and cord compression.

Intubation of patients with rheumatic cervical spine disease is best addressed in an elective, controlled situation after the cervical spine has been assessed. *In an emergency, a patient with a stiff neck should be intubated by the most experienced operator available. Atlantoaxial instability should be assumed, and extremes of head manipulation avoided.*

The spinal cord can be affected by transverse myelitis in SLE, and a number of factors can induce an anterior spinal artery syndrome in patients with rheumatic diseases. The anterior spinal artery is a direct branch of the aorta; dissection of the aorta, vasculitis, or embolism can impair blood supply to the anterior cord and produce a clinical picture distinct from transverse myelitis or metastatic tumor by sparing of posterior column function (position sense and vibration).

The Eye

Temporal arteritis often causes sudden blindness, usually before the condition is diagnosed. Blindness can be prevented, however, if prodromal visual changes and coexistent symptomology are recognized.

Temporal arteritis is a granulomatous arteritis of the thoracic aorta and its branches; the vasculitis and ischemia in this distribution induce characteristic signs and symptoms: new headache, tender scalp, fluctuating vision, diminution or loss of a brachial pulse, pain in the jaw or tongue while chewing or talking, and constitutional symptoms. An

Table 165-6. Examination of Synovial Fluid

Indicator	Normal	Noninflammatory*	Inflammatory†	Hemarthrosis‡
Gross appearance	Transparent, clear	Transparent, yellow	Cloudy, yellow	Bloody
String sign	Normal	Normal	Diminished or absent	
WBC/mm³	< 200	< 200	> 2000	Approaches peripheral
PMN	< 25%	< 25%	> 50%	
Culture	Negative	Negative	> 50% positive	Negative
Crystals	Negative	Negative	± Positive	Negative

* Associated conditions are osteoarthritis, trauma, neuropathic arthritis, SLE, HPOA, rheumatic fever

† Associated conditions are septic arthritis, crystal arthritis, seronegative spondyloarthritis, RA, SLE, PM, acute RF, Lyme disease

‡ For associated conditions, see Table 165-7.

elevated Westergren sedimentation rate (> 50 mm/h), elevated liver function studies (particularly the alkaline phosphatase), and unexplained anemia are common laboratory abnormalities.

Temporal arteritis affects the middle-aged and elderly. Polymyalgia rheumatica, with proximal shoulder and hip girdle morning stiffness and aching, coexists in 10 to 30 percent of these patients. Prodromal changes in vision almost always precede blindness. A high index of suspicion is critical when evaluating anyone older than 50 with a new headache, fluctuating vision, or jaw, tongue, or upper extremity claudication. Diagnosis is established on temporal artery biopsy. If the clinical diagnosis is reasonably certain, steroid therapy should be initiated at a prednisone dosage of 60 mg/day to prevent blindness; this will not obscure pathologic findings if the biopsy is obtained within a week.

Sjögren's syndrome, a lymphocytic infiltration of the lacrimal and salivary glands causing dry eyes and dry mouth, may complicate many rheumatic diseases or occur independently. It predisposes the patient to corneal irritation, ulceration, and superimposed infection.

In RA a red eye requires careful evaluation. Under bright natural light examination can reveal the difference between episcleritis, which is self-limiting, and scleritis, which is an emergency. Episcleritis is a painless injection of the episcleral vessels giving the eye a pink-red appearance; it rarely impairs vision. As it is self-limiting, no therapy is indicated. Scleritis causes exquisite ocular tenderness. The eye has a deep purplish discoloration. Visual impairment and scleral thinning with rupture are feared outcomes. High-dose steroids and intensive ophthalmologic management are required.

The Kidney

Nephritis is a major determinant of morbidity and mortality in patients with SLE and systemic vasculitis. Renal dysfunction secondary to hypertension and microangiopathy occurs in scleroderma. Worsening renal function in the above diseases or new abnormalities in renal function in RA or other diseases should prompt a search for remediable causes of renal dysfunction. Patients with SLE and the nephrotic syndrome can develop renal vein thrombosis, which presents with flank pain and proteinuria. Patients treated with NSAIAs, particularly the elderly, can develop renal insufficiency and fluid retention on the basis of alteration in renal blood flow; this is mediated by prostaglandin inhibition.

Occasionally a patient with florid myositis (as in dermatomyositis or polymyositis) or metabolic muscle disease develops acute renal insufficiency due to rhabdomyolysis. In metabolic muscle diseases muscle pain and breakdown can be triggered by exercise.

Myoglobinuria should be suspected when the urine is brown and the dipstick shows blood but no red blood cells. In contrast to a hemolytic state, the serum is clear, CPK is elevated, and haptoglobin is normal. Patients should be hydrated with normal saline to restore intravascular loss that accompanies muscle necrosis. Lasix and one dose of mannitol to preserve urinary output are also recommended during this early phase.

AMBULATORY EVALUATION

Musculoskeletal complaints frequently bring patients into emergency rooms, and evaluation of the most painful and disabling complaints (trauma, crystal-induced arthritis and septic arthritis) is the physician's first priority.

Aspiration and Examination of Synovial Fluid

Accurate diagnosis of musculoskeletal problems often depends on aspiration and examination of synovial fluid. Aspiration of a joint can clarify whether an acute arthritis is septic, traumatic, or crystal-induced. A large number of tests can be run on synovial fluid, but a few simple indicators suffice to elucidate the etiology of acute joint pain (see Table 165-6).

Children should be sedated prior to aspiration (see Chapter 8). The site to be aspirated should be infiltrated with local anesthetic. Intraarticular injection should be avoided, since anesthetic contamination of synovial fluid can inhibit bacterial growth. Cellulitis or impetigo at the aspiration site are absolute contraindications to aspiration or injection. Septicemia and coagulopathy are relative contraindications, but should not preclude aspiration of a joint to exclude infection. A large-bore needle (18 gauge) facilitates aspiration of thick purulent fluid and promotes drainage of infected fluid under pressure; the joint space should be emptied as completely as possible. Table 165-6 summarizes synovial fluid characteristics in different diseases, and Table 165-7 lists conditions associated with hemarthrosis.

Technique

Some joints such as the knee may be easily aspirated from more than one approach. As a small gauge needle is used to administer the anesthetic superficially, it may be advanced further to locate the joint space and left in place to guide the placement of the larger bore needle for aspiration. With the knee fully extended, the midpoint of either the lateral or medial patella should be identified, skin anesthetized, and needle introduced about 2 cm inferior to the patellar edge at a 45 degree angle. See Fig. 165-1.

The ankle also can be entered medially or laterally, anterior to the malleoli. The major tendons and arteries around the ankle can be easily palpated and thus avoided with the needle. The ankle is best held in a 90 degree angle in relation to the shin; the examiner can stabilize the foot and facilitate the procedure by letting the sole of the foot rest on his/her abdomen. The needle is angled slightly cephalad to enter

Table 165-7. Conditions Associated with Hemarthrosis

Trauma with or without fracture (check fluid for marrow fat droplets)
Coagulopathy (especially hemophilia)
Sickle cell disease
Hypermobility syndromes
Scurvy
Pigmented villonodular synovitis (chocolate synovial fluid)
Popliteal artery aneurysm

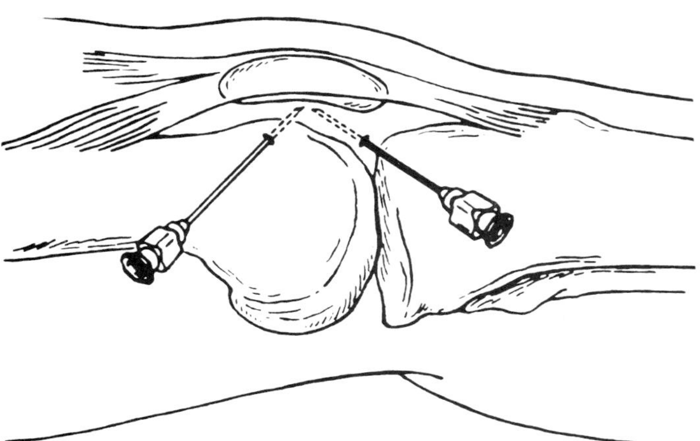

Fig. 165-1. Arthrocentesis of knee (medial approach). (Illustration provided by Dr D Neustadt.)

the tibiotalar space as it passes between the medial malleolus and the tibialis anterior tendon. See Fig. 165-2.

In the shoulder, the subacromial bursa is accessible by palpating the acromion (the lateral bony prominence superior to the humeral head) and passing the needle directly under it (see Fig. 165-3). Injection here bathes the rotator cuff as it passes through this space. The glenohumeral joint may be entered anteriorly by inserting the needle just lateral to the coracoid process. Because of difficulty palpating these landmarks and the remote risk of pneumothorax with this method, a posterior approach is preferable. With the patient sitting upright, the spine of the scapula is palpated at its lateral limit, then a point is identified by moving medially 2 cm along the spine, then inferiorly 2 cm. A 1 1/2 in. needle passed anteriorly to the needle hub, angled toward the coracoid process (also simultaneously palpable with the free hand through a sterile drape over the shoulder), should provide access to the glenohumeral joint.

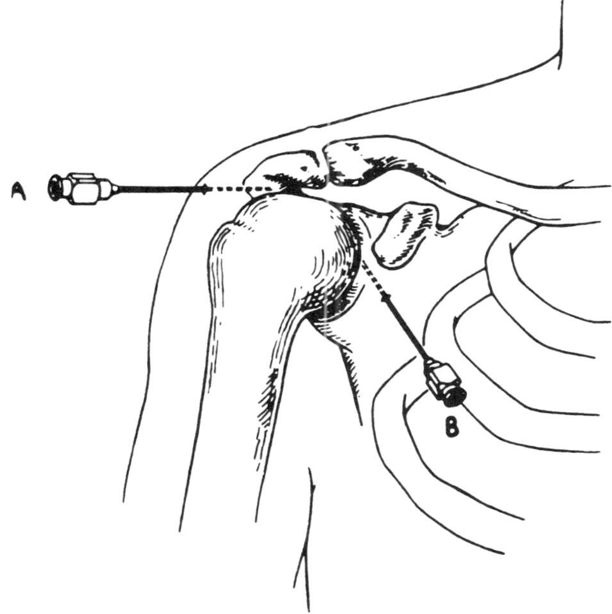

Fig. 165-3. A, Injection of subacromial bursa or supraspinatus tendon; **B,** anterior approach for injection of glenohumeral joint. (Illustration provided by Dr D Neustadt.) [From Schumacher HR (ed.): *Primer on the Rheumatic Diseases,* ed 9. Atlanta, Arthritis Foundation, 1983. With permission.]

The wrist landmarks are palpable with the wrist in a neutral position. The needle should be inserted perpendicular to the skin, just distal to the radial head, slightly ulnar to the anatomic snuffbox. Alternatively, the space between the distal radius and ulna may be entered. See Fig. 165-4.

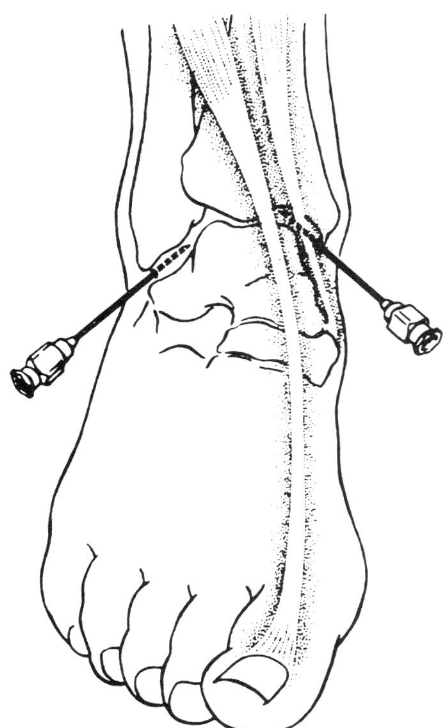

Fig. 165-2. Arthrocentesis of ankle joint (medial and lateral approaches). (Illustration provided by Dr D Neustadt.)

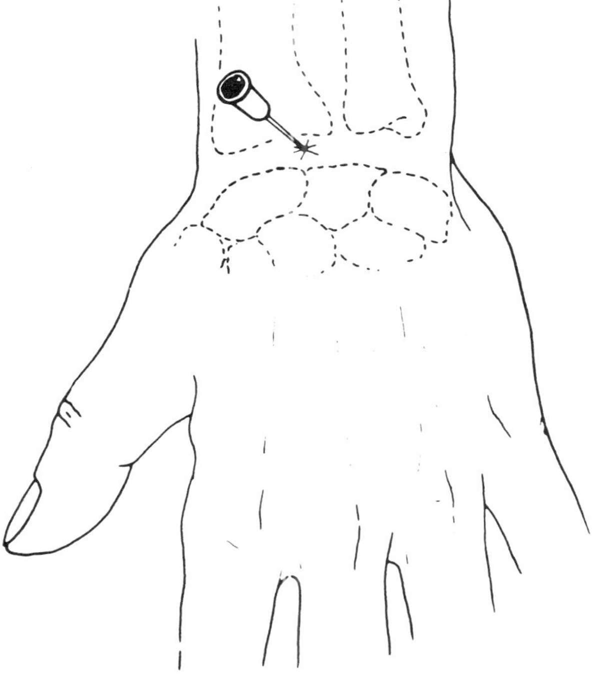

Fig. 165-4. Arthrocentesis of the wrist (radial approach). (Illustration provided by Dr D Neustadt.) [From Schumacher HR (ed): *Primer on the Rheumatic Diseases,* ed 9. Atlanta, Arthritis Foundation, 1983. With permission.]

Traumatic Arthritis

An injury that causes swelling within minutes has a high association with hemarthrosis and internal derangement. Spontaneous bloody effusion usually indicates underlying systemic illness and should trigger a search for primary or secondary coagulopathies. Swelling over hours is consistent with sprain; splinting and pain relief are indicated. With a sprain, children can sustain growth plate fractures, a diagnosis supported by finding tenderness at the end of a long bone.

Septic Arthritis

An infected joint is a medical emergency, as a rampant bacterial infection with a normal inflammatory response can mutilate a joint within hours to days. When one of the usual pyogenic organisms causes septic arthritis (*Staphylococcus, Streptococcus, Haemophilus influenzae*), classic symptomatology is the rule. The involved joint can become exquisitely painful over a few hours. Adults find the discomfort intolerable, and children are troubled by inconsolable night waking and refuse to bear weight or use the affected extremity. On examination, effusions may be scant, but even passive movement is resisted because of splinting. A joint previously injured or affected by arthritis is more susceptible to infection than a normal joint, and flare of a single joint in patients with a history of RA may be indication of infection. Crystalline and septic arthritis may coexist. When in doubt, admit the patient for parenteral antibiotics until synovial culture results are available; delay in treating a septic joint can be catastrophic.

Gonococcal and meningococcal infections have a prodromal phase where migratory arthritis and tenosynovitis predominate before pain and swelling settle in one or more septic joints. Vesiculopustular lesions, especially on the fingers, can be a clue to GC infection in the acute phase. Cultures of the posterior pharynx, urethra, cervix, and rectum prior to antibiotics increase the culture yield in GC, as the synovial fluid is often negative.

More indolent development of symptoms is characteristic of most gram-negative infections. These are rare in healthy children and adults, but are associated with chronic disease (e.g., diabetes), the immunocompromised, the elderly, and intravenous drug abusers. Immunocompromised patients are susceptible to *Mycoplasma* and *Ureaplasma*: synovium rather than synovial fluid must be obtained to detect these organisms. Osteomyelitis and septic arthritis of the foot are more often caused by *Pseudomonas* than by the usual pyogenic organisms. Septic sacroileitis and sternoclavicular septic arthritis are peculiar to intravenous drug abusers. Tenderness and limitation of motion in the absence of radiographic findings are typical diagnostic features.

Intravenous drug abusers are an increasingly important group of patients susceptible to nongonococcal bacterial arthritis, often caused by gram-negative bacilli. The increasing number of outpatients with indwelling catheters for hemodialysis or parenteral medications and nutrition have expanded this vulnerable population. Presumably this increased incidence is due to recurrent bacteremia associated with self-administered injections. Favored sites are the sternoclavicular, sacroiliac, and intervertebral joints. Palpation directly over the involved site frequently elicits tenderness. Because x-rays are usually nearly normal in early septic arthritis, a bone scan may be particularly useful. As precise identification of the offending organism is essential to guide specific therapy, joint aspiration and blood cultures before administration of antibiotics are mandatory wherever possible. A cooperative effort with the orthopedic surgeon and radiologist facilitates a prompt, productive aspiration under fluoroscopic guidance. General anesthesia is strongly encouraged for the sacroiliac joint because it is difficult to access percutaneously. As these infections are often insidious, the emergency physician should maintain a high index of suspicion and proceed with a careful musculoskeletal exam when these patients present with systemic indications of infection but no focal source.

Tubercular and most fungal arthritides tend to smoulder for months before diagnosis is established. Synovial fluid does not reliably yield the organism; synovial biopsy is required. An exception is *Candida*, which presents like a pyogenic arthritis: synovial fluid cultures are usually positive.

Osteomyelitis adjacent to a joint may elicit a sterile sympathetic effusion with a low cell count. Detection of bone tenderness will alert the examiner to the correct diagnosis, and early bone scan or x-rays after 2 weeks of symptoms may be definitive. If there is any suspicion that one is dealing with septic arthritis or osteomyelitis, patients should be admitted for therapy. Intravenous antibiotics are administered and the extremity splinted for patient comfort. The septic joint is aspirated as the effusion recurs; surgical drainage is undertaken if joint fluid is loculated or extremely thick. Table 165-8 summarizes initial management of septic arthritis.

Table 165-8. Recommended Starting Therapy for Septic Arthritis or Osteomyelitis

Patient or Condition	Expected Organisms (Unusual Organisms)	Antibiotics
Neonate	*Staphylococcus*, gram-negative bacteria, Group B *Streptococcus* (*Candida*)	Nafcillin and aminoglycoside
Child < 5 years	*Staphylococcus*, H. *influenzae*	Nafcillin and cefuroxime
Older children and healthy adults	*Staphylococcus, Streptococcus, Neisseria gonorrhoeae* (mycobacteria)	Nafcillin or vancomycin*
Involvement of the foot	*Staphylococcus, Pseudomonas*	Nafcillin and surgical drainage
Susceptible host†	*Staphylococcus*, gram-negative bacteria, mycobacteria, *Candida*	Individualized

* Vancomycin should be employed only for treatment of methicillin-resistant staphylococci.

† The elderly, the immunosuppressed, patients with debilitating diseases (e.g., diabetes, chronic renal failure), and intravenous drug abusers.

Crystal-Induced Synovitis (Gout)

This is primarily an illness of middle-aged and elderly adults. Uric acid (gout) and calcium pyrophosphate (pseudogout) are the two most common culprits. Diagnosis can be easily established by the emergency physician with a joint aspiration during an acute flare. Such documentation enables the primary care physician to proceed with appropriate workup for underlying disease and institute prophylaxis against further attacks.

Joint pain from gout develops over a few hours, whereas pseudogout may evolve over a day. Lower extremities are involved more often than the upper. While the first metatarsophalangeal joint is a classic focus for acute gout, no joint is the exclusive site of involvement by either crystal. Joint aspiration is essential to confirm the inciting crystal, with fluid inspection under a polarizing scope to determine the presence of urate or calcium pyrophosphate. Uric acid crystals appear needle-shaped and blue when the source of light is perpendicular to the crystal ("crossed, urate, blue," or CUB). Calcium pyrophosphate is yellow in this alignment, with a rhomboid shape. Either crystal must be located within a WBC to implicate it as the cause of the arthritis rather than an epiphenomenon. The MTP is difficult to enter even with a small needle, but scant fluid aspirated from adjacent inflamed soft tissues often contains crystals shed from the synovium. Serum uric acid measurements are not helpful in diagnosis of gout because the uric acid level can normalize during an acute exacerbation.

The first priority is exclusion of septic arthritis. If there is doubt, treatment for septic arthritis should be undertaken. When minimal fluid is available for diagnostic studies, it should be sent for bacterial culture and sensitivity: Gram's stain, crystal examination, cell count with differential, and other stains and cultures in decreasing order of importance as quantities allow and as deemed clinically appropriate.

When the diagnosis of gout or pseudogout is established, a NSAIA such as indomethacin, 50 mg tid, is standard first-line therapy if renal function is normal. Rarely is additional treatment necessary for acute pseudogout. Oral colchicine is a reasonable alternative, administered at a dose of 0.6 mg/h until intolerable side effects (nausea, vomiting, diarrhea) or efficacy ensue. Treatment within the first 12 h of symptoms increases the likelihood of its effectiveness. However, because of the excellent response generally obtained with NSAIAs, and because colchicine is associated with serious toxicities such as bone marrow suppression, neuropathy, myopathy, and death, use of colchicine, particularly by the intravenous route, should only be undertaken in consultation with a rheumatologist.

During an acute flare, doses of other medications chronically used to treat a patient's crystalline arthritis should not be adjusted, as this may exacerbate crystal precipitation. When a suspected attack of acute crystalline arthritis has not responded to this regimen, another process, such as a joint infection, should be strongly suspected and evaluated with repeat joint aspiration.

Baker's Cyst in Arthritis of the Knee

Fluid from a chronic inflammatory arthritis of the knee, classically RA, may dissect into a potential popliteal space via a one-way valve, forming a Baker's cyst. Its rupture or dissection into the calf mimics a deep venous thrombosis, causing calf pain and swelling. Helpful discriminating features are (1) swelling that spares the foot, (2) a crescentic, purplish discoloration below the malleoli (crescent sign), due to blood layering at the fascial attachments around the ankle, and (3) the history of a rapid diminution in a knee effusion or popliteal fullness. An arthrogram is the gold standard diagnostic test, but ultrasound in experienced hands may suffice and, with doppler, permits exclusion of a popliteal artery aneurysm. Treatment consists of knee joint aspiration and steroid injection to reduce intraarticular pressure and inflammation.

Bursitis

Because of the proximity of bursae to joints, careful examination is required to differentiate bursitis from arthritis. In the elbow, for example, olecranon bursitis and arthritis will both cause limitation of flexion and extension, but bursitis will not affect pronation or supination. Septic bursitis is usually associated with a puncture or overlying cellulitis. An important point to remember is that in septic bursitis WBC counts are only about 10 percent of that expected in septic arthritis. When a clinical evaluation raises even a remote possibility of infection, the bursa should be drained thoroughly with a large-bore needle. For superficial bursae, the aspiration technique is modified from that used for joint aspiration. The needle should not be inserted perpendicular to the skin directly over the distended bursa; rather, skin should be punctured 1 to 2 cm from the expected pocket of fluid and the needle tunneled through subcutaneous tissue before entering the bursa. This establishes a longer tract between the skin puncture and inflamed bursa, so that as the needle is withdrawn, risk of a chronically draining fistula is minimized.

Tendonitis

Tendonitis and tenosynovitis are almost always caused by overuse. Examination reveals localized tenderness at insertion sites (e.g., the lateral epicondyle in tennis elbow), which is exacerbated by maneuvers which stretch the tendon. These disorders are treated by rest and NSAIAs. Naproxen (250 to 500 mg bid or tid, 10 to 15 mg/kg day), tolmetin (400 to 600 mg tid or qid, 20 to 30 mg/kg per day), or sulindac (75 to 200 mg bid) are good choices. Sulindac is not approved for children.

Corticosteroid Injections

Acute flare of a single joint in RA, JRA, gout, bursitis, or tendonitis may benefit from corticosteroid injection, but injections are associated with complications and repeated injections risk injury to cartilage and tendons. Injection should be undertaken after consultation with a rheumatologist or orthopedist. In the case of overuse syndromes (bursitis and tendonitis) injection should not substitute for cessation or modification of overuse activity. Care should be taken to aspirate as the needle is withdrawn after intraarticular injection to minimize the risk of subcutaneous atrophy at the site. Subcutaneous atrophy is more likely when soft tissues are injected. Injection of a single site should not be repeated more than three times during the growing years.

Limp in the Child

Limp in children may be reflection of disease in the back or pelvis as well as of lower-extremity disease. In the ambulatory setting it is critical to assess quickly for serious osteoarticular injury, infection, or malignancy before planning more elective evaluation for other conditions.

The gait will be antalgic if pain is causing the limp. Locating the cause can be problematic because much lower-extremity skeletal pain is referred. Pain in the back or pelvis can be referred to the abdomen or thigh. In children hip pain is usually referred to the knee or anterior thigh. Gaits that are not antalgic are often associated with leg length discrepancy or neurologic impairment.

Refusal to bear weight is characteristic of fracture, osteoarticular malignancy, osteoarticular infection, and diskitis.

Diskitis

Diskitis is an uncommon musculoskeletal disorder in children. It can present at any age, usually as refusal to walk or sit. Children may complain of back pain or of referred abdominal or leg pain. Children hold themselves rigidly stiff, and any maneuvers which move the spine (e.g., hip flexion) elicit guarding. X-rays may show abnormal lordosis, list, or narrowing of the involved disk space. Later, calcifications appear at the site. Referral to or management with the help of a pediatric orthopedist is recommended.

Toxic Synovitis

Toxic synovitis is a benign self-limited arthritis in young school-age children, affecting primarily the hip and occasionally the sacroiliac joint or knee. There may be low-grade fever. The joint is irritable on movement, but x-rays are normal. The WBC is usually normal and the ESR normal or slightly elevated. Aspiration may be required to exclude septic arthritis and often results in dramatic improvement. Synovial fluid has a normal or low cell count and is often under high pressure. The syndrome resolves in 1 to 2 weeks, but brief recurrences are common. Legg-Calvé-Perthes disease sometimes develops in patients with apparent toxic synovitis.

Trauma

Except in cases of extreme bodily insult (e.g., a cross-body block), trauma is not an explanation for joint swelling in children. Knee swelling in children with pauciarticular JRA often first comes to parental attention after a minor fall and is incorrectly ascribed to injury. The outcome is worse if a child with JRA is immobilized. Injury in the right setting with swelling arising in minutes should raise suspicion of intraarticular bleeding and derangement. Aspiration is indicated, and referral to an orthopedist is recommended. Recurrent hemarthrosis in childhood is seen in cases of hemophilia and internal derangement, and, rarely, in children with intraarticular hemangioma.

Fractures

Type 1 *Salter-Harris fractures* through the growth plate can occur with the sort of injury that would produce a sprain in an adult. This fracture should be suspected in any child with tenderness over the end of a long bone, even if x-rays are normal. Orthopedic evaluation is recommended. The *slipped capital femoral epiphysis,* a chronic fracture similar to Salter-Harris type 1 fractures, presents with the insidious development of thigh or knee pain and a painful limp; hip motion is limited, particularly internal rotation. Anteroposterin and "frog-leg" lateral films of both hips should be obtained for the detection of minor degrees of displacement.

Stress fractures, one manifestation of overuse stress in children, present with a history of discomfort on exertion or weight bearing and localized, tender swelling on examination. Early after onset of pain, stress fractures may not be visible on x-ray; however, differentiation from bone tumor is possible. Films taken after two weeks show callus formation.

Avascular Necrosis

Avascular necrosis of the epiphyses and subchondral bone in children presents with the insidious development of exertional pain and limp. Involvement of the hip (Legg-Calvé-Perthe's disease) usually presents in young boys with limp and pain referred to the knee. Involvement of the medial femoral condyles (osteochondritis dissecans) causes pain and swelling of the knee. Involvement of the bones of the feet (e.g., Kohler's bone disease or Freiburg's disease) is signaled by localized tenderness. X-rays yield the diagnosis if patients have been symptomatic for 2 weeks or more.

Children treated with chronic corticosteroids are at high risk to develop aseptic necrosis.

Osteoarticular Malignancy

Bone tumors present with the insidious development of pain exacerbated by weight bearing; patients are frequently roused from sleep by pain. Leukemia that has infiltrated the joints produces severe pain, inconsolable night walking, and refusal to bear weight. X-rays reveal metaphyseal rarefaction or periosteal elevation. The peak occurrence of leukemia in children is under age 5, and the hemogram usually reveals profound anemia, thrombocytopenia, and leukopenia.

BIBLIOGRAPHY

Cassidy JT, Petty RE: *Textbook of Pediatric Rheumatology.* New York; Churchill Livingstone, 1990.

Kelley WN, Harris ED Jr, Ruddy S, et al: *Textbook of Rheumatology.* Philadelphia; Saunders, 1989.

Rodnan GP, Schumacher HR (eds.): *Primer on the Rheumatic Diseases,* ed. 8. Atlanta, Arthritis Foundation, 1983.

Schumacher HR (ed): *Primer on the Rheumatic Diseases,* ed 9. Atlanta, Arthritis Foundation, 1988.

166 NECK PAIN

Myron M. LaBan

Neck pain has an encyclopedic list of causes including degenerative disease, infections, neoplasms, congenital variations, inflammatory arthritis, and psychic tension as in "You're a pain in the neck!"

Evaluation of this symptom requires an understanding of the anatomy of the cervical spine. The cervical spine consists of seven vertebrae; the fifth through the seventh are alike in shape and size while the first cervical vertebra (atlas) and the second (axis) differ in structure. The lower third through seventh vertebral bodies articulate with each other via their superior and inferior articular processes, allowing limited rotation and lateral flexion. The atlas (C1) supports the occipital condyles and the axis (C2). Its inferior articulations resemble the other inferior vertebral articulations. The dens and its stabilizing horizontal ligament permit rotation between C1 and C2. The transverse processes of each of the cervical vertebrae, except for the atlas, are perforated by a foramen which transmits the vertebral vessels.

The muscles of the neck are compartmentalized into seven fascial planes. These planes normally permit pain-free flexibility of one muscle group on the other. Following acute trauma to the neck, petechial hemorrhages and edema within these same fascial planes can produce limited motion associated with complaints of stiffness, pain, and swelling.

The stable yet flexible cervical spine is linked by both ligaments and disks. Because of major structural differences, the cervical disks are less likely than lumbar disks to prolapse. The cervical spine is more mobile, the superincumbent weight is less, the nucleus pulposis is more anteriorly displaced, and the annulus is posteriorly reinforced in its entire width by the posterior longitudinal ligament.

The eight paired cervical spinal roots exit the intervertebral foramina between the superior and inferior pedicles except for the upper two cervical roots. Unique to the cervical spinal roots, in over half the patients, the ventral and dorsal roots remain discrete at the neural foramina. In these cases isolated irritation of the dorsal (sensory) root posteriorly by an osteophyte may produce only sensory complaints. Similarly, ventral root (motor) compromise by a degenerative disk can produce painless progressive weakness.

The sinuvertebral nerves branch from the dorsal root and reenter the intervertebral foramina to supply sensation to the ligaments of the spinal canal. Anteriorly they supply the posterior longitudinal ligament, and dorsally the ligamentum flavum, meninges, and associated vessels. Ascending and descending branches supply the zygoapophyseal joints, providing position sense.

The cervical portion of the spinal cord is surrounded by spinal fluid and is suspended laterally to the enveloping dura by 20 dentate ligaments. The dura in turn is attached cephalad to the rim of the foramen magnum and within the vertebral spinal canal itself is cushioned from trauma by epidural fat.

HISTORY

A clinical impression of the cause of neck pain can often be obtained by a thorough and searching history. In the vast majority of cases, patients can identify either a singular inciting cause of discomfort or an exacerbating maneuver or position which replicates the discomfort. In traumatic injury, the exact nature of the impact with reference to positioning; accompanying lacerations of the head, neck, or face; the use of restraints; the use of protective sports equipment; associated limb or trunk fractures or contusions; and loss of consciousness or subsequent seizures are all important information. Environmental conditions on the date of injury, preexisting medical conditions, and other contributing factors should also be identified. Finally, the examiner should determine whether litigation has already been initiated by the patient.

As always, a review of systems; age and occupation; antecedent information with respect to systemic illnesses; the character of the pain complaint; and its distribution should be included. Specific neurogenic symptoms should be elicited including extremity weakness, incoordination, sensory aberration, and sphincter and sexual dysfunction. Visual, auditory-vestibular, and pharyngeal-laryngeal symptoms often require direct questioning to elicit complaints. The results of previous laboratory testing, as well as the response to medication and/or physical treatment is useful and may in the patient's response to therapy be diagnostic.

PHYSICAL EXAMINATION

The physical examination may start with an observation of a loss of neck flexibility. Pain may cause splinting of the head on the shoulders during position change. Neck mobility should be tested, both with active and passive movement, including flexion (chin to shoulder) and lateral flexion (ear to shoulder). When localized ipsilateral neck pain is experienced toward the side of head movement, zygoapophyseal joint irritability is suspected. When ipsilateral pain radiates to shoulder or arm (Spurling's sign), a radicular component may be present. Contralateral neck pain suggests either a primary ligamentous or a muscular source of discomfort as these structures are placed on a stretch. Gross shoulder motion both with abduction and with forward flexion should be observed. These maneuvers of both neck and shoulder are normally smooth and symmetric. A break in the rhythm of shoulder motion either at the glenohumeral joint or at the scapulocostal joint, like that of altered asymmetric neck motion, calls attention to the presence of localized abnormality.

Neck palpation of the posterior triangle, the supraclavicular fossa, and the carotid sheaths may demonstrate nodal hypertrophy, or thyroid or salivary gland enlargement. Auscultation of the carotid and the subclavian arteries may demonstrate bruits, in the former instance associated with potential cerebral insufficiency and in the latter with a thoracic outlet or steal syndrome.

Topographically, the first cervical vertebra is located immediately behind the angle of the mandible, the transverse process of the atlas is positioned between the angle of the mandible and the mastoid process, the hyoid bone is anterior to the level of C3, the thyroid cartilage is anterior to C4, and the cricoid cartilage can be felt anterior to the sixth cervical vertebra.

Symptomatic occipital neuralgia can be replicated by firm pressure over the occipital notch, producing scalp numbness or burning dysesthesias in the occipital nerve distribution. Confusing symptoms of temporomandibular joint dysfunction can be recognized by pain or crepitus over this joint, often associated with palpable "weakness" on the symptomatic side of the temporalis muscles in the subzygomatic fossa.

Various compression and distraction maneuvers of the cervical spine are also diagnostically useful. They include vertical skull compression or lateral flexion positions which replicate radicular symptoms, and manual vertical distraction which serves to "unload" the spinal roots and adjacent cervical vertebral joints, thereby reducing pain. In an effort to avoid cervical root distraction by the weight of the dependent arm, a patient may present supporting the extremity with his or her hand on the head (Fig. 166-1).

An evaluation of neck discomfort is incomplete without shoulder and arm examination. Bilateral upper extremity pain complaints invariably originate in the neck as C6 spinal radiculopathies. Localized shoulder abnormality presenting with pain and crepitus includes the glenohumeral joint as well as the sternoclavicular or acromioclavicular joints. A bicipital tendinitis or an acute subdeltoid bursitis can present

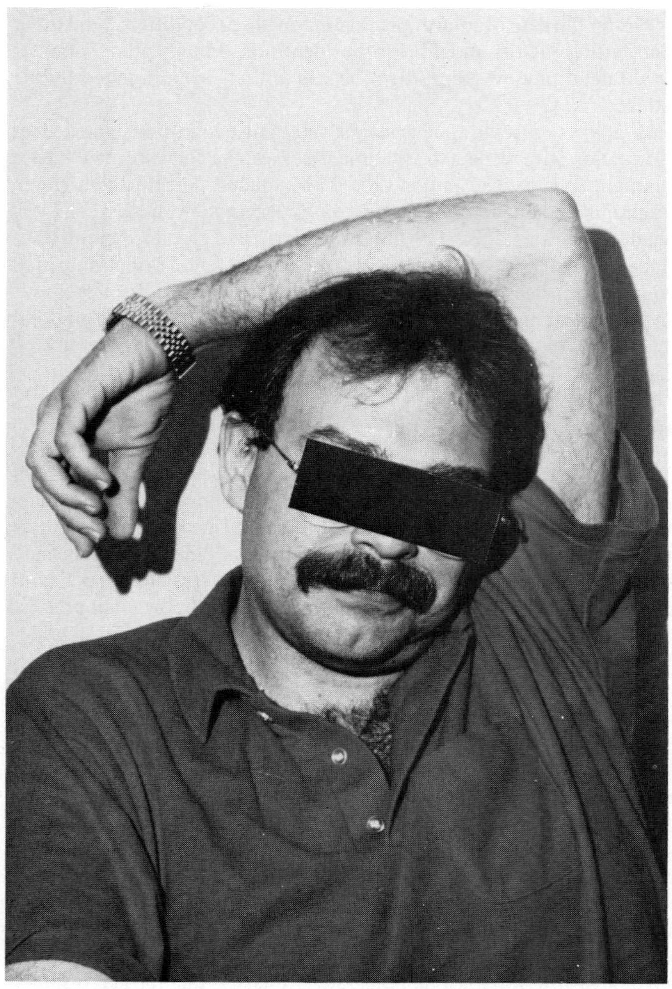

Fig. 166-1. Acute C7 radiculopathy. Arm elevation relieves pain of cervical root distraction.

both with and without capsulitis. In each of these instances localized pain is diagnostic. On occasion, however, subdeltoid bursal syndromes may present as referred pain to the insertion of the deltoid at the deltoid tubercle in the upper one-third of the lateral arm.

A reduction in radial pulse with passive shoulder abduction, particularly when associated with a concomitant bruit over the subclavian artery in either the infraclavicular space or supraclavicular fossa associated with a replication of symptoms, suggests the thoracic outlet syndrome.

Finally, a neurologic examination completes the evaluation (Table 166-1). Gross evidence of muscle atrophy or fasciculations may be patently obvious. A loss of triceps reflex suggests C7 root pathology, a loss of biceps reflex a C5–C6 root syndrome. Manual muscle testing using the "break" maneuver, whereby the patient is given a maximal advantage of position and strength and the examiner "breaks" the muscle comparing one side with the other, is the most useful technique in this regard. The triceps is tested by having the patient extend the elbow and maximally resist the examiner's efforts to flex the elbow against the patient's strength through the long lever of the arm grasped proximal to the wrist. A smooth, asymmetric "give" suggests either a C7–C8, posterior cord, or radial nerve compromise. Similarly, other muscle groups are tested and patterns of weakness are correlated with the clinical history and the symptomatic complaints. A knowledge of peripheral neuroanatomy can clearly delineate both the location and the severity of the lesion.

Local nerve palpation also is a useful adjunct to the examination. The C5–C6 root lesions are often quite tender over the brachial plexus at Erb's point in the supraclavicular fossa, while a C8–T1 root presentation frequently has marked tenderness over the distal ulnar nerve at the elbow. Peripheral nerve entrapment syndromes associated with a positive Tinel's sign to percussion over the lesion and distal weakness may also demonstrate proximal pain radiation. These syndromes may present with only neck and shoulder pain as the primary complaint. Median nerve compromise in the carpal tunnel can present as shoulder pain in this instance, and the ulnar nerve cubital fossa syndromes as a complaint of medial, inferior scapular discomfort.

Sensory symptoms of pain or dysesthesias are difficult to evaluate, particularly when motor signs of nerve compromise are absent. This is all too often the case relative to cervical spinal radiculopathies. The discrete separation at cervical neural foraminal levels of the motor and sensory roots (Fig. 166-2) enhances the opportunity for motor sparing in spite of severe sensory symptoms. An understanding of the known dermatome, sclerotome, and myotome referral distribution of spinal root irritation is essential to diagnosis. Marked cervical root irritability without motor weakness as typically identified in the triceps (radial nerve C7–C8) and in the pronator teres (median nerve C6–C7) can present with the only complaint being aching discomfort at the medial scapular border in its middle one-third, or aching in the myotome distribution to the chest, axilla, or triceps. Severe pectoralis major pain can simulate a myocardial infarction or produce breast discomfort, evoking concerns over a possible malignancy. Numbness or tingling in the C7 dermatome distribution to the middle finger may be the sole symptom of root irritation.

Table 166-1. Signs and Symptoms of Cervical Radiculopathy

Disk Space	Cervical Root	Pain Complaint	Sensory Abnormality	Motor Weakness	Altered Reflex
C1–C2	C1–C2	Neck, scalp	Scalp		
C4–C5	C5	Neck, shoulder, upper arm	Shoulder, thumb	Spinati, deltoid, biceps	Reduced biceps reflex
C5–C6	C6	Neck, shoulder, upper medial scapular area, proximal forearm, thumb	Thumb and index finger, lateral forearm	Deltoid, biceps, pronator teres, wrist extensors	Reduced biceps and brachioradialis reflex
C6–C7	C7	Neck, posterior arm, dorsum, proximal forearm, chest, medial one-third scapula, middle finger	Middle finger, forearm	Triceps, pronator teres	Reduced triceps reflex
C7–T1	C8	Neck, posterior arm, medial proximal forearm, median inferior scapular border, medial hand, ring and little fingers	Ring and little fingers	Triceps, flexor carpi ulnaris, hand intrinsics	Reduced triceps reflex

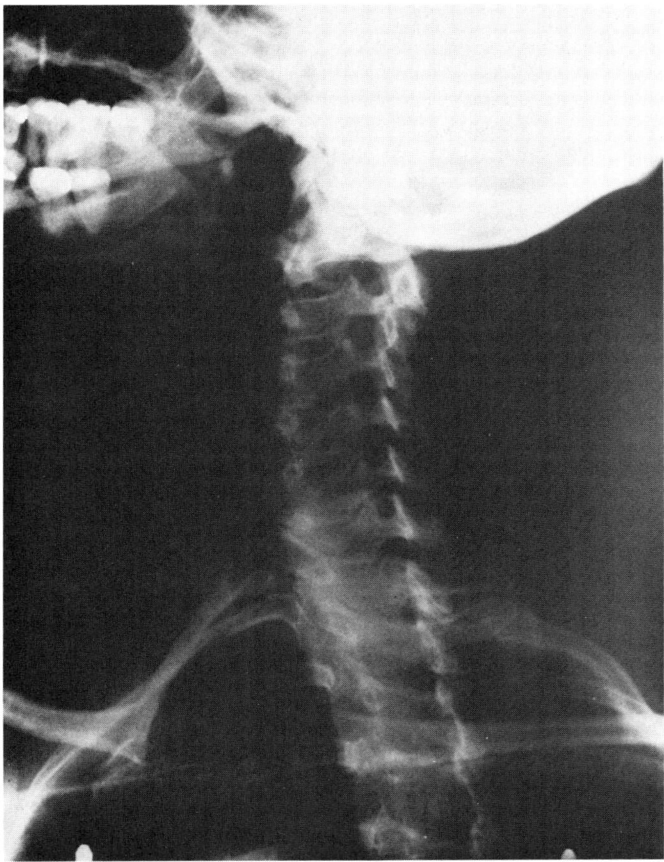

Fig. 166-2. Progressive C7 myotome weakness and atrophy without sensory complaints of dysesthesias or pain. Patient with C6–C7 disk space narrowing improved with cervical traction.

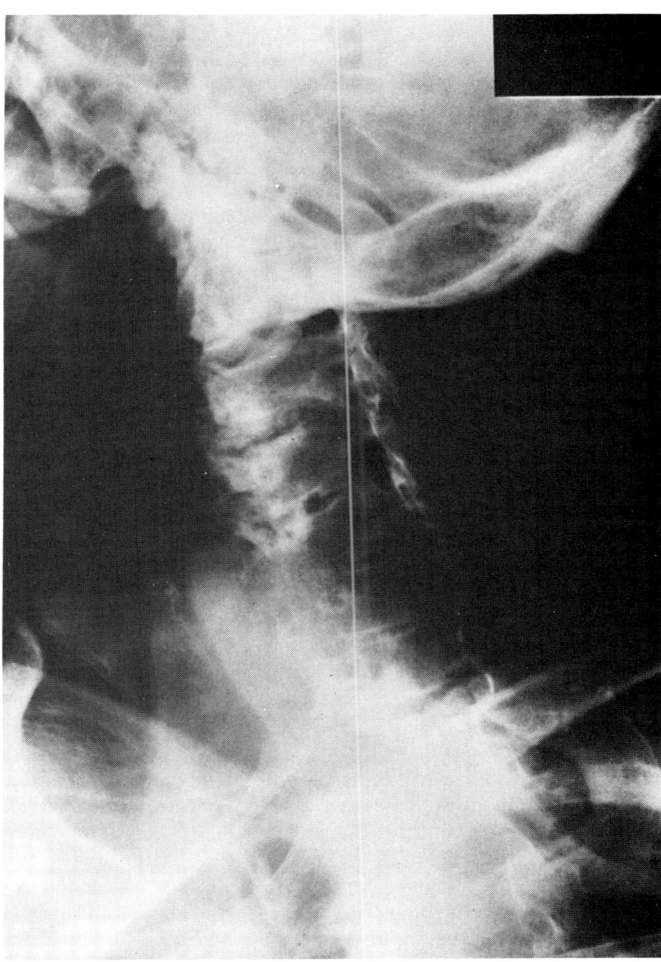

Fig. 166-3. 75-year-old man with acute neck pain and associated myelopathy. Occult epidural prostatic metastasis masked by severe degenerative disk disease.

Early cervical spinal myelopathies can only be recognized if the examiner looks for them. Hyperreflexia with the presence of a Hoffmann's reflex in the upper extremities accompanying neck pain suggests lesions above C5. An absent superficial abdominal skin reflex associated with lower extremity hyperreflexia, an upgoing toe, and sphincter involvement, suggests progressive cervical spinal stenosis or an occult epidural metastasis (Fig. 166-3).

RADIOGRAPHIC EXAMINATION

Radiographic views of the neck should always include oblique views. Both the dens and the lowest cervical and upper thoracic vertebrae should also be visualized. Flexion-extension films are useful if instability is suspected. Neither the CT scan nor nuclear magnetic resonance have been proved superior to cervical myelography in the diagnosis of myelopathy or cervical radiculopathies. An obvious advantage of both, however, is that CT scan and magnetic resonance imaging are noninvasive tests, while myelography is not generally performed unless a surgical lesion is strongly suspected. Of the two, at cervical spinal levels, MRI is the preferred test.

ELECTRODIAGNOSTIC EXAMINATION

Electromyographic studies are useful in ascertaining the presence of neural structure abnormality, assessing both the level and the degree of severity, and providing both a prognostic baseline and an objective means of reassessment. Both electromyography (EMG) and nerve conduction velocity (NCV) testing are particularly useful when the initial presentation is associated with marked degrees of progressive motor impairment or when confusion exists as to the level of neural compromise. As noted previously the actual cervical radicular complaints may be accompanied by peripheral extremity mononeuropathies which may be attributed to the cervical radiculopathy or may in turn be provocative of the neck pain. Unfortunately, with respect to progressive weakness syndromes, acute electromyographic findings lag 2 weeks behind the patient's actual clinical state although the immediate status of motor unit innervation and NCV after an initial 3-day delay can be followed in real time. EMG is a test of motor dysfunction. If the sensory root is solely compromised and the motor root spared, the EMG may be normal.

Cervical spinal evoked potentials are most useful in evaluating the presence of cervical spinal myelopathies and the thoracic outlet syndromes. An asymmetric or slowed response at either cervical or cerebral levels in response to distal upper and lower extremity stimulation may be diagnostic in either instance.

CERVICAL SOFT TISSUE INJURIES

Patients with a history of a cervical hyperextension injury occurring in a motor vehicle accident, sport activity, or accidental fall may endure a great deal of persistent discomfort, often unresponsive to treatment. The frequent lack of discernible objective evidence of injury in the face of persistent disability has given rise to the stereotype spectre of "the whiplash victim" accompanied by both a physician advocate and a guileful attorney. The term *whiplash,* although descriptive, has been abandoned in favor of the more respectable synonym *acceleration flexion-extension neck injury*. When associated with a motor vehicle accident, a vertical component of impact may be added as the cervical spine is compressed when the individual's trunk is lifted by the force of impact. A rear-end collision propels the trunk forward on the pelvis, throwing the head into hyperextension and stretching the anterior structures of the neck. A head-on impact initially produces acute flexion and subsequently a reflex hyperextension, injuring both the anterior and posterior neck structure. Staged automobile accidents using cadavers have demonstrated injuries ranging from muscle and ligament distraction to vertebral dislocations and fractures, as well as occasional herniations of the intervertebral disk. Head-on injuries produce damage to the ventral neck with tears and hemorrhages in the sternocleidomastoid muscles and ruptures of the anterior longitudinal ligament and the ventral parts of the annulus fibrosis. Dorsal injury to the annulus fibrosis with hemorrhage in the paraspinal muscles is more common when trauma occurs from behind.

Elasticity of the cervical spine itself is a major variable, as is the patient's ability to prepare for the impact. Often the site of most serious residual complaint is at that level of the cervical spine with the most significant degenerative change. Passengers forewarned of an impending rear collision can potentially protect themselves by derotating the head and tucking the chin against the chest. A rotated-flexed head potentiates the risk of ligamentous rupture and articular dislocation.

Postinjury complaints are highly variable and may include pain and dysesthesias, visual symptoms, dizziness, tinnitus, dysphagia, and hoarseness. Typically, the pain complaints are initially delayed for a number of hours following the accident. They can present as localized discomfort associated with stiffness, occipital radiation, or a radicular component. Symptoms and signs of either a temporomandibular joint or thoracic outlet syndrome may also be present. Restricted cervical range of motion can be associated with radicular patterns of myotome weakness suggesting cervical root compromise. Blurring of vision and orbital pain may accompany periorbital edema or frank ecchymosis. Spacial instability affecting balance is not uncommon and may be described as the perception of "sliding" or "veering" with changes of direction rather than of a spinning sensation associated with true "vertigo." This rather unique description of spacial instability may be attributable to injury to the zygoapophyseal joints of the neck rather than the inner ear, falsely biasing the cervical righting reflex. Electronystagmography is useful in evaluating these symptoms. Dysphagia can occur as a result of pharyngeal edema or retropharyngeal hematoma. Vocal hoarseness can be attributed to a stretch of the larynx, often associated with marked edema of the sternocleidomastoid muscles and carotid sheaths, potentially increasing neck circumference by one collar size. The symptom complex of tinnitus, vertigo, visual aberrations, ear and eye pain, and headache is termed the syndrome of Leiou-Barré.

Cervical spine x-ray films are of value to exclude vertebral trauma, including avulsion fractures or joint subluxations. The initial roentgenograms may reveal only an initial loss of the normal cervical lordosis, with subsequent studies possibly revealing new evidence of ligamentous ossification. Extension views of the cervical spine can demonstrate vacuum clefts in the anterior surface of the cervical disks, suggesting the presence of an avulsed disk.

Treatment initially consists of bed rest, splinting of the neck with a fitted soft cervical collar fastened in slight flexion, and the use of topical ice packs. Early mobilization exercises starting at 72 h to restore flexibility should be combined with superficial moist heat and a gradual reduction in the use of the soft collar. Early in recovery diathermy and cervical traction should be discouraged as they are likely to aggravate symptoms. However, these modalities are useful later when ligamentous or articular pain persists or for radicular symptoms. In both instances treatment must be predicated on a specific diagnosis. Oral analgesics including narcotics initially are appropriate for pain relief. Muscle relaxants are not effective except as soporifics. With chronic discomfort the oral nonsteroidal anti-inflammatory drugs are useful. On specific occasions where occipital neuralgia or myofascial symptoms predominate as sources of continuing pain, local injections of a mixture of long-acting steroid and 1% lidocaine followed by ice massage and ultrasound can be therapeutic. Formal outpatient therapy can be complemented by instruction in an appropriate home care program, again predicated on an accurate diagnosis.

CERVICAL DISK PATHOLOGY

Cervical disk herniations occur as the nucleus pulposus protrudes through the posterior annulus fibrosis, producing either an acute radiculopathy or occasionally a myelopathy. Chronic cervical degenerative disk disease or cervical spondylosis is associated with a subtle progression of symptoms, including neck stiffness or localized pain, occipital neuralgia, extremity-referred radicular pain, and occasionally clinical manifestions of a progressive myelopathy.

ACUTE CERVICAL DISK HERNIATIONS

Evidence of degeneration of the nucleus pulposus and the annulus fibrosis usually proceeds a cervical disk herniation. These protrusions are usually confined by the posterior longitudinal ligament but can occasionally extrude through this ligament as free fragments. Direct posterior ruptures, although infrequent, can produce progressive myelopathy while the more common posterolateral herniations precipitate the symptoms and signs of an acute cervical radiculopathy. Disk prolapse is $1\frac{1}{2}$ times more common in males, occurring most often in the fourth decade. The levels of most frequent involvement are C6–C7 (C7 root) usually left-sided, and C5–C6 (C6 root) usually right-sided.

The symptoms of an acute cervical disk prolapse include neck pain, headache, sclerotomal referral to the shoulder and along the medial scapular border, myotome pain in the spinal root distribution to the shoulder and arm, and dermatomal sensory dysesthetic complaints to the appropriate finger. Motor signs include fasciculations; atrophy and weakness in the myotome distribution of the spinal root; loss of deep tendon reflexes; and with cervical myelopathy, lower extremity hyperreflexia, Babinski's sign, and, rarely, loss of sphincter control. Cervical hyperextension and lateral flexion to the symptomatic side can replicate the symptoms as can Valsalva maneuvers, while manual cervical distraction in flexion alleviates them. A thorough and searching examination, including muscle testing, easily delineates the level of root involvement (Table 166-1).

Electroneuromyography as an extension of the clinical examination can be complementary in diagnosis and excludes in the process occult peripheral mononeuropathies and confusing acute brachial plexopathies (Parsonage-Turner syndrome). Cervical spine x-ray films are often more useful in these syndromes for what they fail to reveal, rather than what they demonstrate. The presence of degenerative disease may mask a soft cervical disk protrusion. In the younger adult, x-ray films may be normal, failing to reveal a large disk herniation. In this instance myelography or MRI are necessary for diagnosis.

Treatment consists of analgesics sufficient to obtain pain control, a cervical soft collar, and, without evidence of carotid bruits and/or myelopathy, a trial of intermittent cervical traction. If the symptoms and signs of acute cervical root compression fail to respond to conservative treatment or reoccur, surgery can be recommended if visualization procedures demonstrate a prolapsed cervical disk with root compression.

CHRONIC DEGENERATIVE DISK DISEASE

Cervical spondylosis is a progressive condition which can present either as a loss of cervical flexibility or as a primary pain complaint. The pain is associated either with localized zygoapophyseal joint degeneration or with cervical root irritability when occipital, shoulder, and arm pain referral is experienced. The process of progressive cervical spondylosis is initiated by the development of degenerative disk disease which predisposes to progressive osteoarthrosis of the cervical zygoapophyseal joints. A loss of disk height associated with annulus bulging produces cervical segment instability, excessive facet weight bearing, and incongruous joint motion during neck movement, accelerating articular degeneration. Ligamentous strain responses to altered mechanical stresses produce traction osteogenesis with subsequent spur formation. These spurs can encroach posteriorly on the spinal canal, producing cervical myelopathy; laterally on the intervertebral foramen, producing cervical radiculopathy; and anteriorly with esophageal pressure, producing symptoms of dysphagia.

The combination of an extended congenitally narrowed spinal canal further compromised by a vertebral osteophytic bar anteriorly and a buckling ligamentum flavum posteriorly increases the risk of myelopathy as the diameter of the spinal canal is reduced to under 12 mm. Selective impingement of the dorsal spinal root by an osteophyte arising from the zygoapophyseal joint can present with complaints of digital numbness or vague myalgias, which on subsequent appraisal can be related to the known dermatome and myotome distribution of a spinal root. In this regard the C6 myotome encompasses most of the major proximal shoulder muscles. The C6 nerve root emerges between the C5 and C6 vertebrae and is the earliest and most frequent site of a degenerative disk. A complaint of bilateral shoulder pain invariably has an associated element of C6 radiculopathy.

Spurious osteophytes can produce Horner's syndrome, vertebral-basilar symptoms, severe radicular symptoms without associated neck pain, painless upper extremity myotome weakness, and chest pain mimicking angina. Radiographic studies demonstrating typical segmental degenerative changes may in fact bear no relation to the actual spinal root level of the presenting complaint. Foraminal encroachment visible on x-ray views may be more severe at C5–C6, with the patient presenting with both clinical and electromyographic evidence of a progressive C7 radiculopathy arising from the C6–C7 level.

Treatment is predicated on recognizing the exact site of complaint. Localized neck pain and stiffness attributable to arthritis at the zygoapophyseal joint can be treated with cervical collar support, superficial ice massage, ultrasound, flexibility exercises, and nonsteroidal anti-inflammatory drugs. Often in these instances cervical traction therapy aggravates pain. Correspondingly, intermittent cervical traction initially in the formal setting of an outpatient physical therapy facility, followed by ongoing home cervical traction, is an effective approach to cervical radicular pain. In both instances, instruction in appropriate neck biomechanics is helpful in continuing management. Myofascial pain complaints often associated with palpable nodules in the trapezius muscle can be effectively managed in most cases with topical ice, deep kneading massage, stretching exercises, and on occasion localized injections of steroids and lidocaine. The prompt recognition and correction of aggravating factors such as emotional stress, or prolonged postural neck hyperextension related to overly soft seating or to the use of bifocal glasses during reading, may in itself be curative.

The management of neck and shoulder pain requires a continuum of care. Medical conditions often necessitating a clinical reevaluation if they are to be identified early include those with life-threatening potential, i.e., an occult spinal epidural metastasis initially masked by x-ray evidence of cervical degenerative disease, or an apical Pancoast tumor presenting as a subdeltoid bursitis. Often, in these instances as well as in more benign cases, such as polymyalgia with temporal arteritis, rheumatoid arthritis, and infectious diseases, serial reexamination is necessary for correct diagnosis.

BIBLIOGRAPHY

Burney RG, Moore PA, Duncan GH: Management of head and neck pain. *Int Anesthesiol Clin* 21:79, 1983.

Cailliet R: *Neck and Arm Pain*, 2d ed. Philadelphia, Davis, 1981.

Dillin W, Booth R, Cuckler J, et al: Cervical radiculopathy—A review. *Spine* 11:986, 1986.

Gregorius FK, Estrin T, Crandall PH: Cervical spondylotic radiculopathy and myelopathy. *Arch Neurol* 33:618, 1976.

LaBan MM: Electrodiagnosis in cervical radicular and myelopathic syndromes, in Herkowitz HN: *Seminars in Spinal Surgery*. Philadelphia, Saunders, 1989, pp 222–228.

LaBan MM, Meerschaert JR, Taylor RS: Breast pain: A symptom of cervical radiculopathy. *Arch Phys Med Rehabil* 60:315, 1979.

Lieberman JS: Cervical soft tissue injuries and cervical disc disease, in Leek JC, Gershwin ME, Fowler WM (eds): *Principles of Physical Medicine and Rehabilitation in the Musculoskeletal Diseases*. Orlando, Grune & Stratton, 1986, pp 263–286.

MacNab I: Acceleration extension injuries of the cervical spine, in Rothman RH, Simeone FA (eds): *The Spine*, 2d ed. Philadelphia, Saunders, 1982, pp 647–660.

Rothman RH: The pathophysiology of disc degeneration. *Clin Neurosurg* 20:174, 1973.

Simeone FA, Rothman RH: Cervical disk disease, in Rothman RH, Simeone FA (eds): *The Spine*, ed 2. Philadelphia, Saunders, 1982, pp 440–499.

167 THORACIC AND LUMBAR PAIN SYNDROMES

Myron M. LaBan

THORACIC SPINE

Although spine pain complaints are more common at cervical and lumbar levels, thoracic complaints can be as disabling. This region of the spine is comparatively stable and protected both by the rib cage and the orientation of the facet joints. In this region, the spinal cord and paired segmental nerves traverse the narrowest of bony canals and any compromise of the available space can result in rapid and profound neurological deficits.

Thoracic spine fractures occur most commonly at the T10–L2 levels. Vertebral fractures resulting from spinal osteoporosis occur in 8 percent of women over 80 years of age. Such compression fractures are usually wedge shaped and are stable. The presenting symptom is usually severe pain, and myelopathy is rare. However, when long tract signs such as hyperreflexia, Babinski's sign, and urinary incontinence are present, a malignancy metastatic to the spine must be suspected. An epidural metastasis may present similarly as an acute myelopathy with or without pain or abnormal x-rays. Myelography, CT, or magnetic resonance imaging is needed to differentiate the relatively rare thoracic disc protrusion (1 percent of all disc herniations) from a spinal cord tumor. Slowed lumbar spinal evoked potentials can also be diagnostic in confirming thoracic spinal myelopathy.

Localized paravertebral pain can be associated with an acute facet syndrome. Plica entrapped within the thoracic zygoapophyseal joints can produce severe and disabling pain. Radicular pain and localized stiffness associated with osteoarthrosis of these same vertebral joints cause chronic pain, and can result in narrowing of the neural and spinal canals. The latter can lead to signs and symptoms of thoracic spinal stenosis.

Herpes zoster neuralgia can also be associated with acute thoracic radiculopathy. It is difficult to diagnose before vesicles and bullae are evident.

Diabetic thoracic radiculopathy may present as abdominal pain. When this condition is suspected, electromyography demonstrating thoracic paraspinal and abdominal muscle segmental denervation (T7–T12) can be diagnostic.

LUMBAR SPINE

Low back pain is second only to the common cold as a cause of industrial absenteeism and is the number one cause of reduced working capacity. Whenever possible, lumbar pain syndromes both with and without attendant sciatic radiculopathy are managed on an outpatient basis. Admission criteria include intractable pain and loss of function (Table 167-1).

General Considerations

The causes of lumbosacral pain are as diverse as the complex and interrelated anatomic structures of the lumbar spine itself. Additionally, pain of remote origin, outside the spine itself, can present as lumbar pain. Pain of visceral disorders, including that of kidney, pancreas, and gallbladder; duodenal ulcers; colonic diverticulitis; and endometriosis can all mimic primary low back disorders. A history of associated systemic symptoms and a lack of therapeutic response to a trial of initial bed rest, combined with an abnormal abdominal, pelvic, or rectal examination, are usually sufficient to refocus the examination to an appropriate extraspinal diagnosis.

The examiner must give credence to historical fact, age, and circumstances of onset in establishing a diagnosis. For example, an elderly woman with severe midthoracic pain, without a history of trauma, has an osteoporotic vertebral compression fracture until proved otherwise. The onset of lumbosacral pain associated with bilateral leg pain radiation and a sudden loss of bladder control should be presumed to indicate a midline herniated disk with the threat of paraparesis.

Pain from an expanding abdominal aortic aneurysm is constant and aching and can be referred to the lower abdomen and inguinal areas as well as the low back. In the evaluation of low back pain in the elderly, the presence of an abdominal aortic aneurysm must always be considered in the differential diagnosis.

Ambulation producing either lumbar, gluteal, or calf pain may be a manifestation of peripheral vascular disease which is often indistinguishable from that of lumbar spinal stenosis. Both vascular insufficiency and spinal stenosis are aggravated by activity and relieved by rest. Vascular signs in the former instance or neurologic abnormality in the latter can lead to the diagnosis, but arteriography or myelography may be necessary for confirmation.

Lesions within the central nervous system, and in the spinal cord within or above the lumbar area, can also produce both low back pain and radicular leg discomfort. Parasagittal brain tumors and thoracic root lesions, including neurofibromata, can simulate lumbar root syndromes. Pain from thoracic root lesions is usually worse at night while reclining and is relieved by assuming an erect position. Patients may sleep sitting up in a chair, and they may on initial examination demonstrate Babinski reflexes that disappear after a brief period of rest. Distal nerve entrapment syndromes also can present with primary complaints of lumbosacral pain. The most notable example of this situation is tibial nerve entrapment (S1) in the tarsal tunnel behind the medial ankle malleolus.

The physical examination must include both abdominal, vascular, and lower extremity appraisal. Abdominal visceral palpation and auscultation over both the aorta and renal arteries, as well as an assessment of peripheral pulses, color, and temperature, should be routine.

With mechanical dysfunctions of posture or the presence of neurologic signs such as alteration of deep tendon reflexes, weakness, atrophy, restricted or crossed straight-leg-raising (CSLR) signs, and the presence of long tract signs or sphincter dysfunction, the diagnosis of primary spinal-neural pathology becomes self-evident. Establishing a diagnosis in the absence of neurologic signs is more difficult. The examiner must rely to a greater extent on the details of the history, and the ability to replicate and alleviate symptoms by anatomic maneuvers. X-ray examination may or may not be helpful. For example, a herniated disk may well be associated with normal x-rays, while x-ray evidence of osteoarthritis does not assist in the diagnosis of clinically acute sacroiliitis.

In the evaluation of low back syndromes, the examiner's goal is to discriminate between pain of neurogenic and pain of musculoskeletal origin. Although the potential for surgical intervention is by far greater with neurologic than with musculoskeletal involvement, in both instances surgery is indicated in less than 1 percent of all cases. Fortunately, the majority of all lumbosacral syndromes respond to routine symptomatic treatment, including bed rest, superficial heat, and oral analgesics. When seen on a one-time basis in the emergency center, each patient should be given follow-up in the event that the problem is not self-limiting.

Physical Examination

With the patient disrobed, the spine and pelvis should be observed for abnormal spinal curves, pelvic tilts, or the presence of spinal-pelvic lists, all suggesting splinting or guarding in response to pain. The gait should be observed for a loss of normal, symmetric spinal-pelvic rhythm. Asymmetric posturing suggests pain or weakness to which the patient is accommodating. Guarding or splinting can best be dem-

Table 167-1. Admission Criteria for Low Back Pain*

	Admission Criteria	Evaluation
PATIENT SEEN IN OFFICE PRACTICE		
Acute pain; patient requires immediate admission:	Immediate: 1. Paraparesis—paralysis 2. Loss of bowel or bladder function 3. L-S pain and spasticity 4. Cannot stand or sit 5. Sleeping in an upright position 6. Presence of metastatic cancer	1. L-S spine x-ray studies 2. EMG and NCV or evoked potentials 3. Cystometrogram, related to bladder symptoms 4. CBC, SMAC, protein electrophoresis, acid phosphatase, CEA, sedimentation rate 5. Myelogram, CT scan, MRI
Acute pain; observed progression of symptoms requires admission:	With progression: 1. Unilateral paresis with or without pain 2. Absent reflex 3. Atrophy 4. Intractable radicular pain unresponsive to appropriate conservative therapy (pain alone requires 2 weeks or outpatient conservative therapy) 5. Marked restriction of hip and knee extension (bow stringing) 6. Unilateral spasticity 7. Progressive EMG changes	As outpatient: 1. L-S spine x-ray studies, MRI 2. EMG and NCV or evoked potentials 3. "Therapeutic" trial of treatment, i.e., bed rest, physical therapy, corseting 4. If patient experiences the progression of the signs above and symptoms and/or is unresponsive to conservative therapy, oral or injectable medications, the patient is admitted for inpatient evaluation with myelogram, CT scan, or MRI
Chronic pain after surgery:	1. Intractable radicular pain 2. Altered neurologic signs as progressive paresis, loss of straight-leg raising, lateralizing neurologic signs, atrophy 3. Progressive EMG changes 4. Unresponsive to conservative therapy, including physical therapy, corseting, TENS, injections	1. Myelogram 2. CT scan or MRI 3. EMG and NCV or evoked potentials 4. Psychometrics
Chronic pain with surgery:	1. Intractable radicular pain 2. Progressive loss of ambulatory range—vascular vs. neurogenic claudication	1. L-S spine x-ray, CT scan, and MRI studies 2. EMG/NCV/H reflex/evoked potentials 3. Myelogram, CT scan, MRI 4. Abdominal x-ray studies, ultrasound arteriogram 5. CBC, urinalysis, ZSR, protein electrophoresis, SMAC, acid phosphatase, CEA
Chronic pain—no surgery contemplated:	1. Intractable radicular pain	1. Psychometrics 2. Response to analgesics, mood elevators, and TENS 3. Pain clinic referral
ADMISSION THROUGH THE EMERGENCY DEPARTMENT	Essentially the same with the addition of the following admission criteria: 1. Second emergency room visit; 2. Neurologic signs; 3. X-ray film with defects.	

* *Abbreviations:* L-S, lumbosacral; EMG, electromyography; NCV, nerve conduction velocity; CBC, complete blood count; SMAC, complete blood profile; CEA, carcinoembryonic antigen; CT, computed tomography; ZSR, zeta sedimentation rate; TENS, transcutaneous electrical nerve stimulation; MRI, magnetic resonance imaging.

onstrated at slower cadences and can be dramatically accentuated by spinal extension and flexion maneuvers. Extension of the lumbar spine on the pelvis narrows the neural foramina and loads the zygoapophyseal joints on the ipsilateral side. This maneuver will exacerbate radicular pain causing distal sciatic referral, and will also aggravate local articular pain. Similarly, extension and lateral flexion maneuvers to the opposite side reduce the load on the symptomatic joints and open the normal foramina, reducing pain. Flexion maneuvers can demonstrate painful limitations of spinal-pelvic range of motion as measured from fingertips to toes; adjacent spinal segments may be visualized to move as a singular unit in response to localized guarding. Palpation of the paraspinal muscles and the spinal vertebral processes in relation to their relative excursion to each other vividly dramatize this loss of spinal segment mobility. The presence of an acute lumbar radiculopathy associated with a "tethered" root or prefixed spinal root syndrome interjects a precipitous sequence of maneuvers on the painful side in an effort to unload the root: the sequence includes a lateral thrust of the spine, elevation and forward thrust of the pelvis, as well as acute flexion of the hip and knee to reduce tension on the inflamed nerve root.

Localized pain over the ischial tuberosities, greater trochanters, or sciatic notches may suggest localized abnormality, including a bursitis at the tuberosity or trochanter or an entesitis, i.e., inflammation at the tendinous attachment of muscle to bone, at the insertion of the hip abductor and extensor muscle groups. Proximal L5 and S1 root compression is suggested distally by the presence of pain (L5) to palpation over the peroneal nerve at the fibular head and the tibial nerve (S1) in the tarsal tunnel. Percussion pain over the bony spine itself supports the presence of an osseous abnormality, such as compression fracture, metastasis, or disk or vertebral infection. Costovertebral angle percussion pain is invariably associated with retroperitoneal pathology, most often kidney.

Excessive lateral trunk sway to the stance leg during ambulation, a compensated Trendelenberg gait, suggests primary interarticular hip abnormality. On examination, corroborative evidence of an initial loss of hip internal rotation may be associated with medial groin pain and a positive Patrick's sign, which may radiate to the knee. Attempting to "walk around" primary hip disease produces excessive stress at both the ipsilateral sacroiliac joint and the greater trochanter. Each, singly or together, may initially appear to be the salient problem until the loss of hip mobility is identified as the progenitor of the other complaints. Trochanteric bursitis itself can mimic lumbar radiculopathy with distal pain referral along the iliotibial band to the lateral knee.

An inability to walk on either the heels or the toes because of weakness in the foot dorsiflexors or plantar flexors, respectively, suggests an L5 radiculopathy in the former instance, and S1 root involvement in the latter. Similarly, difficulty in assuming or arising from a squatting position may indicate quadriceps weakness associated with L4 root compromise. Manual muscle testing is often the most neglected part of the clinical examination, but it can also be the most rewarding. Weakness of the hip flexors suggests L3 compromise, of the quadriceps L4, the foot dorsiflexors and great toe extensors L5, and the calf S1 radiculopathy. Deep tendon reflexes are tested and compared one side with the other. An absent or reduced knee jerk suggests an L4 radiculopathy, biceps femoris jerk L5, and an asymmetric Achilles reflex an S1 root compression syndrome.

Straight-leg-raising (SLR) testing can be both confusing and diagnostic but must be evaluated with reference to age and the presence or absence of associated CSLR signs. A CSLR sign occurs when contralateral leg elevation produces sciatic pain in the symptomatic leg. A markedly positive SLR in the younger patient is more likely associated with a prolapsed intervertebral disk than in an older patient, particularly when it is associated with a positive CSLR. Similarly, in the more youthful group, a progressive inability to extend the knee on the symptomatic side with bowstringing of the sciatic nerve in the popliteal fossa is highly suggestive of the presence of a prolapsed disk. When noted in conjunction with a painful "strum" sign as the sciatic nerve is plucked behind the knee, it is almost always pathognomonic of the presence of a herniated disk associated with an impacted root. Additional confirmatory maneuvers include an exacerbation of pain with foot dorsiflexion, or with the addition of head flexion with the SLR maneuver held at the symptomatic limit of sciatic pain tolerance. In the older patient, positive SLR or CSLR tests are less specific, but also do suggest a radicular component of involvement.

Hyperreflexia and the presence of upgoing toe signs suggest the presence of a myelopathy with cord compromise above T12–L1, the terminus of the conus medularis. Metastatic lesions, thoracic disk herniations, and on rare occasions, osteoporotic compression fractures at the thoracolumbar junction can present with both low back pain and long tract signs. A sudden loss of bladder and bowel continence with an associated symmetrical, multilevel areflexia and lower extremity weakness may be associated with a midline lumbar disk herniation with compromise of the more distal cauda equina below the clonus medullaris. In this special instance, with rapid progression of paraparesis, emergency decompressive surgery may be required for restoration of function.

Sensory complaints in the presence of radicular syndromes may be useful in localizing root levels of involvement. Complaints of muscular pain in the myotome and sensory dysesthesias in the dermatome distribution of a spinal root may be accompanied by referred pain in the sclerotome distribution. Compromise of S1 and L5 roots can be experienced, respectively, as muscular pain in the calf mimicking a thrombophlebitis, and muscular pain in the anterior tibial compartment simulating "shin splints." Paresthesias in the great toe suggest L5 root involvement, and in the little toe S1 radiculopathy. Discomfort of articular origin, either lumbar zygoapophyseal or sacroiliac joints, can also be recognized by known sclerotome patterns of pain referral. Sacroiliac joint abnormality is commonly referred to the inguinal and anterolateral thigh, as well as the lower abdominal quadrants, often simulating an acute appendicitis or ovarian cyst. Although symptoms of pain and dysesthesias cannot be objectified in the same manner as physical signs, a sophisticated examiner can replicate or reduce the symptoms by initially burdening and then alleviating the complaints by appropriate anatomic maneuvers.

Specific Diagnoses Associated with Lumbar Syndromes

Spinal Degeneration

A rational approach to the diagnosis and treatment of low back pain or sciatica should be predicated on an understanding of the process of spinal degeneration. Initially beginning with an alteration in the hydroscopic quality of the nucleus pulposus, it can progress from annular degeneration of a single disk to multilevel involvement. Sequential disk degeneration with associated zygoapophyseal joint compromise can be associated with relatively infrequent disk prolapses. More often, progressive posterior facet disease is associated with foraminal or spinal canal encroachment, producing symptoms associated with lateral or central spinal stenosis (Fig. 167-1). The combined retrogressive and proliferative changes in the disk anteriorly and in the posterior joints present with both clinical symptoms and roentgenographic changes referred to as combined three-joint complex degeneration. Three distinct stages in the evolution of this process are clinically recognized. The *stage of dysfunction* is associated with complaints of pain and stiffness, often without radiographic or clinical abnormality. Treatment is with oral analgesics and physical therapy.

The *stage of instability* is associated with evidence of spinal segment movement best exemplified by radiographic evidence of the presence of pseudospondylolisthesis (Fig. 167-2) secondary to advanced degenerative disk disease with preservation of the stabilizing pars in-

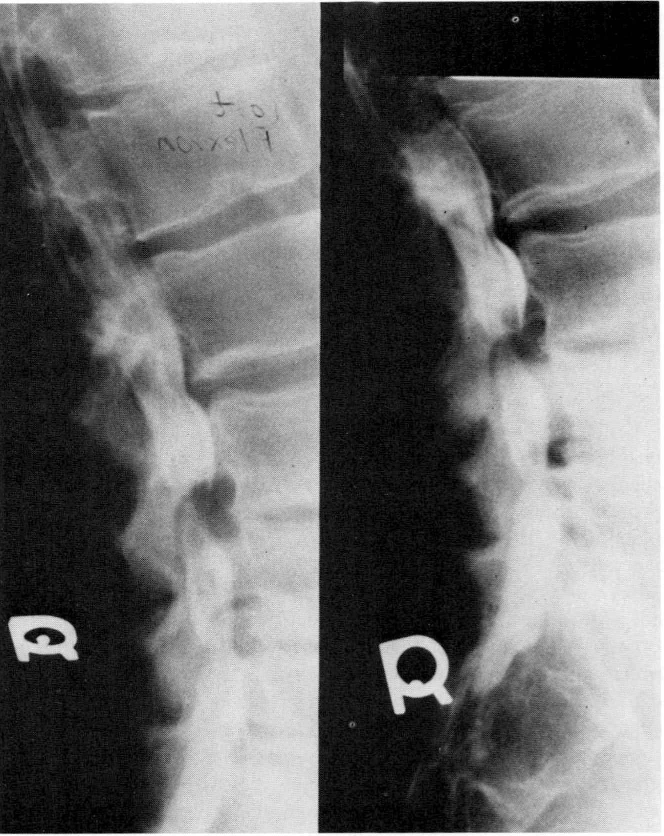

Fig. 167-1. Multilevel evidence of spinal stenosis at lumbar levels with typical hour-glass deformity at disk spaces.

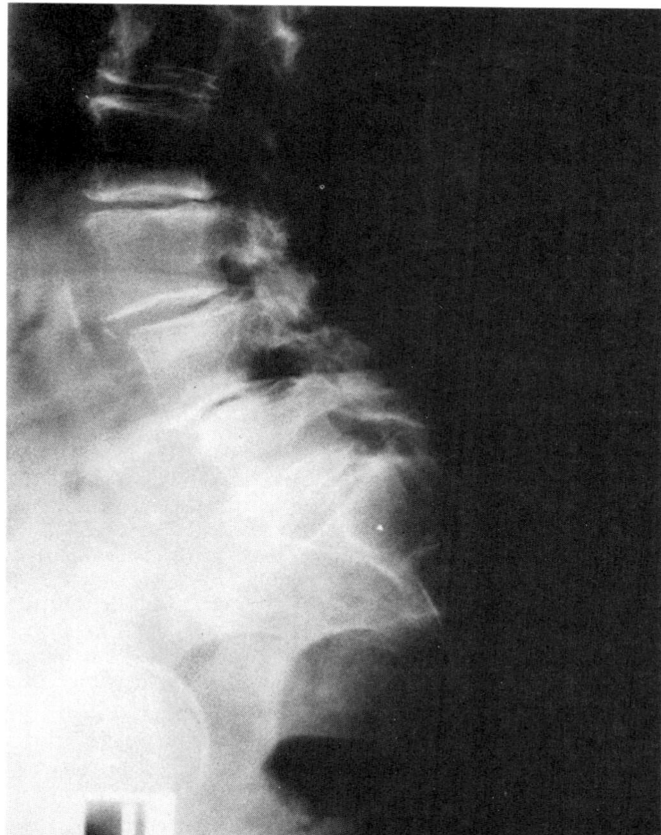

Fig. 167-2. Pseudospondylolisthesis with anterior slip of L4 on L5 associated with neurogenic claudication and night pain.

terarticularis. This phase of spinal degeneration can be clinically recognized by the presence of limited spinal flexibility, a reactive scoliosis, a reduction in the lumbar lordosis, and on occasion, the presence of neurologic abnormality, including alterations in deep tendon reflexes, reductions in muscle strength, and restricted SLR signs. Conservative therapy in this stage is again often successful with the addition of bracing or corseting. When radicular signs and symptoms are preeminent, intermittent pelvic traction is also beneficial.

The final *stage of stabilization* is clinically associated with a marked loss of lumbar flexibility. ''Stiffness'' is a primary complaint which may supersede pain, particularly following periods of immobility. Prolonged standing or walking may precipitate symptoms of localized radicular pain, paresthetic complaints of numbness or tingling, and motor symptoms of ''weakness'' or ''instability'' with or without corroborative motor signs. Articular facet, laminar, and vertebral enlargement associated with osteophytic formation progressing to vertebral fusion are characteristic x-ray features of this stage. The presence of central and lateral lumbar spinal stenosis associated with narrowing of the anteroposterior diameter of the spinal canal with compromise of the dural sac in the former instance, or compression of the spinal nerve root in the intrapedicular, neural canal in the latter case, may be demonstrated by myelography or computed body scans. Patients with spinal stenosis frequently present with severe sciatic radiculopathy and unrestricted SLR, variable lower extremity weakness often directly related to activity, and a ''proximal march of symptoms,'' that is, distal foot numbness progressing proximally with activity.

Conservative therapy appropriate to the earlier stages of degeneration here, too, usually provides symptomatic relief for patients with spinal stenosis. When radicular symptoms are preeminent, heavy intermittent pelvic traction is often palliative. When progressive neurologic defects occur with intractable pain unresponsive to conservative therapy, surgical decompression may be appropriate.

Sacroiliitis

Senescent changes can also occur within the paired sacroiliac joints. Early in this process there may be little or no correlation between symptom severity and radiographic evidence of joint involvement. The pain is usually experienced over the joints themselves, radiating to the anterior lateral or posterior thighs. Usually worse at night, the pain may be bilateral, alternating from side to side. Prolonged standing or sitting, especially on long car trips, exacerbates the discomfort. ''Weakness'' or stiffness, primarily in the morning, is also a predominant symptom of sacroiliitis.

As in the facet joints of the spine, three stages of degeneration can be clinically identified. During the *stage of dysfunction*, although the pain and associated disability can be severe, the x-ray films are often normal. During the secondary *stage of instability*, pelvic x-ray films with alternate leg weight bearing may demonstrate pubic symphysis instability (Fig. 167-3) in excess of 3 mm. Usually the instability is greater on the symptomatic side. Any of the three-joint complex of the pelvis, the paired posterior sacroiliac joints, and the anterior pubic symphysis may be painful or demonstrate concurrent x-ray evidence of progressive degenerative change.

The terminal *stage of immobilization* is associated with anatomic and functional ankylosis of these joints. Paradoxically, osteophytic formation and articular fibrosis with eventual joint fusion present less with pain and more often with complaints of stiffness, particularly in the morning.

Treatment consists initially of bed rest, superficial heat, and oral nonsteroidal antiinflammatory drugs. Bed rest for at least 24 h is to be recommended in a lumbar flexed position, either side lying, prone with a pillow under the abdomen, or supine with hips and knees flexed over a cushion. The topical use of moist heat is useful in preference to dry heat as it is generally better tolerated. In this regard silicon-filled hydrocollator packs which cool from the initial application are to be preferred to electric heating pads which can cause severe burns. In both instances, heat should never be under the patient, but over the painful area. Oral medications include narcotics and nonsteroidal antiinflammatory analgesics. Muscle relaxants as a class are not to be recommended. Their analgesic effects are minimal as they act primarily

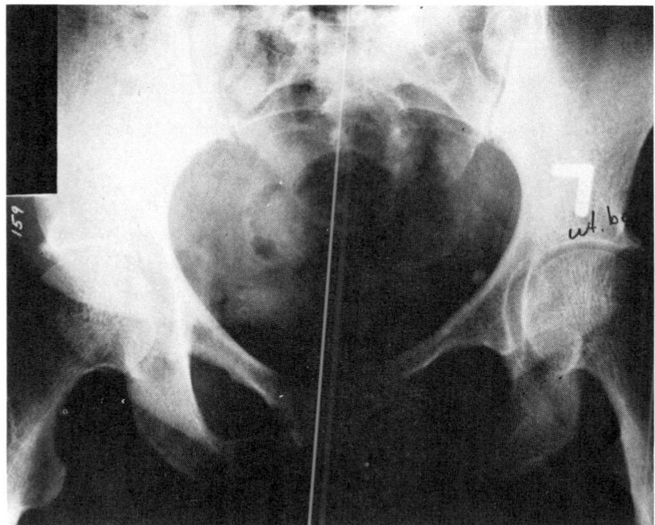

Fig. 167-3. Persistent sacroiliac and pubic symphysis pain 2 years post slip and fall at 3 months of pregnancy. Four millimeters of subluxation at pubic symphysis is demonstrated by alternate leg weight bearing.

as central soporifics with all their attendant risks. Oral narcotic analgesics may be necessary for 24 to 48 h as appropriate to the individual circumstance. Nonsteroidal antiinflammatory medications for the long term are useful, for both their analgesic and their antiinflammatory properties. Their dosage, initially high, should be tapered to a comfortable maintenance level with due concern to water retention and gastric intolerance. Several classes are available. They include fenamates (meclofenamate), indole derivatives (indomethacin, sulindac), phenyl alkonic acids (ibuprofen, naproxen, naproxen sodium), and oxicans (piroxicam). If one group is ineffective, another should be tried. Injecting the symptomatic articulations with a mixture of 1 mL each of both short-acting and long-acting steroids with an additional 1 mL of lidocaine during the acute phase can produce immediate pain relief with a dramatic resolution of a concomitant reactive scoliosis. Later diathermy, weight reduction, lumbar flexibility, and abdominal strengthening exercises combined with corseting are, together, all useful treatment adjuncts.

Referral for continuing outpatient care is absolutely critical. No matter how searching the physical examination, and notwithstanding the experience of the examiner, clinical manifestations can change rapidly, often dramatically, to be recognized only by subsequent evaluations. The use of electromyography, bone scans, myelograms, CT scans and magnetic resonance imaging studies are diagnostic modalities that can be employed at follow-up evaluation.

BIBLIOGRAPHY

Bell GR, Rothman RH: The conservative treatment of sciatica. *Spine* 9:54, 1984.

Bruckner FE, Greco A, Leung AWL: ''Benign thoracic pain'' syndrome: Role of magnetic resonance imaging in the detection and localization of thoracic disc disease. *J R Soc Med* 82:81, 1989.

Khatri B, Baruah J, McQuillen MP: Correlation of electromyography with computed tomography and evaluation of low back pain. *Arch Neurol* 41:594, 1984.

Kirkaldy-Willis WH, Farfan HF: Instability of the lumbar spine. *Clin Orthop* 165:110, 1982.

LaBan MM: ''Vesper's Curse'' night pain—the bane of Hypnos. *Arch Phys Med Rehabil* 65:501, 1984.

LaBan MM: The lumbosacral pain syndrome, in Kaplan PE (ed): *The Practice of Physical Medicine*. Springfield, Charles C Thomas, 1984, pp 107–160.

LaBan MM: Low back pain—Lumbosacral strain—Lumbar disc disease, in Leek JC, Gershwin ME, Fowler WM (eds): *Principles of Physical Medicine and Rehabilitation in Musculoskeletal Diseases*. Orlando, Grune & Stratton, 1986, pp 309–333.

168
ANAPHYLAXIS AND ACUTE ALLERGIC REACTIONS

Joseph A. Salomone III

INTRODUCTION

Allergic reactions can range from mild local eruptions to severe and life-threatening multisystem systemic illnesses. The most common presenting complaints involve the dermatologic and respiratory systems, but gastrointestinal and cardiovascular involvement also occurs frequently. Early recognition, rapid evaluation, and prompt intervention are necessary to prevent potentially fatal outcome. Parenterally administered penicillin and Hymenoptera stings are the two most common etiologies of fatal anaphylaxis.

CLINICAL IMMUNOLOGY

Hypersensitivity is an exaggerated immune system response to presented antigens. Often, on initial contact an antigen produces no obvious clinical response, but sensitizes the immune system so that the next contact produces a clinical response. Immediate hypersensitivity reactions are those that manifest themselves within seconds to minutes after the presentation of the antigen, and an interaction between antigens and antibodies occurs. In humans, these reactions are mediated mostly by IgE, and are responsible for attacks of extrinsic asthma, allergic rhinitis, urticaria, angioedema, and anaphylaxis.

A hapten is a small organic compound that when bound to a protein forms an antigenic complex that can stimulate immune system responses. Antigens that preferentially stimulate the immune system to produce IgE are called allergens, and most are proteins. On initial presentation, these allergens react with B cell precursors and T cells, leading to formation of T helper cells and activated B cells. In turn, memory B cells and plasma cells are created, and the plasma cells then produce specific IgE antibodies.

IgE binds to specific receptors on mast cells and basophils. When antigen binds to the IgE on these cells, it triggers the release of mediators that are responsible for the local and systemic reactions that occur. These biologic mediators cause increased vascular permeability, vasodilation, bronchial constriction, smooth muscle contraction, increased mucous gland secretions, and attraction of inflammatory cells. Clinical manifestations thus depend on the site or sites affected by these mediators. Histamine, bradykinins, platelet-activating factor, heparin, protease, and leukotriens (C_4, D_4, and E_4 or SRS-A) are some of the mediators that are released.

Classically, four types of hypersensitivity reactions are described. However, current research and improved understanding of the complex immune system have defined overlapping and coexisting mechanisms of hypersensitivity. Type I hypersensitivity is an IgE-mediated, and possibly IgG-mediated, reaction to allergens. The binding of allergens to antibodies present on the surface of mast cells and basophils results in the reactions described above.

Type II reactions involve IgG and IgM antibody reactions to antigens on cell surfaces, and involve complement activation and phagocytosis by killer cells. The most frequent clinical manifestations involve blood transfusion reactions, hemolytic anemias, idiopathic thrombocytopenic purpura (ITP), and Goodpasture's syndrome. This appears to be the least common cause for drug-related allergic reactions.

Type III reactions are caused by soluble immune or antigen-antibody complexes that in turn activate the complement system and platelets to form platelet aggregates and IgE complexes. This type of reaction can occur after tetanus toxoid administration in sensitized individuals. Other clinical manifestations include poststreptococcal glomerulonephritis, serum sickness, and systemic lupus erythematosus.

Type IV reactions are cell-mediated reactions not involving complement or antibodies. This reaction is called delayed hypersensitivity and results from the migration of specifically activated T lymphocytes to the area of antigen presentation. Clinical manifestations do not occur for 24 to 48 h after exposure, and include the local reactions seen with skin tests for *Candida,* tuberculosis, and *Trichophyton.*

Persons who exhibit hypersensitivity reactions often have a history of atopic symptoms, as well as familial history of allergy. The duration and quantity of exposure to the precipitating antigen can affect the severity of reaction. Compounds may have similar haptens and thus cause similar sensitization and reactions. Examples of this include the cross reactivity occasionally seen between penicillins and cephalosporins, or sulfonamides and sulfonylurea drugs.

ANAPHYLAXIS

The term *anaphylaxis* was coined by Portier and Richet in 1902, and literally means "removal of protection." Today anaphylaxis describes the clinical syndrome of severe hypersensitivity reaction characterized by cardiovascular collapse and respiratory compromise. A wide variety of substances are now known to produce anaphylactic reactions. Table 168-1 contains a partial list of some of the more common causative agents.

The symptoms associated with anaphylaxis may begin within seconds of exposure to an allergen or may be delayed for up to 1 h. However, the typical response begins within minutes of exposure, and primarily involves the cardiovascular and respiratory systems. The skin and gastrointestinal tract are also commonly involved, and widespread involvement of many organ systems may occur at the same time.

The clinical symptoms of anaphylaxis can vary widely. In patients who have previously suffered from an anaphylactic reaction, an "aura" of impending disaster may occur that warns them of the oncoming reaction. Cutaneous manifestations include generalized erythema, pruritus, progressive urticaria, and angioedema. Angioedema most often involves the head, neck, face, and upper airways. Flushing, chills, and diaphoresis may occur. A vague tightening sensation in the throat and chest progressing to laryngeal and bronchial spasm, manifested as hoarseness, stridor, and wheezing, may progress to severe respi-

Table 168-1. Common Causes of Anaphylaxis and Anaphylactoid and Allergic Reactions

Drugs
Penicillins and related antibiotics
Aspirin
Trimethoprim-sulfamethoxazole
Vancomycin
Nonsteroidal antiinflammatory agents
Foods and additives
Shellfish
Soybeans
Nuts
Wheat
Milk
Eggs
Monosodium glutamate
Nitrates and nitrites
Tartrazine dyes
Other
Hymenoptera stings
Insect parts and molds
Radiographic contrast material

ratory distress. Patients with a previous history of reactive airway disease often have more severe bronchospasm. Nausea, abdominal cramps, vomiting, and diarrhea are frequent complaints. Light-headedness may be the initial manifestation of impending cardiovascular collapse, with resultant tachycardia, hypotension, and typical manifestations of shock. Cardiac dysrhythmias and profound ischemia may occur, which may precipitate a myocardial infarction.

Patients with a prior history of atrophy may be at increased risk for severe anaphylactic reactions. The use of β-blocking agents, particularly in patients at increased risk for anaphylaxis, may predispose patients to more severe reactions. Further, patients who are taking β-blockers and develop anaphylaxis may be refractory to standard epinephrine doses. Drugs such as cimetidine that delay the clearance of β-blockers should also be avoided since they may prolong the activity of the β-blocker and complicate treatment.

The diagnosis of anaphylaxis is often obvious, but in the early stages the potential severity of the reaction may be underestimated. The differential diagnosis will vary depending on whether the predominant symptomatology occurs in a single organ system. Pulmonary embolism, acute myocardial infarction and cardiac dysrhythmias, airway obstruction, tension pneumothorax, acute asthma, hereditary angioedema, volume depletion, and vasovagal reactions are just a few conditions that may need to be considered in the differential diagnosis.

Treatment begins with attention to the airway. A high flow of oxygen via face mask and immediate administration of epinephrine are indicated. If signs of shock are present, intravenous administration of 0.3 to 0.5 mg of a 1:10,000 solution is preferred. If immediate intravenous access cannot be obtained, injection into the venous plexus at the base of the tongue may provide the most rapid access. Endotracheal administration is also an alternative to intravenous access if the airway has been established. Subcutaneous administration of 0.3 to 0.5 mg of a 1:1000 solution is indicated if there is no significant circulatory compromise. Immediate endotracheal intubation may be required, but may be extremely difficult if angioedema or severe laryngospasm is present. Transtracheal jet insufflation or cricothyrotomy may be necessary to control the airway. If the reaction may be due to intravenous solutions, administration should be discontinued. If the patient has sustained recent bite or sting, or received an injection, a tourniquet may be placed proximal to the site to prevent further dissemination of the allergen. To avoid potential injury to the limb, this tourniquet should probably only remain until therapy has begun. Cardiac monitoring should be begun, and an ECG obtained in patients with previous cardiac history or ischemic symptoms. Hypotensive patients should be placed in a head-down position or, at a minimum, have their legs elevated unless respiratory status prevents such positioning. Intravenous fluid therapy with Ringer's lactate or normal saline should be established. Large volumes of crystalloid, 2 to 4 L, may be required in the hypotensive patient. A pneumatic antishock garment (PSAG or MAST) may be beneficial in the initial management of hypotension in both the prehospital setting and the emergency department. Because of the increased vascular permeability, pulmonary edema may develop with or without fluid administration. Patients with severe symptomatology may benefit from CVP or Swan-Ganz monitoring. Administration of antihistamines may be beneficial. Diphenhydramine, 50 mg intravenously, is the most commonly utilized. Inhaled bronchodilators, such as aerosolized albuterol, 0.5 mL in 3 mL saline, can be useful in managing bronchospasm. These can be administered either intermittently or continuously. Aminophylline, initial bolus of 4 to 6 mg/kg followed by a maintenance infusion, may be required for management of severe bronchospasm. Intravenous corticosteroids, such as methylprednisolone, 125 mg, may prevent or lessen delayed reactions. Refractory hypotension may require dopamine, levoterenol, or epinephrine infusions. General anesthesia and neuromuscular blockade may be required to assist ventilation in cases of severe respiratory distress.

All patients with significant generalized reactions should be observed for at least 24 h. Delayed reactions and reoccurrence of symptoms are possible, particularly as the effects of previously administered treatment decrease. Patients may benefit from repeated doses of antihistamines and corticosteroids over the next several days, and these should be prescribed. Oral doses of antihistamines every 4 to 6 h, and oral corticosteroids, should probably be given for at least 72 h. All patients should be referred to an allergy specialist, and advised to carry some form of self-administered epinephrine and antihistamines. Several prefilled syringe kits are available, such as the Epi-pen and Ana-kit.

ANAPHYLACTOID REACTIONS

Anaphylactoid reactions are nonimmunologically mediated systemic reactions that clinically appear very similar to anaphylaxis. Although no immunologic basis is identified, many of the same mediators are involved in these reactions. The most common agent responsible is radiographic contrast media. Other implicated agents include nonsteroidal anti-inflammatory agents, thiamine, and codeine. Recent research has found complement activation or immune-complex-mediated reactions for many agents previously thought to cause anaphylactoid reactions. Treatment is essentially the same as for anaphylaxis.

URTICARIA AND ANGIOEDEMA

Urticaria, or hives, is a cutaneous IgE-mediated reaction marked by the development of pruritic, erythemic wheals of varying size that generally disappear quickly. Erythema multiforme is a more pronounced urticarial variant, characterized by typical target lesions. Angioedema is also an IgE-mediated reaction characterized by edema formation in the dermis, most generally involving the face and neck. These manifestations may accompany many allergic reactions.

As with all allergic manifestations, a detailed history of exposures, ingestions, medications, infections, and family history should be obtained. If an etiologic agent can be identified, future reactions may be avoided. Treatment of these reactions is generally supportive and symptomatic, with attempts to identify and remove the offending agent if it can be identified. Epinephrine, antihistamines, and steroids are most often tried. Oral antihistamines and steroids for several days may be beneficial. The addition of a H_2-receptor agonist, such as cimetidine, may also be useful in more severe cases. Cold compresses to affected areas may be soothing. Referral to an allergy specialist is indicated.

Hereditary angioedema is an autosomal dominant disorder with a characteristic complement pathway deficiency. Reactions often involve the upper respiratory tract and gastrointestinal tract. Minor trauma often precipitates a reaction. Many of the typical treatments of allergic problems, such as epinephrine, steroids, and antihistamines, have been tried, but their effectiveness is not clearly demonstrated.

OTHER COMMON ALLERGIC PROBLEMS

Food Allergy

Hypersensitivity reactions to ingested foods are generally due to IgE-mediated reactions to food components or additives. IgE-coated mast cells lining the gastrointestinal tract react to presented allergens in ingested foods and produce clinical findings associated with the release of biologic mediators, as previously described. Non-IgE-mediated food allergy reactions have also been described. Dairy products, eggs, and nuts are some of the most commonly implicated foods.

A detailed history will provide the best clues to food allergy, with particular attention to other allergic history and prior reactions. Diagnosis is often difficult since the offending food or foods may only occasionally produce symptoms, depending on amount ingested and other foods present.

Symptoms of food allergy include swelling and itching of the lips, mouth, and pharynx; nausea; abdominal cramps; vomiting; and diarrhea. Cutaneous manifestations such as angioedema and urticaria, as well as systemic findings of anaphylaxis, can occur. Treatment is supportive, with the administration of antihistamines to lessen symptomatology. Referral to an allergy specialist is indicated.

Insect Sting Allergy

Insect stings can produce significant and sometimes fatal reactions, particularly in sensitized patients. Approximately 100 patients die annually from insect sting reactions, making insect sting the second most common cause of fatal anaphylaxis. True stinging insects belong to the order Hymenoptera, which includes three families: Apoidea (honeybee), Formicidae (fire ants), and Vespoidae (wasps, yellow jackets, hornets). The venoms of each family are unique, although all have similar types of components, mostly proteins. This difference accounts for the limited cross-reactivity seen. The usual reaction to these stings includes localized pain, pruritus, swelling, and redness. Sensitized individuals may have exaggerated local reactions with or without systemic manifestations. Systemic reactions run from mild nausea and malaise to urticaria, angioedema, or anaphylaxis.

Diagnosis depends on clinical history, with particular attention to past reactions, and an examination to locate the site of the sting. Occasionally, the site of envenomation is overlooked, and predominance of reaction in one organ system can lead to misdiagnosis. Treatment is symptomatic and supportive. Mild local reactions can be managed with application of ice and oral antihistamines. More generalized reactions or local reactions of head and neck may benefit from a short steroid course. Oxygen and inhaled β agonists, and possibly subcutaneous epinephrine, may be indicated for more severe reactions with associated respiratory reaction. Patients with severe reactions should be advised to carry self-administered epinephrine and antihistamines. A referral to an allergy specialist is indicated.

Drug Allergy

Although adverse reactions to drugs are a common clinical problem, true immunologically mediated hypersensitivity reactions probably account for less than 10 percent of these problems. Since most drugs are small organic molecules, they are generally unable to stimulate the immune system alone. However, when a drug or metabolite becomes protein-bound, either in serum or on cell surfaces, this drug-protein complex can become an allergen and stimulate immune system responses. Thus, the ability of a drug or its metabolites to sensitize the immune system depends on the ability to be bound to tissue proteins. Approximately 300 patients yearly die from anaphylactic drug reactions. Penicillin is the drug most commonly implicated in eliciting true allergic reactions, and accounts for approximately 90 percent of all allergic drug reactions. Of those patients who have fatal anaphylactic drug reactions, over 95 percent had reacted to penicillin. Only about 25 percent of patients who die from penicillin anaphylaxis had exhibited allergic reactions during previous courses of the drug. Parenterally administered penicillin was more than twice as likely to produce fatal allergic reactions as orally administered penicillin.

The clinical manifestations of drug allergy are widely varied, and can involve all four types of hypersensitivity reactions. A generalized reaction similar to immune-complex or serum-sickness reactions is very common. Beginning usually in the first or second week after the administration of the drug, this reaction may take many weeks to subside after drug withdrawal. Generalized malaise, arthralgias, pruritus, urticarial eruptions, and fever are common. Drug fever may occur without other associated clinical findings, and may also occur without an immunologic basis. Circulating immune complexes are probably responsible for the lupuslike reactions caused by some drugs. Cytotoxic reactions, such as penicillin-induced hemolytic anemia, can occur. Skin eruptions may include erythema, pruritus, urticaria, angioedema, erythema multiforme, and photosensitivity, and severe reactions, such as those seen in Stevens-Johnson syndrome and toxic epidermal necrolysis, may also occur. Pulmonary complications, including bronchospasm and airway obstruction, can occur. Delayed hypersensitivity reactions may be manifested as a contact dermatitis from drugs applied topically.

Diagnosis is best determined by a careful and thorough history. Treatment is supportive, with oral or parenteral antihistamines, corticosteroids, and β-adrenergic agents as indicated. Immediate drug withdrawal is important; however, reactions can continue or recur after a period of abstinence. Referral to an allergy specialist may be indicated.

BIBLIOGRAPHY

Barach EM, Nowak RM, Tennyson GL, et al: Epinephrine for treatment of anaphylactic shock. *JAMA* 251:2118, 1984.

Bonner JR: Anaphylaxis: I. Etiology and pathogenesis. *Ala J Med Sci* 25:283, 1988.

Bonner JR: Anaphylaxis: II. Prevention and treatment. *Ala J Med Sci* 25:408, 1988.

Cohan RH, Dunnick NR, Bashore TM: Treatment of Reactions to Radiographic Contrast Material. *AJR* 151:263, 1988.

Fath JJ, Cerra FB: The therapy of anaphylactic shock. *Drug Intell Clin Pharm* 18:14, 1984.

Fisher M: Anaphylaxis. *Disease Month*, August 1987, pp. 437–279.

Lucke WC, Thomas H: Anaphylaxis: Pathophysiology, clinical presentations and treatment. *J Emerg Med* 1:83, 1983.

Muelleman RL, Gatz M, Salomone JA, et al: Hemodynamic and respiratory effects of thyrotropin-releasing hormone and epinephrine in anaphylactic shock. *Ann Emerg Med* 18:534, 1989.

Perkin RM, Anas NG: Mechanisms and management of anaphylactic shock not responding to traditional therapy. *Ann Allergy* 54:202, 1985.

Rubenstein E, Federman DD (eds): Clinical immunology, in *Medicine*. New York, Scientific American, 1989, 6, chap. VII.

Sinkinson CA et al (eds): Individualizing therapy for Hymenoptera stings. *Emerg Med Rep* 11:1990.

169 INITIAL APPROACH TO THE TRAUMA PATIENT

Ernest Ruiz

Despite the advent of sophisticated transportation systems and the designation of regional trauma centers, community hospital emergency departments remain the critical link in the resuscitation of a large percentage of trauma victims in this country. Because of weather, distances, and geography, this will continue to be the case. All physicians covering emergency departments should be skilled in trauma resuscitation.

This chapter outlines the process of trauma resuscitation in the prehospital phase and during the first few minutes after arrival in the emergency department. Other chapters will elaborate on the techniques and process of resuscitation when certain injuries are identified.

THE INCIDENCE OF TRAUMA

In the United States, trauma is responsible for more deaths in the 1- to 34-year age group than all other diseases combined and is the leading cause of death up to age 44.

Motor Vehicle Accidents

Motor vehicle accidents account for the largest share of trauma deaths (Fig. 169–1). In 1985 about 50,000 people were killed in crashes. More than half were automobile occupants. Over 50 percent of adult victims were legally classified as intoxicated.

Motorcylist deaths accounted for 10 percent of the highway death toll in 1985. The motorcycle death rate is more than 15 times greater than the automobile death rate.

Bicyclist fatalities in collisions with motor vehicles account for about 2 percent of traffic deaths. Two-thirds of bicyclist deaths occur in the 5- to 14-year age group, with 13-year-old males constituting the largest group.

Pedestrian deaths account for 10 to 15 percent of motor vehicle deaths, making it the second largest category, the largest group of which is the elderly.

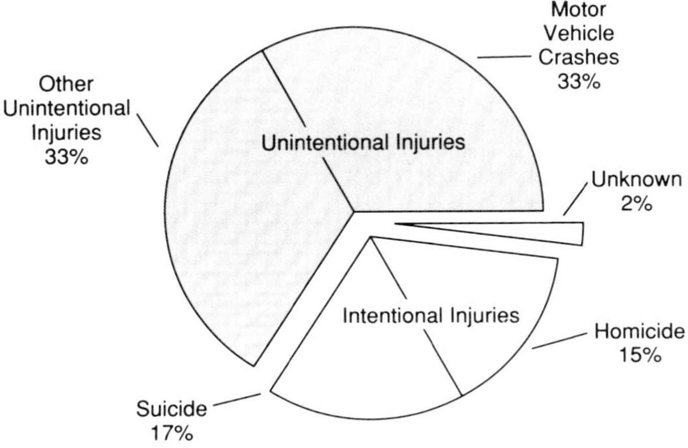

Fig. 169-1. Percent of injury deaths by manner of death, 1980. (*From* Baker SP, O'Neill B, Karpf RS: *The Injury Fact Book*. Lexington, MA. Lexington Books, 1984. Used by permission.)

Other Unintentional Trauma

The leading causes of unintentional trauma fatalities are listed in Table 169-1. More than half of the fatal falls are in the elderly, who account for 4 percent of the population. Fractured hips are the most common type of injury resulting in hospital admission.

Distribution

Overall, 70 percent of trauma fatalities occur in rural areas, even though 70 percent of the population lives in urban areas. There are many logistical explanations for this, including longer times to discovery, response, and delivery to the hospital. However, prehospital care systems and emergency department, operating room, and in-hospital management deserve positive attention. Trauma management in rural areas of the United States has long received too little support from organized medicine, government, and even trauma centers.

PREVENTION

Trauma can be prevented through public education, state and federal legislation, and modification of the physical environment. The latter includes highway improvement, passive restraints, and other measures. The seat belt issue has taught us that although education and physical changes are important, legislation is effective and legislators are receptive to the input of physicians.

Table 169-1. Twenty Leading Causes of Death Due To Unintentional Injury, 1980

Cause	Number of Deaths
Motor vehicle crashes (traffic)	51,930
Falls	13,294
Drowning	7,257
Fires and burns	6,016
Poisoning by solids and liquids	3,089
Firearms	1,955
Aspiration of food	1,943
Airplane crashes	1,494
Machinery	1,471
Aspiration of nonfood material	1,306
Motor vehicle crashes (nontraffic)	1,242
Electric current	1,095
Struck by falling object	1,037
Mechanical suffocation	872
Excessive cold	707
Poisoning by motor vehicle exhaust	611
Pedestrians hit by trains	450
Exposure or neglect	415
Explosions	339
Collision with object or person	318

Source: Baker SP, O'Neill B, Karpf RS: *The Injury Fact Book*. Lexington, MA: Lexington Books, 1984. Used by permission.

PREHOSPITAL CARE

The "load and go" method of managing trauma in the field requires skill and resourcefulness to accomplish safely and rapidly. The objective is to immobilize patients and move them to the hospital as quickly as possible, inserting IV lines while on route rather than at the scene. The receiving emergency department should be contacted early and put on notice that an injured patient is on the way.

RESUSCITATION OF THE TRAUMA PATIENT IN THE EMERGENCY DEPARTMENT

The types of injuries trauma victims can suffer are innumerable, but the ABCs of trauma resuscitation, (airway, breathing, circulation), which are described below, apply to all cases. Table 169–2 outlines the flow of the process.

Table 169-2. A Step-by-Step Procedure for Trauma Resuscitation

1. *Notification by Prehospital Personnel:* The receiving emergency department should be informed about:
   - Airway patency
   - Pulse and respirations
   - Level of consciousness
   - Immobilization
   - Mechanism of injury and blood loss at the scene
   - Anatomic sites of apparent injury
2. *Preparation for Receiving the Trauma Victim*
   - A. Assign tasks to team members
     - Restraints
     - Expose the arms and torso
     - Feel and report the presence of a radial pulse
     - Insert two large-bore arm IVs
     - Draw blood for essential lab tests
     - Obtain O-negative blood
     - Apply cardiac monitor leads
   - B. Check and prepare vital equipment
     - Airway options
     - Blood/fluid warmer
     - Check suction/autotransfusion device
   - C. Summon surgical consultant and other team members not present
3. *Primary Survey.* The most immediately lethal injuries are taken care of as they are identified.
   - A. Airway
     - Clear airway: chin lift, suction, finger sweep
     - Protect airway
       - Depressed level of consciousness or bleeding, tracheal intubation without neck movement
     - Surgical airway
   - B. Breathing
     - Ventilate with 100% oxygen
     - Check thorax and neck
       - Deviated trachea
       - Tension pneumothorax (intervention—needle decompression)
       - Chest wounds and chest wall motion
       - Sucking chest wound (intervention—occlusive dressing)
       - Neck and chest crepitation
       - Multiple broken ribs
       - Fractured sternum
       - Pneumothorax
     - Listen for breath sounds
       - Correct tracheal tube placement?
       - Hemopneumothorax?
         - Chest tube(s)—38 F
         - Collect blood for autotransfusion
   - C. Circulation
     - Apply pressure to sites of external exsanguination
     - Assure that two large-bore IVs established
       - Begin with rapid infusion of crystalloid solution
       - If arm sites unavailable, insert a large central line or perform a saphenous cutdown at the ankle
     - Assess for blood volume status
       - Radial and carotid pulse, BP determination
       - Jugular venous filling
       - Quality of heart tones
     - Beck's triad present?
       - Pericardiocentesis or echocardiogram
       - Decompress tamponade
         - Pericardiocentesis
         - Thoracotomy with pericardiotomy
     - Hypovolemia
       - After 2 L of crystalloid begin blood infusion if still hypovolemic; in children use two 20 mL/kg boluses then 10 mL/kg blood boluses if still unstable
     - Near-term pregnant patient—place roll under right hip
   - D. Disability
     - Brief neurological examination
       - Pupil size and reactivity
       - Limb movement
       - Glasgow Coma Scale
   - E. Continuing Resuscitation
     - Monitor fluid administration
       - Consider central line for CVP monitoring
       - Use fetal heart rate as indicator in pregnant women
       - Record all events
4. *Secondary Survey.* A thorough search for injuries is carried out in order to set further priorities.
   - Trauma series x-rays: lateral cervical spine, supine chest, AP pelvis
   - Head-to-toe examination looking and feeling; quickly bring problems under control as they are discovered
     - Scalp wound bleeding controlled with Raney clips
     - Hemotypanum?
     - Facial stability?
     - Epistaxis tamponaded with balloons if severe
     - Avulsed teeth, broken jaw?
     - Penetrating injuries?
     - Abdominal distension and tenderness?
     - Pelvic stability?
     - Perineal laceration/hematoma?
     - Urethral meatus blood?
     - Rectal examination for tone, blood, and prostate position
     - Bimanual vaginal examination
     - Peripheral pulses
     - Deformities, open fractures
     - Reflexes, sensation
   - Large gastric tube (32 F) inserted
   - Foley catheter inserted
     - Blood?
     - Pregnancy test
   - Deflate the pneumatic trousers sequentially beginning with the abdominal portion if the BP is near normal
   - Log-roll the patient to feel and see the back, flanks, and buttocks
   - Splint unstable fractures/dislocations
   - Assure that tetanus prophylaxis is given
   - Consult with surgeon regarding further tests or immediate need for surgery or preferred IV medications; consider:
     - Emergency thoracotomy to provide aortic compression or cross-clamping
     - Aortogram or upright chest x-ray to r/o ruptured aorta
     - Cystogram if pelvic fracture present or blood in urine
     - IVP or enhanced CT scan of the abdomen
     - Diagnostic peritoneal lavage: open or closed
     - Head CT scan
     - IV mannitol for neurologic decompensation
     - IV steroids for possible spinal cord injury
     - IV antibiotics for possible ruptured abdominal viscus
     - IV antibiotics for perineal, vaginal, or rectal laceration
     - Pelvic arteriogram and embolization for pelvic hemorrhage

Role of Assistants

The physician should assign tasks for assistants prior to patient arrival so that time is not wasted. Before the patient arrives, assistants should do the following:

1. Obtain two units of type O blood if it is known that the patient is hypotensive.
2. Prepare blood tubes and laboratory slips for type and crossmatching, CBC, electrolytes, BUN, glucose, coagulation, and blood alcohol studies. Ideally, a packet of tubes and laboratory slips stand ready at all times already filled out and identified by number so that the blood can be processed as soon as the number is attached to the patient.
3. Have airway and IV equipment at hand.

In hospitals where a trauma surgeon is not on staff, the surgeon on call should be summoned even before the patient arrives.

Once the patient arrives in the emergency department, the assistants should:

1. Restrain the patient's arms and legs.
2. Cut off the clothing on the torso.
3. Palpate the radial or brachial pulse.
4. Place the cart in the Trendelenburg position if the patient's pulse is weak or absent.
5. Insert large-bore (16- or 14-gauge) IV catheters in each arm, and send blood specimens to the laboratory.
6. Infuse lactated Ringer's solution or normal saline at maximum flow rate if the pulse is weak or absent.
7. Apply ECG monitor leads to the chest, avoiding the subclavicular areas, where they would interfere with central venous line placement.

Failure to restrain the patient who appears quiet on arrival frequently results in a struggle when an airway is inserted or an IV line attempted. Personnel are ineffectively used to hold down the patient, delaying IV access and airway management and preventing adequate cervical spine immobilization. A determination of the actual blood pressure is not essential during the first minutes of the resuscitation. The presence of a radial pulse indicates a blood pressure of at least 80 mmHg.

Role of the Team Captain

The resuscitating physician should supervise the placement of the patient on the cart and listen to the report of the ambulance personnel while beginning the primary survey. The assistants should carry out their assigned tasks.

The Primary Survey

A quick look at the patient gives a rough impression as to size, sex, age, body build, color, and alertness, but the first conscious step should be to institute the ABCs. The primary survey rapidly identifies the most immediately lethal injuries and assures that they are managed with the highest priority.

Airway

If the patient is not able to breathe or is not making an effort to breathe, a chin lift or the insertion of an oral or nasal airway may suffice for the moment. Any movement of the neck should be avoided in the usual blunt trauma case. Obtunded or unconscious patients should be tracheally intubated to protect the airway and to provide a means of hyperventilation. Yankauer or dental suction and a transtracheal needle ventilation device should be on hand in case the patient vomits prior to intubation. Log rolling and pharyngeal suction may be necessary if the patient vomits, to prevent aspiration. If the patient is not breathing or if there is severe facial injury, cricothyrotomy or transtracheal needle ventilation may be indicated.

The very agitated trauma patient suffering from head injury, hypoxia, or drug- or alcohol-induced delirium may harbor a cervical spine fracture. A paralyzing agent such as succinylcholine or vecuronium bromide, along with a small dose of diazepam or midazolam, may be necessary to enable safe airway management. Disadvantages of immediate sedation and paralysis are interference with neurological evaluation and the necessity of taking an emergent head CT scan to rule out intracranial bleeding or mass lesion. This is a small price to pay if the victim has been rendered so irrational as to jeopardize survival.

Breathing

With the patient breathing, or now intubated and being ventilated with 100% oxygen, the thorax and neck should be examined and felt to detect abnormalities such as a deviated trachea, crepitation, flail chest, sucking chest wound, fractured sternum, and the absence of breath sounds on one or both sides of the chest. Possible interventions here include (1) insertion of a needle in the chest to relieve a tension pneumothorax; (2) application of an occlusive dressing to a sucking chest wound; (3) withdrawal of the endotracheal tube from the right mainstem bronchus; (4) reintubation of the trachea if no breath sounds are heard; and (5) insertion of large chest tubes (No. 38 French). If blood returns, the blood can be collected in an autotransfusion device. The volume of blood that returns should immediately be noted. If 1500 to 2000 mL of blood comes from the chest tube, thoracotomy may be indicated.

Circulation

Any exsanguinating external hemorrhage should have become apparent by now. Direct pressure should be used to control bleeding. Hemostats can cause injury to adjacent structures. If the bleeding site is on an extremity, a blood pressure cuff can be inflated to a pressure greater than the patient's systolic pressure.

By this time, assistants should have cut off the clothing from the patient's chest and reported the presence or absence of a pulse. Pneumatic trousers should not be deflated until the circulating volume has been sufficiently restored to raise the systemic blood pressure to normal or near normal levels. Two large-bore IV lines should have been established, and blood should have been obtained for the laboratory studies already ordered. If arm veins are not available, a large-bore central line should be inserted. Alternatively, there should be a cut down of the saphenous vein at the ankle and a large cannula inserted. Crystalloid should be infused as rapidly as possible, using manual or pneumatic pressure on the IV bags. If there is no palpable pulse on admission, or no marked improvement after the very rapid infusion of 2 L of crystalloid, O-negative blood should be administered. All team members should be alert to the dangers of iatrogenic air embolism associated with pressure infusion. A blood and fluid warmer should be in use.

The team captain should now listen for heart sounds, observe for neck vein distension, and assess cardiac rhythm on the cardiac monitor. If the clinical findings suggest cardiac tamponade (Beck's triad—low blood pressure, elevated venous pressure, and muffled heart sounds), and if tension pneumothorax has been excluded and the patient is in shock and unresponsive to rapid volume infusion, a pericardiocentesis should be attempted. If pericardiocentesis fails, a left thoracotomy should be performed to directly decompress the pericardial sac. Echocardiography, using a subcostal window, is replacing diagnostic pericardiocentesis in many emergency departments. It is noninvasive, rapid, and accurate.

Disability

An abbreviated neurological evaluation should now be performed, including level of consciousness, pupil size and reactivity, and motor function. The Glasgow Coma Scale (Table 169-3) should be used to quantify the patient's level of consciousness: possible scores range from 3 (no response) to 15 (high response on all measures).

Continuing Resuscitation

At this stage of the primary survey, the blood pressure, pulse pressure, pulse rate, and rectal temperature should be recorded. A narrow pulse pressure is common to both cardiac tamponade and hypovolemia. Ventilation should continue with 100% oxygen. If large volumes are

Table 169-3. The Glasgow Coma Scale Measure of Level of Consciousness

Measure	Response	Score
Eye opening	Opens:	
	Spontaneously	4
	To verbal command	3
	To pain	2
	No response	1
Verbal	Oriented and converses	5
	Disoriented and converses	4
	Inappropriate words	3
	Incomprehensible sounds	2
	No response	1
Motor	Obeys verbal command	6
	To painful stimulus:	
	Localizes pain	5
	Flexion-withdrawal	4
	Abnormal flexion (decorticate rigidity)	3
	Extension (decerebrate rigidity)	2
	No response	1

being infused, trends in central venous pressure should be followed. However, the central venous pressure is sometimes elevated in conditions such as tension pneumothorax and hemothorax, even in the presence of hypovolemia. For very rapid fluid infusion, the guidewire technique can be used to replace a peripheral IV with a No. 8 or 9 French sheath. If there is little or no response to the rapid infusion of 2 L of crystalloid, type O blood should be given if type-specific or fully crossmatched blood is not yet available. Documentation of resuscitative events should be entered on a flow sheet, listing the volumes and type of fluid given, blood pressure and pulse rate, CVP, urine output, gastric suction volume, and neurological status.

Secondary Survey

While resuscitation continues, the team captain should proceed with the secondary survey. The secondary survey is a rapid but thorough physical examination for the purpose of identifying as many injuries as possible. With this information, the resuscitating physician and his or her surgical colleague can set logical priorities for evaluation and management. Frequent assessments of the patient's blood pressure, pulse rate, and central venous pressure should continue.

The examination is conducted in a head-to-toe fashion, beginning with the scalp. Scalp lacerations can bleed profusely. This bleeding can be controlled with plastic Raney clips that grasp the full thickness of the scalp and galea. The tympanic membranes should be visualized to detect hemotympanum, and the pupil examination should be repeated. If epistaxis is a problem, a Foley catheter or a nasal balloon should be inserted to provide posterior tamponade. The examination continues over the neck and thorax. A lateral cervical spine x-ray (if not already obtained), a chest x-ray, and an anteroposterior pelvic x-ray should be obtained while the secondary survey continues. A No. 32 French gastric tube should be inserted into the stomach and connected to suction. When there is facial trauma or basilar skull fracture, the gastric tube should be inserted through the mouth rather than the nose. The clothing at the crotch of the pneumatic antishock trousers is cut away, and the urinary meatus, scrotum, and perineum are inspected for the presence of blood, hematoma, or laceration.

A rectal examination is done, noting sphincter function and whether the prostate is boggy or displaced. Rectal blood indicates rectal laceration. If the prostate is normal and there is no blood at the urethral meatus, a Foley catheter can be placed in the bladder. If a urethral injury is suspected (meatal blood present), a urethrogram (described in Chapter 177) should be obtained prior to passing the catheter. If the prostate is displaced it should be assumed that the urethra is disrupted. Catheterization should not be attempted if the urethra is injured. The urine should be examined for blood. If the patient is a woman of childbearing age, a pregnancy test should be obtained. A bimanual vaginal examination should be performed. If blood is present, a speculum examination will be necessary to identify a possible vaginal laceration in the presence of a pelvic fracture. Palpate all peripheral pulses. The patient should be log-rolled to either side while keeping the neck immobilized, so that every inch of the patient's body is seen and felt. The extremities should be evaluated for fracture and soft tissue injury. Peripheral pulses should be felt. A more thorough neurological examination can now be done, carefully checking motor and sensory function.

If the blood pressure rises and stabilizes with volume replacement, the pneumatic antishock trousers can be sequentially deflated. Start with the abdominal compartment, and then proceed one leg at a time while monitoring the blood pressure. If the pressure falls, the suit should be reinflated.

The three trauma series x-rays—cervical spine, chest, and pelvis—should be carefully read. Every anatomic structure should be checked. Flank stripes (radiopaque lines separating the wall of the colon from the properitoneal fat lines on either flank) signify free fluid in the peritoneal cavity. Diaphragmatic ruptures may be difficult to discern, but if the gastric tube is seen in the left chest, the diagnosis is obvious. If a pelvic fracture is present, a cystogram is useful for outlining the extent of the retroperitoneal hematoma present and for demonstrating an intraperitoneal bladder rupture. The cystogram should be obtained early because it may obviate the need for a diagnostic peritoneal lavage.

If the patient's blood pressure has not responded or stabilized with crystalloid or blood by the end of the secondary survey (which should take only about 10 min in most cases), transfer of the patient to the operating room for abdominal or thoracic exploration should be considered. Ideally, the trauma surgeon will be present during the secondary survey to observe the patient's progress.

On occasion, it will be necessary to perform emergency department thoracotomy to allow tamponade of the aorta at the diaphragm or aortic cross clamping. One indication for thoracotomy—cardiac tamponade—has already been described. Other indications are (1) persistent profound shock despite ventilation and rapid volume and blood infusion and (2) cardiac arrest.

PATIENT DISPOSITION FROM THE EMERGENCY DEPARTMENT

Options include moving the patient to the operating room, admission to the hospital, or transfer to another facility. The primary and secondary survey must have been completed and a gastric tube and a Foley catheter should be in place unless a urethral injury was detected. In most urban hospitals, the trauma surgeon should have been present for the secondary survey and he or she should assume direction of the diagnostic workup and disposition of the case at that time. In rural hospitals that transfer severe trauma cases, the resuscitating physician should relate all of the physical findings discovered during the primary and secondary surveys to the surgeon receiving the patient. Laboratory results, x-rays, and the flow sheet showing blood pressure, pulse, fluids infused, urine output, gastric output, and neurological findings should accompany the patient. If a diagnostic peritoneal lavage was performed, a sample of the lavage fluid should accompany the patient. A patient who is being transported to another facility should be accompanied by personnel capable of administering fluids and monitoring vital signs and pupillary changes. Mannitol should be available if there is neurological deterioration on route.

Pneumatic antishock trousers, as they are commonly used in the field, are inflated to a pressure of about 100 torr. When a patient is left in the trousers for a period of more than 2 to 3 h, the pressure should be reduced to about 20 torr to avoid skin necrosis and compartment syndromes. At this reduced pressure the pneumatic trousers garment is still an effective splint and will tamponade venous and small arterial bleeding. Splinting of long bone fractures and especially pelvic fractures helps prevent continuing blood loss.

FOUNDATIONS OF TRAUMA RESUSCITATION

Time. The primary enemy of the resuscitating physician is elapsing time. The injured patient may harbor continuing hemorrhage or other sources of shock that will kill if not quickly identified and managed. *The most skilled resuscitators make good use of every second of time starting from the moment of notification.* A definite and practiced routine such as outlined here is essential to enable decisive, timesaving leadership.

Go back to the beginning. If, during the course of the resuscitation, the patient reverses course and deteriorates, the resuscitation team must go back to the beginning and repeat the ABCs.

Be thorough. Attention to detail by all team members is critical. Do not compromise patient safety by skipping steps. A central venous line for CVP measurement is essential when large fluid volumes are administered. Do not allow dramatic wounds, such as a limb amputation, to distract you from your systematic search for lethal injuries.

Be skilled. Surgical and nonsurgical airway management, chest tube insertion, venous cannulation and cutdowns, Foley catheter insertion, central venous catheter insertion, and gastric intubation are the basic skills required of resuscitating physicians. The ability to perform emergency thoracotomy, diagnostic peritoneal lavage, and arterial cutdown are also desirable skills.

Be a team player. It is essential that resuscitating physicians and their surgical colleagues work well and closely together. Small minds dwell on who's in charge. The fact that 70 percent of fatal trauma occurs in rural America where trauma surgeons and fully trained emergency physicians are in short supply makes it essential that all physicians who cover emergency departments be well versed in the basics of resuscitation.

Be suspicious. If the mechanism of injury suggests aortic rupture, proceed accordingly. A bent steering wheel or a known high-speed impact should result in referral from a hospital without vascular surgery capabilities to a trauma center. Seat belts, while life-saving, can result in occult abdominal injuries such as "bucket handle" bowel devascularization. An inocuous looking laceration may, in fact, be a bullet or knife wound.

In conclusion, the ABC system of managing the resuscitation of severely injured patients during the first few minutes to 1 hour of arrival offers a proven method of handling the initial approach to the trauma patient. The flow of the process identifies rapidly lethal injuries first and takes steps to reverse them as they are discovered. The process is also painstakingly thorough in order to allow good priority setting. It also saves time by providing a framework for action.

BIBLIOGRAPHY

Asbun HJ, Irani H, Roe EJ, et al: Intra-abdominal seatbelt injury. *J Trauma* 30:189, 1990.

Baker SP, ONeill B, Karpf RS: *The Injury Fact Book.* Lexington, Mass., Lexington Books, 1984.

Committee on Trauma Research: *Injury in America.* Washington, D.C,, National Academy Press, 1985.

Committee on Trauma, American College of Surgeons: *Advanced Trauma Life Support Instructor Manual.* Chicago, American College of Surgeons, 1989.

Niemi TA, Norton LW: Vaginal injuries in patients with pelvic fractures. *J Trauma* 25:547, 1985.

Orsay EM, Dunne M, Turnbull TL, et al: Prospective study of the effect of safety belts in motor vehicle crashes. *Ann Emerg Med* 19:258, 1990.

170
PEDIATRIC TRAUMA
Gary C. Fifield

There is an emotional response to the injured child which separates it from other emergency management problems. Although the priorities of assessment and management are identical in children and adults, there are specific differences in management which result in differences in refinements of care. The objective of this chapter is to point out these differences and to discuss how assessment and management are influenced by them.

In 1988, according to the National Safety Council, 3900 children under 4 years of age, 4400 from 5 to 14 years, and 18,300 from 15 to 19 years died from injuries of all kinds. Motor vehicle–associated accidents are the most frequent cause of death, accounting for 69 percent of the total. Injuries account for 17 percent of hospitalizations and 20 percent of emergency visits in children, as compared to only 8 percent of admissions for those over 20 years of age. It is estimated that 20 percent of all children require at least one emergency room visit because of injury. In 1988, the incidence of injuries resulting in some limitation of activity was 3800 per 10,000 persons under 20 years of age.

Emergency medical personnel are in a unique position to identify and monitor situations, activities, and products which result in an unacceptable risk to children, and should become familiar with the recent literature on injury prevention and become involved in efforts to promote it.

EMERGENCY DEPARTMENT MANAGEMENT

Airway and ventilatory management of the injured child should take into account the unique features of respiratory structure and function in the young. Of course, the airways and the nasopharynx are smaller. Because the work of breathing is related primarily to the radius of the airway, the work of breathing in a child is relatively high. Anything which results in further narrowing or obstruction will compound hypoventilation. Other factors which affect airway management include the relatively large tongue, increased lymphoid tissue, the high position of the glottis in the neck, the shape of the epiglottis, and the anterior and inferior angulation of the vocal cords.

Characteristics of the thorax are important. The chest wall is more compliant. Direct trauma to the ribs may not result in fractures, although underlying structures may be injured. The ribs are oriented in a more horizontal manner. Downward excursion of the diaphragm is limited by the manner of its insertion. These characteristics limit the capacity of the child for respiratory compensation. In addition, the oxygen consumption of the child is relatively higher; thus hypoxia will occur sooner than in the adult. Oxygen by mask should be applied to any child with significant trauma, altered level of conciousness, or respiratory distress.

The traumatized child who requires ventilatory support should receive ventilation with a bag-and-mask apparatus attached to a flow of 100% oxygen. The method of delivery of 100% oxygen will depend on the type of system used. Mask ventilation can usually provide adequate ventilation until more definitive airway management can be accomplished by endotracheal intubation or another method. Details of pediatric intubation are discussed in Chapter 14E, "Pediatric Cardiopulmonary Resuscitation."

For intubation in an awake head-injured child, many authors recommend the use of a rapid-sequence technique which reduces the chance of increased intracranial pressure in response to the procedure. One such procedure, suggested by Mayer, is outlined in Table 170-1. In settings where the physician chooses not to utilize paralytic agents or rapid-acting barbiturates, the use of an intravenous bolus of lidocaine, 1 mg/kg, has been advocated as effective in blunting the rise in intracranial pressure produced by intubation.

When it is judged that airway control is rapidly needed and orotracheal intubation is not possible, transtracheal catheter ventilation (TTCV) may be the best available technique. Experience in our laboratory has persuaded us that the safest procedure in small children is to make a vertical skin incision over the cricothyroid membrane which allows easier localization of the membrane. The catheter can then be placed using the Seldinger technique as follows:

1. A needle with syringe attached is inserted at an angle of about 60° caudad until air is aspirated.
2. The syringe is removed and a flexible guidewire is inserted. The needle is removed.
3. An 18- or 20-gauge end-hole catheter designed for insertion over a wire is threaded into the airway. The wire is withdrawn and the syringe attached to the catheter and aspirated to assure that air is obtained.
4. At this point ventilation can begin with 100% oxygen from the wall and an in-line pressure reducing valve. Wall oxygen is usually about 50 psi pressure. The reducing valve should be set at the lowest effective ventilating pressure.

Such a system can be used to ventilate until endotracheal intubation can be accomplished. The risk of barotrauma increases with time, so TTCV should not be unduly prolonged. If the cricothyroid membrane cannot be located or accessed because of head and neck position, the catheter could be placed with care through the tracheal rings below the cricoid cartilage. If a larger catheter (16 gauge or larger) is placed, it may be possible to ventilate with a bag or oxygen-powered manually triggered device by placing a 15-mm endotracheal tube adapter with a 3.0-mm connecter on the catheter hub. Great care must be exercised in the decision to use this potentially hazardous technique. Orotracheal intubation with head and neck immobilization is the procedure of choice in all but the most desperate situations.

Cricothyrotomy has generally been discouraged in infants and young children because of the danger of a major surgical error in an emergency situation. The technique of cricothyrotomy in elective circumstances has been described in infants without major complications.

Assessment of the circulatory status of the injured child is dependent on observations of the status of the peripheral circulation as well as major organ systems. Skin temperature, capillary refill time, and the quality of the peripheral pulses are the best guides to peripheral perfusion. Prolonged capillary refill (greater than 5 s) over the trunk or forehead indicates shock, requiring rapid volume replacement. The quality of pulses should be assessed beginning distally and proceeding more proximally.

Urine output is the best monitor of renal perfusion, but is difficult to assess early in the care of the injured child. Vital signs must be interpreted in light of the age and the emotional state of the child. The most useful vital sign change is often persistent tachycardia. Tachycardia due to fear may fluctuate while that due to hypovolemia will

Table 170-1. Procedure for Anesthetic Induction for Crash Intubation

100% oxygen by mask for 3 min
Small dose nondepolarizing relaxant (pancuronium 0.01 mg/kg)
Atropine 0.02 mg/kg
Thiopental 1–4 mg/kg or ketamine 1–2 mg/kg
Sellick maneuver
Orotracheal intubation

Source: Mayer T (ed): *Emergency Management of Pediatric Trauma.* Philadelphia, Saunders, 1985, p 73. Used by permission.

respond only to appropriate treatment. Demonstrable hypotension is clear evidence of shock in a late stage and demands very rapid intervention. Normal vital signs for children are discussed in Chap. 14D.

Vascular access in the traumatized child is discussed in Chap. 14C. In situations where shock is profound, multiple access sites should be established with large-bore catheters. In such a circumstance placement of a No. 4 to 5 French introducer catheter in a femoral vessel is an excellent means for administration of large fluid volumes in a short time. In most situations of multiple trauma in children where shock is mild or not present, the secure placement of two 20-gauge catheters in peripheral veins will allow for adequate fluid administration and provide a margin of safety if evidence of further blood loss develops. The superior vena cava may be approached in critical situations via the subclavian vein, which is accessible by supra- or infraclavicular technique. These techniques require significant experience when used in children. Although most investigators have stated that peripheral veins allow the most rapid volume infusion, data from small animal models simulating the pediatric patient indicate that larger central veins may, in fact, be superior. Intraosseous infusion can be used to deliver rapid fluid infusions by using pressure infusion devices or by administering a bolus with a syringe attached to a three-way stopcock. Details of intraosseus infusion are described in Chap. 6.

The initial fluid choice in trauma should be isotonic crystalloid, either lactated Ringer's solution or normal saline. When clinical shock is present, a volume of 20 mL/kg of estimated weight should be infused as rapidly as possible. If signs of shock do not normalize, this volume should be repeated and packed red blood cells obtained for subsequent transfusion. If signs of shock persist, blood should be infused as rapidly as possible and response carefully monitored. The use of O negative or type-specific blood is appropriate when shock is present and when blood is needed before fully crossmatched blood is available.

Neurological status is assessed initially through an abbreviated neurological examination which consists of evaluation of pupillary reflexes, verbal response, eye opening, and motor activity. Evaluation of a child's level of consciousness may be difficult. Uncooperative or combative behavior could be explained by pain, fear, and anxiety or by effects of a head injury or shock. Optimally only one individual should speak to the child, ask questions, give simple commands, and provide reassurance in a calm voice. An experienced examiner can often differentiate the pathological from the situationally induced behaviors. When it is unclear, one should proceed as if the behavior were the result of the injury.

An examination should be done for evidence of cerebrospinal fluid leakage from the ears or nose or other evidence of open head injury. In addition, the vital signs should be assessed for signs consistent with increased intracranial pressure. Infants with an open anterior fontanelle have a readily accessible means of intracranial pressure assessment which should not be ignored.

A good method for quantifying the level of consciousness is the Glasgow Coma Scale (see Tables 169-3, 171-1). However, this form was not designed for pediatric patients and must be adapted for this age group. In infants a cry is considered a normal verbal response, and in older children the evaluation of verbal response is based on age-appropriate criteria.

Mild head injury, that which results in transient or no loss of consciousness, is very common. Children can respond with impressive manifestations of pallor, vomiting, breath holding, lethargy, and irritability. Such children may require admission and observation if the nature or course of the injury is unclear or if a skull fracture is present.

Management of the child with a serious head injury is influenced by the pathophysiology, which differs from that in adults. Space-occupying hematomas occur less frequently in children (approximately 25 to 30 percent versus 40 to 50 percent in adults). On CT scan, evidence of shearing forces upon the brain tissue associated with high-speed injury are more often seen in children than adults.

In children, diffuse brain swelling often occurs following serious head injury. This appears to be associated with increased blood flow. Intervention is designed to blunt this common response to direct brain injury. In addition, shock, hypoxia, and stimuli which may increase intracranial pressure and can result in a further brain injury after the initial trauma must be prevented or corrected.

The most effective method of decreasing intracranial pressure in this setting is hyperventilation. This will require endotracheal intubation in most situations. The goal should be a P_{CO_2} of 25 to 30 mmHg. The head should be positioned to prevent impairment of venous drainage from the brain. If systemic shock has been corrected, the head of the bed should be elevated 30°. Mannitol alone will initially increase cerebral blood flow, but if the child is deteriorating despite hyperventilation, mannitol, 1 g/kg intravenously, should be given rapidly. Diuretics such as furosemide, 1 mg/kg intravenously, have been shown to reduce brain edema without increasing blood flow.

The use of muscle paralyzers (e.g., pancuronium), intravenous anesthetic agents (barbiturates), and sedatives (e.g., diazepam) may be necessary to prevent movement and resultant elevation of the intracranial pressure.

Skull radiography is not as useful as the head CT scan but may have value in identifying patients with fractures over the middle meningeal artery, occipital fractures which extend to the foramen magnum, and fractures over major dural sinuses. Studies validating high yield criteria for skull radiography have been published. These include children under 2 years of age with head injury as moderate risk. The skull is vulnerable to fracture in this age group due to the thin calvarium and the high incidence of direct head trauma from falls, motor vehicles, child abuse, and other mechanisms. Leptomeningeal cysts, or "growing skull fractures," occur in children under 3 years of age.

Although cervical cord injury occurs in only 3 to 5 percent of major trauma victims in childhood, appropriate precautions to limit motion of the head and neck are mandatory. This can be a challenge due to size and children's inability to understand and cooperate with head and neck restraint. "Hard" cervical collars for most sizes are now available. In their absence manual restraint or foam blocks and tape can be utilized.

The assessment of injury to the cervical spine in children has several unique aspects. The developing spine has an appearance very different from that of older patients, and interpretation of radiographs must account for these differences. One of the most troublesome findings is that of the anterior placement of C2 relative to C3, giving the false appearance of traumatic subluxation. There is normal anterior wedging of the vertebral bodies. In infants the prevertebral soft tissues can vary with phases of respiration and produce findings indistinguishable from those of hematoma. Cervical cord injury is less common in younger age groups. When it does occur, it is more often to the high cervical cord. Cervical cord injuries at any level may present with signs and symptoms of cord involvement but no fracture on x-ray.

In children, chest wall compliance allows compression of the chest with underlying visceral injury without fracture of the bony thorax. In addition, the mediastinum is felt to be more mobile in children, and tension pneumothorax produces more shift and may compromise respiratory and cardiovascular function to a greater extent. If thoracic injury produces respiratory dysfunction, hypoxia may supervene more rapidly in children because of their relatively higher metabolic rate and oxygen consumption. The advent of ulse oximetry has provided a noninvasive and cost-effective means to monitor oxygenation and is recommended for any unstable or seriously injured child.

Aerophagia causing gastric distension and a tense, distended abdomen is common, and can result in vomiting withh aspiration. Early placement of a gastric tube through the nose or mouth is important to alleviate these difficulties. The tube should be as large as possible so that it does not become obstructed with partially digested food or other material.

The most commonly injured intraabdominal organs are the liver and the spleen. The retroperitoneal kidneys are also commonly injured.

Nonoperative management of hepatic and splenic injuries is appropriate in the child who (1) has surgical consultation immediately available, (2) can be stabilized with fluids or blood transfusions (less than one-third to one-half of the blood volume transfused), (3) has no evidence of hollow visceral injury, and (4) can be closely monitored in an intensive care setting geared to child trauma victims.

Recent experience has revealed a common pattern of injury associated with automobile lap belt use. The lap belt syndrome includes hollow visceral injury, mesenteric avulsion, lumbar vertebral injury, and abdominal wall contusions. The emergence of this injury pattern is not taken as evidence against the use of lap belts, since they prevent much more serious head injury. Shoulder harness restraints will reduce the occurrence of this new injury pattern.

In addition to physical examination, the noninvasive investigative techniques available include computed tomography, scintigraphy, and sonography. Computed tomography with intravenous and intragastric contrast is the most commonly advocated modality. It is the most accurate of the three techniques. This approach has modified the use of diagnostic peritoneal lavage (DPL) in children. If laparotomy is not anticipated in a child, the finding of blood on DPL is probably not important information. An alternative approach is to perform a peritoneal lavage if indicated by the usual criteria—followed, if positive, by a noninvasive diagnostic study. If the source of hemorrhage is identified by this study, management decisions, including nonoperative management, are based on that information. If the source of bleeding is not identified or DPL indicates hollow visceral injury, operative intervention is indicated.

Pelvic fracture is a relatively common injury in children with serious trauma. A pelvic x-ray is mandatory whenever significant blunt injury has occurred. Management should follow the same principles as used for adults, including careful search for perineal injuries. The use of pediatric pneumatic trousers is an important adjunct to therapy of this injury when significant hemorrhage is suspected or likely.

BIBLIOGRAPHY

Eichelberger M, Randolph J: Pediatric trauma: An algorithm for diagnosis and therapy. *J Trauma* 23:91, 1983.

Guyer B, Gallagher S: An approach to the epidemiology of childhood injuries. *Pediatr Clin North Am* 32:5, 1985.

Kisoon N, Dreyer J, Walia M: Pediatric trauma: Differences in pathophysiology, injury patterns and treatment compared with adult trauma. *Can Med Assoc J* 142:27, 1990.

Krause J, Fife D, Cox P, et al: Incidence, severity, and external causes of pediatric brain injury. *Am J Dis Child* 140:687, 1986.

Mayer T (ed): *Emergency Management of Pediatric Trauma.* Philadelphia, Saunders, 1985.

Mayer T, Walker M, Clark P: Further experience with the modified abbreviated injury severity scale. *J Trauma* 24:31, 1984.

Mayer T, Walker M, Johnson D, et al: Causes of morbidity and mortality in severe pediatric trauma. *JAMA* 245:719, 1981.

Pang D, Wilberger J: Spinal cord injury without radiographic abnormalities in children. *J Neurosurg* 57:114, 1982.

Polley TZ, Coran A: Special problems in the management of pediatric trauma. *Crit Care Clin* 2:775, 1986.

Rachesky I, Boyce WT, Duncan B, et al: Clinical prediction of cervical spine injuries in children. *Am J Dis Child* 141:199, 1987.

Reichard S, Helikson M, Shorter N, et al: Pelvic fractures in children—review of 120 patients with a new look at general management. *J Pediatr Surg* 15:727, 1980.

Schiffman MA: Nonoperative management of blunt abdominal trauma in pediatrics. *Emerg Med Clin North Am* 7:519, 1989.

Stylianos S, Harris BH: Seatbelt use and patterns of central nervous system injury in children. *Ped Emerg Care* 6:4, 1990.

Ward JD: Pediatric head injury: Special considerations, in Becker DP, Gudeman SK (eds): *Textbook of Head Injury.* Philadelphia, Saunders, 1989, pp 319–325.

171 HEAD INJURY

Gaylan L. Rockswold

The leading cause of death in persons up to age 44 years in the United States is trauma, and head injury accounts for approximately half of the deaths related to trauma. The mortality rate from severe head injury is approximately 40 percent, and functional recovery occurs in only 40 to 50 percent of patients with severe head injury.

ANATOMY AND PHYSIOLOGY

Scalp

The scalp consists of five layers: (1) skin, (2) subcutaneous tissue, (3) galea, (4) areolar tissue, and (5) pericranium. The scalp has a very rich blood supply and can be the source of major blood loss. In addition, there is a loose attachment between the galea and the pericranium, allowing for large subgaleal hematomas.

Skull

The skull is a bony container for the brain and provides considerable protection. For practical purposes it is rigid and inflexible, thus contributing to problems with increased intracranial pressure (ICP). Cerebral contusion and contrecoup injuries frequently occur against uneven surfaces of the skull such as the orbital roofs, the sphenoid wing, and the petrous apex.

Brain

The intracranial volume is approximately 1900 mL in the average adult. The brain weighs 1300 to 1500 g and occupies approximately 80 percent of the volume of the intracranial cavity. The brain is partially compartmentalized by attachments of the dura. In the midline, the falx cerebri partially divides the right hemisphere from the left hemisphere of the brain. The tentorium cerebelli partially divides the supratentorial cerebral hemispheres from the brainstem and cerebellum. The cerebral hemispheres are connected to the posterior fossa contents by the midbrain, which occupies the tentorial hiatus. The brain consists of gray and white matter, with the latter consisting primarily of axons and myelin sheaths. Deep in the white matter are nuclei of gray matter. The gray matter also forms the surface of the brain. It consists of nerve cells, and the connecting dendrites and axons of these cells form myriad synapses. The extracellular space is considerably smaller in gray matter than in white matter. The arteries and veins run vertically through the gray and white matter, giving off capillaries at right angles.

Cerebral Blood Flow

Under normal circumstances the blood volume of the brain is approximately 3 to 4 mL/100 g of brain tissue. In the average patient, the average cerebral blood flow (CBF) to the whole brain is about 50 mL/100 g per min, with approximately 75 mL/100 g per min going to the gray matter and 25 mL/100 g per min going to the white matter. Although the brain constitutes only 2 percent of the total body weight, it receives approximately 15 percent of cardiac output and about 20 percent of the oxygen consumed by the body. Variations in arterial P_{CO_3} exert a profound effect on CBF. Hypercapnia causes cerebral vasodilatation, and hypocapnia causes vasoconstriction that can be so marked that brain hypoxia can result. Changes in oxygen tension in arerial blood also influence CBF. As the P_{CO_3} falls below 50 mmHg, there is a marked increase in CBF while hyperbaric oxygen ventilation at 2 atmospheres absolute decreases CBF by 20 to 25 percent.

The brain is unique in the sense that it is autonomous in controlling blood flow within it. This intrinsic property has been labeled *autoregulation,* defined as the tendency of the brain to maintain a constant blood flow despite perfusion changes. Cerebral perfusion pressure (CPP) is defined as the difference between mean systemic arterial blood pressure (SAP) and mean intracranial pressure (ICP) (CPP = SAP − ICP). If autoregulation is intact, CBF remains constant when the CPP ranges between 45 and 160 mmHg. When it falls below 40 mmHg, CBF and cerebral metabolism are critically affected.

Cerebrospinal Fluid

Of the approximate 1900-mL volume of the intracranial cavity, 150 mL is cerebrospinal fluid (CSF), of which 25 to 30 mL is found in the ventricles. The ventricles are ependymal lined cavities deep within the brain. Cerebrospinal fluid is formed primarily by the choroid plexuses within the ventricular system at a rate of 0.35 mL/min or 500 mL/24 h. Cerebrospinal fluid moves from the lateral ventricles through the foramen of Monro into the third ventricle and then via the aqueduct of Sylvius into the fourth ventricle and out through the formina of Luschka and Magendi. Cerebrospinal fluid then flows through the basal cistern and is absorbed in the arachnoid villi along the sagittal sinus and the lateral sinuses. The CSF cushions and buffers the brain and spinal cord against trauma. It also provides a fluid pathway for chemical substances to reach the intercellular spaces of the brain and for metabolites to be returned to the venous system.

PATHOLOGY AND PATHOPHYSIOLOGY

The concept of primary and secondary brain injury due to trauma has become well established. An initial impact injury to the brain produces varying degrees of mechanical neuronal and axonal injury which, at the present state of medical science, cannot be treated. Secondary brain injury occurs from potentially treatable factors such as intracranial hemorrhage, cerebral edema, ischemia, hypoxia, hypercarbia, and increased ICP. Optimal management minimizes the secondary brain injury and decreases the overall mortality and morbidity.

Intracranial Pressure

The craniospinal intradural space is nearly constant in volume, and its contents are relatively noncompressible. Therefore, the sum of the volumes of brain, blood, and CSF remains relatively constant. If there is an increase in volume of one of these three components, it must be offset by an equal decrease in some other component or ICP rises. If the brain were completely incompressible and the cranium unexpandable, the addition of even minimal volume to the intracranial space would lead to dramatic increase in ICP (Fig. 171-1). Initially, as a mass lesion or diffuse edema develops, CSF buffering occurs by the displacement of CSF into the spinal canal. Once CSF buffering becomes exhausted, the elastic properties of the brain tissue itself and its blood vessels play the major buffering role as the pressure begins to elevate rapidly (Fig. 171-1). *Elastance* is the increase in pressure with a given increase in intracranial volume. *Compliance* is the reciprocal of elastance. The elastic properties of the brain are not constant but will depend on the presence of pathological processes such as cerebral edema or a mass lesion. For example, an increase in the arterial pressure stiffens the brain, producing a decreased compliance, whereas a decrease in arterial pressure will have the reverse effect. The pressure-volume curve explains why a patient can appear relatively intact neurologically and then undergo rapid deterioration because of transtentorial herniation.

Increased ICP is defined as CSF pressure greater than 15 mmHg. Following removal of a traumatic intracranial hematoma at least half of comatose patients display an elevated ICP. Approximately a third of patients with diffuse brain injury have elevated ICP. Uncontrollably elevated ICP (defined as an ICP of 20 mmHg or more refractory to

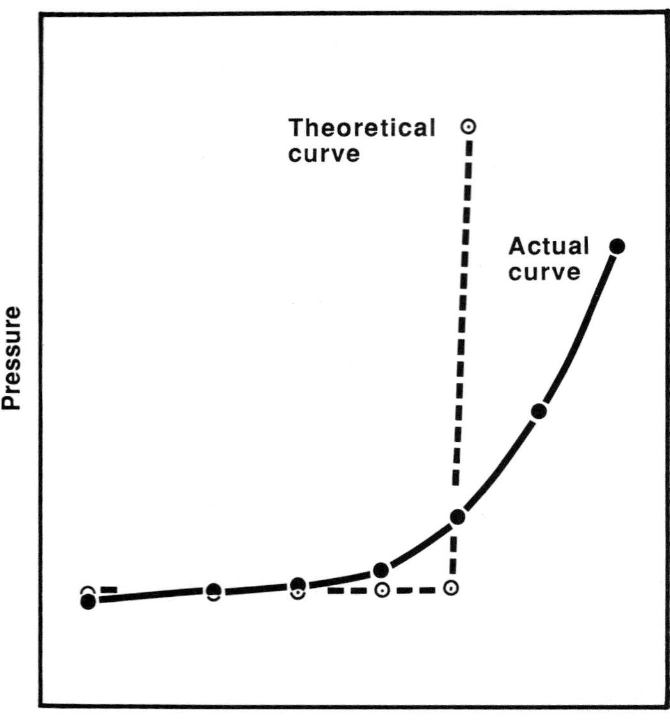

Fig. 171-1. Theoretical pressure-volume curve (broken line) derived if the modified Monro-Kellie hypothesis were strictly true. Acutal pressure-volume curve (solid line).

treatment) is present in over half of all head-injury deaths. If ICP repeatedly elevates to the point where CPP is inadequate, vasoparalysis results, whereupon CBF passively follows systemic arterial pressure. Massive vasodilatation occurs with further elevations in ICP. Autoregulation can be lost in one area and preserved in another. For example, CBF may be markedly lowered in an area of contusion and edema while global ICP and CPP remain relatively normal. Loss of autoregulation leads to the failure of the resistant vessels to constrict normally, and systemic pressure is communicated to the capillaries and veins, resulting in the outpouring of fluid from the intravascular space to the extracellular space (vasogenic edema). The production of lactic acid by anaerobic metabolism may play a role in the loss of CBF autoregulation. The ICP eventually rises to the level of SAP and there is no CPP. Brain death results.

Herniation

Diffusely or focally increased ICP can result in herniation of the brain at several locations. The least important herniation is cingulate or subfalcial, occurring when one cerebral hemisphere is displaced underneath the falx cerebri into the opposite supratentorial space. This is rarely clinically diagnosed. A herniation of major clinical importance in head injury is transtentorial or uncal herniation (Fig. 171-2). A subdural hematoma or temporal lobe mass forces the ipsilateral uncus of the temporal lobe through the tentorial hiatus into the space between the cerebral penduncle and the tentorium. This results in compression of the oculomotor nerve and parasympathetic paralysis of the pupil on the same side, causing it to become fixed and dilated. The cerebral peduncle is simultaneously compressed, resulting in a contralateral hemiparesis. The increased ICP and brainstem compression result in progressive deterioration in the level of consciousness. Occasionally the contralateral cerebral peduncle is forced against the free edge of the tentorium on the opposite side, resulting in paralysis ipsilateral to the lesion—a false localizing sign. The posterior cerebral artery can be compressed against the free edge of the tentorium, resulting in an infarction of the occipital lobe. If the herniation continues untreated, there is progressive brainstem deterioration progressing to hyperventilation and decerebration (extensor response) and then to apnea and death. Uncal herniation can occur bilaterally in cases of diffuse brain swelling or bilateral lesions. Cerebellar tonsillar herniation through the foramen magnum occurs much less frequently in head trauma. Resultant medullary compression causes bradycardia, respiratory arrest, and death.

Diffuse Lesions

Closed-head injuries (CHI) can be divided into diffuse and focal lesions. Diffuse injuries are divided into concussion syndromes and prolonged traumatic coma. Concussion is a transient loss of consciousness that occurs immediately following a nonpenetrating blunt impact to the head. Concussion generally occurs when the head, while moving, strikes or is struck by an object. The duration of unconsciousness is usually short (from seconds to minutes), although it may last for several hours. Loss of consciousness is due to impairment of the reticular activating system, caused by rotation of the cerebral hemispheres on the brainstem. Classically, recovery from concussion was regarded as complete, without pathological lesions of the brain or neurological sequelae. However, persistent headache and problems with memory, anxiety, insomnia, and dizziness can persist in some patients for weeks and sometimes months.

Diffuse axonal injury is a tearing or shearing of nerve fibers occurring at the time of impact. The site and degree of axonal injury are determined by the direction, magnitude and duration of the angular force applied to the head. It results in functional, or physiologic, rather than grossly demonstrable, anatomic abnormalities.

Although diffuse axonal injury has frequently been associated with the severely head injured, it has been demonstrated in patients with mild head injury and can occur either diffusely or focally. Prolonged traumatic coma lasting for at least 6 h appears to result from diffuse axonal injury produced by the accelerating and decelerating forces of the impact. Prolonged coma is present in about one-third of all patients who die from head injury and is associated with poor neurological outcome in survivors.

Focal Lesions

Skull Fractures

Linear nondepressed fractures with the scalp intact do not of themselves require treatment. Severe intracranial bleeding can result if the fracture also causes disruption of the middle meningeal artery or a major dural sinus. Depressed skull fractures are classified as open or closed, if the overlying skin is lacerated or intact respectively.

Basilar skull fractures can occur at any point in the base of the skull, but the typical location is in the petrous portion of the temporal bone. Longitudinal fractures occur much more frequently than do transverse fractures and typically begin with a fracture in the vault extending into the petrous bone. Hemotympanum, otorrhea, disarticulation of the ossicles, and ecchymosis in the mastoid region (Battle's sign) are frequently seen. Transverse fractures of the petrous bone are associated with severe head injury and are secondary to blows to the occiput. Seventh- or eighth-nerve transection can occur.

Contusion

Contusion typically occurs over the crest of gyri, largest at the surface and tapering into the white matter (Fig. 171-3). The area of contusion is usually hemorrhagic and surrounded by edema, with overlying subarachnoid hemorrhage frequently present. Contusions may occur directly under the site of impact or on the contralateral side (a contre-

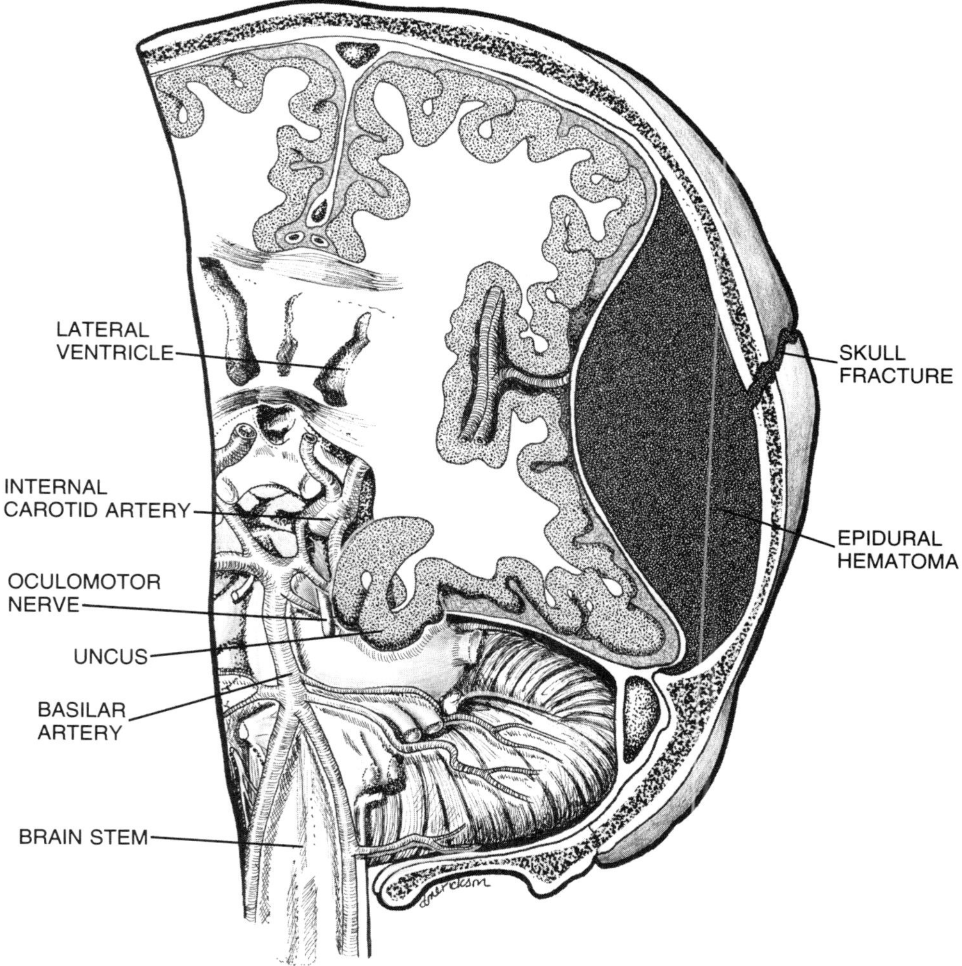

Fig. 171-2. Anterior view of transtentorial uncal herniation caused by a large epidural hematoma. Note skull fracture overlying the hematoma.

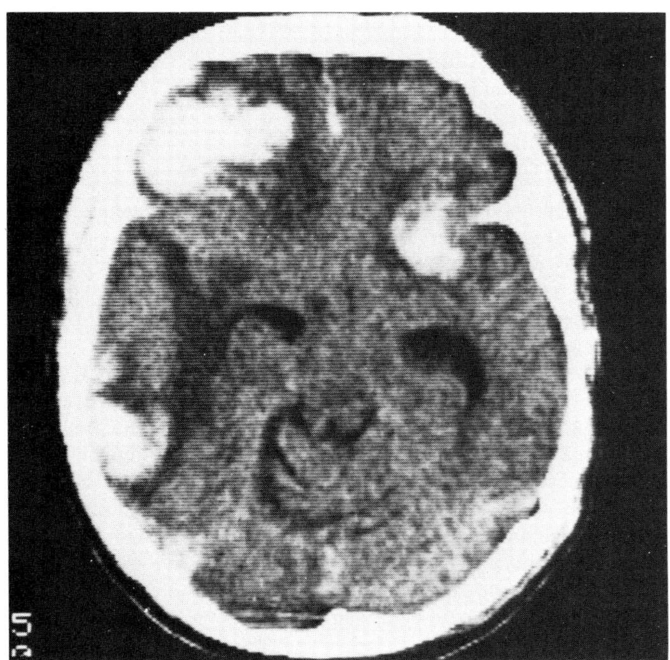

Fig. 171-3. Cerebral contusion with associated hemorrhage occurring subfrontally on the left, superior to the right sphenoid wing, and in the left posterior temporal region. Note the soft tissue swelling in the left frontotemporal region.

coup lesion). Contusions may occur anywhere, but typical locations are the frontal poles, the subfrontal cortex, and the anterior temporal lobes. Movement of the cortical gyri over rough skull surfaces such as the orbital plates or the sphenoid ridge are conducive to contusion.

Intracerebral Hemorrhage

Torn blood vessels can cause parenchymal hemorrhage (Fig. 171-3). Most hemorrhages are delayed for days and only occasionally are seen on the initial computed tomography (CT) scan taken within a few hours of injury. Combined contusion and parenchymal hemorrhage can produce an expanding mass lesion which is particularly treacherous when present in the anterior temporal lobe, since uncal herniation can occur without a diffuse increase in ICP.

Epidural Hematoma

An epidural hematoma is a collection of blood between the inner table of the skull and the dura (Fig. 171-4). Approximately 80 percent of the time, an epidural hematoma is associated with a skull fracture which tears a meningeal artery, usually the middle meningeal. Fracture through a large venous lake or through a major dural sinus can also produce an epidural hematoma. The underlying brain injury is seldom severe. Epidural hematomas are rare in the elderly, presumably because of the very close attachment of the dura to the periosteum of the inner table.

Subdural Hematoma

A subdural hematoma is a collection of blood beneath the dura and overlying the arachnoid and brain (Fig. 171-5). It is usually located

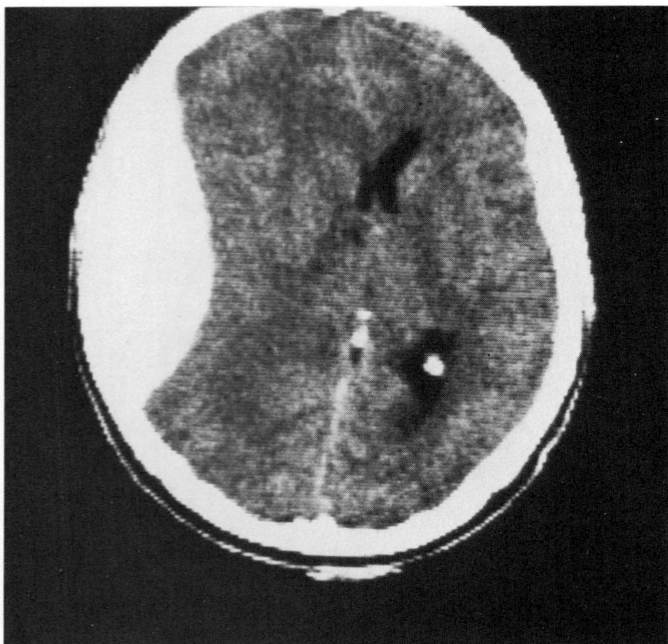

Fig. 171-4. A typical epidural hematoma with a lenticular-shaped configuration.

over the cerebral convexities and results from tears of bridging veins which extend from the subarachnoid space to the dural venous sinuses or from tears in pial arteries. Blood dissects over the cerebral convexities, frequently extending from the sagittal sinus to the floor of the temporal fossa or from the frontal region back to the parietal and occipital lobes. The mechanism of injury is usually acceleration-deceleration. Patients with brain atrophy either due to aging or alcoholism are particularly susceptible to the development of subdural hematomas because the bridging veins span a greater distance and are more easily torn. Acute subdural hematomas become symptomatic within 24 h of injury. These lesions are caused by acceleration-deceleration forces

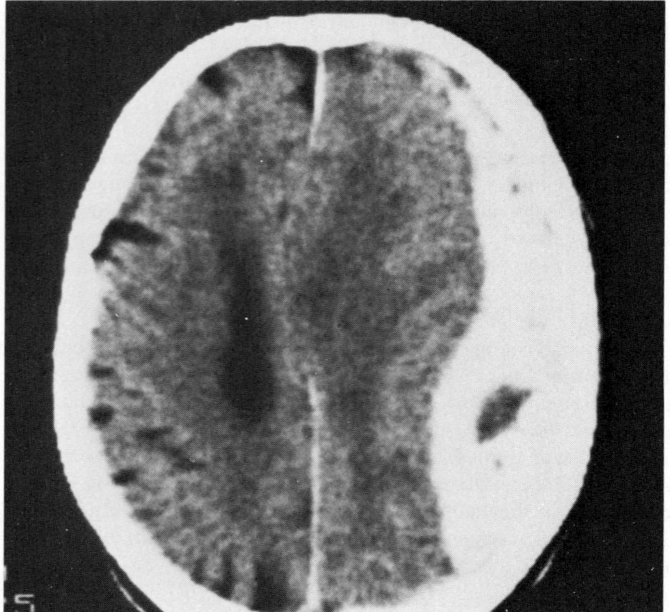

Fig. 171-5. A large acute subdural hematoma with marked midline shift and ipsilateral ventricular collapse.

that cause significant primary impact injury to the brain. Contusions of areas of the brain remote from the site of primary impact also occur. Subacute subdural hematomas become symptomatic from 24 h to approximately 2 weeks after injury. Chronic subdurals become symptomatic 2 weeks or more after injury when the blood clot has liquefied. Occasionally a specific history of trauma cannot be obtained and it is difficult to date the hematoma exactly in terms of the initial trauma. It is important to distinguish this more chronic lesion from the acute subdural hematoma because immediate surgery may not be necessary or advisable.

Brain Laceration

A tear in the brain parenchyma can be produced by a crude penetrating injury or depressed skull fracture. There is frequently associated hemorrhage and necrosis of the brain.

Penetrating Injuries

Penetrating sharp objects and gunshot wounds can result in penetrating injury to the brain. Gunshot wounds inflict injury far beyond their direct penetration of the brain because of the energy exerted as shown by the formula $E = \frac{1}{2}mV^2$ (where E is the energy of the missile, m is its mass, and V is the velocity). The degree of neurological injury will depend on the energy of the missile, whether the trajectory involves a single or multiple lobes or hemispheres of the brain, the amount of scatter of bone and metallic fragments, and whether a mass lesion is present. Hemorrhage can be profuse and life-threatening if a major artery or dural sinus is involved.

ASSESSMENT

History

Prehospital personnel must obtain a history from observers or family regarding the patient's condition immediately after the injury. This includes respiratory effort, duration of unconsciousness, verbalization, and movement of the extremities. In addition, the mechanism of injury, the time of the injury, the presence of a lucid interval, and prior use of drugs and alcohol should be noted. This information should be recorded on the ambulance data sheet and delivered with the patient to the emergency department. Ongoing observations by the prehospital personnel are essential.

Vital Signs

Adequate oxygenation and ventilation are essential to the head-injured patient, since hypoxia and hypercarbia can convert reversible brain injury to irreversible injury. Moderate hypercarbia can cause profound cerebral vasodilatation, resulting in an increased ICP with further ventilatory deterioration. A vicious cycle can ensue whereby the secondary brain injury becomes more profound than the initial primary impact injury.

An elevated systolic blood pressure can reflect a rise in ICP and be part of Cushing's reflex (hypertension and bradycardia). Hypertension is the brain's attempt to maintain CPP. Hypotension is rarely due to head injury except as a terminal event with medullary collapse. Important exceptions are (1) profound blood loss from scalp lacerations and (2) the infant or small child with a relatively small circulating blood volume in whom hemorrhage into the epidural or subgaleal spaces can produce hypovolemic shock. Hypotension in the severely head injured patient can greatly impair neurological function. Blood pressure must be restored before an accurate neurological assessment can be made.

Neurological Examination

The neurological examination is essential in establishing the severity of the head injury and its clinical course. Examination must be adequate to accomplish the goals described above but rapid enough not to delay emergency management of the patient. Repeated examinations are required to determine if the patient is stable, improving, or deteriorating. The level of consciousness is the single most important factor in neurologically assessing the head-injured patient. The Glasgow Coma Scale (GCS) (Table 171-1) as devised by Teasdale and Jennett is a system of examination which can be performed by all levels of medical personnel and is highly reproducible. The scale evaluates three aspects of the patient's responsiveness: (1) eye opening, (2) best verbal response, and (3) best motor response. Each category is described according to a well-defined series of responses that indicate progressive degrees of neurological impairment.

Eye Opening

Spontaneous eye opening suggests that the reticular activating centers are functioning. This does not imply awareness, however. If spontaneous eye opening is not present, verbal stimuli or commands should be used next. If there is no eye opening with verbal stimulation, painful stimulation, such as vigorous pinching or pressure on the nail beds, should be applied.

Verbal Response

Speech suggests a relatively intact central nervous system. Oriented speech implies awareness of oneself and one's environment. A patient should be orientated in all three spheres of name, place, and date. To be characterized as "disoriented and converses," speech should be well articulated and organized but the patient disoriented. Inappropriate words are those which are exclamatory or random only. Incomprehensible speech consists of moaning or groaning but no recognizable words.

Motor Responses

This is the most important and reproducible portion of the GCS. Obeying verbal commands means the ability to move one's limbs readily and without the need for painful stimulation. Localizing pain means that the patient moves a limb sequentially to the location of the painful stimulus in an effort to remove it. Flexion-withdrawal implies that the patient pulls in flexion away from a pain stimulus. Abnormal flexion means a decorticate response which is consistently apparent. An extensor response is decerebration, with abduction and internal rotation of the shoulder and pronation of the forearm. No response is hypotonia or flaccidity, which strongly suggests loss of medullary function. In a head-injured patient who exhibits flaccidity, concomitant spinal cord injury may be present.

Table 171-1. The Glasgow Coma Scale

EYES		
Open:	Spontaneously	4
	To verbal command	3
	To pain	2
No response:		1
BEST VERBAL RESPONSE		
	Oriented and converses	5
	Disoriented and converses	4
	Inappropriate words	3
	Incomprehensible sounds	2
	No response	1
BEST MOTOR RESPONSE		
To verbal command:	Obeys	6
To painful stimulus:	Localizes pain	5
	Flexion-withdrawal	4
	Abnormal flexion (decorticate rigidity)	3
	Extension (decerebrate rigidity)	2
	No response	1
Total		3–15

A maximum score of 15 can be obtained on the GCS, with a low score of 3. Severe head injury is defined as a GCS of 8 or less persisting for 6 h. Moderate head injury is defined as GCS of 9 to 12 and mild head injury, 13 to 15.

Pupil size in millimeters, and reactivity to light, should be carefully recorded. An enlarging pupil in the face of a decreasing level of consciousness is strongly suggestive of uncal herniation with associated oculomotor nerve compression.

Brainstem function can be further tested by checking corneal reflexes with a wisp of Kleenex or cotton. This reflex originates in the pons, with the afferent limb conducted by the ophthalmic branch of the fifth nerve and the efferent limb by the facial nerve. In addition, oculocephalic (doll's eyes) or oculovestibular responses (ice water calorics) are important in testing the integrity of the brainstem. Oculocephalic reflexes should not be tested until the cervical spine has been cleared for the presence of fractures. A lateral cervical spine x-ray alone does not suffice. The presence or absence of a gag reflex and spontaneous respirations will further assess the status of the lower pons and medulla.

Since the diagnosis of basilar skull fracture is primarily clinical, it is important to recognize the physical findings of this entity. They include (1) hemotympanum or bloody discharge from the ear; (2) rhinorrhea or otorrhea; (3) retroauricular ecchymosis (Battle's sign); (4) periorbital ecchymosis ("raccoon's eyes"); and (5) first-, second-, seventh-, and eighth-cranial nerve deficits.

Diagnostic Tests

Approximately 5 percent of patients suffering from severe head injury will have an associated cervical spine fracture. Cervical spine x-rays should be taken in all unconscious patients, in patients with cervical pain, in those with neurological deficits suggesting cervical cord injury, or if the mechanism of injury can produce cervical damage.

Anteroposterior and lateral skull films should be obtained for penetrating wounds of the skull or for suspected depressed skull fracture. Skull x-rays localize the position of a foreign body within the cranium and can determine the amount of bony depression. Skull films also identify significant linear fractures, and if a fracture crosses the vascular groove of the middle meningeal artery or dural sinuses, an epidural hematoma should be anticipated. With an occipital fracture, a contrecoup frontal lobe contusion is likely. The Towne's view reveals fractures of the occiput extending down to the foramen magnum. Anteroposterior and lateral views alone will not demonstrate all fractures. If a CT head scan will be obtained, bone windows can be obtained, eliminating the need for skull films. For patients who have not lost consciousness, and have no focal neurological deficit, no evidence of depressed or basilar skull fracture, no evidence of penetration of the skull, and no indwelling shunt, skull x-rays are not necessary. Intoxicated patients are a particular problem since history is unreliable and drugs or alcohol alter the neurological examination. When there are findings suggesting a blow to the head, skull x-rays are usually indicated.

The main indications for CT scanning in the assessment of head-injured patients are (1) persistent decrease in level of consciousness, (2) clinical neurological deterioration, (3) persistent focal neurological deficit, and (4) skull fractures in the vicinity of the middle meningeal artery or major venous sinuses. The CT scan defines the location and extent of hemorrhage and distinguishes intraparenchymal hemorrhage from brain swelling or edema (Figs. 171-3 to 171-5). The amount of midline shift can be readily determined. CT scanning has been found to be superior to conventional skull x-rays in diagnosing basilar skull fractures but inferior in diagnosing linear skull fractures of the vault.

Laboratory work in all significant head injury should include CBC,

Table 171-2. Concussion-Fracture Patient Flow

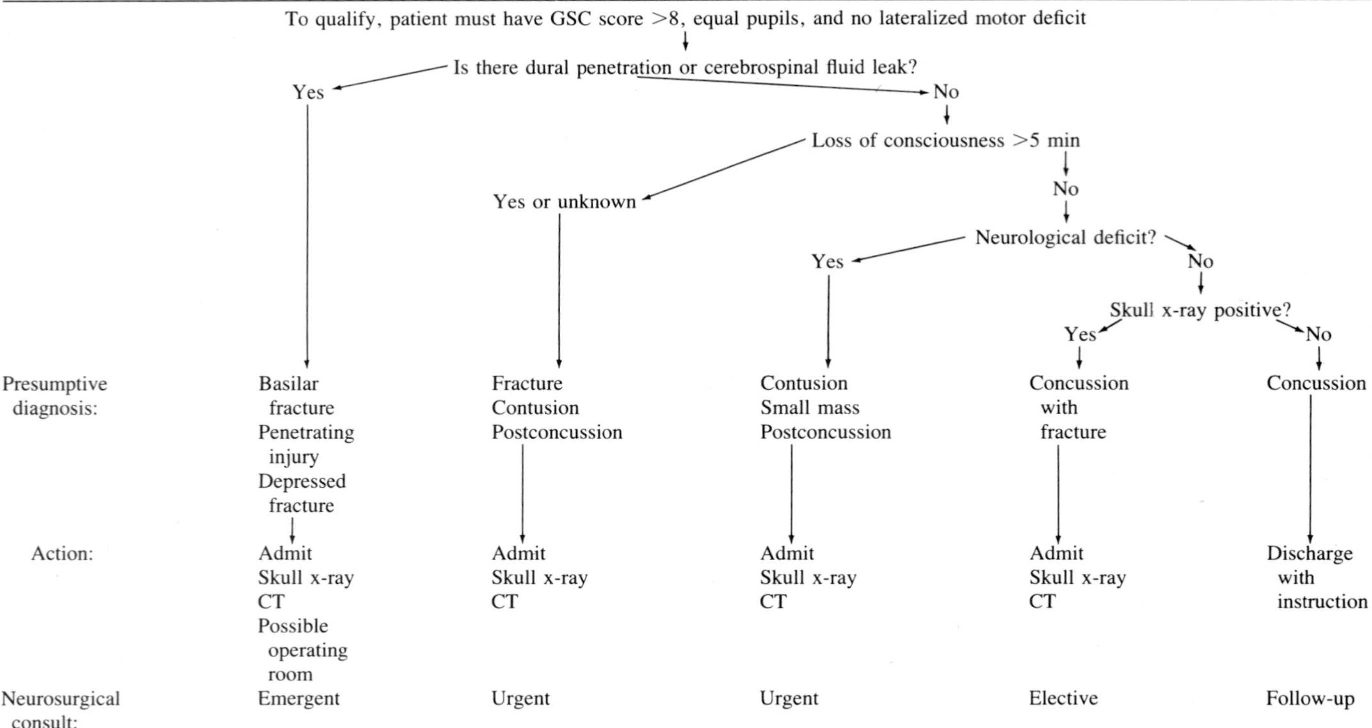

To qualify, patient must have GSC score >8, equal pupils, and no lateralized motor deficit

Is there dural penetration or cerebrospinal fluid leak? → Yes / No

No → Loss of consciousness >5 min → Yes or unknown / No

No → Neurological deficit? → Yes / No

No → Skull x-ray positive? → Yes / No

	Yes (dural penetration or CSF leak)	Yes or unknown (LOC >5 min)	Yes (neurological deficit)	Yes (skull x-ray positive)	No (skull x-ray positive)
Presumptive diagnosis:	Basilar fracture Penetrating injury Depressed fracture	Fracture Contusion Postconcussion	Contusion Small mass Postconcussion	Concussion with fracture	Concussion
Action:	Admit Skull x-ray CT Possible operating room	Admit Skull x-ray CT	Admit Skull x-ray CT	Admit Skull x-ray CT	Discharge with instruction
Neurosurgical consult:	Emergent	Urgent	Urgent	Elective	Follow-up

electrolytes, blood glucose, arterial blood gases, urinalysis, ethanol level, and directed toxicological analysis where indicated. Coagulation parameters, including partial thromboplastin time, prothrombin time, platelets, and fibrinogen level, should be obtained. Blood for type and cross match should be sent immediately. In addition to possible skull x-rays and cervical spine x-rays, a chest x-ray and pelvic x-ray are performed routinely in all cases of severe trauma.

DISPOSITION AND MANAGEMENT

Mild and Moderate Head Injury

The major question is which patient can be safely discharged to home and which patient should be admitted for observation (Table 171-2). The decision depends on the reliability of the patient and the patient's friends or family as well as the degree to which the examining physician is familiar with the patient. For example, a patient who could be observed at home by reliable family members and who is neurologically intact could be discharged home following a relatively minor head injury with a brief loss of consciousness. However, if there is a history of unconsciousness in an unreliable patient or in a patient about whom very little is known, admission to the hospital is advisable. Any patient with a persisting decreased level of consciousness, deterioration in neurological function, focal neurological deficit, seizures, penetrating injuries, or open or depressed skull fractures should be admitted. Seizures should be treated with intravenous phenytoin, 18 mg/kg, at 25 mg/min with cardiac and blood pressure monitoring. Neurological evaluation by the nursing staff should include an assessment and documentation every 15 to 60 min of the level of consciousness, pupillary size and reactivity, movement of the extremities, and vital signs. Any deterioration should be reported immediately to the neurosurgical staff.

Table 171-3. Disposition of Head-Injured Patients

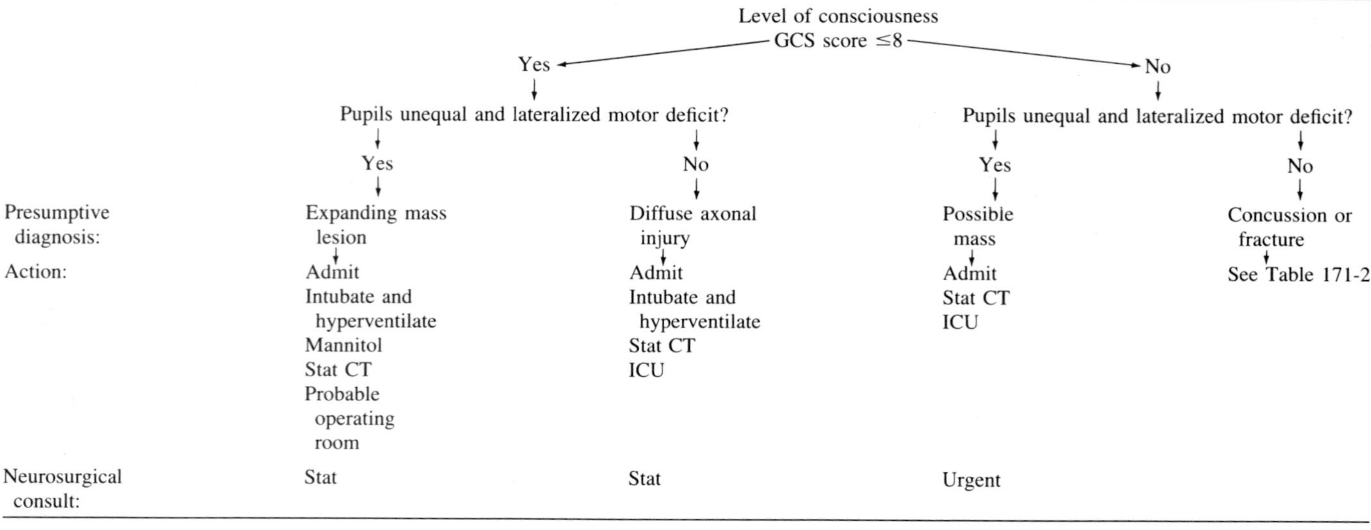

Level of consciousness GCS score ≤8 → Yes / No

Yes → Pupils unequal and lateralized motor deficit? → Yes / No

No → Pupils unequal and lateralized motor deficit? → Yes / No

	GCS ≤8 Yes; pupils/motor Yes	GCS ≤8 Yes; pupils/motor No	GCS ≤8 No; pupils/motor Yes	GCS ≤8 No; pupils/motor No
Presumptive diagnosis:	Expanding mass lesion	Diffuse axonal injury	Possible mass	Concussion or fracture
Action:	Admit Intubate and hyperventilate Mannitol Stat CT Probable operating room	Admit Intubate and hyperventilate Stat CT ICU	Admit Stat CT ICU	See Table 171-2
Neurosurgical consult:	Stat	Stat	Urgent	

Head Injury Referral

In hospitals where neurosurgical care is not available, some patients can be safely observed at the local hospital and some should be referred to a neurosurgical unit (Table 171-3). Patients who have a persisting decreased level of consciousness such that they cannot follow simple commands or utter recognizable words should be referred. Patients who can follow commands or utter recognizable words but who have pupil inequality, lateralized extremity weakness, depressed skull fractures, or basilar skull fractures should be referred. Any patient with neurological deterioration, regardless of the state of consciousness, should be quickly referred. Patients with intracranial hemorrhage of any significance are best observed where neurosurgical care is quickly available. The above categories include the vast majority of patients who sustain acute mortality or significant morbidity.

Prior to transfer, direct communication between the referring physician and the receiving physician should occur. The cardiorespiratory status, the neurological condition, the presence and rate of any neurological deterioration, and the presence of any multiple injuries should be presented. A plan for the best mode of transport, the need for artificial ventilation, the administration of any significant drugs, and the potential need for blood transfusion, especially in the small child or infant, should be determined before the patient leaves the referring institution.

Severe Head Injury

Patients with severe head injuries or those with unequal pupils or lateralizing motor findings, must be treated aggressively (Table 171-3). Establishment of an adequate airway with mechanical hyperventilation is a first priority. Whenever possible, it is important during intubation to use topical nasopharyngeal and laryngotracheal anesthesia. In agitated patients a paralytic agent and sedation may be needed to prevent elevation of ICP, even though these agents will compromise neurological assessment. Nasotracheal intubation is a preferred method for possible cervical spinal injury, unless severe facial fractures or cribriform plate fractures are present. Following intubation, if the cervical spine injury is still suspected and the patient is agitated, the cervical spine must be physically immobilized or the patient then sedated or paralyzed. Patients are artificially ventilated to maintain an arterial P_{CO_2} of 25 to 30 mmHg.

Hypotension can greatly depress neurological function because cerebral perfusion pressure falls and cerebral metabolism is adversely effected. Every attempt must be made to restore adequate blood pressure so that an accurate neurological assessment can be made. Hypertension in conjunction with increased ICP must be treated with caution. Attempts at decreasing the blood pressure may result in inadequate CPP. Also, the blood pressure can be very sensitive to hypertensive medication, resulting in wide swings in the blood pressure. Treatment of hypertension is best directed initially toward reducing increased ICP.

In patients with lateralizing motor findings, pupil inequality, neurological deterioration, or a GCS score of 6 or less, 1 g/kg of intravenous mannitol as a solution of 500 mL of 20% Osmitrol is infused as rapidly as possible through a large-bore intravenous catheter. An indwelling Foley catheter is essential. Mannitol acts as an osmotic diuretic, so significant hypovolemia is a relative contraindication. The agent draws water out of the normal brain by creating an osmotic gradient and can dramatically reduce ICP. An intracranial hematoma can expand somewhat as the brain shrinks, so mannitol should be given only when a definitive study or definitive surgery is to be performed. Although many institutions have discontinued its use, it is our routine practice to give dexamethasone, 1 mg/kg intravenously, as soon as possible after the injury. Dexamethasone is continued at an approximate dose of 10 mg every 6 h for 2 to 3 days and then discontinued. The head of the bed is elevated 30°, and any kinking of the neck is carefully avoided. All patients with focal brain lesions such as extracerebral hematomas, contusions, or intraparenchymal hematomas are given intravenous phenytoin (Dilantin), 18 mg/kg, at 20 mg/min and with cardiac and blood pressure monitoring.

Immediately after stabilization in the emergency department a CT scan of the head is obtained. A high-quality study is ensured by a combination of sedation with intravenous lorazepam (Ativan) 2 mg and pancuronimum bromide (Pavulon) 0.1 mg/kg as needed. Patients with extracerebral or intracerebral hematomas, with 5 mm or more shift of midline structures, and with depressed skull fractures are taken directly to the operating suite. Penetrating foreign bodies should be removed from the skull and brain in the operating room. Patients sustaining gunshot wounds, unless they are moribund, are also taken to the operating room for debridement of their wounds and removal of hematomas and foreign bodies as indicated.

If the original fibrinogen level drawn in the emergency department is less than 250 mg/dL, or if there is intracranial hemorrhage on the initial CT scan, two units of fresh-frozen plasma are administered. Fibrinogen levels are monitored for at least 72 h.

Herniation Syndrome

The patient who develops rapid uncal herniation despite intubation and hyperventilation, and the administration of intravenous mannitol, poses a critical problem. Immediate access to a CT scan and subsequent surgical decompression are required to salvage such a patient. Any delay beyond 15 or 20 min will sometimes preclude survival or a functional recovery. If emergency personnel are adequately trained or if there is a neurosurgeon available in the emergency department, an emergency burr hole over the temporal fossa on the side of the dilated pupil can be done. Some neurosurgeons would prefer to take the patient directly to the operating room. However, approximately 40 percent of such patients will not have an extracerebral hematoma but will have intracerebral hemorrhage, contusion, or edema. If exploratory burr holes are negative, an immediate CT scan should be carried out.

On occasion, chest or abdominal injuries will require immediate attention in the operating suite to prevent exsanguination. If there are focal findings such as pupil asymmetry or lateralizing motor weakness, exploratory burr holes are done simultaneously with the thoracic or abdominal procedure. If the neurological examination is nonfocal, an ICP monitor can be inserted in the operating room so that any increase in ICP can be detected and treated throughout the chest or abdominal procedure. Immediately following the procedure, and while the patient is under the same anesthetic, a CT scan is obtained.

Intracranial Pressure

Management of ICP beginning in the emergency department and continuing throughout the clinical course of the patient is essential to the optimal management of the severely head-injured patient. Intracranial pressure monitoring is routinely instituted in severely injured patients following removal of surgical mass lesions, or in the case of diffuse brain injuries, on admission to the intensive care unit. Patients without focal findings who have purposeful movement of the extremities, and have a normal CT scan, are not monitored. Ventriculostomies are preferred for ICP monitoring because of their accuracy and the ability to remove CSF as a treatment for increased ICP.

If ICP cannot be maintained at less than 20 mmHg with the above routine measures, the following treatments are instituted in a stepwise fashion: (1) hyperventilation is increased to produce an arterial P_{CO_2} of 20 mmHg; (2) cerebral spinal fluid drainage is instituted to the level of the foramen of Monro; (3) mannitol is administered intravenously, to reduce ICP to less than 20 mmHg; (4) pancuronium (Pavulon) is administered intravenously to prevent any movement on the part of the patient; (5) barbiturate coma is initiated if the patient's cardiac status is stable; and (6) repeat craniotomy to remove significant mass lesions is carefully considered in appropriate patients.

In addition, CPP must be maintained and adequate intravascular volume ensured. Not infrequently, barbiturate coma, osmotic dehydration, and sedation can cause hypotension. A Swan-Ganz catheter can be very helpful in ensuring adequate vascular volume and cardiac output.

Seizures

Seizures following trauma are classified as: immediate, early, and late. Immediate seizures are due to traumatic neuronal depolarization and have little morbidity. Early seizures occur the first week after injury, and late seizures occur any time afterward. Five percent of patients sustaining blunt head injury will have an early seizure. Early seizures suggest the presence of focal cerebral contusions, intracranial hemorrhage, hypoxia, or metabolic abnormalities. In addition, early seizures can damage the already injured brain by producing hypoxia, acidosis, and increased ICP, despite adequate controlled ventilation. They also increase the incidence of late seizures from an overall incidence of 5 percent to 25 percent in blunt head injury. The likelihood of late epilepsy is increased by acute intracranial hematomas and depressed fractures.

Early seizures should be treated aggressively. Prophylactic intravenous phenytoin loading at 18 mg/kg should be instituted in all severely head-injured patients with intracranial blood, depressed skull fractures with dural penetration, penetrating wounds, intracranial infections, or early seizures.

PITFALLS TO AVOID IN THE ASSESSMENT AND MANAGEMENT OF THE HEAD-INJURED PATIENT

The following errors should be avoided:

- Inaccurately attributing decreased level of consciousness to alcohol or drugs. Obtain blood alcohol levels and toxicological screens to help with difficult problems.
- Discharging a patient from the emergency department during a "lucid interval." Err on the conservative side when a period of unconsciousness is documented or if unknown.
- Failure to diagnose a cervical fracture or spinal cord injury. Persist with further views or tomograms when in doubt.
- Failure to adequately immobilize an agitated patient with a cervical fracture. When usual restraint systems are inadequate, consider paralyzing the patient.
- Failure to establish an adequate airway. All obtunded or unconscious patients should be intubated and hyperventilated.
- Failure to recognize progressive neurological deterioration. Frequent, documented examinations are necessary.
- Failure to rapidly and correctly manage the patient with uncal herniation. This is an extreme emergency.

PROGNOSIS

Prognosis from mild to moderate severe head injury is usually regarded as good. Mortality rates of patients with head injuries and GCS scores of 10 or greater approach zero unless there has been deterioration to a severe head-injured state. However, a patient who appears to display a good or favorable recovery can exhibit subtle alterations in memory, concentration, and cognition which interfere with function.

The overall mortality rate for severe head injuries is approximately 40 percent with a favorable or functional outcome accounting for another 40 to 50 percent. Even in the functional or favorably recovered patients, formal neuropsychological tests will uncover significant deficits.

The major factors influencing outcome in the severely head-injured patient is the initial GCS score which reflects the severity of the neurological injury and the particular type of lesion causing the neurological deficit. The mortality rate for patients with GCS scores of 3 to 5 is approximately three times that of patients with scores of 6 to 8 (60 vs. 20 percent). Acute subdural hematoma with a GCS score of 3 to 5 will have an approximately 75 percent mortality rate and less than a 10 percent chance for a favorable recovery. On the other hand, diffuse injury without mass lesions with a GCS score of 6 to 8 will have an approximately 10 percent mortality and two-thirds will make a good recovery. Acute subdural hematomas and diffuse injuries associated with coma of longer than 24 h account for 75 percent of head-injury deaths. In addition, bilaterally absent pupillary responses or oculocephalic responses are associated with an approximately 75 percent mortality rate. This is true regardless of whether a surgical or a nonsurgical lesion is present. Increasing age appears to adversely affect the outcome of head injury in general.

Despite improvement in the ability to prognosticate based on the neurological examination and other factors, it is difficult to ascertain the ultimate prognosis in the early phases of treatment. Aggressive stabilization and treatment is indicated in all severely head-injured patients.

DELAYED TRAUMATIC PROBLEMS

Postconcussion Syndromes

The term *postconcussion syndrome* evokes the image of a psychophysiologic reaction in many physicians' minds. This probably is because many of the symptoms such as insomnia, loss of memory, hearing problems, sensitivity to alcohol, depression, and visual disturbances seem, superficially at least, to have no organic basis. There is increasing documentation that the mildly and moderately head-injured patients have evidence of organic brain damage on formal neuropsychological testing. In one study of minor head injury, 34 percent of patients gainfully employed before the accident were unemployed 3 months after the injury. This was felt to be due primarily to problems with attention, concentration, memory, and judgment and also the emotional stress caused by the persistent symptoms. Litigation and compensation may obviously play a role in some cases, but the burden of proof would appear to be on the physician. These patients should be referred for appropriate evaluation if symptoms appear to be legitimately interfering with normal functioning.

Delayed Posttraumatic Cerebral Spinal Fluid Leak

The exact incidence of recurrent posttraumatic CSF leak is difficult to ascertain but is probably as high as 10 percent. Previous head injury with loss of the integrity of the meningeal coverings of the brain is the most common cause of recurrent meningitis in adults. Not all patients having posttraumatic meningitis will necessarily have active CSF leak, although the majority will. Because of this risk of delayed bacterial meningitis, all patients with suspected CSF leak must be referred to a neurosurgeon without delay.

Delayed Posttraumatic Seizures

Delayed posttraumatic seizures, defined as the first seizures occurring after 1 week from the time of trauma, occur in anywhere from 2 to 6 percent of the head-injured population. Eighty-five percent of these seizures occur for the first time within 1 year of the injury. Depressed fractures with tear of the dura or brain associated with intracranial hematomas have a significant increased incidence of posttraumatic seizures. Outpatients with delayed posttraumatic seizures should be loaded with phenytoin as described above and placed on a maintenance dose which should be continued until a 2-year seizure-free interval has passed.

BIBLIOGRAPHY

Adams JH, Graham DI, Murray LS, et al: Diffuse axonal injury due to nonmissile head injury in humans: An analysis of 45 cases. *Ann Neurol* 12:557, 1982.

Gennarelli TA, Spielman GM, Langfitt TW, et al: Influence of the type of intracranial lesion on outcome from severe head injury. A multicenter study using a new classification system. *J Neurosurg* 56:26, 1982.

Mahoney BD, Rockswold GL, Ruiz E, et al: Emergency twist drill trephination. *Neurosurgery* 8:551, 1981.

Mendelow AD, Teasdale G, Jennett B, et al: Risks of intracranial hematoma in head injured adults. *Br Med J* 187:1173, 1983.

Nagib MG, Rockswold GL, Sherman RS, et al: Civilian gunshot wounds to the brain: Prognosis and management. *Neurosurgery* 18:533, 1986.

Narayan RK, Kishore PRS, Becker DP, et al: Intracranial pressure: To monitor or not to monitor? A review of our experience with severe head injury. *J Neurosurg* 56:650, 1982.

Rimel RW, Giordani B, Barth JT: Disability caused by minor head injury. *Neurosurgery* 9:221, 1981.

Seelig, JM, Becker DP, Miller JD, et al: Traumatic acute subdural hematoma. Major mortality reduction in comatose patients treated within four hours. *N Engl J Med* 304:1511, 1981.

172
SPINAL INJURIES

Brian D. Mahoney

It is difficult to imagine an injury more devastating than acute quadriplegia. In 1975, Kraus and coworkers estimated the incidence of new spinal cord injury at 50 per million United States population. This extrapolates to approximately 12,300 new spinal cord injury victims in 1990 in the United States. The typical patient is a man in his early twenties involved in a motor vehicle accident. Motor vehicle accidents (41 percent) are followed in frequency by falls (13 percent), firearms (9 percent), and recreation (5 percent) as sources of spinal cord injury.

PATIENT MANAGEMENT

There are three priorities in the emergency medical management of the patient with a spinal injury. The first is to ensure patient survival by following the ABCDEs of trauma care. The second priority is to preserve residual spinal cord function by stabilizing the injured spinal column and avoiding secondary injury to the spinal cord. The third priority is to initiate treatments aimed at allowing the highest possible chance for the injured cord to recover. After the completion of emergency care, a fourth priority is to restore the bony stability of the spinal column. Even the permanently quadriplegic patient needs bony vertebral stability

The patient suffers the primary injury at the time of impact. Emergency physicians can have the most influence on primary injury by being vocal advocates of public safety issues such as endorsing seat belt usage and penalties for those who drive while intoxicated. Once the patient has sustained primary injury, the critical role of all emergency personnel is to avoid secondary injury. Secondary injury to the cord may occur when there is unnecessary motion of an unstable spinal column, hypoxemia, edema, continued pressure on the cord by an extrinsic mass, or shock that reduces perfusion of the injured cord.

Prehospital Spinal Immobilization

After surveying the scene for hazard and mechanism of injury, the emergency medical technician immediately controls the patient's head and neck. Management of airway, breathing, and circulation follows. Next a semirigid collar and spinal immobilization board are applied. These devices are used to immobilize the spine and not to apply traction, since excessive traction may cause secondary injury. The degree of immobilization provided by a cervical collar varies from minimal with the soft sponge variety to substantial but not complete with semirigid varieties. No collar can adequately immobilize the occiput, C1, and C2. The semirigid collar is an important adjunct to aid in transfer onto the long spinal immobilization board. Immobilization continues until history and physical examination or x-ray studies rule out an acutely unstable spinal column. The semirigid collar may be opened to examine the neck, trachea, and jugular veins but then should be reapplied until the indicated spinal x-rays are cleared. Because a patient is walking at the accident scene does not eliminate the need for proper immobilization.

Emergency Department Assessment and Resuscitation

Maintain spinal immobilization during assessment and management of airway, breathing, circulation, and disability. Airway management is a controversial topic. The apneic patient needs rapid, definitive airway control, since gastric distension followed by regurgitation is likely during unprotected positive-pressure ventilation. Options include orotracheal intubation with in-line immobilization, transtracheal catheter ventilation while x-rays are taken and cleared, or immediate cricothyrotomy. In-line immobilization means immobilization and not traction. During in-line immobilization, pressure on the cricoid cartilage (Sellick's maneuver) will usually allow direct visualization of the vocal cords. For the unconscious patient with adequate spontaneous breathing, the usual approach is supplemental oxygen until completion of x-ray studies. Be prepared to logroll immediately and suction the patient. Leave the patient attached to the backboard so that if he regurgitates he can be rolled with reasonable safety. Unfortunately, logrolling with or without a spinal immobilization board does not completely prevent all spinal column motion. Patient exposure for examination requires temporarily releasing straps, but these should be reattached after cutting and removing the clothing.

Resuscitation involves intravenous access, nasogastric tube, and Foley cathether. Adequate volume resuscitation continues until occult hemorrhage is ruled out or controlled. Next, the critical trauma series of x-ray studies is performed, including lateral cervical spine, chest, and pelvic x-rays.

The secondary survey follows and includes assessment of motor function (graded 0/5 for flaccid, 3/5 for overcoming gravity, and up to 5/5 for normal), perception of pain, reflexes, flaccidity or spasticity of extremities, gross proprioception, diaphragmatic breathing, rectal tone, perirectal sensation and wink, bulbocavernosus reflex, and priapism. A common oversight is to leave out assessment of posterior column function (vibration, gross proprioception, light touch, and motion). Preserved posterior column function is significant in identifying the anterior cord syndrome. The assessment of neurologic loss around the anus is vital to identifying sacral sparing and therefore an incomplete lesion. The absence of reflex activity shows the presence of spinal shock. The level of spinal cord injury can be estimated using Tables 172-1 and 172-2. Information must be accurately and serially recorded. Improvement or loss will have significant impact on the patient's management by the neurosurgeon.

The patient's vital signs may indicate spinal neurogenic shock characterized by hypotension, paradoxical bradycardia, warm dry skin, and adequate urine output. Consider all causes of shock in a patient with possible multiple injuries and vital signs indicative of spinal neurogenic shock. Look for hemorrhagic; mechanical (tamponade, tension pneumothorax); cardiogenic; and, to a lessor extent, septic shock. Complete a thorough search for occult hemorrhage before attributing hypotension to spinal cord injury. Emergency evaluation after physical examination includes chest x-ray, peritoneal lavage or abdominal CT, ECG, echocardiogram, urinalysis, and further x-ray studies as appropriate.

If the patient is still hypotensive after occult blood loss and other causes of shock are controlled, support blood pressure with a dopamine infusion. Patients with otherwise healthy cardiovascular systems tol-

Table 172-1. Muscle Innervation

Root Level	Muscle	Function Lost
C3, C4	Trapezius	Shoulder elevation
C4	Diaphragm	Respiration
C5, C6	Biceps	Forearm flexion
C7	Triceps	Forearm extension
C8	Flexor digitorum	Finger flexion
T1	Interossei	Finger abduction/adduction
T1 to T12	Intercostals and abdominals	Respiration
L1, L2	Iliopsoas	Hip flexion
L3, L4	Quadriceps	Knee extension
L5	Extensor hallucis	Gréat toe dorsiflexion
S1	Biceps femoris	Knee flexion
S1, S2	Soleus and gastrocnemius	Foot plantar flexion
S2 to S4	Rectal sphincter	Sphincter tone

Table 172-2. Sensory Innervation

Root	Sensory Level
C2	Occiput
C4	Shoulder tops
C6	Thumb
C7	Long finger
C8	Little finger
T4	Nipple
T10	Umbilicus
L1	Inginal crease
L2, L3	Medial thigh
L4	Medial calf
L5	Lateral calf
S1	Lateral foot
S2 to S4	Perianal

erate very well the systolic pressures of 80 to 100 common with acute quadriplegia. The optimal blood pressure to maintain is unknown. In animal experiments and theoretically in humans, a pressure nearer normal might aid in perfusing injured areas of the cord. The patient can easily be overhydrated, and a central venous pressure line or Swan-Ganz catheter plus Foley catheter can guide fluid therapy to avoid pulmonary edema.

After completion of the primary survey, resuscitation, trauma series of x-rays, and secondary survey, the presence of spinal column or cord injury should be evident. If the emergency physician is not certain whether a spinal injury is stable or unstable, the patient must remain on the backboard. Consult a neurosurgeon for significant spinal cord or column injuries.

Start very high-dose methylprednisolone as soon as practical after diagnosing spinal cord injury. Bracken and coworkers reported significant improvement of motor, pin, and touch sensation when this treatment began within 8 h of injury. The patient should receive a 30-mg/kg loading dose of methylprednisolone over 15 min in the first hour. Follow this with a 5.4-mg/kg per hour continuous infusion for the next 23 h.

Traction

A key means of preserving and regaining cord function is to remove any extrinsic source of pressure on the spinal cord. The first step is to reduce any displacement of the spinal column. Thoracolumbar injuries usually reduce in the supine position on a rotary bed. For cervical injuries, apply Gardner-Wells tongs and carefully move the patient to a circle or rotary bed. Immobilize the cervical spine by applying 5 to 10 lb of traction to the tongs. Use 2 lb for atlanto-occipital injuries. Add weight in 5- to 10-lb increments every 15 min up to certain weight limits (10 lb with C1 or C2 injuries; 50 lb and sometimes more for the lower cervical segment). Traction must be applied carefully, using serial x-ray films and neurologic examinations as a guide. Excessive traction can permanently destroy cord or nerve root function. Reduction by traction continues until restoration of the anteroposterior (AP) canal diameter to at least two-thirds of normal, there is neurologic deterioration, or an intervertebral disk space exceeds 5 mm, suggesting that distraction may be occurring. Sedation and muscle relaxation may be needed. If reduction cannot be achieved or maintained, surgery follows. After the initial reduction much less weight is required to maintain reduction.

Myelography

After reduction of bony displacement, the patient has an emergent myelogram if (1) there has been a documented loss of function since the first prehospital evaluation, (2) there is an anterior cord syndrome, or (3) the patient has a partial cord syndrome that is not improving. The myelogram identifies bone, disk, or hematoma pressing on the cord. Continued unrelieved pressure on the cord will prevent optimal cord recovery and may lead to continuing deterioration. The myelogram is done via a lateral C1–C2 puncture with the stretcher angled head up. Interpretation involves searching for flattening of the cord, tissue visibly pressing on the cord, swelling of the cord, or inability to pass dye inferior to the lesion showing occlusion. Using CT metrizamide myelography, Allen and coworkers reported that approximately 24 percent of patients (11 of 46) with acute nonpenetrating cervical spinal cord injuries can be shown to have significant continuing spinal cord compression after restoration of adequate alignment.

Disposition

The patient with significant spinal column or cord injury should be managed at a regional trauma center or spinal cord injury center. Transfer should be accomplished when the patient's other injuries allow. If the injured cord progresses in humans in a fashion analogous to that in animal experiments, reduction, decompression, and active experimental interventions must be completed within 4 to 8 h after the injury.

The indications and benefits of early surgery remain controversial. Wagner recommends considering immediate surgery on patients with (1) acute spinal cord injuries with incomplete sensorimotor loss who have undergone a failed attempt at closed reduction, (2) a successful reduction but continued compression proven on myelography, (3) continued bony encroachment despite reduction, or (4) failure to maintain reduction. He does not recommend immediate surgery for patients with incomplete lesions that are improving or for patients with complete lesions despite adequate reduction.

CERVICAL X-RAY STUDIES

Obtain cervical spine x-ray views on all trauma patients with (1) posttraumatic neck pain or tenderness; (2) transient or persistent numbness or paresthesia; (3) loss of consciousness; (4) impaired level of consciousness, such as from intoxication, with evidence of head or neck injury; (5) an examination consistent with cervical cord injury; and (6) other painful, distracting injuries, especially multiple injuries, resulting from high-energy accidents or falls. The minimum views needed are a lateral, AP, and open-mouth odontoid.

The lateral view shows 90 percent of the significant injuries, the open-mouth odontoid 10 percent, and the AP less than 1 percent. Other views add substantial information, but the presence of an injury is usually at least suspected based upon these first three views. In reading an x-ray, it is acceptable to do an initial rapid survey, but this must be followed by an explicit sequence of evaluation, as follows:

1. On the true lateral view, look for all seven cervical vertebrae, including the cervicothoracic junction. If all seven cervical vertebrae plus the upper margin of T1 cannot be seen, then do a repeat lateral with arm traction applied to lower the shoulders, a swimmer's view, or bilateral supine oblique projections. In managing a seriously injured patient, valuable time can be saved by automatically doing the swimmer's view immediately after the lateral view with arm traction applied.
2. Check prevertebral soft tissue; 5 mm or greater down to the C3 to C4 level suggests hematoma secondary to fracture.
3. Check each vertebra for fracture.
4. Check for alignment of the four lordotic curves consisting of the anterior margin of the vertebral body, the posterior margin of the vertebral body, the spinolaminal line, and the tips of the spinous processes. In an adult, up to 3.5 mm of anterior subluxation on a true lateral view taken at 72 in may be normal. Yet to assess ligamentous stability, careful flexion and extension views may be required.
5. Check for abrupt angulation of the cervical column of greater than 11° at a single interspace.

6. Check for fanning of spinous processes, suggesting posterior ligamentous disruption.
7. Check the lateral masses for abrupt change in rotation, suggesting facet dislocation.
8. Check the AP diameter of the spinal canal for congenital stenosis or stenosis due to spondylosis. The actual upper limit of the normal AP diameter of the adult cord is 9.3 mm. Yet, due to the magnification on plain films, if the canal diameter is 13 mm or less, the patient risks cord injury in otherwise minor strain injuries.
9. Check the predental space. If it is greater than 3 mm in adults or 4 mm in children, there may be disruption of the cruciform ligament holding the dens (odontoid) forward against the body of C1.
10. Check the atlanto-occipital relation for dislocation.
11. On the open-mouth odontoid view, look for fracture of the odontoid or body of C2, alignment of the lateral masses of C1 with C2, and symmetry of the C1-to-C2 interspace.

According to a retrospective review by Shaffer and Doris, the lateral view alone failed to show 6 out of 35 cervical spine fractures or dislocations. On 3 more of the 35, the injury was very difficult to see on the lateral view and best seen on the odontoid or AP view. If the patient is unconscious or immobilized so that the patient cannot open his or her mouth, the authors recommend a modified axial supine odontoid process view instead of the open-mouth odontoid view.

If, after obtaining a quality lateral, AP, and open-mouth odontoid view, there is a question about whether a lesion is unstable, CT is the usual next step. If the lesion is most likely stable, then careful lateral flexion and extension views can be made. Take these views with the patient still supine on a stretcher. Use extreme care, with a knowledgeable physician guiding the patient as the patient slowly flexes and later extends his or her neck. If the patient complains of pain or paresthesias, attempt no further motion. Do not do flexion-extension views if the original three views predict an unstable spinal column. In such a case, the neurosurgeon should order and conduct subsequent radiographic examinations.

If there is concern about a lamina, pedicle, facet, or foramen, then order oblique views after interpreting the first three views as stable. Pillar views are for assessing lateral masses. Tomograms add greatly to the accuracy of the diagnosis. CT is indicated in any patient with a neurologic deficit, fracture of the posterior arch, or burst fracture with vertebral fragments retropulsed into the spinal canal, and for equivocal plain films.

SPRAINS AND FRACTURES

Stability

Stability is the ability of the spine to maintain vertebral relations when a load is applied such that there is no damage or irritation to the spinal cord or the nerve roots and no deformity or pain. Trafton has ranked cervical spine injuries according to their degree of instability (Table 172-3). Cervical sprain, that is, damage to ligaments, may lead to dangerous instability and neurologic loss with or without fracture. The atlantoaxial joint is principally maintained by the cruciform ligament. Disruption of this ligament leads to widening of the predental space.

Using CT and Denis' three-column system of categorizing spinal injuries, one can accurately assess spinal stability. The anterior column includes the anterior longitudinal ligament, the anterior two-thirds of the vertebral body, the annulus fibrosus, and the disk. The middle column includes the posterior one-third of the vertebral body, the annulus fibrosus, the disk, and the posterior longitudinal ligament. The posterior column includes all the remaining posterior elements: the pedicles, lateral masses, intertransverse ligaments, facet capsular ligaments, lamina, ligamentum flavum, spinous processes, interspinous and supraspinous ligaments, and ligamentum nuchae. To be unstable, the injury must involve two of the columns.

Table 172-3. The Spectrum of Acute Instability in Cervical Spine Injuries

Most Unstable
1. Rupture of transverse atlantal ligament
2. Fracture of dens
3. Burst fracture with posterior ligamentous disruption (''flexion teardrop'')
4. Bilateral facet dislocation (or equivalent posterior disruption)
5. Burst fracture of vertebral body without posterior ligamentous disruption
6. Hyperextension fracture dislocation
7. Hangman's fracture
8. Extension teardrop fracture (stable in flexion)
9. Jefferson fracture (burst of C1)
10. Unilateral facet dislocation (or equivalent posterior disruption)
11. Anterior subluxation
12. Simple wedge compression fracture without posterior disruption
13. Pillar fracture
14. Fracture of posterior arch of C1
15. Spinous process fracture (clay-shoveler)
Least Unstable

Source: Trafton G: Spinal cord injuries. *Surg Clin North Am* 62:61, 1982. Reprinted with permission.

Some fracture dislocations are obviously unstable, but others, such as severe compression fractures, seat belt fractures, or burst fractures may or may not be unstable, depending on associated ligamentous injury. In such cases, acute stability can be assessed on careful flexion-extension studies. Check for subluxation greater than 3 mm or angulation of one vertebral body over the next greater than 11°. CT avoids the risk of these dynamic studies by more accurately describing the injury.

A principal goal is to identify and protect all patients with acutely unstable spinal columns. There is, in addition, a subset of patients that on initial films including flexion and extension views will have what appears to be a stable column that within 3 weeks will develop subacute instability. This phenomenon is thought to be due to the prevention of subluxation by muscle tension at the initial visit and the occurrence of progressive instability as the muscles relax. It is important that patients with acute cervical strains are referred for follow-up before 3 weeks.

Mechanisms of Injury and Common Fractures

Approximately 39 percent of cervical fractures have associated neurologic injury. Factors that increase the risk of neurologic injury include block vertebrae, spina bifida, os odontoideum, ankylosing spondylitis, rheumatoid arthritis, spinal stenosis, and age-related degenerative changes. Although approximately 20 percent of patients with cervical spine injuries have facial injuries, the converse is not true. People with facial injuries rarely have cervical spine injuries. In a study of 2555 patients with facial fractures severe enough for hospital admission, Davidson found that only 1.3 percent had associated neck injuries. The vast majority of the patients with combined face and neck injuries had multiple-system trauma from motor vehicle accidents.

Harris has classified the various injuries of the cervical spine according to seven mechanisms of injury (Table 172-4). The Jefferson fracture is a burst of the ring of C1 from a vertical compression force. It is most often seen on the open-mouth odontoid view, although tomograms may be necessary. The hangman's fracture is a bilateral fracture through the pedicles of C2. It is often due to hyperextension in a motor vehicle accident. Fortunately, the generous size of the spinal canal at C2 and spontaneous decompression help to limit cord damage. The flexion teardrop fracture refers to the mechanism and shape of the large triangular fragment displaced from the anterior aspect of the involved vertebral body. There is extensive associated posterior and

Table 172-4. Cervical Spine Injuries: Mechanism of Injury

I. Flexion
  A. Anterior subluxation (hyperflexion sprain)
  B. Bilateral interfacetal dislocation
  C. Simple wedge (compression) fracture
  D. Clay-shoveler (coal-shoveler) fracture
  E. Flexion teardrop fracture
II. Flexion-rotation
  A. Unilateral interfacetal dislocation
III. Extension-rotation
  A. Pillar fracture
IV. Vertical compression
  A. Jefferson bursting fracture of atlas
  B. Burst (bursting, dispersion, axial loading) fracture
V. Hyperextension
  A. Hyperextension dislocation
  B. Avulsion fracture of anterior arch of atlas
  C. Extension teardrop fracture of axis
  D. Fracture of posterior arch of atlas
  E. Laminar fracture
  F. Traumatic spondylolisthesis (hangman's fracture)
  G. Hyperextension fracture-dislocation
VI. Lateral flexion
  Uncinate process fracture
VII. Diverse or imprecisely understood mechanisms
  A. Atlantooccipital disassociation
  B. Odontoid fractures

Source: Harris JH, Edeiken-Monroe B, Kopaniky DR: A practical classification of acute cervical spine injuries. *Orthop Clin North Am* 17:15, 1986. Reproduced by permission.

anterior ligamentous disruption and, with it, anterior cord injury. The extension teardrop fracture also has a triangular anterior, inferior fragment, but the mechanism is extension with avulsion of the fragment, leaving the posterior ligaments intact. The burst fracture is a vertical compression injury in which pieces of the comminuted vertebral body are forced posteriorly into the spinal canal. Some authors consider it a variation of the flexion teardrop fracture. The clay-shoveler's fracture is due to avulsion of the spinous process of C7, C6, or T1 (in order of frequency) from a flexion mechanism. It is also caused by direct blows to the spinous process.

Bilateral interfacetal dislocation occurs in flexion. The lesion is unstable, with total ligamentous disruption. On lateral x-ray views, there is anterior displacement of 50 percent or greater of one vertebral body on the next lower body. Unilateral facet dislocation occurs in combined flexion with rotation injuries. It is potentially unstable, depending on ligamentous disruption, and on lateral x-ray views there is anterior dislocation of less than 50 percent of one vertebral body on the next lower body. In addition, the vertebrae inferior to the injury appear in true lateral projection, and above the level of injury there is a sudden change to an oblique view.

THORACOLUMBAR INJURIES

The greatest number of thoracolumbar injuries occur at the junction of the relatively fixed upper thoracic spine (T1–T9) and the relatively mobile thoracolumbar (T10–L5) spine. Because of the buttressing provided by the rib cage, it takes great force to cause a thoracic fracture dislocation. Thoracic fracture dislocations are less common than lower thoracolumbar ones, but when they occur the spinal cord injury is typically more severe for three reasons: the diameter of the thoracic spinal canal is narrow, the thoracic spinal cord fills a larger portion of the canal, and the thoracic cord's blood supply is in a watershed area such that compression on the anterior spinal artery can cause ischemic injury much higher up in the thoracic cord. The great radicular artery of Adamkiewicz enters the spinal canal at L1 but provides circulation as high as T4.

There are four types of thoracolumbar fractures. The first is the wedge, or compression, fracture. It results from axial loading and flexion with failure of the anterior column. Wedge fractures are generally acutely stable. Severe wedge fractures are potentially unstable if the anterior margin of the vertebral body has lost more than 50 percent of its height and there is partial failure of the posterior ligaments. Wedge fractures are particularly common in elderly patients. The order of frequency is L1 > L2 > T12. Neurologic injury is uncommon, and treatment is symptomatic. Patients with acute wedge fractures of greater than 50 percent are often admitted for pain control and in anticipation of an ileus.

The second type of thoracolumbar fracture is the burst. It results from axial loading, causing failure of the anterior and middle columns. The vertebral end-plates fracture, forcing the nucleus pulposus into the vertebral body, resulting in explosion of the body. There is loss of vertebral height both anteriorly and posteriorly. On the AP x-ray the burst may be identified by a widening of the interpedicular distance. In severe burst fractures the posterior portion of the vertebral body explodes into the spinal canal, causing spinal cord compression. CT scan is often necessary to show clearly the true extent of these retropulsed fragments.

The third type of thoracolumbar fracture is a distraction or seat belt injury. In these injuries the seat belt serves as the axis of rotation during distraction, with failure of the spine in its posterior ligamentous and bony components. In the Chance distraction fracture the spine fails entirely in bone, splitting horizontally through the spinous process, laminae, pedicles, and the vertebral body. Abdominal injuries are common with seat belt spinal injuries.

Fracture dislocations involve failure of all three columns. The mechanism is flexion with rotation or shearing from massive blows. These types of injuries are unstable and have the most associated spinal cord injury.

Radiographic Evaluation of Thoracolumbar Injuries

The AP and lateral are the minimum views of the thoracolumbar spine. After initial AP and lateral films identify the level of injury, cone-down views will give more details, especially of the posterior elements. On the lateral radiograph, check the anterior and posterior height of the vertebral bodies, the alignment of the bodies, the posterior bony elements for fracture, and the interspinous distance for evidence of ligamentous disruption. On the AP, check the height of the vertebral bodies, the width between pedicles, and the alignment of the vertebral bodies and follow the spinous processes down the midline. Besides being checked for spinal injury, the AP film should be assessed for associated chest and abdominal injuries. Look for a paraspinal hematoma and for transverse process fractures correlated with trauma to adjacent organs, particularly the kidneys.

Do a CT scan if plain films are equivocal, suggest posterior element injury, or the patient has a neural deficit but no obvious fracture. CT scanning will frequently identify additional injuries, especially injuries of the posterior elements. Do CT myelography if initial x-rays do not explain a neurologic deficit, if the deficit progresses, or if the patient has an unexplained plateau during recovery from a deficit.

SACRAL AND COCCYGEAL INJURIES

Overlying bowel and soft tissue shadows make plain film diagnosis difficult. CT will identify fractures of the sacrum, pelvis, and associated hematoma. Neurologic injury is rare in sacral injuries. When it occurs, it involves damage to sacral nerve roots, impairing bowel, bladder, and sexual functions and motor and sensory function in the posterior legs.

Coccygeal injuries occur due to direct blows and, if severe, may have associated rectal tears. X-rays are not indicated, nor are they helpful in isolated coccygeal injury. Make the diagnosis of coccygeal fracture on rectal examination. Treatment in uncomplicated fractures is symptomatic, with pain medication and a doughnut pillow. Chronic coccydynia occasionally complicates recovery.

SPINAL CORD INJURY SYNDROMES

Severe injury to the spinal cord may cause spinal shock. This is a sudden transient distal areflexia that may last hours to weeks. The patient initially presents with a flaccid quadriplegia. As spinal shock passes (usually within 24 h), segmental reflexes return, and the patient develops a spastic paresis. Spinal neurogenic shock is that part of spinal shock relating to the vasomotor instability that is due to loss of sympathetic tone. The patient typically has a systolic blood pressure of 80 to 100 mmHg. Despite hypotension, the skin is warm, pink, and dry, and there is adequate urine output. In addition, despite the hypotension, there is a paradoxical bradycardia.

The patient also may have other autonomic nervous system dysfunction. Paralysis of the bowel and bladder may lead to paralytic ileus, gastric dilation, and acute urinary retention. Loss of anal sphincter tone leads to fecal incontinence. Priapism may occur and serve as a sign of cord injury. The patient may lose temperature control because of inability to vasoconstrict, vasodilate, shiver, or sweat over a large portion of his or her body. The patient may become poikilothermic and require external thermal control with a warming blanket.

Complete and Partial Cord Syndromes

Cord injury is physiologically complete when all cord function is absent distal to the level of injury. This assessment cannot be made until spinal shock has resolved. The presence of a complete versus an incomplete lesion has tremendous implications for prognosis and treatment. The prognosis of a complete lesion after spinal shock has resolved is for continued quadriplegia. In contrast, partial cord lesions often have at least some degree of recovery. Maynard and coworkers have reported the neurologic prognosis after traumatic quadriplegia among 103 cognitively intact patients. None with complete injury at 72 h were walking at 1 year. Of patients with sensory incomplete function at 72 h postinjury, 47 percent were walking at 1 year, and 87 percent of patients with motor incomplete function at 72 h postinjury were walking at 1 year.

The anterior spinal cord syndrome has been related to compression of the anterior spinal cord itself or compression of the anterior spinal artery with resultant ischemic injury to the cord. There is complete motor paralysis and loss of pain and temperature sensation distal to the lesion. Because the posterior columns are spared, the senses of light touch, motion, vibration, and gross proprioception are preserved. After bony reduction, an emergent CT myelogram is obtained to check for a removable extrinsic mass pressing on the cord.

The central spinal cord syndrome typically occurs with hyperextension injuries in older patients with spondylosis or stenosis. It is a partial cord syndrome characterized by weakness greater in the arms than the legs and worse in the hands than in the proximal upper extremity. There are variable bladder and scattered sensory losses. The cause is unknown, but it is often attributed to buckling of the ligamentum flavum into the cord during extension injury. Ischemic injury primarily to the center of the cord has been found at autopsy. The order of the motor fibers of the corticospinal tract explain the neurologic findings. The motor fibers serving the arms are nearer the injured center of the cord, and those serving the legs more lateral. Treatment usually is nonoperative, and there is a relatively good prognosis.

Brown-Séquard's syndrome involves injury to one side of the cord. There are paralysis and loss of gross proprioception and vibratory sensation on the side of the lesion and loss of pain and temperature sensation on the contralateral side. This crossed lesion is explained by the level of decussation of motor fibers in the medulla and the decussation of pain and temperature fibers two dermatome levels above their point of nerve root entry. This partial cord syndrome is usually due to penetrating wounds, although laterally placed disk protrusion, tumor, or hematoma can cause it.

PENETRATING INJURIES

Acute bony instability is very rare in penetrating wounds of the spine. High-velocity missile wounds can cause direct injury and more remote injury due to concussive forces. Treatment includes antibiotics; tetanus prophylaxis; methylprednisolone; and surgery to remove any extrinsic mass compressing the cord, to repair dural tears, and to debride devitalized tissue.

SPORTS INJURIES

Bruce and coworkers reported that football caused 66 percent of organized-sports-related cervical spine injuries, diving 18 percent, and rugby 9 percent. High school football in the United States causes 20 to 30 quadriplegic injuries per year. C5–C6 is the most common level of injury. Approximately 72 percent of cervical cord injuries occur during tackling, and 50 percent of college football players have experienced a paresthesia at least once.

In rugby, cervical injuries occur primarily when the scrummage collapses in the center and players behind keep pushing. Injuries during tackling are uncommon, since the lack of a helmet leads to different tackling techniques. Although soccer is the most widely played team sport in the world, soccer-related spinal cord injuries are uncommon. In soccer, central nervous system injuries are largely limited to closed head trauma. Wrestling, horseback riding, gymnastics, and trampoline yield a small number of cord injuries.

POSTTRAUMATIC SYRINGOMYELIA

According to Piatt's review, posttraumatic syringomyelia is characterized by progression of neurologic deficits distant from the level of a preceding injury. It occurs in approximately 1 percent of spinal-cord-injured patients but does not show itself for 4 to 9 years. The most common initial complaint is pain with coughing or straining, followed by paresthesias, numbness, weakness, and hyperhidrosis. Physical examination reveals hypesthesia, weakness, and diminished reflexes cephalad from the original lesion. Incomplete cord lesions may progress to spasticity and loss of retained bowel, bladder, and sexual function. It is usually unilateral in onset and remains asymetric over time.

RESEARCH

Allen's animal model for graded spinal cord injury uses a weight dropped a fixed distance through a vented tube onto the exposed spinal cord. Initial impact causes immediate paraplegia without microscopic or pathologic changes. Later, the cord develops a central hemorrhagic lesion. Animal models have shown a 4- to 8-h period in which gray and then white matter necrosis takes place. Therapeutic interventions attempt to halt or limit this ongoing process. Areas of investigation have included corticosteroids, osmotic diuretics, antiadrenergic compounds, naloxone, thyrotropic-releasing hormone, dimethyl sulfoxide, hyperbaric oxygen, and hypothermia. Only methylprednisolone has yet received an adequate trial in human patients. In a double-blind, randomized, controlled clinical trial of very high-dose methylprednisolone-treated patients, Bracken and coworkers reported that patients treated within 8 h of injury showed significantly greater motor function and pin and touch sensation.

Faden has investigated the theory that β endorphins released at the time of spinal cord injury cause a reduction in spinal cord blood flow, allowing secondary injury to occur. Using a cat model he reported that animals treated with naloxone or thyrotropic-releasing hormone showed less damage and significantly improved neurologic recovery than did animals receiving corticosteroids or placebo. Unfortunately, in Bracken and coworkers' multicenter human trial, naloxone showed no evidence of efficacy.

BIBLIOGRAPHY

Allen RL, Perot PL, Gudeman SK: Evaluation of acute nonpenetrating cervical spine cord injuries with CT metrizamide myelography. *J Neurosurg* 63:510, 1985.

Bracken MB, Shepard MJ, Collins WF, et al: A randomized controlled trial of methylprednisolone or naloxone in the treatment of acute spinal-cord injury. *N Engl J Med* 322:20, 1990.

Bruce DA, Schut L, Sutton LN: Brain and cervical spine injuries occurring during organized sports activities in children and adolescents. *Primary Care* 11:175, 1984.

Chilton J, Dagi TF: Acute cervical spinal cord injury. *Am J Emerg Med* 3:340, 1985.

Davidson JS, Birdsell DC: Cervical spine injury in patients with facial skeletal trauma. *Trauma,* 29:9, 1989.

Denis F: Spinal instability as defined by the three-column spine concept in acute spinal trauma. *Clin Orthop Rel Res* 189:65, 1984.

Faden AI: Neuropeptides and central nervous system injury. *Arch Neurol* 43:501, 1986.

Harris JH, Edeiken-Monroe B, Kopaniky DR: A practical classification of acute cervical spine injuries. *Orthop Clin North AM* 17:15, 1986.

Kalsbeek WD, McLaurin RL, Harris BS, et al: The national head and spinal cord injury survey: Major findings. *J Neurosurg* 53:519, 1980.

Kraus JF, Franti CE, Riggins RS, et al: Incidence of traumatic spinal cord lesions. *J Chronic Dis* 28:471, 1975.

Lamont A, Zachary J, Sheldon P: Cervical cord size in metrizamide myelography. *Clin Radiol* 32:409, 1981.

Maynard FM, Reynolds GG, Fountain S, et al: Neurological prognosis after traumatic quadriplegia. *J Neurosurg* 50:611, 1979.

McArdle CB et al: Surface coil MR of spinal trauma: Preliminary experience. *Am J Neuroradiol* 7:885, 1986.

Meyer GA, Berman IR, Doty DB, et al: Hemodynamic responses to acute quadriplegia with or without chest trauma. *J Neurosurg* 34:168, 1971.

Panjabi MM, White AA: Basic biomechanics of the spine. *Neurosurgery* 7:76, 1980.

Riggins RS, Kraus JF: The risk of neurologic damage with fractures of the vertebrae. *J Trauma* 17:126, 1977.

Shaffer MA, Doris PE: Limitation of the cross table lateral in detecting cervical spine injuries: A retrospective analyis. *Ann Emerg Med* 10:508, 1981.

Trafton G: Spinal cord injuries. *Surg Clin North Am* 62:61, 1982.

Wagner FC, Chehrazi B: Spinal cord injury: Indications for operative intervention. *Surg Clin North Am* 60:1049, 1980.

Weir DC: Roentgenographic signs of cervical injury. *Clin Orthoped* 109:9, 1975.

Wilkins RH, Rengachary SS (eds): *Neurosurgery*. New York, McGraw-Hill, 1985.

173
PENETRATING AND BLUNT NECK TRAUMA

Robert Swor

The management of the patient with a direct injury to the neck is a difficult problem in the emergency department. The physician must be concerned with airway patency, control of major hemorrhage, and stability of osseous structures and must also evaluate for other, less apparent but potentially lethal injuries.

The neck is unique in the body in that it has many important visceral structures that are not well protected by bone. It is in part protected by both the face and the chest but is still a region vulnerable to both penetrating injury and, less commonly, blunt trauma.

ANATOMY

The platysma is a major landmark in the discussion of penetrating neck injury, which is defined as any wound that violates the platysma. Along its entire length, this muscle is invested in fascia originating on the clavicle. It inserts on the mandible and extends over the proximal half of the sternocleidomastoid (SCM). It tamponades bleeding from neck injury and makes direct clinical evaluation difficult.

The SCM extends diagonally from the mastoid process of the skull to the superior sternum and clavicle. It divides the neck into the anterior triangle, bounded by the SCM, the midline, and the mandible. It contains most of the major vascular and visceral structures and the airway. The posterior triangle is bounded by the SCM, the trapezius, and the clavicle. It has relatively few structures except at its base. The posterior triangle is further divided by the spinal accessory nerve into a so-called careful region at the base and a carefree region that has a paucity of vital structures (Fig. 173-1).

Major vessels that are frequently injured by both blunt and penetrating injury lie in the anterior triangle. These vessels include carotid arteries, jugular veins, and the thyrocervical trunk. The vertebral arteries are well protected by bone and infrequently injured. The subclavian vessels lie at the base of the posterior triangle and may be injured by a vertical blow to that region.

In penetrating injury, and less commonly in blunt injury, neurologic structures are frequently involved. Understanding their location is important in determining injury to contiguous structures. The sympathetic chain ganglia lie posterior to the carotid sheath and are protected by it (Fig. 173-2). The spinal accessory nerve courses through the midportion of the posterior triangle and is used as an anatomical boundary between areas with vital structures and less worrisome areas.

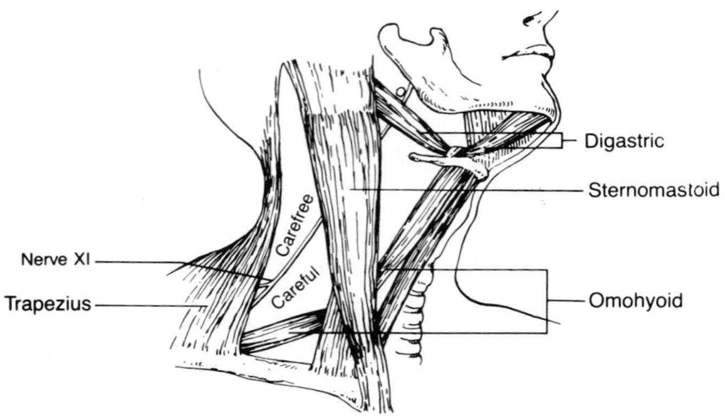

Fig. 173-1. Triangles of the neck.

Fascial planes play a major role in the management of neck trauma. The fascia that invests the platysma serves to tamponade bleeding. The carotid sheath is tough enough to deflect low-velocity missiles such as knives and small-caliber bullets. The cervical visceral fascia envelopes the esophagus and thyroid (Fig. 173-2). It is continuous with the mediastinum and serves as a conduit for mediastinal soilage with esophageal injury.

TYPES OF INJURY

As society becomes more violent, penetrating neck injuries increase in number and severity. Most early experience with such injuries is related to high-velocity missile injury encountered in warfare. Increasing numbers of civilian injuries occur secondary to stab wounds and low-velocity gunshot wounds from handguns.

The majority of injuries after penetrating injury are vascular. These injuries may present with massive hemorrhage or be occult. Both central nervous system (CNS) and peripheral nerve injury are frequent in most series, and bracheal plexus injury can occur with low neck injury. Neurologic injuries are difficult to assess in patients who are intoxicated or in shock. CNS deficits secondary to vascular injury are important to diagnose before surgical intervention. Air embolus secondary to venous injury is a rare but lethal complication. Arteriovenous fisulas are also reported in most series. Cervical spine injury is often overlooked and must be suspected in all neck injuries. Pharyngeal and esophageal injuries are frequently not apparent on initial presentation.

In blunt injury, the force is commonly a direct blow. Common mechanisms for such injury are steering wheel injury to a restrained driver of a car, direct blows during sports, "clothesline"-type injuries to drivers of recreational vehicles (motorcycles, all-terrain vehicles, snowmobiles, etc.), and strangulation. These injuries may cause laryngeal edema or fracture resulting in upper airway obstruction. Laryngotracheal separation has also been reported.

Airway injury is common in blunt trauma because of the anterior and fixed position of the larynx and trachea in the neck. Blunt injury to the vasculature and viscera also occurs. Avulsion of the carotid arteries has been reported after hangings, and cerebrovascular infarcts have also been reported after blunt injury. Perforation of the pharynx and the esophagus, although rare, may occur by the transient increase in intraluminal pressure that occurs during blunt injury.

MAJOR CAUSES OF DEATH

Early death after neck injury occurs by one of three mechanisms: CNS injury, exsanguination, or airway compromise. Most CNS injury occurs at the time of neck injury and is thus not preventable. Exsanguination and airway compromise should be treatable if they are recognized and appropriate emergency care is available. Late deaths occur secondary to sepsis, which may be the the result of missed injury. In a 1977 collective review of penetrating neck injury, Sankaran and Walt stated that approximately 2 percent of patients with penetrating neck wounds died because of iatrogenic error.

RESUSCITATION

Airway

The first priorities in the management of a patient with a neck injury are maintenance of the airway and control of the cervical spine. With both penetrating and blunt neck injuries, cervical spine injury must be assumed until ruled out by examination and cervical radiography. Management of the airway is most difficult because there may be direct damage to the airway itself. For patients in respiratory distress, endotracheal or nasotracheal intubation may be lifesaving. Several caveats, however, are necessary. The neck must be maintained in a neutral position. The patient must not be made to gag or cough, since this could dislodge a clot and produce massive bleeding. The airway itself must be evaluated for possible false passages secondary to the

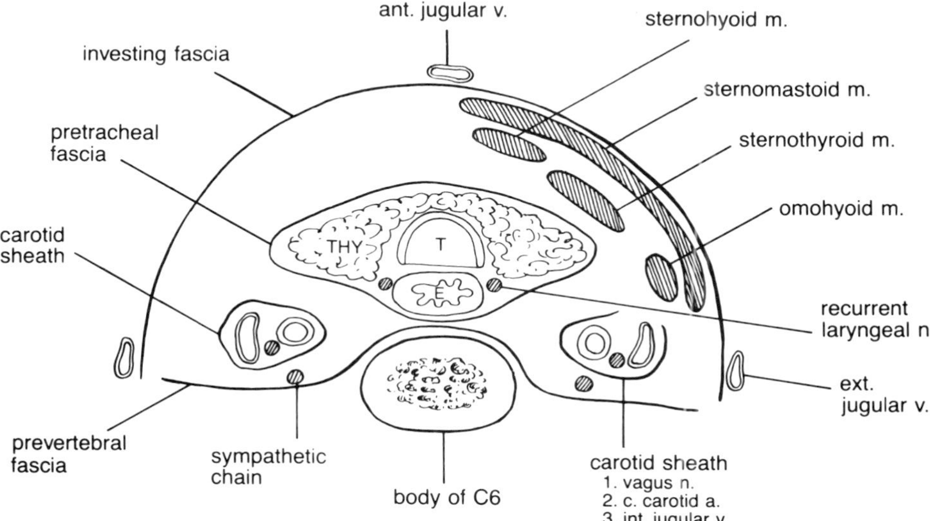

Fig. 173-2. Fascial planes of the neck.

injury. An endotracheal tube or a blind nasotracheal tube introduced into a false channel can cause hemorrhage and airway obstruction. Blunt injury may result in increasing respiratory distress from laryngeal edema or an expanding hematoma.

For many patients with traumatic neck injury, control of the airway from above may not be possible. Intubation without movement of the cervical spine is difficult and might not be technically possible. If the patient has associated maxillofacial injury, profuse emesis, or uncontrolled upper airway bleeding, the patient will require a surgical airway. Cricothyrotomy is the emergency procedure of choice in these cases, and transtracheal jet ventilation is advocated by some as a temporary alternative. Formal tracheotomy should be performed as soon as practical. Tracheotomy, however, is indicated in the setting of a complete laryngotracheal separation, which may occur as a consequence of blunt trauma to the larynx.

Breathing

Because of the proximity of the apex of the lung to the base of the neck, pneumothorox is frequently associated with neck trauma. Most commonly it occurs with penetrating injury, but it may occur secondary to blunt trauma. In both instances, needle decompression and tube thoracostomy may be lifesaving. Subclavian injury with subsequent hemothorax must also be suspected in low neck injury.

Circulation

Priorities that must be simultaneously addressed are control of external hemorrhage, assessment of degree of hemorrhage, and establishment of vascular access. Control of external hemorrhage may be established by direct pressure at the bleeding site without fear of compromising cerebral blood flow. One of the lessons learned during the Vietnam War was that young, healthy brains could tolerate up to 100 min of no flow through a carotid artery without neurologic sequalae. One must not, of course, compromise the airway with direct airway pressure or circumferential bandages about the neck. Attempts to control bleeding, by blind clamping of bleeders is inappropriate and can result in irreversible soft tissue and neurovascular injury. Dissection of a wound to a bleeding site should be done only in the surgical suite, where proximal and distal control of vessels can be obtained.

Vascular access may be done as for any trauma resuscitation, with a few notable differences. Central venous access should not be attempted in the region of an injury, since the resuscitation fluid may merely leak into the surrounding tissues. Similarly, if one suspects injury to the subclavian vessels, at least one intravenous (IV) line should be established in the lower extremity.

Air embolus is potentially fatal. If such injury is suspected, the patient should be kept in Trendelenberg's position.

EVALUATION

The most important part of evaluation is a careful history and physical examination. Injury to the neck produces many incipient injuries and may produce only subtle clues to diagnosis.

This history is focused on complaints related to the aerodigestive systems. Initial complaints of respiratory distress or hoarseness may indicate upper airway injury. Other symptoms suggestive of upper airway injury include neck pain, hemoptysis, or pain with speaking. Pharyngeal or esophageal injury may be indicated by dysphagia, odynophagia, or hematemesis. Complaints regarding neurologic function should also be elicited.

Physical examination must be careful and complete despite the local nature of the injury. One must look carefully for evidence of pneumothorax or hemothorax. A thorough neurologic examination is important (although often difficult in the shocky or intoxicated patient) to establish whether there is peripheral nervous system injury or, more important, CNS injury. The presence of a CNS deficit may be the result of direct CNS trauma or secondary to carotid or vertebral artery injury.

On examination of the neck, look for bleeding, hematoma, drooling, stridor, or tracheal deviation. Normal anatomic landmarks are often lost, especially in a male if there is laryngeal injury. The neck should be palpated for tenderness or crepitation. The neck and upper extremities must be assessed for pulse deficits, thrills and bruits.

Evaluation of the wound itself after a penetrating injury should be limited. The purpose is only to establish whether the platysma has been violated. Further probing can lead to uncontrollable hemorrhage. Full wound evaluation must be reserved for the operating room, where adequate proximal and distal control of vessels can be obtained. Early surgical consultation is mandatory if the platysma is violated.

Radiographic Evaluation

A complete cervical spine series should be obtained for both blunt and penetrating injury, to assess the bony structures, and to evaluate for soft tissue air and swelling. If airway injury is suspected, soft tissue technique should be requested for better airway evaluation. A good-quality chest x-ray must also be obtained to evaluate for the presence of pneumothorax, pneumomediastinum, or hemothorax. These findings suggest esophageal or tracheal injury.

Esophageal injury may be evaluated by the use of barium or gastrograffin esophograms. Most authorities prefer the use of gastrograffin

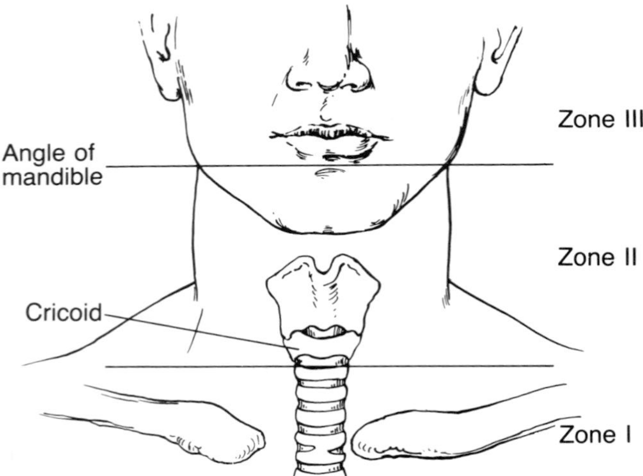

Fig. 173-3. Regions of the neck.

even though it is not as good diagnostically, because it is less irritating to surrounding tissues if extavasated. Regardless of the contrast medium used, this technique has a high false-negative rate (up to 25 percent) and is therefore helpful only if positive.

Interventional Studies

Fiberoptic endoscopy of both the gastrointestinal tract and the respiratory tract have ben used in many series to evaluate for acute injury. Esophagoscopy is a helpful adjunct, but many authors question its accuracy. Bronchoscopy is difficult with a patient in acute respiratory distress secondary to airway injury and may increase edema in an already traumatized airway. If attempted, both techniques should be utilized by an experienced physician and should be done under sedation to minimize trauma.

Arteriography

Early studies of penetrating trauma rarely utilized arteriography as a diagnostic modality. In their review of 20 years' experience in penetrating trauma, Sheely and coworkers report using three arteriograms.

More recently, Roon and Christenson utilized arteriography based on the level of injury to the neck. Dividing the neck into three zones—above the angle of the mandible, below the cricoid cartilage, and between the mandible and the cricoid (Fig. 173-3)—they performed arteriogaphy on all patients with penetrating injury to both high and low zones. The information obtained by arteriogram changed the operative strategy in 29 percent of patients with such injuries. This diagnostic approach has become a standard in most large centers.

Computed Tomography

Computed tomography (CT) has proved to be a valuable adjunct in the evaluation of the airway after blunt trauma, serving to well delineate the type and degree of injury. It is time consuming and should not be attempted in a patient with an acute airway injury.

MANAGEMENT OF PENETRATING INJURY

Management of penetrating neck injury is an area of controversy that continues to be debated in the surgical literature. Some authors argue that all wounds that penetrate the platsyma should have surgical exploration in the operating suite. Others argue that such a radical approach is unnecessary, that these wounds can be evaluated utilizing ancillary modalities, and that exploration can be reserved for unstable patients or those with specific indications.

The rationale for the aggressive approach to penetrating injuries highlights the difficulty in evaluation and the hazards of missed injury.

A. Reasons for exploration:
   1. Fogelman and Stewart reported increased mortality from 6 to 35 percent with delayed exploration. Sheely and coworkers reviewed 20 years' experience in Houston and reported a 4-percent mortality rate for patients with initial negative examination who were observed.
   2. Some series report a large number of patients with clinically negative examinations but positive findings on exploration.
   3. Sankaran and Walt report, in a collective review, a 2-percent mortality rate for esophageal injury with early surgery and a 44-percent mortality rate with delayed operation. Similarly, they report a 15-percent mortality rate with major vascular injury treated with early operation and a 67-percent mortality rate when diagnosis and definitive care are delayed.

B. Reasons for observation:
   1. Rates of negative exploration after mandatory exploration are very high (37 to 63 percent).
   2. Many series report false-negative surgical explorations.
   3. Some wounds, especially posterior triangle injuries, are unlikely to result in significant trauma.
   4. When patients present to the emergency department after significant delay, observation is reasonable.

A number of studies have been designed to address this controversy. Elerding and coworkers established criteria for exploration and prospectively studied all patients with penetrating neck injury who presented to their institution (Table 173-1). All patients were then explored. All patients with significant injury had criteria for exploration, and no patient without criteria had significant injury.

MANAGEMENT OF BLUNT INJURY

Blunt injury to the neck can occur from motor vehicle accidents, sports injuries, or strangulation. Forces that result in injury are direct blows to the airway, hyperextension of the neck, or increase of intraluminal pressure due to thoracic injury or Valsalva maneuvers at the time of injury.

External signs of injury may be limited to soft tissue injury to the anterior portion of the neck, and patient complaints may be minimal. Hoarseness, dysphonia, or dyspnea demand a complete evaluation. Neurologic injury may be the result of blunt vascular injury or injury to the cervical cord. Initial evaluation should include indirect laryngoscopy in the emergency department. Radiographic evaluation may show the presence of soft tissue air or displacement of fracture of the hyoid bond.

Early signs of airway instability require control of the airway, since progression to complete compromise may be rapid. Control of the airway by intubation may not be definitive and may exacerbate injury because of the rare risk of laryngotracheal separation. Close observation

Table 173-1. Indications for Neck Exploration

Vascular
Continued hemorrhage
Unstable vital signs
Diminished or absent pulses
Large or expanding hematoma
Airway
Difficulty breathing
Voice change
Visceral
Difficulty swallowing
Subcutaneous emphysema
Coughing, spitting, or vomiting of blood
Neurologic

of the patient after airway control will ascertain whether a partial airway injury has been worsened by treatment. Some authors argue that laryngotracheal injury is a contraindication to cricothyrotomy and that emergent tracheostomy is the airway procedure of choice.

If laryngeal injury is suspected due to the mechanism of injury or the nature of complaints, the stable airway should be evaluated by CT scanning of the larynx, which is extremely sensitive in identifying subtle injury.

BIBLIOGRAPHY

Beal SL, Pottmeyer EW, Spisso JM: Esophageal perforation following external blunt trauma. *J Trauma* 28:1425, 1988.

Camnitz S et al: Acute blunt laryngeal and tracheal trauma. *Am J Emerg Med* 5:157, 1987.

Carducci B et al: Collective review—penetrating neck trauma: Consensus and controversies. *Ann Emerg Med* 15:208, 1986.

Fogelman MJ, Stewart RD: Penetrating wounds of the neck. *Am J Surg* 91:581, 1956.

Elerding SC, Manart FD, Moore EE: A reappraisal of penetrating neck injury management. *J Trauma* 20:695, 1980.

Gussack GS, Jurkovich GJ: Treatment dilemmas in laryngotracheal trauma. 28:1439, 1988.

Line, WS, Stanley RB, Choi JH: Strangulation: A full spectrum of blunt neck trauma. *Ann Oto Rhinol Laryngol* 94:542, 1985.

Roon AJ, Christianson: Evaluation and treatment of penetrating cervical injuries. *J Trauma* 19:391, 1979.

Sankaran S, Walt AJ: Penetrating wounds of the neck: Principles and some controversies. *Surg Clin North Am* 57:139, 1977.

Sheely CH, Mattox KL, Revl GJ, et al: Current concepts in the management of penetrating neck trauma. *J Trauma* 15:895, 1975.

174
THORACIC TRAUMA
Robert F. Wilson

CHEST WALL, BRONCHI, LUNG, AND DIAPHRAGM

Patients with chest trauma who develop acute severe respiratory distress have a high mortality rate. In Wilson's series, 11 percent of patients admitted with chest trauma required endotracheal intubation almost immediately upon entrance to the emergency department. Of these, 58 percent died. If shock accompanied the respiratory distress, the mortality rate rose to 73 percent. In patients with blunt chest trauma, the most frequent factors associated with acute respiratory distress include shock, coma, multiple rib fractures, and hemopneumothorax. In patients with penetrating trauma, respiratory distress is usually due to severe shock or hemopneumothorax (see Tables 174-1 and 174-2).

Initial Resuscitation, Airway Control, and Ventilation

Diagnosis of the cause of respiratory distress must be made promptly. If the patient is making little or no effort to breathe, central nervous system dysfunction due to head trauma or drugs is the most likely problem. If the patient is attempting to breathe but is moving little or no air, upper airway obstruction should be suspected.

The most common cause of upper airway obstruction in comatose patients is prolapse of the tongue into the pharynx. Other, less frequent causes of upper airway obstruction are dentures, vomitus, or blood clots in the pharynx, larynx, or upper trachea. Occasionally, direct trauma may cause fracture of the larynx or cricotracheal separation. Inspiratory stridor, which is a particularly important sign of upper airway obstruction, does not usually occur unless there is at least a 70-percent occlusion. With any suspected laryngeal injury, cautious endoscopy should be performed in the operating room as soon as possible.

If the patient is attempting to breathe and the upper airway appears to be intact but the breath sounds are poor, thoracic problems such as flail chest, hemopneumothorax, diaphragmatic injury, or parenchymal lung damage should be considered. In all cases of respiratory distress, the airway must be secured while the neck is stabilized. Techniques for airway support are described in detail in Chap. 5. Following airway control, oxygenation and ventilation can be accomplished.

If the patient has poor venous return because of hypovolemia, ventilation with excessive pressures can further reduce venous return and cause cardiac arrest. Hypovolemic patients should probably be ventilated with only 8 to 10 mL/kg tidal volumes at 10 to 14 times a minute until venous return is improved. If there is a lung injury or if there are fragile subpleural blebs, bagging the patient vigorously can also cause a tension pneumothorax to develop rapidly, further reducing venous return.

Any patient with a lung injury, especially with hemoptysis, should be considered at risk for developing a systemic air embolus. Patients with intrabronchial bleeding are also at risk for flooding normal alveoli with blood, causing severe hypoxemia.

Vasovagal responses are rare in injured patients, but they can occur during insertion of endotracheal, nasogastric, or chest tubes. One should be alert for the development of this problem during any invasive procedure if the patient has an inappropriately slow pulse rate that gets even slower as the procedure is being performed. Hyperventilation can cause severe alkalosis, reducing ionized calcium levels and producing serious arrhythmias.

Table 174-1. Causes of Inadequate Ventilation after Chest Trauma

CNS dysfunction	Chest wall injury
Due to trauma	Pain from fractures
Due to drugs	Flail chest
Airway obstruction	Open (sucking) wounds
Pharynx	Pleural collections
Vomitus	Hemothorax
Foreign bodies	Pneumothorax
Relaxed tongue	Simple
Larynx and trachea	Tension
Foreign bodies	Diaphragmatic injuries
Direct trauma	Parenchymal dysfunction
	Contusion
	Aspiration
	Intrabronchial hemorrhage
	Previous pulmonary disease

Relief of Hemopneumothorax

If a hemothorax or pneumothorax is suspected in a patient with acute severe respiratory distress, a "blind" chest tube (a chest tube inserted without waiting for a chest roentgenogram) should be inserted through the fourth or fifth intercostal space in the anterior axillary line on the affected side. Digital examination of the pleural cavity before the chest tube is inserted will reduce the chances of inserting the chest tube into the lung parenchyma (if the lung is stuck to that area by adhesions), through a high diaphragm, or into herniated abdominal viscera.

Once a properly functioning chest tube is in place, it should be connected to 20 to 30 cmH_2O suction. If a tension pneumothorax is present, a large needle can be inserted into the pleural cavity through the second intercostal space in the midclavicular line to produce temporary decompression while a chest tube is being inserted. Use of a stopcock and 50-mL syringe may help remove air from the chest.

Intercostal Nerve Blocks

The severe pain of multiple fractured ribs can greatly impair ventilation. In such circumstances, blocking the intercostal nerves of the fractured ribs plus two ribs above and two ribs below with a long-acting local anesthetic such as 0.5% bupivacaine hydrochloride (Marcaine) mixed with an equal quantity of 1% lidocaine with epinephrine may dramatically relieve pain and improve ventilation for 6 to 8 h or longer. If there are any residual tender spots after the intercostal block, they should also be injected with the local anesthetic.

Ventilatory Support

In patients with chest trauma, impaired ventilation in spite of an open airway, relief of chest wall pain, and drainage of hemopneumothorax is an indication for ventilatory support. Respiratory failure associated with a flail chest is best treated by endotracheal intubation and ventilatory assistance, particularly if there are associated injuries. Ven-

Table 174-2. Injuries Associated with Respiratory Distress after Chest Trauma

Trauma	Incidence (%)
BLUNT	
Intrathoracic	95
Rib fracture/flail chest	75
Hemothorax, pneumothorax	55
Lung contusion	39
Intracranial injury	39
Diaphragmatic injury	9
Spinal cord injury	4
PENETRATING	
Intrathoracic	
Pulmonary damage with hemopneumothorax	55
Cardiac injury	29
Diaphragmatic injury	17
Chest wall defects	7

tilatory assistance should be strongly considered in patients with a flail chest and marginal ventilation if the patient is in shock, has had multiple injuries, is comatose, requires multiple transfusions, is elderly, or has preexisting pulmonary disease. A respiratory rate greater than 30 to 35 breaths per minute, a vital capacity less than 10 to 15 mL/kg, a negative inspiratory force less than 20 to 30 cmH_2O, and an increased respiratory effort can be considered early indications for ventilatory support.

Serial blood gas values are more informative than isolated values. Consequently, an arterial sample should be drawn soon after admission to the hospital and at frequent intervals thereafter. Metabolic acidosis with an arterial P_{CO_2} above 40 mmHg is evidence of a significant reduction in pulmonary function and indicates the need for ventilatory support. If the ventilatory response is adequate, the P_{CO_2} will be less than 35 mmHg if the pH is <7.30, less than 30 mmHg if the pH is <7.20, and less than 25 mmHg if the pH is <7.10.

If the arterial P_{O_2} is less than 50 mmHg while the patient is breathing room air or less than 80 mmHg while the patient is breathing supplemental oxygen (equivalent to an FI_{O_2} of 0.4 or more), the patient should probably be placed on a ventilator.

Continuous pulse oximetry should be part of the initial evaluation of anyone with moderate to severe chest trauma. Pulse oximetry allows one to detect subclinical pulmonary deterioration earlier and to rapidly determine the effect of ventilator or drug changes. When used properly, pulse oximetry can greatly reduce the need for multiple arterial blood gas determinations. Capnometry can also be combined with arterial P_{CO_2} determinations.

Shock

Once adequate ventilation has been attained, efforts should be directed toward rapidly restoring tissue perfusion, particularly if there is any respiratory distress. In our studies, the most frequent causes of shock in patients with blunt chest trauma were pelvic or extremity fractures (59 percent), intraabdominal injuries (41 percent), and intrathoracic bleeding (26 percent). In addition, 15 percent had myocardial contusion, and 7 percent had spinal cord injuries.

In patients with penetrating chest trauma, the cause of shock was intrathoracic injury in 74 percent. The most frequent sources of intrathoracic injuries causing massive bleeding were lung (36 percent), heart (25 percent), great vessels (14 percent), and intercostal or internal mammary arteries (10 percent). In addition, 40 percent of the patients with penetrating chest trauma had extrathoracic injuries contributing to the shock. These included intraabdominal bleeding (14 percent), bleeding from extremity vessels (12 percent), and spinal cord injuries (5 percent).

Treatment

Fluid

Failure to correct hypotension within 15 to 30 min of its onset greatly increases the mortality rate. In previously healthy patients requiring massive transfusions but having hypotension for less than 30 min, the mortality rate has averaged only about 10 percent. However, if the hypotension is present for more than 30 min, the mortality rises to about 50 percent. If the patient has preexisting disease or is over 65 years of age, the mortality with massive transfusions plus prolonged hypotension exceeds 90 percent.

To provide fluids rapidly, one needs at least two large intravenous (IV) catheters. If peripheral veins are not readily available, one may be forced to cannulate the subclavian or internal jugular veins. However, inserting a subclavian vein line on the side opposite a severe chest injury can be very dangerous. If one side of a chest is injured and the other lung is collapsed during insertion of a central IV line, the impaired function of both lungs could be rapidly fatal.

Chest Tube and Thoracotomy

A large hemothorax or pneumothorax can seriously interfere with ventilation and venous return; consequently, it should be evacuated as rapidly as possible. However, if blood is pouring out rapidly through the chest tube, the vital signs should be followed very closely. If the vital signs are improving, the blood can continue to be evacuated. However, if the vital signs deteriorate as the blood is being evacuated in spite of the rapid infusion of IV fluids, the patient may now be exsanguinating into the chest as the tamponading effect of the hemothorax is removed. In these unusual circumstances, the chest tube should be clamped and the patient taken directly to the operating room for an emergency thoracotomy.

Cardiac Arrest

External Massage

In patients with cardiac arrest due to chest trauma, external cardiac massage is generally of no value and is in fact likely to be harmful. Since the trauma patient suffering cardiac arrest is generally hypovolemic, external massage is usually ineffective and may actually cause severe additional injury to the heart, liver, lungs, or great vessels. In one series, major cardiovascular disruption was found in all patients receiving external cardiac compression after truncal trauma. In addition, of the patients receiving forced ventilation and prehospital external cardiac compression, 12 percent died with air emboli in their coronary arteries.

Open cardiac massage is usually performed through an anterolateral incision in the fifth intercostal space on the side of the injury. The pericardium is opened vertically anterior to the phrenic nerve. The thoracic incision allows direct inspection of the heart, control of bleeding sites in the chest, and complete evacuation of any pericardial tamponade or hemopneumothorax. In addition, a left thoracotomy allows the physician to compress or clamp the descending thoracic aorta. Since about 60 percent of the cardiac output normally passes below the diaphragm, clamping the descending thoracic aorta can increase coronary and carotid blood flow almost threefold. If the arterial systolic blood pressure does not rise to 90 mmHg within 5 to 10 min of aortic cross-clamping, further resuscitation will probably be of no avail.

Recently, there has been increased interest in emergency department thoracotomies. It is becoming increasingly clear that emergency department thoracotomy can be helpful in patients with penetrating wounds of the chest, neck, or extremities. However, resuscitative efforts are seldom of benefit in (1) patients requiring cardiopulmonary resuscitation (CPR) for blunt trauma, (2) patients requiring CPR for penetrating abdominal or head injuries, and (3) patients "dead at the scene."

Diagnosis

Symptoms

The most frequent symptoms of thoracic trauma are chest pain and shortness of breath. The pain is usually well localized to the involved area of the chest wall, but not infrequently it is referred to the abdomen, neck, shoulder, or arms. Dyspnea and tachypnea are important symptoms of lung and chest wall damage but are nonspecific and may also be caused by anxiety or pain from other injuries.

Physical Examination

Excessive reliance on chest x-rays may lead to delay in performing life-saving procedures. Unfortunately, many physicians, when confronted with a patient with chest trauma, rely on the chest x-ray and spend relatively little time on the physical examination. After only a brief auscultation of the anterior and lateral chest, they may send the patient directly to the x-ray department. A rather thorough physical examination, however, can be performed rapidly and may provide valuable information to help confirm or rule out any equivocal findings on the x-ray. Tension pneumothorax, in particular, should be diagnosed and treated before obtaining a chest x-ray.

Inspection

Chest Wall

Without careful inspection of the chest wall, one can easily overlook contusions, flail chest, intrathoracic bleeding, and open (''sucking'') chest wounds. In some patients a contusion may be the only external evidence of severe thoracic trauma. The paradoxical motion of a flail chest may be minimal when the patient is first seen, especially if it involves the lateral or posterior thorax, but it will tend to get worse over the next 24 to 48 h.

Although external bleeding is easily recognized, it may be difficult to determine whether the source is intrathoracic or from the chest wall itself. Most chest wounds that communicate with the pleural cavity are readily apparent because of the noise air makes as it passes through the tissue of the chest wall. However, some of these wounds are open only intermittently and may not be discovered until much later when a pneumothorax develops.

Neck

Distended neck veins, especially when the patient is sitting upright, may indicate the presence of pericardial tamponade, tension pneumothorax, cardiac failure, or air embolism. However, the distended neck veins may not appear until hypovolemia has been corrected. If the face and neck are cyanotic and swollen, severe damage to the superior mediastinum, with occlusion or compression of the superior vena cava, should be suspected. Severe subcutaneous emphysema from a torn bronchus or laceration of the lung may cause much swelling of the neck and face, quickly obliterating landmarks and, in some instances, shutting the eyelids.

Abdomen

A scaphoid abdomen may indicate a diaphragmatic injury with herniation of abdominal contents into the chest. Excessive abdominal movement with respiration may indicate chest wall damage that might not otherwise be apparent. A rocking-horse type of ventilation may indicate a high spinal cord injury with paralysis of intercostal muscles.

Palpation

Palpation should begin with determining whether the trachea is in its normal position, which is in the midline or slightly to the right. Palpation of the chest wall may also reveal areas of localized tenderness or crepitation from fractured ribs or subcutaneous emphysema. Well-localized and consistent tenderness over ribs should be considered to be due to rib fractures, even if the initial x-rays appear to be normal.

Motion of a portion of the sternum or severe localized tenderness may be the only objective evidence of a fractured sternum. When a patient is coughing or straining, the physician can sometimes palpate abnormal motion of an unstable portion of the chest wall better than he or she can see it. Sternal fractures can be missed very easily on routine chest x-rays.

Percussion

Percussion of the chest wall can be of great help in differentiating between a hemothorax and pneumothorax. Dullness to percussion over one side of the chest following trauma may be the first evidence that a hemothorax is present; hyperresonance, on the other hand, may indicate the presence of a pneumothorax. A fairly large hemothorax can easily be missed if the chest x-ray is taken while the patient is lying flat.

If the pericardial cavity is greatly distended by an effusion or tamponade, the area of cardiac dullness may extend beyond the midclavicular line on the left or the sternal border on the right. This sign is especially helpful if the point of maximal impulse is located more than an inch inside the left border of cardiac dullness.

Auscultation

Whenever possible, the chest should be auscultated systematically and thoroughly, anteriorly, laterally, and posteriorly at both the bases and apices. If the breath sounds are equal bilaterally, the major bronchi are probably intact. Decreased breath sounds on one side usually indicate the presence of hemothorax or pneumothorax but may also occur if the endotracheal tube is in too far and is ventilating only one lung. Before inserting a chest tube into a patient with acute respiratory distress and decreased breath sounds on one side, one should check the position of the endotracheal tube if one is present. The presence of bowel sounds high in the chest may be the first indication of a diaphragmatic injury. Occasionally, decreased breath sounds on one side are due to a bronchial foreign body or ruptured bronchus.

Injury to the Chest Wall

Soft Tissue Injuries

Bleeding

Probing of penetrating chest wounds to determine their depth or direction can be dangerous because it can damage underlying structures and cause severe recurrent bleeding, pneumothorax, or a sucking chest wound. Bleeding from the larger chest wall muscles can be rather brisk at times and is best controlled initially by local pressure. Later, one can inspect the depths of the wound in the operating room and use ligatures to control the bleeding and carefully close the wound.

Open (Sucking) Chest Wounds

Small open chest wounds can act as one-way valves, allowing air to enter during inspiration but none to leave during expiration, thereby causing an increasing pneumothorax. This not only reduces tidal volume but can also interfere with venous return. With larger chest wall wounds, air may preferentially enter the chest through the wound rather than through the tracheobronchial tree. If the open chest wound exceeds two-thirds the area of the trachea, effective ventilation may cease.

Sucking wounds of the chest should be covered immediately by a sterile airtight dressing, such as a petrolatum gauze, and a chest tube should be inserted at a separate site to relieve the pneumothorax. The chest tube is not inserted through the wound because it is then likely to follow the missile tract into the lung or diaphragm.

Tissue Loss

Injuries caused by close-range shotgun blasts or high-powered rifles may destroy such large quantities of chest wall that it may be impossible to close the chest wall in the usual manner. It is important, however, to cover the lungs and heart and close the diaphragm. For small defects, resection of adjacent ribs and a thoracoplasty may be adequate. With large defects, rotated muscle flaps and/or Marlex mesh may be required.

Subcutaneous Emphysema

Subcutaneous emphysema usually develops because air from lung parenchyma or the tracheobronchial tree has gained access to the chest wall through an opening in the parietal pleura. The air may also reach the chest wall by dissecting back along the bronchi into the hilum and mediastinum and then into the extrapleural spaces. Extensive subcutaneous emphysema should also make one suspect an injury to the pharynx, larynx, or esophagus.

Swelling from subcutaneous emphysema may occasionally reach massive proportions, swelling the eyelids shut and distending the scrotum to several times normal. Although the patient's appearance may be greatly distorted and there may be severe discomfort, the subcutaneous emphysema itself does not usually cause any significant ventilatory or hemodynamic problem unless there is an associated pneumothorax.

Patients with subcutaneous emphysema should be thought to have an underlying pneumothorax even if it is not visible on the chest x-ray. If the patient requires a general anesthetic or is to be placed on a ventilator, a chest tube should be inserted on the involved side(s). If the subcutaneous emphysema is severe, a major bronchial injury should be suspected and sought by bronchoscopy.

If there appears to be any respiratory difficulty that may be due to mediastinal emphysema, a tracheostomy around which the skin and fascia are closed only loosely may serve to maintain adequate ventilation and also allow a route for air to escape from the mediastinum and subcutaneous tissue. Very rarely, linear incisions into the subcutaneous space of the chest wall may be required to relieve massive subcutaneous emphysema. Once the initiating cause is controlled, the subcutaneous emphysema usually disappears gradually over a period of several days.

Bony Injuries

Clavicular Fractures

Isolated clavicular fractures due to blunt trauma are usually relatively harmless. Occasionally, however, direct trauma produces sharp fragments that may injure the subclavian vein and produce a moderately large hematoma or venous thrombosis. Rarely, excess callus forming later at the site of a clavicular fracture may press against the subclavian artery or brachial plexus, producing a thoracic outlet syndrome.

Rib Fractures

Simple Fractures

Rib fractures should be assumed to be present in any patient who has localized pain and tenderness over one or more ribs after chest trauma. Rib fractures are probably the most frequently missed fractures after trauma. Between 10 and 50 percent of rib fractures (especially the anterior and lateral portions of the first four ribs) may not be apparent on x-ray, particularly for the first few days after injury. Furthermore, injuries to the cartilaginous portions of the ribs may never be seen on x-ray.

It is now felt that the principal diagnostic goal with clinically suspected rib fractures is the detection of significant complications, especially hemopneumothorax, pulmonary contusion, or major vascular injury. Of all the available tests, a simple upright posteroanterior (PA) chest x-ray has the greatest yield in detecting fractures and associated injuries or complications.

If there is a suspicion of a pneumothorax that is not seen on the initial chest x-rays, the patient should also have inspiratory and expiratory PA x-rays. As a general rule, a pneumothorax is seen better on expiratory chest films where the pneumothorax space takes up a larger percentage of the involved hemithorax. If the patient had severe trauma, if the rib fractures have sharp fragments, or if the patient had other injuries, serial chest roentgenograms (every 6 to 12 h for 24 to 48 h) should be obtained. Delayed pneumothorax or hemothorax (due to trauma to the lung parenchyma or intercostal vessels by rib fragments) may occasionally develop more than 12 to 24 h after the initial injury.

The pain of rib fractures can greatly interfere with ventilation. Strapping the chest with adhesive tape or a rib belt to relieve the pain may be effective in young athletic individuals with only a few rib fractures; however, in less vigorous patients, strapping may significantly reduce ventilation and cause progressive atelectasis. Probably the best analgesic for mild to moderate chest wall pain is acetaminophen with codeine (Tylenol no. 3) or ibuprofen, 600 to 800 mg every 6 to 8 h as needed. If the patient is admitted, an intercostal nerve block with bupivacaine (Marcaine) may dramatically relieve pain, muscle spasm, and ventilation for 6 to 12 h. Epidural analgesia can work even better but requires admission to an intensive care unit (ICU) or step-down bed for apnea monitoring.

First and Second Rib Fractures

Except with direct trauma, such as with a hammer, it takes great force to fracture the first and second ribs. In a series reported by J. M. Wilson and associates, 40 percent of patients with fractures of the first and second ribs had myocardial contusion, bronchial tears, or major vascular injury.

First rib fractures are usually associated with higher mortalities (15 to 36 percent) than any other rib fractures because of the frequent severe associated injuries. However, in Richardson's series, 49 patients with second rib fractures had a higher mortality (27 percent) than 71 patients with first rib fractures (15 percent). Two-thirds of the deaths were due to head injury or rupture of major vessels.

Multiple Rib Fractures

Severe pain from multiple rib fractures is best controlled with repeated intercostal nerve blocks or epidural analgesia. A chest x-ray should be obtained after each intercostal block, however, to be sure the patient has not developed a pneumothorax.

If a patient with fractured ribs, especially ribs 9, 10, and 11, becomes hypotensive and does not have a large hemothorax or tension pneumothorax, intraabdominal bleeding must be suspected. In one series of 783 patients with blunt chest trauma, 71 percent of the patients admitted in shock had a ruptured intraabdominal viscus.

In general, it is wise to hospitalize patients with fractured ribs for at least 24 to 48 h if they cannot cough and clear their secretions adequately, especially if they are elderly or have preexisting pulmonary disease. Admitting the patient also provides time to observe the patient for associated injuries that might not be apparent initially. Aspiration pneumonitis and fat embolism often do not become apparent clinically for 24 to 48 h.

Flail Chest

Pathophysiology

Segmental fractures (i.e., fractures in two or more locations on the same rib) of three or more adjacent ribs anteriorly or laterally often result in an unstable chest wall, and the phenomenon known as flail chest. This injury is characterized by a paradoxical inward movement of the involved portion of the chest wall during inspiration and outward movement during expiration.

Although the paradoxical motion of the involved chest wall greatly increases the work of breathing, the main cause of the hypoxemia of flail chest is the underlying lung contusion. In the past, pendelluft (a ventilatory phenomenon referring to movement of air back and forth between the injured and uninjured lungs with each breath) was considered to be an important cause of the hypoxemia seen with flail chest. However, pendelluft is probably significant only when the upper airway is partially obstructed.

Immediately after the injury little flail may be apparent. Later, as fluid moves into the area of the pulmonary contusion, lung compliance falls and more pressure is needed to inflate the lungs. The increasing pressure differential between intrathoracic and atmospheric pressure may then overcome the resistance of the muscles attached to the fractured ribs, thereby allowing the involved chest wall to develop increasing paradox. In addition, the patient may fatigue rapidly because of the decreased efficiency of ventilation and increasing muscle effort. Thus, a vicious cycle of decreasing efficiency of ventilation, increasing fatigue, and hypoxemia may develop. In some instances, the increasing fatigue with breathing can result in a sudden respiratory arrest.

Treatment

Initial therapy. A severe flail chest can most quickly be managed initially by applying a sandbag or direct pressure over the unstable portion of the chest wall. Although this reduces vital capacity, it can relieve some of the pain, and it increases the efficiency of ventilation.

Nonventilatory therapy. One of the major advances in the definitive management of severe flail chest has been the use of early ventilatory assistance. Nevertheless, patients with mild to moderate flail chest and little or no underlying pulmonary contusion or associated injuries can often be managed without a respirator.

Trinkle and associates reported a study that indicated that mechanical ventilation is not necessary in many patients with a flail chest and might even be deleterious. Important aspects of his nonventilatory therapy included (1) relief of pain by analgesics or intercostal nerve block, (2) frequent coughing and chest physiotherapy, and (3) restriction of intravenous fluids to prevent fluid overload. He also advised the use of steroids and albumin, but the value of such agents is extremely controversial. His aggressive respiratory therapy kept many patients off the ventilator. However, ventilatory support was provided if, in spite of this regimen, the arterial P_{O_2} remained less than 80 mmHg on supplement oxygen.

Ventilatory support. Our usual indications for early ventilatory support of patients with flail chest include shock, three or more associated injuries, severe head injury, previous severe pulmonary disease, fracture of eight or more ribs, or age greater than 65 years. In our experience, early (prophylactic) ventilatory assistance in patients with flail chest and one or two significant associated injuries is associated with a mortality of only 7 percent. This is in sharp contrast to a mortality rate of 69 percent in similar patients in whom ventilatory assistance is delayed until there is clinical evidence of respiratory failure. Patients with three or more associated injuries have had a high mortality rate even with early ventilatory support.

Ventilated patients seem to do better if intermittent mandatory ventilation (IMV), rather than controlled mandatory ventilation (CMV), is used. In Cullen's series the mean ventilator time of patients treated with IMV and positive end-expiratory pressure (PEEP, 5.1 ± 4.7 days) was significantly less than that of patients treated with standard CMV (11.2 ± 6.2 days).

Sternal Fractures

Sternal fractures are frequently associated with cardiovascular injury, particularly myocardial contusions. In one series, 91 percent (10/11) of patients with a fractured sternum had impaired motion of the anterior heart. Consequently, in patients with a fractured sternum, serial EKGs and creatine phosphokinase isoenzyme (CPK-MB) studies should be done every 8 h for the first 24 to 32 h and a two-dimensional echocardiogram or radionuclide angiogram should be performed on clinically suspicious cases. Transverse, unstable sternal fractures may produce a significant flail and may require ventilator support.

Traumatic Asphyxia

Sudden, severe crushing of the chest, especially by heavy weights, may cause subconjunctival hemorrhage or petechiae together with vascular engorgement; edema; and cyanosis of the head, neck, and upper extremities. This clinical picture appears to be due to an abrupt sustained rise in superior vena caval pressure and concurrent closure of the airway after deep inspiration. Although these patients often look moribund initially, neurologic impairment is usually only temporary, and long-term morbidity is due primarily to associated injuries.

Injury to the Lungs

Pulmonary Contusions

Pathophysiology

The pathologic changes in pulmonary contusion include interstitial edema with capillary damage, resulting in interstitial and intraalveolar accumulations of fluid and extravasation of blood. The increasing interstitial edema and peribronchial extravasation of red blood cells tends to cause a progressive decrease in compliance and an increasing physiologic shunt and hypoxemia for at least 24 to 48 h. If atelectasis and pneumonia can be prevented during that time, the lungs usually improve rapidly thereafter.

Diagnosis

Areas of opacification of the lung following blunt chest trauma are usually considered to be pulmonary contusions. Aspiration pneumonia and fat embolism are not usually seen on the initial chest x-rays. Interestingly, at thoracotomy, autopsy, or CT scan, the extent of the lung injury is usually much larger than suspected on the original chest x-ray. As a general rule, chest x-ray changes tend to lag at least 24 h behind the blood gas changes seen with pulmonary contusions or the adult respiratory distress syndrome (ARDS).

Treatment

Treatment of pulmonary contusions primarily involves maintenance of adequate ventilation of the lungs. Chest physiotherapy, intercostal nerve blocks, epidural analgesia, coughing, and nasotracheal suction are used as needed. If ventilatory assistance is required, ventilation with IMV and PEEP usually provides much better ventilation-perfusion matching, better venous return, and quicker weaning than does standard controlled ventilation.

Although most investigators feel that steroids are of no value in pulmonary contusion, large doses of steroids may reduce the size of experimental pulmonary contusions.

Patients who have a severe unilateral lung injury and are responding poorly to conventional mechanical ventilation may benefit from synchronous independent lung ventilation (SILV) provided through a double-lumen endobronchial catheter. This technique helps prevent overinflation of the normal lung and underinflation of the damaged, poorly compliant lung.

Pulmonary Hematoma

Pulmonary hematomas are rather large parenchymal tears filled with blood. The hematomas generally resolve spontaneously over a few weeks; however, if they become infected, they can form lung abscesses that may be very difficult to manage. The hematomas are more likely to become infected if a thoracotomy is performed or if there is prolonged chest tube drainage of the pleural cavity, especially if the lung is not completely expanded.

Pulmonary Lacerations with Hemopneumothorax

Major hemorrhage from lacerations of the lung following blunt trauma are usually caused by the sharp ends of fractured ribs. Occasionally they may be caused by tearing of the lung at previous pleural adhesions as the lungs move away from the chest wall during rapid deceleration. In some instances, the adhesions themselves are quite vascular, and on rare occasions a torn adhesion will bleed enough to cause shock.

Systemic Air Embolism

In patients with penetrating chest wounds, and particularly those with hemoptysis, positive-pressure ventilation must be used with great care. High ventilatory pressures, especially over 50 cmH_2O, may force air from an injured bronchus into an adjacent injured vessel, producing systemic air emboli. This probably accounts for many of the severe arrhythmias or central nervous system (CNS) changes that occur when patients with penetrating chest wounds are intubated and ventilated.

If systemic air embolism occurs, the head should be lowered and an immediate thoracotomy should be performed to clamp the injured area of lung and then aspirate air from the heart and aorta. Open cardiac massage with clamping of the ascending aorta may help push air through the coronary arteries. Cardiopulmonary bypass should be instituted promptly if it is readily available.

Intrabronchial Bleeding

Intrabronchial bleeding is poorly tolerated and can rapidly cause death from severe hypoxemia by flooding alveoli. Patients with intrabronchial blood tend to die from "drowning" rather than from hypovolemic shock. Relatively small amounts of blood infused into a dog trachea over 30 to 60 min rapidly reduces the P_{O_2} below 60 mmHg with minimal changes in Pa_{CO_2} or airway resistance. The combination of shock and intrabronchial bleeding is highly lethal and can rapidly reduce oxygen transport to less than 25 percent of normal.

In patients with hemoptysis due to trauma, the noninvolved lung must be kept as free of blood as possible, and nasotracheal suction and bronchoscopy should be used as often as necessary. If a thoracotomy is done, it should be performed with the patient supine (through a midsternotomy or anterior thoracotomy) to help prevent the noninvolved lung from being flooded with blood.

If the bleeding is severe, a double-lumen endotracheal (Carlen) tube can be used to confine the bleeding to one lung. If a Carlen or similar tube is not available or cannot be inserted, one may insert an endotracheal tube over a flexible bronchoscope into the left main-stem bronchus. The balloon on the endotracheal tube can then be inflated as needed. If the bleeding is from the left lung, the endotracheal tube prevents blood from passing into the right lung, and ventilation of the right lung may then be maintained either spontaneously or via a mask or another endotracheal tube.

In some instances, the bleeding can only be controlled by occluding the involved bronchus with a Fogarty balloon catheter or by packing it with gauze. Obviously these are temporary measures until the bleeding site can be controlled surgically.

Aspiration

Aspiration of gastric contents is quite common after severe trauma, especially if the patient is unconscious. If it is recognized promptly, immediate bronchoscopy with irrigation of the tracheobronchial tree with buffered saline or a bicarbonate solution may help reduce the severity of the chemical pneumonitis.

Radiologic changes characteristic of aspiration pneumonitis are often delayed for more than 24 to 48 h. Suctioning of food particles, bile-stained fluid, or coffee-ground material from the trachea right after the event should be an indication for urgent bronchoscopy. Although the gastric acid will probably already have caused much of its damage, any remaining food particles can be removed. The use of steroids is controversial.

If an opaque foreign body is aspirated into the tracheobronchial tree, it is usually readily diagnosed. However, radiolucent foreign bodies occasionally can remain lodged in various bronchi, causing repeated pulmonary infections or hemoptysis for years before being discovered. Persistent or recurrent cough, atelectasis, or pneumonia after trauma should be indications for bronchoscopy or bronchography. Inspiratory and expiratory chest films may help diagnosis of a one-way valve effect due to a foreign body by demonstrating failure of one lung to empty properly during expiration.

Hemothorax

Etiology

Hemothorax is most frequently caused by bleeding from lung injuries. However, the compressing effect of the shed blood, the high concentration of thromboplastin in the lungs, and the low pulmonary arterial pressure combine to help reduce bleeding from torn lung parenchyma. Consequently, if there is persistent severe intrathoracic bleeding, it often arises from large lung injuries or from damage to major vessels. Bleeding from intercostal or internal mammary arteries may also be brisk and persistent.

Pathophysiology

Blood in the pleural cavity should be removed as completely and rapidly as possible. Large clots act as a local anticoagulant by releasing fibrinolysins and fibrinogenolysins from their surface. A large hemothorax also restricts ventilation and venous return. Bleeding from multiple small intrathoracic vessels often stops fairly rapidly after the hemothorax is completely evacuated.

Diagnosis

A hemothorax should be suspected following trauma if the breath sounds are reduced and the chest is dull to percussion on the involved side. Fluid collections greater than 200 to 300 mL can usually be seen on good upright or decubitus roentgenograms of the chest. However, if the patient is supine, more than 1000 mL of blood can be missed.

Treatment

Thoracentesis

A very small stable hemothorax does not always have to be removed, but it should be carefully observed. If the hemothorax seems large enough to drain, we have avoided needle aspiration and have relied on chest tubes. Needle aspiration of a hemothorax is usually incomplete and may cause a pneumothorax or infection of the hemothorax.

Chest Tube

Technique. Chest tubes for treatment of traumatic pneumothorax or hemothorax should be inserted in the anterior axillary line just behind the lateral edge of the pectoralis major muscle. For a pneumothorax we tend to place the tube as high and anteriorly as possible. For a hemothorax, the tube is inserted at the level of the nipple and directed posteriorly and laterally.

Once the insertion site is selected, the area around it is painted liberally with an iodophor preparation and then widely draped with a fenestrated sheet. A 22-gauge needle is used to infiltrate the skin, subcutaneous tissue, intercostal muscles, and parietal pleura with 1% lidocaine (Xylocaine) with adrenalin, keeping the total dose below 0.5 mL/kg (5 mg/kg).

A transverse incision 2 to 3 cm in length is then made and extended down to the intercostal muscles. The skin incision for the chest tube should be at least 1 in. below the interspace through which the tube will be placed. A large (Mayo) clamp is then inserted through the intercostal muscles in the next higher intercostal space, with care taken to prevent the tip of the clamp from penetrating the lung. The resulting oblique tunnel through the subcutaneous tissue and intercostal muscles usually closes promptly after the tube is removed, thereby reducing the chances of recurrent pneumothorax.

Once the clamp is pushed through the internal intercostal fascia, it is opened to enlarge the hole to approximately 1.5 to 2 cm. The clamp is then withdrawn, and a finger is inserted through the hole to verify the position within the thorax and to make sure the lung is not stuck to the chest wall. This is particularly important if a chest x-ray has not been taken or if the x-ray does not clearly show that the lung is away from the chest wall.

For a simple pneumothorax, a 24- or 28-French chest tube can be inserted. For a hemothorax, a 32- to 40-French chest tube is preferred. The chest tube is grasped at its tip with the clamp and directed through the hole into the pleural space and advanced in the appropriate direction. The tube is advanced until the last side hole is 2.5 to 5 cm (1 to 2 in.) inside the chest wall. The tube is secured in place with a long, heavy suture (2–0 or 1–0) of nonabsorbable material placed in a U fashion around the tube. The suture is tied so as to pull the soft tissues snugly around the tube and provide an airtight seal. The tails of the suture can be wrapped around the tube in opposite directions approximately half a dozen times and then tied to secure the tube to the chest wall.

The open end of the tube is attached to a combination fluid-collection water-seal suction device, such as the Pleurevac, with 20- to 30-cm H_2O suction. If a significant hemothorax is known to be present or if a large amount of blood starts to drain immediately, consideration should be given to the immediate collection of this blood in a heparinized autotransfusion device so that it can be returned to the patient either directly or after washing the red blood cells in saline solution.

After it appears that the chest tube is correctly situated and working properly, a sterile occlusive dressing is placed over the incision, and additional layers of tape are used to secure the tube to the chest wall so that it will not be accidentally pulled out.

The intrathoracic position of the chest tube and its last hole and the amount of air or fluid remaining in the pleural cavity should be checked with an upright chest film as soon as possible after the tube is inserted. If there is a significant air leak, the chest films are best done as portables at the patient's bedside so as not to risk the development of a tension pneumothorax while the patient is off suction en route to the x-ray department.

If the patient is sent to the radiology department for x-rays, the chest tube should not be clamped because any continuing air leakage can rapidly collapse the lung and/or cause a tension pneumothorax. While the tube is unclamped, the water-seal bottle should be kept 1 to 2 ft lower than the patient's chest.

Serial chest auscultation plus daily chest x-rays and careful recording of the volume of blood loss and the amount of air leakage are important guides to the functioning of the chest tubes. If a chest tube becomes blocked and a significant pneumothorax or hemothorax is still present, the tube should be replaced. This can often be done easily through the same incision that the previous chest tube occupied. Irrigating an occluded chest tube or passing a Fogarty catheter through it in an effort to reestablish its patency seldom works well and almost certainly increases the risk of infection.

If the chest tube is functional and well placed but a decubitus film shows a shift of at least some of the pleural fluid, the hemothorax is partially clotted, and another chest tube placed with ultrasound guidance may be helpful. If a chest tube is inserted because of a pneumothorax, it is left in place on suction for at least 24 h after all air leaks have stopped. If inserted for bleeding, it is left in place until the drainage is serous and less than 100 mL/24 h. However, while the patient is on a ventilator, many physicians would prefer to keep the chest tubes in to act as a safety valve in case a new pneumothorax suddenly develops.

When the tube is to be removed, the patient is asked to take a deep breath and bear down, as in a Valsalva maneuver. While intrathoracic pressure and lung volume are at their maximum, the tube is quickly pulled out and petrolatum or vaseline gauze is immediately applied as an airtight dressing over the chest tube site. It is important that the patient be in full inspiration when the tube is pulled. The involuntary reflex while the tube is being pulled is a quick inspiratory effort because of the pleural pain. This may rapidly suck in several hundred milliliters of air just as the tube is removed, necessitating reinsertion of another tube. Some surgeons put only one throw in their initial chest tube suture so that the ends can be unwound from the chest tube and then tied down to provide an airtight seal of the chest tube hole.

Following removal of the chest tube, a chest x-ray should be obtained to rule out a recurrent pneumothorax. Another chest x-ray should be obtained 24 h later to confirm continued complete expansion of the lungs.

There is much controversy concerning the value of giving prophylactic antibiotics to patients with chest tubes for traumatic hemopneumothorax, but three out of four studies indicate a benefit.

Autotransfusion

In patients with massive bleeding into a body cavity, proper collection and autotransfusion of the shed blood may reduce the need for bank blood and its associated risks. Intrathoracic bleeding is generally ideal for this technique because there is usually no contamination of the blood by bile or intestinal contents.

To use shed blood for autotransfusion, one needs to add citrate or heparin to it as it is removed to keep it from clotting and collect it in a special sterile container. However, in emergency situations with continued shock, attempts at autotransfusion may seem excessively difficult, particularly if adequate type-specific blood is readily available. Furthermore, autotransfused blood may contribute to a tendency for the patient to develop a coagulopathy. If the cells are washed in a cell saver, more autotransfusions can be given, but there is still concern about the coagulopathies. In our own hospital it is generally easier and much faster to use bank blood unless (1) the bleeding is massive and not rapidly controllable by surgery and (2) the blood type is rare.

Thoracotomy

Most patients with intrathoracic bleeding can be treated adequately by intravenous administration of fluids and evacuation of the hemothorax with a chest tube. Only 9 percent of our patients with penetrating chest wounds have required a thoracotomy for continuing hemorrhage. Thoracotomy for intrathoracic bleeding is generally indicated if (1) the patient's vital signs remain or become unstable, (2) more than 1500 mL of blood is lost from the chest tube in the first 12 to 24 h and there is continued bleeding, (3) the drainage of blood from the chest tubes exceeds 200 to 300 mL/h for 4 h, or (4) the chest remains more than half full of blood on x-ray.

Occasionally, when the chest tube is initially inserted, blood emerges at an alarmingly rapid rate. If the patient's condition improves as the blood is being removed, continuing drainage of the blood and observation of the patient are in order. However, if the patient's vital signs deteriorate as the blood is being removed, loss of the tamponading effect of the hemothorax has probably allowed serious bleeding from the lung to recur. Consequently, the chest tube should be clamped and the patient taken directly to surgery.

Pneumothorax

Pathophysiology

Collections of air or blood within the pleural cavity reduce vital capacity and increase intrathoracic pressure, thereby decreasing minute ventilation and venous return to the heart. During inspiration, the negative intrapleural pressure increases the tendency for air or blood to leak into the pleural cavity through any wound in the lung or chest wall. If there is any obstruction of the upper airway or if the patient has chronic obstructive lung disease, additional air may be forced into the pleural cavity during expiration, causing a tension pneumothorax with intrapleural pressures exceeding atmospheric pressure.

Diagnosis

Failure to obtain a chest x-ray soon after admission and again in 4 to 8 h may result in the oversight of significant intrathoracic injuries. The presence of a chest injury is usually readily apparent from the history and physical examination; however, accurate assessment of the damage, especially to the intrathoracic organs, often requires serial chest x-rays.

A pneumothorax is not likely to cause severe symptoms unless it (1) is a tension pneumothorax, (2) occupies more than 40 percent of one hemithorax, or (3) occurs in a patient with shock or preexisting cardiopulmonary disease. If there is a suspicion of a pneumothorax but it is not clearly seen on the first chest roentgenogram, repeat films during expiration may be helpful. Apical-lordotic films may allow better visualization of an apical pneumothorax. Rarely, a pneumothorax after a stab wound is delayed for more than 12 to 24 h. Consequently, serial chest x-rays every 6 to 8 h for 24 h are indicated in selected patients.

One should assume that a tension pneumothorax is present and begin treatment without waiting for a chest x-ray if the patient has (1) severe respiratory distress, (2) decreased breath sounds and hyperresonance on one side of the chest, (3) distended neck veins (if the patient is not hypovolemic), and (4) deviation of the trachea away from the involved side. Insertion of a large needle into the involved side through the second intercostal space in the midclavicular line may help confirm the diagnosis and provide temporary relief while a chest tube is inserted.

If a tension pneumothorax is suspected in an unstable patient, it must be relieved as rapidly as possible. If a chest tube cannot be inserted almost immediately, the pleural cavity should be aspirated anteriorly in the second intercostal space with a needle and syringe.

A small pneumothorax (less than 1.0 cm wide and confined to the upper one-third of the chest) that is unchanged on two chest roentgenograms taken 4 to 6 h apart in an otherwise healthy individual can usually be treated by observation alone. However, in most instances after trauma, a chest tube or small catheter should be inserted as a precautionary measure, especially if the patient cannot be observed closely.

If only a pneumothorax is present, a small- to moderate-sized (24- to 28-French) chest tube may be inserted anteriorly in the second intercostal space in the midclavicular line. However, a high midaxillary tube is generally preferable. Although some physicians insert chest tubes over trocars because it is less painful, especially if the lung is well away from the chest wall, we believe it is safer to avoid the trochar and insert chest tubes using a large hemostat.

Catheter aspiration of a simple pneumothorax (CASP) is not generally suitable for the treatment of traumatic pneumothoraces.

Complications

In general, a small- or moderate-sized pneumothorax does not cause complications unless there is a continuing air leak. Also, a continuing air leak does not usually cause problems if the lung is completely expanded. However, if a combination of pneumothorax and continued air leak is allowed to exist for more than 24 to 48 h, the incidence of empyema and bronchopleural fistula is greatly increased.

The most frequent reasons for failure to evacuate a pneumothorax rapidly and to completely expand the lungs are (1) improper connections in the external tubing or water seal-collection apparatus, (2) improper position of the chest tube(s), (3) occlusion of bronchi by secretions or a foreign body, (4) a tear of one of the larger bronchi, or (5) a large tear of the lung parenchyma. If the lung is not expanded and there is a large air leak, emergency bronchoscopy should be performed to clear the bronchi and identify any damage to the tracheobronchial tree that may need repair. Continued large air leakage and failure of the lung to expand adequately in spite of the measures described above are often indications for early thoracotomy to control the air leak.

Pneumomediastinum

Pneumomediastinum is an important finding in patients with chest trauma. The diagnosis is usually made on the chest x-ray, but it can easily be missed. Subcutaneous emphysema in the neck should make one look closely for a pneumomediastinum. The diagnosis of pneumomediastinum should also be suspected from the presence of a crunching sound (Hamman's sign) over the heart during systole.

Traumatic pneumomediastinum is of itself usually asymptomatic, but one must look closely for an injury to the larynx, trachea, major bronchi, pharynx, or esophagus. Delayed pneumothorax may develop, especially if the patient requires mechanical ventilation.

Tracheobronchial Injury

Lower Trachea and Major Bronchi

Most injuries to major bronchi are due to rapid deceleration and shearing of more mobile bronchi from relatively fixed proximal structures. However, forced expiration against a closed glottis or compression against the vertebral column may also play a role.

Injuries to the trachea or major bronchi should be suspected if there is massive subcutaneous or mediastinal emphysema or if there is a persistent pneumothorax with a continuing large air leak.

Most of these injuries occur within 2 cm of the carina or at the origin of lobar bronchi. On bronchoscopy the usual bronchial injury seen is a transverse tear in the main bronchi or a disruption at the origin of an upper lobe bronchus. The characteristic injury in the trachea is a vertical tear in the membranous portion near its attachment to the tracheal cartilages.

Even if the lung expands and the air leak stops, lacerations of the bronchi involving more than a third of the circumference should be repaired because they tend to eventually cause severe bronchial stenosis with repeated pulmonary infections or complete atelectasis. Untreated tracheal tears may result in severe mediastinitis.

The only patients who survive a tracheal transection generally have their injury in the cervical trachea and have no associated injuries. Intrathoracic tracheal transection is usually associated with two or more major injuries and is almost invariably fatal. Concurrent esophageal injuries occur in almost 25 percent of penetrating tracheobronchial injuries and are easily missed unless esophagoscopy or contrast studies are also performed.

Cervical Tracheal Injuries

Injuries to the cervical trachea from blunt trauma usually occur at the junction of the trachea and cricoid cartilage. This is most frequently caused by striking the anterior neck against the dashboard in an automobile accident or by running on foot or in a snowmobile into a clothesline or wire fence. Evidence of trauma to the neck with subcutaneous emphysema should arouse suspicion of this injury. Inspiratory stridor usually indicates a 70- to 80-percent upper airway obstruction. However, cricotracheal separation is often only suspected when an endotracheal tube or bronchoscope cannot be inserted past the cricoid cartilage.

If the patient has a laceration of the trachea that is small and high, it may be managed simply by performing a tracheostomy below the injury. All lacerations of the trachea should be repaired, especially if they involve more than a third of the circumference.

Diaphragmatic Injury

Etiology

In urban centers, diaphragmatic injuries are caused most frequently by penetrating trauma, particularly gunshot wounds of the lower chest or upper abdomen. Rupture due to blunt trauma is much less frequent and occurs in only 4 to 5 percent of patients hospitalized with chest trauma. If there is a fracture of the pelvis, the incidence increases to about 8 to 10 percent. Because of the protective effect of the liver on the right and the possible increased weakness of the left posterolateral diaphragm, most series report that 80 to 90 percent of the diaphragmatic injuries following blunt trauma occur in that area. However, in Brown's series, in which the right diaphragm was examined very closely, the incidence of right- and left-sided diaphragmatic rupture was almost equal.

Natural History

Since 60 to 70 percent of normal ventilation depends on proper function of the diaphragm, trauma to this structure can cause serious ventilatory problems. However, the initial signs and symptoms are often masked by other injuries. Unless the diaphragmatic lesion is quite large, symptoms due to abdominal viscera in the thoracic cavity usually occur rather late. Over time, sometimes even years, a rather large amount of viscera can gradually work its way up into the chest through rather small diaphragmatic tears because of the negative pressure there. The intrathoracic bowel may then become obstructed or strangulated or cause severe compression of the adjacent lung.

Diagnosis

With penetrating trauma, the diagnosis of diaphragmatic injury is often made only intraoperatively. However, if the entrance wound is in the abdomen and there is evidence of an intrathoracic injury of foreign body, one can assume that the missile or knife has transgressed the diaphragm. In Brown's series, 59 percent of the patients with diaphragmatic injuries had diagnostic chest x-rays. However, eight of nine peritoneal lavages done in these patients were negative. In the only positive lavage, the lavage fluid drained out through a previously placed chest tube.

With blunt trauma, any abnormality of the diaphragm or lower lung fields on chest x-ray should arouse suspicion of a diaphragmatic tear. Occasionally a nasogastric tube is seen to go into the abdomen and then up into the chest because the stomach has passed through a diaphragmatic tear.

Techniques for diagnosing diaphragmatic rupture include (1) peritoneal lavage with a chest tube in place; (2) upper gastrointestinal (GI) series, looking for displacement of viscera into the chest; (3) pneumoperitoneum with carbon dioxide; (4) CT scan with contrast, and (5) intraperitoneal technetium sulfur colloid.

HEART

Penetrating Injury to the Heart

There are many factors affecting survival from penetrating injury to the heart. They include the weapon used, the size of the myocardial injury, the injured cardiac chamber, coronary artery damage, the presence of tamponade, associated injuries, and the time taken to reach the hospital. Every patient with penetrating chest injury and shock on admission should be considered as having a cardiac injury until proven otherwise.

With early aggressive resuscitation and surgery, up to one-third of patients arriving in a trauma center ''in extremis'' with a cardiac injury can be saved. In patients who can be brought to the operating room with signs of life and recordable blood pressure, the survival rate should exceed 70 percent for gunshot wounds and 85 percent for stab wounds. In one series, 23 consecutive patients with isolated penetrating injuries of the heart reaching the operating room alive survived.

Pathophysiology

Penetrating wounds of the heart are usually rapidly fatal, generally because of massive hemorrhage, and less than one-fourth of the patients with this injury reach the hospital alive. Patients surviving more than 15 to 30 min usually have either a small wound or some component of pericardial tamponade. In a sense, pericardial tamponade can be a two-edged sword; although it may prolong life by reducing the severity of the initial blood loss, the tamponade itself can also be fatal by interfering with venous return and diastolic filling of the heart.

Diagnosis

Clinical Features

All patients in shock with a penetrating wound of the chest between the midclavicular line on the right and anterior axillary line on the left should be considered to have a cardiac injury until proven otherwise. If the only problem is tamponade and the patient is not hypovolemic, the Beck I triad may present. This includes distended neck veins, hypotension, and muffled heart tones. The last is the least reliable sign, and even with a large acute pericardial tamponade, which seldom is more than 150 to 200 mL, the heart tones are usually fairly clear. Since patients with penetrating heart wounds are usually hypotensive, the neck veins will generally not distend until the blood volume is at least partially restored. Furthermore, chest injuries can cause the patient to breathe abnormally or strain, thereby raising the central venous pressure and distending the neck veins in the absence of tamponade. Other causes of Beck's triad include tension pneumothorax, myocardial contusion, acute myocardial infarction, and systemic air embolism.

Tamponade may also cause two Kussmaul signs. One is increased distension of neck veins during inspiration, and the other is pulsus paradoxus. Paradoxical pulse is characterized by a drop in systolic blood pressure of more than 15 mmHg during normal inspiration. The amount of paradox may be increased by hypovolemia, and bronchospasm is the most frequent cause of pulsus paradoxus.

Invasive Monitoring

As the volume of blood in the pericardial cavity rises, so also will the diastolic pressures in all of the cardiac chambers. This will produce an equalization of the diastolic pressures in all chambers, which should make one suspicious of tamponade. At the same time, stroke volume will tend to fall. The rise in filling pressure and fall in stroke volume and blood pressure may occasionally be difficult to differentiate from heart failure from other causes. However, the circumstances of the injury and the equalization of the diastolic pressures on both the right and the left sides of the heart should certainly increase suspicion for the diagnosis of tamponade.

One must remember that central venous catheters that are inserted too far can also perforate the heart and cause tamponade. A recent report by Aldridge collected 61 such cases with a mortality rate exceeding 50 percent.

X-Rays

Chest films are of little help in diagnosing acute cardiac injury except in the unusual patient with intrapericardial air. Since the average acute tamponade has only 150 to 200 mL of blood and clots, significant early enlargement of the cardiac shadow is unusual. The x-ray may, however, reveal a hemopneumothorax or mediastinal pathology that might not otherwise be noted and treated.

ECG

Electrocardiography changes following cardiac injury are usually nonspecific. ST-T wave changes may indicate pericardial irritation or may reflect associated ischemia or hypoxia.

Echocardiography

Echocardiography can be helpful in diagnosing the presence or absence of increased pericardial fluid. It may also help localize missile fragments in the pericardium. However, it is usually not immediately available, and occasionally there are false positives and negatives.

Pericardiocentesis

Accuracy

There is an increasing tendency to avoid the use of pericardiocentesis as a diagnostic procedure in acutely injured patients with possible tamponade. In Demetriades' series, the incidence of false-negative pericardiocentesis was 80 percent, and the incidence of false positives was 33 percent. In addition to its inaccuracy, it may injure the heart or cause dangerous delays in needed surgery.

Technique

The paraxiphoid approach is commonly used. An 18-gauge, 10-cm spinal needle attached to a stopcock and then a 20 mL syringe can be used. The pericardiocentesis should be done with continuous ECG monitoring if possible. The ECG monitoring is more sensitive if one attaches the V lead of the ECG to the metal pericardiocentesis needle using an insulated wire with alligator clips on both ends.

The needle is passed upward and backward at an angle of 45° for 4 to 5 cm and advanced slowly until the point seems to enter a cavity. Most authors direct the needle toward the left scapula tip; however, directing the needle toward the right scapula is more likely to parallel the right border of the heart and is less likely to penetrate the right ventricle. One should aspirate frequently as the needle is advanced, and if no blood is obtained, one can insert a stylet or inject 0.5 to 1.0 mL of saline solution at intervals to be certain that the needle is not plugged. The needle is then carefully pushed further, about 1 to 2 mm at a time, until blood is obtained, cardiac pulsations are felt, or the ECG shows an abrupt change.

Generally, a large portion of the blood in the pericardial cavity is clotted. Consequently, one can often remove only 4 to 5 mL of blood without manipulating the needle. If 20 mL of blood can be drawn out easily and rapidly, it usually indicates that the blood is being aspirated from the right ventricle.

If an immediate thoracotomy is not possible in a patient with a positive pericardiocentesis, a plastic catheter (inserted over a needle or Seldinger wire) can be left in place for continuous drainage of intrapericardial blood until the cardiac wound can be surgically repaired.

Complications

The pericardiocentesis needle can perforate the right ventricle or a coronary artery and produce a tamponade. Arrhythmias may also occur. A falsely negative pericardiocentesis may delay necessary surgery.

Subxiphoid Pericardial Window

Another alternative for diagnosis of pericardial tamponade is a subxiphoid pericardial window under local anesthesia. If blood is found, the patient can be given a general anesthetic and the incision can be extended up as a midsternotomy to repair the cardiac wound. However, we believe that this procedure is potentially dangerous and has no clear benefit in most cases. If it is done under local anesthetic on a restless patient, it can be extremely difficult to perform, and massive exsanguination may result.

Treatment

Fluid Replacement

It is essential that patients with penetrating wounds of the chest have two or more large IV lines in place with at least one in a leg vein in the event that the superior vena cava or one of its major branches is injured. It is particularly important to have an adequate or increased blood volume if hypovolemia or tamponade is present. If tamponade is present with an elevated central venous pressure, one should not be reluctant to administer further fluid and blood to improve venous return to the heart while moving the patient to the operating suite.

Pericardiocentesis

Patients who are in shock and may have a cardiac injury should have an emergency thoracotomy as soon as possible. If it is not possible to perform an emergency thoracotomy almost immediately, a pericardiocentesis to relieve the suspected tamponade should be attempted.

Pericardiocentesis is primarily a diagnostic procedure, but removal of as little as 5 to 10 mL of blood from the pericardial sac may increase stroke volume by 25 to 50 percent, with a dramatic improvement in cardiac output and blood pressure. In patients who have small puncture wounds of the heart, pericardiocentesis may be curative, and the patient may not require a thoracotomy as long as the vital signs remain stable for at least 24 to 48 h after the procedure.

Thoracotomy

Occasionally, a highly selected stable patient with a small penetrating cardiac injury may be successfully treated without surgery. However, virtually all patients with shock and a suspected injury to the heart should have emergency thoracotomy to completely relieve the tamponade and to repair any injuries found.

Emergency Department Thoracotomy

In hospitals where adequate facilities, equipment, and trained personnel are present, an emergency department thoracotomy may be life-saving. In Rohman's study, it was felt that emergency department thoracotomy for penetrating cardiac injuries is essential for patients who are (1) clinically dead on arrival in the emergency department but had some signs of life in transit (survival, 32 percent) or (2) deteriorating and have no obtainable blood pressure (survival, 33 percent). Emergency department thoracotomies for patients with no signs of life at the scene are almost invariably futile. Factors that correlate with survival following emergency department thoracotomy include the site of injury, mechanism of injury, signs of life at the scene and on admission to the emergency department, cardiac activity at thoracotomy, ECG activity, systolic blood pressure response to thoracic aortic occlusion, and depth of shock on admission. Prediction of neurological recovery prior to emergency department thoracotomy is more difficult. Cogbill noted a correlation between spontaneous respirations at the time of ambulance pickup and ultimate neurological recovery, while Baker suggests that a response to verbal and noxious stimuli prior to emergency department thoracotomy is an important prognosticator of neurological recovery. Postoperatively, an early return to consciousness within 12 h usually indicates an excellent ultimate neurological outcome.

Incision. Once the patient is intubated, an anterolateral thoracotomy is performed in the left fifth intercostal space, which is one interspace below the male nipple. The incision should be as long as possible, extending from just lateral to the sternum to the midaxillary line in the axilla. In females, the breast is displaced upward, and the incision is made through the breast crease. The incision is extended through the intercostal muscles just above the sixth rib into the pleural cavity, with care taken not to injure the underlying lung or heart. A rib spreader is then inserted and opened widely so that two hands can fit inside the chest. Cutting the intercostal cartilages above and below the incision may help increase the exposure. Not infrequently the internal mammary vessels, which lie about 0.5 to 1.0 cm lateral to the sternum, are cut, and, if so, they must be clamped and tied or suture-ligated.

When the injury is to the right of the sternum, a right thoracotomy is initially performed to control any bleeding sites, but strong consideration should be given to extending the incision across the sternum as a bilateral thoracotomy so as to be able to also control the descending aorta and massage the heart, if needed, more effectively. The right and left anterolateral incisions may be connected by transverse division of the sternum using a Gigli saw or rib cutter. This bilateral anterolateral thoracotomy allows wide exposure of both sides of the heart and the proximal great vessels. In the patient with a cardiac arrest, there is usually minimal bleeding from the thoracotomy incision until the circulation is restored. However, as circulation is restored the incisional bleeding may be quite severe, especially from the internal mammary arteries, which should be suture-ligated if they are injured.

Pericardiotomy. Even when the pericardial sac is not distended with blood, it can be difficult to grasp the pericardium with a forceps. It may be necessary at times to "hook" the pericardium with one blade of a scissors and then grab it with a forceps or clamp. Another technique is to very carefully incise the pericardium near the apex of the heart with a knife to produce a hole just big enough to allow the tip of one blade of a scissors. If a scalpel is used to open the pericardial sac, inadvertent injury to the underlying myocardium or left anterior descending coronary artery can easily occur.

The pericardial sac should then be opened further with a scissors in a longitudinal direction 1 to 2 cm anterior to the left (or right) phrenic nerve. The pericardial incision should extend from the diaphragm below to the great vessels above. If the pericardial sac is still tight around the heart, a transverse cut of the pericardium inferiorly along the central diaphragm may greatly help with exposure. The surgeon should then manually evacuate the liquid blood and clots in the pericardial sac and begin cardiac massage if it is needed.

Clamping the descending aorta. The second maneuver in the patient with severe hypotension or a cardiac arrest is compression or clamping of the descending thoracic aorta to help improve coronary and cerebral arterial flow. Since more than 60 percent of the cardiac output goes through the descending thoracic aorta, cross-clamping it can increase blood flow to the coronary and cerebral arteries two- to threefold.

To expose the descending aorta, an assistant on the right side of the patient lifts the left lung up and almost out of the hemithorax. Then the lower descending thoracic aorta is dissected out. The pleura and fascia in front of the aorta are easily opened, but the tougher posterior tissue between the aorta and the vertebral bodies often has to be incised sharply. When the aorta has been exposed, a finger or a vascular clamp can be hooked around it. In this way, clamping is performed under direct vision, and the chances of intercostal arterial or esophageal injuries are reduced. After the clamp is applied, the time is noted, and the left lung is allowed to drop back into the thorax. To be sure that the clamp is applied properly, one should feel pulsations from the heart or cardiac massage above the clamp but none below. If a nasogastric tube is not in place and there is little or no blood pressure, one can easily mistake the esophagus for the aorta.

Clamping injured lung. If there is an obvious associated lung injury, it should be controlled with a vascular or lung clamp to prevent systemic air embolism and to stop the bleeding and air leak until more definitive control can be accomplished. If there is a large central lung injury, one should put a clamp across the hilum. If the hilar clamp does not control the bleeding because the injury is too close to the heart, one may have to clamp the pulmonary vessels inside the pericardium.

Exposing the heart. Once the heart is in view, inspect the right ventricle and right atrium, which are the chambers that are most commonly injured. If the heart injury cannot be seen, the heart can be swung out laterally and anteriorly into the left hemithorax to allow better examination of all parts of the heart. Lifting the heart straight up can increase the possibility of entry of air into a left-sided or posterior cardiac perforation, resulting in sudden fatal coronary or cerebral air embolism.

Controlling cardiac wounds. Most atrial wounds can be temporarily controlled by the application of a Satinsky vascular clamp and then sewn with a running 3–0 or 4–0 polypropylene suture. Wounds of the ventricles can generally be tamponaded by the operator's finger while pledgeted horizontal mattress sutures of 2–0 silk or Prolene are passed under the finger and tied by an assistant. When a wound lies next to a major coronary artery, the mattress suture is placed beneath the artery so as to avoid ligation or compression of the vessel.

For handling more difficult cardiac wounds, several other techniques are available. The insertion of a 5- or 30-mL balloon Foley catheter into a large or inaccessible (posterior) defect may allow for control of hemorrhage until a purse-string suture can be applied around the hole. Such a catheter can also be used to infuse fluids rapidly.

Wide horizontal mattress sutures placed on either side of a large defect and pulled together may control hemorrhage until cardiopulmonary bypass can be instituted. If cardiopulmonary bypass is not readily available, occlusion of the superior vena cava and inferior vena cava by vascular tapes or clamps slows the heart and finally stops it, allowing for quick repair of a large defect without causing exsanguinating hemorrhage. If the latter technique is used, all air is evacuated from the heart by allowing bleeding through the hole prior to tying the final suture.

Cardiac massage. Once cardiorrhaphy has been completed, internal cardiac massage can be performed as needed by compressing the heart between the palms of two hands or between one palm and the sternum. Warm—preferably 40 to 42.2°C (104 to 108°F)—saline solution poured over the heart may help prevent ventricular fibrillation, which is often associated with the hypothermia of shock and resuscitation. If ventricular fibrillation occurs, defibrillation with internal paddles, starting at 20 to 40 W·s should be performed. Lidocaine and correction of severe acidosis or alkalosis may also help if there is recurrent ventricular fibrillation.

Air embolism. If severe arrhythmias or cardiac arrest develops during endotracheal intubation or while the chest is being opened, aspiration of the cardiac chambers for air should be performed immediately. Air embolism may be a complication of a cardiac or lung wound because air may be "sucked" into low-pressure cardiac chambers or veins, especially in the presence of hypovolemia. Systemic air embolism is most frequently diagnosed by air bubbles in the coronary arteries. This serious complication is seldom mentioned in the literature, but is probably not rare.

Continued care. When the patient develops a satisfactory rhythm, the descending thoracic aorta is gradually declamped as infusions of fluid and blood are administered, with care taken to keep the systolic blood pressure above 90 to 100 mmHg. One should avoid a systolic blood pressure greater than 160 mmHg because it may tear open cardiac repairs, excessively dilate the left ventricle, or cause intracerebral bleeding. The use of vigorous inotropes such as epinephrine should be particularly avoided at this point, as they may cause sudden, severe hypertension and also increase the risk of recurrent ventricular fibrillation.

After the cardiac wounds and all bleeding vessels are controlled and an adequate cardiac output has been obtained, all clot is washed out of the pericardial and pleural cavities. One must look closely to make sure that the internal mammary arteries are intact or carefully suture-ligated. If the heart is edematous or dilated, the pericardium can be left open. Occasionally, the sternum cannot even be closed. In such instances, the skin can usually be sutured. The sternum itself can then usually be closed after several days when the cardiac edema and dilatation have resolved.

Coronary artery injuries. Ligation of the cut ends is the treatment of choice for lacerations of small coronary vessels. Torn proximal coronary arteries may also be ligated if there is no evidence of cardiovascular dysfunction. However, such patients must be observed closely. If a large proximal coronary artery is lacerated and arrhythmias, myocardial infarction, or impaired hemodynamic function develops, an aortocoronary bypass with a saphenous vein graft should be performed.

Ventricular septal defects. Up to 5 percent of patients with penetrating cardiac trauma will be found to have a ventricular septal defect postoperatively. If the patient is in heart failure, emergency cardiac catheterization and surgery may be required. In most instances one can usually wait 2 to 3 months to correct the defect.

Valve injuries. Most valvular injuries detected postoperatively can be corrected 3 to 6 months later on an elective basis after cardiac catheterization. Occasionally, however, severe cardiac failure or dysfunction at the initial procedure will require an emergency valve repair or replacement.

Blunt Injury to the Heart

Etiology and Mechanisms of Injury

The most common cause of blunt cardiac trauma is a high-speed vehicular accident. However, myocardial injury has been documented in accidents involving vehicles going less than 20 mph. Other causes include direct blows to the chest, industrial crush injuries, falls from heights, blast injuries, and athletic trauma. Recently, one study has suggested that use of seat belts may increase the incidence of myocardial contusion in motor vehicle accidents.

The heart seems to be relatively well protected within a bony case formed by ribs, sternum, and vertebrae. However, it is suspended relatively freely within the chest cavity from the great vessels, and this mobility plus its location between the sternum and the thoracic vertebrae makes it susceptible to injury as a result of several mechanisms: (1) sudden horizontal acceleration and/or deceleration, causing the heart to impact against the sternum and vertebrae; (2) a compression between the sternum and vertebrae following a direct, forceful blow to the chest; (3) a sudden increase in intrathoracic and intracardiac pressures, causing disruption of myocardium or cardiac valves; (4) a "hydraulic ram effect," with compression of the abdomen forcibly displacing abdominal viscera against the heart with sudden great force, and (5) strenuous or prolonged cardiac massage, particularly if done through the intact chest wall.

Types of Injuries

Blunt trauma to the heart can cause a wide spectrum of injuries including (1) rupture of an outer chamber wall, with resulting death from tamponade or bleeding, (2) septal rupture; (3) valvular injuries, of which injury to the aortic valve is the most common; (4) direct myocardial injury (contusion); (5) laceration or thrombosis of coronary arteries, and (6) pericardial injury.

Some authors have stressed the differences between myocardial concussion and myocardial contusion. With myocardial concussion, there is no anatomic cellular injury, but there is some functional damage, as demonstrated on a two-dimensional echocardiogram or other wall motion studies. With contusion, there is an anatomic injury, as demonstrated either by elevated myocardial creatine phosphokinase (CPK-MB) enzymes or by direct visualization at surgery or autopsy.

Diagnostic Problems

Blunt cardiac trauma can be difficult to detect. The victim may have experienced severe multiple-system trauma, and the presence of a cardiac injury may be overshadowed by other, more obvious injuries. In addition, the forces that produce blunt cardiac trauma may cause little or no external evidence of injury. Therefore, a history of moderate to severe chest or upper abdominal injury, even without abnormalities on physical examination, should make one suspect cardiac injury.

Cardiac Rupture

Cardiac rupture due to blunt chest trauma is the lesion most frequently found at autopsy in patients dying at the scene of an accident. As with myocardial contusion, the anterior right ventricle is the most susceptible. Also vulnerable is the anterior interventricular septum, which tends to rupture near the apex, especially during end-diastole or early systole when the ventricles are most full.

About 80 percent of patients with cardiac rupture die almost immediately at the scene of the accident. However, with today's rapid transport systems, some patients, especially those with only small tears of the right atrium at its junction with the superior vena cava, may arrive in the emergency department with little or no evidence of hemorrhagic shock or tamponade. Unfortunately, most of these patients suddenly deteriorate a short time later and die before appropriate surgery can be performed.

The diagnosis of cardiac rupture should be suspected when shock exists out of proportion to the degree of recognized injury or when shock persists despite control of hemorrhage elsewhere and rapid volume replacement. An immediate left anterior thoracotomy or median sternotomy, preferably with cardiopulmonary bypass on standby, is required to repair these devastating injuries successfully.

In spite of the poor results in most reports, in Calhool's recent series of ten patients with blunt heart rupture seen in a single emergency center during an 11-year period, seven (70 percent) survived. These excellent results were attributed to prompt performance of a pericardial window with subsequent immediate thoracotomy. Similar results were presented in Getz's report of four survivors out of five patients presenting with tamponade after right atrial rupture.

Septal Defects

Septal defects after blunt chest trauma are rare but should be looked for carefully if there is a murmur plus evidence of myocardial damage. The muscular interventricular septum near the apex is particularly susceptible to perforation after blunt trauma. The triad of chest trauma, systolic murmur, and an infarct pattern on ECG should suggest a ventricular septal defect (VSD). It is also important to suspect septal injury in patients with severe early hypoxemia following chest trauma. Any right-to-left shunt will increase hypoxemia, and mechanical ventilation with high pressure will tend to increase right-to-left shunting. If there is severe heart failure, prompt cardiac catheterization with rapid surgical repair may be required to restore adequate oxygen delivery to the tissues. Although small traumatic VSDs in the muscular septum may close spontaneously, surgical repair, preferably 6 to 8 weeks after the trauma, is the treatment of choice.

Isolated atrial septal defects (ASD) due to blunt trauma are extremely rare, and most of these patients die within minutes of the injury. However, if an ASD is suspected, cardiac catheterization and subsequent repair are appropriate.

Valve Injury

Rupture of the aortic valve is the most common valvular lesion found in patients who survive nonpenetrating cardiac injury. Blunt trauma rarely may also lacerate the papillary muscle or chordae tendineae of the mitral valve. The prognosis for rupture of a mitral papillary muscle or a mitral valve leaflet is grave, and death usually occurs within a few days after injury. The tricuspid valve is rarely involved in blunt trauma, and tricuspid insufficiency does not usually cause a significant hemodynamic problem unless the patient has pulmonary hypertension. Patients with bioprosthetic heart valves are particularly likely to have traumatic valve injury.

Myocardial Contusion

Myocardial contusion following blunt chest trauma has intrigued physicians since its initial description in 1676, and many physicians are still unclear as to how to diagnose and treat this problem.

Pathologic Changes

The pathologic changes include subendocardial hemorrhage and a much larger area of focal myocardial edema, interstitial hemorrhage, myofibrillar degeneration, and myocytolysis with infiltrates of polymorphonuclear leukocytes. This injury may resemble an acute myocardial infarction, but the muscle injury with contusion tends to be patchier, and the boundaries of a contusion are usually more sharply demarcated. The anterior right ventricular wall is the area most frequently involved, with the anterior interventricular septum and anterior-apical left ventricle next.

Additional myocardial injury may occur if there are concomitant coronary arterial problems such as spasm, intimal tears, or compression from adjacent hemorrhage and edema. Indeed, some feel that much of the myocardial injury seen in contusions is due to coronary blood flow redistribution. Very occasionally, transient hypotension may cause complete occlusion of a previously diseased coronary artery.

Usually there is complete clinical recovery with minimal residual scarring within 3 to 6 weeks of a myocardial contusion. However, in rare cases with severe transmural injury, a ventricular aneurysm may develop.

Physiological Changes

In addition to the rhythm and conduction disturbances, myocardial contusion can significantly impair myocardial function. In an otherwise normal individual without severe associated injuries, the hemodynamic impairment may not even be noticed. However, in patients who have preexisting cardiac disease or multiple other injuries or require a prolonged general anesthetic, it may greatly reduce the prognosis.

A significant reduction of cardiac output can be found in most victims. The degree of cardiac depression is directly related to the mass of contused myocardium. This has been confirmed in experimental animal studies and shown to persist for 2 to 3 weeks or longer. Abnormal wall motion and a decreased ejection fraction are commonly seen. Although screening tests, such as the ECG, CPK-MB, and MUGA scan are relatively sensitive in diagnosing myocardial contusion, they do not indicate the severity of the injury, nor are they predictive of major morbidity or mortality.

However, most patients have relatively little problem unless (1) the patient has an arrhythmia, especially premature ventricular contractions (PVCs), atrial fibrillation, or a conduction defect; (2) there is clinical evidence of heart failure; (3) there are multiple other injuries; (4) there is preexisting cardiac disease; or (5) the patient requires a general anesthetic.

Diagnosis

There continues to be much debate about how to diagnose myocardial contusion. The value of various diagnostic tests varies greatly in the large number of papers written on the subject.

Clinical Features

Any patient involved in a motor vehicle accident involving speeds exceeding 35 mph and having any chest symptoms or signs should be suspected of having a myocardial contusion. Rarely, a patient with a myocardial contusion will have angina-like pain that is not relieved by nitroglycerin. Differentiation from an acute myocardial infarction may be difficult under such circumstances.

A tachycardia that is out of proportion to the degree of trauma or blood loss may be the first sign of a myocardial contusion. Aside from evidence of significant chest wall injury, the only other helpful physical signs are a friction rub or abnormality in the heart sounds. Occasionally, an irregular rhythm due to atrial fibrillation or premature atrial or ventricular contractions may be noted.

Radiological Examination

The chest x-ray has its greatest value in the recognition of associated injuries. The closest x-ray correlates of myocardial contusion are pulmonary contusion or fractures of the first two ribs, clavicles, or sternum. Sternal fractures are particularly important. In many series, the presence of a fractured sternum is the clinical finding most significantly associated with myocardial contusion. In Harley's series of 11 patients with sternal fractures studied with radionuclide angiography, 10 (91 percent) had functional defects involving the anterior heart. Interestingly, only 4 of these patients had an ECG abnormality, and none had elevated CPK-MB isoenzymes.

Acute cardiac decompensation may be diagnosed by x-ray evidence of acute pulmonary edema associated with a normal-sized heart. Cardiac tamponade usually does not cause an enlarged cardiac silhouette, but a widened azygous vein is suggestive of this diagnosis. One might be alerted to the presence of severe chest trauma, with or without rupture of the great vessels, by a widened mediastinum.

ECG

Some authors feel that the ECG is the best screening test for an acute myocardial contusion, but this is extremely controversial. Nevertheless, an ECG should be obtained initially and at 24, 48, and 72 h postinjury in anyone suspected of having a myocardial injury. ST-T wave abnormalities may be present on admission or may only develop after 12 or 24 h, but such changes are very nonspecific. New atrial fibrillation, multiple PVCs, or conduction disturbances are much more important and are virtually diagnostic.

ECG changes have been noted in 33 to 88 percent of patients with contusions. In one series of 108 clinically diagnosed myocardial contusions, 12 percent had normal ECGs, 22 percent had ventricular rhythm disorders, 32 percent had other arrhythmias or disturbances of conduction, 61 percent had disturbances of repolarization, and 3 percent had ECG evidence of a myocardial infarction.

It must be emphasized that a normal ECG does not exclude a significant myocardial lesion at autopsy. The initial ECG may be normal, and significant changes may only develop 24 to 72 h later, as occurred in 12 of 52 patients in one series. However, in most series the incidence of new ECG changes developing after 24 h is extremely low. Recently, it has been suggested that sinus node dysfunction due to blunt trauma may be more common than formerly suspected. Development of abnormal Q waves indicates a more severe, transmural injury.

Although many physicians rely heavily on the ECG to help diagnose acute myocardial contusion, many patients with otherwise proven contusions will have normal ECG patterns. Sutherland and coworkers, in particular, found that almost two-thirds of their patients with anterior myocardial dysfunction had a normal ECG. This is partly because the ECG tends to reflect changes in the left ventricle, while contusion tends to primarily involve the right ventricle.

Holter monitoring may reveal far more arrhythmias than the routine ECG or continuous cardioscopic monitoring. Both ventricular and supraventricular arrhythmias have been reported.

Enzymes

SGOT, LDH, and CPK levels are often elevated in patients with severe blunt chest trauma because of associated injuries to the liver, lung, bone, brain, or skeletal muscle. Consequently, they are of little value in diagnosing cardiac injuries. However, myocardial (CPK-MB) isoenzymes should be more accurate. These should be drawn initially when the patient is first seen in the emergency department and at 8, 16, 24, and 48 h postinjury. With myocardial contusions, the CPK-MB should peak at about 18 to 24 h.

Most authors consider a ratio of CPK-MB to total CPK of 5 percent or more to be indicative of myocardial damage. Since CPK-MB enzymes are usually less than 1% M in young normal hearts, this isoenzyme is of little help in young patients. CPK-MB fraction may be elevated from a variety of injuries, but tends to get diluted out if the total CPK is very high. There appears to be no correlation between the severity of cardiac injury and the level of CPK-MB isoenzymes. Likewise, normal CPK-MB levels do not entirely rule out blunt myocardial injury. In Sutherland's study, up to two-thirds of patients with impaired ventricular motion on gated radionuclide angiography had normal CPK-MB levels.

Technetium Pyrophosphate Scan

Myocardial cell death is accompanied by an influx of calcium ions, which bind to the crystalline lattice or hydroxyapatite within the mitochondria. Technetium pyrophosphate (^{99m}Tc PYP) is normally used as a bone scanning agent, and it has also been found to label the hydroxyapatite in infarcted myocardium. However, most investigators feel that ^{99m}Tc PYP is less sensitive than ECG or CPK-MB studies for the identification of myocardial contusion. Brantigan and associates studied 29 patients suspected of having myocardial contusion. Of 13 patients with ECG abnormalities, only two (6.8 percent) had positive PYP scans. Similarly, Potkin and coworkers found positive PYP scans in only 2 percent of their patients suspected of having had a myocardial contusion. None of the five patients who had autopsy-proven myocardial contusions had a positive PYP scan.

There are several reasons why ^{99m}Tc PYP scans lack sensitivity in patients with myocardial contusions. In order for such a scan to be positive, a transmural injury is necessary to bind enough scintigraphic tracer to distinguish the lesion from background noise. The sensitivity of the scan is further hampered because it cannot differentiate a contusion of the right ventricle from an overlying sternal fracture or chest wall contusion.

Radionuclide Angiography

First-pass biventricular radionuclide angiography (RNA), including left ventricular segmental wall motion (LVSWM) analysis can now be performed at the bedside as well as in the radiology department. The study can be performed with the patient in any position, although the 30° RAO is preferable. An IV injection of 15 mg of stannous pyrophosphate is followed by a 15-μCi bolus injection of sodium pertechnetate ^{99m}Tc about 10 to 20 min later. Raw data are transferred from a single-crystal camera to magnetic tape, and the acquisitions are analyzed with a digital computer in an event-to-event mode for 30 s. These acquisitions are processed for both right and left ventricular ejection fractions (RVEF and LVEF) and for right and left ventricular segmental wall motion analysis. The normal LVEF is 62 ± 5 percent (mean ± SD), and the normal RVEF is 50 ± 4 percent. A LVEF less than 50 percent (>2.5 SD below the mean) and a RVEF <40 percent are interpreted as abnormal. Using this technique, Harley and Mena found that 11 of 12 patients with sternal fractures had abnormalities of ventricular contraction and motion; however, only 4 had ECG changes, and none had abnormal CPK-MB. Sutherland and associates had similar findings, with less than a third of the patients with abnormal RNA having ECG or CPK-MB abnormalities.

Thus, gated RNA appears to be a very sensitive technique for assessing cardiac function (left and right ventricular ejection fractions) and wall motion abnormalities. The quality of information is similar to that provided by good two-dimensional echocardiograms.

As a result of recent studies of emergency department patients with first-pass RNA, some authors have recommended the use of RNA on all trauma patients with no other problems except suspected cardiac injury. They feel that patients with normal RNA can be observed in the emergency department for 4 to 6 h and then safely discharged home to be followed as outpatients.

Single Photon Emission Computed Tomography

Recently, another technique, utilizing thallous chloride^{201}Tl, for imaging the heart has been described. Following IV injection of this radioactive potassium analogue, the thallium is extracted from the blood into normally functioning myocardial cells. It has been used effectively for some time in the investigation of a number of myocardial conditions such as ischemia and myocardial infarction. However, conventional thallous chloride ^{201}Tl imaging is unreliable for detecting small, partial-thickness lesions. The ability to acquire thallous chloride ^{201}Tl images of the heart in such a way that they can be processed, reconstructed, and displayed by computer in the form of tomographic slices in different planes of the heart is termed single photon emission computed tomography (SPECT). This has been shown to add significantly to the accuracy of thallous chloride ^{201}Tl myocardial imaging.

In Waxman's series of 48 patients with blunt chest trauma, 23 had normal SPECT studies, and none of these 23 developed any serious arrhythmias. However, 5 of 25 with abnormal or ambiguous studies did develop arrhythmias requiring treatment.

Echocardiography

Two-dimensional echocardiography has many advantages in the diagnosis and subsequent management of acute cardiac contusion. Quantitative and qualitative information can be obtained noninvasively on the status of the cardiac chambers, wall motion abnormalities, functional integrity of the valves, cardiac tamponade, and intracardiac thrombus or shunts. In addition, two-dimensional echocardiography can differentiate right from left ventricular contusions as well as right ventricular contusions from pericardial tamponade, a distinction that has important therapeutic implications. Pandian and coworkers found that contused myocardium could be identified on two-dimensional echocardiogram by (1) increased echo brightness, (2) increased end-diastolic wall thickness, and (3) impaired regional systolic function.

The most common abnormality seen is right ventricular free wall dyskinesia, often with some dilation. In addition, almost half the patients studied in some series have had mural thrombi attached to the contused myocardium. Patients with dysfunction demonstrated by abnormal anterior heart wall motion have a significantly increased incidence of hypotension and arrhythmias, especially during prolonged general anesthesia.

Many authors currently advocate obtaining a two-dimensional echocardiogram on all patients with suspected cardiac injuries, particularly if they have an abnormal ECG or elevated cardiac isoenzymes. This can be done safely and rapidly in the emergency department.

Monitoring of Pulmonary Artery Wedge Pressure and Cardiac Output

A pulmonary artery catheter should be inserted to monitor pulmonary artery pressures and cardiac output in patients with suspected myocardial contusion and hemodynamic impairment, preexisting cardiac disease, or need for a major operative procedure under general anesthesia. Determinations of ventricular function curves with fluid loading have revealed a high incidence of subclinical biventricular dysfunction in patients with severe blunt chest trauma and an associated 40-percent morbidity and mortality. Baseline cardiac output may be relatively normal, but there is often a poor response to fluid loading.

Summary of Diagnostic Approach

Patients with known or clinically suspected cardiac injury should be admitted to a unit that can provide continuous cardioscopic monitoring. If the CPK-MB and ECGs are all negative for 48 h, it is unlikely that a significant cardiac injury exists. Nevertheless, two-dimensional echocardiography or RNA are much more accurate tests and should probably be performed in individuals who have other significant injuries or may require a general anesthetic. Determination of ejection fractions and/or studying the response to a fluid challenge with a pulmonary artery wedge pressure (PAWP) catheter in place provides the best information on the degree of myocardial dysfunction. Cardiac catheterization and coronary angiography should be performed if cardiac symptoms persist for more than a few days.

Treatment

Although Glinz's series of 108 patients with myocardial contusions had 37 patients who required treatment of rhythm or conduction disturbances or heart failure, specific treatment interventions are seldom required. Furthermore, Stoll and associates suggest that cardiac monitoring is only necessary in patients with preexisting cardiac disease, severe associated injuries, or ECG changes suggestive of ischemia or arrhythmias. At this time, however, continuous ECG and noninvasive hemodynamic monitoring are probably prudent. Holter monitoring in selected cases may also be wise.

According to Frazee and coworkers, patients without identifiable CPK-MB changes or wall motion abnormalities on two-dimensional echocardiography or RNA do not require continuous cardioscopic monitoring and cardiac precautions unless indicated by severe associated injuries.

Supplemental oxygen should be administered as needed to maintain the P_{O_2} above 80 mmHg, and analgesics should be given as needed to reduce pain associated with tachycardia or hypertension. Coronary vasodilators should not be used unless patients have suspected preexisting coronary artery disease. Cardiac arrhythmias should be diagnosed early and treated appropriately. Prophylactic treatment of arrhythmias is not indicated. Low cardiac output or hypotension should be treated with fluids or inotropic agents as indicated.

Patients with myocardial contusion can safely undergo surgical procedures if the PAWP and cardiac output are closely monitored. In Snow's series, no operative deaths were recorded in 27 such patients. In Flancbaum's series of 19 patients with myocardial contusion proven by RNA who had surgery for associated injuries, 11 required perioperative inotropic support and 1 needed intraaortic balloom pumping (IABP). However, no patient died or had complications due to the myocardial contusion. Thus, important surgery should not be delayed because of a suspected myocardial contusion unless the patient has arrhythmias or is hemodynamically unstable. However, PAWP monitoring is strongly suggested, and IABP should be available if cardiogenic shock develops. If time is available, two-dimensional echocardiography or RNA may be very helpful in assessing the degree of myocardial dysfunction preoperatively.

If the patient remains in a low-output state despite adequate volume, inotropic support, and correction of any mechanical problems, such as tamponade, an intraaortic balloon counterpulsation device should be inserted. Diastolic augmentation with the IABP was shown by Saunders and Doty to improve cardiac output in a group of dogs with experimentally inflicted cardiac contusions. The intervention was most successful in the group whose cardiac output was reduced 26 to 50 percent below that of controls. These authors found that IABP was most effective if applied as early as possible. Snow and associates used this device in several patients with low cardiac output resulting from cardiac contusion and obtained a significant improvement in circulatory dynamics in all of them.

There is some question as to whether patients with a myocardial contusion and an intramural thrombus on two-dimensional echocardiography should have prophylactic anticoagulation if not otherwise contraindicated. Although five of seven patients with chest trauma in Miller's series had echocardiographically proven right ventricular thrombi, none of the patients had subsequent systemic or pulmonary embolization. Furthermore, anticoagulation is contraindicated in most cases of multiple trauma because of the potential for severe hemorrhage. Anticoagulation might also increase the area of contusion necrosis by promoting intramural bleeding or might cause tamponade by increasing the likelihood of bleeding within the pericardium. However, in the unusual instance of a patient with proven intramural thrombosis in whom there is no contraindication to anticoagulation but there is suspicion of embolization, "mild" to "moderate" heparinization (500 to 800 units/h) could be considered.

Coronary Arterial Injury

Direct injury to the coronary arteries from blunt chest trauma occurs very rarely, but if the patient presents with pericardial tamponade or intrathoracic bleeding, immediate operation is required. Coronary artery thrombosis is also rare but has been reported. In one series of eight patients with documented myocardial contusion, one had a coronary artery occlusion on angiography. In a much larger autopsy series, Parmley and coworkers found coronary lacerations in only 10 of 546 patients with fatal blunt chest trauma.

Several investigators have studied postmortem angiograms of experimental myocardial trauma in dogs and in humans following trauma. In dogs, almost immediately following impact a transmural redistribution of small vessel perfusion to the myocardium distal to the site of injury could be demonstrated. The researchers found no associated coronary artery spasm; in fact, a significant decrease in distal small vessel resistance was noted. When dogs were killed immediately after experimental contusion and postmortem angiographic studies were performed, large collections of contrast material were found accumulated in the terminal branches of small vessels in the area of the damaged muscle. These collections appear to be dilated vascular channels or "giant capillary sinusoids," which are probably a type of arteriovenous communication. It was concluded that these channels, with their associated local arteriovenous shunting, and not impaired coronary artery perfusion, lead to regional myocardial ischemia.

A more common clinical problem causing myocardial ischemia and contusion is preexisting coronary artery disease. In patients with coronary disease who already have a decreased cardiac reserve, the added loss of myocardial contractility from a contusion can severely compromise cardiac output. Cardiac catheterization may play an important role in evaluating such patients.

Pericardial Injury and Effusion

Hemopericardium or pericardial effusion with or without frank tamponade can occur with any evidence of blunt cardiac injury. This condition may develop acutely or be delayed as long as a week or more. As with other causes of pericardial effusion, the rate of fluid accumulation has some effect on the hemodynamic consequences.

Pericardial injury from blunt trauma should be suspected if there is ECG or other evidence of myocardial damage. However, a normal ECG does not rule out traumatic pericarditis. In some instances, only echocardiography or autopsy may provide the diagnosis. Tamponade due to effusions from injured pericardium may occur within minutes or as late as a week or more after the injury. If blood is found on pericardiocentesis following blunt trauma, a thoracotomy should be performed, preferably with cardiopulmonary bypass available.

Small serous or serosanguineous posttraumatic pericardial effusions can be seen with many cardiac injuries following blunt chest trauma. The small effusions are usually of no consequence and generally remain asymptomatic and resolve without any therapy. Nevertheless, in rare instances a patient may develop late constrictive pericarditis, occasionally with extensive calcification of the pericardium. Like chronic hemopericardium, this condition may eventually necessitate pericardiectomy.

Occasionally, severe blunt chest trauma may tear the parietal pericardium. If the hole is large enough and near the apex, the heart may actually herniate out through the defect, causing sudden severe shock or cardiac arrest.

Follow-up

Most patients discharged home after blunt cardiac injury do well. When RNA has been repeated after myocardial contusion, there has been almost uniform significant improvement by 3 weeks. By 1 year, follow-up studies indicate that right and left ejection fractions during maximal work load are essentially the same as other patients with chest injuries who have not had any evidence of cardiac trauma.

Nevertheless, it is important that patients with proven or suspected cardiac injury be closely observed, not only throughout their hospital stay but also later, for undiagnosed injuries or complications. One should look particularly for posttraumatic pericarditis, ventricular septal defect, valvular defects, and ventricular aneurysms. When such problems are found and it appears that the defect endangers the patient's life, cardiac catheterization and surgical repair should be performed as soon as possible. However, if the patient tolerates the lesion well, cardiac catheterization can be performed electively 6 to 8 weeks later.

Postpericardiotomy Syndrome

Etiology and Pathogenesis

The cause of the postpericardiotomy syndrome (PPCS) is still largely unknown but may be a delayed hypersensitivity reaction to the presence of damaged blood, pericardium, or myocardium in the pericardial cavity. This damaged tissue can act as a foreign protein, inducing the production of autoantibodies against similar tissues. In fact, antiheart antibodies can be measured, and their serum concentration varies with the severity of the symptoms. On the other hand, autogenous blood and lipids in the pericardium can set up an intense inflammatory response that may also be a contributing factor.

Diagnosis

PPCS should be suspected in individuals who develop chest pain, fever, and pleural or pericardial effusions 2 to 4 weeks after heart surgery or trauma. These patients may also have friction rubs, arthralgia, and even pulmonary infiltrates. The blood count often shows a lymphocytosis, and the ECG will often show ST-T wave changes consistent with pericarditis.

Treatment

Treatment is primarily symptomatic. Salicylates and rest can often reduce symptoms dramatically within 12 to 24 h. Corticosteroids are occasionally required and will also usually reduce the symptoms within 48 to 72 h. Rarely, drainage of pleural or pericardial fluid may be required to relieve symptoms or rule out other, more serious problems.

PENETRATING TRAUMA TO GREAT VESSELS OF THE CHEST

Of the patients who reach the hospital with penetrating chest wounds and require admission, only 5 to 15 percent require a thoracotomy, but up to 25 percent of these patients have major vascular injury. The survival rate with stab wounds is generally much higher than with gunshot wounds. Small knife wounds are often sealed off quite rapidly by surrounding tissue, especially the vascular adventitia. This limits the amount of blood loss, particularly after hypotension develops. If the knife stays in place, it may temporarily seal the involved vessel. The amount of tissue destruction caused by a bullet is determined largely by the kinetic energy (KE) lost after the missile enters the tissue. This can be calculated as $KE = \frac{1}{2}m(V_1^2 - V_2^2)$. Thus, the tissue destruction is proportional to the mass (m) of the missile and the entering velocity squared (V_2^2) minus the exiting velocity squared (V_2^2) as the bullet leaves the tissue. If the bullet remains in the patient, V_2^2 is zero. Thus, a rifle bullet with a velocity of 3000 ft/s can impart 25 times as much damage to tissue as a pistol bullet of similar weight going at 600 ft/s. A close-range shotgun blast, particularly by 12-gauge shotgun pellets, can be even more destructive.

Types of Vascular Injuries

Simple lacerations of the great arteries of the chest can cause exsanguination, tamponade, hemothorax, or air embolism. Other vascular injuries include arteriovenous (AV) fistulas and false aneurysms. Injuries to a systemic artery and vein lying side by side within a contained hematoma can lead to formation of an AV fistula. As time passes, the fistula enlarges. If more than 25 percent of the cardiac output goes through the AV fistula, high-output cardiac failure is likely to develop.

Pulmonary AV fistulas after penetrating chest trauma are said to be extremely rare because of the small pressure differential that usually exists between the pulmonary arteries and veins. However, injuries to adjacent major pulmonary arteries and veins can lead to AV fistulas, especially if pulmonary arterial pressures are high or rise, as they often do in severe trauma. A high degree of shunting in the lung with a persisting pulmonary density should make one suspect this problem.

A small injury to an artery leading into a contained hematoma will often stop bleeding, and the hematoma will gradually resolve. In some instances, however, the opening into the hematoma remains patent, and the hematoma may develop into a false aneurysm with a pseudoendothelial lining. These false aneurysms tend to enlarge and rupture, usually within a few days, but they may remain relatively stable for many years.

Diagnosis

History

Most penetrating wounds of the chest are quite obvious. However, certain historical facts can be helpful. For example, the amount of time the patient spent at the scene and in transit may be extremely important in considering whether to perform an emergency department thoracotomy on a patient who arrives in cardiac arrest. A "down-time" exceeding 10 to 15 min rarely, if ever, allows one to perform a successful resuscitation with satisfactory neurologic outcome.

The size of a knife, its depth, and the angle of penetration may indicate the vessels or organs most likely to be injured. If there are two skin wounds, it may be helpful to know whether they represent two entrance wounds or an exit and an entrance wound. In some instances, a bullet that entered the chest without exiting is not evident on chest or abdominal x-rays because it is in subcutaneous tissues or has entered a major vessel and embolized. It is also extremely important to know, if possible, the caliber of the bullet and whether it was a high-velocity missile (>1000 ft/s), which tends to cause far more tissue destruction than knives or low-velocity bullets. High-velocity missile injuries usually require much more debridement.

Physical Examination

Small wounds, especially in the axilla or in heavy chest hair, may easily be missed. Although one does not usually probe chest wounds because this may restart severe external or internal bleeding, careful superficial instrumentation may provide important information on the direction of the tract.

A large upper mediastinal hematoma may cause an acute superior vena caval syndrome, tracheal compression, and respiratory distress. Occasionally, a decreased upper extremity pulse may be noted. However, Flint and associates found that 45 (32 percent) of 146 patients with 206 injuries to the major vessels at the thoracic inlet had none of the usual diagnostic signs of significant vascular injury.

Distended neck veins may indicate pericardial tamponade, tension pneumothorax, heart failure, systemic air embolism, or damage to or compression of the superior vena cava. However, neck vein distension often does not become apparent until the hypovolemia is at least partially corrected.

One should auscultate the entire chest for bruits after a penetrating chest injury. A systolic bruit, particularly over the back or upper chest, should make one suspect a false aneurysm involving one of the great vessels. A continuous bruit suggests an AV fistula. A millwheel murmur, thought to be due to the churning of air in the heart, may be diagnostic of air embolism. Loss of a peripheral pulse caused by an embolization of a bullet from a thoracic vascular injury is occasionally seen.

Radiography

Plain Radiographs

Evidence of cervical or supraclavicular swelling or widening of the upper mediastinal silhouette on chest x-ray is often present in patients with injury to the innominate vessels. However, the widened mediastinum noted with innominate artery injury is usually more superior than that seen after aortic injury.

One should not assume that a "fuzzy" foreign body (bullet) on an x-ray film is due to poor radiological technique. Because foreign bodies tend to pulsate when they lie next to major vessels, their margins may appear indistinct on chest films. Therefore, a fuzzy foreign body fragment contiguous with clear mediastinal structures on chest films can be an important x-ray clue to vascular injury. Fluoroscopy showing pulsation of the foreign body may lend additional support to the suspicion of vascular involvement. Even if the angiogram is normal, a fuzzy foreign body should still be considered an indication for surgery because a vascular injury is likely to be present.

Computed Tomography Scan

Computed tomography (CT) scans are rarely performed immediately for penetrating wounds of the chest because of the usually precarious condition of the patient. However, in a stable patient, a CT scan can identify localized hematomas or collections of blood that may not be apparent on routine x-rays. If a persistent "mass" is adjacent to a great vessel and does not move with position changes by the patient, one should assume a contained hematoma is present. IV contrast provides additional help for demonstrating a vascular defect or false aneurysm on the CT scan. CT scans can be very helpful in diagnosing thoracic aorta trauma or dissection, and false-negative CT scans without an adjacent hematoma are unusual. Nevertheless, CT scans should be used primarily for screening rather than for definitive diagnosis.

Arteriogram

Arteriograms may be particularly helpful in identifying major intrathoracic vascular injuries within contained hematomas, especially those resulting from penetrating wounds of the lower neck. Indeed, before exploring penetrating injuries of the thoracic inlet in hemodynamically stable patients, one should obtain a preoperative arteriogram to visualize the arch of the aorta and its major branches.

Venograms

Venograms to identify major vascular injuries in the chest are seldom performed. A patient who is actively bleeding from a major venous injury is usually explored emergently because of unstable vital signs or continued blood loss through chest tubes. However, after a venous injury stops bleeding, the hemorrhage often does not recur, and the damaged vessel will usually not require a thoracotomy.

Contrast Swallows

A contrast swallow may be performed on a stable patient if there is concern about associated esophageal injury. Gastrographin is used first, but may miss up to half of esophageal leaks. Barium swallows have fewer false negatives but aggravate the mediastinitis if a perforation is present.

Endoscopy

With penetrating wounds of the chest or lower neck in hemodynamically stable patients, it may be prudent to perform bronchoscopy and esophagoscopy to rule out an injury to the aerodigestive tract. In some patients with "hemoptysis," the source may not be clear, and such bleeding may result from injury to lung parenchyma, trachea, or a major bronchus. In other instances, it may be unclear as to whether mediastinal air is caused by an esophageal, a pulmonary, or a tracheobronchial injury.

Treatment

Initial Resuscitation

The standard ABCs of initial resuscitation should be followed aggressively if the patient is in shock. These steps include (1) rapid clearing and maintenance of the airway; (2) establishment of adequate ventilation using a respirator, oxygen, and/or chest tubes as necessary; and (3) establishment of adequate circulation using IV fluids and control of bleeding (external or internal). Resuscitative internal cardiac massage may also be required.

Particular problems may be seen with injuries to the vessels in the thoracic outlet. Because of massive mediastinal hematoma formation and lower cervical swelling, tracheal compression and airway obstruction may occur. Consequently, early endotracheal intubation should be performed. Tracheostomy should be avoided in patients with injuries at the thoracic inlet, at least initially, because of the possibility of precipitating massive bleeding from an otherwise controlled hematoma.

If the patient is in shock, two to three veins are cannulated with large-gauge vascular catheters, and fluid is administered very rapidly. If the entrance wound is in the lower neck or upper chest, at least one, and preferably two, of the IVs should be started in the lower extremities.

Our goal is to infuse 3000 mL of balanced electrolyte solution in 10 to 15 min if hypovolemic shock is present. If the shock is persistent in spite of this fluid and there is no neck vein distension or any other apparent cause of the shock, the patient is rushed to the operating room while type-specific blood and further fluid are administered rapidly.

Blood in the pleural cavity should be removed completely and rapidly by tube thoracostomy. If the hemothorax is not removed, it not only restricts ventilation and venous return, but its clots will also release fibrinolytic and fibrinogenolytic substances that can act as local anticoagulants and contribute to continued intrathoracic bleeding.

If the patient is still hypotensive after 3000 mL of fluid is infused in the initial 10 to 15 min and there is no other apparent cause for the shock, the patient is brought immediately to the operating room for an emergency thoracotomy to relieve tamponade and control bleeding. If the patient has or is about to have a cardiac arrest in the emergency department, an immediate thoracotomy should be performed there to control bleeding, provide internal cardiac massage, and cross-clamp the descending thoracic aorta.

Even if the patient's vital signs are relatively stable, one should probably perform a thoracotomy for continued bleeding if (1) a total of more than 1500 mL of blood is lost from the chest within the first 4 to 8 h and the patient is still bleeding, (2) the drainage of blood from the chest tubes continues to exceed 200 to 300 mL/h, or (3) the chest continues to be more than half full of blood on x-ray after the chest tubes are inserted and functioning well.

Acute Complications of Penetrating Thoracic Vascular Trauma

The great majority of deaths are due to exsanguination. Many of these patients arrive with no obtainable blood pressure and, in spite of aggressive resuscitation, arrest in the emergency department or arrive in the operating room with continued severe shock. If rapid control of the bleeding sites and cross-clamping of the descending thoracic aortic arch do not raise the systolic blood pressure to at least 90 mmHg within 5 min, terminal cardiovascular failure is present, and almost all of these patients will die in the operating room. If large doses of epinephrine or dopamine combined with aortic cross-clamping can raise the systolic blood pressure over 90 mmHg, death is still almost invariably the outcome.

Bullets entering large systemic veins or the right heart can embolize to the lungs, whereas bullets entering the pulmonary veins, left heart, or major systemic arteries can embolize to carotid, iliac, femoral, or even popliteal arteries. Some of these emboli cause no symptoms or signs and cannot be found except with multiple x-rays. Fluoroscopy in the operating room can be important in tracing these bullets, especially in the central veins or heart, because they can change position rapidly during the surgery itself.

Blunt Trauma to the Great Vessels in the Chest

Incidence

Approximately 80 to 90 percent of patients with blunt trauma to thoracic great vessels, particularly the aorta, die at the scene of the accident or assault, and up to 50 percent of the remaining patients die within 24 h if not promptly treated. The frequency of these injuries appears to be increasing and is primarily related to the use of high-speed automobiles. Each year at least 5000 to 8000 individuals in the United States suffer traumatic rupture of the thoracic aorta or one of the other great arteries in the chest.

Mechanism of Injury

The mechanical factors responsible for traumatic rupture of the thoracic aorta and its major branches are probably somewhat different for each anatomic area. For the descending aorta at the level of the isthmus, three mechanical factors thought to contribute to rupture are shearing stress, bending stress, and torsion stress. The difference in deceleration between the mobile aortic arch and the relatively immobile descending aorta puts the aortic isthmus under tension, and the resultant shearing stress can lead to rupture opposite the site of fixation. Bending stress is produced as the heart exerts downward traction on the aortic arch, resulting in hyperflexion of the blood-filled aortic arch on a transverse mechanical bar and fulcrum created by the hilar structures of the left lung. Torsion stress occurs when there is anteroposterior compression of the chest with displacement of the heart to the left, with a pressure wave of blood transmitted to the aorta. These three forces can combine to produce maximum stress to the inner surface of the aorta at its point of greatest fixation, the ligamentum arteriosum.

The aortic injury tends to progress from the intima out toward the adventitia. The adventitia, which has the lowest elastic limit, seems to withstand these stresses better than the intima or media. Although the aorta tolerates longitudinal stretch forces less well than lateral forces, a sudden increase in intraluminal pressure also may be a factor in rupture of the aorta.

With vertical deceleration injuries, as from falls involving heights, there is a slightly increased incidence of rupture of the ascending aorta, particularly in those who die immediately. The vertical deceleration produces acute lengthening of the aorta, with resultant development of a pressure wave in the aortic blood column. This water-hammer effect, which is greatest in the ascending aorta, is believed to contribute greatly to rupture in that location.

Rupture of the innominate or left subclavian artery at its origins probably results from the interaction of two forces. One is a compression force that displaces the heart into the left chest and places the brachycephalic vessels under tension at their attachment to the aortic arch. The other force occurs when hyperextension of the neck with rotation of the head to one side places the contralateral subclavian vessels under additional stretch. The resulting tension leads to the development of maximum shearing stresses at the origins of these vessels. Injuries to the subclavian arteries can also occur just over the first rib, and these injuries are probably caused by direct trauma and/or stretching over that structure.

Pathologic Changes

Blunt aortic tears usually extend partially or completely around the vessel in a transverse or spiral direction. Preexisting disease, such as atherosclerosis or medial necrosis, does not appear to predispose to traumatic rupture. When the aortic tear involves all layers of the aortic wall, death by exsanguination is usually almost instantaneous. When the tear does not involve the adventitia and the parietal pleura and the surrounding mediastinal tissues remain intact, a false aneurysm is formed. The false aneurysm tends to expand, and about 50 percent rupture within 24 h. However, these false aneurysms may remain intact and not be detected for 20 years or longer. Although lacerations of the subclavian artery are occasionally followed by the formation of a false aneurysm, subclavian arteries injured by blunt trauma usually just occlude.

It should be emphasized that the small hemothorax that is often present with blunt trauma to the aorta does not result from the aortic injury itself, but rather from tears to adjacent small mediastinal vessels or other structures. Although the widened mediastinum may be partly due to the pseudoaneurysm, much of it is actually caused by bleeding from small mediastinal vessels.

Natural History

Of the estimated 5000 to 8000 patients who have a traumatic rupture of the thoracic aorta annually, 80 to 90 percent die within a few minutes of their injury. Parmley and associates found that, of the patients who reach a hospital and survive for 1 h, 20 to 30 percent die within 6 h, 40 to 50 percent die within 24 h, 60 to 80 percent die within 7 days, 80 to 90 percent die within 4 weeks, and 90 to 95 percent die within 3 months.

Many of the early deaths are caused by associated injuries, but even when the aortic injury is an isolated problem, diagnosis and repair should be accomplished quickly. All too often the patient dies of exsanguination before a definitive repair can be effected. Proper control of blood pressure and prevention of Valsalva maneuvers might have prevented many of these early deaths.

Location

At least 90 percent of blunt aortic injuries in patients who reach the hospital alive occur in the isthmus of the aorta between the left subclavian artery and the ligamentum arteriosum. The next most common great artery injured by blunt thoracic trauma in patients reaching a hospital alive is the innominate artery, usually at its origin. Patients do not usually survive injury to the ascending aorta, but this injury may be seen in up to one-third of the individuals who die at the scene of an accident, especially with vertical deceleration from falls from great heights or plane crashes. Tears in the lower aorta below the ligamentum arteriosum are quite uncommon but tend to occur adjacent to severely comminuted fractures of vertebral bodies.

Diagnosis

History

The single most important factor in establishing the diagnosis of acute traumatic aortic rupture is a high index of suspicion because of the nature of the trauma (Table 174-3). Even if there is no external evidence of chest injury, one must still be acutely aware of the possibility of this injury in anyone who has sustained an accident characterized by sudden severe deceleration. This is particularly true of a motor vehicle striking an immovable object.

Patients with traumatic aortic rupture usually complain primarily of their severe associated injuries and generally have no symptoms related to the aortic injury itself. The most common complaint that may be due to the aortic injury itself is retrosternal or interscapular pain from "stretching" or dissection of the adventitia of the aorta. Recurrence or exacerbation of the pain, particularly if associated with a rise in blood pressure (which may be due to excess fluid administration), may herald an impending rupture of the pseudoaneurysm. Less frequent symptoms, due primarily to pressure from the associated hematoma, include dysphagia, stridor, dyspnea, or hoarseness.

Physical Examination

In many reports, at least one-third of the patients with blunt trauma to the aorta have no external evidence of thoracic injury at the time of the initial physical examination. In fact, Kirsch reported that only 15 (27 percent) of 55 patients with traumatic rupture of the aorta (TRA) sustained identifiable chest wall contusion or rib fractures.

Physical findings that suggest aortic injury include (1) an acute onset of upper extremity hypertension, (2) difference in pulse amplitude between the upper and lower extremities, and (3) the presence of a harsh systolic murmur over the precordium or posterior interscapular

Table 174-3. Clinical Features Suggesting Possible Traumatic Rupture of the Aorta

History of high-speed deceleration injury
Multiple rib fractures or flail chest
Fractured first or second ribs
Fractured sternum
Pulse deficits
Hypertension, especially in the upper extremities
Systolic murmur, especially interscapular
Hoarseness or voice change without laryngeal injury
Superior vena cava syndrome

area. Upper extremity hypertension has occurred in 31 to 43 percent of the patients reported in the literature and has been attributed to compression of the aortic lumen by a periaortic hematoma. Nevertheless, the hypertension may also be secondary to stretching or stimulation of special receptors located in the vicinity of the aortic isthmus. This mechanism could account for the upper extremity hypertension that occurs without aortic narrowing and for the slowly resolving postoperative hypertension that is seen in up to one-third of patients successively repaired.

If the torn intima and media form a flap that acts as a "ball valve," partial or complete aortic obstruction can occur. With partial obstruction, an "acute coarctation syndrome" can develop, with hypertension in the upper extremities and weak pulses or hypotension in the lower extremities. A systolic murmur, thought to be caused by turbulent blood flow across the area of transection, is found in less than 30 percent of the patients with acute aortic rupture. If complete aortic obstruction occurs, anuria and paraplegia can develop almost immediately.

Other, less frequently encountered physical findings include hoarseness, voice change, superior vena cava syndrome, and swelling at the base of the neck, with an increase in collar size. Because the aorta is covered with a periadventitial sheath that extends up to the neck, a partial aortic tear may allow blood to extravasate along the branches of the aorta.

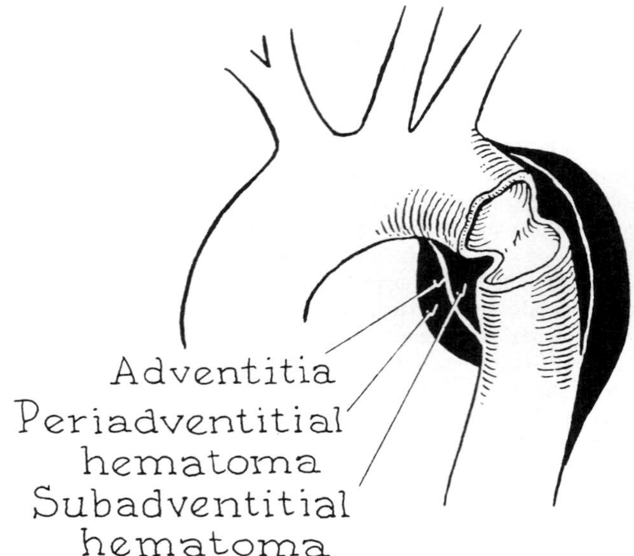

Fig. 174-1. The widening of the mediastinum around a traumatic rupture of the aorta usually results from hematoma in the subadventitial and periadventitial spaces. The periadventitial hematoma may be very large and is due primarily to bleeding from small mediastinal vessels.

Plain Chest X-ray

Although the circumstances of the accident and the physical examination may be helpful, the diagnosis of TRA is usually suspected from findings on routine chest x-ray (Table 174-4). The most frequent radiological finding noted is widening of the superior mediastinum, usually to more than 8.0 to 8.5 cm, caused primarily by subadventitial and periadventitial hematoma (Fig. 174-1). The ratio of the mediastinal width to the width of the chest may provide more accurate measurements but does not seem to be as specific or accurate as just the subjective impression of widening on a good upright chest x-ray.

One of the main reasons that many unnecessary aortograms are performed is a technically poor chest x-ray. The upper mediastinum tends to appear wider than normal if the chest x-ray is taken (1) anteroposteriorly (AP) rather than posteroanteriorly (PA), (2) with the patient less than 100 cm from the origin of the x-ray beam, (3) with the patient lying flat, or (4) with poor inspiration. The optimal chest x-ray is an upright PA chest x-ray taken at a distance of 6 ft with the patient leaning forward about 15°.

The most accurate x-ray radiograph sign of TRA is usually deviation of the esophagus more than 1 to 2 cm to the right of the spinous process of T_4 (Fig. 174-2). In Ayella's series, none of the patients with the esophagus less than 1.0 cm from the midline had a TRA. In a series of 45 patients, Gerlock and associates also noted that none of the patients with a nasogastric tube in normal position had TRA. A deviation of the esophagus more than 2.0 cm to the right after trauma is frequently due to a TRA. Blurring or obscuration of the aortic knob or descending aorta is almost as accurate an indication of TRA. In Marnocha's study of 86 patients with blunt chest trauma, of whom 13 patients had TRA, none with a normal aortic contour and no deviation of the trachea or nasogastric tube to the right on the chest x-ray had TRA.

Table 174-4. Some Chest Radiographic Findings Associated with Traumatic Rupture of the Aorta

Deviation of esophagus to the right at T4 more than 1.0–2.0 cm
Superior mediastinal widening
Obscuration of the aortic knob
Obliteration of the outline of descending aorta
Tracheal deviation to the right
Apical cap
Depression of left main stem bronchus more than 40 degrees
Obliteration of the aortopulmonary window
Obscuration of medial aspect of left upper lobe
Widened paravertebral stripe
Thickened and/or deviated paratracheal stripe
Fracture of first or second ribs
Fractured sternum, especially in younger individuals

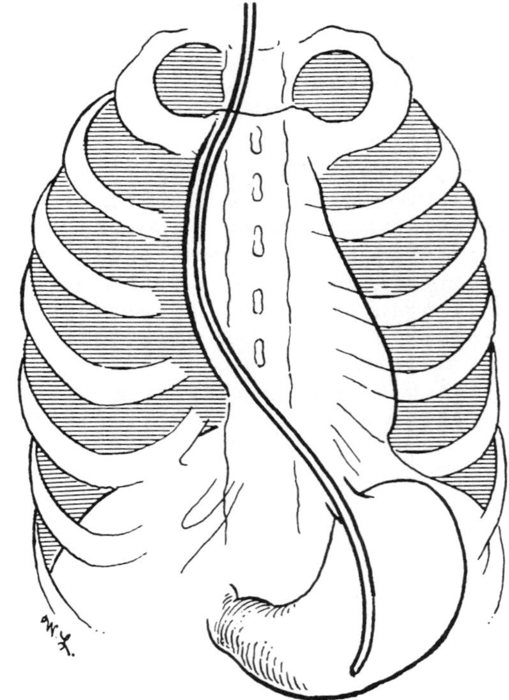

Fig. 174-2. Deviation of the esophagus (nasogastric tube) to the right is generally a very accurate sign of traumatic rupture of the aorta. If the distance from the nasogastric tube to the spinous process of the fourth thoracic vertebra is greater than 2.0 cm, it is almost 100-percent indicative of a torn descending thoracic aorta.

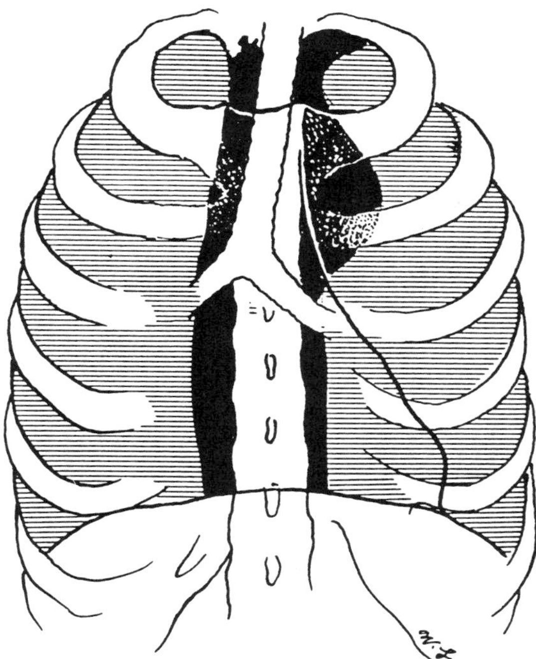

Fig. 174-3. Mediastinal hematomas, indicated by the blackened areas, may widen and displace the paratracheal stripe separating the right side of the tracheal air column from the medial border of the right lung by more than 5 mm. Mediastinal hematomas may also displace the right and left paraspinal lines in the lower thorax rather widely from the lateral edges of the thoracic spine. The paraspinal lines are not readily seen on most x-rays because of overlying structures.

Other chest x-ray signs include a left apical cap, displacement of the left main stem bronchus more than 40° below the horizontal, obliteration of the usual clear space between the aortic knob and the left pulmonary artery, widening of the right paratracheal stripe, and displacement of the right paraspinous interface (Fig. 174-3). In 1975, Simeone and associates stressed the value of the extrapleural left apical cap as a sign of an aortic isthmus tear. However, in 1981, they observed that if no other signs of TRA were present, aortography was not indicated.

The paratracheal stripe is a linear structure to the right of the tracheal air column. It extends from the thoracic inlet to the proximal right bronchus and normally measures less than 5 mm in thickness at a level 2 cm above the azygous vein. If the paratracheal stripe is more than 5 mm wide and/or deviated to the right, this may be another sign of mediastinal hemorrhage.

The right paraspinal line is usually not visible on routine chest x-rays, but if it is seen and is displaced to the right in the absence of spinal or sternal fractures, it may be of some diagnostic value. Peters and Gamsu found this sign in eight of fourteen patients with TRA and in none without this injury. The paraspinal lines lie between the pleura and the lung, projected away from the lateral margin of the thoracic spine. The left paraspinal line may be distinguished from the image of the descending aorta by the fact that it is not continuous with the aortic knob. When displaced more than one-half the distance from the spine to the left margin of the descending aorta without spine or sternal fractures, it was 83-percent specific.

It often takes great force to fracture the first or second ribs or sternum, especially in young patients. Consequently, such fractures tend to be associated with an increased incidence of major intrathoracic injuries. It is now controversial whether fractures of the first or second ribs are associated with an increased incidence of traumatic aortic rupture.

One should not assume that a TRA has been ruled out if the initial chest x-ray is normal. Unfortunately, in up to one-third of patients, widening of the mediastinum and other x-ray changes may not be apparent on the chest x-ray for several hours after the injury. Consequently, serial chest films should be taken in any patient with severe chest trauma at 6- to 8-h intervals during the first day and then daily for at least the next 3 days. However, Gundry and associates reported that up to two-thirds of patients older than 65 years with traumatic aortic rupture may not show mediastinal widening. In such individuals, the circumstances of the accident should be the main indication for ordering an aortogram.

Transesophageal Ultrasound

If transesophageal ultrasound is available and it can be performed on a cooperative patient without excessive gagging or vomiting, it can be a great help in the early diagnosis of intrathoracic problems after severe chest trauma.

Computed Tomography Scans

Although aortography has been considered the ideal method of diagnosing traumatic aortic rupture, there has been recent increasing enthusiasm for performing contrast-enhanced CT scans. In Heiberg's study of ten trauma patients, of whom four had TRA, CT examination provided no false positives or negatives, whereas one of thirteen positive aortograms was falsely positive.

In a recent study by Miller and associates, 10 percent of patients with chest trauma had both CT scans and thoracic aortograms looking for great vessel injuries. Of 67 with "negative" CT scans, 5 (7 percent) had a positive aortogram. A "positive" CT scan (hematoma directly contiguous to a vessel) was noted in 26 patients, but only 6 (23 percent) were positive on aortograms. Eleven had equivocal CT scans (soft tissue density contiguous to the aorta or a great vessel in which hematomas could not be ruled out) but were negative on aortogram.

Subtle changes in the aortic contour indicating transection or a thin filling defect from torn intima and media may be missed between the various CT scanning planes, which are usually 10 mm apart. The presence of a mediastinal hematoma on CT scan is an indication for aortography. We have used the CT scan primarily as a screening tool, and if there is any suspicion at all of an aortic injury on the CT scan, we order an aortogram. We are not aware of a TRA being missed on a properly done and properly read CT scan.

Magnetic Resonance Imaging

The newer generations of MRI may be particularly good for diagnosing dissecting aneurysms and therefore should be ideal for posttraumatic studies of the thoracic vessels if the patient is stable and can lie still long enough.

Aortography

If an aortic rupture is suspected on clinical or radiological grounds, an aortogram should be performed. While waiting for the aortogram or surgery, it is important to ensure that the blood pressure does not rise above 110 to 120 mmHg, as may easily occur with excess pain or IV fluids. It is also important to protect the patient from excessive gagging or straining such as may occur during insertion of a nasogastric tube.

The most common finding on aortogram is a pseudoaneurysm of the isthmus of the aorta. A slight pouching out of the inferior or inner border of isthmus, sometimes referred to as a pseudodiverticulum, is normal but may be confused with a traumatic pseudoaneurysm. Bulging of the aorta laterally is a more reliable indicator of TRA. A linear filling defect caused by torn intima and media is the best evidence that a TRA is present.

The left anterior oblique (LAO) x-ray appears to be optimal for examining the aortic arch and proximal descending aorta. In addition, the entire aorta and its branches, particularly those coming off the arch, should be visualized to rule out the less common ruptures that might otherwise be missed. A patient who is in shock from a suspected traumatic aortic rupture or who has a rapidly expanding mediastinal hematoma should be taken directly to the operating room without undergoing aortography. It should be remembered that occasional false negatives occur with aortography and up to 6 or 7 percent of aortograms cause significant complications.

Intraarterial Digital Subtraction Angiography

In an effort to improve the speed and accuracy of angiography and reduce the dose of contrast material, Mirvis and associates studied 61 consecutive patients with blunt thoracic trauma and obscuration of the aortic knob or mediastinal widening on the chest x-ray using intraarterial digital subtraction angiography (IA-DSA) of the thoracic aorta. Ten of these patients had aortic ruptures diagnosed by IA-DSA. Digital subtraction aortography proved 100-percent accurate, as indicated by results of surgery, conventional arteriography, serial chest x-rays, and clinical follow-up. The method was 50-percent faster than conventional aortography and significantly reduced x-ray film costs. The use of smaller-caliber catheters for the intraaortic injection and a decrease in radiographic contrast media requirements also make this method safer than conventional arteriography.

Treatment

Although it is essential to resuscitate severely injured patients aggressively and to rapidly correct hypotension and hypoxemia, the patient with a TRA should not be allowed to develop a systolic blood pressure over 110 to 120 mmHg or to perform a Valsalva maneuver. Fluid administration should be watched carefully, and administration of sedatives, analgesics, or even vasodilators may be required to keep the patient's systolic blood pressure at safe levels.

Although it is often important to insert a nasogastric tube in patients with multiple injuries, it is essential that the patient with a suspected TRA not perform a vigorous Valsalva maneuver. Sudden gagging or bearing down can cause intraaortic pressure to rise abruptly to well over 200 mmHg and complete the rupture of a partially torn aorta. Similar precautions must be undertaken when inserting an endotracheal tube.

Since the initial report of a successful repair of an acute traumatic thoracic aortic disruption in 1958, emergency operation has become the accepted standard for treatment. However, in selected cases, delays in surgical intervention may be warranted and safe. Such delay should be considered if (1) the patient is stable but the conditions for surgery are not ideal, or (2) the patient represents an extremely high operative risk because of associated injuries or preexisting medical conditions.

Special Considerations in Less Frequent Great Vessel Injuries

Injuries to the Ascending Aorta

Incidence

Very few patients with ascending aortic injury survive long enough for the diagnosis to be established and repair to be carried out. These injuries are frequently associated with cardiac rupture or severe myocardial contusion, and the aortic tears are multiple in up to 15 to 20 percent of these cases. These are not usually simple deceleration injuries. Most victims have been hit by or thrown from moving vehicles or have fallen from great heights.

Diagnosis

Since most ascending aortic tears occur within the pericardium, if there is a small complete tear, there is often evidence of both shock and pericardial tamponade. The chest x-ray findings often show a widened superior mediastinum with or without obscuration of the aortic knob. Aortography must be performed for the diagnosis to be established. The aortogram usually shows a pseudoaneurysm with an intimal tear seen as an irregular filling defect within the lumen. If there is an associated aortic valvular injury, aortic insufficiency of varying magnitude may also be seen.

Injury to the Lower Thoracic Aorta

Thoracic aortic injuries distal to the isthmus should be suspected with severe chest trauma in which a lower thoracic vertebra is severely crushed. Aortography is the diagnostic test of choice.

Other Great Vessel Injuries

Innominate Artery

Incidence

In patients reaching the hospital alive, blunt injuries of the innominate artery are second in frequency only to rupture of the aorta at the isthmus. Associated injuries, such as rib fractures, flail chest, hemopneumothorax, fractured extremities, head injuries, facial fractures, and abdominal injuries, are found in more than 75 percent of these patients.

Diagnosis

The diagnosis of blunt injury to the innominate artery may be difficult because there are no characteristic physical findings except for some diminution of the right radial or brachial pulse, which occurs in about 50 percent of the patients. Signs and symptoms of distal ischemia are uncommon. Occasionally, a systolic murmur may draw attention to a possible lesion in this area.

The chest x-ray findings are quite similar to those seen with TRA (i.e., a widened mediastinum with obscuration of the aortic knob shadow). However, the outline of the descending aorta may be preserved.

Aortography must be performed for the diagnosis to be established. Tears of the innominate artery typically show bulbous dilation of the vessel just distal to its origin, associated with a crescentic line across its base, representing retraction of the torn intima into the lumen of the vessel. Associated injuries in other brachycephalic vessels or the aorta are found in about 10 percent of patients.

Subclavian Artery Injury

Etiology

Although occasionally a subclavian artery is avulsed at its origin because of sudden deceleration, direct trauma to the distal artery with intimal damage and occlusion associated with fractures of the first rib or clavicle are much more likely. Incorrectly applied shoulder restraints that are too loose may be a major factor in causing this injury.

Diagnosis

The most important sign of a subclavian occlusion is absence of a radial pulse. In the patient with only a partial laceration and no occlusion, the radial pulse is usually readily palpable. Other physical findings that are highly suggestive of subclavian artery rupture are a pulsatile mass or a bruit in the root of the neck. Occasionally a patient may develop an acute subclavian steal syndrome if the subclavian artery injury is proximal to the origin of the vertebral artery.

Up to 60 percent of patients with blunt injury to the subclavian artery, especially from motor vehicle accidents, will also have damage to the brachial plexus. Consequently, a complete neurological examination preoperatively is important in these patients. A Horner's syndrome often indicates avulsion of nerve roots from the spinal cord.

The chest x-ray with subclavian artery injuries may show the presence of a widened superior mediastinum without obscuration of the aortic knob shadow. The angiogram usually shows occlusion, but a pseudoaneurysm is occasionally found. Blunt subclavian artery injuries are associated with other major vascular injuries in about 10 percent of patients.

Treatment

The treatment of acute subclavian artery injury is usually immediate repair. However, in certain high-risk patients who are doing poorly, ligation may be the treatment of choice. If the artery is already occluded, observation may be all that is required. The collateral circulation for the distal portions of the vessel is usually very good; however, many of the collateral vessels may be damaged by severe blunt trauma to the shoulder girdle. In Costa's series, 53 percent (8 of 15) of patients with blunt subclavian artery injuries had critical ischemia of the hand. In addition, during World War II, ligation of subclavian arteries resulted in upper extremity gangrene in 29 percent of cases.

BIBLIOGRAPHY

Chest Wall, Bronchi, Lung, and Diaphragm

Bassett JS, Gibson RD, Wilson RF: Blunt injuries to the chest. *J Trauma,* 8:418, 1968.

Brown GL, Richardson JD: Traumatic diaphragmatic hernia. *Ann Thorac Surg* 39:172, 1985.

Cullen P, Modell JH, Kirby RR, et al: Treatment of flail chest: Use of intermittent mandatory ventilation and positive end-expiratory pressure. *Arch Surg* 110:1099, 1975.

Daly RC, Mucha P, Pairlero PC, et al: The risk of percutaneous chest tube thoracostomy for blunt thoracic trauma. *Ann Emerg Med* 14:865, 1985.

LoCurto JL, Swan KG, Tischler CD, et al: Tube thoracostomy and trauma: Antibiotics or not? *J Trauma* 26:1067, 1986.

Mandal A, Montano J, Thadepalli H: Prophylactic antibiotics and no antibiotics compared in penetrating chest trauma. *J Trauma* 25:639, 1985.

Richardson JD, McElvein RB, Trinkle JK: First rib fracture: A hallmark of severe trauma. *Ann Surg* 181:251, 1975.

Trinkle JK, Richardson JD, Franz JL, et al: Management of flail chest without mechanical ventilation. *Ann Thorac Surg* 19:355, 1975.

Washington B, Wilson RF, Steiger Z, et al: Emergency thoracotomy: A four-year review. *Ann Thorac Surg* 40:188, 1985.

Wiencek RG, Wilson RF, Steiger Z: Acute injuries of the diaphragm. *J Thorac Cardiovasc Surg* 92:989, 1986.

Wilson JM, Thomas AN, Goodman PC, et al: Severe chest trauma: Morbidity implication of first and second rib fracture in 120 patients. *Arch Surg* 113:846, 1978.

Wilson RF, Soullier GW, Wiencek RG: Hemoptysis in trauma. *J Trauma* 27:1123, 1987.

Heart

Aldridge HE, Jay AWL: Central venous catheters and heart perforation. *Can Med Assoc J* 135:1082, 1986.

Arbulu A, Thoms N: Control of bleeding from a gunshot of the inferior cava at its junction with the right atrium by means of a Foley catheter. *J Thorac Cardiovasc Surg* 63:427, 1972.

Baker CC, Caronna JJ, Trunkey DD: Neurologic outcome after emergency room thoracotomy for trauma. *Am J Surg* 19:677, 1980.

Baker CC, Thomas ANM, Trunkey DD: The role of emergency room thoracotomy in trauma. *J Trauma* 20:848, 1980.

Brantigan CO, Burdick D, Hoperman AR, et al: Evaluation of technetium scanning for myocardial contusion. *J Trauma* 18:460, 1978.

Calhool JH, Hoffmann TH, Trinkle JK, et al: Management of blunt rupture of the heart. *J Trauma* 26:495, 1986.

Chiu CL, Roelofs JD, Go RT, et al: Coronary angiographic and scintigraphic findings in experimental cardiac contusion. *Radiology* 116:679, 1975.

Cogbill MH, Moore EE, Millikan JS, et al: Rationale for selective application of emergency department thoracotomy in trauma. *J Trauma* 23:453, 1983.

Demetriades D: Cardiac wounds. *Ann Surg* 203:315, 1985.

Doty DB, Anderson AE, Rose EF, et al: Clinical and experimental correlations of myocardial contusion. *Ann Surg* 180:452, 1974.

Flancbaum L, Wright J, Siegel JH: Emergency surgery in patients with post-traumatic myocardial contusion. *J Trauma* 26:795, 1986.

Frazee RC, Mucha P, Farnell MB, et al: Objective evaluation of blunt cardiac trauma. *J Trauma* 26:510, 1986.

Getz BS, Davies E, Steinberg SM, et al: Blunt cardiac trauma resulting in right atrial rupture. *JAMA* 255:761, 1986.

Glinz W: Problems caused by the unstable thoracic wall and by cardiac injury due to blunt injury. *Injury* 17:322, 1986.

Harley DP, Mena I: Cardiac and vascular sequelae of sternal fractures. *J Trauma* 26:553, 1986.

Harner TJ, Oreskkovick MR, Copass MK, et al: Role of emergency thoracotomy in the resuscitation of moribund trauma victims. *Am J Surg* 142:96, 1981.

Hassett A, Moran J, Sabiston DC, et al: Utility of echocardiography in the management of patients with penetrating missile wounds of the heart. *J Am Coll Cardiol* 7:1151, 1986.

Jaszczak RJ, Whitehead FR, Lim CB, et al: Lesion detection with single photon emission computerized tomography (SPECT) compared with conventional imaging. *J Nucl Med* 23:97, 1982.

King RM, Mucha P, Seward JB, et al: Cardiac contusion: A new diagnostic approach utilizing two-dimensional echocardiography. *J Trauma* 23:610, 1983.

Layton TR, Dimarco RF, Pellegrini RF: Rupture of the left atrium from blunt trauma. *J Trauma* 19:117, 1979.

Leidtke J, Allen RP, Nellis SH: Effects of blunt cardiac trauma on coronary vasomotion, perfusion, myocardial mechanics and metabolism. *J Trauma* 20:777, 1980.

Martin LF, Mavroundis C, Dyess DL, et al: The first 70 years' experience managing cardiac disruption due to penetrating and blunt injuries at the University of Louisville. *Am Surg* 52, 1986.

Michelow BJ, Bremner CG: Penetrating cardiac injuries: Selective conservatism—favorable or foolish? *J Trauma* 27:398, 1987.

Michelson WB: CPK-MB isoenzyme determinations: Diagnosis and prognostic value in evaluation of blunt chest trauma. *Ann Emerg Med* 11:562, 1980.

Miller FA, Seward JB, Gersh BJ, et al: Two-dimensional echocardiographic findings in cardiac trauma. *Am J Cardiol* 50:1022, 1982.

Moreno C, Moore EE, Majure JA, et al: Pericardial tamponade: A critical determinant for survival following penetrating cardiac wounds. *J Trauma* 26:821, 1986.

Muwanga CL, Cole RP, Sloan JP, et al: Cardiac contusion in patients wearing seat belts. *J Accident Surg* 17:37, 1986.

Pandian NG, Skorton DJ, Dothy DB, et al: Immediate diagnosis of acute myocardial contusion by two-dimensional echocardiography: Studies in a canine model of blunt chest trauma. *J Am Coll Cardiol* 2:448, 1983.

Parmley LF, Manion WC, Mattingly TW: Nonpenetrating traumatic injury to the heart. *Circulation* 18:371, 1958.

Potkin RT, Werner JA, Trobaugh GB, et al: Evaluation of noninvasive tests of cardiac damage in suspected cardiac contusion. *Circulation* 66:627, 1982.

Rodriguez A, Shatney C: The value of technetium-99m pyrophosphate scanning in the diagnosis of myocardial contusion. *Am Surg* 48:472, 1982.

Rohman M, Ivatury RR, Steichen RM, et al: Emergency room thoracotomy for penetrating cardiac injuries. *J Trauma* 23:570, 1983.

Rothestein RJ: Myocardial contusion: *JAMA* 250:2189, 1983.

Rothstein RJ, French RS, Mena I, et al: Myocardial contusion diagnosed by first-pass radionuclide angiography. *Am J Emerg Med* 4:210, 1986.

Saunders CR, Doty DB: Myocardial contusion: Effect of intraaortic balloon counterpulsation on cardiac output. *J Trauma* 18:706, 1978.

Shimazu S, Clayton HS: Outcomes of trauma patients with no vital signs on hospital admission. *J Trauma* 23:213, 1983.

Snow N, Richardson JD, Flint IM: Myocardial contusion: Implications for patients with multiple traumatic injuries. *Surgery* 92:744, 1982.

Stoll J, Schecter WP, Schlobolm RM, et al: Routine ICU admission for suspected myocardial contusion: Is it indicated? *J Trauma* 25:718, 1985 (abstract).

Sutherland GR, Cheung HW, Holliday RL, et al: Hemodynamic adaptation to acute myocardial contusion complicating blunt chest injury. *Am J Cardiol* 57:291, 1986.

Sutherland GR, Driedger AA, Holliday RL, et al: Frequency of myocardial injury after blunt chest treatment as evaluated by radionuclide angiography. *Am J Cardiol* 52:1099, 1983.

Tenzer ML: The spectrum of myocardial contusion: A review. *J Trauma* 25:620, 1985.

Washington B, Wilson RF, Steiger Z, et al: Emergency thoracotomy: A four-year review. *Ann Thorac Surg* 40:188, 1985.

Waxman K, Soliman MH, Braunstein P, et al: Diagnosis of traumatic cardiac contusion. *Arch Surg* 121:689, 1986.

Great Vessels

Ayella RJ: *Radiologic Management of the Massively Traumatized Patient.* Baltimore, William & Wilkins, 1978.

Barcia TC, Livoni JP: Indications for angiography in blunt thoracic trauma. *Radiology* 147:15, 1983.

Besson A, Saegesser F: *Chest Trauma and Associated Injuries.* Oradell, N.J., Medical Economics Books, 1983, vol 2.

Costa MC, Robbs JV: Nonpenetrating subclavian artery trauma. *J Vasc Surg* 8:71, 1988.

Egan TJ, Neiman HL, Herman RJ, et al: Computer tomography in the diagnosis of aortic aneurysm dissection of traumatic injury. *Radiology* 136:141, 1980.

Flint IM, Snyder WH, Perry MD, et al: Management of major vascular injuries in the base of the neck. *Arch Surg* 106:407, 1973.

Fox S, Pierce WS, Waldhausen JA: Acute hypertension: Its significance in traumatic aortic rupture. *J Thorac Cardiovasc Surg* 75:622, 1979.

Gerlock AJ, Muhletaler CA, Coulam CM, et al: Traumatic aortic aneurysm: Validity of esophageal tube displacement sign. *Am J Radiol* 135:713, 1980.

Graham JM, Feliciano DV, Mattox KL, et al: Management of subclavian vascular injuries. *J Trauma* 20:537, 1980.

Gundry SR, Williams S, Burney RE: Indications for aortography in blunt thoracic trauma: A reassessment. *J Trauma* 22:664, 1982.

Heiberg E, Wolveson MK, Sundaram M, et al: CT in aortic trauma. *Am J Radiol* 140:1119, 1983.

Kirsh MM, Sloan H: *Blunt Chest Trauma.* Boston, Little, Brown, 1977.

Marnocha KE, Maglinte DDT, Woods J, et al: Blunt chest trauma and suspected aortic rupture: Reliability of chest radiograph findings. *Ann Emerg Med* 14:644, 1985.

Mattox KL: Symposium: New approaches in vascular trauma. *J Vasc Surg* 7:725, 1988.

McFadden PM, Jones JW, Ochsner JL: The fuzzy foreign body fragment: A subtle roentgenographic clue to mediastinal vascular injury. *Am J Surg* 149:809, 1985.

Miller FB, Richardson JD, Thomas HA, et al: Role of CT in diagnosis of major arterial injury after blunt thoracic trauma. *Surgery* 106:596, 1989.

Mirvis SE, Pais OS, Gens DR: Thoracic aortic rupture: Advantages of intra-arterial digital subtraction angiography. *Am J Radiol* 146:987, 1986.

Oudkerk M, Overbosch E, Dee P: CT recognition of acute aortic dissection. *Am J Radiol* 141:671, 1983.

Pandian NG, Skorton DJ, Doty DB, et al: Immediate diagnosis of acute myocardial contusion by two-dimensional echocardiography: Studies in a canine model of blunt chest trauma. *J Am Coll Cardiol* 2:488, 1983.

Parmley LF, Mattingly TW, Manion WC: Nonpenetrating traumatic injury of the aorta. *Circulation* 17:1086, 1958.

Peters DR, Gamsu G: Displacement of the right paraspinous interface: A radiologic sign of acute traumatic rupture of the thoracic aorta. *Radiology* 134:599, 1980.

Rich NM, Spencer FC: Injuries of the intrathoracic branches of the aortic arch, in *Vascular Trauma.* Philadelphia, Saunders, 1978, p. 287.

Simeone JF, Deren MM, Cagle F: The value of the left apical cap in the diagnosis of aortic rupture. *Radiology* 139:35, 1981.

Simeone JF, Minagi H, Putman CE: Traumatic disruption of the thoracic aorta: Significance of the left apical extrapleural cap. *Radiology* 117:265, 1975.

Symbas PN, Goldman M, Erbesfeld MH, et al: Pulmonary arteriovenous fistula, pulmonary artery aneurysm, and other vascular changes of the lung from penetrating trauma. *Ann Surg* 191:336, 1980.

Washington B, Wilson RF, Steiger Z, et al: Emergency thoracotomy: A four-year review. *Ann Thorac Surg* 40:188, 1985.

White RD, Dooms GC, Higgins CB: Advances in imaging thoracic aortic disease. *Invest Radiol* 21:761, 1986.

Wilson RF, Arbulu A, Basset J, et al: Acute mediastinal widening following blunt chest trauma: Critical decisions. *Arch Surg* 104:551, 1972.

Wilson JM, Thomas AN, Goodman PC, et al: Severe chest trauma: Morbidity implication of first and second rib fracture in 120 patients. *Arch Surg* 113:846, 1985.

175
ABDOMINAL TRAUMA

Arthur L. Ney
Robert C. Andersen

Abdominal trauma is difficult to evaluate because of the many possible injuries and their varied presentations. The most serious mistake is to delay surgical intervention when it is needed. Most preventable deaths are a result of this mistake. The thrust of the examination and resuscitation should be to recognize surgical lesions, not to diagnose specific injuries. It is only occasionally helpful to know the exact injury preoperatively, and a prolonged examination to pinpoint the exact injury is generally detrimental.

The evaluation of the patient with abdominal trauma must be done in the context of the entire patient, and any injury must be dealt with after determining its priority. This means that a head, cardiac, great vessel, or respiratory injury may take precedence over an abdominal injury.

Peritoneal lavage continues to be the most useful adjunctive diagnostic test in abdominal trauma. In an unstable patient, the diagnostic peritoneal lavage (DPL) remains the "gold standard" in the evaluation of abdominal injury. Retroperitoneal injuries are, however, rarely diagnosed with this test. Computed tomography (CT) scanning has proved to be a valuable examination and in some centers has replaced DPL under certain circumstances. Lavage has the advantage of rapid evaluation of the peritoneal viscera with considerable sensitivity. Both tests have advantages and disadvantages. The choice of examination will depend on local resources. Neither test will eliminate the need for careful clinical evaluation and follow-up to monitor for progression of findings suggesting injury.

PATHOPHYSIOLOGY

Abdominal injuries are frequently divided into two main types on the basis of the wounding mechanism: blunt and penetrating. A fundamental point to be remembered is that combined injuries often occur. For example, a patient that has been stabbed may also have been kicked or beaten. Likewise, a patient in a motor vehicle accident will be expected to have significant blunt injury, but penetration from sharp objects can also occur. This concept of evaluating injuries serves to focus attention on the more likely injuries and to direct further diagnostic maneuvers.

Blunt Trauma

With blunt trauma to the abdomen, diagnostic acumen is necessary to identify injuries quickly. The presentation of injury may vary, depending on the area of the abdomen involved. The main divisions within the abdomen are the peritoneal cavity and the extraperitoneal potential space. The extraperitoneal area includes the retroperitoneum and the extraperitoneal pelvis. The retroperitoneum and extraperitoneal pelvis are difficult to examine. Peritoneal lavage is unreliable and can actually give a false sense of security. Ancillary tests are of the most help in evaluating these injuries. Intravenous pyelography, upper gastrointestinal contrast studies, cystography, angiography, and CT scanning will all be helpful in selected cases. CT scanning with contrast appears to be the most helpful single test in evaluating injury to retroperitoneal organs. Serum amylase is a helpful indicator of potential injury; however, significant pancreatic injury may be present with a normal serum level. A digital rectal examination and stool testing for occult blood are essential. Because of the insidious nature of these injuries, it is essential to maintain a high index of suspicion.

Injuries in the peritoneal cavity usually result in findings on examination of the anterior abdomen. Guarding, rigidity, rebound tenderness, or the presence of a palpable mass all suggest injury. In the absence of these signs, significant injury is unlikely but can occasionally occur, even in the presence of normal neurologic function. When there is doubt, diagnostic peritoneal lavage is extremely sensitive and reliable in evaluating the viscera in this portion of the abdomen.

Penetrating Injuries

Penetrating injuries can be thought of as two main types: those from gunshots and those from stab wounds. Injuries from gunshot wounds should be routinely explored. The only somewhat controversial area is the management of injuries close to the abdominal cavity where it is felt that peritoneal penetration is unlikely but remotely possible. In this situation, peritoneal lavage can help differentiate patients with and without peritoneal penetration. Use of DPL in these cases will need to be done in conjunction with the surgeon caring for the patient. An example is a low chest gunshot wound with hemopneumothorax where there remains a remote possibility that the bullet traversed the diaphragm. Some surgeons favor lavage followed by exploration if any red blood cells are present. Many would, however, routinely explore any patient with a gunshot injury when it is even remotely possible that the abdomen has been entered. High-velocity gunshot wounds may cause intraabdominal injury without peritoneal penetration, and a negative DPL may be misleading.

Penetrating injuries from stab wounds are associated with a high incidence of negative laparotomy if routinely explored. For this reason, these patients are managed in a more selective manner in trauma centers where experienced clinical monitoring and operating rooms are immediately available. There is a group of patients in which it is clear that celiotomy is indicated. This group includes patients with evisceration, peritoneal irritation, or persistent hypotension. We evaluate the remainder by wound exploration under local anesthesia. A positive wound exploration is the finding of penetration of the superficial fascia. It is very difficult, and as a result unreliable, to explore deeper wounds to detect peritoneal penetration in most patients. Sinograms are generally of no value. The next maneuver for evaluating peritoneal penetration is peritoneal lavage with an aliquot of the lavage fluid sent for evaluation. The accepted value for a positive count is still controversial, with trauma surgeons advocating celiotomy for a red blood cell count as low as 1000 cells/mm^3 to a high of 100,000 cells/mm^3. At our institution the positive value is 10,000 cells/mm^3. In patients with fewer or no red blood cells per cubic millimeter, a period of at least 24 h of observation is indicated. It is essential that these patients have a normal neurologic examination before they are discharged. Drug intoxication and head or spinal cord injuries can interfere with an adequate examination to rule out missed injuries.

EMERGENCY DEPARTMENT EVALUATION

History and Physical Examination

A directed history and physical examination are essential. The history should include a brief past medical history in addition to that relative to the wounding mechanism. The paramedical personnel are important sources of information, particularly in neurologically impaired patients. The condition of the vehicle and the status of other passengers in a motor vehicle accident are helpful indicators of the severity of the injuring mechanism. Preexisting conditions, medications, and allergies must be considered, since all can affect the diagnosis, management, and outcome.

Physical examination of the abdomen includes evaluation of the back, lower chest, and perineum, with rectal and vaginal examinations. Such an examination is especially important in patients who require emergent exploratory celiotomy. An injury to the back or perineum is difficult to diagnose at celiotomy, and proper treatment depends on accurate preoperative evaluation.

Resuscitation Room X-Rays

A pelvic x-ray is important in all multiply injured patients but has particular importance in patients with abdominal trauma. Pelvic injuries can result in significant blood loss and are often associated with intraabdominal visceral injury. In the presence of a fracture, DPL should be done through a supraumbilical incision to avoid entering the pelvic hematoma with a resultant false-positive examination. When urethral tear is suspected, a urethrogram should be done before Foley catheter placement. An intravenous pyelogram and a cystogram are helpful in the presence of hematuria and may negate the need for DPL if intraperitoneal bladder rupture is identified. Any x-ray revealing free air, suggesting hollow visceral injury, would also negate the DPL.

Adjunctive Tests

DPL

DPL remains an excellent test for quickly evaluating the abdomen. Advantages of the test include its sensitivity (98 percent in many reports), its availability, and the relative speed with which it can be performed. Problems with the test are related to the potential for iatrogenic injury and its misapplication to the evaluation of retroperitoneal injuries. The fairly high incidence of false-positive examinations has been used as an argument for the superiority of the CT scan. The relative lack of specificity has also been pointed out. When one considers the question of the need for emergency exploratory celiotomy, and not whether an abdominal injury exists, the examination has a high level of sensitivity and specificity.

Indications for DPL in blunt trauma include a history of significant abdominal trauma when the physical examination is equivocal. DPL is especially useful in patients in whom the examination is unreliable, as in patients with a head or spinal cord injury or with drug intoxication. Unexplained hypotension when intraabdominal hemorrhage is a possibility is another indication. Patients who will be unavailable for monitoring by abdominal examination, such as those who will require general anesthesia for other injuries, may also benefit from DPL.

In penetrating injury, lavage should be used when it is not clear that celiotomy is necessary. In stab wounds, this is when clinical signs of peritoneal irritation are absent and local wound exploration indicates that the superficial muscle fascia has been violated. In low-velocity gunshot wounds, there may be some value when peritoneal penetration is unclear and the clinical examination is negative. DPL in tangential wounds or wounds of the low chest may be helpful in confirming a negative examination. In high-velocity gunshot wounds, most surgeons feel exploratory celiotomy should be done when any question of penetration exists.

There are no absolute contraindications to peritoneal lavage, only relative contraindications. It is clearly not necessary in patients in whom indications for surgery are present, since it will delay surgery and does have potential complications. The relative contraindications are in patients for whom the procedure carries a greater risk. In patients who have had previous abdominal surgery or gravid uterus, DPL may be performed with a modified technique. By making the incision away from previous incisions or the uterus and using the open technique, the examination can be done safely. Extensive adhesions may result in loculation and prevent distribution of fluid throughout the entire abdomen. This can result in a false-negative examination. Marked gaseous distension, which may result from external ventilation with a mask, increases the risk of bowel injury. Open lavage should be used if DPL is felt to be necessary.

Three techniques can be used: closed, semiclosed, or open. In all three, the patient should have a Foley catheter and nasogastric tube placed first for drainage. The area should be prepared, draped, and anesthetized with local anesthetic with epinephrine in a concentration of 1 : 100,000. In the closed technique, a skin nick is made, followed by needle placement in the peritoneum. Using the Seldinger technique, a lavage catheter is placed. In the semiclosed technique, the incision is carried down to the fascia, which is visualized prior to peritoneal puncture. In the open technique, the incision is carried down to the peritoneum, which is opened under direct visualization, and a catheter is placed in the peritoneal cavity. The incision is usually made in the midline but can be made paramedianly or supraumbilically, depending on the location of previous incisions or the presence of a pelvic fracture.

After catheter placement, fluid is aspirated, and if more than 5 mL of blood is returned the test is positive. If no blood is aspirated, then 20 mL/kg of lactated Ringer's solution up to 1000 mL is instilled into the peritoneum. The patient's position may be changed or the abdomen massaged to assure complete distribution and sampling throughout the abdomen. Fluid is returned by placing the IV bag below the level of the abdomen. Slight reverse Trendelenburg position may facilitate return. Inadequate return of the lavage fluid is a common problem. Usually this is a result of catheter positioning, but translocation of the fluid into the thorax can occur with diaphragm rupture. An aliquot of the lavage fluid is then examined. The examination is positive if the red blood cell count is >100,000 cells/mm^3, the white blood cell count is >500 cells/mm^3, the amylase level is >200 units/100 mL, or bile is present or if, on microscopic examination, bacteria or vegetable material is seen.

In penetrating injury, the criteria for a positive examination are controversial. Many centers reduce the red blood cell count considered to be a positive test. In gunshot wounds, the use of lavage remains controversial.

In situations where the initial appearance of the fluid is slightly pink, suggesting an equivocal test, or when the patient will be transferred, the catheter may be left in place for a repeat examination later. If the patient is to be transferred, a sample of the lavage fluid should accompany the patient.

CT Scan

The CT scan is an excellent test and complements the DPL. When performed under optimal conditions, the scan has a much greater specificity than DPL. A useful examination requires a cooperative patient and personnel skilled in the examination of trauma patients. For optimal resolution, oral and intravenous contrast material should be given. The oral contrast should be in two boluses. This is generally given by nasogastric tube. The first bolus is 500 mL of 3 percent water-soluble contrast given approximately 30 min before the examination. The second bolus, of 250 mL, is given in the CT suite. The intravenous contrast is given as a bolus at the time of the study. Iodinated contrast material, 100 mL of a 60 percent solution, is used in adults. Studies are now being done to determine the value of contrast by enema to increase the sensitivity in evaluation of colon perforation.

The main advantage of scanning is the ability to better evaluate the retroperitoneum and to more precisely locate injury present preoperatively. In addition, the study may be able to clearly identify lesions that are best managed nonoperatively, for example, liver hematoma (Fig. 175-1). There are conflicting reports as to the sensitivity of the test, but there are multiple reports indicating that surgical lesions have been missed. Jejunal perforations appear to be the most difficult to diagnose. It should be emphasized that both DPL and CT scanning should be evaluated in the context of the clinical status. Neither test is absolute, and each should be used in conjunction with the clinical findings over time.

Arteriography

The evaluation of major vessel injuries may best be accomplished by arteriography. The CT scan with contrast does, however, appear to be replacing the arteriogram as a screening test for renal arterial lesions. In pelvis fractures bleeding sites can be located and there is the potential for control through embolization (Fig. 175-2).

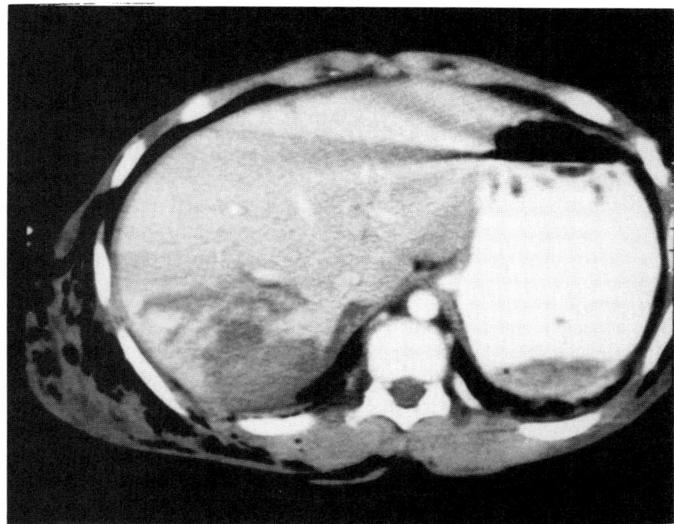

Fig. 175-1. A CT scan of the abdomen revealing an intrahepatic hematoma. This injury was managed nonoperatively.

MANAGEMENT

The approach to the patient with abdominal trauma is not unique. All traumatized patients should have a similar approach. The ABCs are assessed and managed first. The airway is managed with cervical spine control, breathing with ventilatory assistance if necessary, followed by evaluation and resuscitation of circulation. Fluid resuscitation is done with several large-bore IV lines. The rate at which fluid can be delivered is dependent on the caliber of the catheter inserted; when massive fluid replacement is necessary, a 9-French catheter can be placed either peripherally or centrally using the Seldinger technique. At the time of line placement, blood can be drawn for laboratory studies. A routine trauma laboratory series should be obtained, including at least a complete blood count, electrolytes, blood sugar, amylase, type and crossmatch, urinalysis, and toxicology as indicated. Additional evaluation as a baseline in the severely injured should include renal, hepatic, and clotting function tests.

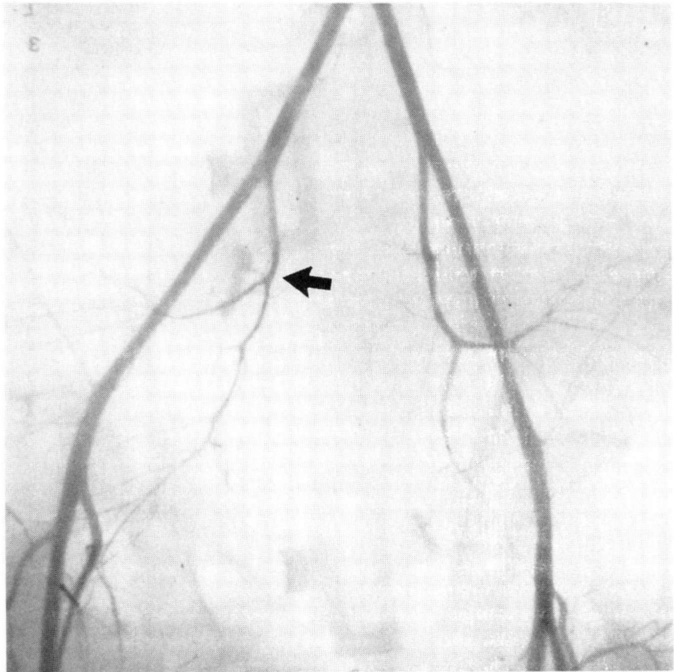

Fig. 175-2. Pelvic arteriogram revealing bleeding from a branch of the right iliolumbar artery (arrow) in a patient with a pelvic fracture. This bleeding vessel was successfully selectively embolized.

A nasogastric tube may be useful for both diagnostic and therapeutic reasons. The presence of bloody gastric aspirate suggests nasopharyngeal or gastrointestinal injury. Patients with trauma frequently have gastric distension, and tube placement will help to prevent aspiration. Nasal placement of the tube is contraindicated in the presence of facial injury with suspected cribriform plate fracture.

Foley catheter placement should follow a urethrogram when there is an injury or findings suggestive of urethral tear. Blood at the urethral meatus or a large perineal hematoma suggests urethral tear. When there is a suspected pelvic fracture, a rectal examination should be done before Foley catheter placement to determine the position of the prostate gland. If the position of the gland is abnormal, a urethrogram should be done. With hematuria, an intravenous pyelogram and cystogram should be considered. In the evaluation of more stable patients, CT scanning with contrast gives better resolution in renal parenchymal injuries.

Subsequent management depends on the findings of the above mentioned examinations. DPL, CT scanning, and exploratory laparotomy may all be indicated under certain circumstances (Table 175-1). In cases where there is a suspicion of bowel injury, antibiotics active against both aerobes and anaerobes should be given preoperatively. Triple antibiotic therapy with intravenous penicillin (ampicillin), gentamycin, and clindamycin is the "gold standard." Alternatively, a single broad-spectrum antibiotic (mefoxin) can be given intravenously.

SPECIFIC ORGAN INJURY

In the evaluation of patients with abdominal injury, it is important to keep in mind the management techniques that will be used for different injuries. A concept of the surgical treatment of different injuries gives perspective to preoperative evaluation and preparation. An obvious example is the case of a low rectal injury. This is easily missed at exploratory laparotomy, and the appropriate treatment of colostomy will not be done if that injury is not detected preoperatively. What follows is a brief discussion of specific injuries and the diagnostic and therapeutic techniques in their management.

Hollow Organs

Injury to these organs has the potential for significant morbidity and mortality as a result of the spillage of the organ contents. Most have a resident bacterial flora that represent a significant risk when spilled into the peritoneum. Injuries to these organs often result in symptoms of peritonitis. Most of these injuries will be detected with DPL, but water-soluble contrast studies are often necessary to document organ disruption. These injuries can be insidious, and it is in this circumstance that they frequently become fatal. Sudden compression by a seatbelt may result in a hollow viscus rupture as a result of "submarining" when only a lap belt is used.

Stomach

The stomach is resistant to blunt injury. In addition, an excellent blood supply makes primary repair the most common technique used, with

Table 175-1. Indications for Exploratory Celiotomy

1. Abdominal trauma and hemodynamic instability
2. Abdominal wall disruption with evisceration
3. Clinical findings of peritoneal irritation
4. Free air in abdomen on x-ray
5. Retroperitoneal air on x-ray
6. Ruptured urinary bladder (intraperitoneal)
7. Positive peritoneal tap or lavage
8. Rectal perforation
9. Surgically correctable lesions suggested by CT scan

generally excellent results. In trauma patients, a distended stomach will increase the chances of injury. Heme-positive nasogastric return is usually present with injury. Confusion occurs when there has been nasopharyngeal trauma either from the original injury or iatrogenically with tube insertion. Contrast studies are on rare occasions necessary to confirm the diagnosis.

Duodenum

The retroperitoneal position of the duodenum makes the diagnosis of injury difficult. Signs and symptoms are often slow to develop and, when present, indicate significant injury. Specific clues as to the presence of duodenal injury include retroperitoneal air (Fig. 175-3) or elevation of the serum amylase level. The definitive test for evaluating duodenal injury is a contrast study showing extravasation. On CT scan the contrast may not adequately distend the duodenum, and formal fluoroscopic examination may be necessary. Duodenal injuries may range in severity from an intramural hematoma to an extensive crush or laceration too severe for simple closure. Hematoma is best managed nonoperatively if the diagnosis can be assured without exploration. If the lesion is found incidentally at surgery, it is difficult to decide how to manage it. The hematoma is usually drained at that point, which carries somewhat higher morbidity.

Small Bowel

Small bowel injuries are similar to stomach injuries in that they are most frequently the result of penetrating injury and generally carry a good prognosis. In most cases, injury to the small bowel will result in peritoneal irritation with significant symptoms. There is, however, the potential for subtle and also delayed injury. A deceleration injury can cause a bucket-handle tear of the mesentery. The bowel can lose its viability over a period of time. Such injuries are often diagnosed late, especially in head-injured patients. DPL is usually positive in these injuries. The majority of small bowel injuries can be repaired primarily after local debridement. In more extensive injuries or those with compromise to the blood supply, resection and anastomosis will be necessary.

Colon

The management of injury to the large bowel is controversial. The number of lesions felt to be amenable to management without stomas is considerable, and some surgeons feel that most lesions should be repaired primarily. This practice is certainly well accepted for right-sided lesions and left-sided lesions found early with minimal contamination. Colostomy is frequently employed in any left-sided lesions with extensive injury or any colonic injury with extensive contamination. Excessive contamination may be the result of delayed surgical treatment. To avoid this situation, colonic lesions must be suspected and specifically searched for. The use of CT scanning with contrast instilled in the rectum is an attempt to address this problem. If there is any doubt, a gastrograffin enema with fluoroscopy remains the optimal test for evaluating colon perforation. Barium, while giving superior contrast studies, is extremely irritating to the peritoneal cavity and causes an intense inflammatory response. When perforation is suspected, water-soluble contrast should be used. If doubt persists, exploration may be prudent.

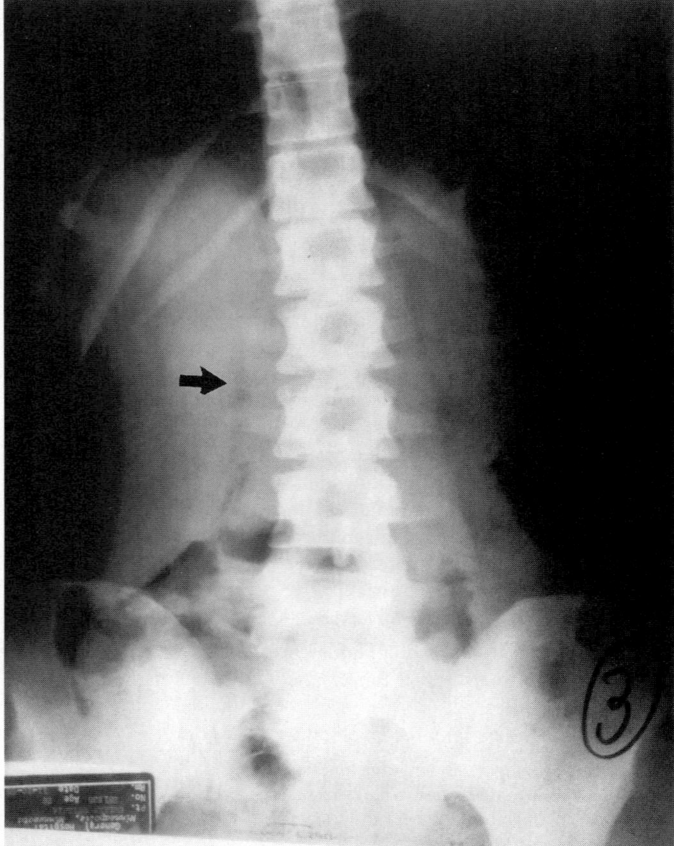

A

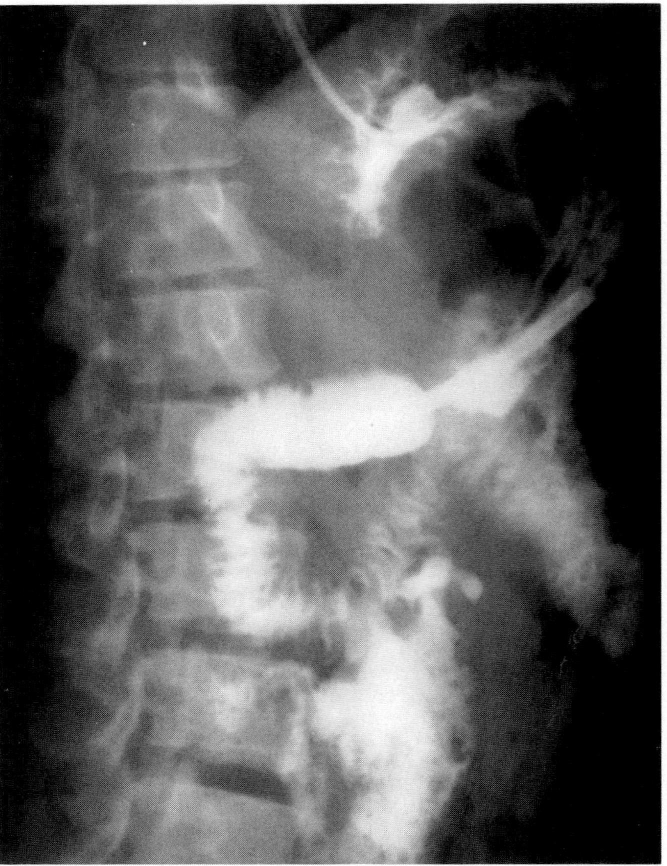

B

Fig. 175-3. A. A flat plate radiograph of the abdomen revealing vertically oriented air bubbles (arrow) over the upper psoas shadow. About 20 percent of patients with duodenal rupture will have this finding. **B.** Gastrograffin study of the same patient showing leakage of duodenal contents into the retroperitoneal space.

Rectum

Injuries to the rectum are especially important to diagnose preoperatively, since diagnosis at surgery is difficult. The rectum is an extraperitoneal organ, and physical findings may be minimal. Careful palpation should be done to search for evidence of bony penetration with a pelvic fracture, and stool should be tested for blood. Undetected, an open pelvic fracture will rapidly develop into overwhelming sepsis. Surgical management of these patients involves both an abdominal and a perineal approach. If the diagnosis is not made before exploratory laparotomy, reoperation with colostomy will be necessary. Management includes preoperative broad-spectrum antibiotics, repair of associated injuries, drainage, and fecal diversion. This usually includes a diverting-end sigmoid colostomy proximal to the rectal injury, washout of the distal rectum with saline solution, and placement of presacral drains through the perineum. This combination of complete diversion and rectal washout has markedly reduced the morbidity and mortality of this injury. Clearly, early accurate diagnosis is essential.

Gallbladder and Biliary Ducts

Injuries to the gallbladder and biliary ducts are rare. Gallbladder injury occurs most frequently as a result of penetrating trauma. Cholecystectomy is the treatment of choice. Common bile duct injury may occur after blunt injury and frequently involves transection at the papilla. This injury is extremely difficult to diagnose preoperatively. It should, however, be found during exploration. Adequate mobilization of the duodenum with a Kocher maneuver and, in rare cases where there is doubt, an intraoperative cholangiogram will help identify these lesions. Bile should be tested for on DPL specimens and is present with these lesions.

Genitourinary Tract

Lesions of the genitourinary tract are addressed more fully elsewhere (see Ch. 177). In the presence of microscopic or gross hematuria, contrast studies are necessary for diagnosis. The contrast CT scan provides an excellent study when time allows. In situations where this is not possible, a rapid cystogram and intravenous pyelogram in the resuscitation area are helpful. When time allows, oblique and lateral views as well as postvoid films improve visualization of subtle injuries. In the hypotensive patient, nonvisualization is common, and an intravenous pyelogram should be obtained after patient stabilization. Occasionally, an intraoperative study is necessary. These studies, although technically inferior, frequently identify extravasation or absence of function, which are the major concerns in these patients. At operation, dyes that are excreted in the urine, such as methylene blue and indigo carmine, may be useful to identify the location of extravasation.

Solid Organs

Injury to the solid organs causes morbidity and mortality primarily as a result of blood loss. The products of secretion are potential sources of morbidity. They are generally sterile and, as such, are less of an early risk. Blood loss may be life-threatening, and immediate surgery to control the bleeding will be critical. Presentation will be with tachycardia and hypotension in addition to the abdominal findings. When the hemorrhage is contained within a fixed space, a mass may develop that can be palpated or found on radiologic examinations. In isolated injuries to the spleen or the liver, autotransfusion at surgery is often of benefit. In some centers, additional personnel will need to be notified to run the equipment.

Liver

The liver is commonly injured in both blunt and penetrating trauma to the abdomen. Most injuries are self-limited, with the bleeding stopped at laparotomy. With CT scanning, lesions are now being identified that can be managed nonoperatively.

In massive liver injury with caval or hepatic vein injury, total vascular isolation of the liver may be necessary. The mortality from this injury is high (50 to 100 percent), with rapid control of bleeding the key to obtaining survival. Control is with a shunt from the lower cava to above the liver. The key to this technique is placement of the shunt quickly. The best access is through the right atrium using a median sternotomy. A Pringle maneuver, clamping of the hilum of the liver, will complete major vascular isolation. In some cases, vascular control (aortic) by thoracotomy before abdominal exploration will prevent the excessive blood loss related to the removal of tamponade before control can be achieved. Liver packing has gained prominence in situations where control cannot be obtained by other techniques.

Late potential complications of liver injury include bile fistula, sepsis (intrahepatic or abdominal), and vascular injury with pseudoaneurysm and hematobilia. Septic foci are usually diagnosed with CT scanning and are treated with drainage. This can be done either surgically or with CT or ultrasound guidance. Hematobilia often presents weeks to months postinjury, and the trauma history may need to be specifically sought. Findings in this syndrome include gastrointestinal bleeding, jaundice, and colicky abdominal pain relieved by hematemesis. Selective angiography is used to make the diagnosis and has been used in reported cases to embolize the fistula. The standard treatment is surgical with interruption of the inflow to the pseudoaneurysm. Bile fistulas usually are noted early postoperatively and will usually close spontaneously if drainage is adequate and there is no distal obstruction.

Spleen

The spleen is the most frequently injured organ in blunt abdominal trauma and is commonly associated with other intraabdominal injuries. The traditional treatment for splenic injuries had been splenectomy, but multiple reports have highlighted the risks of postsplenectomy sepsis, and currently a selective approach is optimal. In some cases, splenectomy is still the treatment of choice, but splenorrhaphy and nonoperative observation are also indicated in some cases.

Symptoms of injury to the spleen include those of blood loss with tachycardia, hypotension, and syncope as a late sign. Kehr's sign, or left shoulder-strap pain, is a classic finding in rupture of the spleen. Abdominal pain and tenderness in the left upper quadrant are usually attendant. Lower rib fractures on the left should suggest injury to the spleen and warrant further evaluation. Diagnosis of splenic injury is made with surgical exploration in patients who require laparotomy or by CT scanning with contrast in those managed nonoperatively. Liver and/or spleen scanning may be helpful. Management after diagnosis depends on associated injuries, hemodynamic stability, and transfusion requirements.

Delayed splenic rupture is a rare injury, which is reported to occur in 1 to 2 percent of cases of abdominal trauma. The rupture may occur at a remote time from the original trauma and not be readily associated with injury by the patient. Symptoms are similar to those in the acute injury, with diagnosis frequently made by scanning techniques.

Late complications associated with splenic injury are related to the treatment modality. With splenorrhaphy or nonoperative management, secondary bleeding episodes or abscess formation occur. With splenectomy, the late development of overwhelming bacterial sepsis is seen in children, and recent reports indicate a definite risk in adults even after polyvalent pneumococcal vaccine prophylaxis. Studies are not conclusive as to the role of prophylactic antibiotics. Patients who require splenectomy should be vaccinated and apprised of the risk of infection, since close monitoring of infections can have a significant positive effect on the outcome of septic episodes.

Pancreas

Pancreatic injury is most common with penetrating trauma. It may also occur as a result of a crushing injury, dividing the pancreas over

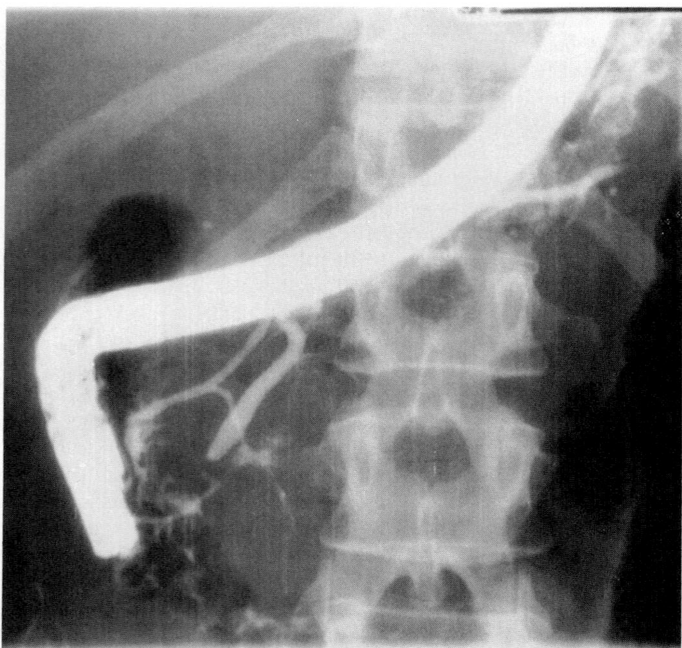

Fig. 175-4. Endoscopic retrograde cholangiopancreatography (ERCP) revealing minor ductal injury managed with drainage alone.

the vertebral column. The classic case is a blow to the mid-epigastrium such as that from a steering wheel or the handlebar of a bicycle. CT scanning has been helpful in the diagnosis of these injuries. Unrecognized, this injury has considerable morbidity and mortality. The exocrine products from the pancreas have an irritative effect on the peritoneum. A form of autodigestion occurs, resulting in an ideal medium for bacterial proliferation. In some situations it is clear that there is a possibility of this injury preoperatively, although most cases are discovered at exploration.

If ductal injury is suspected and if the patient is stable, an ERCP study will help identify the anatomy. The surgical management of these lesions is difficult, since the ducts are small and hard to identify. The "road map" provided by ERCP can be quite helpful. Its greatest value is in documenting the absence of major ductal injury, since these lesions can be managed by drainage alone, without resection (Fig. 175-4). Diagnosis at surgery is usually difficult without opening the duodenum for a contrast study via the papilla. Since this adds risk to the procedure, it is rarely done.

Isolated pancreas injury is rare in blunt trauma. When associated with duodenal or biliary tract injury, management includes many options, and specific treatment will depend on the combination of injuries. Pseudocyst is a late complication possible with any type of pancreatic injury.

Kidney

Renal parenchymal injury usually results in hematuria. Most renal injuries can be managed nonoperatively, but accurate diagnosis is essential. Prior to laparotomy or at surgery, an intravenous pyelogram will identify major lesions. Most contusions and some lacerations can be managed nonoperatively. Renal vascular lesions can be diagnosed with selective angiography or, in many cases, with contrast and CT scanning. Indications for surgery include evidence of continuing blood loss, laceration through Gerota's fascia, or loss of function.

Diaphragm

Diaphragm injuries are often insidious, with the diagnosis made late. In many cases there is no herniation, and the only finding is blurring of the diaphragm or an effusion. With herniation of the abdominal viscera into the chest, the diagnosis is usually clear. Inability to pass a nasogastric tube should suggest this possibility. Diagnosis frequently is made with contrast studies, CT scans, or DPL. This injury is diagnosed most often on the left, although it can occur on the right. Treatment is surgical, with the abdominal approach usually used in acute cases to manage the frequently associated injuries within the abdomen. In chronic cases, presentation may be with symptoms of obstruction or bowel strangulation.

Abdominal Wall

With abdominal wall penetrating injuries, there is the potential for evisceration. In these patients, there is a high incidence of associated intraabdominal visceral injuries, necessitating a complete abdominal exploration and making DPL unnecessary. Repair of the associated lesions is followed by repair of the abdominal wall defect. If necessary, polypropylene mesh is used to cover the defect. In cases where the only organ eviscerated is omentum, confusion may occur, since the appearance is very similar to that of subcutaneous fat. It is important to make the correct diagnosis, since laparotomy is necessary. Any eviscerated organ should be covered with moist sterile dressings and replaced when examined at surgery. Replacement of organs that appear to have vascular compromise is rarely necessary and should be done in consultation with the surgeon who will be caring for the patient. Such replacement is usually done in cases where the patient is being transferred and a delay in exploration is unavoidable.

Vascular Structures

Both abdominal arterial and venous injuries are potentially life-threatening as a result of hemorrhage. As in solid viscera injury, these lesions present with the signs of hypovolemia and occasionally with an abdominal mass. Management is directed at early control of hemorrhage. Military antishock trousers may be particularly helpful in these lesions. Prior to abdominal exploration, thoracotomy to control the proximal aorta or use of the aortic Fogarty balloon can help prevent blood loss with release of the tamponade. The key to the surgical management of all vascular injuries is proximal and distal control of the vessels. In all cases the chest, as well as the upper thighs, should be prepared. This will give exposure for control of thoracic vessels and open cardiac massage should it be necessary and the saphenous vein if grafting is necessary. In isolated injuries to the abdominal vasculature, the use of autotransfusion should be considered, and the appropriate backup for the use of that device should be arranged prior to exploration.

COMPLICATIONS AND IATROGENIC INJURIES

The major problems that result from abdominal injuries are related to either missed injuries or overtreatment of suspected injuries. Most preventable deaths are of patients with surgically correctable injuries in whom the diagnosis was missed or delayed. In missed solid organ and vascular injuries, hemorrhage and the complications of shock predominate. In hollow viscera injury, local or systemic sepsis is the major risk. Negative laparotomy has minimal associated morbidity and is often necessary to be certain that a life-threatening injury is not present. Finding no correctable lesion at surgery does not make this surgery inappropriate, and an acceptable negative laparotomy rate will depend on the initial indications for surgery.

Hypothermia is a major risk to the traumatized patient. These patients often present cold, and the use of blood without warmers and cold crystalloid solution intravenously and in DPL contribute to the problem. These patients need to be disrobed for a complete examination, and this also contributes to heat loss. Temperature needs to be monitored carefully. Fluid warmers, warming blankets, and warm peritoneal lavage help to avoid this problem.

Coagulopathy is a frequent problem and is due to a combination of factors. Dilution from massive transfusion, baseline coagulopathy in patients with alcoholic liver disease, hypothermia, and brain injury can all contribute. Careful monitoring and replacement are necessary.

SUMMARY

Prompt diagnosis and management of surgically correctable lesions is the most important means of avoiding preventable deaths. Initial examination, with documentation of findings, coupled with ongoing examinations is essential to pick up missed injuries or those that develop over time. Abdominal injuries are often insidious, and a high index of suspicion is the key to successful management of these injuries.

BIBLIOGRAPHY

American College of Surgeons Committee on Trauma: *Advanced Trauma Life Support Course* (manual). Chicago, 1984.

Anderson PA, Rivara FP, Maier RV, et al: The epidemiology of seatbelt-associated injuries. *J Trauma* 31:60, 1991.

Ang JGP, Hanslits ML, Clark RA, et al: Computed tomography of abdominal and pelvic trauma. *J Emerg Med* 3:311, 1985.

Cue JI, Miller FB, Cryer HM, et al: A prospective, randomized comparison between open and closed peritoneal lavage techniques. *J Trauma* 30:880, 1990.

Gibson DE: Abdominal trauma. *Trauma Q* 4:11, 1987.

Marx JA, Moore EE, Jorden RC, et al: Limitations of computed tomography in the evaluation of acute abdominal trauma: A prospective comparison with diagnostic peritoneal lavage. *J Trauma* 25:933, 1985.

McAnena OJ, Moore EE, Marx JA: Initial evaluation of the patient with blunt abdominal trauma. *Abdom Trauma* 70:495, 515, 1990.

Moore EE, Marx JA: Penetrating abdominal wounds: Rationale for exploratory laparotomy. *JAMA* 253:2705, 1985.

Thal ER, May RA, Bessinger OD: Peritoneal lavage: Its unreliability in gunshot wounds of the lower chest and abdomen. *Arch Surg* 115:430, 1980.

Wisner DH, Wold RL, Frey CF: Diagnosis and treatment of pancreatic injuries: An analysis of management principles. *Arch Surg* 125:1109, 1990.

176
PENETRATING TRAUMA TO THE POSTERIOR ABDOMEN AND BUTTOCK

Mark D. Odland
Arthur L. Ney

Penetrating trauma to the back, flank, and buttock is most likely to occur from gunshot and stab wounds. The extent of injury can be difficult to assess when extraperitoneal injury occurs and there is a desire to avoid nontherapeutic or diagnostic celiotomy. Due to the increasing sophistication of diagnostic testing, selective management is now possible, at least in some cases. This chapter outlines the evaluation of patients with penetrating trauma to the posterior abdomen and buttock and the rationale for safer selective management.

PENETRATING TRAUMA TO THE POSTERIOR ABDOMEN

Penetrating trauma to the posterior abdomen is a distinct subcategory of penetrating torso trauma. Because of the protection afforded by the pelvis, spine, and thick musculature of the back, intraperitoneal and retroperitoneal contents are less likely to be injured. However, extraperitoneal visceral injury can occur without associated intraperitoneal injury, with minimal physical findings seen on examination. This apparent absence of physical findings will delay the diagnosis of duodenal, colonic, rectal, and pancreatic injuries. Given the morbidity and mortality of such injuries when left untreated, diagnostic accuracy is of the utmost importance.

The posterior abdomen, namely the flank and back, is the area posterior to the anterior axillary line, extending from the tip of the scapula to the iliac crest. The organs most commonly injured by penetrating trauma to this area are the liver, kidney, and colon. With any thoracic injury below the tip of the scapula, diaphragmatic injury and subsequent intraperitoneal injury may occur. Consequently, both the abdomen and chest must be evaluated in all cases of penetrating injury to the posterior abdomen or thorax. The treatment of specific organ injuries is covered in the chapters on abdominal trauma (Chapter 175) and genitourinary tract trauma (Chapter 177).

Routine Evaluation

All patients with penetrating trauma to the posterior abdomen should be evaluated according to a routine regimen. Initial resuscitation should follow the ABCs, as outlined in Chapter 169. The importance of obtaining a complete history and performing a thorough physical examination cannot be overemphasized. Mechanism of injury, description of the wounding object, and time elapsed since wounding are all important to the evaluation of these patients. Baseline hemogram, chest radiograph, urinalysis, and rectal examination are performed on all patients. Physical examination followed by observation was highly accurate in identifying significant injuries in Los Angeles County–USC Medical Center emergency department admissions for injuries of this type. Diagnostic accuracy can be further improved by the use of other diagnostic modalities. False-negative examinations result from the absence of physical findings in cases of hidden retroperitoneal injury. Unrecognized, such injuries can lead to significant morbidity and mortality.

Exploration

If any of the following signs or symptoms exist, immediate celiotomy should be performed:

1. Shock
2. Hemodynamic instability
3. Evisceration
4. Peritonitis
5. Transabdominal missile path
6. Intraperitoneal free air
7. Ongoing blood loss

All intraperitoneal and retroperitoneal organs should be visualized using appropriate operative maneuvers.

Adjunctive Diagnostic Measures

If immediate celiotomy is not indicated, adjunctive diagnostic measures can be used. These measures include wound exploration, diagnostic peritoneal lavage (DPL), and computed tomography (CT).

Local Wound Exploration

In the patient with a history and physical examination consistent with a low probability of visceral injury, wound exploration may be performed. Only on rare occasion should a missile wound be explored. Local wound exploration using sterile technique, adequate anesthesia, good exposure, and hemostasis has been used to decide whether further evaluation or hospitalization is necessary. If the injury does not extend through fascia or muscle, the patient may be treated as an outpatient. With deeper penetrating injuries, exploration can be terminated and other diagnostic studies performed. Wound exploration through deep tissue planes may lead to hemorrhage, further tissue damage, and a false sense of security. More information is obtained from DPL or CT scanning. Wound exploration has a very limited role in evaluating the patient with penetrating trauma to the posterior abdomen.

Diagnostic Peritoneal Lavage

Diagnostic peritoneal lavage is highly accurate in determining whether intraperitoneal injury exists, but poorly detects the presence of retroperitoneal injury. If, on DPL, blood is obtained on aspiration or a red blood cell (RBC) count of $10{,}000/mm^3$ or greater is obtained, it is the authors' custom to perform a celiotomy. Other trauma surgeons use different RBC criteria, ranging from $1000/mm^3$ to $100{,}000/mm^3$. Controversy exists over whether to perform DPL before CT scanning, which more accurately examines the retroperitoneal contents. In the stable patient in whom there is a low suspicion of intraperitoneal injury, the authors perform a CT scan before DPL, to avoid confusion caused by the infused fluid. The unstable patient is taken to the operating room for definitive therapy, without any adjunctive diagnostic testing. DPL is performed after CT scan in hemodynamically stable patients with no indications for immediate celiotomy, but in whom injury to the diaphragm or hollow viscus is suspected.

Computed Tomography

CT scanning has become a valuable adjunct in the evaluation of patients with posterior abdominal penetrating trauma. A diagnostic accuracy of nearly 97 percent has been achieved in some series. Oral and intravenous contrast are necessary for an optimal study, and some centers include rectal contrast. Organ injuries can be visualized and management based on the findings and the type of injury. More commonly, a retroperitoneal hematoma without associated organ injury is found. Angiography is necessary if the hematoma is located near the great vessels or in a perinephric location. If a hematoma is located near a hollow organ, fluoroscopic contrast studies or celiotomy may be required. Free peritoneal fluid suggests intraperitoneal penetration and the need for celiotomy.

Management

Management of penetrating trauma to the posterior abdomen remains controversial. Some have advocated mandatory celiotomy to detect insidious injuries early. With the increasing availability and accuracy of computed tomography, many surgeons now favor close observation of the patient and selective management. Mandatory celiotomy is indicated in gunshot wounds or other missile injuries, since missile wounding results in visceral injury in 80 to 90 percent of cases. If history and physical examination indicate a low likelihood of intraperitoneal injury, as with superficial tangential wounds, then selective management may be entertained. However, cases suitable for selective management are rare. Blast effect does occur, making possible a visceral injury from a missile on an extraperitoneal course; this must be taken into account when evaluating and treating these superficial missile injuries. Selective management is more appropriately applied in cases of stab wounding.

It is the authors' practice to manage penetrating trauma to the posterior abdomen as follows.

1. When the diagnosis of intraperitoneal or vascular injury can be made on the basis of history and physical examination alone, immediate celiotomy is performed.
2. Gross hematuria without other signs and symptoms that warrant immediate celiotomy is further clarified through CT scanning and/or angiography.
3. When there are no signs or symptoms of significant organ injury, other adjunctive diagnostic measures are used to identify hidden injuries. CT scanning with oral contrast, rectally administered contrast, and intravenous contrast is done to identify duodenal, pancreatic, colonic, and renal injuries or hematomas.
4. Further diagnostic workup, such as DPL or angiography, is then performed as indicated.

Management of these patients is directed by the findings. All patients are hospitalized and examined frequently for any changes in their condition. In the authors' experience, this regimen identifies nearly all significant injuries.

PENETRATING BUTTOCK INJURIES

Penetrating trauma to the buttock has the potential to injure multiple organ systems, including the gastrointestinal (GI), genitourinary (GU), and neurologic systems, and evaluation must assess each of these systems. In addition, intraperitoneal injury may be present, necessitating celiotomy. Indications for mandatory celiotomy include shock, intraperitoneal penetration as evidenced by missile trajectory, peritonitis, free air, or evidence of vascular, GU, or bowel injury.

After initial resuscitation, evaluation begins with a thorough history and physical examination and an assessment of the likelihood of visceral injury. Abdominal examination results consistent with peritonitis, hemodynamic instability, or blood within the GI tract all indicate the need for operative therapy. Routine radiologic examination of the pelvis may reveal bony injury, suggesting penetration of the pelvis and possibly the intraperitoneal cavity. Routine proctosigmoidoscopy will accurately identify rectal injuries. If there is blood within the GI tract, contrast enemas may identify colon injury. Hematuria, scrotal hematoma, or penile hematoma could signify lower GU tract injuries, prompting further investigation with retrograde urethrograms, cystograms, and intravenous pyelography. Signs of vascular injury, such as pulselessness, pain, pallor, paresthesias, or paralysis, should prompt operation or further investigation. Hypotension, evidence of ongoing blood loss, and nerve injuries are suggestive of significant vascular injury. CT scanning of the pelvis can determine the presence or absence of a hematoma and indicate any need for further investigation.

The mechanisms of nerve injury include transection, concussion, and stretch injury secondary to hematoma or false aneurysm. With sciatic nerve or femoral nerve injuries, early operative intervention is necessary to assess the nature of the injury and repair the nerve.

Operative therapy for penetrating buttock injuries should follow standard surgical principles for the injured organ system. Debridement and closure of bowel injuries, or colostomy if indicated, are standard operative therapies for small or large bowel injury. Proximal sigmoid colostomy, distal washout, and presacral drainage continue to be the treatment of choice for rectal injuries. Lower GU tract injuries are safely treated with suprapubic cystostomy, debridement, and drainage, as indicated. Vascular injuries are best treated with primary repair or autogenous grafts.

When a patient has sustained a penetrating injury to the buttock and presents with signs or symptoms of organ injury, such as shock, peritonitis, hematuria, or gastrointestinal bleeding, the authors recommend proctosigmoidoscopy to identify rectal injury, followed by celiotomy. In the stable patient without evidence of intraperitoneal or retroperitoneal organ injury, further evaluation is done by proctosigmoidoscopy and cystourethrogram. CT scanning with rectal and intravenous contrast may be done to look for colon, urinary tract, or vascular injury. When the CT scan reveals the presence of a pelvic hematoma, angiography and venography may detect significant vascular injury. If femoral or sciatic nerve deficit exists, nerve exploration is performed.

SUMMARY

Penetrating trauma to the posterior abdomen is a distinct subcategory of penetrating abdominal and thoracic trauma. Insidious injuries may occur; therefore a systematic approach to the evaluation of these injuries is necessary. Because significant retroperitoneal injury can occur without intraperitoneal injury, there may be an absence of physical findings. Left untreated, these injuries can cause significant morbidity and mortality.

Penetrating injuries to the buttock can injure several different organ systems and result in significant morbidity and mortality. The associated visceral injuries are often extraperitoneal and have subtle or minimal physical findings. Successful management requires a thorough, systematic evaluation to identify these injuries early. With appropriate surgical mangement, morbidity and mortality should be kept to a minimum.

BIBLIOGRAPHY

Berne TV: Management of penetrating back trauma. *Surg Clin North Am* 70:671, 1990.

Demetriades D, Rabinowitz B, Sofianos C, et al: The management of penetrating injuries to the back. *Ann Surg* 207:72, 1988.

Fallon WF, Reyna TM, Brunner RG, Cromms C, Alexander RH: Penetrating trauma to the buttock. *South Med J* 81:1237, 1988.

Henneman PL, Marx JA, Moore EE, et al: Diagnostic peritoneal lavage: Accuracy in predicting necessary laparotomy following blunt and penetrating trauma. *J Trauma* 30:1345, 1990.

Meyer DM, Thal ER, Weigelt JA, et al: The role of abdominal CT in the evaluation of stab wounds to the back. *J Trauma* 29:1226, 1989.

Peck JG, Berne TV: Posterior abdominal stab wounds. *J Trauma* 21:298, 1981.

Phillips T, Scalafani JA, Goldstein A, et al: The use of contrast-enhanced CT enema in the management of penetrating trauma to the flank and back. *J Trauma* 26:1226, 1989.

Rao PM, Nallathanbi M, Guadino J, et al: Penetrating gluteal injury. *J Trauma* 22:706, 1982.

177
TRAUMA TO THE GENITOURINARY TRACT

Joe Y. Lee
Alexander S. Cass

In the multiply injured patient the management of life-threatening injuries takes precedence over urologic injury, so that the diagnostic evaluation of genitourinary trauma is usually delayed. However, early diagnosis and surgical management can optimize the restoration of function. The basic processes of obtaining a patient history, performing a physical examination, examining the urine, and properly using and interpreting radiographic imaging are essential for accurate diagnosis and treatment.

The indications for immediate radiological evaluation of the urinary tract following trauma are gross or microscopic hematuria fractures of the transverse processes of the lumbar vertebrae or bony pelvis, high-velocity deceleration injuries, and pain, tenderness, or palpable mass in the side of the abdomen or flank. While almost all major urinary tract injuries are associated with gross hematuria, the degree of hematuria cannot be used as an index of trauma severity with absolute certainty. If the mechanism of injury can produce urinary tract trauma, radiographic evaluation is indicated even with microscopic hematuria. Dipstick testing for blood will be positive in the presence of either myoglobin or hemoglobin. A positive test for blood in the absence of red cells on urine examination suggests myoglobinuria, which can be confirmed by electrophoresis.

When blood is found at the external urinary meatus, a retrograde urethrogram with contrast solution is performed before any instrumentation of the urethra is attempted. This will determine the integrity of the urethra before insertion of a catheter, which could convert a partial rupture into a complete transection.

To perform a urethrogram in the emergency department, introduce approximately 10 mL of radiocontrast solution into the urethral meatus while maintaining traction on the penis. An oblique x-ray of the penis and pelvis is then obtained while the operator (wearing lead gloves) holds the syringe tip in the meatus. The x-ray should be positioned so that the entire length of the urethra will be seen.

A cystogram is performed after bladder catheterization. A 500-mL bottle of contrast is connected to the Foley catheter with tubing designed for this purpose to avoid the spillage that occurs when a funnel system is used. In adults, 400 mL of solution is used, and in children, 5 mL/kg. The bottle should not be raised more than 2 ft above the patient, to avoid excessive pressure. At 2 ft the intravesical pressure generated will be within the physiological range of pressure generated during voiding. Unless the bladder is fully distended, some extraperitoneal ruptures will not be visualized. After the anteroposterior (AP) film is taken, the bladder is emptied of the contrast solution and washed out with saline solution; then another AP film is taken as the "washout film."

Following the cystogram, an intravenous pyelogram (IVP) with 100 mL of 60% iodine-containing solution injected IV is obtained, as long as the patient is not allergic to radiocontrast solution. This is twice the dose used under routine circumstances because of the equipment used, the unprepared colon, and the need to quickly visualize both kidneys. Films of the abdomen are obtained at 5, 10, and 20 min following the injection of contrast if possible. If extravasation, incomplete filling, or delayed visualization is seen, a computed tomographic (CT) scan of the abdomen is obtained. The CT scan displays retroperitoneal anatomy and can define hematomas, renal lacerations, and devascularization. If the IVP or CT scan reveal nonfunction, a renal arteriogram is necessary.

When ordering genitourinary contrast studies in the trauma patient, the following facts must be considered: (1) IV contrast agents can cause false-positive scans for blood; (2) the total quantity of contrast required to obtain all the studies desired may limit choices; especially in shock; (3) hypotensive patients are at risk for developing contrast-induced acute renal failure; and (4) abdominal CT scans reveal more than IVPs but take longer (an IVP is a quick way to determine whether the patient has two functioning kidneys, and this is all the surgeon may need to know prior to emergency laparotomy).

RENAL INJURIES

Renal injuries comprise the most frequent form of genitourinary trauma (Table 177-1).

Gunshot wounds of the flank are explored operatively because of the high incidence of injury to adjacent structures such as bowel, liver, and spleen. An IVP should be obtained to document contralateral renal function.

Stab wounds to the flank (posterior to the anterior axillary line) often do not have associated organ injuries. Radiographic imaging by IVP or CT can discern renal injuries that would necessitate surgical exploration. Associated injuries to other organs would also require exploration.

Blunt injuries are evaluated with radiographic imaging by IVP or CT scan. The kidneys are well protected because of their retroperitoneal location, surrounding bulky musculature and fascia, and the lower rib cage. Considerable force is generally necessary to severely injure them in blunt trauma. Fractured ribs, vertebral transverse process fractures, flank bruises or hematomas, and hematuria are indications for radiographic evaluation.

Renal Contusion

Contusions include bruises or minor tears of renal tissue with an intact renal capsule. Contusions account for 92 percent of renal injuries. The IVP is usually normal. The subcapsular hematoma is limited in extent. Conservative treatment is indicated, consisting of bed rest, monitoring of vital signs and hematocrit, and examining each voided urine specimen for the degree of hematuria present. When gross hematuria has cleared, the patient is mobilized. Renal contusions almost always return to normal unless there is a preexisting renal lesion such as hydronephrosis, cyst, or tumor.

Renal Laceration

Renal lacerations, which constitute 5 percent of renal injuries, are identified when the IVP shows extravasation of contrast adjacent to the kidney. Lacerations are parenchymal disruptions with damage to the renal capsule with or without calyceal disruption. The resulting perirenal hematoma can be large and can fill the perirenal space and displace Gerota's fascia, which acts to tamponade the spread within the flank. The management of renal lacerations is controversial. Some believe that renal lacerations self-heal, while others promote surgical management. Conservative management consists of bed rest and monitoring of vital signs, hematocrit, and hematuria. If the patient becomes

Table 177-1. Incidence of Sites of Genitourinary Injuries 1959–1985, St. Paul Ramsey Hospital and Hennepin County Medical Center

Site	Number	Percent
Kidney	1667	67
Ureter	30	1
Bladder	534	22
Urethra	79	3
Testis	75	3
Penis/scrotum	101	4
Total	2486	100

clinically unstable or septic or requires transfusion for hematuria, surgical exploration is indicated.

Renal Rupture

Rupture is fragmentation or shattering of the kidney and accounts for 1 percent of renal injuries. A large expanding perirenal hematoma accompanies renal rupture and the patient becomes clinically unstable from the continued bleeding. The IVP shows extravasation of contrast or little function. Renal exploration, with preliminary pedicle control with vascular clamps, and nephrectomy is the treatment of choice.

Renal Pedicle Injury

Renal pedicle injuries include tearing or occlusion of the renal vein or artery or their branches as the result of disruption during kidney deceleration in high-velocity injuries or from direct penetrating trauma. Renal pedicle injuries make up 2 percent of all renal injuries. When the renal artery is occluded or divided, the IVP shows nonfunction and an arteriogram reveals renal artery occlusion or bleeding. In blunt trauma the most common renal pedicle injury is thrombosis of the renal artery secondary to an intimal tear with intact adventitial and medial layers. There is bruising surrounding the renal artery but no perirenal hematoma, as in laceration or rupture of the artery or the vein and their branches.

Thrombosis or disruption of the renal artery and vein should be repaired within 12 h of the injury if a viable kidney is to result. If the thrombosis is limited in extent, the involved segment is excised with end-to-end anastomosis of the blood vessel. Otherwise, a saphenous vein graft is used to shunt blood from the aorta to the distal renal artery. Laceration or rupture of the renal vein is repaired by direct suture.

Renal Pelvis Rupture

Rupture of the renal pelvis involves extravasation of urine into the perirenal space and along the psoas muscle. The IVP shows a normally functioning kidney and calyceal system with extravasation of contrast. Renal pelvis rupture is rare and is often misdiagnosed as a small renal laceration. The patient develops high fever and increasing abdominal pain and tenderness as the extravasation of urine continues into the retroperitoneal space. The diagnosis is confirmed by retrograde pyelogram.

URETERAL INJURIES

Ureteral injuries are the rarest of all genitourinary injuries from external trauma. Blunt trauma can induce a rupture at or just below the ureteropelvic junction as a result of hyperextension of the spine with the lower end of the ureter fixed at the trigone of the bladder. With penetrating injuries there can be contusion and partial or complete rupture of the ureter. Gunshot wounds can cause contusion of the ureter when the path of the bullet is beside the ureter, resulting in shock wave damage to the vessels in the ureteral wall, inducing bleeding or thrombosis (Fig. 177-1). On surgical exploration, the path of the bullet is traced beside the ureter and the ureteral wall appears intact or shows slight bruising. If thrombosis of the vessels in the ureteral wall occurs, delayed necrosis with a urinary fistula will result.

BLADDER INJURIES

The bladder is an intraabdominal organ in a child but is situated deep in the bony pelvis in the adult; it is thus protected from all but the most severe injuries to the abdomen and pelvis. Bladder injuries are the second most common injury to the genitourinary tract after renal injury and are usually associated with a fracture of the pelvis.

Bladder contusion is bruising of the bladder wall with hematuria. The cystogram shows an intact bladder outline. With a fractured pelvis there is often a large hematoma inside the bony pelvis, causing displacement of the bladder either superiorly or laterally (Fig. 177-2). Management is conservative, as the bruise will resolve, leaving an intact bladder wall.

Intraperitoneal bladder rupture is usually the result of a deceleration injury to the abdomen or pelvis when the bladder is full, resulting in a large rent in the dome and spillage of urine into the peritoneal cavity. The cystogram will show intraperitoneal extravasation of contrast along both paracolic gutters and between the coils of intestine. Exploration of the abdominal cavity and repair of the rupture in the dome of the bladder are required.

In extraperitoneal rupture of the bladder, the cystogram will show extravasation along the lateral wall of the pelvis and behind the bladder. The washout film is most helpful when the extravasation is predominantly behind the bladder and obscured by contrast in the full bladder film of the cystogram. Until recently, exploration was done with repair

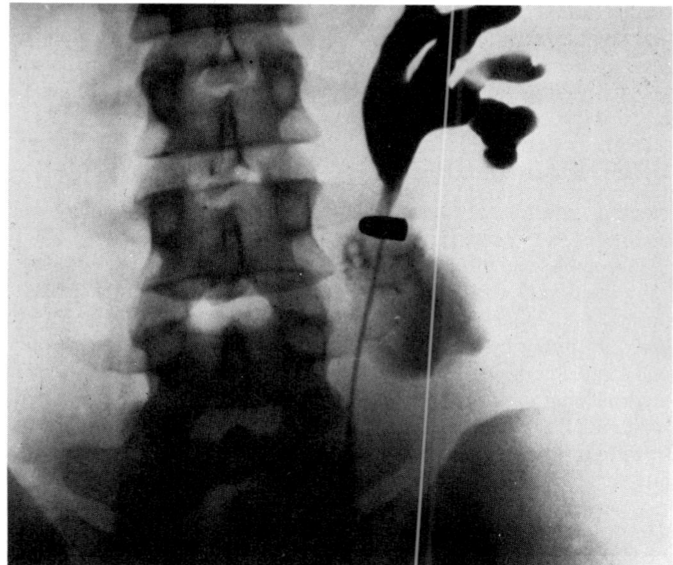

Fig. 177-1. Rare ureteral injury from gunshot wound with extravasation of contrast on retrograde pyelogram.

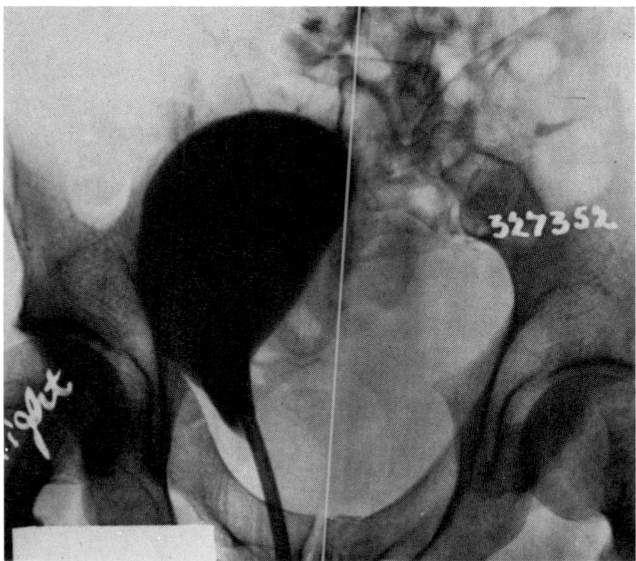

Fig. 177-2. Bladder contusion and displacement from pelvic hematoma.

of the extraperitoneal rupture. With a single extraperitoneal rupture and small extravasation, however, urethral catheter drainage alone has been used successfully. The catheter remains indwelling for 14 days, and the cystogram is repeated to verify healing before pulling the urethral catheter.

URETHRAL INJURIES

Urethral injuries may occur to the posterior (prostatomembranous) urethra or to the anterior (bulbous and penile) urethra.

In complete urethral rupture, the urethrogram will show a large extravasation of contrast at the site of injury with no contrast passing up into the bladder. This injury should be surgically repaired in the anterior urethra by debridement and end-to-end anastomosis. Suprapubic catheter drainage is used to divert the urinary stream and a small urethral stent used to splint the anastomosis.

In partial urethral rupture, the urethrogram will reveal limited extravasation of contrast at the site of injury, with contrast passing up into the bladder. Partial ruptures are managed by an indwelling urethral catheter (placed by a urologist) alone or with suprapubic cystostomy with healing in several weeks.

In urethral contusion, the urethrogram is normal, but there is blood at the external urinary meatus. The contusion heals with conservative management, with or without a urethral catheter.

Posterior urethral injuries are usually associated with fracture of the pelvis, whereas anterior urethral injuries are the result of direct blows (fall-astride injuries, straddle injury, kick). The digital rectal and perineal examinations reveal the presence of a perineal hematoma or high-riding detached prostate that is associated with complete urethral disruption. Visual examination of the perineum may show the classic ''butterfly rash'' caused by a perineal hematoma limited by the attachments of the fascia lata.

When there is a complete rupture of the posterior urethra, controversy exists regarding primary alignment of the ruptured urethra with suprapubic cystostomy or suprapubic cystostomy alone. With primary alignment, the catheter realigns the bladder, prostate, and urethra as the pelvic hematoma resolves in several weeks. A urethrogram is repeated to verify satisfactory healing before removing the catheter. If a suprapubic cystostomy alone is used, the pelvic hematoma resorbs, allowing the prostate to lie in its normal position. The urethra heals, but stricture formation occurs with both of these techniques, and the impotence and incontinence rate are approximately the same.

GENITAL INJURIES

Testicle

The mobility of the testis, cremaster muscle contraction, and the tough capsule of the testis (tunica albuginea) are responsible for the infrequent injury to the testis in the patient injured in a traffic accident. A direct blow with impingement of the testis against the symphysis pubis results in a testicular injury. The injury is either a contusion or a rupture. In both cases the tunica vaginalis sac is filled with blood (hematocele), resulting in a large, tender, blue scrotal mass. Early exploration with evacuation of blood clots and repair of testicular rupture results in a faster return to normal activity than does conservative management, and there are fewer complications of hematoma infection and testicular atrophy. It remains controversial whether scrotal ultrasound imaging is necessary prior to exploration. Penetrating injuries to the scrotum through the tunica vaginalis require exploration.

Denuding of the testicle with loss of scrotal skin is managed by housing the testicle in the remaining scrotal skin even though the reconstruction places the skin under tension. Usually the scrotum will have returned to nearly normal size within a few months.

Penis

Self-inflicted injuries of the penis include vacuum cleaner injuries and blade injuries. Vacuum cleaners cause extensive injury to the glans penis as well as some loss of the urethra, requiring debridement of devitalized tissue and reshaping or recontruction. Blade injuries range from superficial lacerations of the prepuce or the glans penis to complete amputation. Amputation of the penis is managed by replantation or local reshaping measures. Replantation is preferable if the distal penis is available and in good condition, and the ischemia time is less than 18 h.

Traumatic rupture of the corpus cavernosum of the penis or fracture of the penis occurs when the erect penis impacts forcibly on a hard object (sexual partner's pubis or the floor), receives a direct blow, or is subjected to abnormal bending. A cracking sound is heard, followed by penile pain, immediate detumescence, rapid swelling, discoloration, and distortion. This injury is managed by immediate surgical evacuation of blood clot and repair of the torn tunica albuginea of the corpus cavernosum.

Loss of penile skin by avulsion injury or burns is managed by split-thickness skin grafts after the denuded penis is clean and uninfected. The avulsed skin should not be reapplied, for it invariably becomes necrotic and infected and must be subsequently removed.

Zipper injury to the penis is caused when the foreskin is trapped in the trouser zipper. Extraction by manipulation of the zipper is usually prolonged and painful. It is better to use wire-cutting or bone-cutting pliers to divide the median bar (or diamond) of the zipper, which causes the zipper to fall apart.

Contusions of the perineum or penis, which can result from straddle or toilet seat injuries, are treated conservatively with cold packs, rest, and elevation. If the patient is unable to void, catheter drainage is used.

BIBLIOGRAPHY

Cass AS, Susset J, Khan A, et al: Renal pedicle injury in the multiple injured patient. *J. Urol* 122:729, 1979.

Culp DA: Genital injuries: etiology and initial management. *Urol Clin North Am* 4:143, 1977.

Federle MP, Kaiser JA, McAninch JW, et al: The role of computed tomography in renal trauma. *Radiology* 141:455, 1981.

Guice K, Oldham K, Eide B, et al: Hematuria after blunt trauma: When is pyelography useful? *J Trauma* 23:305, 1983.

McAninch JW: Assessment and diagnosis of urinary and genital injuries, in Blaisdell FW, Trunkey DD (eds): *Trauma Management*. New York, Thieme-Stratton, 1985, chap. 1, p. 1.

Palmer JK, Benson GS, Corriere JN: Diagnosis and initial management of urological injuries associated with 200 consecutive pelvic fractures. *J Urol* 130:712, 1983.

Peters PC, Bright TC: Blunt renal injuries. *Urol Clin North Am* 4:17, 1977.

Pokorny M, Pontes JE, Pierce JM: Urological injuries associated with pelvic trauma. *J Urol* 121:455, 1979.

Sagalowsky AI, McConnell JD, Peters PC: Renal trauma requiring surgery. *J Trauma* 23:128, 1983.

Webster GD, Mathes GL, Selli C: Prostatomembranous urethral injuries: A review of the literature and a rational approach to their management. *J Urol* 130:898, 1983.

178
BASIC MANAGEMENT OF FRACTURES AND DISLOCATIONS

Joseph F. Waeckerle

The following is a brief synopsis of the pathophysiology and treatment of fractures and dislocations. Its purpose is to supplement the knowledge of the emergency physician with regard to some orthopedic problems often seen in the emergency department. It is not intended to be a complete discussion of fractures or their treatment. Recommended readings are offered at the end of the chapter.

DEFINITIONS

Fracture—A fracture is a complete or incomplete break in the continuity of a bone.

Complete fracture—A complete fracture is a fracture which extends all the way through the bone and involves both cortexes as well as the medullary system.

Incomplete fracture—An incomplete, torus, buckle, or greenstick fracture is a fracture in which only one cortex and possibly the medullary system is involved but the opposite cortex remains intact.

Closed fracture—A closed fracture does not communicate with the external environment through overlying soft tissue injuries.

Open fracture—An open fracture communicates with the external environment through a soft tissue injury. It may be produced by a force from outside such as a projectile or by the bone itself damaging the soft tissue and puncturing the skin.

Comminuted fracture—A comminuted fracture has three or more fragments.

Impacted fracture—An impacted fracture has one of the fragments driven into the cancellous opposite fragment.

Avulsion fracture—An avulsion fracture, or pull-off fracture, most commonly is due to a ligament or tendons being stronger than the bone and pulling off a fragment of the bone at its attachment.

DESCRIPTION

Fractures may be described in several ways: (1) by anatomic location—that is, whether they occur at the proximal, middle, or distal area of the bone or whether they are supracondylar or subtrochanteric, etc.; (2) by the direction of the fracture line—a transverse line, an oblique line, which is usually less than 45°, and a spiral line, which is an oblique fracture combined with a rotatory component; (3) by the number of fragments present—a linear fracture, two components, or a comminuted fracture, three or more fragments; (4) by complete or incomplete defects in the bone; (5) by the presence of impaction or angulation, i.e., alignment; and (6) by the fact that the fracture is open or closed.

Angulation is often described in terms of the direction of the distal fragment relative to the midline of the body. Angulation away from the midline is called *valgus* deformity, and angulation towards the midline is called *varus* deformity.

CLASSIFICATION OF FRACTURES BY MECHANISM OF INJURY

Direct Trauma

Fractures which are the result of the direct application of a force over the fracture site are divided into three classifications. The first is the *''tapping''* fracture, which is more commonly understood as a nightstick fracture. This is a linear fracture through the bone with little or no soft tissue involvement. The second fracture seen with direct trauma is a *crush* fracture. The bone is usually comminuted or transversely fractured due to such forces. There is also extensive soft tissue injury associated with this fracture. The third fracture encountered with direct forces is *penetrating*. Emergency physicians often see such injuries associated with missile wounds. These projectile injuries are usually classified into high- and low-velocity injuries as determined by the kinetic energy of the bullet, which varies directly with the square of its velocity and with its mass ($\frac{1}{2}\ mV^2$). High-velocity projectiles, greater than 650 to 800 m/s, cause extensive soft tissue injuries due to fragmentation of bone which produces secondary missiles. In contrast, low-velocity missiles produce little in the way of fragmentation of the bone.

Indirect Trauma

Fractures produced by forces acting at a distance from the fracture site are the result of indirect trauma. They are classified into traction or tension, angulation, rotational, and compression fractures, and combinations of the above. *Traction,* or *tension,* fractures are usually transverse fractures which are the result of the bone's being pulled apart. *Angulation* fractures are the result of the long axis of the bone's being bent so that the convex portion is under tension stress and the concave portion is under compression stress. As a result, a transverse fracture occurs with frequent splintering of the cortex under compression. *Rotational* stress, or torque, produces spiral fractures. Pure rotational stress or torque is rare, and it is more commonly associated with an axial load. The result is an oblique fracture which is usually equal to or less than 45°. *Compression* forces act on the longitudinal axis of the bone and produce axial loading.

Any combination of the above forces can be seen. Angulation and axial loading produce oblique fractures with splintering. A common example of this is a butterfly fragment associated with an oblique fracture. Fractures may also be produced by angulation with a rotational load. Such fractures are long and sharp spiral fractures. As mentioned above, rotational fractures are commonly associated with compression injuries and usually cause oblique fractures of less than 45°.

Pathologic Fractures

Pathologic fractures are due to a weakness in the bone secondary to a disease process. They are usually caused by an injury that would not normally fracture bone. When an emergency physician sees a fracture under such circumstances, a pathologic fracture should be considered and the underlying etiology pursued. The etiologies may be divided into general and local causes. Some common examples of general diseases of the bone that cause pathologic fractures are osteoporosis, developmental abnormalities, nutritional and hormonal disorders, hematopoietic diseases, and Paget's disease of the bone. There are many causes for a localized disease of the bone such as cysts, benign and malignant tumors, infections, irradiation, and neurotrophic problems such as syphilis, diabetes, osteomyelitis, and syringomyelia.

Stress Fractures

Another commonly seen fracture in today's athletic society is the *stress* fracture. Repeated or cyclic stresses will cause fatigue on all tissues which bear those forces. As the tissues absorb the forces acting upon them, they must store some of these forces. When the muscle and soft tissue, which are absorbing the loads along with the bone, begin to fatigue, there is a greater concentration of load upon the bone itself. After the bone becomes sufficiently fatigued, it will fail, resulting in a stress fracture. Stress fractures may be difficult to see on x-ray yet are symptomatic. They should be suspected in any person, especially the athlete, who presents with a history of a sudden increase in the frequency, duration, or intensity of training. These fractures frequently are not seen on the first x-ray examination and may require a second examination 10 to 14 days later, or a bone scan.

COMPLICATIONS OF FRACTURES

The immediate complications of fractures are damage to the neurovascular system and associated soft tissue or visceral injuries. All patients who present to the emergency department with possible fractures should have an assessment of the neurovascular status above and below the fracture site recorded on the medical record. An intermediate complication is fat embolism. Long-term sequelae of fractures include nonunion, avascular necrosis, angulation deformities, shortening, overgrowth, infection, joint stiffness, posttraumatic ossification, and posttraumatic arthritis.

HEALING

Primary healing is defined as *union*. Once primary union takes place, consolidation and remodeling, which are determined by the stress loads acting upon the bone, will take place. Healing is affected by a number of conditions. Favorable conditions include fractures through cancellous bone; adequate blood supply, which is especially prevalent at the ends of bones; minimal soft tissue injuries adjacent to the bone; minimal hematoma surrounding the fracture site; impaction, spiral, or oblique fractures with good apposition; and absence of infection.

In contrast, there are unfavorable conditions which retard bone healing. These include poor apposition with separation or distraction of the fragment ends; severe comminution; severe soft tissue damage with large fracture hematomas; shearing or rotatory forces producing the fracture; loss of blood supply to the area; infection of the fracture site; metabolic or systemic disorders which affect the patient's ability to heal; and certain medications. These adverse conditions can result in delayed union, malunion, or nonunion.

CLINICAL FEATURES

The history is of the utmost importance in evaluating any fracture. If the patient is able to recall the mechanism of injury, it is of great help to the physician as it may have diagnostic and therapeutic implications. A seemingly trivial mechanism of injury producing a fracture raises suspicion of a pathologic fracture. An abrupt change in training regimes may signal a stress fracture. The past medical history is helpful in determining whether the patient has had prior injury to the area and has been in good health prior to the injury, and to elicit any known allergies, medical problems, and medications, if any, including the use of aspirin.

The physical examination usually demonstrates some or all of the classic findings associated with fractures. These include local swelling, deformities seen or felt due to muscle spasm or angulation of the bone, ecchymoses, tenderness and pain (provided the patient's neurologic status is intact), loss of function of the extremity secondary to the pain and loss of the lever arm (this is not necessarily seen with greenstick, impaction, or fatigue fractures), crepitance, abnormal mobility, and lastly, the patient's attitude. Crepitance with abnormal mobility is pathognomonic for fractures. The patient's attitude may be very helpful, as the physician can ascertain how the patient guards the injured area and carries himself or herself to protect the injured area. An appropriate clinical evaluation must always include a primary survey with attention to the ABCs of resuscitation to rule out any life-threatening emergencies. A fractured spine, some pelvic fractures, and, rarely, a fractured femur may produce life-threatening emergencies.

Once the primary survey is completed and the patient is stabilized, the secondary survey can be carried out, at which time a careful physical examination of the affected area should be performed to ascertain the presence of a fracture. During the secondary survey, a detailed neurovascular assessment above and below the injured area must be done and documented. Associated soft tissue injuries, especially the presence of an open wound, also should be documented. Any visceral damage, especially when the fractures involve areas such as the scapula, ribs, clavicle, and pelvis, should be ruled out. Lastly, examination of adjacent bone and joints should always be done. If there was enough force produced to fracture one bone, there might have been enough force to fracture other bones or damage the joints. Neighboring fractures or joint injuries are often overlooked, e.g., a fractured femur with a dislocated hip joint or a fractured tibia with a posterior cruciate ligament injury.

RADIOGRAPHIC EXAMINATION

X-rays are essential in the appropriate evaluation of an orthopedic complaint. They aid the physician in detecting fractures and evaluating their seriousness, indirectly assessing ligamentous integrity, looking for complicating factors, and following results of treatment. There are times when the clinical findings and the x-rays are both positive; conversely, there are times when the clinical findings are negative but the x-rays are positive; and there are times when the x-rays are negative but the clinical findings are suspicious enough to warrant therapy. At least two views showing trabecular detail taken at right angles to each other are required to properly assess any bony injury. Special views may be needed to determine the angulation and severity of injury of some fracture sites. Comparison views of the opposite side may be helpful, especially in children with open epiphyses. When x-raying long bones, the joints above and below must be included to have a complete radiographic examination. Often there are associated injuries to the joints when a long bone is fractured. If no fracture is visible but the patient has positive clinical findings, the patient should be treated conservatively and subsequent x-rays ordered after a 7- to 10-day wait to see if a fracture line appears.

In determining primary healing of a bone, that is, bony union, one must evaluate the patient clinically and radiographically. Clinically, there should be no motion, crepitance, or tenderness at the fracture site. On x-ray, the physician should see bony trabeculae across the fracture. Such trabeculation demonstrates that the fracture union is mature. Earlier in the course of healing, a visible callus bridging the fragments is seen. This callus should start to form within 5 to 7 days after the injury but may not be seen on x-ray for several weeks depending on the bone involved.

GENERAL PRINCIPLES OF TREATMENT

Initial Care

The proper handling of a patient with a possible fracture is important. It begins in the field with the maxim "Splint them where they lie" as the basis of therapy. As a general rule, no attempt at reduction of dislocations or grossly displaced fractures should be done in the field unless there is danger of losing life or limb. Rarely, in fact, do circumstances occur in which an injured extremity should even be moved without prior splinting. Adequate splinting prevents further injury to both bone and soft tissues, as well as possible complications, diminishes the patient's pain, and allows easier transportation. Splints themselves should be practical, safe, and efficient. Necessity being the mother of invention, almost anything can be used as a splint, from a newspaper to towels. Most emergency medical service personnel have access to the more conventional splints such as wood, metal, and inflatable splints, along with various appliances designed to splint specific fractures, such as the Thomas, Howard, and Sayre splints. Emergency medical service personnel and emergency physicians should be familiar with the splints and trained in their proper usage.

Definitive Treatment

Once the patient is evaluated and stabilized, the physician is ready to treat the fracture. The physician should attempt to achieve as close to perfect an anatomic alignment of the fracture site as possible with the hope of returning normal function and appearance to the patient within the shortest period of time. As the human body will remodel and reshape with time, accurate apposition of fragments is not always necessary, especially if no angular or rotational deformities exist and shortening is not too great. However, it is essential that the physician attempt to restore the normal planes of functions of the joints above and below the fracture site. It is also important that articular fractures be near-perfectly respositioned. Two other principles should be kept in mind: the reduction should be done as soon as possible without jeopardizing the patient; and the physician should never forcefully manipulate a fracture to attain anatomic alignment.

Closed Reduction

Fractures are reduced by traction or traction and manipulative measures. Traction requires a soft tissue bridge to act as a hinge and hold the fracture site in apposition. Reduction by traction may be obstructed or inhibited if there is a large hematoma present at the fracture site, if some soft tissue is obstructing apposition of the bone, or if the bone has "buttonholed" through the soft tissue. Traction is always in the longitudinal axis of the bone. When one attempts to manipulate a fracture while traction is being applied, the physician should manipulate the distal fragment, which is the fragment that can be moved and controlled, rather than the proximal fragment, which usually cannot be moved or controlled.

Anesthesia is essential for the comfort of the patient and the attainment of an anatomic reduction. There are a number of ways of anesthetizing an area to achieve reduction. These include local infiltration into the fracture hematoma with an anesthetic agent, regional intravenous anesthesia into the extremity, a regional nerve block, and intravenous sedation, which causes some amnesia. General anesthesia may be required, especially in children.

There are certain times when closed reduction is not indicated: when there is no displacement of significance, or when operative intervention is indicated. There are certain instances in which surgery is indicated. General guidelines indicating surgery are fractures in which no reduction is possible because the reduction cannot be held, the fracture is a result of a traction stress, or there is no soft tissue bridge to act as a hinge; displaced articular fractures; fractures associated with arterial injuries; fractures through metastatic lesions; and fractures in patients who should not be confined to bed for prolonged periods of time.

Immobilization

Immobilization of a fracture site, once reduction has taken place, is utilized to maintain the reduction and prevent further stresses on the fracture site. Immobilization should be carried out so that the joints which are not involved are free to move, especially in adults, and so that the patient is able to ambulate and move about as much as possible and as soon as possible. Immobilization of a fracture site may be done by plaster or synthetic casting, traction, or fixation. Only immobilization using plaster or synthetic casting will be discussed in this chapter.

Plaster is a muslin cloth impregnated with dextrose or starch and hemihydrated calcium sulfate. The combination of plaster with water causes crystallization, which is exothermic. The setting time of the plaster is directly proportional to the temperature of the water and to the amount of heat produced by the reaction of the calcium taking on another water molecule. The hotter the water, the shorter the setting time and the more heat produced. Care must be taken because enough heat can be produced to cause discomfort to the patient or thermal burns. These burn injuries are related to too little cast padding, too many layers of plaster, the improper use of fast-drying plasters, hotter water temperatures, and the use of elastic wraps over the plaster without precautions. Such injuries should not occur. Lukewarm water is recommended. The crystallization of the plaster may be retarded by using colder water or adding salt to the water.

There are some basic rules when applying either a circular or a splint cast. Usually one immobilizes the joint above and below a fracture site. Also, one should hold the reduction with the plaster, which requires an appropriately snug fit utilizing stockinet, wadding, and the plaster as the three layers of the cast. More wadding should be utilized if the physician anticipates swelling, and all bony prominences should be well-padded before the plaster is applied.

Application of a Circular Plaster Cast

Following are some helpful hints for applying a circular cast to a patient. Before the physician dips the plaster, the first 2 to 3 in. should be unwrapped so that the end is easily found. Lukewarm water is used in all instances. The plaster roll should be the largest size possible to apply to the affected area. It should be dipped in the water until no bubbles come from the plaster. While it is in the water or once removed, the physician should pinch both ends of the plaster after allowing the excess water to drain, but should not twist the plaster. By pinching the ends, the unwanted "roll off" of the plaster will be inhibited.

The plaster should always be applied in the same direction as the wadding and should be rolled by the dominant hand without taking the roll off the patient at any time. There should be a 50 percent overlap as the physician applies the plaster, and the roll should always be moving. The physician should use the palms and thenar eminences and not the fingers in applying the plaster. As the extremity changes circumference, "tucks" should be used to ensure that there are no irregularities in the plaster. This should be done at the lower border where the circumference change is the greatest and should be done by the nondominant hand. The plaster should be applied with minimal tension, and at no time should the direction of the plaster be reversed. Once a roll is applied it should be smoothed and molded in the opposite direction of the application with the palm and thenar eminences of the hands so that a homogeneous plaster cast is produced.

After the appropriate number of layers is utilized to immobilize the joint, further manipulation of the fracture site to ensure appropriate reduction may be done while the plaster is still wet. As mentioned above, it should be done with the palms and thenar eminences and must be done before crystallization occurs because if the plaster sets up and then is fractured, it will not recrystallize and the benefits of the plaster cast will be lost. The plaster cast should be applied so that it is slightly too long on the patient. It then can be trimmed and cut back to the appropriate length, after which the stockinet may be rolled or turned back and smoothed with one small layer of plaster roll. Once the plaster is applied, manipulated, and smoothed, it must be allowed to set up. Plaster will harden within 15 to 30 min but will not totally set up for approximately 24 h. No weight bearing should be allowed during that time, nor should the cast be made wet after it has set.

Splints

Splints are utilized in certain situations, especially by the emergency physician, to treat fractures. They allow for swelling, allow the area surrounding the fracture site to be visualized and treated as needed, and allow appropriate immobilization without the feared sequelae of neurovascular compromise. There are a number of ways of making a splint, but basically a splint is a layer of stockinet, with or without wadding, and approximately 10 layers of plaster cut to the proper length. The ends of the splint should be molded and smoothed so as to prevent harm to the patient. The splint should be immersed in lukewarm water then applied dripping wet. It is then carefully affixed by a cotton or elastic bandage. The cotton or elastic bandage should not be wrapped too tightly. Careful application will avoid thermal burns and neurovascular compromise. Numerous premade splints are commercially available and useful, if they serve to comfortably immobilize the desired area.

Synthetic Materials

Synthetic casts have been on the market for a period of time. In the past, they have required a special light source or other mechanism to initiate their conforming to the fracture site. New materials are now in use which can be dipped into cold water, rolled similar to plaster, and easily molded. The advantages of a synthetic cast are many: It is light and comfortable, long-wearing and water-resistant, and the patient may bear weight within 30 min of application. It is especially useful as the second cast. Application and use take practice.

Also available are braces that consist of a rigid plastic shell lined with preinflated air cells, foam, or gel components. These products are currently marketed to treat acute ankle injuries and as prophylactic treatment for athletes with ankle problems. The advantages are ease of application, convenience, compression, and excellent lateral and medial support. The disadvantages include cost, lack of anterior and posterior support, and the possibility of an inexact fit if not properly applied.

Complications of Immobilization by Plaster

There are obviously complications with any form of treatment, and the use of plaster is no exception. Any loose-fitting cast which allows movement will produce plaster sores, abrasions, and possibly infection, as well as possible loss of reduction. On the other hand, any tight-fitting cast which does not allow the limb to swell, especially if applied acutely, may compromise neurovascular status, a dreaded complication. The patient should always be instructed to return to the emergency department or call the physician should the area distal to the fracture site or encompassed by the cast hurt an increasing or inordinate amount, or tingle. Moreover, a physician should perform a cast check within the first 24 to 36 h to carefully assess the neurovascular status of the patient, keeping in mind the five P's: pain, pallor, paresthesia, pulselessness, and paralysis. A good rule to follow to avoid such complications is that no circular cast should be applied to a fracture site with excessive swelling or circulatory insufficiency, or to patients with impaired sensation from any cause. The amount of wadding or padding utilized prior to the application of the plaster is somewhat determined by the anticipated swelling, as well as by the need to protect the bony prominences. As the swelling subsides and the second cast is applied, less padding is utilized, so that the immobilization is continued over the fracture area. All fractures, whether splinted or cast, should be elevated, iced, and rested during the first 2 to 3 days.

If a patient presents in the emergency department with evidence of severe swelling causing any neurovascular impingement or hint of neurovascular impingement, the circular cast should be split throughout its entire length. The padding and stockinet are then divided with scissors and the entire cast is spread to decrease the edema and hopefully restore circulation. If the physician must "bivalve" the cast, the cast, wadding, and stockinet are split on opposite sides of the cast. The cast is then bound with cotton elastic bandages.

It is appropriate to inform the patient not only of what to look for in the way of neurovascular compromise should swelling occur, but also that some movement at the fracture site may be experienced until a callus begins to form. Also, it is wise to inform the patient that some itching will occur under the cast during the course of healing: it is dangerous to utilize hangers or wires or other instruments to scratch, as it could induce injury and infection.

Open Fractures

The treatment of the overlying soft tissues is the *sine qua non* of fracture management. If the soft tissue over a fracture is violated, then attention should be paid to this injury first. It should be appropriately cleaned and debrided and a decision made as to whether a primary or secondary closure is required. If the wound communicates with the fracture, surgical irrigation and debridement are required. The decision on prophylactic antibiotics as well as the use of tetanus toxoid and tetanus immune globulin should be made within 3 h of the time of injury so that maximum benefits may be achieved. If a cast is needed to immobilize the fracture, a window may be incorporated into it so that the healing of the soft tissue injury can be monitored. A helpful hint to determine the location of the soft tissue injury is to apply an increased amount of dressing over the soft tissue injury prior to the casting so that a bulge is visible once the cast is completed. This bulge can then be cut out with the cast saw, creating a properly placed window.

Dislocations

A *dislocation* is a complete disruption of a joint so that no articular surfaces are in contact. It should be considered an orthopedic emergency in that a dislocation requires immediate assessment and treatment. A *subluxation,* in contrast, is a partial disruption of the articular surface; it is more commonly associated with a fracture.

Clinical features of dislocation are similar to those of a fracture. The patient experiences pain and loss of normal anatomy and motion as well as guarding the joint. Appropriate evaluation of an injured joint requires radiographic examination. Two views at right angles are especially essential in the correct evaluation of a joint. Neurovascular examination is also very important, as there is an increased incidence of neurovascular injuries with dislocations, especially in the knee and shoulder. Postreduction films, as well as postreduction examination, should be completed and charted.

Children's Fractures

Children's fractures differ from adult fractures. While adults are exposed to a great variety of injuries which can fracture bones, the causes of fractures in children are usually very simple, i.e., direct forces. Bone changes and the outcome of these fractures are usually predictable as long as the basic principles of treatment are followed.

The history, especially the mechanism of injury, is obviously more difficult to obtain in infants and children. Clinical findings do not differ greatly, but the physician should be especially aware of the child's attitude. Infants and children will not assume any painful position and will not move in any way which causes pain.

X-rays are essential but more difficult to interpret in infants and children as ossification may not have occurred. Fractures through the epiphysis (which represent approximately 15 percent of all children's fractures) require expertise in evaluation. It is therefore prudent to x-ray the opposite (hopefully normal), corresponding area for comparison. Any defect is suspicious. A wrinkle or change in contour of the cortex (torus or buckle fracture) may be easily missed if one does not pay careful attention to the x-rays. Moreover, missing an epiphyseal fracture, which may subsequently cause growth disturbances, can produce permanent disability to the patient.

Salter and Harris classified epiphyseal injuries into five types on the basis of radiologic and pathoanatomic patterns of breakage. Their classification of epiphyseal fractures was used to describe the fracture and forces producing it, to define the treatment, and to correlate the injury with subsequent growth disturbances (Fig. 178-1). Type I injures are complete separations of the epiphysis from the metaphysis without any bony fracture. These injuries are due to avulsion or shearing forces. When properly reduced, the prognosis with this injury is excellent. A type II epiphyseal injury is the most common, consisting of a triangular fracture of the metaphysis in combination with an epiphyseal separation. The forces producing this injury are the same as those for type I, and the prognosis is also excellent. Type III fractures are uncommon and require exact treatment to achieve a good prognosis. These fractures involve the articular surface extending from the joint surface to the weak zone of the epiphyseal plate and then run along the plate to its periphery. The type IV fracture is also intraarticular, running from the joint surface through the epiphysis, across the plate, and through a portion of the metaphysis. This complete split requires a perfect reduction to avoid growth disturbances. The rare type V injury is due to severe compression forces applied through the epiphysis onto the plate. The prognosis is poor due to the disruption of the blood supply

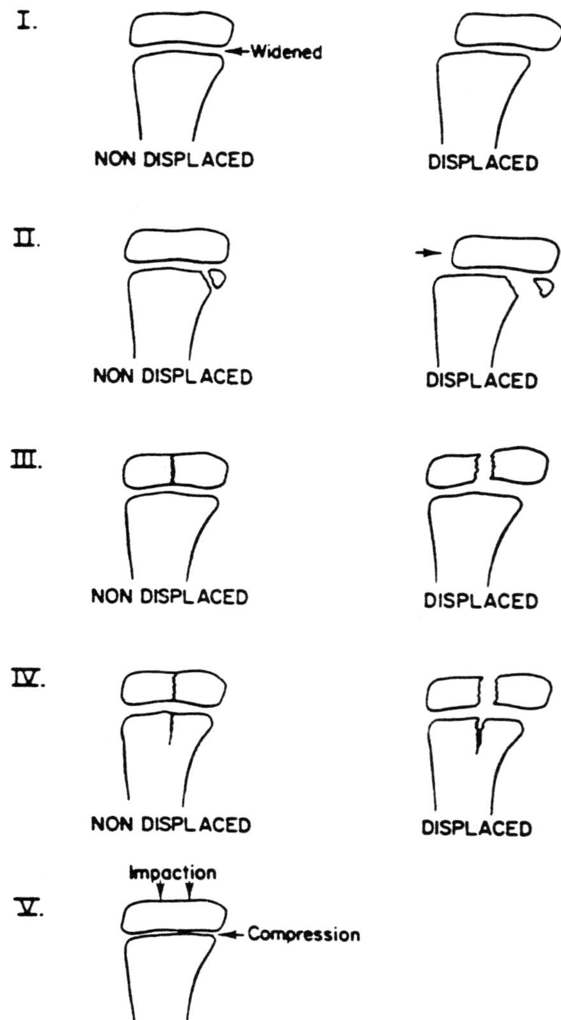

Fig. 178-1. Salter-Harris classification of epiphyseal-metaphyseal fractures. Type I: the epiphyseal line (physis) is widened secondary to some degree of epiphyseal separation. The epiphysis may or may not be displaced. Type II: there is a small or large metaphyseal fracture fragment in association with widening of the epiphyseal line. The epiphysis and fracture fragment may or may not be visibly displaced. Type III: in this type, the fracture occurs through the epiphysis, and the fracture may or may not be displaced. When displacement occurs, often only part of the fractured epiphysis is displaced. Type IV: a fracture exists through the epiphysis and the metaphysis; displacement of the fragments may or may not be present. Type V: an impaction fracture with injury of the epiphyseal plate only is present. No roentgenographic findings other than swelling around the involved epiphyseal-metaphyseal junction usually are present. (From Swischuk LE: *Emergency Radiology of the Acutely Ill or Injured Child,* 2d ed. Baltimore, Williams & Wilkins, 1986, p 318. Used by permission.)

of the plate. While the identification of types I through IV is evident on the initial radiographic films, the diagnosis of type V fracture is retrospective, since it is not identified by radiographic criteria initially. Shapiro demonstrated that this pathoanatomical classification does not predict outcome by itself but combined with a pathophysiologic approach of classifying epiphyseal injuries will aid in the diagnosis, treatment, and prediction of prognosis of these fractures. Orthopedic consultation for suspected epiphyseal injuries in children is recommended.

The principles of treatment for fractures other than those involving the epiphysis are simple, with alignment being the most important factor. Although some angulation is acceptable in children, rotational deformities are not! Children's bones remodel in response to the lines of stress, thus making accurate anatomic reduction less important. The younger the child, the nearer the fracture to the epiphyseal plate, the more remodeling will occur, so more angulation is acceptable. This is especially true when the fracture is near to one of the body's hinge joints. As bone growth is often stimulated, some degree of overriding or side-to-side apposition is desirable in certain age groups, particularly in lower extremity fractures.

Principles of treatment are similar to those for the adult, but techniques do differ. Reduction is always gentle and may require general anesthesia. Immobilization of a child's fracture should be sufficient to prevent any deformity without causing discomfort. Sometimes in children, joints above and below fracture sites need to be immobilized due to the patient's activity. Permanent joint stiffness is virtually unknown in children, in contrast to adults. Therefore, such joint immobilization is acceptable. The period of immobilization is less in children as their bone healing is rapid. Rate of bone healing is inversely proportional to the age. Nonunions in children are uncommon, and open reductions are rarely employed.

If there are clinical findings suggestive of a fracture, but none is seen on the x-ray, it is always wiser to treat the child conservatively with immobilization such as a volar splint. The job of the orthopedic surgeon, family physician, or pediatrician who follows the patient is made easier due to the appropriate immobilization, ice, elevation, and rest.

CONCLUSION

Caring for fractures requires knowledge and experience. Understanding the basics of how fractures occur, how to diagnose and treat such injuries, how bones heal, and reduction and immobilization techniques makes the emergency physician competent and comfortable in evaluating the patient who presents to the emergency department. Moreover, proper evaluation and disposition are what every patient deserves, and our orthopedic colleagues greatly appreciate such competency as well.

BIBLIOGRAPHY

Blount WP: *Fractures in Children.* Baltimore, Williams & Wilkins, 1965, pp 1–8.

Bright RW: Physeal injuries, in Rockwood CA Jr, Wilkins KE, King RE (eds): *Fractures in Children.* Philadelphia, Lippincott, 1984, vol 3, pp 87–173.

DePalma AF: Principles, in *The Management of Fractures and Dislocations,* 2d ed. Philadelphia, Saunders, pp 1–116.

Evarts CM, Mayer PJ: Complications, in Rockwood CA Jr, Green DP (eds): *Fractures in Adults.* Philadelphia, Lippincott, 1984, vol 1, pp 1–126.

Gregory CF, Chapman MW, Hansen ST Jr: Open fracture, in Rockwood CA Jr, Green DP (eds): *Fractures in Adults.* Philadelphia, Lippincott, 1984, vol 1, pp 219–294.

Harkess JW, Ramsey WC, Ahmadi B: Principles of fractures and dislocations, in Rockwood CA Jr, Green DP (eds): *Fractures in Adults.* Philadelphia, Lippincott, 1984, vol 1, pp 1–147.

Salter RB, Harris WR: Injuries involving the epiphyseal plate. *J Bone Joint Surg* 45A:587, 1963.

Shapiro F: Epiphyseal growth plate fracture-separations: A pathophysiologic approach. *Orthopaedics* 5:720, 1982.

Simon RR, Koenigsknecht SJ: *Orthopedics in Emergency Medicine: The Extremities,* 2d ed. New York, Appleton-Century-Crofts, 1987.

Springfield DS, Brower TD: Pathologic fractures, in Rockwood CA Jr, Green DP (eds): *Fractures in Adults.* Philadelphia, Lippincott, 1984, vol 1, pp 295–312.

179
INJURIES AND INFECTIONS OF THE WRIST AND HAND

Robert R. Simon

SOFT TISSUE INJURIES, INFECTIONS, AND DISORDERS

General Principles

The key concept in dealing with hand disorders is to preserve range of motion by early mobilization and splinting in the proper position to maintain function. While in injuries to joints elsewhere in the body, one attempts to preserve stability, in hand injuries the principal goal is to preserve dexterity.

The metacarpophalangeal (MP) joints and their collateral ligaments are lax in extension and taut in flexion. Thus, during immobilization of the MP joints, they should be positioned as close to 90° and no less than 50° of flexion in order to prevent ligament shortening.

Whenever treating an inflammatory process in the hand, the optimal position to promote drainage and preserve motion is with the wrist at 15° of extension, the MP joints at 50° of flexion, and the interphalangeal (IP) joints at 10 to 15° of flexion.

The lymphatics course on the dorsum of the hand; thus, regardless of the site of infection or inflammation, the dorsum of the hand will always swell whenever there is an inflammatory process.

Motions of the Hand

Figure 179-1 shows the motions of the hand. Note that flexion and extension of the thumb are demonstrated by holding the hand open horizontally and moving the thumb in the same plane. Abduction and adduction are demonstrated by raising and lowering the thumb in the vertical plane.

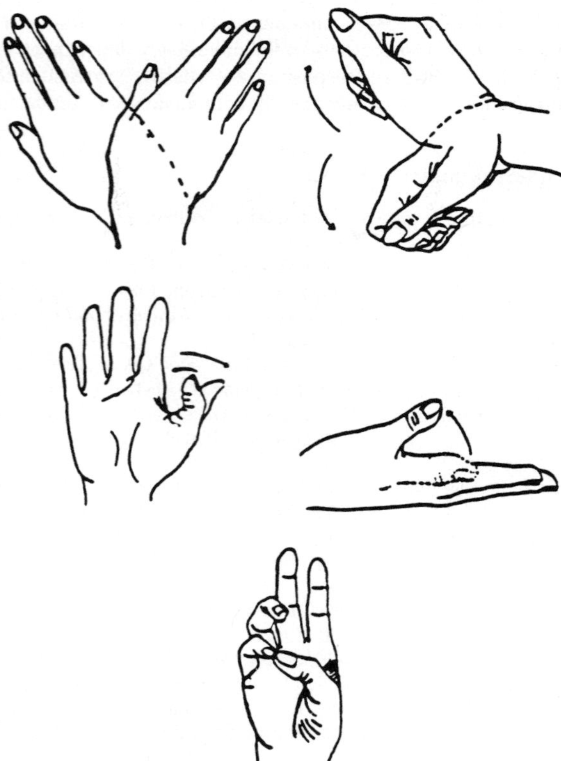

Fig. 179-1. Positions of the hand and digits.

Examination

In examination of the flexor digitorum profundus (Fig. 179-2), the digit should be extended at the MP and proximal interphalangeal (PIP) joints. In testing the flexor digitorum superficialis, one must extend at the MP and IP joints of adjacent digits in order to remove the effect of the profundus (Fig. 179-3).

The extensor carpi radialis longus and extensor carpi radialis brevis are critical tendons to examine because they hold the hand in an extended position necessary for maximum grip strengths. These two tendons are very superficial and easily involved in a laceration on the dorsal surface of the hand.

Tendon Injuries

It is critical to check for both the presence of tendon function as well as strength against resistance. A tendon that is 90-percent lacerated can still have function. However, motion against resistance (strength) is markedly reduced. Determine the position of the hand at the time of injury in order to tell where along its course a tendon was injured.

The site of pain along the course of a tendon correlates with the site of tendon injury in patients with both blunt and penetrating tendon disruption. A negative examination in an uncooperative patient is entirely unreliable in ruling out the presence of tendon injury and must be repeated later.

Treatment

A partial tendon injury can be treated by protective splinting and requires no repair. Complete tendon disruption can be treated by primary, delayed, or secondary repair. A primary repair is optimal when the laceration is clean and incisive. Delayed repair should be used if the wound is dirty or a proper repair cannot be done in a reasonable time limit. Secondary repair is used in wounds that are grossly contaminated, where there is loss of tendon tissue, or when circumstances do not permit primary repair.

Special Tendon Injuries

Mallet Finger

A mallet finger is a disruption of the central slip of the extensor tendon at its attachment to the base of the distal phalanx. When the tendon is not disrupted, an avulsion injury may occur. The fragment of bone is easily seen on x-ray and can be treated conservatively by splinting the distal interphalangeal (DIP) joint or surgically pinning the avulsed fragment.

A tendinous avulsion is easily treated with a dorsal splint that permits

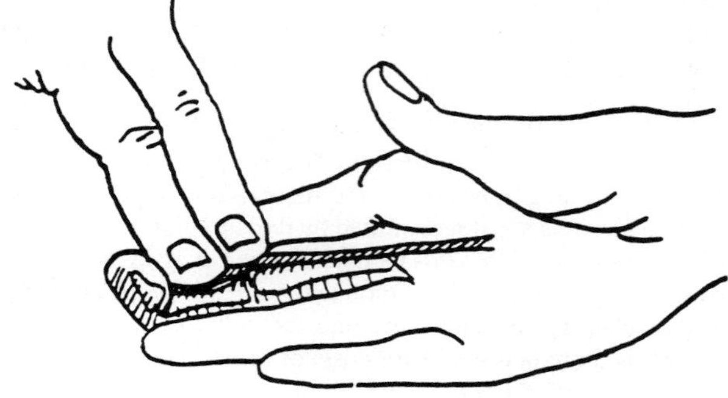

Fig. 179-2. Testing function of flexor profundus.

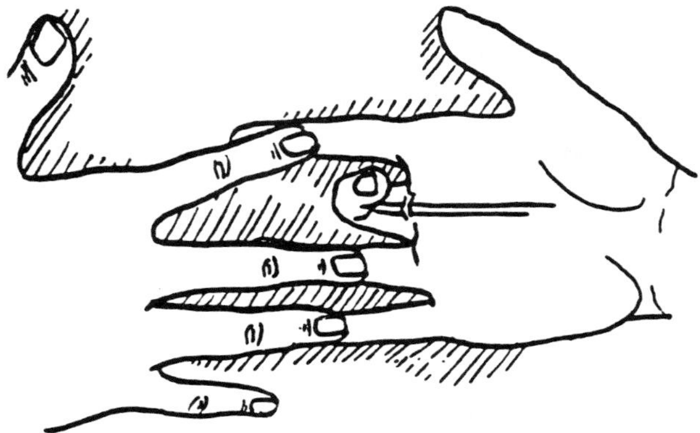

Fig. 179-3. Testing function of flexor superficialis.

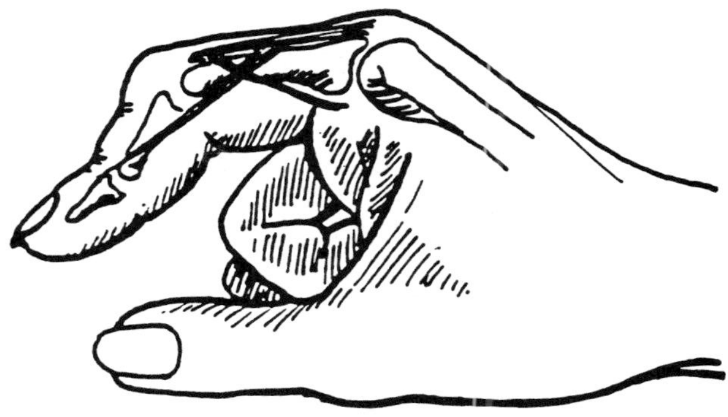

Fig. 179-5. Boutonnière deformity secondary to rupture of extensor apparatus at PIP joint.

motion of the PIP joint but prevents motion at the DIP joint (Fig. 179-4). It is important to maintain immobilization for a period of 6 weeks.

Boutonnière Deformity

A boutonnière deformity results from a disruption of the extensor hood apparatus near the PIP joint. The lateral bands of the extensor hood contract, producing the typical deformity shown in Fig. 179-5.

Injuries to the Collateral Ligaments and Volar Plate

It is critical to understand the functional anatomy of the collateral ligaments and the volar plate. The collateral ligaments and volar plate are interconnected, forming a U-shaped hood around the lateral and volar aspects of the IP and MP joints. These joints are taut in flexion and lax in extension (Fig. 179-6). This is the opposite of collateral ligaments elsewhere in the body, which are taut in extension and lax in flexion. For this reason, the collateral ligaments should be immobilized in flexion following an injury to preserve maximum length and dexterity.

Collateral ligament injuries should be immobilized for the shortest necessary time to prevent stiffness, which is the most common complication following these injuries.

Sprains of the collateral ligaments can be first degree, second degree, or third degree. One can determine the extent of sprain by performing a ''stress test'' perpendicular to the axis of motion of the involved joint. If there is no opening but pain and swelling are present, the patient has a first-degree injury. If there is minimal opening with a firm endpoint, the patient has a second-degree injury. If there is significant opening of more than 3 to 5 mm, the patient has a collateral ligament tear and a volar plate injury. If the volar plate is intact, there cannot be wide opening of the IP joint or MP joint on stress testing. Disruption of both structures should be splinted and referred, since they may need surgical repair.

Treatment of Collateral Ligament Sprains

Never immobilize the MP joint in extension. It should always be immobilized at 50 to 90° of flexion. A partial tear of a collateral ligament of the IP joints can be treated with dynamic splinting (Fig. 179-7). A complete disruption of the collateral ligament with a normal volar plate should be treated in an aluminum splint in the position shown in Fig. 179-8.

Third-degree sprains involving disruption of collateral ligaments of the volar plate should be treated in a gutter splint (Fig. 179-9) or an aluminum splint, and the patient should be referred.

Isolated injuries to the volar plate are secondary to hyperextension forces and can be partial or complete. A digital block should be performed in order to do a proper stress test when pain prevents the test from being done. A hyperextension stress is applied to the involved joint and compared to the normal side. In a partial volar plate injury, the joint should be immobilized in the position shown in Fig. 179-8.

A complete volar plate injury should be referred, since the patient may need surgical repair.

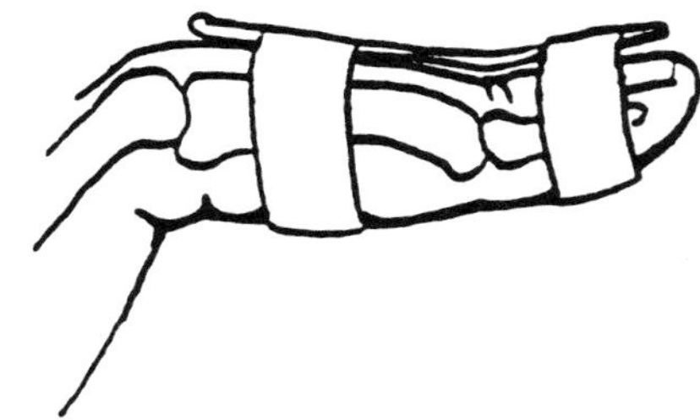

Fig. 179-4. Dorsal splint for extensor rupture.

IP Joint Dislocations

IP joint dislocations are quite common and are usually secondary to a blow to tip of the flexed digit. The most common dislocation is a posterior or dorsal dislocation of the PIP or DIP joint. One should always x-ray the digit involved to be certain it is not a fracture dislocation.

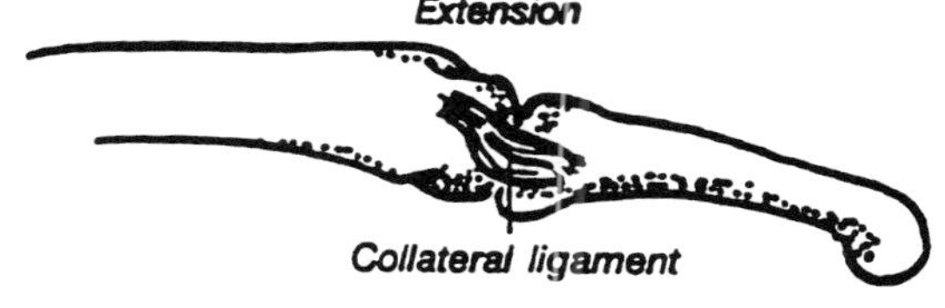

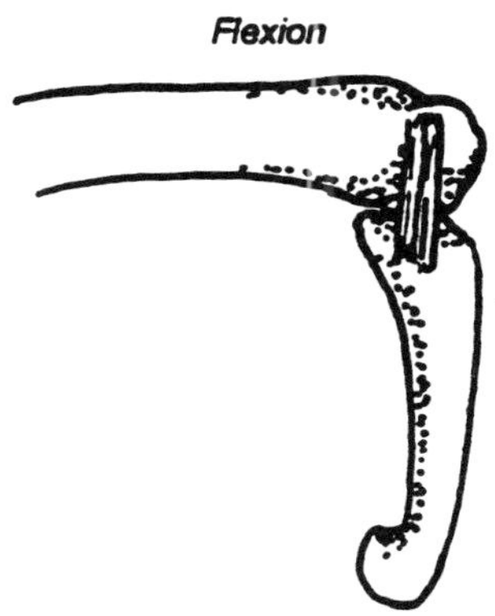

Fig. 179-6. Collateral ligament in flexion and extension.

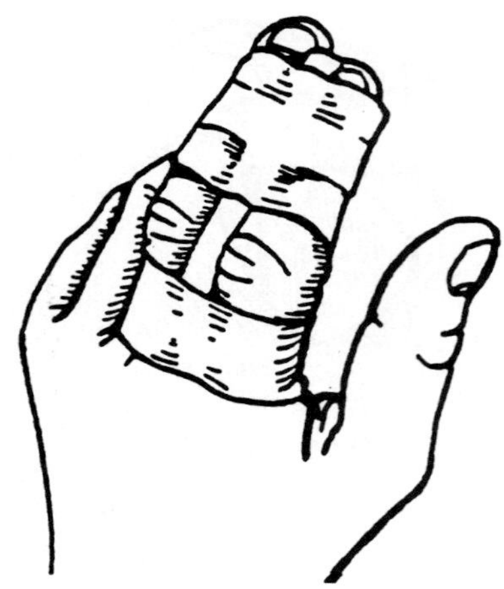

Fig. 179-7. Dynamic splinting of the digits.

PIP or DIP joint dislocations are easily reduced after digital block anesthesia by applying a distracting force along the long axis of the digit while holding the phalanx proximal to the dislocation with the opposite hand.

After distracting the joint, slight hyperextension followed by repositioning of the distal phalanx (DIP joint dislocations) or middle phalanx (PIP joint dislocations) into its anatomic position is easily accomplished. A PIP joint dislocation may be difficult to reduce because of volar plate entrapment. When this occurs, surgical repair is needed.

Following reduction, the examiner should check for collateral ligament injury, which should be treated as indicated above. If there is no collateral ligament disruption, the digit should be splinted to the adjacent digit (dynamic splinting).

MP Joint Dislocations

MP joint dislocations have a mechanism similar to that of IP joint dislocations. Involvement of the volar plate with entrapment in the joint is far more common than in PIP or DIP joint injuries. Thus, unreducible MP joint dislocations are quite common. When this occurs, the MP joint should be splinted and referred for surgical reduction and repair.

Complications of MP and IP Joint Injuries

The most common complication of IP and MP joint injuries, whether they are dislocations or ligamentous sprains, is persistent thickening around the joint and stiffness. Both of these can be prevented or markedly reduced by early immobilization. It is critical that the hand be splinted in the proper position to maintain ligamentous length.

Volar plate injuries are not uncommon, and one should examine for them. If they are present and complete, the patient should be referred.

Occasionally, a small fleck of bone is avulsed with the collateral ligament in an IP or MP joint injury. One should treat this depending upon the degree of ligamentous disruption. However, if the bony avulsion involves more than a 1- to 2-mm fleck of bone, it may require pinning, and the patient should be splinted and referred.

Gamekeeper's Thumb

The ulnar collateral ligament of the MP joint of the thumb is of special significance. When it is completely disrupted, the patient loses the pincer ability to grasp with the thumb. Thus, this is the most critical of all the collateral ligament injuries of the hand.

Complete disruption of the ulnar collateral ligament of the thumb can be determined easily by a stress test following infiltration with analgesia. If the stress test demonstrates laxity with more than 20° of opening compared to the opposite normal side, the patient needs surgical repair. If the opening is less than 20° compared to the opposite side and there is a firm endpoint, the patient may be treated conservatively with a splint similar to that for a collateral ligament injury involving other digits. A thumb spica splint or cast is favored by some.

Nerve Injuries of the Hand

The most common nerve injury of the hand involves a laceration of a digit with partial or complete transection of the digital nerve. Not uncommonly, the median nerve, branches of the radial nerve, or the ulnar nerve may be injured. Ulnar injuries occur proximal to the wrist as the nerve divides into a superficial and deep branch approximately 5 cm proximal to the wrist.

There are three general types of nerve injuries: neuropraxia, a blunt contusion of the nerve; axonotemesis, a more severe contusive injury of the nerve resulting in destruction of the nerve fibers but with pres-

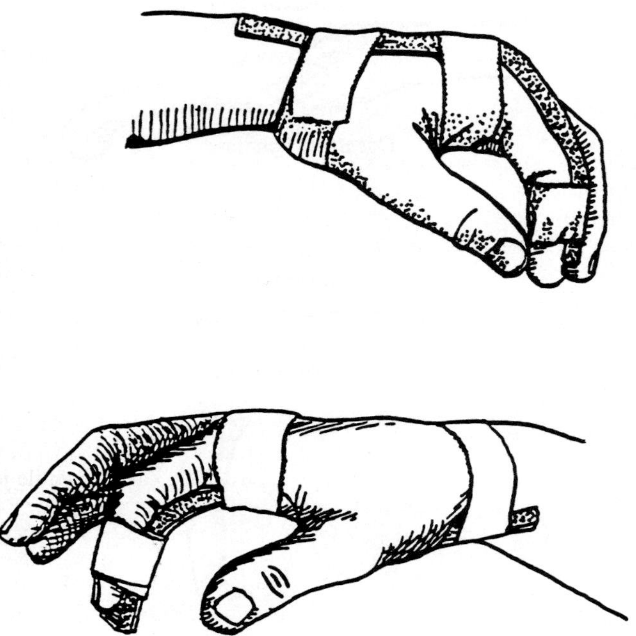

Fig. 179-8. Splints for sprain of PIP, DIP, and MP joints.

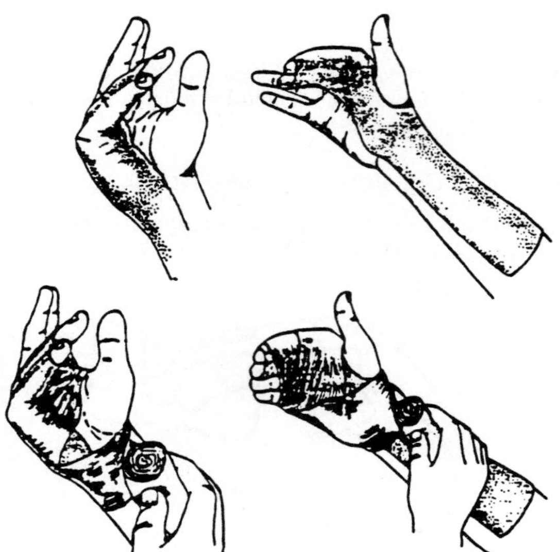

Fig. 179-9. Radial and ulnar gutter splints.

ervation of the myelin sheaths; and neurotemesis, a complete transection of the nerve, which occurs only in penetrating trauma.

Examination

It is important to do two-point discrimination, since this is one of the more sensitive tests for neurologic damage. However, in a patient with digital laceration, two-point discrimination may be entirely normal, and there may still be a partial laceration of the nerve.

If the patient states that he or she has a subjective sensation of numbness distal to a laceration, even if the objective examination is negative, the patient has a partial nerve injury. This injury may later develop a neuroma, and thus the patient should be referred if any problems persist.

Treatment

Complete nerve disruption should be repaired, either primarily or secondarily (contaminated wounds), by a hand surgeon when it involves one of the major nerves supplying the hand or a digital nerve proximal to the PIP joint. This is particularly true when the digital nerve injury involves the radial side of the index finger or ulnar side of the little finger.

Constrictive and Compressive States

DeQuervain's Stenosing Tenosynovitis

DeQuervain's tenosynovitis is a common condition that occurs in patients who have experienced excessive use of the thumb. Often, no good cause can be found. This is a tenosynovitis of the extensor pollicis brevis and abductor pollicis.

The patient presents with pain along the radial aspect of the wrist that may extend into the forearm. The definitive examination that confirms the diagnosis is Finkelstein's test (Fig. 179-10), in which the patient grasps the thumb in the palm of the hand and the examiner ulnar deviates the thumb and hand. This produces sharp pain along the involved tendons.

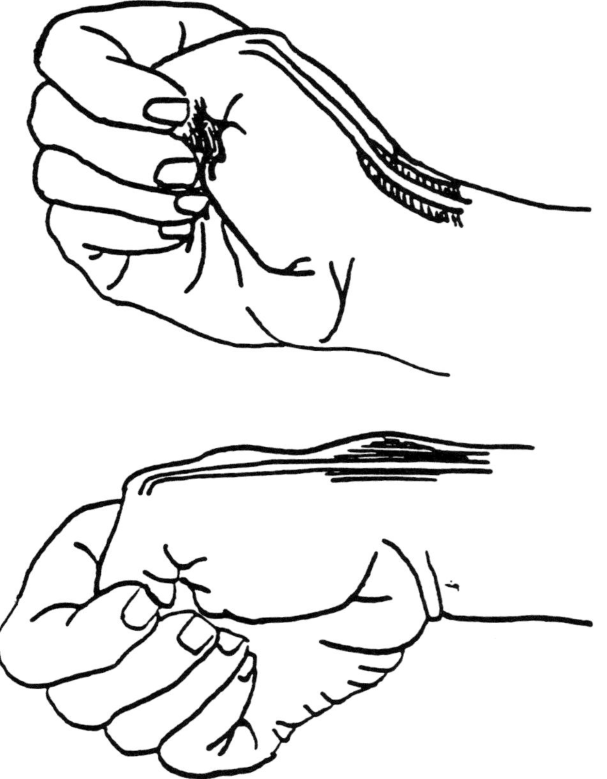

Fig. 179-10. Finkelstein's test.

DeQuervain's tenosynovitis can be treated with injection along the tendon sheath with a marcaine and triamcinalone combination. The thumb should be splinted in a functional position, and the patient should be given anti-inflammatories for a period of approximately 1 week.

Carpal Tunnel Syndrome

Carpal tunnel syndrome involves entrapment of the median nerve in the carpal canal or tunnel, which is covered by the tense transverse carpal ligament. Whenever a condition causes swelling in the carpal tunnel, the median nerve is compressed, causing paresthesias that extend into the index and long finger and along the volar aspect of the thumb. The patient complains of awakening at night with pain in the hand. In addition, patients often complain of numbness when driving a car or using the hand in an extended position for a prolonged period of time.

Tinel's sign confirms the diagnosis and involves tapping the volar aspect of the wrist over the median nerve. This produces paresthesias that extend into the index and long finger. Phalen's sign may be positive and involves flexing the wrist maximally and holding it in this position for at least 1 min. The patient complains of tingling and numbness along the median nerve distribution.

The tourniquet test may also be positive. It involves placing a tourniquet along the arm in the normal position or taking a blood pressure and inflating it to above venous pressure. The tourniquet is usually inflated to between diastolic and systolic blood pressure and left in position for 1 to 2 min. Engorgement of the veins and tissue and the carpal tunnel occurs, producing compression along the median nerve, which in turn produces the symptoms.

Treatment of carpal tunnel syndrome involves placing the patient in a special brace and infiltrating the tunnel with a steroid. If this does not improve the condition, surgical intervention is necessary to release the entrapment. This condition should be diagnosed early, and the patient should be referred to a hand surgeon.

Volkmann's Contracture

Any patient with a compressive dressing or cast of the upper extremity can undergo compromise in circulation to the forearm and hand that will result in Volkmann's ischemic contracture of the forearm muscles. It is critical to prevent this.

Prevention involves early recognition. Whenever a patient complains of increasing pain, a dressing or cast around the arm, forearm, or hand should be removed immediately. Swelling and paresthesia are symptoms that occur later. If the patient has tenderness in the forearm on either the ulnar or dorsal aspect, a fasciotomy may be indicated because of elevated compartment pressures. This syndrome should be suspected in any patient with a fracture around the elbow (supracondylar), severe forearm fractures involving both the ulna and radius, or compressive injuries along the forearm. Early suspicion and referral are essential for preservation of hand function.

Infectious and Noninfectious Inflammatory States of the Hand

All wounds of the hand with drainage should be cultured and Gram-stained. When obtaining a culture, one should take a cotton swab from the depth of the wound. In treating wounds of the hand, pulsatile jet lavage irrigation is the optimal method of irrigating the wound. Debridement should be used judiciously, particularly in dealing with wounds over areas with multiple structures. When dealing with an acute open hand injury, antibiotics should be used, particularly when contamination is expected. Most organisms are susceptible to a cephalosporin or a penicillinase-resistant penicillin analogue. In patients with penicillin allergy, clindamycin or erythromycin may be used.

Felon

A felon is a subcutaneous pyogenic infection of the pulp space of the fingertip. The patient presents with marked throbbing pain. As the pressure within the pulp space increases, perfusion is impaired, which can lead to pulp necrosis, osteomyelitis, and a draining sinus. Occasionally, even pyogenic arthritis or flexor tenosynovitis can occur. The most common organism is *Staphylococcus aureus*.

An anterolateral approach is probably the best incision to use in draining these abscesses. This approach protects the neurovascular bundle. The incision should start 5 mm distal to the distal digital crease and should extend into the pulp space.

Paronychia

Paronychia is an infection of the lateral nail fold and occasionally involves the eponychia. The most common organisms are *S. aureus* and *Streptococcus*. These infections are easily treated by placing a No. 11 blade parallel to and alongside the top of the nail, elevating the epithelium along the lateral nail fold. This will drain the abscess (Fig. 179-11). Warm soaks are continued for a few days. Antibiotics are usually not necessary.

Herpetic Whitlow

Herpetic whitlow is a viral infection in the fingertip involving intracutaneous vesicular bullae. These patients are often thought to have felons. Multiple digital involvement should suggest coxsackievirus. The mainstay of treatment is the prevention of autoinnoculation or transmission of the infection. A dry dressing should be used.

Flexor Tenosynovitis

Flexor tenosynovitis can be diagnosed by the classic clinical findings described by Kanavel. The four cardinal signs are tenderness over the flexor tendon sheet, symmetrical swelling of the finger, pain with passive extension, and flexed posture of the involved digit. The most common organisms are *S. aureus, Streptococcus,* and *Pseudomonas*. These patients require prompt surgical drainage and must be admitted with appropriate antibiotic therapy.

Web Space Infections

Web space infections commonly occur following penetrating injuries in the web space between the digits. These patients present with dorsal and volar swelling of the web space, with separation of the digits. These infections must be treated promptly with intravenous antibiotics and drainage.

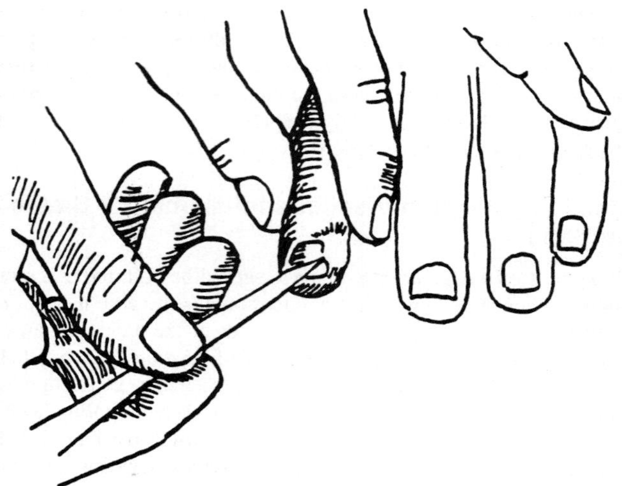

Fig. 179-11. Paronychial abscess drainage.

Mid-Palmar Space Infections

The radial and ulnar bursa that extend into the palm of the hand can become infected, either from extension from a flexor tenosynovitis or from a penetrating wound to the palm. Occasionally, a horseshoe-configuration abscess can be seen because in 50 percent of patients there is communication between both the radial and ulnar bursa. These infections must be diagnosed promptly and treated with incision and drainage in the operating room as well as intravenous antibiotics.

Infections from a Human Bite to the MP Joint

A human bite to the MP joint is often called a clenched fist injury. Infections in the MP joint secondary to a patient's striking an individual's teeth with a clenched fist can be devastating. The skin and extensor tendons may be involved. These infections have the potential of spreading into the dorsal subcutaneous space and involving the tendons of the extensor surface. Pyogenic arthritis and osteomyelitis from contamination of organisms present in human saliva can occur.

Treatment should be initiated immediately with the administration of tetanus prophylaxis. Wound swabs should be sent for Gram's stain and culture of both aerobic and anaerobic organisms. The most common organisms isolated are α- and β-hemolytic *Streptococcus, S. aureus, Eikenella corrodens,* and *Neisseria* species.

The joint should be inspected for cartilage damage in the operating room and should be irrigated with 2 L of saline solution. A drain is left in the joint, and the wound is not closed. Extensor tendon repairs should be delayed for 5 days or until the wound is clean. The original wound should be allowed to heal by secondary intention. When inspecting for tendon injury, put the hand in the fist position in order to bring the tendon into the position it was in when the injury occurred.

Tendinitis and Tenosynovitis

Tendinitis and tenosynovitis can occur involving the flexor and extensor tendons of the hand. These disorders are usually due to an overuse syndrome. Occasionally, a tear in the flexor tendon near the pulley occurs due to repeated friction at that site, leading to deposition of collagenous tissue. This disorder is called a trigger finger.

Simple tendinitis or tenosynovitis can be treated by immobilization for a short time, followed by administration of anti-inflammatory agents. In patients with simple synovitis, injection of a steroid into the synovial sheath is useful but should be done only when one is absolutely certain there is not infection.

FRACTURES OF THE WRIST

The three most common carpal fractures are the scaphoid, dorsal chip, and lunate. All of these occur from falls on the outstretched hand.

Scaphoid Fractures

Scaphoid fractures are the most common of all carpal fractures. The patient presents with tenderness in the anatomic ''snuff box.'' The scaphoid can fracture in four locations. The more proximal the fracture site, the more common is avascular necrosis. Patients with tenderness over the scaphoid should be treated as if a scaphoid fracture is present even if wrist x-rays are normal. Scaphoid views will often demonstrate a fracture that cannot be seen on routine wrist views. These patients should be immobilized in a thumb spica cast. X-rays can be repeated in 2 weeks, when the patient is followed by the orthopedic consultant.

Dorsal Chip Fractures

Dorsal chip fractures are the second most common type of carpal fracture. The most common bone involved is the triquetrum. The patient presents with tenderness dorsally over the ulnar aspect of the wrist. Lateral views of the wrist may demonstrate a small chip of bone on the dorsal aspect of the wrist. Often, the x-ray is negative. If the patient presents with tenderness over the dorsal and ulnar aspect of the wrist following an extension injury, the patient should be treated with a volar splint with the wrist in a neutral position. These fractures heal without compromise, and while most orthopedic surgeons treat them in cast immobilization, a volar splint is adequate.

Lunate Fractures

Lunate fractures are the third most common type of carpal fracture and the most important. The lunate is the most critical and pivotal bone of all the carpals in the proximal row. Since none of the carpals articulate with the ulna and only the scaphoid and lunate articulate with the radius, the lunate occupies two-thirds of the radial surface.

Patients with lunate fractures present with tenderness over the lunate fossa, which is located just distal to the rim of the radius, directly at the base of the long finger metacarpal.

When this condition is suspected, the patient should be treated with a thumb spica cast and referred. Wrist x-rays may or may not demonstrate the fracture. This fracture may be associated with avascular necrosis of the lunate, which is called Keinbach's disease.

Keinbach's disease involves avascular necrosis with collapse of the lunate. This must be prevented at all costs by early detection and proper immobilization. All of these patients should be referred to an orthopedic surgeon.

DISLOCATIONS OF THE WRIST

Lunate Dislocations

Lunate dislocations can occur dorsally or volarly, as shown in Fig. 179-12. Dorsal lunate dislocations are easily diagnosed on the lateral view of the wrist, whereby the lunate is seen dorsal to its normal position within the radial fossa. The lunate is easily palpated over the dorsum of the wrist. Volar dislocations involve displacement of the lunate in the volar direction.

The lunate should be reduced by a hand surgeon. Patients may require surgical intervention for proper reduction and ligamentous stability.

Perilunate Dislocations

Perilunate dislocations involve dislocations of the carpal bones around the lunate. In this dislocation, the lunate remains in its normal position of alignment with the radial head. However, the remainder of the carpal bones are dislocated dorsally or volarly. This can be readily diagnosed on the anteroposterior (AP) and lateral views. Reduction of this dislocation can be accomplished by longitudinal traction using finger traps. However, the patient should be referred to an orthopedic surgeon for early reduction and immobilization.

Scapholunate Dissociation

The normal distance between the lunate and scaphoid on an AP view of the wrist is less than 3 mm. If the space between the scaphoid and lunate is greater than 3 to 5 mL, the patient has a scapholunate dissociation.

This is a very serious injury in that the ligaments connecting the scaphoid and lunate are ruptured and require surgical repair. This must be diagnosed early and referred to a hand surgeon. This condition is one of the most commonly missed diagnoses among emergency department physicians.

Colles' and Smith's Fractures

A Colles' fracture is a fracture of the distal radius at the metaphysis, which is dorsally displaced. This occurs from a fall on the outstretched hand. Typically, this produces a "dinner fork" deformity. One should examine the radiocarpal joint to determine whether the fracture involves that joint. In addition, the radioulnar joint should be examined. Fractures involving the radiocarpal or radioulnar joint predict a much worse prognosis in terms of swelling, persistent pain, and limitation of motion.

Colles' fractures are reduced by placing the patient's hand in a finger trap traction apparatus and a hematoma block followed by reduction of the distal radius.

A Smith's fracture is a reversed Colles' fracture (Fig. 179-13). In a Smith's fracture, there is volar displacement of the distal radius. This fracture is reduced easily in a finger trap traction apparatus, but one must be certain there is no associated median nerve or flexor tendon injury.

A Dorsal dislocation

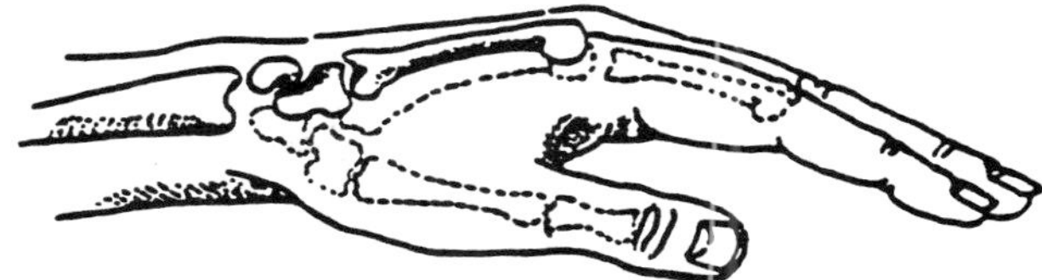

B Volar dislocation

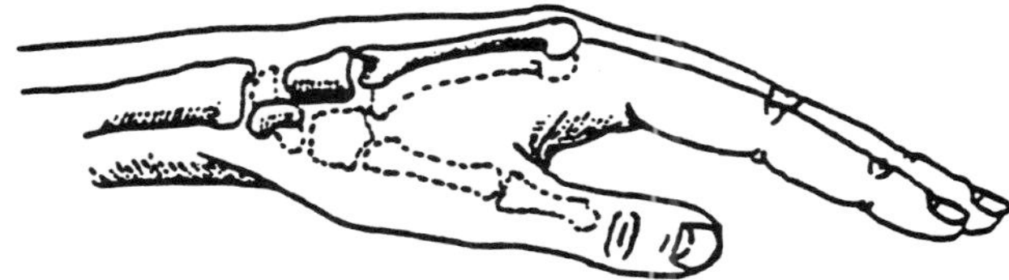

C Dorsal dislocation

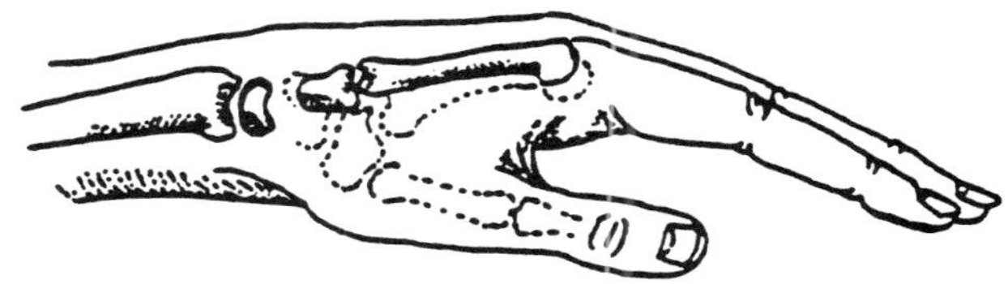

D Volar dislocation

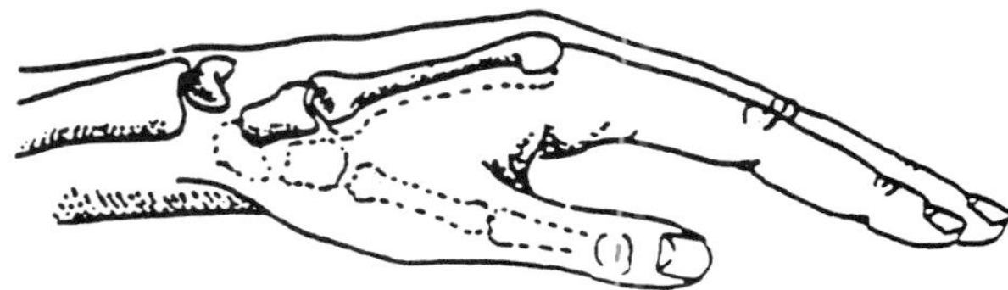

Fig. 179-12. Carpal dislocations.

FRACTURES OF THE HAND

Distal Phalanx

There are five types of fractures of the distal phalanx (Fig. 179-14). The most common distal phalanx fracture is a comminuted fracture, where the comminution involves only the distal tuft. It is often referred to as a "tuft fracture." These fractures are treated in a protective splint.

CLASS A: FLEXION TYPE (SMITH'S FRACTURE)

Type I: Distal radial

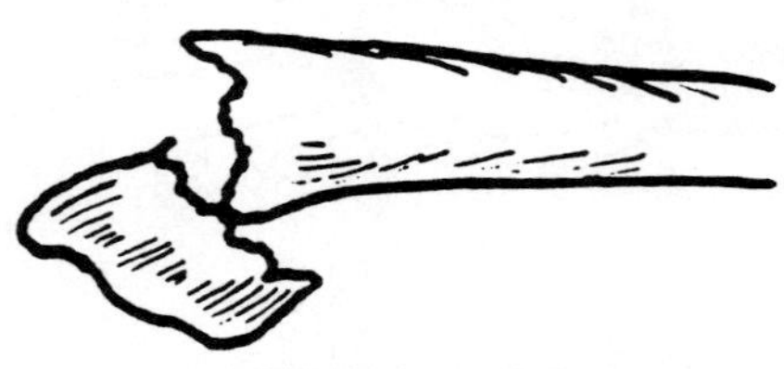

Type II: Distal radial

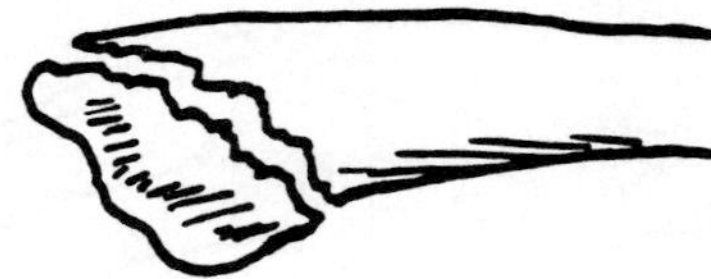

Type III: Distal radial

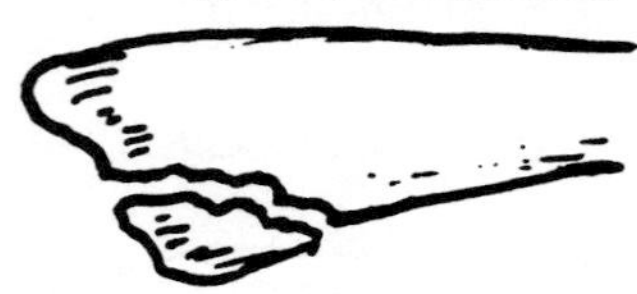

Fig. 179-13. Distal radius fractures.

If a subungual hematoma is present, this should be drained. Transverse fractures with displacement are always associated with a nail bed laceration. The nail bed laceration should be repaired.

Mallet fractures, which involve an avulsion injury at the attachment of the extensor tendon to the distal phalanx, should be treated in an extension splint. If the fragment is large, this may require surgical pinning.

Middle and Proximal Phalanx Fractures

Extraarticular fractures of the middle and proximal phalanx that are not displaced should be treated in an ulnar or radial gutter splint (Fig. 179-9).

An ulnar gutter splint is used in fractures involving the fourth and fifth digits. Fractures of the index and long finger phalanges should be treated in a radial gutter splint. In fractures that are oblique or spiral and in those that are grossly displaced and unstable, a gutter splint can be used temporarily, but the patient should be referred for definitive therapy, which may involve pinning or some other type of surgical intervention.

Fractures involving the articular surface that are nondisplaced can also be treated in an ulnar or radial gutter splint. Displaced fractures involving the articular surface should be reduced anatomically, and this may require surgical intervention. Thus, these patients should be referred.

When applying a radial or ulnar gutter splint for a middle or proximal phalanx fracture, the MP joint should be at 50 to 90° of flexion, the IP joints should be 10 to 15° of flexion, and the wrist should be at 15° extension.

Metacarpal Fractures

Fractures of the metacarpal neck are the most common of all metacarpal fractures. The most common of these is called a boxer's fracture and involves the fifth digit and sometimes the fourth. When fractures of the metacarpal neck involve the second or third metacarpal, the fracture needs to be reduced if the angulation is greater than 15°. The index and long finger metacarpals are relatively stationary bones in the hand, and any angulation or fracture of the metacarpals is poorly tolerated.

CLASS A: EXTRA-ARTICULAR FRACTURES

Type I: Longitudinal

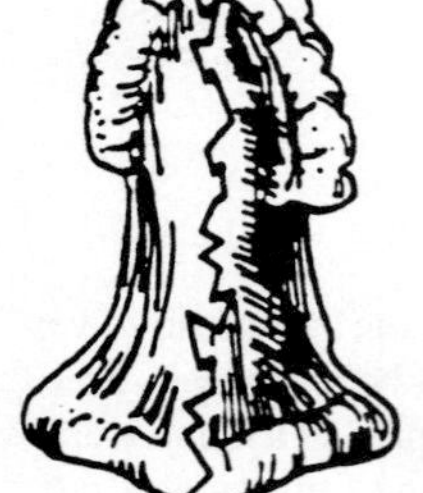

Type II: Transverse

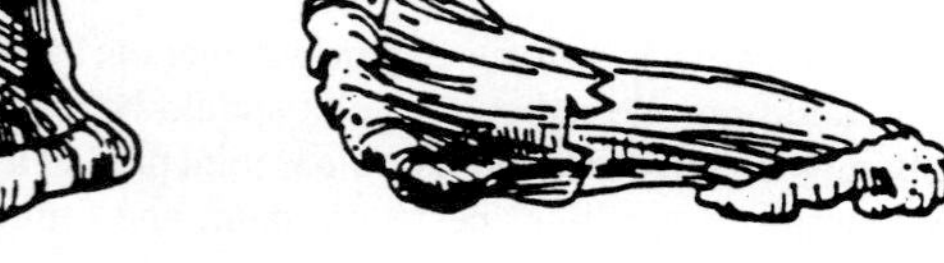

Type III: Comminuted

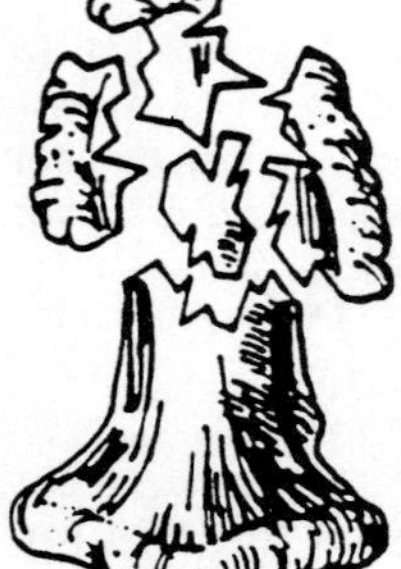

Type IV: Transverse with displacement

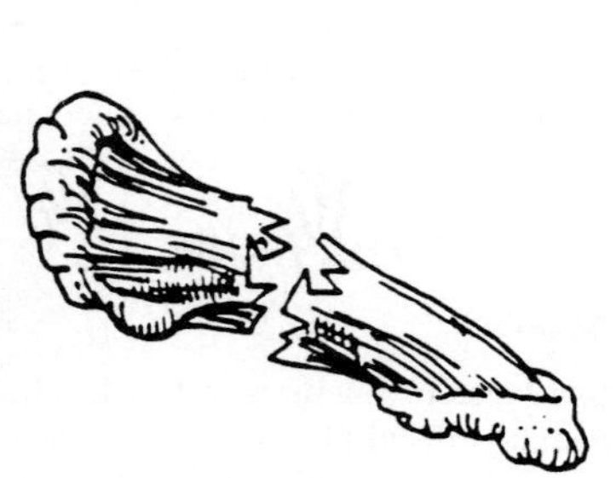

CLASS B: INTRA-ARTICULAR AVULSION FRACTURES

Type I: Dorsal avulsion fracture

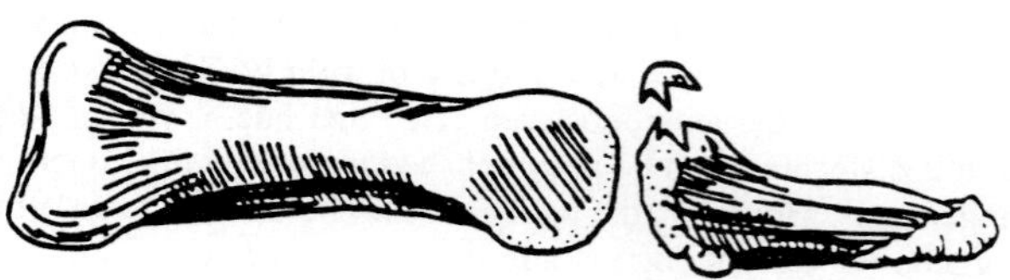

A: "Mallet" fracture (<25% of articular surface)

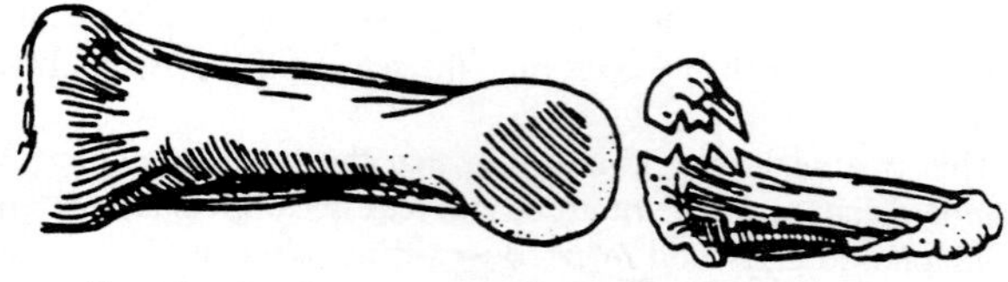

B: "Mallet" fracture (>25% of articular surface)

Fig. 179-14. Distal phalangeal fractures.

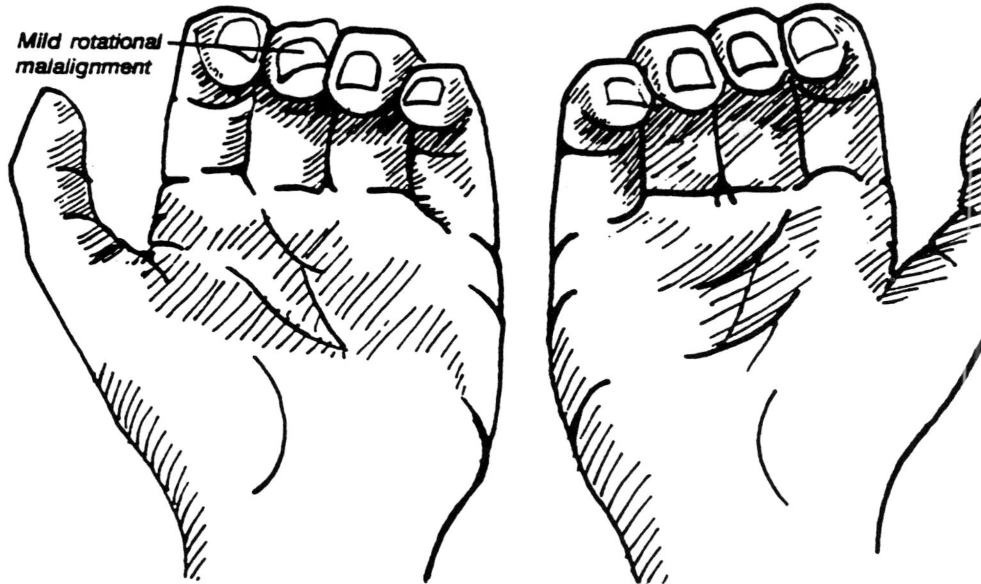

Fig. 179-15. Checking for rotational malalignment.

The name delineates the mechanism, which is basically that of a clenched fist striking an unyielding object. Angulation in a boxer's fracture is usually volar, and if the fracture involves a fourth or fifth digit, one can tolerate up to 30° of volar angulation without reduction.

Fractures of the Metacarpal Shafts

Fractures of the metacarpal shafts can be transverse, oblique, spiral, or comminuted. Oblique and spiral fractures are often angulated or displaced.

Rotational malalignment is a common problem in metacarpal middle and proximal phalanx fractures. It must be detected early, because it is difficult to treat later.

Fractures of the base of the metacarpal are uncommon and often unstable. Displaced fractures of the metacarpal shaft or base should be referred early.

All fractures of the metacarpal neck, shaft, or base can be treated in a gutter splint. In many cases, when the fracture is stable, this therapy can be definitive.

Rotational Malalignment

Rotational malalignment must be detected early and looked for in all patients with middle proximal phalanx and metacarpal fractures. It is very difficult to detect unless one looks for it. One can diagnose rotational malalignment by comparing the plane of the fingernail of

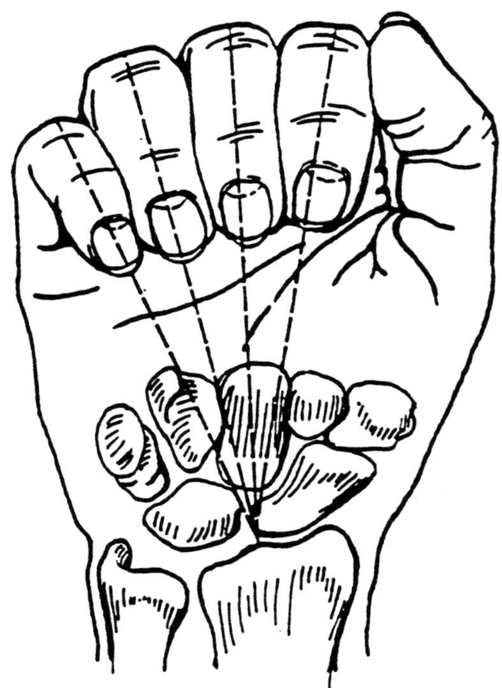

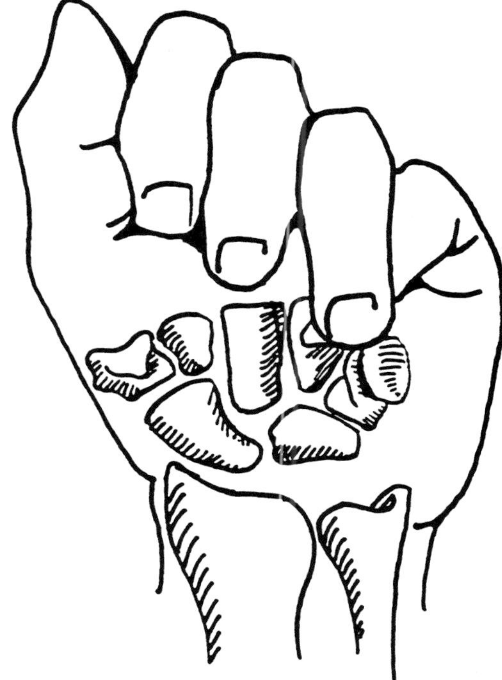

Fig. 179-16. This shows another test for rotational malalignment. See text for discussion.

the partially closed hand in the involved digit, as shown in Fig. 179-15.

Malalignment of the plane of the fingernail indicates rotational malalignment. Another technique that can be used is to close the hand, as shown in Fig. 179-16, and draw a line through the center of the fingernail and carry it to the base of the hand. All of these lines meet unless there is rotational malalignment of the involved digit.

Bennett's Fracture

A fracture of the base of the thumb metacarpal involving the joint is called a Bennett's fracture. It is due to an axial load with a closed hand with the thumb striking an object. This fracture must be anatomically reduced and requires surgical intervention.

BIBLIOGRAPHY

Harris C Jr.: The functional anatomy of the extension mechanism of the finger. J Bone Joint Surg 54(4):713, 1972.

Kettlekamp DB: Traumatic dislocation of extensor tendon. J Bone Joint Surg 53(2):229, 1971.

Kilgore ES, Graham WP: *The Hand.* Lea and Febiger, Philadelphia, 1977.

McConnell CM: Two-year review of hand infections at a municipal hospital. Am Surgeon 61:643, 1979.

Simon RR: The hand and wrist, in *Emergency Orthopedics: The Extremities,* 2d ed. Appleton and Lange, East Norwalk, CT, 1987, pp 294–316.

180
UPPER EXTREMITY TRAUMA

John W. Packer

SHOULDER

The shoulder is made up of the clavicle, scapula, and humerus and is attached to the thorax by the sternoclavicular joint and multiple muscle attachments. The ratio of motion between the glenohumeral joint and the thoracoscapular junction is 2 : 1, so abduction and elevation of the shoulder are carried out as a combination of motions between the shoulder joint and the scapula.

Clavicle Fracture

The clavicle, the most commonly fractured bone at birth, is a bone frequently fractured in children by a fall on the point of the shoulder or on the outstretched arm. In children, the fracture is usually in the middle third of the clavicle, with angulation in a green-stick fashion pointing superiorly. There is sometimes overriding of the fracture fragments with shortening of the clavicle, necessitating a mechanism for pulling the clavicle back to its normal length. Length is restored by application of a figure-of-eight bandage or clavicle strap for protraction of the scapulae. In the adult, the fracture often occurs beyond the coracoclavicular ligaments toward the lateral end of the clavicle. These fractures must be treated quite similarly to an acromioclavicular (AC) dislocation.

Scapula Fracture

When seen early, fractures of the body of the scapula can often be diagnosed by localizing swelling outlining the triangular configuration of the scapula. Rib fractures and pulmonary contusions frequently accompany fractures of the scapula.

Sternoclavicular Joint Dislocation

Sternoclavicular joint dislocations occur in anterior and posterior directions. The anterior dislocation is treated with a clavicle strap and sling. The posterior dislocation can be an emergency because of encroachment upon vital structures in the mediastinum (trachea, esophagus, great vessels). The posterior dislocation can be reduced with retraction of the shoulders using a sandbag between the shoulders, by applying a clavicle strap, or by grasping the clavicle with a towel clip and pulling it forward.

Acromioclavicular Joint Sprain (Dislocation)

Acromioclavicular joint injuries are classified by the degree of injury to the AC and coracoclavicular ligaments. In a first-degree sprain, the AC ligament is partially torn without subluxation of the joint. In a second-degree sprain, the AC joint is torn, allowing subluxation, but the coracoclavicular ligaments are not torn. In a third-degree sprain, both sets of ligaments are torn and there is a complete dislocation of the AC joint (Fig. 180-1).

Acromioclavicular injury can best be diagnosed clinically by localizing tenderness over the AC joint and over the coracoid process. With slight downward traction of the upper arm there is upriding of the clavicle in relation to the acromion. The upriding of the clavicle can be confirmed by anteroposterior (AP) roentgenograms of both clavicles, preferably in the same film, taken while the patient is standing and holding equal amounts of weight in both hands. Measurement between the coracoid process and the clavicle should be the same unless there is upriding of the clavicle. A patient with an AC dislocation can usually be treated with a sling and swath. With marked upriding, special AC splints and straps may be necessary to hold the dislocation reduced, or surgical fixation should be used. Late excision of the distal clavicle will relieve symptoms of AC joint arthritis or excessive upriding of the clavicle.

Shoulder Dislocation

Dislocation of the shoulder is a common injury, particularly in young athletes. The most common direction for dislocation (95 percent) is the anterior or subcoracoid dislocation. The mechanism of injury is usually one that forces the shoulder into marked abduction and external rotation, simultaneously levering the head of the humerus out of the glenoid, tearing the anterior capsule and glenoid labrum with dislocation of the humeral head anteriorly. When the arm is brought to the side, the humeral head rests in a subcoracoid, anteriorly dislocated position. Marked muscle spasm causes pain and prevents easy reduction.

The patient usually has a history of a mechanism of injury that causes abduction and external rotation of the shoulder. There is flattening of the normal contour over the deltoid muscle, and prominence of the acromion, and sometimes the humeral head can be palpable anteriorly.

Roentgenograms show the humeral head in a subcoracoid position (Fig. 180-2). An axillary view and a tangential scapular view confirm that the head is anterior to the glenoid. It should be ascertained whether the greater tuberosity has been avulsed at the time of the dislocation. Any associated fracture, particularly of the surgical neck or humeral head, can complicate attempted reduction. If an associated fracture is recognized, manipulation should be carried out under appropriate general or regional anesthesia to prevent disimpaction of such a fracture.

There is a much higher incidence of recurrent dislocation in young adults who have had severe initial trauma or who have not had adequate initial immobilization. In a patient under the age of 30, the initial treatment should consist of closed reduction and immobilization of the shoulder in adduction and internal rotation by use of a Velpeau's

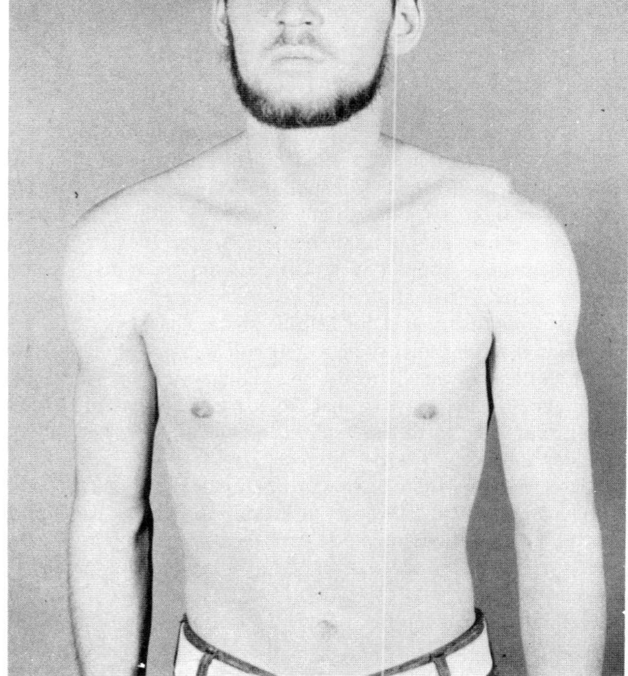

Fig. 180-1. Third-degree sprain of acromioclavicular joint with upriding of the distal clavicle due to complete tear of acromioclavicular and coracoclavicular ligaments.

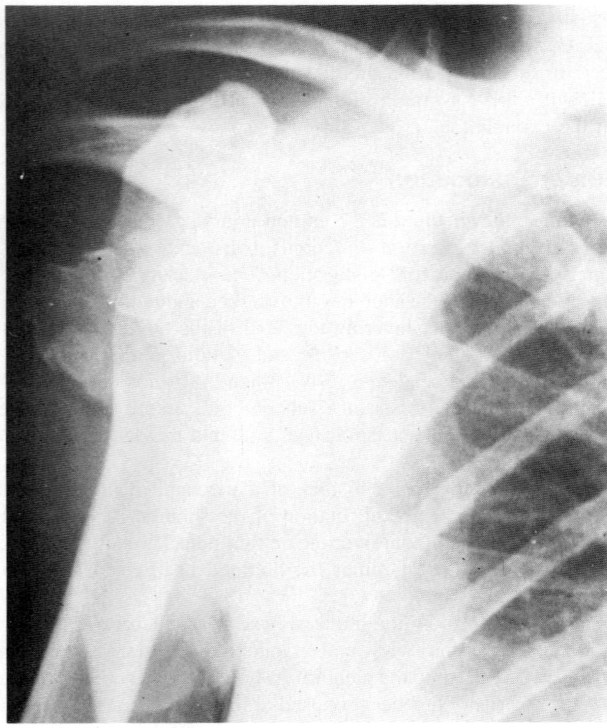

Fig. 180-2. Anterior dislocation of the shoulder. Humeral head is in subcoracoid position. Note the fracture of the greater tuberosity.

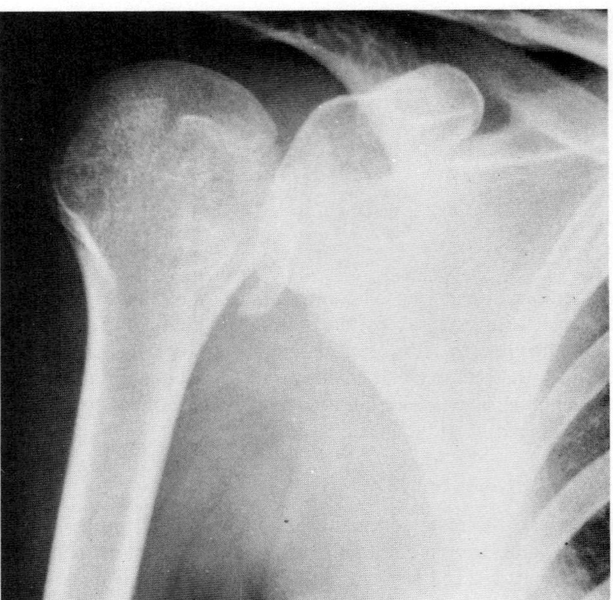

Fig. 180-3. Posterior dislocation of the shoulder. Note the marked internal rotation of the humeral head with the fracture locked on the posterior glenoid rim.

bandage or shoulder immobilizer for at least 4 and usually 6 weeks.

In spite of this treatment, the chance of recurrent dislocation is great if there has been a tear of the glenoid labrum resulting in the Bankart lesion so that the glenid labrum does not reattach to the glenoid rim during the healing process. In recurrent dislocation, the treatment is symptomatic and the long immobilization advised for the initial treatment is not necessary. Once the shoulder has had a recurrent dislocation, the chances of repeated dislocations are so great that surgical repair is advised.

Posterior dislocation of the shoulder is rare. The most common cause is a tonic-clonic seizure with violent internal rotation of the humerus. Posterior dislocation of the shoulder should be suspected in any patient who complains of shoulder pain following a seizure or electric shock phenomenon. Dislocation is often unrecognized because of inadequate radiologic investigation. A true AP film of the scapula should not show overlapping of the humeral head at the glenoid (Fig. 180-3). A tangential scapular view will show posterior displacement of the humeral head in relation to the glenoid. A transthoracic lateral view is often confusing and not helpful in this diagnosis. The best view for demonstrating anterior or posterior dislocation of the shoulder is a good axillary view. Clinically, the patient with a posterior dislocation of the shoulder has pain, inability to passively externally rotate the arm, prominence of the humeral head posteriorly, and relatively flat shoulder anteriorly.

The secret to successful reduction of anterior or posterior dislocation of the shoulder is patient relaxation. A dislocated shoulder can usually be reduced by any of the methods described if the patient is given adequate analgesics, is cooperative, and gives as much voluntary relaxation as possible.

The technique of having the patient lie in a prone position with a weight suspended from the wrist (not held in the hand) is an atraumatic way of reducing the shoulder. Another method is to have an assistant apply countertraction with a sheet and pull from the axilla toward the patient's opposite shoulder. Then the person reducing the shoulder can give gentle constant traction in a longitudinal manner with the shoulder abducted approximately 45°. With prolonged constant traction, this method is usually successful. Occasionally, increasing the abduction to more than 90° while the traction is maintained is necessary to help lever the shoulder back into the proper position. More vigorous methods such as the Kocher maneuver can force the humerus into positions that might result in fracture of the head, neck, or shaft of the humerus. If an associated fracture is noted, a decision whether the patient will need a general anesthetic for maximum muscle relaxation should be made prior to manipulation.

Open reduction and internal fixation are often necessary if the patient has a displaced fracture of the neck of the humerus and a dislocation of the humeral head (Fig. 180-4).

When dislocations of the shoulder are treated, brachial plexus injuries are sometimes evident; however, paralysis of the deltoid and hypesthesia over the deltoid region, as a result of stretching of the axillary nerve, are more common injuries. Prior to any manipulation attempts, the neurologic status of the extremity should be documented, as well as the vascular status, condition of the rotator cuff, or presence of any associated fracture.

Rotator Cuff Tears

Rotator cuff tears result from an indirect force applied to the shoulder. The rotator cuff is made up of tendinous insertions of the subscapularis, supraspinatus, infraspinatus, and teres minor muscles. These tendons blend together and attach to the lesser and greater tuberosities to help initiate abduction and to control internal and external rotation of the shoulder. Many adults over age 50 have degeneration of the rotator cuff. A fall with indirect force applied to the rotator cuff produces a tear that can prevent active abduction of the shoulder. The lesion can occur in younger persons, but greater force is required.

Rotator cuff tendinitis and degeneration are often confused with bursitis or calcific tendinitis but are rarely associated with calcification in the rotator cuff. The radiologic appearance of calcification is a diagnostic sign of calcific tendinitis. The patient with restricted painful motion but without calcification should be considered to have a degenerative tear and tendinitis due to rotator cuff degeneration.

The patient with acute rotator cuff tear has pain, cannot abduct the shoulder at the glenohumeral articulation, is able to shrug the shoulder,

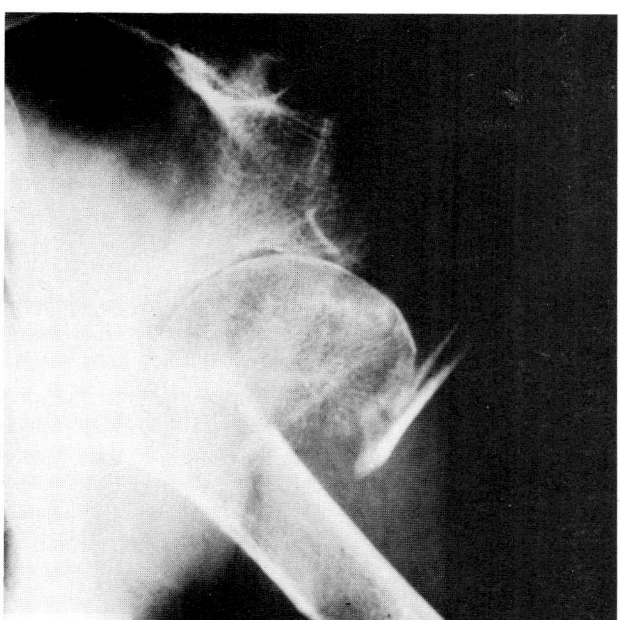

Fig. 180-4. Fracture-dislocation of the proximal humerus. Humeral head is dislocated anteriorly with the shaft displaced. Always obtain a roentgenogram of the shoulder before attempting reduction of a dislocation.

and abducts only at the thoracospacular area. Arthrography of the shoulder is diagnostic of a rotator cuff tear when it demonstrates extravasation of dye from the shoulder joint (Fig. 180-5). Differentiation in the emergency department can often be made by infiltrating a local anesthetic into the area of tenderness in the shoulder. If active abduction can be demonstrated in the resulting absence of pain, the patient does not have a significant rotator cuff tear. If the pain is eliminated and the patient does not have active abduction but has passive abduction, the diagnosis of a rotator cuff tear should be strongly considered. Small rotator cuff tears can often be treated by sling immobilization. Larger rotator cuff tears require surgical repair.

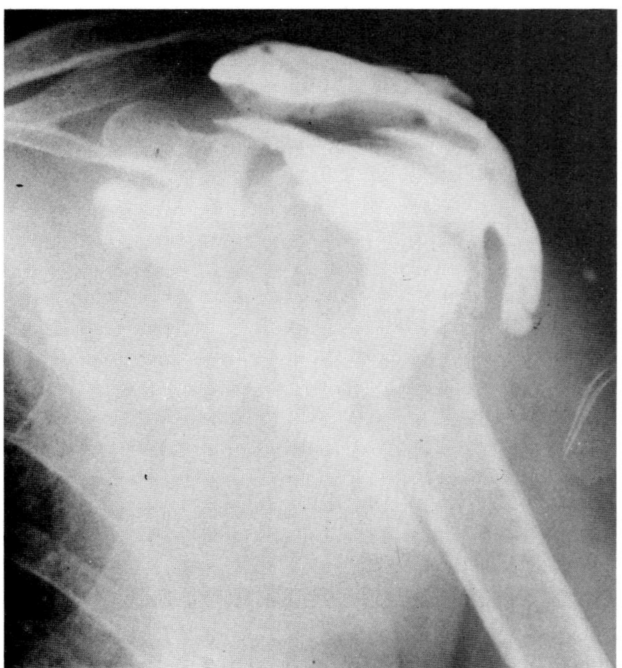

Fig. 180-5. Shoulder arthrogram of rotator cuff tear demonstrating extravasation of contrast material into the subdeltoid bursa.

Tendinitis and Tenosynovitis

Tendinitis and tenosynovitis occur about the shoulder area because of degenerative changes that take place in this relatively avascular tissue, as well as repetitive trauma to which the tendons are subjected. Calcific deposits often form in the reparative process along with inflammatory cells.

Calcific tendinitis occurs most frequently in the supraspinatus tendon. The patient complains of a deep ache in the shoulder, and a painful arc of motion, and has point tenderness over the site of inflammation. Tenosynovitis of the long head of the biceps has similar symptoms with tenderness localized to the bicipital groove anteriorly.

Internal and external rotation films of the shoulder best demonstrate calcification. Lack of calcification should suggest the possibility of a rotator cuff tear.

Nonsteroid anti-inflammatory agents are effective in most cases. For resistant cases, aspiration of the calcification, and injection of a local anesthetic and a steroid into the most tender area, often relieve symptoms.

The patient who does not move his or her shoulders because of conditions that cause pain or because of therapeutic immobility will often develop adhesive capsulitis. This painful condition can be overcome only by exercises to stretch the capsule, restoring its length and allowing the shoulder joint to resume its extensive range of motion.

Humeral Fractures

Proximal humeral fractures. Fractures of the proximal humerus have been classified by C. S. Neer according to displacement (Fig. 180-6). The muscle attachments determine the amount and type of displacement occurring in fractures of the proximal humerus. The lesser and greater tuberosities are separated by the bicipital groove through which the long head of the biceps travels. The subscapularis muscle

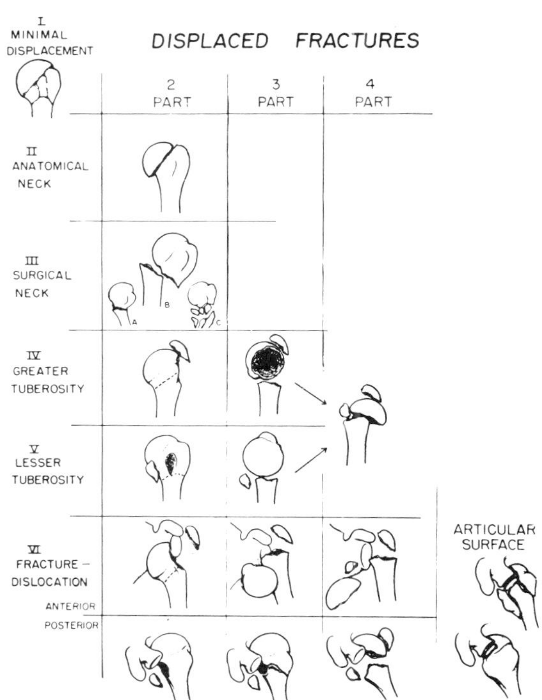

Fig. 180-6. Anatomic classification of displaced fractures of the proximal humerus. (*From* Neer CS II: Displaced proximal humeral fractures. Part I. Classification and evaluation. *J Bone Joint Surg* 52A:1079, 1970. Used by permission.)

attaches to the lesser tuberosity and internally rotates the humerus. The supraspinatus attaches to the greater tuberosity superiorly, resulting in abduction of the humerus. The infraspinatus and teres minor attach posteriorly to the greater tuberosity, initiating external rotation. The deforming force on the shaft of the humerus in a fracture about the surgical neck is the pectoralis major, which pulls the humeral shaft into abduction. Fractures through the anatomic neck cause separation of the humeral head from the shaft. It is left without blood supply or tendinous insertion. Neer's classification shows that fragments can be displaced in predictable directions by the attachment of soft tissue: two-part three-part, or four-part fractures, or anterior or posterior dislocation of the humeral head.

Recognition of fractures of the proximal humerus is important in the emergency department. In those fractures that are not significantly displaced, immobilization by a shoulder immobilizer, a Velpeau's bandage, or sling and swath is usually adequate until rehabilitation is initiated after 1 to 2 weeks. Open reduction and internal fixation are often required if the fracture is significantly displaced or irreducible. The patient should be referred to an appropriate surgeon. Neurovascular status can be impaired in fractures and dislocations about the proximal humerus. The neurovascular status should be documented before and after manipulation of the fracture.

Children with open epiphyses will have significant displacement and angulation of epiphyseal separations in the proximal humeral epiphysis. The anterior angulation accompanying these injuries will usually remodel over a period of 2 to 3 years. If the patient is near skeletal maturity, however, more exact reduction must be carried out.

The possibility of pathologic fractures of the humerus should be considered in the patient who has metastatic carcinoma or multiple myeloma, and in the child with unicameral bone cysts or other bone lesions, because fracture can occur with less than usual violence in these conditions (Fig. 180-7).

Humeral shaft fracture. Closed fractures of the shaft of the humerus are frequently associated with radial nerve paralysis. The nerve is usually stretched, resulting in neuropraxia. Rarely is the nerve lacerated. If the radial nerve paralysis has an onset immediately following the injury, the prognosis for return of function of the nerve is good. Prior to manipulation of a fracture of the shaft of the humerus, documentation of extension of the wrist, thumb, and fingers is mandatory (Fig. 180-8). If, after manipulation, the patient can no longer extend the wrist and fingers, exploration of the fracture with removal of the nerve from entrapment is indicated.

Fractures of the humeral shaft are usually treated in the emergency department by applying a coaptation splint, a hanging arm cast, or another device for external immobilization. Swelling of the elbow and hand are to be expected after this fracture. The patient is more comfortable in a semisitting position so that the fractured humerus is aligned by traction from the weight of the arm. If no distraction occurs, healing is usually complete in 6 to 8 weeks. Fractures of the humerus are frequently associated with delayed union, and they must be immobilized until adequate clinical and roentgenographic union have occurred.

ELBOW

Supracondylar Fracture

The displaced supracondylar fracture in a child is a true emergency. This injury often results in vascular compromise of the musculature in the forearm and hand (Fig. 180-9).

The most common mechanism of injury is a fall on an outstretched arm resulting in a posterior displacement of the supracondylar fragment of the distal humerus and anterior displacement of the knifelife edge of the distal portion of the proximal humeral fragment. Tearing of muscles and occasionally entrapment of the brachial artery or median nerve accompany this injury. Careful assessment of neurovascular status is mandatory.

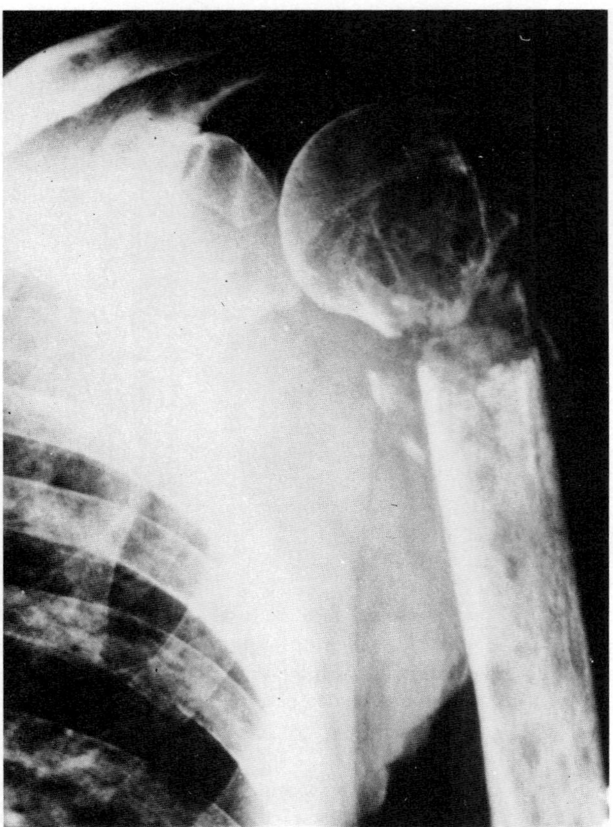

Fig. 180-7. Pathologic fracture of the proximal humerus in multiple myeloma.

Treatment consists of closed reduction under appropriate anesthesia, overhead traction with an olecranon pin, or skin traction in a side-arm position. Hospitalization with close nursing and physician observation is indicated for supracondylar fractures.

Careful monitoring of radial pulse and finger motion prior to definitive treatment is necessary. Prevention of Volkmann's ischemic contracture by timely fasciotomy is occasionally necessary. Maintenance of fracture is sometimes difficult because of the inability to adequately flex the elbow without further compromising circulation. Management of this dangerous and difficult fracture should be in the hands of a well-qualified surgeon.

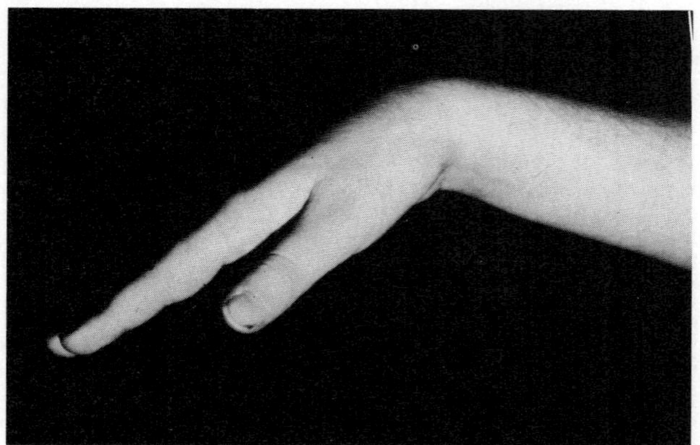

Fig. 180-8. Inability to extend wrist, fingers, and thumb in radial nerve paralysis associated with fracture of the humeral shaft. Do not be fooled by interphalangeal extension by ulnar-innervated interosseous muscles.

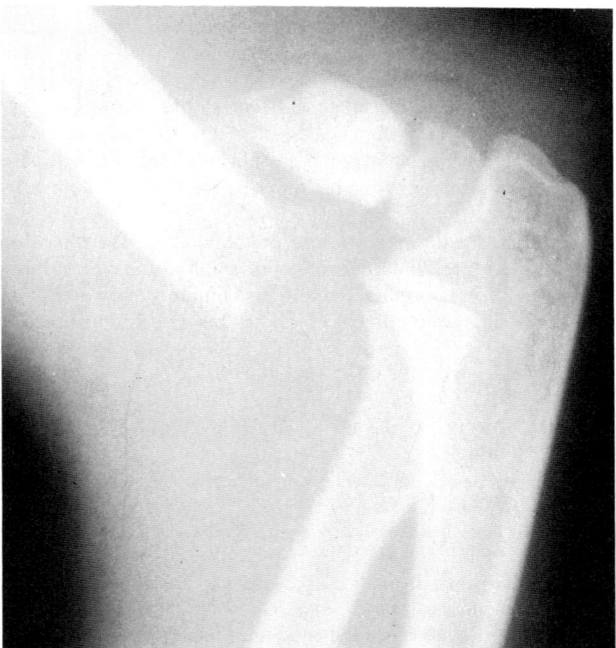

Fig. 180-9. Supracondylar fracture of the distal humerus causes extensive soft tissue damage. Careful monitoring of the neurovascular status is mandatory.

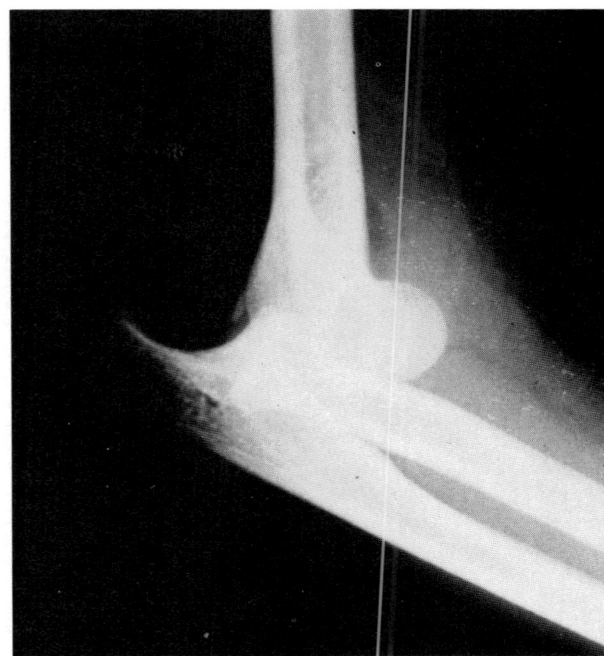

Fig. 180-10. Posterior dislocation of the elbow is best demonstrated on lateral roentgenogram.

Undisplaced supracondylar fractures will often swell a great deal but can be treated on an outpatient basis with adequate flexion of the elbow to prevent further displacement. Close neurovascular observation by responsible parents or medical personnel is essential.

Elbow Dislocation

Dislocation of the elbow joint results from a hyperextension injury. The resulting posterior dislocation can be associated with either medial or lateral displacement. Roentgenograms should include a lateral view of the elbow and an AP view of both the forearm and humerus to prevent distortion of the articular surface due to flexion deformity (Fig. 180-10).

Reduction is accomplished by traction and gentle manipulation. Examination for ligamentous stability will help determine the length of immobilization. Postreduction films are necessary to document complete reduction. If reduction is incomplete, there is usually soft tissue interposition, frequently a nerve. Immobilization in a posterior splint for 2 to 3 weeks is followed by a gradual increase in active motion. Excessive passive motion in the elbow increases the risk of developing myositis ossificans.

Epiphyseal Injuries

Epiphyseal injuries are common in children. Anatomic reduction is mandatory for displaced fractures of the articular surface of the distal humerus. When the lateral epicondyle and capitellum are fractured, they are pulled into a rotated, displaced position by the extensor muscle origin. Medial epicondyle fractures that do not involve the articular surface of the distal humerus can often be left in their displaced position if the displacement is less than 1 cm. Medial epicondyle fractures are occasionally associated with ulnar nerve irritation, requiring exploration, internal fixation, and sometimes anterior transposition of the nerve.

Olecranon and Coronoid Process Fractures

Undisplaced fractures of the olecranon and coronoid processes can be treated by appropriate immobilization in extension or flexion, respectively. Displaced fractures of the olecranon require internal fixation to restore active extension of the elbow.

RADIUS AND ULNA

Radial Head

Fractures of the radial head commonly occur from a fall on the outstretched hand. Most of these fractures are undisplaced or impacted. Aspiration of the hemarthrosis will often give good pain relief and allow early motion. Radial head excision should be considered if there is marked comminution of the fracture, angulation of the articular surface of more than 30°, or more than 2 mm offset in a two-part fracture. The fat pad sign with fat density radiolucency just anterior to the distal humerus is indicative of effusion or hemarthrosis within the elbow joint, and is often a tip-off to an occult radial head fracture. This radiolucency is convex in shape (Fig. 180-10).

Monteggia's Fracture-Dislocation

Monteggia's fracture-dislocation occurs with fracture of the proximal third of the ulna and dislocation of the radial head. In the more common type, there is anterior dislocation of the radial head with anterolateral angulation of the ulna fracture (Fig. 180-11). Posterior dislocation of the radial head is less common. Closed reduction is successful in most children, but open reduction with internal fixation is advised in adults. In any fracture of the proximal half of the ulna, special attention should be paid to the radial head to rule out Monteggia's fracture-dislocation.

Galeazzi's Fracture

An isolated fracture of the shaft of the radius is commonly associated with dislocation of the distal radioulnar joint, Galeazzi's fracture. Both the Monteggia and Galeazzi fractures often require open reduction and internal fixation for stability of the shaft fracture and to maintain appropriate reduction of the accompanying dislocation. Roentgenograms of both the elbow and wrist in fractures of the forearm will ensure that associated dislocation is not overlooked.

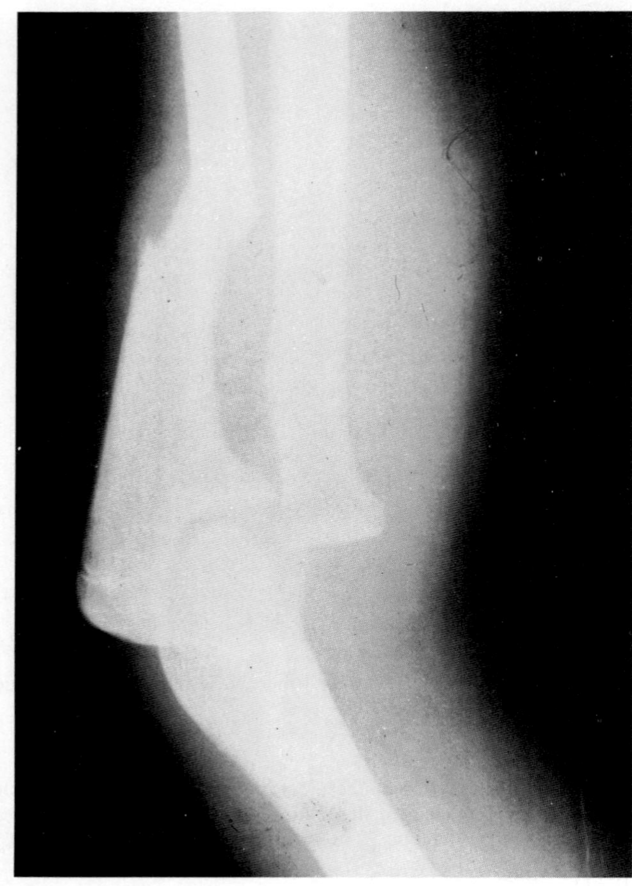

Fig. 180-11. Monteggia's fracture-dislocation: Anterior dislocation of the radial head and fracture of the proximal ulna.

Shaft of Radius and Ulna

Fractures of both bones of the forearm in children are often greenstick fractures with marked deformity and angulation, but they are easily reduced by straightening the angulation and cracking through the intact cortex. Failure to crack through the intact cortex will often result in some recurrence of the deformity. Overriding and displaced fractures frequently require regional or general anesthesia for satisfactory reduction.

Fractures of the shaft of the radius and ulna in adults, when displaced, usually require open reduction and internal fixation with compression plates.

A nightstick fracture, or fracture of the shaft of the ulna from a direct blow, requires immobilization in a long arm cast to prevent rotation of the forearm. This fracture heals quite slowly and must be immobilized until solid clinical union has been accomplished.

BIBLIOGRAPHY

Bruce HE, Harvey JP, Wilson JC: Monteggia fractures. *J Bone Joint Surg* 56A:1563, 1974.

Dameron TB Jr, Reibel DB: Fractures involving the proximal humeral epiphyseal plate. *J Bone Joint Surg* 51A:289, 1969.

Epps CH (ed): *Complications on Orthopaedic Surgery*, ed 2, Philadelphia, Lippincott, 1986.

Heinig CF: Retrosternal dislocation of the clavicle: Early recognition, x-ray, diagnosis, and management. *J Bone Joint Surg* 50A:830, 1968.

McLaughlin HL: Posterior dislocation of the shoulder. *J Bone Joint Surg* 44A:1477, 1962.

Neer CS II: Displaced proximal humeral fractures. Part I. Classification and evaluation. *J Bone Joint Surg* 52A:1077, 1970 (23 refs).

Neer CS II: Displaced proximal humeral fractures. Part II. Treatment of three-part ad four-part displacement. *J Bone Joint Surg* 52A:1090, 1970.

Packer JW, Foster RR, Garcia A, et al: the humeral fracture with radial nerve palsy: Is exploration warranted? *Clin Orthop* 88:34, 1972.

Rockwood CA, Green DP (eds): *Fractures in Adults*, ed 2. Philadelphia, Lippincott, 1984.

Rockwood CA, Wilkins KE(King RE (eds): *Fractures in Children*. Philadelphia, Lippincott, 1984.

Rowe CR, Sakellarides HT: Factors related to recurrences of anterior dislocations of the shoulder. *Clin Orthop* 20:40, 1961.

Smith L: Deformity following supracondylar fractures of the humerus. *J Bone Joint Surg* 42A:235, 1960.

Smith L: Deformity following supracondylar fractures of the humerus. *J Bone Joint Surg* 47A:1668, 1965.

181
TRAUMA TO THE PELVIS, HIP, AND FEMUR

Joseph F. Waeckerle
Mark T. Steele

TRAUMA TO THE PELVIS

Pelvic fractures constitute 3 percent of all skeletal fractures. These fractures and concomitant injuries are a frequent cause of death from blunt trauma sustained in automobile accidents. Fortunately, the mortality has decreased. The treating physician is managing patients with a proactive rather than reactive approach. Most pelvic fractures are secondary to automobile passenger or pedestrian accidents, but about one-third are the result of minor falls in older persons and from major falls or industrial accidents. This chapter discusses the most common fractures of the pelvis, femur, and hip, the mechanisms of injury, radiologic evaluation, and treatment.

Anatomy

The major functions of the pelvis are protection, support, and hematopoiesis. The pelvis consists of the innominate bone, which is made up of the ilium, ischium, and pubis; the sacrum; and the coccyx. The iliopectineal, or arcuate, line divides the pelvis into the upper, or false, pelvis, which is part of the abdomen, and the lower, true pelvis. In addition, this line constitutes the major portion of the femorosacral arch, which, along with the subsidiary tie arch (bodies of pubic bones and superior rami), supports the body in the erect position. In the sitting position the weight-bearing forces are transmitted by the ischiosacral arch augmented by its tie arch, the pubic bones, inferior pubic rami, and ischial rami. When traumatized, the tie arches fracture first, especially at the symphysis pubis, pubic rami, and just lateral to the sacroiliac (SI) joints. Incorporated in the pelvic structure are five joints that allow some movement in the bony ring. The lumbosacral, SI, and sacrococcygeal joints and the symphysis pubis allow little movement. The acetabulum is a ball-and-socket joint that is divided into three portions: the iliac portion, or superior dome, is the chief weight-bearing surface; the inner wall consists of the pubis and is thin and easily fractured; and the posterior acetabulum is derived from the thick ischium.

The pelvis is extremely vascular, a fact that is significant in pelvic fractures. The nerve supply through the pelvis is derived from the lumbar and sacral plexuses. Injury to the pelvis may produce deficits at any level from the nerve root to small peripheral branches.

The lower urinary tract is contained in the pelvis (Fig. 181-1). In the adult, the bladder lies behind the symphysis and pubic bones, and the peritoneum covers the dome and base posteriorly. The location of the bladder and the degree of peritoneal reflection are determined by urine content. The lower gastrointestinal tract housed in the pelvis includes a small portion of the descending colon, the pelvic, or sigmoid, colon, the rectum, and the anus.

Clinical Evaluation

History

The emergency physician should assume that all victims of serious or multiple trauma, or both, have fractures of the pelvis. A patient with a suspected pelvic fracture should be questioned about details of the accident to determine the mechanism of injury and about pre-hospital evaluation and treatment. The patient should be specifically questioned to determine areas of pain, last urination or defecation, present bladder sensation, and the last solid and fluid intake. In addition, the time of the last menses or the presence of pregnancy, current medications, and allergies should be ascertained.

Physical Examination

Symptoms and signs of pelvic injuries vary from local pain and tenderness, especially with walking, to pelvic instability and severe shock. The physician must maintain alertness, perception, and concern (APC) in evaluating these patients. On inspection look for perineal and pelvic edema, ecchymoses, lacerations, and deformities. Look for hematomas above the inguinal ligament or over the scrotum (Destot's sign). Roll the patient over if appropriate and examine the areas overlying the sacrum and coccyx. On palpation feel for irregularities, crepitance, or movement at the iliac crests, pubic rami, and ischial rami. Palpation of a bony prominence or large hematoma or tenderness along the fracture line is possible by rectal examination (Earle's sign). Compress the pelvis lateral to medial through the iliac crests, anterior to posterior through the symphysis pubis, and anterior to posterior through the iliac crests. Compress the greater trochanters and determine the range of motion of the hips. On rectal examination, superior or posterior displacement of the prostate, or rectal injuries are indicative of intraperitoneal and urologic injury. Decrease in anal sphincter tone may suggest neurologic injury. Carefully evaluate neurovascular function. If a pelvic fracture is found, assume intraabdominal, retroperitoneal, gynecologic, and urologic injuries until proved otherwise.

Radiologic Evaluation

Stabilization of the patient takes priority over obtaining x-ray films. Unnecessary movement may produce further injury or cause more blood loss. After stabilization, roentgenographic evaluation of the pelvis is a must in all unconscious patients who have sustained multiple injuries. Lower extremity long bone fractures as well as pelvic symp-

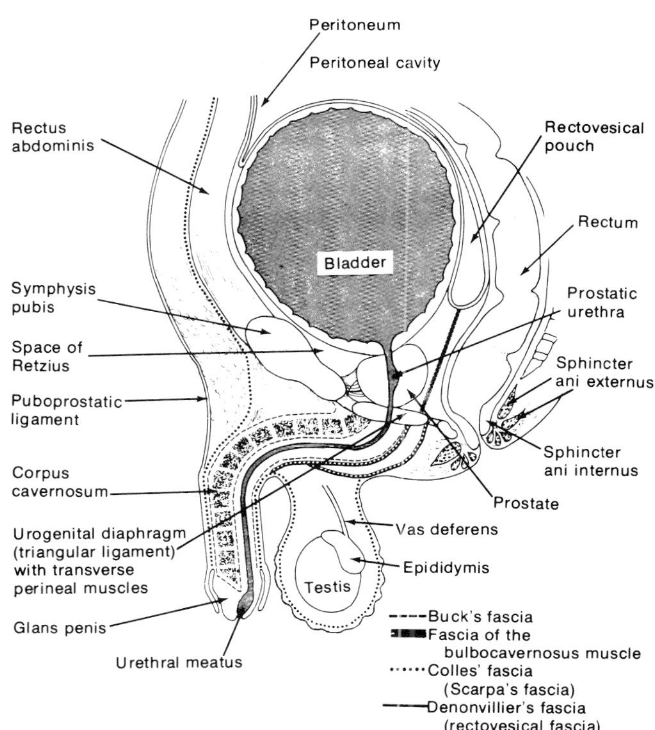

Fig. 181-1. Sagittal section of the male pelvis showing the relation of the full bladder. [From Kane WJ: Fractures of the pelvis, in Rockwood CA Jr, Green DP (eds): *Fractures*, Philadelphia, Lippincott, 1975, vol 2, pp. 916, 917. Used by permission.]

Table 181-1. Classification of Pelvic Fractures

I. Fractures of individual bones without a break in the continuity of the pelvic ring
Avulsion fractures
Anterior superior iliac spine
Anterior inferior iliac spine
Ischial tuberosity
Fracture of the pubis or ischium
Fracture of the wing of the ilium (Duverney)
Fracture of the sacrum
Fracture or dislocation of the coccyx
II. Single break in the pelvic ring
Fracture of two ipsilateral rami
Fracture near or subluxation of the symphysis pubis
Fracture near or subluxation of the SI joint
III. Double breaks in the pelvic ring
Double vertical fractures or dislocation of the pubis or both (straddle fractures)
Double vertical fractures or dislocation or both (Malgaigne)
Severe multiple fractures
IV. Fractures of the acetabulum
Undisplaced
Displaced

Source: Adapted by Kane WJ: Fractures of the pelvis, in Rockwood CA Jr, Green DP (eds): *Fractures in Adults,* ed 2. Philadelphia, Lippincott, 1984, p 1112, from the classification by Key JA, Conwell HE: *The Management of Fractures, Dislocations, and Sprains,* ed 4. St Louis, Mosby, 1946, p 857. Used by permission.

toms or signs are also indications for roentgenograms. A standard anteroposterior (AP) view of the pelvis is the necessary baseline. If additional studies are needed, lateral views, AP views of either hemipelvis, internal and external oblique views of the hemipelvis, or inlet and tilt views of the pelvis may be done. Tomography, CT scans, and special studies may be needed to fully evaluate and manage patients. Angiography or venography may be necessary to determine a source of bleeding. The patient's condition must dictate what is done and when.

Classification of Pelvic Fractures

Fractures of the ilium and ischium comprise about two-thirds of pelvic fractures, while acetabular, coccygeal, and sacral fractures comprise the remainder.

There are many classifications proposed; two commonly used are presented. Pelvic fractures may be classified into types I, II, III, and IV, depending on the degree of disruption of the pelvic ring (Table 181-1 and Fig. 181-2).

Type I Fractures

Type I consists of fractures of individual bones without a break in the pelvic ring (Fig. 181-2). These fractures are usually stable and heal well with bed rest. They make up about one-third of all pelvic fractures.

Avulsion fracture of anterior superior iliac spine. Avulsion occurs because of contraction of the sartorius muscle. Symptoms and signs are local pain, tenderness, and swelling and pain with flexion or abduction of the thigh. There is minimal displacement of the anterior superior iliac spine visible on the AP film of the pelvis.

Avulsion fracture of anterior inferior iliac spine. Avulsion occurs because of forceful contraction of the rectus femoris muscle. Symptoms and signs are sharp pain in the groin, difficulty with ambulation, and inability to flex the hip. The AP film shows downward displacement of the fragment, but this must be differentiated from the epiphyseal line of the os acetabuli.

Avulsion fracture of ischial tuberosity. The mechanism of injury is contraction of the hamstrings, and the fracture is seen in youths whose apophyses are not united. Symptoms and signs include acute or chronic pain with sitting, or upon flexing the thigh with the knee

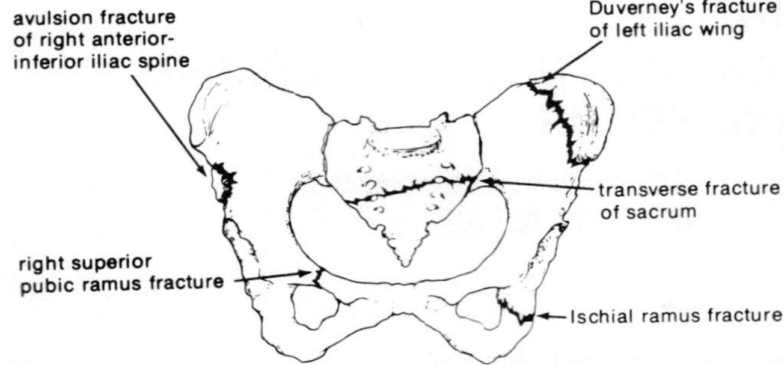

Type I: Fracture of individual bones without break in pelvic ring. Examples shown above.

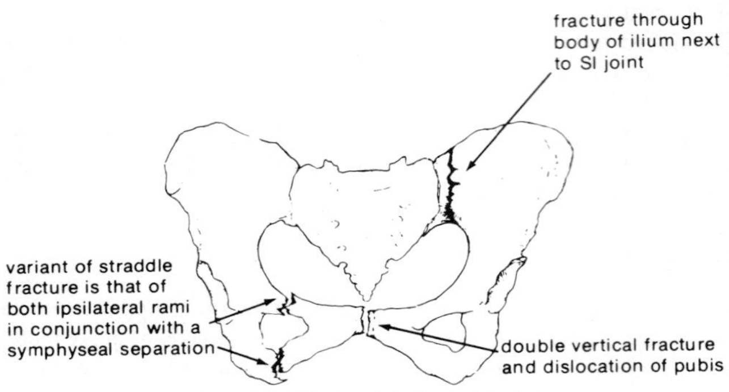

Type II: Single break in the pelvic ring. See examples above.

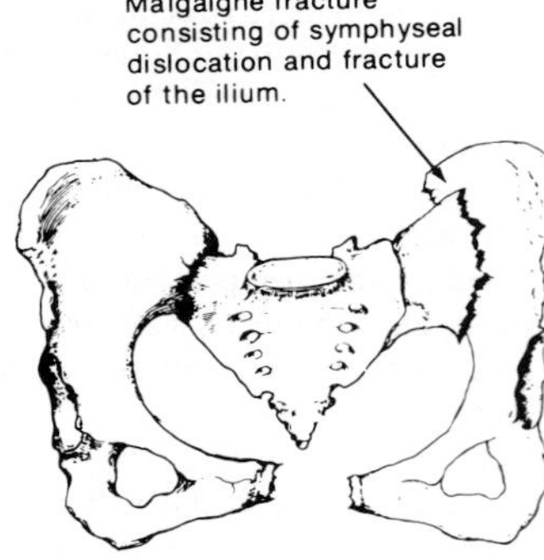

Type III: Double break in pelvic ring.

Fig. 181-2. Pelvic fractures (type I, II, and III) according to classification by Key JA, Conwell HE: *The Management of Fractures, Dislocations, and Sprains,* ed 4, St Louis, Mosby, 1946, p 857, as adapted by Kane WJ: Fractures of the pelvis, in Rockwood CA Jr, Green DP (eds): *Fractures,* ed 2. Philadelphia, Lippincott 1984, vol 2, pp 1133–1142.

extended. Rectal examination reveals tuberosity tenderness. The roentgenogram shows detachment of the apophysis from the ischium with minimal displacement. The apophysis closes between ages 20 and 25.

Fracture of single ramus of pubis or ischium. These injuries are commonly seen in the elderly, and the mechanism of injury is usually a fall with direct trauma. Symptoms and signs include local pain and tenderness and inability to ambulate.

Examination of the pubic bones will usually distinguish a fracture of the pubis from a femoral neck fracture, but a lateral film of the injured hip is recommended to rule out femoral neck injury. The AP roentgenogram of the pelvis shows a nondisplaced fracture of the ramus.

Ischium body fractures. The incidence of ischial body injury is very low. The mechanism of injury is violent, external trauma, such as a fall in a sitting position. Symptoms and signs include local pain and tenderness, and pain with hamstring movement.

The x-ray film shows fracture of the body or tuberosity of the ischium. A large fragment with comminution or a butterfly pattern may be seen on the AP film of the pelvis.

Iliac wing (Duverney) fractures. The mechanism of injury in an iliac wing fracture is direct trauma, usually lateral to medial. Symptoms and signs include pain, swelling, and tenderness over the iliac wing. There is severe pain on ambulation, and Trendelenburg's sign is present. Although accompanying abdominal injuries are infrequent, abdominal rigidity, lower quadrant tenderness, and ileus are common findings. The AP film of the pelvis shows minimal displacement of fragments.

Sacral fractures. Transverse fractures of the sacrum are more common with massive pelvic injuries. The mechanism of injury is direct trauma by a posterior-to-anterior force, producing a transverse fracture. A rectal examination with the other hand on the sacrum causes pain and movement at the fracture site.

Roentgenogram interpretation may be difficult, and exactly aligned AP views are necessary to show the fracture. Look for a transverse fracture line at the level of the lower SI joint, and irregularity, buckling, or sharp angulation of the foramina. Examine the body and wings closely. A lateral view may show displacement anteriorly. Sacral root injury, especially S1 and S2, may be present.

Coccyx fractures. Coccygeal fractures are more frequent in women and are generally caused by direct violence or a fall in the sitting position. Symptoms and signs include pain, tenderness, and swelling and ecchymoses over the lower sacral region. There may be pain upon getting up from a sitting position or straining at stool. The rectal examination reveals pain and movement of the coccyx.

The roentgenogram is of questionable value, but AP and lateral views with sharp flexion of the thighs may demonstrate the fracture.

Type II Fractures

Type II fractures consist of a single break in the pelvic ring (Fig. 181-2). These are by definition stable fractures with little or no displacement and are treated with bed rest. However, about one-fourth of patients with type II fractures have major soft tissue injuries; visceral injuries, especially genitourinary injuries; or hemorrhage.

Fracture of two rami ipsilaterally. The mechanism of injury is direct trauma, but forces through the femur can also cause fractures. Deformity, ecchymoses, and hematoma formation may be detected by palpation, and pain and motion at the fracture site are elicited by compression maneuvers. Flexion, abduction, external rotation, and extension of the hip (Patrick's test, or fabere sign) elicit pain. An AP x-ray film of the pelvis reveals fractures with no or minimal displacement.

Fracture near or subluxation of the symphysis pubis. The mechanism of injury to the symphysis pubis is usually direct AP trauma. These injuries may occur during or after childbirth. Symptoms and signs include severe pain with some external rotation of the lower extremities. Compression and palpation produce displacement pain. Bruising is generally absent.

The x-ray film shows fracture, subluxation, or dislocation. Subluxation may occur in either the sagittal or coronal plane. Dislocation occurs by overlapping in the midline, by superoposterior or inferoanterior displacement of one articulating surface in relation to the other. Complications include genitourinary injuries and SI joint disruption.

Fracture near or subluxation of the SI joint. The mechanism of injury to the SI joint is direct trauma from behind, or from behind and laterally. Symptoms and signs include local pain, pain with ambulation, and pain by compression maneuvers and Patrick's test. The posterior superior iliac spine appears more prominent on the injured side.

Radiologic views of the pelvis, sacrum, and SI joints are required. The films may show fracture through the weak areas of the sacrum (first and second foramina), fracture through the ilium, overlapping of the ilium on the sacrum, or loss of regular joint space. In addition, carefully check for accompanying anterior pelvic ring injuries. CT scans are more informative in many cases.

Type III Fractures

Type III fractures are characterized by a double break in the pelvic ring (Fig. 181-2). They are unstable fractures and are frequently associated with visceral or soft tissue injuries and major hemorrhage.

Double vertical fracture or dislocation of the pubis (straddle fractures). The mechanism of injury in the straddle fracture is direct trauma to the arch, or lateral compression of the pelvis. Symptoms and signs include pain, deformity, bruising, and swelling. The fracture can be seen in the AP view.

Treatment is conservative, but the incidence of complications is high, including genitourinary injuries and visceral abdominal injuries.

Double vertical fracture or dislocation (Malgaigne's fracture). Malgaigne's fracture consists of fractures of the superior and inferior rami, or dislocation of the symphysis in association with sacral or iliac fracture or SI joint dislocation. The mechanism of injury is debatable, but direct AP trauma is probably the most common cause.

Symptoms and signs include pain, crepitance, contusion, swelling, and decreased range of motion of the lower extremity. Middle fragment movement or displacement is seen, and there is pain and movement with compression maneuvers. The ipsilateral leg appears shortened.

Anterioposterior radiologic views may be sufficient, but other views may also be required. All complications associated with pelvic trauma are frequently seen with this injury. Sacroiliac joint reduction is difficult and may result in chronic problems.

Severe multiple pelvic fractures. The mechanism of injury is exceptional trauma to the pelvis with strain on the weakest portion, or anterior tie arches, that causes them to fracture along with the posterior ring. The incidence of sacral fractures ranges from 4 to 74 percent, and the injury is due to forces generated by rotation, leverage, and shearing.

Multiple fractures are easily seen on x-ray, but acetabular and sacral fractures are difficult to see, so special views or CT scans may be necessary. To recognize sacral fractures, compare the distance between the upper and lower borders of the SI joint (the lateral sacral promontory) and the midline on both sides. These should be equal. Also, inspect and compare the sacral foramina.

Complications include genitourinary, gastrointestinal, vascular, and neurologic injuries. Treatment is conservative but requires adequate reduction of the ilium.

Type IV Fractures of the Acetabulum

Type IV acetabular fractures are increasing in frequency with an increase in automobile accidents. They are seen commonly with other pelvic injuries. The roentgenographic anatomy of type IV fractures is shown in Fig. 181-3. There are four anatomic types of fractures, and all are associated with hip dislocations: posterior (Figs. 181-4 and 181-5), ilioischial column (Fig. 181-6), transverse (Fig. 181-7), and iliopubic column (Fig. 181-8). In addition, combinations of any of these fractures can occur.

Posterior fracture. The mechanism of injury in a posterior fracture is direct trauma to a flexed knee and hip. Anteroposterior and lateral radiologic views easily demonstrate the posterior acetabular fracture with the posterior hip dislocation. Complications are sciatic nerve injury and femoral fractures.

Ilioischial column fracture. The mechanism of injury is posteriorly directed force to a knee with the thigh abducted and flexed. The AP

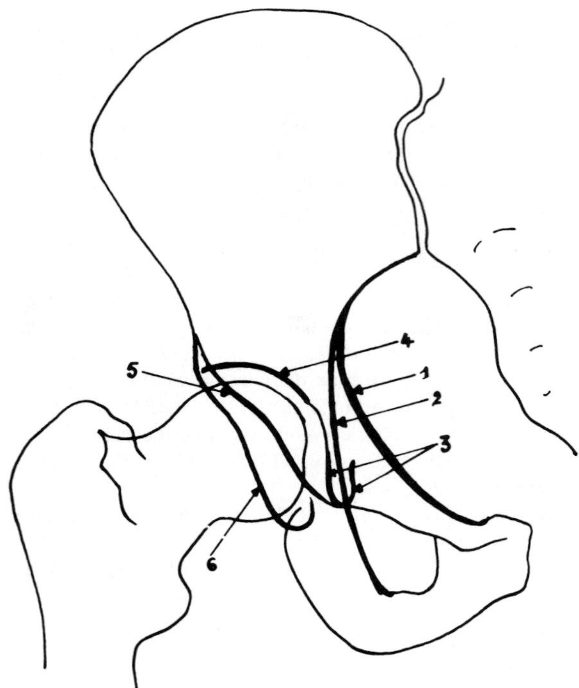

Fig. 181-3. Roentgenographic anatomy of type IV acetabular fractures. The AP view shows (1) arcuate (iliopectineal) line, (2) ilioischial roentgenographic line, (3) roentgenographic U, (4) roof, (5) anterior lip, and (6) posterior lip. (*From* Judet R, Judet J, Letournel E: Fractures of the acetabulum: Classification and surgical approaches for open reduction. *J Bone Joint Surg* 46A:1616, 1964. Used by permission.)

x-ray film demonstrates a large, medially displaced fragment with central dislocation of the femoral head. The most common complication is sciatic nerve injury.

Transverse fracture of acetabulum. The mechanism is force lateral to medial over the greater trochanter, or force posterior to anterior on the posterior pelvis with the hip flexed. An AP x-ray film clearly demonstrates the fracture with a central hip dislocation.

Iliopubic column fracture. The mechanism of injury is a lateral force to the greater trochanter with the hip externally rotated. On roentgenography, there is marked external rotation of the hip. The ilioischial line is disrupted, and the anterior lip is fractured.

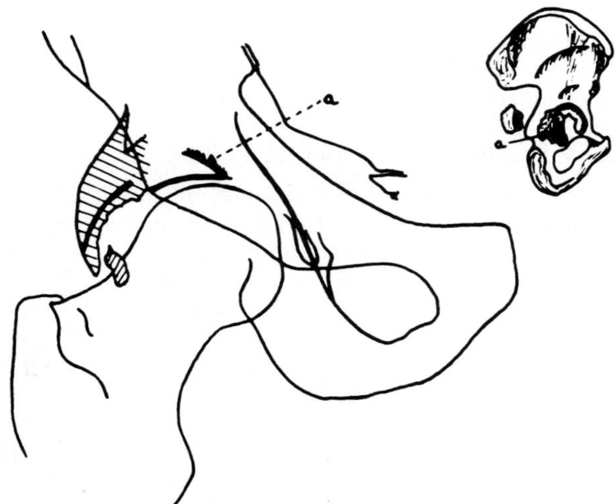

Fig. 181-4. Fracture of posterior lip with some impaction and comminution. (*From* Judet R, Judet J, Letournel E: 1964. Used by permission.)

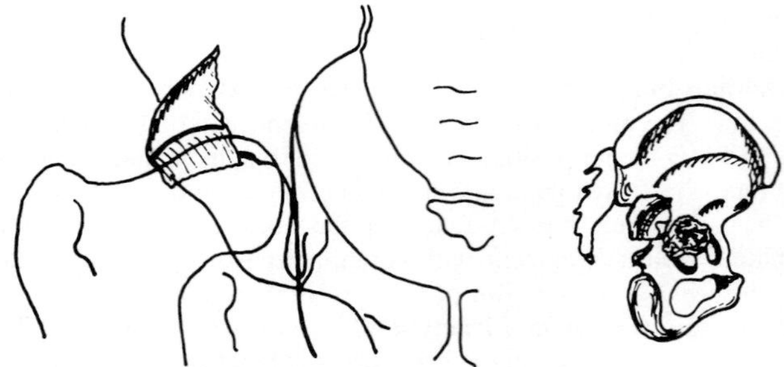

Fig. 181-5. Posterior superior rim fracture. (*From* Judet R, Judet J, Letournel E: 1964. Used by permission.)

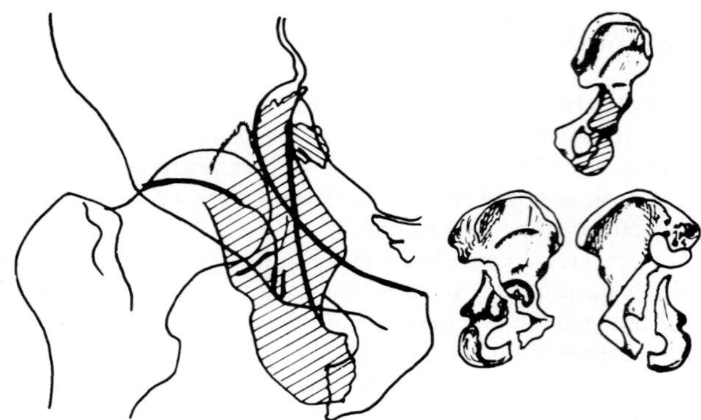

Fig. 181-6. Ilioischial fracture. (*From* Judet R, Judet J, Letournel E: 1964. Used by permission.)

Further discussion on acetabular fractures appears below under "Trauma to the Hip and Femur."

"Shock Trauma" Pelvic Fracture Classification

Another more recent pelvic fracture classification scheme developed at the Shock Trauma Center in Maryland differentiates fracture patterns due to trauma based on mechanism of injury and direction of causative force. Incidence of complications (i.e., urogenital and vascular) is correlated with the fracture pattern, making identification of the type more clinically significant and useful.

Three main types of patterns have been identified. The first and most common mechanism, lateral compression (see Figs. 181-9 to 13), accounts for half the injuries. Motor vehicle accidents in which a car is broadsided or a pedestrian struck from the side are examples. Anteroposterior compression (see Figs. 181-14 to 181-16) is the second

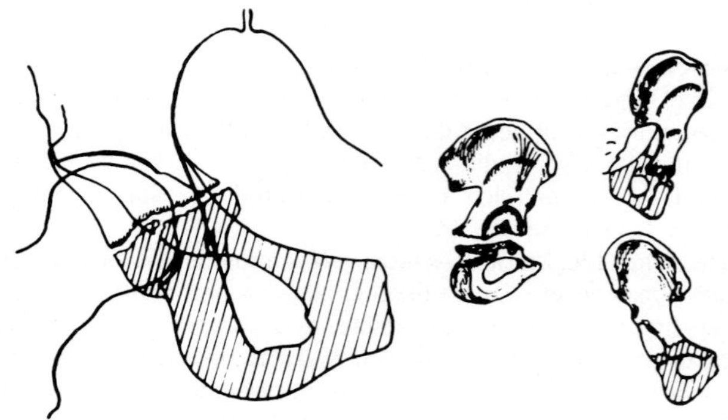

Fig. 181-7. Transverse fracture without displacement. (*From* Judet R, Judet J, Letournel E: 1964. Used by permission.)

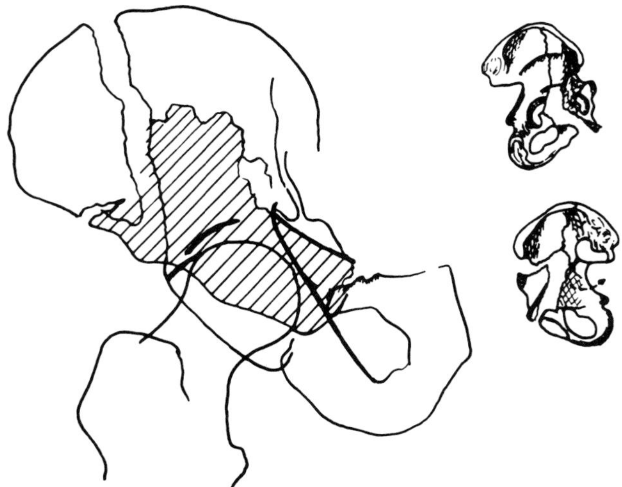

Fig. 181-8. Iliopubic fracture. (*From* Judet R, Judet J, Letournel E: 1964. Used by permission.)

type, accounting for 20 percent of injuries. Head-on type MVAs are the classic example. The least common mechanism was vertical shear (see Fig. 181-17) typified by a fall or jump from a height, accounting for 6 percent of fractures. Mixed patterns of injury make up the other 20 to 25 percent of injuries.

The different injury types may be suggested by history, but can also be differentiated radiographically. The alignment of pubic rami fractures is one such clue to the mechanism and direction of force. Horizontal fractures suggest lateral compression injury whereas vertical ones point to an anteroposterior direction of force. If there is sacroiliac joint diastasis and an associated crush fracture of the sacrum, then the injury is due to lateral compression. Central hip dislocations suggest a lateral compression mechanism whereas posterior dislocation suggests an anteroposterior force. With vertical shear patterns, fractures are vertical in alignment with vertical displacement of fragments. Based on the recognition of the fracture pattern, one can then predict the likelihood of severe hemorrhage or urogenital injury (see Table 181-2).

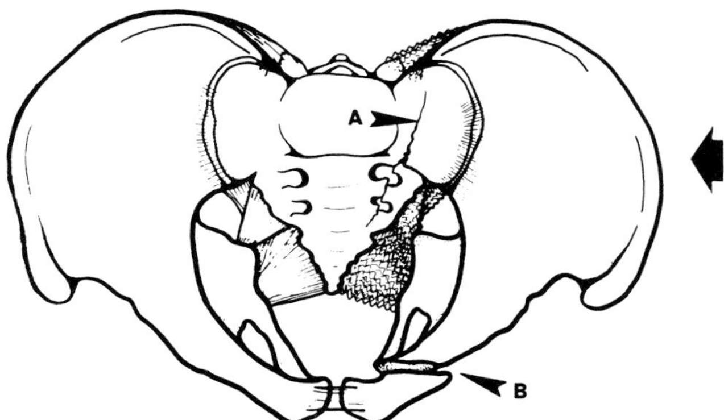

Fig. 181-9. Type I—lateral compression fracture: The lateral force is applied posteriorly (*arrow*). This causes a crush effect on the SIJ: this may be visible radiographically as a sacral fracture (*A*). The characteristic fracture pattern of the pubic rami will be seen (*B*). No ligamentous injury is seen. (*Source:* From Young JWR, Burgess AR: *Radiologic Management of Pelvic Ring Fractures: Systematic Radiologic Diagnosis*. Baltimore, Urban & Schwarzenberg, 1987. Used by permission.)

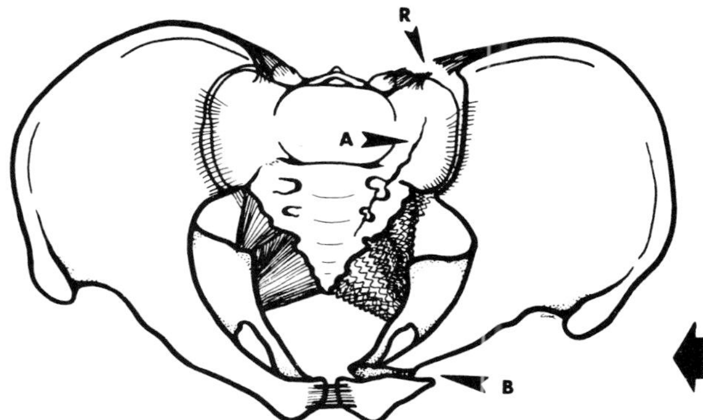

Fig. 181-10. Type II—lateral compression fracture: The force is applied anteriorly (*arrow*), causing the typical anterior pubic rami fractures (*B*). In this case, however, rotation of the pelvis around the anterior sacral margin may occur, causing rupture of the posterior sacroiliac ligaments (*R*). A crush fracture of the sacrum may also be seen (*A*). (*Source:* From Young JWR, Burgess AR: *Radiologic Management of Pelvic Ring Fractures: Systematic Radiologic Diagnosis*. Baltimore, Urban & Schwarzenberg, 1987. Used by permission.)

Treatment

Anatomic restoration is required. If the difficult task of reduction of the femoral head and exact restoration of the displaced fractured acetabulum cannot be done quickly and safely, surgery is indicated. If there is no displacement, bed rest is the treatment of choice. If redislocation occurs, the hip is unstable and surgery is necessary.

Failure to recognize pelvic trauma leads to nonstabilization of the fracture, which, in turn, enhances blood loss and causes further injuries. It may also lead to an incomplete evaluation of pelvic injury.

It is imperative that the physician recognize concomitant injuries, especially those requiring immediate evaluation.

Complications

Complications include hemorrhage, myositis ossificans, infection, thrombophlebitis, and sciatic nerve injuries.

Hemorrhage. Hemorrhage is a major cause of death in pelvic injuries. Hauser and Perry reported that patients with type III fractures require blood replacement 2½ times more often than those with type I, II, or IV and need 2½ times more blood than patients with type I, II, or IV fractures who receive transfusions. Retroperitoneal bleeding is an inevitable complication, and up to 6 L of blood can be accom-

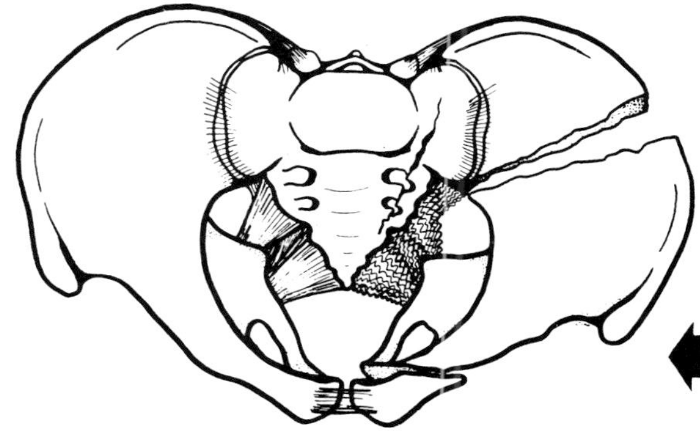

Fig. 181-11. Alternatively (compared to Fig. 181-10), a fracture of the iliac wing may occur, which dissipates the rotational forces and thus leaves the posterior ligaments intact. (*Source:* From Young JWR, Burgess AR: *Radiologic Management of Pelvic Ring Fractures: Systematic Radiologic Diagnosis*. Baltimore, Urban & Schwarzenberg, 1987. Used by permission.)

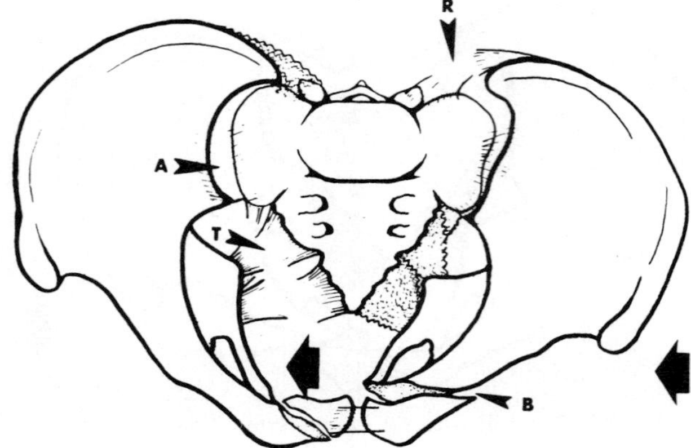

Fig. 181-12. Type III—lateral compression fracture: The force is applied anteriorly (*arrow*), causing internal rotation of the anterior hemipelvis. Continuing through to the contralateral hemipelvis (*arrow*), the force causes it to rotate externally. The result is a pattern of lateral compression on the ipsilateral side, with apparent AP compression on the contralateral side. This results in rupture of the posterior sacroiliac ligaments on the ipsilateral side (*R*) and sacrospinous/sacrotuberous complex (*T*) and anterior ligaments (A) on the contralateral side. Typical public rami fractures (B) are to be expected. (*Source:* From Young JWR, Burgess AR: *Radiologic Management of Pelvic Ring Fractures: Systematic Radiologic Diagnosis.* Baltimore, Urban & Schwarzenberg, 1987. Used by permission.)

modated in this space! Both small and large vessels, especially the superior gluteal and internal pudendal branches of the internal iliac artery, can be disrupted, with hemorrhage disecting from the back to the buttocks.

General resuscitative measures include massive crystalloid, colloid, and blood replacement. Patients may require massive blood replacement.

An antishock garment provides stabilization, may be helpful in controlling bleeding sites, and increases blood pressure by increasing peripheral vascular resistance. Early orthopedic consultation should be considered for placement of external fixator device to help control hemorrhage. Early use of this device has been shown to reduce the incidence of ARDS.

If the patient is exsanguinating, angiography can be done and small bleeding sites controlled. Most authorities agree that aggressive fluid and blood replacement are best. Laparotomy is a last measure.

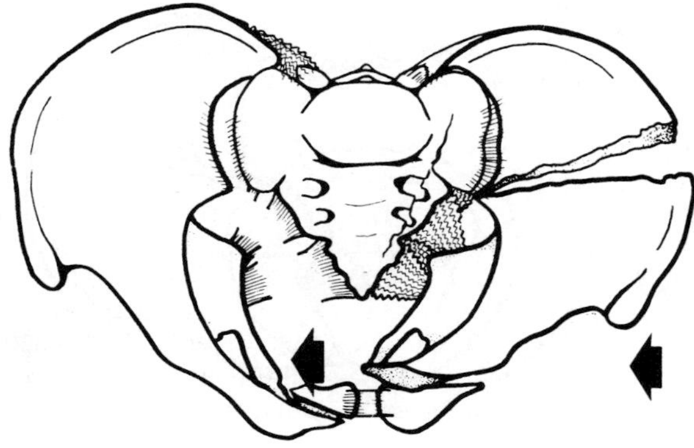

Fig. 181-13. Alternatively (compared to Fig. 181-12), as in type II B fractures (Fig. 181-11), there may be an iliac wing fracture, sparing the posterior SIJ on the ipsilateral side. (*Source:* From Young JWR, Burgess AR: *Radiologic Management of Pelvic Ring Fractures: Systematic Radiologic Diagnosis.* Baltimore, Urban & Schwarzenberg, 1987. Used by permission.)

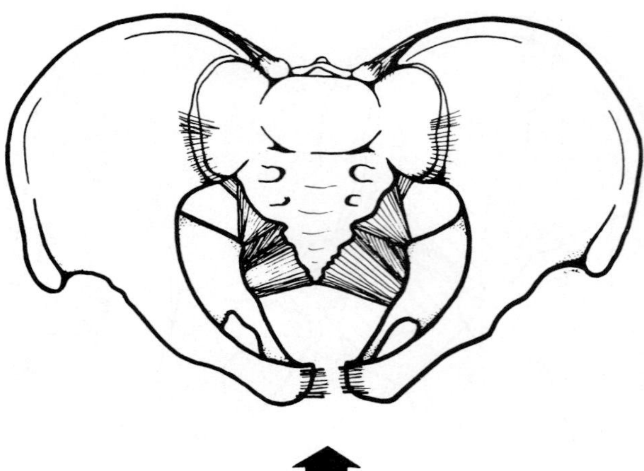

Fig. 181-14. Type I—AP compression fracture: The force is delivered in an AP direction (*large arrow*), tending to "open" the pelvis. This gives rise to mild splaying of the symphysis, due to rupture of the anterior sacroiliac ligaments. (*Source:* From Young JWR, Burgess AR: *Radiologic Management of Pelvic Ring Fractures: Systematic Radiologic Diagnosis.* Baltimore, Urban & Schwarzenberg, 1987. Used by permission.)

Urinary tract injuries. Urinary tract injuries are discussed in Chapter 177, "Trauma to the Genitourinary Tract."

Gynecologic injury. Gynecologic injuries are uncommonly associated with pelvic trauma. Vaginal laceration is the most common injury seen with anterior pelvic fractures. A bimanual pelvic examination should be performed on all women with pelvic fractures. If blood is found in a woman of childbearing age, a speculum examination must be carried out to distinguish menses from laceration. Treatment is irrigation and debridement in the operating room with repair of wounds and antibiotic therapy.

A high fetal death rate is associated with pelvic trauma in pregnancy if the mother is in shock; if there is placental, uterine, or direct fetal injury; or if the mother dies. Immediate cesarean section must be considered.

Rectal injuries. Rectal injuries are uncommon and are usually as-

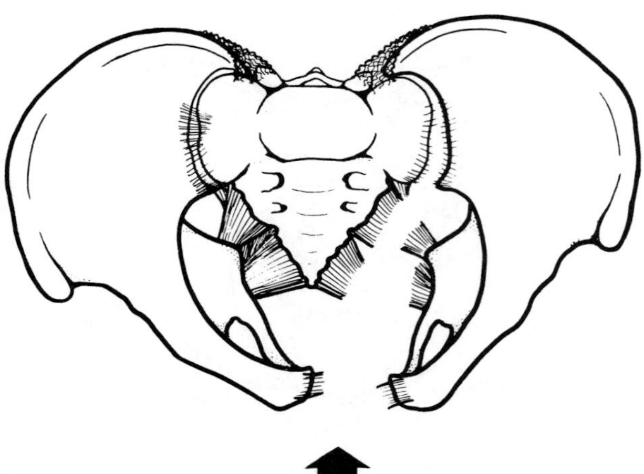

Fig. 181-15. Type II—AP compression fracture: The AP force vector (*large arrow*) has caused further "opening" of the anterior pelvis, with additional rupture of the anterior sacroiliac, sacrotuberous, and sacrospinous ligaments. (*Source:* From Young JWR, Burgess AR: *Radiologic Management of Pelvic Ring Fractures: Systematic Radiologic Diagnosis.* Baltimore, Urban & Schwarzenberg, 1987. Used by permission.)

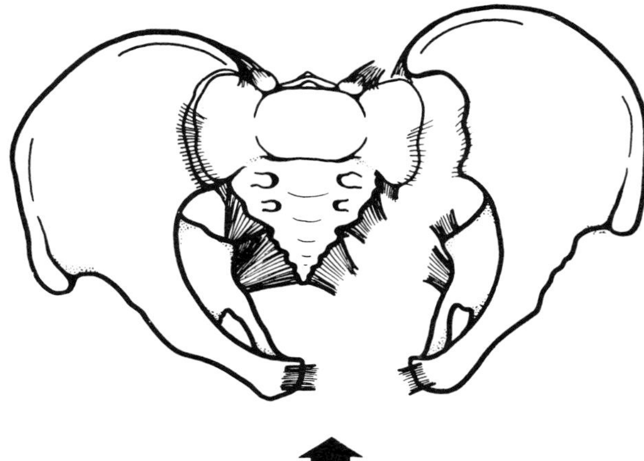

Fig. 181-16. Type III—AP compression fracture: There is total disruption of the SIJ due to wide "opening" of the pelvis. All supporting ligament groups, including the posterior sacroiliac ligaments, may be disrupted. (*Source:* From Young JWR, Burgess AR: *Radiologic Management of Pelvic Ring Fractures: Systematic Radiologic Diagnosis.* Baltimore, Urban & Schwarzenberg, 1987. Used by permission.)

sociated with urinary injuries and ischial fractures. Diagnosis is by rectal examination, whereupon blood is found in the rectum. Treatment includes a diverting colostomy with washout of the distal colon, and presacral space drainage. Antibiotics should be given as soon as the injury is discovered.

Ruptured diaphragm. Ruptured diaphragm associated with fracture of the pelvis may be more common than previously thought. It may be associated with rib injuries. Diagnosis is by physical findings, such as displacement of the heart toward the right, absent breath sounds, presence of bowel sounds in the chest, and a positive chest x-ray film if the defect is large. Diagnosis may be difficult if the defect is small.

Nerve root injury. Nerve root or peripheral nerve injuries can occur because of traction, pressure from hemorrhage, callus or fibrous tissue, and impingement-laceration by bone fragments. The onset of symptoms and signs may be delayed, but deficits usually follow a nerve root pattern. Lumbar nerve root injuries are associated with SI joint dislocation or fracture. Sacral root injuries are associated with sacral fractures, especially fractures of S1 and S2.

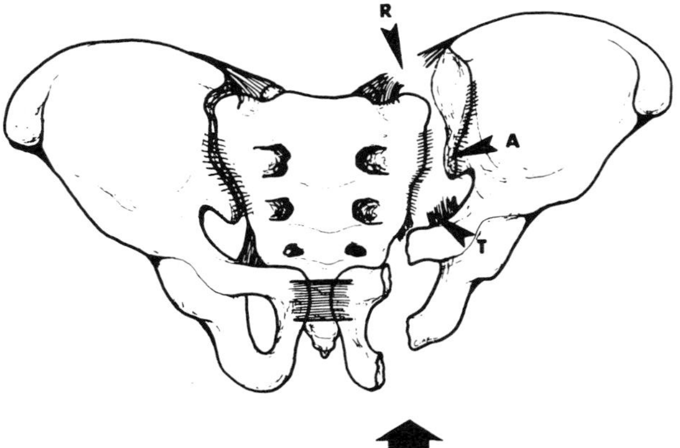

Fig. 181-17. Vertical shear vector: The injury force vector is delivered in a vertical plane (large arrow), causing disruption along this line. Fractures of the pubic rami are usually seen anteriorly, while fractures of the sacrum, SIJ, or iliac wing are usually seen posteriorly. The fractures are vertical and are associated with vertical displacement of fragments. Ligamentous injury to the posterior (*R*) and anterior (*A*) sacroiliac ligaments may be seen, as well to sacrospinous/sacrotuberous (*T*), and (possibly) symphysis ligaments. (*Source:* From Young JWR, Burgess AR: *Radiologic Management of Pelvic Ring Fractures: Systematic Radiologic Diagnosis.* Baltimore, Urban & Schwarzenberg, 1987. Used by permission.)

Table 181-2. Local Associated Injuries

	% OCCURRENCE		
	Severe Hemorrhage	**Bladder Rupture**	**Urethra**
Lateral compression fractures			
Type I	0.5	4.0	2.0
Type II	36.0	7.0	0.0
Type III	60.0	20.0	20.0
AP compression fractures			
Type I	1.0	8.0	12.0
Type II	28.0	11.0	23.0
Type III	53.0	14.0	36.0
Vertical shear fractures	75.0	15.0	25.0
Mixed patterns	58.0	16.0	21.0

Source: From Young JWR, Burgess AR: *Radiologic Management of Pelvic Ring Fractures: Systematic Radiologic Diagnosis.* Baltimore, Urban & Schwarzenberg, 1987. Used by permission.

Pelvic Fractures in Children

Commonly caused by auto-pedestrian accidents, pelvic fractures in children have a high incidence of concomitant injuries because of the smaller protection afforded by the developing pelvis and the significant trauma incurred. Hemorrhage determines mortality. Children in shock who respond poorly to fluid replacement have the highest mortality. Frequent concomitant injuries include head and neck injuries, intraabdominal injuries, and long bone fractures. The incidence of genitourinary injuries is similar to that of adults. Major thoracic injuries are rare but particularly dangerous because they are often overlooked.

Postponement of surgery until stabilization of circulation is recommended unless the patient is exsanguinating despite treatment. If the child does not respond to transfusions equal to the estimated total blood volume (TBV) (88 ml/kg × wt [kg] = TBV) within 1 h, suspect major vascular injury and operate. Both arterial and venous injuries are associated with significant SI joint injury.

TRAUMA TO THE HIP AND FEMUR

Anatomy

The hip is a ball-and-socket joint made up of the acetabulum and the femur (Fig. 181-18). The hip includes the acetabulum and the proximal femur 2 to 3 in. below the lesser trochanter. The functions of the hip are weight-bearing and movement. The fibrous capsule that surrounds the joint on all sides is exceedingly strong. It attaches around the acetabulum proximally and runs to the intertrochanteric line distally on the anterior surface. Posteriorly, it falls short of the intertrochanteric crest and inserts on the neck of the femur. It is weakest posteriorly.

The blood supply of the femoral head is derived from nutrient branches of the obturator, medial femoral circumflex, and superior and inferior gluteal arteries. These course beneath the reflection of the capsule on the neck of the femur, and also along the ligamentum teres. The capsular vessels are much more important than those of the ligamentum teres.

The Physical Examination

The examination of the hip begins with a detailed history and complete examination of the patient. The pelvis and hip are then carefully evaluated. The unclothed, erect patient is inspected for a list, injuries,

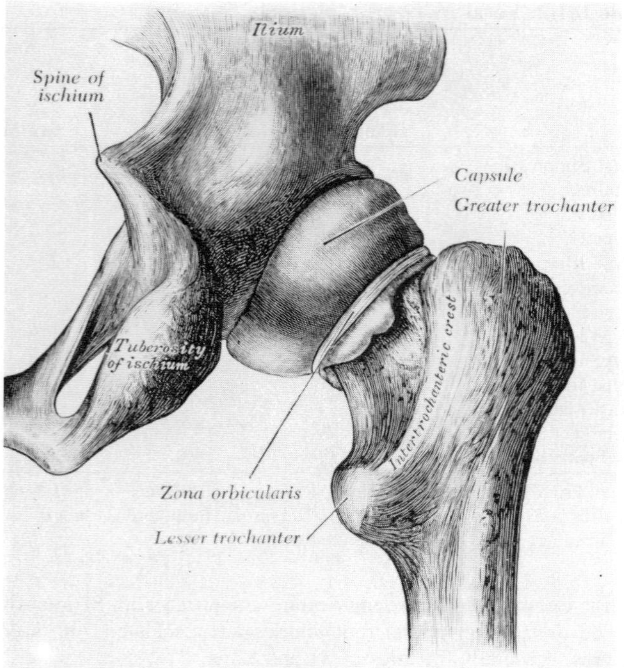

Fig. 181-18. Synovial membrane of capsule of hip joint (distended). Posterior aspect. [*From* Gray H: *Anatomy of the Human Body,* ed 29, Goss CM (ed). Philadelphia, Lea & Febiger, p 344. Used by permission.]

scars, or asymmetry of the muscles. Gait should be tested, if possible.

If the patient is a trauma victim, after primary survey and initial stabilization the physician should observe the position of the extremities, looking for deformities, lacerations, or bruises, and should test for stability and range of motion. On palpation, the physician should feel for irregularities in movement at the iliac crest, pubic rami, and ischial rami. He or she should compress the pelvis lateral to medial through the iliac crest; anterior to posterior through the symphysis pubis; and anterior to posterior through the iliac crest, seeking pain and tenderness. Also, the physician should compress the greater trochanters of the hips.

If no significant abnormalities are found, range of motion of the hips should then be studied. If rotation of the hip with the leg in extension is painful all other maneuvers should be done cautiously. If a hip or pelvic fracture or dislocation is identified in a trauma victim, the physician *must assume* that intraabdominal, retroperitoneal, and urologic injuries have occurred as well until it has been proved otherwise. The physician should always perform a detailed neurovascular examination and a rectal examination, looking for displacement of the prostate in male patients. Associated femoral shaft fractures should be ruled out.

X-Ray Evaluation

Roentgenographic evaluation of the pelvis and hips is a must in all unconscious patients who have sustained multiple injuries. Lower extremity long bone fractures, as well as pelvic symptoms or signs, are also indications for these x-ray examinations. The x-ray evaluation should include a standard AP and a lateral view of the pelvis. If further studies are needed, AP views of either hemipelvis, internal and external oblique views of the hemipelvis as described by Judet et al., or "inlet" and "tilt" views may be done. In certain instances, such views allow better identification and detail of the acetabulum and femoral head and neck. The physician must always inspect not only the hip joint but the femur and knee as well when evaluating hip disorders on x-ray films. Disorders to the knee and the femoral shaft often occur with hip injuries.

Classification of Hip Fractures

Hip fractures are classified as femoral head and neck, trochanteric, intertrochanteric, and subtrochanteric. The prognosis for successful union and restoration of normal function varies considerably with the fracture.

In intracapsular fractures with displacement, the femoral neck vessels are compromised due to a tear or compression secondary to an intracapsular hemarthrosis. The blood supply through the ligamentum teres may not be sufficient to nourish the entire femoral head. Therefore, aseptic necrosis inevitably results unless some of the capsular vessels remain intact. Basilar neck and intertrochanteric fractures below the capsule rarely sever important arteries.

Femoral Head Fractures

Isolated femoral head fractures occur infrequently. They are usually associated with dislocations of the hip. Shear fractures of the superior aspect of the femoral head are associated with anterior dislocations, and shear fractures of the inferior femoral head are associated with posterior dislocations.

In most instances, the symptoms and signs are those of the associated dislocation rather than of the fracture itself. The standard AP and lateral x-ray views usually demonstrate the fragment adequately. When there is an associated dislocation, the postreduction films offer a better view of the fracture fragment.

Treatment by the orthopedic consultant is to reduce the associated dislocation and then attain anatomic reduction of the fracture fragment. Complications are associated with the high-energy trauma which produces the fracture-dislocation, i.e., the more comminuted the fracture, the more severe the dislocation and the greater the severity of trauma to the patient. Life-threatening injuries must then be ruled out.

Femoral Neck Fractures

Femoral neck fractures are commonly seen among older adults, occurring more frequently in women than in men. These fractures are rare among the younger population. The cause of such fractures is usually minor trauma or torsion in the patient with osteoporosis or osteomalacia. In younger patients, the high kinetic energy sustained in the major trauma causes a fracture through normal bone with marked soft tissue disruption and comminution.

The classification of femoral neck fractures is by fragment displacement. The symptoms seen with femoral neck fractures range from complaints of mild pain in the groin or inner thigh in patients with an incomplete fracture to moderate to severe pain in patients with displaced fractures.

Patients who have sustained a fracture without displacement may walk with some limping rather than being unable to bear weight. Their only physical findings are minor pain with movement and minimal muscle spasm limiting range of motion. In contrast, displaced fractures cause severe pain, inability to ambulate, limited range of motion, and no palpable movement of the extracapsular head. The patient lies with the extremity in *slight* external rotation, abduction, and shortening.

X-ray evaluation is essential in any patient suspected of having a femoral neck fracture. Stress fractures, however, may not show up on x-ray for days or weeks, so repeat films in symptomatic patients are done approximately 2 weeks later. The standard AP view should have the patient maximally internally rotated to best demonstrate the femoral neck. The AP view should be inspected for a fracture line starting on the superior surface of the neck. These fracture lines routinely become complete within 10 to 14 days. Also, disruption of Shenton's line may be appreciated on the AP view in some instances. If there is any concern that the patient has sustained a fracture which is not visible on the initial x-ray examination, the patient should be conservatively treated and x-ray films should be made again in 10 to 14 days; or the physician may order a bone scan, which demonstrates the fracture in most instances.

In contrast, displaced fractures are obvious on the AP film, but a lateral view should also be done to ascertain the exact position. The orthopedic surgeon's goal of treatment for femoral neck fractures is anatomic reduction and stability. Treatment for nondisplaced or impacted fractures is somewhat controversial but usually involves a form of internal fixation. Displaced fractures definitely require emergency surgery for fixation, Prosthetic replacements may be required in certain instances. Special note should be made of stress fractures as some are treated in a conservative manner and others are treated with internal fixation, depending upon the type of fracture and the patient's cooperation.

The complications of femoral neck fractures are significant. They include infections, emboli, and avascular necrosis, which is the most feared early complication. Avascular necrosis has an incidence of approximately 15 to 35 percent, with the higher incidence associated with more severe fractures or fractures which are not surgically reduced to anatomic position within 48 h. Nonunion, which occurs in approximately 5 to 15 percent of patients who have been treated properly, is a later complication of such fractures.

Trochanteric Fractures

Greater trochanteric fractures are usually due to avulsions at the insertion of the gluteus medius. In the younger population (7 to 17 years of age), this is a true epiphyseal separation, in contrast to the adult population, in which this is an avulsion fracture with comminution in some instances. The patient presents with pain, especially with abduction and extension, and a limp. Also, there is tenderness to palpation over the greater trochanter.

Standard AP and lateral x-ray views reveal displacement in the superior-posterior area, or comminution. The treatment is controversial but ranges from conservative to surgical fixation, depending on the patient's age and displacement of the fracture. Orthopedic consultation is indicated.

Lesser trochanteric fractures due to an avulsion of the iliopsoas, are commonly seen in children and young athletic adults. These patients present with pain during flexion and internal rotation maneuvers. In most instances, the treatment is bed rest and then gradual weight-bearing to regain full activity.

If greater than 2-cm displacement is seen on the standard AP and lateral views, then screw fixation by the consulting orthopedic surgeon may be indicated.

Intertrochanteric Fractures

These fractures are defined as extracapsular fractures occurring in a line between the greater and lesser trochanters. Intertrochanteric fractures generally occur in the elderly and are more common in women, again due to the high incidence of osteoporosis. The mechanism of injury is usually a fall or occasionally an automobile accident. It is postulated that a rotational component along with the direct trauma is involved in some instances as well.

Symptoms and signs include pain, swelling of the hip, local ecchymosis, and pain with any hip movement or weight-bearing. Moreover, the extremity is markedly externally rotated and shortened, in contrast to the minimal deformities associated with femoral neck fractures. These fractures are classified as stable or unstable. Stable fractures are defined as ones in which the medial cortices of the neck and femoral fragments abut. X-ray evaluation should include AP and lateral views, with the AP view having as much internal rotation as possible to adequately visualize the neck.

The traction splint should be taken off to obtain the best-quality AP view, i.e., the most internal rotation. Severe, life-threatening injuries must be excluded. The consulting orthopedic physician can then admit the patient to the hospital and perform surgical fixation to attain a stable reduction as soon as possible, although this is not an emergency.

The complications and prognosis are related to other associated injuries and prior disease. The overall mortality is approximately 10 to 15 percent. Infection is still a major problem, with an incidence of up to 17 percent. Thromboembolic disease is especially a problem if postoperative mobilization does not occur quickly. Avascular necrosis is rare in these patients, and nonunion is also uncommon. Morbidity is due to the patient's inability to return to prefracture activity.

Subtrochanteric Fractures

Subtrochanteric fractures may be seen in two different populations. They usually occur secondary to falling in the 40- to 60-year old patient with osteoporotic or weakened bone. The second population is young persons who have suffered major trauma with significant kinetic energies directed into the femur. These fractures may be an extension of an intertrochanteric or other isolated fracture and are usually classified as stable or unstable, with stable defined as bony contact of the medial and posterior femoral cortices.

The symptoms and signs are similar to those of trochanteric or femoral fractures, with local pain, deformity, swelling, crepitance, etc. These patients can lose a large amount of blood into the thigh area and may present in hypovolemic shock. Because this injury is due to significant trauma, other, more life-threatening injuries must be excluded prior to treatment of this specific fracture.

Standard AP and lateral x-ray views of the hip are necessary to properly assess the fracture. Moreover, x-ray studies of the pelvis, femur, and knee are indicated to rule out associated fractures.

Treatment consists of immobilization with a traction apparatus and proper evaluation of the entire patient to rule out associated severe injuries. After the patient has stabilized and secondary evaluation has occurred, the orthopedic consultant should determine if this failure is amenable to internal fixation.

The complications are similar to those of intertrochanteric fractures, except that there is a higher incidence of nonunion. Malunion and delayed union occur as well in this population.

Hip Dislocations

Hip dislocations can be classified as anterior, posterior, and central. Acetabular fracture with central hip dislocation has been discussed under type IV pelvic fractures.

Anterior Dislocations

About 10 percent of hip dislocations are anterior, and the majority are secondary to automobile accidents, but they may also result from a fall, or a blow to the back while squatting. The mechanism of injury is forced abduction that causes the femoral head to be levered out through an anterior capsular tear. The affected extremity is in abduction and external rotation. Neurovascular compromise is an unusual, but possible, complication.

An AP film of the pelvis easily demonstrates the femoral head to be inferior and medial to the acetabulum. A lateral view illustrates the anterior dislocation more clearly, although it may be difficult to obtain because of the patient's pain.

Treatment for the dislocation is early closed reduction, usually under general anesthesia. Strong, in-line traction is done while flexion and internal rotation are carried out. Finally, the hip is abducted once the head clears the rim of the acetabulum. The dislocation should be reduced quickly, within a few hours, because the longer the delay in reduction, the higher the incidence of aseptic necrosis.

Posterior Dislocations

Posterior dislocations constitute 80 to 90 percent of hip dislocations. They are caused by force applied to a flexed knee, directed posteriorly.

Acetabular fractures may result as well. On examination, the extremity is found to be shortened, internally rotated, and adducted. Concomitant life-threatening injuries must be ruled out.

Anteroposterior and lateral x-ray films of the pelvis and hip will reveal the dislocation, but further assessment of the acetabulum and femur must be done to rule out fractures. The oblique views of Judet et al. will reveal an acetabular fracture. Also, inferior femoral head fracture will be seen on the AP or oblique view. Hip dislocations are difficult to recognize with femoral shaft fractures, so roentgenograms of the pelvis and hips should be routinely obtained in such cases.

The treatment of posterior dislocation without fracture is closed reduction, preferably under general anesthesia, as quickly as possible and always within 48 h. In-line traction, gentle flexion to 90°, and then gentle internal-to-external rotation is done (Allis maneuver). The Stimson maneuver may prove useful in certain situations.

Complications include sciatic nerve injury in about 10 percent of the patients, and avascular necrosis that increases in direct proportion to the delay in adequate reduction.

Hip Injuries in Children

Fractures and Dislocations

Fractures of the proximal end of the femur are extremely rare in children. Trauma may produce a displaced epiphysis or a fracture of the neck, trochanteric, or subtrochanteric region. Traumatic epiphyseal separation is probably less common than the previously mentioned fractures, but is more common than dislocation. The treatment is anatomic reduction, usually best obtained by surgery. There is a significant complication rate, especially with improper treatment.

Traumatic dislocations in children are rare. They are more common in boys (4:1) and more common between ages 4 and 7, and 11 and 15. The frequency of left versus right is equal, and bilateral dislocations are reportable. Posterior dislocations occur with an 80 to 85 percent frequency. The mechanism of injury and the clinical picture are similar to those seen in traumatic dislocation in the adult. The presence of an associated fracture is rare.

The treatment is closed reduction. Dislocation is an orthopedic emergency, and reductions should be done within 12 h. Delay in reduction past 24 h is associated with a much higher incidence of complications.

Pediatric Disorders of the Hip/Child with a Limp

The differential diagnosis of pediatric disorders of the hip is presented by age. These entities make up the bulk of problems that must be entertained when a toddler or older child or adolescent presents with a limp. (See Ch. 183, "Leg Injuries," for discussion of toddler's fracture—one of the more common causes of limp in a toddler.)

Congenital Hip Dislocations

Roughly 70 percent of congenital hip dislocations occur in the first baby of the family. The incidence is approximately one in every 1000 live births, and it is six times more common in females than in males. Diagnosis is made by examination consisting of the Ortolani and Barlow tests. X-ray studies are not useful in newborns because there is no visible bone to ascertain femoral head position.

The Ortolani test is done to determine if the hip is subluxed or dislocated. Each thigh is grasped with the thumbs over the medial aspect and the middle fingers over the greater trochanter. The thighs are then lifted and abducted. If reduction of the femoral head takes place, a palpable or audible click may be appreciated.

The Barlow exam assesses hip instability by producing dislocation or subluxation of the hip. Each thigh is grasped with the thumbs over the medial aspect and the fingers over the greater trochanter. With the hip and knees flexed to 90 degrees, the thighs are adducted while gentle downward pressure is applied. The femoral head will slip out of the acetabulum if instability is present.

Orthopedic consultation is indicated for any child with suspected subluxation-dislocation of the hip. The complications of missed congenital hip dislocation are poor hip development and occasionally avascular necrosis.

Septic Arthritis

The majority of cases of septic arthritis occur in children under the age of four. It is the most common etiology of a painful hip joint in infants. As a result, any child with a possible hip problem should be assumed to have septic arthritis until proven otherwise. Hematogenous seeding is the most common mode of infection. In older children, local extension from osteomyelitis can occur as well as inadvertent direct needle innoculation when obtaining arterial blood gases. Staphylococcus is the most common organism after infancy. *Staph. epidermidis* and streptococcus species are the next most frequent. *Haemophilus influenzae* is common during the first two years of life and Group B streptococcus during infancy.

Toddlers and older children with septic arthritis generally present with a limp or refusal to ambulate. Infants demonstrate signs and symptoms of infective disorders in general. This includes irritability, fever, and loss of appetite. There can be a delay in the diagnosis in neonates and young infants because of the nonspecific presentation in this age group. Consequently, careful examination of the joints should be performed on all neonates and young infants who are febrile or have evidence of infection elsewhere.

On exam, there is decreased hip range of motion due to pain. The hip typically is held in a flexed, abducted and externally rotated position because this allows for the greatest volume in the swollen hip joint. Laboratory usually shows an increased white blood cell count and increased sedimentation rate. Blood cultures are positive in 50 percent of cases. Definitive diagnosis is confirmed by needle aspiration, which should be done by an orthopedic consultant under fluoroscopic guidance. Differential diagnosis includes transient synovitis. Treatment of septic arthritis includes hospitalization, appropriate intravenous antibiotic therapy, and surgical drainage.

Transient Synovitis

Transient synovitis is probably the most common cause for a painful hip in children. It is most prevalent in males with a peak incidence of five to six years and range of 18 months to 12 years. It is usually unilateral, but can be bilateral. The cause is unknown.

The history of onset may be abrupt, but is more typically gradual. Medical attention is usually sought because of a limp or inability to bear weight. Approximately 50 percent of patients will have a history of minor trauma or antecedent or intercurrent illness. ESR and WBC count are usually normal but may be elevated. As a result, they do not discriminate transient synovitis from septic hip, osteomyelitis or other infectious etiology. Because transient synovitis is a diagnosis of exclusion, orthopedic consultation, hip aspiration, and admission to the hospital are recommended. Transient synovitis is self limiting, usually lasting only 3 to 4 days. Bed rest only is necessary as treatment.

Legg-Calvé-Perthes Disease

This uncommon disease is most often found in males aged 5 to 9. It is an idiopathic avascular necrosis of the femoral head. The onset is insidious, and limp is the most common early sign of disease. Exam reveals decreased hip range of motion and spasm. Laboratory examination is usually normal. Typical x-ray changes consist of necrosis, reabsorption, and regeneration but may take years to develop. X-rays early on may be normal but bone scan is usually positive. Definitive treatment of Legg-Calvé-Perthes disease should be handled by an orthopedic surgeon.

Slipped Capital Femoral Epiphysis

This entity occurs most commonly in adolescents and preadolescents between the ages of 10 and 16 years. It occurs bilaterally in 20 to 40 percent of cases and is five times more common in males. The etiology is unknown. The condition appears to occur more commonly with certain body types, specifically patients with Frohlich's type of obesity with underdeveloped genitalia and in long, slender, rapidly growing adolescents.

With this condition, the onset of symptoms is generally insidious, though sudden development of them can occur. Early symptoms consist of groin discomfort after activity. With progression, hip stiffness and limp may develop. Pain, as with any primary hip complaint, may be referred to the knee.

Radiographic exam including anteroposterior and lateral views of the hip is necessary to make the diagnosis. Initial films may be normal, prompting the need for repeat exam if symptoms persist. A slip of the epiphyseal plate posteriorly is best seen on the lateral view. Emergency Department treatment consists of making the patient non-weight bearing and consulting orthopedics. Definitive therapy utilizes traction and surgical fixation.

Open Hip Injuries

Open wounds to the hip joint should be treated like any other open joint. An initial culture should be done and the wound cleaned by debridement and copious irrigation in the operating room. Primary wound care with secondary closure is suggested by most authorities. Tetanus prophylaxis is ensured by the administration of toxoid and immune globulin if indicated. Prophylactic antibiotics are recommended. Continuous irrigation of the hip may be indicated.

Bursitis

Approximately 18 bursa surround the hip joint. These are derived developmentally from and are physiologically similar to synovium and tendon sheaths. As a result, they suffer from the same inflammatory afflictions which cause problems to the joint itself. Conditions which affect the bursa include traumatic inflammation, which is usually secondary to overuse or excessive pressure; infections; metabolic disorders such as gout; and benign and malignant growths.

Treatment consists of rest, ice, anti-inflammatory medications orally, and occasionally intrabursal injections. Ultrasound physical therapy may help as well. The prognosis for such patients is good as long as associated problems such as infection and low-back disk disease are ruled out. Mechanical problems, especially leg length discrepancies, must be sought and, if found, properly treated so that further trochanteric bursitis does not occur.

Femoral Shaft Fractures

Fractures of the shaft of the femur most often occur in men during their most active period in life. Falls, and industrial and automobile accidents account for the majority of these fractures.

Severe, direct trauma may result in transverse fractures with displacement; oblique or spiral oblique fractures; or badly comminuted segments.

The femur is surrounded by large muscle groups with a rich vascular supply (Fig. 181-19). Therefore, femoral fractures may result in the loss of 1 L or more of blood into the soft tissues of the thigh, producing clinical shock. The initial evaluation should always include careful neurovascular examination of the extremity.

It is best to splint the leg with a traction splint at the time of injury. Hare traction or a Thomas splint can be placed over the trousers, applying traction to a sling around the ankle and forefoot.

In infants and children up to 3 or 4 years of age, fractures of the shaft of the femur are treated by direct overhead traction applied to both legs.

In an older child or adult, the Fisk type of traction by means of a half Thomas ring and Pearson attachment, to allow for flexion of the knee, is satisfactory.

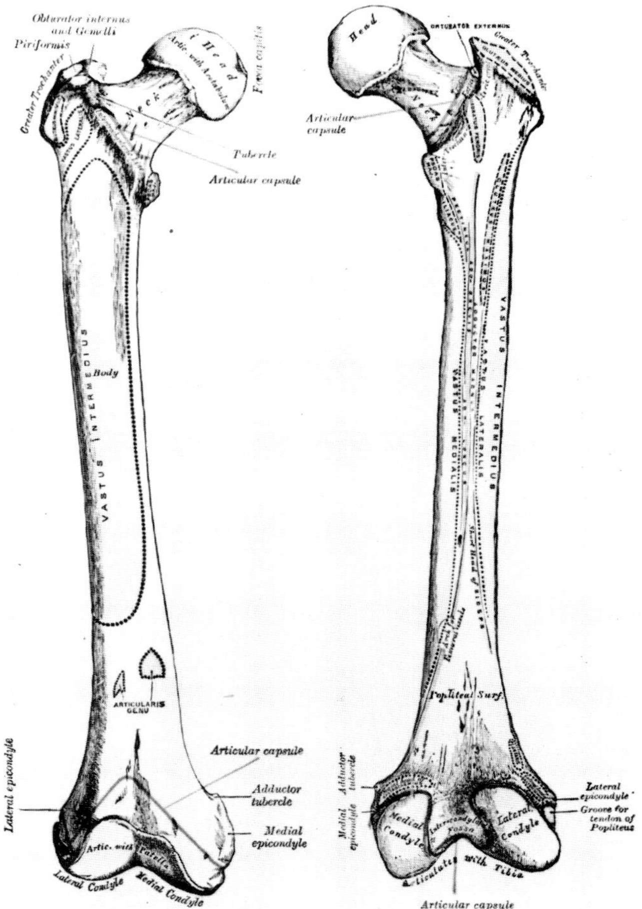

Fig. 181-19. Anterior and posterior surfaces of right femur. [*From* Gray H: *Anatomy of the Human Body,* ed 29, Goss CM (ed). Philadelphia, Lea & Febiger, p 241. Used by permission.]

The intramedullary rod is frequently the method of choice for the treatment of uncomplicated fractures of the midshaft and junction of the upper and middle thirds of the femur, except where comminution is so extensive that stability with the rod cannot be maintained.

In cases where comminution is severe, either dual plating or the use of a compression plate device can result in excellent fixation.

BIBLIOGRAPHY

Trauma to the Pelvis

Antrum RM, Solowkin JS: A review of antibiotic prophylaxis for open fractures. *Orthop Rev* 16:246, 1987.

Brooks DH, Grenvik A: G-suit control of massive retroperitoneal hemorrhage due to pelvic fracture. *Crit Care Med* 1:257, 1973.

Canale ST: Fracture of the pelvis, in Rockwood CA Jr, Wilkins KE, King RE (eds): *Fractures in Children.* Philadelphia, Lippincott, 1984, vol 3, pp 733–782.

Epstein HC: Traumatic dislocations of the hip. *Clin Orthop* 92:116, 1973.

Froman C, Stein A: Complicated crushing injuries of the pelvis. *J Bone Joint Surg* 49B:24, 1976.

Goodell CL: Neurologic deficits associated with pelvic fractures. *J Neurosurg* 24:837, 1966.

Gustilo RB, Merkow RL, Templeman D: The management of open fractures. *J Bone Joint Surg* 72:299, 1990.

Harris WR: Avulsion of lumbar roots complicating fractures of the pelvis. *J Bone Joint Surg* 55A:1436, 1973.

Hauser CW, Perry JF Jr: Massive hemorrhage from pelvic fractures. *Minn Med* 49:285, 1966.

Hawkins L, Pomerantz M, Eiseman B: Laparotomy at time of pelvic fracture. *J Trauma* 10:619, 1970.

Kane WJ: Fractures of the pelvis, in Rockwood CA Jr, Green DP (eds): *Fractures in Adults,* ed 2. Philadelphia, Lippincott 1984, vol 2, pp 1093–1211.

McAvoy JM, Cook JH: A treatment plan for rapid assessment of the patient with massive blood loss and pelvic fractures. *Arch Surg* 113:986, 1978.

Patterson EP, Morton KS: The cause of death in fractures of the pelvis. *J Trauma* 13:849, 1973.

Rothenberger DA, Velasco R, Strate R, et al: Open pelvic fracture: A lethal injury. *J Trauma* 18:184, 1978.

Rothenberger D, Quattlebaum FW, Perry JF Jr, et al: Blunt maternal trauma: A review of 103 cases. *J Trauma* 18:173, 1978.

Trauma to the Hip and Femur

Canage ST, King RE: Fractures of the hip, in Rockwood CA Jr, Wilkins KE, King RE: *Fractures in Children.* Philadelphia, Lippincott, 1984, vol 3, pp 782–845.

DeLee JC: Fractures and dislocations of the hip, in Rockwood CA Jr, Green DP (eds): *Fractures in Adults,* ed 2. Philadelphia, Lippincott, 1984, vol 2, pp. 1211–1357.

Hodges DL, McGuire TJ: Hip pain in children: an anatomic approach. *Orthop Rev* 17:251, 1988.

Hughes RA, Tempos K, Ansell BM: A review of the diagnoses of hip pain presentation in the adolescent. *Br J Rheumatol* 27:450, 1988.

Simon RR, Koenigsknecht SJ: *Orthopaedics in Emergency Medicine: The Extremities,* 2d ed. New York, Appleton-Century-Crofts, 1989.

182
KNEE INJURIES

Joseph F. Waeckerle

Injuries to the knee are becoming increasingly more common in our sports-oriented society. The emergency physician must become familiar with the examination of the normal and abnormal knee to be able to recognize specific injuries and to treat and appropriately refer these injuries. This chapter will deal with examination of the knee and with recognition of fractures and dislocations of the patella; fractures of femoral condyles; fractures of the tibial spines, tuberosity, and plateaus; ligamentous and meniscal injuries of the knee joint; knee dislocation; and osteochondritis dissecans.

As with all orthopedic injuries, the accurate diagnosis of the injured knee is required before proper treatment can be instituted. However, it is particularly important to do a complete and careful examination in a stepwise manner since the knee is essential for ambulation. Radiologic evaluation is a necessary part of the examination. The first examination is usually the easiest to perform, since the patient does not anticipate pain and therefore does not guard, and involuntary muscular spasm causing futher guarding may not yet have occurred.

EXAMINATION

The examination of the knee is divided into five phases: history, observation, inspection, palpation, and stress testing.

History

The mechanism of injury as well as any prior serious problems frequently clarifies subtleties in the examination, allowing a more accurate diagnosis and appropriate treatment.

Observation

The patient should be examined while walking, if possible, and in both the sitting and lying positions. The physician should take note of the gait, muscular development, and functional range of motion at this time.

Inspection

The knee should be inspected for swelling, ecchymoses, effusion, masses, patella location and size, muscle mass, erythema, and evidence of local trauma. Also, the physician should note at this time, with the patient in a supine position, leg lengths (equal or unequal). Lastly, the physician should ask the patient to perform the best possible active range of motion.

Palpation

Initially the neurovascular status of the leg should be noted. As with all orthopedic examinations, the noninjured or normal knee should be compared with the injured knee during all aspects of the examination but especially during palpation and stress testing. When the physician palpates the knee, he or she should begin in the nontender areas and work lastly toward the tender area so that the patient does not guard or become apprehensive. The examiner should always palpate the knee joint in a systematic manner. Effusion, tenderness, increased temperature, strength, sensation, and location of pulses should be noted.

The physician should examine the patella for size, shape, and location with the knee in flexion, while mobility should be checked with the knee in extension. The patella should be compressed to check for pain as well as moved laterally and medially to ascertain possible subluxation. The popliteal space should also be palpated for masses, swelling, and circulation status.

Stress Testing

The final phase of the examination of the knee is stress testing. This is the most difficult aspect of the examination although potentially the most informative. The patient must be reassured and relaxed and made as comfortable as possible. This may require allowing the leg to hang over the side of the bed with the bed supporting the posterior thigh rather than the physician holding the leg, as is usually done during stress testing. The first examination is often the most valid, especially if performed soon after the injury. The patient will not expect to experience any pain during this first examination, nor do the inflammation and effusion associated with an acute traumatic injury cause voluntary or involuntary guarding. The uninjured, hopefully normal, opposite knee should be examined first to determine the patient's normal laxity. A brief summary of the instabilities and tests to demonstrate them are presented in the section on ligamentous and meniscal injuries.

FRACTURES

Fractures of the Patella

Fractures of the patella occur from a direct blow, a fall on the flexed knee, or forceful contraction of the quadriceps muscles. Fractures may be transverse, comminuted, or of the avulsion type (when the quadriceps muscle pulls off a small portion of the patella; Fig. 182-1). Any fracture may be open or closed. A nondisplaced transverse fracture of the patella should be treated with immobilization for 6 weeks. During this time the patient should be encouraged to walk on crutches, with partial weight bearing progressing to full weight bearing as tolerated.

If the transverse fracture is nondisplaced, a cylinder cast may be sufficient, assuming adequate reduction occurs. However, this usually requires open reduction and wire fixation. If the fragments are widely separated, most often there is associated knee joint injury.

Comminuted fractures must be treated surgically by removal of smaller fragments (or all fragments if they are small) and suturing of the quadriceps tendon and patellar ligaments.

All open fractures must be debrided and irrigated.

Fractures of Femoral Condyles

Fractures of the femoral condyles include supracondylar, intercondylar, condylar, and distal femoral epiphyseal fractures (Fig. 182-2). Most often, these injuries are secondary to direct trauma from a fall or blow to the distal femur. Examination reveals pain, swelling, deformity, rotation, and shortening. Although neurovascular injuries are uncommon, the status of distal sensation and pulses must be checked. The space between the first and second toe, innervated by the deep peroneal nerve, should be tested for sensation. In addition, a search for ipsilateral hip dislocation or fractures, and damage to the quadriceps apparatus, must be made. Depending on the type of fracture, closed or open reduction, skeletal traction, and cast immobilization may be necessary. Therefore, orthopedic consultation in essential.

Fractures of the Tibial Spines and Tuberosity

Although isolated injuries of the tibial spine are uncommon, they usually result in damage to the cruciate ligaments. The injury is most often caused by a force directed against the flexed proximal tibia in an anterior or posterior direction, resulting in incomplete avulsion of the tibial spine, with or without displacement, or complete fracture of the spine. Examination shows a painful, swollen knee, secondary to hemarthrosis, inability to extend fully, and a positive Lachman's sign. If the fracture is incomplete or nondisplaced, closed reduction

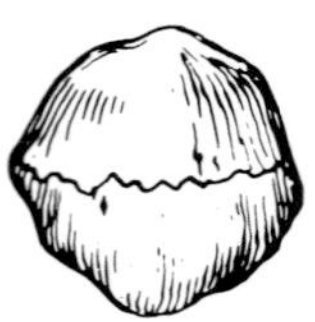

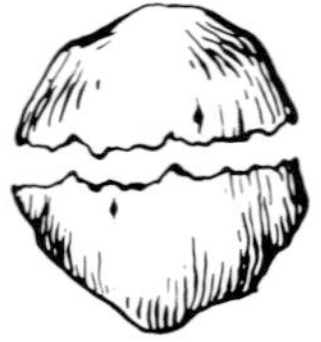

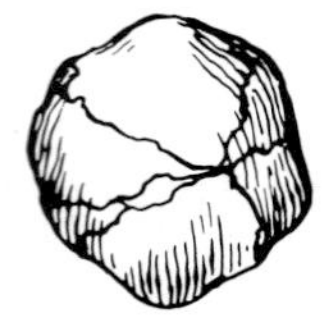

Fig. 182-1. Types of patellar fractures. [From Hohl M, Larson RL: Fractures and dislocations of the knee, in Rockwood CA Jr, Green DP (eds): *Fractures*. Philadelphia, Lippincott, 1975, vol 2, p 1149. Used by permission.]

by an orthopedic surgeon may be attempted. Complete, displaced fractures often need open reduction.

The quadriceps mechanism inserts on the tibial tubercle. A sudden force to the flexed knee with the quadriceps muscle contracted may result in a complete or incomplete avulsion of the tibial tubercle. The fracture line may extend into the joint. Examination reveals pain and tenderness over the proximal anterior tibia with pain on passive or active extension. If the avulsion is small or nondisplaced, the fragment may be maintained in position by immobilization; otherwise, open reduction and internal fixation are necessary.

Fractures of the Tibial Plateaus

Fractures of the tibial plateaus are seen more commonly in the older population and can be very difficult to detect. They are produced by direct force which drives the femoral condyles into the articulating surface of the tibia. Both medial and lateral plateaus may be fractured simultaneously, although the lateral plateau is more often fractured. Direct trauma to the lateral aspect of the knee may account for the preponderance of lateral tibial plateau fractures. The patient presents with painful swelling of the knee and limitation of motion. Radiographs may demonstrate a fracture but often only show a lipohemarthrosis on the lateral view. Careful review of the x-rays is essential. Ligamentous instability may also be demonstrated. If one or both plateaus are fractured but not displaced, treatment in a long leg plaster cast, without weight bearing, should be adequate. Depression of the articular surface necessitates open reduction and elevation of the bony fragment.

RECOGNITION AND MANAGEMENT OF LIGAMENTOUS AND MENISCAL INJURIES

The knee joint depends on ligaments and muscles for support (Fig. 182-3). It is frequently subjected to injuries from traumatic forces while extended or in various stages of flexion. These traumatic forces include abduction, flexion, and internal rotation of the femur on the tibia; adduction, flexion, and external rotation of the femur on the tibia; hyperextension; and anteroposterior displacement. By far the most common are abduction, flexion, and internal rotation of the femur on the tibia, which produce injuries to the medial side of the knee. Injuries to the lateral side of the knee are produced by adduction, flexion, and external rotation. Such forces may result in a strain or rupture of the medial or lateral collateral ligaments, the anterior or posterior cruciate ligaments, the capsular structures, or a tear in the medial or lateral menisci, singularly or in combination. Functional instability of the knee is determined by stress testing, which will demonstrate abnormal laxity when properly done.

Initial stress testing is an abduction or valgus deformity applied to the knee, which is in approximately 30° of flexion, to determine the integrity of the medial joint structures. The medial collateral ligament supplies the majority of restraint to valgus deformities of the knee in all stages of flexion. A varus or adduction force is then applied to the lateral aspect of the knee, again with approximately 30° of flexion, to ascertain the integrity of the lateral structures. The lateral collateral ligament, similar to the medial collateral ligament, is the major restraint to varus laxity on the knee at all positions of flexion. If there is a demonstrated laxity of greater than 1 cm without a firm endpoint as compared to the other knee, there is a complete rupture of the medial or lateral collateral ligament. If there is laxity with a firm endpoint or a laxity of less than 1 cm, an incomplete or partial tear is present. If there is no demonstrated instability but there is pain, the patient has suffered a strain in the ligamentous structures tested. The patient who is unstable with the varus or valgus test performed with 30° of flexion

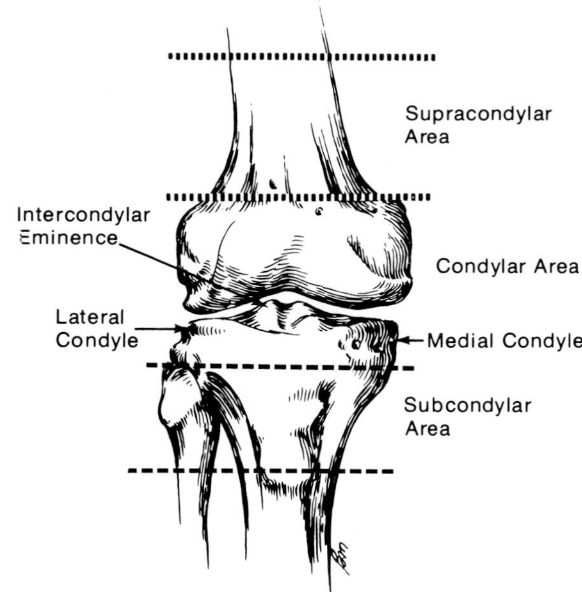

Fig. 182-2. The supracondylar and condylar areas of the femur, and the medial and subcondylar areas of the tibia. [Modified from Hohl M, Larson RL: Fractures and dislocations of the knee, in Rockwood CA Jr, Green DP (eds): *Fractures*. Philadelphia, Lippincott, 1975, vol 2, pp 1132, 1147. Used by permission.]

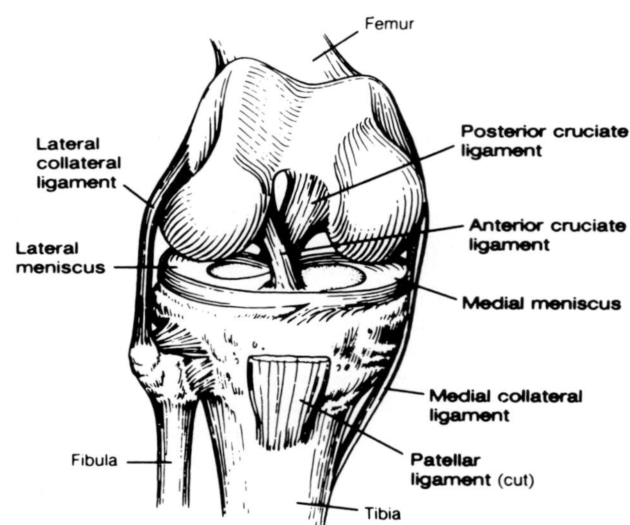

Fig. 182-3. Ligaments of the right knee joint. The articular capsule and the patella have been removed. (From Spencer AP, Mason EB: *Human Anatomy and Physiology*. Menlo Park, Benjamin/Cummings, 1979, p 174. Used by permission.)

should be brought into full extension, if possible, and similar maneuvers carried out. Medial instability in full extension indicates a severe lesion involving the cruciate ligaments and posterior capsule along with the medial ligaments. Lateral instability in extension likewise indicates a severe injury that may involve the posterolateral corner of the knee as well as the cruciate ligaments. Peroneal nerve injuries may also occur in lateral injuries.

Injury to the anterior cruciate ligament may be the most common ligamentous injury today. The mechanism of injury is usually noncontact; a deceleration, hyperextension, or marked internal rotation of the tibia on the femur results in an injury to the cruciate. There may be an associated medial meniscal tear as well. Such a mechanism of injury combined with the presence of a traumatic effusion is very suggestive of a disruption of the anterior cruciate ligament.

The diagnosis of the anterior cruciate ligament injury is ascertained by utilizing the Lachman test, the anterior drawer sign, and the pivot shift. While the anterior drawer sign has been used for a long time, it is not very sensitive. The maneuver is done with 45° flexion at the hip and 90° flexion at the knee. The physician then attempts to forwardly displace the tibia from the femur. A displacement of greater than 6 mm as compared to the normal, opposite knee indicates that there has been an injury to the anterior cruciate ligament. There are false negatives associated with this maneuver. The Lachman test, which is currently more popular, is a much more sensitive test. The examiner places the knee in 20° of flexion by resting it on a pillow and stabilizes the femur above the knee with his or her nondominant hand. The dominant hand is placed behind the leg at the level of the tibial tubercle, and the examiner introduces an anterior force, attempting to displace the tibia forward. If a displacement of greater than 5 mm as compared to the opposite knee occurs or if there is a soft, mushy end point, then a tear in the anterior cruciate ligament has occurred. While this examination is more sensitive than the anterior drawer and able to identify partial tears in the anterior cruciate ligament when the examiner is skilled, it is difficult on patients who have large legs. The pivot shift is the third maneuver by which the examiner can determine the integrity of the anterior cruciate ligament. The pivot shift is easily performed once the examiner is familiar with it, but it may be somewhat painful to the patient. While the patient is supine and relaxed, the examiner lifts the heel of the foot to approximately 45° of hip flexion with the knee fully extended. The opposite hand grasps the knee with the thumb behind the fibular head. The examiner then internally rotates the ankle and knee, applies a valgus force to the knee, and flexes the knee. If an anterior subluxation of the tibia is present, a sudden visible, audible, and palpable reduction of the subluxation occurs at about 20 to 40° of flexion. This indicates a deficit in the anterior cruciate ligament, which is required to stabilize the knee in this position. There are other tests described in the literature to determine the integrity of the anterior cruciate ligament, including the jerk test and dynamic extension testing.

The posterior cruciate ligament can also suffer an isolated injury or be injured in combination with other ligamentous structures of the knee. In contrast to anterior cruciate injuries, isolated posterior cruciate injuries are seen much less frequently. The posterior cruciate ligament provides initial resistance to posterior translation at all angles of flexion of the knee. The mechanism of injury then is usually an anterior to posterior force applied to the tibia or lower leg. Posterior cruciate injuries are seen in association with other ligamentous injuries when a serious injury has occurred to the knee. A deficit in this ligament is determined by the posterior drawer test. The knee is examined with flexion at the hip and at the knee as described for the anterior drawer sign. The physician applies a posterior force to the tibial tubercle. If there is displacement posteriorly, then the examiner can diagnose an injury to this ligament. The physician might also notice a posterior sag or drop back of the tibial tubercle due to loss of integrity of the posterior cruciate when observing the knee with 45° flexion at the hip and 90° flexion at the knee. This test can be misleading, however, if there is a straight anterior instability resulting in a subluxation of the knee forward. This abnormal position would give the physician the false impression of too much posterior play when performing the posterior drawer test because the knee would be reduced to its normal anatomic alignment from the forwardly subluxed position.

Combined instabilities of the knee are often seen by the emergency physician, especially in athletes. Anteromedial and/or anterolateral instability are the two that occur most frequently. They result from external rotation and abduction or adduction forces placed upon the knee. Virtually any combination of medial and lateral instabilities of the knee can occur, however.

One knee injury that is especially difficult to detect is injury to the posterolateral structures. Posterolateral instability usually involves a tear of the popliteus-arcuate complex, which may occur in combination with lateral ligament injury and possible anterior or posterior cruciate ligament injury. Isolated injuries to the popliteus-arcuate complex can occur of themselves but are rare. Isolated posterolateral instability is demonstrated by testing at 0 to 30° of flexion for maximal posterior translation and 90° of flexion for maximal external rotation as compared to the normal opposite knee. Further testing to determine the integrity of the lateral collateral ligament and anterior or posterior cruciates must be done as well.

Most ligamentous injuries of the knee present with hemarthroses. In fact, approximately 75 percent of all hemarthroses are due to disruption of the anterior cruciate ligament. Serious ligament injuries, however, may present with minimal pain and no hemarthrosis due to complete disruption of the ligamentous and capsular fibers, allowing leakage of the blood into the soft tissue spaces. Hemarthrosis can also be due to osteochondral fractures or fractures that extend into the joint line or peripheral meniscal tears. These hemarthroses usually occur within a few hours of injury, in contrast to chronic effusions of the knee due to synovial inflammation, which occur 1 to 2 days after strenuous use of the joint. Usually the physician does not need to tap a sudden effusion associated with a knee injury to determine whether it is bloody. The indications for tapping a knee with a hemarthrosis are to relieve the pressure and pain caused by fluid distension and to see if fat globules are present, indicating a fracture (lipohemarthrosis). The complications of aspirating a joint space include the possibility of contamination and subsequent infection.

Continued refinements in magnetic resonance imaging (MRI) have resulted in high-quality images of the ligamentous and meniscal structures of the knee. The emergency physician can confirm the results of the stress testing by ordering an MRI examination of the knee if the appropriate equipment and personnel are available.

Treatment

Stable injuries involving a single ligament with minor strain can be managed with a knee splint, ice packs, elevation, and ambulation as soon as is comfortable for the patient. More severe but stable ligamentous injuries necessitate ice, elevation, and immobilization. These injuries should be referred to an orthopedic surgeon within the next few days for follow-up examination and definitive management. Unstable injuries necessitate immediate orthopedic consultation so that definitive management can be planned.

Meniscal Injuries

Meniscal injuries of the knee occur of themselves or in combination with ligamentous injuries. For example, anterior cruciate injuries are commonly associated with meniscal injuries. There have been many maneuvers described in the literature to determine whether a meniscus has been injured. Most of these tests, however, have an unacceptable specificity and sensitivity. While the diagnosis of a meniscal tear is difficult to make in certain patients, a combination of a suggestive history and physical findings on examination should lead the emergency physician to entertain the diagnosis. Upon questioning the patient, the physician should ask if the patient experiences locking of the knee joint that is painful and limits further activity. This sign clearly points to the diagnosis of a torn meniscus. Effusions that occur after activity; a sensation of popping, clicking, or snapping; a feeling of an unstable joint, especially with activity; or tenderness in the anterior joint space after excessive activity suggests the diagnosis of a meniscal tear. When performing a physical examination, a physician should attempt to identify atrophy of the quadriceps muscle due to disuse and joint line tenderness, which is very suggestive. Various maneuvers, such as McMurray's test or the grind test, are useful but, as mentioned earlier, are positive only about 50 percent of the time. If a tentative diagnosis of a meniscal tear is entertained, referral to an orthopedic surgeon is warranted.

The patient who presents to the emergency department with a locked knee can experience a great deal of pain along with loss of mobility. The emergency physician can attempt to unlock the knee by positioning the patient with the leg hanging over the edge of the table with the knee in approximately 90° of flexion. After a period of relaxation, the physician can apply longitudinal traction to the knee with internal and external rotation in an attempt to unlock the joint. If this maneuver is unsuccessful, consultation with the orthopedic surgeon is recommended.

Knee Dislocation

Knee dislocation is a result of tremendous ligamentous disruption due to hyperextension, direct posterior force applied to the anterior tibia, force to the fibula or medial femur, force to the tibia or lateral femur, or rotatory force resulting in anterior, posterior lateral, medial, or rotatory dislocation. Very often reduction occurs spontaneously. However, suspicion of the injury is important because of the high incidence of associated complications, including popliteal artery injury and peroneal nerve injury, in addition to ligamentous and meniscal injury. Early reduction of the dislocation is essential; orthopedic and perhaps vascular surgery consultation should be obtained immediately.

Patella Dislocation

Dislocation of the patella usually occurs from a twisting injury on the extended knee. The patella is displaced laterally over the lateral condyle, resulting in pain and deformity of the knee. Reduction is accomplished by hyperextending the knee, flexing the hip, and sliding the patella back into place. This is accompanied by immediate relief of pain, but further soreness from capsular injury persists for a period of time. The patella and knee should be x-rayed to rule out a fracture and the knee should be immobilized after reduction. Recurrent lateral dislocations of the patella and superior, horizontal, and intercondylar dislocations require referral to an orthopedic surgeon for possible surgical intervention.

Osteochondritis Dissecans

Osteochondritis dissecans is a loose body in a knee joint which may cause locking, effusion, and buckling of the knee. X-ray examination may be negative or may reveal a calcified body in the joint.

KNEE INJURIES IN CHILDREN

Although knee injuries do occur in children, they are usually the result of fractures of the bone rather than significant ligamentous injuries. Ligamentous injuries can occur in children but are not common. Careful examination and radiographic evaluation usually reveal that the ligaments are intact and there has been an epiphyseal injury. Meniscal tears also occur in children with a much lower incidence than in adults. The characteristic finding of meniscal tears in children is that they have a more insidious history than in the adult. Patellar fractures are also very infrequent in children. They can be difficult to diagnose because of the difficulty in evaluating the radiographs. The opposite knee should be x-rayed for comparison views to help the physician in the diagnosis of a fracture. Lastly, dislocations are, fortunately, an exteremly rare condition in children. If they occur, however, they have the same ominous complications as in the adult.

Separation of Distal Femoral Epiphysis

In children this is a common epiphyseal injury which can occur in the anterior plane or coronal plane. The anterior separation is usually the result of a hyperextension injury. The more common coronal separation is the result of abduction and adduction forces, most often occurring during sports activities or play. The patient complains of acute injury with inability to bear weight and presents with a flexion deformity. As with most epiphyseal injuries, the examiner finds circumferential tenderness around the entire epiphyseal plate. The standard radiographic views for evaluating the knee are required. The Salter-Harris classification (see Fig. 178-1) is used to classify these fractures, with type II being the most common. The treatment for separation of the distal femoral epiphysis is conservative; closed reduction and immobilization are the basis for therapy.

Separation of Proximal Tibial Epiphysis

The separation of the proximal tibial epiphysis is a rare phenomenon because the tibia is well-protected. The mechanism of injury is usually indirect forces of abduction or hyperextension against a fixed knee. Occasionally this injury is due to a direct force such as encountered in an automobile-pedestrian accident. Again, the classification is the Salter-Harris method. The symptoms and signs are similar to those of all other knee injuries, with pain, swelling, effusion, and a limited range of motion, especially extension-flexion. As with all epiphyseal injuries, there is circumferential tenderness over the injured growth plate. Stress examination reveals instability to the various maneuvers. Standard radiographs to evaluate the knee are recommended, with stress films required if no injury is seen but one is suspected. Careful evaluation looking for an occult fracture line is important. The treatment is immediate reduction and conservative therapy. The complications are similar to those of distal femoral epiphyseal separation.

Injuries to the Tibial Tubercle

Two problems can occur at the tibial tubercle. The first is the acute avulsion of the tibial tubercle; the second is the classic Osgood-Schlatter lesion. Avulsion injuries are usually incurred as an acute event during sports and play. The patient presents with the inability to walk, because of the injury, as well as with localized tenderness and swelling. The lateral radiographic view is most important as it demonstrates both the size of the fracture fragment and the degree of displacement. The treatment for any but the smallest fragment is surgical so that there are minimal complications and a good prognosis. In contrast, Osgood-Schlatter lesions present with a vague history in adolescent boys. The pain is mild and intermittent, allowing the child to continue to participate in sports and play but not at a full level of involvement. Osgood-Schlatter disease is seen bilaterally in approximately 25 percent of the cases. In contrast to patients with avulsion injuries, patients with Osgood-Schlatter lesions experience pain with range of motion, especially range of motion against resistance, and not at rest. The treatment is symptomatic and supportive. There are minimal complications, and the prognosis is good.

Fracture of the Intercondylar Eminence of the Tibia

This fracture is usually encountered in 8- to 15-year-olds, who most often relate a history of a fall from a bicycle. This causes the intercondylar eminence to be avulsed from the tibia, resulting in a painful and acutely swollen knee. The patient has a positive Lachman's test and a drawer sign and may have concomitant medial collateral ligamentous instability to valgus stress testing. Radiographs usually reveal evidence of a fracture on the lateral view with the knee slightly flexed.

The treatment is closed in most instances, as proper positioning can reduce the fracture fragment to its anatomic state. The concomitant injuries to the medial collateral ligament do not often require surgical intervention and can be treated while the patient is recovering from the fracture. The prognosis with proper treatment is good.

Osteochondral Fractures

Osteochondral fractures occur infrequently in children and adolescents. If they do occur, most often in adolescent boys, they are usually fracture fragments from the femoral condyles or the patella. The history is one of an acute injury with a pop or snap, causing severe pain and an acute effusion. The fracture is difficult to see on radiographs, so careful attention should be paid to the femoral condyles as well as to the patella. Treatment is surgical removal of the foreign body so that no sequelae can develop.

SUMMARY

In summary, the knee is a complex joint. Understanding the anatomy and physiology of its motion, understanding the mechanism of the forces producing injuries, and facility in examination of the knee are essential for the emergency physician, who will be confronted relatively often by injuries to this joint. Thorough and careful examination on initial presentation, recognition of significant abnormalities, thoughtful initial care, and appropriate referral are the emergency physician's goals in management of knee injuries.

BIBLIOGRAPHY

Hohl M, Larson RL, Jones DC: Fractures and dislocations of the knee, in Rockwood CA Jr, Green DP (eds): *Fractures in Adults*, 2d ed. Philadelphia, Lippincott, 1984, vol 2, pp 1429–1593.

Roberts JM: Fractures and dislocations of the knee, in Rockwood CA Jr, Wilkins KE, King RE: *Fractures in Children*. Philadelphia, Lippincott, 1984, vol 3, pp 891–983.

Simon RR, Koenigsknecht SJ: *Orthopaedics in Emergency Medicine: The Extremities*. New York, Appleton-Century-Crofts, 1982.

Sisk TD: Knee injuries in Crenshaw AH (ed): *Campbell's Operative Orthopaedics*, 7th ed. St. Louis, Mosby, 1987, vol 3, pp 2305–2335.

183 LEG INJURIES

Joseph F. Waeckerle
Mark T. Steele

Although the fractured tibia is the most common of all long bone fractures, its treatment is varied and sometimes controversial. Because of the many fractures seen and the frequency of open fractures, tibial fractures are associated with a high complication rate. The frequency of fractures, as well as the complication rate, is due to the fact that the tibia, and fibula as well, has minimal protection from surrounding soft tissues.

The leg is susceptible to direct and indirect mechanisms of injury. Direct blows usually cause tibial shaft fractures which are associated with fibular shaft fractures. Because the violence is directly to the bone, soft tissue injury with initial displacement of the fracture site and comminution of the fracture often result. In contrast, indirect forces such as rotation and compression usually cause spiral or oblique fractures of the tibia, sometimes associated with fibular shaft fractures. Isolated fibular shaft fractures are, in fact, uncommon injuries.

ANATOMY

The tibia and fibula run parallel and are tightly connected by the interosseous ligament. The surrounding soft tissue may be divided into three compartments. The first, the anterior compartment, consists of the muscles (tibialis anterior, extensor digitorum longus, extensor hallucis longus, and peroneus tertius), the anterior tibial artery, and the deep peroneal nerve. Because this compartment is bound by the tibia, fibula, and fascia, there is little room for swelling. The second compartment is the lateral compartment, which consists of the peroneus brevis and peroneus longus muscles, along with the superficial peroneal nerve. The superficial peroneal nerve is at risk when an injury occurs high up the fibular shaft or at the neck of the fibula. The third compartment is the posterior compartment, which consists of the soleus, gastrocnemius, tibialis posterior, flexor hallucis longus, and flexor digitorum longus muscles, the posterior tibial nerve, and the posterior tibial artery.

Injuries from swelling to the anterior compartment are more often seen than such injuries to the lateral or posterior compartments. The latter two are also bound compartments, and if a significant amount of swelling occurs, a compartment syndrome may also be seen there.

There are multiple classifications for describing leg fractures. Probably the easiest is to classify tibial fractures as stable or unstable, which helps with regard to treatment. Some classifications, by describing the fractures with regard to displacement, comminution, and soft tissue injuries, can somewhat predict the healing potential.

CLINICAL EVALUATION

As with all orthopedic injuries, the symptoms and signs the patient presents with are directly proportional to the severity of the leg fracture. Pain is usually severe and localized. Crepitance in motion and obvious deformity are often present. Usually the deformity is external rotation and valgus in nature. Local swelling and discoloration and the presence of wounds may aid the physician in diagnosing a fracture. When associated with a leg fracture, any wound which violates the integrity of the skin must be considered an open fracture. Although direct neurovascular injury is not a common complication of leg fractures, neurovascular assessment should always be done and recorded on the chart. This consists of documentation that both the vascular supply to the foot and the motor and sensory supply to the leg, especially the functions of the peroneal nerve, are intact.

In evaluating leg fractures, AP and lateral x-ray views are generally adequate to demonstrate the fracture, as well as the position of the fragments. As always, the x-ray views require good trabecular detail to demonstrate the smaller, nondisplaced fractures, especially those seen in the fibula. Also, the x-ray views should demonstrate both the knee and the ankle articular surfaces.

Treatment

Emergency department management of leg fractures is usually not difficult. Once the initial examination is completed and the fracture is identified and defined, closed reduction, an immobilization long leg splint, and referral are appropriate. Difficulty in managing such fractures in the emergency department occurs when the physician is not able to obtain an adequate reduction or there are severe associated soft tissue injuries with an open fracture. It is emphasized again that it is more important to treat the soft tissue injuries properly than to treat the fracture itself. This requires that the physician gently but thoroughly cleanse the soft tissue by debridement and irrigation and provide appropriate tetanus prophylaxis and antibiotic coverage. The immobilization must allow the physicians treating the patient to view the soft tissue wounds. Occasionally emergency reduction of a fracture may be required because the fracture has compromised vascularity distal to the fracture site. Although this is not common, such reduction might be needed prior to x-ray evaluation when the compromise threatens the limb's blood supply.

Complications

The most common complication associated with leg fractures is the soft tissue injury with secondary infection. As with any orthopedic injury, an infection can be disastrous. Also, as mentioned earlier, the compartment syndrome, seen some 24 to 48 h after injury, can occur. Nerve damage is usually uncommon with leg fractures but may occur if there is an injury to the fibular head. This involves the superficial peroneal nerve. Damage to the vascularity is also not usual but can occur in upper tibial fractures with injury to the anterior tibial artery as it passes through the interosseous membrane. As with all orthopedic injuries, nonunion or delayed union is common if the fracture site is complicated by a severe displacement or comminution. Also, arthritis may occur in some individuals.

Compartment Syndrome

Compartment syndrome occurs when injured muscle enveloped in a fascial sheath swells and causes secondary compression of blood vessels and nerves that traverse the compartment. If unrecognized, this syndrome can result in permanent nerve and muscle damage. The most common sites where this may occur include the four fascial compartments in the leg: peroneal, anterior, deep, and superficial posterior. The volar and dorsal compartments of the forearm and the interosseous muscles of the hand can also be affected. The anterior compartment of the leg is the most common site of compartment syndrome and usually is caused by fractures of the tibia. The causes of skeletal muscle injury are many and varied and include, but are not limited to, trauma, electrical injury, infectious disease (i.e., infectious myositis), hyper- or hypothermia, toxins, snake bite, polymyositis, arterial embolism or injury, seizures, and prolonged immobility that may occur following CVA or drug overdose.

A high index of suspicion is needed to make the diagnosis, particularly in unconscious or uncooperative patients. Time is of the essence since irreversible muscle damage can occur in 4 to 6 hours. A complete neurologic and motor exam of the affected extremity is essential. Tenderness and pain in the affected area are common with active or passive motion. Paresthesias and pain with passive finger or toe movement are early signs. Abnormal two point discrimination or light touch of a traversing nerve are also early indicators of a compartment syndrome. The affected compartment may be tense, indurated and erythematous, but this is a late finding. Initial capillary refill and pulses are usually normal in compartment syndrome. As a result, the finding of normal pulses and capillary refill *does not* rule out the condition.

Laboratory data generally show evidence of rhabdomyolysis, including myoglobinuria and elevated muscle enzyme activity. (CPK levels over 20,000 IV per mL are not unusual.) Renal function should be assessed and may show early deterioration due to the myoglobinuria. Immediate orthopedic consultation and admission is indicated if there is suspicion of compartment syndrome. Compartment pressures should be measured using a Wick catheter or 18 gauge needle and saline manometer. Pressure of 0–8 mmHg is considered normal. Pressure over 30 mmHg can cause ischemia and thus is an indication for emergency fasciotomy.

Fibular Fractures

Isolated fibular fractures, especially of the shaft, are uncommon. The more common injury to the fibula is fracture at the ankle joint, which is addressed in Chapter 184, "Ankle Injuries." Occasionally, however, fractures due to direct and indirect trauma do occur to the fibular shaft. The patient may present with local swelling and tenderness over the fracture site itself and pain on ambulation. Because of the difficulty in sometimes seeing a fracture of the fibula (especially if it is a stress fracture, which is commonly seen in the distal third), x-ray views which show good trabecular detail are required. AP and lateral views are generally adequate.

Treatment of fibular fractures is usually designed to give the patient comfort. Very often the patient does not require immobilization. However, in some instances the patient may be more comfortable in a short leg walking cast and crutches for approximately 2 weeks.

Achilles Tendon Rupture

The gastrocnemius and soleus muscles join in the middle of the calf to form the Achilles tendon. Rupture of the tendon is often missed by the physician on initial exam, the injury frequently mistaken for an ankle sprain. Tendon rupture most often occurs secondary to indirect mechanisms resulting in forceful dorsiflexion of the ankle. Initiating a sprint, slipping on a stair or ladder, or a fall from a height may result in sufficient dorsiflexion to rupture the tendon. Tendon tears can also be caused by direct trauma from blows to a taut tendon or by lacerations from glass or a lawn mower. Most commonly rupture occurs in middle-aged men and the left Achilles is involved significantly more often than the right.

History most often suggests the diagnosis of Achilles tendon rupture. The patient experiences sudden pain, often described as a feeling like someone kicked them in the calf. An audible snap may be heard and the patient subsequently has difficulty stepping off on the foot. Physical exam usually reveals swelling of the distal calf as well as a palpable defect in the tendon 2 to 6 centimeters proximal to its insertion into the calcaneus, the location where rupture most frequently occurs. Plantar flexion of the injured ankle will be weaker when compared to the uninjured side. Active plantar flexion of the injured side *does not*, however, rule out the diagnosis of Achilles tendon rupture because other muscles, including the toe flexors, peroneals, and tibialis posterior, can generate some ankle plantar flexion. Additionally, the calf squeeze or "Thompson's test" will help confirm the diagnosis of complete tendon rupture. A positive Thompson's sign is indicated by failure of the foot to plantar flex against gravity with calf compression when the patient is lying prone and the knee is flexed 90°. X-ray films are generally not helpful in establishing the diagnosis.

Early treatment includes orthopedic consultation and splinting of the lower extremity in a posterior splint in passive equinus (the position the foot assumes when dependent). The patient should remain non-weight bearing and keep the extremity elevated. Definitive treatment is controversial. Conservative therapy consists of short leg-cast immobilization in the equinus position for 8 weeks followed by 4-week use of a 2.5-cm heel lift and exercise program to strengthen the gastrocnemius and soleus. Some studies have found decrease in plantar flexion strength in patients treated conservatively compared with those who underwent surgery. As a result, surgical repair is usually recommended for younger athletic patients who want to optimize their strength in the injured leg.

Calf Strains/Gastrocnemius Rupture

Falls leading to forceful dorsiflexion of the ankle or sudden push-off during athletic events such as tennis or basketball may result in partial rupture of the medial head of the gastrocnemius at the musculotendinous junction. Clinically, the patient localizes pain to the medial midcalf and ambulation and standing on tiptoe are difficult and painful. Soft tissue swelling and ecchymosis are usually present. The calf squeeze or Thompson's sign is negative, differentiating it from complete Achilles tendon rupture. Venous thrombosis must also be considered in the differential diagnosis. Initial treatment consists of immobilization with a posterior splint. Ice, elevation, and oral anti-inflammatory agents are indicated. Protected crutch weight bearing can be initiated within a week along with the use of bilateral heel lifts.

LEG INJURIES IN CHILDREN

Tibial and Fibular Shaft Fractures

Tibial and fibular shaft fractures are the most common lower extremity injuries to bone in children. The mechanism of injury is usually an indirect force, such as occurs from a twist. Rarely, direct trauma causes the injury. The patient presents with pain on walking and a mild limp if there is a fibular fracture, a greenstick fracture, or stress fracture. If, however, both the tibia and fibular are fractured, the patient is unable to walk and has pain at rest. The examining physician may see a deformity, which is usually minimal in contrast to the deformity of adult fractures. Neurovascular involvement is uncommon in these injuries. Radiographic evaluation requires standard AP and lateral views, with the opposite leg for comparison occasionally. Treatment is usually closed and conservative. The complications of these fractures in children are basically deformity types, with leg-length discrepancy and malrotation the most important. Neurovascular complications are rare.

Specific fractures of the tibia and fibula can occur. The toddler fracture can occur in younger children. They are a common cause for a limp or refusal to ambulate. Toddler fractures are usually spiral fractures of the tibia, with no fibular involvement. Bicycle spoke injuries are also seen occasionally. The history is usually that the child's foot was thrust between the spokes of a bicycle wheel, causing a severe compression or crush injury of the soft tissues of the foot and ankle. Special care should be taken in such cases, as the soft tissue problems are significant.

Lastly, stress fractures in children present with a different pattern than in adults. The upper third of the tibia is nearly always affected in children. Boys usually have more problems with this type of fracture because of their activity levels. They present with a painful limp of insidious onset. The pain is relieved when the child is at rest and is increased with activity. There is local tenderness to examination. Radiographic evaluation, as with all stress fractures, may not be helpful initially as the fracture may not show up for a period of time. Bone scan is usually helpful. Treatment is conservative and symptomatic.

Tibial Metaphyseal Injuries

Fractures of the proximal tibial metaphysis are usually due to significant violence. Because of this, they are associated with significant complications. The most important complication for the physician to recognize immediately is arterial involvement associated with valgus deformities. In contrast to proximal tibial injuries, distal tibial metaphyseal fractures are usually greenstick fractures with minimal sequelae and good prognosis.

BIBLIOGRAPHY

Dias LS: Fractures of the tibia and fibula, in Rockwood CA Jr, Wilkins KE, King RE (eds): *Fractures in Children*. Philadelphia, Lippincott, 1984, vol 3, pp 983–1043.

Leach RE: Fractures of the tibia and fibula, in Rockwood CA Jr, Green DP (eds): *Fractures in Adults*. Philadelphia, Lippincott, 1984, vol 2, pp 1593–1665.

Simon RR, Koenigsknecht SJ: *Orthopaedics in Emergency Medicine: The Extremities*, 2d ed. New York, Appleton-Century-Crofts, 1988.

184 ANKLE INJURIES

Joseph F. Waeckerle
Mark T. Steele

The ankle bears as much weight per unit area as any other joint in the body. Its anatomic design and weight-bearing function predispose it to a wide variety of injuries. To recognize and appropriately treat ankle injuries, the physician must understand the anatomy and mechanisms of injury. Treatment should be designed so that no prolonged disability or irreparable damage results.

ANATOMY

The ankle consists of three bones, the tibia, fibula, and talus, which are bonded together by ligaments to form a hingelike joint. Groups of muscles cross the joint and produce movement, mostly through dorsiflexion and plantar flexion.

Bones. Bony stability is provided by the talus being interposed between the tibia and fibula. The talus is wider anteriorly than posteriorly to provide for articulation with the distal tibia and the medial and lateral malleoli. In dorsiflexion, more of the anterior, wider portion of the talus fits into the slightly concave undersurface of the tibia. This tighter fit allows the malleoli of the tibia and fibula to bear more stress if any twisting motion occurs. In plantar flexion, the narrower, posterior portion of the talus occupies the mortise so that there is more play in the ankle joint. It is therefore easier for twisting motions to result in injury with the ankle in plantar flexion. Due to the inherent joint design, dorsiflexion is accompanied by eversion and plantar flexion with inversion.

Ligaments. Three groups of ligaments unify the bony structures of the ankle. The medial collateral, or deltoid, ligament is a thick triangular band that provides medial support to the ankle joint. It consists of a superficial and a deep set of fibers. Both sets of fibers originate from the broad, short, and strong medial malleolus. The superficial fibers run in a sagittal plane and insert on the navicular and talus. Deep fibers run more horizontally and insert on the medial surface of the talus.

The lateral support of the ankle is provided by the anterior talofibular, calcaneofibular, and posterior talofibular ligaments (Fig. 184-1). They originate and insert as their names suggest. Along with the lateral malleolus, these ligaments prevent lateral movement of the talus.

The lower portions of the tibia and fibula are bound together by the ligaments of the syndesmosis. These ligaments consist of the anterior and posterior tibiofibular ligaments, the interosseous ligament, and the inferior transverse ligament. The anterior and posterior tibiofibular ligaments are bands of fibers running between the margins of the tibia and fibula anteriorly and posteriorly. The inferior transverse ligament is a strong group of fibers that supports the posterior inferior portion of the ankle joint. Finally, the interosseous ligament is simply the lower portion of the interosseous membrane. It provides the strongest bond between the tibia and fibula at the joint.

Muscles. There are basically four compartments of muscles that traverse the ankle joint (Fig. 184-2). Anteriorly, the tibialis anterior, extensor digitorum longus, and extensor hallucis longus run over the ankle joint and contribute to dorsiflexion of the ankle. Medially, the tibialis posterior, flexor digitorum longus, and flexor hallucis longus run behind the medial malleolus and contribute to inversion of the foot. Posteriorly, the soleus and gastrocnemius muscles provide plantar flexion. Laterally, the peroneus longus and brevis muscles run in a sheath directly behind the lateral malleolus. These muscles contribute to eversion and plantar flexion.

Nerves and blood supply. The vascular supply to the area of the ankle is a continuation of the external iliac, femoral, and popliteal arterial system. The anterior and posterior tibial arteries as well as the peroneal artery are continuations of the popliteal artery and supply the ankle and foot. Nervous supply is from the sciatic nerve.

In summary, the ankle joint is a ring consisting of the tibia, fibula, and talus bound together by three major groups of ligaments. Almost all injuries to the ankle are due to the abnormal motion of the talus as it sets in the mortise. The talar motion causes direct or indirect stress on the malleoli or lower portion of the tibia, resulting in injury. If there is a single break in the ring, talar shift may not occur because of the ligamentous support. However, if there are two breaks in the ring, a fracture of the malleoli, a fracture of one malleolus and a rupture of one ligament, or a rupture of both ligaments, then integrity of the ring is violated and talar shift will occur. This anatomic fact is important in assessing the stability of any injured ankle.

HISTORY OF INJURY

As with all orthopedic injuries a careful history of the mechanism of injury is essential and should always precede clinical and roentgenographic examination. The physician should attempt to ascertain the position of the foot, the direction of the stresses, and all other pertinent data to reconstruct the injury. This will aid in the determination of what bones or ligaments are most likely to be injured. It is also helpful to ask if during the time of injury there was any noise that might indicate that a ligament popped, a bone subluxed or dislocated, or a tendon snapped. The physician should ask if the onset of pain was immediate, if swelling occurred right after the injury, and if disability was immediate or delayed. A history of previous ankle injury and its treatment may affect physical findings and treatment.

CLINICAL EXAMINATION

A partial clinical examination should always precede roentgenographic examination. If the ankle is grossly deformed, the diagnosis of an unstable joint is obvious and radiologic evaluation should occur after the physician ensures that neurovascular status is not compromised. In the absence of a gross deformity, inspect for local swelling and the loss or prominence of anatomic landmarks. Look for ecchymoses, although subcutaneous bleeding may occur with either fractures or sprains. Palpation can localize the area of maximal tenderness, crepitance, and loss or distortion of anatomic landmarks. Gently put the ankle through a range of motion to evaluate stability and to determine positions that produce or relieve pain. Manipulation must be gentle to avoid further injury. After examining the injured ankle, examine the opposite and hopefully normal joint. This will give an idea of the range of motion and laxity of the normal ankle joints. Again, the physician must keep in mind past history because a prior injury to the uninjured joint will prevent proper comparison.

ROENTGENOGRAPHIC EXAMINATION

Roentgenograms are ordered to detect fractures and evaluate their severity. Although ligamentous injuries are not seen on x-ray films, improper anatomic relationships give a hint that ligamentous injury has occurred. The roentgenogram also allows the physician to look for further complicating factors such as foreign bodies or diseases of the bone. Lastly, the physician can utilize radiologic evaluation to follow the results of treatment of the patient with the ankle injury.

Proper radiologic evaluation of any ankle injury is essential. The examination should consist of an AP film in which the ankle is in 5 to 15° of adduction; a true lateral view that includes the base of the fifth metatarsal; and a 45° internal oblique film with the ankle in dorsiflexion. The roentgenogram should be of sufficient quality that trabecular detail is seen in all views. A comparison view of the opposite side can be helpful, especially in children. Also, a cone-down view or stress view of an area with questionable findings may be helpful. The

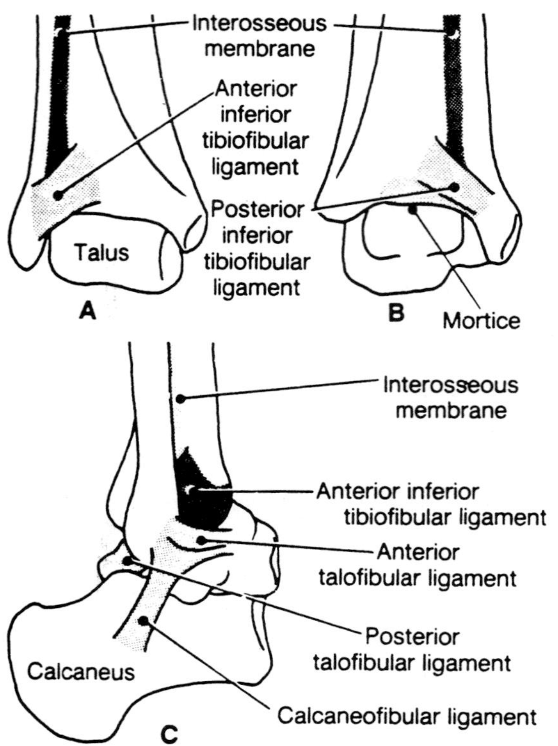

Fig. 184-1. Lateral ligaments of the ankle. **A.** Anterior view. **B.** Posterior view. **C.** Lateral view. (From Ramamurti CP: *Orthopedics in Primary Care.* Tinker RV (ed): Baltimore, Williams & Wilkins, 1979, with permission.)

physician should use the bright light to properly examine the outline of the bony detail and to detect soft tissue swelling.

LIGAMENTOUS INJURIES OF THE ANKLE

Approximately 75 percent of all ankle injuries are sprains. More than 90 percent involve the lateral ligaments, less than 5 percent involve the deltoid ligament, and less than 5 percent involve the anterior or posterior tibiofibular ligament and anterior and posterior capsule (see Figs. 184-1 and 184-2). Of lateral ligament injuries, 90 percent involve the anterior talofibular ligament, with 65 percent of these sprains being isolated, and 25 percent with concomitant injuries to the calcaneofibular ligament. The posterior talofibular ligament, or third component of the lateral collateral ligament, stabilizes against posterior displacement of the talus and is therefore rarely injured except in cases of complete dislocation. Because the anterior talofibular ligament and calcaneofibular ligament are two separate structures, the standard classification of first-degree, second-degree, and third-degree sprains is difficult to apply. Hence, injury to these ligaments is classified as either a single or double ligament injury. Only one ligament may be torn so that the integrity of the joint is weakened in one plane of direction, but it is not necessarily unstable. These ligaments usually tear in sequence from anterior to posterior, so that the anterior talofibular ligament tears first, followed by the calcaneofibular ligament.

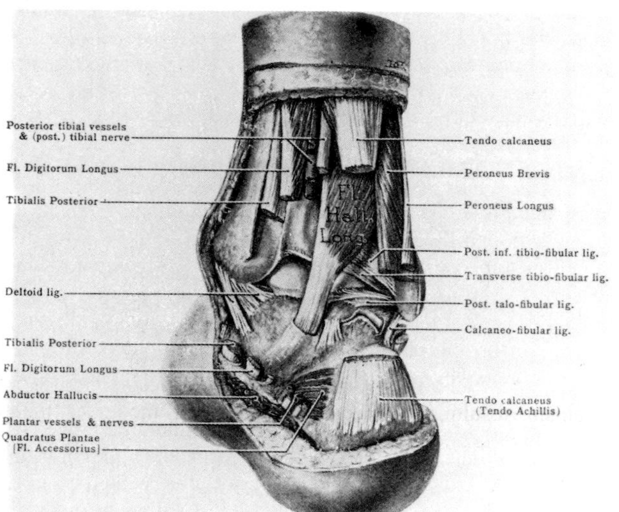

Fig. 184-2. Ankle and heel, posterior view. (From Anderson JE: *Grant's Atlas of Anatomy,* ed 7. Baltimore, Williams & Wilkins, 1978, Plate 4–89. Used by permission.)

Lateral Collateral Ligament Injuries

Laxity of the anterior talofibular ligament may be adequately assessed by physical examination. The most helpful test is the anterior drawer maneuver. If the ligament is torn by an inversion stress the talus will sublux anteriorly and laterally out of the mortise with observable movement and crepitation at the limit of excursion. This maneuver should be performed on all patients with suspected lateral ligamentous injuries.

With one hand, grasp the calcaneus with the finger and thumb behind the malleoli, and with the opposite hand stabilize the extreme distal tibia and fibula. The foot should be slightly plantar flexed and inverted, which is its normal relaxed position. Next, apply a forward anterior force to the calcaneus, keeping the distal tibia and fibula fixed. Movement of the talus anteriorly more than 3 mm *may* be significant, but movement greater than 1 cm *certainly* is significant. There are both false-positive and false-negative results with this test, but the most common difficulty is the physician's unfamiliarity with the examination.

If the tear extends further posteriorly into the calcaneofibular portion of the lateral ligament, talar tilt occurs, since the lateral ankle is now unstable, not only in the anterior posterior plane but in the medial lateral plane as well. Place the foot at 20 to 30° of plantar flexion with slight adduction, and apply inversion stress upon the calcaneal forefoot. Talar tilt or movement of the talus in the mortise is clinically felt because of tilting of the talus in relation to the distal articular surface of the tibia. This is then compared with the normal side.

Good muscle relaxation is important for proper evaluation. If diagnostic maneuvers are painful, voluntary and involuntary muscle contractions to guard against further movement will prevent assessment. The use of ice packs or local anesthetic infiltration can be helfpul.

If the posterior talofibular ligament is involved, the ankle is obviously unstable, with both a positive anterior drawer sign and marked talar tilt. In most posterior talofibular ligament injuries, the ankle is dislocated and neither test need be performed.

Medial Collateral Ligament Injuries

The medial collateral ligament is rarely injured alone. Its injury is usually accompanied by a fracture of the fibula or tear of the tibiofibular ligaments anteriorly or posteriorly. This injury is usually the result of a significant eversion stress. It is almost impossible to tear the deltoid ligament without an accompanying fracture of the fibula or separation of the tibiofibular syndesmosis. Evaluation of the medial collateral ligament is done by stressing the ankle with a medial-to-lateral force which is simply a talar tilt sign.

Tibiofibular Syndesmotic Ligament Injuries

Tibiofibular syndesmotic ligaments are a continuation of the interosseous ligaments at the distal tibia and fibula. Injuries to this ligament system occur secondary to hyperdorsiflexion and eversion. The talus usually pushes superiorly, separates the tibia and fibula, and displaces the fibula laterally, resulting in a partial or complete rupture. Diastasis will not necessarily be evident on radiologic or physical examination because the interosseous membrane above the ligament system will usually keep the tibia and fibula together.

The history is often nonspecific, but frequently the patient reports that he or she felt something pop or give during a movement which caused dorsiflexion and eversion. There is little swelling, and the patient complains of pain over the anterior and posterior superior aspects of the ankle. The patient prefers to walk on the toes. On examination point tenderness over the anterior or posterior ligaments is found. There may be some tenderness over the medial malleolus secondary to a concomitant medial collateral ligament injury. In severe injury, there is also point tenderness over the distal tibia and fibula. Bilateral compression of the malleoli also causes pain as it causes movement in the injured area. Radiologic changes may only include soft tissue swelling at or below the medial malleolus and above the lateral malleous up to the midshaft fibula. This is a serious injury with significant long-term sequelae. A stress test of sorts may be helpful: Dorsiflex the foot with the patient supine or standing. This will cause pain due to separation of the tibia and fibula.

Roentgenographic Findings in Ankle Sprains

The physician should always order standard x-ray views to evaluate an ankle injury, for radiologic findings can be surprising. If the standard views show avulsion or pull-off fracture, oblique or spiral fracture, transverse fracture, diastasis of the tibia/fibula or the interosseous membrane, or a fractured fibular shaft, there is also rupture of the concomitant ligament. In such instances, no stress films are needed. However, stress films are indicated if instability is suspected or demonstrated by abnormal talar positioning, or if the joint line between the talus and mortise of the ankle is not symmetric.

The anterior drawer sign as explained earlier may be done under x-ray or fluoroscopic examination. There is some difficulty in establishing reference points for measuring the movement of the talus anteriorly in relation to the mortise of the ankle. Although different authors have utilized different reference points, the current literature suggests that greater than 3-mm movement of the talus anteriorly to the posterior border of the calcaneus may be significant. Greater than 1 cm is certainly indicative of disruption. If there is some question as to the findings, the opposite ankle should be stressed in a similar manner and measured for comparison, providing the opposite ankle has not been injured in the past.

The talar tilt test, whether done in the medial or lateral ligamentous system, is also not extremely sensitive because there is variability of tilt among normal individuals and even between a pair of normal ankles. Moreover, pain, spasm, and edema may prevent adequate evaluation. As with the anterior drawer maneuver, there is no way to standardize the amount of force used by the physician during the test. However, the test may be positive if there is greater than 5° of talar tilt. If there is greater than 25° talar tilt, the examination is definitely abnormal. A difference of 5 to 10° talar tilt between the injured and uninjured side is probably significant in most instances.

In experienced hands, ankle arthrography is quick and simple to perform. It should be done within 24 to 48 h since clot formation after that time may prevent leakage of dye. Extraarticular leak of contrast material is generally indicative of a tear. However, the flexor hallucis longus and flexor digitorum longus tendon sheath fill in 20 percent of normal individuals, the peroneal tendon sheath fills in 14 percent, and the talocalcaneal joint space fills in 10 percent. Evaluation of the calcaneofibular ligament by standard arthrography techniques is associated with a high incidence of false-negative results.

Classification of Sprains

Ligamentous injuries are classified into first-, second-, and third-degree sprains. A first-degree sprain is stretching or microscopic tearing of a ligament, causing local tenderness and minimal swelling. Weight bearing is possible, and x-ray films are normal.

In a second-degree sprain, there is severe stretching and partial tearing of a ligament, causing marked tenderness, moderate edema, and moderate pain with weight bearing. Radiologic evaluation with standard views will not demonstrate bony abnormality. However, if the ankle is stressed, loss of ligamentous function will be demonstrated by the abnormal relationship of the talus and mortise.

Third-degree sprain is due to complete rupture of ligaments. The patient is unable to bear weight, and there is marked tenderness and swelling, and often an obviously deformed joint. Standard radiologic evaluation reveals an abnormal relationship of the talus and mortise. Usually, stress films are not needed, but with a complete rupture they are almost always positive if the test is performed properly.

Treatment

There is much debate with regard to the treatment of ankle injuries. First-degree sprains may be treated by compression dressings, elevation, ice and immobilization. Fifteen minutes of ice application to produce local anesthesia, followed by range-of-motion exercises to the development of pain, followed again by 15 min of ice application is beneficial. This should be done approximately four times a day until the patient can resume normal function without pain. The decision to institute nonweight bearing or partial weight bearing is an individual one. Plaster or synthetic splints or ankle braces may be used. In the case of an athlete with a first-degree sprain, full athletic activity should not be resumed until that person can sprint without limping, run circles and figures of eight at full speed without pain, and, finally, cut at right angles off the affected joint without pain.

Second-degree sprains of the ankle are best treated with the ice method as described above, and immobilization. If there is extensive edema, a splint, crutches, ice, and elevation are utilized until swelling diminishes; then, immobilization for 2 weeks in a walking cast, followed by 2 weeks in a walking hinge cast, is usually recommended.

The treatment of third-degree sprains of the ankle is debatable. The decision whether to immobilize or to operate is not made easily, and a number of considerations are important. The emergency physician is not usually asked to advise treatment for third-degree sprains because orthopedic consultation should be obtained for such injuries.

It is always prudent to maintain good liaison and communication with the patient's orthopedic surgeon. Patients with ankle injuries need appropriate diagnosis and treatment. Long-term sequelae of misdiagnosis and mistreatment are significant. Appropriate follow-up of ankle injuries is an absolute necessity.

ACHILLES TENDON RUPTURE

The gastrocnemius and soleus muscles join in the middle of the calf to form the Achilles tendon. Rupture of the tendon is often missed by the physician on initial exam, the injury frequently mistaken for an ankle sprain. Tendon rupture most often occurs secondary to indirect mechanisms resulting in forceful dorsiflexion of the ankle. Initiating a sprint, slipping on a stair or ladder, or a fall from a height may result in sufficient dorsiflexion to rupture the tendon. Tendon tears can also be caused by direct trauma from blows to a taut tendon or by lacerations from glass or lawn mower accidents. Most commonly rupture occurs in middle-aged men and the left Achilles is involved significantly more often than the right.

History most often suggests the diagnosis of Achilles tendon rupture.

The patient experiences sudden pain, often described as a feeling like someone kicked them in the calf. An audible snap may be heard and the patient subsequently has difficulty stepping off on the foot. Physical exam usually reveals swelling of the distal calf as well as a palpable defect in the tendon 2 to 6 centimeters proximal to its insertion into the calcaneus, the location where rupture most frequently occurs. Plantar flexion of the injured ankle will be weaker when compared to the uninjured side. Active plantar flexion of the injured side *does not,* however, rule out the diagnosis of Achilles tendon rupture because other muscles, including the toe flexors, peroneals, and tibialis posterior, can generate some ankle plantar flexion. Additionally, the calf squeeze or "Thompson's test" will help confirm the diagnosis of complete tendon rupture. A positive Thompson's sign is indicated by failure of the foot to plantar flex against gravity with calf compression when the patient is lying prone and their knee is flexed 90°. X-ray films are generally not helpful in establishing the diagnosis.

Early treatment includes orthopedic consultation and splinting of the lower extremity in a posterior splint in passive equinus (the position the foot assumes when dependent). The patient should remain non-weight bearing and keep the extremity elevated. Definitive treatment is controversial. Conservative therapy consists of short leg cast immobilization in the equinus position for 8 weeks followed by 4 week use of a 2.5 cm heel lift and exercise program to strengthen the gastrocnemius and soleus. Some studies have found decrease in plantar flexion strength in patients treated conservatively compared with those who underwent surgery. As a result, surgical repair is usually recommended for younger athletic patients who want to optimize their strength in the injured leg.

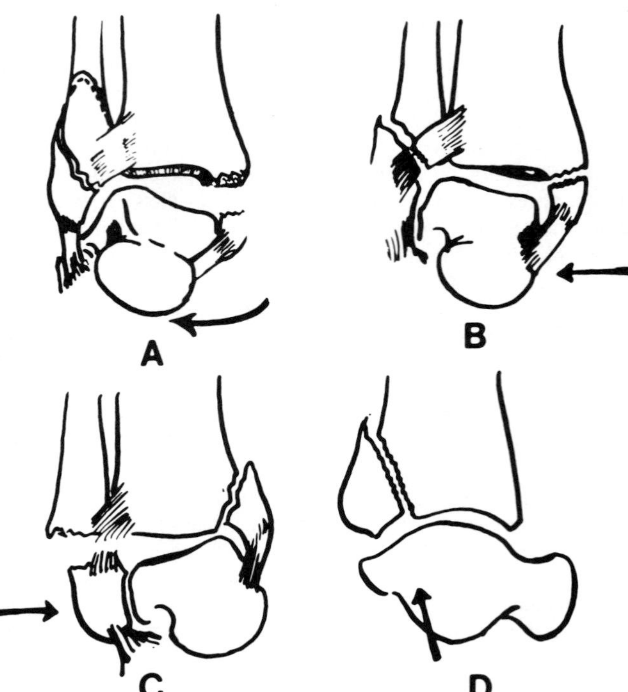

Fig. 184-3. Basic mechanisms of ankle injury with the characteristic fractures produced by each. **A.** External rotation. **B.** Abduction. **C.** Adduction. **D.** Vertical compression. [From Wilson FC: Fractures and dislocations of the ankle, in Rockwood CA Jr, Green DP (eds): *Fractures.* Philadelphia, Lippincott, 1975, vol 2, p 1369. Used by permission.]

ANKLE FRACTURE

Fractures are caused by forces acting upon the ankle joint that produce disruption of the joint ring. After the mechanism of injury has been ascertained, standard roentgenograms are necessary for fracture diagnosis. Ligamentous avulsions will usually cause transverse malleolar fractures or small chip or pull-off fractures of the malleolus below the joint line. Shifting of the talus causes it to strike the opposite malleolus and may cause an oblique fracture, often with comminution on the side of the bone subjected to the compression force. This evidence allows for prediction of the mechanism of injury, which is important because injuring forces must be reversed for fracture reduction.

Ligamentous injuries often occur with fractures and have a more serious prognosis than the fracture itself.

Classification of Fractures

Wilson classifies ankle fractures by mechanism of injury, according to four primary forces: external rotation, abduction, adduction, and vertical compression (Fig. 184-3). Although convenient, this classification is limited in usefulness in that almost all ankle fractures occur as a result of a combination of the four forces.

External rotation. External rotation is usually associated with abduction, but it may be associated with other forces as well. Rotation at the ankle joint causes sequential injuries that are initiated on the medial side and extend laterally. Therefore, the first injury to occur is either a pull-off or a transverse fracture of the medial malleolus or rupture of the deltoid ligament. As the forces continue, the anterior tibiofibular ligament is ruptured. The talus then impacts upon the fibula and fractures it. Finally, the posterior tibial tubercle fractures, and the interosseous, posterior inferior tibiofibular, and the inferior transverse ligaments tear.

Abduction. Injuries to the ankle from abduction alone are less common but do occur. Again, the sequence of injury is medial to lateral but without a rotatory component. The initial injury is either a transverse or pull-off fracture of the medial malleolus or rupture of the deltoid ligament, the latter of which is the rarer of the two. This is followed by either a fracture of the fibula below the syndesmotic ligaments or a rupture of the syndesmotic ligaments. If the ligaments rupture before the fibula fractures, the fibula fractures near the junction of the middle and distal third of the fibula. Therefore, the shaft of the fibula must be visualized upon radiologic evaluation of such an injury.

Adduction. The third primary force is adduction, lateral to medial. This force is frequently an isolated event in contrast to the preceding two. The lateral collateral ligaments rupture, or cause a pull-off or a transverse fracture of the lateral malleolus. With the continuation of the force, the talus impacts upon the medial malleolus and causes a spiral fracture.

Vertical compression. Vertical compression is most often associated with the other forces in the production of ankle fractures; however, it may occasionally cause an isolated fracture. Depending upon the position of the talus in the mortise, vertical compression can cause an anterior or, rarely, a posterior marginal fracture of the tibia. Radiologic evaluation may demonstrate small fractures of the anterior or posterior lip of the tibia due to ligamentous pull-off, or larger vertical fractures through the articular surface of the tibia. Comminution is common with both anterior and posterior fractures, making anatomic reduction very difficult.

Other ankle fractures are intraarticular or osteochondral fractures of the talus, and avulsion fractures of the base of the fifth metatarsal that usually occur on the lateral aspect of the talus. If undetected, intraarticular fractures of the talus or osteochondritis dissecans can lead to loose bodies floating in the joint, and early degenerative arthritis.

Avulsion fractures of the base of the fifth metatarsal are probably one of the most commonly missed fractures. The history is an ankle injury due to plantar flexion and inversion. The peroneus brevis insertion at the base of the fifth metatarsal is stressed, resulting in a pull-off fracture. The base of the fifth metatarsal should be evident in proper radiologic examination of the ankle, but this is not necessarily always the case. The physician may not see the fracture if he or she does not suspect it. The epiphyseal plate of the base of fifth metatarsal can be differentiated from a pull-off fracture since the epiphyseal plate is usually oblique or longitudinal, while the fracture line is transverse.

Treatment

The goals of treatment of all ankle injuries, including fractures, are to restore the anatomic position of the talus in the mortise, return the joint line parallel to the ground, and ensure a smooth articular surface. These goals are achieved by immobilization or surgery. Most ankle injuries can be appropriately and adequately treated by immobilization. The primary indication for operative treatment is the inability to maintain anatomic positioning of the talus in relation to the ankle mortise.

Anatomic reduction is usually done by reversal of the injuring forces. Plantar flexion of the ankle in reduction of medial malleolar injuries should be avoided since the anterior fibers of the deltoid ligament are taut in this position, preventing positioning of the medial malleolus.

OTHER INJURIES OF THE ANKLE

Contusion

Direct trauma can produce contusion of the soft tissues or periosteum with swelling, discoloration, and point tenderness. Radiologic evaluation may demonstrate a cortical fracture in addition to soft tissue swelling. Treatment is symptomatic and consists of ice, a compression dressing, rest and elevation, and analgesics.

Tenosynovitis

Tenosynovitis is usually secondary to direct trauma or overuse of the tendons. The patient has tenderness and swelling in the localized area but may have crepitance of the tendon as it moves through the sheath. X-ray films are negative. Treatment is ice and rest, but partial immobilization and anti-inflammatory medication may be necessary.

Subluxation. Peroneal tendon subluxation or tear may result from a direct blow, with or without dorsiflexion and eversion. The peroneal retinaculum tears, and the tendons slip from their anatomic position. There may be an associated tenosynovitis. The patient usually complains of a clicking, slipping sensation, with pain and tenderness at the posterior lateral malleolus. The examining physician may feel or see displacement of the peroneus musculature upon contraction of the muscle group.

Achilles tendon injuries are common in runners and joggers. They are usually seen in the older individual but may be seen in the young. The patient gives a history of direct trauma or repetitive irritation to the area with symptoms of swelling and tenderness over the Achilles tendon or at its insertion. Treatment is rest, shortening of the Achilles tendon by heel elevation, and anti-inflammatory medication. In the younger individual, the Achilles tendon may rupture due to intense athletic activity. Such an injury is disabling and requires immediate orthopedic consultation and surgery in most instances.

ANKLE INJURIES IN CHILDREN

In adolescents over 15 to 16 years old, epiphyseal plates are closing or have already closed, so the adult types of fractures occur in this population. In children, the ligamentous injuries are rare because the ligaments are stronger than the bone. This causes fractures to occur at the epiphyseal plates. The mechanism of injury usually involves indirect forces, most commonly inversion or eversion. Direct injuries are rare. The Salter-Harris classification is the most common classification utilized to describe these fractures. The patients present with the usual findings associated with fractures. On palpation, the patient is maximally tender over the injured growth plate. Standard x-ray evaluation is important in these patients. More importantly, the entire tibia and fibula should be included in any radiographic evaluation to rule out high fibular fractures. Occasionally, the Salter-Harris type I and II injuries are difficult to see on the radiographs because of minimal displacement. The physician must be careful to inspect the films for soft tissue swelling which would occur over the fracture area. The treatment for the majority of these fractures is conservative, and minimal complications occur. If a complication does occur, it is usually a disturbance of the growth plate, resulting in angular deformities and leg length changes.

COMPLICATIONS

There are a number of complications associated with ankle injuries, especially if they are improperly treated.

Nonunion occurs in 10 to 15 percent of fractures of the medial malleolus treated by a closed method. If it occurs, surgical correction is required.

Malunion can occur at any fracture site. If the patient is symptomatic and arthritic changes are not significant, surgery to correct the malunion may be done. Such surgery is often unsuccessful. Fusion may be the treatment of choice if there is degenerative or traumatic arthritis, or if the surgery has not been successful.

Infections are a complication of open fractures or the surgical treatment of closed fractures.

Traumatic arthritis occurs in 20 to 40 percent of ankle fractures regardless of the methods of treatment, but it is more common in inappropriately treated injuries. Loss of either the anterior or posterior tibial vessels may result in tissue destruction. The best treatment of possible neurovascular injuries is prophylaxis. Sudeck's atrophy secondary to sympathetic dystrophy is a complication of ankle injuries. Synostosis, or ossification of the interosseous membrane, may follow injuries to the syndesmotic ligaments, resulting in stiffness of the ankle joint. Finally, instability of the talus in the mortise is the most feared sequela. The loss of the support function of the ligaments predisposes the patient to recurrent sprains, resulting from progressively less trauma. This is especially disabling in athletes.

BIBLIOGRAPHY

Anderson JE: *Grant's Atlas of Anatomy*, ed 7. Baltimore, Williams & Wilkins, 1978.

Dias LS: Fractures of the tibia and fibula, in Rockwood CA Jr., Wilkins KE, King RE (eds): *Fractures in Children*. Philadelphia, Lippincott, 1984, vol 3, pp 1014–1032.

Simon RR, Koenigsknecht SJ: *Orthopaedics in Emergency Medicine: The Extremities*, 2d ed. New York, Appleton-Century-Crofts, 1989.

Wilson FC: Fractures and dislocations of the ankle, in Rockwood CA Jr, Green DP (eds): *Fractures in Adults*, ed 2. Philadelphia, Lippincott, 1984, vol 2, pp 1665–1703.

185
FOOT INJURIES

Joseph F. Waeckerle

The foot bears the weight of the body, and any injuries to it are magnified because of tremendous stress. The patient with an injured foot becomes debilitated to the point of not being able to bear weight, or to function properly. Loss of mobility of the joints of the foot as well as pain at the fracture site and subsequent arthritis may cause the patient discomfort and disability seemingly out of proportion to the injury sustained. It behooves the physician treating the patient with a foot injury to minimize disability by appropriately treating the bone and soft tissue injuries from the beginning.

The mechanisms of injury resulting in fractures and soft tissue damage to the foot include direct and indirect trauma as well as overuse, or stress, injuries. An adequate history will often help the physician determine the location of the injury and predict what injuries might be seen. This is important because radiographic evaluation of the foot is sometimes very difficult due to the many overlying bony shadows, secondary ossification centers, and sesamoid bones. Comparison views with the opposite foot are often essential to properly evaluate an injured foot.

Classification of the fractured foot is complex, and it is beyond the scope of this chapter to present a detailed classification or complete discussion of all fractures of the foot. The following discussion will touch upon the more common injuries seen. For more detail the reader is referred to the texts which discuss fractures and dislocations.

ANATOMY

The foot consists of the hindpart, which is made up of the calcaneus and talus; the midpart, which is separated from the hindpart by Chopart's joint and consists of the navicular, cuboid, and cuneiforms; and the forepart, which is separated from the midpart by Lisfranc's joint and consists of the metatarsals and phalanges. There are 28 bones, 57 major articular surfaces, and many ligaments as well as tendons and other soft tissues that contribute to the stability and integrity of the foot.

Following are some major points to keep in mind. (1) The long arch of the foot depends upon the position and alignment of the bones and not the soft tissue as commonly believed. (2) Weight bearing on the foot causes an equal distribution of forces between the heel and forepart. (3) The first metatarsal head bears two times as much weight as the other metatarsal heads. This is important because treatment of great toe injuries, especially of the metatarsal head, requires a more conservative approach. (4) Lastly, when a push-off force on the foot occurs, the maximum load is borne by the second metatarsal. With repeated pushing off, stress fractures of the second metatarsal may be seen. Some stress fractures of the third metatarsal may also be seen because, after the second metatarsal, it bears more weight than the others during the push-off, or acceleration, phase.

CALCANEAL FRACTURES

The calcaneus is the largest of the tarsal bones in the foot and functions as the base for locomotion and support of the weight of the body. It is the most often fractured of the tarsal bones, being involved in some 60 percent of such injuries. The difficulty with calcaneal fracture is that there is no optimal treatment, and, therefore, a good result is not often obtained. Calcaneal fractures are usually classified as fractures involving the processes or tuberosity, and fractures involving the body. The mechanism of injury is usually compression.

Because the patient must sustain a significant compression force to fracture the calcaneus, associated injuries are not uncommon; 10 percent of all calcaneal fractures are associated with lumbar compression injuries, and 26 percent are associated with other injuries to the extremity. Thus it is important to get a good history of the mechanism of injury. Also, the physician must examine the patient for injuries associated with the calcaneal fracture, including back, pelvic, hip, and knee injuries. The symptoms and signs associated with calcaneal fractures are directly proportional to the location and severity of the injury to the calcaneus as well as other associated injuries. Generally, the patient will experience swelling, pain, and ecchymoses at the fracture site. Often the fracture site will be exquisitely tender locally, with decreased range of motion and the inability to bear any weight on the fracture.

Standard radiographic views of the foot which consist of three different views may not be sufficient in evaluating calcaneal fractures, but should be ordered initially. Besides the AP, lateral, and axial views, certain "scout films" may be required to specifically delineate various fracture sites of the calcaneus. It is essential that, in evaluating calcaneal fractures, the x-ray films demonstrate good trabecular detail.

Treatment

As with all fractures, the objective in treating the patient is to restore normal anatomy and function as quickly as possible. This requires a great deal of skill and expertise with most calcaneal fractures; therefore, a consultant should be called in early in the management of the case. If the patient has gross swelling or is unstable, conservative treatment with a posterior splint providing immobilization, as well as attention to the soft tissue swelling and injuries, is imperative. In all instances, reduction of the calcaneal fracture to the closest anatomic position should be done as soon as possible by the consultant.

TALUS FRACTURES

Although talus fractures are the second most common foot fracture, they are still relatively uncommon. The talus is held in place by ligaments surrounding it and has no muscular attachments. Because most of the talus is covered by articular cartilage, the blood supply is tenuous and enters by way of the ligamentous and capsular support to the bone. Therefore, fractures of the talus, especially of the neck, associated with body dislocations, may cause avascular necrosis of the bone. The mechanism of injury which produces a talus fracture dislocation is usually hyperextension. The patient complains of intense pain and is unable to bear weight. There is localized swelling, discoloration, and tenderness to palpation. Moreover, there is an obvious loss of the normal contour of the foot. Any range of motion is intensely painful to the patient. X-ray evaluation for suspected talus fractures usually requires routine views of the foot. In certain instances, more detailed and specific x-ray views may be ordered.

Treatment

Treatment of talus injuries depends somewhat upon the extent of the fracture. Simple, nondisplaced minor chips or avulsion fractures require immobilization as well as ice, elevation, and follow-up. These patients do not usually have long-term complications. In contrast, fractures of the neck and body, or fracture dislocation of the talus, may be very difficult to treat, causing extensive problems for both the patient and the physician in the long run. In such instances, besides assessing neurovascular status of the foot and adequately evaluating and immobilizing the injury, the emergency physician should seek consultation for further care.

MIDPART FRACTURES

The midpart of the foot is infrequently fractured, but if it is injured, multiple fractures may occur. This area of the foot is most susceptible to direct trauma because it is the least mobile portion of the foot and includes five tarsal bones and all their articular surfaces and ligamentous support. Due to the many articulating surfaces, injuries to the midpart of the foot are associated with subluxation and/or dislocation. If the physician encounters an isolated midfoot fracture, it is most often of the navicular bone. Injuries to the cuboid and cuneiforms occur in combination with injuries to the navicular or one another and are usually the result of a crushing-type injury. Various classifications are used to describe injuries to the midfoot. Such injuries are divided into those to the navicular and those to the other bones.

Symptoms and signs are similar to those of other orthopedic-type injuries. That is, the patient presents with pain, swelling, and tenderness over the involved area. The standard x-ray views (AP, lateral, and oblique) are generally adequate to demonstrate most injuries in this area.

Treatment

The treatment is ice, elevation, and immobilization if there is no displacement and the anatomic position is acceptable. If not, then consultation for further closed reduction or open reduction-internal fixation are required so that the patient can achieve and maintain as close to anatomic reduction as possible.

TARSAL-METATARSAL FRACTURE/DISLOCATIONS

The tarsal-metatarsal joint is referred to as Lisfranc's joint. Injuries to this area are uncommon and are usually caused by automobile accidents. The mechanism of injury is complicated and varied but is usually a severe hyperextension of the forefoot on the midfoot, causing dorsal dislocation. There may be associated fractures. Such injuries occur because ligamentous support is the stabilizing support to this joint. The keystone of this joint is the second metatarsal; it is the locking mechanism of the midpart of the foot. Therefore, a fracture at the base of the second metatarsal is almost pathognomonic of a disrupted joint. Symptoms and signs are pain, swelling, discoloration, loss of range of motion, loss of weight bearing, and possibly some paresthesia in the midpart of the foot. X-ray views needed are the standard three views, but a comparison view with the opposite side is almost mandatory to properly evaluate the patient.

Treatment

The treatment of this fracture/dislocation is very difficult because complete restoration of position by closed reduction requires strong traction. In fact, correction of this deformity may require open reduction and internal fixation. Therefore, it is important to get the consulting surgeon involved in the case as early as possible.

METATARSAL FRACTURES

The second and third metatarsals are relatively fixed because of their anatomic configuration and are subjected to a great deal of stress, especially during the push-off phase of running or walking. In contrast, the first, fourth, and fifth metatarsals are relatively mobile. The significance of this is that excessive stress over a period of time can result in the development of stress fractures usually occurring in the second and third metatarsals. Other mechanisms of injury to the metatarsals are direct trauma or crush injuries and occasionally indirect force such as twisting-type injury. Because the direct trauma or crush injury is usually fairly significant, frequently more than one metatarsal is fractured. Moreover, associated soft tissue injuries with severe swelling and possible vascular compromise may occur.

Metatarsal fractures are divided into neck fractures and shaft fractures. Specific mention should be made of the pull-off fracture of the base of the fifth metatarsal, which is commonly called the ballet dancer's fracture. This injury is usually due to plantar flexion and inversion, resulting in the peroneus brevis tendon pulling off a portion of the bone where it inserts. This specific fracture may often be confused with a ligamentous injury to the ankle. It behooves the physician, when evaluating lateral ankle injuries, to include in the x-ray views the base of the fifth metatarsal to ensure that this fracture has not occurred.

Patients who experience metatarsal fractures present with typical findings but especially local tenderness. The x-ray evaluation consists of the three standard views of the foot and usually does not require any further x-ray evaluation.

Treatment

Treatment for metatarsal fractures is ice, elevation, analgesics, and noncircumferential immobilization. A cast should not be applied to these patients before 24 to 48 h because severe swelling may be associated with the crushing type injury which caused the fracture. Once the swelling goes down, a short leg cast should be applied for 4 to 6 weeks.

Fractures at Base of Fifth Metatarsal

Fractures at the base of the fifth metatarsal are by far the most common of the metatarsal fractures. These patients will specifically present with local tenderness over the fracture site. As mentioned earlier, this injury is often confused with lateral ligamentous sprain to the ankle, and it is important that the base of the fifth metatarsal be visualized in x-ray views of the ankle to rule out such fracture. Moreover, the physician must keep in mind that this is a secondary growth center or apophysis and that oblique and transverse fractures may be confused with the growth center. The treatment for this fracture is usually conservative and consists of taping, a postoperative or fracture shoe, and crutches for a short period of time.

Special mention should be made of the Jones fracture, which was formerly described as an avulsion fracture of the base of the fifth metatarsal. Recently it has been reported that this is, in fact, a fracture of the diaphysis and not an avulsion-type injury. This is an important distinction because true Jones fractures have a higher incidence of nonunion or delayed union in both children and adults, in contrast to the more common avulsion fracture.

Stress Fractures

Brief mention should be made of stress fractures to the second and third metatarsal; such fractures usually occur proximal to the head. These fractures are usually insidious in onset and may not appear on x-ray films for 2 to 3 weeks after their occurrence. The physician may treat the patient as if he or she has a stress fracture, even though it is not present on x-ray films, and then re-x-ray the patient 2 or 3 weeks later, or perform a bone scan which will usually delineate the fracture site. Treatment for stress fractures is rest or, occasionally, immobilization.

PHALANGEAL INJURIES

Injuries to the phalanx are common and usually result from direct trauma. Such injuries consist of both fractures and fracture dislocations. The majority of phalanx fractures are the result of a direct trauma, such as dropping a heavy object on the toes. An indirect mechanism causing fractures is hyperextension; an indirect mechanism causing dislocations is compression with dorsiflexion of the proximal phalanx.

The patient presents with pain, swelling, and discomfort, especially when wearing shoes and walking, within a few hours after an injury to the phalanx and/or its joints. In some instances when a dislocation or subluxation has occurred there is obvious deformity, but this may not always be the case because swelling may be significant enough to mask the deformity. X-ray evaluation is usually best in the AP and oblique views.

Treatment

Treatment is similar to that of all other fractures; that is, reduction of the subluxation or dislocation and reduction of the fracture to its most anatomically correct position and then ice, elevation, and immobilization. Immobilization can occur through dynamic splinting (so-called buddy taping), a postoperative shoe, or in certain instances a walking boot cast. Because the great toe bears one-third of the body weight of that side, it may need more extensive immobilization such as is provided by the walking boot cast. Displaced phalangeal fractures which are irreducible because of their instability may require internal fixation and, therefore, early referral. Open phalangeal fractures demand adequate soft tissue treatment, and early referral is strongly recommended for them as well. If the injury, whether it be a fracture or dislocation, is resistant to attempts at closed reduction to achieve anatomic position, referral to the orthopedic specialist is recommended because of the possible long-term sequelae.

FOOT INJURIES IN CHILDREN

Fractures of the foot are unusual in children because of the pliability of the bone and cartilage, but they are usually easy to treat. Specific mention will be made of some of the more common injuries.

Talus fractures, although rare, are being recognized more frequently. These usually occur secondary to a forced dorsiflexion-type injury. The symptoms and signs, x-ray views, and treatment are similar to those of adults, but there is a greater incidence of avascular necrosis in children. Calcaneal fractures are not a major problem in children and are associated with minimal complications. Isolated midpart foot fractures are unusual in children. They are usually associated with other injuries of the midpart of the foot, indicating that a major injury has occurred. Tarsal-metatarsal injuries of the foot, while rare, are more common than generally recognized. They occur because of indirect injuries produced by significant forces, usually plantar flexion. The symptoms, signs, x-ray evaluation, and treatment are similar to those of adults. Fractures of the base of the second metatarsal indicate disruption to the tarsal-metatarsal joint, a sign that the patient has suffered a significant injury. The proper treatment is good anatomic reduction, which, in certain instances, may require fixation devices. Metatarsal fractures are common in children. They may be the result of torque-type forces causing fractures of the neck, or direct injuries such as crush forces causing fractures of the shaft. The symptoms, signs, and x-ray evaluation are similar to those of adults. The treatment is closed, and the complications are minimal with an occasional compartment syndrome seen.

Fractures of the base of the fifth metatarsal are relatively common in children. In the past these fractures were felt to be the result of a ''pull-off'' of the peroneous brevis insertion. Recently, however, the abductor digiti minimi and lateral component of the plantar aponeuroses have been implicated in this fracture. On radiographic examination, the fracture is usually seen perpendicular to the longitudinal axis of the bone. It must be distinguished from the apophysis and the sesamoid bone, os vesalianum. The treatment is conservative, and the complications are minimal.

Phalangeal injuries are very uncommon in children, because their bone and cartilage, as well as soft tissues, are very pliable. If they occur, they are usually the result of direct trauma. These fractures should be treated conservatively, with the major goal being to prevent malrotation-type deformities similar to those of phalangeal injuries of the hand.

BIBLIOGRAPHY

Gross RH: Fractures and dislocations of the foot, in Rockwood CA Jr, Wilkins KE, King RE (eds): *Fractures in Children*. Philadelphia, Lippincott, 1984, vol 3, pp 1043–1105.

Heckman JD: Fractures and dislocations of the foot, in Rockwood CA Jr, Green DP (eds): *Fractures in Adults*. Philadelphia, Lippincott, 1984, vol 2, pp 1703–1820.

Simon RR, Koenigsknecht SJ: *Orthopaedics in Emergency Medicine: The Extremities*, 2d ed. New York, Appleton-Century-Crofts, 1989.

186
COMPARTMENT SYNDROMES

Robert R. Simon
Ernest Ruiz

Compartment syndromes are among the most potentially devastating problems presenting to emergency departments. Early diagnosis and treatment are curative, while delay results in permanent and severe disability. An understanding of the pathophysiology and the early signs of the process is crucial if the emergency physician is to intercede appropriately.

PATHOPHYSIOLOGY

Simply stated, compartment syndromes are due to increased pressure within closed tissue spaces which compromises the flow of blood through nutrient capillaries in muscles and nerves. The complex relationships between time, Starling forces, and systemic and venous pressure are not completely understood. The clinical variables of each case make a definitive explanation of how capillary blood flow is compromised a difficult, if not impossible, exercise. A discussion of these variables is beyond the scope of this text, but the reader is encouraged to read the text and articles cited in the bibliography.

Table 186-1. Classification of Acute Compartment Syndromes

I. Decreased compartment size
  A. Constrictive dressings and casts
  B. Closure of fascial defects
  C. Thermal injuries and frostbite
II. Increased compartment contents
  A. Primarily edematous accumulation
    1. Postischemic swelling
      a. Arterial injuries
      b. Arterial thrombosis or embolism
      c. Reconstructive vascular and bypass surgery
      d. Replantation
      e. Prolonged tourniquet time
      f. Arterial spasm
      g. Cardiac catheterization and angiography
      h. Ergotamine ingestion
    2. Prolonged immobilization with limb compression
      a. Drug overdose with limb compression
      b. General anesthesia with knee-chest position
    3. Thermal injuries and frostbite
    4. Exertion
    5. Venous disease
    6. Venomous snakebite
  B. Primarily hemorrhagic accumulation
    1. Hereditary bleeding disorders, e.g., hemophilia
    2. Anticoagulant therapy
    3. Vessel laceration
  C. Combination of edematous and hemorrhagic accumulation
    1. Fractures
      a. Tibia
      b. Forearm
      c. Elbow, e.g., supracondylar
      d. Femur
    2. Soft tissue injury
    3. Osteotomies, e.g., tibia
  D. Miscellaneous
    1. Intravenous infiltration, e.g., blood, saline
    2. Popliteal cyst
    3. Long leg brace

Source. From Mubarak SJ, Hargens AR: *Compartment Syndromes and Volkmann's Contracture*. Philadelphia, Saunders, 1981. Used by permission.

Normal tissue pressure is about zero and usually less than 10 mmHg. Capillary blood flow within the compartment is compromised at pressures greater than about 20 mmHg, and muscle and nerves are at risk for ischemic necrosis at pressures greater than about 30 to 40 mmHg. Of the tissues within the compartments, muscle is most sensitive followed by nerve tissue. Blood flow through arteries, arterioles, and collaterals is not compromised significantly at these pressures. Nevertheless, tissues within the compartment that are dependent on the nutrient capillaries become ischemic and then necrotic if the compartment pressure is not reduced promptly. By the time that distal pulses are reduced, muscle necrosis has occurred. Ischemic muscles hurt, and this pain is exacerbated by active muscle contraction and passive stretching of the muscle.

An increase in compartmental pressure can be caused by (1) compression of the compartment, for example, by burn eschar, a circumferential cast, or a pneumatic pressure garment, and (2) by a volume increase within the compartment due to hematoma and edema. Direct trauma with resulting bleeding and edema is probably the most common cause, but overexertion (shin splints) and limb compression as a result of alcohol or drug overdose are also common causes. Mubarak has developed a classification of the acute compartment syndromes (Table 186-1) listing the myriad of possible causes.

COMPARTMENTS AT RISK

Virtually any muscle mass invested in fascia is at risk given the right conditions. The compartments clinically relevant to the emergency physician are the upper extremity and the lower extremity.

Upper Extremity

The upper arm has an anterior and a posterior compartment. The anterior compartment contains the biceps-brachialis muscle and the

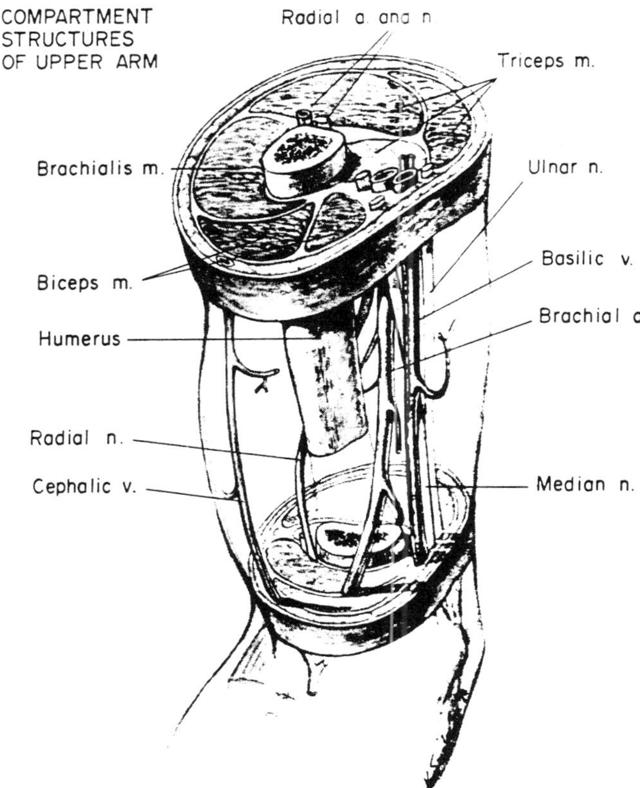

Fig. 186-1. The biceps-brachialis (anterior) and triceps (posterior) compartments of the right arm. (From Mubarak SJ, Hargens AR: *Compartment Syndromes and Volkmann's Contracture*. Philadelphia, Saunders, 1981. Used by permission.)

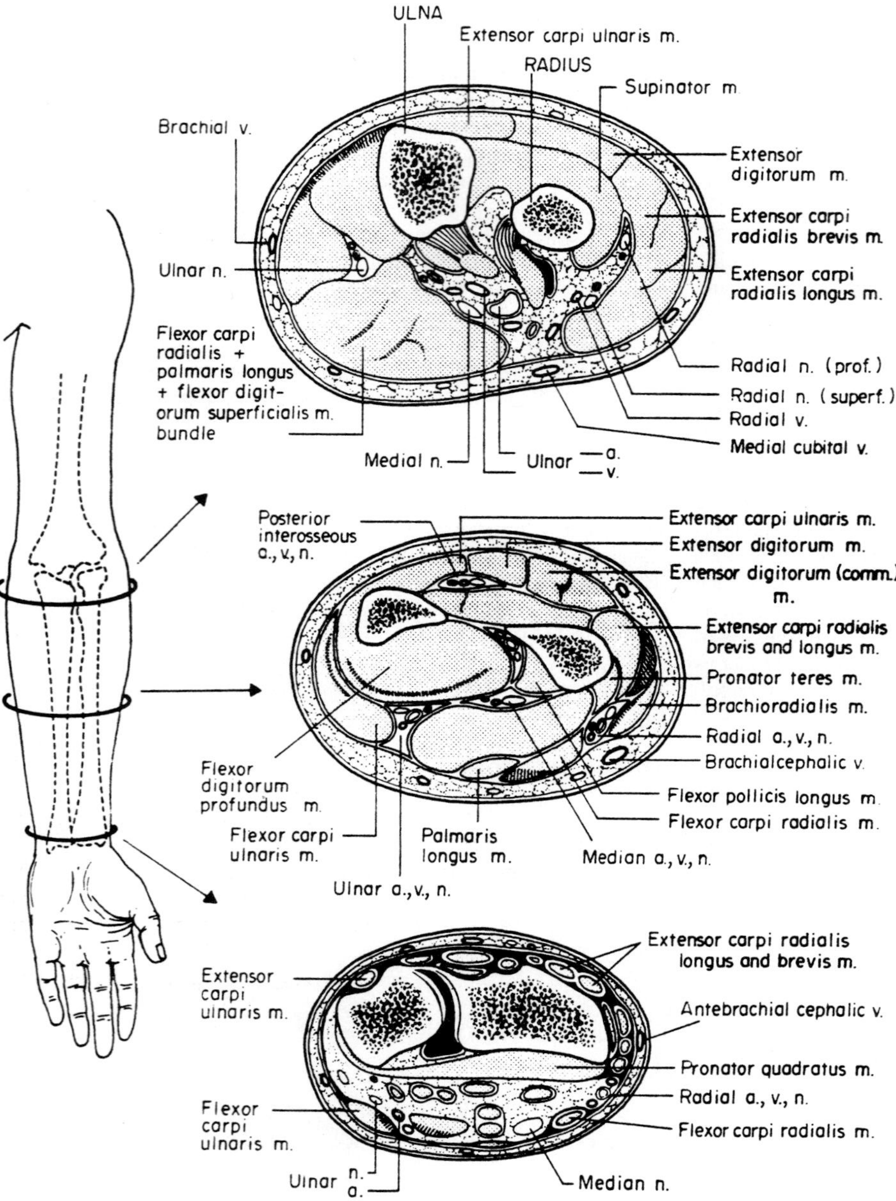

Fig. 186-2. Forearm compartments: transverse sections through the left forearm at various levels. (From Mubarak SJ, Hargens AR: *Compartment Syndromes and Volkmann's Contracture*. Philadelphia, Saunders, 1981. Used by permission.)

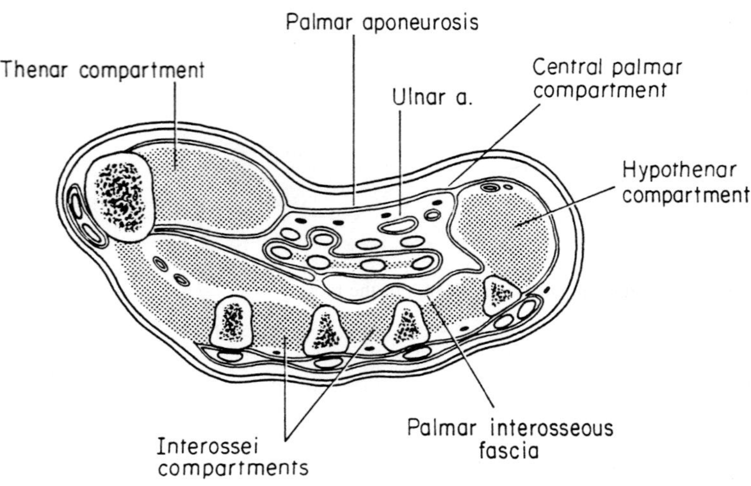

Fig. 186-3. Hand Compartments: transverse section through the right hand. (From Mubarak SJ, Hargens AR: *Compartment Syndromes and Volkmann's Contracture*. Philadelphia, Saunders, 1981. Used by permission.)

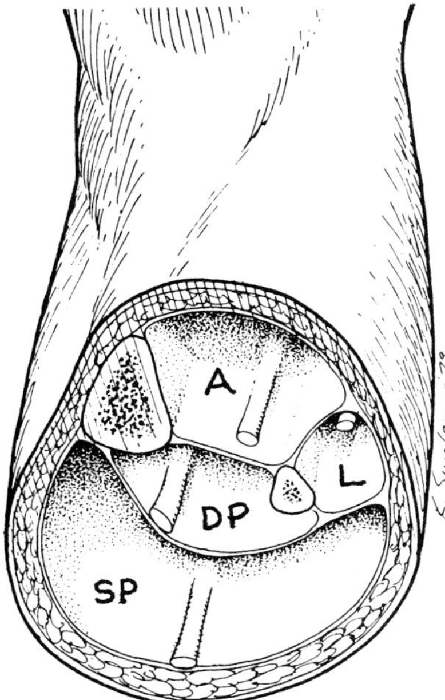

Fig. 186-4. The four compartments of the leg. (From Mubarak SJ, Hargens AR: *Compartment Syndromes and Volkmann's Contracture.* Philadelphia, Saunders, 1981. Used by permission.)

ulnar, median, and radial nerves (Fig. 186-1). The posterior compartment contains the triceps muscle. The forearm has volar and dorsal compartments that are further subdivided into smaller compartments by investing fascia at mid-forearm (Fig. 186-2). The volar compartment contains wrist and finger flexors, and the dorsal compartment contains wrist and finger extenders. The hand has thenar and hypothenar compartments, containing the intrinsic muscles of the thumb and little finger, respectively. The interosseous muscles of the hand are contained in their own compartments (Fig. 186-3).

Lower Extremity

There are three gluteal compartments of the buttocks. One contains the tensor muscle of the fascia lata, another the gluteus medius and minimus, and the third the gluteus maximus. The sciatic nerve lies adjacent to the gluteus maximus and can be compressed by it. The thigh has an anterior compartment containing the quadriceps group and a posterior compartment containing the hamstring group of muscles as well as the sciatic nerve. The leg has four compartments (Fig. 186-4). The anterior compartment, the compartment most frequently involved by this syndrome, contains the tibialis anterior muscle and the extensor muscles of the toes. The lateral compartment contains the evertors of the foot, the peroneous longus and peroneous brevis, and the peroneal nerve. The superficial posterior compartment contains the gastrocnemius and the soleus muscles and the sural nerve. The deep posterior compartment contains the tibialis posterior and the flexors of the toes.

DIAGNOSIS

The history, including mechanism of injury, is very important since many patients at risk for the syndrome are severely ill or injured and cannot relate whether or not they are experiencing pain. Palpation of the compartments in question may or may not reveal tenseness and swelling; when in doubt, the resuscitating physician should measure tissue pressure.

Alert and intact patients will virtually always relate that they are experiencing severe and constant pain over the involved compartment. Palpation of the compartment will also elicit pain. Active contraction of the involved muscles will increase the pain, as will passive stretching of the muscles (Table 186-2). Hypoesthesia resulting from compromise of nerves traversing the involved compartment appears later than muscle weakness and pain.

Possible compartment syndromes associated with injuries such as fractures or penetrating wounds should prompt an immediate surgical consultation, since the presence of a compartment syndrome may influence subsequent treatment choices.

In patients without a clear need for surgical consultation, measuring

Table 186-2. Symptomatology of Acute Compartment Syndromes

UPPER EXTREMITY	
Upper arm	
Anterior compartment	Pain on active and passive flexion and extension of the elbow Hypoesthesia in the distribution of the median, ulnar, and radial nerves
Posterior compartment	Pain on active and passive flexion and extension of the elbow Hypoesthesia over the dorsum of the hand
Forearm	
Volar compartment	Pain on active and passive flexion and extension of the fingers Hypoesthesia over the palm of the hand
Dorsal compartment	Pain on active and passive flexion and extension of the fingers
Hand	
Thenar and hypothenar compartments	Pain on thumb and little finger opposition
Interosseous compartments	Pain on abduction and adduction of the fingers
LOWER EXTREMITY	
Gluteal compartments	Pain on active and passive flexion and extension of the hip Sciatic nerve paresthesias
Thigh compartments	Pain on active and passive flexion and extension of the knee Sciatic nerve paresthesias with posterior compartment involvement
Leg	
Anterior compartment	Pain on active and passive dorsiflexion and plantar flexion of the foot Hypoesthesia of the first web space
Lateral compartment	Pain on active and passive eversion and inversion of the foot Hypoesthesia of the first web space
Superficial posterior compartment	Pain on active and passive plantar flexion and dorsiflexion of the foot Hypoesthesia of the lateral foot
Deep posterior compartment	Pain on dorsiflexing the toes and everting the foot Hypoesthesia of the plantar surface of the foot

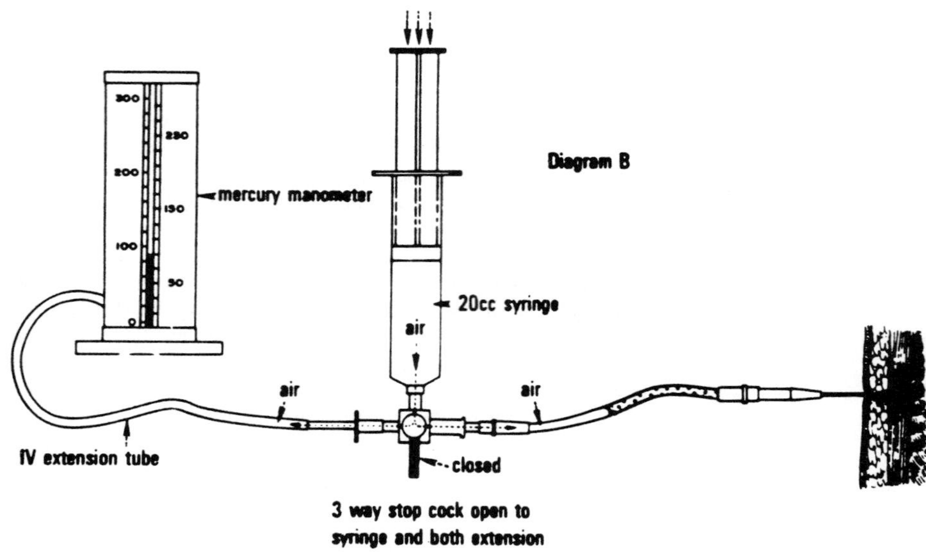

Fig. 186-5. The tissue pressure is measured by determining the amount of pressure within this closed system which is required to overcome the pressure within the closed compartment and inject a minute quantity of saline. (From Whitesides TE, Haney TC, Morimoto K, et al: Tissue pressure measurements as a determinant for the need of fasciotomy. *Clin Orthop* 113:43, 1975. Used by permission.)

the compartment pressures in the emergency department assures safe patient disposition and management. Compartment pressure can be quickly and easily measured using a commercially available battery-powered monitor (Stryker S.T.I.C. Monitor). Pressure is measured after careful aseptic preparation and insertion of an 18-gauge needle into the compartment. Alternatively, compartment pressure can be measured using the following supplies, available in any emergency department: a 20-mL syringe, two IV extension tubes, a three-way stopcock, a small bottle of sterile saline, a mercury manometer, and an 18-gauge needle. They should be assembled as shown in Fig. 186-5. The bottle of saline is vented with an 18-gauge needle and the needle on the apparatus is then inserted into the saline and saline withdrawn until the IV extension is half filled. When removing the needle from the saline bottle, it is important to avoid getting any air in the needle. The needle is then placed in the compartment and the apparatus kept at the level of the needle and the stopcock turned so that it is open in all three directions. Two people are required for this test. One watches the manometer while the other slowly depresses the plunger in the syringe while watching the saline meniscus. When the meniscus moves toward the patient, the operator notifies the manometer watcher, who notes the reading at that instant. In this way, only a minute amount of saline is injected into the compartment. Occasionally, the needle may be inserted into a tendon or investing fascia, resulting in a false high reading. For that reason, the test should be repeated to confirm elevated readings. Low readings are reliable.

MANAGEMENT

Compartment pressures between 15 and 20 are problematic. If the problem is acute and the patient is reliable, the patient can be told to return for repeat measurement if symptoms do not improve. A pressure of 20 mmHg can be damaging if it persists for several hours; therefore, admission or surgical consultation will be needed for unreliable patients. Pressures greater than 20 mmHg demand admission and surgical consultation. A pressure of 30 to 40 mmHg is generally considered grounds for emergent fasciotomy in the operating room. Fasciotomy is accomplished by making a longitudinal skin incision over the compartment. The underlying fascia is then split the length of the compartment, allowing the contained muscle to expand.

BIBLIOGRAPHY

Aprahamian C, Gessert G, Bandyk DF, et al: MAST-associated compartment syndrome (MACS): A review. *J Trauma* 29:549, 1989.

Mubarak SJ, Hargens AR: *Compartment Syndromes and Volkmann's Contracture*. Philadelphia, Saunders, 1981.

Whitesides TE, Haney TC, Morimoto K, et al: Tissue pressure measurement as a determinant for the need for fasciotomy. *Clin Orthop* 113:43, 1975.

187
WOUND BALLISTICS

Jeremy J. Hollerman
Martin L. Fackler

An understanding of wound ballistics allows the physician to evaluate and treat missile wounds without repeating the errors of conventional "wisdom." The medical literature contains many papers suggesting harmful and unnecessary treatment for gunshot wounds based on common misconceptions about wound ballistics. An example of such an unnecessary and harmful recommendation is for mandatory surgical excision of the tissue surrounding the wound tract (the path of the projectile through tissue) anytime an extremity wound is caused by a "high-velocity" bullet. This is based on the belief that these tissues will become necrotic. Clinical experience and research show this to be false.

Common misconceptions about wound ballistics include the following:

1. Missile velocity and missile kinetic energy are erroneously viewed as the main factors that determine the wound produced.
2. Kinetic energy transfer is erroneously believed to be the main mechanism of wounding. It is erroneously thought that all "high velocity" bullets wound mainly by the explosive effect of temporary cavity formation (*tissue stretch*).
3. It is incorrectly thought that there is a constant and fundamental difference between the wound produced by a "high-velocity" bullet and that produced by a "low-velocity" bullet.
4. A common misconception is that one wound path through tissue is much like another in terms of the effect a bullet will produce in tissue. The changes in the wound when the bullet contacts a large bone (versus if it had not) are often ignored. Whether the bullet is "low" or "high"-velocity is incorrectly thought to be the primary determinant of the severity of tissue damage. The properties of the specific tissues traversed and their relationship to the wound produced are often ignored.
5. Some erroneously believe that military bullets are more damaging to tissue than civilian bullets.
6. A frequent error in medical literature is the statement that when an undeformed bullet is present in tissue, its lack of deformation is diagnostic of the bullet's being jacketed.
7. Some erroneously believe that a round fired from a handgun will produce a bullet with the same ballistic properties as if that same round had been fired from a rifle. The influence of barrel length on bullet velocity is often ignored.
8. A common misconception is that rounds of the same caliber (bullet diameter) have the same wounding potential.
9. Some erroneously believe that bullets usually tumble in flight.
10. Some authors have the misconception that wound ballistics research conducted with small animals and spherical projectiles can accurately predict the tissue effect of bullets in humans. Some authors erroneously believe that, when using inanimate material to "catch" the bullet, recording media such as duct sealing compound, clay blocks, and soap blocks are as useful and accurate as properly calibrated ballistic gelatin.

To understand why these are misconceptions, one must understand the two mechanisms by which missiles wound tissue: crushing and stretching.

MECHANISMS OF WOUNDING

Both missile and tissue characteristics determine the nature of the wound. Missile characteristics are partly inherent (mass, shape, and construction) and are partly conferred by the weapon (longitudinal and rotational velocity). Tissue characteristics (elasticity, density, and anatomic relationships) also strongly affect the nature of the wound. The severity of a bullet wound is influenced by the bullet's orientation during its flight through tissue and by whether the bullet fragments or deforms (e.g., into the typical mushroom shape of the expanding hollow-point or soft-point bullet).

Two major mechanisms of wounding occur: the crushing of the tissue struck by the projectile (forming the permanent cavity) and the radial stretching of the projectile path walls (forming a temporary cavity; Fig. 187-1).

In addition, a sonic pressure wave precedes the projectile through tissue. The sonic pressure wave plays no part in wounding.

Crushing of Tissue

A missile crushes the tissue it strikes, thereby creating a permanent wound channel (permanent cavity). If the bullet is traveling with its pointed end forward and its long axis parallel to the longitudinal axis of flight (0° of yaw, which is the angle between the long axis of the bullet and its path of flight), it crushes a tube of tissue no greater than its approximate diameter. When the bullet yaws to 90°, the entire long axis of the bullet strikes tissue, and the amount crushed may be three times greater than at 0° of yaw.

When striking soft tissue with sufficient velocity, soft-point and hollow-point bullets deform into a mushroom shape. This increases surface area and the amount of tissue crushed. For most big-game hunting, such bullets are mandated by law. This is to increase the probability of prompt lethality, rather than creating a disabling but nonlethal wound, causing the animal prolonged suffering. If the mushroomed diameter is 2.5 times greater than the initial diameter of the bullet, the area of tissue crushed by the bullet is 6.25 times greater than the amount that would have been crushed by the undeformed bullet.

Bullet fragmentation also increases the volume of tissue crushed. After bullet fragmentation, surface area is increased, and much more tissue is crushed. For large handgun (e.g., a .44 magnum) and rifle bullets, the striking of bone is one of the causes of early bullet fragmentation.

Comminuted fracture may be created by rifle and large handgun bullets striking bone. Bone fragments can become secondary missiles, crushing tissue. Many handgun bullets are unable to significantly fragment bone. When a large bone is struck, it is likely that the bullet will expend its wounding potential in the patient and will not exit.

Bullet fragments and secondary missiles (bone fragments, teeth, dental fillings, coins, etc.) are likely to increase the severity of the wound. Multiple perforations weaken tissue and create focal points for stress (stress risers), which are particularly vulnerable to the effect of temporary cavitation stretch.

Unjacketed lead bullets cannot be driven faster than about 2000 ft/s (610 m/s) without some of the lead stripping off in the barrel. This is avoided if a jacket made of a harder metal (e.g., copper or a copper alloy) is used to surround the lead.

The jacket of a military bullet completely covers the bullet tip (a full metal jacket). Civilians often use hollow-point or soft-point bullets. Hollow-point bullets have a hole in the jacket at the bullet tip, and soft-point bullets have some of the lead core of the bullet exposed at the bullet tip. These constructions weaken the bullet tip, causing it to flatten on impact. This flattening often greatly exceeds bullet diameter, resulting in a mushroom-shaped projectile. This bullet expansion, termed mushrooming, increases diameter, causing more tissue to be crushed, making a larger hole (the permanent bullet tract) than would the original unexpanded bullet. Bullets of the hollow-point or soft-point variety are also more likely to fragment in tissue than are full metal jacket bullets, adding to tissue disruption. Therefore, the hollow-point and soft-point bullets used by civilians are often more damaging to tissue than military bullets fired from rounds otherwise configured identically. Because of this, wounds produced by civilian hunting rifles, shotguns, and large-caliber handguns are usually more severe than wounds produced by military rifle bullets.

When military full metal jacket bullets break and fragment, they do so as a result of yawing to 90°. The resulting stresses cause flattening of the sides of the bullet as if it had been squeezed in a vise. Full metal jacket bullets do not flatten at the bullet tip, as do soft-point or hollow-point bullets (they do not mushroom). Although the M-193 military bullet of the M16 rifle fragments in soft-tissue wounds with a characteristic pattern depending on range, most other full metal jacket military bullets, such as those fired from the AK-47, the AK-74, and the NATO 7.62-mm rifle (U.S. version), do not fragment unless they strike a large bone.

If a bullet is jacketed, the bullet jacket usually cannot be distinguished from the lead core on standard radiographs, since the entire bullet is metallic density. Occasionally, as the bullet deforms or fragments, the bullet jacket separates from the bullet and is visible on a radiograph.

In extremity wounds, when a radiograph reveals an undeformed bullet lying in the soft tissues and no fracture is present, tissue disruption is usually minor. However, if a major vessel or nerve is divided, even a simple wound can have a severe effect.

Although soft-point and hollow-point bullets from center-fire rifle rounds usually expand into a mushroom shape in tissue, increasing the volume of tissue crushed, even the magnum versions of some soft-point and hollow-point handgun bullets sometimes fail to expand. This is most likely with short-barreled handguns and those of less potent calibers (e.g., .25 and .32) because of slower bullet velocity. Overall, about one-third of soft-point and hollow-point handgun bullets fail to expand in human soft tissue.

The shorter the barrel length, the shorter the time available for bullet acceleration by the expanding gases created by burning gunpowder. Therefore, when identical rounds are fired, the gun with the shorter barrel produces a lower-velocity bullet. Its velocity may be too low to induce mushrooming after impact.

Temporary Cavitation (Tissue Stretch)

Fired from an appropriate and well-designed weapon, a bullet flies in air with its nose pointed forward; it yaws only 1 to 3°. Yaw occurs around the bullet's center of mass. In pointed rifle bullets, the center of mass is behind the midpoint of the bullet's long axis. Although the bullet's most naturally stable in-flight orientation would be with its heaviest part (its base) forward, for aerodynamically efficient flight it must fly point forward.

During flight, a bullet is stabilized against yaw by the spin imparted to it by the spiral grooves (rifling) in the gun barrel. The longer (and heavier) the bullet in relation to its diameter, the more rapidly it must be rotated to avoid significant yaw in flight. Therefore, a gun barrel intended to fire a heavier bullet has rifling that makes a full turn in fewer inches of barrel length than does the rifling in a barrel intended for a shorter, lighter bullet of the same caliber.

Although the bullet's spin is adequate to stabilize it against yaw in its flight through air, it is not adequate to stabilize it in its path through tissue, because of the higher density of the medium. If it does not deform, a pointed bullet eventually yaws to a base-forward position (180° of yaw). Expanding bullets lose the physical stimulus to yaw because after "mushrooming" their heaviest part is forward.

As a bullet passes through 90° of yaw, it is crushing the maximal amount of tissue (unless it fragments, which will crush more). It is slowed down rapidly as its wounding potential is used up moving tissue radially away from its path. This force creates the temporary cavity. This aspect of the wounding process is analogous to the splash of a diver entering the water.

If a diver enters the water very straight and point forward (similar to the point-forward configuration of a bullet at 0° of yaw), the splash may be minimal. If the diver does a belly-flop (similar to a bullet at 90° of yaw), a large splash is induced. In tissue, this splash, the temporary cavity, produces localized blunt trauma.

The maximal size of the temporary cavity occurs several milliseconds after the bullet has passed through the tissue. Because forces follow paths of least resistance, temporary cavitation is likely to be asymmetrical and spread out through tissue planes.

The temporary cavity caused by common handgun bullets is generally too small to be a significant wounding factor in all but the most sensitive tissues (brain and liver). Center-fire rifle bullets and large handgun bullets (e.g., .44 magnum) often induce a large temporary cavity [10–25-cm (4–10-in.) diameter] in tissue. This can be a significant wounding factor, depending on the characteristics of the tissue in which it forms.

Near-water density, less elastic tissue (e.g., brain, liver, or spleen), fluid-filled organs (including the heart, bladder, or gastrointestinal tract), and dense tissue (e.g., bone) may be damaged severely when a large temporary cavity contacts them or forms within them. More elastic tissue (e.g., skeletal muscle) and lower-density elastic tissue (e.g., lung) are less affected by the formation of a temporary cavity. Because of these tissue differences, transmitted blunt trauma from temporary cavitation caused by a bullet traveling 800 to 950 m/s can cause a more severe pulmonary contusion when the bullet traverses the chest wall musculature than the pulmonary contusion it would have caused if passing through the lung.

Although the formation of a large temporary cavity often has devastating effects in the brain or liver, its effect in wounds of the extremities has frequently been exaggerated. Fracture of large bones not hit by the bullet and tearing of major vessels or nerves by the temporary cavity are often mentioned in the literature but are rare in clinical experience. This includes a systematic review of 1400 rifle wounds sustained in the Vietnam conflict and analyzed in the Wound Data and Munitions Effectiveness Team (WDMET) study. Most of the permanent damage done in wounds of the extremities is the result of structures being hit by the intact bullet, bullet fragments, or secondary missiles. As in all blunt trauma, shear forces develop and tear structures at points where one side is fixed and the other side is free to move. The temporary cavity is no exception. In the unlikely event that the blunt trauma of the temporary cavity tears a vessel wall, this is particularly likely to occur at the vessel origin.

BALLISTIC PROPERTIES AND THE WOUND PRODUCED

Recent controlled animal experiments using military rifle bullets have clearly disproved the assertion that all tissue exposed to temporary cavitation is destroyed. These studies also show that, not only does the 14-cm-diameter temporary cavity produced by the AK-74 assault rifle not destroy a great amount of muscle, but the sizable stellate exit wound it causes in an uncomplicated thigh wound ensures excellent wound drainage, which assists healing. A history that the wound was caused by a "high-velocity" bullet does *not* mandate radical excision of the wound path.

The characteristics of the wounded tissue, the thickness of the body part, the point in the path of the bullet at which yaw or fragmentation occurs, and other factors strongly influence the wound produced. Bullets of equal wounding *potential* may produce wounds of quite different severity, depending on which tissues they traverse. The heavier, slower bullet crushes more tissue but induces less temporary cavitation. Most of the wounding potential of the lighter, faster bullet is likely to be used up forming a larger temporary cavity, but this bullet leaves a smaller permanent cavity. The heavier, slower bullet causes a more severe wound in elastic tissue than does the lighter, faster bullet, which uses up much of its potential producing tissue stretch (temporary cavitation). This tissue stretch may be absorbed with little or no ill effect by elastic tissue, such as lung or muscle. In less elastic tissue, such as liver or brain, the temporary cavity produced by the lighter, faster bullet can produce a more severe wound.

Experiments with ballistic gelatin (which reproduces the projectile deformation and penetration depth of living animal muscle) have shown that most full-metal-jacketed rifle bullets yaw significantly only at tissue depths greater than the diameter of human extremities. In the first 12 cm (the average thickness of an adult human thigh) of a soft-tissue wound path, there is often little or no difference between the wounding effect of low- and high-velocity bullets when the high-velocity bullet is of the military full metal jacket type. This is particularly true of the relatively heavier military rifle bullets, such as those fired by the AK-47 and NATO 7.62-mm (U.S. version) rifles. A wound of an extremity caused by an AK-47 bullet that does not hit bone is often similar to a handgun bullet wound. A soft- or hollow-point bullet fired from a civilian rifle deforms soon after entering tissue and produces a much more severe extremity wound. If a high-velocity, heavy bullet does not deform, fragment, or hit a bone, it may exit an extremity with much of its wounding potential unspent. These same bullets are often lethal in chest or abdominal wounds because the trunk is thicker than an extremity and allows the bullet a sufficiently long path through tissue to yaw. Maximal temporary cavitation induced by the AK-47 bullet usually occurs at a tissue depth of 28 cm, much greater than the diameter of a human extremity.

The more recently developed, smaller caliber AK-74 fires a bullet that is lighter than the AK-47 bullet and yaws earlier. Its maximal temporary cavity occurs at a tissue depth of 11 cm. Extremity wounds from the AK-74 can be expected to be more severe than those from the AK-47. The lighter, smaller AK-74 round allows a soldier to carry many more rounds of ammunition. This was the primary motivation for development of the M16 and the AK-74.

Caliber

Caliber (bullet diameter in decimals of an inch or in millimeters) is only one indicator of wounding potential and not a very good one (Fig. 187-1). Although the .22 long rifle bullet (.22 LR) and the M16 bullet (which is .224 caliber) ar similar in diameter (caliber), the M16 bullet is heavier (3.6 versus 2.7 g for the .22 LR bullet), mainly because the M16 bullet is longer. The M16 bullet, which is fired from a center-fire cartridge holding much more gunpowder, travels at much higher velocity than the .22 LR bullet. Because the M16 bullet fragments in tissue, because of its greater bullet mass, and because of its higher velocity [3094 ft/s (943 m/s) as opposed to 1122 ft/s (342 m/s) for the .22 LR bullet], the M16 bullet has the potential to cause a much more severe wound. If it traverses only extremity muscle, does not yaw, does not fragment, and does not hit a bone, the M16 may still produce a relatively minor ice-pick type extremity wound. Usually, the M16 produces a much larger permanent cavity and a much larger temporary cavity than does the .22 LR. The large temporary and permanent cavities formed by the M16 bullet occur mainly from 11 to 30 cm deep in tissue. Remember that the bullet has its highest velocity when it enters the tissue but forms a small wound channel at that point. Only when it fragments or yaws to 90° is its severe wounding effect realized. At that point, it is traveling slower and has less than its maximum velocity. Velocity is only one factor in wounding.

Unfortunately, commonly used weapon and bullet designations are often numerically incorrect. For example, the .38 special and the .357 magnum use bullets that have the same diameter [.357 in. (9.07 mm)]. These bullets are often exactly the same weight. The longer cartridge case of the magnum can hold more powder, giving the bullet higher velocity and greater wounding potential.

Assessment of Missile Type

On a radiograph, assessment of missile caliber is difficult because of magnification and missile deformation. If an undeformed bullet is seen in two views at 90° and its degree of magnification is known, it is possible to determine the approximate caliber of the bullet. The focus-object distance and focus-image distance (also known as the focus-film distance) must be known. This requires knowing the position of the bullet in the patient's body and its location relative to the film. Armed with this knowledge, one usually can distinguish an undeformed .22 from a .25 and a .38 from a .44, but probably cannot distinguish a .357 or .38 from a 9 mm because they are too similar in diameter.

Many radiographs show only fragments of the bullet and do not allow determination of the type of weapon and projectile causing the wound. However, certain bullets fragment in a characteristic pattern (e.g., the M16 military bullet, the .357 magnum 125-grain Remington semijacketed hollow-point, and others). Sometimes the pattern of fragments can be used to identify the bullet. Deformation of large lead shotgun pellets (e.g., 00 buckshot) after contact with bone can cause these to be confused with deformed bullet fragments.

Gunshot Fractures

Handgun wounds of the extremities yield characteristic fracture patterns. Frequently seen are divot fractures of cortical bone, drill-hole fractures, butterfly fractures, and double butterfly fractures. Nondisplaced fracture lines sometimes radiate from these defects. They usually heal well. Unusual spiral fractures proximal or distal to the bony gunshot wound also occur, probably because of stress risers and the fact that the bone was under load or stress at the time of impact. Early fasciotomy to prevent compartment syndrome is important when needed.

In gunshot fractures from rifles and large handguns, a greater extent of comminution may be seen. These fractures often have complications because of the soft-tissue damage these bullets cause. Wound infections are more common in this group.

At some hospitals, outpatient treatment is being used successfully for extremity fractures caused by handguns if no significant neurologic or vascular compromise has occurred.

Trunk Wounds

Bullets are not sterilized by the heat of firing. They can carry bacteria from the body surface or body organs, such as a perforated colon, deep into the wound.

In trunk wounds, an analysis of the bullet path is mandatory to determine whether a laparotomy is needed. Two radiographs at 90°, CT, clinical examination, and peritoneal lavage are all useful. Abdominal CT is more accurate if performed before peritoneal lavage. If peritoneal penetration by a bullet is suspected, laparotomy is indicated. The morbidity and mortality of an exploratory laparotomy that shows no significant intraabdominal injury is low compared with that of missed intestinal injury. CT is useful, especially when an exclusively body wall or retroperitoneal path is suspected. CT has largely replaced excretory urography as the preferred means of evaluating the urinary tract after penetrating trauma.

Any bullet wound below the nipple line should raise the question of whether the diaphragm or abdomen has been penetrated. CT sometimes can be used to make this determination. Laparotomy is required if peritoneal penetration cannot be excluded. As in the rest of the body, because of the skin's elastic properties, a nearly spent bullet is often arrested subcutaneously at the end of the wound path.

Whenever a gunshot wound traverses the midline of the neck or the width of the mediastinum, perforation of the esophagus should be suspected. Esophageal evaluation should not be overlooked after angiographic evaluation of the neck or chest.

Head Wounds

In skull wounds, inward beveling of the calvarial defect at the bullet entrance and outward beveling of the skull at the exit wound are typical,

(A)

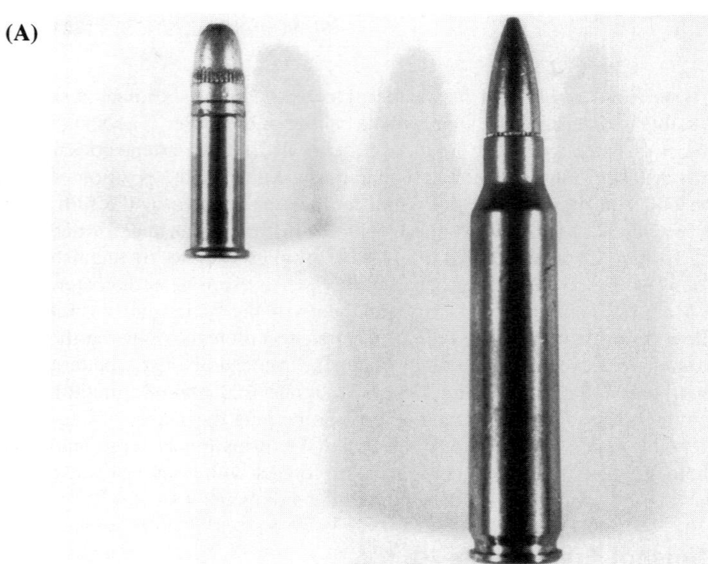

Fig. 187-1 (A). A .22 long rifle round (left) and an M16 round (right). Wound profiles of **(B)** the same .22 long rifle and **(C)** .224 cal M-193 round of the M16A1 rifle. Full metal case (FMC) is a synonym for full metal jacket (FMJ), the type of bullet used in the military. This figure shows that caliber (bullet diameter in decimals of an inch or in millimeters) is only one indicator of wounding potential and not a very good one. Because of much higher velocity [3094 ft/s (943 m/s), as opposed to 1122 ft/s (342 m/s) for the .22 long rifle bullet], because it fragments in tissue, and because of greater bullet mass, the M16 bullet has the potential to cause a much more severe wound if the anatomic part struck is sufficiently thick. Note that both the permanent cavity and the temporary cavity are much larger. As is usual, the temporary and permanent cavities caused by the .22 long rifle bullet are largest when the bullet is at 90° of yaw. (From Hollerman JJ: Gunshot wounds: 1. Bullets, ballistics, and mechanisms of injury. *AJR* 155:685–690, 1990, © by American Roentgen Ray Society. Used by permission.)

(B)

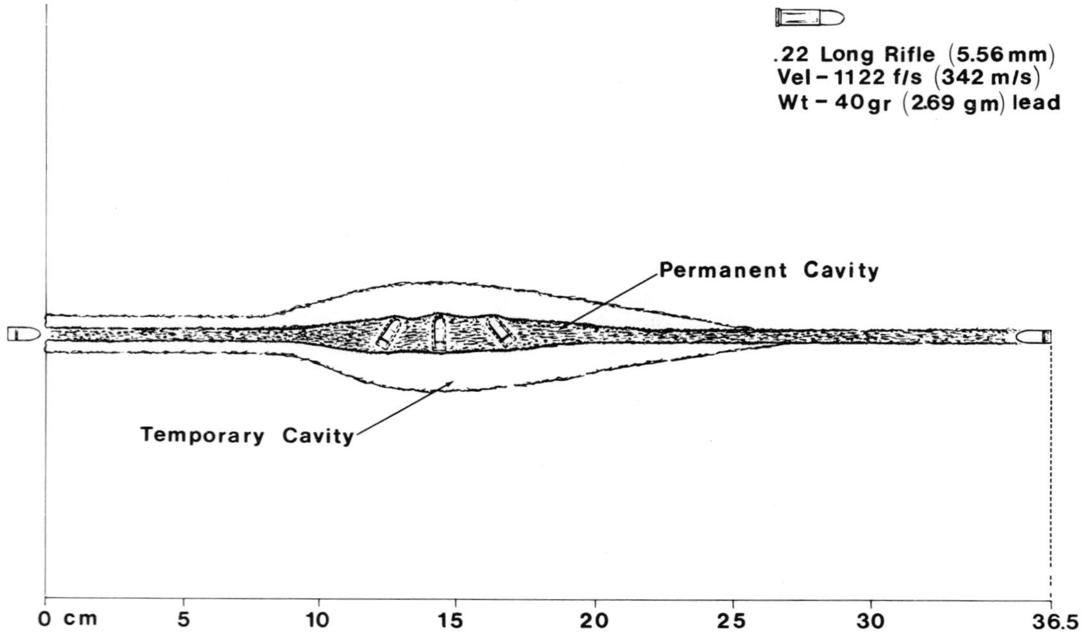

.22 Long Rifle (5.56 mm)
Vel – 1122 f/s (342 m/s)
Wt – 40 gr (2.69 gm) lead

Permanent Cavity

Temporary Cavity

0 cm 5 10 15 20 25 30 36.5

(C)

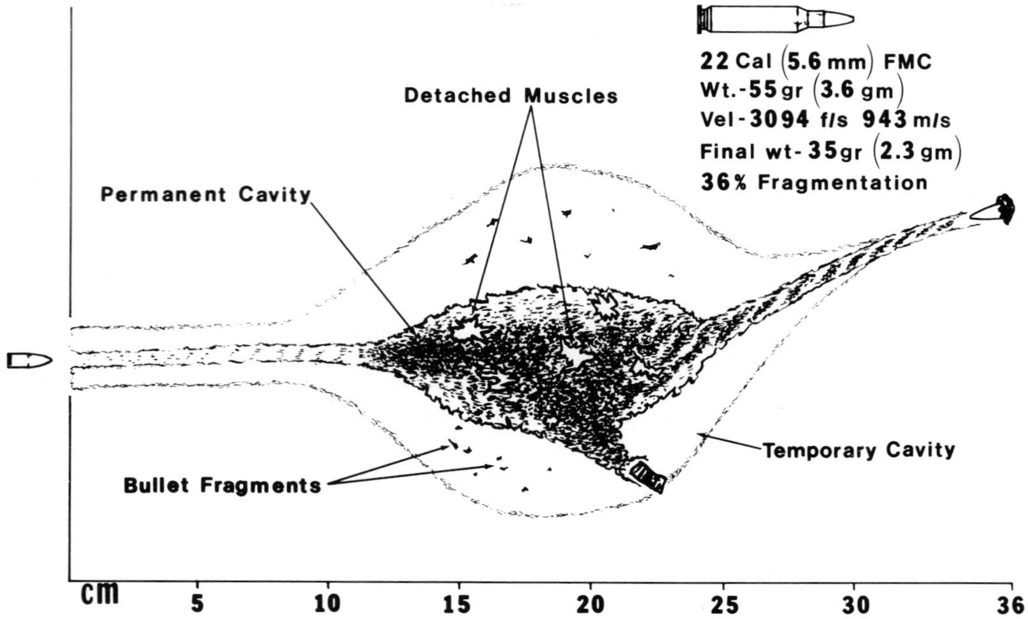

22 Cal (5.6 mm) FMC
Wt.-55 gr (3.6 gm)
Vel-3094 f/s 943 m/s
Final wt-35 gr (2.3 gm)
36% Fragmentation

Detached Muscles

Permanent Cavity

Temporary Cavity

Bullet Fragments

cm 5 10 15 20 25 30 36

due partly to the geometry of the skull and partly to the bullet-bone interaction. Characteristic fracture patterns of the skull can be used to identify entrance and exit wounds. When there is a cranial exit wound, skull fractures propagate across the calvarium faster than the bullet travels through the brain, producing characteristic patterns of fracture sometimes allowing differentiation of entrance and exit wounds.

Brain, whose tissue properties include near-water density, very little elasticity, and poor tissue cohesiveness, is extremely sensitive to temporary cavitation forces. When disrupted by such forces, severe brain injury often results. In addition to the relative lack of elasticity of brain tissue, its enclosure in the rigid cranial vault magnifies brain disruption by temporary cavitation forces.

Pellet Wounds

Compared with the pointed rifle bullet, the spherical pellet slows rapidly in its flight through air or tissue. In tissue, the entire wounding potential of the shot pellet at its entrance velocity is likely to be delivered to the target, often with no exit wound. At close range (less than 3 m), shotgun pellets remain tightly clustered. Therefore, shot pellet size makes little difference, since the entire load of the pellets functions as a unit, with a velocity virtually equal to muzzle velocity. Shotgun wounds at ranges less than 5 m consist of multiple parallel wound channels, which grossly disrupt the blood supply to tissue between the wound channels. The most severe civilian firearm wounds typically seen are those inflicted by a shotgun from close range. After a close-range or contact shotgun wound to the trunk, external examination of the patient, particularly after adequate volume resuscitation, often does not disclose the severity of the internal injuries present. Preoperative angiography of most close-range shotgun extremity wounds is recommended. Major neural injury after shotgun wounding may be more important than fracture or major vascular injury in determining the final outcome. During surgical exploration of a close-range shotgun wound, it is important to search for wadding, casing debris, plastic shot cup, and surface materials carried into the wound (e.g., clothing, glass, or wood). Many of these materials are radiolucent.

Diagnosing long-range injury on the basis of the pattern of pellet spread is sometimes problematic. When shotgun pellets are tightly clustered or widely spread out, close-range or long-range injury (respectively) is usually suspected. However, in close-range injuries, the ''billiard ball'' effect may cause considerable pellet spread. On radiographs, particularly in trunk wounds, this effect can simulate the pellet spread of a longer-range injury. This pitfall can be avoided if the skin physical examination is correlated with the radiologic findings.

Recent BB guns and airguns that fire small pellets have considerably higher muzzle velocity than older guns of this type. Penetrating injuries from these weapons are sometimes fatal. These firearms should not be considered toys.

Localization of a Missile

As in all of radiology, localization requires two views at 90° or a tomographic image. CT of the head and body is often useful for analysis of bullet path. The CT digital scout radiograph can be used for missile localization. It usually can be taken in anteroposterior and lateral projections without moving the patient. The ability to manipulate the display window and level allows visualization of bullets seen through dense structures, such as the shoulders and pelvis.

Missile Embolization

It always must be ascertained whether the path from the entrance wound is consistent with the bullet's current location, as a bullet may have reached its present location by embolization. Arterial and venous embolization of bullets and shotgun pellets as well as bullet movement within the subarachnoid space in the head and spine have been reported. It is generally accepted that a missile freely floating within a cardiac chamber should be removed to prevent embolization. Missiles clearly embedded in chamber walls are relatively safe. In one case reported by Kase and coworkers, a shotgun pellet was probably dislodged from the heart during cardiopulmonary resuscitation and embolized to the intracranial circulation, with a fatal result. Missile size does not seem to be especially important, as all sizes can produce morbidity after embolization. Two-dimensional echocardiography is useful in determining whether a missile is embedded in a chamber wall. CT (particularly high-speed CT) and MRI for nonmagnetic missiles also have a role. On chest radiographs, blurring of the margins of a pericardiac missile or fragment is grounds for suspecting that the missile is in or next to the heart.

Whenever a bullet is not found on radiographs of the body part predicted to contain it based on the entrance wound, the bullet's location is not known, and there is no exit wound, additional radiographs or fluoroscopy to find the bullet is mandatory. Immediately before surgery for removal of a missile, repeat radiographic confirmation of the exact location of the missile is usually indicated.

Interventional radiologic tecnhiques are useful in bullet removal, including the removal of intravascular and intrarenal bullets. Significant deformation of an intravascular bullet is a relative contraindication to retrieval using a transarterial catheter because of potential damage to the intima. Arthroscopy sometimes can be used for removing bullets from joints, especially the knee.

Even in the absence of embolization, bullets, particularly handgun bullets, do not always follow a straight path in the body. They may ricochet off body structures, especially bone, or may follow fascial or tissue planes. However, most bullets do follow fairly straight paths through the body. Bullets traveling less than 1100 ft/s (335 m/s) are the ones most likely to be deflected by anatomic structures or to follow tissue planes. Bullet shape also influences the tendency to be deflected.

Lead Fragments and Lead Poisoning

Lead fragments in soft tissue usually become encapsulated with fibrous tissue and do not cause problems. Lead intoxication occasionally can result from soft-tissue wounds, particularly those containing many lead pellets. Intraarticular, disk space, and bursal locations of bullet fragments are common for bullet-induced lead poisoning. Lead fragments in the brain are usually benign unless they are copper-plated (as are many civilian .22-caliber bullets). Copper-plated lead pellets produced a sterile abscess or granuloma in the brain of cats surgically implanted with missiles of this type. The abscess or granuloma was often associated with downward migration of the missile, resorption of copper from the surface of the missile, progressive neurologic deficit, and often death. These findings were absent in cats whose brains were implanted with uncoated lead pellets.

Intraarticular fragments should be removed to avoid the destructive synovitis lead can cause. Fragments within a joint space may be distributed by joint mechanics such that they create an arthrogram-like effect on radiographs, delineating cartilage surfaces and joint capsule recesses. Significant damage to the articular cartilage visible at surgery may be present as a result of lead synovitis when radiographs remain normal except for bullet fragments. If large fragments are present in the joint, they can cause severe mechanical trauma during motion. This motion can lead to further lead fragmentation. Lead is relatively soluble in synovial fluid.

Whether lead poisoning occurs depends largely on the surface area of the retained lead particles and their location in the body. In several cases, a fibrotic mass containing gray fluid with a high lead content has been observed adjacent to the site of large bullet fragments. Sometimes, the onset of clinical lead poisoning can be quite rapid, but usually it takes years.

CONCLUSION

The common misconceptions about wound ballistics listed in the introduction are discussed in order.

1. The properties of the tissue through which the missile passes (tissue elasticity, density, cohesiveness, and internal architecture); the diameter, shape, mass and velocity of the projectile; whether it fragments or expands; its internal construction; the length of the wound path; and whether it is sufficiently long to allow yaw to 90°, are all primary determinants of wounding. A center-fire "high-velocity" rifle bullet, if it traverses only elastic tissue such as skeletal muscle, does not yaw to 90°, does not fragment or deform, and does not hit a major blood vessel or nerve, usually causes a fairly minor wound. It will exit the extremity with most of its wounding potential unspent. If this same bullet hits a large bone, fragments, and does not exit, it will crush a large volume of tissue; will create secondary missiles, such as bone fracture fragments, which also crush tissue; and is likely to disrupt the neurovascular integrity of the area wounded, expending its wounding potential in the patient and usually producing a severe wound. The amount of tissue crushed by a bullet depends on projectile size and shape and whether it deforms or fragments. If the tissue wounded is relatively elastic and cohesive, the amount of tissue crushed is the primary determinant of wounding, as the tissue stretch of temporary cavitation may have relatively little wounding effect. If an organ is inelastic, near-water density, and not very cohesive, tissue stretch (temporary cavitation) can cause a severe wound. The bullet's mass and velocity, the depth of the organ in the body, and whether the bullet has traveled a long enough tissue path to yaw significantly or fragment at the site of the organ will be the primary determinants of the wound produced. Significant temporary cavitation, blunt trauma forces occur only if the bullet enters the body with sufficient velocity and then deforms, fragments, or yaws to 90°.
2. It is apparent that bullet velocity is only one factor in wounding and in some wounds may be a minor factor. Kinetic energy expended in elastic tissue may produce little damage, since tissue stretch may be well tolerated. Crushed tissue is always damaged. If a rubber ball and a raw egg of equal weight are dropped on a cement floor from the same height, these two missiles of equal kinetic energy will sustain different degrees of damage. Missile mass and velocity establish an upper limit of *possible* tissue damage. Whether or not this tissue damage occurs depends on numerous properties of the tissue, the missile, and its path. Also, collisions between bullets and tissue are not elastic, and kinetic energy is not conserved. Some of the energy, possibly most, is lost as heat.
3. As discussed above, many factors determine wound severity. Some "high-velocity" wounds are minor, and some "low-velocity" wounds are devastating. A stab wound to the brain, heart, spinal cord, aorta, or other vital structure, with properties similar to a small handgun bullet wound, is often lethal. An AK-47 military "assault" rifle wound of an extremity often is like an ice-pick stab wound and may have little effect. Bullet mass has a great deal to do with determining the maximum penetration depth achieved. A light but very high-velocity bullet may cause a substantial but superficial wound, sparing deep vital structures. A heavier, slower bullet may penetrate more deeply, reaching vital structures. It is important to examine each patient and to "treat the wound, not the weapon." Adherence to treatment guidelines, including no primary closure, the administration of prophylactic antibiotics to prevent streptococcal bacteremia, and performance of fasciotomy when necessary to prevent compartment syndrome will serve the patient well. Delayed primary closure or no wound closure is recommended. Never attribute hypesthesia, pallor, or weak pulse to arterial spasm after a gunshot wound, since it is more likely due to thrombus. Appropriate diagnostic evaluation and treatment are required.
4. The length of the tissue wound tract, the sequence of tissues encountered, and their properties are critical in determining whether the wounding potential of the missile will be expended in tissue. The bullet was spinning fast enough (because of the rifling of the barrel) to be stable in air, and it takes some distance in the higher-density medium of tissue for the bullet to become unstable and to yaw. This requires a sufficiently long tissue path. A bullet may yaw little or not at all in a short tissue path, such as an extremity. In trunk wounds, organs deeper in the body, such as in the abdomen or mediastinum, are more likely to experience blunt trauma from temporary cavitation in the region where the bullet yawed to 90°. Hard objects, such as a large bone or a belt buckle, are wound-modifying structures. When these are hit by a bullet, the severity of tissue damage will often increase, as bullet fragmentation or deformation increases the volume of tissue crushed and decreases the likelihood of missile exit.
5. Because civilian bullets deform and fragment much more easily than their full metal jacket military analogs, they cause more tissue crush and tissue stretch at shallower penetration depth. Frequently, this means that the wounding potential of a civilian rifle bullet is expended in the wounded animal, rather than the bullet exiting with wounding potential unspent. Civilian rounds have as much powder in the cartridge case and as much bullet mass as the comparable military round. The difference lies in the bullet jacket.
6. When an undeformed bullet is seen on a radiograph, it is usually not possible to state accurately whether it is fully jacketed. It may not have deformed because it entered the patient with insufficient velocity; it did not strike a structure, causing it to deform; or it is a full metal jacket bullet. Unless the bullet jacket has separated from the bullet, the jacket, if present, is not visible on standard radiographs.
7. A gun with a shorter barrel will generally produce a bullet of lower velocity than would a weapon with a longer barrel when firing the same round. With shorter barrel length, the expanding gasses of the burning gunpowder have less time to accelerate the bullet before they are discharged into the atmosphere. When identical rounds are fired by a rifle and a handgun, bullet velocity is often significantly different because of different barrel length. A .22 long rifle round fired in a rifle will produce a bullet with up to 300 ft/sec more bullet velocity than would the same round fired in a handgun.
8. Caliber alone is a poor indicator of the wounding potential of a round (Fig. 187-1). Bullet caliber does not tell one how much powder is in the cartridge case. The cartridge case may have a different diameter than the bullet and may be any length. Caliber does not reveal bullet mass. The bullet may be any length. Caliber only specifies diameter. The bullet's composition and construction (and therefore tendency to yaw, fragment, or deform) do not relate to caliber.
9. Bullets typically yaw only 1° to 3° in flight when fired from a properly designed weapon. If the bullet strikes an intermediate target, the bullet may yaw, deform, or decelerate as a result, and its wounding properties will be altered.
10. To be useful, wound ballistics research must be conducted using appropriate materials and methods. Erroneous conclusions frequently result from poor experimental design.

In essence, bullet wounds are assessed as is all other trauma. The amount, site, and type of tissue injury, assessed primarily by physical examination and radiologic studies, determine the treatment needed. The history of the episode is usually unreliable and, even if accurate, is usually irrelevant in determining treatment.

BIBLIOGRAPHY

Bowen TE, Bellamy RF: *Emergency war surgery: Second United States Revision of the Emergency War Surgery NATO Handbook,* 2d ed. Washington, D.C.: United States Government Printing Office, 1988; pp 13–238.

Daniel RA Jr: Bullet wounds of the lungs. *Surgery* 15:774, 1944.

DeiPoli G, BaimaBollone PL: An interpretation of the discrepancy between the entry and exit holes made by bullets in the skull. *Panminerva Med* 20:181, 1978.

Deitch EA, Grimes WR: Experience with 112 shotgun wounds of the extremities. *J Trauma:* 600, 1984.

DeMuth WE Jr: Bullet velocity and design as determinants of wounding capability: An experimental study. *J Trauma* 6:222, 1966.

Dixon DS: Exit keyhole lesion and direction of fire in a gunshot wound of the skull. *J Forensic Sci:* 336, 1984.

Dixon DS: Pattern of intersecting fractures and direction of fire. *J Forensic Sci* 29:651, 1984.

Fackler ML: Ballistic injury. *Ann Emerg Med* 15:1451, 1986.

Fackler ML: Wound ballistics: A review of common misconceptions. *JAMA* 259:2730, 1988.

Fackler ML: Wounding patterns of military rifle bullets. *Int Defense Rev* 22:59, 1989.

Fackler ML, Breteau JPL, Courbil LJ, et al: Open wound drainage versus wound excision in treating the modern assault rifle wound. *Surgery* 105:576, 1989.

Fackler ML, Surinchak JS, Malinowski JA, et al: Bullet fragmentation: A major cause of tissue disruption. *J Trauma* 24:35, 1984.

Fackler ML, Surinchak JS, Malinowski JA, et al: Wounding potential of the Russian AK-74 assault rifle. *J Trauma* 24:263, 1984.

Feliciano DV, Burch JM, Spjut-Patrinely V, et al: Abdominal gunshot wounds: An urban trauma center's experience with 300 consecutive patients. *Ann Surg* 208:362, 1988.

Fragomeni LSM, Azambuja PC: Bullets retained within the heart: Diagnosis and management in three cases. *Thorax* 42:980, 1987.

Froede RC, Pitt MJ, Bridgemon RR: Shotgun diagnosis: "It ought to be something else." *J Forensic Sci* 27:428, 1982.

Grogan DP, Bucholz RW: Acute lead intoxication from a bullet in an intervertebral disc space. *J Bone Joint Surg* (Am) 63(suppl A):1180, 1981.

Hampton OP Jr: The indications for debridement of gun shot (bullet) wounds of the extremities in civilian practice. *J Trauma* 1:368, 1961.

Harvey EN, Korr IM, Oster G, et al: Secondary damage in wounding due to pressure changes accompanying the passage of high-velocity missiles. *Surgery* 21:218, 1947.

Hollerman JJ, Fackler ML, Coldwell DM, et al: Gunshot wounds: 1. Bullets, ballistics and mechanisms of injury. *AJR* 155:685, 1990; 2. Radiology. *AJR* 155:691, 1990.

Kase CS, White RL, Vinson TL, et al: Shotgun pellet embolus to the middle cerebral artery. *Neurology* 31:458, 1981.

Leffers D, Changler RW: Tibial fractures associated with civilian gunshot injuries. *J Trauma* 25:1059, 1985.

Linden MA, Manton WI, Stewart RM, et al: Lead poinsoning from retained bullets: Pathogenesis, diagnosis, and management. *Ann Surg* 195:305, 1982.

Lindsey D: The idolatry of velocity, or lies, damn lies, and ballistics (editorial). *J Trauma* 20:1068, 1980.

Messmer JM, Fierro MF: Radiologic forensic investigation of fatal gunshot wounds. *Radiographics* 6:457, 1986.

Moore EE, Moore JB, VanDuzer-Moore S, et al: Mandatory laparotomy for gunshot wounds penetrating the abdomen. *Am J Surg* 140:847, 1980.

Robison RJ, Brown JW, Caldwell R, et al: Management of asymptomatic intracardiac missiles using echocardiography. *J Trauma* 28:1402, 1988.

Ryan JR, Hensel RT, Salciccioli GG, et al: Fractures of the femur secondary to low-velocity gunshot wounds. *J Trauma* 21:160, 1981.

Sclafani SJA, Vuletin JC, Twersky J: Lead arthropathy: Arthritis caused by retained intra-articular bullets. *Radiology* 156:299, 1985.

Selbst S, Henretig F, Fee M, et al: Lead poisoning in a child with a gunshot wound. *Pediatrics* 77:413, 1986.

Sights WP, Bye RJ: The fate of retained intracerebral shotgun pellets: An experimental study. *J Neurosurg* 33:646, 1970.

Smith HW, Wheatley KK Jr: Biomechanics of femur fractures secondary to gunshot wounds. *J Trauma* 24:970, 1984.

Smith OC, Berryman HE, Lahren CH: Cranial fracture patterns and estimate of direction from low-velocity gunshot wounds. *J Forensic Sci* 32:1416, 1987.

Staniforth P, Watt I: Extradural plumboma: A rare cause of acquired spinal stenosis. *Br J Radiol* 55:772, 1982.

Wang ZG, Feng JX, Liu YQ: Pathomorphological observations of gunshot wounds. *Acta Chir Scand* 508(suppl):185, 1982.

Woloszyn JT, Uitvlugt GM, Castle ME: Management of civilian gunshot fractures of the extremities. *Clin Orthop* 226:247, 1988.

SECTION 19
Emergency Wound Management

188
THE EVALUATION OF WOUNDS IN THE EMERGENCY DEPARTMENT

Richard F. Edlich
George T. Rodeheaver
John G. Thacker

When caring for wounds, the ultimate goal is to restore the physical integrity and function of the injured tissue without infection. Treatment of wounds involves a series of decisions that determine if the wound heals or becomes infected.

PREHOSPITAL CARE

In patients with soft tissue injuries, treatment should be initiated by the paramedics under the guidance of the emergency department physician using radio and telemetered communication. The primary survey must evaluate ventilation and circulation, and detect bleeding.

External bleeding almost always can be controlled by a pressure dressing. Before applying the dressing, all skin flaps that are kinked or twisted should be returned to their original position to prevent vascular compromise. Bleeding of an injured extremity that is refractory to direct pressure will stop following inflation of a sphygmomanometer placed proximal to the bleeding site. After the injured extremity is elevated for 1 min, the cuff is inflated to a pressure that is greater than the patient's systolic blood pressure. This measured level of inflation pressure can be maintained for at least 2 h without injury to the underlying vessels and nerves. Once the patient's condition has been stabilized, the secondary survey must follow.

EMERGENCY DEPARTMENT

When the patient arrives in the emergency department, treatment of life-threatening injuries continues to take precedence over management of soft tissue wounds. When a life-threatening injury warrants immediate operative intervention, soft tissue wounds can be repaired simultaneously if there is careful coordination and planning between surgical specialists and anesthesiologists.

Before inspecting the wound, the emergency physician must carefully question the patient regarding the time and mechanism of injury. The time since the accident occurred has considerable influence on surgical decisions. A delay in treatment lasting longer than 3 h is often associated with a proliferation of bacteria to a level that results in the development of infection and limits the therapeutic efficacy of antibiotics.

Mechanism of Injury

The divided edges of the wound are more susceptible to infection than the unwounded tissue. The resistance to infection varies with the mechanism of injury. In most soft tissue injuries, a shearing force is applied by a piece of glass, a metal edge, or a knife, resulting in a linear laceration. The resultant wound exhibits considerable resistance to the development of infection.

If a wound is caused by a collision of two bodies, the mechanism of injury is predominantly compression or tension, rather than shear. The energy requirement for tissue failure as a result of these forces is considerably greater than that for shear forces. The absorbed energy of this impact force disrupts the skin, resulting in a characteristic stellate laceration. Wounds due to compression or tension injuries are 100-fold more susceptible to infection than those caused by shear forces. While antibiotic therapy is clearly beneficial in these wounds, its efficacy is substantially less than that in wounds caused by shear forces that are subjected to a similar level of bacterial inoculum.

Disruption of the vessels in the skin and underlying tissue produces an ecchymosis. Disruption of vessels in the underlying tissue results in a hematoma. Some hematomas resorb, but those that become encapsulated usually require surgical treatment. Left untreated, such hematomas may result in permanent subcutaneous deformity. When still in the currant-jelly stage, a hematoma is best treated by incision and drainage. As further liquefaction occurs, aspiration with a large-bore needle (18 gauge or larger) may be possible.

Firearm injuries cause a considerably higher level of energy absorption per unit volume of tissue than blunt injuries. As tissues are struck by a missile, a combination of shear, tensile, and compressive forces interacts to produce a relatively reproducible amount of destruction. The severity of the wound in the body is related to the amount of kinetic energy deposited in the body. Firearm injuries are discussed in further detail in Chapter 187, "Wound Ballistics."

Wound Contaminants

The environs in which the injury occurred may be predictive of the number of pathogens in the wound. An infective dose of bacteria may be derived from either an exogenous source (e.g., wounding instrument) or the endogenous microflora of the patient. In general, the composition of the skin microflora allows subdivision of the body into three anatomic areas (Table 188-1). Over most of the body surface, trunk, upper arms, and upper legs, the density of the bacterial population is quite low, a few thousand or less per square centimeter. The moist areas of the body, such as the axillae, perineum, toe webs, and intertriginous areas harbor millions of bacteria per square centimeter. The exposed anatomic areas (head, face, hands, and feet) of the body constitute the third anatomic region and display a bacterial density numbering in the millions per square centimeter. No error is more frequent than the habit of generalizing about the microflora in this exposed anatomic region. The dissimilarities in the density and diversity of organisms which inhabit this unique province are truly profound. Normally, the organisms are quite sparse on the palms and

Table 188-1. Composition and Concentration of Skin Microflora

Anatomic Site	Total Bacterial Concentrations	Ratio Aerobe : Anaerobe
Moister areas		
(axillae, perineum)	10^4–10^6	10 : 1
Drier areas		
(trunk, upper arms, and legs)	10^1–10^3	5–10 : 1
Exposed areas		
(head, face, hands, and feet)*	10^4–10^6	5–10 : 1

* Anaerobes may outnumber aerobes in the skin of the cheeks, upper back, and presternum.

dorsa of the hands, numbering in the hundreds per square centimeter. The majority of organisms on the hands reside beneath the distal end of the nail plate or adjacent to the proximal or lateral nail folds. The scalp and the forehead skin also exhibit luxuriant bacterial growth, in the millions per square centimeter.

In most anatomic regions, bacterial colonization of the skin is limited to the horny layer of skin, which is composed of a sloughing mass of dead cells, full of cracks which harbor bacteria. Beneath this horny layer, the stratum corneum, composed of tightly packed cells, provides an effective barrier against bacterial invasion. The horny layer of pilosebaceous appendages that line the infundibulum of hair follicles forms a receptacle for bacteria. However, these bacteria rarely descend any further than the entrance of the sebaceous ducts. Similarly, the depths of apocrine glands and sweat glands are devoid of bacteria. The organisms that reside less than 250 μm beneath the surface are within reach of topically applied antiseptic agents. As a result of topical antisepsis, sterility or near sterility can be achieved in most skin areas of the body.

Lacerations contacting the oral cavity usually are heavily contaminated with facultative species and obligate anaerobes. Within the oral cavity, the largest number of organisms is encountered in the gingival crevices and in plaque on the teeth. The plaque on teeth and the debris removed from the crevices are composed primarily of bacteria in the range of 10^{11} per gram wet weight, a number that is far greater than infective doses of bacteria ($\geq 10^6$ bacteria per gram of tissue) for most soft tissue wounds. This potential source of heavy contamination accounts for the reported high infection rate of wounds resulting from human and animal bites. Feces also possess a luxuriant microflora occurring in a concentration of 10^{11} per gram of passed feces. Approximately 20 to 30 percent of the net weight of stool is a solid mass of bacteria, nearly all anaerobes. Wounds contacted by human or animal fecal contaminants run a high risk of infection despite therapeutic intervention.

A careful history can also predict the likelihood of nonviable foreign bodies being in wounds. In missile injuries, clothing and missile fragments are encountered in the wounded tissue. Soil and dirt frequently are found in lacerations resulting from industrial or farming accidents. Specific infection-potentiating fractions have been identified in the soil; these fractions include its organic components as well as its inorganic clay fractions. For wounds contaminated by these fractions, only 100 bacteria are necessary to elicit infection. Their ability to enhance the incidence of infection appears to be related to their damage to host defenses. In the presence of these fractions, leukocytes are not able to ingest and kill bacteria. This deleterious effect on white blood cell function is a result of direct interaction between the highly charged soil particles and white cells. Soil infection-potentiating fractions also have considerable influence on non-specific humoral factors. Exposure of fresh serum to these fractions eliminates its bactericidal activity. As expected, these fractions, which consist of highly charged particles, react chemically with amphoteric and basic antibiotics, limiting their activity in contaminated wounds.

The concentration of these fractions in soil can be correlated with their location. Environmental conditions in swamps, bogs, and marshes encourage the production of soil composed almost entirely (90 percent) of organic infection-potentiating fractions. The major inorganic infection-potentiating particles are the clay fractions, which reside in heaviest concentration in the subsoil rather than in topsoil. Consequently, traumatic soft tissue injuries occurring in swamps or excavation run a high risk of being contaminated by these fractions, which predispose the wound to serious infection.

A corollary to these observations is that some soil constituents, such as sand grains, are relatively innocuous. The sand fraction, which has a large particle size and a low level of chemical reactivity, exerts considerably less damage on tissue defenses than the infection-potentiating fractions do. Surprisingly, the black dirt on the surface of highways also appears to have minimal chemical reactivity.

Wound Examination

The examining medical personnel should don gloves and wear a mask when inspecting the wound. Powder-free gloves are recommended because the powder on surgical gloves (e.g., corn starch or talc granules) are foreign bodies that damage the host's resistance to infection. The physician's visualization of the wound can be enhanced by magnification loupes. Physicians uniformly prefer a Keplerian lens system over that of the Galilean lens system. The advantages of the Keplerian lens system are its increased field of view and clearer peripheral image. This system allows the physician to visualize the exquisite details of the wound and to perform wound closure using microsurgical techniques. Examination of the injured site must begin by detecting any sensory, motor, and vascular complications or injuries to specialized ducts. When the injury occurs in an extremity, this examination can be conducted in the absence of hemorrhage if a sphygmomanometer proximal to the injury is inflated to a pressure greater than the patient's systolic blood pressure. Palpation of the bone adjacent to the wound may detect tenderness or instability consistent with an underlying bone injury. Roentgenograms of the injured site will confirm this diagnosis. Injuries requiring open reduction of fractures, neurorrhaphy, vascular anastomosis, tendon juncture, or repair of specialized ducts are best treated in the operating room, where good lighting, instruments, and assistance make the procedure safer. In the absence of these underlying injuries, wound treatment can be undertaken in the emergency department. Important considerations in wound management are also the location, configuration, and biomechanical properties of the wound.

Wound Biomechanical Properties

The ultimate appearance and function of a scar can be predicted by the magnitude of the static and dynamic skin tensions on the surrounding skin. The static skin tensions are the forces that stretch the skin over the underlying bony framework when the body remains motionless. These inherent forces are dependent on the natural characteristics of dermal collagen fibers and on the pattern in which they are woven. Clinical evidence of these tensions is the retraction of the edges of the wounds permitting visualization of the underlying tissue.

Static skin forces differ considerably in their magnitude and direction between individuals and at various anatomic sites within the same person. In one human volunteer, the static skin tensions were fivefold greater in his extremities than in his abdominal skin. In some regions of the body there is a directional orientation of static skin tensions. The most aesthetically pleasing scar occurs when the long axis of the scar is in the direction of the maximal skin tension. The pull of the stronger skin tensions at the ends of the wound tends to oppose the weaker forces that are perpendicular to the wound edges, thereby bringing its edges closer together. Following approximation of the wound edges, the static skin tensions continuously pull on the wound edges, resulting in the development of a visible scar. The ultimate width of the scar is proportional to the magnitude of the static skin tensions. Wounds made in skin subjected to strong static skin tensions usually heal with wide, unattractive scars. In contrast, narrow, fine scars often result from repair of wounds in skin with weak static skin tensions.

Clinical observation of the wound in the emergency department is a reliable method of predicting the ultimate appearance of the healing scar after closure. The degree to which the divided skin edges retract provides a rough estimate of the magnitude of static skin tensions. Wounds with marked retraction of their edges (≥ 5 mm) are subjected to strong static skin tensions and heal with wide scars (Fig. 188-1). When there is minimal separation of the wound edges (< 5 mm), wound repair is accomplished with fine scars. This information should be shared with the patients as well as their families so that they can appropriately credit the aesthetic result to the biology of wound repair.

The magnitude of static skin tension per unit length of wound is

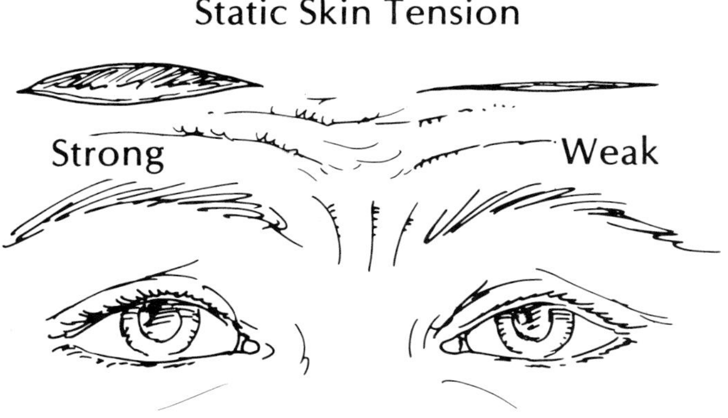

Fig. 188-1. The degree to which the wound edges retract can be correlated with the magnitude of static skin tensions. The wound on the right side of the patient's forehead exhibits marked retraction of its edges (≥5 mm) being subjected to strong static skin tensions. The minimal separation of the edges of the wound (<5 mm) on the left side of the patient's forehead is consistent with the presence of weak static skin tensions.

influenced considerably by the configuration of the wound. In uneven, jagged-edged wounds, the perimeter of the wound is considerably longer than that of a linear incision. Consequently, the magnitude of static tensions per unit length of a jagged-edged wound is less than that of a straight laceration. Plastic surgeons have learned that meticulous reapproximation of the jagged edges of the wound yields a gratifying result with a narrow scar. Those unaware of the biomechanical principles involved in wound repair may elect to convert the jagged wound edges into a straight wound. This decision adds insult to the injury. The ill-conceived debridement eliminates the potential benefits of the long wound perimeter and leaves a lenticular-shaped defect that is considerably wider than the initial wound. Reapproximation of the edges of the debrided wound requires greater closing forces than would have been needed prior to debridement, resulting in a wide, unattractive scar. Faced with this physical deformity, the patient may seek the advice of a plastic surgeon. Six to twelve months after the injury, the plastic surgeon may elect to revise the scar by a W- or Z-plasty. The revised incision usually yields a gratifying result, healing with a narrower scar.

Dynamic skin tensions also have considerable impact on the static skin tensions as well as on the magnitude and extent of scar formation. These changing tensions are caused by a combination of forces that are associated with joint movement or mimetic muscle contraction. The clinical significance of dynamic tensions is particularly apparent in skin of changing dimensions where elasticity is needed for normal function. In general, a linear scar intersecting the transverse axis of a joint or running perpendicular to the wrinkle lines can result in a serious contracture because the scar does not stretch or recoil like uninjured tissue.

The direction of the dynamic skin tensions can be ascertained by rather simple practical measurements (Fig. 188-2A and B). At the ends of the laceration, mark points A and B; then mark points C and D, which are perpendicular to the laceration and equidistant between points A and B. Measure first the distance between points A and B and then the distance between points C and D before and after flexion of the underlying joints or contraction of the muscles of facial expression. The dynamic skin tensions are in the direction of greatest change in dimension. Wounds with their long axes in the direction of dynamic skin tension heal with conspicuous scars that interfere with function and are aesthetically unattractive. If the long axis of the wound is perpendicular to the dynamic skin tension in a site that remains relatively stationary during muscle contraction, the magnitude of the scar formation can be predicted by the inherent static skin tensions.

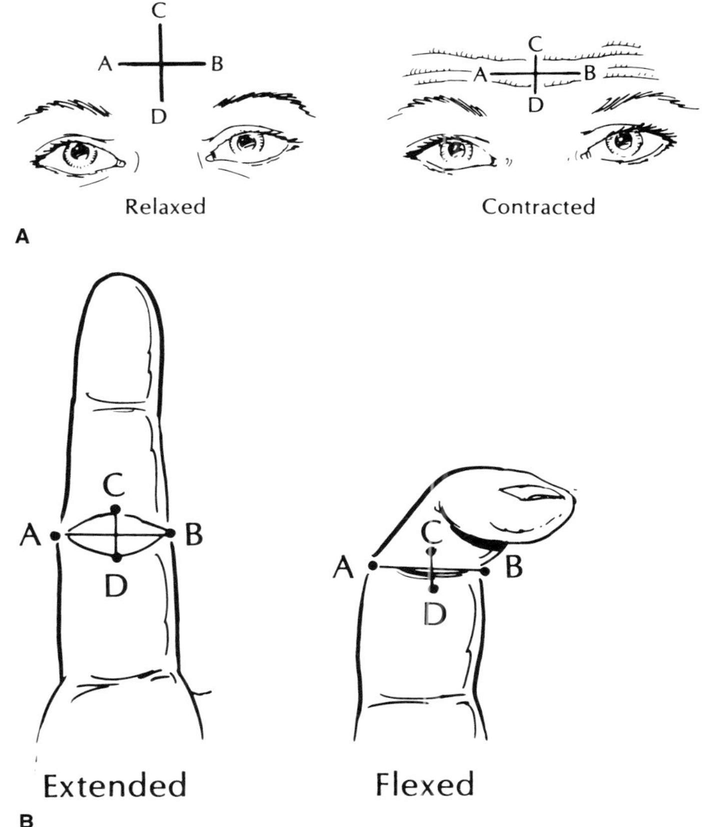

Fig. 188-2. A. Contraction of the frontalis muscle considerably shortens the skin in the direction of dynamic skin tensions (line CD). B. As the proximal interphalangeal joint flexes, the distance along the longitudinal axis of the joint shortens considerably in the same direction as the dynamic skin tension (line CD).

Unfortunately, accidental injuries often result in wounds whose axis parallels the dynamic skin tensions. In such cases, it is imperative to warn the patient of the impending development, and referral to a plastic surgeon for follow-up examination and treatment is recommended. At a later date (6 to 12 months), the directional orientation of the scar can be altered by W- or Z-plasty so that the direction of a portion of the wound is perpendicular to the dynamic skin tensions.

This research was supported by a generous gift from the Texaco Philanthropic Foundation, White Plains, New York.

BIBLIOGRAPHY

Overview

Edlich RF: The biology of wound repair and infection: A personal odyssey (Kennedy Lecture). *Ann Emerg Med* 14:1018, 1985.

Edlich RF, Rodeheaver GT, Morgan RF, et al: Principles of emergency wound management. *Ann Emerg Med* 17:1294, 1988.

Prehospital Care

Edlich RF, Crampton RS, Rockwell DD, et al: Prehospital management of the trauma patient. *EMT J* 5:186, 1981.

Biology of Wound Infection

Edlich RF, Smith QT, Edgerton MT: Resistance of the surgical wound to antimicrobial prophylaxis and its mechanisms of development. *Am J Surg* 126:583, 1973.

Roettinger W, Edgerton MT, Kurtz LD, et al: Role of inoculation site as a determinant of infection in soft tissue wounds. *Am J Surg* 126:354, 1973.

Mechanism of Injury

Cardany CR, Rodeheaver G, Thacker J, et al: The crush injury: A high risk wound. *JACEP* 5:965, 1976.

Fackler ML: Ballistic injury. *Ann Emerg Med* 15:1451, 1986.

Wound Contaminants

Haury BB, Rodeheaver GT, Pettry D, et al: Inhibition of nonspecific defenses by soil infection-potentiating factors. *Surg Gynecol Obstet* 144:19, 1977.

Pecora DV, Landis RE, Martin RE: Location of cutaneous microorganisms. *Surgery* 64:1114, 1968.

Wound Biomechanical Properties

Thacker JG, Iachetta FA, Allaire PE, et al: Biomechanical properties—Their influence on planning surgical excisions, in Krizek TJ, Hoopes PE (eds): *Symposium on Basic Science in Plastic Surgery*. St Louis, Mosby, 1975, vol 15, pp 72–79.

189
LOCAL AND REGIONAL ANESTHESIA FOR WOUND REPAIR

Richard F. Edlich
George T. Rodeheaver
John G. Thacker

Cleansing bacteria and other debris from traumatic injuries and debridement cannot be accomplished without anesthesia. The selection of the anesthetic agent for infiltration anesthesia is based on pharmocologic and toxicologic considerations. The pharmacodynamic properties of these agents include severity of pain elicited by the injection of the agent, onset and duration of anesthetic activity, and frequency of adequate anesthesia. The toxicologic manifestations of local anesthesia agents are almost exclusively local complications (e.g., damage to tissue defenses) because when these agents are absorbed systemically they do not affect organ systems clinically except the peripheral nerves. Because the amide-type local anesthetic agents appear to be relatively free of sensitivity and allergic reactions characteristic of the ester-type agents, emergency physicians usually use lidocaine and bupivacaine for infiltration anesthesia. These anesthetic agents do not damage tissue defenses or promote infection. In addition, the pain of subdermal injection, the onset of anesthesia, and the frequency of satisfactory anesthesia are similar. Clinical studies have demonstrated that the pain of local anesthetic administration can be reduced dramatically by buffering the local anesthetic agents before injection. Because the duration of local anesthesia induced by bupivacaine is nearly four times longer than that by lidocaine, bupivacaine is recommended for infiltration anesthesia or regional nerve blocks in most anatomic sites.

Prolonged anesthesia may not be desirable in some anatomic sites. Anesthesia of the oral cavity is such a case. Disappearance of the anesthetic effect allows the patient to resume activities requiring the use of the mouth, cheek, tongue, and lips without concern about inadvertently biting the anesthetized mucous membranes. This same principle applies to repaired fingertip injuries in which the patient must resume activities requiring normal tactile sensation.

The duration of anesthetic activity of these agents can be enhanced by the addition of the vasoconstrictor epinephrine, which slows the clearance of the agent from the tissue, thereby prolonging the duration of anesthesia. This benefit must be weighed against its deleterious effects on tissue defenses; epinephrine will damage local tissue defenses. The infection-potentiating effect of this powerful vasoconstrictor is proportional to its concentration and results from its vasoactivity. As a result of its local vasoconstrictive action, epinephrine may result in hypoxic conditions that limit white blood cell function. Consequently, the increased infection rate of epinephrine-treated wounds may result from impaired killing of bacterial contaminants by wound leukocytes in the ischemic wounds. This damage to tissue defenses argues against the use of epinephrine in potentially heavily contaminated wounds.

INFILTRATION ANESTHESIA

The simplest and most practical technique of anesthetizing most lacerations is infiltration anesthesia. The subcutaneous branches of the sensory nerves to the wound are anesthetized by injecting 0.5% bupivacaine through a no. 30 needle into intact skin at the periphery of the wound. Injections through the cut edge of the wound may be less painful, but they serve to disseminate bacteria throughout uninvolved tissue around the contaminated wound and, therefore, should be avoided.

The depth and speed of injection are important determinants of the magnitude of discomfort experienced by the patient. Placement of the needle into the superficial dermis is more uncomfortable than needle passage into the subdermal area. Moreover, intradermal injections resulting in superficial wheals are significantly more painful than injections into the subdermal region. Rapid injection of a local anesthetic agent (<2 s) always causes more pain than when the same volume of anesthetic agent is instilled over 10 s. Intracutaneous instillation of lidocaine at 37°C (98.6°F) is no less painful than injection at 21°C (69.8°F). Full anesthesia to pinprick is produced immediately with intradermal injections and is present 5 to 6 min after subdermal injection. A reliable method of minimizing the discomfort of infiltration anesthesia is to use a syringe fitted with a no. 30 needle and to inject the smallest amount of anesthetic agent slowly (≥10 s) into the deep dermal-subcutaneous tissue as the needle is slowly withdrawn.

REGIONAL NERVE BLOCKS

When the nerve supply to the wound is superficial, a regional nerve block is a valuable clinical tool that can be safely mastered by the emergency physician. A distinct advantage of this route of administration over infiltration anesthesia is that it does not distort the wound, facilitating reapproximation of the wound edges. Its clinical value becomes especially apparent when anesthetizing lacerations of the palm of the hand or the sole of the foot. Infiltration of a local anesthetic agent into this exquisitely sensitive skin is unbearable. Fortunately, the nerve supply of these anatomic regions is very susceptible to regional nerve blocks. Such blocks may be accomplished by passage of the needle through more proximal skin, which has a considerably higher threshold to pain than skin of the palm or sole.

Wrist Blocks

For lacerations of the hand, regional blocks at the wrist are performed at the level of the proximal volar skin crease (Fig. 189-1). The median nerve is anesthetized by inserting a no. 27 needle perpendicular to the skin between the tendons of the palmaris longus and flexor carpi radialis muscles. A regional block of the ulnar nerve is accomplished by passage of the needle between the ulnar artery and the flexor carpi ulnaris. Once inserted, the needle is moved fanwise transversely until paresthesias are elicited. When paresthesias occur, the needle is held in place and 5 to 10 mL of 0.5% bupivacaine with epinephrine (1:200,000) is injected slowly. The median nerve innervates the radial side of the palmar surface and the palmar surfaces of the lateral three-and-one-half fingers. The ulnar nerve is distributed to the residual ulnar surface of the palm as well as to the palmar surfaces of the little finger and the ulnar side of the ring finger.

The superficial rami of the radial nerve can be blocked by raising a subcutaneous ring with 5 to 10 mL of 0.5% bupivacaine with epinephrine (1:200,000) beginning at the level of the tendon of the extensor carpi radialis and extending around the radial border of the wrist, dorsal to the styloid process (Fig. 189-2). The radial nerve is the sensory nerve to the radial side of the dorsum of the hand.

Finger Blocks

For an isolated laceration of a finger, the common digital nerves proximal to the finger webs may be anesthetized with 1% lidocaine. A no. 27 needle is introduced into the skin covering the midportion of the base of the proximal phalanx of the involved finger. The needle should be angled around the bone until it induces blanching of the skin on the palmar surface of the web space. As the needle is withdrawn, approximately 2 mL of 1% lidocaine is injected. Before the needle is withdrawn completely from the skin, it should be redirected to the opposite side of the injured finger to inject the local anesthetic agent in a similar manner. The total volume of the injected anesthetic agent should not exceed 4 mL. In these cases, epinephrine must not be used

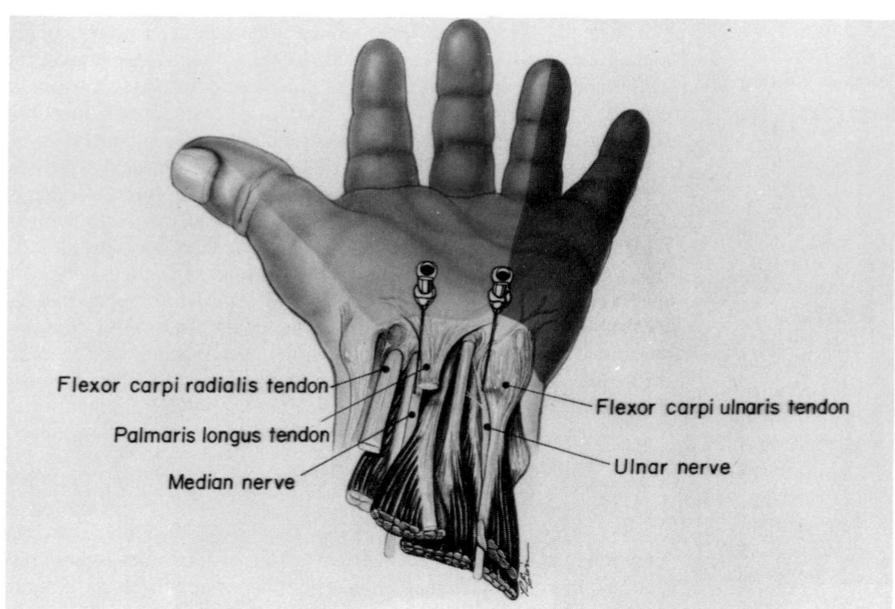

Fig. 189-1. Regional blocks of the ulnar and median nerves.

as an adjunct to lidocaine, because it may result in irreversible ischemic injury to the finger.

Ankle Blocks

A regional nerve block of the tibial nerve results in anesthesia of all of the sole of the foot, except the lateral side of the heel and foot. The tibial nerve is located along the medial aspect of the ankle between the medial malleolus and Achilles tendon, lying just posterior and slightly deeper than the posterior tibial artery (Fig. 189-3). Generally, the nerve divides into the medial and lateral plantar nerves just below the inferior margin of the medial malleolus, giving off the calcaneal branches proximal to this division. The medial plantar nerve supplies muscular and cutaneous branches of the sole of the foot, where its distribution closely resembles that of the median nerve of the hand. The lateral plantar nerve provides muscular and cutaneous branches of the sole of the foot analogous to the distribution of the ulnar nerve. The tibial nerve is anesthetized as it passes behind the medial malleolus. Bupivacaine (0.5%) is injected through a no. 30 needle into the subcutaneous tissue lateral to the tibial artery or, should this be impalpable, immediately anterior to the medial border of the Achilles tendon at the level with the upper border of the medial malleolus (Fig. 189-3). Through this anesthetized skin, a 6- to 8-cm-long no. 22 needle is inserted at right angles to the posterior aspect of the tibia until it is immediately lateral to the posterior tibial artery. The direction of the needle is shifted in a mediolateral direction, often eliciting paresthesias of the tibial nerve, at which time 5 to 10 mL of 0.5% bupivacaine with epinephrine (1:200,000) is injected. If paresthesias are not encountered, 10 to 12 mL of this anesthetic solution is injected against the posterior aspect of the tibia as the needle is drawn back 1 cm. The onset of anesthesia may occur in 5 to 10 min if paresthesias have been elicited, but it takes up to 30 min in their absence.

Toe Blocks

For a laceration of the toe, digital, rather than ankle, nerve blocks are utilized. In these cases, epinephrine must *not* be used as an adjunct to bupivacaine, because it may result in irreversible ischemic injury

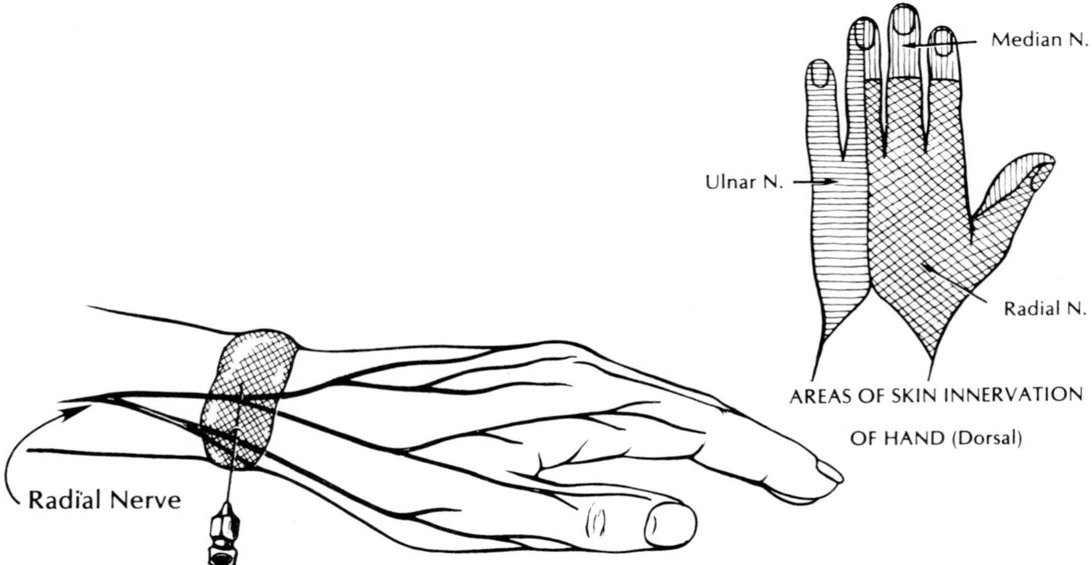

Fig. 189-2. Regional block of several rami of the radial nerve.

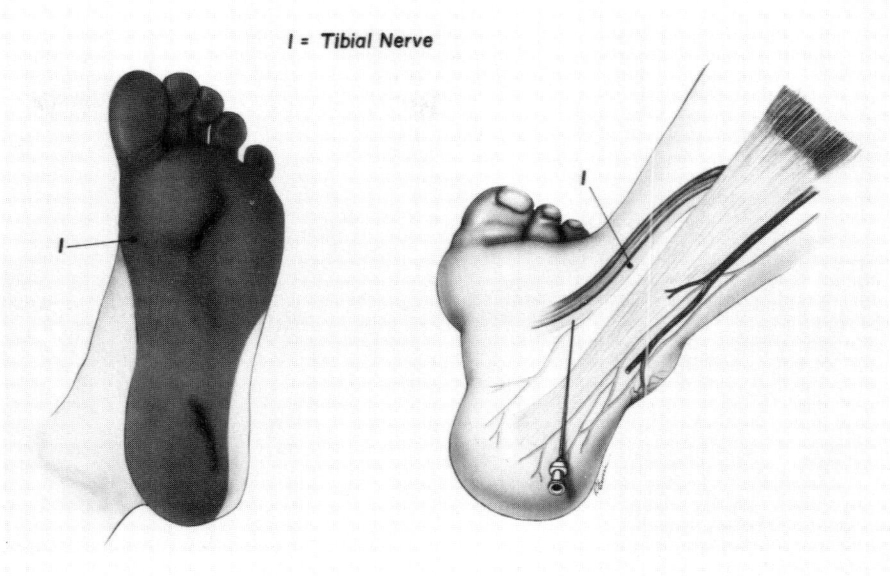

Fig. 189-3. Regional block of the tibial nerve.

to the toe. A no. 27 needle should be introduced through the skin on the dorsal aspect of the base of the midpoint of the involved toe (Fig. 189-4). The needle should be angled around the bone until it induces blanching of the skin on the plantar surface. As the needle is withdrawn, approximately 1.5 mL of 0.5% bupivacaine is injected. Before the needle is withdrawn completely from the skin, it should be redirected to the opposite side of the injured toe to inject the local anesthetic agent in a similar manner. The total volume of the injected local anesthetic agent should not exceed 3 mL.

For the hallux (great toe), a modified collar (ring) block is employed (Fig. 189-4). The no. 27 needle is inserted through the skin on the dorsolateral aspect of the base of the toe until it blanches the plantar skin. As the needle is withdrawn, 1.5 mL of 0.5% bupivacaine is injected into the tissues. Before the needle is removed completely from the skin, the needle is passed under the skin on the dorsal aspect of the toe and 1.5 mL of 0.5% bupivacaine is injected as the needle is withdrawn from the skin. The needle is then introduced through the anesthetized skin on the dorsomedial aspect of the toe and advanced until it produces blanching of the plantar skin, at which time the needle is withdrawn and 1.5 mL of 0.5% bupivacaine is injected. Usually, approximately 4.5 mL of 0.5% bupivacaine is needed to anesthetize the hallux.

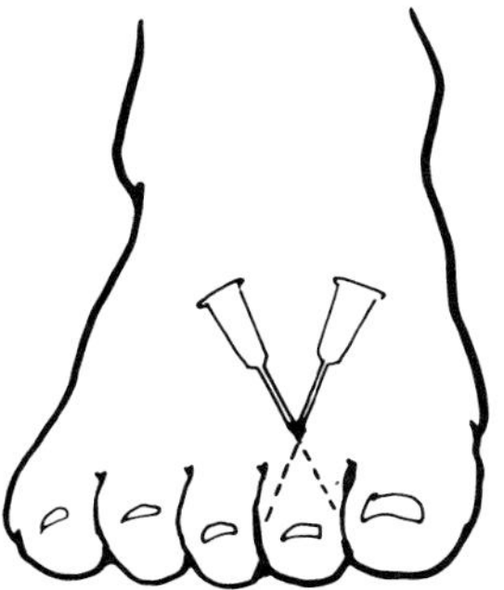
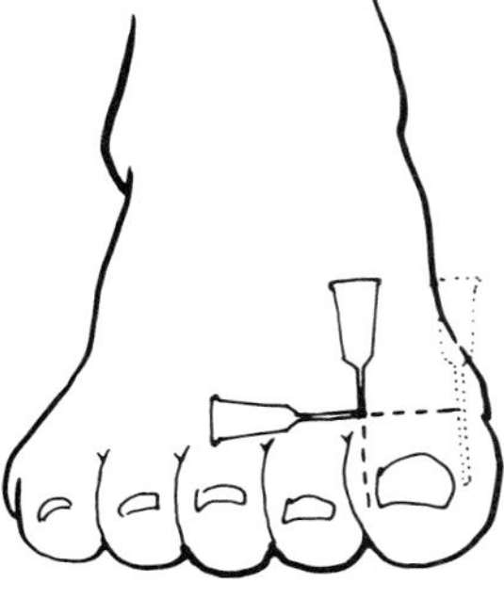

Fig. 189-4. (Left) Regional block of toe. (Right) Regional block of hallux (great toe).

Facial and Oral Blocks

Regional nerve blocks of the supraorbital, supratrochlear, lingual, mental, infraorbital, and greater auricular nerves are other simple and safe techniques worth remembering. A regional nerve block of the forehead is accomplished with 3 to 6 mL of 0.5% bupivacaine by raising a wheal above the nasion, after which the point of the no. 27 needle is advanced under the skin immediately above the entire length of the eyebrow (Fig. 189-5).

A regional block of the lingual nerve is the preferred route for administering anesthetics for patients with a deep laceration of the anterior tongue. It offers distinct advantages over infiltration anesthesia of the exquisitely sensitive moving tongue. The lingual nerve is a

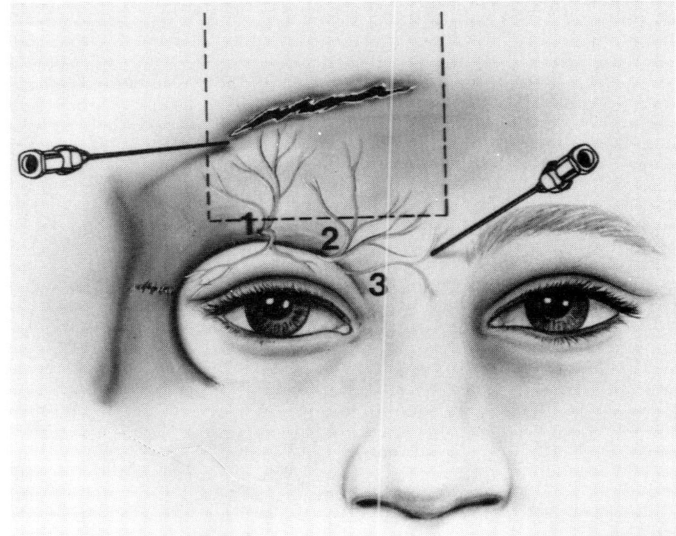

Fig. 189-5. Regional blocks of (1) the lateral branch of the frontal nerve, (2) the medial branch of the frontal nerve, and (3) the supratrochlear nerve. Infiltration anesthesia is an alternative approach to anesthetizing lacerations of the forehead.

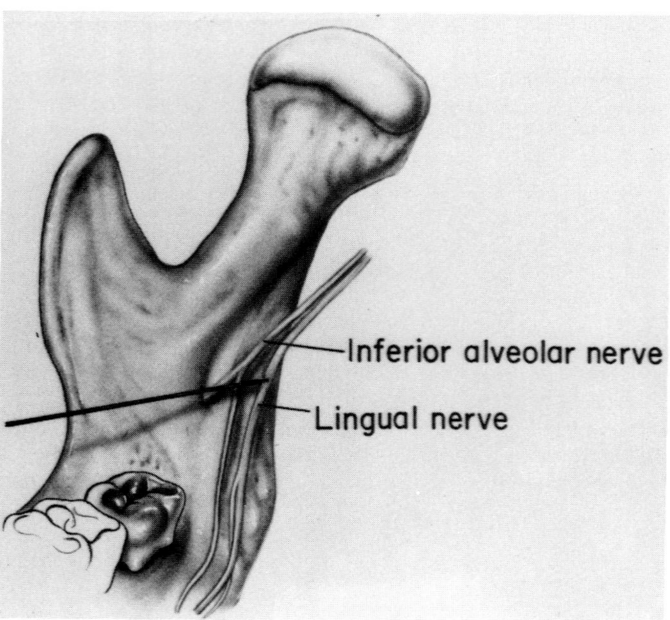

Fig. 189-6. Regional block of the lingual nerve.

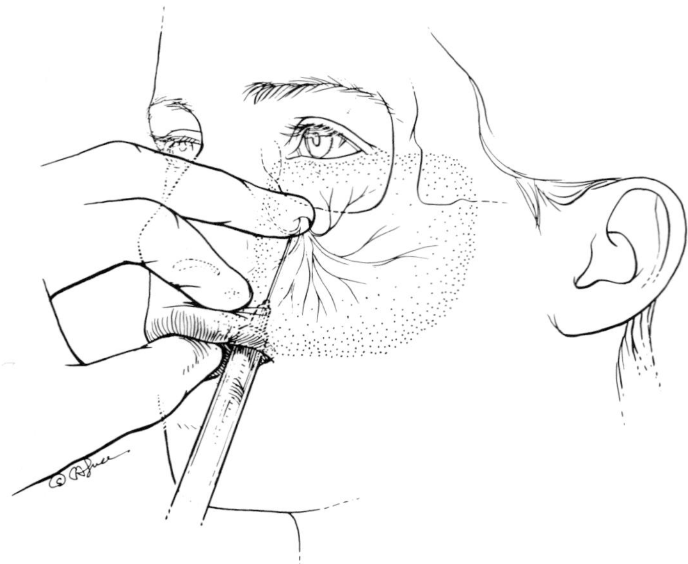

Fig. 189-8. Intraoral approach to regional nerve block of the infraorbital nerve.

general sensory nerve with added taste and secretory fibers from the chorda tympani. It supplies the anterior two-thirds of the ipsilateral tongue, the floor of the mouth, and the gums. It enters the mouth between the medial pterygoid and the mandibular ramus. An intraoral block of the lingual nerve is initiated by first identifying the anterior border of the mandible (the oblique line). The no. 27 needle is then inserted just medial to this line at a point that is approximately 1 cm above the occlusal surface of the third molar (Fig. 189-6). The introduction of a no. 27 needle through the mucosa can be made painless by anesthetizing the mucosa with a topical anesthetic agent. The most effective anesthetic agents on mucous membrane, in order of decreasing activity, are 1% tetracaine, 40% cocaine, and 4% lidocaine. This concentrated form of cocaine is not used clinically. Mixing two drugs does not enhance the duration of activity. After the mucosal injection site is anesthetized, the needle is slowly advanced along the medial side of the ramus to a depth of 2 cm. During the introduction of the needle, the syringe must lie parallel to the body of the mandible and the occlusal surfaces of the teeth of the lower jaw. From 2 to 4 mL of 1% lidocaine with epinephrine (1:100,000) is injected after the syringe is rotated to the premolar region of the opposite side of the mandible, while the needle remains in contact with the ramus of the mandible.

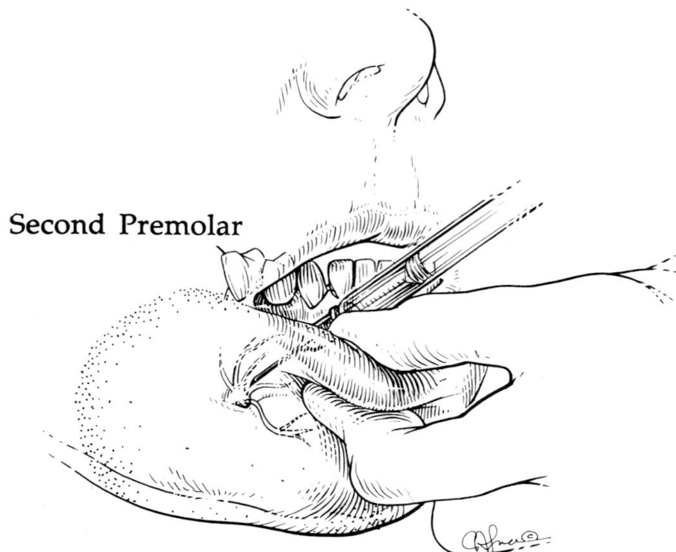

Fig. 189-7. Regional block of the mental nerve.

When anesthetizing the lingual nerve, it is difficult to avoid blocking the inferior alveolar nerve that exists in the mandibular canal as the mental nerve. This nerve supplies the skin and mucous membrane of the ipsilateral lower lip. A regional nerve block of the mental nerve at the mental foramen, however, is a more practical method of anesthetizing lacerations of the lower lip than a regional block of the lingual nerve (Fig. 189-7). A regional block of the mental nerve can be accomplished either extraorally or intraorally. In the latter case, the mucous membrane should be anesthetized by a topically applied local anesthetic agent prior to the introduction of the needle. The mental foramen is located inside the lower lip at its junction with the lower gum, just posterior to the first premolar tooth. The needle is inserted at a point close to the mental foramen, after which 2 mL of 1% lidocaine with epinephrine (1:100,000) is injected. The needle is *not* introduced into the mental foramen to avoid inducing nerve injury with subsequent numbness of the lower lip.

The infraorbital nerve is the continuation of the maxillary nerve. After exiting through the orbital foramen, the infraorbital nerve divides to supply the skin of the lower eyelid, the side of the nose, the upper lip, and the mucous membrane lining the nasal vestibule. A regional nerve block of the infraorbital nerve can be accomplished either extraorally or intraorally. In the latter case (Fig. 189-8), the mucous membrane should be anesthetized by a topically applied anesthetic agent before introduction of the needle. The infraorbital nerve is identified by first palpating the midpoint of the lower border of the orbit with the tip of the long finger, after which it is then advanced caudad 1 cm to the site of the palpable neurovascular bundle that exits through the foramen. With the long finger remaining on the infraorbital foramen, the tips of the thumb and index finger grasp the upper lid and elevate it cephalad. A needle with syringe held in the other hand is introduced into the mucous membrane at its reflection from the upper gum until its point comes to lie under the tip of the long finger. The needle is directed parallel to the long axis of the second bicuspid tooth. The needle is not introduced directly into the infraorbital foramen

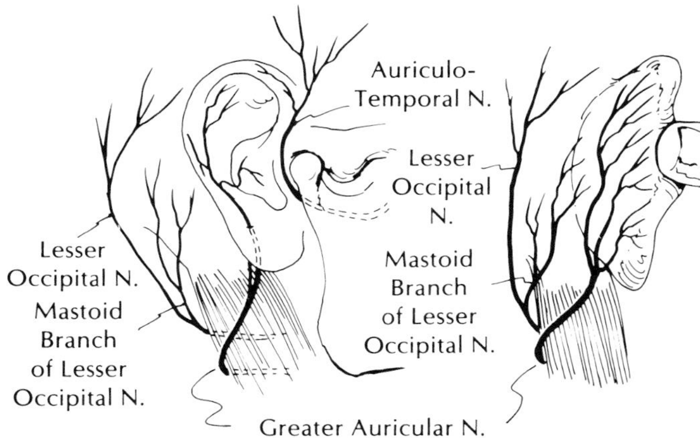

Fig. 189-9. Sensory nerve supply of auricle.

to avoid nerve injury with subsequent numbness of the cheek. Regional anesthesia is accomplished by instilling 2 mL of 1% lidocaine with epinephrine (1:100,000). Care must be taken to avoid injecting the anesthetic agent into the facial artery and vein that are in close proximity to this nerve.

Ear Block

The auricle is also very susceptible to a regional nerve block. Its sensory supply stems mainly from the anterior and posterior branches of the greater auricular nerves, with lesser contributions from the auriculotemporal and lesser occipital nerves (Fig. 189-9). Regional anesthesia of the auricle is accomplished readily by instilling the 0.5% bupivacaine through a no. 27 needle along its base anteriorly and posteriorly (Fig. 189-10). At times, a supplement may be needed at the posterior wall of the external auditory meatus, an area supplied by the auricular branches of the vagal nerve.

SIDE EFFECTS OF ANESTHETIC AGENTS

The side effects of local anesthetic agents can be divided into allergic reactions and systemic toxicity. True allergic reactions to local anesthetic agents are rare. The ester derivatives of para-aminobenzoic acid, such as procaine, were responsible for most allergic reactions;

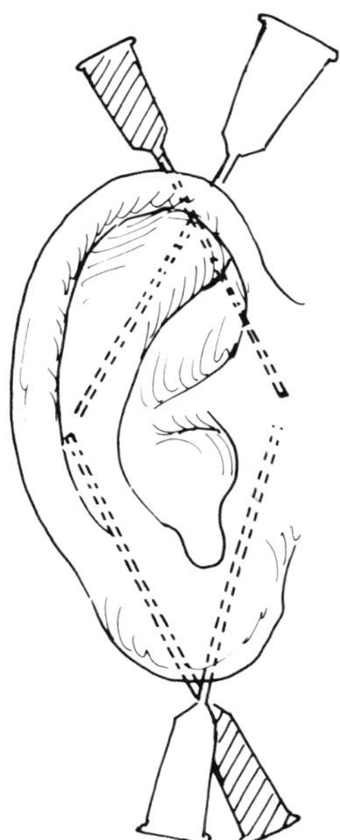

Fig. 189-10. Technique of regional anesthesia of the auricle.

the amide-type local anesthetic compounds have accounted for relatively few. Because the amide-type compounds are believed to be incapable of stimulating antibody formation, true anaphylaxis should not be encountered when these compounds are used. Some patients presumed to be allergic to the amide-type compound had positive skin responses to the preservatives (e.g., methylparaben) or stabilizers added to local anesthetic agents, but not to the anesthetic agent. Because the systemic clinical manifestations of a toxic response to the drug are similar to those of an allergic reaction, it may be difficult to identify a true allergic reaction. Central nervous system (CNS) stimulation by these agents manifested by tachycardia, nausea, vomiting, and seizures may be confused with IgE-mediated response or anaphylaxis. The use of vasoconstrictors, like epinephrine, with the local anesthetic agents may produce system effects that simulate the symptoms of anaphylaxis.

Systemic toxicity is usually due to either a rapid inadvertent intravenous injection, administration of the agent into a highly vascularized area, or injection of an excessive amount of the local anesthetic agent. Adverse reactions involve primarily the CNS and cardiovascular system and can be divided into four stages. The first adverse premonitory signs are CNS symptoms, such as dizziness, tinnitus, periorbital tingling, nystagmus, and fine skeletal muscle twitching. Such systemic reactions can be treated by discontinuing the administration of the anesthetic agent, ensuring a patent airway, providing supplemental oxygen to prevent cerebral hypoxia, and hyperventilation. Overt convulsions of the tonic or clonic type may follow. Most localized or systemic convulsions are self-limiting because of the rapid redistribution to the organ reservoirs, resulting in a decrease in blood levels. When convulsions persist, small incremental doses of diazepam are administered intravenously and repeated cautiously as needed. CNS depression may ensue in which the seizure activity ends and respiratory efforts become shallow. This stage responds to supportive measures that include maintenance of a patent airway, supplemental oxygen, and hyperventilation. Signs and symptoms of cardiovascular collapse are the final stage and require treatment with intravenous fluids and a vasopressor or positive inotropic agent.

Systemic toxicity is treated best by prevention. Rapid injections of the local anesthetic agent should be avoided, and recommended drug dosages should be used. When treating a patient with a convincing history of allergy to an amide-type anesthetic agent, the emergency physician should try a subcutaneous challenge with a local anesthetic agent different from the one causing the previous allergic reaction. An alternative approach is to inject an antihistamine, like 1% diphenhydramine hydrochlorine into the wound, achieving anesthesia for approximately 30 min. The actual mechanism of its anesthetic activity is unclear.

TOPICAL ANESTHESIA

One method of topical anesthesia of lacerations is the use of a topical solution containing 0.5% tetracaine, 1:2000 epinephrine, and 11.8% cocaine (TEC). Advantages are (1) anesthesia without discomfort or tissue swelling and (2) intense vasoconstriction, resulting in a bloodless wound. TEC cannot be used in lacerations involving the ear, penis, and digits because their limited vascularity may be compromised. It also cannot be used on or applied onto mucous membranes, because a toxic reaction to cocaine will result.

In our work, topical application of TEC resulted in an increased incidence of infection and necrosis of the wound edges. Also, the dangers of cocaine toxicity, especially in children, and the necessity of narcotic control are additional hazards to its use.

Another resolved issue involves the medicolegal implications of the use of TEC. It is not commercially available and is prepared in the hospital pharmacy for use in the emergency department. Because TEC is prepared in the pharmacy and is not distributed outside the institution, it is exempt from Food and Drug Administration (FDA) manufacturing regulations. In the absence of regulatory overview, the usual drug testing regimens, such as animal trials, clinical trials, etc., have not been undertaken. It is unclear if this lack of specific FDA approval will result in greater liability in the event that serious toxic consequences occur.

This research was supported by a generous gift from the George Newton Bullard Foundation, Brentwood, Tennessee.

BIBLIOGRAPHY

Adriani J; Etiology and management of adverse reactions to local anesthetics. *Int Anesthesiol Clin* 10:127, 1972.

Adriani J, Zepernigh R: Clinical effectiveness of drugs used for topical anesthesia. *JAMA* 188:711, 1964.

Altman RS, Smith-Coggins R, Ampel LL: Local anesthetics. *Ann Emerg Med* 14:1209, 1985.

Arndt KA, Burton C, Noe JM: Minimizing the pain of local anesthesia. *Plast Reconstr Surg* 72:676, 1983.

Barker W, Rodeheaver GT, Edgerton MT, et al: Damage to the tissue defenses by a topical anesthetic agent. *Ann Emerg Med* 11:307, 1982.

Covino BG, Vassallo HG: *Local Anesthesia, Mechanism of Action and Clinical Use*. New York, Grune & Stratton, 1976, pp 57-95.

Edlich RF, Smith JF, Mayer NE, et al: Performance of disposable needle syringe systems for local anesthesia. *J Emerg Med* 5:83, 1987.

Fariss BL, Foresman PA, Rodeheaver GT, et al: Anesthetic properties and toxicity of bupivacaine and lidocaine for infiltration anesthesia. *J Emerg Med* 5:275, 1987.

Pryor GJ, Kilpatrick WR, Opp DR: Local anesthesia in minor lacerations. Topical TAC versus lidocaine infiltration. *Ann Emerg Med* 9:568, 1980.

Stevenson TR, Rodeheaver GT, Golden GT, et al: Damage to tissue defenses by vasoconstrictors. *JACEP* 4:532, 1975

190 WOUND PREPARATION

Richard F. Edlich
George T. Rodeheaver
John G. Thacker

HAIR REMOVAL

Hair is a source of wound contamination, and removal of hair prevents hair from becoming entangled in suture and the wound during closure. However, the infection rate in surgical wounds following razor preparation of the skin is significantly greatly than that after hair removal by electric clippers.

This increased incidence of infection following razor preparation is probably related to the trauma inflicted by the razor. As a result of the shave, wounded hair follicles provide access to and substrate for bacteria. Surgical electric clippers cut hair close to the skin surface without nicking the skin, and we now employ only electric clippers when it is necessary to remove hair. Recent advances in the design of electric clippers make them especially suitable for hair removal. The clipper blade assembly can be easily removed from its mounting assembly on the electric motor so that it can be cleaned and sterilized. Sterilization of the clipper blade assemblies for the electric clipper eliminates its high level of bacterial contamination.

Hair provides an important landmark for the precise reapproximation of the divided tissue. This is particularly true in the eyebrow, where misalignment of the wound edges may be exceedingly difficult to correct at a later date.

SKIN ANTISEPSIS

Disinfection of the skin around the wound should be initiated without contacting the wound itself. Two groups of antiseptic agents, containing either an iodophor or chlorhexidine, exhibit activity against a broad spectrum of organisms and suppress bacterial proliferation. The superiority of one antiseptic agent over another has not been shown. Although these agents can reduce the bacterial concentration on intact skin, they appear to damage the wound defenses and invite the development of infection within the wound itself. Consequently, inadvertent spillage of these agents into the wound should be avoided.

HEMOSTASIS

During any wounding process, blood vessels will be divided resulting in bleeding into the wound. The magnitude of blood loss is directly related to the size of the divided vessels. Fortunately, most bleeding can be stopped by applying direct pressure to saline soaked lint-free sponges placed within the wound. Rubbing or abrading the wound must be avoided, because this dislodges thrombi and may cause further bleeding. Furthermore, emergency physicians should never resort to hot wet sponges for hemostasis because this treatment results in a hyperthermic injury to tissue that potentiates the development of infection.

Following removal of the gauze sponges, persistent bleeding from vessels whose diameter is less than 2 mm should be stopped by pinpoint electrosurgical coagulation. The use of bipolar coagulation is a more precise method of hemostasis that limits the tissue injury encountered with the more traditional monopolar coagulation. An equivalent current passed through a monopolar electrode causes approximately three times as much necrosis of the surrounding tissue as the use of bipolar coagulation. Bleeding from cut ends of large vessels whose diameter is over 2 mm can rarely be controlled by electrocoagulation. In such cases, hemostasis can be achieved easily with a suture ligature of nonreactive synthetic absorbable braided suture materials. The divided end of the vessel should be isolated over a short length and clamped with a small curved hemostat. This technique is preferred over clamping the retracted vessel along with the contiguous blood stained tissue. In the latter case, the amount of strangulated tissue is about five times greater than with the vessel-isolating technique.

Occasionally, as with a patient with a bleeding diathesis, primary wound closure cannot be accomplished because of persistent bleeding. In such cases, the wound should be packed with type I gauze sponges and elevated, if the anatomic site of the wound allows. The wound should then be reexamined within 24 hours to determine if hemostasis is now sufficient to allow primary closure. Prior to closure, any residual hematoma should be evacuated from the wound because it can serve as a culture medium for bacteria.

SURGICAL DEBRIDEMENT

Debridement removes tissue heavily contaminated by soil infection-potentiating fractions and bacteria and excises devitalized tissues that impair the wound's ability to resist infection. The capacity of devitalized fat, muscle, and skin to enhance bacterial infection is comparable.

Deviatlized soft tissue enhances infection by acting as an anaerobic culture medium promoting bacterial growth, and by inhibiting phagocytosis. Identification of the exact limits of devitalized tissue in wounds remains a challenging problem, especially in muscle. Viability of muscle can be determined by the "4C" guidelines (color, consistency, contraction, circulation). Generations of physicians have identified non-viable muscle by its dark color, its mushy consistency, its failure to contract when pinched with forceps, and the absence of brisk bleeding from its cut surface. These clinical indicators of muscle viability are most accurate when the wound is examined 4 to 5 days after the initial operation.

The viability of skin is considerably easier to judge than that of muscle. At 24 h after injury, a sharp line of demarcation is often apparent between the devitalized and viable skin. In fresh skin wounds in which this demarcation is not precise, the distribution of an intravenously injected flourescein dye within the tissues may prove helpful. Early staining of the injured tissue by fluorescein is evidence of tissue viability. At times, active bleeding from the distal dermal margin may be present and indicates viability.

In some anatomic sites, like the trunk, debridement is best accomplished by more complete excision of the skin and deep tissues. The soft tissues are usually free of specialized tissues, such as nerves or tendons, that perform important physical functions. In these regions, heavily contaminated wounds with serpiginous defects can be converted into clean wounds by more generous tissue excisions.

The adequacy of debridement may be monitored either by forcibly packing the wound with gauze or by coloring the wound surface with a vital dye (Fig. 190-1). Complete excision of the wound, back to a margin of normal tissue, is judged by dissecting in a plane that does not expose the gauze or the blue dye. Suturing the skin edges of the wound prior to excision may further minimize mechanical spread of the wound contaminants into uninjured tissue.

When a heavily contaminated wound contains specialized tissues, such as nerves or tendons, complete excision often is not feasible. In such cases, high-pressure irrigation, followed by excision of all fragments of tissue that are not clearly viable, is indicated. In a compound wound of the hand, selective debridement of nonviable fascia, tendon, fat, etc., is tedious but essential as it constitutes dangerous pabulum for bacteria if left in situ.

A specific exception to the general principle of removing all devitalized tissue is made in treating specialized tissues that perform

This research was supported by a generous gift from the Ira W. DeCamp Foundation, New York, NY.

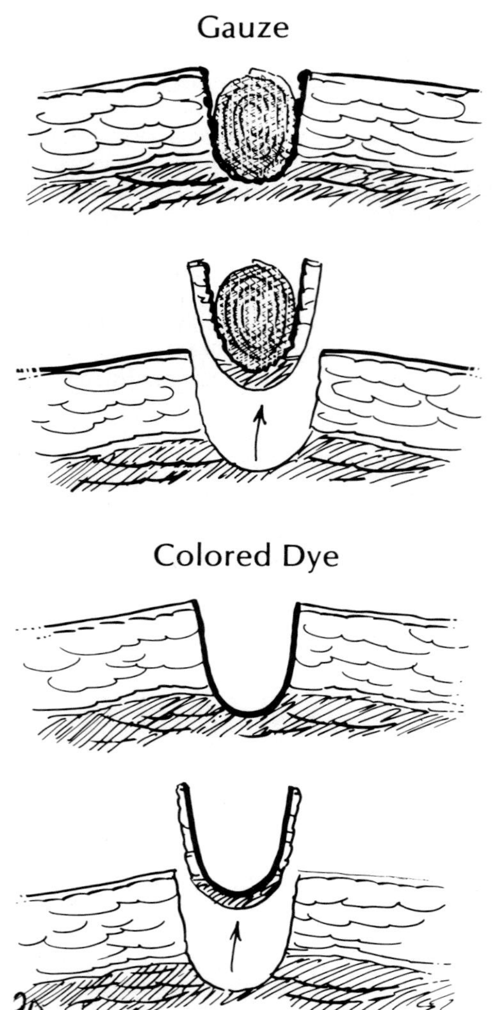

190-1. Monitoring the adequacy of debridement of forcibly packing the wound with gauze (top) or by coloring the wound surface with a vital dye (bottom).

important physical functions, regardless of their viability. Tissues like dura, fascia, and tendon may survive as free grafts without living cells if immediately covered by healthy pedicle flaps. Cells from the wound may then invade the graft as part of the healing process. If these tissues can be rendered surgically clean, they should be left in the wound.

Following debridement, the selection of wound closure technique is dependent on the level of wound contamination and the amount of residual devitalized tissue. In wounds contacted by gross pus or feces, an infective dose of bacteria often remains on the wound surface despite the most aggressive wound cleaning. Infection can be minimized by utilizing delayed primary closure. As the wound heals, it gains increased resistance to infection, premitting closure on or after the fourth postwounding day without subsequent infections.

For high-energy-depositor missile injuries, tissue injury is extensive and difficult to ascertain accurately soon after injury. In these cases, the wound should be explored in the operating theater to remove devitalized tissue and foreign bodies, to rule out damage to vessels and nerves, and to relieve increased compartmental pressure that may follow edema or slow bleeding into a fascia-enclosed muscle compartment. Open wound management is the method of choice.

Civilian traumatic wounds resulting from impact injuries or low-energy-depositor missiles usually contain devitalized tissue that is easily recognized. Debridement, cleansing, and antibiotic treatment usually convert these wounds into clean wounds, which are amenable to primary closure either by direct approximation of the wound edges or by coverage with a flap or graft.

Debridement of skin and underlying tissue leaves a significant soft tissue defect that resists reapproximation. As a result of strong static skin tensions on the edges of the debrided wound, repair is accomplished with a wide scar. In general, extensive wound debridement is best performed in an operating room theater with adequate lighting and surgical instruments.

MECHANICAL CLEANSING

Mechanical forces are employed to rid the wound of bacteria and other particulate matter that are retained on the wound surface by adhesive forces. The two basic modes employed are hydraulic forces and direct contact.

In irrigation, the hydraulic forces of the irrigating stream act on particulate matter in the wound. The magnitude of the hydraulic forces is a function of the relative velocities and the configuration of the particle. When subjected to the same irrigating stream, particles with a smaller frontal surface area experience less force than particles with a similar configuration, but with a greater surface area. Consequently it takes significantly smaller hydraulic pressures to rid the wound of large foreign bodies that it does to remove small particles and bacteria.

The level of hydraulic forces experienced by the particle is also increased considerably as the velocity of the irrigating stream is raised. The simplest and most practical methods of raising the velocity are to increase the pressure within the irrigating syringe and to enlarge the internal diameter of the needle or catheter.

The pressure exerted by fluid delivered through a 19-gauge needle by a 35-mL syring is 8 lb/in^{2}. Irrigation pressure of this magnitude or higher has been classified "high pressure," while irrigation pressure below this level, as with a bulb syringe, has been designated "low pressure." High-pressure irrigation cleanses the wound of small particulate matter, bacteria, and soil infection-potentiating fractions. Low-pressure irrigation, even with large volumes of fluid, does not remove small particles like bacteria or soil infection-potentiating fractions, but easily removes large particles like detached devitalized tissue.

Despite the advantages of high-pressure irrigation, several theoretical objections have been raised against the routine use of this technique. One commonly expressed concern is that foreign bodies on the surface of the wound may be disseminated more deeply into the wound as a result of high-pressure irrigation. On the basis of recent studies, this fear appears to be unfounded. Consequent to high-pressure irrigation, bacteria remain at the surface of the wound even though the irrigant solution may disseminate deeply into the tissues. The tissue penetration of a high-pressure irrigating stream is predominantly in a lateral direction, similar to that encountered with a jet parenteral injection.

However, concern that high-pressure irrigation can damage tissue defenses appears to be justified. Pulsatile or syringe irrigation results in trauma to the tissues that makes the wound more susceptible to experimental infection. Therefore, high-pressure irrigation should be reserved for use in heavily contaminated wounds, where the benefits of this technique outweigh its consequences.

In the clinical setting, high-pressure irrigation is accomplished with an inexpensive disposable irrigation assembly consisting of a 19-gauge plastic needle or catheter attached to a 35-mL syringe (Fig. 190-2). Sterile electrolyte solution (usually 1000 mL of 0.9% sodium chloride) is delivered through a one-way valve attached to the syringe barrel via standard intravenous plastic tubing. The tip of the needle, fastened to the syringe filled with saline, is placed perpendicular, and as close as possible, to the surface of the wound; then the plunger is depressed with maximal force.

An example of direct mechanical contact is scrubbing a dirty wound with a sponge. Although this technique is an effective means of removing bacteria from wounds, tissue trauma inflicted by scrubbing

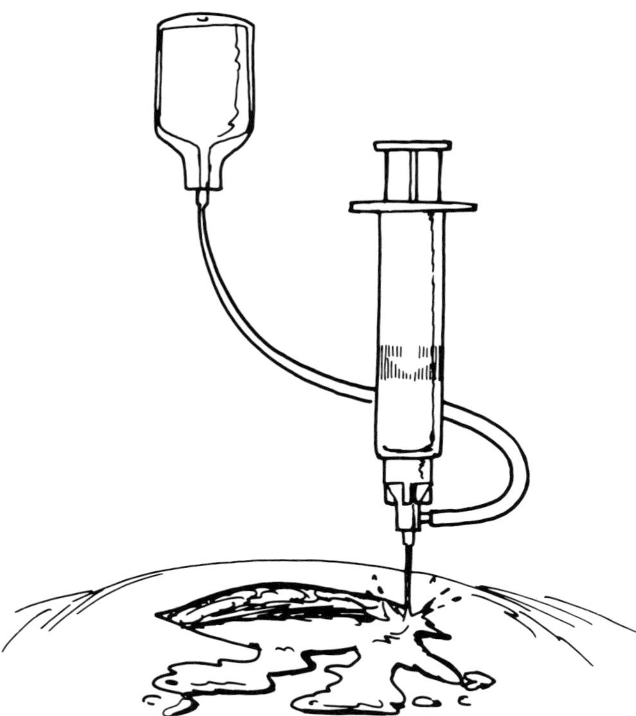

190-2. High-pressure syringe irrigation assembly. Note that the needle is held as close as possible and perpendicular to the surface of the wound during wound irrigation.

impairs the wound's ability to resist infection and allows residual bacteria to elicit an inflammatory response. Sponges with a low porosity are more abrasive and exert more damage to the wound than sponges with a higher porosity. The addition of a nontoxic surfactant, poloxamer 188, to a fine-pore sponge, minimizes the tissue damage it inflicts while maintaining the bacterial removal efficiency of mechanical cleansing.

Poloxamer 188[1] is a member of a family of block copolymers called Pluronic polyols. In contrast to all other commercially available scrub solutions, this surfactant is so innocuous that it can be used to soak an unanesthetized wound without discomfort to the patient. These circumstances offer a distinct advantage over other surgical scrub solutions that evoke considerable pain following contact with the injured tissue. Toxic effects and allergic reactions are very rare, and poloxamer 188 does not alter the wound's resistance to infection and healing, or the cellular components of blood. However, it exhibits no antibacterial activity.

Exposure of the wound to either Hibiclens[2] or Betadine Surgical Scrub Solution[3] causes pain or irritation and damages tissue defenses, inviting infection. In our opinion, a safe and effective surfactant—one that satisfies the dictum "The only solution that should be placed in a wound is one that can be safely poured in the physician's eye"—should replace toxic scrub solutions.

[1]Calgon Corporation, St. Louis, Mo.

[2]Stuart Pharmaceuticals, Wilmington, Del.

[3]Purdue Frederick, Norwalk, Conn.

Embedded foreign debris should be removed as soon as possible. Removal of embedded foreign particles requires either local or regional anesthesia. A natural fiber scrub brush soaked in poloxamer 188 removes the embedded debris from most wounds. Power-driven abraders with stainless steel cylinders coated with tungsten carbide grit can also be used to dislodge these foreign bodies. When isolated foreign bodies are embedded deeply in the deep dermal tissue, a no. 11 scalpel blade can be used as a spud to tease or excise these particles individually. An operating room micriscope enhances visualization of the particles allowing prompt, aggressive, and meticulous removal. While the skin edges are stabilized with fine-tooth eye forceps (Bonn forceps with 0.1-mm teeth), particles are removed from the depth of the wound with a no. 67 Beaver scalpel blade. Any recalcitrant particles are excised with the no. 65 Beaver blade. Wound closure is accomplished with a single 8–0 monofilament synthetic nonabsorbable suture. The debrided wound is covered by fine-mesh gauze (type I) that is impregnated with bacitracin. This antibiotic is reapplied every 6 h for approximately 3 to 4 days, when the gauze spontaneously separates from the underlying healing epidermis. If the foreign debris is not removed immediately, it becomes impossible to trace the paths and remove the individual particles in the depths of the dermis, resulting in a permanent traumatic tattoo.

BIBLIOGRAPHY

Hair Removal

Alexander JW, Fischer JE, Boyajian M, et al: The influence of hair-removal methods on wound infections. *Arch Surg* 118:347, 1983.

Masterson TS, Rodeheaver GT, Morgan RF, et al: Bacteriologic evaluation of electric clipper for surgical hair removal. *Am J Surg* 148:301, 1984.

Skin Antisepsis

Custer J, Edlich RF, Prusak M, et al: Studies in the management of the contaminated wound. V. An assessment of the effectiveness of pHisoHex and Betadine surgical scrub solutions. *Am J Surg* 121:572, 1971.

Kaul AF, Jewett JF: Agents and techniques for disinfection of the skin. *Surg Gynecol Obstet* 152:677, 1981.

Surgical Debridement

Bongard FS, Elings VB, Markison RE: New uses of fluorescence in the management of necrotizing soft tissue infection. *Am J Surg* 150:261, 1985.

Haury B, Rodeheaver G, Vensko J, et al: Debridement: An essential component of traumatic wound care. *Am J Surg* 135:238, 1978.

Mechanical Cleansing

Bryant CA, Rodeheaver GT, Reem EM, et al: Search for a non-toxic surgical scrub solution for periorbital lacerations. *Ann Emerg Med* 13:317, 1984.

Edlich RF, Schmolka IR, Prusak MP, et al: The molecular basis for toxicity of surfactants in surgical wounds. 1. EO:PO block polymers. *J Surg Res* 14:277, 1973.

Rodeheaver GT, Kurtz L, Kircher BJ, et al: A promising new skin wound cleanser. *Ann Emerg Med* 9:572, 1980.

Rodeheaver GT, Smith SL, Thacker JG, et al: Mechanical cleansing of contaminated wounds witha surfactant. *Am J Surg* 129:241, 1975.

Stevenson TR, Thacker JG, Rodeheaver GT, et al: Cleansing the traumatic wound by high pressure syringe irrigation. *JACEP* 5:17, 1976.

Wheeler CB, Rodeheaver GT, Thacker JG, et al: Side-effects of high pressure irrigation. *Surg Gynecol Obstet* 243:775, 1976.

191
ANTIBIOTICS AND DRAINS IN WOUND MANAGEMENT

Richard F. Edlich
George T. Rodeheaver
John G. Thacker

ANTIBIOTICS

The relative success of antibiotic therapy in the prevention of infection in wounds is influenced by the time of administration, the concentration of bacteria in the wound, the presence of soil infection-potentiating fractions, and the mechanism of injury. In laboratory and clinical studies, antibiotic therapy is significantly more effective when the drug is administered preoperatively rather than intraoperatively or postoperatively. Delay in antibiotic treatment diminishes its therapeutic merit. When there is an unavoidable delay in administering these drugs, the length of time during which the wound is left open becomes significant. Exposure causes a sequence of events that substantially limits the therapeutic value of antibiotics.

When any wound is left open, its vessels exhibit a marked increase in vascular permeability. Fluids from the intravascular space extravasate and fill the wound crater. This exudate is rich in a wide variety of proteins, including fibrinogen. Once outside the vessels, much of the protein exudate is reabsorbed and partly polymerizes to form fibrin. This resulting fibrinous coagulum surrounds the bacteria and protects them from contact with the antibiotic. The cause of this exaggerated inflammatory response in the open wound has not been defined. However, it may be related to environmental conditions. The temperature of the emergency department is usually considerably below the systemic body temperature, encouraging loss of heat from the wound. In addition, evaporation of fluid from the wound surface results in further heat loss and cooling of the tissues. A consequence of fluid heat loss from the wound is desiccation. Warming the treatment room or covering the wound with wet sponges should reduce these environmental effects. Paradoxically, the fibrinous wound coagulum, which limits the effectiveness of antibiotics, may be a crucial positive factor in the host's defense against infection. The coagulum may serve as a plug in the open mouths of lymphatics preventing dissemination of bacteria. Occlusion of lymphatics by the coagulum then becomes an obstacle to the invasion of bacteria and, in part, accounts for the resistance of an open wound to systemic sepsis.

This surface coagulum may be disrupted by a variety of mechanisms. Gentle scrubbing of the surface of the wound with a gauze sponge disturbs the fibrinous cover and allows an antibiotic to gain intimate contact with the bacteria. Consequently, the therapeutic effectiveness of antibiotics is measurably enhanced by this treatment. Enzymatic digestion is a less traumatic and more selective means of disrupting the coagulum. The in vitro fibrinolytic capacity of certain enzymes provides an accurate measure of their ability to potentiate antimicrobial activity. Travase, a proteolytic enzyme produced by *Bacillus subtilis,* has the greatest fibrinolytic capacity and is the most effective enzymatic adjunct to antibiotic treatment. Hydrolysis of the protein coagulum can be accomplished within 30 min by the topical application of Travase. This brief exposure does not damage the wound's defenses or its healing capacity.

The presence of wound contaminants can influence the outcome of antibiotic therapy. When the wound is contaminated by an exceedingly large number of organisms (more than 10^9), infection will develop despite antibiotic treatment. This circumstance is encountered when the wound surface is contacted by either pus, feces, vaginal discharge, or saliva. Soil infection-potentiating fractions in wounds also have considerable influence on the efficacy of specific antibiotics. The benefit of antibiotics in the presence of these fractions is predicted by the chemical composition of the antibiotic. The basic antibiotics (e.g., gentamicin) and amphoteric antibiotics (e.g., tetracycline) are inactivated by these negatively charged fractions. The acidic antibiotics, like cephalosporins and penicillin, do not bind with these fractions and thus exert their antibacterial effect in wounds contaminated by them. Finally, impact injuries result in a demonstrable reduction in blood flow to the wound edges, limiting the access of systemically administered antibiotics. Thus the efficacy of antibiotic therapy in impact wounds is substantially less than in wounds caused by shear forces.

Antibiotic Prophylaxis

Antibiotic prophylaxis has theraupeutic merit in seveal clinical settings. Because bacterial endocarditis is associated with significant morbidity and mortality, its prevention by antibiotic treatment has been a universally accepted and worthwhile goal. Patients at risk for developing endocarditis following a transient bacterema include those with prosthetic valves, arteriovenous fistula, patent ductus arteriosus, tetralogy of Fallot, ventricular septal defect, coarction of the aorta, and valvular disease.

Certain general principles provide the basis for antibiotic prophylaxis of bacterial endocarditis. Owning to the uncertainty of antibiotic sensitivity of the circulating organisms, antibiotics that display a broad spectrum of antibacterial activity are recommended. Moreover, the efficacy of a single bactericidal agent or a mixture of bactericidal agents is judged to be superior to that of bacteriostatic agents. Finally, a parenteral regimen that produces a high initial concentration of the agents, followed by a prolonged inhibitory concentration, is preferred. The timing of antibiotic administration appears to have considerable influence on its efficacy. Whenever it can be anticipated that microorganisms might gain access to the circulation of the patient, appropriate antimicrobial chemotherapy should be instituted immediately and during and after the period of risk. When pretreatment is impossible, as in the case of lacerations or infections, intravenous injection of antibiotics should be instituted as soon as possible. The intravenous route is preferred over the intramuscular route because it results in reliable antibiotic concentrations without precipitating intramuscular bleeding in the anticoagulated patient.

Staphylococcus aureus and *S. epidermidis* are the pathogens most often responsible for soft tissue infections resulting in bacterial endocarditis. Because most *S. aureus* isolates, whether community- or hospital-acquired, are resistant to penicillin, the current recommended regimen for preventing infective endocarditis includes either a penicillinase-resistant penicillin, or a cephalosporin (Table 191–1). In patients who are allergic to penicillin, vancomycin is an appropriate alternative. The addition of gentamicin produces a synergistic effect against *S. aureus* in vitro and in experimental staphylococcal endocarditis in rabbits.

The choice of an appropriate regimen to prevent bacterial endocarditis when *S. epidermidis* is the etiologic agent is complicated by the unpredictable and high frequency of multiple methicillin-resistant strains. In some institutions, these resistant strains account for 70 to 90% of the *S. epidermidis* causing bacterial endocarditis. There is probably no satisfactory antimicrobial regimen to prevent infective endocarditis due to methicillin-resistant *S. epidermidis,* but recent in vitro studies suggest that an aminoglycoside with a cephalosporin may be helpful. If the patient is allergic to the cephalosporin, vanocomycin can be used.

Convincing cases of hematogenous infections of arterial grafts (those appearing more than 60 days after surgery) are nearly unknown. Almost all reported infections probably originated from contamination at surgery, from contiguous areas of purulence, or from the development

Table 191-1. Regimen for Prophylaxis of Infective Endocarditis

Adults	Children
PATIENTS NOT ALLERGIC TO CEFAZOLIN	
Cefazolin 2.0 g IV	Cefazolin 30 mg/kg IV
plus	*plus*
Gentamicin 1.5 mg/kg IV	Gentamicin 2.0 mg/kg IV
Give initial dose immediately, then repeat both drugs every 8 h for five additional doses.	Give initial dose immediately, then repeat both drugs every 8 h for five additional doses.
PATIENTS ALLERGIC TO CEFAZOLIN	
Vancomycin 0.5–1.0 g IV infused slowly over 1 h	Vancomycin 20 mg/kg infused slowly over 1 h
plus	*plus*
Gentamicin 1.5 mg/kg IV	Gentamicin 2.0 mg/kg IV
Both drugs may be repeated 12 h later.	Both drugs may be repeated 12 h later.

of a fistula between the graft and the GI tract. Even in hip arthroplasties, the sources of infection have been distant sites of established suppuration, such a tonsillitis, cholecystitis, dental abscess, pyoderma, suppurative parotitis, or cystitis, rather than procedure-induced transient bacteremia. These findings emphasize the importance of prompt and thorough treatment of distant infections in patients with indwelling prosthetic devices.

Lymphedematous patients are especially likely to develop infection. A streptococcus or, less often, a staphylococcus can be isolated from the infected tissue. Each infection produces more lympathic destruction and edema. In patients with lymphedema and recurrent cellulitis, a generally accepted antimicrobial prophylaxis is 1.2 million units of penicillin G. benzathine administered intramuscularly per month. When a minor soft tissue laceration occurs in lymphadematous tissue, antimicrobial treatment should be initiated immediately before wound closure.

Antibiotic prophylaxis should be considered for the immunocompromised patient with a wound. Primary immunodeficiency defects are defects in cellular differentiation and are classified according to whether the prominent defect is in neutrophil or T- or B-cell function. The practicing emergency physician is unlikely to encounter primary immunodeficiency; most immunosuppression in emergency department patients is acquired secondary to disease process (e.g., malnutrition, diabetes, renal failure) or medical interventions (e.g., immunosuppressive medications). Wound infections in such patients are caused by common pathogens such as *S. aureus* and mixed bacterial species. There may, however, be a delayed onset of infection.

Antibiotic treatment of soft tissue lacerations is also advocated when the probability of infection is high (equal to or more than 10%). Several factors have been identified that increase the likelihood of infection. The anatomic site is one of the most important. Wounds of the feet are especially prone to infection, whereas facial and scalp wounds are rarely infected. The appearance of the wound is a reliable index of its risk for infections. Wounds that are judged to be dirty or contaminated exhibit a higher incidence of infection than do clean wounds. Moreover, experimental studies demonstrate that stellate lacerations with abrasions of the skin adjacent to the wound are much more infection prone than are linear lacerations. The weakened local tissue defenses of stellate lacerations make them susceptible to the development of infection by a relatively small inoculum.

The length of the wound may be another important consideration. In our review of clinical studies, the infection rate of long wounds (5 cm or longer) was greater than that of short ones. Another indication for antibiotic treatment of a soft tissue laceration is a delay in wound cleansing and repair for 6 h or more.

Antibiotic treatment is also indicated in a patient with a wound contaminated by either saliva, feces, or vaginal secretions. Antibiotic treatment can reduce the number of bacteria in such heavily contaminated wounds, but a significant number of organisms often persists, resulting in a high incidence of infection. Consequently the most reliable method of preventing the development of infection in such wounds is open wound management.

Antibiotics must be administered to patients with wounds in which the magnitude of tissue injury is extensive and difficult to ascertain accurately soon after injury. In such cases, open wound management is the method of choice with subsequent additional debridement as dictated by the appearance of the wound. It must be emphasized that antibiotic therapy is an adjunct to debridement, rather than a replacement. In all missile injuries, adequate blood levels of penicillin or an antibiotic (cephalosporin) with a similar spectrum of activity should be established as soon as possible after wounding to prevent streptococcal bacteremia. Streptolysin produced by the virulent streptococcal species breaks down the fibrin that has been deposited in the body in an attempt to wall off collections of bacterial pathogens. Since the discovery of antibiotics, streptococcal bacteremia has all but been eliminated in cases of missile injuries.

When antibiotic treatment of soft tissue lacerations is indicated a number of therapeutic guidelines for antibiotic usage must be considered. The immediate selection of the specific antimicrobial agent is based on consideration of the results of direct microscopic examination of a wound biopsy, the normal bacterial flora harbored in different parts of the body, and the pathogens usually encountered in various diseases or conditions. Later, the results of immediate antibiotic sensitivity testing can also influence the emergency physician's choice of antibiotic. Antibiotic sensitivity testing is performed under aerobic conditions directly on the bacterial suspension prepared from the wound biopsy specimen rather than on strains isolated from the tissue. Because soft tissue wounds are contaminated by mixtures of facultative organisms, a broad-spectrum antibiotic must be chosen. The antibiotic should be present in the wound tissue fluid in an effective concentration at the time of wound closure. Consequently, the antibiotics should be administered by an intravenous route that results in high tissue concentrations.

DRAINAGE

Drainage evacuates potentially harmful collections of certain fluids, such as pus and blood, from wounds. In instances in which no definite localized fluid exists, drainage is prophylactic and its potentially harmful effects become more important. Drains act as retrograde conduits through which skin contaminants gain entrance into the wound. Placement of drains within experimental wounds exposed to subinfective inoculations of bacteria greatly enhanced the rate of infection compared with undrained controls. In our experience, both Silastic and Penrose drains dramatically increased the infection rate of soft tissue wounds. The rate of infection when the drain was brought out through the wound was similar to the rate when the drain lay entirely within the wound, suggesting a deleterious effect of the drain per se.

This research was supported by a generous gift from Mr. Alex von Thelen of Charlottesville, Virginia.

BIBLIOGRAPHY

Antibiotics

Edlich RF, Kenney JG, Morgan RF, et al: Antimicrobial treatment of minor soft tissue lacerations: A critical review, *Emerg Med Clin North Am* 4:560, 1986.

Edlich RF, Madden JE, Prusak M, et al: Studies in the management of the contaminated wound. VI. The therapeutic value of gentle scrubbing in prolonging the limited period of effectiveness of antibiotics in contminated wounds. *Am J Surg* 121:668, 1971.

Rodeheaver G, Edgerton MT, Elliott MB, et al: Proteolytic enzymes as adjuncts to antibiotic prophylaxis of surgical wounds. *Am J Surg* 127:564, 1974.

Rodeheaver G, Marsh D, Edgerton MT, et al: Proteolytic enzymes as adjuncts to antimicrobial prophylaxis of contaminated wounds. *Am J Surg* 129:537, 1975.

Talkington CM, Thompson JE: Prevention and management of infected prostheses. *Surg Clin North Am* 62:515, 1982.

Van Scoy RE, Wilkowske CJ: Prophylactic use of antimicrobial agents. *Mayo Clin Proc* 58:241, 1983.

Verklin R, Rodeheaver GT, Hudson R, et al: Rapid antibiotic disk sensitivities of burn eschar and infected wounds. *Surg Gynecol Obstet* 144:507, 1977.

Drainage

Krizek,TJ, Davis JH: The role of the red cell in subcutaneous infection. *J Trauma* 5:85, 1965.

Magee C, Rodeheaver GT, Golden GT, et al: Potentiation of wound infection by surgical drains. *Am J Surg* 131:547, 1976.

Smith M, Enquist IF: A quantitative study of impaired healing resulting from infection. *Surg Gynecol Obstet* 125:965, 1967.

192 PUNCTURE WOUNDS AND MAMMALIAN BITES

George Podgorny

PUNCTURE WOUNDS

Puncture wounds usually occur accidentally and result from penetration of a sharp, elongated object through the skin into the deeper tissues. The elasticity of the skin and the pressure generated by physical activity frequently close the entrance wound, permitting potential entrapment of microorganisms in the deeper level.

Punctures caused by extremely thin items such as needles, pins, or thin wire usually heal without complications. Wounds from thicker penetrating objects such as ice picks, large nails, barbed wire, glass, metal, or wood are much more likely to become infected. Any debris deposited into the depth of a puncture wound will serve as a focus in infection.

If a radiopaque foreign body may have been introduced at the time of injury, an x-ray should be obtained. This is particularly important when the offending item may be a broken needle or pin, wire, glass, or coral. Puncture wounds should be explored for foreign body fragments, copiously irrigated, and cleansed. Application of a cuff tourniquet and excision of a small core of skin at the entrance site may aid in exploration.

There no consensus on the use of prophylactic antibiotics for punctures. Broad-spectrum antibiotics such as cephalosporins may be useful for contaminated wounds. Tetanus prophylaxis is indicated for all puncture wounds.

Puncture wounds of the palmar aspect of the hand can damage tendons, nerves, or arteries, and are especially prone to infection. When the sole of the foot is punctured parts of the sole of the shoe may be driven ahead of the nail into the deeper tissues of the foot. The midsole portion of rubber-soled ''sneaker'' type shoes with synthetic insets may harbor *Pseudomonas aeruginosa,* and puncture wounds of the foot made by nails or glass shards that have penerated through the soles of such shoes may inoculate deep tissues with *P. aeruginosa* bacteria. Such contamination may result in the delayed development of septic arthritis of the tarsal joints, osteomyelitis, or osterchondritis of the calcaneal apophysis. Staphylococci and streptococci have also been isolated from such wounds. Patients should be informed about the possibility of delayed infections. However, routine antibiotic prophylaxis is not currently recommended. If infection develops, ciprofloxacin, amoxicillin-clavulanate, tobramycin, or ceftazidime should be given, with treatment guided by the results of cultures and sensivitity. Cases that do not respond promptly to oral antibiotics should undergo surgical exploration, debridement, and intravenous antibiotic treatment.

HUMAN BITES

In addition to injury of the skin and soft tissues, infection must be considered as a complication in the treatment of a human bite. The human oral cavity is heavily populated with aerobic and anaerobic microorganisms, including fusospirochetes; as a result, infections of human bites are common.

The scalp and the dorsum of the hand are the most common locations of human bites. Scalp bites are frequent in children, while hand bites generally occur from contact between a closed fist of one individual and the open mouth of another. Other common locations of human bites include the penis, scrotum, vulva, breasts, ear, nose and forearm.

Frequently, the injury is not reported as a human bite and is even vociferously denied to have been produced by the human mouth. Therefore, when treating cuts, scratches, and lacerations of the scalp, dorsum of the hand, or genitalia, consider the possibilty that they were produced by a human bite.

A variety of organisms have been recovered from the human mouth and from cutaneous infections caused by human bites. These include aerobic and anaerobic streptococci, *Staphylococcus aureus,* other gram-positive cocci, gam-negative rods, and *Bacteroides* species, among others.

Treatment

A wound due to a human bite should be meticulously cleansed and irrigated with copious amounts of sterile saline solution. Saline or other cleansing fluid should be poured perpendicularly or tangentially over and into the wound. Very small wounds can be irrigated with a syringe, directing the stream into the depth of the puncture wound. Devices are available that generate a steady or intermittent stream for irrigation. After copious irrigation, sterile gauze pads can be used to gently but firmly rub the area of the wound to remove any loosened debris, followed by additional irrigation. Inspect the wound for tooth fragments and, if present, remove them. Sharply debride any loose skin tags or loose underlying soft tissue. If the wound appears minor, antibiotics can be withheld, and the patient instructed to return if signs of infection develop. With more extensive wounds, antibiotics are given because it can be assumed that significant bacterial contamination has occurred.

The decision to perform primary closure of a laceration secondary to a human bite depends on the clinical circumstance. Some physicians prefer to leave all such wounds open. This methodology is certainly acceptable with small lacerations on extremities and genitalia, particularly in males. More extensive or gaping lacerations secondary to a human bite on the face, neck, and hands, particularly in females, present serious cosmetic problems. After adequate cleansing and debriding, loosely close such lacerations with synthetic nonabsorbable sutures (silk should be avoided because a granulomatous reaction may result). Antibiotic coverage should include a penicillinase-resistant penicillin.

If a portion of a finger, ear, or nose is bitten off, instruct emergency medical technicians and law enforcement personnel to bring all tissue to the hospital. Skin from some severed portions of the body can be removed and used for full-thickness grafts. The ear or a portion of it can be denuded and the cartilage buried in the subcutaneous tissue of the abdomen until the basic wound has been healed. The cartilage can then be reimplanted and a full-thickness graft applied. Tetanus prophylaxis is indicated for all bites.

Human bites of the hand represent a different problem because of proximity of the deep structures of the hand to the skin, the importance of the hand, and the ease of infection. All human bites of the hand should be explored. After adequate neurological, vascular, and orthopedic examination of the area, local anesthesia should be provided and the wound should be thoroughly and copiously cleansed and irrigated with saline and with hydrogen peroxide. The hand should be gently bandaged and splinted if necessary, but the wound should be left open as much as possible.

Human bites of the hand and the genitalia frequently require hospitalization for intravenous antibiotic treatment, debridement, and observation. Patients with human bites involving the palmar spaces, joint spaces, or bones of the hand should be admitted.

ANIMAL BITES

Despite the wide variety of animal bites that may be encountered, the management consists of cleansing, debriding and repair of skin and soft tissue injury, and the prevention and treatment of rabies, tetanus, and other specific infections peculiar to the biting animal. Rabies is discussed in Chapter 84 and tetanus in Chapter 83. Remember that with all animal bites adequate protection against tetanus must be assured. It is useful to think of the mnemonic RATS: R for rabies, A for antibiotics, T for tetanus, and S for soap.

Dog Bites

The most common animal bite is a dog bite. Large dogs can inflict serious injuries including crushing injuries of the face, head, and limbs particularly in children. A canine bite, as do those of any carnivore, presents a danger of contamination from flora of the animal's mouth. Various organisms such as streptococci, staphylococci, diphtheroids, clostridia, and even gram-negative organisms have been cultured from animal bite wounds. *Pasteurella multocida* is also a common pathogen It has now been demonstrated that leptospirosis, a disease caused by *Leptospira* and formerly thought to be limited to people with specific occupations, such as sewer, rice, sugarcane, farm, and abattoir workers, can be acquired from family pets. Even a healthy, immunized dog can shed the organisms, and it does not require a bite for transmission.

Closure of a dog bite wound is frequently debated. Small puncture wounds or lacerations can be cleansed and left open. Most lacerations, except those of the hand with potential for joint or tendon involvement, should be closed primarily after meticulous irrigation and debridement. Hand wounds should be cleansed, debrided, and explored. If tendon or joint involvement is suspected, they should be left open, and antibiotics administered. Primary closure of simple hand wounds is still controversial. Following cleansing, debridement, and repair, treatment with a broad-spectrum antibiotic may be instituted. Penicillinase-resistant penicillin, a cephalosporin (ceftriaxone), tetracycline, or amoxicillin-clavulanate can be used initially. Cultures should be obtained if infection develops, but are not needed for initial treatment.

Cat Bites and Scratches

Cats usually injure by scratching, but either a tooth or claws may cause puncture wounds. The contaminating organisms are similar to those in dog bites, and treatment is as outlined for dog bites, although *P. multocida* is more commonly found in cat bite infections. Cat-scratch fever is an ill-understood disease, most likely caused by a virus related to the lymphogranuloma-psittacosis group. It is basically a nonbacterial, chronic, regional lymphadenitis which develops secondary to a primary cutaneous lesion. Biopsy may be necessary to distinguish it from lymphoma. Similar lesions are observed in patients who have scratches from sources such as thorns and fragments of animal bones. Occasionally, the wound may become suppurative, and incision and drainage may be necessary. Tetracycline, penicillin V, amoxicillin-clavulanate, or ceftriaxone can be used.

Miscellaneous Small Animal Bites

Bites by squirrels, rats, chipmunks, bats, raccoons, and mice usually result in puncture wounds. Meticulous cleansing and debridement are required. Rat bites are the most common and usually occur in sleeping infants, children, and intoxicated adults. Recent data suggest that rat bites heal well and have a low rate of infection. However, ampicillin or tetracycline can be used for high-risk wounds.

Large Animal Bites

Bites of lions, tigers, and bears are rare and usually occur in a zoo or animal park setting. Such injuries can be extensive and life-threatening.

Monkey bites are not rare in the United States because of the number of monkeys used for scientific and educational purposes, as well as those that are kept in zoos or as pets. Since the flora of the mouth of the monkey is similar to that of the human, treatment is the same. Herpes simplex virus may be transmitted from Rhesus monkeys.

Cows, horses, and camels occasionally inflict bites. The main consideration of these wounds is their magnitude. In a camel bite, the injured part is usually the victim's face and the cranium. In certain parts of the world, the most common cause of skull fracture is a camel bite.

Injuries caused by large animals are frequently massive and require resuscitation for hemorrhagic shock, followed by major surgical repair.

In cases of bites by any animal, invasion of the joint space is a requirement for surgical exploration, irrigation, and antibiotic treatment. Radiography should be used liberally in examination of hands in particular when animal bites are present.

Larger human and animal bites can be drained after closure for 24 to 48 h. Penrose drains or sterile rubber bands can be used.

BIBLIOGRAPHY

Aghababian RV, Conte JE Jr: Mammalian bite wounds. *Ann Emerg Med* 9:79, 1980.

Baker MD, Moore SE: Human bites in children: A six year experience. *Am J Dis Child* 141:1285, 1987.

Brakenbury PH, Muwanga C: A comparative double-blind study of amoxycillin/clavulanate vs. placebo in the prevention of infection after animal bites. *Ann Emer Med* 6:251, 1989.

Brook I: Human and animal bite infections. *J Fam Prac* 28:713, 1989.

Callaham M: Controversies in antiobiotic choices for bite wounds. *Ann Emerg Med* 17:1321, 1988.

Dreyfuss U, Singer M: Human bites of the hand: A study of 106 patients. *J Hand Surg* 10a:884, 1985.

Edlich R, Morgan RF, Mayer NE, et al: Mammalian bites. *Curr Concepts Wound Care* 15, 1986.

Rest J, Goldstein E: Management of human and animal bite wounds. *Emerg Med Clin North Am* 3:117, 1985.

Trott A: Care of mammalian bites. *Pediatr Infect Dis J* 6:8, 1989.

193
WOUND CLOSURE

Richard F. Edlich
George T. Rodeheaver
John G. Thacker

After wound cleansing, the physical integrity and function of the injured tissue must be restored. The technique of wound closure selected depends on the type of wound. Primary closure can be accomplished with clean wounds without tissue loss. For wounds with associated tissue loss, grafts or flaps are often required to close the defect. These procedures are usually performed in the operating room.

Infected or heavily contaminated wounds, and wounds resulting from high-energy-depositor missile injuries, should be left open until delayed closure can be undertaken. Wounds contaminated by pus, vaginal discharge, feces, or saliva, as well as those in which treatment is delayed longer than 6 h, should also be considered for open wound management.

Open wound management prior to delayed primary closure is accomplished by packing the wound with sterile fine-meshed gauze (type I) that is then covered by a sterile dressing. The wound should not be disturbed for the first 4 days after injury unless the patient develops an unexplained fever. Unnecessary inspection during this period increases the risk of contamination and subsequent infection. On or after the fourth day after wounding, the wound margins can be inspected. In the absence of infection and devitalized tissue, the wound edges can be approximated with minimal risk of infection.

Once it is decided to close the wound, a closure technique must be selected that allows the most accurate and secure approximation of the skin edges. Suturing is the oldest and most popular method. However, specially designed surgical tapes and staples, more recent innovations, have important roles in skin wound closure. The closure method should hold tissue in apposition until the strength of the wound is sufficient to withstand stress.

SUTURES

Important considerations in skin closure are the type of suture, the tying technique, and the configuration of the suture loops. Selection of a suture material is based on its biologic interaction with the wound as well as its mechanical performance in vivo and in vitro. Sutures are divided into two general classes on the basis of their in vivo degradation: (1) Sutures that undergo rapid degradation in tissues, losing their tensile strength within 60 days, are considered "absorbable" sutures. (2) Sutures that maintain their tensile strength for longer than 60 days are "nonabsorbable" sutures. This terminology is somewhat misleading, because some so-called nonabsorbable sutures (e.g., silk, cotton, and nylon) lose some tensile strength during this 60-day interval. Silk loses approximately one-half of its tensile strength in 1 year and has no strength at the end of 2 years. Cotton loses 50 percent of its strength in 6 months, but still has 30 to 40 percent of its strength at the end of 2 years. Nylon loses approximately 25 percent of its original strength over 2 years.

Nonabsorbable sutures can be classified according to their origin. Nonabsorbable sutures made from natural fibers include silk, cotton, and linen. Metallic sutures are derived from stainless steel. There are a variety of synthetic fibers: polyamides (nylon), polyesters (Dacron), polyolefins [polyethylene, polypropylene (PP)], polytetrafluoroethylene (PTFE), and polybutester. Polybutester is a block copolymer that contains poly(butylene)terephthalate (84 percent) and poly(tetramethylene ether)glycol terephthalate (16 percent). The PTFE suture has been expanded to produce a porous microstructure that is approximately 50 percent air by volume. Nonabsorbable sutures may also be classified according to their physical configuration. Sutures constructed from one filament are called monofilament sutures (nylon, PP, polybutester, PTFE and stainless steel); sutures containing multiple fibers are called multifilament sutures (nylon, polyester, stainless steel, silk, and cotton). Only nylon and stainless steel sutures are available as both monofilament and multifilament sutures.

Absorbable sutures are made from either collagen or synthetic polymers. Collagen sutures are derived either from the submucosa of ovine or bovine small intestine (gut suture) or from reconstituted collagen manufactured from bovine tendon collagen (collagen suture). This collagenous tissue is treated in an aldehyde solution which cross-links and strengthens the suture and makes it more resistant to enzymatic degradation. Suture materials treated in this way are called plain gut or plain collagen. If the suture is additionally treated in chromium trioxide, it becomes chromic gut or chromic collagen, which is more highly cross-linked and more resistant to absorption than plain gut or collagen. The shortcomings of collagen and gut sutures include variable strength and unpredictable absorption.

Synthetic substitutes for collagen sutures are produced from polyglactin 910 or polyglycolic acid. These high-molecular-weight polymers are extruded into thin filaments and made into braided sutures which lose their strength in tissues during a 4-week period after implantation.

Two other synthetic absorbable monofilament sutures, polydioxanone and glycolide trimethylene carbonate, retain approximately 70 percent of their breaking strength after implantation for 28 days. The chemical degradation of these synthetic absorbable monofilament sutures is by a predictable and uniform hydrolysis of their ester bonds.

All sutures compromise the local tissue defenses against infection. Several mechanisms are implicated:

1. The trauma of inserting a needle is sufficient to cause an inflammatory response.
2. Sutures tied too tightly impair blood flow and cause tissue necrosis.
3. Sutures that penetrate the intact skin provide an avenue for wound contamination via the perisutural cuff.
4. The quantity of suture and the chemical reactivity of the material affect the susceptibility to infection.

The infection-potentiating effects of suture materials are listed in Table 193-1. The infection-potentiating effect of polybutester suture has not been measured.

The relatively high infection rates encountered with either monofilament or multifilament stainless steel sutures may be the result of their chemical or physical configuration. Stainless steel is not generally as inert as pure polymers and undergoes degradation in vivo. In addition, metallic sutures are so stiff that patient movement induces tissue damage that impairs the wound's ability to resist infection. Sutures made of natural fibers may potentiate infection more than other nonabsorbable sutures, and should be avoided in contaminated wounds. The incidence of infection from monofilament sutures is less than that of multifilament sutures constructed from comparable materials.

There are two techniques for sutural closure of skin: percutaneous and dermal (subcuticular). Percutaneous sutures are passed through the epidermal and dermal layers of skin. Dermal, or subcuticular,

Table 193-1. Infection-Potentiating Effect of Surgical Sutures*

Absorbable	Nonabsorbable
Synthetic absorbable	Nylon, PP, PTFE
Plain gut	Dacron (coated, noncoated)
Chromic gut	Metal
	Silk, cotton

* The least reactive suture materials are listed first.

sutures reapproximate the divided edges of the dermis without penetrating the epidermis. Occasionally, dermal and percutaneous sutures are used together. Either type can be used as a continuous (''running'') suture or as an interrupted suture.

Percutaneous sutures of either monofilament nylon or PP are excellent for skin closure because these materials have the least effect on the wound defenses. Polybutester sutures have unique performance characteristics that may be advantageous for wound closure. With this type of suture, low forces yield significantly greater elongation than with other sutures. In addition, polybutester sutures have superior elasticity, allowing the suture to return to its original length once the load is removed. In a clinical setting in which the tied suture loops are extended by the edema of the wound and yet are expected to return to their original length once the edema disappears, the performance of the polybutester suture would be expected to be superior to that of other sutures. Sutures with less extensibility under low forces, like nylon, PP, polyester, or silk, will frequently lacerate or necrose the encircled tissue, thereby increasing its susceptibility to infection.

Percutaneous sutures are recommended for closure of stellate lacerations resulting from crush injuries. In these wounds, meticulous closure with percutaneous sutures approximates the skin edges more exactly than does tape. Closing these wounds is often like putting together a jigsaw puzzle, and tapes have little practical value. The more accurate approximation of skin edges by skillfully applied sutures leads to a more pleasing cosmetic result.

Because the magnitude of the damage to the local tissue defenses is related to the quantity of the suture within the wound (that is, diameter and length), we use the suture with the narrowest diameter (5–0 or 6–0) whose strength is sufficient to resist disruption of the closure. Approximating the mid-portion and the bisected portions of the unclosed wound with percutaneous sutures allows the least length of suture to be used in the skin closure. An interrupted dermal suture placed in each quadrant of the wound subjected to strong static and dynamic skin tensions provides sufficient strength to permit early suture removal.

It is important to mention that sutural closure of the adipose tissue beneath the skin should be avoided. Obliteration of this potential dead space between the cut edge of adipose tissue by even the least reactive suture increases the incidence of infection.

When wounds of different thickness are to be reunited, the needle should be passed through one edge of the wound and then drawn out before reentry through the other edge. This maneuver ensures that the needle is inserted at comparable levels on each side of the wound. Unless appropriate adjustment of the bite is made on the thinner side, uneven coaptation of the skin will occur, resulting in a step-off scar. During reapproximation of the wound, grasping or crushing of the skin edges by forceps should be avoided.

Dermal sutures can be used alone or as adjuncts to percutaneous sutures in wounds subjected to strong skin tensions, to serve as an added precaution against disruption of the wound. Some emergency physicians prefer a synthetic absorbable suture for dermal closure, while others favor a synthetic nonabsorbable suture. When continuous nonabsorbable sutures are employed, suture removal is recommended before the eighth day after wound closure to prevent the development of needle puncture scars.

Percutaneous sutures should be avoided in favor of dermal sutures in the following circumstances: (1) in infants frightened at the prospects of suture removal, (2) when follow-up appointments will be difficult for the patient to keep, (3) when wounds are covered by casts, and (4) in patiens prone to the development of keloids. When dermal closure alone is used, it is advisable to immediately apply tape skin closures to the wound edges to provide a more accurate approximation of the epidermis.

However useful, the dermal skin closure technique potentiates wound infection more than percutaneous sutures. This increased infection rate appears to be related to the large quantity of suture material that is required for a continuous dermal skin closure. Once infection develops, the collecting purulent exudate spreads preferentially between the divided edges of fat rather than penetrating the tightly sutured skin edges. By the time the infection becomes clinically apparent, it has involved the entire extent of the wound. In contrast, the localized collections of purulent discharge encountered in infected tape-closed wounds first exit between the wound edges before spreading preferentially between the divided layers of adipose tissue.

Despite the immediate aesthetically pleasing appearance of dermal skin closure, it does not improve the ultimate cosmetic appearance of the healing wound. The scar width after dermal skin closure is comparable to the scar width of wounds healing in the absence of dermal sutures. In contrast, galeal sutures limit the width of scalp scars. In fact, the use of nonabsorbable PP galeal suture reduces the postoperative stretching and depth of skin scars more than does the use of polyglycolic acid galeal suture of comparable size. Another effective method of reducing scar width is to undermine the skin edges prior to wound closure, thereby diminishing the static skin tensions. However, this benefit must be weighed against the potential damage to the skin blood supply, which may compromise the host's defenses and invite infection. Consequently, undermining the wound edges of lacerations is not recommended in the emergency department, but is reserved for elective surgery.

The ideal surgical needle should introduce a suture that provides meticulous approximation of the wound edges. It should make a hole in the tissue that is only large enough to allow introduction of the suture. Its body should be designed so that it can be grasped securely by the needle holder. The design specifications for a surgical needle vary considerably and depend on the biomechanical characteristics of the tissue being approximated. Regardless of their design, American Society for Testing Materials (ASTM) stainless steel alloy 45500 is best suited for needle manufacture because it has greater yield and tensile strength than the other alloys.

Cutting edge needles to be used for suturing are ground and honed to provide edges that will pass through the dense, irregular, and relatively thick connective tissue of dermis. The point of the needle has a tapered triangular configuration with its three cutting edges at the apexes of the triangle. Two cutting edges are located at the sides of the needle point, and the third cutting edge is positioned at the apex of the triangular configuration of the needle point. The location of the third cutting edge influences its performance. On the conventional cutting edge needle it is located on the inner concave curvature; it cuts tissue beneath the surface and directs the needle point toward the skin (surface seeking). Because the physician has the tendency to apply greater force toward the concave side of the needle, there is a potential danger of dividing some tissues that ultimately will be encircled by the suture. As the needle passes through the skin, it produces a triangular defect, the apex of which is closest to the incision and is the site for the tied suture ligature. Positioning of the suture ligature at this point may predispose to skin cut-through.

In contrast, reverse cutting edge needles differ from conventional cutting edge needles in that the third cutting edge is located on the outer convex curvature of the needle. This configuration offers the advantage of having the flat surface of the needle closest to the edges of the incision or wound, limiting the opportunity for tissue cutout and directing the point of the needle toward the depth of the wound (depth seeking). The hole in the skin left by the needle leaves a flattened wall of tissue for the suture to be tied against, which should resist suture pull-through.

Other important considerations in the design of cutting edge needles for skin closure involve the geometry of the needle point. When the portion of the needle point that has tapered triangular cutting edges is lengthened, the angle of the needle point becomes smaller, affording superior sharpness and ease of penetration through skin. However, because a significant length of the needle has a cutting edge, it may cut excessively through a thin layer of connective tissue, such as oral mucous membrane. A tapercut needle has been specially developed to prevent excessive cutting of the mucous membrane. This needle combines features of the reverse cutting edge and tapered point needles. Its three cutting edges extend a considerably shorter distance than those of the reverse cutting edge needle before graduating into the round, tapered body. The tapercut point provides smooth passage through oral mucous membrane, yet the round shaft, which has no cutting edges, will not cut through deeper tissues.

The body, or shaft, should be designed so that it can be grasped securely by the needle holder. The inner and outer curvatures of the body should be flattened where the needle is to be grasped. If the body is flattened on the sides into an I-beam configuration, the needle's resistance to bending is enhanced considerably.

The longitudinal part of the body may be straight, half-curved, curved, or compound-curved. Compound-curved needles facilitate skin closure. They have short, straight, sharpened points with reverse cutting edges, followed by curved distal sections. The design of these needles enables the physician to pass them through the skin to a controlled depth and length of bite with a greater accuracy than is afforded by curved cutting edge needles with a single radius of curvature.

The needle should be grasped between needle holder jaws that securely hold the needle without causing irreversible needle bending or deformation. If the needle holder jaws are used for tying sutures, the face of the jaws should be smooth with rounded edges to allow manipulation of monofilament sutures without damage to the sutures. Needle jaws with teeth cause distinct structural damage to monofilament sutures that reduces their breaking strength. The needle holder jaw should grasp only the needle body; clamping the needle point damages the cutting edge and dulls the needle.

To prevent the development of needle puncture scars, skin sutures must be removed before the eighth day after wound closure (Fig. 193-1). Immediately following suture removal, the wound edges should be reinforced with tape skin closure to prevent wound dehiscence.

TAPE

The superior resistance to infection of taped wounds compared with sutured wounds indicates that tape closure is a significant clinical tool. The incidence of infection of contaminated wounds whose edges are approximated even with the least reactive suture is significantly higher than the infection rate of taped wounds subjected to a comparable level of contamination. The ease with which wounds can be closed by tape varies according to the anatomic and biomechanical properties of the wound site. Linear wounds in skin subjected to minimal static and dynamic tensions are easily approximated by tape. The relatively lax skin of the face and abdomen makes it amenable to wound closure by tapes. Contrary to the usual expectation, tape closue without sutures is more easily accomplished in obese patients, and the thick cut edges of adipose tissue tend to evert the skin. The taut skin of the extremities, which is subjected to frequent dynamic joint movements, requires dermal sutures before taping. The copious secretions from the skin of the axilla, palms, and soles discourage tape adherence.

The difficulties encountered in performing sutureless tape closure of wounds subjected to strong tensions can be explained by the deformation of skin at the periphery of the wound. When the skin is cut, its inherent skin tensions retract its edges. As with any elastic membrane, the shrinkage in surface area of the skin is greatest at the wound margin, becoming progressively less as the distance from the wound increases. The extent of these changes is directly related to the magnitude of the static and dynamic forces within the skin. The use of dermal sutures prior to taping stretches the skin to its uninjured dimensions and makes application of tape skin closures considerably easier. In wounds subjected to weak skin tension, tape skin closure can be accomplished without the use of reinforcing dermal sutures. In such cases, the tape skin closure is first attached to the skin at one wound edge. The other wound edge is then pulled toward the taped edge before the remaining portion of the tape skin closure is applied to the skin.

When tape skin closures are properly employed to close linear wounds subjected to weak tensions, cosmetic results are excellent. The discomfort of anesthetic infiltration and of suture removal, and the development of suture puncture scars, are avoided. In the child or woman with glabrous skin, tape skin closures are especially valuable for closing transverse lacerations over the brow, under the chin, or across the malar prominence.

Wound closure tapes will not adhere to wet skin. Drying with a gauze sponge sometimes does not completely remove wet exudate, and the residual fluid continues to impair tape adhesion. Compound benzoin tincture can be applied to the wound edges with applicator sticks prior to tape application. Compound benzoin tincture should not be spilled into the wound, as it increases the likelihood of infection.

STAPLES

With the advent of disposable stapling devices, skin closure by metal staples can be accomplished quickly and economically. In fact, stapling is the fastest method of skin closure. An additional advantage of staples is their low level of tissue reactivity. There is uniform agreement that wounds closed by metal staples exhibit a superior resistance to infection than wounds subjected to the least reactive suture. These advantages of skin staples must be weighed against one notable drawback. The skin staple does not provide the same meticulous coaptation of lacerations with irregular skin edges that skin sutures do. The wound edges must be accurately aligned before wound closure to permit simultaneous implantation of the staple points. Because this accurate prepositioning of the wound edges is very difficult in most lacerations, staple implantation will often result in malapposition of wound edges, an invitation to the development of scar deformity. Consequently, we reserve skin staples for lacerations in anatomic sites in which the healing scar is not readily apparent (e.g., scalp).

A variety of stapling devices are commercially available for use in the emergency department. All staplers implant stainless steel staples, which assume an incomplete rectangular or arcuate shape when fully formed. The selection of a stapler by the emergency physician will be determined by its performance. Ideally, the device should be designed so that it does not obstruct the physician's view of the wound edge. Moreover, the stapler should have a prepositioning mechanism that permits the physician to hold the staple securely during its for-

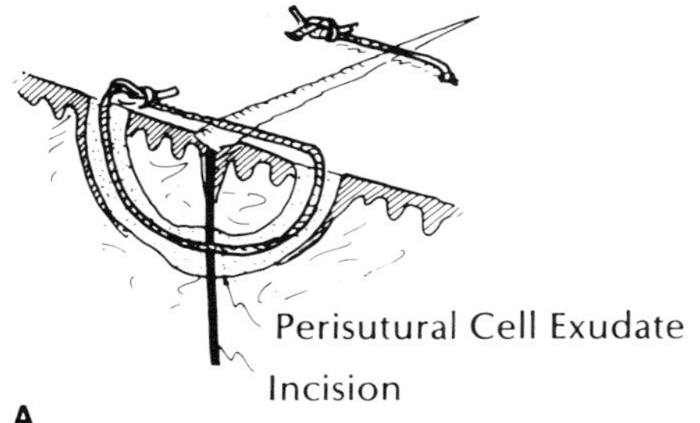

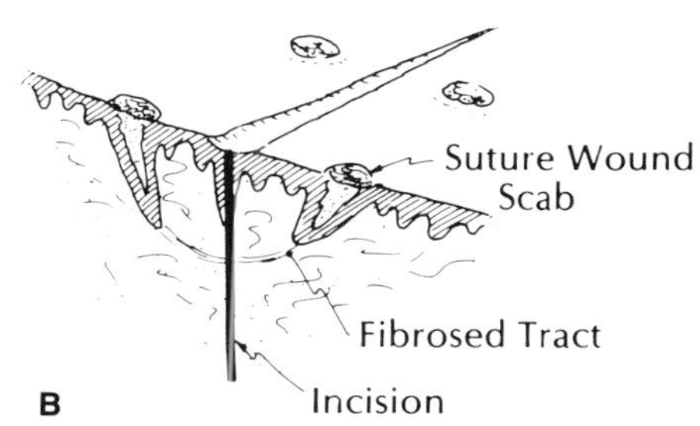

Fig. 193-1. A. Epithelial cells migrate downward, forming a perisutural cuff. **B.** If percutaneous sutures are not removed before the eighth day after surgery, the invasive spurs of epithelium result in needle puncture scars.

mation. The configuration of the stapler should allow the position of its cartridge to be adjusted manually to facilitate placement of the staple. In addition, the stapler should have an ejection spring that automatically releases the staple. Finally, the handling characteristics of the stapler should be such that the physician can easily implant a large number of staples without becoming fatigued.

With the advent of absorbable staples, manufacturers should now consider designing a stapler for closure of the dermis (subcuticular closure). Dermal closure is recommended in all skin wounds subjected to strong static skin tensions. These dermal staples would serve as an added precaution against disruption of the wound and permit early removal of either percutaneous staples or sutures.

This research was supported by a generous gift from Mr. Roger Milliken & Co., Spartanburg, South Carolina.

BIBLIOGRAPHY

deHoll D, Rodeheaver G, Edgerton MT, et al: Potentiation of infection by suture closure of dead space. *Am J Surg* 127:716, 1974.

Edlich RF, Becker DG, Thacker JG, et al: Scientific basis for selecting staple and skin closures. *Clin Plast Surg* 17:571, 1990.

Edlich RF, Panek PH, Rodeheaver GT, et al: Physical and chemical configuration of sutures in the development of surgical infection. *Ann Surg* 177:679, 1973.

Edlich RF, Rodeheaver G, Kuphal J, et al. Technique of closure: Contaminated wounds. *JACEP* 3:375, 1974.

Edlich RF, Rogers W, Kasper G, et al: Studies in the management of the contaminated wound. I. Optimal time for closure of contaminated wounds. II. Comparison of resistance to infection of open and closed wounds during healing. *Am J Surg* 117:323, 1969.

Edlich RF, Tsung MS, Rogers W, et al: Studies in the management of the contaminated wound. I. Technique of closure of such wounds together with a note on a reproducible experimental model. *J Surg Res* 8:585, 1968.

Katz AR, Mukherjee DP, Kaganov AL, et al: A new synthetic monofilament absorbable suture made from polytrimethylene carbonate. *Surg Gynecol Obstet* 161:213, 1985.

Laufman H, Rubel T: Synthetic absorbable sutures. *Surg Gynecol Obstet* 145:597, 1977.

McGuire MF: Studies of the excisional wound: I. Biomechanical effects of undermining and wound orientation on closing tension and work. *Plast Reconstr Surg* 66:419, 1980.

Panek PH, Prusak MP, Bolt D, et al: Potentiation of wound infection by adhesive adjuncts. *Amer Surg* 38:343, 1972.

Rodeheaver GT, Halverson JM, Edlich RF: Mechanical performance of wound closure tapes. *Ann Emerg Med* 12:203, 1983.

Rodeheaver GT, Thacker JG, Edlich RF: Mechanical performance of polyglycolic acid and polyglactin 910 synthetic absorbable sutures. *Surg Gynecol Obstet* 153:835, 1981.

Rodeheaver GT, Thacker JG, Owen J, et al: Knotting and handling characteristics of coated synthetic absorbable sutures. *J Surg Res* 35:525, 1983.

Winn HR, Jane JA, Rodeheaver G, et al: Influence of subcuticular sutures on scar formation. *Am J Surg* 133:257, 1977.

194 POSTOPERATIVE WOUND CARE AND TETANUS PROPHYLAXIS

Richard F. Edlich
George T. Rodeheaver
John G. Thacker

POSTOPERATIVE WOUND CARE

Wound Dressings

The manner in which a dressing functions is determined by its physical and chemical composition. There are eight types of absorbent cotton gauze, each type defined by the number of warp and woof threads per square inch (Table 194-1). The degree of dressing adherence to a wound is directly related to the size of dressing interstices. The larger the interstices, the greater the chance that the dressing will be penetrated by the granulation tissue. If debridement is the objective, the physician should use a dressing with greater interstice size, at least larger than Type I. Absorption of wound exudates is another important function of a dressing. The beneficial effects of absorbency are that (1) the bacteria contained within the absorbed fluid are removed, (2) the exudate itself is removed, depleting the wound of bacterial nutrients, and (3) tissue maceration is prevented. High absorbency is incompatible with nonadhesion because the serous exudate forms a powerful and coherent glue as it dries. Removal of the absorbent dressing disrupts the fibrinous scab and any granulation tissue that has become entrapped in the dressing. Absorbent dressings are therefore useful for the debridement of open wounds.

In primarily closed wounds, the dressing acts as a barrier against exogenous bacteria. Soaking dressings with serum permits passage of bacteria through the dressing. Saturation of a dressing with fluid that wets both inner and outer surfaces of the dressing is called fluid strike-through. As long as its outer surface remains dry, however, a dressing will remain an effective barrier to bacterial contamination.

The length of time that dry dressings should cover the closed wound is based on knowledge of the period during which the wound is susceptible to bacterial penetration. Sutured wounds, as they heal, become increasingly resistant to the development of infection following surface contamination. Swabbing the surface of the wound with either *Staphylococcus aureus* or *Escherichia coli* during the first 48 h after closure can cause localized gross infections. Contamination after the third day may not produce gross infection in the sutured wound. Thus barrier dressings are useful to protect the fresh incision from surface contamination in the first few days. Thereafter, removal of the dressing permits daily inspection and palpation of the wound. Wounds closed with tape have a greater capacity to resist infection than sutured wounds and do not need protective dressings.

Table 194-1. Types of Absorbent Cotton Gauze

	Threads/in^2	
Type	**Warp**	**Woof**
I	41–47	33–39
II	30–34	26–30
III	26–30	22–26
IV	22–26	18–22
V	20–24	16–20
VI	18–22	14–18
VII	18–22	10–14
VIII	12–16	8–12

Another important purpose of some dressings is to exert pressure on the underlying tissues. A pressure dressing minimizes the accumulation of intercellular fluid within the wound and limits dead space. Maximal pressure should be applied to the wound site, as well as distal to it. Proximal to the wound, the pressure applied is decreased to minimize any chance of compromising the venous or lymphatic return.

A pressure dressing, by the very nature of its bulk, immobilizes what it covers. Immobilization of the site of injury is of great value—lymphatic flow is reduced, thereby minimizing the spread of the wound microflora. Furthermore, immobilized tissue demonstrates the best resistance to the growth of bacteria. Whenever possible, the site of injury should be elevated above the patient's heart, to limit the accumulation of fluid in the wound interstitial spaces. The injured wound with little edema proceeds more rapidly to complete rehabilitation than the markedly edematous wound does.

Dressings should also provide a physiologic environment that is conducive to epithelial migration from the wound edges across the surface of the fresh wound. When an area of epidermis is lost, water vapor begins at once to evaporate from the exposed dermal tissue. The exudate on the surface dries and becomes the outer layer of the scab, which does not prevent water from evaporating from the dermis underneath. The surface of the dermis itself progressively dries (within 18 h). This dry scab and dried dermis resist migration of epidermal cells, which must seek the underlying fibrous tissue of the upper reticular layer of dermis where enough moisture remains to support cellular viability. When the wound is covered by a dressing that prevents or delays evaporation of water from the wound surface, the scab and underlying dermis remain moist. Epidermal cells can easily migrate through the moist scab over the surface of the dermis. Under such dressings, epithelialization is more rapid and no dry dermis is sacrificed.

The dressing that delays evaporation of water vapor would seem to be ideal for coverage of primarily closed wounds and has been usefully employed in the treatment of donor sites, meshed grafts, and dermabraded skin. Unfortunately, excessive exudate may make it difficult to keep the fully occlusive dressing in place, and the moist exudate that provides an ideal medium for epidermal repair is also a suitable culture medium for the proliferation of microorganisms.

In our emergency service, primarily closed wounds (with the exception of those located on the face) are covered by nonwoven microporous polypropylene dressings, which are attached to surrounding skin by wide strips of microporous tape with no reinforcing fibers. In facial lacerations the development of blood clots between the edges of the sutured wounds is of more concern than the potential dangers of surface contamination. These clots will be replaced by a healing scar that can easily be avoided by swabbing the wound with half-strength hydrogen peroxide every 6 h until the wound edge is free of blood. Because hydrogen peroxide causes the sutures to lose their color, the decolorized suture becomes a sign of patient compliance with our postoperative wound care regimen.

In abraded skin, this method of suture line care is ineffective. Even if the wound is washed with hydrogen peroxide, it develops a scab which makes suture removal tedious and often painful to the patient. In such cases, we swab the wound and its adjacent edges with a water-soluble ointment, such as polyethylene glycol, that becomes dissolved by wound exudates, thereby encouraging their exodus from the wound. These sutures must be removed before the eighth postoperative day because needle puncture scars can develop. The wound edges should then be supported by sterile, microporous tape skin closures until their adhesive bond weakens.

Abraded skin will develop permanent hyperpigmentation after exposure to the sun. Consequently, abraded skin should be protected with a sun-blocking agent for at least 6 months after injury. Photoprotection against UVA was in the past limited by the restricted range of UVA wavelengths absorbed by available sunscreen agents. With the introduction of Parsol 1789 in combination with padimate 0 (Photoplex), emergency physicians now have a sun block with absorbent effect against the entire ultraviolet spectrum. This sunscreen should prove valuable in helping prevent hyperpigmentation.

TETANUS PROPHYLAXIS

Two-thirds of the recent tetanus cases in the United States have followed lacerations, puncture wounds, and crush injuries. When employing tetanus prophylaxis, we follow the guidelines recommended by the Committee on Trauma of the American College of Surgeons and the Centers for Disease Control.

Pertinent information about the mechanism of injury, the characteristics and age of the wound, previous active immunization status, history of a neurologic or severe hypersensitivity reaction following a previous immunization treatment, and plans for follow-up should be recorded in a permanent medical record. Each patient should receive an appropriate written record that describes the treatment administered and provides follow-up instructions that outline wound care, drug therapy, immunization status, and potential complications. Patients should be referred to designated physicians who will provide comprehensive follow-up care, including completion of active immunization.

Modern immunobiologic agents are extremely safe and effective, but not completely so. Adverse reactions have been reported for all immunobiologic agents. Ideally, the emergency physician should question the patient or other responsible person regarding any adverse effects to the specific toxoids or vaccines that may be used to immunize patients. In addition, the patient or responsible person should be given information on the risks of drugs to be used, as well as on the major benefits of preventing disease both in individuals and in the community. There should be ample opportunity to ask questions before immunization. Important statements that give a risk-benefit analysis of various immunobiologic agents have been developed by different health agencies. Emergency physicians should distribute these or similar materials to their patients.

A wallet-size card documenting immunization received and date of immunization should be given to every wounded patient, who should be instructed to carry the written record at all times and, if indicated, to complete active immunization. Precise tetanus prophylaxis requires an accurate and immediately available history regarding previous active immunization against tetanus or rapid laboratory titration to determine the patient's serum antitoxin level. Serum antitoxin levels above 0.01 IU/mL have been considered protective against tetanus.

Regardless of the active immunization status of the patient, meticulous surgical care with aseptic technique that includes removal of all devitalized tissue and foreign bodies should be provided immediately for all wounds. Such care is essential as part of the prophylaxis against tetanus.

Table 194-2. Clinical Features of Wounds

Clinical Features	Tetanus-Prone Wounds	Non-Tetanus-Prone Wounds
Age of wound	>6 h	≤6 h
Configuration	Stellate wound	Linear wound
Depth	>1 cm	≤1 cm
Mechanism of injury	Missile, crush, burn, frostbile	Sharp surface (e.g., knife)
Signs of infection	Present	Absent
Devitalized tissue	Present	Absent
Contaminants (dirt, feces, soil, saliva)	Present	Absent
Denervated and/or ischemic tissue	Present	Absent

Table 194-3. Guide to Tetanus Prophylaxis

History of Adsorbed Tetanus Toxid (Doses)	TETANUS-PRONE WOUNDS Td[a]	TETANUS-PRONE WOUNDS TIG[b,c]	NON-TETANUS-PRONE WOUNDS Td[a]	NON-TETANUS-PRONE WOUNDS TIG
Uncertain or <3	Yes	Yes	Yes	No
3 or more[d]	No[e]	No	No[f]	No

[a] For children less than 7 years old, diphtheria and tetanus toxoids and pertussis vaccine adsorbed (For Pediatric Use DTP) are preferred to tetanus toxoid alone. Diphtheria and tetanus toxoids (For Pediatric Use DT) are recommended if pertussis vaccine is contraindicated. For persons 7 years old and older, tetanus and diphtheria toxoids adsorbed (For Adult Use Td) are preferred to tetanus toxoid alone.

[b] TIG: Human tetanus immune globulin.

[c] When TIG and Td are given concurrently, separate syringes and separate sites should be used.

[d] If only three doses of fluid toxoid have been received, a fourth dose of toxoid, preferably an adsorbed toxoid, should be given.

[e] Yes, if more than 5 years since last dose. (More frequent boosters are not needed and can accentuate side effects.)

[f] Yes, if more than 10 years since last dose.

The effectiveness of antibiotics for prophylaxis of tetanus is uncertain. Proper immunization plays the most important role in tetanus prophylaxis. Recommendations on tetanus prophylaxis are based on (1) the condition of the wound and (2) the patient's immunization history. Table 194–2 outlines some of the clinical features of wounds that are prone to develop tetanus. A wound with any one of these clinical features is considered tetanus-prone.

A summary guide to tetanus prophylaxis of the wounded patient is displayed in Table 194–3. Passive immunization with TIG (250 units) must be considered individually for each patient. Equine tetanus antitoxin should be administered only if the possibility of tetanus outweighs the potential reactions to horse serum. If the patient is known to be immunosuppressed (e.g, primary or acquired immunodeficiency), the development of active immunization against tetanus is diminished. In such patients, passive immunization with TIG (250 units) should be instituted in conjunction with active immunization. After immunization, test the patient's serum for antitoxin to ensure that the patient has an adequate response to treatment.

Recent clinical studies suggest that many elderly people are inadequately protected against tetanus and that their immunologic response following a tetanus booster is delayed. It has been postulated that those who fail to seroconvert do carry a risk of developing tetanus despite the prophylaxis administered. Consequently, a more liberal approach to the use of TIG is being considered in the situation in which elderly patients with an unknown immunization history and no past military service present to the emergency department with a break in the skin barrier.

Precautions and Contraindications

The only contraindication to tetanus and diphtheria toxoids is a history of neurologic or severe hypersensitivity reaction following a previous dose. Local side effects do not preclude continued use. Local reactions, generally erythema and induration with or without tenderness, are common after the administration of vaccines containing diphtheria, tetanus, and pertussis antigens. These reactions are most common following diphtheria and tetanus toxoids and pertussis vaccine adsorbed (for pediatric use) (DTP) (40 to 70 percent of doses) and are usually self-limited and require no therapy. If a systemic reaction is suspected to represent allergic hypersensitivity, immunization should be postponed until appropriate skin testing is undertaken at a later time. If the use of a tetanus toxoid-containing preparation is contraindicated, passive immunization against tetanus should be considered in a tetanus-prone wound. A history of convulsions following DTP administration is not a contraindication to the receipt of diphtheria and tetanus toxoids.

Contraindications to the receipt of the pertussis vaccine include (1) a personal history of a previous convulsion, (2) hypersensitivity to pertussis vaccine components, (3) presence of an evolving neurologic disorder, and (4) a history of a severe reaction (usually within 48 h) following a previous dose. Severe reactions following receipt of the pertussis vaccine include any of the following: (1) collapse or shocklike state, (2) persistent screaming episodes—prolonged episodes of crying or screaming that cannot be controlled by comforting the infant, (3) high temperature ≥ 40.5°C (104.9°F), (4) convulsion(s) with or without accompanying fever, (5) encephalopathy, with or without convulsions, manifested by bulging fontanel, changes in level of consciousness, and generalized and/or local neurologic signs (the encephalopathy may lead to permanent neurologic deficit), and (6) a systemic allergic reaction. If such definitive contraindications to the receipt of the pertussis vaccine are identified in the infant or young child with a wound, diphtheria and tetanus toxoids adsorbed (for pediatric use) (DT) should be used instead of DPT.

A static neurologic condition, such as cerebral palsy or a family history of a neurologic disease or convulsions, is not a contraindication to giving vaccines containing pertussis antigen. Although hemolytic anemia and thrombocytopenic purpura have previously been considered contraindications, the evidence of a causal link between these conditions and pertussis vaccination is not sufficient to retain them as contraindications.

This research was supported by a generous gift from Carr-Scarborough Microbiologicals, Decatur, Georgia.

BIBLIOGRAPHY

Postoperative Wound Care

Colebrook L, Hood AM: Infection through soaked dressings. *Lancet* 2:682, 1948.

James JH, Watson ACH: The use of Opsite®, a vapour permeable dressing, on skin graft donor sites. *Br J Plast Surg* 28:107, 1975.

Schauerhamer RA, Edlich RF, Panek P, et al: Studies in the management of the contaminated wound. VII. Susceptibility of surgical wounds to postoperative bacterial contamination. *Am J Surg* 122:74, 1971.

Ship AG, Weiss PR: Pigmentation after dermabrasion: An avoidable complication. *Plast Reconstr Surg* 75:528, 1985.

Winter GD: Formation of the scab and the rate of epithelization of superficial wounds in the skin of the young domestic pig. *Nature* 193:293, 1962.

Tetanus Prophylaxis

Committee on Trauma of the American College of Surgeons: Prophylaxis against tetanus in wound management. *Bull Am Coll Surg* 69(10):22, 1984.

Fraser DW: Preventing tetanus in patients with wounds. *Ann Intern Med* 84:95, 1976.

Immunization Practices Advisory Committee (ACIP): Diphtheria, tetanus and pertussis: Guidelines for vaccine prophylaxis and other preventive measures. *MMWR* 30:403, 1981.

Immunization Practices Advisory Committee (ACIP): General guidelines on immunization. *MMWR* 32:1, 1983.

Immunization Practices Advisory Committee (ACIP): Supplementary statement of contraindications to receipt of pertussis vaccine. *MMWR* 33:169, 1984.

195 SOFT TISSUE INJURIES TO THE FACE

Richard F. Edlich

INTRODUCTION

Facial wounds are among the most frequently encountered injuries. All wounds of the face may be divided into two basic groups: (1) injuries of the soft tissues and (2) injuries to the bone. This chapter focuses on soft tissue injuries to the face. The goals of treatment of soft tissue wounds are first to care for all injuries that are an immediate threat to life and second to repair wounds so that there is an optimal return of function and restoration of appearance.

Because facial injuries may be associated with serious injuries to other sites, emergency treatment of life-threatening conditions must take precedence over management of facial injuries. Active bleeding from soft tissue wounds of the face must be treated immediately by a pressure dressing. Because a carefully applied dressing will usually arrest bleeding, shock is not a frequent consequence of hemorrhage from facial trauma. Before applying the dressing, all kinked or twisted flaps of tissue should be returned to their original position to prevent further vascular compromise. Bleeding from the oral cavity, which is not susceptible to control by pressure, can obstruct the airway. In such cases, a patent airway can be maintained, usually by sucking blood from the patient's mouth using a Yankauer tonsil sucker. The patient should be transported immobilized and secured by a backboard. Aspiration can be prevented by turning the patient and backboard as a unit so that the patient is lying on his or her side.

Repair of facial soft tissue injuries requires an understanding of the anatomy of each special site, assessment of the aesthetic and functional deformity, and selection of the appropriate techniques for repair. Because the surgical treatment of the injury to each site of the face is dependent, in part, upon its anatomic configuration, the anatomy of the specific site will be discussed in conjunction with our surgical approaches to wound repair. The technical factors involved in wound care outlined in Section 19, "Emergency Wound Management," are applicable to soft tissue injuries of the face.

SCALP

Anatomy

The scalp and forehead are parts of the same anatomic structure (Fig. 195-1). They are composed of the following five layers: (1) skin, (2) subcutaneous tissue, (3) occipitofrontalis muscle, (4) a layer of loose aponeurosis, and (5) the pericranium (Fig. 195-1A). The first layers are intimately connected and are not easily separated. The scalp skin is very thick and firmly attached to the underlying epicranial aponeurosis (galea aponeurotica) by fibrous septa. It has abundant hair follicles, sebaceous glands, and a rich network of blood vessels. The subcutaneous tissue is divided by the fibrous septa into multiple fat lobules. The septa limit vessel retraction following injury and are responsible for profuse hemorrhage.

The occipitofrontalis muscle has two pairs of muscles connected by a broad aponeurosis, the galea aponeurotica (epicranial aponeurosis). The anterior pair of muscles are the frontalis muscles, attached to the epicranial aponeurosis a little in front of the coronal suture (Fig. 195-1C). The posterior pair of muscles (occipitalis muscles) are attached to the occipital bone above the lateral two-thirds of the nuchal line and to the mastoid process of the temporal bone. The epicranial aponeurosis is attached posteriorly to the external occipital protuberance and anteriorly to the supraorbital margin of the frontal bellies. Laterally, it blends with the fascia covering the temporalis muscle above the level of the zygomatic arch (Fig. 195-1B). It is separated from the periosteum (pericranium) overlying the skull by loose areolar tissue. This subgaleal layer permits free movement of the scalp over the cranium and is the plane where avulsion occurs in scalping injuries. This space is considered the danger zone of the scalp because hematoma and infection can spread easily through it. It is traversed by small arteries that supply the pericranium, and by the emissary veins connecting the intracranial venous sinuses with the superficial veins of the scalp. Thrombosis of the emissary veins may extend to the dural sinuses. The pericranium is adherent at the sutures and thus limits the spread of infection.

The sensory nerve supply to the entire scalp and face is supplied by branches of the trigeminal nerve, except for the skin overlying the posterior portion of the masseter muscle, which is innervated by posterior and anterior branches of the upper cervical nerves. Injuries to these sensory nerves rarely result in permanent anesthesia because of the rich overlapping system of undamaged nerves as well as nerve regeneration.

The scalp has a luxurious blood supply from five arteries on each side of the head. The occipital, superficial temporal, and posterior auricular arteries are branches of the external carotid artery, while the supraorbital and supratrochlear arteries arise from the internal carotid arteries.

Injuries and Treatment

Soft tissue injuries of the scalp can be divided into four groups: lacerations, abrasions, contusions, and avulsions. Over half are due to motor vehicle accidents. The front-seat passenger is most commonly thrown up and forward, sustaining an impact injury to the head caused by the windshield. The construction of the windshield is a key determinant of the type of injury. Automobiles manufactured prior to 1966 had safety-glass windshields that were susceptible to penetration by the occupant's head in an angle of approximately 45 degrees in a 14-mph frontal crash. After the forward momentum had stopped, the passenger was thrown back and down into the front seat. As the victim's face returned past the lower edge of the broken windshield, it tore the brow and forehead, resulting in superiorly based U-shaped flaps. Occasionally, complete avulsion occurred and the tissue was found on the broken windshield.

High-penetration-resistant (HPR) windshields were introduced in 1966 and have changed dramatically the pattern of facial soft tissue injuries. In HPR windshields, the pane is laminated to a plastic interlayer that prevents the occupant's head from penetrating the windshield. After impact, the plastic layer stretches out, cushioning the head against it. The inner glass pane fractures into a typical mosaic pattern of breakage at the site of impact that is responsible for the characteristic soft tissue injuries consisting of numerous small, superficial lacerations and triangular avulsion flaps. Glass particles are often buried in the lacerations. These facial injuries can be avoided by the use of shoulder-lap seat belts and/or air-bag restraint systems.

Total avulsion of the scalp in an occupational hazard for personnel with long hair who work in close proximity to rotary machines. The loose areolar tissue beneath the galea aponeurotica allows the scalp to be pulled off the pericranium. Stringent safeguards have reduced the incidence of industrial accidents of this type.

It must be emphasized that eyebrows should never be clipped or shaved because their delicate contour and form are valuable landmarks for the meticulous reapproximation of the wound edges. After the wound has been cleansed and hemostasis achieved, the base of the wound should always be palpated. Physical examination is often a more accurate technique for diagnosing injuries to the underlying bone than is x-ray examination.

When the edges of a laceration of either the eyebrow or the scalp

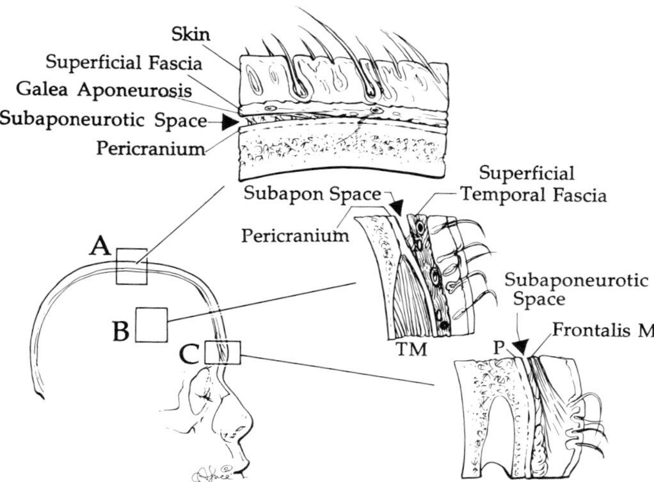

Fig. 195-1. Diagram of five layers of the scalp.

are devitalized, debridement is mandatory. When debriding these sites, the scalpel should cut at an angle that is parallel to that of the hair follicles. If the cut is made vertical to the skin surface, injury to hair follicles adjacent to the cut edge will occur and areas on both sides of the scar will be hairless.

Wound closure should be initiated first with approximation of the galea aponeurotica with buried, interrupted nonabsorbable 4–0 synthetic sutures. Galeal suture closure reduces the depth and width of the overlying skin scar. This beneficial effect of galeal sutures on scar formation is significantly more evident with nonabsorbable sutures than absorbable sutures. Another advantage of galeal suture is that it provides a barrier to the spread of superficial infection into the underlying loose areolar plane. The divided edges of muscle and fascia must also be closed with buried, interrupted, braided absorbable 4–0 synthetic sutures to prevent further the development of depressed scars.

The skin edges of anatomic landmarks should be approximated first with key stitches, using interrupted nonabsorbable monofilament 5–0 synthetic sutures (Fig. 195-2). Accurate alignment of the eyebrow, transverse wrinkles of the forehead, and the hairline of the scalp is essential. It may be necessary to have younger patients raise their

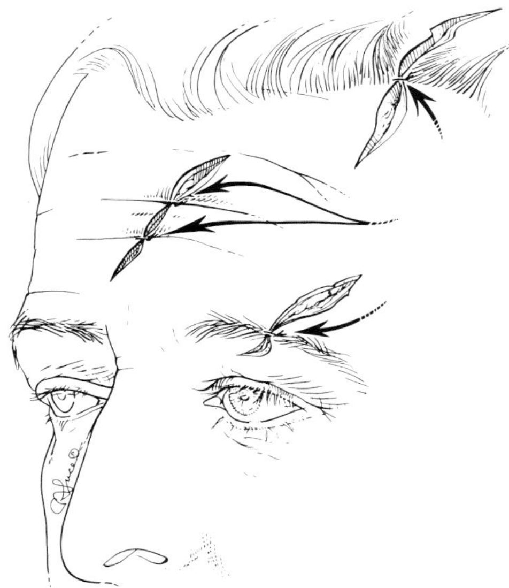

Fig. 195-2. Key stitches in the eyebrow.

eyebrows to create wrinkles, which will guide accurate placement of the key stitches.

An irregular laceration should be put together as it came apart, because it usually heals with a scar whose width is narrower than that of a linear laceration. Moreover, an irregular laceration undergoes less contraction than a linear one.

Z-plasty and flap rotation should never be considered for primary repair because there is no guarantee either that scar contracture will occur or that the repaired wound will not become infected. Scar revisions are always best accomplished when tissue healing and scar maturation are complete, 6 to 12 months after injury.

In forehead and scalp lacerations where underlying muscle and galea are divided, hematomas may form and dissect beneath the galea aponeurotica. A firm pressure dressing placed around the head can close any potential dead space, encourage hemostasis, and prevent hematoma formation. This pressure dressing should be left in place for 48 h.

Contusions of the scalp and forehead heal readily unless there is an underlying hematoma; this may become localized, with subsequent formation of an encapsulated seroma. The seroma can erode into the outer table of the skull to result in Pott's puffy tumor. A hematoma is best evacuated by an incision when still in the currant-jelly stage. As further liquefaction of the blood clot occurs, aspiration with a large-bore needle (No. 16 or larger) may be successful. After evacuation of either a hematoma or seroma, a pressure dressing should be applied to the forehead and scalp for 48 h to close the dead space and prevent reaccumulation of blood or serous exudates.

The objective of treatment of avulsion injuries of the scalp is to achieve proper skin coverage of all denuded areas as soon as possible. In most of these injuries, the pericranium is intact. The most appealing method of reconstruction is microvascular surgical techniques. The entire scalp can be replaced successfully by anastomosing the superficial artery and its paired vein bilaterally. By 6 months, hair growth and frontalis muscle activity can return.

Care of the amputated part requires limited treatment at the scene of injury. Any gross contaminant can be washed off, but lengthy irrigation of the part should not be undertaken because it can make identification of structures more difficult. The amputated part should be placed in a plastic bag in an ice container.

When the avulsed part is not available, treatment will depend on whether the periosteum is present. When the pericranium is intact, coverage of the exposed periosteum with a split-thickness skin graft taken either from the avulsed scalp itself or from the thigh or buttock is recommended in the operating room.

When the pericranium is destroyed, the outer table of the skull loses its blood supply and will not maintain the viability of skin grafts. In this case, coverage with pedicle flaps is recommended. Pedicle flap coverage can be achieved by either a local flap or a free flap in the operating room.

EYELIDS

Anatomy

The upper and lower eyelids are reinforced folds of tissue which form movable curtains. From its superficial to its deep surface, the eyelid is composed of the following structures: (1) skin, (2) subcutaneous tissue, (3) orbicularis oculi muscle, (4) tarsal plate, and (5) conjunctiva. The skin of the eyelid is thinner than at any other anatomic site of the body, and has fine, downlike hairs. It is freely movable over the underlying tissues and can be picked up readily with the finger. There is normally a fold in the upper lid (supratarsal fold) under which the lower portion of the lid disappears when elevated. When the eyelids are opened, they are separated from each other by an elliptical space, the palpebral fissure. The angles of the space are the lateral and medial canthi.

The subcutaneous tissue is relatively free of fat and is penetrated by the superficial fibers of the orbicularis oculi muscle. The muscle can be divided into three parts: orbital, pretarsal and preseptal. The orbital portion forms a muscular ring extending over the orbital margin widely, interdigitating with fibers of the frontalis muscle. Contraction of this orbital portion brings the skin of the forehead and eyelids downward and shades the eyes; it is used to close the lids tightly. The pretarsal portion overlies the tarsus and divides medially into superficial and deep heads. The superficial head joins its counterpart in the opposing lid to form the medial canthal tendon, which inserts above and anterior to the anterior lacrimal crest. The deep head, after joining its counterpart, advances posteriorly to the lacrimal sac and inserts behind the posterior lacrimal crest. The preseptal part of the muscle overlies the septum orbitale and has superficial and deep fibers. Its superficial fibers insert on the orbital margin below the canthal tendon, while its deeper fibers insert on the posterior lacrimal crest just above the deep head of the pretarsal portion. The insertion of the heads of the pretarsal and preseptal parts on the posterior lacrimal crest maintains the eyelids against the ocular globe, and is responsible for the depth of the naso-orbital valley. If the medial canthal tendon is severed, reattachment of the canthal tendon posterior to the lacrimal crest is essential to reestablish the depth of the naso-orbital valley.

Both the pretarsal parts of the orbicularis oculi muscle form a raphe that is attached to the skin of the lateral canthus. The pretarsal muscles of the upper and lower lids have a tendinous insertion (lateral canthal tendon) into the orbital tubercle. The pretarsal and preseptal portions of the orbicularis oculi muscle are able to close the eyelids and are responsible for involuntary blinking. Forced closure of the eye requires the entire muscle to contract. While the temporal branch of the facial nerve innervates the major portion of the orbicularis oculi muscle, the zygomatic branch of this nerve also supplies this muscle.

The orbital septum unites the margins of the tarsal plates to the infraorbital and supraorbital margins and attaches to the medial and lateral canthal tendons. By separating the tissues of the lid from the orbital contents, it contains the orbital structures behind the lids, preventing orbital fat from herniating forward and distorting the surface contour of the lid. An intricate fascial system, known as Lockwood's suspensory ligament, is attached to the orbital walls, forming a sling beneath the eye. It attaches medially to the posterior lacrimal crest and laterally below the lateral orbital tubercle.

The upper eyelid is more movable than the lower; attached to it is the levator palpebrae superioris, which is innervated by the third cranial nerve. Together with the superior rectus muscle, it arises from the small wing of the sphenoid above and in front of the optic foramen, passes with this muscle, and finally separates from it to enter the upper lid as a fan-shaped muscle. The main insertion of the muscle is the upper part of the tarsal plate. Some of its fibers pass through the orbicularis oculi muscles to be attached to the skin of the upper eyelid and the subconjunctival fornix. The expansions of the levator palpebrae superioris, which are attached to the medial and lateral canthal ligaments, are important landmarks when attempting to locate the severed muscles. Injury to this muscle or its nerve supply results in ptosis.

Müller's muscle is a thin muscle in the upper lid which lies closely behind the levator palpebrae superioris, to which it is loosely connected by fine connective tissue fibers as far as its attachment to the superior margin of the tarsus. While the levator palpebrae superioris is striated muscle, Müller's muscle is smooth muscle, receiving innervation from the sympathetic nervous system. Stimulation of the sympathetic nerve supply of Müller's muscle results in elevation of the upper lid by 3 to 4 mm. In the lower lid, Müller's muscle arises from the sheath of the inferior rectus and is inserted on the lower border of the tarsus. Contraction of these fibers results in a lowering of the lower lid. Opening of the palpebral fissure is due to contraction of the levator palpebrae superioris and Müller's muscle in conjunction with relaxation of the orbicularis oculi.

The tarsal plate itself forms the main body of the lower half of the lid. It consists of some elastic tissue in a dense matrix of connective tissue. The upper tarsus is much larger than the lower. Its free border extends to the lid margin. Embedded in the tarsal plate are a number of simple branched alveolar glands, the meibomian glands. They open into the white line just in front of the conjunctival edge of the lid margin. In the lid margin the eyelashes are arranged in three irregular rows. Their follicles extend obliquely into the tarsal plate.

The posterior surface of the eyelid is covered by a transparent membrane, the conjunctiva. This membrane lines the lid as the palpebral conjunctiva and is reflected onto the anterior surface of the eyeball as the bulbar conjunctiva. This reflection forms a deep recess known as the fornix.

The excretory lacrimal duct system begins at the upper and lower puncta, which are positioned at the apex of the lacrimal papilla. Each punctum, which is the beginning of a canaliculus, has a diameter of 0.3 mm and is surrounded by a ring of connective and elastic tissue. The canaliculi are approximately 10 cm long and consist of a 2-cm vertical component and an 8-cm horizontal section. In the horizontal part of the canaliculi, the lumen widens to form the ampulla, which is 2 to 3 mm at its widest diameter. In 90 percent of the population, the canaliculi join to form an internal common canaliculus before entering the lacrimal sac, which is situated in the lacrimal fossa. The lacrimal sac is the membranous extension of the nasolacrimal duct, whose length is approximately 20 mm. The nasolacrimal duct extends 3 to 5 mm above the level of the medial canthus before it becomes the osseous portion of the nasolacrimal duct. This duct opens into the anterior part of the inferior meatus of the nose. The ostium is guarded by a fold of mucosa named Hausner's valve. Tears are propelled into the excretory lacrimal duct system by gravity, the venturi effect in the inferior meatus, and the lacrimal pump.

The lacrimal pump mechanism is involved in the excretory functions of tears into the nose. The superficial and deep heads of the pretarsal muscles furnish the motor power for the lacrimal pump, closing the ampulla and shortening the canaliculi, and forcing fluid into the lacrimal sac. The preseptal muscles, through their intimate connection with the lacrimal diaphragm, also produce negative pressure in the lacrimal sac. The elasticity of the diaphragm returns it to its position of rest, and fluid is forced into the nasolacrimal duct. Closure of the eye shortens the canaliculus and exerts pressure on the lacrimal ampulla. Opening of the eye creates a vacuum within the lacrimal sac and initiates the pump mechanism.

Injuries and Treatment

In treating eyelid injuries, major considerations are to protect the eye and to maintain vision. Preoperative examination of the eye by an ophthalmologist is mandatory. If an ocular injury is detected, treatment of the eye injury must precede repair. During wound repair, the cornea must be protected from desiccation, irritation, and trauma. Desiccation can be prevented by instilling a few drops of 0.9% saline into the conjunctival sac during wound closure. The use of a contact lens is recommended to protect the cornea from injury.

Trauma in this region can be divided into injuries to the upper and lower eyelids, to the canthal tendons, and to the lacrimal system. Injuries to the eyelids are either lacerations or avulsions. In either case, damage to the levator palpebrae superioris may be evident. The lacerations can be classified into two groups according to their depth: lacerations through the skin and lacerations through the lid margins. A superficial laceration of the skin parallel to the lid margin may require no closure, especially if it aligned with the lid fold. If the laceration is not aligned with the skin fold, approximation of the skin edges with a running, subcuticular nonabsorbable monofilament 5–0 synthetic suture is recommended. The suture should be removed 72 h after injury to avoid the development of epithelial cysts at the entrance and exits of the suture. Because the direction of this laceration is perpendicular to that of the dynamic skin tensions, wound repair will usually result in a narrow, aesthetically pleasing scar. In contrast, lacerations through skin whose direction is perpendicular to the lid

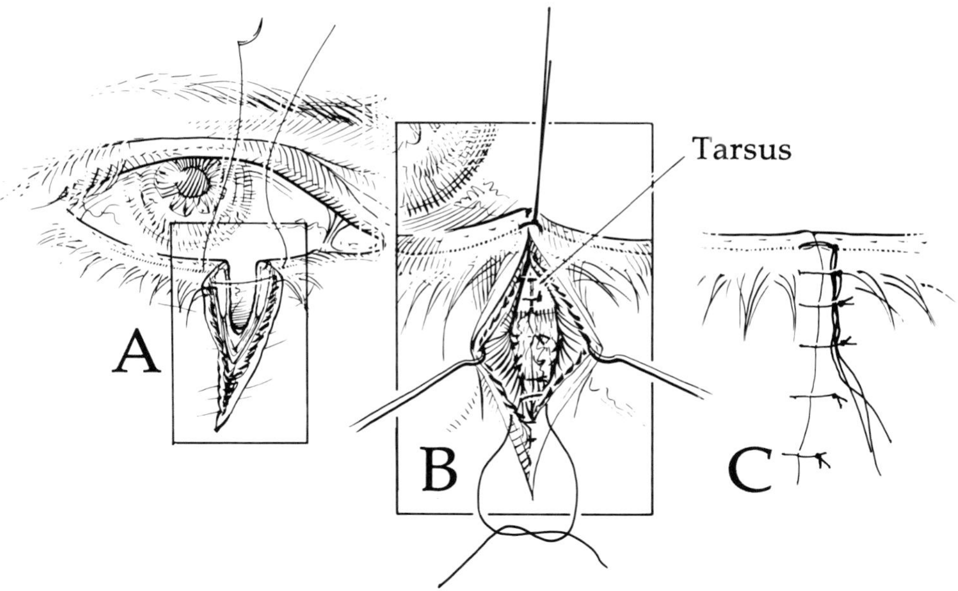

Fig. 195-3. Repair of lacerations through the lid. A scleral lens has been placed in the conjunctival sac. **A.** The first suture is passed through the "gray-line" of the eyelid. **B.** The conjunctiva and tarsal plate are then closed. **C.** A skin suture is tied over the long ends of the marginal suture. (See text for detail.)

margin will heal with a conspicuous scar that often develops a linear contracture causing an upward pull on the lid. A Z-plasty revision of the healing scar 6 to 12 months later will lengthen the contracture and prevent this deformity.

Closure of a laceration that extends through the entire eyelid requires a three-layer closure, with meticulous approximation of each layer (Fig. 195-3). After a protective lens is positioned in the conjunctival sac, closure should begin with a marginal nonabsorbable monofilament 5–0 synthetic suture, aligning and approximating the "gray line," which is the end of a sheet of fascia between the orbicularis oculi muscle and the tarsal plate (Fig. 195-3A). If the "gray line" is not approximated accurately, notching of the eyelid often results, with possible inversion of the eyelashes. Traction of the long untied ends of the marginal suture approximates the wound edges and aligns the anterior and posterior lid margins.

The conjunctiva and tarsal plate are then closed with interrupted, braided absorbable 6–0 synthetic sutures, whose knots are buried so that they do not abrade the cornea (Fig. 195-3B). The orbicularis oculi muscle is approximated by interrupted, braided absorbable 6–0 synthetic sutures. The eyelid skin is closed with interrupted nonabsorbable monofilament 6–0 synthetic sutures whose knots lie on the surface. A skin suture 2 mm from the lashes is tied over the long ends of the marginal suture, which prevents it from irritating the conjunctiva (Fig. 195-3C). The skin and marginal sutures are removed on the fourth postoperative day. In the following 6 months, linear contraction of the vertical scar may be encountered, resulting in a pull on the lid margin. In such cases, lengthening of the skin scar with a Z-plasty corrects the deformity.

Dog bites, human bites, and accidents of varying types may cause avulsion injuries of the eyelid. These avulsions may be classified according to their depth, the eyelid involved, and the size of the resulting defect. Treatment will depend on the type of injury as well as to whether the avulsed tissue specimen is available for reconstruction.

The levator palpebrae superioris is involved frequently in injuries to the upper lid, especially in automobile accidents and injuries from various types of machinery. In all deep transverse lacerations of the eyelid, it is important to verify levator palpebrae superioris function. If the patient cannot raise the upper lid for reasons other than edema, primary suture of the injured muscle must be undertaken in the operating room.

Medial and lateral canthal tendon deformities are usually sequelae of orbital fractures that may be associated with midfacial bone fractures and naso-orbital fractures. Zygomatic fractures are a frequent cause of dislocation of the lateral raphe and lateral canthal tendons. Deep vertical lacerations along the lateral or medial walls of the orbit may occasionally damage the lateral and medial canthal tendons. Division of the medial canthal tendon results in a characteristic deformity with a rounded medial canthus and decreased intercanthal distance (Fig. 195-4). The division of the medial canthal tendon and the inability of the orbicularis oculi muscle to maintain normal muscle tone between the medial and lateral canthal tendons causes a relaxation of the lower eyelid, eversion of the lacrimal puncta, and inadequate evacuation of tears from the lacrimal lake. Interference with the muscle power of the orbicularis oculi muscle also affects the lacrimal pump, and this further hampers the excretory system. This injury is usually complicated by an interruption of the continuity of the excretory lacrimal system.

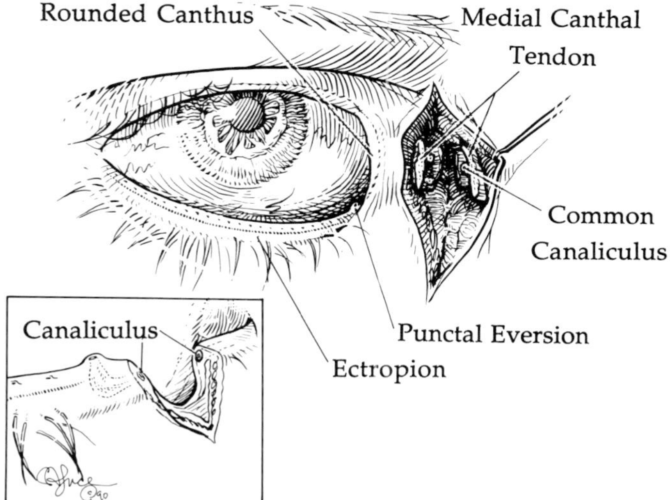

Fig. 195-4. The orbicularis oculi muscle exerts traction in a lateral direction on the medial canthus when the medial canthal tendon is severed. This results in a characteristic deformity with a rounded medial canthus and a decreased distance between the medial and lateral canthi. Insert: Laceration of the lower lid through the lacrimal canaliculus.

Restoration of the integrity of the medial canthal tendon is achieved by reattachment of the divided ends of the tendon with wire sutures in the operating room. After repair of the medial canthal tendon, the continuity of the injured lacrimal system is reestablished. Complete detachment of the lateral raphe and lateral tendon results in a rounded lateral canthus and a diminution of the horizontal dimension of the palpebral fissure. Restoration of the divided ends of these structures can usually be accomplished with the same wire-fixation technique used in repair of severed medial canthal tendons.

Injuries of the lacrimal system occur most frequently in naso-orbital fractures and soft tissue lacerations. They may be difficult to diagnose because of severe ecchymosis of the eyelids. However, the location of the laceration and the physical findings can alert the emergency physician to a possible injury to this system which may be caused by a laceration medial to the punctum caused by a knife, razor, or even a coat hanger (Fig. 195-4, inset). Severance of the lower lacrimal canaliculus results in widening of the palpebral fissure. The orbicularis oculi muscle tends to enlarge the areas of the laceration and produce ectropion. Laceration of either canaliculus displaces the injured lid laterally. Proper management of injuries to this system is necessary to prevent subsequent complications, such as annoying epiphora and dacryocystitis.

While repair of injury to the lacrimal system should be done as early as possible, local edema and hemorrhage may make early operative repair difficult and even hazardous. In such cases, it is prudent to delay surgery for 12 to 24 h, by which time the bleeding will have subsided and some of the edema will have resolved. In addition, the cut ends of the canaliculus tend to evert during this time and are more easily identified. Their divided ends usually appear as small, pearly white rings.

If the cut ends are not readily apparent, there are several techniques to facilitate their identification using an operating room microscope. One technique involves introducing a blunt-ended plastic catheter into the uninjured punctum and injecting either a solution of methylene blue or a 0.5 to 2% fluorescein dye solution. The appearance of the dye from the severed end of the canaliculus reveals its location. Another approach is to instill 0.9% saline into the medial canthal region as the patient lies in a supine position. By injecting air through the blunt-ended needle in the uninjured canaliculus, bubbles will be seen coming from the severed end.

Whenever possible, the injured canaliculus should be repaired in the operating room, even though the other remains intact. The most important principle in repairing the canalicular laceration is to reestablish canalicular patency by direct microsurgical anastomosis, suturing of the severed ends, and endocanalicular support, preferably with silicone tubing. It is important to emphasize that a properly performed repair of the canalicular system by a plastic surgeon or ophthalmologist is successful in nearly 100 percent of cases. However, improper treatment by the inexperienced surgeon leads to distortion of the structures, which may lead to chronic dacryocystitis. In such cases, external dacryocystorhinostomy is necessary.

NOSE

Anatomy

The nose is a triangular pyramid composed of cartilaginous and osseous structures that support the overlying skin and musculature and the underlying mucosa. A median septum divides the pyramid into right and left halves that extend from the columella anteriorly to the nasal choanae posteriorly. The cephalic portion of the dorsal border of the septal cartilage is connected intimately with the cephalic portion of the lateral cartilages.

The supporting framework of the nose consists of a nasal skeleton cephalad and a cartilaginous framework caudad. The nasal skeleton is composed of the frontal processes of the maxillae laterally and the paired nasal bones and the bony nasal septum centrally. The cartilaginous framework is made up of the triangular lateral and alar cartilages laterally and the cartilaginous septum centrally. There is an overlap of about 1 cm between the nasal bones and the lateral cartilages, with an intimate fusion of the periosteum and perichondrium.

The paired, C-shaped alar cartilages form the cartilaginous support for the tip of the nose. Each alar cartilage has a medial and lateral crus. The medial crura curve downward into the columella and then diverge as they approach the base of the columella. The alar and lateral cartilages are connected by aponeurotic tissue. Muscles (procerus, nasalis, and levator labii superioris) cover the entire external surface of the bony and cartilaginous framework, except the alar cartilages where the skin is tightly bound to the cartilage. The skin covering the remaining portion of the nose is thin, supple, and mobile.

The nasal lining in the columella and vestibule is skin. The nasal vestibule is limited posteriorly by the protrusion of the lower border of the upper lateral cartilages, forming folds or internal nares. These folds extend laterally and inferiorly along the pyriform aperture outlining the posterior extent of the vestibule. The lining of the anterior part of the vestibule has thick, long hairs (vibrissae) with which are associated large sebaceous glands. The zone of the vibrissae is succeeded by the transitional zone in the vestibule lined by thick, stratified squamous epithelium. Sweat and sebaceous glands, as well as hair, are absent in the transitional zone. The mucous membrane overlying the remaining portion of the nasal canal is composed of ciliated, pseudostratified columnar epithelium.

Injuries and Treatment

Lacerations of the nose may be limited to skin or may involve the deeper structures (sparse nasal musculature, cartilaginous framework, and nasal mucous membrane). They are repaired by accurate reapproximation of each tissue layer (Fig. 195-5).

When the laceration extends through all tissue layers, closure should begin with a marginal nonabsorbable monofilament 5–0 synthetic suture that aligns the skin surrounding the entrances of the nasal canals, to prevent malapposition and notching of the alar rim (Fig. 195-5A). Traction upon the long, untied ends of the marginal suture approximates the wound and aligns the anterior and posterior margins of the divided

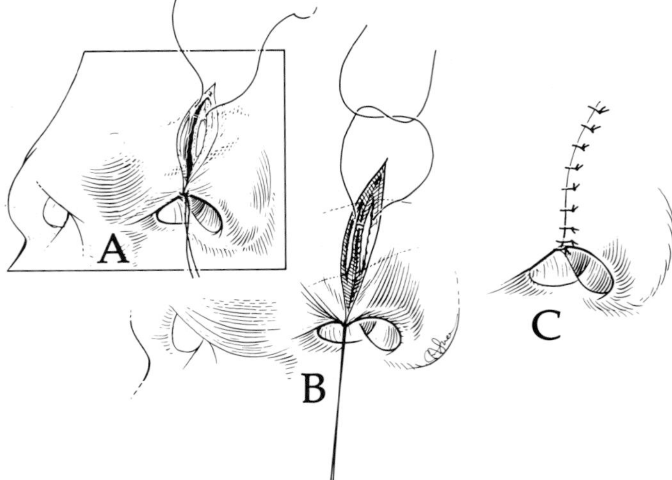

Fig. 195-5. Repair of a linear laceration extending through all tissue layers of the nose. **A.** A marginal suture should be placed through the alar rim to align the nasal canal. Traction should be applied to the marginal suture to align the individual tissue layers. **B.** The divided nasal mucosa and cartilage should be approximated separately. **C.** The skin edges are approximated by interrupted nonabsorbable monofilament 5–0 synthetic sutures.

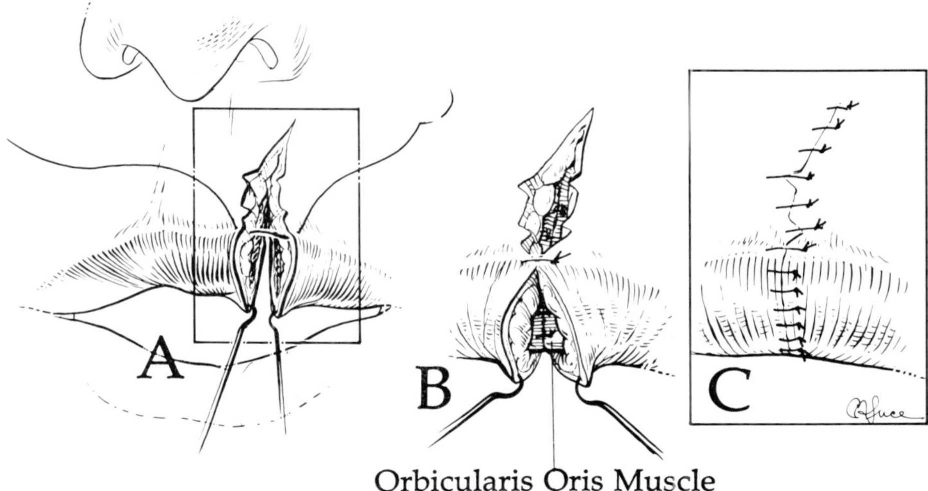

Fig. 195-6. Irregular-edged vertical laceration of the upper lip. **A.** Traction is applied to the lips and closure of the wound is begun first at the vermilion-skin junction. **B.** The orbicularis oris muscle is then repaired with interrupted, braided absorbable 4–0 synthetic sutures. **C.** The irregular edges of the skin are then approximated.

tissue layers. The mucous membrane should then be repaired with interrupted, braided absorbable 5–0 synthetic sutures with their knots buried in the tissue. The divided edges of the cartilage should then be approximated with interrupted, braided absorbable 5–0 synthetic sutures (Fig. 195-5B). The cut edges of the skin, with its adherent musculature, are closed with interrupted nonabsorbable monofilament 5–0 synthetic sutures (Fig. 195-5C). After wound closure, linear lacerations of the alar rim may shorten and result in notching of the rim 3 to 6 months later. A Z-plasty at the alar rim will correct this deformity.

A hematoma develops between the septal mucoperichondrium and the cartilage after either fracture or dislocation of the septum or excessive bending of the septal cartilage. Hematoma is often bilateral because the fractured septum permits passage of blood from one side to the other. If the hematoma is not detected, fibrosis may develop in the hematoma, resulting in permanent thickening of the nasal septum, with partial obstruction of the nasal airway. An untreated septal hematoma also may cause absorption of the septal cartilage, especially if infected, resulting in septal perforation and/or saddle nose deformity. Consequently, the nasal septum should be inspected for hematoma formation using a nasal speculum following any nasal injury. Packing the nose with gauze soaked in a vasoconstrictive agent (4% cocaine) limits nasal bleeding and facilitates the examination.

The presence of bluish swelling in the septum confirms the diagnosis of septal hematoma. Treatment of the hematoma is evacuation of the blood clot. Drainage of a small hematoma can be accomplished by aspiration of the blood clot through a No. 18 needle. A larger hematoma is drained through a horizontal incision through the mucoperichondrial layer along the floor of the nose. In bilateral hematomas, resection of a portion of the septal cartilage in the operating room is recommended to allow communication between both hematomas. Reaccumulation of blood can be prevented by either nasal packing or simple suction catheter drainage (scalp vein cannula and vacuum tube*). Simple suction catheter drainage is preferred over packs because subsequent pack removal is uncomfortable and may precipitate bleeding. By comparison, removal of the catheter is painless and is not accompanied by bleeding. Antibiotic treatment is recommended to prevent infection that predisposes to necrosis of cartilage.

When there is avulsion of components of the nose, it is best to restore the architecture with the avulsed specimen, using microsurgical techniques. If the avulsed tissue is not recovered or not suitable for replantation, the technique of reconstruction will depend on the magnitude and depth of injury.

*Abbot Hospital, Inc., North Chicago, Illinois.

LIPS

Anatomy

The external surfaces of the lips have three distinct regions: the cutaneous area (skin), the vermilion, and the oral mucosa. The vermilion is a relatively thick layer of noncornified stratified epithelium that is deeply indented by vascular connective tissue papillae. Its superficial epithelial cells contain eleidin, making them translucent and permitting the underlying vascular papillae to give the vermilion its color. Glands are absent in this region, except for occasional sebaceous glands. The vermilion is continuous with a mucous membrane that covers the inner surface of the lips. Vascular connective tissue papillae of moderate length indent the epithelial cover, resulting in the pink color of the mucous membrane. Numerous glands of a mixed (mucous and serous) type and a mucous type are present in the underlying submucosal layer.

The skin meets the red-colored vermilion at the ''red line.'' A surface prominence of paler vermilion contiguous with the skin-vermilion junction is called the ''white line.'' Another important anatomic landmark is the junction between the red vermilion and the pink mucous membrane. Superficial landmarks unique to the skin over the upper lip are the philtral hollow, its eminences, and the associated curving of ''white'' and ''red lines'' into cupid's bows.

The orbicularis oris muscle is the voluntary muscle that surrounds the mouth. It is located between the skin and oral mucosa and is responsible for the damming of saliva and the formation of labial sounds. Lip sensation is mediated by the infraorbital and mental branches of the trigeminal nerve. The labial arteries of the upper and lower lips are branches of the facial artery that form anastomosing coronary arteries located beneath the mucosa on the inner surface of the lips, just below their free borders.

Injuries and Treatment

The technique of closure will depend largely on the type of lip wound. There are essentially two types of wound: lacerations and avulsions. Superficial lacerations involve the skin and subcutaneous tissue. Deep lacerations may extend through the muscle and underlying mucosa. Bleeding may be profuse if the labial arteries are involved. Clamping the cut ends of the vessel with a hemostat and tying them with suture ligatures will control bleeding. Each tissue layer of the laceration must be reapproximated meticulously (Fig. 195-6). The vermilion-cutaneous and the vermilion-mucosal margins are important anatomic landmarks that must be apposed by key stitches to prevent the development of a ''step-off'' deformity that is difficult to correct at a later date.

Repair of a laceration through the lip requires a three-layered closure (Fig. 195-6). Using skin hooks, traction is applied to align the anterior and posterior borders of the laceration. Closure of the wound is begun first at the vermilion-skin junction with a nonabsorbable monofilament 6–0 synthetic suture (Fig. 195-6A). The orbicularis oris muscle is then repaired with interrupted, braided absorbable 4–0 synthetic sutures (Fig. 195-6B). The vermilion-mucous membrane junction is approximated with a braided absorbable 5–0 synthetic suture. This suture ligature is constructed so that its knot is buried in the subcutaneous tissue. The divided edges of the mucous membrane and vermilion are then closed using interrupted, braided absorbable 5–0 synthetic sutures with a buried-knot construction. The skin edges of the laceration are usually jagged and irregular, but can be fitted together as the pieces of a jigsaw puzzle using interrupted nonabsorbable monofilament 6–0 synthetic sutures with their knots formed on the surface of the skin (Fig. 195-6C). During healing, a linear wound of the lip may undergo contraction, resulting in notching of the lip. The deformity can be corrected by a Z-plasty revision of the linear scar.

Tissue loss from the lip usually involves either the skin surface or all tissue layers. Defects involving all tissue layers of the lip can be further classified by location into median defects, lateral defects, and complete loss of lip. Tissue loss at the commissure is a distinct entity that deserves special consideration. Reconstruction of these lip deficits should be performed by a plastic surgeon in an operating room. If the avulsed tissue is available, replantation using microsurgical techniques is the optimal method of reconstruction. If the avulsed tissue specimen is either not recovered or not amenable to replantation, the lip defect should be reconstructed with innervated muscle containing tissue with inner and outer epithelial linings.

CHEEKS

Anatomy

The main boundaries of the mouth are partly osseous and partly muscular. The lateral walls are formed by the cheeks and are lined by skin and mucous membrane. Between the linings are a fat pad and facial muscles. The buccinator muscle arises from the alveolar processes of the mandible and maxilla, and the pterygomandibular raphe. It inserts into the orbicularis oris muscle and is responsible for compressing the cheeks and maintaining tone. Important structures within the cheek include branches of the facial nerve, the parotid (Stensen's) duct, and a portion of the parotid gland (Fig. 195-7).

The parotid gland is composed of superficial and retromandibular parts. The gland lies on the masseter muscle, and extends posteriorly to the sternocleidomastoid muscle and to the cartilaginous portion of the external auditory meatus. The parotid duct arises from the most prominent part of the anterior border of the gland, passes forward on the masseter muscle, and then turns around its anterior border to pierce the buccinator muscle. It enters the vestibule of the mouth at the level of the crown of the second upper molar tooth. The course of the parotid duct is deep to a line drawn from the tragus of the ear to the mid-portion of the upper lip (line 2 in Fig. 195-7). Line 1 is a vertical line drawn from the inner canthus. If the peripheral branches of the facial nerve are injured medial to line 1, the nerve does not have to be repaired. However, a facial nerve or its branches injured lateral to this line should always be repaired.

The facial nerve emerges from the stylomastoid foramen, after which it becomes sandwiched or enfolded between the two lobes of the parotid gland. It divides within the substance of the gland into two main subdivisions, temporofacial and cervicofacial. Branches of these subdivisions radiate out from the margins of the gland in five divisions—temporal (T), zygomatic (Z), buccal (B), marginal mandibular (M), and cervical (C)—with multiple intercommunicating, dividing, and reuniting branches (Fig. 195-7).

Knowledge of the various types of branching of the facial nerves is helpful in the identification of the severed ends of the facial nerves in a facial injury. The buccal and zygomatic branches have connections in 80 percent of the cases. The marginal mandibular branches are connected in only 5 to 12 percent.

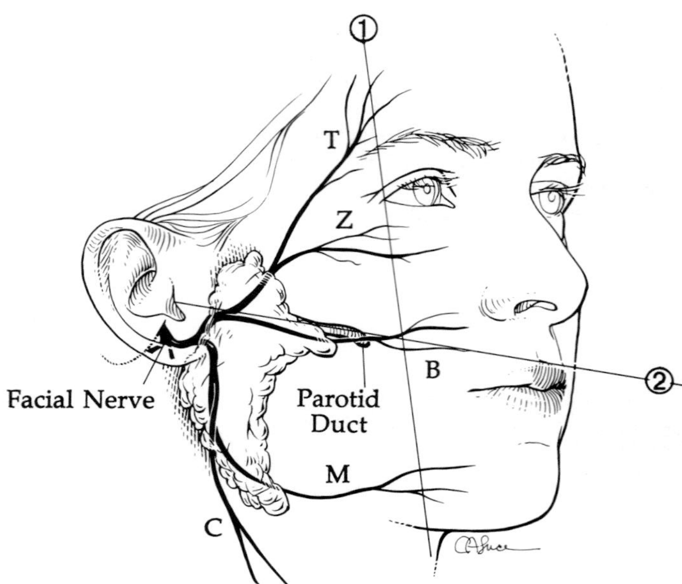

Fig. 195-7. The facial nerve and parotid gland.

Because the facial nerve is mainly a motor nerve governing the muscles of facial expression, facial symmetry in repose and in action (motility) is of paramount importance in detecting functional deficits. Resting tone is less important than motility in this evaluation because it is largely dependent on the smoothness of the skin surface, the thickness of the layer of subcutaneous adipose tissue, and the mass and firmness of the connective tissue. In early injuries to the facial nerve or its branches in children or in patients of pyknic body type, a good resting tone with a high degree of facial symmetry is evident in the absence of muscle function.

The temporal branches innervate the anterior auricular muscles, part of the superior auricular muscles, and the muscles of the forehead, including the major portion of the orbicularis oculi muscle. Division of the temporal branch of the facial nerve results in a unilateral paralysis of the frontalis muscle. The result of this injury is asymmetry of the forehead. The muscle on the unaffected side produces the usual transverse folds across the forehead, which contrast with the smooth surface on the paralyzed side. The patient will be unable to wrinkle the forehead on the affected side.

The zygomatic branches also supply the orbicularis oculi muscles, the muscles around the nares, and the levators of the upper lip. Because of the multiple connections between the nerves that innervate the orbicularis oculi muscle, paralysis is rarely encountered. When the temporofacial subdivision of the facial nerve or both the zygomatic and temporal branches are injured, paresis of the orbicularis oculi is noted with changes in the resting tone and motility of the periocular region. The size of the palpebral fissure on the affected side will be 3 mm wider than on the uninjured side. When the tonus of lower lid on the affected side is poor, ectropion results. The inability to close the eyelids of the affected side either loosely as in sleep or firmly is evidence of abnormal motility in the periocular region.

The buccal branch of the facial nerve traverses the face along the course of the parotid duct and is usually severed if the duct has been lacerated. The buccal nerve innervates most of the muscles around the lip. Of these muscles, the orbicularis oris produces recognizable clinical signs after denervation. The orbicularis oris is a group of muscles arranged in a sphincteric fashion around the mouth. Through its action, this muscle puckers the lips, draws them inward at the commissures, or presses them against the teeth. Injury to the buccal branch limits puckering of the lips, drawing the commissures inward on the affected side. For objective grading, a decrease in the distance between the philtrum and corner of the mouth following pursing the lips is measured. Because of the numerous connections between the buccal and zygomatic branches, gradual spontaneous regeneration is frequent.

The course of the marginal mandibular branch of the facial nerve, being near the posterior facial vein, is always deep to the platysma muscle. Bleeding from this vessel is often associated with injury to the marginal mandibular branch of the facial nerve. In approximately 20 percent of patients, it is located 1 to 1.5 cm below the mandible, between the angle of the jaw and the mandibular notch. In the remaining 80 percent, the marginal mandibular branch lies on the mandible throughout its course. This nerve innervates the lower group of circumoral muscles, consisting of the triangularis, the quadratus labii inferioris, and the platysma; these muscles depress the corner of the mouth and the lower lip. Injury to this branch causes an elevation of the ipsilateral lower lip at rest and an inability to depress it.

Injuries and Treatment

Lacerations of the cheek are of great concern because they may be associated with injury to the facial nerve and/or parotid duct. An early, accurate evaluation of the integrity of the facial nerve must be made before wound closure. Facial nerve injury may be easily missed in the unconscious patient or a patient with a bandaged head. If the functions of the facial nerve are not tested soon after injury, the extent and site of injury may be missed. Damage to the cerebral cortex or corticobulbar fibers can result in upper motor neuron lesions, with loss of movement of the mimetic muscles of the lower part of the contralateral side of the face. Lower motor neuron damage to the facial nerve can occur either intracranially, in the middle ear, or at the mastoid or stylomastoid foramen.

The site of injury to the facial nerve can be assessed accurately by assessing the functionality of its various branches. During its passage through the facial canal, it gives off several important branches: the greater superficial petrosal nerve, the chorda tympani, and the nerve to the stapedius muscle. The greater superficial petrosal nerve, which innervates tear production, can be evaluated by a modification of Schirmer's test. A strip of filter paper is hooked over the lower lid and acts as a wick. The patient is given a whiff of ammonia and the rate of flow along it is compared to that of a similar strip applied to the opposite conjunctival sac. Loss of stapedius muscle function may be detected by an acoustic impedance bridge. The chorda tympani, which supplies the anterior two-thirds of the tongue and innervates the submandibular gland, can be assessed by evaluating taste and salivary production. In cases of facial paralysis following blunt trauma, *without* soft tissue disruption, the prognosis for recovery is good and exploration is generally not needed.

The timing of nerve exploration is critical. If there is no loss of nerve substance, primary repair should be accomplished in the operating room within 5 to 6 days after injury, in a well-vascularized bed that is free of foreign debris, devitalized tissue, and any infective inocula of bacteria. If the wound bed is not acceptable and/or there is loss of nerve substance, it is wiser to achieve adequate skin closure in the operating room and delay the nerve repair. The optimal time for early secondary repair is when the original wound has healed without edema, usually 2 to 6 weeks after wound closure.

The goal of nerve repair is to produce a primary and accurate union of nerve ends with minimal scar formation. If the cut ends are contused or ischemic, or have been approximated under tension, scar formation of the nerve junction will interfere with repair. The chances of good nerve regeneration after nerve repair will be enhanced if the nerve repair is performed by an experienced surgeon using an operating microscope.

Injury to the parotid duct should be suspected if clear fluid is seen emerging from a wound in the cheek. The injury can be readily identified by passing a small silicone catheter into the opening of the parotid duct. After the distal divided end of the duct is identified, the patient is transferred to the operating room for repair of the duct.

Division of the submandibular glands and ducts does not require repair. The glands will drain through a fistula that usually develops after injury to the floor of the mouth. Lacerations of the cheek should be reapproximated with interrupted, nonabsorbable monofilament 5-0 synthetic sutures in a manner similar to that of putting together a jigsaw puzzle. In resurfacing skin loss of the cheek, the defect should be converted in the operating room to one that conforms to the aesthetic unit of the face. Through-and-through defects of the cheeks caused by severe trauma are also best repaired in the operating room.

EAR

Anatomy

The external ear consists of the external auditory canal and auricle. The latter consists of a double fold of skin supported by a fibrocartilaginous framework, which in the vicinity of the lobule is replaced by fibrofatty tissue. The skin layer is more adherent laterally than medially. The configuration of the cartilage on its medial side is fairly smooth, while characteristic elevations and depressions of the auricle are noted on its lateral side. The prominent outer rim of the auricle, the helix, occasionally has a small cartilaginous tubercle, the Darwin tubercle. The helical rim terminates anteriorly in a crus that lies almost horizontally above the external auditory meatus. A second rim of the ear, the antihelix, is adjacent to and almost parallel with the helix. The antihelix diverges into superior and anterior crura, enclosing the triangular fossa. Between the helix and antihelix is a long, deep furrow, the scapha. Within the substance of, and partly surrounded by, the antihelix, a deep cavity, the concha, leads into the external meatus. The conchal cavity, composed of cymba and cavum, arises from a floor that is at least 1 cm deeper than the overlying tragus and antitragus. The most lateral point of the auricle should lie between 1.7 and 2.0 cm from the scalp. Viewed from the front, the helical rim should be visible behind the antihelix.

The auricle has a luxurious blood supply from the superficial temporal and posterior auricular arteries. The sensory nerve supply arises primarily from the anterior and posterior branches of the greater auricular nerve, with lesser contributions from the auriculotemporal and lesser occipital nerves. Regional anesthesia of the auricle is accomplished by instilling an anesthetic solution along its base anteriorly and superiorly. Since the posterior wall of the external auditory canal is supplied by the auricular branches of the vagus nerve, this site must be injected separately.

Injuries and Treatment

Trauma to the ear can be divided into three general types: hematoma, laceration, and avulsion. A common injury in contact sports is auricular hematoma. Within hours after injury, the skin covering the anterior surface of the auricle is raised from the auricle by a hematoma or seroma, which forms in a plane between cartilage and its perichondrium. If drained, the potential space fills with serosanguinous exudate. Unless drainage is maintained, the elevated perichondrium produces neocartilage in the tethered and scarred cauliflower ear.

For the best results, treatment should be initiated within 72 h. Many different therapeutic approaches have been proposed. Most methods for dealing with auricular hematoma depend on evacuation of the hematoma and replacing the perichondrium back on the cartilage. Hematoma drainage has been achieved by repeated aspiration, incision and drainage with pressure dressing, and suction drainage. The concept of closed suction drainage to obtain complete evacuation of the hematoma is appealing in its simplicity because no dressing is required and the patient can resume normal activities.

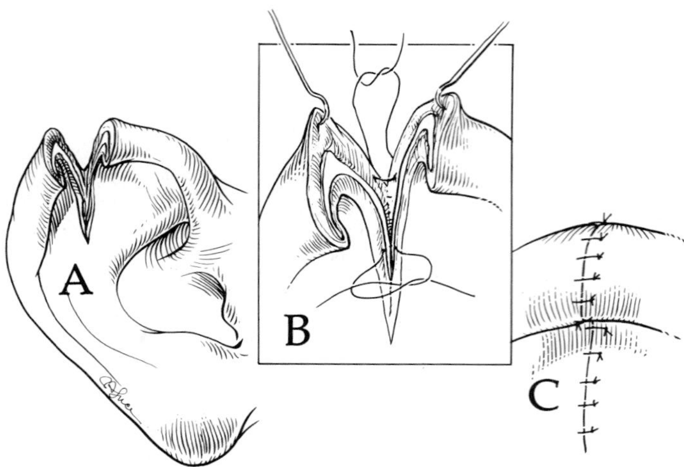

Fig. 195-8. A. Laceration through auricle. **B.** One or two interrupted, braided 6–0 synthetic sutures will approximate divided edges of cartilage. **C.** Interrupted nonabsorbable monofilament 6–0 synthetic sutures approximate the skin edges.

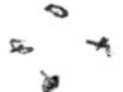

A laceration of the skin on the lateral aspect of the auricle should be subjected to minimal debridement because skin deficits in this site are not easily closed without distortion of the cartilage. In through-and-through lacerations, approximating the skin with minimal cartilaginous suturing will restore contour without numerous buried sutures (Fig. 195-8A, B, and C). Notching of the helical rim can be prevented by a Z-plasty, which is best performed 6 to 12 months after wound closure. Circular lacerations through the external auditory canal should be closed carefully with interrupted nonabsorbable monofilament 6–0 synthetic sutures. After wound closure, the canal should be packed tightly with an impregnated gauze. A prosthetic appliance should be worn for 4 months to prevent the development of stenosis of the canal. One of the most common injuries is laceration of the earlobe caused by traction on an earring in the pierced lobe. The repair is accomplished by resuturing the divided edges together. Incorporating a Z-plasty of the rim that will prevent notching may be performed 6 to 12 months later.

Full-thickness skin loss with intact perichondrium may be resurfaced with a postauricular, supraclavicular, or upper-eyelid full-thickness skin graft. When the perichondrium is missing, a preauricle or postauricular pedicle flap should be used to cover the defect.

A major auricular avulsion presents a challenging surgical problem. Microvascular surgery has played an important role in replanting ears that are amputated along with the scalp in scalping injuries. At least two ear replantations have been successful. Microvascular repair also appears to enhance survival in an incomplete ear amputation.

When the detached auricular tissue is either not available or not suitable for reconstruction, a variety of procedures can be used to reconstruct the ear.

Our research has been supported by a generous gift from Mrs. Ruth E. Tanner, Staunton, Virginia.

BIBLIOGRAPHY

Butt WE: Auricular haematoma: Treatment options. *Aust NZ J Surg* 57:391, 1987.

Carraway JH, Mellow CG: Simple suction drainage: An adjunct to septal surgery. *Ann Plast Surg* 24:191, 1990.

Crawford JS: Intubation of obstructions of the lacrimal system. *Can J Opthalmol* 12:289, 1977.

Davis RA, Anson BJ, Budinger JM, et al: Surgical anatomy of the facial nerve and parotid gland based upon a study of 350 cervicofacial halves. *Surg Gynecol Obstet* 102:384, 1956.

Dingman RO, Grabb WC: Surgical anatomy of the mandibular ramus of the facial nerve based on the dissection of 100 facial halves. *Plast Reconstr Surg* 29:266, 1962.

Edlich RF, Kenney JG: Soft-tissue injuries of the face, in Dudley H, Carter D, Russell RCG (eds): *Operative Surgery. Part 1: Trauma Surgery*. London, Butterworth, 1989, pp 120–149.

Ohlsen L, Skoog T, Sohn SA: The pathogenesis of cauliflower ear. *Scand J Plast Reconstr Surg* 9:34, 1975.

Tachmes L, Woloszyn T, Marini C, et al: Parotid gland and facial nerve trauma: A retrospective review. *J Trauma* 30:1395, 1990.

196 FINGERTIP INJURIES

Richard F. Edlich
Raymond F. Morgan

INTRODUCTION

The fingertip is the part of the hand most frequently injured. The primary treatment consideration in fingertip injury is the functional rehabilitation of the patient. The fingertip is the end organ for touch and is richly supplied with special sensory receptors that enable the hand to perceive, relaying the shape, texture, and temperature of a manipulated object. Fingertip injuries can destroy these receptors, and the primary goal of management after fingertip injuries should be restoration of these special sensory functions whenever possible. Other management goals include (1) preservation of functional length, (2) prevention of symptomatic neuromas, (3) prevention of joint contracture, (4) short morbidity, and (5) early return of the patient to work or play. Fingertip injuries can be divided into four categories: (1) digital tip amputation with skin or pulp loss only, (2) digital tip amputation with exposed bone, (3) injury of the perionychium, and (4) fracture of the distal phalanx. Successful repair of fingertip injuries requires a knowledge of anatomy and techniques of reconstruction, and sound surgical judgment.

ANATOMY

The glabrous skin of the palm and fingertip is specially adapted for pinch and grasp functions (Fig. 196–1). Although there are no sebaceous glands in palmar skin, eccrine sweat glands are abundant and provide pores on elevated ridges. These ridges, along with intervening valleys, make up the irregular, friction-producing surface that exhibits characteristic fingerprint patterns. The palmar skin is stabilized by numerous fibrous septa, including Clelland's and Grayson's ligaments, which anchor the skin to the underlying bone and flexor and tendon sheath. Dorsal hand skin is thinner than palmar skin and loosely adherent with little subcutaneous tissue.

The axial digital arteries and nerves pass through the subcutaneous tissue between Grayson's and Clelland's ligaments, dividing into many small branches within the pulp of the fingertip. The digital nerves trifurcate near the distal interphalangeal joint, sending a dorsal branch to the perionychium, one to the fingertip, and a third to the volar pulp. A dorsal sensory branch of each digital nerve is evident at the level of the midproximal phalanx and innervates the skin over the middle and distal phalanx. The digital nerves are volar to the arteries in the digit. The lateral bands of the extensor mechanism continue distally to insert at the dorsal base of the distal phalanx. The flexor digitorum profundus tendon inserts on the volar base of the distal phalanx.

The perionychium includes the entire complex of the nail plate, nail bed, nail matrix, and surrounding paronychium. It acts as a protective covering and assists in grasping small objects and scratching. The major part of this appendage is the hard nail plate, which is roughly flat and rectangular in shape. The nail plate is like hair, being composed primarily of protein and having a lipid content of less than 5 percent. The nail plate is intimately related to five epidermal components.

Matrix

Most of the nail plate is produced by the nail matrix. The nail plate consists of dead cornified cells derived from the matrix. The cells of the matrix, which are similar to basilar cells, lose their nuclei, flatten, cornify, and are added to already formed nail plate. The nail matrix begins deep within the proximal nail fold beneath the eponychium and extends to the lunula of the nail, the most distal portion of the nail matrix.

Nail Bed

The nail bed extends from the lunula to the hyponychium. There is little doubt that some material is added to the undersurface of the nail plate by the nail bed as it progresses distally, because the distal portion of the nail is thicker than the proximal portion. As additional cells are produced by the matrix, the nail plate progresses distally on the nail bed. The nail plate is loosely attached to the matrix, but densely adherent to the nail bed and eponychium. The nail bed acts as a guiding surface for the advancing nail plate. Linear ridges in the nail bed securely anchor the nail plate to the underlying epithelium. Complete longitudinal nail growth takes approximately 70 to 160 days.

The dermal component of the matrix and nail bed is unique in that it is limited by the underlying phalanx and is closely associated with its vasculature; there is no subcutaneous tissue. Consequently, the nail bed and matrix are between two relatively unyielding structures, the distal phalanx and the nail plate. These structures protect the nail bed and matrix from many moderate forces and require that the actual injuring force to the structures be significant enough to either break the bone on which the nail bed sits or deform the nail plate under which they reside.

Proximal Nail Fold

This fold consists of two layers of epidermis. The dorsal part forms the dorsal portion of the finger epidermis, while its ventral portion overlies the newly formed nail plate. The thin membrane extending from the nail fold on to the dorsum of the nail is the eponychium. The proximal nail fold provides a protective cover for the matrix and adds a thin layer of cells to the surface of the nail. This layer of cells is derived from germinal cells located on its ventral portion and gives the nail a smooth, shiny appearance. If the proximal nail fold is absent, the nail surface will be irregular and dull.

Hyponychium

The hyponychium is the junction of the nail bed and the fingertip skin, beneath the distal free margin of the nail plate. In this region, the nail plate leaves the underlying nail matrix and becomes a free, unattached structure. When the nail bed does not adhere securely to the nail plate, foreign material can enter over the hyponychium and be trapped between the nail bed and nail plate, becoming a source for infection. Like the nail matrix, the hyponychium requires adequate skeletal support. Without this support, the nail plate will follow an abnormally positioned nail bed and hyponychium, resulting in a hook nail deformity.

Paronychium

The paronychium is the lateral nail fold. The nails progress distally because of confinement by these folds. If this fold has abnormal alignment, growth of the nail plate may damage the paronychium, causing irritation, pain, and infection (ingrown nail).

GENERAL PRINCIPLES OF MANAGEMENT

The majority of patients with fingertip injuries can be cared for in the emergency department as outpatients by using digital metacarpal nerve blocks. Severe injuries that required distant flaps or extensive bone fixation should be repaired in the operating room under regional block or general anesthesia. A thorough patient history and examination of the injured finger should be performed prior to initiating treatment. The etiology and time of injury will often influence the method of treatment. The age, sex, occupation, and hand dominance of the patient should also be determined. The relative importance of each finger, from the more important thumb and index finger to the less critical

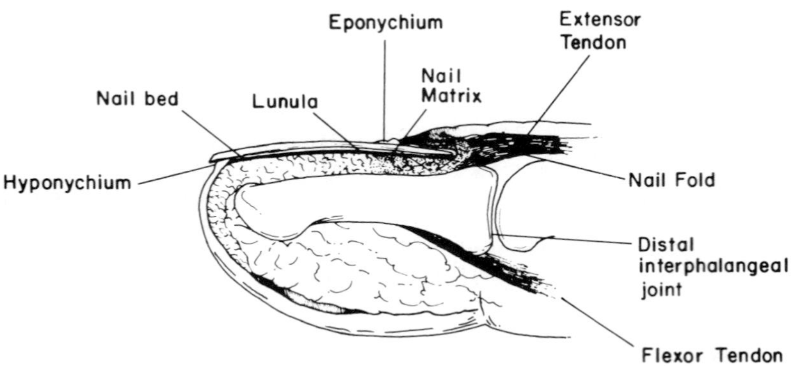

Fig. 196–1. The anatomy of the fingertip is shown in sagittal section.

small finger, as well as the patient's use of the injured finger, should be considered. An office worker's nondominant small fingertip amputation should be regarded differently from a pianist's dominant index fingertip soft tissue amputation. Preoperative x-rays should be taken to identify phalangeal fractures or retained foreign bodies. Appropriate tetanus prophylaxis should be undertaken in each patient. Antibiotic treatment is usually not recommended.

Surgical repair of fingertip injuries must be performed in a bloodless field, created by a tourniquet, after wrapping with an Esmarch's bandage. The tourniquet must be calibrated, at least daily and preferably before each case. The use of a sterile, disposable tourniquet helps prevent the risk of cross-contamination. Several layers of soft cast padding are wrapped around the upper arm. The tourniquet's pneumatic cuff is applied snugly and as close to the axilla as possible. The intact skin is washed with an antiseptic solution (iodophor or chlorhexidine). Before skin antisepsis, a towel is wrapped around the distal edge of the cuff to prevent seepage of the antiseptic solutions beneath the cuff, which may result in a chemical burn.

The arm is elevated and wrapped with a disposable Esmarch's bandage to exsanguinate blood from the arm prior to inflation of the tourniquet. The tourniquet is inflated to a pressure of 250 mmHg, or 20 to 50 mmHg greater than the patient's systolic blood pressure. Slightly greater pressures are required for the person with a particularly muscular or obese arm. A pressure of 150 to 200 mmHg is recommended for children. The tourniquet may be left in place for approximately 2 h without danger of ischemia. However, most patients can tolerate the maximum cuff pressures for only 10 to 20 min before they complain of pain. The administration of pre- or intraoperative sedation or systemic analgesia will extend the limits of tourniquet use significantly.

When a minor procedure is performed on a finger, an elastic constricting device can be placed around the base of the digit as a tourniquet. A broad Penrose drain is safer than a rubber band or narrow catheter. The Penrose drain is wrapped around the base of the finger and clamped with a hemostat. Exsanguination of the digit prior to application of the tourniquet can be accomplished by wrapping the digit from distal end to proximal end with either a 4 by 4 in gauze sponge or a Penrose drain. Although this technique is reasonably safe for short procedures, there are distinct hazards. Because there is no practical way to standardize or measure the pressure beneath a digital tourniquet, compression of the underlying digital nerves may be excessive.

The wound should be thoroughly cleansed using fine-pore cell-size sponge soaked in poloxamer 188 (Calgon, Inc., St. Louis, MO) or normal saline. High-pressure syringe irrigation can also be used to cleanse wounds that have been contaminated. Magnification loupes are essential for visualizing the minute details of the wound that provide the landmarks for repair.

DIGITAL TIP AMPUTATION

Amputation of the fingertip results from either impact or shear forces. Trapping of a fingertip between two objects is the most common cause of this injury, doors being the most frequent impact forces. Saws, lawn mowers, and knives provide sufficient shear forces for fingertip amputation. The age groups most frequently affected are children and young adults.

When the digital tip is amputated, the geometry of the defect dictates the various treatment possibilities. The loss may be transverse or oblique, with more volar skin loss than dorsal skin loss, or the reverse may be true. Some slicing amputations may take skin primarily from the ulnar or radial side of the digit and spare the distal tip.

Skin or Pulp Loss Only

There are a multiplicity of techniques for management of digital tip amputations with skin or pulp loss only. Healing by secondary intention is the simplest. Two other options are replantation of the avulsed tissue as a composite graft and defatting the avulsed tissue before replantation. The use of split-thickness skin grafts has been one of the most popular methods for closure of these injuries. Some surgeons prefer more technically demanding procedures, such as cross-finger flaps or advancement flaps.

There is ample evidence that conservative management of fingertip injuries in children where there is no bone exposed is the preferred method. In children under 12, spontaneous regeneration of the fingertip occurs, usually with excellent cosmetic results. Several alternative forms of conservative treatment have been proposed. They all have in common the use of some nonadhering dressing, which is changed periodically until healing is completed. Recent studies also indicate that conservative management of fingertip injuries in adults yields results comparable to those in children, despite the fact that the regenerative potential of soft tissue in the adult is substantially less than in children.

Patients who have had skin grafts of the fingertip frequently complain about induration and fissuring of the skin, reduced sensibility in the area of the graft, and problems involving the donor site. Tenderness at the site of the graft, and cold sensitivity, are common complaints of individuals who have undergone split-thickness skin grafts. With early coverage by split-thickness skin grafts, symptomatic difficulties are likely to continue.

It is important to emphasize that there is between a 30 and 50 percent chance of having some cold intolerance and approximately 30 percent chance of having some aberration in sensitivity, regardless of what technique is used. These complications are a result of the injury and not the treatment.

Exposed Bone

When bone is exposed in cases of digital tip amputation, the decision-making process is similar to that in cases of digital amputation of pulp alone, but with two additional considerations. Rongeuring a small protruding portion of a phalanx to shorten the fingertip and then allowing healing by secondary intention is another choice. Microsurgical replantation of the amputated part at the level of the distal interphalangeal joint is another alternative.

Conservative management of digital tip amputation with exposed bone is a valuable technique in children less than 12 years old. Their regenerative powers are so great that fingertip regeneration has been reported when the site of amputation is just proximal to the nail. Take of the amputated part as a composite graft at this same amputation site has also been reported in children less than 2 years old.

When the site of amputation is at the level of the distal interphalangeal joint, or proximal to it, microvascular replantation can be successful. Replantation of a sharply amputated single finger at this level in a child should always be considered because the future occupation of the child cannot be predicted. Amputations distal to the superficialis insertion have been found to function well after microvascular replantation because this intact flexor usually provides excellent range of motion of the digit. Because of the thumb's critical importance to hand function, even amputations distal to the interphalangeal joint should be treated by replantation if suitable vessels are found distally.

In adults, the regenerative powers of the fingertip with exposed bone are significantly less than in children. Consequently, shortening the exposed bone by rongeuring and then allowing the wound to heal by secondary intention is an attractive choice for fingertip amputations distal to the distal interphalangeal joint. As surgeons have gained more experience, they have performed fewer local and distant flaps in an effort to cover a small portion of exposed bone. Coverage of exposed bone in the distal phalanx by skin that is hypesthetic, dysesthetic, or tender may lead to a functional amputation of this part so that the patient excludes the tip of the repaired finger from activities.

As with digital tip amputation with skin or pulp loss only, regardless of the treatment modality, there is between a 30 to 50 percent chance of having some cold intolerance and approximately a 30 percent chance of having some aberration in sensitivity.

INJURY OF THE PERIONYCHIUM

The mechanism of most nail bed injuries is impact, with the force of impact dictating the magnitude of injury. Forces that can break the durable nail plate can disrupt the nail matrix and bed. When a relatively sharp object, like a nail, compresses the nail between the nail and bone, a straight or tearing laceration of the nail bed or matrix occurs (Fig. 196–2). Compression of the nail by a wider object, like a hammer or door, results in stellate lacerations of the nail matrix and bed (Fig. 196–3). It is rare to have a truly sharp laceration of the nail bed. When a sharp object strikes the nail bed hard enough to perforate it, it goes through and amputates the tip. Belts or sanders are more likely to avulse portions of the nail matrix, bed, or fingertip.

If the impact forces do not contact the nail plate, they can fracture the terminal phalanx without breaking the nail plate. In such cases, the fracture often disrupts the nail bed and matrix, causing bleeding with hematoma formation beneath the intact nail. Hematomas occurring following fractures or lacerations are painful and cause the patient to seek medical treatment because of the throbbing pain.

When the nail matrix or bed sustains either a linear or stellate laceration, it will heal by scar formation. Because scar does not produce a nail, nail deformity occurs. Scar formation in the matrix results in a split or absent nail. Scars in the nail bed are followed either by a split or nonadherent nail. The magnitude of scar formation can be lessened by the meticulous repair of the injured nail matrix and bed. Because the results of late reconstruction of an injured nail are unpredictable, it is preferable to treat nail injuries as soon as possible after injury. Injuries of the perionychium can be divided into the following four groups: (1) injury with a small hematoma (less than 25 percent of the nail plate), (2) injury with a large hematoma (more than 25 percent of the nail plate), (3) injury associated with fracture of the distal phalanx, and (4) injury with avulsion of the nail bed and matrix.

The question confronting the emergency physician is whether the laceration of the matrix or bed is severe enough to require suturing

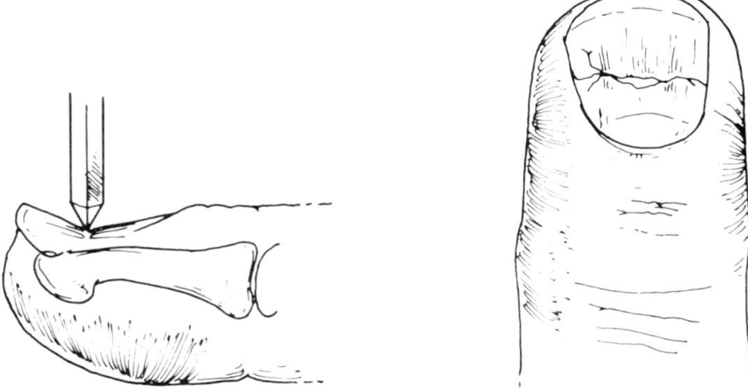

Fig. 196–2. A sharp object, like a nail, applies forces over a small area that usually results in a linear laceration of the nail bed or matrix.

to assure accurate approximation of the nail matrix or bed. The judgment is complicated by the difficulty of assessing the matrix through the nail plate because of the overlying hematoma. Thus examination of patients presenting with nail bed hematomas may require removal of the nail plates for a complete inspection of the nail beds. It is generally agreed that hematomas, which have separated over 25 percent of the nail plate from its underlying matrix or bed warrant surgical exploration.

Small Hematoma

In an injury to the perionychium with a hematoma involving less than 25 percent of the visible nail plate, the pressure of the hematoma beneath the nail plate may cause throbbing pain, necessitating evacuation of the hematoma (Fig. 196–4). A hole must be made in the nail plate that is large enough to allow prolonged drainage. Use of a battery-powered microcautery unit is an excellent way to create the hole in the nail plate. Its heated tip passes through the nail plate, is cooled by the hematoma, and does not injure the nail bed or matrix. A paper clip heated until red hot by either a Bunsen burner or alcohol lamp is an alternate approach. With either of these techniques, after decompression of the hematoma, the nail bed and matrix will heal with minimal scar and nail deformity. Other techniques may produce a small hole that decompresses the hematoma immediately, but does permit continued drainage, allowing formation of another hematoma.

Large Hematoma

If a large hematoma is present, the nail must be removed to permit examination of the injury to the nail bed or matrix (Fig. 196–5A).

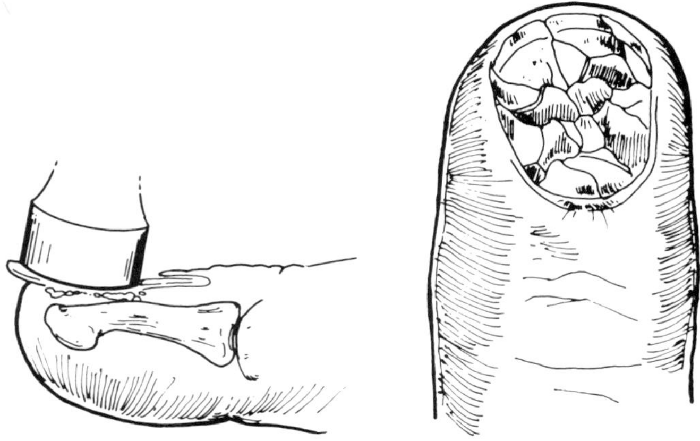

Fig. 196–3. A hammer applies force over a large area, resulting in multiple stellate lacerations of the nail bed and matrix.

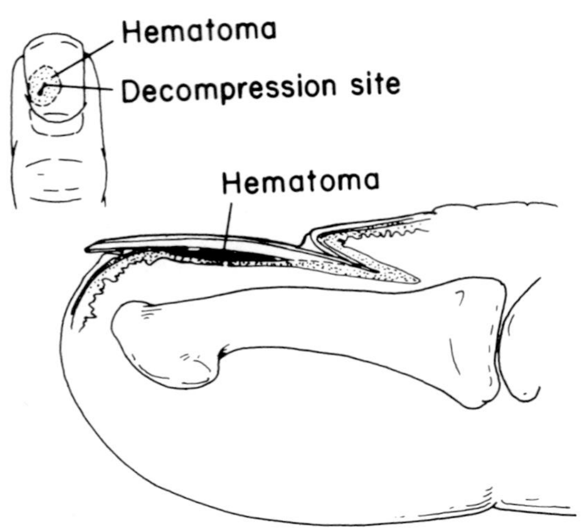

Fig. 196–4. A small hematoma beneath the nail plate is caused by a small laceration of the nail bed or matrix. By drilling a hole through the nail plate, decompression and drainage of the hematoma can be achieved.

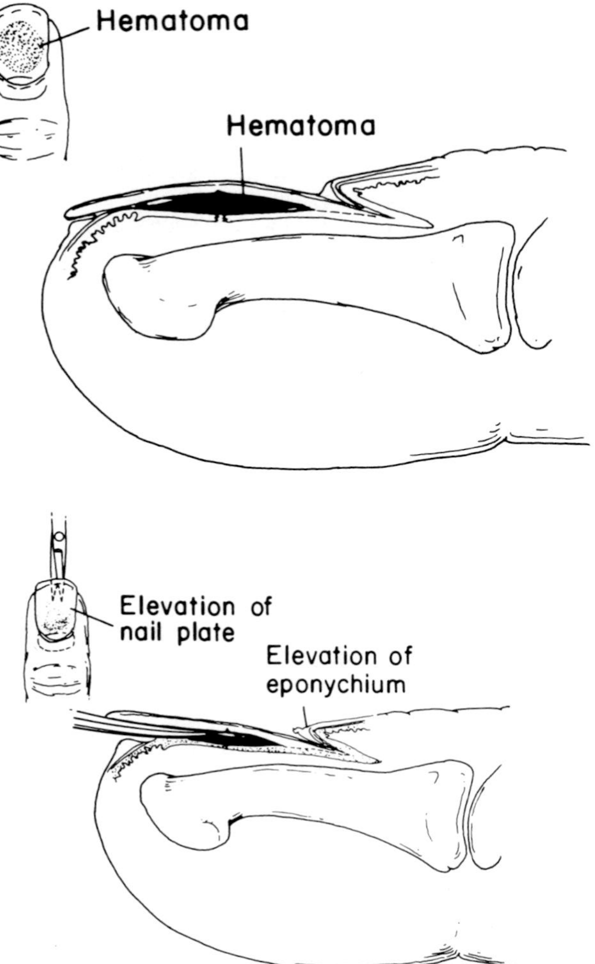

Fig. 196–5. A. A large hematoma involves more than 25 percent of the visible nail plate. **B.** The nail plate must be removed to permit appropriate examination and repair of the nail bed and matrix.

With appropriate anesthesia, the nail is elevated using the blades of Iris scissors (Fig. 196–5B). By opening and closing the blades of the Iris scissors, a cleavage plane is developed between the nail bed and matrix and the nail plate. Using the same technique, a similar plane is developed between the eponychium and nail plate. Once the nail plate is elevated, gentle distal traction on the nail plate will separate the plate from the proximal nail sulcus.

After washing the nail bed and matrix with a fine-pore cell-size sponge soaked in poloxamer 188 or normal saline, the nail bed and matrix are examined for lacerations. The linear and stellate lacerations are approximated with interrupted 7–0 chromic gut sutures, which are double-armed to CS-Ultima-8 (Ethicon, Inc., Somerville, NJ) needles. Because the micropoints of these needles are side-cutting, they are ideally suited to repair thin membranes, such as the nail bed and matrix.

Accurate approximation of the stellate laceration is comparable to putting together a jigsaw puzzle. Meticulous approximation of the lacerations of the nail bed matrix can provide surprisingly good results. Occasionally, such lacerations are associated with partial avulsion of the nail matrix from the sulcus (Fig. 196–6). In such cases, sutures should be passed from the proximal portion of the sulcus into the free margin of the nail matrix, bringing the matrix back into position beneath the nail fold. Visualization of the injured matrix may be enhanced by incisions in the proximal nail folds. The incision should be made perpendicular to the lateral curved margin of the eponychial fold (Fig. 196–7).

After the nail bed and matrix are reapproximated, the nail plate is thoroughly cleansed with poloxamer 188 saline. A hole is burned through the nail plate at a point not over the repair site to allow drainage of any blood or hematoma. The nail plate is then replaced back into the proximal sulcus to serve as a stent and protective cover of the nail bed and matrix. The nail plate is held in place by an interrupted monofilament 5–0 nylon suture attached to a PS2 reverse-cutting-edge needle passed through the distal end of the nail plate to fingertip skin. The fingertip is then dressed with nonadherent gauze, followed by a 2-in. gauze dressing. A volar splint protects the injured part, restricts

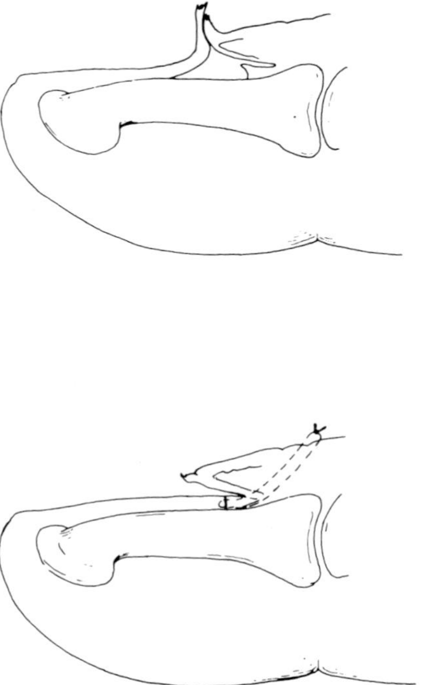

Fig. 196–6. Top. Partial avulsion of the nail matrix from the sulcus. **Bottom.** A horizontal mattress suture, through the proximal nail fold to the avulsed segment of the nail matrix, returns the matrix into the fold.

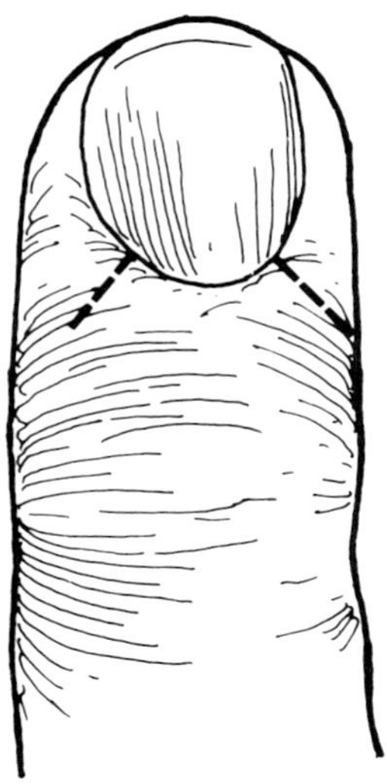

Fig. 196–7. Incisions in the eponychium enhance visualization and repair of injury of the nail matrix.

movement of the distal interphalangeal joint, and alleviates pain. The dressing is removed 5 days later, and the nail checked for evidence of new hematoma formation. The volar splint remains in place for 7 to 10 days to immobilize the joint. If hematoma recurs, the hole is reopened, and the hematoma evacuated. The suture is removed from the nail 3 weeks after injury. The nail plate will frequently adhere to the nail bed and matrix for 1 to 3 months until dislodged by the new growing nail.

If the nail is destroyed or too badly damaged to be used as a splint, several synthetic substitutes have been devised. A nail-shaped sheet of 0.020-in. silicone sheet can be fabricated. A monofilament 6–0 nylon suture is passed through the proximal portion of the proximal nail fold to the proximal part of the nail sulcus and then through the edge of the silicone sheet at each corner as a horizontal mattress suture to keep the silicone sheet in place (Fig. 196–8). The silicone sheet conforms to the configuration of the nail bed and matrix and keeps the nail fold open. These benefits must be weighed against the potential for erosion of bed or fold by the sheeting, mechanical interference with nail plate growth, and increased risk of infection. The use of firmer prosthetic materials, such as polypropylene, does not eliminate these problems, and these materials do not conform to the underlying tissues.

The nail bed and matrix can also be left open and covered by a nail-shaped nonadherent dressing which extends beneath the proximal nail fold and adheres adequately to the underlying tissue until healing has occurred. After dressing the wound, movement of the distal interphalangeal joint should be restricted for 7 to 10 days by the volar splint. The gauze should be removed 5 to 10 days after repair.

It should be explained to the patient that nail plate growth will take 6 to 12 months. It is also anticipated that if the injury is severe, severe nail deformity which may require surgical revision, is likely. The patient should be reminded that the leading edge of the regenerating nail plate will be irregular, and prone to catch on objects. When the nail's leading edge has extended beyond the hyponychium, it should be trimmed and filed.

Lacerations Associated with a Fracture of the Distal Phalanx

Approximately 50 percent of nail bed injuries have an associated fracture of the distal phalanx. When a fracture of the distal phalanx occurs, there may be an associated injury to the nail matrix, often manifested by an avulsion of the nail plate out of the nail sulcus, located above the eponychium and proximal nail fold (Fig. 196–9). If a fracture of the tuft or distal phalanx is present, it must have a stable anatomic reduction. The nail bed and matrix should then be repaired, as previously described. The replaced nail plate, due to proximity to the periosteum, serves as an excellent splint to maintain fracture reduction. If stable anatomic reduction cannot be maintained, fixation with a 0.028-in. Kirschner wire is recommended (Fig. 196–10). If the fracture is not realigned accurately, nail deformity will result.

Avulsion of the Nail Bed

The best tissue for repair of avulsions of the nail bed or matrix is the avulsed tissue. When the nail plate is avulsed, a fragment of the nail bed may remain attached to the nail plate, which can be removed from the nail plate and placed in the wound as a graft (Fig. 196–11). The nail plate should be replaced accurately, serving as a stent. All retrievable fragments unattached to the nail plate should also be replaced as free grafts. A graft 1 cm in diameter or less will often survive by inosculation and ingrowth of circulation from the periphery, even on the bare cortex of the distal phalanx. The nail bed is one of the few areas in which cortical bone will accept a soft tissue graft. As long as bone is attached proximally to a good blood supply, grafting directly on bone is very successful. The graft should be carefully approximated to the nail bed segments using 7–0 chromic sutures. Skin remnants

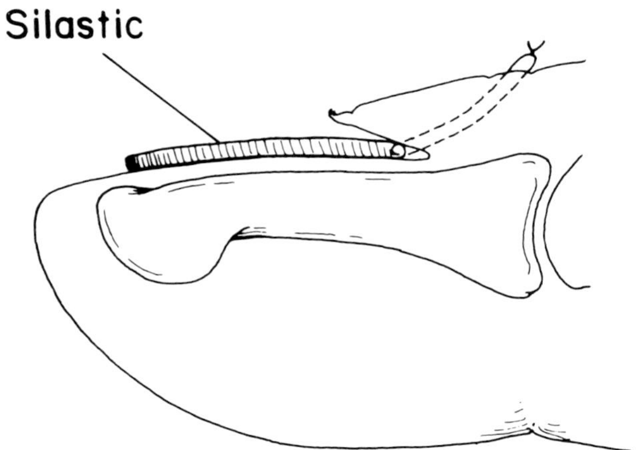

Fig. 196–8. A horizontal mattress suture secures the silicone (silastic) sheet to the proximal nail sulcus.

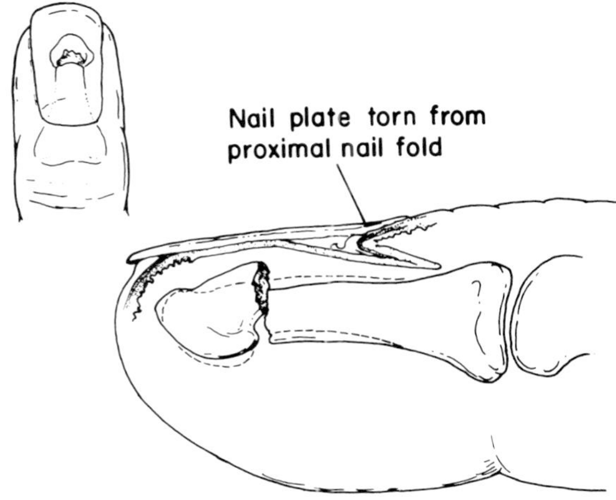

Fig. 196–9. A fracture of the distal phalanx may be associated with injury to the nail matrix. A manifestation of this injury is avulsion of the nail plate out of the nail sulcus.

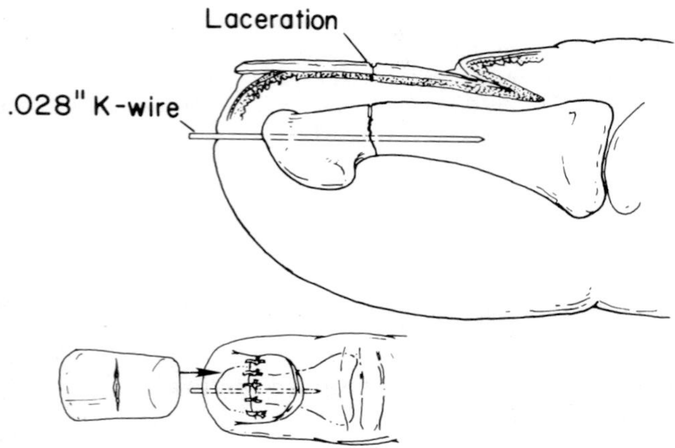

Fig. 196–10. Following nail bed repair, if the fracture fragments are unstable, fixation by a Kirschner wire is recommended. After stabilization, the nail plate should be returned to cover the sutured nail bed and matrix, serving as a stent.

are attached to the skin with monofilament 6–0 nylon. Blood should be eliminated from beneath the graft and a pressure dressing applied to prevent accumulation of blood and serum beneath the graft.

In the absence of retrievable avulsed nail bed and matrix, nail bed grafting is indicated to replace the avulsed tissue. If an adjacent finger has been amputated, or is so severely crushed that it has to be amputated, removal of a full-thickness nail bed graft or a split-thickness nail bed graft is a good choice for coverage of the avulsion. Split-thickness nail bed grafts from the adjacent nail bed of the injured finger or from a toe nail bed provide excellent results, without causing deformities in the donor area. In harvesting a split-thickness nail bed graft, attempt is made to keep the graft so thin that the point of the knife can be seen through the graft; the thickness of such grafts varies from 0.007 to 0.01 in.

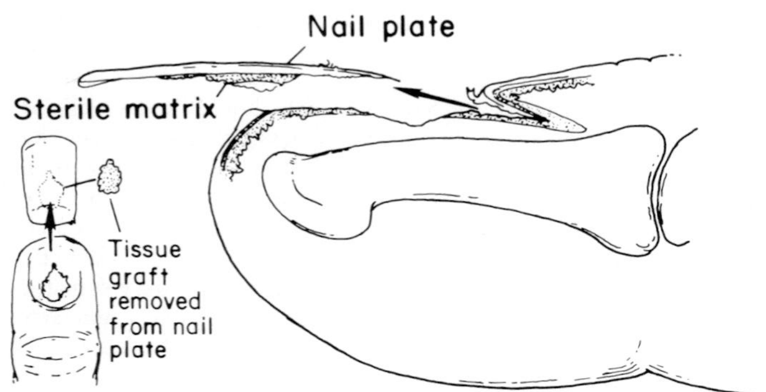

Fig. 196–11. Avulsion of a segment of nail bed and matrix is best treated by retrieving the avulsed tissue and replacing it as a graft. If the avulsed nail bed is not available, grafts of nail bed can be used to repair the nail bed and matrix.

FRACTURES OF THE DISTAL PHALANX

Fractures of the distal phalanx heal without complications for several reasons. There are no tendons spanning the bone that deform the fracture site. In addition, the phalanx is supported dorsally by the nail plate and volarly by pulp with fibrous septa.

Fractures are common radiographic manifestations of a crushed fingertip. When a fracture of the distal phalanx has occurred, there may be an associated injury to the nail bed and matrix, which must be repaired. The excellent soft tissue support of the bone facilitates anatomic alignment of the fracture. Splinting of the fracture is necessary for 10 to 14 days. When soft tissue support is lost, fixation of the fracture with Kirschner wire is required.

Because the epiphyseal plate is weaker than the insertion of the extensor tendon, an epiphyseal separation, rather than a mallet finger, results when the child is struck on the fingertip. While this injury presents clinically as a mallet finger deformity, it is usually an open fracture of the base of the proximal phalanx with the nail plate lying superficial to the eponychium. The extensor tendon inserts on the proximal fragment of the epiphyseal plate, and the flexor profundus tendon flexes the distal fragment. Closed reduction by hyperextension and placing the nail plate back under the proximal nail fold after proper cleansing is recommended.

This research was supported by a generous gift from the Texaco Philanthropic Foundation, White Plains, New York.

BIBLIOGRAPHY

Fingertip Amputations

Elsahy WI: When to replant a fingertip after its complete amputation. *Plast Reconstr Surg* 60:14, 1977.

Rosenthal LJ, Reiner MA, Bleicher MA: Nonoperative management of distal fingertip amputations in children. *Pediatrics* 64:1, 1979.

Suzuki K, Matsuda M: Digital replantations distal to the distal interphalangeal joint. *J Reconstr Microsurg* 3:291, 1987.

Injuries of the Perionychium

Shepard GH: Management of the acute nail bed avulsion. *Hand Clin* 6:39, 1990.

Van Beek AL, Kassan MA, Adson MH, et al: Management of acute fingernail injuries, *Hand Clin* 6:23, 1990.

Zook EG: Anatomy and physiology of the perionychium. *Hand Clin* 6:1, 1990.

SECTION 20
Behavioral Emergencies

197
BEHAVIORAL DISORDERS: CLINICAL FEATURES

Stephen C. Olson
Douglas A. Rund

Psychiatric disorders are common in the emergency department patient population. In a study by Summers et al. in which emergency patients were screened for psychiatric illness, including drug abuse and alcoholism, the prevalence of psychiatric illness was 38 percent. The "after-midnight" group of emergency department patients had significantly more psychiatric illness (56 percent) than did the daytime group (20 percent). In some instances, psychiatric disorders clearly constitute the primary reason for an individual's presentation to an emergency department. In other cases, psychiatric disorders lead to injury and illness. Such conditions then create the need for emergency care. As screening studies have shown, psychiatric disorders may constitute part of the medical history of a patient yet play little direct role in the immediate clinical condition. In studies that report categories of psychiatric illness seen in the emergency department, the most prominent diagnoses are substance abuse, affective disorders, anxiety disorders, antisocial personality disorder, and severe cognitive impairment.

DIAGNOSIS

In the assessment of patients presenting with psychiatric symptoms, as with other medical conditions encountered in the emergency department, it is more crucial for the emergency physician promptly to stabalize the patient's acute condition and evaluate the major complaint immediately. Formulating a specific diagnosis must necessarily follow initial stabilization procedures in this clinical process. The determination that an individual is suicidal and in need of hospitalization, for instance, is more important than deciding whether that person has schizophrenia or psychotic depression.

Nevertheless, provisional psychiatric diagnoses can be made in the emergency department. Recognition of specific behavioral syndromes can assist the emergency physician in evaluating the presenting complaint, pursuing associated symptoms, and determining treatment and disposition. Emergency physicians therefore should be sufficiently familiar with commonly seen psychiatric illnesses to describe their predominant clinical features.

Despite this reasonable expectation, until recently the formulation of a specific diagnosis was not a burning issue even among psychiatrists, who were more concerned with understanding the psychodynamics of the symptoms. Awareness of the unreliability of psychiatric diagnosis was a major impetus to the development in the 1970s of operational criteria for each disorder, allowing both researchers and clinicians to agree consistently on whether a disorder was present or absent. In addition, the criteria are based on observable signs and the patient's report of symptoms, not on unconscious psychic mechanisms. This simplifies the task of diagnosis for emergency physicians and other nonpsychiatrists, since extensive knowledge of pathophysiology and unconscious metal processes is not essential.

Standard Diagnostic Taxonomy

The current official diagnostic nomenclature, published in 1987 by the American Psychiatric Association, is the *Diagnostic and Statistical Manual of Mental Disorders,* third edition-revised, commonly known as DSM-III-R. A copy of DSM-III-R should be available for reference in the emergency department since it contains not only the list of criteria for each disorder, but also additional material on demographics, associated symptoms and syndromes, and differential diagnosis.

Multiaxial Diagnostic System

DSM-III-R diagnoses are made on a multiaxial system in which each axis refers to a different class of information. Axis I disorders comprise the clinical syndromes of mental disorder. Conditions listed on Axis II are the personality disorders and developmental disorders, including mental retardation, which may underlie the more florid Axis I syndrome. Axis III is used to note physical disorders and conditions. Axes IV and V are used to record psychosocial stressors and adaptive functioning. It is generally unnecessary for the emergency physician to make a complete multiaxial diagnosis, but knowledge of this system may facilitate an understanding of medical records and psychiatric consultants' notes. For instance, a patient with previous medical records containing DSM-III-R diagnoses of Axis I: Alcohol Intoxication; Axis II: Antisocial Personality Disorder; Axis III: Scalp Laceration should be recognized as likely to display features of the Axis II personality disorder, although the patient's chief complaint may be a new problem.

PSYCHIATRIC SYNDROMES (AXIS I DISORDERS)

The organization and major categories of Axis I disorders are listed in Table 197-1. A useful strategy for making a DSM-III-R diagnosis is to classify the chief complaint into one of these major categories, consider possible organic etiologies for the complaint, and then utilize one of the decision trees in Appendix B of the DSM-III-R manual to identify the appropriate diagnosis. The decision trees guide the clinician who is unfamiliar with the intricacies of the criteria within a category to identify the features which distinguish closely related conditions.

Table 197-1. Axis I Disorders

Organic brain syndromes
Delirium
Dementia
Organic affective disorders
Organic delusional disorder
Organic hallucinosis
Organic personality disorder
Major psychiatric disorders
Schizophrenic disorders
Paranoid disorders
Affective (mood) disorders
Anxiety disorders
Somatoform disorders
Psychosexual disorders
Dissociative disorders
Substance use disorders
Adjustment disorders

Organic Brain Syndromes and Organic Mental Disorders

The general heading of organic brain syndromes consists of a group of syndromes in which the patient's abnormal behavior is presumed to be the consequence of a physical disease or an exogenous substance interfering with normal brain function. The most common forms of organic brain syndrome are *dementia, delirium, intoxication,* and *withdrawal. Amnestic syndrome,* in which the cognitive disturbance is limited to memory impairment, is relatively uncommon. The other organic brain syndromes, *organic affective disorder, organic delusional disorder, organic hallucinosis,* and *organic personality disorder* are used when an organic etiology is assumed on the basis of examination, history, or laboratory findings, and the psychobehavioral syndrome mimics a functional psychiatric disorder such as depression, schizophrenia, or a personality disorder. Common medical causes of these disorders are covered in Chap. 198.

In the initial evaluation of psychiatric disorders, and organic etiology for the abnormal behavior must be excluded by a thorough history and diagnostic studies. Such studies usually require more time than typically available in the emergency department. However, organic etiologies must be considered for nearly all unexplained abnormalities of thought and behavior.

There are several distinct and relatively common causes of organic brain syndromes in which the causative factor is known. Multiinfarct dementia and alcohol withdrawal delirium, which have specific criteria listed in DSM-III-R, are examples. Such cases, and those in which a particular substance is presumed to be producing the condition, are classified under the more specific heading of organic mental disorders. The common organic brain syndromes are described in more detail below.

Dementia

The essential clinical feature of *dementia* is a pervasive disturbance of cognitive functioning in several areas including memory, abstract thinking, judgment, personality, and other higher cortical functions such as language. If clouding of consciousness is present, then the patient does not have solely a dementing illness, but rather *delirium* or *intoxication.* The presence of global congnitive impairment may be ascertained by a bedside cognitive examination such as the Mini Mental State examination, and additional confirmatory history should be gathered from an informant such as a family member. Memory disturbance is usually the earliest sign to be apparent to others, and unless it is very mild, it can be identified easily by examination.

Patients with dementia may be brought to the emergency department after having been found wandering away from home or an institution. Because the onset of most forms of dementia is slow and gradual, presentation to the emergency department often occurs only when there is some acute worsening of the mental status, which may be the result of a superimposed medical illness, adverse drug effect, or environmental change, to all of which the demented patient is susceptible. The demented patient's diminished intellectual and physiological resources allow abrupt worsening of function with the addition of such stressors.

Especially early in the course of dementia, anxiety, depression, or psychosis may dominate the clinical picture and obscure cognitive dysfunction. For this reason, a high degree of clinical suspicion of dementia should be maintained when evaluating an elderly patient with no prior psychiatric history who presents with new psychiatric problems. Demented persons also are prone to unrecognized physical illness because of inability to perceive or describe symptoms. Careful examination and appropriate laboratory testing always is indicated in the initial and ongoing evaluation of such patients.

It must be noted that dementia is not synonymous with the older designation of chronic organic brain syndrome, which implies irreversibility. Common causes of reversible dementia include metabolic and endocrine disorders, polypharmacy, and depression. Often, especially in elderly patients, a severe depression may mimic dementia, a condition often erroneously labeled pseudodementia, but more accurately called *reversible dementia of depression.* The presence of a relatively acute onset, prominent mood changes, and vegetative disturbances such as loss of appetite and weight, sleep disturbance, or expressions of guilt or suicidal ideation all point to depression as the cause. In these situations, definitive treatment of the mood disorder should result in complete resolution of the cognitive impairment.

Delirium

Like dementia, *delirium* is characterized by global impairment in cognitive function, but it is distinguished from it in two major ways. In delirium, the patient has clouding of consciousness, a reduction in the awareness of the external environment (manifest as difficulty sustaining attention), varying degrees of alertness ranging from drowsiness to stupor, and sensory misperception.

The primary distinguishing feature of delirium is its course, which is typically acute, with rapid deterioration in hours or days, rather than months as in the case of dementia. Also, the severity of delirium tends to fluctuate over the course of hours; the patient may appear relatively normal at one time and wildly agitated a few hours later. Extreme changes in psychomotor activity, ranging from restlessness and hyperactivity to stupor, are frequent in delirium, but uncommon in dementia, except in the later stages when a delirious state may be superimposed. Finally, hallucinations, often visual, are common in delirium. They typically have a vivid quality to which the patient reacts strongly. Such hallucinations contrast with the visual hallucinations seen by psychotic patients, often described and experienced in an indifferent manner.

Intoxication

When recent ingestion of a specific exogenous substance produces maladaptive behavior and impairment of judgment, perception, attention, emotional control, or psychomotor activity, and the patient does not display features of delirium, hallucinosis, or other organic brain syndromes, a diagnosis of *intoxication* is made. When the offending substance is known, it should be specified (e.g., alcohol intoxication or amphetamine intoxication). The specific features of intoxication syndromes commonly seen in the emergency department are described in greater detail in the section "Toxicology."

As a general rule, the diagnosis of intoxication can be rather easy when laboratory analysis reveals the type and amount of intoxicant circulating in the system. The clinical features of alcohol intoxication are familiar to experienced emergency physicians and range from impaired judgment and coordination through ataxia, lethargy, and coma. When repeated episodes of intoxication occur in a brief period of time, the individual by definition has a substance abuse disorder, and the additional diagnosis is made.

Withdrawal

Withdrawal can follow cessation or reduction in use of a substance of abuse. The category signifies a syndrome characteristic of withdrawal from that particular drug, when the clinical syndrome does not satisfy the criteria for delirium or another organic brain syndrome. For example, mild forms of alcohol withdrawal would be classified here, but if the patient is confused, hallucinating, and agitated, a diagnosis of alcohol withdrawal delirium is indicated. The diagnosis is made by identification of the withdrawal syndrome along with evidence of recent use of the substance in a pattern sufficient to produce withdrawal when the amount ingested is decreased. Specific withdrawal patterns depend on the agent customarily used.

Alcohol withdrawal, for instance, includes up to four stages: autonomic hyperactivity (6 to 8 h after cessation of drinking), hallucinations (24 h after withdrawal), major motor seizures (1 to 2 days), and global confusion (3 to 5 days after last use of alcohol). Some withdrawal syndromes, particularly from alcohol or barbiturates, can be life-threatening.

MAJOR PSYCHIATRIC DISORDERS

Major psychiatric disorders are those which cause substantial impairment in social or occupational functioning and are generally considered to include the psychotic, affective, anxiety, and substance-abuse disorders. The distinction is somewhat arbitrary, since other mental conditions also may produce severe impairment, but such a classification is useful as a conceptual framework for understanding these disorders. Major psychiatric disorders are quite common and can be detected in a large proportion of the patients seen in most emergency departments. Patients or their families often are unwilling to seek psychiatric care because of the stigma of mental illness. Their evaluation in the emergency department constitutes their point of entry into the health care system. Also, due to poor judgment, financial considerations, or cognitive impairment, many psychiatric patients do not seek medical attention regularly until an emergency intervenes. They then seek emergency treatment for their medical needs. The most serious manifestations of mental illness (suicide, psychosis, and violent behavior) constitute medical emergencies and consequently are dealt with appropriately in the emergency department. Therefore, emergency physicians require substantial knowledge and skill to be able to recognize psychiatric disorders, perform crisis intervention and stabilization, and refer the patient for psychiatric hospitalization or outpatient care as needed.

Schizophrenic and Delusional Disorders

Schizophrenic and delusional disorders are marked by the presence of psychotic symptoms, primarily delusions and hallucinations. Delusions are defined as fixed false beliefs, which are not amenable to arguments or facts to the contrary and which are not shared by others of similar cultural background. Common delusions are of several types. Persecutory delusions are those in which one believes that one is being attacked, followed, harassed, or conspired against. Grandiose delusions are those that involve themes of special powers or abilities. Bizarre delusions are those with patently absurd content, such as believing that one's thoughts are controlled by extraterrestrial beings. Hallucinations are false perceptions experienced in a sensory modality and occurring in clear consciousness. Auditory hallucinations are the most common, followed in order of prevalence by visual, tactile, olfactory, and gustatory. The most prevalent psychosis is *schizophrenia,* described in detail in the next section. The other psychotic disorders,discussed briefly, are considerably less common. A decision tree helpful in evaluating psychotic symptoms is presented in Fig. 197–1.

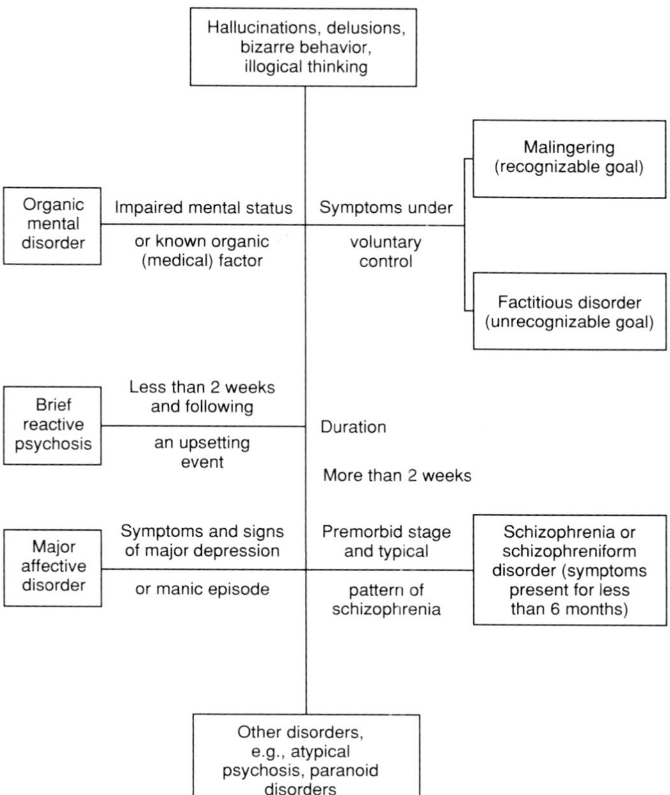

Fig. 197-1. Decision strategies for evaluation of patient with psychotic behavior and thought. (From Rund DA, Hutzler JC: *Emergency Psychiatry*. St. Louis, Mosby, 1983, p 44. Used by permission.)

Schizophrenia

Schizophrenia is one of the most serious public health problems in the world and accounts for 25 percent of admissions to psychiatric hospitals. The essential features are a deterioration in functioning, the presence of hallucinations or characteristic delusions, and the absence of a causal organic factor. Research has established the importance of genetic factors in its cause, and schizophrenia is most likely a group of disorders of varying etiology which share a final common pathway, much as is the case with mental retardation. It is a brain disease, and there is no evidence that psychosocial stressors or poor parenting are responsible for the cause of the illness, although these may have a profound effect on the patient's adaption to this usually chronic disorder.

Schizophrenia usually starts in late adolescence or early adulthood, although the onset can occur at any age. The childhood history of schizophrenics often is marked by shyness, oddness or eccentric behavior, school difficulties, or suspiciousness, but such features are not always present. A prodromal phase, in which a gradual deterioration of function is noted, usually precedes the development of active delusions or hallucinations. Such deterioration usually includes the worsening of social withdrawal or the new onset of social withdrawal, odd behavior or speech, and difficulty in functioning in school or work. Patients or their families rarely seek care until the onset of the active phase of psychosis. Schizophrenics seldom seek care at all because they lack insight; they do not realize that their perception, thoughts, and behavior are abnormal.

Antipsychotic drugs usually reduce the severity of delusions and hallucinations. Other manifestations of schizophrenia less responsive to antipsychotics include negative symptoms (lack of volition, blunting of emotion, anhedonia, and inattention). Such symptoms result in lasting impairment in selfcare, work, and social relations.

Disorganization of thinking and behavior characterizes schizophrenia. Disheveled appearance and grooming, bizarre behavior, poor judgment, and loosening of associations indicate such disorganization. Loosening of associations refers to a loss of the normal logical connections between one thought and the next; thus the schizophrenic's speech is often vague, rambling, disjointed, or nonsensical. Fantastic experiences and bizarre ideas are described in an indifferent manner with unchanging facial expression.

Common reasons for persons with schizophrenia to come to the emergency department include worsening of psychosis resulting from stress or noncompliance with medication, suicidal behavior, assaultiveness (often as a result of paranoid thinking), and extrapyramidal side effects of neuroleptic drugs. Schizophrenics constitute a large share of the chronic homeless population and may be brought in by authorities in a confused state, obviously unable to attend to their basic needs. Their poor judgment and disorganization may lead to disregard for medical problems, so attention must be given to their physical status and their psychiatric problem

Schizophreniform Disorder

Schizophreniform disorder is diagnosed when the patient meets the criteria for schizophrenia, but the symptoms have been present continuously for less that 6 months. A rapid onset over a few days and good premorbid functioning are more common than in schizophrenia.

Brief Reactive Psychosis

Some individuals may become acutely psychotic after exposure to an extremely traumatic life experience. If such a psychosis lasts for less than 2 weeks, it is termed a *brief reactive psychosis*. Precipitants of the psychosis include the death of a loved one or a life-threatening situation such as combat or a natural disaster. Emotional turmoil, confusion, and extremely bizarre behavior and speech are common.

Delusional (Paranoid) Disorder

Delusional disorder is a syndrome distinct from schizophrenia characterized by persistent nonbizarre delusions. Unlike schizophrenia, delusional disorder rarely is characterized by impairment in daily functioning, and the patient may appear outwardly normal aside from the strange ideas expressed. The onset is in middle or late adulthood, and the delusions develop over months or years. Several subtypes have been identified, the most common of which is the persecutory type, in which the delusions follow themes of being conspired against, cheated, followed, poisoned, or harassed. Other types of delusional disorder include delusional jealousy, in which the patient has an unsubstantiated conviction that one's partner is unfaithful, and the somatic type, in which patients believe they emit a foul odor or are infested with parasites.

Emergency medical evaluation may be occasioned by threats or acts of violence directed at the alleged persecutors, by suicidal behavior, or by involuntary commitment. Delusional disorders are rare, and more common causes of this syndrome are psychotic depression or chronic stimulant abuse.

Mood (Affective) Disorders

The affective or mood disorders are the most prevalent of the major psychiatric disorders, affecting about 10 to 15 percent of the general population at some time in their lives. Depressive disorders are the major cause of completed suicide. An unsuccessful attempt may bring the patient to the emergency department. Mood disorders, substance abuse, and anxiety disorders are the most common psychiatric diagnoses in emergency patients.

Mood disorders differ from the normal extremes of sadness and happiness in that characteristic clusters of psychological and vegetative symptoms (depressive or manic syndrome) are present, and functioning is impaired. Any of the features of schizophrenia such as delusions, hallucinations, or disorganization may be present, but if a full depressive or manic syndrome exists, a diagnosis of a psychotic mood disorder is required. Another important characteristic of affective disorders is that they tend to be episodic, with periods of remission and normal function.

Major Depression

The essential feature of *major depression* is a persistent dysphoric (sad) mood or pervasive loss of interest in usual activities, lasting for at least 2 weeks. Associated psychological symptoms include guilt over past deeds, self-reproach, feelings of worthlessness or hopelessness, inability to experience pleasure, and recurrent thought of death or suicide. Vegetative symptoms are those which involve physiologic functioning and include loss of appetite and weight, sleep disturbance, fatigue, inability to concentrate, and psychomotor agitation or retardation. The depression may begin gradually or rapidly but usually will have been present for several weeks before the patient comes for treatment.

In	Interest
S	Sleep
A	Appetite
D	Depressed mood
C	Concentration
A	Activity
G	Guilt
E	Energy
S	Suicide

Fig. 197-2. *In sad cages.* A screening mnemonic for major depression. (From Rund DA, Hutzler JC: *Emergency Psychiatry*. St. Louis, Mosby, 1983, p 144. Used by permission.)

When the patient complains of the full spectrum of depression symptoms, the diagnosis of major depression is easy to make, but when the chief complaint is a single symptom such as insomnia or fatigue, it will be necessary to elicit the other symptoms of major depression to make the diagnosis. Somatic complaints such as vague pain or weakness may be part of major depression, as may generalized anxiety. A useful screening mnemonic is presented in Fig. 197-2.

Major depression is more common in women, persons with a family history of depression or suicide, and individuals with medical or other psychiatric illnesses. When a medical disorder or drug produces a depressive syndrome through a presumed biological effect on the brain, the diagnosis should be organic affective disorder. Major depression is often superimposed on other mental disorders such as substance abuse, personality disorders, and anxiety disorders.

Primary mood disorders tend to display more biological features, are more familial, and respond better to somatic antidepressant treatment than do organic mood disorders. The lifetime risk of suicide is 15 percent, so prompt and aggressive treatment is indicated strongly. Major depression is often recurrent, so certain patients must be maintained on long-term treatment to prevent relapse.

Bipolar Disorder

Bipolar disorder, previously termed *manic-depressive illness,* is characterized by the occurrence of mania. A full manic syndrome is one of the most striking and distinctive conditions in clinical practice. The essential disturbance in mood is one of elation or irritability. Manics feel "on top of the world," expansive, energetic, and precarious but may quickly become argumentative, hostile, and sarcastic, especially when their plans are thwarted.

The vegetative signs of mania are a decreased need for sleep, increased activity, rapid pressured speech, and racing thoughts. Manics may have grandiose ideas, such as unrealistic plans to start a business or run for public office, and if the grandiosity reaches delusional proportions, these patients may believe themselves to be famous, fabulously wealthy, or blessed with special powers and abilities. Poor judgment in spending money and sexual behavior may lead to problems which prompt manics' families to seek treatment for them, as manics usually lack insight into their abnormal condition and deny that anything is wrong. For this reason, reports from informants such as relatives often reveal important information to substantiate the diagnosis. Since patients who have had a manic episode almost invariably have depressions at some time (the other "pole" of bipolar disorder), a history of depression may also help in diagnosis.

The disorder is equally common in men and women, and the onset is usually in the third and fourth decades. Complications include suicide, substance abuse (excessive alcohol use is common during the manic phase), and marital and occupational disruption. The course of bipolar disorder is episodic, with the duration, frequency, and regularity of the episodes varying greatly. Depressive episodes are more frequent than manic episodes.

Dysthymia

Dysthymia is a more chronic and less severe form of depressive illness and was previously termed depressive neurosis. The symptoms must have been present for at least 2 years without any period of more than a few months of normal mood. Psychotic features are not seen, and these patients often have a life-long gloomy, pessimistic outlook. Women are more often affected, and the onset is in childhood, adolescence, or early adulthood. Associated personality disorders and substance abuse are common. When vegetative symptoms are present, they are usually less severe than with major depression. Major depression may be superimposed on dysthymia, often in association with stressful life events. When major depression complicates dysthymia, the patient may be brought in for evaluation because of the severity of symptoms or treatment after a suicide attempt.

Anxiety Disorders

The anxiety disorders are mental disorders in which apprehension, fears, and excessive worry dominate the psychological life of the individual. Pathological degrees of anxiety are accompanied by varying degrees of autonomic activity out of proportion to any real danger or threat. Since anxiety is a ubiquitous condition and frequently is associated with medical illness, depression, organic brain syndromes, and psychoses, a diagnosis of a primary anxiety disorder should be made by exclusion of other causes.

Anxiety disorders are found in 2 to 4 percent of the general population and more often diagnosed in women than men. Because of the physical nature of certain symptoms associated with anxiety disorders, patients often seek treatment and evaluation in medical rather than psychiatric settings.

Panic Disorder

Patients who experience recurrent attacks of severe anxiety are said to have *panic disorder*. A panic attack consists of a sudden extreme surge of anxiety and dread accompanied by autonomic signs, including palpitations, tachycardia, shortness of breath, chest tightness, dizziness, sweating, and tremulousness. The symptoms develop over a few minutes at most and may either be unprovoked or occur with a phobic stimulus, such as a crowded store. After that attacks begin, some patients start to avoid situations which seem to precipitate the panic (phobic avoidance). Such behavior can impair their functioning severely. When activities are severely limited, the complication of *agoraphobia* (literally, fear of the marketplace) is diagnosed. In agoraphobia, the patient tends to avoid situations where ready escape or assistance during an attack are not possible. The frequency and severity of panic attacks wax and wane, but the illness generally is chronic. Unless agoraphobia is severe, most patients are married, employed, and seldom require psychiatric hospitalization unless depression is superimposed on the anxiety disorder.

Because of the very real and frightening nature of the panic attack and its unexpected occurrence, the emergency department is a frequent initial source of medical attention. The presenting complaints may mimic a variety of medical emergencies, and careful exclusion of an organic etiology is mandatory.

Generalized Anxiety Disorder

When anxiety attacks are absent, yet the patient complains of persistent worry, tension, or free-floating anxiety, a diagnosis of generalized anxiety disorder should be entertained. This condition lasts at least 6 months and is characterized by apprehensive worrying, muscle tension, insomnia, irritability, restlessness, jumpiness, or distractibility. Muscle tension may be so severe that the patient actually experiences diffuse muscular pain. Associated autonomic symptoms include the cardiopulmonary, gastrointestinal, and neurological symptoms seen in panic attacks. In generalized anxiety disorder, such symptoms occur more continuously and chronically than in panic disorder.

Phobic Disorders

Phobic disorders, other than agoraphobia, discussed above, are an unusual cause of self-referral to the emergency department. In phobias, the anxiety symptoms are recognized as excessive and occur when the patient is exposed to, or anticipates exposure to, a specific situation which then leads to avoidance of the stimulus to a degree that interferes with the patient's life. In social phobia, the situation involves having the attention of others drawn to the patient. Such activities as public speaking or meeting strangers create a fear that the patient will be embarrassed in some way. Simple phobias are quite common; they involve fear of a very specific stimulus such as animals, heights, the dark, or flying.

Other Anxiety Disorders

Posttraumatic stress disorder is an anxiety reaction to a severely psychosocial stressor, usually life-threatening, such as military combat, a fire, rape, or natural disaster. Symptoms involve repetitive and intrusive memories of the event, nightmares, emotional numbing, survivor guilt, and varying degrees of depression and anxiety. Substance abuse appears to be a frequent complication.

Obsessive-compulsive disorder is a mental disorder in which the patient experiences intrusive thoughts or images which cannot be eliminated from the mind. Typical thoughts involve images of graphic violence to self or others, contamination, or perverse sexual behavior which the patient would not carry out but nevertheless obsessively fantasizes about. To control the obsessive thoughts, the individual may engage in compulsive behavior or rituals such as excessive washing, repetitive checking, or counting. When the obsessions and compulsions occupy a great deal of time, the patient may become significantly disabled and seek psychiatric attention. The sense of helplessness and the impairment can lead to the development of depression which also leads the patient to seek help.

Somatoform Disorders

Many patients have particular complaints or symptoms for which no medical explanation can be identified. When a physical cause has been eliminated and the complaint is not delusional or occurring in the context of a depression or anxiety disorder, somatoform disorders may be considered. When the complaint involves a loss of function, usually in the neurological system (e.g., paralysis, blindness, or numbness) and psychological factors are deemed etiologic, a *conversion disorder* may be present. The term *conversion* reflects Freud's hypothesis that unexpressed emotion associated with a traumatic event or situation could be "converted" into physical symptoms and signs. A popular form of therapy, therefore, included free association or hypnosis to recreate the recollection of the traumatic event, allow appropriate emotion to be expressed, and thus eliminate the clinical disability. Conversion disorders are much more common in culturally and psychologically unsophisticated persons. This diagnosis should be made with extreme caution, if at all, in the emergency department since studies indicate that many patients diagnosed with conversion disorder eventually develop signs of a physical disorder explaining the symptoms. Erroneous attribution to a mental disorder obviously deprives the patient of appropriate medical treatment.

Some patients have a wide variety of complaints and long complicated histories of medical problems which have no apparent medical

Table 197-2. Symptoms of Somatization Disorder*

Gastrointestinal symptoms: Vomiting (other than during pregnancy), abdominal pain, nausea, bloating, diarrhea, food intolerance
Pain symptoms: Pain in extremities, back pain, joint pain, pain during urination, other pain (excluding headaches)
Cardiopulmonary symptoms: Shortness of breath when not exerting oneself, palpitations, chest pain, dizziness
Pseudoneurologic symptoms: Amnesia, difficulty swallowing, loss of voice, deafness, double vision, blindness, fainting or loss of consciousness, seizure or convulsion, trouble walking, paralysis or muscle weakness, urinary retention or trouble urinating
Sexual symptoms: Burning sensation in sexual organs or rectum (other than during intercourse), sexual indifference, pain during intercourse, impotence
Female productive symptoms (judged by patient as more severe than most women): painful menstruation, irregular menstrual periods, excessive menstrual bleeding, or vomiting throughout pregnancy

* At least 13 symptoms are needed to satisfy criteria for somatization disorder. In order to count, symptoms must be medically unexplained, not due to a panic attack, and cause the person to see a doctor, take medication or alter their life style.

cause. Such individuals may have *somatization disorder,* a disorder beginning in the teens and twenties, usually in women, and leading to considerable unnecessary diagnostic and surgical intervention. The prototypical patient is a middle-aged woman who describes a positive review of systems in a dramatic and confusing way. Conversion symptoms, menstrual complaints, multifocal pain, dizziness, and diverse psychiatric symptoms are common findings. The diagnosis is made by asking the patient about the list of symptoms of somatization disorder (Table 197–2) and determining how many symptoms were unexplained by a medical cause, yet resulted in either seeking medical attention or taking medication to relieve the symptom. Symptoms appearing in the table in bold-face type can be used to screen patients quickly for possible somatization disorder; the presence of two or more of these items suggest a high likelihood of somatization disorder.

Hypochondriasis may be diagnosed when the patient claims to be ill yet cannot be assured to the contrary when appropriate examination do not identify a cause. The diagnosis is appropriate when the more pervasive and chronic somatization disorder is absent.

Finally, when pain is the sole complaint and the intensity and secondary disability are unexplained by a known physical ailment, a diagnosis of *somatoform pain disorder* may be considered.

Identification of a somatoform disorder in the emergency department and labeling the patient as such has profound implications on future management that it is advisable to avoid making a firm diagnosis of a hysterical or functional disorder unless a long history of prior similar complaints is documented and no organic disease has become apparent. This wisdom is tempered additionally by the fact that well-established conversion or other psychogenic complaints provide absolutely no protection against the development of a treatable medical disorder; new complaints always warrant careful examination for objective findings. When the physician is sure that no organic disease exists, the patient may be reassured that no serious physical illness is present. Avoid telling the patient that it is "all in your head" since this is not likely to be believed. Regular follow-up with a general internist or family physician is the best management for somatization disorder. Patients with this disorder notoriously resist psychiatric referral and treatment.

Dissociative Disorders

The dissociative disorders are a group of uncommon and poorly understood conditions where the central feature is a sudden alteration in the normal integration of identity and consciousness. The dissociation often occurs under severe stress and may or may not be recurrent, although it is rarely permanent. The forms of dissociative state relevant to emergency practice are *psychogenic amnesia,* a temporary loss of memory for important personal details that is not due to an organic cause, and *psychogenic fugue,* in which a similar loss of memory and assumption of a new identity are accompanied by travel away from home. Dissociative disorders are difficult to distinguish from malingering, in which the individual in pursuit of a clear goal, such as avoiding incarceration or military duty, may consciously feign amnesia. As always, organic causes such as drug intoxication or loss of memory such as that resulting from transient global amnesia must be excluded.

Other conditions in this category include *multiple personality disorder* and *depersonalization disorder.*

PERSONALITY (AXIS II) DISORDERS

Personality refers to an enduring pattern of perceiving, relating to, and reacting to one's environment and interpersonal relations. When a pattern of behavior is lifelong, not limited to periods of illness, and causes significant impairment in social or occupational functioning or considerable distress, a *personality disorder* is present. Some individuals are painfully aware of the consequences of their behavior but are unable to alter these fundamental ways of dealing with their world. Most of the patients who are seen clinically in medical and psychiatric settings who are diagnosed with a personality disorder lack a clear awareness of how their behavior alienates others or aggravates their own stress. Even when such insight is possible, actual personality change is unlikely.

The patient presenting with a personality disorder often may be recognized by the characteristic effect perceived by the physician and medical staff. Antisocial patients, for instance, are disliked immediately. They seem to be in control of their behavior, unlike psychotic or depressed patients, but, nonetheless repeatedly have engaged in maladaptive behavior. The patient may be seen as using the emergency department for some vague, or obvious, goal. These disorders are the most common secondary diagnosis in the malingerer.

The emergency physician seldom needs to decide which of the personality disorders relates appropriately to the patient. General categories of personality disorders are grouped in Table 197–3. When such features are present and seem to be interfering with some important aspect of the patient's life, personality disorder can be suspected. The presenting complaint should be evaluated appropriately, since patients with well-established character disorders still develop bona fide medical illnesses.

The personality disorder which constitutes a disproportionate share of emergency visits is *antisocial personality disorder.* The patient shows a continuous pattern of maladaptive behavior displaying dis-

Table 197-3. Clusters of Behavioral Characteristics that Suggest Various Groups of Personality Disorder Diagnoses

Behavior	Personality Disorder Group
Eccentric, odd, isolated, withdrawn, suspicious, inhibited, no friends, overly sensitive	Paranoid Schizoid Schizotypal
Emotional, dramatic, angry, seductive, impulsive	Antisocial Histrionic Borderline Narcissistic
Anxious, fearful, "nervous," caution	Dependent Avoidant Compulsive Passive-aggressive

Source: Rund DA, Hutzler JC: *Emergency Psychiatry,* St. Louis, Mosby, 1983, p 201. Used by permission.

regard for the rights of others in a variety of ways: criminal behavior, fighting, lying, abuse and neglect of dependents and spouses, financial irresponsibility, recklessness, and inability to sustain enduring attachments to others.

The sociopathic behavior begins before the age of 15, but the diagnosis may not be made until after the age 18. Sociopathy is much more frequent in male patients, in lower socioeconomic classes, and in relatives of alcoholics and sociopaths. Alcohol and drug abuse, imprisonment, multiple divorces, traumatic injury, accidental and violent deaths, and poor medical compliance are common complications.

Management of the antisocial patient in the emergency department is often frustrating, but anger toward the patient can be minimized and the interaction hastened along by setting firm limits on behavior, focusing on the chief complaint, and providing the patient with necessary information about the medical problem at hand. No effective psychiatric intervention can be forced on the patient, although certain patients may benefit from substance abuse treatment, psychotherapy, or organized religion when motivated to make changes in their lives. Fortunately, the most violent and disruptive behavior of many antisocials seems to "burn out" in the late 20s or after, although their adjustment to society often continues to be marginal.

SUMMARY

The official classification of mental disorders, DSM-III-R, provides a framework for understanding the confusing clinical presentation of psychiatric patients. The use of diagnostic criteria and decision trees allows the emergency physician to categorize the syndromes better, therefore improving communication with consultants and suggesting appropriate and specific management.

BIBLIOGRAPHY

American Psychiatric Association: *Disgnostic and Statistical Manual of Mental Disorders,* 3d ed (DSM-III). Washington, DC, 1980.

American Psychiatric Association: *Diagnostic and Statistical Manual of Mental Disorders,* 3d ed, revised (DSM-III-R). Washington, DC, 1987.

Dilsaver S: The mental status examination. *Am Fam Physician* 41:1489, 1990.

Drugs that cause psychiatric symptoms. *Med Lett Drugs Ther* 28:81, 1986.

Gomberg E: Suicide risk among women with alcohol problems. *Am J Public Health* 79:1363, 1989.

Greenstein R, Ness D: Psychiatric emergencies in the elderly. *Emerg Med Clin North Am* 8:429, 1990.

Lowenstein D, Massa S, Rowbotham M, et al: Acute neurologic and psychiatric complications associated with cocaine abuse. *Am J Med* 3:841, 1987.

Rund DA, Hutzler JC: *Emergency Psychiatry*. St. Louis, Mosby, 1983.

Summers WK, Rund DA, Levin ML: Psychiatric illness in a general urban emergency room: Daytime versus nighttime population. *J. Clin Psychiatry* 41:340, 1979.

198 BEHAVIORAL DISORDERS: EMERGENCY ASSESSMENT AND STABILIZATION

Jeffrey A. Coffman
Douglas A. Rund

As shown in Fig. 198–1, the majority of psychiatric patient visits to the emergency department occur at night when psychiatric services are limited; therefore, the hospital must be staffed with adequate personnel adept at handling patients who are suicidal, violent, or otherwise distraught or psychotic.

EMERGENCY AND INTERVENTION APPROACHES TO PSYCHIATRIC ASSESSMENT

Decision-Making in Emergency Practice

A decision strategy for emergency psychiatric assessment should follow this sequence: (1) whether the patient is stable or unstable; (2) whether the patient has a serious medical condition manifest in abnormal behavior or thought processes; (3) whether the condition is primarily "psychiatric" ("functional"), what is its nature and severity, when is psychiatric consultation needed; and (4) when the patient can be forcibly detained for emergency evaluation.

Stabilization

Most situations that require emergency stabilization include actual or potential violence, suicide, and rapidly progressive medical conditions causing disturbed behavior (e.g., hypoglycemia or meningitis).

Disturbances involving actual or threatened violence provide the greatest difficulty for emergency department staff. Such difficulties are imposed in part by fear of injury, and by limitations of the physical facility and immediately available staff.

Actual violent behavior demands immediate restraint. Hospital security forces or police are best equipped and best trained to subdue the patient, with the least chance for staff or patient injury. An initial show of force may be sufficient to induce the patient to accept physical or chemical restraint without further resistance. Under ideal circumstances the emergency department staff should organize themselves to be able to subdue a violent person if security personnel are not immediately available. The approach to the patient usually requires five team members, with one member assigned to each limb and the leader assigned to the head. When approached from different directions and grabbed simultaneously, the violent person can usually be immobilized and restrained. Techniques of restraining the violent or near-violent patient are discussed in the section of this chapter dealing specifically with violent behavior.

Potentially violent behavior requires the summoning of adequate force and the adoption of a nonthreatening attitude by physician and staff. In general, the physician should maintain adequate distance from the patient, avoid excessive eye contact, maintain a submissive posture, avoid blocking a potential escape exit, and allow the patient to ventilate feelings verbally. Setting limits on acceptable behavior and making neutral comments may diffuse a potentially violent situation.

Stabilization of the actively suicidal patient requires adequate suicide precautions. All dangerous objects are removed from the patient and the treatment room. A staff member should be assigned to watch the patient closely and not allow that person to leave the examining room unaccompanied by a staff member.

Patients with actual or potential violent behavior must be disrobed, gowned, and searched for weapons. Seemingly innocuous objects such as belts or belt buckles can be used by the patient to inflict self-injury or injure others. Sone emergency departments have installed metal detectors to prevent highly lethal weapons from entering the department.

Stabilization of a medical condition creating abnormal thought or behavior, of course, depends on the responsible condition. It may be as simple as administering intravenous glucose or as complicated as initiating therapy for acute renal failure.

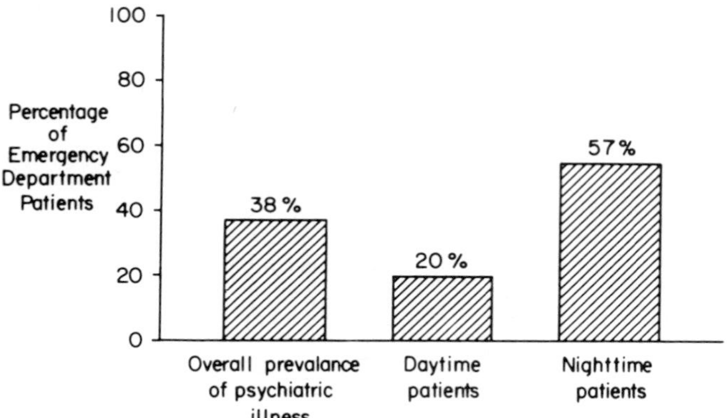

Fig. 198-1. Daytime versus nighttime distribution of psychiatric patient visits to the emergency department.

Initial Evaluation

The most effective tool available for the evaluation of behavioral disorders, particularly where "organic" mental disorders may be involved, is a cogent medical-psychiatric history. The history (including use of medication, alcohol, or other drugs), physical examination, neurological examination, and mental status examination should be incorporated in the early stages of evaluation of an individual with disturbed behavior.

The episode which led to the patient's presentation provides a starting point for inquiry. Sudden onset of major changes in behavior, mood, or thought in an individual who previously had functioned normally may be the result of an urgent medical disorder. Behavioral disorders have resulted from all of the following life-threatening conditions:

Central nervous system (CNS) infection: meningitis or encephalitis
Intoxication
Withdrawal
Hypoglycemia
Hypertensive encephalophathy
Hypoxia
Intracranial hemorrhage
Poisioning
CNS trauma
Seizure disorder
Acute organ failure: renal or hepatic failure

A *sudden* change in behavior, especially in a patient over the age of 40, is potentially important indicator of a new and potentially correctable process. Neurologic symptoms associated with behavioral changes should be explored. Such symptoms include fainting, dizziness, brief periods of disorientation, impairment of speech, confusion, loss of consciousness, headaches, and difficulty performing previously familiar tasks. A history of previous similar episodes may alert the physician to the possibility of seizure disorder or other recurrent disorders.

Particularly important are reports of the patient's behavior gained from family, friends, or other third parties. Such individuals may have observed subtle changes in behavior of which the patient is unaware and may be the only source of information if history is unobtainable from the patient. They may also report substance abuse concealed by the patient. Moreover, the present episode must be assessed against the background of previous functioning. The presence of a history of previous psychiatric illness may or may not aid the evaluation of a new presentation to the emergency department. A previous history of similar problems occurring over the years weighs against the onset of a new ''organic'' process that may offer a correctable solution. However, it is important to weigh available information carefully to avoid a quick assumption that the patient's presentation is due to repeated occurrence of a preexisting disorder.

A full medical history and review of systems is particularly important. The patient should be asked about any recent medical illnesses or symptoms such as infections, head trauma, fever, difficulty in breathing, and dizziness. This information may have to be gathered from the patient's family and friends if the patient is unable or unwilling to provide the information. Such general inquiries should be followed by a review of systems, placing special emphasis on any history of neurologic symptoms. Recent onset of periods of confusion, speech difficulties, fainting, or incontinence could be potentially important indicators of serious brain disease. A history of exposure to toxic substances such as heavy metals, organic solvents, or other occupational hazards may suggest a cause for newly disturbed behavior. To complete the investigation, family and social history may identify stresses in the patient's environment that are either direct cause of changes in behavior or which accentuate any responses to underlying disease.

Prescribed drugs, over-the-counter medications, illicit drugs, and alcohol create disturbed behavior in a significant number of patients in most emergency departments. The examiner should obtain information regarding the use of sedative hypnotics, stimulants, psychotropic agents, anticonvulsants, anticholinergic agents, antiparkinsonian medications, cardiovascular drugs, diuretics, hormones, analgesics, anti-inflammatory drugs, anti-infective agents, and other categories of prescription drugs. Many of these medications have behavioral side effects when taken in high doses, and some do even at therapeutic levels. If the patient is unable to provide an adequate history regarding drug usage, family or friends may be helpful. The physician should ask specifically about over-the-counter drugs because patients rarely consider these medications to be relevant. Chronic use of over-the-counter analgesics containing salicylates may produce delirium with hallucinations, delusions, and other symptoms. Sedative hypnotics may contain scopolamine, antihistamines, or bromides that may induce toxic psychoses or delirium. Scopolamine, in particular, is likely to produce an anticholinergic delirium with psychotic symptoms. Cold and allergy preparations containing phenylpropanolamine have a stimulant effect similar to amphetamines. The patient should also be asked about the use of illicit drugs or alcohol. Illicit drugs including phencyclidine (PCP), LSD, mescaline, amphetamines, or cocaine can produce an acute toxic psychosis. Other drugs of abuse such as barbiturates, benzodiazepines,methaqualone, or glutethimide may produce a confusional state or delirium on intoxication or withdrawal. Many of the sedative hypnotics, particularly those with short durations of action, and alcohol are associated with severe withdrawal symptoms.

According to Rund and Summers, 15 to 20 percent of emergency department patients meet diagnostic criteria for alcohol abuse. The many syndromes associated with alcohol abuse should be recognized by emergency physicians. Such syndromes include intoxication, withdrawal, delirium, hallucinosis, alcohol amnestic disorder, paranoid behavior, and dementia. Blood alcohol tests may be useful in disturbed patients even when the odor of ethanol is not present. Other testing modalities, including breath analyzers and chemically treated paper strips, may be used to screen blood alcohol levels.

Mental Status Examination

An abnormal mental status examination suggests an organic basis for abnormal thought or behavior. A great deal of the information obtainable in mental status examination becomes available to the physician through initial interview with the patient (see Table 198–1). The physician can observe the patient's *behavior* during the examination. Lability of *affect* with frequent changing from crying to jocularity and stages in between, the necessity to repeat simple questions, irritability, and lack of cooperation may be some indications of acute behavioral disturbance attributable to organic factors.

When questioned about the mental status examination, emergency physicians list level of consciousness, spontaneous speech, behavioral observation, physical appearance, relay of history information, attention, and language comprehension as important components of their mental status examination (Zun and Gold). Such data are usually easily perceived during the taking of a history. The more traditional mental status examination relies on assessment of orientation, memory, intellect, judgment, and affect.

The physician should compare direct observations of the patient with reports of family and friends. Documentation of the patient's *orientation* should include an assessment of attention, ability to concentrate on a specific task, and the traditional evaluation of person, place, and time. Impaired *language* performance, including difficulty with speech, reading, writing, and word finding, may indicate a neurologic disorder. *Memory* is often divided into three catagories: immediate, recent, and remote. Immediate memory is tested by asking the patient to repeat a series of digits forward and backward. Recent memory can be tested by asking the patient to repeat three unrelated words immediately and then again after a few minutes of discussion about unrelated topics. The patient may also be asked about events that have occurred in the last few hours for which the examiner has corroborative evidence. Remote memory can be tested by asking about previous addresses, occupations, or historical events from an early period in the patient's life. Tests of memory should include details of significant personal, national, and international historical events. The examiner must be able to verify facts.

The investigation of *higher cognitive functions* usually includes assessment of the patient's general command of information; mental calculation, especially subtraction; and spelling of words forward and backward. Patients with significant brain pathology often have difficulty performing tasks such as spelling backward or serial calculation. The patient's *affect* or outward display of emotion should be evaluated for sadness, euphoria, and anxiety. This may be of particular relevance in determining the distinction between the cognitive disturbance induce by depressive disorders and dementia due to significant cerebral pathology. The examiner can draw some conclusions regarding the patient's *thought processes* during the patient's own relation of history.

Table 198.1. Mental Status Examination in the Emergency Department: An Outline

Behavior
  What is the patient doing?
Affect
  What feelings is the patient displaying?
Orientation
  Does the patient know what is happening, where, and when?
Language
  Is the patient understanding and being understood?
Memory
  Can the patient recall historical details, recent and remote?
Thought content
  Is the patient reporting beliefs that make little sense?
Perceptual abnormalities
  Is the patient experiencing unusual sensory phenomena?
Judgment
  Is the patient able to make rational decisions?

Attention should be given to circumstantial or generally confused thought process. *Thought content* of note includes paranoid or grandiose delusions or fixed false beliefs as well as delusional denial of illness. Such beliefs should be compared with reports from family and friends.

Patients with significant cerebral pathology may experience *perceptual abnormalities* such as hallucinatory phenomena. Visual hallucinations do occur in functional psychotic illnesses (schizophrenia or affective disorder) but more often result from major cerebral pathology. Delirious patients may experience illusions, such as misperceiving a shadow or moving curtain as an intruder entering through the window. Perceptual changes occurring as a result of significant cerebral pathology typically disturb the patient, whereas they may not disturb in functional disorders. *Judgment* may be impaired in patients who are showing disturbed behavior. Historical evidence of faulty judgment is often our best indicator of such a disturbance. The patient may have been walking heedlessly through traffic prior to being brought to the emergency department, for instance. Further insight about the patient's judgment can be gained by asking how one would deal with day-to-day problems such as finding one's way home from the hospital. Finally, the examiner should be alert for the possibility of specific focal cortical deficits including apraxias, agnosias, right-left disorientation, aphasias, denial of half of the body, and inability to follow complex spoken and written commands. They may or may not occur in association with other localizing neurologic signs such as asymmetric reflexes, paresthesia, or paraplegia.

Physical Examination

A problem-oriented physical examination should be conducted on every patient. In most cases, this examination will not differ greatly from that which is conducted in patients without behavioral changes.

Vital signs are a simple physical screening test for patients with altered behavior. Abnormal vital signs, when observed, must not be dismissed as secondary to anxiety or stress. Bradycardia can be seen in patients with hypothyroidism, Stokes-Adams syndrome, or elevated intracranial pressure. Tachycardia may be apparent in patients suffering from hyperthyroidism, infection, heart failure, pulmonary embolus, or alcohol withdrawal. Fever is often associated with extreme hyperthyroidism or thyroid storm, sepsis, vasculitis, alcohol withdrawal, sedative hypnotic withdrawal, meningitis, or various inflammatory processes. Hypothermia is observed in sepsis, dermal disease, hypoendocrine states, CNS dysfunction, and intoxication. Hypotension may be an indicator of shock, Addison's disease, hypothyroidism, or medication side effects. Hypertension may be associated with intracranial space-occupying lesions, by hypertensive encephalopathy, or stimulant abuse. Tachypnea is seen in patients with metabolic acidosis, pulmonary embolus, pneumonia, cardiac failure, or fever. Any such disorders may result in a secondary behavioral disturbance. The limited expense of, and useful information provided by, vital signs justifies their use in all patients.

A general physical examination should ideally be conducted with the patient completely disrobed and gowned. The patient should be carefully checked for signs of trauma. Contusions or abrasions of the head, face, and neck may be common if the patient is bellicose and may suggest the possibility of otherwise unsuspected head injuries. Extremities should be checked for frostbite or other evidence of exposure-related injury. If trauma is demonstrated or suggested by history, the mechanism of injury should be carefully reconstructed. For a variety of reasons, patients may over- or under report the the extent and cause of trauma.

Chest, cardiac, and abdominal examinations should be carefully performed and a careful neurologic examination should be specific for assessment of cranial nerves, motor function, sensory function, normal reflexes, speech deficits, and gait disturbances, as well as emergence of primitive reflexes (glabellar tap and the grasp reflexes) that may suggest diffuse cortical disease. Other neurologic signs, such as bilateral asterixis or multifocal myoclonus, are often associated with delirium.

Laboratory Evaluation

The selection of particular laboratory tests emerges from diagnostic needs suggested by the history, mental status examination, and physical examination. In a review by Purdie, fluid and electrolyte disorders were found in 12 percent of patients with an acute behavioral disturbance. Gleadhill et al. reported a 15-fold greater incidence of hyponatremia in schizophrenics with evidence of acute behavioral change than in nonschizophrenic psychiatric patients. Case finding factors intervene remarkably. For example, Fauman and Fauman found in 500 consecutive psychiatric patients without evidence of delirium or other acute behavioral disturbance attributable to a neuropathological process, that the only useful laboratory studies were blood glucose and white blood cell count. Therefore, screening on grounds of history and physical examination should be done prior to ordering tests, as there exists no universal screening panel.

EMERGENCY SITUATIONS REQUIRING EMERGENCY INTERVENTION

Suicide

Suicide is the ninth leading cause of death in our population and the second leading cause of death in persons under age 24. There seem to be epidemiologic differences between suicide attempters and suicide completers. Suicide completers, for instance, are more likely than attempters to be older, male, living alone, or physically ill. The ratio of attempted suicides to completed suicides is estimated to be about 40:1. The suicide attempter must be protected and evaluated carefully in the emergency department with special attention to those characteristics that are likely to move someone from the suicide attempter category to the suicide completer category.

One of the difficulties in evaluating individuals who attempt suicide is the popular impression that preoccupation with suicide is a common accompaniment of the "downward" portion of the normal mood swings occasionally experienced by everyone. The data show that suicidal ideation (feeling that life was not worth living within the past year), is reported in only 7.8 percent of subjects selected from the general population. In the same study, 2.6 percent had seriously considered taking their lives and 1.1 percent had actually made a suicide attempt. Suicidal ideation has been shown to be more frequent in women than men and to be associated with depression, social isolation, undesirable life events, and early parental loss. Suicidal ideation precedes the actual attempt by up to 1 year in many cases, and follow-up studies suggest that suicidal ideation persists in many patients long after improvement in mental status and in personal relationships.

The conclusion one must make, therefore, is that the suicide attempter must be at least initially taken seriously. The attitude of the staff should be empathetic, suicide precautions should be instituted, and, following medical management, the assessment of suicide risk should be carefully evaluated and documented.

Attitudes toward the suicide attempter among the emergency staff should be empathetic and nonjudgmental. Negative attitudes toward the suicide attempter have been documented in all types of emergency personnel: paramedics, nurses, and emergency physicians. A negative attitude intensifies the patient's already low self-esteem, thus increasing the risk of subsequent suicide and making it difficult to establish a therapeutic relationship with a psychiatrist or mental health worker.

In the early stages of emergency assessment, the suicide attempter should be regarded as a patient with a condition that could cause sudden death if inadequately managed. The decision to hold and hospitalize, transfer, or discharge the patient depends on that individual's psychiatric condition, known risk factors, attitude, and future plans.

Schizophrenia, substance abuse, and depression are psychiatric diagnoses that place a suicidal patient at relatively high risk. Ten percent of schizophrenics eventually kill themselves. Alcoholics have a suicide rate that is 50 times higher than the norm, and as many as 25 percent of all successful suicides are associated with alcohol. Depression is a diagnosis associated with suicide attempts of higher lethality and with those who successfully complete suicide.

Personality disorder and adjustment disorder implying a transient situational disturbance are frequent diagnoses in suicide attempters and are generally associated with relatively lower completion risk than the major psychiatric illnesses noted above. Patients with these disorders still show a higher risk of completed suicide than the general population.

Drug overdose accounts for the overwhelming majority of all contemporary suicide attempts. Drugs used for suicide attempts tend to parallel prevailing prescribing patterns. An increase in the prevalence of suicide attempts observed during the 1960s and early 1970s led to speculation that availability of safer psychotropic agents encouraged wide spread prescription and ultimately contributed to their availability for suicide attempt. The extent of poisoning created by the drugs usually reflects the lethal intent of the patient and thus the relative risk. The patient taking a large dose of amitriptyline would thus be considered at greater risk than someone taking a few antihistamine tablets. Some patients may be relatively unaware of the potential toxicity of their overdose, however, and assessment of such knowledge and their continuing intent to die must be assessed by questions such as ''Were you surprised to find yourself alive after taking the overdose?''

Violent attempts (shooting, jumping, hanging) are generally considered serious and a high risk factor for future attempt unless injury outcome is consistent with another explanation. A number of reports have described a ''wrist cutting syndrome'' in young, attractive, unmarried women whose self-mutilation, although often repetitive, was seldom thought to be serious in intent. Such acts have often been described as carried out in a state of mounting tension or depersonalization followed by relief and indifference to the injury. Investigators studying representative samples of attempted suicides found substantial numbers of men, as well as older men and women, among self-mutilators.

The idea that self-mutilators represent a low-risk group for completing suicide has been contradicted by at least one follow-up study which noted that 3 of 19 wrist slashers, traced 5 to 6 years following initial presentation, subsequently died of suicide.

Certain demographic characteristics have been traditionally useful in determining suicidal intent. As a general rule, the risk of successful suicide rises with advancing age. Men are two to three times more likely than women to *complete* suicide, while women are two to three times more likely than men to *attempt* suicide. Patients who are single, divorced, separated, widowed, or unemployed are statistically at higher risk than those married and employed.

The psychotic patient who attempts suicide must be evaluated by a psychiatrist and hospitalized. Such a patient may respond unpredictably to distorted preceptions or false perceptions in a fearful or driven manner.

Secondary gain specifies that while the primary motive appears to be death, the attempt may meet another need such as attention from parents or lover, or a plea for emotional help. When such needs are met by the attempt, secondary gain is achieved and the risk of subsequent suicide attempt lessened. However, assumptions regarding relative gain are just that and should not be relied on as firm predictors of behavior.

Perhaps the most important part of the assessment of the suicide attempter is a determination of the patient's feelings and thoughts at the time of the attempt and at the time of the interview. The patient who experiences helplessness, exhaustion, overwhelming depression, and a clear expression of intent to die certainly remains at high risk. If the patient expresses continuation of these feelings at the time of the interview, the physician has sufficient evidence that the patient needs psychiatric consultation immediately. Some patients, however, seem to equate self-injury with other forms of emotional discharge such as crying, talking to a friend, or becoming inebriated. They do not perceive the event as an attempt to end their life. When asked about their feelings at the time of the attempt, such patients may indicate that they were angry or vengeful. Attitudes and affect that generally indicate a good prognosis at the time of interview are anger, remorse, or embarrassment. The patient who sits quietly, refusing to provide additional information to the examiner, should be considered at high risk until proved otherwise.

Feelings of hopelessness seem to be among the clearest indicators of long-term suicidal risk in patients hospitalized at one time for depression. Persons expressing feelings of hopelessness, helplessness, or exhaustion must be regarded at high risk for a serious suicide attempt.

Before discharging the patient, the physician must be assured that that person has a good social support system. Such a system usually includes a place to live and some family or close friends who will support the patient emotionally in the absence of clearly pathological features that predispose the patient to subsequent suicide.

The emergency physician can calculate an intuitive risk:rescue ratio by estimating the lethality of the attempt and the likelihood of rescue. When there is a high likelihood of rescue and low lethality, the patient is considered at lower risk than in the reverse situation. The patient who makes a hanging attempt in a desolate wooded area is a greater risk than the person who takes a handful of relatively nontoxic pills in front of witnesses.

Patients who have made previous suicide attempt have traditionally been considered to be a greater risk for future suicide, even though one controlled prospective study did not demonstrate any correlation between previous attempt and successful suicide (Fawcet et al.). Prior attempts seem a particularly ominous sign, however, if the intensity and apparent lethality of the suicide attempts escalate with each subsequent attempt. Bengelsdorf achieved a 97 percent concordance with a crisis triage system to predict the need for inpatient hospitalization. The factors which need to be considered include dangerousness, support system, and motivation or ability to cooperate.

A summary of high- and low-risk suicide profiles is given in Table 198–2.

Clinical Management

High-risk patients whose suicide intent is strong and immediate should be referred for immediate psychiatric hospitalization. Moderate-risk patients are those who present in a serious suicidal crisis but who, because of a positive response to initial intervention and favorable social support, are not judged to be an immediate danger. Hospitalization can often be avoided in such patients, provided practical outpatient treatment can be established immediately; such determinations are most often made in concert with a psychiatric consultant. Available means of suicide, such a firearms or drug caches, should be removed and any psychotropic medication should be used judiciously and prescribed conservatively. It is important to have a family member take charge of the patient's medications.

Low-risk patients frequently present with suicidal threats or minor attempts that occur in the context of a clearly definable external crisis. Social support is usually available and responsive. However, as many attempts that appear trivial on first glance are found to have more serious implications on closer examination, all patients presenting following a suicide attempt should be carefully assessed. If there is question in the physician's mind about the safety of discharging a *suicidal* patient, in the absence of immediate psychiatric consultation, that patient should be hospitalized.

Violence

The reported percentages of psychiatric patients seen in emergency settings or admitted to hospitals for assaultive behavior vary widely

Table 198-2. Evaluation of Risk

	High Risk	Low Risk
Demographic and social profile		
Age	Over 45 years	Below 45 years
Sex	Male	Female
Marital status	Divorced or widowed	Married
Employment	Unemployed	Employed
Interpersonal relationships	Conflictual	Stable
Family background	Chaotic or conflictual	Stable
Health		
Physical	Chronic illness	Good health
	Hypochondriac	Feels healthy
	Excessive drug intake	Low drug use
Mental	Severe depression	Mild depression
	Psychosis	Neurosis
	Severe personality disorder	Normal personality
	Alcoholism or drug abuse	Social drinker
	Hopelessness	Optimism
Suicidal activity		
Suicidal ideation	Frequent, intense, prolonged	Infrequent, low intensity, transient
Suicide attempt	Multiple attempts	First attempt
	Planned	Impulsive
	Rescue unlikely	Rescue inevitable
	Unambiguous wish to die	Primary wish for change
	Communication internalized (self-blame)	Communication externalized (anger)
	Method lethal and available	Method of low lethality or not readily available
Resources		
Personal	Poor achievement	Good achievement
	Poor insight	Insightful
	Affect unavailable or poorly controlled	Affect available and appropriately controlled
	Poor rapport	Good rapport
Social	Socially isolated	Socially integrated
	Unresponsive family	Concerned family

Source: Modified from Adam KS: Suicide and attempted suicide. *Med Clin North Am* 34:3200, 1983. Used by permission.

in the literature: from 4 to 60 percent. The variability undoubtedly reflects concentrations of violence in certain environments and institutions. In general, violence can be considered to result from substance abuse, delirium, neuropsychiatric disturbance, or personality disorder. The evaluation of the violent or near-violent patient, therefore, must proceed carefully as outlined, provided adequate restraint has been applied or can be applied swiftly as the need arises.

The first priority in the evaluation of the violent patient is provision of adequate restraint to prevent injury to the patient or others. In the instance where the patient is brought to the emergency department by police, adequate restraint and removal of weapons may already have been accomplished. In addition, police can often be helpful in maintaining physical restraint of the patient until leather restraints can be applied.

In the event that a patient enters the emergency department without police escort or becomes violent after initial presentation, steps need to be taken by emergency department staff in order to achieve control of the dangerous behavior. When weapons with major capacity for injury are wielded, such as firearms or explosives, emergency department staff are probably best advised to clear the area and rely on police assistance. When violent behavior is confined to wielding of knives or blunt objects, a situation which may arise more acutely, emergency department staff may be forced in intervene directly on their own.

When emergency department staff must intervene on their own with a violent or threatening patient, strength in numbers is well advised. When confronted by 5 to 10 individuals who approach in a manner suggesting that they are willing to contain behavior, the potentially violent patient will often submit to restraint. A form of insurance that can be used in approaching such a patient is to do so behind a mattress and thus using two mattresses to "sandwich" the person and safely institute restraint. Whatever method is used, a calm approach should be taken in moving toward the patient, as well as explanation for the need of restraint, even when such explanation seems not to be understood.

After restraint is achieved, the patient should be searched, as should all clothing, for hidden weapons, drugs, or other injurious material.

The decision to release the patient from physical restraints should be made by the physician or paramedical personnel on the basis of a judgment regarding the patient's condition and behavior and not as a result of the patient's bargains or threats. Restraints should be removed in a stepwise fashion, from four limbs to two, to none.

Pharmacologic restraint of patients should follow gathering of as much information as possible in order to allow provisional diagnostic assessment. Once initial medical history, physical examination, and laboratory information have been obtained, if the patient continues to chafe against restraints and to show uncontrolled behavior, the use of a pharmacological intervention to assist in behavioral control might be considered. Although a variety of medications could be brought to bear in this setting, the only one with a clear advantage over the rest is lorazepam (Ativan), a potent benzodiazepine which has the advantages of the wide therapeutic index of the class, rapid onset of action, and the ease of administration by parenteral or oral routes. Lorazepam is the only benzodiazepine which can be reliably administered intramuscularly, and its oral and parenteral potencies do not greatly differ, allowing for ease in dosage calculation. Alternative medications such as short-acting barbiturates have a much narrower therapeutic index, and neuroleptic medications such as the phenothiazines have the disadvantage that those which are most sedating also cause the greatest difficulty with orthostatic hypotension. Useful dosage levels of lorazepam would be 1 to 2 mg orally or intramuscularly every half hour until an adequate level of sedation is achieved. If this is insufficient, haloperidol can be used. The dose is 5 mg IM in adults and 1–2 mg IM in the elderly. However, haloperidol should not be given to those with Parkinson's disease or other movement disorder.

CONSULTATION AND REFERRAL

In the ideal setting, all emergency department would have psychiatric consultation available at all times. However, in many instances, the physician in the emergency department will be forced to rely on more limited resources. Many psychiatric problems leading to emergency department presentation do not require immediate definitive treatment. In many instances, disposition following initial screening can be made to a variety of secondary sources of evaluation and treatment. Judgments regarding referral depend on assessment of the patient's likelihood of becoming violent toward self or others. Clues that suggest potential violence include hostile behavior, verbal aggressiveness, or statements about violent intent. Such patients need immediate hospitalization. Marked disorientation and confusion require evaluation for organic components. In the absence of such indications, referral can be made to a psychiatrist or a psychiatric facility. It is often helpful to the patient and to the facility to which that patient might be referred for initial medical screening procedures to be completed in the emergency department. Results of the emergency department evaluation should be provided to the consultant.

BIBLIOGRAPHY

Adam G, Adam KS, Bay M, et al: A family-oriented crisis intervention service for attempted suicide, in Sanbrier JP, Vedninne J (eds): *Depression and Suicide: Proceedings of the 11th International Congress for Suicide and Crisis Intervention.* New York, Pergamon, 1983.

Adam KS: Attempted suicide. *Psychiatr Clin North Am* 8:183, 1985.

Beck AT, Steer RA, Kovacs M, et al: Hopelessness and eventual suicide: A 10 year prospective study of patients hospitalized with suicidal ideation. *Am J Psychiatry* 142:559, 1985.

Clinton J, Sterner S, Stelmachers Z, Ruiz, E: Haloperidol for sedation of disruptive emergency patients. *Ann Emerg Med* 16:319, 1987.

Derlet R, Albertson T: Emergency department presentation of cocaine intoxication. *Ann Emerg Med* 18:182, 1989.

Fauman MA, Fauman BJ: The differential diagnosis of organic based psychiatric disturbance in the emergency department. *JACEP* 6:315, 1977.

Fawcet J, Scheftner W, Clark D, et al: Clinical predictors of suicide in patients with major affective disorders: A controlled prospective study. *Am J Psychiatry* 144:35, 1987.

Gleadhill IC, Smith TA, Yium JJ: Hypotentremia in patients with schizophrenia. *South Med J* 75:426, 1982.

Lavoie F, Carter G, Danzl D, et al: Emergency department violence in United States teaching hospitals. *Ann Emerg Med* 17:1227, 1988.

Levy A, Salagnik I, Rabinowitz A, et al: The dangerous psychiatric patient. Part I: Epidemiology, etiology, prediction. *Med Law* 8:131, 1989.

Luna G, Kendall K, Pilcher S, et al: The medical and social impact of nonaccidential injury. *Arch Surg* 123:825, 1988.

Purdie FR, Honigman B, Rosen P: Acute organic brain syndrome. A review of 100 cases. *Ann Emer Med* 10:455, 1981.

Rund DA, Saunders AF, Hutzler JC: The suicide attempt. *Emerg Med Surv* 162:53, 1981.

Rund DA, Summers WK, Levin M: Alcohol use and psychiatric illness in emergency patients. *JAMA* 245:1240, 1981.

Sateia MJ, Gustafson DH, Johnson SW: Quality assurance for psychiatric emergencies: An analysis of assessment and feedback methodologies. *Psychiatr Clin North Am* 13:35, 1990.

Selden B, Schnitzer P, Nolan F: Medicolegal documentation of prehospital triage. *Ann Emerg Med* 19:547, 1990.

Shapiro S, Skinner EA, Kessler LG, et al: Utilization of health and mental health services: Three epidemiologic cathment area sites. *Arch Gen Psychiatry* 41:971, 1984.

Slap G, Vorters D, Chaudhuri S, et al: Risk factors for attempted suicide during adolescence. *Pediatrics* 84:762, 1989.

Summers WK, Rund DA, Levin ML: Psychiatric illness in general urban emergency room: Daytime versus night time population. *J Clin Psychiatry* 41:340, 1979.

Suokas J, Lonnqvist J: Work stress has negative effects on the attitudes of emergency personnel towards patients who attempt suicide. *Acta Psychiatr Scand* 79:474, 1989.

Tardiff K: Management of the violent patient in an emergency situation. *Psychiatr Clin North Am* 11:539, 1988.

Tobias C, Turns D, Lippman S, et al: The violent patient: What to do? *South Med J* 81:640, 1988.

Zun L, Gold I: A survey of the form of the mental status examination administered by emergency physicians. *Ann Emerg Med* 15:916, 1986.

199
PSYCHOTROPIC MEDICATIONS

Kathy E. Shy
Douglas A. Rund

More than one-third of all emergency department patients have diagnosable psychiatric illness, and one out of every five adults in the United States has received a prescription for a psychoactive drug. The emergency physician must be able to administer certain selected psychotropic medications appropriately and recognize and manage side effects, toxicities, and adverse interactions with other medications.

There are five major classes of psychotropic medications: antipsychotics; anxiolytics, sedatives, and hypnotics; heterocyclic antidepressants; monoamine oxidase (MAO) inhibitors; and lithium. Of these, only two, the antipsychotics and the anxiolytics, sedatives, and hypnotics, have undisputed utility on an emergency basis. Heterocyclic antidepressants, MAO inhibitors, and lithium are rarely prescribed by the emergency physician, primarily because they have long latencies of action and multiple side effects and require careful long-term monitoring. Only in exceptional circumstances, in consultation with a psychiatrist who agrees to provide follow-up care, might the emergency physician elect to initiate antidepressant or lithium therapy. Extensive pretreatment evaluation and detailed patient education weigh against prescribing lithium, MAO inhibitors, or heterocyclic antidepressants in the emergency department.

The emergency physician should be familiar with the emergency indications, common side effects, toxic reactions, and common interactions of the psychotropic medications. Caution in prescribing is the rule. Certain cases are bound to be complex, requiring detailed psychiatric evaluation, and serious medical disorders may coexist with psychiatric disorders. Patients with medical disorders, a history of serious side effects with psychotropic medication, or apparent need for more than one psychoactive medication usually require psychiatric consultation. Several excellent references deal in depth with side effects and toxicity of psychotropic medications (Baldessarini and Hyman).

ANTIPSYCHOTICS (NEUROLEPTICS)

Indications

Because antipsychotic medications are symptom-specific (not disease-specific), they are useful in nearly all psychoses, whether "functional," organic, or drug-induced. In the emergency setting, they are most often indicated to control agitated psychotic behavior that constitutes an imminent danger to the patient or others. Antipsychotic medications may also be the agents of choice to control nonpsychotic agitation in patients with acute sedative/hynotic or alcohol intoxication, since there is significant risk of respiratory depression if benzodiazepines are employed. Notable exceptions to these general principles are the regurgitating patient, who may aspirate if sedated, and the patient with anticholinergic psychosis, whose symptoms may worsen with antipsychotics.

A known allergy to a specific antipsychotic medication is a contraindication to its use and to use of other antipsychotic medications of the same class. Most patients who claim to be allergic to antipsychotic medications, however, actually describe a history of acute dystonic reactions when questioned more carefully. A history of malignant neuroleptic syndrome and pregnancy are relative contraindications, and hospitalization is indicated before antipsychotic medications are initiated in these patients.

Guidelines

Low-potency antipsychotics (Table 199-1) such as chlorpromazine (Thorazine) and thioridazine (Mellaril) may cause life-threatening hypotension and thus are rarely used in emergency medicine. High-potency antipsychotics such as haloperidol (Haldol) and fluphenazine (Prolixin) have relatively few anticholinergic and α-blocking effects and are remarkably safe, even at high doses. They are the emergency antipsychotic agents of choice.

Moderate dosages of antipsychotic medications have proven to be at least as effective as the larger dosages previously employed in rapid neuroleptization techniques and are probably safer. Clinical trials using predetermined fixed dosages of antipsychotics have failed to support routine use of dosages of more than 10 to 15 mg of haloperidol a day and suggest that higher dosages may actually be less effective. Optimal pharmacologic management of acute psychotic agitation, therefore, now typically combines antipsychotic medication on a scheduled basis with a PRN benzodiazepine if additional sedation is required. The high-potency antipsychotic and benzodiazepine combination is usually associated with fewer side effects than either agent used independently in higher dosages, and the benzodiazepine may actually offer some protection against neuroleptic side effects. A typical dosing regimen would be 5 mg haloperidol or its equivalent, either intramuscularly (IM) or orally (PO) (using the liquid concentration form) twice a day plus lorazepam, 1 to 2 mg PO or IM every 60 min as necessary. Dosages should be half of those described if the patient is elderly or debilitated.

Side Effects

Antipsychotics block dopamine receptors throughout the central nervous system (CNS). Dopamine receptor blockade in the mesolimbic areas accounts for their antipsychotic properties. Dopamine blockage in the nigrostriatal terminals is responsible for the majority of motor side effects, including acute dystonias, akathisia, and Parkinson's syndrome.

Table 199-1. Commonly Used Antipsychotic Agents

Generic Name	Brand Name	Approximate Equivalent Dose, mg	Relative Potency
	TRICYCLICS		
Phenothiazines			
Aliphatic			
Chlorpromazine	Thorazine	100	Low
Triflupromazine	Vesprine	30	Low
Piperidines			
Mesoridazine	Serentil	50	Intermediate
Thioridazine	Mellaril	100	Intermediate
Piperazines			
Acetophenazine	Tindal	15	Intermediate
Perphenazine	Trilafon	10	Intermediate
Trifluoperazine	Stelazine	5	High
Fluphenazine	Prolixin, Permitil	2	High
Thioxanthines			
Aliphatic			
Chlorprothixene	Taractan	100	Low
Piperazine			
Thiothixene	Navane	4	High
Dibenzapine			
Loxapine	Loxitane, Daxolin	15	Intermediate
	NONTRICYCLICS		
Dihydroindolone			
Molindone	Moban	10	Intermediate
Butyrophenones			
Haloperidol	Haldol	2	High
Droperidol	Inapsine (for injection)	2	High

Acute dystonias, which usually occur in young males during the first few days of antipsychotic treatment, are probably the most common side effect of antipsychotic medications seen in the emergency department. Muscle spasms of the neck, face, and back are the most common dystonias, but oculogyric crisis and even laryngospasm may also occur. When a drug history is not carefully obtained, dystonias are often misdiagnosed as primary neurologic illnesses (seizures, meningitis, tetanus, etc.). Treatment with either 1 to 2 mg of benztropine (Cogentin) intravenously (IV) or 25 to 50 mg of diphenhydramine (Benadryl) IV rapidly corrects the dystonia. Dystonias often recur, even if the antipsychotic is decreased or discontinued, however, unless an antiparkinson drug such as benztropine, 1 mg PO two to four times daily, is administered over the next several days.

Akathisia, a sensation of motor restlessness with a subjective desire to move, can begin several days to several weeks after initiation of antipsychotic treatment. Often misdiagnosed as anxiety or exacerbation of psychiatric illness, akathisia is aggravated by subsequent increases in antipsychotic dosage. Other extrapyramidal effects, such as cogwheel rigidity and shuffling gait, suggest antipsychotic effect, but these signs are not invariably present. Management is difficult. If possible, the dosage of the antipsychotic should be decreased. Antiparkinson drugs, such as benztropine (Cogentin), 1 mg PO two to four times daily, may also afford some relief. In refractory cases, the antipsychotic may need to be changed or an alternative form of therapy tried.

Antipsychotic-induced *Parkinson's syndrome* is particularly common in the elderly and usually begins in the first month of treatment. A complete Parkinson's syndrome, including bradykinesia, resting tremor, cogwheel rigidity, shuffling gait, masked facies, and drooling, can occur, but often only one or two features of the syndrome are obvious. Antipsychotic dosage reduction and/or anticholinergic medication is usually effective.

While antidopaminergic side effects such as acute dystonia, akathisia, and Parkinson's syndrome occur more often with high-potency neuroleptics, anticholinergic and anti-α-adrenergic effects are usually seen with low-potency neuroleptics. Both anticholinergic and α-blocking effects are dose related and much more common in the elderly.

Anticholinergic effects range from mild sedation to delirium. Peripheral manifestations may include dry mouth and skin, blurred vision, urinary retention, constipation, paralytic ileus, cardiac arrhythmias, and exacerbation of narrow-angle glaucoma. The central anticholinergic syndrome is characterized by dilated pupils, dysarthria, and an agitated delirium. Discontinuation of the antipsychotic and institution of supportive measures is the most prudent therapy. Physostigmine, 1 to 2 mg administered slowly IV, may temporarily reverse the syndrome but may be very toxic and should be reserved for life-threatening situations.

Cardiovascular side effects are seen almost exclusively with low-potency antipsychotics. α-Adrenergic blockade and a negative inotropic effect on the myocardium may cause pronounced orthostatic hypotension and, rarely, cardiovascular collapse. Usually the hypotension can be easily managed with IV fluids. In severe cases, agonists, such as metaraminol (Aramine) or norepinephrine (Levophed), may be required.

Neuroleptic malignant syndrome (NMS) is an uncommon idiosyncratic reaction to neuroleptic drugs manifested by rigidity, fever, autonomic instability (tachycardia, diaphoresis, and blood pressure abnormalities), and a confusional state. Elevation of muscle enzymes, such as creatinine phosphokinase (CPK) and aldolase; the white blood cell count; and liver function tests are often seen. While high-potency antipsychotics may be more likely to cause the disorder, all antipsychotics are potential offenders. NMS is a medical emergency and has a mortality rate as high as 20 percent. Management includes immediate discontinuation of the antipsychotic medication and meticulous supportive treatment in an intensive care setting. Medications such as dantrolene sodium or bromocriptine are sometimes used to relieve the rigidity.

Overdose

While antipsychotics are rarely fatal when taken alone, overdose can present some unique management problems. With the exception of thioridazine (Mellaril), antipsychotics are potent antiemetics. The antiemetic effect may interfere with pharmacologic induction of emesis, and gastric lavage is often required. Agents with β-agonist activity such as isopreoterenol (Isuprel) are contraindicated for cardiovascular support because β-stimulated vasodilatation may worsen hypotension. Extrapyramidal effects may also be prominent in antipsychotic overdosage and are best treated with 25 to 50 mg of diphenhydramine (Benadryl) IV.

Clozapine

Clozapine (Clozaril) is a new "atypical" antipsychotic medication that is preferentially more active at limbic than at striatal dopamine receptors and causes little or no extrapyramidal side effects. Unfortunately, it is more likely to produce agranulocytosis than are standard antipsychotic medications, and its use is therefore reserved for patients with schizophrenia unresponsive to standard agents or for those suffering from severe extrapyramidal side effects or tardive dyskinesia with the standard agents. It is strongly sedating and strongly anticholinergic and has considerable hypotensive effects. It also poses a substantial risk for inducing seizures, particularly when higher doses are used. Fatal overdosages have been reported, usually at dosages over 2500 mg. Altered sensorium, delirium, coma, tachycardia, hypotension, respiratory depression, and sialorrhea are the most commonly reported features of overdose.

ANXIOLYTICS

Indications

Severe emotional distress may indicate psychotropic medication even if the patient is not psychotic or an imminent threat to him- or herself or others. While not a substitute for psychotherapy, short-term anxiolytic therapy may be particularly beneficial in the anxious, agitated patient during a psychosocial crisis. Anxiolytics are also indicated for acute pain reactions unresponsive to reassurance.

Anxiolytics also have utility in medical and surgical emergencies. Nonpsychiatric uses include facilitation of cooperation and muscle relaxation during painful procedures; controlling seizures; treating alcohol, sedative, or hypnotic withdrawal; and allaying anxiety when a painful procedure such as surgery has been delayed.

Benzodiazepines are contraindicated in patients with known hypersensitivity to benzodiazepines and in acute, narrow-angle glaucoma. Pregnancy, particularly in the first trimester, is a relative contraindication.

Guidelines

Before prescribing anxiolytics, the emergency physician should try to rule out any serious underlying psychiatric illness. Because agitation and anxiety may indicate incipient psychosis or major affective disorder, anxiolytics should be used with extreme caution in patients with a history of major psychiatric illness. The possibility that a patient may be feigning illness to procure controlled substances should also be considered.

Benzodiazepines are very effective anxiolytics with a high therapeutic index. Nonbenzodiazepine anxiolytics (e.g., barbiturates and propanediols) have low therapeutic indices and high addition potential. Except in the rare case of an allergy to benzodiazepines, nonbenzodiazepine anxiolytics have little use in modern psychopharmacology. Buspirone hydrochloride (BuSpar), an atypical anxiolytic medication that does not interact with the benzodiazepine-GABA receptor complex, has a delayed onset of action of days to weeks, which makes it impractical for use in emergent situations. Since it does not have cross-

Table 199-2. Commonly Used Benzodiazepines

Generic Name	Brand Name	Approximate Half-life, h	Usual Total Oral Dose, mg
	ANXIOLYTICS*		
Alprazolam	Xanax	12	1–6
Chlorazepate	Tranxene	48	15–60
Chlordiazepoxide	Librium	20	15–100
Diazepam	Valium	35	15–60
Lorazepam	Ativan	16	2–6
Midazolam	Versed	2	—‡
Oxazepam	Serax	15	20–60
Prazepam	Centrax	15 + 100†	20–60
	HYPNOTICS		
Flurazepam	Dalmane	2 + 72†	15–30 qhs
Temazepam	Restoril	15	15–30 qhs
Triazolam	Halcion	2	0.125–0.5 qhs

* Anxiolytics are administered in divided doses, usually three or four times daily.

† Flurazepam and prazepam have active metabolites with long half-lives.

‡ Midazolam is available for parenteral use only.

tolerance with other sedative/hypnotics or alcohol, it is not useful in treatment of sedative/hypnotic or alcohol withdrawal.

Certain benzodiazepines have relatively long half-lives (Table 199-2), including diazepam (Valium), chlordiazepoxide (Librium), flurazepam (Dalmane), and prazepam (Centrax). Agents with long half-lives gradually accumulate in the body and thus have a greater potential for causing sedation and confusion, particularly in the elderly. For short-term use, these agents may benefit the young, healthy person in crisis who complains of insomnia but is also anxious during the day. A single bedtime dose both induces sleep and has a mild anxiolytic effect the following day. For the most part, however, with the exception of the use of diazepam in seizures, short-acting benzodiazepines such as lorazepam (Ativan), oxazepam (Serax), and alprozolam (Xanax) are the preferred agents in emergency medicine. Alprozolam (Xanax), 0.25 to 0.50 mg PO, is a particularly effective treatment in acute panic attack. Only midazolam (Versed), a very short-acting agent, and lorazepam (Ativan) have reliable intramuscular absorption. Lorazepam, an agent with very low cardiopulmonary toxicity, is particularly well suited for emergency use. Dosages of 1 to 2 mg PO or IM are usually effective. As with all benzodiazepines, dosage adjustments may be necessary: higher dosages may be required in patients with histories of alcohol or sedative/hypnotic abuse; lower dosages, in patients with hepatic disease or severe debilitation. Because they potentiate other CNS depressants, benzodiazepines should be used with extreme caution in intoxicated patients.

Side Effects

Benzodiazepine side effects are usually mild and easily treated. Drowsiness, decreased mental alertness, sedation, and ataxia are the most common side effects. Such effects can usually be managed conservatively by decreasing the dose and advising the patient to avoid potentially hazardous activities, such as driving or operating dangerous machinery. Infrequent paradoxical responses of insomnia and agitation are more common in the elderly and require discontinuation of the medication. Because benzodiazepines have abuse potential and high street value, the emergency physician should never prescribe more than a week's supply.

Overdose

Benzodiazepines are rarely fatal in overdose unless taken in combination with other drugs or alcohol. Conservative supportive management is the best approach.

HETEROCYCLIC ANTIDEPRESSANTS (HCAs)

Although tricyclic antidepressants (named for their three-ring structure) were first synthesized in the nineteenth century, their antidepressant properties were not recognized until the late 1950s. Since that time, tetracyclic and other "-cyclic" antidepressant agents have been formulated, thus creating need for the more general term *heterocyclic* (Table 199-3). The therapeutic effect of HCAs is believed to be related to their ability to block presynaptic reuptake of norepinephrine and serotonin and thus increase the interneuronal amount of these neurotransmitters in the CNS. HCAs are the drugs of choice for major depression, and they may also be effective for dysthymia, panic disorder, agoraphobia, obsessive compulsive disorder, enuresis, and school phobia. As previously advised, initiation of HCA therapy in the emergency department is not routinely recommended.

Side Effects

HCAs have low therapeutic indices. Side effects are common and often occur with customary dosages, even though serum levels may be within the designated therapeutic range. The majority of side effects are either anticholinergic or cardiotoxic.

Anticholinergic side effects are the most common. They are particularly likely to occur with concomitant use of other drugs with anticholinergic properties, such as low-potency antipsychotics, antiparkinsonian agents, antihistamines, and over-the-counter sleeping remedies. Both peripheral and central effects may occur. Peripheral effects include dry mouth, metallic taste, blurred vision, constipation, paralytic ileus, urinary retention, tachycardia, and exacerbation of narrow-angle glaucoma. Central effects include sedation, mydriasis, agitation, and delirium. Mild to moderately severe anticholinergic effects may be managed by dosage reduction, change to a medication with fewer anticholinergic properties, or addition of urecoline, 10 to 25 mg PO three times daily. For acute urinary retention, urecoline, 2.5 to 5 mg, may be given subcutaneously. With therapeutic doses, anticholinergic effects become life-threatening, physostigmine, 1 to 2 mg administered *very slowly* IV, may be used. If physostigmine toxicities ensue, the effects can be reversed with IV atropine sulfate, 0.5 mg for each 1.0 mg of physostigmine administered.

Cardiac side effects of HCAs may include nonspecific T-wave changes, prolonged QT interval, varying degrees of AV block, and atrial and ventricular arrhythmias. Orthostatic hypotension from α-adrenergic blockage may be significant, particularly in the elderly.

HCA therapy may also be complicated by allergic obstructive jaundice; decreased seizure threshold (especially with maprotiline); and, very rarely, agranulocytosis.

Table 199-3. Commonly Used Heterocyclic Antidepressants

Generic Name	Brand Name	Usual Dose, mg/day
	TRICYCLICS	
Amitriptyline	Amitril, Elavil, Endep	75–200
Amoxapine	Asendin	100–300
Desipramine	Norprammin, Pertofrane	75–200
Doxepin	Adapin, Curetin, Sinequan	75–200
Imipramine	Janimine, Presamine, SK-Pramine, Tofranil	75–200
Nortriptyline	Aventyl, Pamelor	40–150
Protriptyline	Vivactil	15–40
Trimipramine	Surmontil	75–200
	OTHERS	
Maprotiline	Ludiomil	100–150
Trazodone	Desyrel	100–200

Overdose

HCA overdose is potentially fatal and, unfortunately, increasingly common, particularly in younger age groups. In addition to the anticholinergic toxicities previously described, cardiac and CNS toxicities are often severe. Death may occur from hypotension, cardiac arrhythmias, CNS depression, or seizures. Serum levels above 1000 mg/mL and/or QRS complex duration of greater than 0.10 s are ominous.

Therapy of HCA overdose begins with cardiopulmonary stabilization and gastric lavage followed by activated charcoal. The arrhythmogenic effect of tricyclic compounds such as amitriptylie may be attributed to their direct local anesthetic actions in blocking sodium channels in cardiac membranes. Sodium bicarbonate administration seems to result in increased extracellular sodium concentration and diminished local anesthetic effect of such compounds. Alkalinization of the blood using sodium bicarbonate is therefore the initial therapy of choice for cardiac arrhythmias. Approximately 3 mEq/kg of sodium bicarbonate can be given over 1 to 3 min by IV push (although doses of 18 to 36 mEq/kg have been used successfully in animal models). The arterial blood pH should be maintained around 7.45 by continual bicarbonate infusion as needed.

Diazepam and phenytoin are considered the drugs of first choice for HCA-induced seizures. Short-acting barbiturates are contraindicated because of their potential for exacerbating both hypotension and CNS depression.

MONOAMINE OXIDASE INHIBITORS (MAOIs)

MAO catalyzes the oxidation of biogenic amines (tyramine, serotonin, dopamine, and norepinephrine) throughout the body. The therapeutic effect of MAOIs is probably related to their ability to increase norepinephrine and serotonin in the CNS. They are recommended for "atypical" depressions, characterized by hyperphagia, hypersomnolence, reversed diurnal variation (worse in the evening), emotional lability, and rejection hypersensitivity. They are also occasionally useful in selected cases of HCA-refractory major depression and panic disorder (although the latter use is not yet approved by the FDA). Only two agents in this class, phenelzine (Nardil) and tranylcypromine (Parnate), are commonly used in the Untied States. As with HCAs, initiation of therapy in the emergency department is not recommended. The physician who initiates MAOI therapy must have firmly established an appropriate indication for use and provided the patient with extensive counseling about toxic interactions with numerous medications and foods.

Side Effects

In general, MAOIs have fewer side effects than do HCAs. *Orthostatic hypotension,* although occasionally severe, usually responds to supportive therapy. *CNS irritability,* including agitation, motor restlessness, and insomnia, is managed by dosage reduction or addition of a benzodiazepine. Occasionally, MAOIs, like other antidepressant medications, actually precipitate a manic episode. *Autonomic side effects,* such as dry mouth, constipation, urinary retention, and delayed ejaculation, sometimes occur but are usually mild.

MAOIs block oxidative deamination of tyramine and may precipitate a *hypertensive crisis* when certain drugs, such as sympathomimetic amines, L-dopa, narcotics, or HCAs, or tyramine-containing foods are ingested. Common tyramine-containing foods include aged cheese, beer, wine, pickled herring, yeast extracts, chopped liver, yogurt, sour cream, and fava beans. The onset of the crisis is usually heralded by a severe headache. While hypertension is potentially the most serious effect, cardiac arrhythmias, restlessness, diaphoresis, mydriasis, and vomiting may also occur. Mild cases of hypertension may respond to chlorpromazine (Thorazine), 25 to 50 mg IM. In more severe cases, an α antagonist, such as phentolamine 5 mg IV, repeated as necessary, is indicated. β Blocking agents are contraindicated, since they may intensify vasoconstriction and worsen hypertension. Although death may occur from hypertensive intracranial hemorrhage, the vast majority of patients recover completely from the hypertensive episode within a few hours. The MAOI can be restarted the following day after dietary counseling is reinforced.

Drug-drug interactions often complicate MAOI therapy. MAOIs potentiate the actions of sympathomimetics, anticholinergics, and oral hypoglycemics. They also inhibit metabolic degradation of alcohol, barbiturates, and narcotics. When combined with meperidine (Demerol), MAOIs may cause a variety of adverse effects, including hypotension, hypertension, fever, and neuromuscular irritability. While the interactions listed are among the most common, the list is far from exhaustive. More comprehensive accounts may be found in standard references.

Overdose

Deaths, usually from malignant hyperthermia, have been reported from relatively small doses (170 mg of tranylcypromine, 375 mg of phenelzine) of MAOIs. Symptoms, which may also include agitation, delirium, muscular rigidity, tachycardia, and seizures, may be delayed in onset by up to 12 h after ingestion. Therapy is basically supportive, although excretion of tranylcypromine may be enhanced by forced diuresis and urinary acidification.

SECOND-GENERATION ANTIDEPRESSANTS

Two atypical antidepressant medications, fluoxetine (Prozac) and bupropion (Wellbutrin), have recently been introduced.

Fluoxetine

Fluoxetine is a unique cyclic antidepressant that is a potent reuptake inhibitor of serotonin with the strongest serotonergic activity of all available antidepressants. It appears to lack significant anticholinergic effects and the cardiovascular effects seen with other cyclic antidepressants. The most common side effects are nausea, anorexia, anxiety, jitteriness, insomnia, headache, tremor, diarrhea, light-headedness, and drowsiness. Seizures may also occur. Clinical experience with fluoxetine overdose is limited. Nausea, vomiting, agitation, hypomania, insomnia, and tremor are the most commonly reported signs and symptoms. Mild electrocardiographic changes (sinus tachycardia, nonspecific ST-T wave changes, and ST segment depression) and seizures have also been reported. Two patients enrolled in initial clinical fluoxetine trials died of overdoses. Both patients, however, overdosed on a combination of other medications that included HCAs.

Bupropion

Bupropion is an aminoketone, structurally distinct from previous antidepressants. The mechanism of its antidepressant effect is unknown; it has very little effect on serotonin or norepinephrine uptake and few anticholinergic or antihisaminic effects. Its side effect profile is similar to that of fluoxetine. Dry mouth, dizziness, headache, tremor, insomina, and psychomotor agitation are the most commonly reported side effects. Anticholinergic and cardiovascular effects are minimal. Seizures may occur, particularly in bulimic patients. Its use is contraindicated in patients with histories of eating disorders, head trauma, or any other predisposition toward seizures, including medications that could lower seizure threshold. While clinical experience with overdoses has been limited, overdoses of from 900 to 3000 mg have been easily managed without any cardiovascular problems. On the basis of animal studies, it is recommended that seizures associated with overdoses be treated with benzodiazepines.

LITHIUM

Lithium carbonate is indicated for both acute mania and maintenance therapy in bipolar disorder. It also has utility in some cases of major depression (both unipolar and bipolar) and in some disorders characterized by episodic explosive outbursts or self-mutilation. Its mechanism of action is unknown, although it does increase central norepinephrine reuptake and decrease central norepinephrine release. The extensive pretreatment evaluation and long latency of action preclude the use of lithium as an emergency psychotropic medication.

Side Effects

Patients vary widely in susceptibility to lithium side effects. While most of the serious adverse effects are associated with toxic serum levels, mild side effects such as gastrointestinal distress, dry mouth, excessive thirst, fine tremors, mild polyuria, and peripheral edema are often seen even when serum levels lie within the designated therapeutic range. This is particularly common during the first few weeks of therapy. Many of the more chronic side effects, including polyuria, nephrogenic diabetes insipidus, benign diffuse goiter, hypothyroidism, skin rashes and ulcerations, psoriasis, and leukocytosis without a left shift, appear unrelated to serum lithium levels. Underlying neurologic illness, dehydration, salt-restricted diets, and childbirth predispose to both minor and major side effects.

Toxicity and Overdose

The severity of lithium toxicity is related to both the serum lithium level and the duration of the elevated level. Even in acute overdose, symptoms may not be fully apparent for up to 48 h. As a general rule, lithium toxicity is rare at serum levels of less than 2 mEq/L. Early signs of toxicity include nausea and vomiting, dysarthria, lethargy, and a coarse hand tremor. As toxicity worsens, neurologic symptoms increase. Ataxia, myasthenia, incoordination, hyperreflexia, muscle fasciculation, blurred vision, and scotomas may develop. Eventually, confusion, choreoathetosis, myoclonus, and seizures occur, and the patient may finally become comatose. Cardiovascular toxicity is unusual at serum levels of less than 4 mEq/L. In addition to nonspecific T-wave changes, high lithium levels may be associated with hypotension, AV conduction defects, ventricular tachyarrhythmias, and eventually complete cardiovascular collapse.

Because lithium toxicity may cause permanent brain damage, it should be considered a medical emergency. General supportive care, with particular attention to fluid and electrolyte balance, is the foundation of therapy. Lithium excretion may be facilitated by forced saline diuresis and alkalization of the urine with IV sodium lactate. Mannitol, 50 to 100 mg IV, may also be added to promote osmotic diuresis. Aminophylline, 500 mg given slowly IV, also promotes lithium clearance by both suppressing renal tubular reabsorption of lithium and increasing renal blood flow. If the serum level exceeds a 4 mEq/L, the patient should be dialyzed immediately. Dialysis may also be required for serum levels in the range of 2 to 4 mEq/L if the patient's clinical condition is poor.

BIBLIOGRAPHY

Baldessarini RJ: *Chemotherapy in Psychiatry*. Cambridge, MA, Harvard University Press, 1985.

Baldessarini RJ, et al: Significance of neuroleptic dose and plasma level in the pharmacological treatment of psychoses. *Arch Gen Psychiatry* 45:79, 1988.

Bernstein JG: *Handbook of Drug Therapy in Psychiatry*, 2d ed. Littleton, MA, PSG Publishing, 1988.

Boehnert MT, Lovejoy FJ: Value of the QRS duration versus the serum drug level in predicting seizures and ventricular arrhythmias after an acute overdosage of tricyclic antidepressants. *N Engl J Med* 313:474, 1985.

Fauman BS, Fauman MA: *Emergency Psychiatry for the House Officer*. Baltimore, Williams & Wilkins, 1981.

Gelenberg, AJ: Fluoxetine (Prozac) overdose. *Biol Ther Psychiatry Newsl* 12:11, 1989.

Gilman AG, Goodman LS, Rall TW, et al (eds): *Goodman and Gilman's Pharmacological Basis of Therapeutics*, 7th ed. New York, Macmillan, 1985.

Hillard JR (ed): *Manual of Clinical Emergency Psychiatry*. Washington, D.C., American Psychiatric Press, 1990.

Hollister LE, Csernanasky: *Clinical Pharmacology of Psychotherapeutic Drugs*, 3d ed. New York, Churchill Livingstone, 1990.

Hyman SE (ed): *Manual of Psychiatric Emergencies*, 2d ed. Boston, Little, Brown, 1988.

Kaplan HI, Sadock BJ: *Comprehensive Textbook of Psychiatry*, 4th ed. Baltimore, Williams, & Wilkins, 1985.

Rund DA, Hutzler JC: *Emergency Psychiatry*. St. Louis, Mosby, 1983.

Salby AE, Lieb J, Trancredi LR: *The Handbook of Psychiatric Emergencies*, 3d ed. New York, Elsevier, 1986.

Sasyniuk BI, Jhamandas V, Valois W: Experimental amitriptyline intoxication: Treatment of cardiac toxicity with sodium bicarbonate. *Ann Emerg Med* 15:1052, 1986.

Settle EC Jr: Bupropion: A novel antidepressant—update 1989. *Int Drug Ther Newsl* 24:29, 1989.

Tomb DA: *Psychiatry for the House Officer*, 2d ed. Baltimore, Williams & Wilkins, 1984.

Walker JI: *Psychiatric Emergenices*. Philadelphia, Lippincott, 1983.

200
ANOREXIA NERVOSA AND BULIMIA NERVOSA

Alexander H. Sackeyfio
Susan J. Gottlieb

Anorexia nervosa and bulimia nervosa have reached epidemic proportions in the past 10 years. These diseases were once viewed as purely psychological in nature. However, increasing evidence has confirmed that both disorders involve physical complications, and knowledge of and ability to treat the medical complications that accompany eating disorders are crucial for the patient's well-being.

Eating disorders affect between 5 to 10 percent of adolescent girls and young women, and up to 0.10 percent of males. Originally regarded as rich girls' diseases, they are now recognized across all socioeconomic and racial groups, in patients between the ages of 8 and 80. The onset of anorexia is usually between 12 years of age and the mid-thirties, with a bimodal distribution of ages 13 to 14 and 17 to 18. Bulimia usually begins between the ages of 17 and 25. The onset of both disorders has been reported in older persons.

Anorexia, with its resulting starvation syndrome, is more likely to be recognized than bulimia, which is frequently concealed from both family and physician. Table 200-1 lists the signs and symptoms that suggest a diagnosis of anorexia, and Table 200-2 lists the signs and symptoms of bulimia.

Anorexic patients may present with one or all of the following:

1. Refusal to maintain body weight over a minimum normal weight for age and height, for example, weight loss, or failure to make expected weight gain during a period of growth, leading to body weight 15 percent below normal.
2. Intense fear of becoming obese even when underweight.
3. Disturbance in the way in which body weight, shape, or size is perceived. For example, the obviously underweight or even emaciated patient may complain of being fat, or may believe that one area of the body is "too fat."
4. Absence of at least three consecutive expected menstrual cycles (primary or secondary amenorrhea).

A diagnosis of bulimia is suggested by the following:

1. A minimum average of two episodes of binge eating (rapid consumption of a large amount of food in a short period of time) per week for at least 3 months.
2. During the eating binges, there is a feeling of lack of control over the eating behavior.
3. The individual regularly engages in self-induced vomiting, use of laxatives, strict dieting, fasting, or vigorous exercising in order to prevent weight gain.
4. Persistent overconcern with body shape and weight.

Families of patients with eating disorders tend to be outwardly orderly, respectable, and conventional. However, the inner dynamics of the family involve a rigid adherence to secret obligations and stifling prohibitions. Honesty and spontaneity are discouraged, and true autonomy and self-gratification are submerged beneath the adolescent's desire to please and gain approval from other family members.

Table 200-1. Clues to Undiagnosed Anorexia Nervosa

1. Unexplained growth retardation (individual may be actively or passively affected)
2. Unexplained primary amenorrhea
3. Weight loss of unknown origin
4. Unexplained hypercholesterolemia or carotenemia in a thin person
5. Exercise abuse
6. Membership in a vulnerable vocation group (see Table 200-2, item 10)

ETIOLOGY

The onset of anorexia most often occurs during adolescence. Normal physiologic changes which are preparation for the reproductive function, namely an increase in total body fat (up to 200 percent in adolescent females) as well as the accumulation of fat around the chest and hips, are perceived as "fatness," and the adolescent begins to diet to lose the unwanted weight. Various reasons have been proposed for the progression of "normal" dieting into an eating disorder. Some feel that for the anorexic, restriction of eating serves as part of a general need to control impulses and disturbing feelings. Others have suggested that the central problem might be an avoidance of adulthood, an emergent panic related to the challenges of late adolescence and the loss of the security enjoyed by the child and early adolescent.

Bulimics have an intense need for approval, a high self-expectation, and a poor body image. Binging provides escape from boredom, anger, and loneliness and is sometimes a preferred social experience, especially when interpersonal intimacy has been elusive. Purging only adds an already negative self-image. Binge eating in bulimics almost always begins as a response to hunger from dieting and weight loss. Late in the syndrome, binge eating becomes generalized to deal with emotional distress.

DIFFERENTIAL DIAGNOSIS

The differential diagnosis includes both psychiatric and medical disorders. Schizophrenics can present with an aversion to eating and sometimes with eating and purging. In depressive illness, anorexia and hyperphagia can be part of the presenting symptoms. Hysterics, inadequate personality disorders, and patients with borderline personality disorders may also exhibit eating disorders.

A number of medical disorders should be considered, including superior mesentric artery syndrome, inflammatory bowel disease, chronic hepatitis, Addison's disease, diabetes, hyperthyroidism, hyperemesis gravidarum, tuberculosis, and malignancy.

About 20 percent of teenage diabetics also have an eating disorder.

Extremely thin people in professions requiring low weight (such as ballet dancers, models, and jockeys) and obligatory runners may or may not have an eating disorder.

PATHOPHYSIOLOGY

Eating disorders are associated with a number of physiologic changes (Table 200-3). Self-induced vomiting results in various disorders. Dental problems are caused by gastric acid regurgitated into the oral cavity.

Table 200-2. Signs and Symptoms of Bulimia in Adolescents and Young Adults

1. Hypokalemia of unknown cause or complications of hypokalemia (cardiac, renal, CNS)
2. Parotid gland or submandibular gland enlargement; esophagitis; esophageal bleeding or rupture
3. Large unexplained weight fluctuations or weight loss
4. Unexplained elevations of serum amylase
5. Unexplained secondary amenorrhea
6. Extensive loss of dental enamel or onset of many new caries
7. Scars on the knuckles of the hand (from induced vomiting)
8. Presence of juvenile diabetes mellitus
9. Other disorders of impulse control—alcoholism, drug abuse, borderline personality disorder
10. Member of predisposed vocational group—models, ballet students or professionals, wrestlers, jockeys

Table 200-3. Physiologic Changes Associated with Eating Disorders

Hematologic
Normochromic and normocytic anemia
Leukopenia with relative lymphocytosis
Low sedimentation rate
Reduced C3 complement
Biochemical
Hypokalemia
Hyponatremia
Hypomagnesemia
Hypocalcemia
Hypophosphatemia
Carbohydrate metabolism
Low serum insulin levels
High serum glucagon levels
Starvation ketosis and hypoglycemia
Abnormal glucose tolerance due to fasting
Hypercholesterolemia
Endocrine
Normal T4 but low T3
High serum cortisol without diurnal variation
Low serum LH, FSH, and estradiol
Low total urinary estrogens
Increased growth hormone
Pseudo Bartter's syndrome (laxative and diuretic abusers)
Decreased ADH secretion (diabetes insipidus)
Decreased peripheral adrenergic activity with normal adrenomedullary function

In addition, the oral hygiene of most anorexics is poor, and the vigorous brushing often done by bulimics aggravates dental problems. This poor oral hygiene, together with dietary difficiencies and dehydration of the soft tissues of the mouth, can cause gingivitis and dental erosion.

Parotid and submandibular gland enlargement is often seen. Oral lacerations and contusions, and callous formations on knuckles from stimulating the gag reflex, are common. Dysphagia, hematemesis, and rarely rupture of the esophagus, subcutaneous emphysema, or pneumomediastinum can occur following excessive purging. Easy bruising due to loss of bile salts and poor absorption of vitamin K is another complication. Severe hypokalemia and hypovolemia often accompany recurrent vomiting. Ipecac abuse can cause a dermatomyositis-like syndrome and cardiomyopathy. Hyperamylasemia, probably of salivary gland origin, is associated with purging episodes.

Laxative abuse produces weight loss mainly by dehydration and hypokalemia. Common nonspecific complaints of laxative abuse include constipation, diarrhea, abdominal cramping, and bloating. Specific effects include melanosis coli and cathartic colon. In cathartic colon, the colon is converted into an inert tube incapable of propelling the fecal stream without large doses of laxatives. This condition is not entirely reversible and may require colectomy. Brownish grainy hyperpigmented areas on the skin are reported as complications of phenolphthalein-containing laxatives (Correctol, Ex-Lax).

Diuretic abuse results in dehydration and multiple serum abnormalities including hypokalemia, hypercalcemia, hyperuricemia, hypomagnesemia, and hyponatremia.

Binge eating after a period of starvation can result in acute gastric distension and/or pancreatitis. Postbinge pancreatitis has a reported 10 percent mortality rate.

Periods of starvation result in hypoglycemia, which is a poor prognostic indicator. Hypoglycemia is often associated with hypothermia, coma, and infections, and may be fatal. Starvation leads to low insulin levels that are insensitive to both glucose and amino acid infusion. Gastric distension and reduced gastric emptying produce enhanced satiation and prolonged intermeal intervals. Food has been demonstrated to remain in the stomachs of anorexics for up to 24 h.

Starvation causes a decreased hypoxic ventilatory drive decreased vital capacity, tidal volume, and minute ventilation. In addition, the surfactant pool is reduced, resulting in "stiffer" lungs with a greater tendency to collapse. The muscles of ventilation are affected by starvation, causing reduced diaphragm mass and respiratory muscle weakness.

Cardiovascular changes include brady- and tachyarrhythmias due to cardiomyopathy or electrolyte abnormalities. ST-T-wave changes, and Q-T-interval prolongation, may be evident. Decreased peripheral adrenergic activity with normal adrenomedullary function results in bradycardia and orthostatic hypotension.

Dermatologic changes include pedal or pretibial edema, with or without hypoalbuminemia; excessive loss of subcutaneous fat; brittle hair and nails; pellagra or scurvy; and petechiae or purpura.

Peripheral neuropathy, most likely a product of chronic malnutrition, is a notable complication. Localized compression neuropathies secondary to subcutaneous tissue loss can also develop. Some patients experience paresthesias of the fingers and toes. Deep tendon reflexes may be diminished, and gross motor coordination may be impaired.

Anorexics are especially likely to be compulsive exercisers. Stress fractures in the feet, march hemoglobinuria, and various musculoskeletal overuse syndromes have been identified in our institution as complications of compulsive exercise.

Osteoporosis is common in anorexics. It usually affects the femur, radius, and spine in decreasing frequency. Estrogen deficiency is not a major causative factor. Any patient with an eating disorder who has been amenorrheic and low in weight for more than a year should undergo bone density studies. We have seen a femur fracture in a young anorexic who tripped on a rug.

Adolescent diabetics induce ketosis by skipping insulin for a day or two to lose weight; sometimes they overeat and increase insulin in compensation. The abuse of insulin and food can lead to severe metabolic consequences. Young diabetics with frequent hospitalizations should be evaluated for a coexisting eating disorder.

PSYCHOLOGICAL PRESENTATIONS

In addition to the presenting physical symptoms, psychological manifestations may also be detected on emergency evaluation. Depression, including suicidal ideation, is the primary psychological complication of eating disorders. Other psychological manifestions include obsessive-compulsive personality traits, with rumination about food, calories, and weight. Ritualistic eating and exercising behavior are also evident. Perfectionistic striving often results in deterioration of friendships and leisure activities.

Impulse control disorder is a psychological complication of eating disorders more commonly seen in bulimics than anorexics. Behavioral manifestations include shoplifting and stealing, sexual promiscuity, drug and alcohol abuse, and self-mutilation.

PROGNOSIS

As with most illnesses, the earlier the onset, detection, and treatment the better the prognosis. The prognosis for individuals who have engaged in maladaptive eating patterns for years is guarded. Behaviors may remain constant or the patient may improve briefly and return to the eating disorder during stressful times. Chronicity increases the risk of morbidity.

In spite of the advances in the understanding of anorexia and bulimia nervosa, the emergence of multidisciplinary treatment teams, and current research on effective management, eating disorders are still associated with significant long-term morbidity and mortality. Psychological immaturity persists in about 50 percent of the patients, with difficulties in social adjustment, and one-third continue to have problems with eating.

Mortality figures range from 2 to 5 percent to a high of 18 percent. Death may result from suicide, starvation, metabolic catastrophe, infection, and cardiac insufficiency. Agents used to induce weight loss may lead to fatal complications.

TREATMENT

Emergency management of the patient with an eating disorder involves consideration of the complications and effects of the disorder.

Hypokalemia is always coexistent with hypovolemia and other metabolic disturbances. Aggressive replacement with isotopic saline thiamine, multivitamins,and magnesium should also be given. Discharge with potassium supplements is inappropriate. Refeeding for anorexics has to take into account the delayed gastric emptying, the deficiency of lipases and lactases,impaired cholescystokinin production, and the likelihood of refeeding edema.

A period of 48 h in an inpatient setting is essential to determine the extent and severity of the illness and its complications. An eating disorders unit is a place for this evaluation, but a regular medical floor with involvement of a multidisciplinary psychiatric and internal medicine team is advised.

Hospitalization is suggested for the following:

1. Weight loss greater than 30 percent over 3 months
2. Severe metabolic disturbance
3. Depression severe enough to be at risk for suicide
4. Severe binging and purging
5. Failure to maintain outpatient weight contract
6. Psychosis
7. Family crisis
8. Need to confront patient and family denial
9. Need for initiation of therapy (individual, family, and/or pharmacotherapy)
10. Complex differential diagnosis

A trial of outpatient psychological treatment can be attempted if food restriction and weight loss are of less than 3 month's duration, and if there is a very positive family support system. Referral to a local health professional who specializes in the treatment of eating disorders or to a self-help group can be obtained by contacting the following national organizations:

National Association of Anorexia Nervosa and Associated Disorders (ANAD)
P.O. Box 271
Highland Park, IL 60035
(312) 831–3438

Anorexia Nervosa and Related Eating Disorders, Inc.
P.O. Box 5102
Eugene, OR 97405
(503) 344–1144

American Anorexic/Bulimic Association, Inc.
133 Cedar Lane
Teaneck, NJ 07666
(201) 836–1800

National Anorexic Aid Society, Inc.
P.O. Box 29461
Columbus, OH 43229
(614) 895–2009

Center for the Study of Anorexia and Bulimia
1 West 91st Street
New York, NY 10024
(212) 595–3449

BIBLIOGRAPHY

American Psychiatric Association: *Diagnostic and Statistical Manual of Mental Disorders*, 3d ed, revised.

Blinder, Chaitin, Goldstein: *Eating Disorders*, New York, PMA Publishing Corps, 1988.

Brownell, Foreyt: *Handbook of Eating Disorders*, New York, Basic Books, 1982.

Comerci, D: Eating disorders in adolescents. *Pediatr Rev* 10: 1985.

Garner, DM, Garfinkel, PE: *Anorexia nervosa: A Multidimension Perspective*, New York, Bruner/Mazel, 1982.

Keys, A, et al: *The Biology of Human Starvation*. Minneapolis, University of Minnesota Press, 1950, vol 2.

Mackenzie, JR, LaBan, MM, Sackeyfio, AH: Prevalence of peripheral neuropathy in patients with anorexia nervosa. *Arch Phys Med Rehabil*. 70: 1989.

201
PANIC DISORDER

Suck Won Kim

Panic disorder (PD) is a subcategory of anxiety disorders. A basic aspect of the type of anxiety that is acute enough to be classified as a disorder is apprehension, which is defined as "anticipation of unfavorable things: suspicion or fear especially of future evil." Pathological apprehension is a dominant symptom of PDs. A person who is pathologically apprehensive is in a chronic state of hypervigilance, and tends to respond to stimuli, even ordinary life events, with a startle reaction. He or she may appear tense and rigid, and exhibit agitated behavior such as inability to sit still, wringing of the hands, nail biting, etc. Signs of autonomic dysfunction include cold or sweaty hands and trembling.

CLINICAL FEATURES

The early phase of PD is characterized by brief, intermittent episodes that terminate in less than 10 min. Between attacks, most patients appear completely normal during a routine visit to a physician's office, and may not even mention symptoms such as dizziness, difficulty in breathing, numbness, or palpitation until asked about them by their physician.

During the attack, the patient is suddenly overwhelmed by anxiety. Somatic symptoms include tachycardia, tachypnea, dyspnea, chest tightness, weakness, and dizziness. Although panic attacks usually occur without a specific provoking incident, it is not uncommon to find that stressful life events have preceded their development. Once the first attack has occurred, it is likely to be followed by recurrent attacks, all usually of 10-min duration.

It is now believed that agoraphobia develops after repeated panic attacks associated with certain situations. Patients with advanced PD frequently want a companion present to help them in case of emergency, and in severe cases of agoraphobia, the patient may become homebound. Recurrent panic attacks also lead to anticipatory anxiety, secondary depression, and an increased risk of suicide (Fig. 201-1). Eventually, significant social and occupational dysfunction develops.

The natural history of PD with or without agoraphobia is highly variable. Patients with milder forms may have prolonged periods of remission with less frequent and less intense attacks, while others may suffer many panic attacks during the course of a single day. Panic disorder is more common among young women, and the illness tends to prevail through midlife. A recent large-scale epidemiologic survey showed the lifetime prevalence of PD to be about 1% of the population. After the age of 60, the incidence of PD rapidly declines.

PATHOPHYSIOLOGY

Why PD symptoms appear in some individuals but not others is not fully understood. A number of recent studies suggest abnormal biogenic aminergic function in anxiety disorders, especially in the noradrenergic and serotonergic systems. The functional relationship between the central biogenic amine systems and the peripheral autonomic system is not fully elucidated at the present time. But it is clear that patients who have anxiety symptoms usually show evidence of abnormal autonomic function.

Redmond and Huang demonstrated that stimulation of the locus coeruleus causes panic symptoms. Under clonidine (an α_2 agonist) and yohimbine (an α_2 antagonist) challenge, PD patients showed either blunted or overstimulated release of prolactin, growth hormone, or cortisol that is mediated through the α-adrenergic system. These findings support the possible involvement of the noradrenergic system in PD.

Some studies have suggested involvement of the serotonin system in PD. Fluoxetine, a serotonin-reuptake inhibitor, is effective in treating PD. Improvement in panic symptoms is correlated with serum imipramine level and not desipramine level. This is significant because the imipramine binding site is linked to serotinin uptake while the desipramine binding site is linked to the norepinephrine uptake site. The noradrenergic and serotonergic systems are functionally linked, and an alteration of one system causes alterations in the other.

Whether GABA and benzodiazepine receptors are directly involved in the pathogenesis of PDs is not well known. GABA-activity enhancing drugs, like benzodiazepines, may exert their pharmacologic activity partly through the input into the norpinephrine and serotonin systems. Both systems have significant GABA input that has modulating influence upon firing rate and release of monoamines. Benzodiazepine receptor agonists (anxiolytic), antagonists, and inverse agonists (anxiogenic) have been used to study anxiety states. Administration of ethyl β-carboline-3-carboxylate (β-CCE), a benzodiazepine inverse agonist, causes marked agitation and anxiety in rhesus monkeys. FG-7142, another benzodiazepine inverse agonist, has also induced profound anxiety in human subjects. Interested readers can also find studies of lactate infusion and carbon dioxide inhalation in PD.

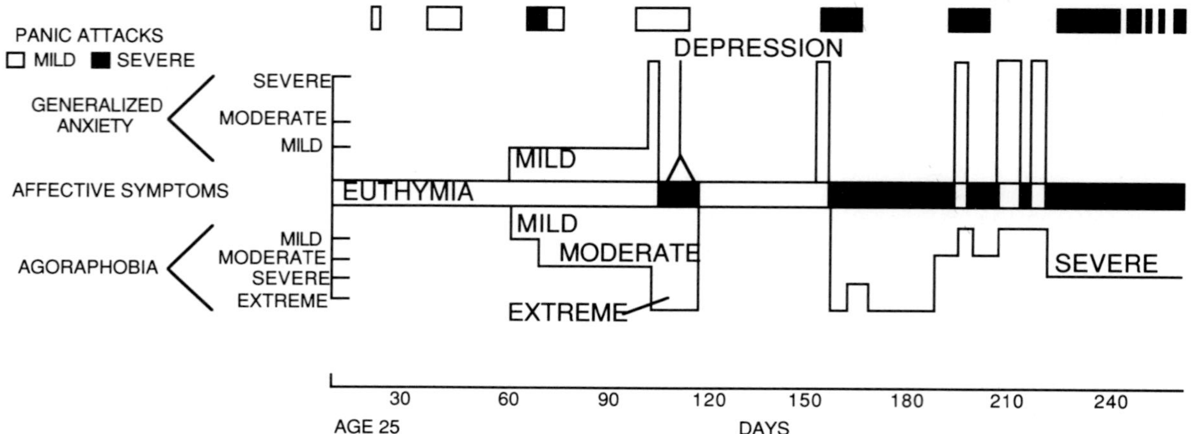

Fig. 201-1. Sequential development of panic attacks, generalized anxiety, agoraphobia, and depression during the first 9 months of illness in a 25-year-old woman. (From Uhde TW, Boulenger JP, Roy-Byrne PP, et al: Longitudinal course of panic disorder: Clinical and biological considerations. *Prog Neuropsychopharmacol Biol Psychiatry*. 9:47, 1985. Used by permission.)

Table 201-1. Medical Disorders That Mimic Panic Symptoms

Acute myocardial infarction
Hypoglycemia
Hyperthyroidism
Pheochromocytoma
Complex partial seizures
Mitral valve prolapse
Alcohol withdrawal
Drug withdrawal
Sleep disorders

Table 201-2. Psychiatric Differential Diagnosis

Generalized anxiety disorder
Depressive disorders
Schizophrenia
Depersonalization disorder
Somatoform disorders
Phobic disorders
Posttraumatic stress disorder

There have been laboratory findings in PD in recent years but their usefulness is limited to research at this time. Reiman and his associates using positron emission tomography (PET) reported increased right parahippocampal blood flow and oxygen metabolism in PD patients. Fontaine and colleagues applied magnetic resonance imaging (MRI) and reported focal abnormalities in the right mesiotemporal area in PD patients. Recent development of radiotracers for various receptor types promises to provide valuable information in this area in the near future.

Other findings include blunted thyroid stimulating hormone (TSH) response to thyrotropin (TRH) in PD patients. Platelet α_2-adrenergic receptor study results are not conclusive. The results of platelet imipramine binding studies in PD are largely normal. Although rapid eye movement (REM) sleep may not be decreased in a PD patient who has nocturnal panic symptoms, the REM latency on the night of the spells is significantly increased compared to nonpanic nights. Further studies of sleep-related panic symptoms will help elucidate the pathophysiology of this disorder.

DIFFERENTIAL DIAGNOSIS

It is not uncommon for patients with PD to consult numerous physicians because of cardiac symptoms (chest pain, tachycardia, irregular heartbeat), gastrointestinal symptoms (epigastric pain), or neurologic symptoms (headache, dizziness, vertigo, syncope, paresthesias). Patients with PD may describe only their physical symptoms or depression while ignoring core panic symptoms. Recently, Katon reported that 89 percent of the PD patients studied had presented only physical symptoms, resulting in misdiagnosis which often continued for months or years. It is essential to inquire about alcohol, drug, and caffeine use. Individuals commonly develop panic symptoms during a period of alcohol withdrawal. Excessive caffeine use can also induce panic symptoms. Recent studies by Uhde and colleagues have shown that an average of 5 cups of coffee will trigger panic attacks in 38 percent of PD patients. Irritable bowel syndrome can also disguise underlying PD.

Physiologic illnesses that can be associated with spells resembling panic attacks are summarized in Table 201-1. Panic attacks may be secondary to a number of psychiatric disorders, which are listed in Table 201-2.

TREATMENT

Generally, treatment is divided into drug and behavior therapy. Traditional psychotherapy is usually ineffective. Many communities now have specialty clinics and support groups. Patients should be guided into one of these programs if necessary. It will be reassuring to patients to find that the physician understands the nature of the symptoms. Careful listening, explanation, and reassurance frequently bring about a positive therapeutic response.

For those patients willing to take medication, imipramine, 10 to 25 mg, may be given at night as a starting dose. If needed, up to 150 mg/day can be given. Duration of treatment is highly individualized. Alcohol and caffeine should be avoided if possible. Some patients will complain of motor restlessness or a "speedy" feeling during the early phase of treatment. If this happens, the dose should be lowered and then increased very slowly as tolerated. Some may not be able to tolerate more than 10 mg/day.

Because imipramine has anticholinergic side effects, individuals with narrow-angle glaucoma or prostatic hypertrophy should not be given this drug. Postural hypotension and sedation are other adverse effects.

Newer drugs such as fluoxetine and clomipramine have been shown to be effective in the treatment of PD. However, these serotonin-reuptake inhibitors are likely to trigger initial drug-induced anxiety and should be used cautiously. Patients should always be informed that "keyed up" or "wired" sensations may develop during the early phase of treatment. Prescribing physicians must be thoroughly familiar with these newer drugs before using them. For example, fluoxetine tends to increase serum levels of other concomitantly prescribed antidepressants up to threefold.

Alprazolam, 1 to 2 mg/day will rapidly relieve panic symptoms in some mildly affected persons, though some patients will require 4 mg/day or more. Larger doses should be reserved for prescription by psychiatrists. Recently, however, withdrawal symptoms, such as anxiety, depression, and/or insomnia, have raised concern about its use, and it is important to rule out drug abuse or alcoholism before the drug is prescribed. If the drug is discontinued, it should be tapered slowly over 1 to 3 months. During the withdrawal period, carbamazepine has been shown to be helpful in mitigating withdrawal symptoms. Clonazepam may also be effective.

Although β blockers were used in the past, they are no longer considered drugs of choice in managing the illness. Clonidine can be effective during the first 4 weeks of treatment, but tachyphylaxis develops and long-term efficacy is in question. Imipramine or desipramine are not associated with tolerance and they are generally considered safe for long-term use. Patients who require monoamine oxidase inhibitors such as phenelzine should be referred to psychiatrists.

BIBLIOGRAPHY

Ballenger JC (ed): Neurobiology of panic disorder, in *Frontiers of Clinical Neuroscience*. New York, Alan R. Liss, 1990, vol 8.

Katon W: *Panic Disorder in the Medical Setting*. National Institute of Mental Health. US Dept of Health and Human Services publication no. (ADM)89-1629. Government Printing Office, 1989.

Klein DF: Anxiety reconceptualized, in Klein DF, Rabkin J (eds): *Anxiety: New Research and Changing Concepts*. New York, Raven Press, 1981.

Murphy DL, Pigott TA: Comparative examination of a role for serotonin in obsessive compulsive disorder, panic disorder, and anxiety. *J Clin Psychiatry* 51(suppl):53, 1990.

Redmond DE Jr, Huang YH, Snyder DR, et al: Behavioral effect of stimulation of the nucleus locus coeruleus in the stump tailed monkey (*Macaca arctoides*). *Brain Res* 116:502, 1976.

Reiman EM, Raichle ME, Robins E, et al: The application of positron emission tomography to the study of panic disorder. *Am J Psychiatry* 143:469, 1986.

Tyrer P (ed): Psychopharmacology of anxiety. British Association for Psychopharmacology monograph No. 11, New York, Oxford University Press, 1989.

Uhde TW, Boulenger JP, Roy-Byrne PP, et al: Longitudinal course of panic disorder: Clinical and biological considerations. *Prog Neuropsychopharmacol Biol Psychiatry* 9:39, 1985.

Uhde TW, Nemiah JC: Anxiety disorders, In Kaplan HI, Sadock DJ (eds): *Comprehensive Textbook of Psychiatry*, ed 5. Baltimore, Williams & Wilkins, 1989.

202
CONVERSION REACTIONS

Gregory P. Moore
Kenneth C. Jackimczyk

DEFINITION

For a diagnosis of conversion reaction to be made the following five criteria must be met: (1) there is a change or loss of physical function suggesting a physical disorder, (2) the patient has undergone a recent psychological stressor or conflict, (3) the patient unconsciously produces the symptom, (4) the symptom cannot be explained by a known organic etiology, and (5) the symptom is not limited to pain or sexual dysfunction.

PATHOPHYSIOLOGY

An illustrative example involves the case of a young wife who is scheduled to visit her debilitated father in the hospital. His recent diagnosis of cancer has left her distraught, and the sight of him depresses her greatly. On the morning of her visit, she suddenly becomes blind.

This example typifies conversion reactions in which conflict is caused by the patient's intense, but psychically unacceptable, urge to avoid a required action (in this case visiting her father). The patient is trapped until the physical symptom (blindness) allows expression of the urge (how can she drive there if she is blind?) without consciously confronting the feelings that led to the wish. At the same time, the symptom imposes morbidity as a punishment for the wish. Often, the presenting symptom will have a symbolic relationship to the conflict but this is not always the case. In this case the sight of her father is distressing and therefore loss of sight is the chief complaint. Conversion reactions are often thought of as nonverbal exertion of control on the environment. Two mechanisms are responsible for the symptoms. The first is "primary gain," in which the symptom allows patients to avoid confronting their uncomfortable feelings. The second is "secondary gain," in which uncomfortable situations are avoided and support is given that might not normally be available. In the above case secondary gain would occur if the patient's husband then stayed home from work to tend to his "blind" wife.

PREDISPOSING FACTORS

Conversion reactions are described as rare, with an annual incidence in outpatient psychiatric settings of 0.01 to 0.02 percent. An incidence of 5 to 16 percent in inpatients with psychiatric consultations has been noted. Most agree that the incidence is declining. Cases predominantly involve neurologic and orthopedic manifestations, and are seen in the military during times of war, in victims of industrial accidents, and in victims of violence. The most common ages of presentation are adolescence or early adulthood, although other age groups are also affected. Conversion reactions are more prevalent in rural, lower socioeconomic, and less educated populations. Other predisposing factors include medical illness, depression, anxiety, schizophrenia, somatization disorder, dependent personality disorder (5 to 21 percent of patients), borderline personality disorder, and passive aggressive personality disorder.

CLINICAL PRESENTATION

Conversion reactions usually present as a single symptom with a sudden onset related to a severe stress. Precise history taking is imperative for making the diagnosis, focusing on how the problem affects the patient and the surrounding events at time of onset. It may be necessary to interview the patient and family separately to confirm diagnostic suspicions. The most reliable diagnostic criterion for conversion reaction is either a previous history of it or a somatization disorder (each found in one-third of cases). Symptoms may vary in cases of recurrence.

Motor complaints, usually involving voluntary muscles, are more common than sensory complaints.

Rarely the autonomic and endocrine systems are involved. Vomiting can be a psychogenic manifestation of disgust, and pseudocyesis (false pregnancy) can represent a wish for or fear of pregnancy.

Classic symptoms of conversion reactions include paralysis, aphonia, seizures, coordination disturbances, akinesia, dyskinesia, blindness, tunnel vision, anosmia, anesthesia, and paresthesia. Pseudoseizures represent 10 to 40 percent of conversion reactions referred to psychiatrists. Patients may describe their condition with surprising lack of concern considering the severity of the symptom (*la belle indifférence*). This was previously thought to be a hallmark of the disorder, but it is absent in 46 to 59 percent of cases and is found just as often in patients with organic disease. It is no longer considered diagnostic.

Diagnosis is made first and foremost by ruling out organic pathology. Absence of a medical condition does not solely support the diagnosis of conversion reaction, since the appropriate psychological criteria must also be met. Suspicion for the disorder should arise when no physical findings related to the symptom are found or the examination is not consistent with known anatomic or pathophysiologic states. Several techniques that can be used in the physical examination are helpful in testing for true neurologic deficits (see Table 202-1). Appropriate laboratory and ancillary studies should be ordered to confirm suspected organic disease. It is important to remember, however, that organic disease may be present concurrently with conversion reaction.

DIFFERENTIAL DIAGNOSIS

A careful history and physical examination should be utilized to rule out significant neurologic disease. A high index of suspicion should be maintained for physical disorders that have a vague onset, such as SLE, MS, polymyositis, etc. Schizophrenia and depression may have associated conversion reactions, and recognition of these is discussed in other chapters. In somatization disorders, the symptoms are more chronic and involve multiple organ systems. With hypochondriasis the patient is usually without loss of function and displays the conviction that some terrible undiscovered illness is present. Hypochondriacal patients will be overly concerned with symptoms. In cases of factitious symptoms, usually associated with malingering, the patient will consciously complain about symptoms to get out of undesirable duty, or receive sympathy or undeserved compensation. These patients rarely have neurologic complaints.

TREATMENT AND PROGNOSIS

In true cases of conversion reaction, if improvement in symptoms is desired, the emergency physician must realize that the patient is not conscious that the symptoms have no organic course. Confronting the patient and insisting that nothing "real" is wrong will do nothing to alleviate the symptoms and may worsen the patient's condition. If the precipitating dilemma is identified, correction of the problem should be attempted. Meanwhile the patient should receive reassurance that no serious medical problem has been identified. It should be suggested to the patient that the symptoms will resolve. Nonspecific supportive therapy should be prescribed. For instance, in the example cited at the beginning of this chapter it could be suggested that the patient visit her father less often, call daily instead, and have her husband accompany her to the hospital. She should expect the blindness to resolve if she follows this course.

Referral is mandatory. Patients with conversion reactions may need repetitive reassurance and suggestion that symptoms will resolve before

Table 202-1. Physical Examination Techniques Used to Distinguish True Neurologic Deficits and Conversion Disorder

Function	Technique
I. Sensation	
Yes-no test	Patient closes eyes and responds "yes" or "no" to touch stimulus. "No" response in numb area favors conversion reaction.
Bowlus and Currier test	Patient extends crossed arms with thumbs pointed down and palms facing together. Fingers (but not thumbs) are interlocked, then hands are rotated inward toward chest. The distortion of body position makes false responses to sensory stimuli difficult.
Strength test	Patient closes eyes. Test "strength" by touching finger to be moved. True lack of sensation would not allow patient to ascertain finger to be moved.
II. Pain	
Gray test	With abdominal pain due to psychological factors, the patient will close eyes during palpation. In pain of organic basis, the patient is more likely to watch examiner's hand in order to anticipate pain.
III. Motor	
Drop test	When lifting limb in patient with paralysis of nonorganic etiology, the affected limb will drop more slowly than normal or fall with exaggerated speed. Additionally, an extremity dropped from above the face will miss it.
Stretch reflex text	The patient contracts a muscle at maximum strength while countertraction is provided. The examiner suddenly jerks the muscle into extension. This will produce a stretch reflex that reveals the patient's true muscle strength.
Thigh adductor test	Examiner places hands against inner thighs of patient. Patient is told to adduct normal leg against resistance. With pseudoparalysis, other leg will adduct.
Hoover test	Examiner's hands encircle both ankles of patient and patient is asked to elevate normal leg. With pseudoparalysis, other leg will push downward.
Sternomastoid test	Patient with nonorganic hemiplegia cannot turn head to weak side.
IV. Coma	
Corneal reflex	Corneal reflexes remain intact in awake patient.
Bell's phenomenon	Eyes divert upward when lids opened, whereas eyes remain in neutral position in true coma.
Lid closing	In true coma, lids when opened close rapidly initially then more slowly as lids descend. Awake patients will have lids stay open, snap shut, or flutter.
V. Seizures	
Corneal reflex	Usually intact in pseudoseizure.
Abdominal musculature	Palpation of abdominal musculature reveals lack of contractions with pseudoseizure.
VI. Blindness	
Opticokinetic drug	Rotating drug with alternating black and white stripes or piece of tape with alternating black and white sections pulled laterally in front of patient's open eyes will produce nystagmus in patient with intact vision.

Source: Adapted from Purcell, TB: The somatic patient. *Emerg Clin North Am* 9(1):137, 1991.

returning to full function. Periodic follow-up is also important to monitor for subtle organic disease. Between 25 and 50 percent of patients diagnosed with conversion reactions later develop serious organic conditions.

Most conversion reactions are of short duration and quickly resolve. Favorable prognostic factors are (1) lack of other psychiatric disorders, (2) sudden severe stress as a precipitating cause, and (3) absence of medical problems. (Some cases are resistant and require hypnosis or amytal interview for resolution. This should be coordinated by the primary care provider.) Approximately 25 percent of patients will have another conversion reaction over the next 1 to 6 years which may involve the same or a new symptom complex.

Some patients develop a chronic form of the disorder with complications including contractures and atrophy of muscle groups. In addition, unnecessary diagnostic tests may lead to iatrogenic complications.

BIBLIOGRAPHY

American Psychiatric Association: *Diagnostic and Statistical Manual of Mental Disorders,* 3d ed, revised. Washington, D.C., 1987.

Dubovsky SL, Weissberg MP (eds.): Hypochondriasis, in *Clinical Psychiatry in Primary Care,* 3d ed. Baltimore, Williams & Wilkins, 1986, pp 1–22.

Fauman B: Conversion reaction, in Tintinalli JE, Rothstein RJ, Krome RL (eds.): *Emergency Medicine: A Comprehensive Study Guide,* 1st ed. McGraw-Hill, 1985, pp. 945–946

Hafeiz HV: Hysterical conversion: A prognostic study. *Br J Psychiatry* 136:548, 1980.

Kaplan HI, Sadock BJ (eds.): Conversion disorder, in *Comprehensive Textbook of Psychiatry,* 5th ed. Baltimore, Williams & Wilkins, 1989, vol 1, pp 1013–1017.

Lazare A: Conversion symptoms. *N Engl J Med* 305:745, 1981.

Purcell TB: The somatic patient. *Emerg Clin North Am* 9(1):137, 1991.

Schecker NH: Childhood conversion reactions in the emergency department: I. Diagnostic and management approaches within a biopsychosocial framework. *Pediatr Emerg Care* 3:202, 1987.

Schecker NH: Childhood conversion reactions in the emergency department: II. General and specific features. *Pediatr Emerg Care* 6:46, 1990.

203 CRISIS INTERVENTION

Zigfrids T. Stelmachers

A crisis is an internally experienced, acute disturbance resulting from an inability to cope with ominous or stressful events or feelings. Crisis intervention is best aimed at normal individuals without psychiatric histories and without current psychiatric symptoms, who have experienced a traumatic event. One of the goals is the prevention of the development of psychiatric symptoms.

Some normal individuals, however, develop abnormal reactions to stressful events, such as severe panic, paranoid reactions, and brief psychotic episodes, which may require traditional psychiatric treatment. The mentally ill often experience crisis situations since they are vulnerable to negative life changes. Finally, when the mentally ill are in a crisis, psychiatric symptoms may exacerbate. In the above instances, crisis intervention coupled with psychiatric treatment may be indicated. An emergency department has to be prepared to offer crisis intervention as well as treatment for psychiatric emergencies.

TYPES OF CRISES

A classification of emotional crises is as follows:

1. Dispositional crises, such as no food or no place to live; acute financial problems; need for information, referral, or advocacy
2. Crises of predictable life stages, such as adolescence, sexuality, marriage, childbirth, "midlife crisis," and retirement
3. Crises due to negative life changes and trauma, such as discovery of a debilitating illness; divorce; victimization; criminal prosecution; loss of job; or death of a loved one
4. Maturational crises, such as dependence/independence conflicts; sexual identity problems; difficulties with emotional intimacy; and value conflicts
5. Crises in which preexisting psychopathology has contributed to the precipitation, presentation, or prognosis of the crisis
6. Acute psychiatric emergencies in which the patient is dangerous to self or others

Not only should the care givers understand several crisis intervention principles and techniques but they need to be familiar with the characteristics of various patient populations and their target symptoms (i.e., rape victims, drug addicts, grief reactions, etc.)

CRISIS DEVELOPMENT

The stressfulness of an event is to a large extent determined by a person's *perception* and *interpretation* of the event rather than its objective and more universal properties. Interpretation depends on personality variables and prior life experiences.

In addition, there are individual repertoires of coping mechanisms—accumulated over time—and mediating variables which act as catalysts in the process of crisis resolution. Examples of such variables are social support, a generally hopeful and optimistic attitude toward life, and a belief in being in control of one's life situation and destiny. Finally, some psychological reactions to traumatic events may develop into chronic maladaptive response patterns, including psychiatric disorders. These reactions, if initially suppressed, may eventually result in delayed reactions with their cause obscured by intervening events. The delayed symptoms include such secondary problem development as increased drinking, interpersonal conflicts, divorce, and loss of job. All these various factors and the general sequence of events are portrayed in Table 203–1.

PATIENT ASSESSMENT

Assessment consists of the following:

1. The patient's current complaints, problems, and symptoms, including their severity, frequency, and duration.
2. The causes of the presenting complaints, including stresses and negative life changes.
3. The effect of the critical events on the patient's overall functioning. Has there been a serious disruption of the patient's interpersonal relationships? Has school or work performance deteriorated significantly? Has personal hygiene been affected?

In addition to changes in the patient's behavior, there may be less visible alterations in the patient's inner emotional and mental state. Changes in mood, affect, emotional control, and thought patterns should be thoroughly investigated.

An information-gathering approach with an emotionally disturbed patient often creates a barrier to establishing good rapport. Some symptoms may need to be "treated" before assessment is completed; in fact, obtaining relevant information may be nearly impossible with agitated or uncooperative patients. Therefore, one cannot neatly separate the interview into an assessment and an intervention phase. Instead, the two have to be flexibly and sensitively intertwined from the very beginning. In order to accomplish this, it is useful to watch for divergent agendas between the care giver and the patient. The former may be mainly interested in obtaining information to arrive at the diagnosis and treatment plan, while the patient's main motivation may be to express anger at an alcoholic and abusive husband. If this divergence of motives is not recognized, a communication breakdown may develop and assessment and treatment efforts will suffer.

Patients differ widely in their readiness to get help. The most elaborate and well-designed treatment plans will not be effective with patients lacking in motivation for such interventions. Much time can be wasted in making complicated treatment and disposition arrangements only to learn too late that the patient has little intention to go through with the plans. It is therefore helpful to assess the patient's motivational strength early on; if motivation is lacking, this should be addressed directly and *before* one gets involved in time-consuming planning.

Precrisis Adjustment

To assess the seriousness of the current crisis reaction, compare it with the patient's usual behavior patterns and mental state. What is described as a crisis situation may sometimes represent relatively continuous or repetitive behavior disturbances best treated by ongoing long-term treatment rather than crisis intervention.

A careful history should be taken of the patient's responses to earlier crisis intervention efforts. The knowledge of what helped and what didn't assists the crisis worker in the formulation of a more effective treatment. Furthermore, the history may reveal that the patient has already developed a repertoire of coping skills as a result of dealing with these earlier crises. It is reassuring to patients to be reminded of their own previous successes, and it encourages them to be self-reliant.

Finally, knowledge of the patient's premorbid vulnerabilities helps identify the stresses which provoked the current crisis.

Crisis Precipitants

It is important to determine what final event motivated the patient to seek help, especially for patients with multiple problems. Longstanding problems may be presented along with acute ones, and severe ones with minor stresses. In an emergency setting it is impractical—often

Table 203-1. The Crisis Kaleidoscope, A Theoretical Model

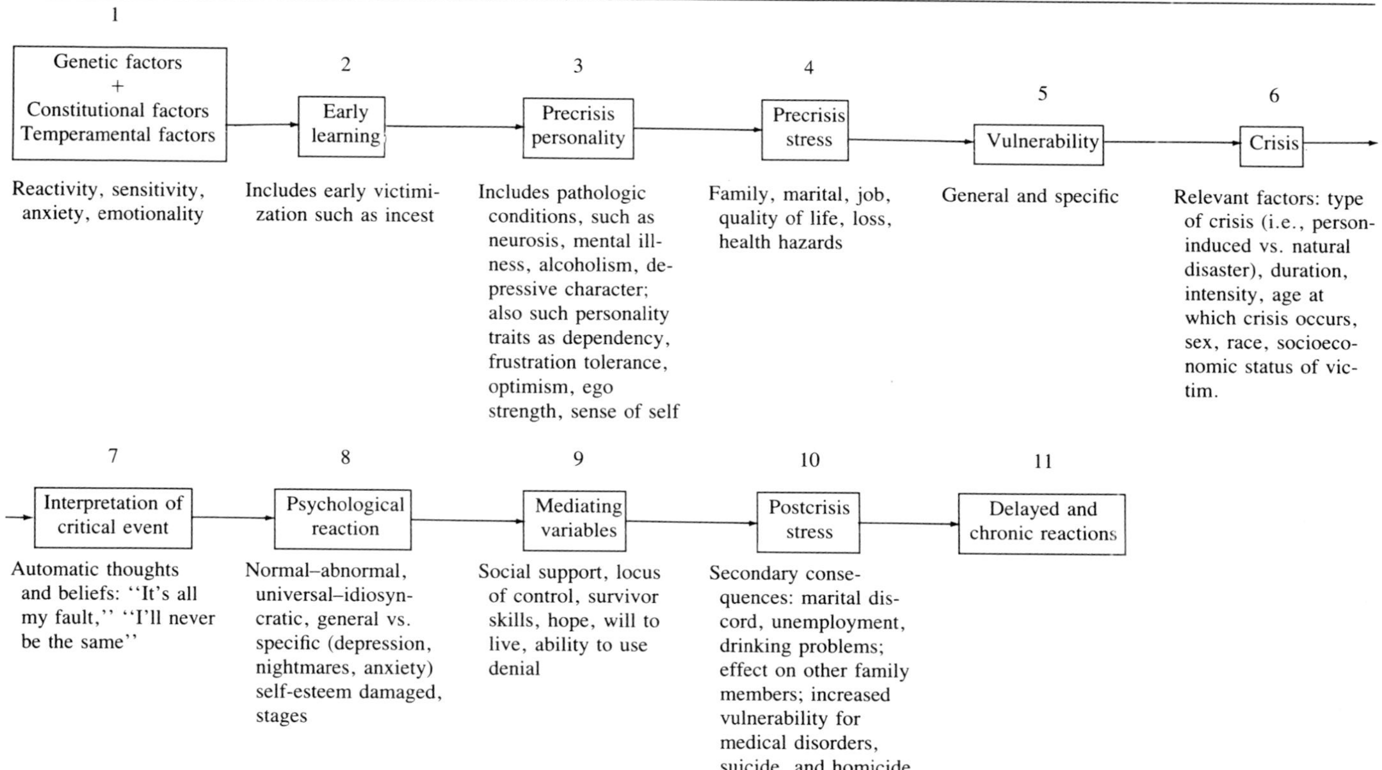
1
Genetic factors + Constitutional factors Temperamental factors
Reactivity, sensitivity, anxiety, emotionality
2
Early learning
Includes early victimization such as incest
3
Precrisis personality
Includes pathologic conditions, such as neurosis, mental illness, alcoholism, depressive character; also such personality traits as dependency, frustration tolerance, optimism, ego strength, sense of self
4
Precrisis stress
Family, marital, job, quality of life, loss, health hazards
5
Vulnerability
General and specific
6
Crisis
Relevant factors: type of crisis (i.e., person-induced vs. natural disaster), duration, intensity, age at which crisis occurs, sex, race, socioeconomic status of victim.
7
Interpretation of critical event
Automatic thoughts and beliefs: "It's all my fault," "I'll never be the same"
8
Psychological reaction
Normal–abnormal, universal–idiosyncratic, general vs. specific (depression, nightmares, anxiety) self-esteem damaged, stages
9
Mediating variables
Social support, locus of control, survivor skills, hope, will to live, ability to use denial
10
Postcrisis stress
Secondary consequences: marital discord, unemployment, drinking problems; effect on other family members; increased vulnerability for medical disorders, suicide, and homicide
11
Delayed and chronic reactions

not necessary—to address an entire cluster of problems. One needs to identify the immediate precipitant because it usually indicates the problem most responsible for the current crisis. Intervention can then concentrate on this main problem area, resulting in effective and economical treatment.

If a specific precipitant cannot be identified, it may be advisable to ask the patient to describe the events of the day just before the decision was made to seek treatment. During such a recounting of events it may be possible to tease out the precipitant even though the patient may not be aware of the connection.

One should also watch for sudden changes in the patient's interactional pattern, such as silences, tearfulness, or anger outbursts, because such changes often signify that a currently active conflict has been touched.

Stages of Response

People often react to stressful events in predictable stages similar to those identified in grief and loss. The sequence starts with a feeling of shock followed by denial, which at some point fails and leads to negative emotions such as anxiety, fright, depression, or regressive dependency. Guilt is almost invariably present because it is quite typical for victims of all kinds of tragedies to blame themselves. The next stage may be obsessiveness about the critical event, often followed by apathy and resignation. Finally, there may be a period of inner- or outward-directed rage.

Although many individuals follow the described general pattern, others skip a stage or two or progress through the stages in a different sequence. For some there are no stages at all but merely a confusing array of constantly changing feelings, an emotional roller coaster with peaks of highly emotional experiences separated by valleys of relative calm. These "waves," at various times, may be composed of different emotions in different proportions and predominance. Some individuals may have a "preferred" and rather persistent emotion perhaps characteristic of their personalities and pretrauma response tendencies to stressful events. Nevertheless, to the extent that at least some patients react in stages, it is useful for the physician to identify the current stage of the patient in order to select the best intervention.

Outside Information

Individuals in a crisis situation are often very emotional, confused, perplexed, anxious, withdrawn, or agitated. These emotional states make them poor and unreliable informants. Data collected under such conditions is often incomplete or distorted. The interview must be supplemented with information from outside sources, such as family members, friends, police officers, therapists, ministers, or apartment managers.

One should not forget that the setting to a large extent determines how people behave, and that a hospital represents a rather artificial environment for the purpose of predicting patients' behavior in their home setting. Therefore, it is inadvisable to dismiss or minimize the observations of a "hysterical mother," an "overreacting therapist," or a "dumb cop" who lacks formal mental health training but has the considerable advantage of having observed the patient during a domestic quarrel. In a supportive and professional setting the patient is likely to be more relaxed and in better emotional control. The stimulus triggering the crisis situation is usually not present, and it is therefore not surprising that the patient is behaving "normally." It would be unwise to conclude from this that a true crisis is not present or that the emergency aspects of the problem have been exaggerated. If under such conditions a patient is released and returns to the irritant, another crisis may quickly develop.

Self-Esteem

It is important to identify the impact of the crisis on the patient's concept of self. Faced with major problems which defy easy solution, some patients experience considerable anxiety or depression and yet are able to preserve a healthy sense of self-worth. Other patients, however, engage in self-blame or self-hate which exacerbates the crisis reaction. The latter patients require a more psychological intervention approach, more reassurance and emotional support in addition to specific treatments, help in problem solving, and a variety of environmental manipulations.

Resources

In order to properly assess the patient's ability to cope one needs to know about the patient's strengths, repertoire of coping skills, "fighting spirit," social and other environmental resources available as well as his weaknesses and deficiencies. Social support is one of the most important mediating variables which significantly influences the crisis outcome. What is important here is not the *quantity* of social support but its *quality:* a few close and caring friends have more positive impact than a larger number of acquaintances, fellow club members, or hostile and rejecting relatives.

Directiveness of Interview

In inquiring about sensitive and potentially embarrassing issues, one should use a matter-of-fact and straightforward approach. Subtle and indirect questioning may not yield the concrete detail necessary for effective intervention and disposition. This is especially true in cases of elevated suicide or violence potential. It is quite appropriate, even desirable, to ask such questions as: "Are you currently so depressed that you have thought of taking your life?" "Do you have a plan?" "Have you selected a method?" "Is it readily available?" "Is the time and place set?" "Have you ever committed acts of violence?" "Did they result in injury?" "Are you in the habit of carrying a weapon?" "Was the violent act provoked, premeditated, indiscriminate, or aimed at a particular person or situation?"

Perhaps surprisingly, many patients are quite willing to share this information without undue defensiveness. And if they are not ready to reveal their inclinations and plans, the chances are that an indirect approach will yield no better results that a straightforward inquiry.

Family Members

Family members and friends who accompany the patient are not only often deeply involved in the patient's problems but themselves may have developed clinical signs and symptoms of crisis. In that sense they become co-patients in need of professional attention. Quite frequently they are more disturbed than the identified patient, expecting the primary patient to receive immediate attention, hospitalization, certain medications, or some other specific disposition. Even though they may appear to be exaggerating the urgency of the primary patient's condition or to be "overinvolved" and, as a result, interfere with clinical decision making and patient care, their needs have to be addressed. In any crisis intervention it is useful to have family members as allies rather than antagonists because one often has to rely on outside resources and support for the implementation of treatment plans.

Successive Assessments

Sometimes a single assessment episode is insufficient to provide a satisfactory formulation of problem and treatment. The patient's current mental state may preclude an adequate evaluation because the patient is guarded, mute, incoherent, or intoxicated. At other times the symptom picture may be confusing or inconsistent. With such patients the final decision can be made only after a succession of assessment episodes separated in time. This way either an increase or a decrease in symptoms can be demonstrated, and the treatment plan modified accordingly. If suicide or violence potential is one of the suspected symptoms, it is most prudent to admit such patients to the hospital, on a legal hold if necessary.

GOALS OF CRISIS INTERVENTION

The goals are usually short-term, although some critical interventions may lead to long-term consequences which are not predictable. Solving the patient's long-standing and severe life problems is seldom necessary for effective crisis resolution; sometimes just changing the patient's *perception* of a particular problem can have very beneficial immediate impact.

Other goals of crisis intervention are to

1. Prevent the development of psychiatric symptoms.
2. Prevent the development of delayed or chronic reactions.
3. Sort, early in treatment, patients into two groups: those requiring a hospital setting and those who can be treated in an outpatient environment.
4. Relieve symptoms.
5. Restore emotional equilibrium.
6. Restore power and control, especially to patients who have been victimized.
7. Return the patient to precrisis or higher level of functioning.

Chronic problems need ongoing therapy and counseling programs.

INTERVENTION STRATEGIES AND COMPONENTS

Intervention Components

Effective crisis intervention, whatever its specific treatment strategies and techniques, always contains the following core elements.(Table 203–2):

1. Mobilize hope.
2. Instill and maintain expectation for improvement.
3. Like and respect the patient.
4. Be enthusiastic.

Sympathetic, Active, and Selective Listening

When patients are asked to identify the one component which was most helpful to them, being listened to is by far the most frequently mentioned one. Listening should be accompanied by positive emotional involvement and genuine concern, but the patient should be discouraged from straying to irrelevant or unmanageable issues.

Emotional Support

Emotional support is not synonymous with an indiscriminate siding with the patient. It is tempting to agree with the patient's perceptions of certain events, but such partiality may encourage the patient to select

Table 203-2. Essential Components of Crisis Intervention

1. Sympathetic, active, and selective listening
2. Emotional support
3. Nonjudgmental acceptance
4. Reassurance
5. Providing information
6. Providing opportunity for ventilation
7. Intellectual clarification
8. Advice and persuasion
9. Confrontation
10. Setting limits
11. Facilitation and advocacy
12. Final disposition and follow-up

an imprudent course of action, or may backfire if the patient has been critical of a significant other whose cooperation turns out to be necessary for the patient's treatment.

Nonjudgmental Acceptance

Accepting the patient's statements should not imply condoning the patient's views. One can listen to what the patient has to say without judging the correctness of the patient's assumptions or the wisdom of his or her actions. Special care should be exercised to not appear to blame the patient even if it is done inadvertently or indirectly by such questions as, "Why did you walk alone in this neighborhood so late at night?"

Suggested responses to victims of rape and other violent crimes include "I'm sorry it happened;" "I'm glad you are alive and well;" and "You did nothing wrong."

Reassurance

It is often important to begin the intervention by reassuring the patient that it was a good idea to come for help. Many patients feel embarrassed and awkward about seeking treatment, may feel that it implies a character weakness or that their problems are too trivial to deserve professional attention. They are also uncertain about the reception they will get ("Will they treat me like a mentally ill person?").

When people are in an acute emotional turmoil, they frequently feel that they may be losing their mind, are "going crazy," will fall apart, will have a nervous breakdown, etc. Quick and unequivocal reassurance to the contrary often has an immediate calming effect and helps establish rapport. The more specific and concrete the reassurance, the more effective it is. "Things are going to be all right" is less effective than, "In the past when you had these symptoms, they were very short-lived and you could function quite adequately even while they were acute."

Providing Information

Patients' problems are often aggravated by misperceptions, misconceptions, and a variety of myths. Factual information, if available and known to the crisis worker, can be very helpful and reassuring to the patient, but must not be permitted to expand into a minilecture.

Providing Opportunity for Ventilation

Emotional expression is very therapeutic for most patients. Notable exceptions are hysterical or emotionally labile individuals who habitually respond to stressful events with intense and dramatic outbursts.

Intellectual Clarification

It is not unusual for patients to be overwhelmed by a confusing array of symptoms, problems, and emotions whose meaning and future implications are far from clear to them. Intellectual understanding, even if it falls short of genuine insight, can provide a sense of order. A seemingly chaotic and ominous situation loses some of its threat once it is "explained."

Advice and Persuasion

If sparingly and cautiously used, advice and persuasion can be effective crisis intervention tools. However, a distinction needs to be made between advice regarding real life circumstances (e.g., "You should get a divorce") and advice regarding treatment issues (e.g., "You should consider medication"). Advice on real life situations is potentially hazardous because it presumes a full understanding of the patient's personality and life situation as well as superior wisdom on the therapist's part. It is much safer to give the second type of advice.

Confrontation

A patient may display considerable denial, rationalization, and repression. It may be tempting to force the patient to face reality, but the patient who is not ready to accept the "truth" will resist a frontal attack and become adversarial. If the patient needs to accept reality as part of the intervention, the approach should be supportive, gentle, and gradual.

Setting Limits

With patients who are dangerous to themselves or others, aggressively act out their conflicts, display excessive dependency, or behave manipulatively or provocatively, limit setting is often necessary. Rules of conduct have to be established and enforced, or, better yet, the patient should be given choices with clearly spelled out consequences attached to them.

Facilitation and Advocacy

Many crises are predominantly the result of external stresses which cannot be readily changed by treating the patient. In such instances, the patient's environment has to be manipulated as part of the crisis intervention. This can take the form of facilitating the solution of some dispositional problem (such as money, no place to live,legal difficulties, etc.). Other patients may be in a crisis because of discrimination and ill treatment accorded to them as a group by various law enforcement, health, and welfare agencies. Victims of various crimes, especially rape and battering, are examples of such groups. Special advocates can assist the primary intervention by pleading the victim's cause before the relevant agencies.

Final Disposition and Follow-Up

Speedy and successful referral is an essential part of crisis intervention. A good referral is more like a transfer from one facility to another. Instead of just sending a patient to another agency, finalize the arrangements, including appointment time, the agency's address and telephone number, and the name of the intake worker or receiving professional. The tighter the arrangements, the harder it is for an ambivalent patient to renege on the treatment commitment. Such "transfers" approximately double the success rate of the usual much looser referrals.

Finally, time permitting, it is advisable to do a very short term follow-up: Did the patient keep the appointment? Was this an appropriate referral? Was the patient accepted for treatment? If the patient chose not to go through with the referral, was it for clinically sound reasons and does he or she need further crisis services (while being put on a waiting list, for instance)?

Strategies for Different Stages

Treatment approaches have to be matched with the needs of patients during different time periods following the critical event. During the first 24 to 48 h, the patient needs *emotional first aid,* which can be provided either at the site of trauma, the patient's home, a shelter, or a hospital emergency department. During this period the patient's safety and physical well-being should be a primary concern, plus massive doses of reassurance and emotional support, in addition to provision of relevant information.

During this period, *crisis management* may be needed for more severely disturbed and intoxicated patients, including such security measures as seclusion and restraint. Intoxicated patients often profit from an overnight stay in the emergency department. During their intoxicated state these patients may be highly suicidal and assaultive and yet may not require hospitalization if managed properly in the emergency department. Most of them no longer exhibit their previous night's behavior disturbance the next morning, so they can be safely discharged with arrangements for further outpatient treatment.

During the next 6 weeks or so, following the initial visit, the treatment of choice for most crisis patients is classic *crisis intervention*. For that time segment, the crisis workers need to have a thorough knowledge of crisis intervention techniques as well as familiarity with specific target symptoms and reactions (i.e., those common in victims of rape, grief,etc.). Patients whose reactions persist beyond 6 weeks or who develop delayed symptoms may require *crisis therapy*, which is more similar to brief psychotherapy. This requires a better knowledge of personality theory and psychotherapeutic principles and techniques.

Use of High Emotional Arousal

During a crisis situation patients display a higher degree of emotional arousal. This usually leads to a higher level of motivation to seek or accept treatment. Thus it provides a unique opportunity to gain access to the patient's more chronic problems which have been neglected during noncritical periods. Patients should be guided to definitive treatment at this very time when they are most ready to make use of it.

STRESS OF CRISIS WORK

Any crisis-oriented service has to be prepared to deal with very difficult, challenging, unpleasant patients; patients chronically in crisis, expecting and demanding immediate services; dependent and clinging patients who use clinical services for human contact; patients who are manipulative and provocative but are unwilling to take responsibility for their behavior; powerless, chaotic, and frustrated patients ready to vent their pent-up anger at anyone who represents the ''system.''

Members of the helping professions are especially vulnerable to these patients because the care givers are impelled to live up to the image of a caring and compassionate individual. The intrinsic reward for this ethic is the feeling of being needed, liked, and appreciated. Such rewards are not forthcoming with the patients described above. Unless the helper recognizes these danger signs it can lead to burnout and compromised patient care.

To help the helpers to protect and take better care of themselves, the following tactics are offered:

1. Try to be aware of your own negative feelings and discharge them in small and harmless dosages instead of suppressing and bottling them up.
2. Recognize the type of patient you have particular problems with because of your own temperament and life experiences.
3. Don't take patients' blaming and hostility personally; most of it represents aimless discharge of frustration, or it may be displaced to you from a more primary source.
4. Be aware that some undesirable behavior may be the direct result of the patient's mental condition and is not under his or her control.
5. Resist overinvolvement and heroic rescue efforts with guilt-inducing, dependent, and demanding patients.
6. If your treatment plan is contrary to the patient's wishes, don't expect cooperation and gratitude.
7. Look for fear, loneliness, and inadequacy under cocky, arrogant, and hostile behavior.
8. Accept your own shortcomings and the limitations of the services you provide; this includes the realization that you don't have something for everyone, even if it seems to be expected of you.

BIBLIOGRAPHY

Barton GM: Standards of care, in Gorton J, Partridge R, (eds): *Practice and Management of Psychiatric Emergency Care*. St Louis, Mosby, 1982.

Butcher JN, Stelmachers ZT, Maudal GR: *Crisis Intervention and Emergency Psychotherapy*. Clinical Methods in Psychology, New York, Wiley, 1983.

Caplan G: *Principles of Preventive Psychiatry*. New York, Basic Books, 1984.

Danto B, Frederick C, Harvey G, et al: *Certification Standards Manual for Crisis Intervention Programs*. American Association of Suicidology, 1984.

Hoff LA: *People in Crisis: Understanding and Helping*, ed 2. Menlo Park, Addison-Wesley, 1984.

Leff-Simon SI, Slaikeu KA, Hansen K: *Crisis Intervention in Hospital Emergency Rooms*. Crisis Intervention, A Handbook for Practice and Research. Boston, Allyn and Bacon, 1984.

SECTION 21
Emergencies in the Disabled Patient

204
INJURY IN THE ELDERLY AND ELDER ABUSE

John F. Brown
Daniel W. Spaite

The elderly are one of the largest growing segments of the American population today. Figures from the Bureau of the Census show that there were 30 million people over age 65 in the U.S. as of 1988, or nearly 13 percent of the overall population. This represents a growth of 31 percent during the 1980s and the number is forecast to increase to 39 million in the next 20 years. The fastest growing subsegment of the elderly population are the very elderly, with over 12 million U.S. citizens now over the age of 75. These facts have placed new demands on health care systems and will have a profound impact on emergency medicine in the future. Compared with 50 years ago, the elderly today are much more geographically mobile, more independent, and functioning at a more active level in society. They are more likely to be living alone and be geographically distant from their offspring. This life-style has increased the utilization of emergency departments by elderly patients and the utilization of emergency medical services systems.

Trauma is the fifth leading cause of death for those over the age of 65. The incidence of trauma suffered by the elderly is equivalent to that of the overall population. However mortality rates for injuries sustained by geriatric patients are markedly increased compared with those for younger patients with similar injuries. In addition, of those elderly trauma victims who do survive an acute event, as many as 88 percent do not return to their previous level of function. These differences are primarily due to the physiologic changes that occur with aging (Table 204-1). Concomitant with these physiologic changes is the higher incidence of chronic diseases which further complicates the body's response to injury and compromises the ability of the patient to recover. Immediate pathophysiologic consequences of traumatic stress include poor renal response to fluid shifts, decreased cardiac index, and reduced lean body mass with the resulting poor ability to accommodate increased catabolism.

The emergency physician must have a high index of suspicion for disease processes that may predispose the elderly patient to trauma. These include acute CNS disease, occult myocardial ischemia or infarction, arrhythmias, hypothermia, and medication interactions or sensitivities. In addition, decompensation of a chronic, but previously stable, condition such as diabetes or malnutrition can lead to significant complications. Neglecting to diagnose such underlying problems may result in increased morbidity or mortality.

The care of geriatric patients in the emergency department setting can be aided by preplanning and special resources. Examples of these measures are social services responsive to emergency department consultation, geriatric consultation services in the disciplines of internal medicine and orthopedics, provision for alternative transportation home from the emergency department, and visiting nurse services to provide necessary follow-up.

MECHANICS AND ANATOMIC ASPECTS OF INJURY

Due to their increasingly active life-styles, the elderly are at risk from multiple sources of trauma. Two recent investigations revealed that while falls account for a majority of injuries in the elderly, other mechanisms such as motor vehicle accidents, pedestrian incidents, assaults, burns, and self-inflicted injuries account for a significant portion of trauma.

The extremities are the most commonly traumatized body region regardless of the mechanism of injury. Head trauma, while not necessarily more common in the elderly than in the younger population, results in a higher morbidity and mortality. In these older patients, severe injuries can often be occult, making late or missed diagnosis more likely. Chest trauma often results in severe injury due to the noncompliance of the chest wall and diminished pulmonary function. Pulmonary and cardiac contusion, major vessel damage (especially in the region of atheromatous plaques), and rib fractures are common and may have serious sequelae. Early invasive monitoring, aggressive respiratory management including intubation and ventilation, and surgical intervention may be warranted. Abdominal trauma can result in significant injury without overt peritoneal signs in the fully alert and conscious geriatric patient. It is interesting to note that abdominal visceral injury is unusual without fractures. Significant skeletal trauma can be occult because the elderly often have diminished pain perception and absence of bony tenderness does not eliminate the possibility of fracture.

Table 204-1. Physiologic Effects of Aging

Organ System	Effects	Consequences
CNS	Decline in number of neurons, impaired memory & learning skills, increased reaction time	Problems with independent living, caring for self, impaired ability to prevent injury
Peripheral nerves	Decreased number of fibers in nerve trunks	Slowness of "righting" reflexes; muscle wasting
Cardiovascular	Increasing atherosclerosis, reduced cardiac reserve	Poor exercise and stress tolerance
Respiratory	Decreased vital capacity, reduced compliance and increased residual volume, poor ciliary function	Poor exercise and stress tolerance, increased susceptibility to infection
Renal	Loss of nephrons, reduced glomerular filtration rate and tubular reabsorption	Elevated BUN, reduced renal reserve
Musculoskeletal	Osteoarthritis, osteoporosis, decreased lean muscle mass	Poor mobility and balance, increased risk of fracture
Skin	Loss of elastic tissue	Increased fragility
Metabolism	Decreased GI absorption, protein binding, and altered excretion	Increased risk of drug side effects; increased incidence of drug interactions; nutritional deficits

Table 204-2. Complications of Elder Trauma

Complication	Potential Causes	Prevention Strategies
Pulmonary edema	Overhydration, cardiac injury, underlying heart disease	Invasive monitoring, meticulous attention to volume status
Pulmonary embolus	Prolonged immobilization	Heparinization, early mobilization
Respiratory failure	Mechanical injury to chest wall, CNS injury	Monitoring, aggressive pulmonary toilet, and early intubation as necessary
Sepsis	Infection from wounds, lungs and invasive procedures	Aggressive wound care, pulmonary toilet, and aseptic technique
Myocardial infarction	Stress to cardiovascular system	Monitoring and aggressive treatment of ischemia
Nonunion of fractures; avascular necrosis	Missed injury with subsequent early use and further damage	Radiography and careful interpretation with appropriate special procedures & consultation
Contractures and joint immobility	Prolonged immobilization	Appropriate consultation and follow-up for early mobilization & physical therapy
Depression & emotional complications	Additional limits to activity, privacy, and autonomy	Address elder's concerns and fears acutely, offer support services as appropriate

Falls account for the majority of traumatic injuries to the elderly, with 8 to 40 percent of all falls resulting in a fracture. While tripping is the most common cause of falls in those aged 65 to 75, other medical conditions, including instability of gait, light-headedness, or syncope are very common and increase in those over age 75. Frequent fractures incurred during falls include the femoral neck, radius/ulna, acetabulum, and pelvic ring. Osteoporosis is common among elderly women, and fractures may not be immediately discernible on radiographs. Confounding factors that impair the physician's ability to evaluate elderly patients include an inability to ambulate, altered level of consciousness, and confusion induced by an unfamiliar environment. In this setting, if plain films are negative and a high index of suspicion remains for fracture, more sensitive testing, such as bone scanning or computed tomography, should be ordered. All elderly patients, regardless of the source or site of their traumatic injury, are prone to complications (Table 204-2).

There are several prevention, assessment, and treatment strategies to be used when dealing with the elderly patient who has sustained trauma. As previously mentioned, having a high index of suspicion for occult injury and ordering appropriate radiographs and special diagnostic studies are of paramount importance. This must be coupled with a lower threshold for admission of these patients. The emergency physician must guard against the tendency to label such admissions as "social." Such a naive attitude exposes the ignorance of some medical personnel with regard to the *medical* and *physiologic* changes in the geriatric population. Examples of this type of age-specific problem potentially requiring admission are the inability to ambulate or use crutches, coexisting medical conditions that impair the patient's ability to provide self-care, decreased cognitive abilities that may be exacerbated by "minor" injuries, and lack of attentive care from the family at home. Whether supportive measures are able to make the home environment as conducive to recovery as inpatient care is controversial. Nonetheless, social service consultation and follow-up are highly desirable and probably improve patient outcome. The ability of the patient or the family to comprehend multiple medication regimens must be evaluated carefully before discharge.

ELDER ABUSE

Elder abuse has become an increasingly recognized problem in our society. Estimates of the prevalence of this phenomenon are that 4 percent of the population at risk, or 1.1 million elderly persons, are victims of abuse. Tragically, this figure has been increasing at the rate of 100,000 estimated cases per year. The great strides that have occurred in the recognition of child abuse have not yet been accomplished for the elderly. Legal intervention for elder abuse falls under the jurisdiction of the states. Reporting requirements, intervention options, and financial support for these interventions vary from state to state. The optimal strategies for combating this problem are unknown.

It is suspected that most elder abuse goes undetected and unreported by both medical and social service personnel. Numerous reasons have been postulated and include: (1) a significant number of home-bound, or "invisible" elderly, who do not have access to potential points of discovery by medical or social service professionals, (2) discriminative attitudes toward the elderly on the part of health and social service professionals, (3) poor or nonexistent medical training specific to geriatric issues, and (4) unwillingness or inability of the elder victim to complain of the abuse due to cognitive impairment or social pressures.

There are several types of elder abuse, including physical abuse (or assault), psychological abuse, neglect, sexual abuse, deprivation of rights, and financial abuse. This discussion will concentrate on physical abuse and neglect, because these problems commonly present to the emergency department and can be immediately life threatening if not recognized and addressed in a timely manner. Table 204-3 summarizes potential indicators of elder abuse that should be recognized by emergency department personnel. In the past, elder abuse was thought to be primarily a problem of the institutionalized elderly. However, it is now found in many settings, including elders who live alone, live with relatives, or are in extended-care facilities. Recent studies have shown

Table 204-3. "Red Flags" and Indicators of Possible Elder Abuse

History
- Elder brought to emergency department by someone other than caregiver.
- Elder with chronic debility found home alone.
- Prolonged interval between injury and presentation for care.
- Medication noncompliance.
- Pattern of emergency department or physician hopping.
- The history does not fit the injury.
- Previous unexplained injuries.

Physical
- Suspicious injuries
  - Unusual fractures, dislocations
  - Lacerations or burns in unusual locations or shapes
  - Injuries to the head with unknown mechanism
  - Contusions in unusual locations or in varying degrees of healing
- Poor hygiene
- Unexplained dehydration
- Signs of medication noncompliance
- Genital complaints, including unexplained sexually transmitted diseases

Observations
- Psychologic state of patient, e.g., unexplained depression, withdrawal, or suicidal ideation
- Interactions between patient and caregiver
  - Patient fearful of caregiver
  - Differing accounts of injury
  - Caregiver indifferent or hostile to patient
  - Caregiver overly concerned with financial aspects of care
  - Caregiver tries to prevent patient interacting privately with physician

that incapacity of elderly patients may play a smaller role in placing them at risk of abuse than problems related to the caregiver. These problems often include dependency on the elder, financial or other exogenous stress, and chemical dependency on the part of the caregiver.

When gathering a history from elderly patients that the physician suspects may be at risk for abuse, it is important that the patient is interviewed alone first and then with the caregiver, if appropriate. Physicians should ask direct questions about the patient's care. Emphasis should be placed on the patient's unmet needs as a way to elicit background information. The patient should always be asked if they feel they are in danger and if they wish to remain at home.

The physical examination should be thorough and complete. The patient should be completely exposed and rolled over to examine the entire body for lacerations, burns, contusions, or pressure sores. Careful assessment of the mental status, hydration status, hygiene, head, and musculoskeletal system should be made. Other aspects of the examination should emphasize other organ systems relevant to the patient's presenting complaint. Documentation of all findings should be meticulous—it may be necessary for use as legal document in potential court proceedings.

The objectives for managing elder trauma patients are

1. Identify the elder who is at risk for abuse.
2. Institute measures to protect the elder from further injury.
3. Provide evaluation for treatment of acute injuries and medical conditions resulting from abuse or neglect.
4. Remain objective and nonjudgmental but effective in protecting the patient.
5. Attempt to establish and maintain an interactive relationship with the family during the patient's visit.
6. Report all suspected cases of elder abuse and/or neglect in accordance with local statutes.

Resources for the treatment and protection of the abused elderly vary by geographic location. They may include social service consultants, visiting nurses, shelters, and extended-care facilities. Some states provide accelerated access to legal resources, such as restraining orders. It is important for each emergency department to establish protocols for appropriate cases. These protocols can be tailored for individual institutions and become a part of the patients' medicolegal record.

A unique and important aspect of elder abuse treatment is the recognition of the elder's right to choose. Once competency of the patient is established, they may decide to stay in a potentially dangerous environment. It is important in these cases to offer support services, provide continued access to the health care system, and carefully document the patient's decision. If the patient is not competent to decide on their treatment and they are in a potentially dangerous environment, consultation and admission with or without caregiver consent may be the wisest choice for patient protection. Emergency physicians should know the legal prerogatives afforded by the laws governing this issue in the state where they practice. Finally, the identification and prevention of elder abuse must be considered a primary responsibility of emergency physicians. Although it requires time, training, and energy to remain attentive to this issue, the potential to decrease pain and suffering among the elderly is enormous if the specialty of emergency medicine will take this responsibility seriously.

BIBLIOGRAPHY

AMA Council on Scientific Affairs: Elder abuse and neglect. *JAMA* 257:966, 1987.

Bloom JS, Ansell P, Bloom MN: Detecting elder abuse: A guide for physicians. *Geriatrics* 44:40, 1989.

Copeland AR: Fatal accidental falls among the elderly–The Metro Dade County Experience, 1981–1983. *Med Sci Law* 25:172, 1985.

Finelli FC, Jonsson J, Chapion HR, et al: A case control study for major trauma in geriatric patients. *J Trauma* 29:541, 1989.

Hogue CC: Injury in late life: Part I. Epidemiology. *J Am Geriatrics Soc* 30: 183, 1982.

Jones J, Doughery J, Schelble D, et al: Emergency department protocol for the diagnosis and evaluation of geriatric abuse. *Ann Emerg Med* 17:1006, 1988.

Martin RE, Teberian G: Multiple trauma and the elderly patient. *Emerg Med Clinics North Am* 8:411, 1990.

O'Malley TA, Everitt DE, O'Malley MA, et al: Identifying and preventing family-mediated abuse and neglect of elderly persons. *Ann Intern Med* 98:998, 1983.

Oreskovich MR, Howard JD, Copass MK, et al: Geriatric trauma: Injury patterns and outcome. *J Trauma* 24:565, 1984.

Perry BC: Falls among the elderly: A review of the methods and conclusions of epidemiologic studies. *J Am Geriatrics Soc* 30:367, 1982.

Pillemer K, Finkelhor D: Causes of elder abuse: Caregiver stress vesus problem relatives. *Am J Orthopsychiatry* 59:179, 1989.

Quinn MJ, Tomita SK: *Elder Abuse and Neglect*. New York, Springer, 1986, pp. 162–163.

Scalea TM, Simon HM, Duncan AO, et al: Geriatric blunt multiple trauma: Improved survival with early invasive monitoring. *J Trauma* 30:129, 1990.

Select Committee on Aging, U.S. House of Representatives: *Elder Abuse: A National Disgrace*. Washington, DC, 1985, Comm Pub. #99-502, pp. 47–49.

Sklar DP, Demarest GB, McFeeley P: Increased pedestrian mortality among the elderly. *Am J Emerg Med* 7:387, 1989.

Spaite DW: Fractures, dislocations and major ligamentous injuries of the thoracic and lumbar spine, *in* Galli R, Spaite DW, Simon RR(eds): *Emergency Orthopedics: The Spine*. Norwalk, Appleton, Century and Crofts, 1989, pp 212–237.

Spaite DW, Criss EA, Valenzuela TD, et al: Geriatric injury: An analysis of prehospital demographics, mechanisms, and patterns. *Ann Emerg Med* 19:1418, 1990.

U.S. Bureau of the Census: *Statistical Abstract of the United States 1990*. Washington DC, 1990, p. 37.

Weingarten MS, Tark Wainwright ST, Sacchetti AD: Trauma and aging effects on hospital costs and length of stay. *Ann Emerg Med* 17:10, 1988.

The views expressed in this chapter are those of the authors and do not reflect the official policy or position of the Department of the Navy, the Department of Defense, or the U.S. Government.

205 ASSESSMENT OF THE NEUROLOGICALLY IMPAIRED PATIENT

David C. Anderson

Evaluation of patients with preexisting neurologic defects for a possible new problem is difficult under the least pressured circumstances. The challenge is even greater in the emergency department. In such patients, the value of both the history and examination may be diminished. A history available from the patient will be unreliable if cognitive deficits are present. Furthermore, interpretation of examination data is likely to be confounded.

In previously normal patients, the neurologic examination is an accurate guide to the nature of a new neurologic problem. A structural process is made unlikely by a normal examination. A focal deficit reflects focal pathology and diffuse deficits, a diffuse process. These generally reliable rules of assessment must be modified or suspended in patients with preexisting neurologic defects (Tables 205-1 and 205-2). An awareness of particular risks that various neurologic diseases pose is helpful but cannot be the only guide. The safest approach is to maintain a high index of suspicion, a low threshold for recommending hospitalization, and a willingness to perform tests.

Table 205-1. Well-Recognized Phenomena when New Processes Occur in Patients with Preexisting Neurologic Deficits

Focal lesions may present with generalized or diffuse neurologic manifestations, e.g., a new stroke may be manifested primarily by confusion in a patient with multiple previous stroke-related deficits.

Generalized neurologic processes may present with reemergence of old compensated focal neurologic deficits, e.g., an old hemiparesis related to a remote crebrovascular event may reappear in a patient with acute hyponatremia.

Normally well-tolerated systemic insults may produce neurologic dysfunction, e.g., increased confusion or even coma may occur in a patient with dementia during an otherwise occult urinary tract infection.

The sensitivity of the neurologic examination in detection of lesions is compromised dramatically when a patient cannot cooperate fully with all its components, e.g., it is not possible to perform reliable tests of the sensory and coordination systems in patients with preexisting dementia.

Table 205-2. Guidelines for Identifying New Problems

Listen to caregivers who have experience with the patient. They have the best sense for what the patient's baseline is, and they know best when something has changed. If they have much experience, they may even know where to look. For example, nursing home personnel may know that the last time a demented patient became more confused he had a fecal impaction.

Be willing to cast a wide net remembering that our usual indications for test ordering (i.e., a computed tomography scan for focal signs and toxicology and metabolic screens for diffuse manifestations) are different in this setting. A scan would be appropriate in an acutely confused patient who has old deficits related to stroke or trauma if other explanations are not immediately forthcoming.

In the same vein, be prepared to look outside of the nervous system for explanations for neurologic deterioration, e.g., a patient with Parkinson's disease may become unable to ambulate because of dehydration.

Be aware of particular risks posed by a preexisting neurologic process, e.g., head injury is a risk in patients with disorders that impair gait stability. Aspiration pneumonia, which may present with confusion, frequently complicates bulbar dysfunction due to brain stem or, more often, bihemispheric lesions.

CHRONIC MENTAL STATUS CHANGES

Results of history and mental status examination define neurologic behavioral syndromes. The onset, duration, and progress of the abnormality is ascertained through the history. Typically, organic or nonpsychiatric brain diseases affecting behavior impair attention, orientation, recent memory, calculations, judgment, language, and constructional tasks like cube drawing. Acquired, chronic, usually progressive impairment across all cognitive aspects is called dementia.

Dementia may present for the first time in emergency circumstances because of complications of self-neglect (e.g., advanced infections), injuries related to impaired judgment (e.g., falls and vehicular accidents), or behavioral complications (e.g., fear and aggressive behavior). Formal mental status assessment will define the cognitive deficit pattern in such circumstances. If memory deficits are severe, however, it may be unclear without a collateral history whether the cognitive deficits are sufficiently long standing to qualify as dementia. Acute confusion or delirium is characterized by the same profile of diffuse cognitive impairment but is differentiated from dementia by its more recent onset. In the absence of definitive information about mode of onset and duration, clinical features sometimes provide a clue. A waxing and waning course, severe impairment in attention, and reduced level of consciousness are typical of the syndrome of acute confusion but not dementia. The distinction between the two syndromes is important in theory because the etiologic concerns are different for the two syndromes. Because confident distinction cannot be established on the grounds of available data, it is often necessary to consider the causes for both syndromes in evaluating a given case.

In those cases when the presence of dementia can be established by history (acquired, chronic, and progressive) and formal mental status testing (across-the-board cognitive deficits), the appropriate goals are to seek out and eliminate treatable causes or contributors. The yield for treatable causes of true dementia is relatively low, but the stakes obviously are high. Structural possibilities like chronic subdural hematoma, benign tumors, and hydrocephalus warrant an imaging study. Chronic metabolic and nutritional abnormalities (e.g., hypothyroidism and vitamin B_{12} deficiency) should be sought. It should be recalled that depression may resemble dementia in some cases. Finally, unexpected but potentially serious incidental medical problems (such as occult urinary tract infections, pneumonia, and gastrointestinal bleeding) are discovered by screening in a significant proportion of individuals presenting with dementia.

In the emergency setting, it is probably more common for a patient with previously documented dementia to present with a possibly related or new problem. Brain disease and cognitive impairment will influence the mode of presentation of the problem and usually interfere with its discovery. Problems remote from the nervous system may present as worsening dementia. On the other hand, new neurologic processes may be camouflaged by the preexisting deficits and the patient's inability to cooperate for careful neurologic examination. Particularly common among the former are urinary tract infections, pneumonia, myocardial infarction, and congestive heart failure. Common complicating neurologic processes in demented patients are subdural hematomas from falls, which are usually unreported by the patient and sometimes unwitnessed, and cerebrovascular disease.

Finally, demented patients are particularly susceptible to the effects of medications. The most seemingly innocent of agents, including over-the-counter medications, may cause profound deterioration of function. Particularly notorious causes of toxic confusion are drugs with anticholinergic actions and sedatives, which sometimes cause a paradoxical agitation. Withdrawal syndromes, especially from benzodiazepines, can result in increased confusion and agitation. Medication may have been suddenly stopped because of confusion or inability to refill a prescription.

OTHER COMMON CHRONIC NEUROLOGIC CONDITIONS

Like chronic cognitive deficits, deficits of other systems may become more severe in the setting of systemic illness. The preexisting abnormalities will interfere with the sensitivity of neurologic examination. Finally, such deficits predispose to problems, especially falls, which may produce intracranial hematomas, and infections (e.g., aspiration pneumonitis and urinary tract infection), which produce neurologic deterioration indirectly. Unfortunately, the clinical manifestations of these two different types of complications are often similar.

Common mechanisms of acquired chronic brain dysfunction are severe head trauma and cerebrovascular disease. In both cases, the specific deficits will depend on the location of the injury. In contrast to the degenerative conditions discussed below, both of these types of injury produce static deficits that may be complicated by seizure disorders.

Multiple sclerosis typically causes visual, motor, sensory, cerebellar, and urinary bladder dysfunction in otherwise healthy young adults. The disease usually follows an exacerbating and remitting course. In extreme examples, patients may be functionally normal one week, neurologically devastated the next, and recovered several weeks to months later. Over the long term, there is often a gradual downhill trend. Flairs may reflect a reactivation of the chronic immunopathologic processes thought to be the etiologic basis of the disease. They may also be due to reappearance of deficits referable to old lesions sustained during remote disease activity. This decompensation typically occurs in the setting of a new infectious process (especially urinary infection). Interference with conduction along diseased tracts by elevated body temperature may be the mechanism of decompensation.

Parkinsonism is manifested by resting tremor, increased tone, a reduction in spontaneous movement, and postural instability. Bulbar dysfunction (e.g., dysarthria, dysphonia, and dysphagia) and autonomic disturbances (e.g., postural hypotension and urinary bladder dysfunction) are common in advanced disease. Dementia develops in some patients with long-standing parkinsonism. Systemic illness may produce an exacerbation of all these features. Inability to walk, for example, may be the mode of presentation for dehydration or urinary infection.

Motor system disease (amyotrophic lateral sclerosis or Lou Gehrig's disease) causes weakness of the bulb (swallowing, articulating, and phonating), limbs, and ventilatory muscles without deficits of other systems (cognition and sensation, for examples, are normal). Features of both upper (toe signs, brisk reflexes, and spasticity) and lower motor neuron involvement (atrophy and fasciculations) are present. Aspiration pneumonitis is a common complication that may precipitate respiratory failure.

Parkinson's disease and motor system disease are examples of system degenerations or abiotrophies in which neurons in specific neurologic functional units die (substantia nigra in the former and upper and lower motor neurons in the latter). The resulting clinical pictures are common and well known. Less common, sometimes familial, degenerative diseases produce different patterns of cell loss pathologically and their own characteristic clinical pictures. The clinical syndromes intermix extrapyramidal, pyramidal, cerebellar, autonomic, sensory, and sometimes cognitive deficits. Like parkinsonism, these deficits predispose to problems (e.g., falls or aspiration) and may be worsened by systemic processes.

COMPLICATIONS OF DRUGS USED IN CHRONIC NEUROLOGIC CONDITIONS

Chronic diseases of the nervous system typically are treated with medications that have characteristic side effects. Ironically, the nervous system itself is often the target of untoward effects.

Anticonvulsants

In addition to the usual anticonvulsant side effects, patients with chronic neurologic disorders may manifest unexpected toxicities. For example, chorea, athetosis, and dystonias may occur with toxic levels of phenytoin or carbamazepine. Stupor or coma may occur in patients treated with valproic acid, usually in conjunction with other anticonvulsants.

Antipsychotic Agents

The anticholinergic effects of some antipsychotics may have the unintended effect of increasing confusion when used in patients with mild dementia complicated by disturbed behavior. Actions on the bladder and bowel may also cause difficulty. Also, patients with underlying brain disease may be at greater risk for the extrapyramidal complications of chronic dopamine blockade. Parkinsonism, chorea, dystonias, akathisia, tardive movements, and the malignant neuroleptic syndrome may result.

Antiparkinsonian Agents

Agents used in treating Parkinson's disease include anticholinergics (confusion, bowel and bladder dysfunction, and heat dysregulation), the dopamine releaser amantadine (confusion, especially in dialysis patients, and fluid retention), L-dopa (confusion, hyperkinetic movement disorders, and postural hypotension), dopamine agonists like bromocriptine (confusion and hyperkinetic movement disorders), and the monoamine oxidase inhibitor deprenyl (confusion).

Antispasticity Agents

The gamma-aminobutyric acid agonist, baclofen, and benzodiazepines act centrally to reduce tone and prevent painful spasms. Both types of drugs may cause sedation. It should be recognized that some patients may depend on spasticity for weight bearing or as a fulcrum for transfers. Consequently, successful reduction in tone may be associated with functional difficulty interpreted as neurologic deterioration. Dantrolene sodium acts on spastic muscles themselves. Hepatic toxicity is common.

SPECIAL PRECAUTIONS IN NEUROLOGICALLY DISABLED PATIENTS

Beyond the caveats and recommendations presented in Tables 205-1 and 205-2, the following are useful guidelines. Use much smaller doses of psychoactive agents in patients with underlying chronic neurologic conditions. For example, when dosing haloperidol, a commonly used sedative in elderly patients, begin at 0.5 mg in patients with underlying dementia. Be wary of physical restraints. Ironically, although applied to prevent injury from falls, they may be an instrument of harm in some patients, for example by causing strangulation. Patients with movement disorders, like chorea and hemiballism, sustain less tissue damage if they are cared for without restraints by applying protective padding to dangerous adjacent surfaces and edges (e.g., bed railings).

BIBLIOGRAPHY

Buchner DM, Larson EB: Falls and fractures in patients with Alzheimer-type dementia. *JAMA* 257:1492, 1987.

Clarfield AM: The reversible dementias: Do they reverse? *Ann Intern Med* 109:476, 1988.

Consensus Conference: Differential diagnosis of dementing diseases. *JAMA* 258:3411, 1987.

Dubin WR, Weiss KJ, Zeccardi JA: Organic brain syndrome: The psychiatric imposter. *JAMA* 249:60, 1983.

Evans LK, Strumpf NE: Tying down the elderly: A review of the literature on physical restraint. *J Am Geriatr Soc* 36:65, 1989.

Irvine P: An approach to the management of medical problems in demented patients. *Clin Geriatr Med* 4:703, 1988.

Larson EB, Reifler BV, Sumi SM, et al: Diagnostic tests in the evaluation of dementia: A prospective study of 200 elderly outpatients. *Arch Intern Med* 146:1917, 1986.

Larson EB, Kukull WA, Buchner D, et al: Adverse drug reactions associated with global cognitive impairment in elderly persons. *Ann Intern Med* 107:169, 1987.

Odenheimer GL: Acquired cognitive disorders of the elderly. *Med Clin North Am* 73:1383, 1989.

Rosebush P, Stewart T: A prospective analysis of 24 episodes of neuroleptic malignant syndrome. *Am J Psychiatry* 146:717, 1989.

Task Force Sponsored by the National Institute on Aging: Senility reconsidered: Treatment possibilities for mental impairment in the elderly. *JAMA* 244:259, 1980.

Waxman HM, Dubin W, Klein M, et al: Geriatric psychiatry in the emergency department. II: Evaluation and treatment of geriatric and nongeriatric admissions. *J Am Geriatr Soc* 32:343, 1983.

SECTION 22
The High Technology Patient

206
PATIENTS WITH ORGAN TRANSPLANTS

Leslie Rocher

The treatment of end-stage organ failure of the kidney, heart, and liver by transplantation is increasing as rapidly as the supply of appropriate organs allows. Once viewed as experimental, results are now sufficiently improved that transplantation of these organs is now an accepted, life-saving, clinical treatment in appropriately selected recipients. In 1989, approximately 9000 renal transplants, 2400 liver transplants, and 2000 heart transplants were performed in the United States. The 1-year success rate for graft function of cadaver donor kidney transplants was 78 percent and for living donor kidney transplants was 89 percent, with 1-year patient survival exceeding 90 percent for both procedures. For heart transplantation, 1-year patient survival is now 80 to 85 percent and 5-year survival approaches 70 percent. Similar success rates are achieved at experienced liver transplant centers. Marrow transplantation, because it is performed for an extremely broad array of indications (such as genetic diseases, aplastic anemia, and a variety of leukemias and lymphomas), has a more variable success rate, which is dependent on several host and donor factors.

Over the next decade, pancreas transplantation, either whole organ or with islet cells alone, and lung transplantation will become more successful and common. In the more distant future, small bowel transplantation, neural transplant, and xenografts (donor recipient pairs of disparate species origin) may be feasible as the science of transplant immunobiology advances.

The emergency physician must be able to recognize the unique array of complications that may occur in this group of individuals and develop appropriate algorithms to evaluate the transplant recipient. Renal-transplant recipients will serve as a model for all whole organ recipients in this chapter. The emergency physician is far more likely to encounter renal rather than extrarenal-transplant recipients, and in general, the complications related to immunosuppression of the renal-transplant recipient may be extrapolated to recipients of other solid organs. Where appropriate, comments about unique features of nonrenal transplant recipients will made.

IMMUNOLOGY OF TRANSPLANTATION

The recipient of a whole-organ allograft is always at risk to reject his or her transplant and must therefore maintain immunosuppression indefinitely. In the case of liver and heart transplantation, this represents the lifetime of the recipient. For the renal transplant recipient, immunosuppression is maintained as long as a renal allograft continues to function. This difference exists because dialysis may serve as an extended treatment of end-stage renal failure if the transplant fails, whereas the only treatment for an irreversibly failing heart or liver graft is retransplantation.

There are three major types of rejection observed in whole-organ transplantation: hyperacute, acute, and chronic. The rarest, most severe, and least treatable is hyperacute rejection, which is mediated by preformed circulating anti-human leukocyte antigen (HLA) antibody in the host directed toward the donor. In the vast majority of cases, it may be prevented by choosing ABO-compatible donor-recipient pairs and performing an immediate pretransplant assay for such anti-HLA antibody (this assay is known as a cross match). If the cross match is positive, the transplant is not performed. This is always the case in renal transplantation, but exceptions may be made in liver and heart transplants. If hyperacute rejection occurs, it does so within a few minutes to hours after surgery and causes irreversible allograft destruction.

Acute rejection is the most common form of rejection. It typically develops from 1 week to 3 months after transplant surgery. It may also occur, albeit with less frequency, at any time thereafter. Acute rejection is the result of disparity between donor and host in the major histocompatibility antigen system (HLA) in humans. This system is extremely polymorphic as evidenced by over 100 known HLA antigens. It is, therefore, not generally possible to completely match donor and recipient for these antigens in the case of cadaver donors. The HLA system encodes two classes of cell-surface structures that usually serve to distinguish self from nonself immunologically and also serve to present processed foreign antigen to appropriate host cells to initiate an immune response. The genetic code for these two classes of molecules resides on the short arm of the sixth chromosome. Class I antigens are found on virtually all nucleated cells and are composed of a heavy chain glycoprotein noncovalently linked to B2 microglobulin. In clinical practice, relevant class I antigens are termed HLA-A and HLA-B. Every person codominantly expresses both parental HLA antigens on each cell, or two HLA-A and two HLA-B antigens. Class II antigens are much more restricted in their distribution and are found on B lymphocytes, activated T lympocytes, macrophages, and cytokine-stimulated endothelial cells and tissue parenchymal cells. Class II antigens are composed of an α- and a β-glycoprotein chain. In clinical practice the relevant class II antigen system is termed HLA-DR. As with class I antigens, each individual codominantly expresses both parentally inherited class II antigens. In general, it is believed that class II antigen disparity is the primary stimulus of the host immune response to an allograft and that class I antigens of donor parenchymal tissue serve as a major target for killer T lymphocytes of host origin.

In current clinical practice, six HLA antigens can be routinely identified (two each at HLA-A, -B, and -DR loci). The more well-matched the donor-recipient pair for the HLA system, the better the chance of long-term successful engraftment. This is best demonstrated in the renal-transplant recipient who has a mean duration of graft function of 6 to 8 years with a cadaver donor (average HLA match, one to two antigens), 10 to 12 years with a semi-identical HLA matched kidney (as from a parental donor, three of six antigens matched), and 25 years with an HLA identical match (HLA identical sibling, six of six antigens). The fact that even recipients of HLA identical sibling kidneys require immunosuppression provides strong argument that other inherited histocompatibility antigen systems, not encoded on the sixth chromosome, are also clinically relevent. Only recipients of grafts from identical twins are spared the need for immunosuppression.

Chronic rejection is the least well understood of the three forms of rejection. It too is the result of HLA donor-recipient disparity. Its course is, however, much more indolent than acute rejection and, once started, is more difficult to interrupt because intervention with short-term intense immunosuppression does not seem to confer benefit.

CLINICAL PRESENTATION AND THERAPY OF ACUTE REJECTION

Of the three forms of rejection described above, diagnosis and treatment of acute rejection is the most critical. Without timely recognition and intervention, allograft function may deteriorate irreversibly in a few days.

The renal-transplant recipient, when symptomatic from acute rejection, will complain of vague tenderness over the allograft (in the left or right iliac fossa, a heterotopic location in contrast to the orthotopic location of liver or heart transplants). The patient also may describe decreased urine output, a rapid weight gain (from fluid retention), a low-grade fever, and a generalized malaise. Physical examination may disclose worsening hypertension, allograft tenderness, and peripheral edema. *The absence of these symptoms and signs, however, does not exclude the possibility of acute rejection.* With improved methods of maintenance immunosuppression (see below), the only clue may be an asymptomatic decline in renal function, as assessed by a rising serum creatinine. Therefore, even small asymptomatic changes in serum creatinine cannot be dismissed as unimportant and must be investigated. Even a change in creatinine from 1.0 mg/dL to 1.2 or 1.3 mg/dL may be important. When such changes in creatinine are reproducible, a careful workup consists of, in addition to a careful history and examination, a complete urinalysis, renal ultrasonography, and a trough level of cyclosporine. It is critical to interpret changes in renal function in the context of prior data (e.g., trends of recent serum creatinines, recent history of rejection, or other causes of allograft dysfunction). The workup should proceed in a manner to consider the multiple etiologies of decreased renal function in the renal transplant recipient as outlined in Table 206-1. The two most common causes, apart from acute rejection causing an increase in creatinine, are volume contraction and cyclosporine-induced nephrotoxicity.

The clinical clues to allograft rejection in the recipient of a liver transplant may also be very subtle and include vague right upper quadrant pain and slight tenderness of the liver to palpation. Increases in the bilirubin and transaminase levels have the same importance in these patients as does the serum creatinine in renal transplant recipients. The cardiac-transplant recipient will not experience chest pain with acute rejection but may manifest symptoms and signs of congestive heart failure late in rejection. In these patients, a routine schedule of right ventricular endomyocardial biopsy is needed to monitor the development of rejection; less invasive means are not sufficiently sensitive or specific.

Table 206-1. Causes of Renal Allograft Dysfunction: The Differential Diagnosis of an Elevated Serum Creatinine

Acute rejection
Prerenal axotemia from volume contraction
Drug-induced renal dysfunction
Cyclosporine
Trimethoprim-sulfamethoxazole
Nonsteroidal antiinflammatory drugs
Aminoglycosides
Urologic complication
Ureteral obstruction
Compression of ureter by lymphocele
Urine leak
Transplant glomerulonephritis
Recurrent disease
De novo glomerulonephritis
Urinary tract infection or pyelonephritis
Systemic infection
CMV disease
Sepsis
Vascular complication
Renal artery stenosis
Transplant renal vein thrombosis
Chronic rejection

Treatment of allograft rejection generally is divided into two phases. The first is high-dose corticosteroids, typically methylprednisolone 250 to 500 mg intravenously, for 3 to 4 consecutive days. Occasionally, oral steroids may be increased to 100 to 200 mg per day and rapidly tapered toward maintenance levels. If allograft function remains unimproved or partially improved, a biopsy is often done to assess if rejection is ongoing. If ongoing rejection is documented, therapy is initiated with antibody preparations directed toward lymphocytes, most commonly with OKT3, a murine monoclonal antibody directed to the CD3 receptor present on all circulating T lymphocytes. Such therapy is highly immunosuppressive and has multiple potential toxicities including fever, pulmonary edema, hypotension, diarrhea, headache, and aseptic meningitis. It is, therefore, undertaken only after adequate exclusion of other causes of persistent allograft dysfunction and with careful monitoring under rigorous protocols defined by the transplant service at each institution.

MAINTENANCE IMMUNOSUPPRESSION

Not all patients experience episodes of acute allograft rejection as discussed above. Maintenance, daily oral immunosuppression is used to prevent such episodes and to mitigate emergence of chronic rejection. Patients are instructed to remain absolutely rigorous and faithful in their dosing of these medications. Interruption of maintenance immunosuppression for even 1 day may be sufficient to induce an episode of acute rejection. Currently, three drugs are used as maintenance immunosuppression: cyclosporine, azathioprine, and prednisone. New drugs currently are being tested and may alter protocols dramatically in the next 5 to 10 years. These include FK506 and rapamycin.

Cyclosporine is a cyclic 11-amino acid fungal metabolite introduced into clinical transplantation in the late 1970s and made generally available in 1983. It is a potent inhibitor of T lymphocyte activity and interferes with the generation of interleukin-2 (IL-2), a necessary factor for propagation of the immune response to the whole-organ allograft. It is highly lipophilic, and its metabolism is almost exclusively hepatic through the cytochrome P_{450} system. Typical doses vary substantially, but are usually 3 to 6 mg/kg/per day as a single dose or in two divided doses. The therapeutic level of cyclosporine is very dependent on the type of assay used and is commonly 75 to 200 ng/mL. Many drugs are known to potentiate the metabolism of cyclosporine and thus to increase to the required dose of the immunosuppressant. Other drugs inhibit its metabolism and therefore may promote high cyclosporine drug levels. Table 206-2 lists some of these drugs. A sudden increase in cyclosporine levels often is accompanied by a decrease in renal function which usually is hemodynamically mediated and reversible if recognized. A sudden decrease in cyclosporine drug levels may open the door to an episode of acute rejection. It is therefore incumbent on any physician treating a patient receiving cyclosporine to check that any addition or withdrawal of drugs or changes in drug doses does not potentially affect cyclosporine metabolism. If a drug from Table 206-2 must be added, deleted, or its dose changed, the patient and the transplant center should be informed of the potential consequences of the maneuver and a follow-up trough cyclosporine level should be obtained in the near future.

Common side effects of cyclosporine include hypertension, hirsutism, and tremulouness. It may produce hyperkalemia, hypomagnesemia, and hyperuricemia. Attacks of gouty arthritis have been attributed to the drug. Less common are glucose intolerance, gingival hyperplasia, and seizures. The most common serious toxicity of the drug is renal insufficiency; this is a particularly vexing problem in the renal-transplant recipient in whom this may be confused with acute rejection. In recipients of heart and liver transplants, the drug has caused end-stage renal failure requiring dialysis or renal transplant. In general,

Table 206-2. Cyclosporine (CsA) Drug Interactions

Drugs augmenting CsA metabolism (dropping CsA levels)
Phenobarbital
Phenytoin
Rifampin
Isoniazid
Drugs interfering with CsA metabolism (increasing CsA levels)
Ketoconazole
Verapamil
Diltiezem
Fluconazole
Erythromycin
Cimetidine

however, cyclosporine nephrotoxicity is a prerenal, vasospastic process that reverses upon lowering of the drug dose. Clearly, a fine line exists between drug-induced renal dysfunction and underimmunosuppression from too low a drug level.

Azathioprine is a derivative of 6-mercaptopurine and interferes with the purine metabolism of rapidly proliferating cells. It is typically given at doses of 1 to 2 mg/kg per day. Its primary toxicity is bone marrow suppression, particularly of neutrophils, but it may also cause anemia and thrombocytopenia. There are no drug levels available in clinical practice, and the white blood cell count is surveyed frequently with the dose adjusted to avoid neutropenia. The most important drug interaction is with allopurinol which inhibits xanthine oxidase-mediated degradation of 6-mercaptopurine, thereby dramatically potentiating the effect of azathioprine. There are case reports of profound and prolonged cytopenias after unmonitored use of allopurinol with azathioprine and consequent secondary fatal superinfections.

Corticosteroids are also an integral part of posttransplant immunosuppression in most patients. The relevant action of corticosteroids in these patients is mediated by interference with synthesis of IL-1 and IL-6. The numerous toxicities of this class of drugs are recognized widely and include hypertension, glucose intolerance, acne, osteopenia, cataract formation, salt retention, obesity, hyperlipidemia, mood swings, myopathy, impaired wound healing, peptic ulcer disease, alopecia, and a dampened febrile response to infection. Typical maintenance doses 3 months after surgery are 10 to 20 mg/day. Occasionally, alternate-day prednisone or even steroid withdrawal may be prescribed in well-matched donor-recipient pairs. It is hoped that, with the introduction of more potent alternatives to currently available immunosuppression, routine use of steroids may be avoided in the future.

The sum effect of maintenance immunosuppression used in the prevention of allograft rejection and intermittent high-dose immunosuppression used to treat acute rejection is a variable depression in cell-mediated immunity and a consequent increase in the risk of opportunistic infections. It is also believed that the vigor of immunosuppression is proportionally associated with an increased risk of malignancy.

POSTTRANSPLANT INFECTIOUS COMPLICATIONS

Infections after transplantation are a common and feared complication. Predisposing factors include ongoing immunosuppression in all patients, and the presence of diabetes mellitus, advanced age, obesity, and other host factors in some. Table 206-3 displays the broad array of potential infections stratified by the time after transplant they are most apt to occur.

Prophylaxis of infections is becoming an increasingly important part of transplant protocols. Pretransplant patients are generally vaccinated with pneumoccocal vaccine and often with hepatitis B vaccine. Posttransplant, most recipients receive trimethoprimsulfamethoxazole for at least 3 months to minimize the risk of *pneumocystis carinii* pneumonia and urinary tract infections. High-dose acyclovir, sometimes in combination with immune globulin, may attenuate the risk of posttransplant cytomegalovirus infection. Nystatin frequently is prescribed during the early transplant period when corticosteroid doses are at their highest to prevent oral candidiasis. Prophylaxis for dental procedures also is prescribed. It should be recognized that some vaccines are contraindicated in the posttransplant period because live attenuated viruses still are potentially too virulent in this population. Such vaccines include the oral poliovirus vaccine and measles, mumps, and rubella vaccines.

Table 206-3. Infectious Complications of Whole-Organ Transplantation

First month posttransplant
Bacterial
Wound infection
Pneumonia
Urinary tract infection
Line-related sepsis
Viral
Herpes simplex
Hepatitis B
Fungal
Candidal pharyngitis, esophagitis, cystitis
Second to 6th months posttransplant
Bacterial
Pneumonia—pneumococcal and other community acquired pneumonitis
Urinary tract infection
Nocardial infection
Listeriosis
Viral
Cytomegalovirus, EBV, HSV, varicella zoster
Adenovirus
Hepatitis A, B, C
Papovavirus
Fungal
Asperigillosis
Candidal pharyngitis, esophagitis, cystitis
Other opportunistic infection
Pneumocystis carinii pneumonia, tuberculosis, toxoplasmosis
Beyond 6th month posttransplant
Bacterial
Pneumonia—pneumococcal and other community acquired pneumonitis
Urinary tract infection
Listeriosis
Viral
Cytomegalovirus chorioretinitis
Varicella zoster
Fungal
Cryptococcal
Other opportunistic infection
Pneumocystis carinii pneumonia

The most common life-threatening infection in recipients of solid organs, and even more so in the case of bone marrow graft recipients, is cytomegalovirus (CMV). Exposure to this double-stranded DNA herpes virus is very common; most people over the age of 35 exhibit detectable IgG antibody to CMV antibody levels. After initial infection of a nonimmunocompromised patient, the virus enters a latent phase and is present in virtually all organs. Hence, an allografted kidney, heart, or liver may transmit the virus. In a transplant recipient without prior CMV immunity, receipt of an organ from a serologically positive donor makes the risk of a primary CMV infection high. This infection may manifest with daily fever and malaise in its mildest form. Progressively more serious disease manifestations include leukopenia, hepatopathy (elevated transaminase enzymes), enteropathy (epigastric pain and diarrhea), and pneumonitis. The mortality associated with CMV pneumonitis exceeds 50 percent. CMV infection occurs most commonly 4 to 12 weeks after transplant surgery. Thus a patient presenting with a febrile illness at that time should have as part of their assessment a complete blood count, chest x-ray, and measurement of liver function tests. Serology (conversion to detectable anti-CMV antibody levels and detectable IgM anti-CMV antibody levels occurs well after the initial presentation and is not immediately helpful in the emergency room setting). During active CMV infection, immunosuppression is maintained at the minimum possible level, and if liver, gut, or pulmonary involvement is documented, intravenous ganciclovir therapy, often in conjunction with immune globulin, is prescribed.

The initial presentation of a potentially life-threatening infectious illness may be quite subtle in transplant recipients. The transplant recipient receiving corticosteroids may not mount an impressive febrile response. A nonproductive cough with little or no findings on physical examination may be the only clue to emerging *P. carinii* pneumonia or CMV pneumonia. The threshold for obtaining chest x-rays in the evaluation of these patients should be quite low. Central nervous system (CNS) infections are much more common in transplant recipients than other patients. Common etiologies include *Listeria monocytogenes* and cryptococci. Therefore complaints of recurrent headaches with or without fever should be investigated vigorously first with a structural study to exclude a mass lesion (CNS lymphomas occur with increased frequency, too) and then with a lumbar puncture. Finally, a significant subset of renal-transplant recipients have undergone intentional splenectomy in an effort to improve allograft survival. While this procedure is no longer routinely practiced, these patients, as in other postsplenectomy patients, are at particularly high risk for overwhelming sepsis due to encapsulated bacteria such as the pneumococci or meningococci. Appropriate vaccines are critical in this subpopulation.

Table 206-4. Noninfectious Complications of Organ Transplantation

Malignancy
Cutaneous (squamous cell, basal cell, melanoma)
Lymphoma (B cell and non B cell, CNS lymphoma)
Cervical and uterine carcinoma, Kaposi's sarcoma, carcinoma of retained native kidneys (in renal transplantation)
Cardiovascular
Hypertension
Ongoing/accelerated atherosclerosis (prominent in diabetics)
Transplant renal artery stenosis (in renal transplantation)
Obliterative atherosclerosis of coronary arteries (in cardiac transplantation
Musculoskeletal
Aseptic necrosis (particularly of femoral head and knees)
Idiopathic polyarthralgia syndrome
Osteopenia
Gout
Electrolyte
Hypercalcemia, hyperkalemia, renal tubular acidosis, hypomagnesemia, hyperuricemia
Endocrine/Metabolic
Glucose intolerance
Hyperlipidemia
Hematologic
Posttransplant erythrocytosis (in renal transplantation), anemia, thrombocytopenia, leukopenia
Genitourinary
Reflux (in renal transplantation), impotence, sexual dysfunction.
Nervous system
Pseudotumor cerebri, CNS lymphoma, neuropathy
Gastrointestinal
Vanishing bile duct syndrome (in liver transplantation), pancreatitis, peptic ulcer disease, diverticulitis, fecal impaction, ileus, hepatitis (noninfectious)
Immune
Graft-versus-host disease (in bone marrow transplantation), recurrent glomerulonephritis (in renal transplantation), de novo glomerulonephritis (in renal transplantation)
Psychiatric
Depression, mania
Ocular
Cataract, pseudotumor cerebri, astigmatism (in corneal transplantation)
Pulmonary
Obliterative bronchiolitis (in heart-lung and lung transplantation)
Other
Recurrence of original disease (in renal, liver, marrow, pancreas, corneal, heart-lung, and lung transplantation)

NONINFECTIOUS COMPLICATIONS OF ORGAN TRANSPLANTATION

The list of potential noninfectious complications after organ transplantation is imposing, as illustrated in Table 206-4. However, it should be remembered that quality of life in the vast majority of recipients is very acceptable, and most are able to return to their full level of activity before their organ failure.

Several of the complications listed in Table 206-4 merit discussion. Malignancies may occur in 4 to 6 percent of transplant recipients, depending on the intensity of immunosuppression to which they are subjected. Careful monitoring with routine skin, node, breast, and prostate examinations, Papanicolaou smears, mammograms, sigmoidoscopy and chest x-rays are warranted. Patients are advised to use sun screens. Smoking should be particularly discouraged.

Cardiovascular complications may result from immunosuppression as in the case of obliterative atherosclerosis of coronary arteries in cardiac-transplant patients or from usual risk factors as in the hyperlipidemic diabetic renal-transplant recipient.

Aseptic necrosis of the hips and knees is most common in renal-transplant recipients who have had lengthy therapy with corticosteroids and who also had secondary hyperparathyoidism associated with chronic renal failure before transplantation. The presentation of aseptic necrosis of the hips often shows referred pain to the knees or to the medial thigh. An MRI scan is the most sensitive roentgenographic study for this lesion.

Finally, while isolated organ transplantation offers enormous potential for the individual with disease of a single organ system, the individual with other more systemic illness, such as diabetes mellitus or autoimmune disease, is at great risk of progression or recurrence of underlying disease activity despite a transplant and its attendant immunosuppression.

BIBLIOGRAPHY

Braun WE: Long-term complications of renal transplantation. *Kidney Int* 37:1363, 1990.

Carpenter CB: Immunosuppression in organ transplantation. *N Engl J Med* 322:1224, 1990.

Cerilli GJ (ed.) : *Organ Transplantation and Replacement.* Philadelphia: Lippincott, 1988.

Flye MW (ed.): *Principles of Organ Transplantation.* Philadelphia, Saunders, 1989.

Morris PJ (ed.): *Kidney Transplantation: Principles and Practice,* 2d ed. Orlando, Grune & Stratton, 1984.

Rocher LL: Approach to the patient with renal transplant, in Kelley WN (ed.), *Textbook of Internal Medicine.* Philadelphia, Lippincott, 1989.

Terasaki PI (ed.): *Clinical Transplants 1988.* California, The regents of the University of California, 1988.

Williams GM, Burdick JF, Solez K (eds.): *Kidney Transplant Rejection: Diagnosis and Treatment.* New York, Marcel Dekker, 1986.

207
COMPLICATIONS OF COMMON MEDICAL DEVICES

Robert A. Rusnak

This chapter will discuss the complications and treatment of various medical devices used to enhance the lives of adult outpatients receiving sophisticated medical therapies.

TRACHEOSTOMY

The tracheostomy is the surgical creation of an opening between the surface of the anterior neck and the lumen of the trachea for the purpose of maintaining an airway. This procedure is usually performed electively on patients who require long-term airway management. The complications of this procedure are listed in Table 207-1.

LONG-TERM HOME OXYGEN THERAPY

In 1970, it was shown that long-term home oxygen therapy could increase the overall survival in patients with chronic obstructive pulmonary disease. There is seldom a risk of oxygen toxicity because the $F_{I_{O_2}}$ is rarely greater than 50 percent in these situations, although hypoventilation and CO_2 retention are theoretical risks of home oxygen therapy in patients with chronic obstructive lung disease who have preexisting CO_2 retention. The goal of oxygen therapy is to reverse or prevent hypoxia and that goal should take precedence over concerns about CO_2 retention. Although this should be closely monitored with arterial blood gases in a controlled situation before prescribing a flow rate for patients, the pH has been advocated as a better guide for following low-flow oxygen therapy than P_{CO_2}. Although warned not to do so, some patients may increase the oxygen flow rate of their oxygen delivery device when they experience a worsening of their chronic obstructive lung disease. This self-treatment may lead to acute respiratory failure or cardiac arrest, and these patients will require appropriate resuscitative measures to reverse these processes.

THE HICKMAN-BROVIAC CATHETER

The Hickman-Broviac catheter is a subcutaneously tunnelled, intravenous, silastic catheter positioned in the superior vena cava or the right atrium via the subclavicular subclavian vein approach. It is used for long-term intravenous access and blood sampling and infusion of intravenous fluids, medications, total parenteral nutrition, blood products, or chemotherapy. The insertion of these double- or triple-lumen catheters involves the creation of a subcutaneous tunnel of varying lengths between entry of the catheter into a vein and the skin exit site containing the catheter ports. The catheter is kept open by periodic injections of heparinized saline through these injection ports. Complications are listed in Table 207-2.

Table 207-1. Tracheostomy

Complications	Diagnosis	Treatment
Hemorrhage, usually occurs between the 1st and 2nd week	Clinical signs	Surgical location and correction of bleeding
Infection (usually tracheitis or pneumonia)	Clinical signs and symptoms	Antibiotics
Obstruction with or without death secondary to plugging with dry crusts or mucus	Clinical signs or symptoms	Relieve obstruction, replace tracheostomy tube
Tube displacement	Clinical signs of airway obstruction	Tube repositioning
Pneumothorax (more common in children)	Chest x-ray	Tube thoracostomy
Atelectasis secondary to crusts or mucous plugs	Chest x-ray	Humidification to prevent dried secretions, control of any bleeding to prevent the development of crusts, suctioning, antibiotics
Tracheal stenosis	Usually presents clinically as dyspnea, stridor, or wheezing	Surgical correction of stenosis, creation of a lower tracheostomy or endotracheal intubation site if airway obstruction imminent
Tracheoesophageal fistula secondary to erosion of the posterior trachea and anterior esophageal walls between cuffed tracheostomy tube and vertebral column	Clinical signs, x-ray studies	Surgical correction, limit duration of cuff inflation to meal times; use non-cuffed tubes whenever possible
Aerophagia/dysphagia	Clinical signs and symptoms, usually occur early after tracheostomy creation	Supportive
Keloid formation	Clinical observation	Surgical removal

Table 207-2. Hickman-Broviac and Porta-Caths

Complications	Diagnosis	Treatment
Infection	Blood cultures	Intravenous antibiotics or catheter removal*
Inability to aspirate blood secondary to (1) clot, (2) thrombosis, or (3) fibrin sheaths	Difficult aspiration or infusion	Declotting with heparin or thrombolytics, catheter removal
Accidental dislodgement	Venogram	Repositioning under fluoroscopy, removal
Catheter migration from original placement site to a smaller vessel or subcutaneously	Venogram	Catheter removal or repositioning
Leakage around infusion or aspiration ports	Observation during use or swelling around entrance site	Repair or removal
Dislodgement due to pendulous breasts	Difficulty with infusion or aspiration, swelling, pain or redness at catheter entrance site	Removal or repositioning
Catheter splitting or ballooning of catheter shaft during infusion	Difficulty with infusion, pain during infusion	Catheter removal

* Sepsis is not an absolute indication for removal of these catheters. In one report, only 18 of 143 catheters required removal because of infection; from Ulz L, Peterson FB, Ford R, et al: A prospective study of complications in Hickman right-atrial catheters in marrow transplant patients. *J Parenter Enteral Nutr* 14:27, 1990.

PORTA-CATHS

The Porta-cath is a subcutaneously implanted intravenous access device that couples a central venous pressure catheter to an implanted subcutaneous injection port that is usually located on the chest wall. These catheters are commonly used in cancer patients undergoing long-term outpatient chemotherapy. Porta-caths are usually inserted via a direct approach of the cephalic vein in the deltopectoral groove and positioned such that the catheter tip lies in the superior vena cava or the high right atrium. In men, the subcutaneous injection port usually lies a few centimeters above the nipple; in women, it usually lies near the clavicle. The injection port is flushed with a heparin saline solution with a special needle (the Huber-Point right-angled needle) after each use. If other types of needles are inserted into the device, it will lose its ability to seal off. Problems such as blocked catheter, subcutaneous extravasation during fluid administration, wound dehiscence, and ulceration of the subcutaneous injection port located in the chest wall are treated as per complications of the Hickman-Broviac catheters noted above (Table 207-2).

CARDIAC PACEMAKER

Implantable cardiac pacemakers have been used in humans since 1958. Currently approximately 300,000 pacemakers are inserted or replaced each year in the United States. After pacing or sensing defects, infection is the most common pacemaker-related problem. These infections may involve the pacemaker electrode or the generator pocket. Patients with electrode infections are generally ill patients, who have systemic signs of infection including fever, chills, rigors, or leukocytosis; two-thirds of these patients have positive blood cultures and should be assumed to have infective endocarditis until proved otherwise. Patients with epicardial pacing systems (usually recognized on chest x-ray as a pair of coiled wire electrodes over the myocardium) may also develop mediastinitis, pericarditis, or bronchopleural cutaneous fistulas. Patients who develop infections of the generator pocket, with or without erosions or abscesses of the overlying skin, generally develop erythema and drainage from the pocket, and have positive cultures or purulent secretions. Treatment of these infections is institution dependent and ranges from local wound care, irrigation with antibacterial solutions, or intravenous antibiotics, to removal of the generator and replacement in an alternate site. Other complications are listed in Table 207-3.

THE AUTOMATIC IMPLANTABLE CARDIOVERTER-DEFIBRILLATOR

These devices are inserted to prevent sudden death in patients with drug refractory arrhythmias. Early postoperative complications include postoperative refractory congestive heart failure, coronary artery erosion, subclavian vein thrombosis, or postoperative stroke. Late complications likely to be seen in the emergency department (as opposed to the early postoperative period) include: infection at the generator site, discharge in the absence of symptoms (secondary to sensed myopotential due to shivering or excessive arm activity, atrial fibrillation with a rapid ventricular response, sinus tachycardia, or nonsustained ventricular tachycardia or unknown factors), lead migration, failure to recognize or terminate arrhythmias, and generator failure (usually occurs 8 to 14 months after initial generator placement). These complications usually can be diagnosed by clinical symptoms or signs and by analysis of the automatic cardioverter-defibrillater generator, using a magnet and an external analyzer device.

HALO PIN TRACTION

Immobilization of the unstable cervical spine with an external cervical immobilizer applied through pins between the metal ring of the halo and inserted into the bony skull has become a common neurosurgical practice. The metal halo and support rods are connected to a special vest, or a cast, worn by the patient over the shoulders and around the chest. Numerous complications of these halo cervical immobilizers have been reported and are listed in Table 207-4.

FOLEY CATHETERS

Latex balloon indwelling urinary catheters have been in use since 1937. Numerous complications are listed in Table 207-5. One of the most nettlesome problems is the inability to remove a Foley catheter because the balloon does not deflate. The following techniques have been described to correct this problem. In women, swab the anterior vagina with antiseptic solution, apply gentle traction to the catheter, moving the balloon to the bladder neck, and insert a 25-gauge spinal needle through the anterior vaginal wall into the balloon. This will cause the water to drain from the balloon through the needle or cause the balloon to rupture. In men, prepare and anesthetize the skin in the suprapubic region just above the symphysis pubis, hold gentle traction on the catheter to position the balloon at the bladder neck, and insert a 25-gauge spinal needle through the abdominal wall into the bladder neck. This will drain the balloon or cause it to rupture. In men, the transrectal approach to the Foley balloon also has been described, using this technique. Another technique describes transsecting the Foley catheter 1 cm distal to the urinary meatus and inserting a well-lubricated No. 26 orthopedic wire suture through the balloon channel of the catheter. This wire suture will almost always pass to the point of obstruction in the balloon channel, allowing water to drain around the wire suture. After the water drains from the balloon, the catheter can be removed by gentle traction.

Table 207-3. Cardiac Pacemakers

Complications	Diagnosis	Treatment
Myocardial perforation and cardiac tamponade secondary to insertion or removal of pacemaker electrode catheter	Clinical signs and symptoms, echocardiography	Pericardial drainage
Pressure dermatitis from an implanted pacemaker generator	Patch testing	Pacemarker generator replacement if local measures are unsuccessful
Runaway pacemaker with or without pacemaker induced tachycardia	Electrogram, clinical signs	Placement of magnet over pacemaker battery Reprogramming the pulse generator to a lower output* Use of external chest wall overdrive stimulation* Connect external pacemaker to the permanent pacing lead after locating and removing implanted pacemaker unit Place transcutaneous pacemaker, then disconnect permanent pacing lead from the pacemaker generator

* Treatment that involves reprogramming the pulse generator or use of external chest wall overdrive stimulation requires an adequate escape rhythm.

Table 207-4. Halo Pins

Complications	Diagnosis	Treatment
Pain	Symptoms	Rule out loose pins, infection, or penetration of the inner table of the skull by pins, before prescribing analgesics
Loosening of pins	Observation	Pin tightening. Consider tangential radiographs to assure that tightened pins do not penetrate inner table of skull.
Pin site infection	Clinical symptoms	Local wound care, antibiotics, radiologic studies to rule out penetration of pins beyond inner table of skull
Pressure sores under vest or cast	Clinical signs	Wound care of pressure sores, cast or vest modification to allow open treatment of pressure sores
Loss of cervical immobilization	Neurologic examination, pain, radiologic studies	Neurosurgical consultation
Osteomyelitis of the skull	Clinical signs or symptoms, drainage from pin site holes, radiologic studies	Neurosurgical consultation
Intradural or extradural abscesses (usually secondary to penetration of the inner table of the skull by pins)	Clinical signs or symptoms, radiologic studies	Neurosurgical consultation

Table 207-5. Foley Catheters

Complications	Diagnosis	Treatment
Infection	Clinical signs and symptoms	Adequate urinary catheter drainage, antibiotics
Penile necrosis (usually occurs in patients with diabetes mellitus)	Local inspection of catheter exit site	Catheter removal, warm soaks, intravenous antibiotics, surgical debridement, prevention of excessive traction on catheter
Intraperitoneal bladder perforation with peritonitis and abdominal free air	Clinical signs and symptoms, abdominal x-ray	Laparotomy, bladder drainage
Penile laceration (usually in elderly, demented patients)	Local inspection	Catheter removal and suprapubic drainage, local treatment with warm soaks and topical antibiotics, prevention of traction on anterior urethra by the weight of a full urine reservoir bag and tubing by taping or bag repositioning
Small bowel obstruction by Foley catheter balloon secondary to vesicoenteric fistula	Clinical signs and symptoms, x-ray studies	Surgical correction
Abrupt removal of catheter with balloon still inflated by agitated, demented, or psychotic patient	Clinical observation, urethral bleeding	Catheter replacement, consider intravenous antibiotics before reinsertion and prophylactically thereafter to prevent infection after posttraumatic removal (with or without documented laceration of anterior urethra)

PEG TUBE

The percutaneous endoscopic gastrostomy tube (a PEG tube) is a nonsurgical percutaneous fluoroscopically or endoscopically guided Seldinger technique used to create a gastrostomy. The tip of the PEG feeding tube is usually placed at the duodenojejunal junction to decrease the incidence of aspiration. Complications are listed in Table 207-6.

GASTROSTOMIES AND FEEDING JEJUNOSTOMIES

Gastrostomies or feeding jejunostomies are usually created to maintain nutritional support in patients who are unable to be fed orally or who have swallowing difficulties. Under general anesthesia, a variously sized Foley catheter (usually No. 16 French to No. 30 French) is placed through a stoma created between the abdominal wall and the stomach

Table 207-6. Peg Tubes

Complications	Diagnosis	Treatment
Aspiration/pneumonia	Chest x-ray	Tube repositioning
Gastrointestinal bleeding	Clinical signs, endoscopy	Supportive measures, conventional treatment of bleeding site
Retroperitoneal perforation	Endoscopy, x-ray contrast studies	Catheter repositioning
Extraluminal catheter migration with infusion of tube feedings into peritoneal cavity	Clinical signs, x-ray studies	Repositioning, surgical consultation
Peritoneal leakage with infection	Clinical signs, x-ray studies	Intravenous antibiotics
Postprocedural myocardial infarction	Clinical signs, symptoms, and laboratory studies	Supportive, consider thrombolytics
Infusion of nutrients into gastrostomy balloon port	Inability to deflate balloon or to infuse nutrients	Endoscopic or fluoroscopically guided balloon rupture and catheter repositioning
Colocutaneous fistula, gastrocolic fistula	Contrast studies through gastrostomy tube	Tube removal or repositioning
Pneumoperitoneum and volvulus of colon	Clinical signs, x-ray contrast studies	Surgery
Tube blockage	Inability to infuse nutrients	Tube irrigation or replacement
Intolerance to feedings	Nausea, vomiting, abdominal pain, distension	Reduced flow rate of nutrients, half-strength feedings, antidiarrheals, stop feedings

Table 207-7. Gastrostomies and Feeding Jejunostomies

Complications	Diagnosis	Treatment
Difficulty with tube feedings	Observation, x-ray contrast studies through tube	Attempt to irrigate feeding lumen, ensure that tube feedings are not being given through the inflation balloon, tube repositioning
Aspiration pneumonia	Clinical signs or symptoms, chest x-ray	Antibiotics, tube repositioning
Tube migration within gut causing intestinal obstructions, acute pancreatitis, obstructive jaundice or gastroesophageal reflux	Clinical and laboratory signs and symptoms, x-ray studies with or without contrast	Tube repositioning, secure placement of tube on abdominal wall
Esophageal rupture (usually in infants)	Chest-x-ray, tube feedings found in chest tube drainage	Surgery
Lost gastrostomy tube	Abdominal x-rays	Allow tube to pass or rupture balloon under fluoroscopic control and allow it to pass spontaneously
Gastric perforation	X-rays with or without contrast through tube	Surgery
Gastropneumatosis with or without gastric outlet obstruction	X-rays with or without contrast through tube	Tube repositioning
Leakage around stoma site	Clinical observation, x-ray contrast studies	Tube repositioning
Extraluminal position of gastrostomy tube	X-ray contrast studies	Tube repositioning
Gastric ulcer	Clinical signs or symptoms, x-ray studies, endoscopy	Ulcer treatment, various options
Gastrointestinal bleeding	Clinical signs or symptoms, x-ray studies, endoscopy	Treatment based on site of hemorrhage
Small bowel intussusception	X-ray contrast studies	Surgery
Sinus or fistula tract formation (with or without malnutrition)	X-ray contrast studies	Tube repositioning

or jejunum and firmly secured to the abdominal wall with tape. While not technically difficult, this procedure has been reported to have a 10 to 35 percent complication rate. These complications are listed in Table 207-7.

Patients commonly are brought to the emergency department for replacement of tubes that have been accidentally pulled out or are nonfunctional. The emergency physician should attempt to replace the tube with a tube of similar configuration and size. If the particular type of tube is not available, using a Foley catheter of the correct size will suffice. The size of the tube is important because the stoma will contract down to the tube, and it will be difficult in the future to restore it to its original size. The trick to replacing the tube is to lubricate it and then slowly insert it with constant forward pressure until it pops into the lumen of the stomach. A common mistake is to use intermittent force that does not allow time for tissue stretching and muscle relaxation. If the original size will not pass without undue trauma, use the next smaller size then try the original size again. This technique generally applies to all forms of tube replacement.

APNEA AND BRADYCARDIA MONITORS FOR INFANTS

Pediatricians commonly recommend apnea and bradycardia monitors for infants that have either suffered a life-threatening apneic or bradycardic event or whose parents have described an episode that may have represented such an event. The parents are given life-support instructions and are instructed to call for help if an event occurs. Most commonly, these devices are not equipped with continuous tape recorders. False alarms are relatively common, but it is usually impossible for the emergency physician to distinguish a false alarm from a true life-threatening event when it was of short duration. The safest course for the physician is to admit the child for monitoring and have the parents bring the home unit to the hospital so that it can be tested in a controlled setting.

VENTRICULOPERITONEAL CEREBROSPINAL FLUID SHUNTS

Inert silicon polymer catheters have made ventriculoperitoneal shunting of cerebrospinal fluid the preferred method of cerebral ventricular decompression. Long-term success with these devices has been achieved preserving intellectual and motor function. Emergency physicians will encounter more of these patients in the future. Complications are shown in Table 207-8.

The most common complication encountered is obstruction or malfunction of the shunt device. The usual signs and symptoms of increased intracranial pressure result from malfunction or obstruction. Nausea, vomiting, headache, lethargy, irritability, and increased seizure activity are encountered. In infants, increasing head circumference or a bulging fontanel also may be found. Papilledema is rarely seen. The rate of rise of intracranial pressure is an important prognostic indicator, with fatal herniation a common result of a rapid rise. The first step in evaluating the shunt is to pump it to see if it is functioning. Some have a single pumping chamber, and others have two chambers. These chambers are located at or within a few centimeters of the site of penetration through the skull. In the case of a single chamber, the chamber should empty with digital pressure then fill rapidly (within 1 to 2 s). When there are two palpable chambers, compress the proximal one and hold while compressing the distal chamber. If the distal chamber does not easily compress, there is distal obstruction. Release the proximal chamber. If it does not rapidly refill, there is proximal obstruction. Proximal obstructions are more common than

Table 207-8. Ventriculoperitoneal Shunts

Complications	Diagnosis	Treatment
Obstruction	Signs and symptoms of increased intracranial pressure. Pump the shunt chamber to see if there is a distal or proximal obstruction. Skull, chest, and abdominal x-ray, CT of the head	Neurosurgical consultation. Pump the chamber to overcome resistance.
Infection	Local erythema, abdominal pain, generalized signs of infection, meningeal signs	Neurosurgical consultation. Intravenous antibiotics

distal obstructions. X-rays of the skull, chest, and abdomen can help detect separation or malposition of the shunt. CT scan of the head can detect increasing ventricular volume. Neurosurgical consultation should be obtained early since sudden decompensation, with cerebellar or transtentorial herniation, is a threat. If signs of herniation appear acutely, the emergency physician may have to puncture the ventricle as a life-saving maneuver if the obstruction is proximal. If the obstruction is distal, puncture of the chamber would be indicated. In an infant with an open fontanel, a 20-gauge spinal needle is inserted 1 cm lateral to the midline along the coronal suture and directed perpendicular to the base of the skull in line with the inner canthus of the ipsilateral eye. The ventricle should be encountered within about 1¼ in. In older children and adults, one conceivably could reverse a rapidly progressing herniation by inserting a 20-gauge spinal needle through the skull opening occupied by the shunt. This would destroy the shunt but could save the patient's life. Fortunately, such rapid herniation occurring in the emergency department is very rare.

Infection of the shunt is the second most common complication. Infection can cause obstruction of the device resulting in signs of increased intracranial pressure. Local infection can result in erythema of the tissues over the shunt. Peritonitis can be caused by primary shunt infection, or it can be caused by erosion of the shunt into the bowel. Infection can ascend in the shunt and cause meningitis or ventriculitis. Other abdominal processes, such as appendicitis, can be confused with shunt infection. Any shunt patient with abdominal symptoms or findings should be evaluated by a neurosurgeon. Most of these patients will require aspiration of their shunts to obtain ventricular fluid for study. The emergency physician should maintain a high index of suspicion when evaluating patients with a shunt as the signs and symptoms of infection may be subtle, nonspecific, and diverse. When infection is suspected, admission with neurosurgical consultation will be needed.

CONCLUSION

New advances in technology have allowed many patients to be medically managed at home or in nursing homes rather than in the hospital. This trend will continue, and emergency physicians will be required to become more knowledgeable about emergencies arising from so-called high-tech equipment failure or misuse.

BIBLIOGRAPHY

Barnes-Snow E, Luchi RJ, Doig R: Penile laceration from a Foley catheter. *J Am Geriatr Soc* 33:712, 1985.

Borbola J, Denes P, Ezri MD, et al: The automatic implantable cardioverter-defibrillator: Clinical experience, complications and follow-up in 25 patients. *Arch Intern Med* 148:70, 1980.

Bui HD, Dang CV: Acute pancreatitis: A complication of Foley catheter gastrostomy. *J Natl Med Assoc* 78:779, 1986.

Chew JY, Cantrell RW: Tracheostomy—complications and their management. *Arch Otolaryng* 96:538, 1972.

Garfin SR, Botte MJ, Triggs KJ, et al: Subdural abscess associated with halo-pin traction. *J Bone Joint Surg* 70A:1338, 1988.

Ghahreman GG, Tsang TK, Vakil N: Complications of endoscopic gastrostomy: Pneumoperitoneum and volvulus of the colon. *Gastrointest Radiol* 12:172–174, 1987.

Gowen GF: The management of complications of Foley feeding gastrostomies. *Am Surg* 54:582, 1988.

Harvey MP, Trent RJ, Joshua DE, et al: Complications associated with indwelling venous Hickman catheters in patients with hemotological disorders. *Aust NZ J Med* 16:21, 1986.

Hessl JM: Removal of Foley catheter when balloon does not deflate. *Urology* 22:219, 1983.

Hicks ME, Suratt RS, Picus D, et al: Fluoroscopically guided percutaneous gastrostomy and gastroenterostomy: analysis of 158 consecutive cases. *AJR* 154:725, 1990.

Ho CS, Yee ACN, McPherson R: Complications of surgical and percutaneous nonendoscopic gastrostomy: Review of 233 patients. *Gastroenterology* 95:1206, 1988.

Huff JP, Rosenblum J, Camara DS: Complications of gastrostomy. *South Med J* 81:1050, 1988.

Kleeman FJ: Technique for removal of Foley catheter when balloon does not deflate. *Urology* 21:416, 1983.

Konda J, Ruggle P: Prolapse of Foley catheter tube causing obstructive jaundice. *Am J Gastroenterol* 76:353, 1981.

Lau JTK: Removal of Foley catheter when balloon does not deflate (letter). *Urology* 22:219, 1983.

Marchlinski FE, Flores BT, Buxton AE, et al: The automatic implantable cardioverter-defibrillator: efficiency, complications, and device failures. *Ann Intern Med* 104:481, 1986.

McDowell GC, Hayden LJ, Wise HA: Penile necrosis secondary to an indwelling Foley catheter. *J Urol* 138:1243, 1987.

Madsen MA: Emergency department management of ventriculoperitoneal cerebrospinal fluid shunts. *Ann Emerg Med* 15:1330, 1986.

Merguerian PA, Erturk E, Hulbert WC, et al: Peritonitis and abdominal free air due to intraperitoneal bladder perforations associated with indwelling urethral catheter drainage, *J Urol* 134:747, 1985.

Mickey H, Anderson C, Nielsen LH: Runaway pacemaker: a still-existing complication and therapeutic guidelines. *Clin Cardiol* 12:412, 1989.

Moorman DW, Horattas MC, Wright D, et al: Hickman catheter dislodgement due to pendulous breasts. *JPEN* 11:502, 1987.

Pessa ME, Howard RJ: Complications of Hickman-Broviac catheters. *Surg Gynecol Obstet* 161:257, 1985.

Saltzberg DM, Anand K, Juvan P, et al: Colocutaneous fistula: An unusual complication of percutaneous endoscopic gastrostomy. *J Parenter Enteral Nutr* 11:86, 1987.

Shaw JHF, Douglas R, Wilson T: Clinical performance of Hickman and Porta-Cath atrial catheters. *Aust NZ J Surg* 58:657, 1988.

Sullivan LP, Davidson PG, Kloss DA, et al: Small bowel obstruction caused by a long-term indwelling urinary catheter. *Surgery* 107:228, 1990.

Tiep BL: Long-term home oxygen therapy. *Clin Chest Med* 11:505, 1990.

Ulz L, Peterson FB, Ford R, et al: A prospective study of complications in Hickman right-atrial catheters in marrow transplant patients. *J Parenter Enteral Nutr* 14:27, 1990.

Valdes-Dapena M, Steinschneider A: Sudden infant death syndrome (SIDS), apnea, and near miss for SIDS. *Emerg Clin North Am* 1:27, 1983.

Wade JS, Cobbs CG: Infections in cardiac pacemakers. *Curr Clin Topics Infect Dis* 9:44, 1988.

Wagman LD, Neifeld JP: Experience with the Hickman catheter: Unusual complications and suggestions for their prevention. *J Parenter Enteral Nutr* 10:311, 1986.

Whitely S, Liu PH, Tellez DW: Esophageal rupture in an infant secondary to esophageal placement of a Foley catheter gastrostomy tube. *Pediatr Emerg Care* 5:113, 1989.

Wilkerson MG, Jordan WP: Pressure dermatitis from an implanted pacemaker. *Dermatol Clin* 8:189, 1990.

Wolf EL, Frager D, Beneventano TC: Radiologic demonstration of important gastrostomy tube complications. *Gastrointest Radiol* 11:20, 1986.

SECTION 23
Newer Imaging Modalities

208
NONINVASIVE VASCULAR STUDIES

Phillip J. Bendick

Acute peripheral vascular problems may be of an arterial or venous nature and require prompt, accurate diagnosis. Such factors, i.e., whether the disease process is acute or chronic; the location, extent and severity of any vascular obstructions present; and the overall functional or hemodynamic significance, are important considerations for initial treatment and ultimate management. While the history and physical examination should *always* be the starting point of any vascular workup, they are subjective in nature and can even be misleading in some cases. Developments in noninvasive evaluation techniques, validated by extensive application in vascular laboratories, now make measurement tools available which give objective, quantitative data for diagnosis.

Most hospitals now have a functional vascular laboratory with personnel familiar with the spectrum of instruments for noninvasive vascular examination. These work very well as a referral source for diagnosing vascular problems, but few of them are available 24 h day, 7 days a week, as is needed in an emergency center. Two primary instruments, however, can (or should) be available as needed whenever patients present. The first of these is the pocket Doppler ultrasound flowmeter, and the second is duplex ultrasound.

The Doppler ultrasound flowmeter is available widely in a variety of pocket or battery-powered portable models. In one form or another, it should be available in every emergency department at all times. In addition, the staff should be familiar with its operation and use. The flowmeter converts the frequency shift of the ultrasound reflected from moving blood (the Doppler shift) to an audible signal suitable for subjective interpretation. Typically, a transducer frequency of approximately 5 MHz is used to provide reasonable sensitivity to blood flow while assuring good tissue penetration in even obese patients. The audible signal itself has obvious differences between the higher pitched, pulsatile sounds of arterial flow and the lower pitched, more constant sound of venous flows. There are also more subtle differences within each vascular system between normal and abnormal sounds, as flows range from a hyperdynamic character to being absent because of occlusions. Practice and experience bring rapid familiarity with these flow signals, and it is possible quickly to develop an "ear" for the normal flows in both the aterial and venous systems by trying the flowmeter out on healthy normal subjects (such as coworkers). Once an appreciation for normal signals has been developed, it is much easier to identify and grade abnormal subjects.

The second technique mentioned, duplex ultrasonography, is much more complicated technologically. It combines high-resolution imaging in real time with simultaneous Doppler capability. Only a few emergency departments have the luxury of a dedicated on-site instrument, but virtually every vascular laboratory or radiology department has one or more, with trained on-call personnel to operate them. It is not necessary for the emergency department staff to develop the skills of a sonographer, but just as in reading radiographs, they should have some of the basic skills of interpretation. The real-time image displays the echo pattern from the interfaces between different tissues. For vascular applications, this is made somewhat easier by the fact that blood is a poor reflector of ultrasound and normally appears anechoic; the surrounding tissues are relatively hyperechoic, providing distinct differentiation. Guided by the image, selective Doppler flow measurements can be made by choosing the placement site of the region of interest, or sample volume, of the flowmeter.

PERIPHERAL ARTERIAL DISEASE

In an emergency department, the majority of applications of noninvasive evaluation techniques in peripheral arterial disease will be to differentiate chronic atherosclerotic occlusive disease from more acute thromboembolic events and determine the hemodynamic significance of the disease. The time course of the patient's symptoms is as helpful as anything else in this regard and again emphasizes the importance of a thorough history in the initial evaluation. The portable Doppler flowmeter can then provide two important functions in completing the diagnosis. The presence or absence of arterial flows assesses vessel patency at the site being examined. If the vessel is patent, the subjective grade of the quality of the flow signal provides additional information regarding any proximal disease. The normal flow signal is considered triphasic, with a sharp systolic signal rapidly increasing and then decreasing in pitch and intensity, and reflected waves comprising the lower-pitched (representing lower flow velocities) diastolic components. As proximal arterial disease becomes more severe, the flow signal becomes monophasic and damped with a weaker, delayed systolic rise, which then slowly fades during diastole. In the case of a total occlusion proximal to the site of interrogation, the quality of the flow signal is related to the adequacy and magnitude of collateral flow.

The second function of the ultrasound flowmeter is that of a Doppler stethoscope in the measurement of limb segmental systolic pressures. With the patient in the supine position, a standard adult blood pressure cuff is wrapped snugly around the ankle just above the malleoli and inflated to suprasystolic pressures. As the cuff pressure is slowly released, either the posterior tibial artery at the ankle or the dorsalis pedis artery on the dorsum of the foot is monitored by Doppler for the return of flow. The cuff pressure noted at the moment that flow is restored has been shown to equate to intraluminal systolic pressure. While this number alone is not diagnostic, when compared with resting brachial artery systolic pressure by calculating the ankle brachial index (ABI), a measure of the severity of any proximal arterial occlusive disease is achieved. A normal ABI is 1.0 or greater. If the ABI falls between 0.5 and 1.0, this usually indicates significant involvement of only a single arterial segment, and the classic presentation by the patient is a history of claudication. If the ABI falls below 0.5, it indicates multiple segment involvement with more severe ischemia likely to cause pain at rest and lead to ulceration and tissue loss. Acute thrombotic occlusions nearly always fall into this category, requiring thromboembolectomy or close continued monitoring during anticoagulation therapy.

Application of duplex ultrasonography to peripheral arterial disease in the emergency department is more limited. Evaluation of the carotid arteries for stenosis or occlusion contributing to symptoms of cerebrovascular ischemia is best done in the more controlled environment of the vascular laboratory or ultrasound department. Upper or lower extremity applications are best reserved for less commonly seen pathologies such as peripheral aneurysmal disease, differentiating hematoma from pseudoaneurysm in a patient presenting with a pulsatile mass, or documenting an arteriovenous fistula, but only if the diagnosis is needed urgently. Generally, duplex ultrasonography is excellent for types of localized arterial disease that do not cause any overall hemodynamic disturbances and thus would not be picked up by more conventional Doppler testing. In cerebrovascular testing, the quality of the examination is likely to be better when not performed at the bedside in the emergency department.

PERIPHERAL VENOUS DISEASE

Peripheral venous disease presents a contrasting picture. Any patient presenting to the emergency department with the signs and symptoms of deep vein thrombosis must be approached with a high index of suspicion because of the life-threatening nature of this disease. There is a degree of urgency to establishing the diagnosis, but with the high potential for bleeding complications related to systemic anticoagulation, there is a corresponding necessity for high accuracy in making the diagnosis. Duplex ultrasonography is the test of choice to exclude deep vein thrombosis. Its accuracy (sensitivity and specificity) is virtually identical to ascending contrast venography for all sites in the lower extremities, including the calves. It is a noninvasive test well suited for screening and follow-up. In addition, it can be performed in the vascular laboratory, the ultrasound department, or by a portable unit at the bedside in the emergency department. Its major drawback is the requirement for an experienced vascular technologist or sonographer to do the study, a skill it would not be reasonable to expect the emergency department staff to perfect. As mentioned above, however, the staff should possess the basic skills of test interpretation, just as they should be capable of reading most radiographs. By directly imaging the venous system, duplex ultrasonography provides an anatomic "road map" similar to venography. The presence or absence of deep vein thrombosis is documented on the basis of echogenicity within the lumen of the vein, an inability to collapse or compress the vein walls with light probe pressure on the surface of the skin, and the absence of flow within the lumen by Doppler. These same criteria also make the diagnosis of superifical thrombophlebitis a straightforward, simple one.

In the event duplex ultrasonography is not available, the Doppler flowmeter can also be helpful in the diagnosis of major acute deep vein thrombosis of the femoropopliteal system, as long as its significant limitations are understood and accepted. The common femoral vein, superficial femoral vein throughout the thigh, and the popliteal vein at the knee can all be evaluated by Doppler. With the patient supine and the head slightly elevated, these sites are interrogated for the magnitude of spontaneous, resting flows; the degree of venous flow augmentation when the distal limb is compressed manually; and the strength of phasic flow variations during the respiratory cycle. If these normal flow characteristics are absent, a strong case for deep vein thrombosis can be made, and numerous studies have shown that with an unequivocally positive examination of this type anticoagulant therapy can be appropriately begun. However, because of the limitations of the Doppler examination a negative or equivocal examination still leaves uncertainty as to the presence or absence of the disease. Well-documented causes of false-negative Doppler studies include the presence of nonocclusive thrombus with no overall hemodynamic significance, thrombosis isolated to the deep veins of the calf without occlusive extension into the popliteal vein, the simultaneous presence of chronic venous disease with overlying acute thrombus, obesity resulting in the loss of a good quality flow signal, anatomic variants such as a dual superficial femoral vein with only one thrombosed,and well-developed collateral channels, particularly in the popliteal space. While a positive test may be unequivocal, it is this rather imposing list of causes of test error that limit the usefulness of the Doppler examination in the emergency setting. Nonetheless because of its extreme portability, the speed with which it can be performed at the bedside, and the relatively little amount of practice required to differentiate clearly abnormal findings, the Doppler test remains a reasonable screening tool, and experienced users can achieve an acceptable level of accuracy in the diagnosis of deep vein thrombosis.

SUMMARY

These established vascular laboratory techniques of noninvasive testing can be applied readily in the emergency department. Some type of portable Doppler flowmeter should be available at all times for use by the staff in screening patients with suspected peripheral vascular disease. Duplex ultrasonography is available widely in most institutions, and while the staff would not necessarily need to have specific imaging skills, basic interpretation can be done within the department itself. These techniques will have the same accuracy and reliability in the emergency department as elsewhere in the hospital and provide increased sensitivity in the diagnosis of the presence and severity of peripheral arterial occlusive diseases and deep vein thrombosis. Once the basics of these techniques and their interpretation have been mastered and they can be applied within the department, a speedier process of diagnosis and quicker implementation of appropriate patient management will result.

BIBLIOGRAPHY

Bendick PJ, Glover JL, Holden RW, et al: Pitfalls of the Doppler examination for venous thrombosis. *Am Surg* 49:320, 1983.

Comerato AJ, Katz ML, Greenwald LL, et al: Venous duplex imaging: Should it replace hemodynamic tests for deep venous thrombosis? *J Vasc Surg* 11:53, 1990.

Cranley JJ: Diagnosis of deep venous thrombosis, in Bernstein EF (ed): *Recent Advances in Noninvasive Diagnostic Techniques in Vascular Disease*. St. Louis, Mosby, 1990, pp 207–212.

Kremkau FW: *Doppler Ultrasound—Principles and Instruments*. Philadelphia, Saunders, 1990, pp 101–120.

Porter JM, Mayberry JC, Taylor LM, et al: Chronic lower-extremity ischemia: Part I. *Curr Probl Surg* 28:29, 1991.

Rutherford RB: Evaluation and selection of patients for vascular surgery, in Rutherford RB (ed): *Vascular Surgery*. Philadelphia, Saunders, 1989, pp 10–16.

Strandness DE Jr: *Duplex Scanning in Vascular Disorders*. New York, Raven, 1990, pp 196–228.

Talbot SR: B-mode evaluation of peripheral arteries and veins, in Zwiebel WJ (ed): *Introduction to Vascular Ultrasonography*, 2d ed. New York, Grune & Stratton, 1986, pp 351–384.

209
EMERGENCY USE OF PELVIC ULTRASONOGRAPHY

Christine Comstock

Ultrasonography has revolutionized the evaluation of the early pregnancy, both normal and abnormal. It is important to understand the following description of the normal ultrasound appearance of a developing pregnancy in order to evaluate the failing pregnancy, both intrauterine and extrauterine, since the radiology resident or attending physician on call may be inexperienced in this area.

TECHNIQUES

There are two types of ultrasound images—static and moving (the latter otherwise known as *real time*). Real-time scanning is the method of choice for obstetric ultrasound examination; the moving image is essential for determining the proper planes in which to measure and for determining fetal viability. A few departments still use static scanners (identified by their long arm), but real-time scanning should always be a part of the examination. Real-time scanning may be done using a linear probe or a sector probe; the image formed by the first is rectangular and by the second pie-shaped.

The full bladder is used as a sonographic window into the pelvis. Air in the bowel reflects sound back to the transducer and allows little or none to reach the pelvic organs. A full bladder pushes the bowel out of the way and gives excellent visualization of the organs below. How full should the bladder be? In nonpregnant women and in early pregnancy, it should always be full enough to cover the entire uterus but not so excessively full that it compresses the uterus and pushes it far posterior. If the posterior wall of the bladder is even with or just above the superior uterine margin, the bladder is perfectly filled. Doubt should be raised about the results of any pelvic ultrasound examination in which the bladder is not full enough to reveal the entire uterus in the sagittal plane or in which it is so full that the uterus looks like a pancake and is pushed far posteriorly.

Scanning through the vagina rather than the abdominal wall is helpful when the patient is unable to or should not (high probability of surgery) drink fluids to fill the bladder and in obese patients in whom the image obtained by transabdominal scanning is markedly downgraded. It is also helpful in any early pregnancy in which the image is so poor that a diagnosis is difficult or impossible. Sometimes even in the normal-weight patient a fetal heartbeat can be seen using a vaginal probe when it cannot be seen transabdominally.

NORMAL EARLY PREGNANCY

The egg is fertilized in the distal Fallopian tube approximately 13 days before the first day of the next expected menstrual period (no matter what the cycle length). The developing embryo travels down into the uterus and implants on the uterine wall 5 days later. Even when the best of eyes and equipment are used, a sac is usually not visible by vaginal ultrasound examination until the serum level of human chorionic gonadotropin (β-HCG assay) has reached 1200 mIU (First International Reference Preparation). Sometimes the decidual reaction or thickening of the endometrium in an ectopic pregnancy can simulate a normal intrauterine sac. However, an intrauterine gestational sac can easily be distinguished from a pseudosac because the intrauterine sac has a double white line around at least a portion of its circumference (Fig. 209-1).

Shortly after the sac appears, usually before 6 weeks from the first day of the last menstrual period, a flickering heartbeat should be seen. As the fetus grows, its length from crown to rump can be measured (Fig. 209-2). This length can estimate fetal age within ± 4 days. This age is understood to represent menstrual age, not conceptual age. By convention all measurements relating to the fetus are expressed as menstrual age (from the first day of the last menstrual period) rather than conceptual age.

FAILING EARLY PREGNANCY

Whatever the location of a pregnancy, either within the uterus or without, the failing early pregnancy will eventually present with bleeding and/or pain.

Intrauterine

Any intrauterine sac of a diameter of 2.5 cm or more should contain a fetus. The sac may continue to get bigger and bigger and the level of β HCG will rise, but if an embryo never develops, or if it is visible but has no heartbeat, a pregnancy is termed an embryonic demise.

If a heartbeat is seen, the pregnancy should be considered viable no matter what the appearance of the sac. However, a low position, decreased amniotic fluid, or a slow heart rate are worrisome.

Ectopic Pregnancy

The term *ectopic pregnancy* refers to any pregnancy outside the normal implantation site in the intrauterine cavity. Ectopic pregnancies can be located in the ovary, cornua, Fallopian tube, cervix, or abdomen.

The primary use of ultrasonography in this case is to establish the presence of an intrauterine pregnancy since this excludes ectopic pregnancy in all but the rare 1 in 30,000 cases in which there are concomitant intrauterine and extrauterine pregnancies. If the patient is at $5\frac{1}{2}$ to 6 weeks menstrual age and has a positive test for urine β HCG of at

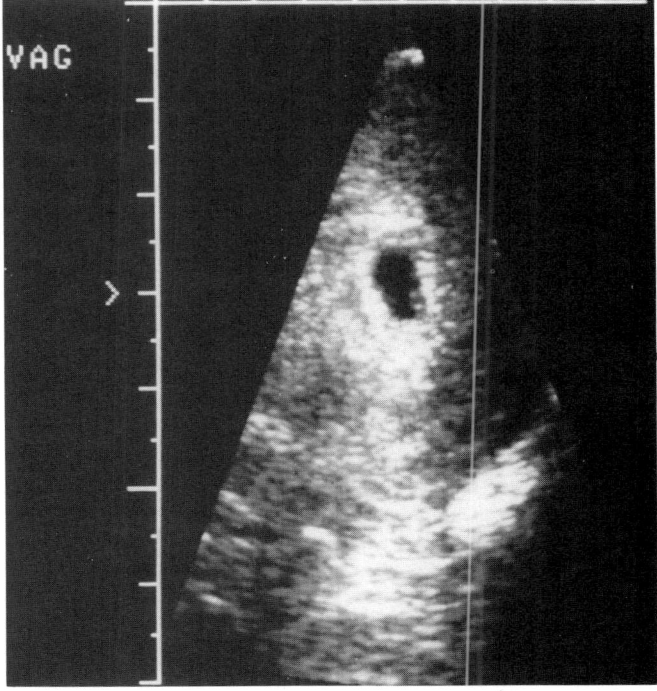

Fig. 209-1. A $5\frac{1}{2}$ week intrauterine gestation seen by vaginal probe. A round yolk sac is seen at 5 o'clock. The bright echo around the dark fluid-filled area represents a combination of the endometrium and gestational sac. The fetus is not yet visible but will develop along the top of the yolk sac. Heart beat should be visible by 6 weeks.

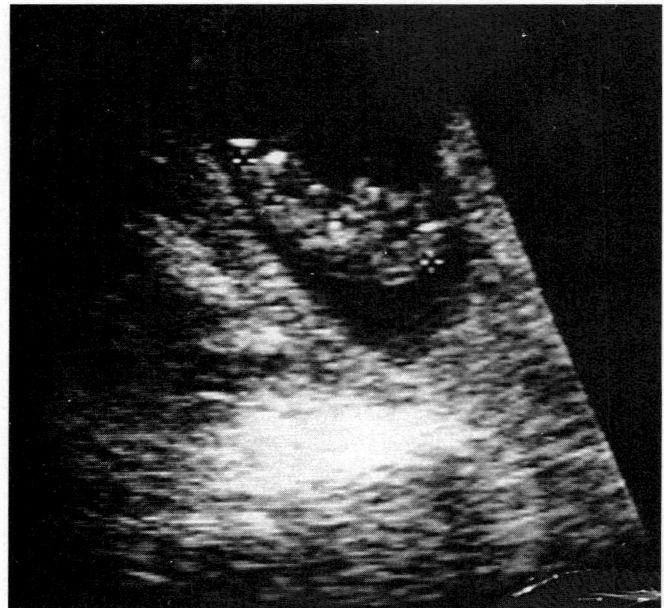

Fig. 209-2. Early fetus. Cross hatches indicate points from which crown-to-rump length is measured.

least 1200 mIU, an intrauterine sac meeting the criteria outlined above should be visualized by vaginal scan. If one is not seen, (1) the pregnancy is less advanced than menstrual dates would suggest, (2) the pregnancy lies outside the uterine cavity, or (3) the patient has just passed an intrauterine pregnancy. If there has been little or no bleeding, the latter is unlikely. *If the serum level of β HCG is greater than 1200 mIU/mL and no sac is seen in the uterus, the likelihood of an ectopic pregnancy is high.*

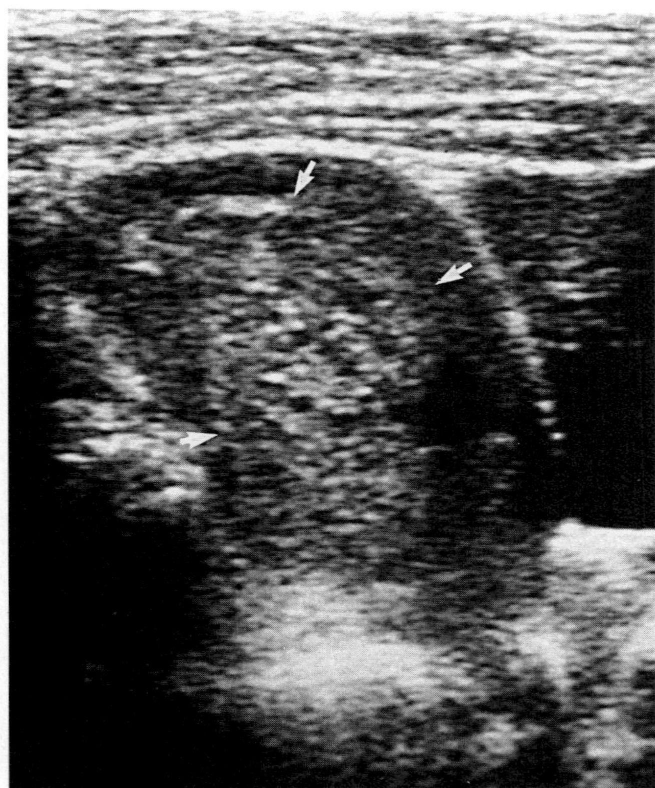

Fig. 209-3. Heterogeneous gray tissue filling the uterus is characteristic of a hydatidiform mole (arrows).

The only absolutely diagnostic ultrasound sign of an ectopic pregnancy is identification of a fetus and/or fetal heartbeat outside the uterus. All other signs, such as complex adnexal mass or free fluid in the cul de sac, can be seen in other entities such as a ruptured or leaking ovarian cyst.

Molar Pregnancy

In a complete hydatidiform mole, the uterus is larger than expected for dates, there is usually spotting, and no fetal heart tones can be heard. The ultrasound scan shows a large uterus with no fetus and abundant placental tissue. The placenta is normally a homogeneous gray, but in a mole there are areas of echolucency and echogenicity mixed in with normal-appearing placenta (Fig. 209-3). Often there are multiple large cysts in the ovary (theca lutein cysts) which have developed in response to abnormally high β HCG levels. A degenerating placenta in a missed abortion may present with the same appearance, so β HCG levels, the presence of theca lutein cysts, or, finally, a dilatation and curettage may be necessary to tell the difference. The evacuation of such a uterus is more complicated than the evacuation of a missed abortion and should be left to someone experienced in dealing with this entity.

THIRD TRIMESTER BLEEDING

Placenta Previa

A patient with more than vaginal spotting in the third trimester *should be assumed to have a placenta previa* unless a previous scan by a very reliable ultrasonographer has shown that the placenta does not cover the internal uterine os (Fig. 209-4). The diagnosis of placenta previa has little meaning before approximately 26 weeks since (1) early in pregnancy many patients have a placenta previa which disappears as the lower uterine segment elongates and (2) a placenta previa is rarely the cause of vaginal bleeding until the third trimester.

Before vaginal examination is attempted, a quick scan should be performed to determine the location of the lower edge of the placenta. The bladder should not be very full since the bladder can deform the lower uterine segment in such a way that a false diagnosis of placenta previa is made (Fig. 209-5). Rather, the bladder should be filled just

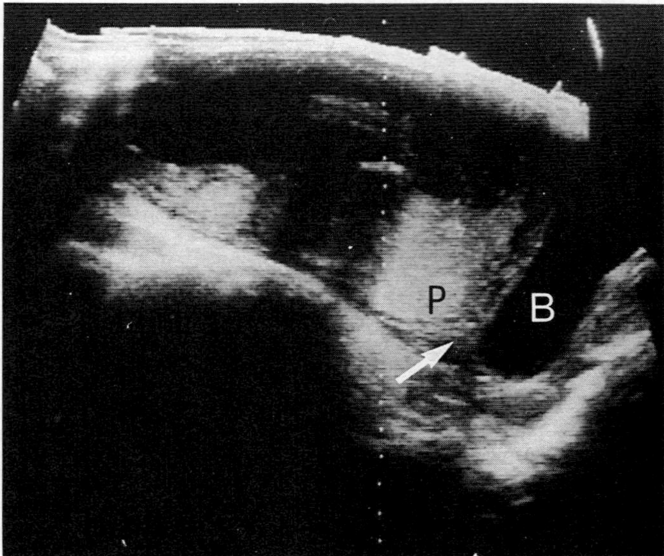

Fig. 209-4. Placenta previa. The placenta (P) covers the internal uterine os (arrow). B = bladder (sagittal).

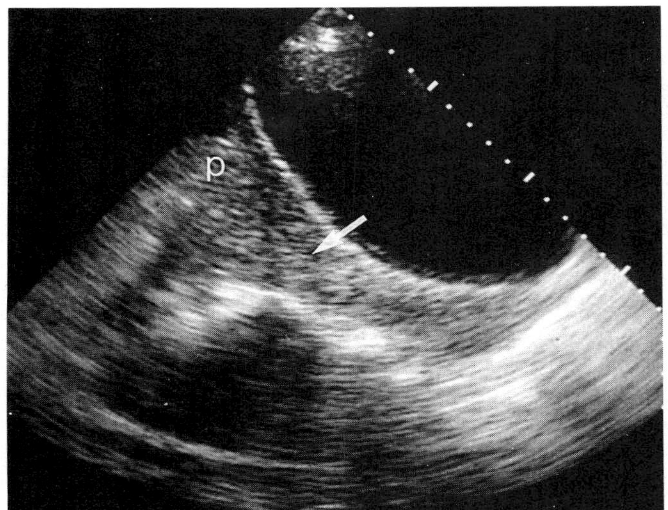

A

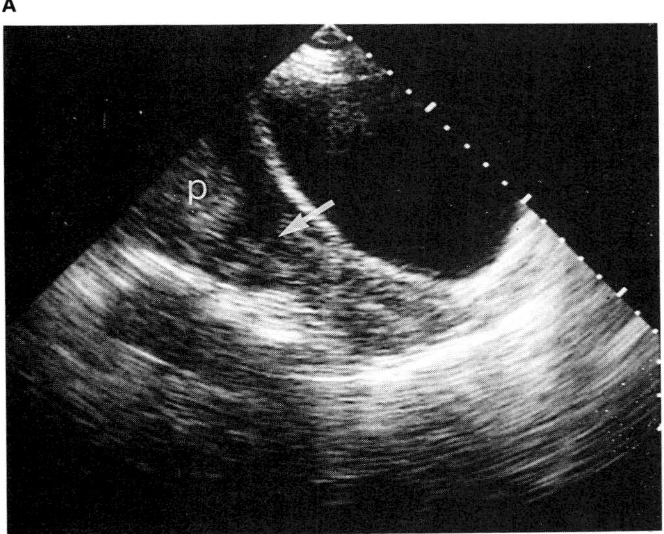

B

Fig. 209-5. A. A very full bladder can push the placenta (p) over the internal os (arrow). **B.** When the bladder is emptied slightly, the placenta falls away from the os (sagittal scans).

enough to allow visualization of the cervix and no more. The scan should clearly show the internal cervical canal and internal os or, if that is not possible, should be done in the plane of the vagina, which is usually exactly midline. If the scan is done to one side or another of midline, a false diagnosis may be made.

Abruptio Placentae

If the patient is bleeding and does not have a placenta previa, the next most likely diagnosis is abruptio placentae, particularly if the patient is having localized uterine pain and/or frequent uterine contractions. *Ultrasound has no role in the diagnosis of abruptio placentae.* Its only role is to exclude placenta previa. The patient without a placenta previa and with the typical clinical findings of abruption constitutes a clinical emergency and should be stabilized and monitored, not taken to the ultrasound department to look for retroplacental collections of blood. These are rarely seen, and their absence does not mean that the patient does not have an abruption.

THE PELVIS IN THE NONPREGNANT WOMAN

The maxim in obstetrics and gynecology is that a woman of reproductive years is pregnant until proved otherwise. Therefore, all women of child-bearing age with lower abdominal complaints should be evaluated for pregnancy.

Ultrasonography of the pelvis does not replace the competent pelvic examination and good clinical judgment; it should not be requested before a pelvic examination has been performed by an experienced clinician. There are many pitfalls in pelvic ultrasonography that may mislead the clinician and result in unnecessary surgery. Bowel can simulate a pelvic mass, as not a few surgeons have discovered unhappily at the time of laparotomy. Pelvic masses can be hidden acoustically behind the bowel. Consequently, the differential diagnosis should be formulated before a scan; this should then answer a specific question and directly influence management. With these caveats in mind, ultrasonography can add valuable information in many situations.

Components of a Satisfactory Scan of the Pelvis

The standard pelvic scan report should contain comments on *both* ovaries and the uterus. It is also the standard of care to scan the abdomen quickly. A vaginal transducer will provide a clearer picture of any pelvic mass (but only at the level of the uterus or lower). A comment should be made about the presence or absence of free fluid. Although there can be 10 to 20 mL of fluid in the normal pelvis, a larger volume is suggestive of a problem in the pelvis or abdomen.

Ultrasound Characteristics of Common Pelvic Masses

Most acute pelvic pain is produced by neoplasms (benign or malignant) of the ovaries or infection of the ovaries or tubes. *Functional cysts* (follicles or corpus luteum) are echolucent with no solid components (Fig. 209-6) unless there is a torsion or hemorrhage within them. They sometimes rupture and can cause significant blood loss. *Dermoids* can be distinguished by the hair or fat in these that produce bright echoes in an otherwise cystic and solid mass (''mixed'' or ''complex''). The ultrasound appearance is often very typical (Fig. 209-7). These are frequently bilateral. *Mucinous cystadenomas* are often very large and septated. They can fill the entire abdomen. Septations with echogenic fluid are characteristic. The more solid the material within, the more

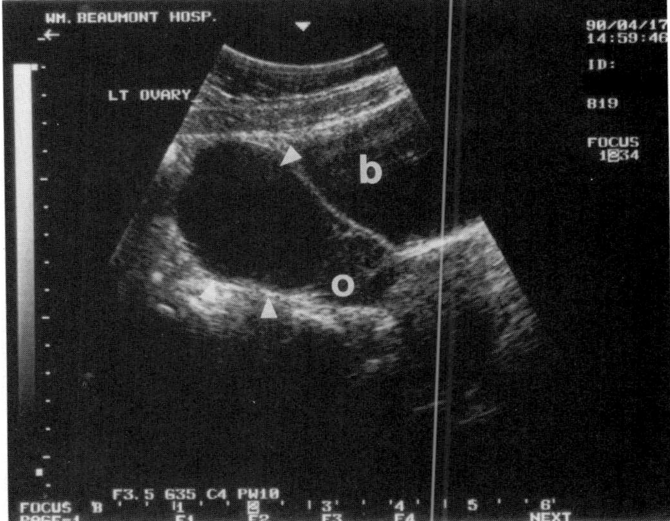

Fig. 209-6. A corpus luteum cyst (arrowheads) appears to contain only fluid. O = ovary, b = bladder.

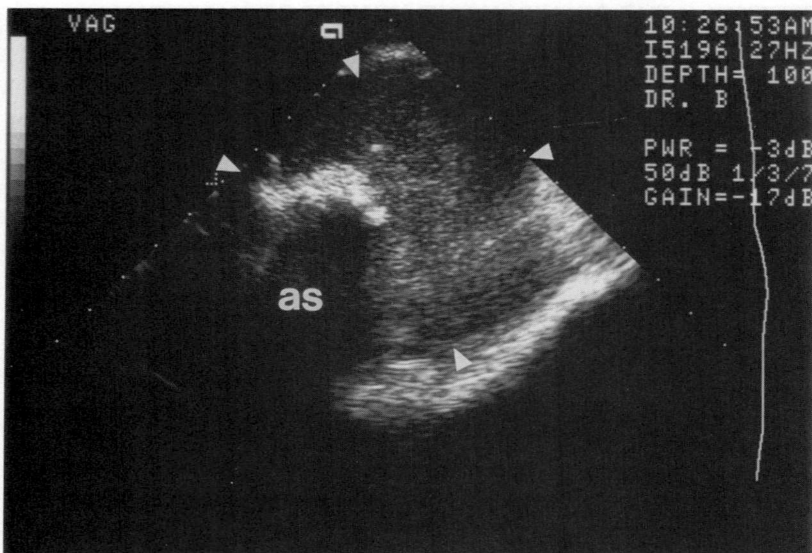

Fig. 209-7. A dermoid (arrowheads) with calcium or fat (arrows) producing very echogenic areas and an acoustic shadow below it (AS).

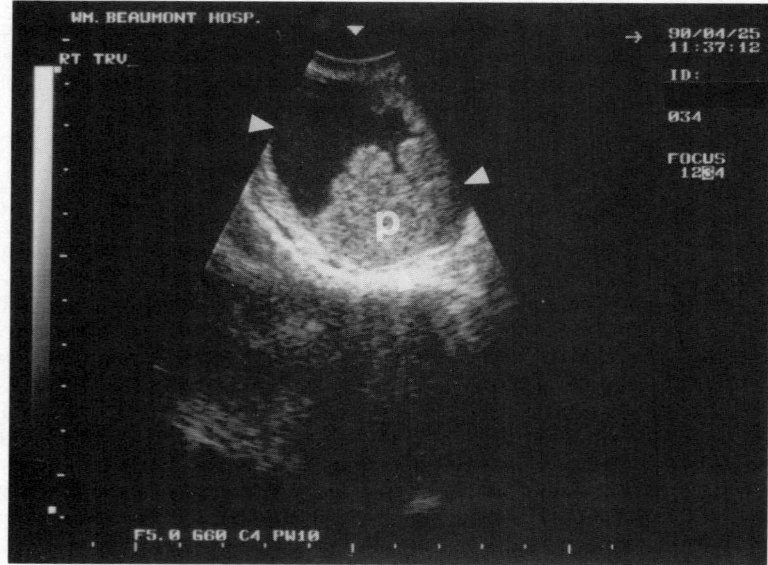

Fig. 209-8. A serous cystadenoma of borderline malignancy (arrowheads) contains considerable papillary solid tissue (P) producing a worrisome ultrasound picture.

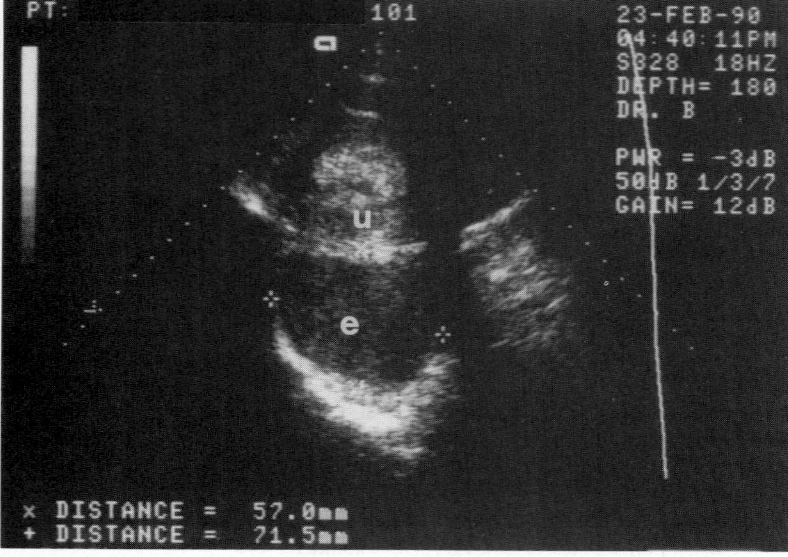

Fig. 209-9. An endometrioma appears solid but is less echogenic than the uterus anterior to it. e = endometrioma, u = uterus.

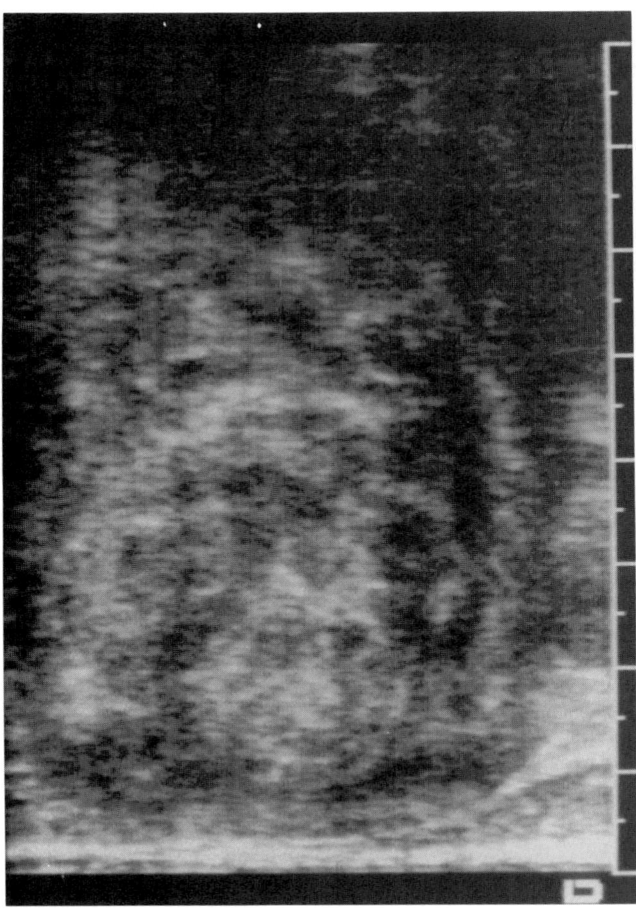

Fig. 209-10. A round mass demonstrates a whorled pattern very characteristic of a uterine fibroid. At the end of the first trimester of pregnancy these can demonstrate internal necrosis.

likely it is to be a cystadenocarcinoma. *Serous cystadenomas* are usually not as large as the mucinous type and may contain only a few septations. The more solid the material is, the more likely it is malignant (Fig. 209-8). *Tuboovarian abscess* is often a complex mass (cystic and solid) with indistinct borders. This diagnosis cannot be made by ultrasonography alone. *Endometrioma* is a solid mass, often homogeneous, originating from ectopic endometrium (Fig. 209-9). *Fibroid* is a solid mass of uterine muscle with a whorled appearance (Fig. 209-10). It can be submucosal, subserosal, or pedunculated. If on a pedicle, it can simulate an ovarian mass. Therefore, it is imperative that a diligent search be conducted for both ovaries. It more often causes acute pain in pregnancy as it outgrows the blood supply at the beginning of the second trimester. *An enlarged uterus* can present as a pelvic mass. Fibroids, uterine carcinoma, or hematocolpos can cause enlargement. However, the most common cause is pregnancy.

All of the above causes of pelvic masses can coexist with an intrauterine pregnancy. The ovaries, particularly if enlarged, can be moved up into the abdomen above the uterus as the pregnancy progresses since they are mobile and there is no extra room in the gravid pelvis. Although the ovaries often cannot be visualized beyond 15 weeks of gestation, a thorough search for them should be made to both sides and above the uterus. Occasionally a large ovarian mass will be found up under the ribs in a woman with advanced gestation. A natural corollary of this is that the ovaries can cause upper abdominal pain in pregnancy.

THE PEDIATRIC PELVIS

In children and adolescents, unlike those of adults, pelvic masses can arise from unusual sources, and, therefore, ultrasound examination is a wise precaution before any surgery is performed. Blood collections in a vagina with a transverse septum, imperforate hymen, pelvic kidneys, or other more unusual anomalies of the genitourinary tract may present as pelvic masses. In addition, cysts of the neural, lymphatic, or gastrointestinal system may present in this age group as a pelvic mass. Serious errors can occur if anatomic relationships are not delineated before surgery.

BIBLIOGRAPHY

Bernuschek G, Rudelstorfer R, Csaicsich P: Vaginal sonography versus serum human chorionic gonadotropin in early detection of pregnancy. *Am J Obstet Gynecol* 158:608, 1987.

Nyberg DA, Filly RA, Mahoney BS, et al: Early gestation: Correlation of HCG levels and sonographic identification. *Am J Radiol* 144:951, 1985.

210 EMERGENCY APPLICATIONS OF ABDOMINAL SONOGRAPHY

Beatrice L. Madrazo

Over the past 30 years, the use of diagnostic ultrasound has increased for a variety of reasons. For example, technological advances have significantly improved image quality; there has been greater acceptance of this technique by both physicians and patients, and its applications have been expanded to include endoscopic techniques, noninvasive vascular imaging, guided punctures and/or biopsies, and so on. It is important to learn to utilize this imaging technique appropriately. Its advantages and disadvantages are well established and are listed in Table 210-1.

The lack of ionizing radiation and of the need for contrast agents allows the widespread use of diagnostic ultrasound from the newborn to the elderly without restrictions. While it is necessary to make contact between the transducer and the area of interest, there are no restrictions as to scanning planes or patient position—hence its great versatility. The introduction of computers for better image processing has significantly improved image quality but has also increased the size of ultrasound scanners. Nevertheless, the systems remain portable. Diagnostic ultrasound has attained the privileged position of being both a high-tech as well as a low-cost method, which are much needed features in this day of economic constraint in medicine.

Despite all these advantages, sonography offers predominantly a morphologic assessment of organs rather than physiologic information. Nevertheless, ongoing research on sonographic contrast agents, for example, may allow determination of the cause of renal failure (i.e., acute tubular necrosis versus prerenal causes of renal dysfunction).

This chapter is divided into areas within the abdomen, including the liver and biliary tree, pancreas, kidneys, and right lower quadrant. It is intended to give the reader an overall view of applications of diagnostic ultrasound in emergency conditions. We do feel, however, that traumatized patients are better assessed with computed tomography (CT), and therefore we will not expand on the topic of abdominal trauma. In addition, suspected aortic dissection is best evaluated by CT.

LIVER AND BILIARY TREE

The right upper quadrant is the best area for evaluation by sonography. The transmission of sound through a compact and good sound transmitter such as the liver allows for excellent portrayal of the liver, gallbladder, biliary tree, pancreas, and right kidney.

The variability in the size and shape of the liver frequently results in the suspicion of a palpable right upper quadrant "mass." This can be readily discriminated using sonography to assess the right upper quadrant. Occasionally, a palpable right renal lower pole is the apparent abnormality. Medical conditions of the liver, such as fatty infiltration and cirrhosis, are prevalent. These conditions present as enlarged livers as well as with elevated liver enzymes. Fat and fibrous tissue deposition in the liver in fatty infiltration and cirrhosis scatters the sound signal, decreasing sound penetration, obliterating the intrahepatic detail, and consequently limiting diagnostic capabilities with this method.

Table 210-1. Advantages and Disadvantages of Sonography

Advantages	Disadvantages
Noninvasive	Morphologic rather than physiologic evaluation
Versatile	Operator dependent
Portable	Inability to penetrate gas
Available	Patient cooperation necessary
Low cost	Limited by patient's body habitus

Liver abscesses can be detected by either sonography or CT. CT may detect smaller lesions; therefore, especially in immunocompromised patients (HIV positive) it is preferred to sonography as an imaging method.

The bile-containing gallbladder is readily identified with sonography due to the strong acoustic impedance mismatch (speed of sound transmission) between the gallbladder and surrounding soft tissues. This sharp delineation of the gallbladder allows for assessment of its walls, intraluminal contents, and pericholecystic spaces. The spatial resolution of sonography (its ability to portray structures without superimposition) results in lack of obscuration of the gallbladder by adjacent bowel loops such as the antrum/duodenum and the hepatic flexure of the colon.

The normal gallbladder wall should be seen as a delicate pencil-thin line measuring no more than 3 mm. Gallstones, due to their strong sound reflectivity, cause a distinct acoustical shadow (lack of sound transmission) posteriorly. The sensitivity, specificity, and accuracy of diagnostic ultrasound in the diagnosis of cholelithiasis is 95 percent. Another important contribution of diagnostic ultrasound is the ability to relate the patient's point of maximal tenderness and precisely evaluate the site of discomfort. Therefore, a positive sonographic Murphy's sign is valuable in confirming acute cholecystitis, especially in the setting of acalculous cholecystitis. Sonography is not as sensitive or specific in diagnosing acalculous cholecystitis as it is with cholecystitis associated with cholelithiasis. In a study comparing primary and secondary signs of acute cholecystitis, Ralles and coworkers found sonography to have a high sensitivity and a specificity when the following were used as criteria: (1) cholelithiasis (99.0 percent), (2) gallbladder wall thickness greater than 3 mm (92.2 percent), and (3) positive sonographic Murphy's sign (98.8 percent). Mirvis and coworkers evaluated the diagnosis of acute acalculous cholecystitis comparing sonography, CT, and scintigraphy retrospectively and found sonography and CT to be highly sensitive (92 and 100 percent, respectively) and specific (96 and 100 percent, respectively). Hepatobiliary scintigraphy was limited by frequent false positives, with a specificity of only 33 percent. Figures 210-1 and 210-2 illustrate cases of cholecystitis with associated cholelithiasis as well as a case of acalculous cholecystitis.

The biliary tree is well evaluated by sonography, both its intrahepatic as well as extrahepatic portions. The biliary ducts lie adjacent to the portal branches, and when dilated present as echo-free areas surrounding these venous structures. They become greater in number and larger in size as they approach the liver hilum. Sound enhancement is present posterior to intrahepatic bile ducts, since the bile is devoid of large particles (e.g., plasma proteins and red blood cells), and therefore no significant sound attenuation takes place. On the other hand, transmission of sound through blood vessels results in sound attenuation caused by scattering of the signal by moving particles such as red blood cells.

The extrahepatic biliary ducts—the common hepatic duct and the common bile duct (CBD)—are seen at the porta hepatis anterior to the hepatic artery and main portal vein. The normal caliber of the common bile duct is 6 mm, being slightly larger in patients 60 years or older. In postcholecystectomy patients, the CBD can measure up to 11 mm. If clinical concern exists regarding a dilated CBD, stimulation of the biliary tree by cholecystokinin and/or oral administration of a fatty meal can be used to assess patency. Decreased caliber of the CBD occurs when there is a normal response, while increased caliber results when obstruction is present. Sonography is not as accurate in diagnosing choledocholithiasis as it is in cholelithiasis, having an accuracy of 75 to 80 percent.

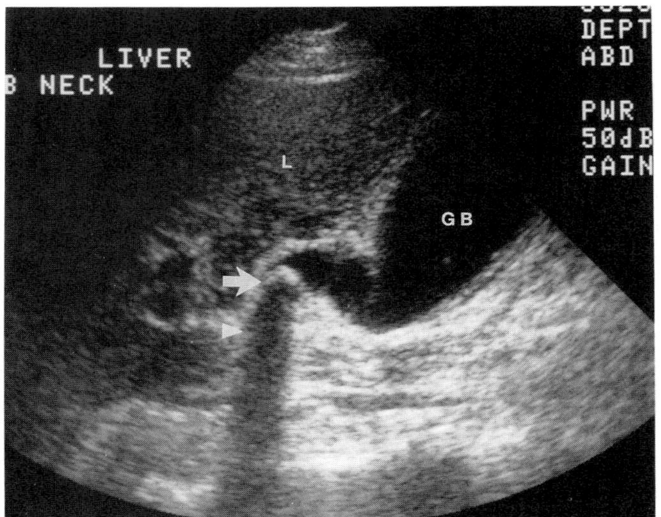

Fig. 210-1. Sagittal sonogram with the patient in the left lateral decubitus position demonstrates the liver (L) and gallbladder (GB). A bright reflector is present in the gallbladder neck/cystic duct region (arrow) consistent with a gallstone. It elicits a posterior acoustical shadow (arrowhead).

PANCREAS

Acute pancreatitis is seen by sonography as an edematous, hypoechoic gland with occasional demonstration of peripancreatic fluid. The pancreas may be diffusely enlarged, have focal enlargement, or be normal in size. Pancreatic pseudocysts are readily identifiable by sonography as either intrapancreatic or peripancreatic fluid collections with internal debris, septations, and so on. In chronic calcific pancreatitis, the gland is noted to contain calcifications that present as bright reflectors with or without associated acoustical shadowing. Failure to visualize the pancreas by sonography in cases of acute pancreatitis is due to an ileus of the transverse colon (sentinel sign) due to the inflammatory changes of the transverse mesocolon caused by pancreatic exudates. As mentioned previously, ultrasound is reflected by gas.

KIDNEY

Upper abdominal discomfort can be secondary to renal disease. The typical clinical presentation of fever, flank pain, and pyuria in cases

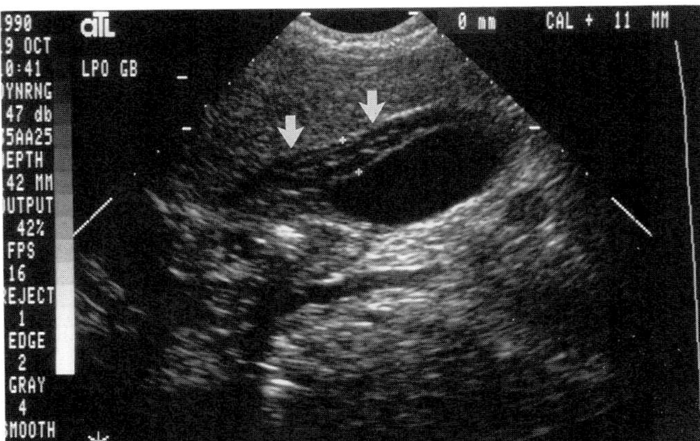

Fig. 210-2. Sagittal sonogram with the patient in a left lateral decubitus position demonstrates a septated fluid collection in the anterior pericholecystic space (arrows). This is seen in acute cholecystitis and is quite helpful in cases of acalculous cholecystitis.

of pyelonephritis makes imaging techniques unnecessary in the evaluation of this group of patients. However, complicated cases of pyelonephritis, such as those where there have been persistent symptoms despite adequate antibiotic therapy, warrant evaluation by sonography. Acute focal pyelonephritis is seen as a focal area of decreased echogenicity with a bulbous configuration of the kidney (lobar nephronia). Renal calculous disease is seen as brightly echogenic foci within the renal parenchyma with associated acoustical shadowing (sound attenuation).

Hydronephrosis is seen as separation of the central renal echo complex by tubular fluid-filled areas. In the setting of acute renal obstruction, excretory urography is the method of choice, since in 41 patients studied by both sonography and excretory urography, Hill and associates found sonography to be only 66-percent sensitive in detecting early obstruction, compared to excretory urography, which detected it in 85 percent.

ACUTE APPENDICITIS

High-resolution gray-scale sonography has been utilized to perform graded compression evaluation of the right lower quadrant. Patients presenting with symptoms related to this abdominal quadrant can be suffering from a variety of conditions, such as (1) Crohn's disease, (2) inguinal hernias, (3) mittleschmerz, (4) ruptured corpus luteum, (5) ectopic pregnancy, (6) renal calculus disease, and (7) appendicitis.

Puylaert and Jeffrey have reported their results using graded compression sonography to diagnose acute appendicitis. The criteria for diagnosing acute appendicitis with this technique include (1) visualization of a noncompressible appendix, (2) measurement of the outer contours of the appendix in excess of 6 mm, (3) demonstration of an appendicolith, and (4) demonstration of focal areas of appendiceal wall thickening or abscess. Jeffrey and associates have evaluated 90 patients clinically suspected of having acute appendicitis. They reported an overall sensitivity of 89 percent, a specificity of 95 percent,

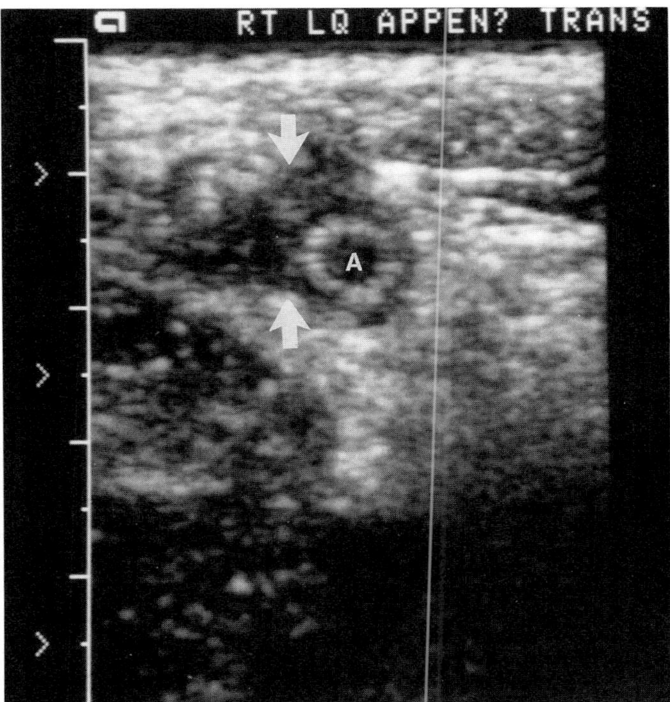

Fig. 210-3. Graded compression of the right lower quadrant demonstrates an enlarged appendix (A; 10 mm). There is thickening of the appendiceal wall (arrows) consistent with acute appendicitis.

and an accuracy of 93 percent. Figure 210-3 illustrates the sonographic findings of acute appendicitis.

The value of Doppler, more specifically color Doppler, as an adjunct to sonographic diagnosis has not yet been fully evaluated. We have noted increased flow (hyperemia) in a variety of acute conditions, such as cholecystitis, pyelonephritis, and appendicitis. Prospective clinical series will be needed to establish the role of Doppler in the evaluation of acute abdominal and pelvic diseases.

BIBLIOGRAPHY

Cronan JJ, Mueller PR, Simeone JF, et al: Prospective diagnosis of choledocolithiasis. *Radiology* 146:467, 1983.

Hill MC, Rich JL, Mardiat JG, et al: Sonography vs. excretory urography in acute flank pain. *Am J Roentgenol* 144:1235, 1985.

Jeffrey RB Jr: *CT and Sonography of the Acute Abdomen*. New York, Raven, 1990.

Jeffrey RB Jr, Laing FC, Lewis FR: Acute appendicitis: High-resolution real-time US findings. *Radiology* 163:11, 1987.

Laing FC, Jeffrey RB Jr, Wing WV, et al: Biliary dilatation: Defining the level and cause by real time. *US Radiol* 160:39, 1986.

Mirvis SE, Vainright JR, Nelson AW, et al: The diagnosis of acute acalculous cholecystitis: A comparison of sonography, scintigraphy and CT. *Am J Roentgenol* 147:1171, 1986.

Mittlestatt CA: *Abdominal Ultrasound*. New York, Churchill Livingstone, 1987.

Puylaert JBCM: Acute appendicitis: US evaluation using grade compression. *Radiology* 158:355, 1986.

Ralles PW, Colletti PM, Lapin SA, et al: Real-time sonography in suspected acute cholecystitis: Prospective in detection of primary and secondary signs. *Radiology* 155:767, 1985.

211 CARDIAC ULTRASOUND IN THE EMERGENCY DEPARTMENT

Andrew M. Hauser

Cardiac ultrasound provides immediate bedside assessment of both cardiac anatomy and function. Direct observation of left ventricular contractility allows accurate detection of myocardial ischemia even in the absence of electrocardiographic abnormalities. Physiologic blood flow information, provided by the complementary Doppler ultrasound examination, rivals the accuracy obtained by invasive means. The echocardiographic identification of pericardial effusions and valvular abnormalities may frequently clarify the etiology of symptoms or physical findings (Table 211-1). Cardiac ultrasound, which requires expertise in both the method of recording and interpretation of data, remains primarily a tool of the cardiologist. Considerably greater technical skill is required to record an echocardiogram than an ECG; however, it is probably easier to obtain basic skills in echocardiographic interpretation than ECG interpretation. Although it may or may not be feasible for noncardiologists to gain sufficient proficiency in echocardiography to use the technique as a screening procedure in the emergency department, emergency physicians should have, at at minimum, sufficient knowledge to know when the technique is applicable to a patient's problem.

TECHNIQUES

The two-dimensional echocardiographic examination provides a cross-sectional image of the beating heart in real time. Because no patient preparation is required, the echocardiographic study may be quickly obtained and even repeated should the patient's condition change. Clinically adequate examinations may even be obtained during CPR. All four cardiac chambers, valves, and the ascending aorta are visualized and recorded with a simultaneous ECG on videotape. Adequate visualization of all cardiac structures may be accomplished by an experienced ultrasonographer in all but approximately 5 to 10 percent of patients. Common limiting factors are inability to position some subjects in the left lateral decubitus position, obesity, and lung hyperinflation due to COPD.

The technique of transesophageal echocardiography employs an ultrasound transducer mounted on a flexible endoscope. Introduction of the transesophageal probe may be performed at bedside with minimal or no sedation and topical anesthetic spray. Since the esophagus is in immediate anatomic proximity to the descending thoracic aorta, this approach is particularly well suited for evaluation of suspected aortic dissections. Imaging success by this method approaches 100 percent.

Doppler ultrasound is a complementary ultrasound technique that provides physiologic information regarding the direction and velocity of moving red blood cells. Laminar flow is readily distinguished from turbulent flow, thereby allowing localization of murmurs and quantification of valvular regurgitation and stenosis. Color-flow Doppler mapping provides a real-time color display of blood flow that, superimposed on the echocardiographic image, yields a vivid representation of intracardiac blood flow. This has been likened to a ''noninvasive angiogram.''

Table 211-1. Etiologies of Symptoms Which May Be Determined by Cardiac Ultrasound

Chest pain	Dyspnea
Myocardial ischemia	Heart failure
Pulmonary embolus	Pulmonary embolus
Pericarditis	Tamponade
Aortic dissection	Pulmonary hypertension
Noncardiac (by exclusion)	Atrial myxoma
Hypotension	Valvular dysfunction
Hypovolemia	
Cardiogenic shock	
Right ventricular infarct	
Pulmonary embolus	

Applications in Ischemic Heart Disease

In the emergency setting, echocardiography is most often used to identify ongoing or recent ischemic events and to quantify global left ventricular function. Localized, or segmental, wall motion abnormalities identify past infarction or recent ischemia and may be apparent even in the presence of a nonspecific ECG tracing. Accordingly, occlusion of a coronary artery will almost invariably result in reduced wall motion localized to the segments perfused by the obstructed vessel. The presence of scar and thinning of the myocardium imply that an infarction has evolved at least several weeks before examination, and their presence or absence may be useful to distinguish recent from past ischemic events (Fig. 211-1). The extent of myocardial segments involved and their degree of abnormality influence global left ventricular function.

Definitive assessment of left ventricular performance in acute infarction is important because prognosis is most closely linked to the extent of functional impairment. Cardiac ultrasound is superior to clinical assessment of Killip classification and to the ECG in predicting death or major complications following acute myocardial infarction. The sensitivity of echocardiography in the identification of myocardial infarction is probably greater than 90 percent. Smaller infarctions, particularly in the distribution of the left circumflex coronary artery, and nontransmural infarctions may, at times, escape detection. Such limited ischemic events tend to be associated with a low frequency of clinical complications. The greater the degree of left ventricular impairment, the greater likelihood of subsequent complications such as heart failure or death. An important application of cardiac ultrasound in the emergency department is the identification of patients at high risk among those who appear initially stable. Such information may assist in decisions regarding triage and therapy. Because the presence of a segmental wall motion abnormality is a sensitive indicator of ischemia and the degree of abnormality is predictive of prognosis, echocardiography is a powerful tool for the diagnosis and triage of

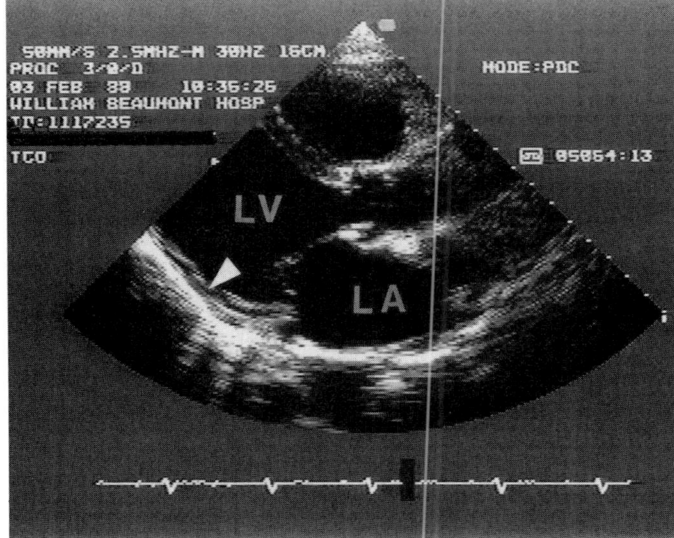

Fig. 211-1 Posterior wall infarct showing localized thinning (arrow) and absent wall motion LV = left ventricle; LA = left atrium.

patients presenting with chest pain to the emergency department. An echocardiographic study displaying normal left ventricular wall motion during chest pain is a strong predictor of a nonischemic etiology and thus, low risk. When symptoms are atypical or the initial ECGs reveal only nonspecific findings, echocardiography may be particularly helpful. Among patients with nonspecific ECG abnormalities in the setting of chest pain presenting to a large community hospital, echocardiography altered the admission diagnosis in 18 percent and disposition plans in 22 percent.

Now that overwhelming evidence indicates that thrombolytic agents reduce patient morbidity and mortality in cases of acute myocardial infarction, never before has emergency decision making been so vitally important in determining their outcome. Because the efficacy of thrombolytic therapy is closely linked to the time from onset of ischemia to treatment, and the administration of such drugs has substantial risks, emergency physicians are under increased pressure to make early and accurate diagnoses. The ECG may not provide an accurate indication of the presence and degree of ongoing ischemia, particularly in the early evolution of an infarction. Thus, echocardiography has a key role in the selection of patients for acute interventions.

Complications of myocardial infarction, including pump failure, mitral insufficiency, septal rupture, right ventricular infarction, and ventricular thrombus, are also readily detected by echocardiographic and Doppler examinations (Fig. 211-2). Clinically important and coexisting myocardial, valvular, and congenital abnormalities may also be identified. The causes of hypotension or dyspnea in patients presenting to the emergency department with unknown cardiac disorders may similarly be clarified by cardiac ultrasound.

Applications in Aortic Dissection

Although the proximal ascending aorta is generally imaged satisfactorily using standard transthoracic imaging technique, the transverse and descending thoracic aorta is generally insufficiently visualized by this method to evaluate most patients with spontaneous or traumatic aortic dissections. The method of transesophageal echocardiography (TEE) is, however, very effective for assessing aortic dissection, especially when biplanar TEE instrumentation is utilized. The results of the European Cooperative Study of Aortic Dissection reported by Erbel and colleagues demonstrated favorable results with TEE when compared with angiography and CT (Table 211-2). Since TEE may be employed at bedside with minimal patient preparation, the earlier time to diagnosis may be lifesaving in this high-risk setting. Additionally, patients may be spared the risk of angiography and contrast dye administration by using TEE in suspected cases of aortic dissection. Using TEE, the intimal flap is readily identified (Fig. 211-3), and the complementary color Doppler examination displays the entry points with greater precision compared to angiographic methods.

Table 211-2. Diagnosis of Aortic Dissection by TEE Compared to Angiography and Computerized Tomography

Technique	Sensitivity %	Specificity %
Angiography	88	94
CT	83	100
TEE	99	98

Source: From Erbel et al: European Cooperative Study Group for Echocardiography: Echocardiography in diagnosis of aortic dissection. *Lancet* 1:457, 1989.

Miscellaneous Applications

Cardiac Tamponade

The identification of a large pericardial effusion in the appropriate clinical setting may identify a correctable cause of hypotension or dyspnea. The presence of diastolic collapse of the right atrium or ventricle may provide further confirmatory echocardiographic data for the presence of tamponade or "pretamponade" (Fig. 211-4). Performance of pericardiocentesis may be often facilitated by echocardiography, which can be used to guide the selection of an appropriate site for needle insertion.

Valvular Heart Disease

Although the identification and quantification of valvular abnormality is generally a nonemergent procedure, identification of a flail leaflet due to myxomatous degeneration or endocarditis may explain the etiology of hypotension or dyspnea in clinical settings when even a significant murmur may be lacking and will guide appropriate medical and surgical measures to stabilize the patient.

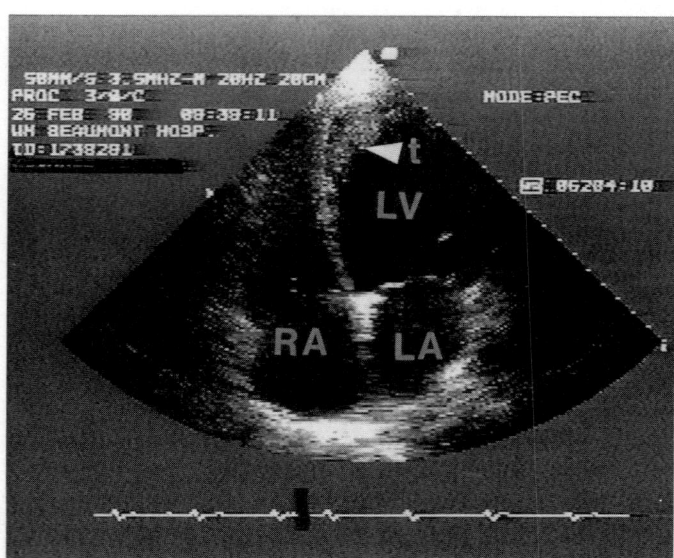

Fig. 211-2. Anteroapical infarct with apical thrombus LV = left ventricle; LA = left atrium; RA = right atrium; t = thrombus.

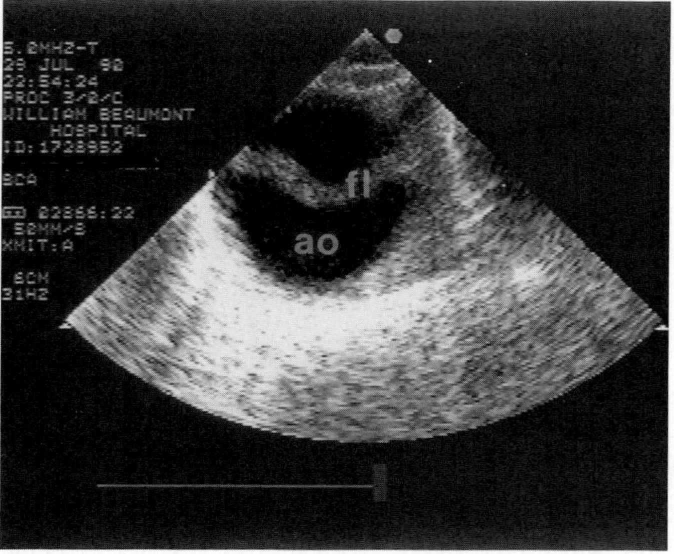

Fig. 211-3. Aortic dissection visualized by transesophageal echocardiography fl = intimal flap; ao = aortic false lumen.

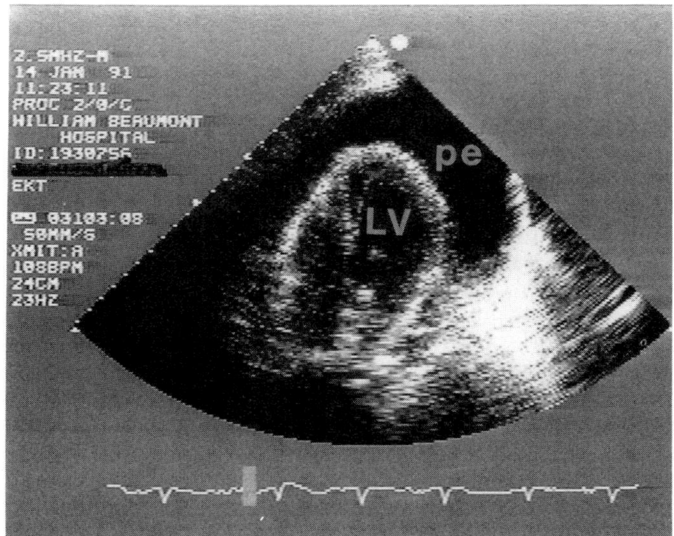

Fig. 211-4. Large pericardial effusion (pe) in patient presenting with cardiac tamponade.

Cardiomyopathy and Intracardiac Masses

Echocardiography may identify hypertrophic cardiomyopathies and intracardiac masses responsible for syncope, dyspnea, or hypotension which are unexplained by other clinical evaluations.

CONCLUSION

Echocardiography is a powerful diagnostic tool that has many emergency department applications. Although the performance and interpretation of cardiac ultrasound exams by emergency physicians is feasible, the practicality of such application has not yet been thoroughly tested. Cardiac ultrasound training in emergency medicine programs is warranted and this is now being offered in some residency training programs and in postgraduate seminars.

The relatively high cost of modern instrumentation may currently prohibit full-time dedication of such units to most centers. However, many hospitals have clinically serviceable instruments made available through displacement by newer units. These instruments, perhaps lacking color Doppler or other sophisticated features, may be sufficient for emergency department screening examinations. The support of an experienced echocardiographer for expert review is essential to maintain quality assurance and ongoing education for emergency personnel who may wish to participate in cardiac ultrasound examinations.

BIBLIOGRAPHY

Bocka JJ, Overton DT, Hauser A: Electromechanical dissociation in human beings: An echocardiographic study. *Ann Emerg Med* 17:450, 1988.

Callahan JA, Seward JB, Tajik AJ, et al: Pericardiocentesis assisted by two-dimensional echocardiography. *J Thorac Cardiovasc Surg* 85:877, 1983.

Erbel R, et al: European Cooperative Study Group for Echocardiography: Echocardiography in diagnosis of aortic dissection. *Lancet* 1:457, 1989.

Hauser AM: The emerging role of echocardiography in the emergency department. *Ann Emerg Med* 18:1298, 1989.

Kloner RA, Parisi AF: Acute myocardial infarction: Diagnostic and prognostic applications of two-dimensional echocardiography. *Circulation* 75:521, 1987.

Oh, JK, Miller FA, Shub GS, et al: Evaluation of acute chest pain syndromes by two-dimensional echocardiography: Its potential application in the selection of patients for acute reperfusion therapy. *Mayo Clin Proc* 62:59, 1987.

Peels KH, Visser CA, Kupper AJF, et al: Value of 2D-echocardiography for immediate detection of coronary artery disease in the emergency room. *Circulation* 78(suppl II):463,1988.

212 COMPUTED TOMOGRAPHY

Jeremy J. Hollerman

Few recently trained clinicians can imagine practicing medicine without the information obtained from computed tomography (CT). CT scanning of the head and body, which was uncommon as recently as 1975, is now routine and is often essential for state of the art patient care.

IMAGE FORMATION

In CT, a section of the head or body with a *slice thickness* defined by the thickness of the x-ray fan beam is scanned then mathematically divided into many tiny blocks of equal volume called *voxels*. Each voxel is assigned a number that corresponds to the degree to which the material in that voxel absorbed the x-ray beam. This absorption is numerically stated as the linear attenuation coefficient. The composition of the material in the voxel (its density and average atomic number) and the quality of the x-ray beam (its average photon energy and energy distribution) determine the linear attenuation coefficient of the voxel. The image is formed by displaying the front face of each voxel (called a *pixel*) with a shade of gray whose darkness is proportional to the linear attenuation coefficient of that voxel.

The length of the voxel is equal to the thickness of the x-ray fan beam, but the *pixel size* (the size of the front face of each voxel cube) is determined mathematically by equations in the computer program. Scan parameters chosen by the CT operator, such as field of view and image matrix size, determine pixel size. The smaller the pixel size and the shorter the voxels, the better the spatial resolution of the image.

Many of the same types of mathematical analysis and data manipulation used for image formation in CT scanning are used to numerically form tomographic images in magnetic resonance imaging (MRI), nuclear medicine single photon emission computed tomography (SPECT), and positron emission tomography (PET) scanning. Many of these mathematical methods depend on Fourier analysis. Mathematical filters consisting of a series of equations are used to remove imaging artifacts, enhancing the visibility of anatomic structures.

CT NUMBERS

The linear attenuation coefficient of each voxel is mathematically normalized to a scale where water is assigned a value of zero. These normalized linear attenuation coefficients are then multiplied by a numerical constant to give the *CT number* In the body, attenuation values cover a range of 4000 CT numbers from air at −1000 to cortical bone at +3000 *Hounsfield units (HU)*. Water has a density of 0 HU. Structures that absorb more of the x-ray beam than does water, such as bone, have positive values, and structures that absorb less of the x-ray beam than does water, such as air and fat, have negative values.

One of the major advantages of CT is its ability to display as different, tissues that have linear attenuation coefficients that are very close together. In general, on conventional roentgenograms (plain x-rays), structures must differ in density by at least 10 percent for it to be possible to recognize them as different densities. The difference in linear attenuation coefficient needed to allow a visible difference in density on CT is much less. For example, intracranial soft tissues vary in density by only 4 percent but are easily distinguished by CT. Gray matter, white matter, and cerebrospinal fluid (CSF) are all easily differentiated. This is achieved by manipulating the CT data display using window and level.

WINDOW AND LEVEL

Window and level are numerical values that are selected to determine the appearance of the image displayed. The same data set of pixels, each pixel assigned a CT number, can appear very different, depending on the values of window and level chosen. The *level* is the point at which the gray scale is centered. Half of the shades of gray available will be used for CT numbers higher than the level and half for CT numbers lower than the level. The *window* is the range of CT numbers to be displayed by the gray scale. Pixels with CT numbers higher than the level plus one-half the window width are displayed as white, and pixels with CT numbers lower than level minus one-half the window width are displayed as black. Values between these numbers are displayed using the gray scale. Up to 256 shades of gray can be displayed by the CT scanner monitor. Many more shades of gray can be displayed on CT films. The human eye can distinguish as different only about 50 shades of gray. If the window width is less than 256 CT numbers, then less than 256 shades of gray will be used in the image display, since no more than one shade of gray can be used per CT number.

The concept of level is easily understood. It is the CT number about which the gray scale is centered. The concept of window is more difficult to grasp. If the window is narrow (such as 100), the range of CT numbers displayed as shades of gray is very limited, and the image will be very *high contrast*. This may or may not be beneficial. If the high-contrast gray scale is centered by the level selected on the range of CT numbers of a specific organ in which subtle differences in density need to be detected (e.g., a narrow window display of the liver to look for a subtle lesion), the high contrast may be beneficial. However, densities outside the narrow range selected will be uniformly too white or too black for evaluation.

A wide window produces a *low contrast* image that displays a large range of CT numbers within the gray scale. This is very useful for evaluation of structures, such as lung or bone, with components of very disparate linear attenuation coefficients (e.g., cortical bone, trabecular bone, and marrow fat (Fig. 212-1). Evaluation of anatomy in parts of the image where adjacent structures are very close in density, such as soft tissue where all parts are very close to water in density, will be limited on wide window settings. A wide window means that large increments of CT numbers are assigned to each shade of gray. Soft tissue structures will appear as an undifferentiated, nearly uniform gray mass (Fig. 212-1A).

One often looks at the data from a particular CT section at several different display settings. For example, an upper abdominal CT section might be viewed at lung settings to look for pneumothorax (Fig. 212-2A), pulmonary infiltrate, pulmonary contusion or mass, or free intraperitoneal air (Fig. 212-3B); viewed at soft tissue settings (Fig. 212-3A) to look for liver, spleen, pancreas, kidney, adrenal, or vascular lesions or adjacent adenopathy; and viewed at a bone window (Fig. 212-1A) to evaluate the vertebrae and ribs. This extensive evaluation can be performed by numerical display manipulation of the same scan data set without exposing the patient to additional radiation from rescanning.

For evaluation of the lung or to look for pneumothorax one uses a wide window (e.g., 1400) and a low level (e.g., −600) to center the gray scale toward air densities. For display of soft tissue structures of the body, one uses a moderate window width (e.g., 350) centered at a level just above water (e.g., +30) to use the gray scale to see a range of tissue densities near water. To evaluate bone, one uses a wide window (e.g., 1500) and a higher level (e.g., +305) to center the gray scale toward denser structures. For brain CT, one uses a narrow window display (e.g., a window width of 90) because the structures to be differentiated are very close in linear attenuation coefficient, and

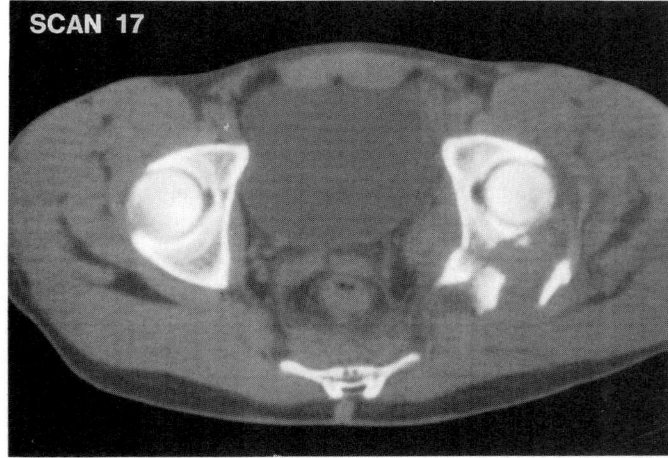

A

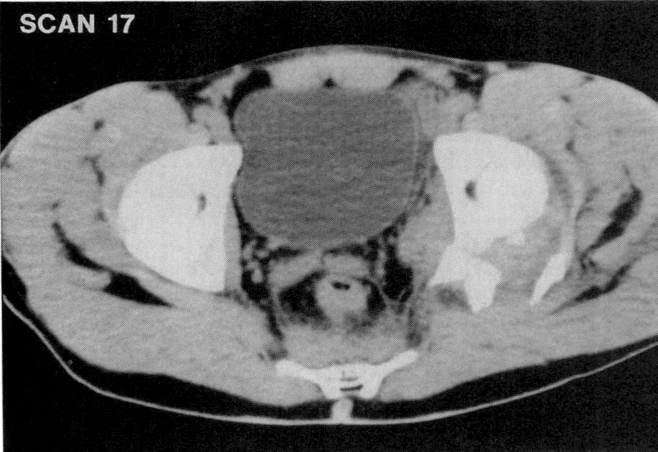

B

Fig. 212-1. The same CT scan displayed at different window and level settings. A posterior wall fracture of the left acetabulum is shown at settings for bone (**A**) and at settings for soft tissue (**B**). The wider window and higher level of the bone settings allow better visualization of bone detail but make all soft tissue structures nearly the same shade of gray. Soft tissue settings allow examination for hemarthrosis and adjacent soft tissue hematoma.

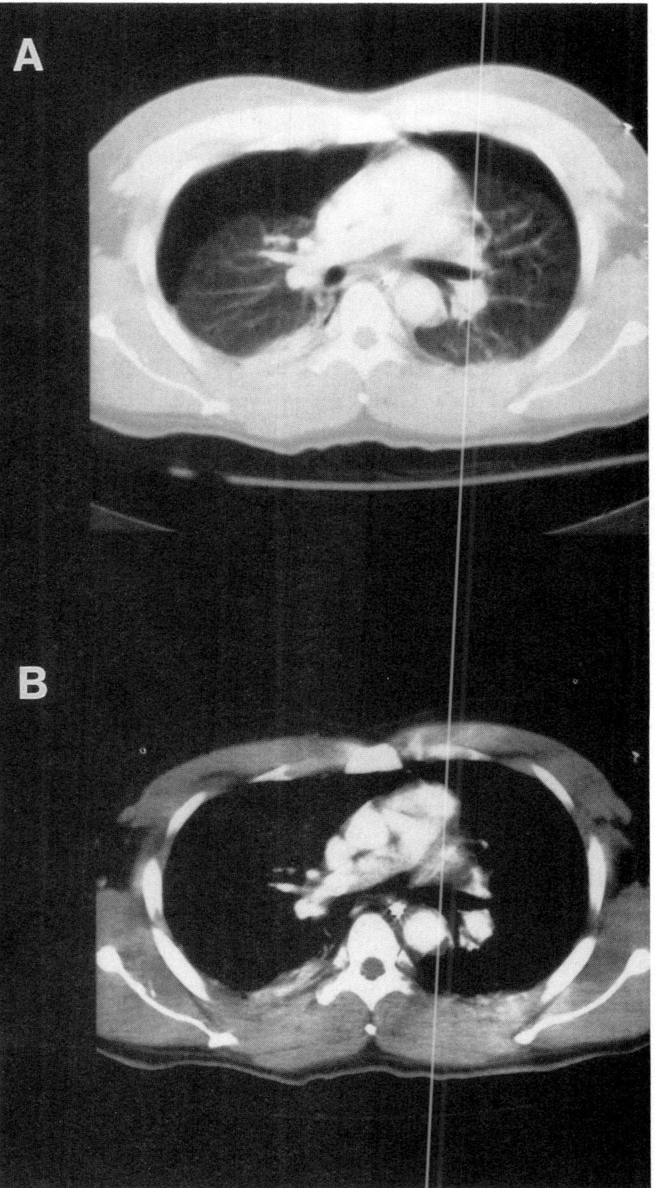

Fig. 212-2. Lung (**A**) and soft tissue (**B**) displays of the same IV contrast-enhanced dynamic scan section. Note how the patient's bilateral pneumothoraces are clearly visible in A but are invisible in B due to different window and level display settings.

one uses a level just above water (e.g., +30) to place the center of the gray scale near the center of the range of CT numbers of the structures to be examined.

FIELD OF VIEW, MULTIPLANAR RECONSTRUCTION, AND THREE-DIMENSIONAL DISPLAY

Many CT scanners can recompute scan data for each slice to a smaller *field of view* with smaller pixel size and higher resolution of an area of interest. Slice thickness cannot be changed without rescanning. Usually, such recomputation must be done on original scan data before image archiving. *Image archiving* is often done at the end of each examination and reduces the size of the data set to be permanently stored. Recomputation to a higher-resolution smaller field of view is especially useful for examination of the spine after acquiring a whole body image or for examination of the pancreas to look for tumor or trauma after examining a whole body image.

Reformatting of scan data for coronal or sagittal section display can also be done. Thin-section (4 mm or thinner) scans provide the best *multiplanar reconstructions* but take longer to acquire than thicker sections and raise patient radiation dose somewhat.

Three dimensional data display, *surface data display*, and other display options now exist. These options are particularly useful to surgeons for operative planning. An example of the use of three-dimensional display is in complex acetabular fractures, where CT scan data can be numerically manipulated to disarticulate and remove the proximal femur from the image of the acetabulum and then create a rotating three-dimensional image of the pelvis. This allows a direct enface view into the fractured acetabulum for reconstructive planning. The three-dimensional image may be rotated in any plane with varying degrees of surface and internal structure shading. All of these options require computer and operator time in addition to that required for usual scanning.

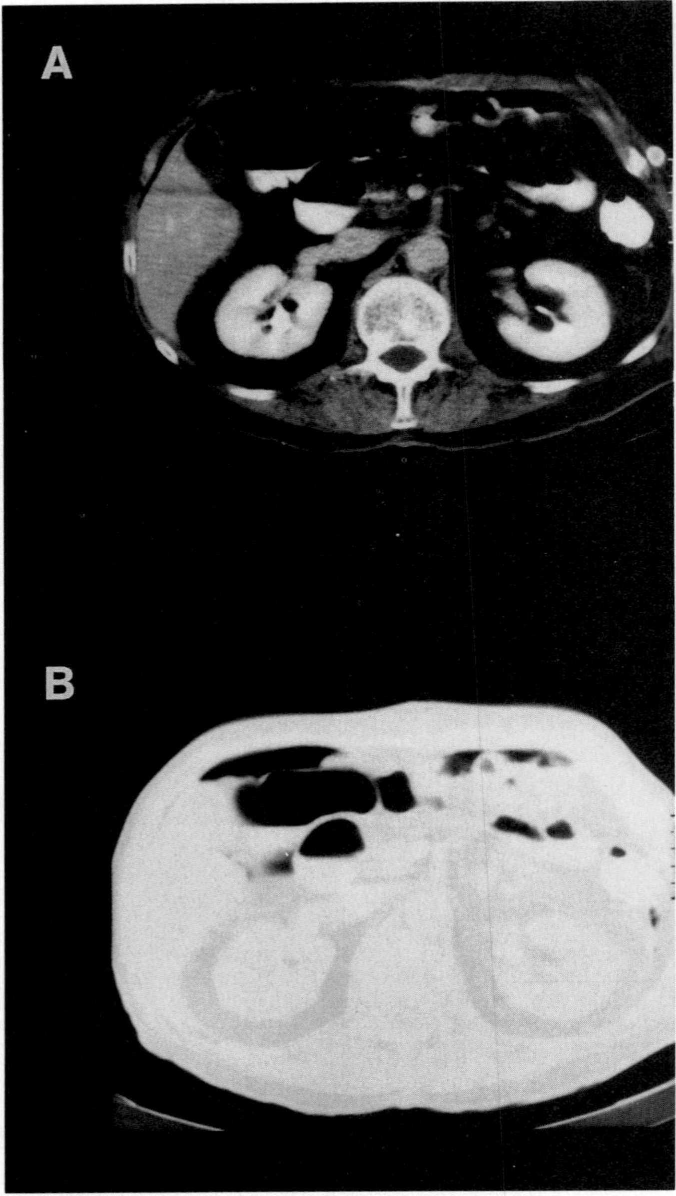

Fig. 212-3. Soft tissue (**A**) and lung window (**B**) displays of the same abdominal scan. Note how the patient's free intraperitoneal air is well shown in B in both the left and right anterior abdomen, anterior to gas-filled intestinal loops. The patient is lying supine on the scan table.

VOLUME AVERAGING

It is important to understand the effect on the image of several CT phenomena. *Volume averaging* is what happens when a voxel only partly overlaps a structure or the structure is smaller than the length of the voxel. This voxel is partly filled with the structure of interest and partly filled with an adjacent structure, which may be very different in density (such as air versus soft tissue). The voxel will be assigned a linear attenuation coefficient and resulting CT number that is the average density within the voxel. The shade of gray assigned may be very different from that which would have been assigned had the entire voxel contained the structure of interest.

Therefore, at the margins of a structure or if a structure is smaller than a voxel, the CT number measured and the shade of gray assigned may be erroneous. If either CT number accuracy or resolution of small structures is of paramount importance, decreasing the scan thickness so that the entire voxel is filled by the structure of interest will improve accuracy.

SLICE THICKNESS, SUBJECT CONTRAST, AND IMAGE NOISE

Like raindrops falling on a roof, x-ray photons are not entirely uniform in distribution. On the basis of random distribution, certain areas get more or less than the average number. This *quantum mottle* is a major source of image noise. One's ability to detect lesions is highly dependent on the signal-to-noise ratio of the data set. Increasing the radiation dose decreases the quantum mottle. However, as in all of radiology and nuclear medicine, for CT we do not select the radiation dose to produce the best image. Rather, we choose the minimum radiation dose that will reliably produce a *diagnostic image*. This image is usually a less perfect depiction of anatomic detail than that which is possible but spares the patient unnecessary radiation.

Increasing the slice thickness improves the detectability of small differences in image contrast by decreasing quantum mottle but worsens volume-averaging artifact. Decreasing the slice thickness reduces volume-averaging artifact but increases image noise, decreasing the detectability of small differences in subject contrast. This can be overcome by using a higher radiation dose for thin sections when necessary. Knowledge of the clinical question to be answered determines the optimum way to perform the CT study. For example, 10-mm contiguous sections are often used to survey the entire chest for pulmonary lesions and mediastinal or hilar adenopathy. If a small pulmonary nodule is found, thin sections of the nodule will provide an accurate measurement of its density to determine whether it is calcified, and because of improved spatial resolution will better depict the nodule's periphery to reveal satellite lesions, spiculation, or pleural extension.

INTRAVENOUS CONTRAST ADMINISTRATION AND DYNAMIC SCANNING

Dynamic scanning is the rapid acquisition of a series of CT images during the bolus phase of intravenous contrast administration. This technique is possible only on relatively newer CT scanners due to improved x-ray tube cooling and enhanced numerical image processing capabilities. As a result, *interscan delay* (the amount of time between scans) is shortened, and scan time itself may also be shortened. Often, a *mechanical (power) injector* is used to administer the IV contrast bolus for this technique. Dynamic scanning allows organ evaluation during the *bolus phase* of IV contrast administration, when organ-to-lesion image contrast is usually at its maximum. The shorter *scan time for acquisition* of each slice decreases the effect of all types of *patient motion,* both voluntary and involuntary. This includes respiratory motion and cardiac pulsations, both of which are transmitted to the abdominal organs. Comatose patients on respirators are unable to hold their breath. The development and use of dynamic scanning is a very significant step in improving the ability of radiologists to accurately assess trauma by CT.

CT done without IV contrast is commonly referred to as *noncontrast* or *C* − CT. CT done during and after the administration of IV contrast is often referred to as *postcontrast, contrast-enhanced,* or *C* + CT.

Increasing the density of a structure by administering elements, such as iodine or barium, that absorb more x-ray photons per unit volume than does soft tissue is called *contrast enhancement.* IV contrast increases the density of the portion of an organ receiving vascular supply. This effect is most pronounced during the bolus phase, when the rapidly administered bolus is circulating in the vascular system and has not yet equilibrated with other fluid compartments (Fig. 212-4). Hematoma, hemoperitoneum, pleural effusion, empyema, abscess, pseudocyst, urinoma, and bileoma do not enhance their avascular portions, and densely enhance their hypervascular portions after IV contrast

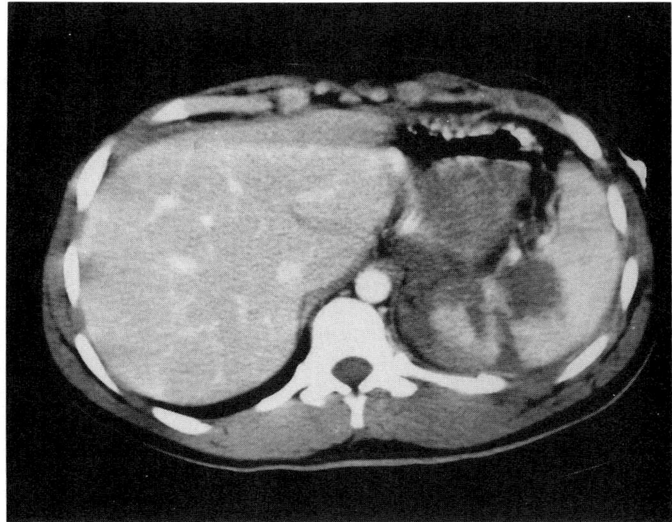

A

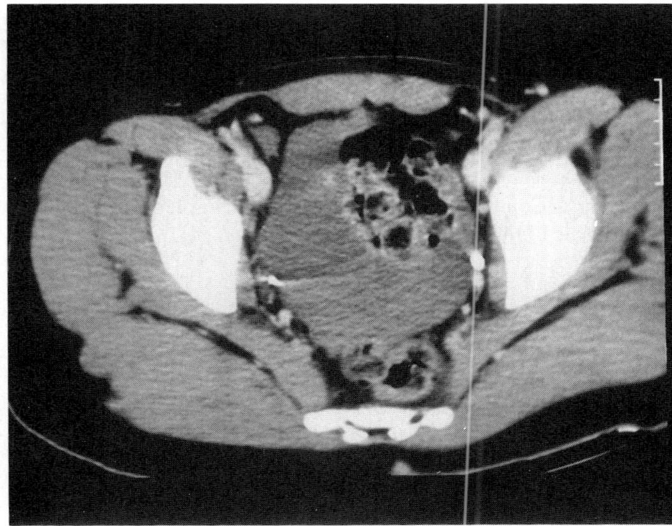

B

Fig 212-4. Images from an IV contrast-enhanced dynamic scan of the abdomen after blunt trauma. The patient's fractured spleen and perisplenic blood clot are well shown in **A**. Free blood in the pelvis surrounding loops of the sigmoid colon is seen in **B**. In the supine patient with hemoperitoneum, the most dependent portions of the abdomen are Morison's pouch (**C**) and the pelvis (**B**). Therefore, hemoperitoneum accumulates in these two sites first. For upper abdominal trauma, it is not adequate to scan only the upper abdomen, since significant pelvic hemoperitoneum will often be missed unless the pelvis is scanned.

administration. This increases their visibility in relation to surrounding tissues (Fig. 212-4).

Most tumors, both primary and metastatic, enhance as if they are hypovascular relative to the organ in which they dwell, but some are hypervascular. Most will be seen best during the bolus phase of contrast enhancement. Some liver metastases of pancreatic endocrine tumors, renal cell carcinoma, carcinoid tumors, pheochromocytoma, and possibly some breast carcinomas will enhance to *isodensity* (the same density) with the surrounding liver during the bolus phase and become invisible. For these tumors, it is important to do precontrast and postcontrast scanning of the liver to look for metastases, since some of their liver metastases will be most apparent before the IV contrast is given.

Use of C−C+CT technique (pre- and postcontrast CT imaging) is also useful in other clinical situations. Among these is the examination of a lesion to differentiate a simple cyst from a tumor, particularly in the kidney or liver. A thin-section CT scan of the lesion is obtained before IV contrast is given. The thin section avoids density measurement error from volume averaging. Then IV contrast is administered, and bolus- and delayed-phase thin-section images of the lesion are obtained. The CT density of the lesion on each image is measured. If the lesion demonstrates any significant contrast enhancement (rise in density determined by CT number and visual assessment), it is not a simple cyst. Simple cysts are avascular and do not enhance. Simple cysts also have an almost imperceptible thin wall and a homogenous near-water-density interior. If contrast enhancement occurs, tumor, abscess, and other processes must be ruled out. Ultrasound imaging is often useful to determine whether the lesion is cystic or solid.

A dense hematoma adjacent to an abdominal organ or viscus, the ''sentinel clot sign,'' may be observed before and sometimes after IV contrast administration on abdominal CT scans for trauma (Fig. 212-5). It is a very useful marker for sites of organ or visceral injury.

Administration of an adequate volume of IV and oral contrast is essential for the performance of state-of-the-art CT imaging of abdominal trauma. Without IV contrast, a hematoma adjacent to an organ is usually slightly denser than the organ (Fig. 212-5), although this difference may sometimes be difficult to detect (Fig. 212-6). Sometimes a blood clot is isodense (has the same CT density) relative to organs such as the spleen or liver, making its detection difficult or impossible (Fig. 212-6A). The isodense or nearly isodense hematoma is one of the most important reasons why IV contrast is used for abdominal trauma CT. Blood may be hyper-, iso-, or hypodense relative to an adjacent organ, depending on whether it is clotted, on the patient's hematocrit, and on the density of the adjacent organ (influenced by the administration of IV contrast material, the presence of fatty infiltration of the liver, hemochromatosis, and other conditions).

Administering too small a dose of IV contrast or administering it too slowly will often enhance a solid organ to isodensity with an adjacent hematoma, making detection of the hematoma difficult or impossible. On older abdominal CT studies where inadequate volumes of IV contrast were administered, often by drip infusion or another nonbolus technique, scans taken before the administration of IV contrast may demonstrate pathology later obscured by organ enhancement to isodensity.

In trauma imaging, the detection efficiency of properly performed IV contrast-enhanced abdominal CT is so superior to abdominal CT performed without IV contrast that the use of noncontrast scanning alone is not recommended.

Administration of an adequate volume of IV contrast by the bolus technique and the use of dynamic scanning maximize CT image quality. For adult patients, a total dose of 40 to 50g of organically bound iodine is used. This may be administered as 150 mL of 60 percent diatrizoate meglumine (ionic) IV contrast or 150 mL of 300 to 320 mg/mL iodine content low-osmolar nonionic contrast; for children the amount is usually 3 mL/kg up to a maximum of 150 mL. With a power injector, an administration rate of 1.5 to 2.0 mL/s is often used. This should not be given through a butterfly-type IV catheter because of the risk of contrast extravasation.

A short delay from the beginning of the IV contrast bolus until the beginning of scanning allows circulation of contrast to the area of interest. If imaging of the arterial vascular phase is sought, as in most chest CT scans, a shorter delay, such as 30 to 45 s, is used. If imaging of the capillary phase of organ enhancemnt is desired on initial scans to maximize organ-to-lesion contrast, as for upper abdominal CT scans, a longer delay, such a 60 to 90 s, is used from the beginning of the IV bolus until the beginning of scanning.

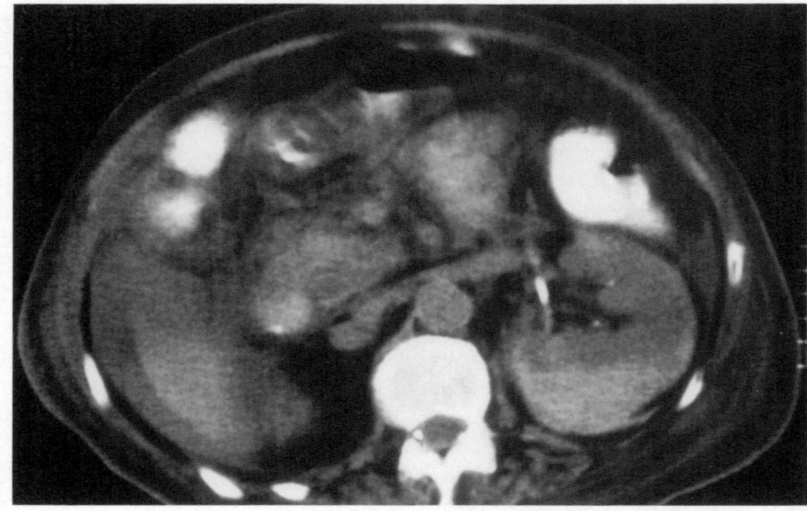

Fig. 212-5. A no-IV-contrast narrow-window display of the abdomen after blunt flank trauma, showing the left perirenal clot well. Subsequent IV contrast-enhanced dynamic scanning of the abdomen and pelvis should be done to evaluate the symmetry of enhancement of the kidneys (to rule out vascular pedicle injury); to examine the renal parenchyma, collecting systems, and ureters for injury; and to examine other organs, including the spleen, for associated injury.

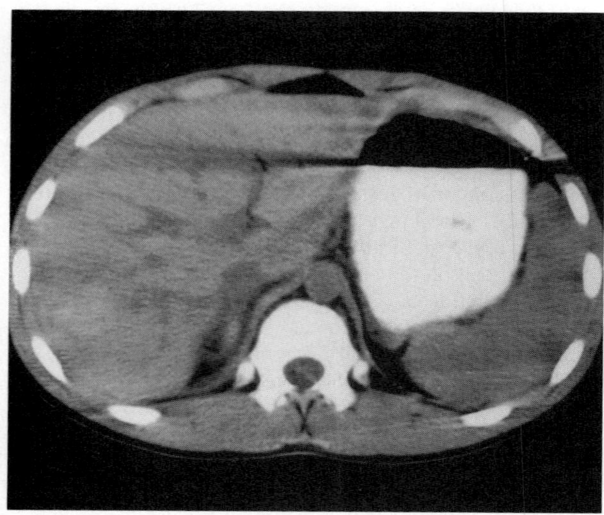

A

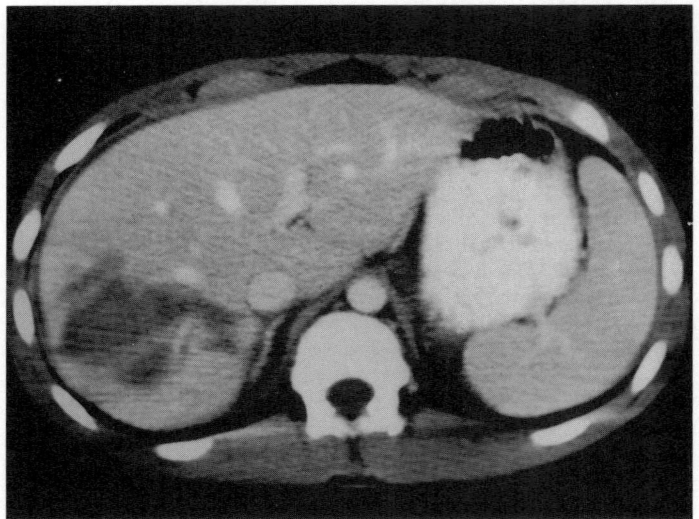

B

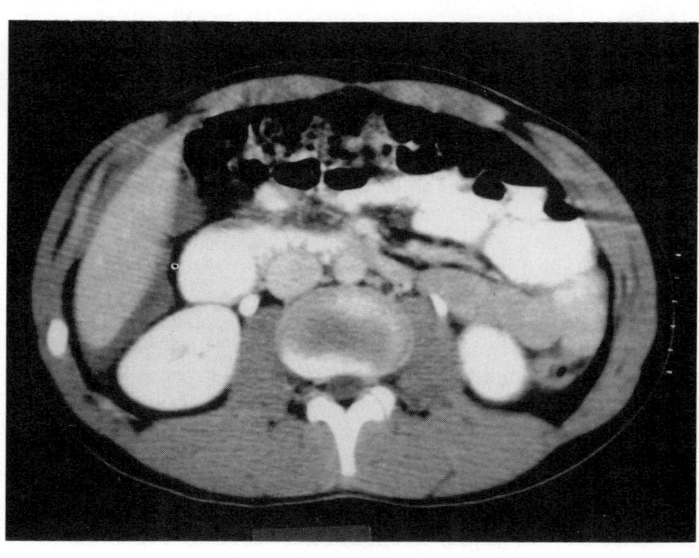

C

Fig. 212-6. Scans of a 16-year-old male after a skiing accident. **A.** A scan before IV contrast bolus enhancement. It is displayed at standard abdominal soft tissue settings, and the intrahepatic clot and laceration are difficult to see. **B.** After bolus IV contrast administration during dynamic scanning, a scan at the same level as **A** shows the hepatic laceration well. It extends immediately behind but does not apparently involve the right hepatic vein. **C.** The upper abdominal component of this patient's relatively small volume hemoperitoneum is seen as blood in Morison's pouch (the right posterior subhepatic space between the liver and kidney). There was also free blood in the pelvis similar to that shown in Fig. 212-4B.

IONIC VERSUS NONIONIC IV CONTRAST

The question of whether to use ionic or nonionic IV contrast is in evolution. Nonionic contrast is approximately 10 times as expensive as ionic contrast. It causes fewer lethal reactions than does ionic contrast. Because the lethal reactions are rare (approximately one severe adverse reaction per 14,000 and one fatal contrast reaction per 40,000 IV contrast procedures using ionic contrast), a great deal of money must be spent to prevent each death. Nonionic contrast also causes some fatal contrast reactions. Very large studies are necessary to gather any meaningful statistics. Nonionic contrast was introduced into widespread use in 1986. Based on currently available studies, the rate of both severe and lethal reactions to nonionic contrast appears to be significantly lower than that for ionic contrast. In one prospective study of 337,647 radiologic procedures in which IV contrast was administered, severe reactions (contrast reactions requiring treatment) were 5.5 times as frequent with ionic contrast than with nonionic contrast (0.22 versus 0.04 percent of patients). A history of a previous reaction to iodine contrast media increased the probability of a severe reaction to subsequent contrast administration by a factor of 4.

Minor reactions to intravenous and intraarterial contrast are much more common than severe or lethal reactions. The overall prevalence of all types of adverse reactions to contrast was 12.7 percent with ionic contrast and 3.1 percent with nonionic contrast in the Katayama study. In patients with a history of allergy, these values were 23.6 and 6.9 percent, respectively. Patients receiving nonionic contrast have less nausea, vomiting, flushing, bradycardia, dizziness, urticaria, injection site pain, and headache. Less pain at the injection site is important for improving examination quality by reducing patient motion when contrast is used intraarterially, as for angiography. The reduction in pain is probably because nonionic contrast is less hyperosmolar relative to blood than is ionic contrast.

Nonionic contrast also appears to induce fewer serious but nonlethal reactions, such as hypotension, bronchospasm, dyspnea, chest pain, cardiac arrhythmia, and angioneurotic edema (particularly of concern when it involves the pharynx). Whether nonionic agents are less nephrotoxic than ionic agents is not settled.

Relative contraindications to the administration of IV contrast include pheochromocytoma (since hypertensive crisis can be precipitated); multiple myeloma and other gammopathies (since contrast-induced precipitation of protein in the renal tubules can cause obstruction and acute tubular necrosis); and a history of previous anaphylactoid reaction to iodine-based contrast (although, because of the idiosyncratic nature of contrast reactions, a previous serious reaction to contrast does not mean that the patient will have the same reaction to the same contrast the next time it is administered). When an IV contrast procedure is absolutely necessary, appropriate pretreatment may include steroids and histamine-blocking agents for patients with severe contrast allergy, α-blocker therapy for patients with pheochromocytoma, and adequate hydration for multiple myeloma patients.

Renal dialysis is not a contraindication to IV contrast administration, since the contrast material is dialyzed off, and renal function is already as impaired as it is going to get.

Patients at higher risk for an adverse reaction to IV administration of iodine-based contrast include patients over 60 years old; patients with heart disease or a history of allergy, asthma, or atopic constitution; patients who have had a previous reaction to iodine-based contrast; severely ill patients; and patients with renal insufficiency, diabetes, or dehydration.

ORAL CONTRAST ADMINISTRATION

The administration of an adequate volume of liquid contrast material into the gastrointestinal (GI) tract is vital for most types of abdominal CT. Oral contrast poses no threat to the kidneys and should be used even in patients with marginal renal function. Either barium-based or iodine-based oral contrast can be used. The amount of iodine absorbed from the GI tract is almost always insignificant to the kidneys, although it can be significant for allergy. Barium is physiologically inert and is not absorbed.

The dense line of oral contrast in the intestinal lumen allows evaluation of bowel wall thickness for hematoma, edema, or mass. Contrast extravasation can be seen in the presence of a full-thickness tear or laceration. In the absence of oral contrast, the gas and stool in the colon provide some natural contrast, making the colon easier to evaluate than the small bowel. The lumen of small bowel loops often contains little or no liquid or gas. Without oral contrast, collapsed small bowl loops can be difficult to differentiate from other soft-tissue-density structures, such as hematoma, abscess, or lymph nodes. The tubular nature of a collapsed small bowel loop assists identification but may be difficult to appreciate when small bowel loops are tightly packed together, particularly in patients with little fat in the mesentery.

Dilated bowel can simulate abscess or free air. When oral contrast is seen in a large gas and air collection in the abdomen, it means that it is either a dilated intestinal loop or and abscess with communication with the GI tract.

Iodine-based CT oral contrast passes through the intestine more quickly than the barium-based oral contrast. This is an advantage in trauma patients in whom quick bowel opacification is necessary. If intestinal perforation or speed of passage through the GI tract is a consideration, we use dilute iodine-based CT oral contrast such as 3 percent Hypaque oral solution (Winthrop) and 97 percent water. This contrast is water-soluble. The barium-based CT oral contrast is a 1.7 percent suspension of barium in water. Both types of CT oral contrast are much more dilute than the contrast used for fluoroscopic radiologic studies, such as upper GI and barium enema studies. Contrast of that density causes metallic star artifacts on CT scans, obscuring anatomy.

For elective abdominal CT, we make an effort to have the patient drink oral contrast intermittently for 2 hours before the procedure so that a total of approximately a liter will have been ingested prior to the CT examination.

For adult patients having abdominal trauma, we use 450 mL of iodine-based CT oral contrast administered via nasogastric (NG) tube in the trauma room immediately when the decision to perform an abdomen CT is made. This is followed by another 250 to 400 mL via NG tube at the time the patient is placed on the CT scan table. This opacifies the stomach, duodenum, and a variable amount of the jejunum and ileum, allowing improved evaluation for intestinal hematoma or laceration.

The only situation in which oral contrast is contraindicated is when the patient is severely allergic to iodine and cannot have barium-based contrast because of possible intestinal perforation or complete colon obstruction. Both are only relative contraindications to barium-based oral contrast. Extravasated barium in the concentration present for CT poses little threat of barium peritonitis. If perforation is present, small amounts of extravasated barium contrast may permanently remain, staining the peritoneum, a situation avoided with iodine-based oral contrast. Complete colon obstruction can allow the formation of a barium stone in the colon proximal to the obstruction if the water in barium-based oral contrast is absorbed by the colon, leaving solid barium. This is a risk only when there is adequate peristalsis to allow the oral contrast to reach the colon and then a sufficient delay before surgery to allow the water to be absorbed. This combination of circumstances is relatively unlikely in a patient with complete colon obstruction.

Because iodine-based CT oral contrast is more than 98 percent water, it is not nearly the inflammatory risk to the lung posed by the undiluted iodine-based oral contrast used for fluoroscopic GI studies. CT oral contrast pulmonary aspiration or extravasation from a torn esophagus, though not desirable, is not the emergency that pulmonary aspiration of full-strength iodine-based oral contrast represents. When aspirated into the lung, full-strength iodine contrast causes a severe inflammatory reaction and induces severe pulmonary edema.

CT OF HEAD TRAUMA

Preparation and Indications for CT

In general, one prefers to perform CT on patients with stable vital signs. Sometimes, CT imaging of an unstable patient is required. This may be for triage decision making, such as for deciding whether a craniotomy or laparotomy is most urgent in a multiply injured hypotensive patient or for lesion localization in a patient with intracranial bleeding and incipient herniation syndrome. Clinical judgment and appropriate consultation between clinician and radiologist are required for the development of the best imaging sequence for the patient.

A secure airway, appropriate control of breathing with a cuffed endotracheal tube and mechanical volume ventilator when required, and adequate vascular access for volume replacement and monitoring (the ABCs of trauma; airway, breathing, and circulation) should be instituted prior to CT scanning. The cervical spine should be cleared or adequately immobilized.

Head CT without IV contrast should be done prior to IV contrast administration for other body CT examinations. IV contrast administration may make appreciation of intracranial hemorrhage or calcifications more difficult.

Indications for head CT after trauma include loss of consciousness, neurologic deficit, protracted vomiting, seizure after head trauma, severe scalp lacerations or hematoma, or skull fracture. These are not mandatory indications but are situations in which head CT will have an increased rate of positive findings. In patients with skull fracture, it is not the fracture, but rather what has happened to the brain and its coverings, that is important.

Intracranial Hemorrhage

Common types of posttraumatic intracranial hemorrhage are subarachnoid hemorrhage, subdural hematoma, epidural hematoma, and intracerebral hematoma.

Subarachnoid Hemorrhage (SAH)

SAH is the most common type of intracranial hemorrhage from trauma. If very minimal, it may not raise the density of the CSF in the subarachnoid space enough to be visible on CT. It can be detected by lumbar puncture and CSF analysis. When the volume of SAH increases, the density of the subarachnoid spaces rises to isodensity with the brain, making the basal cisterns, suprasellar cistern, and portions of the ventricular system invisible. With a greater volume of subarachnoid hemorrhage, these CSF spaces will have areas of hyperdensity relative to brain, due to their blood content. Sulci, the tentorial edges, cisterns, and/or portions of the ventricular system will become hyperdense, depending on the location and extent of the hemorrhage. High-density, bloody CSF may also layer out in the interpeduncular region of the midbrain. The "zipper sign" of SAH may be seen, due to bloody CSF tracking into the interhemispheric fissure and adjacent sulci.

After trauma, SAH is often localized to a few sulci adjacent to sites of injury. If SAH is seen in nearly all sulci and cisterns, consider a ruptured intracranial aneurysm as the cause, with trauma, if present, being subsequent to the physiologic derangement associated with aneurysm rupture.

SAH is most commonly from tearing of the meningeal vessels especially at the vertex, where brain movement is greatest during trauma. After SAH, some patients get arachnoid adhesions. These may cause convexity block of CSF flow pathways, leading to hydrocephalus.

Traumatic intraventricular hemorrhage is not as grave a prognostic sign as previously thought. It usually resolves in 5 to 7 days. It often layers out in the temporal horns and atria of the lateral ventricles.

Subdural Hematoma (SDH)

SDH as a result of trauma is less common than SAH but is several times as common as epidural hematoma (EDH). Usually, SDH is a venous bleed, but it can occasionally be arterial in origin. Because of their usually venous origin and the large potential space (the subdural space) in which they dwell, SDHs develop more slowly than EDH.

SDHs are most often caused by tearing of the bridging veins that connect the cortical veins of the subarachnoid space with the dural venous sinuses. At the time of trauma, there is a shift of the brain, tearing the bridging veins at the point where the veins are fixed as they pass through the dura. They bleed into the subdural space between the dura and the arachnoid. In 25 percent of patients, the SDHs are bilateral. Sagittal violent shaking of children can lead to SDH and retinal detachment. Children are especially vulnerable because they have a large head relative to body size and have poor neck strength to support the head.

SDH is most likely to occur in the elderly, who often have large CSF spaces due to brain atrophy. When trauma causes rapid head motion, the shearing forces developed are greatest in the elderly because of the room available for the brain to move within the skull.

When elderly patients get an SDH, they often tolerate it better than would a younger person. This is because, by resorbing CSF, they can create intracranial space for the mass effect of the blood. In a younger person without cerebral atrophy, there is not substantial intracranial space for a blood collection other than that created by compressing the brain. Therefore, younger patients are less likely to get SDH from trauma, but when they do get SDH they tolerate it more poorly than older patients.

The subdural space is a large potential space between the arachnoid and pia mater. It is not divided at suture margins. SDHs cross suture margins but do not cross the falx or tentorium. Acute SDHs are usually crescent-shaped (like a new moon). Interhemispheric SDHs may be triangular at their anterior or posterior margin, where they separate the cerebral hemispheres by their mass effect. They then continue as a linear interhemispheric density that does not track into adjacent sulci, in contrast to the zipper sign of SAH, in the same location. Tentorial SDHs are oriented obliquely along the course of the tentorium cerebelli. Because of volume-averaging effects, the margin of this obliquely oriented linear blood collection is often fuzzy and looks like ill-defined contrast enhancement of a too thick tentorium.

If not drained or resorbed, when SDHs become chronic they sometimes become biconvex in shape (like a lens, the same shape as an EDH), but they often stay in their original crescent shape. Chronic SDHs can calcify. It is not uncommon for them to be bilateral, especially in elderly patients with cerebral atrophy and repetitive falls.

SDHs go through three phases of density. In patients with a normal hematocrit, *acute SDH* is hyperdense in relation to brain. The density of the blood collection decreases at a variable rate. Usually, some time 1 to 3 weeks after trauma, the SDH is the same density (isodense) as the brain, making it difficult to see without IV contrast enhancement. The mass effect of the isodense SDH will remain evident both without and with IV contrast. This is the *subacute phase of SDH,* during which a portion or all of the SDH is isodense. This phase lasts 2 to 3 weeks from the end of the acute (hyperdense) phase.

The decrease in density of the SDH is often not uniform. The medial portion of the SDH becomes isodense with brain earlier than the lateral portion which remains high density. This can lead to underestimation of the size of the SDH on a head CT exam without IV contrast done during the subacute phase. By three to six weeks after injury the majority of SDH are lower density than normal brain. This is the *chronic phase of SDH.*

After sufficient time, SDHs sometimes become near water density. A very chronic SDH that has had all its cellular elements lysed and absorbed and is near water density must be distinguished from an accumulation of CSF in the subdural space due to an arachnoid tear, a true subdural hygroma.

In response to the SDH, after a period of days to weeks, a very vascular enhancing membrane of granulation tissue forms at the interface between the brain and the SDH. This enhancing membrane is often the source of rebleeding into the SDH. Rebleeding raises the CT density of the SDH. The increased density may be homogenous or inhomogenous. By raising the SDH to isodensity, rebleeding may make it more difficult to appreciate part of all of the SDH. It will cause the SDH to appear less old than it actually is. IV contrast-enhanced CT allows determination of the size of the SDH by making the enhancing membrane visible, marking the margin of the brain.

SDHs often occur from contrecoup forces, especially in the temporal region. Frontal SDHs are often just below the point of impact (coup forces). When SAH is associated with intracerebral hematoma or SDH without a history of trauma, SDH of arterial origin, especially from aneurysm or arteriovenous malformation, should be considered.

After an SDH is surgically drained, especially in elderly patients with chronic SDH, the brain often will not immediately reexpand. This creates a potential space for rebleeding.

Epidural Hematoma (EDH)

There are two layers of the dura mater: the periosteal layer and the meningeal layer. The periosteal layer is attached to the inner table of the skull and is its periosteum. The meningeal layer is inside the periosteal layer. The potential space between the two layers is the location of the dural venous sinuses.

EDHs usually result from arterial bleeding and are usually associated with a skull fracture that tears an epidural vessel, most often a temporal skull fracture tearing the middle meningeal artery. EDHs are biconvex (lenticular) in shape.

The EDH is located between the skull and the periosteal layer of the dura. It strips the dura off the skull. It has the dura as its sharply defined medial margin on CT. EDHs can cross the midline and the tentorium but do not cross intact skull sutures. The dura is tightly adherent to the skull at sutures. If you see an EDH that appears to cross a suture margin, it is probably two adjacent EDHs, or the suture is fractured and the dural attachment disrupted. EDH can elevate a dural venous sinus away from the skull because it is outside the periosteal layer of the dura. Intracranial air is frequently seen with EDH but is uncommon with SDH unless there is an open skull fracture or recent surgery.

EDH is associated with a "lucid interval" in approximately 40 percent of cases. This is the clinical situation where the patient is rendered unconscious from brain concussion, then regains consciousness and becomes lucid for some period of minutes to hours, then becomes obtunded and then unconscious as the mass effect of the EDH causes herniation syndrome.

Intracerebral Hematoma

The intracerebral hematomas seen after trauma are usually irregular in shape and multiple, in contrast to intracerebral hematomas from nontraumatic causes, which are usually solitary and spherical. Both types are often surrounded by a ring of edema. With time, intracerebral hematomas decrease in density from the periphery to the center. They become isodense in 2 to 4 weeks. One to six weeks posttrauma, IV contrast-enhanced head CT usually shows peripheral ring enhancement surrounding each intracerebral hematoma. Three mechanisms account for this: (1.) blood-brain barrier breakdown and extravasation of contrast, (2.) luxury perfusion secondary to loss of cerebral vascular autoregulation, and (3.) formation of hypervascular granulation tissue around the periphery of the hematoma.

Occasionally, a delayed intracerebral hematoma can form up to 2 to 3 days after evacuation of an extracerebral hematoma. This may be due to the loss of the compressive tamponade effect the extracerebral hematoma was having on an injured vessel. A delayed hematoma has a poor prognosis. An excessively high vascular perfusion pressure due to loss of cerebral vascular autoregulation may also be a factor.

Cerebral Edema

Brain swelling after head trauma is from hyperemia and edema. Hyperemia is increased blood flow because of loss of cerebral vascular autoregulation. This and the breakdown of the blood-brain barrier cause *vasogenic edema*. Local trauma also causes dysfunction of cell membranes, including dysfunction of the Na-K pump. This results in *cytotoxic edema*. Plasma leaks into the extracellular space more rapidly than it is absorbed, causing cerebral edema. Children are especially prone to posttraumatic cerebral swelling. The relative contributions of the vasogenic and cytotoxic types of edema vary in different types of cerebral edema (from trauma, tumor, ischemia, toxins, etc.).

Cerebral Contusion

Cerebral contusion is brain bruising or crushing without interruption of the cortex. Punctate hemorrhages (high density), tissue necrosis, and edema (low density) are seen, usually just below the point of impact.

White Matter Shear Injury (Axonal Shear Injury)

These injuries occur in the white matter, usually near the gray-white matter junction. They may be secondary to differential speeds of rotation of different sections of the brain after a torquing injury of the head. The prognosis is grave. Often, small punctate hemorrhages are seen in the corpus callosum, basal ganglia, thalamus, hypothalamus, and upper brainstem, associated with varying degrees of brain swelling. Sometimes the degree of brain swelling that develops is not very severe in spite of the severity of the injury from the point of view of outcome. One or both hemispheres may become uniformly hypodense, mimicking infarction. Subsequently, the cerebrum atrophies. Often the initial head CT scan does not look that bad, with only a few scattered tiny foci of hemorrhage visible in the white matter to mark the severity of the injury.

Basilar Skull Fracture

It is very important to remember that most lateral views of the skull in the trauma room are taken with cross-table lateral technique. The air-fluid level in the sphenoid sinus associated with a basilar skull fracture will be vertical when the x-ray is placed on a viewbox as if the patient were standing. A vertically oriented straight edge in the sphenoid sinus with homogenous fluid density behind it is not incomplete pneumatization of the sphenoid sinus but, rather, an air-fluid level that is a marker for basilar skull fracture after trauma.

Basilar skull fractures often give intracranial air if they communicate with a sinus.

Intracranial Foreign Bodies

After a gunshot wound, metallic bullet fragments and bone fragments are easily seen by CT. Other material that may have been driven into the skull by trauma can be more difficult to recognize. Clothing fragments, wood, plastic, stones, and other relatively radiolucent material can be nearly isodense with brain or may be difficult to identify when surrounded by hemorrhage. In one case, a piece of intracranial wood was mistaken for a pneumatocele on a CT scan. Tampons in the vagina, when not soaked with blood, appear on abdominal CT as air collections distending the vagina. Apparently the same is true of some types of wood, having enough air content and radiolucent material to appear near air density by CT.

Helmet CT

A recent article describes the use of CT for postaccident evaluation of helmet performance and condition. This information can be obtained without destructive dismantling of the helmet into its component layers, a process that may itself create artifactual helmet fractures or other findings not related to helmet performance during the accident.

CHEST TRAUMA

After chest trauma, CT often adds significant finding not seen on chest x-ray. CT and histologic study have disclosed the presence of pulmonary laceration and alveolar hemorrhage in pulmonary contusion, and the role of pulmonary laceration in the etiology of posttraumatic pneumatocele formation, pulmonary hematoma, and late cavitation. CT is more sensitive than chest x-ray for detection of pulmonary contusion and laceration. In one study, 99 lacerations were seen on chest CT scans, when only 5 of them had been prospectively recognized on chest x-rays of the same group of patients.

Chest CT in patients with pulmonary contusion can be helpful in predicting which patients will require a ventilator.

Mediastinal Trauma and Aortic Injury

CT is better than chest x-ray for detecting mediastinal hematoma. Several recent studies suggest that when chest CT shows no evidence of vascular injury or mediastinal hematoma, arch aortogram is not necessary to rule out great vessel transection or laceration. Significant dissenting views exist.

It is usually desirable to image any defect or fracture in a plane perpendicular to the abnormality. CT produces an axial (transverse plane) image of the body. A traumatic aortic laceration typically is also oriented in the transverse plane, parallel to the plane of the CT section, and could be missed. A coronal or sagittal imaging plane would be more sensitive. Many authorities now feel that even if the aortic laceration (rupture, tear, or transsection) itself is not visible on the CT scan, associated abnormalities of pseudoaneurysm, aortic contour deformity, local caliber change, or mediastinal hematoma will be visible on CT and will indicate the need for an aortogram to rule out aortic injury.

An interesting recent finding related to traumatic aortic laceration is the discovery that in some or all cases of blunt chest trauma with aortic laceration near the ligamentum arteriosum, the mechanism of injury may be pinching of the aorta between the spine and anterior bony thorax, rather than the traditional explanation of deceleration shearing forces.

It is important to distinguish aortic laceration from aortic dissection. Aortic dissection is usually associated with atherosclerotic vascular disease or occasionally pregnancy, and not trauma. Up to 11 percent of traumatic aortic lacerations will have significant dissection either antegrade or retrograde, beginning at the site of the tear, due to pulsatile luminal pressure and flow. Such dissections can be in the tunica media but are often subadventitial, in contrast to the dissections of the aorta seen in patients with atherosclerosis or pregnancy, which are usually in the tunica media. Most traumatic aortic lacerations are localized, creating a pseudoaneurysm that does not significantly dissect.

CT OF ABDOMINAL TRAUMA

Several of the important aspects of patient preparation for abdominal CT are covered above, including preparation of the Airway, Breathing, and Circulation (the ABCs); evaluation and immobilization, if necessary, of the cervical spine; administration of water-soluble oral contrast and IV contrast; and use of dynamic scanning. An excellent basic text on CT of trauma is available by Federle and Brant-Zawadzki, and an excellent general text on CT of the body (excluding the head) is by Lee and associates.

Abdominal CT Versus Diagnostic Peritoneal Lavage

CT of the abdomen after blunt abdominal trauma is most appropriate for patients stable enough to avoid physiological compromise during the time required for performance of the examination. This amount of time varies from institution to institution.

When possible, the performance of abdominal CT before or instead of diagnostic peritoneal lavage (DPL) is preferable to doing the abdominal CT examination after DPL. Abdominal trauma CT is useful either before or after DPL; however, DPL introduces fluid and free air, making evaluation for intestinal injury, perception of the "sentinel clot sign," and evaluation of the volume of hemoperitoneum difficult. This increases the problems in determining which patients are candidates for nonoperative management of solid organ injury.

Increased radiologist experience in interpretation of trauma CT examinations and the development of bolus dynamic scanning using a CT power injector for IV contrast administration have significantly improved the sensitivity and accuracy of abdominal CT for evaluation of trauma. At hospitals where state-of-the-art CT is being performed, all published data about the sensitivity and specificity of abdominal trauma CT for detection of solid organ injury is nearly obsolete. Recent CT scanners with improved computer image processing speed and increased x-ray tube cooling can rapidly obtain many scans during the bolus phase of IV contrast administration, markedly improving image quality. Fast scanning techniques decrease motion artifacts.

A recent study comparing CT and DPL for blunt abdominal trauma probably suffers from use of older CT techniques and equipment but still found that CT had similar specificity (99.5 versus 99 percent) and similar accuracy (92.6 versus 98.2 percent) but somewhat lower sensitivity (74.3 versus 95.9 percent) compared to DPL for evaluation of blunt abdominal trauma. The method of IV contrast administration was not specified, and whether they used dynamic scanning was not stated. Two of the patients with negative CT scans required operative treatment of a complication of DPL (out of 301 patients).

Use of CT for evaluation of blunt abdominal trauma decreases the nontherapeutic laparotomy rate. In one study, this decreased from 14 percent with DPL to 5 percent with use of CT.

Solid organ injury (injury to the liver, spleen pancreas, adrenals, and kidneys) in the abdomen is extremely well evaluated by bolus-enhanced abdominal CT (Figs. 212-4 and 212-6). The challenge for radiologists is detection of intestinal and other hollow viscus injury. CT can be quite effective in identifying bowel injury in adult and pediatric patients but is much less sensitive for detection of intestinal injury than for solid organ injury. Missed intestinal injuries are a problem in both adult and pediatric patients.

Nonoperative Management and Occult Intestinal Injuries

Nonoperative management of hemodynamically stable patients with blunt abdominal injury is being used with increasing frequency. In such cases, occult intestinal injuries often are not clinically apparent until several days after the trauma. Morbidity and mortality may increase from such occult intestinal injuries. For this reason, radiologists are increasingly vigilant about evaluation of the intestine on CT examinations, especially after blunt trauma.

Unfortunately, because of limited bowel opacification by oral contrast and the occasional presence of mesenteric hematoma, accurate evaluation for intestinal injury is often difficult on initial examinations after trauma. This is particularly true in adult patients with little intraabdominal fat and in children. Air or fluid introduced by DPL makes evaluation more difficult.

The presence of a focal dense blood clot adjacent to an intestinal loop or other organ is termed the "sentinel clot sign." This sign is particularly useful, when present, to mark sites of probable injury, including intestinal injury. Unfortunately, this sign is often not present at sites of intestinal injury.

For trauma patients, there is usually insufficient time for complete small bowel opacification with oral contrast. Large bowel opacification is usually not necessary, since colon contents create natural contrast.

Iodine-based water-soluble oral contrast should be administered via NG tube in the trauma room as soon as the decision for abdominal CT is made. This will allow maximum time for small bowel transit of oral contrast.

In those patients with intraabdominal injuries treated nonoperatively, the day after admission consideration should be given to the performance of the follow-up abdominal CT examination with complete bowel opacification with oral contrast to search for occult intestinal injury.

CT of Retroperitoneal and Flank Trauma

CT is very accurate for evaluation of the retroperitoneum and flanks. CT may not show every injury but will indicate whether operation is required.

IV contrast-enhanced CT has replaced intravenous pyelography (IVP) as the best method for evaluation and staging of renal trauma (Fig. 212-5). IVP is not very sensitive for detection of renal injuries. CT is much more accurate. Dissenting views are occasionally expressed. However, in one dissenting study, in addition to the added renal findings by CT, 3 of the 60 patients had significant unsuspected extrarenal intraabdominal injuries shown on the CT scan. Two of these patients required laparotomy. Both IVP and CT were performed in this reference for research purposes. The IVP is rarely necessary when CT has been done.

In cases of negative IVP and positive CT, although CT shows the type and extent of renal injury much more accurately than IVP, its additional findings often do not change management from nonoperative to operative, since nonoperative management of most renal trauma is appropriate. The additional findings provided by CT often alter the pattern of follow-up and return to activity recommendations.

Stool usually contains substantial amounts of gas. This and the other gas in the colonic lumen usually allow adequate colon evaluation without additional colon contrast (Fig 212-4B). If a specific portion of the colon is difficult to evaluate by CT, either changing the patient's position to move colon gas to the area of interest or rectal administration of water-soluble CT oral contrast can be performed to create a CT enema. The use of rectal contrast for CT is extremely useful in selected cases. The routine use of rectal contrast for trauma abdominal CT examinations is not necessary and delays the performance of the examination.

Bladder and Diaphragm Injuries

Use of CT to evaluate the contrast-filled bladder can be very helpful when extravasation is shown, indicating bladder rupture or laceration. A negative CT cystogram does not rule out a bladder injury completely, however, and a standard retrograde cystogram is necessary for best evaluation if bladder injury is suspected.

CT has great difficulty diagnosing injuries to the diaphragm. Chest x-ray obtained on admission and repeated soon after, when coupled with a high index of suspicion, is more sensitive than previously thought for diagnosis of traumatic rupture of the diaphragm, particularly on the left side.

Abdominal CT Findings and the Decision for Laparotomy

In both adult and pediatric patients, the extent of hemoperitoneum and the appearance of organ injuries are not the only factors in deciding whether a laparotomy is necessary. Various CT-based grading systems have been tried in an attempt to predict from the CT results alone which patients with abdominal trauma need laparotomy. These studies show that the hemodynamic status of the patient and the results of serial laboratory studies and bedside assessments are necessary in conjunction with the CT results to determine the need for laparotomy.

The flat inferior vena cava sign is very useful in showing that the patient having CT has severe volume depletion and immediately incipient hemodynamic crisis. This is true in both adult and pediatric patients.

In pediatric patients, the experience is the same as that in adult patients. CT is excellent for abdominal injury detection, but the decision for laparotomy is based not only on the extent of injury shown on the CT scan but also substantially on the physiological condition of the child. Some pediatric studies have shown a positive correlation among the volume of hemoperitoneum, the need for laparotomy, and the mortality rate; however, other studies disagree with this assertion.

For patients with gunshot wounds of the chest or abdomen, an analysis of the bullet path to determine whether the peritoneum has been traversed is mandatory. Two radiographs at 90 degrees, CT, clinical examination, and peritoneal lavage are all useful. If peritoneal penetration by a bullet is suspected, laparotomy is indicated. The morbidity and mortality of an exploratory laparotomy that shows no significant intraabdominal injury is low compared with that of missed intestinal injury. CT is particularly useful when an exclusively body wall or retroperitoneal path is suspected.

CT OF SPINE TRAUMA

Plain films should be used to guide the levels to be CT-scanned. An intact vertebra above and below the vertebra suspected of injury on standard radiographs should be included in the CT scan, since a substantial number of occult injuries will be found in these adjacent vertebrae.

Standard radiographs are quite a good guide to the areas suspicious for fracture. In one study, only 1 of 49 patients with cervical fracture visible on CT had completely normal standard radiographs. If there is a strong clinical suspicion of occult injury because of symptoms or signs in spite of negative radiographs, CT of the area of interest can easily be performed.

CONCLUSION

CT has revolutionized the evaluation and treatment of patients with many different types of pathology. Working together, the radiologist and clinician create the best sequence of imaging examinations for each clinical problem. CT is often one of the examinations and is cost- and time-effective. Understanding some of the technical aspects of CT helps the clinician order the appropriate study and use the results for correct decision making. The experience of the radiologist in invaluable for study design, performance, and interpretation. Emergency physicians find the information gained from the CT examination of trauma patients particularly useful for improving patient care.

BIBLIOGRAPHY

Acheson MB, Livingston RR, Richardson ML, et al: High-resolution CT scanning in the evaluation of cervical spine fractures: comparison with plain film examinations. *Am J Roentgenol* 148: 1179, 1987.

Bergen CT, Chan FN, Bodzin JH: Intravenous pyelogram results in association with renal pathology and therapy in trauma patients. *J Trauma* 27: 515, 1987.

Brick SH, Taylor GA, Potter BM, et al: Hepatic and splenic injury in children: role of CT in the decision for laparotomy. *Radiology* 165: 643, 1987.

Brooks AP, Olson LK, Shackford SR: Computed tomography in the diagnosis of traumatic rupture of the thoracic aorta. *Clin Radiol* 40: 133, 1989.

Bulas DI, Taylor GA, Eichelberger MR: The value of CT in detecting bowel perforation in children after blunt abdominal trauma. *Am J Roentgenol* 153: 561, 1989.

Cass AS, Vieira J: Comparison of IVP and CT findings in patients with suspected severe renal injury. *Urology* 29: 484, 1987.

Christensen EE, Curry TS III, Dowdey JE: Computed tomography, in *An Introduction to the Physics of Diagnostic Radiology*, 2d ed. Philadelphia, Lea & Febiger, 1978, 329–360.

Cooter RD: Computed tomography in the assessment of protective helmet deformation. *J Trauma* 30: 55–68, 1990.

Crass JR, Cohen AM, Motta AO, et al: A proposed new mechanism of traumatic aortic rupture: The osseous pinch. *Radiology* 176: 645, 1990.

Demos TC, Solomon C, Posniak HV, et al: Computed tomography in traumatic defects of the diaphragm. *Clin Imag* 13: 62, 1989.

Federle MP, Brant-Zawadzki M (eds.): *Computed Tomography in the Evaluation of Trauma,* 2d ed. Baltimore, Williams & Wilkins, 1986.

Federle MP, Brown TR, McAninch JW: Penetrating renal trauma: CT evaluation. *J Comput Assist Tomogr* 11: 1026, 1987.

Feliciano DV, Burch JM, Spjut-Patrinely V, et al: Abdominal gunshot wounds: An urban trauma center's experience with 300 consecutive patients. *Ann Surg* 208: 362, 1988.

Fletcher TB, Setiawan H, Harrell RS, et al: Posterior abdominal stab wounds: Role of CT evaluation. *Radiology* 173: 621, 1989.

Gelman R, Mirvis SE, Gens D: Diaphragmatic rupture due to blunt trauma: Sensitivity of plain chest radiographs. *Am J Roentgenol* 156: 51, 1991.

Haftel AJ, Lev R, Mahour GH, et al: Abdominal CT scanning in pediatric blunt trauma. *Ann Emerg Med* 17: 684, 1989.

Halsell RD, Vines FS, Shatney CH, et al: The reliability of excretory urography as a screening examination for blunt renal trauma. *Ann Emerg Med* 16: 1236, 1987.

Hauser CJ, Huprich JE, Bosco P, et al: Triple-contrast computed tomography in the evaluation of penetrating posterior abdominal injuries. *Arch Surg* 122: 1112, 1987.

Hofer GA, Cohen AJ: CT signs of duodenal perforation secondary to blunt abdominal trauma. *J Comput Assist Tomogr* 13: 430, 1989.

Jeffrey RB Jr, Federle MP: The collapsed inferior vena cava: CT evidence of hypovolemia. *Am J Roentgenol* 150: 431, 1988.

Jooma R, Bradshaw JR, Coakham HB: Computed tomography in penetrating cranial injury by a wooden foreign body. *Surg Neurol* 21: 236, 1984.

Kadir S: Arteriography of the thoracic aorta, in *Diagnostic Angiography*. Philadelphia, Saunders, 1986, pp. 124–171.

Kane NM, Cronan JJ, Dorfman GS, et al: Pediatric abdominal trauma: Evaluation by computed tomography. *Pediatrics* 82: 11, 1988.

Kane NM, Dorfman GS, Cronan JJ: Efficacy of CT following peritoneal lavage in abdominal trauma. *J Comput Assist Tomogr* 11: 998, 1987.

Katayama H, Yamaguchi K, Kozuka T, et al: Adverse reactions to ionic and nonionic contrast media. *Radiology* 175: 621, 1990.

Kearney PA Jr, Vahey T, Burney RE, et al: Computed tomography and diagnostic peritoneal lavage in blunt abdominal trauma: Their combined role. *Arch Surg* 124: 344, 1989.

Kelly J, Raptopoulos V, Davidoff A, et al: On the value of non-contrast-enhanced CT in blunt abdominal trauma. *Am J Roentgenol* 152: 41, 1989.

Lee JKT, Sagel SS, Stanley RJ (eds.): *Computed Body Tomography with MRI Correlation,* 2d ed. New York, Raven, 1989.

Lowe RJ, Saletta JD, Read DR, et al: Should laparotomy be mandatory or selective in gunshot wounds of the abdomen? *J Trauma* 17: 903, 1977.

Mee SL, McAninch JW, Federle MP: Computerized tomography in bladder rupture: Diagnostic limitations. *J Urol* 137: 207, 1987.

Meyer DM, Thal ER, Weigelt JA, et al: Evaluation of computed tomography and diagnostic peritoneal lavage in blunt abdominal trauma. *J Trauma* 29: 1168, 1989.

Meyer DM, Thal ER, Weigelt JA, et al: The role of abdominal CT in the evaluation of stab wounds to the back. *J Trauma* 29: 1226, 1989.

Miller FB, Richardson JD, Thomas HA, et al: Role of CT in diagnosis of major arterial injury after blunt thoracic trauma. *Surgery* 106: 596, 1989.

Mirvis SE, Kostrubiak I, Whitley NO, et al: Role of CT in excluding major arterial injury after blunt thoracic trauma. *Am J Roentgenol* 149: 601, 1987.

Mirvis SE, Whitley NO, Gens DR: Blunt splenic trauma in adults: CT-based classification and correlation with prognosis and treatment. *Radiology* 171: 33, 1989.

Mirvis SE, Whitley NO, Vainwright JR, et al: Blunt hepatic trauma in adults: CT-based classification and correlation with prognosis and treatment. *Radiology* 171: 27, 1989.

Moore EE, More JB, VanDuzer-Moore S, et al: Mandatory laparotomy for gunshot wounds penetrating the abdomen. *Am J Surg* 140: 847, 1980.

Orwig D, Federle MP: Localized clotted blood as evidence of visceral trauma on CT: The sentinel clot sign. *Am J Roentgenol* 153: 747, 1989.

Palmer FJ: The RACR survey of intravenous contrast media reactions: Final report. *Australas Radiol* 32: 426, 1988.

Parmley LF, Mattingly TW, Manion WC, et al: Non-penetrating traumatic injury of the aorta. *Circulation* 17: 1086, 1958.

Rehm CG, Sherman R, Hinz TW: The role of CT scan in evaluation for laparotomy in patients with stab wounds of the abdomen. *J Trauma* 29: 446, 1989.

Rengachary SS, Szymanski DC: Subdural hematomas of arterial origin. *Neurosurgery* 8: 166, 1981.

Rizzo MJ, Federle MP, Griffiths BG: Bowel and mesenteric injury following blunt abdominal trauma: Evaluation with CT. *Radiology* 173: 143, 1989.

Richardson P, Mirvis SE, Scorpio R, et al: Value of CT in determining the need for angiography when findings of mediastinal hemorrhage on chest radiographs are equivocal. *Am J Roentgenol* 156: 273, 1991.

Sherck JP, Oakes DD: Intestinal injuries missed by computed tomography. *J Trauma* 30: 1, 1990.

Siemens Medical Systems, Inc.: *Somatom DR: Influence of Operating Parameters, Medical Considerations and Physical Factors on Image Quality*. Erlangen, Germany, Siemens Medical Systems, Inc., 1985.

Sivit CJ, Taylor GA, Bulas DJ, et al: Blunt trauma in children: Significance of peritoneal fluid. *Radiology* 178: 185, 1991.

Sorkey AJ, Farnell MB, Williams HJ Jr, et al: The complementary roles of diagnostic peritoneal lavage and computed tomography in the evaluation of blunt abdominal trauma. *Surgery* 106: 794, 1989.

Taylor GA, Fallat ME, Eichelberger MR: Hypovolemic shock in children: Abdominal CT manifestations. *Radiology* 164: 479, 1987.

Taylor GA, Fallat ME, Potter BM, et al: The role of computed tomography in blunt abdominal trauma in children. *J Trauma* 28: 1660, 1988.

Tocino I, Miller MH: Computed tomography in blunt chest trauma. *J Thorac Imag* 2: 45, 1987.

Tsai FY, Teal JS, Hieshima GB: Computed tomography in head trauma, in *Neuroradiology of Head Trauma*. Baltimore, University Park Press, 1984, pp.99–200.

Umlas S-L, Cronan JJ: Splenic trauma: Can CT grading system enable prediction of successful nonsurgical treatment? *Radiology* 178: 481, 1991.

Wagner RB, Crawford WO Jr, Schimpf PP: Classification of parenchymal injuries of the lung. *Radiology* 167: 77, 1988.

Wagner RB, Crawford WO Jr, Schimpf PP, et al: Quantitation and pattern of parenchymal lung injury in blunt chest trauma: Diagnostic and therapeutic implications. *J Comput Assist Tomogr* 12: 270, 1988.

Wagner RB, Jamieson PM: Pulmonary contusion: Evaluation and classification by computed tomography. *Surg Clin North Am* 69: 31, 1989.

Williams AL: Trauma, in Williams AL, Haughton VM (eds.): *Cranial Computed Tomography: A Comprehensive Text*. St. Louis, 1985, pp. 37–87.

ACKNOWLEDGMENTS

I gratefully acknowledge the assistance of Toni Williams and Laura Walsh for aid in literature retrieval, E. Russell Ritenour, Ph.D., for a careful reading of the section on CT technical aspects, and Kim Vojacek of the Minnesota Medical Research Foundation art department for assistance with photographs.

INDEX

Note: With page numbers, "t" indicates a table, "f" a figure.

A,B,C_3, 150
altered mental status and, 151
A/C ventilation (*see* Assist-control ventilation)
Abdomen, muscles of, distinguishing true neurologic deficits from conversion disorder and, 1091t
Abdominal distension, in neonate, 427
Abdominal emergencies, in children, 491–496
diagnosis and management of, 493–496, 494–496f
evaluation of, 491
examination in, 491
in first year of life, 493–495, 494f, 495f
key symptoms in, 491–493, 492t, 493t
2 years of age and older, 495–496, 496f
Abdominal examination:
in altered mental status, 152
in ectopic pregnancy, 390
Abdominal pain, 144–147
analgesia in, 147
in children, 491
in colonic diverticular disease, 333
in Crohn's disease, 328
in females, nongynecologic causes of, 389
history in, 145, 146f
imaging studies in, 146–147
in intestinal obstruction, 323
in irritable bowel syndrome, 333
laboratory evaluation in, 146
laparoscopy in, 147
origins of, 144–145
extraabdominal, 145
intraabdominal, 144–145
metabolic, 145
neurogenic, 145
in perforated viscus, 317
physical examination in, 145–146
referred, 144
somatic (parietal), 144
visceral (splanchnic), 144
Abdominal trauma, 955–961
child abuse and, 500
complications of, 960–961
computed tomography in, 9–10
bladder and diaphragm injuries and, 10
diagnostic peritoneal lavage versus, 9
laparotomy and, 10
nonoperative management and occult injuries and, 9–10
retroperitoneal and flank trauma and, 10
emergency department evaluation of, 955–956
hollow organ injury and, 957–959, 958f
iatrogenic, 960–961
management of, 957, 957t
pathophysiology of, 955
blunt trauma and, 955
penetrating trauma and, 955
to posterior abdomen, 962–963
computed tomography in, 962
diagnostic peritoneal lavage in, 962
evaluation of, 962
exploration of, 962
local wound exploration in, 962
management of, 962–963
during pregnancy (*see* Pregnancy, abdominal trauma during)
solid organ injury and, 959–960, 960f
vascular structures and, 960
Abdominal wall, injury to, 960
ABGs (*see* Arterial blood gases)
ABI (*see* Ankle brachial index)
Abortion, 411
complete, 412
incomplete, 412
induced, complications of, 423–424
inevitable, 412
infected, 391
spontaneous, 391
threatened, 412
Abruptio placentae, 412, 415
pelvic ultrasonography in, 1117
Abrus precatorius, 722, 724
Abscess(es):
in Crohn's disease, 329
intraabdominal, postoperative, 369
in narcotic overdose, 566–567
(*See also specific sites*)
Absence (petit mal) seizures, 804
Absence (petit mal) status, 485
ABU (*see* Asymptomatic bacteriuria)
Abulic state (akinetic mutism; "coma vigil"), 150
Abuse:
of children (*see* Child abuse)
of elders, 1098t, 1098–1099
ABV (*see* Alternobaic vertigo)
Accelerated idioventricular rhythm (AIVR), 95–96, 96f
in acute myocardial infarction, 205
clinical significance of, 96
treatment of, 96
Acceleration flexion-extension neck injury (whiplash injury), 893–894
Acceptance, nonjudgmental, in crisis intervention, 1095
Accessory conduction pathways, verapamil and, 621
Accidents:
diving (*see* Dysbarism, diving casualties and)
drowning (*see* Near drowning)
(*See also specific types of accidents*)
Accommodation, spasm of, 838
Acebutolol (Sectral):
actions of, 111
in angina, 201t
dosage, actions, pharmacokinetics, and indications for, 112t
pharmacology and properties of, 622
Acetabulum, type IV fractures of, 983–984, 984f, 985f
Acetaminophen(s) (APAP; paracetamol), 593–597
in acute mountain sickness, 673
pharmacology of, 593
toxic hepatitis and, 360
Acetaminophen poisoning:
antidotal treatment of, 549t, 596–597
rationale for, 594–596, 595f
clinical toxicity and, 594, 594t
general evaluation and management in, 596
mechanism of toxicity and, 593f, 593–594
prognostic factors for, 594–596, 595f
Acetaminophen with codeine (Tylenol no. 3), in rib fractures, 935
Acetazolamide (Diamox):
in acute angle closure glaucoma, 836
in acute mountain sickness, 673, 673f
in chronic mountain polycythemia, 676
in metabolic alkalosis, 48
ophthalmic, 838
in seizures, in children, 480t
Acetic acid burns, 697
Acetic acid derivatives, overdose of, 628
Acetophenazine (Tindal), 1080t
N-Acetylcysteine (Mucomyst; NAC), in acetaminophen poisoning, 595–597
N-Acetylcysteine (Mucomyst; NAC):
in acetaminophen poisoning, 596
in mushroom poisoning, 719
Achilles tendon rupture, 1005, 1009–1010
Acid(s):
aspiration of, aspiration pneumonia and, 276
burns and, 695–699, 696t
ocular, 699–700, 834
gastric, loss of, metabolic alkalosis and, 47
ingestion of (*see* Caustic ingestions)
inorganic, reduced excretions of, anion gap changes due to, 40
nonvolatile
excretion of, 36
weak, 37

Acid(s) (*Cont.*):
organic, anion gap changes and, 40
volatile (*see* Carbon dioxide)
weak, anion gap changes due to, 40
Acid-base problems, 35–49
alcoholic ketoacidosis and, 740, 741t
anion gap and, 40–42
alkalemia and, 41
analytical errors and, 41–42
changes in, due to artifacts, 40
decreased, 41, 41t
decreased unmeasured anions and, 41
decreased unmeasured cations and, 41
definition of, 39
exogenous anions and, 40
hyperglycemic coma and, 40
increased, 40–41
increased organic acids and, 40
increased unmeasured cations and, 41
increased unmeasured weak acids and, 41
ketoacidosis and, 40
lactic acidosis and, 40, 40t
ratio of change in anion gap to change in plasma bicarbonate and, 42
reduced inorganic acid excretions and, 40
toxic ingestions and, 40
unmeasured cations and anions and, 39, 39t
urinary, 42, 42t
buffers and, 36–37
base excess and, 37
buffer base and, 37
carbon dioxide and
carbon dioxide content and, 38
production, transport, and excretion of, 36
compensatory changes and, 38–39
failure of compensatory mechanisms and, 39
metabolic acidosis and, 38, 43
metabolic alkalosis and, 39
metabolic compensations and, 38t, 39
deficit and, 162
Henderson-Hasselbach equation and, 35
hydrogen ion concentrations and, 35, 35t
in hypothermia, 649
laboratory report consistency and accuracy in, 38
correlation of carbon dioxide content and bicarbonate and, 37
correlation of chloride and bicarbonate levels and, 38
correlation of pH and electrolyte values and, 38
effect of P_{CO_2} and HCO_3^- on pH and, 38
mixed disorders and, 38
nonvolatile acids and
excretion of, 36
weak, 37
pH and, 35
intracellular, 35–36
single disorders and, 38, 38t
terminology for, 35–36
venous studies and, 43
(*See also* Acidosis, metabolic; Acidosis, respiratory; Alkalosis, metabolic; Alkalosis, respiratory)
Acid-fast stain, in meningitis, 828
Acid phosphatase, in female rape victims, 401
Acidosis:
anion gap, 748
in methanol poisoning, 572, 572t, 573t
cerebrospinal fluid, in diabetic ketoacidosis, 737
in children, treatment of, 163
in methanol poisoning, treatment of, 573
renal tubular, in hydrocarbon poisoning, 603
(*See also* Ketoacidosis)
Acidosis, metabolic, 38, 43–46
in carbon monoxide poisoning, treatment of, 706
deficit of, 162
diagnosis of, 44–46
increased anion gap acidosis and, 44–46
normal anion gap (hyperchloremic) acidosis and, 46
in ethylene glycol poisoning, 574
treatment of, 574
etiology of, 43
increased anion gap acidosis and, 43, 43t
normal anion gap (hyperchloremic) acidosis and, 43, 43t
in nonketotic hyperosmolar coma, 745
pathophysiology of, 43–44
in status asthmaticus, in children, 471
treatment of, 46, 218
Acidosis, respiratory, 49
in asthma, 467
diagnosis of, 49
etiology of, 49
pathophysiology of, 49
in status asthmaticus, in children, 471
treatment of, 49–50
ACLS (*see* Advanced cardiac life support; Cardiopulmonary resuscitation)
Acquired immune deficiency syndrome (AIDS):
anorectal infections related to, 342, 342t
cocaine use and, 580
oral manifestations of, 862
Pneumocystis carinii pneumonia and, 272
spontaneous pneumothorax and, 285–286
transplacental infection with, 410
tuberculosis and, 279, 282, 283t
(*See also* Human immunodeficiency virus infection
Acromioclavicular joint sprain, 981, 981f
Actaea rubra, 722, 724
ACTH (*see* Adrenocorticotropic hormone)
Activase (*see* Tissue plasminogen activator)
Activated charcoal, in poisoning, 548
(*See also* Gastrointestinal decontamination)
Activation phase, of disaster response, 193
"Acute coarctation syndrome," 950
Acute disseminated encephalomyelitis (ADE; postinfectious encephalomyelitis), 817, 821
Acute mountain sickness (AMS), 671–673
clinical presentation of, 672
incidence of, 671
pathophysiology of, 672, 672f
prevention of, 673
susceptibility to, 672
treatment of, 672–673, 673f
Acute myocardial infarction (AMI), 201–214
angiography in, preparation for, 213–214
aspirin in, 209
β-blockers in, 210–211
calcium channel blockers in, 210
cardiac enzymes in, 202t, 203
chest pain and, 127, 128, 130
clinical features of, 202
cocaine use and, 579
complications of, 203–207
arrhythmias as, 203–205, 205t
cardiogenic shock as, 206
conduction disturbances as, 205, 205t
left ventricular pump failure as, 206, 206t
mechanical defects as, 206–207
pericarditis as, 207
right ventricular infarction as, 207
thromboembolism as, 207
echocardiography in, 203
in elderly patients
thrombolytic therapy in, 258
treatment of, 258
electrocardiography in, 128–129, 129t, 202, 202t, 204f
heparin in, 209–210
non-Q-wave versus Q-wave, 202
pathogenesis of, 201
pathophysiology of, 201
premature ventricular contractions and, 95
treatment of, 95
radionuclide scans in, 203
reperfusion in, 211
in rheumatic disorders, 884
symptoms other than chest pain in, 128
temporary pacing in, indications for, 211
thrombolytic therapy in, 211–214
anisoylated plasminogen streptokinase activator complex in, 213, 213t
comparison of agents for, 213, 213t
in elderly patients, 258
patient selection for, 211–212
streptokinase in, 212, 213t
tissue plasminogen activator in, 212–213, 213t
urokinase in, 213, 213t
transmural versus nontransmural (subendocardial), 202
treatment of, 112t, 115t, 207–208
triage and prehospital treatment of, 209
Acute necrotizing hemorrhagic encephalomyelitis (ANHE), 817, 821
Acute necrotizing ulcerative gingivitis (ANUG), 861
Acute tubular necrosis (ATN), 372
"Acute urethral syndrome," 377
Acyclovir:
in genital herpes, 396
in herpes progenitalis, 518
in human immunodeficiency virus infections, 521, 521t
Adalat (*see* Nifedipine)
"Adam" ("Ecstasy"; MDMA; 3,4-methylenedioxymethamphetamine), 583, 586
1-Adamantanamine hydrochloride (Amantadine), in pneumonia, viral, 268
Addiction, to benzodiazepines, 625
Addison's disease (*see* Adrenal insufficiency, primary)
ADE (*see* Acute disseminated encephalomyelitis)
Adenocard (*see* Adenosine)
Adenoidectomy, bleeding following, 842
Adenoma(s):
endocrine, multiple, hypercalcemia and, 77
villous, anorectal, 343
Adenosine (Adenocard), 120–121
actions of, 120–121
adverse effects of, 121
dosing and administration of, 121
indications for, 121
in paroxysmal supraventricular tachycardia, 205
pharmacokinetics of, 121
in reentrant supraventricular tachycardia, 93
in Wolff-Parkinson-White syndrome, 105
Adenosine monophosphate (AMP), cyclic, in asthma, 469–470

Adenosine triphosphate (ATP), cerebral ischemia and, 8
Adenylate, cerebral ischemia and, 8
ADH (*see* Antidiuretic hormone)
Adhesions, small bowel obstruction and, 322
Adolescent:
  intoxicated, 576
  vulvovaginitis in, 464-465
Adrenal apoplexy, 760
Adrenal crisis, 759, 760, 762
  clinical presentation of, 762
  treatment of, 762
Adrenal glands, pathophysiology of, 759
Adrenal insufficiency:
  in corticosteroid-treated patients with rheumatic diseases, 885
  diagnosis of, 761
  hypercalcemia and, 78
  in malignancy, 782
  primary (Addison's disease), 759-760
    bilateral adrenal hemorrhage and, 760
    clinical presentation of, 760
    idiopathic, 759, 759t
    infiltrative or infectious, 759-760
    laboratory studies in, 760
  secondary, 760-761, 761t
    clinical presentation of, 761
    treatment of, 762
  treatment of, 761t, 761-762
Adrenaline, 580
  for pediatric analgesia, 512
Adrenergic agents:
  complications of, treatment of, 243
  in hypertensive emergencies, 244
Adrenergic blocking agents, in hypertensive emergencies, 243-244
Adrenocorticotropic hormone (ACTH):
  adrenal insufficiency and, 759
  stimulation and, in secondary adrenal insufficiency, 761
Adult respiratory distress syndrome (ARDS), 287-288
  diagnosis of, 288
  management of, 288-289
  massive blood transfusion and, 777
  pathophysiology of, 287-288, 288f
Advance directives, resuscitation and, 4-5
Advanced cardiac life support (ACLS), 176
  (*See also* Cardiopulmonary resuscitation)
Advanced life support (ALS), 191
  ambulances and, 189
Advice, in crisis intervention, 1095
Advocacy, in crisis intervention, 1095
AEDs (*see* Automatic external defibrillators)
A, E, I, O, and U, in altered mental status, 155, 155t
Aerogastralgia (gas in the gut), 681
Aeromedical transport, 192
Aerophagia, in pediatric trauma victim, 911
Affective disorder, affective, 1068
Affective (mood) disorders, 1070-1071
Afterload, 205, 206
  treatment of, 218
Age:
  gestational, determination of, 418
  oxygenation and ventilation and, 56
  postconceptional, 431
  (*See also* specific age groups)
β_2-Agonists, in asthma, in children, 470, 472, 473
AIDS (*see* Acquired immune deficiency syndrome)
AIDS dementia complex (HIV encephalopathy; subacute encephalitis), 521
AIDS-related complex (ARC), 519
Air:
  alveolar, rate of renewal by atmospheric air, 53
  expired, 54
  inspired, 53, 53t
    humidification of, 53
  (*see also* Blood gases, alveolar gases and)
Air bubbles, arterial blood gases and, 141
Air embolism:
  dysbaric, 681
    treatment of, 684, 684f
  in penetrating injury to heart, 942
  systemic, lung injuries and, 936-937
Air embolization, in blast injury, treatment of, 687
Air leaks, pulmonary, in neonate, 173-174
Air-puff tonometer, 833
Airway:
  advanced airway support and, 10-19
    bag-valve-mask unit and, 10, 10t
    cricothyrotomy and, 15-16, 16f
    esophageal obturator airways and, 10-11, 11f
    extubation and, 19
    fiberoptic laryngoscopy and, 14-15, 15f
    high-frequency ventilation and, 19
    mechanical ventilatory support and, 19
    nasotracheal intubation and, 12-14, 13f
    neuromuscular blockade and, 16-18, 17t
    oral and nasal airways and, 10
    orotracheal intubation and, 11-12
    rapid sequence induction and, 18t, 18-19
    retrograde tracheal intubation and, 15
    suctioning and, 19
    translaryngeal ventilation and, 14, 14f
  assessment of
    in poisoning, 545
    in trauma patient, 907
  establishment of, in organophosphate/carbamate poisoning, 612
  management of
    in barbiturate overdose, 562
    in epiglottitis, in children, 184
    in thoracic trauma, to chest wall, bronchi, lung, and diaphragm, 932-933
  in neck trauma, 928-929
  opening, 2
  protection of, in poisoning, 548
Airway obstruction:
  chronic
    compensated, 298-299
    decompensated, 299-307
  consequences of, asthma and, 291t, 291-292
  in malignancy, 780
  sudden infant death syndrome and, 434
  upper airway and, 842-845
    differential diagnosis of, 843f, 843-845
    management of, 845
    signs and symptoms of, 842-843
AIVR (*see* Accelerated idioventricular rhythm)
Akathisia:
  antipsychotics and, 1081
  neuroleptics and, 555, 556t
Akinetic mutism (abulic state; "coma vigil"), 150
Albendazole, in parasitic infections, 537t
Albumin, 776
Albuterol:
  in allergic reactions, 902
  in asthma, in children, 470, 473
  in bronchiolitis, in children, 474
  in chronic decompensated airflow obstruction, 301
  in status asthmaticus, in children, 472
Alcohol (*see* Alcohol abuse/alcoholism; Ethanol; Ethylene glycol; Isopropanol; Methanol)
Alcohol abuse/alcoholism:
  acetaminophen hepatotoxicity in, 594
  liver disease and (*see* Liver disease, alcoholic)
  myopathy and, 813
  pancreatitis and, 363
  in pregnancy, 410
  psychiatric disorders and, 1075
  suicide attempts and, 1077
  (*See also* Ethanol poisoning)
Alcoholic (Laennaec's) cirrhosis, 361
Alcoholic ketoacidosis, 740-741
  clinical presentation of, 740
  diagnosis of, 740-741
  differential diagnosis of, 741
  laboratory studies in, 740, 741t
  pathogenesis of, 740
  treatment of, 741
Aldosterone, adrenal insufficiency and, 759
Alkalemia, 41
Alkali:
  burns and, 695, 698, 699
    conjunctivitis and, 834
    ocular, 699, 708, 834
  ingestion of (*see* Caustic ingestions)
Alkaline phosphatase, in pregnancy, 414
Alkalosis, metabolic, 39, 47-48
  deficit of, 162
  diagnosis of, 48
    saline-resistant alkalosis and, 48
    saline-responsive alkalosis and, 48
  physiologic effects of, 47-48
  treatment of, 48
    chloride-resistant alkalosis and, 48
    chloride-responsive alkalosis and, 48
Alkalosis, respiratory, 48
  diagnosis of, 48
  etiology of, 48
  physiological effects of, 48
  septic shock and, 138
  treatment of, 48-49
Alkyl mercury compound burns, 699
Allen's test, 25
Allergic neuropathy, 814
Allergic reactions, 901
  anaphylactoid, 902
  anaphylaxis and, 901t, 901-902
  angioedema and, 902
  clinical immunology and, 901
  conjunctivitis and, 834
  to drugs, 903
  to foods, 902-903
  to insect stings, 903
  to milk, in neonate, 427
  to transfusions, 778
  treatment of, 902
  urticaria and, 902
Aloe barbadensis, 722, 724
Alprazolam (Xanax), 1082, 1082t
  in panic disorder, 1089
ALS (*see* Advanced life support)
ALTE (*see* Apparent life threatening event)
Altered mental status, 150-158
  assessment of, guidelines for, 157-158, 158f
  in beta blocker overdose, 622
  chronic changes and, 1100
  confusional states and, 150
  definition of, 150
  history taking in, 152

Altered mental status (*Cont.*):
infratentorial compressive syndromes causing, 157
laboratory studies in, 155, 158
management of, initial, 151
pathophysiology of, 150–151
bilateral cortical disease and, 151
reticular activating system lesions and, 151
patients who appear asleep and, 150
patients who appear awake but are unresponsive and, 150
physical examination in, 152–155
abdominal examination and, 152
breath in, 152
cardiac examination and, 152
cranial nerves in, 153, 154
mental status in, 153
motor testing in, 154
neurological examination and, 152, 152t
ocular movements in, 153–154, 154t
pupils in, 153
reflex status in, 154–155, 155t
respiratory pattern in, 153
sensory examination and, 154
skin in, 152
vital signs in, 152
radiographic studies in, 155, 158
supratentorial focal lesions causing, 156–157
toxic and metabolic disorders causing, 155–156
treatment of
algorithm for, 158, 158f
initial, 151–152
(*See also* Coma; Consciousness)
Alternobaic vertigo (ABV), 681
Altitude, oxygenation and ventilation and, 55–56, 56t
Altitude physiology, 190
Alveolar-capillary (respiratory) membrane, 52
gas diffusion through, 52
Alveolar fractures, 864
mandibular, 850, 851f
Alveolar gas equation, 53
Alveolar mucosa, 860
Alveolar osteitis ("dry socket"), 861
Alveolar ventilation, 51
arterial Pa_{CO_2} and, 54
arterial Pa_{O_2} and, 55
Amantadine (1-adamantanamine hydrochloride), in pneumonia, viral, 268
Amatoxin poisoning:
clinical toxicity and, 717, 717t
pharmacology of, 716, 717t
treatment of, 719–720
Amaurosis fugax, 837
Ambulance, 189–190
transport of maternal patients and, emergency delivery and, 418, 419t
Amebas, 538
American Anorexic/Bulimic Association, Inc., 1087
Aminoglycosides, during pregnancy, 407
Aminophylline (theophylline ethylenediamine):
in allergic reactions, 902
in asthma, in children, 471, 472
in bronchospasm, in Hymenoptera stings, 656
in chronic decompensated airflow obstruction, 300
in lithium overdose, 1084
in pulmonary edema, 218
in status asthmaticus, in children, 471, 472
4-Aminopyridine, in calcium channel blocker overdose, 621
Amiodarone (Cordarone), electrophysiologic actions of, 110t
Amnesia:
psychogenic, 1072
transient global, 796
Amnestic syndrome, 1067
Amniotic fluid, meconium staining of, neonatal resuscitation and, 171
Amobarbital, pharmacology of, 561t
Amoxicillin:
in bacteremia, in children, 454
in Lyme disease, 540
in otitis media, 440, 441
in sinusitis, in children, 449, 449t
in urinary tract infections, 379t
in children, 463
Amoxicillin/clavulanate, in cutaneous abscess, 878t
Amphetamine(s), 582–583
designer, 583, 586
pharmacology of, 582
withdrawal from, 582
Amphetamine toxicity, 582–583
management of, 582
Amphotericin, in pneumonia, in neonate, 428t
Amphotericin B:
in human immunodeficiency virus infections, 521, 521t
in parasitic infections, 537t
Ampicillin:
in acute gastroenteritis, in children, 490
in bacterial pneumonia, 264t
in colonic diverticular disease, 334
in diarrhea, 351t
in epiglottitis, 844
in human immunodeficiency virus infections, 521t
in meningitis, in children, 456
in otitis media, 440
in periorbital/orbital cellulitis, in children, 452t
in pneumonia, in neonate, 428t
in sepsis, in children, 454
in septic shock, 139t
Amputation:
in deep venous thrombosis, massive, 255
of digital tip, 1062–1063
exposed bone and, 1062–1063
skin or pulp loss only and, 1062
Amrinone (Inocor), 124–125
actions of, 124
adverse effects of, 125
in cardiogenic shock, 136
in congestive heart failure, 217
in depressed cardiac output, 206
dosing and administration of, 124–125
indications for, 124
pharmacokinetics of, 124
AMS (*see* Acute mountain sickness)
Amyl nitrite, in cyanide poisoning, 634, 709
Amylase levels, in Reye's syndrome, 476
Amyotrophic lateral sclerosis (Lou Gehrig's disease), 1101
Ana-Kit, in Hymenoptera stings, 657
ANAD (*see* National Association of Anorexia Nervosa Associated Disorders)
Anal crypts, 339
clinical features of, 339
treatment of, 339
Anal fissure (*see* Fissure in ano)
Anal warts (condylomata acuminata), proctitis and, 342
Analgesia:
in abdominal pain, 147
in children, 511–514
for brief, painful procedures, 512–514
infiltrative, 511–512
local, 511–512
for longer, painful procedures, 514
regional nerve blocks and, 512
systemic, 512t, 512–514, 513t
topical, 512
during pregnancy, 407
Analytical errors, anion gap changes due to, 41
Anaphylactoid reactions, 902
Anaphylaxis, 901t, 901–902
Anatomic dead space, 51
Androgen(s):
in adrenal insufficiency, 761–762
adrenal insufficiency and, 759
Anectine (*see* Succinylcholine)
Anemia:
aplastic, in nonsteroidal anti-inflammatory drug overdose, 627–628
dilutional, in pregnancy, 414
hemolytic, in nonsteroidal anti-inflammatory drug overdose, 627–628
normochromic normocytic, in malaria, 531
sickle cell (*see* Sickle cell anemia)
Anemone envenomations, 667–668
Anesthesia:
for closed reduction of fractures, 969
for incision and drainage of cutaneous abscess, 877
maternal, seizures and, 172
in multiple sclerosis, 820–821
ophthalmic, 838
for wound repair (*see* Wound repair, anesthesia for)
Aneurysm(s):
aortic
dissecting (*see* Aortic dissection)
(*See also* Aortic aneurysms)
mycotic, in narcotic overdose, 567
popliteal, symptomatic, 254
Angina pectoris, 200–201
chest pain and, 127, 128, 130
chronic stable, treatment of, 119, 120
treatment of, 112t, 120, 125, 200t, 200–201, 201t
unstable (crescendo or preinfarction), chest pain and, 130
unstable (crescendo; preinfarction), 200
chest pain and, 127
in elderly patients, 258
unstable (crescendo: preinfarction) treatment of, 119
variant (Prinzmetal's), 200
chest pain and, 127, 130
vasospastic, treatment of, 119
Angiodysplasia, gastrointestinal bleeding and, 149
Angioedema, 902
Angiography:
in cerebral vascular accident, 795
digital subtraction, intraarterial, in blunt trauma to great vessels, 952
gastrointestinal, in gastrointestinal bleeding, 148
in myocardial contusion, 945
preparation for, 213–214
pulmonary, in pulmonary embolism, 235
Angioneurotic edema, upper airway obstruction and, 844
Angioplasty, in acute myocardial infarction, in elderly patients, 258
Angle fractures, mandibular, 851

ANHE (*see* Acute necrotizing hemorrhagic encephalomyelitis)
Animal bites, 1043–1044 (*see* Marine animals, trauma and envenomations from; Rabies)
Anion(s), nonresorbable, excretion of, metabolic alkalosis and, 47
Anion gap (*see* Acid-base problems, anion gap and)
Anion gap acidosis, 748
Anisoylated plasminogen streptokinase activator complex (Anistreplase; APSAC; Eminase), in acute myocardial infarction, 213, 213t
Ankle brachial index (ABI), in peripheral vascular disease, 1113
Ankle injuries, 1007–1011
  Achilles tendon rupture and, 1009–1010
  anatomy and, 1007, 1008f
  in children, 1011
  clinical examination in, 1007
  complications of, 1011
  contusions and, 1011
  fractures and, 1010–1011
    abduction, 1010
    adduction, 1010
    classification of, 1010f, 1010–1011
    external rotation fractures and, 1010
    treatment of, 1011
    vertical compression, 1010
  history of, 1007
  ligamentous (sprains), 1008–1009
    anterior talofibular ligament and, 1008
    classification of, 1009
    medial collateral ligament and, 1008
    radiographic studies in, 1009
    tibiofibular syndesmotic ligament and, 1009
    treatment of, 1009
  radiographic studies in, 1007–1008
  tenosynovitis and, 1011
  treatment of, 1011
Annulus fibrosis (atrioventricular ring), 86
Anorectal abscesses, 340
  clinical features of, 340
  treatment of, 340
Anorectal disorders, 336–346
  examination in, 336, 338f
  (*See also* specific disorders)
Anorectal surgery, complications of, 369
Anorectal tumors, 343t, 343–344
  clinical features of, 343
  treatment of, 343–344
Anorectum, anatomy of, 336, 337f
Anorexia, in appendicitis, 320
Anorexia nervosa, 1085t, 1085–1087
  differential diagnosis of, 1085
  etiology of, 1085
  pathophysiology of, 1085–1086, 1086t
  psychological presentation of, 1086
  prognosis of, 1086–1087
  treatment of, 1087
Anorexia Nervosa and Related Eating Disorders, Inc., 1087
Anoscopy, in anorectal disorders, 336, 338f
Ant stings (*see* Insect and spider bites/stings, Hymenoptera stings and)
Antabuse (disulfiram), 576
Antacids:
  metabolic alkalosis and, 47
  in peptic ulcer disease, 313
Anterior approach, to internal jugular vein, 24
Anterior cruciate ligament injury, 1001
Anterior drawer sign, in knee injury, 1001
Anterior drawer test, in anterior talofibular ligament injuries, 1008
Anterior spinal cord syndrome, 926
Anterior supply, 793
Anterior talofibular ligament injuries, 1008
Antiarrhythmic agents, 109–122
  class I, 110–111
    in restrictive cardiomyopathy, 229
  class IB, 110–111
  class II, 111–118
    actions of, 111, 112t
    adverse effects of, 117
    dosing and administration of, 117
    indications for, 111
    pharmacokinetics of, 111, 113–116t
  class III, 118
  class IV, 118–120
  electrophysiologic effects of, 109, 110t
  in premature ventricular contractions, 95
  (*See also specific agents*)
Antiarrhythmics, in theophylline poisoning, 615
Antibiotic therapy:
  during pregnancy, 406–407
  in aortic regurgitation, 224
  in appendicitis, 321
  in asthma, 297
  in caustic ingestions, 608
  in colonic diverticular disease, 334
  in hernia, 327
  in intestinal obstruction, 324
  in perforated viscus, 318
  in Pneumocystis carinii pneumonia, 273–274
  in septic shock, 138, 139t
  in tetanus, 525–526, 526t
  in ulcerative colitis, 330, 331
  in veneral proctitis, 342
  in wound management, 1040–1041
    prophylaxis and, 1040–1041, 1041t
  ophthalmic, 838
  prophylactic, in hypertrophic cardiomyopathy, 228
Anticholinergic(s), 636t, 636–637
  in asthma, 296–297
    in children, 470
  pharmacologic properties of, 636
Anticholinergic effects:
  antipsychotics and, 1081
  heterocyclic antidepressants and, 1082
Anticholinergic poisoning, 586, 636–637
  clinical presentation of, 636–637
  treatment of, 637
Anticholinesterase inhibitors, in myasthenia gravis, 823–824
Anticholinesterase tests, in myasthenia gravis, 823
Anticoagulants:
  in acute myocardial infarction, 207
  in deep venous thrombosis, 367
  in mitral stenosis, 221
  during pregnancy, 407
  pulmonary, 235
Anticonvulsant therapy, during pregnancy, 407
Anticonvulsants:
  adverse effects of, 486
  complications of, 1101
  drug interactions of, 486
  drug levels and, 807
  during pregnancy, 407
Antidepressants:
  cyclic (*see* Cyclic antidepressants)
  second-generation, 1083
Antidiuretic hormone (ADH):
  diabetes insipidus and, 69
  hyponatremia and, 67–68
  in nonketotic hyperosmolar coma, 743
  syndrome of inappropriate secretion of ADH and, 66t, 66–67
Antidotes:
  in poisoning, 547, 549t
  (*See also specific types of poisoning*)
Antiepileptics, in theophylline poisoning, 615
Antihypertensive therapy (*See also* Drug therapy, in hypertensive emergencies)
  in pregnancy, 408–409, 409t
  withdrawal from, 245
Antinauseants, during pregnancy, 407
Antiparkinson drugs, 1081
  complications of, 1101
Antiplatelet agents, in acute myocardial infarction, 207
Antipsychotics (neuroleptics), 1069, 1080–1081
  complications of, 1101
  guidelines for, 1080, 1080t
  indications for, 1080
  overdose of, 1081
  side effects of, 1080–1081
Antipyretics, in fever, 159, 160
Antisocial personality disorders, 1072–1073
Antispasticity agents, complications of, 1101
Antivenin:
  for snake bites, 662–663
    administration and dose of, 663
    coral snakes and, 664
    horse serum sensitivity and, 663
  for stonefish envenomations, 669
Antivenin Index, 664
ANUG (*see* Acute necrotizing ulcerative gingivitis)
Anxiety, vertigo and, 801
Anxiety disorders, 1071
  generalized, 1071
Anxiolytics, 1081–1082
  guidelines for, 1081–1082, 1082t
  indications for, Anxiolytics
  overdose of, 1082
  side effects of, 1082
Aorta:
  ascending, injuries to, 952
  lower thoracic, injuries to, 952
  tears of, blunt, 949
Aortic aneurysms:
  abdominal, abdominal pain and, 144–145
  thoracic, 247–248
    diagnosis of, 248
    etiology of, 248
    management of, 248
    presentation of, 248
    prognosis of, 248
  thoracic, expanding and ruptured, 248–249
    management of, 249
    presentation of, 248
    prognosis of, 249
Aortic dissection:
  acute, 247
    classifications of, 247
    diagnosis of, 247
    etiology of, 247
    management of, 247
    presentation of, 247
  chest pain and, 128, 130, 130t
  thoracic
    hypertension and, 239
    treatment of, 242, 245
  ultrasonography in, 1124, 1124f, 1124t
Aortic injury, computed tomography and, 9
Aortic regurgitation, 223–224
  clinical features of, 223–224

Aortic regurgitation (*Cont.*):
in acute aortic regurgitation, 223
in chronic aortic regurgitation, 223-224
treatment of, 224
Aortic stenosis (AS):
in children, 438
in elderly patients, 260
valvular, 222-223
chest pain and, 131
clinical features of, 222-223
treatment of, 223
Aortic valve, injury to, blunt injury to heart and, 943
Aortography:
in blunt trauma to great vessels, 951-952
in innominate artery injury, 952
in thoracic aortic aneurysms, 248
APAP (*see* Acetaminophen(s); Acetaminophen poisoning)
Apathetic thyrotoxicosis, 753
Apgar Score, 170, 170t
neonatal resuscitation and, 171
Aplastic anemia, in nonsteroidal anti-inflammatory drug overdose, 627-628
Apnea:
central, 434
expiratory, 434
monitoring, 432, 435-436
monitors and, 1110
in neonate, 428, 432, 432t
in pneumonia, in children, 459
sudden infant death syndrome and, 434-436
home monitoring and, 435-436
Apneustic breathing, in altered mental status, 153
Apparent life threatening event (ALTE; "near miss" sudden infant death syndrome), 434
Appendectomy, complications of, 369
Appendicitis, 320-321
in children, 320, 495, 496f
clinical presentation of, 320, 321t
colonic diverticulitis differentiated from, 334
in elderly patients, 320
laboratory studies in, 320-321
radiographic studies and, 321
morbidity and mortality in, 320
in pregnancy, 320, 410
treatment of, 321
ultrasonography in, 1121f, 1121-1122
Appendicoliths, in children, 495, 496f
Apresoline (*see* Hydralazine)
Aprindine, electrophysiologic actions of, 110t
Aprobarbital, pharmacology of, 561t
APSAC (*see* Anisoylated plasminogen streptokinase activator complex)
Arachidonate, cerebral ischemia and, 8
ARC (*see* AIDS-related complex)
ARDS (*see* Adult respiratory distress syndrome)
Arfonad (*see* Trimethaphan camsylate)
Argyria, 141
Arm, compartments at risk for compartment syndromes in, 1007, 1007f, 1008f, 1009
Arrhythmia(s), 86-108, 87-97
in acute myocardial infarction, 201, 203-205, 204t
treatment of, 207
atrial, treatment of, 110
cardiac pacemakers in (*see* Cardiac pacing)
in children, cardiopulmonary resuscitation and, 180, 180t
in chronic renal failure, 374
defibrillation and synchronized cardioversion in, 106
in hydrocarbon poisoning, 603
in hypothermia, treatment of, 650
junctional, 93-94
premature contractions and, 93-94, 94f
normal cardiac conducting system and, 86
normal electrocardiogram and, 86-87, 87f
preexcitation syndromes, 103f, 103-106, 104f
clinical significance of, 104-105, 105f
treatment of, 105-106
preterminal rhythms
electromechanical dissociation, 102, 103f
idioventricular rhythm, 102-103, 103f
supraventricular, 89-93
atrial fibrillation, 91f, 91-92
multifocal atrial tachycardia, 90, 90f
premature atrial contractions, 89-90, 90f
sinus arrhythmia, 89, 89f
sinus bradycardia, 89, 89f
sinus tachycardia, 89, 89f
supraventricular tachycardia, 92f, 92t, 92-93
trial flutter, 90-91, 91f
syncope and, 142, 260
treatment of, 109-112, 113-116t, 117-125, 125t
triggered, 88
ventricular, 94-97
accelerated idioventricular rhythm, 95-96, 96f
in acute myocardial infarction, 204
premature ventricular contractions, 94f, 94-95, 95t
treatment of, 109-111, 117, 118, 122
ventricular fibrillation, 97, 97f
ventricular parasystole, 95, 95f
ventricular tachycardia, 96f, 96t, 96-97
"warning," 95
(*See also* Bradyarrhythmias; Tachyarrhythmias)
Arrhythmias, supraventricular, treatment of, 111, 112, 117
Arsenic poisoning, 640-642
antidote to, 549t
clinical effects of, 641
diagnosis of, 641
differential diagnosis of, 641
management of, 641-642
pharmacology of, 640-641
prognosis and sequelae of, 642
Arsine poisoning, 642
Arterial blood gases (ABGs), 54-59
alveolar-arterial oxygen differences and, 56
arterial Pa_{CO_2} and, 54-55
alveolar ventilation and, 54
carbaminohemoglobin and carbaminoproteins and, 54-55
carbohydrate metabolism and, 54
carbon dioxide dissociation curve and, 55
carbon dioxide transport in blood and, 54
change in blood acidity during carbon dioxide transport and, 55
dead space and, 54
Haldane effect and, 55
respiratory quotient changes and, 55
arterial Pa_{O_2} and, 55-56
age and, 56
altitude and, 55-56, 56t
alveolar ventilation and, 55
fraction of inspired O_2 and, 55, 55t
in asthma, 294, 294t
in children, 468
in carbon monoxide poisoning, 705
in chronic compensated airflow obstruction, 299
in cyanosis, 140-141
in children, 437
in hypothermia, 649
monitoring oxygenation and ventilation and, 55
oxygen availability and, 58-59
oxyhemoglobin saturation and, 56t, 56-57, 57t
physiologic shunting in lung and, 57-58, 58t
in *Pneumocystis carinii* pneumonia, 273
in poisoning, 549
in pregnancy, 414
in pulmonary embolism, 233
respiratory index and, 57
in status asthmaticus, in children, 471, 472
in thoracic trauma, 933
Arterial cannulation, 25-26, 27-29, 29f
assessment and complications of, 25-26
of pulmonary artery, 27f, 27-29, 28t, 29f, 30f
technique of, 26
Arterial occlusion, in mesenteric ischemia, 251
Arterial pressure monitoring, 27-29, 28f
arterial cannulation and, 27, 29f
pulmonary artery and, 27f, 27-29, 28t, 29f, 30f
Arterial probes, systemic, 59
Arterial trauma, 254
diagnosis of, 254
Arteriography:
in abdominal trauma, 956, 957f
in great vessel injuries, 948
in mesenteric ischemia, 251, 252
in neck trauma, 930, 930f
in peripheral vascular disease, 254
thoracic, in aortic dissection, 247
Arteriolar dilators, direct, in hypertensive emergencies, 243
Arteriosclerotic heart disease (ASHD), high altitude and, 676
Arteriovenous (AV) fistulas, 947
Arteriovenous malformations (AVMs), gastrointestinal bleeding and, 149
Arthritis:
of knee, Baker's cyst in, 889
rheumatoid, 883, 884t, 886
in children, 883, 884t, 889
(*See also* Rheumatoid disorders)
septic, 888, 888t
in child, 990
in narcotic overdose, 569
traumatic, 888
Arthropathy, in sickle cell anemia, 774
Artifacts, anion gap changes due to, 39-40
AS (*see* Aortic stenosis)
Ascaris infections, 535-536
ASD (*see* Atrial septal defect)
Aseptic necrosis, following organ transplantation, 1106
ASHD (*see* Arteriosclerotic heart disease)
Asphyxia:
neonatal resuscitation and, 171-172
in tetanus, 879, 880t
traumatic, 936
Aspirate cultures:
in cellulitis, in children, 450-451
in sinusitis, 449
Aspiration:
catheter, in pneumothorax, 285, 286f
in hydrocarbon poisoning, 601-602
lung injuries and, 937
in poisoning, 548
Aspirin:
in acute mountain sickness, 673
in acute myocardial infarction, 209
in cerebral vascular accident, 795

Reye's syndrome and, 160, 475
in thyroid storm, 753
(*See also* Salicylate intoxication; Salicylates)
Assist-control (A/C) ventilation, 19
Asterixis ("liver flap"), in portosystemic encephalopathy, 362
Asthma, 290-297
assessing severity of attacks in, 293-294
profile of high-risk asthmatic patient and, 293
subjective versus objective assessment and, 293
warning signs of severe asthma and, 293-294, 294t
in children, 466-474
clinical findings in, 467
death from, 466
differential diagnosis of, 468-469, 469t
etiology of, 466
laboratory studies in, 467-468
pathophysiology of, 466-467
radiographic studies in, 468
treatment of, 469-473
classification of, 290, 290t
clinical presentation of, 292, 292t
blood and sputum cultures and, 292
electrocardiography and, 292
history taking and, 292
physical examination and, 292
pulmonary function testing and, 292
radiographic studies and, 292
exercise-induced, 466
extrinsic, 290, 466
intrinsic, 290, 466
mixed, 466
pathology of, 292
pathophysiology of, 290-292
bronchial hyperreactivity and, 290-291, 291t, 466
mechanisms of bronchospasm and, 291t, 291-292
during pregnancy, 292-293, 407
management of, 293
severe, 293
status asthmaticus and, 293
treatment of, 294-297
β-adrenergic agonists in, 295, 295t
antibiotics in, 297
anticholinergics in, 296-297
calcium channel blockers in, 297
corticosteroids in, 296
indications for hospital admission and, 294, 294t
mechanical ventilation in, 297
theophylline in, 295-296, 296t
(*See also* Status asthmaticus)
Asymptomatic bacteriuria (ABU), 377
Asystole, treatment of, 113t, 114t, 122, 125
Ataxic breathing, in altered mental status, 153
Atelectasis:
in asthma, in children, 472
postoperative, 366
Atenolol (Tenormin):
actions of, 111
in acute myocardial infarction, 210
in angina, 201t
dosage, actions, pharmacokinetics, and indications for, 112t
Atherosclerosis, of coronary arteries (*see* Coronary artery disease)
Ativan (*see* Lorazepam)
ATN (*see* Acute tubular necrosis)
Atomic weights, 62, 62t
Atopy, 290
ATP (*see* Adenosine triphosphate)
Atracurium, neuromuscular blockade and, 17, 17t
Atrial fibrillation, 91f, 91-92
in acute myocardial infarction, 205
clinical significance of, 91
treatment of, 91-92, 110, 115t, 117, 119, 121, 122
in Wolff-Parkinson-White syndrome, 105-106
Atrial flutter, 90-91, 91f
clinical significance of, 91
treatment of, 91, 110, 115t, 117, 119, 121, 122
in Wolff-Parkinson-White syndrome, 105-106
Atrial septal defect (ASD), blunt injury to heart and, 943
Atrioventricular (AV) block, 99-100
clinical significance of, 100
first-degree, 99, 99f
in acute myocardial infarction, 205
clinical significance of, 99
treatment of, 99
high-grade, in acute myocardial infarction, 205
nodal and infranodal, 99, 100
second-degree Mobitz I (Wenckebach), 99f, 99-100
in acute myocardial infarction, 205
clinical significance of, 100
treatment of, 100
second-degree Mobitz II, 100, 100f
in acute myocardial infarction, 205
clinical significance of, 100
treatment of, 100
third-degree (complete), 100, 100f
in acute myocardial infarction, 205
treatment of, 100
Atrioventricular (AV) dissociation, 98f, 98-99, 99f
clinical significance of, 99
treatment of, 99
Atrioventricular (AV) node, 86
Atrioventricular ring (annulus fibrosis), 86
Atropine, 125
actions of, 111t, 125
adverse effects of, 111t, 125
as antidote to organophosphate/carbamate poisoning, 612
in bradyarrhythmias, 88
in calcium channel blocker overdose, 621
cardiopulmonary resuscitation and, in children, 178t, 179, 180f, 180t
in chronic decompensated airflow obstruction, 301
contraindications and forms of, 111t
in digoxin toxicity, 122
dosing and administration of, 111t, 125
indications for, 111t, 125
in junctional rhythms, 94
in mushroom poisoning, 720
neuromuscular blockade and, 17, 18
ophthalmic uses of, 838
in organophosphate/carbamate poisoning, 634, 709
pharmacokinetics of, 125
poisoning by, antidote to, 549t
in second-degree Mobitz I (Wenckebach) atrioventricular block, 100
in second-degree Mobitz II atrioventricular block, 100
in sinoatrial block, 98
in sinus arrest (pause), 98
in third-degree (complete) block, 100
Attachment apparatus, 860
Auricular wounds, 1059-1060
anatomy and, 1059
avulsion, 1060
hematoma and, 1059
lacerations, 1060, 1060f
treatment of, 1059-1060, 1060f
Auscultation:
in abdominal pain, 145
in pneumonia, in children, 457
in thoracic trauma, 934
Austin-Flint murmur:
in aortic regurgitation, 223
in mitral stenosis, 220
Autisms, in altered mental status, 153
Automatic external defibrillators (AEDs), 33-34, 191
Automatic implantable cardioverter-defibrillator, complications of, 1108
Autonomic nervous system:
asthma and, 290-291, 291t
dysfunction of, in tetanus, treatment of, 526, 526t
Autonomic side effects, monoamine oxidase inhibitors and, 1083
Autopsy, in sudden infant death syndrome, 436
Autotransfusion, 777
in hemothorax, 938
AV (*see headings beginning with term* Arteriovenous)
AV node (*see* Atrioventricular node)
Avascular necrosis, in children, 890
AVMs (*see* Arteriovenous malformations)
Avulsion, of teeth, 863-864, 864f
Axillary vein, venous access and, in children, 168-169
Axonal shear injury (white matter shear injury), computed tomography and, 8
Azathioprine:
in Crohn's disease, 329
in myasthenia gravis, 824
in organ transplantation, 1105

Babesia infections, 538
Babesiosis, 542-543
clinical presentation of, 543
diagnosis of, 543
treatment of, 543
Babinski's sign, 787-788
in acute cervical disk herniations, 894
lumbar spine lesions and, 896
in thoracic spine fractures, 896
Bacillus cereus, diarrhea and, 349
Bacitracin, in pseudomembranous enterocolitis, 331
Back blow technique, 2
Bacteremia:
in children, 159, 454
diagnosis and treatment of, 454
in penumonia, 459
fever and, 158
gram-negative, septic shock and, 136
in infants, 159
occult, 159
in pneumonia, in children, 459
Bacterial infection, wound contaminants and, 1027t, 1027-1028
Bacterial infections:
acute gastroenteritis and, in children, 488
acute toxic neuropathies and, 811-812
diarrhea and, 348-350
treatment of, 348-350, 351t, 352
rashes and, in children, 505-506, 506f
(*See also specific infections*)
Bacterial peritonitis, spontaneous, 362

Bacterial vaginosis (BV; *Corynebacterium* vaginitis; *Gardnerella* vaginitis; *Haemophilus* vaginitis; nonspecific vaginitis), 396
Bacteriuria, 377
  asymptomatic, 377
  in children, 462
    asymptomatic, 463
  diagnosis of, 378
Bactrim (*see* Trimethoprim/sulfamethoxazole)
Bag-valve-mask (BVM) unit, 10, 10t
  children and, 177
"Baggers," 602
Bainbridge reflex, in sinus arrhythmia, 89
Baker's cyst, in arthritis of knee, 889
BAL (*see* British anti-Lewisite)
Balanitis, 384
Balanoposthitis, 384
Ballet dancer's fractures, 1013
Ballistics (*see* Gunshot wounds; Wound ballistics)
Balloon pump, aortic:
  in cardiogenic shock, 136
  in mitral regurgitation, 221
Balloon tamponade:
  adverse reactions to, 148–149
  in gastrointestinal bleeding, 148–149
Barbital, pharmacology of, 561t
Barbiturate coma, 156
Barbiturates, 561–562
  intoxication by, 561–562
    clinical presentation of, 561
    treatment of, 562
  neuromuscular blockade and, 18
  pharmacology of, 561, 561t
  withdrawal from, 562
Barium contrast studies:
  in abdominal pain, 147
  in appendicitis, 321
  in gastrointestinal bleeding, 148
  in great vessel injuries, 948
  in intestinal obstruction, 324
  in ulcerative colitis, 331
Barodontalgia (tooth squeeze), 681
Barosinusitis, 849
Barotitis, 842
Barotitis externa (external ear squeeze), 679
Barotitis media (middle ear squeeze), 679–680
  treatment of, 679–680
Barotrauma, 679–681
  of ascent (reverse squeeze), 680–681, 681t, 682f
  of descent (squeeze), 679–680, 680f
  pulmonary, 284, 681, 681t
Bartholin's cyst, 876
Bartter's syndrome, 48
Base deficit, 37
Base excess, 37
  negative, 37
Basic life support (BLS) ambulances, 189
Basilar artery occlusion, 796
  altered mental status and, 157
Battery ingestion, 310, 311, 311f, 606–607
Bed rest, in high altitude pulmonary edema, 675
Bee stings (*see* Insect and spider bites/stings, Hymenoptera stings and)
Behavior disorders (*see* Psychiatric disorders)
Behavioral abnormalities, in poisoning, 547, 548–549
Bell's palsy, 815, 815t
Bell's phenomenon, distinguishing true neurologic deficits from conversion disorder and, 1091t
Benadryl (*see* Diphenhydramine)
Bends, 683
Bennett's fracture, 980
γ-Benzene hexachloride (GBH; Kwell), in scabies, 658
Benzene poisoning, 603
Benzodiazepines, 624t, 624–625
  abuse and dependence on, 625
  in ethanol withdrawal, 577
  overdose of, 624–625
    clinical features of, 624–625
    management of, 625
  pharmacology of, 624
  withdrawal from, 625
Benztropin (Cogentin), in antipsychotic side effects, 1081
Benzyl penicillin (*see* Penicillin G)
Beryllium, radiation injury and, 713
Beta adrenergic agents, 621–622
  in acute myocardial infarction, 207
  in angina, 200–201, 201t
  in asthma, 295
    β_2-adrenergic drugs and, 295, 295t
    aerosol therapy with, 295
  in atrial fibrillation, 91
  in chronic decompensated airflow obstruction, 301
  in congestive heart failure, 218
    in neonate, 175–176
  in mitral valve prolapse, 222
  overdose of
    clinical presentation of, 622
    disposition/follow-up in, 622
    laboratory studies in, 622
    range of toxicity in, 622
    treatment of, 622
  pharmacology and properties of, 621–622
  in pulmonary edema, 218
Beta adrenergic blockers (*see* Antiarrhythmic agents, class II)
  in acute myocardial infarction, 210–211
  in cocaine intoxication, 581
  in hypertrophic cardiomyopathy, 228
  hypoglycemia and, 732
  in theophylline poisoning, 615
Beta blockers (*see* Beta adrenergic blockers)
Betapace (*see* Sotalol)
Betaxolol (Kerlone):
  in angina, 201t
  dosage, actions, pharmacokinetics, and indications for, 112t
Bezoars, small bowel obstruction and, 322
Bicarbonate:
  correlating with chloride, 38
  correlation with carbon dioxide content, 37
  increased, hypokalemia and, 71
  plasma, ratio of change in anion gap to, 41–42
  (*See also* Sodium bicarbonate
Biliary ducts:
  injury to, 959
  ultrasonography and, 1120
Biliary dyskinesia, 353
Biliary obstruction, postoperative, 369
Biliary scintiscanning, in cholecystitis, 354
Biliary tree, ultrasonography and, 1120, 1121f
Bilirubin, 356
  (*See also* Jaundice)
Binge eating, 1086
Bipolar disorder, 1070–1071
Bites:
  animal, 1043–1044 (*see* Marine animals, trauma and envenomations from)
    rabies and (*see* Rabies)
  human, 1043
    hand infections and, 976
    treatment of, 1043
  insect (*see* Insect and spider bites/stings)
  reptile (*See* Gila monster bite; Snake bites)
  venomous, treatment of, 113t
Bladder, in pregnancy, 414
Bladder injury, computed tomography in, 10
Blakemore intubation, in esophageal disease, 308–309
  anatomic considerations and procedure for, 308–309
  indications for, 308
Blast, 685 (*see also* Dysbarism, blast injury and)
Blast wave, 685, 685f
Blast winds, 685
Bleeding, 765–767
  chest wall injuries and, 934
  in fissure in ano, 339
  gastrointestinal (*see* Gastrointestinal bleeding)
  gynecologic
    early pregnancy complications as causes of (*see* Pregnancy)
    following hysteroscopy, 422
    following laparoscopy, 422
    nonpregnancy, 392–393
    postconization, uterine, dysfunctional, 393
  gynecologicpostconization, 423
  from hemorrhoids, 337, 338
  hemostasis and, 765t, 765–766, 766f
  intrabronchial, lung injuries and, 937
  laboratory studies in, 766t, 766–767
  from oral cavity, 1052
  postadenotonsillectomy, 842
  signs of bleeding diathesis and, 765
  vascular, hemostasis and, 765, 765t
  (*See also* Hemorrhage)
Bleeding disorders, acquired, 768–769
Blepharitis, 835
Blindness, 837
  amaurosis fugax and, 837
  central retinal artery occlusion and, 837
    central retinal vein occlusion and, 837
    eclipse burn (sun gazer's retinopathy) and, 837
    retrobulbar neuritis and, 837
  hysterical, 837
  retinal detachment and, 837
  snow, 676
Blocadren (*see* Timolol)
Blood:
  acclimatization to high altitude and, 670
  acidity of, carbon dioxide transport and, 55
  alkalinization of, in cyclic antidepressant overdose, 553
  carbon dioxide transport in, 54
    blood acidity and, 55
    effect of oxygen-hemoglobin reaction on, 55
  in stool, in infant, 492
  temperature of, arterial blood gases and, 141
  type O universal donor, 777
  volume of, in pregnancy, 414
  warming before infusion, 22
  whole, 775
  (*See also* Red blood cells)
Blood chemistry, in seizures, 806–807
Blood cultures:
  in asthma, 292
  in cellulitis, in children, 450
  in occult bacteremia, 159
  in pneumonia, bacterial, 265
  in septic shock, 138
Blood dyscrasias, oral manifestations of, 862, 862f

Blood flow:
- cerebral
  - anatomy and physiology of, 913
  - during closed-chest massage, 1
- regional, military antishock trouser garment and, 6
- to uterus, in pregnancy, 414

Blood gases, 51-61
- alveolar gases and, 53-54
  - alveolar gas equation and, 53
  - carbon dioxide concentration in alveoli and, 53
  - expired air and, 54
  - humidification of inspired air and, 53
  - inspired, 53, 53t
  - oxygen concentration and partial pressure in alveoli and, 53
  - PA_{O_2} estimation and, 53
  - rate at which alveolar air is renewed by atmospheric air and, 53
- arterial (*see* Arterial blood gases)
- in aspiration pneumonia, 276
- capnography and, 60
- conjunctival oxygen and carbon dioxide measurements and, 60
- cord, acidotic, 170
- in cyanosis, in neonate, 175
- gas pressures and, 51-52
  - diffusion and, 51-52
- mass spectrometry and, 60-61
- pulmonary artery catheters and, 59, 59t
- pulse oximetry and, 59t, 59-60
- systemic arterial probes and, 59
- transcutaneous oxygen and carbon dioxide monitoring and, 60
- ventilation and, 51
  - alveolar, 51
  - dead space and, 51
  - minute, 51
- (*See also* Arterial blood gases)

Blood glucose levels, in Reye's syndrome, 476

Blood pressure:
- diastolic, during closed-chest massage, 1
- in jugular vein, in hypertrophic cardiomyopathy, 228
- military antishock trouser garment and, 6
- monitoring of (*see* Arterial pressure monitoring; Catheterization, central venous)
- in pregnancy, 414
- in tetanus, 879, 880t
- (*See also* Hypertension; Hypotension; Pulmonary artery wedge pressure)

Blood supply, of ankle, 1007

Blood transfusion, 775-779
- autotransfusion and, 777
- blood components and, 775-776
- blood transfusion devices and, 776-777
- delayed reactions and, 778
- emergency release of blood and, 777
- in hemophilia, 770-772, 771t
- in hemorrhagic shock, 134
- immediate transfusion reactions and, 778
  - allergic, 778
  - febrile, 778
  - hemolytic, 778
- infections and, 778-779
- massive, 777
- in peptic ulcer disease, 314
- in sickle cell anemia, 774
- specific factor therapy and, 776

Blood urea nitrogen (BUN):
- in nonketotic hyperosmolar coma, 745
- in pregnancy, 414
- in Reye's syndrome, 476

Blood vessels, age-related changes in, 257

Blowout fracture, orbital, 852

BLS (*see* Basic life support ambulances)

Blue diaper syndrome, hypercalcemia and, 78

Blue spells, in neonate, 428-429

Body fractures, mandibular, 851

Body packers, 580

Body stuffers, 580

Body temperature:
- neonatal resuscitation and, 171
- in poisoning, 545

Boerhaave's syndrome, 309

Bohr effect, 57

Bolus phase, computed tomography and, 3

Bone(s):
- of ankle, 1007
- (*See also* Fracture(s))

Bone pain, in narcotic overdose, 569

Boston exanthem, rash in, in children, 507

Botulism, 811-812, 825-826
- differentiating from diphtheria or Guillain-Barré syndrome, 812
- infant, 812

Boutonnière deformity, 973, 973f

Bowel:
- infarction of, abdominal pain and, 144
- injury to, hysteroscopy and, 422
- ischemia of, abdominal pain and, 144
- malrotation of, in children, 493
- perforation of, in chronic renal failure, 375
- small (*see* Small bowel)
- sterilization of, in Reye's syndrome, 478
- thermal injury to, laparoscopy and, 422
- traumatic injury of, laparoscopy and, 422
- (*See also* Colon; Intestinal obstruction)

Bowel sounds, in perforated viscus, 317

Bowlus and Currier test, distinguishing true neurologic deficits from conversion disorder and, 1091t

Box jellyfish envenomations, 667

Boxer's fracture, 979-980

Boyle's law, 678

BPD (*see* Bronchopulmonary dysplasia)

Bradyarrhythmias:
- mechanisms of, 88-89
- in phenytoin toxicity, treatment of, 565
- in poisoning, 547
- treatment of, 113t, 114t, 124

Bradycardia:
- in children, 180
- sinus, 89, 89f
  - in acute myocardial infarction, 204-205
  - clinical significance of, 89
  - in myxedema coma, 757
  - treatment of, 89
- treatment of, 113t, 114t, 124
- (*See also* Sick sinus syndrome)

Bradycardia monitors, 1110

Brain:
- anatomy and physiology of, 913
- contusion of, 914-915, 915f
- herniation of, head injury and, 914, 915f
- laceration of, 916
- phenytoin toxicity and, 563
- (*See also* Central nervous system: Central nervous system disorders)

Brain abscess, 830-831
- headache and, 791

Brain death, 4

Brainstem:
- intrinsic lesion of, 151
- left, cerebral vascular accident and, 797
- tumors of, altered mental status and, 157

Breast surgery, complications of, 370

Breastfeeding, in acute gastroenteritis, 489

Breath, in altered mental status, 152

Breathing:
- apneustic, in altered mental status, 153
- assessment of, in trauma patient, 907
- cluster, in altered mental status, 153
- evaluation of, in poisoning, 545
- labored, in children, upper respiratory disorders and, 182
- mouth-to-mouth, in children, 177, 177t
- in neck trauma, 929
- neonatal patterns of, 425
- neonatal resuscitation and, 171
- noisy, in neonate, 428
- periodic, in neonate, 428
- rapid, in neonate, 427t, 427-428
- toxic, in altered mental status, 153
- (*See also headings beginning with term* Respiratory)

Brescia-Cimino fistula, problems related to, 375, 376

Bretylium (Bretylol), 118
- actions of, 111t, 118
- adverse effects of, 111t, 118
- contraindications and forms of, 111t
- dosing and administration of, 111t, 118
- electrophysiologic actions of, 110t
- indications for, 111t, 118
- pharmacokinetics of, 118
- in ventricular tachycardia, 97

Brevibloc (*see* Esmolol)

Brevital (*see* Methohexital)

Brief reactive psychosis, 1070

British anti-Lewisite (BAL; dimercaprol):
- in lead poisoning, 640, 642
- in mercury poisoning, 643

4-Bromo-dimethoxyamphetamine (DOB), 583

Brompheniramine maleate, in Hymenoptera stings, 656

Bronchial hyperreactivity, 290-291, 291t, 466

Bronchial stenosis, diagnosis of, 469

Bronchiolar obstruction, in bronchiolitis, 467

Bronchiolitis:
- in children, 428, 466-469, 473-474
  - clinical findings in, 467
  - differential diagnosis of, 468-469, 469t
  - etiology of, 466
  - pathophysiology of, 466-467
  - pneumonia and, 459
  - radiographic studies in, 468
  - treatment of, 473-474
- in neonate, 428

Bronchitis:
- chronic, 298
- high altitude and, 676

Bronchoconstriction, drug-induced, 291

Bronchopulmonary dysplasia (BPD):
- in infant, 469
- in neonate, 431-432, 432t

Bronchoscopy, in neck trauma, 930

Bronchospasm, 290
- in Hymenoptera stings, treatment of, 656
- mechanisms of, 291-292
  - consequences of airflow obstruction and, 291t, 291-292
- in poisoning, 548
- treatment of, 122
- (*See also* Asthma)

Broselow Resuscitation Tape, 178, 179, 179f

Brown-Séquard's syndrome, 926

Brudzinski's sign:
- in meningitis, 159, 827
- in neonate, 426

Bruises, estimating duration of, 500
Buffers, 36–37
  base excess and, 37
  buffer base and, 37
Bulimia nervosa, 1085t, 1085–1087
  differential diagnosis of, 1085
  etiology of, 1085
  pathophysiology of, 1085–1086, 1086t
  prognosis of, 1086–1087
  psychological presentation of, 1086
  treatment of, 1087
Bullous myringitis, 841
Bumetanide (Burinex):
  actions and pharmacology of, 244
  in congestive heart failure, 217
  in hypertensive emergencies, 244
  indications for, 244
  side effects and contraindications to, 244
  use of, 244
BUN (*see* Blood urea nitrogen)
Bupivacaine:
  for pediatric analgesia, 512
  for regional nerve block, 1031–1034
Bupropion, 1083
Burinex (*see* Bumetanide)
Burn(s):
  chemical, 695–700
    acids and, 695–700, 696t
    alkalis and, 695, 698, 699
    alkyl mercury compounds and, 699
    cantharides and, 699
    diquat dibromide and, 699
    DMSO and, 699, 700
    of ear, 842
    general approach to, 695–696
    hydrocarbons and, 698–699, 700
    iatrogenic, 700
    lacrimators and, 699
    mustard gas and, 699
    ocular, 699–700, 834
    pathophysiology of, 695
    potassium permanganate and, 699, 700
    systemic toxicity and, 700
    treatment of, 113t
    white phosphorus and, 699, 700
  from lightning, 702
  radiation, 711, 713
  thermal, 691–693
    of bowel, laparoscopy and, 422
    child abuse and, 500
    in children, treatment of, 164
    cigarette, 500
    criteria for burn center referral and, 691
    of ear, 842
    emergency department care in, 692t, 692–693, 693f
    first-degree, 691
    "glove-and-stocking" pattern of, 500
    outpatient management of, 693
    pathophysiology of, 691f, 691–692, 692f
    prehospital care in, 692
    scald, 500
    second-degree, 691
    third-degree, 691
Bursitis, 889
  of hip, 991
Butabarbital, pharmacology of, 561t
Buticonazole, in vaginitis, *Candida*, 395
Buttock, penetrating injuries of, 963
Button battery ingestion, 310, 311, 311f, 606–607
BV (*see* Bacterial vaginosis)
BVM (*see* Bag-valve-mask unit)

C-reactive protein (CRP) determinations, in meningitis, 829
CABG (*see* Coronary artery bypass grafting)
CAD (*see* Coronary artery disease)
Calan (*see* Verapamil)
Calcaneal fractures, 1012
  in children, 1014
  treatment of, 1012
Calcitonin (Calcimar):
  calcium levels and, 74
  in hypercalcemia, 79, 79t
Calcium, 74–79
  control of levels of, 74
  cytosolic accumulation of, cerebral ischemia and, 8
  functions of, 74
  in hypocalcemia, 77t, 75076
  in hypophosphatemia, 82
  ionized and protein-bound, 74
  massive blood transfusion and, 777
  movement into "sick cells," 75
Calcium argluceptate, actions, indications, dosage and administration, adverse effects, contraindications, and forms of, 113t
Calcium channel blockers, 620–621
  in acute myocardial infarction, 210
  in angina, 201, 201t
  in asthma, 297
  in hypertensive emergencies, 242–243
  overdose of, 620–621
    diagnosis of, 620
    disposition/follow-up in, 621
    management and treatment of, 620–621
    presentation of, 620
    range of toxicity and, 621
    treatment of, 113t
  pharmacology and properties of, 620
Calcium chloride:
  actions, indications, dosage and administration, adverse effects, contraindications, and forms of, 113t
  in calcium channel blocker overdose, 621
  cardiopulmonary resuscitation and, in children, 178t, 180, 180f, 180t
  in hyperkalemia, 73
  in hypocalcemia, 77
  in hypoglycemia, in ethylene glycol poisoning, 574
Calcium gluconate:
  actions, indications, dosage and administration, adverse effects, contraindications, and forms of, 113t
  in calcium channel blocker overdose, 621
  in caterpillar stings, 659
  for emergency delivery, 419t
  in hydrofluoric acid burns, 697–698
  in hyperkalemia, 73
  in hypocalcemia, 77
  in seizures, in children, 482t
  in snake bites, 662
Calcium oxide (lime) burns, 698
Calf squeeze ("Thompson's test"), in Achilles tendon rupture, 1005, 1010
Calf strains, 1005
Camel bites, 1044
Campylobacter fetus, diarrhea and, 349
  treatment of, 351t
$CaNa_2$-EDTA, in lead poisoning, 640
Cancer (*see* Carcinoma; Malignancy; Tumor(s); *specific organs*)
Candida, vaginitis and, 395
Candidiasis:
  in children, 464
  oral
    in children, 429
    in human immunodeficiency virus infections, 523
Cannulation, arterial (*see* Arterial cannulation)
Cantharide burns, 699
Capnography, 60
Capoten (*see* Captopril)
Capsicum annuum, 722, 724
Captopril (Capoten):
  actions and pharmacology of, 244
  in congestive heart failure, 218
  in dilated cardiomyopathy, 227
  in hypertensive emergencies, 244
  indications for, 244
  side effects and contraindications to, 244
  use of, 244
Carbamate poisoning (*see* Organophosphate/carbamate poisoning)
Carbamazepine (Tegretol):
  in headaches due to idiopathic cranial neuralgias, 792
  in seizures, 808t
    in children, 480t
Carbaminohemoglobin, 54–55
Carbaminoproteins, 54–55
Carbenicillin, in bacterial pneumonia, 264t
Carbicarb, in lactic acidosis, 750
Carbohydrate metabolism, arterial Pa_{CO_2}, 54
Carbolic acid (phenol):
  burns and, 697, 700
  poisoning and, 709, 709t
Carbon dioxide:
  carbon dioxide content and, 37
    correlating with bicarbonate, 37
  concentration in alveoli, 53
  conjunctival measurements of, 60
  production, transport, and excretion of, 36
  retention of, in bronchiolitis, 467
  transcutaneous monitoring of, 60
  transport in blood, 54
    blood acidity and, 55
    effect of oxygen-hemoglobin reaction on, 55
Carbon dioxide dissociation curve, 55
Carbon monoxide (CO):
  combination with hemoglobin, 59
  poisoning and, 703–706
    antidote to, 549t
    clinical presentation of, 703–704, 704t
    evaluation and laboratory studies in, 705–706
    pathophysiology of, 703
    sources of, 703
    systemic manifestations of, 704t, 704–705
    treatment of, 706
Carbon tetrachloride poisoning, 603
Carboxygen, in carbon monoxide poisoning, 706
Carboxyhemoglobin level, in carbon monoxide poisoning, 705
Carboxyhemoglobinemia, 141
Carbuncle, 876
Carcinoma:
  altered mental status and, 156
  colorectal, intestinal obstruction and, 322
  gastrointestinal bleeding and, 149
  (*See also* Malignancy; Tumor(s))
Cardene (*see* Nicardipine)
Cardiac arrest:
  in abdominal trauma, in pregnancy, 416
  in chronic renal failure, 374
  lightning injuries and, 701
  in thoracic trauma, 933
    external massage and, 933

treatment of, 114t, 122, 125
Cardiac arrhythmias (*see* Arrhythmia(s))
Cardiac care, emergency medical services and, 191
Cardiac catheterization, in aortic regurgitation, 224
Cardiac compression, external, in children, 177
Cardiac conducting system, normal, 86
Cardiac conduction system (*see* Conduction disturbances)
Cardiac decompensation, treatment of, 124
Cardiac disorders:
antidepressants and, 1082
in beta blocker overdose, 622
in carbon monoxide poisoning, 704, 704t
in cyclic antidepressant overdose, treatment of, 553-554
in hydrocarbon poisoning, 603
in rheumatic disorders, 885, 885t
(*See also* Cardiopulmonary disorders; Cardiovascular disorders; *specific disorders*)
Cardiac enzymes, in acute myocardial infarction, 202t, 202-203, 204t
Cardiac massage:
neonatal resuscitation and, 171
in penetrating injury to heart, 942
Cardiac monitoring, in arsenic poisoning, 641
Cardiac output:
depressed, in acute myocardial infarction, 206
low, acute ischemia of extremities and, 253
oxygen availability and, 58-59
in pregnancy, 414
Cardiac pacing, 29-33, 31f, 106-108, 107f, 107t
in beta blocker overdose, 622
complications of, 1108, 1108t
in digoxin toxicity, 122
external, 88
in calcium channel blocker overdose, 621
internal, 89
pacemaker malfunction and, 107-108
permanent, 106-107
power source for, 106-107
in sinoatrial block, 98
in sinus arrest (pause), 98
temporary, 107
in acute myocardial infarction, 211
in torsade de pointes, 96
transcutaneous, 29-30, 31f, 32, 32f, 107
in second-degree Mobitz II atrioventricular block, 100
transthoracic, 32-33, 33f, 107, 107f
transvenous, 32f, 30-33, 107
in calcium channel blocker overdose, 621
in second-degree Mobitz II atrioventricular block, 100
transvenous ventricular demand, in second-degree Mobitz I (Wenckebach) atrioventricular block, 100
urgent versus emergency, 29-30
ventricular demand
in sick sinus syndrome, 103
in third-degree (complete) block, 100
Cardiac pump theory, 1
Cardiac sounds, in intestinal obstruction, 323
Cardiac tamponade, ultrasonography in, 1124, 1125f
Cardiac tumors, ultrasonography in, 1125
Cardiac ultrasonography (*see* Ultrasonography, cardiac)
Cardiogenic shock (*see* Shock, cardiogenic)
Cardiomegaly:
in myxedema coma, 757
unexplained, differential diagnosis and evaluation of, 229
Cardiomyopathy, 227-229
classification and definition of, 227
dilated, 227, 227t
clinical profile of, 227
treatment of, 227
hypertrophic (idiopathic hypertrophic subaortic stenosis), 227-228, 229
chest pain and, 131
clinical profile of, 227-228, 228t
treatment of, 228
idiopathic, 229
ischemic (*see* Ischemic heart disease)
restrictive, 228t, 228-229
clinical profile of, 228-229
treatment of, 229
ultrasonography in, 1125
Cardiopulmonary bypass, heated, in hypothermia, 650-651
Cardiopulmonary disorders:
in ethylene glycol poisoning, 574
in neonate, 427-429
Cardiopulmonary injuries, from lightning, 701-702
Cardiopulmonary resuscitation (CPR), basic, 1-3
cardiac pump theory and, 1
in children, 176-181
airway and, 176-177
arrhythmias and, 180, 180t
bag-valve mask and, 177
defibrillation and cardioversion and, 180-181, 181t
drug therapy and, 177-180, 178t, 179f, 180f
equipment for, 181, 181t
external cardiac compression and, 177
fluids and, 177
foreign body management and, 176-177
intubation and, 176
management guidelines for, 181, 181t
mouth-to-mouth breathing and, 177, 177t
vascular access and, 177
complications of, 3
cough-CPR, 1
epinephrine in, 122
in hypothermia, 649
in near drowning, 688
neonatal, in sudden infant death syndrome, 429
physiology of closed-chest massage and, 1
hemodynamics and, 1
mechanism of low generation and, 1
technique of closed-chest massage and, 2-3
airway, opening, 2
assistance, obtaining, 2
breathlessness, establishing, 2
compressions, beginning, 3
pulselessness, establishing, 3
unresponsiveness, establishing, 2
ventilation, beginning, 2
terminating, 3
thoracic pump theory and, 1
basic technique of closed-chest massage and, foreign-body obstruction, relieving, 2-3
Cardiopulmonary support, in septic shock, 138
Cardiotocodynamometry, in abdominal trauma, in pregnancy, 416
Cardiovascular collapse, prosthetic heart valves and, 225
Cardiovascular depression, in carbon monoxide poisoning, 703
Cardiovascular disorders:
amphetamines and, 582
in anorexia nervosa, 1086
antipsychotics and, 1081
in heatstroke, 653
in human immunodeficiency virus infections, 523
hypertensive emergencies and (*see* Hypertensive emergencies; Hypertension)
in myxedema coma, 756-757
following organ transplantation, 1106
in phenytoin toxicity, 564
treatment of, 565
in poisoning, management of, 548
poisoning and, 547
salicylate intoxication and, 589
in theophylline poisoning, 614
in thyroid storm, 752
Cardiovascular system:
acclimatization to high altitude and, 671
hyponatremia and, 67-68
phenytoin toxicity and, 563
pregnancy-associated changes in, 414
(*See also* Heart)
Cardioversion, 106
in atrial fibrillation, 205
in children, 180-181, 181t
in digitalis toxicity, 618
in paroxysmal supraventricular tachycardia, 205
in supraventricular tachycardia, in children, 439
synchronized, 106
in atrial fibrillation, 91
complications of, 106
in reentrant supraventricular tachycardia, 93
in ventricular tachycardia, 205
unsynchronized (defibrillation), in ventricular tachycardia, 97
in Wolff-Parkinson-White syndrome, 105
Cardizem (*see* Diltiazem)
Carotid sinus hypersensitivity, syncope and, 143, 259
Carotid sinus massage, in reentrant supraventricular tachycardia, 93
Carpal tunnel syndrome, 815t, 975
Carteolol (Cartrol):
in angina, 201t
dosage, actions, pharmacokinetics, and indications for, 112t
Carvallo's sign, in tricuspid regurgitation, 224
CAs (*see* Cyclic antidepressants)
Casting, in fractures, 969-970
Cat bites and scratches, 1044
Catapres (*see* Clonidine)
Catatonic state (psychogenic unresponsiveness), 150
Catecholamines:
hypertensive emergencies induced by, 239
metabolic acidosis and, 43
Caterpillar stings, 658-659
treatment of, 659
Cathartics:
activated, 548
in poisoning (*see* Gastrointestinal decontamination)
Catheter(s):
pulmonary artery, 59, 59t
pulmonary artery thermodilution, 27, 28f
Catheter-through-needle devices, 23, 24f
Catheterization:
central venous, 22-25

Catheterization (*Cont.*):
 anatomy and, 22–23, 23f
 central venous pressure measurement and, 24–25
 central venous puncture and, 22–25, 23f, 24f
 complications of, 25
 equipment for, 23, 24f
 peripheral sites for, 22
 preparation for, 23–24
 technique of, 24
 venous cutdown and, 25
 in diagnosis of urinary tract infections, 378
 in urinary retention, in males, 388
Cations (*see* Acid-base problems, anion gap and)
Caustic ingestions, 606–608
 classification of caustic substances and, 606, 606t
 clinical evaluation in, 606–607
 complications of, 606
 emergency department treatment of, 608
 incidence of, 606
 management of, 607t, 607–608
 pathophysiology of, 606
CD4 lymphocyte count, in *Pneumocystis carinii* pneumonia, 273
Cecum, sigmoid, 322
Cefaclor:
 in cutaneous abscess, 878t
 in otitis media, 441
Cefadroxil, in urinary tract infections, 379t
Cefamandole, in bacterial pneumonia, 264t
Cefazolin:
 in bacterial pneumonia, 264t
 in periorbital/orbital cellulitis, in children, 452t
 in septic shock, 139t
 in toxic shock syndrome, 404–405
Cefixime (Suprax):
 in otitis media, 441
 in sinusitis, in children, 449t
Cefotaxime:
 in conjunctivitis, in children, 448t
 in pneumonia, in neonate, 428t
 in septic shock, 139t
Cefotetan, in pelvic inflammatory disease, 394t
Cefoxitin:
 in aspiration pneumonia, 278
 in gas gangrene, 880
 in pelvic inflammatory disease, 394t
 in septic shock, 139t
Ceftazidine, in septic shock, 139t
Ceftin (cefuroxime axetil), in otitis media, 441
Ceftriaxone:
 in chancroid, 518
 in gonorrhea, 517
 in pelvic inflammatory disease, 394t
 in periorbital/orbital cellulitis, in children, 452t
 in pyelonephritis, 380
 in septic shock, 139t
 in sinusitis, in children, 449t, 450
Cefuroxime:
 in bacteremia, in children, 454
 in bacterial pneumonia, 264t
 in periorbital/orbital cellulitis, in children, 452t
 in septic shock, 139t
 in sinusitis, in children, 449t, 450
Cefuroxime axetil (Ceftin), in otitis media, 441
Celiotomy, in abdominal trauma, to posterior abdomen, 963
Cell count, in cerebrospinal fluid, in meningitis, 828
Cellular concentrates, 775
 in hemophilia, 771–772
Cellulitis, 880–881
 in children, 450–451
  clinical findings in, 450, 450t
  complications of, 451
  definition of, 450
  diagnosis of, 450–451
  differential diagnosis of, 451
  epidemiology of, 450
  etiology of, 450, 450t
  management of, 451, 451f, 452t
  pathophysiology of, 450
  periorbital/orbital, 451–452
 clinical features of, 880, 881t
 cuff, gynecologic procedures and, 423
 facial, 857–858
 in narcotic overdose, 566
 orbital, in sinusitis, 449
 periorbital, in sinusitis, 449
 of salivary glands, 842
 treatment of, 881
Center for the Study of Anorexia and Bulimia, 1087
Central nervous system (CNS):
 glucose deprivation and, 727
 hypertensive emergencies involving, 238, 238f, 239t
 hyponatremia and, 67
 military antishock trouser garment and, 6
Central nervous system (CNS) disorders:
 cocaine use and, 580
 in cyclic depressant overdose, 551
 in ethylene glycol poisoning, 574
 in human immunodeficiency virus infections, 521
 in hydrocarbon poisoning, 602
 in hypothermia, 649
 infections and
  altered mental status and, 156
  protozoan, in immunocompromised host, 539
  Reye's syndrome versus, 476
 irritability and, monoamine oxidase inhibitors and, 1083
 in isopropanol poisoning, 577
 in mercury poisoning, 642
 in narcotic overdose, 568
 in neonate, cyanosis and, 175
 nonsteroidal anti-inflammatory drug overdose and, 628
 in organophosphate/carbamate poisoning, 611
 in phenytoin toxicity, 564
 in salicylate intoxication, treatment of, 591
 salicylate intoxication and, 589
 in sickle cell anemia, 774
 in thyroid storm, 752
Central pontine myelinosis (CPM), 67, 68
Central retinal artery occlusion, 837
Central retinal vein occlusion, 837
Central spinal cord syndrome, 926
Central venous pressure (CVP):
 measurement of, 24–25
 monitoring, in Reye's syndrome, 477
 (*See also* Catheterization, central venous)
Centrax (Prazepam), 1082t
Cephadrine, in cutaneous abscess, 878t
Cephalexin:
 in cutaneous abscess, 878t
 in impetigo, in children, 448
 in periorbital/orbital cellulitis, in children, 452t
Cephalic vein, venous access and, 21, 21f
Cephalosporin:
 in bacterial pneumonia, 264t
 in colonic diverticular disease, 334
 third-generation, in diarrhea, 351t
Cephazolin sodium, in masticator space infection, 858
Cerebellar testing, 787
Cerebellopontine angle, tumors of, vertigo and, 800
Cerebellum, hemorrhage of, 797
Cerebral artery syndromes, 796
Cerebral blood flow:
 anatomy and physiology of, 913
 during closed-chest massage, 1
Cerebral contusion, computed tomography and, 8
Cerebral edema:
 in carbon monoxide poisoning, treatment of, 706
 computed tomography and, 8
 in diabetic ketoacidosis, in children, 503
 high altitude, 672, 674, 674t
Cerebral embolism, cerebrovascular lesions and, 793–794
Cerebral vascular accident (CVA; stroke), 793–798
 altered mental status and, 156–157
 cerebrovascular lesions and, 793–794
 clinical features of, 794–795
 cocaine use and, 580
 differential diagnosis of, 797–798
  left hemiplegia and, 797–798
  left-sided weakness and numbness and, 798
  right-sided weakness and, 797
 hemorrhagic syndromes and, 796–797
  hypertensive intracerebral hemorrhage and, 797
  subarachnoid hemorrhage and, 796–797
 high altitude and, 674
 incidence of, 794
 ischemic stroke syndromes and, 796
  anterior cerebral artery and, 796
  cerebellar infarcts and, 796
  lacunar infarction and, 796
  middle cerebral artery and, 796
  posterior cerebral artery and, 796
  transient global amnesia and, 796
  vertebrobasilar syndromes and, 796
 pathophysiology of, 793–794
 seizures and, in neonate, 172
 treatment of, 795–796
  in hemorrhagic stroke, 795–796
  in thrombotic and embolic stroke, 795
Cerebrospinal fluid (CSF):
 acidosis of, in diabetic ketoacidosis, 737
 anatomy and physiology of, 913
Cerebrospinal fluid (CSF) examination:
 in cerebral vascular accident, 794–795
 in encephalitis, 830
 in meningitis, 827t, 827–829
  in children, 455
 in multiple sclerosis, 818–819
 in rabies, 528
Cerebrospinal fluid (CSF) leak, posttraumatic, delayed, 920
Cerebrospinal fluid (CSF) rhinorrhea, 847–848
Cerebrovascular circulation, syncope and, 143
Cervical disk disease, 894–895
 acute herniations and, 894
 chronic degenerative disk disease and, 894–895
Cervical spine:
 assessment of injury to, in pediatric trauma victim, 911
 immobilization of, altered mental status and, 151

in rheumatic disorders, 885
Cervix, "strawberry," 395
Cesarean section, postmortem, 413, 416
Cestodes (flatworms), 538
Chalazion, 836
CHAMP, in hydrocarbon poisoning, 603
Chancroid, 518
"Chandelier sign", in pelvic inflammatory disease, 393
Chaotic atrial rhythm (*See* Multifocal atrial tachycardia)
Charcoal, activated, in poisoning, 548
(*See also* Gastrointestinal decontamination)
Charcot-Leyden crystals, asthma and, 292
Charcot's triad, in ascending cholangitis, 353
Cheek wounds, 1058-1059
anatomy and, 1058f, 1058-1059
lacerations, 1059
treatment of, 1059
Chelation therapy:
in arsenic poisoning, 642
in lead poisoning, 640
in mercury poisoning, 643
in radiation injury, 713
Chemical restraints, in poisoning, 548, 549
Chernobyl accident, 714
"Cherry-red skin," in carbon monoxide poisoning, 704
Chest pain, 127-132
in acute pericarditis, 230
ancillary studies in, 128-129, 129t
cocaine use and, 579
diagnostic decision aids in, 129-130
esophageal, 131, 307
in hypertrophic cardiomyopathy, 228
initial evaluation of, 127-128
history in, 127
location and radiation in, 128
onset and duration in, 127-128
quality in, 128
symptom relief in, 128
symptoms other than chest pain and, 128
major causes of, 130-132
acute myocardial infarction, 127, 128-129, 129t, 130
angina pectoris, 127, 128, 130
aortic dissection, 128, 130, 130t
esophageal disorders, 131
hypertrophic cardiomyopathy (idiopathic hypertrophic subaortic stenosis), 131
hyperventilation, 131-132
mediastinitis, 131
mitral stenosis, 131
mitral valve prolapse, 131
musculoskeletal, 131
pericarditis, 130-131
radicular, 131
respiratory (pleuritic), 127
spontaneous pneumomediastinum, 131
spontaneous pneumothorax, 131
unstable (crescendo or preinfarction) angina, 127, 130
valvular aortic stenosis, 131
variant (Prinzmetal's) angina, 127, 130
physical examination in, 128
precordial, in rheumatic disorders, 883
in spontaneous pneumothorax, 284
treatment priority in, 127
Chest retractions, in children, upper respiratory disorders and, 182
Chest thrusts, 3
Chest trauma, computed tomography in, 9
mediastinal trauma and aortic injury and, 9
Chest tube:
in hemothorax, 937-938
in shock, in thoracic trauma, 933
Chest wall injuries, 934-936
bony, 935-936
soft tissue, 934-935
open (sucking), 934
traumatic asphyxia and, 936
Chest wall pain, 127-128
Cheyne-Stokes respirations, in altered mental status, 153
CHF (*see* Congestive heart failure)
CHI (*see* Closed-head injuries)
Chickenpox (*see* Varicella)
Chilblain (pernio), 645
Child abuse, 498-501
interaction between child and parents and, 500
management of, 500-501
neglect and, 498
neonate and, 426
physical, 499-500
reporting, 500-501
sexual, 498-499
spectrum of abuse and neglect and, 498
sudden infant death syndrome and, 435
Child molestation, 399
Child neglect, 498
Children:
abuse of (*see* Child abuse)
acetaminophen poisoning in, 596
acquired immune deficiency syndrome in, 410
ankle injuries in, 1011
appendicitis in, 320
benign paroxysmal vertigo of childhood and, 801
calcium channel blocker overdose in, 621
carbon monoxide poisoning in, 705
clonidine poisoning in, 570
cyanide poisoning in, treatment of, 634, 709
defibrillation in, 106
digital tip amputation in, 1062, 1063
electrical injuries of, 693
foot injuries in, 1014
foreign body of ear in, 842
fractures in, 970-971, 971f
heart disease in (*see* Heart disease, pediatric)
hip fractures and dislocations in, 990
humeral fractures in, 984
Hymenoptera stings in, 656
hypoglycemia in, 733
iron intoxication in, 599
knee injuries in, 1002-1003
lead poisoning in, 639
treatment of, 640
leg injuries in, 1005
limp in (*See* Limp, in child)
mushroom poisoning in, 718
neglect of, 498
nonsteroidal anti-inflammatory drug overdose in, 628
norepinephrine in, dosage of, 123
organophosphate/carbamate poisoning in, treatment of, 634, 709
pelvic fractures in, 987
poisoning in, 545
rectal prolapse in, 343
rheumatoid arthritis in, 883, 884t
sexual misuse of, 398-399, 399t
physical examination in, 399, 400t
swallowed foreign bodies in, 311
thyroid storm in, treatment of, 753
trauma in, 910-912
upper airway obstruction in, foreign bodies and, 843
(*See also* Adolescent; Infant; Neonate; *under specific disorders*)
Chill, 158
Chin lift, 2
Chlamydial infections:
in children, 459
pneumonia and, 270
proctitis and, 342
sexually transmitted, 518
Chloral hydrate:
in bronchiolitis, in children, 474
for pediatric sedation, 513t, 514
Chloramphenicol:
in aspiration pneumonia, 278
in bacterial pneumonia, 264t
in diarrhea, 351t
in meningitis, in children, 456
ophthalmic, 838
in periorbital/orbital cellulitis, in children, 452t
in Rocky Mountain spotted fever, 507, 541
in sepsis, in children, 454
in sinusitis, in children, 449t, 450
Chlorazepate (Tranxene), 1082t
Chlordiazepoxide (Librium), 1082t
Chloride, 82-85
correlating with bicarbonate, 38
normal levels of, 83
role in kidney, 83
Chloroacetophenone, 699
Chlorobenzylidenemalonitrile, 699
Chlorophytum comosum, 722, 724
Chloroquine:
adverse effects, precautions, and contraindications to, 533t
in diarrhea, 351t
in malaria prophylaxis, 533t
in parasitic infections, 537t
Chloroquine phosphate:
in diarrhea, 351t
in malaria, 532t
in malaria prophylaxis, 533t
Chlorpromazine (Thorazine), 1080t
in monoamine oxidase inhibitor side effects, 1083
pharmacokinetics of, 555
for pediatric analgesia, 514
for rapid tranquilization, 1079t
toxic hepatitis and, 360
Chlorprothixene (Taractan), 1080t
Cholangitis, ascending, 353
Cholecystectomy:
in cholecystitis, 354-355
laparoscopic, complications of, 369
Cholecystitis, 353-355
acalculous, 353
acute, 353
clinical features of, 353-354
pathogenesis of, 353
precalculous, 353
in pregnancy, 410
treatment of, 354-355
Cholelithiasis:
in pregnancy, 410
ultrasonography in, 1120
Cholestasis:
extrahepatic, 356
intrahepatic, 356
Cholestyramine (Questran):
in acute gastroenteritis, in children, 490
in Crohn's disease, 329
Cholinergic poisoning, treatment of, 113t
Chorioamnionitis, 408
Chorioretinitis, in infant, seizures and, 481

Christmas disease (hemophilia B), 770
  replacement therapy in, 776
Chromic acid burns, 697, 700
Chronic mountain polycythemia (CMP), 676
Chronic obstructive pulmonary disease (COPD), 298-307
  causes and predisposing factors for, 298
  compensated chronic airflow obstruction and, 298-299
    clinical features of, 298-299
    treatment of, 299
  decompensated chronic airflow obstruction and, 299-307
    clinical features of, 299-300
    treatment of, 300-301
  pathophysiology of, 298
Chrysiasis, 141
Chvostek's sign, in hypocalcemia, 76
CIE (*see* Countercurrent immunoelectrophoresis)
Cigarette burns, 500
Ciguatera fish poisoning, 350
Cimetidine:
  in allergy to contrast media, 214
  in mushroom poisoning, 719
  in peptic ulcer disease, 313-314
Ciprofloxacin:
  in septic shock, 139t
  in urinary tract infections, 379t
Circulation:
  anterior, 793
  assessment of, in trauma patient, 907
  evaluation of, in poisoning, 545
  in neck trauma, 929
  posterior, 793
Cirrhosis, alcoholic (Laennec's), 361
Citrate:
  massive blood transfusion and, 777
  metabolic alkalosis and, 47
CK (*see* Creatine kinase)
Clavicular fractures, 935, 981
Clavulanate, in bacteremia, in children, 454
Clavulanate potassium, in otitis media, 441
Cleansing, of wounds, mechanical, 1038-1039, 1039f
Clindamycin:
  in aspiration pneumonia, 278
  in babesiosis, 543
  in bacterial vaginosis, 396
  in cutaneous abscess, 878t
  in pelvic inflammatory disease, 394t
  in septic shock, 139t
Clonazepam (Colopin; Klonopin), in seizures, in children, 480t, 482t
  status epilepticus and, 485, 485t
Clonidine (Catapres), 570-571
  actions and pharmacology of, 244
  in hypertensive emergencies, 241t, 244
  indications for, 244
  pharmacology and pathophysiology of, 570
    formulations and, 570
    mechanism of action and, 570
    pharmacokinetics and, 570
    toxic dose and, 570
  poisoning and
    antidotes and, 571
    clinical presentation of, 570, 570t
    laboratory studies in, 570
    treatment of, 570-571
  side effects and contraindications to, 244
  in tetanus, 526t
  use of, 244
  withdrawal from, 239, 241, 571
    treatment of, 245
Closed-chest massage (*see* Cardiopulmonary resuscitation)
Closed-head injuries (CHI), 914
Clostridial myonecrosis (*see* Gas gangrene)
Clostridium difficile, diarrhea and, 349
  treatment of, 351t
Clostridium perfringens, diarrhea and, 349
Clotrimazole:
  in human immunodeficiency virus infections, 521t
  in vaginitis, *Candida*, 395
Cloxacillin, in cutaneous abscess, 878t
Clozaril (clozapine), 1081
Cluster breathing, in altered mental status, 153
Cluster headache, 790
CMP (*see* Chronic mountain polycythemia)
CMV (*see* Cytomegalovirus infections)
CNS (*see* Central nervous system)
CO (*see* Carbon monoxide)
Co-trimoxazole:
  in pyelonephritis, 380
  in urinary tract infections, 379t
Coagulation, hemostasis and, 765t, 766, 766f
Coagulation disorders:
  in Reye's syndrome, 477
  septic shock and, 138
Coagulation factors:
  hemostasis and, 765t, 766, 766f
  in pregnancy, 414
Coagulopathy, abdominal injury and, 961
Cobalamin deficiency, multiple sclerosis versus, 820
Cocaine:
  abuse of, in pregnancy, 410
  forms of, 579
  ingestion of, 311
  as ophthalmic anesthetic, 838
  for pediatric analgesia, 512
  pharmacology of, 579
  topical, 580
  for topical anesthesia, 1035
Cocaine intoxication, 579-580
  body packers and stuffers and, 580
  cardiac complications of, 579-580
    central nervous system complications of, 580
    pulmonary complications of, 580
  obstetrical complications of, 580
  presentation and management of, 580-581
  renal complications of, 580
Coccygeal injuries, 925-926
Coccygeal injuries fractures, 983
Coelenterate envenomations, 667-668, 668t
Cogentin (benztropin), in antipsychotic side effects, 1081
Cognitive development, lead poisoning and, 639
"Coiled spring," in intussusception, in children, 495, 495f
Coin ingestion, 311
Colchicine, in gout, 889
Cold agglutinins, in pneumonia:
  in children, 458
  Mycoplasma, 269, 269t
Cold caloric (oculovestibular) testing, in altered mental status, 154, 154t
"Cold diuresis," 649
Cold stress, in neonate, 431
Cold water, facial immersion in, in reentrant supraventricular tachycardia, 93
Colic:
  esophageal, 306
  intestinal, in neonate, 425-426
Colitis:
  ischemic, colonic diverticulitis differentiated from, 334
  pseudomembranous enterocolitis and, 331
  ulcerative, 330-331
    clinical features and course of, 330
    colonic diverticulitis differentiated from, 334
    complications of, 330-331
    diagnosis of, 331
    pathology of, 330
    treatment of, 331
  (*See also* Crohn's disease)
Collagen vascular disease, oral manifestations of, 862
Collateral ligament injuries, 973, 973f
  treatment of, 973, 974f
Colles fracture, 977-978
Colligative properties, 62-63
Colloids:
  in burns, in children, 164
  in shock
    in children, 162
    hemorrhagic, 134
Colon:
  cancer of
    colonic diverticulitis differentiated from, 334
    in ulcerative colitis, 330-331
  diverticular disease of, 333-335
    diagnosis of, 333
    differential diagnosis of, 333-334, 334t
    drug therapy in, 334
    laboratory studies in, 333
    lower gastrointestinal bleeding in, 335
    physical examination in, 333
  injury to, 958
  obstruction of, 322
  perforation of, foreign bodies and, 344
  polyps of, in children, 496
  sigmoid, volvulus of, 322, 323f
Colonic lavage, in hypothermia, 650
Colonoscopy:
  in Crohn's disease, 329
  in gastrointestinal bleeding, 148
  in ulcerative colitis, 331
Color-flow Doppler mapping, 1123
Colorado tick fever, 543
  clinical presentation of, 543
  treatment of, 543
Colostomy, complications of, 368
Coma, 150
  barbiturate, 156
  definition of, 150
  Glasgow Coma Scale and (*See* Glasgow Coma Scale)
  hepatic (*see* Portosystemic encephalopathy)
  hyperglycemic, 40
  lightning injuries and, 702
  myxedema (*see* Myxedema coma)
  in narcotic overdose, treatment of, 566
  nonketotic hyperosmolar (*see* Nonketotic hyperosmolar coma)
  pentobarbital, in Reye's syndrome, 477
  in poisoning, 548
  psychogenic, definition of, 150
  in Reye's syndrome, 478
  (*See also* Altered mental status)
"Coma vigil" (abulic state; akinetic mutism), 150
Communications:
  disaster medical services and, 195
  for emergency medical services, 189
Compartment syndromes, 1007-1010
  compartments at risk for, 1007-1009

in lower extremity, 1009, 1009f
in upper extremity, 1007, 1007f, 1008f, 1009
diagnosis of, 1009t, 1009-1010, 1010f
in leg fractures, 1004-1005
management of, 1010
military antishock trouser garment and, 7
pathophysiology of, 1007, 1007t
Compazine (prochlorperazine), for emergency delivery, 419t
Compensation, acid-base problems and (*see* Acid-base problems, compensatory changes and)
Compensatory mechanisms, in congestive heart failure, 103, 217f
Complete blood count, in Reye's syndrome, 476
Computed tomography (CT), 1-10
in abdominal trauma, 956, 957f
to posterior abdomen, 962
in altered mental status, 155
in aortic dissection, 247
in appendicitis, 321
in blunt trauma to great vessels, 951
in carbon monoxide poisoning, 705-706
in cerebral vascular accident, 794, 795
CT numbers and, 1
in diving accidents, 685
field of view, multiplanar reconstruction, and three-dimensional display and, 2
in great vessel injuries, 947-948
in gunshot wounds, to trunk, 1021
in head injury, 917
in head trauma (*see* Head trauma, computed tomography in)
in headaches, 789
image formation and, 1
intravenous contrast administration and dynamic scanning and, 3-4, 4f, 5f
ionic versus nonionic intravenous contrast and, 6
in maxillofacial trauma, 855-856
orbital and midfacial fractures and, 855-856, 856f
in meningitis, 827
in neck trauma, 930
noncontrast (C-), 3
oral contrast administration and, 6
postcontrast (contrast-enhanced), 3
in Reye's syndrome, 476
in seizures, 807
slice thickness, subject contrast, and image noise and, 3
in thoracic aortic aneurysms, expanding and ruptured, 248
volume averaging and, 3
window and level and, 1-2, 2f, 3f
Concussion, headache following, 791
Conduction block, new (age-indeterminant), in acute myocardial infarction, 205
Conduction disturbances, 86-108, 98-100
in acute myocardial infarction, 205, 205t
atrioventricular block, 99
first-degree, 99, 99f
second-degree Mobitz I (Wenckebach), 99f, 99-100
second-degree Mobitz II, 100, 100f
third-degree (complete), 100, 100f
atrioventricular dissociation, 98f, 98-99, 99f
clinical significance of, 99
treatment of, 99
defibrillation and synchronized cardioversion in, 106
normal cardiac conducting system and, 86
normal electrocardiogram and, 86-87, 87f
sinoatrial block, 98, 98f
clinical significance of, 98
treatment of, 98
sinus arrest (pause), 98, 98f
clinical significance of, 98
treatment of, 98
(*See also* Fascicular blocks; Sick sinus syndrome)
Condyle fractures, mandibular, 851
Condylomata acuminata (anal warts), proctitis and, 342
Condylomata lata, in syphilis, 342
Confidentiality, human immunodeficiency virus infections and, 523
Confrontation, in crisis intervention, 1095
Confusional states, 150
Congenital heart disease, seizures versus, 485
Congestive heart failure (CHF), 216-217
asthma and bronchiolitis versus, 469
clinical features of, 217
in congenital heart disease, in children, 438, 438t
in elderly patients, 260-261
etiology of, 216
in neonate, 175-176
causes of, 175
management of, 175-176
signs and symptoms of, 175
pathophysiology of, 216-217, 217f
treatment of, 109, 121-124, 217-218
Conium maculatum, 722, 724
Conjunctiva, 1054
foreign body of, 835
removal of, 840
injuries to, 1055
Conjunctival monitoring, of oxygen and carbon monoxide, 60
Conjunctivitis ("pink eye"; "red eye"), 834
allergic, 447
bacterial, 834
staphylococcal allergic conjunctivitis and, 834
chemical, 834
acid burns and, 834
alkali burns and, 834
in children, 446-447
clinical findings in, 446
complications of, 446
definition of, 446
diagnosis of, 446
differential diagnosis of, 446
epidemiology of, 446
etiology of, 446, 446t
management of, 103, 447f, 447t, 448t
pathophysiology of, 446
gonococcal, in neonate, 429
in neonate, 429
viral, 834
allergic, 834
epidemic keratoconjunctivitis and, 834
herpes zoster, 834
Consciousness:
altered level of
in phenytoin toxicity, 564
in poisoning, 547, 548
definition of, 150
loss of (*see* Coma; Syncope)
(*See also* Altered mental status; Coma)
Constipation:
following anorectal surgery, 369
in intestinal obstruction, 323
in neonate, 427
Consumer participation, emergency medical services and, 190
Contact lenses, problems with, 840
Continuous positive airway pressure (CPAP), 10, 19
in aspiration pneumonia, 278
in near drowning, 689
in pulmonary edema, 218
Contraception:
history taking and, 389-390
postcoital, in female rape victims, 400
Contrast media:
allergic reaction to
angiography and, 214
intravenous pyelography and, 374
computed tomography and, 1, 3
Control ventilation, 19
Controlled mechanical hypoventilation, in asthma, 297
Convallaria majalis, 722, 724
Conversion reactions, 1071, 1090-1091
clinical presentation of, 1090, 1091t
definition of, 1090
differential diagnosis of, 1090
pathophysiology of, 1090
predisposing factors for, 1090
treatment and prognosis of, 1090-1091
Convulsions (*see* Epilepsy; Seizures)
Coordination, in neurological examination, 787
COPD (*see* Chronic obstructive pulmonary disease)
Coprine poisoning:
clinical toxicity of, 717-718
pharmacology of, 716, 717t
treatment of, 720
Coral cuts, 666
"Coral poisoning," 666
Coral snake, 661
bites of, 664-665
Cordarone (Amiodarone), electrophysiologic actions of, 110t
Corgard (*see* Nadolol)
Cornea:
abrasions of, 838
foreign bodies of, 835
foreign body of, removal of, 840
lacerations of, 838
ulcer of, 835
Corneal reflex:
in altered mental status, 154
distinguishing true neurologic deficits from conversion disorder and, 1091t
Cornelia de Lange's syndrome, 481
"Cornpicker's pupil," 637
Coronary arteries, injury to, 946
Coronary artery bypass grafting (CABG), in acute myocardial infarction, 211
Coronary artery disease (CAD), 199-200
in elderly patients, 258
natural history of, 199-200
Coronary insufficiency, hypertension and, 239
Coronoid process fractures, 985
Corpus luteum, hemorrhagic, 391
Corrigan's (water-hammer) pulse, in aortic regurgitation, 223
Corrosives, 695
upper airway obstruction and, 844
Cortex, cerebral vascular accident and, 797
Cortical disease, bilateral, 151
Corticosteroids:
in asthma, 296
in children, 470-473
in organ transplantation, 1105
in *Pneumocystis carinii* pneumonia, 274
in rheumatic disorders, 889
in status asthmaticus, in children, 472

Corticosteroids (*Cont.*):
  in treatment of diving accidents, 684
Corticotropin-releasing factor (CRF), adrenal insufficiency and, 759
Corynebacterium vaginitis (bacterial vaginosis; BV; *Gardnerella* vaginitis; *Haemophilus* vaginitis; nonspecific vaginitis), 396
Costosternal syndrome, chest pain and, 131
Cotton sutures, 1045
Cotton-wool spots, in human immunodeficiency virus infections, 522
Cough:
  in children, upper respiratory disorders and, 182
  in neonate, 428
Cough-CPR, 1
Coumadin (*see* Warfarin)
"Count of Monte Cristo" syndrome (locked-in syndrome), 150
Countercurrent immunoelectrophoresis (CIE), in meningitis, 829
Counterpulsation, with aortic balloon pump, in cardiogenic shock, 136
Coxsackievirus A9 infection, rash in, in children, 507
CPAP (*see* Continuous positive airway pressure)
CPK (*see* Creatine phosphokinase)
CPM (*see* Central pontine myelinosis)
CPR (*see* Cardiopulmonary resuscitation)
"Crack lung," 580
Cranial nerves:
  in altered mental status, 153, 154
  in neurological examination, 786
  neuropathy and, 814–815
Cranial neuralgias, idiopathic, headache and, 791–792
"Crank," 583
Crassula argentea, 723, 724
Creatine kinase (CK):
  in acute myocardial infarction, 129, 129t, 203
  in syncope, in elderly patients, 259
Creatine phosphokinase (CPK):
  in carbon monoxide poisoning, 705
  MB fraction of, in myocardial contusion, 944
  in Reye's syndrome, 476
Creatinine, in pregnancy, 414
Creola bodies, asthma and, 292
Cresol burns, 700
CRF (*see* Corticotropin-releasing factor)
"Crib death" (*see* Sudden infant death syndrome)
Cricothyrotomy, 15–16
  complications of, 16
  contraindications to, 15
  indications for, 15
  in pediatric trauma victim, 910
  technique of, 15–16, 16f
  in upper airway obstruction, 845
Cricothyrotomy (laryngotomy), in upper airway obstruction, 845
Crisis intervention, 1092–1096
  components of, 1094t, 1094–1095
  crisis development and, 1092, 1093t
  goals of, 1094
  patient assessment and, 1092–1094
    crisis precipitants and, 1092–1093
    directiveness of interview and, 1094
    family members and, 1094
    outside information and, 1093
    precrisis adjustment and, 1092
    resources and, 1094
    self-esteem and, 1093–1094
    stages of response and, 1093
    successive assessments and, 1094
  strategies for different stages and, 1095–1096
  stress of, 1096
  types of crises and, 1092
  use of high emotional arousal in, 1096
Crisis management, 1095–1096
Crisis therapy, 1096
Critical care units, emergency medical services and, 190
Crohn's disease (granulomatous ileocolitis; regional enteritis; terminal enteritis), colonic diverticulitis differentiated from, 334
Crohn's disease (granulomatous ileocolitis; regional enteritis; terminal ileitis), 328–329
  clinical features and course of, 328–329
  complications of, 329
  diagnosis of, 329
  epidemiology of, 328
  etiology and pathogenesis of, 328
  pathology of, 328
  treatment of, 329–330
Cromolyn sodium, in asthma, in children, 473
Crossed straight-leg raising (CSLR) signs, lumbar spine lesions and, 896, 898
Crotamiton, in scabies, 658
Croup, viral, 182, 184–185
Croup syndrome (*see* Stridor)
CRP (*see* C-reactive protein determinations)
Crying, in neonate, 425–426, 426t
Cryoprecipitate, 776
  in hemophilia, 771
Cryotherapy, in snake bite, 664
Cryptitis, 339
  clinical features of, 339
  treatment of, 339
Cryptococcal infections, of central nervous system, in human immunodeficiency virus infections, 521–522
Cryptosporidium, diarrhea and, 350
Crystalloids:
  in neurogenic shock, 138–139
  in shock, in children, 162
  warming, 22
CsA (*see* Cyclosporine)
CSF (*see* Cerebrospinal fluid)
CT (*see* Computed tomography)
CT number, 1
Cuff cellulitis, gynecologic procedures and, 423
Culdocentesis, in ectopic pregnancy, 411
Cullen's sign, in abdominal pain, 145
Curling's ulcers (*see* Ulcer(s), Curling's)
Curschmann's spirals, asthma and, 292
Cushing's ulcers (*see* Ulcer(s), Cushing's)
Cutaneous abscess, 875–878
  bacteriology of, 875, 875t, 876t
  clinical presentation of, 875–876
  gram stains and, 875
  treatment of, 876–877, 877t
    incision and drainage in, 877–878, 878t
CVA (*see* Cerebral vascular accident)
Cyanide poisoning, 632–636, 708–709
  antidote to, 549t
  biochemical toxicity and, 632
  clinical presentation of, 633t, 633–634
  clinical time course of, 632–633
  differential diagnosis of, 634
  laboratory studies in, 635–636
  prognosis of, 636
  sources of exposure and, 632
  treatment of, 634t, 634–635, 635f
    specific antidotes in, 635
Cyanosis, 140–141
  arterial blood gas determination in, 140–141
  central, 140, 140t, 174
    in neonate, 174–175
  in children, upper respiratory disorders and, 182
  in congenital heart disease, in children, 437
  definition of, 140
  differential diagnosis of, 141
  in infants, hospital admission and, 435
  in neonate, 174–175, 428–429
    causes of, 174–175
    central, 174–175
    diagnosis of, 175
    management of, 175
  peripheral, 140, 140t, 174
  pseudocyanosis and, 141
Cyclic antidepressants, 1080, 1082t, 1082–1083
  overdose of, 1083
  side effects of, 1082
  in ventricular tachycardia, 96
Cyclic antidepressants (CAs):
  overdose with, 551–554
    antidote for, 552
    signs and symptoms of, 551
    treatment of, 551–552
    treatment of complications of, 552–554, 553t
  pharmacology of, 551
Cyclopentolate, 838
Cycloplegics, 838
Cyclosporine (CsA):
  in organ transplantation, 1104–1105
  side effects of, 1104–1105
Cyst(s):
  functional, ovarian, 1117, 1117f
  mediastinal, diagnosis of, 469
  of upper respiratory system, 845
Cystadenoma:
  mucinous, ultrasonography in, 1117, 1118f, 1119
  serous, ultrasonography in, 1118f, 1119
Cystic fibrosis:
  asthma and bronchiolitis versus, 469
  in children, treatment of, 164
  in infants, treatment of, 164
Cystourethrography, voiding, in urinary tract infections, 463
Cytochrome A_3, inhibition of, in carbon monoxide poisoning, 703
Cytomegalovirus (CMV) infections:
  blood transfusions and, 778
  in human immunodeficiency virus infections, 520
  following organ transplantation, 1105–1106
  retinitis and, in human immunodeficiency virus infections, 522

DAE (*see* Dysbaric air embolism)
Dalmane (flurazepam), 1082t
Dalton's law, 678–679
Dantrolene, in tetanus, 526t
Daphne mezerium, 723, 724
Dapsone, in *Pneumocystis carinii* pneumonia, 274
Datura, 723, 724
Dawn phenomenon, 730–731
Daxolin (*see* Loxapine)
DCA (*see* Dichloroacetate)
DCS (*see* Decompression sickness)
Dead space, 51
  arterial Pa_{CO_2} and, 54
Death:
  in acute necrotizing hemorrhagic encephalomyelitis, 821
  from asthma, in children, 466
  brain, 4

in cyanide poisoning, 632
determination of, 4
drowning and, 688
dysbaric, 683
hydrocarbon poisoning and, 603
in iron intoxication, 598
jellyfish envenomations and, 667
in neck trauma, 928
of neonate
expected, at home, 432
(*See also* Sudden infant death syndrome)
status epilepticus and, 808
traumatic, of elderly patients, 1097
(*See also* Mortality)
"Death cap," 716
Debridement:
of burn wound, 693
in gas gangrene, 880
of scalp wounds, 1053
in wound preparation, 1037-1038, 1038f
Decabid (*see* Indecainide)
Decadron, in spinal cord compression, in malignancy, 780
Decerebrate rigidity, in altered mental status, 154
Decompression sickness (DCS), 682f, 682-683, 683t
treatment of, 684, 684f
Decontamination:
gastrointestinal (*see* Gastrointestinal decontamination)
in hazardous materials exposure, 707
in radiation injury, 713
in emergency department, 714
prehospital, 714
of skin, in cyanide poisoning, 635
Decorticate posturing, in altered mental status, 154
Deep venous thrombosis (DVT), 255-256
acute, 255
management of, 255
massive, 255
of upper extremity, 255
of lower extremities, 255
postoperative, 367
pulmonary embolism and, 235
thrombolytic therapy in, 255-256
DEET (*see* N, N-Diethylmetatoluamide)
Deferoxamine, in cerebral ischemia, 8-9
Deferoxamine mesylate, in iron intoxication, 598-599
Defibrillation, 106
in children, 106, 180-181, 181t
in ventricular fibrillation, 97
in ventricular tachycardia, 97
Defibrillators, 33-34
automatic external (AEDs), 33-34
implantable, 34
Definitive care, in poisoning, 547, 549t, 549-550
Deglutition, 303
Dehiscence, of wound, 366
gynecologic procedures and, 423
Dehydration, 64
estimating, 161
hypernatremic, 162
fluid volume restoration in, 163
hyperthermia and, 654
hyponatremic, 161-162
fluid volume restoration in, 163
isonatremic, 161
fluid volume restoration in, 163
magnitude of, in children, 161
metabolic alkalosis and, 47
Dehydroemetine, in diarrhea, 351t
Delirium, 1068
in acquired immune deficiency syndrome, 522
Delirium tremens, 577
Delivery (*see* Obstetric delivery)
Delusion(s):
bizarre, 1069
grandiose, 1069
Delusional disorder:
organic, 1068
paranoid, 1070
Dementia, 1068, 1100
in acquired immune deficiency syndrome, 521, 522
of depression, reversible, 1068
Demerol (meperidine), during pregnancy, 407
Dental emergencies, 860-866
anatomy of teeth and, 860
dentoalveolar trauma and, 862-865, 863f, 864f
hemorrhage and, 865-866
postoperative, 866
secondary to extraction, 865
spontaneous, 865
normal periodontium and, 860, 861f
oral and facial pain and, 860-862
odontogenic, 860-861
oral manifestations of systemic disease and, 861-862
oral medicine emergencies and, 861
periodontal emergencies and, 861
(*See also headings beginning with term* Tooth)
Dentoalveolar trauma, 862-865, 863f
alveolar fractures and, 864
fractures and, 862-863
soft tissue injury and, 865
subluxed and avulsed teeth and, 863-864, 864f
Depakene (*see* Valproic acid)
Depakote (*see* Valproic acid)
Depersonalization disorder, 1072
Depression:
in acquired immune deficiency syndrome, 522
major, 1070, 1070f
DeQuervain's stenosing tenosynovitis, 975, 975f
Dermatitis:
diaper, in neonate, 429
exfoliative, 869-871
clinical evaluation and treatment of, 869
differential diagnosis of, 869
etiology and pathogenesis of, 869, 869t
irritant, sponge envenomations and, 667
in lead poisoning, 713
pruritic, sponge envenomations and, 667
seborrheic, in human immunodeficiency virus infections, 521
Toxicodendron, 867-868
clinical features of, 867, 868f
differential diagnosis of, 868
prophylaxis of, 868
treatment of, 868
Dermoid(s), ultrasonography in, 1117, 1117f
DESD (*see* Detrusor-external sphincter dyssynergia)
"Designer drugs," 583, 586
Desmopressin acetate, in hemophilia, 771
Desoxycorticosterone acetate (Percorten), in adrenal crisis, 762
Dessicants, 695
"Destroying angel," 716
Detoxification, in coelenterate envenomations, 668
Detrusor-external sphincter dyssynergia (DESD), in multiple sclerosis, 818
Developmental abnormalities, seizures and, in neonate, 172
Devic's syndrome, 818
Dexamethasone:
in acute mountain sickness, 673
in adrenal crisis, 762
in head injury, severe, 919
in meningitis, in children, 455
in migraine headache, 790
in Reye's syndrome, 477
Dextrose:
in neonatal resuscitation, 171
in status epilepticus, 809
Diabetes insipidus (DI), hypernatremia and, 69
Diabetes mellitus:
anorexia nervosa in, 1086
in children, 502-504
diabetic ketoacidosis and, 502-503
diagnosis of, 502
etiology of, 502
hypoglycemia and, 503-504
incidence of, 502
early, 728
insulin-dependent drivers and, 731
oral manifestations of, 861-862
in pregnancy, 409
rigid versus tight control of, 731
thoracic pain and, 896
type I (IDDM; insulin-dependent), in children, 502-504
Diabetic ketoacidosis (DKA), 44, 735-739
abdominal pain and, 145
in children, 502-503
cerebral edema and, 503
treatment of, 164, 502-503
clinical presentation of, 735-736
complications of, 739
differential diagnosis of, 736f, 736-737
laboratory studies in, 736-737
mortality in, 739
pathogenesis of, 735
precipitating factors for, 735
treatment of, 737-739, 738f
Diagnostic and Statistical Manual of Mental Disorders (DSM-III-R), 1067
Diagnostic image, computed tomography and, 3
Diagnostic peritoneal lavage (DPL):
abdominal computed tomography versus, 9
in abdominal trauma, 955, 956
to posterior abdomen, 962
in appendicitis, 321
in pediatric trauma victim, 912
in perforated viscus, 318
Dialysis:
in acute renal failure, 372
in chronic renal failure, 374
problems related to vascular access and, 375-376
intermittent, in acute renal failure, 372
in iron intoxication, 599
in nonsteroidal anti-inflammatory drug overdose, 629
peritoneal (*see* Peritoneal dialysis)
(*See also* Hemodialysis)
Dialysis disequilibrium, in chronic renal failure, 375
Diamox (*see* Acetazolamide)
Diaper rash, in neonate, 429
Diaphragmatic injury, 939-940, 960
computed tomography in, 10
diagnosis of, 940
etiology of, 939

Diaphragmatic injury (*Cont.*):
natural history of, 939–940
rupture and, in pelvic fracture, 987
Diarrhea, 347–352
in acute gastroenteritis, in children, 488
bacterial
in children, 488
in neonate, 427
bacterial infections and, treatment of, 348–350
bloody
in acute gastroenteritis, 488–489
in children, 492
in neonate, 427
in children, 427, 488, 492, 492t
treatment of, 165
etiology of, 347–350, 348t
bacterial infections and, 348–350
ciguatera fish poisoning and, 350
parasites and, 350
viral infections and, 347–348
in human immunodeficiency virus infections, 523
inflammatory, 347
management of, 350, 351t, 352
in neonate, 427
parasites and, treatment of, 350
parenteral, in neonate, 427
pathophysiology of, 347, 347t
viral, in children, 488
watery, 347, 347t
in acute gastroenteritis, 489
Diazepam (Valium), 1082t
in cyclic antidepressant overdose, 552
for emergency delivery, 419t
in ethanol withdrawal, 577
for pediatric sedation, 513t, 514
in seizures
in children, 455, 482t
in neonate, 173
in status epilepticus, 809
in children, 484, 485, 485t
in tetanus, 526t
Diazoxide (Hyperstat):
actions and pharmacology of, 242
in hypertensive emergencies, 240t, 241t, 242
indications for, 242
side effects and contraindications to, 242
use of, 242
DIC (*see* Disseminated intravascular coagulation)
Dichloroacetate (DCA), in lactic acidosis, 750
Dicloxacillin:
in cutaneous abscess, 878t
in impetigo, in children, 448
in periorbital/orbital cellulitis, in children, 452t
Dicobalt edetate (Kelocyanor), in cyanide poisoning, 635
Dicoumarol, in hypoprothrombinemia, 768
Dieffenbachia, 723, 724
Dientamoeba fragilis, diarrhea and, 350
Diet, 329–330
in acute renal failure, 372
in colonic diverticular disease, 334
in diarrhea, 352
in fissure in ano, 339
high-fat, metabolic acidosis and, 45
N, N-Diethylmetatoluamide (DEET), in malaria prophylaxis, 534
Differential blood count, in Reye's syndrome, 476
Diffuse axonal injury, 914
Diffusion, 51–52
diffusing capacity and, 52
through respiratory membrane, 52
Digibind (*see* Digoxin-specific antibody fragments)
Digitalis:
in congestive heart failure, 217
in cyclic antidepressant overdose, 554
in dilated cardiomyopathy, 227
Digitalis toxicity, 617–618
clinical presentation and evaluation in, 617–618
acute versus chronic toxicity and, 617–618, 618t
laboratory studies in, 617
management of, 618t, 618–619
antidote therapy and, 619
gastrointestinal decontamination and enhanced elimination in, 619
life-threatening conditions and, 618
predisposing factors for, 617
Digoxin (Lanoxin), 121–122
actions of, 121
adverse effects of, 122
in atrial fibrillation, 91, 205
in congestive heart failure, in neonate, 175
dosing and administration of, 121–122
drug interactions of, 122
electrophysiologic actions of, 110t
in heart failure, in aortic regurgitation, 224
indications for, 121
in mitral regurgitation, 221
in mitral stenosis, 221
pharmacokinetics of, 121
in reentrant supraventricular tachycardia, 93
in restrictive cardiomyopathy, 229
in sick sinus syndrome, 103
in supraventricular tachycardia, in children, 439
toxicity of, 122
ectopic supraventricular tachycardia and, 92
junctional rhythms and, 94
paroxysmal atrial tachycardia and, 92
treatment of, 122
in Wolff-Parkinson-White syndrome, 106
Digoxin-specific antibody fragments (Digibind; FAB):
in digitalis toxicity, 619
in digoxin toxicity, 122
in ectopic supraventricular tachycardia, 92
Dihydroergotamine, in migraine headache, 790
Dilantin (*see* Phenytoin)
Diltiazem (Cardiazem), 120
in acute myocardial infarction, 210
in angina, 201
electrophysiologic actions of, 110t
Diluents, in caustic ingestions, 607
Dilution, hyponatremia and, 65
Dilutional anemia, in pregnancy, 414
Dimenhydrinate (Dramamine), for emergency delivery, 419t
Dimercaprol (*see* British anti-Lewisite)
Dimercaptosuccinic acid (DMSA), in lead poisoning, 640, 642
4-Dimethylaminophenol (DMAP), in cyanide poisoning, 635
"Dinner fork" deformity, 977
"Dip-and-plateau" filling pattern, in restrictive cardiomyopathy, 228
Diphenhydramine (Benadryl):
in allergic reactions, 902
in allergy to contrast media, 214
in antipsychotic side effects, 1081
for emergency delivery, 419t
in horse serum sensitivity, 663
in Hymenoptera stings, 656
in movement disorders, 486
Diphenoxylate (Lomotil), in Crohn's disease, 329
Diphenylhydantoin, in seizures, in neonate, 172–173
Diphtheria, 811
pharyngitis and, 443
Diphtheria-tetanus-pertussis vaccine (DTP), 1050–1051
in tetanus, 879, 880t
Diphyllobothrium (fish tapeworm), 538
Diquat dibromide burns, 699
Disability, assessment of, in trauma patient, 907
Disaster management team, 195
Disaster medical services, 193t, 193–197
communications and, 195
disaster management team and, 195
emergency medical services and, 190–191
hospitals and, 195–196
key points in, 197
mass evacuation and, 197
mental health and, 197
National Disaster Medical System and, 196
organizing multiple casualty scenes and, 103, 195f
phases of disaster response and, 193–194
activation phase and, 193
implementation phase and, 193
recovery phase and, 193–194
public relations and, 196
triage and, 194
Disequilibrium, dialysis, in chronic renal failure, 375
Disequilibrium syndrome, 801
treatment of, 803
Diskitis, in children, 889
Dislocations, 970
Disopyramide (Norpace):
electrophysiologic actions of, 110t
hypoglycemia and, 732
in sick sinus syndrome, 103
in ventricular tachycardia, 96
Disseminated intravascular coagulation (DIC), 769
screening for, 767
septic shock and, 138
Dissociative disorders, 1072
Distress signal, universal, 2
Disulfiram (Antabuse), 576
Diuresis:
in barbiturate overdose, 562
in clonidine poisoning, 571
"cold," 649
excessive, metabolic alkalosis and, 46–47
hypokalemia and, 71
osmotic, in acute lithium toxicity, 560
in urinary retention, in males, 388
Diuretics:
abuse of, 1086
in acute renal failure, 372
in aortic regurgitation, 224
in congestive heart failure, 217
in neonate, 175
in dilated cardiomyopathy, 227
in heart failure, in aortic regurgitation, 224
in left ventricular pump failure, 206
loop
in cardiogenic shock, 135, 136
in hypertensive emergencies, 244–245
in mitral regurgitation, 221
in pulmonary vascular congestion, 218
in restrictive cardiomyopathy, 229

in right ventricular infarction, 207
thiazide
in congestive heart failure, 217
hypercalcemia and, 78
Diuril (hydrochlorothiazide), in congestive heart failure, in neonate, 175
Diver's reflex, in supraventricular tachycardia, in children, 439
Diverticulitis, 333
in chronic renal failure, 375
(*See also* Colon, diverticular disease of)
Diverticulosis:
gastrointestinal bleeding and, 149
lower gastrointestinal bleeding in, 335
management of, 335
pathogenesis of, 335
(*See also* Colon, diverticular disease of)
Diverticulum:
Meckel's
in children, 496
gastrointestinal bleeding and, 149
perforation of, 333
(*See also* Colon, diverticular disease of)
Diving casualties (*see* Dysbarism, diving casualties and)
Dizziness, 799
(*See also* Vertigo)
DKA (*see* Diabetic ketoacidosis)
DMAP (*see* 4-Dimethylaminophenol)
DMSA (*see* Dimercaptosuccinic acid)
DMSO burns, 699
iatrogenic, 700
Do not intubate (DNI) orders, 4
Do not resuscitate (DNR) orders, 4
DOB (4-bromo-dimethoxyamphetamine), 583
Dobutamine, 124
actions of, 124
adverse effects of, 124
in cardiogenic shock, 135
in cyclic antidepressant overdose, 553-554
in depressed cardiac output, 206
dosing and administration of, 124
indications for, 124
pharmacokinetics of, 124
in pulmonary edema, 218
Documentation, disaster medical services and, 196
Dog bites, 1044
"Doll's eye maneuver," in altered mental status, 153-154
Donnan equilibrium, 63-64, 64t
Dopamine (Intropin), 123
actions of, 112t, 123
adverse effects of, 112t, 123
in cardiogenic shock, 135
in congestive heart failure, in neonate, 176
contraindications and forms of, 112t
in cyclic antidepressant overdose, 553
in depressed cardiac output, 206
dosing and administration of, 112t, 123
drug interactions of, 123
in hypotension, in Hymenoptera stings, 656
indications for, 112t, 123
pharmacokinetics of, 123
in pulmonary edema, 218
Doppler flow evaluation:
in acute deep venous thrombosis, 255
in peripheral vascular disease, 1113, 1114
Doppler ultrasonography, 1123
in deep venous thrombosis, 367
real-time, in acute deep venous thrombosis, 255
in superficial thrombophlebitis, 255
Doppler ultrasonography:
in appendicitis, 1122
in peripheral vascular disease, 1113, 1114
Dorsal chip fractures, of wrist, 976-977
"Double-bubble sign," in abdominal trauma, 500
Doxycycline:
in chlamydial infections, sexually transmitted, 518
in gonorrhea, 517
in Lyme disease, 540
in malaria, 532t
in malaria prophylaxis, 533t
in pelvic inflammatory disease, 394t
in septic shock, 139t
in urinary tract infections, 379t
2,3-DPG, oxyhemoglobin dissociation and, 57, 57t
DPL (*see* Diagnostic peritoneal lavage)
"DPT" cocktail, for pediatric analgesia, 514
Drainage:
percutaneous, in cholecystitis, 355
surgical, in septic shock, 138
of wounds, 1041
Dramamine (dimenhydrinate), for emergency delivery, 419t
Dressler's (postmyocardial) infarction, 207
Drift:
in headaches, 789
testing for, 786
Drop test, distinguishing true neurologic deficits from conversion disorder and, 1091t
Droperidol (Inapsine), 1080t
in acetaminophen poisoning, 597
Drowning:
"dry," 688
freshwater, 688
near (*see* Near drowning)
saltwater, 688
Drug(s):
allergy to, 903
bronchoconstriction induced by, 291
hyperthermia and, 654
hypocalcemia and, 75, 75t
labyrinthitis and, 800, 800t
lactic acidosis and, 749
methemoglobinemia and, 141
neuromuscular transmission disorders induced by, 825t, 826
nonketotic hyperosmolar coma and, 744, 744t
pancreatitis and, 363, 364t
during pregnancy, 406-407
sulfhemoglobinemia and, 141
toxic hepatitis and, 359-360
weakness and, 814
(*See also* Drug therapy; *specific drugs and drug types*)
Drug abuse:
acute ischemia of extremities and, 253
septic arthritis and, 888
suicide attempts and, 1077
(*See also* Poisoning; *specific substances*)
Drug addiction, in sickle cell anemia, 774
Drug history, in psychiatric disorders, 1075
Drug intoxication, hypothermia and, 648
Drug reactions, in human immunodeficiency virus infections, 523, 524t
Drug screening:
in calcium channel blocker overdose, 620
in poisoning, 549
Drug therapy:
in acetaminophen poisoning, 595-596
in acute angle closure glaucoma, 836
in acute gastroenteritis, in children, 490
in acute mountain sickness, 673, 673f
in acute necrotizing ulcerative gingivitis, 861
in acute pancreatitis, 365
in acute renal failure, 372
in acute stroke syndromes, 238
in adrenal crisis, 762
in adrenal insufficiency, 761-762
in malignancy, 782
in alcoholic ketoacidosis, 741
in allergic reactions, 902
in alveolar fractures, 864
in amphetamine toxicity, 582
in animal bites, 1044
in anticholinergic poisoning, 637
in antidepressant overdose, 1083
in antidepressant side effects, 1082
in antipsychotic side effects, 1081
in aortic dissection, 247
in apnea, in neonate, 435
in appendicitis, 321
in aspiration pneumonia, 278
in asthma, 295-297
β-adrenergic agonists in, 295, 295t
anticholinergics in, 296-297
in children, 470-473
corticosteroids in, 296
during pregnancy, 293
theophylline in, 295-296, 296t
in babesiosis, 543
in bacterial vaginosis, 396
in barbiturate overdose, 562
in benzodiazepine overdose, 625
in beta blocker overdose, 622
for bleeding esophageal varices, 361
in blepharitis, 835
in brain abscess, 831
in bronchiolitis, in children, 473-474
in burns, 693
in calcium channel blocker overdose, 621
cardiopulmonary resuscitation and, in children, 177-180, 178t, 179f, 180f
in caterpillar stings, 659
in caustic ingestions, 607-608
in cellulitis, 881
in children, 451, 452t
in cerebral vascular accident, 795-796
in chancroid, 518
in chemical burns, ocular, 700
in childhood rashes
bacterial, 505, 506
rickettsial, 507
of unclear etiology, 509, 510
viral, 507, 508
in chlamydial infections, sexually transmitted, 518
in chronic compensated airflow obstruction, 299
in chronic decompensated airflow obstruction, 300-301
β-adrenergic agonists in, 301
atropine sulfate in, 301
glycopyrrolate in, 301
methylxanthines in, 300-301
systemic glucocorticoids in, 301
in chronic mountain polycythemia, 676
in chronic neurologic disorders, complications of, 1101
in clonidine poisoning, 571
in cocaine intoxication, 581
in colonic diverticular disease, 334
in congestive heart failure, in elderly patients, 260-261
in conjunctivitis, in children, 447, 448t
in coronary artery disease, in elderly patients, 258
in coronary insufficiency, 239

Drug therapy (*Cont.*):
in Crohn's disease, 329
in cutaneous abscess, 877, 878t
in cyanide poisoning, 634t, 634–635, 635f
in cyclic antidepressant overdose, 551, 552–554, 553t
in deep venous thrombosis, 367
acute, 255
massive, 255
of upper extremity, 255
in diabetic ketoacidosis, 737–739, 738f
in diarrhea, 348–350, 351t, 352
in digitalis toxicity, 618, 619
in disseminated intravascular coagulation, 769
in eclampsia, 239
in elderly patients, 261
in congestive heart failure, 260–261
in coronary artery disease, 258
for emergency delivery, 419t
in encephalitis, 830
in endometritis, 424
in epiglottitis, 844
in erysipelas, 881
in erythema multiforme, 872
in esophageal trauma, 309
in ethanol poisoning, 576
in ethanol withdrawal, 577
in ethylene glycol poisoning, 574
in food impaction, 310–311
in frostbite, 646
in gas gangrene, 880
in genital herpes, 396
in genital warts, 518
in gonorrhea, 517
in gout, 889
in granuloma inguinale, 518
in hallucinogen intoxication, 587
in hazardous materials exposure, 708, 709
in head injury, severe, 919
in headaches due to idiopathic cranial neuralgias, 792
in hemophilia, 772
in *Hemophilus influenzae* pneumonia, 265
in herpes progenitalis, 518
in herpes simplex keratitis, 836–837
in high altitude pulmonary edema, 675
in human immunodeficiency virus infections, 521t, 521–522, 523
in hydrocarbon poisoning, 604
in hydrofluoric acid burns, 697–698
in Hymenoptera stings, 656
in hypercalcemia, in malignancy, 781
in hypertension, in chronic renal failure, 374–375
in hypertensive emergencies, 239–245
adjuvant agents in, 244–245
adrenergic agonists in, 244
adrenergic blocking agents in, 243–244
calcium channel blockers in, 242–243
cardiovascular, 239
catecholamine-induced, 239
cellular physiology and, 240, 240f
complications of, 245
medication options and, 239–240
primary agents for, 240t, 240–242, 241t
renin-angiotensin system modifiers in, 244
secondary agents for, 242
in hypertensive encephalopathy, 238
in hypoglycemia, 732–734, 734t
in hypoprothrombinemia, 768
in hypotension, in chronic renal failure, 375
in hypothermia, 650
in impetigo, in children, 448
in infection, in malignancy, 782
in infection of cannula site, in dialysis patients, 376
in infections caused by marine animals, 666
in insect sting allergy, 903
in intestinal obstruction, 324
in iritis, 836
in iron intoxication, 598–599
in *Klebsiella* pneumonia, 265
in lactic acidosis, 750
in left ventricular failure, 239
in Legionnaires' disease, 272
in Lyme disease, 540–541
in malaria, 532t, 532–534
in masticator space infection, 858
in meningitis, 829
in children, 455, 456
in mesenteric ischemia, 251–252
in methanol poisoning, 573, 573t
in methemoglobinemia, hazardous materials exposure and, 709
in migraine headache, 790
in monoamine oxidase inhibitor overdose, 1083
in multiple sclerosis, 820
in mushroom poisoning, 719–720
in myasthenia gravis, 823–824
in myxedema coma, 757
in narcotic overdose, 566
in near drowning, 689
in nephrolithiasis, 374
in neuroleptic malignant syndrome, 556–557
in nonketotic hyperosmolar coma, 746
in oral hemorrhage, secondary to extraction, 865
in oral lacerations, 865
in oral lesions, 861
in organ transplant rejection, 1104
in organophosphate/carbamate poisoning, 634, 709
in otitis externa, 442
in otitis media, 440–441
in panic disorder, 1088, 1089
in parapharyngeal space infection, 858
in parasitic infections, 537t
in pediatric trauma victim, 911
in pelvic inflammatory disease, 393–394, 394t
in peptic ulcer disease, 313
in perforated viscus, 318
in pericoronal infection, 857
in periodontal abscess, 861
in periorbital/orbital cellulitis, in children, 452
in peripheral vascular disease, 254
in phenol burns, 697
in phenytoin toxicity, 565
in *Pneumocystis carinii* pneumonia, 273–274
in pneumonia
bacterial, 264t, 265, 266
in children, 459–461
Mycoplasma, 268, 269
viral, 268
in portosystemic encephalopathy, 362
in posttransplant infections, 1105
in priapism, 385
in pruritus ani, 345–346
in pulmonary edema, in hazardous materials exposure, 708
in pulmonary effusion, in rheumatic disorders, 883
in pyelonephritis, 380
in radiation injury, 712
in rapidly progressing glomerulonephritis, 373
in relapsing fever, 542
in resuscitation of potential kidney donor, 376
in retropharyngeal abscess, 844
in Reye's syndrome, 477, 478
in rib fractures, 935
in Rocky Mountain spotted fever, 541
in scabies, 658
in schizophrenia, 1069
in seizures, in children, 479, 480t, 481–486, 482t, 485t
in sepsis, in children, 454
in sinusitis, in children, 449t, 449–450, 450t
in snake bite, 662–663, 664
in spinal cord compression, in malignancy, 780
in spinal injuries, 926–927
in sponge envenomations, 667
in spontaneous bacterial peritonitis, 362
in staphylococcal pneumonia, 266
in status epilepticus, 809, 809t
in streptococcal pharyngitis, 444
in streptococcal pneumonia, group A, 266
in *Streptococcus pneumoniae* pneumonia, 265
in superficial thrombophlebitis, 255
in superior vena cava syndrome, in malignancy, 781
in supraventricular tachycardia, in children, 439
in syncope, in elderly patients, 259
in syphilis, 517
in tendonitis, 889
in tetanus, 525–526, 526t, 879, 880t
in thoracic aortic dissection, 239
in thoracic spinal degeneration, 900
in thyroid storm, 753–754
in toxic shock syndrome, 404–405
in *Toxicodendron* dermatitis, 868
in treatment of diving accidents, 684
in trichomoniasis, 518
in tularemia, 542
in ulcerative colitis, 330, 331
in ultraviolet keratitis, 835
in urethral stricture, in males, 387
in urinary tract infections, 379t, 379–380
in children, 463
in vaginitis
Candida, 395
Trichomonas, 395
in vertigo, 802–803, 803t
(*See also* Chelation therapy)
Drug withdrawal, seizures and, in neonate, 172
"Dry drowning," 688
"Dry socket" (alveolar osteitis), 861
DTP (*see* Diphtheria-tetanus-pertussis vaccine)
DTPA in radiation injury, 713
DUB (*see* Dysfunctional uterine bleeding)
Dumping syndrome, 728
Duodenum, injury to, 958, 958f
Duroziez's sign, in aortic regurgitation, 223
Duverney (iliac wing) fractures, 983
DVT (*see* Deep venous thrombosis)
Dwarfs, psychosocial, 498
Dynamic scanning, 3
Dysautonomias, in multiple sclerosis, 818
Dysbaric air embolism (DAE), 681
treatment of, 684, 684f
Dysbarism, 678t, 678–687
barotrauma of descent and, 679–680, 680f
air embolism and, 681
barotrauma of ascent and, 680–681, 681t, 682f
decompression sickness and, 682f, 682–683, 683t
nitrogen narcosis and, 681–682
treatment of, 683–685, 684f
blast injury and, 685–687

blast physics and terminology and, 685, 685f, 685t
management of, 687
primary (type I) blast injury and, 686
secondary (type II) blast injury and, 686
tertiary (type III) blast injury and, 686
type IV blast injury and, 686
diving casualties and, 678t, 678-685
at-depth (bottom) phase and, 684
descent phase and, 684
differential diagnosis of, 684
gas laws and, 678-679, 679t
hyperbaric treatment of, 684-685
immediate management of, 684, 684f
postdive surface phase and, 684
postrecompression evaluation and, 685
predive surface phase and, 684
pressure and, 678, 678t
Dysesthesias, cervical, 892
Dysfunctional uterine bleeding (DUB), 393
Dysphagia, 303-306
cause of, 304, 305t
characteristics of, 304, 305t
definition of, 304
esophageal body, 305-306
transfer, 304-305
Dyspnea:
in congestive heart failure, 216, 217
in mitral stenosis, 220
nocturnal, paroxysmal, 216
Dysthymia, 1071
Dystonia:
acute, antipsychotics and, 1081
neuroleptics and, 556t
Dystonias:
acute, treatment of, 1081
neuroleptics and, 555
Dysuria:
in children, 462
in females, 377
in males, 378

EAI (exercise-induced asthma) (*see* Asthma, exercise-induced)
Ear:
barotrauma and, 679-680
cauliflower (auricular hematoma), 1059
lightning injuries of, 702
trauma to, 841-842
wounds of (*see also* Auricular wounds)
human bites and, 1043
regional nerve block for repair of lacerations and, 1035, 1035f
EBV (*see* Epstein-Barr virus)
Ecchymosis, scrotal, following surgery for inguinal hernia, 369
ECF (*see* Extracellular fluid)
Echocardiography:
in acute myocardial infarction, 203
in acute pericarditis, 230-231
in chest pain, 129
in chronic compensated airflow obstruction, 299
in constrictive pericarditis, 232
in cyanosis, in neonate, 175
in dilated cardiomyopathy, 227
in hypertrophic cardiomyopathy, 228
in myocardial contusion, 945
in penetrating injury to heart, 940
in syncope, 259
transesophageal, 1123, 1124
Echovirus 9 infection, rash in, in children, 507
Eclampsia, 238-239
postpartum, 239
preeclampsia and, 408, 408t
treatment of, 241, 243
(*See also* Hypertension, in pregnancy)
Eclipse burn (sun gazer's retinopathy), 837
ECMO (*see* Extracorporeal membrane oxygenation)
"Ecstasy" ("Adam"; MDMA; 3,4-methylenedioxymethamphetamine), 583, 586
Ectopic beats, treatment of, 117
Ectopic focus, tachyarrhythmias and, 88
Ectopy, ventricular, treatment of, 111
Edema:
angioneurotic, upper airway obstruction and, 844
cerebral, in diabetic ketoacidosis, 503
scrotal, 383
Edentulous fractures, mandibular, 851
EDH (*see* Epidural hematoma)
Edrophonium:
neuromuscular blockade and, 17
in reentrant supraventricular tachycardia, 93
Edrophonium chloride testing, in myasthenia gravis, 823
EDTA, in hypercalcemia, 79, 79t
Effective osmolality (tonicity), 63
EGTA (*see* Esophageal gastric tube airway)
Eight-nerve lesions, vertigo and, 800, 800t
Elbow dislocation, 985, 985f
Elbow trauma, 984-985
Elder abuse, 1098t, 1098-1099
Elderly patients:
acute renal failure in, 372
apathetic thyrotoxicosis in, 753
appendicitis in, 320
cardiovascular changes in, 257, 257t
congestive heart failure in, 260-261
coronary artery disease in, 258
drug therapy in, 261
hypertension in, 257-258
hypoglycemia in, 730
injury in, 1097-1098
mechanics and anatomic aspects of, 1097-1098, 1098t
mushroom poisoning in, 718
syncope in (*see* Syncope, in elderly patients)
thrombolytic therapy in, in acute myocardial infarction, 212
tuberculosis in, 282
valvular heart disease in, 260
Electrical injuries, 693-694
Electrocardiography (ECG):
in aberrant versus ventricular tachyarrhythmias, 97, 98t
in accelerated idioventricular rhythm, 95, 96f
in acute myocardial infarction, 202, 202t, 204f
in acute pericarditis, 230
ambulatory monitoring of, in syncope, 260
in anticholinergic poisoning, 637
in aortic regurgitation, 223
in asthma, 292
in atrial fibrillation, 91, 91f
in atrial flutter, 90, 91f
in atrioventricular block
first-degree, 99, 99f
second-degree Mobitz I (Wenckebach), 99f, 99-100
second-degree Mobitz II, 100, 100f
third-degree (complete), 100, 100f
in atrioventricular dissociation, 98f, 98-99, 99f
in calcium channel blocker overdose, 620
in carbon monoxide poisoning, 705
in chest pain, 128-129, 129t
hyperventilation and, 132
in congestive heart failure, 217
in constrictive pericarditis, 232
in cyanosis, in neonate, 175
in cyclic depressant overdose, 551, 552
in dilated cardiomyopathy, 227
in electromechanical dissociation, 102, 103f
His bundle, in atrioventricular block, 99
in hypercalcemia, 79
in hypertrophic cardiomyopathy, 228
in hypocalcemia, 76
in hypothermia, 648, 649f
in idioventricular rhythm, 102, 103f
in junctional premature contractions, 93-94, 94f
in junctional rhythms, 94, 94f
in mitral stenosis, 220
in mitral valve prolapse, 222
in multifocal atrial tachycardia, 90, 90f
in myocardial contusion, 944
in myocarditis, 229
normal electrocardiogram and, 86-87, 87f
in penetrating injury to heart, 940
in phenytoin toxicity, 563
in preexcitation syndromes, 103f, 103-104, 104f, 105f
in pregnancy, 414
in premature atrial contractions, 89, 90f
in premature ventricular contractions, 94f, 94-95
in primary adrenal insufficiency, 760
in pulmonary embolism, 234, 234t
in pulmonary stenosis, 225
in restrictive cardiomyopathy, 228-229
in Reye's syndrome, 476
in sick sinus (tachycardia-bradycardia) syndrome, 103, 103f
signal-averaged, in syncope, 260
in sinoatrial block, 98, 98f
in sinus arrest (pause), 98, 98f
in sinus arrhythmia, 89, 89f
in sinus bradycardia, 89, 89f
in sinus tachycardia, 89, 89f
in supraventricular tachycardia, 92, 92f
in children, 439
in syncope, in elderly patients, 259, 260
transtelephonic monitoring of, in syncope, 260
in tricuspid regurgitation, 224
in tricuspid stenosis, 224
in unifascicular block
left anterior superior fascicle, 100-101, 101f
left posterior inferior fascicle, 101, 101f
right bundle branch, 101, 102f
in ventricular fibrillation, 97, 97f
in ventricular parasystole, 95, 95f
in ventricular tachycardia, 96, 96f
Electroencephalography (EEG):
in ethanol withdrawal, 577
in seizures, 807
Electrolytes (*see* Fluids and electrolytes; *specific electrolytes*)
Electromechanical dissociation (EMD), 102, 103f
treatment of, 114t, 122
Electromyography (EMG):
in myasthenia gravis, 823
in neck pain, 893
Electroneuromyography, in acute cervical disk herniations, 894
Ellis fractures, 862-863

Embolectomy:
in peripheral vascular disease, 254
pulmonary, 235-236
Embolism, arterial, in mesenteric ischemia, 250
Embolization, missile, 1023
Embolus, differentiating thrombosis from, 253-254
EMD (*see* Electromechanical dissociation)
Emergency medical services (EMS), 189-192
local role in, 189-191
access to care and, 190
communications and, 189
consumer participation and, 190
critical care units and, 190
disaster linkage and, 190-191
facilities and, 190
independent review and evaluation and, 190
manpower and, 189
mutual aid agreements and, 191
public information and education and, 190
public safety agencies and, 190
standard patient record and, 190
training and, 189
transfer of care and, 190
transportation and, 189-190
medical control of, 191-192
aeromedical transport and, 192
emergency cardiac care and, 191
medical and pediatric care and, 191-192
off line, 191
on line, 191
trauma care and, 191
state role in, 189
Emergency medical technician (EMT), training of, 189
Emesis, coffee-ground, 147
EMG (*see* Electromyography)
Eminase (anisoylated plasminogen streptokinase activator complex), in acute myocardia infarction, 212, 212t
Emotional arousal, 1096
Emotional first aid, in crises, 1095
Emotional support, in crisis intervention, 1094-1095
Emotional ventilation, in crisis intervention, 1095
Emphysema:
pulmonary, 298
subcutaneous, chest wall injuries and, 934-935
Empyema, 277-278
of gallbladder, 353
subdural, altered mental status and, 156
treatment of, 278
EMS (*see* Emergency medical services)
EMT (*see* Emergency medical technician)
Enalapril, in dilated cardiomyopathy, 227
Encainide (Enkaid), electrophysiologic actions of, 107t
Encephalitis, 830
clinical presentation in, 830
laboratory studies in, 830
seizures and, in neonate, 172
subacute (AIDS dementia complex; HIV encephalopathy), 521
treatment of, 830
viral, altered mental status and, 156
Encephalomyelitis:
acute necrotizing hemorrhagic, 817, 821
postinfectious (acute disseminated encephalomyelitis; ADE), 817, 821
Encephalopathy:
hepatic (*see* Portosystemic encephalopathy)
human immunodeficiency virus (AIDS dementia complex; subacute encephalitis), 521
hypertensive, 238, 238f
hypoxic-ischemic, seizures and, 172
in lead poisoning, 639
pancreatic, Reye's syndrome versus, 476
portosystemic (*see* Portosystemic encephalopathy)
Udorn, 475
Wernicke's
in alcoholism, 576
altered mental status and, 156
treatment of, 576
Endobronchial intubation, in hemoptysis, 278
Endocarditis, in narcotic overdose, 567
Endocrine system:
altered mental status and, 156
hypoglycemia and, 729
in hypothermia, 649
Endometrioma, ultrasonography in, 1118f, 1119
Endometriosis, 392
Endometritis, 410-411
following induced abortion, 424
following spontaneous abortion, 391
Endoscopy:
in esophageal disease, 308
in gastrointestinal bleeding, 148
in great vessel injury, 948
in neck trauma, 930
Endotoxin:
antiserum to, in septic shock, 138
septic shock and, 136-137
Endotracheal intubation, 11
as alternative to vascular access, in children, 169-170
cardiopulmonary resuscitation and, in children, 176
in epiglottitis, in children, 184
in upper airway obstruction, 845
Endotracheal suctioning, in aspiration pneumonia, 278
Enkaid (*see* Encainide)
Entamoeba histolytica, diarrhea and, 350
treatment of, 351t
Enteric fever, 347, 348
treatment of, 349
Enteritis, regional (*see* Crohn's disease)
Enterobius (pinworm) infections, 536
Enterobius vermicularis, in children, 464
Enterocolitis, necrotizing (*see* Necrotizing enterocolitis)
Enteroviruses, rash and, in children, 507
"Entrance block," 95
Entrapment injuries, penile, 384, 385f
Envenomations:
from insects (*see* Insect and spider bites/stings)
from marine animals (*see* Marine animals, trauma and envenomations from)
Enzyme immunoassays, in meningitis, 829
EOA (*see* Esophageal obturator airways)
Ephedrine:
for emergency delivery, 419t
in neurogenic shock, 139
Epi-Pen, in Hymenoptera stings, 657
Epicardial "fat pad sign," in acute pericarditis, 230
Epidemic keratoconjunctivitis, 834
Epididymis:
anatomy of, 382
appendages of, torsion of, 386
Epididymitis, 386, 386t
Epidural hematoma (EDH), 915, 916f
acute, altered mental status and, 156
computed tomography and, 8
traction headache and, 791
Epiglottitis, 843f, 843-844
in children, 183f, 183-184, 184f
airway management in, 184
diagnosis of, 183f, 183-184, 184f
supportive therapy in, 184
Epilepsia partialis continua, 485
Epilepsy:
altered mental status and, 156
definition of, 479
(*See also* Seizures)
Epinephrine, 122-123
actions, indications, dosage and administration, adverse effects, contraindications, and forms of, 114t
adverse effects of, 122-123
in allergic reactions, 902
in asthma, 295, 295t
cardiopulmonary resuscitation and, in children, 178t, 179, 180f, 180t
in chronic decompensated airflow obstruction, 301
for diagnostic peritoneal lavage, 956
dosing and administration of, 122
for emergency delivery, 419t
in Hymenoptera stings, 656
hypokalemia and, 71
indications for, 122
in neonatal resuscitation, 171
in oral hemorrhage, secondary to extraction, 865
pharmacokinetics of, 122
for regional nerve block, 1031, 1032, 1034
for topical anesthesia, 1035
Epiphyseal injuries, 985
Episiotomy, 419
Epistaxis, 846
anterior, 846
posterior, 846
Epstein-Barr virus (EBV):
blood transfusions and, 778
in children, 508
pharyngitis and, 443
Erysipelas (St. Anthony's fire), 881
in children, 505
clinical features of, 881
treatment of, 881
Erythema infectiosum (fifth disease), in children, 507-508
Erythema multiforme, 870-872, 902
diagnosis and treatment of, 872
differential diagnosis of, 871
pathology and clinical characteristics of, 870f, 870t, 870-871, 871f
Erythema nodosum, in children, 508-509
Erythrocyte sedimentation rate:
in pneumonia, in children, 458
in pregnancy, 414
Erythromycin:
in bacterial pneumonia, 264t, 266
in chancroid, 518
in conjunctivitis, in children, 447, 448t
in cutaneous abscess, 878t
in diarrhea, 351t
in impetigo, in children, 448
in Lyme disease, 540
ophthalmic, 838
in oral lacerations, 865
in oral lesions, 861
in otitis media, 440-441

in pertussis
in children, 460
prophylaxis of, 460
in pneumonia
in children, 461
in neonate, 428t
during pregnancy, 406
in relapsing fever, 542
in septic shock, 139t
in sinusitis, in children, 449t
in tetanus, 526t
in urinary tract infections, 379t
Erythromycin base, in chlamydial infections, sexually transmitted, 518
Escharotomy, 693, 693f
Escherichia coli:
diarrhea and, 348
treatment of, 351t
urinary tract infections and, 377
Esmarch's bandage, fingertip injuries and, 1062
Esmolol (Brevibloc), 117
actions of, 111, 117
in acute myocardial infarction, 211
adverse effects of, 117
in atrial fibrillation, 91
in cardiogenic shock, 136
dosage, actions, pharmacokinetics, and indications for, 112t
dosing and administration of, 117
indications for, 117
pharmacokinetics of, 117
in reentrant supraventricular tachycardia, 93
in Wolff-Parkinson-White syndrome, 105
Esophageal bleeding, 306-307 (*see* Esophageal bleeding)
arterial, 307
capillary, 307
life-threatening or massive, 307
major, 306-307
mild, 306
moderate, 306
venous, 307
Esophageal colic, 306
Esophageal disorders, chest pain and, 131
Esophageal emergencies, 303-309
anatomy and physiology and, 303, 304f
deglutition and propulsion of food bolus and, 303
venous system and, 303, 305f
Blakemore intubation in, 308-309
endoscopy in, 308
extraesophageal manifestations of, 307
chest pain and, 307
pulmonary, 307
starvation and failure to thrive as, 307
nasogastric intubation in, 307-308, 308f
presenting symptoms of, 303-307
in bleeding esophagus, 306-307
in dysphagia, 303-306, 305t
in esophageal colic, 306
in heartburn, 306
in odynophagia, 306
in regurgitation, 306
traumatic, 309
diagnosis of, 309
etiology of, 309
pathogenesis and clinical presentation of, 309
symptoms of laceration and perforation and, 309
Esophageal gastric tube airway (EGTA), 11
Esophageal laceration, 309
Esophageal obturator airways (EOA), 10-11, 11f
Esophageal perforation, 309
foreign bodies and, 310
Esophageal reflux, chest pain and, 128
Esophageal spasm, chest pain and, 127
Esophageal tracheal comitube, 11
Esophageal varices, bleeding, 361
management of, 361
Esophagitis:
gastrointestinal bleeding and, 149
in human immunodeficiency virus infections, 523
peptic, 303
Esophagoscopy, 308, 309
Ethambutol, in tuberculosis, 283t
Ethanol:
alcoholic ketoacidosis and, 44
altered mental status and, 156
in carbon monoxide poisoning, 705
drowning accidents and, 688
in ethylene glycol poisoning, 574
hypoglycemia and, 732
in methanol poisoning, 573, 573t
phenytoin toxicity and, 563
poisoning by, 575-577, 812
clinical findings in, 576
hypothermia and, 648
pathophysiology of, 575-576
treatment of, 576
withdrawal from, 576-577
clinical features of, 576-577
pathophysiology of, 576
seizures in, treatment of, 808
treatment of, 577
Ethics:
human immunodeficiency virus infections and, 523
of resuscitation (*see* Resuscitation, ethics of)
Ethmozine (*see* Moricizine)
Ethosuximide (Zarontin):
adverse effects of, 486
in seizures, 808t
in children, 480t
Ethylene glycol:
metabolic acidosis and, 45
poisoning by, 573-574
antidote to, 549t
clinical findings in, 574, 575f
pathophysiology of, 573, 574f
treatment of, 574-575
Euphorbia pulcherrima, 723, 724-725
Euvolemia, hyponatremia and, 66t, 66-67
Evacuation:
mass, 197
nuclear accidents and, 713-714
hospital evacuation and, 713-714, 714t
Evaluation, of emergency medical services, 190
"Eve" (3,4-methylenedioxyethamphetamine; MDEA), 583
Evisceration, of wound, gynecologic procedures and, 423
Evoked-response testing, in multiple sclerosis, 818
Exanthem(s) (*see* Rashes)
Exanthem subitum (roseola infantum), rash in, 509-510
Exercise(s):
acclimatization to high altitude and, 671
bronchospasm hyperventilation induced by, 291
hypoglycemia and, 730
oxyhemoglobin dissociation and, 57
Exercise-induced asthma (EIA) (*see* Asthma, exercise-induced)
Explosives, 685
External ear squeeze (barotitis externa), 679
Extracellular fluid, volume restoration and, in children, 163
Extracellular fluid (ECF), 63, 63t
hyponatremia and, 65t, 65-67
Extracorporeal membrane oxygenation (ECMO), in diaphragmatic hernias, in neonate, 173
Extracorporeal shock wave lithotripsy, in cholecystitis, 354
Extubation, 19
Eye:
chemical burns of, 699-700, 708
deviation of, cerebral vascular accident and, 797
discharge from, in neonate, 429
examination of, 833
in neonate, 426
opening, in head injury, 917
redness of, in neonate, 429
trauma to, 837-839
from lightning, 702
(*See also* Ocular disorders; Ophthalmologic disorders)
(*See also* Ocular emergencies)
Eye pain, 836-837
in acute angle closure glaucoma, 836
in herpes simplex keratitis, 836-837
in iritis, 836
in open angle glaucoma, 836
Eye patch, 840
Eye shield, 840
Eye strain, headache and, 792
Eyelashes, in eye, 835
Eyelid:
closing of, distinguishing true neurologic deficits from conversion disorder and, 1091t
lacerations of, 837-838
Eyelid wounds, 1053-1056
anatomy and, 1053-1054
lacerations, 1055, 1055f
treatment of, 1054-1056, 1055f

FAB (*see* Digoxin-specific antibody fragments)
"Face mask squeeze," 680
Facet dislocation, cervical, 925
Facial muscles, in altered mental status, 154
Facial nerves, cheek wounds and, 1058-1059
Facial wounds, 1052
regional nerve block for repair of lacerations and, 1033-1034, 1034f
Facilitation, in crisis intervention, 1095
Factor XII (Hageman factor), septic shock and, 137
Failure to thrive (FTT):
child neglect and, 498
esophageal disease and, 307
in neonate, 431
Fainting (vasovagal syncope), 142
Falls, in elderly patients, 1097-1098
Familial essential tremor, treatment of, 117
Family:
crisis intervention and, 1094
of sudden infant death child, 436
Fansidar (*see* Pyrimethamine-sulfadoxine)
Fascial compartment syndrome, in narcotic overdose, 568
Fascicular blocks, 100-102
bifascicular, 101, 102f
trifascicular, 101-102
unifascicular, 100-101, 101f, 102f
FAT (*see* Fluorescent antibody test)
Fatty liver, in pregnancy, 410
FBs (*see* Foreign body(ies))

Febrile transfusion reactions, 778
Fecal impaction:
  following anorectal surgery, 369
  treatment of, 324
Feeding, of neonate, 425
Feeding difficulties, in neonate, 426
Feeding jejunostomy, complications of, 1109-1110, 1110t
Felon, 976
Femoral condyle fractures, 999
Femoral epiphysis:
  capital, slipped, 890, 990-991
  distal, separation of, in child, 1002
Femoral head fractures, 988
Femoral neck fractures, 988-989
Femoral shaft fractures, 991, 991f
Femoral vein, venous access and, 22
  in children, 169, 169f
Fentanyl (Sublimaze):
  for pediatric analgesia, 512-513
  rapid sequence induction and, 18
Fetomaternal hemorrhage (FMH), 415-416
Fetus:
  carbon monoxide poisoning and, 704-705
  lightning injuries and, 702
  postmortem delivery of, 413, 416
Fever:
  in bronchiolitis, 467
  in children, 158-160
    management of, 159-160
    under 3 months of age, 158
    3 to 24 months of age, 158-159, 160f
    over 2 years of age, 159
  in human immunodeficiency virus infections, 520
  in meningitis, in children, 455
  in multiple sclerosis, treatment of, 820
  in neonate, 429
  physiology of, 158
  in pneumonia, in children, 457
  postoperative, 367
  postpartum, 410-411
  seizures and (*see* Seizures, febrile)
  as symptom, 158
  in thyroid storm, 752
FFAs (*see* Free fatty acids)
FFP (*see* Fresh frozen plasma)
Fibrinolysis:
  hemostasis and, 765t, 766
  in peripheral vascular disease, 254
Fibroid(s), ultrasonography in, 1119, 1119f
"Fibroids," 392
Fibula, 1004
Fibular fractures, 1005
  of shaft, in children, 1005
Ficus, 723, 725
Field of view, computed tomography and, 2
Fifth disease (erythema infectiosum), in children, 507-508
Finger:
  human bites of, 1043
  lacerations of, regional nerve block for repair of, 1031
Finger sweeps, blind, in children, dangers of, 177
Fingernails (*see* Fingertip injuries)
Fingertip injuries, 1061-1066
  anatomy and, 1061, 1062f
  distal phalanx fractures and, 1066
    lacerations associated with, 1065, 1065f, 1066f
  general principles of management of, 1061-1062
  perionychial, 1063f, 1063-1066
    avulsion of nail bed and, 1065-1066, 1066f
    lacerations associated with distal phalanx fractures and, 1065, 1065f, 1066f
    large hematoma and, 1063-1065, 1064f, 1065f
    small hematoma and, 1063, 1064f
  pulp amputation and, 1062-1063
    exposed bone and, 1062-1063
    skin or pulp loss only and, 1062
Finkelstein's test, in DeQuervain's stenosing tenosynovitis, 975, 975f
Firearms (*see* Gunshot wounds; Wound ballistics)
First aid, for snake bites, 662, 662t
Fish tapeworm (*Diphyllobothrium*), 538
Fissure in ano (anal fissure), 339-340
  clinical features of, 339
  treatment of, 339-340
Fistula(s):
  in Crohn's disease, 329
  enterocutaneous, postoperative, 368
  of inner ear, barotrauma and, 680
  perirectal, in ulcerative colitis, 330
  rectovaginal, in ulcerative colitis, 330
  tracheoesophageal, in neonate, 173, 428
Fistula in ano, 340, 341f
  clinical features of, 340
  treatment of, 340
Fitz-Hugh-Curtis syndrome, 146, 393
Fixed-wing ambulances, 189-190
  transport of maternal patients and, emergency delivery and, 418, 419t
Flagyl (*see* Metronidazole)
Flail chest, 935-936
  pathophysiology of, 935
  treatment of, 935-936
Flank trauma, computed tomography in, 10
"Flashback" phenomenon, LSD and, 585
Flashover phenomenon, 701
Flatus:
  in aerogastralgia, 681
  decreased, in intestinal obstruction, 323
Flea bites, 658
Flecainide (Tambocor):
  electrophysiologic actions of, 110t
  in premature ventricular contractions, 95
Flexor tenosynovitis, of hand, 976
Flucytosine, in human immunodeficiency virus infections, 521-522
Fluid(s), neutral, aspiration pneumonia and, 276
Fluid and electrolyte therapy:
  in abdominal trauma, 957, 957t
  in acute gastroenteritis, in children, 490
  in acute pancreatitis, 364
  in adult respiratory distress syndrome, 289
  in alcoholic ketoacidosis, 741
  in allergic reactions, 902
  in arsenic poisoning, 641
  in aspiration pneumonia, 278
  in asthma, 294
  in barbiturate overdose, 562
  in barotrauma of descent, 680
  in bronchiolitis, in children, 473
  in burns, 692
  cardiopulmonary resuscitation and, in children, 177
  in cerebral vascular accident, 795
  in children, 160-165
    acid-base disturbances and, 162
    acidosis and, 163
    in burns, 164
    in cystic fibrosis, 164
    in diabetic ketoacidosis, 164
    extracellular fluid volume restoration and, 163
    magnitude of dehydration and, 161
    maintenance requirements and, 161
    oral rehydration and, 164-165
    potassium deficit and, 162
    in pyloric stenosis, 164
    in salicylate intoxication, 164
    in sepsis, 163-164
    shock phase and, 162-163
    in syndrome of inappropriate antidiuretic hormone, 164
    in trauma, 164
    type of dehydration and, 161-162
  in cyclic antidepressant overdose, 553
  in diabetic ketoacidosis, 737
    in children, 502-503
  in ethylene glycol poisoning, 574
  in heat exhaustion, 653
  in hemorrhagic shock, 134
  in hernia, 327
  in hypotension, in chronic renal failure, 375
  in mesenteric ischemia, 252
  in nephrolithiasis, 374
  in nonketotic hyperosmolar coma, 745-746
  in nonsteroidal anti-inflammatory drug overdose, 629
  in pediatric trauma victim, 911
  in penetrating injury to heart, 941
  in peptic ulcer disease, 314
  in perforated viscus, 317, 318
  in pneumonia, in children, 460
  in Reye's syndrome, 477
  in salicylate intoxication, 591
  in sepsis, in children, 454
  in shock, in thoracic trauma, 933
  in status asthmaticus, in children, 471
  in toxic epidermal necrolysis, 873
  in toxic shock syndrome, 404
  in ulcerative colitis, 331
Fluid balance, acclimatization to high altitude and, 670-671
Fluid intake, in congestive heart failure, in neonate, 175
Fluids and electrolytes, 62-85
  atomic weights and, 62, 62t
  correlating pH with, 37-38
  in diabetic ketoacidosis, in children, 503
  in nonketotic hyperosmolar coma, 745-746
  problems of, approach to, 62
  in Reye's syndrome, 476
  water and, 62-64, 63t, 64t
  (*See also specific electrolytes*)
Flukes (trematodes), 537-538
Flumazenil:
  in benzodiazepine overdose, 625
  for pediatric sedation, 514
Fluorescein staining, in conjunctivitis, 447
Fluorescent antibody test (FAT), in rabies, 528
Fluoxetine, 1083
  in panic disorder, 1088
Fluphenazine (Permitil; Prolixin), 556t, 1080t
  for rapid tranquilization, 1079t
Flurazepam (Dalmane), 1082t
Flutter:
  atrial, 90-91, 91f
    clinical significance of, 91
    treatment of, 91, 110, 115t, 117, 119, 121, 122
    in Wolff-Parkinson-White syndrome, 105-106
  ventricular, 96
Fly bites, 657

treatment of, 657
FMH (*see* Fetomaternal hemorrhage)
Foley catheter, complications of, 1108, 1109t
Foley catheter balloon tamponade, in epistaxis, 846
Folinic acid, in methanol poisoning, 573
Food allergy, 902–903
Food bolus, propulsion of, 303
Food impaction, 310–311
Food particles:
aspiration of, asthma and bronchiolitis versus, 469
aspiration pneumonia and, 276
Food poisoning, 347
Aeromonas hydrophila and, 349
Bacillus cereus and, 349
Campylobacter fetus and, 349
ciguatera fish poisoning and, 350
Clostridium perfringens and, 349
Cryptosporidium and, 350
Dientamoeba fragilis and, 350
Entamoeba histolytica and, 350
Escherichia coli and, 348
treatment of, 351t
Giardia lamblia and, 350
treatment of, 351t
management of, 350, 351t, 352
Salmonella and, 348–349
treatment of, 351t
Shigella and, 348
treatment of, 351t
Staphylococcus aureus and, 349
Vibrio cholerae and, 349
Vibrio parahaemolyticus and, 349–350
Yersinia and, 349
Yersinia enterocolitica and, treatment of, 351t
Foot injuries, 1012–1014
anatomy and, 1012
calcaneal fractures and, 1012
treatment of, 1012
in children, 1014
metatarsal fractures and, 1013
at base of fifth metatarsal, 1013
stress, 1013
treatment of, 1013
midpart fractures and, 1012–1013
treatment of, 1013
phalangeal, 1013–1014
treatment of, 1014
regional nerve block for repair of, 1031–1032, 1033f
talus fractures and, 1012
treatment of, 1012
tarsal-metatarsal fracture dislocations and, 1013
treatment of, 1013
Forehead lacerations, regional nerve block for repair of, 1033
Foreign body(ies) (FBs):
cardiopulmonary resuscitation and, in children, 176–177
of ear, 842
in gastrointestinal tract, in children, 496
intracranial, computed tomography and, 8
nasal, 848
obstruction caused by, relieving, 2–3
ocular, 834–835, 838
conjunctival, 834–835
corneal, 835
eyelashes as, 835
removal of, 840
in puncture wounds, 1043
rectal, 344
foreign bodies in, 344
removal from wounds, 1039
swallowed, 310–315
button batteries and, 310, 311, 311f
clinical presentation of, 310
cocaine and, 311
coins and, 311
food impaction and, 310–311
general emergency department care and, 310
pathophysiology of, 310
sharp and pointed objects and, 311
upper airway obstruction and, 843
urethral, in males, 387
vaginal, 397
vulvovaginitis and, in children, 464
Foreign body aspiration:
aspiration pneumonia and, 276
in children, 185–186
clinical manifestations of, 185
diagnosis of, 185, 185f, 186f
management of, 185–186
Formic acid burns, 697, 700
"Fortification scotoma," 838
Fournier's gangrene, 384, 384f
Fracture(s), 967–970
angulation, 967
avulsion, 967
child abuse and, 500
in children, 970–971, 971f
clinical features of, 968
closed, 967
comminuted, 967
complete, 967
complications of, 968
compression forces and, 967
crush, 967
description of, 967
gunshot, 1021
healing of, 968
impacted, 967
incomplete, 967
mechanism of injury and, 967–968
direct trauma and, 967
indirect trauma and, 967
in neonate, 431
open, 967, 970
orbital, blowout, 838
pathologic, 967
of humerus, 984
penetrating, 967
radiographic studies in, 968
rotational stress and, 967
Salter-Harris clarification of, type I and, in children, 890
Salter-Harris classification of, 970–971, 971f
stress, 967–968
in children, 890
"tapping," 967
traction (tension), 967
treatment of, 968–971
closed reduction in, 969
definitive treatment and, 968–970
immobilization in, 969–970
initial care in, 968
(*See also specific sites*)
Frank-Starling relation, 216
Free fatty acids (FFAs), in nonketotic hyperosmolar coma, 743
Free radicals, oxygen-based, cerebral ischemia and, 8
Freiburg's disease, in children, 890
Fresh-frozen plasma (FFP), in hemophilia, 771, 775–776
Friction rub, pericardial, in acute pericarditis, 230
Frostbite, 645–647
clinical features of, 645–646
complications and sequelae of, 647
deep, 646
of ear, 842
prevention of, 647
superficial, 645–646
treatment of, 646–647
Frostnip, 645
treatment of, 646
FTT (*see* Failure to thrive)
Fugue, psychogenic, 1072
Fundoscopic examination, in headaches, 789
Furazolidone, in diarrhea, 351t
Furosemide (Lasix):
actions and pharmacology of, 244
in cardiogenic shock, 136
in congestive heart failure, 217
in neonate, 175
in hypercalcemia, 79, 79t
in malignancy, 781
in hypertensive emergencies, 244
indications for, 244
in left ventricular pump failure, 206
in pediatric trauma victim, 911
in pulmonary edema, 218
in Reye's syndrome, 477
side effects and contraindications to, 244
in superior vena cava syndrome, in malignancy, 781
use of, 244
Furuncle, 876
of ear, 841

Gait, in neurological examination, 787
Galeazzi's fracture, 985
Gallbladder:
cholecystitis and (*see* Cholecystitis)
empyema of, 353
injury to, 959
perforation of, 316–317
ultrasonography and, 1120
Gallium lung scans, in *Pneumocystis carinii* pneumonia, 273
Gallstone(s):
passing, 353–354
small bowel obstruction and, 322
(*See also* Cholecystitis)
Gallstone ileus, 317
Gamekeeper's thumb, 974
Gamma globulin (immune globulin; serum immune globulin), in viral hepatitis, 358–359
Gamma rays, 711
Ganciclovir, in human immunodeficiency virus infections, 521t, 522
Gangrene:
gas (*see* Gas gangrene)
perforated gallbladder and, 317
scrotal, 384, 384f
Gardnerella vaginitis (bacterial vaginosis; BV; *Corynebacterium* vaginitis; *Haemophilus* vaginitis; nonspecific vaginitis), 396
Gas-forming agents, in food impaction, 311
Gas gangrene (clostridial myonecrosis), 880
clinical presentation of, 880
differential diagnosis of, 880
prevention of, 880
treatment of, 880
Gasoline immersion burns, 698, 700
Gastric acid, loss of:
hypokalemia and, 71

Gastric acid, loss of (*Cont.*):
metabolic alkalosis and, 47
Gastric emptying time, in pregnancy, 414
Gastric lavage:
in gastrointestinal bleeding, 148
in hypothermia, 650
in poisoning, 548
(*See also* Gastrointestinal decontamination)
Gastric motility, in pregnancy, 414
Gastric outlet obstruction, in peptic ulcer disease, 314
Gastritis:
erosive, gastrointestinal bleeding and, 149
hemorrhagic, in peptic ulcer disease, 314–315
Gastrocnemius rupture, 1005
Gastroenteritis, in children, 488–490
diagnosis of, 488–489, 489f, 489t
etiology of, 488
pathophysiology of, 488
treatment of, 489–490, 490t
Gastrointestinal bleeding, 147–149
in children, 492–493, 493t, 496
history in, 147
imaging studies in, 148
laboratory studies in, 148
lower, causes of, 149
in diverticulosis, 335
management of, 148–149
primary, 148
secondary, 148–149
physical examination in, 147–148
upper, causes of, 149
Gastrointestinal decontamination:
in acetaminophen poisoning, 596
in acute lithium toxicity, 559
in arsenic poisoning, 641
in barbiturate overdose, 562
in beta blocker overdose, 622
in calcium channel blocker overdose, 620–621
in caustic ingestions, 607
in clonidine poisoning, 571
in cyanide poisoning, 635
in cyclic depressant overdose, 552, 554
in digitalis toxicity, 619
in ethylene glycol poisoning, 574
in hallucinogen intoxication, 587
in hydrocarbon poisoning, 603–604
in iron intoxication, 598, 599
in methanol poisoning, 573
in mushroom poisoning, 719
in neuroleptic overdose, 557
in nonsteroidal anti-inflammatory drug overdose, 629
in organophosphate/carbamate poisoning, 612
in phenytoin toxicity, 565
in poisoning, 547–548
(*See also specific toxic substances under heading* Gastrointestinal decontamination)
poisonous plants and, 721–722
in salicylate intoxication, 590–591
in theophylline poisoning, 615
Gastrointestinal disorders:
amphetamines and, 582
caustic ingestions and, 606–607
in chronic renal failure, 375
in human immunodeficiency virus infections, 523
treatment of, 521t
in hydrocarbon poisoning, 602–603
in lead poisoning, 639
in myxedema coma, 757
in narcotic overdose, 568
in neonate, 426–427
nonsteroidal anti-inflammatory drug overdose and, 626
in primary adrenal insufficiency, 760
protozoan infections and, in immunocompromised host, 539
in theophylline poisoning, 615
in thyroid storm, 752
Gastrointestinal system:
foreign bodies in, in children, 496
pregnancy-associated changes in, 414
Gastroschisis, in neonate, 174
management of, 174
Gastrostomy, complications of, 1109–1110, 1110t
Gastrostomy tubes, complications of, 368
GBH (*see* γ-Benzene hexachloride)
GCS (*see* Glasgow Coma Scale)
Geiger-Müller counters, 711
Genital examination:
in abdominal pain, 145–146
in sexual abuse
of boys, 499
of girls, 499
Genital warts, 518
Genitalia, human bites of, 1043
Genitourinary problems, in males, 382–388
epididymal, 386, 386t
penile, 384–385
physical examination in, 382–383, 384t
scrotal, 383–384
testicular, 385–387
urethral, 387, 387f
urinary retention and, 387–388, 388t
Genitourinary tract:
injury to, 959
in males, anatomy of, 382, 382f, 383f
Gentamicin:
in bacterial pneumonia, 264t
in gas gangrene, 880
in meningitis, in children, 456
ophthalmic, 838
in periorbital/orbital cellulitis, in children, 452t
in pneumonia, in neonate, 428t
in pyelonephritis, 380
in sepsis, in children, 454
in septic shock, 139t
German measles (rubella), rash in, in children, 508
Gestational age, determination of, 418
Gestational tissue:
following induced abortion, 424
retained, 391
Giant cell arteritis (temporal arteritis), headache and, 791
Giardia infections, 538
diarrhea and, 350
Giardia lamblia, diarrhea and, treatment of, 351t
Gila monster bite, 665
Gingiva, 860
Gingival sulcus, 860
Gingival unit, 860
Gingivitis, acute necrotizing ulcerative, 861
Glasgow Coma Scale (GCS), 152, 152t, 907, 908t, 911
in cyclic depressant overdose, 552
in head injury, 917, 917t
prognosis and, 920
near drowning and, 690
Glaucoma:
acute angle closure, 836
acute narrow-angle, headache and, 792
open angle, 836
Globe, perforation of, 838
"Globus hystericus," 304
Glomerulonephritis:
poststreptococcal, 444
rapidly progressing, 373
Glucagon:
in beta blocker overdose, 622
in food impaction, 310–311
in hypoglycemia, 734
Glucocorticoid(s):
in adrenal insufficiency, 761, 761t
in caustic ingestions, 608
in chronic decompensated airflow obstruction, 301
in hypercalcemia, 79, 79t
in thyroid storm, 753
in treatment of diving accidents, 684
Glucose:
in alcoholic ketoacidosis, 740, 741
in altered mental status, 151
central nervous system deprivation of, 727
in cerebrospinal fluid, in meningitis, 828
hypertonic, in Reye's syndrome, 477
in hypoglycemia, 733–734, 734t
in nonketotic hyperosmolar coma, 746
in seizures, in children, 482t
sudden withdrawal of, hypoglycemia and, 732–733
Glucose homeostasis, hypoglycemia and, 727–728
Glucose-6-phosphate dehydrogenase deficiency (G-6-P-D deficiency), 774
Glycerol:
ophthalmic, 839–840
in Reye's syndrome, 477
Glycopyrrolate, in chronic decompensated airflow obstruction, 301
GMP (*see* Guanosine monophosphate)
Gold, poisoning by, antidote to, 549t
Goldman applanation tonometer, 833
Gonorrhea (GC), 517
prepubertal, 464
proctitis and, 342
Goodpasture's syndrome, 373
Goodsall's rule, fistula in ano and, 56
Gout (crystal-induced synovitis), 888–889
G-6P-D deficiency (glucose-6-phosphate deficiency), 774
Graham-Steell murmur, in mitral stenosis, 220
Gram stains, in cutaneous abscess, 875
Granulocytopenia, in malignancy, 782
Granuloma:
hypercalcemia and, 78
pyogenic, oral manifestations of, 862
Granuloma inguinale, 518
Granulomatous diseases, oral manifestations of, 862, 862f
Granulomatous ileocolitis (*see* Crohn's disease)
Graves' disease, thyroid storm and (*see* Thyroid storm)
Gray test, distinguishing true neurologic deficits from conversion disorder and, 1091t
Great toe lacerations, regional nerve block for repair of, 1032–1033, 1033f
Great vessels, injury to, 947–953
blunt trauma and, 948–953
diagnosis of, 947–948
treatment of, 948
types of injuries and, 947
Grey Turner's sign, in abdominal pain, 145
Grind test, in meniscal injuries, 1002
Group A β-hemolytic streptococcus (GABHS), pharyngitis and, 442–444

Grunting, in children, upper respiratory disorders and, 182
Guanethidine, in thyroid storm, 754
Guanosine monophosphate (GMP), cyclic, in asthma, 469–470
Guarding, in abdominal pain, 145
Guided imagery, in children, 511
Guillain-Barré syndrome, 812–813
"Gun barrel" vision (tunnel vision), 838
Gunshot wounds, 1027
 (*See also* Wound ballistics)
Gynecologic emergencies, 389–394
 (*See also specific disorders*)
Gynecologic injury, in pelvic fracture, 986
Gynecologic procedures, complications of, 422–424
 cuff cellulitis and, 423
 hysteroscopy and, 422
 induced abortion and, 423–424
 laparoscopy and, 422
 postconization bleeding and, 423
 ureteral injury and, 423
 urinary retention and, 423
 wound dehiscence and evisceration and, 423
 wound hematoma and, 423
 wound infection and, 422–423
 wound seroma and, 423
Gyromitrin poisoning:
 clinical toxicity and, 717
 pharmacology of, 716, 717t
 treatment of, 720

HACE (*see* High altitude cerebral edema)
Haemophilus influenzae pneumonia, in children, 459–460
Haemophilus vaginitis (bacterial vaginosis; BV; *Corynebacterium* vaginitis; *Gardnerella* vaginitis; nonspecific vaginitis), 396
Hageman factor (factor XII), septic shock and, 137
Hair folliculitis, scrotal, 384
Hair removal, in wound preparation, 1037
Halcion (triazolam), 1082t
Haldane effect, 55
Haldol (*See* Haloperidol)
Hallucinations, 1069, 1076
 poisonous plants and, 722
Hallucinogens:
 background and definitions of, 584
 intoxication by, 584–587
  diagnosis of, 587
  disposition and, 587
  general management strategy for, 587
Hallucinosis, organic, 1068
Hallux lacerations, regional nerve block for repair of, 1032–1033, 1033f
Halo pin tractor, complications of, 1108, 1109t
Haloperidol (Haldol), 556t, 1080, 1080t
 pharmacokinetics of, 555
 for rapid tranquilization, 1079
Halothane, toxic hepatitis and, 360
Hamman's sign, 131
 in pneumomediastinum, 939
Hampton's hump, in pulmonary embolism, 234
Hand:
 human bites of, 1043
 lacerations of, regional nerve block for repair of, 1031, 1032f
Hand and wrist, 972–980
 examination of, 972, 972f, 973f
 hand fractures and, 978f, 977–980, 979f
 hand motions and, 972, 972f
 soft tissue injuries, infections, and disorders of, 972–976, 972–976f
 wrist dislocations and, 977f, 977–978, 978f
 wrist fractures and, 977
Hand, foot, and mouth disease, rash in, in children, 507
"Hanging drop" slide test, in *Trichomonas* vaginitis, 395
HAPE (*see* High altitude pulmonary edema)
Hapten, 901
Hausner's valve, 1054
Hazardous materials exposure, 707–709
 cyanide and, 708–709
 decontamination and, 707
 hydrofluoric acid and, 709
 hydrogen cyanide and, 709
 initial stabilization and, 708
 methemoglobinemia and, 709
 organophosphate/carbamate insecticides and, 709
 patterns of injury and, 707t, 707–708
 phenol and, 709
 planning for, 707
HBcAg (*see* Hepatitis B core antigen)
HBeAg (*see* Hepatitis B e antigen)
HBOT (*see* Hyperbaric oxygen therapy)
HCM (hypertrophic cardiomyopathy) (*see* Cardiomyopathy, hypertrophic)
HCO_3^-, pH and, 38
HDCV (*see* Human diploid cell vaccine)
HDV (*see* Hepatitis, viral, hepatitis D and)
Head injury, 913–920
 anatomy and physiology and, 913
 assessment of, 916–918
  diagnostic tests in, 917–918
  history taking in, 916
  neurological examination in, 916–917, 917t
  pitfalls to avoid in, 920
  vital signs in, 916
 cerebrospinal fluid and, 913
 in child
  mild, 911
  serious, 911
 child abuse and, 500
 closed-head injuries and, 914
 computed tomography in, 7–9
  basilar skull fracture and, 8
  cerebral contusion and, 8
  cerebral edema and, 8
  helmet CT and, 8–9
  intracranial hemorrhage and, 7–8
  preparation and indications for, 7
  white matter shear injury and, 8
 delayed traumatic problems and, 920
 disposition and management of, 918–920
  herniation syndrome and, 919
  intracranial pressure and, 919–920
  in mild and moderate head injury, 918, 918t
  referral and, 918t, 919
  seizures and, 920
  in severe head injury, 919
 gunshot wounds and, 1021, 1023
 pathology and pathophysiology of, 913–916
  diffuse lesions and, 914
  focal lesions and, 914–916
  herniation and, 914, 915f
  intracranial pressure and, 913–914, 914f
 prognosis of, 920
 seizures and, in children, 482–483
 vertigo following, 801
Head lice, 658
Head tilt, 2
Head-up tilt test, in syncope, in elderly patients, 260
Headache, 789–792
 clinical evaluation of, 789
  ancillary tests in, 789
  history taking in, 789
  physical examination in, 789
 hypertensive, 791
 idiopathic cranial neuralgias and, 791–792
 inflammatory, 791
 migraine, 789–790
  classic, 790
  cluster, 790
  common, 790
  hemiplegic, 790
  immediate posttraumatic, seizures versus, 485
  ophthalmic manifestations of, 838
  ophthalmoplegic, 790
  treatment of, 117, 244, 790
 miscellaneous causes of, 792
 pathophysiology of, 789–792
 postconcussive, 791
 tension, 791
 toxic metabolic, 790–791
 traction, 791
 vascular, 789–791
  migraine, 789–790
  nonmigrainous, 790–791
Healing, of fractures, 968
Health care workers, precautions for, human immunodeficiency virus infections and, 523–524
Hearing loss:
 in otitis media with effusion, in children, 441
 sudden, 841
Heart:
 blunt injury to, 942–947
  cardiac rupture and, 943
  coronary artery injury and, 946
  diagnosis of, 943
  etiology and mechanisms of injury in, 942–943
  follow-up and, 946
  myocardial contusion and, 943–946
  pericardial injury and effusion and, 946
  postpericardiotomy syndrome and, 946–947
  septal defects and, 943
  types of, 943
  valve injury and, 943
 examination of, in altered mental status, 152
 penetrating injury to, 940–942
  diagnosis of, 940–941
  pathophysiology of, 940
  treatment of, 941–942
 rupture of
  in acute myocardial infarction, 206
  blunt injury to heart and, 943
 (*See also headings beginning with terms* Cardiac; Cardiopulmonary; Cardiovascular)
Heart disease:
 arteriosclerotic, high altitude and, 676
 congenital
  in neonate, 428
  (*See also* Heart disease, pediatric)
 cyanotic, in neonate, 174–175
 hypertensive, 229
 ischemic, (*See also* Ischemia, myocardial)
 ischemic (ischemic cardiomyopathy), 199–200, 229
 pediatric, 437t, 437–439
  abnormal pulses and, 437
  congestive heart failure and, 438, 438t
  cyanosis and, 437
  hypertension and, 437–438
  murmurs and, 437

Heart disease (*Cont.*):
  syncope and, 438
  tachycardias and, 438–439
 valvular, 220–225, 229
  aortic regurgitation and, 223–224
  aortic stenosis and, 222–223
  in elderly patients, 260
  mitral regurgitation and, 221
  mitral stenosis and, 220–221
  mitral valve prolapse and, 221–222
  prosthetic valve complications and, 225, 225t
  pulmonary regurgitation and, 225
  pulmonary stenosis and, 224–225
  tricuspid regurgitation and, 224
  tricuspid stenosis and, 224
Heart failure:
 in aortic regurgitation, 224
 "high-output," treatment of, 121
 left-sided, 216
 "low-output," treatment of, 121
 right-sided, 216
 unexplained, differential diagnosis and evaluation of, 229
Heart murmurs:
 Austin-Flint
  in aortic regurgitation, 223
  in mitral stenosis, 220
 classification of, 128
 in congenital heart disease, in children, 437
 in dilated cardiomyopathy, 227
 Graham-Steell, in mitral stenosis, 220
Heart rate, in pregnancy, 414
Heart sounds, 128
 splitting of, 128
Heart valves, injury to:
 blunt injury to heart and, 943
 in penetrating injury to heart, 942
Heartburn (pyrosis), 127, 306
Heat, loss of, 652
Heat cramps, 652–653
Heat exhaustion, 653
Heatstroke, 653–654
 drugs associated with, 652t
 treatment of, 654
Heavy metal poisoning, 638t, 638–644
Heimlich maneuver (manual thrust technique), 3
 in children, dangers of, 177
Helicopter ambulance, 190
 transport of maternal patients and, emergency delivery and, 418, 419t
HELLP syndrome, 729
Helminth infections, 535–538
Hematemesis, 147
Hematochezia, 147
Hematologic disorders:
 in heatstroke, 653–654
 in hydrocarbon poisoning, 603
 in lead poisoning, 639
 nonsteroidal anti-inflammatory drug overdose and, 627–628
Hematologic system, pregnancy-associated changes in, 414
Hematoma, 1027
 auricular (cauliflower ear), 1059
 of ear, 841–842
 intracerebral, computed tomography and, 8
 large, perionychial injuries and, 1063–1065, 1064f, 1065f
 pulmonary, 936
 septal, 1057
 small, perionychial injuries and, 1063, 1064f
 of wound, 366
  gynecologic procedures and, 423
Hematuria, in sickle cell anemia, 774
Hemiplegia:
 hypoglycemic, 733
 left-sided, cerebral vascular accident and, 797–798
Hemlock poisoning, 722
Hemodialysis:
 in acute lithium toxicity, 560
 in acute renal failure, 372
 in barbiturate overdose, 562
 in digoxin toxicity, 122
 in ethylene glycol poisoning, 574–575
 heated, in hypothermia, 650–651
 in isopropanol poisoning, 578
 in methanol poisoning, 573
 in salicylate intoxication, 591
 in theophylline poisoning, 615, 615t
Hemodynamics:
 during closed-chest massage, 1
 monitoring, in adult respiratory distress syndrome, 288
 monitoring of, in mesenteric ischemia, 252
Hemoglobin, combination with carbon monoxide, 59
Hemoglobinopathies, in hazardous materials exposure, 708
Hemolysis, mechanical, of red blood cells, by prosthetic heart valves, 225
Hemolytic anemia, in nonsteroidal anti-inflammatory drug overdose, 627–628
Hemolytic transfusion reactions, 778
Hemopathic disorders, snake bites and, 661
Hemoperfusion:
 in mushroom poisoning, 719
 resin, in digoxin toxicity, 122
 in theophylline poisoning, 615, 615t
Hemophilia, 770–772
 Christmas disease (hemophilia B), 770
  replacement therapy in, 776
 classic (hemophilia A), 770
  replacement therapy in, 776
 management of, 770–772
 mild, 770
 moderate and severe, 770
 special considerations in, 772
 von Willebrand's disease and, 770, 770t
Hemophilus influenzae pneumonia, 265
Hemopneumothorax:
 pulmonary lacerations with, 936
 treatment of, 932
Hemoptysis, 277
 treatment of, 278
Hemorrhage:
 (*See also* Bleeding)
 adrenal, insufficiency and, 760
 following anorectal surgery, 369
 cerebellar, acute, altered mental status and, 157
 control of, military antishock trouser garment and, 6
 of corpus luteum, 391
 in Crohn's disease, 329
 fetomaternal, 415–416
 hydrocephalus following, 432
 intracerebral, 915
  hypertensive, 797
 intracranial, cerebrovascular lesions and, 794
 intraventricular, altered mental status and, 157
 in malignancy, 782–783
 in middle ear, barotrauma and, 680
 oral, 865–866
  postoperative, 866
  secondary to extraction, 865
  spontaneous, 865
 in pelvic fracture, 985–986
 in peptic ulcer disease, 314
 pontine, altered mental status and, 157
 of posterior fossa, traumatic, altered mental status and, 157
 postpartum, 413
 pulmonary, in rheumatic disorders, 883
 stroke and, 795–796
 subarachnoid (*see* Subarachnoid hemorrhage)
 subconjunctival, 835
Hemorrhagic shock (*see* Shock, hemorrhagic)
Hemorrhoids, 336–339
 clinical features of, 337, 338t
 external, 337
  treatment of, 338–339
 gastrointestinal bleeding and, 149
 internal, 337
  treatment of, 338–339
 treatment of, 337–339
Hemostasis, 765–766
 coagulation factors and clotting and, 765t, 766, 766f
 endoscopic, in gastrointestinal bleeding, 148
 fibrinolysis and, 765t, 766
 platelets and, 765, 765t
 in vascular bleeding, 765, 765t
 in wound preparation, 1037
Hemothorax, 937–938
 diagnosis of, 937
 etiology of, 937
 pathophysiology of, 937
 resuscitation and, 948
 treatment of, 937–938
Henderson-Hasselbach equation, 35
Hennebert's sign, in labyrinthitis, 800
Heparin:
 in acute myocardial infarction, 209–210
 arterial blood gases and, 141
 in deep venous thrombosis, 367
 in disseminated intravascular coagulation, 769
 pulmonary, 235
 in pulmonary embolism, 235
 in thromboembolism, 207
Hepatic coma (*see* Portosystemic encephalopathy)
Hepatic encephalopathy (*see* Portosystemic encephalopathy)
Hepatic failure, fulminant, Reye's syndrome versus, 476
Hepatitis:
 alcoholic, 360–361
  emergency department management of, 361
  treatment of, 360
 in narcotic overdose, 568
 toxic, 359–360
  treatment of, 360
 viral, 356–359, 357t
  blood transfusions and, 778
  evaluation and management of, 358, 358t, 359t
  hepatitis A (infectious hepatitis) and, 357
  hepatitis B (serum hepatitis) and, 357
  hepatitis D (HDV) and, 358
  hepatitis non-A, non-B (HNANB) and, 357–358
  prevention and prophylaxis of, 358–359, 359t
Hepatitis B core antigen (HBcAg), 357
Hepatitis B e antigen (HBeAg), 357
Hepatobiliary disease, in Crohn's disease, 328–329
Hepatojugular reflex, in congestive heart failure, 217
Hepatomegaly:

in congestive heart failure, in children, 438
in human immunodeficiency virus infections, 523
Hepatorenal syndrome (HRS), 362
"Herald patch," in pityriasis rosea, 509
Hereditary essential tremor, treatment of, 117
Hernia(s), 326-327
Bochdalek's, in neonate, 173
clinical features of, 326-327
diaphragmatic
clinical manifestations of, 173
management of, 173
in neonate, 173
radiographic studies in, 173
double, 326
external, 326
femoral, 322
pathophysiology of, 326
incarcerated, 327
in children, 493-494
in neonate, 426
incarcerated (irreducible), 326
incisional, 326
inguinal
complications of surgery for, 369-370
direct, pathophysiology of, 326, 327f
indirect, pathophysiology of, 326
internal, 322, 326
Morgagni, in neonate, 173
obturator, 322
pathophysiology of, 326
pantaloon, 326
reducible, 326
Richter's, 326, 327
sliding, 326
small bowel obstruction and, 322
spigelian, 326
strangulated, 326
treatment of, 327
umbilical, 322
pathophysiology of, 326
Herniation syndrome, in head injury, 919
Herpangina, rash in, in children, 507
Herpes simplex keratitis, 836-837
Herpes virus infections:
anorectal, 342
cutaneous, with seizures, 481
genital, 396
in human immunodeficiency virus infections, 521
encephalitis and, 522
pneumonia and, 267
Herpes zoster infection, 814
conjunctivitis and, 834
Herpes zoster neuralgia, thoracic pain and, 896
Herpetic whitlow, 976
HES (*see* Hydroxyethyl starch)
Hexobarbital, pharmacology of, 561t
HF (*see* Hydrofluoric acid)
HFV (*see* High-frequency ventilation)
Hickman-Broviac catheter, complications of, 1107, 1107t
Hidradenitis suppurativa, 876
High altitude, 670f, 670-677
acclimatization to, 670-671
blood and, 670
cardiovascular, 671
exercise and, 671
fluid balance and, 670-671
limitations on, 671
sleep at high altitude and, 671
ventilation and, 670, 671t
acute hypoxia and, 671
acute mountain sickness and, 671-673, 672f, 673f
bronchitis and, 676
cerebrovascular syndromes of, 674
chronic mountain polycythemia and, 676
definition of, 670
extreme altitude and, definition of, 670
high altitude cerebral edema and, 674, 674t
high altitude pulmonary edema and, 674-675, 675t
illnesses aggravated by, 676-677
neurologic symptoms of, 673-674
peripheral edema and, 675
pharyngitis and, 676
reentry pulmonary edema and, 675
retinopathy and, 675-676
ultraviolet keratosis and, 676
very high altitude and, definition of, 670
High altitude cerebral edema (HACE), 672, 674, 674t
High altitude pulmonary edema (HAPE), 674-675
clinical presentation of, 674, 675t
epidemiology of, 674
pathophysiology of, 674-675
treatment of, 675
High-frequency ventilation (HFV), 19
High-penetration-resistant (HPR) windshield, 1052
Hip:
aseptic necrosis of, following organ transplantation, 1106
bursitis of, 991
Hip dislocations, 989-990
anterior, 989
in children, 990
posterior, 989-990
Hip fractures, 987-990
anatomy and, 987
in children, 990
of femoral head, 988
of femoral neck, 988-989
intertrochanteric, 989
physical examination in, 987-988
radiographic studies in, 988
subtrochanteric, 989
trochanteric, 989
Hip injuries, open, 991
Hirschsprung's disease, 492
in neonate, 427
Histamine-2 antagonists, in gastrointestinal bleeding, 148
Histamine$_1$ receptor-blockers, in allergy to contrast media, 214
Histamine$_2$ receptor-blockers, in allergy to contrast media, 214
History taking:
abdominal pain and, 145, 146f
in abdominal trauma, 955
in altered mental status, 152
in ankle injuries, 1007
in asthma, 292
in blunt injury to great vessels, 949, 949t
in diving accidents, 683-684
in elder abuse, 1099
in eye examination, 833
in female rape examination, 398
in great vessel injuries, 947
in gynecologic pain and bleeding, 389-390
in head injury, 916
in headaches, 789
in hypertensive emergencies, 237
in jaundice, 356
in knee injuries, 999
in neurological examination, 785
in pelvic trauma, 981
in poisoning, 545
in psychiatric disorders, 1075
in seizures, 805t, 805-806, 806t
in syncope, in elderly patients, 259
in vertigo, 802
Hives (urticaria), 902
HNANB (*see* Hepatitis, viral, hepatitis non-A, non-B and)
Homan's sign, in acute deep venous thrombosis, 255
Homatropine, 838
Homeostasis:
age-related changes in, 257, 257t
glucose, hypoglycemia and, 727-728
lactate, 747
temperature, physiology of, 648
Hookworms, 536
Hoover test, distinguishing true neurologic deficits from conversion disorder and, 1091t
Hopelessness, suicide attempts and, 1077
Hordeolum (stye), 836
Horse serum sensitivity, snake antivenin and, 663
Hospital(s):
disaster medical services and, 195-196
emergency medical services and, 190
evacuation of, nuclear accidents and, 713-714, 714t
transfer between, emergency medical services and, 190
Hospital admission:
for anorexia nervosa and bulimia nervosa, 1087
in anticholinergic poisoning, 637
in asthma
in children, 470
indications for, 294, 294t
in bacterial pneumonia, admission guidelines for, 266
in beta blocker overdose, 622
in bronchiolitis, in children, 474
in calcium channel blocker overdose, 620
child neglect and, 498
in cyclic antidepressant overdose, 554, 554f
in digitalis toxicity, 618
in frostbite, 646
in hallucinogen intoxication, 587
in hazardous materials exposure, 708
in high altitude pulmonary edema, 675
for human bites, 1043
in human immunodeficiency virus infections, 524
in hydrocarbon poisoning, 604
of infants
with apnea, 435
with cyanosis, 435
in lead poisoning, 640
in mercury poisoning, 643-644
in near drowning, 690
in peritonsillar abscess, 844
in poisoning, 550
in pyelonephritis, 380
in retropharyngeal abscess, 844
in theophylline poisoning, 616
trauma patient and, 908-909
in urinary tract infections, in children, 463
Host defense mechanisms, urinary tract infections and, 377-378
Hounsfield units (HU), 1
H_2-receptor antagonists, in peptic ulcer disease, 313-314

HRS (*see* Hepatorenal syndrome)
HTS/Dex (*see* Saline solution, hypertonic, with dextran 70)
HU (*see* Hounsfield units)
"Huffers," 602
"Huffer's rash," 603
Human bites, 1043
  hand infections and, 976
  treatment of, 1043
Human diploid cell vaccine (HDCV), in rabies, 528–529
Human immunodeficiency virus (HIV) infection, 519–524
  blood transfusions and, 778
  clinical presentations and management of, 519–523, 520t, 521t
    cardiovascular complications and, 523
    cutaneous manifestations and, 520–521, 521t
    gastrointestinal complications and, 521t, 523
    neurologic complications and, 521t, 521–522
    ophthalmologic manifestations and, 521t, 522
    psychiatric disorders and, 522
    pulmonary complications and, 521t, 522t, 522–523
    renal manifestations and, 523
    systemic symptoms and, 519–520, 521t
  disposition in, 524
  drug reactions and, 523, 524t
  ethical considerations and, 523
  immunizations in, 523
  multiple sclerosis versus, 819–820
  pathophysiology of, 519
  precautions for health care workers and, 523–524
Human papillomavirus infection, in human immunodeficiency virus infections, 521
Humeral fractures, 983–984
  of humeral shaft, 984, 984f
  proximal, 304, 983f, 984f
Humidification, of inspired air, 53
Hungry-bone syndrome, hypocalcemia and, 75
Hydatiform mole, 412
  pelvic ultrasonography in, 1116, 1116f
Hydralazine (Apresoline):
  actions and pharmacology of, 243
  in congestive heart failure, 218
  in dilated cardiomyopathy, 227
  in eclampsia, 239
  for emergency delivery, 419t
  in hypertension, in pregnancy, 409
  in hypertensive emergencies, 240t, 241t, 243
  indications for, 243
  side effects and contraindications to, 243
  use of, 243
Hydrocarbon(s), 601–604
  classification of, 601, 601t
Hydrocarbon poisoning:
  determinants of toxicity and, 601, 602t
  disposition and, 604
  epidemiology of, 601
  management of, 603–604
  presentation of, 601–603
Hydrocarbons, burns and, 698–699
Hydrocephalus, posthemorrhagic, in neonate, 432
Hydrochloric acid burns, 697
Hydrochlorothiazide (Diuril), in congestive heart failure, in neonate, 175
Hydrocortisone (Solu-Cortef):
  in adrenal crisis, 762
  in adrenal insufficiency, in malignancy, 782
  in allergy to contrast media, 214
  in Hymenoptera stings, 656
  in hypercalcemia, 79t
  in hypothermia, 650
  in myxedema coma, 757
  in status asthmaticus, in children, 472
  in ulcerative colitis, 330
Hydrofluoric acid (HF):
  burns and, 697–698, 700
  poisoning by, treatment of, 709, 709t
Hydrogen ion concentrations, 35
  (*See also* pH)
Hydrogen sulfide odor, in cyanide poisoning, 634
Hydrogen sulfide poisoning, 634, 709
Hydronephrosis, ultrasonography in, 1121
Hydrops, uvular, 844
Hydrosalpinx, 392
  rupture of, hysteroscopy and, 422
Hydrotherapy, in chemical burns, 695
Hydroxocobalamin (vitamin B_{12}), in cyanide poisoning, 635
Hydroxychloroquine, in pulmonary effusion, in rheumatic disorders, 883
Hydroxyethyl starch (HES), in hemorrhagic shock, 134
Hydroxyzine, for incision and drainage of cutaneous abscess, 877
Hymen, in prepubertal girls, 499
Hymenoptera stings (*see* Insect and spider bites/stings, Hymenoptera stings and)
Hyperactivity, amphetamines and, management of, 582
Hyperaldosteronism, hypokalemia and, 71
Hyperbaric oxygen, in cyanide poisoning, 635
Hyperbaric oxygen therapy (HBOT):
  in blast injury, 687
  in carbon monoxide poisoning, 706
  in gas gangrene, 880
  in mushroom poisoning, 719
  in treatment of diving accidents, 684–685
Hyperbilirubinemia, 356
  conjugated, 356
  in neonate, 429
  unconjugated, 356
Hypercalcemia, 77–79
  diagnosis of, 78t, 78–79
  etiology of, 77–78
  in malignancy, 781
  pathophysiologic effects of, 78
  treatment of, 79, 79t
Hypercapnia, metabolic alkalosis and, 47
Hyperchloremia, 84–85
  diagnosis of, 84–85
  etiology of, 84, 84t
  pathophysiology of, 84
  treatment of, 85
Hyperemesis gravidarum, 407
Hyperglycemia:
  in calcium channel blocker overdose, 620
  coma and, 40
  in diabetic ketoacidosis, 735
    in children, 502
  in nonketotic hyperosmolar coma, 743
  phenytoin and, 565
Hyperinflation, in pneumonia, in children, 458
Hyperkalemia, 72–74
  diagnosis of, 73
  in digitalis toxicity, treatment of, 618
  digoxin toxicity and, 122
  etiology of, 72, 72t
  in nonsteroidal anti-inflammatory drug overdose, 626
  physiologic effects of, 72–73
  treatment of, 73t, 73–74, 113t
Hyperkinetic movement disorders, seizures versus, 485
Hyperlipidemia, hyponatremia and, 65
Hypermagnesemia, 80–81
  diagnosis of, 81
  etiology of, 80–81
  physiologic effects of, 81
  treatment of, 81
Hypernatremia, 69–70
  etiology of, 69, 69t
  pathophysiology of, 69–70
  seizures and, in neonate, 172
  treatment of, 70
"Hyperoxia test," in cyanosis, in neonate, 175
Hyperparathyroidism:
  pancreatitis and, 363
  primary
    diagnosis of, 79
    hypercalcemia and, 77, 77t
Hyperphosphatemia, 82
  etiology of, 82, 82t
  physiologic effects of, 82
  treatment of, 82
Hyperpyrexia, 653
Hyperreflexia, 811
Hypersensitivity (*see* Allergic reactions)
  of carotid sinus, syncope and, 143
Hypersensitivity reactions, phenytoin and, 564–565
Hyperstat (*see* Diazoxide)
Hypertensice crisis, monoamine oxidase inhibitors and, 1083
Hypertension:
  amphetamines and, management of, 582
  benign intracranial (pseudotumor cerebri), headache and, 791
  in chronic renal failure, 374–375
  in clonidine poisoning, 570
  cocaine use and, 581
  in congenital heart disease, in children, 437–438
  in elderly patients, 257–258
  intracerebral hemorrhage and, 797
  mild, uncomplicated, 237
  in neonate, 431
  in poisoning, 547, 548
  portal, in children, 496
  in pregnancy, 408–409
    chronic, 408
    preeclampsia and, 408, 408t
    treatment of, 241, 243, 408–409, 409t
  pulmonary
    in mitral stenosis, 220
    in narcotic overdose, 567
  in rheumatic disorders, 885
  transient, 237
  treatment of, 111, 112t, 117–120, 123
  (*See also* Hypertensive emergencies)
Hypertensive crisis, treatment of, 119
Hypertensive emergencies, 237–245
  acute renal complications and, 239
  cardiovascular, 239
  catecholamine-induced, 239
  drug therapy in, 239–245
    adjuvant agents in, 244–245
    adrenergic agonists in, 244
    adrenergic blocking agents in, 243–244
    calcium channel blockers in, 242–243
    complications of, 245
    direct arteriolar dilators in, 243
    medication options and, 239–240, 240f
    primary agents in, 240t, 240–242, 241t

renin-angiotensin system modifiers in, 244
secondary agents in, 242
involving central nervous system, 238, 238f, 239t
patient approach in, 237-238
diagnostic studies and, 237-238
history taking and, 237
physical examination and, 237
pregnancy-induced hypertension and, 238-239
Hypertensive headache, 791
Hypertensive urgencies, 237
treatment of, 241-244
Hyperthermia, 652t, 652-654
altered mental status and, 156
amphetamines and, management of, 582
in hallucinogen intoxication, treatment of, 587
heat cramps and, 652-653
heat exhaustion and, 653
heatstroke and, 652t, 653-654
in multiple sclerosis, 818
in poisoning, 545
Hyperthyroidism:
hypercalcemia and, 78
thyroid storm and (*see* Thyroid storm)
Hypertrophic cardiomyopathy (*see* Cardiomyopathy, hypertrophic)
Hyperventilation, 55
in altered mental status, 153
in bronchiolitis, 467
bronchospasm and, exercise-induced, 291
chest pain and, 131-132
in cyclic antidepressant overdose, 553
syncope and, 143
Hyperventilation syndrome, 801
seizures versus, 805
Hyperviscosity syndrome, in malignancy, 781-782
Hypervitaminosis A, hypercalcemia and, 78
Hypervitaminosis D, hypercalcemia and, 78
Hypervolemia, hyponatremia and, 67
Hyphema, 838
Hypnosis, in children, 511
Hypocalcemia, 74t, 74-77
diagnosis of, 76
in ethylene glycol poisoning, treatment of, 574
etiology of, 75t, 75-76
physiologic effects of, 76, 76t
postoperative, 75
tetany and, treatment of, 113t
treatment of, 76-77, 77t
Hypochloremia, 83-84
diagnosis of, 83-84
etiology of, 83, 83t
physiologic effects of, 83
treatment of, 84
Hypochondriasis, 1072
Hypofibrinogenemia, 769
Hypoglycemia, 727-734
alimentary, 728
altered mental status and, 155-156
in anorexia nervosa, 1086
artifactual, 730
in beta blocker overdose, 622
central nervous system glucose deprivation and, 727
in children, 503-504
treatment of, 162
clinical presentation of, 733
early morning, 730-731
evaluation of, 733
exercise and, 730
fasting, 728, 730
fed (postprandial; reactive), 728, 730
glucose homeostasis and, 727-728
idiopathic, 728
induced, 730-733, 733t
alcohol and, 732
factitious hypoglycemia and, 732
insulin and, 730t, 730-732, 731t
sulfonylureas and, 732
of infancy and childhood, 733
ketotic, 733
in neonate, 431
nocturnal, 730t, 730-731
pathogenesis of, 728t, 728-733
postgastrectomy, 728
in pregnancy, 409
spontaneous, 728-730
starvation, 730
syncope and, 143
treatment of, 733-734, 734t
Hypokalemia, 71-72
in alcoholic cirrhosis, 361
in anorexia nervosa, treatment of, 1087
diagnosis of, 72
digoxin toxicity and, 122
etiology of, 71, 71t
physiologic effects of, 71-72
in theophylline poisoning, 614-615
treatment of, 72
Hypomagnesemia, 79-80
diagnosis of, 80
etiology of, 79-80, 80t
hypocalcemia and, 75
in neonate, treatment of, 172
physiologic effects of, 80, 80t
treatment of, 80
Hyponatremia, 65-69
in alcoholic cirrhosis, 361
diagnosis of, 68
dilutional, 65
etiology of, 65-67
euvolemic, 66t, 66-67
factitious, 65
hypervolemic, 67
hypovolemic, 66
in myxedema coma, 756
pathophysiology of, 67-68
pseudohyponatremia and, treatment of, 68
seizures and, in neonate, 172
treatment of, 68-69
complications of, 68-69
Hyponychium, 1061
Hypoparathyroidism:
idiopathic, hypocalcemia and, 75
primary, nonsurgical, hypocalcemia and, 75
surgery for, hypocalcemia following, 75
Hypophosphatemia, 81-82
in diabetic ketoacidosis, 738-739
diagnosis of, 82
etiology of, 81t, 81-82
physiologic effects of, 82
treatment of, 82
Hypoproteinemia, severe, metabolic alkalosis and, 47
Hypoprothrombinemia, 768
Hypopyon, 835
Hyporeflexia, 811
Hypotension:
in arsenic poisoning, 641
in aspiration pneumonia, 276
in cardiogenic shock, 135
management of, 135
in chronic renal failure, 375
in cyclic antidepressant overdose, 553
in Hymenoptera stings, treatment of, 656
orthostatic, monoamine oxidase inhibitors and, 1083
in poisoning, 547, 548
treatment of, 122, 123
Hypothermia, 648-651
abdominal injury and, 960
"accidental," 648
altered mental status and, 156
in burns, 692-693
in carbon monoxide poisoning, 706
diagnosis of, 649
etiology of, 648, 648t
high-risk patients for, 648
in hypoglycemia, 733
management of, 649-651
massive blood transfusion and, 777
"mild," 648
in myxedema coma, 756
in near drowning, 689
pathophysiology of, 648-649, 649f, 649t
physiology of temperature homeostasis and, 648
in poisoning, 545
prognosis of, 651
Hypothyroidism, 755-757
causes of, 755, 755t
clinical presentation of, 755-756
myxedema coma in (*see* Myxedema coma)
in neonate, 427
primary, 755
secondary, 755
tertiary, 755
Hypoventilation, mechanical, controlled, in asthma, 297
Hypovolemia:
hyponatremia and, 66
perforated viscus and, 316
Hypoxemia:
in alcoholic cirrhosis, 361
in chronic decompensated airflow obstruction, 300
(*See also* High altitude)
Hypoxia:
acute, high altitude and, 671
air transport of maternal patient and, emergency delivery and, 418, 419t
in asthma, in children, 468
in bronchiolitis, 467
in chronic decompensated airflow obstruction, 299
in lactic acidosis, 749
Hysteroscopy, complications of, 422

Ibotenic acid, 585-586
poisoning and
clinical toxicity of, 718
pharmacology of, 716, 717t
treatment of, 720
Ibuprofen:
overdose of, 627
in rib fractures, 935
"Ice," 583
"Ice rink sign," in corneal abrasion, 838
ICF (*see* Intracellular fluid)
ICP (*see* Intracranial pressure)
ICS (*see* Incident Command System)
IDDM (*see* Diabetes mellitus, type I)
Idiopathic hypertrophic subaortic stenosis (IHSS) (*see also* Cardiomyopathy, hypertrophic)
isoproterenol in, 621
Idiopathic thrombocytopenic purpura (ITP), 768
Idioventricular rhythm (IVR), 102-103, 103f
pulseless, treatment of, 114t

Idioventricular rhythm (IVR) (*Cont.*):
treatment of, 114t
Idioventricular tachycardia (*see* Accelerated idioventricular rhythm)
IHSS (*see* Idiopathic hypertrophic subaortic stenosis)
Ileitis, terminal (*see* Crohn's disease)
Ileocolitis, granulomatous (*see* Crohn's disease)
Ileostomy, complications of, 368
Ileum, perforation of, 317
Ileus, 322
adynamic, postoperative, 367–368
dynamic (*see* Intestinal obstruction)
gallstone, 317
paralytic, 322
Ilex, 723, 725
Iliac spine fractures, 982
Iliac wing (Duverney) fractures, 983
Ilioischial column fracture, 983–984
Iliopsoas sign, in abdominal pain, 145
Iliopubic column fracture, 984
IM (*see* Infectious mononucleosis)
Image archiving, computed tomography and, 2
Imaging (*see specific imaging modalities*)
Imaging studies, in abdominal pain, 146–147
Imipramine, in panic disorder, 1089
Immersion foot (trench foot), 645
Immersion syndrome (*see* Near drowning)
Immobilization:
in fractures, 969–970
hypercalcemia and, 77–78
Immune globulin(s) (gamma globulin; serum immune globulin), in viral hepatitis, 358–359, 776
Immunizations:
in human immunodeficiency virus infections, 523
for neonate, 431
against snake bites, 664
against tetanus, 526, 526t
in tetanus, 879, 880t
tetanus and, 1049–1051, 1050t
Immunocompromised patients:
pediatric, pneumonia in, 460
perforated viscus in, 316
protozoan infections in (*see* Protozoan infections, in immunocompromised host)
varicella in, in children, 508
(*See also* Acquired immune deficiency syndrome)
Immunologic reaction, bronchospasm and, 291
Immunosuppressive therapy:
in Crohn's disease, 329
in malignancy, 782
in multiple sclerosis, 820
in myasthenia gravis, 824
in organ transplantation, 1104–1105, 1105t
Immunotherapy, in Hymenoptera stings, 657
Imodium (loperamide), in Crohn's disease, 329
Impedance plethysmography (IPG):
in acute deep venous thrombosis, 255
in pulmonary embolism, 235
Impetigo:
bullous, in children, 505
in children, 447–448, 505, 506f
clinical findings in, 448
complications of, 448
definition of, 447
diagnosis of, 448
differential diagnosis of, 448
epidemiology of, 447
etiology of, 447
management of, 448
pathophysiology of, 448
Impetigo contagiosum, in children, 505, 506f
Implementation phase, of disaster response, 193
IMS (*see* Industrial methylated spirits)
IMV (*see* Intermittent mandatory ventilation)
Inapsine (*see* Droperidol)
Inborn errors of metabolism:
lactic acidosis and, 749
Reye's syndrome versus, 476
Incest, 399
Incident Command System (ICS), 194
Indecainide (Decabid), electrophysiologic actions of, 110t
Inderal (*see* Propranolol)
Indomethacin:
in hypercalcemia, 79t
overdose of, 626, 628
in pulmonary effusion, in rheumatic disorders, 883
Industrial methylated spirits (IMS), in phenol burns, 697
Infalyte, 165
Infant:
acute gastroenteritis in, breastfeeding and, 490
blood in stool of, 492
botulism in, 812
bowel malrotation in, 493
clonidine poisoning in, 570
hypercalcemia in, 78
hypoglycemia in, 730, 733
incarcerated hernia in, 493
intussusception in, 494
pneumonia in, 457, 459
premature, 420–421
Reye's syndrome in, 475
roseola infantum in, 509–510
seizures in, differential diagnosis of, 485
urinary tract infection in, 463
vulvovaginitis in, 464
(*See also* Neonate)
Infantile spasms, 482
Infants (*see also under specific disorders*)
Infarct(s):
cerebellar, 796
cerebrovascular lesions and, 793
lacunar, 796
Infarction:
of bowel, abdominal pain and, 144
(*See also* Acute myocardial infarction)
Infection(s):
adrenal insufficiency and, 759–760
following anorectal surgery, 369
bacterial (*see* Bacterial infections)
blood transfusions and, 778
following breast surgery, 370
of cannula site, in dialysis patients, 376
of central nervous system, altered mental status and, 156
from human bite to hand, 976
following hysteroscopy, 422
following laparoscopy, 422
in leg fractures, 1004
in malignancy, 782
from marine animal trauma and envenomations, treatment of, 666
of mid-palmar space, 976
in narcotic overdose, 566
in neonate, 426
odontogenic, spread of, 857–859
posttransplant, 1105t, 1105–1106
protozoal (*see* Protozoal infections)
pulmonary, in mitral stenosis, 220
rickettsial, rashes and, 505–506
of shunts, in hydrocephalus, 432
of urinary tract (*see* Urinary tract infections)
viral (*see* Viral infections)
of web space, 976
of wound, 366, 369–370
gynecologic procedures and, 422–423
wound contaminants and, 1027t, 1027–1028
Infectious mononucleosis (IM), 443
rash in, in children, 508
Inflammatory bowel disease:
small bowel obstruction and, 322
(*See also* Crohn's disease)
Inflammatory disorders, of hand, 975–976
Inflammatory headache, 791
Influenza vaccine, viral pneumonia and, 268, 268t
Influenza virus:
pneumonia and, 267
Reye's syndrome and, 475
Infraclavicular subclavian approach, to subclavian vein, 24
Infratentorial pressure, 151
Infratentorial syndromes, compressive, altered mental status and, 157
Infusion rate, 21–22
Inhalation injury, in hazardous materials exposure, 707t, 707–708
physical examination in, 708
Inner ear barotrauma, 680
Innominate artery, injuries to, 952
Inocor (*see* Amrinone)
Inotropic agents, 122–125
in congestive heart failure, 217
in pulmonary edema, 218
Insect and spider bites/stings, 655t, 655–659
allergy to, 903
blister beetle stings and, 659
treatment of, 659
caterpillar stings and, 658–659
treatment of, 659
flea bites and, 658
Hymenoptera stings and, 655–657
diagnosis of, 656
long-term management of, 657, 657t
pathophysiology of systemic reaction to, 655–656
treatment of, 656
type of reaction to, 655
inhalant allergy to insects and, 659
kissing bug bites and, 658
treatment of, 658
lice and, 658
mosquito and fly bites and, 657
treatment of, 657
scabies and, 658
treatment of, 658
treatment of, 113t
Insecticide poisoning (*see* Organophosphate/carbamate poisoning)
Inspection:
in knee injuries, 999
in thoracic trauma, 934
Insulin:
abuse of, in anorexia nervosa, 1086
in diabetic ketoacidosis, 735, 738, 738f
in children, 503
hypoglycemia induced by, 730t, 730–732, 731t
in nonketotic hyperosmolar coma, 746
Insulin-dependent diabetes mellitus (IDDM; type I diabetes mellitus), in children, 502–504
Insulinoma, hypoglycemia and, 728–729
Intellectual clarification, in crisis intervention, 1095

Intermittent mandatory ventilation (IMV), 19
in respiratory alkalosis, 48
synchronized (SIMV) (*see* Synchronized intermittent mandatory ventilation)
Interphalangeal (IP) joint dislocation, 973-974
complications of, 974
Interscan delay, 3
Interstitial fluid (ISF), 63-64
characteristics of, 63
Donnan equilibrium and, 63-64, 64t
Intertriginous infections, in human immunodeficiency virus infections, 521
Intertrochanteric fractures, 989
Intestinal colic, in neonate, 425-426
Intestinal hypomotility, in narcotic overdose, 568
Intestinal injury, occult, computed tomography in, 9-10
Intestinal obstruction (dynamic ileus), 322-325, 323f
abdominal pain and, 144
in children, 494, 494f
in chronic renal failure, 375
clinical features of, 323
closed-loop, 322-323
colonic, 322
in Crohn's disease, 329
laboratory studies in, 323-324, 324f
mechanical, 322
in children, 492
pathophysiology of, 322-323
perforation and, 317
postoperative, 367-368
pseudoobstruction and, 324-325
small intestinal, 322
treatment of, 324
Intestinal tubes, in intestinal obstruction, 324
Intoxication, 1068
Intraabdominal abscess, postoperative, 368
Intraabdominal injuries, in pregnancy, 415
Intraarterial digital subtraction angiography, in blunt trauma to great vessels, 952
Intracellular fluid (ICF), 63, 63t, 64
Intracellular shifts, hypokalemia and, 71
Intracerebral hematoma, computed tomography and, 8
Intracerebral "steal" syndrome, 795
Intracranial pressure (ICP):
elevated, in Reye's syndrome, 477
in head injury, 919-920
in child, 911
head injury and, 913-914, 914f
monitoring of, in near drowning, 690
Intraocular lens implants, 840
Intraocular pressure, measurement of, 833
Intrathoracic-extrathoracic pressure gradient, during closed-chest massage, 1
Intravascular volume, in hypothermia, 649
Intravenous pyelography (IVP):
in nephrolithiasis, 373-374
in ureteral injury, 423
Intropin (*see* Dopamine)
Intubation:
in cervical spinal injury, 16
extubation and, 19
nasotracheal (*see* Nasotracheal intubation)
orotracheal (*see* Orotracheal intubation)
retrograde tracheal (RTI), 15
Intussusception, 343
in children, 494-495, 495f
in neonate, 427
Iodide, in thyroid storm, 753
Iodoquinol:
in diarrhea, 351t
in parasitic infections, 537t
IP (*see* Interphalangeal joint dislocation)
Ipecac, in poisoning, 547-548
poisonous plants and, 721-722
(*See also* Gastrointestinal decontamination)
IPG (*see* Impedance plethysmography)
Ipratropium bromide, in asthma, in children, 470
Iritis:
acute, 836
headache and, 792
traumatic, 838-839
Iron, poisoning by, antidote to, 549t
Iron intoxication, 598-600
clinical picture of, 598
pathophysiology of, 598
toxic dose and, 598
treatment of, 598-599
pitfalls in, 599t, 599-600
Irradiation (*see* Radiation; radiation injuries)
Irrigation:
in chemical burns, 695-696
ocular, 699
of wounds, 1038
Irritability, in neonate, 425-426, 426t
Irritable bowel syndrome, colonic diverticulitis differentiated from, 333-334
Irritants, upper airway obstruction and, 844
Ischemia:
of bowel, abdominal pain and, 144
cerebral, 8-9
clinical implications of, 9
early reperfusion phase of, 8-9
ischemic phase of, 8
late reperfusion phase of, 9
syncope and, 143
cerebrovascular lesions and, 793
of extremities, acute, 253-254
intestinal, "nonocclusive," 251
low-output, 250
mesenteric, 250-252
anatomy and pathophysiology of, 250
clinical presentation of, 250-251
diagnostic studies in, 251
treatment of, 251-252
myocardial
abdominal pain and, 145
chest pain and, 127
pathophysiology of, 199, 199f, 199t
symptoms other than chest pain in, 128
syncope and, 142
treatment of, 111, 117
signs and symptoms of (five P's), 254
"silent," chest pain and, 130
thrombotic, cerebrovascular lesions and, 793
Ischemic heart disease, 199-200, 229
natural history of, 199-200
pathophysiology of, 199, 199f, 199t
ultrasonography in, 1123f, 1123-1124, 1124f
(*See also* Ischemia, myocardial)
Ischemic necrosis, in narcotic overdose, 568
Ischemic stroke syndromes, 796
Ischial tuberosity fractures, 982
Ischiorectal abscess, 56
Ischium, fracture of, 982-983
ISF (*see* Interstitial fluid)
Islet-cell tumor of pancreas, hypoglycemia and, 728-729
Isodensity, computed tomography and, 4
Isoetharine, in chronic decompensated airflow obstruction, 301
Isoetharine mesylate, in asthma, 295t
Isoniazid:
in human immunodeficiency virus infections, 521t
in tuberculosis, 283t
Isopropanol (rubbing alcohol) poisoning, 577-578
clinical features of, 577
pathophysiology of, 577
treatment of, 577-578
Isoproterenol (Isuprel), 123-124
actions, indications, dosage and administration, adverse effects, contraindications, and forms of, 114t
actions of, 123
adverse effects of, 124
in bradyarrhythmias, 88
in congestive heart failure, in neonate, 175-176
dosing and administration of, 124
indications for, 124
in neonatal resuscitation, 171
pharmacokinetics of, 124
in second-degree Mobitz I (Wenckebach) atrioventricular block, 100
in sinoatrial block, 98
in status asthmaticus, in children, 472
in third-degree (complete) block, 100
in torsade de pointes, 96
Isoptin (*see* Verapamil)
Isosorbide dinitrate:
in angina, 200t
in congestive heart failure, 218
Isospora belli, diarrhea and, 350
Isuprel (*see* Isoproterenol)
ITP (*see* Idiopathic thrombocytopenic purpura)
Ivermectin, in parasitic infections, 537t
IVR (*see* Idioventricular rhythm)

Jamaican vomiting sickness, 475
James fibers, 103, 103f
Jaundice, 356, 356t
in children, 493, 493t
emergency department evaluation of, 356
history taking in, 356
laboratory studies in, 356
physical examination in, 356
in neonate, 429, 429t
physiologic, in neonate, 429
in pregnancy, 410
(*See also* Hepatitis)
Jaw thrust, 2
Jejunostomy, feeding, complications of, 1109-1110, 1110t
Jejunum:
perforation of, 317
rupture of, 317
Jellyfish (medusae) envenomations, 667
Jequirity bean, 722
Jimson weed, 586, 637
Joint pain, in narcotic overdose, 569
Jones fractures, 1013
JPCs (*see* Junctional premature contractions)
JRA (*see* Juvenile rheumatoid arthritis)
Jugular vein:
external, venous access and, 21, 21f, 22
in children, 167-168, 168f
internal
right, transvenous pacing and, 32
venous access and, 24, 167, 167f
Junctional premature contractions (JPCs), 93-94, 94f
clinical significance of, 94
treatment of, 94
Junctional rhythms, 94, 94f
atrioventricular, paroxysmal, treatment of, 109
clinical significance of, 94
treatment of, 94, 109

Juvenile rheumatoid arthritis (JRA), 883, 884t, 889

Kaposi's sarcoma:
anorectal, 343
in human immunodeficiency virus infections, 521
Kawasaki disease (MLNS; mucocutaneous lymph node syndrome), 884
rash in, in children, 509
toxic shock syndrome versus, 403–404
Kayexalate, in hyperkalemia, 73
Keflex, in colonic diverticular disease, 334
Keinbach's disease, 977
Kelocyanor (dicobalt edetate), in cyanide poisoning, 635
Kent bundles, 103f, 104
Keratitis, herpes simplex, 836–837
Keratoconjunctivitis, epidemic, 834
Kerlone (*see* Betaxolol)
Kernig's sign:
in meningitis, 159, 827
in neonate, 426
Ketamine, for pediatric analgesia, 513t, 513–514
Ketoacidosis, 40, 44–45
alcoholic, 45 (*see* Alcoholic ketoacidosis)
diabetic (*see* Diabetic ketoacidosis)
Ketoconazole, in human immunodeficiency virus infections, 521t, 523
Ketonemia, in diabetic ketoacidosis, 735
Ketones, in alcoholic ketoacidosis, 740
Ketosis, starvation, 45
Khat, 583
Kidney:
hypertension and, 239
injury to, 960
in rheumatic disorders, 886
role of chloride in, 83
ultrasonography and, 1121
(*See also headings beginning with term* Renal)
Kidney disorders:
cocaine use and, 580
in heatstroke, 653
in human immunodeficiency virus infections, 523
in hydrocarbon poisoning, 603
nonsteroidal anti-inflammatory drug overdose and, 626–627
Kidney donor, resuscitation of, 376
Kissing (reduvid) bug (coenose) bites, 538, 658
treatment of, 658
Klebsiella pneumonia, 265, 270
Kleihauer-Bedke test:
fetomaternal hemorrhage and, 415, 416
in gastrointestinal bleeding, in children, 492
Klonopin (*See* Clonazepam)
Knee, aseptic necrosis of, following organ transplantation, 1106
Knee injuries, 999–1003
in children, 1002–1003
dislocation and, 1002
examination in, 999
fractures and, 999–1000, 1000f
ligamentous and meniscal, 1000f, 1000–1002
knee dislocation and, 1002
osteochondritis dissecans and, 1002
patella dislocation and, 1002
treatment of, 1001
Kohler's bone disease, in children, 890
Koplik's spots, in measles, 508
Kostin's syndrome (*see* Temporomandibular joint syndrome)
Kussmaul's sign:
in acute pericarditis, 230
in constrictive pericarditis, 232
in penetrating injury to heart, 940
Kwell (γ-benzene hexachloride; GBH), in scabies, 658

Labetalol (Normodyne; Trandate), 117–118
actions of, 117
adverse effects of, 118
dosage, actions, pharmacokinetics, and indications for, 112t
dosing and administration of, 118
in hypertensive emergencies, 240t, 241, 241t
indications for, 117–118, 241
pharmacokinetics of, 117
side effects and contraindications to, 241
Labetalol (Normodyne; Trendate):
in angina, 201t
pharmacology and properties of, 622
in tetanus, 526t
Labor, preterm, 407–408
emergency delivery and, 420–421
Laboratory evaluation, in abdominal pain, 146
Laboratory studies:
in abdominal emergencies, in children, 491
in acute pancreatitis, 363–364
in alcoholic ketoacidosis, 740, 741t
in altered mental status, 155, 158
in appendicitis, 320–321
in asthma, in children, 467–468
in bleeding, 766t, 766–767
in bronchiolitis, in children, 468
in calcium channel blocker overdose, 620
in child sexual abuse, 499
in clonidine poisoning, 570
in colonic diverticular disease, 333
in cyanide poisoning, 635–636
in diabetic ketoacidosis, 736–737
in children, 503
in digitalis toxicity, 617
in gastrointestinal bleeding, 148
in head injury, 917–918
in hypertensive emergencies, 237–238
in hypoglycemia, 733
in intestinal obstruction, 323–324, 324f
in jaundice, 356
in Legionnaires' disease, 271
in lightning injuries, 702, 702t
in meningitis, in children, 455
in myasthenia gravis, 822–823
in myxedema coma, 757
in near drowning, 689
in nonketotic hyperosmolar coma, 745
in organophosphate/carbamate poisoning, 611
in phenytoin toxicity, 565
in pneumonia
bacterial, 263, 264t, 265
in children, 458
Mycoplasma, 269
in poisoning, 549
in primary adrenal insufficiency, 760
in psychiatric disorders, 1076
in Reye's syndrome, 476
in salicylate intoxication, 591
in seizures, 806–807
in sepsis, in children, 454
in sexual assault, recent advances in, 401–402
in syncope, in elderly patients, 259
in thyroid storm, 752–753
in vertigo, 802
Labyrinthitis, vertigo and, 800, 800t
Lacerations:
antibiotic prophylaxis of, 1041
distal phalanx fractures and, 1065, 1065f, 1066f
(*See also specific sites*)
Lachman test, in knee injury, 1001
Lacrimal duct system, 1054
injury of, 1056
Lacrimators, 699
Lactate:
metabolic alkalosis and, 47
production of, 747
utilization of, 747–748
Lactate dehydrogenase (LDH), in *Pneumocystis carinii* pneumonia, 273
Lactate homeostasis, 747
Lactic acidosis, 40, 40t, 44, 747–750 (*see* Lactic acidosis)
classification of, 748–749, 749t
clinical presentation of, 748
diagnosis of, 748
physiology of, 747–748
treatment of, 749–750
type A, 749
type B, 749
Lactic dehydrogenase (LDH), in acute myocardial infarction, 203
Lactose intolerance, in Crohn's disease, 329–330
Laennec's (alcoholic) cirrhosis, 361
Lambert-Eaton syndrome, 813–814, 824–825
Landry-Guillain-Barré disease, 812–813
Lanoxin (*see* Digoxin)
Lap belt syndrome, 912, 925
in pregnancy, 415
Laparoscopy:
in abdominal pain, 147
complications of, 422
diagnostic, in appendicitis, 321
Laparotomy:
computed tomography and, 10
in mesenteric ischemia, avoidance of, 251
Laportea, 723, 725
Large bowel (*see* Colon)
carcinoma of, perforation in, 317
perforation of, 317
Laryngomalacia:
in children, 182
in neonate, 428
Laryngoscopy, fiberoptic, 14–15, 15f
Laryngotomy, in upper airway obstruction, 845
Laryngotracheobronchitis, membranous (bacterial tracheitis), 184
LASF (*see* Left anterior superior fascicle)
Lasix (*see* Furosemide)
Lateral (posterior) approach, to internal jugular vein, 24
Latex agglutination, in meningitis, 829
Laxative abuse, 1086
LBB (*see* Left bundle branch)
LDH (*see* Lactic dehydrogenase)
Le Fort fractures, 853–855, 854f
Lead, radiation injury and, 713
"Lead bands," 639
Lead burns, 700
Lead colic, treatment of, 113t
Lead poisoning, 638–640, 812
antidote to, 549t
gunshot wounds and, 1023
inorganic lead and, 638–640
clinical effects of, 639, 639t
diagnosis of, 639
differential diagnosis of, 639
management of, 639–640, 640t
pharmacology of, 638
prognosis of, 640
toxicopathology of, 638f, 638–639
organic lead and, 640
Left anterior superior fascicle (LASF), 86
bifascicular block and, 101

trifascicular block and, 101
unifascicular block and, 100-101, 101f
Left bundle branch (LBB), 86
Left posterior inferior fascicle (LPIF), 86
bifascicular block and, 101
trifascicular block and, 101
unifascicular block and, 100, 101, 101f
Left ventricular (LV) diastolic function, in hypertrophic cardiomyopathy, 227
Left ventricular (LV) failure, hypertension and, 239
Left ventricular (LV) pump failure, in acute myocardial infarction, 201, 205-206, 206t
Leg:
compartments at risk for compartment syndromes in, 1009, 1009f
fractures of, 1004-1005
anatomy and, 1004
in children, 1005
clinical evaluation of, 1004
complications of, 1004-1005
treatment of, 1004
Legg-Calvé-Perthes disease:
in children, 890, 990
Legionella pneumonia, 270
Legionnaires' disease, 271-272
clinical presentation of, 271
course and prognosis of, 272
differential diagnosis of, 271-272
extrapulmonic manifestations of, 272
laboratory studies in, 271
radiographic studies in, 271
transmission and incubation of, 271
treatment of, 272
Leiomyomata, pedunculated, 392
Lenegre's disease, 100
Lens, dislocated, traumatic, 838
Lethargy:
definition of, 150
in neonate, 425-426, 426t
Leukemia, oral manifestations of, 862, 862f
Leukocyte esterase test, in urinary tract infections, 378
Leukocytosis, in pregnancy, 414
Leukotrienes, bronchoconstriction and, 291
Levatol (*see* Penbutolol)
Levator palpebrae superioris, 1055
Lev's disease, 100
LGL (*see* Lown-Ganong-Levine syndrome)
LGV (*see* Lymphogranuloma venereum)
Lhermitte's sign:
in multiple sclerosis, 818
in rheumatic disorders, 885
Libermeister's sign, in dysbaric air embolism, 681
Librium (chlordiazepoxide), 1082t
Lice, 658
Liddle's syndrome, 48
Lidocaine (Xylocaine), 110-111
actions of, 110-111, 115t
adverse effects of, 111, 115t
contraindications and forms of, 115t
in coronary artery disease, in elderly patients, 258
in digoxin toxicity, 122
dosing and administration of, 111, 115t
drug interactions of, 111
in ectopic supraventricular tachycardia, 92
electrophysiologic actions of, 110t
for emergency delivery, 419, 419t
indications for, 111, 115t
for inserting chest tube, 937
intubation of child and, 910
in oral hemorrhage, secondary to extraction, 865
for pediatric analgesia, 511-512
pharmacokinetics of, 111
in premature ventricular contractions, 95
in status epilepticus, 809
in children, 485, 485t
in ventricular fibrillation, 205
in ventricular tachycardia, 97, 205
in Wolff-Parkinson-White syndrome, 105
Lidoflazine, in cerebral ischemia, 8
Life support (*see* Advanced cardiac life support; Cardiopulmonary resuscitation; Resuscitation)
Ligament(s):
of ankle, 1007, 1008f
(*See also specific ligaments*)
Ligamentous injuries, of knee, 1001
Light-headedness, ill-defined, 801, 803
Lightning injuries, 701-702
differential diagnosis of, 701
laboratory studies in, 702, 702t
mechanisms of injury and, 701
pathophysiology of, 701
treatment of, 701-702
Lilly Cyanide Antidote Kit, 634, 709
Lime (calcium oxide) burns, 698
Limit setting, in crisis intervention, 1095
Limp, in child, 889-890
avascular necrosis and, 890
congenital hip dislocation and, 990
diskitis and, 889
fractures and, 890
Legg-Calvé-Perthes disease and, 990
osteoarticular malignancy and, 890
septic arthritis and, 990
slipped capital femoral epiphysis and, 990-991
toxic synovitis and, 889
transient synovitis and, 990
trauma and, 889-890
Lindane, in parasitic infections, 537t
Lip lacerations, 865
Lip wounds, 1057-1058
anatomy and, 1057
avulsion, 1058
lacerations, 1057f, 1057-1058
regional nerve block for repair of lacerations and, 1034, 1034f
treatment of, 1057f, 1057-1058
Lipid(s), peroxidation of, cerebral ischemia and, 8
Listening, in crisis intervention, 1094
Lithium, 559-560, 1080, 1084
acute lithium toxicity and, 559-560
clinical presentation of, 559, 559t
treatment of, 559-560
metabolic acidosis and, 45
pathophysiology of action of, 559, 559t
pharmacologic properties of, 559
during pregnancy, 407
side effects of, 1084
toxicity and overdose of, 1084
Lithotripsy:
extracorporeal shock wave, in cholecystitis, 354
in nephrolithiasis, 374
Liver:
acetaminophen toxicity and, 594-596, 595f
biopsy of, in Reye's syndrome, 476
in congestive heart failure, 217
injury to, 959
ultrasonography and, 1120, 1121f
(*See also headings beginning with term* Hepatic)
Liver disease:
alcoholic, 360-361
alcoholic cirrhosis and, 361
alcoholic hepatitis and, 360
clinical features of, 361
complications of, 361-362
emergency department management of, 361
hepatic steatosis and, 360
management of, 361
treatment of, 360
altered mental status and, 156
bleeding in, 768
in heatstroke, 653
in hydrocarbon poisoning, 603
hypoglycemia and, 729
in narcotic overdose, 568
nonsteroidal anti-inflammatory drug overdose and, 628
in pregnancy, 410
in ulcerative colitis, 330
(*See also* Hepatitis)
"Liver flap" (asterixis), in portosystemic encephalopathy, 362
Liver function tests, in Reye's syndrome, 476
Liver transplantation, in mushroom poisoning, 720
Living wills, 5
Locked-in syndrome ("Count of Monte Cristo" syndrome), 150
Lockwood's suspensoru ligament, 1054
Lomotil (diphenoxylate), in Crohn's disease, 329
Lonicera, 723, 725
Loniten (*see* Minoxidil)
Loperamide (Imodium), in Crohn's disease, 329
Lopressor (*see* Metoprolol)
Lorazepam (Ativan), 1080, 1082, 1082t
in head injury, severe, 919
for rapid tranquilization, 1078
in seizures, in children, 482t
in status epilepticus, 809
in children, 484, 485t
Lou Gehrig's disease (amyotrophic lateral sclerosis), 1101
Lown-Ganong-Levine (LGL) syndrome, 103
Loxapine, 556t
Loxapine (Daxolin; Loxitane), 1080t
for rapid tranquilization, 1079t
Loxitane (loxapine), 1080t
for rapid tranquilization, 1079t
LPIF (*see* Left posterior inferior fascicle)
LSD, 584-585
Ludwig's angina, 842, 858-859
treatment of, 859
Lumbar puncture:
in altered mental status, 155
headache following, 791
in headaches, 789
in lead poisoning, 639-640
in meningitis, 827t, 827-828
in children, 455-456
in multiple sclerosis, 819
in Reye's syndrome, 476
Lumbar spine, 896-900, 897t
physical examination and, 896-898
spinal degeneration and, 898f, 898-899, 899f
Lunate dislocations, 977, 977f
Lunate fractures, 977
Lung(s):
"crack," 580
esophageal disease and, 307
lacerations of, with hemopneumothorax, 936
physiologic shunting in, 57-58, 58t

Lung(s) (*Cont.*):
pneumonia and (*see* Pneumonia)
pregnancy-associated changes in, 414
in Reye's syndrome, 478
(*See also* Blood gases)
Lung disorders:
abscess and, 277, 277f
in narcotic overdose, 567
chronic, high altitude and, 676
decompression sickness and, 683
in human immunodeficiency virus infections, 522t, 522-523
in hydrocarbon poisoning, 601-602
in hypothermia, 649
in narcotic overdose, 567-568
in neonate, cyanosis and, 175
nonsteroidal anti-inflammatory drug overdose and, 627
salicylate intoxication and, 589
(*See also* Chronic obstructive pulmonary disease)
Lung injuries, 936-939
Lung scan:
in chronic compensated airflow obstruction, 299
gallium, in *Pneumocystis carinii* pneumonia, 273
ventilation-perfusion (*see* Ventilation-perfusion lung scans)
in pulmonary embolism, 234
LV (*see* Left ventricular pump failure)
Lye (sodium hydroxide), 606
burns and, 698
(*See also* Caustic ingestions)
Lyme disease, 540-541
clinical presentation of, 540
in stage I, 540
in stage II, 540
in stage III, 540
diagnosis of, 540
multiple sclerosis versus, 819
treatment of, 540-541
Lymphadenopathy:
in pneumonia, in children, 458
in rubella, in children, 508
in tularemia, 542
Lymphedema, antibiotic prophylaxis in, wound management and, 1041
Lymphocytic choriomeningitis virus, pneumonia and, 267
Lymphogranuloma venereum (LGV), 340
proctitis and, 342
Lytren, 165

McMurray's test, in meniscal injuries, 1002
Magnesium, 79-81
in ectopic supraventricular tachycardia, 92
metabolic acidosis and, 45
Magnesium chloride, in hypomagnesemia, 81t
Magnesium hydroxide (milk of magnesia), in hypomagnesemia, 81t
Magnesium oxide, in hypomagnesemia, 81t
Magnesium sulfate:
in eclampsia, 239
for emergency delivery, 419t
in hypertension, in pregnancy, 408, 409t
in hypomagnesemia, 81t
in seizures, in children, 482t
in tetanus, 526t
in torsade de pointes, 96
Magnesium toxicity, treatment of, 113t
Magnetic resonance imaging (MRI):
in blunt trauma to great vessels, 951
in knee injuries, 1001
in multiple sclerosis, 818, 819f
in seizures, 807
Mahaim bundles, 103f, 103-104
Malaria, 530-534
clinical manifestations of, 531
diagnosis of, 531-532, 532t
epidemiology of, 530, 531t
etiology of, 530, 530t
in narcotic overdose, 567
pathophysiology of, 531
prevention of, 533
treatment of, 532t, 532-534
Malfaigne's fracture, 983
Malignancy, 780t, 780-783
acute spinal cord compression and, 780
adrenal insufficiency and shock and, 782
granulocytopenia and, 782
hemorrhage and, 782-783
hypercalcemia and, 77, 781
hyperviscosity syndrome and, 781-782
immunosuppression and, 782
infection and, 782
malignant pericardial effusion with tamponade and, 780-781
nonmyasthenic syndromes of, 813-814
following organ transplantation, 1106
superior vena cava syndrome and, 781
syndrome of inappropriate antidiuretic hormone and, 781
thrombocytopenia and, 782
upper airway obstruction and, 780
Mallet finger, 972-973, 973f
Mallory-Weiss syndrome, 149, 309
Mandibular fractures, 850-851
classification of, 850-851, 851f
examination and diagnosis in, 850
treatment of, 851
Manic-depressive illness, 1070-1071
Mannitol:
in acute angle closure glaucoma, 836
in head injury, severe, 919
in lithium overdose, 1084
in meningitis, in children, 455
in pediatric trauma victim, 911
in Reye's syndrome, 477
Manpower, for emergency medical services, 189
Manual thrust technique (Heimlich maneuver), 3
MAO (*see* Monoamine oxidase inhibitors)
Marfan's syndrome, mitral valve prolapse in, 221
Marijuana, 586-587
Marine animals, trauma and envenomations from, 666-669
bacteriology of marine environment and, 666
bites, lacerations, and punctures and, 666-667
coelenterates and, 667-668, 668t
sponges and, 667
stingrays, scorpionfish, sea urchins, and starfish and, 668-669
treatment of infections caused by, 666
Mass evacuation, 197
Mass spectrometry, respiratory gas measurement by, 60-61
MAST (*see* Military antishock trouser garment)
Masticator space infection, 858
clinical features of, 858, 858f
treatment of, 858
Mastitis, 411
Matrix, nail, 1061
Maxillary fractures, 853-855
Le Fort, 853-855, 854f, 855f
Maxillofacial fractures, 850-856
computed tomography in, 855-856, 856f
mandibular, 850-851, 851f
maxillary, 853-855, 854f, 855f
midfacial, 851-853, 852f, 853f
computed tomography in, 855-856, 856f
MDA (3,4-methylenedioxyamphetamine), 583
MDEA ("Eve"; 3,4-methylenedioxyethamphetamine), 583
MDMA ("Adam"; "Ecstasy"; 3,4-methylenedioxymethamphetamine), 583, 586
Measles:
German (rubella), rash in, 508
pneumonia and, 267
rash in, in children, 508
Meat impaction, 310
Mebendazole, in parasitic infections, 537t
Mechanical (power) injector, computed tomography and, 3
Mechanical ventilation, 19
in adult respiratory distress syndrome, 288
in aspiration pneumonia, 278
in asthma, 297
in chronic decompensated airflow obstruction, 300
in flail chest, 936
in resuscitation of potential kidney donor, 376
in Reye's syndrome, 477
in status asthmaticus, in children, 472
in thoracic trauma, to chest wall, bronchi, lung, and diaphragm, 932-933
Meckel's diverticulum:
in children, 496
gastrointestinal bleeding and, 149
Meconium staining, neonatal resuscitation and, 171
Medial canthal tendon, division of, 1055, 1055f
Medial collateral ligament injury, 1008
Medial longitudinal fasciculus (MLF), in altered mental status, 153
Mediastinal irrigation, in hypothermia, 651
Mediastinal shift, foreign body aspiration and, in children, 185, 185f, 186f
Mediastinal trauma, computed tomography and, 9
Mediastinitis, chest pain and, 131
Medical care:
access to, emergency medical services and, 190
emergency medical services and, 191-192
Medical control, of emergency medical services (*see* Emergency medical services, medical control of)
Medical disaster, definition of, 193
Medical response team, at disaster scene, identifying members of, 194
Medroxyprogesterone acetate, in chronic mountain polycythemia, 676
Medusae (jellyfish) envenomations, 667
Mee's lines, in arsenic poisoning, 641
Mefenamic acid, overdose of, 628
Mefloquine:
adverse effects, precautions, and contraindications to, 533t
in malaria, 532t
prophylaxis of, 533t
Megacolon, toxic, in ulcerative colitis, 330
Melena, 147
Mellaril (*see* Thioradazine)
MEN (*see* Multiple endocrine neoplasia)
Meningitis, 827-830
altered mental status and, 156
aseptic, in nonsteroidal anti-inflammatory drug overdose, 628

bacterial, 827
altered mental status and, 156
treatment of, 829
in children, 454–456
clinical presentation of, 455
laboratory studies in, 455
treatment of, 455–456
clinical presentation in, 455, 827, 827t
diagnosis of, 827t, 827–828
headache and, 791
physical signs of, 159
prophylaxis of, 456
search for organisms causing, 828–829
seizures and, in neonate, 172
treatment of, 455–456, 829
tuberculous, in human immunodeficiency virus infections, 522
viral, 827
Menière's disease, 800
treatment of, 803
Meniscal injuries, 1001–1002
Menstruation:
history taking and, 389
pregnancy diagnosis and, 406
narcotic abuse and, 569
Mental health:
disasters and, 197
(*See* also Psychiatric disorders)
Mental status:
altered (*see* Altered mental status; Coma; Consciousness)
in asthma, 294
in neurological examination, 785
in primary adrenal insufficiency, 760
Mental status examination, in psychiatric disorders, 1075t, 1075–1076
Meperidine (Demerol):
in acute myocardial infarction, 207
incarcerated hernia and, in children, 493–494
for incision and drainage of cutaneous abscess, 877
for pediatric analgesia, 513t, 514
during pregnancy, 407
Mephobarbital, pharmacology of, 561t
6-Mercaptopurine, in Crohn's disease, 329
Mercury poisoning, 642–644
antidote to, 549t
clinical effects of, 642, 643t
diagnosis of, 642–643
differential diagnosis of, 643
pharmacology of, 642
prognosis and sequelae of, 644
toxicopathology of, 642
treatment of, 643–644
Mescaline, 585
Mesoridazine (Serentil), 556t, 1080t
for rapid tranquilization, 1079t
Metabolic disorders:
in hydrocarbon poisoning, 603
seizures and, in neonate, 172
in theophylline poisoning, 614–615
Metabolic neuropathy, 812
Metacarpal fractures, 978–979
Metacarpophalangeal (MP) joint dislocations, 974
complications of, 974
Metal burns, 698
Metal poisoning, 638t, 638–644, 812
Metaproterenol:
in asthma, 295t
in children, 473
in chronic decompensated airflow obstruction, 301
Metaraminol, in reentrant supraventricular tachycardia, 93
Metatarsal fractures, 1013
in children, 1014
fractures of base of fifth metatarsal and, 1014
treatment of, 1013
Methamphetamine, 583, 583t
Methanol (wood alcohol):
metabolic acidosis and, 45
poisoning and, 572–573, 812
antidote to, 549t
clinical findings in, 572, 572t, 573t
pathophysiology of, 572, 572t
treatment of, 573, 573t
Methemoglobinemia, 141
hazardous materials exposure and, 709
in neonate, 428
cyanosis and, 175
Methergine (methylergonovine), for emergency delivery, 419t
Methimazole, in thyroid storm, 753
Methohexital (Brevital):
for pediatric sedation, 513t, 514
pharmacology of, 561t
rapid sequence induction and, 18
Methoxamine, in reentrant supraventricular tachycardia, 93
Methyldopa, toxic hepatitis and, 360
Methylene blue:
in cyanosis, 141
in methemoglobinemia, hazardous materials exposure and, 709
Methylene chloride poisoning, 603
3,4-Methylenedioxyamphetamine (MDA), 583
3,4-Methylenedioxyethamphetamine ("Eve"; MDEA), 583
3,4-Methylenedioxymethamphetamine ("Adam"; "Ecstasy"; MDMA), 583, 586
Methylergonovine (Methergine), for emergency delivery, 419t
Methylprednisolone (Solu-Medrol):
in caustic ingestions, 608
in meningitis, in children, 455
in multiple sclerosis, 820
in organ transplant rejection, 1104
in spinal cord compression, in malignancy, 780
in status asthmaticus, in children, 472
in superior vena cava syndrome, in malignancy, 781
in toxic shock syndrome, 405
4-Methylpyrazone (4-MP), in methanol poisoning, 573
Methylxanthines, in chronic decompensated airflow obstruction, 300–301
Metoclopramide (Reglan), in acetaminophen poisoning, 597
Metoprolol (Lopressor):
actions of, 111
in angina, 200–201, 201t
dosage, actions, pharmacokinetics, and indications for, 112t
Metronidazole (Flagyl):
in acute gastroenteritis, in children, 490
in aspiration pneumonia, 278
in bacterial vaginosis, 396
in colonic diverticular disease, 334
in Crohn's disease, 329
in diarrhea, 351t
in parasitic infections, 537t
during pregnancy, 407
in pseudomembranous enterocolitis, 331
in septic shock, 139t
in tetanus, 526t
in trichomoniasis, 518
in vaginitis, *Trichomonas*, 395
Mexitiline (Mexitil), electrophysiologic actions of, 110t
Mezlocillin, in septic shock, 139t
MFAT (*see* Multifocal atrial tachycardia)
MG (*see* Myasthenia gravis)
MHS-5, sexual assault and, 401–402
Miconazole nitrate, in vaginitis, *Candida*, 395
Microaggregates, massive blood transfusion and, 777
Micropore filters, 776
Midazolam (Versed), 1082t
for pediatric sedation, 513t, 514
rapid sequence induction and, 18–19
Midbrain dysfunction, in neurological examination, 786
Middle ear squeeze (barotitis media), 679–680
treatment of, 679–680
Midfacial fractures, 851–852
computed tomography in, 855–856, 856f
of orbital floor, 853
of zygoma or zygomatic-maxillary complex, 852–853
of zygomatic arch, 851–852, 852f
Midpart fractures, of foot, 1012–1013
treatment of, 1013
Migraine headaches (*see* Headache, migraine)
Military antishock trouser (MAST) garment, 6–7
application and removal of, 7
benefits and efficacy of, 6
in hemorrhagic shock, 134
indications and contraindications to, 6–7
physiological effects of, 6
Milk-alkali syndrome, hypercalcemia and, 78
Milk allergy, in neonate, 427
Milk leg (phlegmasia alba dolens), 255
Milk of magnesia (magnesium hydroxide), in hypomagnesemia, 81t
Millirem (mrem), 711
Milrinone, in congestive heart failure, 217
Mineralocorticoids:
in adrenal insufficiency, 761
metabolic alkalosis and, 47
Minipress (*see* Prazosin)
Minoxidil (Loniten):
actions and pharmacology of, 243
in hypertensive emergencies, 241t, 243
indications for, 243
side effects and contraindications to, 243
use of, 243
Minute ventilation, 51
Miotics, 838
Missiles (*see* Gunshot wounds; Wound ballistics)
Mithramycin, in hypercalcemia, 79, 79t
in malignancy, 781
Mitral annular calcification, in elderly patients, 260
Mitral regurgitation, 221
clinical features of, 221
treatment of, 221
Mitral stenosis, 220–221
chest pain and, 131
clinical features of, 220
treatment of, 220–221
Mitral valve injury, blunt injury to heart and, 943
Mitral valve prolapse, 221–222
chest pain and, 131
clinical features of, 222
treatment of, 222
Mittelschmerz, 392

MLF (*see* Medial longitudinal fasciculus)
Müller's muscle, 1054
MLNS (*see* Mucocutaneous lymph node syndrome)
Molindone, 556t
Molindone (Moban), 1080t
Molluscum contagiosum, in human immunodeficiency virus infections, 521
Monitoring:
of arterial pressure (*see* Arterial pressure monitoring)
of central venous pressure, 24-25
(*See also* Catheterization, central venous)
Monkey bites, 1044
Monoamine oxidase (MAO) inhibitors, 1080, 1083
overdose of, 1083
side effects of, 1083
Mononeuritis multiplex, 814
Mononeuropathy, nontraumatic, in narcotic overdose, 568
Monteggia's fracture-dislocation, 985, 986f
Mood (affective) disorders, 1070-1071
Moray eel bites, 666
Moricizine (Ethmozine), electrophysiologic actions of, 110t
Morning glory, 585
Morphine:
in acute myocardial infarction, 207
in burns, 693
in cardiogenic shock, 135-136
for incision and drainage of cutaneous abscess, 877
in left ventricular pump failure, 206
for pediatric analgesia, 513t, 514
during pregnancy, 407
in pulmonary edema, 218
in tetanus, 526t
Mortality:
in anorexia nervosa and bulimia nervosa, 1087
in diabetic ketoacidosis, 739
Mosquito bites, 657
Motion sickness, 801
Motor responses:
in head injury, 917
in neurological examination, 786
Motor system disease, 1101
Motor testing, in altered mental status, 154
Motor vehicle accidents, 905, 905f, 1052
Mountain sickness (*see* Acute mountain sickness)
Movement disorders, seizures versus, 805
MP (*see* Metacarpophalangeal joint dislocations)
4-MP (*see* 4-Methylpyrazone)
mrem (millirem), 711
MS (*see* Multiple sclerosis)
MTB (*Mycobacterium tuberculosis* pneumonia) (*see* Pneumonia, *Mycobacterium tuberculosis*)
Mucocutaneous lymph node syndrome (Kawasaki disease; MLNS), 884
rash in, in children, 509
toxic shock syndrome versus, 403-404
Mucomyst (*see* *N*-Acetylcysteine)
Mucosa, esophageal, 303
Mules, 580
Multifocal atrial tachycardia (chaotic atrial rhythm; MFAT; wandering atrial pacemaker), 90, 90f
clinical significance of, 90
treatment of, 90
Multiplanar reconstruction, computed tomography and, 2
Multiple endocrine adenomas, hypercalcemia and, 77
Multiple endocrine neoplasia (MEN), type I, 728
Multiple personality disorder, 1072
Multiple sclerosis (MS), 817-821
clinical course of, 818
clinical manifestations of, 817-818
diagnostic tests in, 818-819, 819f
differential diagnosis of, 819-820
flairs in, 1101
treatment of, 820-821
vertigo and, 801
Munchausen by proxy, apparent life threatening events and, 435
Murphy's sign:
in abdominal pain, 145
in jaundice, 356
ultrasonography and, 1120
Muscarine poisoning:
clinical toxicity of, 718
pharmacology of, 716, 717t
treatment of, 720
Muscarinic overstimulation, in organophosphate/carbamate poisoning, 610
Muscimol poisoning:
clinical toxicity of, 718
pharmacology of, 716, 717t
treatment of, 720
Muscle(s):
of ankle, 1007, 1008f
determining viability of, 1037
facial, in altered mental status, 154
function of, metabolic acidosis and, 43
Muscle relaxants, in tetanus, 526, 526t
Muscle spasms, in tetanus, 879, 880t
Muscle weakness, in myasthenia gravis, 822
Musculoskeletal disorders:
chest pain and, 131
decompression sickness and, 683
hyponatremia and, 68
lightning injuries and, 702
in narcotic overdose, 568-569
Mushroom(s), hallucinogenic, 585-586
Mushroom poisoning, 716-720
clinical toxicity and, 717t, 717-718
diagnostic evaluation in, 718-719
general management of, 719
mushroom identification and, 718-719
pharmacology of, 716-717, 717t
toxin-specific treatment of, 719-720
Mustard gas burns, 699
Mutual aid agreements, emergency medical services and, 191
Myasthenia gravis (MG), 813, 822-823
clinical manifestations of, 822
diagnostic tests in, 822-823
drug interactions in, 824
pathophysiology of, 822
transitory, 824
treatment of, 823-824
Myasthenic crisis, 822, 823
Mycobacterium tuberculosis pneumonia (*see* Pneumonia, *Mycobacterium tuberculosis*)
Mycologists, 719
Mycoplasma pneumoniae infections (*See also* Pneumonia, *Mycoplasma*)
rash in, in children, 505-506
Mydriasis:
Jimson weed and, 637
traumatic, 839
Mydriatics, 838
Myelitis, transverse:
in multiple sclerosis, 818
in narcotic overdose, 568
Myelography, in spinal injury, 923
Myocardial contusion, 943-946
diagnosis of, 944-945
pathologic changes in, 943
physiological changes in, 944
treatment of, 945-946
Myocardial infarction (*see* Acute myocardial infarction)
Myocardial ischemia (*see* Ischemia, myocardial)
Myocarditis, 229
clinical profile of, 229
definition of, 229, 229t
treatment of, 229
Myoglobinuria, in rheumatic disorders, 886
Myopathy:
in acute periodic paralysis, 813
alcoholic, 813
differentiating neuropathies from, 813
in myasthenia gravis, 813
in polymyositis syndrome, 813
Myopericarditis, 229
Myringitis, bullous, 841
Myringotomy, in otitis media with effusion, in children, 441
Myxedema, 755
Myxedema coma, 756-757
cardiovascular system and, 756-757
clinical presentation of, 756
gastrointestinal system and, 757
hyponatremia in, 756
hypothermia in, 756
laboratory studies in, 757
nervous system and, 757
precipitating factors for, 756
respiratory failure in, 756
treatment of, 757

NAC (*see* *N*-acetylcysteine)
Nadolol (Corgard):
in angina, 201t
dosage, actions, pharmacokinetics, and indications for, 112t
Naegle's rule, 418
Nafcillin, in toxic shock syndrome, 404
Nail bed, 1061
avulsion of, 1065-1066, 1066f
Nail matrix, 1061
Naloxone (Narcan):
in altered mental status, 151-152
as antidote to clonidine, 571
for emergency delivery, 419t
in neonatal resuscitation, 171
in seizures, in narcotic overdose, 566
Naproxen:
in migraine headache, 790
in tendonitis, 889
Narcan (*see* Naloxone)
Narcolepsy, seizures versus, 805
Narcosis, nitrogen, 681-682
Narcotics, 566-569
abuse of, in pregnancy, 410
addiction to, in sickle cell anemia, 774
intoxication and, 566
overdose of, 566
complications of, 566-569
treatment of, 566
withdrawal from, 566
Nasal airways (nasopharyngeal tubes), 10
Nasal congestion, in neonate, 428
Nasal flaring, in children, upper respiratory disorders and, 182
Nasal fractures, 846-848
frontal, 847
lateral, 847-848

Nasal packing, in epistaxis, 846, 847f
Nasal trauma, 846-848
Nasal wounds, 1055-1056
anatomy and, 1056
avulsion, 1057
human bites and, 1043
lacerations, 1056f, 1056-1057
treatment of, 1056f, 1056-1057
Nasogastric intubation:
in abdominal trauma, 957, 957t
in esophageal disease, 307-308
anatomic considerations and, 307-308, 308f
in intestinal obstruction, 324
in perforated viscus, 318
Nasogastric suction:
in colonic diverticular disease, 334
in peptic ulcer disease, 313, 314, 315
in ulcerative colitis, 330
toxic megacolon and, 331
Nasolacrimal duct, 1054
Naso-orbital injuries, 855
Nasopharyngeal tubes (nasal airways), 10
Nasostat hemostatic nasal balloon, 846
Nasotracheal intubation, 12-14
aspiration pneumonia prophylaxis and, 278
complications of, 14
contraindications to, 13-14
indications for, 13
technique of, 12-13, 13f
National Anorexic Aid Society, Inc., 1087
National Association of Anorexia Nervosa Associated Disorders (ANAD), 1087
National Disaster Medical System (NDMS), 196
Nausea, during pregnancy, 407
Navane (thiothixene), 1080t
for rapid tranquilization, 1079t
NCV (*see* Nerve conduction velocity testing)
NDMS (*see* National Disaster Medical System)
Near drowning, 688-690
clinical course in, 688
definitions and, 688
disposition and, 690
epidemiology of, 688
prognosis and cerebral resuscitation in, 690
treatment of, 688-689
hospital care and, 689, 689f, 689t
prehospital care and, 688t, 688-689
Near syncope, 799, 802
Neck pain, 891-895
acute cervical disk herniations and, 894
cervical disk pathology and, 894
cervical soft tissue injuries and, 893-894
chronic degenerative disk disease and, 894-895
electrodiagnostic examination in, 893
history taking in, 891
physical examination in, 891-893, 892f, 892t, 893f
radiographic studies in, 893
Neck rigidity, in neonate, 426
Neck trauma, 928-931
anatomy and, 928, 928f
blunt, management of, 930-931
evaluation of, 929-930
arteriography in, 930, 930f
computed tomography in, 930
interventional studies in, 930
radiographic studies in, 929-930
major causes of death and, 928
penetrating, management of, 930, 930t
resuscitation and, 928-929
types of, 928
Necrosis:
ischemic, in narcotic overdose, 568
of skeletal muscle, in narcotic overdose, 568
Necrotizing enterocolitis, 174
diagnosis of, 174
medical management of, 174
in neonate, 427
signs and symptoms of, 174
surgical management of, 174
Necrotizing fasciitis, in narcotic overdose, 568
Needles, surgical, 1046-1047
Neglect, of children, 498
Nematode (roundworm) infections, 535-537
Neo-Synephrine (*see* Phenylephrine)
Neo-Synephrine (phenylephrine), ophthalmic uses of, 838
Neomycin:
ophthalmic, 838
in Reye's syndrome, bowel sterilization and, 478
Neonatal intensive care unit (NICU), infant discharged from (*see* Neonate, discharged from neonatal intensive care unit)
Neonate, 425-432
(*See also* Infant)
breathing patterns of, 425
cardiorespiratory symptoms in, 427-429
crying, irritability, and lethargy in, 425-426, 426t
diaper rash in, 429
discharged from neonatal intensive care unit, 431-432
apnea and home apnea monitors and, 432, 432t
bronchopulmonary dysplasia in, 431-432, 432t
cold stress in, 431
expected home death of, 432
failure to thrive in, 431
fractures in, 431
hypertension in, 431
hypoglycemia in, 431
immunizations for, 431
posthemorrhagic hydrocephalus in, 432
feeding patterns of, 425
fever in, 429
gastrointestinal tract symptoms in, 426-427
hypoglycemia in, 733
oral thrush in, 429
pneumonia in, 457, 458-459
reasons for emergency department visits and, 425, 425t
resuscitation of, 172-176
complications of asphyxia and, 171-172
drug therapy in, 171
equipment for, 170
meconium staining and, 171
principles of, 170t, 170-172
risk factors for, 170
shock and, 171
steps in, 171
seizures in (*see* Seizures, in neonate)
sepsis in, 429
stool patterns of, 425
sudden infant death and, 429-430
tetanus in, 525
transitory myasthenia gravis in, 824
weight gain in, 425
(*See also* Infant *and under specific disorders*)
Neoplasms (*see* Carcinoma; Malignancy; Tumor(s); *specific organs*)
Nephritis:
acute interstitial, in nonsteroidal anti-inflammatory drug overdose, 626-627
in rheumatic disorders, 886
Nephrocalcinosis, 373
Nephrolithiasis (urinary calculi), 373-374
clinical features of, 373
complications of, 374
differential diagnosis of, 374
management of, 374
emergency therapy and, 374
pathophysiology of, 373
radiographic studies in, 373-374
Nerium oleander, 723, 725
Nerve(s), of ankle, 1007
Nerve block, regional, for wound repair, 1031-1034, 1032-1035f
Nerve blocks:
intercostal, in thoracic trauma, 932
regional, in children, 512
Nerve conduction velocity (NCV) testing, in neck pain, 893
Nerve entrapments, 815t, 815-816
Nerve injuries, of hand, 974-975
Nerve root injury, in pelvic fracture, 987
Neuritis, retrobulbar, 837
Neuroblastoma(s), in children, 496
Neurogenic shock, 138-139
Neuroleptic(s), 555-557 (*see* Antipsychotics)
acute overdose of, 557
clinical findings in, 557
management of, 557
adverse effects of, 555-557, 556t
neuroleptic malignant syndrome and, 556t, 556-557, 557t
pharmacokinetics of, 555
pharmacology of, 555, 556t
therapeutic indications for, 555
Neuroleptic malignant syndrome (NMS), 556t, 556-557, 557t, 1081
Neurologic disorders:
amphetamines and, 582
in carbon monoxide poisoning, 705
chronic coniditions and, 1100-1101
complications of drugs used in, 1101
in chronic renal failure, 375
decompression sickness and, 683
high altitude and, 673-674
in human immunodeficiency virus infections, 521-522
treatment of, 521t
in hydrocarbon poisoning, 602
in hypoglycemia, 733
lightning injuries and, 702
in myxedema coma, 757
in nonketotic hyperosmolar coma, 745, 745t
patient assessment and, 1100t, 1100-1101
chronic conditions and, 1100-1101
in poisoning, management of, 548-549
poisoning and, 547
snake bites and, 661
special precautions in neurologically disabled patients and, 1101
in theophylline poisoning, 614
(*See also* Central nervous system disorders)
Neurological examination, 785t, 785-788
in altered mental status, 152, 152t
in cerebral vascular accident, 794
coordination in, 787
cranial nerves in, 786
in head injury, 916-917, 917t
history taking in, 785
mental status in, 785
motor response in, 786
in neck pain, 892t, 892-893, 893f

Neurological examination (*Cont.*):
of pediatric trauma victim, 911
reflexes in, 787f, 787–788, 788t
in seizures, 806
sensory response in, 786–787
Neuromuscular blockade, 16–18, 17t, 812
in myasthenia gravis, drug interactions and, 824
in tetanus, 526, 526t, 879, 880t
Neuromuscular disease, congenital, in neonate, 428
Neuronitis, vestibular, vertigo and, 800
Neuropathy:
allergic, 814
differentiating myopathies from, 813
of Guillain-Barré, 812–813
metabolic, 812
Neurosyphilis, multiple sclerosis versus, 819
Newborn (*see* Neonate)
Nicardipine (Cardene), 120
actions of, 120
adverse effects of, 120
dosing and administration of, 120
indications for, 120
pharmacokinetics of, 120
Nicosamide, in parasitic infections, 537t
Nicotine, withdrawal from, treatment of, 244
Nicotinic effects, in organophosphate/carbamate poisoning, 610–611
NICU (neonatal intensive care unit), infant discharged from (*see* Neonate, discharged from neonatal intensive care unit)
Nifedipine (Adalat; Procardia), 119
actions and pharmacology of, 242
actions of, 119
in acute myocardial infarction, 210
adverse effects of, 119
in angina, 201
in congestive heart failure, 218
dosing and administration of, 119
in high altitude pulmonary edema, 675
in hypertensive emergencies, 240t, 241t, 242–243
indications for, 119, 242
overdose of, 620
pharmacokinetics of, 119
in pulmonary edema, 218
side effects and contraindications to, 243
use of, 243
Nightstick fracture, 986
Nimodipine (Nimotop), 120
actions of, 120
adverse effects of, 120
dosing and administration of, 120
indications for, 120
pharmacokinetics of, 120
911 emergency telephone number, 189
Nipride (*see* Sodium nitroprusside)
Nitrate urine test, in urinary tract infections, 378
Nitrates:
in angina, 200, 200t
in congestive heart failure, 218
in dilated cardiomyopathy, 227
in mitral regurgitation, 221
in right ventricular infarction, 207
in valvular aortic stenosis, 223
(*See also specific nitrates*)
Nitrendipine (Baypress), 120
actions of, 120
adverse effects of, 120
dosing and administration of, 120
indications for, 120
pharmacokinetics of, 120
Nitric acid burns, 697
Nitrites, poisoning by, antidote to, 549t
Nitrofurantoins:
during pregnancy, 407
in urinary tract infections, 379t
Nitrogen narcosis, 681–682
Nitroglycerin (NTG), 125–126
actions of, 125
in acute myocardial infarction, 207–208
adverse effects of, 126
in angina, 200t
in chest pain, 128
dosing and administration of, 126
indications for, 125
intravenous
actions and pharmacology of, 241
in hypertensive emergencies, 241t, 241–242
indications for, 241
side effects and contraindications to, 242
use of, 242
in left ventricular pump failure, 206
pharmacokinetics of, 125, 125t
in pulmonary edema, 218
Nitroprusside test, in alcoholic ketoacidosis, 740
Nitrous oxide, for pediatric analgesia, 513, 513t
NMS (*see* Neuroleptic malignant syndrome)
No-code (DNI; DNR) orders, 4
Nonketotic hyperosmolar coma, 743–746
clinical presentation of, 743–745
laboratory studies in, 745
pathogenesis of, 743, 744f
precipitating factors for, 744t, 744–745
treatment of, 745–746
Nonparoxysmal ventricular tachycardia (*see* Accelerated idioventricular rhythm)
Nonspecific vaginitis (bacterial vaginosis; BV; *Corynebacterium* vaginitis; *Gardnerella* vaginitis; *Haemophilus* vaginitis), 396
Nonsteroidal anti-inflammatory drugs (NSAIDs), 626–629
adverse drug interactions of, 628
overdose of
differential diagnosis of, 628
mechanism of toxicity and clinical presentation in, 626–628
treatment of, 628–629
for pediatric analgesia, 514
pharmacokinetics of, 626
Norcuron (vecuronium bromide), neuromuscular blockade and, 17, 17t, 18
Norepinephrine, 123
actions of, 123
adverse effects of, 123
dosing and administration of, 123
indications for, 123
pharmacokinetics of, 123
in reentrant supraventricular tachycardia, 93
Norfloxacin, in urinary tract infections, 379t
Normocytic anemia, normochromic, in malaria, 531
Normodyne (*see* Labetalol)
Norpace (*see* Disopyramide)
Nose (*see headings beginning with term* Nasal)
Nose picker's ulcer, 846
NSAIDs (*see* Nonsteroidal anti-inflammatory drugs)
NTG (*see* Nitroglycerin)
Numbness, left-sided, cerebral vascular accident and, 798
Nutmeg intoxication, 586
Nylen-Barany (Hallpike) testing, in labyrinthitis, 800, 800t, 802
Nylon sutures, 1045
Nystagmus:
in phenytoin toxicity, 564
vertigo and, 799
Nystatin, in pneumonia, in neonate, 428t

OA (*see* Osteoarthritis)
Obicularis oculi muscle, 1053–1054
Observation, in knee injuries, 999
Obsessive-compulsive disorder, 1071
Obstetric delivery:
breech, 420–421
emergency, 418–421
immediate postpartum management and, 421
preparation for, 418–419
preterm, 420–421
procedure for, 419–420, 420f
transport of maternal patients and, 418, 419t
hemorrhage following, 413
out-of-hospital, 412–413
postmortem cesarean section and, 413, 416
(*See also* Labor)
Obstetric emergencies (*see* Labor; Obstetric delivery; Pregnancy)
Occipital neuralgia, 891
Occipitalis muscle, 1052
Occipitofrontalis muscle, 1052
Ocular disorders, 833–840
common presenting symptoms in, 834–837
diagnosis of, 839
eye examination in, 833
ophthalmic medications and, 839–840
in rheumatic disorders, 885–886
traumatic, 837–839
treatment techniques in, 840
(*See also* Ophthalmologic disorders)
Ocular movements, in altered mental status, 153–154, 154t
Oculocephalic reflexes, in altered mental status, 153
Oculovestibular (cold caloric) testing, in altered mental status, 154, 154t
Odontalgia (toothache), 860
Odontogenic pain, 860–861
dental caries and, 860
postextraction, 861
tooth eruption and, 860
Odor, of breath, in altered mental status, 152
Odynophagia, 306
chest pain and, 127
OE (*see* Otitis externa)
Oklahoma Poison Control Center, national snake bite index maintained by, 664
Olecranon fractures, 985
Oliguria, 64, 64t
OME (*see* Otitis media, with effusion)
Omphalocele, in neonate, 174
management of, 174
Oncotic pressure, 63
Ophthalmologic disorders:
in carbon monoxide poisoning, 704
in human immunodeficiency virus infections, 522
treatment of, 521t
Ophthalmoplegia, intranuclear, in altered mental status, 154
Opiates:
poisoning by, antidote to, 549t
withdrawal from, treatment of, 244
Optic neuritis, headache and, 792
Optokinetic drugs, distinguishing true neurologic deficits from conversion disorder and, 1091t
Oral airways (oropharyngeal tubes), 10
Oral cavity, bleeding from, 1052

Oral lacerations, 865
bacterial contamination of, 1028
Oral lesions, 861
Oral rehydration therapy, in acute gastroenteritis, in children, 489–490
Oral thrush, in neonate, 429
Orbicularis oculi muscle, 1055
Orbicularis oris muscle, 1057
Orbit, cellulitis of (*see* Periorbital/orbital cellulitis)
Orbital abscess, in sinusitis, in children, 449
Orbital cellulitis, in sinusitis, in children, 449
Orbital fracture, 1055
blowout, 838, 852
computed tomography in, 855–856, 856f
of orbital floor, 853, 853f
Orchitis, 387
Orellanine/orelline poisoning:
clinical toxicity of, 717
pharmacology of, 716, 717t
treatment of, 720
Organ transplants, 1103–1106
complications of
infectious, 1105t, 1105–1106
noninfectious, 1106, 1106t
immunology of transplantation and, 1103
maintenance immunosuppression and, 1104–1105, 1105t
rejection and, 1103–1104
acute, 1103
chronic, 1103
clinical presentation and treatment of, 1104, 1104t
hyperacute, 1103
Organic affective disorder, 1068
Organic brain syndromes, 1068–1069
Organic delusional disorder, 1068
Organic hallucinosis, 1068
Organic mental disorders, 1068–1069
Organic personality disorder, 1068
Organophosphate/carbamate poisoning, 609–613
antidote to, 549t
clinical presentation of, 610–611, 611t
complications of, 613
diagnosis of, 611–612
exposure and, 610
laboratory studies in, 611
management of, 612t, 612–613
pathophysiology of, 609, 609f, 609t, 610t
treatment of, 634, 709
Oropharyngeal tubes (oral airways), 10
Orotracheal intubation, 11–12
aspiration pneumonia prophylaxis and, 278
blind, 12
complications of, 12
technique of, 11t, 11–12
Orthopnea, 216
Oscilloscopia, 799
Osgood-Schlatter disease, 1002
Osmolal gap:
in ethylene glycol poisoning, 574
in methanol poisoning, 572, 572t, 573t
Osmolality, 62–63
effective (tonicity), 63
Osmolarity, 62–63
Osmotic demyelination syndrome, 67, 68
Osteoarthritis (OA):
chest pain and, 131
of temporomandibular joint, 857
Osteochondral fractures, 1003
Osteochondritis dissecans:
in children, 890
of knee, 1002
Osteomyelitis, 888
hematogenous, in narcotic overdose, 569
in narcotic overdose, 569
Osteoporosis, in anorexia nervosa, 1086
Otalgia, 841
Otitis externa (OE), 841
in children, 441–442
clinical findings in, 442
differential diagnosis of, 442
etiology and pathophysiology of, 442
treatment of, 442
otitis media versus, 442
Otitis media, 841
in children, 440–441
clinical findings in, 440
complications and sequelae of, 441
with effusion, 441–442
etiology of, 440
pathophysiology of, 440
recurrent, 441
treatment of, 440–441
with effusion (OME), in children, 441–442
otitis externa versus, 442
Otologic emergencies, 841–842
Ovary(ies):
functional cysts of, 1117, 1117f
torsion of, 392
Overpressure, 685
Oxacillin:
in bacterial pneumonia, 264t
in periorbital/orbital cellulitis, in children, 452t
in sinusitis, in children, 449t, 450
in toxic shock syndrome, 404
Oxalic acid burns, 698, 700
Oxazepam (Serax), 1082t
Oxidizing agents, 695
Oxprenolol (Trasicor), dosage, actions, pharmacokinetics, and indications for, 112t
Oxygen:
altered mental status and, 156
alveolar-arterial differences in, 56
availability of, 58–59
cardiac output and, 58–59
combination of hemoglobin with carbon monoxide and, 59
oxygen content and, 58
oxygen dissociation in tissues and, 59
concentration in alveoli, 53
conjunctival measurements of, 60
delivery and availability of, metabolic acidosis and, 44
inspired, fraction of, 55, 55t
transcutaneous monitoring of, 60
Oxygen-hemoglobin curve, in carbon monoxide poisoning, 703
Oxygen-hemoglobin reaction, effect on carbon dioxide transport, 55
Oxygen reserve, 59
Oxygen therapy:
in acute mountain sickness, 673
in adult respiratory distress syndrome, 288
in aortic regurgitation, 224
in asthma, 294
in barotrauma of descent, 680
in bronchiolitis, in children, 473
in carbon monoxide poisoning, 706
in chronic decompensated airflow obstruction, 300
in cyanide poisoning, 635
in cyanosis, in neonate, 175
in diving accidents, 684
in hazardous materials exposure, 708
in high altitude pulmonary edema, 675
home, long-term, complications of, 1107
in left ventricular failure, 239
in near drowning, 689
in peptic ulcer disease, hemorrhage and, 314
in pneumonia, in children, 460
in pulmonary embolism, 235
Oxygenation, monitoring, 55
Oxyhemoglobin dissociation curve, in hypothermia, 649
Oxyhemoglobin saturation, 56–57
2,3-DPG and, 57, 57t
exercise and, 57
normal relationships and, 56, 56t
P_{CO_2} and, 57
pH and, 56, 57t
temperature and, 57, 57t
Oxytocin, following emergency delivery, 412–413, 419t, 421

P-QRS-T complex, 86, 87f
P wave, 86
p30, sexual assault and, 401
Pacemakers (*see* Cardiac pacing)
Packed red blood cells (PRBCs), 775, 777
PA_{CO_2}, estimating, 53
PACs (*see* Premature atrial contractions)
PAF (*see* Platelet-activation factor)
Pain:
abdominal (*see* Abdominal pain)
in acute ischemia of extremities, 253, 254
adnexal, in females, 392
anorectal abscesses and, 56
in appendicitis, 320
chest (*see* Chest pain)
in children
analgesia and, 511–514, 512t, 513t
assessment of, 511
nonpharmacologic approaches to, 511
in cholecystitis, 353–354
epigastric, in peptic ulcer disease, 314
esophageal colic and, 306
in extremities, in narcotic overdose, 568
in fissure in ano, 339
gynecologic, early pregnancy complications as causes of (*see* Pregnancy)
in joints, decompression sickness and, 683
in mesenteric ischemia, 251
in peptic ulcer disease, 313
perception of, 127
referred, abdominal, 144
relief of, in acute myocardial infarction, 207
somatic, 127
somatoform pain disorder and, 1072
following surgery for inguinal hernia, 370
on swallowing (odynophagia), 306
in thoracic aortic aneurysms, expanding and ruptured, 248
visceral, 127
deep, 127, 128
Palate lacerations, 865
Pallor, in acute ischemia of extremities, 254
Palpation:
in abdominal pain, 145
in headaches, 789
in knee injuries, 999
in neck pain, 891, 892
in perforated viscus, 317–318
of prostate, 383
in thoracic trauma, 934
"Palpitations," in hypertrophic cardiomyopathy, 228
PALS (*see* Pediatric Advanced Life Support Course)
2-PAM (*see* Protopam)
Pancreas, injury to, 959–960, 960f

Pancreatic abscess, in acute pancreatitis, 365
Pancreatic pseudocyst, in acute pancreatitis, 365
Pancreatitis:
  acute, 363t, 363–365
    diagnosis of, 363–364
    treatment of, 364–365
  alcoholic, 363
  "biliary," 363
  etiology of, 363, 363t
  hypocalcemia and, 75
  in hypothermia, 649
  pathophysiology of, 363, 364t
  postoperative, 369
  in Reye's syndrome, 478
  ultrasonography in, 1121
Pancuronium bromide (Pavulon):
  in head injury, severe, 919
  neuromuscular blockade and, 17, 17t
  in Reye's syndrome, 477
  in tetanus, 526t
Panic disorder (PD), 1071, 1088–1089
  clinical features of, 1088, 1088f
  differential diagnosis of, 1089, 1089f
  pathophysiology of, 1088–1089
  treatment of, 1089
Papanicolaou (Pap) smear:
  in female rape victims, 401
  in genital herpes, 396
Papillary muscle:
  dysfunction of, in acute myocardial infarction, 206
  rupture of, in acute myocardial infarction, 206–207
Paracetamol (*see* Acetaminophen(s); Acetaminophen poisoning)
Parainfluenza virus, pneumonia and, 267
Paraldehyde:
  metabolic acidosis and, 45
  in status epilepticus, in children, 485, 485t
Paralysis:
  in acute ischemia of extremities, 254
  in altered mental status, 154
  lightning injuries and, 702
  periodic, acute, 813
  postictal, in children, 483
  tick, 541–542, 812
    clinical presentation of, 541
    diagnosis and treatment of, 542
  of vocal cords, 845
  Volkmann's, 814
Parapharyngeal abscess, upper airway obstruction and, 844, 845
Parapharyngeal space infection, 858, 858f
  clinical features of, 858
  treatment of, 858
Paraphimosis, 384, 385f
Parasitic infections, 535–539
  helminthic, 535–538
  history of, 535, 535t
  protozoan, 538–539
  symptoms of, 535, 536t, 537t
Paraspinal line, right, 951
Parasympathetic nervous system (PSNS), asthma and, 290–291
Parasystole:
  clinical significance of, 95
  treatment of, 95
  ventricular, 95, 95f
Parathormone (PTH), calcium levels and, 74
Paratracheal stripe, 951
Parents, of possibly abused child, 500, 501
Paresthesias, in acute ischemia of extremities, 254
Parkinsonism, 1101
  neuroleptics and, 555, 556t
Parkinson's disease, 1101
Parkinson's syndrome, antipsychotic drugs and, 1081
Parkland formula, 164
Paromomycin, in parasitic infections, 537t
Paronychia, 976, 976f
Parotid gland, 1058, 1059
Paroxysmal atrial tachycardia (PAT), 92, 92t
  in children, 180
  treatment of, 109, 112, 117, 121
Paroxysmal nocturnal dyspnea, 216
Paroxysmal pain, of neuropathic origin, 861
Paroxysmal supraventricular tachycardia (PSVT), 92
  treatment of, 109, 115t, 116t, 119, 121
Paroxysmal supraventricular tachycardia (PVST), in acute myocardial infarction, 205
Parsonage-Turner syndrome, 894
Partial pressure, in alveoli, 53
Partial thromboplastin time (PTT), prolongation of, 766
PASG (*see* Pneumatic antishock garment)
PAT (*see* Paroxysmal atrial tachycardia)
PATC (*see* Pulmonary artery thermodilution catheter)
Patella dislocation, 1002
Patellar fractures, 999, 1000f
Pathologic fractures, 967
Patient autonomy, resuscitation and, 4–5
Patient motion, computed tomography and, 3
Patient records, 190
  emergency medical services and, 190
Patient selection, for thrombolytic therapy, in acute myocardial infarction, 211–212
Pavulon (*see* Pancuronium bromide)
PAWP (*see* Pulmonary artery wedge pressure)
PBT (*see* Pulmonary barotrauma)
PCO (hallucinogenic drug), 584
P_{CO_2}:
  oxyhemoglobin dissociation and, 57
  pH and, 38
PCP (*Pneumocystis carinii* pneumonia) (*see* Pneumonia, *Pneumocystis carinii*)
PD (*see* Panic disorder)
PE (*see* Pulmonary embolism)
Peak expiratory flow rate (PEFR), in asthma, 293–294
  in children, 468
Pedialyte, 165
Pediatric Advanced Life Support Course (PALS), 178
Pediatric care:
  emergency medical services and, 191–192
  (*See also* Children; *specific disorders*)
PEEP (*see* Positive end-expiratory pressure)
PEFR (*see* Peak expiratory flow rate)
PEG (*see* Percutaneous ensoscopic gastrostomy)
PEG 300 (*see* Polyethylene glycol 300)
Pellet wounds, 1023
Pelvic abscess, postoperative, 369
Pelvic examination, in ectopic pregnancy, 390
Pelvic fractures, 981–987, 982f, 982t
  anatomy and, 981, 981f
  in children, 987
  clinical evaluation of, 981–982
  complications of, 985–987
  multiple, severe, 983
  in pregnancy, 415
  "shock trauma" classification of, 984–985, 985–987f, 987t
  treatment of, 985
  type I, 982–983
  type II, 983
  type III, 983
  type IV, 983–984, 984f, 985f
Pelvic inflammatory disease (PID), 393t, 393–394
  colonic diverticulitis differentiated from, 334
Pelvic pain:
  in ectopic pregnancy, 390
  in females
    nongynecologic causes of, 389
    nonpregnancy adnexal accidents as causes of, 392
Pelvic trauma, in children, 912
Pelvic tumors, ultrasonography in, 1117–1119f, 1119
Penbutolol (Levatol):
  in angina, 201t
  dosage, actions, pharmacokinetics, and indications for, 112t
D-Penicillamine:
  in lead poisoning, 640, 642
  in mercury poisoning, 643
D-Penicillamine mobilization test, in arsenic poisoning, 641
Penicillin(s):
  allergy to, 903
  in conjunctivitis, in children, 448t
  in masticator space infection, 858
  in periorbital/orbital cellulitis, in children, 452t
  phenoxymethyl (Penicillin V)
    in alveolar fractures, 864
    in bacterial pneumonia, 264t
    in cutaneous abscess, 878t
    in Lyme disease, 540
    in oral lacerations, 865
    in oral lesions, 861
    in pericoronal infection, 857
    in periodontal abscess, 861
    in streptococcal pharyngitis, 444
  procaine, in bacterial pneumonia, 264t
Penicillin G (benzyl penicillin), 881
  in aspiration pneumonia, 278
  in bacterial pneumonia, 264t
  in gas gangrene, 880
  in mushroom poisoning, 719
  in streptococcal pharyngitis, 444
  in syphilis, 517
  in tetanus, 526t, 879, 880t
Penicillin V-K, in aspiration pneumonia, 278
Penis:
  anatomy of, 382, 382f
  balanoposthitis and, 384
  carcinoma of, 385
  entrapment injuries of, 384, 385f
  fracture of, 384–385
  paraphimosis and, 384, 385f
  Peyronie's disease and, 385
  phimosis and, 384
  priapism and, 385, 385t
Pentamidine isothionate:
  in human immunodeficiency virus infections, 521t, 522
  in parasitic infections, 537t
  in *Pneumocystis carinii* pneumonia, 273–274
Pentanyl, for pediatric analgesia, 513t
Pentazocine, in acute myocardial infarction, 207
Pentobarbital:
  for pediatric sedation, 513t, 514
  pharmacology of, 561t
  in status epilepticus, 809
Pentobarbital coma, in Reye's syndrome, 477
Peptic ulcer disease, 313–315
  clinical features of, 313

complications of, 314
hemorrhage as, 314
obstruction as, 314
perforation as, 314
gastrointestinal bleeding and, 149
pathophysiology of, 313
postoperative, 368
stress ulcers and hemorrhagic gastritis and, 314-315
treatment of, 313-314
Percorten (desoxycorticosterone acetate), in adrenal crisis, 762
Percussion:
in perforated viscus, 317
in thoracic trauma, 934
Percutaneous coronary angioplasty (PTCA):
in acute myocardial infarction, 211
risks of, 213-214
Percutaneous endoscopic gastrostomy (PEG), complications of, 1109, 1109t
Percutaneous translaryngeal ventilation (PTV), 14, 14f
complications of, 14
Perforation:
of diverticulum, 333
esophageal (*see* Esophageal perforation)
in peptic ulcer disease, 314
of viscus, 316-319
clinical features of, 317-318, 318f
gallbladder perforation and, 316-317
large bowel perforation and, 317
pathophysiology of, 316-317
perforated ulcer and, 316
small bowel perforation and, 317
treatment of, 318-319
Perfusion, of vital organs, indicators of, 133, 133t
Perianal abscess, 56
Perianal disorders:
in Crohn's disease, 329
(*See also* Abscess(es), perianal)
Periapical infection, 857
Pericardial effusion:
in blunt injury to heart, 946
malignant, with tamponade, 780-781
Pericardial friction rub, in acute pericarditis, 230
Pericardial injury, 946
Pericardial knock, in constrictive pericarditis, 232
Pericardiocentesis, in penetrating injury to heart, 940-941
Pericarditis, 229-232, 230t
acute, 230-231
ancillary laboratory evaluation in, 231, 231t
echocardiography in, 230-231
electrocardiography in, 230
radiographic assessment in, 230
symptoms and signs of, 230
in acute myocardial infarction, 207
chest pain and, 130-131
constrictive, 229, 231-232
echocardiography in, 232
electrocardiography in, 232
pathology of, 231
radiographic assessment in, 232
symptoms and signs of, 231-232
uremic, 374
Pericoronal infections, 857
treatment of, 857
Pericoronitis, 860
Perilunate dislocations, 977
Periodontal infections, 857
abscess and, 861
treatment of, 857
Periodontium, normal, 860, 861f
Perionychium, 1061
injury of (*see* Fingertip injuries, perionychial)
Periorbital/orbital cellulitis:
in children, 451-452
clinical findings in, 451
complications of, 452
definition of, 451
diagnosis of, 452
differential diagnosis of, 452
epidemiology of, 451
management of, 452
pathophysiology of, 451
in sinusitis, in children, 449
Periosteitis, 861
Peripheral edema, high altitude and, 675
Peripheral nerve lesions, 811t, 811-816
acute myopathies and, 813
acute toxic neuropathies and, 811-812
Guillain-Barré syndrome and, 812-813
metabolic neuropathy and, 812
metallic poisons and, 812
mononeuritis multiplex and, 814
nonmyasthenic syndromes of malignancy and, 813-814
organic compounds and, 812
tick paralysis and, 812
trauma and nerve compression syndromes and, 815-816
Peripheral neuropathy, in anorexia nervosa, 1086
Peripheral perfusion, assessment of, in adult respiratory distress syndrome, 288-289
Peripheral vascular disease, 253-254
acute ischemic of extremities and, 253
arterial, noninvasive vascular studies in, 1113-1114
arterial trauma and, 254
differential diagnosis of, 253-254
initial evaluation in, 253
management of, 254, 254f
pathophysiology of, 253
popliteal aneurysms and, 254
syncope and, 142-143
venous, noninvasive vascular studies in, 1114
Perirectal abscess, 876
in ulcerative colitis, 330
Peritoneal dialysis:
in acute renal failure, 372
in salicylate intoxication, 591
Peritoneal irritation, in pregnancy, 414
Peritoneal lavage:
in acute pancreatitis, 365
diagnostic
in appendicitis, 321
in perforated viscus, 318
in hypothermia, 650
Peritoneal tap, diagnostic, in appendicitis, 321
Peritonitis:
abdominal pain and, 144
bacterial, spontaneous (*see* Hepatorenal syndrome)
in chronic renal failure, 375
pelvic, 393
(*See also* Fitz-Hugh-Curtis syndrome)
Peritonsillar abscess, upper airway obstruction and, 844
Pernia (chilblain), 645
Perphenazine (Trilafon), 1080t
Personality disorders, 1072t, 1072-1073
antisocial, 1072-1073
multiple personality disorder and, 1072
organic, 1068
Persuasion, in crisis intervention, 1095
Pertussis (whooping cough):
catarrhal stage of, 460
in children, 460
convalescent stage of, 460
paroxysmal stage of, 460
prophylaxis of, 460
Pertussis vaccine, contraindications to, 1050-1051
Petechiae, fever and, 159
Petit mal (absence) status, 485
Peyote cactus, 585
Peyronie's disease, 385
PGI_2 (*see* Prostacyclin)
pH:
acid-base problems and, 35
correlating with electrolyte values, 38
intracellular, 35-36
lactate production and, 747
oxyhemoglobin dissociation and, 56, 57t
P_{CO_2} and HCO_3^- and, 38
Phalangeal fractures:
of distal phalanx, 977-978, 978f
of middle and proximal phalanx, 978
Phalangeal injuries, 1013-1014
in children, 1014
distal fractures and, 1065, 1065f, 1066, 1066f
treatment of, 1014
Phalen's sign, in carpal tunnel syndrome, 975
Pharyngitis:
in children, 442-444
diagnosis of, 444
differential diagnosis of, 443
etiology of, 442
streptococcal pharyngitis and, 443-444
treatment of, 444
gonococcal, 443
high altitude and, 676
streptococcal, 443-444
diagnosis of, 443-444
management of, 444
Pharyngotracheal lumen airway (PTL), 11, 11f
Pharynx, 303
Phenelzine, in monoamine oxidase inhibitor overdose, 1083
Phenobarbital:
in cyclic antidepressant overdose, 552
in ethanol withdrawal, 577
pharmacology of, 561, 561t
in seizures, 808t
in children, 480t, 481, 482, 482t, 483
in neonate, 172
in status epilepticus, 809
in children, 485, 485t
Phenol (carbolic acid):
burns and, 697, 700
poisoning and, 709, 709t
Phenothiazine(s):
poisoning and, 812
in ventricular tachycardia, 96
Phentolamine (Regitine):
actions and pharmacology of, 243
adverse effects of, 244
dosage of, 244
in hypertensive emergencies, 240t, 241t, 243-244
indications for, 243
in monoamine oxidase inhibitor side effects, 1083
Phenylephrine (Neo-Synephrine):
in neurogenic shock, 139
ophthalmic uses of, 838
in reentrant supraventricular tachycardia, 93
Phenylpropanolamine (PPA), 583
Phenytoin (Dilantin):
adverse effects of, 486

Phenytoin (Dilantin) (*Cont.*):
  in cyclic antidepressant overdose, 552–553, 553
  in digoxin toxicity, 122
  in ectopic supraventricular tachycardia, 92
  electrophysiologic actions of, 110t
  in head injury, severe, 919
  hyperplasia and, 862
  pharmacokinetics of, 563–564
    absorption and, 563
    distribution and, 563
    free phenytoin fractions and, 563
    metabolism and, 563–564
  during pregnancy, 407
  in seizures, 807, 808t
    in children, 480t, 482, 482t
  in status epilepticus, 809
    in children, 485, 485t
  in Wolff-Parkinson-White syndrome, 105
Phenytoin toxicity, 563t, 563–565
  clinical presentation of, 564–565
    cardiovascular toxicity and, 564
    central nervous system toxicity and, 564
    hypersensitivity reactions and other side effects and, 564–565
    vascular extravasation and soft tissue toxicity and, 564
  differential diagnosis of, 565
  disposition in, 565
  laboratory diagnosis and ancillary studies in, 565
  serum levels and range of, 564
  toxic mechanism and pathophysiology of, 563
    brain and, 563
    cardiovascular system and, 563
    effects of propylene glycol and ethanol diluents and, 563
  treatment of, 565
Pheochromocytoma, 239
  treatment of, 241, 243
Philodendron, 723, 725
Phimosis, 384
Phlebotomy, in pulmonary edema, 218
Phlegmasia alba dolens (milk leg), 255
Phlegmasia cerulea dolens, 255
Phlegmon, scrotal, 384
Phobic disorders, 1071
Phosphate(s):
  in hypercalcemia, 79
  in hypophosphatemia, 82
  overload of, hypocalcemia and, 75
  replacement of, in diabetic ketoacidosis, 738–739
Phosphorus (phosphate), 81–82
Physical abuse, of children (*see* Child abuse)
Physical examination:
  abdominal pain and, 145–146
  in abdominal trauma, 955
  in altered mental status, 152–155
  in ankle injuries, 1007
  apparent life threatening events and, 435
  in asthma, 292
  in blunt injury to great vessels, 949–950
  in cerebral vascular accident, 794
  in child abuse, 499–500
  in child sexual misuse, 399, 400t
  in colonic diverticular disease, 333
  in cyanosis, in neonate, 175
  in ectopic pregnancy, 411
  in elder abuse, 1099
  in eye examination, 833
  in female rape examination, 398
  in fractures, 968
  in gastrointestinal bleeding, 147–148
  in great vessel injuries, 947
  in hazardous materials exposure, 708
  in headaches, 789
  in hip and femoral trauma, 987–988
  in hypertensive emergencies, 237
  in jaundice, 356
  in knee injuries, 999
  in male genitourinary problems, 382–383, 384t
  in mushroom poisoning, 718
  in neck pain, 891–893, 892f, 892t, 893f
  in neck trauma, 929
  in pelvic trauma, 981
  in poisoning, 545
    temperature in, 545
    toxic syndromes and, 545, 546–547t
    vital signs in, 545
  in psychiatric disorders, 1076
  in seizures, 806
  in syncope, in elderly patients, 259
  of thoracic spine, 896–898
  in thoracic trauma, 933–934
  in vertigo, 802, 802t
Physical restraints (*see* Restraints, physical)
Physician(s), air transport and, 190
Physiologic shunting, in lung, 57–58, 58t
Physostigmine:
  in anticholinergic poisoning, 637
  in antidepressant side effects, 1082
  in antipsychotic side effects, 1081
  in cyclic antidepressant overdose, 553, 554
  in mushroom poisoning, 720
Phytolacca americana, 723, 725
Pickwickian syndrome, 49
Picric acid burns, 700
PID (*see* Pelvic inflammatory disease)
Pilocarpine, in acute angle closure glaucoma, 836
Pilonidal abscess, 876
Pilonidal sinus, 344–345
  clinical features of, 344
  treatment of, 344–345
Pindolol (Visken):
  actions of, 111
  in angina, 201t
  dosage, actions, pharmacokinetics, and indications for, 112t
  pharmacology and properties of, 622
"Pink eye" (*see* Conjunctivitis)
Pinworm (*Enterobius*) infections, 397, 536
Piperazine, in parasitic infections, 537t
Pit vipers, 660–661
Pityriasis rosea, in children, 509
Pivot shift, in knee injury, 1001
Pixels, 1
Placenta, following emergency delivery, 421
Placenta previa, 412
  pelvic ultrasonography in, 1116f, 1116–1117, 1117f
Plants, poisonous, 721t, 721–726, 722t
  descriptions and common names of plants and, 724–726
  initial management and, 721–724
Plasma protein fraction, 776
Plasmapheresis:
  in myasthenia gravis, 824
  in rapidly progressing glomerulonephritis, 373
Platelet(s):
  hemostasis and, 765, 765t
  transfusion of, 775
Platelet-activation factor (PAF), asthma and, 467
Platelet count, in Reye's syndrome, 476
Plethysmography, impedance, in pulmonary embolism, 235
Pleural effusion:
  in congestive heart failure, 217
  examination of fluid and (*see* Thoracentesis)
Pleural lavage, in hypothermia, 650
Pleurisy, in rheumatic disorders, 883
PMNs (*see* Polymorphonuclear leukocytes)
Pneumatic antishock garment (PASG), in reentrant supraventricular tachycardia, 93
Pneumocystis carinii pneumonia (*see* Pneumonia, *Pneumocystis carinii*)
Pneumomediastinum, 939
  spontaneous, chest pain and, 131
Pneumonia:
  aspiration, 269, 276–278
    clinical features of, 276
    empyema and, 277–278
    hemoptysis and, 277
    lung abscess and, 277, 277f
    pathophysiology of, 276
    treatment of, 278
  bacterial, 263t, 263–266, 269
    admission guidelines for, 266
    anaerobic, 269
    in children, 461
    complications of, 264t
    empiric therapeutic guidelines for, 266
    gram-negative, 265, 269
    Hemophilus influenza, 265
    Klebsiella, 265
    laboratory studies in, 263, 264t, 265
    in neonate, 427t, 427–428
    staphylococcal, 266
    streptococcal, 458–459
    streptococcal (group A), 266
    Streptococcus pneumoniae, 265
    treatment of, 264t
  in children, 457–461
    chlamydial, 459
    clinical examination in, 457
    clinical history in, 457
    epidemiology of, 457t, 457–458
    group B streptococcal, 458–459
    Haemophilus influenzae, 459–460
    immunocompromised, 460
    laboratory studies in, 458
    management of, 460–461
    Mycoplasma pneumoniae, 460
    radiographic studies in, 458
    respiratory syncytial virus and, 459
    Streptococcus pneumoniae, 460
  chlamydial, 270
    in children, 459
  community-acquired, comparative analysis of, 269t, 269–270
  Klebsiella, 265, 270
  Legionella, 270
  Mycobacterium tuberculosis (MTB), in human immunodeficiency virus infections, 522–523
  Mycoplasma, 268–269
    in children, 460
    clinical manifestations of, 268
    comparative analysis of community-acquired pneumonia and, 269t, 269–270
    complications and extrapulmonary manifestations of, 268–269
    incidence and etiology of, 267, 267t
    laboratory studies in, 269
    management of, 269
    pathology and pathogenesis of, 268
    radiographic studies in, 269
    serology in, 269, 269t
  in neonate, 427t, 427–428

in pertussis, in children, 460
Pneumocystis carinii, 272-274
clinical course and prognosis of, 274
clinical presentation of, 272-273
diagnosis of, 273
differential diagnosis of, 273
extrapulmonary infections and, 273
in human immunodeficiency virus infections, 522
laboratory studies in, 273
prophylaxis of, 274
radiographic studies in, 273
transmission and incubation of, 272
treatment of, 273-274
viral, 267-268
in children, 457-458
comparative analysis of community-acquired pneumonia and, 269t, 269-270
diagnosis of, 267-268
incidence and etiology of, 267, 267t
influenza and parainfluenza viruses and, 267
influenza vaccine and, 268
management and prophylaxis of, 268
pathology and pathogenesis of, 267
(*See also* Legionnaires' disease)
Pneumonitis:
in hydrocarbon poisoning, 602
in lead poisoning, 713
Pneumoperitoneum, in perforated viscus, 318
Pneumothorax, 284-286, 938-939
in asthma, in children, 472
complications of, 939
diagnosis of, 938-939
diving and, 681
iatrogenic, 284-285
treatment of, 285, 286f
pathophysiology of, 938
postoperative, 366
spontaneous, 284
acquired immune deficiency syndrome and, 285-286
chest pain and, 131
clinical features of, 284, 285f
tension, 284, 285f, 939
Pocket, 861
Poisindex, 719
Poison ivy/oak/sumac (*see* Dermatitis, *Toxicodendron*)
Poisoning:
in adults, 545
altered mental status and, 156
anion gap changes due to, 40
in children, 545
cholinergic, treatment of, 113t
complications of, 547
cardiovascular, 547
neurologic, 547
respiratory, 547
"coral," 666
emergency department management of, 547-550
decontamination in, 547-548
definitive care in, 549t, 549-550
diagnostic studies in, 549
disposition and, 550
supportive care in, 548-549
incidence of, 545
metabolic acidosis and, 45
patient evaluation in, 545-547
history taking in, 545
physical examination in, 545, 546-547t
salicylate, treatment of, 164
(*See also* Hazardous materials exposure; *specific toxic substances*)
Poisons, altered mental status and, 156
Poloxamer 188, for wound cleansing, 1039
Polyarteritis nodosa, in rheumatic disorders, 884
Polycythemia:
high altitude and, 676
in neonate, cyanosis and, 175
Polyethylene glycol 300 (PEG 300), in phenol burns, 697
Polymorphonuclear leukocytes (PMNs):
in acute gastroenteritis, in children, 489
in cerebrospinal fluid, in meningitis, 828
Polymyositis, 814
Polymyositis syndrome, 813
steroid-induced, 814
Polyneuritis, in narcotic overdose, 568
Polyneuropathy, peripheral, in hydrocarbon poisoning, 602
Polyps, colonic, in children, 496
Polytetrafluoroethylene (PTFE) sutures, 1045
Pontine dysfunction, in neurological examination, 786
Pontine hemorrhage, 797
Pork tapeworms (*Taenia*), 538
Porta-cath, complications of, 1107t, 1108
Portland cement burns, 698
Portosystemic encephalopathy (hepatic coma; hepatic encephalopathy; PSE), 361-362
clinical features of, 362
treatment of, 362
Portuguese man-of-war envenomations, 667
Positive end-expiratory pressure (PEEP), 19
in adult respiratory distress syndrome, 288
in aspiration pneumonia, 278
in pulmonary edema, 218
in Reye's syndrome, 477
Postcholecystectomy syndrome, 353
Postconceptional age, 431
Postconcussion syndromes, 920
Posterior (lateral) approach, to internal jugular vein, 24
Posterior circulation, 793
Posterior cruciate ligament injury, 1001
Posterolateral instability, knee injury and, 1001
Posthitis, 384
Postmyocardial (Dressler's) syndrome, 207
Postpericardiotomy syndrome (PPCS), 946-947
diagnosis of, 947
etiology and pathogenesis of, 946
treatment of, 947
Posttraumatic stress disorder, 1071
Posttraumatic syringomyelia, 926
Posture, in congestive heart failure, in neonate, 175
Potassium, 70-74
deficit of, in children, 162
depletion of, in nonketotic hyperosmolar coma, 743
in diabetic ketoacidosis, in children, 503
Potassium chloride, in diabetic ketoacidosis, in children, 503
Potassium iodide, in radiation injury, 712
Potassium nitrate burns, 700
Potassium permanganate burns, 699
iatrogenic, 700
Potassium phosphate, in diabetic ketoacidosis, in children, 503
Potassium replacement, in diabetic ketoacidosis, 737
Pott's puffy tumor, 848
in children, 449
PPA (*see* Phenylpropanolamine)
PPCS (*see* Postpericardiotomy syndrome)
PPD test (*see* Tuberculin skin test)
PR interval, 86
Pralidoxime (2-PAM; Protopam), in organophosphate/carbamate poisoning, 612-613, 634, 709
Prazepam (Centrax), 1082t
Praziquantel, in parasitic infections, 537t
Prazosin (Minipress):
actions and pharmacology of, 243
in congestive heart failure, 218
in hypertensive emergencies, 241t, 243
indications for, 243
side effects and contraindications to, 243
use of, 243
PRBCs (*see* Packed red blood cells)
Precordial catch syndrome, chest pain and, 131
Prednisolone, in ulcerative colitis, 330
Prednisone:
in allergy to contrast media, 214
in asthma, in children, 471
in caustic ingestions, 608
in chronic decompensated airflow obstruction, 301
in Crohn's disease, 329
in Hymenoptera stings, 656
in *Pneumocystis carinii* pneumonia, 274
in sponge envenomations, 667
in *Toxicodendron* dermatitis, 868
in ulcerative colitis, 331
Preeclampsia, 410
Preexcitation syndromes, 103f, 103-106, 104f
clinical significance of, 104-105, 105f
treatment of, 105-106
Pregnancy, 406-413
abdominal trauma during, 414-416
cardiac arrest and postmortem cesarean section and, 416
evaluation and management of, 416
abortion and
infected, 391
spontaneous, 391
abruptio placentae and, 412, 415
anatomic and physiological changes associated with, 414
appendicitis in, 320, 410
asthma in, 292-293
management of, 293
bacterial vaginosis in, 396
carbon monoxide poisoning in, 704-705
cholecystitis in, 410
cocaine use and, 580
diabetes mellitus in, 409
diagnosis of, 406, 406t
drug and radiation exposure in, 406-407
ectopic, 390-391, 411, 496
culdocentesis in, 411
differential diagnosis of, 411, 411f
pelvic ultrasonography in, 411, 1115-1116
physical examination in, 411
pregnancy test and, 411
symptoms of, 411
treatment of, 411
in girls, 496
hemorrhagic corpus luteum and, 391
high altitude and, 677
history taking and, 389-390
hyperemesis gravidarum and, 407
hypertensive disorders in, 238-239, 408-409
treatment of, 241, 243, 408-409, 409t
(*See also* Eclampsia)
intrauterine, failing, pelvic ultrasonography in, 1115
lightning injuries during, 702
liver disease in, 410

Pregnancy (*Cont.*):
mastitis following, 411
molar, 412
pelvic ultrasonography in, 1116, 1116f
treatment of, 412
narcotic abuse and, 569
nausea of, 407
necessity of ruling out, 389
normal, pelvic ultrasonography in, 1115, 1115f, 1116f
out-of-hospital delivery and, 412–413
past history of, 389
placenta previa and, 412
postmortem cesarean section and, 413
postpartum fever and, 410–411
postpartum hemorrhage and, 413
premature rupture of membranes in, 408
diagnosis of, 408
treatment of, 408
preterm labor and, 407–408
prophylaxis for, in female rape victims, 400
Rh immunoprophylaxis following, 411
signs and symptoms of, 390
substance abuse in, 410
third trimester bleeding in
abruptio placentae and, 1117
placenta previa and, 1116f, 1116–1117, 1117f
thromboembolism in, 409
urinary tract infection in, 409
uterine incarceration in, 392
vaginal bleeding in, 411–412
verapamil in, 620
viral or protozoal infection in, 409–410
(*See also* Obstetric delivery)
Pregnancy test, 390, 406, 406t
in abdominal pain, 146
in ectopic pregnancy, 411
in female rape victims, 400
Pregnancy tumor, 862, 862f
Prehospital care:
in acute myocardial infarction, 209
of burns, 692
in near drowning, 688t, 688–689
in radiation injury, decontamination and, 713
spinal injuries and, 922
in trauma, 906
in wounds, 1027
(*See also* Emergency medical services)
Preload, 205–206, 216
military antishock trouser garment and, 6
treatment of, 218
Premature atrial contractions (PACs), 89–90, 90f
in acute myocardial infarction, 205
clinical significance of, 89
treatment of, 90
Premature contractions:
atrial (*see* Premature atrial contractions)
junctional, 93–94, 94f
clinical significance of, 94
treatment of, 94
ventricular (*see* Premature ventricular contractions)
Premature rupture of membranes (PROM), 408
diagnosis of, 408
treatment of, 408
Premature ventricular contractions (PVCs), 94f, 94–95
in acute myocardial infarction, 204–205
clinical significance of, 95, 95t
treatment of, 95, 107, 109, 115t
Prepubertal girls:
genital examination in, 499
vulvovaginitis in, 464
Pressure:
injuries due to (*see* Dysbarism)
oncotic, 63
Pressure dressing, 1049
Presyncope, 141
Preterminal rhythms, 102–103
electromechanical dissociation, 102, 103f
idioventricular rhythm, 102–103, 103f
Priapism, 385, 385t
in sickle cell anemia, 774
Primaquine:
adverse effects, precautions, and contraindications to, 533t
in malaria, 532t
in parasitic infections, 537t
Primary survey:
spinal injuries and, 922
trauma patient and, 907–908
Primidone (Mysoline):
pharmacology of, 561t
in seizures, 808t
in children, 480t
Probenecid, in pelvic inflammatory disease, 394t
Procainamide (Pronestyl), 109
actions, indications, dosage and administration, adverse effects, contraindications, and forms of, 115t
actions of, 109
adverse effects of, 109
in atrial fibrillation, 91
dosing and administration of, 109
electrophysiologic actions of, 110t
indications for, 109
pharmacokinetics of, 109
in sick sinus syndrome, 103
in ventricular tachycardia, 96, 97
in Wolff-Parkinson-White syndrome, 105
Procardia (*see* Nifedipine)
Prochlorperazine (Compazine), 556t
in acute mountain sickness, 673
for emergency delivery, 419t
in migraine headache, 790
Procidentia (*see* Rectal prolapse)
Proctitis, venereal, 340–343, 342t
clinical features of, 340, 342, 342t
treatment of, 342–343
Proctoscopy, in gastrointestinal bleeding, 148
Proctosigmoidoscopy, in ulcerative colitis, 331
Proguanil:
adverse effects, precautions, and contraindications to, 533t
in malaria prophylaxis, 533t
Prolixin (*see* Fluphenizine)
PROM (*see* Premature rupture of membranes)
Promethazine, 556t
for incision and drainage of cutaneous abscess, 877
for pediatric analgesia, 514
Pronator syndrome, 815t
Pronestyl (*see* Procainamide)
Propafenone (Rhythmol), electrophysiologic actions of, 110t
Proparacaine, 838
Propionic acid derivatives, overdose of, 628
Propranolol (Inderal), 112, 117
actions and pharmacology of, 245
actions of, 112
adverse effects of, 117
in angina, 200, 201t
in atrial fibrillation, 91, 205
in cardiogenic shock, 136
dosage, actions, pharmacokinetics, and indications for, 112t
dosing and administration of, 117
electrophysiologic actions of, 110t
in hypertensive emergencies, 240t, 245
in hypertrophic cardiomyopathy, 228
indications for, 112, 117, 245
in migraine headache, 790
in mitral stenosis, 221
pharmacokinetics of, 112
pharmacology and properties of, 621, 622
in reentrant supraventricular tachycardia, 93
in sick sinus syndrome, 103
side effects and contraindications to, 245
in thyroid storm, 753
in Wolff-Parkinson-White syndrome, 105
Propylene glycol, phenytoin toxicity and, 563
Propylhexedrine, 583
Propylthiouracil (PTU), in thyroid storm, 753
Prostacyclin (PGI_2), septic shock and, 137
Prostaglandin(s), septic shock and, 137
Prostaglandin E_1, in cyanosis, in neonate, 175
Prostate:
anatomy of, 382
palpation of, 383
Protein(s):
in cerebrospinal fluid, in meningitis, 828
synthesis of, cerebral ischemia and, 9
Proteolytic enzymes, in meat impaction, 310
Prothrombin time (PT):
in hemophilia, 770
prolongation of, 766
Protopam (pralidoxime), in organophosphate/carbamate poisoning, 612–613, 634, 709
Protoplasmic poisons, 695
Protozoan infections, 538–539
in immunocompromised host, 538–539
central nervous system, 539
gastrointestinal, 539
respiratory, 538–539
in pregnancy, 409–410
Proximal nail fold, 1061
Pruritus:
in human immunodeficiency virus infections, 520
sponge envenomations and, 667
Pruritus ani, 345t, 345–346
clinical features of, 345
treatment of, 345–346
Pryantel pamoate, in parasitic infections, 537t
PSE (*see* Portosystemic encephalopathy)
Pseudocyanosis, 141
Pseudocyst, pancreatic, in acute pancreatitis, 365
Pseudohyponatremia, treatment of, 68
Pseudohypoparathyroidism, hypocalcemia and, 75
Pseudoinfarction pattern, in hypertrophic cardiomyopathy, 228
Pseudomembranous enterocolitis, 331
Pseudoobstruction, intestinal, 324–325
Pseudoseizures, seizures versus, 485–486
Pseudotumor cerebri (benign intracranial hypertension), headache and, 791
Psilocin poisoning (*see* Psilocybin/psilocin poisoning)
Psilocybin, 585
Psilocybin/psilocin poisoning:
clinical toxicity of, 718
pharmacology of, 716, 717t
treatment of, 720
PSNS (*see* Parasympathetic nervous system)
PSVT (*see* Paroxysmal supraventricular tachycardia)
Psychiatric disorders, 1067–1091
axis I, 1067t, 1067–1069
axis II, 1072t, 1072–1073

diagnosis of, 1067
multiaxial diagnostic system and, 1067
standard diagnostic taxononomy and, 1067
drug therapy in, 1080–1084
antipsychotics and, 1080–1081
anxiolytics and, 1081–1082
heterocyclic antidepressants and, 1082t, 1082–1083
lithium and, 1084
monoamine oxidase inhibitors and, 1083
second-generation antidepressants and, 1083
emergency assessment and stabilization in, 1074–1079
consultation and referral and, 1079
decision-making in, 1074
initial evaluation and, 1074–1075
laboratory studies in, 1076
mental status examination and, 1075t, 1075–1076
physical examination and, 1076
suicide and, 1076–1077, 1078t
violence and, 1077–1079, 1079t
in human immunodeficiency virus infections, 522
major, 1069–1072
in nonsteroidal anti-inflammatory drug overdose, 628
(*See also specific disorders*)
Psychiatric syndromes, 1067t, 1067–1069
Psychogenic amnesia, 1072
Psychogenic fugue, 1072
Psychogenic unresponsiveness (catatonic state), 150
Psychomotor agitation, hallucinogens and, 587
Psychosis, 1069–1070
in acquired immune deficiency syndrome, 522
brief reactive, 1070
LSD and, 585
suicide attempts and, 1077
Psychosocial dwarfs, 498
Psychotropic drugs, during pregnancy, 407
Psychotropic medications (*see* Psychiatric disorders, drug therapy in; *specific drugs and drug types*)
PT (*see* Prothrombin time)
PTCA (*see* Percutaneous coronary angioplasty)
PTFE (*see* Polytetrafluoroethylene sutures)
PTH (*see* Parathormone)
PTL (*see* Pharyngotracheal lumen airway)
PTT (*see* Partial thromboplastin time)
PTV (*see* Percutaneous translaryngeal ventilation)
Pubic lice, 658
Pubis:
double vertical fracture or dislocation of, 983
fracture of, 982–983
Public education:
about emergency medical services, 190
emergency medical services and, 190
Public information, about emergency medical services, 190
Public relations, disaster medical services and, 196
Public safety agencies, emergency medical services and, 190
Pulmonary air leaks, in neonate, 173–174
signs and symptoms of, 173
treatment of, 173–174
Pulmonary angiography, in pulmonary embolism, 235
Pulmonary artery, cannulation of, 27f, 27–29, 28t, 29f, 30f
Pulmonary artery catheters, 59, 59t
Pulmonary artery thermodilution catheter (PATC), 27–28, 28t, 28–30f
Pulmonary artery wedge pressure (PAWP):
in adult respiratory distress syndrome, 288
in myocardial contusion, 945
Pulmonary barotrauma (PBT), 284, 681, 681t
Pulmonary contusions, 936
diagnosis of, 936
treatment of, 936
Pulmonary disorders (*see* Chronic obstructive pulmonary disease; Lung disorders)
Pulmonary edema, 216
in hazardous materials exposure, treatment of, 708
high altitude (*see* High altitude pulmonary edema)
in narcotic overdose, 567
noncardiogenic, 216
in poisoning, 548
permeability, 287, 287t
(*See also* Adult respiratory distress syndrome)
reentry, 675
sampling and analysis of fluid and, 288
treatment of, 218, 242
Pulmonary effusions:
in pneumonia, in children, 458
in rheumatic disorders, 883
Pulmonary embolectomy, pulmonary, 235–236
Pulmonary embolism (PE), 233–236
arterial blood gases in, 233
chest pain and, 131
chest x-ray in, 234
clinical features of, 233, 233t, 234t
electrocardiography in, 234, 234t
impedance plethysmography in, 235
postoperative, 367
predisposing factors for, 233, 233t
prognosis of, 236
pulmonary angiography in, 235
treatment of, 235–236
anticoagulation in, 235
pulmonary embolectomy in, 235–236
stabilization and, 235
thrombolytic therapy in, 235
vena cava interruption in, 235
venography in, 235
ventilation-perfusion lung scan in, 234
Pulmonary emphysema, 298
Pulmonary function, military antishock trouser garment and, 6
Pulmonary function testing:
in asthma, 292
in children, 468
in chronic compensated airflow obstruction, 299
in narcotic overdose, 568
in *Pneumocystis carinii* pneumonia, 273
Pulmonary regurgitation, 225
clinical features of, 225
treatment of, 225
Pulmonary stenosis, 224–225
clinical features of, 224–225
treatment of, 225
Pulse(s):
in acute ischemia of extremities, 254
bifid (pulsus bisferiens), in hypertrophic cardiomyopathy, 228
biphasic, in hypertrophic cardiomyopathy, 228
in congenital heart disease, in children, 437
Pulse oximetry, 59t, 59–60
Pulsus bisferiens (bifid pulse), in hypertrophic cardiomyopathy, 228
Pulsus paradoxus:
in asthma, 292, 467
in chronic decompensated airflow obstruction, 299–300
Puncture wounds, 1043
Pupil(s):
in altered mental status, 153
unilateral dilated fixed pupil and, 838
Purified protein derivative test (*see* Tuberculin skin test)
Putamen, hemorrhage of, 797
PVCs (*see* Premature ventricular contractions)
Pyelonephritis, 380–381
appendicitis differentiated from, 410
ultrasonography in, 1121
Pyloric obstruction, in peptic ulcer disease, 314
Pyloric stenosis:
in children, 494
treatment of, 164
in infants, treatment of, 164
Pyogenic granuloma, oral manifestations of, 862
Pyosalpinx, 392
Pyracantha, 723, 725
Pyrazinamide:
in human immunodeficiency virus infections, 521t
in tuberculosis, 283t
Pyridostigmine bromide, in myasthenia gravis, 823
Pyridoxine (vitamin B_6):
dependence on, seizures and, 172
in hypoglycemia, in ethylene glycol poisoning, 574
in mushroom poisoning, 720
in seizures
in children, 482t
in neonate, 173
Pyrimethamine:
in human immunodeficiency virus infections, 521t
in parasitic infections, 537t
Pyrimethamine-sulfadoxine (Fansidar):
adverse effects, precautions, and contraindications to, 533t
in malaria, 532t
in malaria prophylaxis, 533t
Pyrogens, 158
Pyrosis (heartburn), 306
Pyruvate, lactate production and, 747
Pyuria, in children, 462

Q fever, 542
Q waves, 87
septal, in hypertrophic cardiomyopathy, 228
QRS complexes, 86–87
wide, 97
QT interval, 87
Quadriplegia, 926
Quantum mottle, computed tomography and, 3
Questran (*see* Cholestyramine)
Quinacrine:
in diarrhea, 351t
in parasitic infections, 537t
Quincke's sign, in aortic regurgitation, 223
Quinidine, 109–110
actions of, 109
adverse effects, precautions, and contraindications to, 110, 533t
in atrial fibrillation, 91
dosing and administration of, 110
electrophysiologic actions of, 110t
indications for, 110
in malaria, 532t

Quinidine (*Cont.*):
  pharmacokinetics of, 109
  in sick sinus syndrome, 103
  in ventricular tachycardia, 96
Quinine:
  adverse effects, precautions, and contraindications to, 533t
  in babesiosis, 543
  in malaria, 532t
  in parasitic infections, 537t

RA (rheumatoid arthritis) (*see* Arthritis, rheumatoid; Rheumatic disorders)
Rabies, 527–529
  clinical presentation of, 527
  diagnosis of, 527–528
  pathophysiology of, 527
  postexposure prophylaxis and, 528, 529f
  reporting, 529
  transmission of, 527
  treatment guidelines for, 528–529
Rabies immune globin (RIG), 528
Rad, 711
Radial head fractures, 985
Radial nerve entrapment, 815t
Radiation:
  dose of, 711, 713, 714
  electromagnetic, 711
  exposure to, during pregnancy, 407
  ionizing, 711
  nonionizing, 711
  particulate, 711
  weakness and, 814
Radiation Emergency Assistance Center/Training Site (REAC/TS), 713, 715
Radiation injuries, 711t, 711–715
  burns and, 711, 713
  Chernobyl accident and, 714
  clinical features of, 711–712, 712t
  decontamination in
    in emergency department, 713
    prehospital, 713
  evacuation and, 713
    of hospital, 713–714, 714t
  pathophysiology of, 711
  special aspects of, 714–715
  treatment of, 712–713
Radiation Management consultants (RMC), 726
Radiographic studies:
  in abdominal trauma, 956
    in pregnancy, 416
  in acute pancreatitis, 364
  in acute pericarditis, 230
  in altered mental status, 155, 158
  in ankle injuries, 1007–1008
    ligamentous, 1009
  in aortic dissection, 247
  in appendicitis, 321
  aspirated foreign bodies and, 469
  in aspiration pneumonia, 276
  in asthma, 292
    in children, 468
  in blunt injury to great vessels, 950f, 950t, 950–951, 951f
  in bronchiolitis, in children, 468
  in calcaneal fractures, 1012
  in carbon monoxide poisoning, 705
  chest x-ray, in chest pain, 129
  in child abuse, 500
  in cholecystitis, 354
  in chronic compensated airflow obstruction, 299
  in congestive heart failure, 217
  in constrictive pericarditis, 232
  in Crohn's disease, 329
  in cyanosis, in neonate, 175
  in dilated cardiomyopathy, 227
  in empyema, 277
  in epiglottitis, 843, 843f
    in children, 183, 183f, 184f
  in foreign body aspiration, in children, 185, 185f, 186f
  in fractures, 968
    in children, 970
  in gastrointestinal bleeding, 148
  in great vessel injuries, 947–948
  in head injury, 917
  in hernia, 327
  in hip and femoral trauma, 988
  in hydrocarbon poisoning, 602
  in hypertrophic cardiomyopathy, 228
  in hypocalcemia, 76
  in intestinal obstruction, 323–324, 324f
  in intussusception, in children, 494–495, 495f
  in lead poisoning, 639
  in leg fractures, 1004
  in Legionnaires' disease, 271
  in lung abscess, 277, 277f
  in mandibular fractures, 850
  in maxillary fractures, 854
  in mesenteric ischemia, 251
  in mitral stenosis, 220
  in myocardial contusion, 944
  in myocarditis, 229
  in narcotic overdose, 567
  in naso-orbital injuries, 855
  in near drowning, 689, 689f
  in neck pain, 893
  in neck trauma, 929–930
  in nephrolithiasis, 373–374
  in orbital floor fractures, 853, 853f
  in pediatric trauma victim, 911
  in pelvic trauma, 981–982
  in penetrating injury to heart, 940
  in perforated viscus, 318, 318f
  in *Pneumocystis carinii* pneumonia, 273
  in pneumonia
    bacterial, 263, 264t
    in children, 458, 459
    Mycoplasma, 269
  during pregnancy, 407
  in pulmonary embolism, 234
  in restrictive cardiomyopathy, 228
  in retropharyngeal abscess, in children, 186, 186f
  in rib fractures, 935
  in seizures, 807
  in sinusitis, in children, 449
  in spinal injuries, thoracolumbar, 925
  in spinal injury, 923–924
  in spontaneous pneumothorax, 284
  swallowed foreign bodies and, 310
  in talus fractures, 1012
  in thoracic aortic aneurysms, 248
  in tuberculosis, 282, 282t
    extrapulmonary, 281, 281f
    miliary, 282, 282f
    reactivation, 280f, 280–281, 281f
  in urinary tract infections, in children, 463
  in wheezing, in children, 469
  in zygoma and zygomatic-maxillary complex fractures, 853
  in zygomatic arch fractures, 852, 852f
Radionuclide scanning:
  in abdominal pain, 147
  in acute myocardial infarction, 203
  in chest pain, 129
  in cholecystitis, 354
  in myocardial contusion, 944–945
  ventilation-perfusion lung scan and, in pulmonary embolism, 234
Radius, trauma to, 985–986
Ranitidine, in theophylline poisoning, 615
Rape (*see* Sexual assault)
Rapid sequence induction (RSI), 18t, 18–19
Rapidly progressing glomerulonephritis (RPGN), 373
Rash, in toxic shock syndrome, 404
Rashes:
  in children, 505t, 505–510
    bacterial, 505–506, 506f
    differential diagnosis of, 505, 505t
    rickettsial, 506–507, 507f
    unclear etiology and, 508–510
    viral, 507–508
  in hydrocarbon poisoning, 603
  phenytoin and, 564
  in rheumatic disorders, 884
RATS, animal bites and, 1044
Rattlesnakes, 660
RBB (*see* Right bundle branch)
RBCs (*see* Red blood cells)
REAC/TS (*see* Radiation Emergency Assistance Center/Training Site)
Reassurance, in crisis intervention, 1095
Recovery phase, of disaster response, 193–194
Rectal examination:
  in abdominal pain, 146
  in anorectal disorders, 336
Rectal prolapse (procidentia), 343
  in children, 343
  clinical features of, 343
  treatment of, 343
Rectovaginal fistula, in ulcerative colitis, 330
Rectum:
  biopsy of, in ulcerative colitis, 331
  foreign bodies in, 344
    treatment of, 344
  injury to, 959
    in pelvic fracture, 986–987
  perforation of, foreign bodies and, 344
Red blood cell scan, in lower gastrointestinal bleeding, in diverticulosis, 335
Red blood cells (RBCs):
  mechanical hemolysis of, by prosthetic heart valves, 225
  packed, 775, 777
  washed, 775
"Red eye" (*see* Conjunctivitis)
"Red strawberry tongue," in scarlet fever, 506
Redline, 1057
Redox state, lactate production and, 747
Reducing agents, 695
Reduvid (kissing) bug (coenose) bites, 538, 658
  treatment of, 658
Reentry, tachyarrhythmias and, 88, 88f
Reflex(es):
  in altered mental status, 154–155, 155t
  Bainbridge, in sinus arrhythmia, 89
  corneal, in altered mental status, 154
  distinguishing true neurologic deficits from conversion disorder and, 1091t
  hepatojugular, in congestive heart failure, 217
  hyperreflexia and, 811
  hyporeflexia and, 811
  in neurological examination, 787f, 787–788, 788t
  oculocephalic, in altered mental status, 153
  pathological, 787–788
Reformatting, computed tomography and, 2
Regional enteritis (*see* Crohn's disease)
Regitine (*see* Phentolamine)

Reglan (metoclopramide), in acetaminophen poisoning, 597
Regurgitation, 306
in neonate, 426
Rehydralyte, 165
Rehydration:
in acute gastroenteritis, in children, 489
in children, 164-165
(*See also* Fluid and electrolyte therapy)
Reissner's membrane, tear in, barotrauma and, 680
Relapsing fever, 542
clinical presentation of, 542
diagnosis of, 542
treatment of, 542
Relaxation techniques, in children, 511
Rem, 711
Renal failure:
acute, 371-373
acute tubular necrosis and, 372
differential diagnosis of, 371, 372t
in elderly patients, 372
etiology of, 371, 371t
management of, 371-372
postrenal, 371
prerenal, 371-372
prevention of, 372-373
prognosis of, 372
chronic, 374-376
blood pressure alterations and, 374-375
cardiac arrest and, 374
cardiac arrhythmias and, 374
gastrointestinal disorders and, 375
neurologic problems and, 375
problems related to vascular access and, 375-376
resuscitation of potential organ donor and, 376
uremic pericarditis and, 374
hypocalcemia and, 75
metabolic acidosis and, 45
oliguric, in ethylene glycol poisoning, 574, 575f
in Reye's syndrome, 478
Renal pelves, dilatation of, in pregnancy, 414
Renal system, hyponatremia and, 68
Renal tubular acidosis, in hydrocarbon poisoning, 603
Reperfusion:
in acute myocardial infarction, 211
in cerebral ischemia
early reperfusion phase of, 8-9
late reperfusion phase of, 9
Reproductive organs, pregnancy-associated changes in, 414
Reserpine, in thyroid storm, 754
Reset osmostat, 66-67
Residual volume, in pregnancy, 414
Resol, 165
Respiratory arrest, lightning injuries and, 701
Respiratory disorders:
cocaine use and, 580
congenital, in neonate, 428
in neonate, with bronchopulmonary dysplasia, 431-432, 432t
in poisoning, management of, 548
poisoning and, 547
protozoan infections and, in immunocompromised host, 538-539
in rheumatic disorders, 883-885, 884t, 885t
Respiratory failure, in myxedema coma, 756
Respiratory index, 57
Respiratory insufficiency:
chronic, in neonate, 428
in sickle cell anemia, 774
Respiratory pattern, in altered mental status, 153
Respiratory quotient (RQ), 55
Respiratory rate, in pregnancy, 414
Respiratory syncytial virus (RSV):
bronchiolitis and (*see* Asthma, exercise-induced)
pneumonia and, 267
in children, 459
Respiratory system, tumors of, 845
Restoril (temazepam), 1082t
Restraints:
chemical
hallucinogens and, 587
in poisoning, 548, 549
in psychiatric disorders, 1074
in violence, 1078-1079, 1079t
for children, 511
physical
hallucinogens and, 587
in neurologically disabled patients, 1101
in poisoning, 548-549
in psychiatric disorders, 1074
trauma patient and, 907
in violence, 1078
Resuscitation:
in acquired immune deficiency syndrome, 523
emergency department, spinal injuries and, 922t, 922-923, 923t
ethics of, 4-5
advance directives and, 4-5
determination of death and, 4
terminal illness and, 4
triage and, 5
in great vessel injury, 948
in neck trauma, 928-929
airway and, 928-929
breathing and, 929
circulation and, 929
neonatal (*see* Neonate, resuscitation of)
in thoracic trauma, to chest wall, bronchi, lung, and diaphragm, 932-933
of trauma patients, in emergency department, 906t, 906-908
(*See also* Cardiopulmonary resuscitation)
Reticular activating system, lesions of, 151
Retinal detachment, 837
traumatic, 838
Retinitis, cytomegalovirus, in human immunodeficiency virus infections, 522
Retinopathy:
high altitude and, 675-676
sun gazer's (eclipse burn), 837
Retrobulbar neuritis, 837
Retroesophageal space, 303
Retrograde tracheal intubation (RTI), 15
Retroperitoneal trauma, computed tomography in, 10
Retropharyngeal abscess:
in children, 186, 186f
upper airway obstruction and, 844
Retropharyngeal space, 303
Reversible dementia of depression, 1068
Review, of emergency medical services, 190
Rewarming:
in frostbite, 646
in hypothermia, 650t, 650-651
Reye's syndrome, 160, 475-478
clinical picture in, 475
complications of, 478
diagnosis of, 475-476
differential diagnosis of, 476
etiology of, 475
laboratory studies in, 476
management of, 477-478
pathologic confirmation of, 476
prognosis of, 478
recovery phase of, 478
staging of, 476-477
Rh immunoprophylaxis, 411
Rh sensitization, fetomaternal hemorrhage and, 415-416
Rhabdomyolysis, cocaine use and, 580
Rheumatic disorders:
ambulatory evaluation in, 886-890
aspiration and examination of synovial fluid and, 886t, 886-887
baker's cyst in arthritis of knee and, 889
bursitis and, 889
corticosteroid injections and, 889
gout and, 888-889
limp in children and, 889-890
septic arthritis and, 888, 888t
tendonitis and, 889
traumatic arthritis and, 888
associated with risk of mortality, 883-884
respiratory system and, 883-884, 884t, 885t
corticosteroid treatment of, adrenal insufficiency and, 885
with high risk of morbidity, 885-886
cervical spine and spinal cord and, 885
eye and, 885-886
hypertension and, 885
kidney and, 886
Rheumatic fever, 884, 884t
prevention of, 444
Rheumatoid arthritis (RA) (*see* Arthritis, rheumatoid; Rheumatic disorders)
of temporomandibular joint, 857
Rhinorrhea, cerebrospinal fluid, 847-848
Rhodanase, in cyanide poisoning, 634, 635f
Rhododendron, 723, 725
Rhythmol (propafenone), electrophysiologic actions of, 108t
Rib fractures, 935
first and second ribs and, 935
multiple, 935
simple, 935
Ribavarin, in pneumonia, in neonate, 428t
Ricelyte, 165
Ricinus communis, 723, 725
Rickettsial infections, rashes and, in children, 506-507, 507f
Rifampin:
in human immunodeficiency virus infections, 521t
prophylaxis of meningitis and, 456
in tuberculosis, 283t
RIG (*see* Rabies immune globin)
Right bundle branch (RBB), 86
bifascicular block and, 101, 102f
trifascicular block and, 101
unifascicular block and, 100, 101, 102f
Right ventricular (RV) infarction, in acute myocardial infarction, 207
Right ventricular (RV) pump function, in acute myocardial infarction, 201
Ringer's solution, lactated:
in burns, in children, 164
in shock, in children, 162
Risk factors, for coronary artery disease, in elderly patients, 258
Risus sardonicus, 812
RMC (*see* Radiation Management consultants)
Rocky Mountain spotted fever (RMSF), 541
in children, 506-507, 507f
clinical presentation of, 541
diagnosis of, 541

Rocky Mountain spotted fever (RMSF) (*Cont.*):
treatment of, 541
Romberg test, 786–787
Root syndromes, 815
Roseola infantum (exanthem subitum), rash in, 509–510
Rotational malalignment, of hand, 979f, 979–980
Rotator cuff tears, 203, 983f
Roundworm (nematode) infections, 535–537
Rovsing's sign, in appendicitis, 320
RPGN (*see* Rapidly progressing glomerulonephritis)
RQ (*see* Respiratory quotient)
RSI (*see* Rapid sequence induction)
RSV (*see* Respiratory syncytial virus)
RTI (*see* Retrograde tracheal intubation)
Rubbing alcohol (*see* Isopropanol poisoning)
Rubella (German measles), rash in, in children, 508
"Rum fits," 577
Rust rings, 835
RV (*see* Right ventricular infarction; Right ventricular pump function)

S tube, 10
SA block (*see* Sinoatrial block)
Sacral fractures, 983
Sacral injuries, 925–926
Sacroiliac joint, fracture near subluxation of, 983
SAH (*see* Subarachnoid hemorrhage)
St. Anthony's fire (erysipelas), in children, 505
Salicylate(s):
hypoglycemia and, 732
metabolic acidosis and, 45
during pregnancy, 407
Salicylate intoxication, 589–592
acute versus chronic, 590
bronchiolitis versus, 469
in children, treatment of, 164
gastrointestinal decontamination in, 590–591
pathophysiology and clinical findings in, 589
toxic doses and salicylate levels in, 589–590, 590f
treatment of, 590–592
dialysis in, 591
intravenous fluids and urine alkalinization in, 591
laboratory studies in, 591
neurotoxicity and, 591
Saline:
in hypercalcemia, 79, 79t
hypertonic
with dextran 70 (HTS/Dex), in hemorrhagic shock, 134
in hyponatremia, 68
in shock, in children, 162
Salivary gland problems, 842
Salmonella, diarrhea and, 348–349
treatment of, 351t
Salpingitis, 393t, 393–394
Salpingo-oophoritis, 393
Saphenous vein:
great, venous access and, in children, 166f, 166–167
superficial, venous access and, 21, 21f
SBP (*see* Spontaneous bacterial peritonitis)
Scabies, 658
treatment of, 658
Scald burns, 500
Scalded skin syndrome (*see* Toxic epidermal necrolysis)
Scalp, anatomy and physiology of, 913
Scalp veins, venous access and, in children, 165–166, 166f
Scalp wounds, 1052–1053
anatomy and, 1052, 1053f
avulsion, 1052, 1053
contusions, 1053
human bites and, 1043
lacerations, 1053
treatment of, 1052–1053, 1054f
Scan time for acquisition, computed tomography and, 3
Scaphoid fractures, 976
Scapholunate dissociation, 977
Scapula fracture, 981
Scar(s), wound biomechanical properties and, 1028–1029, 1029f
Scarlet fever:
rash in, in children, 506
staphylococcal, toxic shock syndrome versus, 404
Schefflera, 723, 725
Schistosoma infections, 538
Schiötz tonometer, 833
Schizophrenia, 1069–1070
suicide attempts and, 1077
treatment of, 1069
Schizophreniform disorder, 1070
Scleroderma, dysphagia and, 305
Sclerotherapy, in gastrointestinal bleeding, 148
SCLR (*see* Crossed straight-leg raising signs)
Scorpion stings, 665
treatment of, 665
Scorpionfish envenomations, 668–669
Scotoma, "fortification," 838
Scribner shunt, 375
Scrotum:
anatomy of, 382, 382f
ecchymosis of, following surgery for inguinal hernia, 369
edema of, 383
Fournier's gangrene and, 384, 384f
hair folliculitis and, 384
phlegmon and, 384
Scrub solutions, for wound cleansing, 1039
SDH (*see* Subdural hematoma)
Sea urchin envenomations, 669
Seat belt injuries, 912, 925
in pregnancy, 415
Secobarbital, pharmacology of, 561t
Secondary gain, suicide attempts and, 1077
Secondary survey:
spinal injuries and, 922
trauma patient and, 908
Sectral (*see* Acebutolol)
Sedation, in children, 514
for brief, nonpainful procedures, 514
for longer, nonpainful procedures, 514
Seizures:
in adults, 804–809
electroencephalography in, 807
history taking and, 805t, 805–806, 806t
laboratory studies in, 806–807
physical examination in, 806
radiographic studies in, 807
status epilepticus and, 808–809
treatment of, 807–808
amphetamines and, management of, 582
in arsenic poisoning, treatment of, 642
aseptic, 628
autonomic, in children, 481
in beta blocker overdose, treatment of, 622
in calcium channel blocker overdose, treatment of, 621
in children, 479–486
breakthrough, 483
differential diagnosis of, 485–486
febrile, 480–481
first, 479–480, 480t
head trauma and, 482–483
pitfalls of emergency management of, 486
problems of anticonvulsant use and, 486
status epilepticus and, 483–485, 484t
classification of, 804t, 804–805
clonic
focal, in neonate, 172
multifocal, in neonate, 172
complex partial, 805
in cyclic antidepressant overdose, treatment of, 552–553
definition of, 479
in ethanol withdrawal, 577
febrile, 159, 480–481
evaluation in, 480–481
treatment of, 481
generalized, 804
grand mal, 804–805
in head injury, 920
delayed, 920
high altitude and, 673–674
infantile spasms and, 482
lightning injuries and, 702
in meningitis, in children, 455
in methanol poisoning, 572
multifocal (fragmentary), in children, 481
myoclonic
in children, 481
in neonate, 172
in narcotic overdose, 568
in neonate, 172–173, 481–482
causes of, 172
diagnosis of, 172
differentiation of, 172
evaluation of, 481
treatment of, 172–173, 481–482, 482t
types of, 172
in nonketotic hyperosmolar coma, treatment of, 746
in nonsteroidal anti-inflammatory drug overdose, treatment of, 629
partial (focal), 805
petit mal, 804
in phenytoin toxicity, 564
treatment of, 565
in poisoning, 547, 548
poisonous plants and, 722
progressive migratory partial (jacksonian), in children, 481
psychogenic, 805–806
subtle, in neonate, 172
in theophylline poisoning, 614
treatment of, 615
tonic, in neonate, 172
treatment of
acute seizures and, 807
alcohol withdrawal seizures and, 808
in patient with first seizure, 808, 808t
in patients with previous seizures, 807–808, 808t
unilateral, in children, 481
Self-esteem, crisis intervention and, 1093–1094
Sellick's maneuver:
orotracheal intubation and, 12
in spinal injuries, 922
Semen, detection of, sexual assault and, 401–402
Sensory examination, in altered mental status, 154

Sensory loss, cortical, cerebral vascular accident and, 797
Sensory response, in neurological examination, 786-787
"Sentinel clot sign," computed tomography and, 4, 5f
Sepsis:
in acute pancreatitis, 365
in children, 454
clinical presentation of, 454
treatment of, 163-164, 454
hypothermia and, 648
in neonate, 429
cyanosis and, 175
Septic shock (*see* Shock, septic)
Septra (*see* Trimethoprim/sulfamethoxazole)
Serax (oxazepam), 1082t
Serentil (mesoridazine), 1080t
for rapid tranquilization, 1079t
Serology:
in myasthenia gravis, 823
in pneumonia, *Mycoplasma*, 269
Seroma, of wound, 366
gynecologic procedures and, 423
Serum glutamic-oxaloacetic transaminase (SGOT), in acute myocardial infarction, 203
Serum immune globulin (gamma globulin; immune globulin), in viral hepatitis, 358-359
Sexual abuse/misuse:
assessing for, in vulvovaginitis, 464
of children, 398-399, 399t, 498-499
physical examination in, 399, 400t
Sexual activity, history taking and, 389
Sexual assault, 398-402
child sexual abuse and, 398-399, 399t
physical examination in, 399, 400t
epidemiology of, 398
female rape examination and, 398
history taking in, 398
physical examination in, 398
laboratory studies in, recent advances in, 401-402
male rape examination and, 398
pregnancy prophylaxis and, 400
sperm survivability and, 401, 401f
treatment of victim of, 400t, 400-401
Sexually transmitted diseases (STDs), 517-518
child sexual abuse and, 499
proctitis and, 340-343, 342t
clinical features of, 340, 342, 342t
treatment of, 342-343
vulvovaginitis and, in children, 464, 465
(*See also specific diseases*)
SGM (status grand mal) (*see* Status epilepticus)
SGOT (*see* Serum glutamic-oxaloacetic transaminase)
Shark attacks, 666
Sharp objects, ingestion of, 311
Shigella, diarrhea and, 348
treatment of, 351t
Shock, 132-139
anaphylactic, treatment of, 114t
cardiogenic, 135-136
clinical presentation of, 135
management of, 135-136, 136t
pathophysiology of, 135
treatment of, 114t
in children, treatment of, 162-163
hemorrhagic, 133-134
clinical presentation of, 133
management of, 133-134
pathophysiology of, 133
hypovolemic
in aspiration pneumonia, 276
treatment of, 114t
in lactic acidosis, 749
in malignancy, 782
in meningitis, in children, 455
metabolic, treatment of, 114t
neonatal, resuscitation and, 171
in neonate, cyanosis and, 175
neurogenic, 138-139
pathophysiology of, 132-133, 133t
septic, 136-138
clinical presentation of, 137-138
management of, 138, 139t
pathophysiology of, 136t, 136-137, 137t
toxic shock syndrome versus, 404
treatment of, 114t
in thoracic trauma, 933
treatment of, 933
(*See also* Toxic shock syndrome)
Shoulder dislocation, 981-982, 982f, 983f
Shoulder trauma, 981-984
Shunt(s):
dialysis and, problems related to, 375-376
ventriculoperitoneal, in hydrocephalus, 432
SIADH (*see* Syndrome of inappropriate secretion of ADH)
Sialolithiasis, 842
Sick sinus (tachycardia-bradycardia) syndrome (SSS), 91, 103, 103f
clinical significance of, 103
treatment of, 103
Sickle cell anemia, 773-774
clinical manifestations and treatment of, 773-774
diagnosis of, 773
doubly heterozygous, 773
heterozygosity (Hb AS), 773
homozygosity (Hb SS), 773
pathogenesis of, 773
screening tests for, 773
sickle cell crises in, 773-774
Sickle cell crises, 773-774
aplastic, 773
hemolytic, 773
thrombotic, 773-774
Sickle cell disease, 773
high altitude and, 677
Sickle cell trait, 773
SIDS (*see* Sudden infant death syndrome)
Sigmoidoscopy:
in anorectal disorders, 336
in gastrointestinal bleeding, 148
in intestinal obstruction, 324
(*See also* Proctosigmoidoscopy)
"Silent bubbles," 683
Silibinin, in mushroom poisoning, 719
Silk sutures, 1045
SIMV (*see* Synchronized intermittent mandatory ventilation)
Single photon emission computed tomography (SPECT), in myocardial contusion, 945
Sinoatrial (SA) block, 98, 98f
clinical significance of, 98
first-degree, 98
second-degree, 98
third-degree, 98
treatment of, 98
Sinus arrest (pause), 98, 98f
clinical significance of, 98
treatment of, 98
Sinus arrhythmia, 89, 89f
clinical significance of, 89
Sinus bradycardia, 89, 89f
clinical significance of, 89
treatment of, 89
Sinus node, 86
Sinus squeeze, 680, 680f
Sinus tachycardia, 89, 89f
in children, 180, 180t, 438
treatment of, 117
Sinusitis, 848f, 848-849, 849f
in children, 448-450
clinical findings in, 449, 449t
complications of, 449
definition of, 448
diagnosis of, 449
differential diagnosis of, 449
epidemiology of, 448
etiology of, 448
management of, 449t, 449-450, 450f
pathophysiology of, 448-449
ethmoid, 848
frontal, 848
headache and, 791
maxillary, 848
Sipple's syndrome, 77
Sissure in ano (anal fissure), incarcerated, in neonate, 426
Sjögren's syndrome, 886
SJS (*see* Stevens Johnson syndrome)
Skeletal injuries, child abuse and, 500
Skin:
antisepsis of, in wound preparation, 1037
bacteria on, 1028
"cherry-red," in carbon monoxide poisoning, 704
decontamination of
in cyanide poisoning, 635
in poisoning, 548
examination of, in altered mental status, 152
Skin disorders:
abrasion and, 1049
abscess and (*see* Cutaneous abscess)
in anorexia nervosa, 1086
in carbon monoxide poisoning, 704
chemical burns and, 695
decompression sickness and, 683
in gastrointestinal bleeding, 147
in hazardous materials exposure, 707, 708
in human immunodeficiency virus infections, 520-521
treatment of, 521t
in hydrocarbon poisoning, 603
in narcotic overdose, 566
in nonsteroidal anti-inflammatory drug overdose, 628
in primary adrenal insufficiency, 760
(*See also* Rashes)
Skull, anatomy and physiology of, 913
Skull fracture, 914
basilar, 152
computed tomography and, 8
Slapped-cheek appearance, in erythema infectiosum, 508
Sleep:
definition of, 150
at high altitude, 671
Slice thickness, computed tomography and, 1, 3
Slipping rib syndrome, chest pain and, 131
Slow-reacting substance of anaphylaxis (*see* Leukotrienes)
Slow ventricular tachycardia (*see* Accelerated idioventricular rhythm)
SLR (*see* Straight-leg raising testing)
Small bowel:
injury to, 958
obstruction of, 322

Small bowel (*Cont.*):
perforation of, 317
Smith's fracture, 978, 978f
Snake bites, 660-664
clinical features of, 661
complications of, 664
consultation service for, 664
coral snakes and, 660, 664
harmless snakes and, 664
identification of indigenous snakes and, 660t, 660-661
immunization against, 664
pit vipers and, 660-661
signs and symptoms of, 662
treatment of, 662t, 662-664
variables influencing severity of
snake and, 661
victim and, 661-662
Sniffing position, orotracheal intubation and, 12
Snow blindness (ultraviolet keratitis), 676, 835
SNS (*see* Sympathetic nervous system)
Social service assessment, in child abuse, 500
Sociopathic behavior, 1072-1073
Sodium, 64-70
in acute lithium toxicity, 559
calculating deficits in, 68
in diabetic ketoacidosis, in children, 503
increased intake of, hypernatremia and, 69
loss of, hyponatremia and, 65
Sodium amytal, for emergency delivery, 419t
Sodium bicarbonate:
in alcoholic ketoacidosis, 741
in antidepressant overdose, 1083
cardiopulmonary resuscitation and, in children, 178t, 179-180, 180f, 180t
in cyclic antidepressant overdose, 553
in diabetic ketoacidosis, 737
in children, 503
for emergency delivery, 419t
in hyperkalemia, 73
in lactic acidosis, 750
in metabolic acidosis, 46, 218
in ethylene glycol poisoning, 574
Sodium hydroxide (*see* Caustic ingestions; Lye)
Sodium nitrate burns, 700
Sodium nitrite, in cyanide poisoning, 634, 635, 709
Sodium nitroprusside:
in cardiogenic shock, 136
in left ventricular pump failure, 206
Sodium nitroprusside (Nipride):
actions and pharmacology of, 240
in hypertensive emergencies, 240t, 240-241, 241t
indications for, 240
side effects and contraindications to, 241
use of, 240
Sodium restriction:
in congestive heart failure, 217
in heart failure, in aortic regurgitation, 224
Sodium sulamyd, in pneumonia, in neonate, 428t
Sodium thiosulfate, in cyanide poisoning, 634-635, 635, 635f, 709
Soft tissue toxicity, phenytoin and, 564
Soil, bacterial contaminants in, 1028
Solanum, 723, 725
Solu-Cortef (*see* Hydrocortisone sodium succinate)
Solu-Medrol (*see* Methylprednisolone)
Solvent abuse (*see* Hydrocarbon poisoning)
Somatization disorder, 1072
Somatoform disorder, 1071-1072, 1072t
Somatoform pain disorder, 1072
Sotalol (Betapace):
dosage, actions, pharmacokinetics, and indications for, 112t
electrophysiologic actions of, 110t
Spasm(s):
of accommodation, 838
infantile, 482
muscular, in tetanus, 879, 880t
SPECT (*see* Single photon emission computed tomography)
Spectinomycin, in gonorrhea, 517
Spectrometry (*see* Mass spectrometry)
Sperm, survivability of, 401, 401f
Spider bites (*see* Insect and spider bites/stings)
Spinal cord compression, 815
in malignancy, 780
Spinal cord injury syndromes, 926
Spinal cord lesions, 797
in multiple sclerosis, 818
in rheumatic disorders, 885
Spinal epidural abscess, in narcotic overdose, 568
Spinal injuries, 922-927
cervical, intubation in, 16
computed tomography in, 10
patient management and, 922-923
disposition and, 923
emergency department assessment and resuscitation and, 922t, 922-923, 923t
myelography and, 923
prehospital spinal immobilization and, 922
traction and, 923
penetrating, 926
posttraumatic syringomyelia and, 926
radiographic studies in, 923-924
research on, 926-927
sacral and coccygeal, 925-926
spinal cord injury syndromes and, 926
sports, 926
sprains and fractures and, 924-925
mechanisms of injury and common fractures and, 924-925, 925t
stability and, 924, 924t
thoracolumbar, 925
radiographic studies in, 925
Spine (*see* Cervical spine; Lumbar spine; Spinal injuries; Thoracic spine)
Spirochete infections, multiple sclerosis versus, 819
Spironolactone (Aldactone), in congestive heart failure, in neonate, 175
Spleen, injury to, 959
Splints, in fractures, 968
Spondyloarthropathies, chest pain and, 131
Spondylosis, cervical, 894-895
Sponge diver's disease, 667
Sponge envenomations, 667
Sponging, in fever, 159
Spontaneous bacterial peritonitis (SBP) (*see* Hepatorenal syndrome)
Sport injuries, spinal, 926
Sprain, of ankle (*see* Ankle injuries, ligamentous)
of collateral ligament, treatment of, 973, 974f
spinal, 924
Spurling's sign, in neck pain, 891
Sputum examination and culture:
in asthma, 292
in lung abscess, 277, 277f
in pneumonia
bacterial, 263, 264t, 265
in children, 458
"Square-root sign," in restrictive cardiomyopathy, 228
Squeeze, reverse (barotrauma of ascent), 680-681, 681t, 682f
Squeeze (barotrauma of descent), 679-680, 680f
SSS (*see* Sick sinus syndrome)
SSSS (*see* Staphylococcal scalded-skin syndrome)
ST segment, 87
Stabilization:
in caustic ingestions, 607, 607t
in clonidine poisoning, 570
in nonsteroidal anti-inflammatory drug overdose, 628-629
Staircase phenomenon (treppe), metabolic acidosis and, 43
Staphylococcal pneumonia, 266
Staphylococcal scalded-skin syndrome (SSSS), 873, 873f
in children, 506
Staphylococcus aureus:
antibiotic prophylaxis against, in wounds, 1040-1041, 1041t
diarrhea and, 349
Staphylococcus epidermidis, antibiotic prophylaxis against, in wounds, 1040-1041, 1041t
Staple(s), wound closure and, 1047-1048
Starfish envenomations, 669
Starling equation, 287
Starvation:
in anorexia nervosa, 1086
esophageal disease and, 307
starvation ketosis and, 44-45
Status asthmaticus, 293
in children, treatment of, 471
Status epilepticus (SGM; status grand mal), 808-809
anticonvulsant drugs in, 809, 809t
in children, 483-485, 484t
effects of, 484
treatment of, 484-485, 485t
in cyclic antidepressant overdose, 553
general measures in, 809
in neonate, 482
treatment of, 173
refractory, 809
in theophylline poisoning, 614
Status grand mal (SGM) (*see* Status epilepticus)
STDs (*see* Sexually transmitted diseases)
Steatosis, hepatic, 360
Stelazine (trifluoperazine), 1080t
for rapid tranquilization, 1079t
Sternal fractures, 936
Sternoclavicular joint dislocation, 981
Sternomastoid test, distinguishing true neurologic deficits from conversion disorder and, 1091t
Steroids:
in adrenal crisis, 762
in allergy to contrast media, 214
in caustic ingestions, 607-608
ophthalmic, 838
in septic shock, 138
Stevens-Johnson syndrome (SJS), 870-871, 871f
in nonsteroidal anti-inflammatory drug overdose, 628
Stibogluconate sodium, in parasitic infections, 537t
Stiffness, in headaches, 789
Sting(s) (*see* Insect and spider bites/stings)
from marine animals (*see* Marine animals, trauma and envenomations from)
scorpion, 665
venomous, treatment of, 113t

Stingray envenomations, 668
"Stocking/glove distribution," sensory response and, 786
Stoma(s), complications of, 368
Stomach:
  injury to, 957–958
  (*See also headings beginning with term* Gastric)
Stonefish envenomations, antivenin for, 669
Stones, urinary (*see* Nephrolithiasis)
Stool, decreased, in intestinal obstruction, 323
Stool cultures, in acute gastroenteritis, in children, 489
Stool patterns, of neonate, 425
Straddle fractures, 983
Straight-leg raising (SLR) testing, lumbar spine lesions and, 898
"Strain pattern":
  in aortic regurgitation, 223
  in pulmonary stenosis, 225
  in valvular aortic stenosis, 223
"Strawberry cervix," 395
Strength test, distinguishing true neurologic deficits from conversion disorder and, 1091t
Streptococcal pneumonia:
  in children, 460
  group A, 266
  group B, in children, 458–459
Streptococcus pneumoniae pneumonia, 265
Streptokinase:
  in acute myocardial infarction, 212, 213t
  in pulmonary embolism, 235
Streptomycin:
  in tuberculosis, 283t
  in tularemia, 542
Stress, of crisis work, 1096
Stress fractures, 967–968
  metatarsal, 1013
Stress hormones, diabetic ketoacidosis and, 735, 736f
Stress testing, in knee injuries, 999–1001
Stretch reflex test, distinguishing true neurologic deficits from conversion disorder and, 1091t
Stridor:
  biphasic, 182
  in children, 182–183, 183t
    congenital causes of, 182, 183t
  inspiratory, 182
  in neonate, 428
Stroke (*see* Cerebral vascular accident)
Strongyloides (threadworm) infections, 536
Stupor, definition of, 150
Stye (hordeolum), 836
Subaortic stenosis, idiopathic hypertrophic (*see* Cardiomyopathy, hypertrophic)
Subarachnoid hemorrhage (SAH), 796–797 (*see* Subarachnoid hemorhage)
  altered mental status and, 156
  computed tomography and, 7
  headache and, 791
  treatment of, 120
Subclavian artery injury, 952–953
  diagnosis of, 952
  etiology of, 952
  treatment of, 952–953
Subclavian steal syndrome, syncope and, 143
Subclavian vein, venous access and, 24
  in children, 168, 168f
Subcortex, cerebral vascular accident and, 797
Subdural hematoma (SDH), 915–916, 916f
  altered mental status and, 156
  in chronic renal failure, 375
  computed tomography and, 7–8
  traction headache and, 791
Subglottic stenosis, in neonate, 428
Sublimaze (*see* Fentanyl)
Subluxation, 970
  of teeth, 863
Submucosa, esophageal, 303
Substance abuse, in pregnancy, 410
Subtrochanteric fractures, 989
Subxiphoid pericardial window, 941
Succinylcholine (Anectine):
  neuromuscular blockade and, 17t, 17–18
  side effects of, 18
  in tetanus, 526t
Suctioning, 19
Sudden infant death syndrome ("crib death"; SIDS), 429–430, 434–436
  apnea and, 434
  clinical picture of, 435
  epidemiology of, 434
  evaluation and, 435
  home monitoring and, 435–436
  "near miss," 434
  pathophysiology of, 434
  victims of, 436
"Sudden sniffing death," 603
Sufentanil (Sufenta), rapid sequence induction and, 18
Suicide, poisoning as attempt at, 545
Suicide attempt, 1076–1077, 1078t
  clinical management of, 1077
  stabilization and, 1074
"Suit squeeze," 680
Sulfacetamide, 838
Sulfadiazine, in human immunodeficiency virus infections, 521, 521t
Sulfamethoxazole:
  in urinary tract infections, 379t
  (*See also* Trimethoprim/sulfamethoxazole)
Sulfasalazine:
  in Crohn's disease, 329
  in ulcerative colitis, 331
Sulfhemoglobinemia, 141
Sulfisoxazole:
  in otitis media, 440–441, 441
  in sinusitis, in children, 449t
  in urinary tract infections, in children, 463
Sulfonamides, during pregnancy, 406
Sulfonylureas, hypoglycemia and, 732
Sulfuric acid burns, 697
Sulindac:
  overdose of, 628
  in tendonitis, 889
Sun gazer's retinopathy (eclipse burn), 837
Superior vena cava syndrome, in malignancy, 781
Superoxide dismutase, in cerebral ischemia, 8
Supportive care:
  in acute lithium toxicity, 560
  in clonidine poisoning, 571
  in epiglottitis, in children, 184
  in hazardous materials exposure, 708
  in myxedema coma, 757
  in poisoning, 547, 548–549
    cardiovascular complications and, 548
    neurologic complications and, 548–549
    respiratory complications and, 548
  in thyroid storm, 753
Supraclavicular subclavian approach, to subclavian vein, 24
Supracondylar fracture, 984–985, 985f
Supratentorial lesions, focal, altered mental status and, 156–157
Supratentorial pressure, 151
Supraventricular arrhythmias (*see* Arrhythmias, supraventricular)
Supraventricular tachycardia (SVT), 92f, 92–93
  in children, 180, 180t, 438–439
  clinical significance of, 92, 92t
  ectopic, 92–93
  paroxysmal, 92
    in acute myocardial infarction, 205
    treatment of, 109, 115t, 116t, 119, 121
  reentrant, 92, 92f, 93
    in Wolff-Parkinson-White syndrome, 105, 105f
  treatment of, 92–93, 109, 112t, 117, 121
Suprax (*see* Cefixime)
Surface data display, computed tomography and, 2
Surgical debridement, in wound preparation, 1037–1038, 1038f
Surgical lesions, in neonate, 426
Surgical needles, 1046–1047
Surgical treatment:
  in acute pancreatitis, 365
  in anorectal abscesses, 56
  in aortic dissection, 247
  in appendicitis, 321
  of breast, complications of, 370
  in burns, 693, 693f
  in cerebral vascular accident, 795
  in cholecystitis, 354–355
    in pregnancy, 410
  complications of, 366–370
    genitourinary, 367
    postoperative fever as, 367
    respiratory, 366
    vascular, 366–367
    of wound, 366
  in coronary artery disease, in elderly patients, 258
  in Crohn's disease, 330
  in cutaneous abscess, 877–878, 878t
  in deep venous thrombosis, massive, 255
  in fissure in ano, 340
  in fistula in ano, 56
  in frostbite, 646–647
  gastrointestinal
    anorectal, 369
    appendectomy and, 369
    biliary, 369
    complications of, 367–370
    gastric, 368
    for inguinal hernia, 369–370
    pancreatic, 369
  for gastrointestinal foreign bodies, in children, 496
  in great vessel injury, 948
  of hemorrhoids, 338–339
  in hemothorax, 938
  in hernia, 327
  in hypertrophic cardiomyopathy, 228
  hypocalcemia following, 75
  in intestinal obstruction, 324
  in malignant pericardial effusion, with tamponade, 781
  in mandibular fractures, 851
  in mesenteric ischemia, 251–252
  in multiple sclerosis, 820–821
  in mushroom poisoning, 720
  in myasthenia gravis, 824
  in neck trauma, 930
  in nephrolithiasis, 374
  in otitis media with effusion, in children, 441
  in parapharyngeal abscess, 845
  in penetrating injuries of buttocks, 963
  in penetrating injury to heart, 941–942

Surgical treatment (*Cont.*):
in peptic ulcer disease, 314
in perforated viscus, 318–319
in peripheral vascular disease, 254
in peritonsillar abscess, 844
in pharyngitis, 444
in pilonidal sinus, 344–345
postadenotonsillectomy bleeding and, 842
postoperative wound care and, 1049
for rectal foreign bodies, 344
in rectal prolapse, 343
in retropharyngeal abscess, 844
in shock
septic, 137
in thoracic trauma, 933
in snake bites, 663–664
in thoracic aortic aneurysms, 248
expanding and ruptured, 249
in thoracic aortic dissection, 239
in ulcerative colitis, 331
in upper airway obstruction, 845
in uremic pericarditis, 374
in zygomatic arch fractures, 852
Sutilans (Travase), in wound management, 1040
Suture(s), 1045t, 1045–1047, 1047f
absorbable, 1045
cotton, 1045
dermal (subcuticular), 1045–1046
nonabsorbable, 1045
nylon, 1045
percutaneous, 1045–1046
polytetrafluoroethylene, 1045
silk, 1045
Suture line care, 1049
SVT (*see* Supraventricular tachycardia)
Swallowing:
dysphagia and (*see* Dysphagia)
pain on (odynophagia), 306
Sweating, in heatstroke, 653
Sympathetic nervous system (SNS), asthma and, 291
Symphysis fractures, mandibular, 851
Symphysis pubis:
fracture near, 983
subluxation of, 983
Synchronized intermittent mandatory ventilation, in respiratory alkalosis, 48
Synchronized intermittent mandatory ventilation (SIMV), 19
Syncope, 141–143, 799
in congenital heart disease, in children, 438
definition of, 141
differential diagnosis of, 142, 142t
in elderly patients, 259–260
ambulatory electrocardiographic monitoring in, 260
head-up tilt test in, 260
history and physical examination in, 259
laboratory studies in, 259
signal-averaged electrocardiography in, 260
transtelephonic monitoring in, 260
evaluation of, 143
incidence of, 141–142
near, 799, 802
orthostatic, 142–143
pathophysiology and causes of, 142t, 142–143
cardiac causes and, 142
cerebrovascular circulation and, 143
peripheral vascular disorders and, 142–143
seizure disorders and, 142
risk for, 143
seizures versus, 485, 805
vasovagal, in elderly patients, 259
vasovagal (common faint), 142
Syndrome of inappropriate secretion of ADH (SIADH), 66t, 66–67
in children, treatment of, 164
in malignancy, 781
Synovial fluid:
aspiration of, technique for, 886–887, 887f
examination of, in rheumatic disorders, 886t, 886–887
Synovitis:
crystal-induced (gout), 888–889
toxic, in children, 889
transient, in child, 990
Syphilis, 517
blood transfusions and, 778–779
primary, 517
proctitis and, 342
secondary, 517
tertiary, 517
Syringomyelia, posttraumatic, 926
Syrup of ipecac, in poisoning, 547–548
(*See also* Gastrointestinal decontamination)
Systemic arterial probes, 59
Systemic lupus erythematosus (SLE), 883, 884t
multiple sclerosis versus, 819
Systolic pump failure, in dilated cardiomyopathy, 227

T wave, 87
TAC, 580
for pediatric analgesia, 512
Tachyarrhythmias:
aberrant versus ventricular, 97, 98t
mechanisms of, 88, 88f
pacemaker-initiated, 107–108
in poisoning, 547, 548
treatment of, 117
ventricular, treatment of, 118
in Wolff-Parkinson-White syndrome, 104
Tachycardia:
antidromic, in Wolff-Parkinson-White syndrome, 105, 105f
atrial
multifocal (*See* Multifocal atrial tachycardia)
paroxysmal, 92, 92t, 112, 117, 121
cocaine use and, 581
in congenital heart disease, in children, 438–439
idioventricular (*see* Accelerated idioventricular rhythm)
junctional, in acute myocardial infarction, 205
reflex, treatment of, 245
sinus, 89, 89f
in acute myocardial infarction, 204
in children, 180, 180t, 438
clinical significance of, 89
treatment of, 89, 117
supraventricular (*see* Supraventricular tachycardia)
ventricular (*see* Ventricular tachycardia)
Tachycardia-bradycardia syndrome (*see* Sick sinus syndrome)
Tachypnea, in children, upper respiratory disorders and, 182
Taenia (pork tapeworm) infections, 538
Talus fractures, 1012
in children, 1014
treatment of, 1012
Tambocor (*see* Flecainide)
Tamponade, malignant pericardial effusion with, 780–781
Tanner scale, 399, 400t, 464
Tannic acid burns, 700
Tape, wound closure and, 1047
Tapeworms:
fish (*Diphyllobothrium*), 538
pork (*Taenia*), 538
Tar, burns and, 698–699
Taractan (chlorprothixene), 1080t
Tardive dyskinesia, neuroleptics and [illegible]5, 556t
Tarsal-metatarsal injuries:
in children, 1014
fracture dislocations and, 1013
treatment of, 1013
Tarsal plate, injuries to, 1055
Tarsal tunnel syndrome, 815t
Taxus, 724, 725–726
TBSA (*see* Total body surface area)
TEC (tetracaine, epinephrine, and cocaine), for topical anesthesia, 1035
TEE (*see* Transesophageal echocardiography)
Teeth:
agenesis of, 860
supernumerary, 860
(*See also* Dental emergencies)
TEF (*see* Tracheoesophageal fistula)
Tegretol (*see* Carbamazepine)
TEL (*see* Tetraethyl lead intoxication)
Temazepam, in acute mountain sickness, 673
Temazepam (Restoril), 1082t
Temperature, oxyhemoglobin dissociation and, 57, 57t
Temperature homeostasis, physiology of, 648
Temporal arteritis (giant cell arteritis):
headache and, 791
in rheumatic disorders, 885–886
Temporomandibular joint:
dislocation of, 856
clinical features of, 856
radiographic studies in, 856
treatment of, 856
internal derangements of, 857
osteoarthritis and, 857
rheumatoid arthritis and, 857
Temporomandibular joint syndrome (Kostin's syndrome), 856–857
clinical features of, 856–857
headache and, 792
radiographic studies in, 857
treatment of, 857
TEN (*see* Toxic epidermal necrolysis)
Tendinitis, 889
of hand, 976
of shoulder, 983
Tendon injuries, of hand and wrist, 972–973
treatment of, 972
Tenesmus, in intestinal obstruction, 323
Tenormin (*see* Atenolol)
Tenosynovitis:
of ankle, 1011
sublixation and, 1011
DeQuervain's stenosing, 975, 975f
flexor, of hand, 976
of hand, 976
of shoulder, 983
Tension headache, 791
Terbutaline:
in asthma, 295, 295t
in children, 470, 473
in chronic decompensated airflow obstruction, 301
for emergency delivery, 419t
in status asthmaticus, in children, 472
Terminal ileitis (*see* Crohn's disease)
Terminal illness, resuscitation ethics and, 4
Testes:
anatomy of, 382, 383f

  appendages of, torsion of, 386
  cancer of, 387
  orchitis and, 387
  torsion of, 385-386, 386f
Tetanus, 525-526, 812, 879
  cephalic, 525
  clinical features of, 879
  clinical manifestations of, 525
  differential diagnosis of, 879
  epidemiology of, 525
  generalized, 525
  local, 525
  management of, 525-526
    active immunization and, 526, 526t
    antibiotics in, 525-526
    autonomic dysfunction and, 526
    muscle relaxants in, 526
    neuromuscular blockade in, 526
    tetanus immune globulin in, 525
  microbiology of, 525
  in narcotic overdose, 567
  neonatal, 525
  prophylaxis of, 525, 526, 526t, 693, 879, 880t, 1050-1051, 1050t
    in gas gangrene, 880
    in mandibular fractures, 851
    precautions and contraindications to, 1050-1051
  treatment of, 879
  wound management in, 879, 880t
Tetanus-diphtheria toxoid (Td), in tetanus, 879
Tetanus immune globulin (TIG), 525, 526t, 1050, 1050t
  in tetanus, 879, 880t
Tetanus toxoid, 526, 526t
  in burns, 693
Tetany, hypocalcemia, treatment of, 113t
Tetracaine, 580, 838
  for pediatric analgesia, 512
  for topical anesthesia, 1035
Tetracycline(s), 407
  adverse effects, precautions, and contraindications to, 533t
  in bacterial pneumonia, 264t
  in chlamydial infections, sexually transmitted, 518
  in diarrhea, 351t
  in granuloma inguinale, 518
  in Lyme disease, 540
  in pelvic inflammatory disease, 394t
  in periodontal abscess, 861
  in relapsing fever, 542
  in Rocky Mountain spotted fever, 541
  in syphilis, 517
  in tularemia, 542
Tetraethyl lead (TEL) intoxication, 640
Tetralogy of Fallot:
  in children, 437, 438
  pulmonary stenosis and, 224
Thalamus, hemorrhage of, 797
Theophylline:
  in apnea, in neonate, 435
  in asthma, 295-296
    in children, 470, 471, 473
  in chronic decompensated airflow obstruction, 300-301
  dosage, 296, 296t
  pharmacology of, 296, 614, 614t
  serum levels of, 296
  in status asthmaticus, in children, 471
Theophylline ethylenediamine (*see* Aminophylline)
Theophylline poisoning, 614-616
  disposition in, 615-616
  prevention of, 616
  toxic effects and, 614-615
  treatment of, 615
    indications for, 615-616
Thiamine:
  in alcoholic ketoacidosis, 741
  in altered mental status, 151
  deficiency of, in alcoholism, 575
  in ethanol poisoning, 576
  in hypoglycemia, in ethylene glycol poisoning, 574
  in lactic acidosis, 750
  in status epilepticus, 809
Thiamylal, pharmacology of, 561t
Thigh adductor test, distinguishing true neurologic deficits from conversion disorder and, 1091t
Thimerosol burns, iatrogenic, 700
Thiobendazole, in parasitic infections, 537t
Thiopental:
  neuromuscular blockade and, 18
  pharmacology of, 561t
  rapid sequence induction and, 18
Thioridazine, 556t (*see* Mellaril)
Thiothixene (Navane), 556t, 1080t
  for rapid tranquilization, 1079t
Thomas shunt, 375
"Thompson's test," in Achilles tendon rupture, 1005, 1010
Thoracentesis:
  in hemothorax, 937
  in pneumonia, bacterial, 265
Thoracic outlet syndrome, chest pain and, 131
Thoracic pump theory, 1
Thoracic spine, 896
  fractures of, 896
Thoracic trauma, 932-953
  chest wall, bronchi, lung, and diaphragm and, 932t, 932-940
  to chest wall, bronchi, lung, and diaphragm
    cardiac arrest and, 933
    diagnosis of, 933-934
    initial resuscitation, airway control, and ventilation in, 932t, 932-933
    shock and, 933
  to great vessels, 947-953
  to heart, 940-947
    blunt injury and, 942-947
    penetrating injury and, 940-942
Thoracolumbar injuries, 925
Thoracotomy:
  in great vessel injury, 948
  in hemothorax, 938
  in penetrating injury to heart, 941-942
  in shock, in thoracic trauma, 933
Thorazine (*see* Chlorpromazine)
Threadworm (*Strongyloides*) infections, 536
Three dimensional display, computed tomography and, 2
Three Mile Island accident, 714
Throat culture, in streptococcal pharyngitis, 443, 444
Thrombin time (TT), in hemophilia, 770
Thrombocytopenia, 768
  dilutional, massive blood transfusion and, 777
  in malignancy, 782
  management of, 768
  septic shock and, 138
Thromboembolism:
  in acute myocardial infarction, 207
  in pregnancy, 409
  prosthetic heart valves and, 225
Thrombolytic therapy, 769
  in acute myocardial infarction, 207 (*see* Acute myocardial infarction, thrombolytic therapy in)
  in deep venous thrombosis, 255-256
  pulmonary, 235
Thrombophlebitis, 254-256
  deep venous thrombosis and (*see* Deep venous thrombosis)
  in narcotic overdose, 567
  pelvic, in pregnancy, 411
  superficial, 255
    postoperative, 366-367
Thrombosis:
  arterial, in mesenteric ischemia, 250, 251
  differentiating embolus from, 253-254
  venous, in mesenteric ischemia, 251
Thromboxane A2 (TXA2), septic shock and, 137
Thrush:
  in human immunodeficiency virus infections, 523
  in neonate, 429
Thymectomy, in myasthenia gravis, 824
Thyroid hormone, in myxedema coma, 757
Thyroid storm, 752-754
  apathetic thyrotoxicosis and, 753
  clinical presentation of, 752
  laboratory studies in, 752-753
  pathogenesis of, 752
  precipitating factors for, 752
  treatment of, 753-754
Thyrotoxicosis:
  apathetic, 753
  "masked," 753
Thyroxine, in myxedema coma, 757
TIA (*see* Transient ischemic attack)
Tibia, 1004
  fractures of, in children, 1005
  intercondylar eminence of, fracture of, 1002-1003
  metaphyseal injuries of, in children, 1005
  vascular access and, in children, 169, 169f
Tibial epiphysis, proximal, separation of, in child, 1002
Tibial plateau fractures, 1000
Tibial spine fractures, 999-1000
Tibial tubercle injuries, in child, 1002
Tibial tuberosity fractures, 999-1000
Tibiofibular syndesmotic ligament injuries, 1009
Tic douloureux (trigeminal neuralgia), 814
Tick-borne disease, 540-543
  prevention of, 543
  (*See also* Lyme disease; Rocky Mountain spotted fever)
Tick paralysis, 541-542, 812
  clinical presentation of, 541
  diagnosis and treatment of, 542
Tidal volume, in pregnancy, 414
Tietze's syndrome, chest pain and, 131
TIG (*see* Tetanus immune globulin)
Tilt test:
  head-up, in syncope, 260
  in hypertensive emergencies, 237
Timolol (Blocadren; Timoptic):
  in acute angle closure glaucoma, 836
  in angina, 201t
  dosage, actions, pharmacokinetics, and indications for, 112t
Tindal (acetophenazine), 1080t
Tinel's sign, in carpal tunnel syndrome, 975
TIPS, in altered mental status, 155, 155t
Tissue hypoxia:
  in carbon monoxide poisoning, 703

Tissue hypoxia (*Cont.*):
cyanosis and, 140
Tissue loss, chest wall injuries and, 934
Tissue perfusion, in metabolic acidosis, 46
Tissue plasminogen activator (Activase; tPA), in acute myocardial infarction, 213, 213t
in pulmonary embolism, 235
TM (*see* Tympanic membrane)
TMG (*see* Transitory myasthenia gravis)
TMP/SMX (*see* Trimethoprim/sulfamethoxazole)
Toadstools (*see* Mushroom(s); Mushroom poisoning)
Tobramycin:
in bacterial pneumonia, 264t
ophthalmic, 838
in periorbital/orbital cellulitis, in children, 452t
Tocainide (Tonocard), electrophysiologic actions of, 110t
Todd's paralysis, postictal, in children, 483
Toe lacerations, regional nerve block for repair of, 1032–1033, 1033f
Tolazoline, as antidote to clonidine, 571
Toluene poisoning, 603
Tongue lacerations, 865
regional nerve block for repair of, 1033–1034, 1034f
Tonicity (effective osmolality), 63
Tono-Pen, 833
Tonocard (tocainide), electrophysiologic actions of, 109t
Tonsillectomy:
bleeding following, 842
indications for, 444
Tooth (*see* Dental emergencies; Teeth)
Tooth Preserving System (TPS), 863, 864f
Tooth squeeze (barodontalgia), 681
Toothache (odontalgia), 860
Torsade de pointes (atypical ventricular tachycardia), 96
treatment of, 96
Torsion, testicular, 385–386, 386f
Total body surface area (TBSA), burns and, 691
Tourniquet(s)
in pulmonary edema, 218
in fingertip injuries and, 1062
Tourniquet test, in carpal tunnel syndrome, 975
Toxic drug screening, in altered mental status, 155
Toxic epidermal necrolysis (scalded skin syndrome; TEN), 873f, 873–874
clinical features of, 873, 873f, 874f
diagnosis of, 873
differential diagnosis of, 873
in nonsteroidal anti-inflammatory drug overdose, 628
staphylococcal, 506, 873, 873f
staphylococcal scalded-skin syndrome versus, 506
toxic shock syndrome versus, 404
treatment of, 873–874
Toxic ingestions (*see* Poisoning)
Toxic megacolon, in ulcerative colitis, 330
treatment of, 331
Toxic metabolic headache, 790–791
Toxic shock syndrome (TSS), 403t, 403–405
clinical presentation of, 404, 405f
differential diagnosis of, 403t, 403–404
epidemiology of, 403
etiology and pathogenesis of, 403
management of, 404–405
nonmenstrual, 405, 405t
recurrences of, 405
sequelae of, 405
Toxic shock syndrome toxin-1 (TSST-1), 403
Toxic syndromes, 545, 546–547t
Toxoplasmosis, in human immunodeficiency virus infections, 521
tPA (*see* Tissue plasminogen activator)
TPS (*see* Tooth Preserving System)
Tracheal stenosis, in neonate, 428
Tracheitis, bacterial (membranous laryngotracheobronchitis), 184
Tracheobronchial injury, 939
Tracheoesophageal airway, 11
Tracheoesophageal fistula (TEF), in neonate, 173, 428
diagnosis of, 173
management of, 173
Tracheostomy:
complications of, 1107, 1107t
emergency, in upper airway obstruction, 845
Traction, in spinal injury, 923
Traction headache, 791
Training, for emergency medical services, 189
Trandate (*see* Labetalol)
Transcutaneous monitoring, of oxygen and carbon monoxide, 60
Transesophageal echocardiography (TEE), 1123, 1124
Transient global amnesia, 796
Transient ischemic attack (TIA), 793
syncope and, 143
vertigo and, 801
Transitory myasthenia gravis (TMG), 824
Transportation:
for emergency medical services, 189–190
aeromedical, 192
of maternal patients, emergency delivery and, 418, 419t
Transtracheal aspiration, in pneumonia, bacterial, 263
Transtracheal catheter ventilation (TTCV), in child, 910
Tranxene (chlorazepate), 1082t
Tranylcypromine, in monoamine oxidase inhibitor overdose, 1083
Trasicor (*see* Oxprenolol)
Trauma, 905–909
abdominal, in pregnancy (*see* Pregnancy, abdominal trauma in)
arterial, 254
diagnosis of, 254
in children
limp and, 889–890
treatment of, 164
distribution of, 905
dysbaric (*see* Dysbarism)
in elderly patients, 1097–1098
emergency department resuscitation and, 906t, 906–908
assistants' roles in, 906–907
primary survey and, 907–908
secondary survey and, 908
team captain's role in, 907–908
esophageal (*see* Esophageal emergencies, traumatic)
foundations of resuscitation in, 909
incidence of, 905
motor vehicle accidents and, 905, 905f
from marine animals (*see* Marine animals, trauma and envenomations from)
to neonate, 426
patient disposition for emergency department and, 908–909
prehospital care in, 906
prevention of, 905
upper airway obstruction and, 844
(*See also* Child abuse; *specific sites of trauma*)
Trauma care, emergency medical services and, 191
Trauma series, 500
Travase (sutilans), in wound management, 1040
Trematodes (flukes), 538
Tremor, familial (hereditary) essential, treatment of, 117
Trench foot (immersion foot), 645
Treppe (staircase phenomenon), metabolic acidosis and, 43
Triage:
in acute myocardial infarction, 209
disaster medical services and, 194
resuscitation ethics and, 5
tagging systems and, 194
Triazolam, in acute mountain sickness, 673
Triazolam (Halcion), 1082t
Trichinosis, 536–537
Trichomonas, vaginitis and, 395
Trichomoniasis, 518
Trichuris trichuria infections, 536
Tricuspid regurgitation, 224
clinical features of, 224
treatment of, 224
Tricuspid stenosis, 224
clinical features of, 224
treatment of, 224
Tricuspid valve injury, blunt injury to heart and, 943
Trifluoperazine (Stelazine), 1080t
for rapid tranquilization, 1079t
Triflupromazine (Vesprine), 1080t
Trigeminal neuralgia (tic douloureaux), 814
headache and, 791–792
Trigger zones, 861
Triiodothyronine, in myxedema coma, 757
Trilafon (perphenazine), 1080t
Trimethadione (Tridione), during pregnancy, 407
Trimethaphan camsylate (Arfonad):
actions and pharmacology of, 242
in hypertensive emergencies, 240t, 242
indications for, 242
side effects and contraindications to, 242
use of, 242
Trimethoprim, in *Pneumocystis carinii* pneumonia, 274
Trimethoprim/sulfamethoxazole (Bactrim; Septra; TMP/SMX):
in acute gastroenteritis, in children, 490
in cutaneous abscess, 878t
in diarrhea, 351t
in human immunodeficiency virus infections, 521t, 522
in otitis media, 440
in parasitic infections, 537t
in urinary tract infections, in children, 463
Trimethoprim/sulfamethoxazole (Bactrim; Septra; TMP/SMZ):
in *Pneumocystis carinii* pneumonia, 273–274
Pneumocystis carinii pneumonia prophylaxis and, 274
in pyelonephritis, 380
in septic shock, 139t
Trismus, in tetanus, 879, 880t
Trochanteric fractures, 989
Tropicamide, 838
Trousseau's sign, in hypocalcemia, 76
Trunk syndromes, 815
Trypanosoma infections, 538
TSS (*see* Toxic shock syndrome)
TSST-1 (*see* Toxic shock syndrome toxin-1)

TT (*see* Thrombin time)
TTCV (*see* Transtracheal catheter ventilation)
Tube thoracostomy, in pneumothorax, 285
Tubercle, 279, 280
Tuberculin skin test (PPD test; purified protein derivative test), 279–280
  in human immunodeficiency virus infections, 522
  in primary tuberculosis, 280
    in tuberculous pleural effusion, 281
Tuberculosis, 279t, 279–283
  acquired immune deficiency syndrome and, 282, 283t
  clinical manifestations of, 280–282
    in elderly patients, 282
    in extrapulmonary tuberculosis, 281f, 281–282
    in miliary tuberculosis, 282, 282f
    in primary tuberculosis, 280, 280f
    in reactivation tuberculosis, 280f, 280–281, 281f, 281t
    tuberculous pleural effusion and, 281
  drug therapy in, 283, 283t
    national consensus of chemotherapy and, 283
  oral manifestations of, 862
  pathogenesis of, 279–280
    initial infection and, 279–280
  pathophysiology of, 279, 279t
  prevention of, 283
  radiographic features of, 280f, 280–282, 281f, 282t
Tuboovarian abscess, ultrasonography in, 1118f, 1119
"Tuft fracture," 978
Tularemia, 542
  clinical presentation of, 542
  diagnosis of, 542
  treatment of, 542
  typhoidal form of, 542
Tumor(s):
  abdominal, in children, 493, 496
  of brainstem, altered mental status and, 157
  cerebral, altered mental status and, 157
  computed tomography and, 4
  cranial nerves and, 786
  extrapancreatic, hypoglycemia and, 729
  mediastinal, diagnosis of, 469
  Pott's puffy tumor and, 848
    in sinusitis, 449
  pregnancy, 862, 862f
  small bowel obstruction and, 322
  traction headache and, 791
  vertigo and, 801
  (*See also specific sites*)
"Tumor polyp," in mitral stenosis, 220
Tunnel vision ("gun barrel" vision), 838
TXA_2 (*see* Thromboxane A_2)
Tylenol, in pyelonephritis, 380
Tylenol no. 3 (acetaminophen with codeine), in rib fractures, 935
Tympanic membrane (TM):
  in barotitis media, 679
  in otitis media, 440
  perforation of, traumatic, 842
  rupture of, lightning injuries and, 702
Tympanocentesis, diagnostic, in otitis media, 440
Tympanometry, in otitis media, 440
Tympanoplasty tubes, in otitis media with effusion, in children, 441
Type O universal donor blood, 777
Tzanck smear, in genital herpes, 396
U wave, 87
Udorn encephalopathy, 475
Ulcer(s):
  corneal, 835
  Curling's
    gastrointestinal bleeding and, 149
    in peptic ulcer disease, 314–315
  Cushing's
    gastrointestinal bleeding and, 149
    in peptic ulcer disease, 314–315
  duodenal
    gastrointestinal bleeding and, 149
    perforated, 316
  gastric
    gastrointestinal bleeding and, 149
    perforated, 316
  nose picker's, 846
  prevention of, in Reye's syndrome, 477–478
  stomal, gastrointestinal bleeding and, 149
  stress
    gastrointestinal bleeding and, 149
    in peptic ulcer disease, 314–315
  in Zollinger-Ellison syndrome, 313
  (*See also* Peptic ulcer disease)
Ulcerative colitis (*see* Colitis, ulcerative)
Ulna, trauma to, 985–986
Ulnar nerve entrapment, 815t
Ultrasonography:
  abdominal, 1120t, 1120–1122
    acute appendicitis and, 1121f, 1121–1122
    kidney and, 1121
    liver and biliary tree and, 1120, 1121f
    pancreas and, 1121
  in abdominal pain, 147
  in appendicitis, 321
  in blunt trauma to great vessels, 951
  cardiac, 1123t, 1123–1125
    in aortic dissection, 1124, 1124f, 1124t
    in cardiac tamponade, 1124, 1125f
    in cardiomyopathy and intracardiac masses, 1125
    in ischemic heart disease, 1123f, 1123–1124, 1124f
    techniques for, 1123–1125
    in valvular heart disease, 1124
  in cholecystitis, 354
  duplex
    in mesenteric ischemia, 251
    in peripheral vascular disease, 1113–1114
  in ectopic pregnancy, 390–391
  in nephrolithiasis, 374
  pelvic, 1115–1119
    in children, 1119
    in ectopic pregnancy, 411
    in failing early pregnancy, 1115–1116, 1116f
    in nonpregnant woman, 1117–1119, 1117–1119f
    in normal early pregnancy, 1115, 1115f, 1116f
    techniques for, 1115
    in third trimester bleeding, 1116f, 1116–1117, 1117f
  in perforated viscus, 318
  in pregnancy, 406
  real time, 1115
  in sinusitis, in children, 449
Ultrastructural injury, cerebral ischemia and, 8
Ultraviolet keratitis (snow blindness), 676, 835
Umbilical artery, catheterization of, neonatal resuscitation and, 171
Umbilical vein:
  catheterization of, neonatal resuscitation and, 171
  venous access and, in children, 169
Union, of fractures, 968
United Nations World Health Organization oral rehydration solution, 165
Universal distress signal, 2
Upper respiratory emergencies:
  in children, 182–186
    physical examination in, 182
  (*See also* Airway obstruction, upper; *specific disorders*)
Urecoline, in antidepressant side effects, 1082
Uremia, altered mental status and, 156
Ureter:
  dilatation of, in pregnancy, 414
  injury of, gynecologic procedures and, 423
Urethra:
  "acute urethral syndrome" and, 377
  in males
    foreign bodies in, 387
    stricture of, 387, 387f
Urinalysis, in Reye's syndrome, 476
Urinary calculi (*see* Nephrolithiasis)
Urinary retention:
  following anorectal surgery, 369
  in females, gynecologic procedures and, 423
  in males, 387–388, 388t
  postoperative, 367
  following surgery for inguinal hernia, 369
Urinary tract, pregnancy-associated changes in, 414
Urinary tract infections (UTI), 377–381
  bacteriology of, 377, 377t
  in children, 462–463
    clinical findings in, 462
    complications of, 463
    diagnosis of, 462
    differential diagnosis of, 462
    incidence of, 462
    management of, 463
    microbiology of, 462
    prophylaxis of, 463
    radiographic studies in, 463
  clinical features of, 378
  diagnosis of, 378–379
  in multiple sclerosis, treatment of, 820
  natural history of, 377, 377f
  normal host defense mechanisms and, 377–378
  postoperative, 367
  in pregnancy, 409
  pyelonephritis and, 380–381
  treatment of, 379t, 379–380
Urine:
  acidification of, in amphetamine toxicity, 582
  alkalinization of
    in acute lithium toxicity, 560
    in barbiturate overdose, 562
    in salicylate intoxication, 591
  anion gap and, 42, 42t
Urine culture, in urinary tract infections, in children, 462
Urine specimen:
  collection of, from children, 462
  midstream, collecting from males, 383
Urokinase:
  in acute myocardial infarction, 213, 213t
  in pulmonary embolism, 235
Urologic dysfunction, in multiple sclerosis, treatment of, 820
Urtica, 723, 725
Urticaria (hives), 902
Uterus:
  blood flow to, in pregnancy, 414
  enlarged, ultrasonography in, 1119

Uterus (*Cont.*):
  incarceration of, 392
  perforation of
    hysteroscopy and, 422
    induced abortion and, 423
  in pregnancy, 414
  rupture of, in pregnancy, 415
Uvular hydrops, 844

Vaccine, for prevention of hepatitis B, 358
Vagal maneuvers, in paroxysmal supraventricular tachycardia, 205
Vagina:
  normal secretions of, 395
  trauma to, 392
Vaginal discharge, in children, 465
Vaginal washings, in female rape victims, 401
Vaginitis:
  atrophic, 397
  Candida, in children, 464
  Gardnerella vaginalis, in children, 464
  Trichomonas, in children, 464
  (*See also* Bacterial vaginosis)
Vaginoscopy, in vulvovaginitis, in children, 464
Vaginosis, bacterial, 396
Valium (*see* Diazepam)
Valproate, in seizures, in children, 483
Valproic acid (Depakene; Depakote):
  adverse effects of, 486
  in seizures, 808t
    in children, 480t
  in status epilepticus, in children, 485t
Valsalva maneuver:
  esophageal trauma and, 309
  in mitral regurgitation, 221
  in reentrant supraventricular tachycardia, 93
Valvular heart disease, ultrasonography in, 1124
Valvular incompetence, prosthetic heart valves and, 225
Vancomycin:
  in acute gastroenteritis, in children, 490
  in bacterial pneumonia, 264t
  in diarrhea, 351t
  in pseudomembranous enterocolitis, 331
  in septic shock, 139t
Vaponefrine, in viral croup, 184–185
Vapor pressure of water, 51
Varicella (chickenpox):
  in pregnancy, 410
  rash in, in children, 508, 509f
  Reye's syndrome and, 475
Varicella immune globulin (VZIG), in human immunodeficiency virus infections, 521
Varicella-zoster infections:
  in human immunodeficiency virus infections, 521
  pneumonia and, 267
Varices:
  esophageal, gastrointestinal bleeding and, 149
  gastric, gastrointestinal bleeding and, 149
Vas deferens, anatomy of, 382
Vascular access:
  cardiopulmonary resuscitation and, in children, 177
  in children, 165–170
    axillary vein and, 168–169
    endotracheal route as alternative to, 169–170
    external jugular vein and, 167–168, 168f
    femoral approach and, 169, 169f
    internal jugular catheterization and, 167, 167f
    intraosseous route as alternative to, 169, 169f
    peripheral veins and, 165
    scalp veins and, 165–166, 166f
    subclavian vein and, 168, 168f
    umbilical vein and, 169
    venous cutdown and, 166f, 166–167
  in chronic renal failure, problems related to, 375–376
  in pediatric trauma victim, 911
Vascular disorders:
  abdominal, 960
  peripheral (*see* Peripheral vascular disease)
  of peripheral nerves, 814
  following surgery for inguinal hernia, 370
Vascular extravasation, in phenytoin toxicity, 564
  treatment of, 565
Vascular reactivity, metabolic acidosis and, 43
Vascular resistance, military antishock trouser garment and, 6
Vascular ring, diagnosis of, 469
Vascular studies, noninvasive, 1113–1114
  in peripheral arterial disease, 1113–1114
  in peripheral venous disease, 1114
Vasoactive agents, 122–125, 122–126
  vasoactive and inotropic agents, 122–125
  vasodilator agents, 125–126
Vasoconstrictors, in reentrant supraventricular tachycardia, 93
Vasodilator therapy, 125t, 125–126
  in cardiogenic shock, 136
  in cerebral vascular accident, 795
  in congestive heart failure, 218
  in depressed cardiac output, 206
  in left ventricular pump failure, 206
  in pulmonary vascular congestion, 218
  in restrictive cardiomyopathy, 229
Vasopressin:
  in gastrointestinal bleeding, 148
  septic shock and, 137
VDRL (*see* Venereal Disease Research Laboratories VD test)
Vecuronium bromide (Norcuron), neuromuscular blockade and, 17, 17t, 18
Vein(s):
  anatomy of, venous access and, 22–23, 23f
  (*See also* Vascular access; Venous access; *specific veins*)
Vena cava interruption, pulmonary, 235
Venereal disease(s) (*see* Sexually transmitted diseases; *specific diseases*)
Venereal Disease Research Laboratories VD test (VDRL), in female rape victims, 400
Venography:
  in acute deep venous thrombosis, 255
  in deep venous thrombosis, 367
  in great vessel injuries, 948
  in pulmonary embolism, 235
Venous access, 21–25
  central venous pressure catheterization and monitoring and (*see* Catheterization, central venous)
  flow rates and, 21–22
  sites for, 21, 21f, 22f
  technique and, 21
  (*See also* Vascular access)
Venous cutdown, 25
  technique of, 25
  venous access and, in children, 166f, 166–167
Venous occlusion, in mesenteric ischemia, 250
Venous studies, acid-base problems and, 43
Venous system, esophageal, 303, 305f
Venous thrombosis, in mesenteric ischemia, 251
Ventilation:
  acclimatization to high altitude and, 670, 671t
  age and, 56
  altitude and, 55–56, 56t
  alveolar, 51
    arterial Pa_{CO_2} and, 54
    arterial Pa_{O_2} and, 55
  in cardiopulmonary resuscitation, 2
    mouth-to-mouth, 2
    mouth-to-nose, 2
  dead space and, 51
    arterial Pa_{CO_2} and, 54
  high-frequency, 19
  intermittent mandatory (IMV) (*see* Synchronized intermittent mandatory ventilation)
    synchronized (SIMV) (*see* Synchronized intermittent mandatory ventilation)
  in metabolic acidosis, 46
  minute, 51
  monitoring, 55
  percutaneous translaryngeal, 14, 14f
    complications of, 14
  (*See also* Mechanical ventilation)
Ventilation-perfusion lung scan:
  in pneumonia, bacterial, 263
  in pulmonary embolism, 234
Ventilatory insufficiency, in poisoning, 548
Ventricular arrhythmias (*see* Arrhythmias, ventricular)
Ventricular ectopy:
  junctional, 205
  treatment of, 111
Ventricular fibrillation, 97, 97f
  in acute myocardial infarction, 205
  clinical significance of, 97
  in hypothermia, treatment of, 650
  treatment of, 97, 109, 111, 113–115t, 118, 122
Ventricular flutter, 96
Ventricular outflow obstruction, syncope and, 142
Ventricular parasystole, 95, 95f
  clinical significance of, 95
  treatment of, 95
Ventricular septal defect (VSD):
  blunt injury to heart and, 943
  in penetrating injury to heart, 942
Ventricular septal rupture, in acute myocardial infarction, 206
Ventricular tachyarrhythmia, treatment of, 118
Ventricular tachycardia, 96f, 96t, 96–97
  alternating, 96
  atypical (torsade de pointes), 96
    treatment of, 96
  bidirectional, 96
  clinical significance of, 96-97
  junctional, 205
  low (*see* Accelerated idioventricular rhythm)
  nonparoxysmal (*see* Accelerated idioventricular rhythm)
  polymorphous, 96
  pulseless, treatment of, 111
  slow (*see* Accelerated idioventricular rhythm)
  treatment of, 97, 109, 111, 113–115t, 117, 118
Ventriculoperitoneal cerebrospinal fluid shunts, complications of, 1110t, 1110–1111
Ventriculoperitoneal (VP) shunt, in hydrocephalus, 432
Verapamil (Calan; Isoptic):
  in acute myocardial infarction, 210
  in angina, 201
  in atrial fibrillation, 205
  in mitral stenosis, 221
  overdose of, 620
  toxicity of, 621
Verapamil (Calan; Isoptin), 118–119

actions, indications, dosage and administration, adverse effects, contraindications, and forms of, 116t
actions of, 118–119
adverse effects of, 119
in atrial fibrillation, 91
dosing and administration of, 119
electrophysiologic actions of, 110t
indications for, 119
pharmacokinetics of, 119
in reentrant supraventricular tachycardia, 93
in sick sinus syndrome, 103
in Wolff-Parkinson-White syndrome, 105
Verbal response, in head injury, 917
Vermilion, 1057
Versed (*see* Midazolam)
Vertebrobasilar syndromes, 796
Vertigo, 799–803
alternobaic, 681
benign paroxysmal, of childhood, 801
central, 799, 801
diagnosis of, 802
history taking and, 802
laboratory studies in, 802
physical examination in, 802, 802t
etiology and clinical manifestations of, 799t, 799–802
pathophysiology of, 799
peripheral, 799–801, 800t
physiologic, 801
positional
benign (Barany's), 800, 803
posttraumatic, 801
posttraumatic
acute, 801
positional, 801
psychogenic, 801
treatment of, 802–803, 803t
Vesicants, 695
Vesicoureteral reflux, in children, 463
Vesprine (triflupromazine), 1080t
Vestibular neuronitis, vertigo and, 800
Vestibular-ocular reflex, vertigo and, 799
Vibrio cholerae, diarrhea and, 349
Vibrio parahaemolyticus, diarrhea and, 349-350
Violence, 1077–1079, 1079t
stabilization and, 1074
suicide attempts and, 1077
Viral croup (*see* Croup, viral)
Viral infections:
acute gastroenteritis and, in children, 488
diarrhea and, 347–348
in pregnancy, 409–410
rashes and, in children, 507–508
Reye's syndrome and, 475
(*See also specific infections*)
Viscus, perforation of (*see* Perforation, of viscus)
Visken (*see* Pindolol)
Visual disorders, in methanol poisoning, 572
Visual loss (*see* Blindness)
Visual threat, in altered mental status, 153
Vital organ perfusion, indicators of, 133, 133t
Vital signs:
in altered mental status, 152
in gastrointestinal bleeding, 147
in head injury, 916
in poisoning, 545
in psychiatric disorders, 1076
in spinal injury, 922
(*See also specific signs*)
Vitamin(s), deficiencies of, in alcoholism, 576
Vitamin A, hypercalcemia and, 78
Vitamin B_6 (*see* Pyridoxine)
Vitamin B_{12} (hydroxycobalamin), in cyanide poisoning, 635
Vitamin D:
calcium levels and, 74
deficiency of, hypocalcemia and, 76
hypercalcemia and, 78
in hypocalcemia, 77
Vitamin K, in hypoprothrombinemia, 768
Vocal cord paralysis, 845
Voiding cystourethrography, in urinary tract infections, in children, 463
Volar plate injuries, 973, 973f
Volatile acid (*see* Carbon dioxide)
Volkmann's contracture, 975
Volkmann's paralysis, 814
Volume averaging, computed tomography and, 3
Volume expanders, in hemorrhagic shock, 134
Volvulus, 322, 323f
cecal, 322
in children, 493
of sigmoid colon, 322, 323f
Vomiting:
bilious, in children, 491–492, 492t
in children, 491–492, 492t
in neonate, 426–427
in perforated viscus, 317
projectile, in neonate, 426–427
von Willebrand's disease, 770, 770t
Voxels, 1
VP (*see* Ventriculoperitoneal shunt)
VSD (*see* Ventricular septal defect)
Vulva, trauma to, 392
Vulvitis, in children, 464
Vulvovaginitis, 395–397
Candida, 395–397
in children, 462, 463t, 463–465
clinical findings in, 463–464
etiology of, 464–465
nonspecific, 464
contact, 397
Trichomonas, 395–397
VZIG (*see* Varicella immune globulin)

Wallenberg's syndrome, vertigo and, 801
Wandering atrial pacemaker (*See* Multifocal atrial tachycardia)
Warfarin (Coumadin):
in hypoprothrombinemia, 768
during pregnancy, 407
Warming systems, for blood transfusion, 776–777
"Warning arrhythmias," 95
Washed red blood cells, 775
Wasp stings (*see* Insect and spider bites/stings, Hymenoptera stings and)
Water, 62–64
daily fluid requirements and, 64
basic needs and, 64
current losses and, 64
deficits and, 64, 64t
decreased intake of, hypernatremia and, 69
excess excretion of, hypernatremia and, 69
extracellular fluid and, 63, 63t
interstitial fluid and, 63–64, 64t
intracellular fluid and, 63, 63t, 64
osmolarity and osmolality and, 62–63
Water-hammer (Corrigan's) pulse, in aortic regurgitation, 223
Water intoxication, 67
Water restriction, in hyponatremia, 68
WBC (*see* White blood cell count)
WCT (*see* Wide QRS complexes)
Weakness:
left-sided, cerebral vascular accident and, 798
right-sided, cerebral vascular accident and, 797
Web space infections, 976
Weight gain, in neonate, 425
"Welders' blindness," 835
Wenckebach phenomenon:
in second-degree Mobitz I (Wenckebach) atrioventricular block, 99
in sinoatrial block, 98, 98f
Wermer's syndrome, 77
Wernicke's disease, hypothermia and, 648
Wernicke's encephalopathy:
in alcoholism, 576
altered mental status and, 156
treatment of, 576
Westermark's sign, in pulmonary embolism, 234
Wheezing, 182
in asthma, 467
upper airway obstruction and, 843
(*See also* Stridor)
"Whiff" test, in vulvovaginitis, in children, 465
Whiplash injury (acceleration flexion-extension neck injury), 893–894
White blood cell (WBC) count:
in bacteremia, in children, 454
in cellulitis, in children, 450
in pneumonia, in children, 458
White line, 1057
White matter shear injury (axonal shear injury), computed tomography and, 8
White phosphorus burns, 699, 700
"White strawberry tongue," in scarlet fever, 506
Whole-bowel irrigation, in lead poisoning, 639
Whooping cough (*see* Pertussis)
Wide QRS complexes (WCT), 97
Williams syndrome, hypercalcemia and, 78
Windage, 685
Window, computed tomography and, 1
Windshields, type of injury and, 1052
Wisdom tooth, 860
Withdrawal (*see specific substances*)
Wolff-Parkinson-White (WPW) syndrome, 104
clinical significance of, 104–105, 105f
treatment of, 105–106, 109, 111, 117, 119
type A, 104, 104f
type B, 104, 104f
type C, 104
Wood alcohol (*see* Methanol)
Wood alcohol (methanol), metabolic acidosis and, 45
Wound, 1027–1029
burn, debridement of, 693
closure of, 1045–1048
scalp wounds and, 1053
staples and, 1048
sutures and, 1045t, 1045, 1047f
tape and, 1047
technique of, 1038
dehiscence of, 366
gynecologic procedures and, 423
following laparoscopy, 422
dressings for, 1049–1050
emergency department management of, 1027–1029
mechanism of injury and, 1027
wound biomechanical properties and, 1028–1029, 1029f
wound contaminants and, 1027t, 1027–1028
wound examination and, 1028
evisceration of, gynecologic procedures and, 423
gunshot (*see* Wound ballistics)
hematoma of, 366

Wound (*Cont.*):
gynecologic procedures and, 423
infection of, 366, 369–370
gynecologic procedures and, 422–423
postoperative care of, 1049–1050
prehospital care of, 1027
preparation of, 1037–1039
hair removal and, 1037
hemostasis and, 1037
mechanical cleansing and, 1038–1039, 1039f
skin antisepsis and, 1037
surgical debridement and, 1037–1038, 1038f
puncture, 1043
seroma of, 366
gynecologic procedures and, 423
Wound ballistics, 1019–1024
ballistic properties and wound produced and, 1020–1023
caliber and, 1021
gunshot fractures and, 1021
head wounds and, 1021, 1023
lead fragments and lead poisoning and, 1023
localization of missile and, 1023
missile embolization and, 1023
missile type and, 1021
pellet wounds and, 1023
trunk wounds and, 1021
mechanisms of wounding and, 1019–1020, 1022f
crushing of tissue and, 1019–1020
temporary cavitation and, 1020
Wound management, 1040–1041
antibiotics in, 1040–1041
prophylactic, 1040–1041, 1041t
drainage in, 1041
in tetanus, 879, 880t
Wound repair, anesthesia for, 1031–1035
infiltration, 1031
regional nerve clock as, 1031–1034, 1032–1035f
side effects of anesthetic agents and, 1035
topical, 1035–1036
WPW (see Wolff-Parkinson-White syndrome)
Wrist:
dislocations of, 977f, 977, 978f
fractures of, 976–977

X-rays, 711
Xanax (*see* Alprazolam)
Xerosis, in human immunodeficiency virus infections, 520
Xylocaine (*see* Lidocaine)

Y-type administration sets, 776
Yawning, in altered mental status, 153
Yersinia enterocolitica, diarrhea and, treatment of, 351t
Yersinia enterocolitis, diarrhea and, 349
Yes-no test, distinguishing true neurologic deficits from conversion disorder and, 1091t
Yohimbine, as antidote to clonidine, 571

Zarontin (*see* Ethosuximide)
Zollinger-Ellison syndrome, ulcers associated with, 313
Zygoma fractures, 852f, 852–853
Zygomatic arch fractures, 851–852, 852f
Zygomatic fracture, 1055
Zygomatic-maxillary complex fractures, 852f, 852–853

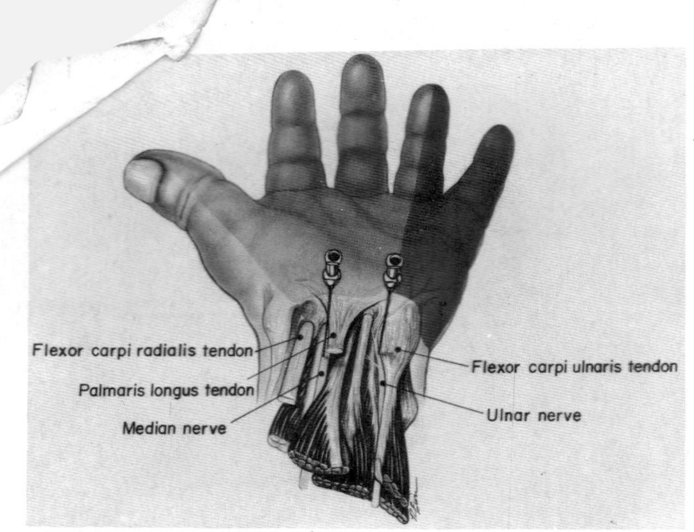

Fig. 189-1. Regional blocks of the ulnar and median nerves.

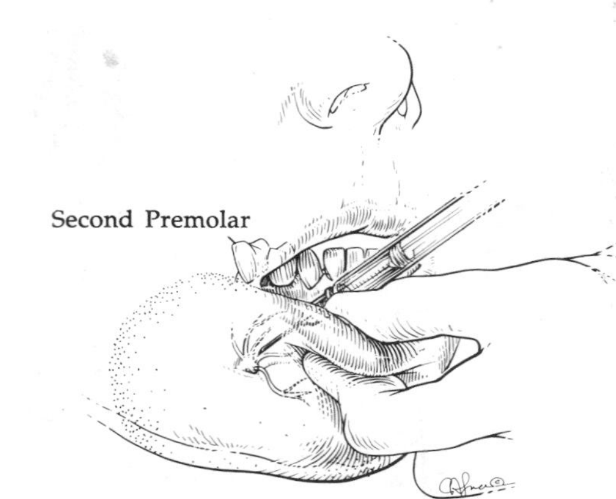

Fig. 189-7. Regional block of the mental nerve.

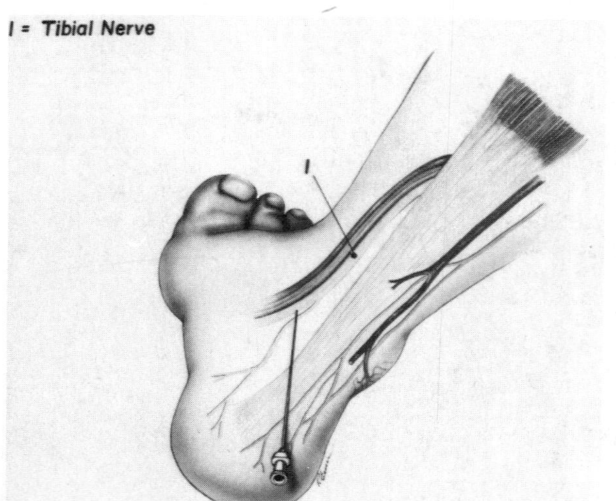

Fig. 189-3. Regional block of the tibial nerve.

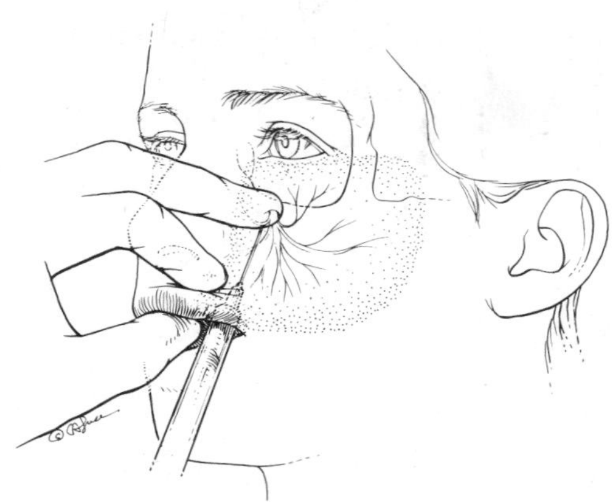

Fig. 189-8. Intraoral approach to regional nerve block of the infraorbital nerve.

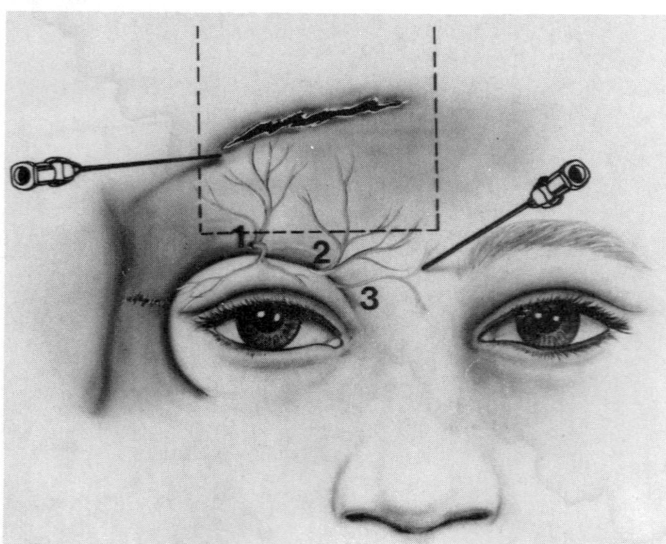

Fig. 189-5. Regional blocks of (1) the lateral branch of the frontal nerve; (2) the medial branch of the frontal nerve, and (3) the supratrochlear nerve. Infiltration anesthesia is an alternative approach to anesthetizing lacerations of the forehead.

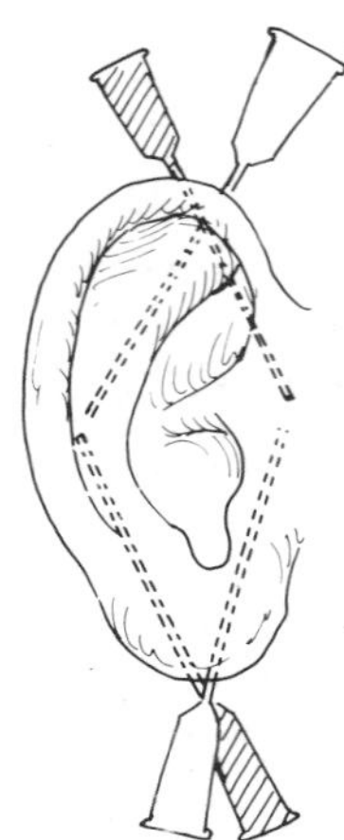

Fig. 189-10. Technique of regional anesthesia of the auricle.

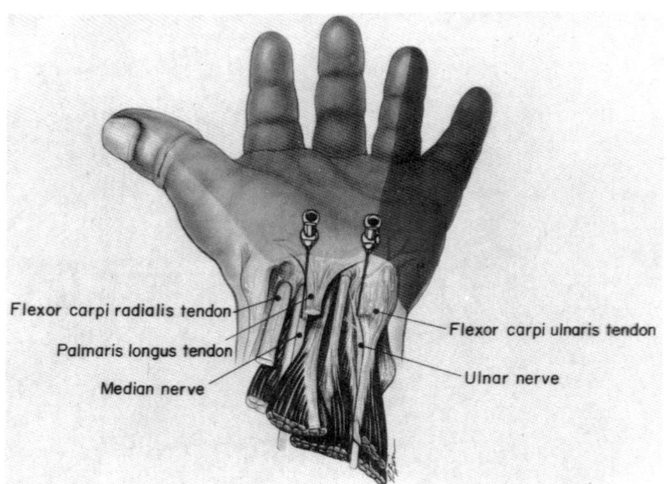

Fig. 189-1. Regional blocks of the ulnar and median nerves.

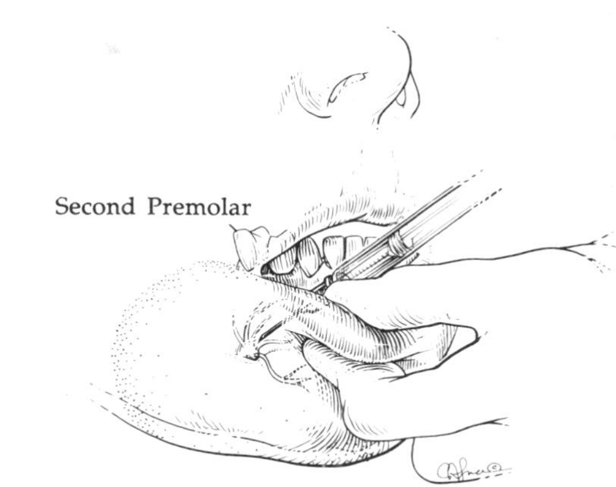

Fig. 189-7. Regional block of the mental nerve.

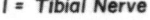

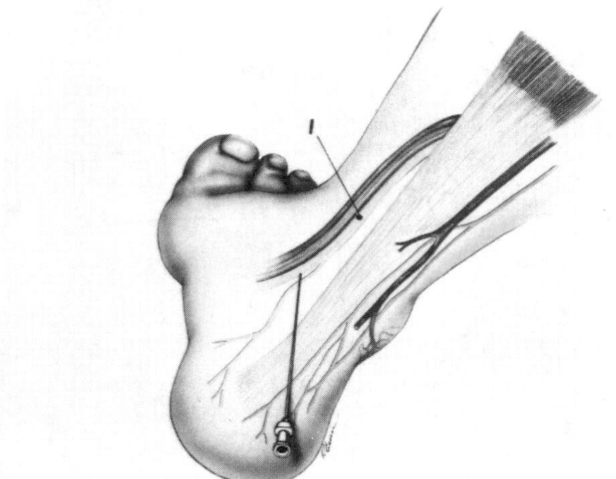

Fig. 189-3. Regional block of the tibial nerve.

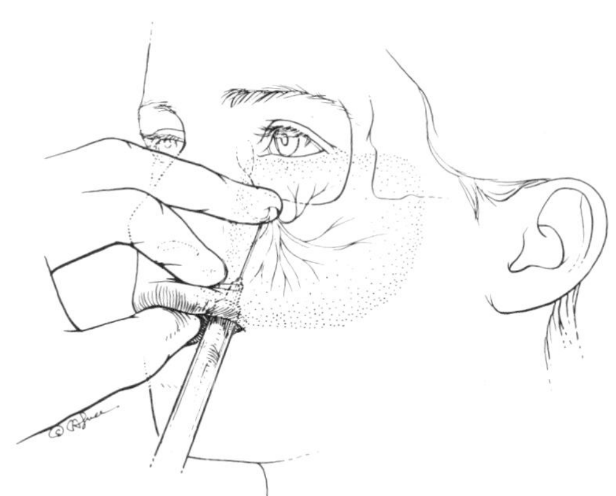

Fig. 189-8. Intraoral approach to regional nerve block of the infraorbital nerve.

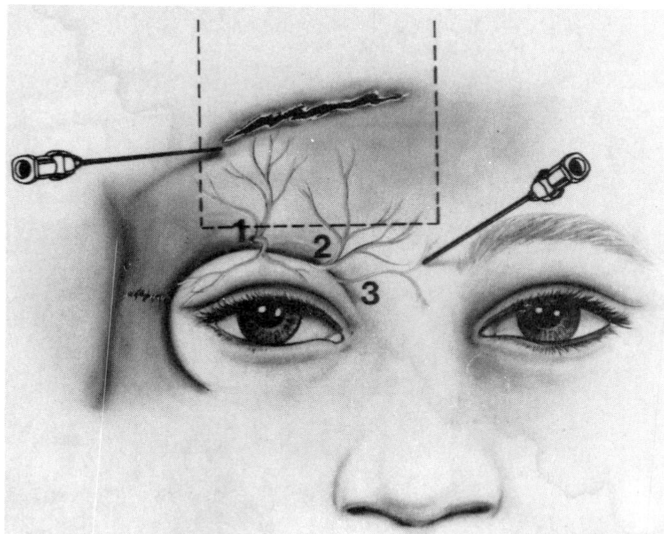

Fig. 189-5. Regional blocks of (1) the lateral branch of the frontal nerve; (2) the medial branch of the frontal nerve, and (3) the supratrochlear nerve. Infiltration anesthesia is an alternative approach to anesthetizing lacerations of the forehead.

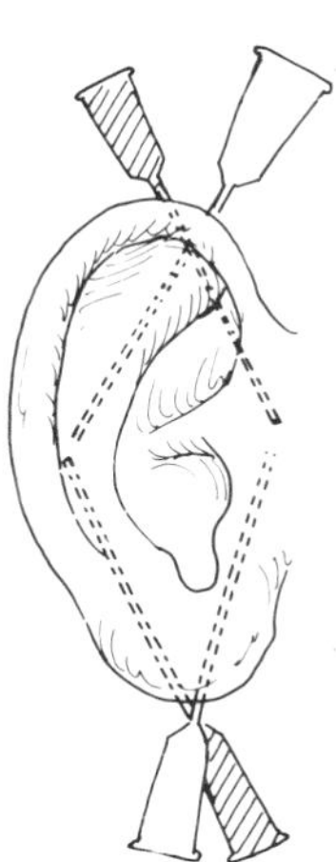

Fig. 189-10. Technique of regional anesthesia of the auricle.